KU-051-939

BRITISH MEDICAL ASSOCIATION

1001218

Oxford Textbook of

Urological Surgery

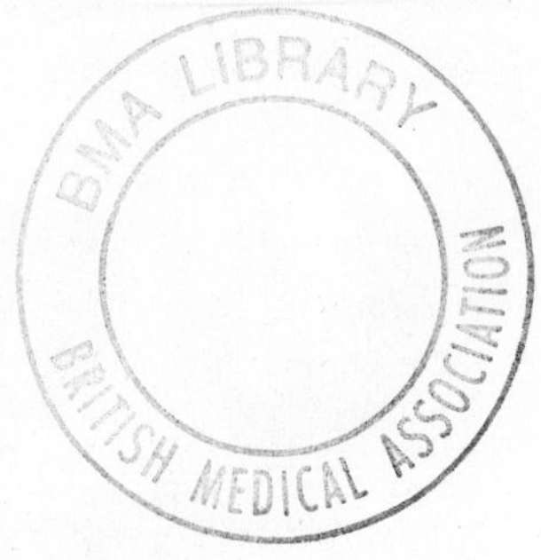

Oxford Textbook of

Urological Surgery

Edited by

Freddie C. Hamdy
Ian Eardley

Section Editors
James W. F. Catto
Christopher R. Chapple
Anthony R. Mundy
Rob Pickard
Rutger Ploeg
David John Ralph
John Reynard
David F. M. Thomas
Michael Weston

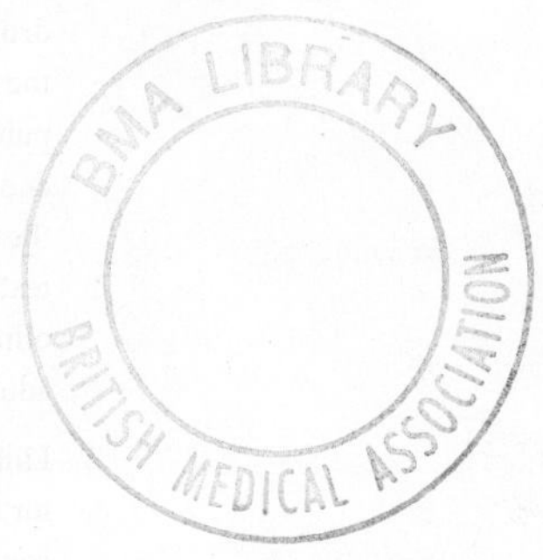

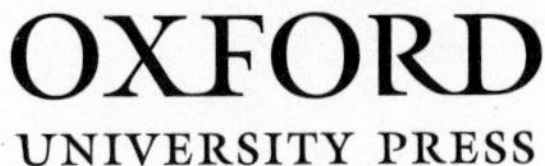

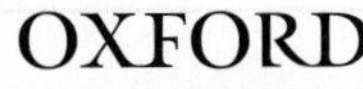

Great Clarendon Street, Oxford, OX2 6DP,
United Kingdom

Oxford University Press is a department of the University of Oxford. It furthers the University's objective of excellence in research, scholarship, and education by publishing worldwide. Oxford is a registered trade mark of Oxford University Press in the UK and in certain other countries

© Oxford University Press 2017

The moral rights of the authors have been asserted

First Edition published in 2017

Impression: 1

All rights reserved. No part of this publication may be reproduced, stored in a retrieval system, or transmitted, in any form or by any means, without the prior permission in writing of Oxford University Press, or as expressly permitted by law, by licence or under terms agreed with the appropriate reprographics rights organization. Enquiries concerning reproduction outside the scope of the above should be sent to the Rights Department, Oxford University Press, at the address above

You must not circulate this work in any other form and you must impose this same condition on any acquirer

Published in the United States of America by Oxford University Press
198 Madison Avenue, New York, NY 10016, United States of America

British Library Cataloguing in Publication Data
Data available

Library of Congress Control Number: 2017934227

ISBN 978–0–19–965957–9

Printed in Great Britain by
Bell & Bain Ltd., Glasgow

Oxford University Press makes no representation, express or implied, that the drug dosages in this book are correct. Readers must therefore always check the product information and clinical procedures with the most up-to-date published product information and data sheets provided by the manufacturers and the most recent codes of conduct and safety regulations. The authors and the publishers do not accept responsibility or legal liability for any errors in the text or for the misuse or misapplication of material in this work. Except where otherwise stated, drug dosages and recommendations are for the non-pregnant adult who is not breast-feeding

Links to third party websites are provided by Oxford in good faith and for information only. Oxford disclaims any responsibility for the materials contained in any third party website referenced in this work.

Series Preface from Professor Sir Peter J. Morris

This is a new development in surgical publishing; the first two editions of the *Oxford Textbook of Surgery* are to be replaced by a series of specialty-specific textbooks in surgery. This change was precipitated by the ever-increasing size of a single textbook of surgery which embraced all specialties (the second edition of the *Oxford Textbook of Surgery* was three volumes), and a decision to adapt the textbooks to meet the needs of the audience; firstly, to suit the requirements of Higher Surgical trainees and, secondly, to make it available online.

Thus, we have produced a key book to deal with the fundamentals of surgery, such as Anatomy, Physiology, Biochemistry, Evaluation of Evidence, and so forth. Then there are to be separate volumes covering individual specialties, each appearing as an independent textbook and available on *Oxford Medicine Online*.

It is planned that each textbook in each specialty will be independent although there obviously will be an overlap between different specialties and, of course, the core book on *Fundamentals of Surgery* will underpin the required scientific knowledge and practice in each of the other specialties.

This ambitious programme will be spread over several years, and the use of the online platform will allow for regular updates of the different textbooks.

Each textbook will include the proposed requirements for training and learning as defined by the specialist committees (SACs) of surgery recognized by the four Colleges of Surgery in Great Britain and Ireland, and will continue to be applicable to a global audience.

This ambitious programme will be spread over several years, and the use of the online platform will allow for regular updates of the different textbooks.

When completed, the *Oxford Textbooks in Surgery* series will set standards for a long time to come.

Professor Sir Peter J. Morris
Nuffield Professor of Surgery Emeritus, and former
Chairman of the Department of Surgery and Director of the
Oxford Transplant Centre, University of Oxford and
Oxford Radcliffe Hospitals, UK

Preface

Urology is a rich, diverse, and varied specialty. For certified urological surgeons, it is becoming increasingly challenging to remain updated in such a wide range of assorted conditions with expanding multidisciplinary treatment options, and it is doubly difficult for the trainee to understand what they need to know, and gain a comprehensive knowledge base which will equip them to become certified specialists.

The welcome initiative by Oxford University Press to create a series of specialty-specific textbooks mapped to the UK postgraduate surgical curricula has directly led to the production of this textbook. The urology curriculum describes the range of knowledge, skills, and behaviours that a trainee is expected to have acquired by the time that they are certified. We have taken the syllabus from within that urology curriculum in the United Kingdom and used it as the template for this textbook, which we hope will serve trainees and established colleagues across the world.

While the syllabus provides the basic architecture of urological surgery, the level of knowledge in each of the chapters goes beyond that which will be required for certification. The *Oxford Textbook of Urological Surgery* will be of value not only to trainees, but also to established urologists who wish to keep up-to-date with advances in urological care in one or more areas specific to their day-to-day practice.

We have recruited able expert section editors with an international reputation in their respective field, who led the development and composition of the varying components of this textbook. They, in turn, have relied on rich contributions from many national and international expert colleagues. The authors were specifically mandated to be concise as well as broadly comprehensive in covering their topic from the basics to the current limits of established knowledge, and to highlight areas of controversy, where they exist. Whereas detail may be lacking at times due to space constraints, the concepts and principles that direct modern urological practice are all included.

Urological science progresses continuously and the extent of knowledge described in this book is only a snapshot in time. However, with modern information technology allowing, we have asked all authors to provide frequent updates of their chapter at regular intervals for an exciting online version of the textbook, as well as future editions. Each chapter is accompanied by a long comprehensive reference list, as well as a short one for those interested in a specific theme.

We are confident that the *Oxford Textbook of Urological Surgery* will provide a novel, easy-to read, and useful source of knowledge and strong foundation both for the practising urologist and for trainees seeking to obtain entry into a wonderful specialty that we both continue to find challenging, fascinating, and enjoyable.

Freddie C. Hamdy
Nuffield Professor of Surgery and Professor of Urology,
Chairman, Nuffield Department of Surgical Sciences,
University of Oxford, Oxford OX3 7DQ,
Director of Surgery & Oncology,
Oxford University Hospitals NHS Foundation Trust,
United Kingdom

Ian Eardley
Consultant Urologist, St James's Hospital,
Leeds Teaching Hospitals NHS Trust,
Former Chairman Joint Committee on Surgical Training,
Vice-President, Royal College of Surgeons of England

Acknowledgements

Delivering a textbook is always an exciting challenge, which one paradoxically relishes and fears to take at the same time. The *Oxford Textbook of Urological Surgery* was no exception, and we are most grateful to our section editors and authors for their generous time and effort in providing such a rich and high-quality series of chapters. We thank Oxford University Press and its staff for helping us to deliver this textbook and for their patience during the lengthy preparation of the final manuscripts. We are particularly grateful to Sir Peter Morris whose vision was to map this series of textbooks to the United Kingdom's established training surgical curricula. We are both honoured to have been invited to deliver this important task, and proud to have completed it in this first edition. Finally, we are indebted to our families for their forbearance for the time that we have spent on this enterprise, most importantly our wives Bettina and Michelle.

Freddie C. Hamdy and Ian Eardley
Oxford and Leeds

Brief contents

Contents

SECTION 3
Functional and female

SECTION 4
Reconstruction

Abbreviations

AAST	American Association for the Surgery of Trauma
ABLC	amphotericin B-lipid complex
ABU	asymptomatic bacteriuria
ACE	angiotensin converting enzyme
ACOG	American Congress of Obstetricians and Gynecologists
ADEM	acute disseminated encephalomyelitis
ADH	antidiuretic hormone
ADPKD	autosomal dominant polycystic kidney disease
AFB	acid-fast bacilli
AHA	acetohydroxamic acid
AIDS	acquired immunodeficiency syndrome
AIS	Abbreviated Injury Scale
AKI	acute kidney injury
ALT	alanine aminotransferase
AMB	amphotericin B
APF	antiproliferative factor
AR	androgen receptor
ARHAI	Antimicrobial Resistance and Healthcare Associated Infection
ART	assisted reproductive techniques
AST	aspartate aminotransferase
ATN	acute tubular necrosis
AUA	American Urological Association
AUR	acute urinary retention
AUS	artificial urethral sphincter
BASICS	British Association for Immediate Care
BAUS	British Association of Urological Surgeons
BCG	Bacille Calmette-Guérin
BCI	bladder contractility index
BMA	bulbomembranous anastomosis
BMI	body mass index
BNC	bladder neck contracture
BOO	bladder outlet obstruction
BOOI	bladder outlet obstruction index
BOOP	bronchiolitis obliterans organizing pneumonia
BPE	benign prostatic enlargement
BPH	benign prostatic hyperplasia
BPO	benign prostatic obstruction
BPS	bladder pain syndrome
BRCA	breast cancer predisposition gene
BTX	botulinum toxin
BUO	bilateral ureteric obstruction
BVE	bladder voiding efficiency
BXO	balanitis xerotica obliterans
CAASB	catheter-associated asymptomatic bacteriuria
cAMP	cyclic adenosine monophosphate
CAUTI	catheter-associated urinary tract infection
CBT	cognitive behavioural therapy
CCD	charge-coupled device
CCU	camera control unit
CDC	disease control and prevention
CDI	clostridium difficile infection
CGH	comparative genomic hybridization
CIPO	chronic idiopathic pseudo-obstruction
cGMP	cyclic guanosine monophosphate
CIS	carcinoma in situ
CISC	clean intermittent self-catheterization
CKD	chronic kidney disease
CKD-EPI	Chronic Kidney Disease-Epidemiology Collaboration
CNF1	cytotoxic necrotizing factor 1
CNS	central nervous system
COLA	cystine, ornithine, lysine, and arginine
COPD	chronic obstructive pulmonary disease
COX	cyclooxygenase
CP/CPPS	chronic prostatitis/chronic pelvic pain syndrome
CPPS	chronic pelvic pain syndrome
CRP	C-reactive protein
CRPC	castration-resistant prostate cancer
CSU	catheter specimen of urine
CT	computed tomography
CTU	CT urography
CUR	chronic urinary retention
DBD	donation after brain death
DBU	double balloon urethrography
DCD	donation after circulatory death
DCS	damage control surgery
DEC	diethylcarbamazine
DGF	delayed graft function
DIT	doxazosin, ibuprofen, and thiocolchicoside
DMSO	dimethylsulphoxide
DRE	digital rectal examination
DSD	disorders of sex development

DTPA	diethyltetrapenta-acetic acid
DVIU	direct vision internal urethrotomy
EAU	European Association of Urology
EBRT	external beam radiotherapy
ED	erectile dysfunction
EEJ	electroejaculation
eGFR	estimated glomerular filtration rate
EHL	electrohydraulic lithotripsy
ELPAT	Ethical, Legal, and Psychosocial Aspects of Transplantation
EMT	epithelial–mesenchymal transition
eNOS	endothelial nitric oxide synthase
EORTC	European Organisation for Research and Treatment of Cancer
EPS	expressed prostatic secretion
ESBL	extended spectrum beta-lactamase
ESRD	end-stage renal disease
ESWL	extracorporeal shock wave lithotripsy
EUCAST	European Committee on Antimicrobial Susceptibility Testing
FAST	focused assessment with sonography for trauma
FDA	US Food and Drug Administration
FG	Fournier's gangrene
FGF	fibroblast growth factor
FGSI	Fournier's Gangrene Severity Index
FNAC	fine needle aspiration cytology
FSH	follicle-stimulatuing hormone
FTSG	full-thickness skin graft
f-URS	flexible ureterorenoscopy
FVC	frequency volume chart
GAG	glucosamine glycan layer
GCS	Glasgow Coma Scale
GFR	glomerular filtration rate
GI	gastrointestinal
GRE	glycopeptide-resistant enterococci
GuF	genitourinary fistulae
GWAS	genome-wide association studies
H&E	haematoxylin and eosin
HAI	healthcare-associated infections
HALDN	hand-assisted laparoscopic donor nephrectomy
HARP	hand-assisted retroperitoneoscopic donor nephrectomy
HA-UTI	hospital-acquired urinary tract infection
HAV	Hepatitis A virus
HBD	heart-beating donation
HCAI	healthcare-associated infections
HES	Hospital Episodes Statistics
HG-NMIBC	high-grade non-muscle invasive bladder cancer
HGPIN	high-grade prostatic intraepithelial neoplasia
HIFU	high-intensity focused ultrasound
HIV	human immunodeficiency virus
HLA	human leukocyte antigen
HlyA	α-haemolysin
HPCR	high-pressure chronic retention
HPV	human papilloma virus
HRPC	hormone-refractory prostate cancer
HRQoL	health-related quality of life
HSV	herpes simplex virus
IBC	intracellular bacterial communities
IC	interstitial cells
ICC	interstitial cells of Cajal
ICIQ	International Consultation on Incontinence Questionnaire
ICP	intracranial pressure
ICS	International Continence Society
ICSI	intracytoplasmic sperm injection
ICU-VS	International Consultation on Incontinence Vaginal Symptoms questionnaire
IDO	idiopathic detrusor overactive
IL-1	interleukin
INH	isoniazid
iNOS	inducible nitric oxide synthase
INR	international normalized ratio
IPP	leak point pressures
IPP	intravesical prostatic protrusion
IPSS	International Prostate Symptom Score
ISC	intermittent self-catheterization
ISD	intrinsic sphincter deficiency
ISS	Injury Severity Score
IUI	intrauterine insemination
IVF	*in vitro* fertilization
IVP	intravenous pyelography
IVU	intravenous urography
JGA	juxtaglomerular apparatus
KTx	kidney transplantation
KTXs	kidney transplants
KUB	kidney, ureter, and bladder
L-AMB	liposomal amphotericin B
LFT	liver function test
LESS	laparoendoscopic single site surgery
LGV	lymphogranuloma venereum
LH	lutenizing hormone
LPCR	low-pressure chronic retention
LPS	lipopolysaccharide
LRP	laparoscopic radical prostatectomy
LSCS	low segment caesarian section
LUT	lower urinary tract
LUTD	lower urinary tract dysfunction
LUTS	lower urinary tract symptoms
MAG3	mercaptoactyl-triglycine
MAP	magnesium ammonium phosphate
MCUG	micturating cystourethrogram
MDRD	modification of diet in renal disease
MDR-TB	multidrug-resistant tuberculosis
MET	medical expulsive therapy
MHRA	Medicines & Healthcare products Regulatory Agency (UK)
MIC	minimum inhibitory concentration
MRHA	mannose-resistant haemagglutination
MLCK	myosin light chain kinase
MRI	magnetic resonance imaging
MRSA	methicillin-resistant Staphylococcus aureus
MRU	magnetic resonance urography
MSA	multiple system atrophy
MSHA	mannose-sensitive haemagglutination
MSM	men having sex with men
MSSU	midstream specimen of urine
MSU	midstream uine

MTOPS	medical therapy of prostatic symptoms
MUCP	maximum urethral closure pressure
MUI	mixed urinary incontinence
MUP	maximum urethral pressure
MVAC	methotrexate, vinblastine, doxorubicin, and cisplatin
NAAT	nucleic acid amplification test
NA	noradrenaline
NADPH	nicotinamide adenine dinucleotide phosphate
NANC	non-adrenergic non-cholinergic
NBI	narrow band imaging
NCCN	National Comprehensive Cancer Network
NCCT	non-contrast computed tomography
NDO	neurogenic detrusor overactivity
NGS	next generation sequencing
NHBD	non-heart-beating donation
NIAID	National Institute for Allergy and Infectious Diseases
NICE	National Institute for Health and Care Excellence
NIDDK	National Institute of Diabetes and Digestive and Kidney Diseases
NIH	National Institutes of Health
NIH-CPSI	National Institutes of Health Chronic Prostatitis Symptom Index
NMIBC	non-muscle invasive bladder cancer
NNIS	National Nosocomial Infections Surveillance
nNOS	neuronal nitric oxide synthase
NNRTI	non-nucleoside reverse transcriptase inhibitors
NO	nitric oxide
NOS	nitric oxide synthase
NOTES	natural orifice transluminal endoscopic surgery
NRTI	nucleoside reverse transcriptase inhibitors
NSAID	non-steroidal anti-inflammatory drug
OAB	overactive bladder
OABS	overactive bladder symptom syndrome
OCC	urothelial cell carcinoma
PAH	p-aminohippuric acid
PAI	pathogenicity islands
PAIR	puncture, aspiration, injection and reaspiration
PAMP	pathogen-associated molecular pattern
PAS	para-aminosalicylic acid
PBP	penicillin-binding protein
PCa	prostate cancer
PCN	percutaneous nephrostomy
PCNL	percutaneous nephrolithotomy
PCR	polymerase chain reaction
PD	peritoneal dialysis
PDD	photodynamic diagnosis
PDE-5	phosphodiesterase type 5
PDT	photodynamic therapy
PET	positron emission tomography
PFDI	Pelvic Floor Distress Inventory
PFS	pressure flow studies
PI	protease inhibitors
PID	pelvic inflammatory disease
PLUTO	percutaneous shunting in lower urinary tract obstruction
PMC	pontine micturition centre
PMD	post-micturition dribble
PN	pneumatic lithotripsy
PNE	percutaneous nerve evaluation
POP	pelvic organ prolapse
POPIQ	POP Impact Questionnaire
PPD	purified protein derivative
PPMT	pre- and post-massage test
PPS	sodium pentosan polysulphate
PSA	prostate-specific antigen
PSF	probability of stone formation
PTB	pulmonary tuberculosis
PTNS	percutaneous tibial nerve stimulation
PUJ	pelviureteric junction
PUJO	pelviureteric junction obstruction
PUV	posterior urethral valve disorder
PVR	post-void residual
PVS	penile vibratory stimulation
PZA	pyrazinamide
QoL	quality of life
RADN	robot-assisted laparoscopic donor nephrectomy
RALP	robotic-assisted laparoscopic prostatectomy
RARP	robotic-assisted laparoscopic radical prostatectomy
RBF	renal blood flow
RCC	renal cell carcinoma
RCT	randomized controlled trial
RI	resistive index
RIRS	retrograde intrarenal surgery
RNA	ribonucleic acid
RP	radical prostatectomy
RPF	renal plasma flow
RRP	robotic radical prostatectomy
RRt	renal replacement treatment
RTA	renal tubular acidosis
RTX	repeats in toxin
RUG	retrograde urethrogram
RVT	renal vein thrombosis
SAT	secreted autotransporter toxin
SCC	squamous cell cancer
SCI	spinal cord injury
SEER	Surveillance, Epidemiology, and End Results programme
SIRS	systemic inflammatory response syndrome
sGC	soluble guanylate cyclase
SJS	Stevens–Johnson syndrome
SLED	slow low-efficiency dialysis
SNARE	sensitive factor attachment protein receptor
SNM	sacral neuromodulation
SPC	suprapubic catheterization
STARR	stapled transanal rectal resection
STI	sexually transmitted infection
STSG	split-thickness skin graft
SUI	stress urinary incontinence
SVI	seminal vesicle invasion
SWL	shockwave lithotripsy
TCC	transitional cell carcinoma
TEAP	transurethral ethanol ablation of the prostate
TEN	toxic epidermal necrolysis
TENS	transcutaneous electrical nerve stimulation
TGF	transforming growth factor
TH	tyrosine hydroxylase

THP	Tamm-Horsfall protein
TIN	testicular intraepithelial neoplasia
TIR	Toll/interleukin receptor
TLR	Toll-like receptor
TNM	tumour-node metastases system
TRUS	transrectal ultrasonography
TUR	transurethral resection
TURB	transurethral resection of the bladder
TURBT	transurethral resection of a bladder tumour
TURP	transurethral resection of prostate
TUU	transureteroureterostomy
TWOC	trial without catheter
UBC	urothelial bladder cancer
UD	urethral diverticula
UDIF	urothelium-derived inhibitory factor
UDT	undescended testis
UE	ureteroscopic endopyelotomy
UGTB	urogenital tuberculosis
UI	urinary incontinence
UICC	Union for International Cancer Control
UK	United Kingdom
UL	ultrasonic lithotripsy
UPEC	uropathogenic *Escherichia coli*
UPJ	ureteropelvic junction
UPOINT	urinary, psychosocial, organ specific, infection, neurological and muscle tenderness
UPOINTS	urinary, psychosocial, organ specific, infection, neurological and muscle tenderness, and sexual dysfunction
UPP	urethral pressure profiles
URS	ureteroscopy
UrVF	ureterovaginal fistula
USS	ultrasound scan
UTI	urinary tract infection
UTUC	upper urinary tract urothelial carcinoma
UUI	urgency urinary incontinence
UVF	urethrovaginal fistula
VAS	visual analogue scales
VCUG	voiding cystourethrography
VEGF	vascular endothelial growth factor
VHL	Von Hippel-Lindau
VIP	vasoactive intestinal polypeptide
VUA	vesicourethral anastomosis
VUF	vesicouterine fistula
VUR	vesicoureteric reflux
VVF	vesicovaginal fistula
WHO	World Health Organization
WIT	warm ischaemia time
XDR-TB	extensively drug-resistant tuberculosis

Contributors

Sally Ager, Leeds Teaching Hospital Trust, UK

Hashim Uddin Ahmed, Division of Surgery, Department of Surgery and Cancer, Faculty of Medicine, Imperial College London, UK

Peter Albers, Department of Urology, University Clinic Düsseldorf Peter Albers, Urologische Klinik, Universitätsklinikum Düsseldorf, Germany

Ased Ali, Department of Urology, Mid Yorkshire Hospitals NHS Trust, UK

Ashraf Almatar, Department of Surgical Oncology, Division of Urology, Princess Margaret Hospital, Toronto, Ontario, Canada

Ines Teles Alves, Department of Urology, Erasmus MC, Rotterdam, the Netherlands

Akwasi Amoako, Department of Urology and Reproductive Medicine, Leeds Teaching Hospitals, Leeds, UK

Daniela E. Andrich, University College London Hospitals NHS Foundation Trust; London Bridge Hospital, both London, UK

Gastón M. Astroza, Duke University School of Medicine, Durham, NC, USA

Aditya Bagrodia, Department of Urology, The University of Texas Southwestern Medical Center, Dallas, USA & Urology Fellow, The David Solit Lab, Memorial Sloan Kettering Cancer Center, NY

Atul Bagul, Endocrine Surgery, Department of General Surgery, Sheffield Teaching Hospitals NHS Foundation Trust, UK

Saba Balasubramanian, Academic Surgical Oncology Unit, University of Sheffield, Royal Hallamshire Hospital, UK

Steve Ball, Department of Endocrinology, Central Manchester University Hospitals and Manchester Academic Health Science Centre, Manchester, UK

Roger Bayston, School of Medicine, University of Nottingham, UK

Mohammed Belal, University Hospitals Birmingham, Edgbaston, Birmingham, UK

Simone Bertz, Institute of Pathology, University Erlangen, Erlangen, Germany

Carlo Bettocchi, Institute of Urology, St. Peter's Hospital, UCH London, UK and University of Bari Aldo Morom, Italy

Anders Bjartell, Department of Urology, Skåne University Hospital, Lund University, Sweden

William Brant, University of Utah, Salt Lake City, Utah, USA

Alberto Briganti, Vita-Salute San Raffaele Hospital, Department of Urology, Milan, Italy

Maree Brinkman, Cancer Epidemiology Centre, Cancer Council Victoria, Melbourne, Australia

Richard J. Bryant, The Nuffield Department of Surgical Sciences, University of Oxford, John Radcliffe Hospital, Headley Way, Oxford, UK

Thomas Bschleipfer, Clinic for Urology, Pediatric Urology and Andrology, Justus-Liebig-University Giessen, Germany

Frank Buntin, Department of General Practice, Katholieke Universiteit Leuven, ACHG-KULeuven, Kapucijnenvoer, Leuven, Belgium

Max Burger, St Josef Medical Centre, Department of Urology of Regensburg University, Regensburg, Germany

Jeffrey A. Cadeddu, Department of Urology, UT Southwestern Medical Center, Dallas, Texas, USA

Fabio Calabrò, Department of Medical Oncology, San Camillo Forlanini Hospital, Rome, Italy

Peter Carroll, University of California, San Francisco, CA, USA

James W.F. Catto, Department of Oncology, The Medical School, Beech Hill Road, Sheffield, UK

Selim Cellek, Anglia Ruskin University, Faculty of Medical Science UK

Christopher R. Chapple, University of Sheffield and Sheffield Teaching Hospitals NHS Foundation Trust, UK

Keith Chapple, Colorectal Surgical Unit, Sheffield Teaching Hospitals NHS Foundation Trust, UK

Liang Cheng, Department of Pathology and Laboratory Medicine, Indiana University School of Medicine, Indianapolis, IN, USA

Noel W. Clarke, The Christie and Salford Royal Hospitals NHS Trusts, Manchester, UK

Pierre Colin, Academic Department of Urology, CHRU Lille, Univ Lille Nord de France, Lille, France

Matthew Cooperberg, Departments of Urology and Epidemiology & Biostatistics, UCSF; Helen Diller Family Comprehensive Cancer Center, San Francisco, CA, USA

Eduardo Cortes, Department of Urogynaecology, Kingston Hospital NHS Foundation Trust, London, UK

David Cranston, The Nuffield Department of Surgical Sciences, University of Oxford, John Radcliffe Hospital, Oxford, UK

Peter Cuckow, Department of Paediatric Urology, Great Ormond Street Hospital NHS Trust, London, UK

Donna Daly, Department of Biomedical Science, University of Sheffield, UK

Ahmed A. Darwish, Ain Shams University, Cario, Egypt and Senior Clinical Fellow Pediatric Surgery and Urology, University Hospital of Wales, Cardiff, UK

Raj Das, Department of Radiology, St. George's Hospital and Medical School, London, UK

Johann De Bono, The Royal Marsden Foundation Trust, The Institute of Cancer Research, UK

Gert De Meerleer, University Hospital of Ghent, Department of Radiation Oncology, Ghent, Belgium

Louise Dickinson, Department of Urology, UCLH NHS Foundation Trust, London, UK

Thorsten Diemer, Pediatric Urology and Andrology, Justus-Liebig-University Giessen, Germany

Rosa Djajadiningrat, Netherlands Cancer Institute - Antoni van Leeuwenhoek Hospital, Amsterdam, the Netherlands

Gert R. Dohle, Department of Urology, Erasmus University Medical Center, Rotterdam, the Netherlands

Frank J.M.F. Dor, Hammersmith Hospital, Imperial College Healthcare NHS Trust, London, UK

Marcus Drake, Bristol Urological Institute, School of Clinical Sciences, University of Bristol, UK

Ian Eardley, Leeds Teaching Hospital Trust, UK

Tim Eisen, Department of Oncology, Cambridge Biomedical Campus, Addenbrooke's Hospital, Cambridge University Health Partners, Cambridge, UK

Julie Ellis-Jones, University of the West of England; and Southmead Hospital, North Bristol Trust, Bristol, UK

Mark Emberton, Division of Surgery and Interventional Science University College London, UK

Stephen Faddegon, University of Texas Southwestern Medical Center, Dallas, USA

Magnus Fall, Department of Urology, Institute of Clinical Sciences, Sahlgrenska Academy at the University of Gothenburg, Sweden

Vincenzo Ficarra, O.L.V. Robotic Surgery Institute, Aalst, Belgium

Mikkel Fode, University of Copenhagen and Department of Urology, Herlev and Gentofte Hospital

Paolo Fornara, Faculty of Medicine, University Hospital, Halle (Saale), Germany

Clare Fowler, University College London, UK; the National Hospital for Neurology and Neurosurgery, Queen Square, London, UK

Simon Freeman, Department of Radiology, Derriford Hospital, Plymouth, Devon, UK

Giulio Garaffa, St Peter's Andrology, University College London Hospitals, London, UK

Mary Garthwaite, James Cook University Hospital, Middlesborough, UK

Tarek P. Ghoneim, Academic Department of Urology, CHRU Lille, University Lille Nord de France, Lille, France

James A. Gilbert, OUH NHS Trust and Clinical Trial Service Unit, Nuffield Department of Population Health, University of Oxford; and Oxford Kidney Unit, Oxford University Hospitals, UK

Inderbir Gill, University of Southern California, Los Angeles, USA

John Goepel, Sheffield Teaching Hospitals, Sheffield, UK

Zachariah G. Goldsmith, Department Urology, St. Luke's Center, USA

Paolo Gontero, University of Torino, Department of Surgival Sciences and Urology, Turin, Italy

Mieke Goossens, Department of General Practice, Katholieke Universiteit Leuven, ACHG-KULeuven, Kapucijnenvoer, Leuven, Belgium

Magnus Grabe, Department of Microbiology, Immunology and Glycobiology (MIG), Lund University, Sweden

Francesco Greco, Department of Urology and Mini-Invasive Centre, Romolo Hospital, Crotone, Italy

Basma Greef, Department of Oncology, Cambridge Biomedical Campus, Addenbrooke's Hospital, Cambridge University Health Partners, Cambridge, UK

Geoffrey I. Hackett, Consultant in Sexual Medicine, Heartlands Hospital, Birmingham, UK; Emeritus Professor of Men's Health and Diabetes, University of Bedfordshire, UK; occasional speaker for Bayer and v Besins Pharmaceuticals.

Simon Harrison, Department of Urology, Pinderfields Hospital, Wakefield, UK

Alice Hartley, Freeman Hospital, Newcastle upon Tyne, UK

Arndt Hartmann, Institute of Pathology, Erlangen University Hospital, Erlangen, Germany; Department of Pathology, Friedrich-Alexander University Medical Centre, Erlangen, Germany

Robert P. Hartman, Department of Radiology, Mayo Clinic School of Medicine, Mayo Clinic, Rochester, MN, USA

Hashim Hashim, Bristol Urological Institute, Southmead Hospital, Bristol, UK

Richard J. Haynes, Clinical Trial Service Unit, Oxford, UK

Susan Heenan, Department of Radiology, St. George's Hospital and Medical School, London, UK

Axel Heidenreich, Department of Urology, RWTH University Aachen, Germany

John Henderson, Churchill Hospital, Oxford

Dennis A. Hesselink, Department of Internal Medicine, Division of Nephrology and Renal Transplantation, Erasmus MC, University Medical Center Rotterdam, Rotterdam, the Netherlands

Christiaan F. Heyns, Formally of Department of Surgical Sciences, Division of Urology, Stellenbosch University, South Africa

Simon Horenblas, Department of Urology, the Netherlands Cancer Institute-Antoni van Leeuwenhoek Hospital, Amsterdam, the Netherlands

Peter Howells, Department of Medical Physics, Leeds General Infirmary, Leeds Teaching Hospitals Trust, Leeds, UK

Kim Hutton, Department of Paediatric Surgery, University Hospital of Wales, Cardiff, UK

Muhammad Waqas Iqbal, Duke University Medical Centre, Durham, North Carolina

Mariam Jafri, School of Clinical and Experimental Medicine, College of Medical and Dental Sciences, Medical and Molecular Genetics, University of Birmingham, UK

Guido Jenster, Department of Urology, Erasmus MC, Rotterdam, the Netherlands

Michael Jewett, Department of Surgical Oncology, Division of Urology, Princess Margaret Hospital, Toronto, Ontario, Canada

Ghalib Jibara, Urology Resident, Division of Urology, Department of Surgery, Duke University Hospital, Durham, NC, USA

Steven Joniau, University Hospital of Leuven, Department of Urology, Leuven, Belgium

Ates Kadioglu, Department of Urology, Medical Faculty of Istanbul, Istanbul University, Turkey

Sajid Kalathil, Department of Diabetes and Endocrine, University of Newcastle, International Centre for Life, Newcastle upon Tyne

R. Jeffrey Karnes, Mayo Clinic, Department of Urology, Rochester, USA

Oliver Kayes, Department of Urology and Reproductive Medicine, Leeds Teaching Hospitals, Leeds, UK

Akira Kawashima, Department of Radiology, Mayo Clinic School of Medicine, Mayo Clinic, Scottsdale, AZ, USA

Steven Kennish, Royal Hallamshire Hospital, Sheffield Teaching Hospitals NHS Foundation Trust, UK

Stephen Keoghane, Portsmouth Hospitals NHS Trust, UK

Timothy J. Key, Cancer Epidemiology Unit, Nuffield Department of Population Health, University of Oxford, UK

Jeannette Kathrin Kraft, Clarendon Wing Radiology Department, Leeds General Infirmary, Leeds Teaching Hospitals Trust, Leeds, UK

Jeff A. Lafranca, Department of Surgery, division of Transplant Surgery, Erasmus MC, University Medical Center Rotterdam, Rotterdam, the Netherlands

Stephen M. Larsen, Rush University Medical Center, Chicago, IL, USA

Andrew J. LeRoy, Department of Radiology, Mayo Clinic School of Medicine, Mayo Clinic, Rochester, MN, USA

Laurence A. Levine, Rush University Medical Center, Chicago, IL, USA

Hans Lilja, Departments of Laboratory Medicine, Surgery, and Medicine, Memorial Sloan Kettering Cancer Center, New York, NY, USA; Nuffield Department of Surgical Sciences, University of Oxford, Oxford, UK; Department of Translational Medicine, Lund University, Malmö, Sweden

Michael E. Lipkin, Duke University Medical Center, Department of Surgery, Division of Urology, Durham, NC, USA

Antonio Lopez-Beltran, Anatomical Pathology Unit, Department of Surgery, Faculty of Medicine and Nursing, University of Cordoba, Cordoba, Spain & Department of Pathology, Champalimaud Clinical Center, Lisbon, Portugal

Yair Lotan, Department of Urology, The University of Texas Southwestern Medical Center, Dallas, USA

Eamonn Maher, School of Clinical and Experimental Medicine, College of Medical and Dental Sciences, Medical and Molecular Genetics, University of Birmingham, UK

Altaf Mangera, Sheffield Teaching Hospitals NHS Trust, Sheffield, UK

Roy Mano, Institute of Urology, Rabin Medical Center, Petah Tikva, and Sackler Faculty of Medicine, Tel Aviv University, Tel Aviv, Israel

Roman Mayr, St Josef Medical Centre, Department of Urology of Regensburg University, Regensburg, Germany

Roberta Mazzucchelli, Università Politecnica delle Marche, Italy

Emma J. McCarty, Department of Genitourinary Medicine, Royal Victoria Hospital, Belfast, UK

Chris G. McMahon, Australian Center for Sexual Health, Sydney, Australia

Richard P. Meijer, Department of Urology, University Medical Centre Utrecht, Utrecht, the Netherlands

Rodolfo Montironi, Section of Pathological Anatomy, Polytechnic University of the Marche Region (Ancona), School of Medicine, United Hospitals, Ancona, Italy

Roland Morley, Imperial College NHS Trust, London, UK

Alexander Mottrie, O.L.V. Robotic Surgery Institute, Aalst, Belgium

Deborah Mukherji, The Royal Marsden Foundation Trust, UK, American University of Beirut Medical Center, Riad El-Solh, Beirut, Lebanon

Anthony R. Mundy, Institute of Urology, University College Hospital, UCLH NHS Foundation Trust Headquarters, London

Asif Muneer, Department of Urology and NIHR Biomedical Research Centre, University College London Hospital, UK

Andreas Neisius, Department of Urology, University Medical Center, Johannes Gutenberg University, Mainz, Germany

Giacomo Novara, University of Padua, Padua, Italy

David Noyes, Consultant in Orthopaedic Trauma Surgery, Oxford University Hospitals NHS Foundation Trust, Oxford, UK

Tim O'Brien, Guys and St Thomas' Hospital, London, UK

Chris A. O'Callaghan, Nuffield Department of Medicine, University of Oxford, UK

Ephrem Olweny, Departments of Urology, Rutgers-Robert Wood Johnson Medical School, New Brunswick, NJ

Aurelius Omlin, The Royal Marsden Foundation Trust, The Institute of Cancer Research, UK

Nadir Osman, Department of Urology, Royal Hallamshire Hospital, Sheffield, UK

Jalesh Panicker, University College London; The National Hospital for Neurology and Neurosurgery; UCL Institute of Neurology, all in London, UK

Amit Patel, Consultant in Urology, Guys and St Thomas' Hospital, London, UK

Nilay Patel, The Nuffield Department of Surgical Sciences, University of Oxford, John Radcliffe Hospital, Oxford, UK

Uday Patel, Department of Radiology, St. George's Hospital and Medical School, London, UK

Carmel Pezaro, The Royal Marsden Foundation Trust, The Institute of Cancer Research, UK

Adrian Pilatz, Clinic for Urology, Pediatric Urology and Andrology, Justus-Liebig-University Giessen, Germany

Hartmut Porst, Private Urological/Andrological Practice, Hamburg, Germany

Glenn M. Preminger, Department of Urologic Surgery, Duke University Medical Center, Durham, NC, USA

Alison J. Price, Cancer Epidemiology Unit, University of Oxford, UK

Samarpit Rai, Division of Urology, University of Miami Miller School of Medicine, Miami, USA

David John Ralph, St Peter's Andrology, University College London Hospitals, London, UK

Ashok Daya Ram, Consultant Paediatric and Neonatal Surgeon, Department of Paediatric Surgery, Norfolk and Norwich University Hospital, Norwich, UK

Yacov Reisman, Urologist, Amstelland Hospital, Laan van de Helende Meesters 8, Amstelveen, the Netherlands

John Reynard, Nuffield Department of Surgical Sciences, University of Oxford, UK

Morgan Roupret, Academic Department of Urology of la Pitié-Salpêtrière Hospital, Assistance Publique-Hôpitaux de Paris, Faculté de Médecine Pierre et Marie Curie, University Paris VI, Paris, France

Antonino Saccà, Department of Urology, Ospedali Riuniti di Bergamo, Bergamo, Italy

Arun Sahai, Department of Urology, Guy's Hospital, Guy's and St Thomas' NHS Trust, King's Health Partners, London, UK

Neveen Said, Department of Radiation Oncology, University of Virginia, USA

Emre Salabaş, Department of Urology, Medical Faculty of Istanbul, Istanbul University, Turkey

Andrea Salonia, University Vita-Salute San Raffaele-Department of Urology, Milan, Italy

Salvatore Sansalone, Department of Urology, School of Medicine Tor Vergata University of Rome, Rome, Italy

Matteo Santoni, Medical Oncology, Università Politecnica delle Marche, Azienda Ospedaliero-Universitaria Ospedali Riuniti Umberto I, GM Lancisi, G Salesi, Ancona, Italy

Charles D. Scales, David Geffen School of Medicine, UCLA

Marina Scarpelli, Università Politecnica delle Marche, Italy

Fritz H. Schröder, Department of Urology, Erasmus University Rotterdam, the Netherlands

Edward Sharples, Oxford University Hospitals NHS Trust, UK

Graham Sleat, Specialty Registar, Trauma & Orthopaedics, Oxford University Hospitals NHS Foundation Trust, Oxford, UK

Jens Sonksen, University of Copenhagen and Department of Urology, Herlev and Gentofte Hospital

Martin Spahn, Inselspital, Department of Urology, Bern, Switzerland

Mark Speakman, Department of Urology, Taunton and Somerset Hospital, Taunton, UK

Marco Spilotros, Institute of Urology, St. Peter's Hospital, UCH London, UK

Roly Squire, Leeds Children's Hospital, Leeds, UK

Henrik Steinbrecher, Department of Paediatric Surgery, Southampton University Hospital, Southampton, UK

Cora N. Sternberg, Department of Medical Oncology, San Camillo Forlanini Hospital, Rome, Italy

Mark Sullivan, The Nuffield Department of Surgical Sciences, University of Oxford, John Radcliffe Hospital, Oxford, UK

Eugene Teoh, Department of Radiology, Churchill Hospital, Oxford University Hospitals NHS Trust, Oxford, and Department of Oncology, University of Oxford, UK

George Thalmann, Department of Urology, University of Bern, Inselspital, Switzerland

Dan Theodorescu, University of Colorado, Comprehensive Cancer Center, Aurora, Colorado, USA

Nikesh Thiruchelvam, Department of Urology, Addenbrookes Hospital, Cambridge, UK; Cambridge University Hospitals NHS Trust, UK

David F.M. Thomas, Leeds Teaching Hospitals NHS Trust, Leeds, UK

Page Toby, Newcastle upon Tyne Hospitals NHS Foundation Trust, UK

Jan Trapman, Erasmus MC, Rotterdam, the Netherlands

Benjamin W. Turney, Department of Urology, Nuffield Department of Surgical Sciences, The Churchill Hospital, Oxford, UK

David Ulmert, Molecular Pharmacology and Chemistry Program, Memorial Sloan-Kettering Cancer Center, NY, USA, and Department of Surgery (Urology), Skåne University Hospital, Malmö, Sweden

Siska Van Bruwaene, University Hospital of Leuven, Department of Urology, Leuven, Belgium

Bas W.G. Van Rhijn, Department of Surgical Oncology, Netherlands Cancer Institute, Antoni van Leeuwenhoek Hospital

Sobhan Vinjamuri, Department of Nuclear Medicine, Royal Liverpool University Hospital, Liverpool, UK

Florian M.E. Wagenlehner, Clinic for Urology, Pediatric Urology and Andrology, Justus-Liebig-University Giessen, Germany

Katherine E. Walton, Department of Microbiology, Newcastle upon Tyne Hospitals NHS Foundation Trust, UK

Wolfgang Weidner, Clinic for Urology, Pediatric Urology and Andrology, Justus-Liebig-University Giessen, Germany

Toby Wells, Department of Radiology, Derriford Hospital, Plymouth, Devon, UK

Sven Wenske, MD. Department of Urology, Columbia University Medical Center, College of Physicians & Surgeons, New York, NY, USA

Michael Weston, Leeds Teaching Hospitals NHS Trust, UK

Christian Winter, Department of Urology, University Clinic Düsseldorf Peter Albers, Urologische Klinik, Universitätsklinikum Düsseldorf, Germany

Han Hsi Wong, Department of Oncology, Cambridge University Hospitals NHS Foundation Trust, Cambridge, UK

Björn Wullt, Department of Microbiology, Immunology and Glycobiology (MIG), Lund University, Sweden

Ofer Yossepowitch, Institute of Urology, Rabin Medical Center, Petah Tikva, Israel

Filiberto Zattoni, University of Padua, Padua, Italy

Maurice P. Zeegers, Nutrition and Translational Research in Metabolism (School NUTRIM), Maastricht University, the Netherlands; Care and Public Health Research Institute (School CAPHRI), Maastricht University, the Netherlands

Pascal Zehnder, Department of Urology, University of Bern, Inselspital, Switzerland

Alexandre R. Zlotta, Division of Urology, Mount Sinai Hospital, Toronto, Canada

SECTION 1

Inflammation

Section editor: Rob Pickard

CHAPTER 1.1

Pathogenesis of urinary tract infection

Ased Ali

Introduction to urinary tract infection

Urinary tract infection (UTI) is one of the most common bacterial infections to affect humans. Its incidence increases with age and the cumulative probability of a woman having had a UTI by the age of 50 is approximately 50%.[1] The normally sterile urinary tract is the site of an ongoing but complex interplay between an evolving pathogen and a highly developed host immune defence system, such that the pathogenesis of a UTI generally requires either greater virulence in the pathogen or deficient host defence. Typically, the process of infection begins with attachment of the uropathogen to the epithelial surface; it subsequently forms colonies, which then disseminate and invade through the urothelial tissue. This dissemination may be associated with ascent up the urinary tract, which may manifest symptomatically as cystitis (in the bladder) or pyelonephritis (in the kidney). Symptomatic infection indicates a powerful immune response and the interplay between pathogen and host will continue, influencing the extent and level of invasion, the duration of infection, and the degree of tissue damage.

An understanding of bacterial pathogenesis and anti-adherence defence mechanisms is important for clinicians so that appropriate strategies for the management and prevention of UTI are used. This section outlines current understanding of the pathogenesis of UTI, with particular emphasis on bacterial virulence and interaction with host defences, together with other factors which increase susceptibility to UTI.

Routes of infection

The ascending route is the commonest mode of infection of the urinary tract with most bacteria originating from the individual's own lower bowel and subsequently colonizing the periurethral tissue before ascending through the urethra and into the bladder.[2] Colonization of the periurethral mucosa with bowel flora is particularly problematic in females, where the shorter urethra provides a convenient conduit for invading pathogens and rapid entry to the lower urinary tract. Even small variations in perineal anatomy in females can increase susceptibility; for example, women with an anal to urethral distance of less than 4.5 cm are at increased risk of UTI.[3] These anatomical risks can be further increased by the influence of external agents such as spermicides, faecal contamination of the perineum, and the use of urethral catheters.[4,5]

Symptomatic UTI is usually confined to the bladder (cystitis), but in up to a half of cases there are signs indicating upper urinary tract involvement such as fever and loin pain.[6] Pyelonephritis is most frequently caused by the ascent of bacteria from the bladder up the ureter and into the renal pelvis, with subsequent invasion of the renal parenchyma through the collecting ducts and disruption of the renal tubules. Certain pathogenic bacterial virulence factors including P-fimbriae and endotoxins can enhance the ability of bacteria to ascend the urinary tract, as can host susceptibility factors such as pregnancy and ureteral obstruction, which inhibit peristalsis.

Haematogenous infection of the urinary tract is uncommon in normal individuals. However, patients with primary foci of infection elsewhere in the body involving *Staphylococcus aureus, Candida spp., Salmonella spp.*, and *Mycobacterium tuberculosis* can suffer secondary kidney infection. The risk of such infection is enhanced when urine drainage from the kidney is obstructed.[7] Infection via the lymphatic route is rare but can be caused by direct invasion of bacteria from adjacent organs in conditions that result in retroperitoneal sepsis and suppuration. The lymphatic route is not thought to play a significant role in the majority of UTIs.

Pathogenic bacterial virulence factors

The interplay between host and pathogen is at the heart of any UTI. Uropathogenic *Escherichia coli* (UPEC) strains for example encode a number of virulence factors, which enable the bacterial clone to colonize the urinary tract and persist in the face of host defences. In recent years, great advances have been made in the understanding of these virulence factors. Prior to their migration, these bacteria will typically have come from a commensal site, such as the bowel. The role of virulence factors is therefore critical in the understanding of how commensals at one site act as pathogens at another.

UPEC strains exhibit a high degree of genetic diversity facilitated by the possession of specialized virulence genes located on specific transferable genetic elements known as pathogenicity islands, which may be as large as 170 kb and can increase the size of the pathogen genome by about 20% over a commensal strain.[8,9] Virulence factors may be broadly divided into two groups according to whether or not they are involved in bacterial adhesion to host epithelium.

Adhesive virulence factors

The presentation of cell surface adhesive organelles (adhesins) by UPEC is one of the most significant determinants of pathogenicity. UPEC may express several adhesins that allow it to attach to urinary tract tissues and contribute to virulence in different ways which include: directly triggering host and bacterial cell signalling pathways; facilitating the delivery of other bacterial products to host tissues; and promoting bacterial invasion.[10] The best characterized group of adhesins are the fimbriae.

Type I fimbriae

Type I fimbriae are the most commonly expressed fimbriae on *E. coli* (Fig. 1.1.1) and are composed of a helical rod with repeating FimA subunits that are bound to a distal tip structure containing the FimH adhesin.[11] Classically these fimbriae (also called type I pili) were shown to mediate haemagglutination of guinea pig erythrocytes[12] and the reaction could be inhibited by the addition of mannose; mannose-sensitive haemagglutination (MSHA).[13,14]

However, while type I fimbriae have been shown to function as virulence factors in animal models of UTI where they facilitate bacterial colonization, their function in human infection is less clear.[10,15–17] This uncertainty arises from the observation that type I fimbriae are expressed in both pathogenic and commensal strains[18,19]; furthermore, there is no significant difference in the Fim gene frequency between more or less virulent strains in the urinary tract.[20] In the mouse model, type I fimbriae bind to the urothelial mannosylated glycoproteins uroplakin Ia (UPIa) and Ib (UP1b) via the adhesin subunit FimH, located at the fimbrial tip.[21] Uroplakins are membrane proteins that are found on the luminal surface of the umbrella cells of bladder epithelium. Interaction between FimH and uroplakins stimulates signalling pathways involved in bacterial invasion and epithelial cell apoptosis and may also contribute to mucosal inflammation.[17,22–24] In humans, the main evidence for the role of type I fimbriae comes from the analysis of urinary bacterial isolates from patients with UTI, which were found to express mannose-sensitive adhesins.[25]

Murine studies show that after binding to the urothelial surface, bacteria with FimH adhesins are quickly internalized within the epithelium as a result of localized actin rearrangement and engulfment of the bound bacterium by the epithelial cell membrane.[26] Within the superficial urothelium, UPEC is able to establish a new niche as a mechanism to avoid host innate immune response.

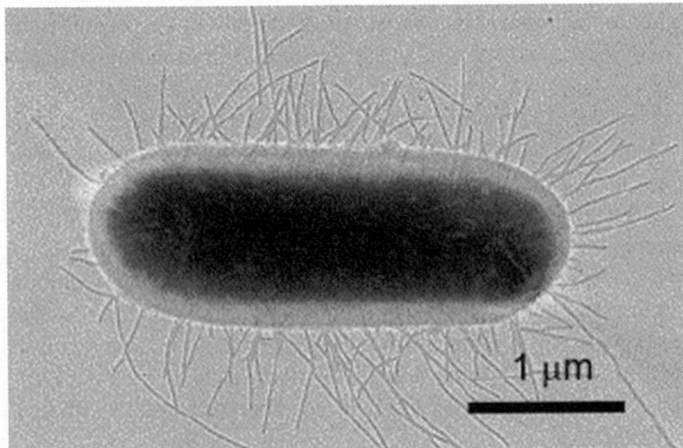

Fig. 1.1.1 Electron micrograph of a uropathogenic *E. coli* cell bearing type 1 fimbriae.

Reprinted from *Microbes and Infection*, Volume 8, Issue 8, Guido Capitani *et al.*, 'Structural and functional insights into the assembly of type 1 pili from Escherichia coli', pp. 2284–2290, Copyright © 2006 Elsevier SAS, with permission from Elsevier, http://www.sciencedirect.com/science/journal/12864579

Within the epithelial cell, UPEC proliferates in the cytosol to form clusters known as intracellular bacterial communities (IBCs).[27] After six to eight hours, the morphology of the bacteria changes to an engulfing biofilm phenotype that further protects the uropathogen from the host immune response.[28] This process has yet to be demonstrated in human cells however.

The biofilm phenotype is characterized by decreased growth rate, allowing the formation of a biofilm matrix. This matrix is able to prevent attack from neutrophils and is also effective at preventing penetration by both host antimicrobials and external antibiotics. Animal models also suggest that bacteria at the edge of IBCs are able to detach and become motile again to re-enter the urine and then re-adhere to the superficial urothelium and reinvade cells to form further IBCs.[29] Ultimately, after a few days, possibly as a result of ongoing immune activity, the invasive bacteria enter a quiescent state, but may persist in a dormant state in IBCs before re-emerging later to cause recurrent infection.[27]

P-fimbriae

P-fimbriae (named from their interaction with P-blood group antigens) mediate haemagglutination of human erythrocytes that is not altered by mannose, which is thus termed mannose-resistant haemagglutination (MRHA). P-fimbriae are believed to play a key role in ascending UTI and pyelonephritis.[30,31] They are heteropolymeric fibres made up of various peptides encoded by the papA-K gene.[32] The adhesin PapG, at the tip of these fimbriae, recognizes kidney glycosphingolipids carrying the α-d-galactopyranosyl-(1–4)-β-d-galactopyranoside determinant on renal epithelia.[30,33,34] The attachment of P-fimbriae leads to the release of ceramide, which acts as an agonist of Toll-like receptor 4 (*TLR 4*), a receptor involved in activation of the innate immune response including antimicrobial peptide and cytokine production.[35] This then activates an inflammatory response cascade producing the symptoms of pyelonephritis.[16]

P-fimbriae may also work synergistically with type I fimbriae by enhancing early colonization of the tubular epithelium, while the latter mediates colonization of the tubular lumen by forming a biofilm. This colony then disrupts tubular filtration, leading to obstruction of nephron and the symptoms of pyelonephritis.[36] P-fimbriae have also been implicated as one of the key virulence factors involved in acute kidney dysfunction in renal transplant patients.[37]

Other adhesins

S-fimbriae and F1C fimbriae have also been shown to play a role in UTI. S-fimbriae bind to sialic acid residues via the SfaS adhesin; this facilitates bacterial dissemination within host tissues and is often associated with *E. coli* strains that cause sepsis, meningitis, and ascending UTIs.[10] F1C fimbriae bind to glycosphingolipids in renal epithelial cells and induce an interleukin-8 inflammatory response.[38] Fimbrial Dr and afimbrial Afa adhesins of *E. coli* are associated with recurrent UTI and UTI during pregnancy.[39–42] Murine models suggest that that Dr and Afa adhesins play a role in the development of chronic kidney infection.[43,44]

Non-adhesive virulence factors

UPEC, in common with other Gram-negative organisms, also has cell wall modifications, motility enhancements, and secreted toxins that further enhance pathogenicity.

Polysaccharides

The bacterial capsule and lipopolysaccharide (LPS) both act as virulence factors. The capsule is a polysaccharide covering for the bacteria that protect it from the host immune system's responses, particularly phagocytic engulfment and complement-mediated attack. Some capsular subtypes, such as K1 and K5 mimic components of host tissue, preventing effective immune response.[45]

LPS is a core component of the cell wall of Gram-negative bacteria, and in UPEC is an important activator of pro-inflammatory epithelial response via the induction of nitric oxide, as well as antimicrobial peptide and cytokine production.[46,47] However, the systemic immune response evoked by UPEC LPS may also have detrimental effects by causing acute kidney injury, particularly in renal transplant patients with UTI.[48,49]

Flagellum

Flagellum, the organelle made up of flagellin protein and responsible for bacterial motility plays a role in the virulence of many UPEC strains for both lower and upper urinary tract infection. Flagella activity may allow bacteria to ascend from the bladder and cause pyelonephritis. These UPEC strains may invade renal collecting duct cells through flagellin acting as an epithelial invasion through interaction with the *TLR 5* receptor.[50] Mice deficient in TLR5 are more susceptible to UPEC infection in both the bladder and the kidney, suggesting that flagellin may be involved in the original ascent into the bladder.[51]

Secreted factors

Secretion of toxins by UPEC and other Gram-negative bacteria is often responsible for inflammatory response and symptoms. The most significant toxin is a lipoprotein called α-haemolysin (HlyA) which is frequently associated with pyelonephritis and renal scarring.[52] α-haemolysin is a pore-forming toxin of the repeats in toxin (RTX) family that are common among Gram-negative pathogens.[53,54] At high concentrations it lyses erythrocytes and host cells, enabling bacteria to cross epithelial barriers, damage immune cells, and gain access to host iron stores.[45,55,56] At low concentrations, it can induce apoptosis of host immune cells and promote the exfoliation of bladder epithelial cells.[57,58] It can also affect intracellular calcium levels in renal epithelial cells, with consequent increases in IL-6 and IL-8 production.[59]

Cytotoxic necrotizing factor 1 (CNF1) is produced by around one-third of all pyelonephritis UPEC strains.[60] Experimental data suggest that CNF1 disrupts the epithelial cell membrane, allowing bacterial invasion.[61] In addition, it has been shown to interfere with polymorphonuclear phagocytosis and cause apoptosis of bladder epithelial cells, thus increasing bladder exfoliation and exposure of vulnerable underlying cells.[62,63]

Other secreted proteins include secreted autotransporter toxin (SAT) and Toll/interleukin (IL-1) receptor (TIR) domain-containing protein (Tcp). *In vitro*, SAT has toxic activity against bladder and kidney cells, suggesting a role in the early pathogenesis of UTI.[64] Recent work has found that Tcp is able to subvert epithelial Toll-like receptor (TLR) signalling, preventing early initiation of the innate immune response, thereby facilitating bacterial survival and kidney infection (Fig. 1.1.2).[65]

Host defences against uropathogenic *Escherichia coli* colonization of the urinary tract

The constant challenge of microbial invasion of the urinary tract epithelium from the host's own bowel has mobilized a variety of host defensive mechanisms to prevent bacterial colonization and survival. The first line of defence is aimed at preventing or limiting bacterial adherence to the epithelium. Once adhesion has occurred, further responses are activated.

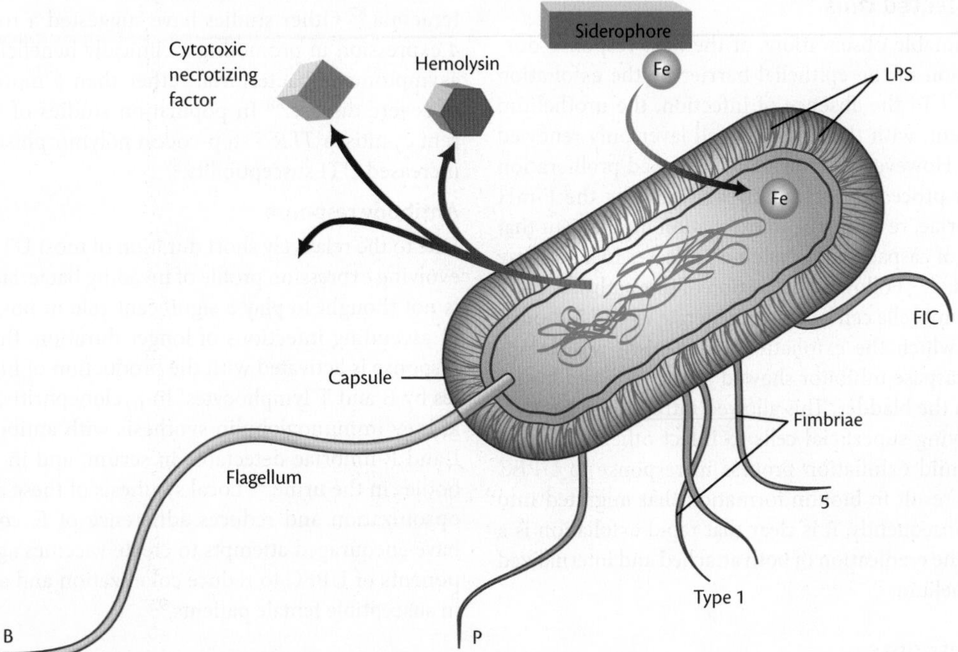

Fig 1.1.2 Diagram of a uropathogenic *E. coli* cell bearing type I fimbriae.

Reproduced from Springer, *The Atlas of Infectious Diseases*, Volume 9, 2004, Chapter 1, Edward S. Wong, Jack Sobel, and Gerald Mandell, Figure: Virulence determinants of uropathogenic *Escherichia coli*, Copyright © 2004. With kind permission from Springer Science+Business Media B.V.

Constitutive defences

The normal urinary tract has a number of constitutive (continually present) physiological and immune defences to prevent or avert bacterial colonization. First is the 'washout' effect of urine flow. This rinses away loosely adherent or non-attached pathogens from the epithelial surface.[66] Adherence is further limited by the secretion of glucosamines by the urothelium, which form a protective layer on the luminal surface. The high urinary osmolality and low pH make it difficult for poorly adapted bacteria to survive.

Within the urine there are also a number of larger proteins, which have been identified as important in innate urinary immune defence. The most characterized is Tamm–Horsfall protein (THP), a glycoprotein secreted by the loop of Henlé epithelium present at high concentrations in the urine. THP acts as an anti-adhesive urinary factor by complexing with UPEC type I fimbriae, which is then cleared by voiding.[67] THP knockout mice have been shown to clear *E. coli* less rapidly and go on to develop chronic bladder wall inflammation suggestive of persistent infection.[68] Other renal epithelial proteins, such as lactoferrin and lipocalin also show antimicrobial activity through the sequestering of iron. Cathelicidin and defensins; small, highly cationic antimicrobial peptides, are also secreted by urothelium in response to pathogens.[47] These peptides work in a non-specific manner by attachment to the anionic phospholipids on the bacterial cell wall—disrupting their cell membrane, increasing cell permeability, and causing cell death.[69]

Activated responses

Bacteria that overcome these initial defences are able to have prolonged contact with the urothelium, resulting in the activation of further host immune defence mechanisms. These include epithelial exfoliation and the induction of a local and systemic inflammatory response.

Exfoliation of infected cells

One of the most notable observations of the host response during UTI is disruption of the epithelial barrier by the exfoliation of infected cells.[70,71] In the absence of infection, the urothelium is relatively quiescent, with the umbrella cell layer only renewed every few months. However, the normally repressed proliferation and differentiation processes are rapidly activated by the FimH component of fimbriae, resulting in an exfoliation mechanism that involves activation of caspases and cysteine proteases in a pathway similar to apoptosis.[72,73] Following activation of this pathway, there is potential for the umbrella cell layer to regenerate within 24 hours.

Experiments in which the exfoliation mechanism was dampened using a pan-caspase inhibitor showed greatly reduced bacterial expulsion from the bladder. This allowed intracellular bacteria to transfer from dying superficial cells to infect other cells.[74] In mouse studies, a mild exfoliation process in response to UPEC was more likely to result in biofilm formation that migrated into deeper layers.[27] Consequently, it is clear that rapid exfoliation is a key mechanism in the eradication of both attached and internalized bacteria from urothelium.

Inflammatory response

Successful bacterial adherence to urothelium triggers a variety of other innate immune responses. These are characterized by the production of a number of pro-inflammatory mediators, including cytokines and chemokines.[75–77] Bladder and kidney epithelial cells appear to be a major source of interleukin-6 (IL-6) and interleukin-8 (IL-8) after infection with UPEC, which are important in the development of local tissue damage.[78–79]

IL-6 possesses a variety of pro-inflammatory functions, including neutrophil recruitment and production of acute phase proteins.[80] IL-8 is also a potent neutrophil chemotactic agent. In humans, induction of IL-8 correlates with appearance of neutrophils in the urine.[75] Neutrophil recruitment to the site of infection has been shown to be critical for bacterial clearance from both the bladder and kidney, and their presence is a clinical diagnostic for UTI. Other immune competent cells, such as macrophages, eosinophils, and natural killer cells are also recruited and granulocytes synthesize nitric oxide, which can kill invading bacteria.[81]

Neutrophil migration to the site of infection is initiated by specific bacterial components, which activate pathogen-associated molecular pattern receptors (PAMPs) such as Toll-like receptors (TLRs).[82,83] This triggers a signalling pathway that initiates epithelial antimicrobial and wider inflammatory responses. The primary receptors expressed on urothelium are *TLR 2, 4,* and *5. TLR 2* is activated by peptidoglycan, part of the cell wall of bacteria. *TLR 4* and its co-receptors (CD14 and MD2) recognize bacterial LPS and *TLR 5* is activated by flagellin. Bacteria can evade these responses by expressing virulence factors such as Tcp to inhibit some *TLR*-activated pathways.[65,84] The importance of these early interactions between bacterium and epithelial cell has been further highlighted by the effect of gene polymorphisms. In mice, polymorphisms of the *TLR 4* gene are associated with reduced sensitivity to LPS, absence of neutrophil recruitment, and delayed clearance of bacteria from the urinary tract.[85] Recently, it was also observed that infected mouse urothelial cells were over time able to expel intracellular *E. coli* via a *TLR 4*-initiated and cyclic AMP-mediated mechanism.[86] In humans, a *TLR 4* polymorphism has been shown to increase susceptibility to septic shock and Gram-negative bacteraemia.[87] Other studies have suggested a role for reduced *TLR 4* expression in promoting a clinically beneficial tolerance state in asymptomatic bacteriuria, rather than a more harmful situation of severe disease.[88] In population studies of women with recurrent cystitis, a *TLR 5* stop-codon polymorphism is associated with increased UTI susceptibility.[89]

Antibody response

Due to the relatively short duration of most UTI and the constantly evolving expression profile of invading bacteria, adaptive immunity is not thought to play a significant role in host defence. However, in ascending infections of longer duration, the adaptive immune response is activated with the production of high-affinity antibodies by B and T lymphocytes. In pyelonephritis, there is serum and kidney immunoglobulin synthesis with antibodies targeting type I and P-fimbriae detectable in serum, and in IgG and SIgA antibodies in the urine.[90] Local synthesis of these antibodies enhances opsonization and reduces adherence of *E. coli*.[91] These findings have encouraged attempts to create vaccines against fimbrial components of UPEC to reduce colonization and ascending infections in susceptible female patients.[92]

Further reading

Ali AS, Townes CL, Hall J, Pickard RS. Maintaining a sterile urinary tract: the role of antimicrobial peptides. *J Urol* 2009; **182**(1):21–8.

Anderson GG, Dodson KW, Hooton TM, Hultgren SJ. Intracellular bacterial communities of uropathogenic Escherichia coli in urinary tract pathogenesis. *Trends Microbiol* 2004; **12**(9):424–30.

Bower JM, Eto DS, Mulvey MA. Covert operations of uropathogenic Escherichia coli within the urinary tract. *Traffic* 2005; **6**(1):18–31.

Foxman B, Barlow R, D'Arcy H, Gillespie B, Sobel JD. Urinary tract infection: self-reported incidence and associated costs. *Ann Epidemiol* 2000; **10**(8):509–15.

Ganz T. Defensins: antimicrobial peptides of innate immunity. *Nat Rev Immunol* 2003; **3**(9):710–20.

Hooton TM, Scholes D, Hughes JP, *et al.* A prospective study of risk factors for symptomatic urinary tract infection in young women. *N Engl J Med* 1996; **335**(7):468–74.

Johnson JR. Virulence factors in Escherichia coli urinary tract infection. *Clin Microbiol Rev* 1991; **4**(1):80–128.

Kaper JB, Nataro JP, Mobley HL. Pathogenic Escherichia coli. *Nat Rev Microbiol* 2004; **2**(2):123–40.

Le Bouguénec C. Adhesins and invasins of pathogenic Escherichia coli. *Int J Med Microbiol* 2005; **295**(6–7):471–8.

Mulvey MA. Adhesion and entry of uropathogenic Escherichia coli. *Cell Microbiol* 2002; **4**(5):257–71.

Oelschlaeger TA, Dobrindt U, Hacker J. Pathogenicity islands of uropathogenic E. coli and the evolution of virulence. *Int J Antimicrob Agents* 2002; **19**:517–21.

Reid G, Sobel JD. Bacterial adherence in the pathogenesis of urinary tract infection: a review. *Rev Infect Dis* 1987; **9**(3):470.

Schilling JD, Mulvey MA, Hultgren SJ. Dynamic interactions between host and pathogen during acute urinary tract infections. *Urology* 2001; **57**(6 Suppl 1):56–61.

Serafini-Cessi F, Malagolini N, Cavallone D. Tamm-Horsfall glycoprotein: biology and clinical relevance. *Am J Kidney Dis* 2003; **42**:658–76.

Song J, Abraham SN. TLR-mediated immune responses in the urinary tract. *Curr Opin Microbiol* 2008; **11**(1):66–73.

Wiles TJ, Kulesus RR, Mulvey MA. Origins and virulence mechanisms of uropathogenic Escherichia coli. *Exp Mol Pathol* 2008; **85**(1):11–9.

References

1. Foxman B, Barlow R, D'Arcy H, Gillespie B, Sobel JD. Urinary tract infection: self-reported incidence and associated costs. *Ann Epidemiol* 2000; **10**(8):509–15.
2. Handley MA, Reingold AL, Shiboski S, Padian NS. Incidence of acute urinary tract infection in young women and use of male condoms with and without nonoxynol-9 spermicides. *Epidemiology* 2002; **13**(4):431–6.
3. Hooton TM, Stapleton AE, Roberts PL, *et al.* Perineal anatomy and urine-voiding characteristics of young women with and without recurrent urinary tract infections. *Clin Infect Dis* 1999; **29**(6):1600–1.
4. Hooton TM, Scholes D, Hughes JP, *et al.* A prospective study of risk factors for symptomatic urinary tract infection in young women. *N Engl J Med* 1996; **335**(7):468–74.
5. Foxman B. Epidemiology of urinary tract infections: incidence, morbidity, and economic costs. *Am J Med* 2002; **113**(Suppl 1A):5S–13S.
6. Busch R, Huland H. Correlation of symptoms and results of direct bacterial localization in patients with urinary tract infections. *J Urol* 1984; **132**(2):282.
7. Smellie J, Edwards D, Hunter N, Normand IC, Prescod N. Vesico-ureteric reflux and renal scarring. *Kidney Int Suppl* 1975; **4**:S65–72.
8. Wiles TJ, Kulesus RR, Mulvey MA. Origins and virulence mechanisms of uropathogenic Escherichia coli. *Exp Mol Pathol* 2008; **85**(1):11–9.
9. Oelschlaeger TA, Dobrindt U, Hacker J. Pathogenicity islands of uropathogenic E. coli and the evolution of virulence. *Int J Antimicrob Agents* 2002; **19**:517–21.
10. Mulvey MA. Adhesion and entry of uropathogenic Escherichia coli. *Cell Microbiol* 2002; **4**(5):257–71.
11. Jones CH, Pinkner JS, Roth R, *et al.* FimH adhesin of type 1 pili is assembled into a fibrillar tip structure in the Enterobacteriaceae. *Proc Natl Acad Sci U S A* 1995; **92**(6):2081–5.
12. Duguid JP, Clegg S, Wilson MI. The fimbrial and non-fimbrial haemagglutinins of Escherichia coli. *J Med Microbiol* 1979; **12**:213–27.
13. Svenson SB, Hultberg H, Källenius G, Korhonen TK, Möllby R, Winberg J. P-fimbriae of pyelonephritogenic Escherichia coli: identification and chemical characterization of receptors. *Infection* 1983; **11**(1):61–7.
14. Reid G, Sobel JD. Bacterial adherence in the pathogenesis of urinary tract infection: a review. *Rev Infect Dis* 1987; **9**(3):470.
15. Hultgren SJ, Porter TN, Schaeffer AJ, Duncan JL. Role of type 1 pili and effects of phase variation on lower urinary tract infections produced by Escherichia coli. *Infect Immun* 1985; **50**(2):370–7.
16. Bergsten G, Wullt B, Svanborg C. Escherichia coli, fimbriae, bacterial persistence and host response induction in the human urinary tract. *Int J Med Microbiol* 2005; **295**(6–7):487–502.
17. Connell I, Agace W, Klemm P, Schembri M, Mărild S, Svanborg C. Type 1 fimbrial expression enhances Escherichia coli virulence for the urinary tract. *Proc Natl Acad Sci U S A*. 1996; **93**(18):9827–32.
18. Hagberg L, Jodal U, Korhonen TK, Lidin-Janson G, Lindberg U, Svanborg Edén C. Adhesion, hemagglutination, and virulence of Escherichia coli causing urinary tract infections. *Infect Immun* 1981; **31**(2):564–70.
19. Duguid JP, Old D. Adhesive properties of enterobacteriaceae. In: *Bacterial Adherence, Receptors and Recognition*, pp. 185–217. Beachey E (ed). London, UK: Chapman & Hall, 1980.
20. Plos K, Lomberg H, Hull S, Johansson I, Svanborg C. Escherichia coli in patients with renal scarring: genotype and phenotype of Gal alpha 1–4Gal beta-, Forssman- and mannose-specific adhesins. *Pediatr Infect Dis J* 1991; **10**(1):15–9.
21. Wu XR, Sun TT, Medina JJ. In vitro binding of type 1-fimbriated Escherichia coli to uroplakins Ia and Ib: relation to urinary tract infections. *Proc Natl Acad Sci U S A* 1996; **93**(18):9630–5.
22. Oelschlaeger TA, Dobrindt U, Hacker J. Virulence factors of uropathogens. *Curr Opin Urol* 2002; **12**(1):33–8.
23. Schembri MA, Klemm P. Biofilm formation in a hydrodynamic environment byel fimh variants and ramifications for virulence. *Infect Immun* 2001; **69**(3):1322–8.
24. Thumbikat P, Berry RE, Zhou G, *et al.* Bacteria-induced uroplakin signaling mediates bladder response to infection. *PLoS Pathog* 2009; **5**(5):e1000415.
25. Ljungh A, Wadstrom T. Fimbriation of Escherichia coli in urinary tract infections: Comparisons between bacteria in the urine and subcultured bacterial isolates. *Curr Microbiol* 1983; **8**:263.
26. Martinez JJ, Hultgren SJ. Requirement of Rho-family GTPases in the invasion of type 1-piliated uropathogenic Escherichia coli. *Cell Microbiol* 2002; **4**:19–28.
27. Anderson GG, Dodson KW, Hooton TM, Hultgren SJ. Intracellular bacterial communities of uropathogenic Escherichia coli in urinary tract pathogenesis. *Trends Microbiol* 2004; **12**(9):424–30.
28. Justice SS, Hung C, Theriot JA, *et al.* Differentiation and developmental pathways of uropathogenic Escherichia coli in urinary tract pathogenesis. *Proc Natl Acad Sci U S A* 2004; **101**(5):1333–8.
29. Schilling JD, Mulvey MA, Hultgren SJ. Dynamic interactions between host and pathogen during acute urinary tract infections. *Urology* 2001; **57**(6 Suppl 1):56–61.
30. Leffer H, Svanborg-Edén C. Glycolipid receptors for uropathogenic Escherichia coli on human erthrocytes and uroepithelial cells. *Infect Immun* 1981; **34**(3):920–9.
31. Vaisanen V, Elo J, Tallgren LG, Mannose-resistant haemagglutination and P antigen recognition are characteristic of Escherichia coli causing primary pyelonephritis. *Lancet* 1981; **2**(8260–8261):1366–9.
32. Hull RA, Gill RE, Hsu P. Construction and expression of recombinant plasmids encoding type 1 or D-mannose-resistant pili from a urinary tract infection Escherichia coli isolate. *Infect Immun* 1981; **33**(3):933–8.

33. Kaper JB, Nataro JP, Mobley HL. Pathogenic Escherichia coli. *Nat Rev Microbiol* 2004; **2**(2):123–40.
34. Lund B, Lindberg F, Marklund BI, Normark S. The PapG protein is the alpha-D-galactopyranosyl-(1----4)-beta-D-galactopyranose-binding adhesin of uropathogenic Escherichia coli. *Proc Natl Acad Sci U S A* 1987; **84**(16):5898–902.
35. Fischer H, Ellström P, Ekström K, Gustafsson L, Gustafsson M, Svanborg C. Ceramide as a TLR4 agonist; a putative signalling intermediate between sphingolipid receptors for microbial ligands and TLR4. *Cell Microbiol* 2007; **9**(5):1239–51.
36. Melican K, Sandoval RM, Kader A, *et al.* Uropathogenic Escherichia coli P and Type 1 fimbriae act in synergy in a living host to facilitate renal colonization leading to nephron obstruction. *PLoS Pathog* 2011; **7**(2):e1001298.
37. Rice JC, Peng T, Kuo YF, *et al.* Renal allograft injury is associated with urinary tract infection caused by Escherichia coli bearing adherence factors. *Am J Transplant* 2006; **6**(10):2375–83.
38. Bäckhed F, Alsén B, Roche N, *et al.* Identification of target tissue glycosphingolipid receptors for uropathogenic, F1C-fimbriated Escherichia coli and its role in mucosal inflammation. *J Biol Chem* 2002; **277**(20):18198–205.
39. Foxman B, Zhang L, Tallman P, *et al.* Virulence characteristics of Escherichia coli causing first urinary tract infection predict risk of second infection. *J Infect Dis* 1995; **172**(6):1536–41.
40. Nowicki B, Labigne A, Moseley S, Hull R, Hull S, Moulds J. The Dr hemagglutinin, afimbrial adhesins AFA-I and AFA-III, and F1845 fimbriae of uropathogenic and diarrhea-associated Escherichia coli belong to a family of hemagglutinins with Dr receptor recognition. *Infect Immun* 1990; **58**(1):279–81.
41. Garcia MI, Gounon P, Courcoux P, Labigne A, Le Bouguénec C. The afimbrial adhesive sheath encoded by the afa-3 gene cluster of pathogenic Escherichia coli is composed of two adhesins. *Mol Microbiol* 1996; **19**(4):683–93.
42. Servin AL. Pathogenesis of Afa/Dr diffusely adhering Escherichia coli. *Clin Microbiol Rev* 2005; **18**(2):264–92.
43. Goluszko P, Moseley SL, Truong LD, *et al.* Development of experimental model of chronic pyelonephritis with Escherichia coli O75:K5:H-bearing Dr fimbriae: mutation in the dra region prevented tubulointerstitial nephritis. *J Clin Invest* 1997; **99**(7):1662–72.
44. Le Bouguénec C. Adhesins and invasins of pathogenic Escherichia coli. *Int J Med Microbiol* 2005; **295**(6–7):471–8.
45. Johnson JR. Virulence factors in Escherichia coli urinary tract infection. *Clin Microbiol Rev* 1991; **4**(1):80–128.
46. Bäckhed F, Söderhäll M, Ekman P, Normark S, Richter-Dahlfors A. Induction of innate immune responses by Escherichia coli and purified lipopolysaccharide correlate with organ- and cell-specific expression of Toll-like receptors within the human urinary tract. *Cell Microbiol* 2001; **3**(3):153–8.
47. Ali AS, Townes CL, Hall J, Pickard RS. Maintaining a sterile urinary tract: the role of antimicrobial peptides. *J Urol* 2009; **182**(1):21–8.
48. Wolfs TG, Buurman WA, van Schadewijk A, *et al.* In vivo expression of Toll-like receptor 2 and 4 by renal epithelial cells: IFN-gamma and TNF-alpha mediated up-regulation during inflammation. *J Immunol* 2002 **1**; **168**(3):1286–93.
49. Samuelsson P, Hang L, Wullt B, Irjala H, Svanborg C. Toll-like receptor 4 expression and cytokine responses in the human urinary tract mucosa. *Infect Immun* 2004; **72**(6):3179–86.
50. Pichon C, Héchard C, du Merle L, *et al.* Uropathogenic Escherichia coli AL511 requires flagellum to enter renal collecting duct cells. *Cell Microbiol* 2009; **11**(4):616–28.
51. Andersen-Nissen E, Hawn TR, Smith KD, *et al.* Cutting edge: Tlr5-/- mice are more susceptible to Escherichia coli urinary tract infection. *J Immunol* 2007; **178**(8):4717–20.
52. Mobley HL, Green DM, Trifillis AL, *et al.* Pyelonephritogenic Escherichia coli and killing of cultured human renal proximal tubular epithelial cells: role of hemolysin in some strains. *Infect Immun* 1990; **58**(5):1281–9.
53. Eberspächer B, Hugo F, Bhakdi S. Quantitative study of the binding and hemolytic efficiency of Escherichia coli hemolysin. *Infect Immun* 1989; **57**(3):983–8.
54. Bhakdi S, Mackman N, Nicaud JM, Holland IB. Escherichia coli hemolysin damage target cell membranes by generating transmembrane pores. *Infect Immun* 1986; **52**(1):63–9.
55. Keane WF, Welch R, Gekker G, Peterson PK. Mechanism of Escherichia coli alpha-hemolysin-induced injury to isolated renal tubular cells. *Am J Pathol* 1987; **126**(2):350–7.
56. Cavalieri SJ, Bohach GA, Snyder IS. Escherichia coli alpha-hemolysin: characteristics and probable role in pathogenicity. *Microbiol Rev* 1984; **48**(4):326–43.
57. Smith YC, Grande KK, Rasmussen SB, O'Brien AD. Novel three-dimensional organoid model for evaluation of the interaction of uropathogenic Escherichia coli with terminally differentiated human urothelial cells. *Infect Immun* 2006; **74**(1):750–7.
58. Russo TA, Davidson BA, Genagon SA, *et al.* E. coli virulence factor hemolysin induces neutrophil apoptosis and necrosis/lysis in vitro and necrosis/lysis and lung injury in a rat pneumonia model. *Am J Physiol Lung Cell Mol Physiol* 2005; **289**(2):L207–16.
59. Uhlén P, Laestadius A, Jahnukainen T, *et al.* Alpha-haemolysin of uropathogenic E. coli induces Ca2+ oscillations in renal epithelial cells. *Nature* 2000; **405**(6787):694–7.
60. Landraud L, Gauthier M, Fosse T, Boquet P. Frequency of Escherichia coli strains producing the cytotoxic necrotizing factor (CNF1) in nosocomial urinary tract infections. *Lett Appl Microbiol* 2000; **30**(3):213–6.
61. Bower JM, Eto DS, Mulvey MA. Covert operations of uropathogenic Escherichia coli within the urinary tract. *Traffic* 2005; **6**(1):18–31.
62. Mills M, Meysick KC, O'Brien AD. Cytotoxic necrotizing factor type 1 of uropathogenic Escherichia coli kills cultured human uroepithelial 5637 cells by an apoptotic mechanism. *Infect Immun* 2000; **68**(10):5869–80.
63. Fiorentini C, Fabbri A, Matarrese P, Falzano L, Boquet P, Malorni W. Hinderance of apoptosis and phagocytic behaviour induced by Escherichia coli cytotoxic necrotizing factor 1: two related activities in epithelial cells. *Biochem Biophys Res Commun* 1997; **241**(2):341–6.
64. Guyer DM, Radulovic S, Jones FE, Mobley HL. Sat, the secreted autotransporter toxin of uropathogenic Escherichia coli, is a vacuolating cytotoxin for bladder and kidney epithelial cells. *Infect Immun* 2002; **70**(8):4539–46.
65. Cirl C, Wieser A, Yadav M, *et al.* Subversion of Toll-like receptor signaling by a unique family of bacterial Toll/interleukin-1 receptor domain-containing proteins. *Nat Med* 2008; **14**(4):399–406.
66. Sobel JD. Pathogenesis of urinary tract infection. Role of host defenses. *Infect Dis Clin North Am* 1997; **11**(3):531–49.
67. Serafini-Cessi F, Malagolini N, Cavallone D. Tamm-Horsfall glycoprotein: biology and clinical relevance. *Am J Kidney Dis* 2003; **42**:658–76.
68. Bates JM, Raffi HM, Prasadan K, *et al.* Tamm-Horsfall protein knockout mice are more prone to urinary tract infection: Rapid communication. *Kidney Int* 2004; **65**: 791–7.
69. Ganz T. Defensins: antimicrobial peptides of innate immunity. *Nat Rev Immunol* 2003; **3**(9):710–20.
70. Fukushi Y, Orikasa S, Kagayama M. An electron microscopic study of the interaction between vesical epitherlium and E. *Coli Invest Urol* 1979; **17**(1):61–8.
71. Mysorekar IU, Mulvey MA, Hultgren SJ, Gordon JI. Molecular regulation of urothelial renewal and host defenses during infection with uropathogenic Escherichia coli. *J Biol Chem* 2002; **277**(9):7412–9.

72. Mulvey MA, Lopez-Boado YS, Wilson CL, *et al.* Induction and evasion of host defenses by type 1-piliated uropathogenic Escherichia coli. *Science* 1998; **282**(5393):1494–7.
73. Klumpp DJ, Weiser AC, Sengupta S, Forrestal SG, Batler RA, Schaeffer AJ. Uropathogenic Escherichia coli potentiates type 1 pilus-induced apoptosis by suppressing NF-kappaB. *Infect Immun* 2001; **69**(11):6689–95.
74. Mulvey MA, Schilling JD, Hultgren SJ. Establishment of a persistent Escherichia coli reservoir during the acute phase of a bladder infection. *Infect Immun* 2001; **69**(7):4572–9.
75. Agace W, Hedges S, Andersson U, Andersson J, Ceska M, Svanborg C. Selective cytokine production by epithelial cells following exposure to Escherichia coli. *Infect Immun* 1993; **61**(2):602–9.
76. Schilling JD, Mulvey MA, Vincent CD, Lorenz RG, Hultgren SJ. Bacterial invasionments epithelial cytokine responses to Escherichia coli through a lipopolysaccharide-dependent mechanism. *J Immunol* 2001; **166**(2):1148–55.
77. Schilling JD, Martin SM, Hunstad DA, *et al.* CD14- and Toll-like receptor-dependent activation of bladder epithelial cells by lipopolysaccharide and type 1 piliated Escherichia coli. *Infect Immun* 2003; **71**(3):1470–80.
78. Hedges S, Anderson P, Lidin-Janson G, de Man P, Svanborg C. Interleukin-6 response to deliberate colonization of the human urinary tract with gram-negative bacteria. *Infect Immun* 1991; **59**(1):421–7.
79. Ko YC, Mukaida N, Ishiyama S, *et al.* Elevated interleukin-8 levels in the urine of patients with urinary tract infections. *Infect Immun* 1993; **61**(4):1307–14.
80. Otto G, Braconier J, Andreasson A, Svanborg C. Interleukin-6 and disease severity in patients with bacteremic and nonbacteremicrile urinary tract infection. *J Infect Dis* 1999; **179**(1):172–9.
81. Jantausch BA, O'Donnell R, Wiedermann BL. Urinary interleukin-6 and interleukin-8 in children with urinary tract infection. *Pediatr Nephrol* 2000; **15**(3–4):236–40.
82. Gabay C. Interleukin-6 and chronic inflammation. *Arthritis Res Ther* 2006; **8**(Suppl 2):S3.
83. Poljakovic M, Persson K. Urinary tract infection in iNOS-deficient mice with focus on bacterial sensitivity to nitric oxide. *Am J Physiol Renal Physiol* 2003; **284**(1):F22–31.
84. Albiger B, Dahlberg S, Henriques-Normark B, Normark S. Role of the innate immune system in host defence against bacterial infections: focus on the Toll-like receptors. *J Intern Med* 2007; **261**(6):511–28.
85. Song J, Abraham SN. TLR-mediated immune responses in the urinary tract. *Curr Opin Microbiol* 2008; **11**(1):66–73.
86. Billips BK, Schaeffer AJ, Klumpp DJ. Molecular basis of uropathogenic Escherichia coli evasion of the innate immune response in the bladder. *Infect Immun* 2008; **76**(9):3891–900.
87. Haraoka M, Hang L, Frendéus B, *et al.* Neutrophil recruitment and resistance to urinary tract infection. *J Infect Dis* 1999; **180**(4):1220–9.
88. Song J, Bishop BL, Li G, Duncan MJ, Abraham SN. TLR4-initiated and cAMP-mediated abrogation of bacterial invasion of the bladder. *Cell Host Microbe* 2007; **1**(4):287–98.
89. Lorenz E, Mira JP, Frees KL, Schwartz DA. Relevance of mutations in the TLR4 receptor in patients with gram-negative shock. *Arch Intern Med* 2002; **162**(9):1028–32.
90. Ragnarsdóttir B, Jönsson K, Urbano A, *et al.* Toll-like receptor 4 promoter polymorphisms: common TLR4 variants protect against severe urinary tract infection. *PLoS One* 2010; **5**(5):e10734.
91. Hawn TR, Scholes D, Li SS, *et al.* Toll-like receptor polymorphisms and susceptibility to urinary tract infections in adult women. *PLoS One* 2009; **4**(6):e5990.
92. Rene P, Dinolfo M, Silverblatt FJ. Serum and urogenital antibody responses to Escherichia coli pili in cystitis. *Infect Immun* 1982; **38**(2):542–7.
93. de Ree JM, van den Bosch JF. Serological response to the P fimbriae of uropathogenic Escherichia coli in pyelonephritis. *Infect Immun* 1987; **55**(9):2204–7.
94. Uehling DT, Hopkins WJ, Dahmer LA, Balish E. Phase I clinical trial of vaginal mucosal immunization for recurrent urinary tract infection. *J Urol* 1994; **152**(6 Pt 2):2308–11.

CHAPTER 1.2

Antimicrobial agents

Katherine E. Walton and Sally Ager

Introduction to antimicrobial agents

Urinary tract infections (UTIs) are common and they are experienced more frequently by women than men.[1] It is estimated that up to half of all women will have at least one UTI during their lifetime.[1] Healthcare-associated infections (HCAI) are recognized as important, potentially preventable causes of morbidity, mortality, and healthcare costs. In a recent prevalence survey, UTIs were the second commonest type of HCAI in English hospitals.[2] *Escherichia coli* is the commonest cause of UTI[3] and the urinary tract is the commonest source for *E. coli* bacteraemia (Fig. 1.2.1).[4]

Important risk factors for the development of UTI include sex, age, structural and functional abnormalities of the urinary tract, and catheterization or urinary tract instrumentation. Safe urological practice therefore relies on an understanding of the prevention and management of UTI, including judicious antimicrobial prescribing.

Antimicrobial agents are substances that kill or inhibit the growth of microorganisms, such as bacteria, fungi, or protozoa. Antibacterial agents affect bacteria. Strictly speaking, the term 'antibiotic' refers to antimicrobials produced by a microorganism, thus excluding synthetic antibacterials, although the terms 'antibiotic', 'antibacterial', and 'antimicrobial' are often used interchangeably.

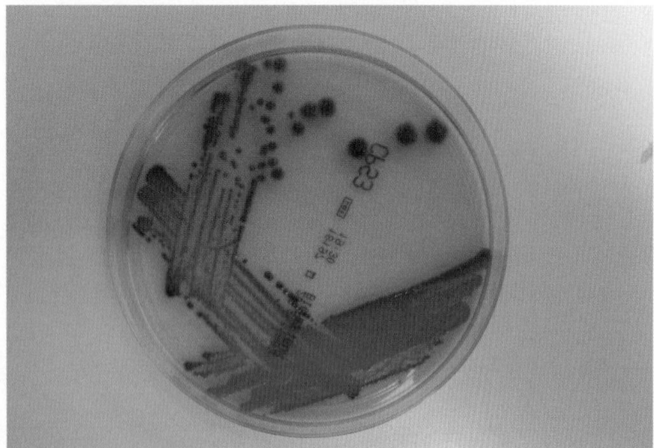

Fig. 1.2.1 *Escherichia coli (E. coli)* growing on chromogenic agar. *E. coli* is the commonest cause of urinary tract infections. Chromogenic media may be used in the laboratory to aid identification of potential uropathogens.
With kind permission of Jesmond IT.

Indications for antimicrobial prescribing

Antimicrobial agents are prescribed for the following reasons:

- Empirical therapy
- Directed therapy
- Prophylaxis

Empirical therapy

Antimicrobials are given based on the most likely causative organism(s) and local resistance patterns, before confirmation of the pathogen's identity. Empirical therapy is required for severe or life-threatening infection; it is important that appropriate, broad-spectrum antibiotics are started quickly, ideally within one hour of the presumptive diagnosis. Whenever possible, relevant diagnostic specimens should be collected prior to starting antimicrobial therapy (Fig. 1.2.2).

Directed therapy

Wherever possible, empirical therapy using broad-spectrum agents should be de-escalated to directed therapy using narrow spectrum antimicrobials once the identity and sensitivities of the pathogen are known. For less severe infections, particularly if the diagnosis is uncertain, it may be appropriate to await culture and sensitivity results before prescribing directed therapy, facilitating targeted treatment with narrow spectrum antimicrobials.

Prophylaxis

Prophylactic antimicrobials are given in circumstances where the risk or consequences of an infection are sufficiently severe to justify preventative action. It should be noted that the use of antibiotics is only part of a range of infection prevention measures.

Surgical prophylaxis

Antimicrobial prophylaxis is recommended for surgical procedures with a recognized risk of infection; generally, clean-contaminated or contaminated operations, and clean surgery involving implantation of prosthetic material.[5–7] Opening of the urinary tract is considered clean-contaminated surgery.[8] Local guidelines are based on the likely organisms associated with the procedure and local antimicrobial susceptibility patterns. Where possible, narrow spectrum agents should be chosen. Many guidelines advise avoidance of agents such as cephalosporins, quinolones, and clindamycin to minimize the risk of *Clostridium difficile* infection.[9]

In order to achieve maximum serum concentration during the procedure, intravenous antimicrobial prophylaxis should be administered at induction of anaesthesia or within 30–60 minutes before the operation starts.[5–8] Single-dose prophylaxis is usually adequate. A second dose may be indicated for significant intraoperative blood loss (more than 1.5 L) or prolonged operations.[5,6,8] Oral agents with good bioavailability can be considered but this may be less reliable and logistically more difficult to administer at the appropriate time.[6,7]

There is good evidence supporting antibacterial prophylaxis for transurethral resection of prostate (TURP) and transrectal prostate biopsy but there have been few studies for other urologic interventions.[10] Nevertheless, antimicrobial prophylaxis is currently recommended for a number of invasive urological procedures (see Table 1.2.1).[6–8,11]

Post-exposure prophylaxis

Post-exposure prophylaxis may be advised for contacts of certain communicable diseases in order to prevent transmission of the infection, for example meningococcal meningitis, pertussis, and tuberculosis.[11]

Prophylaxis of special patient groups

Antibacterial prophylaxis may also be recommended for certain individuals with factors that put them at higher risk for specific infections. For example, asplenic patients may receive phenoxymethylpenicillin in order to prevent pneumococcal infection.[11]

Prophylactic antibacterials may sometimes be prescribed for specific individuals in an attempt to prevent recurrent UTIs, for example in children with vesicoureteric reflux. Prophylaxis should generally only be considered following a risk assessment if other approaches are not possible. Long-term low-dose therapy is administered, basing the choice of agent on previous urinary culture and sensitivity results. Nitrofurantoin or trimethoprim may be considered as options.[11] Long-term antibiotic exposure may result in adverse drug effects and the development of antimicrobial resistance.

Principles of antimicrobial prescribing

Antimicrobial stewardship

Careful consideration must be given before antimicrobial agents are prescribed. They may cause allergic or other adverse reactions, and harm an individual's normal protective microbial flora.[12] Broad-spectrum antibacterial use is associated with the acquisition of resistant organisms such as extended spectrum beta-lactamase (ESBL)-producing Gram-negative bacteria[13,14] or methicillin-resistant *Staphylococcus aureus* (MRSA)[15–18] and the development of *Clostridium difficile* infection (CDI).[9,19–22] Adverse effects can be minimized by the introduction of antimicrobial stewardship programmes such as 'Start smart—then focus'.[23] Antibacterial drugs should not be prescribed unless there is an accepted prophylactic indication or clinical evidence of a bacterial infection requiring treatment. At the same time, patients with severe or life-threatening infections must receive prompt treatment with appropriate, often

Table 1.2.1 Prophylaxis for urological procedures

Procedure	Antibiotic prophylaxis recommended?			Likely pathogens
	EAU	AUA	SIGN	
Transurethral resection of prostate	Yes	Yes	Yes	Enterobacteriaceae and enterococci
Transrectal biopsy of prostate	Yes	Yes	Yes	Enterobacteriaceae and enterococci, possibly anaerobes
Transurethral resection of bladder tumour	No[1]	Yes	No	Enterobacteriaceae and enterococci
Percutaneous nephrolithotomy	Yes	Yes	Yes/No[2]	Enterobacteriaceae, enterococci, and staphylococci
Ureteroscopy for stone removal/fragmentation	Yes/No[3]	Yes	Yes	Enterobacteriaceae, enterococci, and staphylococci
Shock wave lithotripsy	Yes/No[4]	Yes	Yes	Enterobacteriaceae and enterococci
Cystoscopy/urodynamic investigation	No[5]	Yes/No[6]	No[5]	Enterobacteriaceae, enterococci, and staphylococci
Clean open or laparoscopic procedures (urinary tract not opened, e.g. nephrectomy)	No[5]	No[5]	No[7]	Skin organisms, catheter-associated organisms
Clean-contaminated procedures (urinary or gastrointestinal tracts opened, e.g. pyeloplasty, vaginal surgery, cystectomy)	Yes	Yes	Yes	Enterobacteriaceae, enterococci, and staphylococci
Implantation of prosthetic device	Yes	Yes	Yes	Enterobacteriaceae, enterococci, and skin organisms (e.g. staphylococci)
Contaminated open procedures (use of bowel segments)	Yes	Yes	Yes	Enterobacteriaceae, enterococci anaerobes, and skin organisms (e.g. staphylococci)

EAU = European Association of Urology; SIGN = Scottish Intercollegiate Guidelines Network; AUA = American Urological Association.

1: Consider in cases with high risk factors for UTI and for large necrotic tumours; 2: Recommended for stones 20 mm or greater or with pelvicalyceal dilation (one week preoperative fluoroquinolone recommended); 3: Recommended for proximal/impacted stone. Not recommended for uncomplicated distal stone (but consider in high-risk patients); 4: Not recommended for uncomplicated cases. Recommended in cases complicated by stent or nephrostomy catheter; 5: Consider in patients with high risk factors (bacteriuria, indwelling catheters, history of urogenital infection/abnormalities, immunosuppressed/post-transplant patients, diabetes mellitus, long inpatient stay, poor nutritional status, smoking, recent hospitalization, coexistent infection at other sites, older age, obesity); 6: Not if negative urine culture pre-procedure; 7: In children.

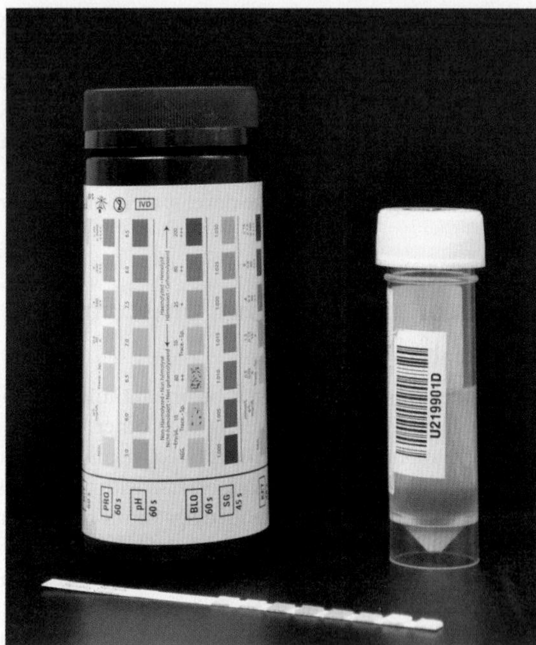

Fig. 1.2.2 Specimen of urine and urine test strip. Near-patient testing of urine samples, including analysis for the presence of leucocyte esterase, nitrites, protein, and blood, may be carried out using urine reagent strips (dipsticks) to give an early indication of the likelihood of urinary infection.
With kind permission of Jesmond IT.

broad-spectrum agents. If indicated, the choice of antimicrobial agent should normally be directed by local or national evidence-based guidelines and, whenever possible, diagnostic specimens should first be collected. Antimicrobial prescriptions should be accompanied by a clear record of the clinical indication, route of administration, duration, and review date. Oral administration is generally preferred, however, if intravenous antimicrobial treatment is required, it should be switched to oral medication as soon as this is safe. The duration of therapy depends on the type and nature of the infection and the clinical response to treatment. Local guidelines should specify standard durations for specific infections and courses should generally be kept to the minimum consistent with safety. Regular review of clinical progress and microbiology results facilitates the de-escalation of therapy, allowing patients who were initially commenced on broad-spectrum agents to be switched to targeted treatment with narrower spectrum antimicrobials. There should be regular review of local antimicrobial guidelines and audit of adherence to the key principles of judicious antimicrobial prescribing.

Antimicrobial choice

Local antimicrobial guidelines should be evidence-based and refer to available national guidelines.[23] Antibacterial choice will depend on the site and severity of the infection, the likely pathogens, and their local antimicrobial resistance patterns. Patient factors should also be considered, including age, clinical status, special factors such as pregnancy or immunosuppression, co-morbidities, allergies, medication which may result in potential drug interactions, previous microbiology results, and antimicrobial treatment history.

Important antimicrobial characteristics include the drug's spectrum of activity, routes of administration, potential side effects, and cost. Pharmacokinetics is the study of the effects of the body on a drug, including absorption, distribution, metabolism, and elimination, while pharmacodynamics is the study of the effect of the drug on the patient. Both factors help to determine optimal dosing regimens. Some antibacterial agents, such as the beta-lactams, are able to kill bacteria (bactericidal), while others only inhibit replication (bacteriostatic), for example sulphonamides. This may be a consideration when choosing therapy. The minimum inhibitory concentration (MIC) provides an assessment of an individual antibacterial agent's activity against a particular organism. Antimicrobials may show time-dependent or concentration-dependent killing. Dosing regimens that expose bacteria to drug concentrations above their MIC for as long as possible are preferred for time-dependent killing (e.g. penicillin therapy). To optimize concentration-dependent killing, peak serum concentrations should exceed the MIC of the target bacterium. This is important for aminoglycoside treatment.

Combination therapy

Treatment with a single antimicrobial agent is generally preferred, however, combination therapy is sometimes indicated. It may provide a broad spectrum of activity for mixed infections or be used for severe infections in immunocompromized patients, empirical treatment of life-threatening infections, or treatment of serious, deep-seated infections, such as prosthetic valve endocarditis. Combination therapy is also indicated for a few specific infections, such as tuberculosis, to prevent the development of resistant bacterial clones.[11]

Therapeutic drug monitoring

Measurement of serum concentration is advisable for some antimicrobials in order to minimize toxicity or determine whether effective concentrations have been achieved.[24] This is particularly important for drugs with a narrow therapeutic index, such as aminoglycosides, where the therapeutic band between effective and toxic concentrations is narrow. The correct timing of the sample is important: pre-dose (trough) concentrations are usually measured, although post-dose (peak) levels may sometime be helpful. Therapeutic drug monitoring is required for courses of parenteral gentamicin and vancomycin as well as other, less frequently used agents.[11,25] Local guidelines should be followed and the advice of a clinical microbiologist or other infection specialist sought in cases of uncertainty.

Prescribing for special patient groups

Patient factors are important when prescribing antimicrobial agents. Examples of special considerations for certain patient groups are given below:

Children

The pharmacokinetics and pharmacodynamics of drugs are often different in children. There may be a greater risk of adverse effects, particularly in the neonate, as a result of reduced drug clearance and different tissue sensitivities to toxins. Certain antimicrobial agents such as tetracyclines are contraindicated in children, while others should be used with caution (e.g. ciprofloxacin). When prescribing for children, the doses of antimicrobial agents must be carefully calculated.[26]

Pregnancy and breast feeding

A risk assessment should be carried out before drugs are prescribed during pregnancy as there may be the potential for teratogenicity or other harmful effects on the embryo or foetus. For example, tetracyclines, quinolones, and aminoglycosides should be avoided throughout pregnancy, trimethoprim should be avoided during the first trimester, and nitrofurantoin should be avoided at term.[11]

It is important to check whether individual antimicrobial agents may be safely prescribed to a breast-feeding mother. Some antimicrobial agents appear only as trace amounts in breast milk, while others reach higher concentrations and are therefore likely to be transmitted to the breast-feeding infant.[11]

The elderly

Serum and tissue concentrations may be increased in the elderly as a result of pharmacokinetic changes, such as reduced renal clearance. Older patients may have several co-morbidities and may also take multiple drugs, increasing the potential for adverse effects and drug interactions.

Hepatic impairment

Hepatic metabolism and elimination of drugs such as metronidazole may be impaired in patients with severe liver disease. In addition, drugs associated with dose-related or idiosyncratic hepatotoxicity may produce their adverse effects more frequently in patients with pre-existing hepatic impairment. For example, flucloxacillin and nitrofurantoin should be used with caution because of the risk of cholestatic jaundice. Monitoring of liver function tests is advised when some antibacterials (e.g. co-amoxiclav) are prescribed for patients with liver disease.

Renal impairment

Dose adjustment is required if reduced renal excretion may lead to drug or metabolite accumulation and toxicity (see Table 1.2.2). Aminoglycosides and glycopeptides should be avoided, or used with caution and careful therapeutic drug monitoring. Some antimicrobial agents, such as nitrofurantoin, will be ineffective for the treatment of UTIs if renal function is impaired because the drug will not achieve therapeutic concentrations in the urine. Expert advice should be sought about the appropriate dosing of antimicrobial agents in patients receiving renal replacement therapy.

The immunocompromized patient

Immunocompromized patients are at greater risk of severe and opportunistic infections. The type and severity of the immunodeficiency or immunosuppression determines the spectrum of likely infections; for example, neutropenic patients are particularly vulnerable to severe bacterial infections, including Gram-negative sepsis. Clinical signs and symptoms of infection may appear atypical as a result of the impaired host immune response. It is therefore important to remain vigilant for evidence of infection, obtain appropriate diagnostic samples, and institute empirical treatment as soon as a clinical diagnosis of severe bacterial infection is made (Fig. 1.2.3). Bactericidal agents are generally preferred for the treatment of severe infections in immunocompromized patients.

Antibiotic allergy

Before prescribing, it is important to ensure that there is no history of drug hypersensitivity. Attempts should be made to establish the nature of the allergic reaction and this should be clearly documented in the medical records. Penicillin allergy is relatively common, occurring in up to 10% of exposed individuals, however anaphylaxis is reported in less than 0.05%.[11] All penicillins should be avoided by patients allergic to one type of penicillin because of the risk of cross-hypersensitivity. Cephalosporins and other beta-lactams should also be avoided if there is a history suggesting an immediate hypersensitivity reaction to penicillins.[11]

Clostridium difficile infection (CDI)

Antibiotic exposure should be minimized, and avoided if possible, in patients with a past history of CDI. The Department of Health of England has advised that the use of some antibacterial drugs, such as cephalosporins, clindamycin, and ciprofloxacin, should be avoided in order to minimize the risk of CDI.[9] If antibacterial treatment must be given, then it is preferable to choose agents other than these and to keep the course as short as possible.

Colonization or infection with multiresistant bacteria

A history of previous colonization or infection with multiresistant organisms such as MRSA, glycopeptide-resistant enterococci (GRE), or multiresistant Gram-negative bacteria including ESBL-producers and carbapenemase-producing Enterobacteriaceae (CPE) should be considered if empirical therapy or prophylaxis is prescribed. It is useful to establish the patient's recent antimicrobial history because prolonged antibacterial therapy or exposure to multiple antibiotics, particularly in the inpatient setting, may predispose to colonization or infection with multidrug resistant bacteria. A travel history should be obtained to ascertain if the patient has travelled to countries or to areas of the UK known to have problems with the spread of CPE, and if they were treated in healthcare premises in these places. In England, hospital admissions must be risk assessed for MRSA and CPE carriage, and high-risk patients should be screened and isolated until screening results are available.[27,28]

Patients colonized with MRSA may be given topical decolonization therapy.[29] Local guidelines will indicate the circumstances under which this should be attempted, and the recommended topical agents. Preoperative screening ensures that appropriate antibacterial prophylaxis may be chosen for MRSA-positive patients and provides the opportunity to administer perioperative decolonization therapy.

Extremes of body weight

The 2015 health survey for England found that 27% of adults were obese, and the prevalence of morbid obesity was 2% in men and 4% in women.[30] Although treatment of patients at extremes of body weight is an increasing occurrence, there is limited data available to guide dosing. The site of infection is important. While the ideal body weight may help guide dosing in some circumstances, calculated doses may be inadequate for optimal treatment of certain severe infections in morbid obesity, particularly those that involve adipose tissue, such as necrotising fasciitis.[31]

Antibacterial agents

Mechanisms of action

Most antibacterial agents affect one of four targets:

- Cell wall synthesis
- Protein synthesis
- Nucleic acid synthesis
- Cell membrane integrity

Table 1.2.2 Antibacterial agents commonly used in urological practice[7,8,11,34]

Antibacterial agent	Usual dosing regimen	Common indications	Notes
Nitrofurantoin	◆ Treatment: 50–100 mg QDS PO or 100 mg BD for the modified-release formulation ◆ Prophylaxis: 50–100 mg PO nocte	Treatment and prophylaxis of lower urinary tract infection	◆ Avoid if creatinine clearance <45 mL/min/1.73 m^2* ◆ Avoid at term in pregnancy (risk of neonatal haemolysis)
Trimethoprim	◆ Treatment: 200 mg BD PO ◆ Prophylaxis: 100 mg nocte PO ◆ Reduce dose in severe renal impairment	Treatment and prophylaxis of lower urinary tract infection	Avoid during the first trimester of pregnancy
Co-trimoxazole	◆ Treatment: 960 mg BD PO ◆ Reduce dose in severe renal impairment	Consider as second-line directed therapy for lower urinary tract infection if pathogen sensitive and there is justification for use in place of trimethoprim	◆ Avoid in first and third trimesters of pregnancy ◆ Coadministration of warfarin and co-trimoxazole may result in a rise in INR
Amoxicillin	◆ 250–500 mg TDS PO or 500 mg–1 g tds IV ◆ Reduce dose in severe renal impairment	Treatment of uncomplicated urinary tract infection where uropathogen is known to be sensitive	
Ampicillin	◆ 250–500 mg QDS PO or 500 mg QDS IV ◆ Reduce dose in severe renal impairment	Treatment of uncomplicated urinary tract infection where uropathogen is known to be sensitive	
Flucloxacillin	◆ 500 mg QDS PO or 500 mg–2 g QDS IV ◆ Reduce dose in severe renal impairment (eGFR <10 mL/min/1.73 m^2)	Treatment of skin and soft tissue infections such as surgical wound infections	
Co-amoxiclav	◆ 375 mg or 625 mg PO 6–8 hourly or 1.2 g 8-hourly IV ◆ In renal impairment (eGFR <30 mL/min/1.73 m^2), give initial dose, then reduce dose	◆ Second-line agent for treatment of simple cystitis caused by bacteria resistant to first-line agents ◆ Consider as treatment for complicated UTIs including pyelonephritis, depending on local antimicrobial sensitivity patterns ◆ Perioperative prophylaxis	
(Piv)mecillinam	◆ 400 mg po initial loading dose then 200–400 mg TDS PO ◆ Reduce dose in renal impairment if prolonged treatment planned	Second-line agent for treatment of lower urinary tract infection caused by uropathogens resistant to first-line agents	Useful option for oral treatment of infections caused by beta-lactamase-producing organisms
Piperacillin-tazobactam	◆ 4.5 g TDS IV ◆ Increase interval between doses to 12-hourly in severe renal impairment (eGFR <20 mL/min/1.73 m^2)	Treatment of complicated UTIs such as pyelonephritis and urosepsis	
Cefalexin	◆ 250 mg qds or 500 mg TDS PO ◆ Reduce dose in renal impairment	Treatment of uncomplicated lower UTIs	Useful option in pregnancy
Cefuroxime	◆ 750 mg–1.5 g TDS IV ◆ Reduce dose in renal impairment (eGFR of less than 20 mL/min/1.73 m^2)	◆ Treatment of complicated UTIs, and urosepsis including pyelonephritis ◆ May be used as prophylaxis for urological procedures	◆ Useful option in pregnancy ◆ May be associated with *Clostridium difficile* infection
Ceftazidime	◆ Treatment: 1–2 g BD or TDS IV ◆ Reduce dose in renal impairment (eGFR less than 50 mL/min/1.73 m^2) ◆ Prophylaxis: 1 g IV	Treatment of serious, complicated urinary infections caused by pathogens resistant to first-line agents	May be associated with *Clostridium difficile* infection

(continued)

Table 1.2.2 Continued

Antibacterial agent	Usual dosing regimen	Common indications	Notes
Ertapenem	◆ 1 g OD IV ◆ Reduce dose in renal impairment	Licensed for abdominal infection, acute gynaecological infections, community-acquired pneumonia, and diabetic foot infections of skin and soft tissue	◆ Not active against *Pseudomonas aeruginosa* ◆ Off-license uses include treatment of severe sepsis, including complicated UTIs, polymicrobial infections, and infections caused by multi-resistant organisms, including ESBL producers
Meropenem	◆ 500 mg–1 g TDS IV ◆ Reduce dose in renal impairment	Treatment of severe sepsis, including complicated UTIs, polymicrobial infections, and infections caused by multiresistant organisms, including ESBL producers	Has antipseudomonal activity
Aztreonam	◆ 1 g TDS IV ◆ Reduce dose in renal impairment (eGFR less than 30 mL/min/1.73 m^2)	Treatment of serious Gram-negative infections, including urosepsis, caused by sensitive pathogens	
Gentamicin	◆ Treatment: 4–7 mg/kg IV OD ◆ Monitor serum levels and adjust dose ◆ To avoid excess dosing in obese patients, use ideal weight for height to calculate dose ◆ For once-daily dosing, a trough level (24-hours post-dose) of <1 mg/L gentamicin is satisfactory ◆ Alternatively, measure serum levels collected between 6 and 14 hours post-dose and use a nomogram to guide subsequent doses ◆ Prophylaxis: 1.5 mg/kg IV	◆ Treatment of complicated UTIs including pyelonephritis and urosepsis ◆ Prophylaxis for urological surgery	◆ Has antipseudomonal activity ◆ Use with caution in patients with renal impairment (reduce dose) ◆ Avoid in pregnancy ◆ Avoid once-daily regimens in patients with burns of >20%, endocarditis, or creatinine clearance of <20 mL/min
Vancomycin	◆ 1–1.5 g bd by slow IV infusion ◆ Monitor serum levels and adjust dose ◆ Maintain pre-dose (trough) levels between 10 and 15 mg/L—higher trough levels of 15–20 mg/L may be required for some specific indications ◆ Reduce dose in renal impairment	◆ Treatment of serious infections caused by resistant Gram-positive bacteria such as MRSA and *Enterococcus faecium* ◆ Second-line Gram-positive treatment for patients with penicillin allergy	
Oral vancomycin	◆ 125 mg PO QDS ◆ Dose may be increased up to 500 mg QDS PO for severe infections	Treatment of severe or recurrent *Clostridium difficile* infection	
Teicoplanin	◆ Weight ≤70 kg: loading dose of 400 mg IV BD for three doses, followed by 400 mg OD IV ◆ Weight >70 kg: loading dose of 6 mg/kg IV BD for three doses, followed by 6 mg/kg OD IV ◆ Reduce dose in renal impairment	◆ Treatment of serious infections caused by resistant Gram-positive bacteria such as MRSA and *Enterococcus faecium*. ◆ Second-line Gram-positive treatment for patients with penicillin allergy	Common indications: Treatment of Clostridium difficile infection
Fidaxomicin	200 mg PO BD for 10 days	Treatment of *Clostridium difficile* infection	Limited clinical data available for use in severe or life-threatening infection therefore caution advised
Ciprofloxacin	◆ 250–750 mg BD PO or 400 mg BD IV ◆ Reduce dose in renal impairment	◆ Second-line treatment of UTIs caused by uropathogens resistant to first-line agents ◆ Treatment of pyelonephritis, prostatitis, and epididymo-orchitis	◆ Has antipseudomonal activity although resistance may develop ◆ Avoid in children and pregnancy ◆ May be associated with *Clostridium difficile* infection

(continued)

Table 1.2.2 Continued

Antibacterial agent	Usual dosing regimen	Common indications	Notes
Colistin	◆ 1–2 million units IV TDS for patients over 60 kg ◆ Reduce dose and monitor levels in renal impairment	Reserve for the treatment of serious Gram-negative infections resistant to other antimicrobial agents	Avoid in pregnancy, especially during second and third trimesters
Linezolid	600 mg BD PO or IV	In UK, licensed for complicated skin and soft tissue infections and pneumonia—usually reserved for treatment of serious infections caused by resistant Gram-positive pathogens such as MRSA or for treatment of patients allergic to first-line agents	◆ A reversible non-selective monoamine oxidase inhibitor (MAOI) ◆ Use not advised while taking, or within two weeks of stopping, another MAOI ◆ Treatment usually limited to 10 days or less to minimize risk of adverse effects
Metronidazole	◆ Treatment: 400–500 mg TDS PO or 500 mg TDS IV ◆ Prophylaxis: 500 mg IV perioperatively ◆ Alternatively, prophylaxis may be given two hours prior to the procedure via the oral route (400 mg PO) or by the rectal administration of a 1 g suppository	◆ Treatment or prophylaxis of anaerobic infections ◆ Treatment of *Clostridium difficile* infection of mild or moderate severity (oral treatment is preferable to IV)	Disulfiram-like reaction if taken with alcohol

BD = 12 hourly; IV = intravenous; eGFR = estimated glomerular filtration rate; TDS = 8 hourly; PO = orally; INR = international normalized ratio; QDS = 6 hourly; nocte = at night; UTI = urinary tract infection.

*Nitrofurantoin may be used with caution in adults with eGFR 30–44 mL/min/1.73 m^2 for a short course only (3–7 days) to treat uncomplicated UTI caused by suspected/proven multiresistant bacteria and only if potential benefit outweighs risk.

Cell wall active agents

These include the beta-lactam agents (penicillins, cephalosporins, carbapenems, and monobactams) and glycopeptides. They competitively inhibit the carboxypeptidase and transpeptidase enzymes (also known as penicillin binding proteins, PBPs) that cross-link the bacterial cell wall polymer, peptidoglycan. This results in cell wall disruption, bacterial lysis, and death.

Inhibitors of protein synthesis

Mammalian and bacterial ribosomes differ in structure and the use of antibacterial agents affecting bacterial protein synthesis exploits

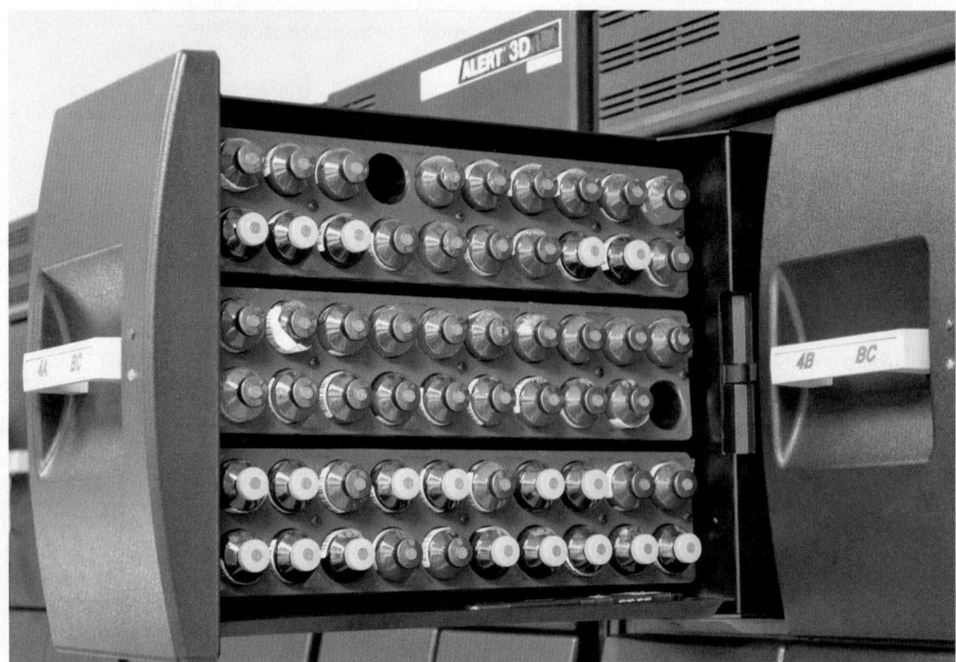

Fig. 1.2.3 Automated blood culture system (BioMerieux BacT/ALERT 3D). Appropriate diagnostic samples, including blood cultures, should be collected from patients presenting with serious urinary infections and urosepsis. Whenever possible, these should be taken before antimicrobial therapy is commenced.
With kind permission of Jesmond IT.

these differences. Aminoglycosides work by blocking the formation of the bacterial initiation complex. Other protein synthesis inhibitors include erythromycin, chloramphenicol, and tetracycline.

Inhibitors of nucleic acid synthesis

Sulphonamides and trimethoprim inhibit DNA synthesis by preventing the formation of purine and thymidine, acting at two different stages in the synthesis of folic acid. Sulphonamides are competitive agonists of para-aminobenzoic acid and trimethoprim inhibits the enzyme dihydrofolate reductase. Fluoroquinolones such as ciprofloxacin inhibit bacterial topoisomerases (DNA gyrases) that are involved in the supercoiling of DNA during nucleic acid synthesis. Metronidazole causes DNA breakage in anaerobic microorganisms.

Cell membrane disruption

Colistin is a polymyxin, which has detergent-like properties. It disrupts bacterial cell membranes, causing cell lysis and death.

Mechanisms of resistance

Bacteria may be intrinsically resistant to certain antimicrobial agents; for example, enterococcal resistance to cephalosporins, or resistance may develop via new mutations or by acquisition of genes from other bacteria. This allows rapid spread of resistance, which is promoted by antimicrobial selection pressure. Individual drugs may be susceptible to inactivation by several resistance mechanisms and some bacteria possess more than one mechanism of resistance.

There are five main mechanisms of antimicrobial resistance:

1. Inactivation or destruction;
2. Inhibition of transport into the cell;
3. Alteration of target site;
4. Bypass of affected metabolic pathway;
5. Active efflux.

Inactivation or destruction of the antimicrobial agent

Beta-lactamases are bacterial enzymes that can inactivate beta-lactam antibiotics by hydrolysis of the beta-lactam ring. There is a wide range of beta-lactamases; their classification is complex, based on spectrum of activity and inhibition or molecular structure. Extended spectrum beta-lactamase (ESBL) enzymes may be produced by some strains of *E. coli* and other coliform organisms, making them resistant to penicillins, aztreonam, and cephalosporins.

Inhibition of transport into the cell

Altered bacterial outer membrane proteins in some strains of *Pseudomonas aeruginosa* affect transport of imipenem into the cell, leading to resistance.

Alteration of antimicrobial target site

MRSA contains a penicillin binding protein (PBP) with a lower affinity for flucloxacillin than the PBP of methicillin-sensitive strains of *S. aureus*. Target site alteration is also a common cause of ciprofloxacin resistance and resistance to antimicrobial agents that act on the bacterial ribosome, such as erythromycin.

Bypass of affected metabolic pathway

Auxotrophs are strains of bacteria with different nutritional requirements from the original or 'wild strain'. These sometimes allow the organism to bypass the adverse effect of an antimicrobial agent. Thymidine-dependent bacteria have lost the enzyme thymidilate synthetase, and therefore require exogenous sources of thymidine for DNA synthesis. Use of pre-formed thymidine bypasses the earlier stages of folic acid production inhibited by trimethoprim and sulphonamides, causing resistance.

Active efflux of antimicrobial agent

Certain bacteria can actively pump antimicrobials, such as beta-lactams and quinolones, out of the cell causing resistance.

Antimicrobial susceptibility testing

Directed therapy requires culture, identification of potential pathogens, and antibacterial susceptibility testing to help to assess the likelihood of the infection responding to treatment with different antimicrobial agents. Disc diffusion testing by internationally standardized methods (e.g. EUCAST[32]) is widely used in diagnostic laboratories, categorizing isolates as sensitive, intermediately sensitive, or resistant to the agents tested (Fig. 1.2.4). The Minimum Inhibitory Concentration (MIC) of an isolate may be determined by the commercial Epsilometer test (Etest), by using automated methods that determine the MICs to a panel of agents (e.g. Vitek®) or occasionally by conventional broth dilution testing. Isolates may also be tested for resistance determinants such as ESBL production.[33]

Common antimicrobial agents used in urological practice

A summary of usual indications and adult doses of antimicrobial agents used in urology and their common or serious adverse effects are shown in Tables 1.2.2 and 1.2.3, respectively.[7,8,11,34]

Nitrofurantoin

Nitrofurantoin affects several different bacterial enzymes, inhibiting ribosomal protein synthesis. It is bactericidal and usually active against a range of Enterobacteriaceae (coliform organisms) such as *E. coli, Klebsiella,* and *Enterobacter* and Gram-positive cocci such as enterococci, including GRE, and staphylococci including MRSA. Some species, such as *Proteus spp.* and *P. aeruginosa*, are intrinsically resistant.

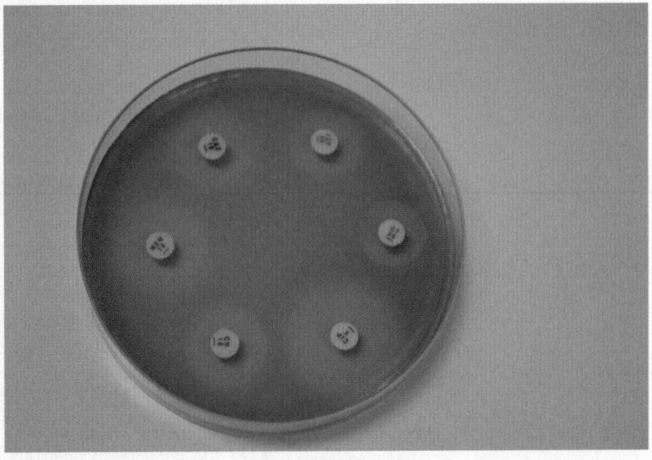

Fig. 1.2.4 Disc diffusion sensitivity tests carried out on an isolate of *Pseudomonas aeruginosa*.
With kind permission of Jesmond IT.

Table 1.2.3 Common and serious adverse events associated with antibacterial agents

Antibacterial agent	Common/serious side effects
Nitrofurantoin	◆ Dose-related GI disturbances (anorexia, nausea, vomiting) ◆ Parotitis ◆ Hypersensitivity reactions (rashes, eosinophilia, fever, anaphylaxis) ◆ Neurological toxicity: headache, confusion, peripheral neuropathy ◆ Pulmonary reactions include pneumonitis, BOOP, and interstitial fibrosis ◆ Hepatotixicity (rare) ◆ Risk of neonatal haemolysis if given to pregnant women at term
Trimethoprim/Co-trimoxazole	◆ GI disturbances: nausea, vomiting, diarrhoea ◆ Hypersensitivity: rash particularly associated with sulphonamide component, including rarely SJS, TEN ◆ Bone marrow depression (inhibition of folic acid pathway), rarely neutropenia/agranulocytosis (sulphonamide-related) ◆ Aseptic meningitis/encephalitis ◆ Hepatotoxicity (rare) ◆ Warfarin interaction; increase in INR ◆ Teratogenic risk in first trimester of pregnancy (trimethoprim) ◆ Neonatal haemolysis and methaemoglobinaemia in third trimester of pregnancy (sulphonamide)
Amoxicillin,* Ampicillin,* Flucloxacillin*, Pivmecillinam*	◆ GI disturbances: nausea, vomiting, diarrhoea ◆ Hypersensitivity reactions (1–10% of exposed patients), ranging from rash to anaphylaxis (less than 0.05%) ◆ Rarely—interstitial nephritis, haemolytic anaemia, neutropenia and, in high doses, encephalopathy with seizures or hepatitis ◆ Cholestatic jaundice or hepatitis may occur up to two months after completion of flucloxacillin treatment ◆ Antibiotic-associated diarrhoea may occur ◆ Pivmecillinam associated with oesophageal stricture formation; advise patients to swallow tablets with plenty of fluid during a meal while sitting or standing
Co-amoxiclav* (amoxicillin/clavulanate)	◆ GI disturbances (nausea, vomiting, diarrhoea) commoner than with amoxicillin alone ◆ Hypersensitivity reactions, ranging from rash to anaphylaxis ◆ Hepatotoxicity (six times more common than with amoxicillin), especially cholestatic jaundice (usually reversible) ◆ CDI ◆ Blood dyscrasias ◆ CNS toxicity (rare, high doses may cause encephalopathy and seizures)
Piperacillin/tazobactam*	◆ GI disturbances, especially diarrhoea ◆ Hypersensitivity: rashes, eosinophilia, fever, pruritis ◆ Abnormal LFTs, jaundice ◆ Blood dyscrasias (neutropenia, haemolytic anaemia, pancytopenia) ◆ CDI (it may be less associated with CDI than many other broad-spectrum antibiotics) ◆ CNS toxicity (rarely, high doses may cause encephalopathy and seizures) ◆ Hepatitis
Cephalosporins*	◆ GI disturbances: nausea, vomiting, diarrhoea ◆ Headache ◆ Hypersensitivity, including rash, anaphylaxis ◆ CDI ◆ Nephrotoxicity rare; may potentiate nephrotoxicity of gentamicin
Carbapenems*	◆ GI upsets: nausea, vomiting, diarrhoea ◆ Hypersensitivity, rashes, eosinophilia, anaphylaxis; there is a low incidence of cross-allergic reactions with penicillins* ◆ Headache ◆ Abnormal LFTs, hepatitis, jaundice ◆ CDI may occur ◆ Ertapenem and imipenem are associated with seizure, rare with meropenem

Table 1.2.3 Continued

Antibacterial agent	Common/serious side effects
Aztreonam*	◆ GI disturbances ◆ Rarely—GI bleeding, thrombocytopenia, neutropenia ◆ Jaundice, hepatitis ◆ Seizures ◆ Flushing, bronchospasm, rash including TEN and erythema multiforme; there is a low incidence of cross-allergic reactions with penicillins*
Aminoglycosides	◆ Ototoxicity, usually only with prolonged high levels; vestibular > cochlear toxicity ◆ Nephrotoxicity (ATN), dose related; less likely with once-daily dosing than multiple daily doses ◆ Neuromuscular blockade ◆ Skin rashes and hypersensitivity reactions are rare
Vancomycin and Teicoplanin	◆ Phlebitis ◆ Hypersensitivity, rashes ◆ Nephrotoxicity at high doses with vancomycin ◆ Ototoxicity is rare; high-frequency hearing loss may occur ◆ Rapid infusion of vancomycin may cause 'red man syndrome' related to histamine release: hypotension, dypnoea, wheeze, pruritis, urticaria, and flushing of the upper body ◆ Both vancomycin and teicoplanin may be associated with leucopenia and thrombocytopenia
Ciprofloxacin	◆ GI disturbances (abdominal pain, nausea, vomiting, diarrhoea) ◆ CNS effects, including headaches, dizziness, seizures (avoid in known epilepsy) ◆ Hypersensitivity reactions; rashes, pruritis, anaphylaxis, photosensitivity ◆ Arthropathy and tendonitis ◆ Renal Impairment, interstitial nephritis ◆ CDI ◆ Haematological side effects (reversible) ◆ Prolonged QT interval
Colistin	◆ Nephrotoxicity ◆ Rash ◆ Parenteral therapy may cause neurotoxicity including apnoea, paraesthesiae (perioral and peripheral), headache, vertigo, muscle weakness ◆ Rarer neurotoxic manifestations include confusion, psychosis, visual disturbances, slurred speech, and vasomotor instability
Linezolid	◆ GI side effects, taste disturbance ◆ Headache ◆ Pancreatitis, hypertension, dizziness ◆ Leucopenia, thrombocytopenia, eosinophilia, pancytopenia ◆ Electrolyte disturbances ◆ Blurred vision, rash, paraesthesia ◆ Rarely—lactic acidosis, pancytopenia, anaemia ◆ Severe optic neuropathy reported rarely on prolonged therapy
Metronidazole	◆ GI disturbances, taste disturbance, anorexia ◆ Very rarely hepatitis, jaundice, pancreatitis, pancytopenia, thrombocytopenia, erythema multiforme ◆ Peripheral neuropathy, seizures, leucopenia reported during prolonged therapy ◆ Patients advised not to drink alcohol because of risk of disulfiram-like reaction

ATN = acute tubular necrosis; BOOP = bronchiolitis obliterans organizing pneumonia; CDI = *Clostridium difficile* infection; CNS = central nervous system; GI = gastrointestinal; INR = international normalized ratio; LFTs = liver function tests; SJS = Stevens–Johnson syndrome; TEN = toxic epidermal necrolysis.

*In patients who have a hypersensitivity or anaphylactoid reaction to penicillin, there is cross-reactivity with all classes of penicillins (aminopenicillins, piperacillin-tazobactam, pivmecillinam) and a low incidence of cross-allergenicity with other beta-lactam antibiotics (cephalosporins, carbapenems, monobactams).

Source: data from the Joint Formulary Committee. *British National Formulary*. 72 ed. London: BMJ Group and Pharmaceutical Press; 2016: 459–546.

Nitrofurantoin is well absorbed after oral administration, but serum levels remain low and therapeutic levels are achieved only in the urine. Consequently, nitrofurantoin is suitable for treatment of simple, uncomplicated lower UTIs. It will not reach therapeutic urinary concentrations and should therefore usually be avoided when the eGFR is less than 45 mL/min/1.73 m^2 (see Table 1.2.2).[11] As development of resistance is relatively rare, and nitrofurantoin is unlikely to affect bowel or vaginal flora, it may be considered as long-term prophylaxis for selected patients suffering from frequent recurrence of UTI caused by susceptible isolates.[7,11] Nitrofurantoin can be given in pregnancy, but should be avoided at term because it may cause neonatal haemolysis.[11]

Trimethoprim and co-trimoxazole

Trimethoprim prevents bacterial DNA replication by inhibiting the enzyme dihydrofolate reductase, which is involved in bacterial folic acid synthesis. Trimethoprim demonstrates synergistic antibacterial activity with sulphonamides, which act earlier in the same metabolic pathway. Co-trimoxazole is a combination drug comprising trimethoprim and the sulphonamide, sulfamethoxazole.

These drugs are active against coliform organisms such as *E. coli* and staphylococci including *Staphylococcus saprophyticus.* Enterococcal UTIs are felt unlikely to be responsive to either agent as they can bypass the inhibition of folate synthesis by utilizing preformed folic acid found in urine.[35] Trimethoprim is only available as an oral formulation, while co-trimoxazole is available as oral and intravenous preparations. Both drugs have high oral bioavailability and reach therapeutic concentrations in the urine.

Trimethoprim is used mainly for the treatment of acute uncomplicated bacterial cystitis but it should not be used empirically in areas with high resistance rates in *E coli.*[36] Trimethoprim penetrates prostatic tissue and a 28-day course may therefore be used for the treatment of acute prostatitis. Long-term, low-dose prophylactic trimethoprim may be considered in selected patients with frequent, recurrent UTIs.[7,11] In the United Kingdom, co-trimoxazole is generally restricted for the treatment of *Pneumocystis jirovecii* (formerly *Pneumocystis carinii*) pneumonia, toxoplasmosis, and nocardia infections because of the risk of serious adverse events including Stevens–Johnson syndrome and blood dyscrasias.[11] As a folate antagonist, trimethoprim poses a risk of teratogenicity and should be avoided during the first trimester of pregnancy.[11]

Amoxicillin and ampicillin

Penicillins are bactericidal drugs that inhibit the formation of cross-links in the peptidoglycan layer of bacterial cell walls, resulting in bacterial lysis. Ampicillin and amoxicillin are semi-synthetic penicillins known as aminopenicillins. They have good activity against streptococci, many enterococci, and some Gram-negative bacilli, including some strains of *E. coli* and *Proteus mirabilis.* However, aminopenicillins are destroyed by bacterial beta-lactamases and are therefore inactive against most staphylococci and many coliform organisms. Amoxicillin and ampicillin are both available as oral, intravenous, and intramuscular preparations. Both drugs are excreted in urine.

Amoxicillin and ampicillin may be used to treat UTIs caused by sensitive uropathogens; however, resistance to these agents is widespread. In one international study, more than half the strains of *E. coli* isolated from patients with uncomplicated UTI were reported to be amoxicillin resistant.[37] For this reason, these agents should not be used empirically.

Penicillin hypersensitivity reactions occur in 1–10% of exposed patients, ranging from rash to anaphylaxis, which occurs in less than 0.05% of treated patients. There is cross-hypersensitivity between aminopenicillins and other penicillins, and a lower cross-hypersensitivity rate with cephalosporins and carbapenems. As a general rule, these agents should all be avoided in patients with a history of anaphylaxis, urticaria, or rash that develops immediately following penicillin treatment.[11]

Flucloxacillin

Flucloxacillin is a semi-synthetic penicillin, which is stable to staphylococcal beta-lactamase. It is active against streptococci and methicillin-sensitive staphylococci including *S. aureus*, but its spectrum of activity does not extend to MRSA, enterococci, or Gram-negative bacteria. Oral and intravenous formulations are available.

Flucloxacillin is used for the treatment of staphylococcal infections including skin and soft tissue infections such as surgical site infections.

Co-amoxiclav

Co-amoxiclav is a combination of amoxicillin and clavulanic acid (a beta-lactamase inhibitor) that protects amoxicillin from enzymatic degradation by many bacterial beta-lactamases, broadening its spectrum of activity. Co-amoxiclav is active against *S. aureus* and many amoxicillin-resistant coliform organisms, although MRSA and *P. aeruginosa* remain resistant. Oral and intravenous formulations are available.

Therapeutic concentrations of both drugs can be achieved in urine. Co-amoxiclav may be used as second-line treatment for simple cystitis caused by uropathogens resistant to narrow spectrum antimicrobial agents. It is also suitable for the treatment of complicated UTIs and some centres use it as perioperative prophylaxis for invasive urological procedures such as cystourethroscopy or ureteroscopy.[7,8]

(Piv)mecillinam

Pivmecillinam is the oral pro-drug of mecillinam, a penicillin that is relatively stable to bacterial beta-lactamases, including ESBLs. Mecillinam is active against a range of coliform organisms, including some multiresistant strains of *E. coli, Klebsiella, Enterobacter,* and *Proteus. Pseudomonas* species are not susceptible; *Morganella* and *Serratia* species are often resistant, and mecillinam has little activity against Gram-positive organisms such as enterococci.

Pivmecillinam is used to treat lower UTIs and may be particularly useful in the outpatient setting for infections caused by beta-lactamase-producing organisms.

Piperacillin-tazobactam

This is a combination of piperacillin, an antipseudomonal penicillin, and tazobactam, a beta-lactamase inhibitor. Piperacillin-tazobactam is an intravenous antibiotic with a broad spectrum of activity against most Gram-negative uropathogens, including *Pseudomonas* species, and many Gram-positive and anaerobic bacteria. MRSA is resistant to piperacillin-tazobactam and some bacteria produce beta-lactamases that are stable to tazobactam, resulting in piperacillin-tazobactam resistance. Piperacillin-tazobactam is used for the treatment of complicated UTIs and urosepsis.

Oral cephalosporins

Cephalosporins are beta-lactam antibiotics, classified into different generations according to their spectrum of activity. The oral cephalosporins include cefalexin and cefradine, which are relatively narrow spectrum first generation cephalosporins, and cefaclor, which is a second generation product. First and second generation cephalosporins are active against *S. aureus* and susceptible strains of coliform organisms such as *E. coli* and *Klebsiella pneumoniae*, but MRSA and *Pseudomonas* species are resistant, as are many *Proteus* and *Enterobacter* species. Enterococci are intrinsically resistant.

Oral cephalosporins are used for the treatment of uncomplicated lower UTIs. Cephalosporins are safe to use in pregnancy and in children. There is a low incidence of cross-hypersensitivity with penicillins (0.5–6.5%);[11] however, cephalosporin use should still be avoided in patients with a history of anaphylaxis, urticaria, or immediate development of rash associated with penicillin treatment.

Cefuroxime

Cefuroxime is a second generation cephalosporin. It has the same basic structure and mechanism of action as the first generation cephalosporins but a broader spectrum of Gram-negative activity. Although it is stable to some beta-lactamases, cefuroxime is inactivated by ESBLs. It has no activity against enterococci, *P. aeruginosa*, or many opportunistic pathogens such as *Acinetobacter* species. Cefuroxime is available in parenteral and oral formulations, although the latter is not well absorbed.

Its uses include treatment of urosepsis and complicated UTIs including pyelonephritis, and is safe to use in children and pregnancy.[11] It may be used as prophylaxis for invasive urological procedures such as transurethral resection of the prostate (TURP).[7,8] The adverse drug reactions of cefuroxime are similar to those of other beta-lactams, however, cefuroxime is associated with a relatively high risk of *C. difficile* infection. Some centres minimize its use for this reason.[9]

Ceftazidime

Ceftazidime is an intravenous third generation cephalosporin. It has a broader spectrum of Gram-negative activity than cefuroxime, including good activity against *P. aeruginosa*, but it is not stable to ESBL-producing bacteria which are becoming increasingly prevalent. Unlike first and second generation cephalosporins, it does not provide good antistaphylococcal cover.

In urology, ceftazidime should be restricted for the treatment of serious UTIs caused by pathogens resistant to first-line agents. It may be considered as prophylaxis for procedures such as TURP in areas with a high prevalence of coliform organisms resistant to first-line prophylactic agents.[7] Side effects of ceftazidime are similar to those of other cephalosporins, and include the risk of promoting *C. difficile* infection. Some hospitals therefore limit its use.[9]

Carbapenems

Carbapenems are broad-spectrum, bactericidal beta-lactams with good activity against the majority of Gram-positive and Gram-negative pathogens, including ESBL-producing bacteria and anaerobes. They are inactive against MRSA and destroyed by carbapenemase-producing bacteria. Carbapenems include ertapenem, imipenem, meropenem, and doripenem. All except ertapenem are active against *P. aeruginosa*. Ertapenem has a long half-life and is therefore suitable for once-daily dosing. Carbapenems are only available in parenteral formulations.

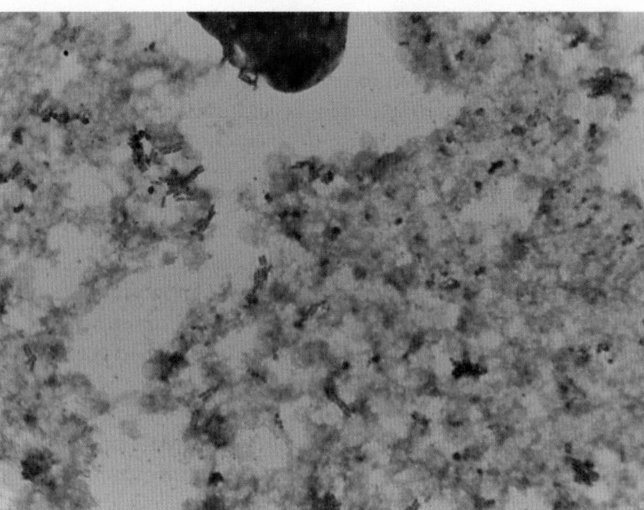

Fig. 1.2.5 Gram-stained preparation of a blood culture showing Gram-negative rods (×1,000 magnification). This blood culture, which subsequently grew *Escherichia coli (E. coli),* was collected from a patient with urosepsis.

As a result of their broad spectrum of activity and stability against bacterial enzymes, carbapenems are indicated for the treatment of severe sepsis, including complicated UTIs, for polymicrobial infections and for the treatment of infection caused by multiresistant bacteria, including ESBL producers (Fig. 1.2.5).

There is a low incidence of cross-hypersensitivity with penicillins, so carbapenems should be avoided if the patient has a history of an immediate hypersensitivity-type reaction to penicillins.[11]

Aztreonam

Aztreonam is a monocyclic beta-lactam agent or monobactam. It inhibits bacterial cell wall synthesis and is bactericidal. Aztreonam is active against a range of Gram-negative bacteria but inhibited by some beta-lactamases including ESBLs and considered to have reduced activity against *Pseudomonas*. Gram-positive and anaerobic bacteria are resistant. It is available only for parenteral administration. Effective serum levels of aztreonam are achieved and the drug is widely distributed in body tissues and urine.

Aztreonam can be used for the treatment of serious Gram-negative infections caused by sensitive pathogens. It is less likely than other beta-lactam agents to cause hypersensitivity reactions in patients with penicillin allergy and may therefore be used with caution.[11]

Aminoglycosides

Gentamicin, tobramycin, and amikacin are bactericidal antibiotics that inhibit bacterial protein synthesis by binding to the 30S ribosomal subunit. They have good activity against coliform organisms, *Pseudomonas* species, and staphylococci, but no activity against streptococci or anaerobes. Amikacin provides a broader spectrum of Gram-negative activity than gentamicin or tobramycin. Aminoglycosides are not absorbed after oral administration and are usually given intravenously.

They are useful for treating complicated UTIs and urosepsis, including infections caused by *P. aeruginosa* and coliform organisms that may be resistant to beta-lactam antibiotics. Single-dose aminoglycoside prophylaxis may be administered for urological procedures.[8] The main adverse drug reactions are dose related. These agents are excreted in the urine; they may accumulate in renal tissue where, in high doses, they can cause acute tubular necrosis.

Once-daily dosing of aminoglycosides reduces the risk of toxicity without reducing the therapeutic response for most infections.[38] Renal function should be assessed prior to the administration of aminoglycosides and regularly during treatment. Therapeutic drug monitoring should be carried out because of the narrow therapeutic index.[11] Aminoglycosides should be avoided in pregnancy and avoided or used with caution in patients with renal impairment.[11] If possible, the concomitant use of other potentially nephrotoxic or ototoxic agents such as furosemide should be avoided and treatment courses should not exceed seven days.

Glycopeptides

The glycopeptides, vancomycin and teicoplanin, are bactericidal drugs that inhibit bacterial cell wall synthesis by binding to cell wall peptidoglycan precursors. They have a broad spectrum of Gram-positive activity covering staphylococci including MRSA, *Clostridium difficile*, and enterococci, although glycopeptide-resistant enterococci are now well recognized. Glycopeptides have no activity against Gram-negative uropathogens. These drugs are not absorbed by mouth and, for systemic use, intravenous administration is required.

The main use of glycopeptides in urology is for the treatment of serious infections caused by resistant Gram-positive bacteria such as MRSA and *Enterococcus faecium*, or as second-line Gram-positive treatment for patients with penicillin allergy. Oral vancomycin is used for the treatment of recurrent or severe *Clostridium difficile* infection including pseudomembranous colitis. Intravenous vancomycin has a narrow therapeutic index and therapeutic drug monitoring is used to monitor levels and guide dosing.[11] Teicoplanin levels are not routinely measured but may be required in order to optimize treatment of certain severe infections.

Ciprofloxacin

Quinolones inhibit the bacterial enzyme DNA gyrase, which is involved in the folding of DNA during nucleic acid synthesis. Ciprofloxacin is the most commonly used fluoroquinolone; oral and intravenous preparations are available. In general, ciprofloxacin has reasonable activity against coliform organisms, *P. aeruginosa,* and many staphylococci, other than MRSA, although ciprofloxacin resistance in both community and hospital settings is an increasing problem. It has limited activity against streptococci and enterococci and most anaerobes are resistant. Oral ciprofloxacin is very well absorbed. Ciprofloxacin penetrates well into tissues including kidney and prostate, and achieves good urine levels in patients with normal renal function.

In urology, ciprofloxacin is used to treat pyelonephritis, prostatitis, epididymo-orchitis, and UTI caused by isolates resistant to first-line agents.[7,11] It should be avoided in children and in pregnancy. Many centres now restrict the use of quinolones in order to minimize the risk of *C. difficile* infection.

Colistimethate sodium (colistin)

Colistin is active against a very wide range of Gram-negative bacteria including *P. aeruginosa* and multiresistant isolates such as ESBL producers, *Acinetobacter baumanii*, and carbapenemase-producing *Klebsiella* species. It has no activity against Gram-positive pathogens. Oral colistin is not absorbed and remains in the bowel. Formulations are available for administration orally, intravenously, or by inhalation of a nebulized solution.

The use of intravenous colistin is usually overseen by a medical microbiologist or other infection specialist and is generally reserved for the treatment of serious Gram-negative infections resistant to other antimicrobial agents. Nebulized colistin may be used as adjunctive topical treatment for patients with cystic fibrosis[39] and oral colistin may be given as part of a bowel decontamination regimen in certain groups of patients in intensive care units.[40]

Linezolid

Linezolid acts by blocking the initiation of bacterial protein synthesis. It is active against a wide range of Gram-positive bacteria including MRSA and GRE, but has no useful Gram-negative activity. Intravenous and oral preparations are available. It is very well absorbed orally, achieving good concentrations in tissue.

In the United Kingdom, linezolid is licensed for the treatment of complicated skin and soft tissue infections and pneumonia.[11] It achieves adequate levels in urine and may sometimes be considered for the off-licence treatment of serious Gram-positive infections, where the use of other agents has been precluded by allergy or multidrug resistance.

Metronidazole

Metronidazole is active against anaerobic bacteria and protozoa. It is metabolized by nitroreductase enzymes to form active compounds that cause DNA breakage. Oral, intravenous, rectal, and topical preparations are available.

Metronidazole is used for the treatment and prophylaxis of anaerobic infections. In urological practice, it is used to provide anaerobic cover for invasive procedures where the colon may be breached, such as transrectal biopsy of the prostate, or cystectomy and bladder reconstruction.[7,8] Oral metronidazole is the treatment of choice for CDI of mild or moderate severity.[9,11]

Antifungal agents

Fungal infections in urology

Candiduria is usually seen in hospital settings where it may reflect contamination of the urine at collection or colonization of a urinary catheter or stent (Fig. 1.2.6).[41] Removal of predisposing factors, such as broad-spectrum antibiotics, urinary catheters, or stents will clear candiduria in almost 50% of asymptomatic patients[42] and few patients require antifungal therapy. Candida species can, however, cause lower UTIs or even invasive upper tract infections, including pyelonephritis, perinephric abscess, and fungal balls.[43,44] Infection is more common in people with diabetes, the immunosuppressed, and patients with indwelling catheters or stents. *Candida albicans* is the most frequently isolated species, but previous antifungal treatment and hospitalization may alter the spectrum of pathogenic yeasts and antifungal susceptibility.[45]

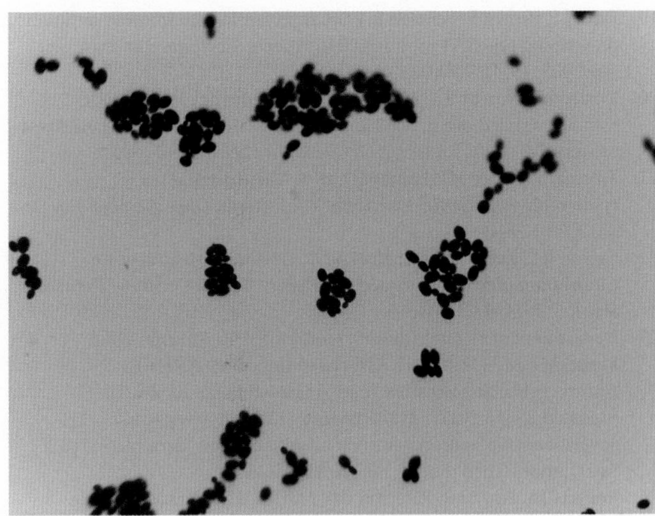

Fig. 1.2.6 Gram stain of *Candida albicans* isolated from a catheter sample of urine (×1,000 magnification).

Antifungal agents

There are four groups of systemic antifungal agent:

1. Azoles
2. Polyenes
3. Echinocandins
4. Flucytosine

Azoles

Azoles are fungicidal, blocking the synthesis of ergosterol, the main sterol in the fungal cell membrane. Fluconazole, itraconazole, voriconazole, and posaconazole are triazoles. While most candida species are susceptible to fluconazole, some are intrinsically resistant and acquired resistance may arise following long-term exposure. Fluconazole is available as oral or intravenous preparations. It has high oral bioavailability and, unlike the other azoles, achieves good urinary concentrations.[46] Fluconazole may be used for the treatment of candidal cystitis, pyelonephritis, and candidaemia. Adverse effects of fluconazole include gastrointestinal upset, rash, and headache. Hepatotoxicity is more common in patients with pre-existing liver abnormalities. Fluconazole inhibits CYP450 isoenzymes in the liver leading to important interactions with some drugs, including warfarin, antiarrhythmics, and calcineurin inhibitors. The dose of fluconazole depends on the clinical indication, and requires adjustment in renal impairment.[11]

Polyenes

Polyenes bind to ergosterol, the main sterol in the fungal cell membrane, causing increased permeability and cell death. Amphotericin B (AMB) has a narrow therapeutic index; liposomal preparations (L-AMB) including amphotericin B-lipid complex (ABLC) and liposomal amphotericin (Ambisome) are less nephrotoxic. Intravenous amphotericin is used to treat systemic fungal infections, usually under the direction of an infection specialist. It should be noted that liposomal preparations do not achieve therapeutic levels in urine. It has a broad spectrum of antifungal activity including *Aspergillus fumigatus* and most yeasts. Acquired resistance is rare.

Adverse effects include infusion reactions (headaches, fever, chills, myalgia), nephrotoxicity, and anaemia. Doses of liposomal amphotericin depend on the formulation chosen. If conventional amphotericin is used, a test dose of 1 mg is followed by a regimen of escalating doses up to a maximum of 1–1.5 mg/kg od by intravenous infusion.[11] Amphotericin should be used with caution in patients with renal impairment.

Echinocandins

These include caspofungin, anidulafungin, and micafungin. Echinocandins cause fungal lysis by inhibiting the synthesis of glucan, a major component of the fungal cell wall. They are active against the majority of candida species, and acquired resistance is rare. Echinocandins may be used for the treatment of systemic candidal infections, but therapeutic levels are not achieved in urine. Adverse effects include gastrointestinal disturbances, rash, flushing, hypokalaemia, and abnormal liver function tests. Echinocandins are given as intravenous infusions. Individual doses should be checked before prescription.[11]

Flucytosine

Flucytosine is a pyrimidine analogue that inhibits fungal DNA synthesis. It is largely excreted unchanged in urine and is active against most yeasts. Flucytosine has a narrow therapeutic index, causing dose-related myelosuppression. It is usually prescribed under the direction of an infection expert and restricted for the treatment of severe life-threatening fungal infections, where it is given in combination with other agents.[11] Short course flucytosine monotherapy may occasionally be considered as treatment for intractable cystitis caused by yeasts resistant to other therapy.[46]

Further reading

Blaser M. Antibiotic overuse: Stop the killing of beneficial bacteria. *Nature* 2011; **476**:393–4.

Joint Formulary Committee. *British National Formulary*. 72 ed. London: BMJ Group and Pharmaceutical Press; 2016: 459–546.

Department of Health Advisory Committee on Antimicrobial Resistance and Healthcare Associated Infection (ARHAI). Antimicrobial Stewardship: 'Start smart—then focus'. London, UK: Department of Health, 2011.

Department of Health and the Health Protection Agency. *Clostridium difficile* infection: How to deal with the problem. London, UK: Department of Health, 2008. Available at: https://www.gov.uk/government/publications/clostridium-difficile-infection-how-to-deal-with-the-problem [Online].

Fisher JF, Sobel JD, Kauffman CA, Newman CA. Candida urinary tract infections-treatment. *Clin Infect Dis* 2011; **52**(Suppl 6):S457–S66.

Grabe M, Bartoletti R, Bjerklund Johansen TE, *et al.* Guidelines on urological infections, 2015 [updated 29 January 2017]. Available at: http://uroweb.org/wp-content/uploads/EAU-Guidelines-Urological-Infections-v2.pdf [Online].

Greenwood D, Barer MR, Slack RCB, Irving WL (eds). Medical Microbiology: A guide to microbial infections: Pathogenesis, Immunity, Laboratory Diagnosis and Control, 18th edition. London, UK: Churchill Livingstone, 2012.

National Institute for Health and Clinical Excellence. NICE clinical guideline 74, Surgical site infections: prevention and treatment. London, UK, 2008. Available at: http://www.nice.org.uk/nicemedia/pdf/CG74NICEGuideline.pdf [Online].

Scottish Intercollegiate Guidelines Network. SIGN 104, Antibiotic prophylaxis in surgery: a national clinical guideline. Edinburgh, UK, 2008. Available at: http://www.sign.ac.uk/pdf/sign104.pdf [Online].

Torok E, Moran E, Cooke F. *Oxford Handbook of Infectious Diseases and Microbiology*, 2nd edition. Oxford, UK: Oxford University Press, 2009.

Wolf JS, Bennett CJ, Dmochowski RR, *et al. Best Practice Policy Statement on Urological Surgery Antimicrobial Prophylaxis. J Urol* 2008; **179**(4):1379–90.

References

1. Foxman B. Epidemiology of urinary tract infections: incidence, morbidity and economic costs. *Am J Med* 2002; **113**:5S–13S.
2. Health Protection Agency. English National Point Prevalence Survey on Healthcare Associated Infections and Antimicrobial Use, 2011: Preliminary data. [updated 17 March 2017]. Available at: http://webarchive.nationalarchives.gov.uk/ 20140714084352/http:/www.hpa.org.uk/Publications/InfectiousDiseases/AntimicrobialAndHealthcare AssociatedInfections/1205HCAIEnglishPPSforhcaiandamu2011prelim/ [Online].
3. Flores-Mireles AL, Walker JN, Caparon M, Hultgren SJ. Urinary tract infections: epidemiology, mechanisms of infection and treatment options. *Nat Rev Microbiol* 2015; **13**(5):269–84.
4. Public Health England. Annual Epidemiological Commentary: Mandatory MRSA, MSSA and *E. coli* bacteraemia and *C. difficile* infection (data 2015/16), 7 July 2016 [updated 28 January 2017]. Available at: https://www.gov.uk/government/uploads/system/uploads/attachment_data/file/535635/AEC_final.pdf [Online].
5. National Institute for Health and Clinical Excellence. NICE clinical guideline 74, Surgical site infections: prevention and treatment, 2008 [updated 29 January 2017]. Available at: https://www.nice.org.uk/guidance/cg74 [Online].
6. Scottish Intercollegiate Guidelines Network. SIGN, Antibiotic prophylaxis in surgery: a national clinical guideline, 2008, [updated 2014; cited 29 January 2017]. Available at: http://sign.ac.uk/guidelines/fulltext/104/index.html [Online].
7. Grabe M, Bartoletti R, Bjerklund Johansen TE, *et al.* Guidelines on urological infections, 2015 [updated 29 January 2017]. Available at: http://uroweb.org/wp-content/uploads/EAU-Guidelines-Urological-Infections-v2.pdf [Online].
8. Wolf JS, Bennett CJ, Dmochowski RR, *et al.* Best Practice Policy Statement on Urological Surgery Antimicrobial Prophylaxis, 2008, [updated 2016, cited 29 January 2017]. Available at: https://www.auanet.org/education/guidelines/antimicrobial-prophylaxis.cfm [Online].
9. Department of Health and the Health Protection Agency. *Clostridium difficile* infection: How to deal with the problem, 2008 [updated 29 January 2017]. Available at: https://www.gov.uk/government/publications/clostridium-difficile-infection-how-to-deal-with-the-problem [Online].
10. Bootsma AM, Laguna Pes MP, Geerlings SE, Goossens A. Antibiotic prophylaxis in urologic procedures: a systematic review. *Eur Urol* 2008; **54**(6):1270–86.
11. Joint Formulary Committee. *British National Formulary*. 72 ed. London: BMJ Group and Pharmaceutical Press; 2016: 459–546.
12. Blaser M. Antibiotic overuse: Stop the killing of beneficial bacteria. *Nature* 2011; **476**:393–4.
13. Livermore DM. Has the era of untreatable infections arrived? *J Antimicrob Chemother* 2009; **64**(Suppl 1):i29–36.
14. Hawkey PM, Jones AM. The changing epidemiology of resistance. *J Antimicrob Chemother* 2009; **64**(Suppl 1):i3–10.
15. Lucet JC, Chevret S, Durand-Zaleski I, Chastang C, Régnier B. Prevalence and risk factors for carriage of methicillin-resistant *Staphylococcus aureus* at admission to the intensive care unit: results of a multicentre study. *Arch Intern Med* 2003; **163**:181–8.
16. Tacconelli E, De Angelis G, Cataldo MA, Pozzi E, Cauda R. Does antibiotic exposure increase the risk of methicillin-resistant *Staphylococcus aureus* (MRSA) isolation? A systemic review and meta-analysis. *J Antimicrob Chemother* 2008; **61**(1):26–38.
17. Dancer SJ. The effect of antibiotics on methicillin-resistant *Staphylococcus aureus. J Antimicrob Chemother* 2008; **61**:246–53.
18. Liebowitz LD, Blunt MC. Modification in prescribing practices for third generation cephalosporins and ciprofloxacin is associated with a reduction in methicillin-resistant *Staphylococcus aureus* bacteraemia rate. *J Hosp Infect* 2008; **69**:328–36.
19. Davey P, Brown E, Fenelon L, *et al.* Interventions to improve antibiotic prescribing practices for hospital inpatients. *Cochrane Database Syst Rev* 2005; **19**(4):CD003543.
20. Wistrom J, Norrby SR, Myhre EB, *et al.* Frequency of antibiotic-associated diarrhoea in 2462 antibiotic-treated hospitalized patients: a prospective study. *J Antimicrob Chemother* 2001; **47**:43–50.
21. Freeman J, Bauer MP, Baines SD, *et al.* The changing epidemiology of *Clostridium difficile* infections. *Clin Microbiol Rev* 2010; **23**:529–49.
22. Nelson RL, Kelsey P, Leeman H, *et al.* Antibiotic treatment for *Clostridium difficile*-associated diarrhea in adults. *Cochrane Database Syst Rev* 2011; **9**:CD004610.
23. Department of Health Advisory Committee on Antimicrobial Resistance and Healthcare Associated Infection (ARHAI). Antimicrobial Stewardship: 'Start smart—then focus'. 2015 [updated 29 Jan 2017]. Available from: https://www.gov.uk/government/uploads/system/uploads/attachment_data/file/417032/Start_Smart_Then_Focus_FINAL.PDF [Online].
24. Roberts JA, Norris R, Paterson DL, Martin JH. Therapeutic drug monitoring of antimicrobials. *Br J Clin Pharmacol* 2012; **73**(1):27–36.
25. Hammett-Stabler CA, Johns T. National Academy of Clinical Biochemistry: Laboratory guidelines for monitoring of antimicrobial drugs. *Clin Chem* 1998; **44**(5):1129–40.
26. Paediatric Formulary Committee. *BNF for Children* 2016–2017. London: BMJ Group, Pharmaceutical Press, and RCPCH Publications, 2016: 281–357.
27. Implementation of modified admission MRSA screening guidance for NHS (2014). Department of Health expert advisory committee on antimicrobial resistance and healthcare associated infection (ARHAI). 2014 [updated 29 Jan 2017]. Available at: https://www.gov.uk/government/uploads/system/uploads/attachment_data/file/345144/Implementation_of_modified_admission_MRSA_screening_guidance_for_NHS.pdf [Online].
28. Public Health England. Acute trust toolkit for the early detection, management and control of carbapenemase-producing Enterobacteriaceae. Dec 2013 [updated 29 Jan 2017]. Available at https://www.gov.uk/government/uploads/system/uploads/attachment_data/file/329227/Acute_trust_toolkit_for_the_early_detection.pdf [Online].
29. Coai JE, Duckworth GJ, Edwards DI, *et al.* Guidelines for the control and prevention of methicillin-resistant *Staphylococcus aureus* (MRSA) in healthcare facilities. *J Hosp Infect* 2006; **63**(Suppl 1):S1–44.
30. Health and Social Care Information Centre. The Health Survey for England 2015 – adult overweight and obesity, 2016 [updated 28 January 2017]. Available at: http://www.content.digital.nhs.uk/catalogue/PUB22610/HSE2015-Adult-obe.pdf [Online].
31. Janson B, Thursky K. Dosing of antibiotics in obesity. *Curr Opin Infect Dis* 2012; **25**(6):634–49.
32. Matuschek E, Brown DFJ, Kahlmeter G. Development of the EUCAST disk diffusion antimicrobial susceptibility testing method and its implementation in routine microbiology laboratories. *Clin Microbiol Infect* 2014; **20**: O255–O266, 2014 [updated 15 January 2017]. Available at: http://www.eucast.org/fileadmin/src/media/PDFs/EUCAST_files/General_documents/Publications/Disk_diffusion_paper_printed_version_March_2014.pdf [Online].
33. Giske CG, Martinez-Martinez L, Cantón R, *et al.* EUCAST guidelines for detection of resistance mechanisms and specific resistances of clinical and/or epidemiological importance. Version 1.0 December 2013. [Updated 29 January 2017]. Available at: http://www.eucast.org/fileadmin/src/media/PDFs/EUCAST_files/Resistance_mechanisms/EUCAST_detection_of_resistance_mechanisms_v1.0_20131211.pdf [Online].
34. Gupta K, Hooton TM, Naber KG, *et al.* International clinical practice guidelines for the treatment of acute uncomplicated cystitis and pyelonephritis in women: A 2010 update by the Infectious Diseases Society of America and the European Society for Microbiology and Infectious Diseases. *Clin Infect Dis* 2011; **52**:103–20.

35. Wisell KT, Kahlmeter G, Giske CG. Trimethoprim and enterococci in urinary tract infections: new perspectives on an old issue. *J Antimicrob Chemother* 2008; **62**(1): 35–40.
36. Gupta K, Stamm WE. Outcomes associated with trimethoprim/sulphamethoxazole (TMP/SMX) therapy in TMP/SMX resistant community-acquired UTI. *Int J Antimicrob Agents* 2002; **19**(6):554–6.
37. Nickel JC. Urinary Tract Infections and Resistant Bacteria: Highlights of a Symposium at the Combined Meeting of the 25th International Congress of Chemotherapy (ICC) and the 17th European Congress of Clinical Microbiology and Infectious Diseases (ECCMID), March 31–April 3, 2007, Munich, Germany. *Rev Urol* 2007; **9**(2):78–80.
38. Freeman CD, Nicolau DP, Belliveau PP, Nightingale CH. Once-daily dosing of aminoglycosides: review and recommendations for clinical practice. *J Antimicrob Chemother* 1997; **39**(6):677–86.
39. Jensen T, Pedersen SS, Garne S, Heilmann C, Høiby N, Koch C. Colistin inhalation therapy in cystic fibrosis patients with chronic *Pseudomonas aeruginosa* lung infection. *J Antimicrob Chemother* 1987; **19**:831–8.
40. de Smet AMGA, Kluytmans JAJW, Blok HEM, *et al.* Selective digestive tract decontamination and selective oropharyngeal decontamination and antibiotic resistance in patients in intensive-care units: an open-label, clustered group-randomised, crossover study. *Lancet Infect Dis* 2011; **11**(5):372–80.
41. Kauffman CA, Fisher JF, Sobel JD, Newman CA. Candida Urinary Tract Infections—diagnosis. *Clin Infect Dis* 2011; **52**(Suppl 6): S452–56.
42. Malani AN, Kauffman CA. Candida urinary tract infections: treatment options. *Expert Rev Anti Infect Ther* 2007; **5**(2):277–84.
43. Kauffman CA, Vazquez JA, Sobel JD, *et al.* Prospective multicenter surveillance study of funguria in hospitalized patients. *Clin Infect Dis* 2000; **30**(1):14–8.
44. Wise GJ, Talluri GS, Marella VK. Fungal infections of the genitourinary system: manifestations, diagnosis, and treatment. *Urol Clin North Am* 1999; **26**(4):701–18, vii.
45. Sobel JD, Fisher JF, Kauffman CA, Newman CA. Candida urinary tract infections- epidemiology. Clin Infect Dis 2011; **52**(Suppl 6):S433–6.
46. Pappas PG, Kauffman CA, Andes DR. IDSA Clinical practice guideline for the management of candidiasis: 2016 update by the Infectious Diseases Society of America. [Updated 19 January 2017]. Available at: http://cid.oxfordjournals.org/content/early/2015/12/15/cid.civ933.full.pdf+html [Online].

CHAPTER 1.3

Hospital-acquired urinary tract infection

Roger Bayston

Introduction to hospital-acquired urinary tract infection

In the United States (USA), over 100,000 hospitalized patients suffer a catheter-associated urinary tract infection (CAUTI) each year, and many sources state that CAUTI is the commonest hospital-acquired infection, accounting for 40% of the total.[1] The corresponding figure for the United Kingdom (UK) is 20% of hospital-acquired infections.[2] However, the distinction between catheter-associated asymptomatic bacteriuria (CAASB) and CAUTI is not consistently made, and the majority of these cases are asymptomatic. Guidelines on diagnosis and treatment of nosocomial urinary tract infections are available, and the principles of prevention of infection, including the role of antimicrobial catheters, have been evaluated. Progress is being driven by governments and health insurers which are reluctant to pay the extra costs associated with hospital-acquired infections that they consider preventable.

Microbiology of urinary tract infection

Uncomplicated urinary tract infection

The spectrum of causative organisms differs in community-acquired or uncomplicated urinary tract infection (UTI), and complicated or catheter-related UTI. Most community-acquired UTI is caused by *Escherichia coli*, with approximately 10% of cases due to *Staphylococcus saprophyticus*.[3–5] Most community-acquired UTI occurs in women. In those infections acquired in hospital, both genders are affected and the bacterial spectrum is more varied. The normal habitat of *E. coli* is the large intestine, but the majority are not intestinal pathogens. Many strains of *E. coli* have an array of fine fibres, or fimbriae, on their surfaces, and these are important in attachment of the bacterial cells to various sites. Uropathogenic *E. coli* strains have specialized fimbriae, which are able to attach to uroepithelium and aid in colonization of the urethra and bladder. *E coli* strains that do not possess uroepithelium-specific fimbriae are mainly associated with asymptomatic bacteriuria. Attachment of fimbriated *E. coli* provokes cytokine release and induces an inflammatory response. Recently, uropathogenic fimbriated *E. coli* strains have been shown to impair ureteric peristalsis, leading to reflux.[6] *S. saprophyticus* also possesses specific adhesins for uroepithelium, but it is also a strong urease producer, increasing urinary pH, and further hampering innate defences.

Catheter-associated urinary tract infection

Urinary catheter use changes the microbial spectrum considerably. In one study of short-term catheterization,[7] many infections were due to mixed organisms, with *Pseudomonas aeruginosa, Klebsiella pneumoniae*, and *E. coli* predominating, alone or together. In another study of short-term catheterization[8] 94% were due to single organisms, with *E. coli* and other enteric bacteria contributing 42% and candida 31%. Candiduria has been associated clearly with antibiotic use.[9] For patients with long-term catheters, *Proteus mirabilis* is more prominent, causing between 30% and 40% of infections.[10,11] A variety of Gram-positive bacteria, notably *Enterococcus spp.*, make up 34% of the remainder. In recent years, enterococci have become a major nosocomial pathogen showing increasing resistance to antibiotics. Catheterization of the urinary tract has been shown to be the strongest risk factor for hospital-acquired UTI, with an estimated 80% reduction in numbers of UTI cases if catheterization were not performed.[12] However, this is not always a realistic option. From the point of view of infection, the process of urethral catheterization can be considered in two groups: short-term and long-term use. The definition of short-term use varies in the literature, but is usually less than 28 days.[13] Intermittent catheterization should also be considered, but this is often not feasible in hospital. Short-term catheters are widely used in hospitals as part of patient care around interventions, particularly those which are surgical. In arthroplasty, they are used mainly for postoperative urinary retention following epidural anaesthesia, and either indwelling or clean intermittent catheterization can be used.[14] Long-term catheters are used when there is no alternative for the management of lower urinary tract dysfunction particularly in the elderly, in those with spinal injuries, especially where loss of upper limb function means that intermittent self-catheterization cannot be used, and after stroke. Though the introduction of closed systems has reduced the infection rate, over 50% of patients with long-term catheters will eventually develop an infection,[15] and all catheters will be colonized within one month[16] with 50% colonized after five days.[17] However, in most cases this is asymptomatic bacteriuria, although 20–30% of bacteriuric patients will go on to develop symptomatic CAUTI.[18]

Pathogenesis of catheter-associated urinary tract infection

The catheter provides a conduit from the environment directly to the bladder, and the normal voiding pattern is converted to continual drainage (unless a valve is used). In each case there is a column of urine in the catheter, and a pool of residual urine in the bladder, providing ideal conditions for bacterial proliferation. Bacteria can be introduced into the bladder from the external meatus, or the gloved fingers of healthcare personnel when the catheter is inserted,[19,20] and while the catheter is *in situ* the risk continues. Bacteria can be introduced into the distal part of the catheter lumen either by sampling from a port, or during bag change. The bag itself also presents a large pool of potentially contaminated urine, and any repositioning of the bag to allow reflux into the catheter, for example when patients are moved from one site to another, must be avoided. Bacteria can also migrate in the catheter-urethral interface. Many enterobacteria are motile by means of whip-like flagella and can swim up the column of urine in the catheter to reach the bladder. However, any bacteria that can attach to a surface will spread over that surface by simple proliferation. Some bacteria such as *Pseudomonas spp.* and particularly *Proteus spp.* can move over both epithelial and catheter surfaces by swarming, forming rafts of cells and, for *Proteus spp.*, increasing the production of urease.[21,22] Urease hydrolyses urea to produce ammonia, which has important implications for uropathogenesis: it raises the pH of the urine to the nucleation point for phosphates of calcium, ammonium, and magnesium[23] causing crystallization in the bladder and in the catheter lumen; and the ammonium ion produced in close proximity to the uroepithelium causes an acute inflammatory response.[24] In addition, CAUTI strains of *P. mirabilis* produce a haemolysin, HpmA, that has been shown to be more cytotoxic than ammonia.[25] The deposition of complex crystalline layers of struvite and apatite interspersed with *Proteus* bacilli and extracellular polymeric substances produced by the bacteria constitutes a biofilm (Fig. 1.3.1). Urease and consequent high ammonia levels are localized within the biofilm, leading to continuing crystal deposition.

Role of biofilms

The bacteria in the biofilm also undergo metabolic change, downregulating cell processes such as cell wall synthesis, protein synthesis, and DNA replication, and the cells enter a dormant phase. This reduces the effectiveness of commonly used antibiotics that target these processes such as beta-lactams, aminoglycosides, and quinolones. Antibiotic concentrations 500–1,000 times the minimum inhibitory concentration (that usually measured in the clinical laboratory) are required to eradicate the dormant bacteria, and even in urine these are usually not achievable. Biofilm formation by any CAUTI pathogen, but particularly by urease-producing bacteria, can be cleared only by catheter removal or change.

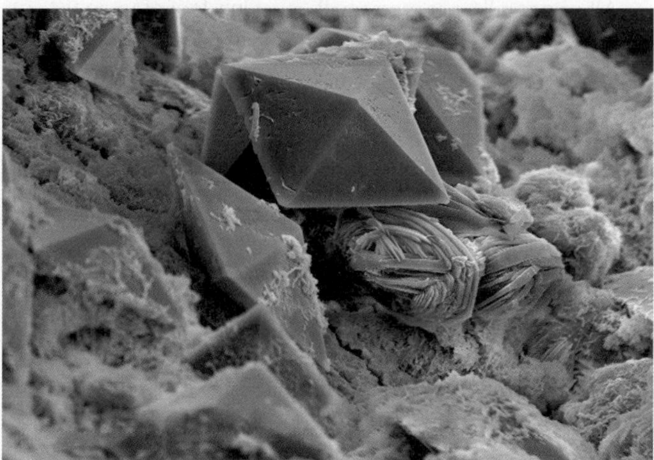

Fig. 1.3.1 Crystals and bacteria in a biofilm from a blocked and encrusted silver hydrogel catheter. The culture grew a mixed population including *Proteus mirabilis*.
Reproduced courtesy of Dr David Stickler, University of Cardiff, UK.

Diagnosis of catheter-associated urinary tract infection

Sampling of urine from the catheter in the absence of symptoms is a pointless waste of resources, except in pregnancy. Urine samples for culture and sensitivity should be taken immediately after catheter change, or by midstream urine sample if the catheter has been removed within the previous 48 hours. Pyuria in the absence of symptoms is not helpful in catheterized patients, even in the presence of significant bacteriuria, unless signs and symptoms suggest UTI. A negative or insignificant semi-quantitative culture in the presence of symptoms is likely to be caused by antibiotic administration, though less likely causes such as tuberculosis must not be forgotten. A significant culture in the absence of symptoms can be due to delay in transit of the sample to the laboratory, and this can also be responsible for reduction in neutrophil count. Pyuria in the absence of symptoms and with an insignificant culture may be found in catheterized patients due to irritation of the bladder mucosa by the catheter. Pyuria with CAASB should not be interpreted as an indication for antimicrobial treatment. The absence of pyuria in a symptomatic patient suggests a diagnosis other than CAUTI. Therefore, any investigations must be driven by clinical indication or suspicion, rather than 'routine' collection.

Catheter-associated asymptomatic bacteriuria and catheter-associated urinary tract infection

Differentiation between symptomatic UTI (CAUTI) and asymptomatic bacteriuria (CAASB) in the catheterized patient is difficult, but the chief determinant should be the presence of urinary tract-related symptoms or signs of infection. These include suprapubic pain or discomfort, but these may be modified in patients with neurogenic bladder dysfunction. Fever >38°C is often cited as a positive sign[26] yet one study found it to be an uncommon occurrence in elderly patients with catheters and significant bacteriuria, and it usually resolved within a few days without treatment.[27] A new onset of fever, or persisting or worsening fever, is more reliable. Renal involvement will be suggested by fever, possibly other systemic symptoms such as malaise and confusion, loin (flank) pain or tenderness, or new haematuria. Once other causes have been excluded, the diagnosis of CAUTI may be supported by urine culture. New onset of confusion, loss of appetite, or behaviour change can also be due to a urinary tract infection in the elderly, even in the absence of fever.[28]

Treatment

Treatment of hospital-acquired symptomatic urinary tract infection

Bacteriuria in pregnancy is often asymptomatic, yet it presents a 20–30 times greater risk of pyelonephritis and should be screened for in early pregnancy and treated promptly.[29,30] Infections are mainly due to *E. coli*. Amoxicillin or a cephalosporin, but not ciprofloxacin, may be used. Nitrofurantoin can also be used but should not be given at or near term (neonatal haemolysis risk); trimethoprim is useful, but should be avoided in the first trimester. For treatment of pyelonephritis, a cephalosporin, ciprofloxacin, or gentamicin should be given intravenously until systemic signs resolve, with conversion to oral therapy as soon as possible and then continued for 10–14 days.[29,31] For treatment of acute prostatitis, ciprofloxacin or trimethoprim should be given for 28 days.[31]

Treatment of catheter-associated urinary tract infection

If CAUTI is suspected, the catheter should be changed, and a urine sample taken from the new catheter for antibiotic susceptibility testing before initiation of antibiotic treatment. The choice of treatment should be according to local guidance to maximize clearance of infection but minimize the risk of inducing multiresistance or *Clostridium difficile* overgrowth. If catheterization can be discontinued, a midstream urine sample should be obtained prior to antimicrobial therapy, to help guide treatment. Such infections often resolve spontaneously without treatment. A three-day course may be considered for women aged ≥65 years with CAUTI.[16,30–32]

Prevention of catheter-associated urinary tract infection

Use of antibiotics

Prophylactic antibiotics have been considered for catheter insertion to reduce CAUTI; at catheter removal or change, to reduce risk of bacteraemia; and during catheterization, again to reduce CAUTI. The European Association of Urology guidelines do not recommend antimicrobial prophylaxis for insertion of urinary catheters[32] though if a symptomatic UTI is already present, then treatment for UTI should begin before catheterization.[33] Many groups of patients undergoing surgical procedures and who are to be catheterized as part of the process of care will receive antibiotic prophylaxis for that procedure, and this has sometimes been associated with a reduction in UTI as an incidental finding.[34] It is recommended that, where feasible, the urinary catheter should be inserted after intravenous antibiotic prophylaxis for surgery has been given. There is no indication to continue surgical 'prophylaxis' for several days until the catheter is removed: the standard of care should be to remove the catheter within 24 hours. Antibiotic use during catheterization has been associated with candiduria[9] and use of ciprofloxacin at catheter removal has been shown to be ineffective and encourages development of resistance.[35] Guidance from the UK National Institute for Health and Clinical Excellence (NICE)[36] states that current evidence does not support administration of antibiotics at change of an indwelling catheter and calls for a randomized controlled trial to clarify the issue. Further NICE guidance[37] states: 'When changing catheters in patients with a long-term indwelling urinary catheter, do not offer antibiotic prophylaxis routinely [but] consider antibiotic prophylaxis for patients who have a history of symptomatic urinary tract infection after catheter change **or** experience trauma during catheterization.'

For patients with long-term catheters, change of catheters has not been found to give rise to significant risk in the absence of CAUTI. In one study of elderly patients,[38] only 4.2% had bacteraemia after catheter change, and bacteria isolated from blood cultures (mainly coagulase-negative staphylococci) did not match those from the removed catheters. No patients experienced systemic infection.

Guidelines and protocols

Several guidelines have been published on the care of catheterized patients to minimize the risk of CAUTI. However, a survey carried out in 719 hospitals in the United States found that over half had no system for monitoring catheterized patients and three-quarters had no system of reminders or logs of duration of catheterization.[39] The following are adapted from North American sources and from the European Guidelines:[32,39]

1. There should be written catheter care protocols, including prompts for catheter removal when no longer needed. Institutions should educate staff about catheter management and indications for catheterization. Practice should be regularly audited. Regular feedback of audit data to all staff closes the audit cycle and reinforces compliance.
2. The use of catheterization and its duration should be reduced to a minimum.
3. Long-term indwelling catheters must be changed if there is any evidence of infection or blockage. Though there is no evidence for timing of pre-emptive catheter change, in practice they are commonly changed after three months.
4. Choice of catheter type should be made carefully, and indwelling catheters should be used only when necessary. They should not be used for the management of urinary incontinence unless all other avenues have been ineffective, or cannot be used in a particular case, such as cognitive impairment; clean intermittent catheterization should be considered when possible.
5. Protocols on hand hygiene must be observed and fresh disposable gloves used for catheter insertion, removal, and sampling.
6. Prior to insertion the meatus should be thoroughly cleaned with soap and water. Use of antiseptics for this purpose is not recommended.
7. A closed catheter system should be used and it should remain closed. Urine samples should always be taken from the catheter port, which should be cleaned with an alcohol swab before use. All urine spills, however small, must be cleaned up as urine is an excellent growth medium for uropathogens.
8. The drainage bag should be handled carefully, especially during ambulation or patient transfer, and must always be kept below the level of the bladder and the connecting tube.
9. Daily toilet of the catheter site with antiseptics is not recommended; if there is obvious soiling, soap and water should be used.
10. Prophylactic antibiotics should not be used at catheter insertion, change, or removal.
11. Antimicrobial prophylaxis should not be used during short-term or long-term catheterization to prevent CAUTI, as evidence shows no benefit and indicates a risk of antibiotic resistance.
12. In most cases, current guidelines do not support the use of antibiotic prophylaxis for catheterized patients undergoing surgical procedures or who have implanted devices, but specific and national guidelines should be consulted.

13. Antiseptics or antibiotics should not be added to the drainage bag as this brings no benefit and selects resistant uropathogens.
14. Catheters should not be irrigated with saline or any other solution to reduce CAUTI or CAASB.
15. The duration of catheterization should be limited postoperatively, and the use of clear protocols for catheter removal has reduced UTI.

Antimicrobial urinary catheters

Because of the widespread problem of bacteriuria associated with catheter use, and particularly because of encrustation, obstruction, and CAUTI in long-term catheterization, attempts have been made to produce an antimicrobial urinary catheter that will significantly reduce these problems. The approaches have included surface modification to reduce bacterial adhesion, such as coating with polytetrafluoroethylene (PTFE), antiseptic or antibiotic coating to kill attached bacteria (such as chlorhexidine or silver alloy), and impregnation of antimicrobials into the latex or silicone catheter material (such as silver and nitrofural). Conflicting results have been found in clinical studies, mainly due to trial design.[40] A properly constructed randomized controlled trial of silver-coated catheters has been called for by numerous authors and health authorities. Recently such a trial has been published, comparing silver-coated and nitrofural-impregnated catheters with a control group consisting of PTFE-coated standard catheters, in over 6,000 patients with short-term catheters.[41] There was no significant difference in outcome (symptoms and antibiotic treatment for clinician-diagnosed UTI within six weeks of catheter insertion) between the silver alloy-coated catheters and the control, and though there was a slight, statistically significant reduction in CAASB and microbiologically proven CAUTI in the nitrofural group, these catheters were associated with increased discomfort and were not considered to be clinically beneficial. The authors were unable to recommend the use of either catheter for short-term use. There are currently no antimicrobial catheters offering reduction of CAUTI in long-term users.

Conclusion

While in many instances asymptomatic bacteriuria is benign and should not be treated, its occurrence in pregnancy is an exception. Symptomatic bacteriuria should be investigated and treated. Catheter use and duration should be kept to a minimum. Bacteriuria in catheterized patients should be treated only when symptomatic, and this should include catheter removal or change. Every healthcare organization should adopt written standards for the management of patients with catheters including strategies to deal with catheter-associated bacteriuria and UTI. These should take into account published and updated local, national, and international guidance documents. Antimicrobial catheters have not been found to be beneficial.

Further reading

Grabe M, Bjerklund-Johansen TE, Botto H, *et al.* Guidelines on Urological Infections. Arnhem, The Netherlands: European Association of Urology, 2011.

Gupta K, Hooton TM, Naber KG, *et al.* International clinical practice guidelines for the treatment of acute uncomplicated cystitis and pyelonephritis in women: A 2010 update by the Infectious Diseases Society of America and the European Society for Microbiology and Infectious Diseases. *Clin Infect Dis* 2011; **52**(5):e103–e20.

Hooton TM, Bradley SF, Cardenas DD, *et al.* Diagnosis, prevention, and treatment of catheter-associated urinary tract infection in adults: 2009 International Clinical Practice Guidelines from the Infectious Diseases Society of America. *Clin Infect Dis* 2010; **50**:625–63.

Hooton TM, Stamm WE. Diagnosis and treatment of uncomplicated urinary tract infection. *Infect Dis Clin North Am* 1997; **11**(3):551–81.

Niel-Weise BS, van den Broek PJ. Urinary catheter policies for short-term bladder drainage in adults. *Cochrane Database Syst Rev* 2005; **20**:CD004203.

Pickard R, Lam T, MacLennan G, *et al.* Antimicrobial catheters for reduction of symptomatic urinary tract infection in adults requiring short-term catheterisation in hospital: a multicentre randomized controlled trial. *The Lancet* 2012; doi.org/10.1016/S0140-6736(12)61380-4.

Saint S, Kowalski CP, SaKaufman SR, *et al.* Preventing hospital-acquired urinary tract infection in the United States: A national study. *Clin Infect Dis* 2008; **46**:243–50.

Tenke P, Kovacs B, Bjerklund-Johansen TE, Matsumoto T, Tambyah PA, Naber KG. European and Asian guidelines on management and prevention of catheter-associated urinary tract infections. *Internat J Antimicrob Ag* 2008; **31S**:S68–S78.

References

1. National Nosocomial Infections Surveillance (NNIS) System Report, data summary from January 1992 through June 2004, issued October 2004. *Am J Infect Control* 2004; **32**:470–85.
2. Smyth ETM, McIlvenny G, Enstone JE, *et al.*, on behalf of the Hospital Infection Society Prevalence Survey Steering Group. Four Country Healthcare Associated Infection Prevalence Survey 2006: overview of the results. *J Hosp Infect* 2008; **69**:230–48.
3. Hooton TM, Stamm WE. Diagnosis and treatment of uncomplicated urinary tract infection. *Infect Dis Clin North Am* 1997; **11**(3):551–81.
4. Svanborg C, Godaly G. Bacterial virulence in urinary tract infection. *Infect Dis Clin North Am* 1997; **11**(3):513–29.
5. Bien J, Sokolova O, Bozko P. Role of uropathogenic escherichia coli virulence factors in development of urinary tract infection and kidney damage. *Internat J Nephrol* 2012; doi:10.1155/2012/681473.
6. Floyd RV, Upton M, Hultgren SJ, Wray S, Burdyga TV, Winstanley C. Escherichia coli–mediated impairment of ureteric contractility is uropathogenic E. coli specific. *J Infect Dis* 2012; DOI: 10.1093/infdis/jis554.
7. Hola V, Ruzicka F, Horka M. Microbial diversity in biofilm infections of the urinary tract with the use of sonication techniques. *FEMS Immunol Med Microbiol* 2010; **59**(3):525–8.
8. Tambyah PA, Maki DG. The relationship between pyuria and infection in patients with indwelling urinary catheters. A prospective study of 761 patients. *Arch Intern Med* 2000; **160**:673–7.
9. Goetz LL, Howard M, Cipher D, Revankar SG. Occurrence of candiduria in a population of chronically catheterized patients with spinal cord injury. *Spinal Cord* 2010; **48**(1):51–4.
10. McLeod SM, Stickler DJ. Species interactions in mixed-community crystalline biofilms on urinary catheters. *J Med Microbiol* 2007; **56**(11):1549–57.
11. Mobley HL. Virulence of Proteus mirabilis. (pp. 245–69) In: Mobley HL, Warren JW (eds). *Urinary Tract Infections: Molecular Pathogenesis and Clinical Management.* Washington DC: ASM Press, 1996.
12. King C, Alvarez L, Holmes A, Moore L, Galletly T, Aylin P. Risk factors for healthcare-associated urinary tract infection and their applications in surveillance using hospital administrative data: a systematic review. *J Hosp Infect* 2012; **82**(4):219–26.
13. Morris NS, Stickler DJ. Encrustation of indwelling urethral catheters by *Proteus mirabilis* biofilms growing in human urine. *J Hosp Infect* 1998; **39**:227–34.

14. van den Brand IC, Castelein RM. Total joint arthroplasty and incidence of postoperative bacteriuria with an indwelling catheter or intermittent catherization with one-dose antibiotic prophylaxis: a prospective randomized trial. *J Arthroplasty* 2001; **16**(7):850–5.
15. Schumm K, Lam TB. Types of urethral catheters for management of short-term voiding problems in hospitalised adults. *Cochrane Database Syst Rev* 2008; **16**:CD004013.
16. Hooton TM, Bradley SF, Cardenas DD, *et al.* Diagnosis, prevention, and treatment of catheter-associated urinary tract infection in adults: 2009 International Clinical Practice Guidelines from the Infectious Diseases Society of America. *Clin Infect Dis* 2010; **50**:625–63.
17. Warren JW. Catheter-associated urinary tract infections. *Infect Dis Clin North Am* 1997; **11**:609–622.
18. Stamm W. Urinary tract infections. In: Bennett J, Brachman P (eds). *Hospital Infection*, 4th edition. Philadelphia PA: Lippincott-Raven, 1998.
19. Barford JMT, Anson K, Yanmin Hu K, Coates ARM. A model of catheter-associated urinary tract infection initiated by bacterial contamination of the catheter tip. *BJU Internat* 2008; **10**(2):67–74.
20. Foxman B, Wu J, Farrer EC, Goldberg DE, Younger JG, Xi C. Early development of bacterial community diversity in emergently placed urinary catheters. *BMC Research Notes* 2012; **5**:332.
21. Stickler D, Hughes G. Ability of proteus mirabilis to swarm over urethral catheters. *Eur J Clin Microbiol Infect Dis* 1999; **18**:206–8.
22. Allison C, Lai H-C, Hughes C. Co-ordinate expression of virulence genes during swarm-cell differentiation and population migration of Proteus mirabilis. *Molecular Microbiol* 1992; **6**:1583–91.
23. Choong S, Whitfield H. Biofilms and their role in urology. *BJU Internat* 2000; **86**(8):935–41.
24. Johnson DE, Russell RG, Lockatell CV, Zulty JC, Warren JW, Mobley HL. Contribution of *Proteus mirabilis* urease to persistence, urolithiasis, and acute pyelonephritis in a mouse model of ascending urinary tract infection. *Infect Immun* 1993; **61**:2748–54.
25. Mobley HL, Chippendale GR, Swihart KG, Welch RA. Cytotoxicity of the HpmA hemolysin and urease of Proteus mirabilis and Proteus vulgaris against cultured human renal proximal tubular epithelial cells. *Infect Immun* 1991; **59**(6):2036–42.
26. Kunin CM, Chin QF, Chambers S. Morbidity and mortality associated with indwelling urinary catheters in elderly patients in a nursing home—confounding due to the presence of associated diseases. *J Am Geriatr Soc* 1987; **35**(11):1001–6.
27. Warren JW, Damron D, Tenney JH, Hoopes JM, Deforge B, Muncie HL. Fever, bacteremia, and death as complications of bacteriuria in women with long-term urethral catheters. *J Infect Dis* 1987; **155**:1151–8.
28. Mouton C, Adenuga B, Vijayan J. Urinary tract infections in long-term care. *Ann Longterm Care* 2010; **18**:35–9.
29. Gupta K, Hooton TM, Naber KG, *et al.* International clinical practice guidelines for the treatment of acute uncomplicated cystitis and pyelonephritis in women: A 2010 update by the Infectious Diseases Society of America and the European Society for Microbiology and Infectious Diseases. *Clin Infect Dis* 2011; **52**(5):e103–e20.
30. Tenke P, Kovacs B, Bjerklund-Johansen TE, Matsumoto T, Tambyah PA, Naber KG. European and Asian guidelines on management and prevention of catheter-associated urinary tract infections. *Internat J Antimicrob Ag* 2008; **31S**:S68–S78.
31. British Medical Association and the Royal Pharmaceutical Society of Great Britain. *British National Formulary*, 63rd edition. UK: BMJ Publishing Group, 2012.
32. Grabe M, Bjerklund-Johansen TE, Botto H, *et al. Guidelines on Urological Infections*. Arnhem, The Netherlands: European Association of Urology, 2011.
33. Ibrahim AI. Hospital acquired pre-prostatectomy bacteriuria: risk factors and implications. *East Afr Med J* 1996; **73**(2):107–10.
34. Boxma H, Broekhuizen T, Patka P, Oosting H. Randomised controlled trial of single-dose antibiotic prophylaxis in surgical treatment of closed fractures: The Dutch Trauma Trial. *The Lancet* 1999; **347**:1133–7.
35. Wazait HD, Patel HR, van der Meulen JH, *et al.* A pilot randomized double-blind placebo-controlled trial on the use of antibiotics on urinary catheter removal to reduce the rate of urinary tract infection: the pitfalls of ciprofloxacin. *BJU Int* 2004; **94**:1048–50.
36. Prevention and control of healthcare-associated infections in primary and community care: NICE Clinical Guideline 139. Available at: https://www.nice.org.uk/guidance/cg139. Issued: March 2012.
37. Urinary incontinence in neurological disease: Management of lower urinary tract dysfunction in neurological disease. NICE Clinical Guideline 148. Available at: https://www.nice.org.uk/guidance/cg148. Issued: August 2012.
38. Bregenzer T, Frei R, Widmer AF, *et al.* Low risk of bacteremia during catheter replacement in patients with long-term urinary catheters. *Arch Intern Med* 1997; **157**:521–5.
39. Saint S, Kowalski CP, SaKaufman SR, *et al.* Preventing hospital-acquired urinary tract infection in the United States: A national study. *Clin Infect Dis* 2008; **46**:243–50.
40. Niel-Weise BS, van den Broek PJ. Urinary catheter policies for short-term bladder drainage in adults. *Cochrane Database Syst Rev* 2005; **20**:CD004203.
41. Pickard R, Lam T, MacLennan G, *et al.* Antimicrobial catheters for reduction of symptomatic urinary tract infection in adults requiring short-term catheterisation in hospital: a multicentre randomized controlled trial. *The Lancet* 2012; doi.org/10.1016/S0140–6736(12)61380–4.

CHAPTER 1.4

Urinary tract infection

Asymptomatic bacteriuria, cystitis, and pyelonephritis in adults

Magnus Grabe and Björn Wullt

Introduction to urinary tract infection

Urinary tract infections (UTI) are among the most frequent infections encountered in the community and hospital environments. Patients with urological anatomical or functional abnormalities are particularly at risk for UTI. This chapter aims to present basic information on epidemiology of bacteriuria and UTI, a current approach to classification and risk factor evaluation, diagnostic tools, and guidelines for the management of different forms of UTI encountered in the general and urological populations.

Epidemiology of bacteriuria and urinary tract infection

Bacteriuria is present in up to 4–5% of the general population.[1,2] The prevalence is 1–3% in school-age girls but much lower in boys. The incidence of asymptomatic bateriuria (ABU) and symptomatic UTI increases in young women following the onset of sexual activity. The prevalence of bacteriuria increases further after the menopause, being between 5–20% in healthy women aged 65–70 years and almost 50% of all women in elderly care homes.[3–5] Almost one in two women will have at least one UTI during their lifetime, and more than one-third of all women will experience a UTI before the age of 24 years, with a substantial number of these experiencing recurrent infections.[1]

Bacteriuria and UTI are uncommon in men up to the age of 50 years. The incidence progressively increases with ageing associated with prostatic enlargement, and other age-related causes of lower urinary tract dysfunction.[1] Younger men on the other hand occasionally suffer from bacterial prostatitis, a condition less frequent than UTI in women, but presenting with similar symptoms.[6,7] Patients with urological diseases often have complicated UTI with underlying risk factors. Urological surgery is associated with the risk of infectious complications and healthcare-associated infections (HAI) are observed in approximately 10% of hospitalized patients in urological wards.[8]

Pathogenesis and pathogens

Pathogenesis

In healthy individuals the urinary tract is generally considered to be sterile or with very low bacterial counts. Pathogens causing UTI mostly originate from the patient's own colonic flora, and predominantly reach the urinary tract by ascending through the urethra.[9] Once the bladder is colonized, the balance between host response and bacterial virulence factors decides the outcome: an acute symptomatic infection of varying severity and localization, or an asymptomatic bacteriuric state (Fig. 1.4.1).[10] Importantly, anatomical and functional urinary tract dysfunctions alter susceptibility to UTI. Females of all ages are more prone to UTIs than males, probably due to their shorter urethra and its close proximity to the vagina and perianal region. Any anatomical or functional reason that impedes normal outflow of urine and subsequently the physical clearing of bacteria increases the risk of UTI, and makes symptomatic infection with less virulent organisms more likely. Severely immunocompromised individuals may get symptomatic infections from normally non-pathogenic strains.[11]

Escherichia coli (E. coli) is the most commonly isolated uropathogen. Virulence factors are encoded by genes clustered on so-called 'pathogenicity islands' (PAI),[12] which include adherence factors mediated by fimbriae and iron-uptake mechanisms. The virulence factors work collectively and may be activated or deactivated during the course of infection. Fimbriae are hair-like organelles expressed on the bacterial surface, that mediate adherence to urothelial cells. P-fimbriae have been shown to be an important virulence factor in pyelonephritis. Type I fimbriae are encoded by virtually all *E. coli* isolates regardless of origin or site of infection and have been proposed as a virulence factor in simple cystitis, but their definitive role in human UTI remains to be defined.[13] Recent experimental data has suggested that *E. coli* during the course of infection penetrate into the urothelium to form intracellular bacterial communities, explaining episodes of relapses in recurrent UTI.[14] However, this concept has not convincingly been demonstrated in human UTI *in vivo*. Biofilm formation, an important bacterial surviving factor in infections involving foreign bodies, may also play a role in human UTI.[15]

The host defence in human UTI is predominantly reliant on innate immune mechanisms. Although specific immune responses with up-regulation of T and B cells and secretion of immunoglobulins do occur, they are not crucial for clearance of the acute infection. The most important cell-surface receptors for triggering an innate immune response are members of the Toll-like receptor family. TLR4 is expressed on uroepithelial surfaces and recognize pathogen-associated molecular patterns specifically on Gram-negative bacteria, such as lipopolysaccharide. In pyelonephritis, the TLR4

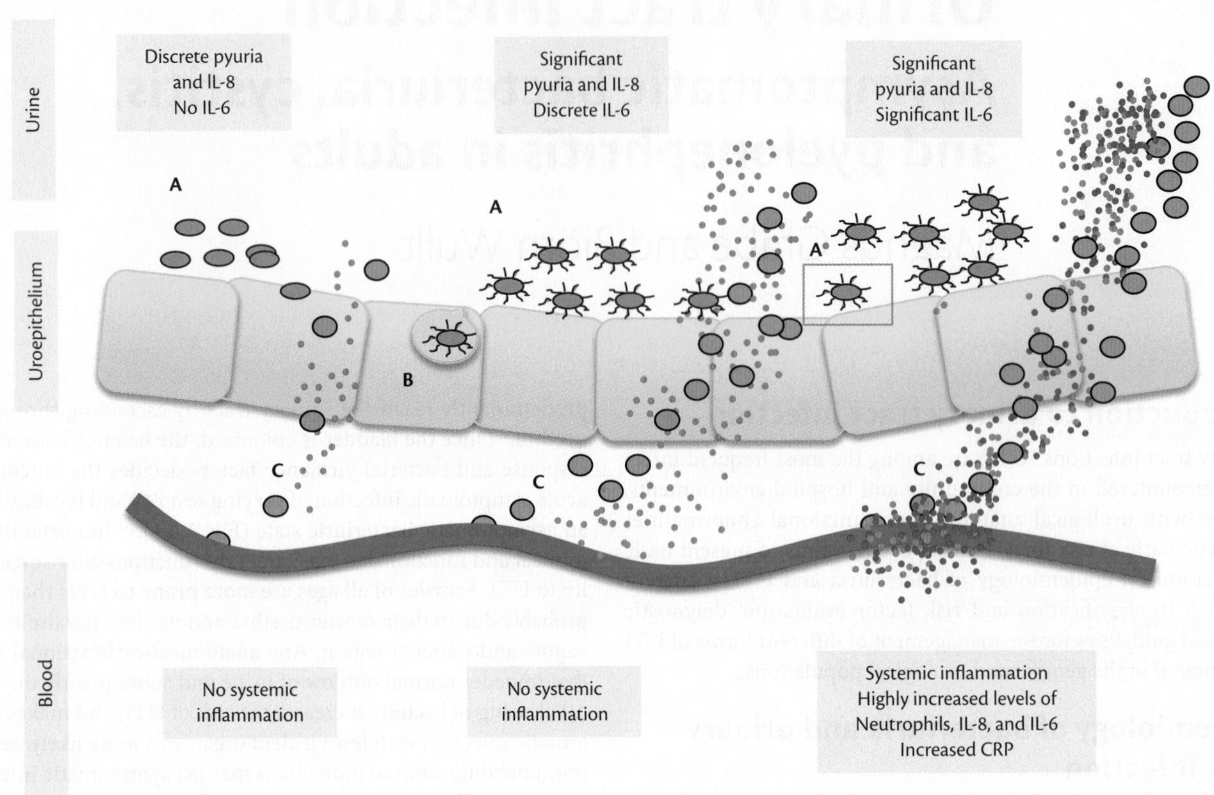

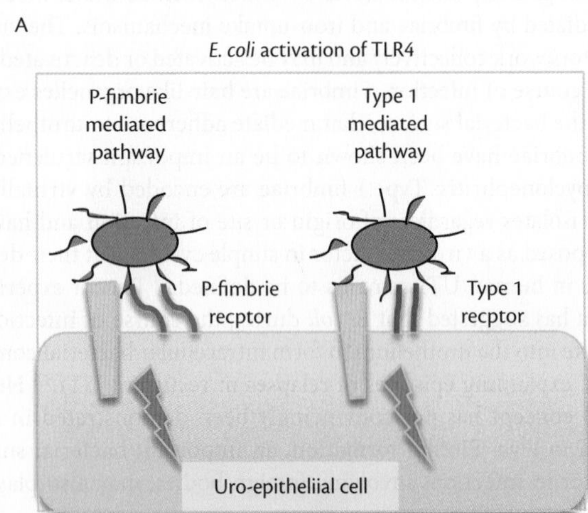

Fig. 1.4.1 Schematic figure outlining bacterial challenge and activation of the host response in urinary tract infections. (A) In ABU there is no or inefficient activation of the uroepithelium. In symptomatic UTI - cystitis and pyelonephritis - bacterial contact with the uroepithelium is mediated by P or Type 1 fimbriae and its receptors on the uroepithelium. Toll-like receptor 4 (TLR4) recognizes the Gram-negative uropathogens, the uroepithelial cell is activated and inflammatory mediators (IL-6 and IL-8) are produced. (B) In recurrent cystitis, intracellular bacterial fabrics have been suggested. (C) Activated neutrophils express the IL-8 receptor (CXCR1) and transmigrate through the tissue following the concentration gradient of IL-8, to the place of infection.

Reproduced from Béla Köves and Björn Wullt, 'The Roles of the Host and the Pathogens in Urinary Tract Infections', *European Urology Supplements*, Volume 15, Issue 4, pp. 88–94, Copyright © 2016, with permission from Elsevier.

Table 1.4.1 The most frequently isolated urinary pathogens and their associated clinical presentation. The individual patient characteristics and results for any previous urine culture are important in predicting potential pathogens to guide empirical antibiotic treatment before the results of urine culture are available

Uropathogen	Association
Gram-negative strains	
Escherichia coli	Most frequent organism in UTI (species consist of many different clones with varying pathogenicity/virulence) Asymptomatic bacteriuria Uncomplicated cystitis and pyelonephritis in women and children
Proteus mirabilis	Infective renal stone formation
Klebsiella, Enterobacter, Serratia, Citrobacter, Pseudomonas	Complicated UTI Healthcare-associated infection Bacteriuria or UTI associated with catheters, stents and nephrostomy tubes, and immunocompromised patients
Gram-positive strains	
Staphylococcus saprophyticus	UTI in sexually active women
Staphylococcus epidermidis	Bacteriuria/UTI associated with catheters, stents, and nephrostomy tubes
Group B Streptococcus (GBS)	Occasionally transient ABU/ contamination
Enterococcus faecalis	Occasionally transient ABU Occasionally causes UTI and febrile UTI (5%) Bacteriuria/UTI associated with catheters, stents, and nephrostomy tubes Kidney transplant patients
Enterococcus faecium	Bacteriuria/UTI associated with catheters, stents, and nephrostomy tubes Complicated UTI/patients with risk factors
Mycobacterium spp.	
Mycobacterium tuberculosis See Chapter 1.6	Renal and urogenital tuberculosis Acquired immunodeficiency syndrome (AIDS)
Fungi	
Candida sp.	Prolonged antibiotic treatment Immunocompromised patients Critically ill patients Patients with diabetes mellitus

mediated cell activation is strongly enhanced by the added effect of P-fimbriae mediated adherence. In the presence of the co-receptor CD14, TLR4 is activated by lipopolysaccharides (LPS) expressed on the cell surface of Gram-negative bacteriae. In the urinary tract, however, type I and P-fimbriae activates TLR4 due to lack of the co-receptor, and this allows the host to fine-tune the response to the particular strain.[16] After TLR4 activation, the uroepithelial cell secretes cytokines such as interleukin 6 (IL-6) and interleukin 8 (IL-8). IL-6 is an inflammatory acute phase reactant and IL-8 is a potent chemoattractant, which recruits neutrophils into the urinary tract tissue. The neutrophil migration in the tissue depends upon the IL8 receptor (CXCR1), which directs the neutrophils towards the IL-8 concentration gradient. The infecting microbes can then be phagocytized at the site of invasion (Fig. 1.4.1).[17]

In clinical practice, it is frequently observed that individuals with or without other urinary tract dysfunctions differ in their susceptibility to symptomatic UTI. Recent research indicates that genetic polymorphisms may play a role in individual susceptibility to UTI. TLR4 gene polymorphism, for example, may increase the risk of development of ABU,[18] and CXCR1 polymorphism may partly explain why some individuals suffer recurrent pyelonephritis and are at risk for renal scarring.[19] We also know that the magnitude of host response to ABU varies between individuals, probably due to individual variation in TLR4 function.[20] Historically, UTI research has focused on the role of bacterial virulence. In the future, we will probably see more research on the variability of host defences between individuals linked to genetic differences and this is covered in greater detail in the chapter about pathogenesis (see Chapter 1.1).[21]

Pathogens

Table 1.4.1 lists the most frequently encountered urinary tract pathogens.[22,23] Primary uropathogens are microorganisms with a proven independent capacity to cause UTI and are typified by *E. coli*, which causes the majority of UTIs, and is also the model organism in UTI research. Among Gram-positive cocci, *Enterococcus faecalis* is the most common cause of UTI. *Staphylococcus saprophticus* is seen frequently in sporadic infections in women of fertile age but rarely in infections in postmenopausal women. Secondary uropathogens are more likely to be found in complicated infections and in urological patients requiring hospitalization, and are frequently components of polymicrobial infections. In recent prevalence studies predominantly involving European urology departments, *E. coli* was found to be the causative organism in 35–60% of patients, while other opportunistic species were identified in proportionally higher frequencies.[8] Fungal infections are also regularly found in hospitalized patients, mainly *Candida* species. *Mycobacterium tuberculosis*, as described in Chapter 1.1, causes chronic infection of the kidneys and may affect the bladder and male genital organs.

UTI is generally an example of strict monocolonization, but sporadically two strains may be isolated such as *Enterococcus faecalis* and a Gram-negative uropathogen. More than two strains are considered an external contamination and a repeat culture is usually recommended. However, in patients with an indwelling catheter, a complicated urological condition, or a colovesical fistula, multiple strains may reflect true colonization or recurrent infections.

In recent years, organisms resistant to several standard antibiotics used in the urinary tract have spread worldwide at an alarming pace. This is particularly true for the extended spectrum

Table 1.4.2 Classification of urinary tract infections (UTI) in relation to anatomical location and presence of risk factors

Risk factor	Organ/space	Type of infection	Symptoms
Uncomplicated UTI No identified risk factor	Urine	Asymptomatic bacteriuria (Location: lower UT)	None
	Urinary bladder	Cystitis (acute, sporadic)	Dysuria, frequency, urgency, bladder tenderness/pain
		Cystitis (recurrent)	
	Kidney	Acute pyelonephritis	Abdominal or flank pain, fever, nausea or vomiting, with or without symptoms of cystitis
Complicated UTI Presence of one or more risk factor (see Table 1.4.3)	Urinary bladder	Cystitis (recurrent with risk factors)	Dysuria, frequency, urgency, bladder tenderness/pain
		Specific infection such as tuberculosis, schistosomiasis	
	Upper urinary tract	Asymptomatic bacteriuria (Location: upper UT)	None
		Febrile UTI	SIRS,[1] fever, systemic illness with or without other symptoms from the urinary tract/abdomen
	Kidney	Acute pyelonephritis Chronic pyelonephritis Abscess of the kidney Emphysematous pyelonephritis Xanthogranulomatous pyelonephritis	Abdominal or flank pain, systemic illness, fever, nausea, or vomiting
		Renal tuberculosis (See chapter 1.6)	Variable, insidious
	Retroperitoneal space	Perinephric abscess	
	Blood stream	Sepsis (urosepsis)	SIRS, systemic symptoms with or without circulatory or organ failure
Male accessory gland infection (interact in male complicated UTI)	Prostate	Acute bacterial prostatitis Abscess of the prostate	Lower abdominal pain, fever, painful prostate, risk for urinary retention
		Chronic bacterial prostatitis	Variable

[1]Systemic inflammatory response syndrome.

UT = urinary tract.

Source: data from Bjerklund-Johansen TE *et al.*, 'Critical review of current definitions of urinary tract infections and proposal of an EAU/ESIU classification system', *International Journal of Antimicrobial Agents*, Volume 38, Supplement, pp. 64–70, Copyright © 2011 Elsevier B.V. and the International Society of Chemotherapy; and European Association of Urology, 'Urological Infections', in *Guidelines of the European Association of Urology 2015*, Copyright © 2015 EAU.

beta-lactamase (ESBL)-producing *Enterobacteriaceae* such as *E.coli* and *Klebsiella spp*. The plasmid-bound ESBL has developed into a subgroup of enzymes with resistance to different antibiotics, including carbapenem ($ESBL_{Carba}$).[24]

Classification of urinary tract infection and terminology

There is no universally accepted classification of UTI. The United States-based Centers for Disease Control and Prevention (CDC) classification is the most often used.[25] Traditionally, UTI have been separated in uncomplicated and complicated UTI, complicated indicating the presence of an anatomical or functional urinary tract anomaly. UTI have also been divided into *upper UTI*, when the infection involves the kidney and the ureter, and *lower UTI*, when located in the bladder or urethra.[26]

Table 1.4.2 illustrates a practical classification of UTI combining the anatomical location, general terminology, and the range of symptoms associated with different types of UTI (phenotype). The European Association of Urology (EAU) working group on urological infections has suggested a slightly different approach to the classification focusing on infections of the urinary tract in a urological perspective combining four different aspects of the infection.[27,28]

1. Site of the infection: the bladder (*cystitis*), the kidney (*pyelonephritis*), the blood stream (sepsis), or unspecified. In urology practice, patients often present with high fever and the presence of inflammatory parameters without distinct clinical signs of pyelonephritis, often referred to as a *febrile UTI*.
2. Assessment of infection severity (Fig.1.4.2): UTI can be seen as a continuum from harmless asymptomatic bacteriuria (ABU) to sepsis with organ failure; the patient's condition can switch from the least severe to the most severe within a short period of time.
3. The presence of risk factors for UTI (Table 1.4.3).
4. Pathogen identification by urine and/or blood culture and its sensitivity to urinary tract antibiotics (Table 1.4.1).

All the information can then be combined into a defined phenotype characterizing the infectious condition.[27]

Other terms

A clinical problem specific to males is differentiating infections of the lower urinary tract and inflammation/infection of the prostate as symptoms overlap (see Chapter 1.6).

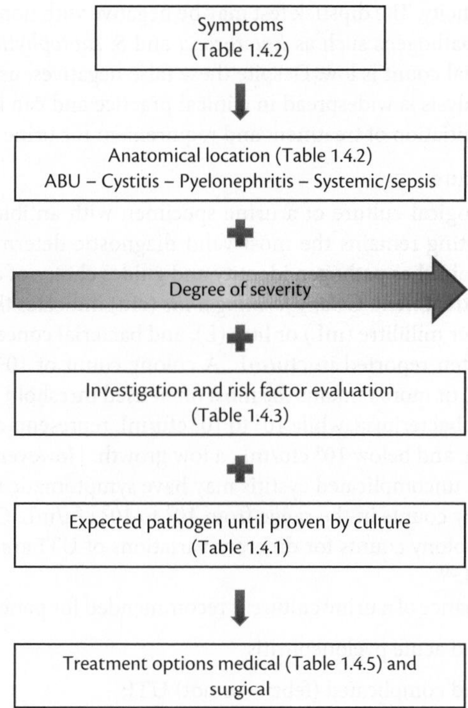

Fig. 1.4.2 The assessment of each individual infection is based on the combination of (i) the symptoms and anatomical localization; (ii) the degree of severity (the patient's general condition); (iii) the evaluation of possible underlying risk factors; and (iv) the expected uropathogen. This assessment is the basis for initiating an empirical antibiotic treatment, supportive treatment, and the need for surgical drainage.

Asymptomatic bacteriuria (ABU) is the microbiologic finding of the presence of bacteria ≥10^5 cfu/mL in two different samples together with the absence of clinical signs or symptoms referable to the urinary tract.[4]

When a kidney infection is combined with obstruction, infected urine stagnates within the renal pelvis creating a *pyonephrosis* and in rare cases *emphysematous pyelonephritis*. This is a highly dangerous condition that easily can turn into *urosepsis* with associated systemic disturbance of vital organ perfusion. In some instances, a *renal abscess* can develop within the kidney. Infected material can also leak outside the kidney, into the confined perirenal space, leading to a *perinephric abscess* (see Chapter 1.5).

Chronic pyelonephritis is a persistent destructive inflammation of the renal parenchyma leading to scars and kidney function loss, and is usually due to stone disease in deformed areas of the kidney. This is in distinction to *reflux nephropathy*, which is a generally stable state of renal scarring resulting from childhood reflux. In rare cases, chronic inflammation of the kidney can progress to *xanthogranulomatous pyelonephritis*.

A *healthcare-associated infection* is an infection arising in association with healthcare provision in a person without identified infection prior to an intervention. For UTI, this most commonly is associated with an indwelling urinary catheter (see Chapter 1.6).[8]

Tuberculosis of the urinary tract, although not frequent, must be recognized. It is a chronic inflammation with progressive destruction of the kidney, ureteral inflammation and cystitis, and can establish in the male genital organs (see Chapter 1.6). Schistosomiasis of the urinary bladder creates an inflammation of the urinary bladder

Table 1.4.3 Risk factors for UTI grouped according to anatomical and functional abnormalities of the urinary tract

Risk factor	Examples
Gender, genetic, and hereditary	Family history of UTI Female gender
Inborn anatomical abnormality	Vesicoureteral reflux Stricture of the pelvoureteric junction Other strictures of the urinary tract Urethra valves Congenital neurological disease
Acquired obstruction of the lower urinary tract	Benign prostate enlargement Residual urine Bladder stone Bladder tumour Stricture of the urethra
Acquired obstruction of the upper urinary tract	Kidney and ureteric stone Ureteric tumour Stricture of the ureter External compression of the ureter (tumour, inflammation) Retroperitoneal fibrosis, previous radiotherapy
Kidney disease	Anatomic abnormality of the kidney (inherited) Polycystic kidney Renal insufficiency Kidney transplant
Concomitant diseases	Diabetes mellitus Dysfunction of immune system (natural, induced) Steroid treatment Connective tissue disorders Circulatory insufficiency Inflammatory disease of the bladder
Spinal cord lesion Other neurological or functional dysfunction	Residual urine Neurological bladder dysfunction Neuromuscular dysfunction of the bladder Incontinence
Catheter treatment	Indwelling urinary catheter Ureteric stent (i.e. double pig tail stent) Nephrostomy tube
Urological surgery	Asymptomatic bacteriuria prior to or at surgery Retrograde endoscopic access to urinary tract Surgery with open urinary tract and/or bowel (i.e. clean-contaminated and contaminated procedures)
Physiological conditions	Pregnancy Postmenopausal oestrogen deficiency Ageing
Behaviour	Sexual activity
Others	Intensive care treatment Long hospital stay

and the ureter, and subsequent fibrosis with formation of scars and strictures.

Risk factors for urinary tract infection

There are a number of factors that increase risk of UTI for an individual from the baseline of spontaneous occurrence. Risk factors can be quantified by the probability that an event occurs in an exposed group compared with an unexposed group. For UTI, they range from genetic and gender-related factors to complicated combinations of medical, functional, and anatomical states. Their identification is essential for the best care of people with UTI and particularly for those undergoing urological surgery.[29]

General risk factors

General risk factors include older age, anatomical abnormalities, poor nutritional status, smoking, altered immune response, diabetes mellitus, long preoperative hospital stay, and coexistent infection at a remote site.

Specific risk factors

Conventional UTI risk factors are listed in Table 1.4.3. An alternative grouping of the different risk factors under the acronym **ORENUC** (**O** = none, **R** = recurrent UTI, **E** = extra-urogenital, **N** = nephropathic, **U** = urological, and **C** = catheter present) based on the underlying location and mechanism has recently been proposed.[27]

Bacteriuria and a previous history of urogenital infection are two critical risk factors for infectious complications related to surgery; where possible, bacteriuria should be controlled or eradicated prior to urologic instrumentation.

Diagnosis of urinary tract infection

Symptoms of UTI are due to the inflammatory response within the target tissue. The most frequently encountered symptoms are presented in Table 1.4.2. It is generally recognized that a UTI is confirmed when at least one of the main symptoms is followed by a urine culture showing bacterial growth of $\geq 10^5$ cfu/mL of a single organism.[30] This threshold potentially misses lower, but clinically relevant bacterial counts (see below and Table 1.4.4). It will therefore sometimes be appropriate to make a clinical diagnosis of UTI based on a combination of symptoms and sound clinical judgement.

Urine analysis

Urine sample collection

To avoid contamination, the urine has traditionally been collected after cleaning of the vulva and the external urethral opening (meatus) in the anterior to posterior direction and caught midstream, avoiding any contact with the surrounding skin. Although some studies have shown that the cleaning might not be necessary, the 'clean catch' technique remains recommended.[31]

Urine reagent strip test

The reagent strip ('dipstick') is a useful test in diagnosing UTI prior to culture. Combining a detection of nitrite test (refecting bacterial conversion of nitrate to nitrite) and of leucocyte esterase as a marker of *pyuria*, dipstick urinalysis has moderate sensitivity, but high specificity. The dipstick test may be negative with non-nitrate-reducing pathogens such as *Enterococci* and *S. saprophyticus*, or if the bacterial count is low. Despite these false negatives, use of dipstick urinalysis is widespread in clinical practice and can be useful to guide initiation of treatment and requirement for urine culture.

Urine culture

Microbiological culture of a urine specimen with antibiotic sensitivity testing remains the most valid diagnostic determinant of UTI. It establishes pathogen identity and guides choice of adequate antibiotic treatment. *Colony forming units* (cfu) indicates the bacterial load per millilitre (mL) or litre (L), and bacterial concentration is most often reported in cfu/mL. A colony count of 10^5 cfu/mL (10^8 cfu/L) or more remains the most often used threshold value for significant bacteriuria, while 10^4 to 10^5 cfu/mL represents a moderate growth, and below 10^4 cfu/mL, a low growth. However, women with acute uncomplicated cystitis may have symptomatic infection with colony counts in the range from 10^3 to 10^5 cfu/mL. Generally accepted colony counts for different variations of UTI are given in Table 1.4.4.[30]

Performance of a urine culture is recommended for patients with:

- suspected acute pyelonephritis;
- suspected complicated (febrile or not) UTI;
- suspected urosepsis (include blood culture);
- suspected UTI in males;
- ABU and suspected UTI in pregnancy;
- recurrent infection symptoms after antibiotic treatment;
- atypical symptoms or unclear diagnosis;
- prior to urological surgery.

Blood analysis

The serum concentration of the biomarker for inflammation, C-reactive protein (CRP), and the leucocyte count in peripheral blood are the most important markers of systemic inflammation in UTI. Serum creatinine will give a hint of acute deterioration in renal function. These parameters will remain at normal baseline levels in lower afebrile UTI, while CRP elevation and leucocytosis are essential diagnostic signs of febrile UTI, pyelonephritis, and urosepsis. Elevation of CRP may take up to 24 hours to develop fully, in contrast to the more immediate rise in leucocyte count.

A carefully taken blood culture avoiding skin organism contamination should be considered at the same time as urine culture, immediately prior to antibiotic administration, in the case of severe systemic symptoms.

Further investigations

It is generally recommended that all patients with complicated UTI should have a negative urine culture confirmed after treatment and, if appropriate, their renal function checked. In patients with febrile UTI or pyelonephritis, a renal ultrasound scan should be performed with further imaging if the ultrasound is abnormal. In older men with UTI, urinary flow rate and residual urine volume should be measured. Rapid investigation to detect impaired urinary tract drainage should be performed in patients who do not promptly improve on adequate treatment, but can otherwise be planned and performed during outpatient follow-up. For otherwise

Table 1.4.4 Bacterial count thresholds for the diagnosis of UTI in relation to the mode of collection of the specimen and the type of infection. This quantitative criterion is valid when one organism is isolated. When a Gram-positive strain or several strains are reported, contamination of the sample should be considered

Type of infection	Colony forming units cfu/mL
Specimen collection	
Usual diagnostic criteria for UTI	$\geq 10^5$
Specimen collected by clean in and out catheter	$\geq 10^2$
Specimen collected with external condom	$\geq 10^5$
Specimen collected by suprapubic aspiration	Any
Chronic indwelling catheter	$\geq 10^5$
Type of infection	
Asymptomatic bacteriuria—women (persistent)	$\geq 10^5$ (two separate samples)
Asymptomatic bacteriuria—male (persistent)	$\geq 10^5$ (gram-negtive strains) No recommendations (Gram-positive strains)
Sporadic uncomplicated cystitis in women	$\geq 10^3$
Acute uncomplicated pyelonephritis	$\geq 10^5$ (>10^4 observed in 5–10% of cases)
Symptomatic UTI in male	$\geq 10^3$
Spinal cord injury (specimen collected by clean intermittent catheterization)	$\geq 10^2$
Urinary diversion	No recommendations but $\geq 10^3$ is reasonably relevant as persistent bacteriuria and clinical UTI

Source: data from Nicolle LE, 'The quantitative urine culture for the diagnosis of urinary tract infection', in Naber KG *et al.* (Eds.), *Urogenital Infections*, European Association of Urology and International Consultations on Urological Diseases, Copyright © 2010.

healthy younger women with an isolated episode of pyelonephritis and normal renal function, only a post-treatment negative urine culture is needed. In the case of recurrence or if *Proteus sp.* are isolated, then renal ultrasound is required to detect urinary tract calculi or dilatation. Further investigation is not necessary for sporadic cystitis.

Management of urinary tract infection

The aims for the management of UTI are:[32]

- effective clinical and antimicrobial treatment;
- prevention of recurrence;
- minimization of risk of development of resistant organisms.

Asymptomatic bacteriuria

Previously, ABU was considered part of the UTI spectrum. Recent knowledge suggests that ABU should be considered as a commensal colonization of the urinary tract, that might even be beneficial for the host by preventing symptomatic infection by more virulent strains.[4,33] It has even been shown that treatment of ABU in adult females results in a higher risk of symptomatic recurrence.[34] ABU prevalence increases with age in women and men presumably as a consequence of the anatomical, hormonal, and functional changes of normal ageing and is more likely to become persistent.

Most guidance recommends no treatment for ABU and avoidance of use of antibiotics for recurrence prevention.[28,35,36] Two exceptions are pregnant women and patients who are due to undergo urological surgery. Evidence is poor for patients undergoing surgical implant insertion.

Acute sporadic uncomplicated cystitis

Acute sporadic uncomplicated cystitis, predominately affecting women, is the most common form of UTI. It is more common among women with a family history of UTI and following the onset of sexual activity or change of sexual partner (*'honeymoon cystitis'*). The natural history is a self-limiting infection that can resolve spontaneously—in some cases within one week[37]—as well as persist and in rare cases progress into an acute episode of pyelonephritis. *E. coli* is the predominant causative pathogen (>75%), with *S. saprophyticus* second (5–10%).[22,23] Other pathogens are uncommon.

The resultant lower urinary tract symptoms are frequency, urgency, dysuria (pain or discomfort passing urine), suprapubic tenderness or pain, urine odour, and occasionally cloudy urine and visible haematuria (Table 1.4.2). Urine analysis usually shows positive nitrite test, leucocyte esterase, and presence of blood cells. There is no requirement for urine culture, although it will be helpful to establish pathogen sensitivity and provide local bacterial ecology information for public health purposes.

A short antibiotic course is usually effective for symptom resolution and clearance of the pathogen (Table 1.4.5). Guidance recommends avoidance of the use of broad-spectrum antibiotics such as cephalosporins and fluoroquinolones due to increasing community *E. coli* resistance levels and overgrowth of gut *Clostridium difficile*.[28,36]

Acute cystitis is uncommon in males. It may also be difficult to differentiate from inflammation of the prostate (see Chapter 1.7) as the symptoms are similar and a raised prostate-specific antigen (PSA) commonly occurs.[6] A urine culture is recommended in males, as well as a careful history of urogenital infections.

Recurrent acute cystitis

Recurrent acute cystitis is common following the initial episode and may severely affect a women's quality of life.[38] It is usually defined as three or more UTIs per year, or at least two in a six-month period. Recurrent UTIs (rUTI) are caused by the re-emergence of the same organism (persistent pathogen) or re-infection by a new strain (recurrent ascending colonization from the bowel flora).

Recurrence is often seen in women with otherwise normal anatomic and functional urinary tracts, but risk factors such as a maternal history of UTI, onset of sexual activity, postmenopausal status, and diabetes may be present. Use of contraceptive pessaries and spermicides, low fluid intake, and infrequent, incomplete bladder emptying are also considered as risk factors.

Urine culture should be repeated regularly to determine the pattern of bacterial strains and antibiotic sensitivities. If recurrences are frequent and bothersome, and particularly where risk factors for more health-threatening disease are present such as visible haematuria or

Table 1.4.5 Most frequent bacterial strains, recommended antibiotics, and treatment regimens for most standard types of UTI

Type of UTI	Pathogens	Antibiotics	Treatment length (days)	Remarks
Uncomplicated UTI				
Asymptomatic bacteriuria (lower UT)	*E. coli* Others spp. (rare)	According to susceptibility	No Individualized when required	No treatment in general Two main exceptions: pregnancy and prior to urological surgery
Acute sporadic cystitis in women	*E. coli* (75–80%) *Proteus* (<5%) *Klebsiella* (<5%) *S. saprophyticus* (5–10%) *Enterococci* (<5%)	Pivmecillinam Nitrofurantoin Cephalosporin (oral) Fosfomycin	3–5	Urine culture not necessary Avoid fluoroquinolones and third generation cephalosporins Trimetoprim usually not recommended due to high resistance
Recurrent cystitis in women	As above	As above	3–7 Individualized	Urine culture essential Avoid fluoroquinolones and third generation cephalosporins as far as possible
Acute sporadic cystitis in males (no risk factors)	Not studied. Probably similar as women except for S. Saprophytics	According to susceptibility	Not well defined As for female	Rare UTI, poorly studied Difficult to differentiate from prostatitis without fever (type II)
Acute uncomplicated pyelonephritis	*E. coli* (75–85%) *Proteus* (<5%) *Klebsiella* (<5%) Others (<10%)	Cephalosporin (third generation) Fluoroquinolone Aminoglycoside	7–14 days Step-down to oral therapy as soon as possible	Urine culture necessary Blood culture in case of severe systemic symptoms High risk for sepsis ESBL-risk evaluation
UTI during pregnancy				
Asymptomatic bacteriuria	As for sporadic infections	Nitrofurantoin Cephalosporin (oral) Pivmecillinam Amoxicillin (high rate of resistance in community)	5–7 days	Surveillance Consider prophylaxis
Acute cystitis			5–7 days	If recurrent: consider prophylaxis
Acute pyelonephritis			7–10 days	Initiate prophylaxis
Complicated UTI				
Febrile UTI (male/women) Acute pyelonephritis Sepsis	*E. coli* (35–60%) *Proteus mirabilis* (6–10%) *Klebsiella, Enterobacter,* Citrobacter, Pseudomonas (up to 25%) *Enterococci* (9–20%)	Cephalosporin Fluoroquinolone Co-trimoxazol Aminoglycoside Piperacillin Carbapenem group	7–14 days	Empirical treatment initiation followed by correction according to susceptibility pattern Investigation of the urinary tract Surgical intervention when necessary ESBL-risk evaluation
Chronic pyelonephritis	Variable	According to urine culture	Not defined	Bacteriuria coming from chronic pyelonephritis or harboured in the kidney is difficult to eradicate. If asymptomatic: avoid treatment
Catheter-associated UTI	*E. coli, Proteus, Enterobacter, Enterococci, S. epidermidis*	According to urine culture	Usually 5–7 days	As short as possible after symptom response
Fungal UTI	*Candida albicans* *Candida glabrata*	Fluconazole Amphotericin B	7–4 days	Only symptomatic infections, and in case of risk of dissemination at instrumentation

loin pain, the urinary tract should be investigated with upper tract imaging generally by ultrasound or CT, cystoscopy and, if indicated, urodynamic studies to detect any dysfunction or abnormality.

The management of recurring UTI (rUTI) should be individualized and decided following a joint discussion with the patient, with careful explanation of the problem and information on available evidence-based and empirical preventive measures. It is important to reassure the patient that symptom-free bacteriuria in the absence of any detected risk factors (ABU) is harmless and should not be treated; a sterile urinary tract should not necessarily be the goal of successful management. Prophylactic antibiotic-based regimens can reduce symptoms and have variable antimicrobial effectiveness, but severe adverse reaction can occur and microbial resistance concerns have limited its use to a highly selected patient group.

It should be considered only after counselling of alternatives and behavioural modifications has been attempted.[28,35,36] Continuous or post-coital prophylaxis should be considered only in women in whom non-antimicrobial measures have been unsuccessful. Self-diagnosis and self-start intermittent treatment with short courses of recommended antibiotics can be used in selected cooperative women.[39] The use of methanamine hippurate, a urine disinfectant, is poorly investigated, but available data from randomized trials suggest that selected women will experience fewer UTI.[40]

Evidence of the effectiveness of preventive advice such as high intake of fluids, regular micturition to avoid large urine volume, post-coital hygiene, and the avoidance of use of spermicides is poor, although much is common sense. In the case of residual volumes above 100 mL, the patient could benefit from behavioural techniques to improve voiding, and clean intermittent catheterization may be considered for larger residual volumes.

Reduced vaginal colonization by lactobacilli related to low local oestrogen levels is also a possible risk factor for rUTI. The use of local oestrogen replacement therapy has been demonstrated to increase lactobacilli growth and to reduce UTI recurrence in postmenopausal women.[41]

Other investigational preventive methods include regular intake of cranberry or pomegranate concentrate-containing proanthocyanidins in high levels, but solid clinical validation is still needed.[42] Oral intake of uropathogenic *E. coli* cell wall constituents for immunization has also shown to reduce infection episodes in female rUTI by approximately one third.[43]

Women with postmenopausal hormonal status are particularly prone to rUTI. Epidemiological studies have shown that approximately 5–20% of healthy women aged 65 to 70 years have bacteriuria. The percentage is even higher in those older than 80 years, reaching 20–50%. Bacteriuria occurs more often in elderly women who are functionally impaired and persistent bacteriuria is frequently observed in women unable to live independently. Risk factors for bacteriuria and UTI are also different in older compared to younger women. These include clinical evidence of local oestrogen deficiency, cystocele, post-void residual urine, urinary and faecal incontinence, and previous urogenital surgery.

For ABU, no treatment is required, and the treatment strategies for clinical UTI are similar to those in premenopausal women.[4,28,36] As for premenopausal women, antibiotic prophylaxis should be reserved for a narrow group of selected patients.

Acute sporadic uncomplicated pyelonephritis

Pyelonephritis is classically associated with fever, chills, nausea, and flank and abdominal pain. However, kidney infection is not the only possible cause of these symptoms. Sometimes, especially in elderly people, kidney infection may have an insidious non-specific onset.

Sporadic uncomplicated pyelonephritis is mainly seen in women and children and is often preceded by lower urinary tract symptoms with urinalysis positive for nitrite, leucocyte esterase, and blood. The urine and, in case of severe systemic symptoms, blood should be cultured, and antibiotic susceptibility tested for isolated pathogens.

Early antibiotic treatment is vital, as a pyelonephritis even in the absence of upper urinary tract obstruction may rapidly progress to life-threatening urosepsis. In the early phase, the treatment can be given orally (if tolerated) using an antibiotic with high intestinal absorption and renal parenchyma distribution, such as a fluoroquinolone. In the presence of systemic symptoms, patients should be admitted to the hospital for intravenous antibiotic treatment. Local guidance should be followed in the choice of initial agent, with subsequent modification according to urine and blood culture results. Step-down to oral therapy should be initiated according to local guidance and continued for 7–10 days. Usually clinical symptoms and signs will improve within two to three days of starting antibiotics, while the normalization of serum markers of inflammation takes a further few days.

There should be a low threshold for imaging of the urinary tract (initially by ultrasound) if there is uncertainty regarding the presence of risk factors for severe infection, or failure to respond to initial treatment. Urinary tract obstruction is the most frequently found complicating factor (see Fig. 1.4.3).

Acute complicated pyelonephritis and febrile urinary tract infection with risk factors

The most frequent risk factor is upper urinary tract obstruction, usually by a ureteric calculus. In addition to symptoms of pyelonephritis, patients may describe pain typical of ureteric colic. Further risk factors that may complicate acute pyelonephritis are listed in Table 1.4.3.[44] It is important to detect these factors and address them if required, for example by drainage of an obstructed urinary tract or close control of blood sugar.

Emphysematous pyelonephritis is an acute necrotizing parenchymal infection caused by a polymicrobial infection including gas-forming uropathogens, such as *E. coli*.[45] The condition occurs mainly in people with diabetes and is more likely if there is urinary tract obstruction. The degree of sepsis is generally severe and urgent drainage or nephrectomy is required to reduce mortality risk (see Fig. 1.4.4).

Possible continued infective consequences to complicated pyelonephristis include renal or perinephric abscess resulting from leakage of infected urine from a ruptured calyx (see Chapter 1.5).

Chronic pyelonephritis

Chronic pyelonephritis is nowadays seen predominately in patients with underlying functional or anatomical urinary tract abnormalities, mainly non-acute stone disease and long-term obstruction. It results in destruction of the renal parenchyma, with scarring and shrinkage of the kidney, and renal function impairment. The inflammatory process can include the whole kidney or may remain localized around calyces, particularly in the lower pole, where drainage is impaired. When bacteriuria is present, it is very difficult to eradicate (see Fig. 1.4.5).

Xanthogranulomatous pyelonephritis is a rare, severe destructive chronic inflammation of the kidney resulting in a non-functioning, enlarged kidney, presenting clinically and on CT as a renal mass, which may be difficult to differentiate from a renal tumour.[46] People with diabetes appear more at risk. It is generally unilateral and associated with nephrolithiasis and obstruction. *E. coli* and *Proteus* are most commonly reported pathogens. A non-functional kidney should be removed.

Sepsis

About 20% of all episodes of systemic sepsis originate in the urinary tract ('urosepsis') and may develop from a community-acquired or a healthcare-associated UTI.[47] A complicating underlying risk factor involving a parenchymatous urogenital organ such as the kidney or the prostate is almost always identified. The systemic inflammatory response syndrome is recognized as the first event in a cascade of events leading to multiple organ failure.[48] Time from admission

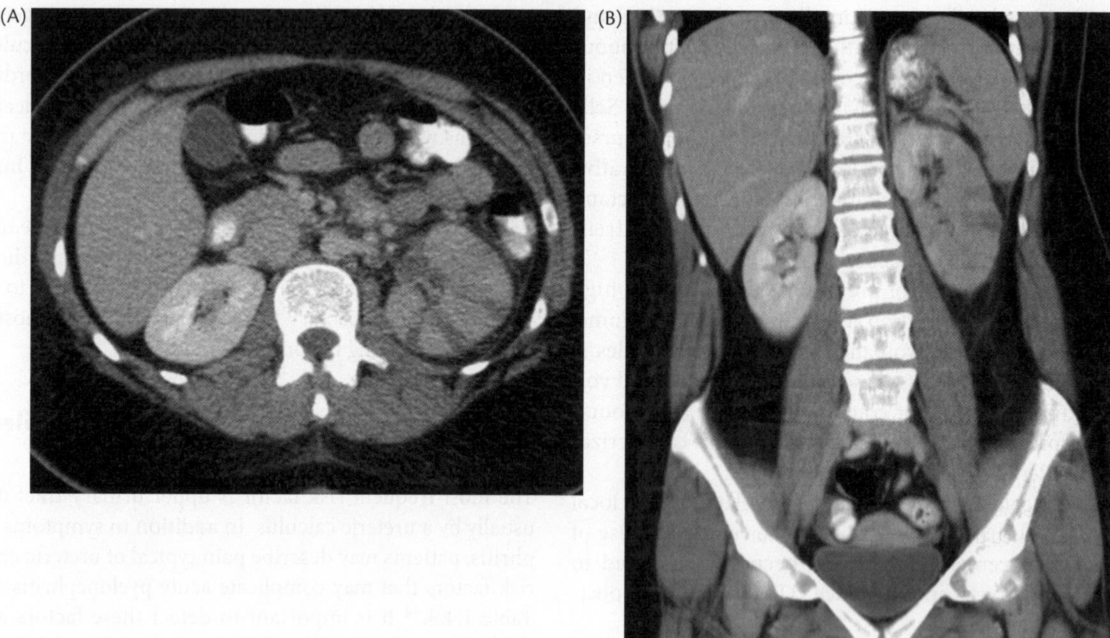

Fig. 1.4.3 Acute pyelonephritis of the left kidney in an otherwise healthy young woman. The computed tomography urography (CT-U) shows the radiological characteristics: the left kidney is larger than the right one, secondary to oedema of the parenchyma. The circulation of the kidney is greatly disturbed and only the upper quarter of the kidney is normally vascularized. Usually, there is also an oedema of the tissue surrounding the kidney. The right kidney is normally vascularized. Recovery and normalization of the circulation is seen after a few weeks of treatment. (A) axial projection; (B) coronal projection.

to treatment is vital for the patient and treatment must be initiated without any delay after urine and blood sampling for culture and inflammatory parameters. Its management consists of:[49]

- Parenteral broad-spectrum beta-lactam antibiotics, often in combination with an aminoglycoside;
- Parenteral antibiotic from the carbapenem group in case of known or suspected ESBL strain;
- Early fluid and oxygen treatment, added by other life supporting care as required;
- Monitoring of vital parameters in intermediary or critical care unit, depending on the severity of the sepsis;
- Early detection of any underlying urological cause, especially obstruction; Drainage should be undertaken by the least invasive way without unnecessary delay.

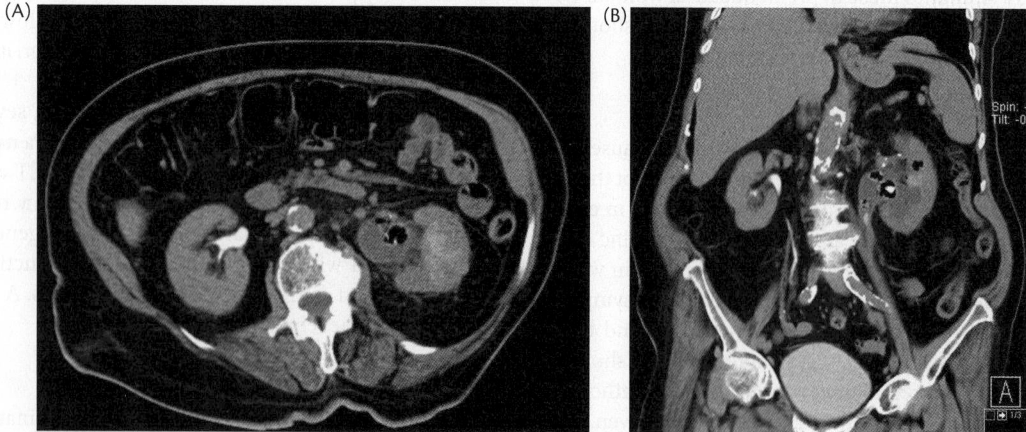

Fig. 1.4.4 Acute emphysematous pyelonephritis in an elderly woman with diabetes mellitus, cardiovascular disease, and kidney stone with post-renal obstruction. The CT-U reveals typical characteristics: the kidney parenchyma is oedematous, the circulation greatly disturbed, and the excretion is delayed. Air bubbles are found in the kidney pelvis and in the parenchyma. *E. coli* was growing in the urinary culture. The infection is life-threatening and in addition to parenteral antibiotic administration and supportive therapy, the kidney must be drained by a nephrostomy tube to control the infection. The percutaneous channel may eventually be used for stone removal. (A) axial projection; (B) coronal projection.

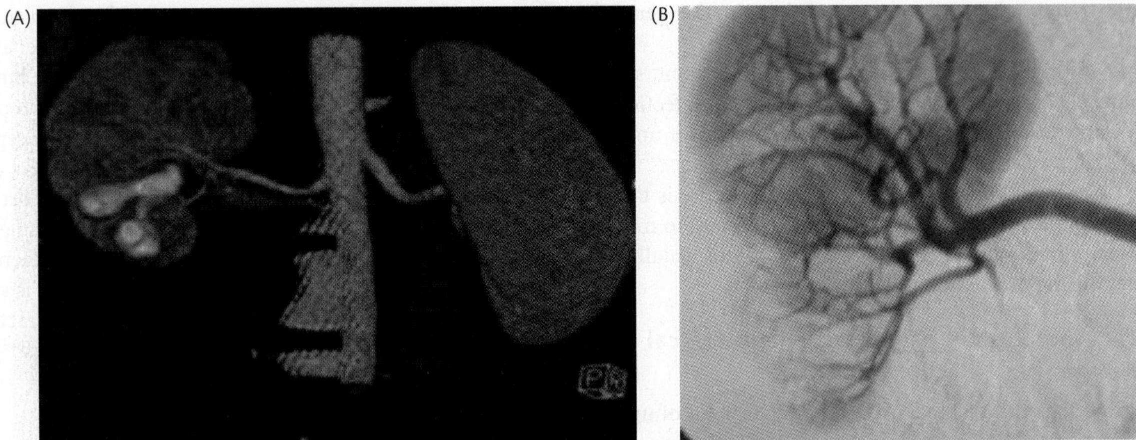

Fig. 1.4.5 Chronic pyelonephritis of the lower section of the left kidney in a middle-aged, otherwise healthy woman. She was previously operated upon with percutaneous stone removal but kidney stone recurred in deformed and scarred lower calyces. The renal parenchyma around the stone burden is reduced. A selective renal angiography confirmed the reduction of parenchyma and the vascular distribution and delimitations to be considered before heminephrectomy, which was eventually performed in the present case. (A) axial projection; (B) coronal projection.

Fungal urinary tract infection

Yeasts such as candida exist as commensals on the external genitalia and are detected in less than 1% of urine cultures. However, the risk of candidal UTI is increased in immunosuppressed patients, critically ill patients, those with uncontrolled diabetes mellitus, and patients with complicated urological conditions. Urological risk factors are the presence of any type of indwelling catheter or stents, and instrumentation. In most cases, candiduria (*C. albicans* and *C. glabrata*) is transient and asymptomatic, and represents a colonization rather than a true infection. It is generally recommended to treat symptomatic infections and to give appropriate prophylaxis to prevent dissemination during urinary tract instrumentation and surgery.[50]

Urinary tract infection in special patient populations

Urinary tract infection and kidney stones

Urease-producing organisms such as *Proteus mirabilis, Klebsiella, Enterobacter, Pseudomonas spp.* and specific intracellular bacteria such as *Ureaplasma urealyticum* are able, in the alkaline environment, to catalyse the degradation of urea to ammonium ions encouraging the development of magnesium-ammonium-phosphate stones (also termed struvite, triple phosphate, or infective stones). These stones are less radio-opaque, harbour bacteria, damage the uroepithelium, precipitate inflammation leading to scar formation (chronic pyelonephritis) and potentially renal failure.[51] Often there is also an underlying anatomical or functional abnormality, particularly neurological dysfunction.

Management consists of a combination of antibiotic treatment and surgery during which all stone material must be removed and drainage ensured to control the infection and prevent recurrence. Patients undergoing surgery for infective stones are at high risk for infective complications in terms of acute kidney infections and systemic sepsis.[52,53] Bacteriuria must be controlled prior to and during stone surgery and continued after in a tentative effort to eradicate infection.[28,54]

Other types of urinary stones such as calcium oxalate and urate may also induce focal inflammation and harbour bacteria.[55] Even apparently small idiopathic stones can induce infective complications and it has been clearly shown that a negative urine culture does not predict the absence of postoperative sepsis. The risk of complications is markedly increased in patients with upper tract obstruction due to 'impacted' ureteral stones.[52,53] The risk for each individual patient must be properly assessed before any intervention for a urinary tract stone and appropriate perioperative prophylaxis considered.

Urinary tract infection in pregnancy

A UTI or unmanaged ABU during pregnancy can harm the developing foetus. Acute pyelonephritis is associated with preterm delivery.[56,57] The urinary tract undergoes physiological modifications following the hormonal changes during pregnancy and pressure from the gravid uterus results in dilatation of the collecting system. Previous pyelonephritis, pre-existing urinary tract abnormalities, renal stones, and painful dilatation of the upper urinary tract are risk factors for pyelonephritis.

ABU is detected in between 4% and 7% of women during pregnancy and pyelonephritis occurs in up to 2%. Guidance recommends that women should be screened for bacteriuria during the first trimester of pregnancy.[28,36] ABU should be eradicated and cystitis treated with short courses of antimicrobial therapy, with agents chosen according to their safety profile (Table 1.4.5) and followed up with urine culture. Pyelonephritis is treated according to standard recommendations for 7–10 days. In the case of recurrent bacteriuria, prophylaxis throughout the pregnancy should be considered. A urine culture is imperative to direct acute effective treatment and prophylaxis.[58]

Urinary tract infection and diabetes mellitus

Between 15% and 25% of women with diabetes have bacteriuria and people with diabetes mellitus have a higher incidence of UTI, which is often more difficult to resolve. The risk of ascending infection is also higher, with greater likelihood of failure to resolve leading to papillary necrosis, renal abscess, and xanthogranulomatous pyelonephritis.[59–62] *E. coli* remains the predominant pathogen, but generally infecting pathogens have a more virulent phenotype.

Candida infection is also more common than in the general population.

Monitoring and control of blood sugar level is important, since it may promote UTI and be elevated during episodes of infection.

Other relevant consequences of diabetes include detrusor underactivity with high post-void residual urine.

In the case of a symptomatic infection, a urine culture is taken and the appropriate antibiotic prescribed. It is important to monitor and control blood glucose levels. ABU should not usually be treated except during pregnancy and prior to surgery.

Urinary tract infection in people with neurological bladder dysfunction

Bladder dysfunction with residual urine and impairment of upper tract drainage occurs following spinal cord lesions including multiple sclerosis, some forms of stroke, and any disturbance of the peripheral nerves, such as in advanced diabetes mellitus. Structural or functional bladder outlet obstruction will compound the problem. The majority of these patients have ABU.[63,64] Gram-negative uropathogens, including *Klebsiella* and *Pseudomonas*, are commonly isolated on urine culture but Gram-positive pathogens such as *Enterococcus faecalis* are also frequently isolated. Highly resistant organisms are frequently encountered, in part due to indiscriminate antibiotic use. These patients will also have a higher frequency of urease-producing bacteria and infective stone formation. UTI is the most common cause of fever for patients with neurological bladder dysfunction, and other consequences of the underlying neurological disease may mask typical UTI symptoms. Patients requiring bladder drainage by indwelling catheter will also be at higher risk of infective complications, and stone formation.

For this patient group it is important, but in practice very difficult, to avoid unnecessary and ineffective use of antimicrobial treatment. Antibiotics should be restricted to severely symptomatic UTI and prior to instrumentation of the urinary tract.[65] Similarly, long-term antibiotic prophylaxis should be avoided, but alternative antimicrobial approaches can be trialled, such as methenamine or cranberry extract.[40,42] Therapeutic colonization of the urinary tract in a cohort of people with neurogenic bladder dysfunction using an ABU *E. coli* strain was effective in reducing the number of episodes of symptomatic UTI, compared to an untreated group.[66]

Catheter-associated urinary tract infection

Placement of an indwelling urinary catheter should be considered as a temporary solution for bladder drainage problems, with alternatives such as condom sheath drainage, pads, or clean intermittent catheterization preferred. However, there are situations when a permanent urethral or a suprapubic catheter is unavoidable. Bacterial urinary colonization is the rule, occurring at a rate of about 5% per day from insertion with almost all patients bacteriuric with *E. coli*, other *Enterobacteriaceae*, or *Enterococci* and other secondary Gram-positive organisms at one month (Table 1.4.1).[9,67]

After short-term catheterization (less than one week), bacteriuria will most often resolve spontaneously. In all cases, the use of antibiotics should be avoided unless there are definite systemic symptoms.

In long-term catheterization, bacterial communities embedded in a secreted extracellular polymeric matrix polyglycan (biofilm) are formed on the catheter and the urinary tract becomes a reservoir of more or less resistant strains hidden from antibiotic or antimicrobial attack.[15,68] The routine change of catheter at standard intervals is a key time for high risk of systemic sepsis, but does not appear to be modified by prior antibiotic treatment/prophylaxis.[69] ABU in catheterized patients should not be treated except prior to surgery. If a patient with an indwelling catheter suffers a symptomatic UTI guidelines[28,36,69] suggest commencing a short course of an appropriate antibiotic together with immediate change of catheter. There is little evidence of any advantage for different catheter materials or surface coatings.[69,70] Although evidence is scanty, the same recommendations are valid for other urinary tract drainage devices, such as nephrostomy tubes and ureteral stents.[69]

Urinary tract infection in urinary diversion

Urinary diversion with ileal conduit, orthotopic bladder substitution, or continent diversion after cystectomy is associated with an increased prevalence of bacterial colonization and ABU.[71] The management is similar to the other described functional lower urinary tract disorders associated with higher UTI risk. Antibiotic prophylaxis should only be given to patients who suffer repeated febrile UTI.

Urinary tract infection and urological surgery

Instrumentation of the urinary tract is followed by infective complications in a substantial number of patients. The underlying causes are related to pre-existing patient risk factors, increased risk associated with the procedure itself, and the risk of HAI. The most important aspects to control infective complications and HAI are:[29]

- Careful preoperative patient assessment and aseptic precautions
- Control of general and specific risk factors (Table 1.4.3)
- Preoperative evaluation of the procedure in terms of level of invasiveness, surgical field contamination level and risk for spillage, duration, and surgical skills
- Adherence to local infection control policies and antimicrobial stewardship programme
- Adherence to perioperative antimicrobial prophylaxis principles
- Clean wards and sterile surgical environment
- Minimization of hospital stay

Conclusions

Urinary tract infections are among the most common infections in the community, in the general hospital environment, and in patients under urological care. They present through a variety of manifestations requiring the clinician to be alert to UTI as a possible diagnosis. It is essential to identify infection and initiate effective treatment recommended by guidelines as early as possible to reduce the risk of progression to severe sepsis. However, it is also important for the safety of the individual patient, their community and the wider population to avoid ineffective, unnecessary, and overuse of antibiotics to reduce the risk of resistance development.

Further reading

Bjerklund-Johansen TE, Botto H, Cek M, Grabe M, Wagenlehner FM, Naber KG. Critical review of current definitions of urinary tract infections and proposal of an EAU/ESIU classification system. *Internat J Antimicrob Agents* 2011; **38S**:64–70.

Bjerklund-Johansen T, Cek M, Naber K, Stratchounski L, Svendsen MV, Tenke P on behalf of PEP-PEAP study group. Prevalence of hospital-acquired urinary tract infections in urology departments. *Eur Urol* 2007; **51**:1100–1112.

European Association of Urology. Urological Infections. In: Guidelines of the European Association of Urology 2015. EAU 6803 AA Arnhem. ISBN 978-90-79754-83-0. Available at: www.uroweb.org/gls/pdf/17_Urological%20infections_LR%20II.pdf [Online].

Foxman B, Brown P. Epidemiology of urinary tract infections: transmission and risk factors, incidence and costs. *Infect Dis North Am* 2003; **17**:227–41.

Fünfstück R, Nicolle LE, Hanefeld M, Naber KG. Urinary tract infection in patients with diabetes mellitus. *Clin Nephrol* 2012; **7**:40–8.

Grabe M, Botto H, Cek M, *et al.* Preoperative assessment of the patient and risk factors for infectious complications and tentative classification of surgical field contamination of urological procedures. *World J Urol* 2012; **30**(1):39–50.

Lichtenberger P, Hooton TM. Antimicrobial prophylaxis in women with recurrent urinary tract infections. *Int J Antimicrobi Agents* 2001; **38**(Suppl):36–41.

Naber KG, Schaeffer AJ, Heyns CF, Matsumotot T, Scoskes DA, Bjerklund-Johansen TE (eds). *Urogenital Infections*. International Consultations on Urogenital Infections and European Association of Urology, 2010 Edition.

Ragnarsdottir B, Lutay N, Grönberg-Hernandez J, Koves B, Svanborg C. Genetics of innate immunity and UTI susceptibility. *Nat Rev Urol* 2011; **8**(8):449–68.

Stapleton A. Urinary tract infections in patients with diabetes. *Am J Med* 2002; **113**(Suppl 1A):80S–4S.

Tenke P, Kovacs B, Bjerklund-Johansen TE, *et al.* European and Asian guidelines on management and prevention of catheter-associated urinary tract infection. *Int J Antimicrob Agents* 2008; **31S**:S68–78.

Wagenlehner F, Naber KG. Treatment of bacterial urinary tract infections: presence and future. *Eur Urol* 2006; **49**:235–44.

Wagenlehner FM, Naber KG. Editorial commentary: asymptomatic bacteriuria—shift of paradigm. *Clin Infect Dis* 2012; **55**(6):778–80.

References

1. Foxman B, Brown P. Epidemiology of urinary tract infections: transmission and risk factors, incidence and costs. *Infect Dis North Am* 2003; **17**:227–41.
2. Lindstedt S, Lindström U, Ljunggren E, Wullt B, Grabe M. Single-dose antibiotic prophylaxis in core prostate biopsy: Impact of timing and identification of risk factors. *Eur Urol* 2006; **50**:832–7.
3. Nicolle LE, SHEA Long-Term-Care-Committee. Urinary tract infections in long-term-care facilities. *Infect Control Hosp Epidemiol* 2001; **22**:167–75.
4. Nicolle LE. Asymptomatic bacteriuria—to treat or not to treat. In: Naber KG *et al.* (eds). *Urogenital Infections*. European Association of Urology and International Consultations on urological diseases, 2010 Edition.
5. Rodhe N, Lofgren S, Matussek Andre M, *et al.* Asymptomatic bacteriuria in the elderly: high prevalence and high turnover of strains. *Scan J Infect Dis* 2008; **40**(10):804–10.
6. Ulleryd P, Zackrisson B, Aus G Bergdahl S, *et al.* Prostatic involment in men with febrile urinary tract infection as measured by serum prostate specific antigen and transrectal ultrasonography. *BJU Int* 1999; **84**(4):470–4.
7. Nicolle LE. Update in adult urinary tract infection. *Curr Infect Dis Rep* 2011; **13**:552–60.
8. Bjerklund-Johansen T, Cek M, Naber K, Stratchounski L, Svendsen MV, Tenke P on behalf of PEP-PEAP study group. Prevalence of hospital-acquired urinary tract infections in urology departments. *Eur Urol* 2007; **51**:1100–1112.
9. Kunin CM. *Urinary Tract Infections: Detection, Prevention and Management*, 5th edition. Baltimore, MA: Williams and Wilkins, 1997.
10. Ragnarsdottir B, Svanborg C. Susceptibility to acute pyelonephritis or asymptomatic bacteriuria: Host-pathogen interaction in urinary tract infection. *Pediatr Nephrol* 2012; **27**(11):2017–29.
11. Johnson J. Virulence factors in Escherichia coli urinary tract infection. *Clin Microbial Rev* 1991; **4**:80–128.
12. Oelschlaeger TA, Dobrindt U, Hacker J. Pathogenicity islands of uropathogenic E. coli and evolution of virulence. *Int J Antimicrob Agents* 2002; **19**(6):517–21.
13. Norinder BS, Koves B, Yadav M, Brauner A, Svanborg C. Do Escherichia coli strains causing acute cystitis have a distinct virulence repertoire? *Microb Pathog* 2012; **52**(1):10–16.
14. Rosen DA, Hooton TM, Stamm WE, Humphrey PA, Hultgren SJ. Detection of intracellular bacterial communities in human urinary tract infection. *PLoSMed* 2007; **4**(12):e329.
15. Tenke P, Kovos B, Nagy K, *et al.* Update on biofilm infections in the urinary tract. *World J Urol* 2012; **30**(1):51–7.
16. Fischer H, Lutay N, Ragnarsdottir B, *et al.* Pathogen specific, IRF3-dependant signalling and innate resistance to human kidney infection. *PLoS Pathog* 2010; **6**(9):e1001109.
17. Wullt B, Bergsten G, Fischer H, *et al.* The host response to urinary tract infection. *Infect Dis Clin North Am* 2003; **17**(2):279–301.
18. Ragnarsdottir B, Jonsson K, Urbano A, *et al.* Toll-like receptor 4 promoter polymorphisms: common TLR4 variants may protect against severe urinary tract infection. *PLoS One* 2010; **5**(5):e10734.
19. Lundstedt AC, McCarthy S, Gustavsson MC, *et al.* A genetic basis of susceptibility to acute pyelonephritis. *PLoS One* 2007; **2**(9):e825.
20. Grönberg-Hernandez J, Sundén F, Connolly J, Svanborg C, Wullt B. Genetic control of the variable innate immune response to asymptomatic bacteriuria. *PLoS One* 2011; **6**(11):e28289.
21. Ragnarsdottir B, Lutay N, Grönberg-Hernandez J, Koves B, Svanborg C. Genetics of innate immunity and UTI susceptibility. *Nat Rev Urol* 2011; **8**(8):449–68.
22. Kahlmeter G. The ECO.SENS Project: a prospective, multinational, multicentre epidemiological survey of the prevalence and antimicrobial susceptibility of urinary tract pathogens. *J Antimicrob Chemother* 2000; **46**(Suppl 1):15–22.
23. Naber KG, Schito G, Botto H, Palou J, Mazzei Teresita. Surveillance study in Europe and Brazil on clinical aspects and antimicrobial resistance epidemiology in females with cystitis (ARESC): Implications for emperic therapy. *Eur Urol* 2008; **54**:1164–78.
24. Carlet J, Colligton P, Goldman D, *et al.* Society's failure to protect a precious resource: antibiotics. *Lancet* 2011; **378**:369–71.
25. Horan TC, Andrus M, Dudeck MA. CDC/NHSH surveillance definition of health care-associated infection and criteria for specific types of infections in the acute care setting. *Am J Infect Control* 2008; **36**(5):309–32.
26. Rubin UH SE, Andriole VT, Davis RJ, Stamm WE, with a modification by a European Working Party (Norrby SR). General Guidelines for the evaluation of new anti-infective drugs for the treatment of urinary tract infections. The European Society of the Clinical Microbiology and Infectious diseases. Taukirchen, Germany 1993:240–310.
27. Bjerklund-Johansen TE, Botto H, Cek M, Grabe M, Wagenlehner FM, Naber KG. Critical review of current definitions of urinary tract infections and proposal of an EAU/ESIU classification system. *Internat J Antimicrob Agents* 2011; **38**(Suppl):64–70.
28. European Association of Urology. Urological Infections. In: Guidelines of the European Association of Urology 2015. EAU 6803 AA Arnhem. ISBN 978-90-79754-83-0. Available at: www.uroweb.org/gls/pdf/17_Urological%20infections_LR%20II.pdf [Online].
29. Grabe M, Botto H, Cek M, *et al.* Preoperative assessment of the patient and risk factors for infectious complications and tentative classification of surgical field contamination of urological procedures. *World J Urol* 2012; **30**(1):39–50.

30. Nicolle LE. The quantitative urine culture for the diagnosis of urinary tract infection. In: Naber KG *et al.* (eds). *Urogenital Infections*. European Association of Urology and International Consultations on urological diseases, 2010 Edition.
31. Lifshitz E, Kramer L. Outpatient urine culture: does collection technique matter? *Arch Intern Med* 2000; **160**(16):2537–40.
32. Wagenlehner F, Naber KG. Treatment of bacterial urinary tract infections: presence and future. *Eur Urol* 2006; **49**:235–44.
33. Wagenlehner FM, Naber KG. Editorial commentary: asymptomatic bacteriuria—shift of paradigm. *Clin Infect Dis* 2012; **55**(6):778–80.
34. Cai T, Mazzoli S, Mondaini N, *et al.* The role of asymptomatic bacteriuria in young women with recurrent urinary tract infections: to treat or not to treat? *Clin Infect Dis* 2012; **55**(6):771–7.
35. Lichtenberger P, Hooton TM. Antimicrobial prophylaxis in women with recurrent urinary tract infections. *Int J Antimicrobi Agents* 2001; **38**(Suppl):36–41.
36. Scottish Intercollegiate Guidelines Network (SIGN). Management of suspected bacterial urinary tract infection in adults. Edinburgh: SIN;2012. (SIGN publication no. 88). (July 2012). Available at: http://www.sign.ac.uk [Online].
37. Ferry SA, Holm SE, Stenlund H, Lunjdholm R, Monsen TJ. The natural course of uncomplicated lower urinary tract infection in women illustrated by a randomised placebo controlled study. *Scan J Infect Dis* 2004; **36**(4):296–301.
38. Bermingham SL, Ashe JF. Systematic review of the impact of urinary tract infections on health-related quality of life. *BJU Int* 2012; **110**(11 Pt C):E830–6.
39. Gupta K, Hooton TM, Roberts PL, Stamm WE. Patient-initiated treatment of uncomplicated recurrent urinary tract infections in young women. *Ann Intern Med* 2001; **135**(1):9–16.
40. Lee BS, Bhuta T, Simpson JM, Craig JC. Methenamine hippurate for preventing urinary tract infections. *Cochrane Database Syst Rev* 2012; **10**:CD003265 [Epub 2012/10/19].
41. Raz R, Stamm WE. A controlled trial of intravaginal estriol in postmenopausal women with recurrent urinary tract infections. *N Engl J Med* 1993; **329**(11):753–6.
42. Jepson RG, Williams G, Craig JC. Cranberries for preventing urinary tract infections. *Cochrane Database Syst Rev* 2012: **10**:CD001321.
43. Naber KG, Cho YH, Matsumoto T, Schaeffer AJ. Immunoactive prophylaxis of recurrent urinary tract infections: a meta-analysis. *Int J Antimicrob Agents* 2009; **33**(2):111–9.
44. Heyns CF. Urinary tract infection associated with conditions causing urinary tract obstruction and stasis excluding urolithiasis and neuropathic bladder. *World J Urol* 2012; **30**(1):77–83.
45. Ubee SS, McGlynn L, Fordham M. Emphysematous pyelonephritis. *BJU Int* 2011; **107**(9):1474–8.
46. Li L, Parwani AV. Xanthogranulomatous pyelonephritis. *Arch Pathol Lab Med* 2011; **135**(5):671–4.
47. Martin GS, Mannino DM, Eaton S, *et al.* The epidemiology of sepsis in the United States from 1979 through 2000. *N Engl J Med* 2003; **348**(16):1546–54.
48. Hotchkiss RS, Karl IE. The pathophysiology and treatment of sepsis. *N Engl J Med* 2003; **248**(2):138–50.
49. Wagenlehner FM, Pilatz A, Weidner W. Urosepsis-from the view of the urologist. *Int J Antimicrob Agents* 2011; **38S**:51–7.
50. Sobel JD, Fisher J, Kauffman CA. Guidelines for the treatment of fungal urinary tract infections. (pp. 903–11) In: Naber KG *et al.* (eds). *Urogenital Infections*. European Association of Urology and International Consultations on urological diseases, 2010 Edition.
51. Griffith DP, Osborne CA. Infection (ureas) stones. *Miner Electrolyte Metab* 1987; **13**(4):278–85.
52. Rao PN, Dube D, Weightman NC, *et al.* Prediction of septicaemia following endourological manipulation for stone in the upper urinary tract. *J Urol* 1991; **146**:955–60.
53. Mariappan P, Smith G, Bariol SV, Moussa SA, Tolley DA. Stone and pelvic urine culture and sensitivity are better than bladder urine as predictors of urosepsis following percutaneous nephrolithotectomy: a prospective clinical study. *J Urol* 2005; **173**:1610–14.
54. Denstedt J, de la Rosette J, (eds). Stone diseases. (Ch. 5, section E). Joint SIU-ICUD international consultations. Glascow, Scotland, October 2014: ISBN:978-0-9877465-8-0.
55. Hugosson J, Grenabo L, Hedelin H, Pettersson S, Seeberg S. Becteriology of upper urinary tract stones. *J Urol* 1990; **143**(5):965–8.
56. Hill JB, Sheffield JS, McIntire DD, Wendel GD. Acute pyelonephritis in prednancy. *Obst Gynecol* 2005; **105**(1):18–23.
57. Millar LK, Cox SM. Urinary tract infections complicating pregnancy. *Infect Dis Clin North Am* 1997; **11**(1):13–26.
58. Smaill F, Vazquez JC. Antibiotics for asymptomatic bacteriuria in pregnancy. *Cochrane Database Syst Rev* **2007**(2):CD000490.
59. Geerlings SE, Stolk RP, Camps MJ, *et al.* Asymptomatic bacteriuria may be considered a complication in women with diabetes. Diabetes Mellitus Women Asymptomatic Bacteriuria Utrecht Study Group. *Diabetes Care* 2000; **23**(6):744–9.
60. Boyko EJ, Fihn SD, Scholes D, *et al.* Diabetes and the risk of acute urinary tract infection among postmenopausal women. *Diabetes Care* 2002; **25**(10):1778–83.
61. Stapleton A. Urinary tract infections in patients with diabetes. *Am J Med* 2002; **113**(Suppl 1A):80S–4S.
62. Fünfstück R, Nicolle LE, Hanefeld M, Naber KG. Urinary tract infection in patients with diabetes mellitus. *Clin Nephrol* 2012; **7**:40–8.
63. De Ruz AE, Leoni EG, Cabrera RH. Epidemiology and risk factors for urinary tract infection in patient with spinal cord injury. *J Urol* 2000; **164**(4):1285–9.
64. Sauerwein D. Urinary tract infection in patients with neurogenic bladder dysfunction. *Int J Antimicrob Agents* 2002; **19**(6):592–7.
65. Garcia Leoni ME, Esclarin De Ruz A. Management of urinary tract infection in patients with spinal cord injuries. *Clin Microb Infect* 2003; **9**(8):780–5.
66. Sundén F, Håkansson L, Ljunggren E, Wullt B. Escherichia coli 83972 bacteriuria protects against recurrent lower urinary tract infections in patients with incomplete bladder emptying. *J Urol* 2010; **184**(1):179–85.
67. Warren JW. Catheter-associated urinary tract infections. *Int J Antimicrob Agents* 2001; **17**(4):299–303.
68. Nicolle LE. The chronic indwelling catheter and urinary infection in long-term-care facility residents. *Infect Control Hosp Epidemiol* 2001; **22**(5):316–21.
69. Tenke P, Kovacs B, Bjerklund-Johansen TE, *et al.* European and Asian guidelines on management and prevention of catheter-associated urinary tract infection. *Int J Antimicrob Agents* 2008; **31**(Suppl):S68–78.
70. Pickard R, Lam T, MacLennan G, *et al.* Antimicrobial catheters for reduction of symptomatic urinary tract infection in adults requiring short-term catheterisation in hospital: a multicentre randomised controlled trial. *Lancet* 2012; **380**(9857):1927–35.
71. Wullt B, Holst E, Stevens K, *et al.* Microbial flora in ileal and colonic neobladders. *Eur Urol* 2004; **45**(2):233–9.

CHAPTER 1.5

Renal and retroperitoneal abscess

Alice E. Hartley and Toby Page

Introduction to renal and retroperitoneal abscess

Infection in the retroperitoneum is often difficult to diagnose due to its non-specific clinical presentation.[1–3] Most occur in people with anatomical abnormalities, malignancy, injury, or infection of the retroperitoneal organs[4,5] but haematogenous spread, lymph node infection, or osteomyelitis can also be causative factors.[5] Despite advances in diagnosis and treatment, it is still important for clinicians to have knowledge of retroperitoneal anatomy in order to understand the origin and spread of infection.

Delayed diagnosis or inadequate treatment of infection in the retroperitoneum and the organs contained within it, such as the kidney, can lead to abscess formation particularly in immunocompromised patients.[3,6,7] Abscess formation results in greater morbidity and, if not drained promptly, appreciable mortality.[8] In well-resourced countries, these risks have been reduced by ready access to computed tomography (CT,) which can rapidly diagnose abscess formation and guide drainage. This advancement, with its associated lower morbidity, may explain the lack of recent literature on retroperitoneal infections and our continued reliance on older studies to guide management.[9]

Anatomy

Altemeier and Alexander (1961) provided a detailed anatomical guide to the retroperitoneum which they defined as '*a potential space between the peritoneum and the transversalis fascia, bordered superiorly by the diaphragm, inferiorly by the pelvic brim and laterally by parietes at the lateral edge of the quadratus lumborum*' (Fig. 1.5.1).[5]

They divided the retroperitoneum into anterior (including the pancreas, colon and duodenum), perinephric (including the adrenals, kidneys, ureters, aorta, and vena cava), and posterior compartments (Fig. 1.5.2) The area posterior to the transversalis fascia, bordered by the psoas fascia, diaphragm, and vertebral column is known as the retrofascial space and includes the psoas muscle.

Superiorly the retroperitoneum is limited by peridiaphragmatic fat. The lack of a limiting anatomical feature inferiorly means that infection can spread from the anterior, perinephric, or posterior compartments across the midline and into the pelvic organs. Posteriorly the transversalis fascia and psoas fascia attach to the iliac crest and iliacus becoming the pelvic fascia.[10] The peritoneum sweeps over the superior aspect of the bladder (and uterus in females) and consequently the bladder, uterus, vagina, and rectum are all retroperitoneal organs. Simons *et al.* (1983) describe four (five in women) pelvic

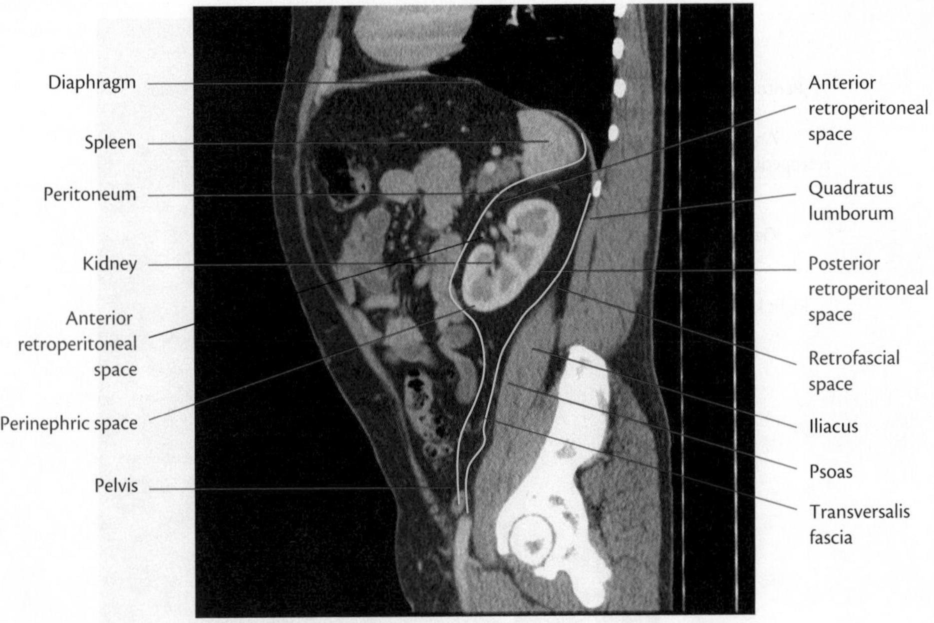

Fig. 1.5.1 A sagittal CT section of the abdomen to demonstrate the retroperitoneum.
Image reproduced courtesy of Dr Ralph Marsh.

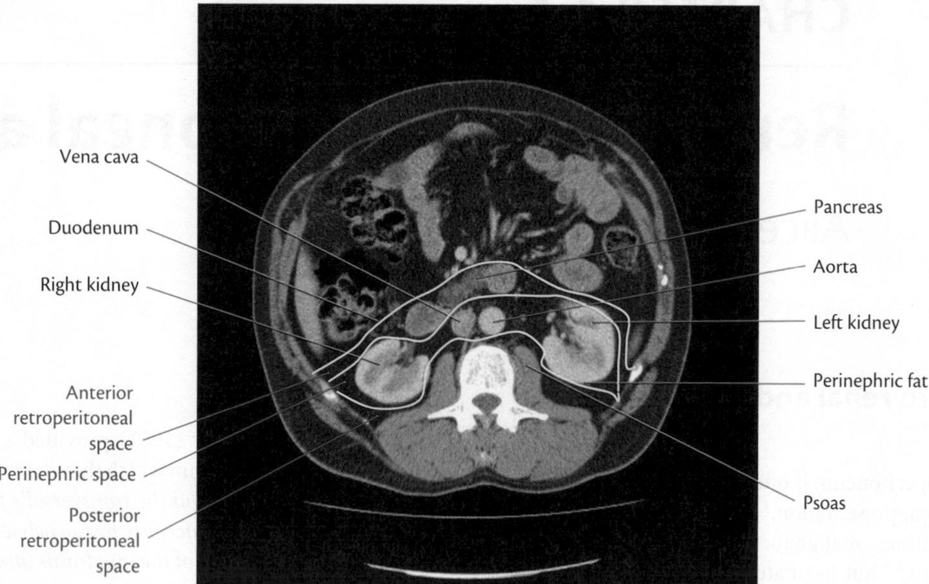

Fig. 1.5.2 A transverse CT image of the abdomen to demonstrate the retroperitoneum.
Image reproduced courtesy of Dr Ralph Marsh.

retroperitoneal spaces in which infection can develop;[10] the prevesical, postvesical, uterorectal, pararectal, and presacral. Infections can arise in any of these spaces, and infections from higher in the retroperitoneum or perineum can track into them.

The *anterior retroperitoneum* is bordered anteriorly by the posterior parietal peritoneum and posteriorly by the anterior renal (Gerota's) fascia (Fig. 1.5.3). On the right this compartment contains the ascending colon, pancreas, and duodenum, and on the left the descending colon and pancreas. The pancreas crosses the midline and therefore unless it is the source, infections do not usually spread from one side to the other.[5,10] The majority of infections in this compartment will originate from the gastrointestinal tract.

The *perinephric retroperitoneum* is contained within Gerota's fascia, which encapsulates the kidneys, adrenals, ureters, and great vessels. The medial connection with the fascia of quadratus lumborum prevents connection between the two sides.[10] Renal and perinephric infections or abscesses usually follow infections or injury of the urinary tract.

The *posterior retroperitoneum* is bound by the posterior layer of Gerota's fascia and the transversalis fascia. Inferiorly, it communicates with the anterior retroperitoneal space and opens into the pelvis. Infections rarely originate in this compartment but infection from the pelvis or other retroperitoneal compartments can track to it.

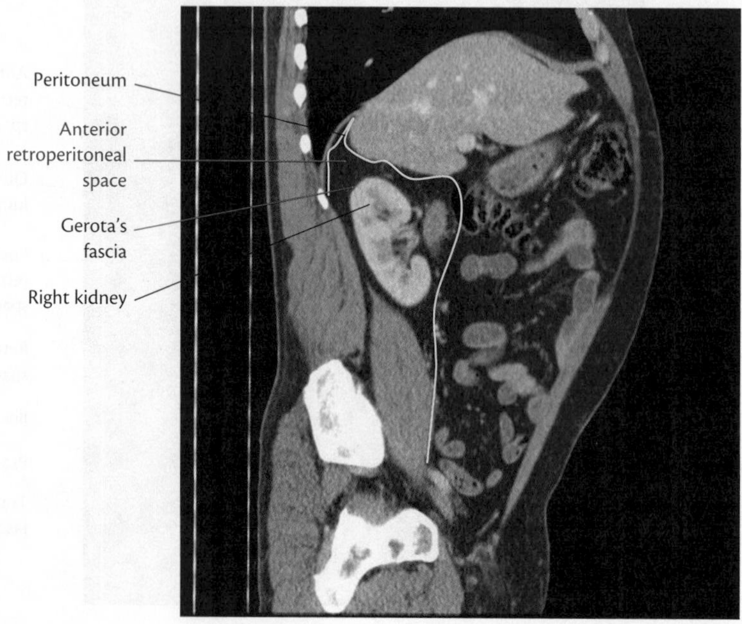

Fig. 1.5.3 A sagittal CT section to show the anterior retroperitoneal space.
Image reproduced courtesy of Dr Ralph Marsh.

The retrofascial space lies posterior to the transversalis fascia outside of the true retroperitoneal space. The lack of inferior limiting margins mean that infection can spread under the inguinal ligament down into the thigh, as well as upwards from the lower limbs and genital tract. It contains the lumbar plexus, resulting in the classical neurological signs related to psoas inflammation.

Clinical presentation

Retroperitoneal infections are most common in the 20 to 70 years age group, and those affecting the perinephric compartment are more common in women.[2,4] Immunocompromised patients, such as those with diabetes, renal, or liver disease, are at higher risk.[4,7,9]

Animal experiments have established that development of retroperitoneal sepsis is an insidious process with a higher rate of chronic abscess if left untreated, in contrast to the rapid development and early death associated with intraperitoneal infection.[11]

This slow time course contributes to the failure to detect retroperitoneal sepsis in patients presenting with chronic non-specific illness, until life-threatening sepsis related to spreading abscess occurs.[1,3,6] Additionally, the retroperitoneum is difficult to examine, with specific clinical signs unusual, and most frequently relate to palpable large abscess present in between 4% and 50% of reported case series.[2,4,6,7,10] Retrospective review following diagnosis confirms the non-specific symptomatology including abdominal pain, fever, and malaise. Referred symptoms, such as hip pain with psoas inflammation, or a mass in the anterior thigh can misdirect investigation.[7] Older studies, prior to widespread availability of CT, suggest an average time from initial presentation to diagnosis of between one and two weeks.[4,6,7,9] Diagnosis of perinephric compartment infections in these historical studies appeared more straightforward than those affecting the anterior compartment.[7]

Source of infection and microbiology

The causative organism(s) will depend on the route of infection, but aerobic and anaerobic organisms often coexist (Table 1.5.1). Several theories have been suggested to explain the coexistence of these organisms, including protection from phagocytosis, growth factor production, or the prevention of oxidizing reactions in the surrounding tissues.[12,13]

In a large case series of patients with retroperitoneal abscess, bacteria were isolated from 84% of specimens despite frequent prior antibiotic treatment. A mean of three organisms were isolated and about 60% of positive cultures grew a mixture of both aerobic (*Escherichia coli, Klebsiella pnemoniae*, Group D *Streptococcus*, and *Staphyloccoccus aureus*) and anaerobic (*Peptostreptococcus sp., Prevotella sp., Bacteroides fragilus, Clostridium perfringens*) organisms. Aerobic organisms were more prevalent in pancreatic abscesses, while anaerobic organisms were more commonly cultured from pelvic abscesses. Mycobacterium species should also be looked for and excluded. In renal and perinephric abscesses, *Escherichia coli, Klebsiella pneumoniae*, and *Staphyloccous aureus* were the most common.[2,4] Recently methicillin-resistant *Staphylococcus aureus* (MRSA) has been isolated, particularly related to prior skin infection.[14]

The likelihood of mixed bacterial populations means that the initial antibiotic regime should cover both aerobic and anaerobic, and both Gram-positive and Gram-negative organisms. To guide more definitive therapy, pus, urine, blood, and tissue should all be cultured where possible.[12]

Table 1.5.1 Anatomical subcompartments of the retroperitoneum, where abscess may occur with the related organs and causes

Compartment	Organ/tissue causing pathology	Predominant cause
Anterior retroperitoneum	Colon Appendix Pancreas	Inflammatory bowel disease Appendicitis Pancreatitis Malignancy
Perinephric	Kidney +/− ureter	Pyelonephritis Stone disease Malignancy Trauma Tuberculosis
Retrofascial	Psoas muscle Vertebrae	*Primary* Trauma Vertebral infections ◆ Discitis ◆ Osteomyelitis ◆ Tuberculosis ◆ Pott's disease ◆ Lymphatic/haematogenous *Secondary* Invasion through the transversalis fascia from other retroperitoneal compartments

Imaging

CT is now widely used in well-resourced countries as part of their early investigation of patients with pyrexia of unknown origin or unresolving abdominal pain (Fig. 1.5.4). Historically, plain abdominal radiographs may have revealed renal stones, retroperitoneal gas, or loss of psoas shadow.[1,3] Intravenous pyelography was previously helpful to detect perinephric extravasation of urine.

Abdominal ultrasound is perhaps more readily available than CT and can be used to locate fluid collections in the retroperitoneum, particularly within or around the kidney. Although the specificity for detecting associated renal and ureteric calculi is lower than CT, the presence of hydronephrosis can be detected in 98–100% of cases[15] and indicates urinary tract obstruction. Nuclear medicine renal scintigraphy (renography using radio-labelled markers such as DMSA or MAG3) can give an estimate of differential renal function and identify non-vascularized segments prior to surgical intervention, although reduced relative function on the affected side may recover following resolution of renal sepsis. Labelled white cell scanning has a limited role in identifying a retroperitoneal source for pyrexia of unknown origin.

Treatment

Early detection and commencement of parenteral antibiotics to cover both aerobic and anaerobic bacteria are essential to limit

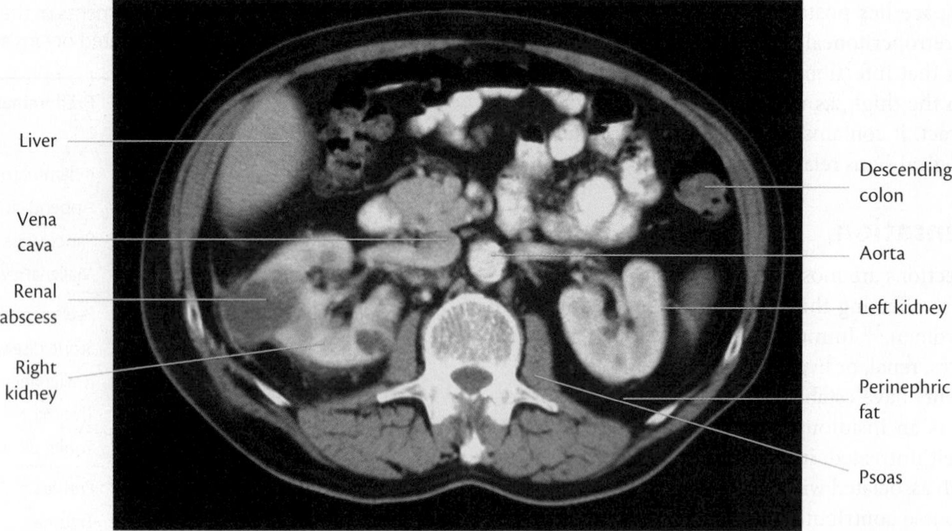

Fig. 1.5.4 A transverse CT cross-section of the abdomen showing abscess in right kidney.
Image reproduced courtesy of Dr Philip Haslam.

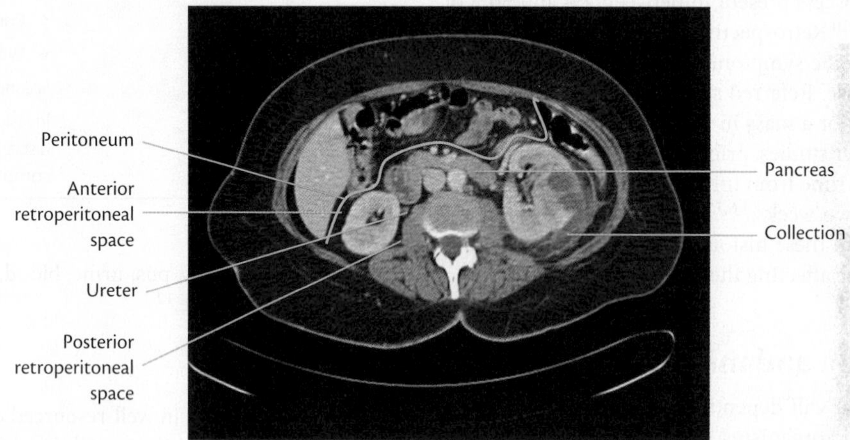

Fig. 1.5.5 A CT scan showing left perinephric collection extending posteriorly.
Image reproduced courtesy of Dr Philip Haslam.

the morbidity and mortality of retroperitoneal infections. Surgical or needle drainage of any subsequently identified abscess, as well as being therapeutic, can identify causative organism to guide definitive therapy. Ideally drainage should be performed percutaneously, rather than by laparotomy to minimize risk of contamination.[3] Untreated, mortality of retroperitoneal infection with abscess approaches 100% (Fig. 1.5.5).[8] Treatment with antibiotics alone may be sufficient for patients with small (<3 cm) perinephric abscess[9] (Fig. 1.5.6) but imaging should be repeated if there is no clinical response and involvement of the microbiology team is essential.[9]

After initial resuscitative treatment, it is important to complete patient assessment to identify and rectify the underlying cause. Most commonly, this will be an obstructing ureteric stone causing an infected urinoma in the retroperitoneum. In the majority of cases, percutaneous drainage or stent insertion is the safest initial option until the patient's condition has normalized. Subsequent stone removal is facilitated by previous drainage from nephrostomy or retrograde stent insertion. For infections that fail to resolve, surgical excision of the infected tissue may be required to allow clearance of the bacterial nidus. For complex renal sepsis such as xanthogranulomatous pyelonephritis, total or partial nephrectomy is indicated, usually via the open route—although laparoscopic

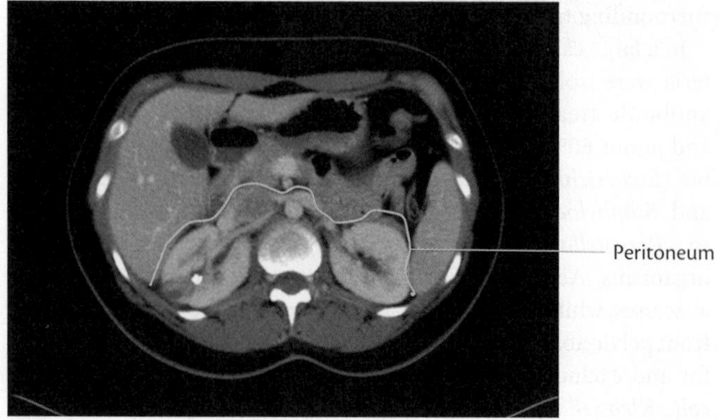

Fig. 1.5.6 A CT scan showing small right renal abscess associated with a calyceal calculus.
Image reproduced courtesy of Dr Philip Haslam.

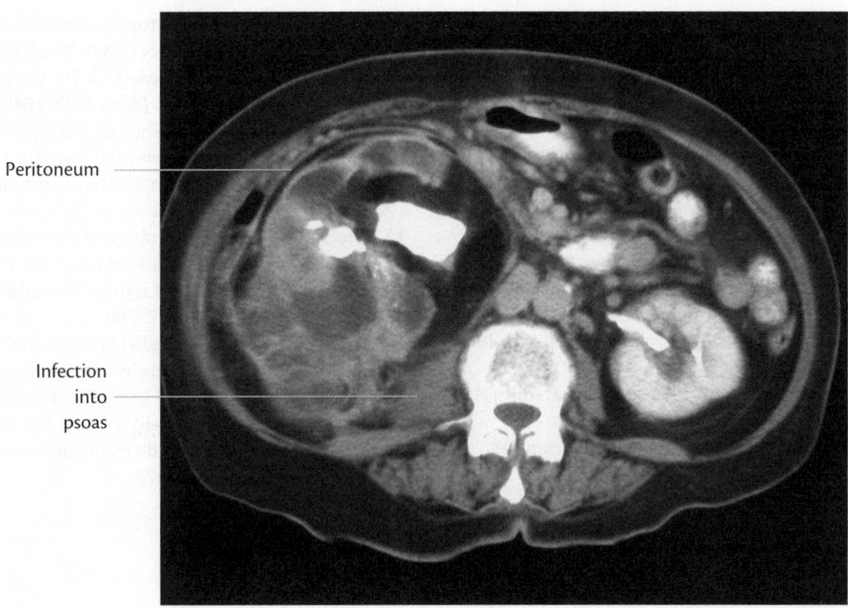

Fig. 1.5.7 A CT scan showing xanthogranulomatous pyelonephritis of the right kidney.
Image reproduced courtesy of Dr Philip Haslam.

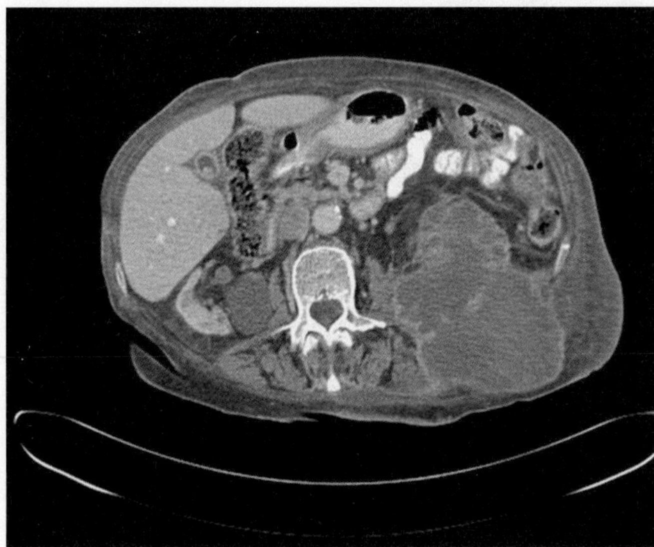

Fig. 1.5.8 A CT scan showing large left renal abscess eroded out through the posterior abdominal wall muscles.
Image reproduced courtesy of Dr Philip Haslam.

series have been described with similar morbidity rates (Fig. 1.5.7). Surgeons should anticipate increased risk of injury to surrounding structures such as bowel, and intraoperative bleeding during mobilization of the renal hilum. Partial nephrectomy to preserve healthy renal tissue is possible but with an increased risk of urine leakage, failure of resolution of sepsis, and bleeding.

Retroperitoneal collections arising from bowel or pancreas pathology are similarly treated with initial percutaneous drainage to allow symptom relief and stabilization of the patient, before definitive treatment by surgical excision of diseased bowel segments, and percutaneous or open necrosectomy.

Summary

The diagnostic possibility of retroperitoneal infection is often not considered in the differential diagnosis of patients with malaise and non-specific abdominal or pelvic symptoms. If untreated, subsequent abscess formation may carry a high risk of morbidity and mortality. Understanding of retroperitoneum compartmental anatomy will help the clinician localize the potential source of infection using ultrasound and CT imaging (Fig. 1.5.8). Following diagnosis and after specimens have been obtained, broad antibiotic coverage should be used initially, with subsequent refinement according to culture and sensitivity testing. Early percutaneous drainage of all but the smallest abscess can reduce the morbidity and mortality associated with this condition and lead to a complete resolution of symptoms, with surgical resection only required to address the underlying pathology, or in complex cases such as xanthogranulomatous pyelonephritis.

Further reading

Altemeier WA, Alexander JW. Retroperitoneal abscess. *Arch Surg* 1961; **83**:512–24.

Brook I, Frazier EH. Aerobic and anaerobic microbiology of retroperitoneal abscesses. *Clin Infect Dis* 1998; **26**(4):938–41.

Coelho RF, Schneider-Monteiro ED, Mesquita JL, Mazzucchi E, Marmo LA, Srougi M. Renal and perinephric abscesses: analysis of 65 consecutive cases. *World J Surg* 2007; **31**(2):431–6.

Crepps JT, Welch JP, Orlando R, III. Management and outcome of retroperitoneal abscesses. *Ann Surg* 1987; **205**(3):276–81.

Daviglus GF, Rush BF, Jr. Retroperitoneal abscess. A clinical study. *Arch Surg* 1961; **83**:322–8.

Meng MV, Mario LA, McAninch JW. Current treatment and outcomes of perinephric abscesses. *J Urol* 2002; **168**(4 Pt 1):1337–40.

Meyer HI. The reaction of the retroperitoneal tissues to infection. *Ann Surg* 1934; **99**(2):246–50.

Sawyer RB, Sawyer KC, Mikolaschek K, Manke WF. Retroperitonitis. *Arch Surg* 1969; **98**(4):534–8.

References

1. Sawyer RB, Sawyer KC, Mikolaschek K, Manke WF. Retroperitonitis. *Arch Surg* 1969; **98**(4):534–8.
2. Coelho RF, Schneider-Monteiro ED, Mesquita JL, Mazzucchi E, Marmo LA, Srougi M. Renal and perinephric abscesses: analysis of 65 consecutive cases. *World J Surg* 2007; **31**(2):431–6.
3. Tunuguntla A, Raza R, Hudgins L. Diagnostic and therapeutic difficulties in retroperitoneal abscess. *South Med J* 2004; **97**(11):1107–9.
4. Shu T, Green JM, Orihuela E. Renal and perirenal abscesses in patients with otherwise anatomically normal urinary tracts. *J Urol* 2004; **172**(1):148–50.
5. Altemeier WA, Alexander JW. Retroperitoneal abscess. *Arch Surg* 1961; **83**:512–24.
6. Daviglus GF, Rush BF, Jr. Retroperitoneal abscess. A clinical study. *Arch Surg* 1961; **83**:322–8.
7. Crepps JT, Welch JP, Orlando R, III. Management and outcome of retroperitoneal abscesses. *Ann Surg* 1987; **205**(3):276–81.
8. Harris LF, Sparks JE. Retroperitoneal abscess. Case report and review of the literature. *Dig Dis Sci* 1980; **25**(5):392–5.
9. Meng MV, Mario LA, McAninch JW. Current treatment and outcomes of perinephric abscesses. *J Urol* 2002; **168**(4 Pt 1):1337–40.
10. Simons GW, Sty JR, Starshak RJ. Retroperitoneal and retrofascial abscesses. A review. *J Bone Joint Surg Am* 1983; **65**(8):1041–58.
11. Meyer HI. The reaction of the retroperitoneal tissues to infection. *Ann Surg* 1934; **99**(2):246–50.
12. Brook I, Frazier EH. Aerobic and anaerobic microbiology of retroperitoneal abscesses. *Clin Infect Dis* 1998; **26**(4):938–41.
13. Brook I. Microbiology of retroperitoneal abscesses in children. *J Med Microbiol* 1999; **48**(7):697–700.
14. Abreu DA, Osorio F, Guido LG, Carvalhal GF, Mouro L. Retroperitoneal infections by community acquired methicillin resistant Staphylococcus aureus. *J Urol* 2008; **179**(1):172–6.
15. Ellenbogen PH, Scheible FW, Talner LB, Leopold GR. Sensitivity of gray scale ultrasound in detecting urinary tract obstruction. *AJR Am J Roentgenol* 1978; **130**(4):731–3.

CHAPTER 1.6

Tuberculosis and parasitic infestations involving the urogenital system

Chris Heyns†

Introduction to tuberculosis

Pathogenesis

Urogenital tuberculosis (UGTB) is caused by *Mycobacterium tuberculosis (MTb)* which is transmitted in droplets from the sputum of individuals with pulmonary tuberculosis (PTB). The organism is inhaled and engulfed by lung macrophages. It has the ability to inhibit phagolysosomal function and slowly multiplies in the cytoplasm of the macrophage. Bacterial antigens stimulate T-lymphocytes to secrete cytokines, which upregulate the macrophage killing mechanisms against *MTb*. An effective cellular immune response prevents dissemination of the organism and leads to healing of the primary focus of infection;[1,2] if ineffective, dissemination, including to the urogenital tract, may occur.

Active UGTB may also arise as a complication of intravesical installation of the attenuated strain of *MTb*, bacille Calmette–Guérin (BCG) used for immunotherapy in urothelial carcinoma.[3,4]

Histologically, the tubercle is a granuloma consisting of macrophages, T and B lymphocytes, and fibroblasts surrounding the infected macrophages. *MTb* may remain viable within the tubercle, resulting in latent (dormant) infection. If the cellular immune response is inadequate, *MTb* spreads via lymphatics and the bloodstream to other organs. Reactivation of dormant TB leads to a chronic inflammatory response with granulomata consisting of lymphocytes, Langhans giant cells, fibroblasts, and central caseous necrosis, eventually followed by fibrosis and dystrophic calcification of necrotic tissue.[5–7] Reactivation of latent TB may occur in conditions which suppress cellular immunity, such as human immunodeficiency virus (HIV) infection, diabetes mellitus, malignancy, steroid treatment or chemotherapy, renal dialysis, and immunosuppressant therapy after organ transplantation.[8–14]

UGTB is the second most common form of extrapulmonary TB (after lymphadenopathy) and, depending on the geographical region, accounts for 14–41% of non-PTB cases.[14] UGTB occurs in 2–10% of cases of PTB in developed (affluent) countries, and in 15–20% of cases of PTB in developing countries.[15]

The routes of dissemination of *MTb* to the urogenital system are:

- haematogenous to the kidneys and adrenals (both sexes), epididymis and prostate (men) and the uterus and fallopian tubes (women);
- endoluminal from the kidney via urine to the ureter and bladder; or from the epididymis in semen via the vas deferens to the seminal vesicles and prostate.[4,16,17]

Haematogenous spread of *MTb* to the kidneys primarily infects the renal cortex.[15,16] Adequate cell-mediated immunity prevents bacterial multiplication, leading to dormant microscopic foci. With reactivation and progression of the disease, tubercles and caseous necrosis extend into the renal medulla. Ulceration of the calyces and sloughing of the papillae enable the organisms to gain access to the collecting system. Areas of caseous necrosis may coalesce to form cavities in the kidney. TB typically heals with fibrosis causing stenosis of the renal infundibula. Extensive granulomata may form a mass lesion (tuberculoma) and there is often calcification of necrotic tissues. Although haematogenous dissemination occurs in both kidneys, clinically active renal TB is usually unilateral.[14,15,18]

The ureter is probably infected by endoluminal spread of *MTb* from renal foci rather than by haematogenous dissemination. TB usually involves the lower ureter, and less commonly the upper ureter and renal pelvis.[19] There is ulceration of the ureteric mucosa and fibrosis of the wall, causing stricture formation or vesicoureteric reflux (VUR).[14] The bladder is usually infected by *MTb* in urine from foci in the kidney, but haematogenous infection may occur without renal involvement. The trigone and ureteric orifices are usually affected first. Tubercles forming in the bladder mucosa typically cause hyperaemic patches and ulceration, while subsequent fibrosis of the bladder wall may cause ureteric obstruction and reduced bladder capacity. Ureteric stenosis is most often unilateral, but may be bilateral, causing obstructive renal failure.[14]

The epididymis is usually infected by haematogenous spread of *MTb* to the cauda (tail) with its more abundant blood supply, but eventually TB involves the whole epididymis.[4] Tubercles with caseous necrosis cause obliteration of the epididymal lumen and may ulcerate through the skin. The testis is involved by direct spread from the epididymis and may be completely replaced by granulomata with caseous necrosis and fibrosis. The vas deferens is involved via endouminal spread of bacteria from the epididymis.[20] The prostate may be infected by haematogenous spread but, also transluminally from urine or semen.[4,21,22] Rarely, TB can be sexually transmitted; to the penis from a female who has TB of the cervix or uterus, or to the female genital organs via infected semen.[23] Anecdotal cases of penile TB have been reported in infants when

† Deceased

circumcision was performed by a person with open PTB who attempted to stop haemorrhage by sucking the penis.[24,25]

Clinical presentation

UGTB is more common in men than women (2:1 ratio) with a mean (range) age of 41 (5–88) years. There is a history of previous PTB in about a third of cases with a mean (range) interval of 22 (1–46) years.[15] The most common presentation (in about 50% of cases) is with cystitis; irritative/storage lower urinary tract symptoms (frequency, nocturia, dysuria, urgency, and urgency incontinence).[4,15] There may be superimposed urinary tract infection (UTI), usually with *Escherichia coli* in 20–40% of all patients and up to 50% of women. Recurrent cystitis with pyuria despite appropriate antibiotic treatment should arouse the suspicion of TB.[15,26] Loin pain occurs in about a third of patients, usually due to hydronephrosis, sometimes with superimposed bacterial infection causing pyelonephritis or pyonephrosis. Ureteric colic may be caused by necrotic papillae, blood clot, or urolithiasis resulting from urinary stasis and recurrent UTI.[15,27,28]

Haematuria is caused by bleeding from papillary necrosis in the kidneys or granulomatous lesions in the bladder or ureteric wall, and occurs in about a third of cases. The haematuria is usually microscopic only, but may be visible. Haematospermia due to involvement of the prostate or seminal vesicles is rare.[27,29] Scrotal swelling due to chronic epididymitis or epididymo-orchitis is present in 10–50% of men with UGTB. It is usually painless and is bilateral in about a third of cases.[15,30] In the early stages, the epididymis is enlarged, firm, and usually non-tender, but later on the whole testis may be involved. A chronic scrotal sinus may also develop. Palpable tubercles and fibrosis along the vas deferens may cause the finding of a 'beaded' vas.[31] Repeated bouts of epididymo-orchitis despite standard antibiotic therapy should arouse the suspicion of TB, particularly when there is sinus formation.

On digital rectal examination, a firm, non-tender nodule in the prostate may mimic prostate cancer.[21,32] Rarely, a uroenteric fistula may develop (e.g. rectoprostatic, vesicoileal, or ureteroileal fistula).[33] The presenting complaint may be infertility due to involvement of the epididymis and vas deferens in the male, and/or the uterus or fallopian tubes in the female.[28,34–36] Penile involvement is rare and usually presents as a chronic ulcer of the glans and prepuce, sometimes with small tubercles under the skin.[37–39] Urethral involvement may cause external meatal stenosis, urethral stricture, or urethrocutaneous fistula.[15,21,31,40] Systemic symptoms such as fever, anorexia, weight loss and night sweats are present in about 20% of patients with UGTB.[15] Bilateral TB necrosis of the adrenals is rare, but invariably causes corticosteroid deficiency (Addison's disease) with generalized weakness.[16]

Diagnosis

A high index of suspicion is required to make the diagnosis of UGTB and it is frequently initially missed, especially in developed countries with low incidence.[16,41] Urinalysis is usually positive for leucocytes; there may also be blood and protein, and nitrites may be present if there is associated bacterial UTI.[42,43] Urine microscopy and culture shows leucocytes with no bacterial growth; sterile pyuria, in up to 90% of cases. However, superimposed bacterial infection, usually with *E coli*, is quite common and may delay diagnosis.[34] Ziehl–Neelsen staining and microscopy for acid-fast bacilli (AFB) in urine specimens has a diagnostic sensitivity of only 42–52%, so urine culture specifically for *MTb* is essential. *MTb* is excreted in the urine intermittently and in low numbers, therefore at least three to six early morning urine specimens should be collected on different days. Detection of *MTb* growth requires special culture media and techniques. The sensitivity of urine culture varies widely from 10–90%, but the specificity is nearly 100%.[15] Recent antibiotic use (especially fluoroquinolones) may lead to false negative TB cultures.

Growth of *MTb* on Löwenstein–Jensen medium may take six to eight weeks.[15,44] A more rapid technique is radiometric detection with the Bactec system, which can provide results in 7–14 days. This involves growth of *MTb* in broth radiolabelled with ^{14}C-palmitate liberating $^{14}CO_2$, which is detected by radiometric analysis.[44–46] Other rapid methods are fluorometric technology to detect O_2 consumption resulting from bacterial growth, or microcalorimetry to detect metabolic heat produced by mycobacterial growth.[47] The polymerase chain reaction (PCR) can be used to amplify and detect small amounts of mycobacterial DNA in urine. The result is available in 24–48 hours and the sensitivity and specificity are both in the range 90–95%.[15,48–51] Inhibitors in the urine may suppress the enzymatic reaction leading to false negative tests.[52] PCR should not be used in isolation to diagnose UGTB, but must be considered together with other findings. PCR will also detect DNA from dead bacteria and therefore cannot be used to determine the effectiveness of treatment.

The tuberculin (Mantoux) skin test makes use of purified protein derivative (PPD) extracted from cultures of *MTb*. A dose of five tuberculin units is injected intradermally into the skin of the forearm. PPD stimulates a T-cell-mediated hypersensitivity reaction leading to local induration which must be read 48–72 hours after the injection. The test is positive after prior exposure to TB and after vaccination or intravesical therapy with BCG, and is therefore not diagnostic of active TB.[53]

Although a non-functioning kidney is present in up to 25% of cases, renal impairment is uncommon.[15,26] Ultrasonography may be useful if there is renal impairment to show hydronephrosis, renal cavitation, hydroureter, and bladder wall changes, but the findings are non-specific.[54–59] A chest X-ray shows fibrosis in the lung apex due to previous (healed) PTB in 25–50% of cases.[18,54] In patients with renal TB, 10–75% may have active PTB, and in patients with active PTB 6–14% may have renal involvement.[55] Abdominal X-ray shows focal calcification in the kidneys in 30–50% of cases. The whole kidney may be replaced with caseous necrosis and calcification, so-called 'putty kidney'.[54] Stone formation may occur secondary to ureteric obstruction and UTI. Calcification of the wall of the ureter or bladder is rare, but may occur in the prostate and seminal vesicle.[4] Intravenous pyelography (IVP) and more recently CT-urography are useful imaging modalities for UGTB. The signs are non-specific, but may include any of the following:[4,18,22,54,56–58]

- Erosion of the renal medulla ('moth eaten' calyces);
- Papillary (medullary) necrosis;
- Hydrocalicosis due to infundibular stenosis (Fig. 1.6.1);
- Cavity formation in the renal parenchyma;
- Calyceal obliteration or amputation (absent or 'phantom' calyx);

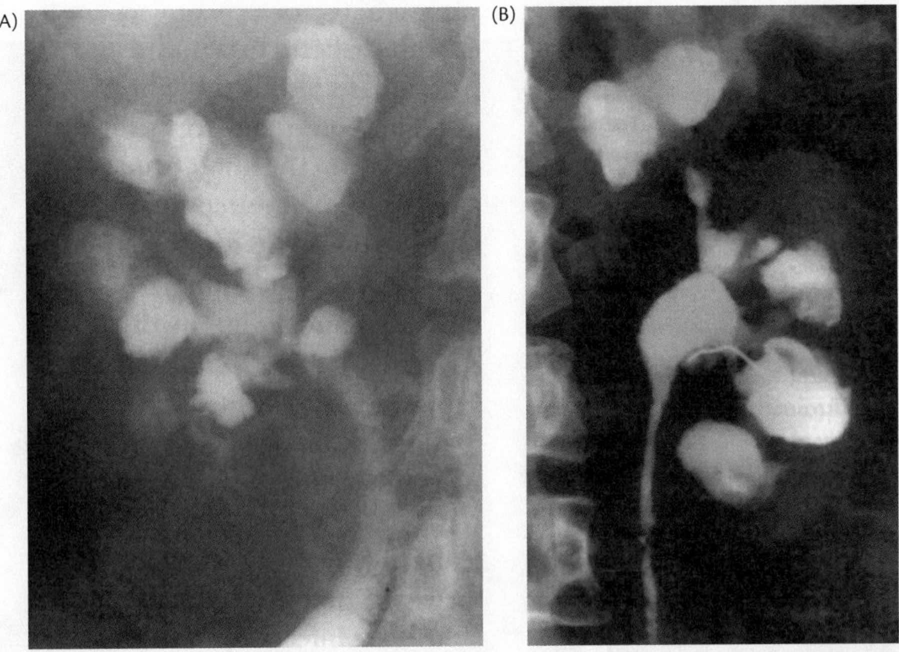

Fig. 1.6.1 (A and B) Intravenous pyelographies (IVPs) of two different patients showing hydrocalyces due to infundibular stenosis, with papillary necrosis and cavity formation in the renal parenchyma, shrunken renal pelvis, and ureteritis cystica.

- Hydronephrosis which may be segmental or total, with irregular margins and filling defects due to caseous debris;
- Pelviureteric junction obstruction (PUJO) usually with a small capacity renal pelvis;
- Non-functioning of the kidney (the term 'autonephrectomy' is a misnomer, because the kidney has not been excised) (Fig. 1.6.2);
- Mucosal irregularity of the ureter ('sawtooth' ureter);
- Straightening, shortening, and medial displacement of the ureter ('pipe-stem' ureter);
- Hydroureter proximal to a stricture, usually in the lower ureter;
- 'Beaded' or 'corkscrew' appearance of the ureter due to multiple strictures;
- Irregularity of the bladder wall (oedema or granulomata);
- Small bladder capacity due to fibrosis of the bladder wall (Fig. 1.6.2).

Ultrasound is a very useful tool to monitor or detect hydronephrosis during treatment as TB heals with fibrosis, which may worsen obstruction. Ultrasound will also differentiate between chronic epididymo-orchitis and testicular tumour in men with scrotal swelling.[4]

Computed tomography (CT) without contrast enhancement is very sensitive in showing calcifications in the kidneys, adrenals, prostate, or seminal vesicles.[54] Contrast-enhanced CT or magnetic resonance imaging (MRI) is useful in showing hydroureteronephrosis, renal mass (tuberculoma), thickening of the walls of the ureter and bladder, or a nodule or abscess in the prostate.[4,54,58,60,61]

Cystoscopy to assess haematuria may show areas of hyperaemia of the trigone and ureteric orifices, mucosal erosion, or ulceration. In florid TB cystitis, the whole bladder may be hyperaemic and haemorrhagic and the ureteric orifices may be impossible to identify. There may be a 'golf-hole' ureteric orifice due to fibrosis, which shortens the ureter. In chronic fibrosis of the bladder wall, the capacity can be severely reduced ('thimble' bladder).[62,63] Retrograde pyelography can be used to assess a non-functioning kidney, obtain a urine sample for TB culture from the upper tract and insert a ureteric stent to improve drainage at diagnosis or during treatment.[64,65]

Percutaneous nephrostomy (PCN) and antegrade stent insertion may be needed if retrograde stent insertion is not possible.[66]

Cystoscopic bladder biopsy is useful to exclude malignancy, but may show TB-related histological findings such as acid-fast bacilli or granulomata in about half of cases.[50,67] There is a small risk of disseminated (miliary) tuberculosis after bladder biopsy or retrograde pyelography.[68,69] In men with scrotal swelling, fine needle aspiration cytology (FNAC) may be diagnostic.[70] About 50–75% of men with genital TB have radiologic abnormalities in the urinary tract; therefore biopsy or excision of the epididymis or testis is only indicated if less invasive studies have failed to establish the diagnosis.[4] Prostate biopsy may be indicated to exclude carcinoma if there is a palpable nodule. Renal biopsy with PCR analysis of the tissues may be considered.[64,71] All patients diagnosed with TB should be tested for HIV infection after appropriate counselling, because TB is one of the conditions defining the acquired immunodeficiency syndrome (AIDS), which will require additional antiretroviral therapy.[72,73]

Treatment

Medical therapy should be given to all patients with UGTB proven by culture. Empirical therapy can be considered, especially in regions with endemic TB, when there is clinical and imaging evidence of UGTB which has yet to be confirmed by culture.[67,74]

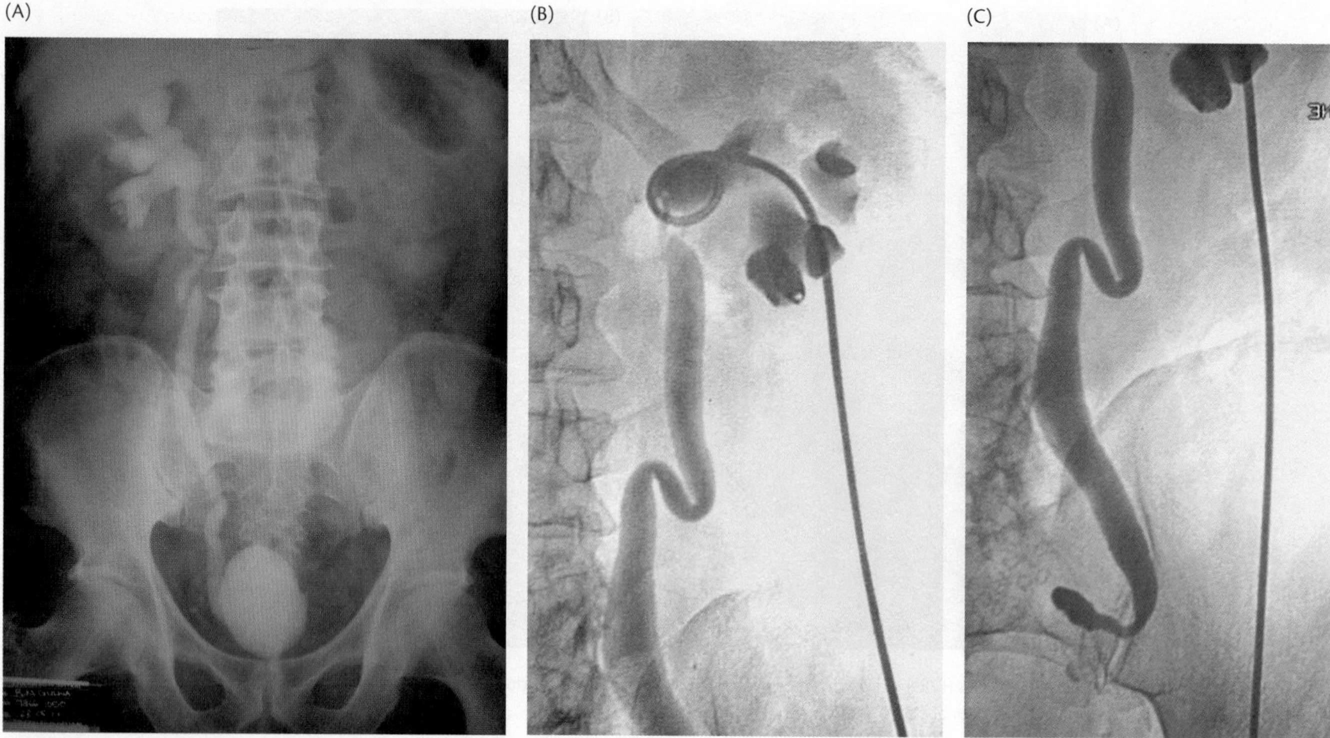

Fig. 1.6.2 (A) IVP showing right hydroureteronephrosis, left non-functioning kidney and small bladder capacity; (B) antegrade left nephrostogram showing pelviureteric stenosis; and (C) complete distal ureteric obstruction.

Multidrug therapy (at least three agents) is essential, because the organisms divide slowly and the drugs have significant differences with regard to tissue penetration, activity at different pH levels in the tissues and urine, and effect on the organism. Resistance develops very rapidly when only one or two drugs are used.[75] UGTB can be managed with short-course chemotherapy (six months) because fewer organisms infect genitourinary tissues and urine, while the available drugs have good tissue penetration and attain high urine levels (Table 1.6.1).[14,15,28,75,76] Guidance varies in different geographical locations but typically first-line therapy consists of rifampicin, isoniazid (INH) and pyrazinamide (PZA) daily for two months, with ethambutol added if drug resistance to INH is suspected. This is followed by four months of treatment with rifampicin and INH two to three times per week. Patients with malnutrition and poor social conditions warrant treatment for nine months or more.[15]

To prevent peripheral neuropathy in patients on INH, pyridoxine (vitamin B_6) 25–50 mg/day can be given. Patient compliance with TB treatment is often poor, so directly observed therapy can be used to improve adherence to the schedule.[77] Monthly monitoring during therapy should include liver function tests, serum creatinine, full blood count, and uric acid levels, direct questioning for visual disturbances, and renal ultrasound for new or worsening hydronephrosis.[19] Relapse occurs in about 5% of cases at a mean (range) of 5 (1 to 27) years after initial urine sterilization, therefore follow-up for 10 years with periodic urine TB cultures is recommended.[15]

In patients with AIDS on retroviral therapy, the dosage of rifampicin should be altered depending on the type of retroviral agent used. If the CD4 count is less than 100 cells/mm^3 TB treatment should be given daily or three times a week (rather than weekly) for at least nine months to prevent the development of drug resistance.[78] Rifampicin induces the hepatic P450 microsomal enzyme and may decrease serum levels of immunosuppressive drugs.[79] Second-line therapy is indicated for cases that fail on first-line therapy. The possible drug options include aminoglycosides (streptomycin), fluoroquinolones (levofloxacin), cycloserine, ethionamide and para-aminosalicylic acid (PAS).[75] There is an increasing incidence worldwide of multidrug-resistant TB (MDR-TB) defined

Table 1.6.1 Typical regimen for first-line therapy of urogenital tuberculosis

Drug	Daily dosage	Intermittent dosage	Adverse effects
Isoniazid (INH)	5 mg/kg (max 300 mg)	15 mg/kg 2–3 times/week	Hepatotoxicity, peripheral neuropathy
Rifampicin	10 mg/kg (max 600 mg)	10 mg/kg 2–3 times/week	Hepatotoxicity, neutropenia
Pyrazinamide (PZA)	20–25 mg/kg (max 1.5 gm)	30–50 mg/kg 2–3 times/week	Hepatotoxicity, hyperuricemia
Ethambutol	15–25 mg/kg	20–50 mg/kg 2–3 times/week	Optic neuritis, visual disturbances

as resistance to INH *and* rifampicin or any other first-line drug. Extensively drug-resistant TB (XDR-TB) is defined as resistance to some of the agents used in second-line therapy. Treatment of MDR-TB requires up to five drugs for at least 18 months and XDR-TB requires treatment according to individual sensitivity.[80]

The rationale for the use of steroids in UGTB is to reduce the inflammatory response and consequent fibrosis. In TB involving the bladder or ureter, steroids may improve symptoms and prevent or limit stricture formation, but this is controversial and steroid-induced adverse effects may outweigh any benefit.[81] Surgery for UGTB should only be performed after four to six weeks of medical treatment, preferably after confirming that the urine TB culture has reverted to negative.[82,83] Ureteric stenting is indicated in patients with hydronephrosis in order to prevent further loss of renal function.[19] and can be performed retrogradely, or antegradely if the ureteric orifices cannot be cannulated. Segmental hydronephrosis due to infundibular stenosis may require multiple stents or neprostomy tubes.[66] Nephrectomy is indicated for a non-functioning kidney as decreased renal blood flow may prevent TB eradication,[81,84] and cause later hypertension.[15,85]

There are a number of options to surgically treat ureteric, pelviureteric junction, and infundibular strictures that persist after successful UGTB treatment. Balloon dilatation or endoscopic incision has a failure rate of up to 50% presumably due to the ischaemic nature and dense fibrosis of TB strictures.[15,86–89] Similarly pyeloplasty may be difficult because of fibrosis and small capacity renal pelvis, making the Foley YV technique most useful. Ureterocalicostomy (anastomosing the ureter to a dilated lower pole calyx) may be required if pyeloplasty is not possible.[90,91] Excision of a ureteric stricture with adequate mobilization to perform tension-free ureteroureterostomy can be performed for upper and middle ureteric strictures.[65] Ureteroplasty can be performed using buccal mucosa as a free graft.[92] Ureteroneocystostomy (reimplantation of the ureter into the bladder) can be performed if there is a strictured lower ureter. The proximal ureter should be healthy and well vascularized.[93] To achieve a tension-free anastomosis, a psoas hitch or Boari flap can be used, provided that bladder capacity is adequate.[94,95] Ileal interposition can be used if there are multiple ureteric strictures involving the upper as well as lower ureter.[81] Alternatively, the ureter can be replaced with a Yang-Monti type of conduit constructed from the terminal ileum.[96] Augmentation or substitution cystoplasty using a segment of terminal ileum, caecum, or sigmoid colon can be performed for a small, contracted ('thimble') bladder,[15,63,82,97] but may be at higher risk of tumour formation.[98]

Transurethral drainage or transperineal aspiration under ultrasound guidance may be indicated for TB abscess of the prostate or seminal vesicles.[99] Epididymectomy may be performed for TB epididymitis that does not resolve on medical therapy.[100,101] Orchidectomy may be indicated for severe epididymo-orchitis or if there is suspicion of testicular malignancy.[102,103]

The prognosis of UGTB is generally good when the disease is detected early, but the mortality may be as high as 26% in some regions.[104]

Schistosomiasis (bilharzia)

Pathogenesis

Schistosomiasis is caused by parasitic trematodes (flatworms) of the genus *Schistosoma* discovered by the German pathologist Theodor Bilharz in 1851. The body of the male schistosome is split by a groove—hence its name, derived from the Greek *skhistos* (divided) and *soma* (body). The female worm is smaller than the male and lies in this cleft, known as the gynaecophoric canal, in a state of permanent copulation, producing 200–500 eggs per day during a lifespan of three to six years.[105–107] Humans are infested through contact with fresh water contaminated with free-swimming cercariae (about 500 micron in length), which penetrate the skin, shed their forked tail, and become schistosomula. They then migrate to the portal veins and in one to four weeks become adult worms (1–3 cm long).[107] Mating adults of *S. haematobium* migrate to the perivesical venous plexuses and predominantly affect the urinary tract, shedding their ova in the urine. The eggs may also be deposited in the seminal vesicles and ejaculatory ducts in men and in the uterus and vagina in women.[108] Other species, *S. mansoni, intercalatum, guineensis, japonicum, and mekongi*, migrate to the mesenteric veins, shed their ova in the faeces and cause gastrointestinal and/or hepatic disease.

The period between penetration of the cercariae and the onset of egg deposition in the tissues is usually two to three months. The ova (70–170 micron in length) hatch after one to three hours in fresh water releasing miracidia (ciliated larvae about 160 micron in length), which penetrate the intermediate host, fresh water snails Bulinis (*S. haematobium*) or Biomphalaria (*S. mansoni*), where they develop as sporocysts over the course of a month or two. Each miracidium produces 20–40 daughter sporocysts, which in turn produce 200–400 cercariae each. The snails release cercariae, which can live for up to four days in fresh water and must penetrate the skin of a human to continue the life cycle. Swallowed cercariae are digested in the stomach and do not cause disease.[105,107]

The ova deposited in tissues elicit cellular and humoral immune responses, leading to eosinophilia and a granulomatous tissue response causing erythematous polypoid masses which project into the lumen of the bladder.[109–112] Granulomata consist of eosinophils, lymphocytes, plasma cells, and giant cells. The ova are destroyed by the host granulomatous response and eventually become calcified. The polypoid lesions are replaced by fibrosis of the bladder wall and ureters. Inactive urinary schistosomiasis (when the adult worms have died) is characterized by the presence of 'sandy patches' consisting of fibrosis and calcification around non-viable ova.[105]

Schistosomiasis affects over 200 million people worldwide (mainly in Africa, the Middle East, and Asia) and causes an estimated 200,000 deaths annually.[113] In endemic areas, children are exposed to water at an early age; therefore, active schistosomiasis usually begins in childhood. In some cultures haematuria in boys is seen as a normal sign of puberty.[106] Schistosomiasis usually affects the lower ureter and bladder wall.[114] Hydroureter is usually asymmetric and may be secondary to fibrotic stricture formation, or ureteric muscular dysfunction. In most cases, ureteric dilatation is not associated with renographic evidence of obstruction.[90,115–117] Obstructive nephropathy can occur and the affected kidney may also suffer glomerulonephritis due to the deposition of immune complexes containing schistosomal antigens.[118] Chronic inflammation of the urothelium leads to squamous metaplasia, which has a greater proliferation rate than normal urothelium and increases the risk of genetic changes leading to carcinogenesis. Chronic infection with *S. haematobium* converts nitrates to nitrites and subsequently to nitrosamines, which are carcinogenic.[106,119,120] Chronic irritation of the urothelium may lead to cystitis cystica and glandularis (intestinal metaplasia), which may lead to adenocarcinoma.[105]

Bladder cancer associated with schistosomiasis is usually squamous cell cancer (SCC) (60–90%) or adenocarcinoma (5–15%) and it occurs in relatively young patients (40–50 years old).[121–124] SCC can be fungating (exophytic) or ulcerative (endophytic), and is often well differentiated or verrucous with a relatively good prognosis if diagnosed early.[125] However, in developing countries it is often diagnosed late and at an incurable stage.[123,126]

Clinical presentation

Penetration of the skin by cercariae may cause an urticarial reaction ('swimmers itch') in previously exposed people. Systemic manifestations with symptoms of fever, urticaria, cough, myalgia, headache, abdominal tenderness, lymphadenopathy, splenomegaly, and eosinophilia may occur 2–12 weeks after infestation (Katayama syndrome).[127,128] Active schistosomiasis usually presents with visible haematuria and terminal dysuria, usually appearing 10–12 weeks after infestation. The haematuria can be severe enough to cause anaemia, ureteric obstruction, or clot retention.[106,129] Involvement of the seminal vesicles and ejaculatory ducts by *S. haematobium* may cause haemospermia or later infertility.[31,130,131] It may also cause scrotal pain or a testicular mass in men, and cervicitis or vaginitis in women.[108]

Added bacterial UTI may occur in up to 50% of patients as a result of obstructive uropathy, urolithiasis, or bladder outlet obstruction. This may cause lower abdominal or pelvic pain, urinary frequency, urgency, and incontinence. Infection caused by non-typhoid *Salmonella* species may occur in some patients, because these organisms reside in the invaginations of the schistosome tegument where they are protected from host defences and antibiotics.[132,133] In the late chronic phase, suprapubic or pelvic pain with dysuria, macroscopic haematuria, and pyuria may be due to bladder ulcers or carcinoma.[106,134]

The chronic inactive phase of the disease may remain asymptomatic despite gross obstructive hydroureteronephrosis.[135] Renal failure is relatively rare, despite severe dilatation of the upper urinary tracts.[105] Patients who develop renal failure are usually in their twenties and have severe disease associated with a heavy egg burden.[136]

Diagnosis

The diagnosis is best established by microscopic detection of ova in filtered urine.[106] The peak excretion of *S. haematobium* ova occurs between 10 a.m. and 2 p.m. and is increased by physical exercise and fluid intake.[137] The ova of *S. haematobium* have a spike at one end (terminal spike) whereas those of *S. mansoni* have a lateral spike. In the chronic inactive phase no ova are excreted, even in patients with severe complications.

Peripheral blood count may show eosinophilia. Serology does not distinguish between active and inactive disease.[107] A plain abdominal X-ray may show linear calcification of the bladder wall, distal ureters, seminal vesicles, and prostate. The ureter is usually dilated and calcification of its wall may cause a 'tram line' appearance.[105] Calcification of the bladder wall usually has an ovoid shape. If the calcification is not complete (circumferential) it should raise suspicion of bladder cancer (Kisner's sign) (Fig. 1.6.3).[138] Contrast imaging with IVU or CT-urogram in the early stage may show striations in the ureter and renal pelvis or filling defects in the bladder or ureter due to polypoid lesions or blood clots.[139] In the later stages, it may show hydroureteronephrosis due to aperistalsis or stenosis of the ureter, non-functioning of the kidney, or a post-void residual if there is bladder neck stenosis. Ureteritis cystica and pyelitis cystica are characterized by air bubble-like filling defects representing ova deposited in the urothelium.[105] In patients with bladder cancer, CT may show a bladder mass with interruption of the calcification where the tumour infiltrates the bladder wall (Fig. 1.6.3). Ultrasonography may show upper tract dilatation, thickening of the bladder wall, and polypoid lesions in the bladder lumen.[140] Radioisotope diuretic renography can be used to determine whether there is obstruction of dilated upper urinary tracts, provided renal function is adequate.[114,141]

Cystoscopy is required to exclude bladder cancer in older patients with haematuria and no ova on urine microscopy.[142] In the acute phase there is hyperaemia and haemorrhage of the bladder wall due to active granuloma formation and there may be bladder ulcers

(A)

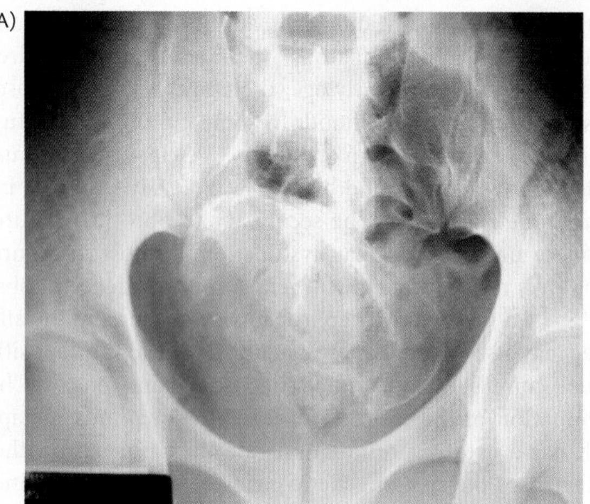

(B)

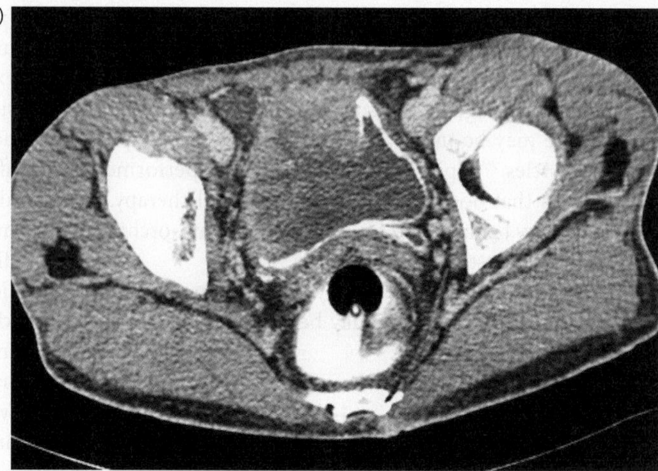

Fig. 1.6.3 (A) Plain abdominal X-ray and (B) CT showing calcification of the bladder wall, which is incomplete on the right side due to an infiltrating squamous cell carcinoma.

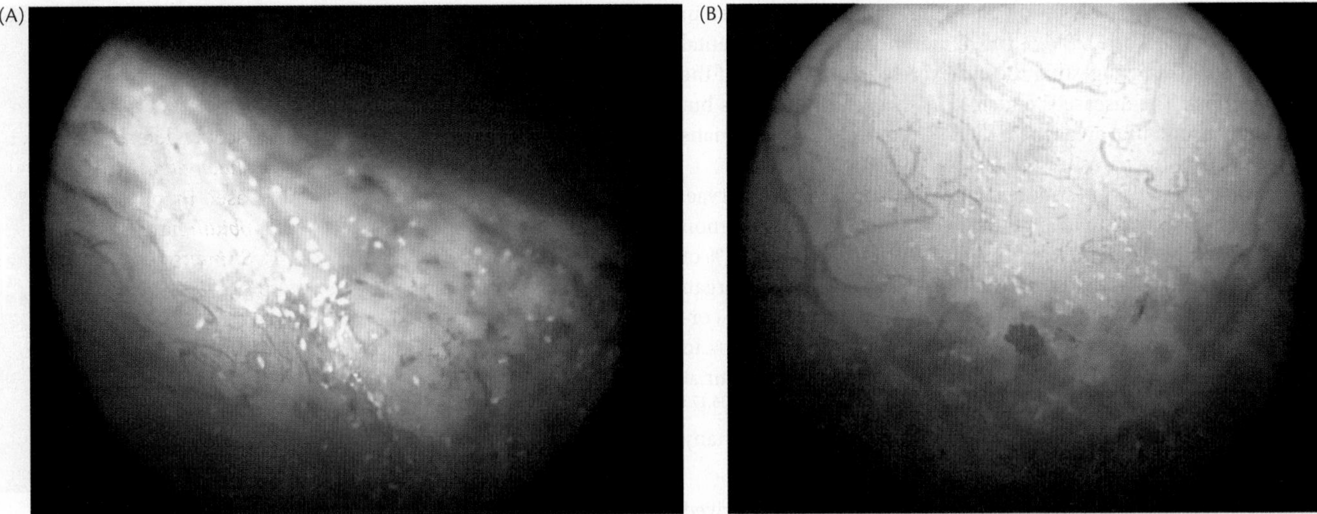

Fig. 1.6.4 Cystoscopic appearance of 'silver sand' (A) and erythematous patches (B) caused by *Schistosoma haematobium* infestation.

due to sloughing of necrotic polyps. The chronic inactive phase is characterized by patches of 'silver sand' appearance on the urothelium due to calcified ova (Fig. 1.6.4).[106] The ureteric orifices may appear dilated ('golf-hole') or stenotic. Bladder ulcers may occur in the chronic inactive stage and may bleed profusely despite fibrosis and ischaemia of the bladder wall. If there is any suspicion of malignancy, transurethral resection or biopsy should be performed.[125]

Treatment

Preventive measures in endemic areas include:

- Education of people to avoid contact with potentially contaminated fresh water;
- Prohibition of water source contamination by human urine or faeces;
- Provision of sanitation and clean water;
- Destruction or biological control of the snail host;
- Repeated antischistosomal drug treatment of susceptible populations (especially children).[113,143–146]

All patients diagnosed with schistosomiasis should receive medical treatment, whether the disease is clinically considered active or inactive. Praziquantel 40 mg/kg as a single oral dose, or two oral doses of 20 mg/kg, should be taken with food. The drug appears to target the schistosome ion channels.[147] It provides cure rates of 73–100% for *S. haematobium*.[110] The success rate is dose-related, increasing from 52% at 40 mg/kg to 91% at 100 mg/kg praziquantel in two divided doses.[148]

Side effects are rare and minor, consisting of gastrointestinal complaints, headache, dizzines, and fever. Urine microscopy should be performed one month after treatment to assess efficacy and patients with viable ova in the urine should be retreated.[106] Repeated treatment during childhood may prevent the development of urinary tract disease in adulthood.[149] A meta-analysis has shown that praziquantel combined with artemisinin derivatives (artemether or artesunate) provides a higher cure rate than praziquantel alone.[148]

Ureteric obstruction in active disease is usually caused by polypoid bladder lesions encircling the intramural ureter and this responds well to medical treatment.[134,136] Recovery of impaired renal function may occur within two months after antischistosomal chemotherapy.[150] Surgery should only be considered after effective medical treatment (i.e. when urine microscopy shows the absence of viable ova). Upper urinary tract obstruction due to a proven ureteric stricture can be managed with luminal dilatation but there is a high recurrence rate.[151–153] Ureteric meatal stenosis can be treated with meatoplasty or transurethral incision of the stenosis. Distal ureteric stricture can be managed with reimplatation, although this may be difficult if the bladder wall is thick and fibrotic.[106,117,154] A long or multisegmental ureteric stricture may require construction of a Boari bladder flap, ileal interposition, or replacement of the ureter by an ileal tube (Yang-Monti procedure).[96,117,155,156] When all surgical options have failed, long-term stenting or nephrostomy drainage may be necessary. Nephrectomy may be indicated if there is recurrent pyelonephritis or stone formation in an obstructed kidney with poor differential function.[157]

Transurethral resection or fulguration of chronic deep bladder ulcers rarely provides symptomatic relief or healing of the ulcer, so partial cystectomy may be indicated. Severely decreased bladder capacity in chronic inactive disease may be managed with hydrodistension, ileocystoplasty, or urinary diversion. Transurethral incision of the bladder neck or resection of the prostate may be considered if there is evidence of functional bladder outlet obstruction.[158] SCC associated with schistosomiasis is best treated with radical cystectomy.[159–161]

Echinococcosis (hydatid disease)

Pathogenesis

Hydatid disease is the larval form of a cestode (tapeworm) of the species *Echinococcus granulosis* or *multilocularis*.[106,162,163] The parasite resides in the intestine of the definitive host, the dog (fox, wolf, or other feral carnivores in some areas). Its ova, excreted in the faeces, contaminate grass or soil and are then ingested by the intermediate host, the sheep or goat (pig, camel, or reindeer in some parts of the world).[164,165] The human becomes an accidental intermediate host by ingesting the ova excreted in the faeces of the definitive host. The disease is endemic in sheep-farming areas but may occur in any rural area where there is contact between humans and the hosts of the parasite.[166,167]

The ova hatch in the intestine and enter the bloodstream as larvae. They are filtered in the liver and lung, which are the most common sites of organ involvement, with the kidney affected in only 2–4% of cases.[168–171] Renal hydatidosis is usually associated with other organ involvement. Renal hydatid cysts are usually single, arise in the cortex, enlarge by one or two centimetres per year and may grow to over 20 cm in diameter.[106,172,173] Rarely, hydatid cysts may occur at other sites (e.g. retrovesical or in the prostate, testis, or ovary).[106,173]

Hydatid cysts develop by slow concentric growth over many years and have three layers:

- Pericyst: outer layer of inflammatory cells and fibroblasts derived from the host tissues, which may calcify;
- Ectocyst: intermediate, non-nucleated layer made up of delicate hyalinized laminations;
- Endocyst: inner germinal layer which gives rise to fluid-filled brood capsules containing large numbers of larvae (scoleces).[166,174–176]

The brood capsules are initially attached by a pedicle to the germinal membrane, but when they detach and move freely in the fluid they are called daughter cysts. Hydatid sand consists of free larvae and daughter cysts.[177,178]

Clinical presentation and diagnosis

Most patients are asymptomatic.[105] Space occupying effects may cause chronic flank or lower back pain.[172,179,180] Microscopic haematuria may occur. Rarely, the cyst may rupture into the collecting system, causing severe colic and passage of debris resembling grape skins in the urine; hydatiduria.[166,172,181]

Eosinophilia may occur in about half of the cases. The Casoni skin test, complement fixation, and other serologic tests are unreliable, but when combined are positive in about 90% of cases.[180,182] There may be a palpable flank or pelvic mass. Plain X-ray may show linear calcification of the cyst wall.[106,181] IVP/CT-urogram may show calyceal distortion or calyectasis due to a cystic mass lesion. If the cyst has ruptured into the collecting system, there may be filling defects (daughter cysts) in the renal pelvis.[176,183] Ultrasound typically shows a multicystic or multiloculated mass, but the appearance may be that of a simple cyst.[184] Changing the position of the patient may show moving echoes ('falling snowflakes') inside the cyst corresponding to hydatid sand.[183,185] CT shows a round, multiloculated cystic mass with a well-defined, enhancing membrane, containing discrete round daughter cysts with a typical peripheral location giving the so-called 'rosette' appearance. CT may also demonstrate ring-like calcification in the cyst wall and involvement of other organs (Fig. 1.6.5).[106,176,183,186–188]

The cyst fluid is highly antigenic and diagnostic aspiration or rupture of the cyst may cause systemic anaphylaxis. Microscopy of the cyst fluid for brood capsules or protoscoleces may be false negative unless the pathologist is alerted to the possible diagnosis of hydatid disease.[189] Serological tests are available, but lack standardization.[190] During surgery, spilling of the cyst content into the peritoneum or bloodstream may lead to metastatic infection.

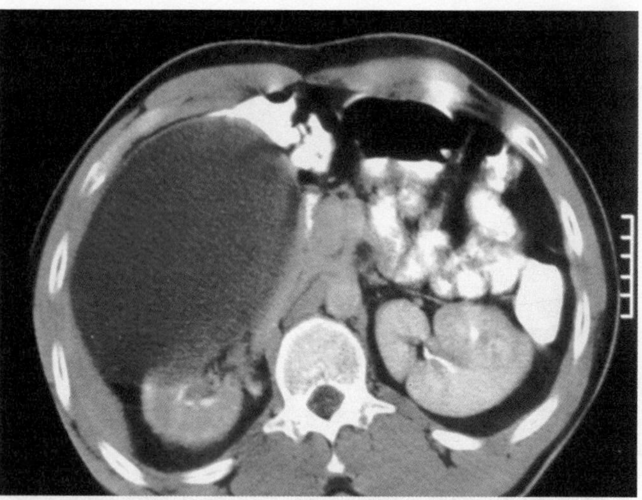

Fig. 1.6.5 Computed tomogram showing hydatid cyst of the right kidney.

Treatment

The primary medical treatment is albendazole 10 mg/kg/day (usually 400 mg twice daily) or mebendazole (40–50 mg/kg given over three days) continued for at least two years.[163] The response rate is 50–60% in cysts <6 cm and 25–50% in cysts >6 cm in diameter, with 40% of cysts still active two years after treatment.[106,190–192] Combining one of these drugs with praziquantel is more effective than either agent alone.[193]

Therapeutic puncture, aspiration, injection and reaspiration (PAIR) is performed under ultrasound guidance with injection of a scolicidal agent (20% sodium chloride, 95% alcohol, 0.5% silver nitrate, 2% formalin or 1% iodine) and reaspiration after 15–20 minutes.[187,190,194] Surgical excision of the cyst may be indicated for pain or obstruction of the collecting system.[195,196] Albendazole should be given for 14–20 days preoperatively and continued for 3–24 months to prevent seeding by daughter cysts.[193] An open or laparoscopic retroperitoneal approach can be used.[197] Renal-sparing surgery (cystectomy plus pericystectomy) is possible in most cases and nephrectomy should be reserved for destroyed kidneys complicated by infection or if malignancy is supected.[170,198,199] If the wall is calcified the larvae are usually dead and surgery is not necessary, unless the cyst is causing symptoms or complications.[106,176]

Filariasis

Pathogenesis

Lymphatic filariasis is caused by nematodes (roundworms) of the species *Wuchereria bancrofti, Brugia malayi*, or *Brugia timori*. The parasite is transmitted by mosquitoes in tropical and subtropical regions.[106,200] Microfilariae in the blood ingested by female mosquitoes become larvae which reside in the salivary glands of the insect and are injected into the skin when the mosquito feeds. In humans, the adult filariae migrate to and inhabit the larger lymph vessels. The infestation elicits both humoral and cellular immune responses. Antifilarial IgE titres rise and eosinophil-mediated killing of microfilariae occurs. Histologically, there are massive granulomas around necrotic filariae.[106,200]

Recent studies have indicated that endosymbiotic bacteria of the species *Wolbachia*, rather than the worm itself, may be the cause of this inflammation-mediated filarial disease.[201–204] Repeated episodes of inflammation over many years lead to scar tissue with obliteration of the lymphatics and the formation of collateral channels which become progressively obstructed, leading to lymphatic dilatation.[204–207] The disease causes acute lymphadenitis, which progresses to chronic lymphadenopathy, lymphatic dilation with hydrocele, oedema of the scrotum and lower limbs (elephantiasis), and chyluria.[208,209]

Clinical presentation and diagnosis

The worms may cause inflammation of the spermatic cord and epididymis (funiculoepididymitis) and even of the testis (orchitis). There may be episodes of pain in the scrotum, simulating torsion or ureteric colic.[210] Cord-like swelling or nodular induration of the spermatic cord or testis may occur, simulating testicular tumour or torsion.[211] The diagnosis can be confirmed by FNAC.[212]

Lymphadenitis with suppuration and abscess formation may occur—the exudate is bacteriologically sterile but may become infected in genital cases.[203,213] Mild scrotal oedema is common during early infection, but penile oedema is rare. Lymph scrotum consists of superficial scrotal lymphangiomatosis which may ooze chyle through the scrotal skin.[31,214] Lymphatic obstruction leads to progressive scrotal oedema and hydrocoele, which can become very large (Fig. 1.6.6).[202,215] The hydrocele fluid may be milky and the tunica vaginalis may be thick and fibrous with cholesterol or calcium deposits. Infestation of the femoral lymphatics leads to massive lymphoedema of the lower limbs resembling the legs of an elephant ('elephantiasis'). Chyluria (lymph in the urine) is caused by obstruction of the renal lymphatics, leading to the rupture of lymph varices into the pyelocalyceal system. It usually occurs in young adults and may lead to severe protein loss, hypoalbuminemia, and generalized oedema.

A blood smear may show eosinophilia. Blood samples to detect microfilariae must be taken when peak microfilaraemia occurs (midnight in the case of *W. bancrofti*). Laboratory tests include immunoassays to detect antifilarial antigens and PCR to detect parasite DNA.[216,217] Plain X-rays may show calcified worms. Ultrasound may show movement of adult filariae in the lymph vessels ('filarial dance sign').[218,219] Lymphangiography is rarely indicated to differentiate the cause of lymphoedema. Histology is pathognomonic when adult worms are observed, but is often false negative.

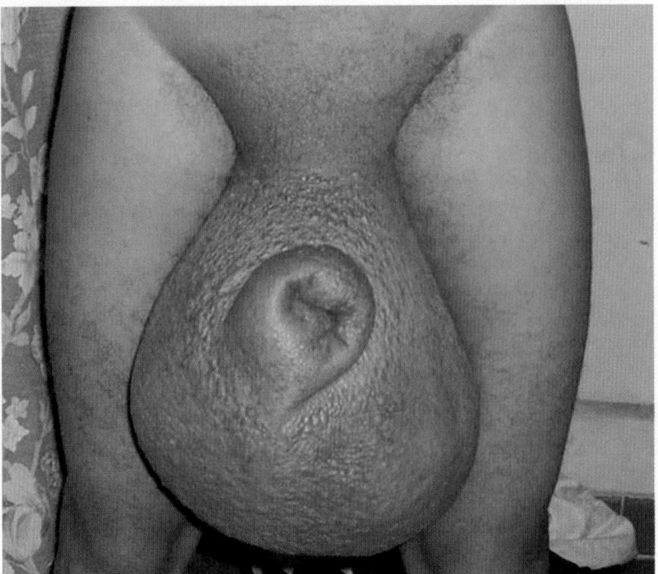

Fig. 1.6.6 Massive hydrocele and genital lymphoedema caused by *Wuchereria bancrofti* infestation.

Treatment

Four drugs can be used alone or in various combinations:[202,220–227]

- Diethylcarbamazine (DEC): effective against adult worms;
- Ivermectin: effective against microfilariae;
- Albendazole: kills both adult worms and microfilariae;
- Doxycycline: kills filariae by eradicating the symbiotic *Wolbachia* bacteria.

Severe immune reactions to the release of antigens by dying filariae can be ameliorated by premedication with steroids or antihistamines.

Filariasis control programmes focus on the prevention of mosquito bites and reduction in mosquito numbers and their breeding sites. Mass prophylactic treatment programmes using DEC or ivermectin and treatment of individual patients to reduce transmission are also carried out.[226,228,229] Hydrocelectomy is indicated for large or symptomatic hydrocoeles, especially those with buried penis.[230,231] Complete excision of the hydrocoele sac and ligation or excision of dilated lymph vessels are recommended.[232] Massive hydrocoele can be treated with excision of redundant tissue and reconstruction of the scrotum using split-thickness skin grafting.[233,234]

The management of chyluria includes:

- Bed rest, which may lead to spontaneous remission;
- Low fat diet supplemented with medium-chain triglycerides;
- Treatment with diethylcarbamazine;
- Diagnostic lymphangiography may sclerose lymphatic fistulas in about 50% of cases[235–237];
- Retrograde ureteropyelography with instillation of a sclerosing agent (0.5% silver nitrate or 5% povidone iodine), repeated if necessary, is successful in 60–70% of cases[238–240];
- Nephrolysis: complete mobilization of the kidney with skeletonization of the renal vessels and ureter and ligation of all lymphatic channels—open or laparoscopic, trans- or retroperitoneal, with omental wrap around the hilum.[106,235,236,239,241]

Further reading

Abbara A, Davidson RN. Medscape. Etiology and management of genitourinary tuberculosis. *Nat Rev Urol* 2011; **8**(12):678–88.

Brunetti E, Junghanss T. Update on cystic hydatid disease. *Curr Opin Infect Dis* 2009; **22**(5):497–502.

Brunetti E, White AC Jr. Cestode infestations: hydatid disease and cysticercosis. *Infect Dis Clin North Am* 2012; **26**(2):421–35.

Burke ML, Jones MK, Gobert GN, Li YS, Ellis MK, McManus DP. Immunopathogenesis of human schistosomiasis. *Parasite Immunol* 2009; **31**(4):163–76.

Burrill J, Williams CJ, Bain G, Conder G, Hine AL, Misra RR. Tuberculosis: a radiologic review. *Radiographics* 2007; **27**(5):1255–73.

Carl P, Stark L. Indications for surgical management of genitourinary tuberculosis. *World J Surg* 1997; **21**(5):505–10.

Ernst JD. The immunological life cycle of tuberculosis. *Nat Rev Immunol* 2012; 13; **12**(8):581–91.

Figueiredo AA, Lucon AM, Junior RF, Srougi M. Epidemiology of urogenital tuberculosis worldwide. *Int J Urol* 2008; **15**(9):827–32.

Kehinde EO, Anim JT, Hira PR. Parasites of urological importance. *Urol Int* 2008; **81**(1):1–13.

Khalaf I, Shokeir A, Shalaby M. Urologic complications of genitourinary schistosomiasis. *World J Urol* 2012; **30**(1):31–8.

Knopp S, Steinmann P, Hatz C, Keiser J, Utzinger J. Nematode infections: filariases. *Infect Dis Clin North Am* 2012; **26**(2):359–81.

Matos MJ, Bacelar MT, Pinto P, Ramos I. Genitourinary tuberculosis. *Eur J Radiol* 2005; **55**(2):181–7.

McManus DP, Gray DJ, Zhang W, Yang Y. Diagnosis, treatment, and management of echinococcosis. *BMJ* 2012; **344**:e3866.

Norões J, Dreyer G. A mechanism for chronic filarial hydrocele with implications for its surgical repair. *PLoS Negl Trop Dis* 2010; **4**(6):e695.

Pfarr KM, Debrah AY, Specht S, Hoerauf A. Filariasis and lymphoedema. *Parasite Immunol* 2009; **31**(11):664–72.

Ross AG, Bartley PB, Sleigh AC, *et al.* Schistosomiasis. *N Engl J Med* 2002; **346**(16):1212–20.

Shebel HM, Elsayes KM, Abou El Atta HM, Elguindy YM, El-Diasty TA. Genitourinary schistosomiasis: life cycle and radiologic-pathologic findings. *Radiographics* 2012; **32**(4):1031–46.

Wise GJ, Marella VK. Genitourinary manifestations of tuberculosis. *Urol Clin North Am* 2003 Feb; **30**(1):111–21.

References

1. Ernst JD. The immunological life cycle of tuberculosis. *Nat Rev Immunol* 2012 **13**; **12**(8):581–91.
2. Kaufmann SH. Protection against tuberculosis: cytokines, T cells, and macrophages. *Ann Rheum Dis* 2002; **61**(Suppl 2):ii54–8.
3. Ströck V, Dotevall L, Sandberg T, Gustafsson CK, Holmäng S. Late bacille Calmette-Guérin infection with a large focal urinary bladder ulceration as a complication of bladder cancer treatment. *BJU Int* 2011; **107**(10):1592–7.
4. Burrill J, Williams CJ, Bain G, Conder G, Hine AL, Misra RR. Tuberculosis: a radiologic review. *Radiographics* 2007; **27**(5):1255–73.
5. Silva Miranda M, Breiman A, Allain S, Deknuydt F, Altare F. The tuberculous granuloma: an unsuccessful host defence mechanism providing a safety shelter for the bacteria? *Clin Dev Immunol* 2012; **2012**:139127.
6. Lowe DM, Redford PS, Wilkinson RJ, O'Garra A, Martineau AR. Neutrophils in tuberculosis: friend or foe? *Trends Immunol* 2012; **33**(1):14–25.
7. Russell DG. Mycobacterium tuberculosis and the intimate discourse of a chronic infection. *Immunol Rev* 2011; **240**(1):252–68. doi: 10.1111/j.1600–065X.2010.00984.x.
8. Gupta A, Kaul A, Tsolaki AG, Kishore U, Bhakta S. Mycobacterium tuberculosis: immune evasion, latency and reactivation. *Immunobiology* 2012; **217**(3):363–74.
9. Pawlowski A, Jansson M, Sköld M, Rottenberg ME, Källenius G. Tuberculosis and HIV co-infection. *PLoS Pathog* 2012 Feb; **8**(2):e1002464.
10. Banerjee D, Bhattacharyya R, Kaul D, Sharma P. Diabetes and tuberculosis: analysis of a paradox. *Adv Clin Chem* 2011; **53**:139–53.
11. Yoshikai Y. Immunological protection against mycobacterium tuberculosis infection. *Crit Rev Immunol* 2006; **26**(6):515–26.
12. el-Agroudy AE, Refaie AF, Moussa OM, Ghoneim MA. Tuberculosis in Egyptian kidney transplant recipients: study of clinical course and outcome. *J Nephrol* 2003; **16**(3):404–11.
13. Hussein MM, Mooij JM, Roujouleh H. Tuberculosis and chronic renal disease. *Semin Dial* 2003; **16**(1):38–44.
14. Eastwood JB, Corbishley CM, Grange JM. Tuberculosis and the kidney. *J Am Soc Nephrol* 2001; **12**(6):1307–14.
15. Figueiredo AA, Lucon AM, Junior RF, Srougi M. Epidemiology of urogenital tuberculosis worldwide. *Int J Urol* 2008; **15**(9):827–32.
16. Abbara A, Davidson RN; Medscape. Etiology and management of genitourinary tuberculosis. *Nat Rev Urol* 2011; **8**(12):678–88.
17. De Backer AI, Mortelé KJ, De Keulenaer BL, Parizel PM. Tuberculosis: epidemiology, manifestations, and the value of medical imaging in diagnosis. *JBR-BTR* 2006; **89**(5):243–50.
18. Gibson MS, Puckett ML, Shelly ME. Renal tuberculosis. *Radiographics* 2004; **24**(1):251–6
19. Shin KY, Park HJ, Lee JJ, Park HY, Woo YN, Lee TY. Role of early endourologic management of tuberculous ureteral strictures. *J Endourol* 2002; **16**(10):755–8.
20. Madeb R, Marshall J, Nativ O, Erturk E. Epididymal tuberculosis: case report and review of the literature. *Urology* 2005; **65**(4):798.
21. Gupta N, Mandal AK, Singh SK. Tuberculosis of the prostate and urethra: A review. *Indian J Urol* 2008; **24**(3):388–91.
22. Lee Y, Huang W, Huang J, Wang J, Yu C, Jiaan B, Huang J. Efficacy of chemotherapy for prostatic tuberculosis-a clinical and histologic follow-up study. *Urology* 2001; **57**(5):872–7.
23. Angus BJ, Yates M, Conlon C, Byren I. Cutaneous tuberculosis of the penis and sexual transmission of tuberculosis confirmed by molecular typing. *Clin Infect Dis* 2001; **33**(11):E132–4.
24. Toledo-Pastrana T, Ferrándiz L, Pichardo AR, Muniaín Ezcurra MA, Camacho Martínez FM. Tuberculosis: an unusual cause of genital ulcer. *Sex Transm Dis* 2012; **39**(8):643–4.
25. Papaevangelou V, Vintila A, Papaparaskevas J, *et al.* Infant penile tuberculosis following circumcision. *J Infect* 2009; **58**(1):83–5.
26. Allen FJ, de Kock ML. Genito-urinary tuberculosis--experience with 52 urology inpatients. *S Afr Med J* 1993; **83**(12):903–7.
27. Wise GJ, Shteynshlyuger A. An update on lower urinary tract tuberculosis. *Curr Urol Rep* 2008; **9**(4):305–13.
28. Lenk S, Schroeder J. Genitourinary tuberculosis. *Curr Opin Urol* 2001; **11**(1):93–8.
29. Wise GJ, Marella VK. Genitourinary manifestations of tuberculosis. *Urol Clin North Am* 2003 Feb; **30**(1):111–21.
30. Gómez García I, Gómez Mampaso E, Burgos Revilla J, *et al.* Tuberculous orchiepididymitis during 1978–2003 period: review of 34 cases and role of 16S rRNA amplification. *Urology* 2010; **76**(4):776–81.
31. Richens J. Genital manifestations of tropical diseases. *Sex Transm Infect* 2004; **80**(1):12–7.
32. Kulchavenya E, Kim CS, Bulanova O, Zhukova I. Male genital tuberculosis: epidemiology and diagnostic. *World J Urol* 2012; **30**(1):15–21.
33. Kumar S, Kekre NS, Gopalakrishnan G. Diagnosis and conservative treatment of tubercular rectoprostatic fistula. *Ann R Coll Surg Engl* 2006; **88**(1):26.
34. Golden MP, Vikram HR. Extrapulmonary tuberculosis: an overview. *Am Fam Physician* 2005; **72**(9):1761–8.
35. Aliyu MH, Aliyu SH, Salihu HM. Female genital tuberculosis: a global review. *Int J Fertil Womens Med* 2004; **49**(3):123–36.
36. Paick J, Kim SH, Kim SW. Ejaculatory duct obstruction in infertile men. *BJU Int* 2000; **85**(6):720–4.
37. Sharma VK, Sethy PK, Dogra PN, Singh U, Das P. Primary tuberculosis of glans penis after intravesical Bacillus Calmette Guerin immunotherapy. *Indian J Dermatol Venereol Leprol* 2011; **77**(1):47–50.
38. Baveja CP, Vidyanidhi G, Jain M, Kumari T, Sharma VK. Drug-resistant genital tuberculosis of the penis in a human immunodeficiency virus non-reactive individual. *J Med Microbiol* 2007; **56**(Pt 5):694–5.
39. Anoop UC, Pavithran K. Genital tuberculosis. *Indian J Dermatol Venereol Leprol* 2002; **68**(3):164–5.
40. Singh O, Gupta SS, Arvind NK. A case of extensive genitourinary tuberculosis: combined augmentation ileo-cystoplasty, ureteric ileal replacement and buccal mucosal graft urethroplasty. *Updates Surg* 2012 Mar 11 [Epub ahead of print].
41. Patterson IY, Robertus LM, Gwynne RA, Gardiner RA. Genitourinary tuberculosis in Australia and New Zealand. *BJU Int* 2012; **109**(Suppl 3): 27–30.

42. Miano R, Germani S, Vespasiani G. Stones and urinary tract infections. *Urol Int* 2007; **79**(Suppl 1):32–6.
43. Rahman NU, Meng MV, Stoller ML. Infections and urinary stone disease. *Curr Pharm Des* 2003; **9**(12):975–81.
44. Sorlozano A, Soria I, Roman J, Huertas P, Soto MJ, Piedrola G, Gutierrez J. Comparative evaluation of three culture methods for the isolation of mycobacteria from clinical samples. *J Microbiol Biotechnol* 2009; **19**(10):1259–64.
45. Scarparo C, Piccoli P, Rigon A, Ruggiero G, Ricordi P, Piersimoni C. Evaluation of the BACTEC MGIT 960 in comparison with BACTEC 460 TB for detection and recovery of mycobacteria from clinical specimens. *Diagn Microbiol Infect Dis* 2002; **44**(2):157–61.
46. Watterson SA, Drobniewski FA. Modern laboratory diagnosis of mycobacterial infections. *J Clin Pathol* 2000; **53**(10):727–32.
47. Bonkat G, Bachmann A, Solokhina A, *et al.* Growth of mycobacteria in urine determined by isothermal microcalorimetry: Implications for urogenital tuberculosis and other mycobacterial infections. *Urology* 2012 Jul 9 [Epub ahead of print].
48. Barnard M, Albert H, Coetzee G, O'Brien R, Bosman ME. Rapid molecular screening for multidrug-resistant tuberculosis in a high-volume public health laboratory in South Africa. *Am J Respir Crit Care Med* 2008; **177**(7):787–92.
49. Piersimoni C, Scarparo C, Piccoli P, *et al.* Performance assessment of two commercial amplification assays for direct detection of Mycobacterium tuberculosis complex from respiratory and extrapulmonary specimens. *J Clin Microbiol* 2002; **40**(11):4138–42.
50. Hemal AK, Gupta NP, Rajeev TP, Kumar R, Dar L, Seth P. Polymerase chain reaction in clinically suspected genitourinary tuberculosis: comparison with intravenous urography, bladder biopsy, and urine acid fast bacilli culture. *Urology* 2000; **56**(4):570–4.
51. Moussa OM, Eraky I, El-Far MA, Osman HG, Ghoneim MA. Rapid diagnosis of genitourinary tuberculosis by polymerase chain reaction and non-radioactive DNA hybridization. *J Urol* 2000; **164**(2):584–8.
52. van Vollenhoven P, Heyns CF, de Beer PM, Whitaker P, van Helden PD, Victor T. Polymerase chain reaction in the diagnosis of urinary tract tuberculosis. *Urol Res* 1996; **24**(2):107–11.
53. Bilen CY, Inci K, Erkan I, Ozen H. The predictive value of purified protein derivative results on complications and prognosis in patients with bladder cancer treated with bacillus Calmette-Guerin. *J Urol* 2003; **169**(5):1702–5.
54. Muttarak M, ChiangMai WN, Lojanapiwat B. Tuberculosis of the genitourinary tract: imaging features with pathological correlation. *Singapore Med J* 2005; **46**(10):568–74; quiz 575.
55. Chijioke A. Current views on epidemiology of renal tuberculosis. *West Afr J Med* 2001; **20**(4):217–9.
56 Matos MJ, Bacelar MT, Pinto P, Ramos I. Genitourinary tuberculosis. *Eur J Radiol* 2005; **55**(2):181–7.
57. Wang LJ, Wu CF, Wong YC, Chuang CK, Chu SH, Chen CJ. Imaging findings of urinary tuberculosis on excretory urography and computerized tomography. *J Urol* 2003; **169**(2):524–8.
58. Engin G, Acunaş B, Acunaş G, Tunaci M. Imaging of extrapulmonary tuberculosis. *Radiographics* 2000; **20**(2):471–88; quiz 529–30, 532.
59. Vijayaraghavan SB, Kandasamy SV, Arul M, Prabhakar M, Dhinakaran CL, Palanisamy R. Spectrum of high-resolution sonographic features of urinary tuberculosis. *J Ultrasound Med* 2004; **23**(5):585–94.
60 Bour L, Schull A, Delongchamps NB, *et al.* Multiparametric MRI features of granulomatous prostatitis and tubercular prostate abscess. *Diagn Interv Imaging* 2012; **15**:pii: S2211-5684(12)00301-4 [Epub ahead of print].
61 Premkumar A, Lattimer J, Newhouse JH. CT and sonography of advanced urinary tract tuberculosis. *AJR Am J Roentgenol* 1987; **148**(1):65–9.
62. Gupta NP, Kumar A, Sharma S. Reconstructive bladder surgery in genitourinary tuberculosis. *Indian J Urol* 2008; **24**(3):382–7.
63. Hemal AK, Aron M. Orthotopic neobladder in management of tubercular thimble bladders: initial experience and long-term results. *Urology* 1999 Feb; **53**(2):298–301.
64. Colbert G, Richey D, Schwartz JC. Widespread tuberculosis including renal involvement. *Proc (Bayl Univ Med Cent)* 2012; **25**(3):236–9.
65. Goel A, Dalela D. Options in the management of tuberculous ureteric stricture. *Indian J Urol* 2008; **24**(3):376–81.
66. Ramanathan R, Kumar A, Kapoor R, Bhandari M. Relief of urinary tract obstruction in tuberculosis to improve renal function. Analysis of predictive factors. *Br J Urol* 1998 Feb; **81**(2):199–205.
67. Chandra S, Chandra H, Chauhan N, *et al.* Male genitourinary tuberculosis—13 years experience at a tertiary care center in India. *Southeast Asian J Trop Med Public Health* 2012; **43**(2):364–9.
68. Salem B. Disseminated tuberculosis following the placement of ureteral stents: a case report. *Cases J* 2008; **1**(1):383.
69. Babanoury AB, Boggs LK. Miliary tuberculosis following retrograde pyelogram. *J Urol* 1966; **96**(1):101–2.
70. Sah SP, Bhadani PP, Regmi R, Tewari A, Raj GA. Fine needle aspiration cytology of tubercular epididymitis and epididymo-orchitis. *Acta Cytol* 2006; **50**(3):243–9.
71. Sun L, Yuan Q, Feng JM, *et al.* Rapid diagnosis in early stage renal tuberculosis by real-time polymerase chain reaction on renal biopsy specimens. *Int J Tuberc Lung Dis* 2010; **14**(3):341–6.
72. Heyns CF, Groeneveld AE, Sigarroa NB. Urologic complications of HIV and AIDS. *Nat Clin Pract Urol* 2009; **6**(1):32–43.
73. Heyns CF, Fisher M. The urological management of the patient with acquired immunodeficiency syndrome. *BJU Int* 2005; **95**(5):709–16.
74. Zarrabi AD, Heyns CF. Clinical features of confirmed versus suspected urogenital tuberculosis in region with extremely high prevalence of pulmonary tuberculosis. *Urology* 2009; **74**(1):41–5.
75. Small PM, Fujiwara PI. Management of tuberculosis in the United States. *N Engl J Med* 2001; **345**(3):189–200.
76. Gow JG, Barbosa S. Genitourinary tuberculosis. A study of 1117 cases over a period of 34 years. *Br J Urol* 1984; **56**(5):449–55.
77. Sia IG, Wieland ML. Current concepts in the management of tuberculosis. *Mayo Clin Proc* 2011; **86**(4):348–61.
78. Nettles RE, Mazo D, Alwood K, *et al.* Risk factors for relapse and acquired rifamycin resistance after directly observed tuberculosis treatment: a comparison by HIV serostatus and rifamycin use. *Clin Infect Dis* 2004; **38**(5):731–6.
79. Khaira A, Bagchi S, Sharma A, *et al.* Renal allograft tuberculosis: report of three cases and review of literature. *Clin Exp Nephrol* 2009; **13**(4):392–6.
80. Johnston JC, Shahidi NC, Sadatsafavi M, Fitzgerald JM. Treatment outcomes of multidrug-resistant tuberculosis: a systematic review and meta-analysis. *PLoS One* 2009; **4**(9):e6914.
81. Carl P, Stark L. Indications for surgical management of genitourinary tuberculosis. *World J Surg* 1997; **21**(5):505–10.
82. Gupta NP, Kumar R, Mundada OP, *et al.* Reconstructive surgery for the management of genitourinary tuberculosis: a single center experience. *J Urol* 2006; **175**(6):2150–4; discussion 2154.
83. Wong SH, Lau WY, Poon GP, *et al.* The treatment of urinary tuberculosis. *J Urol* 1984; **131**(2):297–301.
84. Hemal AK, Gupta NP, Kumar R. Comparison of retroperitoneoscopic nephrectomy with open surgery for tuberculous nonfunctioning kidneys. *J Urol* 2000 Jul; **164**(1):32–5.
85. Flechner SM, Gow JG. Role of nephrectomy in the treatment of non-functioning or very poorly functioning unilateral tuberculous kidney. *J Urol* 1980; **123**(6):822–5.
86. Sinha M, Chacko KN, Kekre NS, Gopalakrishnan G. Tubercular ureteric strictures. *J Pak Med Assoc* 2005; **55**(10):414–6.
87. Hwang TK, Seo SI, Kim JC, Yoon JY, Park YH, Yoon MS. Long-term results of percutaneous endourologic management of renal infundibular stricture. *J Endourol* 1999; **13**(7):495–8.
88. Hwang TK, Park YH. Endocalicotomy in tuberculous renal caliceal stricture. *J Endourol* 1993; **7**(6):493–6.
89. Murphy DM, Fallon B, Lane V, O'Flynn JD. Tuberculous stricture of ureter. *Urology* 1982; **20**(4):382–4.
90. Osman T, Eltahawy I, Fawaz K, Shoeib M, Elshawaf H, El Halaby R. Ureterocalicostomy for treatment of complex cases of ureteropelvic junction obstruction in adults. *Urology* 2011; **78**(1):202–7.
91. Matlaga BR, Shah OD, Singh D, Streem SB, Assimos DG. Ureterocalicostomy: a contemporary experience. *Urology* 2005; **65**(1):42–4.

92. Sadhu S, Pandit K, Roy MK, Bajoria SK. Buccal mucosa ureteroplasty for the treatment of complex ureteric injury. *Indian J Surg* 2011; **73**(1):71–2.
93. O'Boyle PJ, Galli EM, Gow JG. The surgical management of tuberculous lower ureteric stricture. *Br J Urol* 1976; **48**(2):101–5.
94. Png JC, Chapple CR. Principles of ureteric reconstruction. *Curr Opin Urol* 2000; **10**(3):207–12.
95. Motiwala HG, Shah SA, Patel SM. Ureteric substitution with Boari bladder flap. *Br J Urol* 1990; **66**(4):369–71.
96. Ghoneim MA, Ali-El-Dein B. Replacing the ureter by an ileal tube, using the Yang-Monti procedure. *BJU Int* 2005; **95**:455–70.
97. Singh V, Sinha RJ, Sankhwar SN, Sinha SM. Reconstructive surgery for tuberculous contracted bladder: experience of a center in northern India. *Int Urol Nephrol* 2011; **43**(2):423–30.
98. Pickard R. Tumour formation within intestinal segments transposed to the urinary tract. *World J Urol* 2004; **22**(3):227–34.
99. Dewani CP, Dewani N, Bhatia D. Case report: tubercular cold abscess of seminal vesicle: minimally invasive endoscopic management. *J Endourol* 2006; **20**(6):436–42.
100. Lee JY, Park HY, Park SY, *et al.* Clinical characteristics of genitourinary tuberculosis during a recent 10-year period in one center. *Korean J Urol* 2011; **52**(3):200–5.
101. Viswaroop BS, Kekre N, Gopalakrishnan G. Isolated tuberculous epididymitis: a review of forty cases. *J Postgrad Med* 2005; **51**(2):109–11, discussion 111.
102. Paul J, Krishnamoorthy S, Teresa M, Kumar S. Isolated tuberculous orchitis: A mimicker of testicular malignancy. *Indian J Urol* 2010; **26**(2):284–6.
103. Jacob JT, Nguyen TM, Ray SM. Male genital tuberculosis. *Lancet Infect Dis* 2008; **8**(5):335–42.
104. Hsu HL, Lai CC, Yu MC, *et al.* Clinical and microbiological characteristics of urine culture-confirmed genitourinary tuberculosis at medical centers in Taiwan from 1995 to 2007. *Eur J Clin Microbiol Infect Dis* 2011; **30**(3):319–26.
105. Shebel HM, Elsayes KM, Abou El Atta HM, Elguindy YM, El-Diasty TA. Genitourinary schistosomiasis: life cycle and radiologic-pathologic findings. *Radiographics* 2012; **32**(4):1031–46.
106. Kehinde EO, Anim JT, Hira PR. Parasites of urological importance. *Urol Int* 2008; **81**(1):1–13.
107. Ross AG, Bartley PB, Sleigh AC, *et al.* Schistosomiasis. *N Engl J Med* 2002; **346**(16):1212–20.
108. Kjetland EF, Ndhlovu PD, Mduluza T, *et al.* Simple clinical manifestations of genital Schistosoma haematobium infection in rural Zimbabwean women. *Am J Trop Med Hyg* 2005; **72**(3):311–9.
109. Burke ML, Jones MK, Gobert GN, Li YS, Ellis MK, McManus DP. Immunopathogenesis of human schistosomiasis. *Parasite Immunol* 2009; **31**(4):163–76.
110. Leutscher PD, van Dam GT, Reimert CM, Ramarakoto CE, Deelder AM, Ørnbjerg N. Eosinophil cationic protein, soluble egg antigen, circulating anodic antigen, and egg excretion in male urogenital schistosomiasis. *Am J Trop Med Hyg* 2008; **79**(3):422–6.
111. Pearce EJ, MacDonald AS. The immunobiology of schistosomiasis. *Nat Rev Immunol* 2002; **2**(7):499–511.
112. Smith JH, Christie JD. The pathobiology of Schistosoma haematobium infection in humans. *Hum Pathol* 1986; **17**(4):333–45.
113. Salem S, Mitchell RE, El-Alim El-Dorey A, Smith JA, Barocas DA. Successful control of schistosomiasis and the changing epidemiology of bladder cancer in Egypt. *BJU Int* 2011; **107**(2):206–11.
114. Khalaf I, Shokeir A, Shalaby M. Urologic complications of genitourinary schistosomiasis. *World J Urol* 2012; **30**(1):31–8.
115. Bahar RH, Sabha M, Kouris K, *et al.* Chronic urinary schistosomiasis: patterns of abnormalities in radionuclide Tc-99 m DTPA diuretic renogram. *APMIS Suppl* 1988; **3**:54–8.
116. Bahar RH, Sabha M, Kouris K, *et al.* 99mTc DTPA diuretic renography in the evaluation of surgery in chronic schistosomal and non-schistosomal obstructive uropathy. *Br J Urol* 1990; **66**(2):137–43.
117. Al-Shukri S, Alwan MH. Bilharzial strictures of the lower third of the ureter: a critical review of 560 strictures. *Br J Urol* 1983; **55**(5):477–82.
118. Barsoum RS. Schistosomiasis and the kidney. *Semin Nephrol* 2003; **23**(1):34–41.
119. Abol-Enein H. Infection: is it a cause of bladder cancer? *Scand J Urol Nephrol Suppl* 2008;(218):79–84.
120. Michaud DS. Chronic inflammation and bladder cancer. *Urol Oncol* 2007; **25**(3):260–8.
121 Heyns CF, van der Merwe A. Bladder cancer in Africa. *Can J Urol* 2008; **15**(1):3899–908.
122. Bedwani R, Renganathan E, El Kwhsky F, *et al.* Schistosomiasis and the risk of bladder cancer in Alexandria, Egypt. *Br J Cancer* 1998; **77**(7):1186–9.
123. Groeneveld AE, Marszalek WW, Heyns CF. Bladder cancer in various population groups in the greater Durban area of KwaZulu-Natal, South Africa. *Br J Urol* 1996; **78**(2):205–8.
124. Al-Shukri S, Alwan MH, Nayef M, Rahman AA. Bilharziasis in malignant tumours of the urinary bladder. *Br J Urol* 1987; **59**(1):59–62.
125 Shokeir AA. Squamous cell carcinoma of the bladder: pathology, diagnosis and treatment. *BJU Int* 2004; **93**(2):216–20.
126. el-Mawla NG, el-Bolkainy MN, Khaled HM. Bladder cancer in Africa: update. *Semin Oncol* 2001; **28**(2):174–8.
127. Ross AG, Vickers D, Olds GR, Shah SM, McManus DP. Katayama syndrome. *Lancet Infect Dis* 2007; **7**(3):218–24.
128 de Jesus AR, Silva A, Santana LB, *et al.* Clinical and immunologic evaluation of 31 patients with acute schistosomiasis mansoni. *J Infect Dis* 2002; **185**(1):98–105.
129. Mohammed AZ, Edino ST, Samaila AA. Surgical pathology of schistosomiasis. *J Natl Med Assoc* 2007; **99**(5):570–4.
130. Schwartz E, Pick N, Shazberg G, Potasman I. Hematospermia due to schistosome infection in travelers: diagnostic and treatment challenges. *Clin Infect Dis* 2002; **35**(11):1420–4.
131. Corachan M, Valls ME, Gascon J, Almeda J, Vilana R. Hematospermia: a new etiology of clinical interest. *Am J Trop Med Hyg* 1994; **50**(5):580–4.
132. Abruzzi A, Fried B. Coinfection of Schistosoma (Trematoda) with bacteria, protozoa and helminths. *Adv Parasitol* 2011; **77**:1–85.
133. Barnhill AE, Novozhilova E, Day TA, Carlson SA. Schistosoma-associated Salmonella resist antibiotics via specific fimbrial attachments to the flatworm. *Parasit Vectors* 2011; **4**:123.
134. Smith JH, Kelada AS, Khalil A. Schistosomal ulceration of the urinary bladder. *Am J Trop Med Hyg* 1977; **26**(1):89–95.
135. Smith JH, Kelada AS, Khalil A, Torky AH. Surgical pathology of schistosomal obstructive uropathy: a clinicopathologic correlation. *Am J Trop Med Hyg* 1977; **26**(1):96–103.
136. Christie JD, Crouse D, Smith JH, Pineda J, Ishak EA, Kamel IA. Patterns of Schistosoma haematobium egg distribution in the human lower urinary tract. II. Obstructive uropathy. *Am J Trop Med Hyg* 1986; **35**(4):752–8.
137. Doehring E, Feldmeier H, Daffalla AA. Day-to-day variation and circadian rhythm of egg excretion in urinary schistosomiasis in the Sudan. *Ann Trop Med Parasitol* 1983; **77**(6):587–94.
138. Kisner CD. Vesical bilharziasis. Pathological changes and relationship to squamous carcinoma. *S Afr J Surg* 1973; **11**(2):79–87.
139. Hugosson C. Striation of the renal pelvis and ureter in bilharziasis. *Clin Radiol* 1987; **38**(4):407–9.
140. Medhat A, Zarzour A, Nafeh M, *et al.* Evaluation of an ultrasonographic score for urinary bladder morbidity in Schistosoma haematobium infection. *Am J Trop Med Hyg* 1997; **57**(1):16–9.
141. Ibrahim AI, Patil KP, el Tahir MI, Shetty SD, Anandan N. Bilharzial vesicoureteric reflux and bladder neck stenosis: fact or fiction? *Br J Urol* 1991; **68**(6):582–5.
142. Neal PM. Schistosomiasis–an unusual cause of ureteral obstruction: a case history and perspective. *Clin Med Res* 2004; **2**(4):216–27.
143. Fenwick A, Rollinson D, Southgate V. Implementation of human schistosomiasis control: Challenges and prospects. *Adv Parasitol* 2006; **61**:567–622.

144. Doenhoff MJ, Hagan P, Cioli D, *et al.* Praziquantel: its use in control of schistosomiasis in sub-Saharan Africa and current research needs. *Parasitology* 2009; **136**(13):1825–35.
145. Pearce EJ. Progress towards a vaccine for schistosomiasis. *Acta Trop* 2003; **86**(2–3):309–13.
146. Engels D, Chitsulo L, Montresor A, Savioli L. The global epidemiological situation of schistosomiasis and new approaches to control and research. *Acta Trop* 2002; **82**(2):139–46.
147. Doenhoff MJ, Cioli D, Utzinger J. Praziquantel: mechanisms of action, resistance and new derivatives for schistosomiasis. *Curr Opin Infect Dis* 2008; **21**(6):659–67.
148. Liu R, Dong HF, Guo Y, Zhao QP, Jiang MS. Efficacy of praziquantel and artemisinin derivatives for the treatment and prevention of human schistosomiasis: a systematic review and meta-analysis. *Parasit Vectors* 2011; **4**:201.
149. Richter J. The impact of chemotherapy on morbidity due to schistosomiasis. *Acta Trop* 2003; **86**(2–3):161–83.
150. Lehman JS Jr, Farid Z, Smith JH, Bassily S, el-Masry NA. Urinary schistosomiasis in Egypt: clinical, radiological, bacteriological and parasitological correlations. *Trans R Soc Trop Med Hyg* 1973; **67**(3):384–99.
151. El-Nahas AR, Shoma AM, El-Baz M. Bilharzial pyelitis: a rare cause of secondary ureteropelvic junction obstruction. *J Urol* 2003; **170**(5):1946–7.
152. Jacobsson B, Lindstedt E, Narasimham DL, Sundin T, Vijayan P. Balloon dilatation of bilharzial ureteric strictures. *Br J Urol* 1987; **60**(1):28–32.
153. Wishahi MM. The role of dilatation in bilharzial ureters. *Br J Urol* 1987; **59**(5):405–7.
154. Umerah BC. Bilharzial hydronephrosis: a clinicoradiological study. *J Urol* 1981; **126**(2):164–5.
155. Ghoneim MA. Bilharziasis of the genitourinary tract. *BJU Int* 2002; **89**(Suppl 1):22–30.
156. Abdel-Halim RE. Ileal loop replacement and restoration of kidney function in extensive bilharziasis of the ureter. *Br J Urol* 1980; **52**(4):280–4.
157. Ajit MK, Groenewald EA, Speakman M. An unusual presentation of genitourinary schistosomiasis in a Caucasian woman in the UK. *Ann R Coll Surg Engl* 2005; **87**(6):481.
158. Sabha M, Nilsson T. Urodynamic evaluation of calcified bilharzial bladders. *APMIS Suppl* 1988; **3**:50–3.
159. Abdelsalam YM, Mokhtar AA, Kurkar AA, Saleh MA, el-Ganainy EO. Defining patient selection for prostate-sparing cystectomy in squamous cell carcinoma of the urinary bladder associated with bilharziasis: an overview of 236 patients. *Urology* 2011; **78**(6):1351–4.
160. Abol-Enein H, Ghoneim MA. Functional results of orthotopic ileal neobladder with serous-lined extramural ureteral reimplantation: experience with 450 patients. *J Urol* 2001; **165**(5):1427–32.
161. Nabeeh A, Gomha M, Shaaban AA, *et al.* Orthotopic bladder substitutes: histopathologic risk factors. *Scand J Urol Nephrol* 1995; **29**(4):463–7.
162. Brunetti E, White AC Jr. Cestode infestations: hydatid disease and cysticercosis. *Infect Dis Clin North Am* 2012; **26**(2):421–35.
163. Brunetti E, Junghanss T. Update on cystic hydatid disease. *Curr Opin Infect Dis* 2009; **22**(5):497–502.
164. Romig T, Dinkel A, Mackenstedt U. The present situation of echinococcosis in Europe. *Parasitol Int* 2006; **55**(Suppl):S187–91.
165. Jenkins DJ, Romig T, Thompson RC. Emergence/re-emergence of Echinococcus spp.--a global update. *Int J Parasitol* 2005; **35**(11–12):1205–19.
166. Mudholkar VG, Suwarnkar SV, Deshpande SA, Kadam PN. Isolated renal hydatid disease with gross hydatiduria. *Indian J Pathol Microbiol* 2011; **54**(3):640–1.
167. Jenkins DJ. Echinococcus granulosus in Australia, widespread and doing well! *Parasitol Int* 2006; **55**(Suppl):S203–6.
168. Yilmaz Y, Kösem M, Ceylan K, *et al.* Our experience in eight cases with urinary hydatid disease: a series of 372 cases held in nine different clinics. *Int J Urol* 2006; **13**(9):1162–5.
169. Sayek I, Tirnaksiz MB, Dogan R. Cystic hydatid disease: current trends in diagnosis and management. *Surg Today* 2004; **34**(12):987–96.
170. Zmerli S, Ayed M, Horchani A, Chami I, El Ouakdi M, Ben Slama MR. Hydatid cyst of the kidney: diagnosis and treatment. *World J Surg* 2001; **25**(1):68–74.
171. Von Sinner WN, Hellström M, Kagevi I, Norlen BJ. Hydatid disease of the urinary tract. *J Urol* 1993; **149**(3):577–80.
172. Göğüş C, Safak M, Baltaci S, Türkölmez K. Isolated renal hydatidosis: experience with 20 cases. *J Urol* 2003; **169**(1):186–9.
173. Horchani A, Nouira Y, Chtourou M, Kacem M, Ben Safta Z. Retrovesical hydatid disease: a clinical study of 27 cases. *Eur Urol* 2001; **40**(6):655–60.
174. Gottstein B, Hemphill A. Echinococcus multilocularis: the parasite-host interplay. *Exp Parasitol* 2008; **119**(4):447–52.
175. Lewall DB. Hydatid disease: biology, pathology, imaging and classification. *Clin Radiol* 1998; **53**(12):863–74.
176. Migaleddu V, Conti M, Canalis GC, *et al.* Imaging of renal hydatid cysts. *AJR Am J Roentgenol* 1997; **169**(5):1339–42.
177. Arandes AS, Bertomeu FG, Artero JM. Microscopic image of the protoscolex of Echinococcus granulosus on the 'Hydatid Sand'. *Am J Trop Med Hyg* 2010; **82**(6):980.
178. Mahmoud LH, el-Garhy MF. A histochemical study on the hydatid cyst and electron microscopy of the hydatid sand of Echinococcus granulosus. *J Egypt Soc Parasitol* 2002; **32**(2):647–56, 2 p following 656.
179. Yaycioglu O, Ulusan S, Gul U, Guvel S. Isolated renal hydatid disease causing ureteropelvic junction obstruction and massive destruction of kidney parenchyma. *Urology* 2006; **67**(6):1290.e15–7.
180. Kaya K, Gokce G, Kaya S, Kilicarslan H, Ayan S, Gultekin EY. Isolated renal and retroperitoneal hydatid cysts: a report of 23 cases. *Trop Doct* 2006; **36**(4):243–6.
181. Odev K, Kilinc M, Arslan A, *et al.* Renal hydatid cysts and the evaluation of their radiologic images. *Eur Urol* 1996; **30**(1):40–9.
182. Siracusano A, Bruschi F. Cystic echinococcosis: progress and limits in epidemiology and immunodiagnosis. *Parassitologia* 2006; **48**(1–2):65–6.
183. Turgut AT, Odev K, Kabaalioglu A, Bhatt S, Dogra VS. Multitechnique evaluation of renal hydatid disease. *AJR Am J Roentgenol* 2009; **192**(2):462–7.
184. Kilciler M, Bedir S, Erdemir F, Coban H, Sahan B, Ozgok Y. Isolated unilocular renal hydatid cyst: a rare diagnostic difficulty with simple cyst. *Urol Int* 2006; **77**(4):371–4.
185. Polat P, Kantarci M, Alper F, Suma S, Koruyucu MB, Okur A. Hydatid disease from head to toe. *Radiographics* 2003; **23**(2):475–94; quiz 536–7.
186. Parashari UC, Upadhyay D, Khanduri S, Qayyum FA, Bhadury S. Primary renal hydatidosis with associated macroscopic hydatiduria—a computed tomography urography diagnosis with pathological confirmation. *Trop Doct* 2011; **41**(3):187–9.
187. Turgut AT, Akhan O, Bhatt S, Dogra VS. Sonographic spectrum of hydatid disease. *Ultrasound Q* 2008; **24**(1):17–29.
188. von Sinner WN. Imaging of cystic echinococcosis. *Acta Trop* 1997; **67**(1–2):67–89.
189. von Sinner WN, Nyman R, Linjawi T, Ali AM. Fine needle aspiration biopsy of hydatid cysts. *Acta Radiol* 1995; **36**(2):168–72.
190. McManus DP, Gray DJ, Zhang W, Yang Y. Diagnosis, treatment, and management of echinococcosis. *BMJ* 2012; **344**:e3866.
191. Hemphill A, Müller J. Alveolar and cystic echinococcosis: towards novel chemotherapeutical treatment options. *J Helminthol* 2009; **83**(2):99–111.
192. Stojkovic M, Zwahlen M, Teggi A, *et al.* Treatment response of cystic echinococcosis to benzimidazoles: a systematic review. *PLoS Negl Trop Dis* 2009; **3**(9):e524.
193. El-On J. Benzimidazole treatment of cystic echinococcosis. *Acta Trop* 2003; **85**(2):243–52.

194. Akhan O, Ustünsöz B, Somuncu I, Ozmen M, Oner A, Alemdaroğlu A, Besim A. Percutaneous renal hydatid cyst treatment: long-term results. *Abdom Imaging* 1998; **23**(2):209–13.
195. Fazeli F, Narouie B, Firoozabadi MD, Afshar M, Naghavi A, Ghasemi-Rad M. Isolated hydatid cyst of kidney. *Urology* 2009; **73**(5):999–1001.
196. Handa R, Harjai MM. Hydatid cyst of the renal pelvis. *Pediatr Surg Int* 2005; **21**(5):410–2.
197. Agarwal MM, Hemal AK. Surgical management of renal cystic disease. *Curr Urol Rep* 2011; **12**(1):3–10.
198. Mokhtar AA, Al Sayyah A, Al-Hindi H, Seyam RM, Al Khudair W. Isolated renal hydatid disease in a non-endemic country: a single centre experience. *Can Urol Assoc J* 2011 May **1**:1–6 [Epub ahead of print].
199. Zargar-Shoshtari M, Shadpour P, Robat-Moradi N, Moslemi M. Hydatid cyst of urinary tract: 11 cases at a single center. *Urol J* 2007; **4**(1):41–5.
200. Knopp S, Steinmann P, Hatz C, Keiser J, Utzinger J. Nematode infections: filariases. *Infect Dis Clin North Am* 2012; **26**(2):359–81.
201. Genchi C, Kramer LH, Sassera D, Bandi C. Wolbachia and its implications for the immunopathology of filariasis. *Endocr Metab Immune Disord Drug Targets* 2012; **12**(1):53–6.
202. Taylor MJ, Hoerauf A, Bockarie M. Lymphatic filariasis and onchocerciasis. *Lancet* 2010; **376**(9747):1175–85.
203. Pfarr KM, Debrah AY, Specht S, Hoerauf A. Filariasis and lymphoedema. *Parasite Immunol* 2009; **31**(11):664–72.
204. Taylor MJ. Wolbachia in the inflammatory pathogenesis of human filariasis. *Ann N Y Acad Sci* 2003; **990**:444–9.
205. Rajan TV. Natural course of lymphatic filariasis: insights from epidemiology, experimental human infections, and clinical observations. *Am J Trop Med Hyg* 2005; **73**(6):995–8.
206. Figueredo-Silva J, Norões J, Cedenho A, Dreyer G. The histopathology of bancroftian filariasis revisited: the role of the adult worm in the lymphatic-vessel disease. *Ann Trop Med Parasitol* 2002; **96**(6):531–41.
207. King CL. Transmission intensity and human immune responses to lymphatic filariasis. *Parasite Immunol* 2001; **23**(7):363–71.
208. Dreyer G, Norões J, Figueredo-Silva J, Piessens WF. Pathogenesis of lymphatic disease in bancroftian filariasis: a clinical perspective. *Parasitol Today* 2000; **16**(12):544–8.
209. Ramaiah KD, Das PK, Michael E, Guyatt H. The economic burden of lymphatic filariasis in India. *Parasitol Today* 2000; **16**(6):251–3.
210. Pacella M, Corbu C, Naselli A, Quilici P, Carmignani G. Acute scrotum secondary to filarial infection: a case report. *Int Urol Nephrol* 2002; **34**(3):385–6.
211. Di Tonno F, Mazzariol C, Piazza N, Murer B. Filariasis: an emergent cause of acute scrotal pain. *Urologia* 2010; **77**(2):147–9.
212. Kumar B, Karki S, Yadava SK. Role of fine needle aspiration cytology in diagnosis of filarial infestation. *Diagn Cytopathol* 2011; **39**(1):8–12.
213. Olszewski WL, Jamal S, Manokaran G, *et al.* Bacteriologic studies of skin, tissue fluid, lymph, and lymph nodes in patients with filarial lymphedema. *Am J Trop Med Hyg* 1997; **57**(1):7–15.
214. Aguiar-Santos AM, Leal-Cruz M, Netto MJ, Carrera A, Lima G, Rocha A. Lymph scrotum: an unusual urological presentation of lymphatic filariasis. A case series study. *Rev Inst Med Trop Sao Paulo* 2009; **51**(4):179–83.
215. Norões J, Addiss D, Cedenho A, Figueredo-Silva J, Lima G, Dreyer G. Pathogenesis of filarial hydrocele: risk associated with intrascrotal nodules caused by death of adult Wuchereria bancrofti. *Trans R Soc Trop Med Hyg* 2003; **97**(5):561–6.
216. Mishra K, Raj DK, Hazra RK, Dash AP, Supakar PC. The development and evaluation of a single step multiplex PCR method for simultaneous detection of Brugia malayi and Wuchereria bancrofti. *Mol Cell Probes* 2007; **21**(5–6):355–62.
217. Harnett W, Bradley JE, Garate T. Molecular and immunodiagnosis of human filarial nematode infections. *Parasitology* 1998; **117 Suppl**:S59–71.
218. Chaubal NG, Pradhan GM, Chaubal JN, Ramani SK. Dance of live adult filarial worms is a reliable sign of scrotal filarial infection. *J Ultrasound Med* 2003; **22**(8):765–9; quiz 770–2.
219. Amaral F, Dreyer G, Figueredo-Silva J, *et al.* Live adult worms detected by ultrasonography in human Bancroftian filariasis. *Am J Trop Med Hyg* 1994; **50**(6):753–7.
220. Hoerauf A, Pfarr K, Mand S, Debrah AY, Specht S. Filariasis in Africa—treatment challenges and prospects. *Clin Microbiol Infect* 2011; **17**(7):977–85.
221. Horton J. The development of albendazole for lymphatic filariasis. *Ann Trop Med Parasitol* 2009; **103**(Suppl 1):S33–40.
222. Mand S, Pfarr K, Sahoo PK, *et al.* Macrofilaricidal activity and amelioration of lymphatic pathology in bancroftian filariasis after 3 weeks of doxycycline followed by single-dose diethylcarbamazine. *Am J Trop Med Hyg* 2009; **81**(4):702–11.
223. Hoerauf A. Filariasis: new drugs and new opportunities for lymphatic filariasis and onchocerciasis. *Curr Opin Infect Dis* 2008; **21**(6):673–81.
224. Coulibaly YI, Dembele B, Diallo AA, *et al.* A randomized trial of doxycycline for Mansonella perstans infection. *N Engl J Med* 2009; **361**(15):1448–58.
225. Hoerauf A, Mand S, Volkmann L, *et al.* Doxycycline in the treatment of human onchocerciasis: Kinetics of Wolbachia endobacteria reduction and of inhibition of embryogenesis in female Onchocerca worms. *Microbes Infect* 2003; **5**(4):261–73.
226. Bockarie MJ, Pedersen EM, White GB, Michael E. Role of vector control in the global program to eliminate lymphatic filariasis. *Annu Rev Entomol* 2009; **54**:469–87.
227. Bockarie MJ, Tisch DJ, Kastens W, *et al.* Mass treatment to eliminate filariasis in Papua New Guinea. *N Engl J Med* 2002; **347**(23):1841–8.
228. Ottesen EA. Lymphatic filariasis: Treatment, control and elimination. *Adv Parasitol* 2006; **61**:395–441.
229. Erlanger TE, Keiser J, Caldas De Castro M, *et al.* Effect of water resource development and management on lymphatic filariasis, and estimates of populations at risk. *Am J Trop Med Hyg* 2005; **73**(3):523–33.
230. Capuano GP, Capuano C. Surgical management of morbidity due to lymphatic filariasis: the usefulness of a standardized international clinical classification of hydroceles. *Trop Biomed* 2012; **29**(1):24–38.
231. Mante SD, Gueye SM. Capacity building for the modified filarial hydrocelectomy technique in West Africa. *Acta Trop* 2011; **120**(Suppl 1):S76–80.
232. Norões J, Dreyer G. A mechanism for chronic filarial hydrocele with implications for its surgical repair. *PLoS Negl Trop Dis* 2010; **4**(6):e695.
233. Singh V, Sinha RJ, Sankhwar SN, Kumar V. Reconstructive surgery for penoscrotal filarial lymphedema: a decade of experience and follow-up. *Urology* 2011; **77**(5):1228–31.
234. McDougal WS. Lymphedema of the external genitalia. *J Urol* 2003; **170**(3):711–6.
235. Graziani G, Cucchiari D, Verdesca S, Balzarini L, Montanelli A, Ponticelli C. Chyluria associated with nephrotic-range proteinuria: pathophysiology, clinical picture and therapeutic options. *Nephron Clin Pract* 2011; **119**(3):c248–53; discussion c254.
236. Tandon V, Singh H, Dwivedi US, Mahmood M, Singh PB. Filarial chyluria: long-term experience of a university hospital in India. *Int J Urol* 2004; **11**(4):193–8; discussion 199.
237. Gandhi GM. Role of lymphography in management of filarial chyluria. *Lymphology* 1976; **9**(1):11–8.
238. Ramana Murthy KV, Jayaram Reddy S, Prasad DV, Purusotham G. Povidone iodine instillation into the renal pelvis in the management of chyluria: our experience. *Urol Int* 2010; **84**(3):305–8.
239. Zhang X, Zhu QG, Ma X, *et al.* Renal pedicle lymphatic disconnection for chyluria via retroperitoneoscopy and open surgery: report of 53 cases with followup. *J Urol* 2005; **174**(5):1828–31.
240. Goel S, Mandhani A, Srivastava A, *et al.* Is povidone iodine an alternative to silver nitrate for renal pelvic instillation sclerotherapy in chyluria? *BJU Int* 2004; **94**(7):1082–5.
241. Zhang Y, Zeng J, Zhang K, Jin F, Ye J, Wu G, Wang G, Nie Z. Surgical management of intractable chyluria: a comparison of retroperitoneoscopy with open surgery. *Urol Int* 2012; **89**:222–6.

CHAPTER 1.7

Inflammation
Prostatitis syndrome

Florian M.E. Wagenlehner, Adrian Pilatz, Thomas Bschleipfer, Thorsten Diemer, and Wolfgang Weidner

Definition and classification

The prostatitis syndrome is one of the most common entities encountered in urologic practice. The disease classification put forward by the National Institute of Diabetes and Digestive and Kidney Diseases (NIDDK)/National Institutes of Health (NIH) from 1995 is currently applied in both clinical practice and research.[1,2] It is based on the clinical presentation of the patient, the presence or absence of white blood cells in the expressed prostatic secretion (EPS), and the presence or absence of bacteria in the EPS.[3] Depending upon the duration of symptoms, prostatitis is then described as either acute or, if symptoms have been present for at least three months, chronic.[2] This results in four categories of prostatitis; namely acute (type I), chronic bacterial (type II), chronic prostatitis/chronic pelvic pain syndrome (type III), which is further divided into inflammatory and non-inflammatory categories, and finally asymptomatic inflammatory prostatitis (type IV).[2]

Epidemiology

Acute bacterial prostatitis is uncommon but acute urinary tract infections in males might also involve the prostate in an unknown percentage, as indicated by raised serum prostate-specific antigen.[4,5]

Acute bacterial prostatitis may be subdivided into cases that occur spontaneously and those that occur following urological interventions, such as cystourethroscopy or transrectal prostate biopsy.[6]

The incidence of acute and chronic bacterial prostatitis in a population-based study was 1.26 cases per 1,000 men per year.[7] The prevalence of chronic prostatitis/ chronic pelvic pain syndrome (CP/CPPS) symptoms in a managed care population was 11.2%.[8] Approximately 10% of men suffering an episode of acute bacterial prostatitis go on to suffer chronic bacterial prostatitis and similarly 10% progress to CP/CPPS.[9]

Asymptomatic prostatitis defined as the histological finding of prostatic inflammation is found in about 40% of men who undergo transrectal biopsy for prostate cancer diagnosis.[10] In the andrological setting, asymptomatic prostatitis may also be found during investigation for infertility.[11] Elevated reactive oxygen species produced predominantly by leucocytes from the prostate are found in the semen of 40% to 88% infertile men.[12,13]

Aetiology and pathogenesis

Acute bacterial prostatitis

The bacterial spectrum of acute bacterial prostatitis resembles that of complicated urinary tract infections, *Escherichia coli* being the most prevalent occurring in 67% of cases, with *Pseudomonas aeruginosa* in 13%, *Klebsiella sp.* in 6%, and Gram-positive species in 5%.[14] In another study, phylogenetic grouping and molecular characterization of acute bacterial prostatitis showed that most phenotypes were uropathogenic *E. coli* (UPEC) with a marked accumulation of virulence genes characteristic of highly virulent uropathogens.[15]

Chronic bacterial prostatitis

Gram-negative bacteria (especially *E. coli*) are also responsible for the great majority of cases of chronic bacterial prostatitis.[16] More recent epidemiological studies however suggest a preponderance of Gram-positive cocci.[17] However, in these latter series, the median duration of patients' symptoms was only 3.5 weeks and there was some evidence that localization of Gram-positive bacteria was inconsistent in more than 90% of patients.[18] In a reproducible rat model of chronic bacterial prostatitis, prostate colonization and growth studies showed biofilm formation by causative organisms.[19] Support for this mechanism of chronic infection comes from *in vitro* studies where *E. coli* isolates causing prostatitis produced biofilm more frequently than those causing other urinary tract infections.[20]

The role of *Chlamydia trachomatis* in chronic prostatitis continues to be debated and conclusive evidence for a causative role is hampered by possible urethral contamination of collected material for culture. Nevertheless, studies investigating anti-*C. trachomatis* immunoglobulin A (IgA) in the ejaculate of symptomatic men showed that mucosal IgA was detected in 69% of cases, but in none of the controls.[21] This study suggested that mucosal IgA might be a sensitive marker for detection of *C. trachomatis* in the ejaculate.

Chronic prostatitis/chronic pelvic pain syndrome

CP/CPPS in males is a complex disease with a heterogenous and incompletely understood aetiology. Comparable to other chronic pain syndromes, phenomena of peripheral and central sensitization occur, leading to abnormal chronic pain perception from the areas of the pelvis. A variety of causes may be associated with this disease, although cause and effect is always difficult to ascertain.[22] Nevertheless, there is evidence that neurogenic inflammation triggered by mast cells in the prostate might play a role in prostate derived chronic pelvic pain syndrome.[23] Men with chronic pelvic pain syndrome showed increased mast cell tryptase and nerve growth factor in expressed prostatic secretions.[23] The differentiation into inflammatory and non-inflammatory CP/CPPS currently remains, although there is no strong evidence that clinical management differs according to this classification.

Asymptomatic prostatitis

The aetiology of asymptomatic prostatitic inflammation is not well understood. Mouse model data reported increased mast cells, macrophages, neutrophils, and T-lymphocytes in response to elevated endogenous estrogens due to aromatase overexpression.[24] Chronic inflammation, such as proliferative inflammatory atrophy and intraepithelial neoplasia, is also linked to premalignant prostatic lesions.[25] Investigations in benign prostatic hyperplasia strongly suggest that this disease may also have an inflammatory component perhaps linked to autoimmune mechanisms.[26]

Clinical presentation

Men with acute bacterial prostatitis are usually systemically unwell, with fever and systemic signs of inflammation. The most common complications are acute urinary retention and prostatic abscess.

Symptoms experienced by men with chronic bacterial prostatitis do not necessarily differ from those with CP/CPPS. Therefore, NIH categorization cannot be determined from clinical findings alone. The exception is where recurrent febrile or afebrile urinary tract infections are associated with prostatic symptoms suggesting chronic bacterial prostatitis.

The CP/CPPS is characterized by pelvic pain, voiding symptoms and additional individual phenotypic signs, which are however still poorly defined.

In asymptomatic prostatitis, there are by definition no clinical symptoms present.

Diagnosis

Acute bacterial prostatitis

Clinical examination should include palpation of the loin, abdomen, bladder region, scrotal contents, and a careful gentle digital examination of the prostate. The prostate is usually tender and swollen. Accompanying epididymo-orchitis may be present. A tender suprapubic region could be due to severe cystitis or more often due to urinary retention.

A midstream or catheter urine specimen sent for microbiological culture is the only laboratory evaluation of the lower urinary tract required. Prostatic massage should not be performed.

Transrectal ultrasound may be helpful in detecting prostatic abscess, if for example there is a swinging pyrexia and poor response to initial antibiotic treatment.[27] Additionally, residual urine measurement by ultrasound of the bladder should be performed.

Chronic bacterial prostatitis

Quantitative sequential bacteriological localization cultures are essential. The gold standard is the Meares and Stamey 4-glass test, where first voided urine, midstream urine, EPS, and post-prostate massage urine are sampled.[28] A simpler screening test, the 2-glass pre- and post-massage test (PPMT) obtaining a mid stream urine before massage and a first stream urine after, is a reasonable alternative at least for initial evaluation.[29] Semen cultures identify significant bacteriospermia in only about 50% of semen specimens from men with chronic bacterial prostatitis. Therefore, semen culture of the ejaculate alone is not sufficient for diagnosis.[30]

Chronic prostatitis/chronic pelvic pain syndrome

As clinical symptoms do not necessarily differentiate chronic bacterial prostatitis from CP/CPPS, quantitative sequential bacteriological localization cultures are again needed. The prevalence of culture-proven chronic bacterial prostatitis in large cohort studies ranges from 4.2%[31] to 7%, indicating that most men with chronic symptoms will be categorized as CP/CPPS.[16] To further investigate disease phenotype in individual men, multiple tools, including structured symptom assessment that should encompass urinary, pain, sexual and neuropsycological symptoms, and the exclusion of obvious aetiological causes may be used. Practice guidelines tend to recommend use of the National Institutes of Health Chronic Prostatitis Symptom Index (NIH-CPSI).[32]

Asymptomatic prostatitis

Currently no targeted diagnosis for asymptomatic prostatitis is recommended. It is generally an incidental finding from histological examination of prostate tissue or in patients undergoing infertility treatment.

Therapy and management

Acute bacterial prostatitis

Empiric, parenteral administration of high doses of bactericidal antibiotics, such as a broad-spectrum penicillin derivative, a third-generation cephalosporin, or a fluoroquinolone, is recommended until fever and other signs and symptoms of infection subside.[33] After initial improvement, step-down to an oral regimen, such as a fluoroquinolone, if tested susceptible, is appropriate and should be prescribed for at least four weeks with appropriate warnings about adverse effects.[33]

If a prostatic abscess is present, both drainage and conservative therapy strategies appear feasible and effective depending on the size.[34] In one study, conservative treatment was successful if the abscess cavities were smaller than 1 cm in diameter, while larger abscesses were better treated by single aspiration or continuous drainage.[35]

Approximately 10% of men with acute prostatitis will have urinary retention.[36] which can be managed by suprapubic, intermittent, or indwelling catheterization; however, suprapubic cystostomy placement is generally recommended. The use of catheterization without evidence of retention may increase the risk of progression to chronic bacterial prostatitis.[9] Alpha blocker treatment has also been recommended, although clinical evidence of benefit is weak and of low quality.[33]

Chronic bacterial prostatitis

Fluoroquinolones are considered the antibiotic of choice for the treatment of proven chronic bacterial prostatitis because of their favourable pharmacokinetic properties and their broad antimicrobial spectrum, with the best evidence supporting use of ciprofloxacin or levofloxacin.[37–43] The optimal treatment duration is 28 days. Overall, it appears that 60 to 80% of patients with *E. coli* and other enterobacteria can be cured by this regimen. However, prostatitis due to resistant enterobacteria, *P. aeruginosa* and enterococci often fails to respond. In these cases and for patients with pathogens resistant to fluoroquinolones, but susceptible to trimethoprim-sulfamethoxazole, a three-month course of treatment with trimethoprim-sulfamethoxazole can be given. In patients with pathogens resistant to both fluoroquinolones and trimethoprim-sulfamethoxazole, currently no evidence-based recommendation can be given and antibiotic choice should be guided by microbiological advice and local protocols.

Chronic prostatitis/chronic pelvic pain syndrome

Various clinical research studies investigating treatment efficacy with differing designs, duration, and outcomes have been performed in men with CP/CPPS. The heterogeneity in design makes summarization and meta-analysis of the evidence difficult. For this review, studies have been selected according to the following criteria (Table 1.7.1):

1. clearly defined population of CP/CPPS men;
2. randomized placebo-controlled design;
3. validated outcome analyses by NIH-CPSI;
4. English-language journal publication.

Network meta-analysis of 26 studies selected using these criteria[44] showed that alpha blockers, antibiotics (fluoroquinolones and tetracycline), and combinations of these therapies appeared to improve clinical symptom scores compared with placebo, although there was evidence of publication bias. Anti-inflammatory therapies had a lesser but measurable benefit on selected outcomes.

Another recent meta-analysis[45] showed that alpha blockers, antibiotics, and combinations of the two did not show statistically or clinically significant NIH-CPSI reductions. This meta-analysis however found that mepartricin, percutaneous tibial nerve stimulation

Table 1.7.1 Treatment of chronic prostatitis/chronic pelvic pain syndrome (CP/CPPS) in selected studies

Active agent	Reference	Duration of treatment	Patients (n)		Outcome assessment tool	Age mean (SD)	Total NIH-CPSI mean (SD)	Change in NIH-CPSI		Treatment effect
			Active	Placebo				Active	Placebo	
Alpha blocker										
Alfuzosin vs. placebo	Nickel *et al.* 2008[52]	12 weeks	138	134	NIH-CPSI	40.1 (1.4)	24.4 (0.7)	−7.1	−6.5	0.6
Doxazosin vs. placebo	Tugcu *et al.* 2007[53]	24 weeks	30	30	NIH-CPSI	29.1 (5.2)	23.0 (0.4)	−12.4	−1.0	11.4
Tamsulosin vs. placebo	Alexander *et al.* 2004[54]	6 weeks	49	49	NIH-CPSI	44.6 (3.2)	24.8 (1.7)	−4.4	−3.4	1
Tamsulosin vs. placebo	Nickel *et al.* 2004[55]	6 weeks	27	30	NIH-CPSI	40.8 (21–56)	26.3	−9.1*	−5.5	3.6
Terazosin vs. placebo	Cheah *et al.* 2003[56]	14 weeks	43	43	NIH-CPSI	35.5 (20–50)	26.2 (1.6)	−14.3*	−10.2	4.1
Alfuzosin vs. placebo	Mehik *et al.* 2003[57]	24 weeks	17	20	NIH-CPSI	49.5	24.4	−9.9*	−3.8	6.1
Antibiotics										
Ciprofloxacin vs. placebo	Alexander *et al.* 2004[54]	6 weeks	49	49	NIH-CPSI	44.6 (3.2)	24.8 (1.7)	−6.2	−3.4	2.8
Levofloxacin vs. placebo	Nickel *et al.* 2003[58]	6 weeks	35	45	NIH-CPSI	56.1 (36–78)	23.0 (1.7)	−5.4	−2.9	2.5
Tetracycline vs. placebo	Zhou *et al.* 2008[59]	12 weeks	24	24	NIH-CPSI	n.r.	34.3 (1.2)	−18.5	−1	17.5*
Hormonal agents										
Finasteride vs. placebo	Nickel *et al.* 2004[60]	24 weeks	33	31	NIH-CPSI	44.4 (0.5)	n.r.	−3.0	−0.8	2.2
Mepartricin vs. placebo	de Rose *et al.* 2004[61]	8 weeks	13	13	NIH-CPSI	32–34	25.0 (18–45)	−15.0	−5.0	10.0
Anti-inflammatories										
Rofecoxib 25 mg vs. placebo	Nickel *et al.* 2003[62]	6 weeks	53	59	NIH-CPSI	46.8 (2.5)	21.8 (1.1)	−4.9	−4.2	0.7
Rofecoxib 50 mg vs. placebo			49					−6.2		2.0
Prednisolone vs. placebo	Bates *et al.* 2007[63]	4 weks	6	12	NIH-CPSI	40.8 (4.6)	24.3 (3.0)	n.r.	n.r.	No sig. difference
Celecoxib vs. placebo	Zhao *et al.* 2009[64]	6 weeks	32	32	NIH-CPSI	n.r.	24.4 (1.4)	−8.0	−4.0	4.0*

(continued)

Table 1.7.1 Continued

Active agent	Reference	Duration of treatment	Patients (n)		Outcome assessment tool	Age mean (SD)	Total NIH-CPSI mean (SD)	Change in NIH-CPSI		Treatment effect
			Active	Placebo				Active	Placebo	
Phytotherapy										
Pollen extract (cernilton) vs. placebo	Wagenlehner *et al.* 2009[65]	12 weeks	70	69	NIH-CPSI	39.5 (8.1)	19.8 (5.2)	−7.46	−5.37	2.09*
Quercetin vs. placebo	Shoskes *et al.* 1999[66]	4 weeks	15	13	NIH-CPSI	44.9 (5.4)	20.6 (2.1)	−7.9	−1.4	6.5*
Glycosaminoglycan										
Pentosan polysulfate vs. placebo	Nickel *et al.* 2005[67]	16 weeks	51	49	NIH-CPSI	39.2 (21–59)	26.5 (1.6)	−5.9	−3.2	2.7
Neuroleptics										
Pregabalin vs. placebo	Pontari *et al.* 2010[68]	6 weeks	217	104	NIH-CPSI	n.r.	26.1 (5.7)	−6.5	−4.3	2.2*
Antibodies										
Tanezumab 20 mg vs. placebo	Nickel *et al.*[69]	Single IV dose	30	32	NIH-CPSI	n.r.	n.r.	−4.26	−2.83	1.43
Multimodal therapy										
Alpha blocker vs. alpha blocker + anti-inflammatory+ muscle relaxant vs. placebo	Tugcu *et al.* 2007[53]	24 weeks	30	30	NIH-CPSI	29.1 (5.2)	23.0 (0.4)	−12.7	−1.0	11.7
Tamsulosin + ciprofloxacin vs. placebo	Alexander *et al.* 2004[54]	6 weeks	49	49	NIH-CPSI	44.6 (3.2)	24.8 (1.7)	−4.1	−3.4	0.7
Zafirlukast + doxycycline vs. placebo + doxycycline	Goldmeier *et al.*[70]	4 weeks	10	7	NIH-CPSI	35.9 (5.7)	n.r.			No sig. difference
Physical therapy										
Posterior tibial nerve stimulation vs. placebo	Kabay *et al.* 2009[71]	12 weeks	45	44	NIH-CPSI	37.7 (7.4)	n.r.	−13.4	−1.4	12.0*
Acupuncture vs. placebo	Lee *et al.* 2008[72]	10 weeks	44	45	NIH-CPSI	40.9–42.8	24.8–25.2	−10	−6	4*
Electroacupuncture vs. placebo	Lee *et al.* 2009[73]	6 weeks	12	12	NIH-CPSI	36.4–39.8	25.5–26.9	−9.5	−3.5	6*
Extracorporal shock wave therapy vs. placebo	Zimmermann *et al.*[74]	4 weeks	30	30	NIH-CPSI	42–43	23.2–25.07	−3.67	−0.1	3.57*

*significant difference in NIH-CPSI. Verum vs. placebo.

(PTNS), and triple therapy comprising doxazosin, ibuprofen, and thiocolchicoside (DIT) resulted in clinically and statistically significant reduction in NIH-CPSI total score, although these treatment regimens were usually only evaluated by single studies. Approaches treating CP/CPPS by single agents rarely resulted in clinically significant improvements.

Current management and treatment strategies therefore attempt to classify men with CP/CPPS into single or combination phenotypes using six symptom domains: urinary, psychosocial, organ-specific, infection, neurological and muscle tenderness (UPOINT).[46,47] A seventh symptom domain, sexual dysfunction, can be added (UPOINTS).[48] The symptom management approach for individual men then follows this phenotyping and patients might receive multimodal therapy based on their UPOINT(S) phenotype. For example, the presence of urinary symptoms suggests use of alpha blocker or antimuscarinic treatment; psychosocial symptoms may suggest use of antidepressants, or talking therapies. Organ-specific symptoms may indicate trial of phytotherapy. Infection signs (having excluded chronic bacterial prostatitis) may prompt the use of antimicrobials. Neurologic symptoms will indicate further specific neurologic investigations and treatments. Physical therapies can be used for muscle tenderness of muscles:

while sexual dysfunctions may require use of PDE5 inhibitors or other alternatives. Multimodal therapy using the UPOINT(S) system was recently evaluated in a cohort study, which suggested it leads to significant improvement in symptoms and quality of life in 84% of patients treated.[49]

Asymptomatic prostatitis

Active treatment of asymptomatic prostatitis is controversial, with possible indications being prevention of prostate cancer and treatment of subfertility.

TRAMP (transgenic adenocarcinoma of the mouse prostate) mouse models provided evidence that COX-2 inhibition by dietary supplementation with celecoxib at different doses leads to suppression of prostate adenocarcinoma tumour growth in the prostate in a dose-dependent manner, and also further limits the growth of metastatic prostate cancer.[50] There is no evidence at present as to whether this effect seen in laboratory animals is transferable to the clinical situation.

In andrology, it is well known that infection/inflammation accounts for a substantial part of male patient infertility. Therefore anti-inflammatory treatment is of interest. In a clinical study treatment with l-arginine, l-carnitine, acetyl-l-carnitine and ginseng extracts, an anti-inflammatory agent, together with the quinolone, prulifloxacin, improved semen parameters in patients with *C. trachomatis* genital infection and oligoasthenoteratozoospermia, compared to treatment with prulifloxacin therapy alone.[51]

Due to this lack of high level evidence, recommendations regarding the need for active treatment of asymptomatic prostatitis cannot be given.

Summary

There is a consensus on the diagnostic and therapeutic management of bacterial prostatitis (acute and chronic). However, increasing antimicrobial resistance rates for UPEC in respect to quinolones pose problems for the future, especially for therapy of chronic bacterial prostatitis.

In chronic prostatitis/chronic pelvic pain syndrome, the diagnostic approach currently points more and more to an individualized phenotypic assessment, in an effort to direct multimodal management towards improvement of specific symptom domains. Most therapy trials for single agents in CP/CPPS have been negative, therefore stratification by phenotype followed by individualized multimodal treatment seems to be a promising strategy, although good evidence-based data are not available currently to substantiate this.

Consensus regarding the need for treatment of asymptomatic prostatitis is far from being achieved. Therefore, taking the high prevalence of infections and inflammations in different asymptomatic conditions into consideration, further research is urgently needed to address this important field.

References

1. (NIDDK). Workshop Committee of the National Institute of Diabetes and Digestive and Kidney Disease. Chronic Prostatitis Workshop, Bethesda, MD, 7–8 December 1995; 1995.
2. Krieger JN, Nyberg L, Jr., Nickel JC. NIH consensus definition and classification of prostatitis. *JAMA* 1999; **282**(3):236–7.
3. Schaeffer AJ. Prostatitis: US perspective. *Int J Antimicrob Agents* 1999; **11**(3–4):205–11; discussion 13–6.
4. Schaeffer AJ. Clinical practice. Chronic prostatitis and the chronic pelvic pain syndrome. *N Engl J Med* 2006; **355**(16):1690–8.
5. Lee SW, Cheah PY, Liong ML, *et al.* Demographic and clinical characteristics of chronic prostatitis: prospective comparison of the University of Sciences Malaysia Cohort with the United States National Institutes of Health Cohort. *J Urol* 2007; **177**(1):153–7; discussion 8.
6. Millan-Rodriguez F, Palou J, Bujons-Tur A, *et al.* Acute bacterial prostatitis: two different sub-categories according to a previous manipulation of the lower urinary tract. *World J Urol* 2006; **24**(1):45–50.
7. Clemens JQ, Meenan RT, O'Keeffe-Rosetti MC, Gao SY, Calhoun EA. Incidence and clinical characteristics of National Institutes of Health type III prostatitis in the community. *J Urol* 2005; **174**(6):2319–22.
8. Clemens JQ, Meenan RT, O'Keeffe-Rosetti MC, Gao SY, Brown SO, Calhoun EA. Prevalence of prostatitis-like symptoms in a managed care population. *J Urol* 2006; **176**(2):593–6; discussion 6.
9. Yoon BI, Kim S, Han DS, *et al.* Acute bacterial prostatitis: how to prevent and manage chronic infection? *J Infect Chemother* 2012; **18**(4):444–50.
10. Stancik I, Luftenegger W, Klimpfinger M, Muller MM, Hoeltl W. Effect of NIH-IV prostatitis on free and free-to-total PSA. *Eur Urol* 2004; **46**(6):760–4.
11. Schaeffer AJ, Anderson RU, Krieger JN, *et al.* Consensus statement on prostatitis. The assessment and management of male pelvic pain syndrome, including prostatitis. (pp. 343–75) In: Edition MLUTD (ed). 6th International Conference on New Developments in Prostate Cancer and Prostate Diseases. Paris, France: Health Publications, 2006.
12. Lewis SE, Boyle PM, McKinney KA, Young IS, Thompson W. Total antioxidant capacity of seminal plasma is different in fertile and infertile men. *Fertil Steril* 1995; **64**(4):868–70.
13. Rusz A, Pilatz A, Wagenlehner F, *et al.* Influence of urogenital infections and inflammation on semen quality and male fertility. *World J Urol* 2012; **30**(1):23–30.
14. Cho IR LK, Jeon JS. Clinical outcome of acute prostatitis: A multicenter study. American Urological Association Annual Meeting; 2005; San Antonio, TX: *J Urol* 2005.
15. Krieger JN, Dobrindt U, Riley DE, Oswald E. Acute Escherichia coli prostatitis in previously health young men: bacterial virulence factors, antimicrobial resistance, and clinical outcomes. *Urology* 2011; **77**(6):1420–5.
16. Weidner W, Schiefer HG, Krauss H, Jantos C, Friedrich HJ, Altmannsberger M. Chronic prostatitis: a thorough search for etiologically involved microorganisms in 1,461 patients. *Infection* 1991; **19**(Suppl 3):S119–25.
17. Bundrick W, Heron SP, Ray P, *et al.* Levofloxacin versus ciprofloxacin in the treatment of chronic bacterial prostatitis: a randomized double-blind multicenter study. *Urology* 2003; **62**(3):537–41.
18. Krieger JN, Ross SO, Limaye AP, Riley DE. Inconsistent localization of gram-positive bacteria to prostate-specific specimens from patients with chronic prostatitis. *Urology* 2005; **66**(4):721–5.
19. Nickel JC, Olson ME, Costerton JW. Rat model of experimental bacterial prostatitis. *Infection* 1991; **19**(Suppl 3):S126–30.
20. Soto SM, Smithson A, Martinez JA, Horcajada JP, Mensa J, Vila J. Biofilm formation in uropathogenic Escherichia coli strains: relationship with prostatitis, urovirulence factors and antimicrobial resistance. *J Urol* 2007; **177**(1):365–8.
21. Mazzoli S, Cai T, Rupealta V, *et al.* Interleukin 8 and anti-chlamydia trachomatis mucosal IgA as urogenital immunologic markers in patients with C. trachomatis prostatic infection. *Eur Urol* 2007; **51**(5):1385–93.
22. Engeler D BA, Elneil S, Hughes J, *et al.* Guidelines on chronic pelvic pain. (pp. 1–131). European Association of Urology Guidelines 2012 Edition. Arnhem, The Netherlands: European Association of Urology, 2012.
23. Done JD, Rudick CN, Quick ML, Schaeffer AJ, Thumbikat P. Role of mast cells in male chronic pelvic pain. *J Urol* 2012; **187**(4):1473–82.

24. Ellem SJ, Wang H, Poutanen M, Risbridger GP. Increased endogenous estrogen synthesis leads to the sequential induction of prostatic inflammation (prostatitis) and prostatic pre-malignancy. *Am J Pathol* 2009; **175**(3):1187–99.
25. Wagenlehner FM, Elkahwaji JE, Algaba F, *et al.* The role of inflammation and infection in the pathogenesis of prostate carcinoma. *BJU Int* 2007; **100**(4):733–7.
26. Kramer G, Mitteregger D, Marberger M. Is benign prostatic hyperplasia (BPH) an immune inflammatory disease? *Eur Urol* 2007; **51**(5):1202–16.
27. Horcajada JP, Vilana R, Moreno-Martinez A, *et al.* Transrectal prostatic ultrasonography in acute bacterial prostatitis: findings and clinical implications. *Scand J Infect Dis* 2003; **35**(2):114–20.
28. Meares EM, Stamey TA. Bacteriologic localization patterns in bacterial prostatitis and urethritis. *Invest Urol* 1968; **5**(5):492–518.
29. Nickel JC, Shoskes D, Wang Y, Alexander RB, Fowler JE, Jr., Zeitlin S, *et al.* How does the pre-massage and post-massage 2-glass test compare to the Meares-Stamey 4-glass test in men with chronic prostatitis/chronic pelvic pain syndrome? *J Urol* 2006; **176**(1):119–24.
30. Weidner W, Ludwig M, Brahler E, Schiefer HG. Outcome of antibiotic therapy with ciprofloxacin in chronic bacterial prostatitis. *Drugs* 1999; **58**(Suppl 2):103–6.
31. Schneider H, Ludwig M, Hossain HM, Diemer T, Weidner W. The 2001 Giessen Cohort Study on patients with prostatitis syndrome—an evaluation of inflammatory status and search for microorganisms 10 years after a first analysis. *Andrologia* 2003; **35**(5):258–62.
32. Litwin MS, McNaughton-Collins M, Fowler FJ, Jr., *et al.* The National Institutes of Health chronic prostatitis symptom index: development and validation of a new outcome measure. Chronic Prostatitis Collaborative Research Network. *J Urol* 1999; **162**(2):369–75.
33. Grabe M, Bjerklund-Johansen TE, Botto H, *et al.* Guidelines on urological infections. (pp. 1–110) European Association of Urology Guidelines 2012 Edition. Arnhem, The Netherlands: European Association of Urology, 2012.
34. Ludwig M, Schroeder-Printzen I, Schiefer HG, Weidner W. Diagnosis and therapeutic management of 18 patients with prostatic abscess. *Urology* 1999; **53**(2):340–5.
35. Chou YH, Tiu CM, Liu JY, *et al.* Prostatic abscess: transrectal color Doppler ultrasonic diagnosis and minimally invasive therapeutic management. *Ultrasound Med Biol* 2004; **30**(6):719–24.
36. Hua LX, Zhang JX, Wu HF, *et al.* The diagnosis and treatment of acute prostatitis: report of 35 cases. *Zhonghua Nan Ke Xue* 2005; **11**(12):897–9.
37. Pust RA, Ackenheil-Koppe HR, Gilbert P, Weidner W. Clinical efficacy of ofloxacin (tarivid) in patients with chronic bacterial prostatitis: preliminary results. *J Chemother* 1989; **1**(4 Suppl):869–71.
38. Weidner W, Schiefer HG, Dalhoff A. Treatment of chronic bacterial prostatitis with ciprofloxacin. Results of a one-year follow-up study. *Am J Med* 1987; **82**(4A):280–3.
39. Weidner W, Schiefer HG, Brahler E. Refractory chronic bacterial prostatitis: a re-evaluation of ciprofloxacin treatment after a median followup of 30 months. *J Urol* 1991; **146**(2):350–2.
40. Pfau A. The treatment of chronic bacterial prostatitis. *Infection* 1991; **19** (Suppl 3):S160–4.
41. Schaeffer AJ, Darras FS. The efficacy of norfloxacin in the treatment of chronic bacterial prostatitis refractory to trimethoprim-sulfamethoxazole and/or carbenicillin. *J Urol* 1990; **144**(3):690–3.
42. Naber KG, Busch W, Focht J. Ciprofloxacin in the treatment of chronic bacterial prostatitis: a prospective, non-comparative multicentre clinical trial with long-term follow-up. The German Prostatitis Study Group. *Int J Antimicrob Agents* 2000; **14**(2):143–9.
43. Naber KG. Lomefloxacin versus ciprofloxacin in the treatment of chronic bacterial prostatitis. *Int J Antimicrob Agents* 2002; **20**(1):18–27.
44. Anothaisintawee T, Attia J, Nickel JC, *et al.* Management of chronic prostatitis/chronic pelvic pain syndrome: a systematic review and network meta-analysis. *JAMA* 2011; **305**(1):78–86.
45. Cohen JM, Fagin AP, Hariton E, *et al.* Therapeutic intervention for chronic prostatitis/chronic pelvic pain syndrome (CP/CPPS): A systematic review and meta-analysis. *PLoS One* 2012; 7(8):e41941.
46. Shoskes DA, Nickel JC, Dolinga R, Prots D. Clinical phenotyping of patients with chronic prostatitis/chronic pelvic pain syndrome and correlation with symptom severity. *Urology* 2009; **73**(3):538–42; discussion 42–3.
47. Shoskes DA, Nickel JC, Rackley RR, Pontari MA. Clinical phenotyping in chronic prostatitis/chronic pelvic pain syndrome and interstitial cystitis: a management strategy for urologic chronic pelvic pain syndromes. *Prostate Cancer Prostatic Dis* 2009; **12**(2):177–83.
48. Magri V, Wagenlehner F, Perletti G, *et al.* Use of the UPOINT chronic prostatitis/chronic pelvic pain syndrome classification in European patient cohorts: sexual function domain improves correlations. *J Urol* 2010; **184**(6):2339–45.
49. Shoskes DA, Nickel JC, Kattan MW. Phenotypically directed multimodal therapy for chronic prostatitis/chronic pelvic pain syndrome: a prospective study using UPOINT. *Urology* 2010; **75**(6):1249–53.
50. Narayanan BA, Narayanan NK, Pttman B, Reddy BS. Adenocarcina of the mouse prostate growth inhibition by celecoxib: downregulation of transcription factors involved in COX-2 inhibition. *Prostate* 2006; **66**(3):257–65.
51. Cai T, Wagenlehner FM, Mazzoli S, *et al.* Semen quality in patients with chlamydia trachomatis genital infection treated concurrently with prulifloxacin and a phytotherapeutic agent. *J Androl* 2012; **33**(4):615–23.
52. Nickel JC, Krieger JN, McNaughton-Collins M, *et al.* Alfuzosin and symptoms of chronic prostatitis-chronic pelvic pain syndrome. *N Engl J Med* 2008; **359**(25):2663–73.
53. Tugcu V, Tasci AI, Fazlioglu A, *et al.* A placebo-controlled comparison of the efficiency of triple- and monotherapy in category III B chronic pelvic pain syndrome (CPPS). *Eur Urol* 2007; **51**(4):1113–7; discussion 8.
54. Alexander RB, Propert KJ, Schaeffer AJ, *et al.* Ciprofloxacin or tamsulosin in men with chronic prostatitis/chronic pelvic pain syndrome: a randomized, double-blind trial. *Ann Intern Med* 2004; **141**(8):581–9.
55. Nickel JC, Narayan P, McKay J, Doyle C. Treatment of chronic prostatitis/chronic pelvic pain syndrome with tamsulosin: a randomized double blind trial. *J Urol* 2004; **171**(4):1594–7.
56. Cheah PY, Liong ML, Yuen KH, *et al.* Terazosin therapy for chronic prostatitis/chronic pelvic pain syndrome: a randomized, placebo controlled trial. *J Urol* 2003; **169**(2):592–6.
57. Mehik A, Alas P, Nickel JC, Sarpola A, Helstrom PJ. Alfuzosin treatment for chronic prostatitis/chronic pelvic pain syndrome: a prospective, randomized, double-blind, placebo-controlled, pilot study. *Urology* 2003; **62**(3):425–9.
58. Nickel JC, Downey J, Clark J, *et al.* Levofloxacin for chronic prostatitis/chronic pelvic pain syndrome in men: a randomized placebo-controlled multicenter trial. *Urology* 2003; **62**(4):614–7.
59. Zhou Z, Hong L, Shen X, *et al.* Detection of nanobacteria infection in type III prostatitis. *Urology* 2008; **71**(6):1091–5.
60. Nickel JC, Downey J, Pontari MA, Shoskes DA, Zeitlin SI. A randomized placebo-controlled multicentre study to evaluate the safety and efficacy of finasteride for male chronic pelvic pain syndrome (category IIIA chronic nonbacterial prostatitis). *BJU Int* 2004; **93**(7):991–5.
61. De Rose AF, Gallo F, Giglio M, Carmignani G. Role of mepartricin in category III chronic nonbacterial prostatitis/chronic pelvic pain syndrome: a randomized prospective placebo-controlled trial. *Urology* 2004; **63**(1):13–6.
62. Nickel JC, Pontari M, Moon T, *et al.* A randomized, placebo controlled, multicenter study to evaluate the safety and efficacy of rofecoxib in the treatment of chronic nonbacterial prostatitis. *J Urol* 2003; **169**(4):1401–5.
63. Bates SM, Hill VA, Anderson JB, *et al.* A prospective, randomized, double-blind trial to evaluate the role of a short reducing course of oral

corticosteroid therapy in the treatment of chronic prostatitis/chronic pelvic pain syndrome. *BJU Int* 2007; **99**(2):355–9.
64. Zhao WP, Zhang ZG, Li XD, *et al.* Celecoxib reduces symptoms in men with difficult chronic pelvic pain syndrome (Category IIIA). *Braz J Med Biol Res* 2009; **42**(10):963–7.
65. Wagenlehner FM, Schneider H, Ludwig M, Schnitker J, Brahler E, Weidner W. A pollen extract (Cernilton) in patients with inflammatory chronic prostatitis-chronic pelvic pain syndrome: a multicentre, randomised, prospective, double-blind, placebo-controlled phase 3 study. *Eur Urol* 2009; **56**(3):544–51.
66. Shoskes DA, Zeitlin SI, Shahed A, Rajfer J. Quercetin in men with category III chronic prostatitis: a preliminary prospective, double-blind, placebo-controlled trial. *Urology* 1999; **54**(6):960–3.
67. Nickel JC, Forrest JB, Tomera K, *et al.* Pentosan polysulfate sodium therapy for men with chronic pelvic pain syndrome: a multicenter, randomized, placebo controlled study. *J Urol* 2005; **173**(4):1252–5.
68. Pontari MA, Krieger JN, Litwin MS, *et al.* Pregabalin for the treatment of men with chronic prostatitis/chronic pelvic pain syndrome: a randomized controlled trial. *Arch Intern Med* 2010; **170**(17):1586–93.
69. Nickel C, Atkinson G, Krieger J, *et al.* Preliminary assessment of safety and efficacy in a proof-of-concept, randomized clinical trial of tanezumab for chronic prostatitis/chronic pelvic pain syndrome (CP/CPPS). *Urology* 2012; **80**(5):1105–10.
70. Goldmeier D, Madden P, McKenna M, Tamm N. Treatment of category III A prostatitis with zafirlukast: a randomized controlled feasibility study. *Int J STD AIDS* 2005; **16**(3):196–200.
71. Kabay S, Kabay SC, Yucel M, Ozden H. Efficiency of posterior tibial nerve stimulation in category IIIB chronic prostatitis/chronic pelvic pain: a sham-controlled comparative study. *Urol Int* 2009; **83**(1):33–8.
72. Lee SW, Liong ML, Yuen KH, *et al.* Acupuncture versus sham acupuncture for chronic prostatitis/chronic pelvic pain. *Am J Med* 2008; **121**(1):79 e1–7.
73. Lee SH, Lee BC. Electroacupuncture relieves pain in men with chronic prostatitis/chronic pelvic pain syndrome: three-arm randomized trial. *Urology* 2009; **73**(5):1036–41.
74. Zimmermann R, Cumpanas A, Miclea F, Janetschek G. Extracorporeal shock wave therapy for the treatment of chronic pelvic pain syndrome in males: a randomised, double-blind, placebo-controlled study. *Eur Urol* 2009; **56**(3):418–24.

CHAPTER 1.8

Inflammation
Epididymitis and scrotal abscess

Mary Garthwaite

Aetiology and pathophysiology

Epididymo-orchitis and scrotal abscess are most commonly caused by bacterial infection. In men over an approximate age threshold of 35 years, the majority of cases are thought to be due to non-sexually transmitted infection with common enteric Gram-negative uropathogens, such as *Escherichia coli* and *Enterococcus faecium*.[1–3] In this group, infection may also be associated with risk factors such as bladder outlet obstruction, recent instrumentation of the urinary tract, or systemic illness. Among men under 35 years of age, there is clinical consensus that infection is more commonly sexually transmitted and causative organisms include *Chlamydia trachomatis* and *Neisseria gonorrhoeae*. However, men who engage in anal intercourse are also at high risk of infection with enteric uropathogens. It must be noted that the categorization of these groups by age is arbitrary, and a degree of overlap will exist in terms of the likely causative organism.

The pathophysiology of bacterial epididymitis, with or without testicular involvement, usually involves the retrograde spread of urinary pathogens from the urethra and bladder, via the ejaculatory ducts and vas deferens. This leads to bacterial colonization and secondary inflammation of the epididymis. The inflammatory process starts in the tail of the epididymis and then spreads to the body and head of the epididymis. Infection may also reach the epididymis via the lymphatics of the spermatic cord and, in rare cases, organisms from other foci of infection may reach the epididymis via the bloodstream.

Tuberculous epididymitis remains rare even though extrapulmonary tuberculosis (TB) represents 40–45% of TB cases in the UK.[4] It is likely to present in patients from high prevalence countries or with a previous history of tuberculosis, and particularly in patients with immunodeficiency.[5] Tuberculous epididymitis has also been noted as a complication of Bacille Calmette–Guérin (BCG) instillation for treatment of bladder carcinoma.[6]

Viral epididymitis is rare in the adult population, but an increase of mumps epididymo-orchitis has been seen in the United Kingdom due to the 2005 mumps epidemic in a cohort of non-immunized adults born between 1982 and 1986.[7] This complication is thought to occur in up to 40% of post-pubertal males.

Other causes of acute epididymitis include a reversible sterile epididymitis resulting from therapy with the anti-arrhythmic drug amiodarone,[8] and an association with vasculitic processes in Behcet's syndrome and Henock Schonlein purpura.[9–11] The mechanism underlying non-bacterial epididymitis, whether drug-induced or from a vasculitis, is unknown.

Assessment and diagnosis

History and examination

Key diagnostic factors include a history of unilateral scrotal pain and swelling. This may occasionally be associated with storage lower urinary tract symptoms such as frequency and dysuria. Urethral discharge is extremely uncommon. It is important to identify the presence of risk factors in the history. Strong risk factors include a history of unprotected sexual intercourse, bladder outflow obstruction, and recent instrumentation of the urinary tract (including temporary catheterization). Other risk factors include immunosuppression, a history of mumps, and potential or known exposure to *Mycobacterium tuberculosis*.

Signs on examination may include a hot, erythematous, tender hemiscrotum associated with palpable, tender swelling of the epididymis on the affected side. There may be a secondary reactive hydrocele, which can make palpation of the body of the testis difficult. In severe infection, systemic symptoms such as fever and rigours may be reported and intermittent pyrexia may be present. A fluctuant swelling or induration of the scrotal skin may indicate abscess formation, particularly if fever does not resolve after antibiotic treatment.

Differential diagnoses

The most important differential diagnosis is testicular torsion, which is a surgical emergency and should be considered in all patients presenting with acute scrotal pain. Torsion is more likely if the onset of pain is acute and the pain is severe. If it cannot be excluded then scrotal exploration must be performed urgently, as after six hours testicular salvage becomes decreasingly likely. Torsion is more common in children and young men, but it is important to recognize that it can occur at any age but is unlikely over the age of 50 years.

Other differential diagnoses in patients with an acute scrotum include idiopathic scrotal oedema, testicular tumour, infected hydrocele, and strangulated inguinal hernia. Idiopathic scrotal oedema usually affects children, but has been reported in adults.[12] The common presentation is of an acutely swollen, well-demarcated, red hemiscrotum but the condition is usually painless. Testicular tumours are usually painless swellings of gradual onset, but can mimic epididymo-orchitis in some cases. Strangulation of an inguinal hernia that has previously gone unrecognized can result in a 'scrotal' mass that is painful and irreducible and may be confused with epididymo-orchitis or scrotal abscess. There is usually associated nausea and vomiting, and a previous history of an intermittent inguinoscrotal swelling.

Diagnostic tests

Simple urinalysis using a reagent strip (dipstick) may help to identify the presence of urinary tract infection, but it is not diagnostic and should not stop further microbiological investigation in the form of microscopy and culture of a midstream urine specimen. A Gram stain of urethral secretions should be examined by microscopy and will determine the presence of pus cells and/or *Neisseria gonorrhoeae* (Gram-negative intracellular diplococci). Alternatively, a Gram stain of a centrifuged sample of first-pass urine will diagnose urethritis (≥10 polymorphonuclear leucocytes per high power field ×1000). Urethral secretions can also be cultured for *Neisseria gonorrhoeae*. It is now widely recommended that a nucleic acid amplification test (NAAT) be performed on a swab sample of urethral secretions or first-pass urine sample for *Neisseria gonorrhoeae* and *Chlamydia trachomatis*. A blood culture should be performed if bloodstream infection is suspected.

If there is immediate access to colour Doppler ultrasound, this can be used to assess blood flow to the testis, but sensitivity for torsion remains less than 100% and should not replace scrotal exploration if any suspicion of testicular torsion persists (Fig. 1.8.1).[13] An ultrasound scan (USS) may be useful to resolve diagnostic uncertainty in confirming the presence of an infected hydrocele, testicular tumour, or idiopathic scrotal oedema.

If mumps epididymo-orchitis is suspected, mumps IgM/IgG serology should be tested. If tuberculous epididymitis is suspected, then three early morning urine samples should be obtained and tested for alcohol- and acid-fast bacilli. However, a negative result does not exclude the diagnosis. If there is a high index of suspicion, it is recommended that further tests be performed, including renal tract ultrasound scan (USS), urography, epididymal biopsy, and imaging of the chest to detect pulmonary lesions.

Management

The aims of treatment of epididymo-orchitis are to relieve symptoms, eradicate the infection, and prevent complications. In sexually transmitted infection, a further aim is to prevent transmission to others.

Conservative measures such as bed rest, supportive underwear, and simple analgesia, including the use of non-steroidal anti-inflammatory drugs, should be implemented regardless of cause. All patients with suspected bacterial epididymo-orchitis should be commenced on empirical antibiotic therapy before culture or NAAT results are available. The choice of antibiotics and route of administration will depend on illness severity, age, sexual history and other associated risk factors, including recent urinary tract instrumentation, bladder outflow obstruction, systemic disease, or immunosuppression, together with local guidance on antimicrobial use.

If the patient is unwell with signs of systemic sepsis, they will require admission to hospital for intravenous antibiotic and fluid replacement therapy. Surgical incision and drainage, with or without removal of the affected epididymis and testis, is indicated when a scrotal abscess is present, or if signs of active infection do not resolve with antibiotic therapy.

Current guidelines from the United States for the treatment of epididymo-orchitis most probably due to a sexually transmitted pathogen recommend a single dose of ceftriaxone 250 mg, intramuscularly, plus oral 100 mg doxycycline, twice daily for 14 days.[3] If test results are negative for *Neisseria gonorrhoeae* or infection is

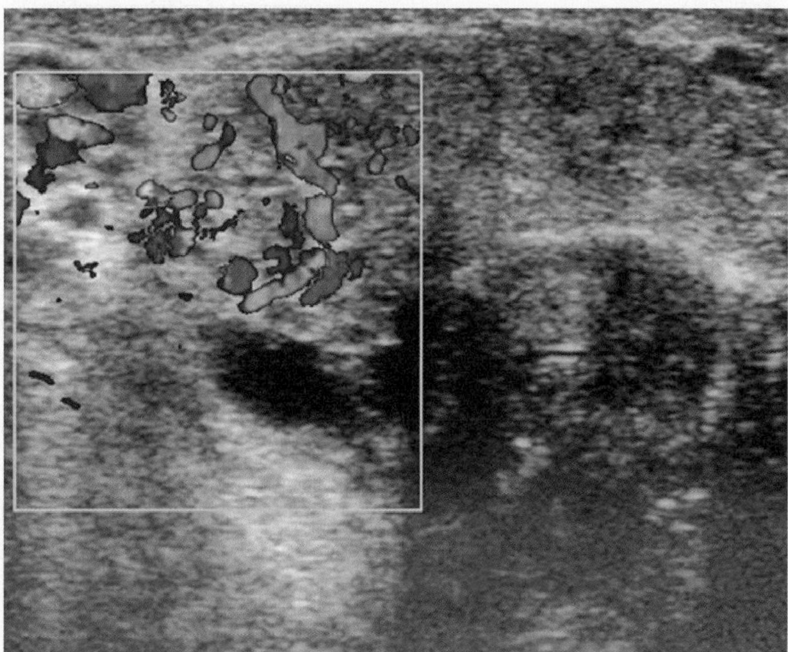

Fig. 1.8.1 Scrotal ultrasound image of testis and head of epididymis. High blood flow is demonstrated within the area of interest (within the white square) localized to rete testis and head of epididymis suggesting the presence of epididymo-orchitis.

Reproduced courtesy of South Tees Hospitals NHS Foundation Trust.

likely to be caused by enteric organisms, empirical therapy with a quinolone is recommended. Guidelines from the United States and Europe suggest either 500 mg levofloxacin orally once daily for 10 days, or ofloxacin 300 mg orally twice a day for 10 days.[3,14] Ciprofloxacin 500 mg twice a day for 10 days is a reasonable alternative. Antibiotic use should conform to local guidance, and step down from intravenous to oral therapy should occur as soon as possible.

If a diagnosis of bacterial epididymo-orchitis has been made but symptoms fail to improve after empirical antibiotic treatment, the patient should be reassessed fully. The persistence or worsening of symptoms may indicate complications such as abscess formation and testicular infarction, or suggest the presence of atypical infections (tubercular or fungal epididymitis) or underlying tumour. USS or surgical exploration should be considered in such cases.

Rare causes of epididymo-orchitis often resolve with conservative measures and treatment of the underlying cause. For example, in drug-induced acute epididymitis due to amiodarone, dose reduction, or discontinuation of the drug should result in rapid resolution of the symptoms. Treatment of tuberculous epididymitis will require specialist referral, as the choice of systemic antibiotics should follow local guidelines given the geographical variability in TB strains and antibiotic resistance patterns. The National Institute for Health and Care Excellence (NICE) guideline recommendation for the treatment of active genitourinary TB is a six-month, four-drug initial regimen (six months of isoniazid and rifampicin, supplemented in the first two months with pyrazinamide and ethambutol). The use of combination tablets is recommended to improve adherence to treatment and prevent accidental or inadvertent single drug therapy which can quickly lead to acquired drug resistance in active TB disease. Combination tablets are usually designed for a daily dosing schedule, which will help minimize side effects.[15]

Complications

The risk of complications is minimized by prompt antibiotic treatment using an appropriate agent with adherence by the patient to the prescribed course.

Scrotal swelling including reactive hydrocele formation is common and will resolve spontaneously, but patients should be made aware that this might take several weeks. Significant abscess formation requires surgical drainage and an infected hydrocele often requires the same intervention.

Infarction of the testicle is a rare complication. It results from occlusion of the testicular blood vessels, either due to involvement of the cord in the inflammatory process or from extrinsic compression by the oedematous epididymis. Ultimately, the testicle will atrophy and this may compromise future fertility. Testicular atrophy is also a recognized complication of mumps epididymo-orchitis. In cases with bilateral orchitis, 13% will have reduced fertility in the future.[7]

If the infection is inadequately treated the inflammatory process can lead to scarring and obstruction of the epididymis, which may result in subfertility or infertility. Although the relationship between epididymo-orchitis and infertility is not fully understood, men who present with obstructive azoospermia are often found to have epididymal obstruction when explored for sperm retrieval. It is thought that such epididymal obstruction is likely to be the consequence of previously unrecognized or incompletely treated infection. The use of corticosteroids in the acute treatment of epididymo-orchitis has not been shown to confer any significant benefit in reducing the risk of developing epididymal obstruction.[16]

The development of chronic pain following acute epididymitis is rare and little is known about its aetiology and pathogenesis.[17] Management is based on reassurance and supportive treatment with analgesics. Epididymectomy is considered only in extreme cases and may not resolve the symptoms.

Summary

In cases of infectious epididymo-orchitis, symptoms often resolve quickly following the initiation of antibiotic therapy, which can lead to non-adherence with treatment and recurrence. Further follow-up is therefore recommended at two weeks to assess treatment adherence, confirmation of causative organism, partner notification, and resolution of symptoms.[18]

Patients with a proven sexually transmitted epididymo-orchitis and those with an indeterminate cause with negative midstream urine (MSU) should be recommended to attend for screening for other sexually transmitted diseases.[18] The evaluation and treatment of all current and recent sexual partners is also recommended in order to prevent illness and complications, and also to prevent re-infection of the index patient.[19]

In cases of non-sexually transmitted epididymitis caused by enteric pathogens, investigation for underlying lower urinary tract pathology, such as bladder outflow obstruction, should be undertaken once the patient has fully recovered. Appropriate investigations include flowmetry, renal tract USS, and possibly flexible cystoscopy.

Further reading

British Association for Sexual Health and HIV. Guidelines for the management of epididymo-orchitis, 2010. Available at: http://www.bashh.org/guidelines [Online].

Dell'Atti L, Fabiani A, Marconi A, *et al.* Reliability of echo-color-Doppler in the differential diagnosis of the "acute scrotum". Our experience. *Arch Ital Urol Androl* 2005; **77**:66–8.

Grabe M, Bjerklund-Johansen TE, Botto H, *et al.* Guidelines on urological infections. European Association of Urology, 2011. Available at: http://www.uroweb.org/guidelines/online-guidelines [Online].

Gupta RK, Best J, MacMahon E. Mumps and the UK epidemic 2005. *BMJ* 2005; **330**:1132–5.

Health Protection Agency. Tuberculosis case reports by site of disease, England 1999–2007. Available at: http://www.hpa.org.uk [Online].

Nicholson A, Rait G, Murray-Thomas T, *et al.* Management of epididymo-orchitis in primary care: results from a large UK primary care database. *Br J Gen Pract* 2010; **60**(579):407–22.

Robinson AJ, Grant JB, Spencer RC, *et al.* Acute epididymitis: why patient and consort must be investigated. *Br J Urol* 1990; **66**(6):642–5.

Workowski KA, Berman S. Centers for Disease Control and Prevention (CDC). Sexually transmitted diseases treatment guidelines, 2010. *MMWR Recomm Rep* 2010; **59**(RR-12):1–110.

References

1. Simms I, Fleming DM, Lowndes CM, *et al.* Surveillance of sexually transmitted diseases in general practice: a description of trends in the Royal College of General Practitioners Weekly Returns Service between 1994 and 2001. *Int J STD AIDS* 2006; **17**(10):693–8.

2. Nicholson A, Rait G, Murray-Thomas T, *et al.* Management of epididymo-orchitis in primary care: results from a large UK primary care database. *Br J Gen Pract* 2010; **60**(579):407–22.
3. Workowski KA, Berman S; Centers for Disease Control and Prevention (CDC). Sexually transmitted diseases treatment guidelines, 2010. *MMWR Recomm Rep* 2010; **59**(RR-12):1–110.
4. Health Protection Agency. Tuberculosis case reports by site of disease, England 1999–2007. Available at: http://www.hpa.org.uk [Online].
5. Viswaroop BS, Kekre N, Goplalkrishnan G. Isolated tuberculous epididymitis: a review of 40 cases. *J Postgrad Med* 2005; **51**(2):109–11.
6. Harada H, Seki M, Shinojima H, *et al.* Epididymo-orchitis caused by intravesically instillated bacillus Calmette-Guerin: genetically proven using a multiplex polymerase chain reaction method. *Int J Urol* 2006; **13**(2):183–5.
7. Gupta RK, Best J, MacMahon E. Mumps and the UK epidemic 2005. *BMJ* 2005; **330**:1132–5.
8. Gabal-Shehab LL, Monga M. Recurrent bilateral amiodarone induced epididymitis. *J Urol* 1999; **161**:921.
9. Kaklamani VG, Vaiopoulos G, Markomichelakis N, *et al.* Recurrent epididymo-orchitis in patients with Behcet's disease. *J Urol* 2000; **163**:487–9.
10. Cho YH, Jung J, Lee KH, *et al.* Clinical features of patients with Behcet's disease and epididymitis. *J Urol* 2003; **170**:1231–3.
11. Lee JS, Choi SK. Acute scrotum in 7 cases of Schoenlein-Henoch syndrome. *Yonsei Med J* 1998; **39**:73–8.
12. Shah J, Qureshi I, Ellis BW. Acute idiopathic scrotal oedema in an adult: a case report. *Int J Clin Pract* 2004; **58**:1168–9.
13. Dell'Atti L, Fabiani A, Marconi A, *et al.* Reliability of echo-color-Doppler in the differential diagnosis of the "acute scrotum". Our experience. *Arch Ital Urol Androl* 2005; **77**:66–8.
14. Grabe M, Bjerklund-Johansen TE, Botto H, *et al.* Guidelines on urological infections. European Association of Urology, 2011. Available at: http://www.uroweb.org/guidelines/online-guidelines [Online].
15. NICE clinical guideline 117. Tuberculosis: Clinical diagnosis and management of tuberculosis, and measures for its prevention and control, March 2011. Available at: https://www.nice.org.uk/guidance/CG117 [Online].
16. Moore CA, Lockett BL, Lennox KW, *et al.* Prednisolone in the treatment of acute epididymitis: a comparative study. *J Urol* 1971; **106**:578–80.
17. Nickel JC. Chronic epididymitis: a practical approach to understanding and managing a difficult urologic enigma. *Rev Urol* 2003; **5**:209–15.
18. British Association for Sexual Health and HIV. Guidelines for the management of epididymo-orchitis, 2010. Available at: http://www.bashh.org/guidelines [Online].
19. Robinson AJ, Grant JB, Spencer RC, *et al.* Acute epididymitis: why patient and consort must be investigated. *Br J Urol* 1990; **66**(6):642–5.

CHAPTER 1.9

Inflammation

Fournier's gangrene

Francesco Greco and Paolo Fornara

Introduction to Fournier's gangrene

Fournier's gangrene (FG) defines a life-threatening, rapidly progressive, necrotizing fasciitis of the external genitalia and perineum, which can extend up to the abdominal wall between fascial planes. It was first described in 1883 by Jean Alfred Fournier, a French dermatologist and venereologist, who reported a series of five men with fatal gangrene of the genitalia.[1]

In current practice, mortality has reduced and most cases occur in elderly men with an identifiable cause such as anorectal sepsis or urogenital trauma associated with infection and an underlying immunodeficiency.[2,3] The number of cases is increasing due to population ageing, the higher prevalence of diabetes, and the wider use of immunosuppressive treatment.

Despite advances in intensive care, FG remains a serious and potentially lethal condition due to progressive and overwhelming infection-related necrosis with mortality rates of 7–45%.[4–6] The heterogeneity of FG presentation makes it difficult to guide clinical practice.[7] Clinicians therefore need to be alert to consider and make the diagnosis, particularly in elderly men presenting with non-specific signs and symptoms.

Epidemiology

Fournier's gangrene is rare, with an approximate overall incidence of 1.6 per 100,000 males per year. A registry study from the United States showed a male:female ratio of 40:1.[6] The lower incidence in females may relate to better drainage of the perineal region through vaginal secretions. The incidence increases with age peaking at 50 years with 3.3 cases per 100,000 males per year.

There is a geographical bias in the United States with the highest incidence in the south, and lowest in the west and midwest. This may be related to prevalence of diabetes with an estimated increase in incidence of FG of 0.2/100,000 males for each 1% increase in diabetes prevalence.[6] Male homosexuals may be at higher risk, especially to resistant bacterial strains.[8] Fournier's gangrene in a patient with acquired immune deficiency syndrome (AIDS) was first reported in 1991 with 12 subsequent case reports.[9] It has been suggested that HIV-induced immunosuppression can contribute to progression from minor perianal infections to FG.[10]

Aetiology

Triggering event

The necrotizing process commonly originates from an infection in the anorectum, urogenital tract, or skin of the genitalia.[11] The triggering event may relate to accidental or surgical trauma, the presence of foreign material, perianal or perirectal abscess, colonic perforation, urethral stricture with urinary extravasation, and epididymo-orchitis.[4] In women cases have been reported related to septic abortions, vulval or Bartholin gland abscess, and hysterectomy, while in children, strangulated inguinal hernia, circumcision, urethral instrumentation, perirectal abscess, systemic infections, and burns have all led to the disease.[8] Poor perineal hygiene or the presence of long-term indwelling catheters, such as in patients with paraplegia, also pose an increased risk.[4,5,8,11]

Microbiology

Fournier's gangrene is typically a polymicrobial infection. *Escherichia coli* is the predominant aerobe, and *Bacteroides spp.* the predominant anaerobe. Other organisms commonly present are Gram-negative rods such as *Proteus sp.*, *Pseudomonas sp.* and *Klebsiella sp.*, and Gram-positive cocci such as *Staphylococcus sp.* (including methicillin-resistant *Staphylococcus aureus* (MRSA)), *Enterococcus sp.*, aerobic and anaerobic *Streptococcus sp.*, together with *Clostridium sp.*[8,11,12]

Predisposition

Any condition resulting in immune deficiency may predispose a patient to the development of FG. Diabetes mellitus is present in up to 60% of cases, and alcoholism, extremes of age, malignancy, chronic steroid use, cytotoxic drugs, lymphoproliferative disease, malnutrition and human immunodeficiency virus (HIV) infection have all been implicated.[8,11]

Pathophysiology

The disease initially causes necrosis of the skin, fascia of the scrotum, penis, and perineum with subsequent spread through fascial planes to the pelvis and abdomen. This process leads to blood stream infection, disturbance of the microcirculation, and circulatory collapse. The aetiologic factors allow the entry of microorganism into the perineum. Compromised immunity provides a favourable environment to initiate the infection, and the virulence of the microorganism promotes the rapid spread of the disease. Bacterial virulence results from the production of toxins or enzymes that create an environment conducive to rapid multiplication and spread along tissue planes amplified by synergistic activity of the mixed bacterial population.[8] These include thrombosis disrupting local blood supply and leading to tissue hypoxia, facilitating further growth of facultative anaerobes and microaerophilic organisms, and lecithinases and collagenases which digest fascial barriers, opening the way to rapid extension of the infection. For this reason, testicular involvement is rare in Fournier's gangrene given its separate blood supply.[13] Severe or fulminant Fournier's gangrene can spread from the fascia, enveloping the genitalia throughout the perineum, into the pelvis, along the trunk, and thighs.

Clinical presentation

Fournier's gangrene typically begins with pruritus and discomfort of the external genitalia. The visible lesion is generally on the penis, scrotum, or perineum (Fig. 1.9.1). It is important to be aware that the appearance of skin overlying the affected region may vary with normal, erythematous, oedematous, cyanotic, blistered, and gangrenous changes all being seen (Table 1.9.1). At the time of presentation to hospital, there is often associated oedema, scrotal pain, crepitus, feculent odour and either fever over 38°C or hypothermia, together with systemic signs of circulatory disturbance.[11]

Diagnosis

Diagnosis of FG is made in a clinical setting, considering the history and findings on examination. Urinalysis and blood investigations can identify associated factors such as diabetes and demonstrate raised inflammatory markers. Bacteriological evaluation of fluid from the lesion, urine, and blood are required to help guide later antibiotic therapy. Imaging can help determine the likely extent of disease, but is not a substitute for surgical exploration. The most useful modality is computed tomography (CT). This can identify soft tissue thickening, fluid collection or abscess, fat stranding around involved structures, and subcutaneous emphysema along fascial planes. The underlying cause may also be demonstrated.[14] Possible alternative diagnoses include scrotal injury, strangulated scrotal hernia, and inflammatory disease.[14]

Multimodality therapy

Immediate resuscitation

Fournier's gangrene is a surgical emergency. Delay in first debridement of a necrotizing tissue infection worsens outcome.[5,15] Early

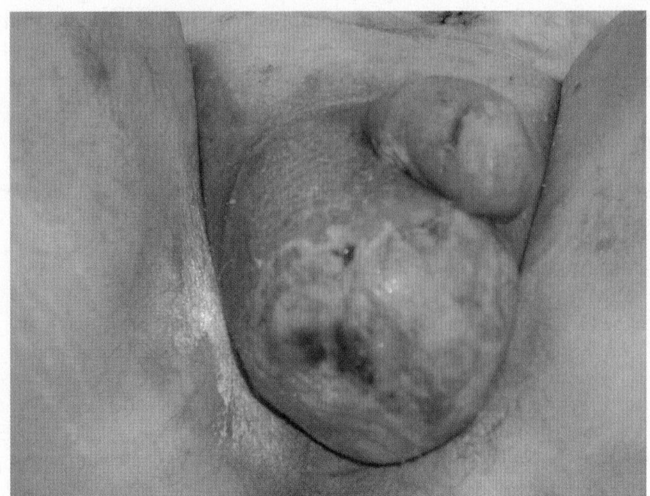

Fig. 1.9.1 Necrosis of the scrotal skin.

Table 1.9.1 Localization and symptoms of Fournier's gangrene

Localization	Percentage of cases (%)
Penis and scrotum	44
Scrotum and perineum	56
Symptoms	
Scrotal oedema	61
Scrotal pain	83
Signs	
Crepitus	53.6
Feculent odour	100
Fever >38°C	26.8
Leucocytosis	85.4

Reproduced with permission from Wagner S *et al.*, 'Is intensive multimodality therapy the best treatment for Fournier gangrene? Evaluation of clinical outcome and survival rate of 41 patients', *Surgical Infection*, Volume 12, Issue 5, pp. 379–83, Copyright © 2011 Mary Ann Liebert, Inc. Publishers, DOI:10.1089/sur.2010.091

admission, rapid diagnosis, and effective treatment are crucial components in achieving a successful outcome. Immediate treatment includes resuscitative measures such as correction of hypovolaemia and hypoperfusion, empirical broad-spectrum parenteral antimicrobial therapy, oxygen, and analgesia.[8] The antibiotic regimen will depend on local guidance but will typically include:

- a penicillin against streptococci;
- metronidazole against anaerobes;
- a cephalosporin combined with gentamicin against Gram-negative organisms.

Surgical debridement

Urinary diversion via a suprapubic cystostomy is appropriate for FG affecting the penis or urethra. Use of catheterization or colostomy should be pragmatic, and guided by the patient's individual cirumstances.[8] Surgical therapy remains the most immediate and necessary step for successful treatment of FG, preferably performed when the disease is still localized, and will involve extensive debridement of the necrotic scrotum and postoperative placement of an occlusive dressing with or without negative pressure drainage (Figs 1.9.2 and 1.9.3).[11] Tissue should be sent for microbiological culture and histology.

A 'second look' under general anaesthesia should be performed within 48 hours and further debridement performed if needed. Orchidectomy can occasionally be required if the testis become gangrenous[3] and similarly, although involvement of the corpora cavernosa is rare, thrombosis and subsequent need for debridement has been described.[16] Repeated debridement should then be continued at appropriate intervals until all necrotic tissue has been removed and the wound is starting to granulate.

Adjunctive therapies

Antibiotic regimen should be refined in the light of culture results and step-down to oral therapy instituted according to local guidance. A number of other adjunctive treatments have been trialled, but there is no high-level evidence to support their routine use.

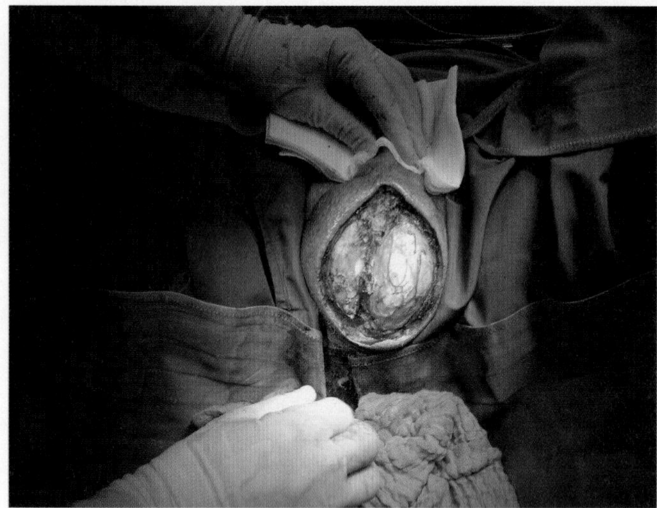

Fig. 1.9.2 Appearance of scrotum after radical debridement.

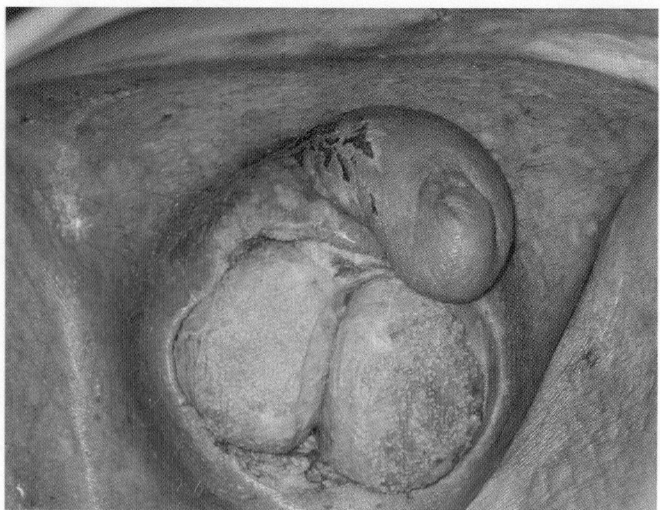

Fig. 1.9.4 Active wound granulation ready for flap or graft reconstruction.

These treatments include hyperbaric oxygen therapy,[3,17–19] which aims to increase tissue oxygenation to inhibit anaerobic bacteria while limiting necrosis and enhancing demarcation of gangrene,[8] and pooled immunoglobulin therapy.

Reconstruction

The often extensive loss of scrotal skin requires primary closure, secondary healing, or more commonly plastic reconstruction using flaps or grafts (Fig. 1.9.4).

Prognosis

Early diagnosis and immediate extensive surgical debridement with broad-spectrum empirical antibiotics and fluid resuscitation represent the main steps in achieving a successful outcome and increasing the chance of patient survival. Mortality risk can be semi-objectively evaluated and patients categorized using the Fournier's gangrene severity index (FGSI), which includes nine metabolic and physiologic parameters and assigns severity scores for abnormal values.[20] In a validation study, the originators identified a value of 9 as being a critical threshold, with scores >9 suggesting a 75% probability of death and scores ≤9 associated with a 78% probability of survival.[20] Subsequent studies were unable to reproduce this predictive value.[5] Other factors associated with poor prognosis include an anorectal source, advanced age, diabetes, extensive disease (involving abdominal wall or thighs), septic shock at presentation, renal failure, and hepatic dysfunction. The mortality of 7–45% usually results from systemic effects such as sepsis, coagulopathy, diabetic ketoacidosis, or acute renal failure leading to multiple organ failure.[3,4,8]

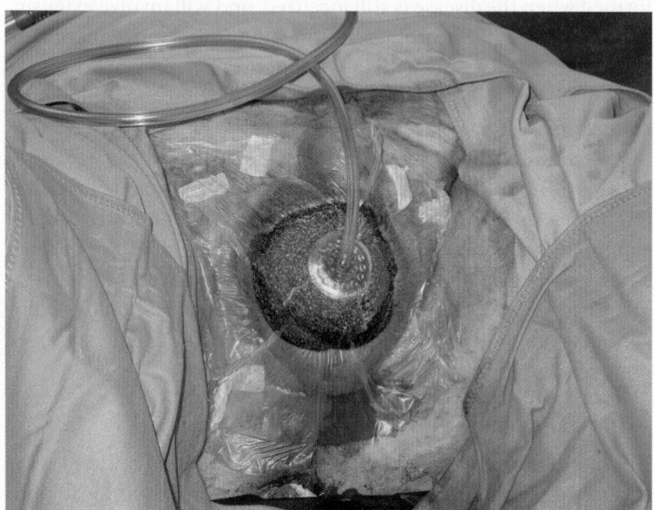

Fig. 1.9.3 Application of negative pressure dressing to debrided wound.

Conclusion

Despite the development of modern intensive care and antibiotic therapy, Fournier's gangrene remains a fulminant and life-threatening disease, with a high mortality. Poor prognosis has been demonstrated in patients with clinical and biochemical evidence of severe sepsis. Early diagnosis and immediate aggressive multimodality therapy with surgical debridement and broad-spectrum empirical antibiotics is crucial to improve survival in patients with necrotizing infections. The role of adjuncts such as hyperbaric oxygen remains unproven.

Further reading

Corcoran AT, Smaldone MC, Gibbons EP, *et al.* Validation of the Fournier's Gangrene Severity Index in a large contemporary series. *J Urol* 2008; **180**:944–8.

Eke N. Fournier's gangrene: A review of 1,726 cases. *Br J Surg* 2000; **87**:718–21.

Grabe M, Bjerklund-Johansen TE, Botto H, *et al.* Guidelines on urological infections. European Association of Urology, 2011. Available at: http://www.uroweb.org/guidelines/online-guidelines [Online].

Laor E, Palmer LS, Tolia BM, *et al.* Outcome prediction in patients with Fournier's gangrene. *J Urol* 1995; **154**:89–92.

Mindrup SR, Kealey GP, Fallon B. Hyperbaric oxygen for the treatment of Fournier's gangrene. *J Urol* 2005; **173**:1975–7.

Sorensen MD, Krieger JN, Rivara FP, *et al.* Fournier's Gangrene: population based epidemiology and outcomes. *J Urol* 2009; **181**:2120–6.

Tuncel A, Aydin O, Tekdogan U, *et al.* Fournier's gangrene: three years of experience with 20 patients and validity of the Fournier's gangrene Severity Index Score. *Eur Urol* 2006; **50**:838–43.

Wagner S, Greco F, Hoda MR, Kawan F, Heynemann H, Fornara P: Is intensive multimodality therapy the best treatment for Fournier gangrene? Evaluation of clinical outcome and survival rate of 41 patients. *Surg Infec* 2011; **12**(5):379–83.

References

1. Fournier JA. Gangrène foudroyante de la verge. *Semin Med* 1883; 3:345–8.
2. Corman JM. Classic articles in colonic and rectal surgery. *Dis Colon Rectum* 1988; **31**:984–8.
3. Eke N. Fournier's gangrene: A review of 1,726 cases. *Br J Surg* 2000; **87**:718–21.
4. Yanar H, Taviloglu K, Ertekin C, *et al.*: Fournier's gangrene: risk factors and strategies for management. *World J Surg* 2006; **30**:1750–4.
5. Tuncel A, Aydin O, Tekdogan U, *et al.* Fournier's gangrene: three years of experience with 20 patients and validity of the Fournier's gangrene Severity Index Score. *Eur Urol* 2006; **50**:838–43.
6. Sorensen MD, Krieger JN, Rivara FP, *et al.* Fournier's Gangrene: population based epidemiology and outcomes. *J Urol* 2009; **181**:2120–6.
7. Chawla SN, Gallop C, Mydlo JH. Fournier's gangrene: an analysis of repeated surgical debridement. *Eur Urol* 2003; **43**:572–5.
8. Eke N, Raphael JE. Fournier's gangrene. (Chapter 4, pp. 37–48) In: Vitin A (ed). *Gangrene—Current Concepts and Management Options*. Rijeka, Croatia: InTech, 2011.
9. Roca B, Cuñat E, Simòn E. HIV infection presenting with Fournier's gangrene. *Neth J Med* 1998; **53**:168–71.
10. Merino E, Boix V, Portilla J, *et al.* Fournier's gangrene in HIV-infected patients. *Eur J Clin Microbiol Infect Dis* 2001; **20**:910–13.
11. Wagner S, Greco F, Hoda MR, Kawan F, Heynemann H, Fornara P: Is intensive multimodality therapy the best treatment for Fournier gangrene? Evaluation of clinical outcome and survival rate of 41 patients. *Surg Infec* 2011; **12**(5):379–83.
12. Grabe M, Bjerklund-Johansen TE, Botto H, *et al.* Guidelines on urological infections. European Association of Urology, 2011. Available at: http://www.uroweb.org/guidelines/online-guidelines [Online].
13. Gupta A, Dalela D, Sankhwar S, *et al.* Bilateral testicular gangrene: does it occur in Fournier's gangrene? *Int Urol Nephrol* 2007; **39**:913–15.
14. Kearney D. Fournier's gangrene: diagnostic and therapeutic considerations (Chapter 2, pp. 19–28) In: Vitin A (ed). *Gangrene—Current Concepts and Management Options*. Rijeka, Croatia: InTech, 2011.
15. Elliott DC, Kufera JA, Myers RAM. Necrotizing soft tissue infections: risk factors for mortality and strategies for management. *Ann Surg* 1996; **224**:672–83.
16. Campos J, Martos J. Synchronous caverno-spongious thrombosis and Fournier's gangrene. *Arch Esp Urol* 1990; **43**:423.
17. Corcoran AT, Smaldone MC, Gibbons EP, *et al.* Validation of the Fournier's Gangrene Severity Index in a large contemporary series. *J Urol* 2008; **180**:944–8.
18. Mindrup SR, Kealey GP, Fallon B. Hyperbaric oxygen for the treatment of Fournier's gangrene. *J Urol* 2005; **173**:1975–7.
19. Pizzorno R, Bonini F, Donelli A, *et al.* Hyperbaric oxygen therapy in the treatment of Fournier's disease in 11 male patients. *J Urol* 1997; **158**:837–40.
20. Laor E, Palmer LS, Tolia BM, *et al.* Outcome prediction in patients with Fournier's gangrene. *J Urol* 1995; **154**:89–92.

CHAPTER 1.10

Sexually transmitted infection

Emma J. McCarty and Wallace Dinsmore

Introduction to sexually transmitted infections

The term venereal disease has been replaced by sexually transmitted infection (STI). These infections frequently present to urology departments. In the United Kingdom, they are usually investigated in genitourinary medicine clinics and in Europe by dermatovenereologists. In the United States, infectious diseases physicians investigate these conditions but the majority of patients are treated in primary care. The aim of this chapter is to outline the major STIs and indicate how they may be relevant to the practice of urologists.

Sexually transmitted infections are extremely common, with approximately 448 million infections being diagnosed globally per year.[1] These include 12 million cases of syphilis, 92 million of chlamydia, 62 million of gonorrhoea, and 174 million of trichomonas. In addition, there were an estimated 34 million people living with human immunodeficiency virus (HIV) in 2010, with approximately 2.7 million new HIV infections diagnosed annually.[2] It is important to note that HIV and syphilis in particular can mimic many other pathological processes and should be included in many urological differential diagnoses. Later consequences of STIs, particularly urethral stricture and infertility, will also require assessment and treatment. A working knowledge of STIs and the ability to take a considered and careful sexual history is therefore essential for all those practising in the field of urology.

Non-specific urethritis

Non-specific genital infection refers to a urethral discharge which is not caused by *Neisseria gonorrhoea* (i.e. non-gonococcal). This is frequently caused by chlamydia (approximately 50%) and a range of various other organisms including ureaplasma, mycoplasma, bacterial vaginosis, candida, and herpes simplex.[3]

Symptoms

A urethral discharge occurs in the majority of males, which may be clear or mucoid. This discharge may be minimal and present only as a slight moistness. It is frequently accompanied by redness of the urethral meatus and dysuria. There may be a history of a new sexual partner within the previous two to three weeks. This condition frequently presents to urology services and will often lead to cystoscopy as part of the investigative pathway for dysuria. A careful sexual history will enable the patient to be more appropriately investigated and managed.

Investigation

A loop may be inserted into the urethral meatus to sample the discharge. A Gram stain is conducted, with the presence of more than five pus cells per high power field (×1,000 magnification) confirming the diagnosis in the absence of *Neisseria gonorrhoea*. Detection of specific DNA segments from *Chlamydia trachomatis* and *Neisseria gonorrhoea* using polymerase chain reaction (PCR) on a urine sample is now part of the standard investigation of this condition. Midstream specimen of urine is frequently taken if urinary tract infection is suspected; however, this is usually negative in non-specific urethritis.

Management

Patients should be advised to abstain from sexual intercourse until the infection is treated in the patient and their partner. All sexual partners should be contacted and are treated empirically regardless of their symptoms or laboratory results. The treatment of choice is azithromycin 1 g as a single oral dose or doxycycline 100 mg twice daily for seven days. In some cases the condition may be persistent or relapsing without a new sexual risk and despite adequate initial treatment. It may be diagnosed by symptoms and the continuing presence of leucocytes on a Gram stain. Recurrence should be treated by azithromycin 500 mg as a single oral dose, followed by 250 mg once daily for six days, together with metronidazole 400 mg twice daily for one week.

Chlamydia trachomatis

Aetiology

Chlamydia trachomatis is the commonest bacterial sexually transmitted infection worldwide. Its prevalence among sexually active individuals in the United Kingdom is 1.6%–12.7%, with the highest incidence in females aged 16–19 and males aged 20–24 years. Risk factors for chlamydial infection are being under 25 years of age, having a new sexual partner in the last year, ethnic minority status, and inconsistent condom use. Transmission of chlamydia after a single episode of unprotected penetrative sex is approximately 10%. It can infect a number of sites including the genitalia, nasopharynx, rectum, and conjunctiva.

Symptoms and signs

Genital infection

- **Female**
  - 70% asymptomatic
  - Symptoms include post-coital/intermenstrual bleeding, lower abdominal pain, increased vaginal discharge, and dysuria
  - Signs may include mucopurulent cervicitis (mucopurulent discharge and friability of cervix) on vaginal speculum examination

- **Male**
  - 50% asymptomatic
  - Symptoms include dysuria and urethral discharge
  - Signs may include cloudy or clear urethral discharge and erythema of urethral meatus

Rectal infection

- Usually asymptomatic but may cause anal discharge and proctitis

Pharyngeal infection

- Usually asymptomatic

Conjunctival infection

- Concomitant anogenital infection in 60–70%
- Usually a unilateral conjunctivitis caused by direct or manual transfer of genital chlamydial infection to the eye

Complications

Pelvic inflammatory disease (PID) will occur in 10–40% of untreated chlamydial infection in women. This can result in infertility, ectopic pregnancy, and chronic pelvic pain syndrome. The risk of PID increases with each episode of chlamydia infection.[3,4]

- Fitz-Hugh-Curtis syndrome (perihepatitis)
- Epididymo-orchitis in men
- Sexually acquired reactive arthritis (Reiter's syndrome)

Investigation

Nucleic acid amplification tests (NAAT) are routinely used for the diagnosis of chlamydia. This method is more sensitive (90–100%) and specific (99%) than the previously available tests, such as culture (Fig. 1.10.1). Testing is non-invasive using a first void urine sample for males and an endocervical swab (or self-taken vulvo-vaginal swab) from females. Other sites which can be swabbed for chlamydia infection using NAAT test include the rectum and throat.

Management

The following are recommended antibiotics for the treatment of chlamydial infection:

First line: Azithromycin 1 g orally single dose*
Doxycycline 100 mg orally twice daily for 7 days

Alternative: Erythromycin 500mg orally twice daily for 10–14 days*
Ofloxacin 200 mg orally twice daily or 400 mg once daily for 7 days

*Recommended treatment in pregnancy

A test of cure is not routinely recommended following treatment, unless the patient is pregnant or there is reason to suspect reacquisition or poor adherence to treatment. Patients should be advised to abstain from sexual intercourse (including oral sex) for one week after both they and their partner are treated. Partner notification is extremely important in the management of chlamydia. In symptomatic males, the look-back period is two weeks or until the last sexual partner. In asymptomatic males and all females, the look-back period for contact tracing is three months, or until the last sexual partner.

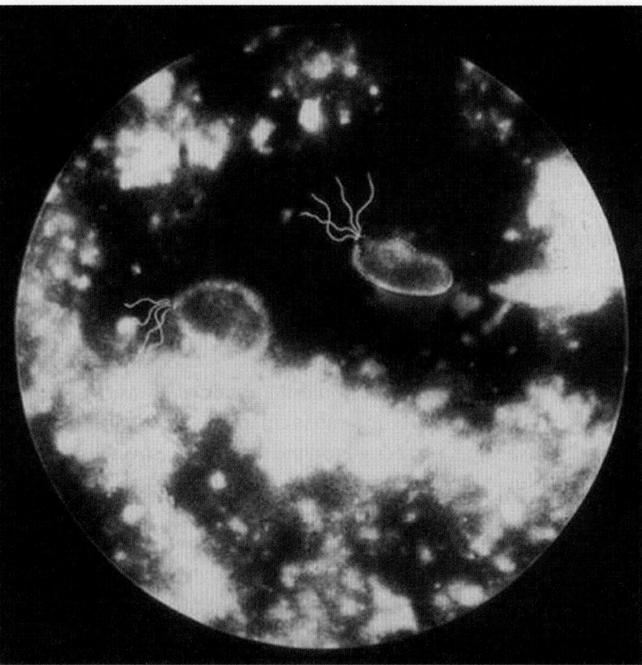

Fig. 1.10.1 Dark-ground trachomatis vaginalis.
Reproduced from Richard Pattman et al. (Eds.), *Oxford Handbook of Genitourinary Medicine, HIV, and Sexual Health, Second Edition*, Plate 8, Oxford University Press, Oxford, UK, Copyright © 2010, with permission from Oxford University Press.

Lymphogranuloma venereum

Aetiology

Lymphogranuloma venereum (LGV) is caused by the invasive serovars (L1-L3) of *Chlamydia trachomatis*. Until 2003, this infection was uncommon outside endemic areas such as South Africa, India, Madagascar, and Caribbean countries. Reports emerged in the last 10 years of outbreaks of LGV proctitis in Europe, primarily among men having sex with men (MSM). These outbreaks tended to occur in white MSMs, often coinfected with HIV. Risk factors included group sex, use of sex toys, and high risk sexual practices such as fisting.

Symptoms and signs

LGV has three clinical stages:

- *Primary*
  A small painless papule appears at the site of inoculation within 3–30 days in 30–50% patients. It may go unnoticed and typically heals without scarring.
- *Secondary* (inguinal syndrome)
  Usually occurs within 1–6 weeks of primary infection, but may be up to 6 months later. The majority (70%) of males with LGV develop unilateral inguinal lymphadenopathy. Only 15–30% females are found to have inguinal lymphadenopathy as lesions in the vulva, vagina, or anus will preferentially drain to pelvic or perirectal nodes. Other symptoms include fever, arthralgia, hepatitis, and skin lesions (erythema nodosum or erythema multiforme).

- *Tertiary* (anorectal syndrome)
  This stage usually occurs in females and MSM as a result of lesions draining into perirectal lymph nodes. Patients present with proctocolitis including rectal discharge, bleeding, pain on defaecation, and constitutional symptoms such as fever and malaise.

Complications

Chronic untreated infection may lead to fistula formation, strictures, abscesses, and scarring. Lymphoedema of the external genitalia may occur and may lead to elephantiasis.

Diagnosis

A swab for chlamydia PCR should be obtained from the relevant site (e.g. rectal, throat). If the swab is chlamydia positive and LGV is clinically suspected, further genotypic testing at a specialist laboratory is conducted to confirm the presence of serovars L1–3.

Management

The recommended antibiotic regime is doxycycline 100 mg twice daily for three weeks or erythomycin 500 mg four times daily for three weeks.

Gonorrhoea

Aetiology

Gonorrhoea is caused by *Neisseria gonorrhoea*; a Gram-negative diplococcus found within polymorphs (Fig. 1.10.2). Infection does not confer future immunity and repeated infections are common. Gonorrhoea is often associated with other sexually acquired infections, particularly chlamydia. It is typically transmitted through sexual exposure, although other routes are possible. Gonorrhoea is particularly infectious, with a 60–80% chance of transmission from male to female and a 20% chance from female to male during one episode of sex. Rates of gonorrhoea are increasing worldwide, partly due to increasing rates of unsafe sex and also due to increased sensitivity of commercially available tests with more rapid and earlier diagnosis.[4]

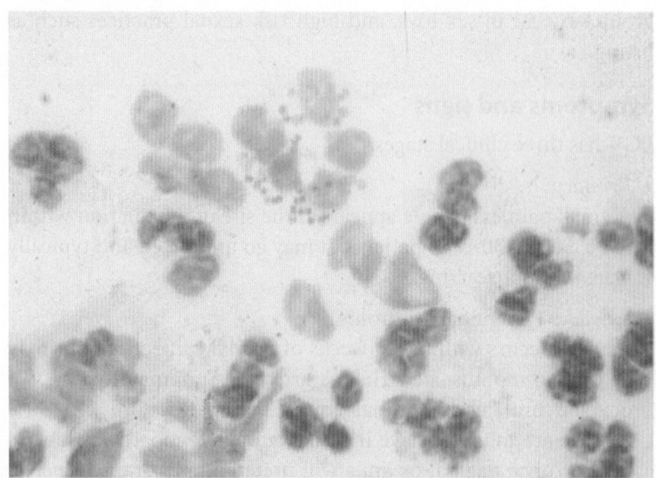

Fig. 1.10.2 Gonorrhoea Gram stain.
Reproduced from Richard Pattman et al. (Eds.), *Oxford Handbook of Genitourinary Medicine, HIV, and Sexual Health, Second Edition*, Plate 6, Oxford University Press, Oxford, UK, Copyright © 2010, with permission from Oxford University Press.

Symptoms and signs

Male:

- Purulent yellow urethral discharge in 80%
- Dysuria in 50–60%
- Symptoms usually occur 2–8 days after sexual exposure

Female:

- Over 50% of females are asymptomatic
- Increased vaginal discharge
- Dysuria
- Lower abdominal pain 20%
- Irregular menstrual bleeding

Other sites for infection include phaynx, rectum, and conjunctiva. Pharyngeal infection is usually asymptomatic and detected through routine screening in high risk groups. Rectal infection will result in symptoms in approximately 15%, including anal discharge, pruritis, tenesmus, and bleeding. Conjunctival infection presents as unilateral or bilateral inflammation and discharge; if untreated, this can lead to blindness.

Diagnosis

In a symptomatic patient, a swab is taken from the relevant site (urethra, endocervix, or rectum), and microscopy following Gram-staining may show classical Gram-negative intracellular (within polymorphs) diplococci. Culture using the appropriate medium will enable antibiotic sensitivities to be obtained. This is particularly important due to increasing worldwide resistance to most antibiotics. More recently, PCR testing using gonorrhoea NAAT has become available. This has much greater sensitivity than culture, particularly for specimens obtained from the pharynx and the rectum. It has resulted in greater ease in testing for gonorrhoea—swabs should be taken from the cervix, throat, and rectum, and a first void specimen of urine to detect urethral infection.

Treatment

The recommended treatment at present is ceftriaxone 500 mg intramuscular.[5] A single dose of 1 g azithromycin orally should also be given regardless of chlamydia detection result. It is important to obtain culture from the site of gonorrhoea prior to antibiotic treatment. A test of cure is carried out at least two weeks after completion of treatment.

Complications

There are numerous complications associated with gonorrhoea infection, including perihepatitis, septic arthritis, prostatitis, urethral stricture, epididymal obstruction, and pelvic inflammatory disease.

Anogenital warts

Aetiology

Genital warts are the most frequently diagnosed STI in developed countries. There are over 100 different genotypes of human papilloma virus (HPV), however subtypes 6 and 11 account for the majority of cases of genital warts. These are non-oncogenic (or 'low-risk') compared with 'high risk' HPV types 16 and 18, which are detected in >95% of cervical neoplasms. Genital HPV DNA may be found in 10–20% of young sexually active adults; however, only approximately 1 in 10 of these individuals will develop genital warts. The lifetime risk of carrying at least one HPV subtype is thought to be as high as 80%. Smoking increases the risk of HPV infection and also results in higher recurrence rates. Transmission of HPV virus is primarily through sexual activity (including non-penetrative contact), however perinatal and digital–genital transmission may occur. The median incubation period is three months, but may be significantly longer. Warts are usually evident in areas where friction or abrasion occurs during intercourse (see Fig. 1.10.3).

Symptoms and signs

Warts do not generally cause discomfort but occasionally itching may be reported. Lesions may be disfiguring and often cause significant psychological distress. The appearance is variable and often depends on the affected site. Soft, fleshy warts (condylomata acuminata) are often seen moist skin such as the glans penis, female introitus, and anal margin. Keratinized warts usually occur on the dry skin of penile shaft, perineum, or perianal area. *Giant condylomata of Buschke and Lowenstein* is an eponymous term for warts which begin as a keratotic papule and progress into a very large cauliflower-shaped lesion. These are diagnosed histologically and should be completely excised, as malignant transformation occurs in up to 50%.

Diagnosis

The presence of genital warts is a clinical diagnosis. If the appearances are atypical and there is uncertainty, a biopsy can be obtained under local anaesthetic for histology.

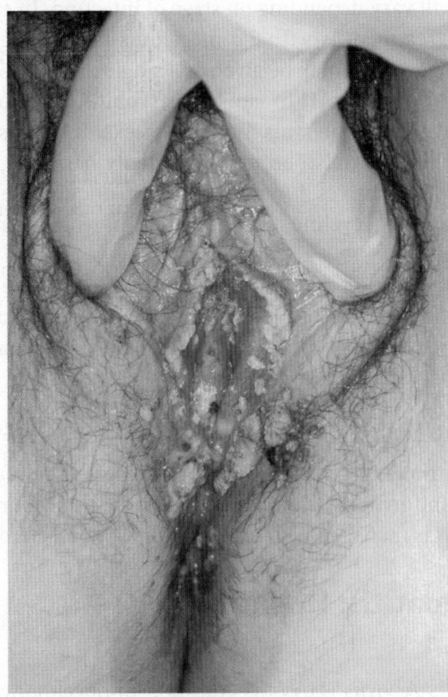

Fig. 1.10.3 Presentation of vulval warts.
Image reproduced courtesy of the CDC/Joe Millar, ID#: 4097, available from http://phil.cdc.gov/phil/quicksearch.asp

Treatment

Treatment is primarily for cosmetic purposes and relapse rates are high. Topical agents such as podophyllotoxin cream or imiquimod 5% are often used in combination with cryotherapy. Other treatment modalities include ablation with cryotherapy, cautery, trichloroacetic acid, or surgical excision. Condom use is recommended while warts are being treated, and for six months after clearance with any new sexual partner or if sex has always been protected with the present partner. No contact tracing is required as HPV is highly prevalent and usually asymptomatic.

Anogenital herpes

The herpes simplex virus (HSV) is a double-stranded DNA virus which is classified as either type I or type II. Traditionally type I causes oral lesions and type II causes genital lesions. The virus is passed usually through sexual intercourse, but may also frequently pass during oral sex from an oral cold sore to the genital area. Genital herpes is a distressing diagnosis because it is often exquisitely painful, associated with relapses, and is likely to result in psychological problems along with the break-up of relationships. In some cases, it can cause infections of the neonate.

Symptoms

The first attack of genital herpes is associated with multiple painful ulcers, which usually occur on the penis or vulva (unlike the classically painless syphilitic ulcer). There is frequently systemic illness, with fever and flu-like illness with headache and photophobia. These symptoms occur 6–12 days after sexual contact or exposure, and last for about 10–12 days. There is frequently tender inguinal lymphadenopathy. Rarely, urinary retention occurs as a result of pain passing urine over the lesions, and this may require suprapubic catheterization. Recurrent lesions are not due to re-infection, but are a consequence of the primary infections. They are more common in HSV2 (90%) than HSV1 (60%). Recurrent attacks tend to be less severe than primary attacks and usually occur a few months after the primary attack.

Diagnosis

The diagnosis is generally a clinical diagnosis supported by a swab for HSV PCR taken from the wet ulcers.

Management

The initial management is with analgesia and saline washes. In rare cases hospitalization is required for urinary retention. Antivirals should be given within five days of lesions appearing and continued for five days. The normal doses are aciclovir 200 mg five times daily, famciclovir 250 mg three times daily, or valaciclovir 500 mg twice daily. Recurrent attacks may necessitate suppressive therapy for 6–12 months if they occur more than six times per year. Usual treatment for recurrent herpes would be aciclovir 400 mg twice daily, famciclovir 250 mg twice daily, or valaciclovir 500 mg twice daily. The condition is frequently associated with emotional issues, particularly if recurrent. Therefore, voluntary bodies that offer support and counselling may play a useful role in dealing with the distress of this condition. The Herpes Association is the largest group for this purpose in the United Kingdom (www.herpes.org.uk).

Syphilis

Syphilis is becoming much more common in the developed world in recent years and is increasingly prevalent among men having sex with men.[3,4] It is caused by the spirochaete bacterium *Treponema pallidum*. The symptoms of secondary syphilis mimic many other diseases and urologists should consider this in many common presentations if the diagnosis is unclear (see Fig. 1.10.4).

Clinical stages

Acquired syphilis is divided into early syphilis (primary, secondary, or early latent) and late syphilis.

Primary syphilis

Primary syphilis has an incubation period of 9–90 days (mean 21 days). An ulcer which is usually solitary and painless appears at the sight of infection. If the ulcer is left untreated it will resolve in 3–10 weeks.

Secondary syphilis

Secondary syphilis usually presents 4–8 weeks after primary syphilis as a maculopapular rash, which may cover the whole body including the palms of the hands and soles of the feet (see Fig. 1.10.5). Pustular lesions and 'snail track' ulcers may appear in genital areas. Condylomata may mimic genital warts in genital areas. Other features may include constitutional symptoms, alopecia, periosteitis, hepatitis, glomerulonephritis, and iritis.

Early latent syphilis

Early latent syphilis is defined as occurring less than two years from the primary infection and is asymptomatic.

Late syphilis

Syphilis infection that has been present for more than two years is referred to as late syphilis. It may be latent, with no symptoms or sequelae, or may affect other systems such as neurosyphilis, cardiovascular syphilis, or gummatous disease.

Diagnosis

Syphilis is diagnosed by serological testing. There are multiple tests available and different tests are used in different laboratories. Advice and interpretation of syphilis tests should be sought from an expert in laboratory aspects of genitourinary medicine.

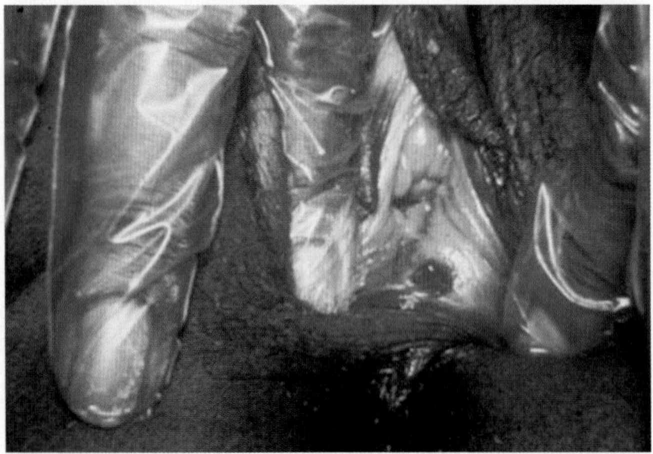

Fig. 1.10.4 Primary syphilitic chancre.
Image reproduced courtesy of the CDC, available from http://phil.cdc.gov/phil/quicksearch.asp

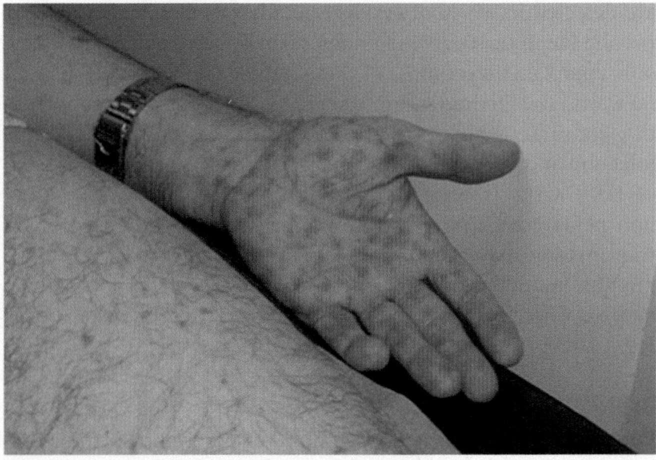

Fig. 1.10.5 Presentation of secondary syphilis.
Reproduced from Richard Pattman et al. (Eds.), *Oxford Handbook of Genitourinary Medicine, HIV, and Sexual Health, Second Edition*, Plate 4, Oxford University Press, Oxford, UK, Copyright © 2010, with permission from Oxford University Press.

In early primary syphilis, *Treponema* may be seen in the serous exudate from the primary ulcer using dark-ground microscopy. In suspected neurosyphilis, cerebrospinal fluid should be obtained and analysed for presence of syphilis. In all cases where there has been a potential exposure to syphilis and initial testing is negative, serology should be repeated at three months to cover the 'window period'.

Treatment

Syphilis infection is sensitive to penicillin which is the first-line treatment, usually by intramuscular injection. Referral should be made to a local genitourinary medicine clinic for management, as treatment will vary depending on stage of infection. In early syphilis, usually treatment is with 2.4 megaunits benzathine penicillin intramuscular, which may be given as a single dose or as two doses repeated one week apart. In late latent syphilis, this dose may be replicated at weekly intervals for three weeks. Intramuscular procaine penicillin may also be used on a daily basis for 17 days as treatment. Alternatives for patients with documented penicillin allergy are doxycycline and azthromycin, which may be given orally.

Partner notification in syphilis is essential. This may be a sensitive area, especially in cases of syphilis diagnosed as part of a dementia screen where children will require testing. This is normally carried out through specialist clinics.

Complications

Jarisch–Herxheimer reaction is a febrile illness with myalgia, rigour, flush, and hypertension, which occurs within hours of initial treatment. It is managed with a short course of oral steroids.

Viral hepatitis: Hepatitis A

Aetiology

The hepatitis A virus (HAV) is common in developing countries with poor sanitation, and immunity approaches 100% in these individuals. Prevalence is much lower in developed countries where the main mode of transmission is usually faeco-oral from contaminated food or water. Outbreaks are known to certain occur in certain populations including MSM, injecting drug users, and those living in institutions. Individuals are infectious for two weeks prior and one week after the onset of symptoms. Lifelong immunity follows resolution of initial infection.

Symptoms and signs

Asymptomatic infection occurs in up to 50% adults. Symptoms usually develop within two to six weeks of exposure and include a prodromal flu-like illness followed by an icteric illness with jaundice, nausea, fatigue, and right upper quadrant pain. Pale stools and dark urine may be reported.

Complications

Fulminant hepatic failure is uncommon (<0.4%) and is more common in those coinfected with hepatitis B or C.

Diagnosis

Serology for HAV IgM will be positive within five days of infection. HAV IgG positivity indicates past infection or immunity from vaccination. Liver transaminases (ALT and AST) and bilirubin may be significantly elevated.

Management

Most individuals can be managed as an outpatient and only require follow-up if liver function tests do not settle within one to two months. General advice should be given to reduce alcohol, abstain from sexual intercourse, and avoid food handling until symptoms settle. Hepatitis A is a notifiable illness and public health will arrange contact tracing of close contacts (household and sexual partners) for testing and vaccination.

Hepatitis B

Aetiology

Hepatitis B virus is endemic in many parts of the world (especially Southeast Asia) where carriage rates are up to 20%. The seroprevalence in non-endemic settings is 0.01–1% and those at risk include MSM, injecting drug users, and those with sexual contacts from areas where the virus is endemic. It is highly transmissible by mucous membrane contact through peno-vaginal or peno-anal sex. In acute adult infection symptoms are present in up to 50%, with approximately 5% becoming chronic carriers. In children, acute infection is uncommon but the majority (90%) become chronic carriers.

Symptoms and signs

Acute infection is similar to hepatitis A infection. In chronic infection, signs of chronic liver disease may be evident.

Complications

Fulminant hepatitis develops in <1%, but is more common in those coinfected with hepatitis C.

Diagnosis

Serum markers

- Hepatitis B surface antigen (HBsAg): positive in acute and chronic infection, usually within three months of acquisition. It becomes negative if or when infection is cleared.
- Hepatitis B extracellular antigen (HBeAg): if positive indicates high infectivity.
- Hepatitis B surface antibody (HBsAb or anti-HBs): marker of successful vaccination, with titres indicating the level of immunity.
- Liver function tests (LFTs): may be normal or may show elevated transaminases.

Management

General advice to avoid unprotected intercourse until partner is tested and successfully vaccinated. Hepatitis B is a notifiable illness and public health will arrange contact tracing of close household contacts and sexual partners. Referral should be made to hepatology for follow-up and treatment if necessary.

Vaccination schedules for hepatitis A and B

Hepatitis A: 0 and 6–12 months

Hepatitis B: 0, 1, 6 months (standard course)
0, 1, 2 months (rapid course)
0, 1, 3 weeks (ultra-rapid course)

Combined hepatitis A and B: standard course as above

Hepatitis C

Aetiology

Hepatitis C affects over 170 million people worldwide. In the United Kingdom, the prevalence is less than 1% of blood donors but up to 80% in injecting drug users. Sexual transmission is uncommon but is associated with high risk sexual practices such as fisting and oro-anal sex.

Symptoms and signs

Hepatitis C has a long incubation period (4–20 weeks). Acute icteric illness occurs in 20% and is associated with an increased likelihood of clearing the virus.

Complications

Acute fulminate hepatitis failure is rare. Chronic carriage occurs in >80% of those infected. Liver cirrhosis is more rapid in those coinfected with HIV or hepatitis B. There is an increased risk of developing hepatocellular carcinoma.

Diagnosis

Hepatitis C antibody test should be sent and if this is positive, further testing should be conducted with hepatitis C PCR for viral RNA. Antibodies may take up to six months to develop; therefore, serology should be repeated six months after a risk to exclude infection.

Management

Hepatitis C is notifiable. General advice should be given about safe sex, avoiding sharing needles, reducing alcohol intake, and so on. Referral should be made to hepatology for treatment and follow-up. No vaccine is available for close contacts.

Human immunodeficiency virus and acquired immunodeficiency syndrome

Background

HIV is one of the most important communicable diseases, affecting more than 33.3 million people worldwide. It was estimated that there were 86,500 people living with HIV in the United Kingdom at the end of 2010.[6] HIV is transmitted through sexual contact, blood-to-blood contact (e.g. sharing needles, transfusion of infected blood products) and vertically from mother to child transmission. In developing countries, transmission is mostly through heterosexual sex; however, in the United States and Europe, the majority of cases occur in men having sex with men. While effective antiretroviral therapy has resulted in a dramatic reduction of HIV-related deaths, there is still significant mortality associated with those presenting late in the course of their infection.

Natural history of human immunodeficiency virus

HIV is a retrovirus that preferentially infects CD4 lymphocytes. There are several stages of infection as defined by symptoms and CD4 count.

1. **Primary HIV infection (seroconversion)**
   Symptoms occur in 50–90% individuals within five days to four weeks of HIV acquisition. These symptoms may vary from a mild flu-like illness to severe multisystem involvement (e.g. aseptic meningitis). During this stage of viraemia, the individual is highly infectious and at high risk of transmitting the virus to others during sexual contact.
2. **Asymptomatic stage**
   The symptoms of primary infection usually resolve within a few weeks and the asymptomatic stage begins. The individual may remain in good health for several years with no obvious clinical signs or symptoms to prompt testing. Over the course of time, the CD4 count will gradually decrease (usually by 50–100 cells/mm^3 per year).
3. **Symptomatic stage**
   If HIV infection remains undiagnosed, eventually the decline in immune function results in various signs and symptoms evolving including constitutional symptoms (such as weight loss, night sweats, and diarrhoea), or widespread lymphadenopathy. Other conditions such as seborrhoeic dermatitis, recurrent herpes simplex infection, or bacterial pneumonia may prompt diagnosis.
4. **Acquired immune deficiency syndrome**
   Acquired immune deficiency syndrome (AIDS) usually occurs when CD4 count falls to below 200 cells/mm^3. It is characterized by the presence of one or more specific 'AIDS-defining illnesses'. These conditions include opportunistic infections (such as pneumocystis pneumonia, cytomegalovirus, toxoplasmosis, cryptosporidium, oesophageal candidiasis), or certain malignancies (such as Kaposi's sarcoma, non-Hodgkin's lymphoma, cervical, or anal cancer). Significant mortality is still associated with this late stage of infection.

Diagnosing human immunodeficiency virus infection

Testing is recommended in all clinical situations where HIV may fall within the list of differential diagnoses. In addition, UK National Guidelines for HIV testing 2008 recommend routine testing for all individuals who fall into higher-risk groups (e.g. MSM, injecting drug users, those from countries of high HIV prevalence) and in all individuals registering in primary care, or admitted to hospital who live in areas where HIV prevalence exceeds 2 in 1,000.[7]

The majority of commercially available HIV assays detect HIV antibodies and p24 antigen. These combined antibody-antigen tests have resulted in the ability to diagnose HIV infection earlier, and may provide a positive result within 28 days of acquisition. It is however still recommended to repeat the HIV test three months after potential exposure in those at high risk. A positive initial result must always be confirmed with a second sample. When offering an HIV test, no specific pre-test counselling is required. Verbal consent is sufficient prior to testing. It is important to ensure accurate contact details are available to the patients and establish how they may wish to receive the result.

Antiretroviral therapy

In the United Kingdom and Europe, antiretroviral therapy is usually commenced when CD4 count falls to less than 350 cells/mm^3. There are currently six classes of antiretroviral drugs available:

- Nucleoside reverse transcriptase inhibitors (NRTI)
- Non-nucleoside reverse transcriptase inhibitors (NNRTI)
- Protease inhibitors (PI)
- Integrase inhibitors
- Fusion inhibitors
- Entry inhibitors

Prior to commencing treatment, a resistance profile is obtained to ensure the virus is susceptible to all classes of drugs. The rate of acquired HIV resistance is approximately 8% in the United Kingdom, with NNRTI resistance being the most common. Each drug regime is tailored individually for each patient, taking into consideration issues such as pill burden and potential side effects to ensure optimal adherence to therapy. It is important to consider other medications (including over-the-counter or recreational drugs) as there may be significant drug interactions with certain antiretrovirals. Typically patients are treated with a combination of three antiretroviral agents—usually two NRTIs with the third agent either a PI or NNRTI. Response to treatment is monitored by serum HIV viral load, which should be undetectable within six months of commencing treatment.

Relevant drug side effects/toxicities

Antiretroviral drugs have evolved over the last decade with improved tolerability and reduced toxicity. Side effect profiles tend to be class-related, although there are often subtle variations within each drug class. Protease inhibitors are often associated with gastrointestinal upset (e.g. nausea, diarrhoea, bloating); however, this tends to improve after several weeks of therapy. In particular, there are reports of darunavir causing pancreatitis and atazanavir has been associated with renal stones. Tenofovir (belonging to NRTI class) may cause renal tubular dysfunction, and as such, monitoring of renal function, phosphate, and urine protein creatinine ratio is recommended.

Further reading

British HIV Association. Available at: http://www.bhiva.org/Publications.aspx [Online].

British Association of Sexual Health & HIV Guidelines. Available at: http://www.bashh.org/guidelines [Online].

- Management of gonorrhoea, 2011
- Management of chlamydia, 2006
- Management of genital herpes, 2007
- Management of syphilis, 2008
- Management of sexually acquired reactive arthritis, 2008
- UK National Guidelines on HIV testing

Further reading

Pattman R, Snow M, Handy P, Sankar KN, Elawad B (eds). *Oxford Handbook of Genitourinary Medicine, HIV and AIDS*. Oxford, UK: Oxford University Press, 2005.

References

1. World Health Organization, Geneva, 2011. Document freely available on the internet. Available at: http://www.who.int/mediacentre/factsheets/fs110/en/index.html [Online] [Accessed March 2013].
2. UNAIDS 2012 Report on the Global AIDS Epidemic, Geneva, 2012. Document freely available on the internet. Available at: http://www.unaids.org/en/resources/campaigns/20121120_globalreport2012/globalreport [Online] [Accessed March 2013].
3. Pattman R, Snow M, Handy P, Sankar KN, Elawad B (eds). *Oxford Handbook of Genitourinary Medicine, HIV and AIDS*. Oxford, UK: Oxford University Press, 2005.
4. Clutterbuck D. *Specialist Training in Sexually Transmitted Infections & HIV*. Edinburgh/London/New York: Elsevier/Mosby, 2004.
5. Bignell C, FitzGerald M. UK National Guidelines for the management of gonorrhoea in adults. British Association for Sexual Health and HIV, 2011. Document freely available on the internet. Available at: http://www.bashh.org/guidelines [Online] [Accessed March 2013].
6. Health Protection Agency. HIV in the United Kingdom: 2012 Report. London: Health Protection Services, Colindale. November 2012. Document freely available on the internet. Available at: http://www.hpa.org.uk/webc/HPAwebFile/HPAweb_C/1317137200016 [Online] [Accessed March 2013].
7. British Association for Sexual Health and HIV. UK National Guidelines for HIV testing 2008. Document freely available on the internet. Available at: http://www.bashh.org/guidelines [Online] [Accessed March 2013].

CHAPTER 1.11

Bladder pain syndrome
Interstitial cystitis

Magnus Fall

Historical introduction to bladder pain syndrome/interstitial cystitis

The term interstitial cystitis (IC) was introduced by Skene in 1887.[1] However, the physician most associated with initial characterization of the syndrome is Hunner. Over 100 years ago, he described a symptom complex of bladder pain associated with a peculiar cystoscopic feature of mucosal lesions, the 'elusive ulcer', later termed Hunner's ulcer.[2] In 1949, John Hand[3] presented a large series of IC patients. He noted that IC did not comprise just one single entity, but this observation did not attract much attention before Messing and Stamey[4] and Fall *et al.*[5] went into more detail about the variation in individual phenotypes. Messing and Stamey believed that there might be an early form of the disease, displaying what is called submucosal glomerulations: small, dotted, submucosal bleeding points, with no similarity to Hunner's ulcers. They postulated that this entity could eventually progress into the well-known classic disease, while Fall *et al.*[5] and Peeker and Fall[6] maintained that there are separate phenotypes, related by similar symptoms and a chronic course. The latter statement was based on the fact that a progression from an 'early form' to the classic ulcerous form has actually never been reported. Since definition of the generic concept, the scope of IC became wider and more varied, and in order to achieve a standard for use in scientific studies, the US National Institute of Diabetes, Digestive and Kidney disorders (NIDDK) defined a number of criteria mainly based on exclusions.[7] The criteria were also utilized clinically, but were found by many to be too restrictive. Subsequently, IC essentially represented a symptom complex with quite varying contents, an evolution resulting in much confusion in research, and even more in the understanding of how to help sufferers gain symptom relief. Current consensus suggests that the ulcerative form is denoted 'interstitial cystitis' (IC) and the non-ulcerative form 'bladder pain syndrome' (BPS). It is acknowledged that there is overlap with other chronic pain syndromes and functional symptom complexes, both in the pelvic area and elsewhere in the body.

Epidemiology

Reports of the prevalence of BPS/IC have varied tremendously. The first systematic study by Oravisto indicated that IC affected approximately 10/100,000 (18/100,000 for women) in Finland,[8] and a similar prevalence was later described in the United States.[9] However, recent studies suggest that these early figures may be underestimates.[10] A report from the United States indicated that up to 30% of young women may be afflicted.[11] Interestingly, 30 years after the Oravisto study, Leppilahti *et al.*[12] found dramatically higher figures in Finland: the prevalence of clinically confirmed probable IC in women was 230/100,000 and that of possible/probable IC was 530/100,000. Their conclusion was that BPS/IC is substantially more common than was previously thought. When comparing all studies, uncertainty remains about the real prevalence due to varying diagnostic criteria and definitions of the populations at risk.

There is a female:male predominance of about 10:1.[3,8,13] It has been proposed that BPS/IC may have a genetic component, but evidence is conflicting.[14,15] BPS/IC has high economic costs, with an estimated healthcare and personal spend of US$750 million per year in the United States.[16]

Symptom analysis

The characteristic symptoms of pain are perceived in the urinary bladder, in the form of urinary frequency and urgency. Symptoms may fluctuate but there appears to be no evidence of a worsening of overall disease severity over a five-year period.[17] Sometimes the onset is sudden, the condition presenting immediately with a full-blown set of signs and symptoms, and sometimes it is gradual. The median time to diagnosis was four to five years in two different reports.[18,19] The long time lag is thought to be due to the failure of clinicians to appreciate and recognize the typical symptoms.[20] There is no doubt that the key to the diagnosis of BPS/IC is a careful history with identification of the characteristic symptoms, especially the character and severity of bladder pain and discomfort. Bacterial cystitis, prostatitis, endometriosis, and chronic pelvic pain are common alternative causes that need exclusion.

Pain can be localized to the bladder, or rather in the area that the patient perceives as the bladder, or in the lower abdomen and pelvis. The classic description is imperative urge on bladder filling with increasing suprapubic pain, which in many instances is severe, relieved by voiding, although soon returning. Other descriptions of the sensation are 'pressure', 'burning', 'sharp', and 'discomfort'. Typically, the pain is felt in, but is not limited to, the suprapubic region; it can be referred to locations throughout the pelvis, including the urethra, vagina, lower abdomen, lower back, medial aspect of the thigh, and the inguinal area in any combination.[21] Consequently, it is not always obvious that the pain is coming from the bladder. Intercourse, cold, and constrictive clothing can exacerbate the pain, which is also the case for some diets, spicy food, coffee, and alcohol.

The degree of symptoms is best illustrated using two- or three-day micturition diaries, registering the volume and time for each void, but also including visual analogue scales to describe the degree of pain. These simple instruments can also be used to assess the result of treatment attempts. More sophisticated instruments include condition-specific and generic health questionnaires, especially useful in the research situation.

Although bladder pain and urinary frequency may be the only or major complaints in some individuals, others have a broader spectrum of problems, including associations of BPS/IC to allergy, fibromyalgia, vulvodynia, chronic fatigue syndrome, anxiety disorders, and depression. Such associations should be acknowledged in the patient's history.

Cystoscopy and physical examination

Cystoscopy under anaesthesia is the cornerstone for the investigation of BPS/IC patients since sufficient distension is required to visualize lesions characteristic of BPS/IC. The BPS/IC patient can tolerate filling with only a very limited volume in their unanaesthetized bladder, irrespective of the true bladder capacity during anaesthesia. Local anaesthetic cystoscopy can still be a useful first step to examine the mucosa, urethral calibre, and determine any local tenderness of the bladder and/or urethra. Abnormal tenderness or heightened sensation of the external and internal genitalia and the various components of the pelvic floor are also noted, including any trigger points. Such physical signs are important for diagnostic completeness and the design of a rational treatment programme. Other possible causes for lower urinary tract pain, such as tumour, stone, inflammation, or mucosal metaplasias can be noted or excluded. The presence of submucosal petechial bleeding, so called glomerulations, after decompression of the previously distended bladder has until recently been regarded as one of the endoscopic hallmarks of the disease.[3,4,22,23] Current data is however casting doubt on the practical usefulness of this finding in patient management[19] (see also Further reading, Wennevik 2016).

Hunner's ulcers can only be fully identified and characterized with cystoscopy under anaesthesisa. The typical lesion is a circumscribed, reddened mucosal area with small vessels radiating towards a central scar, with a fibrin deposit or coagulum attached to this area. On further bladder distension this site ruptures (Fig. 1.11.1), with petechial haemorrhage from the lesion and the mucosal margins in a waterfall manner. A quite characteristic finding at the second filling of the bladder in a patient with this classic type of lesion is a varying degree of oedema, sometimes with peripheral extension.[6,22] The use of a rigid cystoscope is preferred to allow easy and rapid filling and emptying, particularly when bleeding is encountered. Diagnostic hydrodistension should be performed in a standard manner at a pressure of 80 cmH_2O above the level of the patient's bladder.[23] Irrigating fluid (glycine) is allowed to run into the bladder until it stops spontaneously at capacity, as observed when checking the dripping chamber of the fluid reservoir. This volume is then held for two to three minutes with any leakage around the cystoscope sheath controlled by urethral compression. The volume and the degree of bleeding into the bladder fluid are noted when evacuating the bladder. The maximum bladder capacity is often reduced in the classic type of IC, whereas it is normal or only slightly reduced in the non-ulcerative BPS. The bladder is refilled to approximately 20–50% of capacity and again inspected for lesions and haemorrhages, which will not be conspicuous until the bladder is filled for a second time. The changes typically spare the trigone. It is important to be ready to

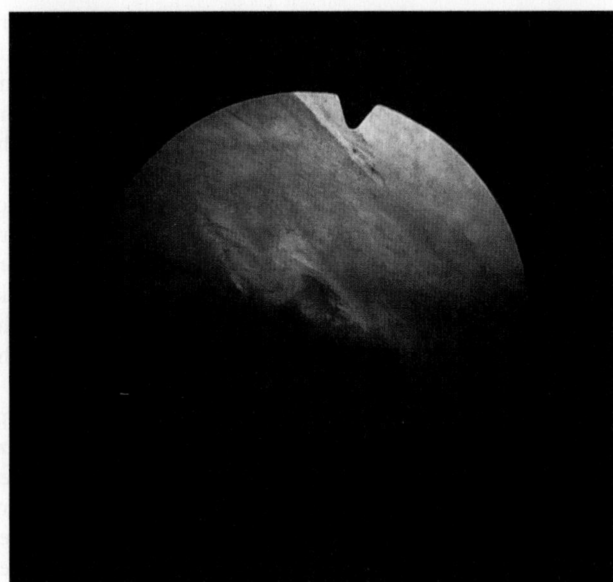

Fig. 1.11.1 Cystoscopic view during bladder distension in a woman with the classic Hunner (ESSIC 3C) type of disease. In the centre of the photo, a deep rupture of the mucosa is seen with the beginning of marginal, petechial bleeding.

note any changes to the bladder mucosa during initial slow bladder filling, since once bleeding occurs it is difficult to inspect the mucosa thoroughly. Repeated bladder flushing can restore vision to detect post-distension mucosal changes essential to objective patient categorization. It should be remembered that although the mucosal findings are diagnostically important, they frequently do not parallel the type or severity of symptoms, nor the subsequent response to treatment.[24,25]

Bumpus[26] first described the possible therapeutic benefit of simple hydrodistension for patients with IC; this remains an intervention that can be offered, although its efficacy is doubtful.

Filling cystometry is helpful should overactive bladder (OAB) be suspected, to estimate bladder capacity, and to record sensations with bladder filling. In females, post-void residual urine volume and cystometry are optional, while in males, a flow rate should be done in all; and if maximum flow is <20 mL/s, a pressureflow study and recording of residual urine volume should be performed.

Histopathology

The primary purpose of obtaining bladder biopsies in BPS/IC is to exclude other causes of bladder pain,[22] principally carcinoma *in situ*.[27] Histopathological examination is also of value in diagnosing BPS/IC. Although the histopathologic features are not distinctive in non-ulcer disease, there are microscopic findings pathognomonic for classic IC. These include urothelial vacuolization and detachment, mucosal infiltrates of lymphocytes, plasma cells, neutrophil and eosinophil granulocytes, as well as an increase of mast cell numbers in all compartments of the bladder wall.[28,29] Granulation tissue is one further feature of the classic disease, speculatively as a result of repeated trauma by bladder filling and stretch of the areas of inflammatory involvement.[30]

In an analysis of pathological findings of more than 200 US patients with IC, three morphology clusters were identified, corresponding to unique pathological groupings. The largest group comprised 90% of patients with no consistent pathological features.

A small second group showed multiple signs of parenchymal damage, including several inflammatory features, while the third group was characterized by complete denudation of the urothelium and variable oedema. This categorization correlated with symptom complexity and severity, indicating a role for histopathology in the predictive modelling of BPS/IC.[31]

Morphological methods continue to evolve using immunohistochemistry, polymerase chain reaction *in situ*, and various immunoblotting and RNA expression array techniques. One relevant example is the application of tryptase staining for mast cells, making the older staining techniques obsolete.[32,33] In this manner, the precision of the diagnosis may be improved in future, reducing the reliance on subjective clinician assessment.

Histopathologic features in BPS/IC may also guide the development of future treatment possibilities. It is reasonable to hypothesize that the various components of the cell infiltrate play various roles, although they are as yet poorly characterized. For example, lymphocytes have one role: studies suggest that T and B-cells are associated with various clinical features of IC and moreover there are marked differences in lymphocyte populations in classic versus non-ulcer disease,[34–36] while macrophages have a possible role in the massive production of nitric oxide (NO) seen in the Hunner-type of disease.[37–39] Special interest has been devoted to the mast cell, supposed to be a major player in this disease complex, involving the diagnosis, development of symptoms, and relation to detrusor fibrosis, to give some examples.[29,32,38–42] Mast cells can be activated by a variety of agents, leading to release of a number of distinct inflammatory mediators, with or without degranulation. How these differential mast cell responses are controlled is still unresolved.[43] Investigating cause and effect in different bladder wall cellular responses is required to be able to reveal the nature of various BPS/IC phenotypes.

The role of markers

Characterization of a predictive urinary or serum biomarker for the diagnosis and likely treatment responsiveness of patients with possible IC/BPS would be a tremendous advance. The problem with IC is that molecular pathways of disease in differing phenotypes and local and systemic responses is largely lacking. The heterogeneity of the syndrome also makes it unlikely that a single biomarker could cover the entire spectrum. The most promising candidate was antiproliferative factor (APF), a component of urine that inhibits urothelial cell proliferation, which appears in higher concentration in IC patients compared to controls.[44] However there is insufficient evidence to support APF as a generally useful diagnostic tool. The many other candidates tested remain confined to the research field.[45]

A further possibility arises from the observation that the formation of urinary NO is increased in patients with the classic Hunner's ulcerative form of IC,[46] possibly related to increased activity of the inducible form of nitric oxide synthase (iNOS).[47] This production may occur in different tissue compartments including the urothelium[37] and in infiltrating inflammatory cells present in IC.[39] A significant advantage is that technology to measure NO evaporation is easy and simple to use, but requires a special device.[46] At this stage, biomarkers have a very limited role in routine diagnosis of BPS/IC, but they do hold promise for the future.

Treatment

No curative conservative treatment has yet been identified. Given the current limited understanding of the aetiology and pathogenesis of BPS/IC, all treatments are given on an empirical (try it and see) basis. Despite this uncertainty, a number of management algorithms have been suggested and these are often based on the observation that several modalities have to be tried before benefit is seen, and that a combination of therapies may give added benefit. Once the diagnosis has been made, the intensity and severity of symptoms will indicate whether to institute therapy or use a policy of supportive care. Initially, if not done before, an empiric course of antibiotics is not unreasonable, preferably using doxycycline or ciprofloxacin. However, if unsuccessful, further antibiotic courses should be strongly discouraged, because in the absence of positive cultures they are unlikely to give benefit and may cause harm. As general measures, stress reduction, physical exercise, warm tub baths, and efforts by the patient to maintain a normal lifestyle can all contribute to maintenance of a good quality of life.

Much epidemiological research points towards a multifactorial aetiology for IC/BPS whereby one or more pathways may be involved, resulting in the typical symptom complex. A number of hypotheses concerning possible pathways have been generated, leading to the popularization of a wide variety of treatment options, which are usually backed by low levels of evidence preventing firm recommendation for their use (Table 1.11.1). Here the principles of treatment and some specific examples are summarized.

The bladder lining as treatment target

One popular theory of pathogenesis is the 'leaky urothelium'; a defect in the bladder glucosamine glycan layer (GAG) allowing noxious urinary constituents to penetrate and affect the underlying sensory innervation.[48] This theory suggests that replenishment of the GAG layer would restore mucosal integrity and alleviate symptoms. Each of the possible treatment can be administered orally or intravesically.

Sodium pentosan polysulphate (PPS), a highly sulphated mucopolysaccaride, is the only oral therapy approved by the US Food and Drug Administration. Up to 50% of selected patients describe an initial symptom benefit, which falls to 30% with continued use and can take up to six months to work.[49,50] The usual dosage is 150–300 mg daily, divided in two or three doses. As an alternative, a variety of other mucopolysaccharide products (chondroitin sulphate, hyaluronate/hyaluronic acid)[51,52] have been used intravesically with the object to get a more direct and prompt effect, with less systemic side effects, but however entailing the significant disadvantage of repeated urethral catheterization. The compounds are typically administered as weekly installations for six weeks, and then monthly maintenance if benefit occurs.

Dimethylsulphoxide (DMSO) is the standard treatment with the longest history, being used for four decades.[53] It is an organic solvent, a by-product of the paper pulp industry, and has analgesic, anti-inflammatory, collagenolytic, and muscle relaxant properties. It is also a scavenger of the intracellular OH radical. It is administered intravesically weekly or every two weeks, sometimes combined in intravesical cocktails with lidocaine, heparin, and sodium bicarbonate. DMSO is the only intravesical therapy approved by the US Food and Drug Administration for BPS/IC.

Chronic bladder inflammation as treatment target

Systemic steroid administration has a long tradition as well; anti-inflammatory treatment using cortisone has been used, although

Table 1.11.1 Compilation of treatments of bladder pain syndrome with levels of evidence and grades of recommendation

A. Evidence statements	
Conclusions	**Level of evidence**
None of the present existing treatments have any effect on all BPS subtypes or phenotypes	4
Conventional analgesics have little efficacy; opioids are effective in controlling BPS pain	2b
Corticosteroids are not recommended as long-term treatment	3
Hydroxyzine has limited efficacy shown in RCT and is effective in associated non-bladder diseases	1b
Limited data exist on effectiveness of cimetidine in BPS	2b
Amitriptyline is effective in pain and related symptoms of BPS	1b
Oral PPS is effective in pain and related symptoms of BPS	1a
Oral PPS plus subcutaneous heparin is effective in pain and related symptoms of BPS especially in patients who are initially low responders to PPS alone	1b
Only limited data exist on the effectiveness of antibiotics in the treatment of BPS	2b
Insufficient data for the effectiveness of prostaglandins in BPS exist; adverse effects are frequent	3
Global response on cyclosporin A was superior to PPS, but associated with more adverse effects	1b
Duloxetin has shown no effect and tolerability is poor	2b
Oxybutynin has limited effect in BPS pain, but data are scant	3
Only insufficient data exist for the effectiveness of gabapentin in BPS	3
Only insufficient data exist for the effectiveness of suplatast tosilate in BPS	3
Preliminary data showed effectiveness of quercetin alone and in multimodal uncontrolled studies	3
Intravesical lidocaine plus sodium bicarbonate is effective in the short term	1b
Intravesical PPS is effective, as based on limited data and may enhance effect of oral treatment	1b
There are limited data on the effectiveness of intravesical heparin	3
Intravesical hyaluronic acid may have long-term effects in BPS patients with positive intravesical modified KCl test	2b
Intravesical chondroitin sulphate may be effective according to non-randomized studies; published RCTs are underpowered	2b
Intravesical DMSO is effective in the treatment of BPS, but side effects have to be considered	1b
Intravesical submucosal BTX-A injection plus hydrodistension has sustained and significantly improved effect over hydrodistension alone	1b
Only limited data exist on the effectiveness of BTX-A injection into detrusor or trigone	3
Data on effectiveness of intravesical vanilloids are contradictory; largest of RCTs without efficacy	1b
Intravesical Bacillus Calmette–Guérin (BCG) is not effective in BPS	1b
Intravesical clorpactin has insufficient data to support effectiveness and high complication rates	3
There is only insufficient data to support effectiveness of bladder distension	3
Scarce data indicate electromotive drug administration may have a beneficial effect in patient subsets	3
Transurethral resection (coagulation and laser) may be effective in BPS type 3C	3
Sacral neuromodulation may be effective in BPS	3
Pudendal nerve stimulation is superior to sacral nerve stimulation for the treatment of BPS	1b
Bladder training may be effective in patients with predominant urinary symptoms and little pain	3
Manual and physical therapy may have limited effects	3
Avoidance of some food and drink avoids pain triggering	3
Acupuncture: data contradictory	3
Psychological therapy may be effective in ameliorating coping with disease	3
No definitive conclusion on the effectiveness of surgical organ removal for BPS can be drawn, as based on large variability results in reported series	3

(*continued*)

Table 1.11.1 Continued

B. Recommendations for clinical practice	
Recommendations	**GRADE**
Subtype and phenotype-oriented therapy for BPS is recommended	A
Multimodal behavioural, physical, and psychological techniques should always be considered alongside oral or invasive treatments for BPS	A
Opioids might be used in BPS in disease flare-ups; long-term application solely if all treatments failed	C
Corticosteroids are not recommended as long-term treatment	C
Hydroxyzine is recommended for use in BPS	A
Consider cimetidine as a valid oral option before invasive treatments	B
Amitriptyline is recommended for use in BPS	A
Oral PPS is recommended for use in BPS	A
Treatment with oral PPS plus subcutaneous heparin is recommended, especially in low responders to PPS alone	A
Antibiotics can be offered when infection is present or highly suspected	C
Prostaglandins are not recommended; insufficient data on BPS, adverse effects considerable	C
Cyclosporin A might be used in PPS, but adverse effects are significant and should be carefully considered	B
Duloxetin is not recommended for BPS treatment	C
Oxybutynin might be considered for the treatment of BPS	C
Gabapentin might be considered in oral treatment of BPS	C
Consider intravesical lidocain plus sodium bicarbonate prior to more invasive methods	A
Consider intravesical PPS before more invasive treatment alone or combined with oral PPS	A
Consider intravesical heparin before more invasive measures alone or in combination treatment	C
Consider intravesical hyaluronic acid before more invasive measures	B
Consider intravesical chondroitin sulphate before more invasive measures	B
Consider intravesical DMSO before more invasive measures	A
Consider intravesical bladder wall and trigonal injection of BTX-A if intravesical instillation therapies failed	C
Consider submucosal injection of BTX-A plus hydrodistension if intravesical instillation therapies failed	A
Intravesical therapy with Bacillus Calmette–Guérin is not recommended in BPS	A
Intravesical therapy with clorpactin is not recommended in BPS	A
Intravesical therapy with vanilloids is not recommended in BPS	C
Bladder distension is not recommendedas atreatment of BPS	C
Electromotive drug administration might be considered before more invasive measures	C
Consider transurethral resection (or coagulation or laser) of bladder lesions, but in BPS type 3C only	B
Neuromodulation might be considered before more invasive interventions	B
Consider bladder training in patients with little pain	B
Consider manual and physical therapy in first approach	B
Consider dietary avoidance of triggering substances	C
Acupuncture is not recommended	C
Consider psychological therapy in multimodal approach	B
All ablative organ surgery should be as last resort for experienced and BPS knowledgeable surgeons only	A

PPS = pentosanpolysulphate sodium; DMSO = dimethyl sulphoxide; BPS = bladder pain syndrome.

Level of evidence classification reference.

Grade of recommendation reference.

Reproduce with permission from Engeler, D., Baranowski, A.P., Elneil, S., Hughes, J., Messelink, E.J., van Ophoven, A., de Williams, A.C.: *EAU Guidelines on Chronic Pelvic Pain*, Copyright © 2012 European Association of Urology.

not as a standard option, in BPS/IC for more than four decades. Efficacy has been demonstrated in the classic ulcerative type of disease, but as the harms of chronic steroid treatment can be very serious and irreversible, it is difficult to justify systemic, long-term use. Another modality is sublesional injection of cortisone, occasionally being reported to be efficacious in the Hunner's ulcer type of BPS/IC.

Mast cells are regarded by many authorities to have a pivotal role in BPS/IC, and a number of treatments are aimed at stopping or minimizing the effects of mast cell activation. Hydroxyzine is a histamine H1 receptor blocker inhibiting neuronal activation of mast cells. Hydroxyzine hydrochloride has been trialled using doses of 25 mg increasing to 75 mg/day. Initial results were promising but a better designed randomized comparison showed no benefit over placebo.[54]

Various immunosuppressants have also been trialled in the IC/BPS patient group. The most recent and promising one according to the literature is cyclosporine A. In a randomized comparison against the control of pentosan polysulphate, 1.5 mg/kg cyclosporine was more effective than 300 mg/day of pentosan over six months.[55] However, there was also a higher rate of symptoms such as gingival pain, paraesthesias, and muscle pain. If cyclosporine therapy is tried, careful frequent follow-up with blood pressure and kidney function testing is mandatory.

Hyperbaric oxygen has been tested in small trials, with repeated sessions of inhalation of 100% O_2 found helpful in a small subgroup of BPS/IC patients.[56] This treatment is limited by high costs, time-consuming care, and restricted availability.

Mucosal ablation of circumscribed Hunner areas of chronic bladder inflammation using transurethral techniques has been advocated.[57] Transurethral resection (TUR) shows favourable results in this patient subgroup, but requires complete resection of all lesions, including the peripheral oedema zone and the underlying superficial detrusor muscle, involving minimum coagulation. A case series of over 100 patients showed long-term symptomatic relief was provided for 90% of patients,[58] while TUR has been suggested to result in symptom improvement by the removal of intramural nerve endings engaged by the inflammatory process. Similar results have been reported following ablation by neodymium YAG laser,[59] but again benefit is limited to those with Hunner's ulcerative subtype only. The excellent symptomatic effect in the majority of patients makes transurethral resection of the bladder (TURB) a first-line treatment for this group, with few comparably effective alternatives.

The pelvic floor as a treatment target

Overactivity in the pelvic floor musculature with possible involvement of joints, ligaments, fasciae, and viscera may cause adverse interactions and painful sensations. Therapeutic approaches include breath work, biofeedback techniques, and soft tissue manipulations to aid in muscle relaxation of the pelvic floor.[60] Especially important seems to be the identification of trigger points, frequently found in the pubococcygeus, piriformis, external oblique, rectus abdominis, hip adductors, and gluteus medius muscles. A number of manipulative but also invasive soft tissue techniques are available to release symptoms related to soft tissue pathology in BPS/IC; but at present, these are not often used in the standard clinical management of patients with these pain syndromes.

The peripheral nervous system as a treatment target

Early reports on the use of intravesical lidocaine in BPS/IC indicate a potential role of such a regimen.[61] Alkalization of lidocaine before instillation improves pharmacokinetics,[62] and in a placebo-controlled, multicentre study, actively treated patients had significant, sustained symptom relief for up to one month. An important limitation is the need to use repeated urethral catheterization, but other ways of administration are now tested.

Vanilloids disrupt sensory neurons, a conceptually attractive approach to control symptoms in BPS/IC. Capsaicin and resiniferatoxin have been trialled, but a significant adverse event was pain on instillation limiting their use. Botulinum toxin (BTX) injections, into the detrusor or the trigone, respectively, are used extensively in frequency, urgency, and urgency incontinence syndromes with varying aetiology. BTX has an antinociceptive effect; decrease in daytime frequency, nocturia, and pain and an increase in functional bladder volume has been demonstrated in BPS/IC. The results reported in the literature are conflicting and are as yet from a low level of evidence, but there seems to be a potential for BTX.[63]

The rationale behind the use of surface or percutaneous electrical nerve stimulation is to relieve pain by stimulation of myelinated afferents, thus activating segmental inhibitory circuits.[64] Suprapubic and tibial nerve sites have been tested, all with some symptom benefit but controlled studies are scant. Patient self-administration makes this a less costly alternative with few harmful effects.

Another off-label therapy is invasive neuromodulation (used for frequency and urgency syndromes), either using the sacral nerve approach or pudendal nerve stimulation, also with favourable preliminary results. In one study, the pudendal positioning of the electrode was the preferred site, and more than 90% of patients stating that they, if needed, would undergo repeated implantation.[65]

The central nervous system as a treatment target

The long-term appropriate and supervised use of analgesic medications forms an integral part of the treatment of a chronic pain condition such as BPS. These can include simple analgesics and neuromodulatory agents, and frequently a combination of both is required for maximal benefit.

Amitriptyline, a tricyclic antidepressant, has a number of properties including muscarinic receptor blockade, inhibition of reuptake of released serotonin and noradrenalin, and blockade of histamine H1 receptors. This drug is standard in chronic pain treatment and can be used alone or in combination with other treatments. It is used in doses starting at 10 mg daily, which are slowly increased over several weeks to up to 50–75 mg daily as tolerated.[66] It tends to diminish pain, increase bladder capacity, block the actions of histamine, act as a mild antimuscarinic, and aid sleep. However 'hangover' effects are common and it is unsuited to those with active occupations. Newer alternatives such as gabapentin and pregabalin are now more often used.

The treatment of pain needs to be addressed directly, and in some instances referral to an anaesthesia/pain specialist clinical service can be the appropriate early step in conjunction with ongoing treatment of BPS. The reason is that in chronic pain it is believed that changes occur within the central nervous system (CNS) throughout the whole neuraxis and that central changes may be responsible for some of the psychological changes that modify pain mechanisms. Core muscles may become hyperalgesic with multiple trigger points. Other organs may also become sensitive, such as the bowel with 'irritable bowel' symptoms. There have been many ideas to explain associations, like neuronal sensitization in spinal segments of common projection,[67] or that the disease progresses from an organ-centred condition to a regional and finally a systemic pain syndrome.[68] A maladaptive coping strategy, such as a catastrophizing personality is associated with greater pain, increased symptoms, and poorer quality of life.[69] Generally, the patient's quality of life can be seriously affected, both from a physical and psychological standpoint. Thus, other components than bladder pain must be identified and deserve attention, too. Involvement of various experts may be needed, like pain specialists and the pain nurse, physiotherapists, clinical psychologists, and rarely psychiatrists. When standard, organ-centred trials of treatment fail, early involvement of the multidisciplinary team is vital. If consultation is delayed, hypothetically there is a risk that CNS patterns of pain processing will be permanently changed, resulting in a chronic pain condition.

When all conservative trials fail: the role of major surgery

Major surgery for BPS is a reasonable alternative for patients with severe symptoms who are long-term failures from multiple trials of standard conservative strategies, and when the disease course suggests that spontaneous remission is not to be expected. There are, however, serious limitations to major surgery requiring the balancing of likely benefits with possible harms, and acceptance of the need for a changed lifestyle. Patients with a small bladder capacity under anaesthesia are less likely to respond to conservative attempts at therapy and have been found to be better candidates for bladder reconstruction. In fact, patients with end-stage Hunner's ulcerative IC and severe bladder contracture have the best results with major surgery. At this stage of the disease process, there is little pain but intolerable urinary frequency. On this indication, subtotal cystectomy and ileocystoplasty has yielded excellent results.[70,71] In contrast, major surgery, irrespective of method, is not likely to benefit sufferers of other presentations of BPS/IC.[71] In non-Hunner BPS patients with debilitating symptoms, the decision is difficult. Here, if one conceptualizes BPS as composed of two main components, one of pain and the other of frequency, it becomes easier for the patient and physician to rationalize the decision. Conduit urinary diversion can be relied upon to resolve the frequency symptoms, and if the patient would consider this alone sufficient, there is reason to seriously consider this option. However, pain may persist; diversion, or cystectomy with diversion, or even more extensive surgery, cannot guarantee a pain-free result,[72] and it is critical for the patient to seriously take this fact into account before the decision to embark to this irreversible step.

Terminology issues

During the last few years, general consensus has evolved that a more sophisticated classification of patients with pain perceived in the bladder and lower urinary tract is needed, with a diagnosis based solely on symptoms not being sufficient as a basis for treatment. International confusion among patients, clinicians, and healthcare providers as to the nature and meaning of descriptive terminology has not helped the proper organization of care for this problem and has also hampered badly needed high quality trials of treatment options and basic scientific research. In order to design a comprehensive classification, the umbrella terms 'painful bladder syndrome'[73] or, more recently, 'bladder pain syndrome' were suggested, incorporating the classic concept of ulcerative IC as a separate phenotype.[22,74] Internationally, there are even differences in ideas on leading symptoms and all these differences have yet to be resolved. An exact and uniform terminology is an indispensable basis for science and precisely directed clinical management.

Conclusion

The key to the diagnosis for people with bladder pain is symptom recognition. Increasing the awareness of BPS by family doctors and other primary care practitioners is an important step. When investigating BPS, relying only on symptoms is not sufficient. Objective recordings are needed to exclude other conditions and to recognize relevant BPS phenotypes, especially the classic Hunner's ulcerative type of disease (now termed ESSIC type 3C), and pelvic floor dysfunction/trigger points, respectively. Such observation may make immediate and successful treatment possible. To help all patients achieve both symptom benefit and a coming to terms with the disease is still difficult, however. Involvement of the multidisciplinary team should always be considered when standard treatments fail. In the future, in order to to move forwards, phenotypes based on well-defined criteria, symptomatic as well as objective, have to be established.

Further reading

Chaitow L, Lovegrove Jones RE. *Chronic Pelvic Pain and Dysfunction. Practical Physical Medicine*. London, UK: Churchill Livingstone Elsevier 2012.

Engeler D, Baranowski AP, Elneil S, *et al.* EAU Guidelines on Chronic Pelvic Pain, 2012. Available at: https://uroweb.org/wp-content/uploads/26-Chronic-Pelvic-Pain_LR.pdf [Online].

FitzGerald M, Brensinger C, Brubaker L, Propert K, Group. IS: What is the pain of interstitial cystitis like? *Int Urogynecol J Pelvic Floor Dysfunct* 2006; **17**(1):69–72.

Gillenwater JY, Wein AJ. Summary of the National Institute of Arthritis, Diabetes, Digestive and Kidney Diseases Workshop on Interstitial Cystitis, National Institutes of Health, Bethesda, Maryland, August 28–29, 1987; *J Urol* 1988; **140**(1):203–6.

Nordling J, Anjum F, Bade J, *et al.* Primary evaluation of patients suspected of having interstitial cystitis (IC). *Eur Urol* 2004; **45**(5):662–9.

Parsons CL, Lilly JD, Stein P. Epithelial dysfunction in nonbacterial cystitis (interstitial cystitis). *J Urol* 1991; **145**(4):732–5.

Peeker R, Aldenborg F, Fall M. Complete transurethral resection of ulcers in classic interstitial cystitis. *Int Urogynecol J* 2000; **11**:290–5.

Rosenberg M, Newman D, Page S. Interstitial cystitis/painful bladder syndrome: symptom recognition is key to early identification, treatment. *Cleve Clin J Med* 2007; **74**(Suppl 3):S54–62.

Rössberger J, Fall M, Jonsson O, Peeker R. Long-term results of reconstructive surgery in patients with bladder pain syndrome/interstitial cystitis: subtyping is imperative. *Urology* 2007; **70**(4):638–42.

van de Merwe JP, Nordling J, Bouchelouche P, *et al.* Diagnostic criteria, classification, and nomenclature for painful bladder syndrome/interstitial cystitis: an ESSIC proposal. *Eur Urol* 2008; **53**(1):60–7.

Wennevik GE, Meijlink JM, Hanno P, Nordling J. The role of glomerulations in bladder pain syndrome: A review. *J Urol* 2016; **195**(1):19–25.

References

1. Skene AJC. *Diseases of Bladder and Urethra in Women*. New York, NY: Wm Wood, 1887: p. 167.
2. Hunner GL. A rare type of bladder ulcer: further notes, with a report of eighteen cases. *JAMA* 1918; **70**:203–12.
3. Hand JR. Interstitial cystitis: Report of 223 cases (204 women and 19 men). *J Urol* 1949; **61**:291–310.
4. Messing EM, Stamey TA. Interstitial cystitis: early diagnosis, pathology and treatment. *Urology* 1978; **12**:381–92.
5. Fall M, Johansson SL, Aldenborg F. Chronic interstitial cystitis: a heterogeneous syndrome. *J Urol* 1987; **137**:35–8.
6. Peeker R, Fall M. Towards a precise definition of interstitial cystitis: further evidence of differences in classic and nonulcer disease. *J Urol* 2002; **167**:2470–2.
7. Gillenwater JY, Wein AJ. Summary of the National Institute of Arthritis, Diabetes, Digestive and Kidney Diseases Workshop on Interstitial Cystitis, National Institutes of Health, Bethesda, Maryland, August 28–29, 1987. *J Urol* 1988; **140**(1):203–6.
8. Oravisto KJ. Epidemiology of interstitial cystitis. *Ann Chir Gynaecol Finn* 1975; **64**:75–7.
9. Held PJ, Hanno PM, Wein AJ, Pauly MV, Cann MA. Epidemiology of interstitial cystitis 2. (pp. 29–48) In: Hanno PM, Staskin DR, Krane JR, *et al.* (eds). *Interstitial Cystitis*. New York, NY: Springer-Verlag, 1990.
10. Curhan GC, Speizer FE, Hunter DJ, Curhan SG, Stampfer MJ. Epidemiology of interstitial cystitis: a population based study. *J Urol* 1999; **161**:549–52.
11. Parsons CL, Tatsis V. Prevalence of interstitial cystitis in young women. *Urology* 2004; **64**(5):866–70.
12. Leppilahti M, Sairanen J, Tammela TL, *et al.* Prevalence of clinically confirmed interstitial cystitis in women: a population based study in Finland. *J Urol* 2005; **174**(2):581–3.
13. Koziol JA. Epidemiology of interstitial cystitis. *Urol Clin North Am* 1994; **21**(1):7–20.
14. Warren JW, Keay SK, Meyers D, Xu J. Concordance of interstitial cystitis in monozygotic and dizygotic twin pairs. *Urology* 2001; **57**(6 Suppl 1):22–5.
15. Altman D, Lundholm C, Milsom I, *et al.* The genetic and environmental contribution to the occurrence of bladder pain syndrome: an empirical approach in a nationwide population sample. *Eur Urol* 2011; **59**(2):280–5.
16. Clemens JQ, Meenan RT, Rosetti MC, Kimes T, Calhoun EA. Costs of interstitial cystitis in a managed care population. *Urology* 2008; **71**(5):776–80.
17. Propert K, Schaeffer A, Brensinger C, Kusek J, Nyberg L, Landis J. A prospective study of interstitial cystitis: results of longitudinal followup of the interstitial cystitis data base cohort. The Interstitial Cystitis Data Base Study Group. *J Urol* 2000; **163**(5):1434–9.
18. Richter B. *Bladder Pain Syndrome: Symptoms, quality of life, treatment intensity, clinical and pathological findings, and their correlations*. Herlev University Hospital, University of Copenhagen, Denmark, 2010.
19. Richter B, Hesse U, Hansen A, Horn T, Mortensen S, Nordling J. Bladder pain syndrome/interstitial cystitis in a Danish population: a study using the 2008 criteria of the European Society for the Study of Interstitial Cystitis. *BJU Int* 2010; **105**(5):660–7.
20. Rosenberg M, Newman D, Page S. Interstitial cystitis/painful bladder syndrome: symptom recognition is key to early identification, treatment. *Cleve Clin J Med* 2007; **74**(Suppl 3):S54–62.
21. FitzGerald M, Brensinger C, Brubaker L, Propert K, Group. IS: What is the pain of interstitial cystitis like? *Int Urogynecol J Pelvic Floor Dysfunct* 2006; **17**(1):69–72.
22. van de Merwe JP, Nordling J, Bouchelouche P, *et al.* Diagnostic criteria, classification, and nomenclature for painful bladder syndrome/ interstitial cystitis: an ESSIC proposal. *Eur Urol* 2008; **53**(1):60–7.
23. Nordling J, Anjum F, Bade J, *et al.* Primary evaluation of patients suspected of having interstitial cystitis (IC). *Eur Urol* 2004; **45**(5):662–9.
24. Messing EM. The diagnosis of interstitial cystitis. *Urology* 1987; **29** (4 Suppl):4–7.
25. Wyndaele JJ, Dyck. v, Toussaint N. Cystoscopy and bladder biopsies in patients with bladder pain syndrome carried out following ESSIC guidelines. *Scand J Urol Nephrol* 2009; **43**(6):471–5.
26. Bumpus HC. Interstitial cystitis: its treatment by over-distension of the bladder. *Med Clin North Am* 1930; **13**:1495–8.
27. Tissot W, Diokno A, Peters K. A referral center's experience with transitional cell carcinoma misdiagnosed as interstitial cystitis. *J Urol* 2004; **172**(2):478–80.
28. Fall M, Johansson SL, Vahlne A. A clinicopathological and virological study of interstitial cystitis. *J Urol* 1985; **133**(5):771–3.
29. Aldenborg F, Fall M, Enerbäck L. Proliferation and transepithelial migration of mucosal mast cells in interstitial cystitis. *Immunology* 1986; **58**:411–6.
30. Johansson SL, Fall M. Clinical features and spectrum of light microscopic changes in interstitial cystitis. *J Urol* 1990; **143**(6): 1118–24.
31. Leiby B, Landis J, Propert K, Tomaszewski J, ICDBS group. Discovery of morphological subgroups that correlate with severity of symptoms in interstitial cystitis: a proposed biopsy classification system. *J Urol* 2007; **177**(1):142–8.
32. Peeker R, Fall M, Enerbäck L, Aldenborg F. Recruitment, distribution and phenotypes of mast cells in interstitial cystitis. *J Urol* 2000; **163**:1009–15.
33. Larsen M, Mortensen S, Nordling J, Horn T. Quantifying mast cells in bladder pain syndrome by immunohistochemical analysis. *BJU Int* 2008; **102**:204–7.
34. Harrington DS, Fall M, Johansson SL. Interstitial cystitis: bladder mucosa lymphocyte immunophenotyping and peripheral blood flow cytometry analysis. *J Urol* 1990; **144**(4):868–71.
35. Christmas T. Lymphocyte sub-populations in the bladder wall in normal bladder, bacterial cystitis and interstitial cystitis. *Br J Urol* 1994; **73**(5):508–15.
36. Ueda T, Tamaki M, Ogawa O, Yamauchi T, Yoshimura N. Improvement of interstitial cystitis symptoms and problems that developed during treatment with oral IPD-1151T. *J Urol* 2000; **164**(6):1917–20.
37. Koskela L, Thiel T, Ehren I, De Verdier P, Wiklund N. Localization and expression of inducible nitric oxide synthase in biopsies from patients with interstitial cystitis. *J Urol* 2008; **180**:737–41.
38. Richter B, Roslind A, Hesse U, *et al.* YKL-40 and mast cells are associated with detrusor fibrosis in patients diagnosed with bladder pain syndrome/ interstitial cystitis according to the 2008 criteria of the European Society for the Study of Interstitial Cystitis. *Histopathology* 2010; **57**(3):371–83.
39. Logadottir Y, Hallsberg L, Fall M, Peeker R, Delbro D. Bladder pain syndrome/interstitial cystitis ESSIC type 3C: High expression of inducible nitric oxide synthase in inflammatory cells. *Scand J Urol Nephrol* 2013; **47**(1):52–6.
40. Pang X, Boucher W, Triadafilopoulos G, Sant GR, Theoharides TC. Mast cell and substance P-positive nerve involvement in a patient with both irritable bowel syndrome and interstitial cystitis. *Urology* 1996; **47**(3):436–8.
41. Larsen S, Thompson SA, Hald T, *et al.* Mast cells in interstitial cystitis. *Br J Urol* 1982; **54**(3):283–6.
42. Sant G, Kempuraj D, Marchand J, Theoharides T. The mast cell in interstitial cystitis: role in pathophysiology and pathogenesis. *Urology* 2007; **69**(4 Suppl):34–40.
43. Theoharides T, Kempuraj D, Tagen M, Conti P, Kalogeromitros D. Differential release of mast cell mediators and the pathogenesis of inflammation. *Immunol Rev* 2007; **217**:65–78.
44. Kim J, Keay S, Freeman M. Heparin-binding epidermal growth factor-like growth factor functionally antagonizes interstitial cystitis antiproliferative factor via mitogen-activated protein kinase pathway activation. *BJU Int* 2009; **103**:541–6.
45. Erickson D, Tomaszewski J, Kunselman A, *et al.* Urine markers do not predict biopsy findings or presence of bladder ulcers in interstitial cystitis/painful bladder syndrome. *J Urol* 2008; **179**(5):1850–6.

46. Logadottir Y, Ehren I, Fall M, Wiklund NP, Peeker R. Intravesical nitric oxide production discriminates between classic and nonulcer interstitial cystitis. *J Urol* 2004; **171**:1148–51.
47. Lirk P, Hoffmann G, Rieder J. Inducible nitric oxide synthase– time for reappraisal. *Curr Drug Targets Inflamm Allergy* 2002; **1**:89–108.
48. Parsons CL, Lilly JD, Stein P. Epithelial dysfunction in nonbacterial cystitis (interstitial cystitis). *J Urol* 1991; **145**(4):732–5.
49. Mulholland SG, Hanno P, Parsons CL, Sant GR, Staskin DR. Pentosan polysulfate sodium for therapy of interstitial cystitis. A double-blind placebo-controlled clinical study. *Urology* 1990; **35**(6):552–8.
50. Nickel JC, Barkin J, Forrest J, *et al.* Randomized, double-blind, dose-ranging study of pentosan polysulfate sodium for interstitial cystitis. *Urology* 2005; **65**(4):654–8.
51. Nickel JC, Egerdie RB, Steinhoff G, Palmer B, Hanno P. A multicenter, randomized, double-blind, parallel group pilot evaluation of the efficacy and safety of intravesical sodium chondroitin sulfate versus vehicle control in patients with interstitial cystitis/painful bladder syndrome. *Urology* 2010; **76**(4):804–9.
52. Kallestrup EB, Jorgensen SS, Nordling J, Hald T. Treatment of interstitial cystitis with Cystistat: a hyaluronic acid product. *Scand J Urol Nephrol* 2005; **39**(2):143–7.
53. Sant GR, LaRock DR. Standard intravesical therapies for interstitial cystitis. *Urol Clin North Am* 1994; **21**(1):73–83.
54. Sant GR, Propert KJ, Hanno PM, *et al.* A pilot clinical trial of oral pentosan polysulfate and oral hydroxyzine in patients with interstitial cystitis. *J Urol* 2003; **170**(3):810–5.
55. Sairanen J, Tammela TL, Leppilahti M, *et al.* Cyclosporine A and pentosan polysulfate sodium for the treatment of interstitial cystitis: a randomized comparative study. *J Urol* 2005; **174**(6):2235–8.
56. van Ophoven A, Rossbach G, Pajonk F, Hertle L. Safety and efficacy of hyperbaric oxygen therapy for the treatment of interstitial cystitis: a randomized, sham controlled, double-blind trial. *J Urol* 2006; **176**:1442–6.
57. Fall M. Conservative management of chronic interstitial cystitis: transcutaneous electrical nerve stimulation and transurethral resection. *J Urol* 1985; **133**:774–8.
58. Peeker R, Aldenborg F, Fall M. Complete transurethral resection of ulcers in classic interstitial cystitis. *Int Urogynecol J* 2000; **11**:290–5.
59. Shanberg AM, Malloy T. Treatment of interstitial cystitis with neodymium:YAG laser. *Urology* 1987; **29**(4 Suppl):31–3.
60. Chaitow L, Lovegrove Jones RE. *Chronic Pelvic Pain and Dysfunction. Practical Physical Medicine*. London, UK: Churchill Livingstone Elsevier 2012.
61. Asklin B, Cassuto J. Intravesical lidocaine in severe interstitial cystitis. Case report. *Scand J Urol Nephrol* 1989; **23**(4):311–2.
62. Henry RA, Patterson L, Nickel C, Morales A. Alkalinized intravesical lidocaine to treat interstitial cystitis: absorption kinetics in normal and interstitial cystitis bladders. *Urology* 2001; **57**(6 Suppl 1):119.
63. Giannantoni A, Mearini E, Del Zingaro M, Proietti S, Porena M. Two-year efficacy and safety of botulinum a toxin intravesical injections in patients affected by refractory painful bladder syndrome. *Curr Drug Deliv* 2010; **7**:1–4.
64. Fall M, Lindstrom S. Transcutaneous electrical nerve stimulation in classic and nonulcer interstitial cystitis. *Urol Clin North Am* 1994; **21**(1):131–9.
65. Peters KM, Feber KM, Bennett RC. A prospective, single-blind, randomized crossover trial of sacral vs pudendal nerve stimulation for interstitial cystitis. *BJU Int* 2007; **100**(4):835–9.
66. van Ophoven A, Pokupic S, Heinecke A, Hertle L. A prospective, randomized, placebo controlled, double-blind study of amitriptyline for the treatment of interstitial cystitis. *J Urol* 2004; **172**(2):533–6.
67. Giamberardino M, De Laurentis S, Affaitati G, Lerza R, Lapenna D, Vecchiet L. Modulation of pain and hyperalgesia from the urinary tract by algogenic conditions of the reproductive organs in women. *Neurosci Lett* 2001; **18**(304):61–4.
68. Nickel JC, Tripp DA, Pontari M, *et al.* Interstitial cystitis/painful bladder syndrome and associated medical conditions with an emphasis on irritable bowel syndrome, fibromyalgia and chronic fatigue syndrome. *J Urol* 2010; **184**(4):1358–63.
69. Rothrock N, Lutgendorf S, Kreder K. Coping strategies in patients with interstitial cystitis: relationships with quality of life and depression. *J Urol* 2003; **169**(1):233–6.
70. Peeker R, Aldenborg F, Fall M. The treatment of interstitial cystitis with supratrigonal cystectomy and ileocystoplasty: difference in outcome between classic and nonulcer disease. *J Urol* 1998; **159**(5):1479–82.
71. Rössberger J, Fall M, Jonsson O, Peeker R. Long-term results of reconstructive surgery in patients with bladder pain syndrome/interstitial cystitis: subtyping is imperative. *Urology* 2007; **70**(4):638–42.
72. Baskin LS, Tanagho EA. Pelvic pain without pelvic organs. *J Urol* 1992; **147**(3):683–6.
73. Abrams P, Cardozo L, Fall M, *et al.* The standardisation of terminology in lower urinary tract function. Report from the Standardisation Sub-committee of the International Continence Society. *Neurourol Urodynam* 2002; **21**:167–78.
74. Fall M, Baranowski AP, Fowler CJ, *et al.* EAU guidelines on chronic pelvic pain. *Eur Urol* 2004; **46**(6):681–9.

SECTION 2

Stones and endourology

Section editor: John Reynard

CHAPTER 2.1

Epidemiology of stone disease

Ben Turney and John Reynard

Introduction to epidemiology of stone disease

The lifetime prevalence of kidney stones is around 10% in developed countries and most commonly affects people of working age.[1–4] After passage of a first stone, the risk of recurrence is around 40% at 5 years and 75% at 20 years.[5] Direct and indirect costs associated with kidney stones have been estimated at more than $5 billion annually in the United States.[6]

The incidence of stone disease is increasing.[4,7,8] In part this is a true increase and in part a consequence of increased detection from radiological investigations done for non-stone symptoms, especially abdominal computed tomography (CT), with its high sensitivity and specificity for detecting stones.[9–12] A recent analysis of CT scans performed for colon cancer screening in asymptomatic Americans demonstrated a prevalence of renal stones in the adult patient population of 7.8%.[13] The 'true' increase in stone incidence probably relates, at least in part, to increased consumption of food with a tendency to promote stone formation combined with low fluid intake.[14–17] The epidemic of obesity and increased incidence of the metabolic syndrome are other likely factors.[15–18] Approximately 25% of stone formers have a family history of kidney stone disease,[19] but only a small minority have a monogenic cause such as cystinuria, Dent's disease, and primary hyperoxaluria. Overall, despite the increasing prevalence of kidney stones, the majority are categorized as idiopathic.

United Kingdom data

Analysis of NHS Hospital Episodes Statistics (HES) data[3] suggests that over the last decade there has been a 63% increase in the number of people in the United Kingdom presenting with a diagnosis of upper urinary tract stones.[7] In 2009–2010 there were over 83,000 hospital attendances in England. The mean age of presentation remained constant at 49 years, but there has been an increase in incidence in all age groups. The incidence of stones in children has increased 19% in the last 10 years, but the numbers remain relatively low at around 400 cases per annum.

As a result of its high prevalence, stone disease is a major contributor to both emergency and elective urological procedures performed in the United Kingdom. The numbers of all stone related procedures have increased significantly in recent years[7]: the number of ureteroscopies performed for stones is now over 14,000 per annum, and the number of lithotripsy treatments over 22,000. The reported number of percutaneous nephrolithotomies (PCNLs) in 2010 was 1,732. Put into context, lithotripsy is being performed almost as frequently as transurethral resection of the bladder (TURP) or transurethral resection of a bladder tumour (TURBT), stone ureteroscopy outnumbers total nephrectomies, prostatectomies, and cystectomies combined, and annual rates of PCNL and cystectomy are now similar.

Since the advent of less invasive endoscopic surgical options, open procedures for stones have declined dramatically. Open stone procedures in England have fallen from 278 cases in the year 2000 to 47 cases in 2010 (83% reduction).

Intrinsic risk factors for stone formation

Intrinsic risk factors include age, gender, genetics, and metabolic syndromes. The incidence of stone disease peaks between the ages of 20 and 60 years. While historically the male to female ratio was around 3:1, the gender gap is closing.[4,20]

An underlying genetic predisposition to stone disease is suggested by a number of observations. A twin study demonstrated that the heritability of the risk for stones was 56%,[21] which indicates that for a population around half of the risk is due to genetic factors and half due to environmental factors. Other studies have demonstrated that 30–40% of stone formers have a first-degree relative with a positive history of stones.[22,23] An Icelandic study suggested that first-time stone formers are 2.25 more likely to have an affected first-degree relative. Recurrent stone formers are 10 times more likely to have an affected first-degree relative.[24]

Extrinsic risk factors

Extrinsic risk factors implicated in the genesis of stones include diet, obesity, and fluid intake; environmental factors (e.g. climate and season); and personal circumstances such as stress, occupation, and affluence.

Obesity has an established association with risk of stone formation.[15,17] Other dietary factors implicated in promoting stone disease are low fluid intake (or high fluid loss through exertion), diets high in protein, salt (sodium) and oxalate, and low in fruit, fibre, and calcium.[14,19,25,26] While it is generally recommended that patients should adopt a lifestyle that minimizes stone risk factors, the impact of such measures on reducing risk of stone formation and stone events is difficult to predict in the individual.[27] For some patients, there may be benefit in medical management to correct metabolic abnormalities with drugs such as potassium/magnesium citrate and thiazide diuretics. Medical treatments can reduce recurrence rates.[28–32]

Further reading

Barcelo P, Wuhl O, Servitge E, Rousaud A, Pak CY. Randomized double-blind study of potassium citrate in idiopathic hypocitraturic calcium nephrolithiasis. *J Urol* 1993; **150**(6):1761–4.

Borghi L, Meschi T, Amato F, Briganti A, Novarini A, Giannini A. Urinary volume, water and recurrences in idiopathic calcium nephrolithiasis: a 5-year randomized prospective study. *J Urol* 1996; **155**(3):839–43.

Borghi L, Schianchi T, Meschi T, *et al.* Comparison of two diets for the prevention of recurrent stones in idiopathic hypercalciuria. *N Engl J Med* 2002; **346**(2):77–84.

Curhan GC, Willett WC, Rimm EB, Stampfer MJ. A prospective study of dietary calcium and other nutrients and the risk of symptomatic kidney stones. *N Engl J Med* 1993; **328**(12):833–8.

Edvardsson VO, Palsson R, Indridason OS, Thorvaldsson S, Stefansson K. Familiality of kidney stone disease in Iceland. *Scand J Urol Nephrol* 2009; **43**(5):420–4.

Ettinger B, Tang A, Citron JT, Livermore B, Williams T. Randomized trial of allopurinol in the prevention of calcium oxalate calculi. *N Engl J Med* 1986; **315**(22):1386–9.

Ettinger B, Pak CY, Citron JT, Thomas C, Adams-Huet B, Vangessel A. Potassium-magnesium citrate is an effective prophylaxis against recurrent calcium oxalate nephrolithiasis. *J Urol* 1997; **158**(6):2069–73.

Goldfarb DS, Fischer ME, Keich Y, Goldberg J. A twin study of genetic and dietary influences on nephrolithiasis: a report from the Vietnam Era Twin (VET) Registry. *Kidney Int* 2005; **67**(3):1053–61.

Jeong IG, Kang T, Bang JK, *et al.* Association between metabolic syndrome and the presence of kidney stones in a screened population. *Am J Kidney Dis* 2011; **58**(3):383–8.

Laerum E, Larsen S. Thiazide prophylaxis of urolithiasis. A double-blind study in general practice. *Acta Med Scand* 1984; **215**(4):383–9.

Romero V, Akpinar H, Assimos DG. Kidney stones: a global picture of prevalence, incidence, and associated risk factors. *Rev Urol* 2010; **12**(2-3):e86–96.

Saigal CS, Joyce G, Timilsina AR. Urologic Diseases in America Project. Direct and indirect costs of nephrolithiasis in an employed population: opportunity for disease management? *Kidney Int* 2005; **68**(4):1808–14.

Scales CD Jr, Smith AC, Hanley JM, Saigal CS. Urologic Diseases in America Project. Prevalence of kidney stones in the United States. *Eur Urol* 2012; **62**(1):160–5.

Taylor EN, Stampfer MJ, Curhan GC. Obesity, weight gain, and the risk of kidney stones. *JAMA* 2005; **293**(4):455–62.

Turney BW, Reynard JM, Noble JG, Keoghane SR. Trends in urological stone disease. *BJU Int* 2012; **109**(7):1082–7.

Worcester EM, Coe FL. Clinical practice. Calcium kidney stones. *N Engl J Med* 2010; **363**(10):954–63.

References

1. Stamatelou KK, Francis ME, Jones CA, Nyberg LM, Curhan GC. Time trends in reported prevalence of kidney stones in the United States: 1976–1994. *Kidney Int* 2003; **63**(5):1817–23.
2. Akoudad S, Szklo M, McAdams MA, *et al.* Correlates of kidney stone disease differ by race in a multi-ethnic middle-aged population: The ARIC study. *Prev Med* 2010; **51**(5):416–20.
3. Hospital Episodes Statistics (HES). NHS Digital. Available at: http://www.hesonline.nhs.uk [Online].
4. Scales CD Jr, Smith AC, Hanley JM, Saigal CS; Urologic Diseases in America Project. Prevalence of kidney stones in the United States. *Eur Urol* 2012; **62**(1):160–5.
5. Worcester EM, Coe FL. Clinical practice. Calcium kidney stones. *N Engl J Med* 2010; **363**(10):954–63.
6. Saigal CS, Joyce G, Timilsina AR; Urologic Diseases in America Project. Direct and indirect costs of nephrolithiasis in an employed population: opportunity for disease management? *Kidney Int* 2005; **68**(4):1808–14.
7. Reynard JM, Noble JG, Keoghane SR. Trends in urological stone disease. *BJU Int* 2012; **109**(7):1082–7.
8. Romero V1, Akpinar H, Assimos DG. Kidney stones: a global picture of prevalence, incidence, and associated risk factors. *Rev Urol* 2010; **12**(2–3):e86–96.
9. Wang JH, Shen SH, Huang SS, Chang CY. Prospective comparison of unenhanced spiral computed tomography and intravenous urography in the evaluation of acute renal colic. *J Chin Med Assoc* 2008; **71**(1):30–6.
10. Smith RC, Rosenfield AT, Choe KA, *et al.* Acute flank pain: comparison of non-contrast-enhanced CT and intravenous urography. *Radiology* 1995; **194**(3):789–94.
11. Miller OF, Rineer SK, Reichard SR, *et al.* Prospective comparison of unenhanced spiral computed tomography and intravenous urogram in the evaluation of acute flank pain. *Urology* 1998; **52**(6): 982–7.
12. Dalrymple NC, Verga M, Anderson KR, *et al.* The value of unenhanced helical computerized tomography in the management of acute flank pain. *J Urol* 1998; **159**(3):735–40.
13. Boyce CJ, Pickhardt PJ, Lawrence EM, Kim DH, Bruce RJ. Prevalence of urolithiasis in asymptomatic adults: objective determination using low dose noncontrast computerized tomography. *J Urol* 2010; **183**(3):1017–21.
14. Borghi L, Meschi T, Amato F, Briganti A, Novarini A, Giannini A. Urinary volume, water and recurrences in idiopathic calcium nephrolithiasis: a 5-year randomized prospective study. *J Urol* 1996; **155**(3):839–43.
15. Taylor EN, Stampfer MJ, Curhan GC. Obesity, weight gain, and the risk of kidney stones. *JAMA* 2005; **293**(4):455–62.
16. Taylor EN, Fung TT, Curhan GC. DASH-style diet associates with reduced risk for kidney stones. *J Am Soc Nephrol* 2009; **20**(10):2253–9.
17. Asplin J. Obesity and urolithiasis. *Adv Chronic Kidney Dis* 2009; **16**(1):11–20.
18. Jeong IG, Kang T, Bang JK, *et al.* Association between metabolic syndrome and the presence of kidney stones in a screened population. *Am J Kidney Dis* 2011; **58**(3):383–8.
19. Curhan GC1, Willett WC, Rimm EB, Stampfer MJ. A prospective study of dietary calcium and other nutrients and the risk of symptomatic kidney stones. *N Engl J Med* 1993; **328**(12):833–8.
20. Scales CD Jr, Curtis LH, Norris RD, *et al.* Changing gender prevalence of stone disease. *J Urol* 2007; **177**(3):979–82.
21. Goldfarb DS, Fischer ME, Keich Y, Goldberg J. A twin study of genetic and dietary influences on nephrolithiasis: a report from the Vietnam Era Twin (VET) Registry. *Kidney Int* 2005; **67**(3):1053–61.
22. Curhan GC, Willett WC, Knight EL, Stampfer MJ. Dietary factors and the risk of incident kidney stones in younger women: Nurses' Health Study II. *Arch Intern Med* 2004; **164**(8):885–91.
23. Ljunghall S, Danielson BG, Fellström B, Holmgren K, Johansson G, Wikström B. Family history of renal stones in recurrent stone patients. *Br J Urol* 1985; **57**(4):370–4.
24. Edvardsson VO, Palsson R, Indridason OS, Thorvaldsson S, Stefansson K. Familiality of kidney stone disease in Iceland. *Scand J Urol Nephrol* 2009; **43**(5):420–4.
25. Meschi T, Maggiore U, Fiaccadori E, *et al.* The effect of fruits and vegetables on urinary stone risk factors. *Kidney Int* 2004; **66**(6):2402–10.
26. Borghi L1, Schianchi T, Meschi T, *et al.* Comparison of two diets for the prevention of recurrent stones in idiopathic hypercalciuria. *N Engl J Med* 2002; **346**(2):77–84.
27. Flagg LR. Dietary and holistic treatment of recurrent calcium oxalate kidney stones: review of literature to guide patient education. *Urol Nurs* 2007; **27**(2):113–22, 143; quiz 123.
28. Ettinger B, Tang A, Citron JT, Livermore B, Williams T. Randomized trial of allopurinol in the prevention of calcium oxalate calculi. *N Engl J Med* 1986; **315**(22):1386–9.
29. Laerum E, Larsen S. Thiazide prophylaxis of urolithiasis. A double-blind study in general practice. *Acta Med Scand* 1984; **215**(4):383–9.
30. Borghi L, Meschi T, Guerra A, Novarini A. Randomized prospective study of a nonthiazide diuretic, indapamide, in preventing calcium stone recurrences. *J Cardiovasc Pharmacol* 1993; **22**(Suppl 6):S78–86.
31. Barcelo P, Wuhl O, Servitge E, Rousaud A, Pak CY. Randomized double-blind study of potassium citrate in idiopathic hypocitraturic calcium nephrolithiasis. *J Urol* 1993; **150**(6):1761–4.
32. Ettinger B, Pak CY, Citron JT, Thomas C, Adams-Huet B, Vangessel A. Potassium-magnesium citrate is an effective prophylaxis against recurrent calcium oxalate nephrolithiasis. *J Urol* 1997; **158**(6):2069–73.

CHAPTER 2.2

Kidney stones

Types and predisposing factors

Ben Turney and John Reynard

General predisposing factors

Factors that predispose to stone formation are both genetic and environmental. Twin studies have suggested the heritability of the risk for stones is 56%, suggesting that around half of stones causation can be attributed to an underlying genetic background risk.[1] A genetic link is supported by epidemiological studies that suggest up to 25% of stone formers have an affected first-degree relative.[2]

Occupational or recreational factors resulting in dehydration lead to concentration of the urine, which increases the risk of crystallization. Supersaturation of urine is a risk factor for all types of stone formation and represents the concentration at which crystals can spontaneously nucleate and grow. Urine also contains substances such as magnesium, citrate, glycosaminoglycans, and Tamm–Horsfall protein (uromodulin) and other proteins that can promote or retard urinary crystallization.[3] The amounts of these substances determine the concentration boundary between the metastable and oversaturated zone (the formation product) (Fig. 2.2.1). At present, of these inhibitory factors. Only citrate concentrations can be manipulated clinically. Maintaining a high fluid intake dilutes the urine, keeps the concentration of solutes low, and prevents crystallization.

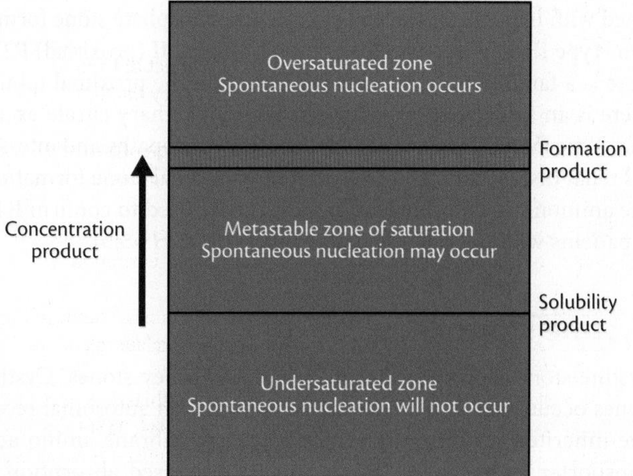

Fig. 2.2.1 Diagram to show the relationship between urinary saturation and nucleation of stones. The formation product boundary is determined by both the concentration of solutes and the balance of inhibitory and promoting factors in urine.

Medical conditions

Medical conditions such as bowel disorders (e.g. Crohn's disease and following bowel resections), gout, renal disease, endocrine conditions (such as hyperparathyroidism and hyperthyroidism) increase risk of stone formation. Trauma, bone fracture, and other conditions that result in immobilization (spinal cord injury) can result in demineralization of bone and hypercalciuria.

Medications

Many medications may alter blood and/or urine biochemistry and predispose to stone formation. Corticosteroids increase absorption of calcium from the gut and cause hypercalciuria. Topirimate (for seizures or migraines), sulphasalazine (for rheumatoid arthritis), diuretics containing triamterene, acetazolamide (for myotonia), antacids containing trisilicate, calcium supplements, vitamin D supplements, vitamin C in high doses, indinavir (for HIV), and some herbal medicines (containing ephedrine) all increase stone risk.

Anatomy

Renal tract anatomical abnormalities, especially those resulting in urinary stasis (e.g. pelviureteric junction obstruction, duplex systems, and horseshoe kidney) predispose to stone formation.

Dietary factors

Dietary factors such as oxalate, animal protein, salt, and strange diets and eating disorders (e.g. anorexia) may alter urine biochemistry and predispose to stone formation.

These risk factors are reflected in the blood and 24-hour urinary profiles of stone formers. Many stone formers have subtle biochemical changes that while individually are within normal quoted ranges, may nonetheless act synergistically to create an overall increase in stone risk. Several algorithms have been developed to incorporate some of these factors (e.g. PSF [probability of stone formation], P_{CaOx}index, EQUIL, Bonn Risk Index).[4–6]

Evaluating causative risk factors should take into account lifestyle, medical history, and medication use, dietary factors, and family history as well as analysis of blood and urine biochemistry to try and determine and thus reduce the risk of stone recurrence.

Calcium oxalate stones

Around 90% of kidney stones contain calcium either as calcium oxalate or calcium phosphate. Nearly 80% of all kidney stones are composed of calcium and oxalate. Calcium oxalate supersaturation is independent of urinary pH. The most common metabolic abnormality found in patients with recurrent stones is hypercalciuria, defined as excretion of >7 mmol of calcium per day in men and >6 mmol per day in women.[7] While most commonly familial and idiopathic, hypercalciuria is strongly influenced by diet. Hypercalciuria can be categorized into three main groups: absorptive (increased intestinal absorption); renal (renal leak of calcium); and resorptive (increased demineralization of bone). Small subsets of patients with hypercalciuria also have hypercalcaemia, and most of these have primary hyperparathyroidism. Stone formation has a higher prevalence in hyperparathyroid patients stones but the urine profiles of those that form stones are indistinguishable from those that do not.[8,9] Thus, stone risk in these patients cannot be attributed to hypercalciuria alone.

Calcium oxalate stones can also form as a consequence of excess amounts of oxalate in the urine (hyperoxaluria). This may be discovered in people with a history of inflammatory disease or surgery of the intestinal tract resulting in changes in the homeostasis of calcium and oxalate (enteric hyperoxaluria). More rarely, primary hyperoxaluria (due to enzyme defects in the liver) results in high urinary oxalate levels. Ascorbic acid and high protein intake also increase oxalate production.

Citrate forms a soluble complex with calcium (chelation), and prevents complexing of calcium with oxalate. Hypocitraturia may be idiopathic or due to rarer disorders such as distal renal tubular acidosis, hypokalaemia, and carbonic anhydrase inhibitors.

Calcium oxalate stones may also precipitate on a urate crystal nidus. Thus, hyperuricosuria may contribute to calcium oxalate stone formation.

Uric acid stones

Around 5–10% of stones are predominantly uric acid (urate). Uric acid is produced from protein breakdown. Unlike birds, humans are unable to convert uric acid (which is relatively insoluble) into allantoin (which is very soluble). Uric acid exists in two forms in urine: uric acid and sodium urate. Sodium urate is 20 times more soluble than uric acid. At a urine pH of 5, <20% of uric acid is present as soluble sodium urate. At a urine pH of 5.5, half the uric acid is ionized as sodium urate (soluble) and half is non-ionized as free uric acid (insoluble). At a urine pH of 6.5, >90% of uric acid is present as soluble sodium urate. Thus, uric acid is essentially insoluble in acid urine and soluble in alkaline urine. Low urinary pH and high levels of urinary uric acid predispose to urate stones. Patients with metabolic syndrome and those who consume high levels of animal protein are particularly at risk. Changes in diet and the obesity epidemic in resource rich countries are translating into increasing numbers of uric acid stones.

Gout is also associated with uric acid stone formation. Around 20% of patients with gout form uric acid stones, and conversely around 50% of patients with uric acid stones have gout. A patient with gout has a risk of stone formation of around 1% per year from the time of the first attack of gout. Myeloproliferative disorders (especially following treatment with cytotoxic drugs) result in a high turnover of cells and release of nucleic acids, which are converted to uric acid. Consequently these patients are at risk of uric acid stones.

Struvite stones (infection stones)

Struvite stones (also known as infection stones, triple phosphate stones, and MAP stones—magnesium ammonium phosphate) are composed of mixtures of magnesium, ammonium, phosphate, and calcium carbonate phosphate crystals. Struvite stones form 2–20% of all stones depending on the country. These stones develop as a consequence of recurrent or chronic urinary tract infection with urease-producing bacteria, which produce ammonia from breakdown of urea (urease hydrolyses urea to carbon dioxide and ammonium), and in so doing, alkalinize urine:

$$NH_2-O-NH_2+2H_2O \Rightarrow 2NH_3+CO_2+H_2O \Rightarrow 2NH_4^+ + HCO_3^- + H^+$$

Struvite stones that occupy the renal pelvis and one or more calyces are known as staghorn stones.

Calcium phosphate stones

Calcium phosphate stones often contain a calcium oxalate component and may form the nidus on which calcium oxalate stones form. Pure calcium phosphate stones are relatively rare and occur in patients with some types of renal tubular acidosis (RTA)—a state of metabolic acidosis with high urinary pH, consequent on an inability to acidify urine. There are several types of RTA. Only types I (distal RTA) and III are associated with renal stones. Approximately 70% of RTA type I patients form stones.

In type I (distal) RTA the distal tubule is unable to maintain a proton gradient between the blood and the tubular fluid. This results in a metabolic acidosis with high urinary pH. Alkaline urine (pH >5.5), supersaturated with calcium and phosphate, and combined with hypocitraturia leads to calcium phosphate stone formation. Type III RTA is a variant of type I. In type II (proximal) RTA, there is a failure of bicarbonate resorption in the proximal tubule. There is an associated protective increase in urinary citrate excretion. Type IV RTA is observed in diabetic nephropathy and interstitial renal disease and is not associated with renal stone formation. The ammonium chloride loading test can be used to confirm RTA in patients with persistently high urinary pH (pH >5.5).

Cystine stones

Cystine stones account for only 1% of all kidney stones. Cystine stones occur only in patients with cystinuria, an autosomal recessive inherited condition in which a transmembrane amino acid transporter is defective. This results in decreased absorption of cystine, ornithine, arginine, and lysine from the gut and proximal tubule of the kidney. Cystine is insoluble, particularly in acidic urine, and precipitates from the proximal tubule.

Further reading

Berger AD, Wu W, Eisner BH, Cooperberg MR, Duh QY, Stoller ML. Patients with primary hyperparathyroidism—why do some form stones? *J Urol* 2009; **181**(5):2141–5.

Curhan GC, Willett WC, Rimm EB, Stampfer MJ. A prospective study of dietary calcium and other nutrients and the risk of symptomatic kidney stones. *N Engl J Med* 1993; **328**(12):833–8.

Goldfarb DS, Fischer ME, Keich Y, Goldberg J. A twin study of genetic and dietary influences on nephrolithiasis: a report from the Vietnam Era Twin (VET) Registry. *Kidney Int* 2005; **67**(3):1053–61.

Laube N, Hergarten S, Hoppe B, Schmidt M, Hesse A. Determination of the calcium oxalate crystallization risk from urine samples: the BONN Risk Index in comparison to other risk formulas. *J Urol* 2004; **172**(1): 355–9.

Rejnmark L, Vestergaard P, Mosekilde L. Nephrolithiasis and renal calcifications in primary hyperparathyroidism. *J Clin Endocrinol Metab* 2011; **96**(8):2377–85.

Robertson WG, Peacock M, Heyburn PJ, Marshall DH, Clark PB. Risk factors in calcium stone disease of the urinary tract. *Br J Urol* 1978; **50**(7):449–54.

Ryall R. Macromolecules and urolithiasis: parallels and paradoxes. *Nephron Physiol* 2004; **98**(2):37–42.

Wilcox WR, Khalaf A, Weinberger A, Kippen I, Klinenberg JR. Solubility of uric acid and monosodium urate. *Med Biol Eng* 1972; **10**(4):522–31.

Worcester EM, Coe FL. New insights into the pathogenesis of idiopathic hypercalciuria. *Semin Nephrol* 2008; **28**(2):120–32.

References

1. Goldfarb DS, Fischer ME, Keich Y, Goldberg J. A twin study of genetic and dietary influences on nephrolithiasis: a report from the Vietnam Era Twin (VET) Registry. *Kidney Int* 2005; **67**(3):1053–61.
2. Curhan GC, Willett WC, Rimm EB, Stampfer MJ. A prospective study of dietary calcium and other nutrients and the risk of symptomatic kidney stones. *N Engl J Med* 1993; **328**(12):833–8.
3. Ryall R. Macromolecules and urolithiasis: parallels and paradoxes. *Nephron Physiol* 2004; **98**(2):37–42.
4. Laube N, Hergarten S, Hoppe B, Schmidt M, Hesse A. Determination of the calcium oxalate crystallization risk from urine samples: the BONN Risk Index in comparison to other risk formulas. *J Urol* 2004; **172**(1): 355–9.
5. Wilcox WR, Khalaf A, Weinberger A, Kippen I, Klinenberg JR. Solubility of uric acid and monosodium urate. *Med Biol Eng* 1972; **10**(4):522–31.
6. Robertson WG, Peacock M, Heyburn PJ, Marshall DH, Clark PB. Risk factors in calcium stone disease of the urinary tract. *Br J Urol* 1978; **50**(7):449–54.
7. Worcester EM, Coe FL. New insights into the pathogenesis of idiopathic hypercalciuria. *Semin Nephrol* 2008; **28**(2):120–32.
8. Rejnmark L, Vestergaard P, Mosekilde L. Nephrolithiasis and renal calcifications in primary hyperparathyroidism. *J Clin Endocrinol Metab* 2011; **96**(8):2377–85.
9. Berger AD, Wu W, Eisner BH, Cooperberg MR, Duh QY, Stoller ML. Patients with primary hyperparathyroidism—why do some form stones? *J Urol* 2009; **181**(5):2141–5.

CHAPTER 2.3

Evaluation of stone formers

Muhammad Waqas Iqbal, Ghalib Jibara, Michael E. Lipkin, and Glenn M. Preminger

Epidemiology

Worldwide epidemiological data show an increase in incidence and prevalence of kidney stone disease. In the United States, stone disease affects approximately 10% of the population, with a 1.4% increase in stone prevalence over the last 20 years.[1] Similar trends have been noted in other developed countries like Germany, where the incidence of stone disease rose from 0.54% to 1.47% over a 10-year period,[2] and Japan where between 1965 and 1995, a significant increase in incidence of stone disease was seen.[3] Although wider availability of more sensitive diagnostic tools like computed tomography (CT) imaging may be partly responsible for this trend, modern-day lifestyle, dietary habits with a notably high salt and high acid ash content (a diet high in animal protein), and a boom in obesity and accompanying insulin resistance are potential factors contributing towards this trend.[4]

Whereas traditionally males were affected two to three times more frequently than females, recent data suggests that female nephrolithiasis prevalence is fast approaching that in males. This finding is especially true for those of African American heritage.[5] Peak occurrence of stone disease occurs in the fourth to sixth decade.[6]

Nephrolithiasis has a higher prevalence in hot or dry climates (mountainous, desert, or tropical regions). Worldwide regions of high stone prevalence include the United States, United Kingdom, Scandinavian, and Mediterranean countries, northern India and Pakistan, northern Australia, central Europe, portions of the Malay peninsula, and China, a region collectively known as the 'Stone Belt'.[7]

The prevalence and incident risk of nephrolithiasis are directly correlated with weight and body mass index (BMI) in both genders, although the magnitude of this association is greater in women than in men.[8,9]

A study from Duke University found that the most common metabolic disturbances in obese patients with body mass index greater than 30 were gouty diathesis (54%) and hypocitraturia (54%), followed by hyperuricosuria (43%).[10] Eisner and associates examined the relationship between BMI and 24-hour urine constituents and found a significant relationship between BMI, increasing urinary sodium and low pH in men, and increasing urinary uric acid, sodium, and decreasing citrate in women.[11]

The geographical distribution of stone disease within the United States is variable, with the southeastern regions having a stone prevalence 50% higher than the northwestern region.[12] It is hypothesized that higher mean annual temperatures 8°C higher in the southeast account for 70% of this variability (by affecting hydration status and urine volumes), while other risk factors such as age, gender, race, diuretic use, and sunlight index account for the rest.[12,13]

It is expected that with global warming, mean annual temperatures will rise further in the United States leading to northwest expansion of the Stone Belt and an increase in prevalence of stone disease. Brikowski has predicted that as the proportion of US population living in high risk stone zones increases from 40% in 2000 to 56% by 2050, and to 70% by 2095, there would be a 30% rise in cases of nephrolithiasis, representing 1.6 to 2.2 million new cases by 2050.[14]

Evaluation of stone formers

The stone recurrence rates among first-time stone formers is as high as 50% over 5–10 years, but with appropriate medical treatment stone remission rates are as high as 80–90%.[15] The principal purpose of biochemical evaluation of stone formers is to prevent stone recurrence in high risk groups and to minimize the growth of any existing stones.[16] The counter-argument to such evaluation is that since 50% of stone formers will not experience a recurrence in their lifetime, why bother with a comprehensive evaluation.[17] However, based on Pak's finding single stone formers to have the same incidence and severity of metabolic abnormalities as recurrent stone formers,[18] we believe that all stone formers, whether single or recurrent, should have a basic evaluation to identify any factors that may predispose to recurrent stone formation. The basic evaluation is reviewed in Box 2.3.1.

History

A focused medical history should be obtained in all stone formers to identify conditions that may require a detailed metabolic evaluation, a history of previous stone episodes, and family history of stone disease (both important predictors of recurrence). While 25% of patients with urolithiasis have a positive family history, the relative risk of stone formation is higher in men with positive family history compared to women.[19]

- Inflammatory bowel disease (Crohns, ulcerative colitis), chronic diarrhoea, tropical spruce, short bowel, blind loop syndromes, gastric bypass surgery, ileostomy, colostomy, or various malabsorption syndromes may lead to dehydration, low urine volumes,

Box 2.3.1 Basic evaluation for all stone formers

History
Physical exam
Serum chemistry

- Chem-7 (serum sodium, potassium, chloride, urea, creatinine, bicarbonate)
- Serum calcium, phosphate
- Serum uric acid
- Parathyroid hormone (intact)

Urine analysis

- pH
- Crystals
- WBC, RBC, Leukocyte esterase, Nitrite

Urine culture
Stone analysis
Urine for qualitative cystine if stone analysis not available
Radiological imaging

- Stone protocol CT scan (CT-KUB)

hypocitraturia, gouty diathesis, or enteric hyperoxaluria, thus increasing the risk of calcium oxalate and uric acid stone disease.

- A history of recurrent urinary tract infections may indicate the presence of struvite stones.
- Abdominal pain, bony pain, polyuria, and polydypsia may indicate primary hyperparathyroidism with hypercalcaemia and possible calcium phosphate stones.
- Malignant tumours and granulomatous lung diseases (sarcoidosis, tuberculosis), may cause hypercalcaemia, and hence stone disease.
- Gout or cancer chemotherapy are associated with uric acid stones.
- Diabetics are more prone to stone disease because of altered ammonia metabolism in the renal tubules and hypocitraturia.
- A focused dietary history should include query about animal protein content, consumption of high oxalate foods, excessive calcium products, and fluid intake.
- Finally, the patients' occupation may identify occupational risk factors for stone disease (e.g. heavily physical labour).

Physical examination

Physical exam may give clues to bony diseases like hypophosphataemic rickets; lymphadenopathy may identify metastatic processes, or haematological or lymphoproliferative disorders. Patients may have undergone gastrointestinal surgery and may have an ileostomy or colostomy, or may appear malnourished secondary to malabsorption syndromes. Immobility may predispose to hypercalciuria and calcium stone disease (spinal cord injury, for example). Patients with neurologic deficits, urinary incontinence, and history of urinary tract infections may have infectious (struvite) stones.

Serum chemistry and haematological tests

A full-blood count may indicate an occult haematological malignancy. Hypokalaemia, hyperchloraemia, and low bicarbonate levels may indicate type I (distal) renal tubular acidosis. High serum calcium levels need to be corrected to albumin levels. If high, a serum parathormone level should be checked. Low serum phosphate levels may indicate type III hypercalciuria.

Urine analysis

The specific gravity of urine is an indicator of hydration status for dehydrated patients having persistently high specific gravity, and for well-hydrated patients having specific gravity around 1,010. A persistently low urinary pH less than 5.5 indicates a gouty diathesis with the resulting risk of calcium oxalate and/or uric acid lithiasis. A persistent pH >6.5 may indicate type I renal tubular acidosis and warrants further investigation. A persistent pH >7.5 may indicate urinary tract infection with urea splitting organisms (*Proteus, Pseudomonas, Klebsiella*, or staphylococcal species), which are associated with formation of struvite stones. The presence of a positive leukocyte esterase, nitrite, and white blood cells may indicate an infection warranting urine culture.

Urine microscopy of sediments may identify various crystal types. The presence of hexagonal crystals indicates cystinuria, while the presence of rectangular coffin lid crystals indicates struvite stones. Tetrahedral envelope-shaped calcium oxalate crystals can be a normal finding in a number of non-stone formers.

Stone analysis

Stone analysis is an important parameter, giving clues not only to potential metabolic disorders predisposing to stone formation, but also determines whether a specific metabolic evaluation is needed in a particular patient. It may even guide the surgeon towards choosing the ideal modality of treatment, or direct future surgical therapy to remove similar stones in the future. Patients with pure uric acid and cystine stones require a modified evaluation, whereas patients with 100% struvite stones do not need a 24-hour urine for evaluation. Patients with calcium phosphate stones may require an ammonium chloride loading test to identify occult renal tubular acidosis.

The generally accepted methods of stone analysis are X-ray diffraction and infrared spectroscopy. Polarization microscopy is also a reliable method, but may only be available in highly specialized centres.

Stone type identification by assessment of Hounsfield readings on CT imaging are unreliable because of significant overlap among various stone types. Recent evidence suggests that dual energy CT may be able to predict *in vivo* stone composition.[20]

Radiological evaluation

Plain abdominal radiography, also referred to as flat plate or KUB radiography ('kidneys, ureter, bladder'), is useful for a rapid assessment of total stone burden, size, shape, composition, and location of urinary calculi in a single image. The majority of upper urinary tract calculi are radio-opaque (since most contain calcium oxalate), but pure uric acid, indinavir, and cystine calculi are relatively radiolucent on plain radiography. Plain abdominal imaging has relatively low sensitivity (40–50%) and specificity for renal and ureteral calculi. Many patients have pelvic calcifications that make specific stone diagnosis difficult. Calcific densities on a KUB radiograph that overlie the course of the ureter may not be a stone.

While not completely extinct in high-income countries, intravenous urography is far less frequently used in the era of the CT-KUB (also known as a non-contrast CT—NCCT), now considered the gold standard for diagnosis of urolithiasis because of its high sensitivity and specificity.[21] The CT-KUB can reliably detect all stone types except indinavir stones, provides detailed anatomic information with regard to atone location and renal anatomy, and can identify obstruction (hydronephrosis, perinephric stranding) without the need for any bowel preparation or intravenous contrast. The radiation dose with modern CT stone protocols is comparable to an intravenous urogram (IVU). In addition, CT can identify non-urological causes of flank pain such as acute appendicitis, diverticulitis, or leaking abdominal aortic aneurysms. CT is considered the imaging modality of choice to document stone-free status after stone intervention.

Ultrasonography avoids radiation exposure, but has considerably poorer sensitivity and specificity for identifying stones. A recent meta-analysis comparing CT to ultrasonography indicated a sensitivity of 44.5% and specificity of 93.8% for ureteric calculi, and 44.7% sensitivity (55.3% false negatives; i.e. more than half of stones not identified) and 87.5% specificity for renal calculi.[22]

The combination of renal ultrasound with X-ray KUB improves sensitivity to 77–96% and specificity to 91–93%.[23,24]

Radiological evaluation in the context of suspected ureteric stone disease

According to the recent American Urological Association (AUA) imaging guidelines for patients presenting with severe flank pain, a non-contrast CT (NCCT) is the preferred initial imaging modality of choice (level A evidence).[25] Low-dose CT (<4 mSv) is preferred for patients with a BMI ≤30, as this imaging study limits the potential radiation exposure while maintaining both sensitivity and specificity at 90% or higher. Low-dose CT is not recommended for those with a BMI >30 due to lower sensitivity and specificity. Renal ultrasonography combined with plain KUB X-ray is a reasonable alternative to NCCT in known stone formers previously known to have had radio-opaque stones. Sensitivities of 58–100% and specificities of 37.2–100% have been reported for this combination of modalities (level C evidence).[26–28]

The AUA imaging guidelines recommend a standard KUB X-ray be performed if the stone is not visible on the CT scout image, so that patients with stones identifiable on the initial KUB X-ray, but not on the CT scout film can be followed by KUB X-ray.[29,30]

The preferred initial imaging modality in children is renal ultrasound, to eliminate radiation risk. Low-dose CT should be considered where a ureteric stone is still suspected but ultrasound is non-diagnostic. For the same reason, renal ultrasonography is the initial imaging modality of choice during pregnancy. In the first trimester where the diagnosis is not established, MRI without contrast should be considered as second-line imaging modality. MRI helps us to identify the level of obstruction and may provide an estimate of stone size. The AUA guidelines further recommend that low-dose CT may be performed for women in the second and third trimesters if ultrasonography is not diagnostic. This recommendation is further endorsed by the American Congress of Obstetricians and Gynecologists (ACOG), which suggests that an exposure of less than 5 rads, a threshold well above the average for a low-dose CT, is not associated with the development of foetal anomalies.[31]

Radiological evaluation in the context of medical expulsive therapy for ureteric stones

The AUA imaging guidelines for ureteral calculi also provide recommendations for follow-up imaging after medical expulsive therapy (MET) or definitive treatment. Patients with a known radio-opaque ureteral calculus on MET can be followed by a combination of ultrasonography and plain KUB. However, for patients who continue to have symptoms, without evidence of stone passage, and where ultrasound and KUB X-ray fail to demonstrate hydronephrosis or a persistent stone, further imaging either with oblique plain radiographs or low-dose NCCT limited to the area of interest is indicated. Patients with known radiolucent stones on MET, who continue to have symptoms without evidence of stone passage, require repeated low-dose NCCT to confirm stone passage.

Radiological evaluation post-stone treatment

Patients who have undergone ureteroscopy with stone fragmentation should undergo follow-up imaging with a ultrasound (for radiolucent stones in an asymptomatic patient) or an ultrasound and KUB X-ray (for radio-opaque stones) to detect any residual fragments and/or hydronephrosis. For patients with an initially radiolucent stone who remain symptomatic or who have hydronephrosis on an ultrasound, a low-dose NCCT to identify obstructing residual fragments is indicated.

For patients treated post-ESWL (extracorporeal shock wave lithotripsy), a follow-up KUB X-ray for radio-opaque stones or renal ultrasound for those with radiolucent stones should be performed. For the asymptomatic patient where the KUB X-ray and ultrasound are negative, no further imaging is required. If hydronephrosis and/or residual fragments are identified, further observation with repeat imaging or secondary treatment are necessary. Patients with radiolucent stones and no hydronephrosis who remain symptomatic or those who are asymptomatic, but have not passed fragments should be further observed with repeat imaging or intervention as indicated.

Metabolic evaluation

There continues to be debate as to which patients should undergo comprehensive metabolic evaluation. In a meta-analysis of randomized trials for medical prevention of calcium oxalate nephrolithiasis versus placebo, Pearle found clinical benefit in terms of reduced stone recurrence rates only in the groups offered *specific* medical therapy targeted at *specific* metabolic defects.[32] Hence, allopurinol was effective only in studies with hyperuricosuria; thiazides worked best in patients with hypercalciuria; potassium citrate was effective only in patients with hypocitraturia.

Conservative therapy alone without comprehensive metabolic evaluation does decrease stone recurrence. Dietary management alone decreases the rate of stone recurrence in 58% of patients with a range of metabolic conditions. A 71% and 47% reduction in stone formation in patients with hypercalciuria and hyperuricosuria while on high fluid intake and avoiding dietary excesses has been reported.[33] That said, several studies report drug therapy to be more cost-effective.[34–37] Of note, the majority of models of cost-effectiveness are based on idiopathic calcium oxalate stone formers.

Cost-effectiveness of metabolic evaluation

Concerns have been raised about the cost of preventive medical therapy versus no such treatment. Chandhoke evaluated the cost of metabolic evaluation, drugs, and doctor office visits with the cost of acute stone management.[38] Data was collected from academic centres in 10 countries, which showed there was great variability in cost of medical and surgical therapies across various countries. For a recurrent stone former, the frequency of stone recurrence, at which medical therapy on the one hand and the cost of managing an acute stone episode on the other becomes equal for calcium stone disease ranged from 0.58 stones/year in the United Kingdom to 4.4 in Germany. In other words—medical prophylaxis becomes cost-effective only if a stone recurs at least once every two years. With less frequent recurrence, the benefits at least in terms of *cost*, of metabolic evaluation combined with medical therapy, are questionable. However, the benefits in terms of enhanced quality of life and time lost from work, neither of which the study addressed, may shift the balance in favour of metabolic evaluation combined with medical therapy. First-time stone formers are keen to pursue stone prevention strategies (metabolic evaluation and preventive therapy),[39] which suggests that stone disease has a very significant impact on quality of life.

Patients requiring comprehensive metabolic evaluation

Patients with non-calcium stones, notably pure uric acid and cysteine stones, have additional significant metabolic abnormalities that require a more extensive metabolic evaluation.

With the caveats noted above, patients with recurrent, multiple, bilateral, or residual calcium stone disease are likely to benefit from metabolic evaluation. Patients with stones that are difficult to treat (e.g. those with spinal deformities, other anatomic abnormalities that make renal access problematic, or morbid obesity) are also likely to benefit from a more thorough metabolic evaluation aiming at a preventive strategy. Box 2.3.2 gives a detailed list of patients at increased risk of stone recurrence, who are more likely to benefit from a comprehensive metabolic evaluation.

Box 2.3.2 Patients at high risk for recurrent stone disease

- History of recurrent stone formation
- Multiple stones
- Bilateral stones
- Children with stones
- Mixed struvite stones
- Uric acid stones
- Cystine stones
- Brushite stones
- Hyperparathyroidism
- Gastrointestinal diseases (inflammatory bowel disease, short bowel, gut diversions, malabsorption syndromes, bariatric surgery)
- Family history of stone disease
- Residual stone fragments (three months after stone therapy)
- Solitary kidney
- Transplanted kidney
- Nephrocalcinosis
- Bone disease
- Renal tubular acidosis type I
- Renal insufficiency
- Metabolic diseases (gout, diabetes mellitus type 2, metabolic syndrome)
- Stones that are difficult to treat because of anatomic abnormalities that make renal access problematic (e.g. spinal deformity, morbid obesity)
- Urinary tract reconstruction, solitary kidney, neuropathic bladder, special professions (e.g. pilots, frequent business travellers)

Metabolic evaluation in patients forming non-calcium stones

Patients with pure uric acid stones should have a 24-hour urine for quantification of uric acid, pH, and creatinine (to assess adequacy of collection). Patients with cystine stones should also complete a 24-hour urine collection because they have an increased likelihood of associated metabolic abnormalities. Pure struvite stones do not require a metabolic evaluation. However, patients with stones with a mixed calcium component should undergo a comprehensive evaluation.

Metabolic evaluation for calcium stone formers

A comprehensive metabolic evaluation currently involves collection of one or two 24-hour urine studies on random diet.[40] The major difference between this evaluation and the original comprehensive evaluation first described by Pak, is that different types of absorptive and renal leak hypercalciuria cannot be differentiated. All patients with normal serum calcium and hypercalciuria are treated with thiazide diuretics.

Prerequisites of 24-hour urine collection

Patients should be on their normal routine of diet and physical activity. Any urinary tract infection should be treated before the collection, as this may lead to abnormally high pH and hypocitraturia. The urine collections should not be performed during an acute stone event, but can be performed four to six weeks after stone passage or a urological intervention. It is not necessary that a patient be stone-free during the collections, but they should not be obstructed or infected. The adequacy of collection can be checked by measuring total creatinine or creatinine/kg and compared to standards.

At Duke University Stone Center in the United States, we perform two 24-hour urine collections on a random diet, followed by dietary or medicinal modification of urinary risk factors. Another 24-hour collection is repeated in four months to confirm compliance, identify the need for dose adjustment, and identify side effects. We repeat the 24-hour collection every six months until urinary risk factors have stabilized, and then yearly thereafter.

Metabolic classification

Once we have the results of metabolic evaluation and stone analysis, urological stone disease may be classified as calcium-based nephrolithiasis and non-calcium stones. Figure 2.3.1 gives the metabolic classification of nephrolithiasis.

Calcium-based nephrolithiasis

This includes calcium oxalate and calcium phosphate stones. Calcium oxalate stones are further classified into monohydrate and dihydrate. Calcium oxalate accounts for 40–60% of stone disease, while calcium phosphate accounts for 2–4% of stones.[41] Patients with calcium-based stones have a variety of metabolic abnormalities on 24-hour urine samples. The most common diagnosis is low urine volume followed by hypercalciuria, hypocitraturia, hyperoxaluria, hyperuricosuria, and gouty diathesis.

Hypercalciuria is defined as a 24-hour urine calcium greater than 250 mg in men and 200 mg in women. This is the most common abnormality found in stone formers. Hypercalciuria may be further classified into absorptive, renal leak, and resorptive hypercalciuria. This categorization is possible only with an extensive metabolic evaluation and the calcium fast and loading tests. Absorptive hypercalciuria results from increased calcium absorption from the intestinal tract, with fasting urinary calcium levels being normal. Patients with absorptive hypercalciuria have normal serum paratharmone levels. The exact aetiology of absorptive hypercalciuria is not clearly defined, as both vitamin D-associated as well as independent processes have been invoked to explain this effect.

Patients with absorptive hypercalciuria type I have increased urinary excretion of calcium despite being on a calcium-restricted diet, whereas in type II, urinary calcium normalizes on diet restricted in calcium, but is high on a regular diet. Type III hypercalciuria is secondary to renal phosphate leak leading to low serum phosphate levels, which in turn stimulate increased vitamin D production, resulting in increased absorption of calcium and phosphate from the intestine.

Renal leak hypercalciuria results from an intrinsic defect in the distal renal tubule leading to increased loss of calcium in urine. These patients have normal serum calcium levels, with mildly elevated levels of serum paratharmone to maintain calcium homeostasis.

Resorptive hypercalciuria results from increased mobilization of calcium from bone as a result of primary hyperparathyroidism. This condition is diagnosed by increased serum calcium, low phosphate and increased intact parathormone levels (i-PTH). Primary hyperparathyroidism causes stone disease only in 1–2% of cases.[42] Increased parathyroid hormone causes increased mobilization of calcium and phosphate from bone as well as increased production of vitamin D3 in kidneys, which in turn leads to increased absorption of calcium and phosphate from the intestine. There is selective

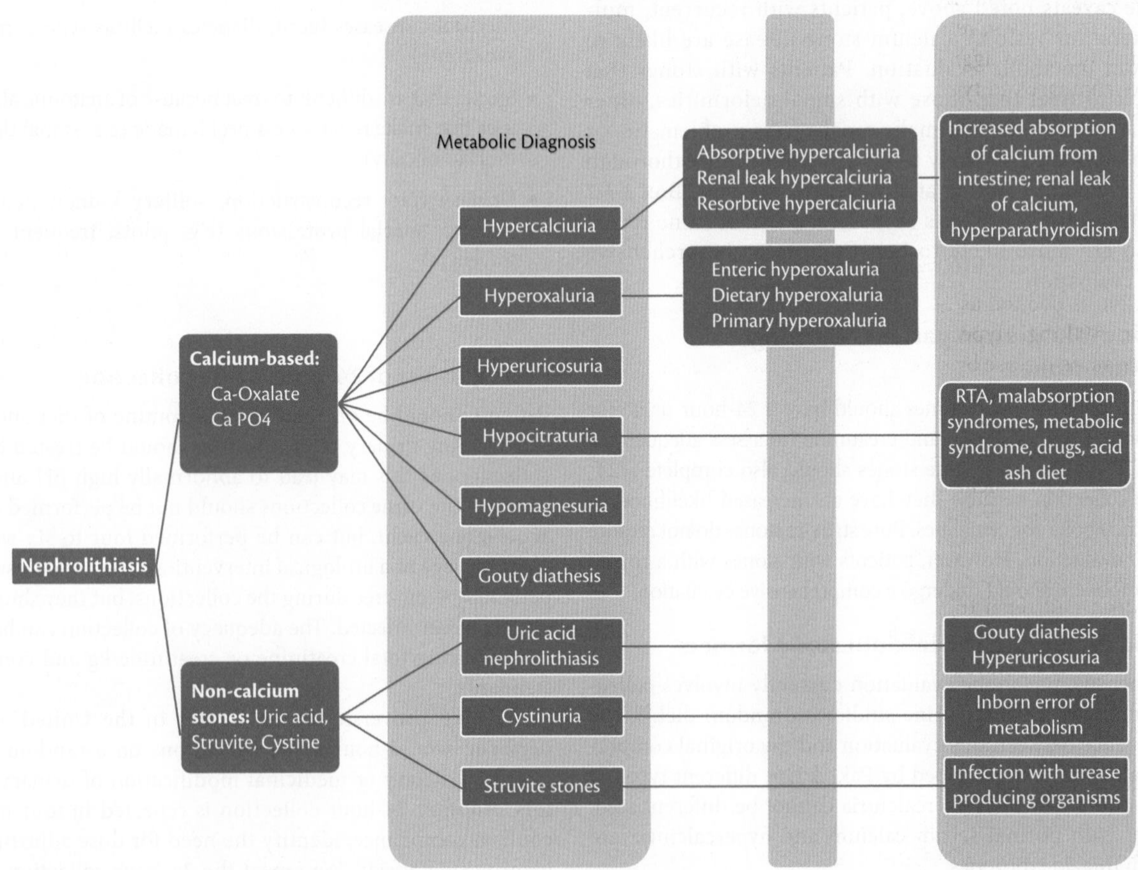

Fig. 2.3.1 Metabolic classification of nephrolithiasis.

loss of phosphate from the kidneys. This action causes elevated serum calcium and low serum phosphate levels.

Hyperoxaluria is defined as urine oxalate levels greater than 40 mg/day. Hyperoxaluria occurs as enteric, dietary, and primary forms. Hyperoxaluria is most commonly due to increased oxalate absorption from the intestine—enteric hyperoxaluria. This defect occurs in conditions leading to intestinal malabsorption. Normally the dietary calcium binds to oxalate to form complexes which are not absorbed. During intestinal malabsorption, excess of fatty acids bind with calcium to form salts, leading to increased availability of free oxalate, which is absorbed from the intestine. Poorly absorbed fatty acids increase the permeability of the colon to oxalate, further increasing oxalate absorption. This action may occur in a number of conditions including inflammatory bowel disease, short gut syndrome, bacterial overgrowth, blind loop syndromes, and so on. Patients with intestinal malabsorption also have a host of other metabolic abnormalities including low urine volumes secondary to intestinal fluid loss, mild metabolic acidosis due to intestinal alkali loss, hypocitraturia, gouty diathesis, and low urinary calcium levels because of complexation with fatty acids. Dietary hyperoxaluria occurs as a result of excessive intake of oxalate-rich foods, especially in the realm of relative calcium restriction; very high doses of vitamin C (>2,000 mg/day) may also cause hyperoxaluria because of conversion of ascorbic acid into oxalate in the liver.

Hyperoxaluria also occurs as autosomal recessive inherited disorder known as primary hyperoxaluria. Type I hyperoxaluria results from deficiency of the enzyme alanine glyoxylate aminotransferase that catalyses conversion of glyoxylate to glycine in liver. Primary hyperoxaluria type II results from deficiency of the enzyme glyoxylate reductase in the liver, resulting in high oxalate levels. Type II hyperoxaluria has a less aggressive course with less occurrence of renal failure compared to type I, however it may lead to hyperoxaluric nephrolithiasis.[43]

Patients with primary hyperoxaluria and end-stage renal failure require a combined kidney and liver transplant to prevent disease recurrence in the graft kidney.

Hyperuricosuric calcium oxalate nephrolithiasis

This condition is defined as 24-hour urine excretion of uric acid of more than 800 mg. Hyperuricosuria can lead to increased calcium oxalate stone disease by providing a nidus for calcium oxalate crystal deposition, a process known as heterogeneous nucleation or epitaxy.[44] Rarely, these patients have a history of hyperuricemia and symptomatic gout. Patients with hyperuricosuria with normal urinary pH may form calcium oxalate stones, whereas those with hyperuricosuria and gouty diathesis (urine pH < 5.5) may form calcium oxalate or pure uric acid stones.[45]

Calcium phosphate stones are commonly associated with hyperparathyroidism and renal tubular acidosis. Such stones occur in two forms—carbonate apatite and brushite. Carbonate apatite crystallization occurs at pH levels of ≥6.8, may be infection related, or may form mixed stones with calcium oxalate. Brushite crystallizes in a very narrow range of pH between 6.5–6.8.

Hypocitraturia

Hypocitraturia is defined as urinary citrate levels less than 450 in men and 550 in women. Citrate is an important inhibitor of calcium nephrolithiasis. It binds with calcium, decreasing availability of ionic calcium to precipitate oxalate or phosphate. It also acts as a direct inhibitor of calcium oxalate crystallization and prevents heterogeneous nucleation of calcium oxalate by monosodium urate.[46] Hypocitraturia has varied aetiologies, but is usually based on acid-base balance within the body such as renal tubular acidosis, hypokalaemia, increased animal protein diet, systemic acidosis, chronic diarrheal states, or thiazide diuretics.

Renal tubular acidosis (RTA) is a heterogeneous disorder characterized by inability of the nephrons to acidify urine. Distal RTA type I is characterized by non-anion gap metabolic acidosis with hyperchloremia, which is hypokalaemia with profoundly low urinary citrate levels.[47] The urinary pH is consistently more than 6.5. Patients may have the complete or overt version with typical metabolic findings. The covert type or incomplete RTA has less profound hypocitraturia and normal urinary pH. This can be diagnosed by ammonium chloride loading test. The first voided urine specimen is sometimes used to identify type I RTA, these patients typically having a morning urinary pH no lower than 5.5. Renal tubular acidosis may also occur as an acquired disorder in conditions such as obstructive uropathy, pyelonephritis, analgesic nephropathy, acute tubular necrosis, renal transplantation, sarcoidosis, and primary hyperparathyroidism.[48]

Hypomagnesuria

Magnesium is an important inhibitor of calcium oxalate stone disease and may be low in conditions such as inflammatory bowel disorders, excessive laxative use, or chronic thiazide use.

Non-calcium nephrolithiasis

These include patients with pure uric acid, cystine, and struvite stones.

Uric acid nephrolithiasis

Uric acid stones are most commonly associated with gouty diathesis, defined as a urine pH less than 5.5. Low urine volumes with a normal acid load from a normal diet may cause significant lowering of urinary pH. The solubility of uric acid depends upon urinary pH, with more than 90% of uric acid being ionized and soluble at a pH of 6.5, but only 50% of uric acid being soluble at a pH of 5.5.[49]

Hyperuricosuria is rare in pure uric acid stone formers. Patients on cancer chemotherapy are predisposed to hyperuricosuria; however, the modern practice of prescribing allopurinol, a xanthine oxidase inhibitor, prevents high levels of uric acid.

Cystinuria

Cystine stones form as a result of an inborn error of metabolism known as cystinuria. It is an autosomal recessive trait resulting in defective transepithelial transport of a number of amino acids at the level of renal tubule including cystine, ornithine, lysine, and arginine (COLA).

In addition to cystinuria, patients with cystine stones often have a number of additional metabolic defects including hypocitraturia, hyperuricosuria, and hypercalciuria in 44.4%, 22.2%, and 18.5%, respectively.[50]

Struvite nephrolithiasis

These stones are composed of magnesium ammonium phosphate. Struvite stones are associated with organisms which produce an enzyme urease, which converts urea, a major metabolite of protein metabolism, into ammonia. The ammonium hydroxide converts the urinary pH to alkaline, with pH levels exceeding 7.5 and ensuing precipitation of magnesium ammonium phosphate.[51,52]

Patients with pure struvite stones do not need a metabolic evaluation, whereas patients with a mixed composition (struvite plus calcium components) may have underlying urinary metabolic abnormalities, which may contribute to stone formation.[50]

Dietary risk factors identified from metabolic evaluation

Low urine volume (<2 litres/24 hours) by increasing the super saturation of solutes may increase risk for calcium or non-calcium nephrolithiasis. This is one of the least expensive and easily modifiable risk factors to prevent recurrent stone formation. Dietary sodium has a significant bearing on urinary calcium levels. Urinary calcium excretion increases by 25 mg for every 100 mmol increase in dietary sodium.[53] Further sodium also reduces citrate excretion and increases cystine excretion.[54] Urinary sodium levels should be maintained under 150 mg /day for optimal results. In patients on thiazide diuretics, the efficacy of hypocalciuric action is significantly affected in the presence of high urinary sodium.

Urinary potassium can be used as a marker to determine compliance for patients on potassium citrate therapy. Moreover, urine potassium may directly impact on urinary citrate levels. Yachantha studied the relationship between serum potassium and urinary citrate levels and found that hypokalaemia may cause hypocitraturia by altering intracellular acid-base milieu.[55]

Urinary magnesium is an inhibitor of stone formation, as the magnesium complexes with oxalate making it unavailable for further interaction. Magnesium may also increase urinary citrate levels by decreasing its tubular reabsorption. Laxative abuse, malabsorption syndromes, and malnutrition may all lead to low magnesium levels.

Further reading

American College of Obstetricians and Gynecologists: guidelines for diagnostic imaging during pregnancy. ACOG Committee Opinion No 299. *Obstet Gynecol* 2004; **104**:647–51.

Brikowski TH, Lotan Y, Pearle MS. Climate-related increase in the prevalence of urolithiasis in the United States. *PNAS* 2008; **105**(28):9841–6.

Chandhoke PS. When is medical prophylaxis cost effective for recurrent calcium stones? *J Urol* 2002; **168**:937–40.

Chandhoke PS. Evaluation of the recurrent stone former. *Urol Clin North Am* 2007; **34**(3):315–22.

Delvecchio FC, Preminger GM. Medical management of stone disease. *Curr Opin Urol* 2003; **13**(3):229–33.

Eisner BH, Eisenberg ML, Stoller ML. Relationship between body mass index and quantitative 24-hour urine chemistries in patients with nephrolithiasis. *Urology* 2010; **75**:1289–93.

Fulgham PF, Assimos DG, Pearle MS, Preminger GM. Clinical effectiveness protocols for imaging in the management of ureteral calculous disease: AUA technology assessment. *J Urol* 2013; **189**(4):1203–13.

Healy KA, Ogan K. Pathophysiology and management of infectious staghorn calculi. *Urol Clin North Am* 2007; **34**(3):363–74.

Johnston R, Lin A, Du J, *et al.* Comparison of kidney-ureter-bladder abdominal radiography and computed tomography scout films for identifying renal calculi. *BJU Int* 2009; **104**:670–3.

Pak CY, Sakhaee K, Moe O, *et al.* Biochemical profile of stone-forming patients with diabetes mellitus. *Urology* 2003; **61**:523–7.

Pak CYC, Peterson R. Successful treatment of hyperuricosuric calcium oxalate nephrolithiasis with potassium citrate. *Arch Intern Med* 1986; **146**:863–8.

Pearle MS, Roehborn CG, Pak CYC. Meta-analysis of randomized trials for medical prevention of calcium oxalate nephrolithiasis. *J Endourol* 1999; **13**:679–85.

Porena M, Guiggi P, Micheli C. Prevention of stone disease. *Urol Int* 2007; **79**(Suppl 1):37–46.

Ray AA, Ghiculete D, Kenneth T. Pace KT, Honey JD'A. Limitations to ultrasound in the detection and measurement of urinary tract calculi. *Urology* 2010; **76**:295–300.

Sakhaee K, Poindexter JR, Pak CY. The spectrum of metabolic abnormalities in patients with cystine nephrolithiasis. *J Urol* 1989; **141**(4):819–21.

Strohmaier WL. Course of calcium stone disease without treatment. What can we expect? *Eur Urol* 2000; **37**:339–44.

Wang AJ, Preminger GM. Distal renal tubular acidosis. *AUA Update series* 2011; **30**: lesson 25.

References

1. Stamatelou KK, Francis ME, Jones CA, Nyberg LM, Curhan GC. Time trends in reported prevalence of kidney stones in the United States: 1976–1994. *Kidney Int* 2003; **63**:1817–23.
2. Hesse A, Brandle E, Wilbert D, Kohrmann KU, Alken P. Study on the prevalence and incidence of urolithiasis in Germany comparing the years 1979 vs. 2000. *Eur Urol* 2003; **44**(6):709–13.
3. Yoshida O, Terai A, Ohkawa T, Okada Y. National trend of the incidence of urolithiasis in Japan from 1965 to 1995. *Kidney Int* 1999; **56**(5):1899–1904.
4. Taylor EN, Curhan GC. Role of nutrition in the formation of calcium-containing kidney stones. *Nephron Physiol* 2004; **98**:55–63.
5. Scales CD, Curtis LH, Springhart WP, *et al.* Changing gender prevalence of nephrolithiasis. *Urol* 2005; **173**(Suppl):298.
6. Hiatt RA, Dales LG, Friedman GD, Hunkeler EM. Frequency of urolithiasis in a prepaid medical care program. *Am J Epidemiol* 1982; **115**:255–65.
7. Finlayson B. Symposium on renal lithiasis: Renal lithiasis in review. *Urol Clin North Am* 1974; **1**:181–212.
8. Curhan GC, Willett WC, Rimm EB, *et al.* Body size and risk of kidney stones. *J Am Soc Nephrol* 1998; **9**:1645–52.
9. Taylor EN, Stampfer MJ, Curhan GC. Obesity, weight gain, and the risk of kidney stones. *JAMA* 2005; **293**:455–62.
10. Ekeruo WO, Tan YH, Young MD, *et al.* Metabolic risk factors and the impact of medical therapy on the management of nephrolithiasis in obese patients. *J Urol* 2004; **172**:159–63.
11. Eisner BH, Eisenberg ML, Stoller ML. Relationship between body mass index and quantitative 24-hour urine chemistries in patients with nephrolithiasis. *Urology* 2010; **75**:1289–93.
12. Chen YY, Roseman JM, DeVivo MJ, Huang CT. Geographic variation and environmental risk factors for the incidence of initial kidney stones in patients with spinal cord injury. *J Urol* 2000; **164**:21–6.
13. Soucie JM, Coates R, McClellan W, Austin H, Thun M. Relation between geographic variability in kidney stones prevalence and risk factors for stones. *Am J Epidemiol* 1996; **143**:487–95.
14. Brikowski TH, Lotan Y, Pearle MS. Climate-related increase in the prevalence of urolithiasis in the United States. *PNAS* 2008; **105**(28): 9841–6.
15. Delvecchio FC, Preminger GM. Medical management of stone disease. *Curr Opin Urol* 2003; **13**(3):229–33.
16. Chandhoke PS. Evaluation of the recurrent stone former. *Urol Clin North Am* 2007; **34**(3):315–22.
17. Strohmaier WL. Course of calcium stone disease without treatment. What can we expect? *Eur Urol* 2000; **37**:339–44.
18. Pak CY. Should patients with single renal stone occurrence undergo diagnostic evaluation? *J Urol* 1982; **127**:855–8.

19. Resnick M, Pridgen DB, Goodman HO. Genetic predisposition to formation of calcium oxalate renal calculi. *N Engl J Med* 1968; **278**:1313–18.
20. Zilberman DE, Ferrandino MN, Preminger, GM, Paulson EK, Lipkin ME, Boll DT. In vivo determination of urinary stone composition using dual energy computerized tomography with advanced post-acquisition processing. *J Urol* 2010; **184**(6):2354–9.
21. Smith RC, Rosenfield AT, Choe KA, *et al.* Acute flank pain: comparison of non-contrast-enhanced CT and intravenous urography. *Radiology* 1995; **194**:789–94.
22. Ray AA, Ghiculete D, Kenneth T. Pace KT, Honey JD'A. Limitations to ultrasound in the detection and measurement of urinary tract calculi. *Urology* 2010; **76**:295–300.
23. Catalano O, Nunziata A, Altei F, *et al.* Suspected ureteral colic: primary helical CT versus selective helical CT after unenhanced radiography and sonography. *AJR Am J Roentgenol* 2002; **178**:379–87.
24. Mitterberger M, Pinggera GM, Pallwein L, *et al.* Plain abdominal radiography with transabdominal native tissue harmonic imaging ultrasonography vs unenhanced computed tomography in renal colic. *BJU Int* 2007; **100**:887–90.
25. Fulgham PF, Assimos DG, Pearle MS, Preminger GM. Clinical effectiveness protocols for imaging in the management of ureteral calculous disease: AUA technology assessment. *J Urol* 2013; **189**(4):1203–13.
26. Dalla PL, Stacul F, Bazzocchi M, *et al.* Ultrasonography and plain film versus intravenous urography in ureteric colic. *Clin Radiol* 1993; **47**:333.
27. Ripollés T1, Agramunt M, Errando J, Martínez MJ, Coronel B, Morales M. Suspected ureteral colic: plain film and sonography vs unenhanced helical CT. A prospective study in 66 patients. *Eur Radiol* 2004; **14**:129–36.
28. Gorelik U, Ulish Y, Yagil Y. The use of standard imaging techniques and their diagnostic value in the workup of renal colic in the setting of intractable flank pain. *Urology* 1996; **47**:637–42.
29. Johnston R, Lin A, Du J, *et al.* Comparison of kidney-ureter-bladder abdominal radiography and computed tomography scout films for identifying renal calculi. *BJU Int* 2009; **104**:670–3.
30. Ege G, Akman H, Kuzucu K, Yildiz S. Can computed tomography scout radiography replace plain film in the evaluation of patients with acute urinary tract colic? *Acta Radiol* 2004; **45**:469–73.
31. American College of Obstetricians and Gynecologists: American College of Obstetricians and Gynecologists: guidelines for diagnostic imaging during pregnancy. ACOG Committee Opinion No 299. *Obstet Gynecol* 2004; **104**:647–51.
32. Pearle MS, Roehborn CG, Pak CYC. Meta-analysis of randomized trials for medical prevention of calcium oxalate nephrolithiasis. *J Endourol* 1999; **13**:679–85.
33. Hosking DH, Erickson SB, Van den Berg CJ, Wilson DM, Smith LH. The stone clinic effect in patients with idiopathic calcium urolithiasis. *J Urol* 1983; **130**(6):1115–18.
34. Tiselius HG. Comprehensive metabolic evaluation of stone formers is cost effective. (p. 349) In: Rodgers AL, Hibbert BE, Hess B, Kahn SR, Preminger GM (eds). *Urolithiasis 2000, Proceedings of the 9th International Symposium on Urolithiasis, Cape Town, South Africa.* University of Cape Town Press: Cape Town, South Africa.
35. Parks JH, Coe FL. The financial effects of kidney stone prevention. Kidney Int 1996; **50**:1706–12.
36. Robertson WG. The economic case for the biochemical screening of stone patients. (p. 403) In: Rodgers AL, Hibbert BE, Hess B, Kahn SR, Preminger GM (eds). *Urolithiasis 2000, Proceedings of the 9th International Symposium on Urolithiasis, Cape Town, South Africa.* University of Cape Town Press: Cape Town, South Africa.
37. Strohmaier WL, Hormann M. Economic aspects of urolithiasis and metaphylaxis in Germany. (p. 406) In: Rodgers AL, Hibbert BE, Hess B, Kahn SR, Preminger GM (eds). *Urolithiasis 2000, Proceedings of the 9th International Symposium on Urolithiasis, Cape Town, South Africa.* University of Cape Town Press: Cape Town, South Africa.
38. Chandhoke PS. When is medical prophylaxis cost effective for recurrent calcium stones? *J Urol* 2002; **168**:937–40.
39. Grampsas SA, Moore M, Chandhoke PS. 10-year experience with extracorporeal shockwave lithotripsy in the state of Colorado. *J Endourol* 2000; **14**:711–14.
40. Pearle MS, Goldfarb, DS, Assimos DG, *et al.* Medical management of kidney stones: *AUA guideline J Urol* 2014; **192**:316–24.
41. Moe OW. Kidney stones: patho physiology and medical management. *Lancet* 2006; **367**(9507):333–44.
42. Broadus AE. Primary hyperparathyroidism. *J Urol* 1989; **141**:723–30.
43. Johnson SA, Rumsby G, Cregeen D, Hulton SA. Primary hyperoxaluria type-2in children. *Pediatr Nephrol* 2002; **17**:597–601.
44. Coe FL. Hyperuricosuric calcium oxalate nephrolithiasis. *Adv Exp Med Biol* 1980; **128**:439–50.
45. Pak CY, Sakhaee K, Moe O, *et al.* Biochemical profile of stone-forming patients with diabetes mellitus. *Urology* 2003; **61**:523–7.
46. Pak CYC, Peterson R. Successful treatment of hyperuricosuric calcium oxalate nephrolithiasis with potassium citrate. *Arch Intern Med* 1986; **146**:863–8.
47. Wang AJ, Preminger GM. Distal renal tubular acidosis. *AUA Update series* 2011; **30**: lesson 25.
48. Buckalew VM Jr. Nephrolithiasis in renal tubular acidosis. *J Urol* 1989; **141**:731–737
49. Gutman AB, Yu TF. Uric acid nephrolithiasis. *Am J Med* 1968; **45**:756–79.
50. Sakhaee K, Poindexter JR, Pak CY. The spectrum of metabolic abnormalities in patients with cystine nephrolithiasis. *J Urol* 1989; **141**(4):819–21.
51. Nemoy NJ, Staney TA. Surgical, bacteriological, and biochemical management of "infection stones". *JAMA* 1971; **215**(9):1470–6.
52. Healy KA, Ogan K. Pathophysiology and management of infectious staghorn calculi. *Urol Clin North Am* 2007; **34**(3):363–74.
53. Heilberg IP, Schor N. Renal stone disease: causes, evaluation, and medical treatment. *Arq Bras Endocrinol Metab* 2006; **50**:823–31.
54. Porena M, Guiggi P, Micheli C. Prevention of stone disease. *Urol Int* 2007; **79**(Suppl 1):37–46.
55. Yachantha C, Hossain, RZ, Yamakawa K, *et al.* Effect of potassium depletion on urinary stone risk factors in Wistar rats. *Urol Res* 2009; **37**:311–16.

CHAPTER 2.4

Prevention of idiopathic calcium stones

Ben Turney and John Reynard

Principles of stone prevention

The main principles of idiopathic calcium oxalate stone prevention are to maintain dilute urine through increasing fluid intake and to reduce calcium and oxalate excretion. The influence of various urinary factors on the risk of stone formation has been quantified mathematically (Fig. 2.4.1). Urine volume and urinary oxalate concentration are most influential on therisk of stone formation, while magnesium concentration contributes a small amount to risk.

Generic advice

The concentration of urinary solutes can be manipulated via appropriate fluid intake, diet, and medical therapy. Fluid intake should be increased to maintain a urine volume greater than 2 L in 24 hours[1] and should take into account occupation and sensible and insensible water loss. Calcium and oxalate secretion can be manipulated to varying degrees by diet alteration. A diet low in sodium (<100 mmol/day), animal protein (<0.8–1 g/kg/day), oxalate (<100 mg/day), and calcium (800–1,000 mg/day) is recommended.[2,3] A diet diary may be useful to identify the foods that contribute to risk. Sodium and animal protein affect urinary calcium and urate levels. Low calcium intake is avoided because of evidence that this increases stone risk.[4]

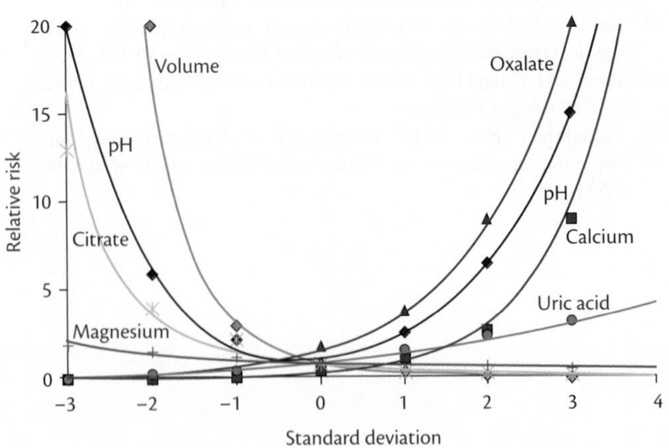

Fig. 2.4.1 Relative contribution of urinary factors to risk of stone formation.
Reproduced with kind permission from Dr William Robertson.

Hypercalciuria

For patients with hypercalciuria, thiazide diuretics (e.g. chlorthalidone 12.5–50 mg/day, indapamide 1.25–2.5 mg/day, hydrochlorothiazide 125–25 mg/twice daily) can reduce urinary calcium concentration by decreasing calcium excretion in the distal convoluted tubule.[5–7] In these placebo-controlled, prospective studies, significant reductions in recurrence rates were observed (greater than 50% additional benefit). Potential side effects include hypokalaemia, hypotension, allergy and sun sensitivity, and hypocitraturia (which tends to promote stone formation).

Hyperoxaluria

Oxalate and calcium bind in the gut and hyperoxaluria may occur when dietary calcium is low (which probably explains why low calcium diets are lithogenic[4]), oxalate intake is high, or uncommonly when oxalate is overproduced. Restriction of dietary oxalate (<100 mg/day) and avoidance of high vitamin C (a precursor of oxalate) intake may limit oxalate excretion.[8] Oxalate is found in high levels in spinach, rhubarb, wheat bran, chocolate, beets, miso, tahini, and most nuts. Significant or resistant hyperoxaluria may be due to one of the primary hyperoxaluria syndromes.

Hypocitraturia

Potassium alkali (usually potassium citrate 10–20 mmol twice or three times a day) chelates calcium and inhibits growth of calcium crystals. It is useful for patients with hypocitraturia[9,10] but can lead to excessive alkalinization of the urine, which may facilitate calcium phosphate stone formation. Patients taking potassium citrate should have their urine pH monitored.

Hyperuricosuria

Hyperuricosuria decreases the solubility of calcium and oxalate, so increasing risk of calcium oxalate stone formation. Allopurinol (100–300 mg/day) has been shown to reduce urinary uric acid levels and stone recurrence in patients with hyperuricosuria who form calcium stones.[11] The benefits are not clear for calcium stone formers that are normouricosuric. A reduction in the intake of animal protein (purines) is also advised.

Calcium phosphate stones

Preventive measures for calcium phosphate stones are similar to those for calcium oxalate stone prevention, with the exception that potassium citrate must be used with caution as it raises urinary pH and can thus increase calcium phosphate supersaturation.

Conclusion

In conclusion, preventive treatment has been shown to reduce stone recurrence in long-term clinical follow-up.[12] However, unless regular monitoring is undertaken, patient compliance falls with time.[13]

References

1. Borghi L, Meschi T, Amato F, Briganti A, Novarini A, Giannini A. Urinary volume, water and recurrences in idiopathic calcium nephrolithiasis: a 5-year randomized prospective study. *J Urol* 1996; **155**(3):839–43.
2. Borghi L, Schianchi T, Meschi T, *et al.* Comparison of two diets for the prevention of recurrent stones in idiopathic hypercalciuria. *N Engl J Med* 2002; **346**(2):77–84.
3. Nouvenne A, Meschi T, Prati B, *et al.* Effects of a low-salt diet on idiopathic hypercalciuria in calcium-oxalate stone formers: a 3-mo randomized controlled trial. *Am J Clin Nutr* 2010; **91**(3):565–70.
4. Curhan GC, Willett WC, Rimm EB, Stampfer MJ. A prospective study of dietary calcium and other nutrients and the risk of symptomatic kidney stones. *N Engl J Med* 1993; **328**(12):833–8.
5. Borghi L, Meschi T, Guerra A, Novarini A. Randomized prospective study of a nonthiazide diuretic, indapamide, in preventing calcium stone recurrences. *J Cardiovasc Pharmacol* 1993; **22**(Suppl 6):S78–86.
6. Ettinger B, Citron JT, Livermore B, Dolman LI. Chlorthalidone reduces calcium oxalate calculous recurrence but magnesium hydroxide does not. *J Urol* 1988; **139**(4):679–84.
7. Laerum E, Larsen S. Thiazide prophylaxis of urolithiasis. A double-blind study in general practice. *Acta Med Scand* 1984; **215**(4):383–9.
8. Massey LK, Liebman M, Kynast-Gales SA. Ascorbate increases human oxaluria and kidney stone risk. *J Nutr* 2005; **135**(7):1673–7.
9. Barcelo P, Wuhl O, Servitge E, Rousaud A, Pak CY. Randomized double-blind study of potassium citrate in idiopathic hypocitraturic calcium nephrolithiasis. *J Urol* 1993; **150**(6):1761–4.
10. Ettinger B, Pak CY, Citron JT, Thomas C, Adams-Huet B, Vangessel A. Potassium-magnesium citrate is an effective prophylaxis against recurrent calcium oxalate nephrolithiasis. *J Urol* 1997; **158**(6):2069–73.
11. Ettinger B, Tang A, Citron JT, Livermore B, Williams T. Randomized trial of allopurinol in the prevention of calcium oxalate calculi. *N Engl J Med* 1986; **315**(22):1386–9.
12. Parks JH, Coe FL. Evidence for durable kidney stone prevention over several decades. *BJU Int* 2009; **103**(9):1238–46.
13. Parks JH, Asplin JR, Coe FL. Patient adherence to long-term medical treatment of kidney stones. *J Urol* 2001; **166**(6):2057–60.

CHAPTER 2.5

Prevention of other non-calcium stones

Muhammad Waqas Iqbal, Ghalib Jibara, Michael E. Lipkin, and Glenn M. Preminger

Introduction to prevention of other non-calcium stones

The primary aim of stone preventive therapy is to minimize future recurrences or prevent growth of any existing stones. Non-specific measures as well as specifically targeted medical therapy can be utilized to decrease future stone-related events. This has been possible with the advancements in understanding of the pathophysiology of urinary stone formation, identification of metabolic risk factors, and availability of selective and non-selective strategies to modify these risks.[1–3]

Non-calcium based stones include uric acid, cystine, and struvite stones. The goal of prevention for uric acid stones is to raise the urinary pH with alkaline therapy. For cystine stone formers, prevention is centred at raising urinary pH to increase the solubility of cystine and reducing urine cystine concentration. The management of struvite stones is founded on complete stone removal. Suppressive antibiotics and acetohydroxamic acid can be used to prevent recurrence.

Non-specific measures

Non-specific dietary management alone can decrease the rate of stone recurrence in 58% patients with a variety of metabolic conditions. Avoiding dietary excesses of sodium and animal protein in addition to increasing fluid intake resulted in 71% and 47% reductions in stone formation in patients with hypercalciuria and hyperuricosuria, respectively.[4]

Non-specific measures include:

Increased urine volume

Prospective randomized trials have shown that increased fluid intake with concomitant increased urine output decreases stone recurrence.[5] Increase in urine volume diluted urinary solutes, leading to decreased crystallization of metabolically active salts. The overall increased urinary flow also washes away the crystals and prevents precipitation. We recommend urine volume greater than 2–2.5 L in a 24-hour period.

Citrus fruits

Citrus juices may play an adjunctive role in stone prevention by virtue of their citrate content. Citrate is an important inhibitor not only of calcium based stone disease, but also prevents uric acid and cystine stones by altering urinary pH. Both orange and lemon juices have been shown to reduce the risk of stone formation.[6,7]

The citrate content of various drinks has been evaluated to estimate their beneficial effect on stone prevention. There appears to be variation in content related to the preparation and possible methodology utilized to measure concentrations. Haleblian[8] assessed the citrate concentrations of various citrate juices and drinks using nuclear magnetic resonance spectroscopy (1H NMR) and found the highest citrate concentrations in grapefruit juice (Florida's Natural® Ruby Red grapefruit juice, 64.7 mmol/L), squeezed lemon juice (47.66 mmol/L), orange juice (Tropicana® Original style, 47.36 mmol/L), pineapple juice (Dole, 41.57 mmol/L), reconstituted lemonade ((Tropicana® 38.65 mmol/L) and lemonade flavoured Crystal Light (Kraft Foods, 38.39 mmol/L).

Penniston[9] evaluated the citric acid content of 21 commercially available juices and juice concentrates using ion chromatography and found fresh lemon or lime juice to contain the highest levels of citrate 45–48 g/L, while ready-to-consume lemonades from various brands contained 1.6–7.3 g/L of citrate. Florida's Ruby Red ready-to-consume grapefruit juice had 25 g/L, while Tropicana ready-to-consume orange juice had 16.9–16.7 g/L, and fresh orange juice from fruit had 9.10 g/L of citrate.

Controversy still exists in the literature as to the best drink available for stone prevention because of variation in their citrate, potassium, oxalate, caloric, sodium, and potential calciuric effects.

Lemonade therapy has been shown to increase urinary citrate and decrease the stone burden in calcium nephrolithiasis, however, it has not been successful in elevating the urinary pH, which is the mainstay for prevention of uric acid stones as well cystine stones. This has been attributed to presence of a proton with citrate, which potentially nullifies the effect of bicarbonate produced from citrate in the liver. The presence of potassium in other citrus juices (e.g. orange) results in the delivery of more bicarbonate to the kidneys leading to an alkaline urinary pH.[10,11]

Kang[7] retrospectively evaluated the impact of long-term lemonade therapy on urinary metabolic parameters and stone formation in patients with hypocitraturic nephrolithiasis. Patients were given 120 mL concentrated lemon juice (5.9 gm citric acid) mixed with 2 L water consumed throughout each day, whereas the control group received 20 mEq of potassium citrate tablets twice daily. At mean follow-up of 42.5 months, almost all patients on lemonade therapy demonstrated increased urinary citrate levels (mean increase of 383 mg per day ($p < 0.05$), while those on potassium citrate therapy demonstrated a mean increase in urinary citrate of 482 mg per day, $p < 0.0001$). No change in urinary oxalate was observed. There was a decrease in mean stone burden in the lemonade group from 37.2 to 30.4 mm^2 (p <0.05). During lemonade therapy, the stone formation rate decreased from 1.00 to 0.13 stones per patient per year (p <0.05). No change in urinary pH was observed in the lemonade therapy group, whereas pH increased from 6.3 to 6.9 in the potassium citrate group.

Orange juice, on the other hand, is known to increase urinary pH as well as citrate levels and hence may be more productive in preventing uric acid and cystine stone disease. Wabner and Pak[12] compared the effect of 1.2 L of orange juice to potassium citrate 60 mEq per day. Orange juice caused a similar increase in urinary pH (6.48 vs. 6.75 from 5.71) and citrate (952 vs. 944 from 571 mg per day). Additionally it decreased urinary undissociated uric acid levels. However, orange juice increased urinary oxalate, which may be counterproductive for calcium oxalate stone disease. Potassium citrate, on the other hand, decreased urinary calcium without altering urinary oxalate. Webner and Pak suggested that orange juice could be beneficial in the control of calcareous and uric acid nephrolithiasis.

In a randomized, cross-over study[11] involving 14 patients comparing the effects of orange juice with those of lemonade (Minute Maid®, 400 mL taken three times daily for one week) and control on acid-base profile and urinary stone risk factors under controlled metabolic conditions, Odvina noted that although the urinary oxalate was modestly and significantly higher for orange juice, it provided a significantly higher urinary pH than lemonade or control. Similarly, the calculated undissociated uric acid was lower in the orange juice phase, compared to lemonade or control phases (77 vs. 181 mg/d). The study also showed that the mean increase in citrate per 240 mL of juice consumed was 88 ± 30 mg for orange and only 11 ± 23 mg for lemonade.

Hönow *et al.*[13] analysed the effect of orange juice on urinary parameters in nine normal healthy subjects. They noted that consumption of 0.5 L of orange juice resulted in an increase in mean urinary pH from 6.08 to 6.42 (p <0.01), whereas citrate excretion also increased from 3.2 to 3.8 mmol/l (p <0.05).

Recently, melon juice, a non-citrus source of potassium, citrate, and malate, has been found to yield equivalent increases in urinary citrate excretion compared to orange juice. Baia *et al.*[14] evaluated the effects of consuming 385 mL of either freshly squeezed orange juice, freshly blended melon juice, or freshly squeezed lime juice on urinary pH, citrate, and other urinary parameters in hypocitraturic stone formers. The urinary pH was significantly higher after both melon and orange juice consumption. It increased to 6.46 ± 0.73 from a baseline of 6.05 ± 0.60 in the orange group, and 6.52 ± 0.50 from a baseline 6.16 ± 0.75 in the melon group. No significant changes were observed for urinary pH in the lime group. There was no difference in urinary citrate excretion among the three groups.

Dietary restrictions

Low salt diet: Increased sodium intake causes increase urinary calcium excretion urine[15] and produces mild metabolic acidosis leading to hypocitraturia. In addition, increased sodium intake causes increased cystine excretion. Therefore, low salt should be encouraged as a general measure to prevent urinary stone disease.

Animal protein: Animal protein with its acid ash content can cause hypocitraturia, gouty diathesis, and hyperuricosuria, thus predisposing to calcium and uric acid stone formation. Animal protein and salt restriction, with a normal calcium intake, decreases stone recurrence rates compared to a simple calcium restricted diet.[2]

Weight loss and low fat diet: Obesity increases the risk of stone disease by predisposing to hypocitraturia, gouty diathesis, and hyperuricosuria. Hence, weight loss and a low fat diet should be encouraged.

Selective medical therapy

Selective medical therapy is available for the prevention of uric acid, cystine, and struvite stones. The primary risk factor for formation of uric acid stones is gouty diathesis or urinary pH ≤5.5. Medical therapy is instituted to increase the urinary pH, thereby increasing the solubility of uric acid. This can be accomplished with potassium citrate or sodium bicarbonate. Cystine stones form from elevated concentration of cystine in the urine. Cystine levels can be reduced by a number of medications including tiopronin, D-penicillamine, and captopril. Cystine is also more soluble at higher urinary pH, so potassium citrate is a useful adjunct in these patients. Finally, struvite stone formation results primarily from urease splitting bacteria. Medical therapy for prevention includes suppressive antibiotic therapy, as well as acetohydroxamic acid (Fig. 2.5.1).

Uric acid nephrolithiasis

Medical therapy should address the three metabolic abberations that lead to uric acid stone formation: acidic urinary pH, low urinary volume, and hyperuricosuria. Persistently low urine pH is associated with uric acid nephrolithiasis. Alkalinization of the urine along with increased hydation is the cornerstone of prevention of uric acid nephrolithiasis.[16–18] With a pKa of uric acid at 5.3, patients with normal uric acid excretion but a low urinary pH can develop uric acid stones, whereas those with a normal or higher urinary pH but excessive urate excretion will not.

Potassium citrate

Potassium citrate is used not only to prevent calcium nephrolithiasis, but also utilized for urinary alkalinization to increase solubility of uric acid and cystine. A number of randomized trials have shown efficacy of potassium citrate in prevention of recurrent calcium stones. Potassium citrate is the treatment of choice to correct gouty diathesis, the most common underlying cause of uric acid nephrolithioasis.[16,17] The goal of therapy is to maintain urinary pH between 6.5–7 to enhance dissolution of uric acid. However a pH above 7.0 may predispose to calcium phosphate stone formation.

A large portion of absorbed citrate is metabolized in the liver to bicarbonate, which provides the alkali load that induces increased citrate excretion by the kidney. A portion of absorbed citrate is excreted in urine providing the citraturic action. A number of studies have demonstrated that potassium citrate is effective in increasing urinary pH.[7,12]

Pak *et al.*[19] described a retrospective review of patients with uric acid nephrolithiasis that underwent long-term treatment (mean of 2.7 years) with potassium citrate (usually 60 mEq/day). This resulted in an increase in urinary pH from 5.30 to 6.19–6.46. Urinary citrate increased from 503 mg/day to 852–998 mg/day. Urinary undissociated uric acid decreased from 204 ± 82 mg/day to 64–108 mg/day. New stone formation rate declined from 1.20 ± 1.68 stones/year to 0.01 ± 0.04 stones/year (p <0.001). Remission was experienced in 94.4% of patients, and the stone formation rate declined by 99.2%

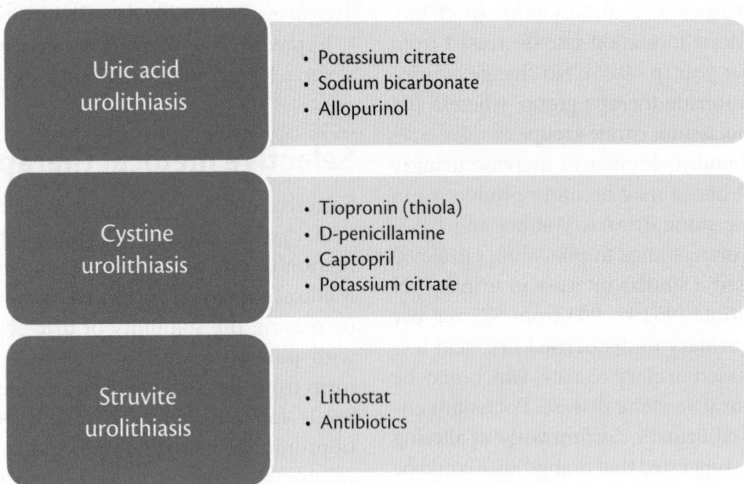

Fig. 2.5.1 Medical therapy options for non-calcium stones.

In a retrospective cohort of 503 patients on potassium citrate therapy for a mean of 41 months (range 6–168), urinary pH increased from 5.9 to 6.46, whereas citrate increased from 470 mg/day to 700 mg/day. The stone formation rate also significantly decreased from 1.89 to 0.46 stones per year (p <0.0001). There was a 68% remission rate and a 93% decrease in the stone formation rate. Of note, 40% of patients in this study had gouty diathesis and 12% hyperuricosuria. The median dose of potassium citrate was 20 mEq twice daily. In 10% of cases, patients were also on allopurinol.[20] Citrate is available as slow release potassium citrate tablets, liquid preparations, and potassium–magnesium citrate, which has the added benefit of having magnesium. The current formulation of potassium citrate embedded within a wax matrix may help alleviate the risk of gastric irritation. Patients are strongly encouraged to take this medication with meals to increase tolerability. The usual starting dose of slow release potassium citrate tablets is 20 mEq PO twice daily; doses as high as 120 mEq/day may be required in certain patients with titration based on urinary pH, citrate levels, and tolerability of medicine. However, potassium citrate shares with other potassium salts the tendency to irritate gastric mucosa, with side effects including ballotment, nausea, or vomiting.[21–24]

Serum potassium needs to be monitored in patients on potassium supplements, especially those with renal insufficiency or taking potassium-sparing diuretics. Patients with hypocitraturia associated with malabsorption may benefit from liquid preparations, as the slow release preparations may not be absorbed and passed intact due to the decreased bowel transit time associated with these conditions.

Sodium bicarbonate

In patients who do not tolerate potassium citrate, have renal insufficiency, or hyperkalaemia, sodium bicarbonate may be given. The usual starting dose of two 650 mg tablets twice daily with meals may need titration to up to four tablets three times daily; doses may go as high as 1.3 g four times a day. The sodium content may, however, cause increased excretion of calcium in urine and promotion of monosodium urate-induced crystallization of calcium oxalate. Caution needs to be exercised as it may predispose to aggravation of congestive cardiac failure or make hypertension control difficult.

Sodium citrate possesses the same alkalinizing characteristics, but like sodium bicarbonate, its sodium content may negate its usefulness.

Hyperuricosuric uric acid lithiasis can be treated with xanthine oxidase inhibitors to decrease uric acid production or alternatively with potassium citrate, which increases its solubility in urine. Allopurinol is preferred in patients with marked hyperuricosuria (>1,000–1,200 mg/day), especially if hyperuricemia coexists.

Allopurinol and febuxotat are inhibitors of xanthine oxidase, the enzyme that catalyses the conversion of hypoxanthine to xanthine and xanthine to uric acid. This decreases the concentration of serum and urine uric acid. An important consideration in patients with acidic pH is to alkalinize the urine to increase uric acid solubility. Allopurinol has a dose range of 100–300 mg once daily. In a randomized placebo-controlled trial involving patients with calcium oxalate stone disease, 75% patients treated with allopurinol had no stone recurrence compared to 45% in the placebo group over a three-year period.[25] The common side effects are rash and hepatotoxicity. The dose needs to be reduced in patients with renal insufficiency.

Febuxostat, a newer agent, is unlike allopurinol, metabolized chiefly in the liver and so it does not need dose readjustment in renal insufficiency. The uric acid lowering capacity of this drug at doses of 80 mg and 120 mg is superior to allopurinol and placebo in randomized controlled trials.[26]

Febuxostat may be used in patients who are allergic to allopurinol or manifest hypersensitivity, and in patients who fail to achieve serum uric acid targets with allopurinol.[27]

Cystine stones

The cornerstone of management of cystinuria is to decrease the concentration of cystine to below its solubility limit (i.e. <200–250 mg/L of urine). Increased fluid intake to increase urine volume and dilute excreted cystine are critical. Urine volumes >3–4 L per 24 hours are optimum. Alkaline pH makes cystine more soluble, however with pKa of 8.3, urinary pH manipulation therapy has a limited role in the management of these patients. The solubility of cystine does not increase significantly until urinary pH is 7.5 or higher and such urine pH levels can predispose to calcium phosphate stone formation. The aim is for a urinary pH of 6.5–7.0. This range is best achieved with the administration of potassium citrate at a dose of 10–20 mEq twice daily. Patients who are intolerant may be given sodium bicarbonate or sodium citrate. Reduction of sodium intake is associated with a reduction in cystine excretion, although the basis for this effect is unclear.[28,29]

When conservative measures fail to achieve target cystine levels, thiols (tiopronin, D-pencillamine, captopril) are indicated. Cystine is a dimer of cysteine linked by a disulfide bridge. Thiol derivatives cleave cystine into two cysteine moieties and combine with a molecule of cysteine to form a highly soluble disulfide compound, decreasing the excretion of poorly soluble free cystine.

Alpha-mercaptopropionylglycine (tiopronin)

Tiopronin or Thiola® (Mission Pharmacal) is considered the first-line treatment for significant cystinuria, being as effective as D-pencillamine but with a much better adverse effect profile. It is better tolerated than D-penicillamine, with 30.6% needing to stop therapy compared to 69.4% taking pencillamine in a non-randomized study.[30] Side effects occur in 64.7% of patients on Thiola compared to 83.7% who suffered toxicity to D-penicillamine. Remission of stone formation was seen in 71% of patients on Thiola, and stone formation rate decreased in 94% of patients. The average dose of Thiola used in the study was 1,193 mg per day, with urinary cystine levels of 350–560 mg per day being achieved. Tiopronin was as effective as D-penicillamine in reducing cystine excretion.

In another study, thiol derivatives were initially prescribed to 15 cases who had failed with conservative measures of hyperhydration and urinary alkalinization. Nine patients were treated with thiols for a mean 12.5 ± 6.8 years. In six patients treated with D-penicillamine and three treated with tiopronin, mean cystine excretion decreased significantly from 789 ± 126 to 517 ± 92 and 1,052 ± 161 to 755 ± 81 mg daily, respectively. The median daily dose for D-penicillamine was 900 mg, while that for tiopronin was 750 mg. No significant difference was noted for cystine excretion in three patients treated with captopril (mean decrease 1,044 ± 57 to 1,039 ± 137 mg). Six patients (40%) on thiols, including 4 on D-penicillamine and 2 on tiopronin discontinued treatment because of adverse events, notably heavy proteinuria in 2, gastric intolerance in 2, pruritus in 1, and suspicion of multiple sclerosis in 1.[31] Another study noted 21 of 43 patients (49%) treated with D-penicillamine had drug-related complications.[32]

Worcester and colleagues[33] treated 52 cystinuric patients with increased fluid intake, potassium alkali, and a thiol as required and demonstrated a significant reduction in the need for stone-removing procedures, from four procedures/patient to 0.9 procedures/patient, over a mean treatment period of 4.3 years. However, the surgical intervention rate was still higher than that for 'routine' stone formers.

Chow determined efficacy of different treatment options given step-wise to correct progressively worsening cystine stone disease in a small cohort of patients. Nine patients were treated with hydration and alkalization (aiming pH >7.5) for a total of 354 months. During treatment, 1.6 stone events occurred per patient-year. Treatment with hydration, alkalization, and D-penicillamine (1–2 gm/d) or tiopronin (800–1,200 mg/d) was utilized in nine patients for a total of 550 treatment months, and this was associated with 0.52 events per patient-year. Hydration, alkalization, and captopril (50 mg three times daily) were used in six patients for a total of 169 months. A stone event rate of 0.71 per patient-year was observed. Five patients were treated by alkalization with thiols and captopril. This represented the most refractory group in the study. During 177 patient-months of treatment for this group, 0.54 events per patient-year were observed.[34]

Pietrow *et al.*[35] evaluated long-term results of medical management in patients with cystinuria. Twenty-six patients with cystinuria were treated with hyperhydration, alkalinization, and tiopronin. The mean treatment duration was 11 years. Average follow-up was 38.2 months. Only 15% achieved and maintained therapeutic success, defined by urine cystine less than 300 mg/l. Patients achieving theraputic success had an average of one stone every other year, those with intermittent compliance had 4.5 stones/ year, while those who never achieved therapeutic results had almost 25 stones/ year. Sixty per cent (60%) of patients reported treatment-related adverse effects with gastrointestinal upset in 25%, joint pain 10%, fatigue 5%, and memory loss 5%.

The usual starting dose of tiopronin is 300 mg twice daily (100 mg tablets) with a dose range of 10–15 mg/kg/day and a maximum dose of 2 g per day.

D-Pencillamine, the first thiol, has efficacy similar to tiopronin but has a much more severe side effect profile including haematologic toxicity, liver dysfunction, anorexia, abnormal taste sensation, nausea, vomiting or diarrhoea, nephrotic syndrome, haematuria, neurotoxicity, thrombocytopenia, pulmonary infiltrates, rash, and drug induced fever.[36,37] Typical doses start at 250 mg per day and are titrated to effect. Pyridoxine deficiency has been reported with the use of thiols and patients are recommended to have pyridoxine supplementation (50 mg/d) during treatment.

Pencillamine is not considered front-line therapy at this time, but may be considered in those not tolerating Thiola or where the latter is ineffective. Patients on thiols should be monitored with serial full blood counts, liver function tests, urine for proteins, and haematuria every six months.

Thiol agents should be avoided during pregnancy, especially during the first trimester, because such agents have been demonstrated to be teratogenic.[38] Pregnant patients should continue on fluid therapy and urinary alkalinization achieved by sodium bicarbonate, as potassium citrate is not recommended in this setting.

Captopril

This is considered third-line therapy and is not as effective as the aforementioned drugs. Before treatment, the mean rate of new stone formation or stone growth was 1.2 events per patient-year for one to three years of observation. With 50 mg of captopril three times daily in addition to standard fluid and alkalinization therapy, stone events declined to 1.03 events per patient-year for 0.5 to 6 years, but statistical significance was not reached.[39]

Captopril is given in daily dose of 75–150 mg. Its side effect profile is much less severe than that of Thiola or D-pencillamine. It has the additional benefits of controlling hypertension, heart failure, or proteinuria if present. It should not be administered to those with hyperkalaemia or allergy to angiotensin converting enzyme (ACE) inhibitors.

Overall, the compliance and longevity of treatment success in patients on cystine stone therapy remains suboptimal.[35,40] Restriction on diets rich in methionine, the precursor of cystine, including meat, eggs, milk, wheat, and cheese have been tried, but have been found impractical and ineffective.

Struvite stones

The aim of treatment is to prevent recurrent infection once a stone-free state is achieved. Pure struvite stone formers can be placed on long-term prophylactic antibiotics, such as macrobid, as well as started on a urease inhibitor acetohydroxamic acid (Lithostat® Mission Pharmacal).

Acetohydroxamic acid (AHA) decreases stone recurrence and growth in randomized double-blind trials involving struvite stone formers. Patients with spinal cord injury having chronic urinary infections with urea-splitting organisms were treated with acetohydroxamic acid and followed for two years. The active drug treatment arm had significantly longer intervals to first stone growth (15 vs. 9 months, $p < 0.005$). There was also a significantly smaller proportion of patients exhibiting stone growth at 12 months for patients on acetohydroxamic acid when compared to patients treated with placebo (33% vs. 60%, $p = 0.017$). At 24 months, AHA appeared better for preventing stone growth than placebo, but the difference was not statistically significant (42% on AHA had stone growth vs. 60% on placebo, $p = 0.26$). Side effects of therapy were reported in 62% of acetohydroxamic acid and 29% of placebo patients. Patient attrition rate was 31% in the placebo group and 62% in the acetohydroxamic acid group, with follow-up of two years.[41]

Griffith reported the efficacy and safety of acetohydroxamic acid in preventing urinary stone disease in a prospective, double-blind, placebo-controlled study. The study involved 94 patients with chronic urinary infection. Stone growth occurred in 17% of the AHA group and 46% of the placebo ($p < 0.005$). Patients on AHA had psychoneurologic and musculo-integumentary side effects, which were reversible. Some 22.2% of patients on AHA had intolerable side effects compared to two (4.1%) in the placebo group.[42]

In another randomized controlled trial involving struvite stone formers, 18 patients received acetohydroxamic acid (15 mg/kg per day, in divided oral doses) for a mean of 15.8 months compared to 19 patients receiving placebo for a mean of 19.6 months. Both groups were treated with suppressive antibiotics throughout the study. Seven patients receiving the placebo had 100% increase in the surface area of their stones. No patient on acetohydroxamic acid had a doubling of stone size ($p < 0.01$). Nine patients receiving the drug and one patient receiving placebo required a decrease in dosage or cessation of treatment because of adverse effects. Side effects associated with therapy were tremulousness in 27.7%, and phlebothrombosis in 16.6%.[43]

The usual dose for Lithostat is 250 mg (one tab) three times daily. The most common side effects are anorexia, nausea, vomiting, tremors, anxiety, headaches, and haemolytic anaemias, rash, hepatotoxicity, and deep venous thrombosis. Additionally, Lithostat is contraindicated in patients with renal insufficiency.[44,45] Administration of AHA induces low-grade intravascular coagulation, consistent with increased levels of fibrinopeptide A and low platelet counts, and perhaps explains the incidence of thrombosis seen in these patients.[46]

Antibiotic prophylaxis

Long-term antibiotic therapy (trimethoprim, nitrofurantoin, and cephalosporins) may be used in patients with infection stones after stone removal. Antibiotic therapy should prevent not only septic complications but also recurrence or re-growth of stones after treatment.[45,47,48] Others have shown struvite calculi may dissolve partially in the presence of sterile urine.[45,48] Antibiotics may not render urine sterile, but they may result in reduction of the bacterial colony count leading to significant decrease in urease production.[49]

Use of antibiotics as the primary treatment modality is considered suboptimal[47] as bacteria can thrive within the stone itself, hence making antibiotics ineffective to eradicate infection unless the patient is a poor surgical candidate.[44,50,51]

Wang and associates[44] have outlined recommendations for antibiotic therapy. Initially, patients are given therapeutic doses of antibiotics for one to two weeks. After confirmation of sterile urine, the dosage is often decreased by half for up to three months, and monthly urine cultures are obtained. If bacteriuria recurs, or the patient becomes symptomatic, then the full dosage is resumed. Antibiotics are discontinued when sterile urine has been present for three months. Subsequent to this, urine cultures are obtained every three months. Several studies have recommended culture-specific antibiotics as prophylaxis against recurrent infections after stone removal.[45,50,51]

Further reading

Barbey F, Joly D, Rieu P, Méjean A, Daudon M, Jungers P. Medical treatment of cystinuria: critical reappraisal of long-term results. *J Urol* 2000; **163**(5):1419–23.

Becker MA, Schumacher HR Jr, Wortmann RL, *et al.* Febuxostat compared with allopurinole in patients with hyperuricemia and gout. *N Engl J Med* 2005; **353**:2450–61.

Cohen TD, Preminger GM. Struvite calculi. *Semin Nephrol* 1996; 4:425–34.

Cohen TD, Streem SB, Hall P. Clinical effect of captopril on the formation and growth of cystine calculi. *J Urol* 1995; **154**(1):164–6.

Goldfarb DS, Coe FL, Asplin JR. Urinary cystine excretion and capacity in patients with cystinuria. *Kidney Int* 2006; **69**:1041–7.

Griffith DP, Gleeson MJ, Lee H, Longuet R, Deman E, Earle N. Randomized, double-blind trial of Lithostat (acetohydroxamic acid) in the palliative treatment of infection-induced urinary calculi. *Eur Urol* 1991; **20**:243–7.

Haleblian GE, Leitao VA, Pierre SA, *et al.* Assessment of citrate concentrations in citrus fruit-based juices and beverages: implications for management of hypocitraturic nephrolithiasis. *J Endourol* 2008; **22**(6):1359–66.

Kang DE, Sur RL, Haleblian GE, Fitzsimons NJ, Borawski KM, Preminger GM. Long-term lemonade based dietary manipulation in patients with hypocitraturic nephrolithiasis. *J Urol* 2007; **177**(4):1358–62.

Pak CY, Fuller C, Sakhaee K, Zerwekh JE, Adams BV. Management of cystine nephrolithiasis with alpha-mercaptopropionylglycine. *J Urol* 1986; **136**:1003–8.

Penniston KL, Nakada SY, Holmes RP, Assimos DG. Quantitative assessment of citric acid in lemon juice, lime juice, and commercially-available fruit juice products. *J Endourol* 2008; **22**(3):567–70.

Pietrow PK, Auge BK, Weizer AZ, *et al.* Durability of the medical management of cystinuria. *J Urol* 2003; **169**(1):68–70.

Rodriguez LM, Santos F, Malaga S, Martinez V. Effect of a low sodium diet on urinary elimination of cystine in cystinuric children. *Nephron* 1995; **71**:416–18.

Sakhaee K, Alpern R, Poindexter J, Pak CY. Citraturic response to oral citric acid load. *J Urol* 1992; **147**:975–6.

Wang LP, Wong HY, Griffith DP. Treatment options in struvite stones. *Urol Clin North Am* 1997; **24**:149–62.

Williams JJ, Rodman JS, Peterson CM. A randomized double-blind study of acetohydroxamic acid in struvite nephrolithiasis. *N Engl J Med* 1984; **311**(12):760–4.

Worcester EM, Coe FL, Evan AP, Parks JH. Reduced renal function and benefits of treatment in cystinuria vs other forms of nephrolithiasis. *BJU Int* 2006; **97**(6):1285–90.

References

1. Sutherland JW, Parks JH, Coe FL. Recurrence after a single renal stone in a community practice. *Miner Electrolyte Metab* 1985; **11**:267–9.
2. Borghi L, Schianchi T, Meschi T, *et al.* Comparison of two diets for the prevention of recurrent stones in idiopathic hypercalciuria. *N Engl J Med* 2002; 34677–84
3. Moe OW. Kidney stones: Pathophysiology and medical management. *Lancet* 2006; **367**:333–44.
4. Osking DH, Erickson SB, Van den Berg CJ, Wilson DM, Smith LH. The stone clinic effect in patients with idiopathic calcium urolithiasis. *J Urol* 1983; **130**(6):1115–18.
5. Borghi L, Meschi T, Amato F, Brganti A, Novarini A, Giannini A. Urinary volume, water and recurrences in idiopathic calcium nephrolithiasis: a 5-year randomized prospective study. *J Urol* 1996; **155**:839–43.
6. Seltzer MA, Low RK, McDonald M, Shami GS, Stoller ML. Dietary manipulation with lemonade to treat hypocitraturic calcium nephrolithiasis. *J Urol* 1996; **156**(3):907–9.
7. Kang DE, Sur RL, Haleblian GE, Fitzsimons NJ, Borawski KM, Preminger GM. Long-term lemonade based dietary manipulation in patients with hypocitraturic nephrolithiasis. *J Urol* 2007; **177**(4):1358–62.
8. Haleblian GE, Leitao VA, Pierre SA, *et al.* Assessment of citrate concentrations in citrus fruit-based juices and beverages: implications for management of hypocitraturic nephrolithiasis. *J Endourol* 2008; **22**(6):1359–66.
9. Penniston KL, Nakada SY, Holmes RP, Assimos DG. Quantitative assessment of citric acid in lemon juice, lime juice, and commercially-available fruit juice products. *J Endourol* 2008; **22**(3):567–70.
10. Sakhaee K, Alpern R, Poindexter J, Pak CY. Citraturic response to oral citric acid load. *J Urol* 1992; **147**:975–6.
11. Odvina CV. Comparative value of orange juice versus lemonade in reducing stone-forming risk. *Clin J Am Soc Nephrol* 2006; **1**:1269–74.
12. Wabner CL, Pak CY. Effect of orange juice consumption on urinary stone risk factors. *J Urol* 1993; **149**(6):1405–8.
13. Hönow R, Laube N, Schneider A, Kebler T, Hesse A. Influence of grapefruit, orange and apple juice consumption on urinary variables and risk of crystallization. *Br J Nutr* 2003; **90**(2):295–300.
14. Baia Lda C, Baxmann AC, Moreira SR, Holmes RP, Heilberg IP. Noncitrus alkaline fruit: a dietary alternative for the treatment of hypocitraturic stone formers. *J Endourol* 2012; **26**(9):1221–6.
15. Bataille P, Achard JM, Fournier A, *et al.* Diet, vitamin D and vertebral mineral density in hypercalciuric calcium stone formers. *Kidney Int* 1991; **39**:1193–205.
16. Henneman PH, Wallach S, Dempsey EF. The metabolic defect responsible for uric acid stone formation. *J Clin Invest* 1962; **3**:537–42.
17. Pak CY, Sakhaee K, Peterson RD, *et al.* Biochemical profile of idiopathic uric acid nephrolithiasis. *Kidney Int* 2001; **60**:757–61.
18. Pak CY, Poindexter JR, Adams-Huet B, Pearle MS. Predictive value of kidney stone composition in the detection of metabolic abnormalities. *Am J Med* 2003; **115**:26–32.
19. Pak CY, Sakhaee K, Fuller C. Successful management of uric acid nephrolithiasis with potassium citrate. *Kidney Int* 1986; **30**(3):422–8.
20. Robinson MR, Leitao VA, *et al.* Impact of long term potassium citrate therapy on urinary profiles and recurrent stone formation. *J Urol* 2009; **181**:1145–50.
21. Spivacow FR, Negri AL, Polonsky A, Del Valle EE. Long-term treatment of renal lithiasis with potassium citrate. *Urology* **2010: 76**(6):1346–9.
22. Barcelo P, Wuhl O, Servitge E, Rousaud A, Pak CY. Randomized double-blind study of potassium citrate in idiopathic hypocitraturic calcium nephrolithiasis. *J Urol* 1993; **150**:1761–4.
23. Hofbauer J, Hobarth K, Szabo N, Marberger M. Alkali citrate prophylaxis in idiopathic recurrent calcium oxalate urolithiasis—a prospective randomized study. *Br J Urol* 1994; **73**:362.
24. Ettinger B, Pak CY, Citron JT, Thomas C, Adams-Huet B, Vangessel A. Potassium-magnesium citrate is an effective prophylaxis against recurrent calcium oxalate nephrolithiasis. *J Urol* 1997; **158**(6):2069–73.
25. Ettinger B, Tang A, Citron JT, Livermore B, Williams T. Randomized trial of allopurinol in the prevention of calcium oxalate calculi. *N Engl J Med* 1986; **315**:1386–9.
26. Becker MA, Schumacher HR Jr, Wortmann RL, *et al.* Febuxostat compared with allopurinole in patients with hyperuricemia and gout. *N Engl J Med* 2005; **353**:2450–61.
27. Jansen TL, Richette P, Perez-Ruiz F, *et al.* International position paper on febuxostat. *Clin Rheumatol* 2010; **29**:835–40.
28. Rodriguez LM, Santos F, Malaga S, Martinez V. Effect of a low sodium diet on urinary elimination of cystine in cystinuric children. *Nephron* 1995; **71**:416–18.
29. Goldfarb DS, Coe FL, Asplin JR. Urinary cystine excretion and capacity in patients with cystinuria. *Kidney Int* 2006; **69**:1041–7.
30. Pak CY, Fuller C, Sakhaee K, Zerwekh JE, Adams BV. Management of cystine nephrolithiasis with alpha-mercaptopropionylglycine. *J Urol* 1986; **136**:1003–8.
31. Barbey F, Joly D, Rieu P, Méjean A, Daudon M, Jungers P. Medical treatment of cystinuria: critical reappraisal of long-term results. *J Urol* 2000; **163**(5):1419–23.
32. Dahlberg PJ, van den Berg, Kurtz SB, Wilson DM, Smith LH. Clinical features and management of cystinuria. *Mayo Clin Proc* 1977; **52**:533–42.
33. Worcester EM, Coe FL, Evan AP, Parks JH. Reduced renal function and benefits of treatment in cystinuria vs other forms of nephrolithiasis. *BJU Int* 2006; **97**(6):1285–90.
34. Chow GK, Streem SB. Medical treatment of cystinuria: results of contemporary clinical practice. *J Urol* 1996; **156**(5):1576–8.
35. Pietrow PK, Auge BK, Weizer AZ, *et al.* Durability of the medical management of cystinuria. *J Urol* 2003; **169**(1):68–70.
36. Sakhaee K. Pathogenesis and medical management of cystinuria. *Semin Nephrol* 1996; **16**(5):435–47.
37. Halperin EC, Thier SO, Rosenberg LE. The use of D-penicillamine in cystinuria: efficacy and untoward reactions. *Yale J Biol Med* 1981; **54**(6):439–46.
38. Solomon L, Abrams G, Dinner M, *et al.* Nenonatal abnormalities associated with D-penicillamine treatment during pregnancy. *N Engl J Med* 1977; **296**(1):54–5.
39. Cohen TD, Streem SB, Hall P. Clinical effect of captopril on the formation and growth of cystine calculi. *J Urol* 1995; **154**(1):164–6.
40. Ahmed K, Khan MS, Thomas K, *et al.* Management of cystinuric patients: an observational, retrospective, single-centre analysis. *Urol Int* 2008; **80**(2):141–4.
41. Griffith DP, Khonsari F, Skurnick JH, James KE. A randomized trial of acetohydroxamic acid for the treatment and prevention of infection-induced urinary stones in spinal cord injury patients. *J Urol* 1988; **140**(2):318–24.
42. Griffith DP, Gleeson MJ, Lee H, Longuet R, Deman E, Earle N. Randomized, double-blind trial of Lithostat (acetohydroxamic acid) in the palliative treatment of infection-induced urinary calculi. *Eur Urol* 1991; **20**:243–7.
43. Williams JJ, Rodman JS, Peterson CM. A randomized double-blind study of acetohydroxamic acid in struvite nephrolithiasis. *N Engl J Med* 1984; **311**(12):760–4.
44. Wang LP, Wong HY, Griffith DP. Treatment options in struvite stones. *Urol Clin North Am* 1997; **24**:149–62.
45. Rodman JS. Struvite stones. *Nephron* 1999; **81**(Suppl l):50–9.
46. Rodman JS, Williams JJ, Jones RL. Hypercoagulability produced by treatment with acetohydroxamic acid. *Clin Pharmacol Ther* 1987; **42**(3):346–50.
47. Griffith DP, Moskowitz PA, Carlton CE Jr. Adjunctive chemotherapy of infection-induced staghorn calculi. *J Urol* 1979; **121**:711–15.
48. Stamey TA. *Infection Stones in Urinary Infections*. Baltimore, MA: Williams and Wilkins, 1972: p. 213.
49. Griffith DP, Osborne CA. Infection (urease) stones. *Miner Electrolyte Metab* **1987: 13**:278–85.
50. Cohen TD, Preminger GM. Struvite calculi. *Semin Nephrol* 1996; **4**:425–34.
51. Segura JW. Staghorn calculi. *Urol Clin North Am* 1997; **24**:71–80.

CHAPTER 2.6

Stone fragmentation techniques
Extracorporeal shock wave lithotripsy

Andreas Neisius, Ghalib Jibara, Micheal E. Lipkin, Glenn M. Preminger, and James F. Glenn

Introduction to stone fragmentation techniques

Used clinically for the first time in 1980, shock wave lithotripsy (SWL)[1] quickly became the treatment of choice for the majority of small intrarenal stones. It continues to be considered first-line therapy for such stones, as well as for many ureteric stones.

This chapter reviews the fundamental principles of SWL, advances in lithotripsy technology and adjuncts to improve SWL efficacy, and current indications and contraindications in the context of the updated AUA/EAU Guidelines.

Fundamental principles of shock wave lithotripsy

Shock waves are high-energy amplitudes of pressure generated in water or air by an abrupt release of energy in a small space. They consist of an initial sharp peak in positive pressure followed by a prolonged negative pressure wave. While they travel unimpeded through substances of similar densities, when a shock wave encounters a boundary between substances of differing acoustic impedance, such as the interface between urine and stone, compressive stresses are generated along the initial surface. In general, the forces contributing to stone fragmentation can be divided into two primary categories: stress waves that act inside the stone, and cavitation that acts in the fluid surrounding the stone.

Spallation

As a shock wave crosses the trailing edge of the stone, part of the energy is reflected, creating tensile stress and fragmentation along the trailing edge. This process is known as spallation—literally the separation of fragments of stone from its surface; in the case of SWL, by generation of tensile stresses as the shock wave is reflected from the trailing edge of the stone (a 'spall' is literally a splinter of rock).[2] Solids are generally weaker when subjected to tensile as opposed to compressive stresses. These stresses lead to a dynamic fracture process consisting of nucleation, coalescence, and growth of microfractures in the stone leading to fragmentation.[3,4]

Cavitation

Cavitation also plays a major role in stone comminution. As a shock wave passes through fluid, bubbles form and grow at the stone surface as a consequence of the negative pressure component of the wave (a positive wave compresses fluid, the negative wave literally pulls it apart, thereby generating a cavity). When the next shock wave arrives, the positive pressure causes these bubbles to violently collapse, releasing a microjet of energy directed towards the stone surface. Cavitation damage is characterized by minute pittings of the stone as a result of localized stress concentration.[5,6] These forces act in conjunction to ultimately fragment a stone.[7,8]

Squeezing and shear stresses

The stone is literally squeezed by the shock wave at its incident surface. Compressive and shear waves propagate within the stone. Stones consisting of layers shear between the layers.

Superfocusing

The curved surfaces of a stone will reflect shock waves from the distal stone surface, thereby effectively focusing ('superfocusing') the shock wave within the stone, and so creating high-stress regions.

Tissue damage from shock wave lithotripsy

While soft tissues have physical properties that limit their susceptibility to damage from shock waves (an acoustic impedance similar to that of water), not surprisingly a shock wave that can fragment a solid stone can cause some collateral tissue damage. SWL-induced renal injury is primarily a vascular event,[9] as is SWL-induced vasoconstriction resulting in ischaemia.[10,11] Two primary mechanisms have been postulated for SWL-induced renal vascular injury: cavitation and shear stress. Cavitation bubble expansion in small blood vessels causes vessel rupture.[12] High-speed photography has demonstrated that cavitation bubbles generated during SWL can cause vessel distension and vessel invagination. Bubble collapse releases high velocity fluid microjets, which can puncture holes in vessels.[13,14] Shear forces from repeated shock wave applications can also lead to vessel damage.[15] This damage to blood vessels leads to localized ischaemia and may result in free radical formation as the final pathway of tissue injury.[16,17]

Shock wave lithotripters: Shock wave generation, localization, and coupling

Shock wave generation and focusing

All shock wave lithotripters require (i) a stone localization system; (ii) an energy source to generate the shock wave; (iii) a focusing device to direct the shock wave at a focal point; and a (iv) a coupling medium.[2]

Stone localization

Fluoroscopy or ultrasonography are used for stone localization. While fluoroscopy is a more familiar imaging modality to most urologists and can localize mid and proximal ureteric stones that ultrasound cannot, it clearly involves a degree of ionizing radiation exposure. Automated fluoroscopic localization has been shown to decrease radiation exposure.[18] For radiolucent stones, intravenous contrast can be administered to aid identification.

Many newer lithotripters utilize ultrasound, which allows stone localization in real time and the identification of radiolucent stones, while avoiding ionizing radiation exposure to. Ultrasound has been shown to be effective in localizing stone fragments as small as 2–3 mm, and may even be superior to routine kidney, ureter, and bladder X-ray (KUB) in assessing residual stone fragments following lithotripsy.[19] Localization of mid-ureteric stones with ultrasound is almost impossible and proximal ureteric stones, especially where there is no dilated ureter above, is challenging.

Energy source to generate the shock wave

There are three common mechanisms of shock waves generation: electrohydraulic, piezoelectric, and electromagnetic.

The *electrohydraulic* generator, exemplified by the original Dornier HM3 lithotripter (Dornier MedTech, Kennesaw, GA, USA), produces shock waves by an electrical spark gap at the base of a water bath located in the focus (F1) of an ellipsoidal reflector. The high-voltage discharge causes the rapid vaporization of water at the tip of the electrodes, thereby producing a shock wave. The acoustic shock wave is focused at a second focal point (F2; where the target stone is located) by the ellipsoidal reflector. Electrohydraulic lithotripters offer the advantage of increased efficacy in fragmenting stones, however the relatively short life of the electrode and the necessity for general anaesthesia are obvious disadvantages.[9]

Piezoelectric shock waves are generated by ceramic elements located on the surface of a sphere, which undergo a sudden expansion when excited by a high frequency, high-voltage energy pulse, thereby generating a shock wave. The spherical dish creates convergence of the shock waves generated from each of the ceramic elements, thus producing a single, high-energy shock wave directed at the focal point of the sphere.[19] The focal point produced by a piezoelectric lithotripter is relatively narrow.[20] Advantages of piezoelectric lithotripters include better focusing, a longer service life, and better patient tolerance because the wide area of skin that the shock wave enters the patient through reduces pain.[9,20] The major disadvantage is the poorer comminution efficacy caused by the decreased power it delivers compared to other lithotripter types.[9]

Nowadays *electromagnetic* devices are the most commonly used. Shock waves are produced when an electrical impulse moves a thin, circular metallic membrane that is housed within a 'shock tube'. The resulting shock wave passes through the water-filled shock tube and is then directed at the focal point by an acoustic lens.[21] Electromagnetic lithotripters introduce the shock wave into the patient's body over a large surface area, reducing the need for anaesthesia while maintaining a high amount of energy at the focus.[9] The relatively small focus with high energy produced by electromagnetic lithotripters may increase the risk of subcapsular haematomas.[9]

Coupling of the shock wave

The original Dornier HM3 utilized a 1,000 L water bath for coupling shock waves to the patient. This remains the best coupling with the smallest loss of energy by minimizing the number of interfaces between the shock wave source and the stone, but it is clearly less practical. Second and third generation lithotripters use water cushions with ultrasound gel as the coupling medium, thereby avoiding the need to submerge the patient in a water bath.[18] The quality of the coupling media impacts significantly on SWL efficacy. Air bubbles trapped in the coupling media reduce the efficiency of the shock waves dramatically.[22,23]

Indications and contraindications to shock wave lithotripsy

SWL is considered first-line treatment for non-lower pole renal stones less than 2 cm, though as stone burden increases, stone-free rates for SWL decrease.[9] The 2016 American Urologic Association/Endourological Society guidelines for the management of ureteral calculi state that SWL is an acceptable first-line therapy for the treatment of ureteral stones.[24]

Active infection, distal obstruction, pregnancy, proximate calcified abdominal aortic or renal artery aneurysms, and bleeding diathesis are absolute contraindications to SWL.[9]

Relative contraindications to SWL are cystine or calcium oxalate monohydrate stones (relatively resistant to fragmentation by SWL), stone size over 2 cm, and obesity. Increasing skin-to-stone distance decreases the efficacy of SWL,[25,26] and a skin-to-stone distance greater than 110 mm has been proposed as a cut-off that predicts SWL failure.[26]

Renal calculi

To decide whether SWL is the appropriate treatment modality for a stone, three factors should be taken into consideration: (i) location, (ii) size, and (iii) composition. Stone location plays a role in determining the efficacy of SWL. Stones less than 2 cm in size in the renal pelvis, upper calyces, and middle calyces can be effectively treated with SWL.[27] For stones located in the lower pole, SWL is less effective. A randomized, prospective trial comparing SWL to percutaneous nephrolithotomy (PCNL) for the treatment of lower pole stones demonstrated markedly decreased stone-free rates for SWL compared to PCNL (37% vs. 95%).[28] Percutaneous nephrolithotomy outperformed SWL even when stratified by stone size. SWL can be used to treat lower pole stones, but is probably best restricted to stones less than 10 mm in diameter.

Stone-free rates achieved with SWL are inversely proportional to stone burden,[29–31] stones less than 10 mm in diameter being associated with improved stone-free rates.[30] Stone-free rates for renal stones less than 10 mm are approximately 80%.[30,32] For stones larger than 2 cm, percutaneous nephrolithotomy (PCNL) is considered first-line treatment,[9,31,33] though clearly there may be certain clinical circumstances that dictate SWL as being preferable to PCNL in select patients with stones larger than 2 cm.

Stone composition also influences SWL outcomes. Cystine, calcium oxalate monohydrate, and brushite stones are relatively resistant to fragmentation with SWL.[34] Cystine stones are ductile, meaning they are able to absorb energy from shock waves by plastic deformation, and this contributes to their resistance to fragmentation.[34] Brushite and calcium oxalate monohydrate stones are hard, which makes them resistant to deformation from shock waves, fracture propagation, and cavitation microjet impact.[34] Measuring Hounsfield units (i.e. density unit of material on computed tomography (CT)) on preoperative CT can predict resistance to fragmentation. Stones with a density greater than 900 Hounsfield units are more resistant to fragmentation with SWL.[26] Dual-energy CT can accurately determine stone composition.[35,36]

Ureteral calculi

In management of ureteral stones less than 10 mm, shock wave lithotripsy is still considered a first-line treatment[24] along with ureteroscopy. Stone composition affects the efficacy of SWL for the treatment of ureteral stones in the same manner as for renal stones. Stone location and size also play a major role in determining SWL efficacy. Patients with proximal ureteral stones treated with SWL show a stone-free rate of approximately 82%,[24] which is comparable to stone-free rates achieved with ureteroscopy. Fragments from ureteral stones treated with SWL typically clear within one to three days, with a mean of 4.6 days to stone-free status.[37] Routine ureteral stenting is not recommended prior to SWL of ureteral stones, as it has not been shown to improve stone-free rates.[24] Medical expulsive therapy with alpha-adrenergic blockers and calcium channel blockers has been shown to improve stone clearance after SWL.[38,39]

For patients with stones in the distal and mid-ureter, the stone-free rate decreases to 74% and 73%, respectively.[24] In such cases ureteroscopy has a clear advantage, with reported stone-free rates of 86% for mid-ureteral stones and 94% for distal ureteral stones.[24] The advantage in stone-free rates with ureteroscopy must be balanced against the requirement for general or regional anaesthesia.

With some of the newer third generation SWL machines, the shock wave head can be used in a so-called overtable position so that the patient can be treated in the supine position. Patients with a distal and juxtavesical stone can be treated in the prone or modified sitting position. Studies have demonstrated >85% stone-free rate with one treatment on the HM-3 lithotripter, with patients positioned in the prone position.[40–42]

A recent Cochrane review comparing ureteroscopy and SWL for the treatment of ureteral stones found that ureteroscopy has a greater stone-free rate, but is associated with a higher complication rate and longer hospital stay. Seven randomized controlled trials with a total of 1,205 patients were included in the review. Stone-free rates were lower in patients who underwent SWL (7 studies, 1,205 participants: RR 0.84, 95% CI 0.73–0.96). Retreatment rates were lower in patients who were treated with ureteroscopy (6 studies, 1,049 participants: RR 6.18, 95% CI 3.68–10.38). SWL patients had less need for auxiliary treatment (5 studies, 751 participants: RR 0.43, 95% CI 0.25–0.74), fewer complications (7 studies, 1,205 participants: RR 0.54, 95% CI 0.33–0.88) and shorter length of hospital stay (2 studies, 198 participants: MD −2.55 days, 95% CI −3.24 to −1.86).[43]

Large calculi/staghorn calculi

While percutaneous nephrolithotomy is considered first-line treatment for staghorn or partial staghorn calculi,[33] SWL has a role as an adjunct to PCNL for some of these larger stones. If SWL is to be used in conjunction with PCNL for the treatment of staghorn calculi, it is recommended that SWL precede PCNL.[33] SWL is also effective at treating small post-PCNL residual fragments. In select patients with smaller staghorn stones and normal collecting system anatomy, SWL can be attempted with renal drainage via either a ureteral stent or nephrostomy tube.[33]

Calyceal diverticular calculi

Calyceal diverticulae are urine-filled cavities connected to the normal collecting system by a narrow isthmus or stenotic infundibulum. They often contain stones. Indications for treating calyceal diverticular calculi include flank pain, recurrent urinary tract infections, or persistent gross haematuria. The primary goal of treating a calyceal diverticular stone is removal of the stone and eradication of the diverticulum.[9,44] Treatment options for calculi within calyceal diverticula are numerous, ranging from SWL to PCNL to ureteroscopy (URS), but clearly SWL cannot obliterate the diverticulum or enhance drainage from it.[44] Stone-free rates reported for the treatment of calyceal diverticular stones with SWL average 21%.[45] Despite poor stone-free rates, the majority of patients with calyceal diverticular stones treated with SWL will have resolution of their symptoms. However, many of these patients will have recurrence of symptoms when followed for longer periods of time.[46] The preferred treatment for calyceal diverticular stones is endoscopic management with either PCNL or ureteroscopy.[44] SWL should only be used for the treatment of diverticular stones if the isthmus is proven, by preoperative imaging with either intravenous pyelogram or CT urography, not to be too narrow.

Advances in shock wave lithotripsy technology

Several groups are investigating ways to improve the safety and efficacy of SWL, based on our current understanding of the role of cavitation in stone fragmentation as well as the role of cavitation, vasoconstriction, and free radical formation in SWL-induced tissue injury. This increasing knowledge of the mechanisms of stone fragmentation and tissue injury contribute to advances in lithotripter designs, and improvement in treatment strategies and the medical adjuncts to improve SWL safety and efficacy.

Lithotripter modifications

A reflector insert has been designed that can be integrated with the original Dornier HM3 reflector, to create a second shock wave immediately after the original shock wave. The superposition of this second shock wave partially cancels the negative tensile component of the original wave, preventing cavitation bubbles from overexpanding in blood vessels, so reducing their chance of rupture. This combination resulted in improved comminution of stones implanted in pig kidneys and decreased renal parenchymal injury compared to the unmodified HM3.[47]

Electrohydraulic lithotripters generate a second direct wave from the source in addition to the focused shock wave, which can induce cavitation prior to the arrival of the focused wave. This may interfere with the cavitation activity of the focused wave. The cavitation activity from the direct wave can be suppressed by installing a direct wave suppressor close to the spark source.[48]

The Storz Modulith SLX-F2 (Storz-Medical, Kreuzlingen, Switzerland), an electromagnetic lithotripter, has a dual focus system that allows the operator to change the focal size depending on requirements.[49] It accomplishes this by modifying the pulse duration from the electromagnetic source.[18] The PiezoLith 3000 (Richard Wolf, Knittlingen, Germany), a piezoelectric lithotripter, utilizes a double layer design to increase shock wave energy.[18]

A further modification is the delivery of a shock wave from two lithotripters to the same focal point. This can be accomplished by placing the shock wave sources at a 90-degree angle from one another.[50] This so-called dual pulse lithotripsy has been shown to increase comminution without increasing tissue injury in animal studies.[51] In clinical trials, patients treated with the dual head device showed minimal changes to the renal parenchyma, despite it delivering twice as many shocks.[52] The long-term effects of dual pulse lithotripsy remain to be assessed.

Treatment strategy modifications

Modification of rate of shock wave delivery and energy also appear to impact on SWL efficacy and safety. A randomized controlled trial showed that reducing the rate of shock wave delivery to 60 shocks per minute compared to 120 shocks per minute significantly improves stone-free rates.[53] The stone-free rate for patients treated with 60 shocks per minute was 60% vs. 28% in patients treated with 120 shocks per minute. Patients treated with the slower rate needed fewer shocks, but the procedure took longer. Other studies have confirmed improved stone-free rates in patients treated with a slower shock wave rate.[54,55] This has also been demonstrated in an *in vivo* study using pigs treated with one of the current third generation lithotripters.[56] Furthermore, the percentage of stone fragments capable of spontaneous passage was significantly higher in the 60 shocks per minute group, compared to the 120 shocks per minute group. A recent meta-analysis looking at randomized controlled trials comparing 60 shocks per minute versus 120 shocks per minute confirmed the findings of improved treatment success with 60 shocks per minute.[57] The utilization of slower shock rates during SWL leads to fewer additional procedures and improved cost-effectiveness when compared to faster rates.[55] Side effects are comparable in both treatment groups.[56]

Improved stone comminution and decreased renal tissue injury has been demonstrated in a number of studies using a treatment strategy that begins with a low energy and gradually increases energy. An *in vitro study* comparing a gradual increase in energy versus a gradual decrease in energy found improved fragmentation efficiency with an increasing energy strategy.[58] These findings were confirmed in an *in vivo* study performed in a pig model.[59] Stones treated with an increasing strategy of 18 kV, 20 kV, and 22 kV for 600, 600, and 800 shocks, respectively, had better fragmentation efficiency than those treated with a decreasing strategy of 22 kV, 20 kV, and 18 kV for 800, 600, and 600 shocks, respectively. Patients treated with an escalating voltage strategy versus those treated with a fixed voltage showed improved stone-free rates, as demonstrated in a recent randomized controlled trial.[60] Pretreatment with low-energy shock waves has also been shown to reduce renal damage.[61,62] The low-energy shock waves induce vasoconstriction during SWL, whereas standard protocols lead to vasoconstriction after SWL.[62] Vascular injury from high-energy shock waves may be prevented, with the early vasoconstriction induced by preconditioning with low-energy shock waves during the treatment. The dictum seems to be, 'start slow and low'.

Different approaches to improve shock wave lithotripsy efficacy and safety

Two recent meta-analyses indicate that medical expulsive therapy, using either a calcium channel blocker or an alpha-adrenergic blocker, improves stone passage and stone-free rates after SWL.[38,39] The calcium channel blocker nifedipine increased the success rate of SWL treatment of ureteral stones in a randomized prospective study.[63] The alpha-adrenergic blocker tamsulosin has also been shown to improve stone-free rates after SWL in a randomized prospective study.[64] Additionally, potassium citrate appears to improve residual fragment clearance after SWL.[65]

Patient selection also impacts on the efficacy of SWL. Preoperative evaluation of patients with CT may be helpful to predict outcomes of SWL, by for example allowing better determination of internal stone architecture.[66] Several studies have demonstrated that determining the Hounsfield units of renal stones on pretreatment, non-contrasted CT may be able to predict stone-free rates of patients treated with SWL.[26,67.] More recently, the use of multidetector CT has been shown to very accurately predict different stone compositions *in vivo*,[36] thereby potentially allowing patients with 'SWL resistant' stones (e.g. calcium oxalate monohydrate or cystine stones) to be identified and treated with ureteroscopy or PCNL. Preoperative CT is also useful in determining skin-to-stone distance. A number of studies have shown decreased efficacy of SWL as skin-to-stone distance increases.[25,26,67]

There is a large body of evidence that suggests free radicals play a role in SWL-mediated tissue injury. Several studies have investigated the role of antioxidants in protecting the renal parenchyma against free radical injury.[68–70] Patients pretreated with mannitol, a known free radical scavenger, have been shown to have reduced urinary β2-microglobulin (which indicates renal cell damage), compared to a control group.[68] Other groups have demonstrated that antioxidants reduce indicators of renal cellular damage in patients undergoing SWL, regardless of whether given pretreatment and post-treatment.[70] Another study has demonstrated, in an *in vitro* model, that vitamin E and citrate reduce shock wave induced increase in free radicals.[69] Patients at high risk of renal damage during SWL may benefit from use of free radical scavengers and periprocedure antioxidants.

Conclusions

Extracorporal shock wave lithotripsy has revolutionized the treatment of renal and ureteric since its introduction in 1980. Though the technology for SWL continues to evolve, the fundamental principles of delivering a shock wave to fragment a stone remain the same. Increasing experience with SWL has enabled better patient and stone selection to improve both safety and efficacy. Modified treatment strategies and medical adjuncts, such as medical expulsive therapy and antioxidants, have further improved stone-free rates and safety. A number of advancements in lithotripter design, such as improved imaging for localization and modified coupling devices, may impact on future efficacy. Future research will be dedicated to modifying lithotripters' design to improve the delivery of shock waves, coupling of the shock wave head to the patient, improving stone localization, and increasing the efficiency while reducing side effects.

Further reading

Aboumarzouk OM, Kata SG, Keeley FX, Nabi G. Extracorporeal shock wave lithotripsy (ESWL) versus ureteroscopic management for ureteric calculi. *Cochrane Database Syst Rev* 2011(12):CD006029.

Albala DM, Assimos DG, Clayman RV, *et al.* Lower pole I: a prospective randomized trial of extracorporeal shock wave lithotripsy and percutaneous nephrostolithotomy for lower pole nephrolithiasis-initial results. *J Urol* 2001; **166**(6):2072–80.

Chaussy C, Schmiedt E, Jocham D, Brendel W, Forssmann B, Walther V. First clinical experience with extracorporeally induced destruction of kidney stones by shock waves. *J Urol* 1982; **127**(3):417–20.

Gillitzer R, Neisius A, Wöllner J, Hampel C, Brenner W, Bonilla AA, Thüroff J. Low-frequency extracorporeal shock wave lithotripsy improves renal pelvic stone disintegration in a pig model. *BJU Int* 2009; **103**(9):1284–8.

Lingeman JE, Matlaga BR, Evan AP. Surgical management of urinary lithiasis. (pp. 1431–507) In: Wein AJ, Kavoussi LR *(eds). Campbell-Walsh Urology.* Philadelphia, PA: Saunders, 2007.

Pace KT, Ghiculete D, Harju M, Honey RJ; University of Toronto Lithotripsy Associates. Shock wave lithotripsy at 60 or 120 shocks per minute: a randomized, double-blind trial. *J Urol* 2005; **174**(2):595–9.

Preminger GM, Assimos DG, Lingeman JE, *et al.* Chapter 1: AUA guideline on management of staghorn calculi: diagnosis and treatment recommendations. *J Urol* 2005; **173**(6):1991–2000.

Rassweiler JJ, Knoll T, Köhrmann KU, *et al.* Shock wave technology and application: an update. *Eur Urol* 2011; **59**(5):784–96.

Seitz C, Liatsikos E, Porpiglia F, Tiselius HG, Zwergel U. Medical therapy to facilitate the passage of stones: what is the evidence? *Eur Urol* 2009; **56**(3):455–71.

Türk CK, Knoll T, Petrik A, Sarica K, Straub M, Seitz C. Guidelines on Urolithiasis. European Association of Urology (EAU) [Guidelines], 2012. Available at: http://uroweb.org/wp-content/uploads/22-Urolithiasis_LR_full.pdf [Online].

Williams JC Jr, Kim SC, Zarse CA, McAteer JA, Lingeman JE. Progress in the use of helical CT for imaging urinary calculi. *J Endourol* 2004; **18**(10):937–41.

Zhong P, Preminger G. Physics of shock wave lithotripsy. (pp. 529–48) In: Coe FL *et al. (eds) Kidney Stones: Medical and Surgical Management.* Lipencott-Raven Publishers: Philadelphia, PA, 1996.

Zhou Y, Cocks FH, Preminger GM, Zhong P. The effect of treatment strategy on stone comminution efficiency in shock wave lithotripsy. *J Urol* 2004; **172**(1):349–54.

Zhu S, Cocks FH, Preminger GM, Zhong P. The role of stress waves and cavitation in stone comminution in shock wave lithotripsy. *Ultrasound Med Biol* 2002; **28**(5):661–71.

Zilberman DE, Ferrandino MN, Preminger GM, Paulson EK, Lipkin ME, Boll DT. In vivo determination of urinary stone composition using dual energy computerized tomography with advanced post-acquisition processing. *J Urol* 2010; **184**(6):2354–9.

References

1. Chaussy C, Schmiedt E, Jocham D, Brendel W, Forssmann B, Walther V. First clinical experience with extracorporeally induced destruction of kidney stones by shock waves. *J Urol* 1982; **127**(3):417–20.
2. Zhong P, Preminger G. Physics of shock wave lithotripsy. (pp. 529–48) In: Coe FL *et al.* (eds). *Kidney Stones: Medical and Surgical Management.* Lipencott-Raven Publishers: Philadelphia, PA, 1996.
3. Lokhandwalla M, Sturtevant B. Fracture mechanics model of stone comminution in ESWL and implications for tissue damage. *Phys Med Biol* 2000; **45**(7):1923–40.
4. Preminger GM. Shock wave physics. *Am J Kidney Dis* 1991; **17**(4):431–5.
5. Zhong P, Chuong CJ. Propagation of shock waves in elastic solids caused by cavitation microjet impact. I: Theoretical formulation. *J Acoust Soc Am* 1993; **94**(1):19–28.
6. Zhong P, Chuong CJ, Preminger GM. Characterization of fracture toughness of renal calculi using a microindentation technique. *J Mater Sci Lett* 1993; **12**(18):1460–2.
7. Coleman AJ, Saunders JE, Crum LA, Dyson M. Acoustic cavitation generated by an extracorporeal shockwave lithotripter. *Ultrasound Med Biol* 1987; **13**(2):69–76.
8. Zhu S, Cocks FH, Preminger GM, Zhong P. The role of stress waves and cavitation in stone comminution in shock wave lithotripsy. *Ultrasound Med Biol* 2002; **28**(5):661–71.
9. Lingeman JE, Matlaga BR, Evan AP. Surgical management of urinary lithiasis. (pp. 1431–507) In: Wein AJ, Kavoussi LR (eds). *Campbell-Walsh Urology*. Philadelphia, PA: Saunders, 2007.
10. Willis LR, Evan AP, Connors BA, Reed G, Fineberg NS, Lingeman JA. Effects of extracorporeal shock wave lithotripsy to one kidney on bilateral glomerular filtration rate and PAH clearance in minipigs. *J Urol* 1996; **156**(4):1502–6.
11. Willis LR, Evan AP, Connors BA, Fineberg NS, Lingeman JE. Effects of SWL on glomerular filtration rate and renal plasma flow in uninephrectomized minipigs. *J Endourol* 1997; **11**(1):27–32.
12. Zhu S, Dreyer T, Liebler M, Riedlinger R, Preminger GM, Zhong P. Reduction of tissue injury in shock-wave lithotripsy by using an acoustic diode. *Ultrasound Med Biol* 2004; **30**(5):675–82.
13. Chen H, Brayman AA, Bailey MR, Matula TJ. Blood vessel rupture by cavitation. *Urol Res* 2010; **38**(4):321–6.
14. Zhong P, Zhou Y, Zhu S. Dynamics of bubble oscillation in constrained media and mechanisms of vessel rupture in SWL. *Ultrasound Med Biol* 2001; **27**(1):119–34.
15. Freund JB, Colonius T, Evan AP. A cumulative shear mechanism for tissue damage initiation in shock-wave lithotripsy. *Ultrasound Med Biol* 2007; **33**(9):1495–503.
16. Delvecchio F, Auge BK, Munver R, *et al.* Shock wave lithotripsy causes ipsilateral renal injury remote from the focal point: the role of regional vasoconstriction. *J Urol* 2003; **169**(4):1526–9.
17. Munver, R., Delvecchio FC, Kuo RL, *et al.* In vivo assessment of free radical activity during shock wave lithotripsy using a microdialysis system: the renoprotective action of allopurinol. *J Urol* 2002; **167**(1):327–34.
18. Rassweiler JJ, Knoll T, Köhrmann KU, *et al.* Shock wave technology and application: an update. *Eur Urol* 2011; **59**(5):784–96.
19. Abernathy BB, Morris JS, Wilson WT, Miller GL. *Evaluation of residual stone fragments following lithotripsy: Sonography versus KUB.* (pp. 247–54) In: Lingeman JE, Newman DM (eds). *Shock Wave Lithotripsy II*, Plenum Press: New York, NY, 1989.
20. Preminger GM. Sonographic piezoelectric lithotripsy: more bang for your buck. *J Endourol* 1989; **3**:321–7.
21. Rassweiler J, Köhrmann U, Heine G, *et al.* 10/20—experimental introduction and first clinical experience with a new interdisciplinary lithotriptor. *Eur Urol* 1990; **18**(4):237–41.
22. Pishchalnikov YA, Neucks JS, VonDerHaar RJ, Pishchalnikova IV, Williams JC Jr, McAteer JA. Air pockets trapped during routine coupling in dry head lithotripsy can significantly decrease the delivery of shock wave energy. *J Urol* 2006; **176**(6 Pt 1):2706–10.
23. Jain A, Shah TK. Effect of air bubbles in the coupling medium on efficacy of extracorporeal shock wave lithotripsy. *Eur Urol* 2007; **51**(6):1680–6; discussion 1686–7.
24. Assimos D, Krambeck A, Miller NL, *et al.* Surgical Management of Stones: American Urological Association/Endourological Society Guideline, PART II. *J Urol* 2016; **196**(4):1161–9.

25. Patel T, Kozakowski K, Hruby G, Gupta M. Skin to stone distance is an independent predictor of stone-free status following shockwave lithotripsy. *J Endourol* 2009; **23**(9):1383–5.
26. Wiesenthal JD, Ghiculete D, D'A Honey RJ, Pace KT. Evaluating the importance of mean stone density and skin-to-stone distance in predicting successful shock wave lithotripsy of renal and ureteric calculi. *Urol Res* 2010; **38**(4):307–13.
27. Wen CC, Nakada SY. Treatment selection and outcomes: renal calculi. *Urol Clin North Am* 2007; **34**(3):409–19.
28. Albala DM, Assimos DG, Clayman RV, *et al.* Lower pole I: a prospective randomized trial of extracorporeal shock wave lithotripsy and percutaneous nephrostolithotomy for lower pole nephrolithiasis-initial results. *J Urol* 2001; **166**(6):2072–80.
29. el-Damanhoury H, Schärfe T, Rüth J, Roos S, Hohenfellner R. Extracorporeal shock wave lithotripsy of urinary calculi: experience in treatment of 3,278 patients using the Siemens Lithostar and Lithostar Plus. *J Urol* 1991; **145**(3):484–8.
30. Elkoushy MA, Hassan JA, Morehouse DD, Anidjar M, Andonian S. Factors determining stone-free rate in shock wave lithotripsy using standard focus of Storz Modulith SLX-F2 lithotripter. *Urology* 2011; **78**(4):759–63.
31. Logarakis NF, Jewett MA, Luymes J, Honey RJ. Variation in clinical outcome following shock wave lithotripsy. *J Urol* 2000; **163**(3):721–5.
32. Clayman RV, McClennan BL, Garvin TJ, Denstedt JD, Andriole GL. Lithostar: An electromagnetic acoustic shock wave unit for extracorporeal lithotripsy. *J Endourol* 1989; **3**:307–13.
33. Preminger GM, Assimos DG, Lingeman JE, *et al.* Chapter 1: AUA guideline on management of staghorn calculi: diagnosis and treatment recommendations. *J Urol* 2005; **173**(6):1991–2000.
34. Zhong P, Preminger GM. Mechanisms of differing stone fragility in extracorporeal shockwave lithotripsy. *J Endourol* 1994; **8**(4):263–8.
35. Ferrandino MN, Pierre SA, Simmons WN, Paulson EK, Albala DM, Preminger GM. Dual-energy computed tomography with advanced postimage acquisition data processing: improved determination of urinary stone composition. *J Endourol* 2010; **24**(3):347–54.
36. Zilberman DE, Ferrandino MN, Preminger GM, Paulson EK, Lipkin ME, Boll DT. In vivo determination of urinary stone composition using dual energy computerized tomography with advanced post-acquisition processing. *J Urol* 2010; **184**(6):2354–9.
37. Resit-Goren M, Dirim A, Ilteris-Tekin M, Ozkardes H. Time to stone clearance for ureteral stones treated with extracorporeal shock wave lithotripsy. *Urology* 2011; **78**(1):26–30.
38. Schuler TD1, Shahani R, Honey RJ, Pace KT. Medical expulsive therapy as an adjunct to improve shockwave lithotripsy outcomes: a systematic review and meta-analysis. *J Endourol* 2009; **23**(3):387–93.
39. Seitz C, Liatsikos E, Porpiglia F, Tiselius HG, Zwergel U. Medical therapy to facilitate the passage of stones: what is the evidence? *Eur Urol* 2009; **56**(3):455–71.
40. Turk TM, Jenkins AD. A comparison of ureteroscopy to in situ extracorporeal shock wave lithotripsy for the treatment of distal ureteral calculi. *J Urol* 1999; **161**(1):45–6; discussion 46–7.
41. Becht E1, Moll V, Neisius D, Ziegler M. Treatment of prevesical ureteral calculi by extracorporeal shock wave lithotripsy. *J Urol* 1988; **139**(5):916–8.
42. Rodrigues Netto Júnior N, Lemos GC, Claro JF. In situ extracorporeal shock wave lithotripsy for ureteral calculi. *J Urol* 1990; **144**(2 Pt 1):253–4.
43. Aboumarzouk OM, Kata SG, Keeley FX, Nabi G. Extracorporeal shock wave lithotripsy (ESWL) versus ureteroscopic management for ureteric calculi. *Cochrane Database Syst Rev* **2011**(12):CD006029.
44. Cohen TD1, Preminger GM. Management of calyceal calculi. *Urol Clin North Am* 1997; **24**(1):81–96.
45. Renner C, Rassweiler J. Treatment of renal stones by extracorporeal shock wave lithotripsy. *Nephron* 1999; **81**(Suppl 1):71–81.
46. Jones JA, Lingeman JE, Steidle CP. The roles of extracorporeal shock wave lithotripsy and percutaneous nephrostolithotomy in the management of pyelocaliceal diverticula. *J Urol* 1991; **146**(3):724–7.
47. Marguet CG, Young MD, Maloney M, *et al.* Improved stone comminution and simultaneously reduced tissue injury with an upgraded electrohydraulic lithotripter: in vivo studies. Paper presented at the American Urological Association Annual Meeting: San Francisco, CA, 2004.
48. Matula TJ, Hilmo PR, Bailey MR. A suppressor to prevent direct wave-induced cavitation in shock wave therapy devices. *JASA* 2005; **118**(1):178–85.
49. De Sio M, Autorino R, Quarto G, *et al.* A new transportable shock-wave lithotripsy machine for managing urinary stones: a single-centre experience with a dual-focus lithotripter. *BJU Int* 2007; **100**(5):1137–41.
50. Sheir KZ, Zabihi N, Lee D, *et al.* Evaluation of synchronous twin pulse technique for shock wave lithotripsy: determination of optimal parameters for in vitro stone fragmentation. *J Urol* 2003; **170**(6 Pt 1):2190–4.
51. Sheir KZ, Lee D, Humphrey PA, Morrissey K, Sundaram CP, Clayman RV. Evaluation of synchronous twin pulse technique for shock wave lithotripsy: in vivo tissue effects. *Urology* 2003; **62**(5):964–7.
52. Sheir KZ, El-Diasty TA, Ismail AM. Evaluation of a synchronous twin-pulse technique for shock wave lithotripsy: the first prospective clinical study. *BJU Int* 2005; **95**(3):389–93.
53. Pace KT, Ghiculete D, Harju M, Honey RJ; University of Toronto Lithotripsy Associates. Shock wave lithotripsy at 60 or 120 shocks per minute: a randomized, double-blind trial. *J Urol* 2005; **174**(2):595–9.
54. Chacko J, Moore M, Sankey N, Chandhoke PS. Does a slower treatment rate impact the efficacy of extracorporeal shock wave lithotripsy for solitary kidney or ureteral stones? *J Urol* 2006; **175**(4):1370–3; discussion 1373–4.
55. Koo VI, Beattie I, Young M. Improved cost-effectiveness and efficiency with a slower shockwave delivery rate. *BJU Int* 2010; **105**(5):692–6.
56. Gillitzer R, Neisius A, Wöllner J, Hampel C, Brenner W, Bonilla AA, Thüroff J. Low-frequency extracorporeal shock wave lithotripsy improves renal pelvic stone disintegration in a pig model. *BJU Int* 2009; **103**(9):1284–8.
57. Semins MJ, Trock BJ, Matlaga BR. The effect of shock wave rate on the outcome of shock wave lithotripsy: a meta-analysis. *J Urol* 2008; **179**(1):194–7; discussion 197.
58. Zhou Y, Cocks FH, Preminger GM, Zhong P. The effect of treatment strategy on stone comminution efficiency in shock wave lithotripsy. *J Urol* 2004; **172**(1):349–54.
59. Maloney ME, Marguet CG, Zhou Y, *et al.* Progressive increase of lithotripter output produces better in-vivo stone comminution. *J Endourol* 2006; **20**(9):603–6.
60. Lambert EH, Walsh R, Moreno MW, Gupta M. Effect of escalating versus fixed voltage treatment on stone comminution and renal injury during extracorporeal shock wave lithotripsy: a prospective randomized trial. *J Urol* 2010; **183**(2):580–4.
61. Willis LR, Evan AP, Connors BA, Handa RK, Blomgren PM, Lingeman JE. Prevention of lithotripsy-induced renal injury by pretreating kidneys with low-energy shock waves. *J Am Soc Nephrol* 2006; **17**(3):663–73.
62. Handa RK, Bailey MR, Paun M. Pretreatment with low-energy shock waves induces renal vasoconstriction during standard shock wave lithotripsy (SWL): a treatment protocol known to reduce SWL-induced renal injury. *BJU Int* 2009; **103**(9):1270–4.
63. Porpiglia F1, Destefanis P, Fiori C, Scarpa RM, Fontana D. Role of adjunctive medical therapy with nifedipine and deflazacort after extracorporeal shock wave lithotripsy of ureteral stones. *Urology* 2002; **59**(6):835–8.
64. Agarwal MM, Naja V, Singh SK, *et al.* Is there an adjunctive role of tamsulosin to extracorporeal shockwave lithotripsy for upper ureteric stones: results of an open label randomized nonplacebo controlled study. *Urology* 2009; **74**(5):989–92.
65. Cicerello E, Merlo F, Gambaro G, *et al.* Effect of alkaline citrate therapy on clearance of residual renal stone fragments after extracorporeal shock wave lithotripsy in sterile calcium and infection nephrolithiasis patients. *J Urol* 1994; **151**(1):5–9.

66. Williams JC Jr, Kim SC, Zarse CA, McAteer JA, Lingeman JE. Progress in the use of helical CT for imaging urinary calculi. *J Endourol* 2004; **18**(10):937–41.
67. Perks AE, Schuler TD, Lee J, *et al.* Stone attenuation and skin-to-stone distance on computed tomography predicts for stone fragmentation by shock wave lithotripsy. *Urology* 2008; **72**(4):765–9.
68. Ogiste JS, Nejat RJ, Rashid HH, Greene T, Gupta M. The role of mannitol in alleviating renal injury during extracorporeal shock wave lithotripsy. *J Urol* 2003; **169**(3):875–7.
69. Delvecchio FC1, Brizuela RM, Khan SR, *et al.* Citrate and vitamin E blunt the shock wave-induced free radical surge in an in vitro cell culture model. *Urol Res* 2005; **33**(6):448–52.
70. Al-Awadi KA, Kehinde EO, Loutfi I, *et al.* Treatment of renal calculi by lithotripsy: minimizing short-term shock wave induced renal damage by using antioxidants. *Urol Res* 2008; **36**(1):51–60.

CHAPTER 2.7

Intracorporeal techniques of stone fragmentation

Gastón M. Astroza, Ghalib Jibara, Michael E. Lipkin, and Glenn M. Preminger

Introduction to intracorporeal techniques of stone fragmentation

The surgical management of nephrolithiasis has undergone dramatic changes over the last 40 years. Developments in radiographic equipment, endourologic devices, and intracorporeal lithotrites have completely changed patient care, thereby providing more effective stone comminution with a significant reduction in operative morbidity compared to the open alternatives.

The use of intracorporeal lithotripsy for the management of larger ureteral and intrarenal calculi has dramatically improved. The small working channel of the semi-rigid and flexible endoscopes has limited the size and usefulness of instruments which can be passed and used for stone removal. Indeed, for larger stones, baskets or grasping forceps are often inadequate and potentially dangerous to accomplish successful stone extraction.

Even with the availability of shock wave lithotripsy (SWL) for the management of urinary tract stones, intracorporeal lithotripsy provides significant advantages in select cases. Since fragmentation is performed under direct vision, the stone can be entirely removed and there is no need to wait for fragments to pass, as with SWL. Although the choice of intracorporeal fragmentation is frequently based on the location and composition of the stone to be treated, the experience of the clinician and availability of equipment often dictates this decision.

Different modalities of intracorporeal lithotripsy are currently available: ultrasonic lithotripsy (UL); pneumatic lithotripsy (PN); combination ultrasonic and pneumatic lithotripsy (combo); electrohydraulic lithotripsy (EHL); and laser lithotripsy.

Electrohydraulic lithotripsy

The principles of electrohydraulic lithotripsy were described and developed by a Russian engineer in 1950.[1] This technology had been used extensively for the destruction of bladder stones and in 1975, reports were published on its use for the fragmentation of ureteral stones.[2,3] The EHL unit consists of a probe, a power generator, and a foot pedal. The probe is made up of a central metal core and two layers of insulation with another metal layer between them. Probes are flexible and available in varying sizes. Commercially available EHL units are manufactured with power up to 120 volts. The electrical discharge is transmitted to the probe, where a spark is generated at the tip. The intense heat production in the immediate area surrounding the tip of the probe results in a cavitation bubble, which produces a shock wave that radiates spherically in all directions.[4] The bubble's collapse causes a second shock wave. These shock waves, repeated at a frequency of 50–100 per second, result in destruction of the stone.

EHL is effective for the fragmentation of all kinds of urinary calculi, including cystine, uric acid, and calcium oxalate monohydrate stones.[5] The primary disadvantage of EHL is its inability to remove stone fragments. All particles need to be washed out during intraoperative irrigation, or grasped with forceps.

Excellent fragmentation of most ureteral calculi is to be expected, and intracorporeal lithotripsy with EHL for both urinary tract and biliary calculi offers an effective and cost efficient modality when small calibre, flexible lithotripsy probes are used. However, according to the most recent American Urological Association guidelines, clinicians should not utilize EHL as the first-line modality for intraureteral lithotripsy due to high risk of ureteral perforation.[6]

Ultrasonic lithotripsy

Ultrasonic energy was first used to fragment kidney stones in 1979. Commercially available units consist of a power generator combined with an ultrasound transducer and a probe that form the 'sonotrode'. A piezoceramic element in the handle of the sonotrode is stimulated to resonate, and this converts electrical energy into ultrasound waves (23,000–27,000 Hz) which are transmitted along the hollow metal probe creating a vibrating action at its tip. When the vibrating tip is brought in contact with the surface of a stone, the stone can be disintegrated. The probe must be rigid since sound waves cannot be transmitted without energy loss along flexible probes. The probes come in varying sizes and are passed through the straight working channel of a rigid endoscope. Suction tubing can be connected to the end of the sonotrode probe thus converting the unit into a 'vacuum cleaner' for stone fragments.[7–9] Smaller 2.5 Fr solid ultrasound probes are available for use through rigid ureteroscopes[10] and these can be utilized for rare cases in which fragmentation of large, distal ureteral calculi with EHL or laser lithotripsy has been ineffective. In all cases, normal saline at body temperature should be used as irrigant.

We continue to utilize ultrasound mainly for the fragmentation of large renal calculi during percutaneous nephrolithotripsy procedures. Ultrasound is used only rarely via an ureteroscopic approach.

Laser lithotripsy

The development of the pulsed dye laser for fragmentation of ureteral calculi was initiated in 1986.[11,12] Significant advances in laser fibres and power generation systems have propelled laser lithotripsy to be the treatment of choice for fragmentation of most ureteral stones. The pulsed dye laser delivers short, one microsecond energy pulsations at 5–10 Hz produced from a coumarin green dye. Instantaneous fluid evaporation causes a plasma at the stone surface, resulting in a highly localized shock wave. The 504 nm wave length produced by the pulsed dye laser is selectively absorbed by the stone, but not the surrounding ureteral wall. As the energy is delivered in short pulses, minimal heat is generated, again protecting the ureteral mucosa. Initial experience yielded stone fragmentation rates ranging from 64% to 95%.[13,14] Failures have been related to equipment malfunction (4–19%) or due to stone composition.

Continued development in laser technology has yielded larger diameter laser fibres that are able to more effectively fragment hard calculi. Newer 300 and 320 micron laser fibres are superior to the original 200 micron fibres for the fragmentation of calcium oxalate monohydrate and cystine stones. Fragmentation rates of greater than 90% have been obtained with these new fibres.

Solid-state lasers have been developed (Q-switched YAG, alexandrite, and holmium lasers) for the fragmentation of bladder calculi. These solid-state systems offer similar efficacy rates as compared to the dye lasers, but are significantly less expensive than the dye lasers and have reduced maintenance costs.[15]

The holmium wavelength is not selectively absorbed and works equally well to fragment stones of varying colour and composition.[16–18] Moreover, the holmium laser has the advantage of being a multipurpose laser system. It can be used for stone fragmentation, and for haemostatic and tissue effects including incision of urinary tract strictures and prostatic resection.[19,20] A potential limitation of this device is its 'drilling action' on hard stones. This can often be time-consuming, particularly when using the smaller holmium fibres.[21,22] Moreover, the tissue effects demand a greater degree of caution, as injury to the urothelium, guidewire, or endoscope can occur during stone fragmentation.

The major advantage of the holmium laser is that these small fibres can be placed through small, flexible ureteropyeloscopes. Both the 200 μ and 365 μ fibres can be placed through a flexible ureterorenoscope, though the 200 μ fibre is preferred when managing intrarenal calculi, since the smaller fibre diameter allows for greater ureteroscopic deflection. The relatively low power required to fragment calculi also allows the use of low-power holmium lasers. These low-power units provide 25–30 watts of power, at a significantly reduced cost as compared to the high-power, 80 watt lasers.

Our own experience with the holmium laser shows it to be ideal for use through all kinds of flexible endoscopes, and we now use it almost exclusively as our fragmentation modality of choice with both semi-rigid and flexible ureteroscopes.

As an alternative to holmium laser lithotripsy, the frequency doubled, double pulse Nd:YAG (FREDDY) laser (World of Medicine, Berlin, Germany) has shown to provide excellent stone fragmentation and minimal stone retropulsion.[23] The FREDDY laser effects stone fragmentation by production of a plasma bubble. Upon bubble collapse, a mechanical shock wave is generated, causing stone fragmentation. This mechanism of action is in contrast to the holmium laser, which cause stone destruction by vaporization.

Thulium laser is another alternative that has been recently developed and tested to use in stone management. Thulium fibre laser beam diameter is 18 μ, allowing easy coupling of the laser radiation into small-core optical fibres. Such small fibres have a great potential use when coupled with flexible endoscopes in demanding applications such as access to the lower pole of the kidney for lithotripsy.[24] In an *ex vivo* study, the stone mass loss with thulium laser was higher than with holmium laser. Further development is necessary to improve the use of thulium laser as a laser lithotripsy.[25]

Pneumatic lithotripsy

Another technique developed for the fragmentation of ureteral, renal, and bladder calculi is pneumatic lithotripsy. The first pneumatic device, the LithoClast, consists of a pneumatically driven piston which will fragment stones by direct contact (Fig. 2.7.1).[26,27] A major advantage of this device is its efficiency in breaking up calculi of all composition. Pneumatic lithotrites utilize a semi-rigid probe and therefore can only be passed through instrumentation with a straight working channel. At the present time, the smallest pneumatic probe is 0.8 mm, which can be used with the small semi-rigid ureteroscopes.

There have been a number of basic science and clinical studies demonstrating the safety and efficacy of the pneumatic device.[28,29] Hofbauer and Marberger performed a randomized prospective trial comparing the fragmentation of distal ureteral calculi with both EHL and pneumatic lithotripsy.[30] While the fragmentation rates for both devices were basically identical (85% fragmentation for EHL and 90% fragmentation for pneumatic lithotripsy), ureteral

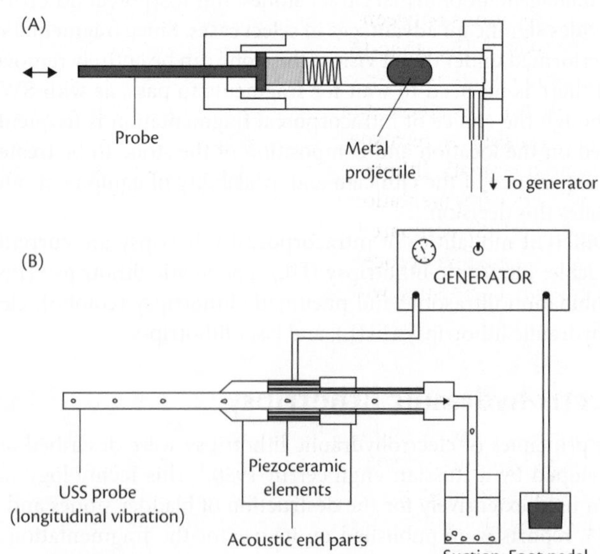

Fig. 2.7.1 The first pneumatic device, the Lithoclast, consists of a pneumatically driven piston that will fragment stones by direct contact.
Reproduced from Walsh PC, Retik AB, Vaughan D, and Wein AJ, *Campbell's Urology, Eighth Edition*, pp. 3395–7, Saunders, Philadelphia, USA, Copyright © 2002, with permission from Elsevier.

perforation was noted in only 2.6% of the patients undergoing pneumatic lithotripsy, while there was a 17% incidence of perforation in the EHL group. In a clinical experience utilizing pneumatic lithotripsy, successful fragmentation of stones of varying composition located in the kidney, ureter, and bladder was achieved, though ureteral stone migration was a problem in a limited number of patients who had significantly dilated proximal ureters.[5]

Recent innovations have expanded the use of pneumatic lithotripsy for the intracorporeal fragmentation of ureteral calculi. A suction device (Lithovac; EMS, Nyon, Switzerland) has been developed to aid in removal of stone fragments during pneumatic lithotripsy and limit the proximal migration of ureteral calculi.[31,32] In addition, flexible pneumatic probes are under development which will allow the use of pneumatic lithotripsy with flexible ureteroscopes.[33–35]

Another device, the LMA StoneBreaker™ (LMA, Durban, South Africa) is a portable, non-electric, contact ballistic intracorporeal lithotripter which is activated by a hand switch. This device weighs around 500 g and requires no extraneous electric or pneumatic connections. It is powered by a detachable cartridge of high pressure CO_2 with a maximum preadjusted operating pressure of 31 bars with a single pulse mode. It has demonstrated its utility in management of ureteral calculi. Some studies have been performed to analyse the use of this lithotripter, and they have showed good fragmentation efficacy and no complications associated with its use.[36] In a prospective randomized multicentre trial, StoneBreaker was compared with Swiss LithoClast® (EMS) during percutaneous nephrolithotripsy and was demonstrated to be an effective tool for intracorporeal lithotripsy, particularly for hard stones. It has also proved easy to set up and use.[37]

Pneumatic lithotripsy is an attractive option for the management of distal ureteral calculi, used through a semi-rigid ureteroscope with a straight working channel. Moreover, the pneumatic devices can be used for the fragmentation of bladder calculi and, in select cases, of renal calculi that do not respond well to UL. In a randomized prospective trial, Salvado *et al.* compared the success rates and complications between LithoClast classic, Ho:YAG laser, and StoneBreaker.[38] The stone-free rate between the three devices was similar and no difference in complications were found.

For proximal ureteral stones, no prospective randomized trials are available. A retrospective comparison between holmium laser and pneumatic lithotripsy in managing upper ureteral stones showed better fragmentation rates for holmium laser-assisted ureteroscopy (URS) compared with the pneumatic LithoClast. The necessity for auxiliary procedures after holmium laser-assisted URS was less when compared with LithoClast.[39]

Electrokinetic lithotripsy

The EMS Swiss Lithobreaker is a portable, electrokinetic lithotripter. Its tip velocity and displacement characteristics have been compared with the LMA StoneBreaker™. The electrokinetic device had significantly higher tip displacement and slower tip velocity. In the same study in a percutaneous model, the electrokinetic device required an average of 484 impulses over 430 s to fragment one BegoStone (BEGO, Lincoln RI), while the pneumatic device required 29 impulses over 122 s to fragment one stone. Both clearance times and number of impulses required for percutaneous stone clearance were significantly different. In an ureteroscopy model, the mean clearance time was 97 s for the electrokinetic lithotripter and 145 s for the pneumatic lithotripter. Comparing the pneumatic device with the electrokinetic device ureteroscopically, there was no significant difference in clearance time. Clinical studies are needed to confirm these findings *in vivo*.

Combination ultrasonic/pneumatic lithotripsy

Lithoclast Master (EMS) is a device which incorporates the fragmentation ability of pneumatic lithotripsy with the efficient stone removal capabilities of UL. This device has been shown during *in vitro* studies to clear artificial stones in a more efficient manner than ultrasonic or pneumatic devices alone.[40] Moreover, the size of fragments created by the combination ultrasonic/pneumatic device are significantly smaller than the standard lithotrites. A prospective randomized trial comparing combined ultrasonic and pneumatic lithotrite with a standard ultrasonic lithotrite for percutaneous nephrolithotomy has shown that stone ablation and clearance rates were similar for both devices. The combined device was more efficient only for harder stones.[41]

Cyberwand® (Olympus, Center Valley, PA) is an intracorporeal lithotripter with a dual-probe ultrasonic design that incorporates coaxial high frequency with low frequency. The inner probe is fixed to the handpiece and the outer probe is free to move in a reciprocating fashion and is pushed outward by a sliding piston driven by the vibration energy of the inner probe. In an *in vitro* study, Kim compared the stone penetration time between CyberWand and LithoClast Ultra® (EMS). The stone penetration time for the first device was significant shorter than the second one.[42]

In a randomized controlled, multicentre clinical trial, the CyberWand was compare to a single-probe lithotrite for percutaneous nephrolithotomy. In this study, no significant difference in stone clearance rate, intraoperative, and postoperative complications and primary stone-free rates were founded.[43]

Intracorporeal lithotripsy: Selection of modality

There are a number of modalities that can be used for intracorporeal lithotripsy of urinary tract calculi. While there is no 'best' device, considerations for choosing a specific technology include efficacy, safety, and cost. However, if a holmium laser is available, then this multipurpose laser offers perhaps the best option for ureteral stones. Both ultrasonic and pneumatic lithotripsy offer the advantage of rapid fragmentation, even with very large or hard stones, but its use is limited to rigid or semi-rigid delivery systems. With these characteristics, they could be the first option to treat large or hard stones.

Further reading

Auge B, Lallas C., Pietrow P, Zhong P, Preminger GM. In vitro comparison of standard ultrasound and pneumatic lithotrites with a new combination intracorporeal lithotripsy device. *Urology* 2002; **60**(1):28–32.

Chew B, Arsovska O, Lange D, *et al.* The Canadian StoneBreaker trial: A randomized, multicenter trial comparing the LMA StoneBreakerTM and the Swiss LithoClastR during percutaneous nephrolithotripsy. *J Endourol* 2011; **25**(9):1415–19.

Denstedt JD, Eberwein PM, Singh RR. The Swiss Lithoclast: a new device for intracorporeal lithotripsy. *J Urol* 1992; **148**:1088–90.

Goodfriend R. Ultrasonic and electrohydraulic lithotripsy of ureteral calculi. *Urology* 1984; **23**:5–8.

Haupt G, van Ophoven A, Pannek J, Herde T, Senge T. In vitro comparison of two ballistic systems for endoscopic stone disintegration. *J Endourol* 1996; **10**:417–20.

Huang S, Patel H, Bellman GC. Cost effectiveness of electrohydraulic lithotripsy v Candela pulsed-dye laser in management of the distal ureteral stone. *J Endourol* 1998; **12**:237–40.

Krambeck AE, Miller NL, Humphreys MR, et al. Randomized controlled, multicentre clinical trial comparing a dual-probe ultrasonic lithotrite with a single-probe lithotrite for percutaneous nephrolithotomy. *BJU Int* 2011; **107**(5):824–8.

Kuo RL, Aslan P, Zhong P, Preminger GM. Impact of holmium laser settings and fiber diameter on stone fragmentation and endoscope deflection. *J Endourol* 1998; **12**:523–7.

Lehman D, Hruby G, Phillips C, *et al.* Prospective randomized comparison of a combined ultrasonic and pneumatic lithotrite with a standard ultrasonic lithotrite for percutaneous nephrolithotomy. *J Endourol* 2008; **22**(2):285–9.

Matlaga BR, Lingeman JE. Surgical management of stones: new technology. *Adv Chronic Kidney Dis* 2009; **16**(1):60–4.

Nerli RB, Koura AC, Prabha V, Kamat G, Alur SB. Use of LMA stonebreaker as an intracorporeal lithotrite in the management of ureteral calculi. *J Endourol* 2008; **22**(4): 641–4.

Raney AM, Handler J. Electrohydraulic nephrolithotripsy. *Urology* 1975; **6**:439–42.

Teh CL, Zhong P, Preminger GM. Laboratory and clinical assessment of pneumatically driven intracorporeal lithotripsy. *J Endourol* 1998; **12**:163–9.

Teichman JM, Rao RD, Rogenes VJ, Harris JM. Ureteroscopic management of ureteral calculi: electrohydraulic versus holmium:YAG lithotripsy. *J Urol* 1997; **158**:1357–61.

Vassar GJ, Chan KF, Teichman JM, *et al.* Holmium: YAG lithotripsy: photothermal mechanism. *J Endourol* 1999; **13**:181–90.

Watson G, Murray S, Dretler SP, Parrish JA. The pulsed dye laser for fragmenting urinary calculi. *J Urol* 1987; **138**:195–8.

References

1. Rouvalis P. Electronic lithotripsy for vesical calculus with "Urat-1". An experience of 100 cases and an experimental application of the method to stones in the upper urinary tract. *Br J Urol* 1970; **42**:486–91.
2. Raney AM. Electrohydraulic lithotripsy: experimental study and case reports with the stone disintegrator. *J Urol* 1975; **113**:345–7.
3. Raney AM, Handler J. Electrohydraulic nephrolithotripsy. *Urology* 1975; **6**:439–42.
4. Zhong P, Tong HL, Cocks FH, Preminger GM. Transient oscillation of cavitation bubbles near stone surface during electrohydraulic lithotripsy. *J Endourol* 1997; **11**:55–61.
5. Teh CL, Zhong P, Preminger GM. Laboratory and clinical assessment of pneumatically driven intracorporeal lithotripsy. *J Endourol* 1998; **12**:163–9.
6. Assimos D, Krambeck A, Miller NL, *et al.* Surgical Management of Stones: American Urological Association/Endourological Society Guideline, PART II. *J Urol* 2016; **196**(4):1161–9.
7. Huffman JL, Bagley DH, Schoenberg HW, Lyon ES. Transurethral removal of large ureteral and renal pelvic calculi using ureteroscopic ultrasonic lithotripsy. *J Urol* 1983; **130**:31–4.
8. Goodfriend R. Ultrasonic and electrohydraulic lithotripsy of ureteral calculi. *Urology* 1984; **23**:5–8.
9. Weinerth JL, Flatt JA, Carson CC 3d. Lessons learned in patients with large steinstrasse. *J Urol* 1989; **142**:1425–7.
10. Chaussy C, Fuchs G, Kahn R, Hunter P, Goodfriend R. Transurethral ultrasonic ureterolithotripsy using a solid-wire probe. *Urology* 1987; **29**:531–2.
11. Watson G, Murray S, Dretler SP, Parrish JA. The pulsed dye laser for fragmenting urinary calculi. *J Urol* 1987; **138**:195–8.
12. Dretler SP, Watson G, Parrish JA, Murray S. Pulsed dye laser fragmentation of ureteral calculi: initial clinical experience. *J Urol* 1987; **137**:386–9.
13. Huang S, Patel H, Bellman GC. Cost effectiveness of electrohydraulic lithotripsy v Candela pulsed-dye laser in management of the distal ureteral stone. *J Endourol* 1998; **12**:237–40.
14. Grasso M, Bagley DH. Endoscopic pulsed-dye laser lithotripsy: 159 consecutive cases. *J Endourol* 1994; **8**:25–7.
15. Pearle MS, Sech SM, Cobb CG, *et al.* Safety and efficacy of the Alexandrite laser for the treatment of renal and ureteral calculi. *Urology* 1998; **51**:33–8.
16. Teichman JM, Rao RD, Rogenes VJ, Harris JM. Ureteroscopic management of ureteral calculi: electrohydraulic versus holmium:YAG lithotripsy. *J Urol* 1997; **158**:1357–61.
17. Zhong P, Tong HL, Cocks FH, Pearle MS, Preminger GM. Transient cavitation and acoustic emission produced by different laser lithotripters. *J Endourol* 1998; **12**:371–8.
18. Santa-Cruz RW, Leveillee RJ, Krongrad A. Ex vivo comparison of four lithotripters commonly used in the ureter: what does it take to perforate? *J Endourol* 1998; **12**:417–22.
19. Razvi HA, Chun SS, Denstedt JD, Sales JL. Soft-tissue applications of the holmium:YAG laser in urology. *J Endourol* 1995; **9**:387–90.
20. Kuo RL, Aslan P, Fitzgerald KB, Preminger GM. Use of ureteroscopy and holmium:YAG laser in patients with bleeding diatheses. *Urology* 1998; **52**:609–13.
21. Kuo RL, Aslan P, Zhong P, Preminger GM. Impact of holmium laser settings and fiber diameter on stone fragmentation and endoscope deflection. *J Endourol* 1998; **12**:523–7.
22. Vassar GJ, Chan KF, Teichman JM, *et al.* Holmium: YAG lithotripsy: photothermal mechanism. *J Endourol* 1999; **13**:181–90.
23. Marguet C, Sung J, Springhart W, *et al.* In vitro comparison of stoneretropulsion and fragmentation of the frequency doubled, double pulse ND:YAGlaser and the Holmium:YAG laser. *J Urol* 2005; **173**(5):1797–800.
24. Matlaga BR, Lingeman JE. Surgical management of stones: new technology. *Adv Chronic Kidney Dis* 2009; **16**(1):60–4.
25. Blackmon RL, Irby PB, Fried NM. Holmium:YAG (lambda = 2,120 nm) versus thulium fiber (lambda = 1,908 nm) laser lithotripsy. *Lasers Surg Med* 2010; **42**(3):232–6.
26. Denstedt JD, Eberwein PM, Singh RR. The Swiss Lithoclast: a new device for intracorporeal lithotripsy. *J Urol* 1992; **148**:1088–90.
27. Hofbauer J, Hobarth K, Marberger M. Lithoclast: New and inexpensive mode of intracorporeal lithotripsy. *J Endourol* 1992; **6**:429–32.
28. Denstedt JD, Razvi HA, Rowe E, Grignon DJ, Eberwein PM. Investigation of the tissue effects of a new device for intracorporeal lithotripsy—the Swiss Lithoclast. *J Urol* 1995; **153**:535–7.
29. Haupt G, van Ophoven A, Pannek J, Herde T, Senge T. In vitro comparison of two ballistic systems for endoscopic stone disintegration. *J Endourol* 1996; **10**:417–20.
30. Hofbauer J, Hobarth K, Marberger M. Electrohydraulic versus pneumatic disintegration in the treatment of ureteral stones: a randomized, prospective trial. *J Urol* 1995; **153**:623–5.
31. Haupt G, Pannek J, Herde T, Schulze H, Senge T. The Lithovac: new suction device for the Swiss Lithoclast. *J Endourol* 1995; **9**:375–7.
32. Delvecchio FC, Kuo RL, Preminger GM. Clinical efficacy of combined lithoclast and lithovac stone removal during ureteroscopy. *J Urol* 2000; **164**(1):40–2.
33. Loisides P, Grasso M, Bagley DH. Mechanical impactor employing Nitinol probes to fragment human calculi: fragmentation efficiency with flexible endoscope deflection. *J Endourol* 1995; **9**:371–4.
34. Tawfiek ER, Grasso M, Bagley DH. Initial use of Browne Pneumatic Impactor. *J Endourol* 1997; **11**:121–4.

35. Zhu S, Kourambas J, Munver R, Zhong P, Preminger GM. Characterization of tip movement of the lithoclast flexible probe. *J Urol* 2000; **163**(4S):318.
36. Nerli RB, Koura AC, Prabha V, Kamat G, Alur SB. Use of LMA stonebreaker as an intracorporeal lithotrite in the management of ureteral calculi. *J Endourol* 2008; **22**(4): 641–4.
37. Chew B, Arsovska O, Lange D, *et al.* The Canadian StoneBreaker trial: A randomized, multicenter trial comparing the LMA StoneBreaker™ and the Swiss LithoClast® during percutaneous nephrolithotripsy. *J Endourol* 2011; **25**(9):1415–19.
38. Salvado J, Mandujano R, Saez I, *et al.* Ureteroscopic lithotripsy for distal ureteral calculi: Comparative evaluation of three different lithotripters. *J Endourol* 2012; **26**(4):343–346.
39. Bapat S, Pai K, Purnapatre S, Yadav PB, Padye AS. Comparison of Holmium laser and pneumatic lithotripsy in managing upper-ureteral stones. *J Endourol* 2007; **21**(12):1425–7.
40. Auge B, Lallas C., Pietrow P, Zhong P, Preminger GM. In vitro comparison of standard ultrasound and pneumatic lithotrites with a new combination intracorporeal lithotripsy device. *Urology* 2002; **60**(1):28–32.
41. Lehman D, Hruby G, Phillips C, *et al.* Prospective randomized comparison of a combined ultrasonic and pneumatic lithotrite with a standard ultrasonic lithotrite for percutaneous nephrolithotomy. *J Endourol* 2008; **22**(2):285–9.
42. Kim SC, Matlaga BR, Tinmouth WW, *et al.* In vitro assessment of a novel dual probe ultrasonic intracorporeal lithotriptor. *J Urol* 2007; **177**(4):1363–5.
43. Krambeck AE, Miller NL, Humphreys MR, *et al.* Randomized controlled, multicentre clinical trial comparing a dual-probe ultrasonic lithotrite with a single-probe lithotrite for percutaneous nephrolithotomy. *BJU Int* 2011; **107**(5):824–8.

CHAPTER 2.8

Kidney stones
Presentation and diagnosis

John Reynard and Ben Turney

Presentation

Renal stones may present in a variety of ways:

- Loin pain
- Haematuria
- Urinary tract infections
    - lower urinary tract infections (specifically recurrent cystitis)
    - renal abscess
    - perinephric abscess
- Incidentally (asymptomatic) during radiological investigation for other intra-abdominal symptoms

Loin pain

Loin pain is a common presentation to the urology outpatient clinic as it is to the emergency department. We know that approximately 50% of patients presenting with loin pain thought (by their attending doctors) to be indicative of a ureteric stone have no evidence of urolithiasis within the ureter or kidneys, or indeed of any other urological pathology on unenhanced computed tomography (CT) scanning. It follows that a substantial proportion (presumably something in the region of 50%) of those with loin pain who present less acutely also do not have evidence of renal or ureteric stone disease.[1]

Even for patients where unenhanced CT scanning confirms the presence of a stone, the only sure way of determining whether or not this is the cause of the loin pain that they complain of is to remove the stone. If their loin pain resolves, then it can be said that the stone was the cause. Not surprisingly, patients who are assured that their loin pain is caused by their stone will be disappointed (as will be their urologist) when their pain persists despite successful stone clearance.

That said, the small non-obstructing calyceal stone assumed, because of its small size, not to be responsible for loin pain, may certainly cause such pain[2] and removal of these stones can improve or resolve pain in a proportion of such patients.[3]

Haematuria

Rarely, visible haematuria (with or without loin pain) may be a presenting symptom of renal stone disease. Other more serious causes of haematuria must be excluded. Dipstick or microscopic (non-visible) haematuria is common though not universal.

Urinary tract infections

Renal stones may be both the cause of recurrent urinary tract infections or UTIs (cystitis) and be caused by them. Not surprisingly, populations at risk of UTI (women; patients with neurological disease such as spinal cord injury[4] and spina bifida; those with urinary diversions; those with congenital urinary tract abnormalities) are more likely to form stones and their stones are more likely to be so-called infection stones (composed of struvite—magnesium ammonium phosphate hexahydrate). Once an infection stone forms, it will harbour vast quantities of bacteria and thus perpetuate episodes of recurrent UTI. Because (obviously) stones are not vascularized, no amount of antibiotics will resolve the recurrent UTIs.

Occasionally renal stones may present with serious upper tract infection in the form of a pyonephrosis (an infected hydronephrosis), a perinephric abscess (arising from rupture of an abscess in the cortex into the perinephric tissues), emphysematous pyelonephritis, or xanthogranulomatous pyelonephritis.

As for loin pain, the proof that recurrent UTIs are caused by the stone is their successful resolution following complete stone removal. It is therefore advisable to warn patients that resolution of UTIs may not follow complete stone clearance.

The incidental (asymptomatic) finding of renal stone disease

Asymptomatic renal stone disease is prevalent: 389 (7.7%) of 5,047 asymptomatic individuals undergoing unenhanced CT colonography over a four-year period have urinary tract stones (mean size 3 mm, range 1–20 mm; mean stone number per patient 2).[5]

Diagnosis

Plain radiography remains a good way of identifying renal stones if calcified, will identify cysteine stones which are relatively radiolucent, but cannot 'see' non-calcium-containing stones (e.g. uric acid, triamterene, indinavir).

The sensitivity of ultrasound for detecting renal calculi is variably reported at between 50–95%.[6]

Unenhanced CT is nowadays regarded as the diagnostic gold standard for identifying renal calculi, for measuring their size

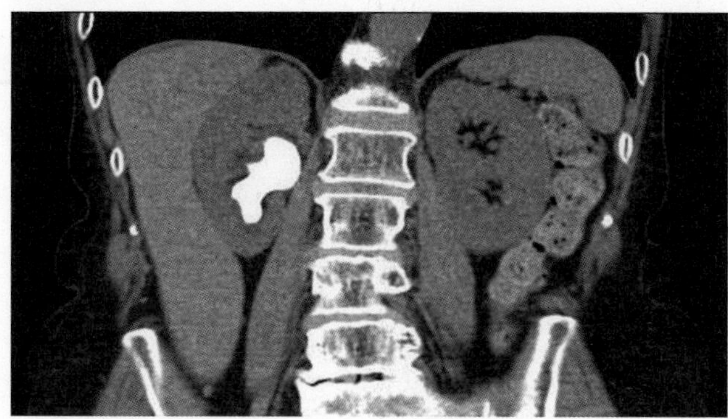

Fig. 2.8.1 A large right renal calculus diagnosed on a CT-KUB.
Image reproduced courtesy of John Reynard

and number and, to a lesser degree, determining their location (Fig. 2.8.1). Where doubt exists over stone location, precise determination requires either CT urography or retrograde ureterorenography. The 'limitation' of CT is its radiation dose, but as a single 'upfront' diagnostic test, there is no substitute.

References

1. Smith RC, Verga M, McCarthy S, Rosenfield AT. Diagnosis of acute flank pain: value of unenhanced helical CT. *Am J Roentgen* 1996; **166**:97–101.
2. Coury TA, Sonda LP, Lingeman JE, Kahnoski RJ. Treatment of painful caliceal stones. *Urology* 1988; **32**:119–23.
3. Taub DA, Suh RS, Faerber GJ, Wolf JS Jr. Ureteroscopic laser papillotomy to treat papillary calcifications associated with chronic flank pain. *Urology* 2006; **67**:683–7.
4. DeVivo MJ, Fine PR, Cutter GR, Maetz HM. The risk of renal calculi in spinal cord injury patients. *J Urol* 1984; **131**:857–60.
5. Boyce CJ, Pickhardt PJ, Lawrence EM, Kim DH, Bruce RJ. Prevalence of urolithiasis in asymptomatic adults: Objective determination using low dose noncontrast computerized tomography. *J Urol* 2010; **183**:1017–21.
6. Haddad MC, Sharif HS, Abomelha ME, Riley PJ, Sammak BM, Shahed MS. Management of renal colic: redefining the role of the urogram. *Radiology* 1992; **184**:35–6.

CHAPTER 2.9

Watchful waiting for stone disease

John Reynard and Ben Turney

Introduction to stone disease

When 5,047 asymptomatic individuals underwent unenhanced computed tomography colonography between 2004–2008, 395 (7.8%) were found to have urinary tract stones (99% renal stones—mean size 3 mm, range 1–20 mm, mean stone number per patient 2; and 1% ureteric or bladder stones).[1] Symptomatic urolithiasis subsequently developed in 36 (9%) of these 395 individuals after an average of 1.3 years from initial stone diagnosis. So, while 9% of screened individuals experienced a stone event, 91% remained asymptomatic for several years afterwards. This is not a unique observation and forms the basis for watchful waiting as a management option, at least for *small* calyceal renal stones. Why intervene if the stone may not do anything?

So what is the risk that symptoms will develop or intervention will be required?

In 63 patients with 80 asymptomatic stones (stone size and number not recorded) and an average follow-up of 7.4 years,[2] 45% experienced an increase in stone size and 51% experienced pain, while 16% of stones passed spontaneously, 40% required surgical intervention, and 38% remained *in situ*.

In Glowacki's study,[3] 70% of 107 initially asymptomatic patients remained asymptomatic over a mean of 2.5 years of follow-up. Meanwhile, 15% developed ureteric colic, 8% required extracorporeal shock wave lithotripsy (ESWL), 6% ureteroscopy, and 3% percutaneous nephrolithotomy (PCNL). Kaplan–Meier analysis predicted the probability of a symptomatic event in 10% at one year, 20% at two years, 30% at three years, 40% at four years, and 50% at five years. Half of symptomatic events required intervention.

As a ballpark figure, these studies from the 1980s suggest that within approximately five to seven years, pain will develop in roughly half of patients with initially asymptomatic stones, and intervention will be required in-between approximately 20–40%.

Can the risk of pain and the requirement for intervention be more accurately predicted for individual patients?

Risk of requirement for intervention versus stone size

In the largest observational study to date, Burger[4] related risk of intervention (ESWL, ureteroscopy, PCNL), development of pain, and increase in stone size to stone size and location. The study must be interpreted with a caveat—the decision to intervene was left to the patient, apparently without physician involvement. Thus, a percentage of patients (but it is not clear from the study how many) may have decided to undergo intervention because of a *perceived* risk of a future stone event (increase in size or sudden ureteric stone migration) without actually knowing the real risk of a stone event. It is not clear how many patients required intervention for actual ureteric stone migration as opposed to the fear of stone migration, and so the study fails to quantify the risk of stone migration—that sudden, very painful, and unpredictable event that presumably all patients want to avoid. Three-hundred men with asymptomatic stones (mean age 63 years) were followed over a mean of 3 years (range 0.2–10 years). Stone size at presentation was <5 mm in 32%, 5–10 mm in 55%, 11–15 mm in 10%, and >15 mm in 3%. Stone location was 26% upper pole, 28% middle pole, 44% lower pole, and 2% renal pelvis.

Intervention was required in 26%, being more likely for stones >4 mm in diameter (Table 2.9.1). Kaplan–Meier analysis predicted a 50% chance of intervention at seven years. An increase in stone size occurred in 47% with upper and middle pole stones, and 61% with lower pole stones.

The most robust data (derived from a prospective randomized controlled trial) for the actual risk of sudden ureteric stone migration is provided by Keeley's ESWL (n = 101 patients) versus observation (n = 99 patients) study[5] of asymptomatic stones <15 mm, with a mean of 2.2 years follow-up for 200 patients (range 1–5 years). Stone-free status was achieved in 17% of the observation group, nine passing their stone spontaneously, and seven were rendered stone-free by intervention (28% of the ESWL patients achieved stone-free

Table 2.9.1 Approximate three-year risk of intervention, pain, or increase in stone size versus stones size, measured as the largest single diameter (where >1 stone present)

	Stone size			
	<5 mm	5–10 mm	11–15 mm	>15 mm
% Requiring intervention	20%	25%	40%	30%
% Causing pain	45%	40%	40%	55%
% Increasing in size	50%	55%	60%	70%

Source: data from Burgher A, Beman M, Holtzman JL, and Monga M, Progression of nephrolithiasis: long-term outcomes with observation of asymptomatic calculi, *Journal of Endourology*, Volume 18, pp 534–9, Copyright 2004 Mary Ann Liebert, Inc. publishers.

Table 2.9.2 The risk of intervention being required for initially asymptomatic small renal calculi (mostly <15 mm in size)

Study	Number of patients followed	Years of follow-up	% of patients requiring intervention (or symptomatic event)
Boyce 2010[1]	395	1 year	Symptomatic stone event 9%
Keeley 2001[5] <15 mm	99	Mean 2.2 years	20%
Burgher 2004[4] majority <15 mm	300	Mean 3 years	25%
Inci 2007[6]	24	Mean 4.3 years	11%
Glowacki 1992[3]	107	At 5 years	25%
Hubner and Porpazcy 1990[2]	63	Mean 7.4 years	40%

Source: data from Boyce 2010[1]; Keeley 2001[5]; Burgher 2004[4], Inci 2007[6]; Glowacki 1992[3]; and Hubner and Porpazcy 1990.[2]

status—a surprisingly small proportion). Additional treatment was required in 21% of the observation group—ESWL in 18 patients, ureteroscopy in six, and stent insertion in four (and in 15% of the ESWL group). There was no difference in quality of life or time off work between the two groups. In this well designed, carefully conducted study, the bottom line thus seems to be that one in five patients with asymptomatic stones who opt to watch and wait will require ESWL, ureteroscopy, and/or stent insertion over 2.2 years.

Inci[6] followed 24 patients with asymptomatic lower pole stones over a mean of 52.3 months. Mean stone diameter at presentation was 8.8 mm (range 2–26 mm). Progression in stone size was demonstrated in 9 of 27 renal units (33.3%) with 2 (11.1%) requiring intervention. Three stones passed spontaneously without any pain, a further three patients developed pain, with two passing a stone spontaneously.

Pain will develop or intervention (ESWL, ureteroscopy, stent insertion) will be required in 10% of patients at 1 year,[1] 20% at 2 years,[5] and 40–50% at 5–7 years[2–4] (Table 2.9.2). The chances of an increase in stone size are highly variable being reported in-between 33–70% of patients, at least partly being related to stone size at the start of observation. An increase in stone size does not necessarily translate into a requirement for intervention.

Who is suitable for watchful waiting?

As a rule of thumb for the asymptomatic stone, the younger the patient and the larger the stone, the more inclined are we to recommend treatment, the perception being that large stones will, if left untreated, be more prone to cause complications over the many years of life ahead of the patient and may (possibly) grow faster. What both urologist and patient need is data on which to base a decision to watch and wait—they need an idea of the *risk* of watchful waiting over a period of time.

How is watchful waiting defined?

The short answer is—it has not been defined. No national or international guidelines exist to inform decision-making or to indicate the appropriate frequency, duration, mode, and logistics of observation (family doctor vs. hospital-based), which remain matters for debate. Too short an observation interval risks more radiation exposure and is onerous and costly for patients and healthcare systems alike, as is follow-up over many years. Too long an interval between imaging risks an increase in stone size beyond the range of less invasive options (ESWL) and into the range where more invasive treatments may be required (f-URS, PCNL). From a medicolegal perspective, it is therefore important to warn patients who elect watchful waiting over immediate stone treatment that they may miss the opportunity for simpler and safer treatment (ESWL) and may require more complex treatment (f-URS, PCNL) if their particular stone grows more rapidly than anticipated in-between imaging studies.

The two groups of patients with small asymptomatic stones suitable for watchful waiting (the never previously symptomatic vs. those who have experienced a previous stone event) may require different (respectively, perhaps less vs. more frequent) follow-up screening protocols, but again no evidence is available to inform follow-up frequency.

Stones that are not suitable for watchful waiting

- Airline pilots cannot fly once diagnosed with an asymptomatic renal calculus. The rules determining when they are allowed to fly again can be found on the CAA (Civil Aviation Authority) website.
- For drivers of heavy goods vehicles, the DVLA (Drivers Vehicle Licensing Agency) gives advice[7] (renal failure, septicaemia, pyonephrosis, perinephric abscess).[8–10] The combination of the neurogenic bladder and staghorn calculus seems to be particularly associated with a poor outcome.[11]

Stones where treatment may be recommended over watchful waiting

- Women considering pregnancy.
- Patients with solitary kidneys.
- Patients with spinal cord injuries where silent (asymptomatic) ureteric stone migration can lead to silent and even complete loss of renal function on the affected side.

References

1. Boyce CJ, Pickhardt PJ, Lawrence EM, Kim DH, Bruce RJ. Prevalence of urolithiasis in asymptomatic adults: Objective determination using low dose noncontrast computerized tomography. *J Urol* 2010; **183**:1017–21.
2. Hubner WA, Porpaczy P. Treatment of calyceal calculi. *Br J Urol* 1990; **66**:9–11.
3. Glowacki LS, Beecroft ML, Cook RJ, Pahl D, Churchill DN. The natural history of asymptomatic urolithiasis. *J Urol* 1992; **147**:319–21.
4. Burgher A, Beman M, Holtzman JL, Monga M. Progression of nephrolithiasis: long-term outcomes with observation of asymptomatic calculi. *J Endourol* 2004; **18**:534–9.
5. Keeley FX, Tilling K, Elves A, *et al.* Preliminary results of a randomized controlled trial of prophylactic shock wave lithotripsy for small asymptomatic renal calyceal stones. *BJU Int* 2001; **87**:1–8.

6. Inci K, Sahin A, Islamoglu E, Eren MT, Bakkaloglu M, Ozen H. Prospective long-term followup of patients with asymptomatic lower pole caliceal stones. *J Urol* 2007; **177**:2189–92.
7. Borley NC, Rainford D, Anson KM, Watkin N. What activities are safe with kidney stones? A review of occupational and travel advice in the UK. *Brit J Urol Int* 2007; **99**:494–6.
8. Blandy JP, Singh M. The case for a more aggressive approach to staghorn stones. *J Urol* 1976; **115**:505–6.
9. Rous SN, Turner WR. Retrospective study of 95 patients with staghorn calculus disease. *J Urol* 1977; **118**:902–4.
10. Vargas AD, Bragin SD, Mendez R. Staghorn calculus: its clinical presentation, complications and management. *J Urol* 1982; **127**:860–2.
11. Teichman JM, Long RD, Hulbert JC. Long-term renal fate and prognosis after staghorn calculus management. *J Urol* 1995; **153**:1403–7.

CHAPTER 2.10

Retrograde intrarenal surgery
Flexible ureterorenoscopy

Gaston M. Astroza, Ghalib Jibara,
Michael E. Lipkin, and Glen M. Preminger

Introduction to retrograde intrarenal surgery

The European Association of Urology (EAU) and the American Urological Association (AUA) have recommended percutaneous nephrolithotomy (PCNL) for the management of kidney stones over 2 cm as a first-line treatment, and retrograde intrarenal surgery (RIRS) in the form of flexible ureterorenoscopy (f-URS) or extracorporeal shock wave lithotripsy (ESWL) for stones under 2 cm.[1,2] This is with the caveat that stones in the *lower pole* between 1.0 and 1.5 cm are best managed by PCNL as first-line treatment given the lower stone-free rate with ESWL[3–5] with a higher residual stone fragment rate, which leads to recurrent stone formation.[6]

However, with technological advances (small calibre, actively deflectable ureterorenoscopes) and improvements in endoscopic techniques, it is becoming apparent that f-URS has stone-free rates equivalent, if nor superior to, ESWL. As a consequence, f-URS is increasingly being recognized as an alternative to ESWL.[7–11]

Indications

Currently, f-URS is recommended as a first-line treatment by both the AUA and EAU guidelines for treatment of patients with with a total non-lower pole renal stone burden ≤20 mm and those with lower pole renal stones ≤10 mm in diameter. Flexible ureterorenoscopy is additionally indicated[12–15]:

- where ESWL has failed to achieve stone clearance;
- in the presence of a bleeding diathesis;
- in cases where body mass index precludes effective ESWL;
- in the presence of musculoskeletal deformities or infundibular stenosis;
- for multiple unilateral intrarenal stones;
- in patients not considered candidates for PCNL where staged f-URS may be offered.

Flexible ureterorenoscopy can be safely performed in the anticoagulated, as demonstrated by Turna's matched pair analysis comparing flexible ureteroscopy outcomes and complications in anticoagulated and non-anticoagulated patients. In either arm, none of the procedures were aborted and there was no difference in stone-free rates, or in intraoperative or postoperative complications, including postoperative haemorrhage and thromboembolic events.[16] Flexible ureterorenoscopy has also been shown to be equally efficacious in terms of stone-free rates in normal, overweight, and obese patients.[17]

The presence of multiple unilateral intrarenal stones is also an indication for f-URS, since the reported stone-free rate of 50% with shock wave lithroscopy (SWL) in this group of patients is lower than in cases of single intrarenal stones.[18–20] In a retrospective review of outcomes with flexible ureteroscopy and laser lithotripsy for multiple unilateral intrarenal stones, Breda[3] found an overall stone-free rate after f-URS of 64.7% with one procedure and 92.2% after two procedures. For patients with multiple intrarenal stones, PCNL has equal or better outcomes than f-URS, but at the expense of a high complication rate. In particular, patients with multiple intrarenal stones who undergo PCNL may require multiple tracts, which increases the risk of complications.[21]

Patient with stone-bearing calyceal diverticula are candidates for f-URS, which allows both stone removal and dilatation, or incision of the diverticula neck, thereby reducing risk of stone recurrence (while ESWL improves symptoms in a proportion of such cases, many patients will experience recurrent symptoms over time).[22] PCNL for calyceal diverticular stones results in higher stone-free rates when compared with f-URS[23,24] at the expense of a slightly higher complication rate.

For the 1 cm or less lower pole renal stone, a prospective randomized trial showed no significant difference in stone-free rates between ESWL and f-URS, but ESWL was associated with a shorter convalescence.[4] In another study that also compared SWL versus f-URS in the treatment of lower pole renal calculi, the stone-free rates and final success rates were similar, but ESWL was more cost-effective.[25]

For the larger renal stones (>2 cm), the stone-free rate of PCNL is better than f-URS and fewer procedures are required, but complication rates are higher though statistically not significantly so.[26–28] In patients with a contraindication to PCNL, such as irreversible coagulopathy, f-URS offers a viable alternative in treating these large stones.

Instrumentation

Innovations in fibre-optic and digital technology have propelled the development of flexible ureterorenoscopes. Modern flexible scopes have up to 270 degrees of active deflection, allowing access the entire upper urinary tract including all of the intrarenal collecting system.[13,29,30] Digital image acquisition (as opposed to conventional fibre-optic systems) has improved visualization of the collecting system, which in turn reduces operative times.[31,32]

Holmium laser fibres for intrarenal collecting system stone fragmentation range in size (diameter as opposed to circumference) from 200 (greater deflection) to 365 microns (less deflection) for use down flexible ureterorenoscopes (Fig. 2.10.1). Modern flexible ureterorenoscopes maintain downward deflection up to 175 degrees, even with a 365 micron holmium laser fibre (representing the minimal deflection needed to access the lower pole).[33]

Nitinol baskets, ranging in size from 1.3 Fr to 2.4 Fr, allow active retrieval of stone fragments from the intrarenal collecting system. Although a 1.9 Fr nitinol basket significantly reduces irrigant flow through the working channel, flow remains high enough for adequate visualization.[34]

Typically, the distal ureter does not need to be dilated prior to f-URS, given the small calibre of flexible ureterorenoscopes. Where the flexible ureterorenoscope will not pass through the distal ureter, a semi-rigid ureteroscope, balloon dilator, or a tapered ureteral dilators can be used to dilate the ureteral orifice and intramural ureter.[35]

Ureteral access sheaths (10/12 Fr to 14/16 Fr) facilitate multiple passages of the ureterorenoscope in and out of the ureter, so allowing more retrieval of stone fragments. They reduce operative times and costs during fURS[36] and can improve stone-free rates (79% vs. 67% for the treatment of intrarenal stones with a ureteral access, compared to treatment without an access sheath).[37] Ureteral access sheaths may also prolong scope life.

Technique

The patient is placed lithotomy or supine with the legs flat in an attempt to 'iron out' the curve of the ureter. The lithotomy position tends to exaggerate the curve of the ureter. A rigid cystoscope is passed to allow passage of the first guidewire and, if the surgeon prefers, a 4–6 Fr open-ended ureteral catheter so that a retrograde pyelogram can be performed to delineate ureteral and intrarenal collecting system anatomy (some surgeons prefer to perform the retrograde pyelogram once the flexible ureterorenoscope is in position within the renal pelvis). A 0.038 inch floppy-tipped 'safety' guidewire (e.g. a Sensor guidewire) (Fig. 2.10.2) is placed through the open-ended catheter up to the kidney under fluoroscopic guidance. Many surgeons pass a dual lumen catheter, to allow both ureteric dilatation and passage of a second 'working' guidewire.

It is our practice to routinely use a 12/14 Fr ureteral access sheath, passed over the working wire (leaving the safety wire outside the sheath), into the proximal ureter. It is often helpful to pass the inner sheath alone first to gently dilate the ureteral orifice and distal ureter. Once the access sheath is in appropriate position, the flexible ureterorenoscope is advanced up into the kidney over the working guidewire.[36] Concerns over the possibility of relative ureteral ischaemia after ureteral access sheath placement, reported in an animal model, do not appear to have translated into any clinical consequences with long-term follow-up.[38] On the positive side, ureteral access sheaths certainly allow easier access to the kidney, prevent the scope coiling within the bladder, improve irrigation flow, hence better visibility, and decreased intrarenal pressure (they 'vent off' the collecting system).[39–40]

The safety guidewire remains located within the renal pelvis until the procedure is completed.

Under direct vision, the holmium laser, stone baskets, grasping forceps, or snares are used to fragment renal calculi and remove the resulting stone fragments under direct vision. During stone basket withdrawal, a distance of a few millimetres is maintained between the entrapped stone and the end of the scope, so allowing the surgeon to ensure that the ureter is not in danger of being avulsed by the stone as it is withdrawn down the ureter.

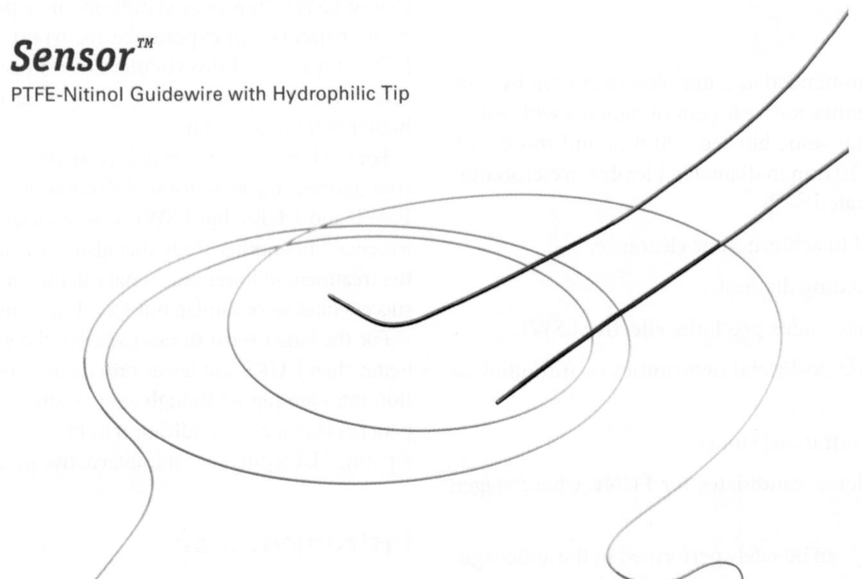

Fig. 2.10.1 A Sensor guidewire combining a Terumo-type tip with a more rigid 'shaft', so allowing ease of manipulation past stones while maintaining ease of handling.
Photographs provided courtesy of Boston Scientific, Copyright © Boston Scientific 2015. Do not copy or distribute. The content of this website is under the sole responsibility of its respective authors and does not represent the opinion of Boston Scientific (BSC). Access to this site does not imply any responsibility for BSC. Please refer to BSC product DFUs for indications, contraindications, precautions and warnings.

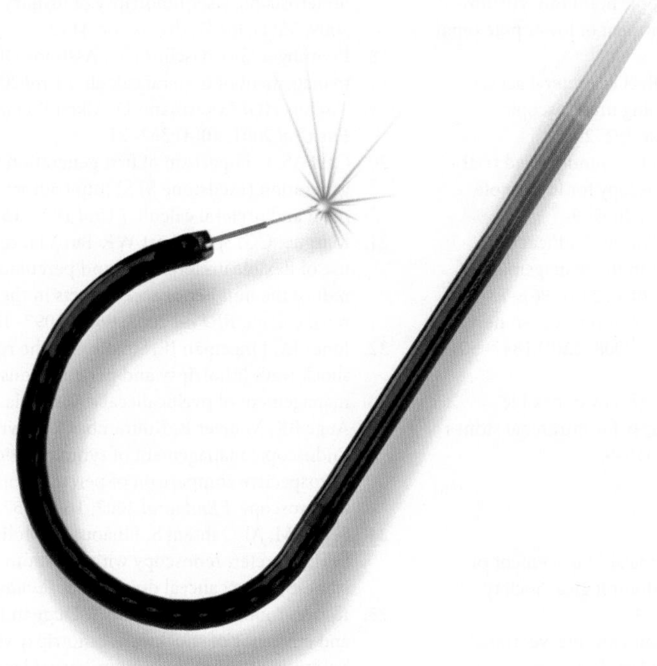

Fig. 2.10.2 200 micron fibres allow complete deflection of the ureterorenoscope.

Photographs provided courtesy of Boston Scientific, Copyright © Boston Scientific 2015. Do not copy or distribute. The content of this website is under the sole responsibility of its respective authors and does not represent the opinion of Boston Scientific (BSC). Access to this site does not imply any responsibility for BSC. Please refer to BSC product DFUs for indications, contraindications, precautions and warnings.

A stent is placed at the discretion of the surgeon. The routine use of double J ureteral stent is non-mandatory, as two meta-analyses have shown no difference in complication rates whether a stent is placed or not at the end of the procedure.[41–42]

Limitations

Inevitably, the reduction in size of ureterorenoscopes, so critical to allowing access to the renal collecting system, has led to a reduction in the size of the working channel to 3.6–4.0 Fr. This limits the instrumentation that can be passed down the channel, as well as restricting irrigant flow and hence visualization. The irrigant flow through a flexible ureterorenoscope with a 3.6 Fr working channel is only 32 mL/min with gravity irrigation—only 40% of the flow that can be achieved through a 13 Fr rigid ureteroscope.[43] With placement of a 3 Fr instrument through a 3.6 Fr working channel, gravity irrigant flow falls to only 2 mL/min. Reducing instrument size to approximately 1 Fr increases irrigant flow to 24 mL/min with gravity irrigation.[43] Raising the irrigant pressure by using a mechanical pump, hand irrigation system, or pressure bag applied to the bag of irrigant fluid significantly increases irrigant flow. However, forceful hand irrigation can raise intrarenal pressures to over 400 mm Hg, a pressure which can cause rupture of the intrarenal collecting system.[43,44]

Conclusions

Flexible ureterorenoscopy is an effective and safe method for the management of intrarenal stones. It has nearly equivalent stone-free rates when compared to percutaneous nephrolithotomy, with fewer complications. However, in the treatment of large stones, it may require multiple procedures. As technology continues to evolve with improved flexible ureterorenoscopes and better instrumentation for stone fragmentation and fragment removal, the indications for f-URS are likely to increase.

Further reading

Akman T, Binbay M, Ozgor F, *et al.* Comparison of percutaneous nephrolithotomy and retrograde flexible nephrolithotripsy for the management of 2-4 cm stones: a matched-pair analysis. *BJU Int* 2012; **109**(9):1384–9.

Breda A, Ogunyemi O, Leppert JT, Lam JS, Schulam PG. Flexible ureteroscopy and laser lithotripsy for single intrarenal stones 2 cm or greater—is this the new frontier? *J Urol* 2008; **179**(3):981–4.

Breda A, Ogunyemi O, Leppert JT, Schulam PG. Flexible ureteroscopy and laser lithotripsy for multiple unilateral intrarenal stones. *Eur Urol* 2009; **55**(5):1190–6.

Bryniarski P, Paradysz A, Zyczkowski M, Kupilas A, Nowakowski K, Bogacki R. A randomized controlled study to analyze the safety and efficacy of percutaneous nephrolithotripsy and retrograde intrarenal surgery in the management of renal stones more than 2 cm in diameter. *J Endourol* 2012; **26**(1):52–7.

Grasso M, Bagley D. Small diameter, actively deflectable, flexible ureteropyeloscopy. *J Urol* 1998; **160**(5):1648–53; discussion 1653–4.

Grasso M. Ureteropyeloscopic treatment of ureteral and intrarenal calculi. *Urol Clin North Am* 2000; **27**(4):623–31.

Knoll T, Jessen JP, Honeck P, Wendt-Nordahl G. Flexible ureterorenoscopy versus miniaturized PNL for solitary renal calculi of 10–30 mm size. *World J Urol* 2011; **29**(6):755–9.

Koo V, Young M, Thompson T, Duggan B. Cost-effectiveness and efficiency of shockwave lithotripsy vs flexible ureteroscopic holmium: yttrium-aluminium-garnet laser lithotripsy in the treatment of lower pole renal calculi. *BJU Int* 2011; **108**(11):1913–6.

L'Esperance JO, Ekeruo WO, Scales CD Jr, *et al.* Effect of ureteral access sheath on stone-free rates in patients undergoing ureteroscopic management of renal calculi. *Urology* 2005; **66**(2):252–5.

Pearle MS, Lingeman JE, Leveillee R, *et al.* Prospective, randomized trial comparing shock wave lithotripsy and ureteroscopy for lower pole caliceal calculi 1 cm or less. *J Urol* 2005; **173**(6):2005–9.

Sejiny M, Al-Qahtani S, Elhaous A, Molimard B, Traxer O. Efficacy of flexible ureterorenoscopy with holmium laser in the management of stone-bearing caliceal diverticula. *J Endourol* 2010; **24**(6):961–7.

Traxer O. Flexible ureterorenoscopic management of lower-pole stone: does the scope make the difference? *J Endourol* 2008; **22**(9):1847–50; discussion 1855.

Turna B, Stein RJ, Smaldone MC, *et al.* Safety and efficacy of flexible ureterorenoscopy and holmium: YAG lithotripsy for intrarenal stones in anticoagulated cases. *J Urol* 2008; **179**(4):1415–9.

References

1. Assimos D, Krambeck A, Miller NL, *et al.* Surgical Management of Stones: American Urological Association/Endourological Society Guideline, PART II. *J Urol* 2016; **196**(4):1161–9.
2. Türk C, Petřík A, Sarica K, *et al.* EAU Guidelines on Interventional Treatment for Urolithiasis. *Eur Urol* 2016; **69**(3):475–82.
3. Breda A, Ogunyemi O, Leppert JT, Schulam PG. Flexible ureteroscopy and laser lithotripsy for multiple unilateral intrarenal stones. *Eur Urol* 2009; **55**(5):1190–6.
4. Pearle MS, Lingeman JE, Leveillee R, *et al.* Prospective, randomized trial comparing shock wave lithotripsy and ureteroscopy for lower pole caliceal calculi 1 cm or less. *J Urol* 2005; **173**(6):2005–9.
5. Kijvikai K, Haleblian GE, Preminger GM, de la Rosette J. Shock wave lithotripsy or ureteroscopy for the management of proximal ureteral calculi: an old discussion revisited. *J Urol* 2007; **178**(4 Pt 1):1157–63.
6. Osman MM, Alfano Y, Kamp S, *et al.* 5-year-follow-up of patients with clinically insignificant residual fragments after extracorporeal shockwave lithotripsy. *Eur Urol* 2005; **47**(6):860–4.
7. Bagley DH, Huffman JL, Lyon ES. Combined rigid and flexible ureteropyeloscopy. *J Urol* 1983; **130**(2):243–4.
8. Preminger GM, Kennedy TJ. Ureteral stone extraction utilizing nondeflectable flexible fiberoptic ureteroscopes. *J Endourol* 1987; **1**:31–35.
9. Traxer O. Flexible ureterorenoscopic management of lower-pole stone: does the scope make the difference? *J Endourol* 2008; **22**(9):1847–50; discussion 1855.
10. Wendt-Nordahl G, Mut T, Krombach P, Michel MS, Knoll T. Do new generation flexible ureterorenoscopes offer a higher treatment success than their predecessors? *Urol Res* 2011; **39**(3):185–8.
11. Hosking DH, Bard RJ. Ureteroscopy with intravenous sedation for treatment of distal ureteral calculi: a safe and effective alternative to shock wave lithotripsy. *J Urol* 1996; **156**(3):899–901; discussion 902.
12. Breda A, Ogunyemi O, Leppert JT, Lam JS, Schulam PG. Flexible ureteroscopy and laser lithotripsy for single intrarenal stones 2 cm or greater—is this the new frontier? *J Urol* 2008; **179**(3):981–4.
13. Grasso M. Ureteropyeloscopic treatment of ureteral and intrarenal calculi. *Urol Clin North Am* 2000; **27**(4):623–31.
14. Grasso M, Bagley D. Small diameter, actively deflectable, flexible ureteropyeloscopy. *J Urol* 1998; **160**(5):1648–53; discussion 1653–4.
15. Wen CC, Nakada SY. Treatment selection and outcomes: renal calculi. *Urol Clin North Am* 2007; **34**:409–19.
16. Turna B, Stein RJ, Smaldone MC, *et al.* Safety and efficacy of flexible ureterorenoscopy and holmium:YAG lithotripsy for intrarenal stones in anticoagulated cases. *J Urol* 2008; **179**(4):1415–9.
17. Natalin R, Xavier K, Okeke Z, Gupta M. Impact of obesity on ureteroscopic laser lithotripsy of urinary tract calculi. *Int Braz J Urol* 2009; **35**(1):36–41; discussion 41–2.
18. Preminger GM, Tiselius HG, Assimos DG, *et al.* 2007 guideline for the management of ureteral calculi. *J Urol* 2007; **178**(6):2418–34.
19. Tiselius HG, Ackermann D, Alken P, *et al.* Guidelines on urolithiasis. *Eur Urol* 2001; **40**(4):362–71.
20. Cass AS. Comparison of first generation (Dornier HM3) and second generation (Medstone STS) lithotriptors: treatment results with 13,864 renal and ureteral calculi. *J Urol* 1995; **153**(3 Pt 1):588–92.
21. Marguet CG, Springhart WP, Tan YH, *et al.* Simultaneous combined use of flexible ureteroscopy and percutaneous nephrolithotomy to reduce the number of access tracts in the management of complex renal calculi. *BJU Int* 2005; **96**(7):1097–100.
22. Jones JA, Lingeman JE, Steidle CP. The roles of extracorporeal shock wave lithotripsy and percutaneous nephrostolithotomy in the management of pyelocaliceal diverticula. *J Urol* 1991; **146**(3):724–7.
23. Auge BK, Munver R, Kourambas J, Newman GE, Preminger GM. Endoscopic management of symptomatic caliceal diverticula: a retrospective comparison of percutaneous nephrolithotripsy and ureteroscopy. *J Endourol* 2002; **16**(8):557–63.
24. Sejiny M, Al-Qahtani S, Elhaous A, Molimard B, Traxer O. Efficacy of flexible ureterorenoscopy with holmium laser in the management of stone-bearing caliceal diverticula. *J Endourol* 2010; **24**(6):961–7.
25. Koo V, Young M, Thompson T, Duggan B. Cost-effectiveness and efficiency of shockwave lithotripsy vs flexible ureteroscopic holmium:yttrium-aluminium-garnet laser lithotripsy in the treatment of lower pole renal calculi. *BJU Int* 2011; **108**(11):1913–6.
26. Akman T, Binbay M, Ozgor F, *et al.* Comparison of percutaneous nephrolithotomy and retrograde flexible nephrolithotripsy for the management of 2–4 cm stones: a matched-pair analysis. *BJU Int* 2012; **109**(9):1384–9.
27. Knoll T, Jessen JP, Honeck P, Wendt-Nordahl G. Flexible ureterorenoscopy versus miniaturized PNL for solitary renal calculi of 10–30 mm size. *World J Urol* 2011; **29**(6):755–9.
28. Bryniarski P, Paradysz A, Zyczkowski M, Kupilas A, Nowakowski K, Bogacki R. A randomized controlled study to analyze the safety and efficacy of percutaneous nephrolithotripsy and retrograde intrarenal surgery in the management of renal stones more than 2 cm in diameter. *J Endourol* 2012; **26**(1):52–7.
29. Bagley DH. Removal of upper urinary tract calculi with flexible ureteropyeloscopy. *Urology* 1990; **35**(5):412–6.
30. Bagley DH. Active versus passive deflection in flexible ureteroscopy. *J Endourol* 1987; **1**:15–18.
31. Zilberman DE, Lipkin ME, Ferrandino MN, *et al.* The digital flexible ureteroscope: in vitro assessment of optical characteristics. *J Endourol* 2011; **25**(3):519–22.
32. Binbay M, Yuruk E, Akman T, *et al.* Is there a difference in outcomes between digital and fiberoptic flexible ureterorenoscopy procedures? *J Endourol* 2010; **24**(12):1929–34.
33. Paffen ML, Keizer JG, de Winter GV, Arends AJ, Hendrikx AJ. A comparison of the physical properties of four new generation flexible ureteroscopes: (de)flection, flow properties, torsion stiffness, and optical characteristics. *J Endourol* 2008; **22**(10):2227–34.
34. Kruck S, Anastasiadis AG, *et al.* Flow matters: irrigation flow differs in flexible ureteroscopes of the newest generation. *Urol Res* 2011; **39**(6):483–6.
35. Elashry OM, Elbahnasy AM, Rao GS, Nakada SY, Clayman RV. Flexible ureteroscopy: Washington University experience with the 9.3F and 7.5F flexible ureteroscopes. *J Urol* 1997; **157**(6):2074–80.
36. Kourambas J, Byrne RR, Preminger GM. Does a ureteral access sheath facilitate ureteroscopy? *J Urol* 2001; **165**(3):789–93.
37. L'Esperance JO, Ekeruo WO, Scales CD Jr, *et al.* Effect of ureteral access sheath on stone-free rates in patients undergoing ureteroscopic management of renal calculi. *Urology* 2005; **66**(2):252–5.
38. Lallas CD, Auge BK, Raj GV, Santa-Cruz R, Madden JF, Preminger GM. Laser Doppler flowmetric determination of ureteral

blood flow after ureteral access sheath placement. *J Endourol* 2002; **16**(8):583–90.
39. Vanlangendonck R, Landman J. Ureteral access strategies: pro-access sheath. *Urol Clin North Am* 2004; **31**(1):71–81.
40. Auge BK, Pietrow PK, Lallas CD, Raj GV, Santa-Cruz RW, Preminger GM. Ureteral access sheath provides protection against elevated renal pressures during routine flexible ureteroscopic stone manipulation. *J Endourol* 2004; **18**(1):33–6.
41. Makarov DV, Trock BJ, Allaf ME, Matlaga BR. The effect of ureteral stent placement on post-ureteroscopy complications: a meta-analysis. *Urology* 2008; **71**(5):796–800.
42. Nabi G, Cook J, N'Dow J, McClinton S. Outcomes of stenting after uncomplicated ureteroscopy: systematic review and meta-analysis. *BMJ* 2007; **334**(7593):572.
43. Wilson WT, Preminger GM. Intrarenal pressures generated during flexible deflectable ureterorenoscopy. *J Endourol* 1990; **4**:135–41.
44. Schwalb DM, Eshghi M, Davidian M, Franco I. Morphological and physiological changes in the urinary tract associated with ureteral dilation and ureteropyeloscopy: an experimental study. *J Urol* 1993; **149**(6):1576–85.

CHAPTER 2.11

Kidney stone treatment
Percutaneous nephrolithotomy

Andreas Neisius, Ghalib Jibara
Michael E. Lipkin, and Glenn M. Preminger

Introduction to kidney stone treatment

In 1941 Rupel and Brown published the first study in which an operatively established nephrostomy tract was used to extract an obstructing renal calculus.[1] Removal of a renal calculus via a percutaneous tract was performed successfully by Fernström in three patients 20 years later.[2] The first large cohort of percutaneous nephrolithotomy (PCNL) was reported by Alken in 1981 and subsequently it has become the preferred treatment method for large and/or complex renal and proximal ureteral calculi.[3]

Contemporary indications and contraindications

Shock wave lithotripsy (SWL) and more recently, retrograde intrarenal surgery (RIRS—or flexible ureterorenoscopy) have had a significant influence on the general indications for percutaneous stone management. These indications are currently well-defined and most are relative, rather than absolute. Several factors affect the choice of treatment for kidney stones including size, location, and stone composition. In their current guidelines, the European Association of Urology (EAU) recommends PCNL as first-line therapy for all renal calculi ≥20 mm and for lower pole stones ≥15 mm. For stones ≥10 and ≤15 mm in the lower pole, the EAU states that RIRS is a feasible option in high-volume centres.[4] In 2001, the lower pole I study group reported a prospective randomized trial comparing PCNL to SWL for lower pole stones and demonstrated that PCNL achieves stone-free rates of 95% in lower pole stones ≥10 mm compared to 21% utilizing SWL, with no difference in complications rates.[5] Lower caliceal stones have a lower stone clearance rate after SWL and stones size for treatment in this location is generally limited to 10 mm for SWL.[5,6] The role of RIRS for lower pole stones >10 mm remains unclear.

According to the American Urologic Association (AUA) guideline for the management of staghorn calculi, 'PNL should be the first-line treatment for most patients'.[7] The meta-analysis performed by the AUA guideline panel found higher stone-free rates for the treatment of staghorn stones when compared to SWL. Indications for PCNL other than staghorn stones include unusual body habitus precluding SWL (including gross obesity such that SWL is not feasible); urinary tract obstruction distal to the stone, cysteine, brushite, or calcium oxalate monohydrate stones; stones associated with upper tract foreign bodies; and large or otherwise complex stones. Currently, indications for PCNL rather than SWL include the presence a proximate calcified aortic or renal artery aneurysm. Clearly where SWL has failed, PCNL is a treatment option.

Currently, the only absolute contraindication to percutaneous stone extraction, SWL, or open stone surgery is an irreversible or uncorrected coagulopathy. RIRS is an alternative approach in these patients as the risk for bleeding is significantly less. Severe obesity is considered a contraindication for SWL due it causing decreased efficacy of SWL, as skin-to-stone distance increases and it being a relative contraindication for PCNL because of lower success rates; thus RIRS is favoured in severely obese patients.[4] With the advance of endourologic technology, RIRS is considered as a reasonable alternative to SWL and PCNL in patients with low stone volume, and even as first-line therapy in particular cases with intermediate stone burden in the lower calyx and/or co-morbidities.[8–12]

Preoperative preparation

Preoperative counselling includes the risks of requiring secondary intervention, transfusion of blood products, infection, or rarely, emergency open operative intervention. The risk of complications is clearly countered by the relatively short hospital stay and period of convalescence, especially compared to open operative intervention.[13–16] Formal cross-matching is generally not necessary, though a 'group and save' ('type and screen') should be done.

Urinary tract infection

According to the current EAU guidelines, all patients should undergo urinalysis and culture before PCNL. Urinary tract infections should be treated before stone removal. In cases of clinically significant infection and obstruction, drainage should be performed for several days, via a stent or percutaneous nephrostomy, before starting stone removal.[4] Bootsma *et al.* reported in a systematic review that there was low evidence for better outcomes utilizing prophylactic antibiotics in endoscopic procedures including PCNL. The amount of irrigation fluid used and the duration of the procedure are significant risk factors for postoperative fever.[17] Fever is correlated with bacterial urine load, severity of obstruction, the presence of bacteria in the calculi, and to stone size (≥20 mm).[18] In a recently published prospective study, Bag *et al.*

demonstrated significant better results for antibiotic prophylaxis with furadantin one week prior to PCNL in patients with stone size ≥25 mm and/or hydronephrosis.[19] Others recommend the routine collection of pelvic urine cultures and stone cultures instead of just bladder urine, because of better sensitivity and higher likelihood for predicting potential urosepsis.[20] Infection following PCNL is common, but only a very few cases progress to urosepsis. Positive preoperative urine, intraoperative urine, and infected stone cultures are predictive factors for the development of postoperative systematic inflammtory response syndrome.[21] Eighty per cent (80%) of the patients in this study who developed septic shock were positive for all cultures, and the other 20% at least for stone cultures.

In accordance with these findings, our patients with positive cultures are treated for approximately one week with culture sensitivity specific antibiotics on an outpatient basis. Patients receive preoperative intravenous antibiotics, which are continued for 24 hours. In general, patients are not discharged home with antibiotics unless they develop fever or signs of infection postoperatively. For patients with a negative preoperative urine culture, patients are given perioperative intravenous antibiotics for prophylaxis. In general, we use ampicillin and gentamicin for perioperative antibiotic prophylaxis.

Imaging

Preoperative imaging is essential to assess feasibility for PCNL and to allow treatment planning. Renal ultrasound, plain abdominal kidney, ureter, and bladder radiograph (KUB), intravenous urogram, and non-contrast computerized tomography (NCCT) are the most common studies performed prior to PCNL, determining stone size and location, grade of obstruction, and anatomic abnormalities.

For diagnosis and staging purposes, renal ultrasound is limited by its low sensitivity,[22] but it is the favoured to method to guide renal puncture for PCNL. Visualization is best in dilated collecting systems, which allows the difference between solid renal parenchyma and fluid in the collecting system to be distinguished. It also allows identification of the overlying bowel and is ideal for gaining access to transplanted kidneys, or after urinary diversions.

KUB X-ray is inexpensive and readily available but limited by low sensitivity (58–62%) and specificity (67–69%). Pure uric acid stones are usually not visualized on plain X-ray films unless they have some calcium component. As KUB provides little information of regarding intrarenal anatomy and surrounding structures, it is of limited value in planning percutaneous access.[23]

IVP (intravenous pyelography) identifies the anatomical relationship between the ribs and the kidney and the configuration of the calyces (including the angle of the infundibulum to the renal pelvis) and the localization and size of the stones in relation to the collecting system.[24–26] IVP is of particular value in cases of complex renal anatomy, such as calyceal diverticulum stones.

NCCT has a reported sensitivity and specificity approaching 100% and 97%, respectively, and as such represents the gold standard for diagnosing renal and ureteral calculi.[27–30] As NCCT is available at most centres and emergency departments, the majority of patients entering via emergency room have already undergone a NCCT before even seeing the urologist, which allows the exclusion of other abdominal pathology.[31] In planning for PCNL, NCCT

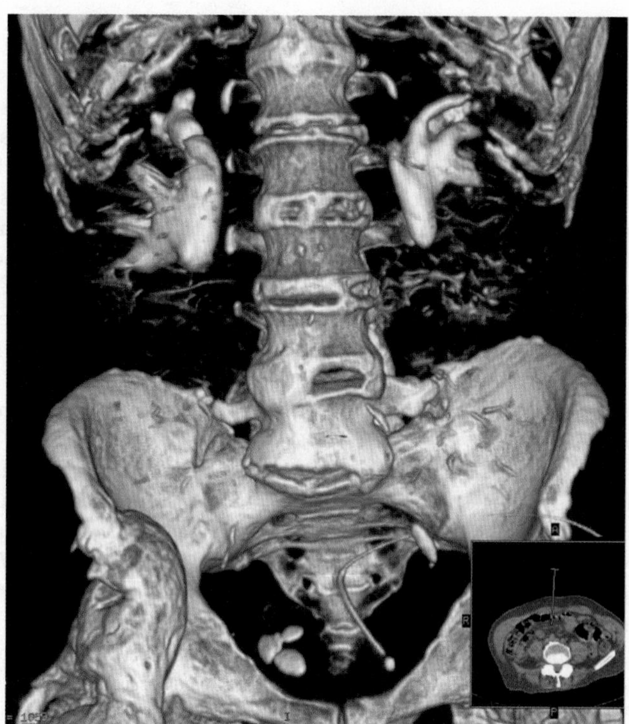

Fig. 2.11.1 A 3D reconstruction of a renal stone prior to percutaneous nephrolithotomy (PCNL).
Image reproduced courtesy of John Reynard.

provides detailed information about number, size, and location of stones, and about any anatomical abnormalities such as horseshoe kidneys or surrounding structures. Knowing the size and location of adjacent organs such as the lung, liver, colon, and spleen can help in gaining safe access to the kidney.[32–33] As adjacent organs around the kidney may move when shifting from supine to prone position and the majority of NCCT scans are routinely provided in supine position, some institutions repeat scans in the prone position. A portion of the colon can be retrorenal on the right side in 13.6% of men and 13.4% of women, and on the left side in 11.9% of men and 26.2% of women.[34] Others have shown that there is no significant change in the orientation of calyces between supine and prone positions, and have concluded that supine CT is adequate for PCNL planning.[35]

With increasing computer power and improved specific software, three-dimensional (3D) CT urography allows a 3D reconstruction of the kidneys and collecting system, and also of the vascular system (Fig. 2.11.1), which may be especially helpful in complex cases (e.g. complex staghorn calculi requiring multiple tracts or patients with severe scoliosis or spina bifida). Higher cost and radiation exposure are important limitations.[36–40]

Technique

The exact technique of percutaneous stone extraction used is specific to the size, location, configuration, presumed composition of the stone, body habitus, anatomical abnormalities and/or previous surgeries. However, the procedure is performed with the same sequential steps that include establishing percutaneous access, dilation of the tract, stone fragmentation, and stone extraction.

Access

Access to the collecting system can be provided by a radiologist or urologist with ultrasound, fluoroscopy, CT, or magnetic resonance guidance (still experimental). Ultrasound-guided access minimizes radiation dose and identifies surrounding organs such as the bowel.[41] This technique is particularly useful in pelvic dystopic kidneys, after renal transplantation, and in patients after urinary diversions.[42–47] Ultrasound imaging is operator dependent and is difficult in non-dilated collecting systems and obese patients.[22] Recent evidence suggests Doppler ultrasound guidance decreases haemorrhagic complications and transfusion rates during PCNL access, by avoiding renal blood vessels with stones >35 mm.[48,49] CT has been used in patients with a high risk of damage to adjacent organs.[50]

Fluoroscopy remains the gold standard technique for achieving access to the collecting system. It is used to puncture the collecting system, pass guidewires, dilators and instruments and to place double J stents (DJ) or nephrostomy tubes (NT) after the procedure. We routinely obtain percutaneous renal access at the time of surgery using fluoroscopy.

To establish access, with the patient in lithotomy, we use a cystoscope to pass a guidewire up the ureter followed (Fig. 2.11.2) by a 6 Fr open-ended ureteral catheter. A Foley catheter is placed into the bladder and the ureteral catheter is secured to the Foley. The patient is then placed in a prone or slightly oblique position with the ipsilateral side elevated to approximately 20 degrees. For patients with rotational anomalies such as horseshoe kidneys, the contralateral side is elevated to allow a more medial rotation of the otherwise anteriorly projected renal pelvis. This allows the posterior infundibula and calices to project more laterally, thus fluoroscopically simulating a more orthotopic position of the kidney. A retrograde air pyelogram is performed through the previously placed open-ended ureteral catheter with injection of approximately 5 mL of air. Air is used, due to it preferentially filling the posterior calyx that provides direct access to the stone, and the fact that air does not obscure the view of the stone[51] (contrast is a perfectly reasonable alternative and is preferred by many urologists and radiologists (Fig. 2.11.3).

An 18-gauge trocar needle is used to obtain access in the selected posterior calyx. This needle is advanced under fluoroscopic guidance during expiration (especially for supracostal punctures to avoid chest complications)[52] into the tip of the calyx to establish initial puncture and introducing a wire antegrade into the ureter.

Ideally for large stones, an upper pole access is utilized that will allow the surgeon to work without torqueing the nephroscope. Using a mid or upper pole access, the surgeon has also excellent access to the ureteropelvic junction and to the ureter if antegrade ureteroscopy needs to be performed. For isolated mid or lower pole stones, a mid or lower pole access is usually performed. Access tracts established over the eleventh rib have in increased risk of complications (e.g. hydro- or pneumothorax). The risk of a hydro- or pneumothorax after PCNL is as high as 12% for access above the twelfth rib and increases up to 35% with access above the eleventh rib.[53,54] In another study, Aron demonstrated that multiple tract access is safe and should be the first option for massive renal staghorn calculi. In 121 renal units in which an upper pole access was performed, hydrothorax occurred in only 2.4%, even with 76% of the accesses being supracostal.[55] For these cases, an intraoperative or immediately postoperative chest X-ray should be performed to identify this complication and solve the issue by placement of a thoracostomy tube while the patient is still under anaesthesia.

At this point, prior to percutaneous stone manipulation, a second wire should be placed as a safety wire utilizing a nine or ten

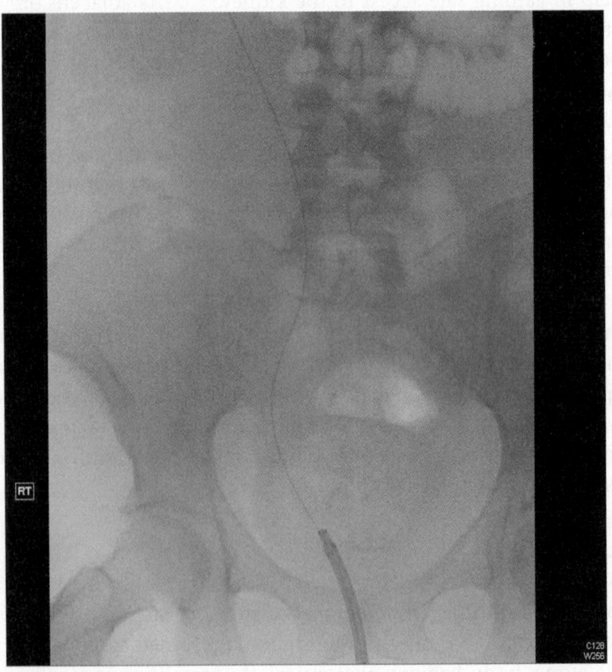

Fig. 2.11.2 Placement of a guidewire into the renal collecting system—the first step in PCNL access by a 6 Fr open-ended ureteral catheter.
Image reproduced courtesy of John Reynard.

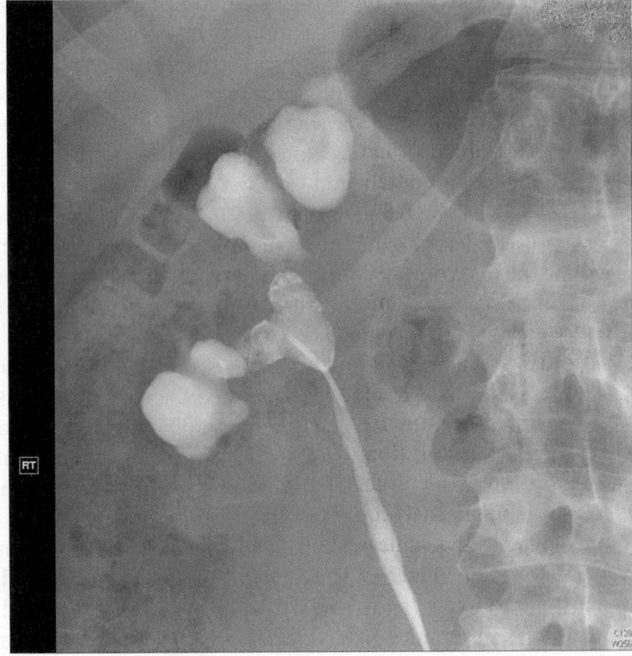

Fig. 2.11.3 Contrast fills the calyces to guide needle puncture.
Image reproduced courtesy of John Reynard.

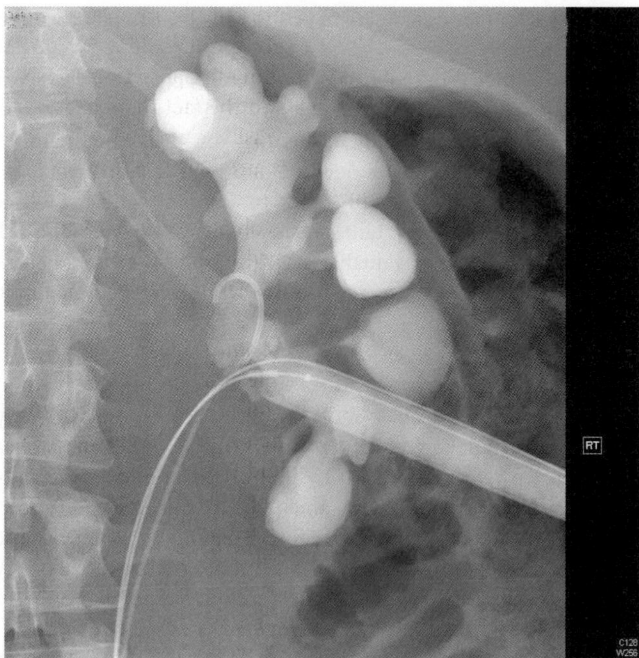

Fig. 2.11.4 The access sheath in place with guidewires prior to stone removal. Image reproduced courtesy of John Reynard.

French introducer set. Over the remaining 'working' wire, the tract is dilated to 30 Fr, utilizing either sequential fascial dilators (Alken or Amplatz) or what we preferably use, a 30 Fr, NephroMax™ high-pressure nephrostomy balloon catheter (Boston Scientific, Marlborough, MA, USA) with a burst pressure of 17 ATM over which is a back-loaded, 30 Fr working sheath. This sheath will stay in place with a safety wire alongside (Fig. 2.11.4). It has been demonstrated that balloon dilation results in less renal parenchymal damage and bleeding compared to metal Alken or Amplatz fascial dilators.[56,57] However, others who use the Alken dilators exclusively stated in contrary that no blood transfusion was required in a series of 315 patients.[58] In a recently published prospective database from the United Kingdom, Armitage showed that for 987 patients undergoing 1,028 PCNL, there was a non-significant trend to higher rates of blood transfusions in patients who had a balloon dilatation (3.2% versus 0.8%, $p = 0.093$).[59]

Stone extraction itself can be accomplished with a variety of techniques. At most centres, percutaneous stone extraction is accomplished utilizing ultrasonic lithotripsy guided by direct vision through a rigid nephroscope. This approach was first described by Alken and Marberger in Germany and Austria[3,60] and subsequently popularized in the United States by Segura[61] and Clayman.[62]

The nephroscope is inserted through the working sheath. Normal saline is used for irrigation.[63] Vision may be obscured by blood clots, which are easily evacuated by adjusting the irrigation and suction from the nephroscope sheath, or by using suction through the ultrasound wand while ultrasonic energy is applied to the clot.

Stones with a diameter <9–10 mm in size are small enough to extract intact through the working sheath. Such stones are simply grasped under direct vision utilizing rigid graspers or endoscopic forceps passed via the working port of the nephroscope. However, as most stones are too large to be extracted intact, intracorporeal lithotripsy is required, most frequently using ultrasonic lithotripsy.[64]

The ultrasound lithotrite with its own suction attachment is introduced via the working channel of a rigid nephroscope. Under direct vision, the tip of the lithotrite is impacted against the stone while suction is applied through the hollow lithotrite, holding the stone in place. This allows the stone pieces to be evacuated via the lithotrite as fragmentation proceeds. Fragments that are too large to pass through the lithotrite, but now measure less than 9 mm, are easily extracted using graspers or baskets via the nephroscope under direct vision. The process of ultrasonic fragmentation with suctioning of fragments or forceps extraction continues until all visible stone fragments have been removed.

For some physically very hard stones like large calcium oxalate monohydrate stones, which often appear extremely dense and homogenous on plain X-rays, and some mixed calcium oxalate/uric acid stones, ultrasonic lithotripsy might not be adequate. In these cases, intracorporeal lithotripsy can be performed effectively with several alternative modalities including electrohydraulic lithotripsy (EHL), which has proven safe and effective in this setting.[60,65] Two more of these alternative modalities, currently in use by many urologists, are pneumatic or combined pneumatic lithotrites, for example the Swiss Lithoclast® (Electro Medical Systems (EMS), Switzerland) and the Ltihoclast Ultra® (Boston Scientific Corporation, Marlborough, MA). The Swiss Lithoclast, the first pneumatic lithotrite, is powered by compressed air like a jackhammer. The Lithoclast Ultra consists of a combination of two handpieces; the pneumatic probe is inserted through the ultrasonic handpiece. Energy levels can also be modulated independently.[66–68] The technique of stone clearance is more or less equivalent to the ultrasound technique described above.

A newer dual probe ultrasound lithotrite (Cyberwand®, Olympus Corporation of the Americas Center Valley, PA, USA) failed to show significantly better stone fragmentation in a multicentre randomized controlled trial compared to the standard ultrasound device Olympus LUS-II (Olympus Corporation of the Americas, Center Valley, PA, USA).[69]

Contemporary alternatives to electrohydraulic, pneumatic, and ultrasonic lithotripsy (which are variations of electromechanical lithotripsy) include the holmium laser, which is widely used with all kinds of flexible instruments.[70]

For infundibular or caliceal calculi lying at acute angles to the percutaneous tract, visualization, fragmentation, and extraction often require flexible nephroscopy.[71,72] Although flexible nephroscopy can be successful when used during the initial percutaneous procedure, even a moderate amount of bleeding may obscure vision due to decreased irrigation through the flexible scope. In either case, a working sheath is again in place and the flexible nephroscope passed through this under direct vision. Fluoroscopic guidance is even more important during flexible rather than rigid procedures to assure proper orientation. When the stone is visualized, a grasping forceps, prongs, or basket can be passed through the working port of the flexible scope, and the stone engaged and withdrawn intact. Alternatively, larger stones can be fragmented with either the holmium laser or EHL, both of which allow intracorporeal lithotripsy via flexible instruments. Once stone fragmentation and removal is complete, the collecting system is completely examined with the flexible nephroscope. Fluoroscopy is also used to determine if there are residual fragments.

At this point, the decision to perform the surgery tubeless or to leave a nephrostomy tube is made. It is our practice to leave a nephrostomy tube in cases of collecting system injury, significant residual stone burden necessitating a second look procedure, significant bleeding, or altered urinary tract anatomy (i.e. patients with urinary diversions). In all other cases, a consideration is made to perform a tubeless procedure. In our institution, more than 85% of all PCNL are performed tubeless (with a temporary open-ended ureter catheter or DJ stent). In general, for patients undergoing tubeless PCNL, we leave the 6 Fr open-ended ureteral catheter in place overnight secured to a 16 Fr balloon catheter (a tubeless, stentless PNL). A DJ stent is left in place in cases where a large proximal ureteral stone is treated and in cases of access above the eleventh rib.

For patients who are left with just the 6 Fr ureteral catheter, at the conclusion of the procedure the safety wires and percutaneous access sheath are removed. Manual pressure is held over the percutaneous tract for five minutes. A 3–0 vicryl suture is used to reapproximate the subcutaneous tissue. A 4–0 monocryl suture is used to close the incision in a subcuticular fashion. The incision is dressed with gauze and tegaderm.

In patients where a DJ stent is left instead, one of the guidewires is back-loaded into the rigid nephroscope. The 6 Fr ureteral catheter is removed under vision. The DJ stent is then placed in an antegrade fashion over the wire through the nephroscope under vision and fluoroscopic confirmation that the proximal end of the stent is in the bladder. The wire is removed and fluoroscopy is again used to confirm an appropriate curl in the bladder. The proximal curl (in the kidney) is confirmed under vision. The remaining safety wire and the percutaneous access sheath are removed. Afterwards, beginning with manual pressure, the remainder of the session is carried out as as outlined above.

If we decide to leave a nephrostomy drain, our preference is to pass a 10 Fr loop nephrostomy tube. The tube is placed over a wire through the working sheath and the position is fluoroscopically confirmed. The remaining safety wire and access sheath is then removed. The nephrostomy tube is secured to the skin using a 2–0 silk drainage stitch.

Specific indications

Body habitus

Patients in whom an unusual body habitus or severe obesity precludes SWL, due to limitations of table capacity and/or focal length,[73] can also be challenging for PCNL. In these patients, both percutaneous access and tract dilation are more difficult, partly because fluoroscopic imaging and instrumentation is compromised. In the last decade, it has been shown that supine positioning is a good alternative approach for patients with severe obesity. Despite the advantages of not having to reposition these patients after placing the open-ended ureteral catheter, ventilation is also improved and operation time is shorter. In a recent Cochrane based meta-analyses, Liu *et al.* compared supine versus prone position and found no difference in terms of stone-free, transfusion, fever, and complication rates, but supine position was in favour for shorter operation times.[74]

Assmy performed a study in 1,121 PCNL patients and demonstrated no significant difference in complication rates, need for auxiliary procedures, and length of hospital stay between different body mass index (BMI) groups.[75] Overall, PCNL seems to be a safe procedure in obese patients, but the need for special instruments and modified patient positioning have to be taken into consideration.[75–77]

Patients with severe scoliosis or body contractures may prevent adequate positioning of the stone for SWL. In these patients, access with PCNL may be also difficult because of the altered anatomy. In some, the kidney may be located in a relatively anterior position, such that prevention of injury to adjacent solid or hollow viscera becomes an important consideration. We have found CT or ultrasound guidance valuable in preventing injury to adjacent organs in patients with severe scoliosis or other related anatomic abnormalities.

Hard stones

Brushite or calcium oxalate monohydrate stones are particularly hard and resistant to fragmentation with SWL. Cysteine stones are also often refractory to SWL due to their homogenous composition. These stones are very amenable to most forms of intracorporeal lithotripsy.[78] At our centre, percutaneous ultrasonic nephrolithotomy remains the preferred approach for the majority of cystinuric patients requiring intervention, though RIRS might be also taken into consideration.[4] For harder stones, such as calcium oxalate monohydrate, intracorporeal pneumatic lithotripsy or combined pneumatic/ultrasonic lithotripsy can potentially provide more rapid stone fragmentation than ultrasound alone.

Upper tract foreign bodies

Retained ureteral stents can present a technical challenge for removal. Often these stents are severely encrusted. If the proximal curl of a retained ureteral stent does not appear to be severely encrusted, an attempt at ureteroscopic management is justified. If ureteroscopic management has failed or if the proximal portion of the stent appears severely encrusted, a percutaneous approach is indicated.[79] Access, instrumentation, lithotrites, and removal of fragments are performed according to the standards described above.

Obstruction

Stone clearance after SWL requires spontaneous passage. As such, obstruction distal to the targeted stone is a contraindication to shock wave lithotripsy as first-line treatment. For most affected patients, distal obstruction will relate to the ureter or ureteropelvic junction (UPJ), though the same principle applies to stones in caliceal diverticula, or those in calices associated with true infundibular stenosis. In these patients, percutaneous management is ideal as it provides an opportunity to remove the stone and provide permanent relief of obstruction.

Stones in caliceal diverticula or in calices drained by long, narrow infundibula, or those in calices associated with true infundibular stenosis are best treated with a percutaneous approach or RIRS.[80–82] Ideally, the access should involve direct puncture of the diverticulum or of the obstructed calyx containing the stone. Working and safety wires can either be coiled within the diverticulum/calyx or occasionally, under fluoroscopic control, passed through the diverticular neck, into the main pyelocaliceal system, and down the ureter. Nephroscopic stone removal proceeds in a standard fashion. After stone removal, the diverticular neck is often better visualized. If a wire has not already been passed across the neck, it can often be done at this time, and the diverticular neck subsequently dilated or incised. When the neck appears wide enough, a nephrostomy tube is left across it into the main pyelocaliceal system for several days. In rare cases, dilute methylene blue may be injected in a retrograde fashion through the ureteral catheter to allow identification of the diverticular neck by nephroscopic visualization. An alternative to dilation of a diverticular neck, especially when it cannot be visualized directly or intubated fluoroscopically, is simple fulguration.[83] A nephrostomy tube is left in place in the diverticulum, but not across the neck. This acts to 'marsupialize' the diverticulum, which does not have secretory urothelium. In contrast to the management of caliceal diverticular necks, a stenotic infundibulum should always be dilated or laser incised, rather than fulgurated, as the calyx does contain secretory urothelium. The infundibulum can be dilated using either sequential fascial dilators, or preferably with a balloon catheter under direct vision, fluoroscopic control, or both. Following stone extraction and dilation of the infundibulum, a large calibre nephrostomy tube is left indwelling across the infundibulum into the renal pelvis.

The association of upper tract stones with UPJ obstruction provides an ideal setting for percutaneous management, as this allows simultaneous extraction of the stones and relief of obstruction.[84] Percutaneous management of the stones is performed in a standard manner with a more superolateral calyx or infundibulum that will allow optimal endoscopic access to the UPJ. To prevent extravasation of irrigant or stone particles during stone fragmentation and removal, stone extraction should precede the actual endopyelotomy incision. At the remainder of the procedure, a relatively large calibre stent is left indwelling for approximately four weeks. Currently, in most cases of intrarenal stones associated with a UPJ obstruction, consideration should be made for a robotic pyeloplasty with concurrent stone removal as the first-line therapy, as it has been shown to have better long-term outcomes than endopyelotomy. Open pyeloplasty and pyelolithotomy have reported success rates of 90% compared to antegrade endopyolotomy with concomitant percutaneuous stone removal with 64–85%.[84–87] In a multi-institutional review, overall long-term successful outcomes from robotic pyeloplasty, including patients with concurrent stone removal, have been demonstrated at 95.7%.[88]

Transplanted and pelvic kidneys

For stones in transplanted kidneys, several caveats pertain. In general, these are solitary kidneys, and retrograde access to the ureter may be impossible following the requisite ureteral reimplantation, which may also cause a relative narrow ureteral orifice aggravating stone clearance after SWL. Keeping this in mind, consideration should be given to percutaneous management for even moderate-sized stones. Percutaneous access to transplanted kidneys is generally straightforward, as the kidney lies at or near skin level, and preferably ultrasound or CT guidance may be used for initial puncture. Once the tract is established, the procedure proceeds as for native kidneys with standard tract dilation, stone manipulation, and internal or external drainage. In contrast to transplanted kidneys, congenital pelvic kidneys are deeper within the pelvis and peritoneal contents, including small and large intestines, may be interposed. In such cases, ultrasound or CT guidance is crucial.

Large or complex calculi

According to the AUA guideline for the management of staghorn calculi, 'PNL should be the first-line treatment for most patients'.[7] This is in conformity with the current European guidelines.[4] As referenced above, Aron demonstrated in a study with 397 tracts in 121 renal units the safety of multiple tract access and concluded that PCNL monotherapy should be considered first-line therapy for renal staghorn calculi. Percutaneous management can be used as a primary approach for 'debulking' prior to adjunctive SWL as part of a planned, combination 'sandwich' approach to increase stone-free rates up to 94%.[55,89] A second look can then be taken via the mature tract or tracts within 24 to 48 hours of the shock wave procedure to hasten clearance of stone fragments and allow early nephrostomy tube removal.[89]

Failed shock wave lithotripsy

Percutaneous management can be used as a 'salvage' procedure for patients who have undergone unsuccessful shock wave lithotripsy. Additionally, remaining ureteral fragments can be extracted in an antegrade or retrograde fashion ureteroscopically using flexible or semi-rigid instrumentation.

Postoperative care

The patients are kept in the hospital overnight in an observation unit. Vital signs are monitored closely, and serial blood counts are obtained as determined by the clinical course. For the first 24 hours postoperatively, intravenous fluids are administered and intravenous antibiotics are continued. For those patients with documented urinary infection associated with stone disease, culture-specific antibiotics are continued intravenously for at least 24 hours while the patient is in the hospital, and then orally for one week. A Foley catheter draining the bladder is left in place. For patients who were left with just a ureteral catheter, the Foley and ureteral catheters are removed the morning of the first postoperative day. Also, patients with a DJ stent typically have their Foley removed on postoperative day one. The stents are generally left in place for one to two weeks, depending on the indication for stent placement. For patients who were left with a NT for bleeding or collecting system injury, the tube is typically clamped on postoperative day two and then removed (if the patient tolerates it clamped). Alternatively, a nephrostogram can be performed prior to NT removal, especially if there is concern for urinary extravasation or obstruction. If there are no residual stones nor any obstruction or extravasation noted on the nephrostogram, the nephrostomy tube is removed. Ureteral obstruction found at this time usually results from blood clots or oedema, either of which should resolve spontaneously within 24–48 hours, or occasionally results from small stone fragments in the ureter, which will often pass spontaneously, or may be managed with antegrade or retrograde manipulation. The patient is then discharged home and allowed to return to full pre-hospitalization activity seven to ten days later. Patients are seen for a postoperative visit two weeks after surgery. The DJ stent is removed with a flexible cystoscope in the clinic one to two weeks after surgery. Imaging is typically obtained at a three-month visit, with either an intravenous pyelogram or non-contrast CT scan.

Complications of percutaneous stone removal

In cases of a significant perforation of the collection system, we recommend the placement of a NT at the end of the procedure. When the injury occurs at the UPJ, it is preferable to have a ureteral stent across the UPJ in addition to the nephrostomy tube. The nephrostomy tube can then be removed as soon as the extravasation is no longer evident and distal patency is assured on nephrostogram.

When there is increased risk for pleural injury (supra eleventh rib puncture), we recommend leaving a DJ stent and possibly a NT.

Bleeding is one of the most significant complications associated with percutaneous stone removal. Bleeding during access usually stops when the sheath is in place and effectively tamponades. The more recent use of balloon dilators may reduce the incidence of bleeding during this step. For cases in which there is significant intraoperative bleeding, the procedure should be suspended and a NT should be left in place. On rare occasions, if brisk bleeding is noted from the nephrostomy tract, 5 mL of FloSeal® gelatin matrix can be instilled followed by manual compression (Baxter, Berkshire, UK).[90]

Bleeding through the nephrostomy tube is often evident at the completion of even a relatively uncomplicated procedure. Successful management in almost all such cases can be achieved by temporarily plugging the nephrostomy tube and allowing the collecting system to tamponade. Several hours later, the NT can be unplugged again. If brisk bleeding occurs during removal of the nephrostomy tube, it should be immediately reinserted; however, when the tract has matured for even 24 hours, fluoroscopic control is generally not required. Delayed haemorrhage, that is, bleeding occurring several days following removal of the nephrostomy tube, is best managed conservatively with close monitoring of vital signs, bedrest, hydration, and transfusion as necessary.

Bleeding at any time that does not respond to conservative measures that include transfusion is best managed by renal angiography, and selective or even superselective arterial embolization. 'Open' operative exploration should be reserved only for failure of all other modalities due to the fact that surgery generally leads to partial, or more likely total, nephrectomy.[91]

Extrarenal organ injury

Injury to a hollow or solid organ other than the kidney (spleen, liver, or colon) have been reported from 0% to 0.4% in large series (>900 patients).[59,75,92] As mentioned above, even with the increasing use of upper pole and supracostal access, the rates for hydro, haemo- or pneumothorax stay surprisingly low, with rates of 16% for supracostal and 4.5% for subcostal access (irrespective of percutaneous approach: 8.3%). Access over the twelfth rib was associated with 10% rates, compared to 35% complication rates for access over the eleventh rib.[93] When possible, it is best to avoid access over the eleventh rib; however, if this access is mandatory, CT-guided or ultrasound-guided access can be considered.[50]

Management of thoracic adverse events depends on the patient's clinical picture. If the patient is completely stable with no ventilatory or respiratory compromise, observation alone may allow spontaneous resolution. A thoracic drain may be required for a few days, however.

If colonic injury occurs, in many cases conservative management may again be successful. A separation of the nephrocolonic communication is needed and consists of withdrawing the nephrostomy tube back to the colon to provide 'percutaneous colostomy' drainage. An internal stent should also be placed into the involved collecting system to separate the colonic and urinary pathways. Conservative management should include the use of intravenous antibiotics and total parenteral nutrition for about a week. If the lesion is extraperitoneal, conservative management is more likely to be successful. This can be determined with a nephrostogram or a CT scan. However, intraperitoneal injuries should be given careful consideration for immediate open operative repair instead of the delayed approach.[94]

Conclusions

Percutaneous nephrolithotomy is considered as first-line therapy for large (>2 cm, >1.5 cm for lower pole with unfavourable factors) and complex kidney stones. PCNL has been demonstrated to be safe and efficacious. On average, while stone-free rates of approximately 70% overall[59] can be achieved at experienced high-volume centres, this rate can approach 100%.[95–97] Furthermore, it has been documented that PCNL can be performed as a tubeless procedure in uneventful cases, in children, in obese patients, and even in patients with supracostal access with similar low complication rates, but significantly reducing the length of hospital stay.[98] In general, morbidity for PCNL is low, even in patients with comorbid medical conditions and complex stones. Clavien 2 complication rates (including blood transfusion and parenteral nutrition) appear in approximately 7%, Clavien 3 complication rates (requiring intervention) in 4.1%, Clavien 4 (life threatening) in 0.6%, and Clavien 5 rates (mortality) in 0.04%, as reported in a recently published comprehensive review including 115 studies.[99] It has been demonstrated that percutaneous nephrolithotomy has little, if any, clinically significant adverse effect on renal function, notwithstanding of pre-existing renal insufficiency or anatomically solitary kidneys.[100–103]

Acknowledgements

Supported by a Ferdinand Eisenberger grant of the Deutsche Gesellschaft für Urologie (German Society of Urology), grant ID NeA1/FE-11 (A. Neisius).

Further reading

Albala DM, Assimos DG, Clayman RV, *et al.* Lower pole I: a prospective randomized trial of extracorporeal shock wave lithotripsy and percutaneous nephrostolithotomy for lower polenephrolithiasis-initial results. *J Urol* 2001; **166**(6):2072–80.

Alken P, Hutschenreiter G, Gunther R, Marberger M. Percutaneous stone manipulation. *J Urol* 1981; **125**(4):463–6.

Armitage JN, Irving SO, Burgess NA. Percutaneous nephrolithotomy in the United Kingdom: Results of a prospective data registry. *Eur Urol* 2012; **61**(6):1188–93.

Chew BH, Arsovska O, Lange D, *et al.* The Canadian StoneBreaker trial: a randomized, multicenter trial comparing the LMA StoneBreaker and the Swiss LithoClast(R) during percutaneous nephrolithotripsy. *J Endourol* 2011; **25**(9):1415–9.

de la Rosette J, Assimos D, Desai M, *et al.* The Clinical Research Office of the Endourological Society Percutaneous Nephrolithotomy Global Study: indications, complications, and outcomes in 5803 patients. *J Endourol* 2011; **25**(1):11–7.

El-Assmy AM, Shokeir AA, El-Nahas AR, *et al.* Outcome of percutaneous nephrolithotomy: effect of body mass index. *Eur Urol* 2007; **52**(1):199–204.

Liu L, Zheng S, Xu Y, Wei Q. Systematic review and meta-analysis of percutaneous nephrolithotomy for patients in the supine versus prone position. *J Endourol* 2010; **24**(12):1941–6.

Mariappan P, Smith G, Moussa SA, Tolley DA. One week of ciprofloxacin before percutaneous nephrolithotomy significantly reduces upper tract infection and urosepsis: a prospective controlled study. *BJU Int* 2006; **98**(5):1075–9.

Preminger GM, Assimos DG, Lingeman JE, *et al.* Chapter 1: AUA guideline on management of staghorn calculi: diagnosis and treatment recommendations. *J Urol* 2005; **173**(6):1991–2000.

Seitz C, Desai M, Hacker A, *et al.* Incidence, prevention, and management of complications following percutaneous nephrolitholapaxy. *Eur Urol* 2012; **61**(1):146–58.

Tiselius HG, Ackermann D, Alken P, *et al.* Guidelines on urolithiasis. *Eur Urol* 2001; **40**(4):362–71.

Van Der Molen AJ, Cowan NC, Mueller-Lisse UG, Nolte-Ernsting CC, Takahashi S, Cohan RH. CT urography: definition, indications and techniques. A guideline for clinical practice. *Eur Radiol* 2008; **18**(1):4–17.

Yoon GH, Bellman GC. Tubeless percutaneous nephrolithotomy: a new standard in percutaneous renal surgery. *J Endourol* 2008; **22**(9):1865–7; discussion 9.

Zilberman DE, Lipkin ME, de la Rosette JJ, *et al.* Tubeless percutaneous nephrolithotomy—the new standard of care? *J Urol* 2010; **184**(4):1261–6.

References

1. Rupel E, Brown R. Nephroscopy with removal of stone following nephrostomy for obstructive calculous anuria. *J Urol* 1941; **46**(2):177–82.
2. Fernström I, Johansson B. Percutaneous pyelolithotomy. A new vextraction technique. *Scand J Urol Nephrol* 1976; **10**(3):257–9.
3. Alken P, Hutschenreiter G, Gunther R, Marberger M. Percutaneous stone manipulation. *J Urol* 1981; **125**(4):463–6.
4. Türk C, Petřík A, Sarica K, *et al.* EAU Guidelines on interventional treatment for urolithiasis. *Eur Urol* 2016; **69**(4):475–82.
5. Albala DM, Assimos DG, Clayman RV, *et al.* Lower pole I: a prospective randomized trial of extracorporeal shock wave lithotripsy and percutaneous nephrostolithotomy for lower pole nephrolithiasis-initial results. *J Urol* 2001; **166**(6):2072–80.
6. Tiselius HG, Ackermann D, Alken P, *et al.* Guidelines on urolithiasis. *Eur Urol* 2001; **40**(4):362–71.
7. Preminger GM, Assimos DG, Lingeman JE, *et al.* Chapter 1: AUA guideline on management of staghorn calculi: diagnosis and treatment recommendations. *J Urol* 2005; **173**(6):1991–2000.
8. Auge BK, Dahm P, Wu NZ, Preminger GM. Ureteroscopic management of lower-pole renal calculi: technique of calculus displacement. *J Endourol* 2001; **15**(8):835–8.
9. Chung SY, Chon CH, Ng CS, Fuchs GJ. Simultaneous bilateral retrograde intrarenal surgery for stone disease in patients with significant comorbidities. *J Endourol* 2006; **20**(10):761–5.
10. Holland R, Margel D, Livne PM, Lask DM, Lifshitz DA. Retrograde intrarenal surgery as second-line therapy yields a lower success rate. *J Endourol* 2006; **20**(8):556–9.
11. Kourambas J, Delvecchio FC, Munver R, Preminger GM. Nitinol stone retrieval-assisted ureteroscopic management of lower pole renal calculi. *Urology* 2000; **56**(6):935–9.
12. Preminger GM. Management of lower pole renal calculi: shock wave lithotripsy versus percutaneous nephrolithotomy versus flexible ureteroscopy. *Urol Res* 2006; **34**(2):108–11.
13. Brannen GE, Bush WH, Correa RJ, Gibbons RP, Elder JS. Kidney stone removal: percutaneous versus surgical lithotomy. *J Urol* 1985; **133**(1):6–12.
14. Brown MW, Carson CC 3rd, Dunnick NR, Weinerth JL. Comparison of the costs and morbidity of percutaneous and open flank procedures. *J Urol* 1986; **135**(6):1150–2.
15. Burns JR, Hamrick LC, Keller FS. Percutaneous nephrolithotomy in 86 patients: analysis of results and costs. *South Med J* 1986; **79**(8):975–8.
16. Preminger GM, Clayman RV, Hardeman SW, Franklin J, Curry T, Peters PC. Percutaneous nephrostolithotomy vs open surgery for renal calculi. A comparative study. *JAMA* 1985; **254**(8):1054–8.
17. Bootsma AM, Laguna Pes MP, Geerlings SE, Goossens A. Antibiotic prophylaxis in urologic procedures: a systematic review. *Eur Urol* 2008; **54**(6):1270–86.
18. Mariappan P, Smith G, Moussa SA, Tolley DA. One week of ciprofloxacin before percutaneous nephrolithotomy significantly reduces upper tract infection and urosepsis: a prospective controlled study. *BJU Int* 2006; **98**(5):1075–9.
19. Bag S, Kumar S, Taneja N, Sharma V, Mandal AK, Singh SK. One week of nitrofurantoin before percutaneous nephrolithotomy significantly reduces upper tract infection and urosepsis: a prospective controlled study. *Urology* 2011; **77**(1):45–9.
20. Mariappan P, Smith G, Bariol SV, Moussa SA, Tolley DA. Stone and pelvic urine culture and sensitivity are better than bladder urine as predictors of urosepsis following percutaneous nephrolithotomy: a prospective clinical study. *J Urol* 2005; **173**(5):1610–4.
21. Lojanapiwat B, Kitirattrakarn P. Role of preoperative and intraoperative factors in mediating infection complication following percutaneous nephrolithotomy. *Urol Int* 2011; **86**(4):448–52.
22. Park S, Pearle MS. Imaging for percutaneous renal access and management of renal calculi. *Urol Clin North Am* 2006; **33**(3):353–64.
23. Knudsen B. New trends in percutaneous nephrolithotomy. *AUA Update series* 2011; **30**: lesson 26.
24. Mutazindwa T, Husseini T. Imaging in acute renal colic: the intravenous urogram remains the gold standard. *Eur J Radiol* 1996;**23**(3):238–40.
25. Weiss A, Price R, Sage M, Barratt L. The intravenous pyelogram in renal colic. *Australas Radiol* 1988; **32**(4):429–33.
26. Yilmaz S, Sindel T, Arslan G, *et al.* Renal colic: comparison of spiral CT, US and IVU in the detection of ureteral calculi. *Eur Radiol* 1998; **8**(2):212–7.
27. Boulay I, Holtz P, Foley WD, White B, Begun FP. Ureteral calculi: diagnostic efficacy of helical CT and implications for treatment of patients. *AJR Am J Roentgenol* 1999; **172**(6):1485–90.
28. Chen MY, Zagoria RJ. Can noncontrast helical computed tomography replace intravenous urography for evaluation of patients with acute urinary tract colic? *J Emerg Med* 1999; **17**(2):299–303.
29. Pearle MS, Watamull LM, Mullican MA. Sensitivity of noncontrast helical computerized tomography and plain film radiography compared to flexible nephroscopy for detecting residual fragments after percutaneous nephrostolithotomy. *J Urol* 1999; **162**(1):23–6.
30. Pfister SA, Deckart A, Laschke S, *et al.* Unenhanced helical computed tomography vs intravenous urography in patients with acute flank pain: accuracy and economic impact in a randomized prospective trial. *Eur Radiol* 2003; **13**(11):2513–20.
31. Ulahannan D, Blakeley CJ, Jeyadevan N, Hashemi K. Benefits of CT urography in patients presenting to the emergency department with suspected ureteric colic. *Emerg Med J* 2008; **25**(9):569–71.
32. Nolte-Ernsting C, Cowan N. Understanding multislice CT urography techniques: Many roads lead to Rome. *Eur Radiol* 2006; **16**(12):2670–86.
33. Van Der Molen AJ, Cowan NC, Mueller-Lisse UG, Nolte-Ernsting CC, Takahashi S, Cohan RH. CT urography: definition, indications and techniques. A guideline for clinical practice. *Eur Radiol* 2008; **18**(1):4–17.
34. Chalasani V, Bissoon D, Bhuvanagir AK, Mizzi A, Dunn IB. Should PCNL patients have a CT in the prone position preoperatively? *Can J Urol* 2010; **17**(2):5082–6.
35. Sengupta S, Donnellan S, Vincent JM, Webb DR. CT analysis of caliceal anatomy in the supine and prone positions. *J Endourol* 2000; **14**(7):555–7.
36. Buchholz NP. Three-dimensional CT scan stone reconstruction for the planning of percutaneous surgery in a morbidly obese patient. *Urol Intern* 2000; **65**(1):46–8.
37. Hubert J, Blum A, Cormier L, Claudon M, Regent D, Mangin P. Three-dimensional CT-scan reconstruction of renal calculi. A new tool for mapping-out staghorn calculi and follow-up of radiolucent stones. *Eur Urol* 1997; **31**(3):297–301.
38. Liberman SN, Halpern EJ, Sullivan K, Bagley DH. Spiral computed tomography for staghorn calculi. *Urology* 1997; **50**(4):519–24.
39. O'Connor OJ, Maher MM. CT urography. *AJR Am J Roentgenol* 2010; **195**(5):W320–4.

40. Silverman SG, Leyendecker JR, Amis ES Jr. What is the current role of CT urography and MR urography in the evaluation of the urinary tract? *Radiology* 2009; **250**(2):309–23.
41. Basiri A, Ziaee AM, Kianian HR, Mehrabi S, Karami H, Moghaddam SM. Ultrasonographic versus fluoroscopic access for percutaneous nephrolithotomy: a randomized clinical trial. *J Endourol* 2008; **22**(2):281–4.
42. Evans HJ, Wollin TA. The management of urinary calculi in pregnancy. *Curr Opin Urol* 2001; **11**(4):379–84.
43. Fabrizio MD, Gray DS, Feld RI, Bagley DH. Placement of ureteral stents in pregnancy using ultrasound guidance. *Tech Urol* 1996; **2**(3):121–5.
44. Francesca F, Felipetto R, Mosca F, Boggi U, Rizzo G, Puccini R. Percutaneous nephrolithotomy of transplanted kidney. *J Endourol* 2002; **16**(4):225–7.
45. Kavoussi LR, Albala DM, Basler JW, Apte S, Clayman RV. Percutaneous management of urolithiasis during pregnancy. *J Urol* 1992; **148**(3 Pt 2):1069–71.
46. Lu HF, Shekarriz B, Stoller ML. Donor-gifted allograft urolithiasis: early percutaneous management. *Urology* 2002; **59**(1):25–7.
47. McAleer SJ, Loughlin KR. Nephrolithiasis and pregnancy. *Curr Opin Urol* 2004; **14**(2):123–7.
48. Lu MH, Pu XY, Gao X, Zhou XF, Qiu JG, Si-Tu J. A comparative study of clinical value of single B-mode ultrasound guidance and B-mode combined with color doppler ultrasound guidance in mini-invasive percutaneous nephrolithotomy to decrease hemorrhagic complications. *Urology* 2010; **76**(4):815–20.
49. Tzeng BC, Wang CJ, Huang SW, Chang CH. Doppler ultrasound-guided percutaneous nephrolithotomy: a prospective randomized study. *Urology* 2011; **78**(3):535–9.
50. Matlaga BR, Shah OD, Zagoria RJ, Dyer RB, Streem SB, Assimos DG. Computerized tomography guided access for percutaneous nephrostolithotomy. *J Urol* 2003; **170**(1):45–7.
51. Lipkin ME, Mancini JG, Zilberman DE, *et al.* Reduced radiation exposure with the use of an air retrograde pyelogram during fluoroscopic access for percutaneous nephrolithotomy. *J Endourol* 2011; **25**(4):563–7.
52. Netto NR Jr, Ikonomidis J, Ikari O, Claro JA. Comparative study of percutaneous access for staghorn calculi. *Urology* 2005; **65**(4):659–62; discussion 62–3.
53. Aron M, Goel R, Kesarwani PK, Seth A, Gupta NP. Upper pole access for complex lower pole renal calculi. *BJU Int* 2004; **94**(6):849–52; discussion 52.
54. Stening SG, Bourne S. Supracostal percutaneous nephrolithotomy for upper pole caliceal calculi. *J Endourol* 1998; **12**(4):359–62.
55. Aron M, Yadav R, Goel R, *et al.* Multi-tract percutaneous nephrolithotomy for large complete staghorn calculi. *Urol Intern* 2005; **75**(4):327–32.
56. Davidoff R, Bellman GC. Influence of technique of percutaneous tract creation on incidence of renal hemorrhage. *J Urol* 1997; **157**(4):1229–31.
57. Traxer O, Smith TG 3rd, Pearle MS, Corwin TS, Saboorian H, Cadeddu JA. Renal parenchymal injury after standard and mini percutaneous nephrostolithotomy. *J Urol* 2001; **165**(5):1693–5.
58. Osman M, Wendt-Nordahl G, Heger K, Michel MS, Alken P, Knoll T. Percutaneous nephrolithotomy with ultrasonography-guided renal access: experience from over 300 cases. *BJU Int* 2005; **96**(6):875–8.
59. Armitage JN, Irving SO, Burgess NA. Percutaneous nephrolithotomy in the United Kingdom: Results of a prospective data registry. *Eur Urol* 2012; **61**(6):1188–93.
60. Marberger M, Stackl W, Hruby W. Percutaneous litholapaxy of renal calculi with ultrasound. *Eur Urol* 1982; **8**(4):236–42.
61. Segura JW, Patterson DE, LeRoy AJ, McGough PF, Barrett DM. Percutaneous removal of kidney stones. Preliminary report. *Mayo Clin Proc* 1982; **57**(10):615–9.
62. Clayman RV, Surya V, Miller RP, *et al.* Percutaneous nephrolithotomy: extraction of renal and ureteral calculi from 100 patients. *J Urol* 1984; **131**(5):868–71.
63. Schultz REH, Wein AJ. Percutaneous ultrasonic lithotripsy: Choice of irrigant. *J Urol* 1953; **130**:853.
64. Clayman RV. Techniques in percutaneous removal of renal calculi. Mechanical extraction and electrohydraulic lithotripsy. *Urology* 1984; **23**(5 Spec No):11–9.
65. Raney AM, Handler J. Electrohydraulic nephrolithotripsy. *Urology* 1975; **6**(4):439–42.
66. Chew BH, Arsovska O, Lange D, *et al.* The Canadian StoneBreaker trial: a randomized, multicenter trial comparing the LMA StoneBreaker and the Swiss LithoClast(R) during percutaneous nephrolithotripsy. *J Endourol* 2011; **25**(9):1415–9.
67. Kuo RL, Paterson RF, Siqueira TM Jr, *et al.* In vitro assessment of lithoclast ultra intracorporeal lithotripter. *J Endourol* 2004; **18**(2):153–6.
68. Denstedt JD, Razvi HA, Rowe E, Grignon DJ, Eberwein PM. Investigation of the tissue effects of a new device for intracorporeal lithotripsy--the Swiss Lithoclast. *J Urol* 1995; **153**(2):535–7.
69. Krambeck AE, Miller NL, Humphreys MR, *et al.* Randomized controlled, multicentre clinical trial comparing a dual-probe ultrasonic lithotrite with a single-probe lithotrite for percutaneous nephrolithotomy. *BJU Int* 2011; **107**(5):824–8.
70. Teichman JM, Rao RD, Glickman RD, Harris JM. Holmium:YAG percutaneous nephrolithotomy: the laser incident angle matters. *J Urol* 1998; **159**(3):690–4.
71. Lange PH, Reddy PK, Hulbert JC, *et al.* Percutaneous removal of caliceal and other "inaccessible" stones: instruments and techniques. *J Urol* 1984; **132**(3):439–42.
72. Reddy PK, Lange PH, Hulbert JC, *et al.* Percutaneous removal of caliceal and other "inaccessible" stones: results. *J Urol* 1984; **132**(3):443–7.
73. Thomas R, Cass AS. Extracorporeal shock wave lithotripsy in morbidly obese patients. *J Urol* 1993; **150**(1):30–2.
74. Liu L, Zheng S, Xu Y, Wei Q. Systematic review and meta-analysis of percutaneous nephrolithotomy for patients in the supine versus prone position. *J Endourol* 2010; **24**(12):1941–6.
75. El-Assmy AM, Shokeir AA, El-Nahas AR, *et al.* Outcome of percutaneous nephrolithotomy: effect of body mass index. *Eur Urol* 2007; **52**(1):199–204.
76. De Sio M, Autorino R, Quarto G, *et al.* Modified supine versus prone position in percutaneous nephrolithotomy for renal stones treatable with a single percutaneous access: a prospective randomized trial. *Eur Urol* 2008; **54**(1):196–202.
77. El-Assmy AM, Shokeir AA, Mohsen T, *et al.* Renal access by urologist or radiologist for percutaneous nephrolithotomy--is it still an issue? *J Urol* 2007; **178**(3 Pt 1):916–20; discussion 20.
78. Chow GK, Streem SB. Contemporary urological intervention for cystinuric patients: immediate and long-term impact and implications. *J Urol* 1998; **160**(2):341–4; discussion 4–5.
79. Troy RB, Streem SB, Zelch MG. Percutaneous management of upper tract foreign bodies. *J Endourol* 1994; **8**(1):43–7.
80. Bellman GC, Silverstein JI, Blickensderfer S, Smith AD. Technique and follow-up of percutaneous management of caliceal diverticula. *Urology* 1993; **42**(1):21–5.
81. Hulbert JC, Reddy PK, Hunter DW, Castaneda-Zuniga W, Amplatz K, Lange PH. Percutaneous techniques for the management of caliceal diverticula containing calculi. *J Urol* 1986; **135**(2):225–7.
82. Shalhav AL, Soble JJ, Nakada SY, Wolf JS Jr, McClennan BL, Clayman RV. Long-term outcome of caliceal diverticula following percutaneous endosurgical management. *J Urol* 1998; **160**(5):1635–9.
83. Monga M, Smith R, Ferral H, Thomas R. Percutaneous ablation of caliceal diverticulum: long-term followup. *J Urol* 2000; **163**(1):28–32.

84. Motola JA, Badlani GH, Smith AD. Results of 212 consecutive endopyelotomies: an 8-year followup. *J Urol* 1993; **149**(3):453–6.
85. Atug F, Castle EP, Burgess SV, Thomas R. Concomitant management of renal calculi and pelvi-ureteric junction obstruction with robotic laparoscopic surgery. *BJU Int* 2005; **96**(9):1365–8.
86. Cassis AN, Brannen GE, Bush WH, Correa RJ, Chambers M. Endopyelotomy: review of results and complications. *J Urol* 1991; **146**(6):1492–5.
87. Meretyk I, Meretyk S, Clayman RV. Endopyelotomy: comparison of ureteroscopic retrograde and antegrade percutaneous techniques. *J Urol* 1992; **148**(3):775–82; discussion 82–3.
88. Mufarrij PW, Woods M, Shah OD, *et al.* Robotic dismembered pyeloplasty: a 6-year, multi-institutional experience. *J Urol* 2008; **180**(4):1391–6.
89. Streem SB, Yost A, Dolmatch B. Combination "sandwich" therapy for extensive renal calculi in 100 consecutive patients: immediate, long-term and stratified results from a 10-year experience. J Urol 1997; **158**(2):342–5.
90. Yoon GH, Bellman GC. Tubeless percutaneous nephrolithotomy: a new standard in percutaneous renal surgery. *J Endourol* 2008; **22**(9):1865–7; discussion 9.
91. Kessaris DN, Bellman GC, Pardalidis NP, Smith AG. Management of hemorrhage after percutaneous renal surgery. *J Urol* 1995; **153**(3 Pt 1):604–8.
92. de la Rosette J, Assimos D, Desai M, *et al.* The Clinical Research Office of the Endourological Society Percutaneous Nephrolithotomy Global Study: indications, complications, and outcomes in 5803 patients. *J Endourol* 2011; **25**(1):11–7.
93. Munver R, Delvecchio FC, Newman GE, Preminger GM. Critical analysis of supracostal access for percutaneous renal surgery. *J Urol* 2001; **166**(4):1242–6.
94. El-Nahas AR, Shokeir AA, El-Assmy AM, *et al.* Colonic perforation during percutaneous nephrolithotomy: study of risk factors. *Urology* 2006; **67**(5):937–41.
95. Bass RB Jr, Beard JH, Cooner WH, Mosley BR, Pond HS, Rutherford CL Jr. Percutaneous ultrasonic lithotripsy in the community hospital. *J Urol* 1985; **133**(4):586–7.
96. Reddy PK, Hulbert JC, Lange PH, *et al.* Percutaneous removal of renal and ureteral calculi: experience with 400 cases. *J Urol* 1985; **134**(4):662–5.
97. Segura JW, Patterson DE, LeRoy AJ, *et al.* Percutaneous removal of kidney stones: review of 1,000 cases. *J Urol* 1985; **134**(6):1077–81.
98. Zilberman DE, Lipkin ME, de la Rosette JJ, *et al.* Tubeless percutaneous nephrolithotomy--the new standard of care? *J Urol* 2010; **184**(4):1261–6.
99. Seitz C, Desai M, Hacker A, *et al.* Incidence, prevention, and management of complications following percutaneous nephrolitholapaxy. *Eur Urol* 2012; **61**(1):146–58.
100. Chandhoke PS, Albala DM, Clayman RV. Long-term comparison of renal function in patients with solitary kidneys and/or moderate renal insufficiency undergoing extracorporeal shock wave lithotripsy or percutaneous nephrolithotomy. *J Urol* 1992; **147**(5):1226–30.
101. Marberger M, Stackl W, Hruby W, Kroiss A. Late sequelae of ultrasonic lithotripsy of renal calculi. *J Urol* 1985; **133**(2):170–3.
102. Schiff RG, Lee WJ, Eshghi M, Moskowitz GW, Levy LM, Smith AD. Morphologic and functional changes in the kidney after percutaneous nephrosto-lithotomy. *AJR Am J Roentgenol* 1986; **147**(2):283–6.
103. Streem SB, Zelch MG, Risius B, Geisinger MA. Percutaneous extraction of renal calculi in patients with solitary kidneys. *Urology* 1986; **27**(3):247–52.

CHAPTER 2.12

Open stone surgery for kidney stones

Gastón M. Astroza, Ghalib Jibara, Michael E. Lipkin, and Glenn M. Preminger

Introduction to open stone surgery for kidney stones

The development of shock wave lithotripsy and minimally invasive therapies (percutaneous nephrolithotomy (PCNL) and ureteroscopy (URS)) have narrowed the indications for open surgery for renal and ureteric calculi.[1–3]

The outcomes associated with other techniques (stone-free rate for staghorn stones with PCNL 78% vs. 71% with open procedures), similar rates of overall significant complications, and lower transfusion rates demonstrate the advantages of shock wave lithroscopy and other endoscopic approaches.[4]

Current indications for open surgery (or alternatively a laparoscopic approach[5–11]) include an associated anatomic abnormality, which would best be managed with open operative intervention at the time of stone removal; a failure of or a contraindication to shock wave lithotripsy, retrograde intrarenal surgery and percutaneous management; or, in the urologist's judgement, a stone so large and complex that a single open operative procedure would more likely render the patient stone-free, with less risk than the option of a complicated percutaneous procedure with or without adjunctive shock wave lithotripsy.

The type of open procedure is determined by stone size, configuration, and pyelocaliceal location.

Pyelolithotomy

Czerny was the first to perform removal of a stone via an incision in the renal pelvis in 1880.[12] In 1913, Lower popularized a vertical pyelolithotomy, which remained the preferred approach for uncomplicated renal pelvic calculi for many years.[13] In 1965, Gil-Vernet advocated a transverse rather than a vertical pyelolithotomy based on his studies of the functional anatomy of the renal pelvic musculature.[14]

Open pyelolithotomy was supplanted almost 20 years ago by the advent of percutaneous and shock wave technology. Currently, the only indications for this procedure are a failure of or contraindication to other techniques, or the presence of an associated abnormality such as pelviureteric junction obstruction (PUJO), the open approach allowing simultaneous pyeloplasty. However, the advent of percutaneous and laparoscopic approaches to correction of PUJO, as well as stone removal has no doubt contributed to the continuing decline in indications for open pyelolithotomy.[5–7] Furthermore, in patients with solitary large renal pelvic stones without an associated abnormality, a laparoscopic approach is a feasible technique associated with a high stone-free rate and a low number of complications.[8–11]

Operative approach to standard open pyelolithotomy

Currently the indications for a standard pyelolithotomy, within the context of the limited indications for open operative intervention, include stones limited to the renal pelvis with minimal or no branching. The procedure is performed through a standard flank incision or through a dorsal lumbotomy. The retroperitoneum is entered and Gerota's fascia opened posteriorly at the lower pole of the kidney. The proximal ureter is identified and surrounded with a vessel loop; this aids dissection and prevents distal stone migration during the procedure. The dissection is then carried proximally along the posterior aspect of the ureter towards the renal pelvis. Once the pelvis is exposed posteriorly, stay sutures are placed in preparation for a transverse pyelotomy. This incision is made well away from the pelviureteric junction and carried as far laterally on the pelvis as is necessary to extract the stone under direct vision. After the stone is removed and the vessel loop is relaxed, a catheter is passed antegrade down the ureter to ensure ureteral patency. The pyelotomy is then closed in a single layer using a running or interrupted a 4–0 absorbable suture, placed full thickness through the renal pelvic wall. An internal ureteral stent and external drainage are recommended.

Extended pyelolithotomy

Extended pyelolithotomy, as advocated by Gil-Vernet in 1965[14] takes advantage of dissection into the renal sinus to gain access to the intrarenal collecting system. In general, its use had been limited to management of relatively large renal pelvic stones with or without extension into one or more infundibula, but without dumbbell-shaped caliceal extensions or associated infundibular stenosis.

The posterior aspect of the renal pelvis is exposed in the same way as that for a standard pyelolithotomy. Dissection is then carried into the renal sinus by incising the fibrous tissue between the posterior hilar lip of renal parenchyma and the renal pelvis itself, and the plane between the renal pelvis and peripelvic fat is entered. Further exposure of the intrarenal collecting system can then be accomplished using vein retractors, or specifically designed Gil-Vernet renal sinus retractors, to elevate the posterior parenchymal lip. Dissection into the sinus then continues using a moist gauze or Kittner sponge. As described by Wulfsohn, temporary occlusion of the renal artery with local hypothermia can serve to soften the renal parenchyma and allow further exposure of the intrarenal collecting system.[15,16] A curvilinear transverse pyelotomy is performed between stay sutures, taking care to avoid the pelviureteric junction. The pyelotomy is then extended along both the upper and lower infundibula, thus creating a renal pelvic flap, which affords access to even large calculi with early branch formation. Any infundibular extensions that remain after extraction of the renal pelvic stone can be removed using Randall's forceps.

For more extensive stones, this approach can be combined with a simple or lower pole nephrotomy, which is best reserved for patients with associated cortical loss and local cortical thinning.

Lower pole infundibulocaliceal extensions of pelvic calculi can be managed by extending the inferior aspect of the pyelotomy incision onto the posterior renal parenchyma itself as a pyeloinfundibulotomy, directly over the involved lower infundibulum.

Upon removal of all visible and palpable stone material, a catheter is passed antegrade down the ureter and the intrarenal collecting system is thoroughly irrigated. If multiple stones have been present, intraoperative images should be taken to exclude residual calculi. The pyelotomy incision is closed as for a standard pyelolithotomy, and an internal stent placed in selected cases.

Caliceal diverticulolithotomy

Caliceal diverticula are transitional epithelium-lined cavities in the renal parenchyma, which communicate with a calix or infundibulum—although that communication may not be demonstrable. Because some caliceal diverticula are associated with localized urinary stasis, they may be a source of stone formation.[17] The indications for intervention for caliceal diverticular stones are the same as for any upper tract stones (recurrent urinary tract infections; pain thought to be caused by the stone). In highly select patients, shock wave lithotripsy can be successful,[18] but ureteroscopic and percutaneous techniques are considered more definitive.[19,20] When these techniques are contraindicated or have failed, open surgery may be considered.

Generally, the diverticulum is readily apparent by inspection, though intraoperative localization may be required with intraoperative fluoroscopy or ultrasound. Localization can be confirmed by aspiration of urine from the diverticulum or by 'sounding' the calculus using a small gauge needle.

When the diverticulum is associated with thinning of the overlying parenchyma, an appropriate management method is marsupialization. If the diverticulum is located deep within the renal parenchyma, the diverticulum can be identified with the aid of intraoperative ultrasound. In such cases, a local wedge resection is more appropriate.

While open caliceal diverticulolithotomy and diverticulectomy should be a part of the urologic armamentarium, many patients with a contraindication to or failure of less invasive techniques can be managed with a laparoscopic approach.[21]

Anatrophic nephrolithotomy

Open operative intervention for staghorn calculi was recommended by the American Urological Association Staghorn Calculi Clinical Guidelines Panel[4] in cases where the stone was so extensive that an unreasonable number of percutaneous (with or without extracorporeal shock wave lithotripsy (ESWL)) would be required to achieve stone-free status. In practice, such cases represent complete, fully branched staghorn calculus with multiple dumbbell-shaped infundibulocaliceal extensions. Multiple areas of true infundibular stenosis would also be a relative indication for open operative intervention, since a narrow infundibulum restricts access to the renal pelvis.

In such cases, the most appropriate open operative approach is generally anatrophic nephrolithotomy, as initially described by Boyce and Smith in 1967.[22] The stones are removed through an incision that is least traumatic to overall renal function (i.e. an incision through a relatively avascular plane in the kidney). The renal artery is temporarily occluded during the procedure to provide a bloodless field, and the kidney must therefore be protected from ischaemia by cooling.

Our preference is a flank approach with resection of the eleventh or twelfth rib, with medial extension of the incision to the lateral border of the rectus muscle and reflection of the peritoneum medially. The kidney is completely mobilized and the renal pedicle isolated (Fig. 2.12.1). The renal artery is surrounded with a vessel loop and 12.5 mg of mannitol is given intravenously for renal protection. Further dissection of the renal artery is accomplished until the anterior and posterior divisional branches are identified.

As described by Brodel in 1901[23] and subsequently by Graves in 1954,[24] an avascular plane exists between the junction of the blood supply to the anterior and posterior segments of the kidney. At the surface of the kidney, this generally lies on the posterior aspect approximately two-thirds of the way from the renal hilum to the true lateral border of the kidney (Fig. 2.12.2). When desired,

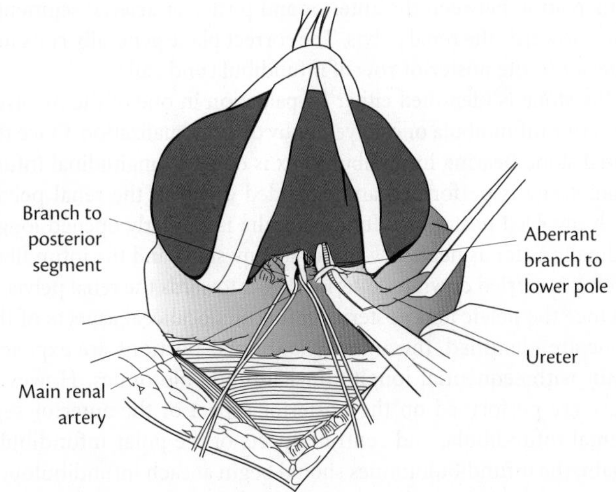

Fig. 2.12.1 Diagram of an anatrophic nephrolithotomy showing slings positioned around the renal vessels.

Reproduced from Jon Reynard et al., *Oxford Handbook of Urological Surgery*, Figure 6.2.7, p. 439, Oxford University Press, Oxford, UK, Copyright © 2008, with permission from Oxford University Press.

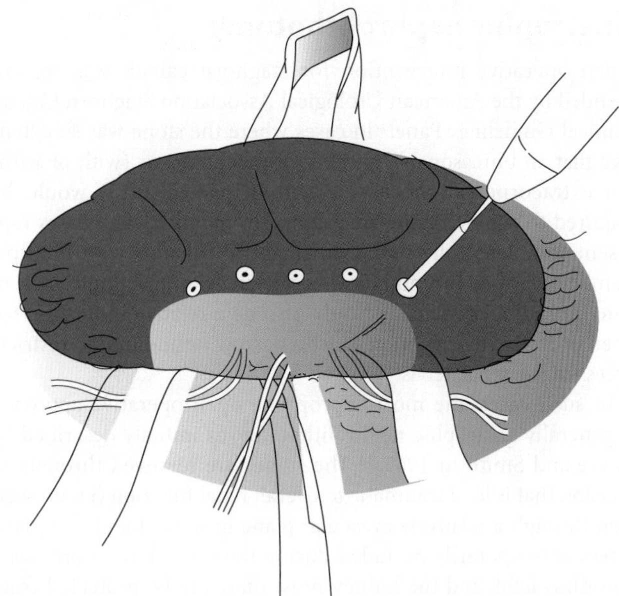

Fig. 2.12.2 Diagram of an anatrophic nephrolithotomy demonstrating Brodel's line—the intersegmental avscular plane.
Reproduced from Jon Reynard et al., *Oxford Handbook of Urological Surgery*, Figure 6.2.7, p. 439, Oxford University Press, Oxford, UK, Copyright © 2008, with permission from Oxford University Press.

this can be further delineated but is not a requisite for a successful 'nephron-sparing' result.[25]

An additional 12.5 mg of mannitol is given, and the main renal artery is then occluded with a vascular clamp. At this point, the renal vein may also be occluded to assure a blood-free surgical field. The kidney is packed with slush with the aim of obtaining a core temperature of 10°C, again as protection from renal ischaemia.

Once the kidney has reached core temperature, the capsule is incised longitudinally between the anterior and posterior segments, but extended only to the apical and basilar renal segments. The incision through the parenchyma continues in a plane along the line of demarcation between the anterior and posterior arterial segments, down towards the renal pelvis. The correct plane generally runs just anterior to the posterior row of infundibula and calices.

The stone is identified either by palpation in one of the involved posterior infundibula or calicyes, or by direct visualization. Once the initial stone-bearing infundibulocalix is open, a longitudinal infundibulotomy is performed and extended down to the renal pelvis. Each involved posterior infundibulocalix is similarly opened longitudinally as far as necessary to extract any stone and the infundibulotomy is carried down its anterior aspect towards the renal pelvis.

Once the pelvic and posterior infundibulocaliceal aspects of the stone are identified, the anterior and polar portions are exposed, again with sequential longitudinal infundibulotomies. However, these are performed on the posterior aspect of the anterior segmental infundibula, and central aspects of the polar infundibula. Again, the infundibulotomies should begin at each infundibulopelvic junction and extend outward towards the calix as far as necessary to provide adequate exposure for stone removal.

Eventually, the entire staghorn calculus is exposed and ready for removal. Once the bulk of the stone is removed, each infundibulocalix is explored to exclude residual fragments. Occasionally, these fragments can be palpated through thin parenchyma, but the infundibulum leading to the stone cannot be visualized. In such cases, a small nephrotomy made over the stone is acceptable. Because an optimal result requires removal of all stone fragments, adjunctive manoeuvres can be performed, including the taking of intraoperative images.

An internal stent is not mandatory and the collecting system is reconstructed using an absorbable suture. In areas of significant infundibular stenosis, infundibulorrhaphy is performed by suturing the adjacent borders of involved infundibula on their mirror image sides, thus converting two or more stenotic infundibulocaliceal systems into one larger portion of the renal pelvis. Alternatively, isolated infundibular stenosis or polar infundibular stenosis can be managed with an individual infundibulorrhaphy that involves horizontal closure of the initial vertical infundibulotomy in a Heineke-Mikulicz fashion. However, when no infundibular stenosis is present, separate closure of the collecting system may not be necessary.[22]

The renal capsule is approximated with running or interrupted absorbable sutures incorporating only a very small portion of renal parenchyma. Perirenal fat can be reapproximated over nephrotomy incisions, and external drainage is placed near any nephrotomy incisions.

Partial nephrectomy

Partial nephrectomy is indicated when stone disease is associated with a localized area of irreversibly poor renal function (e.g. in the setting of chronic obstruction, especially with infection).

Nephrectomy

Nephrectomy is indicated for stone disease associated with a non-functioning or poorly functioning kidney (determined with a renal scintigraphy). Conservative management risks morbidity from recurrent urinary tract infection, pyelonephritis, or sepsis.[26–30]

Laparoscopic surgery

Almost all open stone procedures can be performed laparoscopically with the advantages of less postoperative pain, reduced hospitalization, shorter convalescence period, and better cosmetic outcomes.[31–33] A recent meta-analysis comparing ESWL, URS, and laparoscopic approaches for the management of large proximal ureteral stones reported better stone-free rates with laparoscopic techniques, but increased postoperative pain and length of stay. On this basis, laparoscopic ureterolithotomy currently remains a second-line treatment to URS or ESWL.[34]

Extended pyelolithotomy can be performed robotically (see Badani *et al.*[16]), but is not a suitable technique for patients with complete staghorn calculi.

Laparoscopic and robotic anatrophic nephrolithotomy have also been described with good outcomes. Both of these minimally invasive techniques are less invasive than the traditional open approach.[26–31]

Conclusions

In the era of endoscopic stone surgery, open surgery is a nowadays only rarely required for renal and ureteric calculi. Relative indications for this approach are patients with urinary stones associated with anatomical abnormalities or with a high stone burden. In all cases where open surgery is an option, a laparoscopic approach provides a less invasive, less painful, and as effective an alternative to open surgery.

Further reading

Al-Hunayan A, Khalil M, Hassabo M, Hanafi A, Abdul-Halim H. Management of solitary renal pelvic stone: laparoscopic retroperitoneal pyelolithotomy versus percutaneous nephrolithotomy. *J Endourol* 2011; **25**(6):975–8.

Badani KK, Hemal AK, Fumo M, *et al.* Robotic extended pyelolithotomy for treatment of renal calculi: a feasibility study. *World J Urol* 2006; **24**(2):198–201.

Falahatkar S, Khosropanah I, Allahkhah A, Jafari A. Open surgery, laparoscopic surgery, or transureteral lithotripsy—which method? Comparison of ureteral stone management outcomes. *J Endourol* 2011; **25**(1):31–4.

Giedelman C, Arriaga J, Carmona O, *et al.* Laparoscopic anatrophic nephrolithotomy: developments of the technique in the era of minimally invasive surgery. *J Endourol* 2012; **26**(5):444–50.

Kerbl K, Rehman J, Landman J, Lee D, Sundaram C, Clayman RV. Current management of urolithiasis: progress or regress? *J Endourol* 2002; **16**:281–8.

Matlaga BR, Assimos DG. Changing indications of open stone surgery. *Urology* 2000; **59**:490–3.

Paik ML, Wainstein MA, Spirnak JP, Hampel N, Resnick MI. Current indications for open stone surgery in the treatment of renal and ureteral calculi. *J Urol* 1998; **159**:374–8.

Preminger GM, Assimos DG, Lingeman JE, *et al.* AUA Nephrolithiasis Guideline Panel. AUA guideline on management of staghorn calculi. *J Urol* 2005; **173**(6):1991–2000.

References

1. Paik ML, Wainstein MA, Spirnak JP, Hampel N, Resnick MI. Current indications for open stone surgery in the treatment of renal and ureteral calculi. *J Urol* 1998; **159**:374–8.
2. Kerbl K, Rehman J, Landman J, Lee D, Sundaram C, Clayman RV. Current management of urolithiasis: progress or regress? *J Endourol* 2002; **16**:281–8.
3. Matlaga BR, Assimos DG. Changing indications of open stone surgery. *Urology* 2000; **59**:490–3.
4. Preminger GM, Assimos DG, Lingeman JE, *et al.* AUA Nephrolithiasis Guideline Panel. AUA guideline on management of staghorn calculi. *J Urol* 2005; **173**(6):1991–2000.
5. Salvadó JA, Guzmán S, Trucco CA, Parra CA. Laparoscopic pyelolithotomy: optimizing surgical technique. *J Endourol* 2009; **23**(4):575–8.
6. Atug F, Castle EP, Burgess SV, Thomas, R. Concomitant management of renal calculi and pelvi-ureteric junction obstruction with robotic laparoscopic surgery. *BJU Int* 2005; **96**(9):1365–8.
7. Ball AJ, Leveillee RJ, Patel VR, Wong C. Laparoscopic pyeloplasty and flexible nephroscopy: Simultaneous treatment of ureteropelvic junction obstruction and nephrolithiasis. *JSLS* 2004; **8**(3):223–8.
8. Al-Hunayan A, Khalil M, Hassabo M, Hanafi A, Abdul-Halim H. Management of solitary renal pelvic stone: laparoscopic retroperitoneal pyelolithotomy versus percutaneous nephrolithotomy. *J Endourol* 2011; **25**(6):975–8.
9. Casale P, Grady RW, Joyner BD, Zeltser IS, Kuo RL, Mitchell ME. Transperitoneal laparoscopic pyelolithotomy after failed percutaneous access in the pediatric patient. *J Urol* 2004; **172**(2):680–3; discussion 683.
10. Chander J, Suryavanshi M, Lal P, Singh L, Ramteke VK. Retroperitoneal pyelolithotomy for management of renal calculi. *JSLS* 2005; **9**(1):97–101.
11. Goel A, Hemal AK. Evaluation of role of retroperitoneoscopic pyelolithotomy and its comparison with percutaneous nephrolithotripsy. *Int Urol Nephrol* 2003; **35**(1):73–6.
12. Czerny V. Veber Nierenextripation. *Zentralbl Chir* 1897; **6**:737.
13. Lower WE. Conservative surgical methods in operating for stone in the kidney. *Cleve Med J* 1913; **12**:260.
14. Gil-Vernet J. New surgical concepts in removing renal calculi. *Urol Int* 1965; **20**:255–88.
15. Wulfsohn MA. Extended pyelolithotomy: The use of renal artery clamping and regional hypothermia. *J Urol* 1981; **125**:467–70.
16. Badani KK, Hemal AK, Fumo M, *et al.* Robotic extended pyelolithotomy for treatment of renal calculi: a feasibility study. *World J Urol* 2006; **24**(2):198–201.
17. Hsu THS, Streem SB. Metabolic abnormalities in patients with caliceal diverticular calculi. *J Urol* 1988; **160**:1640–2.
18. Streem SB, Yost A. Treatment of caliceal diverticular calculi with ESWL: Patient selection and extended follow-up. *J Urol* 1992; **148**:1043–6.
19. Hulbert JC, Reddy PK, Hunter DW, Castaneda-Zuniga W, Amplatz K, Lange PH. Percutaneous techniques for the management of caliceal diverticula containing calculi. *J Urol* 1986; **135**:225–7.
20. Shalhav AL, Soble JJ, Nakada SY, Wolf JS Jr, McClennan BL, Clayman RV. Long-term outcome of caliceal diverticula following percutaneous endosurgical management. *J Urol* 1998; **160**:1635–9.
21. Ruckle HC, Segura JW. Laparoscopic treatment of a stone-filled caliceal diverticulum: A definitive, minimally invasive therapeutic option. *J Urol* 1994; **151**:122–4.
22. Boyce WH, Smith MGV. Anatrophic nephrotomy and plastic calyrrhaphy. *Trans Am Assoc Genitourin Surg* 1967; **59**:18–24.
23. Brodell M. The intrinsic blood vessels of the kidney and their significance in nephrotomy. *Bull Johns Hopkins Hosp* 1901; **12**:10–13.
24. Graves FT. The anatomy of the intrarenal arteries and its application to segmental resection of the kidney. *Br J Surg* 1954; **42**:132–9.
25. Morey AF, Nitahara KS, McAninch JW. Modified anatrophic nephrolithotomy for management of staghorn calculi: Is renal function preserved? *J Urol* 1999; **162**:670–3.
26. Giedelman C, Arriaga J, Carmona O, *et al.* Laparoscopic anatrophic nephrolithotomy: developments of the technique in the era of minimally invasive surgery. *J Endourol* 2012; **26**(5):444–50.
27. Zhou L, Xuan Q, Wu B, *et al.* Retroperitoneal laparoscopic anatrophic nephrolithotomy for large staghorn calculi. *Int J Urol* 2011; **18**(2):126–9.
28. Nouralizadeh A, Simforoosh N, Masoudi P, Soltani MH, Javaherforooshzadeh A. Bilateral laparoscopic anatrophic nephrolithotomy for managing staghorn renal calculi. *Urol J* 2010;7(2):133–5.
29. Simforoosh N, Aminsharifi A, Tabibi A, *et al.* Laparoscopic anatrophic nephrolithotomy for managing large staghorn calculi. *BJU Int* 2008; **101**(10):1293–6.
30. Deger S, Tuellmann M, Schoenberger B, Winkelmann B, Peters R, Loening SA. Laparoscopic anatrophic nephrolithotomy. *Scand J Urol Nephrol* 2004; **38**(3):263–5.
31. Hruza M, Schulze M, Teber D, Gozen AS, Rassweiler JJ. Laparoscopic techniques for removal of renal and ureteral calculi. *J Endourol* 2009; **23**(10):1713–8.
32. Falahatkar S, Khosropanah I, Allahkhah A, Jafari A. Open surgery, laparoscopic surgery, or transureteral lithotripsy—which method? Comparison of ureteral stone management outcomes. *J Endourol* 2011; **25**(1):31–4.
33. Skrepetis K, Doumas K, Siafakas I, Lykourinas M. Laparoscopic versus open ureterolithotomy. A comparative study. *Eur Urol* 2001; **40**(1):32–6; discussion 7.
34. Lopes Neto AC, Korkes F, Silva JL 2nd, *et al.* Prospective randomized study of treatment of large proximal ureteral stones: extracorporeal shock wave lithotripsy versus ureterolithotripsy versus laparoscopy. *J Urol* 2012; **187**(1):164–8.

CHAPTER 2.13

Medical therapy (dissolution therapy)

Ben Turney and John Reynard

Introduction to medical therapy of stones disease

Medical therapy of stone disease aims to prevent stones (preventive therapy) or dissolve existing stones (dissolution therapy). Dissolution therapy aims to dissolve stones through the administration of oral agents or by direct chemolysis through renal irrigation. Since dissolution therapy may take weeks to achieve an effect, it is usually used as an adjunct to endourological treatment.

Urate stones are most amenable to dissolution therapy. Stones containing any calcium have a lower chance of successful dissolution.

Irrigating chemolysis

Providing stone composition is known, irrigating chemolysis is an option for patients with large stone burdens who are unsuitable for percutaneous nephrolithotomy (PCNL). In theory, struvite stones can be treated with 10% hemiacidrin (pH3.5–4) or Suby's G solution, but there is a potential risk of death from hypermagnesaemia.[1,2] These solutions may also be used to treat residual brushite stone fragments. Both uric acid and cystine stones can be treated with irrigating solutions of trihydroxymethyl-aminomethan (THAM; 0.3 or 0.6 mol/L) with pH 8.5–9.0, though it takes a long time (1–4 days) to dissolve stones and oral treatment is preferred.[3–8] The European Association of Urology (EAU) guidelines recommend that at least two nephrostomy catheters are used to irrigate the collecting system to maintain a low renal pressure and to prevent chemolytic fluid draining into the bladder.

Oral chemolysis

Oral chemolitholysis can be used to dissolve uric acid stones and is based on alkalinization of urine with oral alkaline citrate (e.g. potassium citrate 30–60 mEq/day) or sodium bicarbonate (650 mg tds or qds). Modifying dose according to self-monitored urine pH, aiming to achieve a urinary pH of 7–7.2 throughout the day, optimizes stone dissolution therapy.

Preventive medical therapy

For uric acid stones, adjuncts to prevent recurrent stones include treatment with allopurinol (100–600 mg/day) which inhibits conversion of hypoxanthine and xanthine to uric acid, maintenance of a high fluid intake, and a diet low in animal protein. Allopurinol is useful in patients forming stones (both uric acid and calcium oxalate) if the uric acid excretion in urine is >4 mmol/day or if the patient has hyperuricaemia (>380 μmol).[9]

Medical therapy has a very significant preventive role in cystinuric patients. Most cystinuric patients excrete about 1g of cystine per day, which is well above the solubility of cystine. Cystine solubility in acid solutions is low (300 mg/l at pH 5,400 mg/l at pH 7).

The aim of treatment is to:

(a) dilute the urine through maintaining a high fluid intake;

(b) reduce cystine excretion through dietary restriction of the cystine precursor amino acid methionine;

(c) reduce sodium intake to <100 mg/day);

(d) increase the solubility of cystine by alkalinization of the urine (>pH 7.5);

(e) use drugs which bind cystine to form a more soluble compound. Cystine binding drugs include D-penicillamine, N-acetyl-d-penicillamine, and mercaptopropionylglycine (Tiopronin) and captopril. All have higher solubility than the relatively insoluble cystine–cystine dimers. The unpleasant and potentially serious side effects of D-penicillamine limit its use (allergic reactions, nephrotic syndrome, pancytopenia, proteinuria, epidermolysis, thrombocytosis, hypogeusia). It is reserved for cases where alkalinization therapy and high fluid intake fail to dissolve the stones.

References

1. Tiselius HG, Hellgren E, Andersson A, Borrud-Ohlsson A, Eriksson I. Minimally invasive treatment of infection staghorn stones with shock wave lithotripsy and chemolysis. *Scand J Urol Nephrol* 1999; **33**(5):286–90.
2. Collins S, Ortiz J, Maruffo F, *et al.* Expedited struvite-stone dissolution using a high-flow low-pressure irrigation system. *J Endourol* 2007; **21**(10):1153–8.
3. Bernardo NO1, Smith AD. Chemolysis of urinary calculi. *Urol Clin North Am* 2000; **27**(2):355–65.
4. Ahlstrand C, Tiselius HG. Treatment of cystine urolithiasis by a combination of extracorporeal shock wave lithotripsy and chemolysis. *J Stone Dis* 1993; **5**(1):32–8.
5. Vandeursen H, Baert L. Combination of chemolysis and extracorporeal shock wave lithotripsy in cystine urolithiasis. *Br J Urol* 1991; **67**(4):435–6.

6. Lee YH, Chang LS, Chen MT, Huang JK. Local chemolysis of obstructive uric acid stone with 0.1 M THAM and 0.02% chlorhexidine. *Urol Int* 1993; **51**(3):147–51.
7. Chugtai MN, Khan FA, Kaleem M, Ahmed M. Management of uric acid stone. *J Pak Med Assoc* 1992; **42**(7):153–5.
8. Moran ME, Abrahams HM, Burday DE, Greene TD. Utility of oral dissolution therapy in the management of referred patients with secondarily treated uric acid stones. *Urology* 2002; **59**(2):206–10.
9. Ettinger B, Tang A, Citron JT, Livermore B, Williams T. Randomized trial of allopurinol in the prevention of calcium oxalate calculi. *N Engl J Med* 1986; **315**(22):1386–9.

CHAPTER 2.14

Ureteric stones
Presentation and diagnosis

Ben Turney and John Reynard

Presentation

Ureteric stones may present in a variety of ways:

- Loin pain
- Strangury (a constant, strong desire to pass urine)
- Haematuria (rare)
- Incidentally (asymptomatic) (very rare)

Loin pain

Ureteric stones classically present with sudden onset, severe loin pain with or without radiation to the groin, testis, or labia majora. Some 50% of patients presenting with loin pain thought (by their attending doctors) to be indicative of a ureteric stone do not have any evidence of urolithiasis, or indeed of any other urological pathology of unenhanced computed tomography (CT) scanning.[1] The range of differential diagnoses is huge. A carefully taken history and examination may identify other probable causes of pain. As a general rule, inflammatory abdominal pathology causing peritoneal irritation or peritonitis (e.g. appendicitis, viscus perforation) causes constant pain exacerbated by movement—the patient lies still—whereas the patient with ureteric colic usually writhes around in agony—they cannot 'get comfortable'.

Strangury

The urgent desire to pass urine, combined with increased urinary frequency and the passage of small voided volumes of urine is suggestive of a vesicoureteric junction stone.

Haematuria

Haematuria as a presenting symptom of a ureteric stone is rare.

Incidentally (asymptomatic) diagnosed ureteric stones

Of 5,047 consecutive adults undergoing routine CT colonography screening, six patients had asymptomatic ureteric stones (four with hydronephrosis implying renal obstruction), giving a prevalence of 0.12%.[2]

Examination and non-radiological diagnostic tests in the patient with suspected ureteric colic

Abdominal examination

This is used more to exclude a diagnosis of a ureteric stone. The identification of abdominal tenderness and guarding argue against a diagnosis of a ureteric stone, by virtue of the fact that ureteric stones do not cause peritoneal inflammation.

Temperature

The most important aspect of examination in a patient with a ureteric stone confirmed on imaging is to measure their temperature. If the patient has a stone and a fever, they may have an infection proximal to the stone. A fever in the presence of an obstructing stone is an indication for urine and blood culture, intravenous fluids and antibiotics; nephrostomy drainage or J stent insertion may be indicated if the fever does not resolve within a matter of hours.

Pregnancy test

A pregnancy test is mandatory in any premenopausal woman presenting with loin pain suggestive of a ureteric stone; firstly to exclude an ectopic pregnancy as the cause of the pain, and secondly to allow diagnostic imaging (unenhanced CT) to be done without fear of exposing a pregnant woman to ionizing radiation.

Dipstick or microscopic haematuria

As a diagnostic test, many patients with ureteric stones have dipstick or microscopic haematuria, but 10–30% do not.[3,4] The sensitivity of dipstick haematuria for detecting acutely presenting ureteric stones is ~95% on the first day of pain, 85% on the second day, and 65% on the third and fourth days.[4] Therefore, roughly one-third of patients with a ureteric stone whose pain started three to four days previously may not have blood detectable in their urine. Dipstick testing is slightly more sensitive than urine microscopy for detecting stones (80% vs. 70%) because blood cells lyse, and therefore disappear, if the urine specimen is not examined under the microscope within a few hours. Both ways of detecting haematuria have roughly the same specificity for diagnosing ureteric stones (~60%).

Bear in mind that blood in the urine on dipstick testing or microscopy may be a coincidental finding from serious, non-stone urological disease (e.g. neoplasm). Conversely, since no abnormality is found in ~70% of patients with microscopic haematuria, and despite full urological investigation, the presence of stones does not mean the haematuria is due to the stones.

Radiological diagnostic tests in the patient with suspected ureteric colic

Plain abdominal (KUB—'kidneys, ureter, bladder') radiography

This has a sensitivity for detecting ureteric stones of 44–77% (so it 'misses' 23–56% of ureteric stones) and a specificity of 80–87%.[5]

Unenhanced CT–KUB in the diagnosis of a suspected ureteric stone

This is nowadays the imaging modality of choice in the acute presentation with loin pain.[6–8] It has greater specificity (92–100%) and sensitivity (94–100%) for diagnosing ureteric stones[6,9,10] than any other imaging test and it has the added advantage of being able to identify non-stone causes of flank pain, of not requiring contrast administration (so avoiding the chance of a contrast reaction). Additionally, it is faster than intravenous urogram (IVU), especially where delayed films are required to identify a stone causing high-grade obstruction, with such delayed films taking hours to identify the precise location of the obstructing stone. In high CT-volume hospitals, costs are equivalent to those of the IVU.[11]

The radiation dose from a CT-KUB is approximately 4.7 mSv compared to 1.5 mSv for an IVU.[12]

Magnetic resonance urography

This is an accurate imaging test for identifying ureteric stones.[13] However, at the present time, cost, restricted availability and limited experience in interpretation of the images by radiologists and urologists limit its usefulness as a routine diagnostic method of imaging in cases of acute flank pain.

Further reading

BAUS Guidelines 2012. BAUS Section of Endourology. Guidelines for acute management of first presentation of renal/ureteric lithiasis, 2012. Available at: http://www.baus.org.uk/_userfiles/pages/files/Publications/RevisedAcuteStoneMgtGuidelines.pdf [Accessed 21 January 2013] [Online].

Heldt JP, Smith JC, Anderson KM, *et al.* Ureteral calculi detection using low dose computerized tomography protocols is compromised in overweight and underweight patients. *J Urol* 2012; **188**:124–9.

Jellison FC, Smith JC, Heldt JP, *et al.* Effect of low dose radiation computerized tomography protocols on distal ureteral calculus detection. *J Urol* 2009; **182**:2762–7.

Smith RC, Coll DM. Helical computed tomography in the diagnosis of ureteric colic. *BJU Int* 2000; **86**(Suppl 1):33–41.

Smith RC, Rosenfield AT, Choe KA, *et al.* Acute flank pain: comparison of non-contrast-enhanced CT and intravenous urography. *Radiology* 1995; **194**:789–94.

Smith RC, Verga M, McCarthy S, Rosenfield AT. Diagnosis of acute flank pain: value of unenhanced helical CT. *Am J Roentgen* 1996; **166**:97–101.

References

1. Smith RC, Verga M, McCarthy S, Rosenfield AT. Diagnosis of acute flank pain: value of unenhanced helical CT. *Am J Roentgen* 1996; **166**:97–101.
2. Boyce CJ, Pickhardt PJ, Lawrence EM, Kim DH, Bruce RJ. Prevalence of urolithiasis in asymptomatic adults: Objective determination using low dose noncontrast computerized tomography. *J Urol* 2010; **183**:1017–21.
3. Luchs JS, Katz DS, Lane DS, *et al.* Utility of hematuria testing in patients with suspected renal colic: correlation with unenhanced helical CT results. *Urology* 2002; **59**:839–42.
4. Kobayashi T, Nishizawa K, Mitsumori K, Ogura K. Impact of date of onset on the absence of hematuria in patients with acute renal colic. *J Urol* 2003; **170**(4 Pt 1):1093–6.
5. Heidenreich A, Desgrandchamps F, Terrier F. Modern approach of diagnosis and management of acute flank pain: review of all imaging modalities. *Eur Urol* 2002; **41**:351–62.
6. BAUS Guidelines 2012. BAUS Section of Endourology. Guidelines for acute management of first presentation of renal/ureteric lithiasis, 2012. Available at: http://www.baus.org.uk/_userfiles/pages/files/Publications/RevisedAcuteStoneMgtGuidelines.pdf [Accessed 21 January 2013] [Online].
7. EAU Guidelines on Urolithiasis 2012. Available at: https://uroweb.org/wp-content/uploads/20_Urolithiasis_LR-March-13-2012.pdf [Accessed 21 January 2013] [Online].
8. Fulgham PF, Assimos DG, Pearle MS, Preminger GM. Clinical effectiveness protocols for imaging in the management of ureteral calculous disease: AUA technology assessment 2012. *J Urol* 2013; **189**(4):1203–13.
9. Niemann T, Kollmann T, Bongartz G.. Diagnostic performance of low dose CT for the detection of urolithiasis. *Am J Roentgen* 2008; **191**:396–401.
10. Worster A, Preyna I, Weaver B, Haines T. The accuracy of non-contrast helical computed tomography versus intravenous pyelography in the diagnosis of suspected acute urolithiasis: a meta-analysis. *Ann Emerg Med* 2002; **40**:280–6.
11. Thomson JM, Glocer J, Abbott C, *et al.* Computed tomography versus intravenous urography in diagnosis of acute flank pain from urolithiasis: a randomized study comparing imaging costs and radiation dose. *Australas Radiol* 2001; **45**:291–7.
12. Fowler JC. Clinical evaluation of ultra-low dose contrast-enhanced CT in patients presenting with acute ureteric colic. *Br J Med Surg Urol* 2011; **4**:56–63.
13. Leyendecker JR, Gianini JW. Magnetic resonance urography. *Abdom Imaging* 2009; **34**:527–40.

CHAPTER 2.15

Ureteric stones

Acute management

Samarpit Rai, Ghalib Jibara, Zachariah G. Goldsmith, Michael E. Lipkin, and Glenn M. Preminger

Introduction to ureteric stones

Ureteral stones are believed to result in increased amplitude of ureteral muscle contraction, decreased frequency of contractions, and an increased ureteral pressure proximal to the stone.[1–2] Relaxation of the ureter in the region of obstruction is thought to lead to improvement of symptoms and facilitate stone passage. Stone size and location are the main factors in determining the likelihood of stone passage.[3] The majority of the small stones (less than 5 mm in size) pass spontaneously without the need for intervention.[4] Of those that do pass, 95% will pass within six weeks.[5] The 2007 joint European Association of Urology and the American Urological Association Guideline Panel for the Management of Ureteral Calculi conducted a meta-analysis of spontaneous passage rates stratified by size.[6] Stones less than 5 mm (224 patients) were found to have a 68% spontaneous passage rate. Stones 5–10 mm (104 patients) demonstrated a 47% spontaneous passage rate.

In this context, the main goals of acute care for a patient presenting with renal colic include symptomatic pain control, facilitating stone passage, and evaluation of the need for urgent urologic intervention. The criteria requiring urgent intervention—including urosepsis, acute renal failure or anuria, unyielding pain, or vomiting—are reviewed in detail in Chapter 2.17. Most patients may be managed conservatively with pain medication and maintenance intravenous hydration. However, as compared to basal rates of hydration, additional fluid bolus of 2 L was demonstrated to result in equivalent rates of spontaneous stone passage and requirement for pain medication, in a small randomized trial.[7] Patients should be instructed to strain their urine at home for several days and bring in any stone that passes for analysis.

According to the EAU/AUA Guidelines for the management of ureteral calculi, observation with periodic evaluation is an option for the initial treatment of a patient that has a newly diagnosed ureteral stone less than 10 mm in size, and medical therapy to facilitate stone passage may be offered as appropriate during the observation period.[6,8] Stones greater than 10 mm in size may be observed or treated with medical expulsive therapy (MET), but in most cases, such stones will require surgical treatment.

Pharmacologic therapy

Several pharmacological therapies have been evaluated to reduce pain during symptomatic stone events (primarily anti-inflammatory and narcotic agents) and to facilitate stone passage as a part of MET (primarily alpha blockers). The pharmacology and clinical evidence supporting the use of each modality is reviewed in detail.

Non-steroidal anti-inflammatory pain control

Non-steroidal anti-inflammatory drugs (NSAIDs) are a major class of drugs used for symptomatic relief in the acute management of ureteral stones. The non-steroidal cyclooxygenase (COX) inhibitors are inhibitors of prostaglandin synthesis. Prostaglandin signalling has been shown to mediate ureteral contraction in animal models (e.g. Sprague-Dawley rats[9]). Both selective COX-2 inhibitors (e.g. diclofenac) and non-selective inhibitors (e.g. ketorolac) have been shown to decrease contractility or tone of porcine, as well as human ureteral segments *in vitro*.[10–14]

In an early randomized, prospective, double-blind trial of 131 patients with acute renal colic, the analgesic effect of diclofenac sodium (75 mg intramuscular) was compared to a placebo. A higher percentage of patients reported complete pain relief in the diclofenac group (59%) compared with the placebo (29%, $p<0.01$).[15] The onset of pain relief was 25 minutes following injection, and no adverse effects were noted. Another randomized, prospective, double-blind study of 47 patients with acute renal colic compared the analgesic effect of indomethacin (50 mg intravenous) to placebo.[16] With this agent as well, a significantly higher proportion of complete pain relief was reported with the NSAID (78% vs. 30%). The efficacy of NSAIDs for treatment of acute renal colic has been evaluated in a meta-analysis which included a total of 19 randomized comparison articles.[17] Among the studies that compared NSAIDs to a placebo, significantly increased rates of total pain relief were observed with NSAIDs (RR: 2.34, 95% CI: 1.79–3.07).

An additional body of work has focused on the comparison of different NSAID agents for pain treatment caused by ureteral stones. In a double-blind prospective trial of 57 patients with acute renal colic, patients were randomized to receive ketorolac (30 mg IV) or diclofenac (75 mg IM).[18] There were no significant differences in patient-reported pain scales at 0, 1, 2, and 6 hours after drug administration. In addition, the number of patients requiring rescue analgesia was equivalent in both treatment groups.

The efficacy of NSAIDs has also been compared to other analgesics, most commonly narcotic agents.[19–22] The results of 16 randomized trials comparing NSAIDs to other analgesic agents were evaluated in a meta-analysis. Similar rates of partial pain relief (RR: 1.07, 95% CI: 1.02–1.12) and complete pain relief (RR: 1.19, 95% CI: 1.03–1.37) were observed between the groups. The authors concluded that NSAIDs are equally effective in treatment of pain from acute renal colic, as compared to alternative analgesics.

Given the positive efficacy demonstrated with intravenous NSAID agents, there is an interest in identifying effective oral agents, which could be administered in an outpatient setting for the management of pain from ureteral stones. In a prospective randomized trial of 53 patients, the efficacy of oral COX-2 inhibitor celecoxib (400 mg followed by 200 mg every 12 hours for 10 days) was compared to a placebo.[22] Notably, no improvements in pain analogue scale, narcotic use, or spontaneous passage rates were observed in this comparison. An additional trial randomized 110 patients to oral rofecoxib (50 mg, single dose), diclofenac (50 mg every eight hours), or placebo.[23] No differences in pain reports or narcotic use were observed between the groups.

Taken together, the safety and efficacy of intravenous NSAIDs for pain management in acute renal colic caused by ureteral stones is supported by level 1a evidence. Despite the advantages of oral administration, including the ease of self-administration of multiple doses over time in an outpatient setting, no improvements compared to placebo have been observed with two small randomized trials. As NSAIDs are metabolized by the kidney, care must be taken to insure adequate renal function and proper hydration prior to prescribing.

Narcotic pain control

Narcotic analgesics are commonly used in the management of pain during acute renal colic. Interestingly, detailed studies characterizing the expression profiles of opioid receptors in the ureter are lacking. In addition, to our knowledge, there are no trials comparing the analgesic effects of narcotics to placebo. Most investigators have focused on the analgesic effects of narcotics compared or combined with non-narcotic agents, especially NSAIDs.

A randomized, double-blind trial of 51 patients with renal colic compared morphine (5 mg IV loading dose and two additional 2.5 mg doses) to indomethacin rectal suppository (100 mg).[20] Self-reported pain scores were significantly lower in the indomethacin group at the 10 minute timepoint ($p = 0.02$). However, there was no significant difference in pain relief between the two groups at 20 minutes or 30 minutes. An additional randomized, double-blind trial of 106 patients with renal colic compared the effects ketorolac (60 mg IV), meperidine (50 mg IV), and combined ketorolac plus meperidine.[19] Fifty per cent (50%) reduction in pain scores were observed in 75% of the ketorolac group and 74% of the combination group, compared with 23% of the meperidine group ($p < 0.001$).

An additional trial focused on the efficacy of combining narcotic with NSAID analgesia. In this prospective, randomized, double-blind trial, 130 patients with acute renal colic received either morphine (5 mg IV), ketorolac (15 mg IM), or a combination of both.[21] Pain scores were assessed at 0 minutes and 40 minutes after administration. The magnitude of pain reduction was significantly greater in the patients receiving combination treatment compared with monotherapy using morphine or ketorolac alone ($p < 0.003$). In addition, patients with combination therapy were less likely to require additional rescue morphine doses compared to the morphine monotherapy group (OR: 0.2, 95% CI: 0.1–0.7, $p = 0.007$).

Major adverse effects of narcotics include nausea, vomiting, pruritus, and dizziness. The prevalence of these adverse effects in the treatment of acute renal colic was well characterized by a meta-analysis of 20 trials including 1,613 patients treated with narcotics or NSAIDs.[22] A trend towards increased prevalence of these events was noted in patients treated with narcotics vs. NSAIDs. In particular, rates of emesis were significantly lower in patients treated with NSAIDs compared to narcotics (OR: 0.35, 95% CI: 0.23–0.53). In addition, the long-term impact of repeat administration of narcotics during acute renal colic on opioid dependency for patients with recurrent nephrolithiasis has yet to be fully characterized.

Medical expulsive therapy

Alpha blockers

Alpha blockers constitute the main category of drugs that are used in MET to facilitate spontaneous stone passage in the setting of an acute stone event. Alpha-stimulatory and beta-inhibitory adrenergic receptors have been well characterized in the ureter.[24–28] Alpha-1 antagonists have been shown to inhibit ureteral contractility in porcine models, both *in vivo* and *ex vivo*. It is believed that reduction in sympathetic tone may facilitate organized ureteral peristalsis, and facilitate stone passage.

The efficacy of alpha blockers in facilitating stone passage was first reported in a study of 104 patients with distal ureteral stones <10 mm.[29] Patients were randomized to treatment with 0.4 mg tamsulosin daily, versus standard care which did not include tamsulosin. Although statistical analysis was lacking, patients receiving tamsulosin appeared to have a higher stone expulsion rate compared to control (80.4% vs. 62.8%). Autorino and colleagues conducted a prospective, randomized study in which 64 patients with ureteral calculi were randomized to receive the group's standard treatment (diclofenac with the vasoactive agent aescin) or standard treatment with the addition of tamsulosin 4 mg daily.[30] The rate of stone expulsion was significantly higher in the group of patients receiving tamsulosin as compared to the control (88% vs. 60%, $p = 0.01$). In addition, the mean time required for stone expulsion was 4.8 days in the tamsulosin group, significantly lower than the mean time in the control group, 7.4 days ($p = 0.005$). Additionally, the patients receiving the treatment with tamsulosin had a significantly lower incidence of analgesic use ($p = 0.003$) and a significantly lower hospitalization rate for recurrent colic ($p = 0.01$), as reported by the same authors in a subsequent randomized study.

In another randomized, double-blind, placebo-controlled study, the authors evaluated the efficacy of alfuzosin in facilitating stone passage, and found that in a population of 69 patients, the mean time before spontaneous passage of the stone was significantly lower in patients receiving alfuzosin (5.2 days) as compared to patients receiving placebo (8.5 days).[31] In addition, patients receiving alfuzosin had a greater decrease in pain scores measured during follow-up, after the initial presentation to the emergency room.[32] Interestingly, the difference in overall rate of spontaneous stone passage among both groups was shown to be equivalent (73.5% for alfuzosin and 77.1% for placebo, $p = 0.83$).

In a meta-analysis incorporating 11 trials including 911 patients, alpha blocker therapy was shown to increase the rate of stone expulsion by 44% as compared to conservative therapy (RR = 1.44,

95% CI 1.31–1.59, p <0.001).[33] In another meta-analysis of nine trials and 693 patients, a pooled analysis of four studies using alpha blockers showed a significantly greater likelihood of stone passage compared to control, with a reported risk ratio of 1.54 (95% CI 1.29–1.85, p <0.0001).[34] Yet another meta-analysis with 29 trials and 2,419 patients reported on the use of alpha blocker therapy to facilitate stone expulsion. Pooled analysis demonstrated an increased rate of stone expulsion with alpha blocker therapy as compared to control (RR = 1.45, 95% CI 1.34–1.57).[35] Despite the concordance in findings among these thee independent analyses, most studies included were small, single-institution, non-blinded studies.

Clinical trials have also compared the efficacy of different formulations of alpha blockers used in MET. A prospective, randomized trial compared the efficacy of terazosin, tamsulosin, and doxazosin in facilitating stone passage.[36] A total of 114 patients were divided into four groups and randomized to the control group or to receive one of the three alpha blockers. There was no significant difference found between the time required for stone expulsion when comparing tamsulosin and terazosin (p = 0.568), tamsulosin and doxazosin (p = 0.612), or terazosin and doxazosin (p = 0.756), confirming the similar efficacy of all three agents in MET.

The use of alpha blockers for the treatment of ureteral stones up to 10 mm in size is supported by increased rates of stones passage, relative safety, and reduction in pain, as supported by level 1a evidence. Although there is sufficient evidence to support the use of alpha blockers, many of these studies are small, single-centre, and are underpowered. Furthermore, a recent multi-center randomized, placebo-controlled trial failed to show benefits of MET in patients with ureteral stones.[37] Urologists should be aware of this potential off-label use for alpha blockers, depending on their regulatory status, and counsel patients appropriately.

Other classes of drugs

Calcium channel blockers

The critical role of calcium influx in mediating muscle contraction is well established. Calcium channel blockers have been used in studying ureteral physiology. Nifedipine treatment has been shown to reduce contractility of human ureteral explants exposed to different chemical stimulants.[38] More recently, in a series of experiments using porcine ureteral explants, it has been demonstrated that the inhibitory effect of nifedipine is more potent than that obtained with tamsulosin.[39] Intraluminal application of verapramil has been shown to induce proximal ureteral dilation in porcine ureters *in vivo*.[40]

The efficacy of nifedipine in mediating stone passage has been studied in a number of randomized trials. Patients with ureteral stones less than or equal to 15 mm in size were randomized to either receive 16 mg methylprednisolone plus nifedipine or a placebo plus methylprednisolone.[41] Patients receiving nifedipine had a significantly higher stone passage rate as compared to placebo, 87% vs. 65% (p = 0.021). Additionally, the mean time before stone expulsion was 11.2 days in patients receiving nifedipine, significantly less than the placebo group at 16.4 days (p = 0.036). In a meta-analysis of nine studies and 686 patients, pooled data analysis showed a 49% increase in the likelihood of stone expulsion with the use of nifedipine as compared to control (risk ratio 1.49, 95% CI: 1.33–1.66).[42] Additionally, six of the nine studies reported a decreased average time (between 2.7 and 12 days) required for stone expulsion in patients treated with nifedipine.

A prospective, randomized, controlled trial with 3,189 patients comparing the efficacy of an alpha blocker (tamsulosin) and nifedipine in MET for distal ureteral stones in patients with renal colic reported that the spontaneous stone expulsion rate was significantly higher in patients receiving tamsulosin, as compared to patients who received nifedipine, 95.86% vs. 73.51% (p < 0.01).[43] Additionally, the patients receiving tamsulosin had a significantly lower average time required for stone passage as compared to those treated with nifedipine, 78.35 hours vs. 137.93 hours (p < 0.01). Also, the number of patients receiving tamsulosin required significantly less pain relief therapy than those on nifedipine, 1.53% vs. 4.84% (p < 0.01).

The use of calcium channel blockers as part of MET is well established and supported by level 1a evidence. However, alpha blockers have been shown to be more effective than calcium channel blockers in terms of higher rates of stone expulsion, less time required for stone expulsion, and lesser requirement for rescue analgesia, as supported by level 1 evidence.

Corticosteroids

The transcriptional activity of multiple genes coding for pro-inflammatory proteins such as COX-2 and phospholipase A2 are inhibited by corticosteroids.[44–46] Given this mechanism, hydrocortisone has been shown to decrease the contractility of porcine ureteral segments *in vitro*.

A number of clinical trials evaluating MET for ureteral colic have included the use of corticosteroids as adjuncts to alpha blockers or calcium channel inhibitors. In a prospective clinical study including 114 patients,[47] the authors evaluated the efficacy of using corticosteroids as an adjunct therapy with alpha blockers as compared with each agent given alone and a control group receiving only analgesics. The group receiving tamsulosin (0.4 mg daily) and deflazacort (30 mg daily) had a significantly higher rate of stone expulsion (84.8%) compared to tamsulosin monotherapy (60%), deflazacort monotherapy (37.5%), and control (33.3%), with a p value of less than 0.001. Dellabella and colleagues evaluated the additional benefit of corticosteroids given with alpha blockers as part of MET in a randomized, prospective study.[48] Sixty patients were randomized to either receive tamsulosin alone (0.4 mg daily) or deflazacort (30 mg daily) plus tamsulosin. The stone expulsion rate was similar in both groups, 90% vs. 96.7%, respectively (p = 0.612). However, the patients receiving corticosteroids as adjunct therapy had a significantly lesser mean time required for stone expulsion as compared to the patients receiving tamsulosin alone, 103.3 hours vs. 139.2 hours (p = 0.036). Additionally, two patients in the group receiving corticosteroids were reported to have experienced a high degree of dyspepsia.

Taken together, although corticosteroids have been included as adjuncts in multiple MET trials, their exact role in medical management for ureteral stones has yet to be fully defined.

Conclusions

Renal colic due to ureteral stones is a common cause of presentation at the emergency department. The main goals for the management of renal colic in the acute setting includes symptomatic relief, pain control, facilitating stone passage, and evaluation of the patient for the requirement of urgent urologic intervention. According to the AUA/EAU guidelines, observation with periodic evaluation is an option for the initial treatment of a newly diagnosed ureteral stone less than 10 mm in size, with the use of MET to facilitate stone passage as and when deemed appropriate by the physician. Stones greater than 10 mm in size may also be managed conservatively or treated with MET, but in most cases they require surgical intervention.

NSAIDs and narcotics are the mainstay of treatment for analgesic relief in the treatment of acute renal colic. The use of both classes of drugs has been evaluated comprehensively and is supported by multiple meta-analyses (level 1a evidence). For MET, the main class of drugs used is the alpha blockers. Multiple randomized controlled trials and meta-analyses have established the efficacy of alpha blockers in facilitating stone passage in acute renal colic. Other classes of drugs, such as calcium channel blockers (nifedipine) have also been proven to be effective in MET, but evidence suggests that alpha blockers such as tamsulosin are more effective than calcium channel blockers in MET.

Further reading

Dellabella M, Milanese G, Muzzonigro G. Medical-expulsive therapy for distal ureterolithiasis: randomized prospective study on role of corticosteroids used in combination with tamsulosin-simplified treatment regimen and health-related quality of life. *Urology* 2005; **66**(4):712–5.

Holdgate A, Pollock T. Systematic review of the relative efficacy of non-steroidal anti-inflammatory drugs and opioids in the treatment of acute renal colic. *BMJ* 2004; **328**:1401.

Hollingsworth JM, Rogers MA, Kaufman SR, *et al.* Medical therapy to facilitate urinary stone passage: a meta-analysis. *Lancet* 2006; **368**:1171–9.

Nakada SY, Jerde TJ, Bjorling DE, Saban R. Selective cyclooxygenase-2 inhibitors reduce ureteral contraction in vitro: a better alternative for renal colic? *J Urol* 2000; **163**(2):607–12.

Preminger GM, Tiselius HG, Assimos DG, *et al.* 2007 guideline for the management of ureteral calculi. *J Urol* 2007; **178**:2418–34.

Seitz C, Liatsikos E, Porpiglia F, Tiselius HG, Zwergel U. Medical therapy to facilitate the passage of stones: what is the evidence? *Eur Urol* 2009; **56**:455–71.

Springhart WP, Marguet CG, Sur RL, *et al.* Forced versus minimal intravenous hydration in the management of acute renal colic: a randomized trial. *J Endourol* 2006; **20**:713–6.

Weiss RM, Bassett AL, Hoffman BF. Adrenergic innervation of the ureter. *Invest Urol* 1978; **16**(2):123–7.

References

1. Stamatelou KK, Francis ME, Jones CA, Nyberg LM, Curhan GC. Time trends in reported prevalence of kidney stones in the United States: 1976–1994. *Kidney Int* 2003; **63**:1817–23.
2. Stewart C. Nephrolithiasis. *Emerg Med Clin North Am* 1988; **6**:617–30.
3. Miller OF, Kane CJ. Time to stone passage for observed ureteral calculi: a guide for patient education. *J Urol* 1999; **162**:688–90.
4. Coll DM, Varanelli MJ, Smith RC. Relationship of spontaneous passage of ureteral calculi to stone size and location as revealed by unenhanced helical CT. *AJR Am J Roentgenol* 2002; **178**:101–3.
5. Parekattil SJ, Kumar U, Hegarty NJ, *et al.* External validation of outcome prediction model for ureteral/renal calculi. *J Urol* 2006; **175**:575–9.
6. Preminger GM, Tiselius HG, Assimos DG, *et al.* 2007 guideline for the management of ureteral calculi. *J Urol* 2007; **178**:2418–34.
7. Springhart WP, Marguet CG, Sur RL, *et al.* Forced versus minimal intravenous hydration in the management of acute renal colic: a randomized trial. *J Endourol* 2006; **20**:713–6.
8. Assimos D, Krambeck A, Miller NL, *et al.* Surgical Management of Stones: American Urological Association/Endourological Society Guideline, PART II. *J Urol* 2016; **196**(4):1161–9.
9. Mastrangelo D, Iselin CE. Urothelium dependent inhibition of rat ureter contractile activity. *J Urol* 2007; **178**(2):702–9.
10. Cole RS, Fry CH, Shuttleworth KE. The action of the prostaglandins on isolated human ureteric smooth muscle. *Br J Urol* 1988; **61**:19–26.
11. Nakada SY, Jerde TJ, Bjorling DE, Saban R. Selective cyclooxygenase-2 inhibitors reduce ureteral contraction in vitro: a better alternative for renal colic? *J Urol* 2000; **163**(2):607–12.
12. Wen CC, Coyle TL, Jerde TJ, Nakada SY. Ketorolac effectively inhibits ureteral contractility in vitro. *J Endourol* 2008; **22**(4):739–42.
13. Chaignat V, Danuser H, Stoffel MH, Z'brun S, Studer UE, Mevissen M. Effects of a non-selective COX inhibitor and selective COX-2 inhibitors on contractility of human and porcine ureters in vitro and in vivo. *Br J Pharmacol* 2008; **154**(6):1297–307.
14. Lee SY, Lee MY, Park SH, *et al.* NS-398 (a selective cyclooxygenase-2 inhibitor) decreases agonist-induced contraction of the human ureter via calcium channel inhibition. *J Endourol* 2010; **24**(11):1863–8.
15. Vignoni A, Fierro A, Moreschini G, *et al.* Diclofenac sodium in ureteral colic: a double-blind comparison trial with placebo. *J Int Med Res* 1983; **11**:303–7.
16. Holmlund D, Sjodin JG. Treatment of ureteral colic with intravenous indomethacin. *J Urol* 1978; **120**:676–7.
17. Labrecque M, Dostaler L-P, Rouselle R, Nguyen T, Poirier S. Efficacy of non-steroidal anti-inflammatory drugs in the treatment of acute renal colic. *Arch Intern Med* 1994; **154**:1381–7.
18. Cohen E, Hafner R, Rotenberg Z, Fadilla M, Garty M. Comparison of ketorolac and diclofenac in the treatment of renal colic. *Eur J Clin Pharmacol* 1998; **54** (6):455–8.
19. Cordell WH, Wright SW, Wolfson AB, *et al.* Comparison of intravenous ketorolac, meperidine, and both (balanced analgesia) for renal colic. *Ann Emerg Med* 1996; **28**:151–8.
20. Cordell WH, Larson TA, Lingeman JE, *et al.* Indomethacin suppositories versus intravenously titrated morphine for the treatment of ureteral colic. *Ann Emerg Med* 1994; **23**:262–9.
21. Udén P, Rentzhog L, Berger T. A comparative study on the analgesic effects of indomethacin and hydromorphinechloride-atropine in acute, ureteral-stone pain. *Acta Chir Scand* 1983; **149**:497–9.
22. Holdgate A, Pollock T. Systematic review of the relative efficacy of non-steroidal anti-inflammatory drugs and opioids in the treatment of acute renal colic. *BMJ* 2004; **328**:1401.
23. Safdar B, Degutis LC, Landry K, Vedere SR, Moscovitz HC, D'Onofrio G. Intravenous morphine plus ketorolac is superior to either drug alone for treatment of acute renal colic. *Ann Emerg Med* 2006; **48**:173–81.
24. Malin JM Jr, Deane RF, Boyarsky S. Characterisation of adrenergic receptors in human ureter. *Br J Urol* 1970; **42**(2):171–4.
25. Weiss RM, Bassett AL, Hoffman BF. Adrenergic innervation of the ureter. *Invest Urol* 1978; **16**(2):123–7.
26. Caine M, Raz S. Some clinical implications of adrenergic receptors in the urinary tract. *Arch Surg* 1975; **110**(3):247–50.
27. Danuser H, Weiss R, Abel D, *et al.* Systemic and topical drug administration in the pig ureter: effect of phosphodiesterase inhibitors alpha1, beta and beta2-adrenergic receptor agonists and antagonists on the frequency and amplitude of ureteral contractions. *J Urol* 2001; **166**(2):714–20.
28. Nakada SY, Coyle TL, Ankem MK, Moon TD, Jerde TJ. Doxazosin relaxes ureteral smooth muscle and inhibits epinephrine-induced ureteral contractility in vitro. *Urology* 2007; **70**(4):817–21.
29. Cervenàkov I, Fillo J, Mardiak J, Kopecný M, Smirala J, Lepies P. Speedy elimination of ureterolithiasis in lower part of ureters with the alpha 1-blocker—tamsulosin. *Int Urol Nephrol* 2002; **34**:25–9.

30. Autorino R, De Sio M, Damiano R, *et al.* The use of tamsulosin in the medical treatment of ureteral calculi: where do we stand? *Urol Res* 2005; **33**:460–4.
31. De Sio M, Autorino R, Di Lorenzo G, *et al.* Medical expulsive treatment of distal-ureteral stones using tamsulosin: a single-center experience. *J Endourol* 2006; **20**:12–16.
32. Pedro RN, Hinck B, Hendlin K, Feia K, Canales BK, Monga M. Alfuzosin stone expulsion therapy for distal ureteral calculi: a double-blind, placebo controlled study. *J Urol* 2008; **179**:2244–7.
33. Parsons JK, Hergan LA, Sakamoto K, Lakin C. Efficacy of alpha-blockers for the treatment of ureteral stones. *J Urol* 2007; **177**:983–7.
34. Hollingsworth JM, Rogers MA, Kaufman SR, *et al.* Medical therapy to facilitate urinary stone passage: a meta-analysis. *Lancet* 2006; **368**:1171–9.
35. Seitz C, Liatsikos E, Porpiglia F, Tiselius HG, Zwergel U. Medical therapy to facilitate the passage of stones: what is the evidence? *Eur Urol* 2009; **56**:455–71.
36. Yilmaz E, Batislam E, Basar MM, Tuglu D, Ferhat M, Basar H. The comparison and efficacy of 3 different alpha1-adrenergic blockers for distal ureteral stones. *J Urol* 2005; **173**:2010–2.
37. Pickard R, Starr K, MacLennan G, *et al.* Medical expulsive therapy in adults with ureteric colic: a multicentre, randomised, placebo-controlled trial. *Lancet* 2015; **386**:341–9.
38. Forman A, Andersson KE, Henriksson L, Rud T, Ulmsten U. Effects of nifedipine on the smooth muscle of the human urinary tract in vitro and in vivo. *Acta Pharmacol Toxicol (Copenh)* 1978; **43**(2):111–8.
39. Troxel SA, Jones AW, Magliola L, Benson JS. Physiologic effect of nifedipine and tamsulosin on contractility of distal ureter. *J Endourol* 2006; **20**(8):565–8.
40. Ames CD, Weld KJ, Dryer ST, *et al.* Pharmacologic manipulation of the porcine ureter: Acute impact of topical drugs on ureteral diameter and peristaltic activity. *J Endourol* 2006; **20**(11):943–8.
41. Borghi L, Meschi T, Amato F, *et al.* Nifedipine and methylprednisolone in facilitating ureteral stone passage: a randomized, double-blind, placebo-controlled study. *J Urol* 1994; **152**:1095–8.
42. Singh A, Alter HJ, Littlepage A. A systematic review of medical therapy to facilitate passage of ureteral calculi. *Ann Emerg Med* 2007; **50**:552–63.
43. Ye Z, Yang H, Li H, *et al.* A multicentre, prospective, randomized trial: comparative efficacy of tamsulosin and nifedipine in medical expulsive therapy for distal ureteric stones with renal colic. *BJU Int* 2011; **108**:276–9.
44. Goppelt-Struebe M. Molecular mechanisms involved in the regulation of prostaglandin biosynthesis by glucocorticoids. *Biochem Pharmacol* 1997; **53**(10):1389–95.
45. Masferrer JL, Seibert K. Regulation of prostaglandin synthesis by glucocorticoids. *Receptor* 1994; **4**(1):25–30.
46. Bandi G, Wilkinson EA, Cary-Coyle TL, Jerde TJ, Nakada SY. Third prize: Effect of hydrocortisone on porcine ureteral contractility in vitro. *J Endourol* 2008; **22**(6):1169–73.
47. Porpiglia F, Vaccino D, Billia M, *et al.* Corticosteroids and tamsulosin in the medical expulsive therapy for symptomatic distal ureter stones: single drug or association? *Eur Urol* 2006; **50**(2):339–44.
48. Dellabella M, Milanese G, Muzzonigro G. Medical-expulsive therapy for distal ureterolithiasis: randomized prospective study on role of corticosteroids used in combination with tamsulosin-simplified treatment regimen and health-related quality of life. *Urology* 2005; **66**(4):712–5.

CHAPTER 2.16

Ureteric stones
Indications for intervention

Charles D. Scales

Indications for intervention

Indications to relieve obstruction or remove a ureteral stone broadly fall into two categories: acute indications, typically requiring immediate intervention, and subacute indications, where interventions may be performed on a more elective basis.

Acute indications

Patients with a ureteral stone and signs or symptoms of an obstructed, infected upper urinary tract should undergo immediate (within hours, allowing for the time required to access the operating theatre or interventional radiology suite) intervention to relieve the obstruction (by JJ stent or nephrostomy). While thresholds for intervention may vary, typically patients with a white blood cell count above 15,000 per microlitre, or a fever >38.5°C, should undergo immediate intervention.[1] Failure to intervene promptly can result in life-threatening sepsis. Following culture of urine and blood specimens, broad spectrum antibiotics should be initiated to cover appropriate genitourinary organisms. After drainage, patients with suspected obstructed pyelonephritis should be monitored and continue to receive empiric antibiotic therapy. Cultures of urine proximal to the stone should be obtained at the time of drainage, and these results may be used to tailor antibiotic therapy. Urine obtained from the bladder should also be cultured, but often the offending organism is only identified in urine proximal to the stone.

Patients with a solitary kidney should also undergo immediate (within hours) intervention, particularly if they are anuric, signalling a completely obstructed renal unit. Even in those patients who do not have evidence of complete obstruction, immediate drainage should be strongly considered. When patients possess two functioning kidneys, the urgency for intervention is typically lower. In this situation, measurement of the patient's renal function using serum creatinine should drive decision-making. When considering impaired renal function as an indication for intervention, comparison to the baseline serum creatinine may be helpful. Given that nausea, vomiting, and decreased oral intake frequently occur in patients with obstructing ureteral stones, dehydration can be another cause for mild deterioration in renal function. In this case, renal function typically responds rapidly to gentle fluid resuscitation. When a patient's renal function does not promptly respond to rehydration, drainage of the affected renal unit should occur urgently in order to avoid permanent damage to the kidney.

Finally, uncontrolled pain can be considered an acute, relative indication for drainage. Non-steroidal anti-inflammatory drugs (NSAIDs), are very effective in relieving pain from ureteral obstruction. NSAIDs inhibit the release of prostaglandins, and therefore can decrease ureteral contraction and renal pressure.[2] Opioid analgesics are excellent adjunctive medications for symptom management, or as monotherapy in those patients who are unable to tolerate or have contraindications to NSAIDs. Emerging evidence also suggests that alpha blockers used for medical expulsive therapy may also decrease pain through inhibition of ureteral contraction.[3] However, in some patients pharmacologic therapy will fail to control symptoms of pain, and therefore intervention is indicated. Patients should be cautioned about discomfort due to nephrostomy tubes and/or ureteral stents following placement; alternatively, in the absence of infection, it may be most effective to simply fragment and/or remove the obstructing stone, and potentially decrease the number of required procedures for the patient.

Subacute indications

Patients with no signs of infection, normal renal function, and well-controlled pain are eligible for a trial of observation and spontaneous stone passage, potentially assisted by medical expulsive therapy, according to AUA/ES guidelines.[4] Randomized controlled trials suggest that alpha blockers can dramatically increase the probability of passage for distal ureteral calculi <10 mm in size. Patients should be counselled that this is an 'off-label' use of these medications. In patients electing observation, periodic monitoring of hydronephrosis, renal function, and patient symptoms should occur. After four to six weeks, if a stone has not passed, then intervention to remove the stone is reasonable. In addition, ureteral stones >10 mm in size are very unlikely to pass spontaneously, and therefore these patients should be considered for fragmentation and removal of the stone on an elective basis, unless signs of urinary infection are present.

Interventions for urinary drainage

Options for renal drainage include percutaneous nephrostomy tube and internal ureteral stent. Percutaneous drainage is typically accomplished by placement of an 8- or 10-French (Fr) pigtail catheter through the flank into the renal pelvis. Ultrasound and/or fluoroscopic guidance is typically used during the procedure to localize the renal pelvis, avoid surrounding structures, and confirm appropriate position of the nephrostomy tube. If infection is suspected, then culture of the urine obtained from the renal pelvis should be performed. Risks of the procedure include infection, bleeding, and injury to adjacent structures (such as the colon), although these complications are typically rare. In septic patients, an acute exacerbation of their condition can occur following instrumentation of the renal system—a risk that applies to both percutaneous nephrostomy and retrograde ureteral stent placement.

A retrograde ureteral stent is usually placed endoscopically. A guidewire is advanced through the ureter, proximal to the obstructing stone, and then an open-ended ureteral catheter advanced over the wire to obtain urine for culture. The wire is replaced through the ureteral catheter, and the indwelling stent placed over the wire. Performance of a retrograde pyelogram, particularly in the patient with suspected infection or sepsis, is controversial. Many surgeons elect not to perform a retrograde pyelogram when infection is suspected, so as not to increase intrarenal pressure and potentially force bacteria or endotoxins into the blood stream through pyelovenous backflow. If a retrograde pyelogram is required in the potentially septic patient, it should be performed with gentle pressure and the minimum amount of contrast necessary to confirm location of the ureteral stent. Risks of retrograde ureteral stent placement include injury to the urethra, bladder or ureter, infection, and bleeding. As with percutaneous nephrostomy placement, instrumentation of the upper urinary tract in the infected or septic patient can result in an acute haemodynamic deterioration, so anaesthesiologists and surgeons should be alert for signs of decompensation.

The results of two randomized controlled trials suggest that little difference exists in the efficacy of percutaneous nephrostomy tubes or ureteral stents for achieving urinary drainage.[4,6] In one study, patients with nephrostomy tubes had a greater requirement for narcotic analgesia following placement, although the cost of retrograde ureteral stent placement was higher.[5] The results of these two studies suggest that choice of intervention for a single obstructing ureteral stone should be tailored according to the patient's clinical condition, preferences, and local practice.

Interventions for stone removal

Two primary interventions to remove ureteral stones exist, both of which are covered in detail elsewhere in this textbook (See Chapter 2.17). Briefly, retrograde ureteroscopy (potentially with laser lithotripsy) and shock wave lithotripsy both are considered first-line options for removing ureteral calculi, according to AUA/EAU guidelines for ureteral stone management.[7] The guidelines panel meta-analysis suggests that stone-free rates following ureteroscopy are generally higher than for shock wave lithotripsy, depending on stone size and location. For example, the stone-free rate for distal ureteral stones is 94% for ureteroscopy, as compared with 74% following shock wave lithotripsy monotherapy.[7] Stone-free rates for mid-ureteral stones are more comparable, at 86% for ureteroscopy as compared to 73% for shock wave lithotripsy.[7] For proximal ureteral calculi, ureteroscopy, and shock wave lithotripsy stone-free rates are very comparable, at just over 80%.[7] However, shock wave lithotripsy (non-invasive) may be preferred by patients over a minimally invasive approach. In addition, ureteral injury and stricture rates (based on historical data) appear to be higher following ureteroscopy. It is unclear if recent advances in ureteroscopic technology have reduced these risks.

Potential complications from both procedures include infection (urinary tract infection and/or sepsis), bleeding, and steinstrasse. Ureteral stricture and ureteral injury are also possible following either procedure, although seem to be more common following ureteroscopy than shock wave lithotripsy. According to AUA/EAU guidelines, routine ureteral stent placement is not indicated prior to shock wave lithotripsy. Moreover, randomized controlled trials suggest that there is little benefit to routine stenting after uncomplicated ureteroscopic cases. Placement of a ureteral stent does have risks and can negatively impact quality of life in the postoperative period. Patients with ureteral stents frequently experience irritative urinary tract symptoms, and are at risk for urinary tract infection, stent encrustation, and a retained ureteral stent, if the patient fails to come back for stent removal. Ureteral injury, stricture, solitary kidney, renal failure, and residual stone burden are considered indications for ureteral stent placement following ureteroscopy.[7]

Summary

Important indications exist for immediate or urgent intervention to assure urinary drainage or to remove obstructing ureteral calculi. In the case of infection, the consequences of failure to relieve the obstructed ureter can include severe sepsis and death. For both emergent and urgent indications for urinary drainage, a ureteral stent or percutaneous nephrostomy tube may be considered first-line options. For those patients that require intervention to fragment and remove a ureteral stone, ureteroscopy, and shock wave lithotripsy are acceptable options. Appropriate application of these techniques will minimize adverse consequences and maximize quality of life in patients with obstructing ureteral stones.

Further reading

Pearle MS, Pierce HL, Miller GL, *et al.* Optimal method of urgent decompression of the collecting system for obstruction and infection due to ureteral calculi. *J Urol* 1998; **160**(4):1260–4.

Preminger GM, Tiselius HG, Assimos DG, *et al.* 2007 guideline for the management of ureteral calculi. *J Urol* 2007; **178**(6):2418–34.

References

1. Pearle MS. Management of the acute stone event. *AUA Update series* 2008; **27**: lesson 30.
2. Moody TE, Vaughn ED Jr, Gillenwater JY. Relationship between renal blood flow and ureteral pressure during 18 hours of total unilateral uretheral occlusion. Implications for changing sites of increased renal resistance. *Invest Urol* 1975; **13**(3):246–51.
3. Pedro RN, Hinck B, Hendlin K, Feia K, Canales BK, Monga M. Alfuzosin stone expulsion therapy for distal ureteral calculi: a double-blind, placebo controlled study. *J Urol* 2008; **179**(6):2244–7; discussion 2247.
4. Assimos D, Krambeck A, Miller NL, *et al.*: Surgical Management of Stones: American Urological Association/Endourological Society Guideline, PART II. *J Urol.* 2016; **196**(4):1161–9.
5. Pearle MS, Pierce HL, Miller GL, *et al.* Optimal method of urgent decompression of the collecting system for obstruction and infection due to ureteral calculi. *J Urol* 1998; **160**(4):1260–4.
6. Mokhmalji H, Braun PM, Martinez Portillo FJ, Siegsmund M, Alken P, Kohrmann KU. Percutaneous nephrostomy versus ureteral stents for diversion of hydronephrosis caused by stones: a prospective, randomized clinical trial. *J Urol* 2001; **165**(4):1088–92.
7. Preminger GM, Tiselius HG, Assimos DG, *et al.* 2007 guideline for the management of ureteral calculi. *J Urol* 2007; **178**(6):2418–34.

CHAPTER 2.17

Surgical treatment options for ureteric stones
Techniques and complications

Zachariah G. Goldsmith, Ghalib Jibara, Michael E. Lipkin, and Glenn M. Preminger

Shock wave lithotripsy

Since the first patient was successfully treated with shock wave lithotripsy (SWL) in 1980, its rapid acceptance and widespread use have made this form of stone therapy a treatment of choice for many patients undergoing intervention for renal and ureteral calculi. Although the basic principles of SWL remain unchanged, a myriad of technological advances and modifications in currently available lithotripters has significantly expanded the clinical applications of lithotripsy. Following the initial success of the first generation lithotripter (Dornier HM3), more than 20 different models of second generation lithotripters (utilizing various energy sources, focusing schemes, coupling media, and stone localization techniques)[1–2] and third generation lithotripters (characterized by their dual imaging and variable power capabilities),[3–6] have also been developed. These advances in lithotripsy technologies have generally led to improved safety, and in some cases, the cost-efficiency, of urolithiasis treatment.

All lithotripters share four main features: an energy source; a focusing device; a coupling medium; and a stone localization system. The objectives for using different types of energy sources include: maximum efficacy (the overall stone-free rate) and maximum efficiency (cost-effectiveness including need for secondary treatments). The two basic types of energy sources for generating shock waves are point sources (electrohydraulic) and extended sources (including piezoelectric and electromagnetic). Shock waves must be focused in order to concentrate their energy on a target calculus, and the the type of shock wave generation dictates the method of focusing used. Coupling with the original Dornier HM3 machine utilizes a 1,000 L water bath to transmit the shock waves to the patient. Second generation lithotripters were designed to alleviate the physiologic, functional, and economic problems of the large water bath, and current models utilize an enclosed water cushion, or a totally contained shock tube, to allow simplified positioning and 'dry' lithotripsy.

Stone localization during lithotripsy is accomplished with either fluoroscopy or ultrasonography. Fluoroscopy provides the urologist with a familiar modality and has the added benefit of effective ureteral stone localization. However, fluoroscopy requires more space, carries the inherent risk of ionizing radiation to both the patient and medical staff, and is not useful, without adjunctive contrast injection, in localizing radiolucent calculi. Sonography-based lithotripters offer the advantages of stone localization with continuous monitoring, and effective identification of even radiolucent stones, without radiation exposure.[3] Additionally, ultrasound has been documented to be effective in localizing stone fragments as small as 2–3 mm, and is as good or better than routine kidney, ureter, and bladder X-ray (KUB) to assess patients for residual stone fragments following lithotripsy.[7] The major disadvantages of ultrasound stone localization include the basic mastery of the use of ultrasonic techniques by the urologist, and difficulty in localizing minimally or non-obstructing ureteral stones. 'Third generation' lithotripters incorporate dual imaging capability—both fluoroscopic and sonographic localization systems available in the same machine—as well as variable shock wave power.

Anaesthesia requirements

Three factors contribute to the need for anaesthesia during shock wave lithotripsy: shock wave pressure (power); area of the shock wave at its skin entry site; and size of the shock wave focal point. The intensity of the shock wave is determined by the type of generator used and the amount of power (usually electrical charge) supplied to the shock wave generator. The original electrohydraulic design delivers the most powerful shock waves, but also causes the greatest amount of discomfort for the patient. Therefore, either general, regional, or local anaesthesia is used in the original spark-gap machines. Recent studies have demonstrated the ability to reduce anaesthesia requirements with the first generation electrohydraulic devices.[8]

The size of the focal point, as well as the area of shock wave entry at the skin are both determined by the configuration of the focusing device. The increased area of skin entry and diminished focal size has lessened the need for general or regional anaesthesia in patients treated on second or third generation lithotripters. Currently, variable power electrohydraulic lithotripters provide the advantage of a wide range of shock wave intensity to allow for either a reduction in anaesthesia requirements, or for increased fragmentation efficacy with higher power under general or regional anaesthesia. Using the lower power setting, however, causes the overall stone-free rate to decrease, while increasing the number of shocks required per treatment, and the retreatment rate. Therefore, in order to achieve an anaesthesia-free status, one must expect the number of secondary treatments to increase. Therefore, the efficiency of that lithotripter will be diminished.

Contraindications to shock wave lithotripsy

Not all ureteral stones are amenable to SWL, and clinical studies have demonstrated that the size and composition of the calculi, along with location and ureteral anatomy, all significantly impact on successful stone fragmentation and clearance. Absolute contraindications to SWL include pregnancy, uncontrolled hypertension, uncontrolled coagulopathy, and obstruction distal to the stone. Relative contraindications may include large stone size, most cystine stones, active infection, and proximate calcified abdominal aortic or renal artery aneurysms.[9] Concerns exist regarding the use of SWL for distal ureteral stones in women of childbearing age, due to theoretical risk of damage to reproductive organs. However, surveys of women treated with SWL for distal ureteral stones have not revealed any significant fertility problems.

Results: According to stone size and location

The first generation Dornier HM3 represents the 'gold standard' in terms of efficacy (overall stone-free rate) in stone fragmentation. As the shock wave pressure and focal point area of second and third generation machines have been reduced, so has the requirement for anaesthesia or analgesia. However, the price paid for anaesthesia-free lithotripsy is an increase in the secondary treatment rates, and a subsequent reduction in efficiency. While there is a compromise in efficiency with the piezoelectric lithotripters, the decreased efficiency may be balanced by the fact that each treatment is an 'office' procedure, without anaesthesia or analgesia. Electromagnetic lithotripsy, usually performed with intravenous or oral sedation, has been found to require a mean of approximately 3,600 shock waves per treatment, with stone-free rates of 69–80% and retreatment rates of 7–21%. The recent large meta-analysis focusing on ureteral stones, conducted by the joint EAU and AUA Nephrolithiasis Guidelines Panel, revealed overall stone-free rates of 74–84%, with the lowest stone-free rates observed for mid-ureteral stones.[10]

With increased stone volume, the efficacy of all lithotripters decreases significantly. In the Nephrolithiasis Guidelines Panel meta-analysis, stones <10 mm demonstrated stone-free rates of 84–90%, while stones >10 mm diameter demonstrated stone-free rates of 68–76%.[10]

Stone location in the ureter is another important determinant of the outcome of shock wave lithotripsy. When stratified by size, stones <10 mm managed with SWL demonstrated stone-free rates of 86%, 84%, and 90% for the distal, mid, and proximal ureter, respectively.[10] For stones >10 mm, observed stone-free rates were 74%, 76%, and 68% in each location, respectively.

Results: According to stone composition

As the stone composition varies, so does the efficacy of shock wave lithotripsy. 'Harder' stones such as calcium oxalate monohydrate and cystine require an increased number of shock waves at higher intensity levels to achieve adequate fragmentation. Even at these higher settings however, results with cystine calculi have been inferior to those with calcium oxalate stones.[11] Most investigators advocate against the use of SWL for large cystine calculi.[12]

Complications of shock wave lithotripsy

Most SWL complications are believed to be minor and self-limiting. Overall rates of major and minor complications have been reported at 0.36% and 5.8%, respectively.[13] Minor complications include transient haematuria, pain, nausea, and vomiting. Steinstrasse, or 'road of stone', can develop when multiple post-SWL fragments become obstructed along the ureter. Most SWL complications are not specific to ureteral calculi, but recent data have focused specifically on complication rates following SWL for ureteral calculi. Rates of Steinstrasse have been reported in 3% patients with ureteral stones <10 mm, and up to 9.5% with 10–20 mm stones.[14] In the large Nephrolithiasis Panel meta-analysis, rates of Steinstrasse were observed to be 4–8%.[10] Obstructing fragments can often be managed with repeated SWL sessions, and stent insertion if necessary. Infectious complications from SWL include urinary tract infection, fever, and sepsis. Rates of sepsis following SWL were observed to be 3–5%.[10]

Conclusions for managing ureteral calculi using shock wave lithotripsy

Shock wave lithotripsy has revolutionized the treatment of urinary calculi, and this modality is an acceptable first-line treatment for most ureteral stones. Major advantages to SWL are its non-invasive nature, low rates of complications, and the ability to perform under sedation. While overall stone-free rates for ureteral stones are approximately 75–85%,[10] superior stone-free rates can be achieved with ureteroscopy (URS), as detailed in the subsequent section.

Ureteroscopy

The advent of ureteroscopy has significantly impacted the management of ureteral calculi. Semi-rigid ureteroscopy can be used in conjunction with pneumatic, ultrasonic, or laser probes to successfully fragment ureteral calculi.[15–17] Flexible, actively deflectable ureteroscopes have made access to the upper ureter and intrarenal collecting system a safer, and at times, less tedious procedure.[18–20] These instruments can be advanced under direct vision or fluoroscopic guidance directly to the level of the stone, which may be fragmented or, when especially small, extracted intact.

Ureteroscopy is a versatile technique that can be used to treat stones throughout the urinary tract,[21–22] though a small working channel often limits the size and usefulness of adjunctive instrumentation which is used for actual stone retrieval. This limitation on available instrumentation has necessitated the use of intracorporeal lithotripsy for the management of most ureteral calculi. Various modalities for intracorporeal stone fragmentation include the holmium laser, and ultrasonic, pneumatic, and electrohydraulic lithotripters. Each class of intracorporeal lithotripter is reviewed in detail elsewhere in this text.

Semi-rigid ureteroscopy

The technique of rigid transurethral ureteroscopy has undergone significant refinements. Early ureteroscopes were large, fixed-lens systems which, although smaller than the cystoscopes of the day, were still cumbersome to use due to their large (11–13 Fr) size, and ureteral dilation was often required for instrument insertion.[23] The current generation of 'semi-rigid' ureteroscopes incorporate fibre-optic light and image bundles into small metal frames.[24–26] This miniaturization of the ureteroscope often obviates the need for ureteral dilation, which saves time and allows the visualization of ureteral mucosa unaltered by the trauma of dilation.

Semi-rigid ureteroscopes utilizing fibre-optic image and light bundles were introduced in the late 1980s. These mini-ureteroscopes were initially designed to use with laser lithotripsy of ureteral calculi. Initial ureteroscope design employed two 2.1 Fr channels for both irrigation and instrument passage. Although these channels were too small to allow use of 'standard' 3 Fr ureteroscopic accessories, they would easily accept laser lithotripsy fibres and guidewires. Since the first mini-ureteroscope was introduced, a number of other semi-rigid fibre-optic ureteroscopes have been developed that utilize either one or two working channels. All share the benefits of significantly reduced outer diameter, and increased ease of passage.

Semi-rigid ureteroscopy: Indications

Semi-rigid mini-scopes are ideally suited for both diagnostic and therapeutic manoeuvres performed in the lower half of the ureter. The semi-rigid mini-scopes are somewhat easier to manipulate in the distal portion of the ureter and therefore allow more rapid ureteroscopic procedures. However, the flexible ureterorenoscope is the ideal instrument to access the proximal half of the ureter, as well as lesions within the renal collecting system. Therefore, a combination approach with both instruments appears to allow easy and safe access to the entire upper urinary tract.

Semi-rigid ureteroscopy: Technique

The standard technique involves passage of a 0.038 inch floppy-tipped guidewire under both cystoscopic and fluoroscopic guidance at the outset of the procedure. The semi-rigid ureteroscope is then passed under direct vision alongside the guidewire to the level of interest. If the ureteral orifice will not accept the ureteroscope, ureteral dilation is performed with a 10 Fr 'introducing' (dual lumen) catheter (Fig. 2.17.1), or if necessary, a standard 15–18 Fr ureteral dilating balloon (Fig. 2.17.2).[27–29] Instruments used with the semi-rigid mini-ureteroscopes include stone baskets and laser lithotripsy fibres.

Flexible deflectable ureteroscopy

Innovations in fibre-optic technology have propelled the further development of flexible ureteroscopes. The widespread use of these new instruments has enabled diagnostic and therapeutic procedures to be performed routinely within the upper ureter and kidney. With the addition of active deflection capabilities, these newer endoscopes are often able to access to the entire upper urinary tract, including all of the intrarenal collecting system,[30–32] and even lesions or stones located in the lower pole or extremely lateral calyces can now be reached.

In addition to the more conventional uses of flexible, deflectable ureteroscopes, many special applications of these instruments have and will be employed to take advantage of their unique capabilities. However, many of the attributes that make flexible ureteroscopy a useful and effective tool can lead to potential complications, as discussed later in this chapter.

Flexible ureteroscopy

Introduction of the flexible ureteroscope

The most difficult aspect of flexible ureteroscopy is the introduction of the instrument into the distal ureter, because the flexibility of these small instruments, which allows their manipulation throughout the entire upper tract, means they flex when they meet even the slightest resistance in the ureter. Dilatation of the intramural ureter may help its subsequent passage. Several techniques

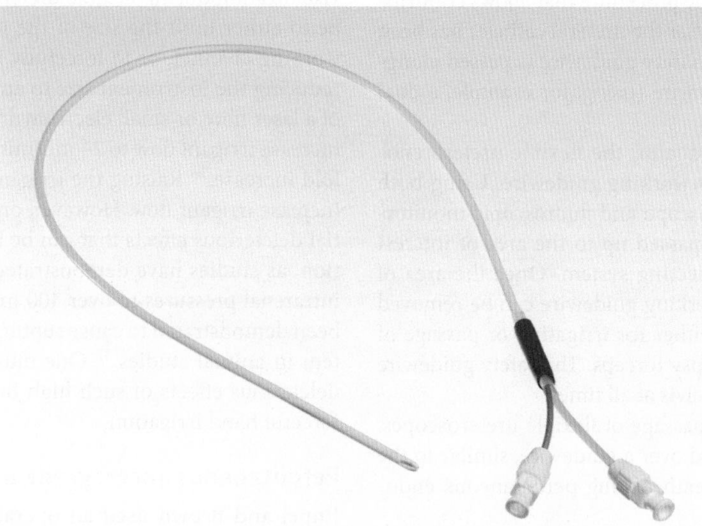

Fig. 2.17.1 A dual lumen catheter both dilates the ureteric orifice and allows rapid placement of a second working wire alongside the initial safety wire.
Courtesy of Boston Scientific.

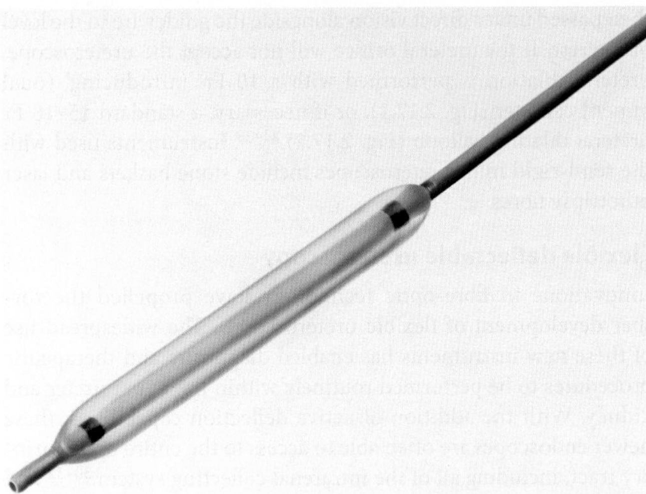

Fig. 2.17.2 A uromax ureteric balloon dilator.
Photographs provided courtesy of Boston Scientific, Copyright © Boston Scientific 2015. Do not copy or distribute. The content of this website is under the sole responsibility of its respective authors and does not represent the opinion of Boston Scientific (BSC). Access to this site does not imply any responsibility for BSC. Please refer to BSC product DFUs for indications, contra indications, precautions and warnings.

can be utilized to pass the flexible ureterorenoscope into the distal ureter. The scope can be passed directly over a guidewire that has been placed between the bladder and the renal collecting system. The instrument is 'followed' fluoroscopically, while the guidewire is held by an assistant to prevent coiling of the wire, and hence the scope in the bladder.

Flexible ureteroscopy: Technique

Our current procedure for passage of an actively deflectable, flexible ureteroscope entails initial placement of a 0.038 inch floppy-tipped wire up to the renal pelvis, usually employing a 6 Fr open end ureteral catheter to help guide the floppy guidewire into the ureteral meatus. Intermittent fluoroscopic monitoring during the entire case is an integral part of the procedure that allows confirmation of ureteroscopic position. After the ureteral catheter has been removed, a second guidewire, or safety guidewire is passed alongside the original (working) guidewire (using, for example, a dual lumen catheter).

After removal of the balloon dilator, the flexible ureterorenoscope is passed directly over the working guidewire. Using both direct vision through the ureteroscope and fluoroscopic monitoring, the flexible ureteroscope is passed up to the area of interest either in the ureter or renal collecting system. Once the area of interest has been reached, the working guidewire can be removed and the working port used for either for irrigation or passage of laser fibres, stone baskets, or biopsy forceps. The safety guidewire remains coiled within the renal pelvis at all times.

Ureteral access sheaths assist passage of flexible ureteroscopes. These sheaths can be easily placed over a guidewire, similar to the placement of a nephroscopy sheath during percutaneous endoscopic procedures.[33–34]

Whatever method is employed, it is strongly recommended that fluoroscopy and a safety guidewire be utilized in every case. Fluoroscopy allows monitoring of the procedure whenever required, and the safety wire provides access to the renal pelvis should a problem occur during the procedure, thereby allowing placement of a ureteral stent if and when required.

Flexible deflectable ureteroscopy: Current applications

The most frequent indication for flexible ureteroscopy is for removal of symptomatic calculi located throughout the ureter or within the intrarenal collecting system. Under direct vision, various intracorporeal lithotripsy devices, stone baskets, grasping forceps or snares can be manipulated to fragment or entrap ureteral or renal calculi, or fragments under direct vision with fluoroscopic monitoring. During withdrawal, distal progression of the scope is monitored fluoroscopically and with visual documentation of the moving ureteral mucosa. This helps assure that the ureter is not entrapped as the stone or fragment is being extracted.

Flexible ureteroscopy: Limitations

With the development of flexible deflectable ureteroscopes, ureteral and renal calculi can often be accessed successfully. However, a major limiting factor in using these smaller endoscopes to manage urinary stones is the small size of the working channel, as the currently available flexible deflectable ureteroscopes have working ports ranging from only 3.6–4.0 Fr in diameter. Current instrumentation to be used through the working ports of these instruments include a wide range of baskets, graspers, electrodes, and laser fibres.

The limited size of the working channels of flexible deflectable ureteroscopes not only limits the instrumentation which can be utilized, but also severely restricts irrigant flow, and this will have a negative impact on visualization during the actual therapeutic procedure. Studies have demonstrated that irrigant flow through a flexible, deflectable ureteroscopes with a 3.6 Fr working channel is only 32 mL/min with gravity irrigation, which is only 40% of the total flow that can be achieved through a 13 Fr rigid ureteroscope.[35] Moreover, when placing a 3 Fr instrument through the 3.6 Fr working channel, the gravity irrigant flow will be reduced to only 2 mL/min, which will significantly impact visualization.

Two potential ways to augment irrigant flow, and thereby enhance visualization during flexible ureteropyeloscopic procedures, would be to either limit the size of the instrument utilized through the working channel, or to forcefully inject irrigant fluids. Indeed, by reducing the instrument size to approximately 1 Fr (about the size of a laser fibre or small electrohydraulic lithotripsy probe), one can increase irrigant flow to 24 mL/min with gravity irrigation, a 1,200-fold increase.[36] Raising the irrigant pressure can also significantly increase irrigant flow. However, one should be aware of the potential deleterious effects that can be induced by forceful hand irrigation, as studies have demonstrated that this manoeuvre can raise intrarenal pressures to over 400 mm Hg, and these pressures have been demonstrated to cause rupture of the intrarenal collecting system in animal studies.[37] One must be cognizant of the potential deleterious effects of such high intrarenal pressures generated by forceful hand irrigation.

Percutaneous antegrade ureteroscopy

Rupel and Brown used an operatively established nephrostomy tract to extract an obstructing renal calculus in 1941.[38] Nearly 15 years later, Goodwin and associates reported the use of percutaneous nephrostomy drainage to provide relief of obstruction and infection.[39] Antegrade URS via percutaneous access

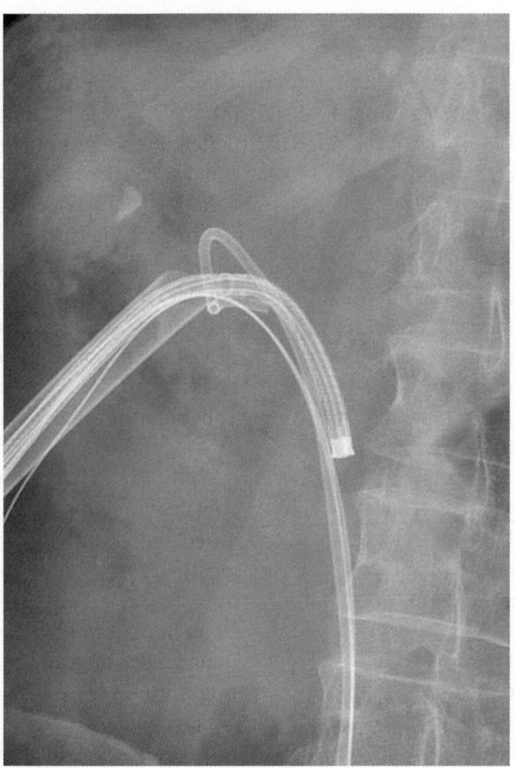

Fig. 2.17.3 Antegrade ureteroscopy to inspect the upper ureter for stones.
Image reproduced courtesy of John Reynard.

to the upper tract can be considered for treatment of very large (>15 mm) impacted stones in the proximal ureter (Fig. 2.17.3).[10] In addition, it is an acceptable approach for concomitant removal of large intrarenal stones, or in patients with lower urinary tract diversion, or other anatomic features which would preclude retrograde access.

The exact technique of percutaneous stone extraction used is specific to the size, location, configuration, and presumed composition of the stone. However, the procedure is always performed with the same four sequential steps employed for percutaneous nephrolithotomy: establishing percutaneous access; dilation of the tract; stone manipulation with fragmentation and extraction; and post-extraction drainage and tamponade of the tract. Techniques of percutaneous access are addressed elsewhere in this volume (Chapter 2.11).

Results: Ureteroscopy

The 2007 joint EAU/AUA Nephrolithiasis Panel Guidelines constitutes the largest review on efficacy of URS for ureteral stones. Overall stone-free rates for ureteral stones treated with URS were 81–94%.[10] As previously described with SWL, efficacy of URS is dependent upon the size and location of the stone. Stones <10 mm demonstrated stone-free rates of 80–97%, while stones >10 mm demonstrated stone-free rates of 79–93%. When stratified by stone location, stones <10 mm demonstrated stone-free rates of 97%, 91%, and 80% the distal, mid, and proximal ureter, respectively. Stone-free rates were 93%, 78%, and 79% in the distal, mid, and proximal ureter, respectively, for stones >10 mm.

Recommending an SWL versus URS approach is a frequent treatment dilemma in the management of ureteral stones. In 2011 the Cochrane Collaboration conducted a meta-analysis of seven trials, in which 1,205 total patients were randomized to SWL versus URS for treatment of ureteral stones.[40] Overall, SWL demonstrated lower stone-free rates versus URS (RR 0.84, 95% CI 0.73–0.96).

An additional outcome metric which appears to differentiate URS from SWL is fewer number of treatments required to achieve stone-free status. In the Nephrolithiasis Panel review, it was not possible to test for a significant difference in procedure counts between SWL and URS due to lack of variance data reported in available clinical trials. Significantly higher rates of retreatment were identified with SWL in the Cochrane review.[40]

Complications of ureteroscopy

Complications of ureteroscopy are usually minor, and in most cases can be treated with placement of an indwelling ureteral stent.[41] The most common complication to develop during ureteroscopy is ureteral perforation, which has been reported in 2–6% of contemporary cases.[42] The perforation is usually a result of stone fragmentation (EHL or laser lithotripsy) as opposed to passage of the ureteroscope. Occasionally, stone material may migrate through a ureteral perforation. Several studies have suggested that there are no long-term sequele if a non-infection-related stone has migrated completely through the wall of the ureter.[43–46] However, if stone fragments remain within the wall, a ureteral granuloma with subsequent stricture formation may result.[47–49]

The most significant complication of ureteroscopic stone retrieval is ureteral avulsion. This complication is usually a result of basketing a stone that is too large to be extracted intact. When in doubt, intracorporeal stone fragmentation should obviate the possibility of avulsion. Although endourologic techniques have been used to manage ureteral avulsion, essentially all these significant complications will require ureteral reconstruction.[50–52]

The joint 2007 AUA/EAU Nephrolithiasis Guidelines Panel examined rates of complications for ureteric stones, including sepsis, Steinstrasse, stricture, ureteral injury, and urinary tract infection.[10] More severe complications, including death and loss of a kidney, were observed to be so rare as to preclude accurate estimate of occurrence. Overall sepsis rates ranged from 2–4%. Steinstrasse ranged from 0–4%, and appeared lower than observed following SWL. Rates of ureteral stricture or injury were reported in 1–4% and 3–6%, respectively. In the Cochrane review, rates of overall complications were significantly lower for SWL, compared to URS (RR 0.54, 95% CI 0.33–0.88).[40]

Ureteroscopy: Conclusions

Technologic advances in endoscope design, digital imaging, intracorporeal lithotripters, and endoscopic accessory devices have revolutionized URS. URS is an acceptable first-line treatment for most ureteral stones.

Adjunctive ureteral stent placement

The efficacy of, and indications for, the use of ureteral stenting as an adjunct to SWL (preoperative) and URS (postoperative) for ureteral stones, is an area of controversy. Internal ureteral stents are associated with high rates of morbidity. When surveyed, up to 80% of patients with double J ureteral stents report bothersome lower urinary tract symptoms and adverse effects on quality of life.[53–54] Patients with an indwelling internal ureteral stent typically report storage symptoms, including frequency, and urgency with or without incontinence. Dysuria, haematuria, and sexual dysfunction are also reported.[53–55] Pain is described most commonly in the groin and flank (60%), followed by bladder (38%), and genitalia (32%). Ureteral stent placement following semi-rigid URS has been associated with increased postoperative flank pain, bladder pain, urinary symptoms, overall pain, and total narcotic use.[56] Given the frequency of these symptoms, a number of investigators have sought to define the utility of ureteral stent placement as an adjunct to SWL and URS.

Pre-shock wave lithroscopy stent placement

The utility and complications for ureteral stent placement prior to SWL have been reviewed in a recent meta-analysis.[57] The results of eight randomized controlled trials of stented versus stentless patients (total n = 876) were analysed. Stone-free rates were equivalent in the stented and stentless group (78.1% vs. 83.0%, $p = 0.27$). Incidence of Steinstrasse appeared to be similar in each group overall, although a significantly higher rate was observed in stentless patients from one study included in the analysis. Notably, the need for auxiliary treatments was equivalent in each group. The only significant difference was identified for incidence of lower urinary tract symptoms, which was significantly higher in the stented group (RR 4.10, 95% CI 2.21–7.61, $p < 0.00001$). Taken together, these results indicate that stent placement prior to SWL may reduce incidence of Steinstrasse, but is associated with a high rates of lower urinary tract symptoms (LUTS), and does not improve stone-free status. Based on these data, the 2016 AUA Guidelines Panel concluded that routine stenting is not recommended as part of SWL.[58]

Post-ureteroscopy stent placement

The effects of postoperative stent placement following uncomplicated URS has been reviewed by a recent meta-analyses. Nabi and colleagues reviewed nine randomized trials of stented versus stentless patients (total n = 831).[59] No significant differences were identified in postoperative analgesia, infection, or stone-free rates. Rates of ureteral strictures were also equivalent in the groups. Incidence of lower urinary tract symptoms were significantly higher in the stented group. However, a trend towards decreased likelihood of unplanned medical visits or hospital admissions was noted with the stented patients, although this did not achieve statistical significance.

The 2016 AUA Guidelines Panel concluded that stenting following uncomplicated URS is optional.[58] The 2007 panel listed the following as clear indications to place a stent following URS: ureteral injury, stricture, solitary kidney, renal insufficiency, or large residual stone burden.

Improving stent discomfort

For patients meeting criteria for stent placement following URS, methods exist to minimize stent-related morbidity. Such manoeuvres include proper selection and placement of the stent, and adjunctive medical therapies.

A number of innovations in stent design have been developed in an attempt to minimize patient discomfort. Currently, no ideal stent material or design has been developed to eliminate morbidity.[60–63] In general, randomized trials have demonstrated equivalent degrees of stent discomfort among stents of different diameters and materials.[64–67] In contrast to stent diameter and material, stent position as well as stent length have been consistently associated with patient discomfort. Multiple studies have identified an association with the presence of the distal stent coil that crosses the midline, or the presence of an incomplete distal coil, with worsened stent symptoms.[68–70] These observations have actually been confirmed in a prospective trial in which 120 patients were randomized to placement of a longer stent (26–28 cm), with the distal coil located across the midline of the bony pelvis and proximal coil in the upper calyx, versus shorter stents (22–24 cm) with a distal coil that did not cross midline, and the proximal coil within the renal pelvis.[71] A significantly increased number of patients reported moderate to severe dysuria, urgency, and worsened quality of life in the group with the longer midline-crossing stents.

Oral agents may be offered to reduce stent morbidity. Extensive level-one evidence supports the use of alpha blockers (tamsulosin 0.4 mg daily, or alfuzosin 10 mg daily) as medical adjuncts in reducing stent-related morbidity. In a meta-analysis by Yakoubi and colleagues, reviewing four randomized trials (with a total of 341 patients), significant decrease in urinary symptoms and pain, and significant improvement in general health with alpha blocker use was observed.[72] An additional meta-analysis again noted a significant reduction Ureteral Stent Symptoms Questionnaire (USSQ) score for urinary symptoms (mean reduction 8.4 [95% CI, 5.6–11.1]) and body pain (mean reduction 7.2 [95% CI, 2.5–11.8]). In addition, a significant benefit was observed with the anticholinergic tolterodine extended release (4 mg daily) in a single randomized trial. When offered to reduce stent-related morbidity, patients should be counselled on the off-label use of these medications.

Evidence-based guidelines for management of ureteric stones

In 2007, the joint EAU and AUA Nephrolithiasis Guidelines Panel developed a guideline for the management of ureteric calculi.[10] Relevant literature documenting stone-free rates, number of procedures performed, spontaneous passage rates, and complications were stratified by stone size and locations, and reviewed in a detailed meta-analysis. For proximal ureteric stones <10 mm, SWL had higher stone-free rates than URS (90% vs. 80%). For proximal ureteric stones >10 mm, URS demonstrated superior stone-free rates (79% vs. 68%). In addition, URS demonstrated significantly superior stone-free rates for distal ureteral stones for all size categories, and a trend towards superiority for mid-ureteral stones. Superior stone-free rates with URS versus SWL were also demonstrated in the 2011 Cochrane review.[40] In addition, higher rates of retreatment were demonstrated for SWL versus URS.

From the 2007 and 2016 Guideline Panel review, the following selected list of treatment guidelines was generated for the management of ureteric stones in the index patient:

- For patients requiring stone removal, both SWL and URS are acceptable first-line treatments
- Patients with bacteriuria should be treated with appropriate antibiotics
- Blind basket extraction without endoscopic visualization should not be performed
- Routine stenting is not recommended as part of SWL
- Stenting following uncomplicated URS is optional

Taken together, for SWL, overall stone-free rates for ureteral stones are approximately 75–85%, and superior stone-free rates can be achieved with URS for most ureteral stones (including distal and mid-ureteral stones of any size, and proximal ureteral stones >10 mm). A notable exception is proximal ureteral stones <10 mm, which demonstrate a 90% stone-free rate with SWL compared to 80% with URS. Compared with SWL, URS achieves a greater stone-free rate for most ureteral stones. Although overall complication rates are low, they appear to be higher than SWL, and this procedure is associated with longer hospital stay.

Further reading

Aboumarzouk OM, Kata SG, Keeley FX, Nabi G. Extracorporeal shock wave lithotripsy (ESWL) versus ureteroscopic management for ureteric calculi. *Cochrane Database Syst Rev* 2011 Dec 7; (12):CD006029.

Chew BH, Lange D. Ureteral stent symptoms and associated infections: a biomaterials perspective. *Nat Rev Urol* 2009; **6**(8):440–8.

Chuong CJ, Zhong P, Preminger GM. Acoustic and mechanical properties of renal calculi: implications in shock wave lithotripsy. *J Endourol* 1993; **7**:437–44.

Fabrizio MD, Behari A, Bagley DH. Ureteroscopic management of intrarenal calculi. *J Urol* 1998; **159**:1139–43.

Joshi HB, Okeke A, Newns N, Keeley FX Jr, Timoney AG. Characterization of urinary symptoms in patients with ureteral stents. *Urology* 2002; **59**(4):511–16.

Preminger GM, Tiselius HG, Assimos DG, *et al.* 2007 Guideline for the management of ureteral calculi. *Eur Urol* 2007; **52**(6):1610–31.

References

1. Preminger GM. Sonographic piezoelectric lithotripsy: More bang for your buck. *J Endourol* 1989; **3**:321–7.
2. Rassweiler J, Henkel TO, Kohrmann KU, Potempa D, Junemann KP, Alken P. Lithotripter technology: Present and future. *J Endourol* 1992; **6**:1–13.
3. Lingeman JE, Newman DM. Dornier MFL 5000 and compact lithotriptors. *Semin Urol* 1991; **9**:225–9.
4. Klein FA. Storz Modulith SL-20: the new optimal acoustic source for extracorporeal lithotripsy. *Semin Urol* 1991; **9**:269–74.
5. Saltzman B. Direx Tripter X-1. *Semin Urol* 1991; **9**:222–4.
6. Bierkens AF, Hendrikx AJ, de Kort VJ, *et al.* Efficacy of second generation lithotriptors: a multicenter comparative study of 2,206 extracorporeal shock wave lithotripsy treatments with the Siemens Lithostar, Dornier HM4, Wolf Piezolith 2300, Direx Tripter X-1 and Breakstone lithotriptors. *J Urol* 1992; **148**:1052–7.
7. Abernathy BB, Morris JS, Wilson WT, Miller GL, Preminger GM. Evaluation of residual stone fragments following lithotripsy: Sonography versus KUB. (pp. 247–54) In: Lingeman JE Newman DM (eds). *Shock Wave Lithotripsy II*. New York, NY: Plenum Press, 1989.
8. Monk TG, Bouré B, White PF, Meretyk S, Clayman RV. Comparison of intravenous sedative-analgesic techniques for outpatient immersion lithotripsy. *Anesth Analg* 1991; **72**:616–21.
9. Streem SB. Contemporary clinical practice of shock wave lithotripsy: A re-evaluation of contraindication. *J Urol* 1997; **157**:1197–203.
10. Preminger GM, Tiselius HG, Assimos DG, *et al.* 2007 Guideline for the management of ureteral calculi. *Eur Urol* 2007; **52**(6):1610–31.
11. Chuong CJ, Zhong P, Preminger GM. Acoustic and mechanical properties of renal calculi: implications in shock wave lithotripsy. *J Endourol* 1993; **7**:437–44.
12. Chow GK, Streem SB. Contemporary urologic intervention for cystinuric patients: Immediate and long term impact and implications. *J Urol* 1998; **160**:341–4; discussion 344–5.
13. Kijvikai K, Haleblian GE, Preminger GM, de la Rosette J. Shock wave lithotripsy or ureteroscopy for the management of proximal ureteral calculi: an old discussion revisited. *J Urol* 2007; **178**(4 Pt 1):1157–63.
14. Soyupek S, Armağan A, Koşar A, *et al.* Risk factors for the formation of a steinstrasse after shock wave lithotripsy. *Urol Int* 2005; **74**(4):323–5.
15. Lyon ES, Kyker JS, Schoenberg HW. Transurethral ureteroscopy in women: a ready addition to the urological armamentarium. *J Urol* 1978; **119**:35–6.
16. Huffman JL, Bagley DH, Lyon ES. Treatment of distal ureteral calculi using rigid ureteroscope. *Urology* 1982; **20**:574–7.
17. Perez-Castro Ellendt E, Martinez-Pineiro JA. Ureteral and renal endoscopy. A new-approach. *Eur Urol* 1982; **8**:117–20.
18. Bagley DH, Huffman JL, Lyon ES. Combined rigid and flexible ureteropyeloscopy. *J Urol* 1983; **130**:243–4.
19. Aso Y, Ohtawara Y, Fukuta K, *et al.* Operative fiberoptic nephroureteroscopy: removal of upper ureteral and renal calculi. *J Urol* 1987; **137**:629–32.
20. Preminger GM, Kennedy TJ. Ureteral stone extraction utilizing nondeflectable flexible fiberoptic ureteroscopes. *J Endourol* 1987; **1**:31–5.
21. Segura JW, Preminger GM, Assimos DG, *et al.* Ureteral Stones Clinical Guidelines Panel summary report on the management of ureteral calculi. *J Urol* 1997; **158**:1915–21.
22. Fabrizio MD, Behari A, Bagley DH. Ureteroscopic management of intrarenal calculi. *J Urol* 1998; **159**:1139–43.
23. Blute ML, Segura JW, Patterson DE. Ureteroscopy. *J Urol* 1988; **139**:510–12.
24. Dretler SP, Cho G. Semirigid ureteroscopy: a new genre. *J Urol* 1989; **141**:1314–16.
25. Huffman JL. Experience with the 8.5 French compact rigid ureteroscope. *Semin Urol* 1989; 7:3–6.
26. Ferraro RF, Abraham VE, Cohen TD, Preminger GM. A new generation of semirigid fiberoptic ureteroscopes. *J Endourol* 1999; **13**:35–40.
27. Clayman RV, Elbers J, Palmer JO, Wassynger W. Experimental extensive balloon dilation of the distal ureter: Immediate and long-term effects. *J Endourol* 1987; **1**:19–22.
28. Huffman JL, Bagley DH. Balloon dilation of the ureter for ureteroscopy. *J Urol* 1988; **140**:954–6.
29. Jarrett TW, Lee CK, Pardalidis NP, Smith AD. Extensive dilation of distal ureter for endoscopic treatment of large volume ureteral disease. *J Urol* 1995; **153**:1214–17.
30. Bagley DH. Removal of upper urinary tract calculi with flexible ureteropyeloscopy. *Urology* 1990; **35**:412–16.
31. Bagley DH. Active versus passive deflection in flexible ureteroscopy. *J Endourol* 1987; **1**:15–18.
32. Grasso M, Bagley D. Small diameter, actively deflectable, flexible ureteropyeloscopy. *J Urol* 1998; **160**(5):1648–53; discussion 1653–4.
33. Spirnak JP, Fleischmann JD. Finlayson ureteral access system: review of 32 cases. *J Endourol* 1991; **5**:237–40.
34. Aslan P, Malloy B, Preminger GM. Access to the distal ureter after failure of direct visual ureteroscopy. *Br J Urol* 1998; **82**:290–1.
35. Wilson TW, Eberhart RC, Preminger GM. Flow, pressure, and deflection characteristics of flexible deflectable ureterorenoscopes. *J Endourol* 1990; **4**:283–9.
36. Wilson WT, Preminger GM. Intrarenal pressures generated during flexible deflectable ureterorenoscopy. *J Endourol* 1990; **4**:135–41.
37. Schwalb DM, Eshghi M, Davidian M, Franco I. Morphological and physiological changes in the urinary tract associated with ureteral dilation and ureteropyeloscopy: an experimental study. *J Urol* 1993; **149**:1576–85.
38. Rupel E, Brown R. Nephroscopy with removal of stone following nephrostomy for obstructive calculous anuria. *J Urol* 1941; **46**:177.
39. Goodwin WE, Casey WC, Woolf W. Percutaneous trocar (needle) nephrostomy in hydronephrosis. *J Am Med Assoc* 1955; **157**:891–4.
40. Aboumarzouk OM, Kata SG, Keeley FX, Nabi G. Extracorporeal shock wave lithotripsy (ESWL) versus ureteroscopic management for ureteric calculi. *Cochrane Database Syst Rev* 2011 Dec 7;(12):CD006029.

41. Harmon WJ, Sershon PD, Blute ML, Patterson DE, Segura JW. Ureteroscopy: current practice and long-term complications. *J Urol* 1997; **157**:28–32.
42. Kramolowsky EV. Ureteral perforation during ureterorenoscopy: treatment and management. *J Urol* 1987; **138**:36–8.
43. Moretti KL, Miller RA, Kellett MJ, Wickham JE. Extrusion of calculi from upper urinary tract into perinephric and periureteric tissues during endourologic stone surgery. *Urology* 1991; **38**:447–9.
44. Evans CP, Stoller ML. The fate of the iatrogenic retroperitoneal stone. *J Urol* 1993; **150**:827–9.
45. Kriegmair M, Schmeller N. Paraureteral calculi caused by ureteroscopic perforation. *Urology* 1995; **45**:578–80.
46. Lopez-Alcina E, Broseta E, Oliver F, Boronat F, Jimenez-Cruz JF. Paraureteral extrusion of calculi after endoscopic pulsed-dye laser lithotripsy. *J Endourol* 1998; **12**:517–21.
47. Dretler SP, Young RH. Stone granuloma: a cause of ureteral stricture. *J Urol* 1993; **150**:1800–2.
48. Grasso M, Liu JB, Goldberg B, Bagley DH. Submucosal calculi: endoscopic and intraluminal sonographic diagnosis and treatment options. *J Urol* 1995; **153**:1384–9.
49. Roberts WW, Cadeddu JA, Micali S, Kavoussi LR, Moore RG. Ureteral stricture formation after removal of impacted calculi. *J Urol* 1998; **159**:723–6.
50. Wise KL, Carson CC. Ileocecal substitution in the treatment of severe ureteroscopy-related ureteral trauma: Report of three cases. *J Endourol* 1990; **4**:143–8.
51. McQuitty DA, Boone TB, Preminger GM. Lower pole calicostomy for the management of iatrogenic ureteropelvic junction obstruction. *J Urol* 1995; **153**:142–5.
52. Postoak D, Simon JM, Monga M, Ferral H, Thomas R. Combined percutaneous antegrade and cystoscopic retrograde ureteral stent placement: an alternative technique in cases of ureteral discontinuity. *Urology* 1997; **50**:113–16.
53. Joshi HB, Okeke A, Newns N, Keeley FX Jr, Timoney AG. Characterization of urinary symptoms in patients with ureteral stents. *Urology* 2002; **59**(4):511–16.
54. Joshi HB, Stainthorpe A, MacDonagh RP, Keeley FX Jr, Timoney AG, Barry MJ. Indwelling ureteral stents: evaluation of symptoms, quality of life and utility. *J Urol* 2003; **169**(3):1065–9; discussion 1069.
55. Hao P, Li W, Song C, Yan J, Song B, Li L. Clinical evaluation of double-pigtail stent in patients with upper urinary tract diseases: report of 2685 cases. *J Endourol* 2008; **22**(1):65–70.
56. Borboroglu PG, Amling CL, Schenkman NS, *et al.* Ureteral stenting after ureteroscopy for distal ureteral calculi: a multi-institutional prospective randomized controlled study assessing pain, outcomes and complications. *J Urol* 2001; **166**(5):1651–7.
57. Al-Awadi KA, Abdul Halim H, Kehinde EO, Al-Tawheed A. Steinstrasse: a comparison of incidence with and without J stenting and the effect of J stenting on subsequent management. *BJU Int* 1999; **84**(6):618–21.
58. Assimos D, Krambeck A, Miller NL, *et al.* Surgical Management of Stones: American Urological Association/Endourological Society Guideline, PART II. *J Urol* 2016; **196**(4):1161–9.
59. Nabi G, Cook J, N'Dow J, McClinton S. Outcomes of stenting after uncomplicated ureteroscopy: systematic review and meta-analysis. *BMJ* 2007; **334**(7593):572.
60. Beiko DT, Watterson JD, Knudsen BE, *et al.* Double-blind randomized controlled trial assessing the safety and efficacy of intravesical agents for ureteral stent symptoms after extracorporeal shockwave lithotripsy. *J Endourol* 2004; **18**(8):723–30.
61. Chew BH, Lange D. Ureteral stent symptoms and associated infections: a biomaterials perspective. *Nat Rev Urol* 2009; **6**(8):440–8.
62. Haleblian G, Kijvikai K, de la Rosette J, Preminger G. Ureteral stenting and urinary stone management: a systematic review. *J Urol* 2008; **179**(2):424–30.
63. Dellis A, Joshi HB, Timoney AG, Keeley FX Jr. Relief of stent related symptoms: review of engineering and pharmacological solutions. *J Urol* 2010; **184**(4):1267–72.
64. Candela JV, Bellman GC. Ureteral stents: impact of diameter and composition on patient symptoms. *J Endourol* 1997; **11**(1):45–7.
65. Erturk E, Sessions A, Joseph JV. Impact of ureteral stent diameter on symptoms and tolerability. *J Endourol* 2003; **17**(2):59–62.
66. Damiano R, Autorino R, De Sio M, *et al.* Does the size of ureteral stent impact urinary symptoms and quality of life? A prospective randomized study. *Eur Urol* 2005; **48**(4):673–8.
67. Joshi HB, Chitale SV, Nagarajan M, *et al.* A prospective randomized single-blind comparison of ureteral stents composed of firm and soft polymer. *J Urol* 2005; **174**(6):2303–6.
68. El-Nahas AR, El-Assmy AM, Shoma AM, Eraky I, El-Kenawy MR, El-Kappany HA. Self-retaining ureteral stents: analysis of factors responsible for patients' discomfort. *J Endourol* 2006; **20**(1):33–7.
69. Rane A, Saleemi A, Cahill D, Sriprasad S, Shrotri N, Tiptaft R. Have stent-related symptoms anything to do with placement technique? *J Endourol* 2001; **15**(7):741–5.
70. Giannarini G, Keeley FX Jr, Valent F, *et al.* Predictors of morbidity in patients with indwelling ureteric stents: results of a prospective study using the validated Ureteric Stent Symptoms Questionnaire. *BJU Int* 2011; **107**(4):648–54.
71. Al-Kandari AM, Al-Shaiji TF, Shaaban H, Ibrahim HM, Elshebiny YH, Shokeir AA. Effects of proximal and distal ends of double-J ureteral stent position on postprocedural symptoms and quality of life: a randomized clinical trial. *J Endourol* 2007; **21**(7):698–702.
72. Yakoubi R, Lemdani M, Monga M, Villers A, Koenig P. Is there a role for alpha-blockers in ureteral stent related symptoms? A systematic review and meta-analysis. *J Urol* 2011; **186**(3):928–34.

CHAPTER 2.18

Management of ureteric stones in pregnancy

Ben Turney and John Reynard

Introduction to management of ureteric stones in pregnancy

Renal colic is the most common non-obstetric cause for abdominal pain and hospitalization during pregnancy.[1] Ureteric stones occur in about 1 in 2,000 pregnancies,[2–4] most (>80%) in the second and third trimesters.[5] Primary management concerns are diagnostic foetal radiation exposure and the potential for adverse perinatal events arising either from the stone or from intervention.

Physiology

During pregnancy, lithogenic and stone inhibitory processes are broadly in balance. Increased renal plasma flow and glomerular filtration rate resulting in hypernatruria, hypercalciuria, and hyperuricosuria[6] combine with a physiological hydroureteronephrosis (partly due to the inhibitory action of progesterone on smooth muscle but mostly due to the mass effect of the gravid uterus[1]) to promote stone formation. They are countered by an increase in urinary levels of stone inhibitors (e.g. magnesium and citrate). Consequently, the incidence of symptomatic nephrolithiasis is comparable to the non-pregnant population.

While previous studies suggested that stone composition in pregnancy is the same as for non-pregnant patients,[7,8] recent papers suggest calcium phosphate stones are more prevalent in pregnant women compared to age-matched non-pregnant women.[9,10]

Symptoms

Pregnant women present with the usual symptoms of renal colic, but distinguishing stone pain from other obstetric and non-obstetric causes of abdominal pain is a diagnostic conundrum.

Risk of perinatal events

Several small case series and some larger observational studies have associated nephrolithiasis with an increased risk of preterm labour, preterm delivery, and premature rupture of membranes, but the data on this is not consistent.[11] Recent large retrospective studies have not found associations between the majority of perinatal events[12–14] and the presence of ureteric stones, and so treatment is directed principally at relieving pain (assuming there is no infection). This goal must be balanced against the risk of inducing premature labour following intervention.

Imaging

Radiation exposure of the foetus should be avoided if possible, but teratogenic risk is low even with computed tomography (CT) and the risks of radiation exposure must be balanced against the risks of failure of or delay in diagnosis of stone disease.[15] Up to 50 mGy has been suggested to be safe in pregnancy. Nonetheless, ultrasound assessment remains the first-line investigation. The physiologically hydronephrotic kidney will inevitably produce diagnostic confusion, but ureteric jets in the bladder and resistive index may help improve accuracy.[16] A resistive index (RI) of 0.7 (sensitivity 45%; specificity 91%; accuracy 87%) or a change in RI more than 0.06 (sensitivity 95%; specificity 100%; accuracy 99%) may be useful in diagnosing a ureteric stone.[17] Transvaginal ultrasound may improve visualization of the distal ureter. IVU, CT, MRI, and renograms have all been evaluated but are not in widespread use currently. Of these, MRI is the most promising as it provides detailed anatomical information without radiation. MR urography may be used when ultrasound fails to obtain a diagnosis. However, in our experience magnetic resonance urography is used so infrequently that radiologists frequently struggle to be able to confirm or refute the presence of a ureteric stone.

Management

Management must optimize safety for the mother and foetus. Infected obstructed systems must be drained. The risks of premature rupture of membranes and preterm labour/delivery must be balanced against the risks of intervention.

Expectant management

As with the non-pregnant patient, conservative management should be first-line. Around 70–80% of stones will pass spontaneously,[5,9,18] although this may be an overestimate due to the limitations of imaging in pregnancy resulting in an overdiagnosis. Loin pain and physiological hydronephrosis seen on ultrasound may be incorrectly attributed to a stone.[10] The patient should be adequately hydrated and pain control optimized with paracetamol and opiate analgesia. In exceptional cases, epidural analgesia may be useful. Non-steroidal anti-inflammatories (NSAIDs) are contraindicated in pregnancy, and the safety and efficacy of medical expulsive therapy is unknown and therefore not recommended. Urinary tract infection is found in up to 50% of pregnant women with stones[2] and is treated depending on sensitivities with an antibiotic that is safe in pregnancy.

Active treatment

Indications for intervention are the same as for the non-pregnant patient, but are influenced by obstetric circumstances. Active treatment options may be temporizing (stent or nephrostomy) or definitive (ureteroscopic stone extraction). Historically, temporizing measures were the only recommended treatment option. However, potential problems associated with temporary drainage mechanisms include recurrent obstruction, infection, nephrostomy displacement, encrustation, infection, and pain. These factors may impact on pregnancy. In recent years, advances in surgical technology and technique have permitted definitive ureteroscopic management of stones during pregnancy.[15] Recent retrospective meta-analysis suggest that ureteroscopy in specialist centres is safe with no evidence of obstetric complications,[15] but small sample size and case selection bias may limit the application of these results to non-specialist centres.[19] Absolute contraindications to ureteroscopy in the pregnant population include the presence of sepsis/infection, inadequate equipment, or experience and a large stone burden necessitating a prolonged ureteroscopy. Of note, lithotripsy is contraindicated in pregnancy due to negative effects on intrauterine growth in animal models and potential risk of foetal death.[20] PCNL is not practical during pregnancy and should be deferred until after delivery.

Further reading

Bánhidy F, Acs N, Puhó EH, Czeizel AE. Maternal kidney stones during pregnancy and adverse birth outcomes, particularly congenital abnormalities in the offspring. *Arch Gynecol Obstet* 2007; **275**(6):481–7.

Burgess KL, Gettman MT, Rangel LJ, Krambeck AE. Diagnosis of urolithiasis and rate of spontaneous passage during pregnancy. *J Urol* 2011; **186**(6):2280–4.

Rosenberg E, Sergienko R, Abu-Ghanem S, *et al.* Nephrolithiasis during pregnancy: characteristics, complications, and pregnancy outcome. *World J Urol* 2011; **29**(6):743–7.

Semins MJ, Matlaga BR. Management of stone disease in pregnancy. *Curr Opin Urol* 2010; **20**(2):174–7.

Srirangam SJ, Hickerton B, Van Cleynenbreugel B. Management of urinary calculi in pregnancy: a review. *J Endourol* 2008; **22**(5):867–75.

Swartz MA, Lydon-Rochelle MT, Simon D, Wright JL, Porter MP. Admission for nephrolithiasis in pregnancy and risk of adverse birth outcomes. *Obstet Gynecol* 2007; **109**(5):1099–104.

References

1. McAleer SJ, Loughlin KR. Nephrolithiasis and pregnancy. *Curr Opin Urol* 2004; **14**(2):123–7.
2. Butler EL, Cox SM, Eberts EG, Cunningham FG. Symptomatic nephrolithiasis complicating pregnancy. *Obstet Gynecol* 2000; **96**(5 Pt 1):753–6.
3. Swanson SK, Heilman RL, Eversman WG. Urinary tract stones in pregnancy. *Surg Clin North Am* 1995; **75**(1):123–42.
4. Drago JR, Rohner TJ, Chez RA. Management of urinary calculi in pregnancy. *Urology* 1982; **20**(6):578–81.
5. Stothers L, Lee LM. Renal colic in pregnancy. *J Urol* 1992; **148**(5):1383–7.
6. Biyani CS, Joyce AD. Urolithiasis in pregnancy. I: pathophysiology, fetal considerations and diagnosis. *BJU Int* 2002; **89**(8):811–8; quiz i–ii.
7. Coe FL, Parks JH, Lindheimer MD. Nephrolithiasis during pregnancy. *N Engl J Med* 1978; **298**(6):324–6.
8. Horowitz E, Schmidt JD. Renal calculi in pregnancy. *Clin Obstet Gynecol* 1985; **28**(2):324–38.
9. Meria P, Hadjadj H, Jungers P, Daudon M; Committee MotFUAU. Stone formation and pregnancy: pathophysiological insights gained from morphoconstitutional stone analysis. *J Urol* 2010; **183**(4):1412–6.
10. Burgess KL, Gettman MT, Rangel LJ, Krambeck AE. Diagnosis of urolithiasis and rate of spontaneous passage during pregnancy. *J Urol* 2011; **186**(6):2280–4.
11. Cormier CM, Canzoneri BJ, Lewis DF, Briery C, Knoepp L, Mailhes JB. Urolithiasis in pregnancy: Current diagnosis, treatment, and pregnancy complications. *Obstet Gynecol Surv* 2006; **61**(11):733–41.
12. Rosenberg E, Sergienko R, Abu-Ghanem S, *et al.* Nephrolithiasis during pregnancy: characteristics, complications, and pregnancy outcome. *World J Urol* 2011; **29**(6):743–7.
13. Bánhidy F, Acs N, Puhó EH, Czeizel AE. Maternal kidney stones during pregnancy and adverse birth outcomes, particularly congenital abnormalities in the offspring. *Arch Gynecol Obstet* 2007; **275**(6):481–7.
14. Swartz MA, Lydon-Rochelle MT, Simon D, Wright JL, Porter MP. Admission for nephrolithiasis in pregnancy and risk of adverse birth outcomes. *Obstet Gynecol* 2007; **109**(5):1099–104.
15. Srirangam SJ, Hickerton B, Van Cleynenbreugel B. Management of urinary calculi in pregnancy: a review. *J Endourol* 2008; **22**(5):867–75.
16. Andreoiu M, MacMahon R. Renal colic in pregnancy: lithiasis or physiological hydronephrosis? *Urology* 2009; **74**(4):757–61.
17. Parulkar BG, Hopkins TB, Wollin MR, Howard PJ, Lal A. Renal colic during pregnancy: a case for conservative treatment. *J Urol* 1998; **159**(2):365–8.
18. Semins MJ, Matlaga BR. Management of stone disease in pregnancy. *Curr Opin Urol* 2010; **20**(2):174–7.
19. Smith DP, Graham JB, Prystowsky JB, Dalkin BL, Nemcek AA. The effects of ultrasound-guided shock waves during early pregnancy in Sprague-Dawley rats. *J Urol* 1992; **147**(1):231–4.
20. Streem SB. Contemporary clinical practice of shock wave lithotripsy: a reevaluation of contraindications. *J Urol* 1997; **157**(4):1197–203.

CHAPTER 2.19

Bladder stones

John Reynard and Ben Turney

Pathology of bladder stones

The majority of bladder stones in Western practice are secondary to underlying pathology—bladder outlet obstruction due to benign prostatic enlargement in men[1] and urethral obstruction from pelvic prolapse or cystocele in women,[2,3] chronic infection in the neuropathic or augmented bladder,[4] or in the neobladder.

As the number of bladder augmentations and neobladders fashioned in women has increased, so the ratio of male:female incidence of stones has fallen.[5,6] The chronically catheterized neuropathic patient has a one in four risk of developing a bladder stone over five years (the same risk whether urethral or suprapubic location of the catheter),[7] with the annual risk of bladder stone formation being 4% when compared with just 0.2% for patients established on intermittent self-catheterization.

The majority of bladder stones arise within the bladder rather than arising from migration of renal stones, as evidenced firstly by very few patients with bladder stones reporting a prior episode of ureteric colic, and secondly by the absence of a calcium oxalate nucleus within the majority of bladder stones.[8]

Secondary bladder stones are composed of struvite if the aetiology is infection and, where the aetiology is obstructive, struvite (indicating the presence of infection related to BOO), calcium phosphate, calcium oxalate, and uric acid.

Foreign body encrustation with calcium oxalate is another aetiological factor, especially in women who have undergone previous gynaecological surgery in the form of sling or mesh procedures, which are either inadvertently passed through the bladder during the initial procedure, or erode into the bladder at a later date.

Primary bladder stones (defined as those without any functional, anatomical, or infectious aetiology) are still common in children in Thailand, Indonesia, North Africa, the Middle East, and Burma, and are usually composed of a combination of ammonium urate, calcium oxalate, uric acid, and calcium phosphate.[9,10] The aetiology is: (a) a diet low in protein and phosphate (breast milk and polished rice or millet) resulting in high peaks of ammonia excretion in the urine (hyperammonuria), which promotes calcium oxalate and ammonium urate precipitation; (b) consumption of oxalate-rich tampala and bamboo shoots; (c) relative dehydration (and hence urine supersaturation with stone-forming elements) from diarrhoea and low fluid intake (as a consequence of inadequate supplies of clean drinking water).

Presentation of bladder stones

The symptoms of primary bladder stones include passage of 'sand' in the urine, abdominal pain, pain on voiding (dysuria), with urinary frequency and haematuria. An unusual symptom (said to be pathognomonic) is pulling of the penis by young boys, a symptom indicative of strangury (painful irritation of the bladder leading to a strong desire to urinate).

Secondary bladder stones may be symptomless especially in the neuropathic patient (an incidental finding on kidney, ureter, and bladder (KUB) X-ray, bladder ultrasound, or on cystoscopy) who has limited or no bladder sensation. In the neurologically intact patient, symptoms include suprapubic or perineal pain, haematuria, urgency, and/or urge incontinence, recurrent urinary tract infection, and hesitancy and poor flow if the stone obstructs the urethra during attempted voiding.

Diagnosis of bladder stones

Most bladder stones are visible on a plain KUB X-ray (Fig. 2.19.1). Many may be seen on a bladder ultrasound if the bladder contains urine at the time of the scan (but not if it is catheterized and therefore empty).

Treatment of bladder stones

The technique of stone removal is determined by the size of the conduit through which access to the bladder is gained. The urethra will accommodate large instruments. Mitrofanoff stomas, if the

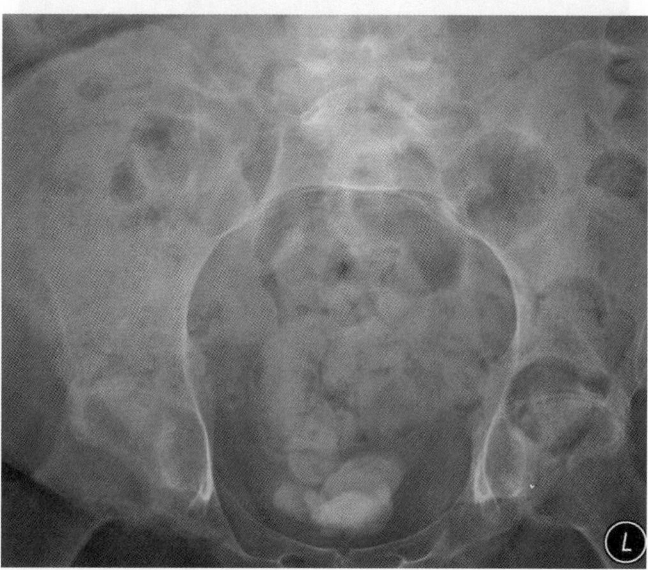

Fig. 2.19.1 Obviously visible bladder stones on a plain abdominal X-ray.
Image reproduced courtesy of John Reynard.

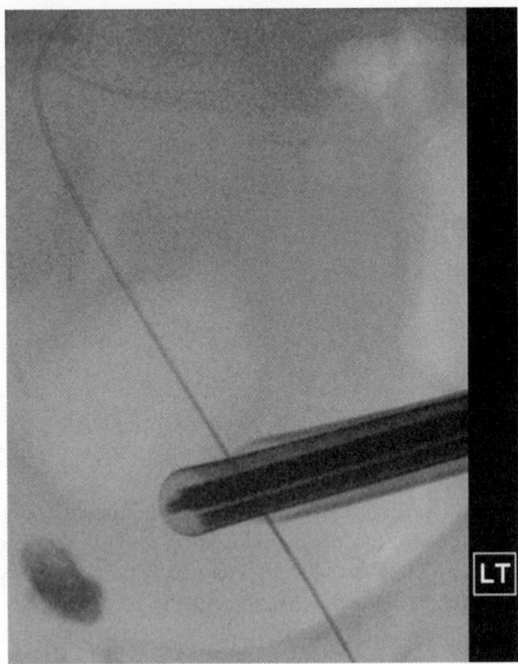

Fig. 2.19.2 Large stones, especially in a neobladder with Mitrofanoff conduit access, only usually require percutaneous or open surgical removal.
Image reproduced courtesy of John Reynard.

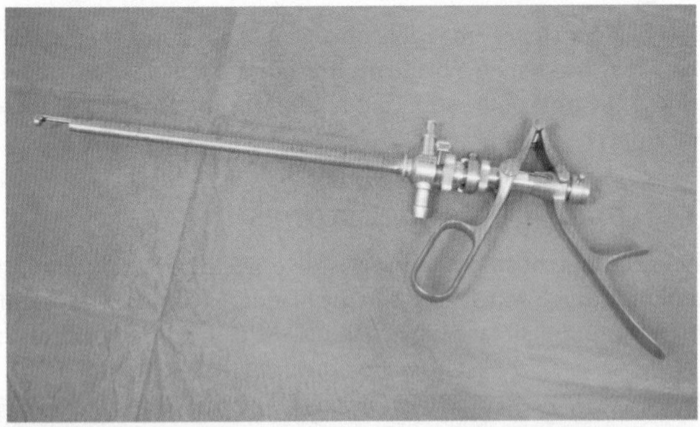

Fig. 2.19.3 The Mauermeyer stone forceps for bladder stone fragmentation.
Image reproduced courtesy of John Reynard.

only route into the bladder (e.g. if the bladder neck has been closed), will only accommodate flexible ureterorenoscopes and small laser fibres. In the augmented or neobladder, mucus and debris may so obscure the view that effective stone fragmentation can be difficult or impossible, and removal of stone fragments, especially where the stone burden is large, may be problematic. Large stones, especially in the augmented or neobladder where access is limited by a narrow Mitrofanoff conduit (Fig. 2.19.2), usually require removal by a percutaneous technique (akin to percutaneous nephrolithotomy).[4,11–16]

Where the urethra can be accessed, most stones are small enough to be removed cystoscopically (endoscopic cystolitholapaxy), using stone-fragmenting forceps for stones that can be engaged by the jaws of the forceps (Fig. 2.19.3). For the larger stone, electrohydraulic lithotripsy (EHL) is still available in some hospitals. However, equipment manufacturers are no longer selling or repairing EHL machines and so EHL will soon no longer be a treatment option. Pneumatic and laser lithotripsy are other options for fragmenting stones too large to be engaged in the jaws of the lithotrite.

Further reading

L'Esperance JO, Sung J, Marguet C, *et al.* The surgical management of stones in patients with urinary diversions. *Curr Opin Urol* 2004; **14**:129–34.

Ord J, Lunn D, Reynard J. Bladder management and risk of bladder stone formation in spinal cord injured patients. *J Urol* 2003; **170**:1734–7.

Schwartz BF, Stoller ML. The vesical calculus. *Urol Clin North Am* 2000; **27**:333–46.

Woodhouse CRJ, Lennon GN. Management and aetiology of stones in intestinal urinary reservoirs in adolescents. *Eur Urol* 2001; **39**:253–9.

Woodhouse CRJ, Robertson WG. Urolithiasis in enterocystoplasties. *World J Urol* 2004; **22**:215–21.

References

1. Smith JM, O'Flynn JD. Vesical stone: the clinical features of 652 cases. *Ir Med J* 1975; **22**:85–9.
2. Schwartz BF, Stoller ML. The vesical calculus. *Urol Clin North Am* 2000; **27**:333–46.
3. Nieder AM, Chun TY, Nitti VW. Total vaginal prolapse with multiple vesical calculi after hysterectomy. *J Urol* 1998; **159**:983.
4. Woodhouse CRJ, Robertson WG. Urolithiasis in enterocystoplasties. *World J Urol* 2004; **22**:215–21.
5. Terai A, Okada Y, Ohkawa T, *et al.* Changes in the incidence of lower urinary tract stones in Japan from 1965 to 1995. *Int J Urol* 2008; **7**:452–6.
6. Yasui T, Iguchi M, Suzuki S, *et al.* Prevalence and epidemiologic characteristics of lower urinary tract stones in Japan. *Urology* 2008; **72**:1000–5.
7. Ord J, Lunn D, Reynard J. Bladder management and risk of bladder stone formation in spinal cord injured patients. *J Urol* 2003; **170**:1734–7.
8. Douenias R, Rich M, Badiani G, *et al.* Predisposing factors in bladder calculi: review of 100 cases. *Urology* 1991; **37**:240–5.
9. Teotia M, Teotia SP. Endemic vesical stone: nutritional factors. *Indian Pediatr* 1987; **12**:1117–21.
10. Ali SH, Rifat UN. Etiological and clinical patterns of childhood urolithiasis in Iraq. *Pediatr Nephrol* 2005; **10**:1453–7.
11. Aron M, Goel R, Gautam G, *et al.* Percutaneous versus transurethral cystolithotripsy and TURP for large prostates and large vesical calculi: refinement of technique and updated data. *Int Urol Nephrol* 2007; **39**:173–7.
12. Demirel F, Çakan M, Yalçinkaya F, *et al.* Percutaneous suprapubic cystolithotripsy approach: for whom? Why?. *J Endourol* 2006; **20**:429–31.
13. Wollin TA, Singal RK, Whelan T, *et al.* Percutaneous suprapubic cystolithotripsy for treatment of large bladder calculi. *J Endourol* 1999; **13**:739–44.
14. DeFoor W, Minevich E, Reddy P, *et al.* Bladder calculi after augmentation cystoplasty: risk factors and prevention strategies. *J Urol* 2004; **172**:1964–6.
15. L'Esperance JO, Sung J, Marguet C, *et al.* The surgical management of stones in patients with urinary diversions. *Curr Opin Urol* 2004; **14**:129–34.
16. Woodhouse CRJ, Lennon GN. Management and aetiology of stones in intestinal urinary reservoirs in adolescents. *Eur Urol* 2001; **39**:253–9.

CHAPTER 2.20

Upper urinary tract obstruction

Mark Sullivan, John Henderson, Inderbir Gill, and Nilay Patel†

Introduction to upper urinary tract obstruction

Urologists are frequently faced with upper tract dysfunction in adults and children. Upper urinary tract obstruction results in obstructive uropathy and nephropathy. The uropathy causes structural and functional changes in the genitourinary tract proximal to the point of obstruction, whilst unrelieved obstruction causes functional and biochemical alterations in the renal parenchyma (nephropathy), which may in turn lead to renal impairment and failure.

Aetiology, pathophysiology, and clinical features

A number of pathologic conditions impair the normal flow of urine from the kidney to the bladder (Table 2.20.1). Obstruction is one of the most common entities in urology. It can occur anywhere from the pelviureteric junction to the meatus, and be either intra- or extraluminal, and acute or chronic. The main consequence of obstruction is urinary stasis and increase in intraluminal ureteral and/or renal pelvicalyceal pressure.

In acute obstruction, such as that seen with ureteral calculi, there will be elevation of the intrarenal hydrostatic pressure. If this persists, it can damage the kidneys, but is initially compensated for by pyelovenous and pyelolymphatic backflow. Urinary extravasation may also occur via calyceal rupture with acute obstruction. Coexistant urinary infection with endotoxin production can further impair ureteral peristalsis.

Long-term obstruction to urinary flow in the ureter will lead to proximal dilatation of the ureter. With dilatation of the ureter, ureteral wall coaptation is inhibited and the dilated ureter becomes inefficient in providing functional contractility. Superadded bacterial infection and endotoxin release will further inhibit smooth muscle activity in the ureter and increase urinary stasis. Following decompression (nephrostomy or stenting) of the upper urinary tract, the renal pelvis and ureter may regain normal tone and function, depending on the duration and degree of obstruction. Radiographic appearances of the upper urinary tract tend to normalize within three to six months unless the obstruction occurred early in foetal development or was long-standing, causing permanent distortion of the ureter and renal collecting system.

† Deceased

Table 2.20.1 Possible causes of obstructive nephropathy

Renal	
Congenital	Polycystic kidney, renal cyst, parapelvic cyst, pelviureteric junction obstruction
Neoplastic	Wilms tumour, renal cell carcinoma, collecting system, transitional cell carcinoma, multiple myeloma
Inflammatory	Tuberculosis, *Echinococcus* infection
Metabolic	Calculi
Miscellaneous	Sloughed papillae, trauma, renal artery aneurysm
Ureter	
Congenital	Stricture, ureterocoele, obstructing megaureter, retrocaval ureter, prune belly syndrome
Neoplastic	Ureteric transitional cell carcinoma, metastatic carcinoma
Inflammatory	Tuberculosis, amyloidosis, schistosomiasis, abscess, ureteritis cystica, endometriosis
Miscellaneous	Retroperitoneal fibrosis, pelvic lipomatosis, abdominal aortic aneurysm, radiation therapy, lymphocoele, trauma, urinoma, pregnancy, radiofrequency ablation
Bladder and urethra	
Congenital	Posterior urethral valves, phimosis, hydrocolpos
Neoplastic	Bladder carcinoma, prostate carcinoma, urethral carcinoma, penile carcinoma
Inflammatory	Prostatitis, paraurethral abscess
Miscellaneous	Benign prostatic hypertrophy, neurogenic bladder, urethral stricture

Obstructive nephropathy also affects renal haemodynamic variables and glomerular filtration. However, these changes depend on the extent and severity of obstruction, unilateral or bilateral obstruction, and whether the obstruction has been relieved or persists.

The differences in uni- or bilateral obstruction were classified based on animal experiments.

Unilateral ureteric obstruction

In unilateral obstruction (UUO), there is a triphasic pattern of renal blood flow (RBF) and ureteral pressure changes. In the first one to two hours, RBF increases together with high renal tubular hydraulic pressure and collecting system pressure. In phase 2, lasting three to four hours, the pressure parameters remain increased, but RBF begins to decline. The third phase, beginning at five hours

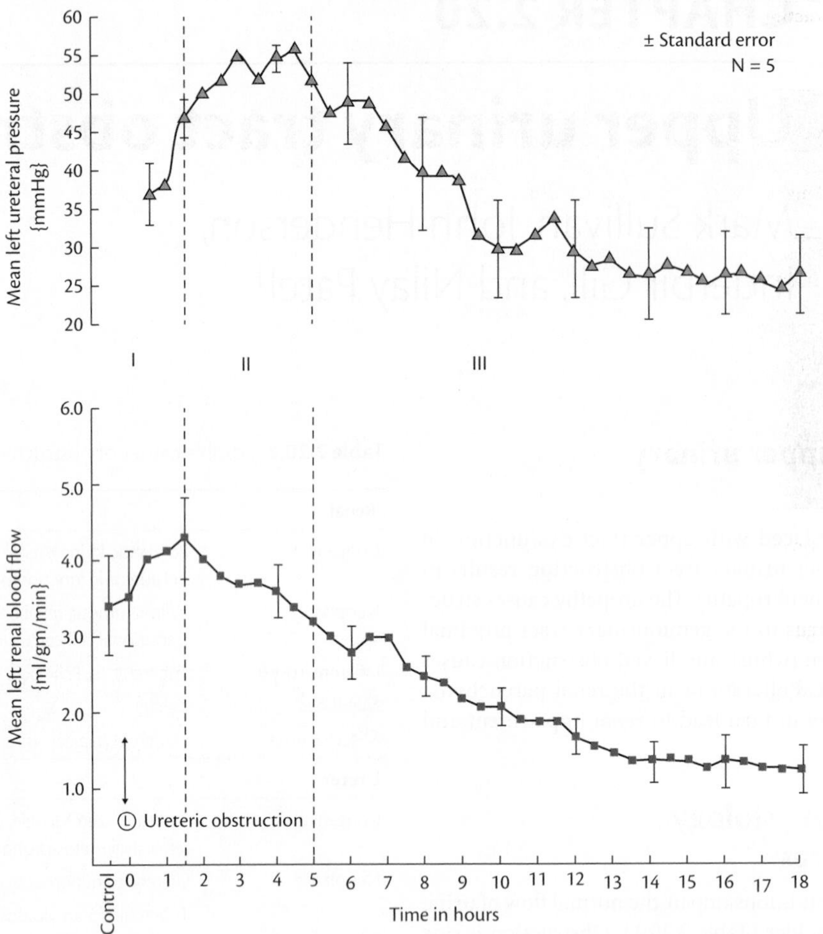

Fig. 2.20.1 Triphasic changes in renal blood flow and ureteral pressure after unilateral obstruction in dogs. Phase I RBF and IPP increase together, phase II RBF decreases while IPP remains high, and phase III RBF and IPP decrease.

Reprinted from *Investigative Urology*, Volume 13, Issue 3, Moody TE *et al.*, Relationship between renal blood flow and ureteral pressure during 18 hours of total unilateral uretheral occlusion: Implications for changing sites of increased renal resistance, pp. 246–51, Copyright Elsevier © 1975.

post-onset of obstruction, characterized by a further reduction in RBF but also the tubular and collecting system pressures.

In the first phase, glomerular filtration rate (GFR) is steady, counterbalanced by tubular pressure increases reducing GFR and renal vasodilatation (mediated via PGE_1 and nitric oxide—NO) increasing GFR. The RBF redistributes itself to the juxtamedullary regions, leaving large regions of the cortex under or non-perfused.

In phase 2, GFR and RBF progressively decline due to reduced glomerular perfusion secondary to afferent vasoconstriction and reduced glomerular capillary pressure. Angiotensin II, thromboxane A2, and endothelin also probably play a role in the reduced RBF in phases 2 and 3 (Fig. 2.20.1).[1]

Bilateral ureteric obstruction

The changes seen here or in a solitary kidney differ from UUO. In the first 90 minutes of bilateral ureteric obstruction (BUO) there is a modest increase in RBF, which is then followed by a profound and prolonged decrease. The early maintenance of renal haemodynamics is probably mediated by NO, while the subsequent profound reduction in RBF is likely mediated via increased renorenal reflex activity. Endothelin, angiotensin II, and thromboxane also probably contribute to the RBF changes. The shift of the blood flow is the opposite to UUO, with increased cortical and reduced medullary flow (Fig. 2.20.2).

Ureteral pressures are higher in BUO than UUO. In the first four to five hours, the ureteral and tubular pressures are increased in both UUO and BUO. Following this, the ureteral pressure remains elevated for at least 24 hours in BUO, while it drops back to preocclusion pressure within 24 hours in UUO. The initial preglomerular vasodilatation followed by prolonged postglomerular vasodilatation maintains the raised ureteral pressures in BUO. In UUO, the initial preglomerular dilation and shortlived postglomerular vasoconstriction are followed by prolonged preglomerular vasoconstriction that will counter the elevations in tubular and glomerular capillary pressures.

If the obstruction is relieved, the diuresis seen in BUO is much greater because of volume expansion, urea, and other osmolytes, and a natriuresis is stimulated probably by atrial natriuretic peptide. In UUO, diuresis is unusual because the contralateral kidney upregulates ion transporters, in particular those controlling sodium balance, to compensate for the changes in the other kidney.[1,2]

Following complete ureteral obstruction in dogs, GFR returns to normal 2 weeks after relief of 7 days of unilateral obstruction, 70% recovery after 14 days of UUO, 30% after 4 weeks, and no recovery after 6 weeks of UUO.[3]

Obstruction	Unilateral			Bilateral		
	IPP	RBF	Total GFR	IPP	RBF	Total GFR
Pre-obstruction	6 mmHg	Normal	↔	6 mmHg	Normal	↔
Early (0–90 mins)	↑ 50–70 mmHg	↑↑ (aff v/d)	↔	↑	↑ then ↓ (aff v/d)	↓
Mid 90–4 hours	↑ 50–70 mmHg	↓ (aff v/c)	↓	↑	↓↓ (eff v/c)	↓
Late 24 hours +	↔ 6 mmHg	↓ (50% of normal)	↓	↑ 12 mmHg	↓↓	↓↓
Blood flow	↓ outer cortex ↑ inner cortex			↑ outer cortex ↓ inner cortex		

Fig. 2.20.2 Summary of changes in intrarenal pressure and renal blood flow in unilateral and bilateral renal tract obstruction. Pressure values are approximate.

In partial ureteric obstruction, similar but slower changes to acute obstruction are seen. In neonates, this has potentially deleterious effects on tubule and glomerulus formation, compromising (though not usually causing complete loss of) renal function.

In adults (dogs), Leahy showed partial obstruction for 14 days was completely reversible; 31% recovery of function was seen after 28 days of partial obstruction and only 8% function was recovered after 60 days of partial obstruction.[4]

Obstruction leads to defects in urinary acidification, mainly in the distal nephron. There is a shift from oxidative metabolism to anaerobic respiration reducing renal ATP, and increasing ADP and AMP.[1]

Histological changes in obstructed kidneys include tubulointerstitial fibrosis, tubular atrophy, apoptosis, and interstitial inflammation.[1]

Clinical presentation

With the routine use of antenatal ultrasound scanning, obstructive uropathy in early life may be suggested by the finding of urinary tract dilatation. This should prompt further investigations and treatment. In a young child, the first presentation of obstruction may be with urinary infection or failure to thrive. In the older child, pain may be a presenting complaint.

Acute obstruction, such as with a renal calculus passing into the ureter, often manifests with severe colicky pain. The location of the pain can correlate with the site of urinary obstruction from proximal obstruction causing loin pain, to vesicoureteric junction obstruction causing isolated scrotal or vulval pain.

Chronic progressive obstruction may be silent and found incidentally on radiological imaging or serum creatinine measurement. A patient with bilateral obstruction, or obstruction of a functionally or anatomically single kidney may describe oliguria, anuria, or uraemic symptoms.

Dietl's crisis, first described in 1864, refers to episodic abdominal pain in association with intermittent renal pelvic obstruction. It is often misdiagnosed and may be accompanied by a palpable mass.

To understand and successfully manage upper tract obstruction, a clear distinction must be made between anatomical and functional studies. *Hydronephrosis* is the finding of renal pelvic and calyceal dilatation. When accompanied by ureteric dilatation, the term *hydroureteronephrosis* is used. It is an anatomical finding suggesting the presence of functional obstruction. The majority of imaging modalities rely on the anatomic finding of hydroureteronephrosis to suggest obstruction. The biochemical findings of increased serum creatinine and decreased GFR may further contribute. However, dilatation of the renal pelvis may be found in the physiological conditions of high urine flow or pregnancy.

Imaging options in upper urinary tract obstruction

Ultrasound (kidneys, ureters, and bladder)

This is a mainstay option, but is an anatomic assessment. It is non-invasive with no radiation exposure and therefore suitable in pregnancy and paediatric patients. It is suitable for patients with renal failure and contrast allergies.

A significant problem is that hydronephrosis is an anatomical finding and not a functional diagnosis. Studies have shown a 35% false negative rate in acute upper tract obstruction.[5] Prior to the routine use of antenatal ultrasound scanning, obstructive uropathy would often present with pain or urinary tract infection. The finding of antenatal urinary tract dilatation should prompt a follow-up ultrasound in the first few weeks after birth to distinguish transient dilatation from more significant disease. Mild dilatation is a common finding and may resolve spontaneously. The anteroposterior diameter of the renal pelvis is an important diagnostic tool and a diameter of greater than 50 mm is almost always associated with significant pathology. The postnatal ultrasound may give clues as to the aetiology, including whether the dilatation is unilateral or bilateral, whether the dilatation includes just the renal pelvis or the ureter and bladder, and whether there is any bladder thickening. Lower urinary tract obstruction accounts for approximately 10% of prenatally detected uropathies. Depending on the likely aetiology, further investigation with diuresis (^{99m}Tc MAG3) or static renography and voiding cystourethrography (VCUG) may be indicated.

Renal resistive indexes measured using Doppler ultrasound may help in diagnosing obstruction but suffers from an inconsistent definition of obstruction in terms of the index figure.[6] Ultrasound can demonstrate crossing vessels at the pelviureteric junction (PUJ).

Intravenous urography

Previously the 'gold standard', this test reveals a delayed nephrogram and pyelogram on the affected side when obstruction is present. Delayed films will eventually reveal the anatomic level of the obstruction. The test relies on GFR and the concentrating ability of the kidney, and is of limited or no use in patients with renal insufficiency. The risk of contrast nephropathy increases with increasing serum creatinine levels and this test should not be used in patients with renal insufficiency. Contrast reaction is also a risk.

Retrograde pyelography

This test is reserved for patients with renal insufficiency or contrast allergy risks or where the anatomy of the upper tract has not been well delineated with other imaging studies. Similarly a loopogram can be performed in people with an ileal conduit or other cutaneous urinary diversion.

Antegrade pyelography

This is used when all other tests have not been possible or have failed, and requires a percutaneous needle or nephrostomy and antegrade contrast injection.

Whitaker test

Reported in 1973,[7] this test involves measurement of the renal pelvic pressure while saline or contrast is infused into the pelvicalyceal system via a percutaneous needle or nephrostomy at a steady rate of 10 mL/min. At the same time, intravesical pressure is monitored via a catheter with transducer tip.

The real value is the renal pressure minus the bladder pressure:

- Pressures <15 cm H_20 = normal;
- 15–22 are indeterminate;
- >22 = obstruction.

The clinical use of this test is limited, however, since it is invasive and the sensitivity and specificity of the test has been reported as low as 79% and 50%, respectively. Individualized infusion rates might improve the sensitivity of the test. For this reason, it is rarely used.

Renal nuclear scans

Renal nuclear scans can be divided into dynamic studies used to investigate function and drainage (e.g. MAG renography) and static studies, which are used to quantify functioning tubular mass (e.g. DMSA scans). The most commonly used radionuclide is metastable 99-Technetium (^{99m}Tc). It emits only gamma rays with an energy level of 140 keV and has a half life of six hours.

Dynamic studies like diuresis renography are important in the diagnosis and follow-up of upper tract obstruction. Mercaptoacetyltriglycine 3 (MAG3) is labelled with ^{99m}Tc, which is filtered at the glomerulus (10%) and secreted in the tubule (90%). The patient is asked to attend well hydrated and normal medication can be continued. Metal objects should be removed from pockets but they may otherwise remain dressed and are asked to void pre-test. A dose of 50–100 Megabecquerels (MBq) MAG3 is given intravenously and images are taken every 20–30 seconds with a gamma camera. Regions of interest are drawn around each kidney and from this, a background region is subtracted to give the final renogram. After 20 minutes, a 0.5 mg/kg bolus of furosemide is given (Fr + 20) if there has not been adequate drainage of either kidney.

The renogram can be divided into the vascular (I), uptake (II) and excretory (III) phases.[8] The vascular phase reflects renal blood flow and split function can be derived from this using a variety of techniques, such as the Rutland method. The normal renogram is obtained after a bolus injection of radionuclide; however, the Rutland method is a mathematical technique which assumes a constant infusion of radionuclide from which differential uptake can be calculated.

There are five characteristic renographic patterns shown in Figure 2.20.3.

If an equivocal response to diuretic is found (type IIIb), the renogram may be refined by giving furosemide 15 minutes before the start (F-15). This reduces the rate of equivocal from 17% to 3%.[6] The type IV curve has a secondary peak called the Homsey's sign. This suggests obstruction occurring only at high urinary flow rates.

These tests involve the use of technetium (99m Tc) labelled agents to provide functional assessment of the upper urinary tract. 99m Diethyl tetra pentacetic acid (DTPA) is a glomerular filtration agent with 20% renal uptake and is also used for dynamic renography.

Both tests have been used to diagnose obstruction. Obstruction can be assessed by the appearance of the clearance curves as above or calculating the time taken to clear half of the radiopharmaceutical from the pelvicalyceal system (the so-called 'half time').

- Half time of <10 minutes = normal.
- 10–20 minutes is equivocal; 20 minutes is obstructed.
- False postive results can be created by renal insufficiency, vesicoureteric reflux, and renal immaturity in neonates.
- Bladder catheterization may be needed in bladder outflow obstruction, neurogenic or non-compliant bladder or low lying pelvic kidneys (where the renal signal can be obscured by tracer in the bladder).
- MAG3 renograms are presently the 'gold standard' imaging test to demonstrate upper urinary tract obstruction.

Computerized tomography

Non-contrast computed tomography (CT) is the most sensitive imaging test for upper tract stones and the test of choice in patients with renal colic type symptoms. It is also superior over ultrasound and intravenous urogram (IVU) in revealing other pathologies which may be relevant (e.g. lymph nodes, retroperitoneal fibrosis, extrinsic malignancies).

Signs of obstruction on CT include ureteral dilatation, nephromegaly, decreased parenchymal density of the involved kidney (compared with other kidney) and perinephric stranding or fluid. These signs have a positive predictive value of 99% and negative predictive value of 95% for acute ureteral obstruction.[9]

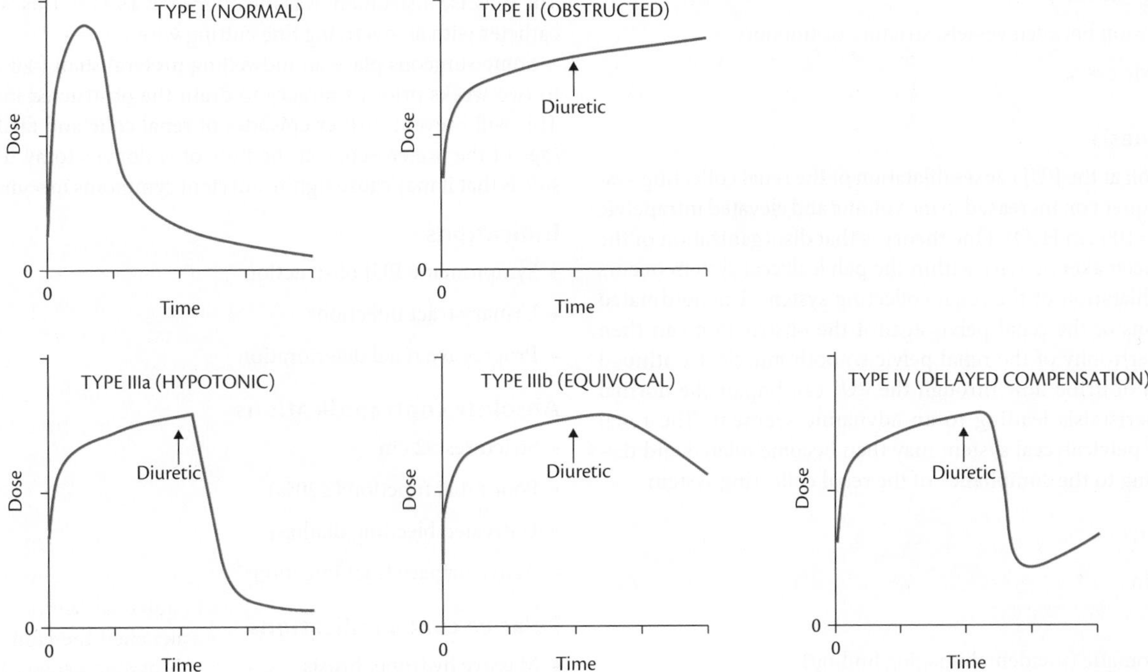

Fig. 2.20.3 The five classic renogram patterns.

Adapted from Rahim Taghavi et al., 'Diuresis Renography for Differentiation of Upper Urinary Tract Dilatation From Obstruction F+20 and F-15 Methods', *Urology Journal*, Volume 4, Number 1, pp. 36–40, Copyright © 2007, under a Creative Commons Attribution 3.0 License. Source: data from O'Reilly PH *et al.*, 'Diuresis renography in equivocal urinary tract obstruction', *British Journal of Urology*, Volume 50, Issue 2, pp. 76–80, Copyright © 1978; and O'Reilly P et al., 'Consensus on diuresis renography for investigating the dilated upper urinary tract. Radionuclides in Nephrourology Group: Consensus Committee on Diuresis Renography', *Journal of Nuclear Medicine*, Volume 37, Number 11 pp. 187–206, Copyright © 1996 Society of Nuclear Medicine and Molecular Imaging.

Contrast-enhanced CT has an increased sensitivity for demonstrating the cause of obstruction compared to an IVU. Triple phase CT's are also very sensitive (97%) for identifying crossing vessels.[10]

Magnetic resonance imaging

The of MRI in upper urinary tract imaging and obstruction has been advanced by a number of developments.

Static MRI imaging (MRU) can be performed either with a static fluid approach relying on the T2 weighted spin echo or using gadolinium enhancement and producing dynamic excretion images. The T2 weighted images produced have been further improved by fast spin echo techniques and post-processing maximum intensity projection. Gadolinium enhancement imaging has been improved using hydration and diuretics, while sensitivity for stones is 93% for T2 weighted spin echo images. Diuretic MRU has been reported to have 100% accuracy for non-calculus obstruction, and 93% for those with obstructing stones.

The use of gadopentoate-DTPA allows both dynamic functional assessment of the pelvicalyceal system comparable to dynamic nuclear scans and much greater anatomical detail than nuclear scans. Differential GFRs can also be calculated from post-imaging processing and contrast washout measured to differentiate dilated non-obstructed from obstructed units.[11] MR angiography (MRA) has a sensitivity for crossing vessels of 95%.[12] Nephrogenic systemic fibrosis has been reported in some patients with renal impairment (GFR <30 mL/min) receiving gadolinium agents and is contraindicated in this group.[13]

Presently, the level of evidence does not support MRI as the preferred imaging modality over CT or ultrasound for the routine evaluation of obstructive uropathy.

Decompression of obstructed upper urinary tracts

Upper urinary tract obstruction that is symptomatic and uncontrolled by analgesia, complicated by infection, bilateral, or causing renal failure requires urgent drainage of the affected side(s). Either percutaneous nephrostomy placement or insertion of internal ureteric stents are options. Certain clinical settings may favour one over the other:

- Percutaneous nephrostomy should be strongly considered if pyonephrosis is suspected and if ureteric stenting is performed, a large diameter stent should be placed.
- No difference is apparent for stone related problems.
- Ureteral stenting may not be as effective for extrinsic ureteric obstruction.[14] Cancer, metastatic disease requiring chemotherapy or radiotherapy, and renal impairment have been shown to be predictors of stent failure (42%) and this failure often (43%) occurs within a week of the stent insertion.[15] Other studies have suggested renal failure alone is the only risk factor for stent failure.[16,17]
- Encrustation increases the risk of stent failure and has been reported to be associated with pregnancy, urinary tract infection (UTI), stasis, dehydration, renal impairment, prolonged dwelling time, and a history of stone disease.[18]

Pelviureteric junction obstruction in adults

Possible causes of PUJ obstruction include:

- congenital malformation;
- calculi;

- crossing vessels;
- compression between vessels, stricture or tumour;
- parapelvic cysts.

Pathogenesis

Obstruction at the PUJ causes dilatation of the renal collecting system consequent on increased urine volume and elevated intrapelvic pressure (>100 cm H_2O). One theory is that disorganization of the normal pacemaker activity within the pelvicalyceal system occurs with the dilatation of the renal collecting system. Uncoordinated contractions of the renal pelvis against the obstruction can then cause hypertrophy of the renal pelvic smooth muscle. Continued disruption of urine flow through the PUJ can impair the normal ureteral peristalsis leading to an adynamic segment. The renal pelvis and pelvicalyceal system may then become dilated and distorted owing to the compliance of the renal collecting system.

Symptoms

- Loin pain
- UTIs
- Asymptomatic (incidental imaging finding)

Investigations

- Urea and electrolytes (U&Es)
- CTKUB + MAG3 renogram

Indications for intervention

- Symptoms due to obstruction
- Impairment of renal function
- Progressive deterioration of split function of affected kidney
- Stone production or infections
- Hypertension (rare)

Numerous treatment options for PUJ obstruction have developed over the last century.

History

1886 Trendelenberg's first description of open repair

1903 Albarran's *ureterotome externe*—the first attempt at endosurgical repair[19]

1943 Davis's intubated ureterotomy[20]

1983 Wickham and Kellett's endoscopic pyelolysis[21]

1984 Ramsay's antegrade endopyelotomy[22]

Retrograde endopyelotomy

This procedure has evolved over the last decade with the development of ureteroscopic and fluoroscopic techniques. It has clear advantages over the antegrade approach, as percutaneous access is not required. Retrograde endopyelotomy can be performed in one of three ways:

1. Using a rigid ureteroscope and a cold/hot/laser incision
2. Flexible ureteroscope with hot/laser incision
3. Using the Acucise device

The Acucise instrument was introduced in 1993.[23] This is a balloon catheter with an overlying fine cutting wire.

Some surgeons place an indwelling ureteral stent (4.8–7 Fr) one to two weeks prior to surgery to drain the obstructed kidney.[24–25] This will prevent further episodes of renal colic and facilitate passage of the ureteroscope at the time of endopyelotomy. The downside is that it may cause significant stent symptoms in some patients.

Indications

- Symptomatic PUJ obstruction
- Urinary tract infections
- Progressive renal deterioration

Absolute contraindications

- Strictures >2 cm
- Poor renal function (≤20%)
- Untreated bleeding diathesis
- Active urinary tract infection[25–27]

Relative contraindications

- Massive hydronephrosis
- High insertion of ureter at PUJ
- Renal anomalies
- Crossing vessels (controversial)[28,29]

Immediate preoperative preparation

- Informed consent—this should include surgeons' results
- Preoperative urine cultures checked—control bacteriuria for 3–5 days if present at preop
- Preoperative clotting screen checked
- Patient side marked and signed by surgeon
- Patient imaging on screen in theatre
- Prophylactic intravenous antibiotics: gentamicin (3 mg/kg) plus cefuroxime (1.5 g) at induction
- Prophylactic heparinization: unfractionated heparin 5,000 international units twice a day or fractionated heparin once a day until discharge
- C-arm in theatre with radiation protection gowns for use

Patient positioning

- Dorsal lithotomy with legs in supports

Operative technique

(i) Advance a stiff guidewire into the kidney under fluoroscopic guidance and place an open-ended ureteral catheter (5 Fr) over the wire. This allows irrigation and protection of the ureter from the electrocautery or laser. Advance the rigid or flexible ureteroscope up the ureter over a separate second guidewire under fluoroscopic control. Once at the PUJ, inspect for pulsations visually. Make a lateral incision with electrocautery or the holmium laser (1–1.5 joule setting). The incision needs to be full-thickness down to the periureteral fat and along the whole length of the stricture. Balloon dilate the PUJ to 24 Fr and place a stent of the surgeons choice over the guidewire and leave *in situ* for four weeks.[25]

(ii) Acucise endopyelotomy also requires initial placement of a stiff guidewire (0.035 inch). Railroad a ureteral catheter over the wire and drain residual urine in the renal pelvis.

(iii) Replace the guidewire. Prealign the Acucise device for a lateral incision and then place over the guidewire and advance to a position just distal to the stricture. Attach the Sureseal II (Applied Medical Resources, Rancho, Santa Margarita, CA) over the guidewire to the centre port of the Acucise catheter and perform a retrograde pyelogram with dilute contrast. Do not use normal saline as the irrigation fluid, and dilute the contrast with sterile water or glycine.

(iv) Advance the Acucise catheter slowly until the radioopaque markers straddle the PUJ. This can be checked by rotating the C-arm laterally. Inflate the balloon partially to confirm correct placement and keep the cautery on standby mode at this point. When the position is correct, inflate the balloon to 2.2cc and apply 75 watts (pure cut) of cautery for three to five seconds. Inflate the Acucise balloon to maximum and leave for 10 minutes to tamponade. Full-thickness incision can be monitored by observing disappearance of the balloon waist or extravasation of contrast. Place a 7 Fr stent or 10 Fr endopyelotomy stent over the guidewire and leave for four to six weeks. Place a Foley catheter initially to monitor active bleeding. The patient can usually be discharged the same day or following morning.[25]

(v) Signs of bleeding after endopyelotomy include haemodynamic instability, a flank mass, ecchymosis, haematuria, and decreased haematocrit.

(vi) Remove the stent between four to six weeks.

Outcomes and complications

Ureteroscopic endopyelotomy (UE) success rates have been reported in 73–90%[30–34] and Acucise in 66–84%.[23,28,35–40] Operative duration is 33–100 minutes with UE and 90.2–180 minutes with Acucise. Hospital stay is 0.38–6 days with UE and 0.52–5 days with Acucise. Both procedures are associated with lower opiate use, hospital stay, and convalescence when compared to antegrade endopyelotomy, open and laparoscopic pyeloplasty.

Complications occur in 2.5–21% of UE and 0–13.6% of Acucise patients. Average drops in haemaglobin are 1.8 mg for both. However, transfusions are reported in 1–9% with transcatheter embolization performed in 4%. UTIs occur in 2% and stent symptoms in 3–5%.

Follow-up is generally required for two years. Most failures have been reported within seven months of surgery, though 13% of failures have been reported in the second year of follow-up. Succesful outcomes ideally require the patient to be completely asymptomatic with normal MAG3 renograms or intravenous pyelography (IVP) postoperatively. Preoperative imaging is required.

No clear difference between UE and Acucise outcomes has been demonstrated and the decision should rest with the surgeon's preference and experience.[23,28,31–40]

Percutaneous endopyelotomy

Percutaneous management of PUJ obstruction was first described by Whitfield and Wickham in 1983.[22] The term 'endopyelotomy' was first coined by Smith *et al.* in 1986.[41] It is specifically indicated for patients who have failed an open approach and is also suited in patients with pyelocalyceal stones that can be managed at the same time.

Indications

- Symptomatic PUJ obstruction
- Urinary tract infections/stones
- Progressive renal deterioration
- Causal hypertension (rarely)

Absolute contraindications

- Strictures >2 cm
- Poor renal function (≤20%)
- Untreated bleeding diathesis
- Active urinary tract infection[26–28]

Relative contraindications

- Massive hydronephrosis
- High insertion of ureter at PUJ
- Renal anomalies
- Crossing vessels (controversial)[29–30]

Immediate preoperative preparation

- Informed consent—this should include surgeons' results
- Preoperative urine cultures checked—control bacteriuria if present for 3–5 days preop
- Patient side marked and signed by surgeon
- Patient imaging on screen in theatre
- Prophylactic intravenous antibiotics: gentamicin (3 mg/kg), plus cefuroxime (1.5 g) at induction
- Prophylactic heparinization: unfractionated heparin 5,000 international units twice a day, or fractionated heparin once a day until discharge
- C-arm in theatre with radiation protection gowns for use

Patient positioning

- Prone position

Operative technique

(i) Access is needed across the PUJ obstruction initially to allow for a safe endopyelotomy. Place an initial hydrophilic guidewire into the kidney under fluoroscopic guidance and then place an open-ended ureteral catheter (5 Fr) over the wire. Remove the wire and then use the catheter for contrast injection to guide percutaneous access. Percutaneous access follows the description under percutaneous nephrolithotomy (PCNL) (Chapter 2.11).[42]

The original description[22] of the technique of endopyelotomy involved a cold knife under direct vision. With two guidewires in place across the PUJ, a direct vision 'endopyelotome' is used. This is a hook-shaped cold knife which can completely incise the full thickness of the PUJ from lumen out to periureteral and peripelvic fat. Extend the incision several millimetres into the normal ureter.

Although a lateral incision is recommended, the ureter does sometimes insert into the renal pelvis on the anterior or posterior wall. In these cases, an anterior or posterior incision may be required, marsupializing the proximal ureter into the renal pelvis. The direct vision allows the crossing vessels to be seen and avoided.

Following complete incision, place a 14/7 Fr endopyelotomy stent over the guidewire in an antegrade fashion. Position the large diameter end of the stent across the PUJ. If this stent is difficult to place, use a standard 8 Fr internal stent. Some authors recommend placing a nephrostomy tube for 24–48 hours, though tubeless percutaneous endopyelotomies have been reported.[43] Place a Foley catheter initially to monitor active bleeding.

Variations of this technique have been described. These include a stent first/hot knife technique.[42] This involves placing the stent in position first with the potential advantages of (i) obviating concern about avulsing the PUJ during stent placement after the endopyelotomy and (ii) better definition of the PUJ allowing more precise incision.

Use a bugbee electrode or Collins knife on a 24 Fr resectoscope to marsupialize the proximal ureter into the renal pelvis. In high-insertion PUJ, extend the incision all the way to the dependent renal pelvis under vision. If stones are present, they should be removed prior to the endopyelotomy so that stone fragments do not migrate into the periureteral and pelvic tissues. Then leave the stent for four to six weeks, and the patient must avoid strenuous exercise for eight to ten days. The use of prophylactic antibiotics for the period of stenting is controversial. Follow-up involves repeat imaging (IVP and MAG3) at one month post stent removal and then 6, 12, and 24 monthly. The duration and timing of imaging follow-up is controversial, but two years is a common period.

Outcomes and complications

Success rates range from 57–100% (mean 73.5%) with follow-up between 2–96 months.[44] More contemporary series report 85–90% success rates and these apply to both primary and secondary PUJ obstruction.[45–47]

Complications are the same as those reported for percutaneous nephrolithotomy (Chapter 2.11). Haemorrhage is slightly less than with PCNL, possibly due to the thinner renal cortex experienced in PUJ obstruction.

Open dismembered pyeloplasty

Kuster described the first pyeloplasty in 1891.[48] Fenger then applied the Heineke-Mickulicz principle to reconstruction of the PUJ.[49] Schwyzer introduced flap techniques in 1923[50] and these were successfully modified by Foley.[51] Culp and DeWeerd reported their spiral flap in 1951,[52] followed by the vertical flap of Scardino and Prince in 1953.[53] In 1949, Anderson and Hynes described the dismembered pyeloplasty.[54]

The dismembered pyeloplasty is generally accepted as the treatment of choice. It can be universally applicable for repair of PUJ obstruction. It has the advantage of being applicable to high ureteral insertions as well as dependent. Reduction of the redundant pelvis or straightening of a lengthy or tortuous ureter. It also allows transposition of the PUJ when crossing vessels are present.

It has become clear with time that whichever technique is used, the anastomosis needs to be widely patent, watertight without tension, and the reconstructed PUJ allows a funnel-shaped transition between pelvis and ureter with dependent drainage.

Indications

- Symptomatic PUJ obstruction
- Urinary tract infections/stones
- Progressive renal deterioration
- Causal hypertension (rarely)
- Impaired renal function in a solitary kidney or bilateral disease

Contraindications

- Lengthy or multiple proximal ureteral strictures
- PUJ obstruction in a small inaccessible intrarenal pelvis

Immediate preoperative preparation

- Informed consent—this should include surgeons' results, ideally including success rates
- Patient side marked and signed by surgeon
- Patient imaging on screen in theatre
- Prophylactic antibiotics: gentamicin (3 mg/kg) plus cefuroxime (1.5 g) at induction
- Prophylactic heparinization: unfractionated heparin 5,000 international units twice a day or fractionated heparin once a day until discharge. There is some controversy with regards to this approach as compressions boots may provide a similar level of protection against thrombosis with fewer haemorrhagic events
- Shave in theatres
- Initial cystoscopy, retrograde pyelogram, and JJ stent insertion (6 Fr, 28 cm) on affected side. We prefer to do this as a final check for stones and stricture as this can alter the surgery required. The stent can be placed antegrade during the pyeloplasty, but we do it at cystoscopy to be certain of its position and to aid in ureteric identification in difficult cases during the pyeloplasty. The stent is 28 cm, as this allows the J at the renal end to lie well above the anastomosis and not potentially cantilever on it, leading to urine leak and loosening of sutures. A JJ stent is placed for dismembered pyeloplasty and all the flap techniques described below
- Catheterize patient—12–14 Ch catheter

Patient positioning

The retroperitoneal approach involves placing the patient in the flank position (lateral decubitus position) with the affected side upwards. Use a flank position with table broken so that lumbar support is raised to maximum height. It is vital to carefully pad soft tissues and bony sites to minimize the risk of neuropraxia, particularly the downside shoulder (axillary roll and posterior back support), hip, knee, and ankle (we prefer a pillow between the legs, buttock support posteriorly, and gel ankle supports). Body warming devices and compression boots are also recommended.

Operative technique

Various incisions have been described, including an anterior extraperitoneal and posterior lumbotomy. An anterior transperitoneal approach may also be of value when there have been previous flank incisions, or when bilateral PUJ obstructions exist. The retroperitoneal approaches allow direct exposure to the PUJ with minimal mobilization of the renal pelvis and proximal ureter, and is our preferred route.

Make a subcostal or supra twelfth rib incision. Cut the various muscle down to the retroperitoneum. Identify the proximal ureter lying on the psoas muscle and dissect it proximally to the renal pelvis. Care needs to be taken not to strip the periuereteral tissue as this may compromise the ureteric blood supply and a successful outcome. Place a stay suture in the ureter distal to the level of obstruction to aid with the anastomosis and orientation. Two stay sutures are then placed at the medial and lateral aspects of the dependent portions of the pelvis. Excise the pelviureteric junction and if the renal pelvis is particularly large, redundant pelvis can also be removed with the PUJ. Spatulate the lateral aspect of the ureter with Potts scissors. Bring the apex of the spatulated ureter to the inferior border of the lateral renal pelvis and bring the medial portion of the ureter to the superior edge of the pelvis. Perform the anastomosis with a fine interrupted or running suture such as 4-0 vicryl. Place the suture full-thickness in a watertight fashion.

If a crossing vessel is present at the PUJ, the dismembered pyeloplasty can be transposed to the other side of the vessel. Lastly, place a 20 Fr Robinson drain in the renal bed.

Postoperatively, remove the urinary catheter when the drain is dry and the drain 24 hours later if there has been no further drainage. The JJ stent is removed via flexible cystoscopy at four weeks post-treatment and the first MAG3 renogram performed at three months.

Other flap techniques

Foley Y-V plasty

This was originally designed for PUJ obstruction with high ureteric insertion. It is contraindicated when transposition is required and pelvic reduction is needed.

Tissue mark a wide-based triangular or V-shaped flap. Position the base of the V on the dependent medial aspect of the renal pelvis and the apex at the pelviureteric junction. Carry the incision from the apex of the flap on to the lateral aspect of the ureter and extend distally beyhond the stenosis and several millimetres onto normal calibre ureter. The initial incision is with a scalpel and then developed with Potts scissors. Bring the apex of the pelvic flap to the apex of ureteric incision distally and suture with 4-0 vicryl. Close the posterior and anterior walls with 4-0 vicryl interrupted sutures.

Culp-DeWeerd spiral flap

This technique is best suited to large extrarenal pelvis with the ureter inserted in the dependent position. It is best suited to a long segment of proximal ureteric narrowing/stricture.

Outline the flap with a broad base situated obliquely on the dependent renal pelvis. The base needs to be lateral to the PUJ (between ureteric insertion and renal parenchyma) to preserve blood supply to the flap. The flap can be spiralled posterior to anterior or vice versa. The length of flap is determined by the length of ureter needed to be bridged, but the ratio of flap length to width should not exceed 3:1 to preserve vascular integrity. It is wise to outline the flap longer than what is perceived to be needed, as flap shrinkage tends to occur when the pelvis is incised. Any excess can be removed. Continue the medial aspect of the flap incision down the ureter beyhond the obstructed segment. Rotate the apex of the flap down to the apex of the ureterotomy and close the posterior and anterior walls with 4-0 vicryl interrupted sutures.

Scardino–Prince vertical flap

This has a limited use today for relatively long areas of proximal ureteral narrowing when the ureter is situated at the medial margin of a large box-shaped extrarenal pelvis. It cannot bridge the same gap as a spiral flap. The flap is similar to the spiral, except the base is situated more horizontally on the dependent aspect of the renal pelvis. Form the flap from straight incisions, which converge from the base vertically to the apex superiorly on the posterior or anterior aspect of the pelvis. The length of the flap is determined by the length of the ureter to be bridged. Continue the medial incision down the ureter beyhond the stricture. Develop the flap with Potts scissors, rotated down, and sutured with a 4-0 vicryl interrupted to the inferior aspect of the ureterotomy. Then close the flap with 4-0 vicryl interrupted sutures.

Outcomes and complications

Mean success rates are 92.6% for dismembered pyeloplasty, and 80.5% for flap techniques. Complication rates are low at 6%. Urinary leak is reported in 5–12.5%, infection in 1.5%, and ileus in 4.6%.[55–59]

Laparoscopic dismembered pyeloplasty

Reconstructive techniques followed quickly after ablative procedures in urological laparoscopy. A variety of pyeloplasty techniques were initially described, although there now appears to be consensus that a dismembered pyeloplasty represents the technique of choice.[60–66] Controversy still exists with respect to crossing vessels and the need for transposition. Laparoscopic pyeloplasty is now an accepted technique, with some authors stating it should be the standard of care in expert hands.[64] Both retro- and transperitoneal approaches have been described.

Indications

- Symptomatic PUJ obstruction
- Urinary tract infections/stones
- Progressive renal deterioration
- Causal hypertension (rarely)
- Impaired renal function in a solitary kidney or bilateral disease

Relative contraindications

- Previous surgery
- Renal inflammation

Immediate preoperative preparation

- Informed consent—this should include surgeons' results, ideally including access injuries, success rates, and conversion rates
- Patient side marked and signed by surgeon
- Patient imaging on screen in theatre
- Prophylactic antibiotics: gentamicin (3 mg/kg) plus cefuroxime (1.5 g) at induction

- Prophylactic heparinization: unfractionated heparin 5,000 international units twice a day or fractionated heparin once a day until discharge. There is some controversy with regards to this approach, as compressions boots may provide a similar level of protection against thrombosis with fewer haemorrhagic events
- Shave in theatres
- Initial cystoscopy, retrograde pyelogram and JJ stent insertion (6 F, 28 cm) on affected side. We prefer to do this as a final check for stones and strictures, as this can alter the surgery required. The stent can be placed antegrade during laparoscopy, but we do it at cystoscopy to be certain of its position and aid in ureteric identification in difficult cases during the laparoscopic pyeloplasty. The stent is 28 Fr as this allows the J at the renal end to lie well above the anastomosis and not potentially cantilever on it, leading to urine leak and loosening of sutures. The stent can be placed or changed (if one has been placed previously) during the laparoscopic procedure being placed in an antegrade direction over a guidewire using the superior port
- Catheterize patient—12–14 Ch catheter

Patient positioning

- Transperitoneal and retroperitoneal approaches: As per laparoscopic simple nephrectomy

Operative technique

(i) *Transperitoneal:* The initial port placement and dissection is the same as for transperitoneal simple nephrectomy, except an 11 cm port replaces the 12 cm port. The proximal ureter is identified lying on psoas with the gonadal vein in close proximity. The proximal ureter is dissected out, being careful not to skin it too much and risk devascularization. The dissection continues proximally to the pelviureteric junction and the pelvis. If a crossing vessel is seen, it will normally lie on the medial aspect of the pelviureteric junction. We prefer to transpose the pelvis and ureter if a vessel is found, and if this is the case, the crossing vessel needs to be dissected out and freed off the peripelvic tissue. The pelvis also needs to be mobilized to allow a tension-free anastomosis. The pelviureteric junction is then incised carefully avoiding cutting the stent. The pelvis and ureter are spatulated at opposing sides. Pelvic reduction can be performed, though is not absolutely necessary. The pelvis and ureter are transposed and an interrupted 3 mg/kg vicryl anastomosis performed intracorporeally. We prefer this to a running suture, which is potentially more ischaemic and if the suture loosens the whole anastomosis can be affected.

The operative site is irrigated with normal saline and a tube drain placed to lie close to but not on the anastomosis and brought out via one of the port sites. Wound closure is as per simple nephrectomy and we remove the catheter on day 2 postoperatively. If there is no further significant drainage from the tube drain in the next 24 hours, this is removed on day 3, the day of discharge.

Patient returns for a flexible cystoscopy and removal of the JJ stent four weeks postoperatively. A MAG3 renogram is performed three months postoperatively.

(ii) *Retroperitoneal:* The initial port placement and dissection is the same as for retroperitoneal simple nephrectomy except an 11 cm port replaces the 12 cm port. The Gerota fascia is opened near psoas transversely. The cut upper leaflet of Gerota is retracted superiorly using a fan retractor and the perinephric fat is swept superiorly and inferiorly to reveal the kidney. The lower pole of the kidney is mobilized and then retracted superiorly. The tissue lying inferior to the lower pole is then dissected carefully by blunt dissection, revealing the renal pelvis and ureter. The same steps as per the transperitoneal approach are followed at this stage with the same postoperative care.

Outcomes and complications

Complication rates are low at 5%. Conversion rates are around 5%, though appear to improve with experience. Success rates based on symptoms and renograms postoperatively are around 94%, comparable with open pyeloplasty results. Mean duration of surgery is two and a half hours and mean hospital stay is three days. These results are all comparable with open pyeloplasty and certainly provide a better cosmetic outcome. Transposition adds 30 minutes to the procedure and there appears to be no significant differences related to the approach. This is however a relatively difficult procedure laparoscopically and it is not presently clear how reproducible the initial results from centres of excellence are.[60–66]

In the elderly, with or without significant co-morbidity, who are experiencing significant complications from their PUJ obstruction, a JJ stent may be an accepted alternative treatment. This can be done under local anaesthetic, although requires six-monthly changes. Poorly functioning renal units (probably <15%) will be best served with nephrectomy.

Pyeloplasty (open/laparoscopic or robotic) has the highest success rates and is considered the gold standard. It is the procedure of choice in patients with gross hydronephrosis, reduced split renal function in the affected kidney, and failed endourological procedures. However, minimally invasive procedures should be offered and have significantly reduced hospital stay and postoperative recovery.

Management of ureteric strictures

Ureteral strictures are relatively rare and occur in a number of benign and malignant conditions:

- Congenital
- Infection (e.g. tuberculosis, schistosomiasis)
- Iatrogenic (e.g. ueteroscopy, gynaecological, or other pelvic surgery)
- Radiation
- Malignancy
- Stones

Symptom

- Loin pain
- UTIs
- Asymptomatic (incidental imaging finding)

Investigations

- U&Es
- IVP/retrograde pyelogram or computed tomography urography (CTU) can define the site and length of the ureteral stricture. CTU will also delineate the anatomy

- Ureteroscopy with biopsy should be performed where aetiology of the stricture is uncertain
- MAG3 renogram will provide split renal function and confirm obstruction. This is important, as the endourological treatments for stricture disease generally need a minimum 25% split function of the affected side to have reasonable success rates[67]

Indications for intervention

- Need to rule out malignancy
- Pain associated with obstruction
- Impairment of renal function
- Recurrent UTIs/pyelonephritis

Ureteric strictures are an uncommon cause of acute obstructive uropathy with the exception of surgical ligatures. They tend to develop slowly, causing chronic obstructive uropathy.

Not all these require surgical intervention. In dealing with ureteral strictures, it is helpful to divide the ureter into proximal, mid, and distal parts. Most strictures occur in the distal ureter due to iatrogenic, malignant, and infective causes.

Nephrostomies or JJ stents can be used both palliatively (i.e. to relieve symptoms) and restore renal function or therapeutically. Therapeutically JJ stents can be used to intubate ureters that have been ligated during other pelvic surgery. The injury has not been recognized during the pelvic surgery and only becomes evident postoperatively. JJ stenting will be therapeutically successful in 50% of cases.

Nephrostomy tracts can be used therapeutically as part of an antegrade approach to a ureteral stricture. Three endoscopic techniques exist to treat ureteral strictures: catheter dilatation, balloon dilatation, and endoincision. These techniques are the same as for the retrograde approach described for PUJ obstruction earlier. Most strictures occur in the distal ureter during endoscopic or pelvic surgery.

The first end-to-end anastomosis of a divided ureter was described in 1885 by Tauffer. Boree reported cutting the ureteric ends obliquely to reduce the chance of stenosis. Transureteroureterostomy was performed in this same time period also. Boari described his bladder flap operation in 1894[68] and ureterointestinal anastomosis was performed by Sir John Simon in 1852. The psoas hitch was popularized by Turner-Warwick and Worth in 1969.[69] Endoscopic procedures to treat or palliate ureteric strictures have been a very recent development and are still undergoing scrutiny.

Conservative management

Specific mention needs to be made of infective causes of ureteric strictures due to tuberculosis and schistosomiasis. In both of these cases, chemotherapy may suffice. The disease needs to be treated when inflammation and oedema rather than fibrosis is present.

With tuberculosis, the lower third of the ureter is most commonly affected. Anti-tuberculous treatment is initiated and weekly full shot IVUs are performed. If there is no improvement after four weeks, prednisolone is added to the regimen. If no further improvement is seen in the subsequent four weeks, surgical intervention is required. An alternative approach to this is to place a JJ stent in combination with the chemotherapy. This may improve outcomes, both in terms of initial success but also subsequent surgery if chemotherapy fails.[70]

Ureteric strictures occur in 25% of cases of urinary schistosomiasis, with 80% of these strictures being in the lower third of the ureter. Medical treatment is the initial approach with or without a JJ stent, and if this fails, surgical intervention.

Endoscopic techniques

Four general endosurgical techniques exist for treating ureteral strictures: JJ stent insertion, catheter dilatation, balloon dilatation, and endoincision.[71,72]

Indications

- Benign ureteric strictures <1 cm
- Palliation of malignant ureteric strictures <1 cm[73–76]

Contraindications

- Stricture length >1 cm[73,75,76]

Relative contraindications

- Ischaemic or radiation-induced strictures
- Mid-ureteric location[73,74,77,78]

Immediate preoperative preparation

- Informed consent—this should include surgeons' results and possible need to do an open surgical repair
- Preoperative urine cultures checked—control bacteriuria for 3–5 days preop
- Patient side marked and signed by surgeon
- Patient imaging on screen in theatre
- Prophylactic intravenous antibiotics: gentamicin (3 mg/kg) plus cefuroxime (1.5 g)
- Prophylactic TED stockings and compression boots
- C-arm in theatre with radiation protection gowns for use

Patient positioning

- Dorsal lithotomy with legs in supports

Operative technique

The first step is to pass a guidewire beyhond the stricture with the tip placed into the kidney under fluoroscopic guidance. A terumo (0.035 inch) guidewire is usually the easiest to place, as its hydrophilic coating facilitates passage through the stricture. Then place an open-ended ureteral catheter (5 Fr) over the wire and exchange the terumo for a stiffer guidewire, such as a Bentson or Amplatz superstiff.

In cases where a suture has been tied around the ureter, if a ureteric stent can be placed this can be definitive treatment and should be left for three months. Following removal, an IVU should be performed four weeks later and if normal, three months on.[79]

For all other cases, catheter or balloon dilatation or retrograde incision via a ureteroscopic or fluoroscopic approach can be performed. Retrogradely, these techniques are similar for those described for PUJ obstruction.

Similarly, a percutaneous approach to upper or mid-ureteric strictures can be performed following the same description of an antegrade endopyelotomy. The incision in the mid-ureter is made laterally, except over the iliac vessels where it is placed anteromedially.

An endoincision also uses the same modalities as endopyelotomy, such as cold knife, endosurgical probe, or laser (Nd:YAG, KTP, or Ho:YAG). The incision needs to be full-thickness. Retroperitoneal fat will be seen usually in the upper, mid, and proximal distal ureter. Retroperitoneal fat may not be seen in marked fibrosis and if the periureteric fat has been seen, no further incision should be made due to the risk of haemorrhage.

Then place a stent (14 Fr nephrostent, 7 or 8 Fr double pigtail, or 10 Fr nephrostomy (for antegrade approach)). Leave a urethral catheter *in situ* for 24–36 hours. If a nephrostomy is in place, perform a nephrostogram after 48 hours and cap the nephrostent. Remove the nephrostent or internal JJ stents after four to six weeks.

If the stricture has caused complete obstruction, it will not be possible to perform a retrograde approach as neither a guidewire or contrast will pass.[80,81] The limits of the stricture need to be ascertained from a combined nephrostogram and retrograde ureterogram. If the occlusion is <1 cm an endosurgical approach can be tried, but if >1 cm then open surgery is recommended.[81]

If the complete obstruction is in the proximal or middle ureter, the technique described for approaching the completely obstructed PUJ is followed. The indwelling stent should be left for 12 weeks.[81]

If the distal ureter is the site of complete obstruction, place a nephrostomy tube. A purely fluoroscopic or combined fluoroscopy and endoscopic incision can then be followed.

In the fluoroscopic approach, introduce a stiff guidewire via the nephrostomy antegrade to the proximal level of the stricture. Fill the bladder with contrast. Use the C-arm to position the guidewire tip, pointing directly at the bladder in both anteroposterior and lateral views.

Introduce a cystoscope and forcibly advance the guidewire into the bladder. Once the guidewire enters the bladder, grasp it, and bring it out through the urethral meatus. Pass a 4–8 mm balloon dilator antegrade into the stricture and dilate for 10 minutes. Then place either a nephrostent or an indwelling ureteric stent with a nephrostomy. If a nephrostomy is placed, a nephrostogram is performed on day 3 after surgery and removed if no extravasation is seen. The stents are left for 6–12 weeks.

The second option is to place an antegrade guidewire to the proximal level of the stricture, followed by a flexible ureteroscope over the wire. Introduce a resectoscope with a Collings knife attached, or an optical urethrotome urethrally. Position the cystoscope so it lies next to the flexible ureteroscope using the C-arm.

Turn off the cystoscope light and theatre lights and make the incision to the bright light coming from the ureteroscope. Once the ureteroscope is uncovered, retrieve the guidewire, and place a nephrostent or indwelling stent, plus nephrostomy and a urethral catheter left *in situ*.

If a nephrostomy is placed, a nephrostogram is performed on day 3 after surgery and removed if no extravasation. If perivesical fat is seen at the time of incision, a cystogram is performed at 7–10 days and the catheter removed if no leak is seen. The urethral catheter is removed on day 2 after surgery otherwise. The stent remains in place for 4–6 weeks.[82]

An alternative for totally obstructed ureters if the above fail is a nephrovesical stent.[82] This involves inserting one end of the stent in the renal pelvis via a percutaneous nephrostomy puncture. The body of the stent is then tunnelled subcutaneously towards the bladder. The distal end of the stent is then placed into the bladder via a percutaneous puncture. The stent needs to be changed every four months using a combined cystoscopic and percutaneous cut-down technique.

Outcomes and complications

Ureteric stent insertion for ligatures will succeed in 50% of patients, while balloon dilatation is successful in 55% (range 45–80) of cases. Endoureterotomy has been reported to achieve patency in 70% (range 55–80). The wide variability is down to differences in technique, data collection, and type of stricture. However, the length of stricture is the most important determinant, with those >1 cm rarely responding to an endosurgical approach. Ischaemic strictures (40% success) do less well than non-ischaemic ones (58% success).

Strictures in the upper and lower ureter that can be marsupialized at their upper border into the renal pelvis or bladder, respectively, do better tha mid-ureteric and those bounded by normal ureter on either end, 80% versus 25%. The duration of the stricture has not been shown to clearly influence the outcome.[70–84]

Metallic stents have also been used to treat unfavourable ureteric strictures. Numerous stents have been described: Wallstents, Palmer-Schatz, Accuflex, Memokath. The first three are meshed stents which allow urothelial ingrowth and are incorporated into the ureter. If complications occur their removal is often impossible.

Management of retroperitoneal fibrosis

First described in 1905 by Albarran,[85] in this rare condition sheets or plaques of collagenous fibrous tissue are deposited on the posterior abdominal wall. The fibrosis can trap the ureters, compressing them and pulling them medially. The ureteric wall cannot stretch due to the fibrosis which prevents urine bolus transmission and leads to subsequent upper tract obstruction. Men are affected twice as often as women, with a mean age of presentation at 50–60 years.

Causes

- Idiopathic (two-thirds of cases)
- Inflammatory aortic aneurysms (15%)
- Intraperitoneal sepsis
- Drugs (e.g. beta-blockers), ergot (methysergide, LSD), chemotherapy, analgesics, dopamine agonists
- Urinary extravasation
- Haemorrhage
- Trauma
- Radiation
- Inflammatory bowel disease
- Collagen disorders
- Fat necrosis

- Malignancy (e.g. carcinoid, Hodgkins/non-Hodgkins lymphoma, sarcomas, carcinomas of colon, prostate, breast, stomach)
- Infection (e.g. tuberculosis, histoplasmosis, actinomycosis)
- Surgery (e.g. lymphadenectomy, colectomy, hysterectomy, aortic aneurysmectomy)

Treatment is usually surgical to relieve ureteral obstruction except with inflammatory aneurysms, where corticosteroids may be indicated as first-line treatment. Patients with significant renal impairment benefit from drainage of the upper urinary tracts, either with JJ stents or nephrostomy. This should be performed prior to definitive surgery as it will improve renal function, fluid and electrolyte balance, and acid-base balance.

Indications

- Retroperitoneal fibrosis due to all causes other than inflammatory aortic aneurysms and malignancy, where stenting and treatment of the malignancy is first line
- Failed medical treatment of retroperitoneal fibrosis

Relative contraindications

- Retroperitoneal fibrosis secondary to inflammatory aortic aneurysms
- Elderly or debilitated patients

Immediate preoperative preparation

- Informed consent—this should include surgeons' results, ideally including access injuries, transfusion rates, and conversion rates
- Patient side marked and signed by surgeon
- Patient imaging on screen in theatre
- Prophylactic intravenous antibiotics: cefuroxime (1.5 g) at induction
- Prophylactic heparinization: unfractionated heparin 5,000 international units twice a day or fractionated heparin once a day until discharge; plus TED stockings and compression boots intraoperatively
- Abdominal shave in theatres
- Catheterize patient—12–14 Ch catheter

Patient positioning

- Supine

Operative technique

The principles of surgery are threefold:

- Ureterolysis
- Lateralization
- Omental wrapping

If JJ stent(s) have not been previously placed, they should be at the beginning of surgery. They will help to protect and identify the ureter(s) during ureterolysis.

Although the fibrotic process may present with unilateral obstruction, it is recommended that bilateral procedures are performed, as later involvement of the contralateral ureter is almost inevitable.

First, make a midline laparotomy incision. Incise the posterior peritoneum in the midline between the duodenum and the inferior mesenteric vein, and develop flaps of posterior peritoneum exposing both ureters in the retroperitoneum. It is usually easiest to identify the ureters proximally where they are dilated and may not be encased in the fibrous plaque. Alternatively, mobilize the ascending and descending colons and sweep medially. Incise the posterior peritoneum over the ureters and dissect off the ureters medially.

Ureterolysis is then performed. It is relatively straightforward once the correct plane is found. An initial sharp dissection is often required to enter this plane, but following this, blunt dissection frees up the ureter. Perform this along the whole of the involved segment. Biopsy the fibrous tissue for histological assessment.

Once the ureters are completely lysed, they can be managed in one of several ways. Either (i) transplanted intraperitoneally; (ii) transposed laterally and retroperitoneal fat interposed between the ureters and the fibrosis; or (iii) wrapped in omental fat.

In (i), the freed ureter is brought anterior to the posterior peritoneal flap. The flap is then tacked laterally onto psoas or the lateral abdominal side wall so the ureters now lie intraperitoneally.

With (ii), retroperitoneal fat is interposed between ureter and the fibrotic plaque.

The omental wrap (iii) involves four steps.[86] Firstly, liberate the hepatic and splenic flexures by dividing the hepatocolic and splenocolic ligaments and fully mobilize the ascending and descending colons medially. With the second step, detach the greater omentum from the transverse colon along its bloodless line of adhesion. Thirdly, divide the omentum in the midline and free each half from the greater curvature of the stomach by dividing some of the short gastric vessels on either side of the midline. The right half of the omentum receives its arterial blood supply from the gastroepiploic branch of the pancreaticoduodenal artery and the left side by the middle colic artery. Wrap the omental flaps completely around each ureter, extending from the hilum of the kidney to the point where the ureter crosses the common iliac artery.

The fibrosis can invade the ureter, though usually only a short segment is involved. Resection of the ureter and ureteroureterostomy is necessary, or if extensive ureteral invasion is present, an ileal ureter may be required.

Outcomes

Recurrent obstruction is reported in 10–50% of cases.[87–90] Development of obstruction in the apparently uninvolved kidney in unilateral obstruction occurs in 20–40%.[87,88] Mortality is between 5–28% in some series, however many of these occur years after surgery and appear to be related to age, the degree of renal impairment preoperatively, and co-morbidity.[87] Ureteric leak is seen in 14–17%,[88–89] intestinal obstruction in up to 14%,[81] ileus in 6%,[82] recurrent UTI in 17%,[82] aortic thrombosis in 6%,[82] wound infection in 11%, and deep vein thrombosis in 10–11%.[88,89]

Ureteric reimplantation

Various open surgical techniques to treat ureteral strictures have been described and which is adopted depends on the position and length of ureteric defect to be bridged, but intraoperative flexibility is required. Ureteric reimplantation can also be used for distal ureteric injuries either occurring intraoperatively or secondary to trauma, or for distal ureteric tumours following local excision.

Ureteroureterostomy

This technique can only be used for short defects, as tension on the anastomosis will nearly always lead to an anastomotic stricture. The determination of whether adequate mobility can be achieved is often only possible intraoperatively.

Indications

- Ureteric stricture ≤2–3 cm in upper/mid-ureter[90–91]

Contraindications

- Ureteric strictures >3 cm
- Lower third ureteric stricture[90–91]

Immediate preoperative preparation

- Informed consent
- Patient side marked and signed by surgeon
- Patient imaging on screen in theatre
- Prophylactic intravenous antibiotics: Cefuroxime (1.5 g) plus gentimicin (3 mg/kg) at induction
- Prophylactic heparinization: unfractionated heparin 5,000 international units twice a day or fractionated heparin once a day until discharge, plus TED stockings and compression boots intraoperatively
- Abdominal shave in theatres
- Catheterize patient—12–14 Ch catheter

Patient positioning

- Lateral (loin incision, upper ureter), supine (Gibson incision, mid-ureter).

Upper ureter

Operative technique

A subcostal incision is made. Skin, connective tissue, and muscle layers opened as previously discussed.

Develop the retroperitoneal space with the peritoneum mobilized and retracted medially. The ureter is attached to the posterior peritoneum and is usually most easily identified as it crosses the common iliac vessels. Mobilize the ureter using a right angle. Care needs to be taken to preserve the adventitia, which loosely attaches the blood supply to the ureter. The ureter is mobilized as the clinical setting dictates, and this equates to avoiding tension on the anastomosis once the strictured area has been excised. Minimal handling of the ureter with non-toothed forceps is recommended. Correctly orientate the ureter and then spatulate the two ends for 5–6 mm. Perform the spatulation in both ureteral ends at 180 degrees to each other. Place a 4-0 vicryl suture in the corner of one ureteral segment and the apex of the other. Suture the opposite corner and apex similarly. Run interrupted sutures up each side of the anastomosis. Place a JJ stent before completion of closure (methylene blue is put into the bladder via the catheter and visualization of the refluxing methylene blue at the anastomotic site indicates correct positioning of the stent in the bladder). Mobilize retroperitoneal fat or omentum to surround the anastomosis. Place a 20 Fr Robinson drain close but not over the anastomosis. The Foley catheter can usually be removed after 1–2 days.

Then remove the drain can when there has been 24–48 hours of minimal drainage (<50 mL) post catheter removal. If drainage persists, the fluid should be sent for creatinine assessment which will determine if it is urine or serous fluid. Finally, endoscopically remove the JJ stent via a flexible cystoscope at four weeks.

Outcomes

Success rates are 90%[92]—fistula have been reported in up to 4%.

Ureteroneocystostomy

Indications

- Ureteric stricture ≤4–5 cm in lower ureter
- Lower third ureteric injuries <5 cm from bladder due to intraoperative injury or trauma[90,91]
- Laparoscopic and robotic approaches have been described for these procedures

Contraindications

- Lower ureteric strictures >5 cm[90,91]

Immediate preoperative preparation

- Informed consent
- Patient side marked and signed by surgeon
- Patient imaging on screen in theatre
- Prophylactic intravenous antibiotics: Cefuroxime (1.5 g) plus gentimicin (3 mg/kg) at induction
- Prophylactic heparinization: unfractionated heparin 5,000 international units twice a day or fractionated heparin once a day until discharge, plus TED stockings and compression boots intraoperatively
- Abdominal shave in theatres
- Catheterize patient—12–14 Ch catheter

Patient positioning

- Supine

Operative technique

This involves an extravesical Lich-Gregoire reimplantation[85,86] via a lower midline or Pfannensteil incision. An extraperitoneal approach is adopted ideally. Identify the ureter as it crosses the common iliac arteries and proximally mobilize. Take care not to skeletonize the ureter and thereby preserving its adventitia and blood supply. Excise the affected length of ureter. Perfom a direct ureteroneocystostomy if a tension-free anastomosis is possible. Fill the bladder with saline via the catheter until it is moderately full. Dissect the peritoneum off the posterior aspect of the bladder where implantation is intended. Preserve major blood vessels (e.g. superior vesical artery) during perivesical dissection. Open the serosal and muscular layers of the detrusor along a straight course cephalad to the ureterovesical junction and the opening continued through the bladder mucosa. Placement in the more mobile lateral bladder wall is discouraged, as this may result in ureteral kinking. It is not necessary to tunnel the ureter and the ureter is placed intraluminally. JJ stents are controversial, but Foley catheters are placed urethrally. The detrusor is then closed over the ureter with 3-0 PDS or vicryl sutures. A 20 Robinson drain is placed in the perivesical space, and the Foley catheter is removed at 7–10 days and JJ stent at 6–8 weeks if placed.

Outcomes

Incidence of complications after the repair of an iatrogenically injured ureter is not reported. Complication rates after repair of traumatic injuries is 25%.[93–96] Prolonged leakage at the anastomosis is the commonest genitourinary complication, presenting as urinoma, abscess, or peritonitis. Drain placement at the time of surgery minimizes this risk and allows its earlier identification. Delayed complications include ureteral stricture and retained ureteral stent leading to stone formation.

Ureteroneocystotomy plus psoas hitch

This procedure was first described by Zimmerman *et al.* in 1960.[97] It has the advantage of maintaining urothelial continuity. It also avoids compromising the function of a normal contralateral ureter and avoids the risks of chronic urinary tract infections and electrolyte abnormalities, problems associated with transureteroureterostomy and ileal substitution, respectively.

Indications

- Ureteric stricture ≤6–10 cm in lower ureter[90,91] (up to pelvic brim generally)
- Lower third ureteric injuries <10 cm from bladder due to intraoperative injury or trauma
- Distal ureteral fistulas
- Distal ureteric tumours
- Failed ureteroneocystostomy[90,91]

Contraindications

- Lower ureteric strictures >10 cm
- Small, contracted bladder[90,91]

Operative technique

The initial operative preparation and patient position is the same as for a neocystostomy. Make a lower midline or Pfannensteil incision. Develop the space of Retzius and mobilize the bladder, dividing the contralateral obliterated umbilical artery, freeing the peritoneal attachments, and dividing the vas deferens or round ligaments. This will usually provide adequate bladder mobility to bridge the ureteral defect, but if not, the urachus, ipsilateral obliterated umbilical artery, and superior vesical artery can also be divided.

Identify the affected ureter is as it crosses the iliac vessels and mobilize it down to the diseased segment. Divide the ureter just proximal to the diseased segment. Place a fine stay suture on the normal proximal ureter. Fill the bladder with 200 mL normal saline and then enter the bladder via an anterior or oblique anterior cystotomy. Place the surgeon's finger directly into the bladder, advancing the ipsilateral bladder to the psoas muscle. Fix the bladder to the psoas tendon using two to four zero PDS sutures. The sutures are placed vertically to avoid injury to the genitofemoral nerve and not too deep, to avoid branches of the femoral nerve. The bladder is fixed prior to the reimplantation to avoid kinks in the distal ureter. Then reimplant the ureter using either a non-refluxing submucosal tunnel or a refluxing-type direct reanastomosis. Place a JJ stent and close the bladder with full-thickness running 20 vicryl sutures. A 20 F Robinson drain is placed in the perivesical space. Lastly, remove the JJ stent at 7–14 days.

Outcomes

Success rates are >95%. The commonest complications are urinary fistulas and ureteral obstruction. A direct refluxing anastomosis does not appear to carry greater complications when compared to non-refluxing.

Ureteroneocystotomy plus Boari flap

First described by Boari in 1894, this technique is required for lower ureteric strictures between 125 cm long[90,91] or to bridge lower ureteric defects 10–15 cm long. A spiralled Boari flap can reach the renal pelvis in some circumstances. Bladder outlet obstruction and neurogenic dysfunction should ideally be addressed preoperatively.

Indications

- Ureteric stricture ≤15 cm in lower and mid-ureter[90,91]
- Lower third ureteric injuries <15 cm from bladder due to intraoperative injury or trauma
- Distal ureteral fistulas
- Distal ureteric tumours

Contraindications

- Lower and mid-ureteric strictures >15 cm
- Small, contracted bladder[90,91]

Operative technique

The initial operative preparation and patient position is the same as for a neocystostomy. Make a lower midline or Pfannensteil incision. A midline incision however allows easier access to the upper ureter. Develop the space of Retzius and mobilize the bladder, dividing the umbilical ligaments, freeing the peritoneal attachments, and dividing the vas deferens or round ligaments and contralateral superior vesical artery. Mobilize the upper ureter down to the diseased or injured portion taking care to preserve the adventitia.

Identify the ipsilateral superior vesical artery or one of its branches as the posterolateral bladder flap is outlined based on this vessel. Fill the bladder with 200 mL normal saline.

Mark out the base of the flap at least 4 cm in width. Continue the flap obliquely across the anterior bladder wall with the tip of the flap being at least 3 cm in width. The flap length should equal the estimated ureteral defect plus 3–4 cm if a non-refluxing anastomosis is desired. An open-ended ureteric catheter can be placed in the contralateral ureter at this point to protect it during the surgery and removed prior to closing the bladder.

Secure the distal end of the flap to the psoas minor tendon or psoas major muscle with two to four 20 vicryl sutures. Deliver the ureter through the posterior flap and spatulate anteriorly. Perform a standard mucosa to mucosa anastomosis with interrupted 4-0 vicryl, making sure there is no tension. Some authors propose routine placement of a JJ stent in the affected ureter, though this remains controversial.[6] The flap is then rolled anteriorly and closed using a continuous 2-0 vicryl suture. The ureteral adventitia can be secured to the distal aspect of the flap with 4-0 vicryl and the base of the flap secured to the psoas with 3-0 vicryl. Close the bladder in one or two layers with 2-0 vicryl. The bladder is drained with a urethral catheter. A Robinson or similar drain is placed in the pelvis adjacent to the Boari flap.

A cystogram is performed two weeks postoperatively and if the bladder is healed, the urethral catheter can be removed.

Outcomes

Successful outcomes are seen in 85% of patients. Recurrent stricture formation is the commonest complication (A tunnelled and cuff anastomosis rather than an end-to-end anastomosis reduces this complication significantly). Early complications of wound and urinary sepsis occur in 20% and 10%, respectively.[98–100]

Repair of ureterocoele

Ureterocoeles are cystic dilatation of the terminal ureter. They occur more frequently in females (4:1) and almost exclusively in whites; 10% are bilateral and 80% arise from upper poles of duplicated systems. Single system ureterocoeles (often referred to as simple ureterocoeles) are usually seen in adults and tend not to have the severe obstructive and dysplastic problems associated with duplex systems. They can however be complicated by stones and infection. Under these circumstances, surgery may be required, and for single system intravesical ureterocoeles, this can be achieved endoscopically.

Indications

- Single system intravesical ureterocoeles[101]

Relative contraindications

There is continuing controversy with regards to

- Ectopic ureterocoeles
- Duplex collecting systems[101]

Operative technique

The initial operative preparation and patient position is the same as for a cystoscopy. The bladder is assessed cystoscopically. The ureterocoele is (i) incised or (ii) punctured. Keep the bladder relatively empty.

(i) Make a transverse full-thickness incision distally on the ureterocoele as close to the bladder as possible without rupturing the bladder. A Collins knife, cold knife, or metal stylet of a ureteral catheter can be used. If a Collins knife is used, set the cautery to cutting at 150 watts.

(ii) Perform the puncture with a 3 Fr Bugbee electrode. Set the cutting current to 150 watts. Place the Bugbee electrode low on the front ureterocoele wall and puncture. Apply flank pressure to visualize urine efflux post puncture, confirming adequate drainage.

Successful decompression of the upper tract can be documented by a kidney, ureter, and bladder ultrasound one month postoperatively.

Outcomes

No data is available from adult endoscopic incision. Data from paediatric series show reoperation rates of 0–100% for all cases of endoscopic incision/puncture. For intravesical single systems, the rates are lower (7–50%) than for ectopic ureterocoeles. Successful decompression is common (94%) and the incidence of recurrent urinary tract infections appears to be reduced.[101–103]

Further reading

Cendron M, Sant GR, Klauber GT. Ureteral pathophysiology. (pp. 61–92) In: *Pathophysiologic Principles of Urology*. Oxford, UK: Blackwell Scientific Publications, 1996.

O'Reilly PH. Standardization of the renogram technique for investigating the dilated upper urinary tract and assessing the results of surgery. *BJU Int* 2003; **91**(3):239–43.

Reynard J, Mark S, Turner K, Armenakas N, Feneley M, Sullivan M. Laparoscopic urological surgery and Surgery for upper tract obstruction and other ureteric surgery. In: Reynard J, Mark S, Turner K, Armenakas N, Feneley M, Sullivan M (eds). *Urological Surgery*. Oxford, UK: Oxford University Press, 2010.

Whitaker RH, Buxton-Thomas MS. A comparison of pressure flow studies and renography in equivocal upper urinary tract obstruction. *J Urol* 1984, **131**:446–9.

References

1. Cendron M, Sant GR, Klauber GT. Ureteral pathophysiology. (pp. 61–92) In: *Pathophysiologic Principles of Urology*. Oxford, UK: Blackwell Scientific Publications, 1996.
2. Moody TE, Vaughn ED, Gillenwater JY. Relationship between renal blood flow and ureteral pressure during 18 hours of total unilateral uretheral occlusion. Implications for changing sites of increased renal resistance. *Invest Urol* 1975; **13**(3):246–51.
3. Vaughan ED Jr, Gillenwater JY. Recovery following complete chronic unilateral ureteral occlusion: Functional, radiographic and pathologic alterations. *J Urol* 1971; **106**:27–35.
4. Leahy AL, Ryan PC, McEntee GM, *et al.* Renal injury and recovery in partial ureteric obstruction. *J Urol* 1989; **142**:199–203.
5. Laing FC, Jeffrey RB jr, Wing VW. Ultrasound vs excretory urography in evaluating acute flank pain. *Radiology* 1985; **154**:613–6.
6. Tublin ME, Bude RO, Platt JF. Review. The resistive index in renal Doppler sonography: where do we stand? *AJR Am J Roentgenology* 2003; **180**(4):885–92.
7. Whitaker RH, Buxton-Thomas MS. A comparison of pressure flow studies and renography in equivocal upper urinary tract obstruction. *J Urol* 1984, **131**:446–9.
8. O'Reilly PH. Standardization of the renogram technique for investigating the dilated upper urinary tract and assessing the results of surgery. *BJU Int* 2003; **91**(3):239–43.
9. Smith RC, Verga M, McCarthy S, Rosenfield AT. Diagnosis of acute flank pain: value of unenhanced helical CT. *AJR Am J Roentgenol* 1996; **166**(1):97–101.
10. El-Nahas AR, Abou-El-Ghar M, Shoma AM, *et al.* Role of multiphasic helical CT in planning surgical treatment for pelvi-ureteric junction obstruction. *BJUI* 2004; **94**:582–7.
11. Chu WC, Lam WW, Chan KW, *et al.* Dynamic gadolinium-enhanced magnetic resonance urography for assessing drainage in dilated pelvicalyceal systems with moderate renal function: preliminary results and comparison with diuresis renography. *BJUI* 2004; **93**(6):830–4.
12. El- Nahas AR, Abou-El-Ghar M, Refae HF, *et al.* Magnetic resonance imaging in the evaluation of pelvi-ureteric obstruction: an all in one approach. *BJUI* 2007; **99**(3):641–5.
13. Broome DR, Girguis MS, Baron PW, *et al.* Gadodiamide-associated nephrogenic systemic fibrosis: why radiologists should be concerned. *AJR Am J Roentgenol* 2007; **188**(2):586–92.
14. Docimo SG, Dewolf WC. High failure rate of indwelling ureteral stents in patients with extrinsic obstruction: experience at 2 institutions. *J Urol* 1989; **142**:277–9.
15. Chung SY, Stein RJ, Landsittel D, *et al.* 15 year experience of management of extrinsic ureteral obstruction with indwelling ureteral stents. *J Urol* 2004; **172**(2):592–5.
16. Rosevear HM, Kim SP, Weizler DL, *et al.* Retrograde ureteral stents for extrinsic ureteral obstruction: nine years experience at the University of Michigan. *Urology* 2007; **70**(5):846–50.

17. McCullough TC, May NR, Metro MJ, Ginsberg PC, Jaffe JS, Harkaway RC. Serum creatinine predicts success in retrograde ureteral stent placement in patients with pelvic malignancies. *Urology* 2008; **72**(2):370–3.
18. Singh I, Gupta NP, Hemal AK, *et al.* Severely encrusted polyurethane ureteral stents: management and analysis of potential risk factors. *Urology* 2001; **58**(4):526–31.
19. Albarran J. Operations plastiques et anastomoses dans la traitment des retentions de veim. These Paris, 1903.
20. Davis DM, Strong GH, Drake WM. Intubated ureterotomy: A new operation for ureteral and ureteral pelvic strictures. *Surg Gynaecol Obstet* 1943; **76**:513–23.
21. Wickham JEA, Kellet MJ. Percutaneous pyelolysis. *Eur Urol* 1983; **9**:122–4.
22. Ramsay JWA, Miller RA, Kellett MJ, *et al.* Percutaneous pyelolysis: Indications, complications, and results. *Br J Urol* 1983; **56**:586–8.
23. Chandoke PS, Clayman RV, Stone AM, *et al.* Endopyelotomy and endoureterotomy with the Acucise ureteral cutting balloon device: preliminary experience. *J Endourol* 1993; **7**:45–51.
24. Thomas R, Monga M, Klein EW. Ureteroscopic retrograde endopyelotomy for management of ureteropelvic junction obstruction. *J Endourol* 1996; **10**:141–5.
25. Nakada SY, Johnson M. Ureteropelvic junction obstruction: Retrograde endopyelotomy. *Urol Clin N Am* 2000; **27**(4):677–84.
26. Badlani GH, Karlin G, Smith AD. Complications of endopyelotomy: Analysis in series of 64 patients. *J Urol* 1988; **140**:473–5.
27. Kim FJ, Herrell SD, Johoda AE, *et al.* Complications of Acucise endopyelotomy. *J Endourol* 1998; **12**:433–6.
28. Preminger GM, Clayman RV, Nakada SY, *et al.* A multicentre clinical trial investigating the use of a fluoroscopically controlled cutting balloon catheter for the management of ureteral and ureteropelvic junction obstruction. *J Urol* 1997; **157**:1625–9.
29. Shalhav AL, Giusti G, Elbahnasy AM, *et al.* Endopyelotomy for high-insertion ureteropelvic junction obstruction. *J Endourol* 1998; **12**:127–30.
30. Van Cangh PH, Wilmart JF, Opsomer RJ, *et al.* Long-term results and late recurrence after endoureteropyelotomy: A critical analysis of prognostic factors. *J Urol* 1994; **151**:934–7.
31. Clayman RV, Basler JO, Kavoussi LR, *et al.* Ureteronephroscopic endopyelotomy. *J Urol* 1990; **144**:246–52.
32. Conlin MJ, Bagley DH. Ureteroscopic endopyelotomy at a single setting. *J Urol* 1998; **159**:727–31.
33. Meretyk I, Meretyk S, Clayman RV. Endopyelotomy: Comparison of ureteroscopic retrograde and antegrade percutaneous techniques. *J Urol* 1992; **148**:775–83.
34. Thomas R, Monga M, Klein EW. Ureteroscopic retrograde endopyelotomy for management of ureteropelvic junction obstruction. *J Endourol* 1996; **10**:141–5.
35. Nadler RB, Rao GS, Pearle MS, *et al.* Acucise endopyelotomy: Evolution of a less-invasive technology. *J Urol* 1996; **156**:1094–7.
36. Faerber GJ, Richardson TD, Farah N, *et al.* Retrograde treatment of ureteropelvic junction obstruction using the ureteral cutting balloon catheter. *J Urol* 1997; **157**:454–8.
37. Gelet A, Combe M, Ramackers JM, *et al.* Endopyelotomy with the Acucise cutting balloon device. *Eur Urol* 1997; **31**:389–93.
38. Kim FJ, Herrell SD, Johoda AE, *et al.* Complications of Acucise endopyelotomy. *J Endourol* 1998; **12**:433–6.
39. Gill HS, Liao JC. Pelvi-ureteric junction obstruction treated with Acucise retrograde endopyelotomy. *Br J Urol* 1998; **82**:8–11.
40. Cohen TD, Gross MB, Preminger GM. Long-term follow up of Acucise incision of ureteropelvic junction obstruction and ureteral strictures. *Urology* 1996; **47**:317–23.
41. Badlani G, Karlin G, Smith AD. Percutaneous surgery for ureteropelvic junction obstruction (endopyelotomy): technique and early results. *J Urol* 1986; **135**:26–8.
42. Streem SB. Percutaneous endopyelotomy. *Urol Clin N Am* 2000; **27**(4):685–93.
43. Bellman GC, Davidoff R, Candela J, *et al.* Tubeless percutaneous renal surgery. *J Urol* 1997; **157**:1578–82.
44. Gerber GS, Lyon ES. Endopyelotomy: Patient selection, results and complications. *Urology* 1994; **43**:2–10.
45. Kletscher BA, Segura JW, LeRoy AJ, *et al.* Percutaneous antegrade endoscopic pyelotomy: Review of 50 consecutive cases. *J Urol* 1995; **155**:701–3.
46. Motola JA, Badlani GH, Smith AD. Results of 212 consecutive endopyelotomies. An 8 year follow up. *J Urol* 1993; **149**:453–6.
47. Shalhav AL, Giusti G, Elbahnasy AM, *et al.* Adult endopyelotomy: Impact of aetiology and antegrade versus retrograde approach on outcome. *J Urol* 1998; **160**:685–9.
48. Kuster: Ein fall von resection des ureter. *Arch Klin Chir* 1892; **44**:850.
49. Fenger C. Operation for the relief of valve formation and stricture of the ureter in hydro or pyonephrosis. *JAMA* 1894; **22**:335.
50. Schwyzer A. New pyeloureteric plastic operation for hydronephrosis. *Surg Clin North Am* 1923; **3**:1441.
51. Foley FEB. New plastic operation for stricture at the ureteropelvic junction. Report of 20 operations. 1937. *J Urol* 2002; **167**(2 Pt 2):1075–95; discussion 1096.
52. Culp OS, DeWeerd JH. A pelvic flap operation for certain types of uretero-pelvic obstruction. Preliminary report. *Mayo Clin Proc* 1951; **26**:483–8.
53. Scardino PL, Prince CL. Vertical flap ureteropelviplasty: Preliminary report. *South Med J* 1953; **46**:325–31.
54. Anderson JC, Hynes W. Retrocaval ureter: A case diagnosed preoperatively and treated successfully by a plastic operation. *Br J Urol* 1949; **21**:209–14.
55. Graversen HP, Tofte T, Genster HG. Uretero-pelvic stenosis. *Int Urol Nephrol* 1987; **19**:245–51.
56. Guys JM, Borella F, Montfort G. Ureteropelvic junction obstructions: prenatal diagnosis and neonatal surgery in 47 cases. *J Paediatr Surg* 1988; **23**:156–8.
57. Mikkelson SS, Rasmussen BS, Jensen TM, *et al.* Long-term follow up of patients with hydronephrosis treated by Anderson-Hynes pyeloplasty. *Br J Urol* 1992; **79**: 121–4.
58. Nguyen DH, Aliabadi H, Ercole CJ, *et al.* Non-intubated Anderson-Hynes repair of uretero-pelvic junction obstruction in 60 patients. *J Urol* 1989; **142**:704–6.
59. Eden CG. Treatment options for pelvi-ureteric junction obstruction: implications for practice and training. *Br J Urol* 1997; **80**:365–7.
60. Kavoussi LR, Peters CA. Laparoscopic pyeloplasty. *J Urol* 1993; **150**:1891–4.
61. Janetschek G, Peschel R, Altarac S, *et al.* Laparoscopic and retroperitoneoscopic repair of ureteropelvic junction obstruction. *Urology* 1996; **47**:311–6.
62. Moore RG, Averch TD, Schulman PG, *et al.* Laparoscopic pyeloplasty: experience with the initial 30 cases. *J Urol* 1997; **157**:459–62.
63. Bauer JJ, Bishoff JT, Moore RG, *et al.* Laparoscopic versus open pyeloplasty: assessment of objective and subjective outcome. *J Urol* 1999; **162**:692–5.
64. Moon DA, El-Shazly MA, Chang CM, Gianduzzo TR, Eden CG. Laparoscopic pyeloplasty: evolution of a new gold standard. *Urology* 2006; **67**(5):932–6.
65. Davenport K, Minervini A, Timoney AG, Keeley FX Jr. Our experience with retroperitoneal and transperitoneal laparoscopic pyeloplasty for pelvi-ureteric junction obstruction. *Eur Urol* 2005; **48**(6):973–7.
66. Inagaki T, Rha KH, Ong AM, Kavoussi LR, Jarrett TW. Laparoscopic pyeloplasty: current status. *BJU Int* 2005; **95**(Suppl 2):102–5.
67. Wolf JS jr, Elashry OM, Clayman RV. Long term results of endoureterotomy for benign ureteral and ureteroenteric strictures. *J Urol* 1991; **158**(3):759–64.

68. Boari A. *La Uretero-cisto-neostomia*. Rome, Italy: Societa Editrice Dante Aligghieri, 1989.
69. Turner-Warwick RT, Worth PHL. The psoas bladder-hitch procedure for the replacement of the lower third of the ureter. *Br J Urol* 1969; **41**:701–9.
70. Shin KY, Park HJ, Lee JJ, *et al.* Role of early endourologic management of tuberculous ureteral strictures. *J Endourol* 2002; **16**:755–8.
71. Glanz S, Gordon PH, Butt K, *et al.* Percutaneous balloon dilatation of the ureter. *Radiology* 1983; **149**:101–4.
72. Smith AD. Management of iatrogenic ureteral strictures after urological procedures. *J Urol* 1988; **140**:1372–4.
73. Meretyk S, Albala DM, Clayman RV, *et al.* Endoureterotomy for treatment of ureteral strictures. *J Urol* 1992; **147**:1502–6.
74. Preminger GM, Clayman RV, Nakada SY, *et al.* A multicentre clinical trial investigating the use of a fluoroscopically controlled cutting balloon catheter for the management of ureteral and ureteropelvic junction obstruction. *J Urol* 1997; **157**:1625–9.
75. Netto Nr jr, Ferreira U, Lemos GC, *et al.* Endourological management of ureteral strictures. *J Urol* 1990; **144**:631–4.
76. Chang R, Marshall FF, Mitchell S. Percutaneous management of benign ureteral strictures and fistulas. *J Urol* 1987; **137**:1126–31.
77. Lang EK. Antegrade ureteral stenting for dehiscence, strictures and fistulae. *AJR* 1984; **143**:795–801.
78. O'Brien WM, Maxted WC, Pahira JJ. Uretral stricture: Experience with 31 cases. *J Urol* 1988; **140**:737–40.
79. Cormio L, Battaglia M, Traficante A, Selvaggi FP. Endourological treatment of ureteric injuries. *Br J Urol* 1993; **72**:165–8.
80. Bagley DH, Huffmann J, Lyon E, *et al.* Endoscopic ureteropyelotomy: Opening the obliterated ureteropelvic junction with nephroscopy and flexible ureteropyeloscopy. *J Urol* 1985; **133**:462–4.
81. Bagley DH. Endoscopic ureteroureterostomy. *J Urol* 1990; **143**:235a.
82. Cubelli V, Smith AD. Transurethral ureteral surgery guided by fluoroscopy. *Endourology* 1987; **2**:8.
83. Desgrandchamps F, Cussenot O, Bassi S, *et al.* Percutaneous extra-anatomic nephrovesical diversion. Preliminary report. *J Endourol* 1993; **7**:323–6.
84. Albarran J. Retention renale par perl externe de l'uretere. *Proces verbaus de Francaise d'Urologie* 1905; **9**:511–7.
85. Tresidder GC, Blandy JP, Singh M. Omental sleeve to prevent recurrent retroperitoneal fibrosis the ureter. *Urol Int* 1972; **27**:144–8.
86. Baker LRI, Mallinson WJW, Gregory MC, *et al.* Idiopathic retroperitoneal fibrosis. A retrospective analysis of 60 cases. *Br J Urol* 1987; **60**:497–503.
87. Tiptaft RC, Costello AJ, Paris AMI, *et al.* The long-term follow-up of idiopathic retroperitoneal fibrosis. *Br J Urol* 1982; **54**:620–4.
88. Cooksey G, Powell PH, Singh M, *et al.* Idiopathic retroperitoneal fibrosis. A long-term review after surgical treatment. *Br J Urol* 1982; **54**:628–31.
89. Osborn DE, Rao PR, Barnard RJ, *et al.* Surgical management of idiopathic retroperitoneal fibrosis. *Br J Urol* 1981; **53**:292–6.
90. Hinman F. Ureter. (pp. 636–93) In: Hinman F (ed). *Reconstruction Atlas of Urologic Surgery*. Philadelphia, PA: WB Saunders Company, 1989.
91. Galal H, Lazica A, Lampel A, *et al.* Management of ureteral strictures by different modalities and effect of stents on upper tract drainage. *J Endourol* 1993; **7**:411–7.
92. Gregoir W, Van Regermorter GV. Le reflux vesico-ureteral congenital. *Urol Int* 1964; **18**:122–36.
93. Lich R, Howerton LW, Goode LS, *et al.* The ureterovesical junction of the newborn. *J Urol* 1964; **92**:436–8.
94. Elliott SP, McAninch JW. Ureteral injuries from external violence: the 25-year experience at San Francisco General Hospital. *J Urol* 2003; **170**:1213–6.
95. Bright TC 3rd, Peters PC. Ureteral injuries due to external violence: 10 years experience with 59 cases. *J Trauma* 1977; **17**:616–20.
96. Ghali AM, El Malik EM, Ibrahim AI, *et al.* Ureteric injuries: diagnosis, management, and outcome. *J Trauma* 1999; **46**:150–8.
97. Zimmerman IJ, Precourt WE, Thompson CC. Direct uretero-cysto-neostomy with the short ureter in the cure of ureterovaginal fistula. *J Urol* 1960; **83**:113–5.
98. Motiwala HG, Shah SA, Patel SM. Ureteric substitution with Boari bladder flap. *Br J Urol* 1990; **66**:369–71.
99. Cukier J. L'operation de Boari. *Acta Urologica Belgica* 1966; **34**:15–28.
100. Bowsher WG, Shah PJR, Costello AJ *et al.* A critical appraisal of the boari flap. *Br J Urol* 1982; **54**:682–5.
101. Byun E, Merguerian PA. A meta-analysis of surgical practice patterns in the endoscopic management of ureterocoeles. *J Urol* 2006; **176**:1871–7.
102. Monfort G, Morisson-Lacombe G, Guys JM, *et al.* Simplified treatment of ureterocoeles. *Chir Pediatr* 1985; **26**:26–30.
103. Hagg MJ, Mourachov PV, Snyder HM, *et al.* The modern endoscopic approach to ureterocoele. *J Urol* 2000; **163**:940–3.

CHAPTER 2.21

The principles of endourology

Stephen Keoghane and Mark Sullivan

Introduction to the principles of endourology

Many urological chapters have been written on the principles behind the subspecialty of endourology; the authors will outline the salient features behind some of these principles.

History

In 1806, Philipp Bozzini constructed the 'lichtleiter' for direct inspection and treatment of the uterus and bladder.[1] These early endoscopes were cumbersome and impractical, made of hollow examining tubes with illumination by candle light directed by a mirror.

1853 Desormeaux performed the first true endoscopic procedure, extracting a papilloma from the urethra through a urethroscope.

1873 Trouve moved the light source from the outside to the inner tip of the endoscope using a glowing hot platinum wire.[1]

1874 Bottini first performed blind electrosurgery of the prostate.

1877 The first major improvement in optics was made by Nitze using a series of precisely aligned thin lenses within a tube.[1]

1897 Albarran introduces a lever allowing the ability to control the electrode.

1900 Freudenber uses an endoscope for visualization.

1910 Beer introduced high-frequency current revolutionizing the field of therapeutic endoscopic procedures.

1912 Hugh Hampton Young performed the first ureteroscopic procedure using a paediatric cystoscope in a two-month-old child with posterior urethral valve.[2]

1926 First resectoscope constructed by Stern.

1931 McCarthy modified the resectoscope with the addition of a lever to move the cutting loop. This basic design is still used today for modern resectosopes.

1960 Harold Hopkins developed the rod lens.[3]

1960s Introduction of fibre-optic cables enabling the transmission of light from an outside source.

1960 Marshall developed the 3 mm flexible fiberoscope.[4]

1968 Takayasu and Aso developed the first flexible pelviureteroscope with an operating channel.[5]

1977 Lyon performed the first rod–lens ureteroscopy to explore the distal ureter with a 11 Fr paediatric cystoscope.[6]

1979 Original ureteroscope constructed by Richard Wolf Medical Instruments (Vernon Hills, IL).[7]

1980 and **1981** The first practical ureteroscopes designed by Enrique Perez-Castro and the Karl Storz Company (Culver City, CA).[8]

Endoscopes

Optics

The postgraduate trainee urologist would be expected to have an understanding of the groundbreaking work of Harold Hopkins[3] and Karl Storz and to be familiar with a longitudinal section of a rigid rod lens cystoscope.

Urologic endoscopes are generally of two optical designs: the rigid, rod-lens system described by Hopkins, while fibre-optic imaging bundles are used in both rigid and flexible endoscopes (Fig. 2.21.1). The rod–lens system consists of a series of glass rods with polished ends with the key feature of air gaps that act as a lens. Light is carried efficiently along the rod, resulting in a clear and bright image.

Fibre-optic bundles are composed of individual two-layer glass fibres that carry light from one end to the other. To achieve an accurate optical image, the fibres need to be oriented identically at each end of the bundle. Fibre-optic bundles can be manufactured for both a flexible endoscope and small diameter rigid systems (ureteroscopes).

Fibre-optic bundles however have spaces between the round fibres and lose optical information, resulting in an image that may not be as clear and bright compared with the rod–lens system.

Cystoscopes

Rigid or flexible cystoscopes range from 8 to 12 Fr (1 Fr = 3 mm) for paediatric endoscopes and 16 to 25 Fr for adult endoscopes. The trainee should be aware of the useful 19 Fr cystoscope sheath for the tight urethra.

Rigid cystoscopes have a rod–lens system, a metal sheath, and a bridge. The sheath is the outer cover through which the rod–lens system is inserted. The sheath remains in the bladder when the rod–lens system is removed or needs to be exchanged. The sheath also has a port for the infusion of irrigation fluids, a necessary requirement to maintain continuous visualization. The sheath can be inserted into the bladder 'blind' using an obturator with an atraumatic tip or using visual obturators, where there is a lumen for the lens allowing safer direct visualization of the passage of the cystoscope. The sheath also attaches to a bridge, which also contains an opening for the rod–lens system and a working

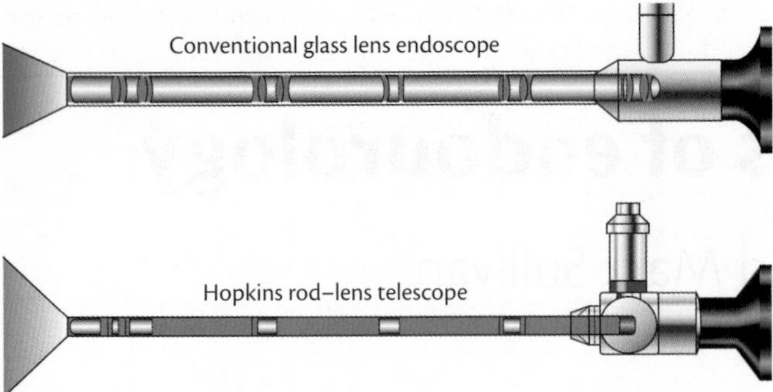

Fig. 2.21.1 The conventional endoscope (above) and the Hopkins® telescope design (below). The glass rods in the Hopkins telescope provide a larger image, greater light transmission, and improved clarity of vision.
Image Copyright © KARL STORZ—Endoskope, Germany.

channel through which instruments such as biopsy forceps, hand held graspers, guidewires, ureteric catheters, and diathermy probes may be inserted. A deflecting Albarran bridge allows more precise deflection of flexible instruments as they pass through the distal part of the cystoscope.

Lenses are designed at different angles (0, 12, 25 or 30, 70, 110–1,200 degrees) and the image can be viewed directly through the eyepiece, but contemporary practice uses a camera attached to the eyepiece transmitting the image to a monitor.

Rigid cystoscopes have the advantage of using larger sheaths to improve irrigation and a larger working channel allowing procedures such as bladder biopsy and retrograde ureteropyelography to be performed with ease under general or regional anaesthesia. Local anaesthetic rigid cystoscopy is feasible in the female, ensuring the bladder is not over distended.

Flexible cystoscopes have small, soft, flexible shafts, a working channel (6.4–7.5 Fr) and an irrigation port. There are a wide variety of long, flexible instruments that can be passed through the working channel, including grasping forceps, biopsy forceps, lithotripsy and electrocautery probes, and basket entrapping devices. The optics consist of either fibre-optic bundles or a distal sensor (either a complementary metal oxide sensor or charge-coupled device). Flexible cystoscopes can be deflected by up to 220 degrees using a thumb-operated lever.

Rigid and semi-rigid ureteroscopes

These are available in a wide range of sizes; however, a 6/7.5 Fr tapered ureteroscope with fibre-optic imaging system and multiple working channels no larger than 4 Fr has become standard. These endoscopes may be short (the distal and lower middle ureter in men and the renal pelvis in women may be accessed using a 31 cm ureteroscope), and long versions (a 40 cm ureteroscope may be needed to reach the renal pelvis in male patients). Although the latter can reach the renal pelvis, it is not generally considered an appropriate instrument for intrarenal procedures.

Most of the available semi-rigid ureteroscopes have round or oval tip designs, but endoscopes with smooth, triangular tips have more recently become available, designed to ease insertion into the ureteral orifice. Ureteroscopes with one large channel for both instrumentation and irrigation, or two channels to separate instrumentation and irrigation are available from most suppliers.

A single, straight, large working channel is possible in ureteroscopes with an offset eyepiece. In contrast, two channel scopes allow passage of a working instrument without diminution in the flow of the irrigant fluid. They usually have a 3.4 Fr working channel that can accommodate a standard 3 Fr instrument and a 2.1–2.4 Fr irrigation channel.

The trainee should have a working knowledge of the endoscopes used in their department.

Flexible ureterorenoscopes

These endoscopes have revolutionized endourology, allowing intrarenal procedures; 7–9 Fr-sized instruments are standard for fibre-optic imaging. The working channel is 3.6 Fr (exception is the Wolf 9 Fr ureteroscope that has a 4.5 Fr working channel). Because the single channel is used for both passage of instruments and irrigation, an instrument in the channel will reduce the irrigant flow rate. The loss of flow may be compensated by pressurizing the irrigant fluid and the use of smaller, less than 1.9 Fr calibre instruments. The 200 μ laser fibre may have the least deleterious effects on the flow rate, whereas the 3.0 Fr basket causes a significant reduction in irrigant flow rate.

Tip deflection is usually via a thumb-controlled handle and may be designed with intuitive or counterintuitive deflection directions. The degree of deflection varies between 130 and 270 degrees, depending on the manufacturer.

Flexible ureteroscopes also contain a passive deflecting segment; it is a more flexible segment, several centimetres proximal to the active deflectable segment. This passive segment, when used with the active deflection, allows the endoscope to curl upon itself when the tip is reflected from the medial aspect of the renal pelvis for manoeuvres into the lower pole infundibulum. The angle of active and passive deflection can become severely restricted by the presence of instruments in the working channel (365 μ laser fibre causing the most restriction, and the 2.2 Fr nitinol basket the least).[9] This effect on the angle of deflection can also be lessened with newer, smaller, and more malleable instruments. Various techniques have been described to limit the impact of instruments in the working channel, including the use of an unsheathed (bare naked) nitinol basket to reduce its diameter (Fig. 2.21.2).[10–11]

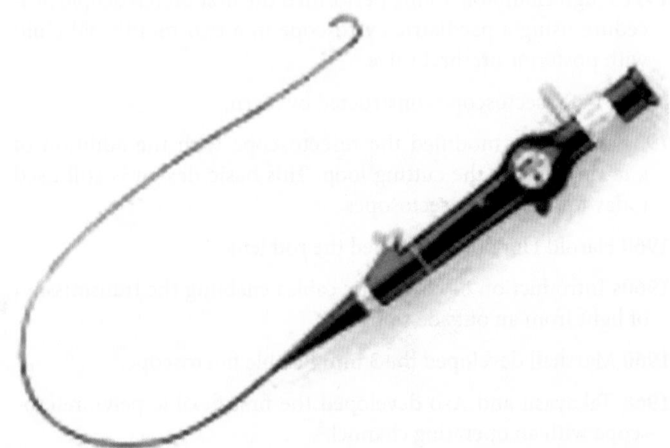

Fig. 2.21.2 Flexible ureterorenoscope (AUR™-7).
Image reproduced courtesy of Olympus Medical.

The angle of visualization may be zero or nine degrees, and instruments exit the endoscope at varying positions according to manufacturer. The tip of the instrument may be flush, or bevelled and triangular which may facilitate insertion into the ureteral orifice and decrease ureteral trauma.

These bevelled tip endoscopes also allow the manufacturers to claim a smaller tip diameter, which rapidly enlarges to the distal shaft size, whereas an instrument with a flush tip maintains the small distal diameter for several millimetres.

Channel size and flow, durability, deflection, service/repair provision, and high image resolution are, in no particular order the factors to consider when investing in flexible endoscopes. The lumen of the working channel may vary in position according to manufacturer.

Video flexible ureterorenoscopes using a charge-coupled device (CCD) chip on the tip may reduce the requirement for frequent repair and allow excellent visualization of the upper urinary tract. Disposable flexible endoscopes may or may not survive the rapid changes in urological technology.

Care and sterilization

Although these modern flexible ureteroscopes are capable of accessing the most difficult areas in the upper urinary tract, they are fragile and require major repair after an average of 6 to 15 uses.[12] Common reasons for repair are broken fibre-optic fibres, a damaged working channel, and reduced or loss of deflection. Currently, the durability and cost of maintenance is the main limiting factor against incorporation of these delicate instruments in most general urology practices.[13–14]

Rigid and semi-rigid ureteroscopes are considerably more durable than their flexible counterparts because of their outer metal casing. However, proper handling by holding near the eyepiece at the base while supporting the shaft should be emphasized. Cleansing with warm water and a non-abrasive detergent, as well as irrigation of the working channels, following each use is important. These instruments can be sterilized by gas (ethylene oxide) or by soaking; some may be autoclaved.

The more fragile flexible ureteroscopes should also be cleaned initially by rinsing and irrigating with warm water and a non-abrasive detergent, and then sterilized by gas or soaking. These delicate scopes are prone to damage during cleaning from bending or trauma to the distal tip or the eyepiece. Every effort should be made to maintain them in a straight orientation during cleansing and use. In addition, the flexible ureteroscopes require venting during gas sterilization, either by manually opening a vent near the irrigation port near the light post, or some may have an automatic, patented, *Autoseal* system.

Liquid sterilization may be accomplished by soaking in 2.4% glutaraldehyde (i.e. Cidex, Advanced Sterilization Products, Irvine, CA) or 35% peroxyacetic acid (i.e. Steris, Mentor, OH). Peroxyacetic acid has been demonstrated to be associated with higher flexible cystoscope repair costs.[15]

The durability of the flexible ureteroscope may also be affected by the technique and number of personnel involved in the cleaning and maintenance rather than the technical demands of the procedure and the endoscopists' technique.[16] The routine use of newer ureteroscopic accessories, such as ureteral access sheaths, nitinol devices, and 200 μ holmium laser fibres can decrease the strain on the flexible ureteroscopes and significantly increase the longevity.[13]

Rigid and flexible nephroscopes

Rigid nephroscopes have undergone little change since the advent of percutaneous nephrolithotomy. They provide excellent visualization with a rod–lens system and an offset eyepiece to allow passage of large, straight instruments for stone fragmentation, such as the ultrasonic lithotripter or the lithoclast. Various lengths are available, ranging from 17.5 to 30 cm, to accommodate a variety of patient body habitus. Sheaths range from 15 to 27 Fr in size; 'mini- and ultra-mini nephroscopes' with a smaller, Fr diameter, which can be used as a compact cystoscope are also available. A flexible cystoscope may be used as a nephroscope when needed.

Disposable equipment

Endourology is an 'all or nothing' specialty. Every variety of disposable device should be accessible in the operating theatre. Halfway through a prolonged flexible upper tract procedure is not the time to find out you have no nitinol basket.

The components of a surgical video system include the light source, video camera, video processor, and display unit (Fig. 2.21.3). These should be lightweight and easily portable, requiring minimal set up, and can be cleaned with alcohol wipes and disinfectant.

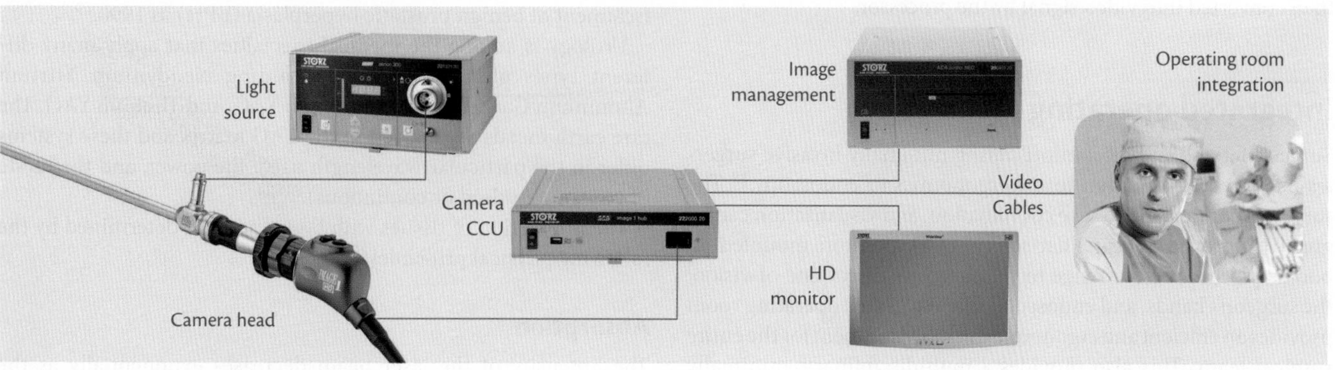

Fig. 2.21.3 An endourology stack.
Image Copyright © KARL STORZ—Endoskope, Germany.

Light source

The most desirable features are a long Xenon lamp life, approaching 500 hours with a minimum of 300 watts. The white balance and manual brightness controls should be accessible from within the sterile field.

Monitor

Most monitors are now LCD (liquid crystal display) flat screens with a minimum size of 22 inches, demonstrating high resolution and HD quality with a minimum of 1,680 × 1,050 pixels.

The response time should be less than 8 m/second with a contrast ratio of 400:01:00. The lower the response time, the less of a blurring effect there will be on the screen, referred to as 'ghosting'. The *contrast ratio* is the difference in brightness from the darkest to the brightest portion on the screen. This can change throughout the screen due to variations in the lighting behind the panel.

High definition television

The most popular high definition television (HDTV) format is 1,080 i, or 1,080 lines interlaced, which produces images by painting the odd lines first, then the even lines in a second pass. The alternative HDTV format is 720 lines progressive scan, or 720 p, which has fewer lines of resolution, but paints all lines in one pass. 720 p is predominantly used for video containing fast-moving content where image jitter is less likely to occur.

To summarize, 1,080 i image reproduction is sharp, highly detailed, and exhibits less pixelation, even at high magnification, than the 720 p HDTV format, but the 720 p may be more stable with less flicker.

Processor

The stand-alone HD processor should be compatible with fibre, rigid, and flexible video endoscopes, demonstrating adequate connectivity to a hospital intranet with outputs to external media storage with the ability to capture images for both clinical and research use. A hard disc drive is an option on modern processors.

Camera head

The camera head should contain both optical zoom and white balance controls. Most modern cameras will contain three CCDs or *charge-coupled devices*, which are composed of tiny photoelectric elements arranged in a grid (pixels) that allow an electronic response from the reflected light from the surgical field, which is then converted into video signal by the processor.

Integrated operating theatres

Surgeon fatigue and discomfort during minimally invasive surgeries has directed attention to the ergonomics of endoscopy.[17] The surgeon's comfort, hand–eye coordination, and visualization can be greatly improved by using flat-screen, LCD monitors mounted on booms placed in close range to the surgeon's direct line of vision, the surgeon's hands, and endoscope. The integrated operating room provides an efficient and ergonomic work environment for the entire surgical team. This also provides a multidisciplinary, minimally invasive surgical suite. Single flat-screen monitors accommodate laparoscopic surgery, whereas the triple flat-screen monitors, on a single boom, provide simultaneous endoscopic and fluoroscopic visualization during endoscopy. The occupational hazards of urological minimally invasive surgery should not be underestimated, especially back problems, and attention should routinely be paid to the surgeon's operating position and the position of the monitor (which ideally should be at eye level or just below, not above).

Narrow band imaging

Narrow band imaging (NBI) is an optical filter technology that radically improves the visibility of capillaries, veins, and other subtle tissue structures, by optimizing the absorbance and scattering characteristics of light. NBI uses two discrete bands of light: one blue at 415 nm and one green at 540 nm. Narrow band blue light displays superficial capillary networks, while green light displays subepithelial vessels and when combined offer an extremely high contrast image of the tissue surface (Fig. 2.21.4).

Blue light technology

Photodynamic diagnosis (PDD) in the urothelium is an exciting recent development, which allows the precise diagnosis of flat *carcinoma in situ* of the urinary bladder, and small satellite malignant lesions. These can be difficult to visualize using white light, and PDD offers the additional advantage of defining tumour borders. Imaging relies on the introduction of a photosensitive marker (5 ALA or HAL) transurethrally into the bladder, where it converts to protoporphyrin IX. As the pigment is absorbed by normal urothelium, it accumulates in cancer cells, emitting red fluorescence under blue excitation illumination. Normal urothelium remains blue, thus helping delineation of the abnormal areas for sampling and resection. This can be performed using the bipolar TURis-B, which reduces the risk of TUR syndrome and accidental obturator nerve stimulation, thus avoiding the risk of bladder wall perforation. (Fig. 2.21.5)[18]

Lasers

Laser is an acronym for *Light Amplification by Stimulated Emission of Radiation*. It is now defined as a device which emits light through optical amplification, based on the stimulated emission of photons.

In urology, Parsons in 1966 experimentally used a pulsed-ruby laser in the canine bladder. Pioneer applications of the laser in urology included the use of a CO_2-laser for condylomata in 1980, photodynamic therapy (PDT) for bladder carcinoma in 1982, the pulsed-dye laser for urolithiasis in 1987,[19] and the Nd:YAG laser for prostatic carcinoma in 1984.[20] The modern era of lasers in urology begins with the use of side-firing fibres and their application in the treatment of benign prostatic hyperplasia (BPH) in 1990.[19]

Urology is among the medical specialties that apply many different types of laser systems including Neodynium Yttrium Aluminium Garnet (YAG), Holmium YAG, and Thulium YAG. The rare earth metals are housed in the YAG matrix and these systems differ in the particular wavelength used, the power, and the mode of emission (pulsed or continuous).[21–24]

The interaction of tissues with laser energy is determined by the following physical principles[25,26]:

Absorption

The 'intensity of the laser beam decreases exponentially as the absorbing medium increases in density. Absorbed laser radiation is converted into heat, causing a local rise in temperature. Depending

(A)

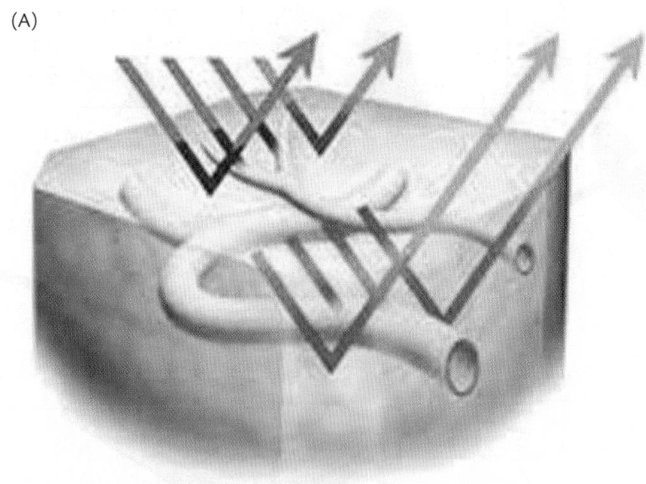

(B)

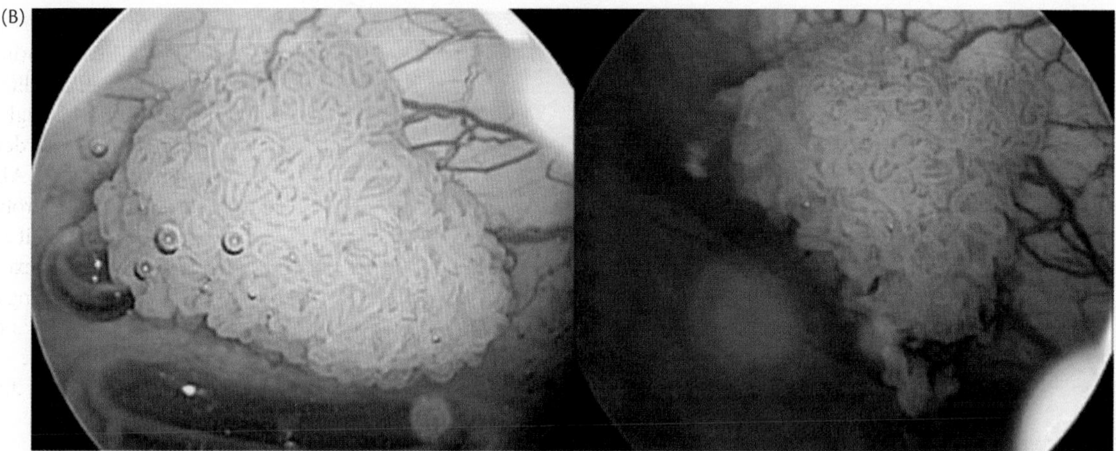

Fig. 2.21.4 (A) Narrow band blue light displays superficial capillary networks, while green light displays subepithelial vessels and when combined offer an extremely high contrast image of the tissue surface. (B) Narrow band imaging (NBI): detection of a papillary bladder tumour with white light on the left and NBI on the right.
(A,B) Image reproduced courtesy of Olympus Medical.

on the amount of heat produced, tissue will coagulate or even vaporize. Heat is more likely to be generated next to the tissue surface because of the exponential decrease in beam intensity as it passes into the tissue and the immediate action of the absorption process.'[26]

'However, absorption can only occur in the presence of a chromophore'; a 'chemical group capable of absorbing light at a particular frequency and thereby imparting colour to a molecule. Examples of body chromophores are melanin, blood and water.'[26]

Reflection

'When the laser beam encounters tissue, a percentage of the beam is reflected by the boundary layer and may therefore heat and damage surrounding tissue. Reflection mainly depends on the optical properties of the tissue and the irrigant surrounding it'[26] but has little clinical impact.

Scattering

'The heterogenous composition of tissue causes the laser beam to scatter … diverting part of the beam away from its intended direction and therefore its intended purpose. The amount of scatter depends on the size of the particles and the wavelength of the laser. Shorter wavelengths are scattered to a much higher degree than longer wavelengths, i.e. blue laser radiation is scattered more than green, green more than red, and red more than infrared.'[26]

Transmission

When energy is not fully absorbed, but rather penetrates tissue there is less transfer of energy.

Extinction length

'The *extinction length* defines the depth of tissue up to which 90% of the incident laser beam is absorbed and converted into heat. An extinction length is equal to 2.3 absorption lengths.'[26]

'Haemoglobin and water are widely used as chromophores for surgical lasers. For a short time after absorption of a circular laser beam, the generated heat is confined in a cylindrical-shaped volume, which has the height of the laser beam's extinction length and the approximate diameter of the laser fibre. The density of the absorbed energy determines the effect of the laser on tissue.'[26]

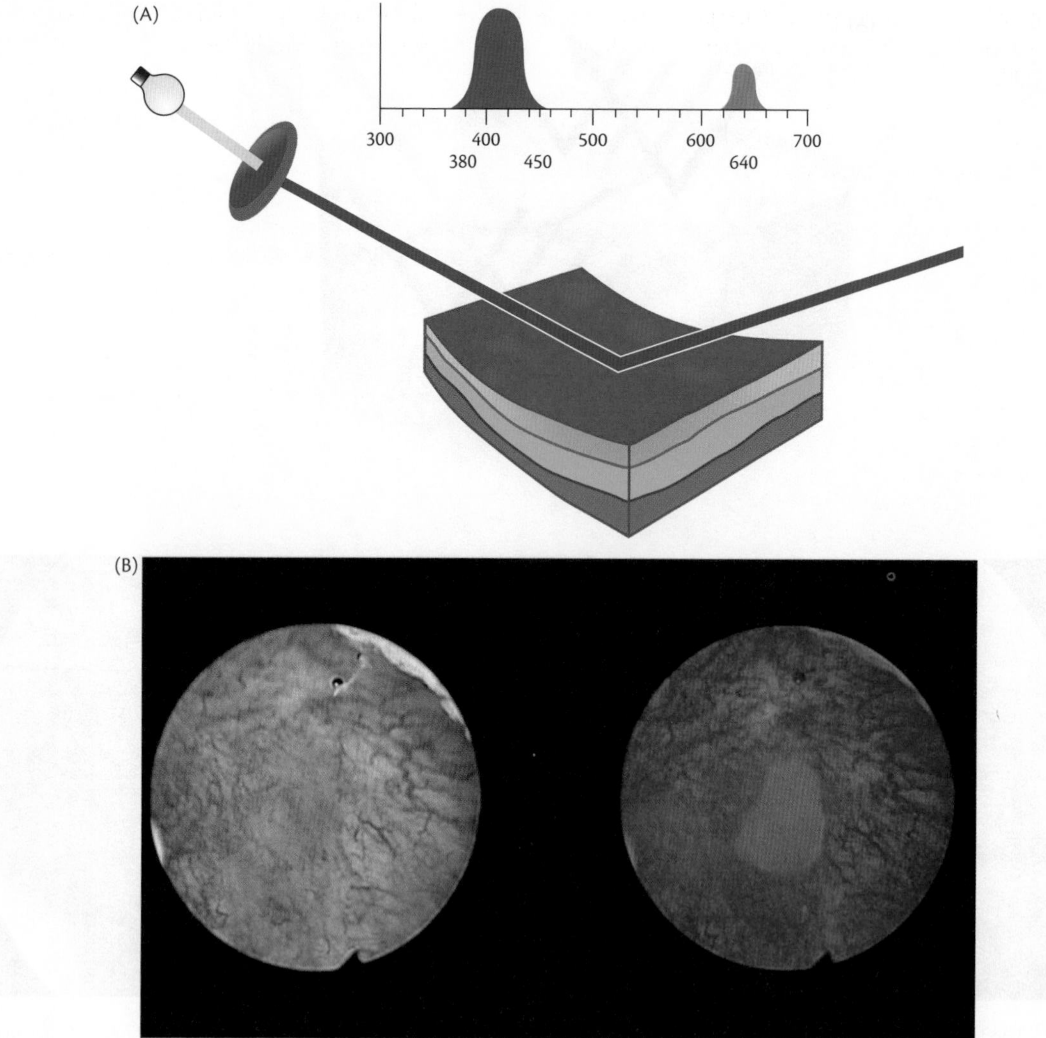

Fig. 2.21.5 (A) To perform photodynamic diagnosis (PDD) observation, the dedicated photosensitive marker (5-ALA or HAL) is first instilled in the bladder. About 90 to 120 minutes later, the endoscopic examination is started. (B) History (left: white light | right: PDD). A slightly uneven surface in white light cystoscopy that was intensely fluorescent in blue light was collected by cold-cup biopsy.

(A,B) Image reproduced courtesy of Olympus Medical.

'It is important to match the achieved effect along the extinction length with the intended surgical effect. At the same power wattage, a laser wavelength with a long extinction length may create a deep necrosis, whereas a laser wavelength with a much shorter extinction length will produce an increase in temperature above boiling point and immediate vaporization of tissue.'[26]

The contact of laser energy with various tissues is accompanied by one or more of the following effects.

There may be a *thermal effect*, whereby when energy is absorbed it is transformed to heat and consequently the temperature of the tissue increases, with various biological effects. These effects are: at >40°C, protein denaturation; at >60°C, protein coagulation; at 100°C vaporization of tissue water; at >250°C, carbonization; and at >300°C, tissue vaporization. The extent of the thermal effect is determined by the wavelength of the laser light, the power density, and particular optical and thermal features of the tissue.

In the infrared region of the spectrum (the CO_2 laser emits at 10 600 nm), there is almost complete energy absorption, resulting in heat generation with carbonization and vaporization. In the near-infrared region (the Nd:YAG laser, at 1,060 nm), there is less absorption and more penetration of energy, resulting in tissue coagulation at considerable depth.

There may be a *mechanical effect*; the application of pulsed laser energy to the surface of a urinary stone results in fragmentation of the latter. The very high power density, which can be altered with recent technological advances, imposed at the stone's surface results in the freeing of a column of electrons and the formation of a 'plasma' bubble. The expansion of this 'plasma' bubble changes the ultrastructure of the stone, disrupting it along stress lines.

There may be a *photochemical effect*, based on the selective photoactivation of a specific drug and its transformation to a toxic compound(s). The laser is an ideal source of light for photoactivation, because of its power and specific wavelength. The formation of toxic metabolites results in cellular death through the intracellular production of singlet oxygen, which generates free radicals and peroxides that damage cellular elements such as DNA and mitochondria.

Finally, there may be a *tissue welding effect*. All the previous effects are destructive and accomplish their therapeutic aim through the ablation of biological material.

Laser tissue welding aims to reconstruct anatomical structures by tissue re-approximation, through the application of focused thermal energy.[27] This energy induces the interdigitation of collagen (biological 'glue') with minimal peripheral tissue destruction. Advantages over conventional surgery include decreased operative duration, improved healing with minimal scar formation and adequate tensile strength, maintenance of luminal continuity with reduced fistula formation, and an immediate watertight seal. The disadvantages include accumulating training and experience, the high cost, and the subjectivity of determining the end point of welding. Adding a proteinaceous material (50% human albumin, i.e. a tissue solder), energy can be focused more selectively at the wound edges, resulting in improved tensile strength on welding, with a simultaneous decrease in peripheral thermal tissue destruction. The addition of a specific dye to the soldering material (chromophore) results in a more selective energy absorption at a given wavelength and consequently less peripheral tissue injury.

Combinations of dyes/laser wavelength are: indocyanine green/805 nm diode laser; iron oxide or fluorescein/532 nm KTP laser; and India ink/1064 nm Nd:YAG laser. In urology, the applications of laser tissue welding include vasovasostomy, urethral reconstruction (hypospadias, stricture, diverticulum or fistula), pyeloplasty, bladder augmentation, and continent urinary diversion.

Theatre ergonomics

Patient positioning

The pelvic tilt induced by the traditional lithotomy position has led to many urologists adopting the Lloyd Davies position for endoscopy.

For anything other than a cystoscopy, the authors favour a disposable transurethral resection (TUR) drape with attached polythene funnel and filter. The end of the filter should be removed to avoid the weight of fluid pulling the drape inferiorly.

For upper tract endoscopy, the affected leg should be lowered, thus flattening the pelvis. This is particularly important for semi-rigid ureteroscopy.

Antibiotics

The use of antibiotic prophylaxis for endourological procedures should follow one or a combination of guidance given in the AUA Best Practice Policy statement on Urologic Surgery Antimicrobial Prophylaxis (http://www.auanet.org/common/pdf/education/clinical-guidance/Antimicrobial-Prophylaxis.pdf),[28] and the EAU Guidelines on Urological Infections 2016 (http://uroweb.org/wp-content/uploads/EAU-Extended-Guidelines-2016-Edn-pdf).

E. coli, Proteus mirabilis, Klebsiella, and *Enterococcus faecalis* represent the majority of urological pathogens and will be adequately covered by prophylactic gentamicin and amoxicillin/cefuroxime. Local microbiological advice should also be sought as local resistence patterns can vary.

The urology resident is expected to have a working knowledge of the principles behind venous thromboembolic prophylaxis and should follow NICE guidance (http://guidance.nice.org.uk/CG92/NICEGuidance/pdf/English).[29] The WHO checklist should be followed for all surgical procedures (http://www.who.int/patientsafety/safesurgery/ss_checklist/en/).[30]

What is the aim of this endourological procedure?

Urinary tract drainage, tumour treatment, or complete or partial stone clearance. It is worth explaining the time-consuming and complexity of upper tract endoscopy to patients and balancing the day case/office nature of these treatments against the need for multiple procedures.

Acknowledgements

Text extracts from Olympus, Resection with Photodynamic Diagnosis (PDD), Copyright © 2013 Olympus Europa SE & CO. KG, available from http://www.olympus-europa.com/medical/en/medical_systems/applications/urology/bladder/photodynamic_diagnosis__pdd_/photodynamic_diagnosis__pdd_.html reproduced with permission from Olympus Medical

Text extracts from A Merseburger *et al.*, (chair), *Guidelines on Lasers and Technologies, European Association of Urology*, Copyright © EAU 2014, reproduced with permission of the European Association of Urology, available from http://www.baus.org.uk/_userfiles/pages/files/professionals/sections/EAU2015-Laser.pdf

'Video systems' section adapted from John Reynard *et al.*, *Oxford Specialist Handbook in Urological Surgery*, Oxford University Press, Oxford, UK, Copyright © 2008, with permission from Oxford University Press.

Further reading

Floratos DL, De La Rosette. Lasers in urology. *BJUI* 1999; **84**:204–11.

Hopkins H, Kapany N. A flexible fiberscope using static scanning. *Nature* 1954; **173**:39–41.

Reuter MA, Reuter HJ. The development of the cystoscope. *J Urol* 1997; **159**:638–40.

References

1. Reuter MA, Reuter HJ. The development of the cystoscope. *J Urol* 1997; **159**:638–40.
2. Young HH, Mckay RW. Congenital valvular obstruction of the prostatic urethra. *Surg Gynecol Obstet* 1929; **48**:509–12.
3. Hopkins H, Kapany N. A flexible fiberscope using static scanning. *Nature* 1954; **173**:39–41.
4. Marshal VV. Fiberoptics in urology. *J Urol* 1964; **91**:110–13.
5. Takagi T, Go T, Takayasu N, Aso Y. A small caliber fiberscope for the visualization of the urinary tract, biliary tract, and spinal canal. *Surgery* 1968; **64**:1033–6.
6. Lyon ES, Kyker JS, Schoenberg HW. Transurethral ureteroscopy in women: A ready addition to the urological armamentarium. *J Urol* 1978; **119**:35–8.
7. Lyon ES, Banno JJ, Schoenberg HW. Transurethral ureteroscopy in men using juvenile cystoscopy equipment. *J Urol* 1979; **122**:152–5.
8. Perez-Castro EE, Martinez-Piniero JA. Transurethral ureteroscopy- a current urological procedure. *Arch Esp Urol* 1980; **33**:445–8.
9. Abdelshehid C, Ahlering MT, Chou D, *et al.* Comparison of flexible ureteroscopes: deflecting, irrigant flow and optical characteristics. *J Urol* 2005; **173**(6):2017–21.
10. Monga M, Dretler SP, Landman J, Slaton JW, Conradie MC, Clayman RV. Maximizing ureteroscope deflection: "Play it straight". *Urology* 2002; **60**:902–5.

11. Landman J, Monga M, El Gabry EA, *et al.* Bare naked baskets: Ureteroscope deflection and flow characteristics with intact and disassembled ureteroscopic nitinol stone baskets. *J Urol* 2002; **167**:2377–9.
12. A fane JS, Olweny EO, Bercowsky E, *et al.* Flexible ureteroscopes: A single center evaluation of the durability and function of the new endoscopes smaller than 9 Fr. *J Urol* 2000; **164**:1164–8.
13. Landman J, Lee DI, Lee C, Monga M. Evaluation of overall costs of currently available small flexible ureteroscopes. *Urology* 2003; **62**:218–22.
14. Pietrow PK, Auge BK, Delvecchio FC, *et al.* Techniques to maximize flexible ureteroscope longevity. *Urology* 2002; **60**:784–8.
15. Fuselier Jr., HA, Mason C. Liquid sterilization versus high level disinfection in the urologic office. *Urology* 1997; **50**:337–40.
16. McDougall EM, Alberts G, Deal KJ, Nagy JM 3rd. Does the cleaning technique influence the durability of the <9 flexible ureteroscope? *J Endourol* 2001; **15**:615–18.
17. Wolf SJ Jr, Marcovich R, Gill IS, *et al.* Survey of Neuromuscular injuries to the patient and surgeon during urologic laparoscopic surgery. *Urology* 2000; **55**:831–6.
18. Olympus. Resection with Photodynamic Diagnosis (PDD), 2013. Available at: http://www.olympus-europa.com/medical/en/medical_systems/applications/urology/bladder/photodynamic_diagnosis__pdd_/photodynamic_diagnosis__pdd_.html [Online].
19. Floratos DL, De La Rosette. Lasers in urology. *BJUI* 1999; **84**:204–11.
20. Sander S, Beisland HO. Laser in the treatment of localized prostate cancer. *J Urol* 1984; **132**:280–1.
21. Smith JA Jr. Urologic laser surgery. (pp. 2923–41) In: Walsh PC, Retik AB, Stamey TA, Vaughan ED (eds). *Campbell's Urology*, 6th editon. Philadelphia, PA: WB Saunders Co, 1992.
22. Watson GM, Murray S, Dretler SP, Parrish JA. The pulse-dye laser for fragmenting urinary calculi. *J Urol* 1987; **138**:195–8.
23. Jung P, WolC JM, Mattelaer P, Jakse G. Role of lasertripsy in the management of ureteral calculi: experience with Alexandrite laser system in 232 patients. *J Endourol* 1996; **10**:345–8.
24. Wollin TA, Denstedt JD. The holmium laser in urology. *J Clin Laser Med Surg* 1998; **16**:13–20.
25. van Hillegersberg R. Fundamentals of laser surgery. *Eur J Surg* 1997; **163**: 3–11.
26. Herrmann TR, Liatsikos EN, Nagele U, Traxer O, Merseburger AS; EAU Guidelines Panel on Lasers, Technologies. EAU Guidelines on Lasers and Technology 2014. *Eur Urol* 2012; **61**(4):783–95.
27. Scherr DS, Poppas DP. Laser tissue welding. *Urol Clin North Am* 1998; **25**:123–35.
28. AUA Best Practice Policy Statement On Urologic Surgery Antimicrobial Prophylaxis. Available at: https://www.auanet.org/education/guidelines/antimicrobial-prophylaxis.cfm [Online].
29. NICE guidance. Available at: https://www.nice.org.uk/guidance/cg92/evidence [Online].
30. The WHO checklist. Available at: http://www.who.int/patientsafety/safesurgery/ss_checklist/en/ [Online].

CHAPTER 2.22

Principles of laparoscopic and robotic urological surgery

Mark Sullivan, Nilay Patel†, and Inderbir Gill

Introduction to principles of laparoscopic and robotic urological surgery

Laparoscopic surgery has successfully been adopted into adult and paediatric urological practice. In principle, laparoscopy can provide a superior visual field, a reduction in the stress response to surgery, reductions in postoperative pain, shorter postoperative recovery time, and superior cosmetic results compared with open surgery. In the field of paediatric urology, the adoption of laparoscopy has been a more gradual process, possibly because of the excellent long-term outcomes of open surgery and relatively modest reduction in postoperative morbidity following paediatric laparoscopic surgery. In addition, current laparoscopic equipment is not ideally suited to the smaller working spaces in children, a factor that contributes to the significant learning curve associated with laparoscopic surgery in children, particularly with regards to reconstructive procedures.

The past decade has also seen the rapid uptake of robotic-assisted surgical platforms such as the da Vinci robot (Intuitive Surgical, Sunnyvale, CA) in urological surgery. These devices have been developed to help overcome some of the inherent disadvantages of conventional laparoscopy. Robotic-assisted paediatric urological surgery has emerged as a valid and reliable surgical therapy, which maintains the advantages of the minimally invasive approach, but avoids the difficulties and disadvantages of laparoscopic surgery.

Laparoscopic urological surgery

General principles

Laparoscopy has been a relatively recent development to treat urologic pathology.

History

1991 First laparoscopic nephrectomy and nephroureterectomy, Clayman, USA[1,2]

1991 First laparoscopic pelvic lymphadenectomy, Schuessler, USA[3]

1992 First laparoscopic cystectomy, Parra, USA[4]

1993 First laparoscopic pyeloplasty, Schuessler, USA[5]

1997 First laparoscopic radical prostatectomy, Schuessler USA[6]

Some of these procedures have clear benefits in comparison to open surgery, but some do not, though may prove to with time. A surgeon must recognize his or her limitations with these procedures and more complex cases may need additional support from more experienced laparoscopic urologists.

Appropriate patient selection is essential and each case treated on its merits with careful consideration of each patient's expectations. Pain, though less, does occur, and requires postoperative analgesia and convalescence. General anaesthesia is required and some patients, for example those with severe cardiopulmonary disease, may not be able to undergo laparoscopy. Patients with mild to moderate chronic obstructive pulmonary disease may struggle to compensate for the hypercarbia associated with insufflation and the insufflation pressures may need to be reduced.[7] Laparoscopy is contraindicated in patients with severely dilated bowel from functional or obstructive ileus, uncorrected coagulopathy, untreated infection, or hypovolaemic shock.[8] As a general rule though, patients who are fit enough to undergo anaesthesia for open surgery are also deemed fit for laparoscopic/robotic surgery. Care needs to be taken in patients who have had previous retro- or transperitoneal surgery. Adhesions are more likely and an open access approach is recommended. Obese patients can present problems with trocar placement, masked anatomic landmarks, and difficulty acquiring an adequate intra-abdominal pressure, thereby limiting the workspace. However, it should be noted that laparoscopic/robotic surgery in the reoperative setting and in obese patients are now being routinely performed at centres with experience in minimally invasive surgery.

Informed consent must be obtained with discussion of all complications, including quoting the surgeon's own experience. Patient preparation is discussed in relation to each procedure.

Basic laparoscopic equipment

Video systems

The laparoscopic image is created through combining a laparoscope with the video system. The video system consists of a video camera, light cable, light source, a video processor (often referred to as the camera control unit (CCU)) and video display (monitor).[9]

The laparoscope usually has a 0 or 30 degree lens and is most commonly 10 mm in size (range 2.7–12 mm). Larger laparoscopes give a wider field of vision, better optical resolution, and brighter image. The camera is locked to the eyepiece in its correct position with 0 degree laparoscopes, while with 30 degree laparoscopes it is loosely attached allowing the laparoscope to rotate. The camera

† Deceased

assistant needs to hold the camera in the true upright position while rotating the laparoscope to allow a wider and more complete field of vision. This is especially helpful around vascular structures. However, inexperienced camera assistants can easily disorientate the view with 30 degree laparoscopes, with potentially disastrous effects on correct identification of anatomy.

The camera head contains charge-coupled devices (CCDs) composed of minute photoelectrical elements (pixels) arranged in a rectangular grid allowing image acquisition. Reflected light from the surgical field is focused on the pixels by the endoscope lens system, producing an electronic response from the pixels, which is transmitted by wire to the video processor for conversion to a video signal.

Video cameras contain either one CCD or three CCDs; called one chip and three chip cameras; three chip cameras provide higher resolution and better colour reproduction. Video processors are usually designed to accept input from either a one chip or a three chip camera but not both; however, there are exceptions.

Video monitors are available in various sizes, with higher resolution images being obtained with smaller screens. One monitor will suffice with pelvic procedures, while two are needed with upper tract surgery to allow clear views to surgeons, assistants, scrub nurses, and anaesthetist.

Integrated operating theatres

Integrated operating theatres (ORs) are theatre suites which provide interactive monitoring and centralized control from a single operator panel and have speaker-independent voice control that enable devices such as cameras, lights, video conferencing units, picture archiving and communication systems (PACS), high frequency equipment, room functions, and the operating table to be operated from the sterile area. Examples include the OR 1TM system by Karl Storz or the EndoalphaTM Centralized OR system by Olympus (Melville, NY).

All the equipment including cables is boom mounted, and therefore safer. It is easier for staff to move around the theatre, which is a health and safety aspect. Monitors can be positioned where they are required. Fewer staff are required due to the central control; however, the system requires more training and increases the dependence on a team effort.

Insufflation system

To achieve satisfactory working space in either the peritoneum or retroperitoneum insufflation is required. Usually CO_2 is used via tubing attached to the initial hasson port or veress needle. Flow is initially at 1 L/min to assess safe entry and can then be increased to high flow (20–40 L/min). In patients with chronic respiratory disease, the accumulation of CO_2 in the blood can be dangerous and helium has been used as an alternative insufflation gas.

Laparoscopic trocars

Numerous disposable and reusable trocars are available in various sizes (2 mm, 5 mm, 10 mm, 12 mm, and 15 mm) (Fig. 2.22.1). The trocar tip can be bladed or blunt. The larger ports (10, 12, and 15 mm) have a valve or reducer system to allow the passage of smaller instruments without gas leakage. Longer trocars are also available for morbidly obese patients. BAUS now recommends the use of non-bladed, radially dilating trocars to minimize the risk of trocar injury during insertion.

Handpieces

A huge range of these exist, both reusable and disposable, and the choice is an individual one.

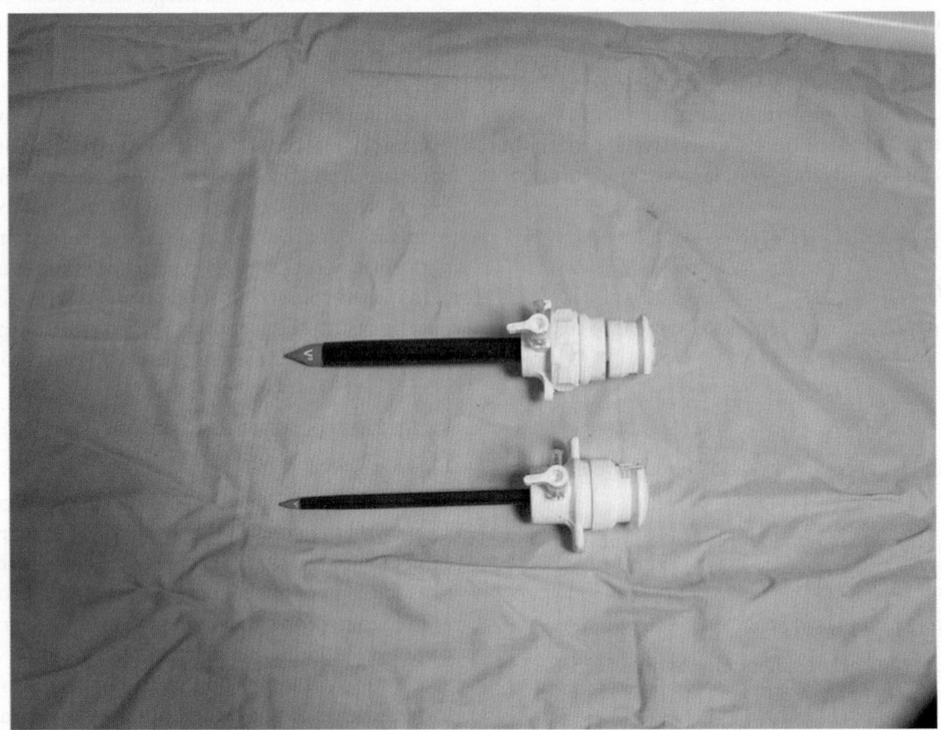

Fig. 2.22.1 12 mm and 5 mm disposable ports (Covidien).

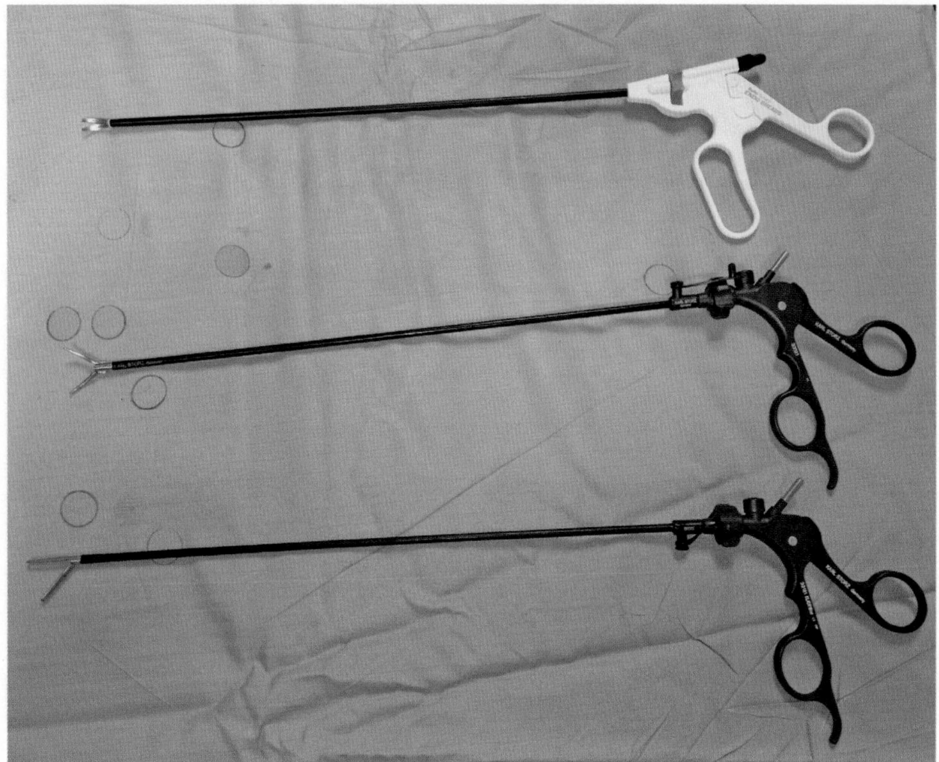

Fig. 2.22.2 Cutting scissors (top), Maryland graspers (middle), and Johann graspers (bottom).

Grasping instruments

These instruments are traumatic or atraumatic, locking or unlocking, single or double action, and come in various sizes (2–12 mm). Reusable instruments are modular allowing attachment of different tips to different handles with varying shaft lengths (Fig. 2.22.2).

Cutting instruments

Straight or curved scissors are available with attachment for electrosurgical leads to deliver monopolar diathermy. The coagulation is set at 30–55 W and cutting at 35 W. The J hook can also be used to dissect through tissues using monpolar diathermy and is very precise around vascular structures. Bipolar devices also exist that will coagulate the tissue but then need to be cut with another device (Fig. 2.22.3).

Needle holders

Many of these exist and the surgeon needs to try each out and select his own. Numerous devices have also been developed to facilitate both intra and extracorporeal suturing. These may help the novice laparoscopist, but we believe freehand intracorporeal suturing allows the greatest flexibility and versatility.

High-energy dissectors

Numerous devices, for example Harmonic (Ethicon), Ligasure (Covidien), hydrodissector, and argon beam have been introduced for laparoscopic tissue cutting and haemostasis (Fig. 2.22.4).

Ultrasonic energy allows tissue cutting and coagulation at lower temperatures (50–100°C) reducing scatter and charring. Ligasure seals vessels ≤7 mm in diameter reliably and reduces charring,[10] and while the Harmonic ACE scalpel can seal vessels up to 5 mm, this is not a consistent event.[10–11] The Harmonic ACE device was superseded by the Harmonic ACE+7 device (Fig. 2.22.5) which now reliably seals vessels up to 7 mm using the Advanced Hemostasis model.

The argon beam coagulator is good for haemostasis on superficial bleeding surfaces such as liver, spleen, kidney, and muscle. There is no forward scatter from this device, but it can cause a very rapid rise in intra-abdominal pressure. One of the trocars should be continuously vented to avoid this.[11] Newer energy devices include Sonicision (Coviden), the first cordless ultrasonic dissection device, and Thunderbeat (Olympus), the first integrated instrument that delivers both advanced bipolar and ultrasonic energy in a single device. All these devices are potentially financially restrictive.

Clips and staplers

These devices are vital to control medium and large calibre vessels. The clips are either made from titanium or plastic and may or may not interlock. The titanium clips are applied through manual- or self-loading applicators and need to be evenly spaced and non-crossing when applied. The interlocking plastic clips allow visualization of complete encirclement of the vessel and are our preferred method. Various sizes now exist to ensure complete encirclement of different size vessels, including the renal vein (Fig. 2.22.6).

Endoscopic staples are used mainly for large calibre vessels, such as the renal vein. They are of a linear GIA type, applying six rows of staples, and cutting between rows 3 and 4. Newer devices can also reticulate and articulate allowing a greater range of angles for application. Different cartridge sizes (30, 45, and 60 mm) and heights (2-, 2.5-, and 3 mm) are available. The staples cannot be applied over clips and care must be taken here.

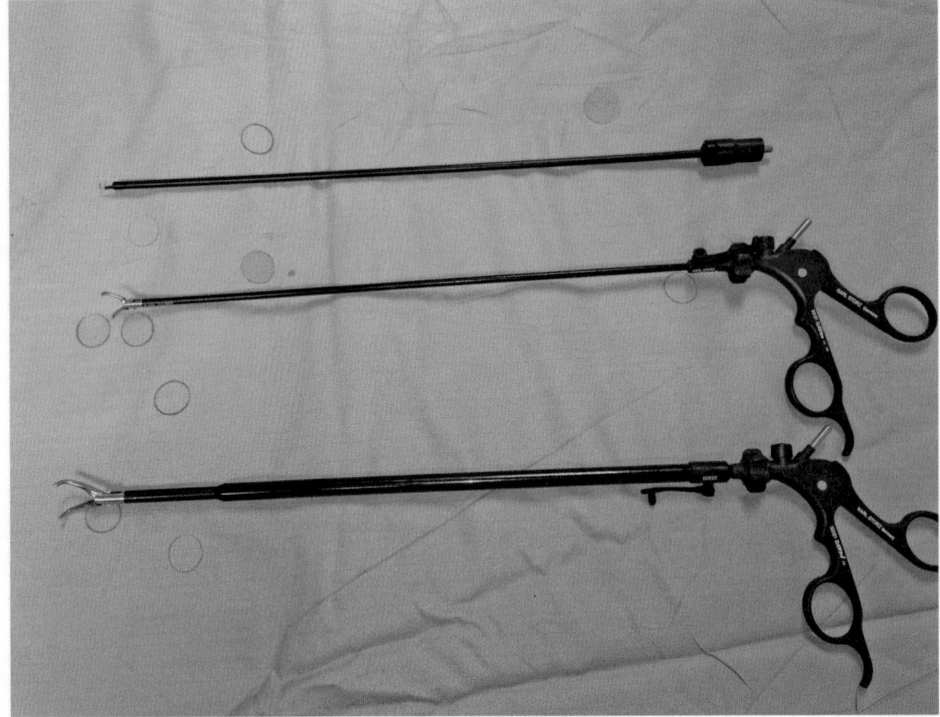

Fig. 2.22.3 Diathermy hook (top), short right-angle (middle), and large right-angle (bottom).

Aspiration and irrigation instruments

A variety of these devices exist both reusable and disposable. The aspirator is either a 5 or 10 mm metal or plastic tube with suction controlled via a stop-cock or spring-controlled valve. The irrigation works via the same mechanism. Normal saline or Ringers solution are the usual irrigants and may need to be delivered under pressure (Fig. 2.22.7).

Laparoscopic access

Accessing the space to perform the relevant laparoscopic procedure is fundamental to a successful outcome. If this step is not achieved correctly, problems from air leakage and a subsequently inadequate operating space to trocar injuries can lead to a disastrous attempt at laparoscopic surgery and possible early conversion.

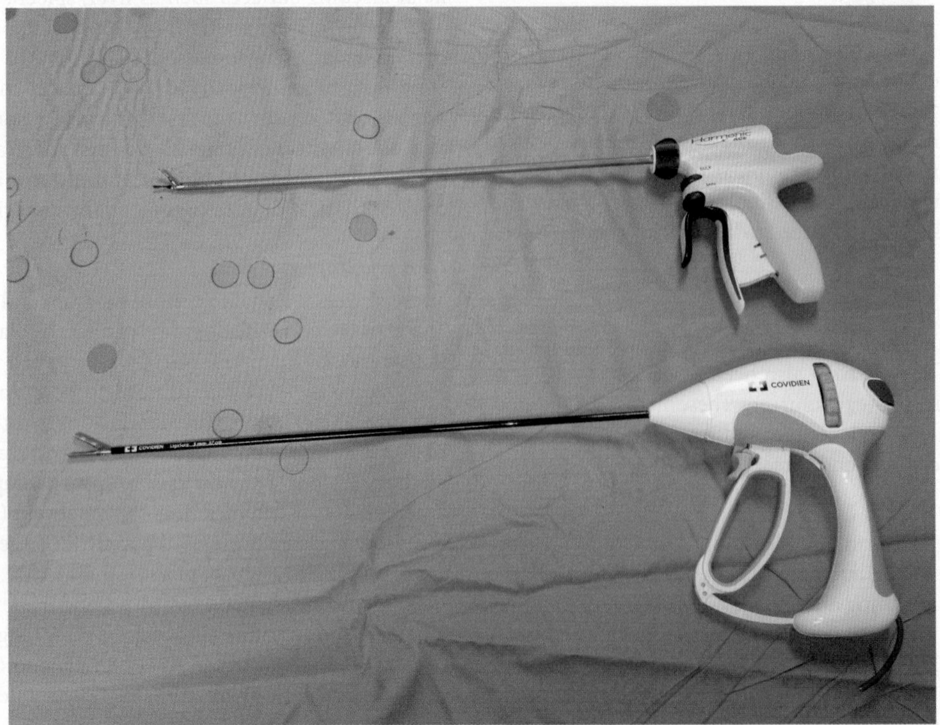

Fig. 2.22.4 Harmonic scalpel (Ethicon) (top) and ligasure device (Covidien) (below).

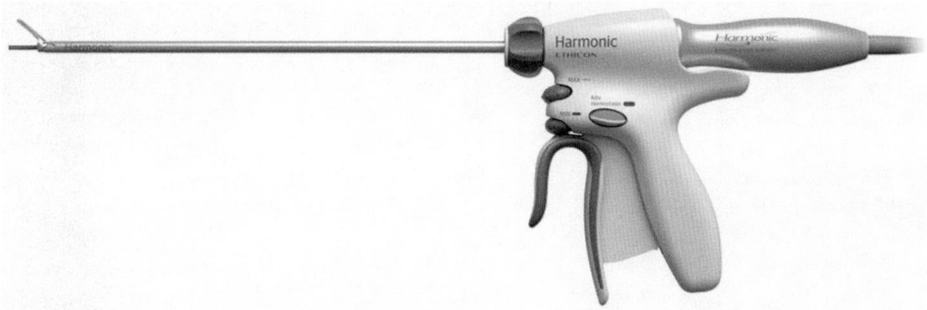

Fig. 2.22.5 Harmonic ACE+7 device.
Image reproduced courtesy of Ethicon Energy.

With transperitoneal approaches, both open and closed access techniques have been described.

Open access (Hasson technique)

A 2.5 cm incision is made usually at the position of the laparoscope port site. The incision continues down through the various abdominal wall layers. We now place two '0' PDS stay sutures into the rectus fascia, which aid closure at the end of the procedure particularly in obese patients and can improve the seal around the port. On reaching the peritoneum, it is grasped with a toothed forceps, clip or right-angle, palpated to check no bowel has been caught and opened sharply. A finger is introduced into the peritoneal cavity to check correct positioning. Obtaining an air tight seal is now critical to prevent insufflation leakage. A Hasson blunt tip cannula can be used and inserted into the peritoneal cavity and secured with the previously placed fascial sutures. Alternatively a blunt tip balloon cannula can be used, which allows the abdominal wall to be cinched between an inflated balloon and sponge on the cannula and this provides an excellent seal.[12]

Closed access using a Veress needle

A Veress needle is placed percutaneously into the peritoneal cavity again via the laparoscope port site. The needle consists of a metallic needle with a retractable protective blunt tip. The blunt tip retracts when the tip of the Veress needle presses against a

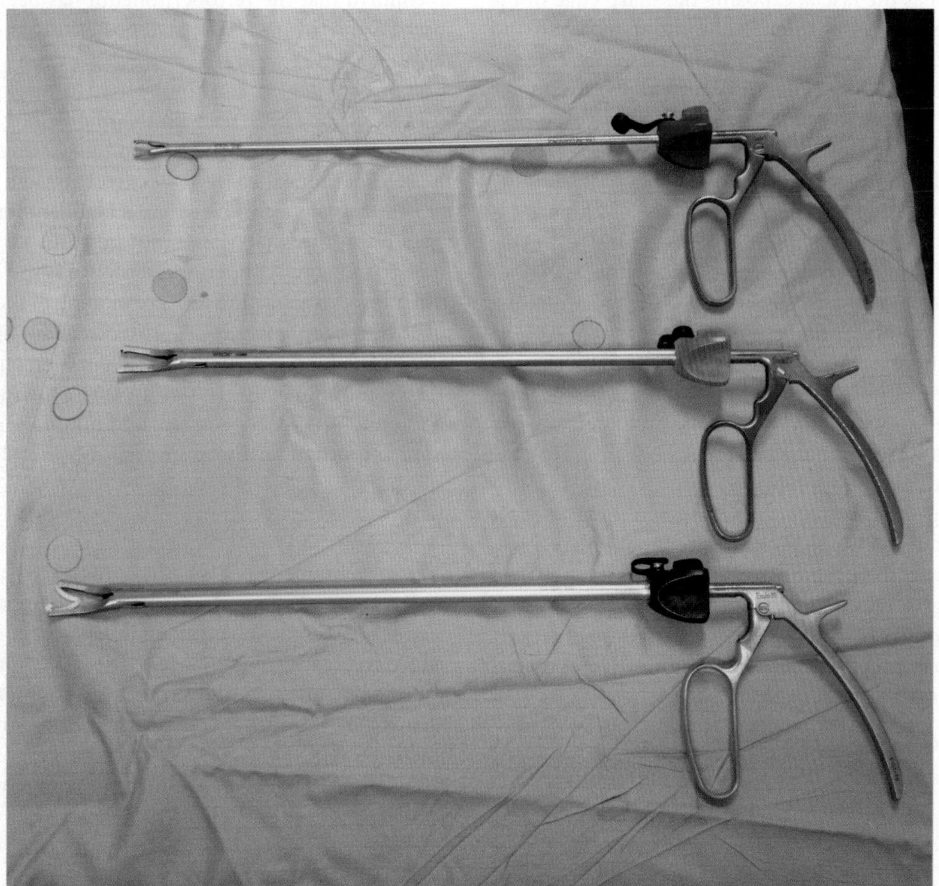

Fig. 2.22.6 Small (top), medium (middle), and large (bottom) clip appliers (Weklok).

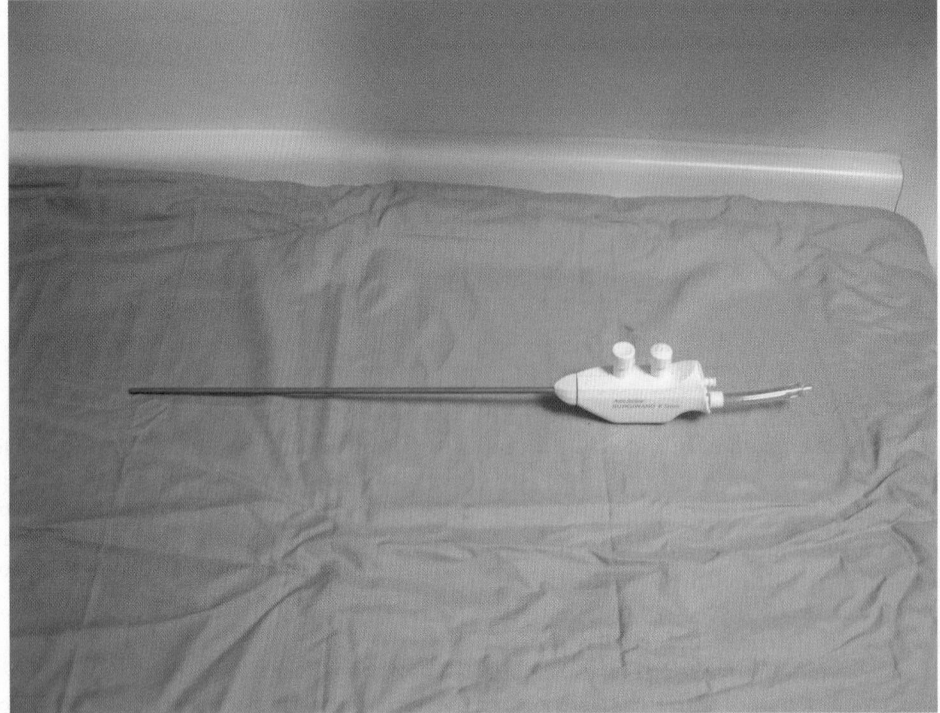

Fig. 2.22.7 Example of irrigation sucker (Covidien).

tough structure such as the fascia, exposing the sharp edge of the needle. Once the needle passes through the abdominal wall and into the peritoneal cavity, the blunt tip is deployed, protecting the abdominal viscera. The cannula is hollow, which allows peritoneal insufflation.[13]

Two distinct sensations of giving way are noticed during passage of the needle: one at the level of the external oblique/rectus fascia, and the second at the transversalis fascia/peritoneum. Once through these layers, the needle is aspirated to rule out blood or bowel contents and correct placement is further confirmed by injecting a small volume of saline and watching the meniscus drop rapidly. A final confirmation is achieved by observing a low intra-abdominal pressure after initiating insufflation at a low flow (1 L/min). Once confirmed, the insufflation rate can be increased to maximum. When the abdomen is maximally inflated (intra-abdominal pressure 15–20 mm Hg) the first trocar is placed, via an appropriate skin incision (to minimize skin gripping on the trocar). With pelvic laparoscopic procedures, the bladder needs to be emptied, patient placed in a Trendelenberg tilt, and the needle directed towards the pelvis to avoid injury to the great vessels.

Once the primary port has been placed, the additional trocars are placed under laparoscopic visualization, minimizing inadvertent vascular or visceral injury.

Retroperitoneal access is usually via an open technique

The initial incision is just below the tip of the twelfth rib. The skin, subcutaneous layer, and external oblique fascia are incised with scissors or diathermy. The fibres of internal oblique and transverses are separated bluntly with langebeck retractors revealing the thoracolumbar fascia. This fascia is divided sharply and the retroperitoneum is entered. Fat oftens pouts when the fascia is incised, and to confirm that the retroperitoneum has been entered, a finger is inserted and the psoas palpated posteriorly and the lower pole kidney superiorly.[14]

Numerous devices can now be used to develop the working space. A 22 Fr silicone catheter with the middle finger of a surgical glove attached is an inexpensive and in our view effective way to dilate the retroperitoneal space.[15] Between 500 and 600 mL of saline or air can be easily introduced via a bladder syringe. Although visualization of the dilatation is not possible we have not found this to be a problem. A superior alternative is the PDB balloon dilator. This allows visualization and positioning of the balloon to precisely dilate the space between the posterior abdominal wall and the kidney. The balloon is dilated up to 800 mL incrementally.

A 10 mm blunt tip balloon trocar is then inserted through the incision to provide a good seal and minimize gas leak. This is even more important in the retroperitoneum, where a more limited working space generally exists.

Basic laparoscopic skills

Skills development is a steadily progressive acquisition of surgical dexterity and spatial orientation. There now exists an urgent need for surgeons to be trained in laparoscopic/robotic skills until judged to be proficient by peers. Especially for the new generation of urologic surgeons, the surgical psychomotor skills needed for laparoscopy/robotics are readily learned and mastered by repetitive practice.

Recommendations for acquiring basic laparoscopic/robotic skills involve:

1. attending basic skills courses and live animal courses followed by working with a mentor when doing one's clinical cases; or
2. undergoing a laparoscopic/robotic fellowship.

Aspects of both of these approaches have been shown to reduce a surgeon's learning curve. However, tools to assess competency are presently not in place and these need to be developed with a sense of urgency.

A significant issue is the lack of an easy laparoscopic urological procedure to allow for high-volume, repetitive practice. There is no urologic cholecystectomy! This problem may be overcome by simulation. This includes bench models, animal simulation, and cadaveric simulation. Developments are awaited in this area; teleconferencing may also provide a novel approach to mentoring.

Robotic urological surgery

Telerobotic surgery involves placing a computer between the patient and the surgeon. The surgeon's hand movements are digitized to improve dexterity. The system also has three-dimensional stereoscopic visualization and is intuitive for the surgeon.

The da Vinci Surgical Robotic system (Intuitive Surgical, Sunnyvale, CA) represents the major technical advance in robotics. It is a master–slave telemanipulation system consisting of a remote console where the operating surgeon (master) controls the robotic surgical arms (slave) via a telerobotic videoscopic link. The surgeon controls the robotic arms with master handles which are located in a virtual three-dimensional space below the visual display. Foot controls are used to activate electrocautery, repositioning the master handles, and focusing. The master handles also control endoscope selection and motion-scaling ratio, as well as filtering tremor in the surgeon's hands and arms. In addition, tactile and force feedback—otherwise known as haptic feedback—can provide useful guidance to the surgeon.

The robotic arm cart holds three or four robotic arms on a central tower. One arm holds the videoscope, while the others are used to attach instrument adaptors connected to robotic instrumentation through the trocars. Stereoscopic vision is provided via a 0 or 30 degree three-dimensional endoscope.

Currently the robotic device utilized in the paediatric and adult population is identical, utilizing 12 mm camera ports and 8 mm working ports.

Access is achieved in the same way as for laparoscopy. Most robotic urological procedures (though not all) are performed transperitoneally, so a pneumoperitoneum is usually created as per laparoscopy. However a significant difference between laparoscopic and robotic port placement is the need for three or four ports for the robotic arms and procedure dependent one or two assistant ports. Port placement is even more critical in robotics as rotation of the operating table, bringing into use gravity as a natural retractor, is effectively lost without dedocking the robot.

Following docking of the robot, various instruments, driven by surgeon preference and operation type, are placed into the operative field. The robotic instruments have both an elbow and wrist joint, allowing seven degrees of freedom and two degrees of axial rotation mimicking natural motions of open surgery.

The remote surgeon at the consul proceeds with the surgery. This is the next significant difference, that is, the remote presence of the surgeon with a single bedside assistant. For this reason alone, the reliance on the assistant is usually greater during robotic compared with conventional laparoscopy. The Si da Vinci robot has two consuls (dual consul capability). Surgeons can exchange control of the instrument arms and endoscope using the surgeon touchpad, while a built-in intercom system facilitates communication. The addition of a second console enables two surgeons of the same or different specialties to collaborate on a single case; an immersive environment for training new *da Vinci* surgeons; a platform for existing *da Vinci* surgeons to more efficiently refine techniques, and learn new procedures directly from their peers.

The second potentially important development on the Si is the TilePro™ multi-input display. This allows the surgeon and the OR team to view 3D video of the operative field, along with up to two additional video sources such as ultrasound and computed tomography. This can be particularly helpful where repeated viewing of the images is required, for example during a partial nephrectomy. The latest Da Vinci robot, the Xi, uses a new overhead instrument arm architecture. This allows flexibility of laparoscope use on any arm and may improve access to certain anatomical sites.

Robotic surgeons take advantage of the three-dimensional vision, the facile articulating robotic wrist, and the lack of tremor. It is recognized that the da Vinci system is expensive, and prospective data attesting to improved outcomes over standard laparoscopy are not available. Yet, robotics does have a shorter learning curve compared to conventional laparoscopy, which has led to its widespread adoption over a rather short period of time in the United States.

Factors which have limited the uptake of robotic surgery in the paediatric population include the limited number of patients and indications for minimally invasive urologic surgery, the lack of paediatric sized ports, and the smaller working space compared to the adult population.

Acknowledgement

'Video systems' section adapted from John Reynard *et al.*, *Oxford Specialist Handbook in Urological Surgery*, Oxford University Press, Oxford, UK, Copyright © 2008, with permission from Oxford University Press.

Further reading

Capelouto CC, Kavoussi LR. Complications of laparoscopic surgery. *Urology* 1993; **42**: 2–12.

Clayman RV, Kavoussi LR, Soper NJ, *et al.* Laparoscopic nephrectomy: initial case report. *J Urol* 1991; **146**:278–82.

Gill IS, Rassweiler JJ. Retroperitoneoscopic renal surgery: our approach. *Urology* 1999; **54**:734–8.

Klingler CH, Remzi M, Marberger M, Janetschek G. Haemostasis in laparoscopy. *Eur Urol* 2006; **50**(5):948–56.

References

1. Clayman RV, Kavoussi LR, Soper NJ, *et al.* Laparoscopic nephrectomy: initial case report. *J Urol* 1991; **146**:278–82.
2. Clayman RV, Kavoussi LR, Figenshau RS, Chandhoke PS, Albala DM. Laparoscopic nephoureterectomy: initial case report. *J Laparoendosc Surg* 1991; **1**:343–9.
3. Scheussler WW, Vancaillie TG, Reich H, *et al.* Transperitoneal endosurgical lymphadenectomy in patients with localised prostate cancer. *J Urol* 1991; **145**: 988–91.
4. Parra RO, Andrus CH, Jones JP, *et al.* Laparoscopic cystectomy: initial report on a new treatment for retained bladder. *J Urol* 1992; **148**:1140–4.
5. Scheussler WW, Grune MT, Tecuanhuey LV, *et al.* Laparoscopic dismembered pyeloplasty. *J Urol* 1993; **150**:1795–9.

6. Scheussler WW, Schulam PG, Clayman RV, *et al.* Laparoscopic radical prostatectomy: initial short term experience. *Urology* 1997; **50**:854–7.
7. Monk TG, Weldon BC. Anaesthetic considerations for laparoscopic surgery. *J Endourol* 1992; **6**:89.
8. Albqami N, Janetschek G. Indications and contraindications for the use of laparoscopic surgery in renal cell carcinoma. *Nature Clin Prac Urol* 2006; **3**(1):32–7.
9. Kourambas J, Preminger GM. Advances in camera, video and imaging technologies in laparoscopy. *Urol Clin North Am* 2001; **28**(1):5–14.
10. Newcomb WL, Hope WW, Schmeizer TM, *et al.* Comparison of blood vessel sealing among new electrosurgical and ultrasonic devices. *Surg Endosc* 2009; **23**:90–6.
11. Klingler CH, Remzi M, Marberger M, Janetschek G. Haemostasis in laparoscopy. *Eur Urol* 2006; **50**(5):948–56.
12. Hasson HM. Open laparoscopy: 29 years experience. *Obstet Gynecol* 2000; **96**:763–6.
13. Peter CA. Complications in pediatric urologic laparoscopy: Results of a survey. *J Urol* 1996; **155**:1070–3.
14. Gill IS, Rassweiler JJ. Retroperitoneoscopic renal surgery: our approach. *Urology* 1999; **54**:734–8.
15. Gaur DD, Rathi SS, Ravandale AV, Gopichand M. A single-centre experience of retroperitoneoscopy using the balloon technique. *BJU Int* 2001; **87**:602–6.

SECTION 3

Functional and female

Section editor: Christopher R. Chapple

CHAPTER 3.1

Anatomy, neurophysiology, and pharmacological control mechanisms of the bladder

Donna Daly and Christopher R. Chapple

Anatomy

The bladder

The bladder is a hollow muscular organ, lined on its inner aspect by an epithelium and on its outer aspect by a serosa. The thick detrusor muscle wall is formed by smooth muscle cells, which are controlled by central and peripheral neural inputs. Being a highly distensible organ, the anatomical position of the bladder varies depending on the degree of distension. The empty bladder is an entirely extraperitoneal pelvic organ and lies behind the symphysis pubis in the shape of a flattened tetrahedron (three-sided pyramid). Anteriorly, the apex of the tetrahedron points towards the superior edge of the pubic symphysis (Fig. 3.1.1) and is anchored to the umbilicus by the median umbilical ligament. The superior surface is covered by peritoneum, behind which the sigmoid colon and small intestine usually rest.

In females, the anteverted uterus lies against the posterosuperior surface (Fig. 3.1.2). With increasing distension, the bladder rises in the shape of a dome well above the symphysis pubis and becomes an abdominal organ which can be palpated and percussed in the suprapubic region. As the bladder distends, the parietal peritoneum is stripped upwards from behind the rectus abdominus, thus access to the bladder (such as for suprapubic catheter insertion) is possible without violating the peritoneal cavity.

In males, the triangular base of the bladder faces posteriorly towards the rectum. Only the uppermost part of the posterior surface is covered by visceral peritoneum, forming the rectovesical pouch. Below this level, the ductus deferens and seminal vesicles are adherent to the posterior surface, and the space between the bladder and rectum contains Denonvilliers' rectovesical fascia.

Bladder neck and trigone

The lowest part of the bladder where the inferolateral surfaces meet the base is called the bladder neck. The lowest part of the neck is the triangular trigone. The two ureters each insert obliquely into the bladder posteroinferiorly, approximately 5 cm apart. The oblique external insertions are an important antireflux mechanism. The trigone is histologically and embryologically different from the rest of the bladder and contains a rich plexus of neuronal tissue; it is also the least mobile part of the bladder and is firmly adherent to the underlying muscle.

The bladder is composed of three distinct layers:

- *Serosa*—an outer adventitial connective tissue layer.
- *Detrusor muscle*—a smooth middle muscle layer, comprising interlacing muscle fibres running randomly in all directions. Only close to the internal urethral meatus do the fibres orientate themselves into three specific layers (inner—longitudinal, middle—circumferential, outer—longitudinal).
- *Urothelium*—an innermost lining comprised of transitional cell epithelium that provides an elastic barrier that is impervious to urine. Immediately beneath this lies a suburothelial layer, which is metabolically active.

The male urethra

The total length of the male urethra is approximately 20 cm and is comprised of four sections: the short prostatic and membranous sections form the 'posterior' urethra, and the longer (approximately 15 cm) bulbar and penile sections form the 'anterior' urethra. The anterior urethra is entirely enclosed within the corpus spongiosum and is sometimes termed the 'spongy' urethra.

A continuation of the circular smooth muscle fibres from the detrusor forms the involuntary internal urethral sphincter at the level of the bladder neck and proximal urethra. This mechanism is sometimes termed the pre-prostatic sphincter and is important in preventing retrograde ejaculation of semen and in maintaining urinary continence. This sphincter is often injured during bladder neck or prostatic surgery, frequently resulting in retrograde ejaculation. However, incontinence occurs less commonly due to the presence of the voluntary external urethral sphincter composed of striated muscle, which surrounds the membranous urethra and is a further powerful anti-incontinence mechanism.

The female urethra

The female urethra is much shorter than the male urethra and is usually only about 4 cm in length. The urethra passes below the pubic symphysis embedded in the anterior vaginal wall, and it curves slightly forward during its course from the bladder neck (internal urethral meatus) to the external urethral meatus.

A longitudinal layer of smooth muscle, continuous with the inner longitudinal layer of detrusor muscle surrounds a submucosa. This is surrounded by a thicker layer of circular smooth muscle, which

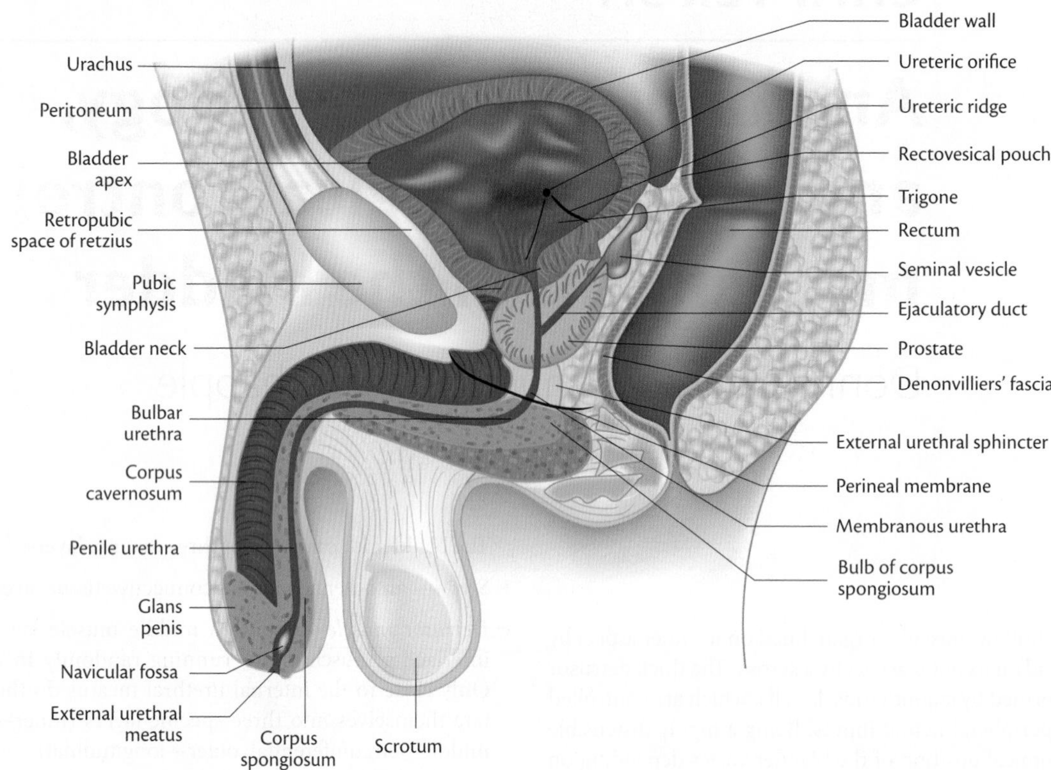

Fig. 3.1.1 Median sagittal section of male pelvis, showing the lower urinary tract.

is continuous with the external detrusor muscle at the bladder neck. These smooth muscle layers form the involuntary urethral sphincter; however, compared to the male, the involuntary urethral mechanism at the bladder neck is poorly developed. Surrounding the involuntary muscle in the middle-third of the urethra is the circular voluntary striated muscle, which forms the external urethral sphincter. This external sphincter is horseshoe-shaped and is thicker at the sides and ventrally. In contrast to males, the involuntary bladder neck and voluntary external sphincters are not distinct structures and both sphincters are much less powerful in females.

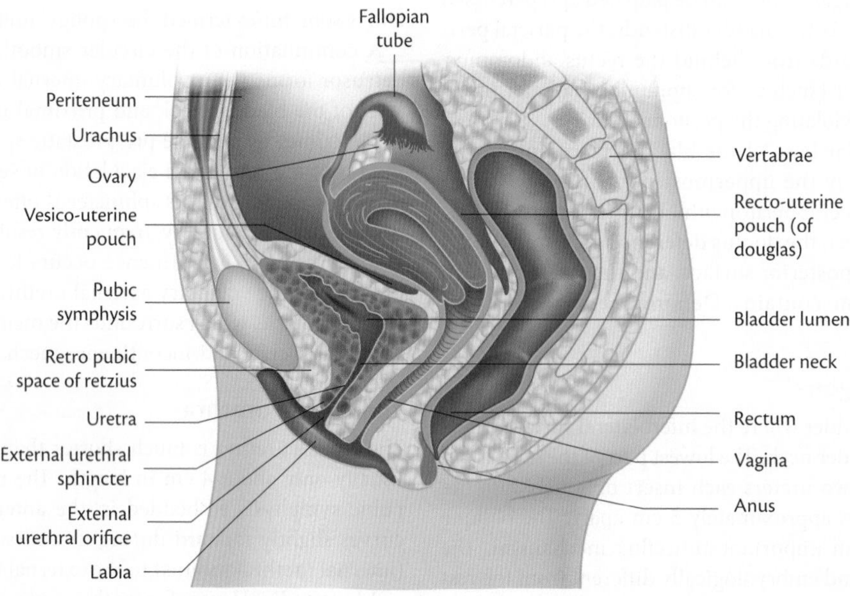

Fig. 3.1.2 Median sagittal section of female pelvis, showing the lower urinary tract.

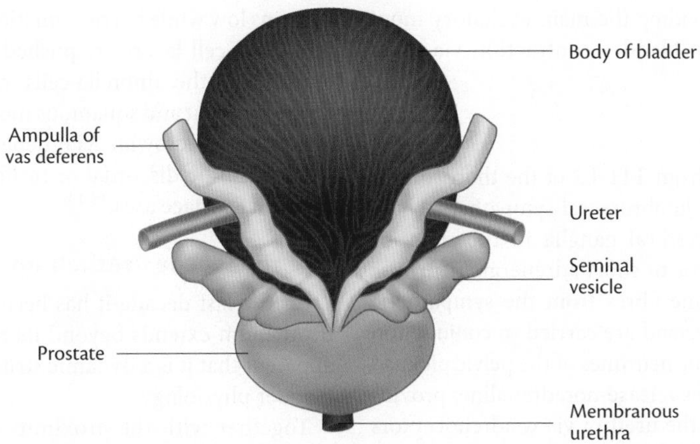

Fig. 3.1.3 Posterior view of bladder and prostate, showing relations of adherent structures.

The weaker sphincter mechanisms, coupled with the much shorter urethra may predispose to urinary incontinence. In addition, the urethra, sphincters, and their innervation along with the pelvic floor muscles may be injured during childbirth, further predisposing women to urinary incontinence.

The prostate

The prostate is an ovoid-shaped (walnut-sized), fibromuscular (30%), and glandular organ (70%). It weighs approximately 20 g and produces about 30% of the volume of seminal fluid, much of the remainder being produced by the seminal vesicles. Beneath the true capsule are circularly orientated smooth muscle fibres and collagenous tissue, forming an involuntary sphincter (Fig. 3.1.3). Deep in this layer is the prostatic stroma of connective and elastic tissues, smooth muscle fibres, and epithelial glands. The prostatic urethra is lined with transitional epithelium.

The prostate lies entirely behind the pubic symphysis and is enclosed within a true capsule of strong connective tissue. Outside this is a layer of pelvic fascia forming a 'false capsule'. The base of the prostate is the superior surface of the organ and is fused to the neck of the bladder. The urethra emerges inferiorly from the base as the membranous urethra. The posterior surface of the prostate is separated from the lower rectum by the two layers of Denonvilliers' fascia. This surface is readily palpable via the rectum. The seminal vesicles and the vas deferens join to form the ejaculatory ducts; these ducts pierce the prostate superior-posteriorly (where the prostate and bladder fuse) and pass obliquely through the gland.

Formally the prostate was classified as consisting of lobes; although these did not correspond with histologically defined structures. The two lateral lobes are separated by a median sulcus which is palpable rectally. A median lobe (between the two ejaculatory ducts) may protrude into the bladder neck and act as a valve, causing obstruction during voiding.

Neurophysiology of the bladder

Afferent innervation

Bladder afferent nerves play a central role in spinal voiding reflexes and convey information to the central nervous system (CNS) about bladder function. Afferent projections from the bladder and urethra travel in the pelvic, hypogastric, and pudendal nerves and pass into discreet regions of the dorsal horn in the lumbrosacral spinal cord (T11-L2 and S2-S4). These afferents consist of myelinated Aδ fibres and unmyelinated C fibres, which convey information about the extent of bladder wall distension, volume, and stretch, and the presence of noxious agents to the brain. Ascending afferent projections travel via the lateral funiculs or the dorsal funiculs and terminate in a number of regions, including the preiaqueductal grey matter[1,2] where they convey information to the pontine micturition centre to initiate the micturition reflex.[3]

Previous studies have classified bladder afferents according to their neurochemical coding (peptidergic vs. non-peptidergic), their sensitivity (mechanosensitivity vs. chemosensitivity), or by their threshold for mechanical activation (low threshold vs. high threshold).[4,5] However, more recent assessments of these nerves classify afferents according to the location of the receptive field (mucosal vs. muscle), the anatomy of the afferent terminal and physiological properties. Currently four functionally distinct classes of bladder afferents have been described. These include the stretch-sensitive 'muscle mechanoreceptors' and 'muscle-mucosal mechanoreceptors' and the stretch-insensitive 'mucosal mechanoreceptors and chemoreceptors'.[6]

Efferent innervation

Autonomic innervation to the bladder is conveyed by hypogastric and pelvic nerves and somatic innervation of the external urethra is conveyed via the pudendal nerve. Autonomic nerves fibres innervating the bladder are broadly classified as either sympathetic (adrenergic) or parasympathetic (cholinergic).

Parasympathetic efferent fibres

Sacral parasympathetic preganglionic neurones supplying the bladder and urethra are in the intermediolateral region of the sacral spinal cord (S2-S4 laminae v-vii) and pass to peripheral ganglia via the pelvic nerve where they synapse in either the pelvic plexus, or the autonomic ganglia located in the detrusor wall. These intramural ganglia convey (and can modulate) information from the preganglionic parasympathetic fibres to the smooth muscle.[7] Postganglionic neurons richly innervate the musculature of the bladder dome and urethra and are predominantly excitatory. Terminal regions of the parasympathetic postganglionic nerves have vesicle-filled varicosities, which release neurotransmitters such as acetylcholine (ACh), providing the main excitatory input to the bladder body resulting in bladder contraction via muscarinic receptors.

Sympathetic efferent fibres

Sympathetic pathways originate from T11-L2 of the thorocolumber spinal cord and pass into the lumbrosacral sympathetic chain ganglia, and then to the preverterbral ganglia in the superior hypogastric and pelvic plexuses, or to short adrenergic neurones in the bladder and urethra.[1] Some fibres from the sympathetic chain may pass to the pelvic nerve and are carried in conjunction with parasympathetic preganglionic neurones of the pelvic plexus.[8] Sympathetic postganglionic nerves release noradrenaline, providing the main excitatory input to the urethra via α-adrenoceptors and an inhibitory input to the bladder body via β-adrenoceptors.[9]

Somatic efferent fibres

The somatic innervation of the urethra arises from Onufs nucleus located in the ventral horn of the spinal cord (S2-4) and projects via the pudendal nerve to the external sphincter muscles, which it excites the muscle via acetylcholine release.[10]

The detrusor muscle

The bladder is largely a muscular organ made up of smooth muscle called the detrusor, a term derived from the Latin word meaning 'to drive out'. Muscular tone and contraction are controlled by complex mechanisms involving interactions between the CNS and local release and degradation of transmitters related to adrenergic, cholinergic, and non-adrenergic non-cholinergic mechanisms (NANC). The detrusor is a highly compliant muscle which can stretch and accommodate without a significant increase in tone, a property that is termed 'receptive relaxation', and which is essential to maintain low intravesical pressure during bladder filling. This is achieved due to the innate elastic properties of the muscle and to relaxation as a result of stimulation of sympathetic beta-adrenoreceptors.

The urothelium

The epithelial layer of the urinary bladder and the underlying laminar propria layer is a specialized lining called the urothelium. The epithelium is typically five to seven cells thick and consist of three layers: a basal cell layer (10 μm diameter cells) attached to a basement membrane; an intermediate layer (10–25 μm diameter cells); and an apical layer made from large specialized polyhedral cells, termed umbrella cells (25–250 μm diameter cells).[11]

Barrier function

The primary function of the apical layer is to protect the underlying tissue from damage or irritation by components of the urine contained in the bladder lumen and to control the passage of water and ions across the epithelial surface. The barrier function is maintained by several properties of the apical cell layer. The cells have special lipid membranes and contain plaques known as uroplakins, which cover 90% of the cell surface; this reduces the permeability of the urothelium to small molecules such as water, urea, or protons. The apical layer is also extensively interconnected by high resistance tight junctions, which limit the movement of ions and solutes between cells.[12]

In the empty bladder, the urothelium is highly pleated and folded in to rugae. During filling and storage, the urothelium undergoes conformational changes to ensure that intravesical pressure remains low while barrier function is maintained. The intermediate and basal cell layers are pushed laterally to unfold the urothelial surface and the umbrella cells transform from a roughly cuboidal shaped to a flat and squamous morphology. This transitional change is accompanied by an ATP-dependent fusion of subapical vesicles (which can be discordal or fusiform shaped), which increases the epithelial surface area.[11,13]

The role of the urothelium in sensation

Over the last decade it has become clear that the function of the urothelium extends beyond its role as a passive barrier. It is now apparent that it is a dynamic structure which plays an active role in bladder physiology.

Together with the proximity of sensory nerve terminals, the urothelium is in the ideal location to monitor bladder filling and influence nerve activity. An array of ion channels and receptors normally associated with neurotransmission have been located on urothelial cells (some highlighted in Table 3.1.1) and studies have shown that the urothelium releases a host of excitatory and inhibitory signalling molecules in response to stretch, distension,[14–18] and noxious stimulation (such as acidic conditions).[19] These molecules act downstream at the afferent terminal to modulate and control afferent nerve activity. The most well-recognized example is the graded release of ATP from the urothelium during bladder filling, which activates puringeric receptors (P2X2 and P2X3) located on nerve terminals to induce afferent nerve activity.[20] This has led to the concept that bladder afferent transmission is a multifactorial process involving cross-talk between the urothelium and the sensory nerves, which work together to form a sensory web.[21]

The role of the urothelium in bladder tone

In addition to modulating sensory function, the urothelium may also modulate bladder smooth muscle tone via the release of transmitters, which diffuse to the underlying smooth muscle. Most notably ACh, NO, and ATP are released by the urothelium in response to stretch and have been shown to modulate contractility of bladder smooth muscle strips in *in vitro* studies. Interestingly, there is also evidence of an unidentified inhibitory mediator, released by the urothelium in response to muscarinic and electrical stimulation.[22–37]

Contraction of isolated feline bladder strips were augmented when the urothelium was removed, suggesting that the urothelium releases an inhibitory mediator which affects the tone or contractile ability of the underlying smooth muscle.[38] A similar inhibitory factor was also identified by Foveus *et al.* (1999), who found an endogenously released mediator from the rat bladder could inhibit the contractile response to the denuded rat aorta. This mediator was unaffected by the presence of a cycoloxygenase inhibitor, indomethacin, or a nitric oxide synthase inhibitor. However, in contrast to the factor suggested by Levin *et al.* (1995), it was not believed to be urothelially derived since the relaxatory response was unaffected by removal of the urothelium. Hawthorn *et al.* (2000) also identified a similar mediator in the pig bladder, which was believed to be a diffusible inhibitory mediator of urothelial origin. Whether these studies have identified the same factor is unclear, however consistent with the findings of Foveus *et al.* (1999), release of this factor was unaffected by inhibition of the nitric oxide pathway or by blockade of catecholamine and cyclooxygenase. The factor now termed the 'urothelium-derived inhibitory factor' (UDIF) inhibits the contractile response

Table 3.1.1 Receptors expressed in the urothelium

Receptor/ stimulus	Subtype expression on the urothelium	Species/evidence	
Purinergic	$P2X_5$, $P2X_6$, $P2X_7$	Rat	Lee *et al.* (2000)[22]
	$P2X_3$	Rat and human	Elneil *et al.* (2001)[23]
	$P2X_{1-7}$ and $P2Y_{1,2,4}$	Cat	Birder *et al.* (2004)[24]
TRP	TRPV1	Rat and mouse and human	Lazzeri *et al.* (2004); Birder *et al.* (2001)[25,26]
	TRPM8	Human and rat	Stein *et al.* (2004)[27]
	TRPV4	Rat and human	Birder *et al.* (2007)[28]
Muscarinic	M_1-M_5	Human and mouse	Zarghooni *et al.* (2007); Bschleipfer *et al.* (2007); Mansfield *et al.* (2005)[29–31]
Nicotinic	α3, α7, α5, β3–4	Rat	Beckel *et al.* (2006)[32]
	α7,α9,α10	Human	Bschleipfer *et al.* (2007)[30]
	α2,4,5,6,7,9 &10	Mouse	Zarghooni *et al.* (2007)[29]
Bradykinin	BK2	Rat	Chopra *et al.* (2005)[33]
Noradrenaline	α1d	Rat	Ishihama *et al.* (2006)[34]
	β-adrenergic	Human	Harmon *et al.* (2005)[35]
Amiloride sensitive Na^+ channel	ENac	Rat and rabbit	Burton *et al.* (2002); Watanabe *et al.* (1999)[36,37]

of the bladder smooth muscle by up to 50% *in vitro*.[39,40] Whether this mediator contributes to normal contractile function and tone *in vivo* is unclear. Some investigators have disputed this idea, suggesting that the plexus of blood vessels which forms in the suburothelium, between the urothelial cells and the muscle, would act as a diffusion barrier. However, if identified, the UDIF could be a promising future target for the treatment of various lower urinary tract conditions.

Interstitial cells

Interstitial cells (ICs) of the bladder were first described by Smett and Jonavicius in 1996. It is now known that bladder ICs are structurally similar to the well-characterized interstitial cells of Cajal (ICC) located in the gut (see[41,42]). They are widely distributed throughout the lower urinary tract and form two distinct plexus; one which lies beneath the urothelium, and the other within the smooth muscle layers.[43–47]

The ICCs of the gut have a well-described pacemaker function, drive peristaltic activity, and act as intermediaries in transmitting signals from the nerve to the muscle; however, the function of bladder ICs has yet to be fully established. Studies to date suggest that the two plexus of bladder ICs have distinct physiological properties and may have distinct functional roles, with the suburothelial ICs participating in amplification and transduction of signals between the urothelium and sensory nerves, and muscle ICs acting as modulators of detrusor smooth muscle spontaneous contractile activity. While more research is still required to fully understand how ICs contribute to normal function and pathophysiology of the lower urinary tract, these unique cells may be an attractive target for the future treatment of lower urinary tract disorders.

Micturition

For the bladder to be effective at storing and voiding in a controlled and efficient manner, all myogenic and neurogenic components need to function in a coordinated manner. This is achieved in a regulated cycle of events known as the micturition cycle. During bladder filling, urine is transferred to the bladder via the ureters at low pressure in a continuous fashion and at a rate dictated by renal urine production. Sympathetic stimulation initiates the release of noradrenaline, which acts via β-adrenoreceptors (predominantly the β3-adrenoreceptors in humans) to relax detrusor smooth muscle, and via α1-adrenoreceptors located on the muscle of the urethral outlet to contract the urethral sphincter mechanism. During the filling phase, the bladder accommodates to the increase in volume without a significant rise in intraluminal pressure. This compliance is dependent on both the spinal reflex mechanisms and the passive electrical properties of the musculature in the wall. During filling, afferent nerve firing frequency gradually increases in response to stretch, distortion, and increased tension, furthermore influenced by the additional non-neuronal release of neurotransmitters; transmitting signals to the brain, via the lateral spinalthalamic tracts and sacral cord (Fig. 3.1.4). This activity initiates the 'desire to void' and a switch from the filling to voiding phase occurs. This is either voluntarily (in the adult) or involuntarily (in the infant) by a release of the negative inhibition imposed by the higher centres on the pontine micturition centres, resulting in parasympathetic stimulation of the detrusor muscle and inhibition of the sympathetic and somatic pathways. This switch inhibits the excitatory input to the striated urethral sphincter, and the muscle of the internal urethral sphincter is relaxed by a release of nitric oxide from the parasympathetic nerves.[48] Simultaneously, parasympathetic nerves innervating the dome and body of the bladder release ACh, eliciting an acute bladder contraction via muscarinic receptor stimulation (Fig. 3.1.4). The contraction of the muscle causes an increase in intravesical pressure and a flow of urine though the urethra.[49]

Pathology and lower urinary tract symptoms

Any physiological disruption in the micturition cycle can give rise to a number of lower urinary tract symptoms (LUTS). These

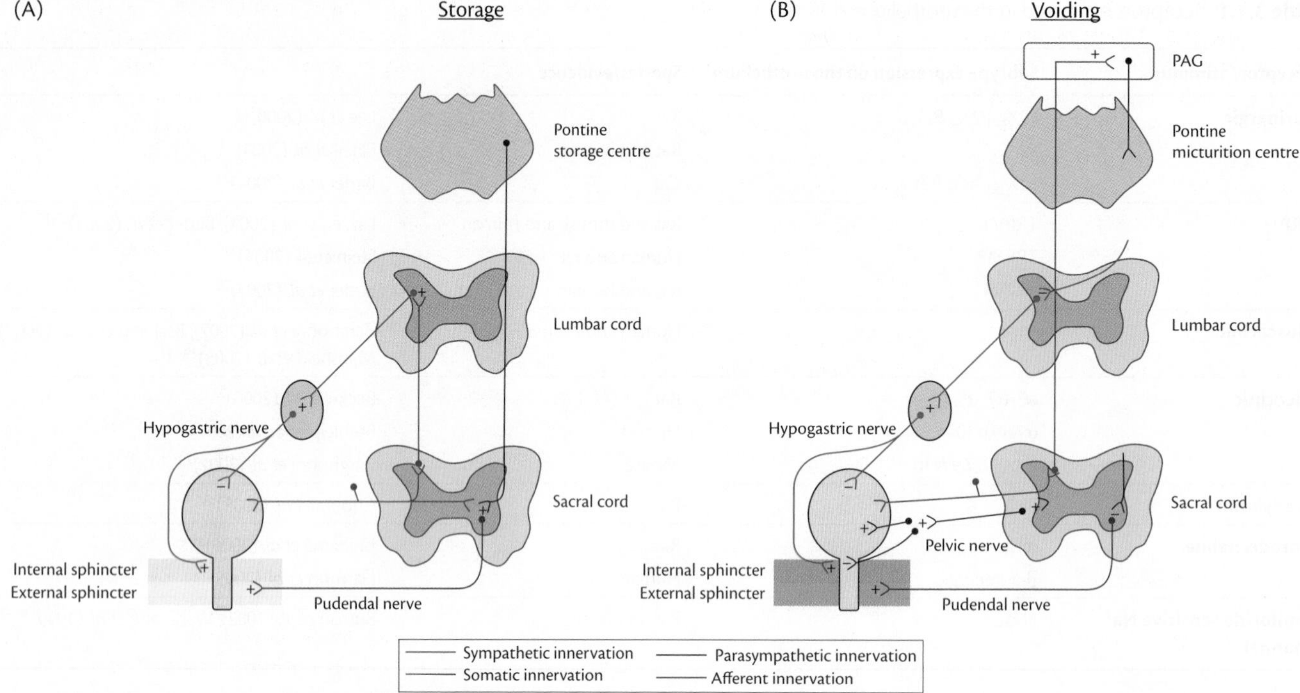

Fig. 3.1.4 (A) Bladder storage pathways. During filling, distension of the bladder activates low-level afferent nerve activity. This activates sympathetic outflow in the hypogastric nerve (resulting in inhibition of the detrusor muscle and activation of the internal urethral sphincter) and activation of pudendal innervation to the external urethral sphincter (resulting in contraction). (B) Bladder voiding pathways. High-level afferent firing activates spinobulbospinal reflex pathways that pass through the pontine micturition centre. This activates parasympathetic nerves resulting in contraction of the detrusor muscle and inhibition of the internal sphincter, and inhibition of the pudendal outflow to the external urethral sphincter.

Adapted by permission from Macmillan Publishers Ltd: *Nature Reviews Neuroscience*, Volume 9, Issue 6, Clare J. Fowler et al., 'The neural control of micturition', pp. 453–466, Copyright © 2008.

disorders can be broadly subdivided into storage disorders (such as overactive bladder symptom syndrome) comprising frequency, nocturia, urgency, and urgency incontinence (OABS), bladder pain syndrome (BPS), and voiding disorders (such as premicturition delay, poor stream, and incomplete bladder emptying).

Storage disorders

During bladder storage, it is essential for the urethral outlet to remain closed, the detrusor muscle to accommodate to increasing volumes, and the afferent nerve activity to remain low (below the level of conscious sensation). This ability can be compromised by a reduction in bladder capacity (either functional due to infection or detrusor overactivity, or anatomical as a consequence of a reduced bladder capacity due to fibrosis such as follows chronic infection c.f. tuberculosis or surgery or radiotherapy), altered functional capacity caused by increased sensation (due to OABS, lower urinary tract infections, or BPS) or neurourological disorders (such as diabetic neuropathy, spinal injury, and multiple sclerosis). Symptoms of storage dysfunction include:

- *Urgency*—the sudden compelling desire to empty the bladder, which is difficult to defer.
- *Frequency*—frequent urination defined emptying the bladder > 8/day (50).
- *Nocturia*—waking in the night to empty the bladder resulting in sleep disturbance, each void preceded and followed by sleep.
- *Urinary incontinence*—involuntary loss of urine, which can be continuous or intermittent.
- *Enuresis*—involuntary loss of urine during the night.
- *Bladder pain during filling*—once infection or other intravesical pathology has been excluded, this is a characteristic feature of BPS.

Bladder pain syndrome

Bladder pain syndrome is a condition of unknown aetiology and is a diagnosis by exclusion of other significant intravesical pathology (see also Chapter 1.11). BPS is disorder which leads to an increase in urinary frequency (± urgency, ± bladder pain) in which cystometry fails to demonstrate a rise in the filling detrusor pressure, suggestive of detrusor overactivity. Urinary frequency is a prominent symptom and bladder pain, rather than impending incontinence, is the trigger. Urgency may also occur but incontinence is not usually present. Nocturnal frequency is often less than diurnal frequency in hypersensitive bladders. Bladder pain, when present, is usually relieved by voiding. Dysuria may be a symptom and suggests the presence of inflammation in the urethra. Strangury is suggestive of trigonal inflammation. Dyspareunia, or painful intercourse, is common in patients with bladder hypersensitivity and haematuria is present in 20–30% of cases.

The symptoms are of BPS are chronic. Typically, the onset of BPS can be traced back to a previous probable urinary tract infection, but often a urine culture has not been performed. The patient receives a course of antibiotics and the symptoms disappear for a while. However, the urine is proved sterile by urine cultures, antibiotics do not work, and the symptoms persist. Women often report improvement at the end of their menstrual cycle and many will have had previous hysterectomy, perhaps for lower abdominal pain, but no obvious gynaecological pathology. Examination may be unremarkable but attention should be paid to the urethral meatus, which may be inflamed or show mucosal prolapse. There may also be bladder tenderness, both suprapubically and on vaginal examination. A gentle bimanual examination will identify other pelvic pathology.

All patients require urinalysis and culture; urine cytology is recommended in selected cases. X-ray studies are generally not useful in the evaluation of patients with bladder hypersensitivity, although pelvic ultrasound may be helpful in excluding gynaecological disease. All cases of hypersensitive bladder should undergo cystoscopy preferably combined with bladder hydrodistension (at a presure of 80 cm water for two minutes) and bladder biopsies. A proportion of patients are improved symptomatically following this procedure, often combined with a urethral recalibration.

Treatment of patients with bladder hypersensitivity is directed at the underlying disease process, but unfortunately this is not always known or understood. Subsequently, therapy is entirely empirical, as the evidence base for the efficacy of all therapy is limited at present. A commonly utilized therapy is to instil protein solutions intravesically with the intention of 'relining' the bladder urothelium, as it is a commonly held view that a significant causative problem is loss of the lining proteinaceous glucosamine glycan layer (GAG) layer in the bladder. All pharmacologically active therapy is entirely empirical and directed at the relief of pain.

Overactive bladder syndrome

The most common storage disorder of the bladder is overactive bladder syndrome (OABS).[50] OABS is characterized by the International Continence Society[51] as urgency, with or without urinary incontinence (roughly one-third of patients exhibit urinary incontinence), frequency, and nocturia in the absence of a proven infection or obvious pathological condition. OABS is reported to have an overall prevalence of 11.8%, comprising 10.8% in males and 12.8% in females.[52,53] The condition affects all ages, but the prevalence of OABS significantly increases with age. Overactive bladder (OAB) has a severe impact on quality of life, negatively affecting work productivity, self-esteem, emotional well-being, and social interaction. Approximately 70% of patients with OABS have urodynamically proven detrusor overactivity (DO). DO is a urodynamic observation that manifests as involuntarily contractions of the detrusor muscle, which occur during the bladder filling phase. DO may be either idiopathic, which is the case for the majority of cases classified as having OABS, or as a result of neurogenic detrusor overactivity.

Neurogenic detrusor overactivity

Neurogenic detrusor overactivity (NDO) is defined as bladder overactivity which results due to neurological dysfunction, or degeneration of the neural pathways controlling micturition. Neurogenic OAB can be caused by supraspinal, suprasacral, or infrasacral lesions.

- *Supraspinal*: Lesions occurring above the pontine micturition centre leading to a loss of voluntary voiding, the pontine micturition centre is still intact; thus the micturition reflex is still coordinated, but voluntary control is lost.
- *Suprasacral*: Spinal cord trauma above the sacral region of the spinal cord leads to a loss of feedback to higher centres. Immediately following a spinal trauma, there is a 'spinal shock' where there is little neurological activity for a period of time. The spinal reflexes gradually recover, but are uninhibited due to a loss of control from the higher centres. Sphincter and detrusor contractions are also uncoordinated due to a loss of input from the pontine micturition centre, known as so-called detrusor sphincter dyssynergia.
- *Infrasacral*: Damage to motor or sensory neurones results in a loss of nervous input to the bladder.

Idiopathic detrusor overactivity

Idiopathic detrusor overactivity (IDO) is defined as bladder overactivity with no identifiable cause and most cases of OAB fall into this group. The mechanisms involved in the pathophysiology of OAB are likely to be complex and involve a combination of peripheral and central components including sensory neural pathways, efferent activity, and the detrusor muscle.

Detrusor overactivity versus overactive bladder?

OABS is a symptomatic diagnosis, whereas DO is a urodynamic observation. Urgency and the other symptoms associated with OABS are generally correlated with the presence of DO, however the two are not synonymous to each other and studies suggest only 65% of OAB patients had identifiable DO.[54] The exact cause of DO is unclear in the absence of a recognized neurological history, however there are currently three hypotheses proposed to explain the basis of DO.

1. *A myogenic hypothesis for detrusor overactivity.*

The myogenic hypothesis for detrusor overactivity suggests that DO arises due to changes in smooth muscle function resulting in hyperexcitability of smooth muscle cells and/or increased electrical coupling resulting in uncontrolled spontaneous contractions. In support of this hypothesis, studies have identified increased spontaneous contractile activity in bladder strips taken from DO patients with bladder outflow obstruction,[55,56] changes in electrical coupling of the detrusor,[57,58] and alterations in calcium handling.[59]

2. *A neurogenic hypothesis for detrusor overactivity.*

The neurogenic hypothesis for detrusor overactivity suggests that DO arises due to changes in peripheral and central neural mechanisms resulting in loss of voluntary or supraspinal control of the bladder. This hypothesis suggests that injury or damage to the descending inhibitory pathways from the higher centres evokes reorganization, sensitization, neuroplasticity, and spouting of nerves to give rise to nerve-mediated excitation of the detrusor muscle.[1]

3. *An integrative hypothesis for detrusor overactivity.*

The integrative hypothesis for detrusor overactivity suggests that DO arises due to changes in the function of other cells types such as the IC cells, the urothelium, and peripheral afferent nerves, leading to enhancement of autonomous contractions.[60]

While the exact pathogenesis of OABS is not yet understood the cardinal symptom of OABS is urgency, which is presumed to arise from increased sensory nerve activity, enhancing the sensation of fullness and triggering the premature onset of micturition. However, whether this is caused by direct alterations in afferent neural traffic due to peripheral factors (such as altered morphology and function of the nerve terminal), or is secondary to alterations in other components (such as the urothelium and detrusor), or due to changes in the central control mechanisms (with a change in the negative inhibition of the pontine micturition centre) is at present not clearly established.

Some studies have suggested that DO elicits an increase in mechanosensory nerve activity and that this results in urgency. There are also studies suggesting that urgency is caused by changes in urothelial-afferent interactions or altered IC cell function. As bladder function is dependent on the complex integration of a number of myogenic and neurogenic components, it seems likely that the pathogenesis of OABS is multifactorial, changes over time, and varies between patients. This is exemplified by the finding that only a proportion of OABS patients exhibit DO and that not all OABS patients have urinary incontinence. However, there is an obvious increase in the prevalence of OABS with increasing age and both central and peripheral mechanisms are likely to be of importance, although clearly their relative role will vary in individual patients.

Voiding disorders

To ensure efficient bladder emptying, without residual urine remaining, the detrusor muscle must contract effectively and the urethral sphincters must open to reduce outlet resistance and allow urine passage. This is achieved by the parasympathetic release of acetylcholine onto the muscle from the efferent nerve terminals and a concomitant relaxation of the urethral outlet (the urethral sphincter in the female, the bladder neck, prostate, and the distal urethral sphincter in the male). It is important to note that the female bladder neck is poorly formed anatomically, is often weak, and has questionable functional significance. Normal voiding can be compromised by a reduction in the power of the detrusor to contract (due to muscle atrophy or detrusor failure, which can be myogenic and/or neurogenic in aetiology), or increased outlet resistance (due to enlargement of the prostate).

Symptoms of voiding dysfunction include:

- *Poor stream*—reduced urine flow
- *Hesitancy*—difficulty in initiating voiding resulting in a delay in the onset of voiding
- *Straining*—abdominal straining to initiate or maintain bladder empting

Detrusor failure

Degeneration of the detrusor smooth muscle or damage either to the muscle or its neural control mechanisms may result in detrusor failure, resulting in incomplete bladder emptying, which may result in chronic urinary retention. Overdistension of the bladder can also result in myogenic failure, which may persist following relief of any underlying obstruction. Sensory and autonomic neuropathy, such as that consequent upon diabetes, can impair bladder emptying due to reduced sensation and impaired bladder function.

Bladder pharmacology and therapeutic options for lower urinary tract symptoms

Muscarinic receptors

ACh is unarguably the most important neurotransmitter in the bladder. At the point of bladder emptying, it is released from parasympathetic efferent nerve terminals to elicit contraction of the body of the bladder. ACh activates muscarinic receptors on detrusor myocytes, causing an increase in intracellular calcium either via extracellular calcium influx, or mobilization of calcium from intracellular stores (Fig. 3.1.5). There are five muscarinic receptor subtypes (M1-M5), and while all are present in the bladder, the detrusor muscle predominantly expresses M2 and M3 subtypes,[61,62] with the density of the M2 receptors being threefold greater than that of the M3 receptor.[63] Despite this difference in receptor number, it is widely accepted that the M3 receptor is functionally predominant. When activated by ACh, M3 receptors couple to G proteins and activate phospholipase C (PLC), causing production of diacyglycerol (DAG) and inositol triphosphate (IP3), resulting in increased cytosolic calcium via extracellular influx through L-type calcium channels and intracellular release from stores. This elevated cytosolic calcium produces contraction of the smooth muscle. The role of the M2 receptor is controversial, but some studies suggest that the M2 receptor may play a role in indirectly mediating bladder contraction via a synergistic mechanism involving the M3 receptor and/or inhibition of cyclic cAMP-mediated relaxatory pathways (Fig. 3.1.5).

Antimuscarinics (Figure 3.1.5)

Antimuscarinics are the first-line therapy for patients with OAB and DO. There are several antimuscarinic drugs currently recommended for treatment and these include oxybutynin, trospium, propiverine, and tolteradine, widely prescribed worldwide, and newer compounds such as solifenacin, fesoteradine, and darifenacin. In general, these drugs are reasonably well tolerated and clinical studies report a significant reduction in urinary frequency, urgency, and urinary incontinence,[64] and significant improvements in health-related quality of life.

For many years, it was presumed that antimuscarinic drugs inhibit muscarinic receptors located on the detrusor to inhibit bladder contraction; however, this being the sole mechanism of action has become increasingly controversial. At licensed doses antimuscarinic drugs appear to work during the filling phase of the micturition cycle where there is no ongoing parasympathetic ACh release, they have efficacy at treating the sensory symptoms of OAB such as urgency, and have little effect on detrusor contraction force during voiding.[65] This has led to the suggestion that antimuscarinics might work via another mechanism of action.

Antimuscarinics and sensory pathways

All five muscarinic receptors have been detected in the urothelium and suburothelium[29] with the M2 receptor predominant in number. Several studies have identified the ACh synthesis and degradation enzymes in the urothelium[66] and studies from the Yoshida laboratory have shown that in response to stretch, the urothelium releases ACh from a non-neuronal source.[18] It has been suggested that urothelially released ACh acts in a paracrine manner on muscarinic and nicotinic receptors in the urothelium to evoke the release of secondary mediators such as ATP (Fig. 3.1.5), which then acts downstream at the afferent terminal to modulate sensory nerve activity. This has led to the suggestion that these mechanisms are disrupted in disease states such as OABS and that antimuscarinic drugs work by inhibiting muscarinic receptors in the urothelium. Moreover, experimental studies conducted in rodents have shown that the antimuscarinics oxybutynin and darafenicin can inhibit sensory nerve firing during bladder filling.[67] Together this has led to the speculation that clinical treatment with antimuscarinic may work by inhibiting sensory nerve activity either via a direct

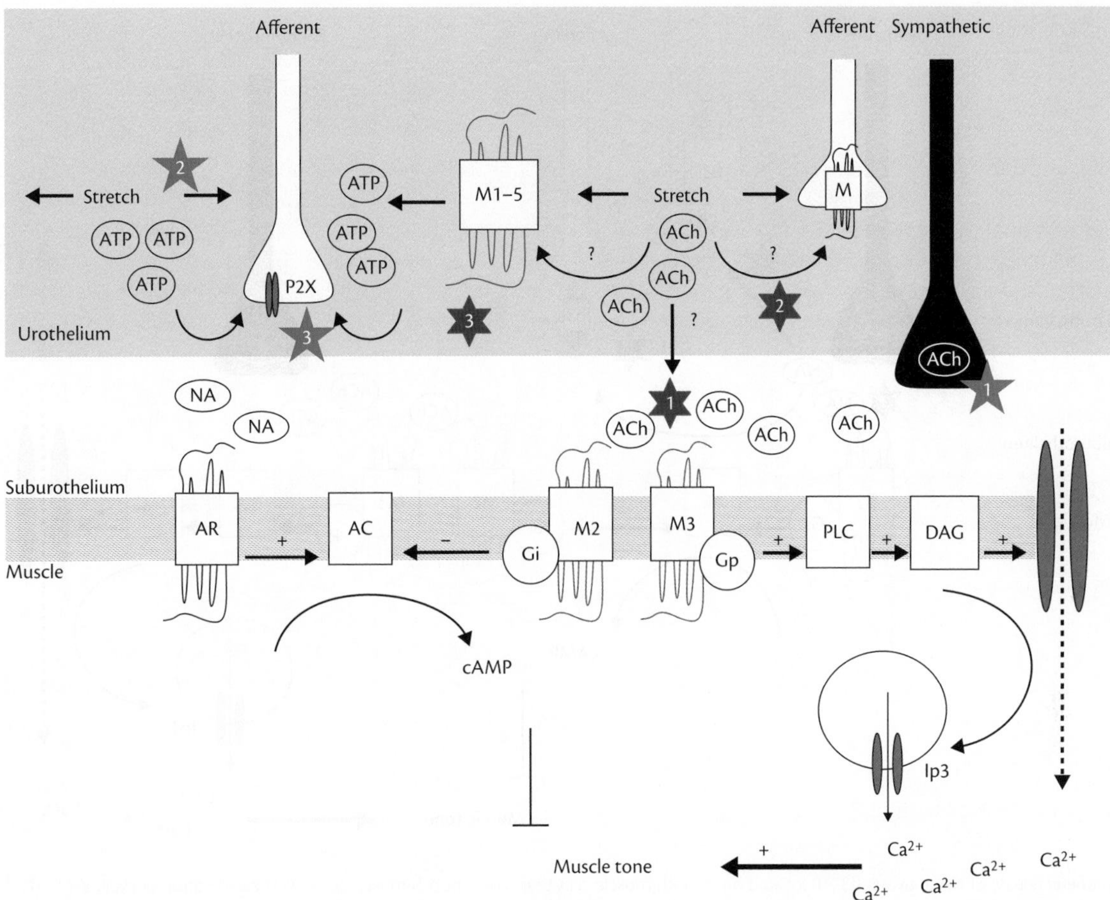

Fig. 3.1.5 Schematic diagram showing the potential site of action of antimuscarinic drugs in the bladder. Parasympathetic release of ACh activates M3 receptors located on smooth muscle cells to elicit influx of extracellular calcium via L-type calcium channels and mobilisation of calcium from intracellular stores. Anti-muscarinic drugs primarily work by inhibiting ACh mediated contraction of the detrusor (1), however more recent studies suggest that they may also inhibit afferent nerve activity either directly by blocking muscarinic receptors on afferent nerve terminals (2) or by altering the release of mediators from the urothelium (3).

ATP: adenosine triphosphate; P2X: purinoreceptor 2 subtype X; NA: noradrenaline; M1–5: muscarinic receptors 1-5; AR: adrenoreceptor; AC: adenylyl cyclase; Gi: G protein subunit I; Gp: G protein subunit; PLC: phospholipase C; DAG: Diacylglycerol; Ip3: Inositol trisphosphate; ACh: Acetylcholine; cAMP: cyclic adenosine monophosphate..

action at the afferent terminal, or in a mechanism involving the urothelium to prolong bladder filling, thus reducing frequency and attenuating urgency. However, much of the previous research was conducted using animal models and this mechanism of action has yet to be confirmed in humans.

Beta-3 agonists (Figure 3.1.6)

The urinary tract is innervated by both the parasympathetic and sympathetic nervous systems. In order to store increasing volumes of urine without a significant rise in intraluminal pressure, the beta-adrenoreceptors (βARs) located in the bladder dome and body mediate relaxation of smooth muscle during the bladder filling phase, in response to sympathetically mediated release of the neurotransmitter noradrenaline (Fig. 3.1.6). All three of the known isoforms of the βAR family have been identified in the bladder smooth muscle (β_1ARs, β_2ARs, and β_3ARs), with the β_3-AR subtype being the most abundant isoform and the most prominent for relaxation of the human detrusor. Several β_3-AR agonists have been shown to relax human detrusor muscle strips and supress spontaneous contractions *in vitro*, and in rodent studies, β_3-AR agonists increase bladder capacity without altering micturition pressure.[68,69] Thus β_3-ARs have been hailed as a potential treatment option for bladder storage disorders for several years. Mirabegron is the first β_3-AR agonist to be developed as a treatment for bladder dysfunction. It has recently completed phase 3 registration trials and is approved as a new oral agent for the treatment of OAB. The clinical evidence shows mirabegron to be a safe, well tolerated, and effective treatment option for urinary frequency, urgency, and incontinence symptoms associated with OABS.[70]

Beta-3 agonists and the urothelium

In a recent experimental study, β3-ARs have also been identified in the urothelium. Stimulation of these receptors with two β3-AR agonists, TAK-677 and BRL37344, inhibited voiding frequency suggesting that β3-AR may have a role in sensory transmission (Fig. 3.1.6).[71] This idea has also been supported by two studies which show that stimulation of β3-AR with intravenous administration of the selective β3-AR agonist CL316243 or mirabegron significantly inhibits afferent nerve firing in the rat, suggesting that β_3-AR agonists could improve the symptoms of urgency and frequency via an action on the sensory nerves.[72,73] Until recently it was assumed that the periphery was the main site of action of these drugs, however Fullhase *et al.* identified β_3-AR in the spinal cord and showed that intrathecal administration of the β_3-AR agonist BRL37344 inhibits

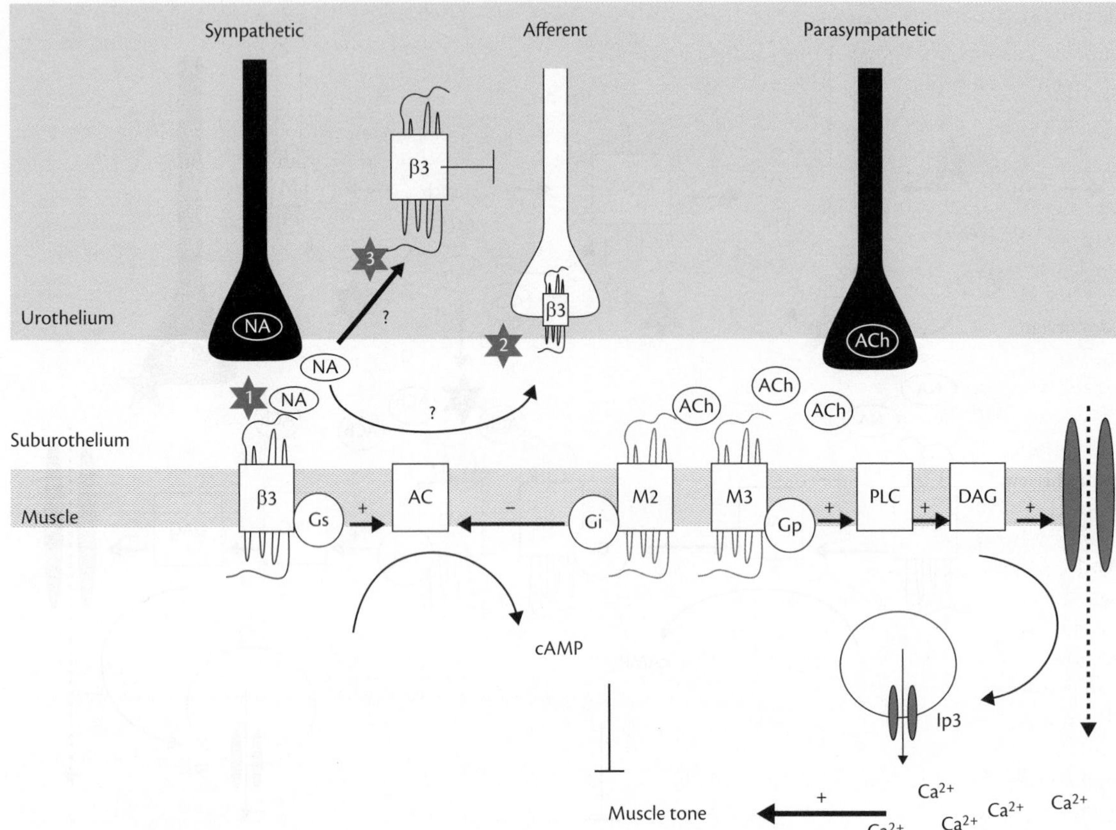

Fig. 3.1.6 Sympathetic release of NA activates β3-AR located on smooth muscle cells to inhibit smooth muscle tone via the generation of cyclic AMP. β3-AR antagonists primarily work by inhibiting contraction of the detrusor (1), however more recent studies suggest that they may also inhibit afferent nerve activity either directly at the afferent nerve terminal (2) or by altering the release of mediators from the urothelium (3).
M2: muscarinic receptors 2; M3: muscarinic receptors 3; Gi: G protein subunit I; Gp: G protein subunit; PLC: phospholipase C; DAG: Diacylglycerol; Ip3: Inositol trisphosphate; ACh: Acetylcholine; cAMP: cyclic adenosine monophosphate.

reflex voiding in the rat, raising the possibility that β_3-AR agonist could have a central site of action.[74] Studies are still required to fully understand the mode of action of these drugs in the human bladder.

Botulinum toxin A

The botulinum toxins are the most potent toxins known to man. They are renowned for their ability to specifically target and disrupt neurotransmission. There are seven distinct isoforms (BoNT type A-G) produced by the bacteria *Clostridium botulinum*. These toxins are now used to treat a host of medical conditions such as strabismus, blepharospasm, nystagmus, facial spasms, and dystonia. Over the past decade, BoNTA (marketed as Botox or OnabotulinumtoxinA (OnaBotA), and Dysport or abobotulinumtoxininA) injected into several distinct sites in the bladder wall, has emerged as a potent and effective treatment for many bladder conditions. Initially OnaBotA was used to treat detrusor sphincter dyssynergia associated with spinal cord injury.[75] However it has subsequently been reported to improve symptoms of idiopathic and neurogenic DO. Currently there are anecdotal reports about its use for treating symptomatic LUTS in men following injection into the prostate and in the management of PBS.

BoNTs consists of a light chain and a heavy chain that are linked by a disulphide bond. The heavy chain is responsible for the binding and transport of the toxin into the neuronal cytosol at various points in the peripheral nervous system. The light chain performs cleavage of intracellular proteins, preventing the endocytic release of neurotransmitters. In the neuromuscular junction of striated muscle, BoNTA binds to a specific high affinity binding site, synaptic vesicle protein 2 (SV2) and enters the neuronal cytosol. It cleaves the SNARE protein synaptosomal-associated protein 25 (SNAP-25) preventing docking and fusion of ACh-filled vesicles into the synapse.[76] In the bladder, BoNTA is believed to work by this mechanism. Clinical studies treating NDO and IDO have shown that BoNTA increases bladder capacity and reduces voiding contractile force, significantly reducing incontinence episodes.[77] The effect has been reported to last six to eight months, have no loss of potency with repeated treatment, and cause no loss of tolerance for up to 10 years (Schurch personal communication). Because of its potent effect on the detrusor, bladder retention is a well-recognized feature of this therapy and patients need to be counselled relating to this before use. An increased incidence of urinary tract infections has been reported as a common adverse effects associated with BoNTA treatment, the exact mechanism for the genesis of this remains unknown.

As BoNTA has also been shown to improve urgency symptoms and have optimal safety/efficacy ratios at lower doses than initially thought,[78] this has led to the speculation that BoNTA may also have some impact on the sensory nerves and the urothelium. Much of the evidence for this idea comes from experimental studies in rodents, which have shown that treatment with OnaBotA inhibits transmitter release from the urothelium and attenuates afferent nerve responses to stretch *in vitro*.[79–82] However, the exact mechanism has not been identified.

Alpha-1-adrenoreceptors

Alpha-1-adrenoreceptors (α1-ARs) are activated by adrenaline and noradrenaline, and mediate smooth muscle contraction via a complex second messenger cascade. Following ligand binding, α1-ARs couple to the Gq11 family of G proteins, generating phospholipase C, and activating diacyglycerol (DAG) and inositol-3-phosphate (IP3). This results in calcium mobilization from intracellular stores and subsequent contraction. Alpha-adrenoreceptors have been extensively characterized by radioligand binding and molecular approaches and three α1-AR subtypes have been cloned, $\alpha1_A$-AR, $\alpha1_B$-AR, and $\alpha1_D$-AR. Some expression of the $\alpha1_B$-AR and $\alpha1_D$-AR has been identified in the lower urinary tract; however, the $\alpha1_A$-ARs predominate with expression on the proximal urethra, the prostate, the vas deferens, ureters, the detrusor, and on the central and spinal innervation.

Benign prostatic hyperplasia (BPH), is a highly prevalent disorder affecting more than half of men over 50. The aetiology of BPH is not known, but studies suggest that somal and glandular cells in the prostate proliferate due to age and long-term androgen exposure. This growth can result in prostate enlargement and eventually constriction of the urethra, leading to bladder outlet obstruction (BOO). In addition, $\alpha1_A$-AR expression in the prostate is increased, leading to an increase in prostatic tone and further urethral constriction. BPH and BOO causes storage and voiding symptoms of the lower urinary tract including premicturition delay, weak stream, incomplete emptying, and are also associated with OABS (nocturia, urgency, and frequency). Bladder contraction against a closed or obstructed urethra can cause a noxious rise in intraluminal pressure, potentially leading damage to the bladder and serious complications such as acute urinary retention, renal failure, bladder stones, and infection. Current traditional pharmacotherapy for LUTS in men, is based on standard therapy for OABS, as noted above where this is the predominant problem; alternatively, alpha-adrenergic blockade or inhibition of the intraprostatic conversion of testosterone to dihydotestosterone using 5 alpha reductase inhibitors (sARI) can also be used.

Alpha-1-adrenoreceptor blockers

α1-ARs antagonists are the mainstay for first-line male LUTS treatment. They work by inhibiting $\alpha1_A$-AR mediated contraction of the prostate, thereby relieving urethral constriction and obstruction of the bladder outlet. The currently prescribed α1-AR antagonists include terazosin, doxazosin, alfuzosin, tamsulosin, and silodosin. Terazosin, doxazosin, alfuzosin are non-selective α1-AR antagonists, whereas tamulosin is (10–15-fold) selective for the $\alpha1_D$-AR, exhibiting higher affinity for the prostate compared to the aorta, reducing cardiovascular side effects. Silodosin is even more selective for the $\alpha1_A$-AR, exhibiting a selectivity of approximately 162-fold. However, all of these α1-ARs antagonists exhibit a similar efficacy for treating the LUTS associated with BPH and BOO. The main importance of the $\alpha1_A$-AR selectivity relates to better cardiovascular tolerability.

In addition to relieving the obstructive symptoms of BPH such as the low urinary flow rate, more recent findings indicate that some of the therapeutic effects of α1-ARs antagonists are due to improvements in the storage symptoms of outlet obstruction such as urgency, suggesting that they could potentially work by another mechanism involving bladder afferents. $\alpha1_A$-AR expression has recently been identified in the urothelium and on sensory neurones innervating the bladder[83,84] and electrophysiological studies in rodents have reported inhibited bladder afferent firing following intravesical application of tamulosin.[85] Moreover, acute intraventricular and intrathecal administration of tamulosin significantly inhibited reflex voiding in normal non-obstructive rats,[86] and chronic systemic treatment with two different α1-AR antagonists inhibited reflex voiding in a rat model of BOO.[87] Though more investigation is required in this area, the current data indicate that that the α1-ARs may be involved in normal and pathological regulation of the micturition reflex via the afferent system.

Phosphodiesterase 5 inhibitors (Figure 3.1.7)

Nitric oxide (NO) is an important NANC transmitter in the central and peripheral nervous system. NO mediates relaxation of the bladder outflow region[48] and modifies afferent neurotransmission from various parts of the urogenital tract.[88] NO is generated intracellularly from the amino acid L-arginine by the action of a nitric oxide synthase enzyme (NOS), which also generates nicotinamide adenine dinucleotide phosphate and oxygen as cosubstrates. Two types of NOS activity have been described: constitutive, calcium-sensitive NOS activity; and inducible, calcium insensitive NOS activity. There are three identified isoforms of NOS. Two constitutive isoforms termed endothelial NOS (eNOS) and neuronal NOS (nNOS) were first described in large vessel endothelial cells and have since been identified in several cell types, including neurons. There is one inducible isoform termed iNOS that was originally identified in active murine macrophages and is induced by inflammatory mediators. Once generated, NO mediates relaxation of smooth muscle via soluble guanylate cyclase (sGC), which catalyses the production of guanosine triphosphate (GTP) to cyclic guanosine monophosphate (cGMP). The increase in cGMP triggers a signal transduction cascade, resulting in cyclic nucleotide dependent kinases, phosphorylation of actin and myosin complexes, and inhibition of calcium channels and ATP-driven calcium pumps on the sarcoplasmic reticulum. This cascade ultimately reduces cytosolic calcium concentrations and initiates relaxation of the muscle (Fig. 3.1.7). Cyclic nucleotides such as cGMP are degraded by a group of hydrolytic enzymes known as the phosphodiesterases (PDE). Inhibition of PDE leads to accumulation of cGMP, increasing the effect of nitric oxide. PDE5 inhibitors have been used for many years as therapy for erectile dysfunction.

There are 11 members of the PDE family (PDE1–11), 8 of which have been identified in the human prostate with PDE4 and PDE5 localized to the stromal and glandular tissue of the transitional zone. In organ bath studies, alpha-1-adrenoreceptor mediated contraction of prostate strips was reduced following application of a PDE5 inhibitor.[89] The PDE5 enzymes play an essential role in relaxation of erectile tissue in the penis; this has led to the use of PDE5s such as sildenafil citrate in the treatment of erectile dysfunction. However, in recent years there has been growing evidence that PDE5 inhibitors may also have a beneficial effect for the treatment of BPH/BOO.

Randomized controlled trials with PDE5 inhibitors (such as sildenafil) report significant improvements in LUTS, increased urinary flow rates, reduction in storage symptoms, and increased patient quality of life.[90] Recently, one agent (tadaalafil) has been granted a licence for the treatment of LUTS in men. It appears to have similar efficacy to alpha blockers independent of any indirect effect by improving erectile dysfunction and without any consistent effect on urodynamic parameters.[91]

PDE5 inhibitors have also been suggested as a potential treatment option for DO and OAB. Data from experimental studies have

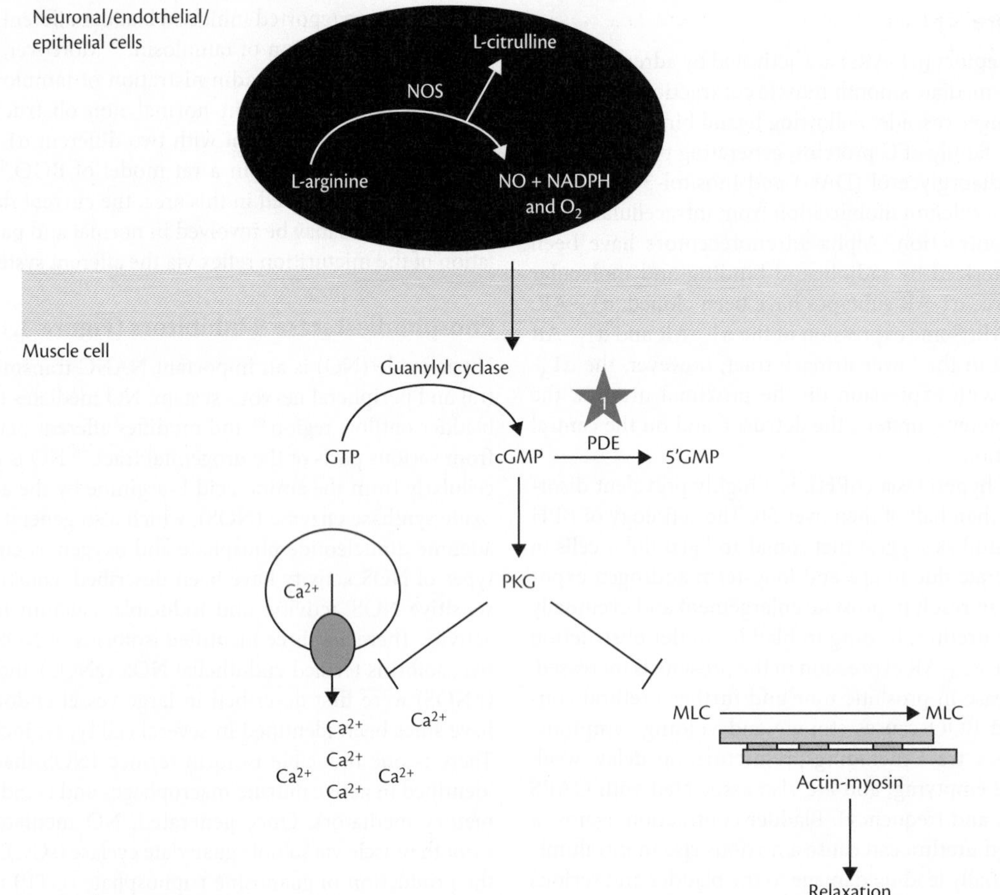

Fig. 3.1.7 NO is generated intracellularly from the amino acid L-arginine by the action of a nitric oxide synthase enzyme (NOS) which also generates nicotinamide adenine dinucleotide phosphate (NADPH) and oxygen as co-substrates.

Once generated, NO mediates relaxation of smooth muscle via soluble guanylate cyclase (sGC) which catalyses the production of guanosine triphosphate (GTP) to cyclic guanosine monophosphate (cGMP). cGMP results in activation of cyclic nucleotide dependent kinases, phosphorylation of actin and myosin complexes, and inhibition of calcium channels and ATP driven calcium pumps on the sarcoplasmic reticulum, reducing cytosolic calcium and initiating relaxation of the muscle. PDE5 inhibitors prevent the conversion of cGMP to 5'GMP (1) which increases cGMP levels and enhances the inhibition of smooth muscle tone. cAMP: cyclic adenosine monophosphate..

identified the presence of PDE5, cGMP, and sGC in the detrusor, however little effect on bladder tone *in vitro* has been observed in response to stimulation of the NO signalling pathway. Moreover, clinical studies using tadalafil show little effect on urodynamic properties, but provide improvements in sensation symptomology, such as urgency. Components of the NO-cGMP cascade have also been identified in the urothelium and rodent studies have shown that PDE5 inhibitors can inhibit single afferent nerve activity, raising the possibility that NO signalling could play a role in afferent transmission.

Further reading

Abrams P, Cardozo L, Fall M, *et al.* The standardisation of terminology of lower urinary tract function: report from the Standardisation Sub-committee of the International Continence Society. *Neurourol Urodyn* 2002; **21**(2):167–78.

Andersson KE, Arner A. Urinary bladder contraction and relaxation: physiology and pathophysiology. *Physiol Rev* 2004; **84**(3):935–86.

Beckel JM, Holstege G. Neuroanatomy of the lower urinary tract. (pp. 99–117) In: Andersson KE, Michel M (eds). *Urinary Tract.* Berlin, Germany: Springer, 2011.

Chapple C. Overview of the lower urinary tract. (pp. 1–15) In: Andersson KE, Michel M (eds). *Urinary Tract.* Berlin, Germany: Springer, 2011.

Chapple C, Khullar V, Gabriel Z, Dooley JA. The effects of antimuscarinic treatments in overactive bladder: a systematic review and meta-analysis. *Eur Urol* 2005; **48**(1):5–26.

Chapple CR. beta3-agonist therapy: a new advance in the management of overactive bladder? *Eur Urol* 2012; **62**(5):841–2.

Chapple CR. Monotherapy with alpha-blocker or phosphodiesterase 5 inhibitor for lower urinary tract symptoms? *Eur Urol* 2012; **61**:926–7.

Chapple CR, Kaplan SA, Mitcheson D, *et al.* Randomized double-blind, active-controlled phase 3 study to assess 12-month safety and efficacy of mirabegron, a beta(3)-adrenoceptor agonist, in overactive bladder. *Eur Urol* 2013; **63**:296–305.

Choppin A, Eglen RM. Pharmacological characterization of muscarinic receptors in mouse isolated urinary bladder smooth muscle. *Br J Pharmacol* 2001; **133**(7):1035–40.

de Groat W, Booth AM, Yoshimura N. Neurophysiology of micturition and its modifications in animal models of human disease. (pp. 227–89) In: Maggi CA (ed). *The Autonomic Nervous System: Nervous Control of the Urogenital System.* London, UK: Harwood, 1993.

Elliot C, Payne C. Evaluation and treatment of male lower urinary tract symptoms. In: Potts J (ed). *Essential Urology*, 2nd edition. Berlin, Germany: Springer, 2012.

Fowler CJ, Griffiths D, de Groat WC. The neural control of micturition. *Nat Rev Neurosci* 2008; **9**:453–66.

Korstanje C, Krauwinkel W. Specific pharmacokinetic aspects of the urinary tract. *Handb Exp Pharmacol* 2011; (**202**):267–82.

Mangera A, Andersson KE, Apostolidis A, *et al. Contemporary management of lower urinary tract disease with botulinum toxin A: a systematic review of botox (onabotulinumtoxinA) and dysport (abobotulinumtoxinA). Eur Urol* 2011; **60**(4):784–95.

Michel MC, Chapple CR. Basic mechanisms of urgency: preclinical and clinical evidence. *Eur Urol* 2009; **56**:298–307.

Patel AK, Chapple CR. Anatomy of the lower urinary tract. *Surgery (Oxford)* 2008; **26**:127–32.

References

1. de Groat WC. A neurologic basis for the overactive bladder. *Urology* 1997; **50**(6A Suppl):36–52; discussion 3–6.
2. de Groat W, Booth AM, Yoshimura N. Neurophysiology of micturition and its modifications in animal models of human disease. (pp. 227–89) In: Maggi CA (ed). *The Autonomic Nervous System: Nervous Control of the Urogenital System*. London, UK: Harwood, 1993.
3. Blok BF, Willemsen AT, Holstege G. A PET study on brain control of micturition in humans. *Brain* 1997; **120**(Pt 1):111–21.
4. Rong W, Spyer KM, Burnstock G. Activation and sensitisation of low and high threshold afferent fibres mediated by P2X receptors in the mouse urinary bladder. *J Physiol* 2002; **541**(Pt 2):591–600.
5. Sengupta JN, Gebhart GF. Mechanosensitive properties of pelvic nerve afferent fibers innervating the urinary bladder of the rat. *J Neurophysiol* 1994; **72**(5):2420–30.
6. Zagorodnyuk VP, Gibbins IL, Costa M, Brookes SJ, Gregory SJ. Properties of the major classes of mechanoreceptors in the guinea pig bladder. *J Physiol* 2007; **585**(Pt 1):147–63.
7. Sullivan MP, Yalla SV. Physiology of female micturition. *Urol Clin North Am* 2002; **29**(3):499–514, vii.
8. de Groat WC, Booth AM. Inhibition and facilitation in parasympathetic ganglia of the urinary bladder. *Fed Proc* 1980; **39**(12):2990–6.
9. Andersson KE, Arner A. Urinary bladder contraction and relaxation: physiology and pathophysiology. *Physiol Rev* 2004; **84**(3):935–86.
10. de Groat WC, Fraser MO, Yoshiyama M, *et al.* Neural control of the urethra. *Scand J Urol Nephrol Suppl* 2001; (207):35–43; discussion 106–25.
11. Apodaca G. The uroepithelium: not just a passive barrier. *Traffic* 2004; **5**(3):117–28.
12. Lewis SA. Everything you wanted to know about the bladder epithelium but were afraid to ask. *Am J Physiol Renal Physiol* 2000; **278**(6):F867–74.
13. Hwang SJ, Oh JM, Valtschanoff JG. Expression of the vanilloid receptor TRPV1 in rat dorsal root ganglion neurons supports different roles of the receptor in visceral and cutaneous afferents. *Brain Res* 2005; **1047**(2):261–6.
14. Birder LA, Apodaca G, De Groat WC, Kanai AJ. Adrenergic- and capsaicin-evoked nitric oxide release from urothelium and afferent nerves in urinary bladder. *Am J Physiol* 1998; **275**(2 Pt 2):F226–9.
15. Ferguson DR, Kennedy I, Burton TJ. ATP is released from rabbit urinary bladder epithelial cells by hydrostatic pressure changes—a possible sensory mechanism? *J Physiol* 1997; **505** (Pt 2):503–11.
16. Khan MA, Thompson CS, Mumtaz FH, Jeremy JY, Morgan RJ, Mikhailidis DP. Role of prostaglandins in the urinary bladder: an update. *Prostaglandins Leukot Essent Fatty Acids* 1998; **59**(6):415–22.
17. Masunaga K, Yoshida M, Inadome A, Iwashita H, Miyamae K, Ueda S. Prostaglandin E2 release from isolated bladder strips in rats with spinal cord injury. *Int J Urol* 2006; **13**(3):271–6.
18. Yoshida M, Inadome A, Maeda Y, *et al.* Non-neuronal cholinergic system in human bladder urothelium. *Urology* 2006; **67**(2):425–30.
19. Sadananda P, Kao FC, Liu L, Mansfield KJ, Burcher E. Acid and stretch, but not capsaicin, are effective stimuli for ATP release in the porcine bladder mucosa: Are ASIC and TRPV1 receptors involved? *Eur J Pharmacol* 2012; **683**(1–3):252–9.
20. Burnstock G. Purines and sensory nerves. *Handb Exp Pharmacol* 2009; (194):333–92.
21. Birder L. Role of the urothelium in bladder function. *Scand J Urol Nephrol Suppl* 2004; (215):48–53.
22. Lee HY, Bardini M, Burnstock G. Distribution of P2X receptors in the urinary bladder and the ureter of the rat. *J Urol* 2000; **163**(6):2002–7.
23. Elneil S, Skepper JN, Kidd EJ, Williamson JG, Ferguson DR. Distribution of P2X(1) and P2X(3) receptors in the rat and human urinary bladder. *Pharmacology* 2001; **63**(2):120–8.
24. Birder LA, Ruan HZ, Chopra B, *et al.* Alterations in P2X and P2Y purinergic receptor expression in urinary bladder from normal cats and cats with interstitial cystitis. *Am J Physiol Renal Physiol* 2004; **287**(5):F1084–91.
25. Lazzeri M, Vannucchi MG, Zardo C, *et al.* Immunohistochemical evidence of vanilloid receptor 1 in normal human urinary bladder. *Eur Urol* 2004; **46**(6):792–8.
26. Birder LA, Kanai AJ, de Groat WC, *et al.* Vanilloid receptor expression suggests a sensory role for urinary bladder epithelial cells. *Proc Natl Acad Sci U S A* 2001; **98**(23):13396–401.
27. Stein RJ, Santos S, Nagatomi J, *et al.* Cool (TRPM8) and hot (TRPV1) receptors in the bladder and male genital tract. *J Urol* 2004; **172**(3):1175–8.
28. Birder L, Kullmann FA, Lee H, *et al.* Activation of Urothelial-TRPV4 by 4{alpha}PDD contributes to altered bladder reflexes in the rat. *J Pharmacol Exp Ther* 2007; **323**(1):227–35.
29. Zarghooni S, Wunsch J, Bodenbenner M, *et al.* Expression of muscarinic and nicotinic acetylcholine receptors in the mouse urothelium. *Life Sci* 2007; **80**(24–25):2308–13.
30. Bschleipfer T, Schukowski K, Weidner W, *et al.* Expression and distribution of cholinergic receptors in the human urothelium. *Life Sci* 2007; **80**(24–25):2303–7.
31. Mansfield KJ, Liu L, Mitchelson FJ, Moore KH, Millard RJ, Burcher E. Muscarinic receptor subtypes in human bladder detrusor and mucosa, studied by radioligand binding and quantitative competitive RT-PCR: changes in ageing. *Br J Pharmacol* 2005; **144**(8):1089–99.
32. Beckel JM, Kanai A, Lee SJ, de Groat WC, Birder LA. Expression of functional nicotinic acetylcholine receptors in rat urinary bladder epithelial cells. *Am J Physiol Renal Physiol* 2006; **290**(b):F103–10.
33. Chopra B, Barrick SR, Meyers S, *et al.* Expression and function of bradykinin B1 and B2 receptors in normal and inflamed rat urinary bladder urothelium. *J Physiol* 2005; **562**(Pt 3):859–71.
34. Ishihama H, Momota Y, Yanase H, Wang X, de Groat WC, Kawatani M. Activation of alpha1D adrenergic receptors in the rat urothelium facilitates the micturition reflex. *J Urol* 2006; **175**(1):358–64.
35. Harmon EB, Porter JM, Porter JE. Beta-adrenergic receptor activation in immortalized human urothelial cells stimulates inflammatory responses by PKA-independent mechanisms. *Cell Commun Signal* 2005; **3**:10.
36. Burton TJ, Edwardson JM, Ingham J, Tempest HV, Ferguson DR. Regulation of Na+ channel density at the apical surface of rabbit urinary bladder epithelium. *Eur J Pharmacol* 2002; **448**(2–3):215–23.
37. Watanabe S, Matsushita K, McCray PB Jr, Stokes JB. Developmental expression of the epithelial Na+ channel in kidney and uroepithelia. *Am J Physiol* 1999; **276**(2 Pt 2):F304–14.
38. Levin RM, Wein AJ, Krasnopolsky L, Atta MA, Ghoniem GM. Effect of mucosal removal on the response of the feline bladder to pharmacological stimulation. *J Urol* 1995; **153**(4):1291–4.
39. Hawthorn MH, Chapple CR, Cock M, Chess-Williams R. Urothelium-derived inhibitory factor(s) influences on detrusor muscle contractility in vitro. *Br J Pharmacol* 2000; **129**(3):416–9.
40. Templeman L, Chapple CR, Chess-Williams R. Urothelium derived inhibitory factor and cross-talk among receptors in the trigone of the bladder of the pig. *J Urol* 2002; **167**(2 Pt 1):742–5.
41. Hirst GD, Edwards FR. Role of interstitial cells of Cajal in the control of gastric motility. *J Pharmacol Sci* 2004; **96**(1):1–10.
42. Ward SM, Sanders KM. Physiology and pathophysiology of the interstitial cell of Cajal: from bench to bedside. I. Functional

development and plasticity of interstitial cells of Cajal networks. *Am J Physiol Gastrointest Liver Physiol* 2001; **281**(3):G602–11.

43. Smet PJ, Jonavicius J, Marshall VR, de Vente J. Distribution of nitric oxide synthase-immunoreactive nerves and identification of the cellular targets of nitric oxide in guinea-pig and human urinary bladder by cGMP immunohistochemistry. *Neuroscience* 1996; **71**(2):337–48.
44. Pezzone MA, Watkins SC, Alber SM, *et al.* Identification of c-kit-positive cells in the mouse ureter: the interstitial cells of Cajal of the urinary tract. *Am J Physiol Renal Physiol* 2003; **284**(5):F925–9.
45. Klemm MF, Exintaris B, Lang RJ. Identification of the cells underlying pacemaker activity in the guinea-pig upper urinary tract. *J Physiol* 1999; **519** Pt 3:867–84.
46. Van der Aa F, Roskams T, Blyweert W, De Ridder D. Interstitial cells in the human prostate: a new therapeutic target? *Prostate* 2003; **56**(4):250–5.
47. Lagou M, De Vente J, Kirkwood TB, *et al.* Location of interstitial cells and neurotransmitters in the mouse bladder. *BJU Int* 2006; **97**(6):1332–7.
48. Persson K, Andersson KE. Nitric oxide and relaxation of pig lower urinary tract. *Br J Pharmacol* 1992; **106**(2):416–22.
49. Chancellor M, Yoshimura N. Physiology and pharmacology of the bladder and urethra. (pp. 829–1734) In: Walsh PC, Retik AB, Darracott Vaughan E Jr, *et al.* (eds). *Campbell's Urology*: Philadelphia, PA: Saunders Publishing, 2002.
50. Wein AJ, Rovner ES. Definition and epidemiology of overactive bladder. *Urology* 2002; **60**(5 Suppl 1):7–12.
51. Abrams P, Cardozo L, Fall M, *et al.* The standardisation of terminology of lower urinary tract function: report from the Standardisation Sub-committee of the International Continence Society. *Neurourol Urodyn* 2002; **21**(2):167–78.
52. Milsom I, Abrams P, Cardozo L, Roberts RG, Thuroff J, Wein AJ. How widespread are the symptoms of an overactive bladder and how are they managed? A population-based prevalence study. *BJU Int* 2001; **87**(9):760–6.
53. Stewart WF, Van Rooyen JB, Cundiff GW, *et al.* Prevalence and burden of overactive bladder in the United States. *World J Urol* 2003; **20**(6):327–36.
54. Hashim H, Abrams P. Is the bladder a reliable witness for predicting detrusor overactivity? *J Urol* 2006; **175**(1):191–4; discussion 4–5.
55. Brading AF. A myogenic basis for the overactive bladder. *Urology* 1997; **50**(6A Suppl):57–67; discussion 8–73.
56. Mills IW, Greenland JE, McMurray G, *et al.* Studies of the pathophysiology of idiopathic detrusor instability: the physiological properties of the detrusor smooth muscle and its pattern of innervation. *J Urol* 2000; **163**(2):646–51.
57. Christ GJ, Day NS, Day M, Zhao W, *et al.* Increased connexin43-mediated intercellular communication in a rat model of bladder overactivity in vivo. *Am J Physiol* 2003; **284**(5):R1241–8.
58. Haferkamp A, Mundhenk J, Bastian PJ, *et al.* Increased expression of connexin 43 in the overactive neurogenic detrusor. *Eur Urol* 2004; **46**(6):799–805.
59. Fry CH, Sui GP, Severs NJ, Wu C. Spontaneous activity and electrical coupling in human detrusor smooth muscle: implications for detrusor overactivity? *Urology* 2004; **63**(3 Suppl 1):3–10.
60. Drake MJ, Harvey IJ, Gillespie JI, Van Duyl WA. Localized contractions in the normal human bladder and in urinary urgency. *BJU Int* 2005; **95**(7):1002–5.
61. Choppin A, Eglen RM. Pharmacological characterization of muscarinic receptors in mouse isolated urinary bladder smooth muscle. *Br J Pharmacol* 2001; **133**(7):1035–40.
62. Hegde SS, Choppin A, Bonhaus D, *et al.* Functional role of M2 and M3 muscarinic receptors in the urinary bladder of rats in vitro and in vivo. *Br J Pharmacol* 1997; **120**(8):1409–18.
63. Wang P, Luthin GR, Ruggieri MR. Muscarinic acetylcholine receptor subtypes mediating urinary bladder contractility and coupling to GTP binding proteins. *J Pharmacol Exp Ther* 1995; **273**(2):959–66.
64. Chapple C, Khullar V, Gabriel Z, Dooley JA. The effects of antimuscarinic treatments in overactive bladder: a systematic review and meta-analysis. *Eur Urol* 2005; **48**(1):5–26.
65. Finney SM, Andersson KE, Gillespie JI, Stewart LH. Antimuscarinic drugs in detrusor overactivity and the overactive bladder syndrome: motor or sensory actions? *BJU Int* 2006; **98**(3):503–7.
66. Hanna-Mitchell AT, Beckel JM, Barbadora S, Kanai AJ, de Groat WC, Birder LA. Non-neuronal acetylcholine and urinary bladder urothelium. *Life Sci* 2007; **80**(24–25):2298–302.
67. Iijima K, De Wachter S, Wyndaele JJ. Effects of the M3 receptor selective muscarinic antagonist darifenacin on bladder afferent activity of the rat pelvic nerve. *Eur Urol* 2007; **52**(3):842–7.
68. Badawi JK, Seja T, Uecelehan H, *et al.* Relaxation of human detrusor muscle by selective beta-2 and beta-3 agonists and endogenous catecholamines. *Urology* 2007; **69**(4):785–90.
69. Biers SM, Reynard JM, Brading AF. The effects of a new selective beta3-adrenoceptor agonist (GW427353) on spontaneous activity and detrusor relaxation in human bladder. *BJU Int* 2006; **98**(6):1310–4.
70. Chapple CR. beta3-agonist therapy: a new advance in the management of overactive bladder? *Eur Urol* 2012; **62**(5):841–2.
71. Kullmann FA, Downs TR, Artim DE, *et al.* Urothelial beta-3 adrenergic receptors in the rat bladder. *Neurourol Urodyn* 2011; **30**(1):144–50.
72. Aizawa N, Igawa Y, Nishizawa O, Wyndaele JJ. Effects of CL316,243, a beta 3-adrenoceptor agonist, and intravesical prostaglandin E2 on the primary bladder afferent activity of the rat. *Neurourol Urodyn* 2010; **29**(5):771–6.
73. Aizawa N, Homma Y, Igawa Y. Effects of mirabegron, a novel beta3-adrenoceptor agonist, on primary bladder afferent activity and bladder microcontractions in rats compared with the effects of oxybutynin. *Eur Urol* 2012; **62**(6):1165–73.
74. Fullhase C, Soler R, Westerling-Andersson K, Andersson KE. Beta3-adrenoceptors in the rat sacral spinal cord and their functional relevance in micturition under normal conditions and in a model of partial urethral obstruction. *Neurourol Urodyn* 2011; **30**(7):1382–7.
75. Schurch B. Botulinum toxin for the management of bladder dysfunction. *Drugs* 2006; **66**(10):1301–18.
76. Baldwin MR, Barbieri JT. Association of botulinum neurotoxins with synaptic vesicle protein complexes. *Toxicon* 2009; **54**(5):570–4.
77. Mangera A, Andersson KE, Apostolidis A, *et al.* Contemporary management of lower urinary tract disease with botulinum toxin A: a systematic review of botox (onabotulinumtoxinA) and dysport (abobotulinumtoxinA). *Eur Urol* 2011; **60**(4):784–95.
78. Dmochowski R, Chapple C, Nitti VW, *et al.* Efficacy and safety of onabotulinumtoxinA for idiopathic overactive bladder: a double-blind, placebo controlled, randomized, dose ranging trial. *J Urol* 2012; **184**(6):2416–22.
79. Lucioni A, Bales GT, Lotan TL, McGehee DS, Cook SP, Rapp DE. Botulinum toxin type A inhibits sensory neuropeptide release in rat bladder models of acute injury and chronic inflammation. *BJU Int* 2008; **101**(3):366–70.
80. Smith CP, Gangitano DA, Munoz A, *et al.* Botulinum toxin type A normalizes alterations in urothelial ATP and NO release induced by chronic spinal cord injury. *Neurochem Int* 2008; **52**(6):1068–75.
81. Smith CP, Vemulakonda VM, Kiss S, Boone TB, Somogyi GT. Enhanced ATP release from rat bladder urothelium during chronic bladder inflammation: effect of botulinum toxin A. *Neurochem Int* 2005; **47**(4):291–7.
82. Khera M, Somogyi GT, Kiss S, Boone TB, Smith CP. Botulinum toxin A inhibits ATP release from bladder urothelium after chronic spinal cord injury. *Neurochem Int* 2004; **45**(7):987–93.
83. Trevisani M, Campi B, Gatti R, *et al.* The influence of alpha1-adrenoreceptors on neuropeptide release from primary sensory neurons of the lower urinary tract. *Eur Urol* 2007; **52**(3):901–8.
84. Yanase H, Wang X, Momota Y, Nimura T, Kawatani M. The involvement of urothelial alpha1A adrenergic receptor in controlling the micturition reflex. *Biomed Res* 2008; **29**(5):239–44.

85. Nagabukuro H, Degenhardt A, Villa KL, *et al.* Correlation between pharmacologically-induced changes in cystometric parameters and spinal c-Fos expression in rats. *Auton Neurosci* 2010; **156**(1–2):19–26.
86. Yoshizumi M, Matsumoto-Miyai K, Yonezawa A, Kawatani M. Role of supraspinal and spinal alpha1-adrenergic receptor subtypes in micturition reflex in conscious rats. *Am J Physiol Renal Physiol* 2010; **299**(4):F785–91.
87. Yazaki J, Aikawa K, Shishido K, *et al.* Alpha1-adrenoceptor antagonists improve bladder storage function through reduction of afferent activity in rats with bladder outlet obstruction. *Neurourol Urodyn* 2011; **30**(3):461–7.
88. Hedlund P. Nitric oxide/cGMP-mediated effects in the outflow region of the lower urinary tract—is there a basis for pharmacological targeting of cGMP? *World J Urol* 2005; **23**(6):362–7.
89. Uckert S, Kuthe A, Jonas U, Stief CG. Characterization and functional relevance of cyclic nucleotide phosphodiesterase isoenzymes of the human prostate. *J Urol* 2001; **166**(6):2484–90.
90. Laydner HK, Oliveira P, Oliveira CR, *et al.* Phosphodiesterase 5 inhibitors for lower urinary tract symptoms secondary to benign prostatic hyperplasia: a systematic review. *BJU Int* 2011; **107**(7):1104–9.
91. Chapple CR, Montorsi F, Tammela TL, Wirth M, Koldewijn E, Fernandez Fernandez E. Silodosin therapy for lower urinary tract symptoms in men with suspected benign prostatic hyperplasia: results of an international, randomized, double-blind, placebo- and active-controlled clinical trial performed in Europe. *Eur Urol* 2011; **59**(3):342–52.

CHAPTER 3.2

Urodynamics

Julie Ellis Jones and Hashim Hashim

Introduction to urodynamics

History of urodynamics

Urodynamics can trace its roots to the 1800s, when instrumentation was first developed and described for the measurement of bladder pressure and urine flow rate. Dubois in 1876 was the first to measure intravesical pressure. In 1882, Mosso and Pellacani did experimental work on pressures and in 1897, Rehfisch described an apparatus used for the simultaneous measurement of vesical pressure and urinary volume, and recorded the timing of onset and finish of micturition. Bonney in 1923 reported crude measurements of urethral function.[1]

D.K. Rose is often considered the father of cystometry. In 1927 he coined the term 'cystometer' and described its development and clinical usefulness. However, it was not until 1933 that Denny-Brown and Robertson used a specially designed double catheter and a photographic recording method to measure pressure in the bladder, urethra, and rectum. In 1937, Kennedy measured urethral resistance in women. In 1948, Talbot was the first person to use the terms 'stable' and 'unstable' bladder detrusors in the urological literature. Also, in the same year, Willard Drake, Jr. pioneered the development of the uroflowmeter.

The 1950s saw the infancy of urodynamics. In 1953, Karlson, reported the successful simultaneous measurements of pressure in the urinary bladder and internal and external urinary sphincters in women. The term 'urodynamics' was coined by Davis in 1954 and Von Garrelts, in 1956, used a transducer to convert changes in pressure of urine collected onto a photokymograph. In the late 1950s and early 1960s, Lapides performed extensive animal and clinical investigations on the urinary sphincter. In 1962, Gleason and Lattimer reported the use of cystometry and uroflowmetry in combination. Miller, in 1967, popularized the use of cinefluoroscopy in conjunction with lower urinary tract urodynamic studies. Then in 1969, Brown and Wickham reported urethral pressure profiles, to measure the pressure exerted by the urethral wall.

The term 'urodynamics' was first used in the *Journal of Urology* in 1962. In 1965 the Urodynamics Society was formed in North Carolina, USA, and in 1971, the International Continence Society was founded in Exeter, England by Eric Glen, with Patrick Bates and David Rowan.

What is urodynamics?

Urodynamics is a study that allows the direct assessment of lower urinary tract (LUT) function by the measurement of relevant physiological parameters. This assessment includes several types of studies including bladder diaries, free uroflowmetry, and post-void residual measurement, pad weight tests, filling cystometry, and voiding pressure/flow studies.

Types of urodynamics

Based on the above definition, urodynamics can therefore be divided into two main types:

(i) Non-invasive

(ii) Invasive

Non-invasive urodynamics includes bladder diaries, pad weight testing, and free uroflowmetry. These are cheap, easy to do, and most importantly non-invasive, therefore do not cause any side effects to patients. They also form part of the basic assessment of patients presenting with lower urinary tract symptoms (LUTS), in addition to a full thorough history, including assessment of the effects on quality of life, focused clinical examination, and a urinalysis to look for infection, blood, glucose, and so on. These will not be discussed in this chapter as they have been discussed in Chapter 3.4.

It is important to mention that although pad weight testing, to categorize the severity of urinary incontinence, may be a useful tool, it is not recommended by NICE,[2] as there is no consensus as to what a specific increase in pad weight implies and whether it would affect the treatment decision. Also, there is no agreement as to what constitutes mild, moderate, or severe incontinence, and it does not correlate with an invasive urodynamic diagnosis, and therefore has no implication on the decision of the type of surgical management. The International Continence Society (ICS) has standardized the methodology for a short one-hour pad test with <2 g urine loss being a negative test.[3] There are also longer pad tests lasting 24 hours or more.

The focus of this chapter is on invasive urodynamics, which can be divided into:

1. Basic
   (a) filling cystometry
   (b) voiding pressure/flow studies
2. Complex
   (a) videourodynamics
   (b) urethral function studies
3. Advanced
   (a) ambulatory urodynamics
   (b) neurophysiological testing

Principles of good urodynamic practice

Urodynamics should start by formulating a urodynamic question, for example why are you doing the test and what are you looking for? Before urodynamic studies are undertaken, it is recommended that a detailed history is taken, allowing the experienced clinician to tailor the investigation to the needs of the patient.

Clinical assessment includes neurological testing, abdominal palpation, and rectal and vaginal examination (in women). With these findings established, the most appropriate urodynamic investigation can be selected.

Good urodynamic practice depends on:

- Having the appropriate indications for the test
- Performing the correct type of urodynamic test
- A first-rate technique ensuring good quality control
- Good and accurate interpretation of the results
- Conveying the important results in an accurate and relevant manner through good reporting, which could be understood by others and used in the future for comparison purposes in patients who may need repeat invasive urodynamics

Aims of invasive urodynamics

The main aim of urodynamics is to reproduce the patient's symptoms with a view to giving more information about the function of the bladder and urethra, or a diagnosis, on which management depends. In other words, the test should only be performed if it is going to change the management of a patient's condition and should not be conducted unless conservative and medical therapy has been tried.

The aims of the test include:

- Defining bladder and urethral function
- Providing a precise diagnosis
- Defining the most significant abnormality
- Allowing selection of the most appropriate treatment
- Predicting potential postoperative problems
- Assessing the results of treatment

Indications for invasive urodynamics

- Equivocal and/or uninterpretable flow rates
- Incontinence not responding to conservative and medical therapy with a view to proceeding to more invasive treatments
- Diabetic and neurological patients to assess the compliance of the bladder and assess LUT function in greater detail to allow appropriate management
- Children and young patients who suffer with lower urinary tract dysfunction (LUTD) and not responding to conservative or medical therapy
- Large residuals, to try to define the cause of the residuals (i.e. is it the bladder or the urethra causing the problem and if there is any treatable cause)
- Persistent bothersome LUTS not responding to conservative or medical treatment
- Postoperative LUTD, such as bothersome incontinence after insertion of a mid-urethral sling
- When things don't add up! For example, if a patient is complaining of incontinence, but is unable to distinguish between stress or urgency incontinence with no response to medical treatment

Physics of urodynamics

Urodynamic studies aim to look at four things:

- How the bladder is behaving during storage and voiding
- How the urethra is behaving during storage and voiding

Before understanding the physics of urodynamics, it is important to understand what normal LUT function is.

During bladder filling, continence should be maintained, and this depends on detrusor relaxation and continuous urethral closure despite intravesical pressure changes. Detrusor muscle relaxation starts at the end of voiding and requires a normal bladder wall composition, which depends on the viscoelastic properties of the detrusor muscle and the inhibitory effect of the sympathetic nerves on the parasympathetic ganglion. Urethral closure is maintained by the bladder neck (proximal sphincter), distal sphincter mechanism, and voluntary pelvic floor contraction. During filling, there is relaxation of the inner longitudinal smooth muscle, contraction in the intraurethral striated muscle with periurethral support from the striated muscles of the pelvic floor and collagen of the endopelvic fascia.

For efficient voiding to occur, there needs to be urethral relaxation with normal urethral geometry and adequate expulsive force by bladder contraction. The urethra relaxes during voiding due to pelvic floor relaxation, relaxation of the urethral rhabdosphincter (intraurethral striated muscle), urethral shortening (contraction of inner longitudinal muscle), and funnelling of the bladder neck. There should also be a sustained detrusor contraction to generate the pressure to void. Sometimes voiding is achieved by the straining of abdominal wall muscles and the diaphragmatic muscle.

In simple terms, flow takes place when the driving pressure exceeds the opposition to flow. Abnormalities in this function could lead to dysfunction of the LUT, which may or may not cause bothersome symptoms. Therefore, flow rate alone is not enough to diagnose these problems and you need to measure bladder pressure as well, both while the patient is filling up (to detect overactivity), and when they are voiding (to measure bladder contraction).

To measure the flow rate (Q) and voided volume (VV), a flow meter is used. VV is usually measured in millilitres (mL), while Q is measured in millilitres per second (mL/s). Pressure in the bladder is measured using a pressure transducer, which converts a pressure to an electrical signal.

Since the bladder is not readily accessible to the outside world, the transducer is allied to a catheter. The most used systems are the fluid-filled catheters with external transducers.

The pressure in the bladder (vesical pressure, p_{ves}) has contributions from the bladder detrusor muscle (p_{det}) and from the abdominal pressure (p_{abd}). It is not possible to measure p_{det} directly, and therefore to determine the pressure due to the bladder muscle alone (p_{det}), it is necessary to subtract the abdominal contribution. Abdominal pressure (p_{abd}) is normally measured in the rectum, but can also be measured in the vagina, or via a stoma. The measurements are done during both bladder filling and voiding.

Equipment

Multichannel cystometry requires a urine flow meter, two (or three) transducers, an electronic subtraction unit to derive $p_{det} = (p_{ves}-p_{abd})$, a recorder with a printout, and an amplifying unit (Fig. 3.2.1).

Pascal is the SI unit for pressure but is tiny by physiological standards, therefore in urodynamics, all pressure measurements are in cmH_2O (approximately 100 Pascals equal one cmH_2O). The pressures involved are typically in the range of 0 to 250 cmH_2O, which are convenient sizes to handle and the fluid infused is saline.

The bladder pressure can be measured using a:

- Fluid-filled line (a double lumen or single lumen epidural catheter is inserted into the bladder and connected to an external pressure transducer). This is the most commonly used method.
- Solid micro-tip pressure transducer (a transducer is mounted on the tip of a solid 7 Fr catheter and hence is an internal pressure transducer system). This catheter-mounted transducer eliminates artefacts arising from the fluid-filled system, which needs to be connected to an external transducer. The catheter-tip transducer is not used much nowadays due to expense and the need for chemical sterilization, which has its own problems. For example, 2% glutaraldehyde (Cidex), does not kill all atypical mycobacteria and can cause irritation to the skin, eyes, and so on.
- Air-filled catheters have been marketed recently, but the evidence for their use, in terms of recording accuracy, has not yet been established and they are undergoing clinical trials to assess the efficacy and quality of the recordings.

Abdominal pressure is measured with a 4.5 Fr rectal (or occasionally vaginal in women) catheter which is inserted into the rectum to approximately 10–15 cm above the anal margin. Previously, a 6 Fr manometer tubing covered with a fingerstall obtained from a non-sterile surgical rubber glove to prevent blockage by faeces has been used. However, in the United Kingdom, it is no longer allowed to modify and use equipment from their original licensed use, and therefore commercially available special rectal catheters with a balloon at the end must be used, which are more expensive.

It is important to make sure that a small cut is made in the balloon before use to allow expulsion of fluid during flushing (Fig. 3.2.2). If this is not present, then the pressure measured will be that of the water-filled balloon and not of true rectal pressure. The rectal line is taped to the patient's buttock, close to the anal verge to prevent any slippage during the test. The tubing must be flushed from the transducer end before recording is commenced.

The reference height for all measurements is taken as being level with the superior aspect of symphysis pubis and the transducers are zeroed to atmospheric pressure. A double lumen (Fig. 3.2.3) filling catheter (6 Fr) is inserted into the bladder via the urethra (or, occasionally, by the suprapubic route). Alternatively, a single lumen (8 Fr) filling catheter with a 16 G catheter (Fig. 3.2.4) inserted alongside it can be used instead of the double lumen catheter. The two-catheter combination is a cheaper alternative that gives similar results and is our preferred method in most patients. Some centres use a 4.5 Fr bladder pressure catheter in preference to a 16 G one. The single lumen filling catheter is pulled out just before voiding and the 16 G catheter is left in the bladder and used to measure pressure.

The advantage of the double lumen catheter is that the patient's bladder can be filled and refilled multiple times should the test require it, and the post-void residual (if any) can easily be drained

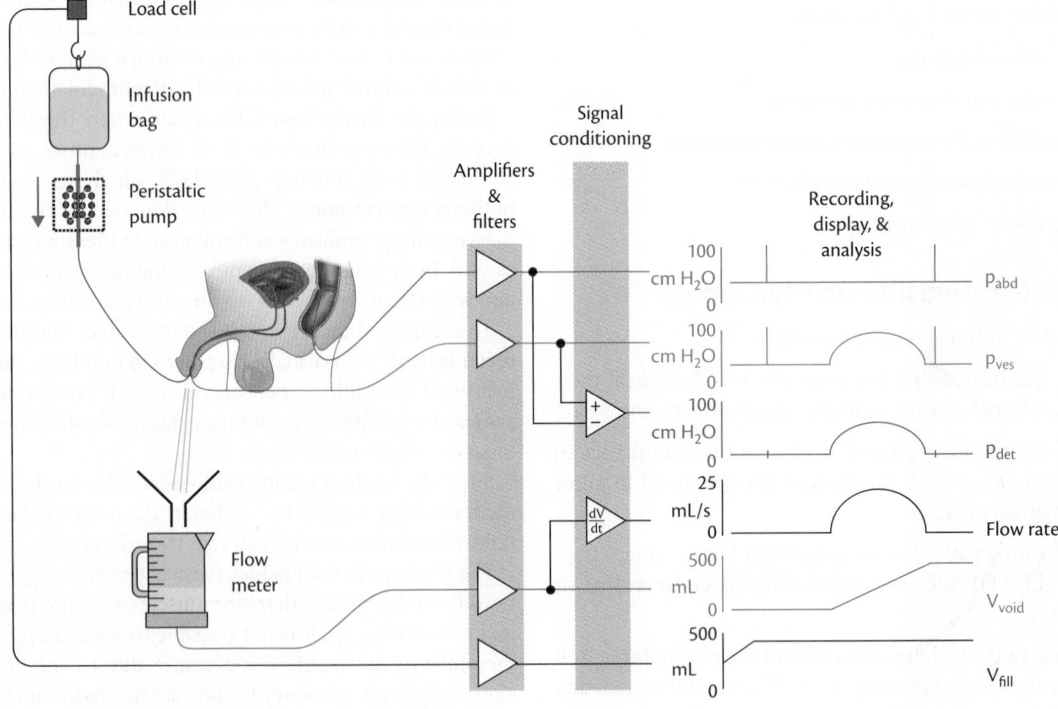

Fig. 3.2.1 Components of an invasive urodynamics test.

Republished with permission of Taylor and Francis Group, LLC, a division of Informa plc, from John G. Webster, *The physiological measurement handbook*, Taylor and Francis Group LLC Books, Copyright © 2015; permission conveyed through Copyright Clearance Center, Inc.

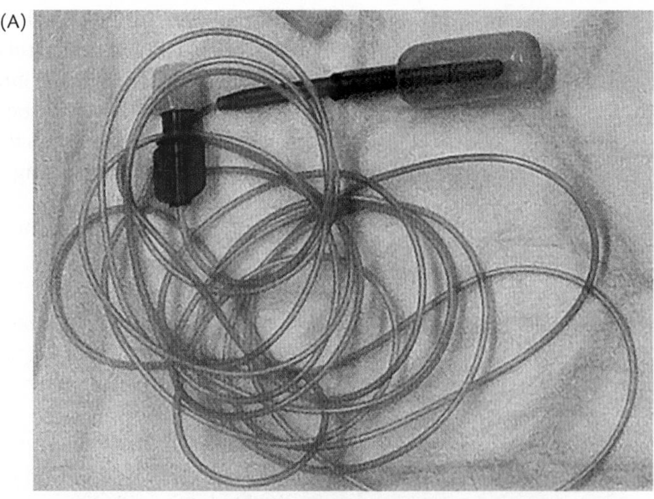

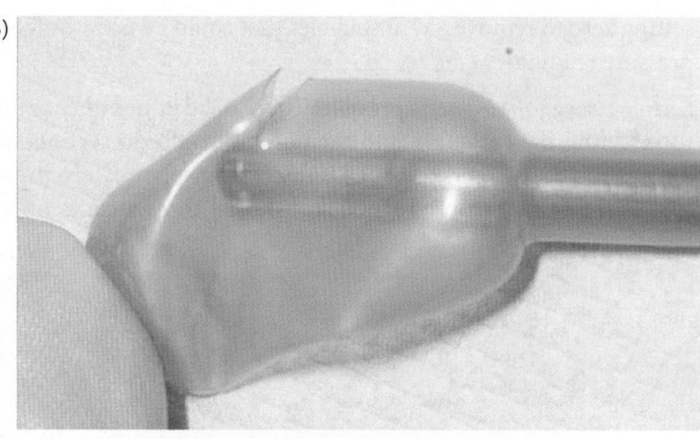

Fig. 3.2.2 (A) Rectal catheter with a hole in the balloon at the end of the catheter; (B) close-up view.

and measured through it; however, it is more expensive to use. The two-catheter technique has the advantage of leaving the 16 G catheter *in situ* to measure pressure at the end of filling and removing the 8 Fr filling catheter. Therefore, the risk of the catheter causing an obstruction during voiding is less than with a double lumen catheter, and when asking the patient at the end of filling to cough and look for stress incontinence, it is less obstructive.

The catheters are fixed in place by tape close to the external urethral meatus on the medial aspect of the thigh in women and around the penis in men.

Filling cystometry

After examining the patient, the rectal tube (p_{abd}) is inserted initially for convenience, and then the urodynamicist washes their hands and wears sterile gloves for the remaining part of the procedure. The bladder is then catheterized urethrally using special filling catheters while in the supine position.

Before initiating the test, the quality of the recording needs to be established. Quality control is vital to allow accurate, reproducible, and interpretable pressure readings, and to allow identification of artefacts. The ICS has defined these steps in the 2002 Good Urodynamics Practices report[4]:

- *Flushing*: The manometer tubing connecting the transducers needs to be fully primed and flushed with sterile water before

Fig. 3.2.3 Double lumen catheter to measure vesical pressure.

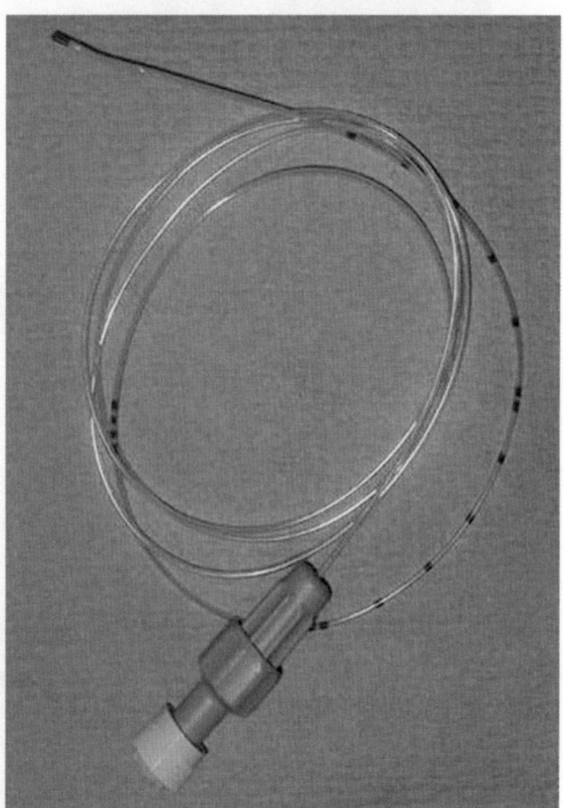

Fig. 3.2.4 16 G catheter to measure vesical pressure.

setting zero to remove any air bubbles that could give low or false pressure readings.

- *Setting zero at atmospheric pressure*: This can be done either prior to inserting the catheters into the patient or after insertion, as long as the transducers are open only to atmosphere. Zero pressure is the value recorded when an external transducer is open only to the environment (the other two sides of a three-way tap are closed) or when the open end of a connected, fluid-filled tube is at the same vertical level as the transducer before insertion into the patient (Fig. 3.2.5). It is advisable to use two three-way taps for each transducer to allow zeroing to atmosphere, even with the catheter being in the patient, and to help with troubleshooting.

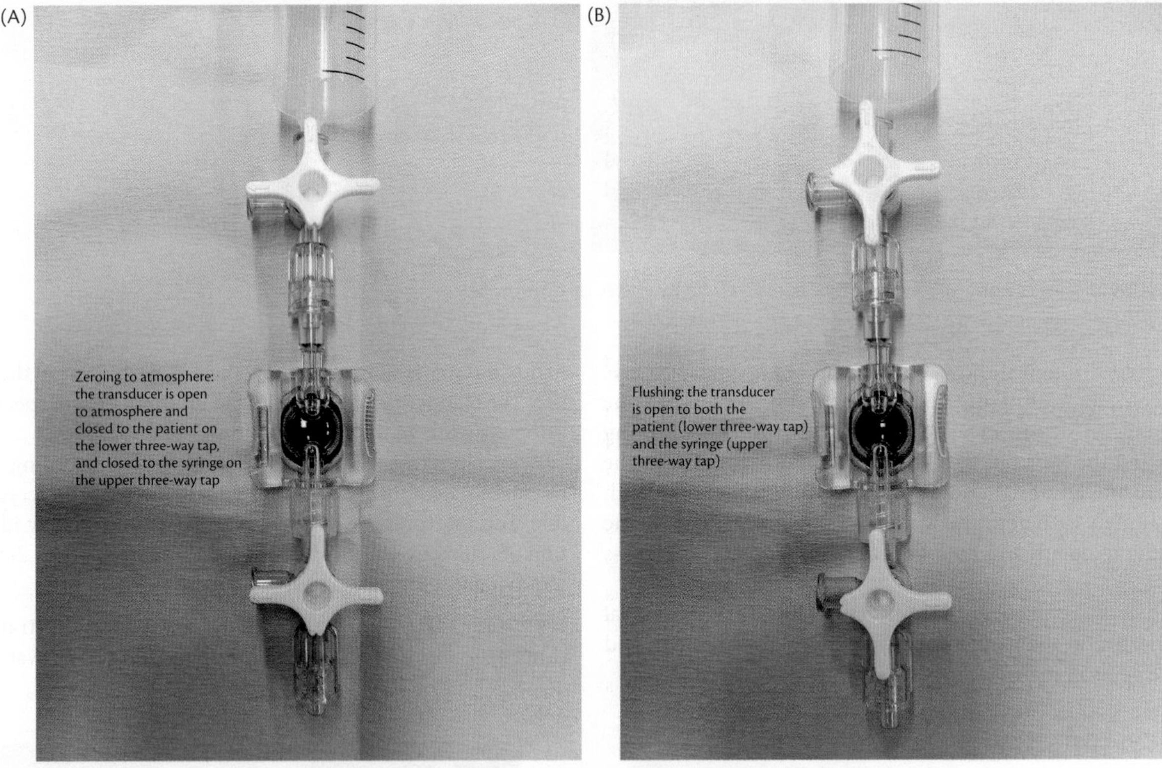

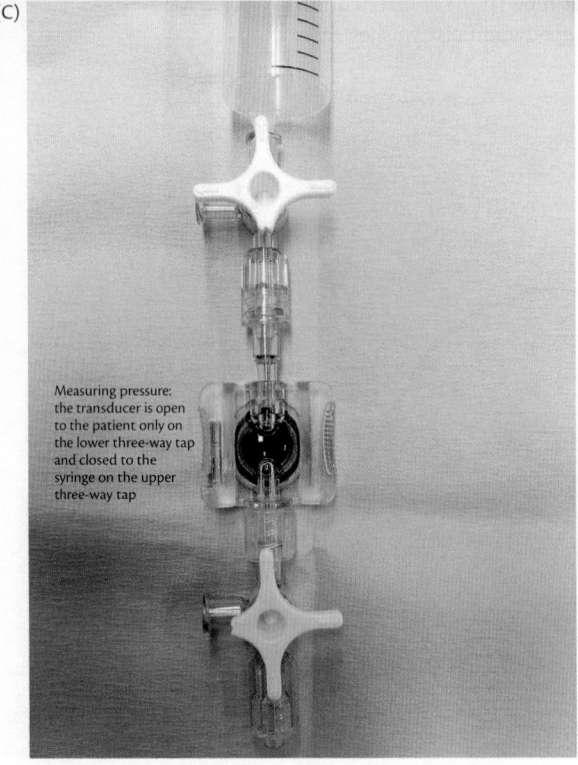

Fig. 3.2.5 Position of three-way taps while zeroing to atmosphere (A), flushing (B) and measuring pressure (C).

- *Checking the calibration of the transducers*: The calibration of the transducers should be checked periodically, ideally daily if performing daily tests, and should be calibrated in the range from 0 to +100 cmH_2O. Full calibration of the transducers and system checks should only be undertaken by trained personnel. Normal resting pressures in the intravesical bladder (p_{ves}) and intra-abdominal rectal (p_{abd}) lines should be in the positive range +5 to +50 cmH_2O (depending on body position and habitus); the resting detrusor pressure (p_{det}) should be between 0 and +10 cmH_2O; however, in clinical practice it can usually range from −5 to +10 cmH_2O.[5]
- *Establishing a reference level for pressure:* The superior border of the symphysis pubis is the fixed reference level for external and fluid-filled catheter systems; the transducers should be levelled to this horizontal plane, so that all measurements have the same hydrostatic component.

During the investigation, quality control is ensured by asking the patient to cough at regular (e.g. 1 minute) intervals. Before recording is started, the patient is asked to cough and the p_{ves} and p_{abd} traces are observed. An equal rise in the two pressure lines must be observed and a complete subtraction of these two pressures should result in no change of the p_{det} line. Sometimes a small artefactual biphasic blip is seen on p_{det}, but this also indicates acceptable subtraction. The biphasic blip occurs due to different speeds of transmission of impulses between the bladder and rectal lines, mainly in older urodynamic systems. The two blips of the biphasic wave should be equal in size; if they are not equal in height, then this indicates poor quality control. The patient should cough before and after voiding to reconfirm quality control and that no displacement of catheters has occurred. During filling, the p_{ves} and p_{abd} lines should not decline and they should not fall below zero (Fig. 3.2.6).

Patient position

Filling cystometry should be done in the upright position, because (i) this is the physiological position, and (ii) because most patients complain of symptoms when upright and active. Women are therefore filled sitting on a commode with a flow meter situated below it to measure any leakage of urine during the test, and because most women void when sitting down. Men, on the other hand, are filled standing with the penis hanging over the flow meter, but not touching it. Filling patients in the supine position might miss detrusor overactivity in at least 30% of patients.[6] Whenever the patient's position is altered, the position of the transducer must be readjusted to the pressure reference level of the upper border of the symphysis pubis, or alternatively the trace is annotated with an event marker to mark the time of position change.

With the catheters in position, the filling catheter is connected to a suitable filling medium. The rest of the equipment should be close to the patient for convenience and, if a computer screen is available, this should be in a position viewable by the patient so that explanations can be given during the test.

If there is severe detrusor overactivity that prevents filling, even at a reduced rate (10–20 mL/min), then the patient can be moved to the supine position so that useful information can be gathered from cystometry and to allow adequate filling of the bladder. Reduced mobility or severe disablement of patients (e.g. by neurological disease) may also necessitate cystometry in the supine position.

Resting values for abdominal (p_{abd}) and intravesical (p_{ves}) pressures are in the typical ranges below, depending on position:

- supine 0–20 cmH_2O
- sitting 15–40 cmH_2O
- standing 30–50 cmH_2O.

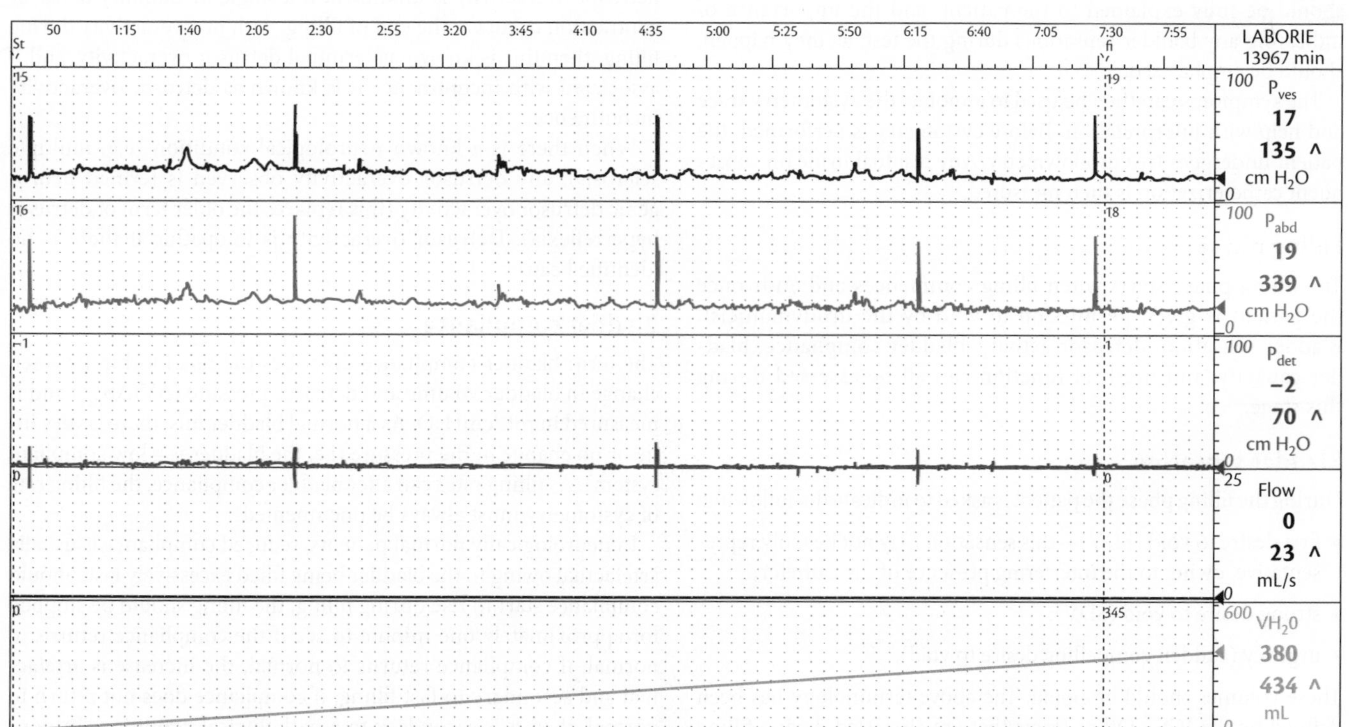

Fig. 3.2.6 Good quality urodynamic trace showing the biphasic blips and regular coughs.

Filling medium

Water and 0.9% (normal) saline are the fluids most frequently used as they are cheap, convenient, and mimic urine in consistency. The fluid is commonly used at room temperature (22°C); however, body temperature (37°C) may be more physiological. It is known that ice-cold infusion fluid can stimulate bladder contraction at low bladder volumes, and therefore should not be used in routine cystometry.

Filling rates

Previously, three filling rates were defined by the ICS:

- Slow-fill: cystometry up to 10 mL/min
- Medium-fill: cystometry between 10 and 100 mL/min
- Fast-fill: cystometry when the rate is greater than 100 mL/min

The ICS no longer divides filling rates into slow, medium, or fast. Currently, the term 'non-physiologic filling rate' is being used, and the precise filling rate should be stated. We recommend a filling rate of 50 mL/min, which, although convenient in the setting of a busy urodynamic unit, is not so fast as to be grossly unphysiological; it also allows time to discuss symptoms with the patient and to assess whether those symptoms have been successfully reproduced. In a patient with very marked detrusor overactivity, the rate can be reduced to 30 mL/min or lower.

The upper limit of physiological filling is defined as:

$$\text{Filling rate (in mL/min)} = \text{Body mass (in kg)} \div 4$$

Slower filling rates are indicated in patients with neurogenic bladders. Rapid filling is rarely used but can be a further provocative test for detrusor overactivity.

The test and all side effects (e.g. risk of urinary tract infection) should be fully explained to the patient, and the importance of indicating any bladder sensations during the test, as they happen, should be emphasized.

The symptoms can then be used to annotate the cystometry trace and help with interpretation. Before cystometry is performed, the patient undergoes free uroflowmetry. Any residual urine on subsequent catheterization is then measured.

Filling phase

The filling phase starts when filling commences and ends once the patient is given permission to void by the urodynamicist. Bladder sensation, detrusor activity, bladder compliance, bladder capacity, and urethral function can all be assessed during this stage.

Bladder sensation

During the filling phase the patient is asked to indicate the following:

- first desire to void (FDV)—this sensation may not be truly representative, owing to the interfering presence of the catheter;
- strong desire to void (SDV);
- urgency (sudden compelling desire to void).

These volumes should be noted. The above terminology has been defined by the ICS.[7] Other terms that are also used during filling cystometry and related to bladder sensation include first sensation of bladder filling, bladder pain, and bladder sensation, which can be categorized as increased, normal, reduced, absent, or non-specific (seen mainly in neurological patients).

Bladder hypersensitivity is a term that has been used in the past and found to be helpful. It was defined as a condition where there is an early FDV at less than 100 mL and this persists and worsens, limiting the bladder cystometric capacity to 250 mL. This term has now been replaced with the term 'increased bladder sensation', which is an early first sensation of bladder filling (or an early desire to void) and/or an early strong desire to void, which occurs at low bladder volume and persists. The new term is subjective and thus it is not possible to quantify volumes.

Detrusor activity

Detrusor activity is described as either 'normal' or 'overactive'. A normal detrusor allows bladder filling with little or no change in pressure, with no involuntary phasic contractions occurring during cystometry, despite provocation.

The presence of involuntary phasic detrusor contractions, occurring throughout filling, is diagnosed by detecting a rise in the detrusor pressure line (there is no lower limit for the amplitude of an involuntary detrusor contraction) and a similar rise in the vesical line with no rise in the abdominal line during filling cystometry. The patient should be asked whether there is any associated urgency and if the sensation mimics the one that is normally experienced and causes problems. Precipitating factors such as coughing or running water, used to provoke symptoms, may also induce detrusor overactivity, and should be annotated on the trace (Fig. 3.2.7).

If the detrusor is shown during cystometry to contract spontaneously or with provocation, then it is said to have phasic detrusor overactivity. Some patients will not experience any symptoms at the time of these contractions, in which case the significance of detrusor overactivity is unknown. If a single involuntary detrusor contraction occurs at the end of filling, with no overactivity during filling, then this is known as terminal detrusor overactivity, and if associated with incontinence it is known as detrusor overactivity incontinence.

When there is a known neurological condition (e.g. multiple sclerosis), any detrusor overactivity observed is termed neurogenic detrusor overactivity (this replaces the older term of detrusor hyperreflexia). Detrusor overactivity is idiopathic if there is no identified cause.

Bladder compliance

The term bladder compliance describes the relationship between change in bladder volume and detrusor pressure ($\Delta V/\Delta p_{det}$) and is measured in mL/cmH_2O. As a normal bladder fills, there is very little or no change in the pressure (i.e. the bladder is a low compliant system). As filling rates can alter bladder compliance, the filling rate of cystometry must always be documented.

In neurologically normal patients, reduced compliance is usually artefactual owing to the bladder being filled excessively fast. Should compliance start to rise during filling, the filling should be stopped for approximately one minute to see if the compliance returns to normal: if compliance returns to normal, the increase is artefactual and secondary to fast filling; if compliance does not return to normal, then it is secondary to a pathological condition. In non-neurological patients, up to 1 cmH_2O detrusor pressure increase

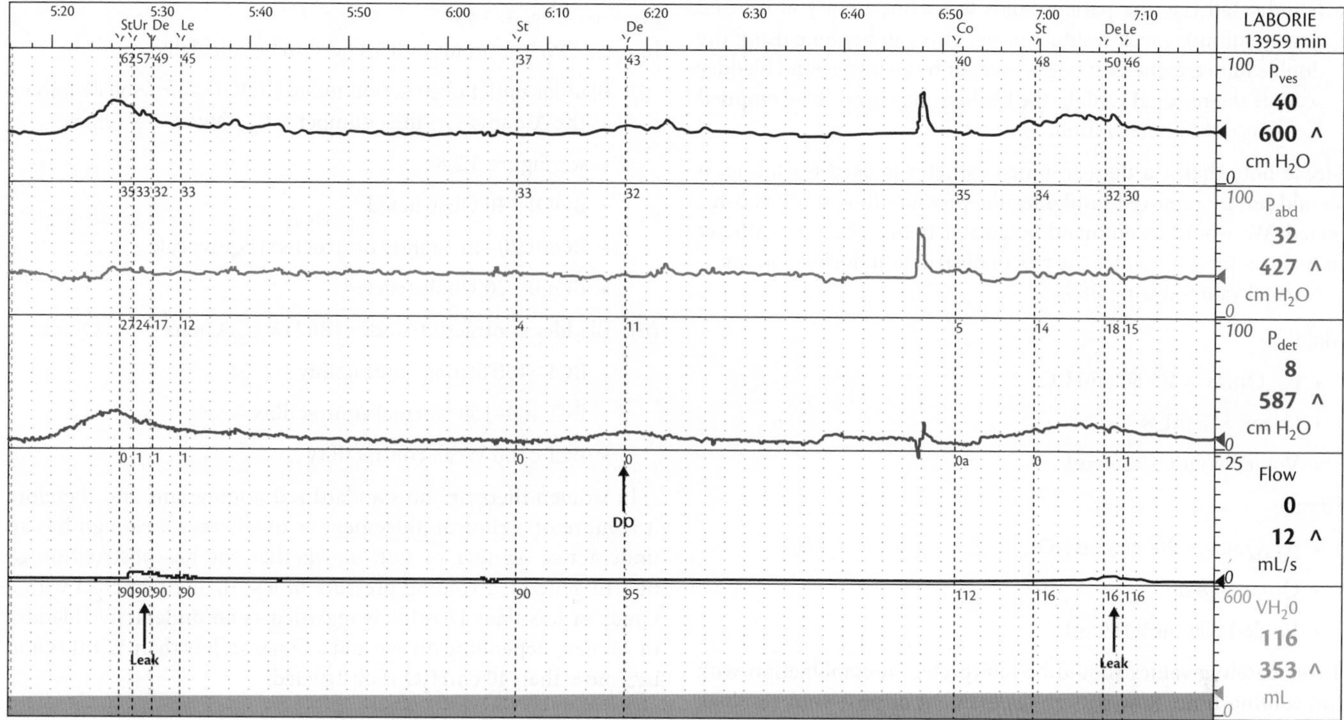

Fig. 3.2.7 Urodynamic trace showing detrusor overactivity with incontinence.

per 40 mL is acceptable, and in neurological patients up to 20 mL/ cmH_2O is acceptable.

Urethral function

During the filling phase, in normal patients, the urethral closure pressure remains positive (i.e. it is greater than the intravesical pressure), even at times of increased intra-abdominal pressure; hence, continence is maintained. To allow voiding, closure pressure falls as the urethra relaxes. If involuntary loss of urine is observed without detrusor overactivity, then the urethral closure mechanism is said to be incompetent.

A diagnosis of urodynamic stress incontinence can be made if leakage is associated with an increase in intra-abdominal pressure that causes the intravesical pressure to exceed the intraurethral pressure in the absence of a detrusor contraction. When filling volume reaches 200 mL, filling is stopped, and the patient is asked to strain (Valsalva manoeuvre) and then to cough to observe any leakage. These two manoeuvres increase intra-abdominal pressure above urethral closure pressure, and if there is an incompetent urethra, the patient will leak.

Voiding pressure/flow studies

Voiding pressure flow studies (PFS) are done at the end of the filling phase, when the patient is given permission to void. All patients should have an attempt at voiding if they are undergoing filling cystometry. PFS are most useful in the assessment of:

- Bladder outlet obstruction
- Dysfunctional voiding
- Preoperatively, for assessment of the voiding phase in patients having surgery for stress incontinence
- Incomplete bladder emptying/large post-void residuals
- Neurological lower urinary tract dysfunction

Two key elements are assessed during voiding PFS:

- Detrusor pressure at maximum flow ($p_{det}Qmax$)
- Maximum urine flow rate (Qmax)

To assist near physiological normal voiding values, it is recommended that male patients void in the standing position, and women void in the seated position.

Technique

- The bladder is filled to normal capacity (when the patient says the bladder is full). This should be done in conjunction with the bladder diary/frequency volume chart, for normal average voided volumes during the day.
- Remove the single lumen filling catheters prior to voiding, leaving the single lumen pressure line or 16 G catheter *in situ* (p_{ves}). If the double lumen catheter is used, then there is no need to remove it prior to voiding (see point below).
- Ask the patient to perform a single cough (quality control check) just before voiding to make sure the pressure line (p_{ves}) has not been displaced during catheter removal at the end of filling.
- Permission is then given to void—it is normal practice to leave the room at this point to allow the patient privacy. Voiding can sometimes be inhibited if the patient is not left alone to void.
- Ask the patient to do a single cough (quality control check) after voiding to make sure the pressure recording is accurate.
- Remove the pressure lines (p_{ves} and p_{abd}).

- If indicated (i.e. the patient voids less urine than you infused during filling), check residual urine. This can be done using the double lumen catheter if one is used, or by an ultrasound bladder scan. If the residual is high, the bladder may need to be emptied by an in/out catheterization.

Please note that if a double lumen catheter is used for filling, it should not be removed until after the pressure flow study is completed. We would recommend no greater than a size 6 Fr catheter in male patients to reduce the risk of obstruction during voiding.

Normal values during PFS:

Male

- $p_{det}Qmax = 40–60\ cmH_2O$
- Qmax >15 mL/s
- Voided volume >150 mL

Female

- $p_{det}Qmax = 20–40\ cmH_2O$
- Qmax >18 mL/s
- Voided volume >150 mL

These baseline values should be interpreted in combination with the voiding time, flow pattern, assessment of post-void residual, and patient's age.

Complications and difficulties

- Patient unable to void—may be related to environment or overfilling the bladder
- Catheter voided before Qmax is reached—PFS may need to be repeated
- Difficulty in removing vesical pressure (p_{ves}) line
- Technical difficulties with equipment (e.g. poor pressure transmission)
- Infection (2–3%): antibiotics are not routinely indicated
- Bleeding
- Discomfort from the catheters

Pressure flow analysis

In men, two important indices need to be calculated:

(i) Bladder outlet obstruction index (BOOI)—previously known as the Abrams-Griffiths number = $p_{det}Qmax–2 \times Qmax$
- see Figure 3.2.8
- BOOI >40 Obstructed
- BOOI 20–40 Slightly obstructed (Equivocal)
- BOOI <20 Unobstructed

(ii) Bladder contractility index (BCI) = $p_{det}Qmax + 5 \times Qmax$
- BCI >150 Strong contractility
- BCI 100–150 Normal contractility
- BCI <100 Weak contractility

In women there are no standardized nomograms and therefore it is more of a clinical judgement as to whether a woman has an underactive bladder or not, or whether she has obstruction or not. In general, a voiding pressure of less than 20 cmH_2O with a Qmax of less than 12 mL/s is regarded as an underactive bladder in women, depending on age and a Qmax of less than 12 mL/s and p_{det} more than 40 cmH_2O is obstructed.

Advanced urodynamics

Videourodynamics

Videourodynamics (VUDS) are usually undertaken in specialist regional centres that have experienced advanced urodynamic practitioners who are skilled in performing the investigations, as well as the interpretation of the results. VUDS give more detailed anatomical information about the urethra, bladder, and upper urinary tracts, combined with measurement of pressure. Its indications include:

- Neurological patients including dysfunctional voiding
- Incontinence following anti-incontinence surgery (e.g post-colposuspension)
- Urinary incontinence after radical prostatectomy in men
- Anatomical abnormalities

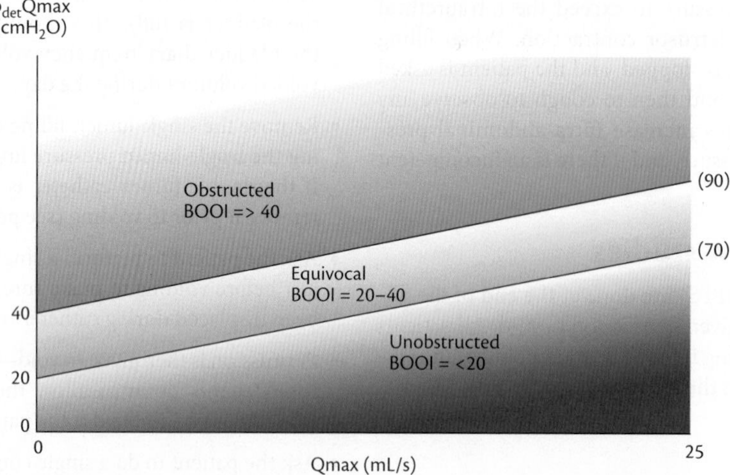

Fig. 3.2.8 Bladder outlet obstruction index nomogram.

Reproduced with permission from P. Abrams, 'Bladder outlet obstruction index, bladder contractility index and bladder voiding efficiency: three simple indices to define bladder voiding function', *BJU International*, Volume 84, Issue 1, pp. 14–15, Copyright © 1999 John Wiley and Sons.

- Paediatric patients
- Young men (<50 years old)—as they are unlikely to have benign prostatic obstruction

However, complications of VUDS include allergic reaction to contrast medium (iodine), while its contraindications include pregnancy.

Again, the principles of good urodynamics practice apply. Some modifications include the use of contrast medium to fill the bladder and the technique must comply with the ionizing radiation (medical exposure) regulations.

Several types of imaging can be used, including X-ray, ultrasound, and MRI. X-ray is the commonest and easiest to use. Screening needs to be done at regular intervals and for short periods of time to avoid large amounts of radiation.

The main advantages of VUDS are that it provides combined structural and functional information and can be used for review in meetings and teaching. The disadvantages include radiation exposure (0.7 mSv = 4/12 background radiation), cost (initial and running), and being an unnatural voiding environment.

VUDS can be used to classify stress incontinence radiologically according to the Blaivas classification,[8] and hence is used in some centres to differentiate between intrinsic sphincter deficiency and urethral hypermobility in women. Types I and II indicate urethral hypermobility of various severity, and type III is consistent with intrinsic sphincter deficiency (ISD).

- Type 0: Vesical neck and proximal urethra are closed at rest and situated at or above the lower end of the symphysis pubis. They descend during stress, but incontinence is not seen.
- Type I: Vesical neck is closed at rest and is well above the inferior margin of the symphysis. During stress, the vesical neck and proximal urethra open and descend <2 cm. Incontinence is seen.
- Type IIa: Vesical neck is closed at rest and is above the inferior margin of the symphysis. During stress the vesical neck and proximal urethra open and descend >2 cm. Incontinence is seen.
- Type IIb: Vesical neck is closed at rest and is at or below the inferior margin of the symphysis. During stress, there may or may not be further descent but as the proximal urethra opens, incontinence is seen.
- Type III: Vesical neck and proximal urethra are open at rest. The proximal urethra no longer functions as a sphincter. There is obvious urinary leakage with minimal increases in intravesical pressure.

Blaivas classification reprinted from *The Journal of Urology*, Volume 139, Issue 4, Blaivas JG and Olsson CA, 'Stress incontinence: classification and surgical approach', pp. 727–731, Copyright © 1998 American Urological Association, with permission from Elsevier, http://www.sciencedirect.com/science/journal/00225347/160

In our centre, we use urethral function studies to help us differentiate between the two types of stress urinary incontinence to avoid irradiating women unnecessarily, and we use VUDS in recurrent stress urinary incontinence.

Urethral function tests

The aim of these is to assess urethral function and they can be performed in the following patient groups:

- Dysfunctional voiding
- Neurological
- Incontinence (e.g. prior to stress incontinence surgery or in post-prostatectomy patients)

There are two main urethral function tests: urethral pressure profiles (UPPs) and leak point pressures (LPP). LPP is the detrusor pressure or the intravesical pressure (p_{det} or p_{ves}) at which involuntary expulsion of urine from the urethral meatus is observed.

Most UPPs are undertaken using the Brown and Wickham technique, which involves slow fluid perfusion (2 mL/min) through a single lumen urethral pressure profile catheter. Resting bladder pressure is continuously monitored, either through a bladder pressure line (preferable option) or a pseudo-pressure abdominal or vaginal line. The UPP catheter is withdrawn at a rate of 1 mm/sec. Continuous pressure measurement is taken to record the following pressure measurements (Fig. 3.2.9):

- Maximum urethral closure pressure (MUCP) = maximum urethral pressure (MUP) minus resting bladder (p_{ves}) pressure
- Functional profile length—this is the urethral length from the start of the UPP to the MUP in men, and the full length of the profile (start to end of UPP) in women.

UPP depends on patient position, volume of fluid in the bladder, pressure recording catheter used, and its orientation within the urethra.

There are two main types of leak point pressures: detrusor (DLPP) and abdominal (ALPP). DLPP is the lowest pressure at which urine leakage occurs in the absence of either a detrusor contraction or increased abdominal pressure and applies mainly in patients with low compliance bladders. ALPP is the intravesical pressure at which urine leakage occurs due to increased abdominal pressure in the absence of a detrusor contraction. ALPP can be divided into Valsalva (VLPP) or cough (CLPP) leak point pressures.

The methodology of performing UPPs and ALPPs has not been standardized. In our centre, we perform UPPs with the patient lying down after catheterizing them with the bladder empty, repeat the process twice, and take the average of the two readings of the MUCP.

ALPP is performed during filling cystometry with the patient in the upright position, once the bladder is filled to 200 mL. The patient is asked to cough and perform Valsalva manoeuvres with increasing pressures by increments of 20 cmH_2O, starting from 40 cmH_2O up to 120 cmH_2O. If the patient does not leak, ALPPs are performed every 100 mL after that until capacity. If the patient fails to leak and they are complaining of stress urinary incontinence, the filling line is removed at capacity and they are asked to perform different provocative manoeuvres such as jumping, squatting, running on the spot, and so on to try to make the patient leak and reproduce their symptoms.

In women who suffer with stress urinary incontinence, the normal value for MUCP is 92—age. An MUCP of less than 20 cmH_2O is indicative of ISD. This low MUCP is equivalent to an ALPP of less than 60 cmH_2O. If ALPP is greater than 90 cmH_2O, then that indicates stress incontinence secondary to urethral hypermobility.

There is level 2 evidence, with grade B recommendation, for the use of UPPs and LPP. They can be helpful in certain circumstances, particularly in distinguishing between ISD and urethral hypermobility, in women with stress urinary incontinence. This may then allow the clinician to decide as to what type of anti-incontinence procedure the patient should have. UPPs could also be helpful in patients

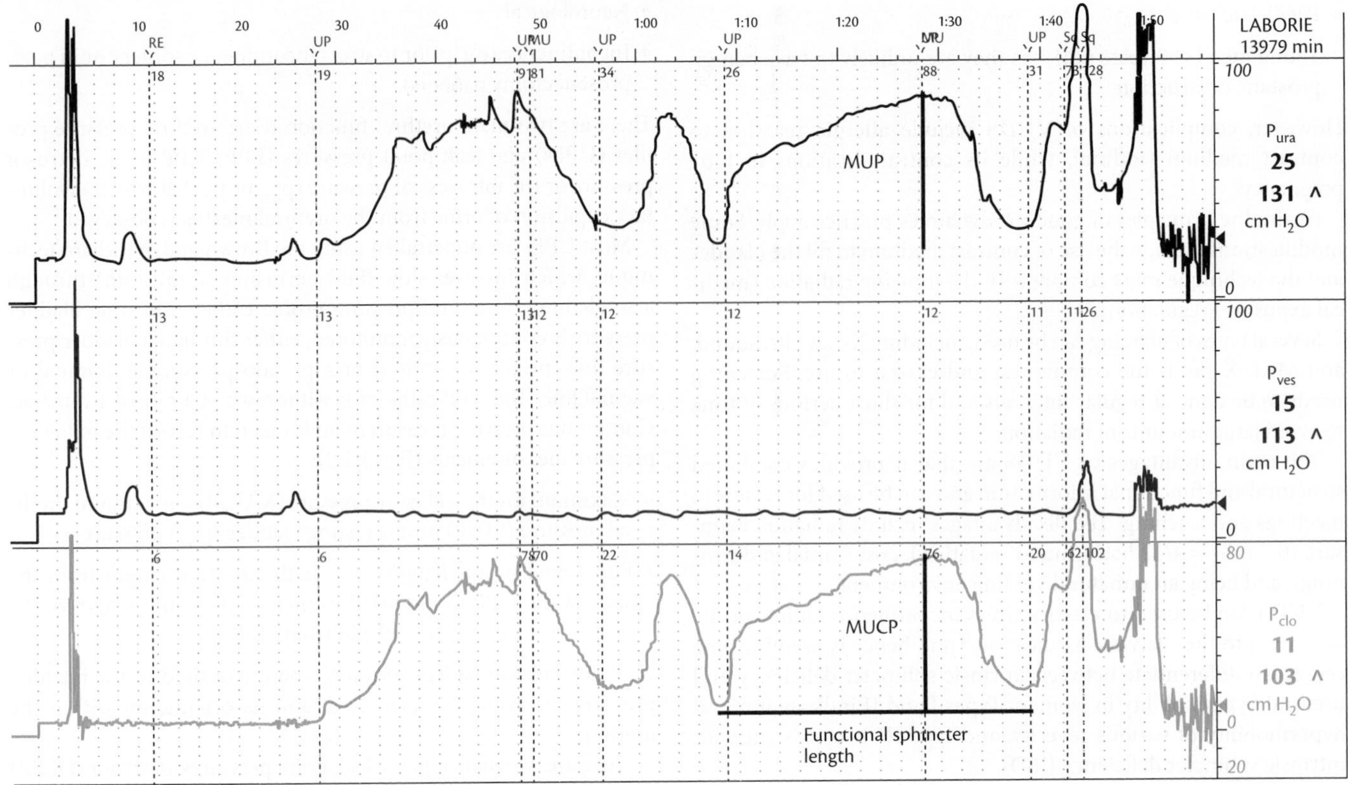

Fig. 3.2.9 Urethral pressure profiles in women (MUP = maximum urethral pressure; MUCP = maximum urethral closure pressure).

with an artificial urinary sphincter to measure the closure pressure of the device and see if it is still the same as when it was implanted, and in patients who complain of leakage after sphincter insertion.

Nonetheless, UPPs and LPPs should not be used as single factors on their own to grade the severity of incontinence, and their results should be judged in relation to other urodynamic tests (such as filling cystometry) and to the clinical examination. They may help to judge the severity of incontinence, or to further 'subcategorize' patients with stress (predominant) incontinence.

The ICS have produced a standardization document on how UPPs should be done and measured.[9]

Ambulatory urodynamics

Ambulatory urodynamics (AUDS) is any functional test of the lower urinary tract, usually performed outside the clinical setting, predominantly utilizing natural filling, and reproducing the subject's normal activity.[10]

'Ambulatory' refers to the nature of monitoring, rather than the mobility of the subject, and 'natural' refers to the natural production of urine to fill the bladder rather than an artificial medium; 'normal activity' refers to the everyday activities of the subject during which their urinary symptoms are most likely to occur.

AUDS are indicated if routine/standard or VUDS fail to reproduce the patient's symptoms, or provide a satisfactory answer to the original urodynamic question. They have also been used in clinical trials to monitor the efficacy of new medical therapies. AUDS usually lasts between two and six hours, with natural filling of the bladder rather than artificial filling through a bladder catheter.

The advantages of AUDS are that it can capture more realistic and/or more physiological observations, such as attempts to increase sensitivity by providing a longer time for detrusor overactivity to manifest itself (up to 17% on conventional cystometry in normal subjects vs. 69% on AUDS), and detects more actual incontinence than conventional cystometry.[11]

The disadvantages are that it is time-consuming, expensive, can cause discomfort in patients having the catheter for long periods of time, may present difficulties in quality control with increased patient movement, and needs experienced staff to interpret the results.

AUDS requires specialized equipment (Fig. 3.2.10) and includes:

- Abdominal and vesical pressure lines
- Pad for urine loss measurement
- Urinary diary
- Host computer
- Lightweight portable recording device with
  - event markers
  - adequate battery capacity
  - fast frequency response

Technique:

- Patients are asked to drink at regular intervals (every 30 minutes).
- Patients are catheterized with a bladder pressure line (p_{ves}) and abdominal line (p_{abd}), which are then attached to a small portable monitoring device, which is worn on a waist belt for the duration of the test.
- Once the test has started the patient can leave the department and perform normal activities such as walking, running, climbing

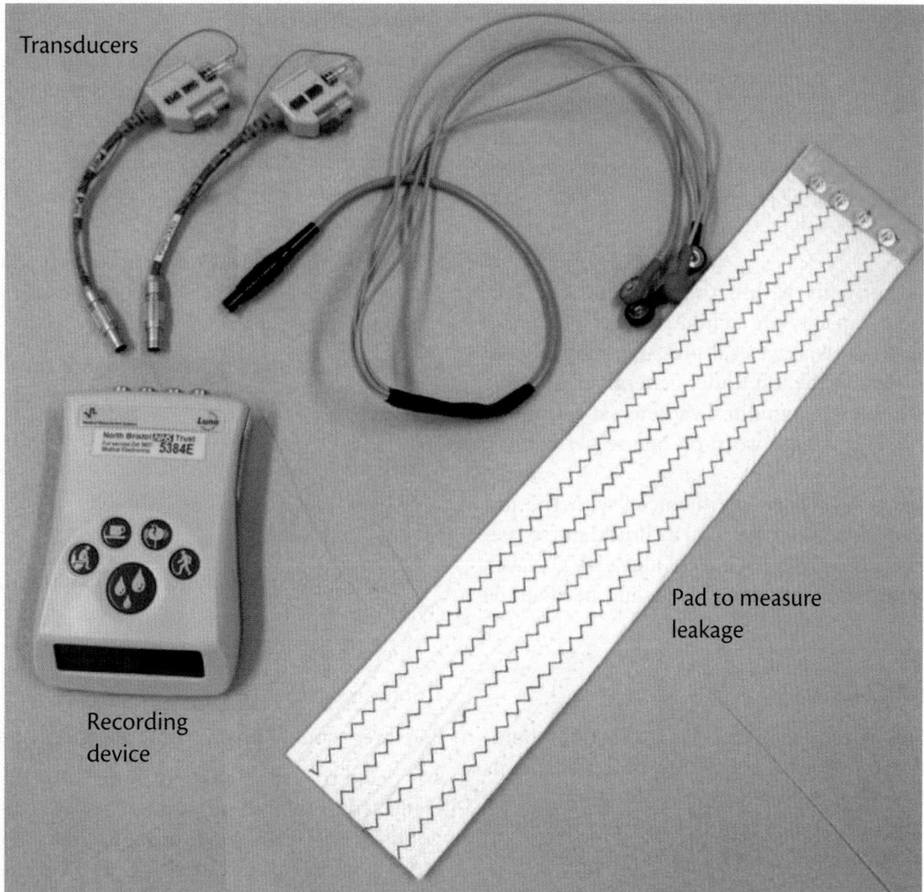

Fig. 3.2.10 Ambulatory urodynamic equipment.

stairs, or any other activity that is a known trigger to reproduce their urinary symptoms in their day-to-day life.

- As symptoms occur during the test, the patient is asked to press a key/button on the portable recording device that will mark it as an event as soon as it occurs (e.g. urgency, leakage).
- The patient completes two fill and void cycles. Sometimes a third is performed if symptoms have not been performed.
- Interpretation of the test is ongoing throughout the test period, events can be clarified with the patient as they occur, and the urodynamicist running the investigation completes the final interpretation and writing of the report.

Neurophysiological testing

Electromyography (EMG) is the commonest neurophysiological urodynamic test performed. The aim of EMG during a urodynamic study is to determine whether the external urethral sphincter complex is coordinated or uncoordinated with the bladder during voiding. This can be done using either surface or needle electrodes.

Surface electrodes are placed on the perineum to detect general striated muscle activity. It is technically difficult to ensure a good quality EMG signal from the appropriate muscle during this procedure. Therefore, this has been abandoned in most major centres around the world.

Needle electrodes, on the other hand, can isolate electrical activity from specific muscle fibres and therefore are more interpretable, but more invasive. The tip of the needle electrode can be either monopolar, concentric, or single fibre in type, varying in dimensions, and the type of metal that is used.

The use of EMG generally, and needle electrodes specifically, is reserved for only selected patients with neurogenic bladder dysfunction, or those with behavioural voiding dysfunction (e.g. Fowler's syndrome).

Specialized patient groups

Urodynamic investigations in paediatric and neurological patients are usually undertaken in specialist centres with experienced advanced urodynamic practitioners skilled in performing the investigations and interpretation of the results. The same principles of good urodynamic practice apply, as above, with some modifications.

Neurological patients

Filling is normally started at the lower rate of 10 mL/minute to assess bladder compliance. This rate can be gradually increased to 50 mL/minute (in minute intervals) if there is no significant change in detrusor pressure or detrusor overactivity during filling.

The patients may have to be filled lying down as they are unable to stand up. Monitoring for autonomic dysreflexia is important and the test may need to be done in a latex-free room with the availability of a hoist. Voiding may also have to be done while the patient is lying down or on their side with a long tube going into the flow meter.

If the patient has large residuals, then the standard teaching is not to empty the bladder and to fill above the patient's baseline residual, as the aim is to see mimic the patient's symptoms. The other reason for not emptying the patient completely is that the residual may be very high and it may take longer to fill them. If the patient self-catheterizes and normally has an empty bladder, then it is important to empty the bladder before the test.

Paediatric patients

Filling in children is normally within the range of 2–5 mL/min. The normal bladder capacity for a child is [(age × 2) + 30]. A suprapubic catheter, to measure vesical pressure, may have to be inserted before the start of the test under general anaesthetic, if the child is unable to tolerate a urethral catheter. It is important that the anaesthetic effects have worn off before performing the test.

In our centre, we have several people involved with the test including a radiographer, a paediatrician, and a clinical nurse specialist. The room is especially equipped with toys and a DVD player, as the test can take up to two hours to complete and needs to be child-friendly.

Interpretation of results

Interpretation of urodynamics is performed using the standardized ICS guidelines for good urodynamic practice and its associated terminology for lower urinary tract function.[4,7] The interpretation of urodynamic traces requires skilled knowledge and analysis of normal trace characteristics, which is based on the following key factors:

- Cough signal—p_{ves} and p_{abd} should be equal and rise (positive pressure) simultaneously. The trace is checked at the start of filling and then every minute throughout the duration of the filling period.
- Quality control—check for regular cough signal every minute, and then before and after voiding.
- Scale—check scales are equal (p_{ves}, p_{abd}, p_{det}). These are normally set at the range 0–100 cmH_2O. Check the scale for flow rate, usually set at 0–25 mL/s.
- Time—check the time scale interval on the trace: seconds or minutes.
- Check the accurate placing of bladder event markers throughout the investigation (e.g. urgency, detrusor overactivity, urinary leakage/type, first desire, normal desire).

It can be difficult to analyse a urodynamic trace if these factors are not adhered to and should be used in conjunction with the resting bladder (p_{ves}) and abdominal (p_{abd}) pressures at the start of filling, throughout filling, and at the end of filling to check for any corresponding rise or fall in pressure. This enables the interpreter to cross check that the recorded values during filling and voiding are accurately recorded, and that the overall quality of the urodynamic trace is of an acceptable and reliable standard.

There is no standardized way of interpreting traces, but the most important tip is to look at all three pressure lines during both filling and voiding and see if there are any changes in them, remembering that a change in the detrusor pressure could be due to a change in the abdominal or vesical lines.

Troubleshooting

Common problems with tests are usually related to the unequal transmission of pressures. If there is unequal transmission of pressure, it is usually caused by one of the following:

- Air in the system, which can cause a 'dampened' signal on the trace, resulting in a slow response to a cough transmission of pressure.
- Check for any loose connections in the taps, luer-locks, transducers, catheters—this will cause a loss of pressure (negative) or negative pressure drift.
- Incorrect set-up of domes and connecting tubing—check that it is fluid-filled and that the set has been fully primed with fluid.
- Kinking of any of the tubing—check for any blockages or kinks in the connecting pressure lines; for example, women may be sitting on the p_{abd} line and cause kinking.

Less frequently:

- Damaged/broken equipment—check transducer domes and connecting cables.
- Operator error.
- Software/hardware failure.

Pressures should remain within the acceptable range:

- p_{ves} and p_{abd} should be positive: 5–50 cmH_2O. This can also be affected by the patient position and weight—a higher body mass index (BMI) can result in higher than normal pressure range. If p_{ves} and/or p_{abd} start at 0 cmH_2O, it means that the pressure lines have been zeroed in the bladder and not to atmosphere. Therefore, the test would be of 'bad' quality.
- There should be a corresponding p_{det}: 0–6 cmH_2O in 80% of cases.

Most problems that occur can be rectified by flushing the lines—normally 2–5 mL is sufficient. After each flush, ask the patient to repeat a cough to check the pressure transmission. It is always worth repeating this if the first attempt does not work. Developing a systematic approach to troubleshooting is an important aspect of good urodynamic practice.

If transducer failure is suspected, it is worth checking zero during the test. A test can be paused (stop filling) while this is being done. Turn the transducer off to the patient and open to atmosphere—pressure should always return to zero at any point during the test. If it does not return to zero, the transducer should be re-zeroed and filling can then be restarted. Most urodynamic software will allow you to do this; if it doesn't, you may need to restart the test again. This is the main advantage of using two three-way taps for each transducer.

Conclusions

Urodynamics needs to be performed interactively, with the patient, by trained personnel[12] to the highest quality according to the ICS good urodynamics protocol, with continuous observation of signals as they are collected and artefacts corrected where possible. The aim is to reproduce the patient's symptoms in order to answer the urodynamic question formulated at the beginning of the test.

Further reading

Abrams P, Cardozo L, Fall M, *et al.* The standardisation of terminology of lower urinary tract function: report from the Standardisation Sub-committee of the International Continence Society. *Neurourol Urodyn* 2002; **21**(2):167–78.

Ionising radiation (medical exposure) regulations, 2000. Available at: http://www.dh.gov.uk/en/Publicationsandstatistics/Publications/PublicationsPolicyAndGuidance/DH_4007957 [Online].

Lose G, Griffiths D, Hosker G, *et al.* Standardisation of urethral pressure measurement: report from the Standardisation Sub-Committee of the International Continence Society. *Neurourol Urodyn* 2002; **21**(3):258–60.

Rosier PF, Schaefer W, Lose G, *et al.* International Continence Society Good Urodynamic Practices and Terms 2016: Urodynamics, uroflowmetry, cystometry, and pressure-flow study. *Neurourol Urodyn* 2016; doi: 10.1002/nau.23124. [Epub ahead of print].

Schafer W, Abrams P, Liao L, *et al.* Good urodynamic practices: uroflowmetry, filling cystometry, and pressure-flow studies. *Neurourol Urodyn* 2002; **21**(3):261–74.

Singh G, Lucas M, Dolan L, Knight S, Ramage C, Hobson PT. Minimum standards for urodynamic practice in the UK. *Neurourol Urodyn* 2010; **29**(8):1365–72.

van Waalwijk van DE, Anders K, Khullar V, *et al.* Standardisation of ambulatory urodynamic monitoring: Report of the Standardisation Sub-Committee of the International Continence Society for Ambulatory Urodynamic Studies. *Neurourol Urodyn* 2000; **19**(2):113–25.

References

1. Perez LM, Webster GD. The history of urodynamics. *Neurourol Urodyn* 1992; **11**:1–21.
2. NICE CG040. Urinary Incontinence: The Management of Urinary Incontinence in Women, 2006. Available at: https://www.nice.org.uk/guidance/cg40?unlid=7533731292016484351. [Online].
3. Abrams P, Blaivas JG, Stanton SL, Andersen JT. The standardisation of terminology of lower urinary tract function. The International Continence Society Committee on Standardisation of Terminology. *Scand J Urol Nephrol Suppl* 1988; **114**:5–19.
4. Schafer W, Abrams P, Liao L, *et al.* Good urodynamic practices: uroflowmetry, filling cystometry, and pressure-flow studies. *Neurourol Urodyn* 2002; **21**(3):261–74.
5. Sullivan J, Lewis P, Howell S, Williams T, Shepherd AM, Abrams P. Quality control in urodynamics: a review of urodynamic traces from one centre. *BJU Int* 2003; **91**(3):201–7.
6. Al-Hayek S, Belal M, Abrams P. Does the patient's position influence the detection of detrusor overactivity? *Neurourol Urodyn* 2008; **27**(4):279–86.
7. Abrams P, Cardozo L, Fall M, *et al.* The standardisation of terminology of lower urinary tract function: report from the Standardisation Sub-committee of the International Continence Society. *Neurourol Urodyn* 2002; **21**(2):167–178.
8. Blaivas JG, Olsson CA. Stress incontinence: classification and surgical approach. *J Urol* 1988; **139**(4):727–731.
9. Lose G, Griffiths D, Hosker G, *et al.* Standardisation of urethral pressure measurement: report from the Standardisation Sub-Committee of the International Continence Society. *Neurourol Urodyn* 2002; **21**(3):258–260.
10. van Waalwijk van DE, Anders K, Khullar V, *et al.* Standardisation of ambulatory urodynamic monitoring: Report of the Standardisation Sub-Committee of the International Continence Society for Ambulatory Urodynamic Studies. *Neurourol Urodyn* 2000; **19**(2):113–25.
11. Cassidenti AP, Ostergard DR. Multichannel urodynamics: ambulatory versus standard urodynamics. *Curr Opin Obstet Gynecol* 1999; **11**(5):485–7.
12. Singh G, Lucas M, Dolan L, Knight S, Ramage C, Hobson PT. Minimum standards for urodynamic practice in the UK. *Neurourol Urodyn* 2010; **29**(8):1365–72.

CHAPTER 3.3

Urinary incontinence principles

Nadir I. Osman and Christopher R. Chapple

Introduction

Urinary incontinence (UI) is a common and bothersome condition that frequently impacts upon the quality of life of individuals. It is defined by the International Continence Society (ICS) as 'the complaint of involuntary loss of urine'[1] and is broadly divided into three main categories of stress urinary incontinence (SUI), urgency urinary incontinence (UUI), and mixed urinary incontinence (MUI). SUI is defined as 'the complaint of involuntary leakage on effort or exertion or on sneezing or coughing',[1] while UUI is defined as 'the complaint of involuntary leakage accompanied by or immediately preceded by urgency'.[1] In this context, urgency is described as the 'compelling desire to pass urine which is difficult to defer'. MUI is defined as 'the complaint of involuntary leakage associated with urgency and also with exertion, effort, sneezing or coughing'.[1] This must be differentiated from mixed symptoms (MS), which is SUI with accompanying urgency. Other types of UI include nocturnal enuresis 'the complaint of loss of urine during sleep'[1] and continuous or 24-hour incontinence, which is the constant leakage of urine.[1] Overflow incontinence is urinary leakage due to an overly full bladder. UI occurring under certain circumstances is termed situational incontinence and includes giggle incontinence and coital incontinence. Post-micturition dribble (PMD) is the leakage of urine occurring immediately following voids.

Epidemiology

Most epidemiological data on UI is derived from patient self-reporting on questionnaires or surveys which include some measure of symptom frequency, severity, and impact on quality of life. Prevalence estimates of UI vary widely in the literature due to the lack of consistency in the definitions used, the wide variety of populations studied, and the different survey methodologies.[2] UI is more common in females and overall around 30–60% of women report suffering any UI with an increasing prevalence with age. In women in middle to later life, 5–15% experience daily episodes of UI.[3] Approximately half of those with UI have SUI followed by MUI, with the smallest proportion having UUI.

The epidemiology of UI in males is less well studied, with reported prevalence ranging widely from 1–39%, but is generally around half as common as in females.[3] As in women, there is an age-related increase in prevalence. In older men, any UI occurs in 11–34%, whereas 2–11% suffer UI on a daily basis.[3] In terms of type of UI, a direct reversal to that observed in women is seen, with UUI being the most common (40–80%), followed by MUI (10–30%), and SUI (<10%). This reflects the differences in anatomy and pathophysiological mechanisms of UI between the sexes. PMD is typically encountered in ageing men, although it may also be seen in younger men with either bladder neck obstruction or urethral strictures. While UUI is mainly seen in women, it does occur in men with increased age, associated in this context with detrusor overactivity (DO) and is a notable problem after prostatectomy.

UI often impacts upon other aspects of an individual's health and quality of life. There is an association with depression,[4] falls in the elderly independent of other risk factors,[5] as well as an increased risk of nursing home admission.[6] UI with an urgency component (MUI, MS, and UUI) is generally more bothersome for individuals than pure SUI.[7] Despite the bother, patients often do not seek treatment believing the problem to be a normal part of ageing, that there are no treatments, or simply being too embarrassed to see their doctor.

The economic costs of UI to the individual and wider society are legion. Cost is incurred in terms of healthcare expenditure to treat UI or associated conditions such as depression, as well as through lost productivity. A study in the United States found the direct costs of UI to be $16.3 billion per annum.[8] In the United Kingdom, the annual cost of treating storage symptoms in women alone was estimated to be £233 million.[9] The source of these costs includes containment devices (e.g. pads), drug therapy, hospital visits (e.g. physiotherapy, outpatient reviews), and surgical intervention.

A multitude of modifiable and non-modifiable risk factors have been implicated in the aetiology of UI (Fig. 3.3.1).[2,3]

Aetio-pathophysiology

Control of urinary incontinence is dependent upon a highly complex interplay between the bladder, the urethral sphincter, the pelvic floor, and the central and peripheral nervous systems.[3] The neural control of storage and voiding function is discussed before focusing on the common pathophysiological mechanisms at play in male and female UI, broadly considered under the headings of urethral sphincter dysfunction and bladder dysfunction.

Neural control mechanisms

During the storage phase of the micturition cycle, there is inhibition of the parasympathetic innervation to the detrusor muscle preventing contraction, while simultaneously there is stimulation of the smooth and striated elements of the urethral sphincter, via the hypogastric and pudendal nerves, respectively, which ensures a closed outlet (Fig. 3.3.2).[10] This process is facilitated by a spinal reflex mechanism, termed the 'guarding reflex', which is initiated

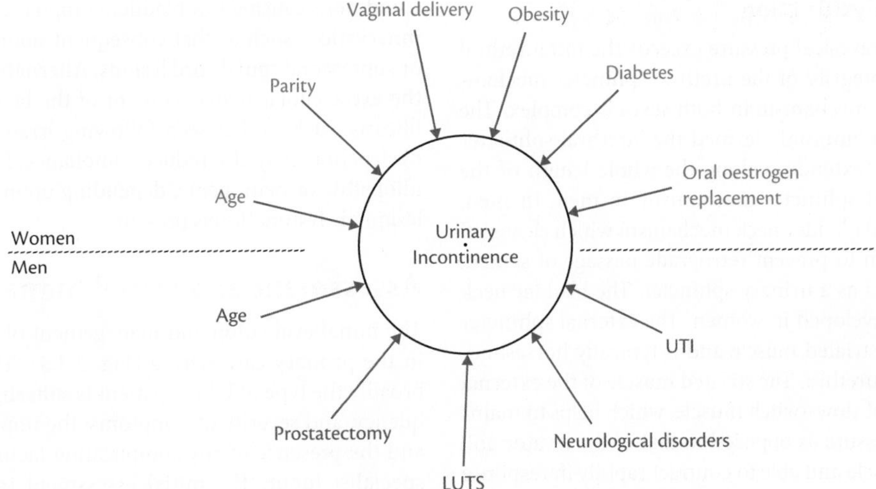

Fig. 3.3.1 Confirmed risk factors for urinary incontinence in women and men (UTI = urinary tract infection; LUTS = lower urinary tract symptoms).

through the low-level afferent activity that occurs as the bladder wall is distended due to filling. Additionally, an area in the lateral pons termed the 'pontine storage centre' is likely to have a role in non-volitional striated sphincter control.[11]

The micturition reflex is initiated by the pontine micturition centre (PMC) in the brain stem, once the negative control of this is released by the central nervous system. During voiding, bladder afferent activity passes centrally to PMC through a spinobulbospinal reflex pathway (Fig. 3.3.2); descending pathways lead to urethral striated muscle relaxation (via inhibition of the guarding reflex), which is followed by parasympathetic activation causing detrusor contraction and urethral smooth muscle relaxation. The entrance of urine is sensed by urethral afferents and triggers a further reflex that potentiates detrusor contraction ensuring bladder emptying.[12]

The timing of voiding is normally under strict volitional control and is influenced by factors such as emotional state,[13] social situation and perception of bladder fullness. Central to this process is thought to be the periaqueductal grey matter (PAG), which has connections to multiple higher brain centres and the PMC. In terms of afferent signals, these are relayed to higher centres by the PAG, leading to the conscious perception of bladder fullness.[11] The PAG also receives projections from higher brain centres, such as the pre-frontal cortex, which is thought have a role in the tonic suppression of voiding until socially appropriate.

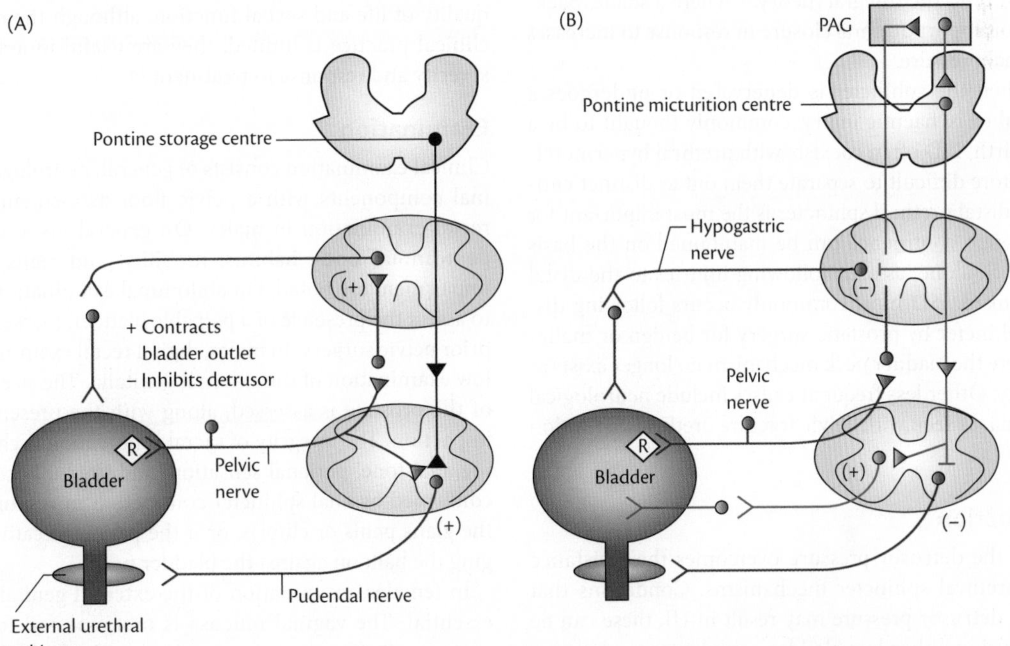

Fig. 3.3.2 Neural control mechanism in storage and voiding: (A) storage reflexes; (B) voiding reflexes (spinobulbospinal reflex pathways in blue, parasympathetic outflow to bladder and urethral smooth muscle in green, and sympathetic outflow to urethral sphincter in red).

Reprinted by permission from Macmillan Publishers Ltd: *Nature Review Neuroscience*, Fowler CJ *et al.*, 'The neural control of micturition', Volume 9, Issue 6, pp. 453–456, Copyright © 2008.

Urethral sphincter dysfunction

UI results when the intravesical pressure exceeds the intraurethral pressure, making the integrity of the urethral sphincter mechanism vital. The sphincter mechanism in both sexes is complex. The external component is commonly termed the 'urethral sphincter mechanism' in women (extending along the whole length of the urethra), and the 'distal sphincter mechanism' in men. In men, there is also the powerful bladder neck mechanism which closes off during seminal emission to prevent retrograde passage of semen, but which also functions as a urinary sphincter. The bladder neck mechanism is poorly developed in women. The external sphincter is composed mainly of striated muscle and is typically horseshoe-shaped, arcing over the urethra. The striated muscle of the external sphincter is comprised of slow-twitch muscle, which helps to maintain urethral resting pressure as opposed to that of the levator ani, which is fast-twitch muscle and able to contract rapidly in response in sudden increases in intra-abdominal pressure.

Under resting conditions, the urethra remains closed due to pressure exerted by a combination of urethral smooth and striated muscle tone, along with mucosal factors which aid coaptation.[14] The muscles and connective tissues of the pelvic floor provide external support to the bladder and urethra, assuming a greater role in maintenance of continence during times of increased stress. Therefore, UI may result due to a functional deficit of the sphincter itself, termed intrinsic sphincter deficiency (ISD), or loss of anatomical urethral support, termed urethral hypermobility.

In women, urethral hypermobility occurs as a consequence of the loss of extrinsic urethral support (it was originally thought that the position of the urethra was the important factor). It was postulated that with urethral descent on increased intra-abdominal pressure, pressure is transmitted to the bladder but not the urethra, and that this imbalance predisposes to leakage.[15] More recently, theories have been based on concepts of urethral support, such as the hammock hypothesis[16] and the Integral theory,[17] where a stable 'backplate' is needed to support urethral closure in response to increases in intra-abdominal pressure.

ISD results when the sphincter is denervated or undergoes a direct mechanical or ischaemic injury, commonly thought to be a sequela of childbirth. ISD often coexists with urethral hypermobility and it is therefore difficult to separate them out as distinct entities. In men, the distal urethral sphincter is the most important for continence, although continence can be maintained on the basis of the bladder neck alone, as seen following injuries to the distal sphincter mechanism. ISD most commonly occurs following disruption of the sphincter by prostatic surgery for benign or malignant disease, where the bladder neck mechanism no longer exists as a functional entity. Other less frequent causes include neurological disease and trauma, as seen with pelvic fracture urethral disruption injuries.

Bladder dysfunction

UI occurs when the detrusor pressure overcomes the resistance exerted by the urethral sphincter mechanisms. Conditions that lead to increased detrusor pressure may result in UI; these can be categorized as causing either low bladder compliance or detrusor overactivity (DO). Low bladder compliance is typified by an abnormal rise in detrusor pressure during filling whereas DO is the occurrence of non-voluntary contractions during bladder filling. Conditions causing low bladder compliance include damage to the innervation, such as that consequent upon radical pelvic surgery, or suprasacral spinal cord lesions. Alternatively, processes that alter the extracellular matrix content of the bladder wall by producing fibrosis, such as that seen following irradiation or bladder outlet obstruction, may also reduce compliance. DO can be categorized as idiopathic or neurogenic, depending upon whether a neurological lesion or dysfunction is present.

Assessment and initial management

The initial evaluation and management of UI may be undertaken in the primary care setting (Fig. 3.3.3). The aim is to determine broadly the type of UI the patient is suffering from; the timing, frequency, and severity of symptoms; the impact upon quality of life; and the presence of any complicating factors[2] that usually require specialist input. The initial assessment includes history taking, physical examination, and urinalysis ± urine microscopy and culture. Following this, management is usually empirical, and may consist of lifestyle measures, physical and behavioural therapies, and pharmacotherapy. Patients are either then managed in primary care if initial measures suffice, or referred for specialist investigation and management (Fig. 3.3.4).

History

The important aspects of history taking include an evaluation of the nature of symptoms, timing, frequency, severity, and associated symptoms. The presence of co-morbidities that may lead to incontinence, particularly in the elderly, should be identified. In both men and women, it is important to determine the nature of any previous genitourinary or pelvic surgery or prior pelvic irradiation. A medication history is also essential to exclude drugs that may cause or worsen UI (Table 3.3.1). Several questionnaires are available that assess the bothersomeness of symptoms and impact on quality of life and sexual function; although their use in everyday clinical practice is limited, they are useful in assessing symptom severity and response to treatment.[18]

Examination

Clinical examination consists of general, neurological, and abdominal components with a pelvic floor assessment in females and rectal examination in males. On general inspection, the general demeanour, body habitus, mobility, and signs of neurological impairment are noted. On abdominal examination, it is important to assess the presence of a palpable bladder, masses, and scars from prior pelvic surgery. In males, digital rectal examination should follow examination of the external genitalia. The size and consistency of the prostate is assessed, along with the presence of any faecal impaction. The integrity of sacral innervation is checked by assessing anal tone, perianal sensation, and the bulbocavernosus reflex, confirmed by anal sphincter contraction in response to squeezing the glans penis or clitoris, or if the patient is catheterized, by tugging the balloon against the bladder neck.

In females, examination of the external genitalia and vagina is essential. The vaginal mucosa is first assessed for signs of poor oestrogenization such as atrophy, a pale epithelium, and loss of rugae. Next, with the patient's bladder comfortably full and the examiner observing the urethral meatus, the patient is asked to cough to demonstrate any stress leakage. The Q-tip test may also

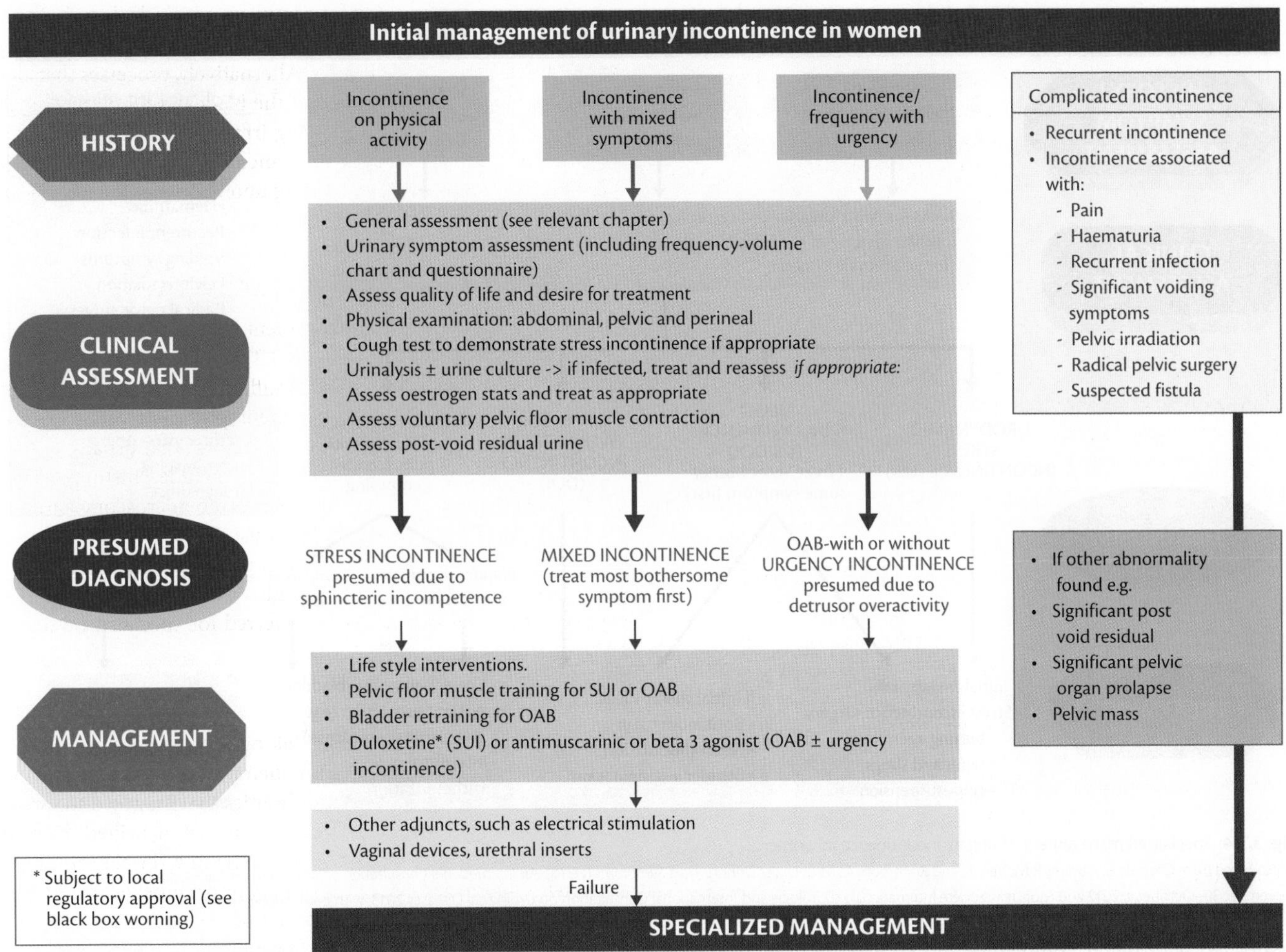

Fig. 3.3.3 Initial management of urinary incontinence in women.
Reproduced from Chapple C, Abrams P, McVary K, and Roehrborn C, *Male Lower Urinary Tract Symptoms (LUTS): An International Consultation on Male LUTS*, Fukuoka, Japan, September 30–October 4, 2012 and Montreal, Société Internationale d'Urologie and International Consultation on Urological Diseases 2013, with permission of the authors.

be performed to assess for the urethral hypermobility, but is not thought to be particularly reliable. Pelvic floor muscle strength is evaluated by inspection and palpation. Finally, an assessment for pelvic organ prolapse with a speculum is performed; where prolapse is present, manual reduction by gentle digital elevation of the urethra can be performed prior to coughing to counteract any pelvic floor mobility and to assess the potential response to any potential surgery.

Urinalysis

Urinalysis is essential to exclude infection. Haematuria may be a sign of malignancy and warrants further investigation. Glycosuria is a useful screening test for diabetes mellitus. Urine microscopy and culture is warranted if the presence of blood or infection is indicated on urinalysis.

Urodynamics

Urodynamics is the collective term given to both the invasive and non-invasive tests that help to confirm the underlying cause of the patient's UI and guide its subsequent management. By collecting objective information on the filling and voiding phases of the micturition cycle, urodynamics has two main aims: (i) to reproduce the patient's symptoms during the test; and (ii) to provide a pathophysiological explanation by correlating the patient's symptoms with urodynamic findings.[19]

Bladder diary

The bladder diary provides valuable information on the frequency and nature (stress or urgency) of incontinence episodes.[20] For the clinician, the diary gives an indication of functional bladder capacity (usually 300–600 mL) and corroborates the severity of symptoms, while determining the presence of underlying polyuria (production of >40 mL of urine/kg/hr in a 24-hour period) or nocturnal polyuria (producing more than 33% of the 24-hour production after retiring to bed), which may exacerbate symptoms. Additionally, it permits for a more accurate assessment of fluid intake pattern,[20] which may allow patients to realize adverse drinking habits.[20] The usual format involves the patient recording the times of voids, voided volumes, and incontinence episodes over a 24-hour period for a minimum period of three days and up to seven days, with a record of fluid intake in terms of volume and type (e.g. cup of tea, or glass of water). Shorter diaries are in fact

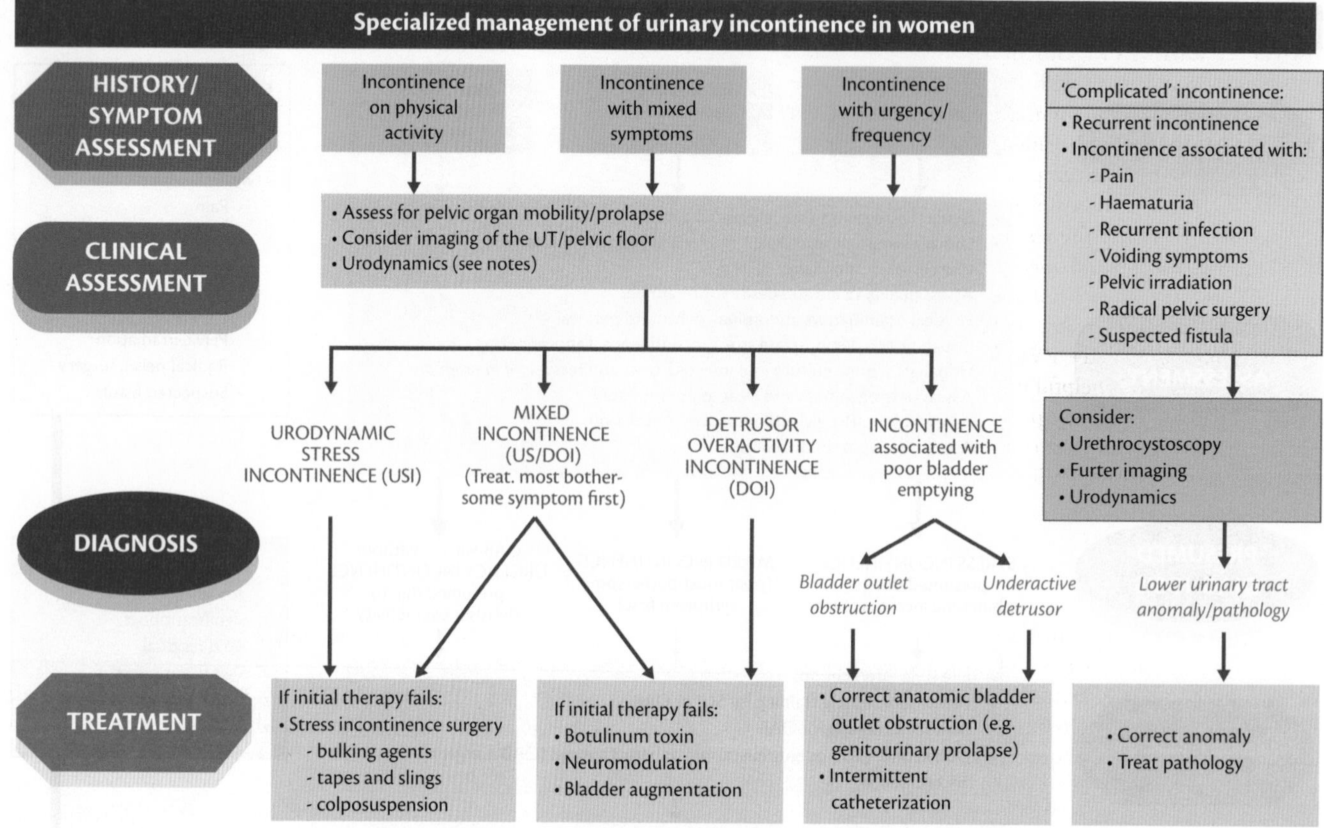

Fig. 3.3.4 Specialized management of urinary incontinence in women.
Reproduced from Chapple C, Abrams P, McVary K, and Roehrborn C, *Male Lower Urinary Tract Symptoms (LUTS): An International Consultation on Male LUTS*, Fukuoka, Japan, September 30–October 4, 2012 and Montreal, Société Internationale d'Urologie and International Consultation on Urological Diseases 2013, with permission of the authors.

associated with better compliance and so may be more accurate than their longer counterparts.[21]

Pad testing

Pad testing is a semi-objective measure of the severity of UI, but does not distinguish between types of UI. When combined with the bladder diary, it provides useful information on the amount and timing of leakage. It involves the patient wearing an incontinence pad(s), which is weighed before and after use thereby gaining an estimation of how much the patient has leaked. It is particularly useful in proving the presence of incontinence when not demonstrable by other means.[19] Different tests have been described; varying mainly by the length of time the pad is worn. The one-hour pad test is recommended by the ICS and involves the patient drinking 500 mL of fluid and within 15 minutes undertaking a series of standardized exercises lasting one hour.[22] An increase in pad weight of 1 g or more is considered diagnostic of UI.[3] Pad testing may also be conducted over longer lengths of time to provide a more realistic picture of UI severity in everyday life. Pads are collected in resealable bags before being weighed with an overall increase of more than 8 g considered diagnostic.[23] A limitation of the test is the change in weight of the pad(s) may be accounted for by increased vaginal secretions or sweating.

Table 3.3.1 Examples of pharmacotherapies associated with UI

	Mechanism	Examples
Drug causing overflow incontinence	Anticholinergic effect	Antidepressants, sedative antihypnotics, antihistamines
	Bladder outflow obstruction	Alpha-adrenoceptor agonists
Drug causing stress incontinence	Urethral relaxation (in women)	Alpha-adrenoceptor antagonists
Drugs exacerbating incontinence	Increasing urine production	Diuretics, Caffeine, alcohol
	Decreased central inhibition	Sedatives, hypnotics, alcohol

Free flow measurement (uroflometry)

Free flow measurement is the simplest urodynamic test and is quick, non-invasive, and inexpensive while providing useful information on voiding function.[24] In men with incontinence, it is useful as a screening test for bladder outlet obstruction (BOO) and is similarly useful in women with prolapse or previous incontinence surgery, who are at increased risk of BOO. In those women with uncomplicated stress incontinence, a 'fast void' may be seen. The obvious limitation of free flow measurement is the inability to distinguish between a low flow due to BOO or detrusor underactivity, which requires pressure flow studies.[19]

Post-void residual

Post-void residual (PVR), although not a urodynamic test as such, is often performed along with free flow measurement. A residual volume of urine may remain in the bladder due to detrusor underactivity, where the patient's bladder was not able to generate an adequate pressure in order to empty, either in the presence or absence of BOO. There is no consensus on what exactly constitutes a pathologically high PVR and the test is known to have poor test-retest reliability, therefore should only be repeated if an abnormal result is found.[25] Generally, any PVR associated with symptoms or urinary infection and/or PVR greater than 40% of the functional bladder capacity (volume voided+ PVR) should be considered clinically significant. The PVR is helpful in identifying men and women with chronic retention who may present with overflow incontinence. When considering antimuscarinic therapy in men at risk of BOO, checking and monitoring PVR is sensible.

Pressure flow studies

Invasive pressure flow studies (PFS) are a valuable diagnostic test in both male and female UI. PFS may confirm UI and the likely cause, assess detrusor function during filling and voiding, and evaluate sphincter weakness and pelvic floor function. When combined with fluoroscopy (videourodynamics), dynamic correlation of anatomy and function is possible, specifically aiding assessment of bladder neck opening and descent/hypermobility. Additionally, in complex situations such as suspected fistula or urethral diverticula, videourodynamics can be of diagnostic use.

The indications for PFS in UI include:

(i) Failure to demonstrate UI with simpler methods

(ii) Failure of conservative measures

(iii) Prior to operative intervention

(iv) Known or suspected neurological disease

(v) Prior incontinence surgery

(vi) Incontinence following pelvic surgery/irradiation[26]

Whether PFS are essential preoperatively in the female with a clear history of SUI remains controversial and is the subject of current study. The concern is with missing an important alternative diagnosis, such as DO; a retrospective analysis from Bristol found that 26.1% of women with clinically diagnosed 'pure' SUI had important alternative diagnoses on PFS.[27] PFS are certainly essential if there is a prior history of failed incontinence surgery. SUI is far less common in men and occurs most commonly due to iatrogenic sphincter injury during prostatectomy. It is considered essential to perform PFS in this setting to exclude BOO, DO, or poor bladder compliance as the cause of UI before operative planning.

In terms of UUI, the typical picture is of leakage occurring in association with a non-voluntary detrusor contraction. Often DO will show a progressively increasing phasic pattern until a terminal contraction occurs, at which point the patient feels they cannot delay voiding any longer otherwise leakage will occur.[24] Alternatively UI may follow provocative manoeuvres such as coughing, which videourodynamics will clearly confirm as occurring due to DO rather than stress.

In patients with MUI, it is essential to combine both the symptomatic and urodynamic assessment to ascertain which is the predominant and most troublesome component. In general, DO when present is treated first. An important point to note in performing PFS in women with MUI is that due to the poor resistance of the outlet, the significance and severity of DO may be underestimated. After outlet surgery, this may then emerge as more pronounced and contribute to an unsatisfactory outcome.

Cystourethroscopy

Cytsourethroscopy is performed in the presence of complicating factors, especially haematuria, but is not a standard part of the assessment of UI. In women, it may be helpful in identifying ostia when diverticula are suspected or when evaluating fistulae. In men, it will allow the exclusion of bladder neck stenosis or urethral stricture, especially in the post-prostatectomy patient where anastomotic stricture can arise and impact upon any subsequent surgery, such as artificial sphincter implantation.

Conclusions

UI is a common and bothersome condition with a diverse aetiology. In women SUI is most frequent, whereas in men UUI predominates. The initial assessment entails a comprehensive history, examination, and urinalysis, following which patients are either initially managed with conservative measures including containment devices, pharmacotherapy, and physical or behavioural therapies. Patients are referred onward for specialist care if complicating factors are present or conservative measures fail. The specialist assessment entails a bladder diary, PVR measurement, and urodynamic studies, which aim to reproduce the incontinence and identify the underlying pathophysiology.

Further reading

Abrams P CL, Wein A, Khoury S. Incontinence: 4th International Consultation on Incontinence. Paris, France: Health Publications, 2009.

Abrams P, Cardozo L, Fall M, *et al.* The standardisation of terminology of lower urinary tract function: report from the Standardisation Sub-committee of the International Continence Society. *Neurourol Urodyn* 2002; **21**(2):167–78.

Chapple CRM, S. Patel, A. *Urodynamics Made Easy*, 3rd edition. London, UK: Churchill Livingstone, 2009.

Fowler CJ, Griffiths D, de Groat WC. The neural control of micturition. *Nat Rev Neurosci* 2008; **9**(6):453–66.

Nitti VW, Blaivas JG. Urinary incontinence: Epidemiology, pathophysiology, evaluation, and management overview. (p. 2046) In: Wein AJ, Kavoussi LR (eds) *Campbell-Walsh Urology*, 9th edition. Philadelphia, PA: Saunders, 2007.

References

1. Abrams P, Cardozo L, Fall M, *et al.* The standardisation of terminology of lower urinary tract function: report from the Standardisation Sub-committee of the International Continence Society. *Neurourol Urodyn* 2002; **21**(2):167–78.
2. Thuroff JW, Abrams P, Andersson KE, *et al.* EAU guidelines on urinary incontinence. *Eur Urol* 2011; **59**(3):387–400.
3. Abrams P CL, Wein A, Khoury S. *Incontinence: 4th International Consultation on Incontinence*. Paris, France: Health Publications, 2009.
4. Nygaard I, Turvey C, Burns TL, Crischilles E, Wallace R. Urinary incontinence and depression in middle-aged United States women. *Obstet Gynecol* 2003; **101**(1):149–56.
5. Brown JS, Vittinghoff E, Wyman JF, *et al.* Urinary incontinence: does it increase risk for falls and fractures? Study of Osteoporotic Fractures Research Group. *J Am Geriatr Soc* 2000; **48**(7):721–5.

6. Nuotio M, Tammela TL, Luukkaala T, Jylha M. Predictors of institutionalization in an older population during a 13-year period: the effect of urge incontinence. *J Gerontol A Biol Sci Med Sci* 2003; **58**(8):756–62.
7. Coyne KS, Zhou Z, Thompson C, Versi E. The impact on health-related quality of life of stress, urge and mixed urinary incontinence. *BJU Int* 2003; **92**(7):731–5.
8. Wilson L, Brown JS, Shin GP, Luc KO, Subak LL. Annual direct cost of urinary incontinence. *Obstet Gynecol* 2001; **98**(3):398–406.
9. Turner DA, Shaw C, McGrother CW, Dallosso HM, Cooper NJ. The cost of clinically significant urinary storage symptoms for community dwelling adults in the UK. *BJU Int* 2004; **93**(9):1246–52.
10. Birder L, de Groat W, Mills I, Morrison J, Thor K, Drake M. Neural control of the lower urinary tract: peripheral and spinal mechanisms. *Neurourol Urodyn* 2010; **29**(1):128–39.
11. Fowler CJ, Griffiths D, de Groat WC. The neural control of micturition. *Nat Rev Neurosci* 2008; **9**(6):453–66.
12. Bump RC. The urethrodetrusor facilitative reflex in women: results of urethral perfusion studies. *Am J Obstet Gynecol* 2000; **182**(4):794–802; discussion 802–4.
13. Holstege G. Micturition and the soul. *J Comp Neurol* 2005; **493**(1):15–20.
14. Ashton-Miller JA, DeLancey JO. Functional anatomy of the female pelvic floor. *Ann N Y Acad Sci* 2007; **1101**:266–96.
15. Enhorning G. Simultaneous recording of intravesical and intra-urethral pressure. A study on urethral closure in normal and stress incontinent women. *Acta Chir Scand Suppl* 1961; Suppl 276:1–68.
16. DeLancey JO. Structural support of the urethra as it relates to stress urinary incontinence: the hammock hypothesis. *Am J Obstet Gynecol* 1994; **170**(6):1713–20; discussion 20–3.
17. Petros PE, Ulmsten UI. An integral theory of female urinary incontinence. Experimental and clinical considerations. *Acta Obstet Gynecol Scand Suppl* 1990; **153**:7–31.
18. International Consultation on Incontinence Modular Questionairre (ICIQ), 2012. Available at: http://www.iciq.net/ [Online].
19. Abrams P. *Urodynamics,* 3rd edition. London, UK: Springer, 2006.
20. Newman D, Wein A. *Managing and Treating Urinary Incontinence,* 2nd edition. Towson, MA: Health Professions Press, 2009.
21. Groutz A, Blaivas JG, Chaikin DC, *et al.* Noninvasive outcome measures of urinary incontinence and lower urinary tract symptoms: a multicenter study of micturition diary and pad tests. *J Urol* 2000; **164**(3 Pt 1):698–701.
22. Abrams P, Blaivas JG, Stanton SL, Andersen JT. The standardisation of terminology of lower urinary tract function. The International Continence Society Committee on Standardisation of Terminology. *Scand J Urol Nephrol Suppl* 1988; **114**:5–19.
23. Lose G, Jorgensen L, Thunedborg P. 24-hour home pad weighing test versus 1-hour ward test in the assessment of mild stress incontinence. *Acta Obstet Gynecol Scand* 1989; **68**(3):211–5.
24. Chapple CRM, S. Patel, A. *Urodynamics Made Easy,* 3rd edition. London, UK: Churchill Livingstone, 2009.
25. Griffiths DJ, Harrison G, Moore K, McCracken P. Variability of post-void residual urine volume in the elderly. *Urol Res* 1996; **24**(1):23–6.
26. Nitti VW, Blaivas JG.Urinary incontinence: Epidemiology, pathophysiology, evaluation, and management overview. (p. 2046) In: Wein AJ, Kavoussi LR (eds). *Campbell-Walsh Urology*, 9th edition. Philadelphia, PA: Saunders, 2007.
27. Agur W, Housami F, Drake M, Abrams P. Could the National Institute for Health and Clinical Excellence guidelines on urodynamics in urinary incontinence put some women at risk of a bad outcome from stress incontinence surgery? *BJU Int* 2009; **103**(5):635–9.

CHAPTER 3.4

Assessment of urinary incontinence

Marcus Drake

Introduction to urinary incontinence

Urinary incontinence is defined by the International Continence Society (ICS) as any involuntary loss of urine.[1] It is a high prevalence problem, which can affect any age group. Prevalence increases with age, reflecting the multifactorial underlying pathophysiology, increasingly manifest because of the accumulation of contributory factors with senescence. Incontinence is a specific subtype of lower urinary tract symptom (LUTS), and assessment of incontinence needs to take into context the LUTS and wider medical issues. Particular emphasis needs to be placed on the desire for treatment on the part of the patient. Deriving a treatment strategy requires an insight into the extent to which the patient is bothered, the underlying contributory factors, and potential co-morbidities, which could complicate the likelihood of a satisfactory treatment outcome.

Sometimes the pathophysiology is relatively straightforward and predictable. For example, pelvic floor ligamentous support may be impaired in a parous woman, resulting in urethral hypermobility as the commonest basis of female stress incontinence. At the other end of the spectrum, neurological disease or people with previous pelvic surgery can have varied and unpredictable pathophysiology, which is difficult to establish from symptomatology. Both circumstances mandate a comprehensive evaluation, to avoid misplaced presumption and consequent misguided intervention. Certain history or examination findings should prompt specialized input.[2] These include the presence of haematuria, previous pelvic surgery or radiotherapy, constant leakage suggesting a fistula, severe voiding difficulty (particularly if the bladder is palpable after voiding), or suspected neurological disease.

History and examination

Key points in the history are listed in Table 3.4.1. The context in which incontinence arises needs to be categorized into stress, urgency, or mixed urinary incontinence, as defined by the ICS.[1]

- Stress urinary incontinence (SUI) is the complaint of involuntary leakage on effort or exertion, or on sneezing or coughing.
- Urgency urinary incontinence (UUI) is the complaint of involuntary leakage accompanied by or immediately preceded by urgency.
- Mixed urinary incontinence (MUI) is the complaint of involuntary leakage associated with urgency and also with exertion, effort, sneezing, or coughing.

Table 3.4.1 Key points in the history and examination of incontinence

History	Examination
Type of incontinence: SUI, UUI, MUI, continuous, giggle, intercourse-related	Occult neurology screening: gait, tremor, coordination, lower back
PMH: medical, surgical, radiotherapy, neurological, medication	Abdominal: scars, palpable bladder, genitalia
Lower urinary tract: LUTS (voiding, post-micturition, storage), UTIs, fluid intake (volume, type)	Pelvic (women): vaginal anatomy and epithelium, urethral hypermobility, SUI, pelvic floor muscles, pelvic mass
Pelvic: parity, gynaecological, sexual, POP, bowel symptoms	Pelvic (men: anal tone, perianal sensation, prostate, masses)

- Other types of urinary incontinence may be situational, for example the report of incontinence during sexual intercourse, or giggle incontinence.

SUI is reported in association with physical exertion, and can have a positional element; for example, it may be more noticeable when walking downhill. A large proportion of women with SUI can be identified primarily from their history.[3] UUI is often described by phrases like 'when I have to go, I *have* to go', to denote the urinary urgency, and 'sometimes I don't make it' to denote the incontinence. MUI means that both types of incontinence are present at different times in the same person. Stimulation of urethral receptors in an SUI episode can give a urinary urgency feeling; this is a form of SUI, which must not be confused with UUI or MUI. Some patients with UUI may have overactive bladder activity elicited by exertion; this can cause stress-provoked UUI, and is a form of UUI, which must not be confused with SUI. Giggle incontinence and intercourse-associated incontinence are not well understood, and there is insufficient research-based evidence to derive insights into pathophysiology. Thus, they are categorized separately from SUI, UUI, or MUI.

Contributory factors need to be considered. For women, this particularly comprises previous childbirth and any difficulties with delivery, such as perineal tears. For both men and women, previous pelvic and abdominal surgery needs to be documented. Because neurological disease can underlie incontinence or sudden onset urgency, some simple screening questions should be considered to exclude undiagnosed (occult) neurological disease. These include new-onset tremor, coordination problems, reduced mental faculties, and erectile dysfunction in men. The medical history should also cover previous surgery, or medical conditions leading to co-morbidity which would influence the selection of certain treatment options. Factors affecting mobility should be considered. A person with urgency is more likely to have UUI if their mobility is impaired. Conversely, if mobility is temporarily impaired, SUI could become more problematic as mobility recovers. Anticipating future changes, and assessing the potential to optimize practical arrangements for toileting, may then be appropriate.

Presence of a history of urinary tract infection (UTI) should be recognized, ascertaining whether the site of infection suggests cystitis or pyelonephritis. It should also be established whether bacteriological confirmation of UTI was obtained. In the history, all aspects of pelvic floor dysfunction should be considered, including urinary bowel prolapse and sexual symptoms.

Urinary leakage may need to be distinguished from sweating or vaginal discharge. In anyone with continuous leakage, the possibility of a fistula or congenital abnormality causing 'pseudo-incontinence' should be considered. A patient with a recent history of surgery, or previous pelvic malignancy could be at risk of a urethrovaginal, vesicovaginal, or ureterovaginal fistula, or a combination. Relevant congenital abnormalities include an ectopic ureter. Classically, the distal end of the upper moiety of a duplex system can rarely insert below the urethral sphincter.[4] There have been case reports of other variants, for example insertion of a ureter from a non-duplex system into the vagina[5] and crossed fused ectopia.[6] For a unilateral ectopic ureter, normal voiding will be present as well as continuous dribbling if there is a functioning contralateral kidney with eutopic ureter.

Lower urinary tract symptoms

In patients reporting incontinence, the presence of coexisting LUTS needs to be recognized. Voiding LUTS, comprising poor stream, hesitancy, terminal dribbling, or post-micturition dribble can occur in either gender, but are more common in men as a consequence of benign prostate enlargement. ICS standardized definitions are[1]:

- Slow stream is reported by the individual as his or her perception of reduced urine flow, usually compared to previous performance or in comparison to others.
- Splitting or spraying of the urine stream may be reported.
- Intermittent stream (intermittency) is the term used when the individual describes urine flow which stops and starts, on one or more occasions, during micturition.
- Hesitancy is the term used when an individual describes difficulty in initiating micturition, resulting in a delay in the onset of voiding after the individual is ready to pass urine.[1]
- Straining to void describes the muscular effort used to initiate, maintain or improve the urinary stream.[1]
- They can often be associated with post-micturition LUTS, namely post-micturition dribble, and the sensation of incomplete emptying.
- Feeling of incomplete emptying is a self-explanatory term for a feeling experienced by the individual after passing urine.[1]
- Post-micturition dribble is the term used when an individual describes the involuntary loss of urine immediately after s/he has finished passing urine, usually after leaving the toilet in men, or after rising from the toilet in women.[1]

Storage LUTS compromise nocturia, urgency, and sensation of increased daytime frequency. ICS standardized definitions are[1]:

- Increased daytime frequency is the complaint by the patient who considers that s/he voids too often by day.
- Urgency is the complaint of a sudden compelling desire to pass urine which is difficult to defer.
- Nocturia is the complaint that the individual has to wake at night one or more times to void.[7] For nocturia, each void is preceded and followed by sleep. The nocturnal frequency includes these and those nocturnal voids which were not preceded and/or followed by sleep. In nocturnal enuresis, the patient fails to wake when passing urine. *'Nocturnal polyuria is present when an increased proportion of the 24-hour output occurs at night (normally during the 8 hours whilst the patient is in bed).'*[1]

The presence of urinary urgency underpins the diagnosis of overactive bladder (OAB), defined as urinary urgency, usually with frequency and nocturia, with or without incontinence. OAB can also be called urgency-frequency syndrome.[1] If nocturia is present it is important to seek systemic conditions,[8] which may alter fluid regulation or renal function, leading to increased overnight urine production, or global polyuria. In people with storage LUTS it is sensible to categorize the nature, volume, and timing of fluid intake, and to recognize that substantial amounts of fluid may be contained in foods such as salad or pasta.

Symptom scoring questionnaires

Clinicians and patients differ in their perception of symptoms,[9] and the subjective patient perception of the condition is crucial to management of the condition. Accordingly, it is now recognized that measuring the patient perspective of the condition using self-completion questionnaires is substantially beneficial.[10] Questionnaires are generally self-administered by the patient and do not add greatly to the burden of assessment. Development of the questionnaires needs to meet key psychometric properties (validity, reliability, and responsiveness)[11] and caution is needed, as sometimes the core properties are not met by specific tools.[12] Symptom assessment questionnaires have been developed to quantify the severity and bother of lower urinary tract symptoms, including questionnaires specific to the context of incontinence. The range of questionnaires available is extensive; generic and gender-specific tools are available for incontinence, and others cover related situations, such as lower urinary tract symptoms, pelvic organ prolapse, and anal incontinence. From the practical perspective, short form questionnaires providing a rapid insight into the severity of specific problems and the bother resulting from each symptom provide the most pragmatic benefit. More detailed questionnaires are valuable in the research setting, and bring additional insights of value in specialized units.

The International Consultation on Incontinence Questionnaires (ICIQ)[13,14] have been developed specifically to quantify the severity and bother of the individual symptoms in a range of pelvic floor disorders, and this can be useful in guiding treatment towards the most bothersome symptoms present. ICIQ tools are available specifically for use in LUTS, pelvic organ prolapse, faecal incontinence, and urinary incontinence, cataloguing quality of life and the other pertinent issues. The International Prostate Symptom Score is the most widely applied in the context of male LUTS,[15] however it does not evaluate incontinence. Questionnaires undoubtedly aid the comprehensive evaluation of individual patients, though evidence to support overall improvement in treatment outcomes on a population basis for incontinence is lacking.[2]

Examination

Physical examination (Table 3.4.1) requires a general examination to consider the possibility of occult neurological disease. Simple screening observations such as abnormality of gait, tremor, dyscoordination, or speech abnormality should be noted. Examination of the back could reveal spinal abnormalities, for example altered curvatures or sacral dimples, the latter potentially suggesting spina bifida occulta. Abdominal examination is required to detect a palpable bladder or abdominal scars. Genital examination can reveal penile abnormalities or altered vaginal oestrogenization. Rectal examination is required in men to examine prostate enlargement or potential malignancy.

Pelvic examination in women

Vaginal examination should be undertaken to evaluate anatomical abnormalities, urethral hypermobility, pelvic floor muscle contraction, pelvic organ support, the oestrogenization of the vaginal epithelium, and the presence of any pelvic mass. Most pelvic floor defects can be visualized during evaluation with a half speculum. Bladder neck mobility can be assessed by visual inspection. When the patient is in lithotomy position, the anterior vagina rotates posteriorly on straining, deflecting the meatus distally and anteriorly. This signifies reduced bladder neck support. The Q-Tip test involves placing a cotton bud into the urethra and asking the patient to strain.[16,17] If the axis of the cotton bud increases by more than 30 degrees from horizontal during the strain, the test is described as positive and signifies hypermobility. It is not a widely used test, due to discomfort and inconsistent findings. A cough stress test when the bladder is reasonably full can be used to confirm the presence of stress incontinence. It is usually initially undertaken in the lithotomy position. If no leakage is observed, the cough stress test should be repeated in the standing position. Sometimes, a single cough will fail to elicit stress incontinence, in which case, a series of coughs may be required. Leakage should occur immediately with the coughing, since coughing can provoke an overactive detrusor contraction which might subsequently lead to urgency incontinence soon afterwards. Such cough-provoked urgency incontinence should not be confused with stress incontinence. The Bonney stress test initially was used to demonstrate urinary leakage during coughing[18]; subsequently, it was developed by adding in digital support of the urethrovesical junction during coughing to see if stress incontinence is reduced or eliminated. It provides some indication of mechanism of stress incontinence being due to hypermobility, but it does not predict the outcome of treatment.

A correct pelvic floor muscle contraction is characterized by an anterior and cephalad movement. Vaginal palpation is needed to evaluate muscle strength, noting the tone at rest and the strength of a maximum voluntary contraction, where the woman attempts to recruit as many muscle fibres as possible to develop force. Factors to be assessed include strength, duration, movement, and repeatability. An overall impression of strong, weak, or absent can be made, but pelvic floor muscle strength rating scales, such as the modified Oxford Grading Scale[19] (Table 3.4.2), provide better objective documentation.[20]

Table 3.4.2 Grading schemes for pelvic flooor muscle strength and for pelvic organ prolapse

Grade	Modified Oxford Scale of pelvic floor muscle strength[1]	Baden-Walker classification of POP[2]
0	No contraction	Normal, no prolapse
1	Flicker	Prolapse is halfway to the introitus
2	Weak	Prolapse is to the introitus
3	Moderate	Prolapse is partly through the introitus
4	Good	Prolapse is completely past the introitus
5	Strong	Not applicable

(1) With kind permission of Springer Science and Business Media: Laycock J., 'Clinical evaluation of pelvic floor muscles' pp. 42–48, in Schussler B, Laycock J, Norton P, and Stanton S, (Eds.) *Pelvic floor re-education: principles and practice*, Springer-Verlag, London, UK, Copyright © 1994; and (2) Reproduced from Baden WF and Walker T., 'Fundamentals, symptoms and classification' p. 14 in Baden WF and Walker T, (Eds), *Surgical repair of vaginal defects*, J.B. Lippincott, Philadelphia, USA, Copyright © 1992, with permission from Lippincott Williams & Wilkins.

Pelvic organ prolapse (POP) often coexists with incontinence, even though the conditions are distinct. Significant anterior POP (cystocoele) (Table 3.4.3) can obstruct voiding and potentially can obscure incontinence. Accordingly, failure to demonstrate incontinence in a woman with POP requires the reduction of prolapse, and potentially the maintenance of reduction with a pessary while undertaking evaluation for incontinence. Documentation of POP should use a quantification system, such as the pelvic organ prolapse quantification (POP-Q) system.[21,22] In the POP-Q test, six specific vaginal sites and the vaginal length are assessed according to position from vaginal introitus (Fig. 3.4.1).[23] The length of the genital hiatus and perineal body are also measured. Anterior vaginal wall prolapse is defined as descent of the anterior vagina, so that the urethrovesical junction is less than 3 cm above the plane of the hymen. Apical segment prolapse is defined as any descent of the cervix (or vaginal cuff scar in women who have had hysterectomy) below a point 2 cm less than the total vaginal length above

Table 3.4.3 Terminology of pelvic organ prolapse

Cystocoele	Prolapse of the posterior bladder wall into the anterior vaginal wall
Urethrocoele	Bulging of the urethra through the anterior vaginal wall
Rectocoele	Bulging of the anterior rectal wall into the posterior vaginal wall
Enterocoele	Bulging of the bowel through the posterior cul-de-sac and posterior wall
Uterine prolapse	Descent of the uterus through the pelvic floor into the vaginal canal
Vault prolapse	Descent of the vaginal walls in a patient with a previous hysterectomy

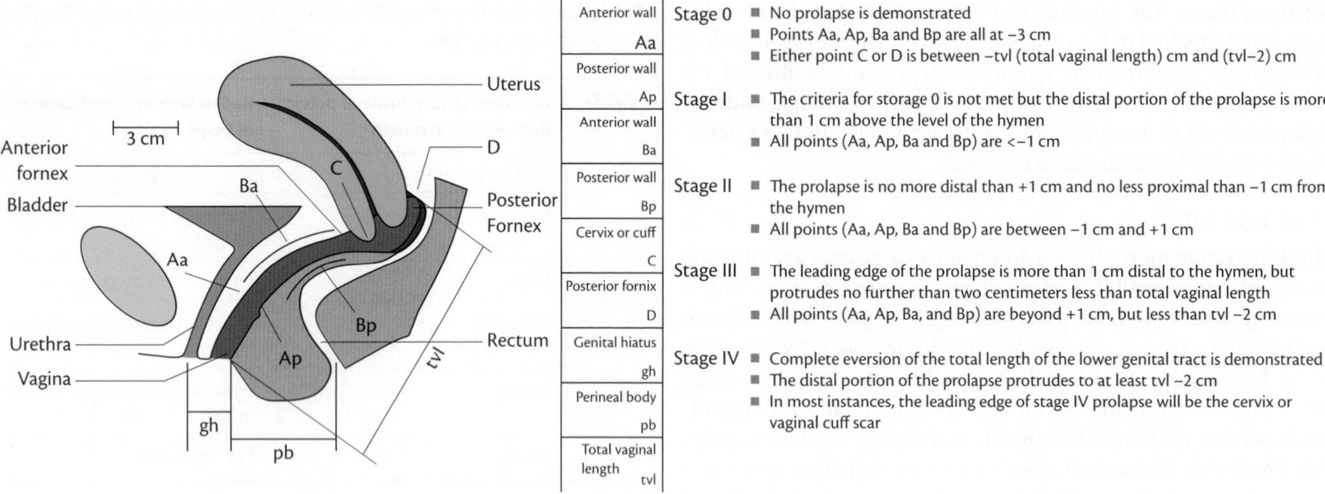
3 cm
Anterior fornex
Bladder
Urethra
Vagina
Ba
Aa
C
Ap
Bp
gh
pb
tvl
Uterus
D
Posterior Fornex
Rectum
Anterior wall Aa
Posterior wall Ap
Anterior wall Ba
Posterior wall Bp
Cervix or cuff C
Posterior fornix D
Genital hiatus gh
Perineal body pb
Total vaginal length tvl
Stage 0
No prolapse is demonstrated
Points Aa, Ap, Ba and Bp are all at −3 cm
Either point C or D is between −tvl (total vaginal length) cm and (tvl−2) cm
Stage I
The criteria for storage 0 is not met but the distal portion of the prolapse is more than 1 cm above the level of the hymen
All points (Aa, Ap, Ba and Bp) are <−1 cm
Stage II
The prolapse is no more distal than +1 cm and no less proximal than −1 cm from the hymen
All points (Aa, Ap, Ba and Bp) are between −1 cm and +1 cm
Stage III
The leading edge of the prolapse is more than 1 cm distal to the hymen, but protrudes no further than two centimeters less than total vaginal length
All points (Aa, Ap, Ba, and Bp) are beyond +1 cm, but less than tvl −2 cm
Stage IV
Complete eversion of the total length of the lower genital tract is demonstrated
The distal portion of the prolapse protrudes to at least tvl −2 cm
In most instances, the leading edge of stage IV prolapse will be the cervix or vaginal cuff scar

Fig. 3.4.1 The POP-Q scheme to categorize nature and severity of pelvic organ prolapse.
Adapted from *American Journal of Obstetrics and Gynecology*, Volume 1, Issue 8, Richard C. Bump *et al.*, 'The standardization of terminology of female pelvic organ prolapse and pelvic floor dysfunction', pp. 10–17, Copyright © 1996 Mosby, Inc., with permission from Elsevier, http://www.sciencedirect.com/science/journal/00029378

the plane of the hymen. Posterior vaginal wall prolapse is defined as any descent of the posterior vaginal wall over the midline point on the posterior vaginal wall, 3 cm above the level of the hymen, or if any posterior point proximal to this lies less than 3 cm above the plane of the hymen.

The Baden-Walker system (Table 3.4.2) is another grading scheme, in which POP is graded between 0 and 4, stage 0 support indicating the absence of prolapse, while stage 4 is extreme prolapse with complete descent of the uterus outside the vagina. Stage 2 prolapse, at which the leading edge of the prolapse extends beyond the hymenal ring, appears to be associated with the greater degree of symptomatic involvement.

Urinalysis

Incontinence occurs more commonly in women with urinary tract infections, and can arise in the immediate aftermath of an acute UTI.[24] Accordingly, urinalysis is an appropriate evaluation for assessment of incontinence in patients who complain of dysuria. Asymptomatic bacteriuria differs from UTI, in that it does not appear to contribute to infection or any other morbidity. Accordingly, findings on urinalysis need to be interpreted according to symptomatic context.

Dipstick urinalysis may be appropriate as a general screening approach in incontinence. If abnormality is present on urinalysis, a formal microscopy and culture may be warranted. Dipstick urinalysis can provide initial pointers towards the presence of bacteriuria. Nitrites are only present if bacteria are present—though not all bacteria produce nitrites in urine. The presence of leukocytes suggests an inflammatory reaction. Thus, the presence of both nitrites and leukocytes strongly suggests UTI; formal microbiological examination of the urine should then be arranged. The presence of protein or blood may arise in the presence of infection. Proteinuria can also be generated in the presence of renal disease. Haematuria can be present in renal disease or urinary tract malignancy. The presence of glucose is likely to signify poorly controlled diabetes mellitus.

Post-void residual volume

Physiologically, complete bladder emptying is expected with voiding. The presence of any urine still within the bladder immediately after a void suggests incomplete emptying. Generally, completeness of emptying is measured immediately after a void with a bladder scanner or ultrasound—though in-and-out catheterization may give the same information. The remaining volume can be expressed as a post-void residual (PVR). Alternatively, the 'bladder voiding efficiency' (BVE) can be used, which is the amount of urine expelled expressed as a proportion of overall volume.[25] PVR can be measured with a non-invasive scanner, or by catheterization; neither method is entirely accurate. A PVR can give a sensation of incomplete emptying, though this may be absent in people with impaired sensory nerve function. PVR may also predispose to UTI or incontinence. If bladder compliance is impaired or reflux is present, the possibility of future dysfunction of the upper urinary tract needs to be considered.

Inefficient bladder emptying may represent the manifestation of bladder outlet obstruction or detrusor underactivity, so a PVR can be evident in people with voiding LUTS. Accordingly, PVR measurement is an important part of incontinence assessment, even though there is no agreed standardization of what constitutes a significant PVR, and the PVR needs to be interpreted according to the clinical circumstances. Most clinicians regard a PVR of less than 100 mL in an asymptomatic patient as not being clinically significant. Most women without LUTS have a PVR of less than 100 mL.[26] In 10% of women with urgency urinary incontinence, the PVR can be greater than 100 mL.[27] PVR can also be elevated in the presence of pelvic organ prolapse.

Expert opinion generally supports the use of PVR measurement in assessing incontinence,[2] but the evidence base is weak and non-standardized. Nonetheless, when planning surgical intervention for incontinence, an elevated PVR prior to intervention could deteriorate after intervention, and this needs to be considered when counselling patients, given the possibility that intermittent self-catheterization could be necessary as a consequence of treatment.

Flow rate testing

Flow rate assessment is a non-invasive urodynamic test which evaluates the synchronous functioning of the bladder and outlet. It is often combined with PVR measurement. The two most common systems for measuring flow rate are:

(i) Gravimetric; flow rate is calculated from the rate of change of weight in the collecting jar.

(ii) Spinning disc; as the urinary stream falls onto a rotating disc, the flow rate machine monitors the additional power needed to keep the disc spinning at the same rate.

The maximum flow rate (Q_{max}) and pattern of flow are the key parameters. Most flow rate machines measure additional parameters, for example average flow rate, voiding time, flow time, and time to maximum flow. However, there is no formal consensus on their utility for decision-making.

Since hydration status alters bladder contractility,[28] the patient should be well hydrated for a flow rate test, but avoid excessive fluid intake. Q_{max} is subject to within-subject variation[29,30]; thus two or three voids ideally should be obtained, since a single reading could affect the conclusions drawn.[31] Bladder volume at start of voiding affects Q_{max}[32,33] but the relationship differs between individuals.[34] Thus, the voided volume is also documented, since a low voided volume (in the absence of a PVR) may indicate that a low Q_{max} could have been artefactually reduced as a consequence of an underfilled bladder at time of testing.[32] Nonetheless, conclusions can be drawn regardless of low voided volume.[35] Overfilling also impairs bladder contractility.[36]

Normal ranges of Q_{max} have been worked out from asymptomatic individuals. For both men and women, the Liverpool nomograms are a well-known example.[33] The Siroky nomogram is also in use for men.[32,37] Q_{max} significantly below normal (two standard deviations below the expected on a nomogram) may be caused by:

- Bladder outlet obstruction (BOO)
- Reduced bladder contractility
- Low voided volume
- Anxiety ('bashful voider')
- Equipment problem (failure to record properly, or inaccurate calibration)

Since Q_{max} may signify the presence of BOO,[38] or reduced detrusor contractility, or both, it is insufficient in isolation as a diagnostic test for BOO. Where Q_{max} is normal, BOO cannot be excluded on flow rate testing alone, as physiological compensatory processes can increase bladder contractility to maintain flow despite outlet resistance.

Pattern of flow is important in potentially giving an indication of mechanism, and in excluding an artefact which might mislead interpretation of Q_{max}. Objective parameters for describing flow patterns have been described.[39] A normal flow curve (Fig. 3.4.2) should have a rapid upstroke, a curve with a clear Q_{max}, and decline quickly to end cleanly; while this is sometimes described as 'bell shaped', the trace is rarely so symmetrical. Abnormal patterns may present as follows.

- Men with benign prostatic enlargement may have a flow curve characterized by a slow upstroke, reduced Qmax, and prolonged downstroke, often with terminal dribbling.[40]

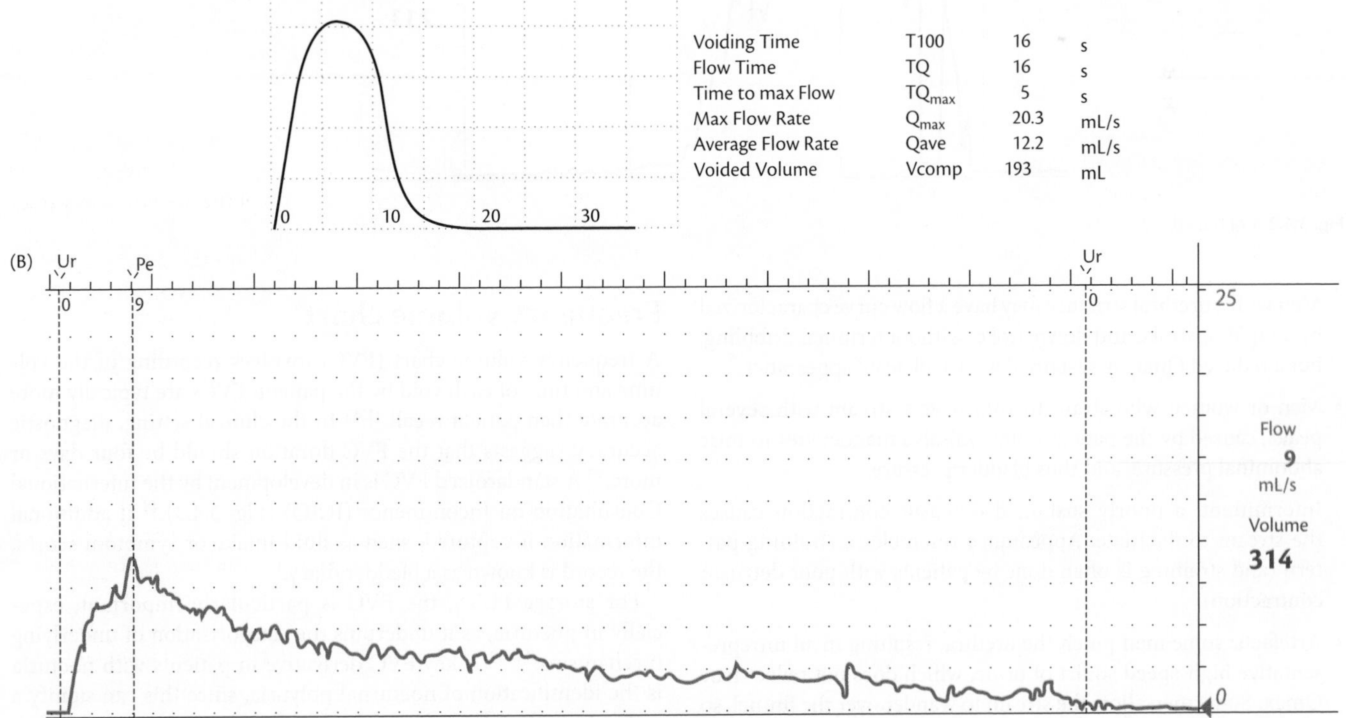

Fig. 3.4.2 Flow rate patterns: (A) normal; (B) 'prostatic'; (C) 'plateau', suggestive of urethral stricture; (D) intermittent; and (E) 'squeeze artefact'—temporary occlusion of the distal urethral with a rapid spike immediately after the compression is released.

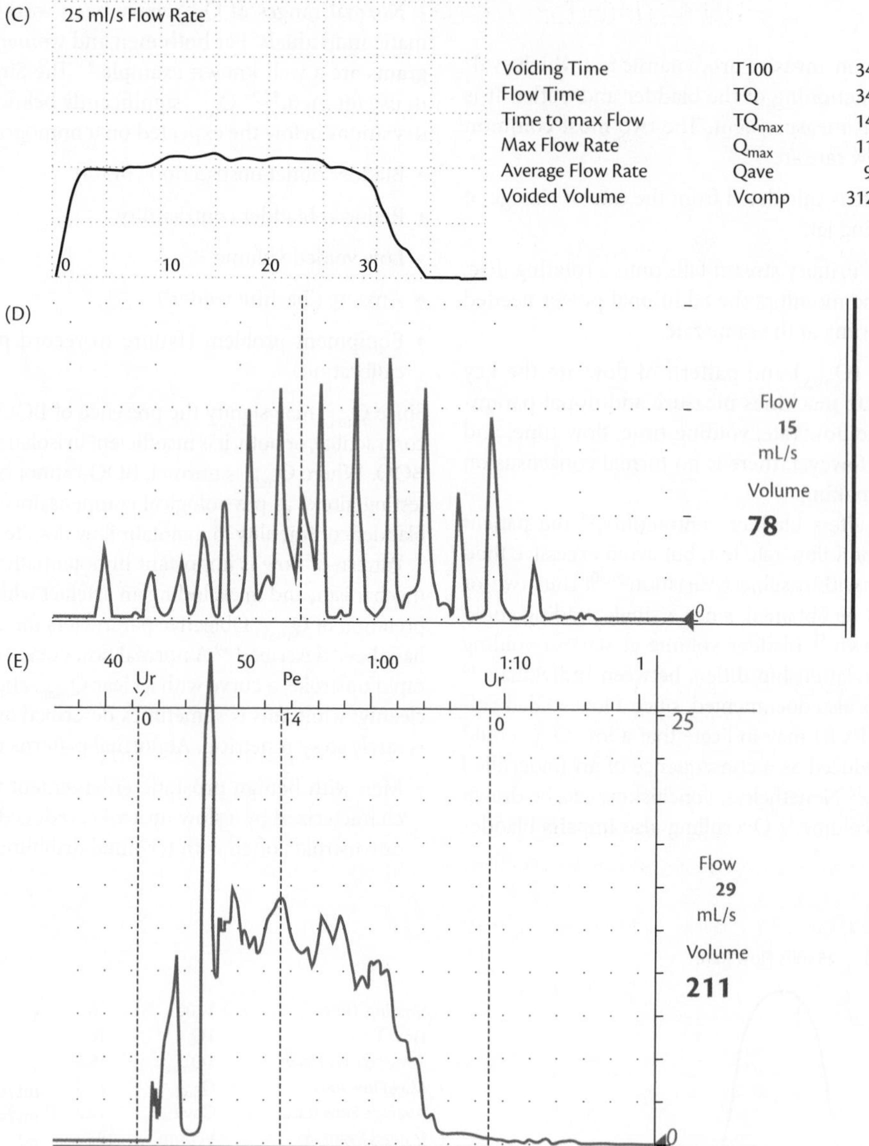

Fig. 3.4.2 Continued.

- Men with a urethral stricture may have a flow curve characterized by a rapid upstroke and downstroke, without terminal dribbling, but a reduced Qmax is sustained with a 'plateau' appearance.
- Men or women who strain to void have a stream with several peaks, caused by the patient doing Valsalva manoeuvres to raise abdominal pressure, and thus bladder pressure.
- Intermittent: a poorly sustained detrusor contraction causes the stream to fluctuate. Appearance resembles a straining pattern (and straining is often done by patients with poor detrusor contraction).
- Artefacts: some men pinch the urethra, resulting in an unrepresentative high-speed squirt of urine, which does not reflect true Qmax. Some men allow the stream to wander over the funnel, so the stream is not evenly delivered to the spinning disc.

Frequency volume chart

A frequency volume chart (FVC) involves recording of the volume and time of each void by the patient. FVCs are typically more accurate than patient recall.[41,42] In the clinical setting, diagnostic accuracy suggests that the FVC duration should be four days or more.[43] A standardized FVC is in development by the International Consultation on Incontinence (ICIQ) (Fig. 3.4.3).[44] If additional information is captured, such as fluid intake or symptom scores, the record is known as a bladder diary.[1]

For storage LUTS, the FVC is particularly important, especially in nocturia, as it underpins the categorization of underlying mechanisms.[45–47] A key FVC derivative in patients with nocturia is the identification of nocturnal polyuria, since this can signify a systemic medical basis for nocturia.[8] The parameters derived from

DEPARTMENT OF UROLOGY – BLADDER DIARY

Name: ____________________

Date of Birth: ☐☐ ☐☐ ☐☐ Are you: Male ☐

DAY MONTH YEAR Female ☐

Please complete this **four day** bladder diary. Enter the following in each column against the time.
You can change the specified times if you need to.

1. Drinks

Write the amount you had to drink and the type of drink you had.

2. Urine output

Enter the amount of urine you passed in millilitres (mls) in the urine output column, day and night. Any measuring jug will do. If you passed urine but couldn't measure it, put a tick in the urine output column. If you leaked urine at any time write **LEAK** in the urine output column.

3. Bladder sensation

Write a description of how your bladder felt when you went to the toilet using the following codes;

***0** - if you had no sensation of needing to pass urine, but passed urine for "social reasons", for example, just before going out, or unsure where the next toilet is.*

***1** - if you had a normal desire to pass urine and no urgency. Urgency is different from normal bladder feelings and is the sudden compelling desire to pass urine which is difficult to defer, or a sudden feeling that you need to pass urine and if you don't you will have an accident*

***2** - if you had urgency but if passed away before you had to visit the toilet.*

***3** - if you had urgency but managed to get to the toilet, still with urgency but did not leak urine.*

***4** - if you had urgency and could not get to the toilet in time so you leaked urine.*

4. Write **BED** when you went to bed and **WOKE** when you woke up in the time column.

Here is an example of how to complete the diary:

Time	Drinks		Urine Output (mls)	Bladder sensation
	Amount	Type		
6am WOKE			350ml	2
7am	Cup	Tea		
8am			✓	
9am				
10am	300ml	Water	Leak	
11am			Leak	3

Fig. 3.4.3 The validated frequency volume chart developed by the International Consultation on Incontinence Questionnaire (ICIQ). The chart is self-completed, and covers four days (only two illustrated).

Reprinted from *The Journal of Urology*, Volume 188, Issue 1, 'The International Prostate Symptom Score Overestimates Nocturia Assessed by Frequency-Volume Charts', pp. 211–215, Copyright (2012), with permission from Elsevier.

a FVC include: daytime urinary frequency; volume of individual voids (mean and maximum); total voided volume; and indices related to nocturia (Table 3.4.4).[48] Polyuria, 'defined as the measured production of more than 2.8 litres of urine in 24 hours in adults',[1] can also be identified.

Pad testing

Attempts to quantify severity of urinary incontinence have used pad tests, in which a pad is weighed before and after a defined period of use, sometimes with standardized physical exertion.

Name ____________________

DAY 1 DATE: ____/____/________

Time	Drinks		Urine Output (mls)	Bladder sensation
	Amount	Type		
6am				
7am				
8am				
9am				
10am				
11am				
Midday				
1pm				
2pm				
3pm				
4pm				
5pm				
6pm				
7pm				
8pm				
9pm				
10pm				
11pm				
Midnight				
1am				
2am				
3am				
4am				
5am				

DAY 2 DATE: ____/____/________

Time	Drinks		Urine Output (mls)	Bladder sensation
	Amount	Type		
6am				
7am				
8am				
9am				
10am				
11am				
Midday				
1pm				
2pm				
3pm				
4pm				
5pm				
6pm				
7pm				
8pm				
9pm				
10pm				
11pm				
Midnight				
1am				
2am				
3am				
4am				
5am				

0 – did not need to go, went just in case

1 – normal desire to pass urine

2 – had urgency but it passed away

3 – had urgency but got to the toilet before leaking

4 – had urgency and leaked

Fig. 3.4.3 Continued.

Short duration tests (e.g. one hour), are generally undertaken under standardized office conditions. Longer tests (e.g. 24 hours) are often done at home. A weight gain of at least 1 g is usually considered positive for a one-hour test, while 4 g is positive for a 24-hour test. Evidence is varied in relation to reliability under retest conditions.[49–52] Longer duration tests tend to be more consistent on repeated testing. Correspondence between short and long duration tests is unreliable.

Overall, the lack of standardized assessment and uncertainty regarding retest reliability, along with practical issues, means that pad tests are not widely employed in the basic clinical diagnosis or assessment of severity of incontinence.

Imaging and cystoscopy

Imaging the lower urinary tract during investigation of urinary incontinence seeks to observe the leakage from the bladder and descent of the bladder neck.[3] Ultrasound and MRI scanning had been used to evaluate dynamic function of the pelvic floor in incontinence. Extensive research has been undertaken, but there

Table 3.4.4 Definitions in classification and aetiology of nocturia

NUV (nocturnal urine volume)	Nightly voided volume, plus first morning voided volume
FBC (functional bladder capacity)	Largest single recorded voided volume from FVC
Nocturia index (Ni)	NUV/FBC
ANV (actual number nightly voids)	Recorded from FVC
PNV (predicted number nightly voids)	Ni − 1
Nocturnal bladder capacity index (NBCi)	ANV − PNV
Nocturnal polyuria index (NPi)	NUV/24 h total voided volume

Reprinted from *The Journal of Urology*, Volume 175, Issue 3, Nocturia: "Do the Math", pp. S16–S18, Copyright © 2006, with permission from Elsevier, http://www.sciencedirect.com/science/journal/00225347

is currently little on which to base recommendations for imaging in incontinence assessment. It is unclear whether imaging can aid selection of appropriate surgical procedures and stress incontinence. Studies have looked at the relationship between sphincter volume and continence function in women. Evaluation of bladder neck mobility using ultrasound or MRI has not yielded predictive information related to urinary incontinence. MRI can provide an overall pelvic floor assessment, including assessment of prolapse, defecation, and integrity of the pelvic floor supports. However, the findings have not been generalized between institutions. Furthermore, correspondence between imaging findings and physical examination in POP is questioned.[53] Accordingly, imaging is not included as routine practice in guideline recommendations.[2]

Cystoscopy is not specifically indicated for incontinence alone. However, if haematuria is also present, guidelines for haematuria assessment should also be followed. For people with recurrent UTIs, cystoscopy is common practice. For women with previous incontinence surgery, especially if haematuria, leukocyturia, or proteinuria is present, cystoscopy should be considered to exclude abnormality such as a migrated paraurethral suture, or intrusion of surgical mesh into the bladder. Cystoscopy should be considered in persistent refractory UUI, as there are anecdotal reports of important conditions, such as bladder cancer, being misdiagnosed as overactive bladder. For men with post-prostatectomy incontinence, cystoscopy is used by some surgeons as part of the work-up for a transobturator sling.

Conclusions

People with incontinence require comprehensive assessment to identify underlying mechanisms and potential risk factors. For women with SUI, a large proportion can be identified primarily from their history, but due care should be taken to ensure that the minority of women with more complex underlying mechanisms are properly identified before irrevocable treatment is instigated. Symptom bother needs to be assessed alongside severity, to ensure therapy focused on the patient's quality of life; this is most effectively and simply captured with validated questionnaires. Coexisting conditions such as POP and systemic medical problems need to be considered. Physical examination needs to cover general aspects, such as the patient's mobility and possibility of occult neurological disease, along with abdominal and pelvic examination. Basic investigations include a frequency volume chart, urinalysis, post-void residual measurement, and flow rate testing. These assessments then empower the clinician to recommend conservative therapy options. Additional testing, such as pad tests or imaging are legitimate, but not currently in general use.

Acknowledgements

Text extracts reproduced from Abrams *et al.*, 'The standardisation of terminology of lower urinary tract function: report from the Standardisation Sub-committee of the International Continence Society', *Neurourology and Urodynamics*, Volume 21, Issue 2, pp. 167–178, Copyright © 2002 Wiley-Liss, Inc., with permission from John Wiley and Sons.

Further reading

Abrams P, Cardozo L, Fall M, *et al.* The standardisation of terminology of lower urinary tract function: report from the Standardisation Sub-committee of the International Continence Society. *Neurourol Urodyn* 2002; **21**:167–78.

Avery KN, Bosch JL, Gotoh M, *et al.* Questionnaires to assess urinary and anal incontinence: review and recommendations. *J Urol* 2007; **177**:39–49.

Bo K, Sherburn M. Evaluation of female pelvic-floor muscle function and strength. *Phys Ther* 2005; **85**:269–82.

Bright E, Drake MJ, Abrams P. Urinary diaries: evidence for the development and validation of diary content, format, and duration. *Neurourol Urodyn* 2011; **30**:348–52.

Lucas MG, Bosch RJ, Burkhard FC, *et al.* EAU Guidelines on Assessment and Nonsurgical Management of Urinary Incontinence. *Eur Urol* 2012; **62**:1130–42.

Martin JL, Williams KS, Abrams KR, *et al.* Systematic review and evaluation of methods of assessing urinary incontinence. *Health Technol Assess* 2006; **10**:1–132, iii–iv.

Persu C, Chapple CR, Cauni V, Gutue S, Geavlete P. Pelvic Organ Prolapse Quantification System (POP-Q)—a new era in pelvic prolapse staging. *J Med Life* 2011; **4**:75–81.

Van Kerrebroeck P. Standardization of terminology in nocturia: commentary on the ICS report. *BJU Int* 2002; **90**(Suppl 3):16–7.

References

1. Abrams P, Cardozo L, Fall M, *et al.* The standardisation of terminology of lower urinary tract function: report from the Standardisation Sub-committee of the International Continence Society. *Neurourol Urodyn* 2002; **21**:167–78.
2. Lucas MG, Bosch RJ, Burkhard FC, *et al.* EAU Guidelines on Assessment and Nonsurgical Management of Urinary Incontinence. *Eur Urol* 2012; **62**:1130–42.
3. Martin JL, Williams KS, Abrams KR, *et al.* Systematic review and evaluation of methods of assessing urinary incontinence. *Health Technol Assess* 2006; **10**:1–132, iii–iv.
4. Gu B, Wang X, Xu Y. Long-term outcome of duplex kidney with ectopic ureter treated by antireflux ureterocystic reimplantation. *Urol Int* 2012; **88**:438–40.
5. Solinas A, De Giorgi F, Frongia M. Embolization of a hypoplastic kidney with a vaginal ectopic ureter in a case of pseudo-incontinence. *Arch Ital Urol Androl* 2004; **76**:117–8.
6. Lin VC, Weng HC, Kian-Lim E, Lin IC, Yu TJ. An atrophic crossed fused kidney with an ectopic vaginal ureter causing urine incontinence. *Urology* 2010; **76**:55–6.
7. Van Kerrebroeck P. Standardization of terminology in nocturia: commentary on the ICS report. *BJU Int* 2002; **90**(Suppl 3):16–7.

8. Gulur DM, Mevcha AM, Drake MJ. Nocturia as a manifestation of systemic disease. *BJU Int* 2011; **107**:702–13.
9. Litwin MS, Lubeck DP, Henning JM, Carroll PR. Differences in urologist and patient assessments of health related quality of life in men with prostate cancer: results of the CaPSURE database. *J Urol* 1998; **159**:1988–92.
10. Aaronson NK. Quality of life assessment in clinical trials: methodologic issues. *Control Clin Trials* 1989; **10**:195S–208S.
11. Donovan J, Bosch R, Gotoh M, *et al.* Symptom and quality of life assessment. (pp. 519–84) In: Abrams P, Cardozo L, Khoury S, Wein A (eds). *Incontinence,* 3rd edition. Proceedings of the Third International Consultation on Incontinence. Plymouth, UK: Health Publications, 2005.
12. Avery KN, Bosch JL, Gotoh M, *et al.* Questionnaires to assess urinary and anal incontinence: review and recommendations. *J Urol* 2007; **177**:39–49.
13. Abrams P, Avery K, Gardener N, Donovan J. The International Consultation on Incontinence Modular Questionnaire: www.iciq.net. *J Urol* 2006; **175**:1063–6; discussion 1066.
14. Avery K, Donovan J, Peters TJ, Shaw C, Gotoh M, Abrams P. ICIQ: a brief and robust measure for evaluating the symptoms and impact of urinary incontinence. *Neurourol Urodyn* 2004; **23**:322–30.
15. Barry MJ. Evaluation of symptoms and quality of life in men with benign prostatic hyperplasia. *Urology* 2001; **58**:25–32; discussion 32.
16. Crystle CD, Charme LS, Copeland WE. Q-tip test in stress urinary incontinence. *Obstet Gynecol* 1971; **38**:313–5.
17. Karram MM, Bhatia NN. The Q-tip test: standardization of the technique and its interpretation in women with urinary incontinence. *Obstet Gynecol* 1988; **71**:807–11.
18. Bonney V. On diurnal incontinence of urine in women. *J Obstet Gynaecol Brit Emp* 1923; **30**:358–65.
19. Messelink B, Benson T, Berghmans B, *et al.* Standardization of terminology of pelvic floor muscle function and dysfunction: report from the pelvic floor clinical assessment group of the International Continence Society. *Neurourol Urodyn* 2005; **24**:374–80.
20. Bo K, Sherburn M. Evaluation of female pelvic-floor muscle function and strength. *Phys Ther* 2005; **85**:269–82.
21. Lemos N, Korte JE, Iskander M, *et al.* Center-by-center results of a multicenter prospective trial to determine the inter-observer correlation of the simplified POP-Q in describing pelvic organ prolapse. *Int Urogynecol J* 2012; **23**:579–84.
22. Persu C, Chapple CR, Cauni V, Gutue S, Geavlete P. Pelvic Organ Prolapse Quantification System (POP-Q)—a new era in pelvic prolapse staging. *J Med Life* 2011; **4**:75–81.
23. Bump RC, Mattiasson A, Bo K, *et al.* The standardization of terminology of female pelvic organ prolapse and pelvic floor dysfunction. *Am J Obstet Gynecol* 1996; **175**:10–7.
24. Moore EE, Jackson SL, Boyko EJ, Scholes D, Fihn SD. Urinary incontinence and urinary tract infection: temporal relationships in postmenopausal women. *Obstet Gynecol* 2008; **111**:317–23.
25. Abrams P. Bladder outlet obstruction index, bladder contractility index and bladder voiding efficiency: three simple indices to define bladder voiding function. *BJU Int* 1999; **84**:14–5.
26. Gehrich A, Stany MP, Fischer JR, Buller J, Zahn CM. Establishing a mean postvoid residual volume in asymptomatic perimenopausal and postmenopausal women. *Obstet Gynecol* 2007; **110**:827–32.
27. Tseng LH, Liang CC, Chang YL, Lee SJ, Lloyd LK, Chen CK. Postvoid residual urine in women with stress incontinence. *Neurourol Urodyn* 2008; **27**:48–51.
28. Schmidt F, Shin P, Jorgensen TM, Djurhuus JC, Constantinou CE. Urodynamic patterns of normal male micturition: influence of water consumption on urine production and detrusor function. *J Urol* 2002; **168**:1458–63.
29. Kranse R, van Mastrigt R. Causes for variability in repeated pressure-flow measurements. *Urology* 2003; **61**:930–4; discussion 4–5.
30. Jorgensen JB, Jensen KM, Mogensen P. Age-related variation in urinary flow variables and flow curve patterns in elderly males. *Br J Urol* 1992; **69**:265–71.
31. Matzkin H, van der Zwaag R, Chen Y, Patterson LA, Braf Z, Soloway MS. How reliable is a single measurement of urinary flow in the diagnosis of obstruction in benign prostatic hyperplasia? *Br J Urol* 1993; **72**:181–6.
32. Siroky MB, Olsson CA, Krane RJ. The flow rate nomogram: I. Development. *J Urol* 1979; **122**:665–8.
33. Haylen BT, Ashby D, Sutherst JR, Frazer MI, West CR. Maximum and average urine flow rates in normal male and female populations—the Liverpool nomograms. *Br J Urol* 1989; **64**:30–8.
34. Sonke GS, Robertson C, Verbeek AL, Witjes WP, de la Rosette JJ, Kiemeney LA. A method for estimating within-patient variability in maximal urinary flow rate adjusted for voided volume. *Urology* 2002; **59**:368–72.
35. Reynard JM, Yang Q, Donovan JL, *et al.* The ICS-'BPH' Study: uroflowmetry, lower urinary tract symptoms and bladder outlet obstruction. *Br J Urol* 1998; **82**:619–23.
36. Pernkopf D, Plas E, Lang T, *et al.* Uroflow nomogram for male adolescents. J Urol 2005; **174**:1436–9; discussion 1439.
37. Siroky MB, Olsson CA, Krane RJ. The flow rate nomogram: II. Clinical correlation. *J Urol* 1980; **123**:208–10.
38. Idzenga T, Pel JJ, van Mastrigt R. Accuracy of maximum flow rate for diagnosing bladder outlet obstruction can be estimated from the ICS nomogram. *Neurourol Urodyn* 2008; **27**:97–8.
39. Nishimoto K, Iimori H, Ikemoto S, Hayahara N. Criteria for differentiation of normal and abnormal uroflowmetrograms in adult men. *Br J Urol* 1994; **73**:494–7.
40. Reynard JM, Lim C, Peters TJ, Abrams P. The significance of terminal dribbling in men with lower urinary tract symptoms. *Br J Urol* 1996; **77**:705–10.
41. Blanker MH, Bohnen AM, Groeneveld FP, Bernsen RM, Prins A, Ruud Bosch JL. Normal voiding patterns and determinants of increased diurnal and nocturnal voiding frequency in elderly men. *J Urol* 2000; **164**:1201–5.
42. van Haarst EP, Bosch JL, Heldeweg EA. The international prostate symptom score overestimates nocturia assessed by frequency-volume charts. *J Urol* 2012; **188**:211–5.
43. Bright E, Drake MJ, Abrams P. Urinary diaries: evidence for the development and validation of diary content, format, and duration. *Neurourol Urodyn* 2011; **30**:348–52.
44. Bright E, Cotterill N, Drake M, Abrams P. Developing a validated urinary diary: phase 1. *Neurourol Urodyn* 2012; **31**:625–33.
45. Cornu JN, Abrams P, Chapple CR, *et al.* A contemporary assessment of nocturia: definition, epidemiology, pathophysiology, and management—a systematic review and meta-analysis. *Eur Urol* 2012; **62**:877–90.
46. Weiss JP. Nocturia: "do the math". *J Urol* 2006; **175**:S16–8.
47. Weiss JP, Ruud Bosch JL, Drake M, *et al.* Nocturia Think Tank: Focus on Nocturnal Polyuria: Report from the ICI-RS 2011. *Neurourol Urodyn* 2012; **31**(3):330–9.
48. Weiss JP, Blaivas JG, Stember DS, Chaikin DC. Evaluation of the etiology of nocturia in men: the nocturia and nocturnal bladder capacity indices. *Neurourol Urodyn* 1999; **18**:559–65.
49. Kinn AC, Larsson B. Pad test with fixed bladder volume in urinary stress incontinence. *Acta Obstet Gynecol Scand* 1987; **66**:369–71.
50. Fantl JA, Harkins SW, Wyman JF, Choi SC, Taylor JR. Fluid loss quantitation test in women with urinary incontinence: a test-retest analysis. *Obstet Gynecol* 1987; **70**:739–43.
51. Sutherst J, Brown M, Shawer M. Assessing the severity of urinary incontinence in women by weighing perineal pads. *Lancet* 1981; **1**:1128–30.
52. Klarskov P, Hald T. Reproducibility and reliability of urinary incontinence assessment with a 60 min test. *Scand J Urol Nephrol* 1984; **18**:293–8.
53. Broekhuis SR, Kluivers KB, Hendriks JC, Futterer JJ, Barentsz JO, Vierhout ME. POP-Q, dynamic MR imaging, and perineal ultrasonography: do they agree in the quantification of female pelvic organ prolapse? *Int Urogynecol J Pelvic Floor Dysfunct* 2009; **20**:541–9.

CHAPTER 3.5

Stress urinary incontinence

Christopher R. Chapple and Altaf Mangera

Definitions of incontinence

The standardization of lower urinary tract symptoms (LUTS) and dysfunction (LUTD) terminology has been undertaken by the International Continence Society.[1] The committee has described urinary incontinence as the complaint of involuntary leakage of urine. When the leaking is accompanied or preceded by urgency, it is labelled as urgency urinary incontinence. Involuntary leakage on effort, exertion, coughing, or sneezing is termed stress urinary incontinence (SUI). When an individual complains of both of the above, they are said to have mixed urinary incontinence. Enuresis is a term synonymous with incontinence and may be preceded by the adjective 'nocturnal', which describes loss of urine during sleep. Overflow urinary incontinence occurs in association with an overdistended bladder and continuous urinary incontinence is the complaint of continuous urine leakage. Unconscious urinary incontinence is the unperceived loss of urine. Finally, situational urinary incontinence occurs only in specific situations such as with giggling or during intercourse. The remainder of this chapter will concentrate mostly on SUI.

Anatomy/physiology of continence

The bladder is a hollow muscular organ. Its two main functions are to store urine at low pressure and allow its expulsion at an appropriate time and place. The bladder spends 99% of its time in the storage phase. Receptive relaxation of the bladder allows the accommodation of urine without an appreciable rise in pressure. Concomitantly, the bladder outflow mechanisms retain sufficient resistance to maintain continence. The urinary continence mechanisms are different in males and females, and are best considered separately.

In males, there are two important sphincteric mechanisms which contribute to continence: a *proximal bladder neck mechanism*, and a *distal urethral mechanism* at the apex (distal end) of the prostate. The sphincters are such that continence should be maintained in the absence of either sphincter. The proximal sphincter is composed of an inner layer of circular muscle fibres, which continue from the bladder trigone into the inner longitudinal layer of smooth muscle in the urethra. This muscle is richly innervated by adrenergic fibres, which when stimulated produce closure of the bladder neck.

The distal urethral sphincter extends from the distal 3–5 mm of the prostate into the membranous urethra and is composed of extrinsic striated muscle capable of sustained contraction in order to maintain continence. This sphincter also contains a smooth muscle component as shown in Figure 3.5.1. The striated urethral sphincter is longer anteriorly and extends higher up the prostate

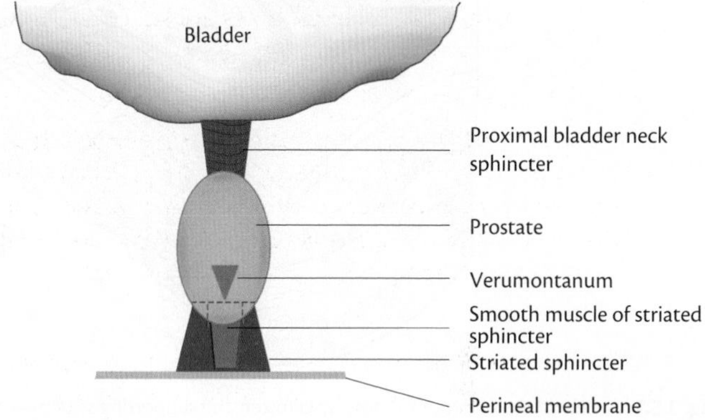

Fig. 3.5.1 Diagrammatic representation of the urinary continence mechanisms in the male.

here.[2] Hence it is easier to inadvertently cut into this anterior portion when performing endoscopic prostatectomy.

In females, the bladder neck sphincter is far weaker than in the male and is absent in 40% of women. Therefore, urinary continence relies upon the integrity of the distal sphincter, which is composed of longitudinal intrinsic urethral smooth muscle and a larger extrinsic striated muscle component. The horseshoe-shaped striated sphincter is most developed in the middle-third of the urethra, with the muscle fibres present ventrally and laterally. It is composed of type I slow-twitch fibres surrounded by collagen. Given the lack of a proximal sphincter, during a cough, urine will enter the proximal urethra. In addition, in the middle and distal thirds of the urethra, a richly vascular submucosa supports the urethral epithelium and contributes significantly to urethral closure pressure.

In order for the urethral sphincter to correctly function in the female, the pelvic floor support mechanism must also be intact. The levator ani muscles, in combination with the endopelvic fascia create an important part of the continence mechanism in women, forming a hammock-like layer which provides support to the posterior bladder neck and urethra (Fig. 3.5.2). Contraction of the levator ani, in particular the pubococcygeus muscle, pulls the vagina against the posterior surface of the urethra, thus closing it. This theory is known as the *hammock hypothesis* and was proposed by DeLancey. Another theory, proposed by Ulmsten and Petros and known as the *integral theory*, states that it is weakness in the anterior wall of the vagina leading to laxity in the posterior urethra which leads to SUI. If the posterior supporting ligaments are weak, then stress incontinence results. This model is analogous to compression of a hose pipe beneath the foot while it is lying on supported and unsupported ground. If the ground is firm good compression may

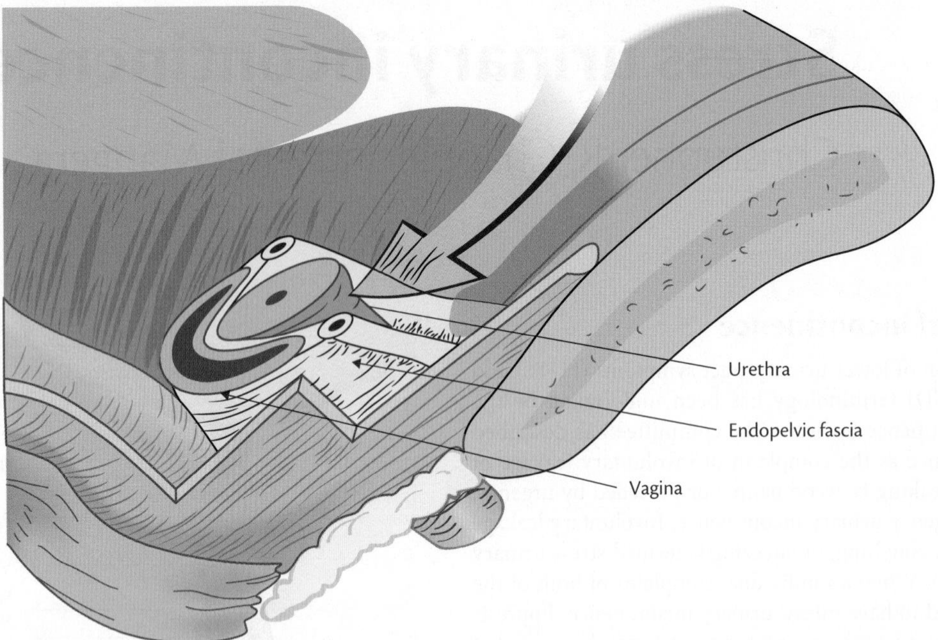

Fig. 3.5.2 A view of the hammock theory by Ulmsten, the supporting structures to the urethra provide a backboard upon which the urethral contraction may be stabilized.

Reproduced with permission from A. J. Wein *et al*, *Campbell-Walsh Urology, Ninth Edition*, Saunders, an imprint of Elsevier Inc., Philadelphia, USA, Copyright © 2006.

be obtained, whereas soft ground will lead to inadequate compression. All women with stress incontinence are thus likely to have a degree of *intrinsic sphincteric deficiency* with a variable degree of *urethral hypermobility* (pelvic floor laxity). In practice, however, there is no absolute method to quantify these two different components accurately.[3]

Neuronal control of the lower urinary tract is under a complex series of coordinated peripheral and central pathways. Generally, storage is under sympathetic control and voiding parasympathetic. Sensory afferents travel in the hypogastric nerves (sympathetic T10–12), pelvic nerves (parasympathetic S2–4), and pudendal nerves (Somatic S2–4). The somatic nerves arise from the nucleus of Onufrowicz (S2–4). The sympathetic nerves arise as postganglionic fibres from the T10-L2 spinal level and the parasympathetic nerves as preganglionic fibres from the S2-S4 level. Hypogastric (sympathetic) and pudendal (somatic) nerve stimulation leads to contraction of the sphincteric smooth and striated muscles, while the pelvic nerve leads to relaxation of both sphincters. In contrast, the detrusor muscle is relaxed by the sympathetic system and contracted by the parasympathetic. Centrally, the pontine micturition centre (PMC) and suprapontine areas of the brain are responsible for coordinating micturition.

Epidemiology and risk factors

In a meta-analysis of 48 studies, the prevalence of urinary incontinence was reported at 16% for women younger than 30 years and 29% for women aged 30 to 60 years.[4] The authors found SUI to be more common than urgency urinary incontinence, with 78% of women having SUI versus 51% with urgency urinary incontinence, and 27% of them having mixed urinary incontinence. Each year, an estimated 135,000 women undergo surgery for urinary incontinence in the United States alone.[5]

The recognized risk factors for SUI include: female gender; age up to 50 years; high body mass index; smoking; pregnancy; vaginal delivery; pelvic surgery; diabetes mellitus; and connective tissue disorders. By far the most common mechanism in these cases may be the effect of the loss of muscle tone, long-term effects of denervation injuries sustained during childbirth, or changes in hormonal status leading to alterations in collagen in paravaginal tissues.[6,7] However, it has proved difficult to show a link between natural menopause and increasing risk of SUI.[8,9] Also the evidence for hormone replacement therapy does not show it to reduce the risk of the development of SUI as evidenced by two RCTs.[10–12]

Symptoms

SUI is very embarrassing for a patient to deal with. It is imperative that a careful history is undertaken and the patient encouraged to describe when and how their incontinence occurs. A qualitative report of the situation in which stress incontinence occurs (i.e. with minimal exercise or strenuous activity, and so on) gives a good indication of severity, as well as the frequency of incontinence episodes with the amount of leakage. Caution should be applied when interpreting pad usage, because some women change their pad at the first sign of moisture compared to others who only change when they are soaked through, and therefore one must ask why the pads are changed and in what condition. The presence of other LUTS is also important in guiding a clinician to any concomitant pathology.

After it has been established that the incontinence is stress-related, one should assess the presence of any of the risk factors described above. Due to the strong sphincteric mechanisms in the male, stress incontinence is uncommon except following radical prostatectomy. Transient causes of incontinence such as delirium, urinary tract infection, polyuria, pharmacological, psychological, stool impaction, and restricted mobility should also be ruled out. Finally, the degree of bother should be ascertained to help guide therapy. There are many questionnaires which may be used to quantify the severity and impact of stress urinary incontinence, such as the ICIQ-UI SF, UDI, and Sandvik severity indices. These are however mostly used as research tools.

Examination

The physical examination should concentrate on detecting anatomic and neurologic abnormalities which may contribute to urinary incontinence. Examination should include palpation of any abdominal masses including a distended bladder along with the external genitalia. The prostate, anal tone, and sensation should be assessed in the male. In the female, the vaginal epithelium should be thick, pink, and contain transverse rugae. Ideally a vaginal examination should be performed with a full bladder (to perform a stress test and assess for pelvic organ prolapse) and empty bladder (to examine the pelvic organs). However, this may be difficult in clinical practice.

The *stress test* is performed in the lithotomy position with the clinician's fingers parting the labia to allow direct visualization of the urethral orifice. For the test, bladder volume, number, and force of coughs should be standardized. However, currently no standards exist. Therefore, the test is performed in the presence of a 'full bladder', during which the patient is asked to cough and leakage is observed. At the same time, a *Bonney test* may be performed by lifting the bladder neck in to the vagina and asking the patient to cough. This test was thought to show whether the urethra had prolapsed out of the abdominal cavity; however, it has been found to be unreliable and it is more likely that the lifting finger obstructs the urethra rather than lifting it back into the abdominal cavity.[13] The *Q-tip test* involves the insertion of a thin sterile cotton tipped applicator into the bladder via the urethra. The applicator is withdrawn up to the point of resistance, which is the level of the bladder neck. The resting angle is recorded. The patient is then asked to strain and the degree of rotation assessed. A resting or straining angle greater than 30 degrees from the horizontal is defined as urethral hypermobility. This test has also been shown to have limited usefulness in a clinical setting.

The vaginal examination should systematically examine all walls of the vagina and assess uterine position or vault position in women post-hysterectomy. An anterior prolapse (cystocele) may need to be reduced to show *occult incontinence*. In the prolapsed state, the cystocele can cause compression of the urethra and prevent incontinence from occurring; this consequently may occur on correction of the prolapse.

Investigation

Urinalysis is a simple test which should be performed in all patients with LUTS. It is not diagnostic, but should be used to screen for haematuria, glycosuria, leukocyte esterase, and nitrates. These may be indicative of carcinoma, diabetes, and infection, respectively, all of which may be associated with incontinence. Similarly, *post-void residual* estimation using an ultrasound bladder scanner is simple and non-invasive. It should be used to exclude overflow incontinence.

A frequency volume chart or bladder diary may be used to quantify the frequency of incontinence episodes and also to obtain an individual's pattern of voiding. The daily voided volume may indicate polyuria, which is defined as the passage of more than 2.8 L urine per 24 hours. The format and duration of the diary has not been standardized. Three different formats exist: *micturition time* charts record the number of voids (and incontinence episodes) in 24 hours; *frequency volume* charts also include the voided volume; and *bladder diaries* record additional information such as number and type of incontinence episodes, pad usage, fluid and food intake, and degree of urgency. The length of time the chart is utilized is also unstandardized. Clearly, a balance needs to be sought between greater accuracy with lengthening the test period and patient compliance. Also, complex bladder diaries are less likely to be completed correctly. Therefore, most commonly a frequency volume chart is used for three to four days.[14] The parameters obtained from a frequency volume chart are described in Chapter 3.4.

Pad tests may detect incontinence but do not shed light on its cause. They can be used for long periods (72 hours) and short periods (one hour). The one-hour test should be performed under fixed conditions of bladder fullness and exercise. The International Continence Society has defined a gain in pad weight of >1 g over one hour or 8 g >24 hours as significant.[1] Any less than this can be due to natural sweating or vaginal secretions. The proposed International Continence Society (ICS) protocol for the one-hour test involves a patient drinking 500 mL over 15 minutes, followed by simple walking around for 30 minutes, and finally provocation manoeuvres for 15 minutes. Patients are disallowed from voiding for the duration of the test. If a more precise 'real life' test is desired, a 24-hour or longer test is preferred.

Urodynamics: Urodynamic studies assume a variety of forms and need to be considered to represent a hierarchical series of progressively complex tests. The frequency volume chart and pad test come as first line under the umbrella of urodynamics, followed by uroflowmetry, which is detailed further in Chapter 3.4. In addition to a flow test, a post-void residual estimation should also be undertaken to exclude overflow incontinence masquerading as SUI. The procedure is simple and can be undertaken in an outpatient department. The full bladder is scanned with an ultrasound probe, the patient voids into the flow meter in private, and a post-voiding scan is carried out to assess bladder residual. One should ensure that the patient has a subjectively full bladder prior to carrying out the study to provide a representative result.

Most often, however, the term urodynamics is used to describe *cystometry*. Cystometry is the method by which the pressure/volume relationship of the bladder is measured. Synchronous cystography with cystometry is termed video urodynamics, and should be considered in complex patients, since this methodology allows a combined anatomical and functional evaluation of lower urinary tract function. In particular, radiological screening provides valuable additional anatomical information on the appearance of the bladder, the presence of vesicoureteric reflux, the degree of support to the bladder base during coughing, and by itself is more than adequate for the diagnosis of sphincteric competence, and/or the level of any outflow obstruction in the lower urinary tract on the voiding phase. This is offset by the need for radiological facilities, extra cost, and doses of radiation, all of which need to be justified.

Cystometry involves the insertion of one small catheter with a pressure transducer into the bladder and one into the rectum. The former also contains a channel which fills the bladder on the urodynamicist's request. The intravesical pressure (P_{ves}) is a consequence of the intrabdominal (P_{abd}) and detrusor pressures (P_{det}). Therefore, the detrusor muscle pressure (P_{det}) may be extrapolated from subtraction of the abdominal pressure (P_{abd}) from the intravesical pressure (P_{ves}) (Fig. 3.5.3).

The cystometry protocol has been standardized by the ICS.[1] The finer details of this procedure can be found in Chapter 3.2 or in a dedicated urodynamics text book.[15] Briefly, the procedure commences with a void in a flow meter, followed by assessment of post-void residue. The patient then has a catheter with a transducer inserted in to the rectum and bladder. The bladder is filled at a rate of 25–50 mL per minute using a peristaltic pump. This is termed the storage phase. The patient is asked to stand during filling to assess this phase.

Throughout the study continuous rectal pressure, total bladder pressure, and electronically subtracted detrusor pressure measurements are recorded at a predetermined rate (usually one Hertz) and the results displayed on the video display unit. During the filling phase, the patient is asked to cough periodically to assess subtraction, which acts as quality control (Fig. 3.5.3). In addition to this the patient is asked to report bladder sensations such as the first sensation, first desire to void, normal desire to void, and severe desire to void, as well as any urgency which they might develop. These sensations and their significance are considered further in Chapter 3.2. The patient is also asked to strain by doing the Valsalva manoeuvre and also to cough, to assess for stress incontinence. The volume of bladder filling at which SUI occurs and the amount of fluid lost during SUI are recorded.

At this juncture, concomitant cystography gives additional information over cystometry alone. Filling the bladder with contrast solution and screening during a cough should allow the differentiation of *intrinsic sphincteric deficiency* from *urethral hypermobility*. The latter is seen as a greater than average movement of the urethrovesical unit during a cough. Some movement is necessary and an experienced urodynamicist can usually distinguish between normal movement and hypermobility. In contrast, with intrinsic sphincteric deficiency, a rectangular-shaped incompetent bladder neck is seen. The urethra does not spring back and continued leaking occurs after the stress event. It must be noted, to some extent, that women will have a combination of urethral hypermobility and intrinsic sphincteric deficiency and experience is necessary to interpret their relative functional significance.

The urodynamic definition of SUI is 'the involuntary leakage of urine during increased intra-abdominal pressure, in the absence of a detrusor contraction'. Detrusor contractions are involuntary contractions of the detrusor muscle during bladder filling and may be associated with urgency. They are considered in more detail in Chapter 3.7. An inexperienced urodynamicist may be caught out by *cough induced detrusor overactivity*. One may assume that the cough is leading to stress incontinence; however, immediately after the cough, the detrusor trace shows a contraction which then leads to incontinence. This is an important finding as the two conditions are treated entirely differently.

If more precise measurements of urethral function are required, then urethral pressure profilometry is undertaken. The pressure is recorded along the urethra consecutively, forming a urethral pressure profile. The intravesical pressure also needs to be recorded to exclude a simultaneous detrusor contraction. At rest the urethra is closed and this must be recognized when interpreting the results of urethral pressure studies. The urethral pressure is described as the fluid pressure required to just open the urethra and the urethral closure pressure profile is calculated by subtracting the intravesical pressure from urethral pressure. The maximum urethral pressure is

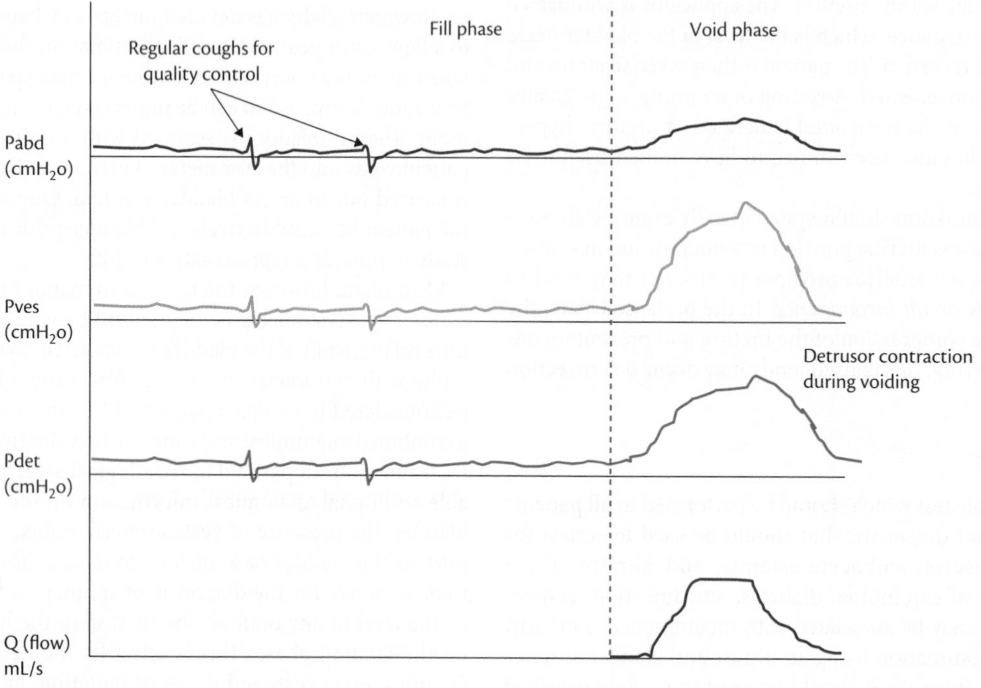

Fig. 3.5.3 A normal cystometry trace showing the storage and voiding phases.

the maximum pressure of the measured profile and the maximum urethral closure pressure is the maximum difference between the urethral pressure and the intravesical pressure. Abdominal leak point pressure is the intravesical pressure at which urine leakage occurs due to increased abdominal pressure in the absence of a detrusor contraction. Detrusor leak point pressure is defined as the lowest detrusor pressure at which urine leakage occurs in the absence of either detrusor contraction or increased abdominal pressure.

Although urethral pressure profilometry has the potential to be highly informative, the test does not comprise routine practice. Principally this is because there is a large overlap in values obtained from normal and symptomatic patients. In addition, it does not discriminate SUI from other urinary disorders, provide a measurement of the severity of the condition, or predict a return to normal urinary function following successful intervention with any sensitivity. However, in certain cases it may be helpful to obtain this information such as when considering a transobturator tape or an autologous sling procedure, which is discussed later in this chapter.

Finally, electromyography can be used to assess nerve abnormalities to the urethral sphincter. Needles are placed into a muscle mass, or surface electrodes are used to record electrical action potentials generated by depolarizing muscle. These have a characteristic waveform and therefore abnormalities may be recognized. These are seldom used outside specialist centres (see Chapter 3.2).

In conclusion, urodynamics is not a technique which should be restricted to a few specialists. In most cases, the principles are simple and well-formulated questions, obtained from a thorough history and examination, are useful in selecting the appropriate test to undertake. The results should always be interpreted in light of the clinical findings. It is useful to view the urinary tract as a sequence of conduits, within which urine movement is dictated by chamber pressures and resistance to flow, with intervening sphincters controlling flow. It is advisable to avoid jargon terms and use the nomenclature of the International Continence Society as presented in this chapter.

Management

The first-line management of SUI should include lifestyle changes such as weight loss and supervised pelvic floor exercises. The long-term evidence for the efficacy of these interventions is questionable and success relies to a great extent on patient motivation.

Pharmacotherapy has principally been used to try and increase urethral pressure in women with SUI. Urethral tone is maintained by the release of noradrenaline onto the alpha-adrenoreceptors and many different alpha-adrenoreceptor agonists have been used to treat SUI. The most widely used have been ephedrine and phenylpropanolamine, but the literature has shown only limited benefit for these and their use has been abandoned because of safety issues, since they can cause hypertension as well as the lack of efficacy. Duloxetine, a serotonin/noradrenaline reuptake inhibitor has also been licensed for use in SUI. Both noradrenaline and serotonin are postulated to lead to enhanced contraction of the urethral rhabdosphincter. A Cochrane review has shown significant improvements in SUI symptoms with duloxetine compared to placebo.[16] SUI episodes have been shown to be halved in up to 64% of women, but the drug was discontinued by 15% due to side effects including nausea and psychiatric disturbances. Given these difficulties and poor cost-effectiveness, pharmacotherapy is not routine practice in the management of SUI.

Bulking agents can be injected intramurally into the urethra to provide bulk and support to the urethral sphincter mechanism. Different urethral bulking agents have been used ranging from collagen, autologous fat, carbon particles, calcium hydroxyapetite, ethylene vinyl calcohol copolymer, dextranomer, and silicone. The implants either become encapsulated or are absorbed by the body, depending on their constitution. Although success rates of cure plus improvement have been reported in up to 46% to 88%, complications related to these procedures include polymer migration, erosion, urinary retention, and embolism. Given that this therapy is costly with cure rates lower than those reported with surgery, most surgeons do not use bulking agents as first-line treatment, except in young female patients who have not completed their family or the elderly; and if used as a first-line treatment, many note an adverse effect on subsequent surgical intervention.

Surgery is often the treatment modality of choice for SUI. There are five main categories of repair:

Paravaginal repair with bladder buttress—this is used when concomitant prolapse exists. A paravaginal repair of the prolapse is performed along with buttressing of the bladder to provide support and/or elevation of the urethra. Meta-analysis has reported the success rate of this procedure to be in the region of 67.8–72%.[17] However, the long-term success rates have been found to decline to 37%.[18] A variant of this procedure is the *vaginal obturator shelf* procedure. The anterior wall and supporting endopelvic fascia of the bladder neck is elevated and sutured to the internal obturator muscle. The premise for this is that there should be no restriction to the intrinsic sphincteric function due to paraurethral tethering. There are, however, limited data to support this technique.

Burch colposuspension is a long-standing effective treatment for SUI. The top of the vagina is lifted and fixed with permanent stitches into the space behind the pubic bone. At five years, Ward and Hilton report a 90% negative pad test among women in the colposuspension arm of a large randomized controlled trial.[19] Complications reported from this study showed a rate of 39.8% of pelvic organ prolapse after this procedure and reoperation rates for incontinence of 3.4%. However, due to the emergence of less invasive techniques, as discussed later, the Burch colposuspension is used less often these days.

Needle suspension procedures use suspending sutures to suspend the bladder neck, usually from bone anchors placed in the pubic bone. These are, however, seldom used due to high failure rates.

Autologous sling procedures—the first pubovaginal sling was described in 1933 by Price, who used autologous rectus fascia. The sling was placed beneath the bladder neck and attached via sutures to the pubic symphysis which was later called the 'sling on a string' procedure. The rectus fascia sling has a success rate of approximately 80% depending on the level of patient selection and follow-up. However, the procedure carries the risk of donor site morbidity. Therefore, researchers have investigated the use of acellular biological matrices as a replacement. The early results have not been as good as that of autologous rectus fascia due to encapsulation or degradation of the biological grafts.

Autologous tissue carries a negligible risk of urethral erosion. It is thought to have greater success in women where there is predominantly intrinsic sphincteric deficiency, as the sling can be placed tighter on the urethra thus increasing sphincteric pressure. These autologous slings are usually used as treatment for intrinsic sphincter deficiency. Caution must be applied when tightening the sling, as there is a risk of urinary retention.

Tape procedures: a synthetic tape is placed beneath the mid-urethra without tension. There are three main methods of positioning the tape, depending on its length. A full-length tape passes through the retropubic space, underneath the urethra to the other side, and is fixed by sutures to the anterior abdominal wall, this is known as the tension-free vaginal tape (TVT). Shorter tapes, known as 'mini slings', are attached by suspending sutures at each end of the tape to the anterior abdominal wall; their use remains investigational at present since their results are not as good as a standard full-length sling. The tape can also be brought around through to the obturator internus muscle and out of the obturator foramen, termed the transobturator tape (TOT) (Fig. 3.5.4). If the transobturator tape is inserted from inside the vagina and taken out of the groin (i.e. inside-out technique), then it is termed a TOT; and if the reverse is true and the tape is inserted from the groin into the vagina, then the proprietary kit is a TVT-O.

More than two million tapes have been placed worldwide, making the tension-free tape the procedure of choice for SUI. The proposed mechanism of action of these tapes is to induce fibrosis in the suburethral tissue, thus forming a tough backboard upon which the urethra can contract. An updated meta-analysis has shown cure rates of 60–80% at five years.[20] The TOT procedure was also shown to carry less risk of intraoperative bladder perforation compared to the TVT due to the course of the tape away from the bladder, but with similar efficacy.

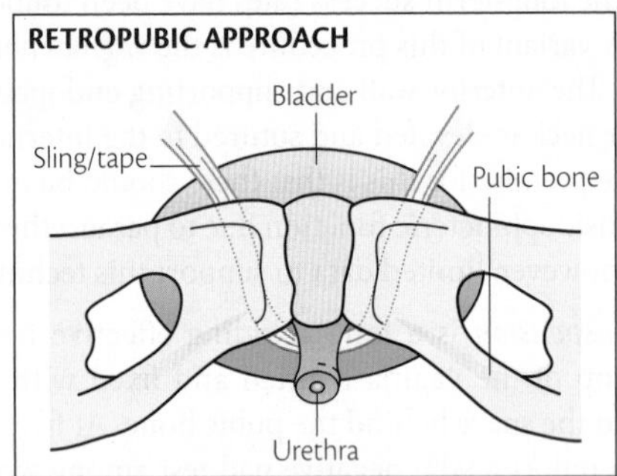

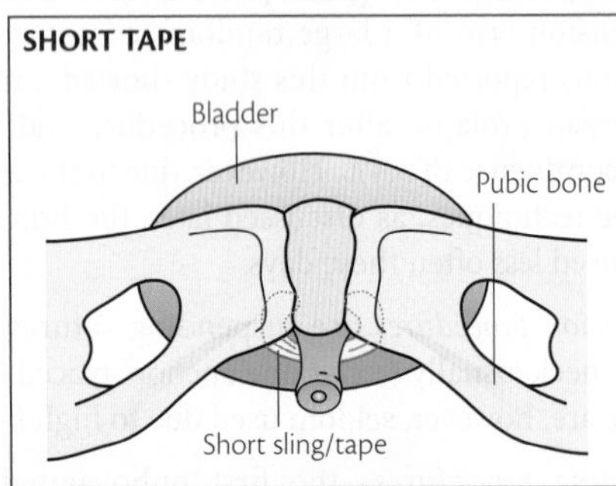

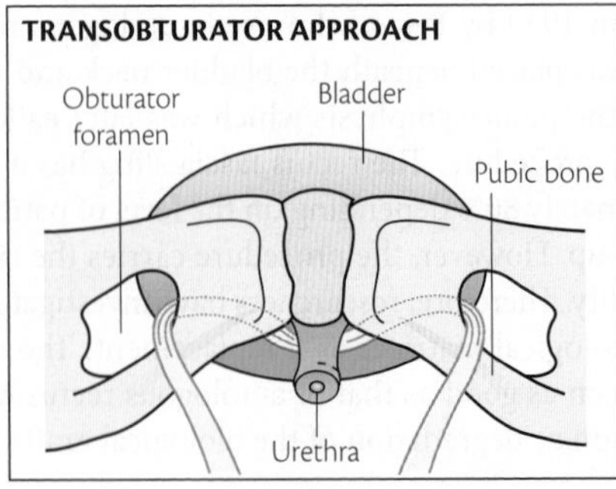

Fig. 3.5.4 Variations of the sling/tape procedure. 1-TVT, 2-mini sling, 3-TOT.

The TVT procedure has been shown to work better in women with a lower mean urethral closure pressure compared to the TOT procedure. This may be due to some tensioning due to tape position and mesh contraction as part of the host inflammatory response. The risk of bladder outflow obstruction is also reported at 10% and may require long-term self catheterization. Urgency and urgency incontinence occur in approximately 10% of cases. More serious complications include extrusion which is exposure of mesh into the vagina or erosion into the urinary tract, which combination occurs in up to 5–6% of patients in existing long-term studies, although this is likely to increase in prevalence with increasing duration of follow-up of patients. In addition, the fibrotic response to the mesh may lead to chronic pain and dyspareunia in a small proportion of women.

In an attempt to reduce the complications of erosion and pain, researchers have tried to limit mesh to the suburethral region (mini sling) and fix this with sutures. Unfortunately, as noted above, the success of these mini slings has not been as great as the longer tapes.[21]

An *artificial urinary sphincter* may be utilized in women who have continuing incontinence after any or a combination of the above surgery. Female artificial urinary sphincters, as first-line therapy, have not been used in women due to their cost and the technical difficulty compared to the other techniques described above, resulting in poor results when this approach is used as second-line therapy. However, a few studies arising from a few specialist centres where the artificial sphincter has been used as first-line therapy have reported excellent mid- to long-term results.[22] Women with urodynamic proven severe intrinsic sphincteric deficiency are postulated to benefit most from this surgery.[23]

The artificial sphincter consists of a cuff, which is placed around the bladder neck that applies pressure to the urethra keeping it closed. This is connected to a reservoir (balloon) and a pump, similar to that in the male. Release of the pump allows the movement of fluid from the cuff in to the reservoir which allows urine out of the bladder. The reservoir has elastic recoil properties and the fluid slowly returns to the cuff after a few minutes thus closing the urethra again.

Mixed incontinence

Mixed urinary incontinence is a term that describes the presence of both urgency urinary incontinence and stress urinary incontinence. Owing to the high prevalence of both conditions individually in the female population, it is not surprising that a proportion of women will have both. The important facts to elucidate in the history are the bother caused by each of the components of incontinence. These women should undergo cystometry if surgical treatment is contemplated and treatment should be directed at the most bothersome complaint. However, the patient must be counselled that by treating one complaint, the other may be made worse. Therefore, a careful balance of effects and side effects is required in these patients.

Post-prostatectomy incontinence

Primary SUI in men is extremely rare. It is mostly secondary to a neurological disorder, prostatic surgery (usually for malignant disease) or chronic retention. It is therefore imperative to obtain the details of any bladder outflow obstruction procedures undertaken and also to assess for any signs of incomplete bladder emptying. Abdominal examination may reveal a palpable bladder or a lower midline scar for a radical prostatectomy; however, many centres perform radical prostatectomy laporoscopically or even robotically and therefore the scars are less conspicuous. A transurethral resection of the prostate (TURP) or laser resection/enucleation leaves no scars.

The risk of SUI post TURP is reported at less than 1%. It may occur due to a pre-existing weak distal urethral sphincter or due to inadvertent prostatic resection distal to the verumontanum. The risk of SUI is higher with radical prostatectomy. It is transient phenomenon in many men, but can be a persistent clinical problem in up to 10% of cases with symptoms subsiding over several months. Bulky disease, previous prostatic surgery, or radiotherapy are additional risk factors.

Three-quarters of patients with post-prostatectomy incontinence will have a damaged sphincter, of which half will also have concomitant detrusor overactivity. Therefore, cystometry is important in this group of patients. In cases of true sphincteric damage, physiotherapy for the pelvic floor muscles may lead to symptomatic improvement but there is a limited literature supporting its use. Intramural urethral bulking agents have not shown any significant success rates and are therefore seldom used. Male sling procedures are advocated in milder forms of sphincteric weakness, particularly when there is no nocturnal leakage—suggesting a milder degree of sphincteric weakness. Modern male slings have only been developed recently and are currently under evaluation. The medium-term evidence shows that they may be more effective in patients with mild to moderate incontinence, but are less effective following radiotherapy or in patients with severe incontinence. They have a reported cure rate of 66% at four years, with a further 20% being improved but not cured.[24] Revision/explantation is required in up to 3%.

The gold standard in this cohort of men remains the artificial urinary sphincter. Its mechanism of action has been described above. Continence rates, long term, have been reported at 90%. The sphincter has a revision rate of 17% at 5 years and 34% to 80% at 10 years.[25,26] The infection rate after initial artificial urethral sphincter (AUS) surgery is 1% to 3%. Sphincters certainly have longer follow-up over slings, and are more likely to result in complete continence, especially in severe cases.

Overflow incontinence

This occurs when a patient develops chronic urinary retention due to incomplete bladder emptying. This is most commonly seen in elderly men with an enlarged obstructive prostate, however younger men with urethral strictures may also develop this. The bladder distends with chronic retention due to incomplete emptying and this may cause back pressure on the ureters and kidneys affecting renal function. SUI occurs due to the increased intra-abdominal pressure on a bladder already under great pressure. Chronic retention must be treated by catheterization. If bladder contractility is preserved (as determined by cystometry) then a bladder outflow procedure, such as a TURP, may be undertaken. If bladder contractility is diminished, then long-term catheterization or, if sufficiently dexterous, intermittent self catheterization will need to be performed.

Continuous incontinence

Continuous incontinence is often due to a fistula, occurring most commonly in developed countries following surgery or obstetric injury. The presentation may include leakage of urine from the vagina (vesicovaginal fistula), while its treatment involves surgical repair of the fistula. Good surgical technique and adequate soft tissue coverage is essential (most commonly the omentum when repairing vesicovaginal fistulae) to ensure good healing and reduce the risk of recurrence. Finally, extraurethral causes, such as an ectopic ureter, may be responsible for the continuous leakage of urine. The treatment of choice here would be reimplantation of the ureter into the bladder.

Further reading

Abdel-Fattah M, Ford JA, Lim CP, Madhuvrata P. Single-incision mini-slings versus standard midurethral slings in surgical management of female stress urinary incontinence: a meta-analysis of effectiveness and complications. *Eur Urol* 2011; **60**(3):468–80.

Abrams P, Cardozo L, Fall M, *et al.* The standardisation of terminology of lower urinary tract function: report from the Standardisation Sub-committee of the International Continence Society. *Neurourol Urodyn* 2002; **21**:167–78.

Chapple CR, MacDiarmid S. *Urodynamics Made Easy*, 3rd edition. London, UK: Churchill Livingstone, 2009.

Guimaraes M, Oliveira R, Pinto R, Soares A, Maia E, Botelho F, Sousa T, Pina F, Dinis P, Cruz F. Intermediate-term results, up to 4 years, of a bone-anchored male perineal sling for treating male stress urinary incontinence after prostate surgery. *BJU Int* 2009; **103**(4):500–4.

Novara G, Artibani W, Barber MD, *et al.* Updated systematic review and meta-analysis of the comparative data on colposuspensions, pubovaginal slings, and midurethral tapes in the surgical treatment of female stress urinary incontinence. *Eur Urol* 2010; **58**(2):218–38.

Venn SN, Greenwell TJ, Mundy AR. The long-term outcome of artificial urinary sphincters. *J Urol* 2000; **164**(3 Pt 1):702–6.

Ward KL, Hilton P. Tension-free vaginal tape versus colposuspension for primary urodynamic stress incontinence: 5-year follow up. *BJOG* 2008; **115**(2):226–33.

References

1. Abrams P, Cardozo L, Fall M, *et al.* The standardisation of terminology of lower urinary tract function: report from the Standardisation Sub-committee of the International Continence Society. *Neurourol Urodyn* 2002; **21**:167–78.
2. Brooks JD, Chao WM, Kerr J. Male pelvic anatomy reconstructed from the visible human data set. *J Urol* 1998; **159**(3):868–72.
3. Smith PP, van Leijsen SA, Heesakkers JP, Abrams P, Smith AR. Can we, and do we need to, define bladder neck hypermobility and intrinsic sphincteric deficiency? ICI-RS 2011. *Neurourol Urodyn* 2012; **31**(3):309–12.
4. Hampel C, Wienhold D, Benken N, Eggersmann C, Thuroff JW. Definition of overactive bladder and epidemiology of urinary incontinence. *Urology* 1997; **50**:4–14.
5. Subak LL, Waetjen LE, van den Eeden S, Thom DH, Vittinghoff E, Brown JS. Cost of pelvic organ prolapse surgery in the United States. *Obstet Gynecol* 2001; **98**:646–51.

6. Nitti VW. The prevalence of urinary incontinence. *Rev Urol* 2001; 3(Suppl 1):S2–S6.
7. Nygaard I, Barber MD, Burgio KL, *et al.* Prevalence of symptomatic pelvic floor disorders in US women. *JAMA* 2008; **300**:1311–16.
8. Swithinbank LV, Donovan JL, du Heaume JC, *et al.* Urinary symptoms and incontinence in women: relationships between occurrence, age, and perceived impact. *Br J Gen Pract* 1999; **49**:897–900.
9. Sommer P, Bauer T, Nielsen KK, *et al.* Voiding patterns and prevalence of incontinence in women. A questionnaire survey. *Br J Urol* 1990; **66**:12–15.
10. Brown JS, Grady D, Ouslander JG, Herzog AR, Varner RE, Posner SF. Prevalence of urinary incontinence and associated risk factors in postmenopausal women. Heart & Estrogen/Progestin Replacement Study (HERS) Research Group. *Obstet Gynecol* 1999; **94**:66–70.
11. Steinauer JE, Waetjen LE, Vittinghoff E, *et al.* Postmenopausal hormone therapy: does it cause incontinence? *Obstet Gynecol* 2005; **106**:940–5.
12. Hendrix SL, Cochrane BB, Nygaard IE, *et al.* Effects of estrogen with and without progestin on urinary incontinence. *JAMA* 2005; **293**:935–48.
13. Bhatia NN, Bergman A. Urodynamic appraisal of the Bonney test in women with stress urinary incontinence. *Obstet Gynecol* 1983; **62**(6):696–9.
14. Bright E, Drake MJ, Abrams P. Urinary diaries: evidence for the development and validation of diary content, format, and duration. *Neurourol Urodyn* 2011; **30**(3):348–52.
15. Chapple CR, MacDiarmid S. *Urodynamics Made Easy*, 3rd edition. London, UK: Churchill Livingstone, 2009.
16. Mariappan P, Ballantyne Z, N'Dow JM, Alhasso AA. Serotonin and noradrenaline reuptake inhibitors (SNRI) for stress urinary incontinence in adults. *Cochrane Database Syst Rev* 2005 Jul 20;(3):CD004742.
17. Jarvis GJ. Surgery for genuine stress incontinence. *Br J Obstet Gynaecol* 1994; **101**:371–4.
18. Bergman A, Elia G. Three surgical procedures for genuine stress incontinence: five-year follow-up of a prospective randomized study. *Am J Obstet Gynecol* 1995; **173**:66–71.
19. Ward KL, Hilton P. Tension-free vaginal tape versus colposuspension for primary urodynamic stress incontinence: 5-year follow up. BJOG 2008; **115**(2):226–233.
20. Novara G, Artibani W, Barber MD, *et al.* Updated systematic review and meta-analysis of the comparative data on colposuspensions, pubovaginal slings, and midurethral tapes in the surgical treatment of female stress urinary incontinence. *Eur Urol* 2010; **58**(2):218–38.
21. Abdel-Fattah M, Ford JA, Lim CP, Madhuvrata P. Single-incision mini-slings versus standard midurethral slings in surgical management of female stress urinary incontinence: a meta-analysis of effectiveness and complications. *Eur Urol* 2011; **60**(3):468–80.
22. Costa P, Poinas G, Ben NK, *et al.* Long-term results of artificial urinary sphincter for women with type iii stress urinary incontinence. *Eur Urol* 2012; **63**(4):753–8.
23. Chung E, Cartmill RA. 25-year experience in the outcome of artificial urinary sphincter in the treatment of female urinary incontinence. *BJU Int* 2010; **106**(11):1664–7.
24. Guimaraes M, Oliveira R, Pinto R, Soares A, Maia E, Botelho F, Sousa T, Pina F, Dinis P, Cruz F. Intermediate-term results, up to 4 years, of a bone-anchored male perineal sling for treating male stress urinary incontinence after prostate surgery. *BJU Int* 2009; **103**(4):500–4.
25. Venn SN, Greenwell TJ, Mundy AR. The long-term outcome of artificial urinary sphincters. *J Urol* 2000; **164**(3 Pt 1):702–6.
26. Fulford SC, Sutton C, Bales G, Hickling M, Stephenson TP. The fate of the 'modern' artificial urinary sphincter with a follow-up of more than 10 years. *Br J Urol* 1997; **79**(5):713–16.

CHAPTER 3.6

Pelvic organ prolapse

Eduardo Cortes, Mohammed Belal, Arun Sahai, and Roland Morley

Introduction to pelvic organ prolapse

Pelvic organ prolapse (POP) is the downward descent of the pelvic organs through or at the introitus. Prolapse can involve the anterior, middle (apical), or posterior compartment, or a combination of all of them. The anterior compartment (anterior vaginal wall) is the commonest form of POP, and involves the descent of the bladder (cystocoele) and/or urethra (urethrocoele). The middle compartment includes the uterus or the vaginal vault post-hysterectomy. This may involve the small bowel (enterocoele) or large bowel (sigmoidocoele). The posterior compartment represents the rectum (rectocoele), which can also involve the small bowel (rectoenterocoele).

The goal of reconstructive surgery is to restore normal vaginal anatomy in order to address any compartment dysfunction and relieve prolapse symptoms. The estimated lifetime risks of POP surgery have been suggested to be 7% with reoperation rates of up to 30%.[1] A recent study suggested that the lifetime risk of having surgery for POP was 11.8% at 80 years.[2] There are currently controversies regarding the use of mesh in pelvic floor surgery. On the one hand, when using mesh the literature tends to suggest lower prolapse recurrence rates compared to native repairs, but on the other their use has been associated with more complications such as erosion and dyspareunia. There is a paucity of randomized controlled trials in this area. Both the FDA and MHRA have issued guidance on the matter and have encouraged careful patient selection, surgery being performed by appropriately trained surgeons, rigorous patient counselling, regular auditing of procedures, encouraging reporting of adverse events through the different online databases provided by the different professional bodies for each subspecialty.

This chapter will focus on the classification as well as the anatomy, aetiology, presentation, investigations, and management of prolapse affecting the three different compartments. Several techniques of repair are possible in each compartment and therefore the chapter will highlight the principles of surgery, rather than be an exhaustive text of every operation available.

Classification and epedimiology

Grading systems

Several classification methods and grading systems are available to define the extent of the prolapse. Any classification of POP should be reproducible with good interobserver and test-retest reliability. The type of POP can be classified at the site of anatomical prolapse; as an urethrocoele, cystocoele, uterine, or vault enterocoele and rectocele, respectively. The advantage of this classification is its simplicity; however, it is not always clear what viscera underlies the prolapse, especially in the case of previous hysterectomy (vault prolapse). A modification of this classification is to divide the prolapse into anatomical compartments, as defined by whether it is the anterior, apical, or posterior vaginal wall prolapse. The terms are defined in Table 3.6.1 according to the International Continence Society Standardisation Committee.[3]

The stage of prolapse also needs to be established. A commonly used grading system is the Baden-Walker system.[4] This defines the degree of prolapse in relation to a fixed point of the hymen (Fig. 3.6.1). Its simple and easy to use system has led to its common use worldwide, especially in the clinic setting. However, it lacks the degree of precision necessary for use in research.

The POP-Q scoring system was first introduced by the International Continence Society (ICS) to standardize the grading of urogenital prolapse with an objective, reproducible site-specific system. Nine measurements (in cm) are made of the position of the midline vaginal structures in relation to the hymenal ring. These are measured while the patient performs a Valsalva manoevre and

Table 3.6.1 International Continence Society (ICS) definitions of pelvic organ prolapse

	ICS definitions
Pelvic organ prolapse	Descent of one or more of: the anterior vaginal wall, the posterior vaginal wall, and the apex of the vagina (cervix/uterus) or vault (cuff) after hysterectomy
Anterior vaginal wall prolapse	Descent of the anterior vagina so that the urethrovesical junction (a point 3 cm proximal to the external urinary meatus) or any anterior point proximal to this is less than 3 cm above the plane of the hymen
Prolapse of the apical segment of the vagina	Descent of the vaginal cuff scar (after hysterectomy) or cervix, below a point which is 2 cm less than the total vaginal length above the plane of the hymen
Posterior vaginal wall prolapse	Descent of the posterior vaginal wall so that a midline point on the posterior vaginal wall 3 cm above the level of the hymen or any posterior point proximal to this, is less than 3 cm above the plane of the hymen

Reprinted from the *American Journal of Obstetrics and Gynecology*, Volume 187, Issue 1, Abrams P, *et al.*, The standardisation of terminology of lower urinary tract function: Report from the Standardisation Sub-committee of the International Continence Society, pp. 116–2, Copyright © 2002 Wiley-Liss, Inc. This material is used by permission of Wiley-Liss, Inc, a subsidiary of John Wiley & Sons, Inc. Published by Mosby, Inc. All rights reserved., with permission from Elsevier, http://www.sciencedirect.com/science/journal/00029378

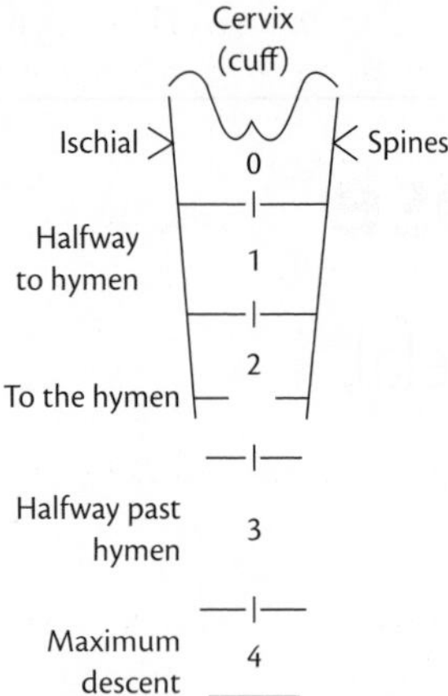

Fig. 3.6.1 Baden-Walker halfway system. Consists of four grades: grade 0—no prolapse; grade 1—halfway to hymen; grade 2—to hymen; grade 3—halfway past hymen; grade 4—maximum descent.

Reproduced with permission from Baden WF, Walker TA, Lindsey JH. The vaginal profile. *Texas Medicine*. 1968 May; 64(5):56–8. PubMed PMID: Copyright © 1968 Texas Medical Association.

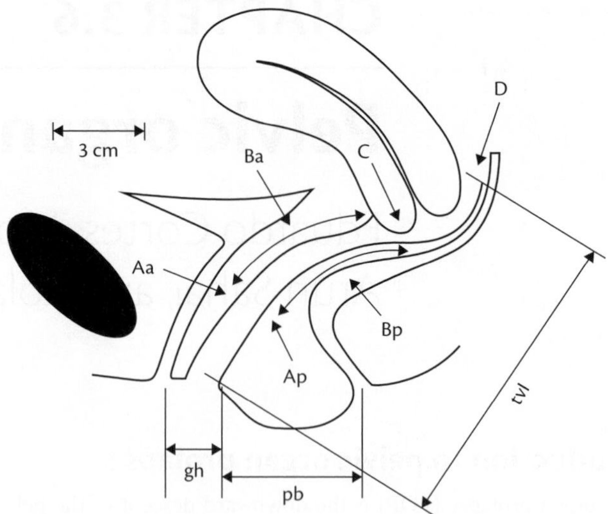

Fig. 3.6.2 Points and landmarks for POP-Q system examination.

Point description range of values

Aa anterior vaginal wall 3 cm proximal to the hymen -3 cm to +3 cm
Ba Most distal position of the remaining upper anterior vaginal wall -3 cm to +tvl
C Most distal edge of cervix or vaginal cuff scar
D Posterior fornix (N/A if post-hysterectomy)
Ap Posterior vaginal wall 3 cm proximal to the hymen -3 cm to +3 cm
Bp Most distal position of the remaining upper posterior vaginal wall -3 cm to + tvl
Genital hiatus (gh) Measured from middle of external urethral meatus to posterior midline hymen
Perineal body (pb) Measured from posterior margin of gh to middle of anal opening
Total vaginal length (tvl) Depth of vagina when point D or C is reduced to normal position

POP-Q staging criteria

Stage 0 Aa, Ap, Ba, Bp = −3 cm and C or D ≤—(tvl—2) cm
Stage I Stage 0 criteria not met and leading edge <-1 cm
Stage II Leading edge ≥-1 cm but ≤1 cm
Stage III Leading edge >+1 cm but <+ (tvl—2) cm
Stage IV Leading edge ≥+ (tvl—2) cm

Reprinted from *American Journal of Obstetrics and Gynecology*, Volume 1, Issue 8, Richard C. Bump *et al.*, 'The standardization of terminology of female pelvic organ prolapse and pelvic floor dysfunction', pp. 10–17, Copyright © 1996 Mosby, Inc., with permission from Elsevier, http://www.sciencedirect.com/science/journal/00029378

recorded in a three-by-three table.[5] This has become the standardized tool for documenting and communicating clinical findings and surgical outcomes (Fig. 3.6.2). However, its use is not yet routine as it is perceived as time-consuming, leaving its main role as a research tool when developing or comparing different surgical techniques. The different stages of the POP-Q are defined in Table 3.6.2.[6]

Risk factors

The prevalence of POP as defined by a sensation of a lump within the vagina is approximately between 5% to 10% in population-based studies. The most common vaginal prolapse is the anterior compartment, followed by the posterior and apical compartments.[7]

Under physiological conditions (pre-prolapse) the levator ani muscles and the endopelvic fascia provide support by forming a dome-like configuration, which prevents the descent of the pelvic viscera. The aetiology of POP is multifactorial and can be attributed to both predisposing and triggering factors. Predisposing factors include neuropathic and muscular conditions, congenital prolapse, abnormal collagen, obesity, and postmenopause. Triggering factors include pregnancy, vaginal delivery, and obstetric injury, chronic conditions increasing intra-abdominal pressure (constipation, chronic obstructive pulmonary disease), and physical activities requiring heavy lifting.[8] Patient awareness of the risk factors may contribute to prevent or delay the onset of prolapse symptoms.

Anterior vaginal wall prolapse

Anatomy and physiology

The vagina is a fibromuscular cylinder, of variable length, between 7 to 10 cm providing anatomical support for urination, defecation, coital, and reproductive functions. The middle of the anterior vagina is normally in opposition with the posterior wall. The anterior wall is shorter than the posterior wall by a few centimetres, with the cervix making the shortfall.

The different pelvic viscera supported by the vagina are kept in place by a combination of pelvic muscles and fascia, and their attachments to the pelvic side wall. The most relevant muscle structure in the pelvis is the levator ani muscle (LAM). This is divided into three different groups (iliococcigeous, pubococcigeous, and puborectalis) and is attached laterally to the obturator internus through the arcus tendineous levator muscle. The anterior vaginal wall is supported by an underlying fascia called the pubocervical

Table 3.6.2 Pelvic organ prolapse quantification system (POP-Q)

Stage	Definition
0	No prolapse
1	Most distal portion of prolapse greater than 1 cm above hymen
2	Most distal portion of prolapse less and equal to 1 cm proximal or distal to hymen
3	Most distal portion of prolapse greater than 1 cm below hymen but less than 2 cm of total vaginal length
4	Complete eversion of total vaginal length

Reprinted from the *American Journal of Obstetrics and Gynecology*, Volume 175, Issue 6, Hall AF *et al.*, Interobserver and intraobserver reliability of the proposed International Continence Society, Society of Gynecologic Surgeons, and American Urogynecologic Society pelvic organ prolapse classification system, pp. 1467–70, Copyright © 1996 Mosby, Inc., with permission from Elsevier, http://www.sciencedirect.com/science/journal/00029378

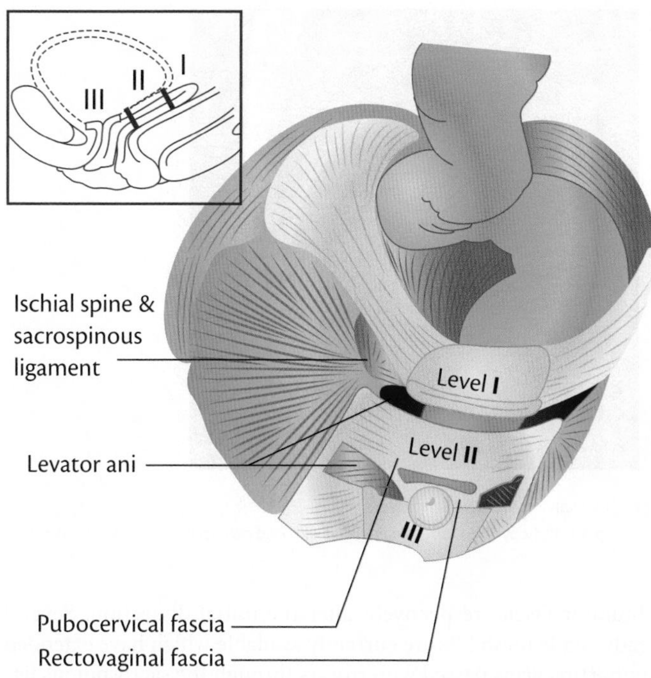

Fig. 3.6.3 Levels of support expressed as DeLancey's biomechanical levels: level I, proximal suspension; level II, lateral attachment; level III, distal fusion.

Reprinted from the *American Journal of Obstetrics and Gynecology*, Volume 6, Issue 1, DeLancey J. O., 'Anatomic aspects of vaginal eversion after hysterectomy', pp. 1717–24, Copyright © 1992 Mosby, Inc., with permission from Elsevier, http://www.sciencedirect.com/science/journal/00029378

fascia, which is a downward extension of the endopelvic fascia containing elastin fibres, collagen, and smooth muscle. It can be divided into perivesical (bladder base) and periurethral fascia (bladder neck). Its lateral insertion to the pelvic side wall is through the arcus tendineous fascia pelvis (ATFP).

Advances in imaging of the pelvis over the past two decades have contributed to a better understanding of the female pelvic anatomy. DeLancey has described three levels of support within the vagina (Fig. 3.6.3).[9] The apical support of the vagina is provided by the endopelvic fascia, and the cardinal and uterosacral ligaments (level I support). The middle anterior vagina wall is attached laterally to the pelvic side wall through the ATFP as described above (level II support). Finally, level III provides the urethral support and is formed of fascia and muscular attachments. The fascial attachments connect the periurethral tissues and anterior vaginal wall to the ATFP, while the muscular attachments connect the periurethral tissues to the medial border of the LAM. This configuration of muscles and fascia are responsible for keeping the bladder neck in its physiological position (3 cm above the inferior aspect of the pubic bone). Damage to any of the supporting structures will lead to anterior vaginal wall prolapse, which can be associated with stress urinary incontinence when level III is also affected.

Aetiology

Damage to any of the structures involved directly or indirectly in the provision of anterior vaginal wall support will lead to prolapse. This can carry within it the herniation of the bladder and urethra, associated with or without urethral hypermobility and stress urinary incontinence. Defects in the pubocervical fascia have been described as attenuation defects (distension injury), tears (central, apical, or lateral), or a combination of both. In the presence of intact lateral supports, surgical repair of an attenuation injury is usually achieved by performing an anterior colporrhaphy. When a tear in the pubocervical fascia is identified, usually by the loss of epithelial rugae, the surgeon will perform a site-specific repair in an attempt to close the anatomical defect. This particular technique has been approached both vaginally and laparoscopically.

Symptoms and presentation

Like any other vaginal prolapse, patients can present with both anatomical and/or functional symptoms. However, the only consistent and specific symptom associated with POP is the sensation of a vaginal bulge, while urinary symptoms can include overactive bladder symptoms, urinary stress incontinence, voiding difficulties, or a combination of these.

Evaluation

The most important aspect of the clinical assessment is to perform a pelvic examination to determine the site and extent of the prolapse. This traditionally is performed in the left lateral position with the use of a Sims speculum. During the examination, the posterior compartment is retracted to assess the anterior vagina wall descent during a Valsalva maneouvre. This can also be repeated for the assessment of the posterior vaginal wall by retracting the anterior vaginal wall. The apical compartment can also be assessed with a Cusco speculum, which is gradually withdrawn as the patient performes a Valsalva maneuvre. Stress urinary incontinence needs to be assessed with a full bladder, asking the patient to cough at the time of examination. In the presence of bladder overactivity, the patient should be assessed using a bladder diary, urine dipstick, and post-void residuals if voiding difficulties are also present. It is recommended that patients presenting with any vaginal compartmental prolapse associated with urinary symptoms (both stress urinary incontinence (SUI) and/or overactive bladder) should undergo urodynamic investigations to establish a preoperative diagnosis. In cases where a degree of urethral kinking is suspected by the prolapse (grade 3 and 4), urodynamics should be performed with a ring pessary in situ to assess for occult urodynamic stress incontinence.

Overactive bladder in the absence of significant post-void residuals should be treated empirically before considering urodynamics. If symptoms persist despite treatment, urodynamic tests are recommended. The use of imaging (both ultrasound and MRI) is limited but can play a role in patients with recurrent and complex prolapse (vault prolapse), as it can help identify the prolapsing viscera (Fig. 3.6.4).

Management

Conservative treatment

Common to any mild pelvic floor prolapse, pelvic floor exercises (PFE) and topical oestrogens may be indicated for symptom relief.[10] While the evidence for the use of PFE is limited, it remains a reasonable initial step. Vaginal pessaries are an alternative to surgery for more severe prolapse with a wide variety of shapes, sizes, and textures available. Generally, the use of vaginal pessaries is also indicated for those patients medically unfit for surgery or who require temporary relief during the postnatal period or prior to surgery. Pessaries can be either supportive (e.g. ring peassary) or space occupying (e.g. Gelhorn), with the former being the most commonly used, while the latter is usually indicated in severe multicompartmental prolapse with increased genital hiatus.

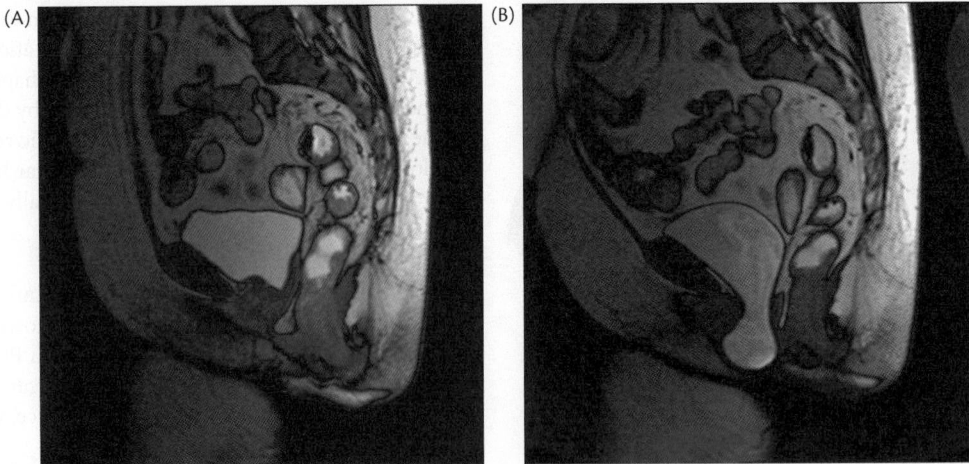

Fig. 3.6.4 MRI pelvis demonstrating anterior compartment prolapse: (A) at rest; and (B) with Valsalva maneuvre employed.

Figures first appeared in Belal M, Morley R., Pelvic Organ Prolapse Repair, *Urology News*, Volume 16, Issue 1, pp. 10–12, Copyright © 2011. Reproduced with kind permission of Pinpoint Scotland Ltd and Miss Tamsin Greenwell.

Contraindications for pessary insertion include the presence of a vaginal fistula and ureterovaginal erosions. The patient should be aware that there could be limitations during sexual intercourse, although younger patients usually can learn to remove and self-insert the ring pessary. The patient should be able to void and carry out normal activities without discomfort or spontaneous expulsion. The pessary should be initially reviewed at three months and then at six-monthly intervals to check for vaginal erosions or other complications. Any vaginal bleeding occurring while using a vaginal pessary should be promptly investigated to rule other sources of bleeding (endometrial, cervical). The evidence about the effectiveness of ring pessaries for the management of vaginal prolapse is limited. A Cochrane review in 2004 did not find any randomized trials of pessary use in women.[11]

Techniques for surgical repair

Indications

The main indications for surgical management include symptomatic POP and failure of conservative measures. Young patients should complete their family ideally prior to POP repair as future pregnancy could disrupt the restored anatomy and function.

Anterior colporrhaphy

This is the treatment of choice for anterior repair in a published survey of gynaecologists in the United Kingdom.[7] All vaginal surgery requires the patient in the lithotomy position with good field exposure (either by using a lone star retractor or at least two assistants). Hydrodissection of the anterior vaginal wall is performed with a mixture of local anaesthesia and adrenaline. A vertical incision is made between the bladder neck down to the vagina apex or cervix. The vagina is dissected from the pubocervical fascia with a combination of sharp and blunt dissection using a wet gauze. This is performed laterally to the vaginal sulci and proximally to the cervix or vaginal vault. Fascial plication with multiple mattress sutures or a purse string is performed with 2/0 to 0 disolvable sutures. A post-procedure cystoscopy is performed in large prolapse or when there are any concerns about the ureters in the plication.

Biological/synthetic mesh

Anterior colporrhaphy with graft (biological or synthetic) sutured to the cardinal, uterosacral ligaments, endopelvic fascia, and obturator fascia, respectively, after the initial dissection. Several ready-made mesh kits are currently available which have extended supporting arms passed with trocars through the sacrospinous ligament and obturator foramen. A recent Cochrane review update suggested that native tissue repair was associated with more failures than polypropylene mesh, but there were no differences in subjective outcomes, quality of life, reoperation rates, or rates of de novo dyspareunia/stress urinary incontinence between groups.[12] However, due to the recent statements by the FDA and MHRA, raising concerns about the indiscrimanate use of prosthetic mesh repairs in vaginal surgery is uncertain.

Paravaginal repair

Paravaginal repair can be approached laparoscopically, abdominally, or vaginally. The abdominal approach is usually a Pfannesteil or lower midline incision. The retroperitoneal space of Retzius is opened and lateral dissection of the bladder from the pelvic side wall is performed. A suture is passed through the anterolateral vagina to the obturator fascia at the arcus tendinous fascia pelvis. This restores the level II support.

Complications

Complications include bleeding (with increased risk if other procedures are taking place concomitantly); infection (increased risk with biological and mesh material); bladder/ureteric/urethral injury (cystoscopy is advised if there are any concerns); dyspareunia; erosion (if mesh used); and lower urinary tract symptoms (de novo storage and voiding symptoms).

Results and evidence base

Anterior colporrhaphy has published success rates that vary considerably from 57% in randomized controlled trials to 100% in case series.[13] What determines success is highly variable in the published literature. The success rates are likely to lie between these two figures. Due to the significant recurrence rate with anterior colporrhaphy, there has been a trend towards the use of mesh. Indeed, the use of polyglactin mesh has been shown to reduce failure rate compared to anterior colporrhaphy alone.[14] However, significant mesh-associated complications have positioned their role mainly into recurrent anterior vaginal prolapse in the United Kindom, where currently mesh is being used in 11% of primary repairs and 56% in recurrent prolapse.[15] The fourth International Consultation on Incontinence has stated that despite level I evidence that the use of polypropylene mesh overlay results in better anatomical reconstruction than traditional repairs, it should be tempered with level II and III evidence of significant functional issues.[8] The FDA stated 'serious complications associated with surgical mesh for transvaginal repair of POP are not rare'. This is a change from what the FDA previously reported on in 2008. Furthermore, it is not clear that transvaginal POP repair with mesh is more effective than traditional non-mesh repair in all patients with POP and it may expose patients to greater risk. Paravaginal surgery success rates quoted are from 67% to 100%, but with a relatively higher complication rate than anterior colporrhaphy via the vaginal approach. A recently published Cochrane review (2016) on the use of mesh versus native tissue concluded that although there are lower recurrent prolapse rates after mesh surgery, these patients are more likely to require further surgery due to urinary incontinence problems or mesh exposure.[16]

The value of prophylactic continence procedures in continent patients with POP on the evidence currently available remains uncertain. This decision must be made with careful counselling of the patient. The Cochrane review on POP surgery stated that continence surgery at the time of prolapse surgery in continent women did not significantly reduce the rate of postoperative SUI.[17] A randomized controlled trial of the use of a mid-urethral tape at the time of anterior compartment repair demonstrated a reduction of incontinence at 12 months (27% vs. 43%), but at the cost of increased adverse events.[18]

Conclusion

The surgical repair of anterior wall prolapse requires careful clinical assessment. Modifiable risk factors need to be addressed with preoperative counselling, and the appropriate surgical technique used for the type of prolapse to be corrected. Mesh use in the vagina remains controversial, and in most of the United Kingdom (with the exception of Scotland where they have been completely withdrawn) it is more often used in the setting of recurrent POP following careful discussion with patients about potential intra- and postoperative complications. Practice in this regard widely differs around the world.

Posterior vaginal wall prolapse

Anatomy and physiology

The posterior vaginal wall is formed by a complex network of muscles, fascia, and nerve supply, interconnected to provide support to the pelvic viscera as well as the necessary control during defecation. The rectovaginal septum (RVS), also known as Denonvillier's fascia is the main anatomical structure inter-connecting these three levels of the posterior vaginal wall. It has been described as a dense layer of tissue present between the rectum and vagina, consisting of elastin fibres, collagen, and smooth muscle, consistent with its endopelvic fascia origin.[19,20] At the most apical aspect (level I) of the vaginal support, the RVS is attached to the cervical ring and endopelvic fascia through the cardinal and uterosacral ligaments. Laterally (level II) is attached to the fascia overlying the LAM (arcus tendineous fascia pelvis). Inferiorly (level III), the RVS is attached to the perineal body,[21] a pyramidal structure allocated between the vagina and anus. Like the hub of a wheel, this serves as a confluence point for the superficial perineal muscles, the bulbocavernosus muscle, the puborectalis part of the LAM, and the external anal sphincter (see Fig. 3.6.5).

The LAM, as the main muscle structure embracing the three vaginal compartments, is formed by three portions: ileococcigeous,

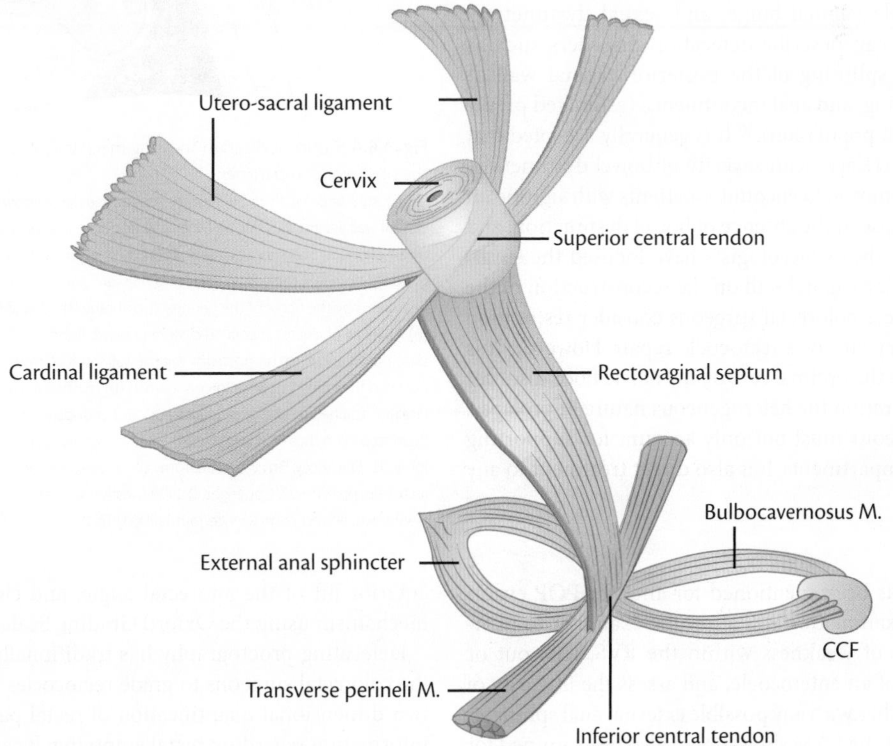

Fig. 3.6.5 Rectovaginal septum and its attachments.

pubococcigeous, and puborectalis, and provides essential anatomical and functional stability to the posterior vaginal wall.[22,23] Its innervation has been dually described between branches of the pudendal nerve and direct nerve supply from the S2-5 spinal roots, known as the levator ani nerve.[24] Contraction of its fibres has two direct actions on the posterior compartment: it provides the horizontal plane (levator plate) on which the pelvic viscera lie; and it contributes, in combination with the RVS, to form a flap valve mechanism which provides the upper level of continence of the external anal sphincter complex.[23] During resting, the puborectalis muscle closes the genital hiatus creating a nearly 90 degree angle between the anal and rectal canals (anorectal angle),[25] also contributing to anal continence. This is summarized in Figure 3.6.6.

Aetiology

Injury to the above structures, whether it is the result of an acute episode (pregnancy, childbirth, or obstetric injury), or cumulative as a result of chronic increase of intra-abdominal pressure (chronic obstructive pulmonary disease, obesity, or chronic constipation) or the combination of both, may lead to anatomical prolapse and/or bowel dysfunction. Herniation of the rectum through the lower aspect of the posterior vaginal wall (usually resulting from the detachment of the RVS from the perineal body), or a peritoneal sac at a higher level containing sigmoid colon or small bowel (where the RVS is attached to the cervical ring) may originate a rectocoele or an enterocoele, respectively, or a combination of both (rectoenterocoele).

Symptoms and presentation

It is important at this stage for clinicians to differentiate between motility disorders and obstructive conditions, as the former will respond better to biofeedback and dietary changes. Patients can present with a history of widening of the genital hiatus, perineal laxity/descent, palpable vaginal bulge, and sexual dysfunction. Additionally, patients can describe defecation disorders such as chronic constipation, splinting of the posterior vaginal wall or digitations, stool trapping, and anal incontinence (estimated prevalence of 7% in the adult population).[26] It is generally accepted that severity of prolapse correlates with severity of bowel dysfunction. However, it is not uncommon to encounter patients with significant posterior vaginal prolapse in the absence of bowel dysfunction, and vice versa.[27] Traditionally, gynaecologists have focused the surgical repair of the posterior vaginal wall on the reconstruction of the altered anatomy, whereas colorectal surgeons consider restoration of function the primary aim of a rectocoele repair. However, it is currently accepted that the optimal care of any pelvic floor disorder must take into consideration the heterogeneous nature of prolapse. Therefore, pelvic surgeons must not only account for supporting defects in different compartments, but also direct treatment to any associated symptoms.

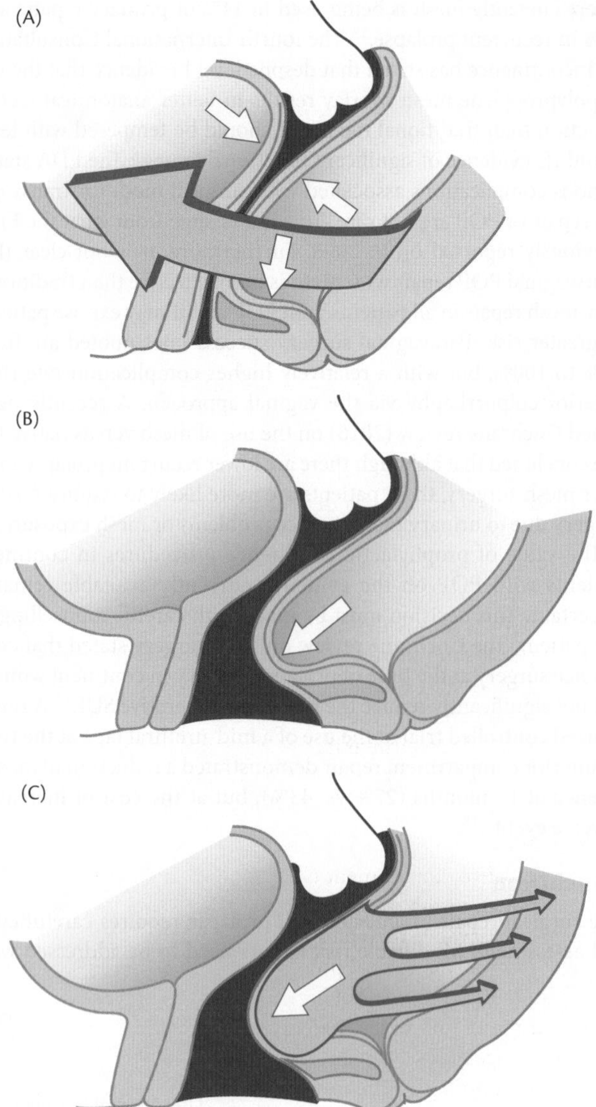

Fig. 3.6.6 Concept diagram showing mechanics of support and continence of the posterior compartment.

(A) Closure of pelvic floor by puborectalis muscle (large arrow) that compresses posterior vaginal wall against anterior wall. Increases in abdominal pressure result in balanced pressure on anterior and posterior vaginal walls (arrows) so that no net force on support results. Caudally, however, there is no balancing pressure, and force results (dashed arrow), which must be resisted by the fibres of the perineal membrane (shaded area) of perineal body.

(B) Absence of levator-mediated closure of pelvic floor. Increases in rectal pressure are unopposed and force on posterior vaginal wall results (arrow).

(C) Level II supports oppose force shown in (B) (dashed arrow) by their upward dorsal tension (arrows attached to posterior vaginal wall and endopelvic fascia).

Reprinted from the *American Journal of Obstetrics and Gynecology*, Volume 180, Issue 4, John O.L. DeLancey, 'Structural anatomy of the posterior pelvic compartment as it relates to rectocele', pp. 815–23, Copyright © 1999 Mosby, Inc., with permission from Elsevier, http://www.sciencedirect.com/science/journal/00029378

Evaluation

In addition to what has been mentioned for anterior POP evaluation, a rectovaginal examination will allow the examiner to identify defects and areas of weakness within the RVS, rule out or confirm the presence of an enterocoele, and assess the integrity of the perineal body together with any possible external anal sphincter defects. The integrity of the LAM sling should also be examined for tone of the muscle complex, duration of contraction (endurance), anterior lift of the anorectal angle, and closure of the flap valve mechanism using the Oxford Grading Scale (see Table 3.6.3).

Defecating proctography has traditionally been used mainly by the colorectal surgeons to grade rectocoeles anteriorly. It provides a two-dimensional quantification of rectal parameters and dynamic information regarding rectal emptying. It can also be used to investigate rectal intussusception or pelvic dyssynergy. Traditionally,

Table 3.6.3 Muscle strength grading scale (Oxford scale)

0/5	No contraction
1/5	Visible/palpable muscle contraction but no movement
2/5	Movement with gravity eliminated
3/5	Movement against gravity only
4/5	Movement against gravity with some resistance
5/5	Movement against gravity with full resistance

Reproduced from Laycock, J & Holmes, D, The place of physiotherapy in the management of pelvic floor dysfunction, *The Obstetrician & Gynaecologist*, 2003, Vol 5 No 4, with permission from Wiley and Sons.

surgical repair has been advocated when the radiographic rectocele exceeds 3 cm in depth, if there is significant barium trapping, or there is digital assistance to defecate.[28,29] However, several studies have shown poor correlation between outcome of rectocoele repair, symptoms, and extent of barium trapping.[30,31] Dynamic MRI defecography has more recently become an alternative to defecography, as it provides a broader anatomical evaluation of the different pelvic floor compartments and their interaction, it is less invasive, and avoids radiation exposure. However, when both tests have been compared, the use of dynamic MRI defecography did not change clinical decision-making, despite costing ten times more.[32]

Management

Conservative treatment

The conservative management of a posterior vaginal wall prolapse will be guided by the presence or absence of bowel dysfunction. Whereas conservative therapies play a very limited role in the management of pure anatomical prolapse, this is not the case in bowel dysfunction. In the absence of bowel dysfunction, pelvic floor exercises, and the use of topical oestrogen in the presence of atrophic vaginal changes may provide some degree of symptom relief in cases of mild prolapse. The use of ring pessaries (both supportive and space occupying) is restricted to those with larger prolapse who are not suitable for surgery, or to evaluate symptom improvement prior to surgery. In the presence of bowel dysfunction associated with pelvic outlet symptoms, biofeedback is the first-line treatment option, although there is still controversy over the criteria and testing that should be used when selecting patients. However, some studies have suggested that the patient's compliance, motivation, and success with biofeedback is mostly dependent on the skill of the therapist.[33,34]

Techniques for surgical repair

Several surgical techniques have been advocated to anatomically restore the posterior vaginal compartment.

Posterior colporrhaphy

Posterior colporrhaphy with or without plication of the LAM in the midline is the most commonly performed procedure. Following a vertical incision of the posterior vaginal wall, dissection of the RVS is first carried out laterally to the medial margins of the puborectalis muscle. At this point, the RVS is plicated in the midline using dissolvable sutures. It was not until 1987 that this surgical technique was evaluated for bowel dysfunction,[35] with anatomical cure results being reported in the range of 70–90%.[36] However, for functional

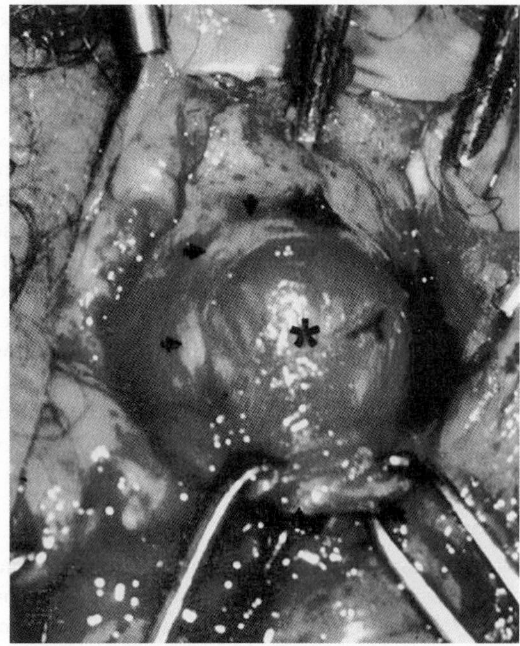

Fig. 3.6.7 A surgical photograph showing a central defect in the rectovaginal septum (asterisk) and the margin of the septum all around (arrowheads). The inferior edge of the septum is grasped with Allis forceps.

Reprinted from K. Singh, E. Cortes, and W. Reid, 'Evaluation of the Fascial Technique for Surgical Repair of Isolated Posterior Vaginal Wall Prolapse', *Obstetrics and Gynecology*, Volume 101, Issue 2, pp. 320–324, Copyright © 2003, with permission from Wolters Kluwer Health.

improvement the results are less encouraging, with de novo dyspareunia (17%) being an important postoperative complication.[37]

Site-specific repair of fascial defects has gained acceptance within the last decade. Although the initial technique is similar to classical colporrhaphy, the main aim of the surgery is to identify and repair any tears present in the RVS (Fig. 3.6.7). These are usually identified at the insertion of the RVS with the perineal body, cervical ring, or on their lateral attachments to the levator muscles. Plication of the levator muscle is avoided, as interposition of the levators between the vagina and rectum is perceived as non-anatomical, whereas perineorrhaphy is performed concomitantly in the presence of a deficient perineum. Anatomical success has been reported at 80–90%, with improvement in bowel function and lower rates of de novo dyspareunia.[38,39]

The Transanal rectocoele repair, mainly associated with obstructed defecation, was first described in the 1960s[40] and is mostly performed by colorectal surgeons as many of their patients have additional anorectal pathology such as haemorrhoids. It is designed for low or distal anterior rectocoeles as described by defecography studies and should be avoided in the presence of an enterocoele. The surgical technique involves a U-shaped or T incision made transanally just above the dentate line. A mucosal flap is raised, dissected from the RVS, and excised. Plication of the RVS from the rectal side includes the anterior rectal musculature, with the mucosa and submucosa being closed in a separate layer. One of the main complications of this technique is *de novo* faecal incontinence, reported as high as 38%, although the aetiology behind it is not clear.[35] More recently, treatment of obstructive defecation in the presence of rectoanal intussusception using stapled transanal rectal resection (STARR) has been advocated as an alternative to the traditional transrectal approaches.[41]

Laparoscopic ventral rectopexy has gained acceptability for the treatment of obstructed defecation/intussusception with or without prolapse. It involves opening the rectovaginal space and dissecting inferiorly to the perineal body. The RVS defects can be repaired and then resutured to the perineal body. A prosthetic mesh is then fixed to the deep ventral aspect of the rectum. The posterior vaginal fornix is also attached to the mesh, which is fixed beneath the sacral promontory with either sutures, screws, staples, or a tacking device. It facilitates addressing adjuvant problems such as perineal descent, vault prolapse, and enterocoele at the same time, and the patient experiences a more rapid recovery. Complications described include faecal impaction (4%), wound infection (2%), bleeding (2%), leak (1%), and retention (1%).[42] Disadvantages of this procedure include the need for surgical expertise in minimal access surgery, an extended learning curve, and increased operating time.

Conclusion

Posterior vaginal wall prolapse is an evolving area for pelvic floor surgeons. Predicting those patients who may benefit from conservative and/or surgical treatment remains a challenge for clinicians who require a detailed understanding of the anatomy of the posterior compartment, as well as the differential diagnosis of defecatory and sexual dysfunction. The literature available to date is mainly comprised of retrospective cases and usually with small numbers. Research is needed to assess the pre-and postoperative clinical changes from both anatomical and functional perspectives overall.

Apical compartment prolapse

This section will discuss uterine prolapse and post-hysterectomy vaginal vault prolapse, in addition to associated descent of the apical compartment of the vagina. It is less common for there to be an isolated apical defect in contrast to multicompartment defects. In recent times, there has been a move towards uterine preservation. However, there are several important factors which will influence the type of procedure performed for symptomatic apical prolapse, such as concomitant pathology, age, completion of family, sexual function, patient choice, and hysterectomy risk of early menopause, vaginal access, and previous surgery. Occasionally an obliterative procedure (colpocleisis) can be considered for those patients too fragile to tolerate surgery or with repeated prolapse surgery failure, who are not sexually active.

Anatomy and aetiology

The anatomy of the supporting structures of the vagina has already been discussed in detail in this chapter. Loss of integrity in level I support, as described by DeLancey, is instrumental in the development of apical compartment prolapse. In the case of vaginal vault prolapse, this is related to attenuation of the cardinal/uterosacral ligament complex following excision during hysterectomy, separation of the pubocervical fascia from the rectovaginal fascia, and separation of these fascia from the cardinal/uterosacral ligament complex.[9] The apex is the centrepiece of pelvic organ support and thus this must be assessed, regardless of the presence or absence of the uterus. In the absence of the normal support structures to the uterus or the vaginal cuff, the anterior and posterior compartments of the vagina are exposed to intra-abdominal forces that may lead to other compartmental prolapse.[13] Anterior compartment prolapse is strongly associated with apical prolapse, and surgery for anterior defects usually requires concomitant repair of the apex.[43]

The anatomy of the sacrospinous ligament and its surrounding structures are required in order to safely perform sacrospinous fixation. The sacrospinous ligament runs from the ischial spine to the lower part of the sacrum/coccyx. Pudendal nerves and vessels lie medial and posterior to the ischial spine, while superiorly and behind the ligament are the inferior gluteal vessels and the hyogastric venous plexus.

Similarly, one must take precaution when placing the mesh over the sacrum during sacrocolpopexy. The anatomy in this area must be understood to prevent potentially life-threatening haemorrhage. The left common iliac vein, which lies medial to the artery, as well as the presacral veins and the median sacral artery and vein are at risk during mesh fixation. Further knowledge of the pathway of the ureters—particularly the right ureter—is required. During surgery, this needs to be identified to avoid inadvertent injury.

Symptoms and presentation

Similar to all POP, apical compartment prolapse can present with symptoms related to pressure, pain, or an obvious bulge. Furthermore, depending on the extent of POP interference with the bowel, urine, and sexual function may occur. To help in its management, one must determine the degree of bother or quality of life impact of the POP. This information can be obtained from a careful history or by using validated questionnaires such as the Pelvic Floor Distress Inventory (PFDI), POP Impact Questionnaire (POPIQ), or the International Consultation on Incontinence Vaginal Symptoms questionnaire (ICI-VS).

Evaluation

Apical or middle compartment prolapse (both uterine and vault prolpase) can represent the most challenging compartment prolapse to identify. For example, it is rare that the anterior vaginal compartment presents as a sole compartment prolapse because it is frequently attached to a degree of prolapse of the middle compartment. Missing this at the time of examination leads to a partial repair of the problem, contributing to the high recurrence rates seen following a single anterior compartment prolapse repair. It can be helpful to look for the hysterectomy scar in cases of vault prolapse. Furthermore, with the aid of the examiner's fingers placed at the apex during a Valsalva maneuvre, one can try and reproduce what was found during speculum examination. The apex is best visualized using a Cusco speculum and asking the patient to perform Valsalva while it is slowly removed from the vagina. As previously described with the anterior compartment, an enterocoele (protrusion of the small intestines and peritoneum into the vaginal canal) is not typically treated as a separate disorder, because most patients with enterocoele also have significant prolapse of other compartments. An isolated enterocoele repair rarely corrects all prolapse symptoms and usually additional support procedures are needed.

It is important to assess for SUI and other lower urinary tract symptoms. In patients with symptomatic SUI, a concomitant continence procedure can be performed. However, in cases where no SUI or even if occult SUI is demonstrated, some surgeons would prefer to perform prolapse surgery first and then later assess whether significant SUI has developed before considering a second-stage continence procedure. This is a controversial area and preoperative urodynamics will help in the decision-making process and help to counsel patients.

Management

Conservative treatment

Conservative measures include weight reduction, PFE (Kegel's exercises), and pessaries. The type of pessary used will depend on two main factors: the degree of apical prolapse, and the integrity of the pelvic outlet. In cases of mild prolapse, a ring pessary is suitable. However, in those with more significant prolapse or a poorly supported introitus, a space-filling pessary is more suitable such as a Gelhorn or Cube.[44]

Techniques for surgical repair

The goals of reconstructive pelvic surgery are to restore anatomy, maintain or restore normal bowel and bladder function, and maintain vaginal capacity for sexual intercourse, if desired.[45]

Vaginal hysterectomy

This is performed for symptomatic and significant uterine prolapse. One of the advantages of the vaginal approach as opposed to the abdominal one is the possibility of performing the surgery under regional anaesthetic block. Indirectly this has made the operation more accessible to women regardless of age and associated medical co-morbidities. The technique itself involves a pericervical incision, access to the peritoneal cavity either through the Pouch of Douglas or through the uterovesical fold, and the division of the different supportive and vascular uterine pedicles in a down-upwards fashion. In order to prevent a future vaginal vault prolapse, the surgeon usually performs a McCall culdoplasty at the same time (see below). Another advantage of the vaginal approach is the possibility to repair any other concomitant vaginal prolapse identified at the time of surgery.

The postoperative recovery from surgery is significantly shorter compared to other gynaecological surgeries, with 60% of women reporting normal activities within a week of their operation.[46] Women also report an increase in their sexual activity (20%) and a reduction in overactive bladder symptoms (50%). Severe intraoperative and postoperative complications are rare (3%) and mainly in the form of intra-abdominal bleed or vaginal vault haematoma. However, it is not uncommon to develop urinary stress incontinence following vaginal hysterectomy, and surgeons are advised to rule out occult SUI in the presence of urinary symptoms prior to surgery.

McCall's modified culdoplasty

This technique involves running sutures from one uterosacral ligament, through the posterior peritoneum, and then to the contralateral uterosacral ligament. A further absorbable suture is run in a similar fashion, but through the posterior vaginal wall. When the sutures are tied, it results in a high closure of the peritoneal cul-de-sac and the associated enterocoele with an attachment of the vaginal apex to the distal endopelvic fascia, which provides apical support and an increase in vaginal length.[45] The procedure helps to prevent future vault prolapse and was the procedure of choice in one study comparing three different techniques after hysterectomy.[47] The ureters tend to be placed 1–2 cm lateral to the uterosacral ligaments at the level of the cervix, and so caution must be taken not to take or kink the ureter with the sutures.

Sacrospinous fixation

This is the commonest apical suspension procedure performed through the vagina and is typically performed for vault prolapse post-hysterectomy and vaginal enterocoele. However, it can be performed with vaginal hysterectomy, or as a unilateral or bilateral hysteropexy. The procedure involves the placement of two to four sutures through (as opposed to around) the sacrospinous ligament and 3 cm medial to the ischial spine to avoid vessel or nerve injury. The placement of sutures can be helped with the use of a suture deploying device. The type of suture is debatable, but can be slowly absorbing or non-absorbable. The procedure is often accompanied by anterior or posterior compartment repairs and reduction of enterocoele. The dissection is typically through a posterior approach, but can be anterior. The procedure is depicted in Figure 3.6.8.

Anterior recurrence is more common than apical recurrence and success rates in relatively modern series are 69–87%.[13] Complications include buttock pain, rectal injury, and sacral/pudendal neurovascular injury. A variation of this approach is the sacrospinous hysteropexy where following the same approach, the uterus is preserved. Complication rates are similar to the sacrospinous ligament fixation; however, the overall failure rates appear to be higher.

Abdominal/laparoscopic sacrocolpopexy

This procedure is used for both vault and uterine prolapse and involves the use of mesh between the vaginal apex and the sacral promontory to correct the underlying prolapse (see Fig. 3.6.9). Traditionally it was performed open, but can now be performed using minimally invasive techniques such as laparoscopy or be robotically assisted. Typically, the mesh utilized is polypropylene but biological material has also been used. In addition to the apical prolapse being fixed, the mesh arms can be extended to treat the prolapse of other compartments. In cases of significant rectocoele and defecatory dysfunction, placement of the mesh posteriorly with dissection of the RVS down to the perineum is warranted, as for ventral mesh rectopexy.

Outcomes of surgery depend on how success is measured but varies between 64–100%.[13] The use of minimally invasive techniques has several advantages including less bleeding, pain, hospital stay, and quicker time to recovery, and can lead to equivalent outcomes.[48] The use of robotic assistance has the potential for easier transition from open surgery to minimal invasion compared with laparoscopy. There are, of course, significant costs associated with robotic-assisted laparoscopy, and in the absence of randomized controlled trials in this area the benefits and pitfalls need to be carefully weighed up.

In a recent update of a Cochrane review, when compared with sacrospinous fixation for the treatment of apical prolapse, open or laparoscopic sacrocolpopexy had less recurrent prolapse and dyspareunia but had longer operating times and was more costly.[12] The CARE trial at two-year follow-up, where patients were randomized to Burch colposuspension in addition to sacrocolpopexy, has suggested the apex was well supported in 95% and those with the additional stress incontinence procedure were less likely to have a positive cough test or an additional SUI procedure.[49] However, a recent meta-analysis assessing the impact of continence surgery at the time of prolapse surgery revealed that concurrent continence surgery did not significantly reduce the rate of postoperative SUI.[12]

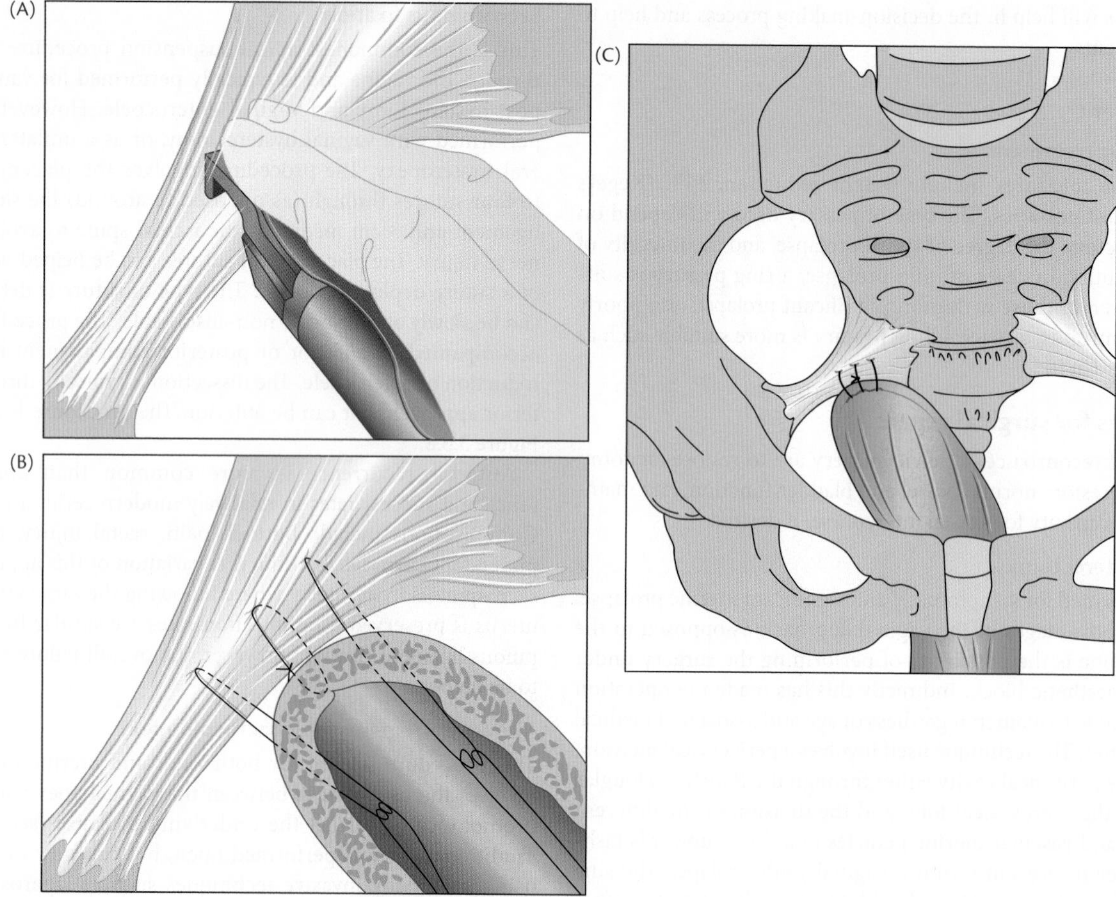

Fig. 3.6.8 (A), (B), and (C) Sacrospinous ligament fixation using a suture deploying device.
Reprinted from Walters MD and Ridgeway BM, Surgical treatment of vaginal apex prolapse, *Obstetrics and Gynecology*, Volume 121, Issue 2, Part 1, pp. 354–74, Copyright © 2013 with permission from Wolters Kluwer Health.

Complications include haemorrhage, particularly over the sacrum where troublesome bleeding can be encountered either from inadvertent damage to the left common iliac vein or more likely from the presacral venous plexus. Bowel, ureteric, rectal and bladder injury, bowel obstruction, mesh erosion, and infection are other risks. Discitis and osteomyelitis involving the sacrum have been reported but are much rarer.

Abdominal/laparoscopic sacrohysteropexy

Over the past decade there has been a move towards preservation of the uterus at the time of prolapse repair.[50] This is partly due to the patient's choice (specially in the younger patients) but is also supported by the evidence that the uterus itself plays no role in the aetiology of prolapse. The technique and evaluation of this new approach has gradually been incorporated by most units in the United Kingdom and ongoing RCTs (such as the Vue trial[51]) are currently looking at the long-term outcomes, as well as intra- and postoperative complications compared to other apical prolapse repair tecniques. Nonetheless, based on the evidence to date, sacrohysteropexy is a safe operation with similar outcomes and risks as seen with the more conventional sacrocolpopexy. Limiting factors include the availability of surgical expertise and pregnancy. Patients still of reproductive age are usually recommended to avoid pregnancy following the surgery. However, there have been cases of successful pregnancies delivered by caesarean section.

At the level of the sacrum, the surgical technique is identical to the traditional sacrocolpopexy with the exposure of the anterior ligament of the sacral promontory and retroperitoneal dissection. The novel aspect of this surgery involves the dissection of the uterovesical fold with bilateral piercing of the broad ligament at the level of the uterocervical junction. Once this is performed, a bifurcated (Y shaped) polypropelene flat mesh is inserted bilaterally through the broad ligament posteriorly and secured anteriorly to the uterine cervix using permanent sutures. The uterus is then lifted and tacked to the sacral promontory using titanium staples. Aditional anterior and/or posterior repair may be needed vaginally at the end of the abdominal procedure. Apart from the risk of bladder injury (particularly in women with a previous caesarean section) and broad ligament vessel injury, other intraoperative risks are similar to those described for the colposacropexy.

Obliterative procedures

These are procedures are generally reserved for the frail elderly, in whom a less invasive procedure is more appropriate and vaginal intercourse is not planned in the future. Partial colpocleisis (for vaginal vault prolapse) or LeFort colpocleisis (for uterine prolapse) involve excision of rectangles of vaginal epithelium from the prolapsed vagina. The vagina is inverted incrementally by purse string sutures and closed with sutured skin edges. The procedure is less commonly performed nowadays, but in a well-selected and

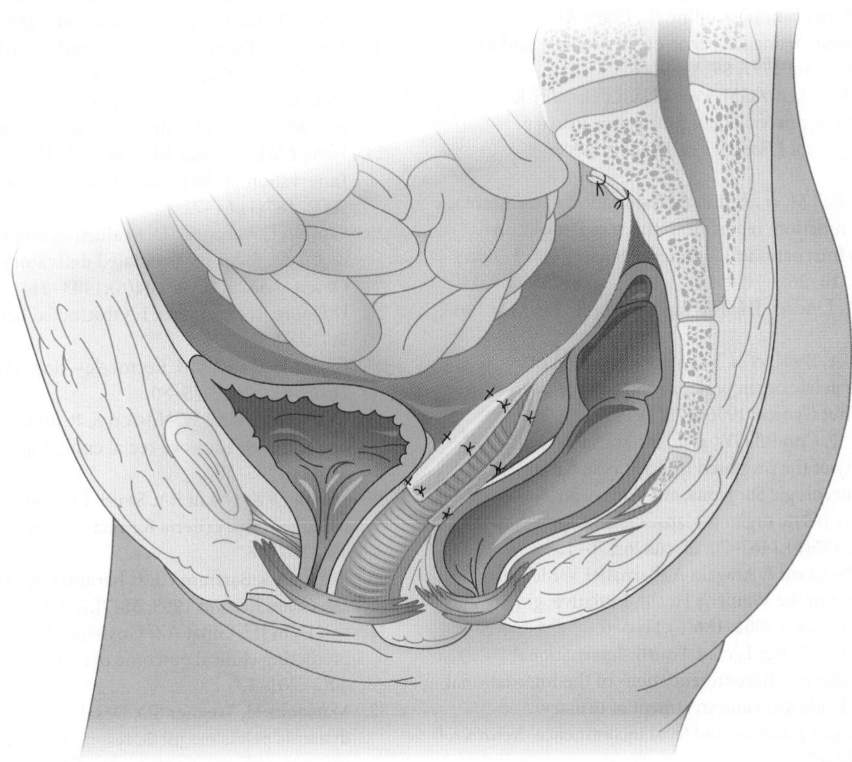

Fig. 3.6.9 Lateral view of sacrocolpopexy at the end. Graft material length is tailored to the individual (i.e. if the patient has a significant rectocoele with defecatory dysfunction, the mesh placement posteriorly may extend to the perineum). In cases with significant uterine prolapse, fenestrations are made in the broad ligament and mesh limbs are placed through them to the sacral promontory.

Reprinted from Walters MD and Ridgeway BM, Surgical treatment of vaginal apex prolapse, *Obstetrics and Gynecology*, Volume 121, Issue 2, Part 1, pp. 354–74, Copyright © 2013 with permission from Wolters Kluwer Health.

appropriately counselled patient may offer effective treatment. In one study of 152 patients with mean age 79 (+/–6) years, 82% and 73% had POP stage < or = 1 at 3 and 12 months, respectively. All pelvic symptom scores and related bother significantly improved at 3 and 12 months, and 95% said they were either 'very satisfied' or 'satisfied' with the outcome of their surgery.[52]

Conclusion

Support of the vaginal apex is critical in the prevention of uterine and vault prolapse, but also plays a significant role in the development of other compartment prolapse. Surgeons involved in POP surgery should not underestimate the need for diagnosing apical defects and the need for concomitant apical support. Obliteration of dead space and uterosacral ligament suspension after hysterectomy cannot be overemphasized in the prevention of vault prolapse. Several techniques exist for apical suspension and in our opinion transvaginal procedures are best reserved for the more elderly patients, those with significant co-morbidity as such that an abdominal approach may put the patient at increased risk, and for those with primary POP.

Further reading

Abrams P, Cardozo L, Fall M, *et al.* The standardisation of terminology of lower urinary tract function: report from the Standardisation Sub-committee of the International Continence Society. *Am J Obstet Gynecol* 2002; **187**(1):116–26.

Brubaker L, Nygaard I, Richter HE, *et al.* Two-year outcomes after sacrocolpopexy with and without burch to prevent stress urinary incontinence. *Obstet Gynecol* 2008; **112**(1):49–55.

Brubaker LGC, Jacquentin B, Maher C, *et al.* Surgery for pelvic organ prolapse. (pp. 1273–320) In: Abrams PCL, Khoury S, Wein A (eds). *Incontinence*, 4th edition. Paris, France: Health Publications Ltd, 2009.

Bump RC, Mattiasson A, Bo K, *et al.* The standardization of terminology of female pelvic organ prolapse and pelvic floor dysfunction. *Am J Obstet Gynecol* 1996; **175**(1):10–7.

DeLancey JO. Structural anatomy of the posterior pelvic compartment as it relates to rectocele. *Am J Obstet Gynecol* 1999; **180**(4):815–23.

Rabin JM. Conservative management of pelvic organ prolapse: Biofeedback and pessaries. (pp. 277–99) In: Badlani GH DG, Michel M, de la Rosette JJ (eds). *Continence: Current Concepts and Treatment Strategies.* Paris, France: Springer-Verlag, 2009.

Maher CM, Feiner B, Baessler K, Glazener CM. Surgical management of pelvic organ prolapse in women: the updated summary version Cochrane review. *Int Urogynecol J* 2011; **22**(11):1445–57.

Olsen AL, Smith VJ, Bergstrom JO, Colling JC, Clark AL. Epidemiology of surgically managed pelvic organ prolapse and urinary incontinence. *Obstet Gynecol* 1997; **89**(4):501–6.

Walters MD, Ridgeway BM. Surgical treatment of vaginal apex prolapse. *Obstet Gynecol* 2013; **121**(2 Pt 1):354–74.

Wei JT, Nygaard I, Richter HE, *et al.* A midurethral sling to reduce incontinence after vaginal prolapse repair. *New Engl J Med* 2012; **366**(25):2358–67.

References

1. Olsen AL, Smith VJ, Bergstrom JO, Colling JC, Clark AL. Epidemiology of surgically managed pelvic organ prolapse and urinary incontinence. *Obstet Gynecol* 1997; **89**(4):501–6.
2. Fialkow MF, Newton KM, Lentz GM, Weiss NS. Lifetime risk of surgical management for pelvic organ prolapse or urinary incontinence. *Int Urogynecol J Pelvic Floor Dysfunct* 2008; **19**(3):437–40.
3. Abrams P, Cardozo L, Fall M, *et al.* The standardisation of terminology of lower urinary tract function: report from the Standardisation Sub-committee of the International Continence Society. *Am J Obstet Gynecol* 2002; **187**(1):116–26.
4. Baden WF, Walker TA, Lindsey JH. The vaginal profile. *Tex Med* 1968; **64**(5):56–8.
5. Bump RC, Mattiasson A, Bo K, *et al.* The standardization of terminology of female pelvic organ prolapse and pelvic floor dysfunction. *Am J Obstet Gynecol* 1996; **175**(1):10–7.
6. Hall AF, Theofrastous JP, Cundiff GW, *et al.* Interobserver and intraobserver reliability of the proposed International Continence Society, Society of Gynecologic Surgeons, and American Urogynecologic Society pelvic organ prolapse classification system. *Am J Obstet Gynecol* 1996; **175**(6):1467–70; discussion 70–1.
7. Hendrix SL, Clark A, Nygaard I, Aragaki A, Barnabei V, McTiernan A. Pelvic organ prolapse in the Women's Health Initiative: gravity and gravidity. *Am J Obstet Gynecol* 2002; **186**(6):1160–6.
8. Abrams P, Andersson KE, Birder L, *et al.* Fourth International Consultation on Incontinence Recommendations of the International Scientific Committee: Evaluation and treatment of urinary incontinence, pelvic organ prolapse, and fecal incontinence. *Neurourol Urodyn* 2010; **29**(1):213–40.
9. DeLancey JO. Anatomic aspects of vaginal eversion after hysterectomy. *Am J Obstet Gynecol* 1992; **166**(6 Pt 1):1717–24; discussion 24–8.
10. Belal M, Morley R. Pelvic organ prolapse repair. *Urology News* 2011; **16**(1):10–2.
11. Adams E, Thomson A, Maher C, Hagen S. Mechanical devices for pelvic organ prolapse in women. *Cochrane Database Syst Rev* 2004; (2):CD004010.
12. Maher CM, Feiner B, Baessler K, Glazener CM. Surgical management of pelvic organ prolapse in women: the updated summary version Cochrane review. *Int Urogynecol J* 2011; **22**(11):1445–57.
13. Brubaker LGC, Jacquentin B, Maher C, *et al.* Surgery for pelvic organ prolapse. (pp. 1273–320) In: Abrams PCL, Khoury S, Wein A (eds). *Incontinence*, 4th edition. Paris, France: Health Publications Ltd, 2009.
14. Sand PK, Koduri S, Lobel RW, *et al.* Prospective randomized trial of polyglactin 910 mesh to prevent recurrence of cystoceles and rectoceles. *Am J Obstet Gynecol* 2001; **184**(7):1357–62; discussion 62–4.
15. Maher C, Feiner B, Baessler K, Christmann-Schmid C, Haya N, Marjoribanks J. Transvaginal mesh or grafts compared with native tissue repair for vaginal prolapse. *Cochran Review*. Available at: http://www.cochrane.org/CD012079/MENSTR_transvaginal-mesh-or-grafts-compared-native-tissue-repair-vaginal-prolapse [Online].
16. Jha S, Moran P. The UK national prolapse survey: 5 years on. *Int Urogynecol J* 2011; **22**(5):517–28.
17. Maher C, Baessler K, Glazener CM, Adams EJ, Hagen S. Surgical management of pelvic organ prolapse in women: a short version Cochrane review. *Neurourol Urodyn* 2008; **27**(1):3–12.
18. Wei JT, Nygaard I, Richter HE, *et al.* A midurethral sling to reduce incontinence after vaginal prolapse repair. *New Engl J Med* 2012; **366**(25):2358–67.
19. Milley PS, Nichols DH. A correlative investigation of the human rectovaginal septum. *Anat Rec* 1969; **163**(3):443–51.
20. Richardson AC. The rectovaginal septum revisited: its relationship to rectocele and its importance in rectocele repair. *Clin Obstet Gynecol* 1993; **36**(4):976–83.
21. Leffler KS, Thompson JR, Cundiff GW, Buller JL, Burrows LJ, Schon Ybarra MA. Attachment of the rectovaginal septum to the pelvic sidewall. *Am J Obstet Gynecol* 2001; **185**(1):41–3.
22. Lefevre R, Davila GW. Functional disorders: rectocele. *Clin Colon Rectal Surg* 2008; **21**(2):129–37.
23. DeLancey JO. Structural anatomy of the posterior pelvic compartment as it relates to rectocele. *Am J Obstet Gynecol* 1999; **180**(4):815–23.
24. Barber MD, Bremer RE, Thor KB, Dolber PC, Kuehl TJ, Coates KW. Innervation of the female levator ani muscles. *Am J Obstet Gynecol* 2002; **187**(1):64–71.
25. Cundiff GW, Fenner D. Evaluation and treatment of women with rectocele: focus on associated defecatory and sexual dysfunction. *Obstet Gynecol* 2004; **104**(6):1403–21.
26. D'Hoore A, Penninckx F. Obstructed defecation. *Colorectal Dis* 2003; **5**(4):280–7.
27. Carter D, Gabel MB. Rectocele—does the size matter? *Int J Colorectal Dis* 2012; **27**(7):975–80.
28. Karlbom U, Graf W, Nilsson S, Pahlman L. Does surgical repair of a rectocele improve rectal emptying? *Dis Colon Rectum* 1996; **39**(11):1296–302.
29. Murthy VK, Orkin BA, Smith LE, Glassman LM. Excellent outcome using selective criteria for rectocele repair. *Dis Colon Rectum* 1996; **39**(4):374–8.
30. Halligan S, Bartram CI. Is barium trapping in rectoceles significant? *Dis Colon Rectum* 1995; **38**(7):764–8.
31. van Dam JH, Ginai AZ, Gosselink MJ, *et al.* Role of defecography in predicting clinical outcome of rectocele repair. *Dis Colon Rectum* 1997; **40**(2):201–7.
32. Matsuoka H, Wexner SD, Desai MB, *et al.* A comparison between dynamic pelvic magnetic resonance imaging and videoproctography in patients with constipation. *Dis Colon Rectum* 2001 Apr;**44**(4):571–6.
33. Jones KR HS, Whitehead WE. Biofeedback for anorectal disorders. (pp. 313–25) In: Drutz HP HS, Diamant NE (eds). *Urogynaecology and Reconstructive Pelvic Surgery*. London, UK: Springer-Verlag, 2003.
34. Koutsomanis D, Lennard-Jones JE, Roy AJ, Kamm MA. Controlled randomised trial of visual biofeedback versus muscle training without a visual display for intractable constipation. *Gut* 1995; **37**(1):95–9.
35. Arnold MW, Stewart WR, Aguilar PS. Rectocele repair. Four years' experience. *Dis Colon Rectum* 1990; **33**(8):684–7.
36. Mellgren A, Anzen B, Nilsson BY, *et al.* Results of rectocele repair. A prospective study. *Dis Colon Rectum* 1995; **38**(1):7–13.
37. Boccasanta P, Venturi M, Calabro G, *et al.* Which surgical approach for rectocele? A multicentric report from Italian coloproctologists. *Tech Coloproctol* 2001; **5**(3):149–56.
38. Porter WE, Steele A, Walsh P, Kohli N, Karram MM. The anatomic and functional outcomes of defect-specific rectocele repairs. *Am J Obstetr Gynecol* 1999; **181**(6):1353–8; discussion 8–9.
39. Singh K, Cortes E, Reid WM. Evaluation of the fascial technique for surgical repair of isolated posterior vaginal wall prolapse. *Obstet Gynecol* 2003; **101**(2):320–4.
40. Marks MM. The rectal side of the rectocele. Diseases of the colon and rectum. 1967; **10**(5):387–8.
41. Pechlivanides G, Tsiaoussis J, Athanasakis E, *et al.* Stapled transanal rectal resection (STARR) to reverse the anatomic disorders of pelvic floor dyssynergia. *World J Surg* 2007; **31**(6):1329–35.
42. Slawik S, Soulsby R, Carter H, Payne H, Dixon AR. Laparoscopic ventral rectopexy, posterior colporrhaphy and vaginal sacrocolpopexy for the treatment of recto-genital prolapse and mechanical outlet obstruction. *Colorectal Dis* 2008; **10**(2):138–43.
43. Rooney K, Kenton K, Mueller ER, FitzGerald MP, Brubaker L. Advanced anterior vaginal wall prolapse is highly correlated with apical prolapse. *Am J Obstet Gynecol* 2006; **195**(6):1837–40.
44. Rabin JM. Conservative management of pelvic organ prolapse: Biofeedback and pessaries. (pp. 277–99) In: Badlani GH DG,

Michel M, de la Rosette JJ (eds). *Continence: Current Concepts and Treatment Strategies*. Paris, France: Springer-Verlag, 2009.
45. Walters MD, Ridgeway BM. Surgical treatment of vaginal apex prolapse. *Obstet Gynecol* 2013; **121**(2 Pt 1):354–74.
46. Pakbaz M, Mogren I, Lofgren M. Outcomes of vaginal hysterectomy for uterovaginal prolapse: a population-based, retrospective, cross-sectional study of patient perceptions of results including sexual activity, urinary symptoms, and provided care. *BMC Womens Health* 2009; **9**:9.
47. Cruikshank SH, Kovac SR. Randomized comparison of three surgical methods used at the time of vaginal hysterectomy to prevent posterior enterocele. *Am J Obstet Gynecol* 1999; **180**(4):859–65.
48. Ross JW, Preston MR. Update on laparoscopic, robotic, and minimally invasive vaginal surgery for pelvic floor repair. *Minerva Ginecol* 2009; **61**(3):173–86.
49. Brubaker L, Nygaard I, Richter HE, *et al.* Two-year outcomes after sacrocolpopexy with and without burch to prevent stress urinary incontinence. *Obstet Gynecol* 2008; **112**(1):49–55.
50. Rahmanou P, Price N, Jackson S. Laparoscopic hysteropexy: a novel technique for uterine preservation surgery. Int Uro J. Available at: http://www.oxfordgynaecology.com/Publications/Laparoscopic%20hysteropexy%20a%20novel%20technique%20for%20uterine%20preservation.pdf [Online].
51. The VUE trial. Available at: http://www.abdn.ac.uk/hsru/research/assessment/interventional/vue/ [Online].
52. Fitzgerald MP, Richter HE, Bradley CS, *et al.* Pelvic support, pelvic symptoms, and patient satisfaction after colpocleisis. *Int Urogynecol J Pelvic Floor Dysfunct* 2008; **19**(12):1603–9.

CHAPTER 3.7

Urgency incontinence and overactive bladder

Christopher R. Chapple and Altaf Mangera

Definitions

The standardization of lower urinary tract symptoms and dysfunction (LUTD) terminology has been undertaken by the International Continence Society (ICS).[1] The committee has described *urinary incontinence* as the complaint of involuntary leakage of urine. When the leaking is accompanied or preceded by urgency, it is labelled as *urgency urinary incontinence*. *Urgency* itself is a sensory symptom and is the defining symptom of overactive bladder symptom syndrome (OAB). It is described as a 'sudden and compelling desire to void which is difficult to defer'. This definition does not discriminate between a discrete or continuous phenomenon and therefore may be problematic to interpret. Urgency must be differentiated from *urge*, which is the normal desire to void when the bladder is reaching fullness. Attempts have been made to grade urgency which has relied on the time from the onset of urgency to actual leak, or the patient's actual subjective assessment of urgency severity. These have, however, not been adopted by the ICS. Moreover, a compelling desire to void is arguably felt by normal individuals if the bladder is sufficiently full and therefore the circumstances of the urgency are also important and should be in a state where urgency would not be expected (i.e. no explanatory cause).

Overactive bladder symptom syndrome (OAB) is a symptom-based syndrome defined as 'urinary urgency with or without urgency incontinence, usually accompanied by urinary frequency and nocturia in the absence of an explanatory cause'. If urgency incontinence is present, then the term OAB-wet may be used whereas there is no urgency incontinence with OAB-dry. Detrusor overactivity is a urodynamic observation of an involuntary characteristic waveform during filling cystometry.

Nocturia is defined as the number of voids during sleep (i.e. each void must be preceded and followed by sleep). The *nocturnal urine volume* is described as the volume of urine produced during sleeping hours, which excludes the last void before bed and includes the first void on waking. The proportion of nocturnal volume over the 24-hour urinary volume is used to calculate nocturnal polyuria. *Nocturnal polyuria* is defined generally, as more than one-third of urine production occurring during nocturnal hours.

Anatomy/physiology of lower urinary tract storage and dysfunction

The bladder is a hollow muscular organ with two principle functions: to store urine at low pressure, and to generate sufficient pressure to allow expulsion of urine at a convenient time and place. The bladder is highly distensible and its most sensitive portion, the *trigone*, is demarcated between the urethra and two ureteric orifices. This is histologically and embryologically different to the rest of the bladder and contains a rich plexus of neuronal tissue. The remainder of the bladder is composed of three distinct layers: the serosa, the outer adventitial connective tissue layer; the detrusor, a smooth muscle layer comprising a randomly arranged syncytium of interlacing muscle bundles; and the urothelium, an impervious inner layer lined by transitional cell epithelium. The urothelium is supported by the suburothelium, which has a high metabolic rate, is richly innervated, and is involved in sensing bladder fullness.

Neuronal control of the lower urinary tract involves coordination of the central and peripheral nervous systems. The somatic nerves arise from the nucleus of Onufrowicz (*Onuf's nucleus*) from the S2-S4 level (spinal micturition centre) and allow control of the external urinary sphincter. The detrusor muscle is under autonomic control from the postganglionic T10-L2 (sympathetic) nerves and preganglionic S2-S4 (parasympathetic) nerves (Fig. 3.7.1). Sympathetic stimulation leads to relaxation of the detrusor muscle and contraction of the bladder neck sphincter. Once a sensory threshold of bladder fullness is reached, the afferent nerves carry impulses to the spinal micturition centre which then activates the efferent arm, leading to detrusor contraction and sphincter relaxation. The pontine micturition centre (PMC) and suprapontine areas of the brain, however, are responsible for coordinating micturition. The PMC communicates with the periaqueductal grey area in the midbrain, which in turn modulates activity in the spinal micturition centre. This importantly delays micturition by inhibiting premature detrusor contractions (sympathetic) until it is convenient to void.

While the pathophysiology of detrusor overactivity remains poorly understood, several theories have been proposed as possible underlying mechanisms to explain the genesis of patients' symptoms in the context of associated OAB. Brading originally proposed it was due to increased myogenic excitability in the detrusor myocytes, caused by localized detrusor contraction spreading across the whole bladder.[2] Alternatively, a neurogenic aetiology has been put forward.[3] Suprapontine nerves involved in the limbic system (associated with emotion) have been shown to have an inhibitory impact on the PMC. Therefore, interruption to these higher centres may allow the return of primitive reflexes, such as detrusor contractions. Alternatively, damage to spinal axons has been suggested

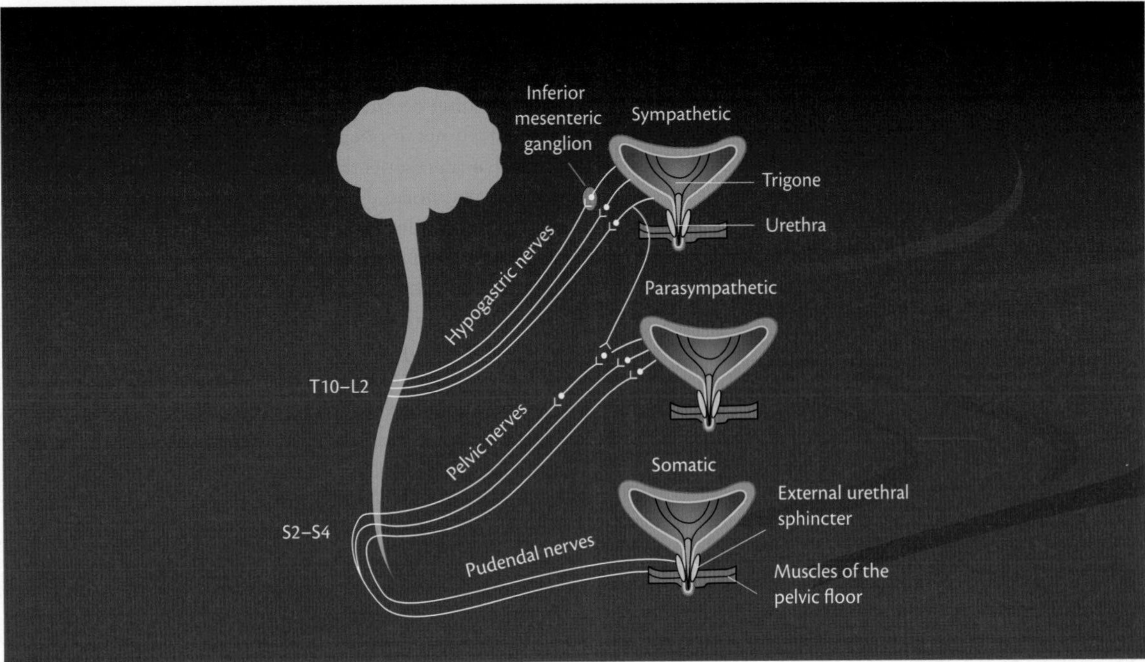

Fig. 3.7.1 Innervation of the lower urinary tract.
Reprinted from Chapter 60, 'Urinary incontinence; Epidemiology, pathophysiology, evaluation and management overview', in Alan J. Wein *et al.*, *Campbell-Walsh Urology, Ninth Edition*, Saunders an imprint of Elsevier Inc., Copyright © 2006, with permission from Elsevier.

to lead to a greater role for unmyelinated C fibres in the reflex arc, which may increase detrusor excitability. These mechanisms have all attempted to address the motor component of OAB. However, the cardinal symptom (of urgency) is sensory in nature. Therefore, much research in recent years has concentrated on the afferent system. The urothelium was once considered an inert barrier but it is now thought to have an important role in sensation, transduction, and modulation of mechanical and chemical stimuli. Evidence has shown that the urothelial cells have purinergic receptors, muscarinic receptors, TRPV1 receptors and additionally, signalling molecules such as ATP, NO, and acetylcholine, which are secreted by the urothelium in response to mechanical (stretch) and chemical stimuli.[4]

Epidemiology and risk factors

Multiple population-based studies have demonstrated the high prevalence of OAB. The European Prospective Investigation into Cancer and Nutrition (EPIC) study surveyed 19,165 adults in four European countries and Canada and found an overall prevalence of OAB in 10.8% in males and 12.2% in females, rising to 13.1% and 14.6% in those over 40.[5] Incontinence was present in 44.5% of females and in 28.0% of males, with over half of patients experiencing trouble from their symptoms. A longitudinal study of 4,072 men has shown that the prevalence increased from 15.6% to 44.4% over 11 years.[6] A systematic review of seven longitudinal studies showed OAB symptom severity was sustained or progressed over time in the majority of individuals, showing that OAB may be a progressive condition.[7] Besides age and female gender, the other risk factors which have been proposed for OAB include obesity, low physical activity, pelvic organ prolapse, and smoking.

Symptoms

It is essential that a complete urological and medical history are taken from patients with suspected OAB. As described above the cardinal symptom is urgency, which is a sudden uncontrollable desire leading to a fear of leaking. Patients will usually describe how long they have to 'make it' and may also plan their daily activities around being in close proximity to toilet facilities. Thereafter dietary habits, particularly caffeine intake, should be recorded. A voiding diary to establish baseline daily and nocturnal frequency should also be documented over at least a three-day period. In certain patients, particularly the elderly male, storage symptoms (OAB) may be present in conjunction with bladder outflow obstruction and therefore accompanied by symptoms such as hesitancy, poor flow, straining, and incomplete bladder emptying.

Thereafter, other obvious pathological causes must be excluded. This involves the use of urinalysis to exclude infection and non-visible haematuria. The latter should prompt further investigation to exclude malignancy. Finally, it is also important to recognize the impact the symptoms are having on a patient's quality of life. For this purpose, questionnaire's such as the OAB-q or ICIQ-OAB may be utilized and can be found at www.ICIQ.net/.

Examination

Examination should be focused towards excluding underlying pathology. The abdomen, external genitalia, and prostate should be examined, as well as the neurological system. A palpable bladder is indicative of chronic retention and incomplete emptying. A neurological examination may be helpful in explaining patient symptoms and may point towards a neurogenic bladder.

Investigation

As described in 'Symptoms', investigation for OAB symptoms should commence with urinalysis to exclude a urinary tract infection and haematuria. A flow rate and post-void residual estimation should be performed in those who describe a poor flow or difficulty with voiding, and is almost routine in all elderly males.

As noted above, a frequency volume chart or bladder diary may be used to quantify the frequency of incontinence episodes and also to obtain an individual's pattern of voiding. The different types and formats of a voiding diary are described in Chapter 3.4. Table 3.7.1 lists the parameters which may be obtained from a voiding diary, how to calculate them, and their normal values. The daily voided volume may indicate 24-hour polyuria which is defined as the passage of more than 2.8 L urine per 24 hours. This may explain frequency in a small cohort of patients who drink excessively or have an underlying endocrine disorder.

The excessive production of urine during sleep hours is termed *nocturnal polyuria*. Generally, over the age of 50 less than one-third of urine production should occur during the sleep hours. It must be noted that when calculating nocturnal urine production, the last void before sleep is excluded but all voids during sleep and the first void on waking are included. This gives the only accurate estimation of nocturnal urine production.

In patients who are resistant to behavioural and pharmacological management, cystometry may be undertaken. The procedure is described in detail in Chapter 3.2, therefore only the parameters which should be documented when undertaking this procedure to evaluate potential bladder filling dysfunction in patients with OAB will be discussed in this section. During the filling phase of cystometry, a number of filling sensations should be sought from the patient; these include the first sensation of filling, first desire to void, normal desire to void, and desperate desire to void. These occur in all normal individuals; however, they may occur with lesser volumes in patients with OAB. Modern urodynamic computer systems allow these sensations to be marked on the program while performing the study, but it is essential when interpreting such data that artefacts are excluded by the investigator with review of the electronic trace. The normal compelling desire to void occurs under normal circumstances but can be controlled in the presence of a full bladder, and therefore is different from urgency. Urgency is a compelling desire to void that is difficult to defer, which particularly in women if not acted upon will lead to urgency incontinence. This also represents the maximum cystometric capacity which varies between normal individuals, but is approximately 400–500 mL.

As the bladder fills, there should be no appreciable increase in the detrusor pressure in a conscious cooperative individual who is trying to inhibit voiding. Any increase of more than 10 cmH_2O over 400 mL of filling represents poor detrusor compliance and is seen as an upward slope (Fig. 3.7.2). The presence of urgency and the volume of filling at which this occurs during filling should also be documented. Involuntary detrusor overactive contractions (Fig. 3.7.3) may be noticed at the same time as the urgency. In addition, the patient may have urgency incontinence at this time. While filling the bladder, provocation manoeuvres such as running a tap or asking the patient to bounce up and down on their toes may be used to provoke detrusor overactivity. Detrusor overactivity is demonstrated in approximately 69% of men and 44% of men with OAB-dry and 90% of men and 58% of women with OAB-wet.[8]

Finally, the voiding phase with synchronous pressure flow measurements is important to assess in these groups of patients. Firstly, because OAB symptoms may be associated with incomplete bladder emptying but also some of the treatments used to treat OAB may have an impact on flow rate and bladder emptying. The urodynamic features to assess the void phase are discussed in more detail in Chapter 3.2.

Management

The first-line management for OAB should include lifestyle changes, such as attention to fluid intake and toileting habits. Patients should be encouraged to reduce excessive fluid and caffeine intake, and to spread fluid intake out over the day rather than concentrate it in the evening. Clinicians need to be aware that significant fluid intake can occur in patients consuming large amounts of fruit and vegetable matter. In conjunction with this, patients are asked to void by

Table 3.7.1 Table of frequency volume chart parameters, their calculation, and normal definitions

Diary parameter	Calculation	Definition of normal
Daily frequency	Frequency per 24 hrs	2–10
Nocturnal frequency	Frequency while asleep (does not include last void before sleep nor first void on waking)	<1–2 (age dependant)
24-hour voided volume	Volume of urine produced in 24 hrs	<2.8 L/24 hrs or <36 mL/kg/24 hrs
Nocturnal volume	Volume of urine produced during sleep (does not include last void before sleep but DOES include first void in day)	<900 mL
% nocturnal volume/24-hour volume	24-hour volume/nocturnal volume × 100	<33%
Functional bladder capacity	Largest voided volume recorded	300–600 mL
Urgency episodes per day	Urgency episodes in 24 hrs	0
Incontinence episodes related to urgency per day	Incontinence episodes in 24 hrs that occurred at the same time as urgency	0
Incontinence episodes NOT related to urgency per day	Incontinence episodes in 24 hrs NOT related to urgency	0
Longest duration between voids (not an average)	Longest time between voids	>3 hrs

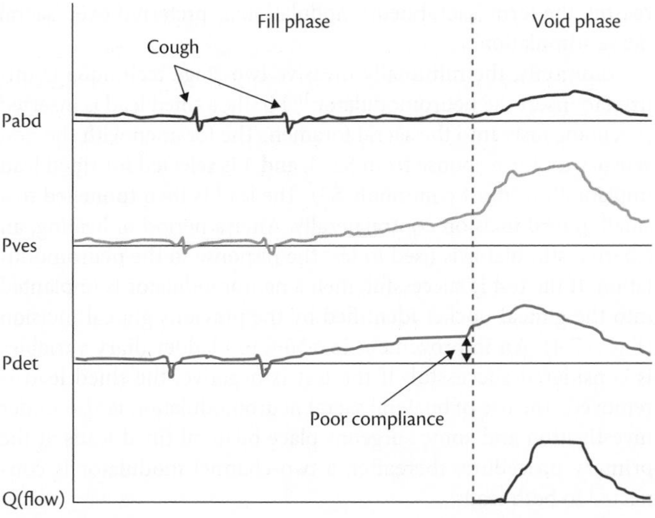

Fig. 3.7.2 Simplified cystometrogram demonstrating poor compliance.

the clock and to try and 'hold on' for longer time periods. In these situations, a bladder diary is very helpful, to facilitate this 'bladder training'.

Pharmacological treatment

Anticholinergics, more specifically antimuscarinics, form the mainstay of therapy after conservative measures fail. They act on the parasympathetic (efferent) system principally through the post junctional M_3 receptor.[9] Although the M_2, M_4, and M_5 receptors are known to exist in the bladder, their roles have not been fully defined. Moreover, muscarinic receptors such as the M_1 predominate in the central nervous system, M_1 and M_3 are present in the salivary glands, M_2 and M_3 in the gastrointestinal smooth muscle, M_3 and M_5 in the eyes, and M_2 in the heart.[10] Therefore, side effects of these drugs can include cognitive impairment, dry mouth, constipation, dry eyes, and pruritus, depending upon the receptor selectivity of the formulation utilized. Contraindications to the use of these drugs include closed angle glaucoma and urinary retention. It was previously feared that the use of antimuscarinics in men with concomitant bladder outflow obstruction could precipitate urinary retention. However, there is no evidence to this effect and it is considered safe to commence antimuscarinics in men with a post-void residual less than 200 mL. In this group of patients, combination of an alpha antagonist with an antimuscarinic may be the treatment of choice.

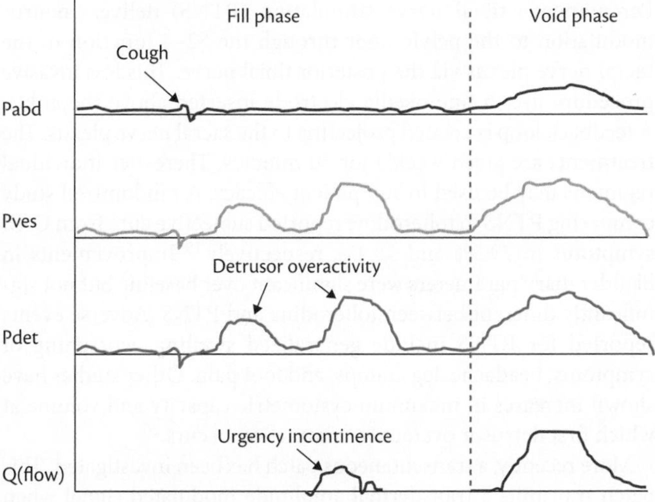

Fig. 3.7.3 Simplified cystometrogram demonstrating detrusor overactivity and urgency incontinence.

Two large meta-analyses have reviewed antimuscarinic use in OAB.[11,12] In total, seven different formulations were included. These drugs have been shown to significantly reduce frequency and incontinence episodes and also increase mean voided volume, first desire to void, and maximum cystometric capacity in patients with OAB. Quality of life improvements have also been reported. Besides immediate release oxybutynin, which has been shown to be inferior to the newer antimuscarinic preparations, there is little to choose between the available preparations as they have not been assessed in head-to-head studies. Nevertheless, different subreceptor affinities means that if one preparation fails, another may be successful. All preparations come in a once-daily formulation and also have variable doses which suit many patients. Of interest to some patients may be the use of antimuscarinic patches or transdermal gels. Although clinical trials, which mostly last 12 weeks, have shown good efficacy and tolerability, long-term marketing data has shown that long-term discontinuation rates are high with antimuscarinic agents.

The urothelium and detrusor muscle also contain β-1, 2, and 3 adrenoreceptors, which when stimulated lead to increases in cyclic AMP levels leading to detrusor relaxation. In humans, detrusor relaxation is mediated by the B_3 subtype. Mirabegron is a specific B_3 agonist which may provide an alternative to antimuscarinics. Three recent phase III trials have provided evidence for its safety and efficacy. Fifty milligrams has emerged as the most efficacious dose. Significant improvements have been shown over placebo for urgency, frequency, and micturition episodes per day.

In a study assessing safety in two groups of 444 patients divided into mirabegron 50 or 100 mg and tolterodine ER 4 mg. The number of adverse events was similar between the groups. The most common adverse events reported for mirabegron were hypertension, urinary tract infection, nasopharyngitis, and constipation. In terms of dry mouth, the incidence was 8.6% for tolterodine, and 2.8% and 2.3% for mirabegron 50 and 100 mg, respectively.

Botulinum toxin

When pharmacotherapy fails, botulinum toxin (BTX) may be injected into the bladder. BTX is produced by the bacterium *clostridium botulinum*, which is known to decrease Acetyl-choline (Ach) from pre-synaptic nerve terminals, thereby blocking transmission of nerve impulses wherever Ach is the neurotransmitter. It was first described in urology to treat detrusor sphincter dyssynergia. Thereafter it was used to treat detrusor overactivity in neurogenic patients followed by OAB patients. More recently, it has also been investigated in painful bladder syndrome and interstitial cystitis.[13]

It was proposed that BTX worked through the efferent neural pathway by reducing involuntary detrusor smooth muscle contraction, which is characteristic of detrusor overactivity. This is achieved by disruption of the SNARE (Soluble N ethylmaleimide-sensitive factor attachment protein receptor) complex leading to a highly specific neuromuscular blockade of vesicular Ach release at somatic and autonomic pre-synaptic nerve terminals. However, evidence is gathering for a more complex picture because urgency with OAB and pain in painful bladder syndrome are sensory symptoms. Therefore, other neurotransmitters such as ATP, calcitonin gene related peptide, and substance P, as well as nerve growth factors may be involved.

There are seven serotypes of BTX (from A-G), with BTX-A being the most commonly used. Even with BTX-A there are different preparations. Due to different isolation, extraction, purification, and formulation processes the dosing, efficacy, and safety are entirely different and therefore these preparations have been given new names by the Food and Drug Administration (FDA). Botox® is now 'onabotulinumtoxinA', Dysport is 'abobotulinumtoxinA', and Xeomin 'incobotulinumtoxinA'.

OnabotulinumtoxinA is the only preparation, at the time of writing, which has a licence for use. Many randomized trials have assessed it in an OAB population. Improvements have been shown in urgency by 53%, frequency by 35%, and incontinence episodes by 68% per day. In addition to this, the maximum cystometric capacity has been shown to increase by 58% and mean detrusor pressure to decrease by 39%. In patients who were incontinent, total continence resumes in 57%. Improvements have also been shown in quality of life. The median duration of effect is nine months.

The early studies all utilized 200 iu (international units) onabotulinumtoxinA. However, a dose ranging study has shown 100 iu was sufficient to have a significant impact on symptoms, bladder diary parameters, and quality of life (QoL).[14] Doses greater than 150 iu did not significantly add to the improvements in symptoms. The authors also found a dose related risk of increased post-void residual (PVR), with 100 iu leading to a PVR >200 mL in 14.5% of patients and 200 iu leading to a risk of 28.8%. Therefore, a more balanced dose of onabotulinumtoxinA to commence patients on may be 100 iu. In patients who develop voiding difficulty and raised post-void residue, intermittent self-catheterization may need to be instigated. This increases the risk of urinary tract infection which ranges 13–40%.

Other adverse events which are reported include dry mouth, muscular weakness, impaired vision, and dysphagia. These are all rare however, and are increased when using higher doses of the toxin. Contraindications to the use of BTX include allergy, infection of proposed injection site, pregnancy, breastfeeding, and myasthenia gravis. Drug interactions include aminoglycosides, penicillamine, quinine, calcium channel antagonists, and muscle relaxants.

The use of flexible cystoscopy has made the delivery of BTX in to the bladder an outpatient procedure. Most commonly, 1 mL containing 10 µ is administered per injection site. The number of injection sites and volume per injection needs further investigation. The depth of the injection (i.e. the detrusor or suburothelium) has not been shown to make a significant difference. It was also feared that injection into the trigone may precipitate ureteric reflux, but in two different studies this has not been shown to be the case, and in fact the trigone injection group showed greater improvements. The rich neural supply of the trigone probably makes it a key site for injection.

Sacral Neuromodulation

Neuromodulation is another technique which may be used in patients with severe OAB, especially if incontinence is present. There are many techniques which include transcutaneous, percutaneous, and sacral approaches. The latter was developed in the 1980s by Tanagho and Schmidt.[15] The proposed mechanism of action is not well understood, but is thought to involve modulation of spinal cord reflexes and higher centres rather than direct stimulation of the efferent (motor) nerves to the detrusor muscle. For this reason, the term 'sacral neuromodulation' is preferred over 'sacral nerve stimulation'.

Commonly, the minimally invasive two-stage technique is utilized to insert the neuromodulator.[16] Firstly, a tined lead is inserted percutaneously into the sacral foramen. The foramen with the best sensory motor response from S2, 3, and 4 is selected for tined lead implantation (most commonly S3). The lead is then tunnelled to a small gluteal incision contralaterally. After a period of healing, an external stimulator is used to test the response to the neuromodulation. If the test is successful, then a neuromodulator is implanted into the gluteal pocket identified by the previous gluteal incision (Fig. 3.7.4). An improvement in >50% in bladder diary variables is considered successful. If the test is negative, the tined lead is removed. The use of bilateral sacral neuromodulation is also under investigation and some surgeons place bilateral tined leads at the primary procedure; thereafter, a two-channel modulator is connected to both leads.

Cautions one should apply in a patient with a neuromodulator include the use of high frequency monopolar diathermy, extracorporeal shock wave lithotripsy, and radiotherapy over the device. Sacral neuromodulation needs to be discontinued in pregnancy and should be turned off if an MRI scan is required. Surgeons should also be aware that the device may be placed in the loin or abdominal wall. Problems include infection, battery failure, lead migration, and loss of efficacy—this can usually be resolved with reprogramming the stimulation parameters, or by insertion of a contralateral lead.

Multicentre trails have shown statistically significant improvements in frequency episodes, urgency episodes, voided volumes, and quality of life parameters over placebo.[17] Switching off the stimulators led to the return of symptoms in patients who subsequently regained efficacy after reactivation of the devices. Five-year success rates are reported in 56–68% of patients.[18] More recent studies have looked at non-continuous neuromodulation (i.e. switching on the device when symptoms are present and off when they have subsided). The intended benefits are that patients are given more autonomy over their condition, a longer battery life, and reduced adaptation of the nervous system to stimulation.

Percutaneous tibial nerve stimulation

Percutaneous tibial nerve stimulation (PTNS) delivers neuromodulation to the pelvic floor through the S2–4 junction of the sacral nerve plexus via the posterior tibial nerve. This less invasive procedure uses a fine needle electrode inserted above the ankle. A feedback loop is created projecting to the sacral nerve plexus. The treatments are given weekly for 30 minutes. Thereafter individual regimens may be used to suit patient efficacy. A randomized study comparing PTNS to tolterodine reported subjective cure from OAB symptoms in 79.5% and 58.4%, respectively.[19] Improvements in bladder diary parameters were significant over baseline but not significantly different between tolterodine and PTNS. Adverse events reported for PTNS include generalized swelling, worsening of symptoms, headache, leg cramps, and foot pain. Other studies have shown increases in maximum cystometric capacity and volume at which first detrusor overactive contraction occurs.[20]

More recently, a transcutaneous patch has been investigated. This patch transmits a transdermal amplitude modulated signal when placed on the skin over the sacrum. After one week of treatment, 50% of patients reported at least 50% reduction in urgency incontinence episodes. The results thereafter were quite mixed, with some

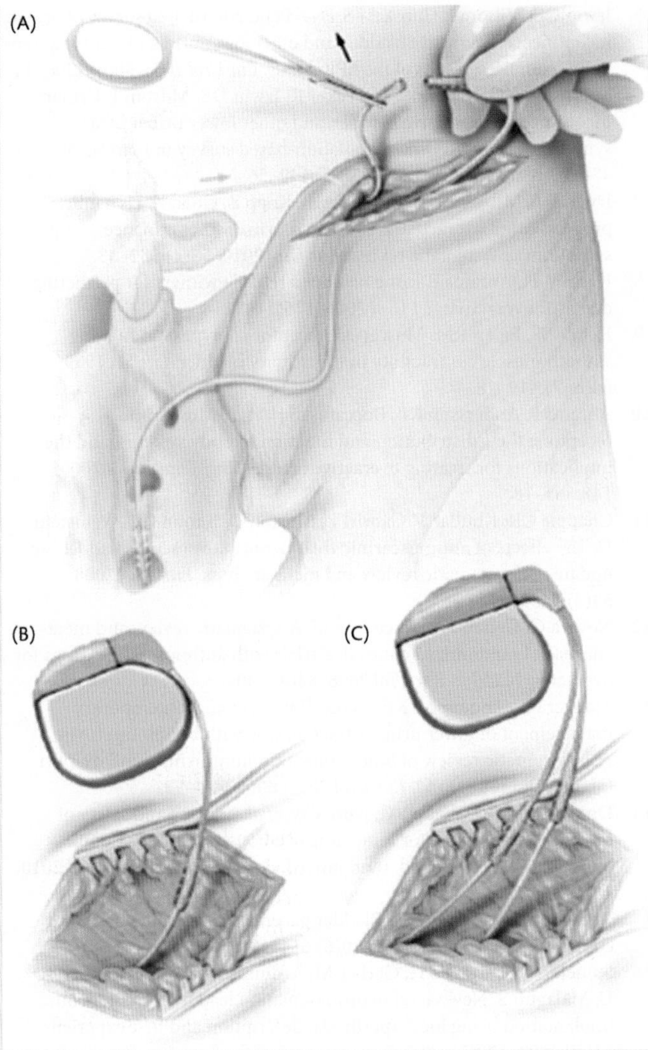

Fig. 3.7.4 Image showing the attachment of the sacral neuromodulator and implantation into the gluteal space: (A) connection tined lead to external stimulator for test phase; (B) single lead connected to single channel neuromodulator; (C) bilateral leads connected to dual channel neuromodulator.
Reproduced from Jens Wöllner *et al*., 'Sacral neuromodulation', *BJU International*, Volume 110, Issue 1, pp. 146–159, Copyright © BJU International 2012, with permission from John Wiley and Sons.

patients doing very well and other less so. This form of therapy clearly requires more investigation.

Cystodistension is occasionally used in patients with OAB. There is little evidence for its use in this group of patients and the technique has not yet been standardized.[21] It is postulated to be more beneficial for smaller capacity bladders. Surgery for refractory incontinence has also been described in severe cases. If the resting detrusor pressure is high or the bladder capacity is severely reduced, then cystoplasty may be utilized to increase capacity. However, this is more routine for a neuropathic bladder. Rarely, a urinary diversion may be required for refractory detrusor overactivity.

Nocturia

Nocturia is a symptom commonly encountered by urologists. Although the definition of OAB proposed by the International Continence Society includes nocturia, the symptom may be due to several other causes. It is therefore important for a urologist to understand these and can manage these appropriately. In addition, nocturia may lead to a large reduction in QoL, work productivity, and increases the risk of falls and mortality in elderly people. It may also be a symptom of serious underlying illness.

In patients with nocturia, global polyuria should be excluded via a frequency volume chart. The causes of polyuria include excess fluid intake (polydipsia), diabetes mellitus, and diabetes insipidus. Polydipsia may be primary or secondary to diabetes. Central diabetes insipidus is caused by a deficiency of antidiuretic hormone (ADH) and nephrogenic diabetes insipidus by the kidneys' inability to respond to ADH.

Thereafter it is important to exclude nocturnal polyuria as a cause of nocturia, as its aetiology and treatment are mostly medical. As described above, the frequency volume chart is fundamental in delineating this symptom. Although generally, >33% of the daily urine production occurring at night is taken as the cut off, in younger individuals 20% may be more appropriate. Recognized causes of nocturnal polyuria include excessive evening fluid intake, heart failure, diabetes mellitus, hypoalbuminemia, venous insufficiency, long-acting diuretics, and obstructive sleep apnoea.

Many of its causes are due to redistribution of third space fluid when the patient lies down, leading to excessive urine production during sleep hours. The treatment for this is mostly medical. Obstructive sleep apnoea is interesting and it is postulated that closure of the soft tissues of the larynx leads to increased intrathoracic pressure, resulting in a reflex tachycardia and right heart strain, which in turn produces atrial naturetic peptide. This increases sodium and water excretion from the kidneys, resulting in nocturnal polyuria. The use of continuous positive airways pressure has been shown to reduce nocturia in these patients.

Other causes of nocturia include incomplete bladder emptying secondary to bladder outflow obstruction or detrusor failure, nocturnal detrusor overactivity, decreased bladder capacity, painful bladder syndrome, bladder or ureteral calculi, urogenital neoplasia, anxiety, poor sleep, psychological disorders, and drugs. In patients with a reduced bladder capacity or dipstick haematuria, a cystoscopy and abdominal ultrasound scan should be undertaken to exclude bladder calculi, neoplasms of the bladder, cystitis, and extrinsic compression of the bladder from prolapse, fibroids, or other masses.

Reducing evening fluid intake, especially caffeine and alcohol, may help patient symptoms and is the first line in conservative therapy. Logically, the use of compression stockings during the day may shift third space fluid and reduce nocturnal polyuria, although evidence is lacking for this it seems a sensible suggestion. To reduce further, third space fluid diuretics may also be employed. Their use in the late afternoon (six hours before bedtime) has been shown to improve nocturia by shifting excess fluid before sleep.[22]

Antimuscarinic agents may be used in patients with nocturia. Although they have been shown to have significant benefits over placebo in randomized controlled trials, this may not be clinically significant.[23] Certainly in patients with urgency and OAB, they may be beneficial and they also show more clinical benefit in those with a higher frequency of nocturia. Asking a patient why they wake and why they go to void, and whether this is due to urgency may help identify those who may attain benefit from antimuscarinics.

Alpha antagonists and 5-alpha reductase inhibitors have been shown to lead to reductions in nocturia in men with other symptoms of bladder outflow obstruction. Their success in men without symptoms of bladder outflow obstruction and poor flow rates is not well documented. Similarly, surgery to relieve bladder outflow obstruction such as transurethral resection of prostate may help reduce nocturia frequency if it is due to bladder outflow obstruction, but not if there is another underlying cause. Therefore, in selected cases it would certainly be worth considering.

If after the causes of nocturia are adequately treated and symptoms persist, then desmopressin is indicated. Desmopressin is a selective vasopressin-2 receptor agonist and is a synthetic analogue of ADH. Desmopressin has been shown to have a significant benefit in patients with nocturia and nocturnal polyuria. The patient must be warned to take only one tablet prior to sleep and not more than one in any 24 hours. It is mandatory to measure serum sodium at three days, one week, and in the long term following ingestion of therapy, especially in elderly patients.

Further reading

Abrams P, Andersson KE, Buccafusco JJ, *et al.* Muscarinic receptors: their distribution and function in body systems, and the implications for treating overactive bladder. *Br J Pharmacol* 2006; **148**:565–78.

Abrams P, Cardozo L, Fall M, *et al.* The standardisation of terminology of lower urinary tract function: report from the Standardisation Sub-committee of the International Continence Society. *Neurourol Urodyn* 2002; **21**:167–78.

Chapple CR, Khullar V, Gabriel Z, Muston D, Bitoun CE, Weinstein D. The effects of antimuscarinic treatments in overactive bladder: an update of a systematic review and meta-analysis. *Eur Urol* 2008; **54**(3):543–62.

Irwin DE, Milsom I, Chancellor MB, Kopp Z, Guan Z. Dynamic progression of overactive bladder and urinary incontinence symptoms: a systematic review. *Eur Urol* 2010; **58**(4):532–43.

Mangera A, Andersson KE, Apostolidis A, *et al.* Contemporary management of lower urinary tract disease with botulinum toxin A: a systematic review of botox (onabotulinumtoxinA) and dysport (abobotulinumtoxinA). *Eur Urol* 2011; **60**(4):784–95.

Novara G, Galfano A, Secco S, *et al.* A systematic review and meta-analysis of randomized controlled trials with antimuscarinic drugs for overactive bladder. *Eur Urol* 2008; **54**(4):740–63.

Smith AL, Wein AJ. Outcomes of pharmacological management of nocturia with non-antidiuretic agents: does statistically significant equal clinically significant? *BJU Int* 2011; **107**:1550–4.

References

1. Abrams P, Cardozo L, Fall M, *et al.* The standardisation of terminology of lower urinary tract function: report from the Standardisation Sub-committee of the International Continence Society. *Neurourol Urodyn* 2002; **21**:167–78.
2. Brading AF, Turner WH. The unstable bladder: towards a common mechanism. *Br J Urol* 1994; **73**(1):3–8.
3. de Groat WC. A neurologic basis for the overactive bladder. *Urology* 1997; **50**(6A Suppl):36–52.
4. Birder LA, Ruggieri M, Takeda M, *et al.* How does the urothelium affect bladder function in health and disease? ICI-RS 2011. *Neurourol Urodyn* 2012; **31**(3):293–99.
5. Irwin DE, Milsom I, Hunskaar S, *et al.* Population-based survey of urinary incontinence, overactive bladder, and other lower urinary tract symptoms in five countries: results of the EPIC study. *Eur Urol* 2006; **50**(6):1306–14.
6. Malmsten UG, Molander U, Peeker R, Irwin DE, Milsom I. Urinary incontinence, overactive bladder, and other lower urinary tract symptoms: a longitudinal population-based survey in men aged 45–103 years. *Eur Urol* 2010; **58**(1):149–56.
7. Irwin DE, Milsom I, Chancellor MB, Kopp Z, Guan Z. Dynamic progression of overactive bladder and urinary incontinence symptoms: a systematic review. *Eur Urol* 2010; **58**(4):532–43.
8. Hashim H, Abrams P. Is the bladder a reliable witness for predicting detrusor overactivity? *J Urol* 2006; **175**(1):191–4.
9. Hegde SS, Eglen RM. Muscarinic receptor subtypes modulating smooth muscle contractility in the urinary bladder. *Life Sci* 1999; **64**(6–7):419–28.
10. Abrams P, Andersson KE, Buccafusco JJ, *et al.* Muscarinic receptors: their distribution and function in body systems, and the implications for treating overactive bladder. *Br J Pharmacol* 2006; **148**:565–78.
11. Chapple CR, Khullar V, Gabriel Z, Muston D, Bitoun CE, Weinstein D. The effects of antimuscarinic treatments in overactive bladder: an update of a systematic review and meta-analysis. *Eur Urol* 2008; **54**(3):543–62.
12. Novara G, Galfano A, Secco S, *et al.* A systematic review and meta-analysis of randomized controlled trials with antimuscarinic drugs for overactive bladder. *Eur Urol* 2008; **54**(4):740–63.
13. Mangera A, Andersson KE, Apostolidis A, *et al.* Contemporary management of lower urinary tract disease with botulinum toxin A: a systematic review of botox (onabotulinumtoxinA) and dysport (abobotulinumtoxinA). *Eur Urol* 2011; **60**(4):784–95.
14. Dmochowski R, Chapple C, Nitti VW, *et al.* Efficacy and safety of onabotulinumtoxinA for idiopathic overactive bladder: a double-blind, placebo controlled, randomized, dose ranging trial. *J Urol* 2010; **184**:2416–22.
15. Tanagho EA, Schmidt RA. Bladder pacemaker: scientific basis and clinical future. *Urology* 1982; **20**(6):614–19.
16. Spinelli M, Giardiello G, Gerber M, Arduini A, van den Hombergh U, Malaguti S. New sacral neuromodulation lead for percutaneous implantation using local anesthesia: description and first experience. *J Urol* 2003; **170**(5):1905–7.
17. Hassouna MM, Siegel SW, Nyeholt AA, *et al.* Sacral neuromodulation in the treatment of urgency-frequency symptoms: a multicenter study on efficacy and safety. *J Urol* 2000; **163**(6):1849–54.
18. van Kerrebroeck PE, van Voskuilen AC, Heesakkers JP, *et al.* Results of sacral neuromodulation therapy for urinary voiding dysfunction: outcomes of a prospective, worldwide clinical study. *J Urol* 2007; **178**(5):2029–34.
19. Peters KM, Macdiarmid SA, Wooldridge LS, *et al.* Randomized trial of percutaneous tibial nerve stimulation versus extended-release tolterodine: results from the overactive bladder innovative therapy trial. *J Urol* 2009; **182**(3):1055–61.
20. Klingler HC, Pycha A, Schmidbauer J, Marberger M. Use of peripheral neuromodulation of the S3 region for treatment of detrusor overactivity: a urodynamic-based study. *Urology* 2000; **56**(5):766–71.
21. Mahendru AA, Al-Taher H. Cystodistension: certainly no standards and possibly no benefits—survey of UK practice. *Int Urogynecol J* 2010; **21**(2):135–9.
22. Reynard JM, Cannon A, Yang Q, Abrams P. A novel therapy for nocturnal polyuria: a double-blind randomized trial of frusemide against placebo. *Br J Urol* 1998; **81**:215–18.
23. Smith AL, Wein AJ. Outcomes of pharmacological management of nocturia with non-antidiuretic agents: does statistically significant equal clinically significant? *BJU Int* 2011; **107**:1550–4.

CHAPTER 3.8

Urinary fistula

Nadir I. Osman and Christopher R. Chapple

Introduction to urinary fistula

Genitourinary fistulae (GuF) are a global public health problem afflicting two to three million women worldwide, most of whom are in developing nations.[1,2] The burden of GuF is significant due to associated stress, psychological upset, and socioeconomic consequences.[3,4] A fistula is defined as an abnormal communication between two or more epithelial surfaces. The close embryological development and anatomic proximity of the genital and urinary tracts predisposes them to associated injuries. Most commonly, fistulation occurs between the bladder and vagina, known as vesicovaginal fistula (VVF). Less commonly, fistulae can form between the urethra and vagina, known as urethrovaginal fistula (UVF); between the ureter and vagina as ureterovaginal fistula (UrVF); and rarely between the bladder and uterus as vesicouterine fistula (VUF).

Historically, in the developed world neglected obstructed labour was the major cause of GuF but with advancements in obstetric care this has now given way to gynaecological surgery, particularly hysterectomy,[5] where it is estimated to occur in 1 in 788 cases.[6] Obstetric injury remains the primary cause in developing countries.

Aetiology, pathogenesis, and risk factors

Vesicovaginal fistula

Vesicovaginal fistula (VVF) is the most prevalent GuF worldwide. In developed countries, the most common cause is pelvic surgery, particularly hysterectomy for benign conditions, which accounts for 50% of all cases.[7] The remainder of causes show an even split between radiation, malignancy, and miscellaneous causes. General risk factors for fistula formation include prior pelvic surgery, irradiation, endometriosis, diabetes, malnutrition, and steroid use.

Post-hysterectomy VVF are usually located above the interureteric bar in the region of the upper vaginal vault. They typically result as consequence of unrecognized bladder injury around the vaginal cuff during the mobilization of the bladder off the anterior vaginal wall, more likely to occur with blunt as opposed to sharp dissection.[8] A urinoma then forms which may spontaneously discharge via the vagina, while ongoing leakage is a sign that a fistula tract has formed. Alternatively, the bladder may be injured due to excessive electrocautery or injudicious suture placement to control bleeding resulting in tissue ischaemia, necrosis, and fibrosis, predisposing to the development of a fistula tract.[9] Pelvic haematoma or local infection also increase the risk of fistula formation.

Pelvic irradiation may result in fistulation years or even decades after treatment and is the primary cause of delayed fistulae. Rates of VVF after radiotherapy for cervical cancer range from 0.6% to 2%.[10] Radiation induces ulceration and fissuring of the bladder epithelium, fibrosis in the bladder wall, and obliterative arteritis leading to tissue ischaemia, necrosis, and atrophy, which predispose to the formation of fistula.[11] It may also be the case that the fistula tract signifies disease recurrence. Primary locally advanced tumours may result in VVF, particularly gynaecological malignancies. Advanced cervical carcinoma with bladder invasion is associated with VVF formation in between 4–48% of cases[12,13] and may be more common in smokers where pre-existent arteriosclerosis may augment radiation-induced vascular injury.[14] It is essential in all cases of VVF where there is a precedent history of cancer to conduct appropriate staging investigations to exclude recurrence, prior to carrying out fistula repair.

Prolonged obstructed labour is the most common cause of VVF in the developing world, representing over 90% of cases.[15] Prolonged impaction of the foetal head against the anterior vaginal wall results in pressure-induced tissue ischaemia and ultimately necrosis of the vaginal wall extending to the bladder, bladder neck, and/or urethra, depending on the level the foetal head descent arrested. Post-partum, sloughing of the necrotic tissue will result in a fistulous tract. Risk factors for obstetric fistula include labouring before physical maturity and malnutrition, both common scenarios in developing countries; this coupled with a lack of obstetric care results in prolonged obstructed labour. Obstetric VVF often occurs simultaneously with injuries to the gastrointestinal, neurological, and musculoskeletal systems due to 'field' ischaemic injury, termed 'the obstetric labour injury complex'.[16]

Miscellaneous causes of VVF include forgotten pessaries, trauma, and infective and inflammatory diseases of the pelvis. Obstetric, gynaecologic, or urological instrumentation may infrequently lead to fistulation.

Urethrovaginal fistula

Urethrovaginal fistula occurs less commonly than VVF and has important differences in aetiology and treatment. In developed countries, UVF occurs most frequently after surgery for stress incontinence, urogenital prolapse, and urethral diverticula. Obstetric labour accounts for most cases in developing countries, where the extensive nature of defects and poor quality of tissue may mean incontinence persists despite closure of the fistula. Less common causes include vaginal malignancy, irradiation, prolonged catheterization, and pelvic fracture. In the last decade, the increased use of artificial slings as treatment for stress urinary incontinence has led to an increase in UVF coupled with sling erosion. Management of these cases involves excision of the fistula tract, as well as excision of the eroded sling.

In general, the management of all UVF is complicated by a high risk of subsequent stress urinary incontinence due to associated sphincteric weakness consequent upon sphincteric damage associated with the fistula.

Ureterovaginal fistula

Ureterovaginal fistula (UrVF) occurs most frequently secondary to iatrogenic injury during hysterectomy, colorectal, or vascular surgery. The ureter is usually injured in its distal segment, either by direct ureterotomy or by inadvertent ligation leading to necrosis and subsequent extravasation of urine, which passes along the path of least resistance to the vaginal suture line to leak externally.

Vesicouterine fistula

Vesicouterine fistula (VUF) is extremely rare and accounts for 1% of fistulas in most series.[17] It represents an abnormal communication between the anterior uterus and posterior bladder wall and is associated with low segment caesarian section (LSCS). The usual scenario is following failed trial of labour in patients who have previously undergone LSCS; where the prior scar acts as the focus for a tear of the tissues at the area of vesicouterine apposition, resulting in a fistula tract forming. Alternatively, VUF may form after a LSCS due to the inadequate mobilization of a bladder adherent to the anterior vaginal and lower uterine walls, resulting in inadvertent cystotomy and incorporation of the bladder into the suture line during closure of the uterus.

Clinical presentation

VVF's typically present days to weeks following surgery, with continuous urinary leakage during day and night that is typically not associated with stress, change in posture, or urgency. In UVF, the presentation depends on the size and location of the fistula.[18] Continence may be preserved when fistulae occur in the distal third of the urethra, with patients experiencing vaginal voiding. Proximal and mid-urethral fistulas may present with intermittent or positional leakage. Other symptoms include perineal skin irritation, vaginal fungal infections, and recurrent urinary tract infections. UrVF presents with constant urinary leakage days to weeks following pelvic surgery which may be preceded by flank pain and fever due to urinoma and/or upper tract obstruction. The patient may also continue to void normally as the bladder fills as usual from the contralateral ureter. VUF may present with urinary incontinence, cyclical haematuria, amenorrhoea, secondary infertility, or first trimester miscarriage. Incontinence is usually seen early following LSCS, whereas haematuria and amenorrhoea can occur months or years later.

Evaluation

A thorough evaluation is central to the successful management of GuF, and in all patients detailed evaluation of both the upper and lower tracts is essential. With lower tract fistulae, precise delineation of the number, location, and size of fistulous tracts, in addition to an assessment of the quality of tissues, function of the urethral sphincter, and any associated ureteric injuries is crucial. This entails a vaginal examination (with speculum) which may identify fistulous tracts (Fig. 3.8.1) and an assessment of any associated prolapse or leakage per urethra on coughing. Additionally, larger fistulae may be palpable on bimanual examination, which is also used to assess for pelvic malignancy.

The three-sponge test can help to confirm the presence of fistula when not apparent on examination.[19] Three gauze sponges are placed in the vagina (Fig. 3.8.2). A dyed solution, such as methylene blue or indigo carmine, is instilled in to the bladder after which the catheter is removed. The sponges are then removed ten minutes later. The results are interpreted as follows: (a) if only the uppermost sponge is stained, it suggests a VVF; (b) if the top sponge is wet (with urine) but unstained while the lower two are unstained, this suggests a UrVF; (c) staining of the lowermost sponge only is suggestive of a urethral origin, potentially either a UVF or back-tracking of urine, associated with concomitant stress incontinence due to a urethral sphincter weakness.

Cystourethroscopy is important to identify fistulae and assess anatomy in relation to the vagina and ureteric orifices. A fistulous opening may appear as an area of hyperaemia, a dimple, or a frank ostium (Fig. 3.8.1) in cases where the fistula tract is more mature. Cannulation with a ureteric catheter or guidewire will help identify fistula anatomy in relation the vagina. In this, it is often easier to identify the fistula by the use of synchronous vaginoscopy using the cystoscope, as the fistula opening in some smaller fistulae is more evident on vaginal examination.

Contrast studies are helpful in confirming the diagnosis and are essential to assess the upper urinary tract (intravenous urography, contrast computed tomography, or MRI). A cystogram will usually

(A)
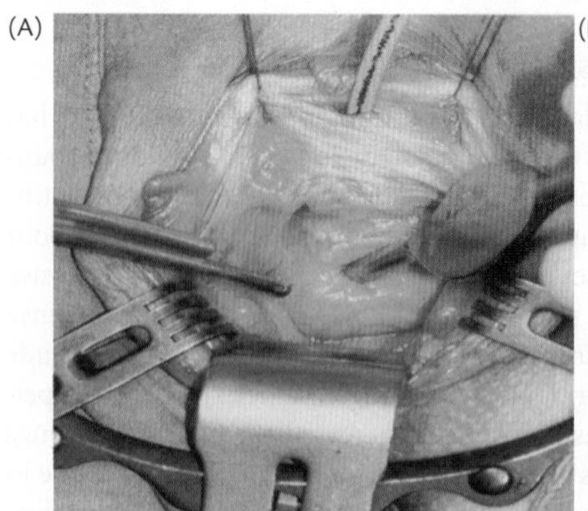
(B)
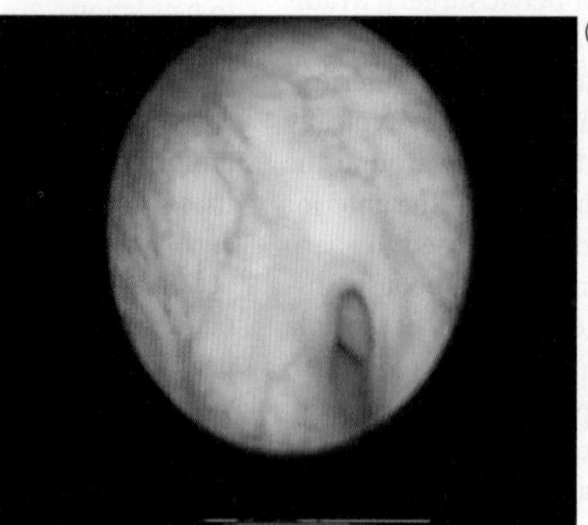
(C)
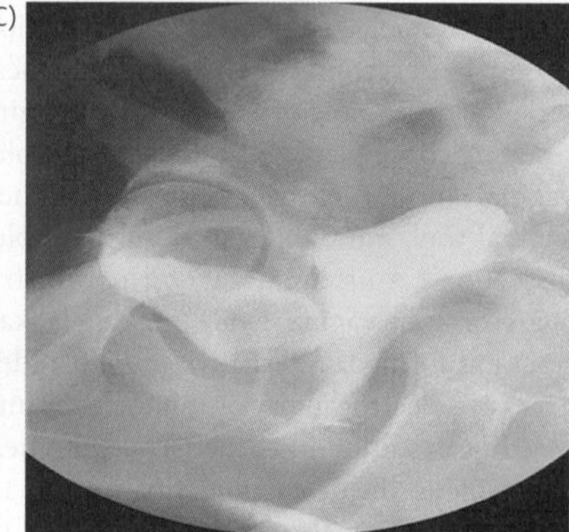

Fig. 3.8.1 Vesicovaginal fistula (VVF): (A) VVF at operation cannulated by a urethral sound; (B) cytsoscopic image of a VVF ostium; and (C) oblique cystogram demonstrating leakage of contrast into the vagina through a VVF.
Images reproduced courtesy of Professor Chapple.

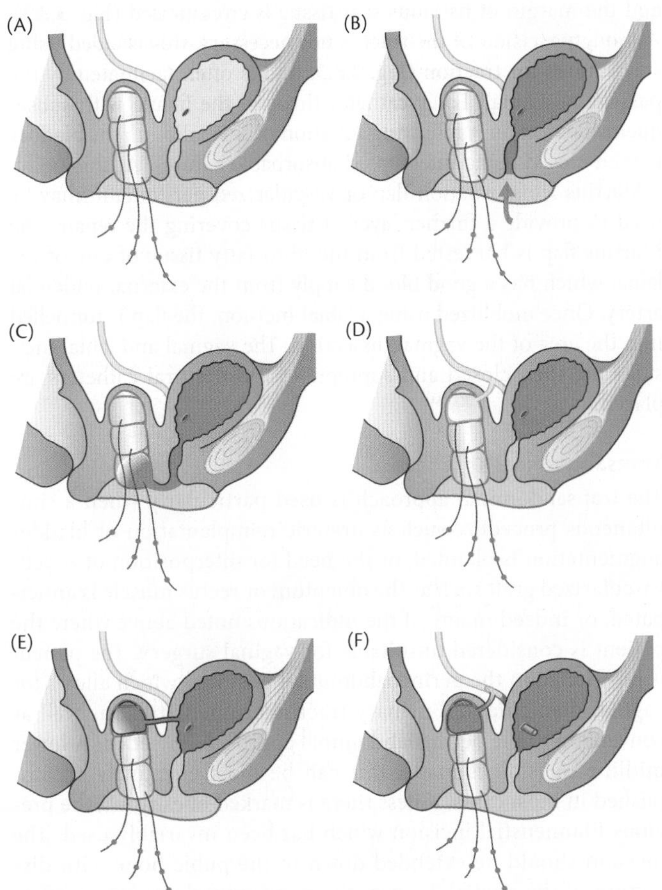

Fig. 3.8.2 The three-sponge test. (A) Three sponges are inserted into the vaginal canal. (B) Dyed solution (e.g. aqueous methylene blue) is instilled into the bladder. The sponges are then removed after 10 minutes. (C) If only the lower most sponge is stained, the cause is either a low UrVF or back tracking from the urethral meatus. (D) If none of the sponges are stained but the top-most sponge is wet with urine, this suggests a UVF. (E) If only the upper sponge is stained, this suggests a VVF. (F) Rarely, staining of the uppermost sponge can be due to reflux of the dye from the bladder into the ureter, then leaking from a UVF.
Images reproduced courtesy of Professor Chapple.

demonstrate clear leakage of contrast into the vagina (Fig. 3.8.1) and voiding phase images may identify smaller fistula and UVF; these are more easily seen in lateral or oblique views. Videourodynamics will additionally provide an assessment for stress incontinence, bladder capacity, and detrusor function. Intravenous urography or retrograde studies will determine the presence of ureteric injury or upper tract obstruction. Cross-sectional imaging is essential to the evaluation of suspected malignancy. When recurrent malignancy is suspected, the tract must also be biopsied.

Classification

Currently there are no universally accepted classification systems for GuF, although many have been proposed.[20] Most classification systems are based on descriptions of the size and location of fistula but do not reliably predict difficulty of repair or chance of successful outcome, limiting their utility in clinical practice. Nevertheless, the adoption of a standardized classification for GuF is essential for interpretation and comparison of series of GuF repair, particularly in the developing world.

Management

The incontinence associated with GuF is often debilitating and so all patients initially should be provided with incontinence pads and advised how to manage their symptoms until definitive treatment.

Conservative

In the postoperative setting, a VVF and UVF diagnosed early (within the first two to three weeks) should not be managed conservatively. Beyond this 'watershed' period, with VVF, if an indwelling catheter results in dryness then providing continuous drainage may result in spontaneous healing of smaller fistulae. UVF are often best managed conservatively in the first instance with a delayed repair being carried out. With conservative management, if there has been no improvement after 30 days resolution is unlikely[21]; however, since this is only used after the watershed period has passed it is continued until definitive interventional surgery. Alternatively, if the fistula tract is deemed small, endoscopic fulguration with an electrode has been suggested, however this may result in necrosis and enlargement of the tract if performed overzealously.[22] Occlusion using fibrin glue may be useful providing a support containing growth and angiogenic factors allowing ingrowth of fibroblasts and the formation of connective tissue; the results reported with this approach are however limited in number.

UrVF should always be managed actively, with either nephrostomy drainage and/or ureteric stenting being instituted at an early stage. Ureteric stenting when the ureter is patent may result in spontaneous resolution.

Surgical

General considerations

The first consideration is the timing of repair, which has been a source of some controversy. Traditionally, a delay of three to six months was advocated as an extrapolation from obstetric fistula practice and to allow inflammation, tissue oedema, and friability to resolve. More recently earlier repair has been advocated, especially in the post-hysterectomy setting, where the fistula results from clean localized surgical trauma as opposed to the wide ischaemic injury seen in obstetric practice.[23] In most cases, contemporary consensus favours a delay of at least six weeks once the initial two to three-week watershed has been passed.

The principles of fistula repair were first described by Simms 150 years ago as:

(i) The excision of all scar tissue

(ii) The approximation of healthy wound edges

(iii) Closure without overlapping suture lines

In most cases it is not necessary to excise the tract, particularly in cases where doing so would create a large defect that would be more difficult to close. Interpositional grafts and flaps should be used to provide additional tissue coverage to repairs.

Preoperatively, patients should be optimized nutritionally, any infection treated with antibiotics, and blood sugar levels controlled in diabetics. Vaginal oestrogen cream can be given to those with atrophic vaginitis. Antibiotic prophylaxis should be administered and continued into the postoperative period. Both a suprapubic and urethral catheter should be placed at operation, to protect the repair should one become blocked. A cystogram at 10–14 days will confirm closure, following which the urethral catheter can be removed and suprapubic catheter clamped.

Each fistula is unique and requires an individualized approach. A detailed exposition of the different approaches for GuF is beyond the scope of this chapter, but the principles of the common reconstructive techniques are discussed. The contemporary principles can be summarized as:

(i) Define anatomy
(ii) Tension-free closure
(iii) Avoid haematoma
(iv) Interpose vascularized tissue wherever possible
(v) Defunction bladder for two to three weeks and confirm success with a contrast study

Vesicovaginal fistula

Surgical repair of non-complicated vesicovaginal fistula is associated with successful outcomes in over 90% of cases.[24] A transvaginal or transabdominal approach may be used, the choice depending on the specific situation and the route which the surgeon is most comfortable with.

Transvaginal approach

The vaginal approach is generally considered to be preferable due to the shorter operating time, reduced blood loss, and shorter hospital stay. The main contraindications are the presence of multiple fistula or fistula to other organs, concomitant ureteric injury, anatomy that would make the approach difficult (e.g. vaginal stenosis, a high fistula) or leg contractures. The patient is positioned in lithotomy or modified Sims position (prone) (Fig. 3.8.3). The ureters are catheterized and should be subsequently stented if they are near the fistula tract, as postoperative oedema will lead to impaired drainage from the upper tract. The vaginal opening of the fistula is identified and the margin of fistulous scar tissue is circumcised (Fig. 3.8.3). Although excision of the tract is not necessary, this is aided using stay sutures for traction (Fig. 3.8.3) and is often facilitated by the passage of a small Foley catheter through the fistula with subsequent traction on it following inflation of the balloon. The bladder is then closed using interrupted absorbable sutures. At this point, a Martius labial rotation flap or vascularized peritoneum may be used to provide a further layer of tissue covering the repair. The Martius flap is harvested from the fibro-fatty tissue of one of the labia, which has a good blood supply from the external pudendal artery. Once mobilized using a labial incision, the flap is tunnelled into the area of the vaginal dissection. The vaginal and labial incisions are then closed and suprapubic and urethral catheters are placed.

Transabdominal approach

The transabdominal approach is used particularly when a simultaneous procedure such as ureteric reimplantation or bladder augmentation is planned, or the need for interposition of a well-vascularized graft such as the omentum or rectus muscle is anticipated, or indeed in any of the indications noted above where the patient is considered unsuitable for vaginal surgery. The patient is positioned in the perineoabdominal position, which allows for vaginal manipulation, urinary tract instrumentation, as well as conversion to the perineoabdominal approach if needed. A lower midline incision is made; this can be most effectively accomplished in most cases, unless there is marked obesity, via the previous Pfannenstiel incision which has been invariably used. The incision should be extended down to the pubic bone with dissection of the medial 2 cm of the rectus muscle insertion off of the pubic bone. The bladder is bivalved to the level of the fistula. The ureteric orifices are identified and stented. The fistula tract is then excised and bladder and vagina are closed separately in

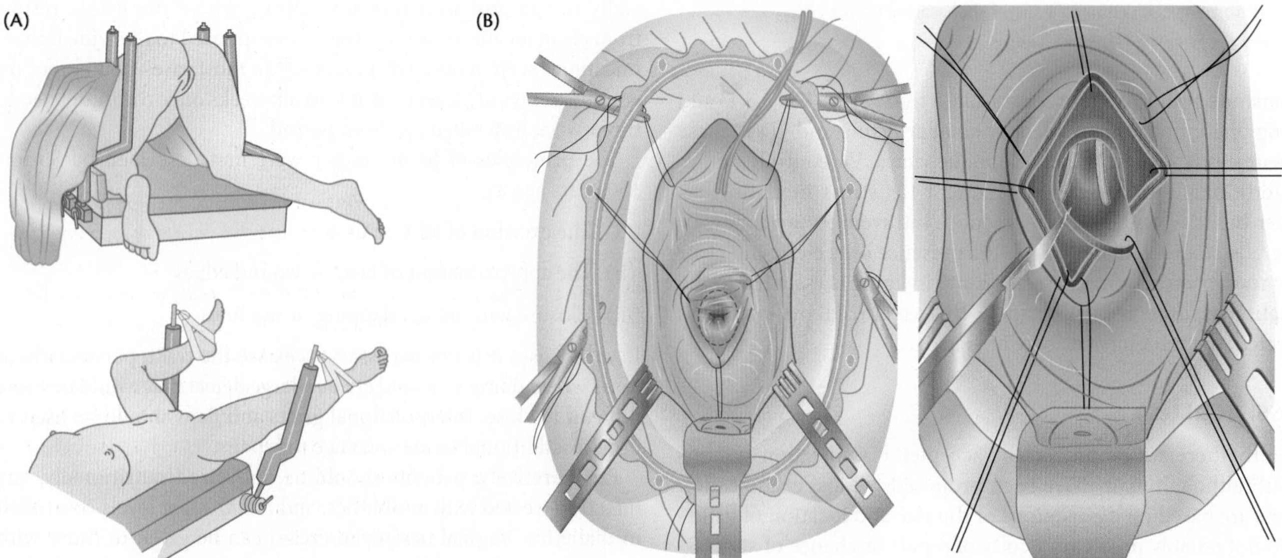

Fig. 3.8.3 Surgical approaches: (A) prone (Simm's) position (top) and lithotomy prepared for abdominopernineal progression (bottom); (B) circumferential incision around VVF tract (left) with the aid of stay sutures (right).
Images reproduced courtesy of Professor Chapple.

layers using interrupted absorbable sutures. A space can then be developed for interposition of mobilized omentum (along its right gastroepiploic pedicle) between the closures of the bladder and vagina. The excellent vascular supply and ability to respond to inflammation and infection makes omentum the ideal tissue support for repair.

Urethrovaginal fistula

In developed countries, urethrovaginal fistulae are more commonly associated with iatrogenic injury from incontinence and prolapse surgery. Patients with mid or proximal UVF should be warned of the risk of postoperative stress incontinence. UVF are approached transvaginally, with the utmost care to avoid excessive dissection of the perifistula tissue, to avoid excessive damage to the urethral sphincter mechanism. The urethra is best closed in a tension-free fashion using interrupted figure-of-eight sutures to facilitate sphincter reconstruction and reduce the risk of stenosis. A Martius flap should also be interposed between the urethral and vaginal closures. UVF due to obstetric injury are usually more extensive, which may necessitate some form of urethral reconstruction using a tubularized vaginal graft/flap or a bladder wall flap. The use of a Martius flap also facilitates the subsequent use of an autologous sling should stress incontinence result and require treatment.

Ureterovaginal fistula

With an acute injury, provided there is little loss of ureter, a direct anastomotic ureteroplasty can be carried out. However, in the majority of cases, where stenting has failed, and the procedure is being carried out after the development of a significant ureteric stenosis, this is not possible. The traditional approach to repair for the lower third is uretero-neocystomy as the extensive fibrotic reaction makes separation of the ureter from the vagina difficult. The ureter should be divided as distally as possible and reimplanted into the bladder, with the aid of a psoas hitch or boari flap if needed. For more proximal injuries, then ileal interposition or transureteroureterostomy can be considered. An alternative is renal autotransplantation into the pelvis. When the kidney on the affected side is functioning poorly, nephrectomy may be a better option.

Vesicouterine fistula

In vesicouterine fistula, management largely depends on the whether the patient still desires to conceive or has completed her family.[25] In the former the tract can be excised and bladder and uterus closed; in the latter excision may be coupled with a hysterectomy.

Urinary diversion

Around 5% of fistulas are deemed incurable; such cases include those where multiple repairs have failed, or where fistulae are deemed so extensive that reconstruction is impossible.[26] In these situations urinary diversion is usually the only option. In developed countries, the most feasible and safest method is an ileal conduit, whereas in developing countries continent diversions such as the ureterosigmoidostomy are more common due to the lack of need for expensive stoma appliances (although these are associated with a higher risk of long-term complications). Percutaneous nephrostomy is an option, albeit a less than desirable one for patients who are not fit for surgery.

Conclusion

GuF are one of the most distressing complications of pelvic surgery. The diagnosis is made commonly after the patient presents with constant urine leakage days to weeks postoperatively. A careful evaluation is needed to establish the number and nature of fistulous tracts, as well as any associated injuries. Approximation of healthy tissue is essential to repair and when there is doubt regarding the potential success of a repair, tissue interposition, using a Martius or omental flap, provides additional tissue support.

Further reading

Chapple C, Turner-Warwick R. Vesico-vaginal fistula. *BJU Int* 2005; **95**(1):193–214.

Hilton P, Cromwell D. The risk of vesicovaginal and urethrovaginal fistula after hysterectomy performed in the English National Health Service—a retrospective cohort study examining patterns of care between 2000 and 2008. *BJOG* 2012; **119**(12):1447–54.

Hilton P. Urogenital fistula in the UK: a personal case series managed over 25 years. *BJU Int* 2012; **110**(1):102–10.

Pushkar DY, Dyakov VV, Kosko JW, Kasyan GR. Management of urethrovaginal fistulas. *Eur Urol* 2006; **50**(5):1000–5.

Rovner ES. Urinary tract fistulae. (pp. 415–21) In: McDougal SWA, Kavoussi L, Novick A, Partin A, Peters C (eds). *Campbell-Walsh Urology*, 10th edition. Philadelphia, PA: Saunders, 2012.

References

1. Wall LL. Obstetric vesicovaginal fistula as an international public-health problem. *Lancet* 2006; **368**(9542):1201–9.
2. Waaldijk K, Au Y. The obstetric fitula: A major public health problem still unsolved. *Int Urogynecol J Pelvic Floor Dysfunct* 1993; **4**:126–8.
3. Roush KM. Social implications of obstetric fistula: an integrative review. *J Midwifery Womens Health* 2009; **54**(2):e21–33.
4. Ahmed S, Holtz SA. Social and economic consequences of obstetric fistula: life changed forever? *Int J Gynaecol Obstet* 2007; **99** (Suppl 1):S10–5.
5. Hilton P. Urogenital fistula in the UK: a personal case series managed over 25 years. *BJU Int* 2012; **110**(1):102–10.
6. Hilton P, Cromwell D. The risk of vesicovaginal and urethrovaginal fistula after hysterectomy performed in the English National Health Service—a retrospective cohort study examining patterns of care between 2000 and 2008. *BJOG* 2012; **119**(12):1447–54.
7. Symmonds RE. Incontinence: vesical and urethral fistulas. *Clin Obstet Gynecol* 1984; **27**(2):499–514.
8. Cornella JL. Diagnosis and management of genito-urinary fistula. *CME J Gynecol Oncol* 2002; **7**:78–90.
9. Garthwaite M, Harris N. Vesicovaginal fistulae. *IJU* 2010; **26**(2):253–6.
10. Perez CA, Grigsby PW, Lockett MA, Chao KS, Williamson J. Radiation therapy morbidity in carcinoma of the uterine cervix: dosimetric and clinical correlation. *Int J Radiat Oncol Biol Phys* 1999; **44**(4):855–66.
11. Pushkar DY, Dyakov VV, Kasyan GR. Management of radiation-induced vesicovaginal fistula. *Eur Urol* 2009; **55**(1):131–7.
12. Million RR, Rutledge F, Fletcher GH. Stage IV carcinoma of the cervix with bladder invasion. *Am J Obstet Gynecol* 1972; **113**(2):239–46.
13. Moore KN, Gold MA, McMeekin DS, Zorn KK. Vesicovaginal fistula formation in patients with Stage IVA cervical carcinoma. *Gynecol Oncol* 2007; **106**(3):498–501.
14. Eifel PJ, Jhingran A, Bodurka DC, Levenback C, Thames H. Correlation of smoking history and other patient characteristics with major complications of pelvic radiation therapy for cervical cancer. *J Clin Oncol* 2002; **20**(17):3651–7.

15. Wall LL, Karshima JA, Kirschner C, Arrowsmith SD. The obstetric vesicovaginal fistula: characteristics of 899 patients from Jos, Nigeria. *Am J Obstet Gynecol* 2004; **190**(4):1011–9.
16. Arrowsmith S, Hamlin EC, Wall LL. Obstructed labor injury complex: obstetric fistula formation and the multifaceted morbidity of maternal birth trauma in the developing world. *Obstet Gynecol Surv* 1996; **51**(9):568–74.
17. Iloabachie GC, Njoku O. Vesico-uterine fistula. *Br J Urol* 1985; **57**(4):438–9.
18. Pushkar DY, Dyakov VV, Kosko JW, Kasyan GR. Management of urethrovaginal fistulas. *Eur Urol* 2006; **50**(5):1000–5.
19. Chapple C, Turner-Warwick R. Vesico-vaginal fistula. *BJU Int* 2005; **95**(1):193–214.
20. Arrowsmith SD. The classification of obstetric vesico-vaginal fistulas: a call for an evidence-based approach. *Int J Gynaecol Obstet* 2007; **99**(Suppl 1):S25–7.
21. Zimmern PE, Hadley HR, Staskin D, Raz S. Genitourinary fistulas: vaginal approach for repair of vesicovaginal fistulas. *Clin Obstet Gynaecol* 1985; **12**(2):403–13.
22. Stovsky MD, Ignatoff JM, Blum MD, Nanninga JB, O'Conor VJ, Kursh ED. Use of electrocoagulation in the treatment of vesicovaginal fistulas. *J Urol* 1994; **152**(5 Pt 1):1443–4.
23. Wang Y, Hadley HR. Nondelayed transvaginal repair of high lying vesicovaginal fistula. *J Urol* 1990; **144**(1):34–6.
24. Angioli R, Penalver M, Muzii L, *et al.* Guidelines of how to manage vesicovaginal fistula. *Crit Rev Oncol Hematol* 2003; **48**(3):295–304.
25. Rovner ES. Urinary tract fistulae. (pp. 415–21) In: McDougal SWA, Kavoussi L, Novick A, Partin A, Peters C (eds). *Campbell-Walsh Urology*, 10th edition. Philadelphia, PA: Saunders, 2012.
26. Arrowsmith SD. Urinary diversion in the vesico-vaginal fistula patient: general considerations regarding feasibility, safety, and follow-up. *Int J Gynaecol Obstet* 2007; **99**(Suppl 1):S65–8.

CHAPTER 3.9

Urethral diverticula

Nadir I. Osman and Christopher R. Chapple

Introduction to urethral diverticula

Urethral diverticula (UD) can be defined as focal out-pouchings of the urethra into the surrounding periurethral tissues. They occur almost exclusively in adult females, usually in the third to fifth decade. The true incidence has been impossible to define but historically has been placed between 1–6%[1] in the general population, rising to up 40% in women with lower urinary tract symptoms (LUTS).[2] By contrast, UD in males are exceedingly rare and may be congenital or associated with urethral stricture, trauma, or surgery. However, we consider female UD in this chapter.

Aetio-pathogenesis

Acquired

UD in adults are considered as acquired phenomena with a primary infectious aetiology. Over a century ago, Routh proposed that UD arose from the paraurethral glands (or Skene's glands).[3] Paraurethral glands are tuboalveolar structures that are positioned posterolaterally along the whole length of the urethra, but are more common in the distal two-thirds, with most ducts draining into the distal third of the urethra. They secrete mucin, which is thought to act as a urethral sealant contributing to continence. UD are hyothesized to occur due to acute infection of the paraurethral glands, which leads to obstruction of the duct and paraurethral abscess formation. Relapsing or persistent infection then causes weakening of the urethral wall adjacent to the affected gland, resulting in rupture into the urethral lumen and epithelialization of the tract. The end result is a cyst-like appendage with a connection to the urethra called the neck (or ostia). The distribution of UD follows the anatomical location of the periurethral glands, with the majority being found at 3 or 9 o'clock position in the middle and distal third of the urethra.[4] The ostia are classically located at the 6 o'clock position. UD may also be compound and have complex configurations extending partially around the circumference of the urethra ('saddlebag') or wrapping entirely around it.[5] An alternative aetiological factor is urethral trauma resulting from childbirth, catheterization, or previous surgery.

Congenital

Congenital urethral out-pouchings have rarely been described in the paediatric population, although they are thought to represent a distinct pathoanatomic entity possibly arising from remnants of Gartner's ducts, Müllerian or cloacagenic cell rests, or aberrant union of primordial folds.[6] Some authors do not consider these to be true UD.

Complications

The long-term sequelae of untreated UD include neoplastic transformation, which may be benign (nephrogenic adenoma) or very rarely malignant (60% adenocarcinoma, 30% transitional cell carcinoma, and 10% squamous cell carcinoma) and formation of calculi (up to 10%) due to urinary stagnation.

Clinical presentation

UD present with a wide array of non-specific symptoms.[7] As such, patients are frequently misdiagnosed as having bladder pain syndrome, recurrent urinary tract infections (UTIs), vulvovaginitis, and other conditions. This often leads to significant delays in diagnosis, with patients seeing more than one consultant before a diagnosis is reached; one study found an average time from presentation to diagnosis of nine months.[8] A high index of suspicion is initially required, after which relevant investigations can be undertaken to confirm and evaluate anatomical configuration.

The classic triad (three Ds) of symptoms—dysuria, dyspareunia, and dribbling—is uncommonly seen. The most frequent symptoms are storage LUTS, dysuria, dyspareunia, and pelvic pain. One-third of patients may present with recurrent urinary tract infection probably to due urine stasis in the diverticulum. Other presentations include stress or urgency incontinence, voiding LUTS, urinary retention, anterior vaginal wall pain and swelling, urethral discharge, or urethral bleeding, which may signify the presence of a diverticular stone or malignant change. A salient feature of symptomatic UD is the relapsing remitting course of symptoms caused by the onset and resolution of acute infective exacerbations. Nevertheless, bearing in mind the relatively high prevalence of UD and the relative rarity with which patients present clinically, most UD are likely to be entirely asymptomatic.

Examination may reveal an anterior vaginal wall mass just proximal to the introitus. During an acute exacerbation, palpation will usually elicit tenderness, antegrade 'milking' of the mass may produce urine or purulent discharge. Hardness and induration associated with bleeding may of course signify malignant change; but this is extremely rare. The differential diagnosis for anterior vaginal lumps includes Müllerian remnant cysts, Gartner's duct cysts, ureterocele, abscess, and neoplasms. Additionally, examination should include an assessment for stress urinary incontinence, urethral hypermobility, and the presence of pelvic organ prolapse, which are important considerations in later surgical planning.

Evaluation

Following history taking and examination, urinalysis ± urine microscopy and culture should be undertaken to assess for infection or haematuria. The choice of diagnostic imaging techniques largely depends on the particular clinical presentation and availability of expertise with particular imaging modalities. While traditionally voiding cystourethrography and double balloon positive pressure urethrography were used, in recent years, magnetic resonance imaging (MRI) scanning has become the gold standard evaluation, although in experienced hands transvaginal ultrasound is equally sensitive.

Urethroscopy

Endoscopic examination of the urethra may allow visualization of a mucosal defect or ostia in up to 60% of cases.[9] A zero-degree lens will optimize visualization and if a palpable mass is present, compression may enhance localization by expelling the contents into the urethral lumen. Occlusion of the proximal urethra and withdrawal of the cystoscope distally while instilling irrigation fluid will allow positive pressure to cause distention and may also aid visualization.

Imaging

Voiding cystourethrography

Voiding cystourethrography (VCUG) was previously considered the study of choice for diagnosis of UD with a reported diagnostic accuracy of around 65%. It relies upon adequate flow being generated for contrast to enter the ostia and distend the diverticulum during the voiding phase of micturition. This may fail if the ostium is stenotic, occluded by debris, or the diverticulum is already partially filled. Additionally, patients may suffer pain or embarrassment, and consequently fail to generate adequate urinary flow. VCUG can be performed as part of a videourodynamic assessment to exclude other causes of symptoms such as urgency or stress urinary incontinence (Fig. 3.9.1). Many patients have paradoxical incontinence (loss of urine from diverticulum with Valsalva manoeuvres) and this can be difficult to differentiate from true stress incontinence.[10] VCUG has been largely abandoned as it is time-consuming, technically difficult, and invasive.[6]

Double balloon urethrography

Double balloon urethrography (DBU) was a popular imaging technique in the mid-twentienth century. A specialized double balloon catheter is inserted into urethra to obstruct the bladder neck and urethral meatus, effectively isolating the urethra. Contrast is then injected at high pressure into the urethra with aim of opening up the ostia and delineating the site and anatomy of UD. Although sensitivity compared favourably to VCUG, this technique is now considered obsolete with the advent of transvaginal ultrasonography and MRI scanning.

Ultrasound

In a variety of approaches, ulltrasound (US) has been advocated in the evaluation of UD. It is widely available, rapidly performed, and inexpensive. Transabdominal US is considered inadequate to assess for small lesions, and therefore not recommended. Transvaginal US provides better detail on the size and location of UD although may inadvertently compress the urethra and miss smaller UD.[11] Transurethral US has been developed more recently and shows good sensitivity and anatomic detail, yet is more invasive, and risks UTI and urethral damage so is not widely used. Although techniques are evolving, currently US requires particular expertise to define the surgical anatomy that is required for preoperative planning. MRI scanning is easier for most clinicians to interpret.

Magnetic resonance imaging

MRI is widely considered to represent the gold standard in imaging of UD. It provides exceptional resolution and multiplanar imaging

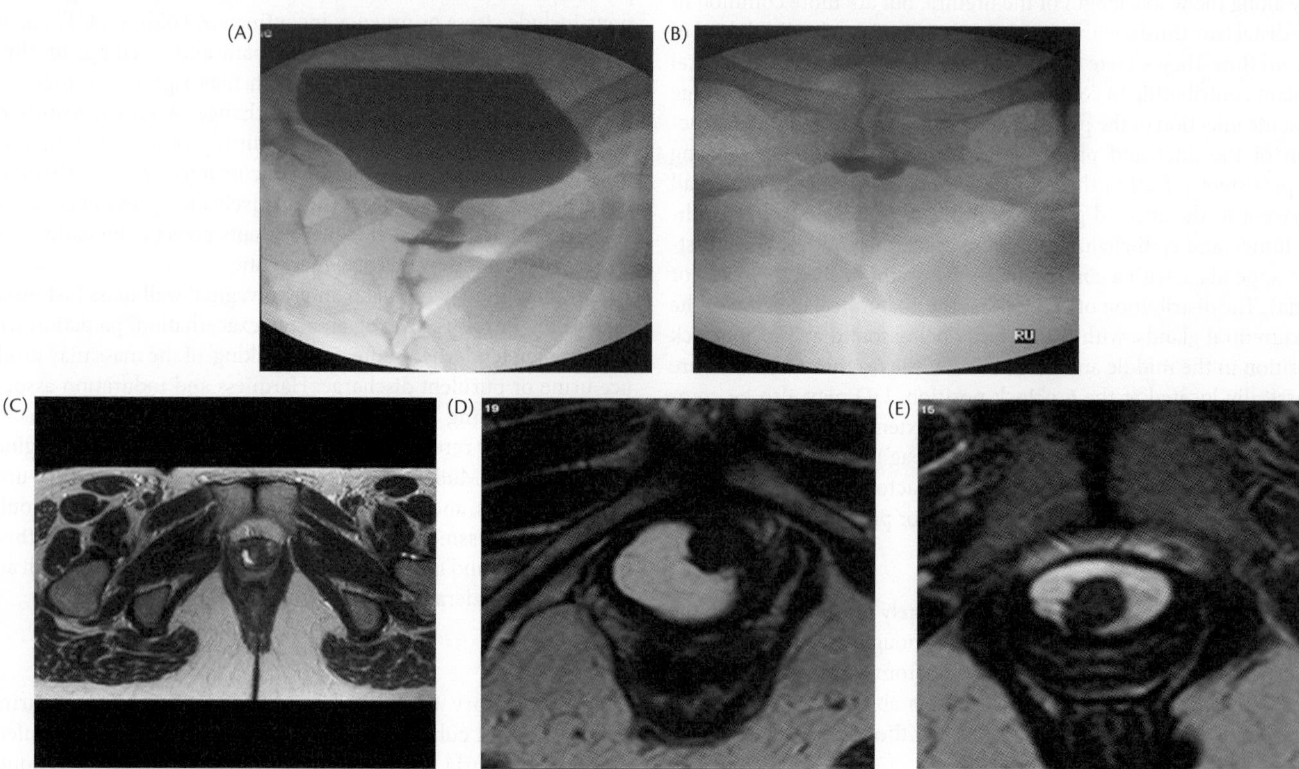

Fig. 3.9.1 Imaging of urethral diverticula (UD). Voiding cystourography: (A) oblique X-ray demonstrating filling of UD during voiding; (B) residual contrast in UD post-voiding. MRI imaging: (C) simple UD; (D) saddlebag UD; and (E) circumferential UD.

Images reproduced courtesy of Professor Chapple.

Table 3.9.1 LNSC3 classification system of UD

L	Location	◆ Site of diverticulum: distal, mid, or proximal urethra ◆ With or without extension behind bladder neck
N	Number	Single or multiple
S	Size	In centimetres
C1	Configuration	◆ Single, multiloculated, or saddle-shaped
C2	Communication	◆ Site of communication with urethra: distal, mid, or proximal
C3	Continence	◆ Is stress incontinence present or not

Reprinted from Gary E. Leach et al., L N S C3: A Proposed classification system for female urethral diverticula, *Neurourology and Urodynamics*, Volume 12, Issue 6, pp. 523–531, Copyright © 1993 Wiley-Liss, Inc., A Wiley Company, with permission from John Wiley and Sons.

Table 3.9.2 Urodynamic findings in UD Urodynamic findings in 55 women with urethral diverticula

Findings	***n***	**Percentage**
Abnormal	33	60
Stress incontinence alone	18	32.5
Stress incontinence with detrusor instability	8	14.5
Detrusor instability alone	5	9
Sensory urgency	1	2
Myogenic decompensation	1	2
Normal	22	40

Reprinted from Gary E. Leach et al., L N S C3: A Proposed classification system for female urethral diverticula, *Neurourology and Urodynamics*, Volume 12, Issue 6, pp. 523–531, Copyright © 1993 Wiley-Liss, Inc., A Wiley Company, with permission from John Wiley and Sons.

of UD and is considered to be more sensitive than VCUG or DBU while avoiding urethral catheterization and the need for voiding.[12] MRI may be performed using the standard surface coil or endoluminal coils (placed in rectum or vagina) which provide an improved signal-to-noise ratio and greater resolution imaging.[13] T2-weighted MRI is the preferred modality, which shows increased signal intensity in diverticulum that contrasts well to the surrounding tissues (Fig. 3.9.1). MRI provides the most detailed anatomic evaluation for surgical planning. It is important not only to request sagittal as well as coronal views, but also to stress that the MRI scan should be performed as a post-voiding study; failure to do so will result in a number of diverticula being 'missed'.

Classification

Two classification systems for UD have been proposed. The simpler of the two divides UD into two classes based on the integrity of the periurethral fascia.[14] The aim is to identify patients with deficient fascia (associated with prior incontinence surgery) who in fact have pseudo-diverticlulae and hence may require a different reconstructive approach. The other classification is more detailed and aims to aid preoperative planning by staging UD based on location, number, size, site of connection with urethra, configuration, and continence state, termed the L N S C3 system (Table 3.9.1).[15]

Management

Conservative

Asymptomatic UD should be treated conservatively and left alone. Conservative management is appropriate in those with minimal symptoms and those declining surgery. Conservative measures, in addition to just observation, include milking the diverticulum after voids to avoid urinary stagnation, and low dose prophylactic antibiotics to prevent infections.

Surgical

A variety of surgical approaches for UD have been described[16] including excision, transurethral incision,[17] open marsupialization in to the vagina,[18] and obliteration with cellulose or Teflon injection.[19] None of these are recommended in contemporary practice. Where intervention is felt to be appropriate, the most common approach is transvaginal excision with reconstruction of the urethra. This should only be carried out in experienced hands as future continence will depend on the integrity of the sphincter mechanism. The surgery requires good exposure and can be a technical challenge due to the significant vascularity and lack of clear tissue planes due to fibrosis from recurrent infection. In general, surgery is best delayed until an acute exacerbation has been treated with antibiotics.

Counselling of patients preoperatively regarding the significant risk of postoperative incontinence is recommended. Conversely the surgery may correct existing urinary incontinence, consequent upon either sphincteric weakness resultant from the diverticulum (stress incontinence), or due to pooling of urine in the diverticulum (paradoxical incontinence). The use of videourodynamics is recommended to define baseline lower urinary tract function. An extensive series of case studies reported in the literature clearly defines the associated pathological conditions, which may be seen preoperatively in these patients (Table 3.9.2).[15]

Patients should be warned about the potential risks of surgery including fistula formation, dyspareunia, and postoperative incontinence. While traditionally patients are operated on in the lithotomy position, we would recommend that with more proximal or complex diverticula, the prone surgical position should be used (Fig. 3.9.2), which provides excellent surgical access. In addition, we have a low index for using a synchronous Martius flap; this in our experience has prevented any fistulae forming in cases where we considered there to be a significant risk of this occurring. Furthermore, where we have considered there to be a significant risk of postoperative stress incontinence, a Martius flap facilitates the subsequent insertion of a fascial sling. Patients should be adequately counselled about the potential for both of these procedures preoperatively.

The general principles of excision can be summarized to include:

(i) Mobilization of well-vascularized vaginal skin flap(s);

(ii) Complete excision of the urethral communication and diverticulum;

(iii) Preservation of urethral anatomy and function;

(iv) Watertight tension-free closure of urethra;

(v) Closure in multiple layers with non-overlapping suture lines.

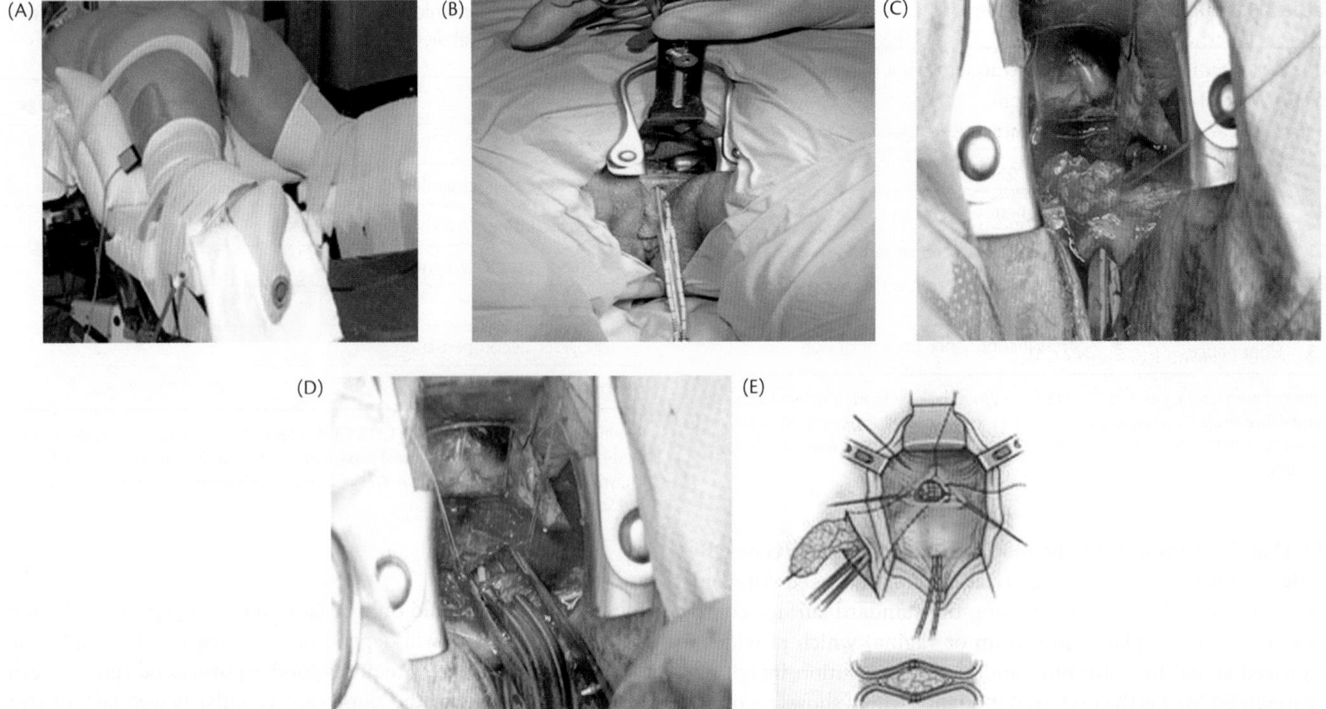

Fig. 3.9.2 Surgical approach to a proximal UD. (A) Patient placed in prone position. (B) Patient draped with ureteric and urethral catheters in place and vaginal walls retracted. (C) Diverticulum being excised. (D) Following removal of diverticulum, showing defect in urethra with exposed urethral catheter. (E) Martius flap and closure.
Images reproduced courtesy of Professor Chapple.

Postoperatively, the bladder is drained with a urethral catheter and a suprapubic catheter. These are left *in situ* for three weeks. The results of excision are generally very good with cure rates of over 70% reported.[6] In our experience, good cure rates have also been described (Fig. 3.9.3).[20] An important preoperative consideration is the presence of stress incontinence (found in up to 50% of patients).[21] Some advocate concomitant incontinence surgery,[22] whereas we favour a staged approach as resolution of symptoms may occur after excision and also as sling placement risks erosion.[5] Stress incontinence develops in up 16% of patients postoperatively.[23] It is associated with the excision of larger, circumferential or saddlebag lesions, probably due to the risk of sphincter injury. Urethrovaginal/vesicovaginal fistula occurs in up to 5% and is more likely if surgery is performed during active infection.[24] Recurrence of UD may be associated with incomplete initial excision. Ureteric injury may occur during excision of large proximal UD, therefore ureteric stenting is advisable before excision of such lesions. Other complications include haematoma, urinary tract infection, and urethral stricture.

Conclusion

UD are an infrequently diagnosed (despite their apparently high prevalence) but important cause of LUTS in the female population.

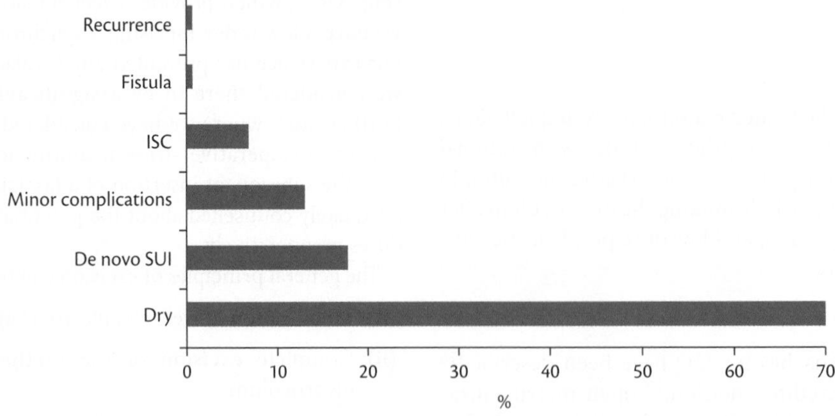

Fig. 3.9.3 Outcomes of UD repair in a series of 69 patients.
Reprinted from *European Urology Supplements*, Volume 10, Issue 2, F.A. Reeves et al, '956 Management of Symptomatic Urethral Diverticula—Single Centre Experience', pp. 289–299, Copyright © 2011 European Association of Urology, with permission from Elsevier, http://www.sciencedirect.com/science/journal/03022838

The presenting features are easily confused with other lower urinary tract pathologies, making diagnosis difficult; as such, a high index of suspicion is required to instigate the relevant investigations. A post-voiding MRI is currently the optimal method of characterizing UD and provides excellent detail for preoperative planning. Excision with reconstruction is the recommended surgical approach and has good functional outcomes but is associated with a risk of significant complications, such as fistula formation and stress incontinence.

Further reading

Chou CP, Levenson RB, Elsayes KM, *et al.* Imaging of female urethral diverticulum: an update. *Radiographics* 2008; **28**(7):1917–30.

Handel LN, Leach GE. Current evaluation and management of female urethral diverticula. *Curr Urol Rep* 2008; 9(5):383–8.

Lee JW, Fynes MM. Female urethral diverticula. *Best Pract Res Clin Obstet Gynaecol* 2005; **19**(6):875–93.

Patel AK, Chapple CR. Female urethral diverticula. *Curr Opin Urol* 2006; **16**(4):248–54.

Rovner ES. Urethral diverticula: a review and an update. *Neurourol Urodyn* 2007; **26**(7):972–7.

Rovner ES. Campbell-Walsh Urology. (pp. 422–6) In: Wein *et al.* (eds). *Campbell-Walsh Urology*, 10th edition. Philadelphia, PA: Saunders, 2012.

References

1. Andersen MJ. The incidence of diverticula in the female urethra. *J Urol* 1967; **98**:96–8.
2. Stewart M, Bretland PM, Stidolph NE. Urethral diverticula in the adult female. *Br J Urol* 1981; **53**(4):353–9.
3. Routh A. Urethral diverticula. *BMJ* 1890; **1**:361–2.
4. Rovner ES. Urethral diverticula: a review and an update. *Neurourol Urodyn* 2007; **26**(7):972–7.
5. Handel LN, Leach GE. Current evaluation and management of female urethral diverticula. *Curr Urol Rep* 2008; **9**(5):383–8.
6. Lee JW, Fynes MM. Female urethral diverticula. *Best Pract Res Clin Obstet Gynaecol* 2005; **19**(6):875–93.
7. Patel AK, Chapple CR. Female urethral diverticula. *Curr Opin Urol* 2006; **16**(4):248–54.
8. Rufford J, Cardozo L. Urethral diverticula: a diagnostic dilemma. *BJU Int* 2004; **94**(7):1044–7.
9. Saito S. Usefulness of diagnosis by the urethroscopy under anesthesia and effect of transurethral electrocoagulation in symptomatic female urethral diverticula. *J Endourol* 2000; **14**(5):455–7.
10. Ganabathi K, Leach GE, Zimmern PE, Dmochowski R. Experience with the management of urethral diverticulum in 63 women. *J Urol* 1994; **152**(5 Pt 1):1445–52.
11. Keefe B, Warshauer DM, Tucker MS, Mittelstaedt CA. Diverticula of the female urethra: diagnosis by endovaginal and transperineal sonography. *AJR Am J Roentgenol* 1991; **156**(6):1195–7.
12. Neitlich JD, Foster HE, Jr., Glickman MG, Smith RC. Detection of urethral diverticula in women: comparison of a high resolution fast spin echo technique with double balloon urethrography. *J Urol* 1998; **159**(2):408–10.
13. Daneshgari F, Zimmern PE, Jacomides L. Magnetic resonance imaging detection of symptomatic noncommunicating intraurethral wall diverticula in women. *J Urol* 1999; **161**(4):1259–61; discussion 61–2.
14. Leng WW, McGuire EJ. Management of female urethral diverticula: a new classification. *J Urol* 1998; **160**(4):1297–300.
15. Leach GE, Sirls LT, Ganabathi K, Zimmern PE. L N S C3: a proposed classification system for female urethral diverticula. *Neurourol Urodyn* 1993; **12**(6):523–31.
16. Rovner ES. Campbell-Walsh Urology. (pp. 422–6) In: Wein *et al.* (eds). *Campbell-Walsh Urology*, 10th edition. Philadelphia, PA: Saunders, 2012.
17. Davis BL, Robinson DG. Diverticula of the female urethra: assay of 120 cases. *J Urol* 1970; **104**(6):850–3.
18. Roehrborn CG. Long term follow-up study of the marsupialization technique for urethral diverticula in women. *Surg Gynecol Obstet* 1988; **167**(3):191–6.
19. Mizrahi S, Bitterman W. Transvaginal, periurethral injection of polytetrafluoroethylene (polytef) in the treatment of urethral diverticula. *Br J Urol* 1988; **62**(3):280.
20. Reeves FA, Chapple, CR, Inman RD. Poster 256-Management of symptomastic Urethral Diverticula-Single centre experience. *Eur Urol Suppl* 2011; **10**(2):298.
21. Bass JS, Leach GE. Surgical treatment of concomitant urethral diverticulum and stress incontinence. *Urol Clin North Am* 1991; **18**(2):365–73.
22. Swierzewski SJ 3rd, McGuire EJ. Pubovaginal sling for treatment of female stress urinary incontinence complicated by urethral diverticulum. *J Urol* 1993; **149**(5):1012–4.
23. Porpiglia F, Destefanis P, Fiori C, Fontana D. Preoperative risk factors for surgery female urethral diverticula. Our experience. *Urol Int* 2002; **69**(1):7–11.
24. Mackinnon M, Pratt JH, Pool TL. Diverticulum of the female urethra. *Surg Clin North Am* 1959; **39**(4):953–62.

CHAPTER 3.10

Faecal incontinence

Keith Chapple

Introduction to faecal incontinence

Faecal incontinence is a common yet vastly under-reported condition with immense physical, psychological, and social impact on a patient's quality of life. The stigma associated with the condition means problems are frequently not volunteered, yet it frequently coexists with urinary incontinence and patients with both urinary and faecal incontinence will be commonly encountered in the urology clinic.

Definition

The condition is characterized by involuntary loss of solid faeces, liquid faeces, or flatus. It is subdivided into either passive incontinence (the passage of stool or flatus without the patient being aware) or urge incontinence (whereby a patient is aware of the need to defecate but cannot prevent the passage of faeces). 'Urgency' refers to the state whereby a patient senses an immediate desire to defecate, with resultant urge incontinence if a toilet is not available. Lastly, 'soiling' (often also referred to as 'seepage' or 'leakage') refers to the passage of a small amount of faecal material from an individual who is otherwise predominantly continent.

Epidemiology

The condition is much under-reported. Although men and women may be equally affected,[1] within surgical practice the condition is predominantly seen in women. There is a point prevalence of 2%[1] in the general population, with the incidence rising to 6–7% in the elderly and up to 20% in nursing and residential care homes.[2]

Aetiology

Continence of faeces depends on a number of factors including stool consistency, capacity, and compliance of the rectum; integrity and function of the anal sphincter mechanism (comprising the involuntary internal anal sphincter and the voluntary external anal sphincter); normal sensation of the anorectum and a normal rectoanal inhibitory reflex (the 'sampling' reflex). Disruption of any of these factors (neatly summarized as 'brain, bowels, and bottom') can lead to incontinence. A wide range of causes have been described and a full list is beyond the requirements of the practising urologist. In practical terms, the commonest causes are obstetric injury, pudendal nerve damage, and iatrogenic injuries from previous anal surgery. Ultrasound evidence of anal sphincter defects has been noted in 30% of women undergoing vaginal delivery[3] and up to 80% of women undergoing forceps delivery.[4] Trauma to the pudendal nerve is commonly seen in conjunction with sphincter injury and results in denervation of the external anal sphincter and pelvic floor.[5] Haemorrhoids may be associated with faecal incontinence, although incontinence problems following haemorrhoid surgery are not uncommon[6] and a history of anal surgery should be elicited in all patients. Pelvic floor dysfunction is common to both urinary and faecal incontinence. Patients aged over 55 years, diabetics, and those who have stress urinary incontinence or detrusor instability are at the highest risk for coexisting faecal incontinence.[7]

Clinical features

History

The type of incontinence (passive or urge) helps to ascertain the likely cause—passive incontinence is suggestive of internal anal sphincter dysfunction, while urgency and urge incontinence are more suggestive of an external anal sphincter defect or reduced rectal capacity. The degree of soiling is commonly ascertained by the number of pads or clothing changes. A symptom diary is often helpful. The effect of the incontinence in the patient's social functioning is vital, as what is a minor degree of soiling to one patient may be devastating to another. Scoring systems such as the Cleveland Clinic system (see Table 3.10.1) have their limitations, but can be helpful in enabling an objective assessment of the incontinence severity and response to treatment.

A recent change in bowel habit to a looser stool, rectal bleeding, or weight loss is suggestive of serious bowel pathology. Other important aspects include an obstetric history, especially with respect to tears or the use of instrumentation, previous pelvic radiotherapy, previous anal or pelvic surgery, and a drug history, as many commonly used drugs (metformin being a frequent culprit) are associated with diarrhoea and reduced anal function.

Examination

Following an abdominal examination, the patient is examined in the left lateral position with the perineum firstly observed at rest, then with the patient straining and subsequently squeezing the anal sphincter. Sphincter tone is assessed by inspecting for the presence of any 'gape' at rest. Digital rectal examination enables an assessment of whether the patient is constipated and has 'overflow diarrhoea', and also allows a further estimation of the resting anal tone, the length of the anal canal, and the presence and location of any sphincter defects. Squeezing the gloved finger gives an assessment of the function of the external anal sphincter. Proctosigmoidoscopy is then performed to assess for anorectal pathology such as prolapse, malignancy, inflammatory bowel disease, or haemorrhoids.

Table 3.10.1 The Cleveland Clinic (Wexner) scoring system for faecal incontinence: five parameters of faecal incontinence and their frequency are assessed, and the sum of these scores gives an indication of the degree of incontinence

	Never	Rarely (less than once a month)	Sometimes (less than once a week)	Usually (less than once a day)	Always (every day)
Incontinence to gas	0	1	2	3	4
Incontinence to liquid	0	1	2	3	4
Incontinence to solid	0	1	2	3	4
Need to wear pad	0	1	2	3	4
Lifestyle alteration	0	1	2	3	4

Reprinted from Springer and *Diseases of the Colon and Rectum*, Volume 36, Issue 1, pp. 77–97, J. Marcio N. Jorge, 'Etiology and management of fecal incontinence', Copyright © 1993 American Society of Colon and Rectal Surgeons with kind permission from Springer Science and Business Media.

Investigations

Although a flexible sigmoidoscopy or colonoscopy is often performed to exclude conditions such as inflammatory bowel disease or malignancy, the majority of patients can be treated without the use of specialized investigations. However, for those patients who fail to respond to initial measures, endoanal ultrasound provides a helpful assessment of anal sphincter anatomy and accurate identification of any associated defects. It is commonly performed as a three-dimensional image (see Fig. 3.10.1). Anorectal physiology complements the ultrasound and provides an assessment of the functional capability of the anal sphincters and rectum. Common measurements include anal canal resting pressure and maximal squeeze pressures (indirect assessments of the internal and external anal sphincters respectively), the rectal capacity, and the presence of the rectoanal inhibitory reflex (which is absent in Hirschsprung's disease). Assessment of the function of the pudendal nerve can also be performed using pudendal nerve terminal motor latency, although the accuracy of this is debatable and the measurement is less useful than previously thought. A defecating proctogram has not been part of the routine investigation of the faecally incontinent patient. However, it is useful in the assessment of intrarectal intussusception, as some groups have proposed the importance of its finding as a cause of faecal incontinence.[8]

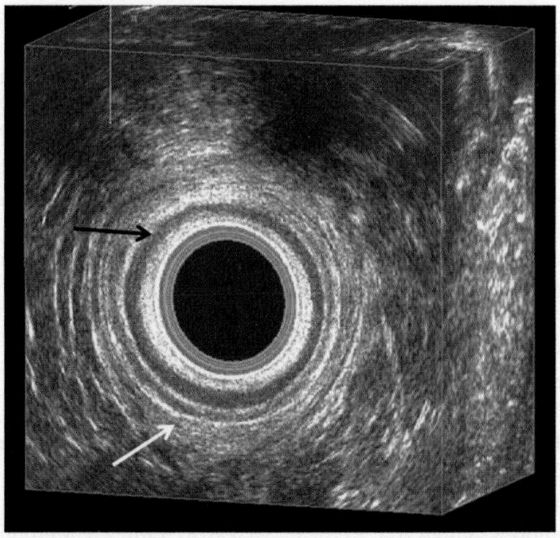

Fig. 3.10.1 Normal three-dimensional endoanal ultrasound image. The internal anal sphincter (black arrow) and external anal sphincter (white arrow) are shown. This investigation provides excellent detail of both normal anal canal anatomy and any associated defects in the anal sphincters.

Images reproduced courtesy of Mr K Chapple.

Treatment

Most patients undergo initial conservative intervention followed by surgery only when conservative options have been exhausted. There unfortunately remains only a limited evidence base supporting the various treatment options. In part, this is because of the difficulty in assessing a successful outcome. Patients with the same objective outcome may have very different views on the success, or otherwise, of the treatment, and it is vital that outcome is assessed using a combination of continence scores, quality of life, and overall patient satisfaction.

Conservative

Lifestyle changes are an obvious target for treatment but often prove unhelpful in providing effective long-term treatment. Obesity is a common risk factor, yet the limited studies investigating the effect of weight reduction on continence have yielded disappointing results.[9] Likewise, increased exercise is only of benefit in nursing home residents.[10] Dietary change is often advocated by clinicians, although the evidence of benefit is limited.[9] 'Biofeedback' encompasses a wide range of therapies and the actual techniques involved vary from centre to centre. Patients are trained on a sessional basis using anal manometry feedback to increase the strength of their anal sphincters. Pelvic floor exercises may also be incorporated into the programme. Although a commonly used intervention and having the undoubted benefit of allowing time with an understanding nurse/physiologist, its overall efficacy is uncertain.[11]

An antidiarrhoeal agent, such as loperamide, is used for patients with a loose stool and has the added effect of increasing anal sphincter tone. It is often also helpful to add in a fibre supplement, as the anal sphincter may better control a large bulky motion than a loose, fluid stool. If urgency is a particular problem, low-dose amitriptyline helps by reducing rectal hypersensitivity. Ensuring an empty rectum is a common-sense method to alleviate faecal incontinence and in its simplest form involves the use of a suppository (commonly glycerine or bisacodyl) after defecation. Rectal irrigation involves the introduction of a plastic tube into the rectum, through which tap water is irrigated to clear the rectum and distal colon of faeces. While it has efficacy in all faecally incontinent patients, its main advantage is seen in spinal injury patients.[12]

As well as its use in patients with overactive bladder, posterior tibial nerve stimulation has recently been used in faecal incontinence. Stimulation of the tibial nerve via a percutaneous electrode is performed over 12 sessions of 30 minutes each. Early results indicate a degree of efficacy,[13] although the long-term effect is unknown.

Surgical

Repair of a damaged external anal sphincter, commonly after obstetric injury, is still performed although concerns exist regarding its long-term efficacy. Primary repair is performed immediately after childbirth and involves apposition of the disrupted sphincter muscle with an end-to-end repair. Patients with an external anal sphincter defect greater than 90 degrees who present later (either due to a missed injury or failed primary repair) may undergo an elective repair, which is invariably performed using an overlapping technique. Short-term outcomes from both techniques are excellent.[14] Although there is a significant deterioration in continence scores over time, most patients remain satisfied with their outcome.[15] Pelvic floor repair involves plication of the levator muscles and external anal sphincter. Although infrequently performed, individual centres have reported excellent results.[16] The Malone antegrade continence enema is particularly valuable in those patients with poor colonic motility, particularly after neurogenic injury.[17] The appendix is mobilized to create an appendicostomy, which is concealed in the umbilicus and through which the patient can irrigate to empty the colon. Passive faecal incontinence caused by internal anal sphincter dysfunction can be effectively treated by injections of anal bulking agents.[18]

For those patients with severe faecal incontinence, creation of an anal 'neosphincter' may be considered. Dynamic graciloplasty involves mobilization of the gracilis muscle which is then used to encircle the anal canal. The muscle is stimulated via an implanted stimulator and continence controlled using an external magnet to allow evacuation. Experience with artificial anal sphincters has been variable. A balloon is placed around the distal rectum and inflation/deflation controlled by a subcutaneous reservoir activated by the patient. There is considerable morbidity and explantation of the device due to infection is a commonly encountered problem.[19]

Sacral neuromodulation has provided the biggest impact into the management of faecal incontinence in recent years. Identical to the procedure used in urological practice, it provides an improvement in symptoms and quality of life for the majority of faecally incontinent patients.[20] Originally used only for patients with an intact anal sphincter, indications have widened with good results achievable despite the presence of pudendal neuropathy,[21] external anal sphincter defects of up to 120 degrees,[22] or previous anal sphincter repair.[21] Lastly, a stoma is often (and wrongly) seen as a last resort or even as a failure of other treatment modalities. However, for the patient with severe, disabling faecal incontinence, it provides successful control of symptoms, resumption of normal activities, and an improved quality of life.[23,24]

Conclusion

Patients with faecal incontinence are common and will be frequently be encountered by the urologist. The condition carries more of a social stigma than urinary incontinence and the problem will often not be volunteered by the patient and must be actively sought. A wide and increasing range of treatments are available, with improvements in continence levels and quality of life possible in all patients.

Further reading

Abrams P, Andersson KE, Birder L, *et al.* Fourth international consultation on incontinence recommendations of the international scientific committee: evaluation and treatment of urinary incontinence, pelvic organ prolapse, and fecal incontinence. *Neurourol Urodyn* 2010; **29**(1):213–40.

Boyle R, Hay-Smith EJ, Cody JD, Mørkved S. Pelvic floor muscle training for prevention and treatment of urinary and faecal incontinence in antenatal and postnatal women. *Cochrane Database Syst Rev* 2012 Oct; 17(10):CD007471.

Brown SR, Wadhawan H, Nelson RL. Surgery for faecal incontinence in adults. *Cochrane Database Syst Rev* 2010 Sep 8; (9):CD001757.

Leroi AM. The role of sacral neuromodulation in double incontinence. *Colorectal Dis* 2011; **13**(Suppl 2):15–8.

Tjandra JJ, Dykes SL, Kumar RR, *et al.* Practice parameters for the treatment of fecal incontinence. *Dis Colon Rectum* 2007; **50**:1497–1507.

References

1. Perry S, Shaw C, McGrother C, *et al.* Prevalence of faecal incontinence in adults aged 40 years or more living in the community. *Gut* 2002; **50**(4):480–4.
2. Tobin GW, Brocklehurst JC. Faecal incontinence in residential homes for the elderly: prevalence, aetiology and management. *Age Ageing* 1986; **15**(1):41–6.
3. Sultan A, Kamm M, Hudson C, Thomas CM, Bartram CI. Anal-sphincter disruption during vaginal delivery. *N Engl J Med* 1993; **329**:1905–11.
4. Sultan AH, Kamm M, Bartram CI, Hudson CN. Third degree obstetric anal sphincter tears; risk factors and outcome of primary repair. *BMJ* 1994; **308**:887–91.
5. Snooks SJ, Swash M, Henry MM, Setchell MM. Risk factors in childbirth causing damage to the pelvic floor innervation. *Int J Colorectal Dis* 1986; **1**:204.
6. Holzheimer RG. Haemorrhoidectomy: indications and risks. *Eur J Med Res* 2004 26; **9**(1):18–36.
7. Chang TC, Chang SR, Hsiao SM, Hsiao CF, Chen CH, Lin HH. Factors associated with fecal incontinence in women with lower urinary tract symptoms. *J Obstet Gynaecol Res* 2013; **39**(1):250–5.
8. Collinson R, Harmston C, Cunningham C, Lindsey I. The emerging role of internal rectal prolapse in the aetiology of faecal incontinence. *Gastroenterol Clin Biol* 2010; **34**(11):584–6.
9. Norton C, Whitehead WE, Bliss DZ, Harai D, Lang J. Management of fecal incontinence in adults. *Neurourol Urodyn* 2010; **29**:199–206.
10. Schnelle JF, Alessi C, Simmons SF. Al-Samarrai NF, Beck JC, Ouslander JG. Translating clinical research into practice: a randomised clinical trial of exercise and incontinence care with nursing home residents. *J Am Geriatr Soc* 2002; **50**:1476–83.
11. Norton C, Cody JD. Biofeedback and/or sphincter exercises for the treatment of faecal incontinence in adults. *Cochrane Database Syst Rev* 2012 Jul 11; **7**:CD002111.
12. Christensen P, Krogh K. Transanal irrigation for disordered defecation: a systematic review. *Scand J Gastroentrol* 2010; **45**(5):517–27.
13. Findlay JM, Maxwell-Armstrong C. Posterior tibial nerve stimulation and faecal incontinence: a review. *Int J Colorectal Dis* 2011; **26**(3):265–73.
14. Fernando R, Sultan AH, Kettle C, Thakar R, Radley S. Methods of repair for obstetric anal sphincter injury. *Cochrane Database Syst Rev* 2006; **19**(3):CD002866.
15. Glasgow Sc, Lowry AC. Long-term outcomes of anal sphincter repair for fecal incontinence: a systematic review. *Dis Colon Rectum* 2012; **55**(4):482–90.

16. Abbas SM, Bissett IP, Neill ME, Parry BR. Long-term outcome of postanal repair in the treatment of fecal incontinence. *ANZ J Surg* 2005; **75**(9):783–6.
17. Teichman JM, Zabihi N, Kraus SR, Harris JM, Barber DB. Long-term results for Malone antegrade continence enema for adults with neurogenic bowel disease. *Urology* 2003; **61**(3):502–6.
18. Watson NF, Koshy A, Sagar PM. Anal bulking agents for faecal incontinence. *Colorectal Dis* 2012; **14**(Suppl 3):29–33.
19. Wong WD, Congliosi SM, Spencer MP, *et al.* The safety and efficacy of the artificial bowel sphincter for fecal incontinence: results from a multicenter cohort study. *Dis Colon Rectum* 2002; **45**(9):1139–53.
20. Uludaq O, Melenhorst J, Koch SM, van Gemert WG, Dejong CH, Baeten CG. Sacral neuromodulation: long term outcome and quality of life in patients with faecal incontinence. *Colorectal Dis* 2011; **13**(10):1162–6.
21. Brouwer R, Duthie G. Sacral nerve neuromodulation is effective treatment for fecal incontinence in the presence of a sphincter defect, pudendal neuropathy, or previous sphincter repair. *Dis Colon Rectum* 2010; **53**(3):273–8.
22. Chan MK, Tjandra JJ. Sacral nerve stimulation for fecal incontinence: external anal sphincter defect vs. intact anal sphincter. *Dis Colon Rectum* 2008; **51**(7):1015–24.
23. Madoff RD. Surgical treatment options for fecal incontinence. *Gastroenterology* 2001; **126**:S48–54.
24. Norton C, Burch J, Kamm MA. Patients' views of a colostomy for fecal incontinence. *Dis Colon Rectum* 2005; **48**:1062–9.

CHAPTER 3.11

Urinary retention in women

Clare J. Fowler and Jalesh N. Panicker

Introduction to urinary retention in women

If a young woman in complete urinary retention is investigated and all urological and neurological investigations are found to be normal, the commonest diagnosis then made is 'Fowler's syndrome' (FS). Described by Fowler *et al.* in 1987, the original syndrome comprised of complete urinary retention with the finding of a particular pattern of electromyographic (EMG) activity recorded with a concentric needle electrode from the striated urethral sphincter, in a young woman with clinical features of polycystic ovaries.[1] Prior to this, much had been written about 'psychogenic urinary retention in women' and medical opinion was that urinary retention in young women was due to 'hysteria'.[2–4] Twenty-five years on, the situation now seems to be that if neither the neurologist nor urologist can discover an underlying abnormality, the woman may be told she has Fowler's syndrome without any positive identification of that condition. However, in a series of women presenting with retention and investigated in the Department of Uro-Neurology at The National Hospital for Neurology and Neurosurgery, University College London Hospitals (UCLH), only about one-third are confirmed as having FS (Fig. 3.11.1).[5] The remainder of this chapter amplifies the clinical features, describes the laboratory investigations that are used to confirm the diagnosis, and discusses the differential diagnosis of FS.

Clinical features of Fowler's syndrome

Table 3.11.1 presents the characteristic features of FS.[6] The typical description is of a young woman postmenarche who is unable to void, presenting with painless urinary retention. Women with the condition are often found to have post-void residual volumes exceeding 1 L at some stage and although they may experience pain rarely do they report urgency, which would be expected at such a large bladder capacity. For this reason, they can go for long intervals without emptying their bladder. Straining while attempting to void does not help with bladder emptying.

Women with FS often report an antecedent event prior to the onset of urinary retention. This can often be an obstetric, gynaecological, or urological surgical procedure using regional or general anaesthesia. The procedure may be distant from the pelvis, and relatively minor such as a tooth extraction, suggesting that the general anaesthetic may be the significant factor. Some women report a history of poor voiding including an interrupted flow before the onset of retention, with women noticing it takes them longer to pass urine than others. Although not a troublesome feature it is an important part of the history as it is indicative of a pre-existing abnormality. It is unclear why a transient event such as a general anaesthetic triggers off urinary retention which then remains unresolved, however this has undoubtedly been the source for litigation.

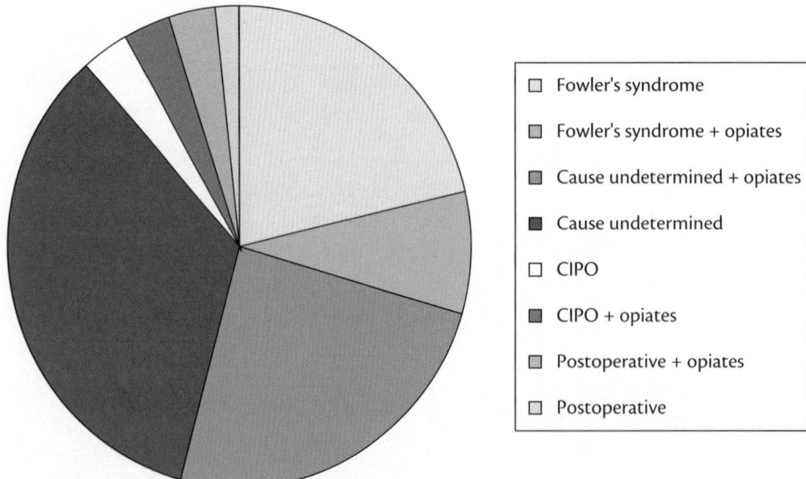

Fig. 3.11.1 Causes for urinary retention in a series of women presenting in the Department of Uro-Neurology at The National Hospital for Neurology and Neurosurgery, University College London Hospitals.

Reprinted from *The Journal of Urology*, Volume 188, Issue 2, Panicker JN *et al.*, 'The Possible Role of Opiates in Women with Chronic Urinary Retention: Observations from a Prospective Clinical Study', pp. 480–484, Copyright © 2012, with permission from Elsevier, http://www.sciencedirect.com/science/journal/00225347

Table 3.11.1 Essential features of Fowler's syndrome

Key features	Comments
Female	The condition has never been found in young men with retention
Aged between onset of menarche and menopause	The peak age of onset is 26
No evidence of urological, gynaecological, or neurological disease	It is important that other possible causes of urinary retention have been excluded by a urologist and/or neurologist, ideally by a cystoscopy and an MRI of the brain and spinal cord
Retention with a volume more than >1,000 mL	Retention of volumes less than 1 L are unlikely to turn out to be due to Fowler's syndrome
No sense of urinary urgency despite high bladder volumes	This is a striking feature of the condition, despite having more than 1 L in the bladder these girls do not have the sense of urgency one might expect. There may be extreme discomfort, but not urgency
Straining does not help emptying	This is also a key feature of the condition. Most girls have tried 'bearing down' but not found it helped emptying
Sense of 'something gripping' or difficulty on removing the catheter which has been used for urinary drainage	This probably contributes to the discomfort of self catheterization, which can be quite a problem for girls with FS
No history of urological abnormalities in childhood or associated abnormalities of the urinary tract	A history of bladder troubles going back into childhood needing urethral reimplants and so on probably indicates some other underlying abnormality of the bladder and urinary system. Possibly 'amyopathy', although this has not been proved yet
Association with polycystic ovarian syndrome and endometriosis	Clinical features of PCO (i.e. hirsutism and acne) were quite prominent in some of the early cases, and although this association does not seem to be inevitable, it was this observation that gave rise to the concept that the problem is hormonally determined

FS: Fowler's syndrome.

Adapted from Fowler's Syndrome, *What is Fowler's Syndrome*, Copyright © Professor Clare J. Fowler, available from http://www.fowlersyndrome.co.uk/01-what-is-fowlers-syndrome, with permission from Professor Clare J. Fowler.

When introduced to clean intermittent self catheterization, women often find this painful, particularly on withdrawing the catheter, and may complain of a sensation of 'something gripping'. The reader is referred to the website http://www.fowlersyndrome.co.uk/ which provides more information about FS.[7]

Investigations

Filling cystometry most often demonstrates a large capacity bladder with delayed or absent sensations. Filling is often stopped at 500 mL on grounds of safety, although the women's capacity is much greater. The patient is then unable to pass urine and so the conclusion is reached from the urodynamics that the woman has an 'acontractile' or 'areflexic' detrusor.

Sphincter electromyography

Concentric needle EMG of the urethral sphincter is diagnostic, and detects characteristic abnormal activity. The EMG activity may sound superficially like myotonia, however detailed analysis shows that the characteristic sound is due to a decelerating component of a complex repetitive discharge.[8] The sound from a number of generators of this type of activity is likened to that of underwater recordings of whale songs. Complex repetitive discharges may be recorded without deceleration, and produce a sound similar to helicopters over the audio-amplifier of the EMG machine. Jitter is so low when components of the complex repetitive discharges are analysed, suggesting that it must be due to ephaptic transmission between muscle fibres which is generating repetitive and circuitous self-excitation.[9] It is thought that this abnormal activity prevents sphincter relaxation, causes an abnormally high urethral pressure, and results in voiding dysfunction or urinary retention.[7]

Urethral pressure profile

The maximum urethral closure pressure (MUCP) is typically found to be elevated with resting values above 100 cm of water measured in women with FS.[9] The formula of 92-age (in years) is used to derive the expected pressure.[7,10]

Urethral ultrasound

Transvaginal ultrasonography may be used to measure the volume of the sphincter and may detect the hypertrophy of the muscle resulting from sustained overactivity, however the test is highly subjective.[11,12] The test does allow the opportunity for the sphincter and urethra to be carefully examined and possibly identify other causes for retention such as a urethral diverticulum.[7]

Association with polycystic ovary

Many of the women reported in the original description of FS, were observed to be hirsute, obese, and to have menstrual irregularities, and it was thought there was a clinical association with polycystic ovaries.[1] The extent of this association is still poorly understood, and although the coincidence of polycystic ovary (PCO) and retention is by no means inevitable, a hormonal basis for the EMG abnormality seems likely.[7]

Sacral neuromodulation

The only treatment that has been found to restore voiding in women with FS is sacral neuromodulation (SNM). Of a cohort of 60 women undergoing percutaneous nerve evaluation and subsequent implant, 70% were voiding spontaneously when followed up, with a mean interval of seven years.[13] This is in line with the findings from other centres of the longer-term efficacy of SNM as a treatment for non-obstructive retention; van Voskuilen *et al.* showing 76.2% efficacy at 70.5 months[14] and Elhilali *et al.* showing efficacy of 78% at 77 months.[15] De Ridder and colleagues showed that women with urinary retention and having an abnormal result in the sphincter EMG test had a better outcome with SNM at five years.[16]

The mechanism of action is uncertain; however, it is thought that stimulation reinforms sensory parts of the brain and allows the bladder to be 'switched on' again. Using functional brain imaging it was possible to show using both PET (position emission tomography) and fMRI (functional magnetic resonance imaging) that the periaqueductal grey (PAG) in the midbrain, a centre that receives sensory signals from the bladder, becomes activated in women with Fowler's syndrome when the stimulator is switched on. This seems to be linked to the patient's report of a return of sensations of bladder fullness.[7,17]

Opiates, Fowler's syndrome, and response to neuromodulation

Recently, a strong association with opiates and the onset of urinary retention is something that has become apparent. An increasing number of young women with urinary retention were taking prescription opiates for pain relief and indeed, in a series of 62 women coming to our clinic with retention, about one-third—see Figure 3.11.1—were taking some form of opiate pain killer,[5] including tramadol, pethidine, morphine (Morphgesic SR, MXL, Zomorph, MST, MXL, Sevredol, Oramorph), or Fentanyl. The common scenario was the prescription of the medication at a pain clinic for chronic back pain and or some other skeletal or pelvic pain, often attributed to endometriosis. Of all the women in this series, one-third did have FS but a quarter of the women were taking opiate medications.[7]

Hypothesis—is Fowler's syndrome the result of spinal cord intoxication by enkephalins?

The abnormal sphincter EMG activity (cause unknown) is likely causing neurotransmitter changes in the spinal cord, which are brought about by the effect of naturally occurring opiates—the body's endorphins or enkephalins. Endorphins play an important role in neural signalling throughout the nervous system and play a role in bladder control. The most recent hypothesis is that Fowler's syndrome is the result of spinal cord intoxication by enkephalins (Fig. 3.11.2). These have the effect of suppressing sensations from the bladder and inducing detrusor areflexia. In fact, the bladder of a woman with FS shares many characteristics with the effects observed in individuals taking opiates.[7]

The response to sacral neuromodulation of urinary retention in FS has been found to be good—and recent analysis somewhat surprisingly showed the response was equally good whether the women had pure FS, had opiate induced retention, or had laboratory features of FS and also taking opiates. The logical conclusion from this observation is that sacral neuromodulation counteracts the excessive spinal levels of endorphins through release of a counteracting and as-yet unidentified neurotransmitter. This probable explanation has resulted in the widespread practice of using the first stage of sacral neuromodulation to assess whether or not the patient's retention is responsive to the procedure without further investigations.

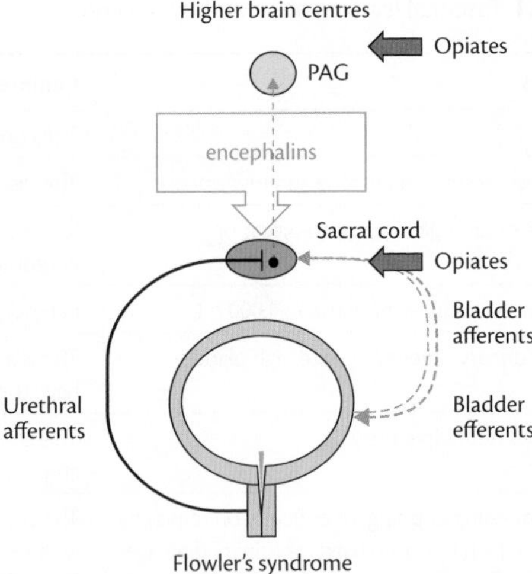

Fig. 3.11.2 Most recent hypothesis that Fowler's syndrome is the result of spinal cord intoxication by enkephalins.

Reproduced from Fowler's Syndrome, *Spinal Cord Intoxication by Encephalins*, Copyright © Professor Clare J. Fowler, available from http://www.fowlersyndrome.co.uk/09-spinal-cord-intoxication-by-encephalins/, with permission from Professor Clare J. Fowler.

Other causes of urinary retention

Table 3.11.2 lists the causes for urinary retention in women. Structural causes for urinary retention are rare in women. Bladder outlet obstruction is extremely rare, however extrinsic lesions can result in urethral obstruction, including diverticula, uterine and cervical fibroids, and cysts of the vaginal wall.

Functional urinary retention is associated with neurological disease, and in most instances, urinary symptoms are accompanied by other neurological symptoms and signs. Spinal cord disease usually manifests with the combination of incomplete emptying of the bladder and detrusor overactivity, and urgency incontinence is usually the prominent symptom. Retention may occur, however, following acute spinal cord injury during the stage of 'spinal shock' that results in detrusor acontractility, lasting some weeks. However, other neurological features will readily be apparent in the clinical examination, or tests such as MRI of the spine and lower limb-evoked potentials. Voiding difficulties, and urinary retention, are a prominent feature in patients with lesions of the conus medullaris, or following damage to the cauda equina. Small nerve fibre involvement occurs in diabetic or amyloid neuropathy, resulting in incomplete bladder emptying or complete retention. Retention may occur in the condition of pure autonomic failure, or following surgical damage to the ganglia and postganglionic fibres during radical pelvic surgery.

Incomplete bladder emptying is a feature of one of the Parkinson-plus syndromes, multiple system atrophy. An increasing post-void residual volume is demonstrated as the disease progresses and patients may go into complete retention.[18]

Medications are an important cause, especially opiates, as already discussed.[5] Chronic idiopathic pseudo-obstruction (CIPO) is a rare syndrome characterized by the gross distension of (predominately) the small bowel without any anatomical or mechanical obstruction, and bladder dysfunction has been reported in up to 10–69% of patients.[19–21] Urodynamic tests reveal changes, including detrusor hypocontractility.[7,19]

Table 3.11.2 Causes for urinary retention in women

Structural	Tumours	Leiomyomas, vaginal wall, or urethral cysts
	Urethral diverticulum	
	Urogenital prolapse	
Functional		
Neurological causes		
	Detrusor external sphincter dyssynergia and poorly sustained detrusor contraction	Spinal cord disease
	Detrusor areflexia or hypocontractility	Multiple system atrophy
		Lesion of conus medullaris or spinal roots (conus medullaris)
		Pure autonomic failure
		Radical pelvic surgery
		Small fibre neuropathy: diabetes, amyloidosis
		Meningitis retention syndrome
Non-neurological causes		
	Primary failure of urethral sphincter relaxation	Fowler's syndrome
	Medication	Opiates
		Drugs with anticholinergic activity
	Chronic idiopathic pseudo-obstruction (CIPO)	

Reprinted with permission from Clare J. Fowler, Jalesh N. Panicker and Anton Emmanuel, (Eds.), *Pelvic Organ Dysfunction in Neurological Disease*, Cambridge University Press, Cambridge, UK, Copyright © 2010 Cambridge University Press.

Acknowledgements

The work was undertaken at UCLH/UCL Institute of Neurology and is supported in part by funding from the United Kingdom's Department of Health National Institute for Health Research (NIHR) Biomedical Research Centres funding scheme.

Further reading

De Ridder D, Ost D, Bruyninckx F. The presence of Fowler's syndrome predicts successful long-term outcome of sacral nerve stimulation in women with urinary retention. *Eur Urol* 2007; **51**(1):229–33; discussion 33–4.

Kavia R, Dasgupta R, Critchley H, Fowler C, Griffiths D. A functional magnetic resonance imaging study of the effect of sacral neuromodulation on brain responses in women with Fowler's syndrome. *BJU Int* 2010; **105**(3):366–72.

Panicker JN, Game X, Khan S, *et al.* The possible role of opiates in women with chronic urinary retention: observations from a prospective clinical study. *J Urol* 2012; **188**(2):480–4.

Swinn MJ, Wiseman O, Lowe E, Fowler CJ. The cause and natural history of isolated urinary retention in young women. *J Urol* 2002; **167**:151–6.

Wiseman OJ, Swinn MJ, Brady CM, Fowler CJ. Maximum urethral closure pressure and sphincter volume in women with urinary retention. *J Urol* 2002; **167**(3):1348–51; discussion 51–2.

References

1. Fowler CJ, Christmas TJ, Chapple CR, Parkhouse HF, Kirby RS, Jacobs HS. Abnormal electromyographic activity of the urethral sphincter, voiding dysfunction, and polycystic ovaries: a new syndrome? *BMJ* 1988; **297**(6661):1436–8.
2. Margolis GJ. A review of literature on psychogenic urinary retention. *J Urol* 1965; **94**(3):257–8.
3. Allen TD. Psychogenic urinary retention. *South Med J* 1972; **65**(3):302–4.
4. Barrett DM. Psychogenic urinary retention in women. *Mayo Clin Proc* 1976; **51**(6):351–6.
5. Panicker JN, Game X, Khan S, *et al.* The possible role of opiates in women with chronic urinary retention: observations from a prospective clinical study. *J Urol* 2012; **188**(2):480–4.
6. Swinn MJ, Wiseman O, Lowe E, Fowler CJ. The cause and natural history of isolated urinary retention in young women. *J Urol* 2002; **167**:151–56.
7. Fowler CJ, Panicker JN, Emmanuel A (eds). *Pelvic Organ Dysfunction in Neurological Disease*. Cambridge, UK: Cambridge University Press, 2010.
8. Fowler CJ, Kirby RS, Harrison MJ. Decelerating burst and complex repetitive discharges in the striated muscle of the urethral sphincter, associated with urinary retention in women. *J Neurol Neurosurg Psychiatry* 1985; **48**(10):1004–9.
9. Wiseman OJ, Swinn MJ, Brady CM, Fowler CJ. Maximum urethral closure pressure and sphincter volume in women with urinary retention. *J Urol* 2002; **167**(3):1348–51; discussion 51–2.
10. Edwards L, Malvern J. The Urethral Pressure Profile: Theoretical considerations and clinical application. *Brit J Urol* 1974; **46**:325–36.
11. O'Connell HE, Hutson JM, Anderson CR, Plenter RJ. Anatomical relationship between urethra and clitoris. *J Urol* 1998; **159**(6):1892–7.
12. O'Connell HE, DeLancey JO. Clitoral anatomy in nulliparous, healthy, premenopausal volunteers using unenhanced magnetic resonance imaging. *J Urol* 2005; **173**(6):2060–3.
13. Datta SN, Chaliha C, Singh A, *et al.* Sacral neurostimulation for urinary retention: 10-year experience from one UK centre. *BJU Int* 2008; **101**(2):192–6.
14. Van Voskuilen AC, Oerlemans DJ, Weil EH, van den Hombergh U, van Kerrebroeck PE. Medium-term experience of sacral neuromodulation by tined lead implantation. *BJU Int* 2007; **99**(1):107–10.

15. Elhilali MM, Khaled SM, Kashiwabara T, Elzayat E, Corcos J. Sacral neuromodulation: long-term experience of one center. *Urology* 2005; **65**(6):1114–7.
16. De Ridder D, Ost D, Bruyninckx F. The presence of Fowler's syndrome predicts successful long-term outcome of sacral nerve stimulation in women with urinary retention. *Eur Urol* 2007; **51**(1):229–33; discussion 33–4.
17. Kavia R, Dasgupta R, Critchley H, Fowler C, Griffiths D. A functional magnetic resonance imaging study of the effect of sacral neuromodulation on brain responses in women with Fowler's syndrome. *BJU Int* 2010; **105**(3):366–72.
18. Ito T, Sakakibara R, Yasuda K, *et al.* Incomplete emptying and urinary retention in multiple-system atrophy: when does it occur and how do we manage it? *Mov Disord* 2006; **21**(6):816–23.
19. Lapointe SP, Rivet C, Goulet O, Fekete CN, Lortat-Jacob S. Urological manifestations associated with chronic intestinal pseudo-obstructions in children. *J Urol* 2002; **168**(4 Pt 2):1768–70.
20. Mousa H, Hyman PE, Cocjin J, Flores AF, Di Lorenzo C. Long-term outcome of congenital intestinal pseudoobstruction. *Dig Dis Sci* 2002; **47**(10):2298–305.
21. Vargas JH, Sachs P, Ament ME. Chronic intestinal pseudo-obstruction syndrome in pediatrics. Results of a national survey by members of the North American Society of Pediatric Gastroenterology and Nutrition. *J Pediatr Gastroenterol Nutr* 1988; 7(3):323–32.

CHAPTER 3.12

Spinal cord injury

Simon C.W. Harrison

Introduction to spinal cord injury

Estimates of the incidence of spinal cord injury (SCI) for Europe are between 10 and 30 per million population per year.[1] Added to this number are patients with spinal cord damage resulting from medical catastrophes such as acute intervertebral disc prolapse, spinal abscess, and spinal cord vascular accident. An injury to the spinal cord has a profound, life-changing impact on the affected person. The SCI will affect mobility, dexterity (if the lesion is high), and sensation but will also impact on urinary, bowel, and sexual function in the large majority of cases.

Over the last 70 years there has been a transformation in the prognosis for a person who sustains SCI from a situation where there were almost no long-term survivors to one where life expectancy for a 25-year-old, who is rendered a complete tetraplegic, is over 30 years; the equivalent figure for a paraplegic is nearly 40 years.[2,3] The introduction of holistic care in spinal cord injury centres, pioneered by Munro and Guttmann, was a key factor in the improvement in outcomes.[2] Progress in urinary tract management has been the result of many developments which include: access to effective antibiotics; improvements in catheter and appliance design and manufacture; the introduction of clean intermittent self-catheterization (CISC); the development of a urodynamic-based understanding of the pathophysiology of SCI; and the use of urinary tract surveillance within long-term follow-up regimes.

Successful management of SCI includes the minimization of secondary spinal cord damage, treatment of the injury to the vertebral column, treatment of associated injuries (head, chest, abdominal, pelvic, and limb), the prevention of secondary complications, and rehabilitation. Rehabilitation has been defined as 'an active, time-limited collaboration of a person with disabilities and professionals, along with other relevant people, to produce sustained reductions in the impact of disease or disability on daily life'.[4] The management of urinary tract, bowel, and sexual dysfunctions should be integrated into the overall care of the SCI patient through multidisciplinary collaboration.

Pathophysiology

The lower urinary tract (LUT) and genital tract receive their innervation from autonomic and somatic centres in the spinal cord but are dependent on the interaction of these spinal centres with the brain in order to function normally.[5] Spinal tracts connect the spinal centres with the brain. Injuries to the spinal cord will have different impacts on urinary and sexual function, depending on whether the spinal centres themselves are destroyed or whether the centres are preserved but the connecting pathways to higher centres are damaged.

It is important to appreciate that some spinal cord injuries lead to the complete destruction of the cord across one or more spinal levels (a complete SCI) while other injuries are incomplete, with preservation of some of the spinal tracts and therefore some sensation and/or voluntary motor function. Consideration can now be given to the effects of different injury patterns to the spinal cord.

Complete injury involving the conus medullaris

The conus medullaris (conus) is the region at the tip of the spinal cord that includes the sacral segments of the cord. It lies at the thoracolumbar region of the vertebral column, with the cord itself ending at the L1, 2 vertebral level. The S2, 3, 4 segments contain the sacral parasympathetic nucleus and Onuf's nucleus; the latter contains the anterior horn cells supplying the striated muscle of the external urethral sphincter (rhabdosphincter). Somatic sensory and motor nerves enter and exit the spinal cord from the pudendal nerve, while the pelvic nerve carries sensory and motor parasympathetic nerves.

Destruction of the conus can arise from direct trauma or because of an injury higher in the spinal cord causing infarction distally. The effects of such a lesion are:

- Loss of sensation in the sacral dermatomes, including the perianal area.
- Flaccid paralysis of the pelvic floor musculature and reduced anal tone. There will be absent conus reflexes which include the anal skin reflex and bulbo-anal reflexes, which are elicited by stimulating the perianal skin or glans penis and observing a contraction of the anal sphincter.
- The detrusor is areflexic with neither voluntary nor reflex contractions being seen.[6,7]
- Reduced bladder compliance is seen in some cases due to a loss of receptive relaxation of the detrusor (Fig. 3.12.1).[6,7]
- The normal sense of bladder filling is lost although some awareness of a full bladder is often present.
- The striated element of the external urethral sphincter is paralysed. Stress incontinence is usually present, but complete incontinence is generally avoided due to the residual tone in the smooth muscle component of the external urethral sphincter (termed 'non-relaxing urethral sphincter obstruction') (Fig. 3.12.2).[8]
- There is loss of urethral sensation.
- Reflex erections and ejaculation in response to penile stimulation are absent.[9–11]
- Psychogenic erection and psychogenic emission may be present if the spinal level is below L2 because the sympathetic innervation to the genitalia is intact.[11,12]

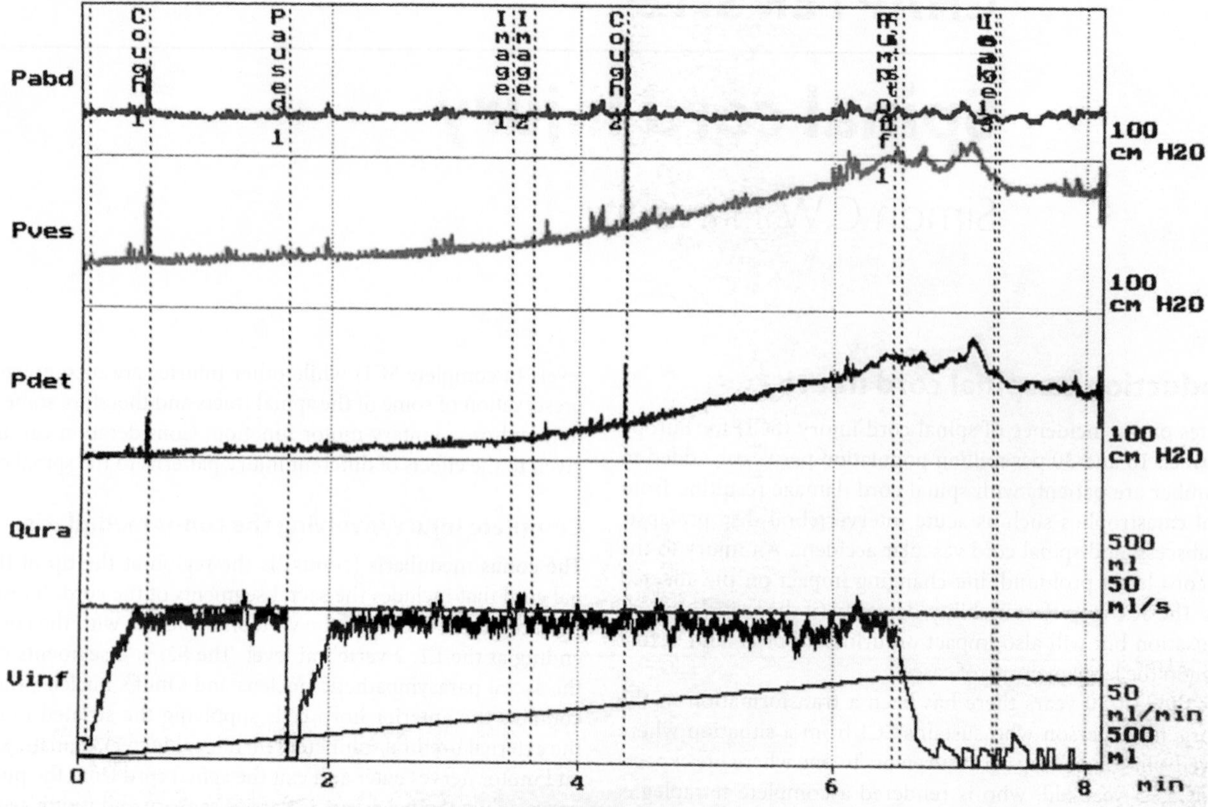

Fig. 3.12.1 Urodynamic trace showing reduced bladder compliance (the black trace records the filling rate). There is a progressive increase in detrusor pressure (Pdet) with filling, which stops immediately as filling ceases.

Complete injury with intact conus medullaris (supraconal injury)

If there is a complete spinal cord transection above the level of the conus and the conus remains intact, the distal segment of the cord is functional but disconnected from the brain (the distal autonomous cord). This allows the LUT and genitalia to exhibit activity based on spinal reflexes. Typical features of an established supraconal SCI are:

- Loss of sensation below the SCI level which will include the sacral dermatomes.

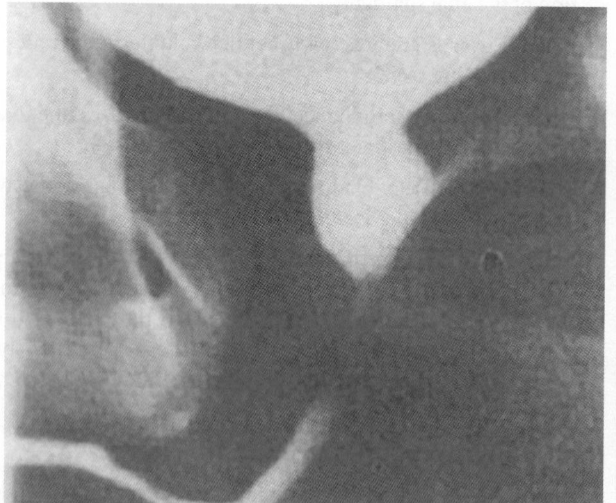

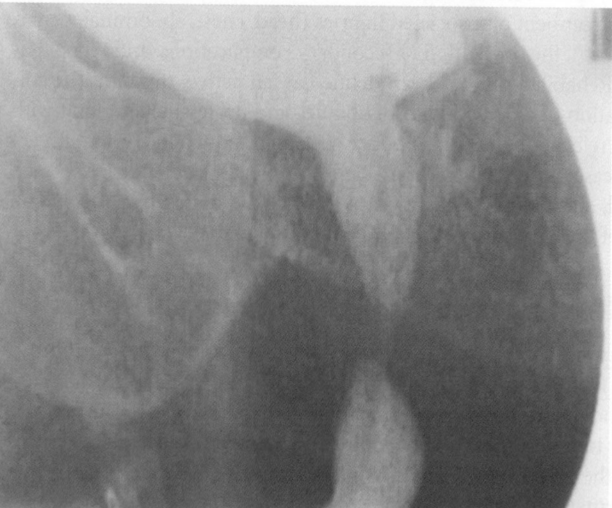

Fig. 3.12.2 Videourodynamic images showing the appearance of detrusor sphincter dyssynergia (left) with a long segment of urethral closure due to contraction of the rhabdosphincter; the prostatic urethra bulges open above the obstruction. On the right is an example of the short length of urethral occlusion seen with non-relaxing urethral sphincter obstruction where the occlusion is due to residual activity in the external urethral sphincter's smooth muscle component.

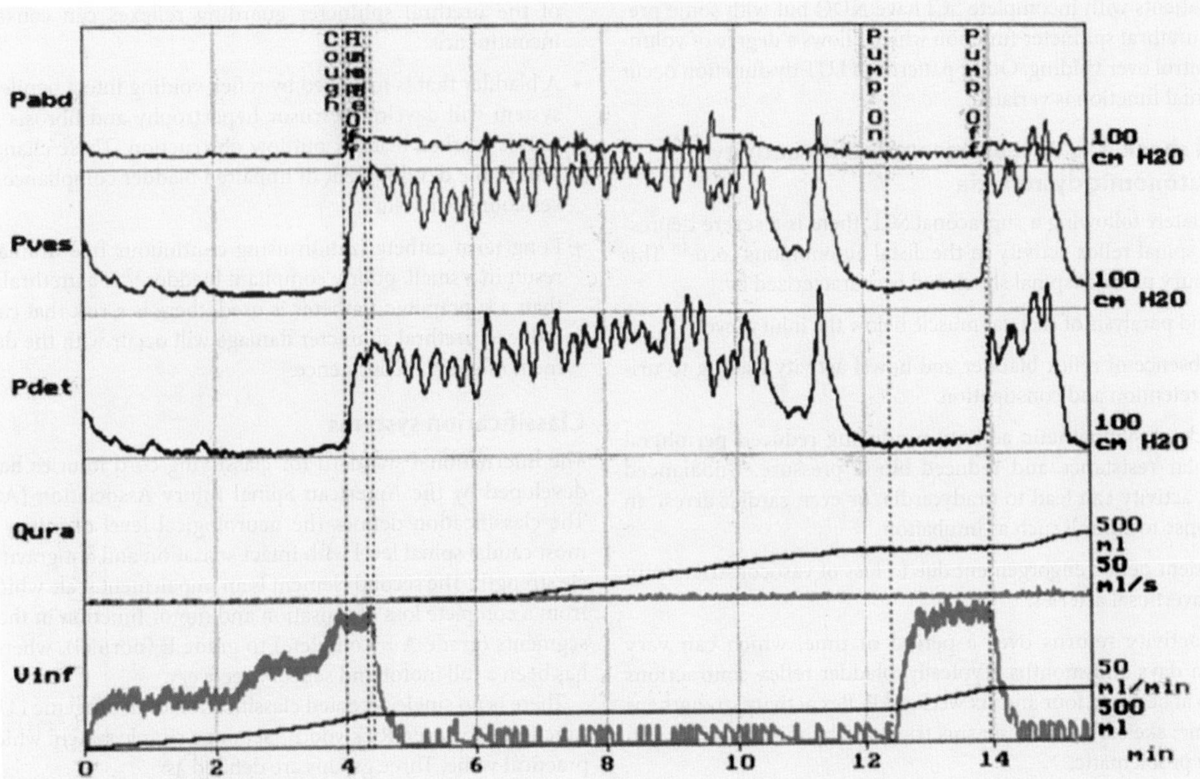

Fig. 3.12.3 Urodynamic trace showing onset of neurogenic detrusor overactivity at four minutes with a prolonged saw-tooth pattern that is typical of detrusor sphincter dyssynergia. The second fill at 14 minutes produced a much shorter period of bladder contraction (the thick red trace is the filling rate).

- Spastic paralysis of skeletal muscle below the injury level with increased muscle tone and brisk reflexes. Anal tone will be normal and conus reflexes will be intact.
- A bladder which contracts in a reflex manner in response to filling (neurogenic detrusor overactivity, NDO).[6,7] Bladder compliance is usually normal.
- A loss of the normal sensation of bladder filling but some awareness of a full bladder is often present.
- The bladder neck and urethral sphincters are competent during bladder filling; urethral guarding reflexes prevent stress incontinence from occurring. Active contraction of the striated sphincter occurs in response to reflex bladder contractions (detrusor sphincter dyssynergia, DSD) (Figs 3.12.2 and 3.12.3).
- There is loss of urethral sensation.
- Reflex erections will occur in response to physical stimulation of the penis but are lost as soon as stimulation is discontinued. Psychogenic erections can also occur if the level of SCI is below L2.[9–11]
- Reflex ejaculation can occur if the lesion is above T11 but will often only occur with a strong penile stimulus (e.g. provided by a medical-grade vibrator).[11]

Incomplete spinal cord injury lesions

The majority of patients who sustain damage to the spinal cord have incomplete cord lesions with some preservation of sensory or motor function distal to the level of injury. While some such patients will have a return to essentially normal LUT and sexual function, most will not.[13] Importantly, some patients who consider themselves to have no significant LUT symptoms are found to have grossly abnormal function on urodynamic assessment.

Many patients with incomplete SCI have a patchy preservation of both sensory and motor function below their injury level. However, others have a functional pattern which corresponds to a specific clinical syndrome:

- An anterior spinal cord syndrome is seen where there is an injury that leads to infarction of a segment of cord in the distribution of the anterior spinal artery. This spares the dorsal columns and leads to a complete motor lesion with preservation of touch sensation and proprioception.
- True hemi-section of the cord is only seen with penetrating injuries but features of the Brown-Séquard syndrome are also seen in patients whose SCI is markedly asymmetrical. The syndrome comprises loss of motor power, touch, and proprioception on the ipsilateral side to the cord lesion with loss of pain and temperature sensation on the contralateral side. Voluntary voiding may be preserved.
- A central cord syndrome is typically seen in an older person who suffers a hyperextension injury to the neck, often without a vertebral fracture. The cord is 'nipped' in a spinal canal that is already narrowed by degenerative changes. This leads to damage to the central part of the cord and results in marked sensory and motor deficits in the upper limbs with better preservation of lower limb function. Such patients may have relatively normal LUT function.

Most patients with incomplete SCI have NDO but with some preserved urethral sphincter function which allows a degree of voluntary control over voiding. Other patterns of LUT dysfunction occur and sexual function is variable.

Spinal shock, the development of reflex activity, and autonomic dysreflexia

Immediately following a supraconal SCI, there is a severe depression of spinal reflex activity in the distal autonomous cord.[14] This post-injury phase is spinal shock and is characterized by:

- Flaccid paralysis of skeletal muscle below the injury level.
- An absence of reflex bladder and bowel activity leading to urinary retention and constipation.
- A lack of sympathetic activity producing reduced peripheral vascular resistance and reduced blood pressure. Unbalanced vagal activity can lead to bradycardia, or even cardiac arrest, in response to stimuli such as intubation.
- Transient penile engorgement due to loss of vasoconstriction in the cavernosal arteries.

Reflex activity returns over a period of time, which can vary between days and months. Typically, bladder reflex contractions develop at between four and six weeks.[14] Reflex activity strengthens over time; skeletal muscle spasms triggered by minor stimuli can become problematic.

The development of autonomic reflexes within the distal autonomous cord affects control over peripheral vascular resistance. The syndrome of autonomic dysreflexia is a potentially fatal product of disordered spinal sympathetic reflex activity.[15] A noxious stimulus, which can be somatic or visceral, feeding into the distal autonomous cord results in a mass sympathetic reflex response and consequent vasoconstriction. In low spinal lesions, the increased peripheral resistance can be compensated by vasodilatation in the body that is normally innervated above the injury level. However, with a spinal lesion at T6 and above, the vascular system that is subject to sympathetic overactivity includes the splanchnic venous bed. Vasoconstriction leads to increased venous return which raises cardiac output to an extent that cannot be compensated, for example by vagally induced bradycardia. Acute hypertension is the inevitable result.

Autonomic dysreflexia can result in dramatic increases in blood pressure with symptoms of headache and anxiety. Its treatment involves removal of the triggering stimulus (for example, by draining a distended bladder), which results in a rapid resolution of the crisis. If a surgical procedure is to be carried out on a patient who is at risk of autonomic dysreflexia, a spinal anaesthetic will eliminate the risk, while a general anaesthetic will provide a measure of control over blood pressure fluctuations.

Secondary changes to urinary tract function

The pathophysiological effects of an SCI on LUT function depend on the primary changes in neurological control, which have been discussed above, and the impact of secondary changes. Examples of such changes include:

- Secondary neurological changes such as those caused by post-traumatic syringomyelia. A descending syrinx that extends into the conus has the capacity to disrupt sacral reflex activity with a loss of reflex erections and bladder contractions.[16] Disruption of the urethral sphincter guarding reflexes can cause stress incontinence.
- A bladder that is managed by reflex voiding into a penile sheath system will develop detrusor hypertrophy and fibrosis if DSD causes marked bladder outflow obstruction. These changes can lead to the development of impaired bladder compliance and/or vesicoureteric reflux.
- Long-term catheterization using continuous free drainage can result in a small, poorly compliant bladder.[17] If a urethral, rather than a suprapubic, catheter is used, there is a risk that catheter-induced urethral sphincter damage will occur with the development of stress incontinence.

Classification systems

The international standard for classifying cord injuries has been developed by the American Spinal Injury Association (ASIA).[18] The classification defines the neurological level of injury as the most caudal spinal level with intact sensation and antigravity muscle strength. The second element is an impairment scale which runs from a complete loss of sensation and motor function in the sacral segments (grade A = complete) to grade E (normal), where there has been a full motor and sensory recovery.

There is no single accepted classification of neurogenic LUT dysfunction. However, Rickwood[19] set out a simple system which is of practical value. Three groups are defined as:

- *Contractile bladder*: neurogenic detrusor overactivity is present and there is no urodynamic stress incontinence. This group includes patients with supraconal SCI.
- *Acontractile bladder*: neurogenic detrusor overactivity is not present but some degree of urodynamic stress incontinence is present. Patients with complete conus SCI fall in this group.
- *Intermediate bladder*: neurogenic detrusor overactivity and urodynamic stress incontinence are present in combination. A small number of SCI patients with incomplete SCI that involve the conus fall in this group but intermediate bladder dysfunction is common in patients with myelomeningocoele.

Reprinted from Rickwood AMK, 'Neuropathic bladder in childhood', in Mundy AR, Stephenson TP, and Wein AJ. (Eds.), Urodynamics: Principles, Practice and Application, Churchill Livingstone, UK, Copyright © 1994, with permission from Elsevier.

Early urological management

Following an SCI there is almost inevitably a phase of urinary retention either due to spinal shock or conus damage, depending on injury level. An indwelling urethral catheter is used to prevent bladder overdistension. Particular care is needed in managing the catheter as absent genital sensation can mean that tension on a catheter goes unnoticed, allowing urethral erosion to occur with the associated risk of urethral sphincter damage (Fig. 3.12.4). A urethral catheter may remain in place during the first weeks following injury while the patient's spinal trauma is being treated either by surgical spinal stabilization or by immobilization; other injuries may also require attention because of head, chest, or limb trauma.

Once the patient's condition is stable, a decision is made, in discussion with the patient, about the next phase of LUT management. There are three options that can be considered:

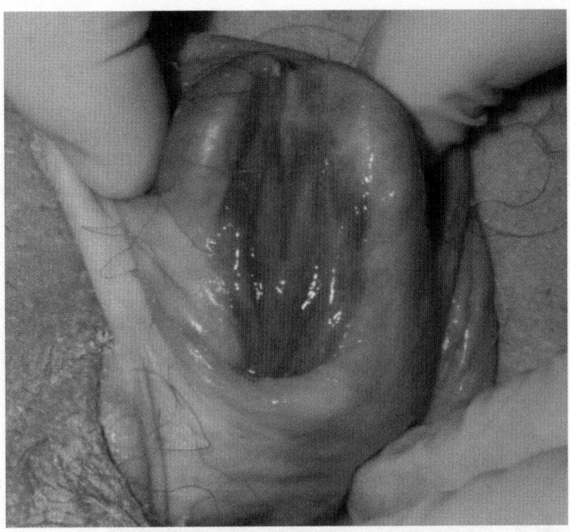
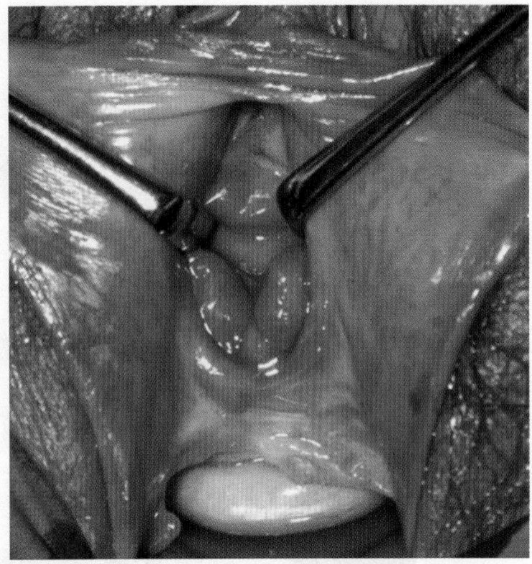

Fig. 3.12.4 Damage caused by a urethral catheter with catheter-induced hypospadias in the male (left) and complete urethral destruction of the female urethra (right); the retractors are positioned in the bladder neck which is wide open.

- *Trial without catheter (TWOC).* For patients with an incomplete SCI, there may be sufficient preserved neurological function to suggest that there will be retained voluntary control over the LUT. A TWOC is undertaken once the patient is mobilizing.
- *Intermittent catheterization (IC).* This can be introduced with one of two aims. Firstly, in patients who are likely to be able to manage CISC, the aim will be to establish the patient on IC with the option of using CISC as long-term management or converting to another management system. Secondly, nurse-performed IC can be introduced in men who will not be able to manage CISC but who are likely to develop reflex voiding and may go on to use a penile sheath collection system.
- *Suprapubic catheterization.* For patients who will require long-term indwelling catheterization, such as women with tetraplegia, a suprapubic catheter (SPC) is inserted at an early stage to prevent urethral complications. The option of using a catheter valve is discussed with the patient.

As the patient progresses through rehabilitation, additional interventions might be needed. For example, a patient on CISC might start to develop incontinence due to reflex bladder contractions (NDO) and be treated with antimuscarinic drugs, or a patient with a SPC might need treatment for recurrent catheter blockages.

Urodynamic investigations

Towards the end of a patient's SCI rehabilitation (usually between four and nine months post-injury), videourodynamic investigations are performed in order to inform discussions about long-term LUT management and to identify patients who might be at a high risk of developing renal complications.

Urodynamic studies in SCI patients are carried out with attention to specific technical issues:

- Radiological screening is aided by the patient standing if they are able; otherwise the test is carried out supine using a pipe to carry urine to the flow meter (Fig. 3.12.5).
- Consider giving prophylactic antibiotics.[20]
- Only drain the residual urine if the patient is known to empty their bladder fully (e.g. they are on CISC).
- Fill rates may need to be modified. Slow fill (10 mL/min) in small capacity bladders, otherwise use medium fill (e.g. 40 mL/min).
- Demonstrating stress incontinence can be difficult as patients may not be able to cough or strain; use suprapubic pressure if necessary.

The result of the urodynamic assessment allows a list of management options to be drawn up and discussed with the patient. This process is discussed below.

Urodynamic investigations also have a role in assessing the risk of renal deterioration from hydronephrosis or scarring. However, there is no substantial data in adult patients that allows the risk from a particular urodynamic finding to be defined. For example, a single fill-void cycle may not be representative of the patient's usual LUT function. This is particularly true of NDO and DSD where a prolonged bladder contraction with high detrusor pressures due to persistent DSD may be seen on one void, but not after a second fill. Furthermore, in patients with reduced bladder compliance, the calculated value (in mL/cmH_2O) will vary with fill rate and at different points on the detrusor pressure trace. Despite these limitations, urodynamic studies do provide some indication as to whether a patient is at added risk of complications and in need of a change in management or closer surveillance. Features that are suggestive of upper tract risk include:

- Reduced bladder compliance where the patient is exposed to prolonged periods of raised detrusor pressure as a result of their management regime. A patient in whom the pressure only starts to increase towards the end of a 400 mL fill is unlikely to be at risk if they empty fully with CISC and rarely hold more than 400 mL. However, if the same patient often fills to 600 mL and empties by straining, leaving a residual of 200 mL, they will be at risk of developing hydronephrosis.
- High-pressure NDO (e.g. over 60 cmH_2O) with prolonged episodes of DSD has the potential to cause hydronephrosis in the patient who is using reflex voiding into a penile sheath system.

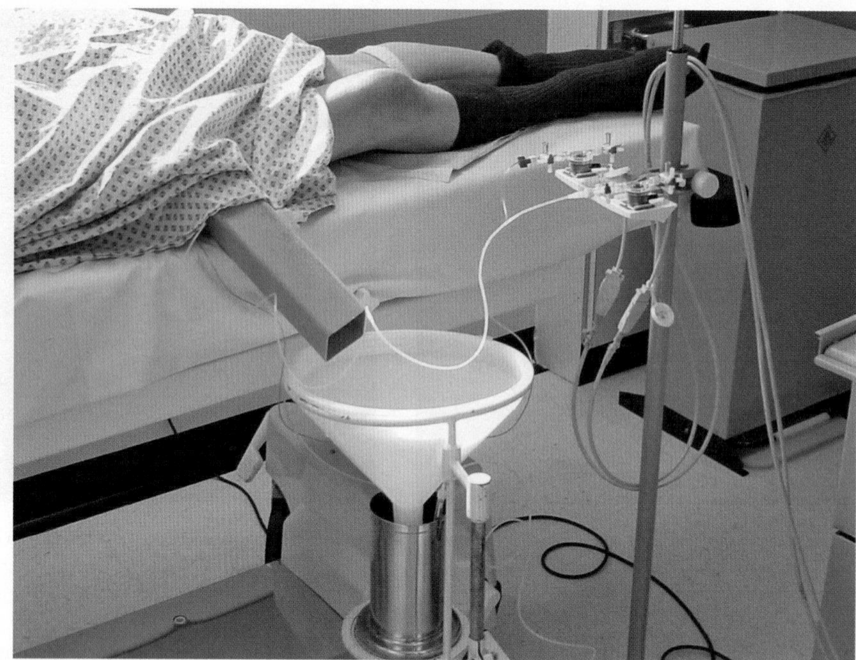

Fig. 3.12.5 A length of drainage pipe can be used to carry urine from the penis to the flow meter during urodynamic studies that must be performed in the supine position.

- Vesicoureteric reflux can be associated with the development of hydronephrosis or renal scarring, particularly if there are episodes of increased detrusor pressure during bladder filling or emptying.[21]

Long-term care: Urological management systems

On completion of rehabilitation and, for supraconal injury patients, when spinal reflex activity is fully established, the patient and clinical team will be in a position to make decisions regarding long-term management of the urinary tract. From the patient's perspective, this revolves around how they are to empty their bladder:

- *Voiding under voluntary control.* This option is likely to be used by two groups of patients. Firstly, those with an incomplete SCI and sufficient sensation and preservation of coordinated micturition to return to normal or near-normal LUT function. They might require additional treatments if they have symptoms. For example, urgency due to NDO might be managed with antimuscarinic drugs and incomplete bladder emptying by occasional CISC. Secondly, patients with conus injuries may be able to empty by straining. This is acceptable if straining is not excessive and if their urethral sphincter weakness enables them to empty effectively, but is not so severe that stress incontinence becomes troublesome.
- *Intermittent self-catheterization.* In practical terms, this is an option that is available to paraplegic patients and highly motivated tetraplegics who have some residual hand function. If urethral catheterization is impractical due to limited hand function, problems with toilet transfers or discomfort, the option of creating a continent, catheterizable abdominal conduit for CISC can be considered.[22] The patient who uses CISC to empty their bladder will wish to be reliably continent and to have adequate storage function to avoid overly frequent catheterization. Many patients will need to have additional treatment for NDO, reduced compliance, or stress incontinence in order to satisfy these requirements.
- *Containment of incontinence.* This approach is most commonly applied to men with supraconal lesions whose bladders empty well as a result of reflex contractions (NDO) and who can successfully use a penile sheath system. If DSD is excessive, an external urethral sphincterotomy can be undertaken.[23] Alternatively, incomplete bladder emptying can be managed by a combination of penile sheath collection and CISC. In SCI, containment of severe incontinence using pads is rarely used as a long-term management option.
- *Indwelling catheterization.* The risk of urethral erosion from chronic urethral catheterization means that all patients who choose to be managed by indwelling catheterization should be advised to undergo placement of an SPC. For tetraplegic women, an SPC is usually the only practical way of managing the LUT. For other patient groups, there is always an alternative approach available, although many patients will regard the use of an SPC as a relatively convenient and reliable way of dealing with their LUT dysfunction.[24] In patients with adequate storage function, the use of a catheter valve should be considered; there are theoretical benefits from the use of catheter valves in terms of preserving bladder capacity and limiting catheter blockages through the 'flushing' effect of intermittent drainage.
- *Sacral anterior root stimulation.* The use of an implantable prosthesis to empty the bladder in patients with a complete supraconal SCI was pioneered by Brindley. Good long-term results are described but the implant's use is restricted to specialist units.[25] It is usual to divide the dorsal roots of S2, 3, 4 at the time of

implantation to abolish NDO and provide high-volume bladder storage capacity. Electrodes are placed around the ventral roots of S2, 3, 4, so that electrical stimulation will produce a contraction of both the urethral sphincter and the detrusor. In response to a burst of stimulation, the smooth muscle of the detrusor produces a sustained contraction, while the striated urethral sphincter muscle rapidly switches on and off. Intermittent bursts of stimulation are produced by the device which allows voiding to occur in the gaps between the bursts, during which the detrusor is continuing to contract but the rhabdosphincter is relaxed.

- *Urinary diversion.* Ileal conduit diversion is a useful salvage procedure which is used occasionally for SCI patients, notably those who are catheter intolerant due to recurrent infections or other complications. If a urinary diversion is undertaken, consideration should be given to carrying out a simultaneous cystectomy in order to prevent pyocystis.

When considering these management options with the patient, discussion has to include the day-to-day practicalities of the systems, any additional treatments that will be needed in order to optimize management and the risks of complications that are associated with the different approaches. This counselling process can be complex and input from specialist nurses is useful. Discussions about long-term risks are hampered by a lack of reliable comparative data, although indwelling urethral catheterization is associated with unsatisfactory outcomes.[26]

The urological toolkit

In many cases, an SCI patient's LUT is not intrinsically suited to a management system that the patient wishes to use. For example, a paraplegic with a supraconal injury might want to use CISC for bladder emptying but has NDO; suppression of the NDO will be needed if they are to be reliably continent. The urologist uses a toolkit of treatment options to manage the various urodynamic abnormalities that may be present:

Impaired urine storage due to neurogenic detrusor overactivity or reduced bladder compliance

Antimuscarinic drugs are capable of controlling symptoms such as incontinence in many patients with NDO and are generally used as first-line therapy. Botulinum toxin type A (BTA) injections into the bladder wall have established a role in managing patients who are refractory to antimuscarinic drugs.[27,28] BTA controls symptoms in about 60% of cases and continues to provide benefit over repeated cycles of use.[29] However, there is uncertainty as to whether either antimuscarinic drugs or BTA have a useful effect on the bladder with reduced compliance or are capable of controlling NDO sufficiently reliably to be safely used in cases where high bladder pressures are causing hydronephrosis to develop. Patients in these situations, or with unresponsive symptoms, are managed by augmentation cystoplasty.[30] Ileum is generally used to augment the bladder although the colon is an alternative; detrusor myectomy has been explored as an alternative but has not established a role.[31]

Neurogenic stress incontinence

Neurogenic stress incontinence (NSI) is seen in patients with an SCI that involves the conus and damages Onuf's nucleus; stress incontinence is also seen in patients where the urethral sphincter has been damaged through catheter trauma. Treatment of NSI is needed in patients who wish to use intermittent self-catherization (ISC) or a suprapubic catheter with a catheter valve.

In men, the artificial urinary sphincter is the mainstay for managing NSI and will restore continence in over 90% of cases.[32] In neurogenic cases, the cuff is usually implanted around the distal prostate or bladder neck as a bulbar urethral cuff does not always produce complete continence. Patients will need to use CISC in order to empty the bladder. In patients with both impaired bladder storage and NSI, a simultaneous augmentation cystoplasty and artificial sphincter implantation can be undertaken.[33]

The artificial sphincter can also be used in women but the use of an autologous fascial pubovaginal sling is an alternative that produces generally satisfactory results without the same need for revision surgery. A wide range of other procedures have been used to treat NSI with satisfactory results being described with some. However, there is no role for the routine use of injectable bulking agents or for synthetic slings and tapes. NSI is the result of intrinsic sphincter deficiency rather than vaginal hypermobility so that tension has to be applied to a sling in order to overcome incontinence; there is concern that applying tension to a synthetic tape will risk erosion into the urethra.[26]

In cases where there is severe damage to the urethra and its sphincter mechanism, a decision may need to be made to formally close the urethra. In women, although an abdominal approach can be used, a vaginal approach is likely to be associated with less morbidity.[34] Closure of the male urethra can be undertaken by an abdominal approach to the bladder neck, or a bulbar urethra closure can be undertaken using perineal access.[35]

Impaired bladder emptying

Incomplete bladder emptying can be a problem for patients who are managing their neurogenic LUT by voluntary voiding, in which case ISC can be used either on a regular or as-required basis. The other group of patients who are affected by this problem are those who are using reflex bladder contractions to empty into a penile sheath system. For these patients, DSD and poorly sustained bladder contractions can lead to incomplete bladder emptying. An external urethral sphincterotomy will usually improve bladder emptying by abolishing DSD but cannot guarantee complete resolution of the problem as bladder contractions can remain poorly sustained.[23] Alternatives to sphincterotomy include the use of botulinum toxin injections into the rhabdosphincter[36] or the use of urethral stents,[37,38] although long-term follow-up data is limited.

For patients who have difficulty with urethral ISC, a continent catheterizable abdominal conduit can be constructed using the appendix (usually elongated with a caecal cuff) or ileum (using the Monti technique).[22]

Vesicoureteric reflux

Videourodynamic testing will demonstrate the presence of reflux in some SCI patients. However, there is uncertainty as to whether intervention to control reflux is of benefit. Reimplanting a ureter into a thick-walled neuropathic bladder is not recommended as the result is likely to be either an obstructed system or persistent reflux. However, injecting a bulking agent under the ureteric orifice can be considered in cases, such as those with active bladder contractions and recurrent urinary tract infection (UTI), where treatment is judged to be appropriate.[21]

Management of sexual dysfunction and infertility

Sexual dysfunction as a result of SCI can have a devastating effect on the couple. Sexual rehabilitation is important and should not be neglected; even patients with tetraplegia report satisfying sex lives provided they adapt to their circumstances.[39] Both males and females with incomplete or low injuries may be orgasmic. Counselling is needed and should cover the avoidance of problems such as incontinence during intercourse.

Men with some preserved erectile function, reflex or psychogenic, respond well to 5-phosphodiesterase inhibitors; penile injection therapy with alprostadil is often effective for non-responders, while penile prostheses or vacuum tumescence devices are required for others.[40] Many couples opt for an active but non-penetrative sex life.

Female fertility is, in general, not affected by SCI. However, during pregnancy, UTIs need to be treated promptly and urinary tract management adapted; for example, CISC may become impractical as the pregnancy advances. Delivery may require collaboration between obstetrician and urologist.

Approximately 5% of SCI men retain natural fertility; for the remainder, ejaculatory failure is the principle cause of infertility. In patients with spinal lesions above T10, the ejaculatory reflex pathway may be intact and can be activated using a strong vibratory stimulus applied to the penile frenulum. If this is effective, some couples are able to use this approach at home along with intravaginal insemination. However, the large majority of SCI men who father children do so with a combination of sperm harvesting using vibrator-induced ejaculation, electroejaculation, or direct sperm harvesting from the testis and assisted conception techniques.[41] Electroejaculators use a rectal probe to provide direct stimulation to the pelvic structures to produce seminal emission (Fig. 3.12.6).

Complications and follow-up

General complications

A SCI patient remains at risk of developing complications related to the SCI. Clinicians who are involved in their care need to take steps to provide:

- Skin protection with a turning regime and suitable mattress.
- Physiotherapy to prevent chest complications.
- An environment which helps maintain a normal body temperature.
- A bowel management routine to prevent constipation or incontinence.
- Prevention or treatment of episodes of autonomic dysreflexia.

Urinary tract complications

There are a number of important urinary tract problems that can lead to morbidity and even mortality in the SCI patient. Important among these are:

- *Urinary tract infection.* UTI is a common problem among SCI patients. If UTI develops as a new problem, or the pattern of infections intensifies, investigation with urinary tract imaging and cystoscopy is indicated. If a treatable cause is not identified, management may include the use of self-start antibiotics or low-dose antibiotic prophylaxis to minimize the frequency and intensity of attacks.
- *Autonomic dysreflexia.* Patients who complain of symptoms of autonomic dysreflexia require urgent investigation in order to identify the cause of the problem. Urinary tract imaging and urodynamic investigation may be included in the diagnostic pathway.
- *Incontinence.* Incontinence can be due to NDO and/or sphincter weakness. If simple measures do not resolve the issue, urodynamic investigations are indicated.
- *Urinary tract stones.* The risk of renal stone formation is highest within three months of injury, and by ten years 7% of patients

(A)

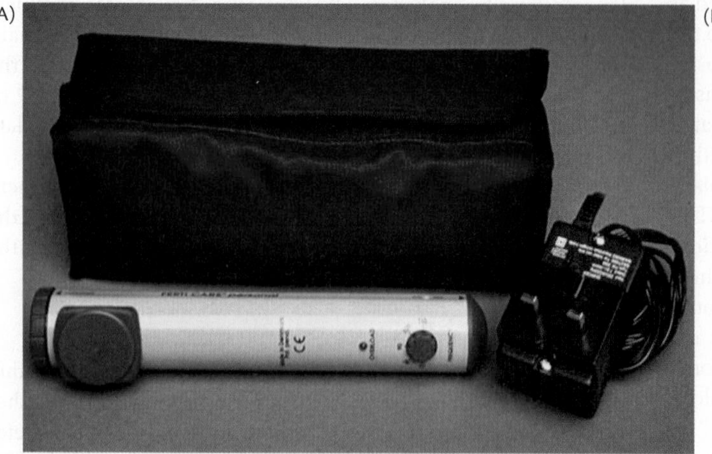

(B)

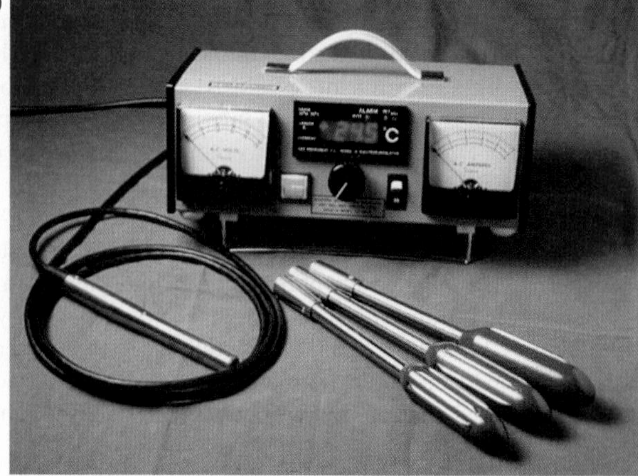

Fig. 3.12.6 Devices used to induce ejaculation in spinal cord-injured patients. (A) A vibrator that can be used by a couple at home. (B) An electroejaculator with an assortment of three rectal probes.

Image reproduced courtesy of Paul Tophill.

will have developed a renal stone.[42] Bacterial colonization of the urinary tract is an important factor in the formation of renal and bladder stones, although metabolic kidney stones are common in SCI patients.[43]

- *Hydronephrosis.* Upper tract dilatation is most commonly caused by high bladder storage pressure, which is demonstrated by the resolution of the hydronephrosis with insertion of an indwelling catheter. However, other possible causes include ureteric calculi, vesicoureteric reflux, and pelviureteric junction obstruction.
- *Renal scarring.* Pyelonephritic scarring is a common finding on follow-up ultrasound scans and is not confined to one system of bladder management. Fortunately, such scarring rarely progresses to the extent that renal replacement therapy is needed.[44] In patients who are being managed by indwelling catheters, the explanation for the development of scarring probably lies in a combination of residual bladder contractile activity, vesicoureteric reflux, and bacteriuria.[45]
- Catheter problems. These include difficulties with catheter changes, recurrent UTI, catheter bypassing, and catheter blockage. The last two of these problems can be difficult to distinguish at times; if incontinence resolves for a few days after a catheter change, then it is likely that the problem is blockage rather than bypassing due to NDO or NSI. Repeated catheter blockage is best investigated by cystoscopy because bladder stones can underlie the problem and are not reliably detected by X-ray or ultrasound scan.
- *Bladder cancer.* Estimates of the risk of bladder cancer in patients with SCI have varied widely and it is unclear whether the probable increased risk is greater with one management system compared with another.[46] Unfortunately, when bladder cancer arises, the tumour is usually a squamous carcinoma and the prognosis poor.

Surveillance policies

Spinal injuries units have traditionally offered lifelong follow-up to their patients on the basis of the range of difficulties that patients may experience and the changing requirements for care with ageing. Continuing care usually includes an element of urinary tract surveillance, which amounts to a screening programme for a high-risk population. There is a consensus that annual or biannual ultrasound scanning of the kidneys is a reasonable approach.[47,48] However, there is no requirement to offer more comprehensive screening investigations, as the value of regular urodynamic investigation, GFR measurement, and cystoscopy is uncertain.[47]

Acknowledgement

I am grateful to Mr Paul Tophill (Consultant Urologist) for providing some of the illustrations as well as helpful comments on the text of this chapter. My insight into SCI urology has been greatly enhanced by our long-standing collaboration as trainers in neurourology.

Further reading

Abrams P, Cardozo L, Fall M, *et al.* The standardisation of terminology of lower urinary tract function: report from the Standardisation Subcommittee of the International Continence Society. *Neurourol Urodyn* 2002; **21**:167–78.

Brindley GS, Polkey CE, Rushton DN, Cardozo L. Sacral anterior root stimulators for bladder control in paraplegia: the first 50 cases. *J Neurol Neurosurg Psychiatry* 1986; **49**:1104–14.

De Groat WC. Integrative control of the lower urinary tract: preclinical perspective. *Br J Pharmacol* 2006; **147**:S25–40.

Everaert K, de Waard WIQ, Van Hoof T, Kiekens C, Mulliez T, D'herde C. Neuroanatomy and neurophysiology related to sexual dysfunction in male neurogenic patients with lesions to the spinal cord or peripheral nerves. *Spinal Cord* 2010; **48**:182–91.

Guttmann L, Frankel H. The value of intermittent catheterisation in the early management of traumatic paraplegia and tetraplegia. *Paraplegia* 1996; **4**:63–84.

International Consultation on Urological Diseases, 2009. Incontinence, 4th Edition, Committee 10: Neurological urinary and faecal incontinence. Available at: www.icud.info/publications.html [Online].

Lapides J, Diokno C, Silber S, Lowe B. Clean, intermittent self-catheterization in the treatment of urinary tract disease. *J Urol* 1972; **107**:458–61.

NICE Clinical Guideline 148: Urinary incontinence in neurological disease. (2012) Available at: www.nice.org.uk [Online].

Schurch B, Stöhrer M, Kramer G, Schmid DM, Gaul G, Hauri D. Botulinum-A toxin for treating detrusor hyperreflexia in spinal cord injured patients: a new alternative to anticholinergic drugs? Preliminary results. *J Urol* 2000; **164**:692–7.

References

1. Wyndaele M, Wyndaele J-J. Incidence, prevalence and epidemiology of spinal cord injury: what learns a worldwide literature survey? *Spinal Cord* 2006; **44**:523–9.
2. Donovan WD. Spinal cord injury—past, present and future. *J Spinal Cord Med* 2007; **30**:85–100.
3. Strauss DJ, De Vivo MJ, Paculdo DR, Shavelle RM. Trends in life expectancy after spinal cord injury. *Arch Phys Med Rehabil* 2006; **87**:1079–85.
4. Royal College of Physicians. Medical rehabilitation in 2011 and beyond. Report of a working party. London: RCP, 2010. Available at: http://bookshop.rcplondon.ac.uk [Online].
5. De Groat WC. Integrative control of the lower urinary tract: preclinical perspective. *Br J Pharmacol* 2006; **147**:S25–S40.
6. Kaplan SA, Chancellor MB, Blaivas JG. Bladder and sphincter behavior in patients with spinal cord lesions. *J Urol* 1991; **146**:113–17.
7. Weld KJ, Dmochowski RR. Association of level of injury and bladder behavior in patients with post-traumatic spinal cord injury. *Urology* 2000; **55**:490–4.
8. Abrams P, Cardozo L, Fall M, *et al.* The standardisation of terminology of lower urinary tract function: report from the Standardisation Subcommittee of the International Continence Society. *Neurourol Urodyn* 2002; **21**:167–78.
9. Bors E, Comarr AE. Neurological disturbances of sexual function with special reference to 529 patients with spinal cord injury. *Urol Surv* 1960; **10**:191–222.
10. Steers WD. Neural pathways and central sites involved in penile erection: neuroanatomy and clinical implications. *Neurosci Behav Rev* 2000; **24**:507–16
11. Everaert K, de Waard WIQ, Van Hoof T, Kiekens C, Mulliez T, D'herde C. Neuroanatomy and neurophysiology related to sexual dysfunction in male neurogenic patients with lesions to the spinal cord or peripheral nerves. *Spinal Cord* 2010; **48**:182–91.
12. Kuhr CS, Heiman J, Cardenas D, Bradley W, Berger RE. Premature emission after spinal cord injury. *J Urol* 1995; **153**:429–31.
13. Patki P, Woodhouse J, Hamid R, Shah J, Craggs M. Lower urinary tract dysfunction in ambulatory patients with incomplete spinal cord injury. *J Urol* 2006; **175**:1784–7.
14. Ditunno JF, Little JW, Tessler A, Burns AS. Spinal shock revisited: a four-phase model. *Spinal Cord* 2004; **42**:383–95.

15. Khastgir J, Drake MJ, Abrams P. Recognition and effective management of autonomic dysreflexia in spinal cord injuries. *Expert Opin Pharmacother* 2007; **8**:945–56.
16. El Masry WS, Biyani A. Incidence, management, and outcome of post-traumatic syringomyelia. In memory of Mr Bernard Williams. *J Neurol Neurosurg Psychiatry* 1996; **60**:141–6.
17. Weld KJ, Marshall JG, Dmochowski RR. Differences in bladder compliance with time and associations of bladder management with compliance in spinal cord injured patients. *J Urol* 2000; **163**:1228–33.
18. Kirsblum SC, Burns SP, Biering-Sørensen F, *et al.* International standards for neurological classification of spinal cord injury (revised 2011). *J Spinal Cord Med* 2011; **34**:535–46.
19. Rickwood AMK. Neuropathic bladder in childhood. In: Mundy AR, Stephenson TP, Wein AJ (eds). *Urodynamics: Principles, Practice and Application.* Edinburgh, UK: Churchill Livingstone, 1994.
20. Pannek J, Nehiba M. Morbidity of urodynamic testing in patients with spinal cord injury. Is antibiotic prophylaxis necessary? *Spinal Cord* 2007; **45**:771–4.
21. Foley SJ, McFarlane JP, Shah PJR. Vesico-ureteric reflux in adult patients with spinal injury. *Br J Urol* 1997; **79**:888–91.
22. Gowda BD, Agrawal V, Harrison SCW. The continent, catheterisable abdominal conduit in adult urological practice. *BJU Int* 2008; **102**:1688–92.
23. Pan D, Troy A, Rogerson J, Bolton D, Brown D, Lawrentschuk N. Long-term outcomes of external sphincterotomy in a spinal injured population. *J Urol* 2009; **181**:705–9.
24. Feifer A, Corcos J. Contemporary role of suprapubic cystostomy in treatment of neuropathic bladder dysfunction in spinal cord injured patients. *Neurourol Urodyn* 2008; **27**:475–9.
25. Kutzenberger J, Domurath B, Sauerwein D. Spastic bladder and spinal cord injury: seventeen years of experience with sacral deafferentation and implantation of an anterior root stimulator. *Artif Organs* 2005; **29**:239–41.
26. NICE Clinical Guideline 148: Urinary incontinence in neurological disease. (2012) Available at: www.nice.org.uk [Online].
27. Cruz F, Herschorn S, Aliotta P, *et al.* Efficacy and safety of onabotulinumtoxinA in patients with urinary incontinence due to neurogenic detrusor overactivity: a randomised, double-blind, placebo-controlled trial. *Eur Urol* 2011; **60**:742–50.
28. Herschorn S, Gajewski J, Ethans K, *et al.* Efficacy of botulinum toxin A injection for neurogenic detrusor overactivity and urinary incontinence: a randomized, double-blind trial. *J Urol* 2011; **185**:2229–35.
29. del Popolo G, Filocamo MT, li Marzi V, *et al.* Neurogenic detrusor overactivity treated with English botulinum toxin A: 8-year experience of one single centre. *Eur Urol* 2008; **53**:1013–20.
30. Gurung PM, Attar KH, Abdul-Rahman A, Morris T, Hamid R, Shah PJ. Long-term outcomes of augmentation ileocystoplasty in patients with spinal cord injury: a minimum of 10 years of follow-up. *BJU Int* 2012; **109**:1236–42.
31. Stohrer M, Kramer G, Goepel M, Lochner-Ernst D, Kruse D, Rubben H. Bladder autoaugmentation in adult patients with neurogenic voiding dysfunction. *Spinal Cord* 1997; **35**:456–62.
32. Patki P, Hamid R, Shah PJ, Craggs M. Long-term efficacy of AMS 800 artificial urinary sphincter in male patients with urodynamic stress incontinence due to spinal cord lesion. *Spinal Cord* 2006; **44**:297–300.
33. Catto JW, Natarajan V, Tophill PR. Simultaneous augmentation cystoplasty is associated with earlier rather than increased artificial sphincter infection. *J Urol* 2005; **173**:1237–41.
34. Zimmern PE, Hadley HR, Leach GE, Raz S. Transvaginal closure of the bladder neck and placement of a suprapubic catheter for destroyed urethra after long-term indwelling catheterization. *J Urol* 1985; **134**:554–7.
35. Hall J, Thomas DG. Surgical closure of the bulbar urethra for the treatment of intractable incontinence in the paralysed patient. *Br J Urol* 1998; **82**:912.
36. Chen SL, Bih LI, Chen GD, Huang YH, You YH. Comparing a transrectal ultrasound-guided with a cystoscopy-guided botulinum toxin a injection in treating detrusor external sphincter dyssynergia in spinal cord injury. *Am J Phys Med Rehabil* 2011; **90**:723–30.
37. Mehta SS, Tophill PR. Memokath® stents for the treatment of detrusor sphincter dyssynergia (DSD) in men with spinal cord injury: The Princess Royal Spinal Injuries Unit 10-year experience. *Spinal Cord* 2006; **44**:1–6.
38. Abdul-Rahman A, Ismail S, Hamid R, Shah J. A 20-year follow-up of the mesh wallstent in the treatment of detrusor external sphincter dyssynergia in patients with spinal cord injury. *BJU Int* 2010; **106**:1510–13.
39. Biering-Sørensen I, Hansen RB, Biering-Sørensen F. Sexual function in a traumatic spinal cord injured population 10–45 years after injury. *J Rehabil Med* 2012; **44**(11):926–31.
40. Deforge D, Blackmer J, Garritty C, *et al.* Male erectile dysfunction following spinal cord injury: a systematic review. *Spinal Cord* 2006; **44**:465–73.
41. Sønksen J, Ohl DA. Penile vibratory stimulation and electroejaculation in the treatment of ejaculatory dysfunction. *Int J Androl* 2002; **25**:324–32.
42. Chen Y, DeVivo MJ, Roseman JM. Current trend and risk factors for kidney stones in persons with spinal cord injury: a longitudinal study. *Spinal Cord* 2000; **38**:346–53.
43. Matlaga BR, Kim SC, Watkins SL, Kuo RL, Munch LC, Lingeman JE. Changing composition of renal calculi in patients with neurogenic bladder. *J Urol* 2006; **175**:1716–19.
44. Edhem I, Harrison SCW. Renal scarring in spinal cord injury: a progressive process? *Spinal Cord* 2006; **44**:170–3.
45. Jamil F, Williamson M, Ahmed YS, Harrison SCW. Natural-fill urodynamics in chronically catheterized patients with spinal-cord injury. *BJU Int* 1999; **83**:396–9.
46. Subramonian K, Cartwright RA, Harnden P, Harrison SCW. Bladder cancer in patients with spinal cord injuries. *BJU Int* 2004; **93**:739–43.
47. Cameron AP, Rodriguez GM, Shomer KG. Systematic review of urological followup after spinal cord injury. *J Urol* 2012; **187**:391–7.
48. Abrams P, Agarwal M, Drake M, *et al.* A proposed guideline for the urological management of patients with spinal cord injury. *BJU Int* 2008; **101**:989–94.

CHAPTER 3.13

Non-traumatic neurourology

Jalesh N. Panicker and Clare J. Fowler

Introduction to non-traumatic neurourology

Lower urinary tract (LUT) dysfunction is common in neurological disease and its importance to patient health and quality of life is now widely recognized. This chapter reviews bladder disturbances in non-traumatic neurological conditions and provides an approach to the evaluation and management.

Neurogenic lower urinary tract dysfunction

Lesions of the nervous system result in characteristic patterns of LUT dysfunction depending upon the level of the lesion in the neuraxis. Accordingly, neurological lesions can be categorized as being suprapontine, infrapontine/suprasacral, or infrasacral and each results in a characteristic clinical profile which becomes evident during the evaluation of the patient (Table 3.13.1).[1] Storage functions of the bladder are affected in diseases at most levels and results in involuntary contractions of the detrusor muscle, known as *detrusor overactivity*. Voiding functions are particularly affected following lesions below the pons. Following spinal cord damage, simultaneous contraction of the external urethral sphincter and detrusor muscle, known as *detrusor sphincter dyssynergia*, results in incomplete bladder emptying and abnormally high bladder pressures. Lesions of the conus medullaris and cauda equina result in voiding dysfunction due to either an underactive detrusor or non-relaxing urethral sphincters.[2]

Cortical lesions

Anterior regions of the frontal lobes are critical to bladder control; the seminal work of Andrew and Nathan in the 1960s provided considerable insight into the effects of frontal lobe lesions on LUT control.[3] A variety of frontal lobe lesions may result in LUT symptoms such as intracranial tumours, ruptured aneurysms, traumatic brain injury, and surgeries such as prefrontal leukotomy. The clinical presentation of frontal lobe incontinence is that of severe urgency and frequency, and urge incontinence; the patient is socially aware and embarrassed by the incontinence. Micturition is normally coordinated, though a few case reports of patients with right frontal lobe disorders having urinary retention which improved after the frontal lobe disorder was treated successfully have been reported.[2,4]

Urinary incontinence may occur after stroke. Commonly, urodynamics demonstrates detrusor overactivity (DO), though patients with haemorrhagic stroke are more likely to have detrusor underactivity.[5] Lesions more anteriorly placed in the brain are more likely to result in LUT symptoms, though it is not possible to demonstrate a correlation between specific lesion sites and urodynamic findings. It is known however that urinary incontinence at seven days following stroke predicts poor survival, disability, and institutionalization independent of level of consciousness.[6] Incontinence in such cases is often the result of a more severe general loss of functions; moreover, incontinent persons may be less motivated to recover both continence and general function.[2]

Table 3.13.1 Results of the diagnostic evaluation for patients with suspected neurogenic bladder dysfunction according to the site of neurological lesion

	Suprapontine lesion e.g. Cortical lesions, stroke, Parkinson's disease	**Infrapontine suprasacral lesion** e.g. spinal cord injury, multiple sclerosis	**Infrasacral lesion** e.g. conus medullaris tumour, cauda equina syndrome, peripheral neuropathy
History/ bladder diary	Urgency, frequency, urgency incontinence	Urgency, frequency, urgency incontinence, hesitancy, interrupted stream	Hesitancy, interrupted stream
Post-void residual urine	PVR < 100 mL	± Elevated PVR	PVR > 100 mL
Uroflowmetry	Normal flow	Interrupted flow	Poor/absent flow
Urodynamics	Detrusor overactivity	Detrusor overactivity Detrusor sphincter dyssynergia	Detrusor underactivity, Sphincter insufficiency

PVR: Post-void residual urine.

Reproduced from *Practical Neurology*, 'The bare essentials: UroNeurology', Jalesh N Panicker and Clare J Fowler, Volume 10, Issue 3, pp. 178–185, Copyright © 2010 British Medical Journal Publishing Group, with permission from BMJ Publishing Group Ltd. Source: data from Panicker, Jalesh N., Clare J. Fowler, and Ranan DasGupta, 'Neurourology' in Robert B. Daroff *et al.* (Eds.), *Bradley's Neurology in Clinical Practice, Sixth Edition*, Elsevier Saunders, Philadelphia, USA, Copyright © 2012 by Saunders, an imprint of Elsevier Inc.

The small perforating vessels of the brain may be affected, resulting in ischaemia to the white matter (small vessel disease, leukoaraiosis). Clinically, patients present with the triad of memory impairment, gait disorder, and urgency incontinence. This is increasingly becoming known as a cause for incontinence in the otherwise functionally independent elderly.[7]

Incontinence is a common problem in patients with dementia. In a study of patients with dementia, incontinence was observed to occur early in the course of patients with dementia with Lewy bodies, as in the more advanced stages of Alzheimer's disease.[8] Normal pressure hydrocephalus is not as common a cause for dementia, however incontinence may be a cardinal feature.[9] This condition belongs to the list of treatable causes for dementia and symptoms improve following drainage of cerebrospinal fluid either by lumbar puncture or a shunt, including overactive bladder symptoms and even urodynamic parameters. Solifenacin is effective in the treatment of overactive bladder symptoms in patients who have undergone ventriculoperitoneal shunt surgery.[10]

Parkinson's disease and related conditions

Parkinsonism encompasses a number of conditions including Parkinson's disease (PD) and various Parkinson-plus syndromes such as multiple system atrophy (MSA), progressive supranuclear palsy, and corticobasal degeneration (CBD).[11]

Parkinson's disease

Although predominantly a movement disorder, PD is often associated with non-motor symptoms, including sleep alterations, neuropsychiatric disturbances, and dysautonomia, with nocturia as the commonest symptom. The incidence of lower urinary tract symptoms (LUTS) in PD varies according to the study quoted and ranges from 38% to 71%.[12,13] Storage symptoms such as nocturia are commonly reported (in more than 60% of patients) and have a considerable impact on quality of life.[14–16] The causes for nocturia are poorly understood, although it has a significant impact on sleep and quality of life in individuals with PD. Detrusor overactivity is the commonest finding on urodynamics.[15] Dopaminergic receptor stimulation through the D1 receptor is known to inhibit the micturition reflex in health,[17] and it is thought that degenerative changes characteristic of PD results in disinhibition of this reflex, resulting in DO.

Additional co-morbidities may contribute to LUT symptoms in PD. Benign prostate obstruction is common in this age group, and transurethral prostate resection can be successfully carried out in properly selected cases.[18] Additional co-morbidities such as cervical spondylosis with cord compression or vascular disease of the brain, or medical conditions such as congestive heart failure, diabetes mellitus, pedal oedema, or medications such as diuretics, and poor mobility or cognitive impairment may be factors contributing to incontinence. Sleep disturbances and disturbed circadian rhythm may be closely associated with nocturia.[19–21] Bradykinesia of the pelvic floor muscles (known as 'pseudo-dyssynergia') has been reported, though significant voiding dysfunction is uncommon in PD.[11]

Levodopa is the most important medication used in managing PD and its effects on overactive bladder (OAB) symptoms are variable. Some patients may improve whereas in others, OAB symptoms may worsen.[22] Deep brain stimulation (DBS) is a well-accepted treatment option in advanced PD and the effects of DBS on LUT symptoms may be variable, with worsening reported in some studies and improvement in others.[11,23–26] Patients with advanced PD on subthalamic nucleus (STN) DBS have reported less nocturia.[24]

Multiple system atrophy

The syndrome previously known as Shy Drager syndrome and olivopontocerebellar atrophy are now classified as MSA-P (parkinsonism predominant) or MSA-C (cerebellar predominant), respectively. This condition is suspected when urogenital symptoms predominate, or predate other symptoms such as parkinsonism or ataxia. The reader is referred to the website http://www.msatrust.org.uk/ for more information about MSA. Some 41% of patients with MSA present initially with LUT symptoms and 97% report symptoms during the course of the disease.[27–30] Symptoms include daytime frequency (45%, 43%; percentage in men and women, respectively), nocturia (65%, 69%), urinary urgency (64% of men), and incontinence (75%, 66%).[31]

In the absence of any gold standard tests, distinguishing PD from MSA is difficult, even for an experienced neurologist. Evaluating urogenital dysfunction may help (Table 3.13.2) and LUTS are more severe and occur much earlier in MSA compared to in PD. Voiding dysfunction is common in MSA and patients are more likely to have an elevated post-void residual (>100 mL).[32,33] Urodynamics may demonstrate detrusor sphincter dyssynergia and an open bladder neck at the start of bladder filling (videocystometrogram).[34] EMG of the anal sphincter may sometimes be useful to distinguish the two conditions, to specifically look for findings of reinnervation.[11,35–37]

Table 3.13.2 Comparison of lower urinary tract dysfunction (LUTD) in multiple system atrophy (MSA) versus Parkinson's disease (PD)

	MSA	PD
Onset	Symptoms may precede other neurological deficits	Usually follows onset of disease and more common in advanced PD
Symptomatology	◆ Urinary frequency and urgency ◆ Early and severe incontinence ◆ As disease advances—chronic urinary retention	◆ Nocturia and urgency ◆ Overactive bladder symptoms, however less severe incontinence
Bladder scan	Elevated post-void residual (>100 mL) as the disease advances	Normal
Urodynamics	Initially detrusor overactivity. Detrusor acontractility later in the course of disease Open bladder neck may be seen at the start of bladder filling in the videocystometrogram	Detrusor overactivity

Multiple sclerosis and related conditions

Estimates of the number of patients with multiple sclerosis (MS) who have LUTS vary according to the severity of the neurological disability; however, a figure of 75% is frequently cited.[38] The most common symptoms are storage symptoms (37–99%), followed by voiding symptoms (34–79%). Commonly, a combination of both types of disorders coexist (51–59%).[39] Urinary incontinence is considered to be one of the worst aspects of the disease, with 70% of a self-selected group of patients with MS responding to a questionnaire as classifying the impact bladder symptoms had on their life as 'high' or 'moderate'.[40] A strong association exists between the presence of bladder symptoms and the presence of clinical spinal cord involvement, such as paraparesis and upper motor neuron signs in the lower limb.[41] In a systematic review of the literature, De Sèze *et al.*[42] found that the duration of disease was one of the principal factors that influenced the frequency of lower urinary tract dysfunction (LUTD). No correlation has been established between the site of MS lesion on MRI and clinical LUTS.[2,43–46]

MS is a progressive condition and with progression, the bladder dysfunction may become more difficult to treat. However, in contrast to LUT dysfunction consequent to spinal cord injury (SCI), progressive neurological disorders such as MS are rarely reported to result in upper urinary tract damage or renal failure. De Sèze *et al.* reviewed the literature and found that duration of MS, presence of an indwelling catheter, and the finding of high detrusor pressures were risk factors of upper urinary tract complications.[42] An epidemiological study has not demonstrated an increased risk of renal failure in people with multiple sclerosis compared to the general population.[47] The reason for sparing of the upper urinary tract is uncertain, but it does mean that in such patients, management should emphasize symptom relief.[2,4]

LUTD is common following other demyelinating conditions. In a consecutive series of 61 patients with acute disseminated encephalomyelitis (ADEM), a third of patients demonstrated evidence for LUTD,[48] and symptoms seem to be as common and severe as in MS.[49] An association has been recognized between LUT symptoms and the finding of lower limb pyramidal involvement.[48]

Urinary tract infections may lead to exacerbation of neurological symptoms in MS. As the disease progresses, it is not uncommon for recurrent infections to result in deficits which accumulate and lead to progressive neurological deterioration.[50] This means that arrangements for treatment of confirmed urinary tract infection (UTI) must be prompt and timely.[51] Urinary dipstick testing allows for rapid and safe management of patients before high-dose corticosteroid treatment for an acute MS relapse.[52]

Management of neurogenic lower urinary tract dysfunction

Recent guidance from the National Institute of Clinical Excellence (NICE) provides a framework for managing urinary incontinence in patients with neurological disease.[53] Urine dipstick is advisable for all patients presenting with new bladder symptoms. While its negative predictive value for excluding UTI is high (>98%), positive predictive value for confirming UTI is only 50%.[54] The necessity to perform a complete urodynamic study in all patients with a suspected neurogenic bladder has been addressed in the NICE guidance. Urodynamics (filling cystometry and pressure-flow studies) should not be offered routinely.[53] Patients diagnosed with spinal cord injury, spina bifida, and possibly advanced MS should undergo investigations such as cystometry because of the increased risk for upper tract damage and renal impairment. However, in most progressive neurological conditions, it is recommended to restrict the initial evaluation to non-invasive tests as the risk for upper urinary tract damage is less.[51]

The aims for treatment of neurogenic bladder dysfunction are to protect the upper urinary tract, to improve urinary continence, restore lower urinary tract functions, and improve quality of life.[55]

General measures

Conservative strategies are generally effective in the early stages when symptoms are mild. The fluid intake should be individualized—between one to two litres a day is suggested—however, it is important to assess fluid balance by means of a bladder diary.[56] Caffeine reduction may reduce symptoms of urinary urgency and frequency. A behavioural management programme, including timed voiding or bladder retraining, aims to restore a normal pattern of micturition.[53] Pelvic floor exercises, with or without neuromuscular stimulation, may play a role in addressing overactive bladder symptoms.[2,57,58]

Antimuscarinics

Antimuscarinics form the mainstay of conservative management of overactive bladder in the neurological patent. Table 3.13.3 lists the currently available medications in the United Kingdom. In a prospective, open-label study of solifenacin for the treatment of OAB in MS patients, van Rey *et al.* demonstrated a significant improvement in urinary frequency, pad use, and severity of urgency compared to baseline following eight weeks of treatment.[59] A recent systematic review suggests that the uses of these medications are associated with improvement in symptoms and significant reduction of maximum detrusor pressure in urodynamics. There appears to be no significant difference between antimuscarinics or the different doses and preparations and the choice of medication should be guided by their side effect profile.[60] The adverse effects include dryness of the mouth, blurring of vision for near objects, constipation, and tachycardia, which arise due to their non-specific antimuscarinic action. Of concern in the patient with neurological disease are their effects on central muscarinic M1 receptors, resulting in impaired cognition and sensorium in susceptible individuals. Medications which have low selectivity for the M1 receptor, such as darifenacin, or whose permeability across the blood brain barrier is restricted, such as trospium chloride, are expected to have less central side effects, however there are only limited studies evaluating their use in patients with cognitive impairment. The post-void residual urine may increase following treatment and should be monitored in individuals reporting short-term or limited benefits. In patients with additional voiding dysfunction, the judicious use of antimuscarinic medication together with intermittent catheterization often proves to be the most effective management strategy (Fig. 3.13.1).[2,51]

Desmopressin

Desmopressin is a synthetic analogue of arginine vasopressin and temporarily reduces urine production by promoting water reabsorption at the distal and collecting tubules of the kidney. It is useful for the treatment of nocturia, especially in patients with MS,

Table 3.13.3 Antimuscarinic medications available in the United Kingdom (presented alphabetically)

Generic name	Trade name	Dose (mg)	Frequency
Darifenacin	Emselex	7.5–15	od
Fesoterodine	Toviaz	4–8	od
Oxybutynin IR	Ditropan, cystrin	2.5–20	bd—qds
Oxybutynin ER	Lyrinel XL	5–20	od
Oxybutynin transdermal	Kentera	36 mg (3.9 mg/24 hours)	One patch twice-weekly
Propantheline	Pro-banthine	15–120	tds (one hour before food)
Propiverine	Detrunorm	15–60	od—qds
Solifenacin	Vesicare	5–10	od
Tolterodine IR	Detrusitol	2–4	bd
Tolterodine ER	Detrusitol XL	4	od
Trospium	Regurin	20–40	bd (before food)

Reproduced from *Practical Neurology*, 'The bare essentials: UroNeurology', Jalesh N Panicker and Clare J Fowler, Volume 10, Issue 3, pp. 178–185, Copyright © 2010 British Medical Journal Publishing Group, with permission from BMJ Publishing Group Ltd.

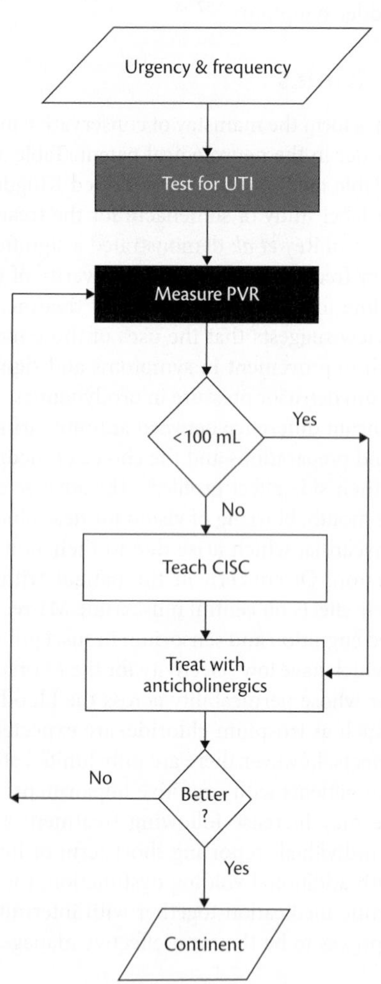

Fig. 3.13.1 Management algorithm for patients with multiple sclerosis presenting with urinary tract intermittent self-catheterization).

Reproduced from *Journal of Neurology, Neurosurgery and Psychiatry*, 'A UK consensus on the management of the bladder in multiple sclerosis' C J Fowler *et al.*, Volume 80, Issue 5, pp. 470–77, Copyright © 2009 British Medical Journal Publishing Group, with permission from BMJ Publishing Group Ltd.

providing symptom relief for up to six hours.[61] Desmopressin is also useful in patients found to have nocturnal polyuria, which is characterized by excessive urine production at night. This may be seen in patients with orthostatic hypotension as part of a more generalized autonomic dysfunction. The feared complication is hyponatraemia and therefore desmopressin should not be used in patients above the age of 65 or with evidence of fluid overload such as dependent leg oedema, and should be used no more than once in 24 hours.[2]

Cannabinoids

Cannabis-based medicinal extracts have been used to ameliorate overactive bladder symptoms, based upon the identification of the cannabinoid receptor in animals and human bladder preparations, and positive anecdotal reports of the effect of cannabis in controlling bladder symptoms in patients MS.[2] In a large placebo-controlled study of 647 patients with MS, an oral cannabis extract of delta-9-tetrahydrocannabinol (THC) reduced urge incontinence episodes and pad weight significantly more than placebo.[62] A multicentre double-blind, placebo-controlled trial specifically studying LUTS in patients with advanced MS used a sublingual spray containing delta-9-THC and cannabidiol (CBD) in a 1:1 ratio found a significant improvement in daytime frequency, nocturia, and the Patient's Global Impression of Change.[63] A cannabis-based medicine has been licensed for treating spasticity in MS; however, this does not cover bladder dysfunction.[2]

Botulinum toxin

The discovery by Schurch, Stohrer, and colleagues[64,65] that intradetrusor injections of botulinum neurotoxin type A (BoNT/A) resulted in a significant improvement in neurogenic detrusor overactivity and incontinence is having far-reaching consequences. Originally proposed on the basis that BoNT/A would block the presynaptic release of parasympathetic acetylcholine mediating detrusor contraction, it seems to be highly probable that BoNT/A also modulates intrinsic bladder reflexes through a multimodal effect on sensory pathways.[66] Intradetrusor injections of BoNT/

A is a minimally invasive treatment that can be performed in an outpatient setting under local anaesthesia using a flexible cystoscope.[67] Exceptional efficacy of BoNT/A treatment has been shown for patients with SCI and MS.[68,69] A small study in patients with Parkinson's disease showed that botulinum toxin was effective in ameliorating symptoms, though its use was associated with the risk of incomplete bladder emptying and need for catheterizing.[70] The effect lasts for 9 to 13 months and it significantly improves storage symptoms and quality of life,[69] despite most patients needing to perform clean intermittent self-catheterization afterwards. Preliminary studies seem to suggest that patients receiving botulinum toxin injections have fewer symptomatic urinary tract infections[71] and reduced catheter bypassing if using an indwelling catheter. NICE recommends its use in patients with spinal cord disease (spinal cord injury or MS) with symptoms of an overactive bladder and in whom antimuscarinics have proven to be ineffective or poorly tolerated.[53]

Neuromodulation

The first use of sacral neuromodulation (SNM) in the management of neurogenic voiding dysfunction was reported by Bosch and colleagues.[72] Since then, a growing body of evidence has accumulated that suggests sacral neuromodulation is effective and safe for the treatment of neurogenic LUTD,[73–75] especially in the short term. In the long term, however, the results of SNM in patients with progressive neurological conditions may be altered by the evolution of the underlying disease, and efficacy may be lost as the disease advances.[75] Furthermore, conditions such as MS may require repeat MRIs as part of their neurological follow-up and the presence of a stimulator precludes this. Thus, in patients with neurological disease, SNM is a viable option only in highly selected patients who present with a stable, indolent course of neurological disease.

The use of tibial nerve stimulation in the management of MS-related OAB symptoms appears to be promising. There is evidence to suggest that stimulation of the tibial nerve is effective in managing OAB symptoms and improved urodynamic parameters.[76] Studies have shown that percutaneous tibial nerve stimulation (PTNS)[76] and transcutaneous tibial nerve stimulation[77] are effective and safe in the management of the overactive bladder in MS.

Surgery

The role of surgery in the management of neurogenic LUTD in patients with a non-traumatic neurological condition has become limited following the advent of less invasive treatment options such as botulinum toxin. If detrusor overactivity is intractable to treatment, then urinary diversion, such as by an ileal conduit[78,79] or bladder augmentation surgery can be considered.[80] However, these are major surgical procedures and not without their own complications, and patients should receive appropriate and realistic preoperative counselling. Patients with predominant stress incontinence should first be offered the various treatment options available for that condition.

Management of voiding dysfunction

The post-void residual volume is measured either by in-out catheterization or a bladder scan. A consensus is lacking regarding the figure of residual volume at which intermittent catheterization should be initiated. However, considering that patients with a neurogenic bladder often have reduced bladder capacity, a residual volume of greater than 100 mL, or more than one-third of the bladder capacity, is generally agreed to be likely to contribute to bladder dysfunction.[51] Incomplete bladder emptying can predispose to urinary tract infections, and can also exacerbate the symptoms associated with detrusor overactivity.

The use of intermittent catheterization has greatly improved the management of the neurogenic bladder. A sterile technique was first introduced in the 1960s, however subsequently a clean technique was found to be adequate. The patient should be taught by someone experienced such as continence advisors. Neurological impairments such as hand weakness, tremor, spasticity, impaired visual acuity, or significant cognitive impairment can influence the success of self-catheterization.[2]

Suprapubic vibration through a mechanical 'buzzer' has been shown to be effective in bladder emptying in patient with MS, however its effect is limited.[81,82] There is limited evidence to show that alpha blockers improve bladder emptying,[83,84] though their use is not recommended.[53] Crede manoeuvre is usually not recommended.[51]

Permanent indwelling catheters

The use of an indwelling catheter should be limited to individuals who are unable to perform self-catheterization or in cases where incontinence is refractory to management. The immediate solution is a urethral indwelling catheter, however the long-term side-effects are well known and therefore a preferred alternative is a suprapubic catheter, though the evidence base for this is lacking.[85] Extreme care is required with their insertion, as patients often have contracted bladders and this contributes to the risk of bowel perforation during catheter placement. Specific instances of this are thought to occur each year.[86]

Urinary tract infections

The presence of asymptomatic bacteriuria alone in a patient performing intermittent self-catheterization should not be an indication for antibiotics.[51] Rather, the antibiotics are usually indicated in the presence of associated local or systemic symptoms. Antibiotic prophylaxis should not be routinely offered. In patients with recurrent urinary tract infections, the catheterization technique should be reviewed and causes such as incomplete bladder emptying or a bladder stone excluded. Antibiotic prophylaxis should be considered in patients with a recent history of frequent or severe infections.[53] The value of cranberry preparations in preventing urinary tract infections in neurological patients is debatable.

Further reading

Araki I, Kitahara M, Oida T, Kuno S. Voiding dysfunction and Parkinson's Disease: urodynamic abnormalities and urinary symptoms. *J Urol* 2000; **164**:1640–3.

de Sèze M, Ruffion A, Denys P, Joseph PA, Perrouin-Verbe B. The neurogenic bladder in multiple sclerosis: review of the literature and proposal of management guidelines. *Mult Scler* 2007; **13**:915–28.

Fowler CJ, Panicker JN, Drake M, *et al.* A UK consensus on the management of the bladder in multiple sclerosis. *J Neurol Neurosurg Psychiatry* 2009; **80**:470–7.

Jamison J, Maguire S, McCann J. Catheter policies for management of long term voiding problems in adults with neurogenic bladder disorders. *Cochrane Database Syst Rev* 2011:CD004375.

Kabay S, Kabay SC, Yucel M, *et al.* The clinical and urodynamic results of a 3-month percutaneous posterior tibial nerve stimulation treatment in patients with multiple sclerosis-related neurogenic bladder dysfunction. *Neurourol Urodyn* 2009; **28**:964–8.

Kessler TM, La Framboise D, Trelle S, *et al.* Sacral neuromodulation for neurogenic lower urinary tract dysfunction: systematic review and meta-analysis. *Eur Urol* 2010; **58**:865–74.

Madhuvrata P, Singh M, Hasafa Z, Abdel-Fattah M. Anticholinergic drugs for adult neurogenic detrusor overactivity: a systematic review and meta-analysis. *Eur Urol* 2012; **62(5)**:816–30.

NICE. Urinary incontinence in neurological disease. Clinical guideline [CG148]. London, UK: National Institute for Clinical Excellence, 2012. Available at: https://www.nice.org.uk/guidance/cg148?unlid=523578585201588322 [Online].

Panicker JN, Kalsi V, de Sèze M. Approach and evaluation of neurogenic bladder dysfunction. In: Fowler CJ, Panicker JN, Emmanuel A (eds). *Pelvic Organ Dysfunction in Neurological Disease: Clinical Management and Rehabilitation.* Cambridge, UK: Cambridge University Press, 2010.

Pannek J, Stohrer M, Blok B, *et al.* Guidelines on Neurogenic Lower Urinary Tract Dysfunction. In: European Association of Urology Guidelines, 2011. Available at: https://uroweb.org/wp-content/uploads/20_Neurogenic-LUTD_LR.pdf [Online].

Roth B, Studer UE, Fowler CJ, Kessler TM. Benign prostatic obstruction and parkinson's disease—should transurethral resection of the prostate be avoided? *J Urol* 2009; **181**:2209–13.

Sakakibara R, Kishi M, Ogawa E, *et al.* Bladder, bowel, and sexual dysfunction in Parkinson's disease. *Parkinsons Dis* 2011; **2011**:924605.

Sakakibara R, Shinotoh H, Uchiyama T, *et al.* Questionnaire-based assessment of pelvic organ dysfunction in Parkinson's disease. *Auton Neurosci* 2001; **92**:76–85.

Tadic SD, Griffiths D, Murrin A, Schaefer W, Aizenstein HJ, Resnick NM. Brain activity during bladder filling is related to white matter structural changes in older women with urinary incontinence. *Neuroimage* 2010; **51**:1294–302.

Tison F, Arne P, Sourgen C, Chrysostome V, Yeklef F. The value of external anal sphincter electromyography for the diagnsosi of multiple system atrophy. *Movement Disorders* 2000; **15**:1148–57.

References

1. Panicker JN, Kalsi V, de Sèze M. Approach and evaluation of neurogenic bladder dysfunction. In: Fowler CJ, Panicker JN, Emmanuel A (eds). *Pelvic Organ Dysfunction in Neurological Disease: Clinical Management and Rehabilitation.* Cambridge, UK: Cambridge University Press, 2010.
2. Panicker JN, Fowler CJ, DasGupta R. Neurourology. In: Daroff RB *et al.* (eds). *Bradley's Neurology in Clinical Practice*, 6th edition. Philadelphia, PA: Elsevier Saunders, 2012.
3. Andrew J, Nathan PW. Lesions on the anterior frontal lobes and disturbances of micturition and defaecation. *Brain* 1964; **87**:233–62.
4. Fowler CJ. Neurological disorders of micturition and their treatment. *Brain* 1999; **122** (Pt 7):1213–31.
5. Han KS, Heo SH, Lee SJ, Jeon SH, Yoo KH. Comparison of urodynamics between ischemic and hemorrhagic stroke patients; can we suggest the category of urinary dysfunction in patients with cerebrovascular accident according to type of stroke? *Neurourol Urodyn* 2010; **29**:387–90.
6. Wade DT, Hewer RL. Outlook after an acute stroke: urinary incontinence and loss of consciousness compared in 532 patients. *Q J Med* 1985; **56**:601–8.
7. Tadic SD, Griffiths D, Murrin A, Schaefer W, Aizenstein HJ, Resnick NM. Brain activity during bladder filling is related to white matter structural changes in older women with urinary incontinence. *Neuroimage* 2010; **51**:1294–302.
8. Ransmayr GN, Holliger S, Schletterer K, *et al.* Lower urinary tract symptoms in dementia with Lewy bodies, Parkinson disease, and Alzheimer disease. *Neurology* 2008; **70**:299–303.
9. Sakakibara R, Uchiyama T, Kanda T, Uchida Y, Kishi M, Hattori T. [Urinary dysfunction in idiopathic normal pressure hydrocephalus]. *Brain Nerve* 2008; **60**:233–9.
10. Chung JH, Lee JY, Kang DH, *et al.* Efficacy and safety of solifenacin to treat overactive bladder symptoms in patients with idiopathic normal pressure hydrocephalus: An open-label, multicenter, prospective study. *Neurourol Urodyn* 2012; **31**:1175–80.
11. Amit Batla, Jalesh N. Panicker, Lower urinary tract dysfunction in Parkinson's disease and multiple system atrophy. Universimed. Available at: http://universimed.com/node/97340 [Online].
12. Andersen JT. Disturbances of bladder and urethral function in Parkinson's disease. *Int Urol Nephrol* 1985; **17**:35–41.
13. Berger Y, Blaivas JG, DeLaRocha ER, Salinas JM. Urodynamic findings in Parkinson's disease. *J Urol* 1987; **138**:836–8.
14. Sakakibara R, Shinotoh H, Uchiyama T, *et al.* Questionnaire-based assessment of pelvic organ dysfunction in Parkinson's disease. *Auton Neurosci* 2001; **92**:76–85.
14. Araki I, Kitahara M, Oida T, Kuno S. Voiding dysfunction and Parkinson's Disease: urodynamic abnormalities and urinary symptoms. *J Urol* 2000; **164**:1640–3.
16. Campos-Sousa RN, Quagliato E, da Silva BB, de Carvalho RM Jr, Ribeiro SC, de Carvalho DF. Urinary symptoms in Parkinson's disease: prevalence and associated factors. *Arq Neuropsiquiatr* 2003; **61**:359–63.
17. Yoshimura N, Kuno S, Chancellor MB, De Groat WC, Seki S. Dopaminergic mechanisms underlying bladder hyperactivity in rats with a unilateral 6-hydroxydopamine (6-OHDA) lesion of the nigrostriatal pathway. *Br J Pharmacol* 2003; **139**:1425–32.
18. Roth B, Studer UE, Fowler CJ, Kessler TM. Benign prostatic obstruction and parkinson's disease—should transurethral resection of the prostate be avoided? *J Urol* 2009; **181**:2209–13.
19. Gomez-Esteban JC, Zarranz JJ, Lezcano E, *et al.* Sleep complaints and their relation with drug treatment in patients suffering from Parkinson's disease. *Mov Disord* 2006; **21**:983–8.
20. Cochen De Cock V, Abouda M, Leu S, *et al.* Is obstructive sleep apnea a problem in Parkinson's disease? *Sleep Med* 2010; **11**:247–52.
21. Menza M, Dobkin RD, Marin H, Bienfait K. Sleep disturbances in Parkinson's disease. *Mov Disord* 2010; **25**(Suppl 1):S117–122.
22. Uchiyama T, Sakakibara R, Hattori T, Yamanishi T. Short-term effect of a single levodopa dose on micturition disturbance in Parkinson's disease patients with the wearing-off phenomenon. *Mov Disord* 2003; **18**:573–8.
23. Seif C, Herzog J, van der Horst C, *et al.* Effect of subthalamic deep brain stimulation on the function of the urinary bladder. *Ann Neurol* 2004; **55**:118–20.
24. Winge K, Nielsen KK, Stimpel H, Lokkegaard A, Jensen SR, Werdelin L. Lower urinary tract symptoms and bladder control in advanced Parkinson's disease: effects of deep brain stimulation in the subthalamic nucleus. *Mov Disord* 2007; **22**:220–5.
25. Finazzi-Agro E, Peppe A, D'Amico A, *et al.* Effects of subthalamic nucleus stimulation on urodynamic findings in patients with Parkinson's disease. *J Urol* 2003; **169**:1388–91.
26. Herzog J, Volkmann J, Krack P, *et al.* Two-year follow-up of subthalamic deep brain stimulation in Parkinson's disease. *Mov Disord* 2003; **18**:1332–7.
27. Sakakibara R, Kishi M, Ogawa E, *et al.* Bladder, bowel, and sexual dysfunction in Parkinson's disease. *Parkinsons Dis* 2011; **2011**:924605.
28. Sakakibara R, Uchiyama T, Yamanishi T, Kishi M. Genitourinary dysfunction in Parkinson's disease. *Mov Disord* 2010; **25**:2–12.
29. Sakakibara R, Uchiyama T, Yoshiyama M, Hattori T. [Disturbance of micturition in Parkinson's disease]. *No To Shinkei* 2001; **53**:1009–14.

30. Sammour ZM, Gomes CM, Barbosa ER, *et al.* Voiding dysfunction in patients with Parkinson's disease: impact of neurological impairment and clinical parameters. *Neurourol Urodyn* 2009; **28**:510–15.
31. Yamamoto T, Sakakibara R, Uchiyama T, *et al.* Questionnaire-based assessment of pelvic organ dysfunction in multiple system atrophy. *Mov Disord* 2009; **24**:972–8.
32. Hahn K, Ebersbach G. Sonographic assessment of urinary retention in multiple system atrophy and idiopathic Parkinson's disease. *Mov Disord* 2005; **20**:1499–1502.
33. Ito T, Sakakibara R, Yasuda K, *et al.* Incomplete emptying and urinary retention in multiple-system atrophy: when does it occur and how do we manage it? *Mov Disord* 2006; **21**:816–23.
34. Sakakibara R, Hattori T, Uchiyama T, Yamanishi T. Videourodynamic and sphincter motor unit potential analyses in Parkinson's disease and multiple system atrophy. *J Neurol Neurosurg Psychiatry* 2001; **71**:600–6.
35. Palace J, Chandiramani VA, Fowler CJ. Value of sphincter electromyography in the diagnosis of multiple system atrophy. *Muscle Nerve* 1997; **20**:1396–403.
36. Tison F, Arne P, Sourgen C, Chrysostome V, Yeklef F. The value of external anal sphincter electromyography for the diagnsosi of multiple system atrophy. *Movement Disorders* 2000; **15**:1148–1157.
37. Kirby R, Fowler C, Gosling J, Bannister R. Urethro-vesical dysfunction in progressive autonomic failure with multiple system atrophy. *J Neurol Neurosurg Psychiatry* 1986; **49**:554–62.
38. Marrie RA, Cutter G, Tyry T, *et al.* Disparities in the management of multiple sclerosis-related bladder symptoms. *Neurology* 2007; **68**:1971–8.
39. Blanc F, Froelich S, Vuillemet F, *et al.* [Acute myelitis and Lyme disease]. *Rev Neurol (Paris)* 2007; **163**:1039–47.
40. Hemmett L, Holmes J, Barnes M, *et al.* What drives quality of life in multiple sclerosis? *QJM* 2004; **97**:671–6.
41. Betts CD, D'Mellow MT, Fowler CJ. Urinary symptoms and the neurological features of bladder dysfunction in multiple sclerosis. *J Neurol Neurosurg Psychiatry* 1993; **56**:245–50.
42. de Sèze M, Ruffion A, Denys P, Joseph PA, Perrouin-Verbe B. The neurogenic bladder in multiple sclerosis: review of the literature and proposal of management guidelines. *Mult Scler* 2007; **13**:915–28.
43. Araki I, Matsui M, Ozawa K, Takeda M, Kuno S. Relationship of bladder dysfunction to lesion site in multiple sclerosis. *J Urol* 2003; **169**:1384–7.
44. Grasso MG, Pozzilli C, Anzini A, Salvetti M, Bastianello S, Fieschi C. Relationship between bladder dysfunction and brain MRI in multiple sclerosis. *Funct Neurol* 1991; **6**:289–92.
45. Pozzilli C, Grasso MG, Bastianello S, *et al.* Structural brain correlates of neurologic abnormalities in multiple sclerosis. *Eur Neurol* 1992; **32**:228–30.
46. Ukkonen M, Elovaara I, Dastidar P, Tammela TL. Urodynamic findings in primary progressive multiple sclerosis are associated with increased volumes of plaques and atrophy in the central nervous system. *Acta Neurol Scand* 2004; **109**:100–5.
47. Lawrenson R, Wyndaele JJ, Vlachonikolis I, Farmer C, Glickman S. Renal failure in patients with neurogenic lower urinary tract dysfunction. *Neuroepidemiology* 2001; **20**:138–43.
48. Panicker JN, Nagaraja D, Kovoor JM, Nair KP, Subbakrishna DK. Lower urinary tract dysfunction in acute disseminated encephalomyelitis. *Mult Scler* 2009; **15**:1118–122.
49. Sakakibara R, Hattori T, Yasuda K, Yamanishi T. Micturitional disturbance in acute disseminated encephalomyelitis (ADEM). *J Auton Nerv Syst* 1996; **60**:200–5.
50. Buljevac D, Flach HZ, Hop WC, *et al.* Prospective study on the relationship between infections and multiple sclerosis exacerbations. *Brain* 2002; **125**:952–60.
51. Fowler CJ, Panicker JN, Drake M, *et al.* A UK consensus on the management of the bladder in multiple sclerosis. *J Neurol Neurosurg Psychiatry* 2009; **80**:470–7.
52. Rakusa M, Murphy O, McIntyre L, *et al.* Testing for urinary tract colonisation before high-dose corticosteroid treatment in acute multiple sclerosis relapses: prospective algorithm validation. *Eur J Neurol* 2013; **20**(3):448–52.
53. NICE. Urinary incontinence in neurological disease. Clinical guideline [CG148]. London, UK: National Institute for Clinical Excellence, 2012. Available at: https://www.nice.org.uk/guidance/cg148?unlid=523578585201588322 [Online].
54. Fowlis GA, Waters J, Williams G. The cost effectiveness of combined rapid tests (Multistix) in screening for urinary tract infections. *J R Soc Med* 1994; **87**:681–2.
55. Pannek J, Stohrer M, Blok B, *et al.* Guidelines on Neurogenic Lower Urinary Tract Dysfunction. In: European Association of Urology Guidelines, 2011. Available at: https://uroweb.org/wp-content/uploads/20_Neurogenic-LUTD_LR.pdf [Online].
56. Hashim H, Abrams P. How should patients with an overactive bladder manipulate their fluid intake? *BJU Int* 2008; **102**(1):62–6.
57. McClurg D, Ashe RG, Marshall K, Lowe-Strong AS. Comparison of pelvic floor muscle training, electromyography biofeedback, and neuromuscular electrical stimulation for bladder dysfunction in people with multiple sclerosis: a randomized pilot study. *Neurourol Urodyn* 2006; **25**:337–48.
58. Vahtera T, Haaranen M, Viramo-Koskela AL, Ruutiainen J. Pelvic floor rehabilitation is effective in patients with multiple sclerosis. *Clin Rehabil* 1997; **11**:211–19.
59. van Rey F, Heesakkers J. Solifenacin in multiple sclerosis patients with overactive bladder: a prospective study. *Adv Urol* 2011; **2011**:834753.
60. Madhuvrata P, Singh M, Hasafa Z, Abdel-Fattah M. Anticholinergic drugs for adult neurogenic detrusor overactivity: a systematic review and meta-analysis. *Eur Urol* 2012; **62**(5):816–30.
61. Bosma R, Wynia K, Havlikova E, De Keyser J, Middel B. Efficacy of desmopressin in patients with multiple sclerosis suffering from bladder dysfunction: a meta-analysis. *Acta Neurol Scand* 2005; **112**:1–5.
62. Freeman RM, Adekanmi O, Waterfield MR, Waterfield AE, Wright D, Zajicek J. The effect of cannabis on urge incontinence in patients with multiple sclerosis: a multicentre, randomised placebo-controlled trial (CAMS-LUTS). *Int Urogynecol J Pelvic Floor Dysfunct* 2006; **17**:636–41.
63. Kavia RB, De Ridder D, Constantinescu CS, Stott CG, Fowler CJ. Randomized controlled trial of Sativex to treat detrusor overactivity in multiple sclerosis. *Mult Scler* 2010; **16**:1349–59.
64. Schurch B, Stohrer M, Kramer G, Schmid DM, Gaul G, Hauri D. Botulinum-A toxin for treating detrusor hyperreflexia in spinal cord injured patients: a new alternative to anticholinergic drugs? Preliminary results. *J Urol* 2000; **164**:692–7.
65. Schurch B, Schmid DM, Stohrer M. Treatment of neurogenic incontinence with botulinum toxin A. *N Engl J Med* 2000; **342**:665.
66. Apostolidis A, Dasgupta P, Fowler CJ. Proposed mechanism for the efficacy of injected botulinum toxin in the treatment of human detrusor overactivity. *Eur Urol* 2006; **49**:644–50.
67. Harper M, Popat RB, Dasgupta R, Fowler CJ, Dasgupta P. A minimally invasive technique for outpatient local anaesthetic administration of intradetrusor botulinum toxin in intractable detrusor overactivity. *BJU Int* 2003; **92**:325–6.
68. Cruz F, Herschorn S, Aliotta P, *et al.* Efficacy and safety of onabotulinumtoxinA in patients with urinary incontinence due to neurogenic detrusor overactivity: a randomised, double-blind, placebo-controlled trial. *Eur Urol* 2011; **60**:742–50.
69. Kalsi V, Gonzales G, Popat R, *et al.* Botulinum injections for the treatment of bladder symptoms of multiple sclerosis. *Ann Neurol* 2007; **62**:452–57.
70. Giannantoni A, Rossi A, Mearini E, Del Zingaro M, Porena M, Berardelli A. Botulinum toxin A for overactive bladder and detrusor muscle overactivity in patients with Parkinson's disease and multiple system atrophy. *J Urol* 2009; **182**:1453–7.
71. Game X, Castel-Lacanal E, Bentaleb Y, *et al.* Botulinum toxin A detrusor injections in patients with neurogenic detrusor overactivity significantly decrease the incidence of symptomatic urinary tract infections. *Eur Urol* 2008; **53**:613–18.
72. Bosch JL, Groen J. Treatment of refractory urge urinary incontinence with sacral spinal nerve stimulation in multiple sclerosis patients. *Lancet* 1996; **348**:717–19.

73. Lombardi G, Del Popolo G. Clinical outcome of sacral neuromodulation in incomplete spinal cord injured patients suffering from neurogenic lower urinary tract symptoms. *Spinal Cord* 2009; **47**:486–91.
74. Wallace PA, Lane FL, Noblett KL. Sacral nerve neuromodulation in patients with underlying neurologic disease. *Am J Obstet Gynecol* 2007; **197**(96):e91–5.
75. Kessler TM, La Framboise D, Trelle S, *et al.* Sacral neuromodulation for neurogenic lower urinary tract dysfunction: systematic review and meta-analysis. *Eur Urol* 2010; **58**:865–74.
76. Kabay S, Kabay SC, Yucel M, *et al.* The clinical and urodynamic results of a 3-month percutaneous posterior tibial nerve stimulation treatment in patients with multiple sclerosis-related neurogenic bladder dysfunction. *Neurourol Urodyn* 2009; **28**:964–968.
77. de Sèze M, Raibaut P, Gallien P, *et al.* Transcutaneous posterior tibial nerve stimulation for treatment of the overactive bladder syndrome in multiple sclerosis: results of a multicenter prospective study. *Neurourol Urodyn* 2011; **30**:306–11.
78. Guillotreau J, Panicker JN, Castel-Lacanal E, *et al.* Prospective evaluation of laparoscopic assisted cystectomy and ileal conduit in advanced multiple sclerosis. *Urology* 2012; **80**:852–7.
79. Legrand G, Roupret M, Comperat E, Even-Schneider A, Denys P, Chartier-Kastler E. Functional outcomes after management of end-stage neurological bladder dysfunction with ileal conduit in a multiple sclerosis population: a monocentric experience. *Urology* 2011; **78**:937–41.
80. Zachoval R, Pitha J, Medova E, *et al.* Augmentation cystoplasty in patients with multiple sclerosis. *Urol Int* 2003; **70**:21–26; discussion 26.
81. Prasad RS, Smith SJ, Wright H. Lower abdominal pressure versus external bladder stimulation to aid bladder emptying in multiple sclerosis: a randomized controlled study. *Clin Rehabil* 2003; **17**:42–7.
82. Dasgupta P, Haslam C, Goodwin R, Fowler CJ. The 'Queen Square bladder stimulator': a device for assisting emptying of the neurogenic bladder. *Br J Urol* 1997; **80**:234–7.
83. O'Riordan JI, Doherty C, Javed M, Brophy D, Hutchinson M, Quinlan D. Do alpha-blockers have a role in lower urinary tract dysfunction in multiple sclerosis? *J Urol* 1995; **153**:1114–16.
84. Panicker JN, Fowler CJ. The bare essentials: uro-neurology. *Pract Neurol* 2010; **10**(3):178–85.
85. Jamison J, Maguire S, McCann J. Catheter policies for management of long term voiding problems in adults with neurogenic bladder disorders. *Cochrane Database Syst Rev* 2011:CD004375.
86. Minimising risks of suprapubic catheter insertion (adults only): National Patient Safety Agency, 2009. Available at: http://www.nrls.npsa.nhs.uk/resources/?EntryId45=61917 [Online].

SECTION 4

Reconstruction

Section editors: Anthony R. Mundy

CHAPTER 4.1

Principles of reconstructive urology

Anthony R. Mundy and Daniela E. Andrich

Introduction to principles of reconstructive urology

From a urological perspective, the fundamental properties of the urinary tract are that it is capable of holding urine for a sufficient duration to allow its owner to empty it voluntarily at a time and place of his or her choosing, with unobstructed flow from the distal convoluted tubules of the kidney through the external meatus to the outside world. Under normal circumstances this urinary tract 'system' is internal, its control is natural and spontaneous, and its lining is impermeable; the need to empty it is only occasional and there is no need for any extraneous 'kit'. In disease, if all else fails or is inappropriate, an ileal conduit urinary diversion into an external collecting appliance satisfies most of these criteria. Indeed, for many years following its introduction by Bricker in the 1950s,[1] the ileal conduit was highly regarded as an alternative to ureterosigmoidostomy, which was the only form of salvage surgery then available for the absent or hopelessly incontinent urinary tract in the earlier part of the twentieth century. During the 1960s and 1970s, a large number of patients were treated by ileal conduit urinary diversion, principally those having a cystectomy for bladder cancer in adult life, or for those with unexplained upper urinary tract problems as a consequence of congenital anomalies of the lower urinary tract in childhood. These included problems that are still difficult to treat nowadays such as neuropathic bladder dysfunction, and major congenital structural abnormalities such as exstrophy/epispadias; and, more importantly, conditions that were poorly understood at the time such as severe vesicoureteric reflux and posterior urethral valves, which are now treated quite differently because their nature is now understood to a much greater degree.

As a consequence of this greater understanding and the general improvements in medical and surgical care in the 1980s and 1990s which made for safe major surgery for benign conditions, the pendulum swung the other way and a large number of patients with ileal conduit urinary diversions were undiverted and reconstructed, largely under the influence of Hendren in the United States. He (and others) developed and refined surgical techniques to reconstruct the ureters and reimplant them into the bladder and to restore a more normal appearance to the urinary tract.[2] Likewise, patients undergoing cystectomy for bladder cancer were being offered a bladder substitution rather than an ileal conduit urinary diversion, largely under the influence of Camey in France. Camey, although not the first to consider a substitution cystoplasty using bowel, was the first to use it as a matter of routine for replacing the bladder after a cystectomy for bladder cancer.[3]

The two critical developments that allowed the development of reconstructive urological surgery in particular were the introduction of clean intermittent self-catheterization (CISC) to provide emptying of the bladder[4]; and the development of an effective artificial urinary sphincter (AUS) to produce continence.[5] Until these two became available the only way of producing both continence and adequate emptying was by a 'controlled obstruction' of the bladder outlet—sufficient to give continence most of the time but allowing bladder emptying by straining and expression when required. This was very hit and miss; was rarely achieved; and, when it was, it was more by good luck than by good management and very rarely sustained in the long term. Although not every patient who undergoes a reconstructive procedure these days will require CISC or an AUS, the mere fact that they are available means that many patients can be offered reconstructive surgery in the knowledge that they are there as a reserve should they be necessary.

These comments apply to reconstructing the urinary tract as a whole. More commonly, reconstruction is required for localized areas of the urinary tract—typically to correct the obstructed ureter or urethra due to trauma or stricture. Urethral strictures and trauma have a very long history going back thousands of years, and urethral dilatation in particular has been used uninterruptedly at least since the age of the Pharaohs.[6] Ureteric strictures and trauma are a much more recent entity because they were undetectable until the development of imaging; most trauma, sufficient to damage the ureter, would probably have been fatal in the days before surgical trauma and gynaecological surgical trauma became causes of such problems. It is only in the last 100 years that surgeons have developed urethroplasty techniques for urethral strictures and trauma—and only in the last 40 years that have they been used with any frequency; similarly, on a smaller scale, for ureteric surgery. Those techniques that had been developed were based on the empirical use of local tissue flaps such as the Thiersch-Duplay procedure for hypospadias (Fig. 4.1.1),[7] or based on the principle of the 'buried strip' technique in which a buried epithelial strip is allowed to develop into a tube around a catheter (Fig. 4.1.2),[8] in just the same way that an accidentally buried fragment of epithelium develops into a dermoid cyst.

Modern concepts of urethral and ureteric surgery are based on an understanding of the vascularization of tissue and the way in which it can be moved around safely and effectively rather than empirically;

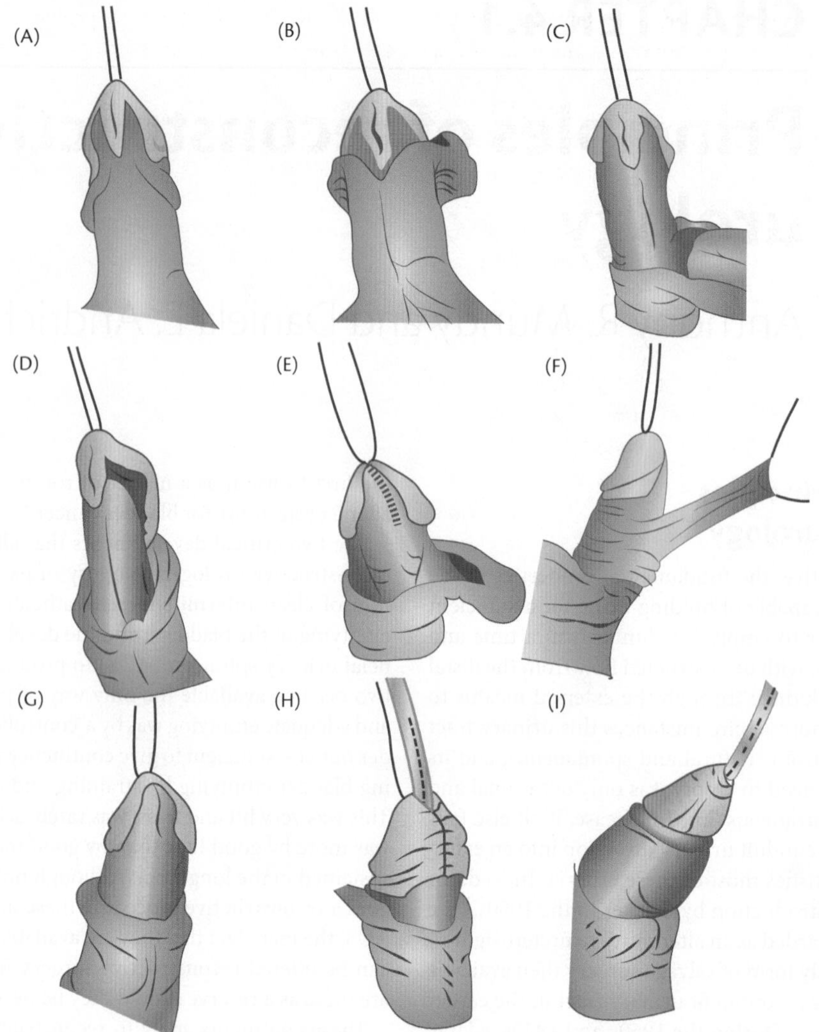

Fig. 4.1.1 The Thiersch-Duplay approach—rolling up the penile shaft skin to form a tube, followed by wide mobilization of the skin on either side to allow it to be closed over the neourethra. (A) The dotted line indicates the incision around the meatus and then, more proximally, as a circumcision to de-glove the penis in (B) and (C). (D) Glans 'wings' are undermined to allow them to be wrapped around the glanular urethra when the para-meatal skin has been sutured to create that glanular urethra. (E) The para-meatal skin has been sutured to create a glanular urethra. (F) The dartos has been separated from the inner aspect of the skin. (G) The dartos layer has been sutured over the neourethra. (H) The glans 'wings' have been sutured together over the dartos layer. (I) The circumcision has been closed.

Reprinted from *The Journal of Urology*, Volume 162, Issue 3, Ross M. Decter *et al.*, 'Distal Hypospadias Repair by the Modified Thiersch-Duplay Technique with or without Hinging the Urethral Plate: A Near Ideal Way to Correct Distal Hypospadias', pp. 1156–1158, Copyright © 1999, with permission from Elsevier, http://www.sciencedirect.com/science/journal/00225347

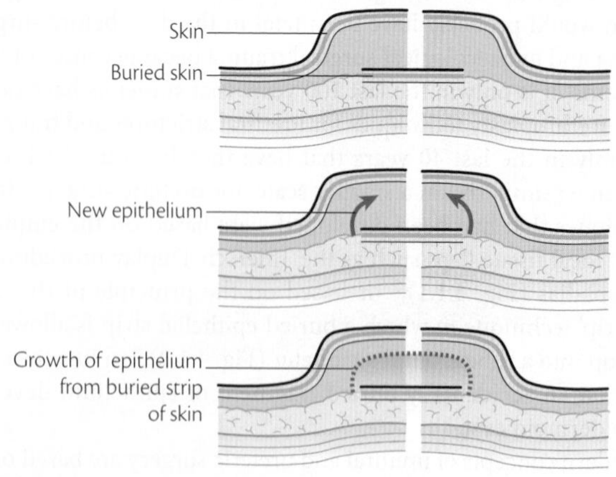

Fig. 4.1.2 The 'buried skin strip' principle.

and an understanding of the use of grafts and flaps as a means of tissue transfer for repair. Using these various methods, we can achieve direct closure of a urethral or ureteric defect with rapid and accurate restoration of calibre as distinct from the slow erratic process associated with the development of a tube from a buried strip of epithelium.

The nature of reconstructive problems in clinical practice

The main causes of problems with which reconstructive urology is associated are congenital and traumatic. Congenital causes include hypospadias, exstrophy, epispadias, and the other major structural birth defects, of which hypospadias is much the most common. Trauma may be iatrogenic or non-iatrogenic ('external'), in which case it might be closed or penetrating. Iatrogenic trauma is much the most common.

The site of the reconstructive problems might be the kidney, ureter, bladder, or urethra in either sex; the prostate in men or the vagina in women. It may involve other organ systems such as the rectum in both sexes; or it may involve more than one other organ system such as, for example, when there has been irradiation damage to the whole pelvis as in the treatment of carcinoma of the cervix, leaving the patient with a vesicovaginorectal fistula.

Thus, in theory, problems such as pelviureteric junction obstruction and its treatment by pyeloplasty may be regarded as reconstructive. In practice this is not generally considered to be the case. For the specific purposes of this textbook, hypospadias surgery will be considered in the section on paediatric urology and gynaecological fistulae will be considered in the section on female urology, although these are certainly reconstructive problems. In the next few chapters we will consider reconstructive problems of the ureter, bladder, and male urethra with particular reference to ureteric trauma, functional problems of the bladder, and urethral strictures and trauma.

General principles of reconstructive urology: grafts and flaps

The general principles of reconstructing the ureter or urethra are similar. One either finds a way of bridging a gap between the two ends of healthy ureter or urethra on either side of the area of pathology, or finds a way of replacing the affected segment in its entirety or, alternatively, of augmenting its calibre if part of the circumference is healthy enough for it to be worth preserving and building upon.

The principles of urethral reconstruction, given that strictures and trauma are most common in the bulbar urethra, are that a defect after trauma or excision of a stricture, up to a certain critical length, may be bridged by virtue of the elasticity (or, to be more accurate, the 'stretchability') of the bulbar urethra and the ability to straighten out its naturally curved course; or otherwise that the calibre of a strictured segment can be augmented to restore a normal calibre with a patch of extraneous epithelialized tissue, which may be in the form of either a graft or a flap. Alternatively, particularly in the penile urethra where the principles of elasticity/stretchability do not apply, the urethral circumference may be replaced in its entirety, when augmentation with a patch is not possible, by a substitution procedure in one or more stages.[9]

In the ureter, there is little elasticity/stretchability because there is no equivalent of the corpus spongiosum but, nonetheless, there is some scope for bridging a gap by extensive mobilization of the ureter on either side of a defect. Otherwise the ureter, along with its blood supply, is mobilized to be reimplanted into a similarly mobilized bladder to bridge a gap. The bladder may be mobilized as a whole, as with the psoas-hitch procedure, or in part, as with a Boari flap procedure. Alternatively, the ureter may be transposed across the posterior abdominal wall for anastomosis to the other ureter in transureteroureterostomy.[10]

Because the ureter is of small calibre it is much less amenable than the urethra to augmentation if it is structured, and its relative inaccessibility makes a staged substitution repair impossible. Thus, when the 'bridging' techniques referred to in the last paragraph are either impossible or inappropriate, the only alternative is interposition of a segment of bowel. In theory, this could be between any two ends of the ureter but in practice, because of the marked disparity of size between the ureter and the bowel, it is best done by constructing an 'ileal ureter' from the renal pelvis to the bladder. In theory, transplantation of the kidney into the pelvis to allow direct anastomosis of the renal pelvis to the bladder is another way of bridging a long ureteric defect—but for a variety of practical reasons, this is often not possible.

With the bladder, the only problems that arise are the need to augment the physically small or functionally abnormal bladder, typically for neuropathy, or otherwise to replace it as after cystectomy for bladder cancer, and to ensure as near normal drainage of the ureters as possible—always without obstruction and preferably (but not necessarily) without vesicoureteric reflux. The general principle of bladder surgery is to produce a structure which is of good volume and low pressure, accepting that CISC may be necessary to empty, although often hoping that the individual will be able to empty adequately, if not completely, by straining.[10]

Grafts

A graft is a piece of tissue which is raised from its normal location—the donor site—and transferred to a new location—the recipient site—where it is expected to pick up a new blood supply from the local circulation. The most commonly used tissues for grafting in urology are skin and oral mucosa although others, such as bladder mucosa and dermis have been used, and are still used occasionally in certain circumstances. A skin graft may be either full thickness or partial thickness. An oral mucosa graft is a full-thickness graft.

Whether or not a graft 'takes' in its new location ultimately depends upon it establishing a blood supply, and this is achieved by forming direct connections between exposed blood vessels on the surface of the recipient site and the under surface of the graft itself. In a split-thickness skin graft (STSG) this is the intradermal plexus; in a full-thickness skin graft (FTSG) it is the subdermal plexus (Fig. 4.1.3). The intradermal plexus is almost always denser than the subdermal plexus, which makes a STSG more likely to 'take' than a FTSG, particularly as a STSG is substantially thinner and there is therefore a much smaller volume of grafted tissue to be kept alive and revascularized.[11,12]

Given that the dermis at the donor site is retained, a large amount of STSG can be taken and the donor defect will still regenerate. The disadvantage of a FTSG is not only that the subdermal plexus is less dense than the intradermal plexus and the volume of the graft substantially greater than a STSG, and therefore that the graft 'take' is more hazardous, but also that there is a limit to the amount of skin that can be harvested as the donor site should be closed primarily or grafted itself.

On the other hand, a STSG, while it has better 'take' and is less demanding for the donor site, is poor in dermal collagen and consequently the graft itself tends to contract and become unsightly. Whereas a FTSG, although it 'takes' less well and is more demanding on the donor site, is rich in dermal collagen and so there is little or no contraction of the graft. This is because dermal collagen inhibits the myofibroblasts at the recipient site which cause fibrosis and graft contracture. The absence of contraction makes FTSGs much more useful than STSGs in reconstructive urology except to provide genital skin cover after trauma or surgery.[11,12]

Mucosal grafts behave like FTSG, but have the advantage that instead of separate intradermal and subdermal plexuses there is a single pandermal plexus throughout the dermal layer, which is dense and therefore gives the advantage over a FTSG of 'taking' more readily (Fig. 4.1.4). Oral mucosal grafts have therefore largely superseded FTSG in reconstructive urology and specifically for use in stricture surgery.[13]

Oral mucosa can be divided into buccal mucosa from the inside of the cheek, labial mucosa from the inside of the lower lip, and lingual mucosa from the underside of the tongue. Buccal mucosa is more plentiful but labial and lingual mucosa are thinner and this may be an advantage in certain situations such as in grafting the inside of the fossa navicularis in a patient with a small glans. None of the donor sites need to be closed primarily; although some

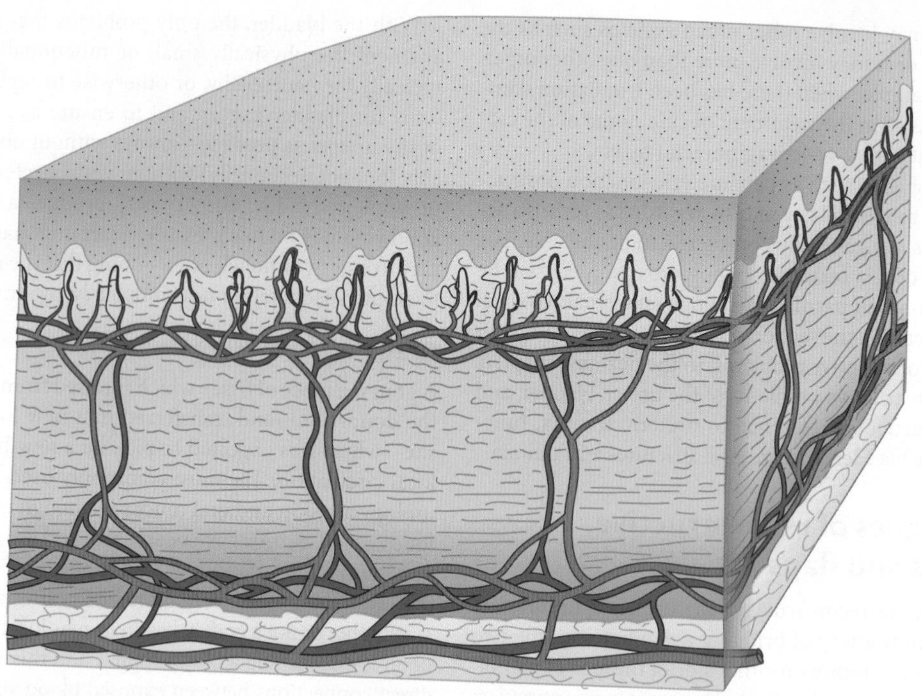

Fig. 4.1.3 Diagrammatic cross section of skin to show the intradermal and subdermal vascular plexuses.
Reproduced from Mundy AR and Andrich DE, 'Urethral Strictures', *BJU International*, Volume 107, pp. 6–27, Copyright © 2011 BJU International, with permission from John Wiley and Sons Ltd.

surgeons prefer to do so, they can be left to heal by second intention. In fact, a labial donor site should never be closed because of the deformity it would cause. Evidence suggests that closure of the donor site of a buccal mucosal graft is not only unnecessary, but may actually cause more swelling and discomfort than leaving it to heal by second intention.[14] A lingual donor site is routinely closed.

A graft 'takes' at the recipient site by two initially simultaneous processes: imbibition and inosculation.[11,12] Imbibition is the process by which oxygen and nutrients are absorbed by osmosis from the fibrin layer between a graft and the recipient bed. In this way, a graft can survive for about 48 hours. Inosculation is the process of neovascularization, which causes a physical linkage between the microvasculature of the recipient bed and the microvasculature on the under surface of the graft. This starts during the phase of imbibition and takes a further 48 hours or so to develop to a degree that the graft will survive thereafter. Providing the graft is kept still

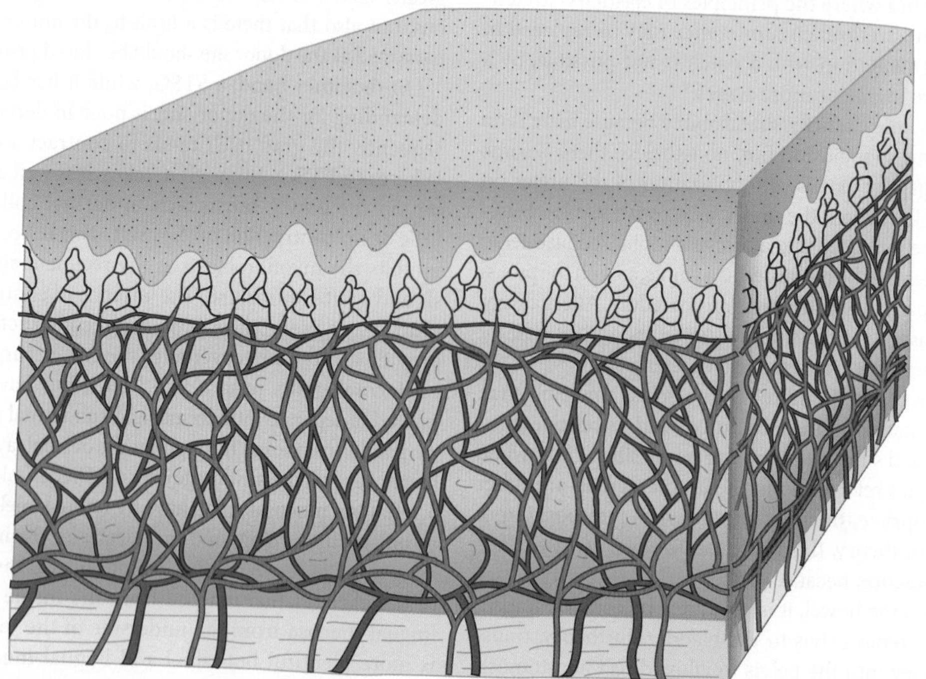

Fig. 4.1.4 Diagrammatic cross section of buccal mucosa to show the pandermal plexus.
Reproduced from Mundy AR and Andrich DE, 'Urethral Strictures', *BJU International*, Volume 107, pp. 6–27, Copyright © 2011 BJU International, with permission from John Wiley and Sons Ltd.

and there is no haematoma between the graft and its bed so that this process can physically happen; and if there is no infection by haemolytic streptococci or similar organisms that can destroy a graft, then a graft will 'take' in four days or so. At this stage the graft tends to be rather swollen and unhappy-looking because the blood supply is tenuous and there is no lymphatic drainage. Over the course of the next few months the process of neovascularization of the graft from the recipient bed, including development of the lymphatic circulation, will progress to completion, which will allow the grafted tissue to return to a normal appearance.

When harvesting a graft, it is important to remember that there is a degree of elastic contraction as soon as the graft is harvested. Thus, the harvested graft will instantly be 10–30% smaller than it was *in situ*. This is as distinct from contracture once graft 'take' has completed. Elastic contraction of 10–30% should be anticipated in the planning process by harvesting a graft that is apparently larger than is needed for its intended purpose. Then afterwards, FTSG contract hardly at all. Oral mucosal grafts contract a little on exposure to the atmosphere. STSGs contract considerably.

Flaps

Flaps are commonly classified according to either their method of elevation or by their method of vascularization.[11,12] The three main types of flap by elevation are: peninsula flaps where there is a full-thickness connection with the surrounding tissue; an island flap where the skin itself is disconnected but the underlying fascia or muscle layer provides vascularization according to the area where the flap is raised; or a free flap in which the blood supply is disconnected and re-established by vascular anastomosis at the recipient site (Fig. 4.1.5). In all types of surgery, a peninsular flap is the most widely used, as is a Z-plasty for revising an untidy scar. An island flap is widely used in urethroplasty or cystoplasty when a skin flap

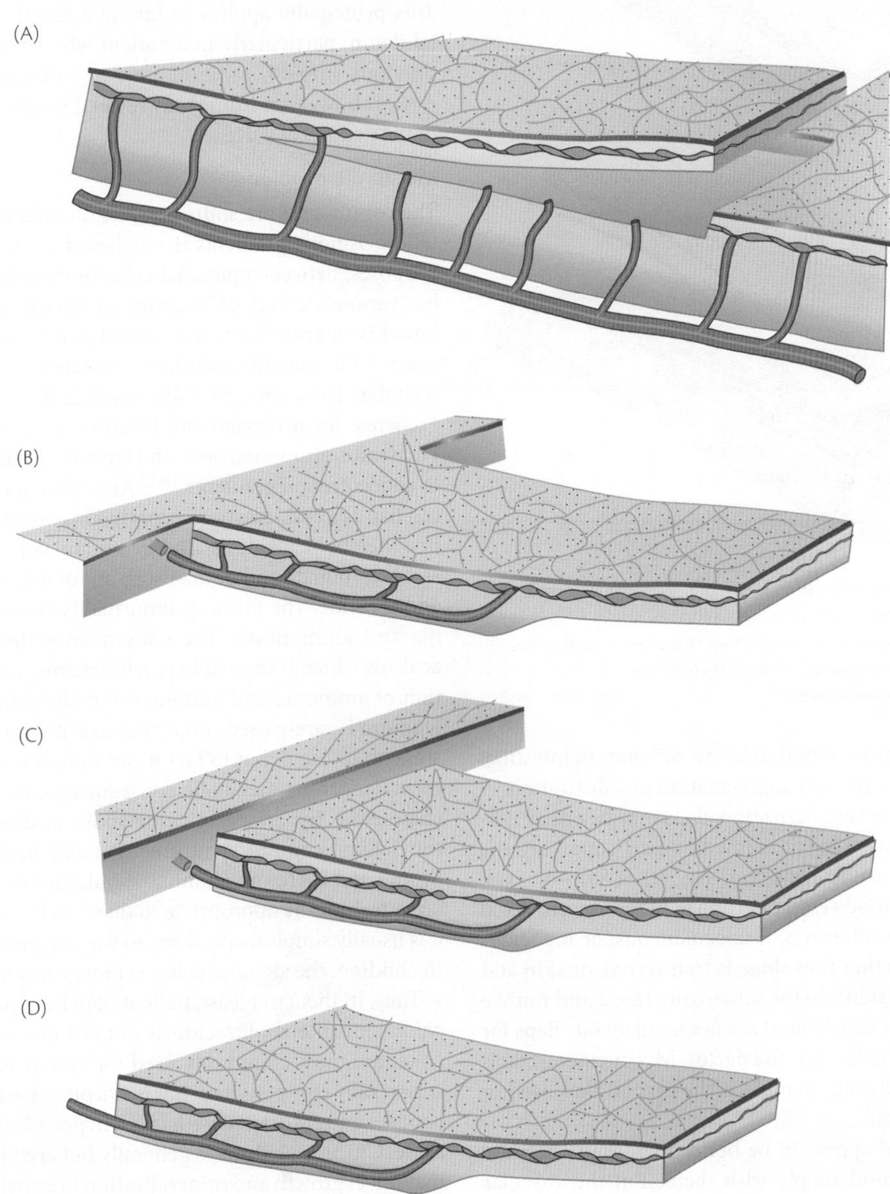

Fig. 4.1.5 Types of flap according to their method of elevation: (A) and (B) peninsula flaps; (C) an island flap; and (D) a free flap.
'Plastic Surgery for the Urologist: Tissue Transfer, Wound Healing, and Tissue Handling' was published in *AUA Update Series*, 2002, Volume 21, Jordan GH, pp 98–103, Copyright © American Urological Association Inc.

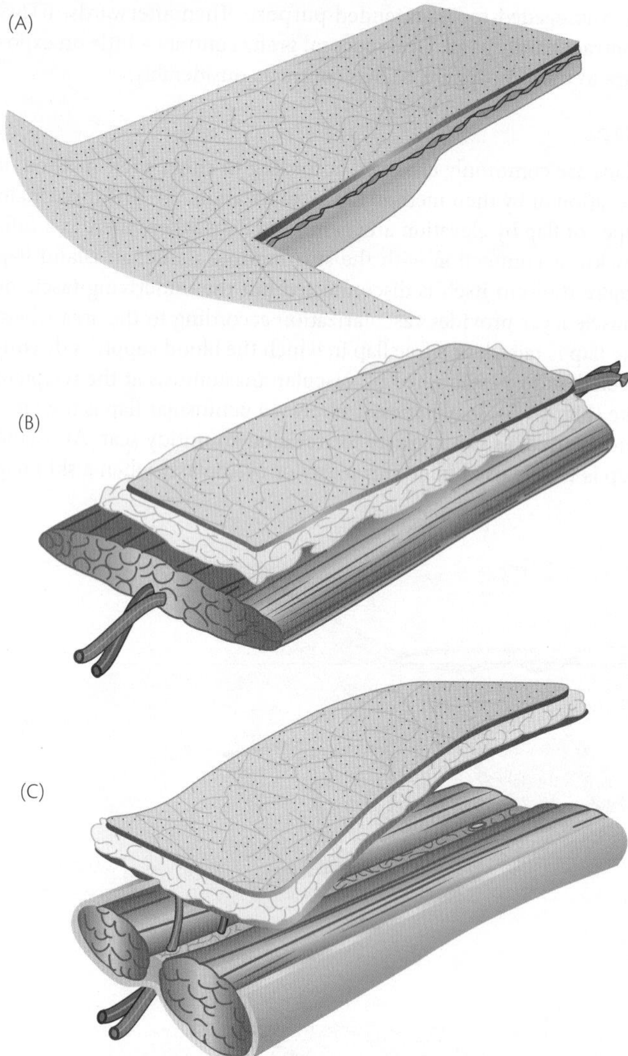

Fig. 4.1.6 Types of axial flap according to their vascularity: (A) cutaneous flap; (B) musculocutaneous flap; and (C) fasciocutaneous flap.

'Plastic Surgery for the Urologist: Tissue Transfer, Wound Healing, and Tissue Handling' was published in *AUA Update Series*, 2002, Volume 21, Jordan GH, pp. 98–103, Copyright © American Urological Association Inc.

is transferred for repair of a urethral stricture, or when an intestinal segment is transferred for bladder augmentation or substitution.

When classified by their vascularization, flaps may be either random when there is no specific (or 'named') vessel supplying the tissue—as in most peninsular flaps (e.g. Fig. 4.1.5(A))—or axial when there is a specific blood vessel or group of blood vessels. Axial flaps (Fig. 4.1.6) may be cutaneous, fasciocutaneous, or myocutaneous depending on whether skin alone is transferred, or skin and the underlying fascia, or skin and the underlying fascia and muscle are transferred. The most widely used are fasciocutaneous flaps for urethroplasty in which the fascia is the dartos. Myocutaneous flaps are only used occasionally: an example is the gracilis flap used in some types of fistula repair.

Intuitively, flaps would appear to be better than grafts because they carry their own blood supply with them. But the vascular pedicle that carries the blood supply is fragile and vulnerable and the range of usefulness of the flap is limited by the axis of rotation of the vascular pedicle—except, of course, for free flaps. Grafts therefore have a wider range of usefulness but are limited in their use when the recipient bed is ischaemic as, for example, after previous surgery or radiotherapy. In such circumstances, flaps are generally more reliable. Both grafts and flaps may be adversely affected by microvascular disease as in diabetics or smokers.

Intestinal flaps in urology

Although we tend to think of flaps as being composed primarily of skin, fascia or muscle, intestinal flaps used for cystoplasty and for ileal conduit urinary diversion are also 'flaps' and, outside of urethroplasty, are probably the most widely used flaps in urology. As a consequence of incorporating intestinal flaps into the urinary tract, there are five main potential problems to be considered—the consequences of removing the gut from its natural site, metabolic problems, infection, stones, and malignant transformation.[12]

Consequences of removing the gut from its natural site

This principally applies to taking a length of the absorptive distal ileum, particularly in a patient who has been compromised by previous surgery, radiotherapy, or inflammatory bowel disease. A short bowel syndrome may result. Diarrhoea may also follow loss of the ileocaecal valve.

Metabolic problems

The commonest are shifts of water and electrolytes. Water tends to follow osmotic gradients through and, particularly for our present purposes, between epithelial cells. In this latter respect, epithelium has various degrees of 'leakiness'. Stomach is the most leaky, small bowel is intermediate, and colon tends to absorb rather than leak water.[15] On the other hand, most electrolyte shifts are mainly transcellular. These are generally coupled: thus, sodium is excreted in exchange for hydrogen and bicarbonate in exchange for chloride. Potassium, ammonia, urea, and creatinine move passively according to concentration gradients.[16,17] As a consequence, the use of a stomach flap as a cystoplasty or a conduit may tend to cause hypochloraemic metabolic alkalosis. The ileum and colon both secrete sodium and bicarbonate and both absorb ammonia, ammonium, hydrogen, and chloride. The primary abnormality is the absorption of ammonia and ammonium. The consequence therefore is a metabolic acidosis which is termed hyperchloraemic, even though the absorption of ammonia and ammonium is the primary abnormality.[18,19] Jejunum is rarely used simply because it does not usually occur to a surgeon to use it, but in fact it can cause the most complicated and most dangerous metabolic consequences: a hyponatraemic, hyperchloraemic, hyperkalaemic, metabolic acidosis.[12] This is known as the 'jejunal conduit syndrome'. Patients have died from this syndrome and therefore jejunum should not be used even if it might seem technically appropriate to do so. When ileum cannot be used, it is usually simplest and safest to use a segment of transverse colon. In children, the sigmoid colon is more commonly used.

Thus, in theory at least, patients can be expected to have a hyperchloraemic metabolic acidosis in most instances, because ileum or colon are most commonly used for cystoplasties or conduits. This is generally compensated, but is uncompensated in about a third of patients and associated with frank hyperchloraemia in about half of these. Chronic acidosis is generally buffered in bone and in theory may affect growth and mineralization in growing children, although how far it actually does so is debatable.[18,20] Hypocalcaemia, hyperkalaemia, hypomagnesaemia, and hyperammonaemia may occur in some. There is always, however, an obligatory water loss of about

0.5–1.5 litre per day associated with an ileal conduit or an augmentation ileocystoplasty (more in a substitution cystoplasty) due to the 'leakiness' of the epithelium; and some degree of absorption of some of the constituents of the urine—which may, in some circumstances, be clinically significant.

In practice the incidence and severity of the metabolic abnormality relates to the size of the bowel segment in contact with urine, renal function, respiratory function, the presence or absence of sepsis, the patient's general health, and how the metabolic abnormality is looked for. In elderly patients with a ureterosigmoidostomy after a cystectomy for bladder cancer, with the whole colon exposed to urine and reflux of faecal material into the upper urinary tracts, and if the metabolic abnormality is looked for by arterial blood gas analysis, the incidence is almost universal. In a young fit healthy adult having an augmentation cystoplasty for benign disease, having a routine venous blood sample the incidence is negligible.

Infection

Eighty per cent (80%) of patients with gut segments incorporated into the urinary tract have bacteriuria. Consequently, 5–20% of them suffer septic episodes each year, particularly in the first year after surgery. The normal bowel is in symbiosis with its bacterial flora and most of the time bacteriuria is not a problem if it is asymptomatic. But urine in a sustitute bladder has a lower concentration of urea and a higher pH which make it less bacteriostatic than in a normal bladder which has, in any case, inherent defences against bacterial infection. If the bowel is distended, whether it is in its normal position or in the urinary tract, bacterial translocation through the bladder wall can occur which may in turn cause septic problems, particularly if the bowel is distended sufficiently for it to have become ischaemic. Therefore, a patient with a cystoplasty should not be left in chronic retention—hence an underappreciated reason of the importance of regular bladder drainage, as well as an explanation of why septic episodes can occur.[12]

Stones

There are several factors that contribute to stone disease in patients with a cystoplasty such as stasis of urine (as a consequence of poor emptying), allowing mucus to accumulate in the presence of bacteriuria. Indeed 86% of stones in a cystoplasty are infective stones.[21] But the urine is also more alkaline and there is typically a higher sodium concentration and proteinuria, a lower calcium and citrate excretion, and commonly foreign material in the bladder as well, as when staples have been used for the construction of the neobladder or cystoplasty.[22] Dietary factors may also be important—stone formers generally have a higher dietary magnesium and phosphate intake. Thus, cystoplasty patients are more prone to stone formation than are normal patients for a number of reasons, but the most important appear to be stasis in the presence of mucus and bacteriuria—another good reason for making sure the bladder is emptied regularly and completely.[21]

Malignant transformation

Cancer as a consequence of urine in a bowel segment was first noted in patients with a ureterosigmoidostomy as this was the first form of urinary diversion using bowel to be widely used.[23] Forty per cent (40%) of ureterosigmoidostomy patients develop polyps at the site of ureteric reimplantation into the sigmoid colon or rectum but more importantly there is a 500–7,000-fold increased incidence of cancer amounting to a 6–29% (mean 11%) incidence of cancer generally, varying according to whether the ureterosigmoidostomy was performed in children or in adults, and was for a benign or a malignant condition.[24] The lag time before the development of the tumour is usually 10–20 years. Importantly it carries a 35% mortality—higher than the 'natural' mortality of colon cancer arising spontaneously.[25]

These tumours tend to occur precisely at the site of implantation of the ureters into the bowel in ureterosigmoidostomy patients, and close to the suture line between the urinary tract and the bowel in patients with cystoplasties, with 85% being adenocarcinomas of bowel origin.[26] There are a number of histological markers of premalignant change, including keratinizing squamous metaplasia and abnormal transitional epithelial mucin distribution, as can be found in patients with polyposis coli who are also prone to develop bowel cancer. The aetiology of the tumours is unknown. It has been postulated that it may be due to the production of nitrosamines by the contact of urine with bowel mucosa, superoxide radicals, or to the increased expression as something such as epidermal growth factor receptors. Nitrosamines in the urine, urinary infection, and histological abnormalities associated with premalignant change are closely correlated.[27]

For all these reasons, there has been considerable debate about how to follow-up these patients.[28] The relative incidence of tumours seems to mirror the natural incidence of cancer in that part of the bowel that the intestinal segment was harvested from and so patients with ureterosigmoidostomy or colocystoplasties should be followed up routinely by annual endoscopy. Otherwise, patients with ileocystoplasties should be advised to return for endoscopy if they have haematuria or develop recurrent urinary infection.[29] MRI may be an alternative to endoscopy. Gastrocystoplasty should probably be avoided if possible.

Other problems

Hyperammonaemia can be a problem in patients with cirrhosis. Glucose re-absorption from the urine may be a problem in diabetics. Altered drug metabolism, notably with phenytoin and methotrexate and other anti-metabolites (in chemotherapy), may be a problem because of absorption of the drugs from the urine.[12]

These principles will be expanded in the following chapters, but one other principle of primary importance is always to consider the patient's best interests. Reconstructive urology is often concerned with the care of patients who have had a complication of previous surgery or other treatment and they want to be returned to normality, immediately, as if nothing had happened. The timing and nature of revisional surgery in their best interests may not always match their desires and reconciling their wishes with their best interests—from a surgical perspective—is sometimes difficult.[12]

References

1. Bricker EM. Bladder substitution after pelvic evisceration. *Surg Clin North Am* 1950; **30**:1511–21.
2. Hendren WH. Reconstruction of previously diverted urinary tracts in children. *J Pediatr Surg* 1973; **8**:135–50.
3. Camey M, Le Duc A. L'Entero-cystoplastie après cystoprostatectomie totale pour cancer de vessie. *Annales d'Urologie (Paris)* 1979; **13**:114–23.
4. Lapides J, Diokno AC, Silber SJ, Lowe BS. Clean, intermittent self catherisation in the treatment of urinary tract disease. *J Urol* 1972; **107**:458–61.

5. Scott FB, Bradley WE, Timm GW. Treatment of urinary incontinence by an implantable prosthetic urinary sphincter. *J Urol* 1974; **112**:75–80.
6. Mundy AR, Andrich DE. Urethral strictures. *BJU Int* 2011; **107**:6–26.
7. Duplay S. 1880, referred to and illustrated (p. 455). In: Murphy LJT (ed). *The History of Urology*. Springfield, IL: Charles C. Thomas, 1972.
8. Davis JS, Traut HF. The production of epithelial lined tubes and sacs: An experimental study. *JAMA* 1926; **86**:339–41.
9. Andrich DE, Mundy AR. What is the best technique for urethroplasty? *Eur Urol* 2008; **54**:1031–41.
10. Mundy AR. *Urodynamic and Reconstructive Surgery of the Lower Urinary Tract*. London, UK: Churchill Livingstone, 1993: Chapter 15.
11. Jordan GH. Principles of wound healing and tissue transfer techniques useful for genitourinary reconstructive surgery. *Semin Urol* 1987; **4**:219–27.
12. Andrich DE, Mundy AR. Tissue transfer in urology (Chapter 31). In: Mundy AR, Fitzpatrick JM, Neal DE, George NJR (eds). *Scientific Basis of Urology*, 3rd edition. London, UK: Informa Healthcare, 2010.
13. Markiewicz MR, Lukose MA, Margarone JE 3rd, Barbagli G, Miller KS, Chuang SK. The oral mucosa graft: a systematic review. *J Urol* 2007; **178**:387–94.
14. Wood DN, Allen SE, Andrich DE, Greenwell TJ, Mundy AR. The morbidity of buccal mucosal graft harvest for urethroplasty and the effect of non-closure of the graft harvest site on postoperative pain. *J Urol* 2004; **172**:580–3.
15. McDougal WS, Koch MO. Accurate determination of renal function in patients with intestinal urinary diversions. *J Urol* 1986; **135**:1175–8.
16. Castro JE, Ram MD. Electrolyte imbalance following ileal urinary diversion. *Br J Urol* 1970; **42**:29–32.
17. Boyd SD, Schiff WM, Skinner DG, Lieskovsky G, Kanellos AW, Klimaszewski AD. Prospective study of metabolic abnormalities in patient with continent Kock pouch urinary diversion. *Urology* 1989; **33**:85–8.
18. Nurse DE, Mundy AR. Metabolic complications of cystoplasty. *Br J Urol* 1989; **63**:165–70.
19. Koch MO, McDougal WS. The pathophysiology of hyperchloremic metabolic acidosis after urinary diversion through intestinal segments. *Surgery* 1985; **98**: 561–70.
20. Mingin G, Maroni P, Gerharz EW, Woodhouse CR, Baskin LS. Linear growth after enterocystoplasty in children and adolescents: a review. *World J Urol* 2004; **22**:196–9.
21. Nurse DE, McInerney PD, Thomas PJ, Mundy AR. Stones in enterocystoplasties. *Br J Urol* 1996; **77**:684–7.
22. Hamid R, Robertson WG, Woodhouse CR. Comparison of biochemistry and diet in patients with enterocystoplasty who do and do not form stones. *BJU Int* 2008; **101**:1427–32.
23. Stewart M, Macrae FA, Williams CB. Neoplasia and ureterosigmoidostomy: a colonoscopy survey. *Br J Surg* 1982; **69**:414–6.
24. Zabbo A, Kay R. Ureterosigmoidostomy and bladder exstrophy: a long-term followup. *J Urol* 1986; **136**:396–8.
25. Husmann DA, Spence HM. Current status of tumour of the bowel following ureterosigmoidoscopy: a review. *J Urol* 1990; **144**: 607–10.
26. Barrington JW, Fulford S, Griffiths D, Stephenson TP. Tumors in bladder remnant after augmentation enterocystoplasty. *J Urol* 1997; **15**:482–5.
27. Creagh TA, Picramenos D, Smalley ET, Walters CL, Mundy AR. The source of urinary nitrosamines in patients with enterocystoplasties. *Br J Urol* 1997; **79**:28–31.
28. Hamid R, Greenwell TJ, Nethercliffe JM, Freeman A, Venn SN, Woodhouse CRJ. Routine surveillance cystoscopy for patients with augmentation and substitution cystoplasty for benign urological conditions: is it necessary? *BJU Int* 2009; **104**:392–5.
29. Husmann DA. Enterocystoplasty: What is the risk of malignancy? State of the Art lecture. American Urologic Association Annual Meeting, Sunday 26 April 2009.

CHAPTER 4.2

Upper urinary tract reconstruction

Anthony R. Mundy and Daniela E. Andrich

Introduction to upper urinary tract reconstruction

We referred in the last chapter to the exclusion of pelviureteric junction obstruction and pyleoplasty, and similar problems affecting the renal pelvis infundibula and calices as being outside the scope of reconstructive urology for the purposes of this text book. In this chapter, we will consider strictures and particularly trauma of the ureter—trauma being much more common, in the developed world at least.

Aetiology

Ureteric strictures may occur as a result of tuberculosis or schistosomiasis.[1] Tuberculous strictures may occur at either end of the ureter; schistosomal strictures occur primarily in the distal ureter. Treatment is medical with the appropriate drug regime—followed, when necessary, by surgical correction if an adequate trial of medical therapy is unsuccessful. In patients with tuberculous strictures, a short course of oral steroids at the same time as the initiation of the specific drug treatment of the disease may reduce oedema at the site and consequently reduce the degree of obstruction at that site while that treatment takes effect.

Ureteric stones are another cause of stricture formation and these tend to occur at the common sites of impaction of a stone; therefore, particularly just above the pelvic brim and just outside the bladder.

Trauma is much more common and is mainly iatrogenic.[2] These days the commonest form of trauma is urological endoscopy for the treatment of stone disease or ureteroscopy for other purposes.[3] Until the development of the ureteroscope, the commonest form of ureteric trauma was during a caesarean section or a hysterectomy or other gynaecological procedure for the treatment of gynaecological cancer, particularly squamous cell carcinoma of the cervix, and particularly when the patient had also had external beam radiotherapy.[4–6]

Besides gynaecological surgery, ureteric injury is associated with colorectal surgery, particularly during a difficult sigmoid colectomy, and vascular surgery, particularly during difficult surgery for an abdominal aortic aneurysm, when the common iliac arteries are also involved.[7]

External trauma to the ureter is rare and usually involves the renal pelvis or pelviureteric junction, particularly in children. Such injuries are discussed in a later chapter. Otherwise, ureteric trauma is mainly to the upper ureter and due to a penetrating injury, and is usually associated with bowel or vascular injuries.[8–10]

In all instances of open iatrogenic trauma, the injury may be a contusion, a transection (partial or complete), or a suture/ligation injury. Intraluminal injuries are usually contusions, but penetrating injuries during laser ureteroscopy or simple ureteroscopy do occur (in about 7%), as do occasional avulsion injuries (in about 0.5%) during stone extraction. With external trauma contusions, partial ruptures and complete ruptures are possible complications.

Diagnosis

The clinical features of a ureteric stricture are usually loin pain, coupled with features of bladder involvement from the underlying disease if present.

In patients with iatrogenic trauma after abdominopelvic surgery, the history of the procedure is the best guide to the nature of the problem in a patient who has developed loin pain or abdominal pain following the procedure. Loin pain is typical with an obstructed ureter, abdominal pain with a partially or completely transected ureter and urinary extravasation, but neither symptom is pathognomonic and both may be present. Indeed, both obstruction and transection may coexist. Haematuria is usual but is absent in up to 30% of patients and, in any case, does not localize the trauma to the ureter.[11] Urine leakage from the wound or from a drain is usual with transection is usual but may take time to develop: after a caesarean section or a hysterectomy, urovaginal fistulation is another type of presentation.

The diagnosis of iatrogenic ureteric injury is generally made on ultrasound scanning in the first instance and further assessment depends on the urgency of the situation. In an urgent situation with, for example, complete ureteric obstruction, the ultrasound scan (Fig. 4.2.1) may lead to the placement of a percutaneous nephrostomy by an interventional radiologist (Fig. 4.2.2), which is both diagnostic and—temporarily—therapeutic. Once a percutaneous nephrostomy has been placed, further investigation becomes elective.

In the elective situation, whether or not there has been a radiological intervention, investigation will usually include computed tomography (CT) scanning and specifically a CT urogram. Extravasation of contrast on a CT scan is diagnostic (Fig. 4.2.3). A MAG3 scan with lasix washout assesses obstruction and possible loss of renal function (Fig. 4.2.4). In patients with percutaneous nephrostomy, an antegrade ureterogram will demonstrate the site

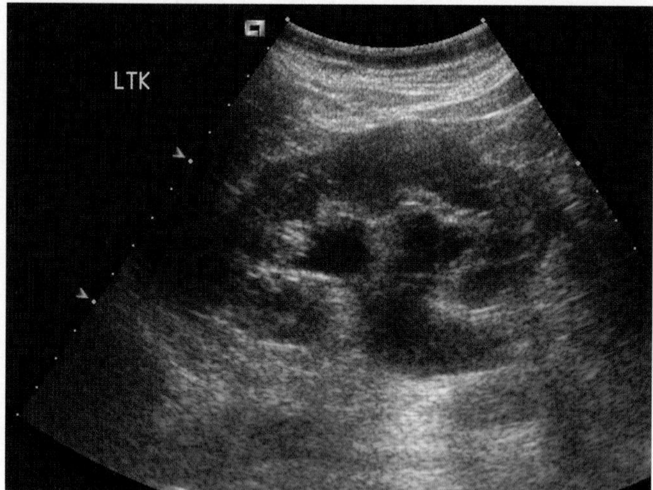

Fig. 4.2.1 An obstructed left kidney on ultrasound after a sacrocolpopexy.

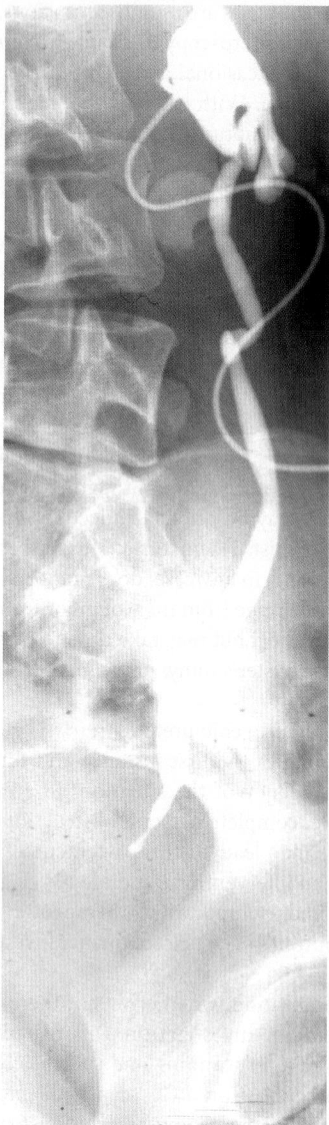

Fig. 4.2.2 A percutaneous nephrostomy relieves the obstruction and an antegrade contrast study shows the obstruction and a leak at that site.

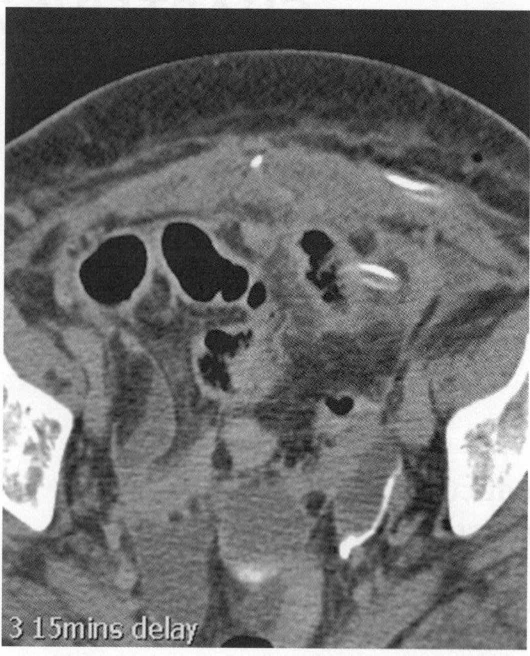

Fig. 4.2.3 Contrast leak shows on the computed tomography (CT) scan.

and nature of the trauma (Fig. 4.2.2). In partial injuries, or chronic long-standing conditions, particularly if a nephrostomy or a ureteric stent have been in place for some time, clamping the nephrostomy to allow renographic evaluation of kidney function may be helpful.

One type of iatrogenic trauma is commonly associated with another type, so when one ureter has been damaged, the other ureter should be assessed; and if the ureter has been ligated, it could have been transected as well, either completely or incompletely, either above or below the ligature.

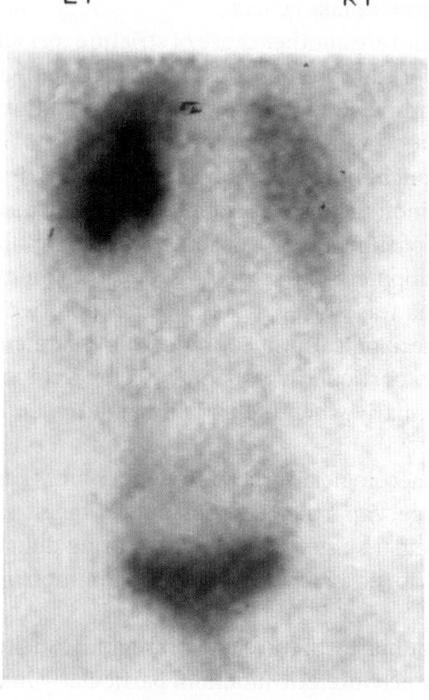

Fig. 4.2.4 A MAG3 scan with lasix washout.

Ureteric injury is rarely considered as a specific diagnosis after external trauma, but should always be suspected and excluded or demonstrated by a CT urogram. As in any situation, extravasation of contrast is diagnostic of ureteric injury. Unfortunately, ureteric injury is easily missed even on careful radiological evaluation.[12]

Treatment

Immediate management

Intraluminal iatrogenic injuries during ureteroscopy are usually identified at the time and, excepting avulsion injuries, can usually be managed by passing a guidewire past the traumatized area and into the renal pelvis, and then passing a stent over it and leaving it for a few weeks.

If an iatrogenic injury is noted during open surgery, then it might be possible to deal with it. Damage to the distal ureter, deep in the pelvis, just outside the bladder, is best dealt with by a psoas hitch or Boari flap or both, with ureteric reimplantation. Direct end-to-end anastomosis is difficult at this site, even if the nature of the injury makes it otherwise possible, because access is limited. At the pelvic brim or above a partial injury might be repaired over a ureteric stent. A short complete rupture may be dealt with by ureteric mobilization on either side and then an overlapping spatulated anastomotic repair over a ureteric stent—if conditions, and particularly access, allow this. Under adverse circumstances, the safest option is an intubated ureterostomy *in situ*—passing an 8 Fr infant feeding tube or some similar stent up the ureter into the renal pelvis, through the site of the injury and bringing the other end out through the abdominal wall. If possible and appropriate it is helpful to tack the two ends of the ureter to the posterior abdominal wall with a coloured non-absorbable suture, as close together as possible to facilitate identification for definitive surgical treatment in the future.

External trauma to the ureter is dealt with in the same way. All types of emergency ureteric surgery are best covered with a suprapubic catheter, a wound drain, and an appropriate antibiotic.

Many instances of iatrogenic abdominopelvic injury to the ureter are not noticed until a day or two afterwards or later. The immediate management depends on the acuity of the situation and in an acute situation, placement of a percutaneous nephrostomy is the emergency treatment of choice. Thereafter, further treatment depends on the general health of the patient. When a ureter has been ligated and the patient is healthy and in a good physical condition, it may be appropriate to take the patient straight back to the operating theatre as soon as possible and explore the operative site with a view to removing the offending ligature. With a completely obstructed kidney on ultrasound, either demonstrable ureteric obstruction on antegrade ureterography through a percutaneous nephrostomy, an inability to pass a ureteric catheter, or perform a retrograde ureterogram at cystoscopy is diagnostic.

When the ureter has been transected, the patient is more likely to be too sick for immediate surgery because of extravasation and associated sepsis, but immediate exploration should nonetheless be considered with a view to definitive treatment. Surgery within the first 48 or 72 hours may be relatively easy and will eliminate the problem rather than waiting for interval surgery weeks or months later.

When there is evidence of a partial injury—either a partial obstruction or partial transection—then the important points are to provide urinary drainage and to prevent extravasation. Drainage will be provided by a percutaneous nephrostomy, but when there is extravasation this may continue despite the presence of a nephrostomy. An antegrade or retrograde placement of a ureteric stent may reduce the degree of extravasation and hasten recovery (Fig. 4.2.5).[13,14] A partial obstruction from a ligature may, in theory at least, improve in time if it is an absorbable ligature but this is by no means to be expected.

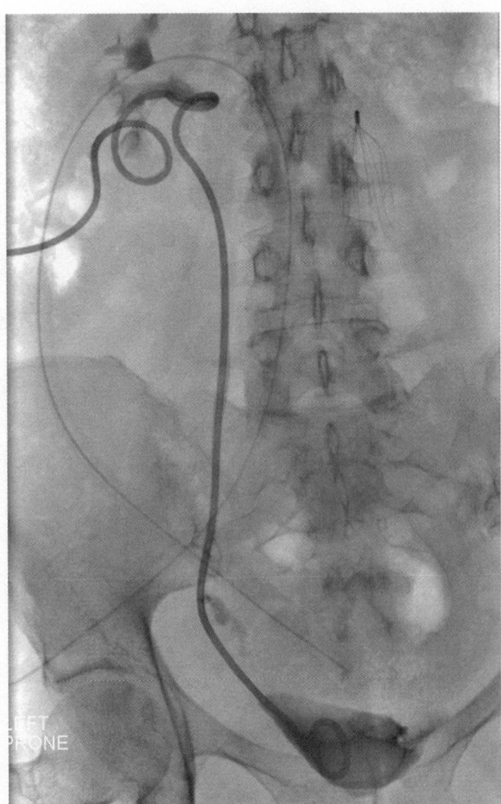

Fig. 4.2.5 A JJ stent has been passed through the site of the injury.

It is important to state at this stage (and we will emphasize both points later on in this chapter) that passage of a stent is rarely curative in patients with a significant ureteric injury,[15] although it may make for excellent short-term management; and that whatever the nature of the injury, a percutaneous nephrostomy is rarely, if ever, 'curative' of a ureteric injury—how could it be?—it too is merely an excellent minimally invasive temporizing procedure to provide drainage and limit extravasation.

In a patient who has passed the emergency and acute phase, with or without a stent, the next step, six weeks or so after the injury and the placement of the percutaneous nephrostomy, is to re-evaluate by antegrade ureterography to look for signs of continuing extravasation or obstruction. An indwelling ureteric stent is best removed with the percutaneous nephrostomy still on drainage. With the stent removed, the nephrostomy is clamped, and the patient is assessed symptomatically and with a MAG3 renogram with lasix washout, to have objective evaluation of outflow obstruction.

If, at three months, there is still objective evidence of outflow obstruction (Fig. 4.2.6), it is not likely to improve any further and arrangements should be made for definitive correction of the problem. Delayed treatment is associated with a worse outcome and the longer the delay the worse the outcome.[15] If the patient appears to

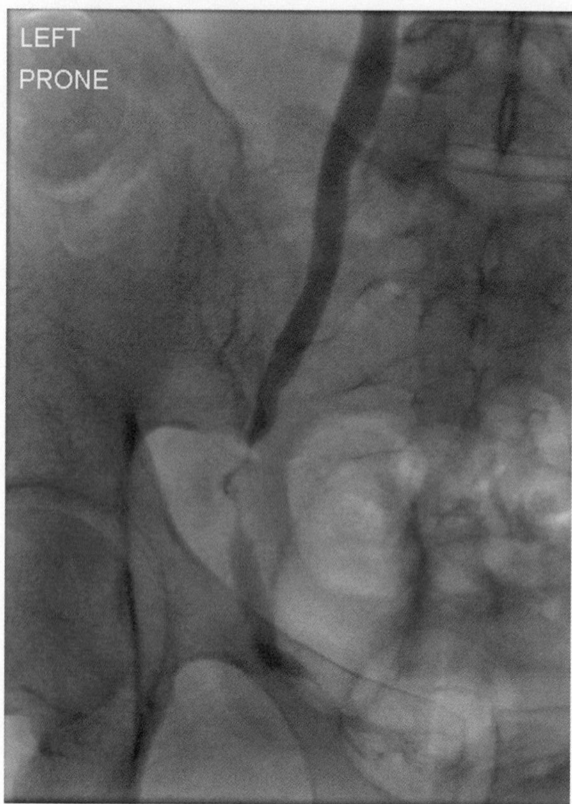

Fig. 4.2.6 Three months later, after removal of the stent, there is a stricture at the site of the injury.

be unobstructed the percutaneous nephrostomy can be removed, but it is sensible to re-evaluate the patient three months later and then six months after that before finally concluding that there is no likelihood of further trouble.

Occasionally patients present simply with a ureteric stricture 1–6 months after the causative injury. A more difficult problem is the patient who has had previous irradiation for carcinoma of the cervix who develops a delayed and commonly bilateral ureteric obstruction, usually 2–3 years after treatment was given, but sometimes many years later. The ureter is the most radio-sensitive abdominal organ[16] and damage from radiotherapy is maximal 4–6 cm proximal to the ureteric orifices, at the base of the broad ligament.[17] Ureteric strictures occur in about 1% of patients (probably more in our opinion) after radiotherapy alone,[18] rising to more than 5% after the combination of surgery and radiotherapy.[19] Such patients commonly present with loin pain, or more generalized back pain, sometimes with recurrent urinary infection, or otherwise the condition is picked up on routine imaging studies done as part of the follow-up of the cervical cancer itself. The question is always whether this is long-term fibrosis or recurrent tumour causing extra-mural ureteric obstruction. It has been suggested that the timing of the onset of the obstruction may be relevant, but this is not a useful guide. In practice the diagnosis can only be made histologically, although a PET CT scan may be highly suggestive of a tumour if it is sufficiently 'hot'.

Post-radiotherapy obstruction of the ureters also requires careful assessment of the bladder as many of these patients, whether they have malignant obstruction or not, will be considered for reimplantation of the ureter into a psoas hitch or Boari flap to relieve their obstruction. This may be difficult if not impossible if the bladder is severely affected by irradiation cystitis causing a small capacity, thick-walled bladder. The state of the bladder is rarely a factor in the surgical correction of the consequences of ureteric trauma in women, except after irradiation as they tend to have bladders that are larger and with a thinner wall than do their male counterparts. Men, particularly with advancing age, may have a small capacity and thick-walled bladder due to age-related change or bladder outflow obstruction.

For all these reasons, radiotherapy—like the degree of ureteric damage and delay in definitive treatment—is an adverse prognostic feature.[15]

Definitive surgical treatment

It should be stressed that when there has been significant ureteric damage, the presence of a stent or a percutaneous nephrostomy or both will not stop a stricture from developing. It may stop it from being manifest but it will not stop it from developing. Also that by three months the die is cast. Thus, if there is evidence of obstruction on removing the stent at three months, there is no point in replacing the stent in the hope that a longer period of stenting will eliminate the stricture. It simply increases the complication rate of long-term stenting, not to mention the commonly associated discomfort, which is sometimes crippling. The longer the ureteric problem remains untreated, the more likely the patient is to end up having a nephrectomy, which tragically occurs all too often.[15] The presence of the stent makes surgery more difficult by causing the ureter to become thick and relatively much more difficult to work with than a ureter that has not been stented.

Definitive treatment of the ureteric injury depends on the location. The two commonest sites are firstly just outside the bladder after gynaecological surgery in women; or at the pelvic brim after radiotherapy for gynaecological cancer in women or after colorectal or vascular surgery in either sex. Occasional uncommon causes, such as penetrating trauma or following a right hemicolectomy for Crohn's disease tend to occur in the abdominal segment of the ureter. In most instances, the damage is over a relatively short segment.[20] Relatively longer segmental damage is more likely to follow ureteric endoscopy, which may prove relatively difficult to treat because of the length itself.

In both male and female patients with a normal bladder, damage to the distal ureter below the level of the pelvic brim is relatively (and we do mean relatively!) easily treated by a psoas hitch supplemented, where necessary, by a Boari flap, coupled with ureteric reimplantation.

When the middle-third of the ureter is involved just above the pelvic brim, it may still be possible to do this in women because of their relatively larger and thinner-walled bladders, but is unusual to be able to do this in a man. However, in both male and female patients there is usually still enough of the upper-third of the ureter to allow a transureteroureterostomy (TUU). The real problem is a stricture for injury of the upper third of the ureter, where there is insufficient ureteric length above the diseased/damaged area to allow a TUU even when that is coupled with medial mobilization of the 'recipient' ureter. In such circumstances, some surgeons have resorted to so-called autotransplantation, in which the kidney is detached from its normal location and transferred down to the pelvis where the renal vessels are anastomosed, as if this was an allograft transplant procedure, and the ureteric remnant or renal pelvis can be anastomosed directly to the bladder. Unfortunately, however attractive this might seem for the surgical enthusiast, it is often difficult (if not impossible) because the process which has led to ureteric damage that high up will usually have caused sufficient damage to the kidney or the surrounding tissues and particularly the tissues surrounding the origin of the main vessels to make the 'nephrectomy' component of the autotransplant procedure difficult if not frankly dangerous. For this reason, the authors usually prefer to create an ileal ureter in which a segment of ureter is mobilized and isolated and sutured directly to the renal pelvis and to the bladder. In theory, a segment of ileum could be interposed between two ends of ureter, but the size disparity makes a total replacement ileal ureter easier and less prone to complications.

Direct end-to-end anastomosis—ureteroureterostomy

Occasional short segment injuries, such as following external penetrating trauma or surgery (e.g. a right hemicolectomy for Crohn's disease) may be amenable to direct ureteroureterostomy. The ability to stretch the ureter to allow an overlapping spatulated anastomosis is somewhat limited, even with full mobilization of both ends of the ureter and mobilization of the kidney as well in order to shift it downwards to help reduce tension. Nonetheless, it should always be considered for high ureteric problem; whereas for distal ureteric problems a psoas hitch is probably more secure however short the ureteric defect appears to be.

Psoas hitch, Boari flap, and ureteric reimplantation

The psoas hitch[21] and Boari flap[22,23] procedures are often regarded as two alternatives for dealing with the same problem. Whereas this may be a perfectly reasonable approach, we prefer to regard them as complementary in providing a step-wise approach to bringing up a suitable extension of the bladder from its normal position to allow a tension-free reimplantation of the ureter (Fig. 4.2.7).

The idea of the psoas-hitch procedure is that the bladder is mobilized all the way around on its anterior and lateral aspects so that it is freely mobile and no longer attached by the superior hypogastric wing of peritoneum and fascia on each side and attached only by the lateral pedicles of the bladder and posteriorly between the two lateral pedicles. In most patients, male and female, with a normal bladder, it is then usually possible to manoeuvre the dome of the bladder so that it reaches the psoas major muscle or psoas minor tendon—preferably—if present. When the bladder can be fixed by sutures to the psoas minor tendon, or to the psoas major muscle if the psoas minor tendon is absent, then it will be apparent if the ureter can be implanted into the psoas hitch without tension. If there is tension or a significant gap, a Boari flap is raised, of adequate width as well as adequate length, to reach up to the ureter, or even, in some females, to the renal pelvis in extreme circumstances.

Occasionally, because the bladder is a sphere and the psoas hitch is an attempt to convert it to a flat plate, as far as it is possible to achieve this, the longitudinal cystostomy incision may allow only a restricted access to the inside of the bladder, or even a restricted degree of bladder mobilization. In this case, a series of short transverse incisions on each side will allow the bladder to be stretched upwards more easily.

Then, from within the bladder, the bladder epithelium can be incised at an appropriate point for a ureteric reimplantation and a subepithelial tunnel created. The ureter can then be pulled into the bladder to create an antireflux subepithelial tunnel of suitable length. A particular advantage of an antireflux type reimplantation into the bladder is not so much that it prevents reflux (although this may be desirable), but to provide a more secure anastomosis of the ureter to the bladder than a simple direct anastomosis can achieve.

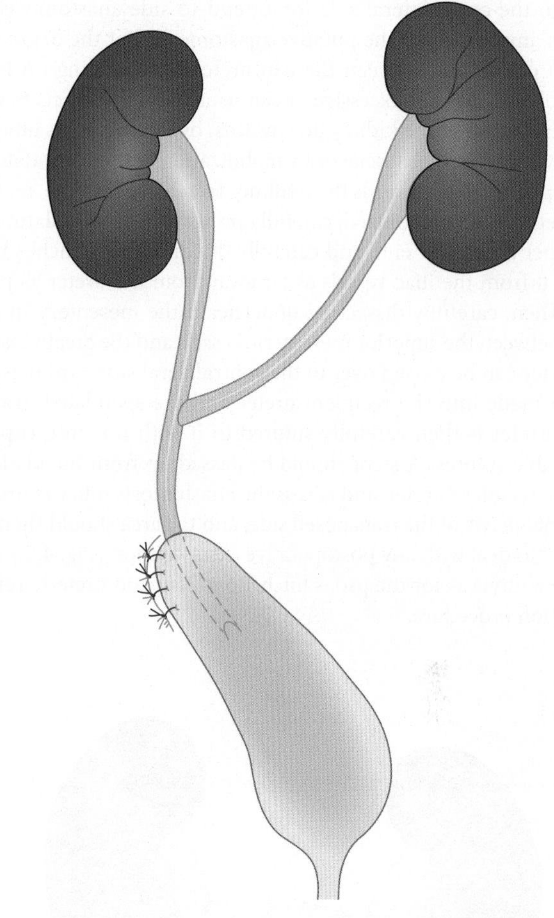

Fig. 4.2.7 A left to right transureteroureterostomy and a tunnelled reimplantation of the right ureter into the bladder with a psoas hitch.
Reprinted from A. R. Mundy, *Urodynamic and Reconstructive Surgery of the Lower Urinary Tract*, Churchill Livingstone, UK, Copyright © 1993, with permission from Elsevier.

A ureteric stent is then generally placed and the bladder closed over a suprapubic catheter. The stent (we use an infant feeding tube or a small-calibre Ryle's tube), is brought out alongside the suprapubic catheter. An internal JJ stent can be used but this has the disadvantage of having to be removed by a further subsequent procedure. We simply get a 'stentogram' at 8–10 days postoperatively to show that there is no leakage at the anastomosis. Then we remove the stent and clamp the suprapubic catheter for a trial of voiding and remove the suprapubic catheter the following day. A follow-up MAG3 renogram with lasix washout at three months and then at one year assures a satisfactory result.

Transureteroureterostomy

The damaged ureter is mobilized up to the renal pelvis. This will involve mobilization of the ascending or descending colon up as far as the hepatic or the splenic flexure depending on the side. Having mobilized the damaged ureter, it is usually apparent whether it will reach to the contralateral side for an end-to-side anastomosis. If there is any tension at the putative anastomosis, but the degree of tension or the gap between the two ureters—depending on how you look at it—is not excessive, it can usually be made acceptable by mobilization of the kidney downwards, by freeing up its attachments within Gerota's fascia; or by mobilization of the contralateral or 'recipient' ureter towards the midline. To achieve this, the 'recipient' ureter is fully mobilized, carefully preserving its vasculature at the upper and lower end, and carefully dividing the branches that run to it from the iliac vessels as far away from the ureter as possible. Then, carefully dissecting underneath the mesentery in the plane between the superior mesenteric vessels and the great vessels, the ureter can be passed over to the contralateral side. An incision is then made into the recipient ureter and the spatulated, transposed ureter is then carefully sutured to it with fine interrupted absorbable sutures. A stent should be passed up from the bladder into the recipient ureter, and across the anastomosis into the ureter and renal pelvis of the transposed side; and the area should then be drained to deal with any postoperative extravasation (Fig. 4.2.7).[24]

Follow-up is as for the psoas hitch/Boari flap and ureteric reimplantation procedure.

The ileal ureter

This was originally developed for use in severe stone disease particularly when associated with infundibular stenosis of the lower pole calyx. An incision was made through the inferior aspect of the renal pelvis, through the renal parenchyma and infundibulum and into the lower pole calyx; and an ileal segment was then interposed between it and the bladder to allow free drainage of both urine and calculous material. When used as an ileal ureter to replace a long defect of the upper ureter—leaving an upper end that is too short for a TUU—it is best to abandon the remaining ureter and anastomose the upper end of a segment of ileum directly to the renal pelvis and the lower end directly into the bladder. It is possible to tailor the ileal segment and attempt a tunnelled reimplantation into the bladder, but there seems little point in doing this. In certain unusual circumstances (e.g. in bilateral urothelial tumours of the upper urinary tract), the ureter and renal pelvis can be excised well into the renal sinus on each side and a longer segment of ileum run from one side (end-to-end) across to the other side (end-to-side) and then down to the bladder (Fig. 4.2.8), or to a substitution cystoplasty if a cystectomy is being performed simultaneously, or simply brought out as an 'ileal conduit'.[25]

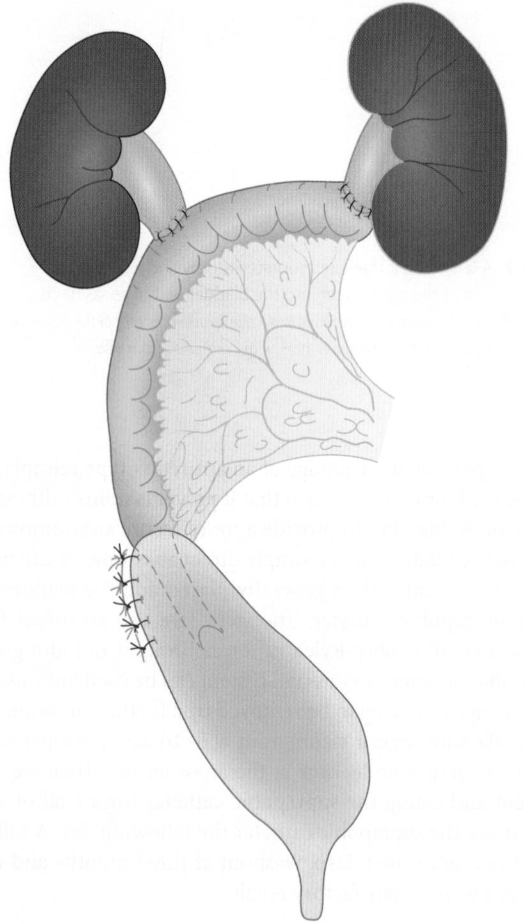

Fig. 4.2.8 An ileal ureter.

Reprinted from A. R. Mundy, *Urodynamic and Reconstructive Surgery of the Lower Urinary Tract*, Churchill Livingstone, UK, Copyright © 1993, with permission from Elsevier.

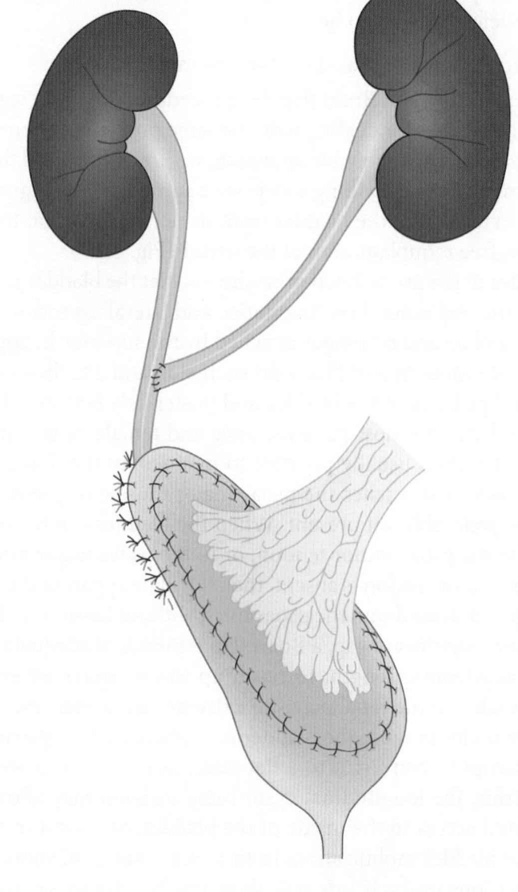

Fig. 4.2.9 Combining a psoas hitch and ureteric reimplantation with an augmentation cystoplasty in a patient with a small bladder—for whatever reason.

Reprinted from A. R. Mundy, *Urodynamic and Reconstructive Surgery of the Lower Urinary Tract*, Churchill Livingstone, UK, Copyright © 1993, with permission from Elsevier.

The irradiated bladder coupled with ureteric obstruction

Sometimes the only reasonable solution is an anterior exenteration removing the bladder and any gynaecological remnants (or even a total pelvic exenteration) and an ileal conduit urinary diversion, or a continent diversion such as a Mitrofanoff procedure.

Occasionally the bladder may be relatively normal and a psoas hitch or Boari flap may be possible, but even in mild irradiation cystitis this is unlikely to be achievable. Between the two extremes, there may be a bladder which is worth preserving because it has some useful capacity and the patient has a functioning sphincter mechanism and is continent. In such patients, an augmentation cystoplasty may allow preservation of normal voiding as well as allowing anastomosis of the healthy ureter(s) to the bladder. One possibility is to use the entire native bladder as a flat plate-type of psoas hitch/Boari flap and close the bladder by onlaying a patch of ileum opened on its antimesenteric border (Fig. 4.2.9). The alternative is to do a subtotal cystectomy and substitution cystoplasty using the right colon and reimplanting the affected ureter, or both ureters, directly into the cystoplasty or, together, to the ileal tail.

Most female patients will be able to void spontaneously, as it is usual to have a degree of sphincter weakness, which will allow voiding by straining and expression. All patients should however be counselled that clean intermittent self-catheterization may be necessary and it would be unwise to proceed with this sort of surgery unless the patient has not only consented to self-catheterization but has also proved that she can do it. In male patients, the procedure is rarely indicated but the need for self-catheterization is much greater.

References

1. Goel A, Dalela D. Options in the management of tuberculous ureteric stricture. *Indian J Urol* 2008; **24**:376–81.
2. Santucci RA, Bartley JM. Urological trauma guidelines: a 21st century update. *Nat Rev Urol* 2010; 7:510–19.
3. Al-Awadi K, Kehinde EO, Al-Hunayan A, Al-Khayat A. Iatrogenic ureteric injuries: incidence, aetiological factors and the effect of early management on subsequent outcome. *Int Urol Nephrol* 2005; **37**:235–41.
4. Bauman J, Solomons E, Levin EJ, Baron J. A pyelographic study of ureteric injuries sustained during hysterectomy for benign conditions. *Surg Gynecol Obstet* 1960; **111**:41–8.
5. St. Martin EC, Trichel EE, Campbell JH, Locke CM. Ureteral injuries in gynecologic surgery. *J Urol* 1953; **70**:51–7.
6. Symmonds RE Ureteral injuries associated with gynecologic surgery: prevention and management. *Clin Obstet Gynecol* 1976;**19**:623–44.
7. Coburn M. Ureteral injuries from surgical trauma. (pp. 181–97) In: McAninch JW (ed). *Traumatic and Reconstructive Urology*. Philadelphia, PA: WB Saunders, 1996.
8. Elliott SP, McAninch JW. Ureteral injuries from external violence: the 25-year experience at San Francisco General Hospital. *J Urol* 2003; **170**:1213–16.
9. Palmer LS, Rosenbaum RR, Gershbaum MD, *et al.* Penetrating ureteral trauma at an urban trauma centre: 10-year experience. *Urology* 1999; **54**:34–6.
10. Perez-Brayfield MR, Keane TE, Krishnan A, *et al.* Gunshot wounds to the ureter: 1 40-year experience at Grady Memorial Hospital. *J Urol* 2001; **166**:119–21.
11. Medina M, Lavery R, Ross SE, Livingston DH. Ureteral trauma: preoperative studies neither predict injury nor prevent missed injuries. *J Am Coll Surg* 1998; **186**:641–4.
12. McGinty DM, Mendez R. Traumatic ueteral injuries with delayed recognition. *Urology* 1977; **10**:115–17.
13. Cormio L, Ruutu M, Traficante A, Battaglia M, Selvaggi FP. Management of bilateral ureteric injuries after gynaecological and obstetric procedures. *Int Urol Nephrol* 1993; **25**:551–5.
14. Turner WH, Cranston DW, Davies AH, Fellows GJ, Smith JC. Double J stents in the treatment of gynaecological injury to the ureter. *J R Soc Med* 1990; **83**:623–4.
15. Cormio L, Ruutu M, Selvaggi FP. Prognostic factors in the management of ureteric injuries. *Ann Chir Gynaecol* 1994; **83**:41–4.
16. Hoekstra HJ, Mehta DM, Oosterhuis JW, Westra P, van den Dungen J, Dijkstra RG. The short- and long-term effect of single high-dose intraoperative electron beam irradiation of retroperitoneal structures—an experimental study in dogs. *Eur J Surg Oncol* 1990; **16**:240–7.
17. Gillette SL, Gillette EL, Powers BE, Park RD, Withrow SJ. Ureteral injury following experimental intraoperative radiation. *Int J Radiat Oncol Biol Phys* 1989; **17**:791–8.
18. Rhamy RK, Stander RW Pyelographic analysis of radiation therapy in carcinoma of the cervix. *Am J Roentgenol Radium Ther Nucl Med* 1962; **87**:41–3.
19. Shingleton HM, Fowler WC Jr, Pepper FD Jr, Palumbo L Ureteral strictures following therapy for carcinoma of the cervix. *Cancer* 1969; **24**:77–83.
20. Cormio L, Ruutu M, Traficante A, Battaglia M, Selvaggi FP. Management of bilateral ureteric injuries after gynaecological and obstetric procedures. *Int Urol Nephrol* 1993; **25**:551–5.
21. Turner-Warwick R, Worth PHL. The psoas-hitch procedure for the replacement of the lower third of the ureter. *Br J Urol* 1969; **41**:701–9.
22. Boari A. *La Uretro-cisto-neostomia*. Rome, Italy: Societa Editrice, Dante Aligheri, 1899.
23. Ockerblad NF. Reimplantation of the ureter into the bladder by a flap method. *J Urol* 1947; **57**:845–7.
24. Noble JG, Lee KT, Mundy AR. Transuretero-ureterostomy: a review of 253 cases. *Br J Urol* 1997; **79**:20–3.
25. Wolff B, Chartier-Kastler E, Mozer P, Haertig A, Bitker MO, Rouprêt M. Long-term functional outcomes after ileal ureter substitution: a single-center experience. *Urology* 2011; **78**:692–5.

CHAPTER 4.3

Lower urinary tract reconstruction

Anthony R. Mundy and Daniela E. Andrich

Introduction to lower urinary tract reconstruction

For the purposes of this chapter, we will refer to the lower urinary tract as the combination of the bladder and the sphincter-active urethra, in both sexes, as a single functional unit. We will concentrate on the surgical management of the neuropathic bladder, or the small capacity bladder for whatever other reason, by augmentation cystoplasty; the management of the lower urinary tract after total or subtotal cystectomy by substitution cystoplasty; the role of the artificial urinary sphincter (AUS) in general and in these latter two situations; the posterior urethral complications of the treatment of prostate cancer with comments on the lower urinary tract that has been impaired by trauma, disease, congenital anomaly or surgery; and on lower urinary tract reconstruction after surgery, chemotherapy, and radiotherapy to the pelvis including post-irradiation fistulae in both sexes.

Abnormalities of the female urethra and bladder, such as vesicovaginal fistulae are dealt with in the section on female urology; we will only comment on post-irradiation problems. The problems of urethral stricture disease are dealt with in the next chapter and of urethral trauma in a later chapter. Congenital problems such as exstrophy/epispadias, are discussed in the section on paediatric urology but will be referred to here insofar as they may cause persistent problems in later life that require reconstructive urology.

Augmentation cystoplasty

Neuropathic bladder

The neuropathic bladder is dealt with in detail in preceding chapters, but there are some aspects relating to surgical treatment that deserve discussion here. These patients present with incontinence and some will have recurrent urinary infection. Historically, impaired renal functional or frank renal failure was a common presenting feature but most patients these days are diagnosed and treated early by (clean intermittent self) catheterization and significant loss of renal function is relatively unusual, although always a risk. Most patients will have had ultrasound screening of their upper tracts and videourodynamic evaluation of the bladder. Most will have had a trial of at least one anticholinergic drug together with prophylactic antibiotics, when indicated; and failure of response to anticholinergic drugs will have led to a trial of intradetrusor Botox injections in some, although the short-term benefit to be gained by this in patients who are clearly going to have a lifelong problem means that some surgeons will regard Botox as a waste of time and will proceed directly to more definitive surgery.

In these patients, the problem in pathophysiological terms is a variable combination of uncontrollable overactivity of the bladder, a loss of coordination between the bladder and the sphincter, a loss of normal bladder sensation, and sphincter weakness. The result is a bladder that behaves as if it has a small functional capacity, and a spectrum of impaired urinary control between frequency, urgency, and urge incontinence at one end of the spectrum and total insensible incontinence at the other—although other patterns, such as chronic retention with overflow, are sometimes seen.

In such patients, the bladder may be small, thick-walled, and trabeculated from long-standing, untreated functional obstruction due to detrusor-sphincter dyssynergia; but from the patient's point of view and from a treatment perspective, the actual size of the bladder is not the problem—the problem is the absence of control. Treatment in these patients by augmentation cystoplasty works, not simply by increasing bladder capacity (although this may be valuable in some), but by splitting the bladder more or less completely into two halves so that it can no longer contract in a coordinated fashion. It will therefore be incapable of emptying involuntarily, the patients relying on clean intermittent self-catheterization (CISC) to empty voluntarily thereafter—although some patients may be able to empty by straining or expression. In this way, the patient gains control of bladder emptying. CISC is the price to be paid for continence; it is not a side effect or adverse effect of a cystoplasty, it is an inevitable consequence of the acontractile bladder that augmentation cystoplasty is intended to cause. Patients with neuropathic bladder dysfunction rarely regard this as a major disadvantage because overall they are so much better off with control of continence.

Other problems

In patients with a small capacity bladder as a result of trauma or surgery, or a congenital anomaly such as exstrophy/epispadias, or a disease such as tuberculous cystitis, the situation is different. The problem is purely and simply the size of the bladder—although in congenital anomalies (commonly) and after trauma or surgery (occasionally), there may be sphincter incompetence as well. Loss of voluntary control is not otherwise a problem because the patient has sensation and is capable of instigating a voluntary detrusor contraction. In these patients, an augmentation cystoplasty is specifically to enhance bladder capacity and the (potential) loss of the ability to void spontaneously and the consequent need for CISC are significant disadvantages to them, because the overall degree of improvement in the quality of life is less dramatic than it is in neuropathic bladder dysfunction.

Evaluation

The fundamental issues, as always, are the ability of the bladder to hold and to empty urine before surgery coupled with an evaluation of the patient's likely ability to hold and empty urine after treatment. Specifically, the ability of the sphincter mechanism to provide continence should be assessed before undertaking a cystoplasty on the grounds that if an AUS is going to be necessary, it might be appropriate to implant it or at least the cuff at the same time as performing the cystoplasty. This most commonly applies to patients with neuropathic lower urinary tract dysfunction. It is equally important in the patient with pelvic fracture-related urethral injuries associated with bladder neck injury and in congenital anomalies such as exstrophy/epispadias, bilateral single ectopic ureters, and ectopic ureterocoeles that open below the bladder neck, because they will almost inevitably have had previous surgery and sometimes repeated surgery. To implant an artificial sphincter around the bladder outlet after having added a cystoplasty to the previous post-surgical scarring may prove impossible, whereas at the time of the cystoplasty it might still be possible.

In short, the surgeon must plan the whole of the patient's treatment with an eye on the end goal, rather than concentrating just on the successive stages to achieve it.

As always, CISC is likely to be necessary, or at least a possibility, so the patient should be counselled and consented preoperatively and shown how to do the technique so that they, in turn, can show their carers they are able to perform it. In patients with congenital or post-traumatic problems, the condition of the urethra and therefore its catheterizability is often in doubt, and it is therefore sensible to cystoscope them. This will allow a check of the urethra and an assessment of the capacity and appearance of the bladder.

Clean intermittent self-catheterization

Catheterization may be traumatic and a cause of lower urinary tract infection, particularly when performed in an unsterile environment. The genius of Jack Lapides was to realize that the risk of poor bladder emptying as a cause of urinary tract infection and of upper urinary tract obstruction were greater than the risks of unsterile catheterization, and that CISC would help resolve the symptoms of a number of causes of voiding dysfunction, neurological and non-neurological, and also give patients a substantial degree of independence from their medical and nursing carers.[1] Since then, we have learned to appreciate the distinction between symptomatic urinary tract infection and asymptomatic bacteriuria and the value of prophylactic antibiotics in the management of recurrent urinary tract infection; atraumatic self-lubricating catheters have been developed; and the use of CISC has been extended as a consequence, for example in the management of urethral strictures.

The details of CISC vary from patient to patient but, generally speaking, self-lubricating hydrophilic catheters are best; a calibre of 12–16 Fr suits most patients except young children; and catheters can be kept clean and used several times—for as long as a week—before discarding them. A catheter less than 12 Fr drains very slowly; 12–14 Fr drains clear urine but not mucus-containing urine (e.g. after a cystoplasty); a 16 Fr catheter can drain cystoplasty urine and bloody urine but not clots—and is best for CISC in the palliation of urethral strictures.

Technique of augmentation cystoplasty

The fundamental principles of augmentation cystoplasty are:

- To mobilize an intestinal segment of an appropriate length on an adequate vascular pedicle that will allow the intestinal segment to reach comfortably down into the pelvis for anastomosis to the bladder remnant.
- To recognize when the bladder remnant is not sufficient to allow augmentation cystoplasty and when substitution cystoplasty should be considered as an alternative.
- To avoid, in preparing the bladder, the risk that the intestinal segment used as a cystoplasty will be 'extruded', as it were, to become a diverticulum.
- To ensure, whenever possible, that when ureteric reimplantation is required, the ureters are reimplanted into bladder rather than into bowel.

The reasons for emphasizing these last two points are:

- because voiding inefficiency is not a side effect of cystoplasty—it is an inevitable consequence of cystoplasty, which is why self-catheterization is so commonly required;
- because producing a single anatomical and functional unit from the bladder remnant and the cystoplasty is the best way of ensuring adequate emptying whether by straining or by CISC;
- because the risk of 'extrusion' of the intestinal segment to effectively become a diverticulum of the bladder is high unless care is taken to prevent it, and this may cause difficulty in bladder emptying by CISC;
- and because ureteric reimplantation into the bladder remnant whenever possible is, in the long term, by which we mean decades, the best of way of avoiding stenosis leading to loss of renal function.

In theory, any segment of bowel can be used for augmentation cystoplasty but in practice the ileum is most commonly used. In children, on opening the abdomen, it is the sigmoid colon that usually presents itself and consequently this is more commonly used in that age group.

The first step is to expose the bladder and then divide it subtotally in the coronal or sagittal plane almost around to the bladder neck on either side (Fig. 4.3.1); hence the use of the term 'clam' cystoplasty.[2,3] Then the cut edge of the bladder is measured and an ileal segment of that measured length is mobilized on its vascular pedicle, 25 cm or so away from the ileocaecal valve to avoid limiting the absorptive capacity of the small bowel. Intestinal continuity is restored by enteroanastomosis. The mobilized segment is opened on the antimesenteric border to create a patch, and the patch is then sewn into the bladder to close it up (Fig. 4.3.2).

When the procedure is being performed for functional bladder disorders, as in neuropathic bladder dysfunction, the intestinal segment, like the circumference of the bladder at the time of the incision, is about 25 cm because in most patients with neuropathic bladder dysfunction, the bladder is not actually anatomically small; the reduction in capacity is functional. When it is being performed for a small capacity bladder because of trauma, surgery, or disease, the bladder is prepared in the same way but the cystoplasty segment will, of necessity, be somewhat longer than the measured circumference of the bladder because the bladder really is small. In these cases, during stitching of the gut segment into the bisected bladder, the procedure will be completed by suture of the gut margins

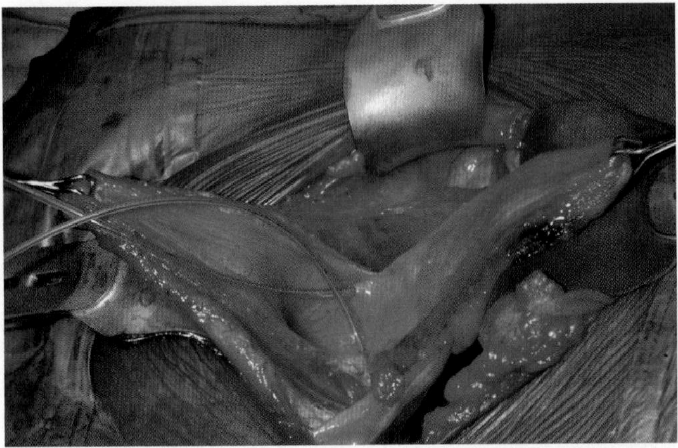

Fig. 4.3.1 Augmentation cystoplasty 1. The bladder has been bisected in the coronal plane. The ureters have been catheterized for clarity.

together at the upper end on each side to produce a pouch of adequate capacity. It is in this group of patients that the patient might decide that it is actually better to excise the rest of the bladder and perform a subtotal cystectomy and substitution cystoplasty—as described below—instead of an augmentation.

In some instances, when the ureters are to be implanted as well, as in undiversion, it might be best to convert the bladder into a single flat plate which is sutured to the psoas to fix it open, with reimplantation of the ipsilateral ureter and transureteroureterostomy (TUU) of the contralateral ureter and then suturing an augmentation cystoplasty of appropriate size on to this bladder plate as described and illustrated in the last chapter.

Substitution cystoplasty

Indications

The other common category of patients undergoing lower urinary tract reconstruction are those patients with bladder cancer, most commonly transitional cell carcinoma of the bladder, in whom

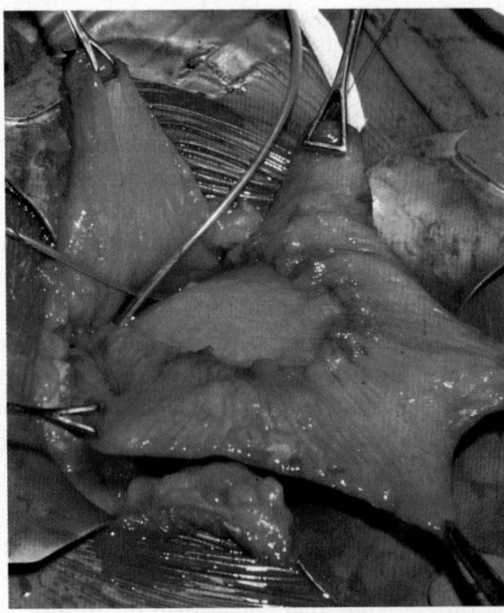

Fig. 4.3.2 Augmentation cystoplasty 2. An appropriately sized patch of ileum has been sutured to the posterior bladder wall. It will now be flipped over to suture the other edge to the anterior bladder wall.

substitution cystoplasty is being considered rather than ileal conduit urinary diversion. Other suitable candidates include occasional patients with interstitial cystitis and those with such severe benign disease—as described above—that an augmentation cystoplasty is unrealistic and substitution cystoplasty is the only realistic option.[4]

Rarely, there are patients with unusual bladder tumours such as an adenocarcinoma in a urachal remnant involving the dome of the bladder, where a wide local excision of the bladder and augmentation cystoplasty may be appropriate. Patients undergoing partial cystectomy as part of a bowel resection for a primary bowel cancer are other potential candidates for augmentation cystoplasty. In most patients, the 'wide local excision' is often a subtotal cystectomy, and so the cystoplasty becomes a substitution rather than an augmentation.

Thus, we need to consider substitution cystoplasty for patients undergoing cystectomy and otherwise for 'end-stage bladders'. These are similar as far as the cystoplasty is concerned but two separate problems as far as preparing the 'recipient site'. Patients undergoing cystectomy for transitional cell carcinoma of the bladder will be having a radical cystoprostatectomy, in which the bladder neck will be removed and the integrity of the urethral sphincter is at risk, whereas the others will be having a simple cystectomy preserving the trigone, bladder neck, prostate, and urethral sphincter.

Technique of substitution cystoplasty

Principles

The principles are, for all practical purposes, much the same as for augmentation cystoplasty except that there is no question of the substitution cystoplasty becoming extruded as a diverticulum after a radical cystectomy, because there is no bladder remnant to extrude it. The other difference is that there is no question of reimplanting the ureter into the bladder remnant; the ureters must, of necessity, be anastomosed to the bowel.

After a simple or subtotal cystectomy, there is a risk of diverticularization because there is a significant, albeit small bladder remnant; but, on the other hand, the ability to retain the smallest bladder remnant allows the ability to retain the normal vesicoureteric junctions and so the surgeon must decide how much bladder remnant to leave behind to minimize the risk of the former without compromise to the latter.

As always, patients should be counselled about CISC and taught the technique, and they must show that they are able to perform it. In practice, most men will not need to undergo CISC but most women will, and it is not predictable in either sex.

The cystectomy

Total cystectomy or cystoprostatectomy for bladder cancer

In males, the important point is to preserve the urethral sphincter mechanism as far as possible by performing a cystoprostatectomy in much the same way as one would perform a nerve-sparing radical prostatectomy (RP) for prostate cancer. In this way, not only is the sphincter preserved but the neurovascular bundles are also preserved, which maximizes the changes of continence and also might preserve potency as well—although complete preservation of normal potency is rare (Fig. 4.3.3).[5]

In females, the proximal urethra will need to be transected immediately below the bladder neck to preserve the sphincter-active urethra. This requires preservation of, and careful dissection from, the anterior vaginal wall.

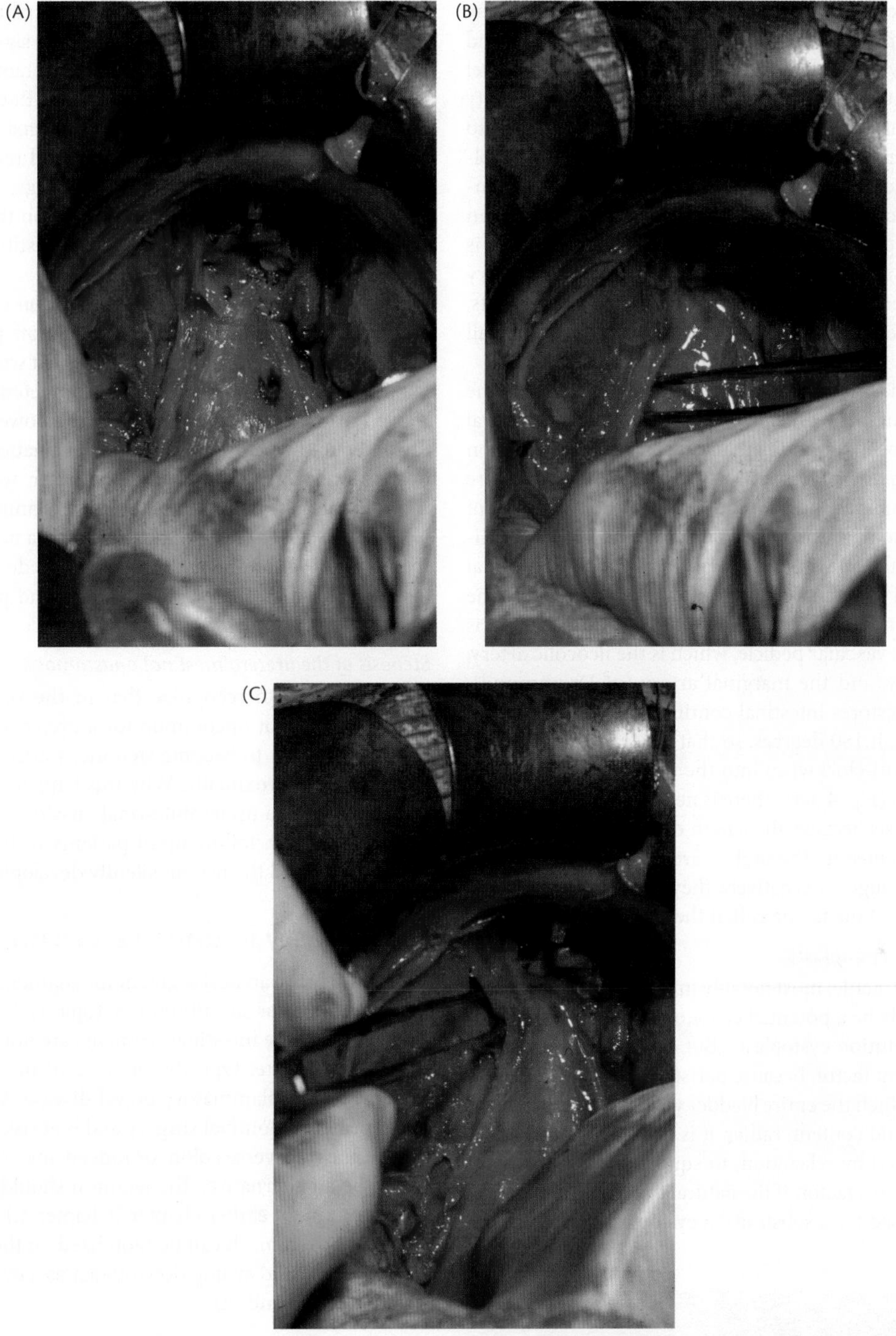

Fig. 4.3.3 (A) The appearance of the stump of the urethra and the pelvic floor after cystoprostatectomy. (B) The neurovascular bundles are identified in the middle, and (C) the pubourethral sling of levator ani on the right.

These points serve to emphasize the importance of careful assessment of patients of either sex for this approach to the management of their bladder cancer.

Simple or subtotal cystectomy for benign disease

If the bladder does not need to be excised, there is an obvious advantage in preserving the bladder base, thereby preserving the bladder neck sphincter mechanism, trigonal sensation, and the vesicoureteric junctions—assuming they are all normal and useful, which is by no means always the case. At the very least, preserving this area reduces the scale of the surgery and its complications. The important point is to remove the bladder as close to these anatomical landmarks as possible—mainly to avoid the risk of diverticularization of the cystoplasty, but also because in some conditions, such as the Hunner's ulcer type of interstitial cystitis, preservation of the trigone risks persistence of symptoms.

The substitution cystoplasty

An intestinal segment of appropriate capacity is mobilized on its vascular pedicle and deployed into the pelvis for anastomosis to the urethral stump. There are several ways in which this could be done and two, in particularly, have been popularized by Hautmann[6] and by Studer.[7] Both rely on mobilizing a section of the small bowel then reconfiguring it in such a way as to maximize its capacity and minimize its contractility. The ureters are then reimplanted to reduce the risk of reflux from the neobladder into the ureters. Abol-Enein[8] has developed a type of cystoplasty with a ureteric reimplantation that is specifically designed to prevent reflux. A problem with the Hautmann pouch, Studer, and Abol-Enein procedures is that they all reply on adequate length of the small bowel mesentery which, in our experience, cannot be guaranteed. In 10% of patients, in our experience, the mesentery is just too short to allow the small bowel to comfortably reach to the urethral stump.

We have developed a much simpler approach that is based on the premise that if you put in a segment with a sufficiently large natural capacity, there is no need to modify it and that if you use the colon rather than the ileum, the adverse effects on intestinal function are minimized. This simplifies the procedure and reduces the risk of complications. We mobilize the right colon from the last few centimetres of the terminal ileum around to the junction of the proximal and middle-thirds of the transverse colon—at the point where the middle colic artery and its bifurcation run into it.[5] This segment is then mobilized on its vascular pedicle, which is the ileocolic artery, the right colic artery, and the marginal artery (of Drummond). Enteroanastomosis restores intestinal continuity. The gut segment is then rotated through 180 degrees, so that the transverse colonic end rotates down (anti-clockwise) into the pelvis for anastomosis to the urethral stump (Fig. 4.3.4). There is never any hint of tension in such an anastomosis because the length of the segment and the axis of rotation guarantee it. The ureters are then anastomosed to the ileal stump—although, alternatively, they could be individually reimplanted into one of the taenia coli, if the surgeon prefers.

Detubularization of a cystoplasty

Normal bowel is contractile, most notably in the form of peristalsis, and this can obviously be a potential cause of postoperative incontinence after a substitution cystoplasty. But contractility of itself is not the only important factor, because peristalsis is not like a bladder contraction, in which the entire bladder wall contracts synchronously to expel its fluid content; rather, it is a wave of contraction, preceded and followed by relaxation, to squeeze its solid content onward. Volume is also a factor. If the natural capacity of an intestinal segment being used for a substitution cystoplasty is well over a litre—as is the right colon, as we have described here—then a urine volume of, say, 500 mL will hardly cause significant distension. If the natural capacity of the segment is substantially less, as it is with ileum in the Hautmann, Studer, or Abol-Enein pouches, then the same volume will cause considerable distension. In such situations, detubularization of the ileal segment and reconfiguration of it as a pouch serves to increase its capacity significantly. The need for detubularization is therefore dependant on the natural capacity of the intestinal segment to be used for substitution cystoplasty and not an absolute prerequisite.[9]

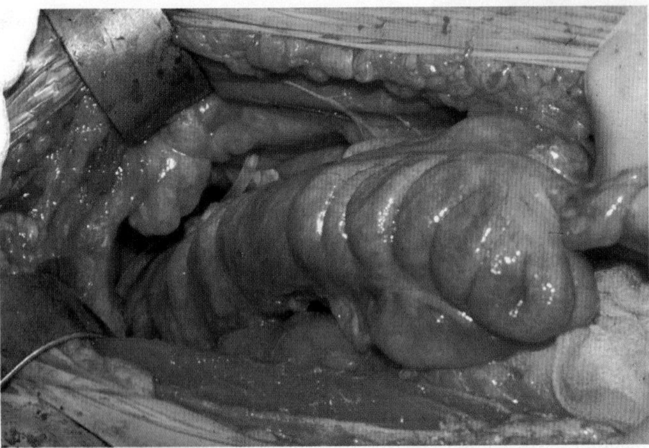

Fig. 4.3.4 The appearance after a substitution cystoplasty using the right colon.

Every now and then after a substitution cystoplasty (and after a continent diversion using a Mitrofanoff procedure) a patient becomes incontinent and one is always left wondering whether this is due to sphincter weakness (or incompetence of the Mitrofanoff 'valve') or excessive contractility of the bowel segment. This confusion is not helped by urodynamic evaluation which often shows both bowel contractility and sphincter weakness (or leakage through the Mitrofanoff catheterizable channel). Suffice to say that it may be necessary to go back and 'patch' a non-detubularized segment to restore continence but the need to do so, in our experience, is no greater than the need to go back and patch a detubularized substitution cystoplasty.

Stenosis of the ureterointestinal anastomosis

It is important to recognize that in the very long term—10 to 20 years—it is not uncommon for a ureter that is anastomosed to a bowel segment to become stenotic, starting at the anastomosis, and extending proximally. Why this happens is not clear but slow deterioration of a ureterointestinal anastomosis is not uncommon and so long-term follow-up of patients with such anastomoses is essential to avoid the patient silently developing renal failure.

Cystoplasty in unusual circumstances

We routinely use an ileal segment for augmentation cystoplasty and the right colon for substitution cystoplasty, but there are occasions when either these intestinal segments are not available or their use is not appropriate, typically because of previous surgery, radiotherapy, or of inflammatory bowel disease. When the patient has had repeated abdominal surgery and is at risk of a short bowel syndrome, the transverse colon, or indeed any other part of the colon, would be an alternative. The jejunum should not be used for reasons given in an earlier chapter (Chapter 4.1). When all else fails, a segment of stomach can be mobilized on the right gastroepiploic artery pedicle and swung down to act as a cystoplasty (or tubularized to form a conduit).

Cystoplasty in unusual conditions

Most of the unusual clinical conditions can be treated in the 'usual' sort of way. So, the small bladder due to congenital anomalies such as exstrophy/epispadias or bilateral single ectopic ureters, or the end-stage bladder with interstitial cystitis (the Hunner's ulcer type, not the non-Hunner's type) can be treated by routine augmentation or substitution cystoplasty.

Follow-up after augmentation and substitution cystoplasty

There are a number of potential complications associated with enterocystoplasty,[10] which mean that some patients need to be followed up. The commonest is urinary infection; the most serious is the potential risk of cancer (this was discussed in Chapter 4.1). In short, the evidence suggests that patients with colocystoplasties and gastrocystoplasties should be followed up by annual endoscopy. Patients with ileocystoplasties should be told to come for follow-up if they develop haematuria, whether associated with urinary tract infection or not, and if they develop *de novo* recurrent urinary tract infection, but do not need routine follow-up.

The artificial urinary sphincter

As we mentioned at the beginning of this chapter, the two fundamental principles are that the reconstructed urinary tract should hold an adequate volume of urine, requiring an adequate continence mechanism, and should be capable of complete emptying. The ultimate backup emptying mechanism is CISC; the ultimate backup continence mechanism is an AUS.

For all practical purposes, the AUS refers to the AMS 800® device produced by American Medical Systems and developed from the original design reported by Scott, Bradley, and Timm in the 1970s.[11] Other devices exist[12–16] with varying degrees of sophistication, but none have stood the test of time, whatever their potential advantages.

It is important to remember that the artificial sphincter is precisely that; it is a sphincter and it is artificial. It is a sphincter and not a means of compensating for abnormal bladder function; indeed, one of the critical features for the success of an AUS implant is to ensure that any associated bladder dysfunction is controlled before implantation. It is artificial and can be expected to give continence under sedentary or moderate activity, assuming that any bladder dysfunction is controlled, but any abdominal pressure surge, particularly when the bladder is full, will cause a degree of leakage which may be minor but could be embarrassing for the individual. In particular, a golf swing, a tennis service, lifting a heavy object, coughing and sneezing, or even just getting out of a low comfortable chair or out of a car, may be associated with a degree of leakage, at least with the AMS 800.

Principles of the artificial urethral sphincter

The AMS 800 consists of three parts—a cuff, a pressure regulating balloon, and a control pump—which are filled with isotonic fluid and connected to each other by kink-proof tubing (Fig. 4.3.5). The device works on the principle that a fluid-filled inflatable cuff is wrapped around a chosen part of the bladder outflow and produces compression of it to hold urine in the bladder. This compression is produced by the hydrostatic pressure generated by the pressure regulating balloon, to which the cuff is connected by means of the control pump. The control pump has two parts: a valve mechanism, which includes a locking mechanism to deactivate the device; and a pump which lies between the inlet and the outlet of the valve mechanism. This pressure in the system is maintained constantly by the pressure regulating balloon, through the control pump, to the cuff—except when the pump is squeezed. With each squeeze of the pump, 0.5 mL or so of the contained fluid is emptied into the balloon. This creates a vacuum in the pump that sucks fluid out of the cuff into the pump, thereby emptying the cuff of that amount and so reducing the compression of the urethra proportionately. In a well-fitting system, the cuff holds about 1–1.5 mL, and so two or three squeezes of the pump will empty the cuff through the pump and valve mechanism into the pressure regulating balloon.

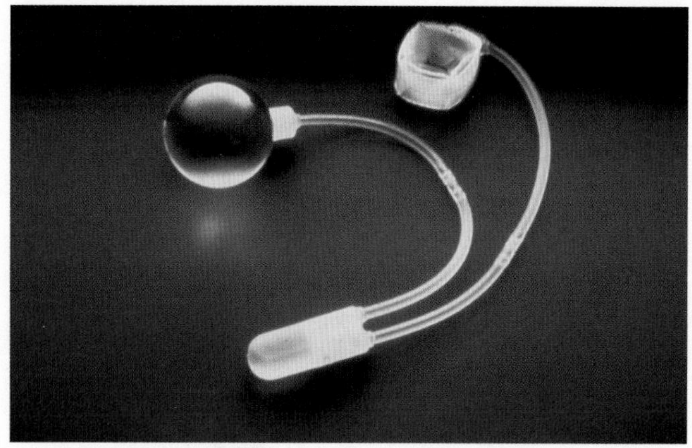

Fig. 4.3.5 The AMS 800 artificial urinary sphincter.
Reprinted from A. R. Mundy, *Urodynamic and Reconstructive Surgery of the Lower Urinary Tract*, Churchill Livingstone, UK, Copyright © 1993, with permission from Elsevier.

The fluid immediately starts to flow back from the balloon to the cuff but this is slowed by the valve mechanism in the control pump to give the patient one to two minutes to empty the bladder to completion before compression of the bladder outflow is restored (Fig. 4.3.6). It is this slow refill of the cuff from the balloon through the valve mechanism which means that the device is unable to compensate for sudden surges in intra-abdominal pressure as described above. This is an inherent disadvantage of the device but, on the other hand, makes for simplicity in its design and function. Other disadvantages[17] include the lack of adjustability of the cuff and the pressure regulating balloon. There is a range of cuff lengths and of balloon pressures to choose from, although in practice these are easy to decide and there seems little doubt that the simplicity of the device has been responsible for its durability over the 40 years or so of its existence.

Ultimately, as long as the device does not get infected at the time of implantation and as long as the area of the bladder outflow within the cuff can withstand the compression without being ischaemic (and assuming the patient was appropriately selected and the procedure performed competently) its durability is only limited by eventual degradation of the material it is made of. This usually presents as perforation of the cuff. When material degradation will occur is unpredictable but, in our experience, the life expectancy of the AMS is about 10–15 years. In practice, this means that if a man with post-prostatectomy incontinence—for example—has a device that is working satisfactorily three months or so after implantation, then it will probably last for the rest of his life.

The pressure within the pressure regulating balloon is determined by the tension in the wall of the balloon in relation to the volume of fluid that it is filled with. When expressed graphically, this pressure–volume relationship is an 'S-shaped' curve. As the balloon is filled from its initial collapsed state, there is little or no rise in pressure for the first 5 mL or so, and the curve is flat. As it fills from about 5–16 mL, there is a steady rise in pressure. During this rising phase of the curve, the pressure inside the balloon is directly related to the filling volume until a plateau phase is reached where a constant pressure is exerted despite further filling—at least up to a point. The pressure regulating balloon is specifically intended to work within the plateau phase in which there is very little pressure change for a relatively large change in volume (17–24 mL). If, for

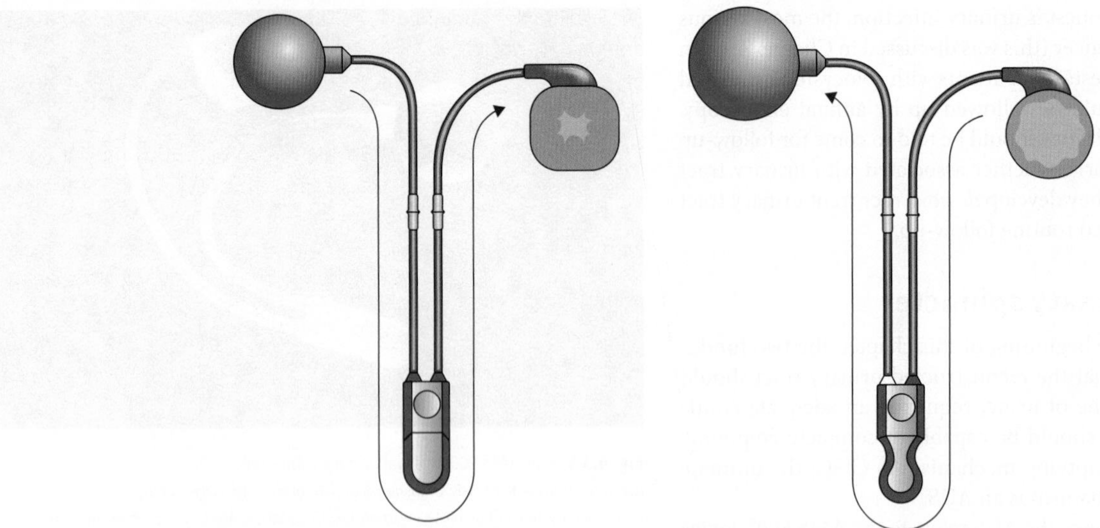

Fig. 4.3.6 The direction of fluid flow and pressure in the AMS 800 at rest and on squeezing the pump to empty the cuff and therefore initiate voiding.
Reprinted from A. R. Mundy, *Urodynamic and Reconstructive Surgery of the Lower Urinary Tract*, Churchill Livingstone, UK, Copyright © 1993, with permission from Elsevier.

any reason, the volume within the pressure balloon drops below a certain critical level, which is around 16 mL, the pressure will start to fall rapidly for very small changes in volume as the pressure–volume relationship drops out of the plateau phase into the ascending limb phase. This brief introduction to the physics of the device is relevant in troubleshooting the device in a patient with postoperative problems.

Patient selection

Patients who are suitable for an artificial sphincter are those who have pure sphincter weakness incontinence. The best examples are men with post-prostatectomy incontinence, with iatrogenic sphincter damage but with no detrusor dysfunction, and women with genuine stress incontinence. Other suitable cases include sphincter weakness incontinence due to trauma. Sphincter weakness incontinence in women is almost always treated by standard antistress incontinence procedures—these days, mainly slings, as described elsewhere in this volume—but these fail in some patients and the AUS may be used for salvage. In these patients, as after trauma, there is usually considerable scarring around the bladder outflow which makes the implantation more difficult and the results less satisfactory than in post-prostatectomy incontinence.

More commonly, a patient with neuropathic bladder dysfunction may be suitable for implantation of an AUS to correct sphincter weakness incontinence after the bladder dysfunction has been corrected. Bladder dysfunction usually dominates the clinical picture, even when significant sphincter weakness incontinence is present. This may require anticholinergic medication or intradetrusor injection of Botox or an augmentation cystoplasty to correct bladder overactivity and clean intermittent self-catheterization to provide bladder emptying. These need to be implemented before an AUS is implanted.

Urodynamic evaluation may be helpful in patients with non-neuropathic dysfunction to identify bladder dysfunction but is not essential in those without symptoms of frequency, urgency, or voiding difficulty. It is, however essential in patients with neuropathic dysfunction in whom multiple urodynamic problems are the rule and symptoms are unreliable.

Preoperative preparation

Critical factors are to make sure that bladder dysfunction has been identified and corrected and to make sure that the risk of infection of the device is reduced to an absolute minimum. We have already referred to bladder dysfunction but the patient with post-prostatectomy incontinence may also have a bladder neck contracture and this needs to be excluded by imaging or endoscopy. Urinary infection is excluded by culture within a week of the planned implantation. To reduce the risk of postoperative perineal contamination, a rectal washout before surgery is helpful. Bathing in an antibacterial solution immediately before surgery is also helpful.

There are a variety of ways of implanting the device according to the surgeon's inclinations, but there are essentially only two approaches: the approach for implantation of the cuff around the bulbar urethra in males; and the approach for implantation around the bladder neck in either sex.

Implantation of a bulbar urethral artificial sphincter

The commonest indication for implantation of an AUS is post-prostatectomy incontinence and here the cuff is almost always implanted around the bulbar urethra.[18]

Ideally one would be able to put all the components of the artificial sphincter in through one incision but this is fraught with problems, even in expert hands. We prefer to use two separate incisions: a midline perineal incision to place the cuff around the bulbar urethra; and a right groin incision to implant the pressure regulating balloon intra-abdominally, extraperitoneally in the right iliac fossa, and the control pump into a dartos pouch in the scrotum on that side (Fig. 4.3.7).

A midline perineal incision is extended down to and through the bulbospongiosus muscle. The urethra is then mobilized by division of Buck's fascia on either side to allow the creation of a plane around the urethra. A purpose-designed measuring tape is placed snugly around the urethra and the circumference is measured. This will usually be 4.5 cm, sometimes 4 cm, occasionally 5 cm, and rarely 5.5 cm. Even if the urethra seems to measure to 4 cm or less, the authors will place a 4.5 cm cuff, as many of these patients will

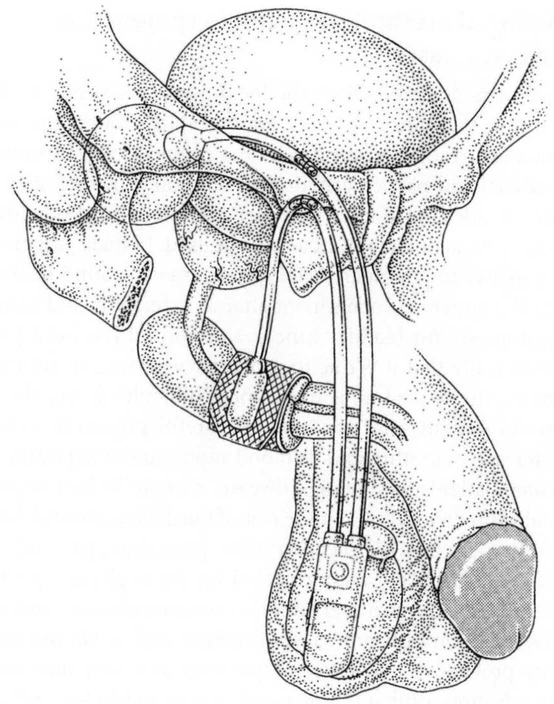

Fig. 4.3.7 The position of the AMS 800 after implantation in a man with post-prostatectomy incontinence.
Reprinted from A. R. Mundy, *Urodynamic and Reconstructive Surgery of the Lower Urinary Tract*, Churchill Livingstone, UK, Copyright © 1993, with permission from Elsevier.

require catheterization or endoscopy at some stage in the future and a 4.5 cm cuff will comfortably allow any form of lower urinary tract endoscopy.

A cuff of the correct size is then flushed with fluid to remove the air from the system. This fluid should be isotonic so that there will be no osmotic fluid shift after implantation. The empty cuff is then implanted at the chosen location. The wound is repeatedly washed with copious amounts of antibiotic solution (we use a mixture of gentamicin and rifampicin) even though the AMS 800 is coated with antibiotics—what AMS call the 'Inhibizone'.

A short skin crease incision is made over the right internal inguinal ring, through which the rest of the components will be placed and all the connections made. This is deepened down to the external oblique aponeurosis, which is incised over the internal inguinal ring and then deepened to create an extraperitoneal space of a size sufficient to accommodate the pressure regulating balloon. A 61–70 cmH_2O balloon is usually used. The balloon is flushed free of air, as with the cuff, dipped in antibiotic solution (the balloon is not coated with Inhibizone) and passed through the internal ring into the extraperitoneal space created for it. It is then filled with 20–25 mL of contrast solution. By putting the balloon in empty and then filling it, rather than putting it in already filled, the incision in the inguinal canal can be kept as small as possible to reduce the risk of subsequent hernia development.

A subcutaneous tunnel is then made from the inguinal canal to the scrotum by blunt dissection, keeping the dissection within the scrotum between the skin and the dartos layer, to create a subcutaneous dartos pouch for the control pump, which is filled in the usual way. The device is then deactivated by pressing the deactivation button. Finally, the tubing is trimmed to an appropriate length and connected with the purpose-made connectors.

Retropubic placement of an artificial urethral sphincter cuff in a male

This mainly applies to patients with neuropathic bladder dysfunction. There are two sites where the cuff might be placed: either above the level of the ejaculatory ducts, around the bladder neck in patients where the preservation of antegrade ejaculation is desirable; or around the membranous urethra when antegrade ejaculation is not an important consideration, when a cystoplasty is being performed at the same time, or is likely to be performed at some stage in the future. The more distal site keeps the cuff away from the cystoplasty. Because of the common need for a cystoplasty in patients with neuropathy we prefer the membranous urethra site for those patients.

Either way, the first step is to open the retropubic space to expose the bladder, the prostate, and endopelvic fascia of the pelvic floor. The endopelvic fascia and pubo-prostatic ligaments are then incised to expose the prostate and subprostatic urethra lying in the pubourethral sling of the levator ani. A curved instrument such as a Satinsky clamp is passed around the subprostatic urethra to create a plane for the cuff, the calibre of the urethra is measured, and a cuff of the appropriate size is implanted.

For a bladder neck placement, the layer of fascia that encloses the bladder neck, prostate, and genital structures must be broken through to allow the cuff to be passed between the bladder neck anteriorly, and the ejaculatory ducts, ampullae, and vesicles posteriorly. A Satinsky clamp can then be insinuated into this plane. When there is any difficulty performing this manoeuvre, it is helpful to open the bladder to allow the bladder neck and trigone to be seen and felt while the clamp is being manipulated through. The cuff is then placed and the procedure completed in the usual way.

As the retropubic space is open, implanting the pressure regulating balloon is straightforward but for a retropubic cuff we use a 71–80 cmH_2O balloon. The rest of the procedure is as described above for a bulbar urethral implant.

Retropubic placement of an artificial urethral sphincter cuff in a female

As in the male, the first step is to open the retropubic space to expose the bladder, bladder neck, proximal urethra, and the endopelvic fascia of the pelvic floor. The endopelvic fascia and pubourethral ligaments are then incised to expose and define the region of the bladder neck and the fascia around it and between it and the anterior vaginal wall. A plane is created for the cuff between the fascia and the anterior vaginal wall with a Satinsky clamp, as in the male. The rest of the implant proceeds as described above for the male except that the control pump is placed in a labial fat pad rather than a dartos pouch, and it is sensible to ensure that the pressure regulating balloon is placed outside the true pelvis to avoid problems during pregnancy and childbirth.

Postoperative management

The timing of activation is debatable. Obviously sufficient time should be allowed for the control pump to be manipulated comfortably and we therefore activate our patients about four to six weeks after the date of implantation. Activation is achieved by a firm squeeze of the pump to dislodge the deactivating valve. The patient is then taught how to use the device. The two points to emphasize are: firstly, to squeeze the pump as many times as it takes until it no longer refills promptly—to ensure that the cuff has been emptied completely—rather than to squeeze it a certain number of times; and, secondly, to avoid deactivating the device by pressing the deactivation button on the control pump accidentally.

Complications

These include: infection of the device; erosion, either internal or external; stress incontinence; device malfunction; or symptoms related to abnormal bladder behaviour.[19–21]

Infection and erosion are the most serious complications, as the device will have to be explanted. As the one inevitably leads to the other, it is often difficult to know which came first. Infection/erosion of the device occurs in about 2–4% of patients, which is about the same as for any implant. It rarely occurs, except as a result of contamination during implantation. It is therefore usually an early complication, which presents with redness, thickening, and tenderness of the tissues around the cuff and pump and around the incisions. It may be difficult, at first, to distinguish from a simple wound infection but this will settle completely with antibiotic treatment over a week or so. Although the clinical features may improve with antibiotics, true infection of the AUS is rarely, if ever eradicated, and it will be necessary to remove the device and reimplant another one three to six months later. If there is any doubt, an ultrasound scan or MRI of the device will usually settle the question. If there is any question of erosion internally, endoscopy and examination under an anaesthetic will resolve the issue.

Other problems are usually difficult to define from the clinical presentation. Nonetheless, examination may show features of local infection/erosion, that the device has been deactivated accidentally, or that the pump can only be squeezed once and then refills only very slowly, in which case there has been a leak of fluid from the system which can be confirmed radiologically. If clinical examination suggests that the device is working normally then it almost certainly is and there will be some other explanation for the patient's problems. Stress incontinence and abnormal bladder behaviour are usually apparent from the history and are confirmed by videourodynamics.

As discussed above a degree of stress incontinence is likely in all patients. Indeed, it is intrinsic in the design of the device that stress incontinence is not compensated for. The valve system of the control pump is specifically designed to slow down filling of the cuff from the balloon to allow adequate time for voiding after the pump has been squeezed, whereas rapid transmission would be necessary to compensate in time for surges in intra-abdominal pressure. If the patient is more than usually active and the degree of persistent leakage is troublesome, then the 61–70 cmH_2O pressure regulating balloon can be changed for a 71–80 cmH_2O balloon.

Device malfunction is rare until the device is at least a few years old. The commonest cause is a leak from a perforation in the cuff. The usual reason for this is that creases develop in the cuff with long-term use and this leads ultimately to perforation. A leak due to a perforation tends to progresses rapidly to complete loss of fluid from the system. As a result, a patient who has been continent for years suddenly becomes incontinent again over a period of a day or two. The leak is revealed by a plain X-ray which shows a deflated balloon if the device was filled with contrast.

The artificial urethral sphincter in conjunction with a cystoplasty

This is contraindicated when the local tissue has been irradiated and cannot, therefore, be used, for example, around the female urethra after irradiation for carcinoma of the cervix. In unirradiated patients and particularly in the commonest situation of neuropathic bladder dysfunction, or after cystectomy and substitution cystoplasty, an artificial sphincter can be used. In male patients, it is an easy matter to put an artificial sphincter cuff around the bulbar urethra if a patient is incontinent after a cystectomy and substitution cystoplasty for bladder cancer, assuming it has been proven urodynamically that it is due to sphincter weakness incontinence. In females, the procedure is much more difficult—hence the need for careful patient selection and for careful preservation of the sphincter-active urethra and its blood supply and innervation.

In some patients with benign disease, it might be best to put the artificial sphincter cuff, if not the rest of the device, around the urethra at the time of their reconstructive procedure, particularly in patients who are being reconstructed for exstrophy/epispadias or bilateral single ectopic ureters or other unusual circumstances who may have had multiple previous procedures and in whom a further separate procedure to implant a sphincter at a later date may be very much more difficult. Our practice is to put in the cuff on its own (which minimizes expense as well as the risk of infection) and then to put in the remainder of the device three months or so later if necessary having cystoscoped the patient to ensure that there are no problems of infection or erosion.

Lower urinary tract reconstruction for complications of the treatment of prostate cancer

There are a number of complications of the treatment of prostate cancer of which the best known and most frequently encountered are erectile dysfunction and sphincter weakness incontinence. Erectile dysfunction is discussed in detail elsewhere in this volume. Five other problems concern us here: sphincter weakness incontinence; bulbo-membranous urethral strictures after either radical prostatectomy or radiotherapy; bladder neck contracture after radical prostatectomy; prostatic urethral stenosis after radiotherapy; and urorectal fistula after either surgery or radiotherapy.[22]

Sphincter weakness incontinence

Most patients have a degree of sphincter weakness incontinence (SWI) after RP but not to a degree they find troublesome; maybe just enough for them to wear a small pad or just some tissue paper in their underpants as a precautionary measure. Some patients will tolerate even a substantial amount of incontinence without complaint whereas others will find any degree of urinary leakage as unacceptable. In other words, 'troublesome' means different things to different people. Assessment and treatment of an individual patient must take account of this. Other important factors include the measured volume of incontinence; the presence of frequency, urgency, and urge incontinence before treatment; the same symptoms since; the nature of the treatment and particularly whether any radiotherapy was given; and the time elapsed since treatment.

There is no effective medical treatment although some patients feel a degree of benefit from duloxetine particularly combined with physiotherapy to the pelvic floor musculature, especially in the early months while the incontinence may improve spontaneously.[23] Likewise, injections of materials such as macroplastique or collagen can give some temporary benefit particularly in mild degrees of incontinence after RP.[24,25] Essentially there are two effective treatments—the AUS and the male sling[26]—although the effectiveness of the male sling and the relative roles of the two procedures are controversial.[27,28]

If a patient is totally incontinent one year after a RP as sole treatment for his prostate cancer, having been completely asymptomatic beforehand, such that he may be completely continent all night (or otherwise when lying down) but has to squeeze his penis to get to the toilet to void first thing in the morning, and is then totally incontinent while he is up and around for the rest of the day, and is otherwise in good health, then he is an ideal candidate for an AUS. But if any of these factors varies significantly, then treatment becomes controversial. The controversy is relatively minor if the patient has had urge symptoms at any stage, or has had radiotherapy or other non-surgical treatment, or is in poor general health because these are adverse features for any treatment. It is in milder cases of SWI that the controversy exists. At this stage, it is true to say that an AUS is the gold-standard of treatment but for minor degrees of incontinence, the male sling may be just as effective with the advantage that there is no manipulation needed for it to function. The three questions to be answered for the male sling are: firstly, at what volume of leakage does the sling become unable to cope and only an AUS will be effective; secondly, are there any other reliable predictors of success or failure; and, thirdly, what is its long-term effectiveness. At present, there is only data up to three years of follow-up for the male sling, compared to more than 10 years for the AUS.

Bulbo-membranous urethral strictures

Urethral strictures are common in men in the age range of those being treated for prostate cancer and so some will inevitably have a stricture coincidentally. Equally some will develop a catheter stricture postoperatively whatever the surgery. But in both these situations it is likely to be an isolated bulbar stricture. The stricture problem that concerns us here are bulbo-membranous (so-called) 'sphincter strictures' which, by involving the sphincter mechanism, may compromise continence as may their treatment. Such patients are best managed by urethral dilatation, as this carries the lowest risk of further damage to the sphincter, supplemented where necessary by CISC to help maintain both outflow patency and sphincteric competence.[29]

Subsphincteric strictures, distinct from the sphincter, may require urethroplasty. This is controversial. Some surgeons advocate a traditional excision and end-to-end anastomosis for short strictures, as most surgeons would in normal circumstances. We feel that with a stricture so close to the vesicourethral anastomosis, a transection of the full thickness of the urethra and the corpus spongiosum is unwise because of the degree of damage to the vascularity this would cause. The safest approach in our view is a non-transecting approach: either a non-transecting excision and end-to-end anastomosis or a stricturotomy and patch procedure, both of which are described in Chapter 4.4.

Irradiation strictures are more complicated. After external beam radiotherapy (EBRT) alone, strictures are short, and are not commonly obliterative. They are relatively straightforward to treat, as described above, but with a lower success rate. After the combination of brachytherapy (BT) and EBRT, the average stricture length is significantly longer and nearly half of the strictures are obliterative.[30] They are therefore much more difficult to treat with correspondingly poorer results.

Bladder neck contracture

The anatomy of the bladder neck after a radical prostatectomy is sometimes difficult to determine but conceptually the whole of the membranous urethra will have been carefully preserved up to the level of the verumontanum. This is part of the prostatic urethra and it is to this point, or just below, that the bladder will be sutured to create a new bladder neck. Thus, in theory at least, there will be, postoperatively, from above down, the vesicourethral (VUA) anastomosis or bladder neck, a short length of inframontanal prostatic urethra, the sphincter-active membranous urethra, and the bulbar urethra. These may be difficult to distinguish radiologically in health because of the typically funnelled appearance of the VUA down to the physiologically contracted area of the sphincter, but they can be distinguished when a bladder neck contracture (BNC) is present if the contracture is restricted to the VUA and has not spread too far distally (as it commonly does) (Fig. 4.3.8).[22]

BNC is realtively common. It seems to be more common after removal of a large prostate when there is a longer gap to bridge with the VUA; and it is more common when there has been postoperative bleeding and haematoma formation, which tend to cause disruption of the anastomosis. Urinary extravasation from the anastomosis will obviously compound the problem.

Mild contractures can often be managed by instrumentation and more substantial contractures by either bladder neck incision or resection but the failure rate is high, indeed 27% are reported to

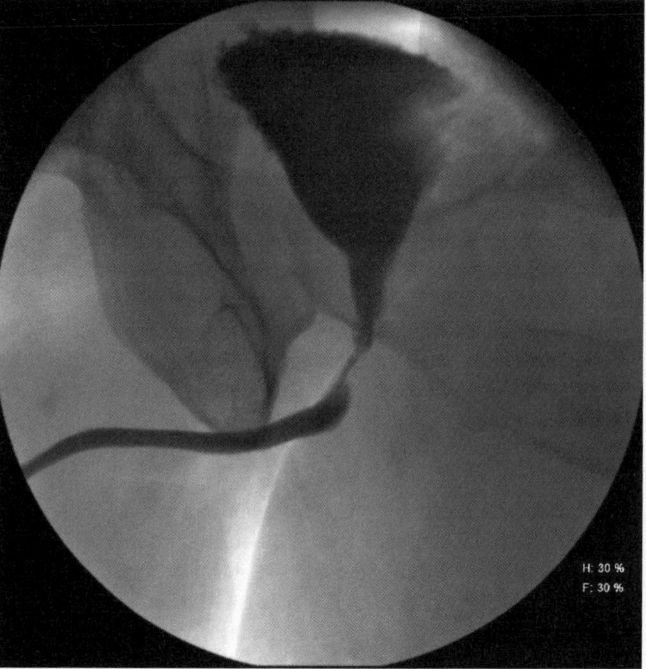

Fig. 4.3.8 The funnelled appearance of the bladder base, bladder neck, and vesicourethral anastomosis (VUA) after a radical prostatectomy (USM = urethral sphincter mechanism).

be refractory to three or more attempts at endoscopic treatment.[31] Some patients will either require repeated instrumentation or a long-term suprapubic catheter or surgical revision of the VUA. This has been infrequently reported but the results would seem to justify its more widespread use.

Several authorities have reported success with urethrotomy combined with implantation of a UroLume stent, coupled, when necessary, with implantation of an AUS to restore continence.[32] Long-term follow-up has dampened enthusiasm for this approach and a realistic view would be that it should be considered in those who wish to avoid major reconstructive surgery, or who are unfit for it, as long as they are prepared to accept repeated endoscopic intervention to deal with complications related to the stent. Thus, the only prospect for a cure for patients with a BNC refractory to a trial of instrumental treatment is revision of the VUA.[22,33]

Many patients have coexisting sphincter weakness incontinence but whether or not they had it before revision of their VUA, they have a very high risk of it afterwards. All patients should therefore be counselled that they should expect to have a two-stage procedure with revision of the VUA first and then implantation of an artificial urinary sphincter three to six months later.

Revision of the VUA is preformed through a transperineal incision. The bulbo-membranous urethra is mobilized up to the site of the obliteration and transected; all scarred tissue needs is excised until a relatively healthy 'bladder neck' can be defined or created. This is generally far forwards in the anterior triangle of the perineum and so consequently it is usual to have to separate the crura for access and common to have to perform an inferior wedge pubectomy to gain the access necessary to create an adequate 'bladder neck'. The urethra is then anastomosed to the 'bladder neck'. This is not an easy procedure. Indeed, we find that revision of a VUA is substantially more difficult than performing a bulbo-membranous anastomotic urethroplasty for a pelvic fracture urethral injury, which seems, at first sight, to be a very similar undertaking.

Prostatic urethral stenosis

This can occur after EBRT, brachytherapy, cryotherapy, or high-intensity focused ultrasound (HIFU) particularly when used sequentially. The obstructive problem is compounded in many patients by a small contracted bladder due to irradiation cystitis.

These patients often do not tolerate suprapubic catheters because of the irradiation cystitis, but they are often poor candidates for surgery because of significant co-morbidities as well as being prone to poor healing. However, if the stenosis is limited to the prostatic urethra, the bladder capacity is 250 mL or more, and the patient is fit and motivated, then we would advise a salvage radical prostatectomy.

Urorectal fistula

Urorectal fistula (URF)[22,34] is the least common but the most incapacitating of all the complications of the treatment of prostatic disease. There has been a considerable rise in the reported incidence of URF in recent years presumably because RP is much more commonly performed and because there is an increasing use of multimodality salvage treatment particularly, but not exclusively, with radiotherapy. Indeed, before 1997, 3.8% of URF were associated with radiation treatment; since then the percentage has risen to 49.6%.

The diagnosis of URF is straightforward: the patients present with urine leakage through the rectum. Some also have pneumaturia and/or faecaluria but this is very much less common. When faecaluria is present, it is an adverse prognostic feature.

Urorectal fistula following RP

This usually follows a direct injury to the rectum at the time of the robotic radical prostatectomy (RRP) and is reported to occur in 1%.[35] If a rectal injury is recognized and repaired at the time then in many, if not most instances, the repair heals, and a URF does not develop. If the injury goes unrecognized or if an attempted repair breaks down, a URF may result. This usually becomes apparent within two to three weeks. The first sign is usually urine leakage from the rectum. Faecaluria is much more serious as this indicates that the leak is large and less likely to be contained leading to local infection and abscess formation and, in more severe cases, to sepsis, and to Fournier's gangrene.[36] With prompt surgical attention, including wound drainage, suprapubic and urethral catheterization, and a defunctioning ileostomy or colostomy, spontaneous healing will occur in 50–75%.

Minor cases with an early postoperative 'leak', without constitutional symptoms, may heal spontaneously—usually within three months, before the track has epithelialized. In such circumstances a colostomy or ileostomy is unnecessary: the patient can be managed expectantly with catheterization alone. After three months the patient should be reinvestigated; an established URF which has epithelialized will never heal spontaneously.

A post-surgical URF is usually small and sometimes only apparent as an area of tethering on rectal examination. It is usually found to arise from the base of the bladder close to the posterior quadrant of the anastomosis, rather than from the anastomosis itself. The diagnosis is usually obvious clinically and is confirmed by a combined ascending urethrogram and micturating cystogram (Fig. 4.3.9). A cystoscopy and examination under general anaesthetic is often helpful in planning treatment.

A variety of techniques have been described to treat URF but there are three main approaches: the transperineal repair[37]; the York Mason transanorectal sphincter-splitting approach[38]; and the Parks per-anal rectal advancement flap.[39] The success rates of all three approaches are high, approaching 100%. Needless to say, not everybody who may be suitable for surgery wants it and there are reports of patients who manage for years with conservative management.[40]

The advantages of the transperineal approach are that the urinary tract and the rectum can be separated and both sides of the fistula closed independently; and that a tissue flap—usually the gracilis muscle—can be interposed to minimize the risk of recurrence when necessary. Access to the rectum is excellent and the rectal defect is relatively easily closed in two layers. The bladder base defect is more difficult to close because there is less flexibility of the tissues and it can often only be closed in one layer.

The disadvantages of both the Parks and the York Mason procedures are that access to the urinary component of the fistula is poor and that the exposure does not allow an interposition flap. An additional incision is necessary for this. The specific disadvantage of the York Mason procedure is the risk of anocutaneous fistulation and anal sphincter incompetence as a consequence of its division, which is at least part of the reason why the York Mason procedure is otherwise obsolete.

With all of these procedures, a covering colostomy is usually performed either at the time of the repair or, more commonly, beforehand and then closed a few weeks or months later. This means that

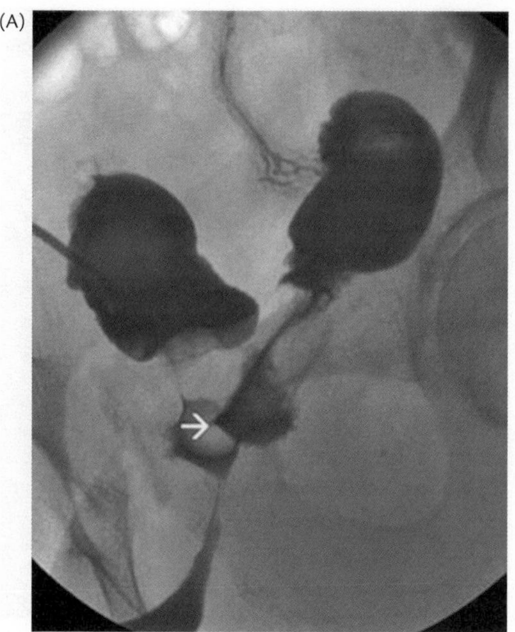

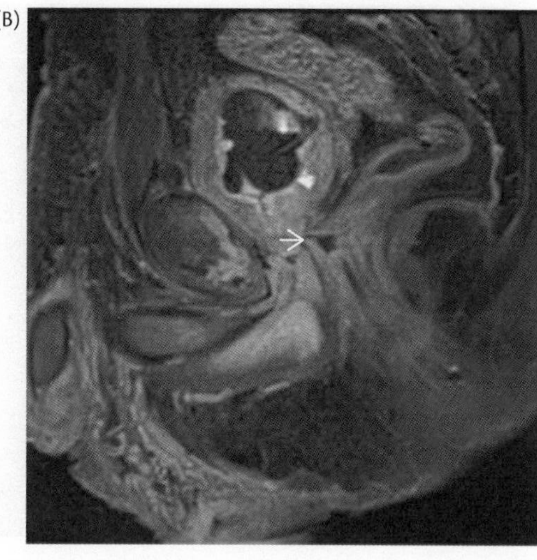

Fig. 4.3.9 (A) A urorectal fistula following radical prostatectomy (white arrow). (B) There is a direct communication without an intervening cavity clearly seen on both the urethrogram and the MRI scan.

for many, if not most patients, these are three-stage procedures, although experience shows that if it was not necessary acutely at its onset, a covering colostomy is unnecessary for the definitive repair. We certainly do not use one as a matter of routine although it is always safe to do so.

Urorectal fistula after radiotherapy, cryotherapy, or HIFU

This group is entirely different, if only because they often still have active disease.[22,41,42] The incidence is up to 10 times higher than in non-irradiated patients and is higher still in those who have combinations of treatment, approaching 100% when EBRT and BT are followed by salvage HIFU. The URF is generally larger, usually about 2 cm, with palpable fibrosis around it on rectal examination. Other complicating factors include irretrievable damage to the anal sphincter and severe anal stenosis, but this is rare.

The fistula usually develops 18 months to 3 years after radiotherapy and typically follows a biopsy of the anterior rectal wall. This should therefore be avoided if at all possible, although close surveillance of the rectum is clearly important because of the significant risk of rectal cancer in irradiated patients. The onset is much less dramatic than in post-surgical URF and is rarely associated with life-threatening sepsis. A faecal diversion is therefore rarely required except for postoperative patients after salvage RP following previous failed EBRT.

Two distinct subgroups can be identified on MRI and retrograde urethrography: those with a fistula causing a direct communication between the prostatic urethra and the rectum, without an intervening cavity and with a definable if small prostatic remnant; and those with an intervening cavity (Fig. 4.3.10), generally made up of those who had had salvage cryotherapy, or HIFU in addition to EBRT who have no discernible prostate.

Even in the patients without cavitation, the urinary tract defect is far less amenable to direct closure than in the post-surgical patient because of both its size and the limited tissue flexibility. Thus, some authors have used a buccal mucosal graft, supported by a gracilis flap, to close the defect. We prefer salvage RP if the prostate is still present because it is more reliable and because the cancer is still active in a significant percentage of patients.

The rectal defect is then closed with inverting interrupted mattress sutures; the omentum is mobilized as an interposition flap; and the VUA is then performed.

In patients with a cavity, the wall of the cavity and the material contained within it is excised transperineally or abdominoperineally and a gracilis or omental flap, respectively, is mobilized and deployed to obliterate the cavity, or abdomino-perineally using the omentum rather than the gracilis to obliterate the cavity and support the VUA.

The postoperative recovery is slow in all these patients. Healing of the VUA may take two to three months and they often require protracted wound drainage and up to 12 weeks of catheterization before complete healing is shown radiologically and the catheters can be removed. Most have limited bladder capacity and poor bladder compliance, and therefore have a degree of frequency of urination in order to stay socially dry. An AUS for sphincter weakness incontinence is necessary in about 50%. Interestingly, we have never (yet) had an instance of failed closure of the rectal effect; the problem, if any, is always with the VUA.

Omental wrap

On most occasions, there is no particular concern about any anastomosis during the types of procedures described but in those patients with more unusual conditions or after repeated surgery or radiotherapy, the vascularity of the operative field may be impaired, or the potential risk of infection or extravasation may need to be mitigated, or a potential dead space may need to be filled. These problems are best addressed by wrapping the anastomosis with the omentum. Omental wrapping will almost certainly mean the extension of a midline abdominal incision up to the xiphisternum, mobilizing the omentum from the transverse colon and the greater curvature of the stomach on its right gastroepiploic arcade and redeploying it around any anastomosis so that the risk of infection and extravasation may be minimized.

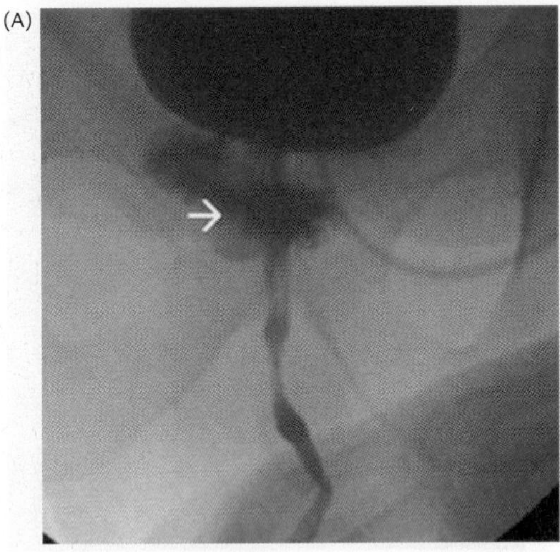

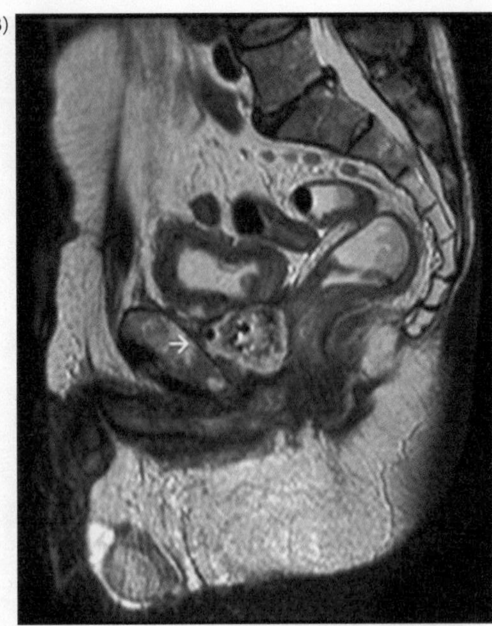

Fig. 4.3.10 (A) A urorectal fistula following external beam radiotherapy and salvage high-intensity focused ultrasound (white arrow). (B) There is an intervening cavity clearly seen on both the urethrogram and the MRI scan.

Lower urinary tract reconstruction for complications of gynaecological or rectal cancer treatment

In both situations, affected patients are not only susceptible to the complications of surgery, putting the ureters, bladder, and urethra at risk, but also to the complications of chemoradiation, which both groups commonly receive. Irradiation cystitis and proctitis are common and can be incapacitating and are probably more common than urologists believe.[43] The problem cases that present urologically are those in which there is fistulation, particularly those that are due primarily to radiotherapy, whether or not surgery may be an associated factor.

In women after treatment for cervical cancer, this normally manifests itself as vesicovaginal or vesicovaginorectal or, less commonly, rectovaginal fistulation. The problems, other than the symptoms and other adverse effects of the fistula, such as skin excoriation, are chronic pelvic sepsis, a small contracted bladder, a similarly affected rectum and vagina; possible compromise of the urinary and faecal sphincter mechanisms; the possibility of irradiation enteritis affecting other parts of the bowel within the irradiated area; and, especially, at least some degree of compromised healing if surgical intervention is contemplated.

In patients of either sex after anterior resection of the rectum,[44] fistulation from the coloanal anastomosis is also a potential problem—prostatorectal in men and rectovaginal in women. Women are relatively protected from complications after abdominoperineal resection of the rectum because the faecal stream is diverted by the end sigmoid colostomy and because of the presence of the uterus and vagina. In men, damage to the base of the bladder or, more commonly, to the prostatic or membranous urethra may leave a fistula through to the perineal wound with an intervening cavity in the pre-sacral space, which may be extensive. This cavity is commonly chronically infected and painful (Fig. 4.3.11).

The state of the bowel is particularly important because the bowel is commonly used for surgical salvage of such problems—whether as a cystoplasty, a conduit, or a continent diversion. In such circumstances, adequate evaluation of the structure and the function of the bowel is therefore important, particularly by radiological contrast studies and colonoscopy. These may indicate where segments of bowel are diseased even if they look macroscopically normal at laparotomy. When exploring such patients, it is commonly necessary to do intestinal resections because of the cause of irradiation enteritis as well as having to reconstruct the urinary tract.

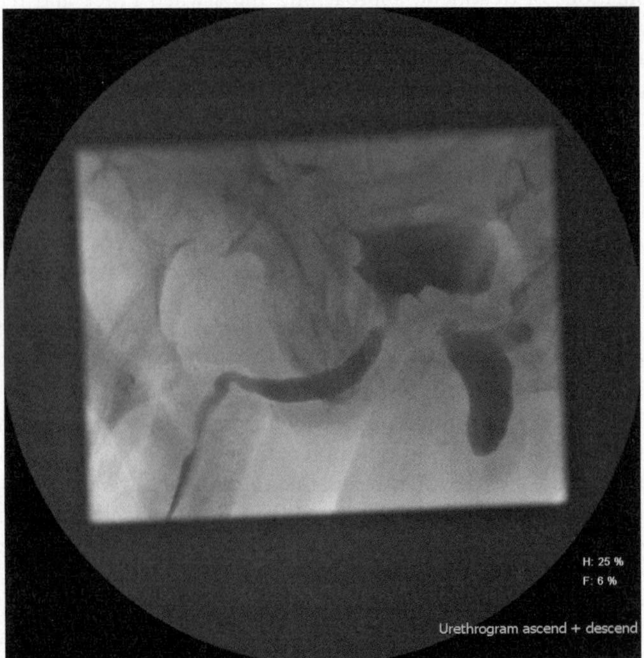

Fig. 4.3.11 A cavity behind the bladder and urethra after chemoradiation and an abdominorectal excision of the rectum for rectal cancer.

The principles of treatment are, first and foremost, to be realistic and to be honest about the risks of poor healing. Many patients with faecal fistulation will already have had a defunctioning colostomy or, more commonly these days, ileostomy and will be relatively happy with it. So, if a rectal reconstruction fails or is inappropriate they will have lost nothing. Urine leakage, one way or another, coupled with chronic sepsis, is the usual indication for operation. The problem, in women, is the potential for curing a vesicovaginal fistula by major surgery, and then finding postoperatively that they are nearly as wet from sphincter weakness incontinence. Careful preoperative evaluation, although essential, may not be very helpful in guarding against the risk of this.

In both sexes, careful excision of heavily irradiated tissue, the use of healthy tissue for repair and the liberal use of omental wrapping to support anastomoses and eliminate dead space are critically important. Equally important is the management of the postoperative period, which can regularly take up to three months, with careful use of catheters, drains and, when necessary, faecal diversion.

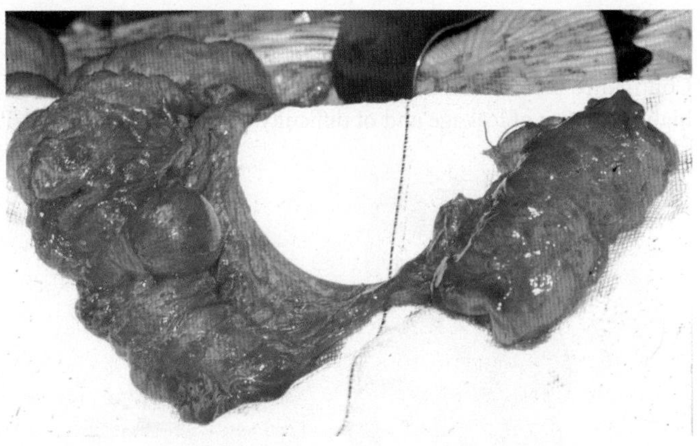

Fig. 4.3.12 Colocysto/vaginoplasty. The right colon and the proximal transverse colon have been mobilized on the marginal artery. The bowel has been divided into two parts, carefully maintaining the continuity of the vascular pedicle. The proximal two-thirds will be anastomosed to the bladder remnant as a substitution cystoplasty. The distal third will be sutured to the introitus as a substitution vaginoplasty.

Vaginoplasty

Occasionally there is a need to augment or substitute the vagina for congenital or acquired conditions, including those just discussed, either as an individual problem or as part of a more generalized pelvic reconstruction. In such cases a segment of colon can be mobilized, either from the sigmoid colon or as described for substitution cystoplasty. Indeed, a suitably long segment of colon can be split—maintaining vascular continuity—in order to use the bulk of it for substitution cystoplasty and the remainder of it for substitution vaginoplasty (Fig. 4.3.12).

Continent urinary diversion—the Mitrofanoff procedure

Some patients are simply not reconstructable or are not sufficiently healthy to withstand a reconstruction. Simply bypassing the lower

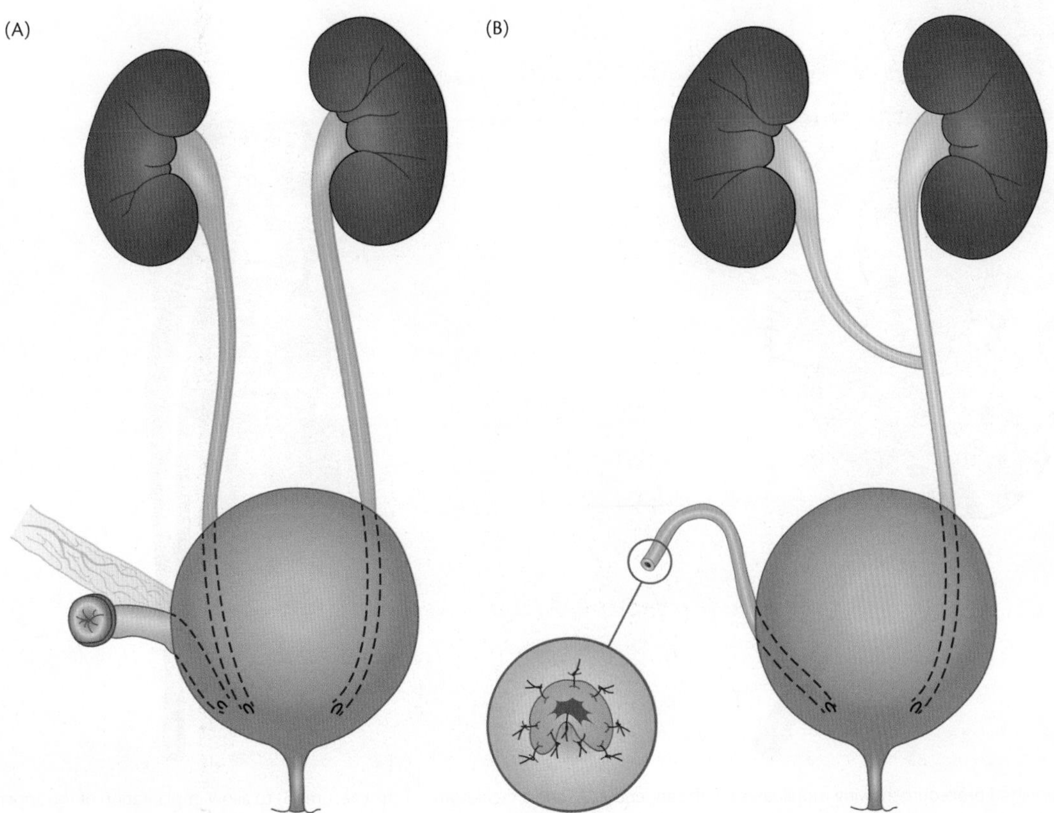

Fig. 4.3.13 The 'classic' Mitrofanoff procedure using either the appendix (A) or the ureter (B) as the continent catheterizable channel.
Reprinted fromA. R. Mundy, *Urodynamic and Reconstructive Surgery of the Lower Urinary Tract*, Churchill Livingstone, UK, Copyright © 1993, with permission from Elsevier.

urinary tract and performing a Mitrofanoff procedure is an alternative, albeit one which we would regard as very much second best. Continence after a Mitrofanoff procedure is unreliable; there is a high incidence of leakage and of difficulty in catheterization and a consequent need for revision. There is also a high incidence of stone disease and recurrent infection in such bladders and these adverse effects steer us away from the Mitrofanoff procedure when there is a reconstructive alternative. Nonetheless, if the choice is between a

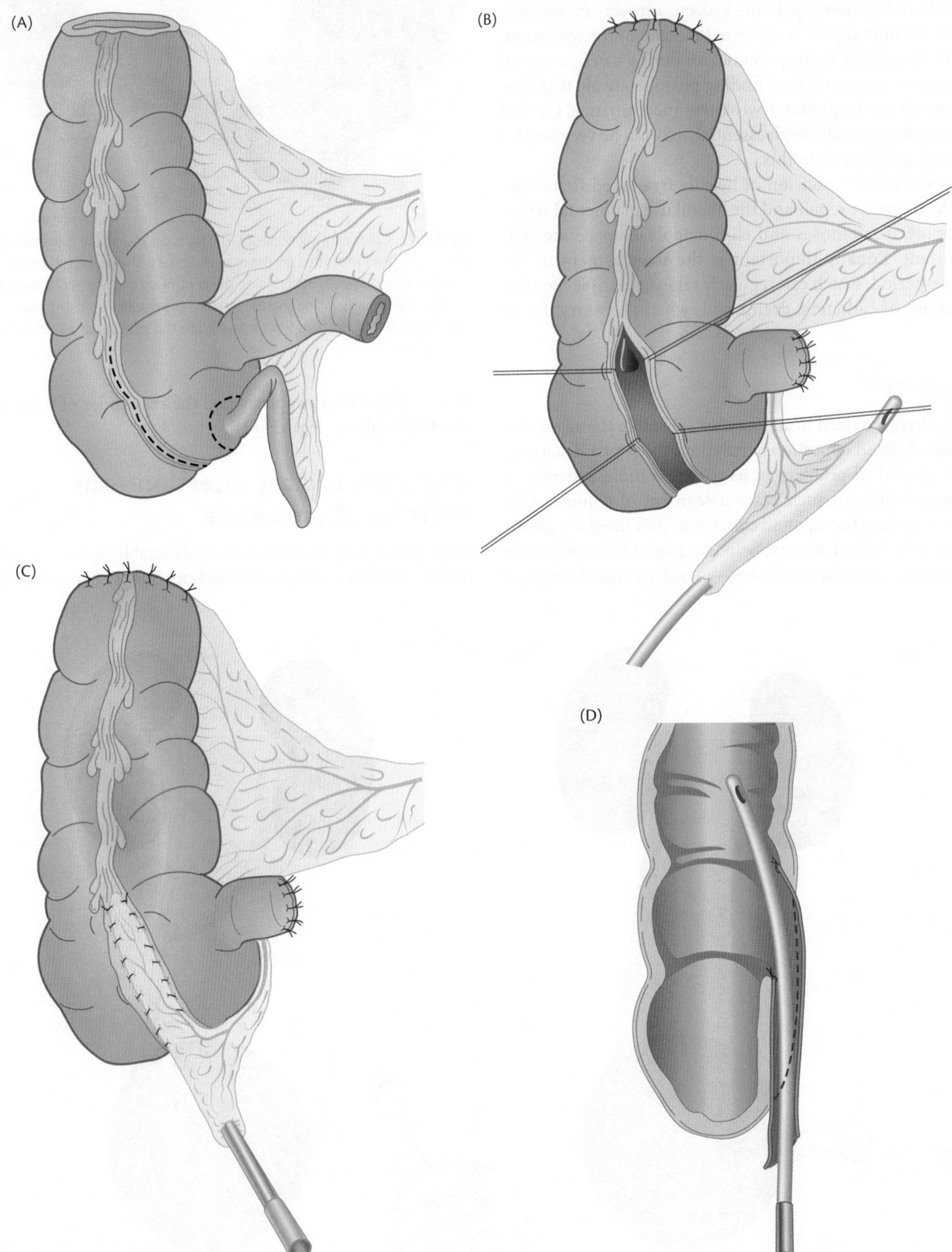

Fig. 4.3.14 A Mitrofanoff procedure showing mobilization of the appendix (A) and a taeniotomy of the caecum (B) to allow implantation of the appendix into the trench (C), thereby creating a catheterizable channel into the colon (D), which will be used, in this case, as a neobladder. The reimplantation technique creates a valve mechanism which acts as a continence mechanism.

Reprinted from A. R. Mundy, *Urodynamic and Reconstructive Surgery of the Lower Urinary Tract*, Churchill Livingstone, UK, Copyright © 1993, with permission from Elsevier.

Mitrofanoff and a conduit urinary diversion, we would go with the patient's wishes if s/he preferred the superior 'body image' that goes with a Mitrofanoff.[45–47]

If the bladder is normal or relatively normal and the problem is with the outflow tract, then a 'standard' Mitrofanoff procedure is suitable and gives good, if not very good results (Fig. 4.3.13). A continent catheterizable channel is created either by creating a channel from the abdominal wall to the bladder using the appendix implanted into the bladder using a tunnel technique to make it continent; or, if the appendix is unavailable or unsuitable, the distal ureter on one side can be brought out to the skin as the channel using the natural ureterovesical junction as the 'continence mechanism'. When the bladder is compromised, some sort of cystoplasty is necessary. In those patients who have a useful capacity to their native bladder, then an augmentation cystoplasty and the creation of a continent catheterizable channel anastomosed to native bladder gives the best outcome in our experience. When the bladder has to be removed or has no useful capacity, it will have to be replaced by a neobladder. We tend to use the right colon for the neobladder in a Mitrofanoff, in the same way as we do in any other patient requiring a substitution cystoplasty. In such circumstances, it seems reasonable to use the native appendix, whenever possible, as the continent catheterizable channel (Fig. 4.3.14).

When the appendix is inadequate or absent, we prefer the Monti-type continent catheterizable channel to any alternative. Where possible we tend to bring it out through the umbilicus, partly for its better cosmetic result but also because the shorter the passage through the abdominal wall, the less prone the continent catheterizable channel is to kinking, and therefore of difficulties with catheterization.

Ileal conduit urinary diversion

If all else fails or is inappropriate, conduit urinary diversion may be in the patient's best interests. Indeed, in the elderly or frail individual or for those who are relatively unconcerned with cosmetic issues, an ileal conduit urinary diversion may be the simplest, quickest, and easiest way to resolve their problem. It is not without its problems and, in the long term, the need for revision of a retracted stoma, or for a parastomal hernia or for a poorly draining loop, is substantial. By and large, these are relatively easy to rectify compared with the complications of an inappropriately advised major reconstructive procedure in an elderly or frail individual for whom major surgery is always going to be an unrealistic option.

References

1. Lapides J, Diokno AC, Silber SJ, Lowe BS. Clean, intermittent self catherisation in the treatment of urinary tract disease. *J Urol* 1972; **107**:458–61.
2. Bramble FJ. The treatment of adult enuresis and urge incontinence by enterocystoplasty. *Br J Urol* 1982; **54**:693–6.
3. Mundy AR, Stephenson TP. "Clam" ileocystoplasty for the treatment of refractory urge incontinence. *Br J Urol* 1985; **57**:641–6.
4. Mundy AR. *Urodynamic and Reconstructive Surgery of the Lower Urinary Tract*. London, UK: Churchill Livingstone, 1993: Chapter 15.
5. Mundy AR, Nurse DE, Dick JA, Murray KHA. Continence and potency preserving cystoprostatectomy and substitution cystoplasty for patients with bladder cancer. *Br J Urol* 1986; **58**:664–8.
6. Hautmann RE, Egghart G, Frohneberg D, Miller K. The ileal neobladder. *J Urol* 1988; **139**:39–42.
7. Studer UE, Casanova GA, Zingg EJ. Bladder substitution with an ileal low-pressure reservoir. *Eur Urol* 1988; **14**(Suppl 1):36–40.
8. Abol-Enein H, Ghoneim MA. A novel uretero-ileal reimplantation technique: the serous lined extramural tunnel. A preliminary report. *J Urol* 1994; **151**:1193–7.
9. Thomas PJ, De Sousa NM, Mundy AR. The effects of detubularisation and outflow competence in substitution cystoplasty. *Br J Urol* 1996; **78**:681–5.
10. Greenwell TJ, Venn SN, Mundy AR. Augmentation cystoplasty. *BJU Int* 2001; **88**:511–25.
11. Scott FB, Bradley WE, Timm GW. Treatment of urinary incontinence by an implantable prosthetic urinary sphincter. *J Urol* 1974; **112**:75–80.
12. Knight SL, Susser J, Greenwell T, Mundy AR, Craggs MD. A new artificial urinary sphincter with conditional occlusion for stress urinary incontinence: preliminary clinical results. *Eur Urol* 2006; **50**:574–80.
13. Staerman F, G-Llorens C, Leon P, Leclerc Y. ZSI 375 artificial urinary sphincter for male urinary incontinence: a preliminary study. *BJU Int* 2013; **111**(4 Pt B):E202–6.
14. Vilar FO, Araujo LA, Lima SV. Periurethral constrictor in paediatric urology: long-term follow-up. *J Urol* 2004; **171**:2626–8.
15. Valerio M, Jichlinski P, Wieland M, *et al.* New concept of artificial muscle for urinary incontinence treatment. *Eur Urol Suppl* 2010; **9**:327 (Abstract 1045).
16. Chung E, Ranaweera M, Cartmill R. Newer and novel artificial urinary sphincters (AUS): the development of alternatives to the current AUS device. *BJU Int* 2012; **110**(Suppl 4):5–11.
17. Nurse DE, Mundy AR. One hundred artificial sphincters. *Br J Urol* 1988; **61**:318–25.
18. Mundy AR, Andrich DE. Artificial urinary sphincter. In: Austoni E (ed). *Atlas of Reconstructive Penile Surgery*. Pisa, Italy: Pacini Editore Medicina, 2010.
19. Venn SN, Greenwell TJ, Mundy AR. The long-term outcome of artificial urinary sphincters. *J Urol* 2000; **164**:702–7.
20. Montague DK. Artificial urinary sphincter: long term results and patient satisfaction. *Adv Urol* 2012; **2012**:835290.
21. Van der Aa F, Drake MJ, Kasyan GR, Petrolekas A, Cornu JN. Young Academic Urologists Functional Urology Group. The artificial urinary sphincter after a quarter of a century: A critical systematic review of its use in male non-neurogenic incontinence. *Eur Urol* 2013; **63**:681–9.
22. Mundy AR, Andrich DE. Posterior urethral complications of the treatment of prostate cancer. *BJU Int* 2012; **110**:304–25.
23. Filocamo MT, Li Marzi V, Del Popolo G, *et al.* Pharmacologic treatment in postprostatectomy stress urinary incontinence. *Eur Urol* 2007; **51**:1559–64.
24. Kylmala T, Tainio H, Raitanen M, Tammela TL. Treatment of postoprative male urinary incontiennce using transurethral macroplastique injection. *J Endourol* 2003; **17**:113–15.
25. Westney OL, Bevan-Thomas R, Palmer JL, Cespedes RD, McGuire EJ. Transurethral collagen injections for male intrinsic sphincter deficiency: the University of Texas-Houston experience. *J Urol* 2005; **174**:994–7.
26. Rehder P, Gozzi C. Transobturator sling suspension for male urinary incontinence including post-radical prostatectomy. *Eur Urol* 2007; **52**:860–7.
27. Bauer RM, Bastian PJ, Gozzi C, Stief CG. Postprostatectomy incontinence: all about diagnosis and management. *Eur Urol* 2009; **55**:322–33.
28. Comiter CV. Male incontinence surgery in the 21st century: past, present and future. *Curr Opin Urol* 2010; **20**:302–8.
29. Mundy AR, Andrich DE. Urethral strictures. *BJU Int* 2010; **107**:6–26.
30. Elliott SP, Meng MV, Elkin EP, McAninch JW, Duchane J, Carroll PR, CaPSURE Investigators. Incidence of urethral stricture after primary treatment for prostate cancer: Data from CaPSURE. *J Urol* 2007; **178**:529–34.
31. Elliott SP, McAninch JW, Chi T, Doyle SM, Master VA. Management of severe urethral complications of prostate cancer therapy. *J Urol* 2006; **176**:2508–13.

32. Anger JT, Raj GV, Delvecchio FC, Webster GD. Anastomotic contracture and incontinence after radical prostatectomy: A graded approach to management. *J Urol* 2005: **173**:1143–6.
33. Pfalzgraf D, Beuke M, Isbarn H, *et al.* Open retropubic reanastomosis for highly recurrent and complex bladder neck stenosis. *J Urol* 2011; **186**:1944–7.
34. Mundy AR, Andrich DE. Urorectal fistulae following the treatment of prostate cancer. *BJU Int* 2011; **107**:1298–303.
35. McClaren RH, Barrett DM, Zincke H. Rectal injury occurring at radical retropubic prostatectomy or prostate cancer. *Urology* 1993; **42**:401–5.
36. Eke N. Fournier's gangrene: a review of 1726 cases. *Brit J Surg* 2000; **87**:718–28.
37. Kilpatrick FR, Mason AY. Postoperative recto-prostatic fistula. *Br J Urol* 1969; **41**:649–54.
38. Parks AG, Motson RW. Peranal repair of rectoprostatic fistula. *Br J Surg* 1983; **70**:725–6.
39. Venkatesan K, Zacharakis E, Andrich DE, Mundy AR. Conservative management of uro-rectal fistulae. *Urology* 2013; **81**(6):1352–6.
40. Lane BR, Stein DE, Remzi FH, Strong SA, Fazio VW, Angermeier KW. Management of radiotherapy induced rectourethral fistula. *J Urol* 2006; **175**:1382–8.
41. Samplaski MK, Wood HM, Lane BR, Remzi FH, Lucas A, Angermeier KW. Functional and quality-of-life outcomes in patients undergoing transperineal repair with gracilis muscle interposition for complex rectourethral fistula. *Urology* 2011; **77**:736–41.
42. Zinman L. The management of the complex recto-urethral fistula. *BJU Int* 2004; **94**:1212–3.
43. Turina M, Mulhall AM, Mahid SS, Yashar C, Galandiuk S. Frequency and surgical management of chronic complications related to pelvic radiation. *Arch Surg* 2008; **143**:46–52.
44. Hayne D, Vaizey CJ, Boulos PB. Anorectal injury following pelvic radiotherapy. *Br J Surg* 2001; **88**:1037–48.
45. Mitrofanoff P. Cystostomie continente trans-appendiculaire dans le traitement dess vessies neurologiques. *Chirurgie Pediatrie (Paris)* 1980; **21**:297–305.
46. Duckett JW, Snyder HM 3rd. The Mitrofanoff principle in continent urinary reservoirs. *Semin Urol* 1987; **5**:55–62.
47. Leslie B, Lorenzo AJ, Moore K, Farhat WA, Bägli DJ, Pippi Salle JL. Long-term followup and time to event outcome analysis of continent catheterizable channels. *J Urol* 2011; **185**:2298–302.

CHAPTER 4.4

Urethral strictures

Anthony R. Mundy and Daniela E. Andrich

Introduction to urethral strictures

A urethral stricture is a constriction of the lumen of the urethra caused by the development of a circumferential scar of the corpus spongiosum. By consensus, the term stricture only applies to the anterior urethra—that is to say, anatomically speaking, the spongiose urethra. By the same consensus, constrictions of the lumen of the posterior urethra are called stenoses or contractures.

Urethral strictures have always been common and the history of the subject stretches back to 3,000 BC. Urethral dilators have been found in the tombs of the pharaohs so that they might be able to catheterize themselves or dilate their own strictures in the afterlife.[1]

The treatment of strictures has hardly changed since 3,000 BC. In the early part of the first century AD, urethrotomy was developed for more recalcitrant strictures. Urethroplasty has only been in use for the last 100 years or so and only in the last 40 years with any regularity.[1]

Incidence and aetiology

In the nineteenth century, it was estimated that 30–50% of the adult male population had a urethral stricture.[1] The estimated prevalence in the United Kingdom at the moment is about 40 per 100,000, rising with age from about 10 per 100,000 in young adults to over 100 per 100,000 in the elderly.[2]

Historically strictures were due either to gonococcal urethritis or to fall-astride injuries. Gonococcal urethral strictures are still prevalent in many parts of the world and trauma is increasing everywhere. Most strictures these days in the developed world occur for no apparent reason (Table 4.4.1).[3] They typically occur at the junction of the proximal and middle-thirds of the bulbar urethra, are found in young adults and have a typical membrane-like appearance—radiologically and at the time of surgery (Fig. 4.4.1). Whether these are simply idiopathic or whether they have a congenital basis is not clear. However, there is a body of opinion that suggests that these are congenital, occurring, as they do, at the junction of that part of the urethra that is common to both sexes and is derived from the urogenital sinus, with that part of the urethra that is only found in males and is derived from the urethral folds, where normal continuity between the two develops in the foetus due to rupture of the urogenital membrane.[4]

That aside, the other causes of urethral strictures include lichen sclerosis (LS), scarcely recognized 40 years ago[5] and, in the trauma category, iatrogenic trauma—the new scourge. Iatrogenic strictures of the urethra typically follow instrumentation and the greater the degree of instrumentation the greater the likelihood of strictures. Thus, passage of a large calibre resectoscope for transurethral resection of the prostate has the highest incidence but any form of instrumentation of the urethra, including catheterization, may be associated with stricture formation.

Table 4.4.1 Aetiology of urethral strictures

Penile	
Idiopathic	15%
Iatrogenic	40%
Inflammatory	40%
Traumatic	5%
Bulbar	
Idiopathic	40%
Iatrogenic	35%
Inflammatory	10%
Traumatic	15%

Reproduced from Mundy AR and Andrich DE, 'Urethral strictures', *BJU International*, Volume 107, Issue 1, pp. 6–26, Copyright © 2011 BJU International, with permission from John Wiley and Sons Ltd.

The stricture process associated with LS typically starts at the external meatus and spreads proximally up the penile urethra. Fall-astride injuries typically occur in the middle and proximal thirds of the bulbar urethra. Iatrogenic strictures due to instrumentation typically affect the meatus, the penoscrotal junction, and the sphincter mechanism, spreading more proximally from there. The other sites of iatrogenic trauma are related directly to the nature of the underlying problem. Thus, strictures following hypospadias occur in the distal penile urethra and those arising from anterior resection of the rectum, or following radiotherapy for prostate cancer typically occur in the posterior urethra.

Pathology

The cause of strictures and their pathogenesis have not been widely studied. In many instances, it is probably ischaemia that is the single commonest factor in the development of a stricture, particularly with catheter strictures, which have been described as 'pressure sores' of the urethra. When strictures have been studied histologically, the underlying cause seems to be a local change in the lining epithelium from its typical pseudo-stratified columnar epithelium to a stratified squamous epithelium.[6] This is a more fragile type of

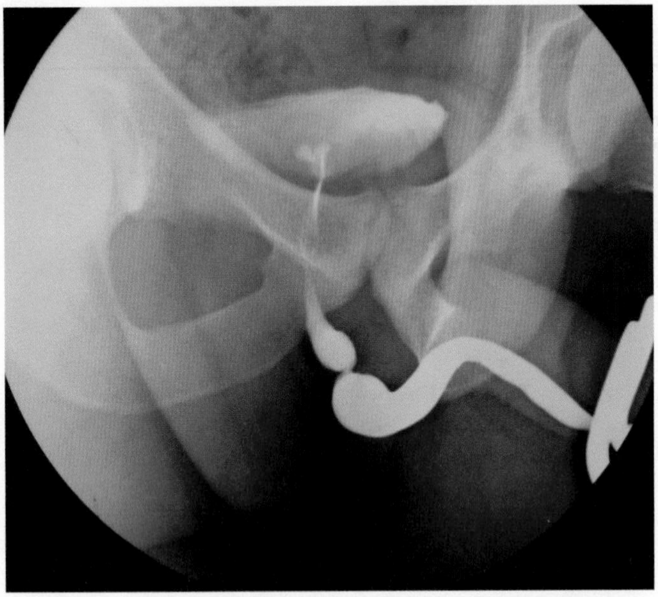

Fig. 4.4.1 A typical idiopathic stricture of the bulbar urethra—short, sharp, and at the junction of the proximal and middle-thirds—putatively congenital.
Reproduced from Mundy AR and Andrich DE, 'Urethral strictures', *BJU International*, Volume 107, Issue 1, pp. 6–26, Copyright © 2011 BJU International, with permission from John Wiley and Sons Ltd.

epithelium and tends to split, leading to microscopic foci of fibrosis. The epithelium of the spongiose (anterior) urethra has, in any case, no subepithelial support to it comparable to the muscularis mucosae in the intestine. As a result, when the epithelium is breached, there is immediate exposure of the subepithelial spongy tissue and, because of the pressure of voiding, extravasated urine is forced into the corpus spongiosum under pressure exacerbating the fibrosis.

With the passage of time, and with repeated episodes of the underlying cause (such as gonorrhoea), these microscopic foci of fibrosis coalesce, and if they become circumferential may lead to stricture formation by constriction of the lumen of the urethra. They then become obstructive—and obstruction in itself may cause squamous metaplasia as described above, thereby potentially extending the stricture process proximally (Fig. 4.4.2).

In experimental animal models, using electrocautery as a model of iatrogenic injury, a similar appearance is found of local fibrosis of the corpus spongiosum made worse by urinary extravasation.[7] When the urine is infected, the fibrosis spreads more widely and more quickly, giving the histological appearance of thrombophlebitis.

The metaplastic change proximal to the definitive stricture accounts for the so-called 'wash-leather' appearance of the urethra at operation when these strictures are explored. Squamous metaplasia may be reversible when the underlying cause is treated or in abeyance, but this reversibility cannot be expected.

At a more detailed level of investigation, it would appear that the fibrosis of stricture disease is not the same as in wound healing elsewhere. It is apparent that there is an unusually high proportion of type 1 collagen compared with type 3 collagen, which is usually prominent in a scar elsewhere.[8]

In LS, the pathology is different.[9] This condition used to be called balanitis xerotica obliterans, and it is still commonly known as this

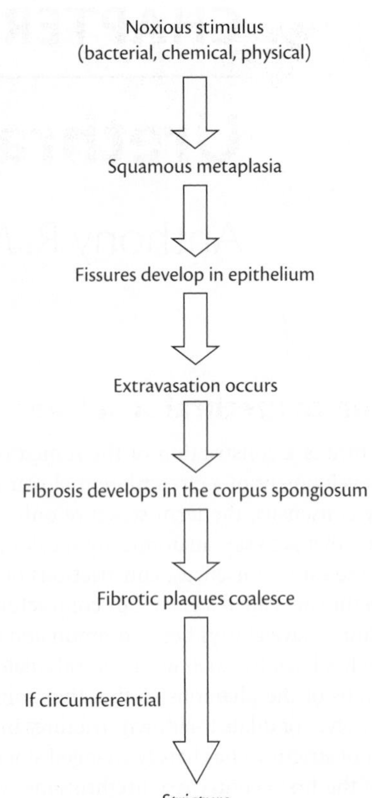

Fig. 4.4.2 Pathology of urethral stricture.
Reproduced from Mundy AR and Andrich DE, 'Urethral strictures', *BJU International*, Volume 107, Issue 1, pp. 6–26, Copyright © 2011 BJU International, with permission from John Wiley and Sons Ltd.

in the form of its initials BXO. LS/BXO is an atrophic rather than a proliferative fibrosis. The cause is not known for sure but there are features that suggest an autoimmune cause, although an infective cause has been proposed. It typically starts as a patch of whiteness on the glans or the prepuce and, as these patches coalesce, so phimosis may result. Left to itself, the local skin changes of LS progress (Fig. 4.4.3). Circumcision is thought to be curative of both the prepucial and the glans lesions. When the prepuce is removed, the glans 'dries out'. Scarring of the glans, around the meatus, if allowed to progress, leads to meatal stenosis, and this meatal stenosis spreads proximally up the urethra—possibly by propagation of the LS itself or alternatively by causing obstruction and then the squamous metaplasia and progressive fibrosis described above. It typically affects only the penile urethra and stops at the junction of the bulbar urethra (Fig. 4.4.4).

In our view, it is best to consider trauma, particularly external trauma, as being an entirely separate condition from stricture disease—particularly in the anterior urethra. The pathology is entirely different and although the type of surgery for trauma is similar to the surgery for stricture disease, the scope and scale are entirely different. Comparing an anastomotic repair for a bulbar urethral stricture with the same procedure for a straddle injury; or the surgery for an iatrogenic sphincter stricture with that for a pelvic fracture urethral injury is like comparing chalk with cheese. The pathology and treatment of urethral trauma will be considered in Chapter 4.8.

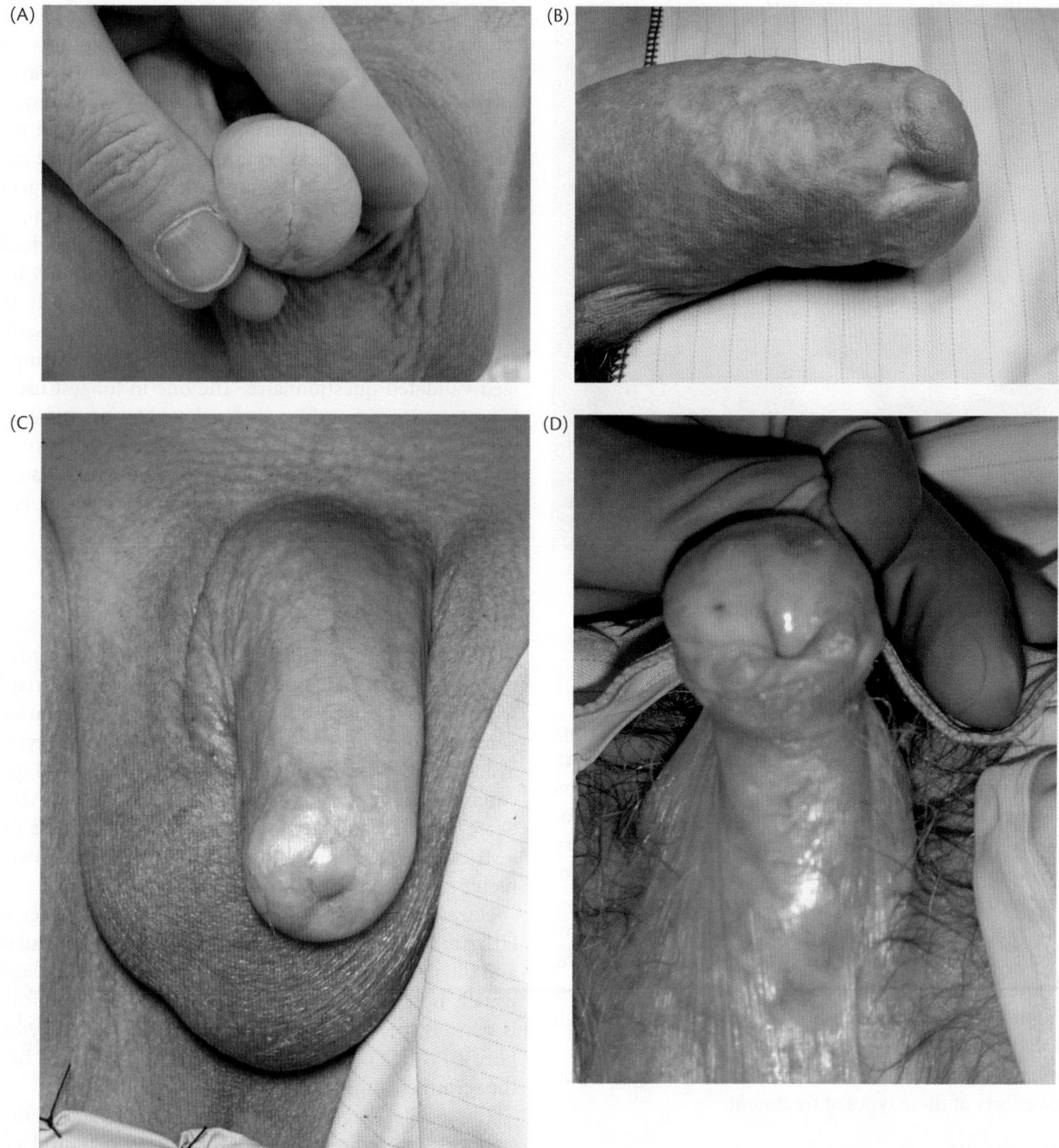

Fig. 4.4.3 The clinical appearance of worsening degrees of lichen sclerosis: (A) a white rim to the meatus (pathognomonic); (B) loss of the normal contour of the glans and the coronal sulcus and meatal regression in a circumcised patient; (C) fusion of the foreskin to the glans in an uncircumcised patient; and (D) as with (C), but with oedema and ulceration of the glans.

Reproduced from Mundy AR and Andrich DE, 'Urethral strictures', *BJU International*, Volume 107, Issue 1, pp. 6–26, Copyright © 2011 BJU International, with permission from John Wiley and Sons Ltd.

Clinical features and natural history

The progressive obstruction of the urethral lumen causes voiding dysfunction and, ultimately, secondary effects further up the urinary tract. Voiding dysfunction presents as hesitancy, pain, or discomfort on voiding, a poor stream, terminal dribbling and, importantly, a feeling of incomplete bladder emptying. All these symptoms may be present and a poor stream is typical but the sensation of incomplete bladder emptying is the symptom that is most closely linked to urethral stricture disease. Haematuria and urinary tract infection may be associated, as may discomfort on voiding, but these are less frequent.[1]

As the degree of obstruction progresses (Table 4.4.2), so the incidence of urinary tract infection increases as residual urine in the obstructed bladder becomes more common. Haematuria or urinary tract infection may lead to acute retention in patients with particularly tight strictures. Even a very small blood clot can obstruct a tightly constricted lumen as can urinary tract infection, by causing oedema.

With progressive long-standing outflow obstruction, the bladder tends to become thick-walled and trabeculated, and residual urine develops. With recurrent infection, epidydimo-orchitis or prostatitis may develop, and stone formation in the obstructed bladder is common. When associated with recurrent infection, fistulation

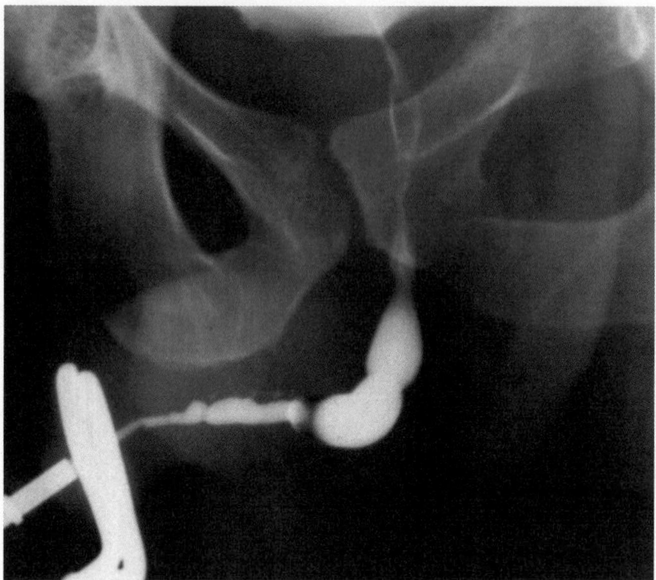

Fig. 4.4.4 The typical appearance of a penile urethral stricture in a patient with lichen sclerosus, but not pathognomonic.
Reproduced from Mundy AR and Andrich DE, 'Urethral strictures', *BJU International*, Volume 107, Issue 1, pp. 6–26, Copyright © 2011 BJU International, with permission from John Wiley and Sons Ltd.

through the urethra and into the periurethral tissues may develop, which may ultimately lead to the so-called watering can perineum.

With increasingly prolonged and severe outflow obstruction, upper urinary tract emptying is affected and so hydroureteronephrosis develops and ultimately the same problems with the lower urinary tract can develop in the upper urinary tract with distension, infection, and stone formation, as well as simple loss of renal function.

Traditional treatment of urethral stricture disease is with urethral dilatation or urethrotomy; both may cause progression of the urethral stricture disease with longitudinal extension of the fibrosis along the length of the urethra, and horizontal extension through the urethral wall and into the periurethral tissues.

Septicaemia and haematuria, or frank urethral bleeding, are also common side effects of these types of treatment.

Clinical assessment

Patients normally present with obstructed voiding. Although strictures can present at any age, they become increasingly common with age. Therefore, in many patients over the age of 50, the prostate may be considered as the source of symptoms rather than a urethral stricture, but a urethral stricture should always be borne in mind—particularly in younger patients. When trauma is the cause, this is usually obvious from the patient's history. In those with an iatrogenic cause the details may be forthcoming, but many patients have no memory of, for example, hypospadias surgery as a child and only their parents, if still alive, may be able to supply any detail. Nonetheless, scarring from surgery will be visible if looked for.

On physical examination, the important points to notice are the stigmata of previous treatment or alternatively the features, often undramatic, of LS. Occasionally patients present with acute retention. Symptomatic assessment is best made using a standardized validated questionnaire. The one in longest use is the AUA Symptom Score, but this was developed for use in benign prostatic hyperplasia. However valuable it may have been shown to be with stricture disease in the past, a purpose-designed patient-reported outcome measure (PROM) which has been developed specifically for urethral stricture disease is better.[10]

Table 4.4.2 Complications of untreated urethral strictures

Thick-walled, trabeculated bladder	85%
Acute retention	60%
Prostatitis	50%
Epidiymo-orchitis	25%
Periurethral abscess	15%
Stones (bladder, urethra)	10%
Hydronephrosis	20%

Reproduced from Mundy AR and Andrich DE, 'Urethral strictures', *BJU International*, Volume **107**, Issue 1, pp. 6–26, Copyright © 2011 BJU International, with permission from John Wiley and Sons Ltd.

Investigation

The next step in assessment is a urinary flow rate study. Here a distinction from benign prostatic hyperplasia (BPH) may be possible when this is the likely alternative diagnosis. BPH causes a slow and generally intermittent stream. A urethral stricture typically causes a slow steady stream with a 'plateau' appearance (Fig. 4.4.5). The combination of a poor score with a PROM (or AUA Symptom Score) and a plateau-type flow rate is more or less diagnostic of a stricture. The combination is also useful for following up treatments after treatment.

Ultrasound is a useful way of assessing the bladder and particularly in looking for a thick-walled bladder trabeculated bladder and the presence of residual urine. More detailed evaluation is not usually necessary, but if the bladder shows any abnormality then it is sensible to scan the kidneys as well to look for hydroureteronephrosis. If this is present, then the next step would be to measure the serum creatinine.

The specific diagnostic technique is retrograde urethrography. In a retrograde urethrogram (RUG), the urethra is displayed by injecting contrast retrograde from the meatus upwards and into the bladder. It is important that the study should show the full length of the urethra up to and through the urethral sphincter mechanism into the prostatic urethra and bladder. The best images are produced with the patient in an oblique position and as steeply obliquely as possible to show the full length of the urethra. In the anteroposterior plane, the urethra is foreshortened and a stricture may be missed or otherwise underestimated in length.

Many patients with lower urinary tract symptoms undergo cystoscopy, particularly flexible cystoscopy, at the time of the initial consultation. This is very helpful in diagnosing the presence of a stricture and even its site, but because the scope cannot be passed any further is not very helpful at determining the length or any abnormalities associated with the stricture as described above. Many urologists will go no further then a flexible cystoscopy, typically because for them the treatment is inevitably going to be urethrotomy and so a urethrogram is not performed. However, it is the authors' view that a urethrogram should always be performed to give the detail necessary for proper evaluation.

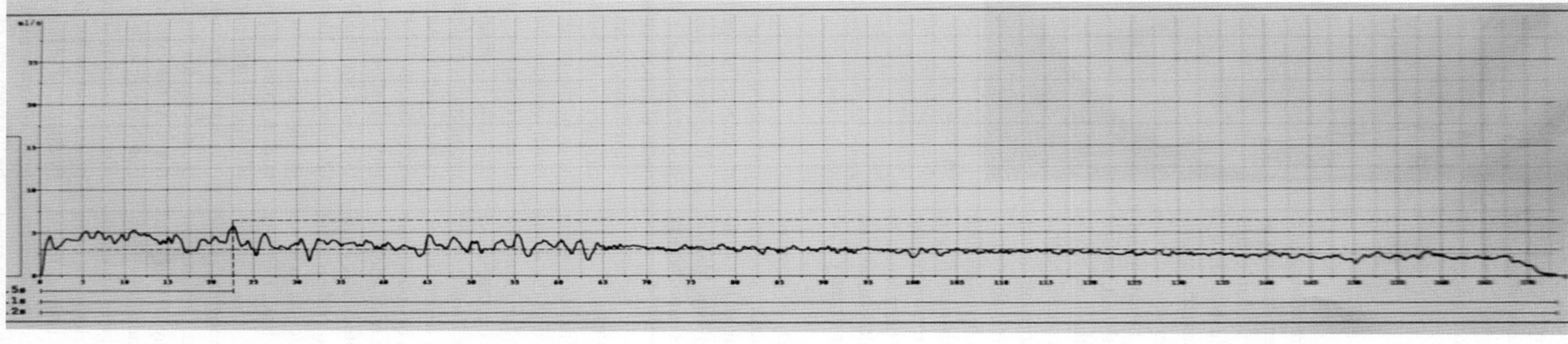

Fig. 4.4.5 The typical 'plateau' appearance of the flow curve in a patient with a stricture.
Reproduced from Mundy AR and Andrich DE, 'Urethral strictures', *BJU International*, Volume 107, Issue 1, pp. 6–26, Copyright © 2011 BJU International, with permission from John Wiley and Sons Ltd.

Some urologists favour the use of ultrasound of the stricture itself. Our view is that although ultrasound may produce impressive images of the stricture, they tend to be less satisfactory the more proximally in the urethra that the stricture is located. Unfortunately, the proximal bulbar urethra is the commonest site where strictures develop.

Treatment

Evaluation with a view to treatment

In the absence of complications, treatment is for symptoms and if the patient's symptoms are not troublesome, treatment may not be necessary. However, symptoms alone are not always reliable. It is in this situation that the flow rate is particularly valuable. Thus, if the patient has obstructive symptoms, without haematuria or urinary infection, and a flow rate more than 15 mL per second with no abnormality on ultrasound of the bladder, then he can be followed prospectively by watchful waiting, repeating the ultrasound and flow rate studies every six months or a year. If the flow rate is reduced to 10–15 mL per second, then he should be counselled that this is abnormal and that regular review becomes more important. Between 5 and 10 mL per second, whether or not there is abnormality of bladder ultrasound study, the patient should be counselled that he is likely to need intervention in the relatively near future. With flow rates below 5 mL per second, a definitive treatment plan should be made. When there is urinary infection or haematuria or urethral bleeding, an abnormality on the bladder ultrasound, and particularly if there are abnormalities on the upper urinary tract then there should be early definitive treatment.

In patients who present with acute retention it may be possible, with the passage of a catheter, to get through the stricture and provide drainage, otherwise a suprapubic catheter is placed. It is common experience that catheterization will allow both the bladder and the urethra to settle down and improve. Why this improvement occurs is not entirely clear.

Instrumental treatment of urethral strictures

Traditional treatment of a urethral stricture is by dilatation using metal dilators. These are metal rods that are curved at the distal end. They come in a graded set usually measured in the French or Charriere scale—in which the number refers to the circumference in millimetres—from something in the region of six French (6 Fr) up to something in the region of 32 French (32 Fr) depending on the exact type used. Typically, these urethral dilators or 'sounds' are passed from smaller to larger size with the intention of dilating the urethral stricture gently. Some surgeons have advocated more forcible dilatation at different times in history. There is no evidence that either gentle or forcible dilatation produce better outcome in terms of cure but forcible dilatation would, intuitively at least, be more likely to cause complications.

The alternative to dilatation is urethrotomy. Although available for nearly 2,000 years urethrotomy was initially blind. Urethrotomy these days means direct vision internal urethrotomy (DVIU) and was introduced by Sachse in 1978.[11] In DVIU, an endoscope identifies the site of the stricture and allows the passage of an endoscopic blade alongside the telescope, through the stricture to open it up. This may be opened in any plane, but dorsally is the thinnest part and ventrally is the thickest part of the corpus spongiosum, and it seems more sensible to cut into the thickest part to avoid perforation of the urethra and damage to the anatomically related structures, and specifically, the corpus cavernosum.

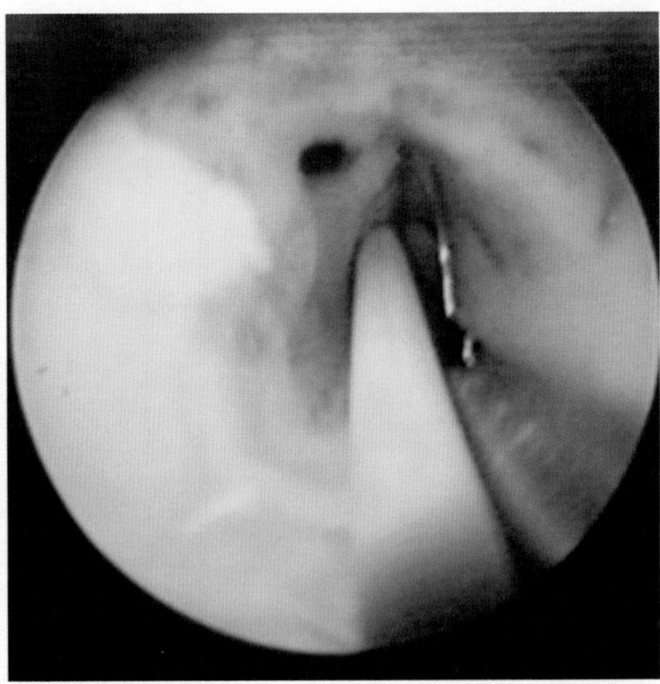

Fig. 4.4.6 Endoscopic photograph of a direct vision internal urethrotomy (DVIU) through a stricture (with an associated false passage) with a fine ureteric catheter (as an alternative to a guidewire) through the stricture to show the way.
Reproduced from Mundy AR and Andrich DE, 'Urethral strictures', *BJU International*, Volume 107, Issue 1, pp. 6–26, Copyright © 2011 BJU International, with permission from John Wiley and Sons Ltd.

It is safest to pass a guidewire or a ureteric catheter through the stricture first as it is remarkably easy to lose one's way out of the urethral lumen without such a guide (Fig. 4.4.6).

Urethrotomy and dilatation are equally effective for a short sharp stricture of the bulbar urethra. For longer strictures and for strictures in the penile urethra or elsewhere in the urethra, they are much less effective. Thus, about 50% of patients with short bulbar strictures may be 'cured' by a single urethrotomy or dilatation. The cure rate is considerably less in other parts of the urethra and if urethrotomy or dilatation need to be repeated a second time in the bulbar urethra. After two attempts, any further instrumentation is never curative.[12–14] Repeated dilatation may be perfectly satisfactory palliation as long as it is infrequent and causes no complications and specifically septicaemia or bleeding. A minor degree of bleeding is not likely to be troublesome, but even a minor degree of infection can be troublesome, and serious septic episodes can be fatal. A course of prophylactic antibiotics at the time of instrumentation is therefore sensible.

Palliation by instrumentation may be particularly valuable for the elderly, for the unfit, and when the stricture is in certain locations. At the external meatus, the patient can perform the dilatation himself with a purpose-designed dilator, a bit like a golf tee. More proximal strictures—so-called 'sphincter strictures' after a prostatectomy for BPH or for prostate cancer—are best managed by dilatation in order to maintain continence.[1,15] When the sphincter is compromised by stricture formation, then a dilatation may be the only way of maintaining both an unobstructed outflow and reasonable sphincter function without resorting to a staged form of surgery—firstly to excise the stricture and perform an end-to-end anastomosis, and then subsequently to implant an artificial urinary sphincter to take care of the inevitable incontinence that follows the excision of the stricture and the end-to-end anastomotic repair, the urethral sphincter being the only remaining sphincter mechanism after a prostatectomy.

Self-dilatation, typically by the passage of a self-lubricating catheter of 12–16 Fr calibre is, of course, dilatation by any other name.[16] Nonetheless, this might be useful to a patient who wishes to avoid surgery and particularly for patients who live in difficult locations where there is no easy availability of medical care. Self-catheterization therefore makes the patient independent of medical care, providing all goes well.

Stents

Another alternative to urethrotomy and dilatation with or without subsequent self-catheterization is implantation of an intraurethral stent. There are two urethral stents that have been used in patients with urethral strictures. The first is the Wallstent or UroLume® (Pfizer Inc, UK) and the Memokath® (Engineers and Doctors A/S Ltd, Hornbaek, Denmark). The UroLume is implanted after the stricture has been opened up by DVIU and it then becomes incorporated, in time, into the urethral wall. The Memokath is also placed after a DVIU, but is not incorporated into the urethral wall. There is quite a lot of information in the literature about the UroLume but not much about the Memokath.[17] There was a great deal of enthusiasm about the initial results of the UroLume,[18] but unfortunately the initial enthusiasm has not been borne out in the long term.[19] Patients suffer discomfort; it is particularly uncomfortable in the bulbar urethra to sit on and it makes using a bicycle almost impossible; and there is also a marked degree of postmicturition dribbling and a corresponding reduction in ejaculation. In theory, both can be removed if they are ineffective. In practice, the Memokath can usually be removed fairly simply, but that is not always the case; and removing a UroLume usually requires open surgery and, very often, a difficult and sometimes staged repair.

In short, if a DVIU or urethral dilatation fail or are inappropriate for a stricture and if the patient is fit enough and wishes to have further treatment that treatment will be a urethroplasty.

There are a few patients who have undergone repeated surgery or for whom surgery would be too much of an undertaking for whom perineal urethrostomy might be a more satisfactory alternative.[20]

Urethroplasty

As with any tube in the human body, there are three possible approaches for dealing surgically with a stricture. Either the strictured segment can be excised and an end-to-end anastomosis performed; or it can be excised and replaced; or it can be incised and patched to restore urethral calibre.[1]

The procedure of choice, currently, is excision and an end-to-end anastomosis, as this restores the urethra more closely to normal and gives the most satisfactory results in terms of patency and durability with the least adverse effects.[21] Unfortunately, it can only be used for short strictures in the bulbar urethra; short because of the limited length of the urethra, and in the bulbar urethra because excision of a segment of the penile urethra would cause penile buckling on erection. Excision and end-to-end anastomosis is also possible in the posterior urethra. This will be covered in the section on posterior urethral trauma in Chapter 4.5.

When excision and end-to-end anastomosis is not possible because of the length or location of the stricture, the next question is whether it is appropriate to preserve the strictured segment, open it, and then patch it to restore its calibre; or whether to excise it and replace it. There is, at the moment, no possibility of replacing it with some 'off-the-shelf' segment of artificial urethra. It can only be replaced using the patient's own tissues and generally because tubed grafts and tubed flaps do not take well, a circumferential reconstruction must be done in stages.[22] As a consequence of this—if for no other reason—a stricturotomy and patch is preferred in most instances where an excision and end-to-end anastomosis is not possible because of the length or location of the stricture. Excision and circumferential repair is only performed when the affected segment of the urethra has to be excised and when the staged approach and the inevitable consequences of that are acceptable.

Bulbar urethroplasty

Bulbar urethral strictures are the most common type of stricture and in the untreated patient, or the patient who has failed to respond to only one or two instrumentations, the stricture is usually short and to be found at the junction of the proximal and middle-thirds of the urethra. Such patients are usually amenable to excision and end-to-end anastomosis.

Anastomotic urethroplasty

The principles of anastomotic urethroplasty are illustrated in Figure 4.4.7. The bulbar urethra is exposed through a midline perineal incision and mobilized from its attachment to the corpora cavernosa dorsally, by dividing Buck's fascia on either side, and from its attachment to the perineal body posteriorly. Passing a catheter then identifies the strictured segment. The urethra is transected at this point and the stricture excised. The two ends are then spatulated and an overlapping anastomosis performed.[1,23]

Augmented anastomotic urethroplasty

In some circumstances, the two ends of the urethra can be brought together end-to-end without tension but cannot be spatulated and overlapped without tension. In such circumstances, an augmented anastomotic urethroplasty can be performed. Both ends are spatulated dorsally and sutured around a buccal mucosal graft quilted onto the tunica albuginea (Fig. 4.4.8). The two ends are then sutured together ventrally.[1,22,24]

Augmentation urethroplasty—the 'stricturotomy and patch' procedure

The anastomotic procedure is possible because of the 'stretchability' (a more accurate term than elasticity) of the bulbar urethra. It is limited by the degree to which the urethra can be stretched, spatulated, and brought together without tension after excision of the stricture.

If the length of the stricture is too long, then a stricturotomy and patch procedure is performed. The stricturotomy may be dorsal, lateral, or ventral[25] in the proximal bulbar urethra—but a dorsal stricturotomy is preferred by many (including ourselves[26]) because the stricturotomy is then through the thinnest and least vascular segment of the bulbar urethra, and the patch can be quilted onto the tunica albuginea to fix it in place and stabilize more easily. A ventral stricturotomy is also possible in the bulbar urethra because of the thickness of the ventral corporal spongiosum but it is more difficult to fix the graft into position in this segment.

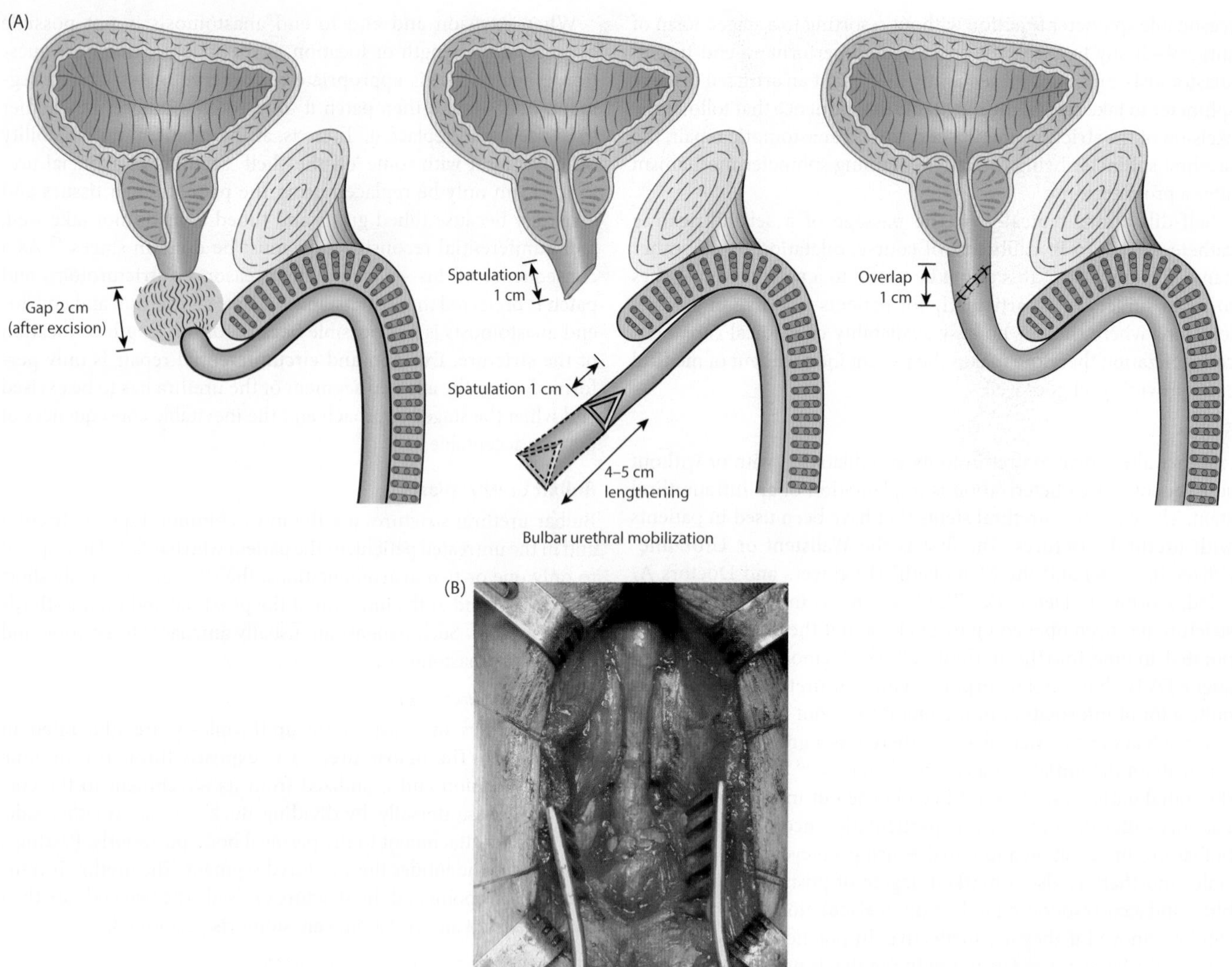

Fig. 4.4.7 (A) The principles of a bulbar anastomotic urethroplasty and (B) the postoperative appearance.
Reproduced from Mundy AR and Andrich DE, 'Urethral strictures', *BJU International*, Volume 107, Issue 1, pp. 6–26, Copyright © 2011 BJU International, with permission from John Wiley and Sons Ltd.

The procedure is shown diagrammatically in Figure 4.4.9. The urethra is mobilized in much the same way as for an anastomotic urethroplasty and a dorsal stricturotomy is then made, opening into normal calibre, healthy-looking urethra at either end. The 'patch' to hold the stricturotomy open thereafter is a graft. Traditionally, skin was used as the graft but skin is fastidious and does not take as readily as does buccal mucosa harvested from the inside of the cheek, so this is now the material of choice.[27] Some surgeons close the donor site but others feel that this tends to cause more swelling and discomfort than leaving the donor site to heal by second intention,[28] although this is controversial.

Having harvested the graft, it is trimmed of extraneous tissue and then quilted on to the tunica albuginea in the region of the stricturotomy. The margins of the urethra are then sewn to the margins of the graft.

Follow-up after bulbar urethroplasty

After either form of bulbar urethroplasty, a catheter of 14 Fr or 16 Fr calibre is left in the urethra for two to three weeks to allow healing and can then be removed. It is safest to perform a pericatheter urethrogram before removing the catheter to be sure that the suture lines are completely healed.

Patients are followed up postoperatively according to an individual surgeon's protocols—there is no proven means of follow-up. We prefer to follow-up the patient with a flow rate and a PROM three months after operation and a flow rate, a PROM, and a urethrogram six months after that. Then, if all is well, the patient can be discharged.

Penile urethroplasty

As mentioned above, excision and end-to-end anastomosis is inappropriate in the penile urethra as this would cause buckling of the penis and this is uncomfortable at rest let alone on erection. Thus, strictures of any length must be treated by a stricturotomy and patch procedure unless the urethral segment must be excised for whatever reason, in which case a staged repair is performed. Excision and circumferential reconstruction is occasionally required for conditions such a condition such as amyloidosis, or an arteriovenous malformation or tumour, but it is very much more commonly required because of severe LS or failure of previous hypospadias surgery.

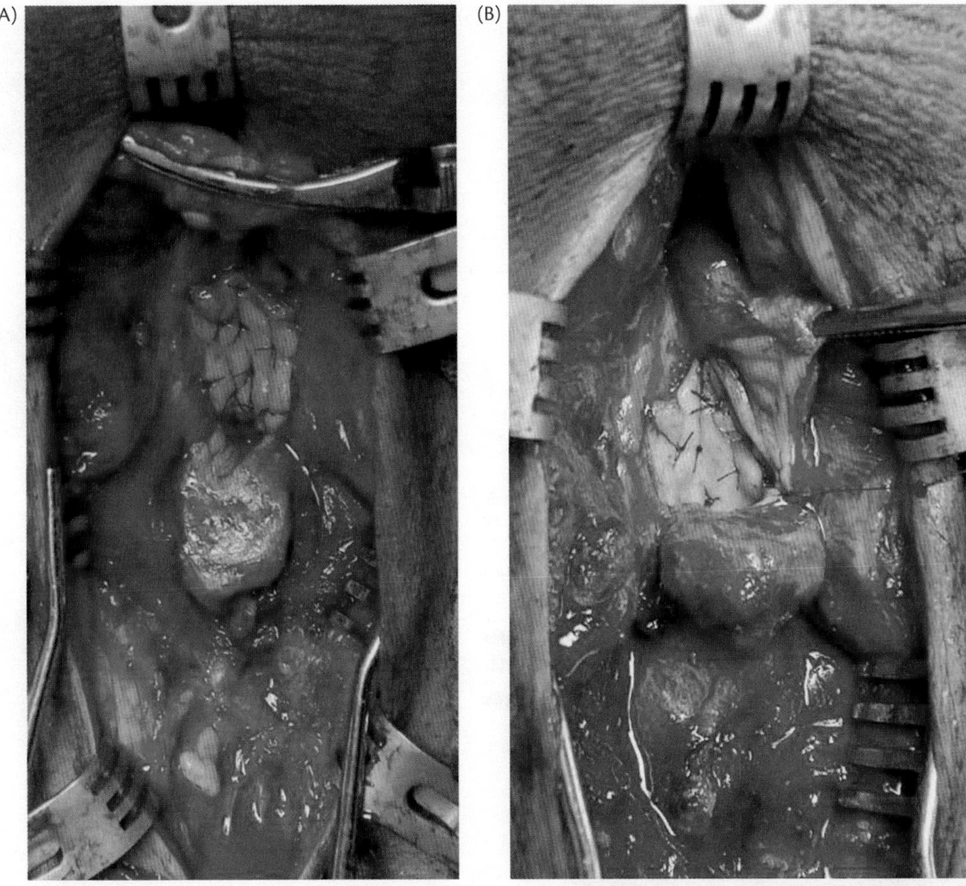

Fig. 4.4.8 The augmented anastomotic repair. The stricture has been excised and both ends spatulated dorsally. A buccal mucosal graft (BMG) has been harvested and quilted to the tunica albuginea of the penis (A). The proximal spatulated end of the urethra is beginning to be sutured to the proximal end of the BMG. The distal spatulated end of the urethra is retracted with a bulldog clamp (B). When the proximal part of the anastomosis is complete, the distal half is sutured—shown here half-finished.

Reproduced from Mundy AR and Andrich DE, 'Urethral strictures', *BJU International*, Volume 107, Issue 1, pp. 6–26, Copyright © 2011 BJU International, with permission from John Wiley and Sons Ltd.

Simple strictures—the 'stricturotomy and patch' procedure

Simple strictures, suitable for a stricturotomy and patch repair are uncommon and usually due to catheterization or instrumentation. The best form of procedure for these simple strictures is probably the Orandi procedure[29] (Fig. 4.4.10) in which the stricturotomy is performed ventrally and a flap of ventral penile shaft skin is rotated in to close the defect. A period of two to three weeks postoperative catheterization follows.

Occasionally, milder cases of LS stricture disease may be amenable to a stricturotomy or patch, but here the penile urethra is mobilized dorsolaterally on one side and a buccal mucosal graft quilted in. This technique may, in fact, be used to perform a full-length urethroplasty from the fossa navicularis up into the proximal bulbar urethra.

Complex strictures—the staged circumferential repair

For hypospadias salvage, or for more severe forms of penile urethral LS, the damaged segment of urethra is excised and replaced circumferentially in two stages. At the first stage, the penile shaft skin is incised ventrally and the affected segment excised.[30] A buccal mucosal graft or grafts are then harvested and then sutured in place to the tunica albuginea to eventually replace the urethral circumference along this length. This completes the first stage. It is important to ensure that the grafts are at least 2.5–3 cm wide, so that the neourethra will be of normal calibre when the grafted area is subsequently rolled up to form a tube at the second stage (Fig. 4.4.11A). This is performed three to six months later—when the appearance is satisfactory (Fig. 4.4.11B).

Modern approaches to urethroplasty

Currently there is enthusiasm for the idea of avoiding transection of the urethra when performing a urethroplasty to preserve the blood supply of the urethra should further surgery be necessary at any stage in the patient's life.[31–33] This 'non-transecting urethroplasty' is finding an increasing number of adherents.[34] The procedure is in fact remarkably similar to a normal anastomotic or patch repair, but without transection of the bulk of the corpus spongiosum and the bulbar arteries within it, thus considerably reducing the degree of surgical trauma to the urethra.

In the penile urethra, the Orandi procedure is, as previously discussed, being progressively replaced by the dorsolateral stricturotomy and patch procedure, as for the bulbar urethra, in patients with non-obliterative LS or catheter-related strictures.[35] And for hypospadias or LS-related problems involving just the meatus and fossa navicularis, the excision and circumferential graft repair is increasingly being done in one stage if circumstances are favourable.

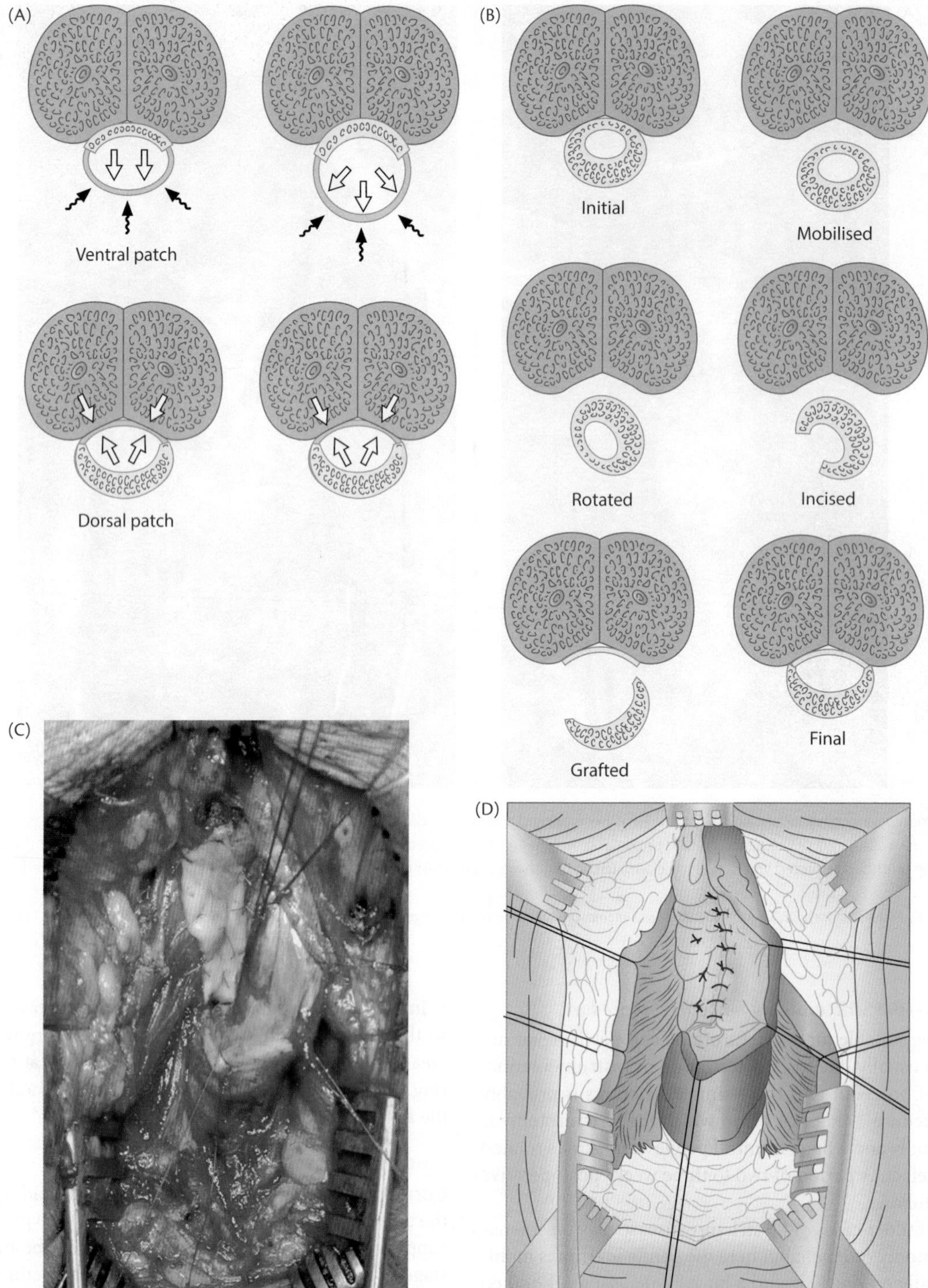

Fig. 4.4.9 The principles of the dorsal stricturotomy and patch procedure: (A) dorsal so that diverticularization of the patch on voiding does not occur; (B) diagrammatic representation of the procedure; and (C) operative appearance and accompanying diagram (D) of the BMG quilted in place before stitching the margins of the urethra to the margins of the graft.

Reproduced from Mundy AR and Andrich DE, 'Urethral strictures', *BJU International*, Volume 107, Issue 1, pp. 6–26, Copyright © 2011 BJU International, with permission from John Wiley and Sons Ltd.

Complex problems

Complexity is usually related to the length of the stricture and whether or not a substantial part of the circumference of the urethra needs to be excised. This particularly applies to LS. Until recently there was some enthusiasm for excising the epithelium and the fibrotic area of the stricture itself in preserving as much of the corpus spongiosum as possible and replacing it with a bladder mucosal graft or a graft of colonic mucosa, using the remaining corpus spongiosum, within its tunica, to provide vascularization. This has been more or less replaced by the extended dorsolateral stricturotomy and patch repair described above.[35] Should there be a shortage of buccal mucosa, then lingual mucosa, from the

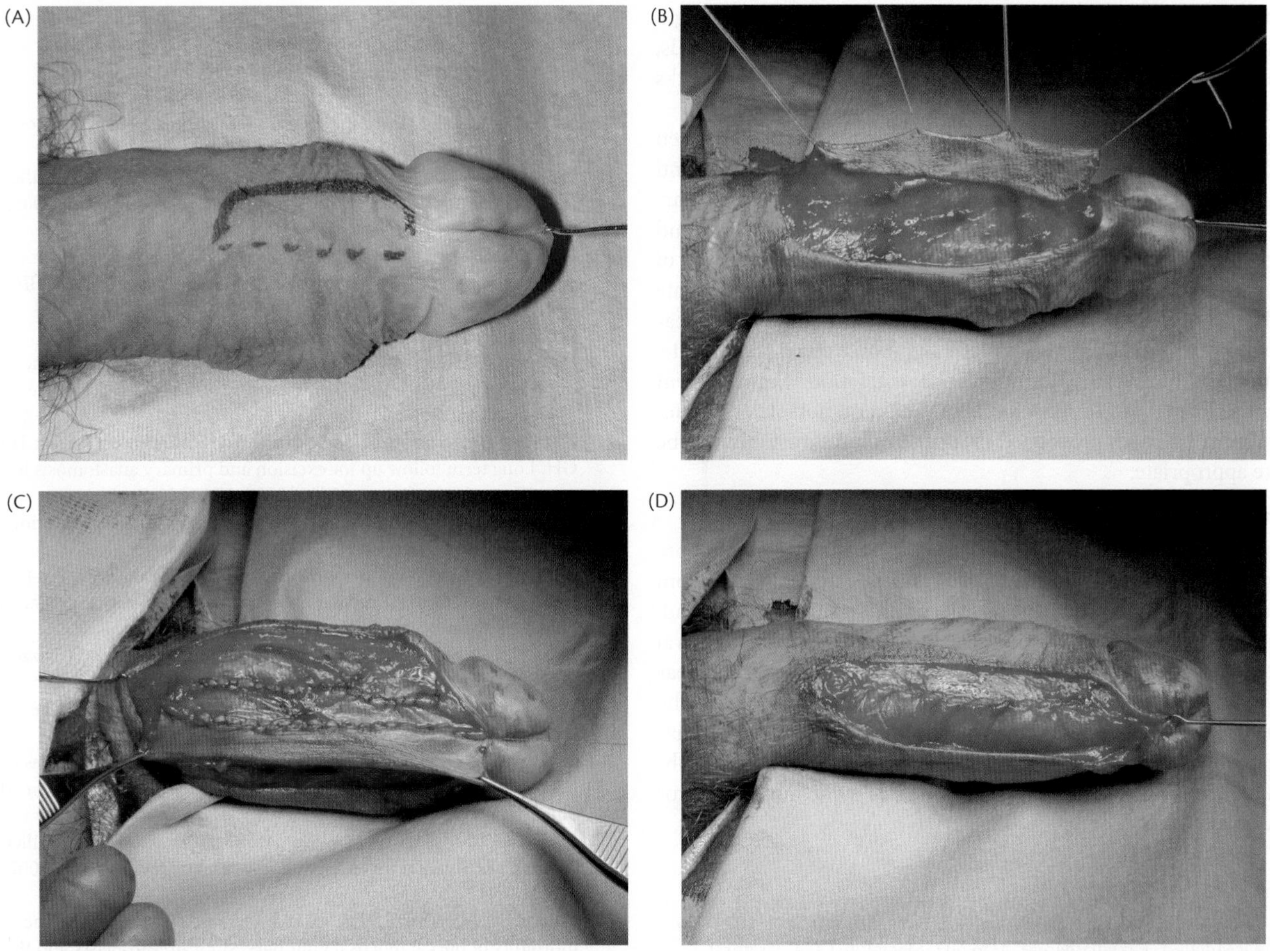

(A) (B) (C) (D)

Fig. 4.4.10 The Orandi procedure for a simple penile urethral stricture; the original flap repair: (A) the skin incision through skin and dartos (solid line) and through skin alone (dotted line); (B) the dartos vascular pedicle developed; (C) the leading edge of the skin paddle sutured to the urethra; and (D) the following edge of the urethra sutured to the other side of the urethra to close it.

Reproduced from Mundy AR and Andrich DE, 'Urethral strictures', *BJU International*, Volume 107, Issue 1, pp. 6–26, Copyright © 2011 BJU International, with permission from John Wiley and Sons Ltd.

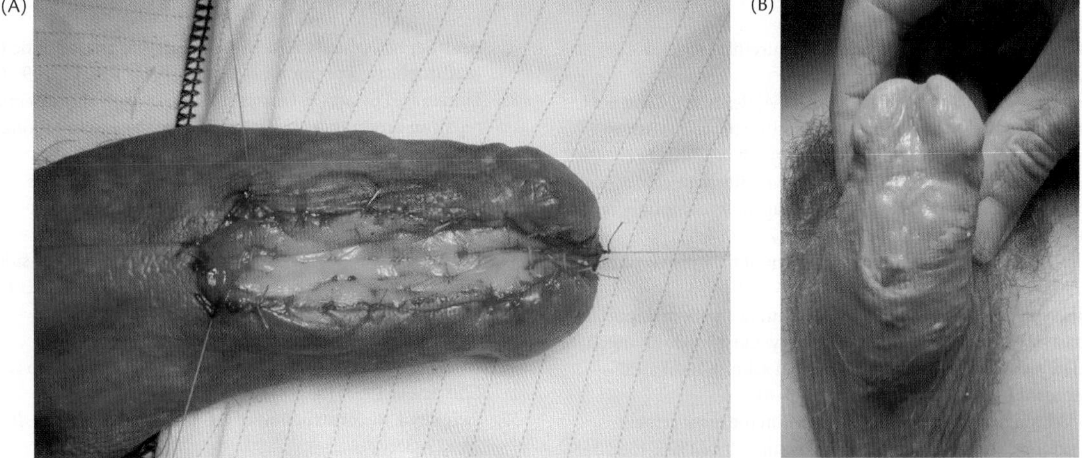

Fig. 4.4.11 The first stage of a staged repair: (A) the diseased urethra has been excised, a glans cleft created, and a BMG quilted in place. (B) Three months later, the graft is ready to be rolled up and closed.

Reproduced from Mundy AR and Andrich DE, 'Urethral strictures', *BJU International*, Volume 107, Issue 1, pp. 6–26, Copyright © 2011 BJU International, with permission from John Wiley and Sons Ltd.

underside of the tongue on each side, will usually provide enough. When the urethra does not have to be excised—in other words, when it is not completely replaced by fibrosis—then this works very well.

In otherwise unsalvageable situations there has, in the past, been recourse to the approach originally described by Johanson[36] and Swinney,[37] in which the strictured urethra is opened up and marsupialized to the surrounding skin. Then, in due course, at a second stage, it is rolled up to form a neourethra incorporating as much of the marsupialized skin as necessary to give a urethra of adequate calibre. This has only very rare indications these days but is occasionally still useful, although it has a significant complication rate, particularly of diverticulum formation, fistulation, and recurrent stricture formation. In most situations, either a dorsolateral stricturotomy and patch procedure, or a perineal urethrostomy will be more appropriate.

Future prospects

It is likely that there will be 'off-the-shelf' grafts available before long.[38,39] Currently, sheets of buccal mucosa can be created from pinch-grafts taken from the inside of the mouth beforehand. Alternatively, it might be possible to actually harvest urethral epithelium in a similar way by a preliminary biopsy from near the stricture site. How far this will replace autografting with the patients' own oral mucosa remains to be seen, except when this has already been extensively harvested. A full-thickness urethral substitute including spongiosal tissue as well as epithelium may provide an alternative.

References

1. Mundy AR, Andrich DE. Urethral strictures. *BJU Intl* 2011; **107**:6–26.
2. McMillan A, Pakianathan M, Mao NH, Macintyre CCA. Urethral stricture and urethritis in men in Scotland. *Genitourin Med* 1994; **70**:403–5.
3. Lumen N, Hoebeke P, Willemsen P, De Troyer B, Pieters R, Oosterlink W. Etiology of urethral stricture disease in the 21st century. *J Urol* 2009; **182**:983–7.
4. Netto NR, Martucci ES, Goncalves ES, Freire JGC. Congenital stricture of male urethra. *Int Urol Nephrol* 1976; **8**(1):55–61.
5. Das S, Tunuguntla HS. Balantis xerotica obliterans—a review. *World J Urol* 2000; **18**:382–7.
6. Chambers RM, Baitera B. The anatomy of the urethral stricture. *Br J Urol* 1977; **49**:545–51.
7. Meria P, Anidjar M, Brouland JP, Teillac P, LeDuc A, Berthon P, Cussenot O. An experimental model of bulbar urethral stricture in rabbits using endoscopic radiofrequency coagulation. *Urology* 1999; **53**:1054–7.
8. Baskin LS, Constantinescu SC, Howard PS, *et al.* Biochemical characterisation and quantification of the collagenous components of urethral stricture tissue. *J Urol* 1993; **150**:642–7.
9. Depasquale I, Park AJ, Bracka A. The treatment of balantis xerotica obliterans. *BJU Int* 2000; **86**:459–65.
10. Jackson MJ, Sciberras J, Mangera A, *et al.* Defining a patient-reported outcome measure for urethral stricture surgery. *Eur Urol* 2011; **60**:60–8.
11. Sachse H. Die sichturethrotomie mit scharfem schnitt, indikation—technik—ergebnisse. *Urologie A* 1978; **17**:177–81.
12. Pansadoro V, Emiliozzi P. Internal urethrotomy in the management of anterior urethral strictures: long term follow-up. *J Urol* 1996; **156**:73–5.
13. Steenkamp JW, Heyns CF, De Kock MLS. Internal urethrotomy versus dilatation as treatment for male urethral strictures: a prospective, randomised comparison. *J Urol* 1997; **157**:98–101.
14. Heyns CF, Steenkamp JW, De Kock ML, Whitaker P. Treatment of male urethral strictures: is repeated dilation or internal urethrotomy useful? *J Urol* 1998; **160**:356–8.
15. Mundy AR. The treatment of sphincter strictures. *Br J Urol* 1989; **64**:626–8.
16. Lawrence WT, MacDonagh RP. Treatment of urethral stricture disease by internal urethrotomy followed by 'low friction' self-catheterisation: preliminary report. *J R Soc Med* 1988; **81**:136–9.
17. Staios D, Shergill I, Thwani A, Junaid I, Buchholz NP. The Memokath stent. *Expert Rev Med Devices* 2007; **4**:99–101.
18. Milroy EJG, Chapple CR, Eldin A, Wallsten H. A new stent for the treatment of urethral strictures, Preliminary report. *Br J Urol* 1989; **63**:392–6.
19. Hussein M, Greenwell TJ, Shah J, Mundy AR. Long-term results of a self expanding Wallstent in the treatment of urethral stricture. *BJU Int* 2004; **94**:1037–9.
20. Peterson AC, Palminteri E, Lazzeri M, Guanzoni G, Barbagli G, Webster GD. Heroic measures may not always be justified in extensive urethral stricture due to lichen sclerosus (balantis xerotica obliterans). *Urology* 2004; **64**:565–8.
21. Eltahawy EA, Virasoro R, Schlossberg SM, McCammon KA, Jordan GH. Long term follow up for excision and primary anastomosis for anterior urethral strictures. *J Urol* 2007; **177**:1803–6.
22. Greenwell TJ, Venn SN, Mundy AR. Changing practice in anterior urethroplasty. *BJU Int* 1999; **83**:631–5.
23. Mundy AR. Anastomotic urethroplasty. *BJU Int* 2005; **96**:921–44.
24. Iselin CE, Webster GD. Dorsal onlay graft urethroplasty for repair of bulbar urethral stricture. *J Urol* 1999; **161**:815–8.
25. Barbagli G, Palminteri E, Guazzoni G, Montorsi F, Turini D, Lazzeri M. Bulbar urethroplasty using buccal mucosal grafts placed on the ventral, dorsal or lateral surface of the urethra: are results affected by the surgical technique. *J Urol* 2005; **174**:955–8.
26. Andrich DE, Leach CJ, Mundy AR. The Barbagli procedure gives the best results for patch urethroplasty of the bulbar urethra. *BJU Int* 2001; **88**:385–9.
27. Markiewicz MR, Lukose MA, Margarone JE 3rd, Barbagli G, Miller KS, Chuang SK. The oral mucosa graft: a systematic review. *J Urol* 2007; **178**:387–94.
28. Wood DN, Allen SE, Andrich DE, Greenwell TJ, Mundy AR. The morbidity of buccal mucosal graft harvest for urethroplasty and the effect of non-closure of the graft harvest site on postoperative pain. *J Urol* 2004; **172**:580–3.
29. Orandi A. One-stage urethroplasty. *Br J Urol* 1968; **40**:717–19.
30. Andrich DE, Greenwell TJ, Mundy AR. The problems of penile urethroplasty with particular reference to 2-stage reconstructions. *J Urol* 2003; **170**:87–9.
31. Jordan GH, Eltahawy EA, Virasoro R. The technique of vessel sparing excision and primary anastomosis for proximal bulbous urethral reconstruction. *J Urol* 2007; **177**:1799–802.
32. Andrich DE, Mundy AR. Non-transecting anastomotic bulbar urethroplasty: a preliminary report. *BJU Int* 2012; **109**:1090–4.
33. Lumen N, Poelaert F, Oosterlinck W, *et al.* Nontransecting anastomotic repair in urethral reconstruction: surgical and functional outcomes. *J Urol* 2016; **196**:1679–84.
34. Ivaz S, Bugeja S, Frost A, Andrich D, Mundy AR. The nontransecting approach to bulbar urethroplasty. *Urol Clin N Am* 2017; **44**; 57–66.
35. Kulkarni S, Barbagli G, Sansalone S, Lazzeri M. One-sided anterior urethroplasty: a new dorsal onlay graft technique. *BJU Int* 2009; **104**:1150–5.
36. Johanson B. Reconstruction of the male urethra in strictures: Application of the buried intact epithelium technic. *Acta Chir Scand* 1953; (Suppl)**176**:1–4.
37. Swinney J. Reconstruction of the urethra in the male. *Br J Urol* 1952; **24**:229–35.
38. Bhargava S, Chapple CR, Bullock AJ, Layton C, MacNeil S. Tissue-engineered buccal mucosa for substitution urethroplasty. *BJU Int* 2004; **93**:807–11.
39. Sievert K-D, Amend B, Stenzl A. Tissue engineering for the lower urinary tract: a review of a state of the art approach. *Eur Urol* 2007; **52**:1580–9.

CHAPTER 4.5

Upper urinary tract trauma

Anthony R. Mundy and Daniela E. Andrich

Introduction to upper urinary tract trauma

Trauma is the main cause of death in patients under the age of 45. Urinary tract trauma occurs in about 10% of patients with abdominal trauma and the kidney is the most frequently involved urological organ. Renal trauma occurs in about 1–5% of all trauma patients and the kidney is the most commonly injured abdominal organ.[1]

Ureteric trauma is mainly iatrogenic and injuries due to external trauma are rare. It is discussed in detail in an earlier chapter (Chapter 4.1).

Iatrogenic injury of the kidney is rare but does occur, mainly during percutaneous renal surgery. The vast majority of injuries due to external violence are from blunt injuries, occurring in 80–95%. Injuries generally occur as a result of road traffic accidents (RTAs), or otherwise as the result of 'recreational' trauma during, for example, sport. Falls or industrial accidents with heavy machinery are other causes. RTAs are the commonest cause of serious blunt injuries, accounting for about 50% overall, and here the most important factor is deceleration injury and particularly the rate of deceleration.[2] This is because rapid deceleration leads to vascular trauma and specifically to renal artery thrombosis, renal vein disruption, or even avulsion of the entire renal pedicle. Nonetheless, the majority of blunt injuries are minor and are managed conservatively. Only 2–3% of patients require surgical management.[3]

The remainder 5–20% of injuries are penetrating injuries, either stab or gunshot wounds—low velocity or high velocity. The latter are associated with particularly severe trauma and most commonly associated with other intra-abdominal injuries.[4] By contrast with blunt injuries, about 55–60% of stab wounds and 75–80% of gunshot wounds require surgery.[5] The ratio of blunt to penetrating injuries is partly environmental: penetrating injuries are rare in rural areas and much commoner in big cities.[6]

The results of the treatment of renal injuries have improved considerably in recent years, mainly as a consequence of the improvement in quality of computed tomography (CT) imaging and of selective angioembolization, and because of improvement in the general quality of critical care.[7] Guidelines have been produced by the American Association for the Surgery of Trauma (AAST)[8] and more recently by the European Association of Urology (EAU).[9] Santucci has recently provided a critical assessment of the EAU Guidelines.[1]

Clinical evaluation

History

Ideally the patient will be conscious and able to give a history; otherwise information about the accident itself may be gleaned from an eyewitness and about the patient's medical history from a relative.

In RTAs, it is helpful to know whether the patient was a passenger or a pedestrian and the speed at impact; in a penetrating injury, the nature of the assault weapon; and after a fall, the height. These are all guides to the severity of the injury.

A history of pre-existing renal disease may be present in 4–22% of injured patients.[10] It is particularly important if there is any suggestion that there might be a solitary kidney. Obviously in such circumstances, every step should be taken to try and preserve the function of that kidney. Otherwise pre-existing renal disease may manifest itself as an elevated baseline serum creatinine. Other important factors are a history of something such as pelviureteric junction (PUJ) obstruction, or its treatment, which may predispose to rupture of the PUJ.

The cardinal feature in the history of a patient after renal trauma is haematuria—either gross haematuria or microscopic haematuria—in the presence of shock. However, even microscopic haematuria may be absent in vascular trauma and particularly in children.[11] It is important, when haematuria exists, to carefully monitor the visual progress of haematuria.

Physical examination

The most important feature is the haemodynamic stability of the patient and specifically whether the systolic blood pressure has ever, at any stage, dropped below 90 mmHg.[1,3,9,10] In those with a low blood pressure or other evidence of haemodynamic instability, the response to resuscitation is important to note. This particularly applies to those with serious injuries. The response to the first two units of transfused blood may make the difference between conservative management and emergency surgery.[1,12,13]

The patient should be examined for entry and exit wounds indicating penetrating trauma and for bruising in the flank, signs of rib fractures, abdominal or flank pain and tenderness and, of course, signs of other injuries (Fig. 4.5.1).

Investigation

CT with contrast is the gold standard. This will show the location of any injury and will specifically identify contusions; devitalized segments; or haematomas or extravasations (Fig. 4.5.2).[1,9] A CT angiogram will be the next step for suspected severe injuries (Fig. 4.5.3).[1,9]

Not all patients need CT imaging—only those with haematuria and haemodynamic instability.[12] If patients have only haematuria—particularly microscopic haematuria with no evidence of haemodynamic instability—then CT scanning is unnecessary, except in penetrating injuries, and perhaps in children in whom injuries are easily missed.

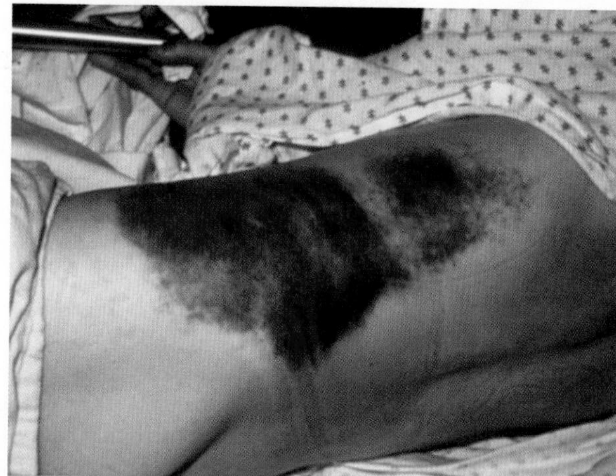

Fig. 4.5.1 Haematoma and general bruising of the left flank in a patient with a renal injury.

(A)

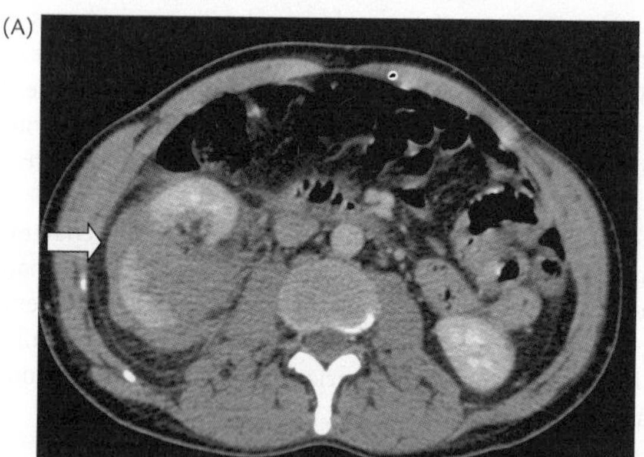

(B)

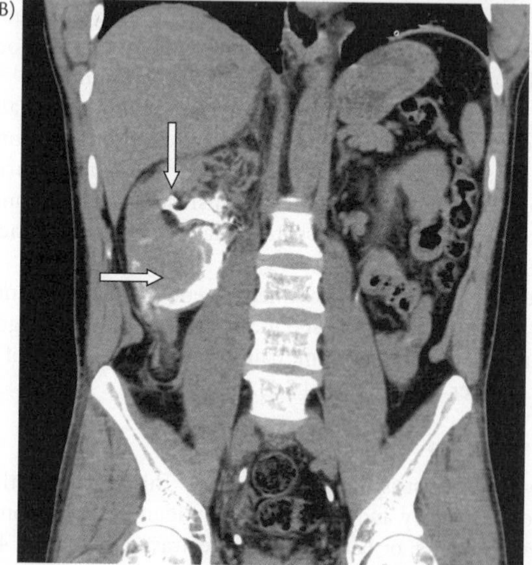

Fig. 4.5.2 Computed tomography (CT) scan showing grade 4 renal trauma to the right kidney. (A) Cross-section showing the parenchymal injury and haematoma; and (B) coronal section showing contrast in the collecting system (upper arrow) and extravasated (lower arrow).

Images reproduced courtesy of Miles Walkden and Alex Kirkham.

(A)

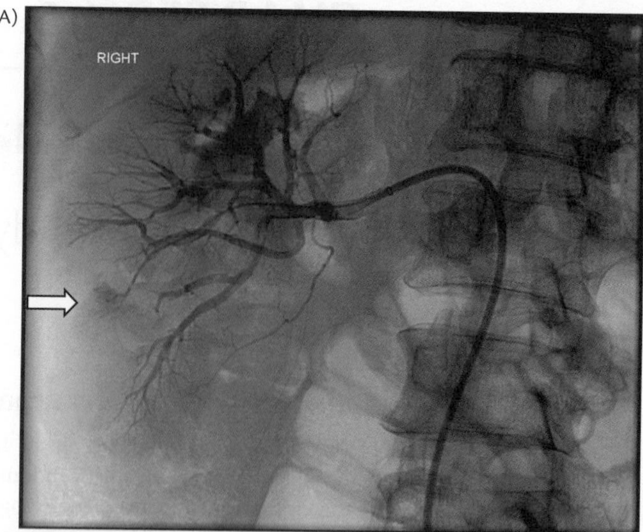

(B)

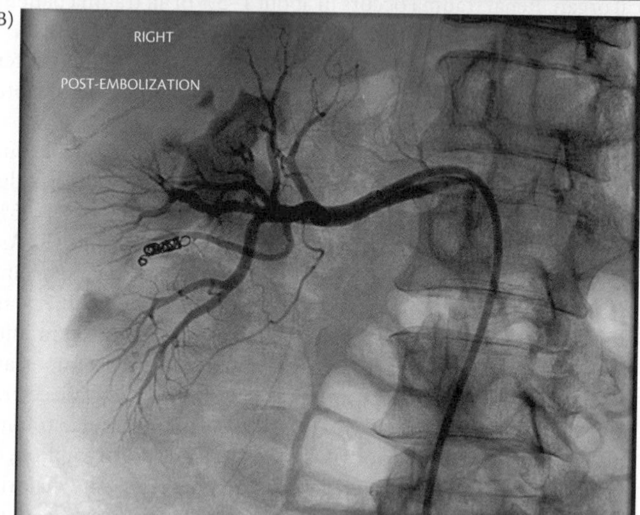

Fig. 4.5.3 Endovascular intervention for significant renal bleeding following a blunt injury. (A) Selective angiogram showing pooling of contrast from active bleeding; and (B) post-embolization image showing pool of previously leaked contrast, but now no flow to area of bleed.

Images reproduced courtesy of Miles Walkden and Alex Kirkham.

Ultrasound scanning is of value in the serial evaluation of stable injuries but of little value in the acute situation.[14] It is quick, non-invasive, cheap, and avoids radiation and contrast. It is good at identifying lacerations, but not very good at demonstrating their depth and severity. It is also good at identifying fluid collections. Unfortunately, it is difficult to find a good acoustic window to scan the kidney in a severely or multiply injured patient, which is just when you need the information.

An intravenous urogram (IVU) is valuable if CT is unavailable—particularly to look for non-visualization or otherwise for extravasation. It is still of value in the emergency situation, even when CT is available, when a patient with severe haemodynamic instability is going to proceed straight to laparotomy. An on-table IVU—one shot, 10 minutes after injecting 2 mL per kilogramme of contrast—will indicate a non-viable, non-functioning, or absent kidney.[15]

An MRI scan is only of value in those patients with an iodine allergy or otherwise, in the longer term, in unusual circumstances.

Urinalysis is also important, in many ways as important as imaging. In those patients with gross haematuria consecutive samples of urine should be kept to monitor the degree of haematuria. For microscopic haematuria,[11] progress can be monitored with dipstick testing. Equally importantly, the haemoglobin and haematocrit should be monitored to look for any signs of continued bleeding, particularly in those with more serious and potentially vascular injuries when gross haematuria is absent.

Classification

The standard form of classification used is that of the American Association for Surgical Trauma (AAST)[8] (Fig. 4.5.4). This was developed in 1989 and has been updated recently by McAninch's group in San Francisco.[16]

AAST classification, updated by Buckley and McAninch

Grade 1 injuries are contusions and subcapsular haematomas. Grade 2 injuries are minor lacerations, a centimetre or less, in the renal cortex and therefore without extravasation but with a stable perirenal haematoma. Grade 3 injuries are more substantial lacerations, more than a centimetre deep, in the renal cortex but still without extravasation. Grade 4 injuries are major lacerations, single or multiple (the so-called 'shattered kidney') through the corticomedullary junction into the collecting system with the potential for extravasation; or segmental renal vascular injuries. Grade 5 injuries are lacerations, avulsions, or thromboses of the main renal artery or vein, or both.

The importance of this classification is that it can be used to define treatment.[17] Almost invariably grades 1, 2, and 3 can be treated conservatively. Until recently, the treatment of grade 4 injuries has been controversial with some patients being surgically treated, but these days this is increasingly uncommon. Part of the problem is that exploring the kidney will sometimes, if not frequently, lead to nephrectomy because it is technically difficult to do a repair, rather than because a nephrectomy is necessary; hence the trend towards conservatism and avoiding surgery whenever possible. Currently about one-third of those patients undergoing exploration for stage 4 trauma will have a nephrectomy[18] and it is possible that in fact none of these nephrectomies are actually necessary.

Indeed, until recently, all patients with stage 5 trauma would undergo surgery with a view to renorrhaphy or nephrectomy. However, it has been shown that 50% can be managed conservatively if they respond to resuscitation and specifically if they show a good response to the transfusion of two units of blood. These are mainly the patients with shattered kidneys, previously graded as grade 5, hence the reason for regrading these injuries as grade 4.[18–20]

Thus, for the vast majority, the treatment will be conservative—up to and including endovascular intervention—excepting only those patients with life-threatening renal bleeding and haemodynamic instability, or those having laparotomy for other injuries who

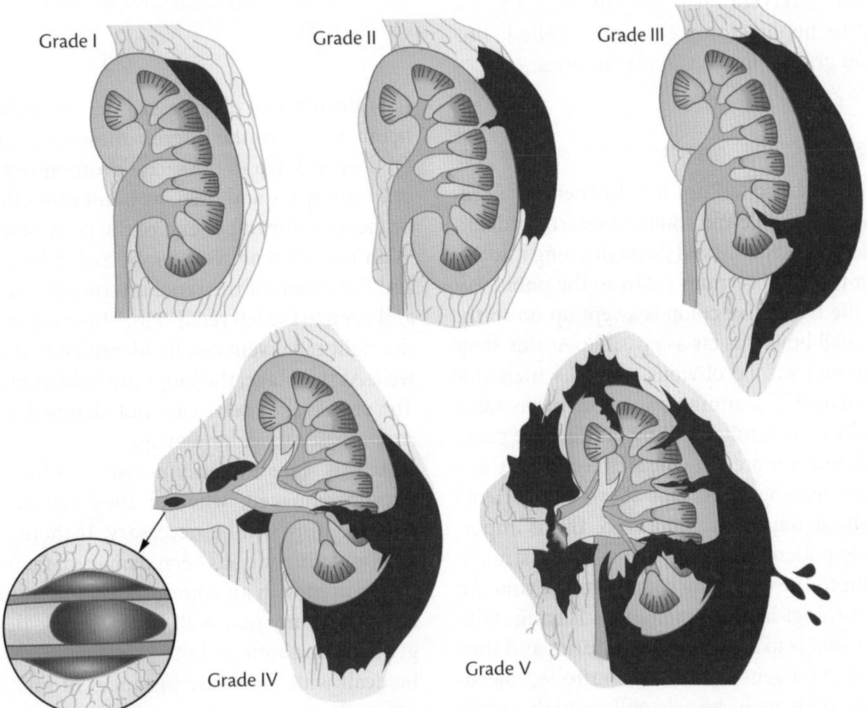

Fig. 4.5.4 The American Association for the Surgery of Trauma (AAST) classification of renal trauma.
Reproduced with permission from Lippincott Williams and Wilkins/Wolters Kluwer Health: Moore EE *et al.*, 'Organ injury scaling: spleen, liver, and kidney', *The Journal of Trauma and Acute Care Surgery*, Volume 29, Issue 12, pp. 1664–6, Copyright © 1989 Williams.

are found, intraoperatively, to have an expanding or pulsatile retroperitoneal haematoma. These are mainly patients with penetrating injuries and specifically high velocity gunshot wounds.

Conservative treatment, as described above, avoids the need for nephrectomy and is usually successful with careful monitoring. Indeed, some authorities report a 99% success rate with conservative management and specifically, in the at-risk group of patients with haemodynamic instability, using the response of the first two units of transfused blood as the guide to whether conservative management can be followed.[21]

It used to be said that patients being managed conservatively should be reassessed with CT scanning within 48–72 hours. However, these days it is generally believed that if the patient is stable, further follow-up scans should only be undertaken for those suspected of continued bleeding, or of sepsis due to infected extravasated urine.[22,23]

Treatment

Endovascular intervention

This is essentially a treatment for bleeding that is significant but not critical or life-threatening to a degree that immediate surgical intervention is required. CT angiography or routine arteriography will identify a specific bleeding point and then, using selective or super-selective angioembolism, the bleeding point is arrested by injection of clot or coils or other thrombogenic material. These days this will deal with most grade 4 injuries and even some grade 5 injuries.[24] If necessary, if a first procedure helps but is not completely successful, the procedure can be repeated.[25]

Essentially endovascular intervention is steadily reducing the indications for surgery to nephrectomy for uncontrolled, life-threatening bleeding from grade 5 major vascular injuries.

Surgery

Vascular control

Almost always surgery is for serious, if not life-threatening bleeding, and so consequently it is sensible and routine to start by identifying the main renal vessels. This is achieved through a long midline abdominal incision from the xiphisternum down to the pubis.[26,27] Through this approach, the transverse colon is swept up on to the chest together with the small bowel, as far as possible. At this stage a retroperitoneal haematoma will be obvious, as will which side the bleeding is if preliminary CT scanning has not demonstrated it. The bleeding can usually be controlled just by putting wet packs over the retroperitoneum and compressing the affected kidney and its blood supply by simply leaning on it. This allows the patient's haemodynamic status to be stabilized and improved. This is important, particularly, in those patients who have been taken straight from the emergency room to the operating room without time for a full assessment of their urological or other injuries. Having stabilized the patient, the next step is to look for other injuries and then prioritize their treatment. As a general rule, uncontrolled bleeding from the kidneys and their main vessels will be high on the priority list.

It is likely that with haemodynamic instability and a large expanding retroperitoneal haematoma, the aorta itself will not be palpable but the inferior mesenteric vein will usually be visible as it is attached to the peritoneum and rises off on the surface of the haematoma, along with the peritoneum itself. The duodenal-jejunal

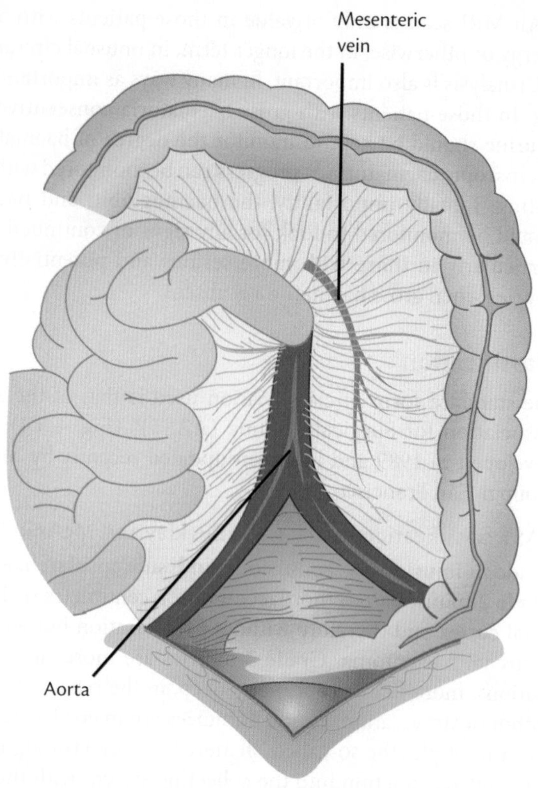

Fig. 4.5.5 The approach to the renal vessels.
Reproduced with permission from Lippincott Williams and Wilkins/Wolters Kluwer Health: McAninch JW, 'Surgery for Renal Trauma' pp. 234–239 in Novick AG *et al.* (Eds.), *Stewart's Operative Urology, Second Edition*, Williams and Wilkins, Baltimore, USA, Copyright © 1989.

(DJ) flexure will also be visible. An incision through the peritoneum medial to the inferior mesenteric vein (Fig. 4.5.5), from the DJ flexure down to the sacral promontory, will open up the retroperitoneal space and then, by blunt dissection, the left renal vein can be found at the upper end of the peritoneal incision and mobilized. With the left renal vein mobilized, a loop can be placed around it and the origin of the renal arteries can be identified; slightly distal and deep to the left renal vein. These two can also be looped. Finally, the right renal vein can be identified and a loop put around that as well. At this stage, the loops are held in place with clips (Fig. 4.5.6). The vessels themselves are not clamped, unless it is essential to do so for major vascular damage.

At this stage the only decision to be made is if the vessels are overtly damaged, whether they can be repaired, or whether a nephrectomy will be necessary. If there are two functioning kidneys and one side has been damaged, then the vascular damage will be repaired with an appropriately fine suture, if possible. However, a nephrectomy may well be necessary, depending on the patient's general condition and the presence or absence of other injuries to be dealt with. In severe instances of multiple injuries, it would be generally unwise to attempt to repair vascular injury of the main vessels or in the hilum of the kidney, and safer to proceed directly to nephrectomy—as long as the surgeon can be sure that there is a contralateral normal kidney—in order to do all the surgery that is necessary and to maximize the patient's chance of survival.

If there is only one functioning kidney, every effort should be made to repair the injury. For this, a degree of vascular clamping

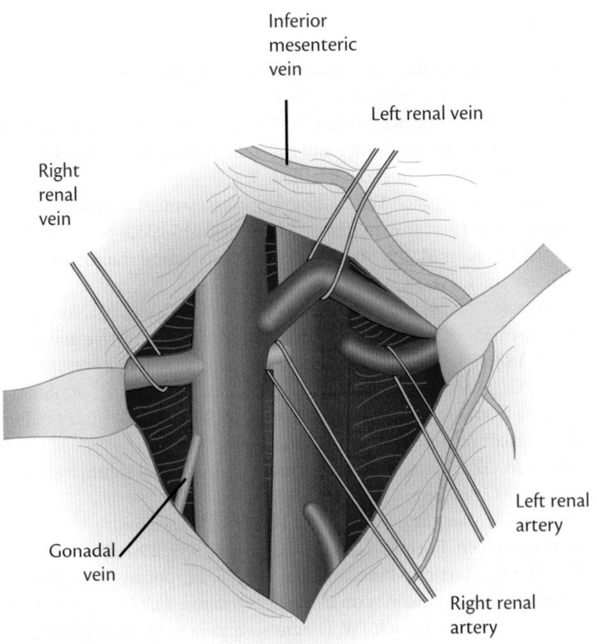

Fig. 4.5.6 Vascular control.
Reproduced with permission from Lippincott Williams and Wilkins/Wolters Kluwer Health: McAninch JW, 'Surgery for Renal Trauma' pp. 234–239 in Novick AG *et al.* (Eds.), *Stewart's Operative Urology, Second Edition*, Williams and Wilkins, Baltimore, USA, Copyright © 1989.

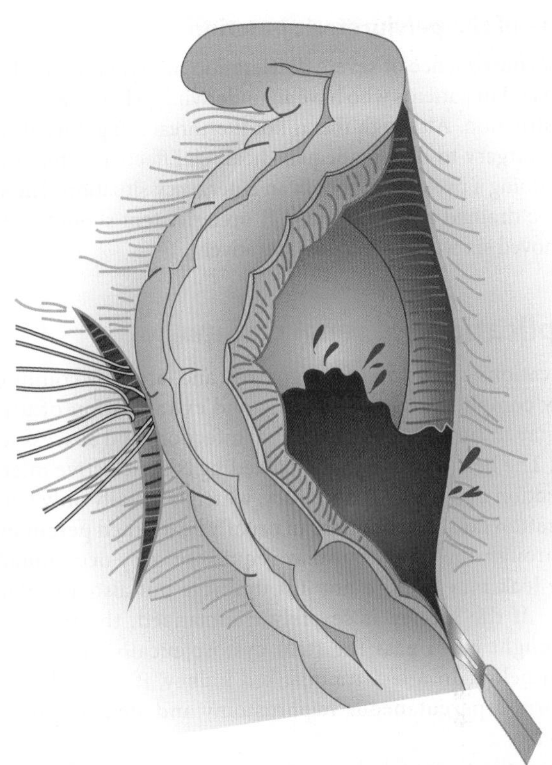

Fig. 4.5.7 Exposing the kidney with the major vessels identified.
Reproduced with permission from Lippincott Williams and Wilkins/Wolters Kluwer Health: McAninch JW, 'Surgery for Renal Trauma' pp. 234–239 in Novick AG *et al.* (Eds.), *Stewart's Operative Urology, Second Edition*, Williams and Wilkins, Baltimore, USA, Copyright © 1989.

will probably be necessary. Ideally this should be limited to less than 30 minutes. In the presence of vascular damage, it is common to lose a considerable amount of blood preoperatively—something in the region of 3–4 L—and so it is particularly important not to begin the exposure of the vessels, and then exposure of the kidney and the subsequent surgery until the patient's haemodynamic status has been stabilized and the extent of the injuries have been assessed, and until there is enough surgical assistance and equipment to deal with it.

Once proximal vascular control has been secured, the next step is to expose the kidney on the affected side by reflecting the colon on that side medially (Fig. 4.5.7). For trauma to the left kidney, an incision is made in the left paracolic gutter along the white line of Toldt. The left colon is then mobilized medially. It is sometimes necessary to mobilize not just the colon but also the pancreas, spleen and, with them, the stomach medially to have full access to the left kidney and the major vessels, in which case the incision along the paracolic gutter must be extended upwards and over the spleen on the under surface of the diaphragm. To expose the right kidney, an incision is made in the right paracolic gutter along the white line of Toldt, up and over and hepatic flexure, and then into the lesser sac. The duodenum is then mobilized ('Kocherized'), and the incision extended downwards around the caecum, and up along the small bowel mesentery as far as is necessary to expose the kidney adequately.

Debridement and reconstruction

One-third of one kidney is enough for a patient to survive without dialysis. In other words—however bad the kidney might look after injury, it is almost always worth trying to salvage it. Indeed, in the absence of major vascular trauma requiring a nephrectomy, the kidney can almost always be salvaged.[28] It may be necessary to clamp the renal vessels to get a good enough view, but if it is possible at any stage and for any length of time to release the clamping then that opportunity should be taken. It may only be necessary to clamp the artery and not the vein; and if both are clamped, then the artery should be clamped first and the vein released first to reduce the risk of rebleeding.

Bleeding points are controlled by suture-ligation using 4/0 or 5/0 absorbable sutures (we use Vicryl) on a round-bodied half-circle needle. When the bleeding is adequately controlled, the collecting system is closed first using the same type of suture material and then the parenchyma is approximated by closing the capsule and as much as is necessary of the underlying parenchyma.

If there is dead or dying tissue, then it should be excised. It is sometimes helpful to use a haemostatic agent during closure of lacerations in the renal parenchyma and often helpful to wrap the repaired kidney in omentum to help secure haemostasis and restrict extravasation.

At the end of the repair, a drain should be left to the operative site and kept there for as long as necessary. The time that any clamping of the renal artery lasted should be noted.

In the patient with multiple intra-abdominal injuries, it is surprising how well renal repair works despite the presence of leakage from the bowel, stomach, pancreas, or liver. Repairing these organs provides even more reason for draining of the operative site but the results are usually just as good.

Rupture of the pelviureteric junction

This is a consequence of severe deceleration injury, particularly in children and in patients who have an underlying pelviureteric junction obstruction. Although this is not life-threatening, this always requires surgery to obtain adequate healing. Effectively this is the same as doing a pyeloplasty, but in an emergency situation. The site should be drained and an internal JJ ureteric stent should be left and removed six weeks or so postoperatively.

Complications of renal trauma

Complications can be divided into early and late. The commonest early complications are bleeding and extravasation of urine which may in turn lead to a urinoma, infection, and abscess formation. The best way of handling bleeding is by selective microembolization or surgery if necessary, which is usually only when embolization fails. A urinoma can usually be drained percutaneously through the flank, but may require surgery occasionally. A urine leak may require not just drainage but also a ureteric stenting. If the kidney is severely traumatized, the preferred option might be to pass the stent cystoscopically up the ureter from below. In a less traumatized kidney, it might be best to perform a percutaneous nephrostomy and stent the ureter from above.

Late complications include a persistent urine leak, which again is best treated by percutaneous nephrostomy and stenting. Vascular complications are not commonly seen but include hypertension, arteriovenous fistulae, and pseudoaneurysm formation.[29] These are usually associated with haematuria. In all instances arteriography identifies the cause of the problem and also, in the case of arteriovenous (AV) fistulae of pseudoaneurysms, provides an opportunity to treat them by embolization.

Hydronephrosis is a consequence of stricture of the pelviureteric junction, which is encountered occasionally, and is treated in the usual way.

There is always concern that renal trauma will lead to loss of renal function and this is certainly a possibility following vascular injury. Aside from patients with significant vascular injury, there is not much evidence of how many patients lose renal function in the long term, because these patients are notoriously difficult to follow up. What information there is suggests that a 'significant percentage' have an elevated serum creatinine or azotaemia, or even acute renal failure at some stage during their inpatient stay following the trauma. However, in the majority of these instances the patients recover their normal renal function if they don't succumb to their injuries.[30]

It also appears to be the case that once patients have recovered from their injuries and have been discharged from hospital, then long-term problems with loss of renal function are rare.

Acknowledgements

Text extracts from Jill C. Buckley and Jack W. McAninch, 'Revision of Current American Association for the Surgery of Trauma Renal Injury Grading System', *The Journal of Trauma and Acute Care Surgery*, Volume 70, Issue 1, pp. 35–37, Copyright © 2011 Wolters Kluwer Health, reproduced with permission from Lippincott Williams and Wilkins/Wolters Kluwer Health.

References

1. Santucci RA, Bartley JM. Urological trauma guidelines: a 21st century update. *Nat Rev Urol* 2010; **7**:510–19.
2. Bjurlin MA, Fantus RJ, Mellett MM, Goble SM. Genitourinary injuries in pelvic fracture morbidity and mortality using the National Trauma Data Bank. *J Trauma* 2009; **67**:1033–9.
3. Miller KS, McAninch JW. Radiographic assessment of renal trauma: our 15-year experience. *J Urol* 1995; **154**:352–5.
4. Baniel J, Schein M. the management of penetrating trauma to the urinary tract. *J Am Coll Surg* 1994; **178**:417–25.
5. Moolman C, Navsaria PH, Lazarus J, Pontin A, Nicol AJ. Nonoperative management of penetrating kidney injuries: a prospective audit. *J Urol* 2012; **188**:169–73.
6. Lloyd GL, Slack S, McWilliams KL, Black A, Nicholson TM. Renal trauma from recreational accidents manifests different injury patters than urban renal trauma. *J Urol* 2012; **188**:163–8.
7. Shenfeld OZ, Gnessin E. Management of urogenital trauma: state of the art. *Curr Op in Urol* 2011; **21**:449–54.
8. Moore EE, Shackford SR, Pachter HL, *et al.* Organ injury scaling: spleen, liver, and kidney. *J Trauma* 1989; **29**:1664–6.
9. Lynch TH, Martinez-Piñero L, Plas E, *et al.* European Association of Urology. EAU guidelines on urological trauma. *Eur Urol* 2005; **47**:1–15.
10. Santucci RA, McAninch JW. Diagnosis and management of renal trauma: past, present, and future. *J Am Coll Surg* 2000; **191**:443–51.
11. Chandoke PS, Mcaninch JW. Detection and significance of microscopic haematuria in patients with blunt renal trauma. *J Urol* 1988; **140**:16–18.
12. Mee SL, McAninch JW, Robinson AL, Auerbach PS, Carroll PR. Radiographic assessment of renal trauma: a 10-year prospective study of patient selection. *J Urol* 1989; **141**:1095–8.
13. Hammer CC, Santucci RA. Effect of an institutional policy of nonoperative treatment of grades I to IV renal injuries. *J Urol* 2003; **169**:1751–3.
14. Pollack HM, Wein AJ. Imaging of renal trauma. *Radiology* 1989; **172**:297–308.
15. Morey AF, McAninch JW, Tiller BK, Duckett CP, Carroll PR. Single shot intraoperative excretory urography for the immediate management of renal trauma. *J Urol* 1999; **161**:1088–92.
16. Buckley JC, McAninch JW. Revision of current American Association for the Surgery of Renal Injury grading system. *J Trauma* 2011; **70**:35–7.
17. Shariat SF, Roehrborn CG, Karakiewicz PI, Dhami G, Stage KH. Evidence-based validation of the predictive value of the American Association for the Surgery of Trauma kidney injury scale. *J Trauma* 2007; **62**:933–9.
18. Shariat SF, Jenkins A, Roehrborn CG, *et al.* Features and outcomes of patients with grade IV renal injury. *BJU Int* 2008; **102**:728–33.
19. Buckley JC, McAninch JW. Selective management of isolated and non-isolated grade IV renal injuries. *J Urol* 2006; **176**:2498–502; discussion 2502.
20. McGuire J, Bultitude MF, Davis P, *et al.* Predictors of outcome for blunt high grade renal injury treated with conservative intent. *J Urol* 2011; **185**:187–91.
21. Brewer ME Jr, Strnad BT, Daley BJ, *et al.* Percutaneous emobilsation for the management of grade 5 renal trauma in hemodynamically unstable patients: initial experience. *J Urol* 2009; **181**:1737–41.
22. Davis P, Bultitude MF, Koukounaras J, *et al.* Assessing the usefulness of delayed imaging in routine follow up for renal trauma. *J Urol* 2010; **184**:973–7.
23. Malcolm JB, Derweesh IH, Mehrazin R, *et al.* Nonoperative management of blunt renal trauma is routine early follow-up imaging necessary? *BMC Urol* 2008; **3**:8–11.
24. Breyer BN, McAninch JW, Elliott SP, Master VA. Minimally invasive endovascular techniques to treat acute renal haemorrhage. *J Urol* 2008; **179**:2248–52.
25. Huber J, Pahernik S, Hallescheidt P, *et al.* Slective transaarterial embolisation for posttraumatic and renal haemorrhage: a second try is worthwhile. *J Urol* 2011: **185**:1751–5.

26. McAninch JW, Carroll PR. Renal trauma: kidney preservation through improved vascular control—a refined approach. *J Trauma* 1982; **22**:285–90.
27. McAninch JW. Surgery for renal trauma. (pp. 234–9) In: Novick AG, Pontes JE, Streem SB (eds). *Stewart's Operative Urology,* 2nd edition. Baltimore, MA: Williams and Wilkins, 1989.
28. Meng MV, Brandes SB, McAninch JW. Renal trauma: indications and techniques for surgical exploration. *World J Urol* 1991; **17**:71–7.
29. Peterson NE. Complications of renal trauma. *Urol Clin North Am* 1989; **16**:221–36.
30. Tasian GE, Aaronson DS, McAninch JW. Evaluation of renal function after major renal injury: correlation with the American Association for the Surgery of Trauma Injury Scale. *J Urol* 2010; **183**:196–200.

CHAPTER 4.6

Lower urinary tract trauma

Anthony R. Mundy and Daniela E. Andrich

Introduction to lower urinary tract trauma

The commonest form of lower urinary tract trauma is iatrogenic trauma. This is largely urological iatrogenic trauma as the result of instrumentation and endoscopic surgery. That aside, lower urinary tract trauma is uncommon.

Trauma to the bladder

The commonest type of bladder trauma is the result of transurethral resection of bladder tumours. In women, gynaecological surgery—specifically, caesarean section, hysterectomy, and sling surgery—is also a common cause. Iatrogenic trauma aside, blunt trauma is the cause of most bladder injuries, particularly road traffic accidents causing pelvic fracture in the presence of a distended bladder.

Broadly speaking, bladder trauma can be divided into extraperitoneal and intraperitoneal rupture. The consequences of gynaecological surgery affecting the bladder may be more chronic and present as vesicovaginal fistulation.

The clinical features of bladder trauma are usually those of the underlying cause. After a pelvic fracture, gross haematuria is usual; clear urine virtually excludes a ruptured bladder. With a ruptured bladder, whether it is extraperitoneal or intraperitoneal, catheterization reveals little or no urine in the bladder or blood-stained urine and the definitive diagnosis is made on imaging. A cystogram may show the rupture (Figs 4.6.1 and 4.6.2) and indicate its site very clearly, but these days a computed tomography (CT) urogram as part of a CT trauma series, to look for other injuries, is likely to be the commonest way in which the diagnosis is made. Both are very sensitive for the diagnosis of bladder rupture, as long as the bladder is sufficiently distended to 300–350 mL.

Management

If an extraperitoneal bladder rupture is diagnosed as an isolated injury because of transurethral perforation of the bladder, or after external injury, then it is usually safe to use an indwelling catheter and await spontaneous healing over the next two to three weeks. If the patient requires surgery for any other reason, usually after external trauma, and particularly after pelvic fracture, then the rupture should be repaired with a suprapubic and a urethral catheter and a drain to the site of the repair. Causes would include a bone fragment sticking into the bladder following a fractured pelvis. Only if there are no signs of spontaneous healing—manifest as inadequate

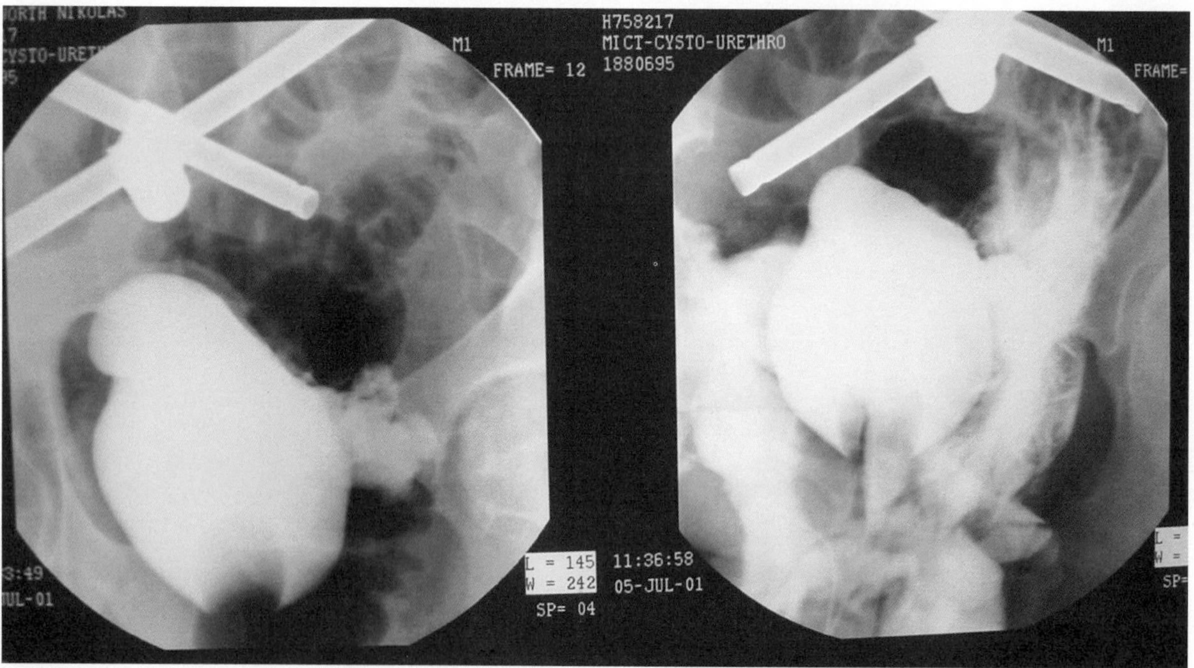

Fig. 4.6.1 Extraperitoneal rupture of the bladder on cystography.

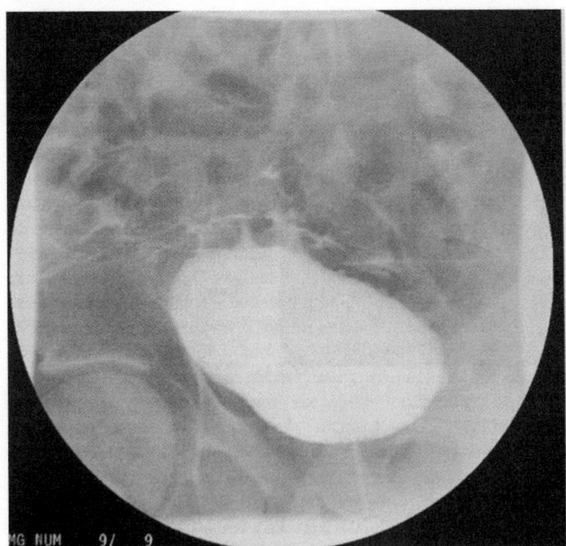

Fig. 4.6.2 Intraperitoneal rupture of the bladder on cystography, with contrast visible between loops of bowel.

urinary drainage coupled with signs of sepsis due to infection of the extravasated urine after iatrogenic injury—would exploration otherwise be necessary.

With intraperitoneal rupture, the standard of care is still to explore the injury and repair the bladder over a suprapubic catheter. This is because of the possibility of bowel prolapse through the rupture site and of urinary peritonitis. In fact, with small ruptures, it is perfectly possible to leave an indwelling catheter and await spontaneous healing, and to explore and repair as above if there is a continuing cause for concern. With small iatrogenic ruptures, a laparoscopic approach may be possible. All penetrating injuries should be explored.

The management of vesicovaginal fistulation and the complications of sling surgery are beyond the scope of the chapter and are discussed in the section on female urology. It is suffice to say that in the short term, vaginal leakage of urine after gynaecological surgery should be managed by urethral catheterization. In some instances, the leaking will cease in a few days and the fistula will heal without further difficulty. If the problem persists, then the fistula should be repaired.

Urethral injury

Any part of the urethra may be injured by iatrogenic or non-iatrogenic trauma and, as with bladder trauma, iatrogenic trauma is the much the commonest type, particularly associated with urethral catheterization.[1,2] Non-iatrogenic trauma of the urinary tract accounts for about 1.5% of all trauma and urethral trauma accounts for about 4% of this, which is equivalent to one case per 1,125,000.[3]

Although iatrogenic trauma is the most common, non-iatrogenic trauma is far more serious if only because the force needed to cause it is so severe. Because of this, about 80% or so of patients have associated injuries. There are three common sites of external trauma to the urethra in the adult male. The commonest is pelvic fracture urethral injury of the posterior urethra, which is about four times commoner than straddle injuries of the bulbar urethra, which is about five times more common than injuries to the penile urethra, which are generally the result of sexual misadventure. Penetrating trauma anywhere is rare but is increasingly common in military injuries with the increasing use of improvised explosive devices.

In the developing world and in children, straddle injuries are about as common as pelvic fracture urethral injuries.

The nature of urethral injury

Anatomically, the urethra is described as being in three parts—the prostatic, the membranous, and the spongiose. Anatomists do not distinguish between the anterior and posterior urethra nor between the bulbar and penile urethra. Furthermore, they regard the membranous urethra as being a misnomer as the 'genitourinary membrane' (or urogenital diaphragm as it is more commonly known) has been shown not to exist.[4]

The urological division is between an anterior and posterior urethra. The anterior urethra consists of the bulbar and penile components the bulbar being that part of the spongiose urethra surrounded by the bulb of the corpus spongiosum and the bulbospongiosus muscle. The posterior urethra is divided into the prostatic and membranous components.

Anatomically, the prostatic urethra is well fixed in position, particularly posteriorly through the lateral ligaments and to Denonvillier's fascia between them. At the apex of the prostate, just above the origin of the membranous urethra, the pubo-prostatic ligaments fix it anteriorly. The membranous urethra is fixed posteriorly by the rectourethralis, which runs from the apex of the prostate to the perineal membrane. The bulbar urethra is fixed to the crura of the penis. The penile segment of the urethra is completely mobile. These relative points and degrees of fixation explain the nature of urethral injury. Prostatic injury is rare because it is firmly fixed in place. The membranous urethra is vulnerable as it runs down to the perineal membrane and is particularly vulnerable at that point. The bulbar urethra is firmly fixed and only amenable to crush injuries. The penile urethra is freely mobile and avoids most injuries except those of a sexual nature.

Endoluminal injury is particularly common at and just below the perineal membrane where the urethra is fixed in its position, and at the point of curvature of the urethra as it runs up into the pelvis.

Posterior urethral injury

There is a strong association of posterior urethral injury with fractures of the pelvis and specifically with those fractures associated with disruption of the pelvic ring; in other words, associated with fracture or fracture dislocation of the sacroiliac joint as well as fracture of the anterior bony ring of the pelvis.[5] The injury to the urethra itself typically occurs at the bulbomembranous junction at the perineal membrane in adults.[6]

Pelvic ring disruptions are typically classified by the degree of instability they produce. The best known is the classification devised by Tile.[7] Type A disruptions are stable; type B show rotational instability; type C show both rotational and vertical instability. Urological injury does not occur with type A disruptions, and mainly occurs with type B rotational disruptions.[6] These are typically one of two types—a so-called 'open book' injury or a lateral compression fracture—and urethral trauma is particularly associated with lateral compression type B injuries. The type C injury, with is both vertically and rotationally unstable, is particularly associated with complete disruptions of the urethra and with complicated injuries such as bladder neck injury.[6]

Occasionally a so-called 'switchblade' injury, in which a bone fragment slices through the urethra, is a cause of urethral injury, rather than a disruption of the pelvic ring. When this occurs, it is usually the bulbar urethra that is affected and a longer and more serious injury results.

These injuries may be partial or complete, while partial appears to be commoner. This has implications for treatment as discussed below.

The commonest cause is a road traffic accident, which account for 65–85% of injuries; falls from a height which account for 20–25% of injuries; or crushing lateral compression injuries, such as a fall from a horse. Young men are usually affected with a mean age of 33.

Interestingly, only 5–10% of ruptures of the pelvic ring are associated with pelvic fracture urethral injuries. It was originally thought that the problem occurred as a result of shearing of the urethra at the junction of the prostatomembranous junction.[8] It was then hypothesized that it was an avulsion rather than a shearing injury—rather like plucking an apple and its stem off the branch of a tree.[9] This was given as the explanation of so-called distraction injuries, as these were thought to be at the time. Nowadays, it is known that these injuries occur at the bulbomembranous junction and contemporary wisdom has it that this is a consequence of the way the pelvic ligaments of the pelvic ring behave, rather than the bone themselves.[6]

Andrich *et al.*[6] have shown that when these pelvic ring disruptions occur, the most likely explanation for involvement of the urinary tract is the way in which the pubo-prostatic ligaments and the perineal membrane behave. Ligaments may rupture either mid-substance or they may tear from their attachment at each end—and, in the case of these ligaments, that means at their bony attachment at one end or their visceral attachment to the urethra at the other. It is only in the latter instance that urethral injury occurs. When ligaments rupture mid-substance or tear away from their bony attachment there will be no urethral injury. Hence the explanation as to why urethral injury may not occur, as well as to why it may occur. Occasionally, with either open book injuries or with type C injuries, there is a vertical tear of the prostate in addition to a tear of the membranous urethra, and as a secondary consequence of tearing of the prostate, a bladder neck injury occurs.[10] In children, before development of the prostate, it is more common to find transverse injury through the prostate or through the bladder neck or in combination with a ruptured urethra.[11] This can also happen following particularly severe injuries in adults.[10]

In females, there is a tendency for the proximal urethra and bladder neck to be ruptured in the same way that the prostate is torn in adults.[12]

Anterior urethral injuries

The epithelium of the spongiose (anterior) urethra has no supporting subepithelial layer comparable to the muscularis mucosae in the intestine. Thus, when the epithelium is breached there is immediate exposure of the subepithelial spongy tissue and, because of the pressure of voiding, extravasated urine is forced into the corpus spongiosum under pressure. Extravasated urine within the corpus spongiosum is initially contained by the fibrous capsule of the corpus spongiosum and by Buck's fascia[13] that surrounds it (Fig. 4.6.3). It is then constrained, should Buck's fascia rupture by Colles' fascia[14] (Fig. 4.6.4). Further extravasation directs the extravasated blood and urine anteriorly from the scrotum towards the penis and then up onto the anterior abdominal wall around the spermatic chords. Extravasated urine is toxic whether it is infected or not.[15] It causes thrombophlebitis and obliterative endarteritis, which progresses to subcutaneous ischaemia and eventually gangrene. Super-added infection is inevitable; indeed, after two weeks it is certain. With super-added infection, the normal fascial barriers break down and spread of the infected extravasated blood and urine can occur in any direction regardless of anatomical layers.

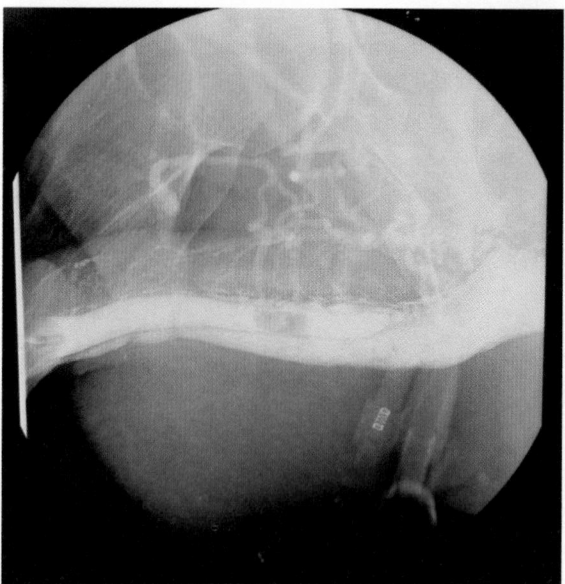

Fig. 4.6.3 Extravasation within the corpus spongiosum after a urethral contusion—constrained by Buck's fascia.

Reproduced from Mundy AR and Andrich DE, 'Urethral trauma: Part I: Introduction, history, anatomy, pathology, assessment and emergency management', *BJU International*, Volume 108, Issue 3, pp. 310–327, Copyright © 2011 the Authors and BJU International, with permission from John Wiley and Sons.

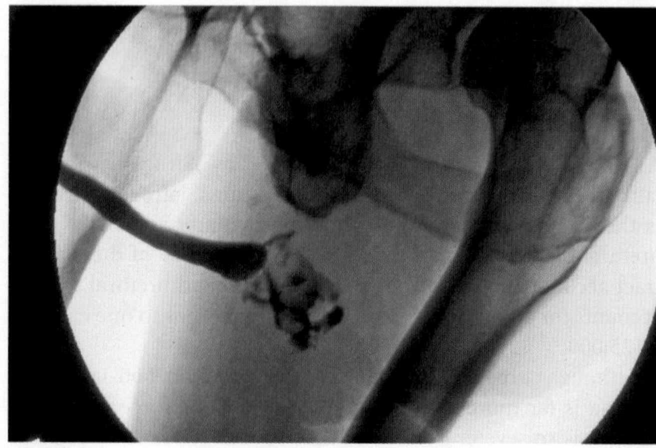

Fig. 4.6.4 Extravasation outside Buck's fascia after a straddle injury to the bulbar urethra—constrained by Colles' fascia.

Reproduced from Mundy AR and Andrich DE, 'Urethral trauma: Part I: Introduction, history, anatomy, pathology, assessment and emergency management', *BJU International*, Volume 108, Issue 3, pp. 310–327, Copyright © 2011 the Authors and BJU International, with permission from John Wiley and Sons.

This infection can lead to bacterial necrotizing fasciitis usually due to the synergistic affect of several bacteria. This ultimately leads to death from sepsis usually coupled with uraemia, because of the failure to excrete urine properly.[16] The aim of treatment of these injuries is to prevent this cycle of events.

Other than intraluminal trauma, which may be due to instrumentation or sexual self-gratification, the causes of injury in the penile urethra is usually a penile fracture. This is described in Chapter 4.7. Associated rupture of the penile urethra is uncommon but occurs in 10–20%. In the bulbar urethra, the usual causes are straddle or fall-astride injuries.[1] This is a crushing injury of the bulbar urethra as it is fixed in position on the crura of the penis. This crush can lead to rupture of the urethra or simple ischaemic necrosis. The crura may rupture as well or suffer ischaemic necrosis, leading to gangrene, and disruption of the corpus spongiosum or corpora cavernosa at this point.

Experimental studies of urethral trauma

It has been shown experimentally that a partial rupture of the urethra can heal completely in all layers. A complete injury cannot because the epithelium retracts on either side of the injury and the space fills with fibrosis. Even if apparent healing does occur across the fibrotic segment, the epithelium is not urethral epithelium, but metaplastic; and the lumen is therefore a false passage in which stricture formation is inevitable.[17–19]

For healing to occur, it is not sufficient to have apposition of the two ruptured ends of the urethra over a catheter—there must be apposition of the epithelium by suture to provide continuity around at least part of the circumference for normal healing to occur through all layers.

The presence of a stenting catheter across urethral injury makes no difference to the outcome. A partial injury may still heal completely, regardless of its presence and a complete injury will not.

Types of injury

There are three main types of injury—contusions, partial ruptures, and complete ruptures (Fig. 4.6.5). Contusions are incomplete ruptures of part of the circumference of the urethra. Partial injuries are complete ruptures of part of the circumference of the urethra and complete injuries are complete ruptures of the complete circumference of the urethra. It can be extremely difficult to distinguish between these, particularly between partial and complete injuries, using retrograde urethrography (for radiological reasons described below) or endoscopy—or even at open surgery, because of the distortion produced by the injury.

In the absence of retrograde urethrography or when imaging is inconclusive, the only way in which different types of injury can be distinguished is by catheterizability of the urethra. A catheterizable urethra may be contused or partially ruptured. It is very unlikely that it will be possible to pass a catheter through a completely ruptured urethra. Historically, and indeed in most parts of the world today, this is how partial and complete ruptures are distinguished.

Clinical features

The cardinal clinical features are urethral bleeding and voiding difficulty, or retention due to so-called 'reflex retention'. All clinical features are time-related and, specifically, it commonly takes at least an hour for a ruptured urethra to cause bleeding that is apparent at the external meatus.[20] Internal bleeding leading to perineal haematoma formation and the typical 'butterfly haematoma' characteristic of straddle or fall-astride injuries takes a day or two to develop (Fig. 4.6.6) and it may take even longer to cause the displacement of the prostate and bladder base (which may or may not be palpable on rectal examination) associated with a pelvic fracture urethral injury.

In situations where a patient may be brought to an emergency department very quickly, there may be no obviously clinical features—certainly when this happens in less than an hour. It is therefore important that a urethral injury is suspected and all patients suspected of having a pelvic ring disruption. The council of perfection is therefore to perform a retrograde urethrogram,[21] typically after a CT 'trauma series'. However, a catheter is often passed in the emergency room as part of monitoring fluid replacement and resuscitation, and sometimes the diagnosis is therefore made on 'catheterizability'. There is often a concern that catheterization in such patients may risk making the situation worse either by worsening the trauma or by causing infection.[22] This does not seem to be borne out in practice after only one attempt at passing a soft catheter under antibiotic cover.

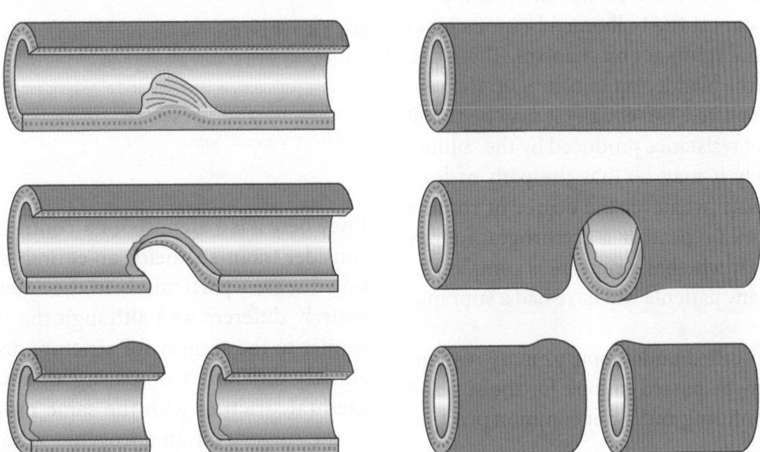

Fig. 4.6.5 Types of urethral injury—contusion, partial, and complete.

Reproduced from Mundy AR and Andrich DE, 'Urethral trauma: Part I: Introduction, history, anatomy, pathology, assessment and emergency management', *BJU International*, Volume 108, Issue 3, pp. 310–327, Copyright © 2011 the Authors and BJU International, with permission from John Wiley and Sons.

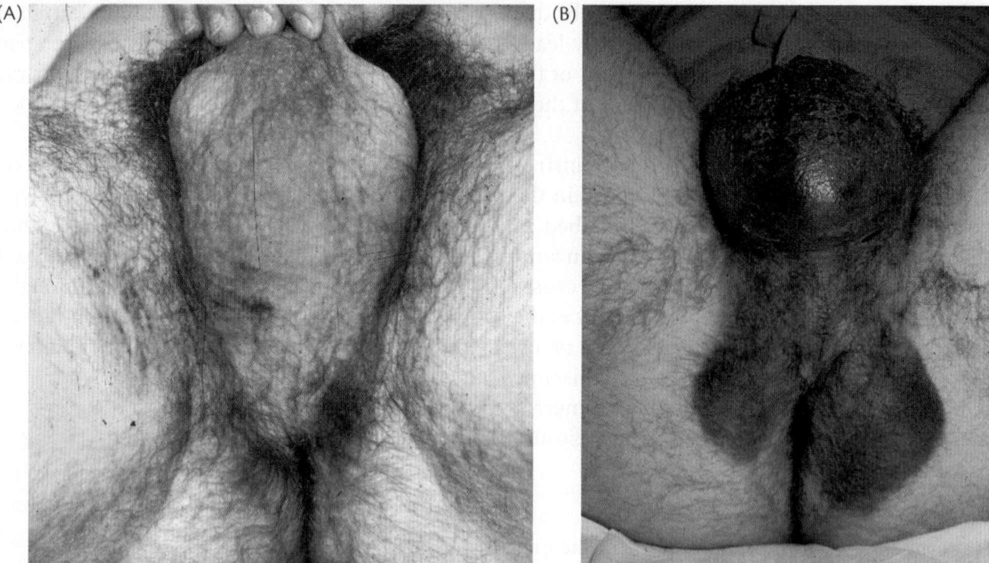

Fig. 4.6.6 Butterfly haematoma at two hours and two days after a straddle injury. (A) Two hours and (B) two days.
Reproduced from Mundy AR and Andrich DE, 'Urethral trauma: Part I: Introduction, history, anatomy, pathology, assessment and emergency management', *BJU International*, Volume 108, Issue 3, pp. 310–327, Copyright © 2011 the Authors and BJU International, with permission from John Wiley and Sons.

Investigation

Catheterizability may distinguish partial from complete injuries, the latter being uncatheterizable, but this is unreliable (and it does not distinguish between contusions and partial injuries) because a partial injury itself may be uncatheterizable. Depending on the urologist's perspective, this may not matter because the standard of care is to proceed immediately to suprapubic catheterization to divert the urine and thereby to provide a means of monitoring fluid replacement, as well as to provide a way of ensuring that retention is relieved and extravasation does not occur.[21] On the other hand, an inability to distinguish between these types of injury makes classification extremely difficult, and therefore makes the interpretation of reported data difficult, if not impossible.

A retrograde urethrogram will show the site of the injury,[23] but it often does not distinguish between complete and incomplete lesions although contusions should be clearly distinguishable. The reason for failing to distinguish between a partial and a complete lesion is because the injury occurs at the bulbomembranous junction below the site of the urethral sphincter mechanism. Therefore, contrast may not pass up into the bladder on injection up the urethra because it is completely ruptured; but equally it may be that it cannot pass through the zone of resistance produced by the sphincter mechanism; or alternatively it may be that the path of least resistance is simply to extravasate, whatever the degree of rupture (Figs 4.6.7 and 4.6.8). Sometimes repeating a urethrogram a day or so later will show more clearly whether a rupture is complete or incomplete, but by this time many patients will have had a suprapubic catheter passed anyway.

With increasing interest in so-called 'endoscopic primary realignment', a flexible cystoscope may be passed to look for the site and type of injury but this can be confusing and is not common practice.

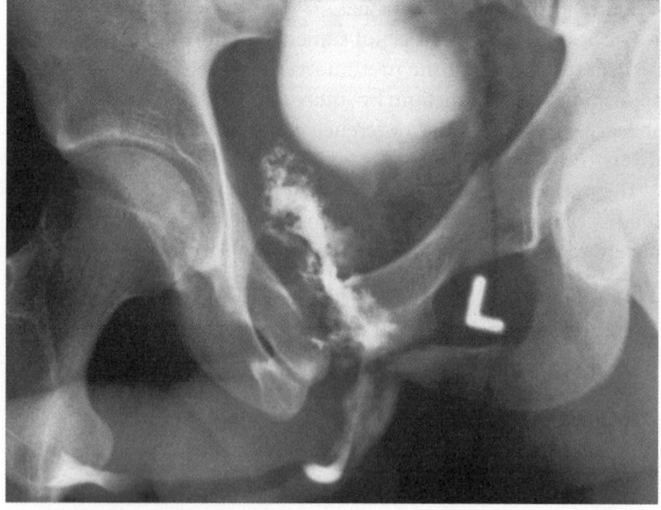

Fig. 4.6.7 Partial injury—contrast passes into the bladder.
Reproduced from Mundy AR and Andrich DE, 'Urethral trauma: Part I: Introduction, history, anatomy, pathology, assessment and emergency management', *BJU International*, Volume 108, Issue 3, pp. 310–327, Copyright © 2011 the Authors and BJU International, with permission from John Wiley and Sons.

Classification

Terminology

By consensus, the term applied to a constriction of the lumen of the anterior or spongiose urethra is a stricture, whatever the cause. Elsewhere it is a 'stenosis' or a 'contracture'.[23] In our view it is best to consider trauma as being an entirely separate condition from stricture disease—particularly in the anterior urethra. The pathology is entirely different and although the type of surgery for trauma is similar to the surgery for stricture disease, the scope and scale are entirely different. Comparing an anastomotic repair for a bulbar urethral stricture with the same procedure for a straddle injury; or the surgery for an iatrogenic sphincter stricture with that for a pelvic fracture urethral injury is like comparing chalk with cheese.

Classification systems

There are several classification systems such as those developed by Colapinto and McCallum,[24] by Goldman *et al.*,[25] by the American

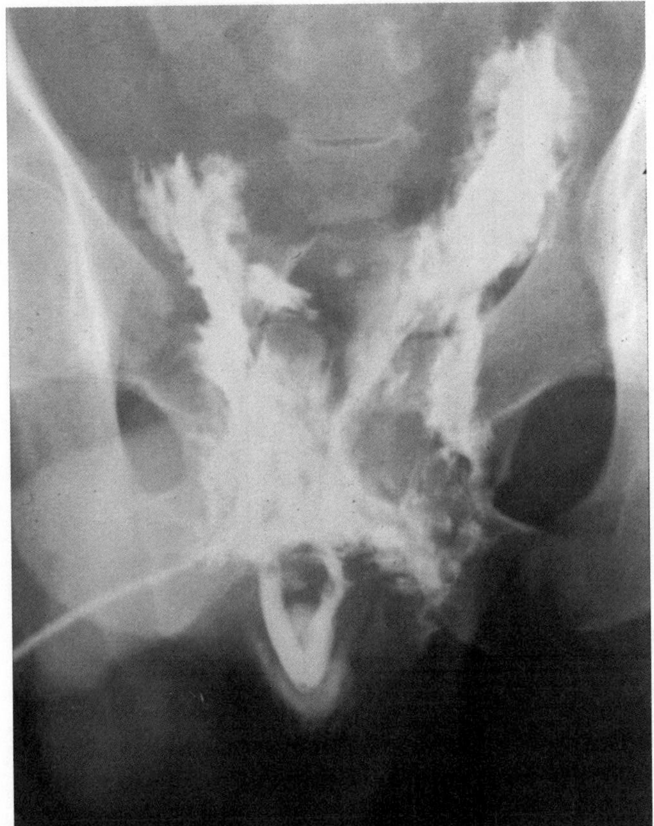

Fig. 4.6.8 A presumed complete injury, because no contrast passes into the bladder.

Reproduced from Mundy AR and Andrich DE, 'Urethral trauma: Part I: Introduction, history, anatomy, pathology, assessment and emergency management', *BJU International*, Volume 108, Issue 3, pp. 310–327, Copyright © 2011 the Authors and BJU International, with permission from John Wiley and Sons.

Box 4.6.1 The EAU classification of urethral injury[21]

- Type 1. Stretch injury. Elongation of the urethra without extravasation on urethrography
- Type 2. Contusion. Blood at the urethral meatus; no extravasation on urethrography
- Type 3. Partial disruption of anterior or posterior urethra. Extravasation of contrast at injury site with contrast visualized in the proximal urethra or bladder
- Type 4. Complete disruption of anterior urethra. Extravasation of contrast at injury site without visualization of proximal urethra or bladder
- Type 5. Complete disruption of posterior urethra. Extravasation of contrast at injury site without visualization of bladder
- Type 6. Complete or partial disruption of posterior urethra with associated tear of the bladder neck or vagina

Thus clinical management can be advised accordingly:

- Type 1. No treatment required
- Types 2 and 3 can be managed conservatively with suprapubic cystostomy or urethral catheterization
- Types 4 and 5 will require open or endoscopic treatment, primary, or delayed
- Type 6 requires primary open repair

Reprinted from *European Urology*, Volume 47, Issue 1, Thomas H. Lynch *et al.*, 'EAU Guidelines on Urological Trauma', pp. 1–15, Copyright © 2004 Elsevier B.V., with permission from Elsevier, http://www.sciencedirect.com/science/journal/03022838

Association of Trauma Surgeons,[26] and by the European Association of Urology (EAU)[21]—but they all flounder on the problem of distinguishing between partial and complete lesions on radiological (or any other) grounds. Consequently, none of the classification systems are of value because they are incapable of giving the necessary definition of the injury that leads to a useful algorithm of management, although the EAU classification comes closest (Box 4.6.1).

Emergency management

The principles of emergency management are to provide urinary drainage to prevent or relieve urinary retention; to prevent or treat urinary extravasation; and to provide the best possible conditions for recovery of the injury.[1]

If a urethral catheter cannot be passed, then a suprapubic catheter may be placed. In the elective situation, this may be placed percutaneously preferably under ultrasound guidance or, if the injury is iatrogenic and identified preoperatively or the patient is to have a laparotomy or other surgery for other injuries, then it can be placed open.

The only other indications for emergency treatment are following external trauma, particularly a pelvic fracture-related urethral injury; an associated bladder injury, which should be repaired; an associated anorectal injury, requiring a defunctioning colostomy and drainage of the pre-sacral space; and a perineal degloving injury, which requires repair and drainage. All of these, if left unattended, may have serious adverse consequences.

The question is what to do next once urinary drainage has been secured, which depends on the nature of the underlying cause and on whether it is iatrogenic and diagnosed at the time of injury or open penetrating trauma or a closed injury of the penile, bulbar, or posterior urethra.

Iatrogenic trauma

This is very common. It is commonly thought to be due to urological surgery and particularly instrumentation but it can occur without this, such as with the kippering of the urethra that one sees with an indwelling catheter (Fig. 4.6.9), or the damage to the shaft of the penis and the urethra within caused by protracted condom drainage. It can be seen after a circumcision or hypospadias repair or following radiotherapy, in all of which circumstances the patient presents electively for care (this is described elsewhere within this volume). Of more immediate concern is intraluminal trauma caused by catheterization or urethral dilatation; or by losing the lumen during direct vision internal urethrotomy. If any iatrogenic trauma during urological intervention is recognized at the time, this is best dealt with by attempting to pass a guidewire through the site and leaving a catheter in—or if this fails, by suprapubic catheterization.[27]

More critically, is damage to the posterior urethra or bladder base during anterior resection of the rectum for rectal cancer.

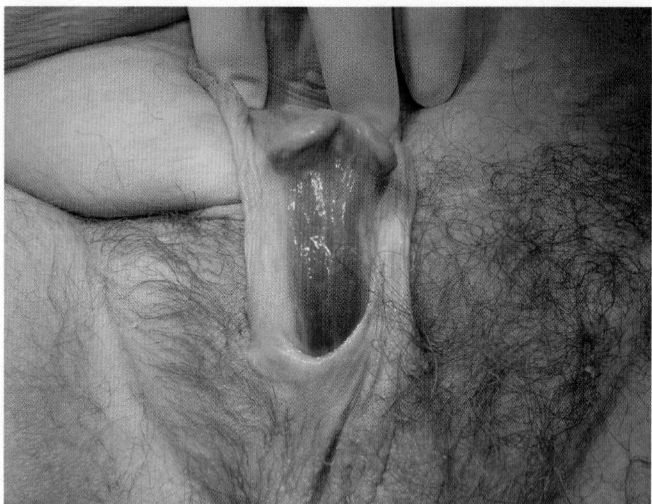

Fig. 4.6.9 Complication of catheterization—a 'kippered' urethra.
Reproduced from Mundy AR and Andrich DE, 'Urethral trauma: Part II: Types of injury and their management', *BJU International*, Volume 108, Issue 5, pp. 630–650, Copyright © 2011 the Authors and BJU International, with permission from John Wiley and Sons.

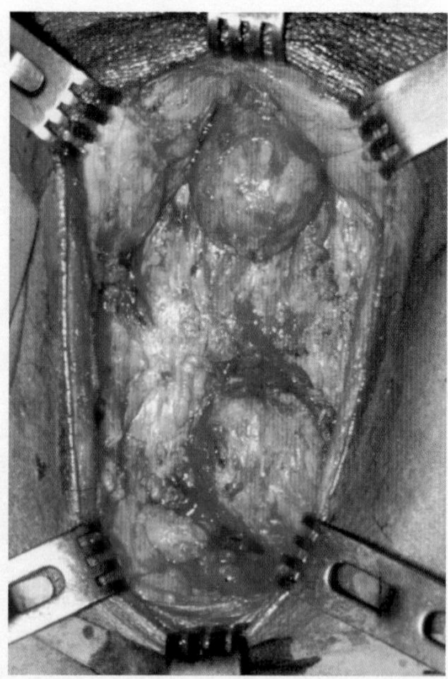

Fig. 4.6.10 Operative photograph of a severe crush injury of the bulbar urethra with ischaemic necrosis of a segment and a gap between the two ends (arrowed).
Reproduced from Mundy AR and Andrich DE, 'Urethral trauma: Part II: Types of injury and their management', *BJU International*, Volume 108, Issue 5, pp. 630–650, Copyright © 2011 the Authors and BJU International, with permission from John Wiley and Sons.

In the latter circumstances, the defect is repaired as far as possible and drained. The omentum should then be mobilized and packed into the space between the injured area of the urinary tract and the area of colorectal surgery, and the patient left with both a urethral and suprapubic catheter to maximize drainage. In the absence of radiation, this may lead to a complete healing of the area. In the irradiated patient—increasingly commonly associated with surgery for colon cancer—this may not suffice.

Penetrating trauma

Open penetrating injury, generally speaking, should be explored in all instances, debrided if necessary, and repaired if possible.[28] However, these principles are coming into question because there is now an increasing trend to manage renal penetrating trauma (the most common form of penetrating trauma) expectantly, subject to careful monitoring. Nonetheless, the general rule now is that penetrating urethral trauma should be explored. Debridement is by no means always necessary because the urethra throughout is well vascularized, the penile and posterior urethra in particular, and so debridement should be limited to obvious serious damage and the removal of foreign material. When a repair is performed, it should only be suture closure. There should be no 'clever' surgery—the use of grafts and flaps in particular—at the time of emergency surgery.[27]

The patient should always be left with at least a urethral catheter, and at best with a urethral and a suprapubic catheter, while the area of injury should be drained.

Closed trauma

Closed penile urethral injuries

Intraluminal trauma from attempted sexual gratification occurs from time to time, and strictly speaking this is a penetrating injury. More dramatic, albeit also uncommon, is a urethral rupture associated with a penile fracture. The penile fracture is usually obvious and its management is described in Chapter 4.7. A urethral rupture is usually an indication for emergency repair of both the penile fracture and the urethral rupture, although in fact both can be managed conservatively if the patient can be catheterized and if bleeding and urinary extravasation are minimal. These points are discussed in Chapter 4.7. This is the one instance in which a cystoscopy may be the best way of making a diagnosis of a urethral injury.

Closed bulbar urethral injuries

Most bulbar urethral injuries are crush injuries leading ultimately, in severe cases, to ischaemic necrosis and gangrene, associated with complete loss of substance (in other words rupture) of the corpus spongiosum, and sometimes of one or both corpora cavernosa as well (Figs 4.6.4 and 4.6.10).

The patient should be managed with a suprapubic catheter and only explored if there is an open wound or expanding haematoma or infection. A urethral catheter should not be placed. Without a urethral catheter, 90% of these urethral injuries will heal without a stenosis. With a catheter, the rate of failure to heal increases from 10% to 65%. Sixty per cent (60%) of these injuries are incomplete and of the 40% that are complete, 75% progress to urethral stenosis without a urethral catheter present—this rate increases to 100% with a urethral catheter.[29,30]

Thus, the best form of management is to leave a suprapubic catheter in place for about three weeks and then clamp it off for a trial of voiding. If there is going to be a stenosis, it will almost certainly be present at this stage or will develop quite quickly thereafterwards. It is only in comparatively unusual circumstances that a stenosis will take six months or more to develop.

For an established stenosis, the best form of treatment is excision and end-to-end, overlapping, and spatulated anastomosis after full mobilization of the urethra on either side. This may require opening of the intercrural plane to allow a tension-free anastomosis. For more severe crush injuries, an augmented anastomotic urethroplasty will be required; that is when the two ends of the urethra may be brought together end-to-end without tension, but cannot be spatulated and overlapped without tension. In order to get a spatulated anastomosis, a buccal mucosal graft will be placed on the dorsal aspect. These procedures are described and illustrated elsewhere.[27]

Although pelvic fracture urethral injuries are commonly regarded as being the most difficult types of injury to repair, a severe crush injury of the bulbar urethra, in our experience, can be even more challenging.

Closed posterior urethral injuries

The early management of these injuries is controversial for several reasons. Having established emergency suprapubic catheter drainage, the question is if anything further can be done in order to make the patient's subsequent recovery easier. Historical experience from when accurate reports started to be kept in the nineteenth century was that the characteristic consequence of a pelvic fracture urethral injury was posterior displacement of the upper end, creating an 'S-bend' malformation at the site of the injury with healing, as well as stricture formation at that site (Fig. 4.6.11). As urethral dilatation was the only form of treatment available for the stricture, this was a problem because the S-bend deformity made instrumentation extremely difficult. Thus, at the beginning of the twentieth century, alternatives were sought, and the first alternative to be tried was primary repair.[31] Primary repair was a big undertaking in such patients at that time and as a consequence of that, in the 1930s, so-called 'realignment' was developed—actually based on a procedure described in 1759—in which, through a suprapubic cystostomy, a catheter was manoeuvred down through the site of injury from above and into the perineum, and then out through a perineal incision to the external meatus.[32] This had rather poor results and consequently it was discontinued in the 1960s in favour of simple suprapubic catheterization.[22,33] By then, urethroplasty had begun to be developed. All alternative management of posterior urethral injuries was developed before the development of urethroplasty.

Contemporaneous with the development of urethroplasty was the development of endoscopy and particularly of high quality rod–lens endoscopy and subsequently of fibre-optic flexible cystoscopy. Consequently, hitherto open realignment came to be performed endoscopically by so-called 'endoscopic primary realignment' (EPR).

Now, 50 years on, the debate falls into two schools of thought. The non-interventionists favour a simple suprapubic catheter and a wait-and-see policy on the grounds that a bulbomembranous anastomotic urethroplasty is performed three to six months after the injury when the patient is fully recovered, and therefore when the operation is performed under ideal conditions, gives such good results that nothing should be done early on to prejudice the outcome. They feel that manipulating the urethra in the early post-traumatic period runs the risk of doing more harm than good.

The interventionists, on the other hand, argue that by so-called 'realignment' the need for a subsequent urethroplasty is reduced; and that if a subsequent urethroplasty is necessary, then it is made easier by the realignment process.

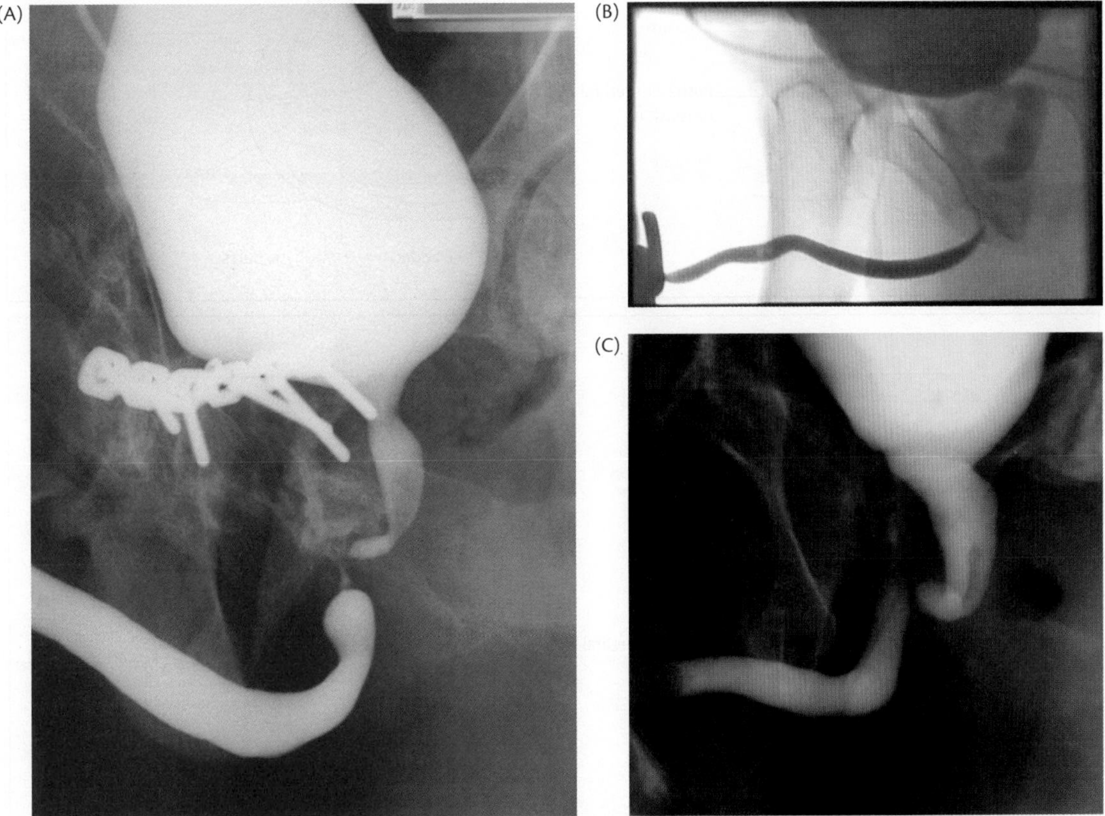

Fig. 4.6.11 (A) S-bend deformity as a result of posterior displacement of (B) the prostate and (C) membranous urethra.

Reproduced from Mundy AR and Andrich DE, 'Urethral trauma: Part II: Types of injury and their management', *BJU International*, Volume 108, Issue 5, pp. 630–650, Copyright © 2011 the Authors and BJU International, with permission from John Wiley and Sons.

This discussion is highly contentious and not least because there are different concepts or definitions of 'success' and different end points. At the present time, there is no definitive objective and uncontroversial evidence that EPR makes a substantial difference. Therefore, the gold standard remains as suprapubic catheterization and interval urethroplasty.[34]

This historical development of the early phase of management of pelvic fracture-related urethral injury has recently been described in some detail elsewhere.[1,27]

Endoscopic primary realignment

There are various techniques of EPR of which the simplest, obviously is simply to pass a urethral catheter in the usual way. In most instances, the technique involves a simultaneous retrograde rigid cystoscopy and an antegrade flexible cystoscopy passing a flexible cystoscope through the bladder neck down to the site of the injury and the retrograde rigid cystoscope up to the site of the injury—and then passing a guidewire between the two so that a catheter can then be passed over the guidewire (Fig. 4.6.12).[35] Various other techniques have been used in the past, typically involving interlocking sounds of some sort or another, but these are largely redundant.

The technique presupposes that realignment—straightening out of the otherwise S-bend deformity back to its natural straight configuration—actually occurs, but there is no evidence that this is so. The haematoma will reabsorb in any case and the urethra tends to adopt its 'S-bend' deformity in any case and in some instances the haematoma does not reabsorb completely whether the 'aligning' catheter is present or not and so a gap remains.

Nonetheless, the protagonists for intervention continue to produce series which show impressive results in maintaining luminal patency and avoiding urethroplasty, except that urethroplasty is avoided at the expense of continuing urethral dilatation or other endoscopic manipulation. Hence the problem mentioned earlier of defining the end points of management. The protagonists of EPR typically use the avoidance of urethroplasty as their end point,

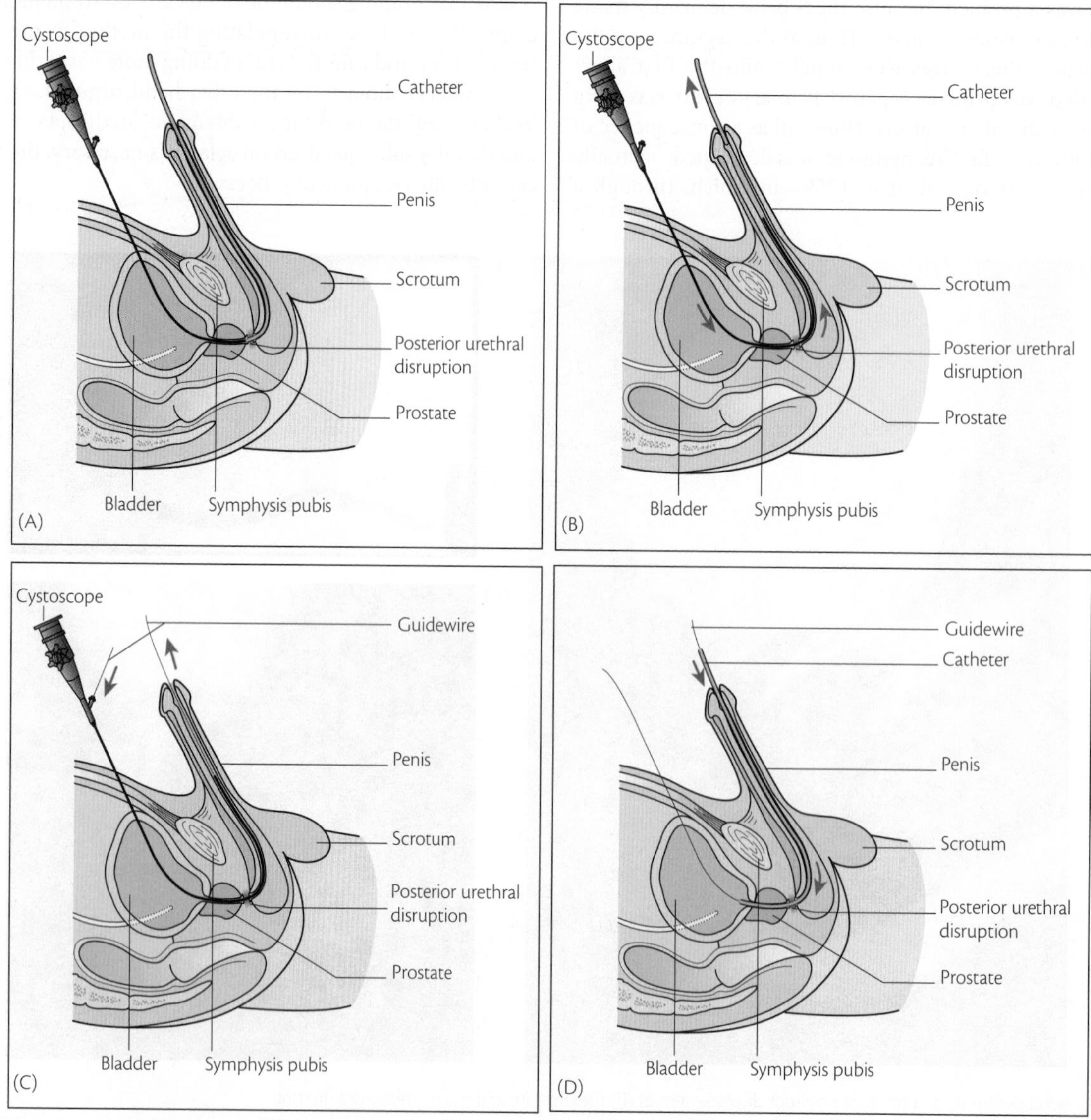

Fig. 4.6.12 Endoscopic primary realignment. (A to D) The basic technique illustrating the principles.

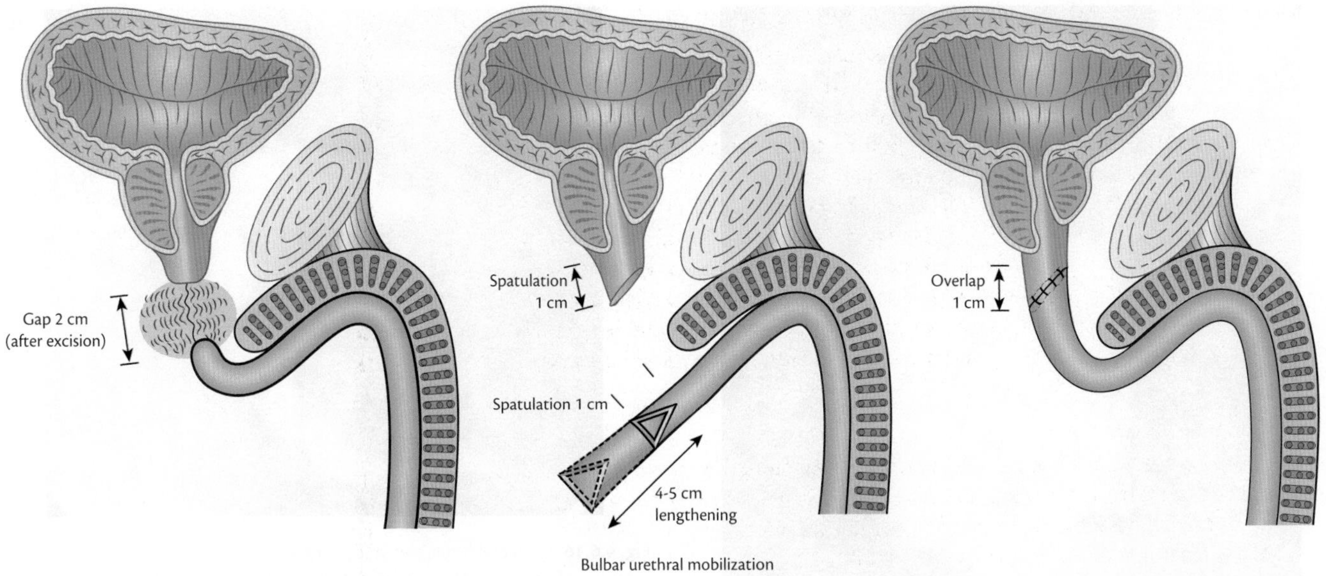

Fig. 4.6.13 Principles of bulbomembranous anastomosis (BMA)—1. The bulbar urethra can stretch.

Reproduced from Mundy AR and Andrich DE, 'Urethral trauma: Part II: Types of injury and their management', *BJU International*, Volume 108, Issue 5, pp. 630–650, Copyright © 2011 the Authors and BJU International, with permission from John Wiley and Sons.

whereas the anti-interventionists use the success rate of the definitive urethroplasty as their's. It therefore seems unlikely that this controversy will ever be resolved.[27,35–39]

Interval urethroplasty

This is typically performed three to six months after the initial injury when the patient has recovered from all other injuries. The procedure involves excision of the injured segment and the associated fibrosis and anastomosis of healthy bulbar urethra below to healthy membranous urethra above—bulbomembranous anastomotic urethroplasty (BMA).[27,40] It is performed, typically, in a step-wise approach based on two principles. The first principle is that the urethra is stretchable (this is a more accurate term than elastic). Thus, an overlapping spatulated anastomosis can be performed and a defect bridged, up to a certain point, just by mobilization alone. This is the same as with bulbo-bulbar anastomosis for a short sharp stricture, or for a relatively short post-traumatic stenosis (Fig. 4.6.13).

The other principle of BMA is that the urethra from the penoscrotal junction to the apex of the prostate is curved around the fused corpora cavernosa and the underlying pubic symphysis. Thus, if the crura are separated and the inferior pubic arch is resected, the urethra can be straightened out and so an even longer defect can be overcome (Fig. 4.6.14).

The procedure can usually be performed transperineally but occasionally it proves difficult if not impossible to identify the apex of the prostate from below and an abdominoperineal approach is necessary. This may also be necessary when other surgery needs to be performed such as, for example, a bladder neck repair.

Bladder neck injuries

Bladder neck injuries[41] are best repaired as soon as they are diagnosed. The injury is a rupture of the prostatic urethra that spreads

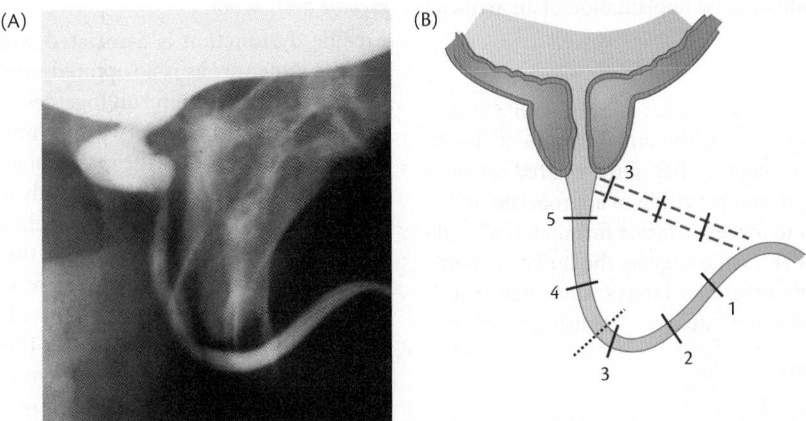

Fig. 4.6.14 Principles of BMA—2. (A) Radiograph and (B) diagram showing the natural course of the bulbar urethra as a curve which can be straightened out.

Reproduced from Mundy AR and Andrich DE, 'Urethral trauma: Part II: Types of injury and their management', *BJU International*, Volume 108, Issue 5, pp. 630–650, Copyright © 2011 the Authors and BJU International, with permission from John Wiley and Sons.

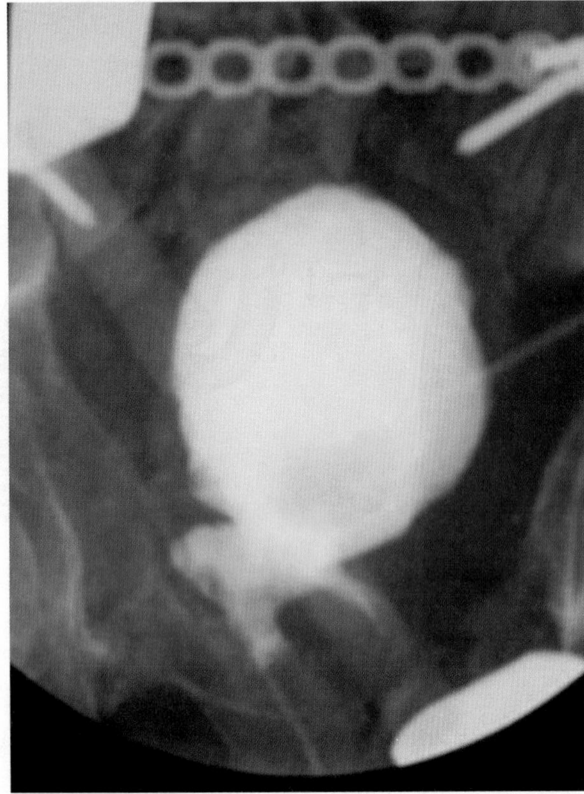

Fig. 4.6.15 A ruptured prostate and bladder neck.
Reproduced from Mundy AR and Andrich DE, 'Urethral trauma: Part II: Types of injury and their management', *BJU International*, Volume 108, Issue 5, pp. 630–650, Copyright © 2011 the Authors and BJU International, with permission from John Wiley and Sons.

upwards. Because of the contraction of the smooth muscle of the bladder neck sphincter mechanism, which pulls the bladder neck open, it never closes spontaneously and a cavity forms which becomes chronically infected (Fig. 4.6.15). This, coupled with the risk to continence as the bladder neck is often the only remaining sphincter mechanism as the initial trauma may have damaged the urethral sphincter, mandates bladder reconstruction at the earliest opportunity. Delayed repair may be successful in restoring continence and is certainly worthwhile as the alternative is management of the inevitable incontinence by implantation of an artificial sphincter.

Urorectal fistulation

This is an unusual event and is associated, typically, with a simultaneous anorectal injury (Fig. 4.6.16). The initial treatment should be by covering colostomy, tacking together of the injured segment if not formal reconstructing it, and provision of appropriate drainage. This is usually sufficient to prevent a fistula forming. If a fistula forms, it can be repaired at the same time as the bulbomembranous anastomotic urethroplasty and an interposition flap placed between the two repairs to stop the fistula re-establishing itself.[42]

Postoperative complications

Incontinence

Incontinence is usually due to an associated bladder neck injury and is corrected as described above. Occasionally the bladder neck is not actually traumatized but the innervation of the bladder neck

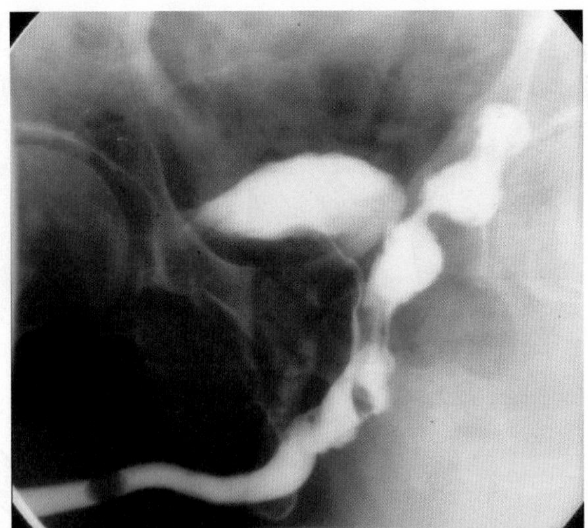

Fig. 4.6.16 Urorectal fistula shown by X-ray.
Reproduced from Mundy AR and Andrich DE, 'Urethral trauma: Part II: Types of injury and their management', *BJU International*, Volume 108, Issue 5, pp. 630–650, Copyright © 2011 the Authors and BJU International, with permission from John Wiley and Sons.

is damaged by a sacral nerve root injury due to the pelvic fracture itself or due to a pelvic plexus traction injury. The bladder neck is undamaged but non-functional and incontinence results.[27]

Occasionally, paradoxically, decentralization of the bladder by pelvic plexus injury leaves the patient with an acontractile bladder and voiding difficulty as a consequence, tending to chronic retention and overflow incontinence. These symptoms are usually thought to be due to a recurrent stenosis. This can be disproved (or proved) endoscopically. Such patients require self-catheterization to void.

In those patients with neuropathic bladder neck dysfunction or a failed bladder neck reconstruction after trauma, implantation of an artificial sphincter is the treatment of choice. In the absence of bladder neck damage, the cuff is best placed around the bladder neck as the urethra has already had its blood supply disrupted by the trauma itself and the subsequent surgery. When the bladder neck has been reconstructed or has been damaged, then the risks of implantation of the cuff of the artificial sphincter should be accepted with the cuff around the bulbar urethra.

Erectile dysfunction

Erectile dysfunction is associated with fracture of the pelvis in just the same way as is a ruptured urethra. The nerves and vessels responsible for erection run together for most of their course, and so it is difficult to be sure whether impotence is a consequence of damage to the nerves or the vessels or a combination of the two. The general opinion is that this is mainly a vascular problem. Erectile dysfunction during the first few weeks after the injury may recover and if there are signs of recovery by three to six months, then there is a good chance that recovery will be complete or, at the least, that it will be complete when supplemented using PDE5 inhibitors such as sildenafil, tadalafil, or vardenafil. These patients are best assessed by clinical evaluation, nocturnal penile tumescence studies, and by Doppler studies of penile blood flow with and without injection of a vasoactive substance such as Quadrimix or Caverject. When there is no evidence of blood flow to the penis the patient usually has as a cold feeling numb penis and this combination of Doppler findings and clinical evaluation is an indication for formal arteriography. Some authorities feel that penile revascularization may be of value although the results of surgery for this situation are often disappointing.[43,44]

Injuries in children

These injuries are not very common in children and when they do occur, they are commonly at a higher level than in adults—through the prostate or through the bladder neck. The treatment is the same, but is more difficult because of the reduced stretchability and underdevelopment of the bulbar urethra. The prognosis for both continence and potency should be guarded until after puberty.[12,45]

Injuries in women

Injuries in women are comparatively uncommon because of the protection afforded by the vagina. When trauma does occur, it may be a transverse rupture as with males and may also be associated with rupture of the vagina and rectum, so that all of the pelvic viscera are ruptured transversely from their anatomical openings—the urethra meatus, the introitus, and the anal canal.[46]

Equally commonly, if not more so, there is a longitudinal rupture of the urethra. Indeed, this may be overlooked at the time of injury and identified during recovery, and thereafterwards as persistent and recalcitrant incontinence.

When identified, it should be repaired early. When established, delayed repair may still be of value. The more complex transverse complete ruptures are a formidable reconstructive challenge.

References

1. Mundy AR, Andrich DE. Urethral trauma: part 1. *BJU Int* 2011; **108**:310–27.
2. Kashefi C, Messer K, Barden R, Sexton C, Parsons JK. Incidence and prevention of iatrogenic urethral injuries. *J Urol* 2008; **179**:2254–8.
3. Bariol SV, Stewart GD, Smith RD, McKeown DW, Tolley DA. An analysis of urinary tract trauma in Scotland: impact on management and resource needs. *Surgeon* 2005; **3**:27–30.
4. Federative Committee on Anatomical Terminology. *Terminologica Anatomica: International anatomical terminology*. New York, Stuttgart: Thieme, 1998: p. 70.
5. Andrich DE, Day AC, Mundy AR. Proposed mechanisms of lower tract injury in fractures of the pelvic ring. *BJU Int* 2007; **100**:567–73.
6. Andrich DE, Mundy AR. The nature of urethral injury in cases of pelvic fracture urethral trauma. *J Urol* 2001; **165**:1492–5.
7. Tile M. *Fractures of the Pelvis and Acetabulum*. Baltimore, MA: Williams and Wilkins, 1984.
8. Pokorny M, Pontes JE, Pierce JM Jr. Urological injuries associated with pelvic trauma. *J Urol* 1979; **121**:455–7.
9. Jordan GH. Management of membranous urethral distraction injuries via the perineal approach. (pp. 393–409) In: McAninch JW (ed). *Trauma and Reconstructive Urology*. Philadelphia, PA: Saunders, 1996.
10. Mundy AR, Andrich DE. Pelvic fracture-related injuries of the bladder neck and prostate: their nature, cause and management. *BJU Int* 2009; **105**:1302–8.
11. Venn SN, Greenwell TJ, Mundy AR. Pelvic fracture injuries of the female urethra. *BJU Int* 1999; **83**:626–30.
12. Singla M, Muruganandam S, Jha K, *et al.* Posttraumatic posterior urethral strictures in children—management and intermediate-term follow-up in tertiary care center. *Urology* 2008; **72**:540–4.
13. Buck G. A new feature in the anatomical structure of the genitor-urinary organs not hitherto described. *Tr Am Med Ass* 1848; **1**:367–73.
14. Colles A. Anatomy of perinaeum. (pp. 174–180) In: Colles A (ed). *A Treatise on Surgical Anatomy*. Dublin, Ireland: Gilbert and Hodges, 1811.
15. Wolfer JA. Urinary extravasation. *Surg Gyn Obs* 1918; **26**:296–302.
16. Eke N. Fournier's gangrene: a review of 1726 cases. *Brit J Surg* 2000; **87**:718–28.
17. Weaver RG, Schulte JW. Clinical aspects of urethral regeneration. *J Urol* 1965; **93**:247–54.
18. McRoberts JW, Ragde H. The severed canine posterior urethra: A study of two distinct methods of repair. *J Urol* 1970; **104**:724–9.
19. Raney AM, Scott MP, Brownstein MD, Bogder JH. Urethral injury. Experimental study. *Urology* 1977: **9**:281–3.
20. Lim PHC, Chng HC. Initial management of acute urethral injuries. *Brit J Urol* 1989; **64**:165–8.
21. Lynch TH, Martínez-Piñeiro L, Plas E, Serafetinides E, Türkeri L, Santucci RA, Hohenfellner M; European Association of Urology. EAU guidelines on urological trauma. *Eur Urol* 2005; **47**:1–15.
22. Mitchell JP. Injuries to the urethra. *Brit J Urol* 1968; **40**:649–69.
23. Chapple CR, Barbagli G, Jordan GH, *et al.* Consensus on genitourinary trauma. Consensus statement on urethral trauma. *BJU Int* 2004; **93**:1195–202.
24. Colapinto V, McCallum RW. Injury to the male posterior urethra in fractured pelvis: a new classification. *J Urol* 1977; **118**:575–9.
25. Goldman SM, Sandler CM, Corriere Jr HN, McGuire EJ. Blunt urethral trauma: a unified anatomical mechanical classification. *J Urol* 1997; **157**:85–9.
26. Moore EE, Cogbill TH, Jurkovich GJ, *et al.* Organ injury scaling. III: chest wall, abdominal vascular, ureter, bladder and urethra. *J Trauma* 1992; **33**:337–9.
27. Mundy AR, Andrich DE. Urethral trauma: part 2. *BJU Int* 2011; **108**:630–50.
28. Marberger M, Stackl W, Dinstl K, Holle J. Reconstructive surgery after perforating trauma of the lower urinary tract. *World J Urol* 1987; **5**:50–6.
29. Park S, McAninch JW. Straddle injuries to the bulbar urethra: Management and outcomes in 78 patients. *J Urol* 2004; **171**:722–5.
30. Elgammal MA. Straddle injuries to the bulbar urethra: Management and outcome in 53 patients. *Int Braz J Urol* 2009; **35**:450–8.
31. Young HH. Treatment of complete rupture of the posterior urethra, recent or ancient, by anastomosis. *J Urol* 1929; **21**:417–49.
32. Ormond JK, Cothran RM. A simple method of treating complete severance of the urethra complicating fracture of the pelvis. *JAMA* 1934; **102**:2180–1.
33. Morehouse DD, Belitsky P, Mackinnon K. Rupture of the posterior urethra. *J Urol* 1972; **107**(2): 55–8.
34. Chapple CR, Barbagli G, Jordan GH, *et al.* Consensus on Genitourinary Trauma. Consensus statement on urethral trauma. *BJU Int* 2004; **93**:1195–202.
35. Gelbard MK, Heyman AM, Weintraub P. A technique for immediate realignment and catheterisation of the disrupted prostatomembranous urethra. *J Urol* 1989: **142**:52–5.
36. Webster GD, Mathes GL, Selli C. Prostatomembranous urethral injuries: a review of the literature and a rational approach to their management. *J Urol* 1983; **130**: 898–902.
37. Mouraviev VB, Coburn M, Santucci RA. The treatment of posterior urethal disruption associated with pelvic fractures: Comparative experience of early realignment versus delayed urethroplasty. *J Urol* 2005; **173**:873–6.
38. Husmann DA, Wilson WT, Boone TB, Allen TD. Prostatomembranous urethral disruptions: management by suprapubic cystostomy and delayed urethroplasty. *J Urol* 1990; **144**:76–8.
39. Levine J, Wessells H. Comparison of open and endoscopic treatment of posttraumatic posterior urethral strictures. *World J Surg* 2001; **25**:1597–1601.
40. Mundy AR. Surgical Atlas: Anastomotic Urethroplasty. *BJU Int* 2005; **96**:921–44.
41. Mundy AR, Andrich DE. Pelvic fracture-related injuries of the bladder neck and prostate: their nature, cause and management. *BJU Int* 2010; **105**:1302–8.
42. Xu YM, Sa YL, Fu Q, Zhang J, Jin SB. Surgical treatment of 31 complex tramatic posterior urethral strictures associated with urethrorectal fistulas. *Eur Urol* 2010; **57**:514–20.

43. Armenakas NA, McAninch JW, Lue TF, Dixon CM, Hricak H. Post-traumatic impotence: magnetic resonance imaging and duplex ultrasound in diagnosis and management. *J Urol* 1993; **149**:1272–5.
44. Anger JT, Sherman ND, Dielubanza E, Webster GD. Erectile function after posterior urethroplasty for pelvic fracture-urethral distraction defect injuries. *BJU Int* 2009; **104**:1126–9.
45. Boone TB, Wilson WT, Husmann DA. Postpubertal genitourinary function following posterior urethral disruptions in children. *J Urol* 1992; **148**:1232–4.
46. Venn SN, Greenwell TJ, Mundy AR. Pelvic fracture injuries of the female urethra. *BJU Int* 1999; **83**:626–30.

CHAPTER 4.7

Genital trauma

Daniela E. Andrich and Anthony R. Mundy

Introduction to genital trauma

Genital trauma accounts for one to two-thirds of all genitourinary trauma. Eighty per cent (80%) of it is blunt trauma but 35% of all penetrating urological injuries are genital injuries.[1,2]

Iatrogenic trauma does occur but most trauma is blunt or penetrating external non-iatrogenic trauma. The commonest type of significant blunt trauma is penile fracture due to sexual intercourse or masturbation. Scrotal trauma causing a ruptured testis or haematocele is less common. Penetrating trauma can occur as a result of animal or human bites, or as a result of amputation, other sharp injury, or as a result of gunshot wounds or other military injuries.

Blunt trauma

Penile fracture (see also Chapter 7.14)

This is the commonest serious injury and occurs as a consequence of acute bending of the erect penis during sexual intercourse, particularly when the female partner is on top.[3] It may occur during masturbation and masturbation-related injury is commoner in the Mediterranean and Middle Eastern countries.[3,4] It only affects the erect penis distal to the suspensory ligament and does so because of the marked thinning of the tunica albuginea on erection, from about 2 mm thick in the flaccid state down to 0.25–0.5 mm on erection.[3] Only one corporal body is affected in most instances.

The characteristic clinical features are a cracking or popping sound associated with pain and detumescence during the sexual act.[3,5,6] A haematoma is a common result causing a so-called aubergine or egg-plant appearance of the penis (Fig. 4.7.1).

The rupture of the tunica albuginea is generally on the ventral or the lateral aspect of the penis. Urethral injury occurs in 10–25% of these patients, usually at the same site as the cavernosal tear.[7] These are usually partial injuries.

If the presentation is delayed due to the patient's embarrassment or otherwise due to a more minor injury, then it may present, additionally, with a butterfly-like haematoma in the perineum (Fig. 4.7.2).

The diagnosis is generally made clinically.[6] The site of rupture of the tunica albuginea is usually palpable. Ultrasonography, cavernosography, and magnetic resonance imaging (MRI) scanning have been used, but clinical diagnosis is normally sufficient. The most reliable way of diagnosing associated urethral injury is by cystoscopy.

Conservative management is possible if there is a minimal haematoma and extravasation,[8] but there is an increased risk of postoperative complications and particularly of pain, erectile dysfunction, or a Peyronie's-like deformation of the penis with conservative management; and for these reasons, and because it gets the patient out of hospital and back to work much quicker, surgical repair is preferred.[3–7,9,10]

The penis is best explored by a degloving incision with a circumcision if necessary to reduce the risk of problems of postoperative oedema and swelling of the foreskin. This incision gives the best exposure to both the corpora cavernosa and the corpus spongiosum, which are repaired with absorbable sutures.

Ruptured suspensory ligament

This occurs from a similar mechanism during sexual intercourse as for penile rupture. It is less common and typically is associated with pain without, necessarily, detumescence. There is a palpable defect on physical examination where the suspensory ligament should be. In the longer term, this is associated with chronic pain and instability of the penis on erection and is best treated by repair of the ligament.

Ruptured testis

Given their relatively exposed location, testicular trauma is not particularly common. Even when circumstances allow the testis to be crushed against the pubis, it takes a considerable force to do so.[11]

A ruptured testis after blunt injury is usually the result of a kick or a blow with a blunt object or, most commonly, a sporting injury.[11] A scrotal haematoma makes clinical examination difficult and the diagnosis is usually made by ultrasound assessment of the testis (Fig. 4.7.3).[12] If there is any suggestion of a rupture or if ultrasound is equivocal then it is sensible to explore the testis.[12–14] Any testicular damage should be debrided and the tunica repaired (Figs 4.7.4, 4.7.5, and 4.7.6). Prompt treatment almost always gives a satisfactory result, whereas delayed treatment reduces the chance of salvage and increases the need for orchidectomy.

Haematocele

If an ultrasound scan after scrotal injury shows a large haematocele then it is usually best drained, even if there is no sign of testicular rupture, to facilitate recovery. In short, after any blunt trauma to the scrotum, the safest approach is to explore it.

High-flow priapism

One of the consequences of perineal or genital trauma is high-flow priapism. This is uncommon and is usually distinguishable from low-flow priapism because of its gradual onset and because it is not painful. It typically follows perineal trauma and rupture of the perineal artery causing an arteriolacunar (the equivalent of an arteriovenous) fistula. Typically, on aspiration of the penis, the blood is bright red and has a normal pH—unlike the colour and pH of low-flow priapism.[3,15]

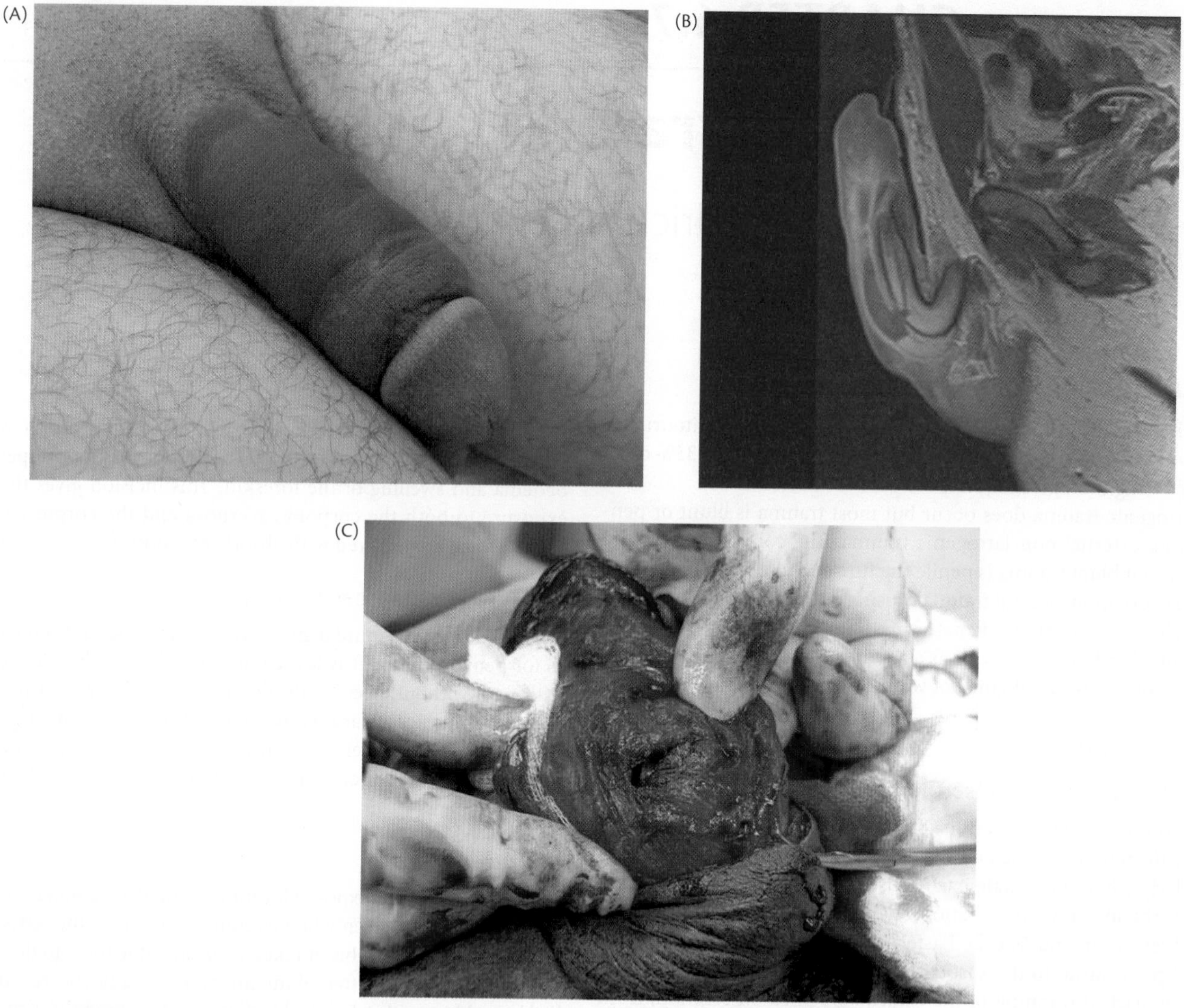

Fig. 4.7.1 Penile fracture associated with urethral injury. (A) Clinical photograph; (B) magnetic resonance imaging (MRI) scan; and (C) operative appearance.
Images reproduced courtesy of Mr David Ralph.

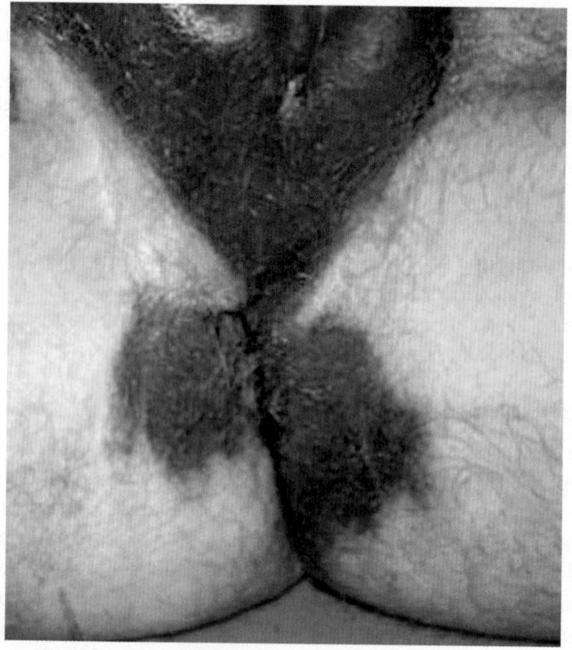

Fig. 4.7.2 Perineal 'butterfly' haematoma associated with late presentation of a penile fracture.

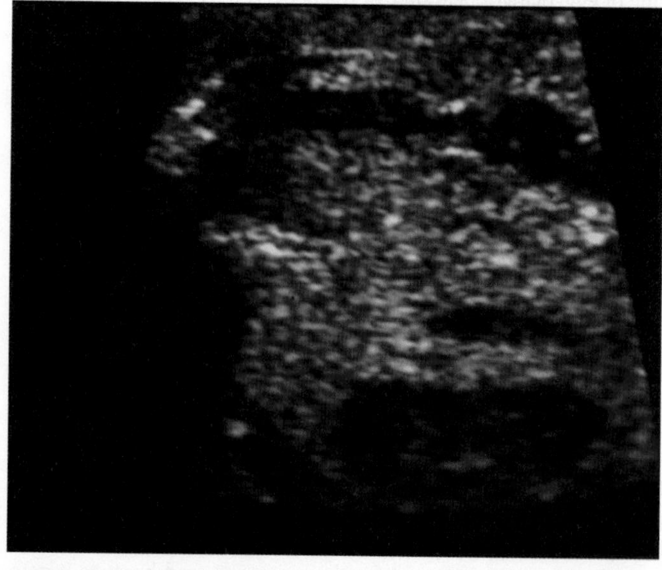

Fig. 4.7.3 Ultrasound scan of a ruptured testis.

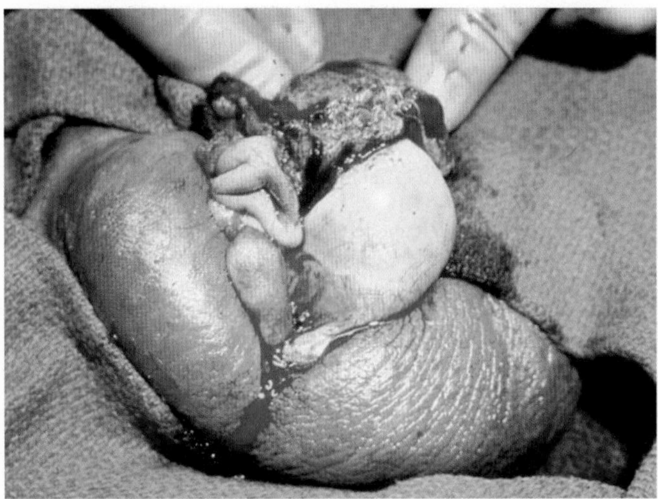

Fig. 4.7.4 Exploration of a ruptured testis.

Ice packs to the penis may reduce or eliminate the priapism; otherwise, arteriography should be performed with a view to embolization (see also Chapter 7.11).

Penetrating injury

Bites

Animal or human bites are not particularly common. Often the patient is embarrassed and does not present himself until late. Whatever the timing of presentation, co-amoxiclav, for the commonest type of infection, *Pasteurella multicida*, should be given. When an animal bite is the cause, one should consider rabies vaccination and a tetanus booster, or vaccination should be given to all patients.[16–19]

The genitalia have an extremely generous blood supply but nonetheless it is sensible to explore, debride, and clean the wound. Damage to the urethra may lead to stricture formation or fistulation.

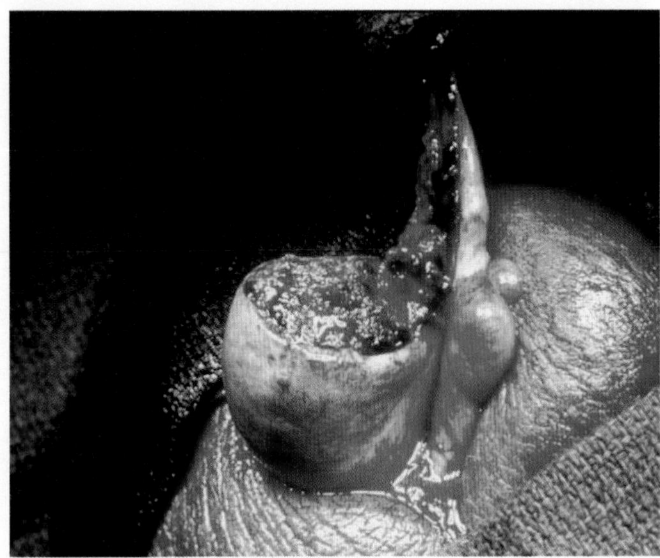

Fig. 4.7.5 Debridement of the testis.

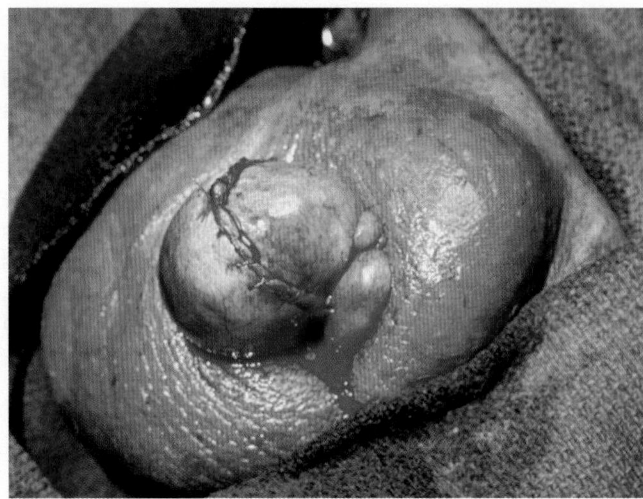

Fig. 4.7.6 Repair of the tunica albuginea.

Stab wounds, gunshot wounds, and other penetrating injuries

Penetrating injuries should always be explored, debrided if necessary, and repaired if possible. In civilian practice, debridement and repair are usually straightforward[2,20]—quite the reverse in a military setting.[21] In either case, these are not usually isolated injuries and associated injuries are the rule. Antibiotic cover and a tetanus booster or vaccination should be given to all patients.

The risk to healthcare personnel of contracting hepatitis B and particularly C appears to be higher than usual in treating patients with penetrating genital trauma, in whom the incidence of these conditions has been reported to be as high as 38%.

Amputation

This may occur for a number of reasons. For some reason or another, women in Thailand in the 1970s started to perform amputation of the penis on their unfaithful husbands. As a result of this, Thai surgeons developed some experience of the management of penile amputation, whether by the patients themselves or by their partners.[22] Self-amputation, nowadays, is more common. This usually occurs in the acutely psychotic patient or in a patient with a psychotic history who is inebriated or otherwise 'affected' at the time. Fifty per cent (50%) are schizophrenic, 20% are psychotically depressed, and a significant number of the remainder have personality or transsexual disorders.

It is clearly important to manage the psychosis—if necessary by sedation. In the meantime, amputations should be treated, if possible, by replanting the penis. The amputated penis, pending replantation, should be wrapped in clean saline gauze and kept on ice. Microsurgical treatment is first to anastomose the dorsal arteries (the cavernosal arteries are much smaller and much more difficult to reanastomose). Attention is then directed to the dorsal veins and the tunica albuginea, and then to the urethra and finally the skin. Anastomosis of the dorsal nerves is usually attempted but whether this leads to an improvement in postoperative erectile function is debatable. Some patients will need a penile prosthesis subsequently.

If the amputated penis has been lost or if it is too late after the injury, then a phalloplasty should be considered as described elsewhere in this volume. These days a free-forearm flap phalloplasty is the procedure of choice anastomosing the donor artery to the inferior epigastric artery and the donor vein to the saphenous vein and the donor nerves to the ilioinguinal nerve. Urethral fistulae and urethral strictures and the difficulties of providing a penile implant are a significant problem in the phalloplasty group, making replantation a better option when possible.

Accidental damage to the penis occurs from time to time for other reasons whether as a result of penetrating trauma, such as military trauma, or mundane causes such as damage to the glans during circumcision. In all instances, the best policy is to explore, debride, and repair where possible, and to cover the procedure with antibiotics. Circumcision should be considered when there is likely to be or already is postoperative swelling and oedema.

References

1. Santucci RA, Bartley JM. Urological trauma guidelines: a 21st century update. *Nat Rev Urol* 2010; **7**(9):510–19.
2. Phonsombat S, Master VA, McAninch JW. Penetrating external genital trauma: a 30-year single institution experience. *J Urol* 2008; **180**:192–5.
3. Mumtaz F, Hellawell G, Ralph D. Penile trauma. (Chapter 9; pp. 165–80) In: Mumtaz F, Woodhouse CRJ, McAninch JW, Conlin DL (eds). *Management of Urological Emergencies*. London, UK: Taylor & Francis, 2004.
4. Zargooshi J. Penile fracture in Kermanshah, Iran: the long-term results of surgical treatment. *BJU Int* 2002; **89**:890–4.
5. Eke N. Fracture of the penis. *Brit J Surg* 2002; **89**:555–65.
6. Koifman L, Barros R, Junior RA, *et al.* Penile fracture: diagnosis, treatment and outcomes of 150 patients. *Urology* 2010; **76**:1488–92.
7. Tsang T, Demby AM. Penile fracture with urethral injury. *J Urol* 1992; **147**:466–8.
8. Muentener M, Suter S, Hauri D, Sulser T. Long-term experience with surgical and conservative treatment of penile fracture. *J Urol* 2004; **172**:576–9.
9. Ibrahiem al-HI, El-Tjoloth HS, Mohsen T, *et al.* Penile fracture: long-term outcome of immediate surgical intervention. *Urology* 2010; **75**:108–11.
10. Yapanoglu T, Aksoy Y, Adanur S, *et al.* Seventeen years' experience of penile fracture: conservative vs. surgical treatment. *J Sex Med* 2009; **6**:2058–63.
11. Wasko R, Goldstein AG. Traumatic rupture of the testicle. *J Urol* 1966; **95**:721–3.
12. Micalir M, Ahmad I, Ramesh N, Nurley M, McInnerney D. Ultrasound features of blunt testicular injury. *Injury* 2001; **32**:23–6.
13. Corrales JG, Corbel L, Cipolla B, *et al.* Accuracy of ultrasound diagnosis after blunt testicular trauma. *J Urol* 1993; **150**:1834–6.
14. Fourner GR, Laing FC, McAninch JW. Social altrasonography and the management of testicular trauma. *Urol Clin North Am* 1989; **16**:377–85.
15. Riccardi R, Bhatt GM, Cynamon J, Bakal CW, Melman A. Delayed high flow priapism. Pathophysiology and management. *J Urol* 1993; **149**:119–21.
16. Donovan JF, Kaplan WE. The theraphy of genital trauma by dog bite. *J Urol* 1989; **141**:1163–5.
17. Presutti RJ. Prevention and treatment of dog bites. *Am Fam Physician* 2001; **63**:1567–72.
18. Presutti RJ. Bite wounds. Early treatment and prophylaxis against infectious complications. *Postgrad Med* 1997; **101**:243–54.
19. Talan DA, Citron DM, Abrahamian FM, Moran GJ, Goldstein EJ. Bacteriologic analysis of infected dog and cat bites. Emergency Medicine Animal Bite Infection Study Group. *N Engl J Med* 1999; **340**:85–92.
20. Perovic SV, Djinovic RP, Bumbasirevic MZ, *et al.* Severe penile injuries: a problem of severity and reconstruction. *BJU Int* 2009; **104**:676–87.
21. Najibi S, Tann ST, Latini JM. Civilian gunshot wounds to the genitoruiary tract: incidence, anatomic distribution, associated injuries, and outcomes. *Urology* 2010; **76**:977–81.
22. Bhanganda K, Chayavatana T, Pongnumkuk C, *et al.* Surgical management of an epidemic of penile amputations in Siam. *Am J Surg* 1983; **146**:376–82.

CHAPTER 4.8

General principles of trauma

Graham Sleat and David Noyes

Introduction to general principles of trauma

Aetiology, incidence, and costs of trauma

Trauma is a major public health problem worldwide, causing substantial morbidity and mortality. It was estimated that in 2015, 5.2 million people will have died as a result of traumatic injuries[1]; and for each person who dies from an injury, many survive, often with long-term physical and/or mental disability. Within England and Wales, traumatic injury is the leading cause of death of people from the ages of 1 to 44,[2] and disproportionately affects people when they are in the most economically active part of their lives, with some estimates placing the cost of major trauma to the economy at £3.7 billion annually.[3] Three times as many men are affected than women and trauma is also seen to have an increased incidence in the more deprived sections of society.[4]

Most serious traumatic injuries seen in England and Wales are due to blunt force trauma, in most cases caused by either falls or road traffic collisions. These result in serious injuries, mainly to the lower limbs (40%) and head (20%), and in up to a third of patients, results in a stay in intensive care.[5]

Injury severity scoring

Traumatic injuries can be graded according to the Injury Severity Score (ISS).[6] This is an anatomical scoring system that gives an overview of the severity of all the injuries a patient has sustained and correlates with patient mortality. The ISS can range from 1 to 75, and by convention major trauma is a score of more than 15, and patients with a score above 8 are felt to have serious injuries.

The score is calculated using the Abbreviated Injury Scale (AIS), where each injury in the body is graded from 1 (minor) to 6 (injury incompatible with life) and the body is divided into regions with only the most severe injury being counted from each region. The squared AIS scores for the most seriously injured three body regions are summed to give the ISS. However, any area which scores an AIS of 6 automatically results in an ISS of 75 as scores of 6 are viewed as incompatible with life.

Models of trauma care

International history of trauma care

Advances in trauma care have often come with the harsh experiences gained in major military conflicts. Step changes in clinical practice have followed conflicts such as the First and Second World Wars and Vietnam in the twentieth century, and more recently Iraq and Afghanistan in the twenty-first century. As with many innovations, it takes a long time for the lessons learnt in one area to be translated into others. This has been the case with the care of the seriously injured.

The first movement towards a structured system of trauma care for the civilian population was seen in the 1970s in the United States, where it was recognized that seriously injured patients required prompt and appropriate care in centres which had a specialist interest in trauma care with the aim of reducing mortality. This was triggered by the National Academy of Sciences/National Research Council (NAS/NRC) Report on Accidental Death in 1966 and led to the development of nascent trauma centres in some areas of the United States, including Florida and Illinois.[7]

Further impetus to change in the USA came from a study by West *et al.*[8] that demonstrated that San Francisco, which had a trauma system, had a lower mortality rate than that seen in neighbouring Orange County. This study resulted in changes not just in Orange County, but throughout the USA. Ultimately this resulted in the system of trauma care seen in the United States today, with the designation by the American College of Surgeons, of level one and two trauma centres.[9]

Subsequently, a systematic review has shown that seriously injured patients treated in a trauma centre as part of a trauma system have a 15% lower mortality than those treated outside of this system.[10] This improvement applies not just to multisystem trauma, but also to injuries such as isolated head injuries, where mortality was found to be significantly higher in England and Wales with no trauma system in place, when compared with Victoria, Australia, which has a well-established trauma system.[11] In addition, trauma systems have been shown to reduce the length of stay in hospital and increase the proportion of those living independently at six months after injury.[12]

Other countries have taken on the American model and are operating trauma systems where the most seriously injured patients are taken directly to major trauma centres, bypassing hospitals with facilities that are inadequate for their needs. Canada and Victoria State in Australia have long established major trauma centres and associated networks that are proven to improve care and reduce mortality.

In parallel with this change in systems of healthcare management for trauma patients, the American College of Surgeons developed the Advanced Trauma Life Support Course®,[13] which has been adopted by many countries worldwide and teaches doctors in the safe and systematic management of trauma patients. Completion of this course or an equivalent is now a mandatory requirement for those coming to apply for their Certificate of Completion of Training in many surgical specialties, although not urology.

United Kingdom history of trauma care and current trauma organization

In the United Kingdom, it has been recognized for many years that the system of care for the seriously injured was inadequate. The standard of care that patients would receive was dependent upon when and where they were injured, as the usual practice for the ambulance services was to take the patient to the nearest hospital's accident and emergency department, irrespective of the availability of specialist care and rehabilitation services. As has been already discussed, there has been increasing worldwide evidence that taking patients directly to the hospital best suited to their needs, even if that means bypassing the nearest hospital with an emergency department, is the most appropriate pathway of care.

The Royal College of Surgeons of England first highlighted the deficiencies in trauma care in 1988 in their report 'The Management of Patients with Major Injuries'. As a result, a pilot major trauma centre was set up at North Staffordshire Royal Infirmary; however, when assessed this only showed modest mortality benefit.[14] This is now thought to be due to the lack of integration of the whole trauma care pathway in this pilot, but the results reduced the momentum for change in the United Kingdom.

As such, trauma was allowed to fall by the wayside and was not seen as a priority despite the accumulating evidence. Finally, following a report by National Confidential Enquiry into Patient Outcome and Death (NCEPOD)—'Trauma: Who cares?' in 2007, the government of the day committed to improving the care provided to trauma patients and appointed the first National Clinical Director for Trauma Care in 2009, Professor Keith Willett, who was tasked with setting up regional trauma networks across England. This task was aided by a critical National Audit Office Report on Major Trauma in 2010 which gave the government a final push towards funding the implementation of major trauma systems across England.

An NHS Clinical Advisory Group was set up as part of this process to assess all the evidence relating to optimal care of the seriously injured; their report is valuable reading for those interested in this field.[15]

In parallel to this work, Lord Darzi's reforms to healthcare in London also involved improving treatment by centralizing care for conditions when this was indicated by the available evidence. This included major trauma and the first three Major Trauma Centres in London (and the United Kingdom) went live in April 2010 at the Royal London Hospital, King's College Hospital, and St George's Hospitals, joined by a fourth (St Mary's Hospital) the following year.

The rest of England now has trauma networks that went live in 2012, with each network covering a population of between 1.5 and 5 million. Currently there are 22 adult major trauma centres (MTC) and associated networks in NHS England, with some combined centres that cater for children as well, and four specialist children's major trauma centres (Fig. 4.8.1).

Since going live, patients who sustain serious injuries within a 45-minute available transit time to an MTC are diverted directly to the MTC and bypass local emergency departments. Pathways have also changed for patients who do not need immediate transfer to the MTC but need urgent specialist care, such as pelvic or acetabular reconstruction, with a target being set for these patients to be transferred within 48 hours.

The impact of the introduction of trauma systems has already been seen with an early audit of major trauma patients, showing that one in five who would have died before the networks were implemented now survive. In addition, it is predicted that for every extra survivor, three will make an enhanced recovery, hopefully allowing an earlier return to work.[16]

In the remainder of the United Kingdom, there are moves to implement similar measures for patients. However, at the time of writing no formal designation of major trauma centres or trauma networks has been made in Wales, Scotland, or Northern Ireland.

Pre-hospital management of trauma care

There is a trimodal distribution of deaths that occur following serious trauma, with the first peak occurring almost immediately after the time of injury, the second peak in the initial hours and days, and the third within the first few weeks following injury. The management of trauma victims cannot address the first peak, but early treatment can prevent death and reduce the morbidity in the other two groups. As such, it is recognized that the treatment of trauma patients needs to begin at the scene of the accident.

Different countries have developed varying setups for treating patients at the scene of any trauma. In the United Kingdom, traditionally ambulance technicians and paramedics have been the mainstay of the management of these patients, unlike some other countries where physicians have been routinely sent out to serious incidents. A large number of voluntary organizations, such as the British Association for Immediate Care (BASICS) and the multiple air ambulance charities have filled the gap, and there has been a growing recognition that pre-hospital care should be an integrated part of the pathway for the seriously injured patient. As such, there is now a specialty of pre-hospital care approved by the General Medical Council in the United Kingdom, and there are an increasing number of doctors being appointed to roles that involve some element of pre-hospital duty. There are also specially trained paramedics such as critical care paramedics and other healthcare professionals, who are able to provide an enhanced level of care (enhanced care team) at the scene to bring some aspects of hospital care directly to the patient.

Different philosophies have held sway in pre-hospital trauma care over the years, but one aspect which is essential when dealing with any trauma situation is triage. Many of the causes of serious injury by their nature mean that multiple casualties may be expected and it is important that any healthcare professional in the pre-hospital field is able to establish safety at the scene, and then rapidly and effectively triage patients so that the needs of patients are prioritized. This may under certain circumstances, particularly if resources are scarce, involve identifying those who are too seriously injured to help. In addition, with trauma networks now in place, those at the scene need to be able to decide when to activate the major trauma pathway, and triage tools are in place to help those on the scene decide whether the patient in front of them needs to go directly to the MTC.

Evidence from organizations such as the London Helicopter Emergency Medical Service (HEMS) has shown that bringing advanced resuscitative care to the patient at the scene saves lives, and it is recognized that certain targeted interventions can be key to preventing secondary injury, saving life, and reducing morbidity. Such

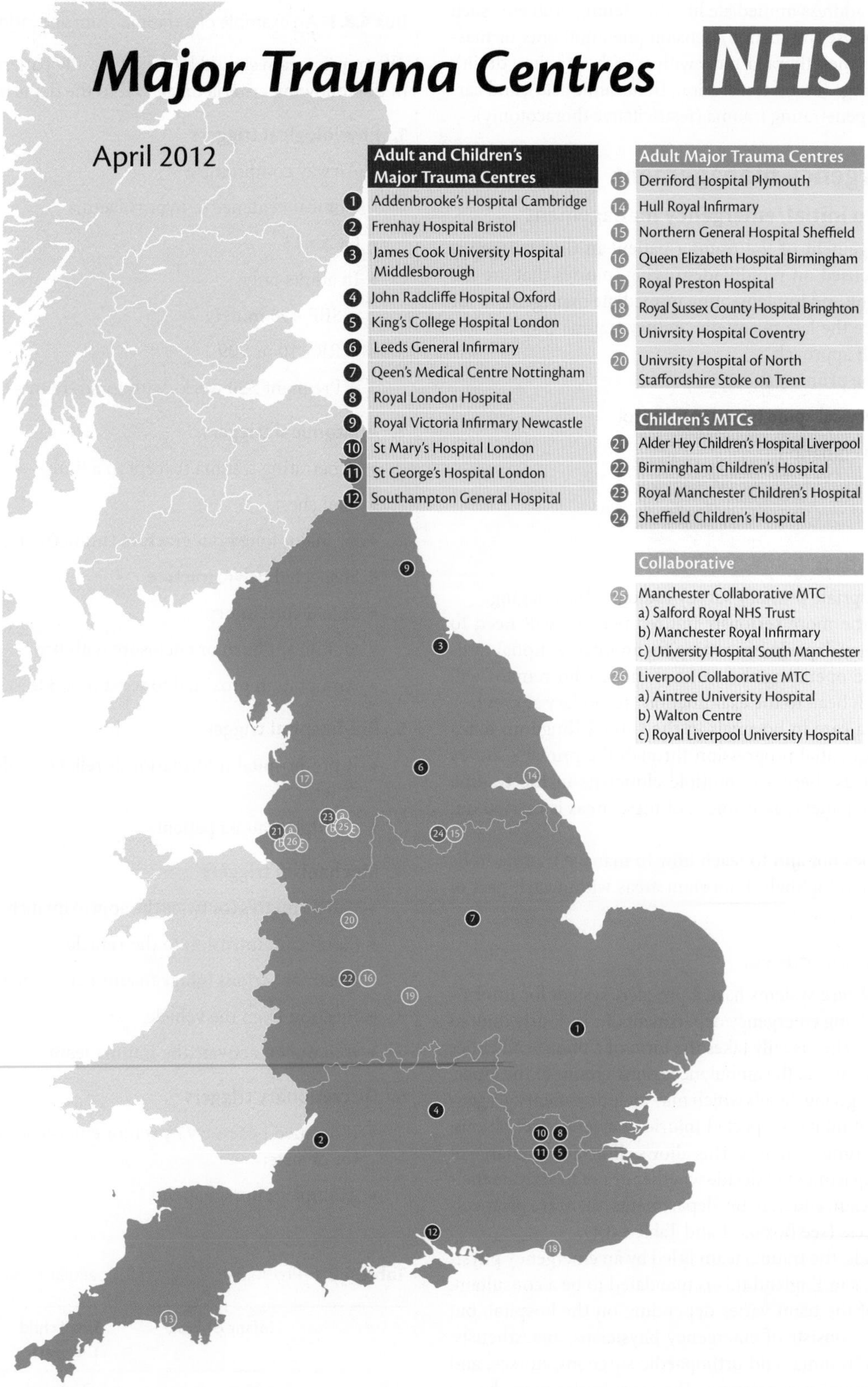

Major Trauma Centres

April 2012

Adult and Children's Major Trauma Centres

1. Addenbrooke's Hospital Cambridge
2. Frenhay Hospital Bristol
3. James Cook University Hospital Middlesborough
4. John Radcliffe Hospital Oxford
5. King's College Hospital London
6. Leeds General Infirmary
7. Qeen's Medical Centre Nottingham
8. Royal London Hospital
9. Royal Victoria Infirmary Newcastle
10. St Mary's Hospital London
11. St George's Hospital London
12. Southampton General Hospital

Adult Major Trauma Centres

13. Derriford Hospital Plymouth
14. Hull Royal Infirmary
15. Northern General Hospital Sheffield
16. Queen Elizabeth Hospital Birmingham
17. Royal Preston Hospital
18. Royal Sussex County Hospital Bringhton
19. Univrsity Hospital Coventry
20. Univrsity Hospital of North Staffordshire Stoke on Trent

Children's MTCs

21. Alder Hey Children's Hospital Liverpool
22. Birmingham Children's Hospital
23. Royal Manchester Children's Hospital
24. Sheffield Children's Hospital

Collaborative

25. Manchester Collaborative MTC
    a) Salford Royal NHS Trust
    b) Manchester Royal Infirmary
    c) University Hospital South Manchester
26. Liverpool Collaborative MTC
    a) Aintree University Hospital
    b) Walton Centre
    c) Royal Liverpool University Hospital

Fig. 4.8.1 Map of major trauma centres in England (April 2012).
Reproduced courtesy of NHS Choices, www.nhs.uk

interventions can address immediate life-threatening problems such as airway compromise (intubation); tension pneumothorax or massive haemothorax (chest thoracostomy with or without a chest drain); massive haemorrhage (blood transfusion, tranexamic acid); and cardiac arrest due to penetrating trauma (resuscitative thoracotomy).

Initial/emergency management

Introduction to initial/emergency management

The initial management of the trauma patient in the emergency department is focused on rapidly identifying injuries that are life or limb-threatening and implementing immediate management for those found. Since the late twentieth century trauma care has followed the ABCDE approach.

This involves the primary survey:

- Airway with cervical spine (C-spine) control
- Breathing and ventilation
- Circulation
- Disability
- Exposure

followed by appropriate primary survey radiographic imaging.

At this point, the more seriously injured patients will need to leave the emergency department setting for an interventional radiology suite or the operating theatre, but those who remain will require a thorough head to toe examination (secondary survey).

Modern trauma care in hospitals in the United Kingdom tends not to involve sequential progression through the primary survey algorithm; rather as there are multiple clinicians in the trauma team to assess the patient, assessment of these areas is carried out simultaneously.

This section does not aim to teach how to manage trauma in its entirety, but aims to highlight important areas within each part of initial trauma management.

Preparation and handover

Most pre-hospital care systems have a pre-alert system for informing the likely receiving emergency department of a seriously injured patient coming in. This usually takes the form of a phone call either directly from scene or via the ambulance control room to the emergency department giving details which may include patient age, gender, mechanism of injury, suspected injuries, current observations, and an estimated time of arrival. This allows clinicians in charge of the emergency department to decide whether or not to activate their hospital trauma team, and in many departments, there are protocols to guide this process (see Box 4.8.1 and Table 4.8.1).

In most hospitals, the trauma team is led by an emergency physician, and in MTCs in England this is mandated to be a consultant. The remainder of the team varies depending on the hospital, but the core typically consists of emergency physicians, anaesthetists, general surgeons, trauma, and orthopaedic surgeons, nurses, and operating department practitioners. The team leader may choose to involve other specialties at an early stage, such as urologists and neurosurgeons, should a relevant injury be suspected either from the pre-alert or initial assessments.

At the time of arrival in the department, the handover typically follows the 'ATMIST' sequence:

- Age of patient
- Time of incident

Box 4.8.1 An example of a trauma team activation protocol

The trauma team should be called for any patients who meet one of the following criteria on arrival to the department.

1. **Physiological triggers**
   - Airway compromise
   - Clinical evidence of hypovolaemia
   - GCS <13
   - In adults only:
     - SBP <90 mmHg
     - RR <10 or >29
     - Pregnant >20 weeks with torso trauma
2. **Anatomical triggers**
   - Penetrating trauma (except in a limb)
   - Flail chest
   - >1 major long bone fracture (humerus/femur/tibia)
   - Suspected pelvic fracture
   - Spinal cord injury
   - Significant burn or enclosure with fire
   - Amuptation proximal to wrist or ankle
3. **Pre-hospital triggers**
   - If pre-hospital information is reliable and fulfils the above criteria
   - Multiple trauma patients
4. **Mechanism triggers**
   - Fall >3 metres (or twice the approximate height of the child)
   - Significant intrusion to the vehicle
   - Death or serious injury to another occupant of the vehicle
   - Ejection from the vehicle
   - If in doubt, activate the trauma team
5. **Discretionary triggers**
   - If deemed necessary by senior emergency department doctor or sister
   - Multiple trauma patients

Table 4.8.1 Physiological triggers for paediatric patients

	Infant <1 year	Small child 1–8 years	Large child 9–15 years
RR	<20 or >50	<20 or >35	<15 or >25
Systolic BP	<70 mmHg	<70 mmHg	<80 mmHg
Pulse	<90 or >170	<75 or >130	<60 or >120
GCS	<13		
Sats	<90%		
Skin	Cool, pale, clammy		

- Elderly (>55 years) or multiple co-morbidities
- If in doubt, activate

Consultant attendance within five minutes of patient arrival (see Table 4.8.1)

Glossary

GCS Glasgow Coma Scale

SBP systolic blood pressure

RR respiratory rate

Sats oxygen saturations

Reproduced courtesy of the Emergency Department, Nottingham University Hospitals NHS Trust.

- Mechanism of injury
- Injuries (top to toe)
- Vital Signs
- Treatment rendered

Airway and C-spine control

Major trauma patients are generally removed from the scene on a long board or scoop with three-point immobilization with head blocks, neck collar, and tape. Should these not be in place for any reason, it is imperative that the cervical spine is protected as soon as is practicable. Difficulties can arise, for example with a combative patient, however this may be a sign that the patient is hypoxic and it is vital that the cause of any irritability is addressed as this will allow safe management of the C-spine. Hard long spinal immobilization boards can rapidly cause pressure sores and should be removed as soon as possible as part of a log roll and examination of the back. In line immobilization of the C-spine and the rest of the spine should be maintained until injury has been ruled out (either clinically or radiologically).

Generally, within the hospital environment the airway is managed by emergency physicians and anaesthetists, but surgeons may be involved should a surgical airway be required. High-flow oxygen is applied to all patients when they first arrive in the department and those who cannot maintain their own airway will require a definitive airway, usually in the form of a cuffed endotracheal tube.

Breathing and ventilation

A rapid assessment of the patient's breathing and ventilation to include screening for any immediately life-threatening injuries is essential. Patients may demonstrate unequal chest rise, tracheal deviation, unequal or absent breath sounds, or changed percussion note. All of these may be signs of immediately life-threatening injuries. These injuries need immediate intervention (e.g. chest tube thoracostomy) in the case of massive haemothorax, along with appropriate resuscitation and treatment of the underlying cause (Table 4.8.2).

Circulation

Patients may present in shock with symptoms and signs as in Table 4.8.3. Haemorrhagic shock is by far the commonest type of shock in trauma patients, but other non-haemorrhagic causes such as cardiac tamponade and neurogenic (spinal cord injury) should be considered. Major haemorrhage is one of the main reasons for death in trauma patients and common sites for haemorrhage causing shock are abdominal (e.g. from splenic rupture) and pelvic (e.g. secondary to pelvic fracture causing arterial bleeding). A focused examination may locate likely sources of bleeding, but manoeuvres such as 'springing' the pelvis are contraindicated. Patients who are suspected to have a pelvic fracture should have a pelvic binder applied; this is often done in the pre-hospital environment (Figs 4.8.2 and 4.8.3). Patients who

Table 4.8.2 Immediately life-threatening chest injuries

Injury	Key signs	Immediate management
Tension pneumothorax	• Tachycardia • Tracheal deviation away from side of lesion • Hyperresonant percussion note on side of lesion • Decreased breath sounds on side of lesion • Breathlessless and hypoxia	Immediate decompression with wide bore cannula inserted into second intercostal space mid-clavicular line, followed by chest tube thoracostomy
Massive haemothorax	• Hypoxia • Hypotension and tachycardia • Dull percussion note on side of lesion	Resuscitate including tranfusion. Chest tube thoracostomy. If significant initial (>1,500 mL) or ongoing (>200 mL/hour) blood loss will require cardiothoracic review and possible thoracotomy
Open pneumothorax	• Obvious chest wall wound with air sucked in on inspiration • Hypoxia	Occlude opening with impermeable dressing secured on three sides for flutter valve effect, followed by chest tube thoracostomy
Flail chest and pulmonary contusion	• Asymmetrical chest wall movement • Crepitations on palpation suggestive of multiple rib fractures • Hypoxia	Supportive. Ensure adequate oxygenation and ventilation, resuscitation. Provide adequate analgesia including possibly an intercostal nerve block. May require high dependency care

Table 4.8.3 Grades of shock with clinical features

Class of haemorrhagic shock	Blood loss	Clinical features
1	0–15% (<750 mL)	Anxious, but normal observations
2	15–30% (750–1,500 mL)	Tachypnoeic, tachycardic, narrowed pulse pressure, decreased urine output
3	30–40% (1,500–2,000 mL)	Markedly tachypnoeic, tachycardic, and hypotensive. Confused
4	>40% (>2,000 mL)	Worsening of features seen in class 3 plus worsening conscious level, bradycardia, and anuria

Source: data from American College of Surgeons Committee on Trauma, *Advanced Trauma Life Support® (ATLS) Student Manual, Ninth Edition*, American College of Surgeons, Chicago, USA, Copyright © 2012; and Louis Solomon et al., *Apley's System of System of Orthopaedics and Fractures, Ninth Edition*, CRC Press, Taylor & Francis, Florida, USA, Copyright © 2010.

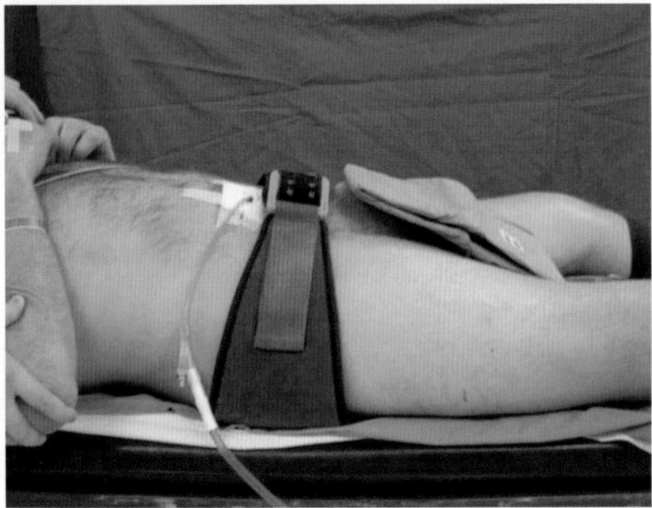

Fig. 4.8.2 Pelvic binder correctly applied.
Image courtesy of Mr Tim Chesser.

have a pelvic fracture and are suspected to have a urological injury should be managed according to the recently published joint British Orthopaedic Association and British Association of Urological Surgeons standards.[17]

Emergent resuscitative measures are necessary to restore and maintain the circulating blood volume and stabilize the patient, but there is also a need for this to be balanced to reduce the risk of dislodging a clot that may lead to further catastrophic haemorrhage. All trauma patients should receive two wide bore intravenous cannulae. Traditionally, they would receive a litre of warmed crystalloid with their response to this being divided into non-responders (surgery required), transient responders (usually surgery required), and responders (serial observation). Knowledge gleaned from military medicine has now influenced the resuscitative phase of treatment and early use of blood products in the seriously injured is recommended. The exact ratio of packed red blood cells to fresh frozen plasma and platelets may vary by institution but most centres now have a massive transfusion protocol that guides the management of trauma patients with suspected major haemorrhage (see Fig. 4.8.4).

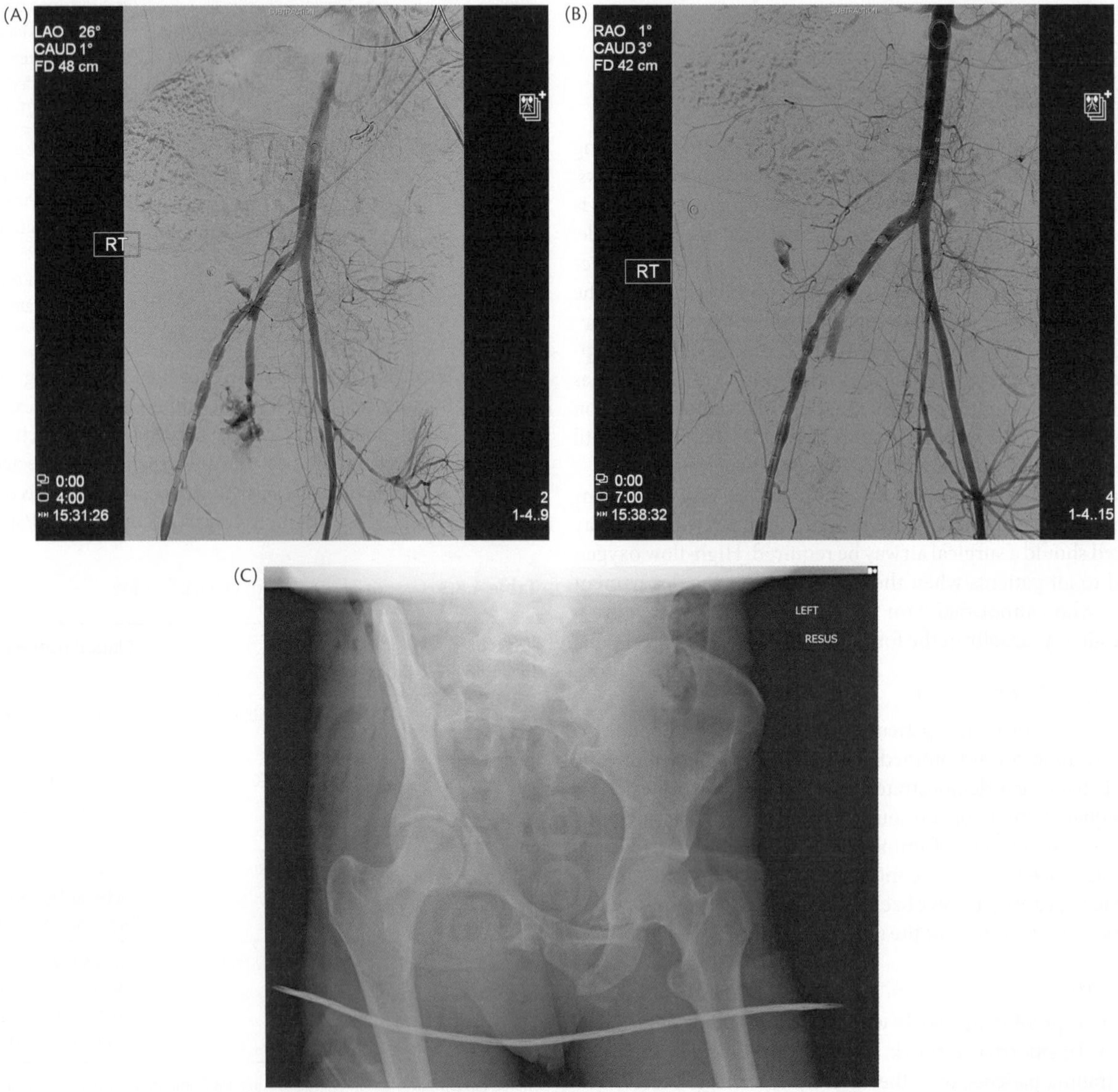

Fig. 4.8.3 (A to C) Open book pelvic fracture XR +/− angioembolization.

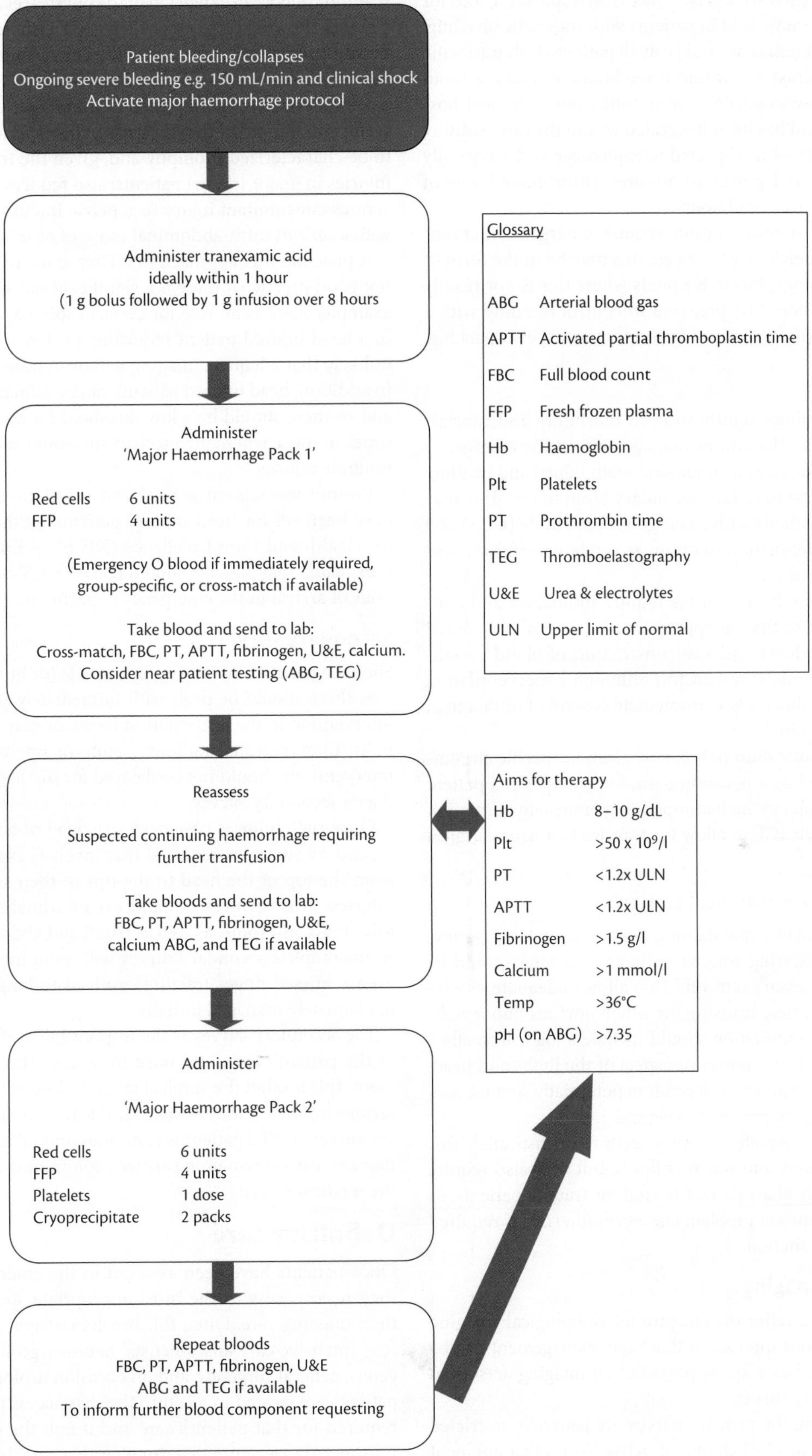

Patient bleeding/collapses
Ongoing severe bleeding e.g. 150 mL/min and clinical shock
Activate major haemorrhage protocol

↓

Administer tranexamic acid
ideally within 1 hour
(1 g bolus followed by 1 g infusion over 8 hours

↓

Administer
'Major Haemorrhage Pack 1'

Red cells	6 units
FFP	4 units

(Emergency O blood if immediately required, group-specific, or cross-match if available)

Take blood and send to lab:
Cross-match, FBC, PT, APTT, fibrinogen, U&E, calcium.
Consider near patient testing (ABG, TEG)

↓

Reassess

Suspected continuing haemorrhage requiring further transfusion

Take bloods and send to lab:
FBC, PT, APTT, fibrinogen, U&E,
calcium ABG, and TEG if available

↓

Administer

'Major Haemorrhage Pack 2'

Red cells	6 units
FFP	4 units
Platelets	1 dose
Cryoprecipitate	2 packs

↓

Repeat bloods
FBC, PT, APTT, fibrinogen, U&E
ABG and TEG if available
To inform further blood component requesting

Glossary

ABG	Arterial blood gas
APTT	Activated partial thromboplastin time
FBC	Full blood count
FFP	Fresh frozen plasma
Hb	Haemoglobin
Plt	Platelets
PT	Prothrombin time
TEG	Thromboelastography
U&E	Urea & electrolytes
ULN	Upper limit of normal

Aims for therapy

Hb	8–10 g/dL
Plt	>50 x 10^9/l
PT	<1.2x ULN
APTT	<1.2x ULN
Fibrinogen	>1.5 g/l
Calcium	>1 mmol/l
Temp	>36°C
pH (on ABG)	>7.35

Fig. 4.8.4 An example of a major haemorrhage protocol.
Reproduced courtesy of Oxford University Hospitals NHS Trust.

Evidence from the CRASH-2 trial[18] has clearly shown a role for administering tranexamic acid in patients with traumatic bleeding. It has been shown to reduce mortality in all patients with traumatic bleeding when administered within three hours of injury without any apparent increase in adverse thrombotic events. In most hospitals, tranexamic acid has been integrated within the care pathway of all trauma patients with suspected haemorrhage and is typically given intravenously as 1 g over 10 minutes within three hours of injury, and then 1 g over eight hours.

Non-responders to resuscitation require emergent intervention. In the case of pelvic haemorrhage this may be in the form of interventional radiology, but in hospitals where this is not readily available surgeons should be prepared to control bleeding with a combination of external fixation and extraperitoneal pelvic packing.

Disability

Head injuries contribute significantly to morbidity and mortality following trauma. The aim of management in the emergency department is to recognize any traumatic brain injury, and institute management that aims to reduce secondary brain injury. This may involve intubating patients with a Glasgow Coma Scale (GCS) of 8 or less, controlling ventilation to optimize cerebral perfusion, and early neurosurgical review.

Patients with severe head injuries require intubation and control of pCO_2 to ensure that an appropriate balance is maintained between cerebral oedema and vasoconstriction of blood vessels. Generally, normocapnia is aimed for, although hyperventilation may be indicated in those where immediate control of intracranial pressure (ICP) is required.

Mannitol (an osmotic diuretic) may be given in specific circumstances when advised by a neurosurgeon, for example in a patient with a severe brain injury who has impending brainstem herniation to acutely reduce their ICP to allow for transfer to a neurosurgical centre.

Exposure and environmental control

Adequate exposure, while maintaining normal body temperature, is essential when assessing trauma patients. Clothing should be removed and, if necessary, cut off. This allows adequate assessment of any deformities, bruising, or other obvious abnormalities on inspection. Examination should include a log roll to allow inspection of the back and posterior aspect of the limbs and head. Omitting any part of exposure will result in potentially serious injuries being missed (e.g. posterior stab wounds).

At the same time, adequate warming needs to be instituted. This may consist of blankets and warmed fluids, but may also require the use of a warm air blanket. This is vital for trauma patients, as haemorrhage is a common problem and normothermia is required for normal clotting function.

Primary survey imaging

Modern trauma care relies on the prompt radiological imaging of patients with serious injuries so that their management can be appropriately planned as soon as possible. All imaging acts as an adjunct to the primary survey.

Radiographs during the primary survey are generally restricted to anterior to posterior (AP) chest and pelvis X-rays that augment clinical assessment of immediately life-threatening injuries. In addition, focused assessment with sonography for trauma (FAST) scanning acts as an extension of the physical examination in trauma patients allowing rapid assessment for free fluid in four areas (perihepatic, perisplenic, pelvis, and the pericardium).

Most centres now assess the most seriously injured patients with a computerized tomography (CT) trauma series that involves a CT scan from the vertex to symphysis pubis. This allows major injuries to be characterized promptly and, given the frequency of multiple injuries in major trauma patients, also reduces the risk of missing a serious concomitant injury (e.g. pelvic fractures may be associated with a serious intra-abdominal cause of bleeding in up to 40%).

A pick and mix approach to CT scanning of patients is generally not good practice if there is a significant mechanism of injury. For example, there is no role for cervical spine X-rays rather than CT in a head injured patient requiring a CT scan of the head as it is unlikely that adequate imaging will be obtained with plain X-rays. In addition, head injured patients can be difficult to assess clinically and so there should be a low threshold for a complete trauma CT series in those where the mechanism would suggest a likelihood of multiple injuries.

Prompt assessment is vital and target times for CT scanning have been set for head injured patients by the National Institute for Health and Care Excellence (NICE) in England and Wales. It is expected that patients should receive a CT head scan within one hour of arrival in the emergency department.

Secondary survey

Should a patient have any significant life (or limb) threatening injuries, these should be dealt with immediately. This may involve an intervention in the resuscitation room, or may involve a procedure in an interventional radiology suite or operating theatre. These interventions should not be delayed for further imaging or to conduct a secondary survey.

Once such injuries have been managed or ruled out, a thorough secondary survey is required that involves examining the patient from the top of the head to the tips of their toes looking for any injuries. This involves eye and ear examination, palpation of all four limbs and spine, as well as trunk and abdominal examination. An incomplete secondary survey will result in missed injuries, and even a missed finger fracture can lead to long-term morbidity if inadequately managed initially.

The secondary survey is the responsibility of the team in charge of the patient's care, and once they leave the emergency department, this is often the surgical team dealing with the patient's most serious injuries. It may not be possible to fully complete the secondary survey until a patient is conscious and talking, and so it is vital that any aspects remaining are well communicated to colleagues via the medical record.

Definitive care

Once patients have been assessed in the emergency department, they need access to the most appropriate specialists to manage their ongoing care. Often this involves several different specialties (e.g. intensive care anaesthetists, neurosurgeons, orthopaedic surgeons, general surgeons, and on occasion urologists). It is vital that patients are treated in a centre that has access to all the specialties required for that patient's care and if not, the patient needs to be transferred to a centre that can offer that care. In areas covered by a trauma network, this is facilitated by either direct admission to an MTC, or by an early transfer from a trauma unit to an MTC.

As discussed in the previous section, patients with life- or limb-threatening injuries often require immediate intervention in the form of surgery. However, in those patients with multiple injuries it is now recognized that dealing definitively with all their injuries in one sitting is potentially dangerous as it can lead to physiological deterioration. This is because the major traumatic episode itself represents a significant insult to the body and prolonged surgery too early following this is a further insult that can result in the lethal triad of coagulopathy, hypothermia, and metabolic acidosis.

This has now been recognized and has resulted in the principles of damage control surgery (DCS) where major injuries are operated on in a staged fashion, with the initial surgery aiming to stabilize the patient by stopping haemorrhage and preventing further injury or harm. Patients are then transferred to intensive care and are returned to theatre within a few days (or when in an improved physiological state) for definitive procedures. The key is to time the definitive procedures so that they do not lead to a worsening systemic inflammatory response syndrome (SIRS) that can lead to multiorgan dysfunction and potentially death.

Examples of DCS include the external fixation of long bone fractures in polytrauma patients and damage control laparotomy where haemorrhage is controlled, damaged bowel resected, and the abdomen temporarily closed.

Rehabilitation and re-enablement

In the past, the rehabilitation phase of a patient's journey following a serious traumatic injury was often forgotten about until the patient was nearing discharge from the acute ward. This attitude is slowly changing and the management of the seriously injured patient must be multidisciplinary involving multiple physicians and surgeons, nurses, physiotherapists, and occupational therapists.

There are a growing number of major trauma centres who employ a director of rehabilitation who is responsible for ensuring the patient receives the rehabilitation and re-enablement services they require; not just in hospital, but extending into the community. This is aided by rehabilitation prescriptions which are a statement of rehabilitation needs that the patient requires to help them along the journey towards a full recovery.

Rehabilitation is not simply about getting a patient back to mobility, but requires a holistic approach. This involves assessing the patient's physical needs, and also any psychological and social needs that require addressing to get them back to as close to normal function as possible. Trauma creates a large financial burden on the nation, and ultimately once a patient's life has been saved, it is vital that they are returned, if possible, to being a productive member of society. For some, this is by enabling rapid return to work, but for others this may not be possible. In those cases, all clinicians need to work together to enable patients to reach their full potential, taking into account the injuries they sustain.

Conclusions

Trauma is the leading cause of death of young adults and children in the world. It is also responsible for a significant incidence of long-term disability. By acquiring knowledge of the key concepts in trauma management, surgeons can help to reduce the long-term impact of traumatic injuries in terms of both morbidity and mortality.

Significant changes in emergent care in recent years include the use of major transfusion protocols and the use of tranexamic acid for those suspected of having traumatic bleeding. The concept of damage control surgery is also vital to ensuring the survival of the most seriously injured. In the future, the areas of rehabilitation and re-enablement will require increasing focus if we are to improve the number of patients able to return to their previous levels of function.

Further reading

American College of Surgeons Committee on Trauma. *Advanced Trauma Life Support® ATLS Student Manual*, 9th edition. Chicago, IL: American College of Surgeons, 2012.

CRASH-2 Collaborators. Effects of tranexamic acid on death, vascular occlusive events, and blood transfusion in trauma patients with significant haemorrhage (CRASH-2): a randomised, placebo-controlled trial. *Lancet* 2010; **376**:23–32.

NHS Clinical Advisory Group. Regional networks for major trauma. NHS Clinical Advisory Groups Report. Available at: http://www.excellence.eastmidlands.nhs.uk/welcome/improving-care/emergency-urgent-care/major-trauma/nhs-clinical-advisory-group/. [Accessed 30 September 2013] [Online].

References

1. World Health Organization. Global burden of disease. Available at: http://www.who.int/topics/global_burden_of_disease/en/. [Accessed on 30 September 2013] [Online].
2. Office for National Statistics. Deaths registered in England and Wales 2012. Available at: http://www.ons.gov.uk/ons/taxonomy/index.html?nscl=Deaths. [Accessed on 30 September 2013] [Online].
3. National Audit Office. *Major Trauma Care in England*. London, UK: The Stationery Office, 2010.
4. Court-Brown CM, Aitken SA, Duckworth AD, Clement ND, McQueen MM. The relationship between social deprivation and the incidence of adult fractures. *JBJS Am* 2013; **95**(6):e321–7.
5. Christensen MC, Ridley S, Lecky FE, Munro V, Morris S. Outcomes and costs of blunt trauma in England and Wales. *Crit Care* 2008; **12**:R23
6. Baker SP, O'Neill B, Haddon W, Long WB. The injury severity score: a method for describing patients with multiple injuries and evaluating emergency care. *J Trauma* 1974; **14**(3):187–96.
7. Mullins RJ. A historical perspective of Trauma System development in the United States. *J Trauma* 1999; **47**(3):S8–S14.
8. West JG, Trunkey DD, Lim RC. Systems of trauma care. A study of two counties. *Arch Surg* 1979; **114**(4):455–60.
9. American College of Surgeons. Verified trauma centers. Available at: http://www.facs.org/trauma/verified.html. [Accessed 30 September 2013] [Online].
10. Celso B, Tepas J, Langland-Orban B, *et al*. A systematic review and meta-analysis comparing outcome of severely injured patients treated in trauma centers following the establishment of trauma systems. *J Trauma* 2006; **60**(2):371–8.
11. Gabbe BJ, Lyons RA, Lecky FE, *et al*. Comparison of mortality following hospitalisation for isolated head injury in England and Wales, and Victoria, Australia. *PLoS ONE* 2011; **6**(5):e20545.
12. State Government Victoria. Victorian State Trauma Registry 2007–08: Summary Report. Available at: http://docs.health.vic.gov.au/docs/doc/76E8679B9E6BCC9ECA257B7100209763/$FILE/0708vstorm-sumrep.pdf. [Accessed 30 September 2013] [Online].
13. American College of Surgeons Committee on Trauma. *Advanced Trauma Life Support® ATLS Student Manual*, 9th edition. Chicago, IL: American College of Surgeons, 2012.
14. Nicholl J, Turner J. Effectiveness of a regional trauma system in reducing mortality from major trauma: before and after study. *BMJ* 1997; **315**:1349–54.

15. NHS Clinical Advisory Group. Regional networks for major trauma. NHS Clinical Advisory Groups Report. Availabe at: http://www.excellence.eastmidlands.nhs.uk/welcome/improving-care/emergency-urgent-care/major-trauma/nhs-clinical-advisory-group/. [Accessed 30 September 2013] [Online].
16. NHS England News. Independent review of major trauma networks reveals increase in patient survival rates. Available at: http://www.england.nhs.uk/2013/06/25/incr-pati-survi-rts/. [Accessed 30 September 2013] [Online].
17. British Orthopaedic Association. BOAST 14: The Management of Urological Trauma Associated with Pelvic Fractures. Available at https://www.boa.ac.uk/wp-content/uploads/2016/09/BOAST-14-Urological-Injuries.pdf. [Accessed 12 December 2016] [Online].
18. CRASH-2 Collaborators. Effects of tranexamic acid on death, vascular occlusive events, and blood transfusion in trauma patients with significant haemorrhage (CRASH-2): a randomised, placebo-controlled trial. *Lancet* 2010; **376**:23–32.

SECTION 5

Benign prostatic hyperplasia

Section editor: Christopher R. Chapple

CHAPTER 5.1

Bladder outflow obstruction

Christopher R. Chapple and Altaf Mangera

Aetiology of bladder outflow obstruction

It is not possible to diagnose bladder outlet obstruction on a history alone. It can be suspected based on the use of a flow rate but can only be diagnosed using pressure flow urodynamics. Although clearly premicturition delay, a poor stream, and a feeling of incomplete bladder emptying all suggest the diagnosis, detrusor underactivity or drugs may lead to the same symptoms as bladder outlet obstruction (BOO). With this in mind, men with lower urinary tract symptoms (LUTS), should not be assumed to have a voiding disorder/prostatic disease based on the history alone. If there is any doubt as to the diagnosis, then pressure/flow cystometry is necessary to differentiate and definitively confirm obstruction.

Mechanical causes of BOO include phimosis, posterior urethral valves, urethral strictures, urethral diverticulum, prostate carcinoma, pelvic masses such as fibroids, urethral kinking as a consequence of a cystocele, and bladder neck stenosis. Due to anatomical differences between the genders, the aetiology of BOO differs between the sexes (Table 5.1.1). In younger men, bladder neck obstruction is the most likely cause if a urethral stricture has been excluded. In elderly men, the most common cause of BOO is an enlarged prostate; and therefore, if a patient is proven to have obstruction caused by the prostate, they are said to have benign prostatic obstruction (BPO). Besides BPO, there are also other causes of BOO. These include detrusor sphincter dyssynergia, which is the simultaneous contraction of the urethral striated muscle or pelvic floor muscles at the same time as the detrusor muscle. If this occurs in neurologically normal individuals, then it is termed dysfunctional voiding, but in all cases it is essential to exclude an underlying neurological abnormality. Both lead to staccato voiding due to intermittent sphincter contraction and relaxation. Certainly, if a neurological abnormality is identified, non-relaxing urethral sphincter obstruction is said to occur, which is characterized by a reduced flow.

Voiding difficulty is far less common in females and when it occurs, it should be thoroughly investigated with anatomical and functional investigations. Most female patients with voiding difficulty have a neuropathic disorder affecting the bladder, but a functional obstruction of the bladder outlet/urethra or detrusor muscle failure must be excluded. Fowler's syndrome occurs in women after menarche, presenting with high volume painless retention in the absence of obvious neurological or pharmacological precipitating factors.[1] These women have high maximum urethral closure pressures and find catheterization extremely painful.

History

The history should be directed at helping the clinician elucidate the underlying cause of BOO. Therefore, important questions include length and progression of symptoms, previous abdominal, gynaecological or urological surgery, and degree of bother. A detailed neurological and drug history is also mandatory as many drugs and neurological conditions will affect detrusor and sphincter coordination, and bladder contractility. Patients may also describe incomplete emptying and secondary frequency +/– urgency. A gynaecological and obstetric history should also be

Table 5.1.1 Causes of voiding difficulty in men and women

	Anatomical	Functional	Detrusor muscle failure
Men	Prostatic obstruction	Detrusor sphincter dyssynergia	Primary
	Bladder neck obstruction	Dysfunctional voiding	Secondary to outflow obstruction
	Urethral stricture	Non-relaxing urethral sphincter	Previous pelvic surgery
	Phimosis		
	Posterior urethral valves		
	Prostatic carcinoma		
Women	Compression from prolapse	Detrusor sphincter dyssynergia	Primary
	Compression from tumour	Dysfunctional voiding	Post parturition
	Urethral stenosis	Non-relaxing urethral sphincter	Secondary to outflow obstruction
	Overcorrection from tape surgery	Fowler's syndrome	Previous pelvic surgery

taken from women, as a pelvic mass may lead to BOO by causing physical obstruction of the bladder outlet and prior pelvic surgery could lead to detrusor underactivity. Objective quantification of BOO symptoms in men should include the International Prostate Symptom Score (IPSS) questionnaire, which measures seven symptom domains scored from 0–5 and has a final quality of life (QoL) question.[2] No similar questionnaire is available for the assessment of voiding symptoms in women.

Examination

Examination for BOO includes an abdominal, digital rectal, per vaginal, and focused neurological examination. Abdominal examination should assess for a palpable bladder and for other abdominal masses. Per vaginal examination should also examine for masses, particularly a vaginal prolapse. The digital rectal examination should assess perianal sensation, anal tone, prostate size, and for any prostatic irregularity. In both genders, the external urethral orifice should be visualized and any stenosis excluded. A phimosis needs to be excluded in men with a prepuce; conversely, a circumcised penis may indicate previous lichen sclerosis, which may point to urethral stricture disease.

Investigations

The term 'the bladder is an unreliable witness' was first coined with the knowledge that LUTS may not be disease specific and can be reported or documented inaccurately by the patient or investigator, respectively. Therefore, further investigations may be necessary to shed light on the underlying abnormality. Lower urinary tract function may be separated into two distinct yet interrelated functions; storage and voiding. BOO arises as a consequence of an abnormality in voiding function.

There are several investigations which may help clarify the underlying cause of apparent BOO and help in differentiating this from poor detrusor contractility. It is best to view these investigations individually. The history is clearly important and should be supplemented by a questionnaire in the male, such as IPSS.

Creatinine and abdominal ultrasound scan

Creatinine estimation and renal ultrasound scan are not routine investigations in patients with suspected BOO. However, if there is a high post-void residual >200 mL or a pelvic mass is suspected, then these should be undertaken.

Uroflowmetry

This is a simple test which can be performed in most outpatient departments with a flow meter and an ultrasound bladder scanner. There are many important parameters which may be obtained from uroflowmetry (Fig. 5.1.1, Fig. 5.1.1A). These include the *voided volume*, which is the total volume of micturition. This must be greater than 150 mL if the flow rate is to be considered representative. The maximum flow rate *(Qmax)* is the flow rate at the peak of the curve after correction for artefacts. The *flow time* is the time over which measureable flow occurs and excludes interruptions when no flow

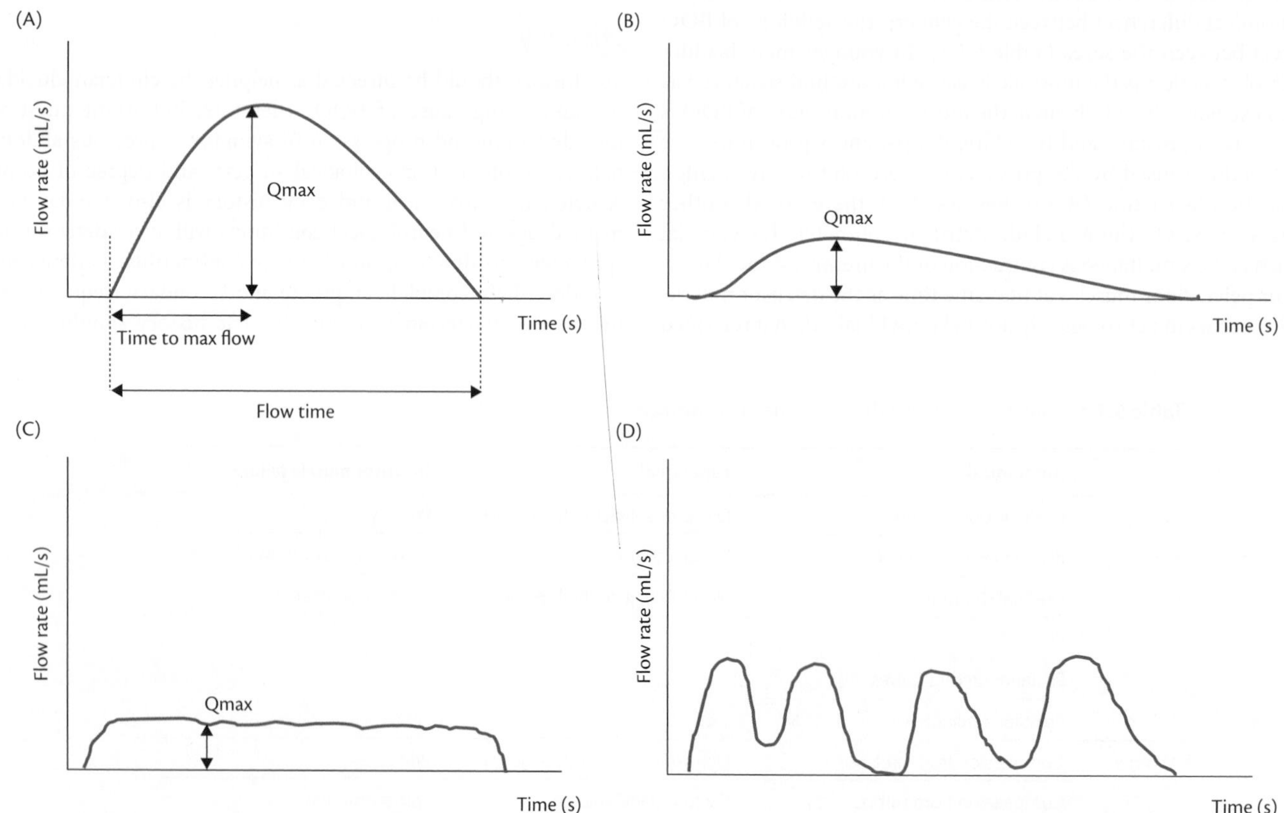

Fig. 5.1.1 (A) Normal flow rate recording showing parameters which may be interpreted. (B) A typical flow rate pattern for a patient with BPO: note the reduced Qmax, and prolonged flow time and time to Qmax. (C) A typical flow rate pattern for a patient with a urethral stricture (note the reduced Qmax and flat plateau flow pattern). (D) A typical flow rate pattern for a patient with detrusor sphincter dyssynergia: note the intermittent flow pattern.

Table 5.1.2 The proportion of patients with BOO for the corresponding Qmax categories

Qmax	Patients with BOO
<10 mL/s	90%
10–14 mL/s	67%
>14 mL/s	30%

is recorded. The *voiding time* is the total time taken for voiding regardless of interruptions. The *average flow rate* is calculated by dividing the voided volume by the flow time. *Time to maximum flow* is the time from onset of flow to Qmax. The typical flow pattern in a male with BPO is described as 'prolonged' and is shown in Fig. 5.1.1B. The characteristic flow pattern for a urethral stricture is shown in Fig. 5.1.1C and is described as 'flat'. Inappropriate sphincteric contraction during voiding will lead to an intermittent flow (Fig. 5.1.1D) and is seen in detrusor sphincter dyssynergia.

Generally speaking, the Qmax in young healthy males is 30–40 mL/s and is 40–50 mL/s in females. With age the Qmax lessens and in men aged >60 years, a Qmax of 15 mL/s may be acceptable and leads to no discernible symptoms. The post-void residue in a normal individual should be minimal (<50 mL). A flow rate will not be able to differentiate between high detrusor pressure with low flow or low detrusor pressure with low flow—this distinction is important because many patients who have an unsatisfactory result following previous prostatic surgery often have low-pressure, low-flow voiding dysfunction.

In male patients, uroflowmetry in general (Qmax in particular) is certainly useful but lacks specificity for a reliable urodynamic diagnosis of the cause of abnormal voiding as shown in Table 5.1.2.

Cystoscopy

Cystoscopy is not routinely utilized in the investigation of BOO and is principally undertaken if a urethral stricture is suspected. In men >60 years with the appropriate history, examination, and flow rate findings, a cystoscopy is seldom required. Treatment for benign prostatic obstruction can be commenced without cystoscopic evidence of obstruction, the only indication being a suspected bladder pathology in the context of marked storage symptoms, haematuria or abnormal urinalysis.

Cystometry (see Chapter 3.2)

The use of cystometry (also called pressure/flow urodynamics) in men with clear obstructive symptoms and a classical flow rate patterns is not necessary, prior to instituting pharmacotherapy. Its utility is more often reserved for patients with either mixed LUTS or chronic retention when detrusor overactivity and underactivity are questioned. In addition, patients who have failed bladder outflow obstruction surgery may undergo these studies. Nevertheless, in many centres it is considered useful as a preoperative diagnostic modality prior to surgery, although the evidence base for a predictive role in determining outcome of surgery is not yet proven.

Cystometry is therefore the method by which the pressure/volume relationship of the bladder is assessed. The term is taken to mean the measurement of detrusor pressure during filling and voiding. Put simply, a catheter with a transducer tip is inserted in to the bladder and another similar catheter is inserted in to the

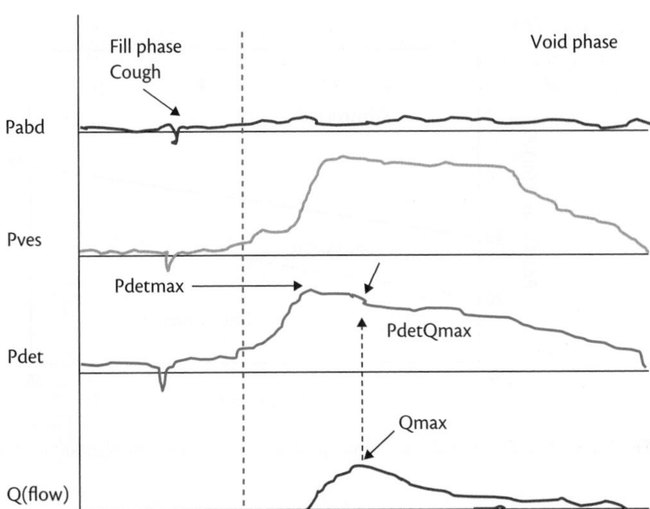

Fig. 5.1.2 Simplified cystometrogram demonstrating the calculation of PdetQmax: note the void phase is usually longer, but has been omitted for clarity.

rectum. The intravesical pressure is a consequence of the detrusor pressure and the abdominal pressure. Therefore, subtraction of the abdominal pressure from the intravesical pressure gives the detrusor pressure (Fig. 5.1.2).

The remainder of this chapter will discuss the changes in the voiding phase of cystometry as the storage phase has been discussed elsewhere. The void phase produces a flow pattern as well as a detrusor pressure trace (Fig. 5.1.2). The flow patterns have been described above. The urodynamicist should also look at the pattern of detrusor contraction. This should rise, be sustained for a period to allow voiding, and fall as shown in Figure 5.1.2. One must be wary that the detrusor pressure is a calculated (subtracted) and any artefacts in the abdominal or intravesical lines may lead to erroneous interpretation of the detrusor pressure. Correctly subtracting cystometry lines should take account for abdominal straining without affecting the detrusor pressure.

The detrusor pressure at the time of maximum flow is known as the PdetQmax. This is important because it allows the calculation of the bladder outlet obstruction index (BOOI). The BOOI has been validated in a male population. The BOOI = PdetQmax–(2*Qmax).[3] If the BOOI >40 cmH_2O then the patient is obstructed. BOOI 20–40 cmH_2O is equivocal and BOOI <20 cmH_2O suggests detrusor underactivity, rather than obstruction.

Similarly, the voiding trace can be plotted on an Abrams-Griffiths or International Continence Society nomogram.[3] These are pre-plotted scatter graphs where the Qmax is plotted on the x-axis and PdetQmax on the y-axis (Fig. 5.1.3, Fig. 5.1.3A). The patient's void phase is plotted on the graph by the urodynamics machine and the furthest point on the x-axis is equivalent to the PdetQmax. The graph contains a BOOI >40 cmH_2O cut off for each Qmax value to signify obstruction, a BOOI<20 cmH_2O for unobstructed, and a 20–40 cmH_2O range for equivocal results. This methodology requires less calculation by the urodynamicist and is therefore sometimes preferred over the calculation of the BOOI but is essentially the same.

Bladder contractility has also been defined by the International Continence Society. 412 PdetQmax +5Qmax. BCI>150 cmH_20 reflects strong bladder contractility, 100–150 cmH_2O is normal and

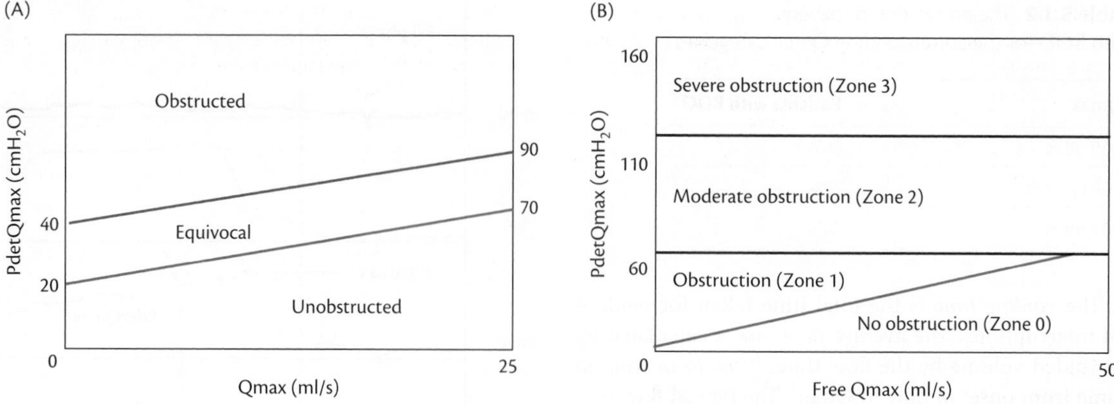

Fig. 5.1.3 (A) International Continence Society nomogram for the bladder outlet obstruction index; and (B) the Blaivas-Groutz nomogram for female obstruction.

<100 cmH_2O is reduced.[3] Similarly, a bladder contractility nomogram may be used. Calculating the above two parameters assists the clinician in differentiating between BOO and reduced detrusor contractility in male patients. An obstructed patient will have a high BOOI and BCI, whereas, a patient with detrusor impairment will have a low BOOI and BCI.

The above definitions and nomograms do not apply in women due to their different voiding characteristics. Men generally, have a high-flow, high-pressure voiding system, while women have a high-flow, low-pressure voiding system. This is due to the differing resistance of the infravesical urinary tract in both genders. The definition of BOO in women is therefore not as well defined as in men. Blavias and Groutz have created a nomogram for female obstruction (Fig. 5.1.3B).[4] In their analysis, BOO was defined as a free Qmax <12 mL/s (i.e. during uroflowmetry without a catheter) and a Pdetmax >20 cmH_2O (this is the maximum detrusor pressure generated and different to the PdetQmax). Another proposed definition was the inability to void in the presence of a sustained detrusor contraction of >20 cmH_2O.

Videocystometry

Cystometry may be combined with concurrent fluoroscopic imaging of the bladder outlet which may help with the diagnosis.[5] The urodynamicist looks at the bladder neck and urethra during a sustained detrusor contraction. This investigation gives a level for the obstruction, which guides the clinician to what may be causing the obstruction, which can be confirmed by appropriate other investigations.

Non-invasive cystometry

Due to the invasiveness of cystometry, a number of non-invasive urodynamic investigations have been proposed. These provide either traditional cystometric measures in a non-invasive manner, or they provide a surrogate marker of obstruction. Indirect isovolumetric bladder pressure may be assessed with the use of a penile cuff[6] or a condom catheter.[7] Alternatively, measures such as bladder wall thickness/bladder weight[8] and bladder vascular resistance[9] as assessed by ultrasound have been reported as proxies to BOO. At the time of writing, all of these techniques are still considered investigational and have not entered routine practice. Ambulatory urodynamics has also been suggested as a potential diagnostic approach, particularly in patients with so-called 'bashful voiding', who cannot void during a urodynamic study, but also remains investigational at present.

Urethral pressure profilometry and electromyography

Both of these two modalities have been evaluated but are not widely used in routine practice for male patients. These tests are reserved for women where neurological, iatrogenic, and local causes of BOO have been excluded. They are not essential and a diagnosis of Fowler's syndrome can be made based on the history and cystometric findings. These women have high maximum urethral closure pressure, increased sphincteric volume, and characteristic striated urethral sphincter abnormalities.[1]

Further reading

Abrams P, Cardozo L, Fall M, *et al.* The standardisation of terminology of lower urinary tract function: report from the Standardisation Sub-committee of the International Continence Society. *Neurourol Urodyn* 2002; **21**(2):167–78.

Abrams P. Bladder outlet obstruction index, bladder contractility index and bladder voiding efficiency: three simple indices to define bladder voiding function. *BJU Int* 1999; **84**(1):14–15.

Blaivas JG, Groutz A. Bladder outlet obstruction nomogram for women with lower urinary tract symptomatology. *Neurourol Urodyn* 2000; **19**(5):553–64.

Chapple CR, MacDiarmid SA, Patel A. *Urodynamics Made Easy*, 3rd edition. London, UK: Churchill Livingstone Elsevier, 2009.

DasGupta R, Fowler CJ. The management of female voiding dysfunction: Fowler's syndrome—a contemporary update. *Curr Opin Urol* 2003; **13**(4):293–9.

Jones C, Hill J, Chapple C. Management of lower urinary tract symptoms in men: summary of NICE guidance. *BMJ* 2010; **340**:c2354.

Nitti VW, Tu LM, Gitlin J. Diagnosing bladder outlet obstruction in women. *J Urol* 1999; **161**(5):1535–40.

Sciarra A, D'Eramo G, Casale P, *et al.* Relationship among symptom score, prostate volume, and urinary flow rates in 543 patients with and without benign prostatic hyperplasia. *Prostate* 1998; **34**(2):121–8.

References

1. DasGupta R, Fowler CJ. The management of female voiding dysfunction: Fowler's syndrome—a contemporary update. *Curr Opin Urol* 2003: **13**(4):293–9.

2. Sciarra A, D'Eramo G, Casale P, *et al*. Relationship among symptom score, prostate volume, and urinary flow rates in 543 patients with and without benign prostatic hyperplasia. *Prostate* 1998: **34**(2):121–8.
3. Abrams P. Bladder outlet obstruction index, bladder contractility index and bladder voiding efficiency: three simple indices to define bladder voiding function. *BJU Int* 1999: **84**(1):14–15.
4. Blaivas JG, Groutz A. Bladder outlet obstruction nomogram for women with lower urinary tract symptomatology. *Neurourol Urodyn* 2000; **19**(5):553–64.
5. Nitti VW, Tu LM, Gitlin J. Diagnosing bladder outlet obstruction in women. *J Urol* 1999; **161**(5):1535–40.
6. Harding C, Robson W, Drinnan M, *et al*. The penile cuff test: A clinically useful non-invasive urodynamic investigation to diagnose men with lower urinary tract symptoms. *Indian J Urol* 2009; **25**(1):116–21.
7. Huang Foen Chung JW, Spigt MG, Knottnerus JA, van Mastrigt R. Comparative analysis of the reproducibility and applicability of the condom catheter method for noninvasive urodynamics in two Dutch centers. *Urol Int* 2008; **81**(2):139–48.
8. Huang T, Qi J, Yu YJ, *et al*. Predictive value of resistive index, detrusor wall thickness and ultrasound estimated bladder weight regarding the outcome after transurethral prostatectomy for patients with lower urinary tract symptoms suggestive of benign prostatic obstruction. *Int J Urol* 2012; **19**(4):343–50.
9. Wada N, Watanabe M, Kita M, Matsumoto S, Kakizaki H. Analysis of bladder vascular resistance before and after prostatic surgery in patients with lower urinary tract symptoms suggestive of benign prostatic obstruction. *Neurourol Urodyn* 2012; **31**(5):659–63.

CHAPTER 5.2

Urinary retention in men

Mark Speakman

Introduction to urinary retention

Urinary retention continues to be a significant burden for both the patient and healthcare services in the United Kingdom and around the world. It is associated with a significant reduction in patients' quality of life. In acute urinary retention (AUR), the impact of the pain may be equivalent to renal colic or childbirth; this is due to the sudden onset with the stretching of the bladder causing considerable pain.[1,2] In chronic urinary retention (CUR), the onset is usually so slow that there may be no pain.

Retention remains a complex subject, presenting in various ways as a result of numerous pathological processes. The abundance of definitions of retention in the literature, particularly for chronic retention, makes this more difficult to comprehend.[3,4]

In the past (20–30 years ago) urinary retention was regarded as an immediate indication for surgery and in older reports, 25% to 30% of men who underwent transurethral prostatectomy (TURP) had AUR as their main indication.[5] With the introduction of medical treatments and changes in practice for the management of retention, these rates have changed significantly.[6]

Definitions

Let's start with the basics; retention literally means the act or an instance of retaining (Oxford English Dictionary [OED]); from the Latin *retinere* to hold back or withhold. It does not, in essence, mean the inability to pass (urine); although this tends to be the medical usage of the term. While this medical definition works well for acute retention, the proper formal definition works better for chronic retention.

Urinary retention is the inability of the bladder to empty to completion. This may be acute, chronic, or acute-on-chronic. AUR is the sudden painful inability to void. In CUR however, voiding is usually preserved until acute-on-chronic retention prevails which only occurs in a relatively small percentage of these patients. CUR is defined by the International Continence Society (ICS) as a non-painful bladder, which remains palpable or percussable after the patient has passed urine.

In AUR, the volumes are typically between 500 mL and 1 L, while in CUR the retained volumes could be anywhere between 450 mL and 4.5 L, or even more. Abrams chose a residual urine volume of >300 mL to define CUR as the minimum volume at which the bladder becomes palpable suprapubically.[4] Caution needs to be exercised in the study of CUR, as much of the knowledge comes from studies of the management of men with lower urinary tract symptoms (LUTS) undergoing medical or surgical treatments and these trials typically exclude men with large residual volumes or chronic retention.[4]

There are several international coding systems that code retention. The main two are:

- The MeSH—Medical Subject Headings classification; a comprehensive listing for the indexing scientific submissions in the life sciences and this records urinary retention as D016055.
- The ICD-9 and ICD-10, the ninth and tenth editions of the International Classification of Diseases code urinary retention as 788.2 and R33, respectively.

Epidemiology

The epidemiology of urinary retention can be studied from two principal sources;

- Firstly, the population-based longitudinal studies of untreated men—community-dwelling men with or without LUTS; and
- Secondly, from studies of men diagnosed with LUTS and entered into the placebo arms of randomized controlled trials for the treatment of LUTS.

Most of the epidemiological data in the literature is for AUR; data for chronic retention is relatively sparse.[3,4] Older studies showed widely varying incidences of retention from 4 to over 100 per 1,000 person-years.[7,8] More recent and better-controlled studies have shown that the incidence rate per 1,000 person-years is more constant around the world; in the order of 5 to 25/1000 person-years or 0.5% to 2.5% per year. In the classic Olmsted County paper by Jacobsen and colleagues, it was 6.8/1000 person-years and in the famous Medical Therapy of Prostatic Symptoms (MTOPS) study, in the placebo arm it was a remarkably similar 2.4% over four years or 0.6% per year.[9,10] However, in a review of placebo-controlled trials by Emberton and colleagues, it was reported that the rate of AUR in placebo-treated men in studies of 12–48 months' duration was 0.4–6.6%.[11]

The explanation for these variations is that the risk of retention is not the same for all men (Box 5.2.1). It grows with increasing age and in men with markers for more significant disease such as increased symptoms or larger prostates.

The Olmsted paper[9] showed that AUR is relatively rare in younger men and in men with mild LUTS (AUA score 7 or less; broadly equivalent to the newer International Prostate Symptom Score [IPSS]). In this study, the incidence of AUR increased from 2.6/1,000 person-years among men 40–49 years old to almost four times commoner in men 70–79 years old (9.3/1,000 person-years). More significant symptoms at baseline were also a significant risk factor for greater progression to retention. The rate in men with moderate to severe symptoms (AUA score >7) increased from 3.0/1,000 person-years for men 40 to 49 years old to more than 10-fold

Box 5.2.1 Factors that have been identified as predictors of acute urinary retention (and lower urinary tract symptom-related surgery)

Baseline variables

- Age
- Severe lower urinary tract symptoms (LUTS)
- Bother score
- A low peak flow rate
- Increased post-void residual urine volume (PVR)
- Prostate size
- Serum prostate-specific antigen (PSA) levels
- Prior acute urinary retention (AUR)
- Inflammation

Dynamic variables

- Worsening symptoms
- Increasing post-void residual volumes in untreated men
- Non-response to medical treatment (IPSS stable or worsening and increasing bother)

greater at 34.7/1,000 person-years among men 70 to 79 years old. This shows that the impact of age and symptom severity together has a much greater impact than either risk factor alone. These authors also showed that flow rate and prostate volume would also predict for AUR risk with men having a maximum urinary flow rate <12 mL/s being at four times the risk of AUR compared with men with flow rates >12 mL/s, and that men with a prostate >30 mL had a 3-fold increase in risk compared with those with smaller prostates.[9] While in the important Proscar Long-Term Efficiency and Safety Study (PLESS) study, analysis of the placebo arm revealed that the predictors of AUR were prostate volume, serum prostate-specific antigen (PSA) levels, and symptom severity.[12]

Subsequent analysis by both Emberton and Roehrborn has added further understanding to this issue with greater clarity of the risk factors for LUTS/benign prostatic hyperplasia (BPH) progression and the increasing risk of retention, including PSA >1.4 and non-response to medical treatments.[11,13] Marberger in particular showed in an analysis of the placebo arms of three finasteride randomized controlled trials (RCTs) that benign prostatic enlargement (BPE) patients with larger prostate volumes and higher PSA levels have an increased risk of developing AUR. He suggested therefore that they might derive the greatest benefit from the risk reduction seen with finasteride therapy.[14] He showed that PSA had an even greater predictive value than prostate volume in calculating the risk of retention.

In addition, dynamic variables such as worsening symptoms and increasing post-void residual volumes in untreated men serve as good predictors of AUR in men with LUTS.[15] Also non-response to medical treatment (IPSS stable or worsening and increasing bother) predicts a greater risk of AUR, or needing prostate surgery.[16]

One retrospective cohort study in the Netherlands of 56,958 males showed that the incidence rate of AUR overall was very low at 2.2/1,000 man-years. However, AUR was the first symptom of LUTS in half (49%) of the 149 AUR cases that occurred. The risk of AUR was 11-fold higher in patients newly diagnosed with LUTS (RR 11.5; 95% CI: 8.4–15.6) with an overall incidence rate of 18.3/1,000 man-years (95% CI: 14.5–22.8).[17]

The incidence of retention has changed over time and one study using data from the Hospital Episode Statistics (HES) database of the Department of Health in England from 1998 and 2003, based on the ICD10 coding system analysed data from 165,527 men who were identified to have been hospitalized with AUR in the study period.[18] The incidence of primary AUR was 3.06/1,000 men yearly. It was spontaneous in 65.3% of cases. The incidence of AUR decreased from 3.17/1,000 men yearly in 1998 to 2.96/1,000 yearly in 2003. Surgical treatment following spontaneous AUR decreased by 20% from 32% in 1998 to 26% in 2003. This trend coincided with a 20% increase in the rate of recurrent acute urinary retention.[18] These authors suggested that the slight decrease in the incidence of AUR may be due to the increased use of oral drug treatments, and the subsequent move away from initial surgical treatments for LUTS has not resulted in an increase in AUR. However, they suggest that the increase in recurrent AUR indicates that the observed decrease in surgery after AUR may have put more men at risk for AUR recurrence.[18] The 2010 HES for England alone recorded 18,000 admissions with AUR. Interestingly, urinary retention appears to be significantly more common in the colder winter months than the warmer months;[19] and in one community-based study, men who currently smoke may be at a modestly reduced risk of AUR.[20]

Inflammation has also been shown to be an important putative risk factor for retention. In a subgroup analysis of the MTOPS study, not a single patient who did not have inflammation on their baseline biopsies developed AUR in the four years of the study.[21] Further support for this hypothesis came from an epidemiological study in men with rheumatoid arthritis, where a group that needed to take daily non-steroidal anti-inflammatory drugs (NSAIDs) were compared with a control group who did not. The rate of LUTS, poor flow and even the risk of an enlarged prostate were all significantly lower in the arthritis group taking regular NSAIDs.[22] The use of NSAIDs therefore may reduce the risk of AUR, although properly constructed RCTs are required to test this hypothesis.

Overall, it was calculated by Roehrborn that a 60-year-old man would have a 23% probability of experiencing AUR if he were to reach the age of 80.[13] Retention is over ten times more common in men than in women and AUR is rare in male children and is then usually associated with infection, with or without phimosis, or occurs postoperatively.[23,24]

More recently, the resistive index of the prostate capsular arteries measured by colour Doppler transrectal ultrasound has been shown to be both a good predictor of retention and to correlate very accurately with urodynamic obstruction. This may become a good predictor of risk in certain patient subgroups.[25,26]

There is, however, the potential for bias when the placebo arms of clinical trials are used to characterize the natural history of the LUTS disease compared with the outcomes in community-dwelling men. One study comparing the Olmsted County data with the placebo data from the MTOPS study showed that the rates of AUR and those for symptom progression were, perhaps surprisingly, higher in the community patients than the placebo-treated patients, while the likelihood of any surgical intervention was almost double in the clinical trial group.[27] In the Olmsted County study, incidence rates per 1,000 person-years were 8.5 (95% CI, 6.4–11.2) for AUR; 97.1 (95% CI, 88.7–106.0) for symptom progression, 6.6 (95% CI, 4.8–9.0) for any surgery; and 105.1 (95% CI, 96.4–114.4) for any outcomes for all men. For the smaller cohort who would have met the MTOPS trial inclusion criteria, incidence rates were higher at 18.3, 86.5, 16.8, and 109.4, respectively. By comparison, incidence rates per 1,000 person-years for the placebo arm of the MTOPS study were 6 for AUR, 36 for symptom progression, and 45 for any outcome. Extrapolation therefore from one study to another must be done with care.[27]

Aetiology

Aetiology is the understanding of why things occur—the factors that come together to cause the abnormality or illness. It is derived from the Greek αἰτιολογία, aitiologia.

Essentially most causes of retention are due to delayed voiding from a variety of causes, leading to overdistension of the bladder thereby reducing the ability of the bladder to contract normally, resulting in retention. Overdistension may lead to detrusor decompensation if it is prolonged. This was suggested a long time ago and is frequently forgotten.[28]

Acute retention

Acute urinary retention is usually characterized by the sudden, painful inability to void; painless AUR is rare and when it occurs is often associated with neurological abnormalities. AUR may be further subdivided into precipitated or spontaneous retention.[1,3,6] Precipitated AUR follows a triggering event such as anaesthesia, surgery, or the use of drugs with a sympathomimetic effect (see Box 5.2.2). All other AUR events with no prior triggering event should be classified as spontaneous. Spontaneous retention is most frequently associated with LUTS and BPE, and is regarded as a sign of disease progression.

Urinary retention has been described with the use of drugs with anticholinergic activity (e.g. antipsychotic drugs, antidepressant agents, and anticholinergic respiratory agents), opioids and anaesthetic agents, alpha-adrenoceptor agonists, benzodiazepines, NSAIDs, detrusor relaxants, and calcium channel antagonists.

The differentiation between precipitated and spontaneous retention is clinically important because prostate surgery is less commonly needed in patients with precipitated AUR; as they are more likely to have a successful trial without catheter (TWOC).

Box 5.2.2 Factors that can trigger precipitated acute urinary retention

Precipitated acute urinary retention may be triggered by:

- Bladder overdistension
- Surgery with either general or regional anaesthesia
- Excessive fluid intake
- Alcohol consumption
- Urinary tract infections
- Prostatic inflammation
- Use of drugs with sympathomimetic, anticholinergic, or antihistamine effects

In addition, the likelihood of recurrent AUR is more likely in the spontaneous group.

The exact initiating cause of the retention may be unclear in many cases but the following mechanisms have been suggested:

(i) Increased resistance to flow of urine (obstructive); either mechanical (e.g. urethral stricture, clot retention) or dynamic obstruction (e.g. increased α-adrenergic activity, prostatic inflammation)

(ii) Bladder overdistension (myogenic); (immobility, constipation, drugs inhibiting bladder contractility)

(iii) Neuropathic causes in the sensory input or the motor output of the detrusor muscle (e.g. spinal disease, diabetic cystopathy)

Postoperative retention

Although this could be seen as just one of the many causes of AUR or sometimes CUR, it merits consideration separately as well. Its rate is highly variable.[29] It is more common after pelvic surgery; for example, anorectal, gynaecological, or urological, as well as after perineal and anal surgery, and of course after surgery of the lower urinary tract, particularly with traumatic instrumentation. Many factors can contribute to this risk, including[30,31]:

- major laparotomy especially if the period of anaesthesia is greater than 60 minutes;
- muscle paralysis and ventilation and cases that were reversed by atropine and neostigmine;
- opiate analgesia, particularly if used intravenously;
- excessive intravenous fluids resulting in bladder distension;
- diminished awareness of bladder sensation;
- pre-existing increased bladder outlet resistance;
- postoperative pain (nociceptive inhibitory reflex);
- prolonged immobilization in the postoperative period.

Patient age and sex may be less important, other factors being equal. Perhaps one of the greatest tragedies is post-partum retention. Once again, bladder distension secondary to decreased awareness of bladder sensation may be more important than local pain or anxiety.

Chronic retention

The aetiology of chronic retention (CUR) is more complex but can usefully be divided into high-pressure chronic retention (HPCR) and low-pressure chronic retention (LPCR).[32–34] The terms 'high' and 'low' refer to the subtracted detrusor pressure, during urodynamic studies, at the end of micturition (i.e. at the start of the next filling phase).[33,34] Bladder outlet obstruction usually exists in HPCR and the voiding detrusor pressure is high, but is associated with poor urinary flow rates. The persistently high bladder pressure in HPCR during both the storage and voiding phases of micturition results in retrograde pressure on the upper tract and leads to bilateral hydronephrosis and varying degrees of renal dysfunction. However, other patients may have large-volume retention in a very compliant floppy bladder with no evidence of hydronephrosis and normal renal function, and these are said to have LPCR. Pressure flow studies in these men with LPCR reveal poor flow rates, low detrusor pressures, and very large residual volumes. The LUTS in both types of CUR, however, are usually mild especially in the early stages of their condition, until typically the onset of nocturnal enuresis, resulting from the drop in urethral resistance during sleep, which is overcome by the maintained high bladder pressure causing incontinence—sometimes inappropriately called overflow incontinence.[33,34]

Some authors like to break the causes of retention into anatomical, myogenic, pharmacological, functional, and psychogenic, but in practice the cause is usually multifactorial and therefore this is not always of much benefit in real life practice.

In young male adults in particular, the use of psychoactive substances, such as stimulants like MDMA (ecstasy) and amphetamine should not be overlooked. The condition of paruresis or shy bladder syndrome, where there is the inability to urinate in the presence of others (such as public toilets), should not be forgotten.[35,36]

Pathogenesis

The pathogenesis of a condition or disease is the description of the underlying mechanism that causes the disease. It comes from the Greek for pathos, 'disease', and genesis, 'creation'. The evidence base for pathogenesis is less robust than that for the aetiology.

Pathology and pathogenesis

Five factors have been implicated in pathogenesis:

(i) Prostatic infarction

(ii) Prostatic inflammation

(iii) Increased α-adrenergic activity

(iv) Decrease in the stromal: epithelial ratio

(v) Neurotransmitter modulation

Prostatic infarction

The finding of prostatic infarction caused by infection, instrumentation, and thrombosis, is far more common in prostatectomy specimens after AUR than in TURP specimens for LUTS alone. This has been suggested in many studies as an underlying cause of retention. In a study of 100 patients, Spiro and colleagues found evidence for infarction in 85% of prostates removed for AUR, compared with only 3% in prostates of men having surgery for LUTS alone.[37] They suggested that the infarction resulted from distortion of the prostatic intraglandular blood supply. Other possible causes would include infection stasis, thrombosis, atherosclerosis, and embolization.[23,38] This may develop because of the accumulation of activated lymphocytes and up-regulation of pro-inflammatory cytokines resulting in tissue destruction and subsequent tissue rebuilding perhaps contributing to these prostatic infarcts.[23,39] A newer hypothesis is that the prostatic infarction may also lead to neurogenic disturbance in the prostatic urethra, preventing relaxation of the prostatic urethra, leading to a rise in urethral pressure and subsequent AUR.[23] This finding appears to be more common in spontaneous than in precipitated AUR.

Prostatic inflammation

Much of the pathophysiology of BPH development involves an underlying inflammatory disorder with a strong association with non-insulin dependant diabetes and metabolic syndrome.[39] There is a statistically significant association between inflammation and both BPH severity and progression to AUR. Kramer and Marberger also reported that inflammation was associated with larger prostates, higher PSA levels, and a greater risk of AUR.[40] Truncel and colleagues reported an increased incidence of prostatic inflammation in men with AUR compared with men with LUTS.[41] More recently in another study, chronic inflammation was more commonly found in the prostate from resections for AUR than in those specimens from men operated upon for LUTS alone.[42] This is further supported by evidence suggesting that prostatic inflammation may be a predictor of BPH progression.[43,44]

In a British study of TURP, 374 patients were studied regarding the finding of acute or chronic inflammation in the resection specimens. Seventy per cent (70%) of men undergoing TURP for retention against only 45% of men undergoing TURP for LUTS alone were found to have inflammation.[45] Regarding logistic regression, the pathological factors associated with TURP for acute retention compared to that for LUTS were more powerful for the presence of acute or chronic inflammation than for prostate volume, using increasing resection weight as a proxy for prostate volume.[45]

Increased α-adrenergic activity

Some cases of AUR are associated with a rise in the prostatic intraurethral pressure through an increase in α-adrenergic stimulation (e.g. stress, cold weather, sympathomimetic agents used in cold remedies, and so on). Prostatic infarction or prostatitis may contribute to this process. Bladder overdistension also leads to increased sympathetic adrenergic tone.[46]

The overdistension can lead to ischaemic injury of the detrusor muscle. Prolonged bladder overdistension leads to a temporary neurogenic detrusor dysfunction, which is associated with decreased or absent bladder sensation; therefore patients do not complain, and management is delayed.

A decrease in the stromal: epithelial ratio

This has been noted in AUR. This may in part explain the effect of the agents finasteride and dutasteride, which are known to act mainly on the epithelial component of the prostate, thereby increasing the stromal:epithelial ratio and may explain how they are able to reduce the risk of retention. Choong and Emberton suggested that it was feasible to bring these three mechanisms together by postulating that changes in epithelial/stromal growth in BPH may result in prostate infarction through changes in the prostatic blood flow. This in turn leads to a rise in urethral pressure indirectly increasing adrenergic tone resulting in increasing obstruction.[23]

Neurotransmitter modulation

Alterations in the non-adrenergic, noncholinergic transmitters (e.g. vasoactive polypeptide (VIP), neuropeptide Y (NPY), substance P) has been postulated as another underlying cause. These may act by influencing the release of acetylcholine and noradrenalin, and will also impact on bladder wall blood flow.[47]

In conclusion, bladder outlet obstruction if present leads to hypertrophy of detrusor smooth muscle cells, leading to detrusor wall thickening and increase in bladder mass, increased collagen synthesis, and deposition. In parallel, the bladder overdistension leads to high intravesical pressures that cause detrusor ischaemia, this leads to the release of neurotransmitters like ATP, NO, and prostaglandin from the urothelium. The obstruction may also lead to partial denervation of the detrusor, supersensitivity of muscarinic receptors to acetylcholine,[48] reorganization of the spinal micturition reflex, neurotramsmitter imbalance, and changes in the electrical properties of detrusor smooth muscle cells. Consequently, this leads to deterioration of bladder contractility and reduced compliance. This multiplicity of factors will decide whether changes are reversible or irreversible.[46,49–51]

Presentation, initial assessment, and investigation

Acute retention

The most common presentation is a patient with lower abdominal pain, an inability to pass urine (or passing only very small amounts of urine), and a palpable mass arising from the pelvis, which is dull to percussion. Although it is usually stated that patients with AUR did not have previous LUTS, it is more likely that many of these patients had not recognized or complained of these symptoms before. That is, they may have either not recognized their significance or assumed them to be an inevitable consequence of ageing. Examination should include a digital rectal examination noting the size and texture of prostate, anal tone, and the presence or absence of constipation. Although AUR is primarily a clinical diagnosis, a bladder volume scan (if available) will further confirm the diagnosis before catheterization. The volume drained is usually less than 1 L. If the volume drained is 1 L or more, this can be used as a distinction between acute and acute-on-chronic retention, particularly if associated with less pain (a finding that is more typical of CUR.[24]

Chronic retention

CUR occurs when patients retain a substantial amount of urine in the bladder after each void. As already stated, a defined volume for CUR is difficult and the finding of persistent residual volumes of >300 mL (some authors suggest >500 mL) after voiding is often used as evidence of chronic retention; some patients however may present with many litres in their bladders. Patients may be asymptomatic or describe low volume micturition, increased frequency, or difficulty initiating and maintaining micturition. Other features of CUR include nocturnal incontinence, a palpable but painless bladder, and signs of chronic renal failure. LUTS are less common and generally less bothersome.

Assessment

In both types of retention, urinalysis should always be performed and a catheter specimen of urine sent if there are signs of infection: urinary infection should be treated. Urea, creatinine and electrolytes, and an eGFR should be checked; this is especially important in (high pressure) CUR. Renal ultrasound is indicated in patients with high-volume retention and in patients with abnormal renal function. Prostate-specific antigen testing is best avoided during the acute episode, since retention and any instrumentation of the prostate leads to a spurious rise in PSA.[52,53]

Bladder volume per se will not separate LPCR from the more serious HPCR. In the author's unit within the last three months, two contrasting men with chronic retention were admitted. One had 1.3 L in the bladder, a creatinine of over 900 and bilateral hydronephrosis; and another patient a few days later with 6.5 L in the bladder and a normal creatinine, and only the slightest degree of hydronephrosis.

Differential diagnosis

This is not usually difficult, but diverticulitis or a diverticular abscess, perforated or ischaemic bowel, or an abdominal aortic aneurysm are all recognized as potentially more serious conditions that can be referred into hospital as 'acute retention'. Urinary retention may also occur secondary to any of the above conditions; it is therefore important for the patient to be re-examined soon after catheterization to confirm that the symptoms and signs have resolved. In addition, any patient with an abdominal mass should be considered for catheterization to exclude a distended bladder prior to further examination or investigation. Occasionally, an obese patient with renal failure may be mistaken for a case of AUR.

Management

Acute retention

The treatment of acute retention is urgent catheterization. This may be urethral or suprapubic catheterization, and this decision is usually based on a combination of factors. Whether patients are catheterized at home by a GP or district/practice nurse, in an accident and emergency department, or in a surgical/urology ward depends mainly on local circumstances, as does the decision to admit or send the patient home after catheterization. If patients are kept in hospital awaiting definitive treatment, this results in an overall longer total hospital stay.[6]

The initial urine volume, typically drained in the first 10–15 minutes following catheterization, must be accurately recorded in the patient's notes, to enable a distinction between acute and

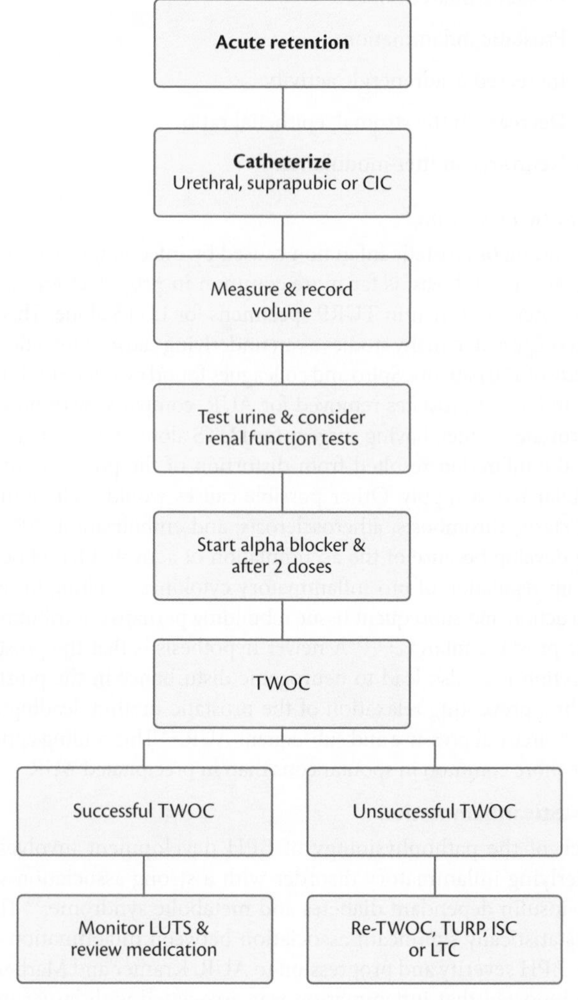

Fig. 5.2.1 Acute retention.

acute-on-chronic retention to be made. This has important clinical implications (Fig. 5.2.1).

Chronic retention

The management of CUR is more complex. Catheterization is less urgent as the condition is generally less painful or painless. Early catheterization is indicated if there is renal dysfunction or upper tract dilatation; both signs of HPCR. These patients with HPCR must be monitored for a postobstructive diuresis. They may pass many litres of urine in the first few days following catheterization (Fig. 5.2.2). The diuresis is due to:

- off-loading of retained salt and water (retained in the weeks prior to the episode of retention);
- loss of the corticomedullary concentration gradient. This is caused by reduced urinary flow through the chronically obstructed kidney;
- osmotic diuresis caused by the high urea level.

In about 10% of cases, the diuresis is excessive and could require careful fluid balance and replacement. Daily weighing can be an accurate way of monitoring fluid output. After the first 24 hours, fluid replacement should not religiously follow the output, which would simply perpetuate the diuresis. Potassium levels, which are often high, should be monitored and will usually (but not always) fall with the diuresis. Catheterization is often followed by haematuria; this is caused by renal tract decompression and not usually by the catheter itself.

If patients present with chronic retention electively through the outpatient department, the indications for catheterization before TURP in cases of CUR are again renal impairment and water and salt retention; otherwise it is best to avoid catheterization to avoid infection and bladder shrinkage before TURP, but the patients should be listed for early surgery once their renal function is stable. Many patients with LPCR do poorly after TURP, frequently failing to void completely after surgery, even after prolonged periods of catheterization; this is primarily due to detrusor decompensation.[32,54,55] Intermittent self-catheterization should be considered in this group.

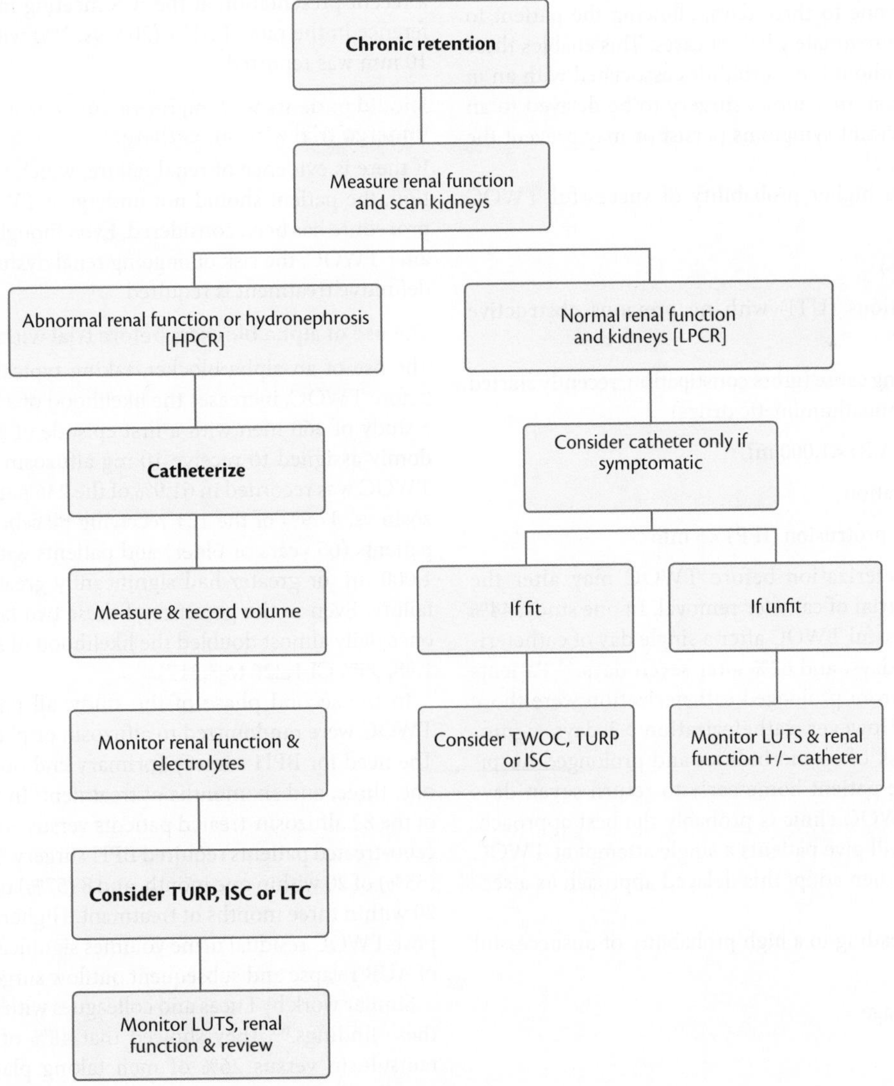

Fig. 5.2.2 Chronic retention.

What should be the speed of bladder emptying?

Rapid emptying of an extended bladder in urinary retention is often considered dangerous because of the risk of haematuria or circulatory collapse. Therefore, many papers and textbooks advise the use of gradual drainage of the bladder. A recent German RCT of rapid or gradual emptying of 260 men has been performed to address this issue.[56] Haematuria occurred in similar numbers in each group (11%), only half of whom required further treatment for this reason. There were no cases of circulatory collapse in this study. Reduction in blood pressure and pulse rate were not clinically significant in either group. In conclusion, the practice of slow decompression is unnecessary and haematuria usually settles after 48–72 hours.[56]

A trial without catheter

The increased morbidity and mortality associated with emergency surgery, particularly when performed shortly after AUR, and the potential morbidity associated with prolonged catheterization (bacteriuria, fever, urosepsis) has led to an increasing use of a TWOC. It is now considered a standard of care in most countries around the world and is utilized in most patients with acute retention, and in a significant number of patients with LPCR.[6,55] The catheter is usually removed after one to three days, allowing the patient to successfully void in approximately half of cases. This enables these patients to go home without the morbidities associated with an *in situ* catheter. In addition, this allows surgery to be delayed to an elective setting if significant symptoms persist or may prevent the need for surgery in some[1,57].

Factors leading to a higher probability of successful TWOC include[1,57]:

- Lower age (<65 years)
- Urinary tract infections (UTI) with no previous obstructive (voiding) symptoms
- Identified precipitating cause (gross constipation, recently started anticholinergic or sympathomimetic drugs)
- Post-void residual (PVR) <1,000 mL
- Prolonged catheterization
- Intravesical prostatic protrusion (IPP) <5 mm

The duration of catheterization before TWOC may alter the chance of a successful trial of catheter removal. In one study, 44% of patients had a successful TWOC after a single day of catheterization, 51% after two days, and 62% after seven days.[23] Patients most likely to benefit from prolonged catheterization were those with a greater PVR. However, catheterization >3 days significantly increases the risk of co-morbidities and prolonged hospitalization. Sending the patient home early to return seven days later to a dedicated TWOC clinic is probably the best approach, although many units will give patients a single attempt at TWOC after 24–48 hours and then adopt this delayed approach as a second option.

Conversely, factors leading to a high probability of unsuccessful TWOC include:

- patients >75 years of age
- drained volume >1 L
- previous LUTS
- voiding detrusor contraction (on urodynamics) of <35 cmH_2O[1,5,22]
- intravesical prostatic protrusion >10 mm

However, even if an initial TWOC is successful, half of these men will experience recurrent AUR over the next year and a third will require surgery within the following six months. Patients with PVR>500 mL, no precipitating factor for AUR, and maximum flow rate <5 mL/s were at increased risk of further retention.[58] In the ALFAUR study, most of the patients requiring surgery after a successful TWOC were due to recurrent AUR.[59] This emphasizes the importance of follow-up in patients with risk factors for recurrent AUR, despite initial successful TWOC.[1,57]

In one study of AUR, intravesical prostatic protrusion predicted for failure of TWOC, with the likelihood of failure being greater for an IPP >10 mm.[60] Also in the Olmsted County study, IPP correlated significantly with greater prostate volume, lower peak flows, and higher obstructive symptoms, thereby suggesting that it may have clinical usefulness in predicting the need for treatment.[61] In another study of IPP in 100 men with AUR, only 33% of men with an IPP greater than 10 mm had a successful TWOC, while 64% of men with IPP from 1 to 5 mm had a successful one,[62] and in a recent presentation at the ICS meeting in Beijing, a 10-fold difference in the rate of AUR (20% vs. 2%) with an IPP either side of 10 mm was reported.[63]

Should patients with high-pressure chronic retention undergo trial without catheter?

If there is evidence of renal failure, which settles with catheterization, the patient should not undergo a TWOC before a definitive procedure has been considered. Even though they might void again after TWOC, the risk of ongoing renal dysfunction is too great and definitive treatment is required.

The use of alpha blockers before trial without catheter

The use of an alpha blocker, taking typically two or more doses before TWOC, increases the likelihood of a successful outcome. In a study of 360 men with a first episode of spontaneous AUR randomly assigned to receive 10 mg alfuzosin or placebo, successful TWOC was recorded in 61.9% of the 236 patients treated with alfuzosin vs. 47.9% of the 121 receiving placebo ($p = 0.012$).[59] Elderly patients (65 years or older) and patients with a drained volume of 1,000 mL or greater had significantly greater chances of TWOC failure. Even in the presence of these two factors, 10 mg alfuzosin once daily almost doubled the likelihood of successful TWOC (OR 1.98, 95% CI 1,226 to 3,217).

In the second phase of the study, all patients with successful TWOC were randomized to alfuzosin or placebo for six months.[64] The need for BPH surgery (primary end point) was assessed after one, three, and six months of treatment. In this phase, 14 (17.1%) of the 82 alfuzosin-treated patients versus 20 (24.1%) of the 83 placebo-treated patients required BPH surgery, 5 (36%) of 14 versus 13 (65%) of 20 within one month, and 8 (57%) of 14 versus 17 (85%) of 20 within three months of treatment. Higher PSA values and larger post-TWOC residual urine volumes significantly increased the risk of AUR relapse and subsequent outflow surgery.

Similar work by Lucas and colleagues with tamsulosin confirmed these findings.[65] They showed that 48% of their patients taking tamsulosin versus 26% of men taking placebo did not require recatheterization ($p = 0.011$; odds ratio 2.47).

Five randomized clinical trials of alpha blockers before TWOC were reviewed in a Cochrane systematic review in 2009.[66] Four trials used alfuzosin and one tamsulosin. In four, the alpha blocker was used for 24–72 hours before TWOC and in one study for eight days. Overall rates of successful TWOC favoured alpha blockers over placebo (RR 1.39, 95% CI 1.18–1.64) irrespective of the alpha blocker used (alfuzosin: RR 1.31, 95% CI 1.10–1.56; tamsulosin: RR 1.86, 95% CI 1.17–2.97).[66] In real life practice, the Reten-World survey revealed that 82% of patients received an α1-blocker before catheter removal; TWOC success was greater in those receiving α-blockers, regardless of age.[57]

This policy allows more patients to return home without a catheter *in situ*, thereby perhaps reducing the subsequent perioperative complications of prostate surgery. This should contribute to decrease the morbidity and mortality associated with emergency surgery and avoids the discomfort and potential morbidity associated with an *in situ* catheter.

Increased mortality in retention patients

Mortality is increased after retention. The rate within the year following an AUR episode is significantly higher than in the general population, especially in younger patients. Mortality in men admitted to hospital with AUR is strongly correlated with age and co-morbidity. Men with AUR have a high risk of developing complications and a greater risk of death after prostatectomy than men having surgery for LUTS alone.[67] In a study of one hundred thousand men who presented with spontaneous AUR,[68] Armitage and colleagues reported that the one-year mortality was 4.1% in men aged 45–54 and 32.8% in those aged 85 and over. In another 75,979 men with precipitated AUR, mortality was higher at 9.5% and 45.4%, respectively. One-year mortality was considerably higher in those patients (aged 75–84) with co-morbidities. Meanwhile, in men with spontaneous AUR it was 12.5% in men without co-morbidity and 28.8% in men with co-morbidity and 18.1% and 40.5%, respectively, in those with precipitated retention. Compared with the general population however, the highest relative increase in mortality was in men aged 45–54 (standardized mortality ratio 10.0 for spontaneous and 23.6 for precipitated acute urinary retention) and the lowest for men aged 85 years and over (1.7 and 2.4, respectively). The mortality was higher in patients with precipitated rather than spontaneous retention, perhaps because precipitated retention occurs after a triggering event that is unrelated to the prostate, and therefore a further indication of co-morbidity. It was suggested therefore that patients would benefit from a multidisciplinary approach to identify and treat co-morbid conditions before surgery. The current main morbidities include diabetes, hypertension, cardiovascular disease, and metabolic syndrome.

It was also shown by the UK National Prostatectomy Audit that immediate surgery after AUR was associated with a greater perioperative morbidity and death rate after surgery at 30 days (RR 26.6) and 90 days (RR 4.4) when compared with elective prostatectomy for symptoms alone.[67] In a more recent study of over 400 men in Taiwan, the rates of recatheterization, septicaemia, and shock were highly significantly more common in the TURP after AUR group, than in those having TURP for symptoms alone.[69] The AUR group also had more UTIs.

Hospitalize versus send home

The decision regarding whether to admit patients to hospital or send them home from accident and emergency or a surgical assessment unit is based more on local resources and preferences than any evidence-based protocol. A UK survey found that most urologists (65.5%) preferred to admit their patients, with only 1 in 5 urologists admitting only in the presence of abnormal renal function.[70] Admission is essential if the patient is: unwell with urosepsis; has abnormal renal function needing investigation and fluid monitoring; has acute neurological problems; or cannot take care of the catheter.[53] A recent publication from China showed that the establishment of an ambulatory care programme for patients presenting to their emergency department with AUR reduced the hospital admission rate and reduced cost without jeopardizing the TWOC success rate and patient safety.[71]

Urethral versus suprapubic catheterization

Apart from specific indications, such as after urethral trauma and for long-term catheterization for bladder dysfunction, suprapubic catheterization (SPC) has perceived advantages for the management of retention. The principal advantages of SPC are reduction in UTIs, less stricture formation, and the fact that it permits TWOC without catheter removal.[72–74] Patients therefore frequently express a preference for SPC because of its increased comfort, and the ability to maintain active sexual function is important to some patients. As a significant number of patients will fail their TWOC, patients will often have to undergo repeat catheterization with all the consequent discomfort. Many studies have shown the benefits of SPC in AUR. It could therefore be regarded as the preferred route of catheterization. However, the suprapubic approach is often overlooked when deciding on the mode of catheterization. In the Reten-World survey, it was reported that a majority of urologists performed urethral catheterization (>80%) with suprapubic catheters inserted for urethral catheter failures.[57] This survey also reported similar complication rates for both types of catheter. Surprisingly, there was no difference in asymptomatic bacteriuria, lower urinary tract infection, or urosepsis between the two catheter types. This may have been due to the fact that this was not an RCT, but rather a study of real life practice, and the indications for the type of catheterization were not standardized. Urethral catheters however were associated with an increased incidence of urinary leakage. Disadvantages associated with SPC insertion are that it is a more complex procedure, which not all health professionals are adequately skilled to perform. Serious complications, such as bowel perforation, posterior bladder wall injury, and peritonitis have been reported.[74,75] SPC safety will have reduced with the introduction of the safer Seldinger technique SPC catheter, which replaces the traditional blind insertion of the trocar and cannula with SPC insertion over a guidewire.[75–77] Wherever possible this should be performed under ultrasound guidance,[75,78] as per the recommended advice of the British Association of Urological Surgeons' (BAUS) guideline.[78] This technique has been shown in a small study to be associated with increased patient satisfaction and clinician confidence.[77] This, together with the use of simulation and models, should in the future support the training of junior doctors, thereby allowing the use of SPC insertion in the emergency setting to become more widespread.[79]

The role of clean intermittent self-catheterization

Clean intermittent self-catheterization (CISC) is a viable alternative to an indwelling catheter. It is a safe, simple, and generally well-accepted technique by patients that results in fewer infections than indwelling urethral catheterization. Without any external devices, maintenance of sexual activity is possible. It may also increase the rate of subsequent successful spontaneous voiding. CISC can be used either instead of an indwelling catheter after an episode of AUR or CUR, or in patients who fail to void following a prostatectomy. This is can be particularly valuable in patients with neurological bladder dysfunction. A period of CISC prior to TURP may be useful in patients with low-pressure CUR, as it may allow recovery of bladder contractility. A retrospective analysis of over 500 patients showed that in-out catheterization for the treatment of AUR was as effective as indwelling catheterization and was likely to be particularly successful for younger men and those with lower residual volumes.[80]

In a randomized study of men with CUR and preoperative urodynamics before TURP, a low detrusor voiding pressure was associated with a poor TURP outcome.[81] Preoperative CISC rather than indwelling urethral catheterization was associated with a significant improvement in voiding and end-filling pressures, indicating some recovery of bladder function. The authors concluded that a preliminary period of CISC before TURP for men with CUR and low voiding pressure might be valuable.[81]

Prevention of acute urinary retention

If one considers the pain and discomfort from AUR, the considerable healthcare costs involved, and the increased mortality from both presentation with retention and the increased risk from prostatic surgery, then the case for primary prevention of AUR should be clear. The benefits however are only accrued by the at-risk group. The risk factors for AUR have already been listed in the epidemiology section (Box 5.2.1). The more of these risk factors that are present the greater the benefit, and the more cost-effective the treatment.[82,83]

The 5-alpha reductase inhibitors

The PLESS, MTOPS, and the CombAT studies were designed to look at the risk reduction of AUR with 5-alpha reductase inhibitor (5-ARI) medical therapy.[10,12,84] The first two studied finasteride and the third dutasteride.

The PLESS was a four-year study of finasteride versus placebo in over 3,000 men.[12] The overall risk of AUR was 6.6% on placebo and 2.8% on finasteride—a risk reduction of 57%. The risk reduction for both spontaneous and precipitated AUR from finasteride treatment varied by both serum PSA and prostate volume at baseline. Stratified by PSA tertiles, the reduction ranges from 7% to 77% for spontaneous and from 35% to 66% for both types of AUR, compared with the placebo-treated patients.[85]

The MTOPS study evaluated doxazosin, finasteride, and combination therapy in 3,047 men followed for a mean of 4.5 years.[10] Combination therapy decreased the risk for AUR by 81% versus placebo (p <0.001), and the risk reduction with finasteride alone was 68% (p <0.001). Doxazosin monotherapy did not significantly decrease the risk for AUR versus placebo (34% risk reduction, p = NS).

Similar results were seen with the 5-ARI, dutasteride.[86] In three phase 3 two-year RCTs including 4,325 men, AUR was reported in 4.2% patients receiving placebo, versus 1.8% patients receiving dutasteride; a relative risk reduction of 57% (hazard ratio: 0.43; 95% CI 0.29–0.62; p <0.001).[86]

In the CombAT study, in which there was no placebo arm, AUR were seen less frequently with dutasteride compared with tamsulosin.[84] The cumulative incidence of AUR at four years was 2.7% (44 events in 1,623 patients) with dutasteride versus 6.8% (109 events in 1,611 patients) with tamsulosin treatment. Also, in the four-year REduction by DUtasteride of prostate Cancer Events (REDUCE) trial, the incidence of acute urinary retention or BPH-related surgery was significantly less in the dutasteride group (2.5%) than in the placebo group (9%) overall (p <0.001), and in each baseline prostate volume quintile (p <0.01).[87]

Assessments of the relative efficacy of these 5-ARIs in non-randomized studies have suggested that dutasteride-treated patients may be less likely to develop AUR than finasteride-treated patients.[88,89] In a retrospective review of data from a large, national healthcare database, the rate of AUR was substantially lower in 1992 BPH patients aged ≥50 years treated with dutasteride versus finasteride for 5–12 months (19 [5.3%] vs. 135 [8.3%], respectively; p = 0.0207)[88], while in a retrospective analysis of medical and pharmacy claims data from 5,090 men aged ≥65 years with enlarged prostate, AUR was reported in 305 (12.0%) and 374 (14.7%) men on dutasteride and finasteride, respectively (odds ratio: 0.79; p = 0.0042)[89]. In an American study, Medicare medical claims data were analysed to determine comparative differences on rates of AUR and prostate-related surgeries among patients over 65 years treated with either dutasteride or finasteride. Patients treated with dutasteride were significantly less likely to experience AUR and prostate-related surgery than finasteride patients. The monthly expenditure over one year covering drug costs, hospital visits, and periods of care in hospital were analysed, and they concluded that the dutasteride-treated patients overall incurred lower costs per month than the finasteride patients, despite the higher drug costs.[90]

The alpha blockers

It is likely that the alpha blockers delay the time to retention without statistically reducing the overall risk. The effects of alfuzosin on AUR appear to be inconsistent. In one six-month study, alfuzosin appeared to significantly reduce the risk of AUR, while in another study there was no reduction in risk.[91,92] In the MTOPS study, doxazosin did not significantly reduce the incidence of AUR over four years versus placebo (9 [1%] vs. 18 [2%] events). However, doxazosin did delay the time to occurrence of AUR episodes.[10] The effect of tamsulosin on AUR has not been investigated in a placebo-controlled study; however, results from the four-year CombAT study showed reduced rates of AUR with tamsulosin in combination with dutasteride (2.2%) compared with tamsulosin monotherapy (6.8%) or dutasteride monotherapy (2.7%).[84]

Caution should always be advised against making direct comparisons of AUR incidence across different trials, because of differences in study design, inclusion and exclusion criteria, baseline characteristics such as prostate volume and PSA, discontinuation rates, and follow-up after discontinuation.[85]

Conclusions

Urinary retention continues to be a significant burden for both the patient and healthcare services in the United Kingdom and around the world. The management of this condition should begin with recognizing and then modifying risk factors for developing AUR. 5-ARI treatment is effective in reducing the risk of retention but the difference between relative and absolute risk should always be borne in mind and only those men with significant risk offered preventive therapy. In men at considerable risk of retention, elective surgical intervention should be considered. Urethral catheterization followed by a TWOC has become a standard of care worldwide and the use of alpha blockade prior to TWOC significantly increases the chances of successful TWOC.

Delay of surgery to treat associated co-morbidities is worthwhile in certain patients to reduce the risk of perioperative morbidity and mortality, as well as allowing the bladder to recover its contractility in those with prolonged overdistension. Ongoing research is needed, especially into the underlying mechanisms of retention—namely the specific inflammatory pathways to reduce the risk, and perhaps even develop new treatments, for retention.

Further reading

Scorer C. The suprapubic catheter. A method of treating urinary retention. *Lancet* 1953; **265**:1222–5.

References

1. Fitzpatrick J, Kirby R. Management of acute urinary retention. *BJUI* 2006; **97**(Suppl 2):16–20.
2. Thomas K, Oades G, Taylor-Hay C, *et al.* Acute urinary retention: what is the impact on patients' quality of life? *BJUI* 2005; **95**:72–6.
3. Kaplan S, Wein A, Staskin R, *et al.* Urinary retention and post void residual urine in men: separating truth from tradition. *J Urol* 2008; **180**:47–54.
4. Negro CL, Muir GH. Chronic urinary retention in men: How we define it, and how does it affect treatment outcome. *BJU Int* 2012; **110**:1590–4.
5. Holtgrewe HL, Mebust WK, Dowd JB, *et al.* Transurethral prostatectomy: practice aspects of the dominant operation in American urology. *J Urol* 1989; **141**:248–53.
6. Fitzpatrick JM, Desgrandchamps F, Adjali K, *et al.* Management of acute urinary retention: a worldwide survey of 6074 men with benign prostatic hyperplasia. *BJU Int* 2012; **109**(1):88–95.
7. Ball AJ, Feneley RC, Abrams PH. The natural history of untreated "prostatism." *Br J Urol* 1981; **53**:613–16.
8. Hunter DJ, Berra-Unamuno A, Martin-Gordo A. Prevalence of urinary symptoms and other urological conditions in Spanish men 50 years old or older. *J Urol* 1996; **155**:1965–70.
9. Jacobsen SJ, Jacobson DJ, Girman CJ, *et al.* Natural history of prostatism: risk factors for acute urinary retention. *J Urol* 1997; **158**(2):481–7.
10. McConnell JD, Roehrborn CG, Bautista OM, Medical Therapy of Prostatic Symptoms (MTOPS) Research Group. The long-term effect of doxazosin, finasteride, and combination therapy on the clinical progression of benign prostatic hyperplasia. *N Engl J Med* 2003; **349**(25): 2387–98.
11. Emberton M, Cornel E, Bassi P, Fourcade O, Gómez M, Castro R. Benign prostatic hyperplasia as a progressive disease: a guide to the risk factors and options for medical management. *Int J Clin Pract* 2008; **62**(7):1076–86.
12. McConnell JD, Bruskewitz R, Walsh P, *et al.* The effect of finasteride on the risk of acute urinary retention and the need for surgical treatment among men with benign prostatic hyperplasia. Finasteride Long-Term Efficacy and Safety Study Group. *N Engl J Med* 1998; **338**(9):557–63.
13. Roehrborn CG. The epidemiology of acute urinary retention in benign prostatic hyperplasia. *Rev Urol* 2001; **3**(4):187–92.
14. Marberger MJ, Andersen JT, Nickel JC, *et al.* Prostate volume and serum prostate-specific antigen as predictors of acute urinary retention. Combined experience from three large multinational placebo-controlled trials. *Eur Urol* 2000; **38**(5):563–8.
15. Emberton M. Definition of at-risk patients: dynamic variables. *BJU Int* 2006; **97**(Suppl 2):12–15; discussion 21–2.
16. Emberton M, Elhilali M, Matzkin H, *et al.* Alf-One Study Group. Symptom deterioration during treatment and history of AUR are the strongest predictors for AUR and BPH-related surgery in men with LUTS treated with alfuzosin 10 mg once daily. *Urology* 2005; **66**(2):316–22.
17. Verhamme KM, Dieleman JP, van Wijk MA *et al.* Low incidence of acute urinary retention in the general male population: the triumph project. *Eur Urol* 2005; **47**(4):494–8.
18. Cathcart P, van der Meulen J, Armitage J, *et al.* Incidence of primary and recurrent acute urinary retention between 1998 and 2003 in England. *J Urol* 2006; **176**(1):200–4.
19. Keller JJ, Lin CC, Chen CS, Chen YK, Lin HC. Monthly variation in acute urinary retention incidence among patients with benign prostatic enlargement in Taiwan. *J Androl* 2012; **33**(6):1239–44.
20. Sarma AV, Jacobson DJ, St Sauver JL, *et al.* Smoking and acute urinary retention: the Olmsted County study of urinary symptoms and health status among men. *Prostate* 2009; **69**(7):699–705.
21. Roehrborn C, Kaplan SA. Biopsy inflammation on the risk of clinical progression. *J Urol* 2005; **173**:(S4)346.
22. Sauver JL, St, Jacobson DJ, McGree ME, *et al.* Protective association between nonsteroidal antiinflammatory drug use and measures of benign prostatic hyperplasia. *Am J Epidemiol* 2006; **164**(8):760–8.
23. Choong S, Emberton M. Acute urinary retention. *BJUI* 2000; **85**:186–201.
24. Kalejaiye O, Speakman MJ. Management of acute and chronic retention in men. *Eur Urol* 2009; S8:523–9.
25. Shinbo H, Kurita Y, Takada S, *et al.* Resistive index as risk factor for acute urinary retention in patients with benign prostatic hyperplasia. *Urology* 2010; **76**(6):1440–5.
26. Zhang X, Li G, Wei X, *et al.* Resistive index of prostate capsular arteries: a newly identified parameter to diagnose and assess bladder outlet obstruction in patients with benign prostatic hyperplasia. *J Urol* 2012; **188**(3):881–7.
27. Roberts RO, Lieber MM, Jacobson DJ, *et al.* Limitations of using outcomes in the placebo arm of a clinical trial of benign prostatic hyperplasia to quantify those in the community. *Mayo Clin Proc* 2005; **80**(6):759–64.
28. Powell PH, Smith PJ, Feneley RC. The identification of patients at risk from acute retention. *Br J Urol* 1980; **52**:520–22.
29. Stallard S, Prescott S. Postoperative urinary retention in general surgical patients. *Br J Surg* 1988; **75**:1141–3.
30. Petros JG, Rimm EB, Robillard RJ, Argy O. Factors influencing postoperative urinary retention in patients undergoing elective inguinal herniorrhaphy. *Am J Surg* 1991; **161**:431–3.
31. Mohammadi-Fallah M, Hamedanchi S, Tayyebi-Azar A. Preventive effect of tamsulosin on postoperative urinary retention. *Korean J Urol* 2012; **53**(6):419–23.
32. Ghalayini IF, Al-Ghazo MA, Pickard RS. A prospective randomized trial comparing transurethral prostatic resection and clean intermittent self-catheterization in men with chronic urinary retention. *BJU Int* 2005; **96**:93–7.
33. Abrams P, Dunn M, George N. Urodynamic findings in chronic retention of urine and their relevance to results of surgery. *BMJ* 1978; **2**:1258–60.
34. George N, O'Reilly P, Barnard R, *et al.* High pressure chronic retention. *BMJ* 1983; **286**:1780–3.
35. Bryden AA, Rothwell PJ, O'Reilly PH. Urinary retention with misuse of "ecstasy". *BMJ* 1995; **310**(6978):504.
36. Soifer S, Nicaise G, Chancellor M, *et al.* Paruresis or shy bladder syndrome: an unknown urologic malady? *Urol Nurs* 2009; **29**(2):87–93.
37. Spiro LH, Labay G, Orkin LA. Prostatic infarction. Role in acute urinary retention. *Urology* 1974; **3**:345–7.
38. Anjum I, Ahmed M, Azzopardi A, *et al.* Prostatic infarction/infection in acute urinary retention secondary to benign prostatic hyperplasia. *J Urol* 1998; **160**:792–3.

39. Briganti A, Capitanio U, Suardi N, Gallina A, Salonia A. Benign prostatic hyperplasia and its aetiologies. *Eur Urol* 2009; S8:865–71.
40. Kramer G, Mitteregger D, Marberger M. Is benign prostatic hyperplasia (BPH) an immune inflammatory disease? *Eur Urol* 2007; **51**:1202–16.
41. Truncel A, Uzun B, Eruyar T, Karabulut E, Seckin S, Atan A. Do prostatic infarction, prostatic inflammation and prostate morphology play a role in acute urinary retention? *Eur Urol* 2005; **48**:277–84.
42. Asgari SA, Mohammadi M. The role of intraprostatic inflammation in the acute urinary retention. *Int J Prev Med* 2011; **2**(1):28–31.
43. Nickel JC. The overlapping lower urinary tract symptoms of benign prostatic hyperplasia and prostatitis. *Curr Opin Urol* 2006; **16**(1):5–10.
44. Nickel JC, Roehrborn CG, O'Leary MP, Bostwick DG, Somerville MC, Rittmaster RS. Examination of the relationship between symptoms of prostatitis and histological inflammation: baseline data from the REDUCE chemoprevention trial. *J Urol* 2007; **178**:896–900.
45. Mishra VC, Allen DJ, Nicolaou C, *et al.* Does intraprostatic inflammation have a role in the pathogenesis and progression of benign prostatic hyperplasia?. *BJU Int* 2007; **100**(2):327–31.
46. Madersbacher H, Cardozo L, Chapple C, *et al.* What are the causes and consequences of bladder overdistension? ICI-RS 2011. *Neurourol Urodyn* 2012; **31**(3):317–21.
47. Lasanen LT, Tammela TL, Liesi P, Waris T, Polak JM. The effect of acute distension on vasoactive intestinal polypeptide (VIP), neuropeptide Y (NPY) and substance P (SP) immunoreactive nerves in the female rat urinary bladder. *Urol Res* 1992; **20**(4):259–63.
48. Speakman MJ, Brading AF, Dixon JS, Gosling J. Bladder outflow obstruction—a cause of denervation supersensitivity. *J Urol* 1987; **138**:1461–6.
49. Oelke M, Baard J, Wijkstra H, de la Rosette JJ, Jonas U, Höfner K. Age and bladder outlet obstruction are independently associated with detrusor overactivity in patients with benign prostatic hyperplasia. *Eur Urol* 2008; **54**(2):419–26.
50. Speakman MJ. Lower urinary tract symptoms suggestive of benign prostatic hyperplasia (LUTS/BPH): More than treating symptoms? *Eur Urol Suppl* 2008; **7**:680–9.
51. Yamaguchi O, Nishizawa O, Takeda M, *et al.* Clinical guidelines for overactive bladder. *Int J Urol* 2009; **16**(2):126–42.
52. Pruthi R. The dynamics of prostate-specific antigen in benign and malignant diseases of the prostate. *BJUI* 2000; **86**:652–58.
53. Kuppusamy S, Gillatt D. Managing patients with acute urinary retention. *Practitioner* 2011; **255**(1739):21–3, 2–3.
54. Bates T, Sugiono M, James E, Stott M, Pocock R. Is the conservative management of chronic retention in men ever justified? *BJUI* 2003; **92**:581–3.
55. Desgrandchamps F, De La Taille A, Doublet JD; RetenFrance Study Group. The management of acute urinary retention in France: a cross-sectional survey in 2618 men with benign prostatic hyperplasia. *BJU Int* 2006; **97**(4):727–33.
56. Boettcher S, Brandt AS, Roth S, Mathers MJ, Lazica DA. Urinary retention: benefit of gradual bladder decompression—myth or truth? A randomized controlled trial. *Urol Int* 2013; **91**(2):140–4.
57. Emberton M, Fitzpatrick J. The Reten-World survey of the management of acute urinary retention: preliminary results. *BJUI* 2008; **101**(S3):27–32.
58. McNeill A, Rizvi S, Byrne D. Prostate size influences the outcome after presenting with acute urinary retention. *BJUI* 2004; **94**:559–62.
59. McNeill SA, Hargreave TB; members of the ALFAUR study group. Alfuzosin once daily facilitates return to voiding in patients in acute urinary retention. *J Urol* 2004; **171**:2316–20.
60. Mariappan P, Brown DJ, McNeill AS. Intravesical prostatic protrusion is better than prostate volume in predicting the outcome of trial without catheter in white men presenting with acute urinary retention: a prospective clinical study. *J Urol* 2007; **178**(2):573–7.
61. Tan YH, Foo KT. Intravesical prostatic protrusion predicts the outcome of a trial without catheter following acute urine retention. *J Urol* 2003; **170**:2339–41.
62. Lieber M, Jacobson D, McGree M. Intravesical prostatic protrusion in men in Olmsted County, Minnesota. *J Urol* 2009; **182**(6):2819–24.
63. Elashry O. *Neurourol Urodyn* 2012: **31**(6):746–7.
64. McNeill SA, Hargreave TB, Roehrborn CG; Alfaur study group. Alfuzosin 10 mg once daily in the management of acute urinary retention: results of a double-blind placebo-controlled study. *Urology* 2005; **65**(1):83–9.
65. Lucas MG, Stephenson TP, Nargund V. Tamsulosin in the management of patients in acute urinary retention from benign prostatic hyperplasia. *BJU Int* 2005; **95**(3):354–7.
66. Zeif HJ, Subramonian K. Alpha blockers prior to removal of a catheter for acute urinary retention in adult men. *Cochrane Database Syst Rev* 2009; (4):CD006744.
67. Armitage JN, Sibanda N, Cathcart PJ, Emberton M, van der Meulen JH. Mortality in men admitted to hospital with acute urinary retention: database analysis. *BMJ* 2007; **335**(7631):1199–202.
68. Pickard R, Emberton M, Neal DE. The management of men with acute urinary retention. National Prostatectomy Audit Steering Group. *Br J Urol* 1998; **81**:712–20.
69. Chen JS, Chang CH, Yang WH, Kao YH. Acute urinary retention increases the risk of complications after transurethral resection of the prostate: a population-based study. *BJU Int* 2012; **110**(11 Pt C):E896–901.
70. Manikandan R, Srirangam S, O'Reilly P, Collins G. Management of acute urinary retention secondary to benign prostatic hyperplasia in the UK: a national survey. *BJUI* 2004; **93**:84–8.
71. Teoh JY, Kan CF, Tsui B, *et al.* Ambulatory care program for patients presenting with acute urinary retention secondary to benign prostatic hyperplasia. *Int Urol Nephrol* 2012; **44**(6):1593–9.
72. Abrams P, Gaches C, Green N. Role of suprapubic catheterisation in retention of urine. *J R Soc Med* 1980; **73**:845–8.
73. Horgan A, Prasad B, Waldron D, O'Sullivan D. Acute urinary retention. Comparison of suprapubic and urethral catheterisation. *Br J Urol* 1992; **70**:149–51.
74. Ahluwalia R, Johal N, Kouriefs C, Kooman G, Montgomery B, Plail R. The surgical risk of suprapubic catheter insertion and long-term sequelae. *Ann R Coll Surg Engl* 2006; **88**:210–13.
75. Jacob P, Rai BP, Todd AW. Suprapubic catheter insertion using an ultrasound-guided technique and literature review. *BJU Int* 2012; **110**(6):779–84.
76. Mohammed A, Khan A, Shergill IS, Gujral SS. A new model for suprapubic catheterization: the MediPlus Seldinger suprapubic catheter. *Expert Rev Med Devices* 2008; **5**(6):705–7.
77. Vasdev N, Kachroo N, Mathur S, Pickard R. Suprapubic bladder catheterisation using the Seldinger technique. *Int J Urol* 2007; **5**(1):DOI: 10.5580/511.
78. Harrison SC, Lawrence WT, Morley R, Pearce I, Taylor J. British Association of Urological Surgeons' suprapubic catheter practice guidelines. *BJU Int* 2011; **107**(1):77–85.
79. Shergill IS, Shaikh T, Arya M, Junaid I. A training model for suprapubic catheter insertion: the UroEmerge suprapubic catheter model. *Urology* 2008; **72**(1):196–7.
80. Ko YH, Kim JW, Kang SG, *et al.* The efficacy of in-and-out catheterisation as a way of trial without catheterisation strategy for treatment of acute urinary retention induced by benign prostate hyperplasia: variables predicting success outcome. *Neurourol Urodyn* 2012; **31**(4):460–4.
81. Ghalayini IF, Al-Ghazo MA, Pickard RS. A prospective randomized trial comparing transurethral prostatic resection and clean intermittent self-catheterisation in men with chronic urinary retention. *BJU Int* 2005; **96**(1):93–7.

82. Khastgir J, Khan A, Speakman M. Acute urinary retention: medical management and the identification of risk factors for prevention. *Nat Clin Pract Urol* 2007; **4**(8):422–31.
83. Emberton M. Definition of at-risk patients: dynamic variables. *BJU Int* 2006; **97**(Suppl 2):12–5.
84. Roehrborn CG, Siami P, Barkin J, *et al.* The effects of combination therapy with dutasteride and tamsulosin on clinical outcomes in men with symptomatic benign prostatic hyperplasia: 4-year results from the CombAT study. *Eur Urol* 2010; **57**(1):123–31.
85. Roehrborn CG. Acute urinary retention: risks and management. *Rev Urol* 2005; **7**(Suppl 4):S31–41.
86. Roehrborn CG, Boyle P, Nickel JC, Hoefner K, Andriole G. Efficacy and safety of a dual inhibitor of 5-alpha-reductase types 1 and 2 (dutasteride) in men with benign prostatic hyperplasia. *Urology* 2002; **60**(3):434–41.
87. Roehrborn CG, Nickel JC, Andriole GL, *et al.* Dutasteride improves outcomes of benign prostatic hyperplasia when evaluated for prostate cancer risk reduction: secondary analysis of the REduction by DUtasteride of prostate Cancer Events (REDUCE) trial. *Urology* 2011; **78**(3):641–6.
88. Issa MM, Runken MC, Grogg AL, Shah MB. A large retrospective analysis of acute urinary retention and prostate-related surgery in BPH patients treated with 5-alpha reductase inhibitors: dutasteride versus finasteride. *Am J Manag Care* 2007; **13**(Suppl 1):S10–6.
89. Fenter TC, Davis EA, Shah MB, Lin PJ. Dutasteride vs finasteride: assessment of differences in acute urinary retention rates and surgical risk outcomes in an elderly population aged > or =65 years. *Am J Manag Care* 2008; **14** (5 Suppl 2):S154–9.
90. Naslund M, Eaddy MT, Kruep EJ, Hogue SL. Cost comparison of finasteride and dutasteride for enlarged prostate in a managed care setting among Medicare-aged men. *Am J Manag Care* 2008; **14**(5 Suppl 2):S167–71.
91. Jardin A, Bensadoun H, auche-Cavallier MC, Attali P. Alfuzosin for treatment of benign prostatic hypertrophy. The BPH-ALF Group. *Lancet* 1991; **337**(8755):1457–61.
92. Roehrborn CG. Alfuzosin 10 mg once daily prevents overall clinical progression of benign prostatic hyperplasia but not acute urinary retention: results of a 2-year placebo-controlled study. *BJU Int* 2006; **97**(4):734–41.

CHAPTER 5.3

Benign prostatic hyperplasia

Nikesh Thiruchelvam

Introduction to benign prostatic hyperplasia

Male lower urinary tract symptoms (LUTS) are very common and with an ageing population, are likely to increase. Previously it was thought that LUTS were due solely to the mass effect of an enlarged prostate which had grown due to benign prostatic hyperplasia (BPH) (see Fig. 5.3.1). It is now clear that male LUTS aetiology is complex and may be related to benign growth of the prostate, as well as a result of age-related bladder dysfunction, malignant prostatic disease, urethral disease, and medical conditions such as polyuria and sleep disorders (see Fig. 5.3.2). It is important that the reader is aware of this while reading this chapter, which focuses on benign prostatic hyperplasia of the prostate. LUTS are now typically categorized into storage symptoms (frequency and urgency), voiding symptoms (poor flow, hesitancy, straining), and post-voiding symptoms (post-micturition dribbling). BPH is typically associated with and results in bladder outflow obstruction (BOO) and voiding symptoms. Terminology has also confused the issue. In simple terms, LUTS (previously called prostatism) may result from BOO due to benign prostatic obstruction (BPO), usually from benign prostatic enlargement (BPE), which is usually due to histological BPH. This chapter describes the basic science of BPH, the natural history of BPH, its complications and assessment, and medical and surgical therapy of BPH.

Basic science of benign prostatic hyperplasia

Prostate biology

The prostate is composed of epithelial components and stromal components with a glue-like matrix (connective tissue) binding these cells together (see Table 5.3.1).[1]

It is the stromal compartment that responds to cholinergic stimulation, with demonstrated selectivity for α1A adrenoceptor.[2] Growth and maintenance of the prostate is affected by hormones and growth factors. Key to this is testosterone (primarily from Leydig cells of the testis) which is converted to the more potent dihydrotestosterone (DHT) within the prostate by 5α-reductase enzymes (type 1 and the more clinically relevant type 2[3]); DHT exerts its action by binding to the androgen receptor within stromal, epithelial, and matrix compartments. In addition, prostatic growth and function, and later, benign and malignant prostatic disease development, is also mediated by a complex interaction between the stroma and epithelial components of the prostate.[4] This occurs by direct cell–cell interactions and also by hormones and growth factors (e.g. fibroblast growth factors, epidermal growth factors) acting in paracrine, autocrine, and intracrine ways.

BPH is a histological diagnosis and is characterized by an increased number (and not size) of epithelial cells and stromal

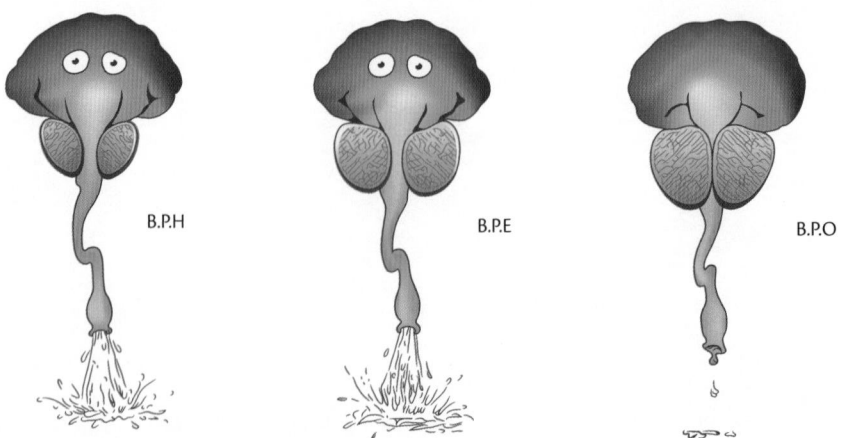

Fig. 5.3.1 Benign prostatic hyperplasia (BPH), bladder outlet obstruction (BOO), and the bladder.

Reproduced from Springer, *Urodynamics, Third Edition*, 2006, Chapter 5 'Urodynamics in Clinical Practice', Paul Abrams, Figure 5.4, Copyright © Springer-Verlag London 2007, with kind permission from Springer Science and Business Media.

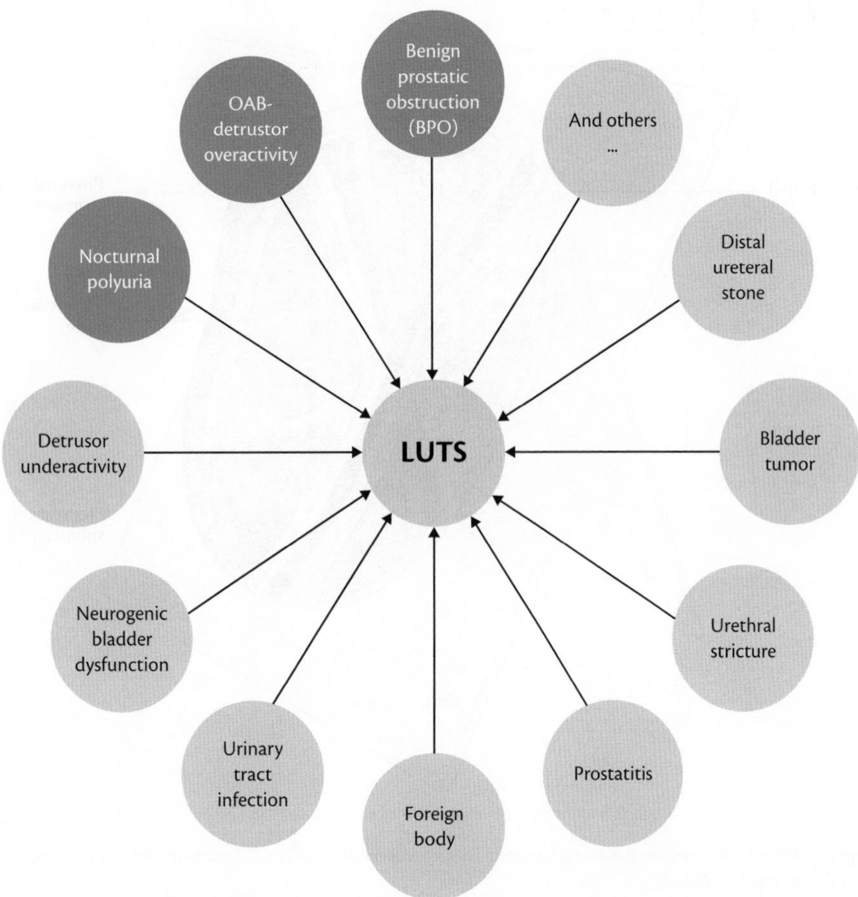

Fig. 5.3.2 Multifactorial aetiology of lower urinary tract symptoms (LUTS).
Reproduced with permission of European Association of Urology (EAU) Guidelines Office, M. Oelke (chairman), A. Bachmann, A. Descazeaud *et al.*, *Guidelines on the Management of Male Lower Urinary Tract Symptoms (LUTS), incl. Benign Prostatic Obstruction (BPO)*, Copyright © European Association of Urology 2012.

cells within the periurethral area of the prostate. The cause of this hyperplasia is unclear but is likely a result of increased cellular proliferation and/or reduced cell death. These cellular processes are mediated by several factors.

Androgens play a role in normal prostatic development as described above, but the role of testosterone and DHT in BPH is not clear. Type 2 5α-reductase is important in BPH development, primarily within stromal cells; and as such, DHT works on stromal cells in an autocrine fashion and on epithelial cells in a paracrine fashion to activate the androgen receptor.

Table 5.3.1 Cellular components of the prostate

Epithelial cells (90%)	Stromal cells (10%)	Tissue matrix
Basal epithelial stem cells	Smooth muscle cells	Extracellular matrix
Intermediate cells	Fibroblasts	Collagen
Neuroendocrine cells	Endothelial cells	Elastin
Columnar luminal secretory cells		Glycosaminoglycans
		Cytomatrix
		Nuclear matrix

Source: data from De Marzo AM *et al.*, 'Stem cell features of benign and malignant prostate epithelial cells', *The Journal of Urology*, Volume 160, Issue 6, Part 2, pp. 2381–92, Copyright © 1998 American Urological Association, Inc. Published by Elsevier Inc. All rights reserved.

Oestrogens possibly play a role in sensitizing prostate to androgens by activating oestrogen receptors within prostatic stromal and epithelial cells.[5]

Growth factors are likely to play a part in proliferation (via promoters such as fibroblast growth factors, vascular endothelial growth factor, and insulin-like growth factor, and inhibitors such as transforming growth factor-β).[6]

Inflammation and autoimmunity inflammatory mediators, and associated signalling pathways have been indentified in BPH and could play an aetiological role.[7]

Family history is an inheritable component to BPH, as shown by a higher percentage of first-degree male relatives needing bladder outlet surgery,[8] although a gene for BPH has not been identified.

Pathophysiology and zonal anatomy of the prostate

BPH nodules first develop in the transition zone of the prostate, which sit around the urethra[9] with further development of BPH within the more proximal periurethral zone. Subsequent growth of these areas (within a constraining outer prostatic capsule) result in compression of the prostatic urethra and contribute to male LUTS. Initially, transition zone nodules consist of proliferation of glandular tissue with a relative reduction in stroma. Over time, there is a slow growth of these nodules and then a later increase in large nodules, with glandular nodules increasing preferentially over stromal nodules. BPH is also characterized by an increase in the volume of

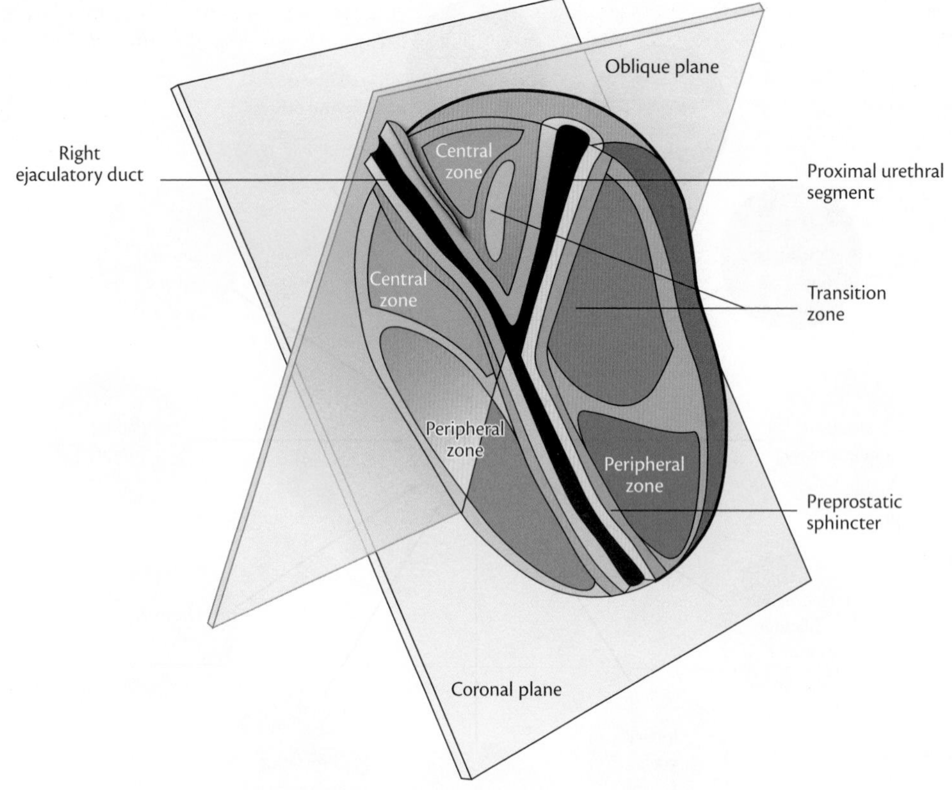

Fig. 5.3.3 Zonal anatomy of the prostate.

Reprinted by permission from Macmillan Publishers Ltd: *International Journal of Impotence Research*, Volume 20, Issue S3, C G Roehrborn, 'Pathology of benign prostatic hyperplasia', pp. S11–18, Copyright © 2008, Rights Managed by Nature Publishing Group.

prostatic smooth muscle[10] with adrenergic stimulation, resulting in an increase in prostatic urethral resistance, primarily acting via the α1A adrenoceptor.[2] Further regulation of prostatic smooth muscle occurs via the kallikrein-kinin[11] and cAMP pathways,[12] the latter pathway being phosphodiesterase-dependent (see Fig. 5.3.3).

Epidemiology of male lower urinary tract symptoms

Epidemiology and natural history of lower urinary tract symptoms

Autopsy studies[13] have shown that BPH develops from the age of 30 and slowly increases with age to a peak of almost 90% of men aged over 80. Also seen was an increase in prostate size from approximately 25 mL in men aged thirty, to 35 mL in men in their seventies. Prevalence and progression of LUTS and BPH has also been studied in depth by population studies (EpiLUTS[14]), longitudinal community-based studies (Olmsted County Study[15] and Health Professionals Follow-Up Study[16]) and by examining the placebo arms of therapeutic studies (Proscar Long-Term Efficacy and Safety Study PLESS,[17] The Medical Therapy of Prostate Symptoms MTOPS,[18] and The Alfuzosin 10 mg Once Daily Long-term Efficacy and Safety Study ATLESS[19]). It is important to note that these studies infer BPH from obstructive LUTS (i.e. from symptoms).

EpiLUTS found that obstructive urinary symptoms (suggestive of BPH) were highly prevalent in all men (aged over 40) with almost a half of men complaining of terminal dribbling, a quarter of men suffering from a weak stream, and a fifth of men having hesitancy. A high prevalence of voiding LUTS in a quarter of all men was also found in a further population study (EPIC[20]). Similar rates were also found in the Boston Area Community Health (BACH) population study.[21] The Olmsted County Study found that a quarter of men aged 40–49 had moderate to severe LUTS, which had increased to almost a half of men aged 70–79; a corresponding fall in flow rate was also observed, from 21 mL/s to 14 mLs/s in the same age groups.

Examining progression of symptoms and risk of acute urinary retention (AUR) has confirmed growth of the prostate over time. The Health Professional Follow-up Study found that the risk of AUR although low, increased over time (0.2% in 40–49 year olds to 3% in men aged >80). Similar progression of AUR risk was observed in the Olmsted County study with the rate increasing from 1% of men 50–59 years old to 9% of men aged over 70. Interestingly the PLESS study found that in men with moderate to severe LUTS, taking placebo did alter the flow rate or risk of AUR over four years. However, MTOPS showed that in the placebo group, the risk of AUR was 2% per year over four years in a group of men with moderate to severe symptoms and also showed a corresponding 24% increase in prostate size over five years. Similarly, ATLESS showed that in moderate and severely affected men with LUTS taking placebo, 2% per year developed AUR over two years. More recently, significant increases in PSA[22] and prostate volume (by approximately 2% per year)[22,23] have been observed in the same group of men over a 14–15-year period.

Risk factors for the development of BPH are poorly understood. EpiLUTS found that obstructive urinary symptoms were more often found in those that also suffered from arthritis, asthma, anxiety, depression, diabetes, heart disease, hypertension, and sleep apnoea.[24] A similar link of LUTS and heart disease, hypertension, diabetes, and depression was also found in the BACH population study.[25] An association has also been discovered between conditions related with the metabolic syndrome (diabetes, hypertension, and obesity) and the development of BPH, as defined by prostate volume.[26] Given that all these conditions increase with age, it is very difficult to prove a causal link to BPH.

Despite anatomical associations and increasing prevalence with age, BPH does not lead to prostate cancer. Although a quarter of prostate cancers arise in the transition zone, the majority of cancers arise in the peripheral zone, whereas BPH arises in the periurethral tissue. In an unscreened population, the chance of detecting prostate cancer during BPH surgery is low, at around 3%.[27]

The obstructed bladder

Inference from animal studies, LUTS, and urodynamic changes suggest that the bladder's response to obstruction is variable and not necessarily predictable.

- Initial response to obstruction is smooth muscle hypertrophy.
- This is followed by smooth muscle dysfunction from a change in contractile protein expression, impaired mitochondrial function and calcium signalling, ischaemia, and increased collagen deposition.[28]
- This is observed clinically; urinary symptoms can continue after surgical deobstruction because of detrusor overactivity or failure.[29]
- The above bladder pathology may also occur to some extent due to the normal ageing processes.

Complications of benign prostatic hyperplasia

The following points may refer to complications of BOO, as well as due to BPH. As above, mechanisms and aetiology remain unknown.

Bladder stones. Autopsy studies show that bladder stones are more common in men with BPH than in controls.[30] However, only 1 in 276 men on surveillance with moderate LUTS developed a bladder stone and only 50% with bladder calculi have urodynamic BOO[31]; indeed, 10% of men with bladder calculi in this latter study had detrusor underactivity.

Urinary tract infections. Incidence rate is low at 0.1 UTI/100 patient-years.[18]

Bladder failure. Aetiology of this and when best to intervene in BOO is not clear. Signs of bladder failure (e.g. bladder fibrosis, poor contracility) occur in both sexes with advancing age. Studies show both improvement in symptoms if undergoing early transurethral resection of prostate (TURP) rather than surveillance and later TURP,[32] and also a high chance of bladder failure despite TURP.[33]

Incontinence. Can occur with overflow incontinence and overdistension, from detrusor overactivity, and from part of the ageing process. The rate of incontinence with BPH has been recorded as low as 0.3/100 patient-years.[18]

Obstructive uropathy. Although older series report rates as high as 14%, contemporary studies report lower rates of <1%.[32]

Haematuria. It is common acceptance that the prostate is the cause of bleeding when other causes have been excluded, and further acceptance due to the benefits of finasteride in treating haematuria caused by prostatic bleeding.[34]

AUR. Precipitated retention occurs after an event such as surgery, catheterization, drugs, and anaesthesia. Patients with spontaneous retention (i.e. no cause, often preceded by LUTS) have a higher chance of recurrence of AUR than with precipitated retention.[35] Risk factors for AUR are increasing age, higher prostate-specific antigen (PSA), and higher prostate volumes.

Erectile dysfunction. Previously it was thought that both male LUTS/BPH increase with age, as does sexual dysfunction. However, over the past decade, it has become apparent that there may be a direct causal effect of one on the other. Higher rates of ED and ejaculatory dysfunction have been observed in men with LUTs as compared to no LUTS,[36] and in men with higher LUTS symptoms scores.[37]

Investigation of male lower urinary tract symptoms

Initial investigation

Clinically, BPH may present as LUTS, detrusor overactivity, poor bladder emptying, AUR, UTI, haematuria, and obstructive uropathy. This section deals with the investigation of LUTS.[38]

History. Detailed history is necessary to aid discussion on treatment options.

Examination. In particular, external genitalia (meatal stenosis), digital rectal examination (prostate and rectal malignancy), focused neurological examination (to aid diagnosis of a neuropathic bladder).

Urinanalysis. To exclude UTI, haematuria, diabetes, and renal disease.

Serum creatinine. Not routinely recommended, but required if in retention, if planning imaging with contrast agents, and prior to surgery.

PSA. Levels increase with prostate cancer, BPH, prostatitis, UTI, and catheterization. After appropriate counselling, men should be offered a PSA test if their LUTS are suggestive of bladder outlet obstruction secondary to BPE, if their prostate feels abnormal on DRE, or they are concerned about having prostate cancer. A high PSA (and high prostate volume) are predictors of BPH progression.[18]

International Prostate Symptom Score. This questionnaire consists of seven symptom questions (previously known as the American Urological Association Symptom Score) and one quality of life question. This score is useful for baseline assessment and assessing response to therapy. The maximum score is 35 (0–7 = mildly symptomatic; 8–19 = moderately symptomatic; 20–35 = severely symptomatic) (see Table 5.3.2).

Frequency-volume chart. Records time and volume of each void. This is defined as a bladder diary if fluid intake and incontinence episodes are also calculated. This is a simple chart (see Fig. 5.3.4) but can yield very useful information:

- Normal frequency and voided volumes.
- Increased frequency and high volumes—an increased 24-hour production of urine, suggesting a high fluid intake from diabetes mellitus, diabetes insipidus, or habitual.

Table 5.3.2 International Prostate Symptom Score

INTERNATIONAL PROSTATE SYMPTOM SCORE (IPSS)						
	Never	**About 1 time in 5**	**About 1 time in 3**	**About 1 time in 2**	**About 2 times in 3**	**Almost always**
1. Over the past month, how often have you had a sensation of not emptying your bladder completely after you finished urinating?	0	1	2	3	4	5
2. Over the past month, how often have you had to urinate again less than two hours after you finished urinating?	0	1	2	3	4	5
3. Over the past month, how often have you found you stopped and started again several times when you urinated?	0	1	2	3	4	5
4. Over the past month, how often have you found it difficult to hold back urinating after you have felt the need?	0	1	2	3	4	5
5. Over the past month, how often have you noticed a reduction in the strength and force of your urinary stream?	0	1	2	3	4	5
6. Over the past month, how often have you had to push or strain to begin urination?	0	1	2	3	4	5
	None	1 time	2 times	3 times	4 times	5 or more times
7. Over the past month, how many times did you most typically get up to urinate from the time you went to bed at night until the time you got up in the morning?	0	1	2	3	4	5
				Total IPSS Score S =		

QUALITY OF LIFE DUE TO URINARY SYMPTOMS							
	Delighted	Pleased	Mostly satisfied	Mixed about equally satisfied and dissatisfied	Mostly dissatisfied	Unhappy	Terrible
1. If you were to spend the rest of your life with your urinary condition just the way it is now, how would you feel about that?	0	1	2	3	4	5	6
			Quality of life assessment index L =				

Copyright 1992, International—Prostate Symptom Score © (I-PSS©) Michael J Barry. All rights reserved. Reproduced with permission.

- Reduced volumes with minimal variation in the volume voided—suggesting bladder wall pathology, such as carcinoma *in situ* or painful bladder syndrome or carcinoma *in situ*.
- Reduced volumes with variation in the volume voided—suggestive of detrusor overactivity.
- Increased nocturnal production—suggestive of fluid-retaining states, hormonal fluid balance abnormality, or idiopathic in origin. Typically, this is due to abnormal physiology rather than lower urinary tract pathology (NB: nocturnal polyuria is defined as night-time output of more than 35% of the 24 hr output).

Secondary care investigation

Pad tests. Useful in the assessment of incontinent men. Variability in recordings within the same patient.

Urinary flow rate. Using a flow meter, the quantity of fluid (volume or mass) voided per unit of time is measured and expressed in millilitres per second (mL/s). Flow meters measure the flow rate by using a spinning disc, a weight transducer, or by measuring capacitance. The flow rate can produce characteristic tracings of BOO and urethral stricture disease (see Fig. 5.3.5), but it is important that in a representative study, the patient voids at least 150 mL. Men under 40 years generally have maximum flow rates (Qmax) over 25 mL/s, while men over 60 years of age with no BOO usually have maximum flow rates over 15 mL/s.

Post-void residual (PVR). Using ultrasound, there is wide variability in this reading in any one patient; in addition, there is no consensus as to what constitutes a significant post-void residual. PVR is useful in patients with non-painful retention and monitoring patients who are on medical therapy for their LUTS (especially with antimuscarinic therapy).

Urodynamics (UDS). This is the only test to confirm BOO as opposed to male LUTS from detrusor failure or detrusor overactivity.[39] However, it is not necessary on every male patient with LUTS. It is useful in planning surgery when the diagnosis of

Bladder Diary

Name:________________________

IN: Measure the fluid, and please note in this column everything that you drink.

OUT: Measure the amount of urine you pass, and note it in the OUT column. If unable to measure, please tick.

LEAK: Place tick in this column each time you leak.

	Date:			Date:		
	IN	OUT	LEAK	IN	OUT	LEAK
6am						
7am						
8am						
9am						
10am						
11am						
Noon						
1pm						
2pm						
3pm						
4pm						
5pm						
6pm						
7pm						
8pm						
9pm						
10pm						
11pm						
12pm						
1am						
2am						
3am						
4am						
5am						
TOTAL:						

Fig. 5.3.4 A bladder diary.

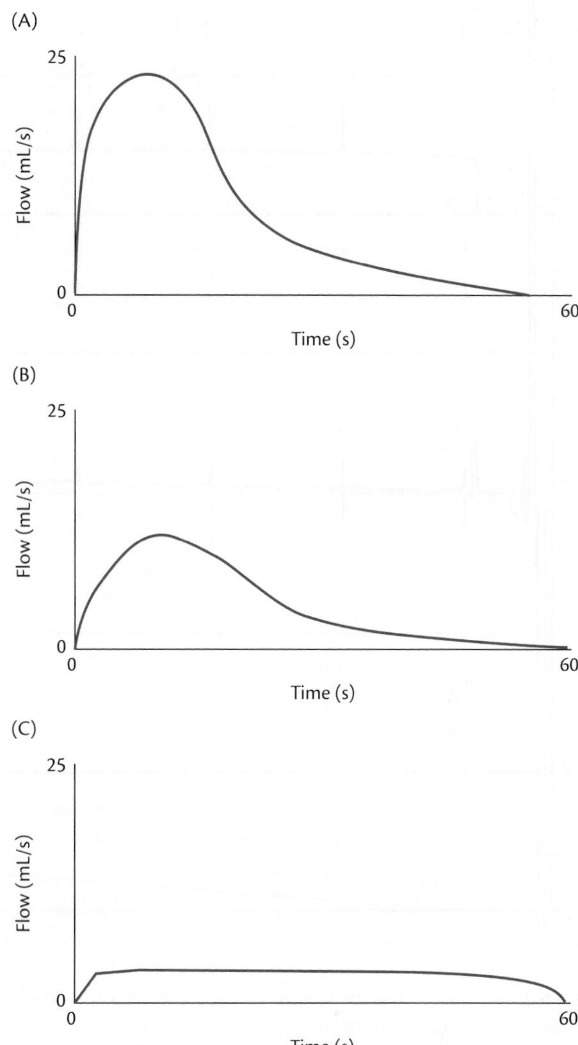

Fig. 5.3.5 Typical flow rate patterns. (A) Normal flow rate; (B) obstructed flow rate; and (C) urethral stricture flow rate.

BOO cannot be ascertained by the above investigations, or when the diagnosis may be in doubt. UDS has been shown to reduce the subjective failure rate of bladder outlet surgery from TURP from 28% to 12%.[29] Accepted indications are:

- LUTS in a man under 50
- LUTS in a man over 80
- LUTS in the presence of neurological disease
- Ongoing symptoms after bladder outflow tract surgery
- Cannot void >150 mL

UDS involves the placement of fluid-filled catheters attached to pressure transducers or catheter-tip pressure transducers placed into the bladder and the rectum. Pressures are then recorded during filling (Fill phase) and then voiding while recording the flow rate. By subtracting the pressure from the line in the rectum (Pabd) from the pressure in the bladder (Pves), the pressure developed by the detrusor muscle can be derived (Pdet) (see Fig. 5.3.6 for a UDS trace of BOO). The maximum detrusor pressure during the maximum flow rate (Qmax) can be used to define bladder outflow obstruction; this can be plotted in a variety of nomogram (e.g. Abrams-Griffiths nomogram, Fig. 5.3.7).

Flexible cystoscopy (FC). This is not routinely recommended in investigation of LUTS or BOO; there is no correlation with the visual extent of prostatic occlusion on cystoscopy and BOO confirmed on UDS. FC is warranted if there is any haematuria, suggestion of urethral stricture disease on history or flow rate, and prior history of bladder cancer, recurrent UTI, sterile pyuria, and painful voiding.

Imaging. Ultrasound is not routinely recommended but is of value if there is a suspicion of chronic retention, haematuria, recurrent infection, sterile pyuria, pain, and significant symptoms.

Benign prostatic hyperplasia and prostate-specific antigen

DRE is not accurate at measuring prostate volume and given that the latter is a marker of BPH, of BPH progression, and is associated with BOO, it would be reasonable to determine post-void (PV) in patients. This would be most accurately performed by TRUSP or cross-sectional imaging, but this is not practical. PSA has been shown to correlate with prostate volume (see Fig. 5.3.8).[40] In

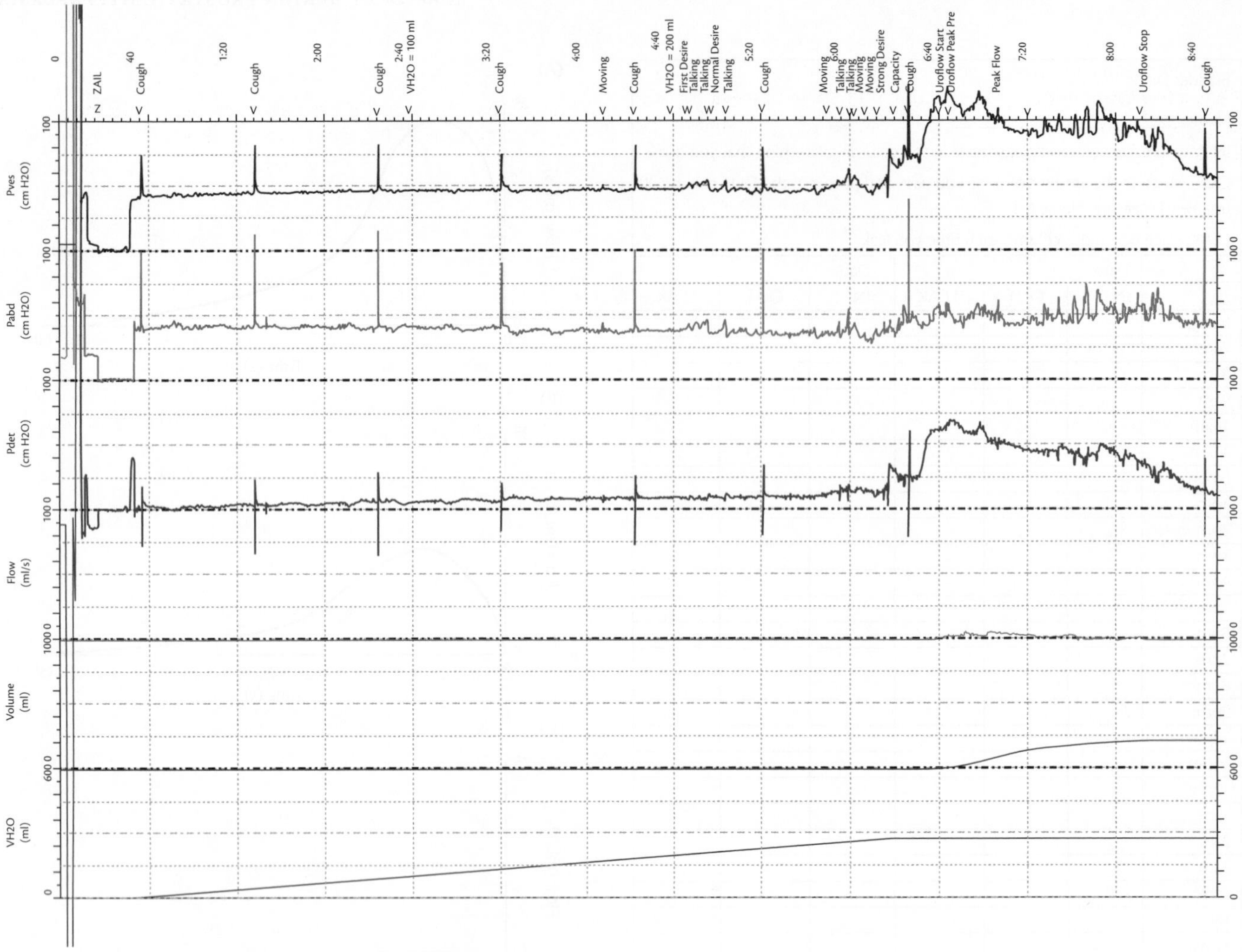

Fig. 5.3.6 Urodynamic tracing shows high-pressure and lowflow BOO (from top down, vesical pressure line Pves, abdominal pressure line Pabdo, detrusor pressure line Pdet, flow, volume voided, and volume instilled).

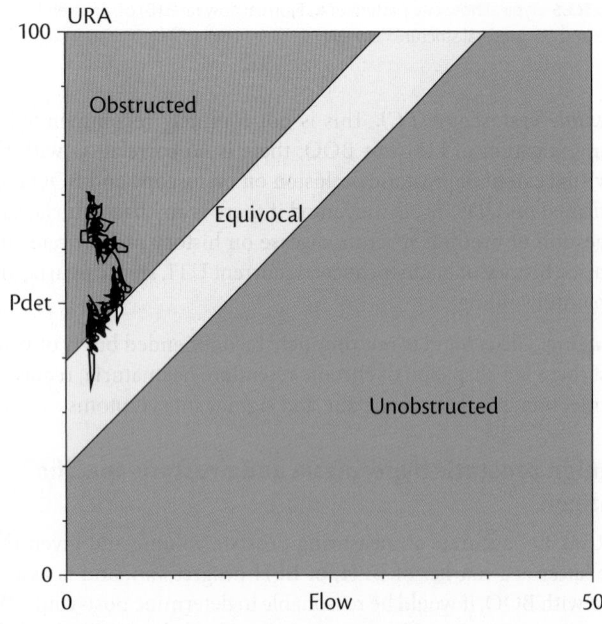

Fig. 5.3.7 Abrams-Griffith nomogram. The voiding detrusor pressure is plotted against the urinary flow. The chart is divided into three zones: the upper obstructed zone; the intermediate equivocal zone; and the lower unobstructed zone. This trace is from the same patient as in Figure 5.3.5 and confirms BOO.

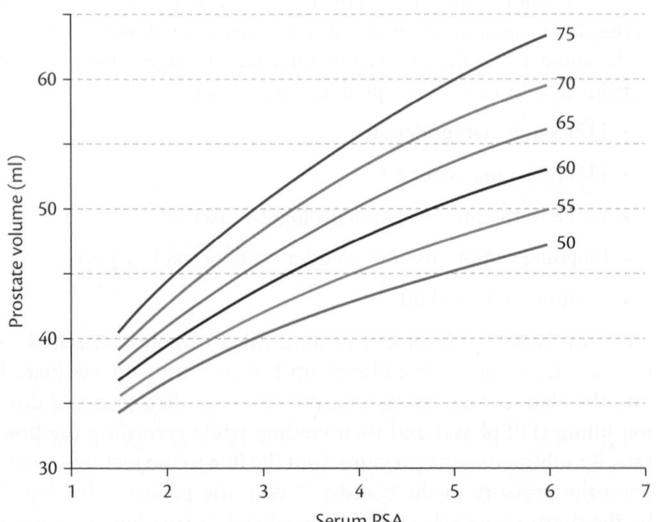

Fig. 5.3.8 Relationship of prostate-specific antigen (PSA) and prostate volume.

Reprinted from *Urology*, Volume 53, Edition 3, Claus G. Roehrborn *et al.*, 'Serum prostate-specific antigen as a predictor of prostate volume in men with benign prostatic hyperplasia', pp. 581–9, Copyright © 1999 Elsevier Science Inc. All rights reserved., with permission from Elsevier, http://www.sciencedirect.com/science/journal/00904295

addition, PSA is useful as a predictor of BPH and BPH progression. Over a five-year period, men with higher PSAs will have faster rates of prostate growth, worse symptom progression, and higher risk of AUR and need for BPH surgery than men with lower PSAs.[17,18] These papers also show that medical therapy is more effective in men with lower PSAs.

Treatment of male lower urinary tract symptoms secondary to benign prostatic hyperplasia

Conservative therapy

Left untreated, most men with BPH will not suffer from the complications of BPH outlined earlier.[41] It is difficult to determine which patients are suitable for surveillance of their symptoms. It does appear clear that those with moderate and severe symptoms do better with earlier intervention with TURP than those that continue surveillance and have later TURP.[32]

Successful watchful waiting techniques include education, reassurance of no cancer, and monitoring of symptoms; these techniques have been shown to improve symptom control and quality of life.[42] Consensus also dictates that lifestyle modification as suggested below will help with symptoms:

- reducing fluid intake for convenient time periods;
- avoidance of caffeine and alcohol;
- double-voiding;
- urethral milking to help with post-micturition dribbling;
- bladder retraining.

Containment may also be a suitable option in some men with BPH and severe LUTS. These products, such as pads, bedpants, penile sheaths, and clamps, should ideally be used in conjunction with local continence services. For those that are not suitable for therapy or because of patient choice, catheterization, either in the form of clean intermittent self-catherization or long-term urethral or suprapubic catheterization, is a reasonable option. Due to easier hygiene, easier catheter changes, facilitation of sexual intercourse, and for prevention of traumatic filleting to the distal penis, a long-term suprapubic catheter is more favourable than a urethral catheter.

Medical therapy

Medical therapy has superceded surgical treatment as the primary choice for most men with BPH and LUTS due to reversibility of treatment, and fewer side effects. Over a 13-year period to 2000, a 55% reduction in TURP has been documented.[43] Some patients demonstrate clear indications for surgical therapy and should not be offered medical therapy as first choice treatment—these are:

- obstructive uropathy
- recurrent retention
- recurrent UTIs

Alpha blockers

As described earlier in the chapter, smooth muscle makes up a major component of the prostate. In 1975, investigators were able to show that human prostrate contracts with the α-adrenergic agonist noradrenaline[44] and subsequently, the α1 receptor has been identified as the main agonist receptor,[45] with the majority within the prostatic stroma. Clinical utility was then described by improvements in peak flow rate (in men with symptomatic BPH) who received the α-adrenergic antagonist terazosin.[46]

Since then, α–adrenergic blockers have continued to evolve. Phenoxybenzamine was first available for symptomatic control for LUTS, but had a high incidence of side effects related to its non-selectivity. Subsequently, α1 receptor blockers (prazosin, alfuzosin, indoramin) and then long-acting α1 receptor blockers (terazosin, doxzosin, and alfuzosin) became available. Some of these agents require dose-titration to be effective. By demonstrating mediation of prostate smooth muscle tension by α1 A activation (there are three subtypes α1 A, α1 B, α1 D), with further refinement, we now have selective α1 A receptor antagonists, tamsulosin, silodosin, naftopidil, and long-acting tamsulosin MR. Tamsulosin has a moderately higher affinity for α1 A than for α1 D; silodosin has a very high selectivity (162:1) for α1 A versus α1 B; and naftopidil is relatively selective for α1 D. These latter two newer agents appear to show equal symptomatic improvement and peak flow rate improvement to tamsulosin.

Tamsulosin remains a very popular α-blocker because of its selectivity; it is well tolerated with modest adverse events (of anejaculation, dizziness and asthenia) and produces rapid and reasonable symptomatic improvement (IPSS score improvement of around 35%). This is in distinction to efficacy trials using tamsulosin (and indeed, all α-blockers) which show modest improvement in peak flow rates (mean difference from placebo of up to 2.6 mL/s). In fact, the picture remains unclear as to how α-blockers fully exert their effects in LUTS. Given that α-blockers result in minimal changes to urodynamically-proven BOO,[47] it is possible that their beneficial effect may also occur due to action on blood vessels, extra-prostatic smooth muscle, within the spinal cord and/or the brain.

α-blockers need to be used with caution in the elderly because of the risk of orthostatic hypotension and dizziness, and subsequent higher risk of falls. There is some benefit of these adverse events in those that suffer from hypertension. In addition to the prostate, α1 A is the major receptor subtype in the iris dilator muscle in the eye. As such, tamsulosin (and less so with other α-blockers) can result in intraoperative floppy iris syndrome that can complicate cataract surgery and make it more difficult to deal with. Clinically, the syndrome results in poor preoperative pupil dilatation, iris billowing and prolapse, and progressive intraoperative miosis. It remains unclear how long before planned surgery α–blockade should be stopped to allow for safer operating.

α–blockers have been shown to improve the success of trial without catheter after AUR. This was first demonstrated with alfuzosin[48] and then later with tamsulosin. In the former ALFAUR study, nearly 50% of men successfully passed their trial without catheter (TWOC) after three days of placebo. This rate was improved to 62% after the use of alfuzosin.

5-α reductase inhibitors

As prostate growth is androgen dependent, surgical castration resulted in symptomatic improvement in LUTS. In brief, non-specific androgen suppression has been tried, with gonadotropin-releasing hormone analogues, progestational agents, and antiandrogens, but due to their side effects and mode of administration, were not popular agents. The 5-α reductase inhibitors, finasteride, and dutaseride, work by reducing levels of DHT (by inhibition of type 1 and type 2 5-α reductase, thereby blocking the enzymatic conversion of testosterone to DHT). This results in reduction of the epithelial components of the prostate and ultimately prostate size. This has then led to a reduction in BOO, presumably from BPH, with a subsequent improvement in LUTS (after approximately six months of treatment).

Finasteride is a selective inhibitor of the type 2 5-α reductase isoenzyme. Castrate levels of DHT are not achieved because of type 1 isoenzymes within the skin and liver. The North American Finasteride Trial[49] was able to show an improvement in peak flow rate (by 1.85 mL/s) and symptom score and a reduction in prostate volume (by 12 cm^3) with the use of 5 mg finasteride for 12 months, as compared to placebo. Following further similar trials and efficacy results, the PLESS study[50] showed that efficacy of finasteride over placebo was maintained at four years; no masking of the detection of prostate cancer was noted, despite the 50% reduction that occurs in PSA measurements. Dutasteride inhibits both type 1 and type 2 isoenzymes and subsequently lowers serum DHT further by 90% as compared to a 70% reduction with finasteride. However, this greater reduction in DHT levels does not translate to clinical improvement with a similar reduction observed with both agents in symptom scores and prostate volumes and improvements in flow rates in randomized placebo-controlled trials.[51] This may be due to the similar 70% intraprostatic reduction in DHT observed in both agents.

Both finasteride and dutaseride result in loss of libido and erectile dysfunction, although this typically occurs early in treatment and then subsides. The agents should be used in men with moderate to severe LUTS and prostates >40 mL or with PSA levels >1.4. Finasteride has also been shown to reduce blood loss during TURP, possibly due to a reduction in prostate vascularity,[52] and as such, is often offered to men with recurrent haematuria secondary to prostatic bleeding.

Combination therapy

Early combination studies did not show large advantages of using dual therapy. The Veterans Affairs study,[53] the ALFIN study,[54] and the Prospective European Doxazosin and Combination Therapy (PREDICT) study[55] showed no advantage of an α-blocker over a combination of an α-blocker and a 5-α reductase inhibitor at up to one year in peak flow rates and symptom scores.

However, the MTOPS trial[18] and subsequent CombAT trial[56] have shown not only an improvement in peak flow rates and LUTS symptom scores but prevention of BPH progression (as determined by IPSS rise >4, a 50% rise in serum creatinine, AUR, recurrent UTIs or incontinence, or BPH surgery rates). MTOPS showed that a combination of doxazosin and finasteride resulted in improvements in symptom scores and peak flow rates and reduced disease progression (primarily as symptom scores) as compared to placebo or monotherapy. CombAT showed that combination therapy with tamsulosin and dutasteride was more effective at reducing BPH progression and improved symptom scores than monotherapy alone. This latter study also showed that combination therapy was superior to tamsulosin monotherapy only at reducing the relative risk of AUR or surgery. This latter aspect has also been highlighted previously in the SMART study,[57] which showed that the use of an alpha blocker and a 5-α reductase inhibitor can be used to provide rapid symptom relief and then subsequent cessation of the alpha blocker after six months allows ongoing symptom control. Further analysis of these studies has led to guideline proposals[38,58] that long-term combination therapy should be offered to men with moderate to severe LUTS with prostates >40 mL, PSA >1.4 ng/nl, and reduced maximum peak flow rates.

Phosphodiesterase type 5 inhibitors

There is a link between erectile dysfunction and LUTS; both occur as men age and an early report highlighted an improvement in LUTS in men treated with Viagra.[59] Hypotheses for mechanism of improvement in LUTS include changes to pelvic atherosclerosis, autonomic hyperactivity, interaction with the Rho-kinase pathway and alterations to nitric oxide levels. Randomized studies[60–62] show no improvement in peak flow rates despite improvements in LUTS (in both storage and obstructive scores) which suggest that improvements occur because of changes to bladder function rather than changes to the prostate or BPH. Despite FDA approval for a phosphodiesterase inhibitor to be used for LUTS (although confusingly referred to as BPH or an enlarged prostate), it is unknown what are the long-term effects of once daily use of this class of drug.

Phytotherapy

Plant extracts, from roots, seeds, bark or fruits, are used to improve LUTS. These compounds consist of a variety of chemicals (such as phytosterols, plant oils, trepenoids) and various production techniques, and therefore careful scientific appraisal and comparison is difficult. Potential mechanisms of action include anti-inflammatory, hormonal, and growth factor pathways. Popular and common agents include *Serenoa repens* (saw palmetto berry extract) and *Pygeum Africanum* (from African Plum). Until further clarity is obtained from higher quality studies,[63] the current body of evidence[64,65] does not favour treatment with these compounds.

Surgical therapy for benign prostatic hyperplasia

Prostate stents

The type and indication for intraprostatic stents is constantly evolving. Early stents were utilized for medically unfit patients instead of a urinary catheter and can be fitted under a local anaesthetic. However, they remain problematic and may be difficult to reposition or remove. Complications are high with haematuria, perineal pain, encrustation, migration, breakage, stress incontinence, and UTIs. Spiral stents can be self-retaining (Prosta coil) or malleable and heat-expandable (Memokath). Using the latter, IPSS reduction can be maintained up to seven years' follow-up[66,67] but there was high rate of repositioning and removal. Epithelial hyperplasia and ingrowth can be problematic. A variety of polyurethane stents are available and have been used as temporary measures to keep the prostatic lumen open during the heating effects of thermotherapy treatment for the prostate, and to prevent post thermotherapy retention. Equally, biodegradable stents have been used as a temporary relieving stent following laser ablative techniques on the prostate. Finally, permanent stents have been tried to treat

BPH in medically unfit patients. UroLume is a metallic stent that allows epithelialization over the stent. It has been used with success in unfit patients who have presented with AUR,[68,69] or as an alternative to TURP.[70] Further complications encountered include irritative LUTS and painful ejaculation. One study showed that at up to 12 years' follow-up, 47% had to be removed.[71] Memotherm is an another thermoexpandable metal stent that is reportedly easy to remove, as traction unravels the single wire. Again, complication rates remain high with a significant incidence of urinary symptoms, UTI, and urethral stricture disease. Overall, prostatic stents are infrequently used in clinical practice.

Minimally invasive therapy

Transurethral microwave thermotherapy (TUMT) is also undergoing evolution and higher energy techniques have been used. In theory, by producing heat variation in the periurethral prostatic tissue, and by causing resultant coagulative necrosis, nerve degeneration, and inducing apoptosis, improvements are observed in LUTS. The prostate is heated using microwave energy with simultaneous cooling of the urethra. Despite lack of improvement in objective parameters such as peak flow rates, considerable improvements in IPSS can be observed. Equally important however is the large number of unpredictable non-responders, even in the higher energy studies. As results are less favourable to TURP over the long term,[72] currently this technique is considered experimental.

Transurethral needle ablation of the prostate (TUNA) also delivers heat to the prostate, via radiofrequency energy delivered by needles placed into the prostate, with resultant necrosis to prostatic tissue. There may also be a neuromodulatory effect. As the needles are placed within the prostate, the prostatic urethra is spared. Treatment efficacy is less comparable to TURP, with very little data on follow-up at greater than one year.[73] Complication rates are low, with the most common adverse events being bleeding (30%), temporary AUR (up to 40%), UTI (7%), and urethral stricture disease (2%). TUNA results in less sexual dysfunction than TURP. As above, this is not a recommended standard technique for BPH management. The technique is associated with a high reoperation rate (14–20% within two years).

Heat delivery between the above methods differ slightly. With microwaves, heat is applied more broadly and deeply than with TUNA. The central temperature is therefore kept lower to protect the capsule and surrounding tissues; as such, treatment takes longer with TUMT. With TUNA, heat generation is faster and hotter, but to a smaller area. Similarities are that both can be done in an outpatient setting with minimal sedation and hence maybe suitable for unfit patients. Both procedures result in marked postoperative irritative urinary symptoms because of postoperative necrosis and subsequent sloughing of prostatic tissue over a number of weeks.

Heat delivery has also been tried with high-intensity focused ultrasound (HIFU). This procedure is a low morbid option with a resultant improvement in symptoms scores.[74–76] However due to complications of AUR and even rectourethral fistula, and a very high rate of early reoperation with TURP (up to 44%), this technique has been abandoned. Hot water-induced thermotherapy involves an extracorporeal heat source and a proprietary closed-loop catheter system. Water, heated to 60°C, is circulated through the catheter to a treatment balloon, which conducts thermal energy to targeted prostatic tissue. Catheters are left in for a minimum of one week. Symptom scores are improved following treatment,[77–79] but due to complications of dysuria, bleeding, AUR, and high retreatment rates, this technique is no longer used.

Transurethral ethanol ablation (TEAP) involves endoscopic injection of up to 13 mL dehydrated ethanol (98% concentration) at four to eight sites in the prostate either transurethrally (most common), transperineally, or transrectally. This results in coagulative necrosis and subsequent prostate gland volume reduction. Symptom scores and flow rates do improve but again, a high reintervention rate is observed. Single-centre series with short follow-up only have been described.[80–82] A further option evaluated in medically unfit patients is injection of botulinum toxin into the prostate. Following transperineal ultrasound guided injection (transurethral and transrectal routes have also been described), short-term improvement is observed in symptom scores in medically unfit patients.[83–86] It is unclear how the toxin exerts its effects (either locally or centrally, via muscle relaxation, or by prostate apoptosis and longer term volume reduction); it is also unclear what are the potential adverse effects of the need for repeated injection into prostate tissue; hence, currently this therapy is experimental. In an early investigational study, radiofrequency energy has also been used clinically for BPH using a pulsed electromagnetic field[87] with promising early results.

Transurethral Prostatectomy (TURP)

Monopolar TURP remains the gold standard treatment for the surgical management of BPH and BOO. This is despite the lack of randomized controlled trial (RCT) evidence to support its introduction. TURP rates have declined over the past two decades. This is primarily related to the beneficial effects of medical therapy of BPH and to a lesser extent on the evaluation of alternative surgical techniques. Indications for TURP include:

- Moderate to severe LUTS (either not controlled with medical therapy or by patient choice)
- AUR
- Recurrent UTI
- Recurrent haematuria
- Obstructive uropathy

It is of value to remind the reader that BOO can only be diagnosed by urodynamic studies; symptoms, flow rates, post-void residual urine measurements, and cystoscopic findings can only infer BOO by BPH. Surgical resection of the prostate can occur by monopolar (standard) or more recently, by bipolar resection. The resection involves a step-wise approach to resect the three lobes of the prostate by resecting the prostatic tissue in small slices and washing out the prostate chips; haemostasis is completed using rollerball diathermy (see Fig. 5.3.9). The urinary catheter may or may not be irrigated and can be removed after 24–48 hours. The reduction in symptoms score and improvement in QoL scores remain high after this operation and currently has not been bettered by any endoscopic technique. The large national prostatectomy audit[88] outlined that that most men underwent TURP because of one of the indications above, rather than for symptoms, and that TURP was effective in reducing symptoms and symptom bother (although not all men experienced a good reduction in symptoms; 4% were worse, 10% were the same, and a quarter experienced only slight improvement). Six per cent (6%) had problematic incontinence (this is less than 2% in contemporary series), two-thirds had retrograde ejaculation, and

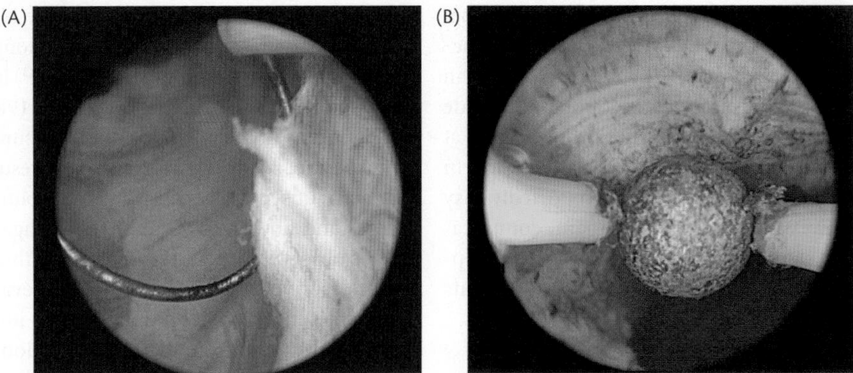

Fig. 5.3.9 (A) Endoscopic view during transurethral resection of prostate (TURP) resection; (B) diathermy.

a third reported erectile dysfunction (it is important to stress that the natural history of impotence in elderly men remains unknown). Mortality risk is low with this operation.[89] Results remain durable with published data up to 22 years.[90] Reoperation, usually with another TURP, is around 1–2% per year. The risk of transurethral resection (TUR) syndrome (dilutional hyponatraemia from fluid absorption) has dramatically decreased (better awareness, reduced operating times, and better perioperative assessment and care) and is less than 1%. Risk factors associated with TUR syndrome are excessive bleeding and an open venous sinus, prolonged operation time, large prostates, and smoking. Postoperative transfusion rates remain low at 2%. Younger men with BOO may benefit from an incision at the bladder neck (BNI or transurethral incision of the prostate, TUIP), usually at the 5 and 7 o'clock positions[91] rather than undergoing a complete TURP.

To improve haemostasis, length of catheterization, and reduce TUR syndrome, bipolar TURP has become popular. The technique uses a specialized resectoscope loop, which contains both the active and return electrodes and allows resection during saline irrigation. Prostate tissue is heated indirectly by the heat from the ignition of the spark that occurs between the electrode loops. The move to this resection technique has occurred, despite the lack of long-term evidence. Studies to date would point to a trend in lower rates of clot retention, catheterization, operating time, irrigation and TUR syndrome with other surgical outcomes (IPSS scores, reoperation rates, and so on) comparable to monopolar TURP in short-term follow-up.[92] At up to five years, results appear to be durable and comparable to monopolar TURP.[93] Prostate enucleation has also been described using bipolar energy.[94]

Transurethral vaporization of the prostate (TUVP) involves vaporization by steam at high heat at the leading edge of the probe and subsequent desiccation to dry out the prostatic tissue at the trailing edge of the probe with resultant coagulation (see Fig. 5.3.10). Generators need to be effective at altering power in response to resistance of the prostatic tissue, which varies depending on the level of hydration. This is a bipolar technique allowing surgery with saline irrigation. There are many electrode designs available; for example, a rollerball, rollerbar, and various loop configurations. At one year, complication rates are similar to TURP, but catheterization, haematuria, and transfusion rates are lower with TUVP[95–97] albeit with longer operating times for the procedure. Similar to TURP, vaporization-resection of the prostate has also been described.

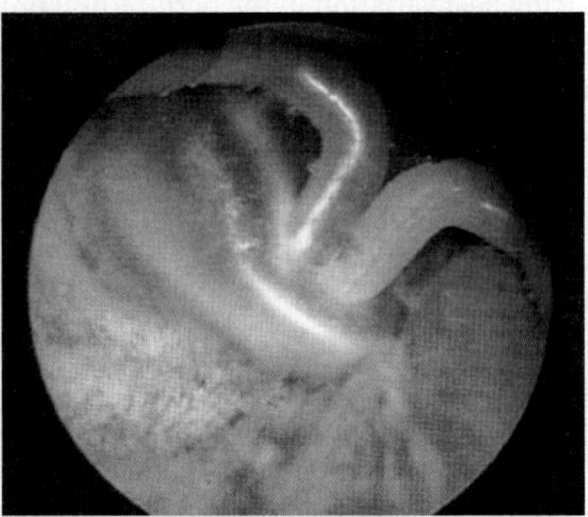

Fig. 5.3.10 Endoscopic view of transurethral vaporization of the prostate (TUVP). Reproduced courtesy of Dr Bogdon Geavlete, Assistant Professor, "Saint John" Emergency Clinical Hospital, Department of Urology, Bucharest, Romania.

Laser surgery

There are currently four groups of lasers used for BPH surgery by either coagulating, vaporizing, or enucleating the prostate:

- Potassium titanyl phosphate (KTP); neodymium yttrium aluminium garnet (Nd-YAG); and lithium borate (LBO)
- Diode lasers
- Holmium (Ho): YAG (HoLEP)
- Thulium (Tm): YAG (ThuLEP or ThuVEP)

KTP lasers have been used for photoselective vaporization of the prostate (PVP). Initially 60 W lasers were used,[98] subsequently 80 W lasers and then more recently the 120 W laser is being used. Two RCTs comparing TURP and PVP with 80 W KTP have been published. One showed equivalent results to TURP at one-year follow-up[99]; the second showed superior flow rate results with TURP at 6 months' follow-up.[100] KTP PVP with 80 W has also shown comparative results with open prostatectomy.[101] LBO PVP has shown similar short-term equivalence to TURP and appears to be quicker than KTP PVP. Both KTP and LBO emit green light and have been shown to reduce intraoperative blood loss and have reduced postoperative blood transfusion rates as compared to TURP. Stricture, retrograde ejaculation, and retreatment rates appear similar to TURP.

Much of the data on diode lasers refer to the 980-mn laser diode. These prospective studies with follow-up to one year show

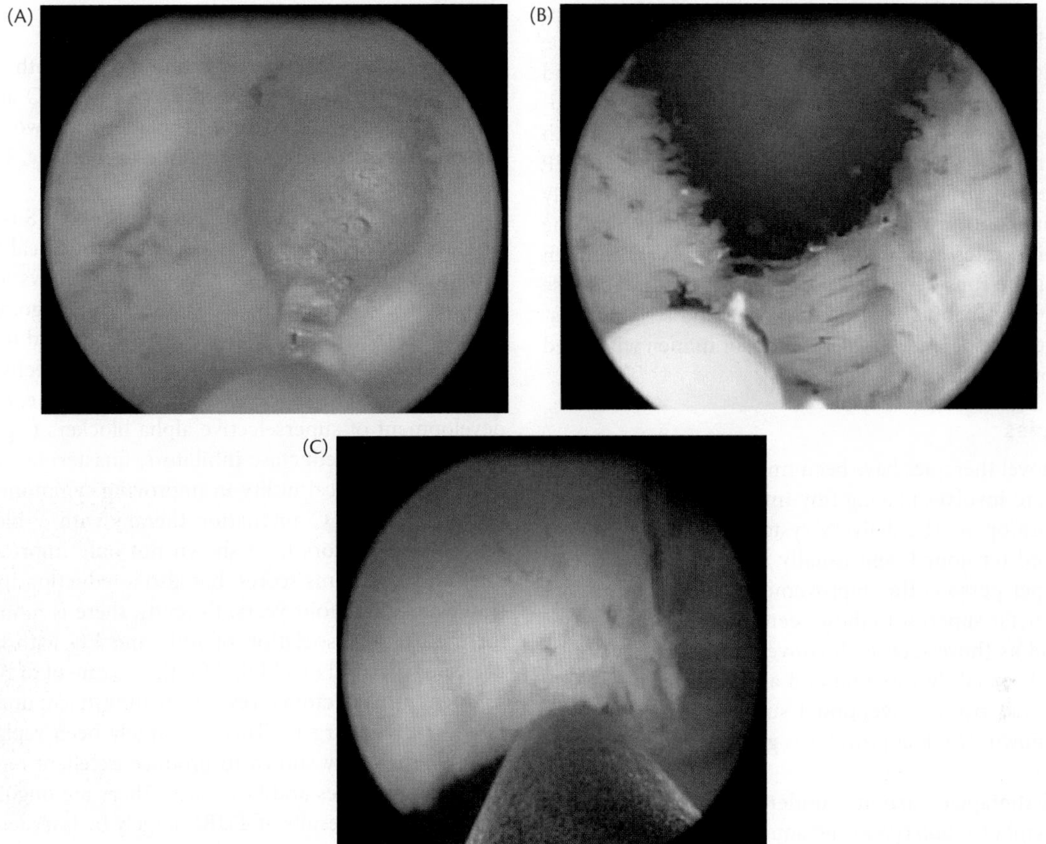

Fig. 5.3.11 (A) Endoscopic views during holmium (Ho): YAG (HoLEP) laser surgery, prostatic incision; (B) just prior to prostate lobe detachment and; (C) during morcellation.
Reproduced courtesy of Mr Tev Aho, Consultant Urologist, Cambridge, UK.

improvement in flow rates and a reduction in PVRs and PSA.[102,103] Worryingly, this technique is associated with higher rates of bladder neck stricture or obstruction from necrotic tissue and as such, this type of BOO surgery is not recommended.

In HoLEP, high temperatures generated by the holmium laser create bubbles of steam which tears tissue apart with excellent haemostasis (see Fig. 5.3.11). Initially holmium lasers were used to vaporize or ablate the prostate (HoLAP), which resulted in urodynamic improvements similar to TURP but with a smaller reduction in prostate volume at short-term follow-up. Holmium was then used to resect the prostate (HoLRP), much like TURP. This technique has now progressed onto HoLEP with enucleation of the entire lobes, which are then pushed into the bladder and then morcellated (see Fig. 5.3.9).[104] There have been six RCTS comparing HoLEP with TURP and one comparing HoLEP with open prostatectomy. Essentially there is no statistically significant difference between HoLEP and TURP in improving symptom scores and quality of life scores at up to seven years.[105–107] HoLEP showed greater improvement in flow rates at one year but not at seven years. Less blood loss and transfusion rates have been observed with HoLEP.[108] HoLEP has a significantly longer operating time than TURP but this may be offset by shorter catheterization or hospital stay in some centres. At five years' follow-up, HoLEP is also comparable to open prostatectomy.[109]

Thulium laser allows better tissue vaporization than holmium. Similar to the evolution of the technique with holmium lasers, thulium lasers have been used to treat BPH by vaporization, vaporesection (ThuVARP), vapoenucleation and laser enucleation (ThuVEP). At one-year follow-up, there seems to be no difference in outcome or complication rates between TURP and ThuVARP.[110] Equally there seems to be no difference between HoLEP and ThuVEP[111] or ThuLEP.[112]

Laser techniques for treating BPH appear to have equivalent results to TURP. They are superior to TURP in anticoagulated patients with lower risks of bleeding and the need for postoperative blood transfusion.[113,114] As with bipolar TURP, saline irrigation can be used and this limits the development of hyponatraemia (this is still possible following use of large volumes of irrigant, inappropriate post-op fluid management, and inappropriate SIADH release). Shorter periods of catheterization and length of stay need to offset the higher operating costs (in terms of equipment and operating time); as such, TURP remains a cost-effective modality for BPH surgery.[115]

Open prostatectomy

Open prostatectomy is still relevant in today's medicine; it involves enucleation of the hyperplastic prostatic adenoma. It was first performed for many centuries via a perineal approach. Later descriptions include Freyer's suprapubic transvesical approach,[116] Millin's retropubic transcapsular prostatectomy,[117] and more recently laparoscopic[118] and robotic-assisted[119] approaches. Prostatectomy still holds a strong place in many developing countries where resources, endourological equipment, and expertise may be lacking. It is clear that simple prostatectomy provides good functional outcome with excellent long-term improvements in flow rates, post-void residuals, and symptom scores.[27,120,121] This has to be weighed up against a longer operating time, hospital stay and recovery, the need for a lower midline incision, and higher postoperative bleeding potential. The common view is that this approach should be reserved for larger prostates. In these patients, HoLEP is a reasonable endourological alternative allowing a minimally invasive alternative to prostate enucleation; functional outcome and complication rates appear the same.[109] However, the open approach should be considered in men with prior urethral disease (e.g. following hypospadius repair and/or ongoing stricture disease), in the presence of large bladder calculi, or in men with fixed hips that do not allow flexion.

Novel therapies

A number of novel therapies have been investigated recently. The Urolift procedure involves placing tiny implants that stretch the prostatic urethra open. The delivery system allows the implant to be placed and tensioned, and usually requires an average of four implants per person. The improvements in symptom score and flow rate are far superior to those seen with medical therapy, but not as good as those seen with conventional surgery. There is no associated sexual dysfunction and although recovery time is superior to that from conventional surgery, long-term outcomes are unknown. NICE approval was granted in 2014 for this procedure.

Other novel therapies currently under investigation include prostate artery embolization (PAE) and aquablation of the prostate. During PAE, an interventional radiologist, using a percutaneous transfemoral approach, performs super-selective catheterization of small prostatic arteries and embolizes them by introducing microparticles of polyvinyl alcohol or gelatin sponge. Aquablation involves using image-guided high-velocity waterjet technology to resect and remove prostate tissue.

Bladder outlet obstruction surgery

Although there seems to be clear indications for BOO surgery, many questions remain in this area.[122] We do not know what specific elements of BOO result in damage to the urinary tract (e.g. bladder pressure at rest or during voiding, the role of compliance in BOO), or to what extent BPH contributes to BOO and to what extent should PV be reduced by surgery to reduce BOO and its complications.[123] It is however clear that in the long term, the bladder plays a central role in the symptoms of men with BPH. BOO surgery is more successful in men who suffer from confirmed BOO.[124] However, untreated BOO does not result in long-term loss of bladder function or greatly alter LUTS.[125] In addition, BOO surgery in men provides no advantage to bladder function or symptoms as compared to surveillance if they suffer from detrusor underactivity.[126] Finally, those with underactivity prior to surgery continue to suffer from long-term underactivity[33] despite surgical deobstruction.

The effect of BOO surgery on erectile dysfunction is unclear. Large scale trials would suggest a detrimental effect on ejaculatory function and potency, regardless of technique.[127,128] However, more detailed examination confirms a high rate of sexual inactivity prior to BOO surgery, and no detrimental (and in some cases a positive) effect of BOO surgery on those men that were sexually active prior to surgery.[129]

Conclusions

BPH affects many men, is very common, and with an ageing population, is a worldwide problem. BPH and BOO are one of many causes of LUTS. The natural history of BPH would suggest that complications from BOO, including haematuria, UTIs, and AUR, occur infrequently.

Simple evaluation of treatment of male LUTS is encouraged in primary care. Following GP assessment, medical therapy can be commenced. Secondary care assessment allows accurate definition of BOO (by urodynamic studies). The ongoing development of medical therapy for obstructive LUTS has led to a reduction in surgical therapy for BPH. Following clinical effectiveness observed in the use of alpha blockade within the prostate, there is ongoing development of superselective alpha blockers (e.g. silodosin and naftopidil). 5-α reductase inhibitors, finasteride, and dutasteride, have shown clinical utility in improving symptoms and reducing prostate volume. Combination therapy with α–blockers and 5-α reductase inhibitors have shown not only improvement in flow rates and symptoms scores, but also a reduction in BPH progression events over four years. Recently, there is mounting evidence for the causal association of BPH and ED with the subsequent licensing approval of a PDE5i for the treatment of BPH.

Open prostatectomy results in long-term durable effectiveness for BOO surgery. This has largely been replaced by TURP, which has equally shown to produce excellent long-term results in symptom scores and flow rates. There are ongoing attempts to improve on the results of TURP, largely by laser techniques which are undergoing constant evolution with higher energy delivery to allow faster prostate volume reduction with lowered catheterization and hospital stay. Many options remain intuitively as good as or better than TURP, but because of difficulties in recruiting to and performing high quality randomized controlled trials in surgery, TURP remains the gold standard deobstructing procedure.

The choice of treatment of BPH will remain under the influence of several factors; this includes findings at assessment in primary and secondary care, treatment choice, and expectations of the patient for onset of symptom control, efficacy, side effects, and disease progression. As patients age, BPH increases, and medical therapy is often superseded by surgical treatment of BPH.

Further reading

Berry SJ, Coffey DS, Walsh PC, Ewing LL. The development of human benign prostatic hyperplasia with age. *J Urol* 1984; **132**(3):474–9.

Bruskewitz R, Girman CJ, Fowler J, *et al.* Effect of finasteride on bother and other health-related quality of life aspects associated with benign prostatic hyperplasia. PLESS Study Group. Proscar Long-term Efficacy and Safety Study. *Urology* 1999; **54**(4):670–8.

Coyne KS, Sexton CC, Thompson CL, *et al.* The prevalence of lower urinary tract symptoms (LUTS) in the USA, the UK and Sweden: results from the Epidemiology of LUTS (EpiLUTS) study. *BJU Int* 2009; **104**(3):352–60.

European Association of Urology. EAU Guideline on Male LUTS, including BPO, 2012. Available at: https://uroweb.org/wp-content/uploads/12_Male_LUTS_LR-May-9th-2012.pdf [Online].

Herrmann TR, Liatsikos EN, Nagele U, Traxer O, Merseburger AS. EAU guidelines on laser technologies. *Eur Urol* 2012; **61**(4):783–95.

Homma Y, Gotoh M, Takei M, Kawabe K, Yamaguchi T. Predictability of conventional tests for the assessment of bladder outlet obstruction in benign prostatic hyperplasia. *Int J Urol* 1998; **5**(1):61–6.

Irwin DE, Milsom I, Hunskaar S, *et al.* Population-based survey of urinary incontinence, overactive bladder, and other lower urinary tract

symptoms in five countries: results of the EPIC study. *Eur Urol* 2006; **50**(6):1306–14; discussion 14–5.
Lee KL, Peehl DM. Molecular and cellular pathogenesis of benign prostatic hyperplasia. *J Urol* 2004; **172**(5 Pt 1):1784–91.
Marker PC, Donjacour AA, Dahiya R, Cunha GR. Hormonal, cellular, and molecular control of prostatic development. *Dev Biol* 2003; **253**(2):165–74.
McConnell JD, Roehrborn CG, Bautista OM, *et al.* The long-term effect of doxazosin, finasteride, and combination therapy on the clinical progression of benign prostatic hyperplasia. *N Engl J Med* 2003; **349**(25):2387–98.
McNeill SA, Hargreave TB, Roehrborn CG. Alfuzosin 10 mg once daily in the management of acute urinary retention: results of a double-blind placebo-ontrolled study. *Urology* 2005;**65**(1):83–9; discussion 9–90.
National Institute of Clinical Health and Excellence. Clinical guideline [CG97] Lower urinary tract symptoms in men: management, 2010. Available at: https://www.nice.org.uk/guidance/cg97 [Online].
Oelke M, Burger M, Castro-Diaz D, et al. Diagnosis and medical treatment of lower urinary tract symptoms in adult men: applying specialist guidelines in clinical practice. *BJU Int* 2012; **110**(5):710–18.
Reich O, Gratzke C, Stief CG. Techniques and long-term results of surgical procedures for BPH. *Eur Urol* 2006; **49**(6):970–8; discussion 8.
Roehrborn CG, Siami P, Barkin J, *et al.* The effects of combination therapy with dutasteride and tamsulosin on clinical outcomes in men with symptomatic benign prostatic hyperplasia: 4-year results from the CombAT study. *Eur Urol* 2010; **57**(1):123–31.

References

1. De Marzo AM, Nelson WG, Meeker AK, Coffey DS. Stem cell features of benign and malignant prostate epithelial cells. *J Urol* 1998; **160**(6 Pt 2):2381–92.
2. Lepor H, Tang R, Meretyk S, Shapiro E. Alpha 1 adrenoceptor subtypes in the human prostate. *J Urol* 1993; **149**(3):640–2.
3. Silver RI, Wiley EL, Davis DL, Thigpen AE, Russell DW, McConnell JD. Expression and regulation of steroid 5 alpha-reductase 2 in prostate disease. *J Urol* 1994; **152**(2 Pt 1):433–7.
4. Marker PC, Donjacour AA, Dahiya R, Cunha GR. Hormonal, cellular, and molecular control of prostatic development. *Dev Biol* 2003; **253**(2):165–74.
5. Barrack ER, Berry SJ. DNA synthesis in the canine prostate: effects of androgen and estrogen treatment. *Prostate* 1987; **10**(1):45–56.
6. Lee KL, Peehl DM. Molecular and cellular pathogenesis of benign prostatic hyperplasia. *J Urol* 2004; **172**(5 Pt 1):1784–91.
7. Kramer G, Mitteregger D, Marberger M. Is benign prostatic hyperplasia (BPH) an immune inflammatory disease? *Eur Urol* 2007; **51**(5):1202–16.
8. Sanda MG, Beaty TH, Stutzman RE, Childs B, Walsh PC. Genetic susceptibility of benign prostatic hyperplasia. *J Urol* 1994; **152**(1):115–9.
9. McNeal JE. The zonal anatomy of the prostate. *Prostate* 1981; **2**(1):35–49.
10. Shapiro E, Becich MJ, Hartanto V, Lepor H. The relative proportion of stromal and epithelial hyperplasia is related to the development of symptomatic benign prostate hyperplasia. *J Urol* 1992; **147**(5):1293–7.
11. Srinivasan D, Kosaka AH, Daniels DV, Ford AP, Bhattacharya A. Pharmacological and functional characterization of bradykinin B2 receptor in human prostate. *Eur J Pharmacol* 2004; **504**(3):155–67.
12. Waldkirch E, Uckert S, Sigl K, *et al.* Expression of cAMP-dependent protein kinase isoforms in the human prostate: functional significance and relation to PDE4. *Urology* 2010; **76**(2):515 e8–14.
13. Berry SJ, Coffey DS, Walsh PC, Ewing LL. The development of human benign prostatic hyperplasia with age. *J Urol* 1984; **132**(3):474–9.
14. Coyne KS, Sexton CC, Thompson CL, *et al.* The prevalence of lower urinary tract symptoms (LUTS) in the USA, the UK and Sweden: results from the Epidemiology of LUTS (EpiLUTS) study. *BJU Int* 2009; **104**(3):352–60.
15. Chute CG, Panser LA, Girman CJ, *et al.* The prevalence of prostatism: a population-based survey of urinary symptoms. *J Urol* 1993; **150**(1):85–9.
16. Meigs JB, Barry MJ, Giovannucci E, Rimm EB, Stampfer MJ, Kawachi I. Incidence rates and risk factors for acute urinary retention: the health professionals followup study. *J Urol* 1999; **162**(2):376–82.
17. Bruskewitz R, Girman CJ, Fowler J, *et al.* Effect of finasteride on bother and other health-related quality of life aspects associated with benign prostatic hyperplasia. PLESS Study Group. Proscar Long-term Efficacy and Safety Study. *Urology* 1999; **54**(4):670–8.
18. McConnell JD, Roehrborn CG, Bautista OM, *et al.* The long-term effect of doxazosin, finasteride, and combination therapy on the clinical progression of benign prostatic hyperplasia. *N Engl J Med* 2003; **349**(25):2387–98.
19. Roehrborn CG. Alfuzosin 10 mg once daily prevents overall clinical progression of benign prostatic hyperplasia but not acute urinary retention: results of a 2-year placebo-controlled study. *BJU Int* 2006; **97**(4):734–41.
20. Irwin DE, Milsom I, Hunskaar S, *et al.* Population-based survey of urinary incontinence, overactive bladder, and other lower urinary tract symptoms in five countries: results of the EPIC study. *Eur Urol* 2006; **50**(6):1306–14; discussion 14–5.
21. Kupelian V, Wei JT, O'Leary MP, *et al.* Prevalence of lower urinary tract symptoms and effect on quality of life in a racially and ethnically diverse random sample: the Boston Area Community Health (BACH) Survey. *Arch Int Med* 2006; **166**(21):2381–7.
22. Fukuta F, Masumori N, Mori M, Tsukamoto T. Natural history of lower urinary tract symptoms in Japanese men from a 15-year longitudinal community-based study. *BJU Int* 2012; **110**(7):1023–9.
23. Lieber MM, Rhodes T, Jacobson DJ, *et al.* Natural history of benign prostatic enlargement: long-term longitudinal population-based study of prostate volume doubling times. *BJU Int* 2010; **105**(2):214–9.
24. Coyne KS, Kaplan SA, Chapple CR, *et al.* Risk factors and comorbid conditions associated with lower urinary tract symptoms: EpiLUTS. *BJU Int* 2009; **103**(Suppl 3):24–32.
25. Kupelian V, McVary KT, Kaplan SA, *et al.* Association of lower urinary tract symptoms and the metabolic syndrome: results from the Boston Area Community Health Survey. *J Urol* 2009; **182**(2):616–24; discussion 24–5.
26. Hammarsten J, Hogstedt B, Holthuis N, Mellstrom D. Components of the metabolic syndrome-risk factors for the development of benign prostatic hyperplasia. *Prostate Cancer Prostatic Dis* 1998; **1**(3):157–62.
27. Gratzke C, Schlenker B, Seitz M, *et al.* Complications and early postoperative outcome after open prostatectomy in patients with benign prostatic enlargement: results of a prospective multicenter study. *J Urol* 2007; **177**(4):1419–22.
28. Levin RM, Haugaard N, O'Connor L, *et al.* Obstructive response of human bladder to BPH vs. rabbit bladder response to partial outlet obstruction: a direct comparison. *Neurourol Urodyn* 2000; **19**(5):609–29.
29. Abrams PH, Farrar DJ, Turner-Warwick RT, Whiteside CG, Feneley RC. The results of prostatectomy: a symptomatic and urodynamic analysis of 152 patients. *J Urol* 1979; **121**(5):640–2.
30. Grosse H. [Frequency, localization and associated disorders in urinary calculi. Analysis of 1671 autopsies in urolithiasis]. *Zeitschrift fur Urologie und Nephrologie* 1990; **83**(9):469–74. Frequenz, Lokalisation und Begleiterkrankungen der Harnsteine. Analyse von 1671 Urolithiasis-Obduktionen.
31. Millan-Rodriguez F, Izquierdo-Latorre F, Montlleo-Gonzalez M, Rousaud-Baron F, Rousaud-Baron A, Villavicencio-Mavrich H. Treatment of bladder stones without associated prostate surgery: results of a prospective study. *Urology* 2005; **66**(3):505–9.
32. Flanigan RC, Reda DJ, Wasson JH, Anderson RJ, Abdellatif M, Bruskewitz RC. 5-year outcome of surgical resection and watchful waiting for men with moderately symptomatic benign prostatic hyperplasia: a Department of Veterans Affairs cooperative study. *J Urol* 1998; **160**(1):12–6; discussion 6–7.

33. Al-Hayek S, Thomas A, Abrams P. Natural history of detrusor contractility—minimum ten-year urodynamic follow-up in men with bladder outlet obstruction and those with detrusor. *Scand J Urol Nephrol Suppl* 2004; (215):101–8.
34. Donohue JF, Hayne D, Karnik U, Thomas DR, Foster MC. Randomized, placebo-controlled trial showing that finasteride reduces prostatic vascularity rapidly within 2 weeks. *BJU Int* 2005; **96**(9):1319–22.
35. Roehrborn CG, Bruskewitz R, Nickel GC, *et al.* Urinary retention in patients with BPH treated with finasteride or placebo over 4 years. Characterization of patients and ultimate outcomes. The PLESS Study Group. *Eur Urol* 2000; **37**(5):528–36.
36. Rosen RC, Wei JT, Althof SE, Seftel AD, Miner M, Perelman MA. Association of sexual dysfunction with lower urinary tract symptoms of BPH and BPH medical therapies: results from the BPH Registry. *Urology* 2009; **73**(3):562–6.
37. Vallancien G, Emberton M, Harving N, van Moorselaar RJ. Sexual dysfunction in 1,274 European men suffering from lower urinary tract symptoms. *J Urol* 2003; **169**(6):2257–61.
38. National Institute of Clinical Health and Excellence. Clinical guideline [CG97] Lower urinary tract symptoms in men: management, 2010. Available at: https://www.nice.org.uk/guidance/cg97 [Online].
39. Homma Y, Gotoh M, Takei M, Kawabe K, Yamaguchi T. Predictability of conventional tests for the assessment of bladder outlet obstruction in benign prostatic hyperplasia. *Int J Urol* 1998; **5**(1):61–6.
40. Roehrborn CG, Boyle P, Gould AL, Waldstreicher J. Serum prostate-specific antigen as a predictor of prostate volume in men with benign prostatic hyperplasia. *Urology* 1999; **53**(3):581–9.
41. Ball AJ, Feneley RC, Abrams PH. The natural history of untreated "prostatism". *Br J Urol* 1981; **53**(6):613–6.
42. Brown CT, Yap T, Cromwell DA, *et al.* Self management for men with lower urinary tract symptoms: randomised controlled trial. *BMJ* 2007; **334**(7583):25.
43. Wasson JH, Bubolz TA, Lu-Yao GL, Walker-Corkery E, Hammond CS, Barry MJ. Transurethral resection of the prostate among medicare beneficiaries: 1984 to 1997. For the patient outcomes research team for prostatic diseases. *J Urol* 2000; **164**(4):1212–5.
44. Caine M, Raz S, Zeigler M. Adrenergic and cholinergic receptors in the human prostate, prostatic capsule and bladder neck. *Br J Urol* 1975; **47**(2):193–202.
45. Hieble JP, Caine M, Zalaznik E. In vitro characterization of the alpha-adrenoceptors in human prostate. *Eur J Pharmacol* 1985; **107**(2):111–7.
46. Shapiro E, Hartanto V, Lepor H. The response to alpha blockade in benign prostatic hyperplasia is related to the percent area density of prostate smooth muscle. *Prostate* 1992; **21**(4):297–307.
47. Kortmann BB, Floratos DL, Kiemeney LA, Wijkstra H, de la Rosette JJ. Urodynamic effects of alpha-adrenoceptor blockers: a review of clinical trials. *Urology* 2003; **62**(1):1–9.
48. McNeill SA, Hargreave TB, Roehrborn CG. Alfuzosin 10 mg once daily in the management of acute urinary retention: results of a double-blind placebo-ontrolled study. *Urology* 2005; **65**(1):83–9; discussion 9–90.
49. Gormley GJ, Stoner E, Bruskewitz RC, *et al.* The effect of finasteride in men with benign prostatic hyperplasia. The Finasteride Study Group. *New Engl J Med* 1992; **327**(17):1185–91.
50. McConnell JD, Bruskewitz R, Walsh P, *et al.* The effect of finasteride on the risk of acute urinary retention and the need for surgical treatment among men with benign prostatic hyperplasia. Finasteride Long-Term Efficacy and Safety Study Group. *New Engl J Med* 1998; **338**(9):557–63.
51. Roehrborn CG, Marks LS, Fenter T, *et al.* Efficacy and safety of dutasteride in the four-year treatment of men with benign prostatic hyperplasia. *Urology* 2004; **63**(4):709–15.
52. Donohue JF, Sharma H, Abraham R, Natalwala S, Thomas DR, Foster MC. Transurethral prostate resection and bleeding: a randomized, placebo controlled trial of role of finasteride for decreasing operative blood loss. *J Urol* 2002; **168**(5):2024–6.
53. Lepor H, Williford WO, Barry MJ, *et al.* The efficacy of terazosin, finasteride, or both in benign prostatic hyperplasia. Veterans Affairs Cooperative Studies Benign Prostatic Hyperplasia Study Group. *New Engl J Med* 1996; **335**(8):533–9.
54. Debruyne FM, Jardin A, Colloi D, *et al.* Sustained-release alfuzosin, finasteride and the combination of both in the treatment of benign prostatic hyperplasia. European ALFIN Study Group. *Eur Urol* 1998; **34**(3):169–75.
55. Kirby RS, Roehrborn C, Boyle P, *et al.* Efficacy and tolerability of doxazosin and finasteride, alone or in combination, in treatment of symptomatic benign prostatic hyperplasia: the Prospective European Doxazosin and Combination Therapy (PREDICT) trial. *Urology* 2003; **61**(1):119–26.
56. Roehrborn CG, Siami P, Barkin J, *et al.* The effects of combination therapy with dutasteride and tamsulosin on clinical outcomes in men with symptomatic benign prostatic hyperplasia: 4-year results from the CombAT study. *Eur Urol* 2010; **57**(1):123–31.
57. Barkin J, Guimaraes M, Jacobi G, Pushkar D, Taylor S, van Vierssen Trip OB. Alpha-blocker therapy can be withdrawn in the majority of men following initial combination therapy with the dual 5alpha-reductase inhibitor dutasteride. *Eur Urol* 2003; **44**(4):461–6.
58. European Association of Urology. EAU Guideline on Male LUTS, including BPO, 2012. Available at: https://uroweb.org/wp-content/uploads/12_Male_LUTS_LR-May-9th-2012.pdf [Online].
59. Sairam K, Kulinskaya E, McNicholas TA, Boustead GB, Hanbury DC. Sildenafil influences lower urinary tract symptoms. *BJU Int* 2002; **90**(9):836–9.
60. McVary KT, Monnig W, Camps JL Jr, Young JM, Tseng LJ, van den Ende G. Sildenafil citrate improves erectile function and urinary symptoms in men with erectile dysfunction and lower urinary tract symptoms associated with benign prostatic hyperplasia: a randomized, double-blind trial. *J Urol* 2007; **177**(3):1071–7.
61. McVary KT, Roehrborn CG, Kaminetsky JC, *et al.* Tadalafil relieves lower urinary tract symptoms secondary to benign prostatic hyperplasia. *J Urol* 2007; **177**(4):1401–7.
62. Stief CG, Porst H, Neuser D, Beneke M, Ulbrich E. A randomised, placebo-controlled study to assess the efficacy of twice-daily vardenafil in the treatment of lower urinary tract symptoms secondary to benign prostatic hyperplasia. *Eur Urol* 2008; **53**(6):1236–44.
63. Lee JY, Foster HE Jr, McVary KT, *et al.* Recruitment of participants to a clinical trial of botanical therapy for benign prostatic hyperplasia. *J Altern Complement Med* 2011; **17**(5):469–72.
64. MacDonald R, Tacklind JW, Rutks I, Wilt TJ. Serenoa repens monotherapy for benign prostatic hyperplasia (BPH): an updated Cochrane systematic review. *BJU Int* 2012; **109**(12):1756–61.
65. Barry MJ, Meleth S, Lee JY, *et al.* Effect of increasing doses of saw palmetto extract on lower urinary tract symptoms: a randomized trial. *JAMA* 2011; **306**(12):1344–51.
66. Perry MJ, Roodhouse AJ, Gidlow AB, Spicer TG, Ellis BW. Thermo-expandable intraprostatic stents in bladder outlet obstruction: an 8-year study. *BJU Int* 2002; **90**(3):216–23.
67. Armitage JN, Rashidian A, Cathcart PJ, Emberton M, van der Meulen JH. The thermo-expandable metallic stent for managing benign prostatic hyperplasia: a systematic review. *BJU Int* 2006; **98**(4):806–10.
68. Chapple CR, Milroy EJ, Rickards D. Permanently implanted urethral stent for prostatic obstruction in the unfit patient. Preliminary report. *Br J Urol* 1990; **66**(1):58–65.
69. McLoughlin J, Jager R, Abel PD, el Din A, Adam A, Williams G. The use of prostatic stents in patients with urinary retention who are unfit for surgery. An interim report. *Br J Urol* 1990; **66**(1):66–70.
70. Bajoria S, Agarwal SA, White R, Zafar F, Williams G. Experience with the second generation UroLume prostatic stent. *Br J Urol* 1995; **75**(3):325–7.
71. Masood S, Djaladat H, Kouriefs C, Keen M, Palmer JH. The 12-year outcome analysis of an endourethral wallstent for treating benign prostatic hyperplasia. *BJU Int* 2004; **94**(9):1271–4.

72. Hoffman RM, Monga M, Elliot SP, Macdonald R, Wilt TJ. Microwave thermotherapy for benign prostatic hyperplasia. *Cochrane Database Syst Rev* 2007; (4):CD004135.
73. Bouza C, Lopez T, Magro A, Navalpotro L, Amate JM. Systematic review and meta-analysis of Transurethral Needle Ablation in symptomatic Benign Prostatic Hyperplasia. *BMC Urol* 2006; **6**:14.
74. Sullivan L, Casey RW, Pommerville PJ, Marich KW. Canadian experience with high intensity focused ultrasound for the treatment of BPH. *Can J Urol* 1999; **6**(3):799–805.
75. Lu J, Hu W, Wang W. Sonablate-500 transrectal high-intensity focused ultrasound (HIFU) for benign prostatic hyperplasia patients. *J Huazhong Univ Sci Technolog Med Sci* 2007; **27**(6):671–4.
76. Madersbacher S, Schatzl G, Djavan B, Stulnig T, Marberger M. Long-term outcome of transrectal high- intensity focused ultrasound therapy for benign prostatic hyperplasia. *Eur Urol* 2000; **37**(6):687–94.
77. Muschter R. Conductive heat: hot water-induced thermotherapy for ablation of prostatic tissue. *J Endourol* 2003; **17**(8):609–16.
78. Corica FA, Cheng L, Ramnani D, *et al.* Transurethral hot-water balloon thermoablation for benign prostatic hyperplasia: patient tolerance and pathologic findings. *Urology* 2000; **56**(1):76–80; discussion 1.
79. Corica AG, Qian J, Ma J, Sagaz AA, Corica AP, Bostwick DG. Fast liquid ablation system for prostatic hyperplasia: a new minimally invasive thermal treatment. *J Urol* 2003; **170**(3):874–8.
80. Magno C, Mucciardi G, Gali A, Anastasi G, Inferrera A, Morgia G. Transurethral ethanol ablation of the prostate (TEAP): an effective minimally invasive treatment alternative to traditional surgery for symptomatic benign prostatic hyperplasia (BPH) in high-risk comorbidity patients. *Int Urol Nephrol* 2008; **40**(4):941–6.
81. Sakr M, Eid A, Shoukry M, Fayed A. Transurethral ethanol injection therapy of benign prostatic hyperplasia: four-year follow-up. *Int J Urol* 2009; **16**(2):196–201.
82. El-Husseiny T, Buchholz N. Transurethral ethanol ablation of the prostate for symptomatic benign prostatic hyperplasia: long-term follow-up. *J Endourol* 2011; **25**(3):477–80.
83. Chuang YC, Chiang PH, Yoshimura N, De Miguel F, Chancellor MB. Sustained beneficial effects of intraprostatic botulinum toxin type A on lower urinary tract symptoms and quality of life in men with benign prostatic hyperplasia. *BJU Int* 2006; **98**(5):1033–7; discussion 337.
84. Brisinda G, Cadeddu F, Vanella S, Mazzeo P, Marniga G, Maria G. Relief by botulinum toxin of lower urinary tract symptoms owing to benign prostatic hyperplasia: early and long-term results. *Urology* 2009; **73**(1):90–4.
85. Sacco E, Bientinesi R, Marangi F, *et al.* Patient-reported outcomes in men with lower urinary tract symptoms (LUTS) due to benign prostatic hyperplasia (BPH) treated with intraprostatic OnabotulinumtoxinA: 3-month results of a prospective single-armed cohort study. *BJU Int* 2012; **110**(11 Pt C):E837–44.
86. Hamidi Madani A, Enshaei A, *et al.* Transurethral intraprostatic Botulinum toxin-A injection: a novel treatment for BPH refractory to current medical therapy in poor surgical candidates. *World J Urol* 2013; **31**(1):235–9.
87. Giannakopoulos XK, Giotis C, Karkabounas S, *et al.* Effects of pulsed electromagnetic fields on benign prostate hyperplasia. *Int Urol Nephrol* 2011; **43**(4):955–60.
88. Emberton M, Neal DE, Black N, *et al.* The National Prostatectomy Audit: the clinical management of patients during hospital admission. *Br J Urol* 1995; **75**(3):301–16.
89. Holman CD, Wisniewski ZS, Semmens JB, Rouse IL, Bass AJ. Mortality and prostate cancer risk in 19,598 men after surgery for benign prostatic hyperplasia. *BJU Int* 1999; **84**(1):37–42.
90. Reich O, Gratzke C, Stief CG. Techniques and long-term results of surgical procedures for BPH. *Eur Urol* 2006; **49**(6):970–8; discussion 8.
91. Orandi A. Transurethral incision of prostate. Seven-year follow-up. *Urology* 1978; **12**(2):187–9.
92. Mamoulakis C, Ubbink DT, de la Rosette JJ. Bipolar versus monopolar transurethral resection of the prostate: a systematic review and meta-analysis of randomized controlled trials. *Eur Urol* 2009; **56**(5):798–809.
93. Xie CY, Zhu GB, Wang XH, Liu XB. Five-year follow-up results of a randomized controlled trial comparing bipolar plasmakinetic and monopolar transurethral resection of the prostate. *Yonsei Med J* 2012; **53**(4):734–41.
94. Liao N, Yu J. A study comparing plasmakinetic enucleation with bipolar plasmakinetic resection of the prostate for benign prostatic hyperplasia. *J Endourol* 2012; **26**(7):884–8.
95. Patel A, Fuchs GJ, Gutierrez-Aceves J, Andrade-Perez F. Transurethral electrovaporization and vapour-resection of the prostate: an appraisal of possible electrosurgical alternatives to regular loop resection. *BJU Int* 2000; **85**(2):202–10.
96. Poulakis V, Dahm P, Witzsch U, Sutton AJ, Becht E. Transurethral electrovaporization vs transurethral resection for symptomatic prostatic obstruction: a meta-analysis. *BJU Int* 2004; **94**(1):89–95.
97. Nuhoglu B, Balci MB, Aydin M, *et al.* The role of bipolar transurethral vaporization in the management of benign prostatic hyperplasia. *Urologia Int* 2011; **87**(4):400–4.
98. Malek RS, Barrett DM, Kuntzman RS. High-power potassium-titanyl-phosphate (KTP/532) laser vaporization prostatectomy: 24 hours later. *Urology* 1998; **51**(2):254–6.
99. Bouchier-Hayes DM, Anderson P, Van Appledorn S, Bugeja P, Costello AJ. KTP laser versus transurethral resection: early results of a randomized trial. *J Endourol* 2006; **20**(8):580–5.
100. Horasanli K, Silay MS, Altay B, Tanriverdi O, Sarica K, Miroglu C. Photoselective potassium titanyl phosphate (KTP) laser vaporization versus transurethral resection of the prostate for prostates larger than 70 mL: a short-term prospective randomized trial. *Urology* 2008; **71**(2):247–51.
101. Skolarikos A, Papachristou C, Athanasiadis G, Chalikopoulos D, Deliveliotis C, Alivizatos G. Eighteen-month results of a randomized prospective study comparing transurethral photoselective vaporization with transvesical open enucleation for prostatic adenomas greater than 80 cc. *J Endourol* 2008; **22**(10):2333–40.
102. Chen CH, Chiang PH, Chuang YC, Lee WC, Chen YT. Preliminary results of prostate vaporization in the treatment of benign prostatic hyperplasia by using a 200-W high-intensity diode laser. *Urology* 2010; **75**(3):658–63.
103. Ruszat R, Seitz M, Wyler SF, *et al.* Prospective single-centre comparison of 120-W diode-pumped solid-state high-intensity system laser vaporization of the prostate and 200-W high-intensive diode-laser ablation of the prostate for treating benign prostatic hyperplasia. *BJU Int* 2009; **104**(6):820–5.
104. Fraundorfer MR, Gilling PJ. Holmium:YAG laser enucleation of the prostate combined with mechanical morcellation: preliminary results. *Eur Urol* 1998; **33**(1):69–72.
105. Tan A, Liao C, Mo Z, Cao Y. Meta-analysis of holmium laser enucleation versus transurethral resection of the prostate for symptomatic prostatic obstruction. *Br J Surg* 2007; **94**(10):1201–8.
106. Lourenco T, Pickard R, Vale L, *et al.* Minimally invasive treatments for benign prostatic enlargement: systematic review of randomised controlled trials. *BMJ* 2008; **337**:a1662.
107. Gilling PJ, Wilson LC, King CJ, Westenberg AM, Frampton CM, Fraundorfer MR. Long-term results of a randomized trial comparing holmium laser enucleation of the prostate and transurethral resection of the prostate: results at 7 years. *BJU Int* 2012; **109**(3):408–11.
108. Martin AD, Nunez RN, Humphreys MR. Bleeding after holmium laser enucleation of the prostate: lessons learned the hard way. *BJU Int* 2011; **107**(3):433–7.
109. Kuntz RM, Lehrich K, Ahyai SA. Holmium laser enucleation of the prostate versus open prostatectomy for prostates greater than 100 grams: 5-year follow-up results of a randomised clinical trial. *Eur Urol* 2008; **53**(1):160–6.

110. Xia SJ, Zhuo J, Sun XW, Han BM, Shao Y, Zhang YN. Thulium laser versus standard transurethral resection of the prostate: a randomized prospective trial. *Eur Urol* 2008; **53**(2):382–89.
111. Bach T, Xia SJ, Yang Y, *et al.* Thulium: YAG 2 mum cw laser prostatectomy: where do we stand? *World J Urol* 2010; **28**(2):163–8.
112. Zhang F, Shao Q, Herrmann TR, Tian Y, Zhang Y. Thulium laser versus holmium laser transurethral enucleation of the prostate: 18-month follow-up data of a single center. *Urology* 2012; **79**(4):869–74.
113. Hauser S, Rogenhofer S, Ellinger J, Strunk T, Muller SC, Fechner G. Thulium laser (revolix) vapoenucleation of the prostate is a safe procedure in patients with an increased risk of hemorrhage. *Urol Int* 2012; **88**(4):390–4.
114. Tyson MD, Lerner LB. Safety of holmium laser enucleation of the prostate in anticoagulated patients. *J Endourol* 2009; **23**(8):1343–6.
115. Lourenco T, Armstrong N, N'Dow J, *et al.* Systematic review and economic modelling of effectiveness and cost utility of surgical treatments for men with benign prostatic enlargement. *Health Technol Assess* 2008; **12**(35):iii, ix–x, 1–146:69–515.
116. Freyer PJ. Total enucleation of the prostate: A further series of 550 cases of the operation. *BMJ* 1919; **1**(3031):121–0 2.
117. Millin T. Retropubic prostatectomy; a new extravesical technique; report of 20 cases. *Lancet* 1945; **2**(6380):693–6.
118. Mariano MB, Tefilli MV, Graziottin TM, Morales CM, Goldraich IH. Laparoscopic prostatectomy for benign prostatic hyperplasia—a six-year experience. *Eur Urol* 2006; **49**(1):127–31; discussion 31–2.
119. Sotelo R, Clavijo R, Carmona O, *et al.* Robotic simple prostatectomy. *J Urol* 2008; **179**(2):513–5.
120. Tubaro A, Carter S, Hind A, Vicentini C, Miano L. A prospective study of the safety and efficacy of suprapubic transvesical prostatectomy in patients with benign prostatic hyperplasia. *J Urol* 2001; **166**(1):172–6.
121. Varkarakis I, Kyriakakis Z, Delis A, Protogerou V, Deliveliotis C. Long-term results of open transvesical prostatectomy from a contemporary series of patients. *Urology* 2004; **64**(2):306–10.
122. Oelke M, Kirschner-Hermanns R, Thiruchelvam N, Heesakkers J. Can we identify men who will have complications from benign prostatic obstruction (BPO)? ICI-RS 2011. *Neurourol Urodyn* 2012; **31**(3):322–6.
123. Abidi SS, Feroz I, Aslam M, Fawad A. Elective hemi transurethral resection of prostate: a safe and effective method of treating huge benign prostatic hyperplasia. *J Coll Physicians Surg Pak* 2012; **22**(1):35–40.
124. Thomas AW, Cannon A, Bartlett E, Ellis-Jones J, Abrams P. The natural history of lower urinary tract dysfunction in men: minimum 10-year urodynamic followup of transurethral resection of prostate for bladder outlet obstruction. *J Urol* 2005; **174**(5):1887–91.
125. Thomas AW, Cannon A, Bartlett E, Ellis-Jones J, Abrams P. The natural history of lower urinary tract dysfunction in men: minimum 10-year urodynamic follow-up of untreated bladder outlet obstruction. *BJU Int* 2005; **96**(9):1301–6.
126. Thomas AW, Cannon A, Bartlett E, Ellis-Jones J, Abrams P. The natural history of lower urinary tract dysfunction in men: the influence of detrusor underactivity on the outcome after transurethral resection of the prostate with a minimum 10-year urodynamic follow-up. *BJU Int* 2004; **93**(6):745–50.
127. Zong HT, Peng XX, Yang CC, Zhang Y. The impact of transurethral procedures for benign prostate hyperplasia on male sexual function: a meta-analysis. *J Androl* 2012; **33**(3):427–34.
128. Frieben RW, Lin HC, Hinh PP, Berardinelli F, Canfield SE, Wang R. The impact of minimally invasive surgeries for the treatment of symptomatic benign prostatic hyperplasia on male sexual function: a systematic review. *Asian J Androl* 2010; **12**(4):500–8.
129. Mishriki SF, Grimsley SJ, Lam T, Nabi G, Cohen NP. TURP and sex: patient and partner prospective 12 years follow-up study. *BJU Int* 2012; **109**(5):745–50.

SECTION 6

Oncology

Section editor: James W.F. Catto

CHAPTER 6.1

Epidemiology of prostate cancer

Alison J. Price and Timothy J. Key

Introduction to the epidemiology of prostate cancer

Prostate cancer is the second most common malignancy and the sixth most common cause of cancer death for men worldwide.[1] Aside from age, ethnicity, and family history of disease, the risk factors are not well understood. This chapter aims to give a description of the geographical and temporal trends in prostate cancer incidence and mortality, and an outline of the risk factors possibly involved in the aetiology of the disease, with an emphasis on the role of hormonal and dietary factors.

The nature of the evidence

Much of the literature pertaining to the aetiology of prostate cancer is derived from epidemiological investigations, both observational (ecological, case–control, and cohort studies) and interventional (randomized controlled trials), of associations between biological, physical, and chemical exposures, and risk for prostate cancer diagnosis or death. Studies of animal models and cell cultures are used to explore findings at a mechanistic and functional level, but these will not be discussed here.

The natural history of prostate cancer is complex as it can take many years to present clinically and, while some men develop an aggressive, lethal form of the disease, many men develop cancer that remains small and undetected, and ultimately these men die with the disease, rather than from it.[2] Differentiating non-aggressive from aggressive disease is known to be crucial for determining the best treatment approach (and preventing men undergoing invasive treatments for cancers that may never become life-threatening), and it may also be important for determining possible aetiological differences. However, determining if identified risk factors are associated more with malignant transformation or tumour progression is difficult, because the duration between onset of asymptomatic disease and clinical symptoms has been estimated to be up to 12 years[3]), and some men will develop a form of disease that has little impact on health even in the absence of treatment.[4] Indeed, autopsy studies have shown microscopic, well-differentiated tumours of the prostate gland in 10–14% of men between the age of 40 and 50 years[5]) and 30–40% of men aged over 50 years.[2] By 80 years of age, it is estimated that 80% of all men have asymptomatic prostatic carcinoma.[6]

A further complication for understanding the aetiology of prostate cancer is the increased use of prostate-specific antigen (PSA) testing in some populations, as it has led to much earlier detection of asymptomatic disease (by as much as 10 years in men aged 55 years[7]), decreased numbers of advanced cancers, and a concomitant increase in the proportion of early localized cancers (of which many may never progress to clinical disease).[8]

While future research may identify diagnostic and prognostic biomarkers of prostate cancer that provide a clear differentiation between aggressive and non- aggressive disease, there are currently no such validated biomarkers in general use, and so disease aggressiveness is determined by stage and grade. The prostate cancer tumour staging system (TNM)[9] and the Gleason score,[10] devised over 40 years ago, are the standard benchmarks for determining the clinical and pathological stages and the histological grade of prostate cancer. However, diagnostic practices and criteria have evolved during this time with implications for the interpretation of stage and grade information. In years, ultrasound-guided needle biopsy tissue (collected at diagnosis) has become widely used for grading disease, whereas previously this information was derived mostly from tissue collected during radical prostatectomy or from transurethral resection of the prostate. A change in pathologists' interpretation of biopsy specimens over time has also been evident, with a trend toward allocation of higher grades to cancers that would have previously been classified as less aggressive forms of the disease.[9,11,12] To accommodate heterogeneous patterns of early disease (detected by PSA testing) that were not apparent when the Gleason criteria were first devised, scoring recommendations have also been updated.[13] In the original system the two predominant Gleason scores were used to grade prostate cancers; however, the current recommendation can be based on the most predominant score and the tertiary score, thereby contributing further to the upward trend in grade allocation over time.[12]

An important consequence of changes in diagnostic practices that alter disease classification during the follow-up period of longitudinal studies is partial misclassification of the outcome. This may obscure aetiological relations between exposures and risk for disease. To address this issue, some prospective observational studies and clinical trials have standardized prostate cancer grade[14] and stage[15] data and collected detailed information on a participant's PSA screening history.[16] However, this may not be feasible for large, international and/or multicentre studies. Furthermore, for studies without information on prostate cancer screening, it becomes difficult to ascertain the likely lead time associated with an individual's diagnosis and to account for this in the analytical methodology.

In summary, the complex natural history of prostate cancer and the use of PSA testing means that incident prostate cancer represents a heterogeneous group of cancers which may impede aetiological investigations. While information on stage and grade of disease may help to differentiate risk factors for disease initiation and progression, this remains a relatively imprecise tool. The totality of the evidence from epidemiological research of risk factors for prostate cancer should be interpreted with these caveats in mind.

Prostate cancer incidence and mortality

Geographic trends

Prostate cancer is the second most common malignancy and the sixth leading cause of cancer death among men worldwide. There were an estimated 1,111,700 new cases and 307,500 new deaths in 2008.[1] The worldwide prostate cancer burden is expected to grow to 1.7 million new cases and 499,000 new deaths by 2030 simply due to the growth and ageing of the global population.[1] Although prostate cancer is the most common type of cancer diagnosed in men in most Western countries,[1] there are large differences between countries in the age standardized incidence rate of the disease (Fig. 6.1.1). The highest age standardized incidence rates of prostate cancer are reported in Western Europe, North America, and Australia, with rates per 100,000 men ranging from 85 to 112 per year, while the lowest rates, between 4.5 and 11.2 per 100,000 men per year, are reported in Northern Africa and South-Central, Eastern, and Southeastern Asia.[17] It is important to acknowledge that although incidence rates can provide useful information about the distribution and frequency of cancer, a reliable calculation requires adequate health infrastructure, including a sophisticated healthcare system, universal access to a diagnosis, good health records, and consistent and timely reporting of new cases to a population-based cancer registry. Differences in healthcare delivery or uptake and reporting of cancers, either between populations or over time, distort temporal and population comparisons, and the wide variation in international prostate cancer incidence rates and trends is in part due to the substantial differences worldwide in the diagnosis of latent cancers through PSA testing of asymptomatic individuals, as well as during prostate surgery.

In comparison with the very wide variation in incidence of prostate cancer between economically developed and developing countries, there is less variation in mortality rates, although this is still substantial (Fig. 6.1.2). Age-standardized mortality rates for prostate cancer are highest in the Caribbean and sub-Saharan Africa (more than 24 per 100,000 men per year), and moderately high in Western countries (between 9 and 15 per 100,000 men per year).[1] The lowest age standardized mortality rates are experienced in parts of Asia, especially South-Central Asia, with less than three prostate cancer deaths per 100,000 men per year.[1] Mortality rates are less sensitive than incidence rates to diagnostic practices, and so provide a more accurate reflection of the true underlying variation in rates of prostate cancer between countries. For example, despite a nearly 30% higher incidence rate among white men in the United States compared with the United Kingdom, 2012 age-adjusted mortality rates in these two countries show a higher mortality rate in the United Kingdom than the United States with 13.1 and 9.8 deaths per 100,000 men per year, respectively.

Temporal trends

Much of the observed geographic variation in prostate cancer incidence may be due to differences in screening practices and the prevalence of PSA testing, which increases early detection of tumours and latent disease.[18] Following the introduction of widespread PSA testing in the United States in the late 1980s, prostate cancer incidence increased by 100% over a seven-year period, reaching a peak incidence in 1992 (in excess of 100 cases

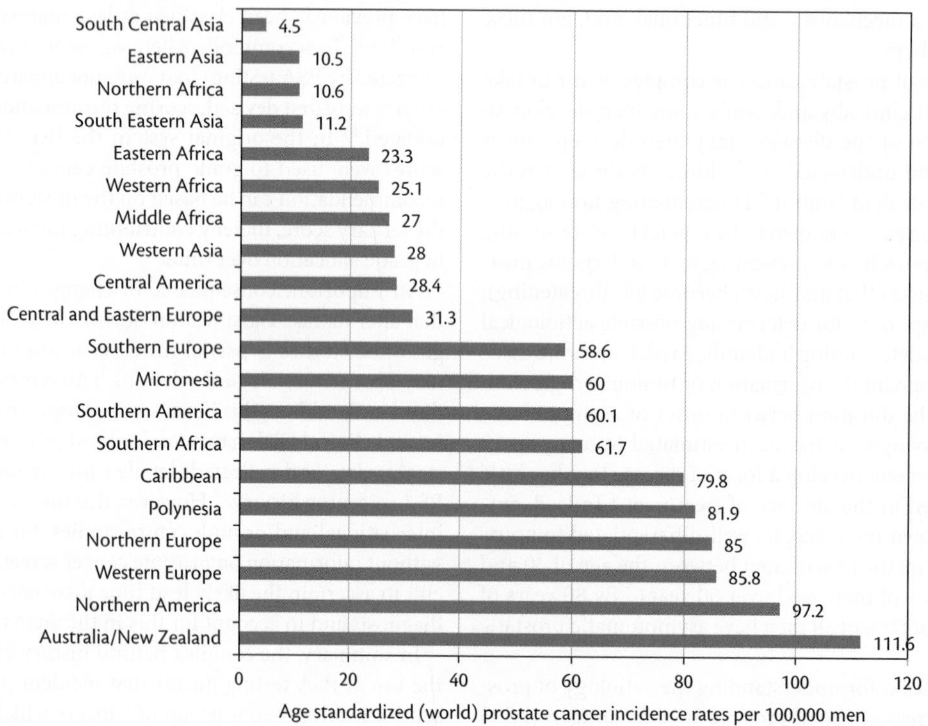

Fig. 6.1.1 Age standardized prostate cancer incidence rates by world area.

Source: data from *GLOBOCAN 2012 Estimated Cancer Incidence, Mortality and Prevalence Worldwide*, International Agency for Research on Cancer (IARC) Cancer. Lyon, France, Copyright © 2017 IARC.

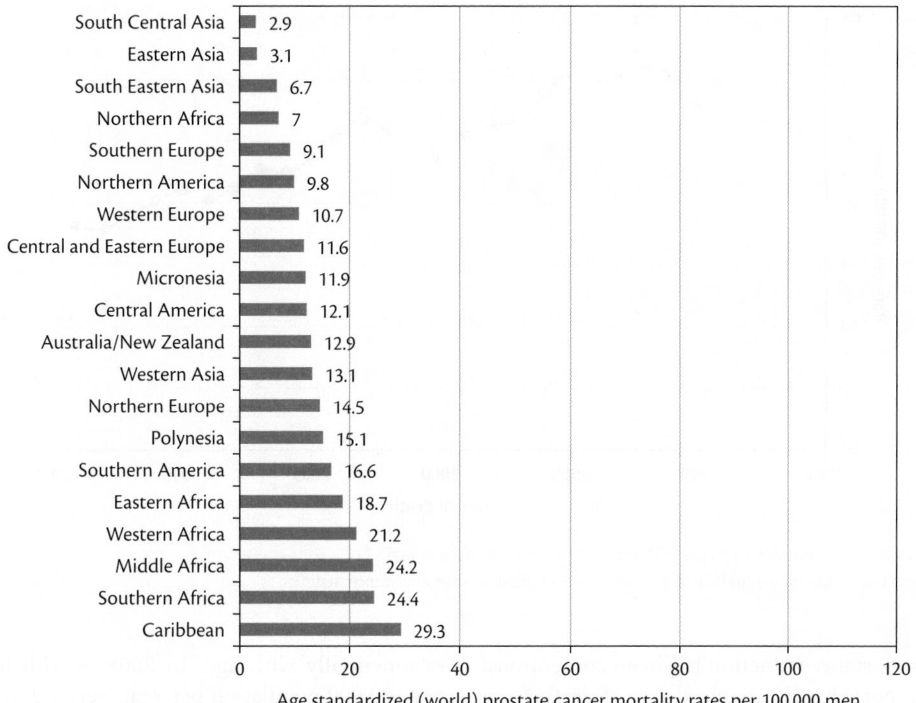

Fig. 6.1.2 Age standardized prostate cancer mortality rates by world area.

Source: data from *GLOBOCAN 2012 Estimated Cancer Incidence, Mortality and Prevalence Worldwide*, International Agency for Research on Cancer (IARC) Cancer. Lyon, France, Copyright © 2017 IARC.

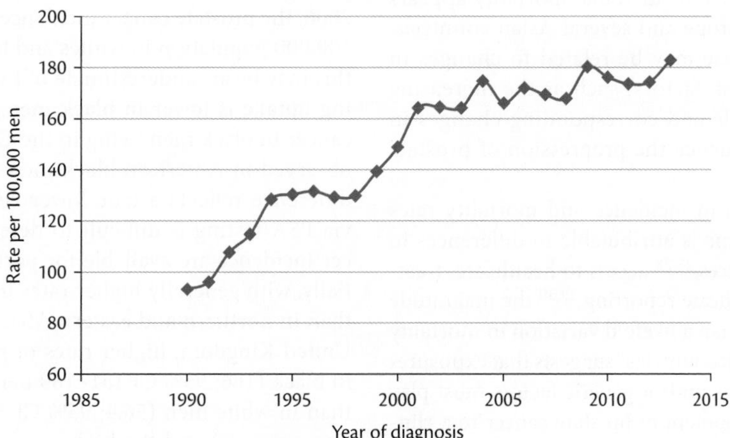

Fig. 6.1.3 European age standardized incidence rates per 100,000 men in the United Kingdom.

Source: data from Cancer Research UK, available from http://www.cancerresearchuk.org/health-professional/cancer-statistics

per 100,000 population per year[19]) and subsequently declined to 85 cases per 100,000 population per year in 2008, as the proportion of prevalent cases diminished.[17] Similar incidence trends have been observed in countries with high uptake of PSA testing, such as Australia and Canada. In the United Kingdom, incidence rates increased more gradually between 1993 and 2009, which may reflect the lower prevalence of PSA testing, with only 6% of men aged 45–84 years tested in 2002[20] compared with 57% in the United States,[21] and 34% in Canada[22] in 2001 (see Fig. 6.1.3 for the temporal trend in prostate cancer incidence in the United Kingdom).

Prostate cancer mortality in most developed countries has been decreasing over the past 10 years,[1] as illustrated for the United Kingdom in Figure 6.1.4. The reasons for this decrease are not well understood, and may include general improvements in treatment and medical care, as well as earlier diagnosis of disease. The

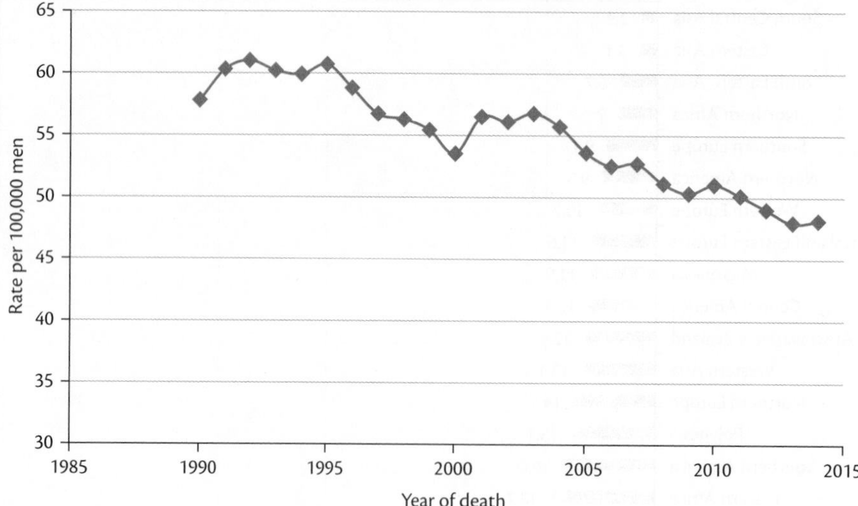

Fig. 6.1.4 European age standardized mortality rates per 100,000 men in the United Kingdom.
Source: data from Cancer Research UK, available from http://www.cancerresearchuk.org/health-professional/cancer-statistics

role of PSA testing in mortality reduction has been contentious; a European trial[23,24] reported a 20% reduced rate of death from prostate cancer in the arm screened with PSA, which was maintained after extended follow-up. In contrast, a large randomized controlled trial in the United States[25] reported no reduction in mortality with PSA testing after 10 years of follow-up, but had low power to detect an effect of organized screening because of high rates of PSA testing in the control arm of the trial. In contrast to the downward trend observed in Northern America, Western and Northern Europe, and Australia, mortality appears to be increasing in Eastern Europe and several Asian countries, including Japan.[26] This increase may be related to changes in exposure to environmental risk factors, such as the increasing adoption of a Western lifestyle and corresponding changes in dietary habits which may influence the progression of prostate cancer.

While some of the variation in incidence and mortality rates between countries and over time is attributable to differences in screening and diagnostic practices,[27,28] access to healthcare, treatment practices, and death certificate reporting,[29,30] the magnitude of the difference (with a more than a fivefold variation in mortality rates between high- and low-risk countries) suggests that exposures to either lifestyle, environmental, and/or genetic factors must play an important part in the development of prostate cancer to a clinical and ultimately fatal form.

Risk factors

Established risk factors for prostate cancer

Advanced age,[31] African ethnic origin,[32,33] a family history of disease,[34–41] and genetic factors[42] are the only well-established risk factors for prostate cancer. Nonetheless, there is much interest in the role of endogenous hormones, diet, and other lifestyle factors in relation to prostate cancer risk.

Age

Worldwide, very few cases of prostate cancer occur in men aged less than 50 years, but incidence and mortality rates increase exponentially with age. In 2008, worldwide age-specific rates per 100,000 population per year were 1.2 in men aged 40–44 but rose to 4.9, 19.1, 51.8, 114.6, 204.6, 293.2 for each successive five-year age group, with the highest rate of 392.1 in men 75 years or older.[43]

Ethnicity

The incidence of prostate cancer in American black men is 50–60% greater than that for American white men.[44] Between 2002 and 2006, the prostate cancer incidence was 146.3 and 231.9 cases per 100,000 population in whites and blacks, respectively,[45] although this may be an underestimate of the difference because PSA testing uptake is lower in black men.[46] Incidence rates of prostate cancer in black men living in the Caribbean are lower than those observed in American black men—but the extent to which this difference reflects a true lower risk or less case ascertainment via PSA testing is difficult to determine. Data on prostate cancer incidence are available for parts of Africa and vary substantially, with generally higher rates in western and southern Africa than in northern and eastern Africa. In a study conducted in the United Kingdom, higher rates of prostate cancer were observed in black (166; 95% CI 151–180 per 100,000 population per year) than in white men (56.4; 95% CI 53.3–59.5 per 100,000 population per year) and the higher risk in black men compared with white men was more apparent in younger age groups (p heterogeneity <0.0001).[32]

Prostate cancer mortality rates are generally high in predominantly black populations, with age standardized mortality rates of 26 and 18 per 100,000 population per year in the Caribbean and sub-Saharan Africa, respectively, while rates less than 4 per 100,000 per year are observed in eastern Asia.[44] Furthermore, the CONCORD study of global cancer mortality found that among 628,000 men in 31 countries diagnosed with incident prostate cancer during 1990–1994 and followed until 1999, the age standardized five-year survival rate for prostate cancer was lower in blacks (85.8%) than in whites (92.4%).[47] In the United States, this disparity may reflect to some extent inequality in access to and uptake of healthcare, as black men are less likely to be diagnosed with localized prostate cancer than white men.[45]

The mechanisms underlying these differences between ethnic groups are unclear. A range of lifestyle factors has been examined, but so far the difference in observed risk for prostate cancer between whites and blacks has not been shown to be explained by lifestyle, including diet.[48] However, genetic susceptibility may vary between ethnic groups. For example, an increased genetic susceptibility and different levels of androgen hormone activity within the prostate may contribute to the increased risk in black men,[32] and a genome-wide association study (GWAS) detected a marker of increased risk for prostate cancer on chromosome 17q21 that appears specific to men of African ancestry.[49] Furthermore, a GWAS of prostate cancer in a Japanese population[50] identified five new susceptibility loci (not identified in white populations) on chromosomes 2p24, 5p15, 6p21, 6q22, and 13q22. While these findings highlight the potential heterogeneity of prostate cancer susceptibility between ethnic groups, the biological contribution of these alleles to prostate cancer risk is not well understood.

Family history and genetic factors

There is clear evidence from studies of familial aggregation of cancer that inherited genes are important in the development of prostate cancer.[38–41] Evidence from twin studies suggests that the heritability of prostate cancer is approximately 40%, which is high compared to other types of cancer.[37]

Men with a first-degree relative (e.g. father, brother) with prostate cancer have incidence rates at least 2.5 times greater than men without a first-degree relative with the disease, and risk appears to increase with an increasing number of affected family members.[38,39] Furthermore, family history of prostate cancer is associated with a higher relative risk in men aged less than 65 years than in men aged 65 years or older at diagnosis.[38–41] There is also some evidence to suggest that having a brother with prostate cancer confers a higher risk than a father with disease,[38] although differences in detection rates may cause some bias in these studies because men with a family history of prostate cancer have increased diagnostic activity.[51]

It is likely that genetic susceptibility to prostate cancer is related to the presence of a few rare inherited genetic variants that confer high risk and of multiple common low to moderate risk polymorphisms.[52] As yet, the single genetic risk factor for prostate cancer with the largest magnitude of effect is a rare deleterious germline mutation of the *BRCA2* gene, first identified in families with a history of early-onset of breast cancer, which confers an 8-fold increased risk of prostate cancer,[53] although due to its low frequency this mutation only explains a small proportion of the genetic susceptibility. Germline mutation in *BRCA1*, another of the breast cancer susceptibility genes, is also associated with an increased risk of prostate cancer, albeit of a smaller magnitude (3.5-fold) and is present in less than 1% of sporadic prostate cancer cases. There are also other rare mutations reported in the *HOXB13*, *NBS1*, and *CHEK2* genes which are associated with an increase in risk for prostate cancer.[42,52]

The association between common genetic variation and prostate cancer risk has been extensively investigated in GWAS and subsequent meta-analyses of GWAS data, and more than 100 common single nucleotide polymorphisms (SNPs) have been indentified that are each associated with a modest increase in prostate cancer risk.[42,54] For men who carry large numbers of these variants, this genetic variation may result in substantially higher risk; based on the combined risks of known susceptibility loci, it has been estimated that men in the top 1% of the risk distribution have a 4.7-fold increased risk of the disease compared to the population average. Among the common genetic factors identified, notable loci include at least three distinct loci on chromosome 8 (8q24) in the vicinity of the C-MYC oncogene, and a SNP on chromosome 10 located near to microseminoprotein-β, a seminal protein that is reduced or absent in prostate cancer.[42,55–61] Few of the SNPs identified to date however are associated differentially with risk for a diagnosis of aggressive disease, so while a score based on the combined risks associated with the known susceptibility loci predicts risk for prostate cancer overall, it does not facilitate population risk stratification for aggressive disease.[53]

Estimates suggest that the genetic variants identified so far can explain about 30% of the familial risk of prostate cancer.[49,50,56–60,62] Thus, there appears to be considerable missing heritability, for which postulated explanations include: rarer variants with greater penetrance that are not adequately captured using existing genotyping arrays; gene–gene interactions; and shared environmental determinants among relatives that are not adequately measured.[63]

Putative risk factors for prostate cancer

Sex hormones

It has long been suspected that variation in lifetime exposure to endogenous androgen sex hormones might contribute to inter-individual and ethnic differences in prostate cancer risk. Sex hormones are known to play an essential role in normal prostate development and growth[64] and use of finasteride or dutasteride, treatments which block the conversion of testosterone to its more active form, dihydrotestosterone (DHT), leading to lower levels DHT in the prostate, reduces prostate cancer incidence by up to 25% (although this reduction is only for low-grade disease, not high-grade disease).[65,66] This evidence strongly suggests a role for androgens in prostate cancer development. However, in epidemiological studies, results from a pooled analysis of prospective data of the association of circulating sex hormones and prostate cancer risk do not support an association with mid-adulthood circulating androgen concentrations, within the normal physiological range.[67] Furthermore, evidence from investigations of polymorphisms of the candidate genes that influence androgen metabolism and action do not shown any clear associations.[68–70] Although the available epidemiological studies have not demonstrated a link between androgens and prostate cancer risk, further data are required to examine whether there may be some reduction in the risk in men with particularly low androgen levels.

Insulin-like growth factor-I

Insulin-like growth factors (IGFs) and their associated binding proteins have been the subject of considerable investigation in relation to cancer because of their role in the regulation of cell proliferation, differentiation, and apoptosis.[71] A pooled analysis of individual participant data found that high IGF-I concentrations (within the normal physiological range) are associated with increased risk of

IGF-I and prostate cancer risk (Roddam *et al*, 2008).

IGF-I (fifth)	Cases/ Controls	RR (95% CI)	RR & 95% CI	χ^2_1 for trend
1	577/909	1.00		
2	593/891	1.07 (0.92–1.24)		
3	690/890	1.25 (1.08–1.45)		25.67
4	716/874	1.34 (1.15–1.55)		$p < 0.001$
5	723/872	1.38 (1.19–1.60)		
			0.75 1.0 1.5 2.0	

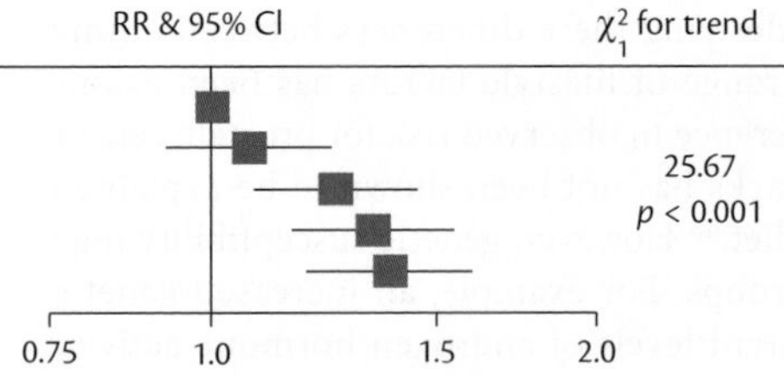

Fig. 6.1.5 Odds ratios for IGF-I and risk of prostate cancer.

Reproduced from Gerald L. Andriole *et al.*, 'Prostate Cancer Screening in the Randomized Prostate, Lung, Colorectal, and Ovarian Cancer Screening Trial: Mortality Results after 13 Years of Follow-up', *Journal of the National Cancer Institute*, Volume 104, Issue 2, pp. 125–32, Copyright © 2012, by permission of Oxford University Press.

prostate cancer (OR 1.38; CI 95% 1.19–1.60; *p* trend <0.001; in the highest vs. lowest quintile)[72] as shown in Figure 6.1.5. The association between higher IGF-I concentration and prostate cancer risk does not differ significantly by cancer stage which supports a role for IGF-I in the progression of prostate cancer, conceivably via established mitogenic and anti-apoptotic mechanisms.[73] There was no significant difference in the association of IGF-I with prostate cancer by grade of disease, although the results suggested that risk might be restricted to low-grade disease,[72] which is consistent with more findings from two further large prospective studies[74]; however, these results should be interpreted with caution due to small numbers of cases in the high-grade subgroup and the potential for misclassification error due to changes in grading practices over time.[11–13]

IGF-I appears to be important for the development of prostate cancer, but more research is needed to clarify the nature of the relationship. Most of the IGF-I circulating in the blood is bound to six binding proteins, but the influence of these binding proteins is not fully understood. There may also be differences in the relationship according to the method of detection of prostate cancer. For example, while the pooled meta-analysis of prospective studies showed a clear association of IGF-I with risk, a large case–control study of approximately 3,000 screen detected cases and 3,000 controls in the United Kingdom found no association between total IGF-I concentration and the risk for PSA-detected prostate cancer.[75] It is possible that the differences between the results of the meta-analysis and those of this study of screen detected prostate cancer[75] reflect a role of IGF-I in disease progression rather than initiation.

Diet

The hypothesis that a Western-style diet may be a risk factor for prostate cancer emerged in the 1970s, as it was evident that the incidence of several cancers (colorectal, breast, endometrial, and prostate) was greater in Western countries than in Asian countries where diets were much lower in animal products, fat, and sugar.[76] There is also some evidence from migrant studies[77–79] that prostate cancer rates in successive migrant generations shift upwards in the direction of the prevailing rates in the host country. However, the absence of significant differences in latent prostate cancer rates between Hawaiian Japanese and those living in Japan, suggested that the role of diet (and other environmental factors) in cancer development may concern cancer progression rather than initiation of disease.[6]

Subsequently, prospective studies have examined the role of diet in risk for prostate cancer but definite associations for specific foods, nutrients, or other dietary factors have not been established. Many studies have examined the possible roles of animal products including meat and dairy foods. The results have generally not implicated meat, but there is a moderate amount of evidence suggesting that high intakes of milk and other dairy foods might increase risk.[80] Further research is needed on this, because high intakes of milk can increase circulating IGF-I,[81] which itself is positively associated with prostate cancer risk (see Fig. 6.1.5). Dairy foods are also a rich source of calcium, and of a branched-chain fatty acid, phytanic acid, which has been suggested as a possible risk factor for prostate cancer, although the sparse data on this fatty acid do not clearly support this hypothesis.[82]

Prospective studies and a few clinical trials have also investigated the possible roles of several micronutrients and other plant constituents. These chemicals have been hypothesized to influence the risk of prostate cancer through various mechanisms, such as through protecting against oxidative damage to the DNA, or improving the integrity of DNA. Overall the results from this area of research are somewhat inconsistent and no convincing associations have yet emerged. For carotenoids, randomized controlled trials have provided substantial, consistent evidence that supplements of β-carotene do not alter the risk for prostate cancer. Lycopene, a carotenoid which is not a vitamin and is primarily obtained from tomatoes, has been associated with a reduced risk in some observational studies, but the data overall do not show a definite association. For B vitamins, the results of observational studies of folic acid are inconclusive and a meta-analysis of randomized controlled trials of folic acid supplements showed no effect on prostate cancer incidence in the folic acid supplement groups.[83] There has been considerable interest in whether vitamin D might have a general anti-cancer effect, but this hypothesis has now been examined for prostate cancer in several observational studies and the results overall are so far null.[84] For vitamin E and selenium, some early studies suggested that there might be protective effects, but a trial has shown no benefit of supplementation with selenium and vitamin E,[85] and another trial demonstrated no effect of vitamin E (or vitamin C) on risk of prostate cancer.[86]

Alcohol

Alcohol is a major cause of many cancers, alongside tobacco, obesity, and chronic infections,[87] with a linear dose-response relation evident for oral, laryngeal, and oesophageal cancers.[88] Alcohol might affect the risk for prostate cancer through various mechanisms, such as the potentially mutagenic metabolite acetaldehyde or through hormonal effects, but extensive evaluation of the association between alcohol intake and risk for prostate cancer by more than 20 cohort studies does not show convincing evidence of a relation.[89]

Tobacco

Tobacco smoking is an established risk factor for many cancers in both men and women, but there is no convincing evidence for an association between tobacco smoking and prostate cancer incidence. In excess of 20 prospective cohorts have examined the association between current smoking and risk for prostate cancer and the majority report a null association. However, there is some evidence to suggest that high tobacco consumption (greater than a pack per day) via smoking increases the risk of death related to prostate cancer.[15,90,91]

Anthropometric measures

Many studies have investigated whether anthropometric factors such as height and body mass index (a measure of fatness) are related to prostate cancer risk. For height, studies are fairly consistent in showing a small positive association, with a slightly higher risk of prostate cancer among taller men than shorter men.[92] There is also some evidence that the increased risk in taller men is greater for high-grade prostate cancer. The mechanism for this association is not known, but it might involve taller men having a larger prostate with more cells at risk for cancer, and/or taller men having greater exposure over their lifetime to growth promoting factors such as IGF-I.[93]

Obesity increases the risk for several types of cancer; for cancers of the breast and endometrium in women, the mechanism is probably increased oestrogen production, whereas for other cancers the mechanism is not clear. For obesity and prostate cancer, individual studies have appeared somewhat inconsistent but meta-analysis has shown that, on average, obesity is very weakly associated with an increased risk of prostate cancer. The risk is, on average, around 10% higher in obese men than in non-obese men[94] and the risk in obese men appears to be particularly for diagnosis with advanced cancer.[95] While the reason for this weak association with risk for advanced cancers is not known, it is possibly partly due to the effect of a later diagnosis in obese men.

Physical activity

High levels of physical activity might reduce cancer risk by various mechanisms, such as hormonal changes, as well as by reducing obesity. For prostate cancer, although there is some evidence suggesting that relatively high levels of physical activity may reduce risk,[96] expert review panels have concluded that the evidence is not sufficient to show a definite effect.[80] Even a modest reduction in risk could be important for public health, therefore more research is required on this topic and on possible mechanisms through which physical activity may alter risk.

Sexual activity and sexually transmitted infections

Sexual activity has been hypothesized to play a role in the development of prostate cancer, but epidemiological data are mainly from case–control studies which are prone to bias, particularly for recall of sexual behaviour in men with prostate cancer and for participation of healthy men as controls.[97] To date, prospective data have not shown any clear association between sexual activity and risk for prostate cancer.[98] As with sexual activity, most of the data on sexually transmitted infections and risk of prostate cancer are from case–control studies and subject to the limitations of this design. While a meta-analysis of 29 case–control studies found a significantly higher risk of prostate cancer for men with a history of any sexually transmitted infection,[99] further investigation is needed on this topic, by using prospectively collected data and blood samples to better understand the nature of the association. So far, studies based on serological evidence of previous infection with agents such as human papillomavirus or Trichomonas vaginalis have not shown clear evidence of an association with prostate cancer risk.[100,101]

Vasectomy

The biological hypothesis for a role of vasectomy in prostate cancer development relates to the possible effects the procedure may have on circulating sex hormone levels, although there is no conclusive evidence from prospective studies to support any significant differences in hormone levels between vasectomized and non-vasectomized men. Although a few studies have shown a higher risk for prostate cancer in men who had had a vasectomy than men who had not,[102,103] the bulk of the evidence has shown no association.[104–106]

Diabetes

Many studies have suggested that, while diabetes has been associated with an increase in the risk for several types of cancer, men with diabetes might have a slightly reduced risk of prostate cancer. In a meta-analysis, the results from 29 cohort studies showed a statistically significant 13% lower risk of prostate cancer in men with diabetes than in non-diabetics.[107] The reason for this association is not clear. It is possible that hormonal changes in diabetes cause a lower risk for prostate cancer, but it is also possible that the association is due to confounding by other factors, such as a lower detection rate in diabetes due to a lower level of PSA.[108]

Conclusions

Prostate cancer risk rises sharply at older ages, is high in men with black African ancestry, and is high in men with a family history of the disease and with a number of inherited genetic markers. None of these factors can be modified, and epidemiological studies of potentially modifiable risk factors for prostate cancer have produced few clear findings. Perhaps the most promising finding is the observation that men with relatively high circulating levels of IGF-I have a moderate increase in risk, although more research is needed on this hormone and related hormonal markers, and on the possibility that dietary composition might affect risk through insulin-like growth factor-I. Factors which are well known to increase the risk for many other types of cancer, and for other serious diseases, such as smoking, excessive alcohol intake, and obesity, appear to have little effect on prostate cancer risk. However, with future research focused on determining the relationships of environmental factors with the risk for clinically significant prostate cancer it is possible that important modifiable risk factors will be discovered.

Further reading

Chan JM, Gann PH, Giovannucci EL. Role of diet in prostate cancer development and progression. *J Clin Oncol* 2005; **23**(32):8152–60.

Hsing AW, Chokkalingam AP. Prostate cancer epidemiology. *Front Biosci* 2006; **11**:1388–413.

Leitzmann MF, Rohrmann S. Risk factors for the onset of prostatic cancer: age, location, and behavioral correlates. *Clin Epidemiol* 2012; **4**(1):1–11.

Sutcliffe S, Platz EA. Inflammation and prostate cancer: A focus on infections. *Curr Urol Rep* 2008; **9**(3):243–9.

Wolk A. Diet, lifestyle and risk of prostate cancer. *Acta Oncol* 2005; **44**(3):277–81.

References

1. Center MM, Jemal A, Lortet-Tieulent J, *et al.* International variation in prostate cancer incidence and mortality rates. *Eur Urol* 2012; **61**(6):1079–92.
2. Breslow N, Chan CW, Dhom G. Latent carcinoma of prostate at autopsy in seven areas. *Int J Cancer* 1977; **20**(5):680–8.
3. Etzioni R, Cha R, Feuer EJ, Davidov O. Asymptornatic incidence and duration of prostate cancer. *Am J Epidemiol* 1998; **148**(8):775–85.
4. Stattin P, Holmberg E, Johansson JE, Holmberg L, Adolfsson J, Hugosson J. Outcomes in localized prostate cancer: National prostate cancer register of Sweden follow-up study. *J Natl Cancer Inst* 2010; **102**(13):950–8.
5. Sánchez-Chapado M, Olmedilla G, Cabeza M, Donat E, Ruiz A. Prevalence of prostate cancer and prostatic intraepithelial neoplasia in Caucasian Mediterranean males: An autopsy study. *Prostate* 2003; **54**(3):238–47.
6. Akazaki K, Stemmermann GN. Comparative study of latent carcinoma of the prostate among Japanese in Japan and Hawaii. *J Natl Cancer Inst* 1973; **50**(5):1137–42.
7. Draisma G, Etzioni R, Tsodikov A, Mariotto A, Wever E, Gulati R, *et al.* Lead time and overdiagnosis in prostate-specific antigen screening: Importance of methods and context. *J Natl Cancer Inst* 2009; **101**(6):374–83.
8. Platz EA, De Marzo AM, Giovannucci E. Prostate cancer association studies: Pitfalls and solutions to cancer misclassification in the PSA era. *J Cell Biochem* 2004; **91**(3):553–71.
9. Schröder FH, Hermanek P, Denis L, Fair WR, Gospodarowicz MK, Pavone-Macaluso M. The TNM classification of prostate cancer. *Prostate* 1992; **20**(Suppl 4):129–38.
10. Gleason DF. Histologic grading of prostate cancer: A perspective. *Hum Pathol* 1992; **23**(3):273–9.
11. Albertsen PC, Hanley JA, Barrows GH, *et al.* Prostate Cancer and the Will Rogers Phenomenon. *J Natl Cancer Inst* 2005; **97**(17):1248–53.
12. Epstein JI, Allsbrook WC Jr, Amin MB, *et al.* The 2005 International Society of Urological Pathology (ISUP) consensus conference on Gleason grading of prostatic carcinoma. *Am J Surg Pathol* 2005; **29**(9):1228–42.
13. Schmidt C. Gleason Scoring System Faces Change and Debate. *J Natl Cancer Inst* 2009; **101**(9):622–9.
14. Mitrou PN, Albanes D, Weinstein SJ, Pietinen P, Taylor PR, Virtamo J, *et al.* A prospective study of dietary calcium, dairy products and prostate cancer risk (Finland). *Int J Cancer* 2007; **120**(11):2466–73.
15. Giovannucci E, Liu Y, Platz EA, Stampfer MJ, Willett WC. Risk factors for prostate cancer incidence and progression in the health professionals follow-up study. *Int J Cancer* 2007; **121**(7):1571–8.
16. Park S, Murphy SP, Wilkens LR, Stram DO, Henderson BE, Kolonel LN. Calcium, vitamin D, and dairy product intake and prostate cancer risk: The multiethnic cohort study. *Am J Epidemiol* 2007; **166**(11):1259–69.
17. Torre LA, Bray F, Siegel RL, Ferlay J, Lortet-Tieulent J, Jemal A. Global cancer statistics, 2012. *CA Cancer J Clin* 2015; **65**(2):87–108.
18. Etzioni R, Penson DF, Legler JM, *et al.* Overdiagnosis due to prostate-specific antigen screening: Lessons from U.S. prostate cancer incidence trends. *J Natl Cancer Inst* 2002; **94**(13):981–90.
19. Hsing AW, Tsao L, Devesa SS. International trends and patterns of prostate cancer incidence and mortality. *Int J Cancer* 2000; **85**(1):60–7.
20. Melia J, Moss S, Johns L. Rates of prostate-specific antigen testing in general practice in England and Wales in asymptomatic and symptomatic patients: A cross-sectional study. *BJU Int* 2004; **94**(1):51–6.
21. Sirovich BE, Schwartz LM, Woloshin S. Screening Men for Prostate and Colorectal Cancer in the United States: Does Practice Reflect the Evidence? J Am Med Assoc 2003; **289**(11):1414–20.
22. Beaulac JA, Fry RN, Onysko J. Lifetime and prostate specific antigen (PSA) screening of men for prostate cancer in Canada. *Can J Public Health* 2006; **97**(3):171–6.
23. Schröder FH, Hugosson J, Roobol MJ, *et al.* Screening and prostate-cancer mortality in a randomized european study. *New Engl J Med* 2009; **360**(13):1320–8.
24. Schröder FH, Hugosson J, Roobol MJ, *et al.* Prostate-cancer mortality at 11 years of follow-up. *New Engl J Med* 2012; **366**(11):981–990.
25. Andriole GL, Levin DL, Crawford ED, *et al.* Prostate cancer screening in the Prostate, Lung, Colorectal and Ovarian (PLCO) Cancer Screening Trial: Findings from the initial screening round of a randomized trial. *J Natl Cancer Inst* 2005; **97**(6):433–8.
26. Baade PD, Youlden DR, Krnjacki LJ. International epidemiology of prostate cancer: Geographical distribution and secular trends. *Mol Nutr Food Res* 2009; **53**(2):171–84.
27. Hankey BF, Feuer EJ, Clegg LX, *et al.* Cancer surveillance series: Interpreting trends in prostate cancer—Part I: Evidence of the effects of screening in prostate cancer incidence, mortality, and survival rates. *J Natl Cancer Inst* 1999; **91**(12):1017–24.
28. Collin M, Martin RM, Metcalfe C, *et al.* Prostate-cancer mortality in the USA and UK in 1975-2004: an ecological study. *Lancet Oncol* 2008; **9**(5):445–52.
29. Shavers VL, Brown ML. Racial and ethnic disparities in the receipt of cancer treatment. *J Natl Cancer Inst* 2002; **94**(5):334–57.
30. Ward E, Jemal A, Cokkinides V, *et al.* Cancer disparities by race/ethnicity and socioeconomic status. *CA Cancer J Clin* 2004; **54**(2):78–93.
31. Ferlay J, Bray B, Pisani P, and Parkin DM. GLOBOCAN 2002: Cancer Incidence, Mortality and Prevalence Worldwide IARC CancerBase No. 5. version 2.0, IARCPress, Lyon, 2004. 2004; Available at: http://www-dep.iarc.fr/, 2009 [Online].
32. Ben-Shlomo Y, Evans S, Ibrahim F, *et al.* The Risk of Prostate Cancer amongst Black Men in the United Kingdom: The PROCESS Cohort Study. *Eur Urol* 2008; **53**(1):99–105.
33. Parkin DM, Bray F, Ferlay J, Pisani P. Global cancer statistics, 2002. *CA Cancer J Clin* 2005; **55**(2):74–108.
34. Cannon L, Bishop DT, Skolnick M, Hunt S, Lyon JL, Smart CR. Genetic epidemiology of prostate cancer in the Utah Mormon genealogy. *Cancer Surv* 1982; **1**:47–69.
35. Steinberg GD, Carter BS, Beaty TH, Childs B, Walsh PC. Family history and the risk of prostate cancer. *Prostate* 1990; **17**(4):337–47.
36. Carter BS, Beaty TH, Steinberg GD, Childs B, Walsh PC. Mendelian inheritance of familial prostate cancer. *Proc Natl Acad Sci U S A* 1992; **89**(8):3367–71.
37. Lichtenstein P, Holm NV, Verkasalo PK, *et al.* Environmental and heritable factors in the causation of cancer: Analyses of cohorts of twins from Sweden, Denmark, and Finland. *New Engl J Med* 2000; **343**(2):78–85.
38. Kiciński M, Vangronsveld J, Nawrot TS. An epidemiological reappraisal of the familial aggregation of prostate cancer: A meta-analysis. *PLoS ONE* 2011; **6**(10):e2713.
39. Johns LE, Houlston RS. A systematic review and meta-analysis of familial prostate cancer risk. *BJU Int* 2003; **91**(9):789–94.
40. Bruner DW, Moore D, Parlanti A, Dorgan J, Engstrom P. Relative risk of prostate cancer for men with affected relatives: Systematic review and meta-analysis. *Int J Cancer* 2003; **107**(5):797–803.
41. Zeegers MPA, Jellema A, Ostrer H. Empiric risk of prostate carcinoma for relatives of patients with prostate carcinoma. *Cancer* 2003; **97**(8):1894–903.

42. Ferlay J, Shin HR, Bray F, Forman D, Mathers C, Parkin DM. GLOBOCAN 2008 v1.2, Cancer Incidence and Mortality Worldwide: IARC CancerBase No. 10 [Internet]. Lyon, France: International Agency for Research on Cancer; 2010. Available at: http://globocan.iarc.fr, accessed on 23/02/2012 [Online].
43. Jemal A, Center MM, DeSantis C, Ward EM. Global patterns of cancer incidence and mortality rates and trends. *Cancer Epidemiol Biomarkers Prev* 2010; **19**(8):1893–907.
44. Jemal A, Siegel R, Xu J, Ward E. Cancer statistics, 2010. *CA Cancer J Clin* 2010; **60**(5):277–300.
45. Etzioni R, Berry KM, Legler JM, Shaw P. Prostate-specific antigen testing in black and white men: An analysis of medicare claims from 1991–1998. *Urology* 2002; **59**(2):251–5.
46. Coleman MP, Quaresma M, Berrino F, *et al.* Cancer survival in five continents: a worldwide population-based study (CONCORD). *Lancet Oncol* 2008; **9**(8):730–56.
47. Mordukhovich I, Reiter PL, Backes DM, *et al.* A review of African American-white differences in risk factors for cancer: Prostate cancer. *Cancer Causes Control* 2011; **22**(3):341–57.
48. Haiman CA, Chen GK, Blot WJ, Strom SS, Berndt SI, Kittles RA, *et al.* Genome-wide association study of prostate cancer in men of African ancestry identifies a susceptibility locus at 17q21. *Nat Genet* 2011; **43**(6):570–3.
49. Takata R, Akamatsu S, Kubo M, *et al.* Genome-wide association study identifies five new susceptibility loci for prostate cancer in the Japanese population. *Nat Genet* 2010; **42**(9):751–4.
50. Bratt O, Garmo H, Adolfsson J, *et al.* Effects of prostate-specific antigen testing on familial prostate cancer risk estimates. *J Natl Cancer Inst* 2010; **102**(17):1336–43.
51. Goh CL, Schumacher FR, Easton D, *et al.* Genetic variants associated with predisposition to prostate cancer and potential clinical implications. *J Intern Med (GBR)* 2012; **271**(4):353–65.
52. Kote-Jarai Z, Leongamornlert D, Saunders E, *et al.* BRCA2 is a moderate penetrance gene contributing to young-onset prostate cancer: Implications for genetic testing in prostate cancer patients. *Br J Cancer* 2011; **105**(8):1230–4.
53. Benafif S, Eeles R. Genetic predisposition to prostate cancer. *Br Med Bull* 2016; **120**(1):75–89.
54. Liu H, Wang B, Han C. Meta-analysis of genome-wide and replication association studies on prostate cancer. *Prostate* 2011; **71**(2):209–24.
55. Al Olama AA, Kote-Jarai Z, Giles GG, *et al.* Multiple loci on 8q24 associated with prostate cancer susceptibility. *Nat Genet* 2009; **41**(10):1058–60.
56. Eeles RA, Kote-Jarai Z, Giles GG, *et al.* Multiple newly identified loci associated with prostate cancer susceptibility. *Nat Genet* 2008; **40**(3):316–21.
57. Yeager M, Orr N, Hayes RB, *et al.* Genome-wide association study of prostate cancer identifies a second risk locus at 8q24. *Nat Genet* 2007; **39**(5):645–9.
58. Gudmundsson J, Sulem P, Gudbjartsson DF, *et al.* Genome-wide association and replication studies identify four variants associated with prostate cancer susceptibility. *Nat Genet* 2009; **41**(10):1122–6.
59. Gudmundsson J, Sulem P, Manolescu A, *et al.* Genome-wide association study identifies a second prostate cancer susceptibility variant at 8q24. *Nat Genet* 2007; **39**(5):631–7.
60. Gudmundsson J, Sulem P, Rafnar T, *et al.* Common sequence variants on 2p15 and Xp11.22 confer susceptibility to prostate cancer. *Nat Genet* 2008; **40**(3):281–3.
61. Whitaker HC, Kote-Jarai Z, Ross-Adams H, *et al.* The rs10993994 risk allele for prostate cancer results in clinically relevant changes in microseminoprotein-beta expression in tissue and urine. *PLoS One* 2010; **5**(10):e13363.
62. Eeles RA, Kote-Jarai Z, Al Olama AA, *et al.* Identification of seven new prostate cancer susceptibility loci through a genome-wide association study. *Nat Genet* 2009; **41**(10):1116–21.
63. Manolio TA, Collins FS, Cox NJ, *et al.* Finding the missing heritability of complex diseases. *Nature* 2009; **461**(7265):747–53.
64. Marker PC, Donjacour AA, Dahiya R, Cunha GR. Hormonal, cellular, and molecular control of prostatic development. *Dev Biol* 2003; **253**(2):165–74.
65. Thompson IM, Goodman PJ, Tangen CM, *et al.* The influence of finasteride on the development of prostate cancer. *New Engl J Med* 2003; **349**(3):215–24.
66. Andriole GL, Bostwick DG, Brawley OW, *et al.* Effect of dutasteride on the risk of prostate cancer. *New Engl J Med* 2010; **362**(13):1192–202.
67. Roddam AW, Allen NE, Appleby P, Key TJ. Endogenous sex hormones and prostate cancer: A collaborative analysis of 18 prospective studies. *J Nat Cancer Inst* 2008; **100**(3):170–83.
68. Ntais C, Polycarpou A, Ioannidis JPA. Association of the CYP17 gene polymorphism with the risk of prostate cancer: A meta-analysis. *Cancer Epidemiol Biomarkers Prev* 2003; **12**(2):120–6.
69. Chu LW, Reichardt JKV, Hsing AW. Androgens and the molecular epidemiology of prostate cancer. *Curr Opin Endocrinol Diabetes Obes* 2008; **15**(3):261–70.
70. Lindström S, Ma J, Altshuler D, Giovannucci E, Riboli E, Albanes D, *et al.* A large study of Androgen Receptor germline variants and their relation to sex hormone levels and prostate cancer risk. results from the National Cancer Institute Breast and Prostate Cancer Cohort Consortium. *J Clin Endocrinol Metab* 2010; **95**(9):E121–7.
71. Jones JI, Clemmons DR. Insulin-like growth factors and their binding proteins: Biological actions. *Endocr Rev* 1995; **16**(1):3–34.
72. Roddam AW, Allen NE, Appleby P, *et al.* Insulin-like growth factors, their binding proteins, and prostate cancer risk: Analysis of individual patient data from 12 prospective studies. *Ann Intern Med* 2008; **149**(7):461–71.
73. Grimberg A. Mechanisms by which IGF-I may promote cancer. *Cancer Biol Ther* 2003; **2**(6):630–5.
74. Nimptsch K, Platz EA, Pollak MN, *et al.* Plasma insulin-like growth factor 1 is positively associated with low-grade prostate cancer in the Health Professionals Follow-up Study 1993-2004. *Int J Cancer* 2011; **128**(3):660–7.
75. Rowlands MA, Holly JM, Gunnell D, *et al.* Circulating insulin-like growth factors and igf-binding proteins in psa-detected prostate cancer: The Large Case-Control Study ProtecT. *Cancer Res* 2012; **72**(2):503–15.
76. Armstrong B, Doll R. Environmental factors and cancer incidence and mortality in different countries, with special reference to dietary practices. *Int J Cancer* 1975; **15**(4):617–31.
77. Haenszel W, Kurihara M. Studies of Japanese migrants. I. Mortality from cancer and other diseases among Japanese in the United States. *J Natl Cancer Inst* 1968; **40**(1):43–68.
78. Whittemore AS, Kolonel LN, Wu AH, *et al.* Prostate cancer in relation to diet, physical activity, and body size in blacks, whites, and asians in the United States and Canada. *J Natl Cancer Inst* 1995; **87**(9):652–61.
79. Shimizu H, Ross RK, Bernstein L, Yatani R, Henderson BE, Mack TM. Cancers of the prostate and breast among Japanese and white immigrants in Los Angeles County. *Br J Cancer* 1991; **63**(6):963–66.
80. World Cancer Research Fund/American Institute for Cancer Research. *Food, Nutrition, Physical Activity and the Prevention of Cancer: A Global Perspective,* 1st edition. Washington, WA: American Institute for Cancer Research, 2007.
81. Crowe FL, Key TJ, Allen NE, *et al.* The association between diet and serum concentrations of IGF-I, IGFBP-1, IGFBP-2, and IGFBP-3 in the European prospective investigation into cancer and nutrition. *Cancer Epidemiol Biomarkers Prev* 2009; **18**(5):1333–40.
82. Price AJ, Allen NE, Appleby PN, *et al.* Plasma phytanic acid concentration and risk of prostate cancer: Results from the European prospective investigation into cancer and nutrition. *Am J Clin Nutr* 2010; **91**(6):1769–76.
83. Vollset SE, Clarke R, Lewington S, *et al.* Effects of folic acid supplementation on overall and site-specific cancer incidence during the randomised trials: Meta-analyses of data on 50 000 individuals. *Lancet* 2013; **381**(9871):1029–36.

84. Gilbert R, Martin RM, Beynon R, *et al.* Associations of circulating and dietary vitamin D with prostate cancer risk: A systematic review and dose-response meta-analysis. *Cancer Causes Control* 2011; **22**(3):319–40.
85. Lippman SM, Klein EA, Goodman PJ, *et al.* Effect of selenium and vitamin E on risk of prostate cancer and other cancers: The selenium and vitamin E cancer prevention trial (SELECT). *J Am Med Assoc* 2009; **301**(1):39–51.
86. Gaziano JM, Glynn RJ, Christen WG, *et al.* Vitamins E and C in the prevention of prostate and total cancer in men: The physicians' health study II randomized controlled trial. *J Am Med Assoc* 2009; **301**(1):52–62.
87. Boffetta P, Hashibe M. Alcohol and cancer. *Lancet Oncol* 2006; **7**(2):149–56.
88. Baan R, Straif K, Grosse Y, *et al.* Carcinogenicity of alcoholic beverages. *Lancet Oncol* 2007; **8**(4):292–3.
89. Leitzmann MF, Rohrmann S. Risk factors for the onset of prostatic cancer: Age, location, and behavioral correlates. *Clin Epidemiol* 2012; **4**(1):1–11.
90. Hsing AW, McLaughlin JK, Schuman LM, *et al.* Diet, tobacco use, and fatal prostate cancer: Results from the Lutheran Brotherhood Cohort study. *Cancer Res* 1990; **50**(21):6836–40.
91. Rohrmann S, Linseisen J, Allen N, *et al.* Smoking and the risk of prostate cancer in the European Prospective Investigation into Cancer and Nutrition. *Br J Cancer* 2012; **108**(3):708–14.
92. Zuccolo L, Harris R, Gunnell D, *et al.* Height and prostate cancer risk: A large nested case-control study (ProtecT) and meta-analysis. *Cancer Epidemiol Biomarkers Prev* 2008; **17**(9):2325–36.
93. Farwell WR, Lourenco C, Holmberg E, *et al.* The association between height and prostate cancer grade in the Early Stage Prostate Cancer Cohort Study. *Cancer Causes Control* 2011; **22**(10):1453–9.
94. MacInnis RJ, English DR. Body size and composition and prostate cancer risk: Systematic review and meta-regression analysis. *Cancer Causes Control* 2006; **17**(8):989–1003.
95. Discacciati A, Orsini N, Wolk A. Body mass index and incidence of localized and advanced prostate cancer-a dose-response meta-analysis of prospective studies. *Ann Oncol* 2012; **23**(7):1665–71.
96. Orsini N, Bellocco R, Bottai M, *et al.* A prospective study of lifetime physical activity and prostate cancer incidence and mortality. *Br J Cancer* 2009; **101**(11):1932–8.
97. Dennis LK, Dawson DV. Meta-analysis of measures of sexual activity and prostate cancer. *Epidemiology* 2002; **13**(1):72–9.
98. Leitzmann MF, Platz EA, Stampfer MJ, Willett WC, Giovannucci E. Ejaculation frequency and subsequent risk of prostate cancer. *J Am Med Assoc* 2004; **291**(13):1578–86.
99. Taylor ML, Mainous AG III, Wells BJ. Prostate cancer and sexually transmitted diseases: A meta-analysis. *Fam Med* 2005; **37**(7):506–12.
100. Stcliffe S, Alderete JF, Till C, *et al.* Trichomonosis and subsequent risk of prostate cancer in the Prostate Cancer Prevention Trial. *Int J Cancer* 2009; **124**(9):2082–7.
101. Sutcliffe S, Viscidi RP, Till C, *et al.* Human papillomavirus types 16, 18, and 31 serostatus and prostate cancer risk in the prostate cancer prevention trial. *Cancer Epidemiol Biomarkers Prev* 2010; **19**(2):614–8.
102. Holt SK, Salinas CA, Stanford JL. Vasectomy and the risk of prostate cancer. *J Urol* 2008; **180**(6):2565–8.
103. Siddiqui MM, Wilson KM, Epstein MM, *et al.* Vasectomy and risk of aggressive prostate cancer: A 24-year follow-up study. *J Clin Oncol* 2014; **32**(27):3033–8.
104. Smith Byrne K, Castano JM, Chirlaque MD, *et al.* Vasectomy and prostate cancer risk in the European Prospective Investigation into Cancer and Nutrition. *J Clin Oncol* 2017; in press.
105. Dennis LK, Dawson DV, Resnick MI. Vasectomy and the risk of prostate cancer: A meta-analysis examining vasectomy status, age at vasectomy, and time since vasectomy. *Prostate Cancer Prostatic Dis* 2002; **5**(3):193–203.
106. Jacobs EJ, Anderson RL, Stevens VL, Newton CC, Gansler T, Gapstur SM. Vasectomy and prostate cancer incidence and mortality in a large US Cohort. *J Clin Oncol* 2016; **34**(32):3880–5.
107. Bansal D, Bhansali A, Kapil G, Undela K, Tiwari P. Type 2 diabetes and risk of prostate cancer: a meta-analysis of observational studies. *Prostate Cancer Prostatic Dis* 2012; **16**(2):151–8, S1.
108. Pierce BL. Why are diabetics at reduced risk for prostate cancer? A review of the epidemiologic evidence. *Urol Oncol Semin Orig Invest* 2012; **30**(5):735–43.

CHAPTER 6.2

Molecular biology of prostate cancer

Ines Teles Alves, Jan Trapman, and Guido Jenster

Introduction to the molecular basis of cancer

The functional unit of life is the cell and the genetic information is transferred to daughter cells via its DNA. This is also true in tumours, which derive from an abnormal cell by accumulated DNA mutations, transferring these mutations to progeny cells. Cancer is a disease of DNA and RNA. Each human cell contains about two times 3.2 billion base pairs, divided over the 22 chromosome pairs and two X chromosomes in females or X, Y in males. About 30,000 genes encoded by the human genome are responsible for the various cellular functions, mainly executed by the proteins encoded by the ~21,000 protein coding genes.[1] About 40% of the genome consists of genes, but only ~1.5% of the genome (the exons) will be transcribed to mRNAs and subsequently translated to proteins. It is unlikely that a random single change in a base pair will influence the properties of the host cell. The chance of effective mutations in the right combination of genes needed for tumour initiation is extremely small. However, with a lifelong accumulation of DNA damage and 10–50 billion cells in our body, in the long term the development of a tumour seems inevitable.

There are various types of DNA changes (mutations) that affect the function or expression of genes:

- *Deletion.* Loss of one copy of the DNA (in one copy of a chromosome pair) is referred to as loss of heterozygosity (heterozygosity is the presence of two different copies of a genomic region in the two chromosomes). Complete loss of two copies of a specific chromosomal region is called a homozygous deletion.
- *Amplifications.* This can vary between short or long duplications of a chromosomal region to tens of additional copies (high-level amplification).
- *Translocations* refer to exchange of DNA fragments within or between chromosomes.
- *Insertions.* Additional base pairs can be inserted due to replication mistakes, but also viral DNA or genomic integration of amplified DNA are covered by this term.
- *Base pair changes* are defined when one or more bases are different without loss or gain. If the same base pair change is observed in >1% among normal healthy individuals, it is called a common variant single nucleotide polymorphism (SNP). If it is less frequent, it is named a rare variant. The change is called a mutation if it is unique for the genome of a tumour, and not present in the DNA from healthy cells of the same individual.

The type of DNA change can have specific effects on the properties of the mutated genes. The genes that cause cancer are classically divided into two types:

- *Oncogenes* are genes generally encoding tumour growth stimulating proteins. A single mutation in one gene copy is enough to activate its oncogenic function. Amplifications are typically associated with oncogenes, but base pair changes and translocations can also cause activated oncogenes or oncogenic fusion genes.
- *Tumour suppressor genes* generally encode proteins that inhibit tumour growth. In order to stop full activity of inhibitory functions, it is almost always necessary to inactivate both gene copies. The type of DNA change typical for tumour suppressor genes is DNA deletion. Often, one copy is lost by deletion, while the second copy might be inactivated by base pair changes. Genetic alterations that predispose to tumour development are found in some hereditary cancer syndromes such as Li-Fraumeni syndrome (P53 mutations), hereditary breast and ovarian cancer syndrome (*BCRA1/2* mutations), Cowden disease (*PTEN* mutations), and Von Hippel-Lindau disease (*VHL* mutations). In these syndromes, one copy of an inactivated tumour suppressor gene is present in the genome of all cells (germline) and therefore inherited, greatly increasing the chance of developing cancer.

The DNA changes described above are permanent alterations. However, chemical base pair modification can also occur and although reversible, can be quite stable and copied from parent to daughter cell (known as epigenetic alterations). An important epigenetic modification associated with cancer is DNA methylation. The frequent addition of a methyl group to cytosine in cytosine-guanine rich regions (referred to as CpG islands) located in promoter regions, will typically inhibit transcription of these genes.[2,3] DNA methylation is therefore an alternative mechanism to turn off tumour suppressor genes.

Hallmarks of cancer

Overcoming a series of cellular and bodily processes is thought to be necessary for the progression from a normal cell to a cancer cell. These may arise through genetic (mutation etc.) or epigenetic (e.g. DNA methylation, histone modification) means and include[4]:

- Self-sufficiency in growth signals
- Insensitivity to anti-growth signals
- Resistance to cell death
- Tissue invasion and metastases

- Limitless potential to replicate
- Inducing angiogenesis
- Evading the immune system

Late stage tumours have acquired all of these hallmarks. The methods used to acquire each hallmark will vary between cancers and in individuals, and reflect inherited or acquired pro-carcinogenic events and individual features for each cancer. The pathway of acquiring these hallmarks is often called the Vogelstein model, after one of the first proponents (Fig. 6.2.1).[5] Almost all cells in our body are fully differentiated, and specialized to perform a limited number of tasks. These terminally differentiated cells have usually lost their potential to grow and so are unlikely to be the cells from which tumours develop. Tissue stem cells and precursor cells (to the differentiated mature cells) possess the capacity to divide and may be the origin of cancer. Except for the sporadic stem cells, all other cell types can only divide about 10–30 times when activated. During each DNA replication cycle, the chromosome ends (telomeres) are shortened. Only stem cells and cancer cells can repair this by expressing the enzyme telomerase. In the absence of support factors, normal cells will stop dividing and become dormant (often by a process referred to as senescence) before they eventually die, in response to shortening telomeres. Many processes in the cell including the cell cycle, DNA damage response, protein expression, and energy metabolism include checkpoints to monitor potential harmful changes. Upon a challenge (e.g. DNA damage, too many incorrectly folded proteins), normal cells halt ongoing processes (stop dividing, stop transcription and translation, and so on) to start repair mechanisms, and if repair is impossible, initiate a programmed cell death programme (apoptosis). Through random mutation and selection, cancer cells have typically mutated genes involved in these checkpoints to circumvent senescence and avoid apoptosis.

In prostate cancer (PCa), many common gene mutations are directly linked to adaptation of the hallmarks (Fig. 6.2.1). The androgen receptor (AR) pathway becomes and remains the major growth stimulatory and anti-apoptotic cascade, partly by regulating the *TMPRSS2-ERG* fusion gene. Self-sufficient growth and resistance to cell death is further accomplished by loss of the tumour suppressor *PTEN* and amplification of the *c-MYC* oncogene. The tumour suppressor P53 can be altered to eliminate cell cycle arrest and prevent apoptosis.[6]

Major signalling pathways affected in prostate cancer

Major pathways targeted by mutations in PCa

In years, the knowledge of molecular mechanisms of prostate cancer (PCa) growth and the role of individual genes and signalling pathways in this process has rapidly increased. This knowledge is crucial for improvement of diagnosis and prognosis, and to offer patients more specific therapies. Like other cancers, PCa development and progressive growth is driven by an accumulation of variable numbers of genetic alterations in the cancer cell genome (Fig. 6.2.1).[7] Moreover, it is becoming increasingly clear that epigenetic events, including the microenvironment of tumours, contribute substantially to regulation of tumour growth.

Approximately 5% of PCa cases have a familial history. Until it was hardly possible to identify the hereditary alterations in the DNA, which are associated with tumour development. However, novel molecular technologies can now be instrumental to investigate this problem. Genetically, sporadic PCa shows a characteristic pattern of chromosomal alterations. Most frequent changes are loss of the complete, or part of the short arm of chromosome 8 (8p), and losses of large regions of chromosome arms 6q, 13q, and 16q. Additionally, in late-stage PCa amplification of 8q is frequently observed. In the affected chromosomal regions, many candidate tumour suppressor genes and oncogenes are located. In most cases, it is difficult to pinpoint exactly which of the genes or combination of genes are most important in tumour

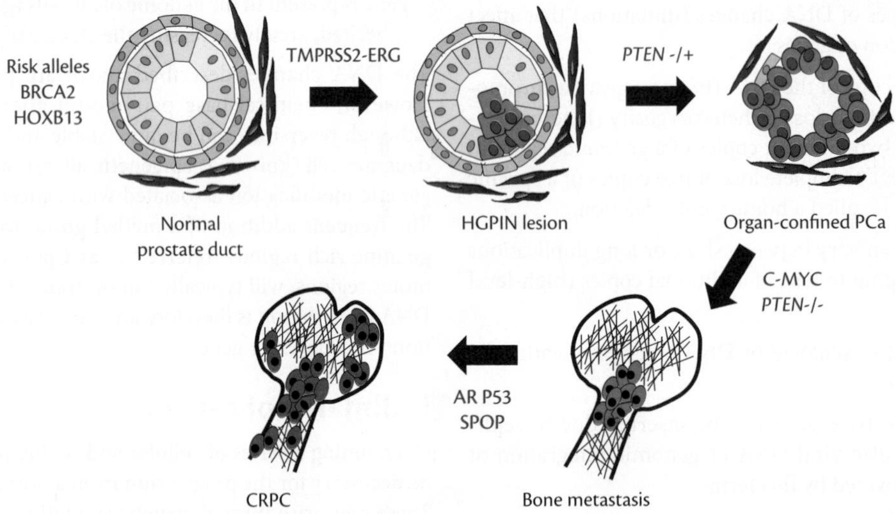

Fig. 6.2.1 Evolution of prostate cancer. The development of high-grade prostatic intraepithelial neoplasia (HGPIN) and subsequent organ-confined prostate cancer is driven by genomic mutations. The presence of germline risk alleles such as *BRCA1/2* and gene polymorphisms increase the chance of developing prostate cancer. One of the first genomic events observed in the cancer cells is the fusion between *TMPRSS2* and *ERG* in about 50% of all tumours. Subsequent mutations include the loss of one *PTEN* allele and amplification of c-MYC on chromosome 8q24. In late stage tumours, the second *PTEN* allele is lost and P53 mutations are observed. After hormone therapy, androgen receptor (AR) amplification and mutations are observed in castration-resistant prostate cancer (CRPC). Recently, sequencing efforts identified *SPOP* as a mutated gene in late-stage cancers.

development, but it is well established that overexpression of *c-MYC* oncogene on 8q is involved in a large percentage of late stage prostate cancers.

Additional to large chromosomal regions, three small genomic regions on 10q, 21q, and Xq, respectively, are frequently altered in PCa. Here, the genes important in PCa can easily be identified. These are the tumour suppressor gene *PTEN*, the *TMPRSS2-ERG* fusion gene, and the AR.

In early stage PCa, one copy of *PTEN* is frequently lost; in late-stage cancer both copies of the gene can be inactivated. *PTEN* is a phospholipid phosphatase that counteracts phosphoinositol-3-kinase (PI3K).[8] PI3K is activated by receptor tyrosine kinases, and following PI3K activation the phospholipid PIP2 can be modified to PIP3. *PTEN* catalyses the opposite conversion, PIP3 to PIP2. High concentrations of PIP3 in the cell lead to activation of the kinase AKT. Activation of this important PI3K/AKT signalling pathway affects many molecular and biological processes in the cell, including protein synthesis, cell proliferation, apoptosis, polarity, and metabolism. The PI3K/AKT pathway cannot only be activated by *PTEN* inactivation, but also by direct activation of PI3K or AKT. Remarkably, although occurring frequently in other tumour types, these alterations are rare in PCa (Fig. 6.2.2).

The androgen receptor pathway in prostate cancer

Dihydrotestosterone (DHT) is essential for development, maintenance of the structure, and function of the prostate. DHT is synthesized in the prostate by metabolism of testosterone (T) by the enzyme 5-alpha-reductase. DHT mediates its function by activation of the AR, a member of the family of nuclear receptors, which are ligand-dependent transcription factors. Upon binding of DHT the androgen receptor (AR) translocates from the cytoplasm to the nucleus. There it modulates gene expression by binding to specific DNA sequences, androgen response elements, in the promoter/enhancer regions of target genes (Fig. 6.2.2).

In the normal prostate, AR expression is high in the luminal epithelial cells and absent in the basal epithelial cells. In stromal cells, the level of AR expression is variable. It is generally accepted that AR in stromal cells is most important during prostate development, and AR in luminal cells for prostate function. Hundreds or even thousands of genes in the prostate are regulated by the activated AR. PSA (prostate-specific antigen; official symbol KLK3), which is exclusively expressed in the luminal epithelial cells, is considered as the prototype of a tightly androgen-regulated gene. Castration has a dramatic effect on the normal prostate and results not only in modified gene expression, but also in enhanced apoptosis.

The *TMPRSS2-ERG* gene fusions in prostate cancer

The AR is vital for the development and function of the normal prostate and for growth of PCa. For a long time, it was unknown which AR-regulated genes were involved in tumour growth. In 2005, Tomlins *et al.* showed the presence of unique recurrent gene fusions between the *TMPRSS2* gene and *ETS* family members *ERG* and ETV1 in prostate cancer.[9] Due to the gene fusion, the androgen-regulated *TMPRSS2* now controls the expression of the *ERG* or *ETV1* oncogene, having a large impact on androgen-dependent growth and survival of prostate cancer.

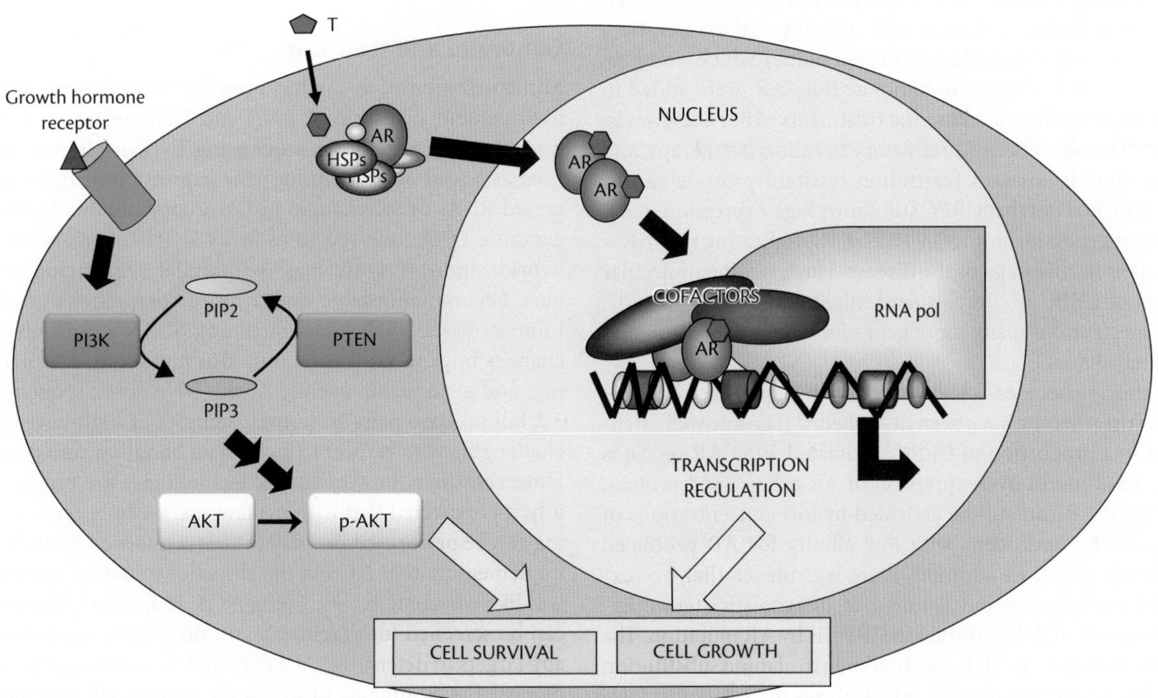

Fig. 6.2.2 The *PTEN/PI3K/AKT* and AR pathways. Prostate cancer (PCa) development and progression is driven by many different pathways of which two play a dominant role. The AR is activated by the androgens testosterone (T) and dihydrotestosterone, after which the AR binds as a dimer to promoter and enhancer regions of target genes. One of the target genes is *TMPRSS2*, which is frequently fused to *ERG* in PCa, thereby regulating the *ERG* oncogene in an androgen-dependent manner. The *PTEN/PI3K/AKT* pathway is activated by various growth factors. At the inner cell membrane, activated *PI3K* eventually results in phosphorylation and activation of *AKT* (*p-AKT*). Loss of *PTEN* results in an increased and persistent activation of *AKT*. Both cascades support cell survival and cell growth and mutations (frequent *PTEN* loss, rare *PI3K* and *AKT* mutations, AR amplification and mutations, *TMPRSS2-ERG* fusion) affect these pathways frequently.

TMPRSS2 and *ERG* are located on chromosome 21 approximately 3 Mb apart and have the same gene orientation. Mostly, *TMPRSS2–ERG* fusions are frequently accompanied by loss of the entire chromosome 21 sequence between *TMPRSS2* and *ERG* genes (interstitial deletion).[10] *TMPRSS2-ERG* has been found as the most common type of *ETS* gene fusion in PCa, with a frequency of approximately 50% across more than 1,500 organ-confined PCa samples.[11] In the PCa precursor lesion, high-grade prostatic intraepithelial neoplasia (HGPIN), the frequency was approximately 20%.[12,13] Additional *ETS* gene fusions have subsequently been identified involving not only *ERG* and *ETV1* but also *ETV4*,[14] *ETV5*,[15] and *FLI1*.[16] The frequency of these variants is much lower compared to *ERG* rearrangements, but still accounts for 2–5% of all ETS gene fusions found in PCa. In the normal situation, members of the *ETS* transcription factor family bind specific DNA sequences regulating the expression of nearby genes. They are believed to play a role in self-renewal-associated proliferation and normal morphogenesis.[17,18] The presence of *ETS* gene rearrangements in precursor lesions such as HGPIN suggests that *ETS* gene fusions have a causal role in the initial steps of PCa development.[19] Still, it is not yet understood how *ETS* gene rearrangements are indeed capable of initiating prostate tumorigenesis, whereas its role in mediating progression towards more aggressive disease is well accepted.[20,21]

Therapeutic targeting the androgen receptor pathway

More than 70 years ago, the beneficial effect of androgen ablation by castration on advanced PCa was described.[22] Medical or surgical castration, aiming at inhibition of T and DHT production, has been the treatment of choice of metastatic PCa. Additional to castration, antiandrogens (e.g. flutamide and bicalutamide) which compete with DHT for AR binding, but do not activate AR, were added to the large panel of different endocrine treatments. After a few years, essentially all tumours become refractory to endocrine therapy, and a resistant tumour emerges (castration-resistant prostate cancer (CRPC)). It turned out that CRPC still shows high expression of AR and AR target genes, including *TMPSS2-ERG*, indicating that AR is still important in this stage of the disease. However, the molecular mechanism of CRPC is complex, and might additionally to *ERG*, include a spectrum of many more genes for which the AR regulation has been altered.[23]

During the last decades, a wide variety of mechanisms of escape from endocrine therapy have been described.[24] It is now well established that in a proportion of CRPC (estimated 30%) AR on Xq is amplified, resulting in overexpression of AR mRNA and protein. Overexpressed AR can still be activated by low concentrations of androgens, or by androgens with low affinity for AR produced by the adrenal gland. In addition, there is evidence that overexpressed AR can function independent of an agonistic steroid ligand. Another way of AR activation in CRPC is by AR mutation. The best-known mutation in AR is the threonine to alanine substitution in the AR ligand-binding domain, which allows the antagonist OH-Flutamide to display agonistic activity. More it was postulated that in CRPC constitutive active AR variants lacking the ligand-binding domain are present and can modify AR regulated gene expression. Moreover, evidence was provided that CRPC cells itself are able to synthesize T and DHT or are able to convert adrenal androgens to DHT.

In years, two novel endocrine therapies have been approved for CRPC treatment.[25] One of the compounds marketed, enzalutamide or MDV3100, is related to more classical antiandrogens. Like other antiandrogens, it blocks AR function by competing with DHT for AR binding. However, enzalutamide also delays nuclear transport of AR. Although enzalutamide has been approved for treatment of CRPC patients following chemotherapy with docetaxel, at the moment there is no reason to believe that it is not effective in earlier stages of PCa. The second novel therapeutic compound is abiraterone acetate. This molecule inhibits the function of CYP17A1, a key enzyme of the DHT synthesis pathway. Abiraterone acetate not only inhibits T synthesis in the testis but also the synthesis of adrenal androgens. Abiraterone acetate is beneficial in late-stage PCa patients resistant to docetaxel therapy. Abiraterone acetate is given in combination with prednisone to reduce its side effects, which seem more severe than for enzalutamide.

Technology developments and emerging markers

Increasing knowledge of the molecular biology of PCa and breakthroughs in various technologies form the basis of the discovery of novel markers and therapy targets. The technologies advanced tremendously in the ability to measure more of the DNA, RNA, and protein content of each individual tumour (high-content) and allow analysis of more samples at the same time (high-throughput). These type of studies are referred to as '-omics'; for DNA, RNA, and protein analyses, genomics, transcriptomics, and proteomics, respectively.

Genomics and transcriptomics

Miniaturization of assays has been the main driving force for the high-content detection of RNA and DNA using array technologies and next generation sequencing (NGS). Microarrays can be used as a read-out system for gene expression by hybridizing processed RNAs or for changes in DNA copy number by hybridizing genomic DNA, referred to as array CGH (comparative genomic hybridization).[26] Only massive parallel sequencing techniques have become affordable and a more comprehensive alternative to array-based analyses. Sequencing of RNA not only identifies changes in gene expression, but also mutations, alternative splicing, and gene fusion events. At the DNA level, sequencing of all 3.2 billion base pairs in human samples at high coverage is still challenging with respect to costs, data handling, and processing.[27] However, since the sequencing technologies are progressing rapidly, it is expected that within a few years, whole genome sequencing can be performed in a day for a few hundred pounds. If so, the implementation of NGS in the clinic for mutation analysis of PCa will likely become reality. Using NGS, individual prostate samples can be screened for diagnostic and prognostic markers and therapy targets to determine on a personal basis the significance of the disease, the treatments to which the patient will respond, and the optimal order of therapies.[28,29]

Proteomics

Large-scale research on proteins is much more complex than genomics and transcriptomics. Instead of the four bases, proteins are build-up by 20 different amino acids that can also be modified in many different ways (e.g. phosphorylation, glycosylation). Proteins cannot be amplified like RNA and DNA using the polymerase chain reaction (PCR) and protein detection technologies, mainly based on antibodies, often lack sensitivity and specificity. The breakthrough in protein detection came with the advancements of mass spectrometry (MS). This technology can accurately measure the mass of proteins and protein fragments and also allows for determining the amino acid sequence of a selected protein fragment.[30] With some effort, hundreds to thousands of different proteins can be identified in tissue extracts or body fluids such as serum or urine. However, low abundant proteins in complex mixtures are typically difficult to detect using MS and in general, blood-based cancer markers other than PSA are present in low quantities. The implementation of MS technologies for marker research has not resulted in a wide range of novel clinically useful protein markers. Reasons are the limitations of MS to detect low abundant proteins and the huge variability in protein composition of body fluids between individuals. MS technology is nowadays slowly improving the detection of low abundant proteins and high-throughput measurements and eventually, MS is expected to become a technique operational in a clinical setting for the detection of protein biomarkers.

Current and new markers and targets based on our knowledge of prostate cancer biology

For the diagnosis of PCa, a limited number of markers are commonly in use. These include family history, serum PSA (see Chapter 6.4), digital rectal examination (DRE) and imaging technologies (e.g. MRI) that provide an indication of prostate abnormalities including cancer. The final diagnosis is established by histopathological examination of prostate needle biopsies. The biopsies provide information for prognosis which includes an estimate of the extent of the cancer (number of positive cores and % cancer area in each core) and particularly the differentiation state of the cancer cells, which is graded using the Gleason score (see Chapter 6.3). Both the diagnosis and prognosis of PCa are far from perfect and there is a strong clinical need for additional markers.

Since *ETS* gene fusions are the most frequent genetic abnormalities found in PCa, there is considerable interest in using *ETS* fusion transcripts as diagnostic and prognostic markers.[18] *ETS* fusion events are unique to cancer and their detection has high diagnostic value. Molecular tests to measure *TMPRSS2-ERG* transcripts in urine after DRE have been developed and are in the final stages of clinical testing. With respect to their prognostic value, conflicting studies report that *ERG* fusions are associated with no, favourable, and unfavourable clinical outcomes.[21] It is unlikely that *ERG* overexpression by itself will be a useful prognostic marker.

Diagnostic RNA markers

Besides *TMPRSS2-ERG*, other transcript markers are making their way into the clinic. PCA3, a long noncoding RNA was discovered in 1999 as a prostate-specific molecule, upregulated in PCa.[31] A commercial test has been developed (Progensa) to measure *PCA3* and PSA mRNA levels in whole urine after DRE. The *PCA3* score is calculated as the ratio of *PCA3*/PSA mRNA ×1,000. The diagnostic role of *PCA3* has been studied in the setting of predicting biopsy outcome, mainly to prevent unnecessary repeat biopsies of men with previous negative biopsies but persisting elevated PSA levels. It was shown that *PCA3* scored better than PSA alone and complements established PCa risk factors such as age, PSA, DRE, and prostate volume, making *PCA3* a strong candidate to add to existing risk calculators.[32]

As a prognostic marker, *PCA3* has been limited in its ability to predict PCa stage and aggressiveness beyond established markers.[32] Since PCa is a very heterogeneous and often multifocal disease, combining different cancer markers, such as *TMPRSS2-ERG* and *PCA3*, is expected to improve diagnostic accuracy. Overall, combining new urine biomarkers that are in the pipeline with the *PCA3* score might significantly improve predictability of biopsy outcome.[32]

Prognostic RNA markers

Many initiatives are being undertaken to identify and validate prognostic RNA markers. Based on knowledge of changes in cell cycle genes in cancer, a cell cycle progression score, created from expression levels of 31 transcripts was tested and validated.[33] This profile requires RNA extracted from cancer tissue and should be performed on positive biopsies. Expression profiling of RNA isolated from whole blood has also been shown to separate men with CRPC in groups with long versus short median survival.[34,35] These whole blood profiles most likely reflect changes in blood cells and not in the rare circulating tumour cells (CTCs) or tumour-derived RNAs. Whether the prognostic power of any of these mRNA profiles persist in large independent validation cohorts still needs to be determined.

Another type of RNA that received much attention for its regulatory role in cancer are short (~22 nt) RNAs, referred to as microRNAs (miRNAs). These miRNAs are rather stable and resistant to sample treatments (e.g. fixation, long term storage) and therefore attractive candidate markers. Several studies have successfully indicated miRNAs as diagnostic and prognostic markers in tissue and blood.[36,37] Like for mRNAs mentioned above, a tissue profile of four miRNAs ((miR-96 × miR-183)/(miR-145 × miR-221)) was shown to improve accuracy and outperform PSA-based diagnosis and predict PCa aggressiveness.[38]

Emerging markers from -omics studies

Recent large-scale NGS projects provided an overview of mutations in PCa.[39–41] As expected, most frequently detected mutated genes were known as part of the AR pathway, *PTEN/AKT* axis or cell cycle regulatory genes. However, tens of novel mutated genes were identified that have a very low occurrence rate (1–3%) in PCa and a few new mutated genes that are more commonly affected (4–15%). One previously unknown common mutated gene is *SPOP*, encoding a protein that is involved in protein degradation and may modulate transcriptional repression. For many of these newly discovered mutated genes, the research on their role as markers and therapy targets has now been initiated.

Exosomes

As described above, on protein level, candidate markers have been discovered in PCa tissue, urine, and serum using mass spectrometry.[42] Thorough independent validation of almost all of these candidate markers still needs to be performed. One of the interesting findings from MS experiments on proteins secreted by cancer cells, is the finding that many of these proteins are secreted via small vesicles, often referred to as exosomes.[43,44] This exosomal secretory pathway is completely different from the well known endoplasmic reticulum-Golgi route that proteins such as PSA follow to

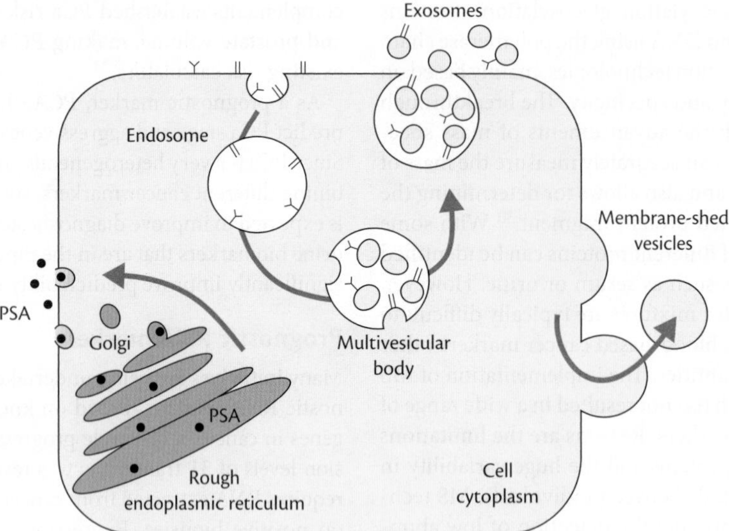

Fig. 6.2.3 Overview of different secretion mechanisms. Proteins with an N-terminal signal peptide are translated at the rough endoplasmic reticulum and transported via the Golgi apparatus to the cell membrane for secretion into the milieu.

be released from cells (Fig. 6.2.3). Exosomes are small (50–100 nm) vesicles which are formed by inward budding of cytoplasmic endosomes.[45] An endosome containing exosomes is called a multivesicular body (MVB) and when the MVB fuses with the cellular membrane, the exosomes are secreted. Exosomes are secreted by most cell types, and also the normal prostate produces large quantities of exosome-like vesicles called prostasomes.[46] Exosomes contain the proteins and RNAs from the cytoplasm of the cell of origin.[47,48] This provides the unique opportunity to study the presence and molecular properties of cancer cells by analysing the protein and RNA content of cancer-derived exosomes. As for PSA, the presence of prostasomes in blood is a marker for PCa.[49]

Genome-wide association studies and genetic variation

It has been known for a long time that approximatey 5% of prostate cancers are clearly linked to a family history. Genome-wide association studies (GWAS) using an enormous number of SNPs have postulated approximately 40 different chromosomal regions associated with hereditary PCa, indicating the presence of a gene (or genes) important for cancer development in these regions.[50,51] So far, however, the number of genes convincingly associated with hereditary PCa is very small. Mutations in the *BRCA2* gene that is very important in hereditary breast cancer are associated with a very small percentage of hereditary prostate cancer.[52] Recently, however, it has been discovered that a specific mutation in *HOXB13* (*HOXB13-G84E*) is associated with approx. 5% of hereditary PCas.[53] The mutation is also present in less than 1% of PCa patients without a known family history. The mutation is approximtely 10-fold more common in PCa patients than in normal controls. Importantly, now that rapid and affordable whole genome sequencing is possible, more common genomic polymorphisms in hereditary PCa and in patients without a family history are expected to become available soon. Hopefully, this will lead to the identification of novel genes that at low- or high-penetrance predispose to the development of high-risk prostate cancer.

Further reading

1000 Genomes Project Consortium, Abecasis GR, Auton A, *et al.* An integrated map of genetic variation from 1,092 human genomes. *Nature* 2012; **491**(7422):56–65.

Attard G, Richards J, de Bono JS. New strategies in metastatic prostate cancer: targeting the androgen receptor signaling pathway. *Clin Cancer Res* 2011; **17**(7):1649–57.

Baca SC, Garraway LA. The genomic landscape of prostate cancer. *Front Endocrinol (Lausanne)* 2012; **3**:69.

Catto JW, Alcaraz A, Bjartell AS, *et al.* MicroRNA in prostate, bladder, and kidney cancer: a systematic review. *Eur Urol* 2011; **59**(5):671–81.

Choudhury AD, Eeles R, Freedland SJ, *et al.* The role of genetic markers in the management of prostate cancer. *Eur Urol* 2012; **62**(4):577–87.

Desai AN, Jere A. Next-generation sequencing: ready for the clinics? *Clin Genet* 2012; **81**(6):503–10.

Duijvesz D, Luider T, Bangma CH, Jenster G. Exosomes as biomarker treasure chests for prostate cancer. *Eur Urol* 2011; **59**(5):823–31.

Hanahan D, Weinberg RA. Hallmarks of cancer: the next generation. *Cell* 2011; **144**(5):646–74.

Huggins C. Effect of orchiectomy and irradiation on cancer of the prostate. *Ann Surg* 1942; **115**(6):1192–200.

Jansen FH, Krijgsveld J, van Rijswijk A, *et al.* Exosomal secretion of cytoplasmic prostate cancer xenograft-derived proteins. *Mol Cell Proteomics* 2009; **8**(6):1192–205.

Nakagawa H, Akamatsu S, Takata R, Takahashi A, Kubo M, Nakamura Y. Prostate cancer genomics, biology, and risk assessment through genome-wide association studies. *Cancer Sci* 2012; **103**(4):607–13.

Roychowdhury S, Iyer MK, Robinson DR, *et al.* Personalized oncology through integrative high-throughput sequencing: a pilot study. *Sci Transl Med* 2011; **3**(111):111ra121.

Tomlins SA, Bjartell A, Chinnaiyan AM, *et al.* ETS gene fusions in prostate cancer: from discovery to daily clinical practice. *Eur Urol* 2009; **56**(2):275–86.

Tomlins SA, Rhodes DR, Perner S, *et al.* Recurrent fusion of TMPRSS2 and ETS transcription factor genes in prostate cancer. *Science* 2005; **310**(5748):644–8.

Yates JR, Ruse CI, Nakorchevsky A. Proteomics by mass spectrometry: approaches, advances, and applications. *Annu Rev Biomed Eng* 2009; **11**:49–79.

References

1. Harrow J, Frankish A, Gonzalez JM, *et al.* GENCODE: the reference human genome annotation for The ENCODE Project. *Genome Res* 2012; **22**(9):1760–74.
2. Jones PA, Baylin SB. The epigenomics of cancer. *Cell* 2007; **128**(4):683–92.
3. Sandoval J, Esteller M. Cancer epigenomics: beyond genomics. *Curr Opin Genet Dev* 2012; **22**(1):50–5.
4. Hanahan D, Weinberg RA. Hallmarks of cancer: the next generation. *Cell* 2011; **144**(5):646–74.
5. Fearon ER, Vogelstein B. A genetic model for colorectal tumorigenesis. *Cell* 1990; **61**(5):759–67.
6. Oren M, Rotter V. Introduction: p53--the first twenty years. *Cell Mol Life Sci* 1999; **55**(1):9–11.
7. Shen MM, Abate-Shen C. Molecular genetics of prostate cancer: new prospects for old challenges. *Genes Dev* 2010; **24**(18):1967–2000.
8. Song MS, Salmena L, Pandolfi PP. The functions and regulation of the PTEN tumour suppressor. *Nat Rev Mol Cell Biol* 2012; **13**(5):283–96.
9. Tomlins SA, Rhodes DR, Perner S, *et al.* Recurrent fusion of TMPRSS2 and ETS transcription factor genes in prostate cancer. *Science* 2005; **310**(5748):644–8.
10. Hermans KG, van Marion R, van Dekken H, Jenster G, van Weerden WM, Trapman J. TMPRSS2:ERG fusion by translocation or interstitial deletion is highly relevant in androgen-dependent prostate cancer, but is bypassed in late-stage androgen receptor-negative prostate cancer. *Cancer Res* 2006; **66**(22):10658–63.
11. Kumar-Sinha C, Tomlins SA, Chinnaiyan AM. Recurrent gene fusions in prostate cancer. *Nat Rev Cancer* 2008; **8**(7):497–511.
12. Cerveira N, Ribeiro FR, Peixoto A, *et al.* TMPRSS2-ERG gene fusion causing ERG overexpression precedes chromosome copy number changes in prostate carcinomas and paired HGPIN lesions. *Neoplasia* 2006; **8**(10):826–32.
13. Perner S, Mosquera JM, Demichelis F, *et al.* TMPRSS2-ERG fusion prostate cancer: an early molecular event associated with invasion. *Am J Surg Pathol* 2007; **31**(6):882–8.
14. Tomlins SA, Mehra R, Rhodes DR, *et al.* TMPRSS2:ETV4 gene fusions define a third molecular subtype of prostate cancer. *Cancer Res* 2006; **66**(7):3396–400.
15. Helgeson BE, Tomlins SA, Shah N, *et al.* Characterization of TMPRSS2:ETV5 and SLC45A3:ETV5 gene fusions in prostate cancer. *Cancer Res* 2008; **68**(1):73–80.
16. Paulo P, Barros-Silva JD, Ribeiro FR, *et al.* FLI1 is a novel ETS transcription factor involved in gene fusions in prostate cancer. *Genes Chromosomes Cancer* 2012; **51**(3):240–9.
17. Sashida G, Bazzoli E, Menendez S, Liu Y, Nimer SD. The oncogenic role of the ETS transcription factors MEF and ERG. *Cell Cycle* 2010; **9**(17):3457–9.
18. Rosen P, Sesterhenn IA, Brassell SA, McLeod DG, Srivastava S, Dobi A. Clinical potential of the ERG oncoprotein in prostate cancer. *Nat Rev Urol* 2012; **9**(3):131–7.
19. Clark J, Attard G, Jhavar S, *et al.* Complex patterns of ETS gene alteration arise during cancer development in the human prostate. *Oncogene* 2008; **27**(14):1993–2003.
20. Carver BS, Tran J, Chen Z, *et al.* ETS rearrangements and prostate cancer initiation. *Nature* 2009; **457**(7231):E1; discussion E2–3.
21. Tomlins SA, Bjartell A, Chinnaiyan AM, *et al.* ETS gene fusions in prostate cancer: from discovery to daily clinical practice. *Eur Urol* 2009; **56**(2):275–86.
22. Huggins C. Effect of orchiectomy and irradiation on cancer of the prostate. *Ann Surg* 1942; **115**(6):1192–200.
23. Sharma NL, Massie CE, Ramos-Montoya A, *et al.* The androgen receptor induces a distinct transcriptional program in castration-resistant prostate cancer in man. *Cancer Cell* 2013; **23**(1):35–47.
24. Lamont KR, Tindall DJ. Minireview: Alternative activation pathways for the androgen receptor in prostate cancer. *Mol Endocrinol* 2011; **25**(6):897–907.
25. Attard G, Richards J, de Bono JS. New strategies in metastatic prostate cancer: targeting the androgen receptor signaling pathway. *Clin Cancer Res* 2011; **17**(7):1649–57.
26. Dufva M. Introduction to microarray technology. *Methods Mol Biol* 2009; **529**:1–22.
27. Wong KM, Hudson TJ, McPherson JD. Unraveling the genetics of cancer: genome sequencing and beyond. *Annu Rev Genomics Hum Genet* 2011; **12**:407–30.
28. Desai AN, Jere A. Next-generation sequencing: ready for the clinics? *Clin Genet* 2012; **81**(6):503–10.
29. Roychowdhury S, Iyer MK, Robinson DR, *et al.* Personalized oncology through integrative high-throughput sequencing: a pilot study. *Sci Transl Med* 2011; **3**(111):111ra121.
30. Yates JR, Ruse CI, Nakorchevsky A. Proteomics by mass spectrometry: approaches, advances, and applications. *Annu Rev Biomed Eng* 2009; **11**:49–79.
31. Bussemakers MJ, van Bokhoven A, Verhaegh GW, *et al.* DD3: a new prostate-specific gene, highly overexpressed in prostate cancer. *Cancer Res* 1999; **59**(23):5975–9.
32. Auprich M, Bjartell A, Chun FK, *et al.* Contemporary role of prostate cancer antigen 3 in the management of prostate cancer. *Eur Urol* 2011; **60**(5):1045–54.
33. Cuzick J, Swanson GP, Fisher G, *et al.* Prognostic value of an RNA expression signature derived from cell cycle proliferation genes in patients with prostate cancer: a retrospective study. *Lancet Oncol* 2011; **12**(3):245–55.
34. Ross RW, Galsky MD, Scher HI, *et al.* A whole-blood RNA transcript-based prognostic model in men with castration-resistant prostate cancer: a prospective study. *Lancet Oncol* 2012; **13**(11):1105–13.
35. Olmos D, Brewer D, Clark J, *et al.* Prognostic value of blood mRNA expression signatures in castration-resistant prostate cancer: a prospective, two-stage study. *Lancet Oncol* 2012; **13**(11):1114–24.
36. Casanova-Salas I, Rubio-Briones J, Fernández-Serra A, López-Guerrero JA. miRNAs as biomarkers in prostate cancer. *Clin Transl Oncol* 2012; **14**(11):803–11.
37. Catto JW, Alcaraz A, Bjartell AS, *et al.* MicroRNA in prostate, bladder, and kidney cancer: a systematic review. *Eur Urol* 2011; **59**(5):671–81.
38. Larne O, Martens-Uzunova E, Hagman Z, *et al.* miQ-A novel microRNA based diagnostic and prognostic tool for prostate cancer. *Int J Cancer* 2012; **132**(12):2867–75.
39. Grasso CS, Wu YM, Robinson DR, *et al.* The mutational landscape of lethal castration-resistant prostate cancer. *Nature* 2012; **487**(7406):239–43.
40. Baca SC, Garraway LA. The genomic landscape of prostate cancer. *Front Endocrinol (Lausanne)* 2012; **3**:69.
41. Barbieri CE, Baca SC, Lawrence MS, *et al.* Exome sequencing identifies recurrent SPOP, FOXA1 and MED12 mutations in prostate cancer. *Nat Genet* 2012; **44**(6):685–9.
42. Goo YA, Goodlett DR. Advances in proteomic prostate cancer biomarker discovery. *J Proteomics* 2010; **73**(10):1839–50.
43. Jansen FH, Krijgsveld J, van Rijswijk A, *et al.* Exosomal secretion of cytoplasmic prostate cancer xenograft-derived proteins. *Mol Cell Proteomics* 2009; **8**(6):1192–205.
44. Cocucci E, Racchetti G, Meldolesi J. Shedding microvesicles: artefacts no more. *Trends Cell Biol* 2009; **19**(2):43–51.
45. Duijvesz D, Luider T, Bangma CH, Jenster G. Exosomes as biomarker treasure chests for prostate cancer. *Eur Urol* 2011; **59**(5):823–31.
46. Ronquist G. Prostasomes are mediators of intercellular communication: from basic research to clinical implications. *J Intern Med* 2012; **271**(4):400–13.
47. Valadi H, Ekström K, Bossios A, Sjöstrand M, Lee JJ, Lötvall JO. Exosome-mediated transfer of mRNAs and microRNAs is a novel mechanism of genetic exchange between cells. *Nat Cell Biol* 2007; **9**(6):654–9.
48. Simpson RJ, Jensen SS, Lim JW. Proteomic profiling of exosomes: current perspectives. *Proteomics* 2008; **8**(19):4083–99.

49. Tavoosidana G, Ronquist G, Darmanis S, *et al.* Multiple recognition assay reveals prostasomes as promising plasma biomarkers for prostate cancer. *Proc Natl Acad Sci U S A* 2011; **108**(21):8809–14.
50. Marchini J, Donnelly P, Cardon LR. Genome-wide strategies for detecting multiple loci that influence complex diseases. *Nat Genet* 2005; **37**(4):413–7.
51. Choudhury AD, Eeles R, Freedland SJ, *et al.* The role of genetic markers in the management of prostate cancer. *Eur Urol* 2012; **62**(4):577–87.
52. Castro E, Eeles R. The role of BRCA1 and BRCA2 in prostate cancer. *Asian J Androl* 2012; **14**(3):409–14.
53. Ewing CM, Ray AM, Lange EM, *et al.* Germline mutations in HOXB13 and prostate-cancer risk. *N Engl J Med* 2012; **366**(2):141–9.

CHAPTER 6.3

Prostate cancer
Pathology

Rodolfo Montironi, Liang Cheng, Antonio Lopez-Beltran, Roberta Mazzucchelli, Matteo Santoni, and Marina Scarpelli

Introduction to the pathlogy of prostate cancer

The incidence of prostate cancer (PCa) has risen dramatically in the last years. This event may be partially explained by the employment of digital rectal examination (DRE), serum prostate-specific antigen (PSA), and transrectal ultrasonography.[1] In developed countries, PCa is the most frequent non-skin malignancy in males.[1] It is estimated that 1 in 6 males will be diagnosed with PCa during their lifetime, the risk of death due to metastatic PCa being 1 in 30.[2] Multiple factors contribute to the development of PCa as well as to its progression to an androgen-independent state[2]: dietary factors, inherited susceptibility factors, gene defects, and androgens and their receptors.[3]

The chapter will discuss the following topics: high-grade prostatic intraepithelial neoplasia (PIN), atypical small acinare proliferation, morphological criteria for the identification of PCa, reporting of PCa biopsies, prognostic factors in radical prostatectomies (RPs) specimens.

High-grade prostatic intraepithelial neoplasia and intraductal carcinoma of the prostate

PIN refers to the atypical cellular proliferations of the epithelial lining of prostatic atypical ductal and acinar cells.[4,5] PIN is classified into low- and high-grade, based on cytological cell characteristics (Fig. 6.3.1). The nuclei of cells composing low-grade PIN is characterized by the presence of cells with enlarged nuclei with various size, normal or slightly increased chromatin content, and small or inconspicuous nucleoli. Otherwise, High-grade PIN (HGPIN) is composed by cells with large nuclei of relatively uniform size, increased and likely irregularly distributed chromatin content, and prominent nucleoli (similar to those of carcinoma cells). HGPIN are characterized by frequent disruptions in the basal cell layer, which is intact or rarely interrupted in low-grade lesions. The architecture of PIN varies from a flattened epithelium to a florid cribriform proliferation.[4,5] HGPIN is identified in 2–16.5% of needle biopsies and represents the most likely precursor of PCa.

The clinical relevance of identifying isolated HGPIN is due to its correlation with the evidence of PCa in re-biopsies. The strength of this association has weakened in years as contemporary prostate biopsy practice has moved to more extensive prostate sampling. Consequently, the predictive likelihood of PCa following a diagnosis of HGPIN has dropped from 36% to 22%, although it remains high for men with HGPIN in ≥3 cores (~40%).[6,7] Unfortunately, clinical parameters, PSA values and DRE/TRUS findings do not identify men with HGPIN on needle biopsy who are more candidate to have cancer in subsequent biopsies.[8]

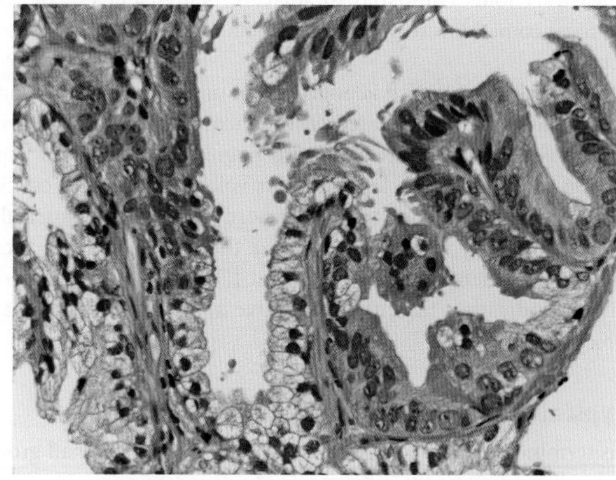

Fig. 6.3.1 High-grade prostatic intraepithelial neoplasia, showing partial involvement of a prostatic gland.

Intraductal carcinoma of the prostate (IDC-P) is defined as a lumen expansile proliferation of secretory cells within prostatic ducts and acini that show marked architectural and cytologic atypia. Morphologic criteria have been proposed to distinguish IDC-P from HGPIN, which is characterized by a significantly different cancer predictive value. In addition to the presence of malignant epithelial cells filling large acini and prostatic ducts with preservation of basal cells, the set of criteria for diagnosing IDC-P includes the presence of (i) a solid cribriform pattern (Fig. 6.3.2), with punched-out luminal spaces accounting for <50% of the central cellular mass; or (ii) marked nuclear atypia, with wider nuclei

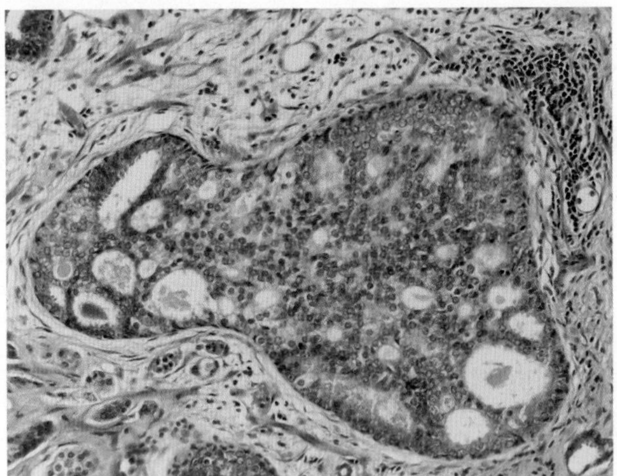

Fig. 6.3.2 Intraductal carcinoma of the prostate with dense cribriform pattern.

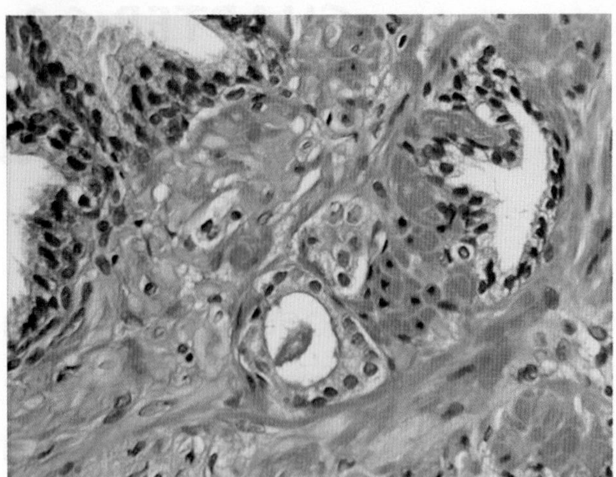

Fig. 6.3.3 Atypical small acinar proliferation suspicious for but not diagnostic of malignancy. The suspicious focus consists of two small acini with adjacent benign glands.

(at least six folds compared to adjacent benign nuclei); or (iii) non-focal comedonecrosis (i.e. intraductal carcinoma with central necrosis).[9]

The detection of IDC-P is not frequent in prostate biopsies, and is even rarer if not associated with concomitant PCa. However, IDC-P is markedly correlated with aggressive PCa, with high Gleason score, and with large tumour volume. Thus, it is crucial for the pathologists to identify and record these lesions, especially in prostate biopsy reports, to optimize the management of these patients. The identification of isolated IDC-P in biopsies represents an indication for either definitive approach or immediate re-biopsy.[10,11]

Atypical small acinar proliferation

This terminology is used to describe the presence of a small group of glands suspicious for a diagnosis of adenocarcinoma in a needle biopsy, without sufficient cytological and/or architectural atypia to definitively identify PCa (Fig. 6.3.3).[12] Atypical small acinar proliferation may encompass benign lesions that mimic malignant glandular lesions and small foci of adenocarcinoma harbouring unsufficient features for a definitive diagnosis of PCa. Notably, atypical small acinar proliferation is not a distinct diagnostic entity, different from HGPIN, and is found in approximately 5% of needle biopsy pathology reports (range 0.7–23.4%).[12,13] The risk to detect carcinoma on needle core re-biopsy is around 40% (reported range: 17–60%).

Clinical parameters have only a limited predictive meaning for cancer on subsequent biopsy.[14] Initial mean PSA levels were higher in patients with atypical small acinar proliferation who had cancer in re-biopsies compared to those with subsequent negative biopsies. Park *et al.* reported that age and digital rectal examination were independent predictors of cancer in 45 patients with 'atypia'[15]; otherwise, several studies reported that serum PSA levels and DRE did not predict cancer on re-biopsies.[16–18]

The association of HGPIN and atypical small acinar proliferation suspicious for malignancy, also called PINATYP, can be observed occasionally on a prostate biopsy. The mean cancer detection rate is higher in patients with an atypical focus and HGPIN (53%) compared to patients with an isolated atypical focus.[19]

Morphological criteria for the identification of prostate cancer

The diagnosis of carcinoma is based on combined architectural and cytological findings. The light microscopic features are usually sufficient, but cases with small suspicious foci may be candidate for immunohistochemical analyses.

Features pathognomonic of cancer

The following four features are considered pathognomonic of cancer, even when present to a very limited extent in a small cancer focus: mucinous fibroplasia (collagenous micronodules), glomerulation, perineural invasion, and extracellular mucin extravasation.[20] The incidence of these four features is as follows: mucinous fibroplasia: 1–2%; glomerulation: 3–15%; perineural invasion: 11–37%; an extracellular mucin extravasation: <1%.[21] Mucinous fibroplasia is a microscopic nodular masse of paucicellular eosinophilic fibrillar material impinging on acinar lumen. It is generally present in mucin-producing PCa and consists of extravasating of acidic mucin into the stroma. Glomerulation is defined as a cribriform not transluminal growth, with a single point of attachment superficially resembling a renal glomerulus. Perineural invasion is defined as the presence of PCa spreading along, around or within a nerve.

Features favouring cancer

Major and minor criteria are included in this group.[21] The major criteria are: infiltrative growth pattern, absent basal cells, and nuclear atypia. The minor criteria are basophilic mucinous secretions (18–52%), pink dense secretions (53–87%), intraluminal crystalloids (21–41%); mitotic figures (rare), and amphophilic cytoplasm (30–60%). Although not specific for PCa, minor criteria are useful in prompting in-depth study of the glands harbouring these changes, with a view towards assessing the major diagnostic criteria.

Architectural features

Architectural features are usually detected at low-medium power magnification, focusing on spacing, size, and shape of acini.[22] The arrangement of the acini is useful for the diagnosis and is the basis of the Gleason grade. Malignant acini have an irregular, haphazard arrangement, randomly localized in clusters, or singly in the stroma. Wide variation in the spacing between malignant acini are frequent. Acinar size may vary, and this represents a useful criterion for cancer diagnosis, particularly when small, irregular, abortive acini with primitive lumens are found at the periphery of a focus of well-differentiated carcinoma.

In suspicious foci, the acini are generally small or medium in size, with irregular contours that contrast with the typical smooth contours of benign and hyperplastic acini. Comparison with the adjacent benign prostatic acini is always useful for the diagnosis of cancer. Well-differentiated carcinoma and the large acinar variant of Gleason grade 3 carcinoma are particularly difficult to distinguish from benign acini in needle biopsies, due to the uniform size and spacing of acini. In these cases, major attention should be placed on the cytologic characteristics, immunohistochemical features, and the presence of smaller acini at the edge of the focus.

The basal cell layer is not present in PCa, differently from benign acini. This is an essential diagnostic feature that may be difficult to assess in routine tissue sections due to false negative results with atrophy and other mimics of cancer. Compressed stromal fibroblasts may resemble basal cells but are usually found only focally at the periphery of acini. Notably, small foci of adenocarcinoma may cluster around or infiltrate near larger benign acini with an intact basal cell layer.[22]

Cytological features

The cytological characteristics of adenocarcinoma comprehend nuclear and nucleolar enlargement, occurring in most malignant cells. Every cell has a nucleolus, so 'prominent' nucleoli with a diameter of at least 1.50 μm are observed.[22] Pathologists do not routinely measure nucleoli for diagnosis; this assessment relies on the comparison with benign epithelial cells elsewhere in the specimen.

Artefacts often obscure the nuclei and nucleoli, and overstaining of nuclei by haematoxylin constitutes one of the most frequent and challenging problems in the identification of suspicious cells. Differences in fixation and handling of biopsy specimens influence nuclear size and chromasia. Many pathologists prefer pale staining with eosin, but this strategy fails to accentuate nucleoli, which are commonly enlarged (Fig. 6.3.4). In specimens with nuclear hyperchromasia and pale eosinophilic staining, increasing the light source and magnification of suggestive foci can help to identify hidden enlarged nucleoli.[22]

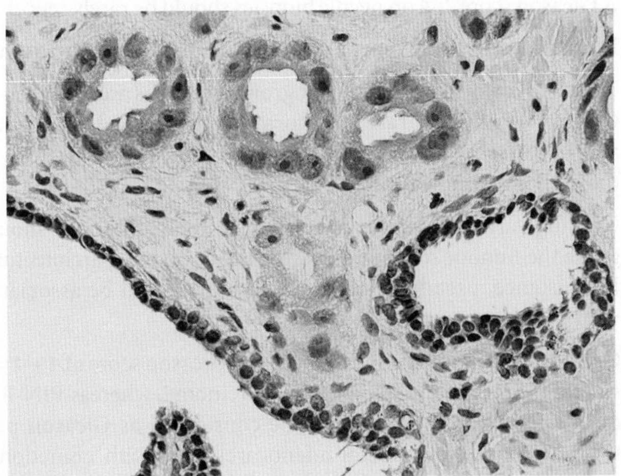

Fig. 6.3.4 Nuclear enlargement and nucleolar prominence in prostate cancer.

Luminal findings

Crystalloids are sharp, needle-like eosinophilic structures often found in the lumens of well/moderately differentiated carcinomas.[23] They are not cancer-specific and can be present also in other conditions. The crystalloids found in the secondary deposits of unknown origin may be suspected for the prostatic origin of the neoplasia.[24] Special stains, as trichrome, toluidine blue, and the Mallory, can show the presence of crystalloids that the light microscopy alone may not highlight.[24] The pathogenesis of crystalloids is unknown, however; they probably arise from the altered metabolism of both protein and mineral in the prostatic acini.

Under the light microscopy, the lumen of the neoplastic acini is often characterized by an amorphous, threadlike, and faint basophilic secretions. This mucin stains with Alcian blue and is best displayed at pH 2.5, while normal prostatic epithelium contains periodic acid Schiff-reactive mucin that is neutral. Acidic mucin is not carcinoma-specific and may be reported in HGPIN, atypical adenomatous hyperplasia (adenosis), sclerosing adenosis and, more rarely, nodular hyperplasia.[25] Occasionally, PCa may show the presence of intraluminal corpora amylacea. These are usually seen in normal ducts and acini, adenosis, and verumontanum mucosal gland hyperplasia.

Stromal findings

The stroma in cancer frequently contains young collagen, which appears lightly eosinophilic, although desmoplasia may be prominent. Muscle fibres in the stroma can be split or distorted. However, this is a difficult report to detect and cannot be relied upon due to the resemblance of the stroma associated with benign acini.[22]

Features against cancer

The following features should make the pathologist hesitate to make a diagnosis of cancer: lobularity, branching glands, larger glands, similar nuclear changes to adjacent benign glands (ruling out (r/o) adenosis), prominent nucleoli yet adjacent PIN (r/o tangential section or out-pouching of PIN), nuclear atypia with inflammation (r/o reactive atypia), atrophic cytoplasm, pale-clear cytoplasm, papillary infoldings, and corpora amylacea.

Ancillary diagnostic studies

In difficult cases, using monoclonal antibodies directed against high molecular weight cytokeratin (i.e. clone 34ßE12) may be employed to evaluate the basal cell layer.[20,21] We use this infrequently and only as an adjunct to the light microscopic findings. The results with this immunohistochemical stain should not be the sole basis to diagnose malignancy, especially in small suggestive foci. Antikeratin 34ßE12 stains nearly all of the normal prostatic basal cells, while no staining occurs in the secretory and stromal cells.

Since the uniform absence of a basal cell layer in prostatic acinar proliferations is a crucial diagnostic finding of invasive carcinoma, and basal cells may be inapparent by haematoxilin-eosin (H&E) stain, basal cell specific immunostains may be used to distinguish invasive prostatic adenocarcinoma from benign small acinar cancer-mimics which retain their basal cell layer (e.g. glandular atrophy, post-atrophic hyperplasia, atypical adenomatous hyperplasia, sclerosing adenosis, and radiation induced atypia).[26]

Sometimes a small group of benign glands may present an interrupted or not demonstrable basal cell layer. The complete lack of a basal cell layer in a small acinar proliferation cannot be considered alone as a sole criterion of malignancy; rather, it should be considered supportive in the diagnosis of invasive carcinoma only in acinar proliferation which shows suspicious cytological and/or architectural characteristics on H&E stain. On the contrary, early invasive prostatic adenocarcinoma may have residual basal cells when it arises in association with high-grade prostatic intraepithelial neoplasia. Residual basal cells can be detected in intraductal spread of invasive carcinoma and in entrapped benign glands. In rare circumstances, the prostatic adenocarcinomas contain scattered neoplastic cells which are immunoreactive for 34βE12, yet these have not the typical distribution of the basal cells. The use of antibodies direct against the basal cells (i.e. 34ßE12) is especially helpful for the diagnosis of what appears deceptively a variant of PCa.

The prostate adenocarcinoma shows negative staining for both cytokeratins 7 and 20. The immunohistochemistry for cytokeratins 7 and 20 can be useful in the differential diagnosis with transitional cell carcinoma.[20]

p63, a member of the *p53* family (a tumour suppressor gene), is a nuclear protein encoded by a gene on chromosome 3q27–29. It has been shown that *p63* affects growth and development of the epithelium of the skin, cervix, breast, and urogenital tract. Specific isotype of *p63* is expressed in basal cells of the prostate. In the diagnosis of prostatic adenocarcinoma, a monoclonal antibody of the *p63* can be utilized in paraffin-embedded tissue following antigen retrieval, as well as the high molecular weight cytokeratins, but with some advantages:

- is easier to interpret because of its strong nuclear staining intensity;
- the staining is less affected by the cautery artefact present in some specimens (i.e. TURP); and
- stains a subset of 34βE12 negative basal cells.

Interpretative limitations associated with the presence or absence of basal cells in small numbers of glands for 34βE12 apply to *p63*, and requires correlation with morphology.[27] Prostatic adenocarcinomas have occasional *p63* immunoreactive cells, that mostly represent entrapped benign glands or intraductal spread of carcinoma with residual basal cells.

AMACR (α-Methyl-CoA Racemase) mRNA was identified as overexpressed in prostatic adenocarcinoma by high throughput RNA microarray analysis. This mRNA was reported to encode a racemase protein, for which polyclonal and monoclonal antibodies active in formalin-fixed, paraffin-embedded tissues have been produced. Immunohistochemical studies with an antibody directed against *AMACR* (P504S) demonstrated that over 80% of prostatic adenocarcinomas are labelled.[28] Certain subtypes of PCa, including foamy gland carcinoma, atrophic carcinoma, pseudohyperplastic and treated carcinoma show lower *AMACR* expression. However, *AMACR* is not specific for PCa and is found in nodular hyperplasia (12%), atrophic glands (36%), HGPIN (>90%), and atypical adenomatous hyperplasia (17.5%).[29,30] *AMACR* may be employed as a confirmatory stain for prostatic adenocarcinoma, in addition with H&E morphology and a basal cell specific marker (Fig. 6.3.5).[29]

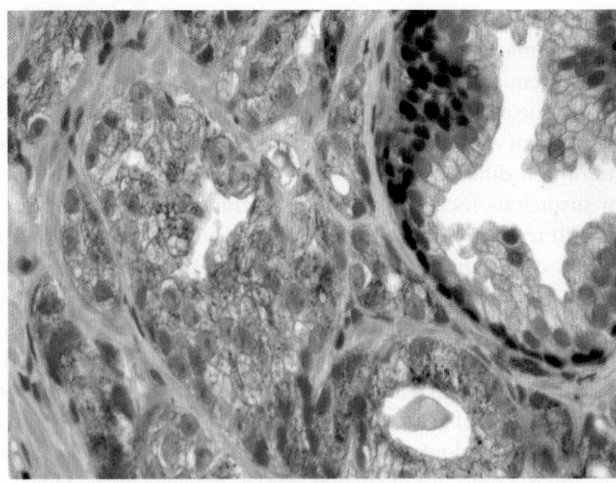

Fig. 6.3.5 Neoplastic epithelial cells with intense cytoplasmic granular staining by an antibody against racemase, whereas the adjacent benign gland shows basal cells stained with an antibody directed against the nuclear protein p63, the secretory cells being negative. (Antibody cocktail against racemase and p63; the reaction of both antibodies is revealed by a brown colour.)

2005 International Society of Urological Pathology-modified Gleason grading system

Histological grading is the clinically most useful tissue-based predictor of prognosis of PCa. In the last years, a gradual shift of how the Gleason grading system is applied has been observed, with a general trend towards upgrading. In 2005, the International Society of Urological Pathology (ISUP) consensus conference aimed to standardize both the perception of histological patterns and the way to compile and report the grade information. Here is a brief summary of the ISUP modified Gleason grading system.[31–33]

- The Gleason score is the sum of the first and second most predominant Gleason grades. In needle biopsies, this definition is modified to include any component of higher grade.
- A Gleason score of 1 + 1 = 2 should not be diagnosed regardless to the type of specimen, with extremely rare exceptions.
- A Gleason score 2–4 on needle biopsies should be rarely reported.
- Individual cells would not be permitted within Gleason pattern 3.
- The wide majority of cribriform growth patterns are classified as Gleason 4 with only rare cribriform lesions defined as for cribriform pattern 3 (see section 'Subsequent 2016 modifications of the ISUP grading system').
- Grading variations of adenocarcinoma: the pathologist should grade the tumour solely considering the underlying architecture. For instance, pseudohyperplastic tumour should be associated with a Gleason score of 3 + 3 = 6.
- Grading variants of adenocarcinoma. A Gleason score of 4 + 4 = 8 should be assigned to ductal adenocarcinoma, whereas PIN-like ductal adenocarcinoma should be considered as Gleason pattern 3. In addition, ductal adenocarcinoma with comedonecrosis should be classified as Gleason pattern 5, while retaining the diagnostic term of 'ductal adenocarcinoma' to identify their

unique clinical and pathological features. Otherwise, there is no consensus on how to grade mucinous (colloid) carcinoma. Several authors suggested that all mucinous carcinomas should be diagnosed as Gleason score of 8, whereas other authors sustained that the extracellular mucin should be ignored, assessing tumour grade based on the underlying architectural pattern. The grading of glomeruloid glands is another controversial point in the modified Gleason system. A Gleason grade should not be given to small cell carcinoma. The appropriateness of the Gleason grading system for sarcomatoid carcinomas is uncertain. In general, a Gleason grade is not given to the sarcomatoid component, whereas the glandular component is graded in the usual fashion.

- Reporting secondary patterns of lower grade in the setting of high-grade cancer should be ignored if the lower grade patterns represent less than 5% of the tumour area.
- As suggested by Egevad *et al.*: 'Reporting secondary patterns of higher grade when present even if with limited extent. High-grade tumour of any quantity on needle biopsy should be included within the Gleason score'.[31]
- As suggested by Egevad *et al.*: 'Tertiary Gleason patterns. The typical situation with tertiary patterns on biopsy includes tumours with patterns 3, 4, and 5 in various proportions. Such tumours should be classified overall as high grade (Gleason score 8–10) given the presence of high-grade tumour (patterns 4 and 5) on needle biopsy. On needle biopsies with patterns 3, 4, and 5, both the primary pattern and the highest grade should be recorded'.[31] For a RP specimen, the assignment of the Gleason score is based on the primary and secondary patterns with a comment as to the tertiary pattern.
- Per cent pattern 4–5. To date, it is not clear whether or not the actual percentage of 4–5 pattern tumour should be included in the report. Therefore, meaningful discriminatory cut-off points for percentage of pattern 4–5 should be defined. It remains an option if one wants to add this information to the routine Gleason score.
- Needle biopsy with distinct cores showing different grades. The pathologist should give an individual Gleason score to separate cores providing they are submitted in separate containers, or the cores are in the same container yet specified by the urologist as to their location (i.e. by different colour inks). In addition to assigning separate cores individual Gleason scores, one may also choose to give an overall score at the end of the case. If more than one core contained cancer in the setting of multiple cores per container, some authors suggest to separately grade each core, while other authors propose to give an overall grade for the involved cores per specimen container. In cases where a container includes multiple pieces of tissue, one should only assign an overall score for that container.[31,32]

Gleason grade migration or upgrading may occur in both needle biopsies and RP specimens. The upgrading in the Gleason score can have clinical consequences, such as the choice of therapy in an individual patient with PCa.[33] As an example, active surveillance should be discouraged in patients with high-grade tumours in the biopsy.

The correlation with patient outcome represents the true test of the validity of the 2005 ISUP modified Gleason system. Uemura *et al.* found that the 2005 ISUP modified Gleason score of needle biopsy specimens was significantly associated with biochemical recurrence-free survival after RP.[34] They found that the ISUP system is clinically useful to determine the most appropriate therapy for patients with early stage PCa.[34] However, further studies with sufficient follow-up periods are needed to confirm these findings.

Subsequent 2016 modifications of the ISUP grading system

It has been recommended that all cribriform patterns be diagnosed as Gleason pattern 4 rather than 3.[35,36] Glomerulations most likely represent an early stage of cribriform pattern 4 and should likely be graded as pattern 4 (2016 ISUP/WHO Gleason system).[36]

As suggested by Epstein *et al.*, 'Based on these clinical outcomes and the excellent prognosis for patients with low Gleason scores, we recommend Gleason grades incorporating a prognostic grade grouping which accurately reflect prognosis and are clearly understood by physicians and patients alike'.[37] This is a 5-tiered grading prognostic system whose use is supported by the WHO and ISUP.[36]

Reporting of prostate biopsies with cancer

The information provided in the surgical pathology report of a prostate needle biopsy with carcinoma has become fundamental for the management and prognostication of these tumours. The surgical pathology report should thus be comprehensive and yet succinct in providing relevant information consistently to urologists, radiation oncologists, and oncologists and, thereby, to the patient.

Site of sampling (specific location of the biopsy)

While obtaining multiple systematic biopsies is relatively standard in urologic practice, the submission of needle cores in two containers (left and right side) or individual containers for each site (site-specific labelling, e.g. right apex, right mid, right base, and so on) remains a matter of urologist/institutional preference. The potential importance of knowing the specific location of the biopsy and, by extension, the location of cancer may be summarized as follows:

- *Correlation with digital rectal examination and imaging studies.*
- *Prognostic importance.* Tumour involvement of base biopsies may influence bladder neck sparing RP; extensive cancer in base biopsies correlates with extraprostatic extension (EPE); and dominant side of prostate biopsy correlates with ipsilateral positivity of surgical margins and EPE.
- *Importance in planning therapy.* Mapping distribution of the cancer in needle biopsies may help plan the field of radiotherapy or may influence nerve sparing or bladder neck sparing during RP.
- *Importance in subsequent patient sampling.* In a patient with atypical glands without cancer, knowledge of site allows for more focused repeat biopsies.
- *Importance in subsequent prostate gland sampling.* Biopsy samples with site-specific labelling usually contain only one or two cores, which is advantageous for block and slide preparation and allows for complete visualization of cores and detection of small foci of cancer. Knowledge of cancer location may help target additional tissue or block sampling in cases without apparent cancer in RP sections.
- *Technical superiority in needle biopsy material examination.* Limited number of cores in site-specific labelled specimens

reduces fragmentation, thereby allowing for more confident assessment of number of cores involved.

- *Knowledge of biopsy site helps recognize potential diagnostic pitfalls.* This includes seminal vesicle epithelium or central zone epithelium, mostly reported in base biopsies and the rare Cowper's glands in apex biopsies.

Histological type

Since acinar adenocarcinoma is the overwhelming histological type of cancer in needle biopsy specimens, it is not necessary specifying such cancer as acinar or conventional type in pathology reports.

Carcinomas of the prostate with architectural or cytological variations such as atrophic, pseudohyperplastic, hypernephroid, and so on, are descriptive terms employed to describe variations in PCa. This may help the pathologists in recognizing diagnostic pitfalls but have no prognostic significance. They may be commented in a microscopic description and should not be mentioned in the final diagnosis.

Several variants of PCa have been characterized. This list includes ductal, mucinous, signet ring cell, adenosquamous, small cell carcinoma, and sarcomatoid carcinoma.[38] The former three can be diagnosed only on examination of RP or transurethral resection specimens. If observed in needle biopsy specimens, the diagnostic terminology used must be: adenocarcinoma of prostate with ductal features; adenocarcinoma of prostate with signet ring cell features; and adenocarcinoma of prostate with mucinous differentiation. Small cell carcinoma, sarcomatoid carcinoma, and adenosquamous carcinoma may be diagnosed on needle biopsies. There are no formal studies that have shown that the presence of these histological variants in needle biopsies may be prognostic or predictive, although the often-aggressive outcome correlated with these tumours supports the value of this exercise.

Cancer grade

The Gleason grading system and the prognostic grade groups are recommended as the international standard for grading PCa.[31–36] The World Health Organization (WHO) nuclear grading system could be employed in addition to the Gleason scheme, but is rarely or never reported.[39]

Extent of involvement of needle core (tumour volume)

The amount of tumour in prostate needle cores is an essential pathologic parameter that must be reported in needle biopsies (Fig. 6.3.6). The extent of tumour involvement of needle cores has been shown to be associated with the Gleason score, tumour volume, surgical margins, and pathologic stage in RP specimens.[40,41] The extent of needle core involvement including bilateral involvement has also been shown as a predictor of biochemical recurrence, post-prostatectomy progression, and radiotherapy failure

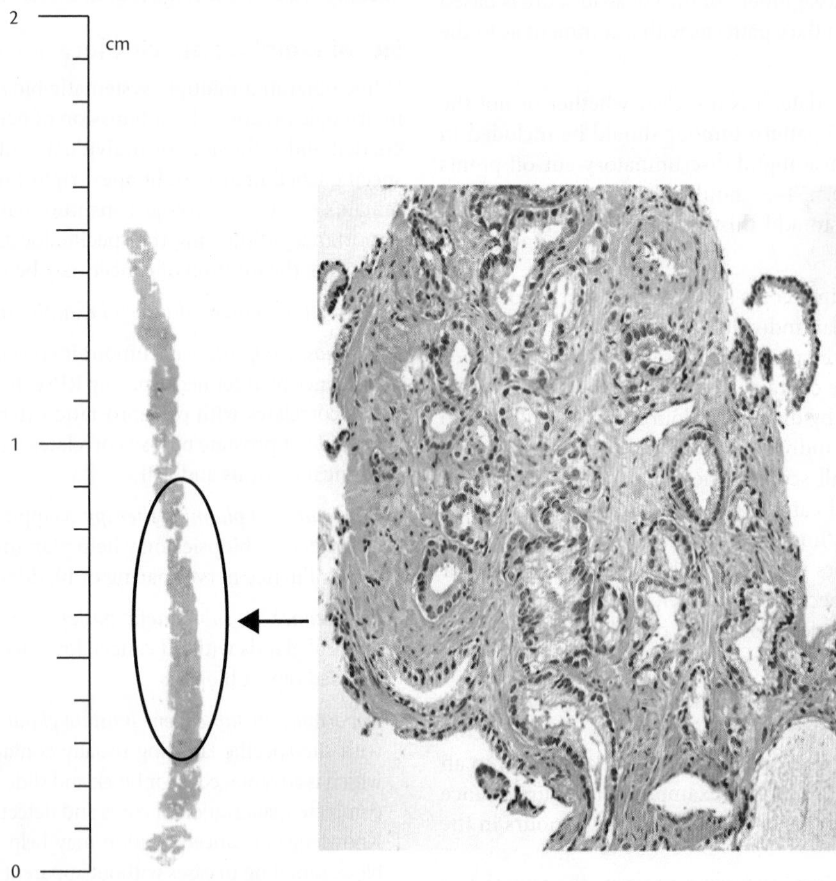

Fig. 6.3.6 Extent of involvement by cancer of a needle core. The length of the core, measured with a ruler on the surface of the slide, is 1.5 cm. The circled area contains cancer. The linear measurement of the cancer is 6.5 mm (i.e. 43% of the core).

at univariate and often at multivariate analyses.[40,41] It is a parameter included in some nomograms designed to predict pathologic stage and seminal vesicle invasion after RP and radiotherapy failure.[41,42]

The amount of cancer in a biopsy specimen depends on many factors, including prostate volume, cancer volume and distribution, technical procedures, number of biopsy cores, and cohort of evaluated patients.

The report should include the number of involved cores (if possible it should include % of cores involved). Moreover, one or both of the following tumour extent methods should be performed. One method is to report the linear length of cancer in mm (total tumour length in all biopsies; longest single length of tumour). The other method consists in estimating a percentage of involvement for each of the cores derived by visual estimation (overall % of cancer in all biopsies, % of each core involved; reporting the percentage of cancer involvement in increments of 5 or 10% is recommended). While high tumour burden in needle biopsies is directly related to a worse outcome, low tumour burden in needle biopsies is not always an indicator of low volume and low-stage in the prostatectomy specimen.

One problem encountered with this otherwise straightforward method is when there is extreme fragmentation of the needle biopsy specimen, making difficult the assessment of the number of cores and of the percentage of cancer within each core. In case of highly fragmented tissue this may be overcome by providing a composite (global) percentage of cancer involvement in all needle biopsy tissue, and this may more accurately correlate with the amount of cancer in the prostate gland.[43]

Bilateral cancer, which indicates multifocality, indirectly suggest a greater tumour volume. This parameter can be easily deduced from the pathology reports of each of the cores submitted and represents a crucial factor to assign a 'pathologic stage' in patients not subsequently treated by RP.

Local invasion

Routine biopsy sampling may occasionally contain extraprostatic fat or seminal vesicle tissue. If it is noted that cancer involves these structures, this would indicate pT3 disease. The invasion of seminal vesicles or the involvement of extraprostatic fat in the biopsy correlates with similar findings at RPs. Extraprostatic fat invasion at needle biopsy is a significant predictor of biochemical recurrence (79% compared to 43% failure rate in cases with EPE not detected by needle biopsy).

Only rarely does fat present within the normal prostate. Hence, tumour in adipose tissue in a needle biopsy specimen can safely be interpreted as EPE.[44,45] Ganglion cells and skeletal muscle involvement by tumour is not equivalent to EPE and they may both be found frequently within the prostate.

The seminal vesicle epithelium and ejaculatory duct epithelium may be impossible to distinguish in limited samples. Occasionally, the seminal vesicle can present a smooth muscle wall, which may help in the diagnosis. On the contrary, ejaculatory duct epithelium presents a rim of fibrous tissue that is rich in thin blood vessels. The distinction between seminal vesicle tissue/ejaculatory duct is not feasible, allowing the use of diagnostic terminology such as 'adenocarcinoma of the prostate with invasion of seminal vesicle/ejaculatory duct tissue'.

In seminal vesicle or extraprostatic fat-targeted biopsies, beyond diagnosing cancer, it is also fundamental to assess whether or not the targeted tissue is represented. In a positive biopsy, if the intended tissue is not present and its absence not specified in the report, there is a high likelihood of misinterpretation of locally advanced disease, which is not present. Also, seminal vesicle-containing/targeted biopsies should demonstrate tumour within the muscular wall.

Perineural invasion

Perineural, circumferential, or intraneural invasion is defined as the presence of PCa juxtaposed intimately along, around, or within a nerve. Extensive (multifocal) perineural invasion and greater nerve diameter constitute significant prognostic factors. Involvement of extraprostatic nerves within the adipose tissue by cancer indicates EPE and deserves notation in the pathology report when present.[42]

Although perineural invasion in needle biopsy specimens does not independently predict the prognosis when the Gleason score, serum PSA and extent of cancer are factored in, most studies indicate that its presence correlates with EPE (38–93%).[46,47] Recent data suggests that perineural invasion may be an independent predictor of lymph node metastasis and post-surgical progression.[46] This parameter may also be employed to plan nerve-sparing surgery.[48] Some of the data from the radiation oncology literature suggest that perineural invasion is an independent predictor of worse outcome after external beam radiotherapy. Furthermore, adjuvant hormonal therapy or dose escalation has been sustained in patients with high Gleason score and perineural invasion.[46,49]

Lymphovascular invasion

Lymphovascular invasion (LVI) consists of tumour cells within endothelial-lined spaces. We do not distinguish between vascular and lymphatic channels, due to the difficulty and lack of reproducibility among different observers by routine light microscopic examination. LVI may be confounded with fixation-associated retraction artefact of acini. Immunohistochemical stains directed against endothelial cells, such as factor VIII-related antigen, CD31, or CD34, may increase the detection rate.

Since LVI as studied in RP specimens is associated with lymph node metastases, biochemical recurrence, and distinct metastases, its presence can play a similar role in the needle biopsies. This feature is very rarely reported in needle biopsy specimens.[42]

Prognostic factors in radical prostatectomy specimens

The pathology report should detail clinically relevant information derived from the macroscopic and microscopic evaluation of the RP specimens.[50,51]

Histological type of cancer

In years, a number of new and unusual histological variants or subtypes have been identified. These variants represent the spectrum of changes which can occur in adenocarcinoma. The biological behaviour of many of these variants may differ from typical adenocarcinoma and their proper clinical management depends on accurate diagnosis and separation from tumours arising in other sites. It is recommended that subtypes, such as small cell, ductal, and mucinous, should be reported if they are noted histologically. Mixtures of distinct histological types should be reported.[38]

Histological grade of cancer

The Gleason score assigned to the tumour is the best predictor of progression following RP (see sections on '2005 International Society of Urological Pathology-modified Gleason grading system' and 'Subsequent 2016 modifications of the ISUP grading system').[31–36]

Staging

The protocol recommends the use of the TNM staging system for carcinoma of the prostate by the American Joint Committee on Cancer (AJCC) and the International Union Against Cancer (UICC).[52,53] The most revision was published in 2009. Clinical classification (cTNM) is usually carried out by the physician during pretreatment clinical evaluation or when pathologic classification is not possible. The prefix symbol 'p' refers to the pathologic classification of the TNM (pTNM). Pathologic classification relies on gross and microscopic examination. Based on AJCC/UICC convention, the designation 'T' in the TNM classification refers only to the first resection of a primary tumour. Therefore, pT requires a resection of the primary tumour or biopsy adequate to assess the highest pT category; pN entails an adequate removal of nodes to identify lymph node metastases; pM implies microscopic examination of distant lesions.

Residual tumour in a resection specimen following previous neoadjuvant therapy of any type (radiotherapy, chemotherapy, or any combined approach) is classified by the TNM using a prescript 'y' to indicate the post-treatment status of the tumour (e.g. ypT1). The assessment of residual disease may be a significant predictor of postoperative outcome. Moreover, the ypTNM classification allows a standardized and accurate evaluation of new neoadjuvant therapies. Tumour with local recurrence after a documented disease-free interval after surgical resection is defined according to the TNM system but modified with the prefix 'r' (e.g. rpT1).

The 2009 International Society of Urological Pathology Consensus Conference in Boston, gave recommendations concerning the necessity to standardize pathology reports of RP specimens.[50]

Tumour multifocality

PCa is multifocal in up to 80% of cases. Typically, there is a dominant focus. This is the largest cancer focus and in most cases has the worse pathological differentiation. This dominant focus can be tremed the index tumour and appears the most important for prognosis. Secondary foci are usually smaller and better differentiated. Noguchi *et al.* found the index tumour volume, and not total tumour volume, was the best independent predictor of tumour progression.[54] The concept of an index tumour was discussed at the ISUP consensus conference, without finding an agreement about an appropriate definition for this. Notably, no consensus was obtained regarding which parameter should have priority for defining the index tumour when there is a conflict between highest grade, stage, or volume between separate tumour foci.

T2 substaging

Staging category pT2 includes tumours that are confined within the prostate gland. Among controversies relating to tumours that present in this staging category, critical issues are represented by the value of substaging, the reporting of multifocal tumours and the prognostic relevance of tumour size.[50,55]

The pathological substaging of pT2 currently mirrors clinical T2 substaging of PCa. A pT2a tumour is defined as a unilateral tumour, affecting less than half of one lobe, a pT2b tumour is unilateral, occupying more than 50% of one lobe, while a pT2c tumour is bilateral. There are several problems with this classification. Stage pT2b is a very rare finding, as most tumours that are larger than one lobe of the prostate gland grow across the midline and are rarely organ-confined. Tumours classified as pT2b are thus large and have less favourable outcome than pT2c tumours. The definition of pT2c is unclear and it is uncertain if the presence of separate, but minute foci of tumour in the contralateral lobe is sufficient to classify a tumour as pT2c, or if the main tumour focus must cross the midline before being considered pT2. There is also debate as to why extension across the midline of the gland should be considered an important prognostic feature. In line with this, many the delegates present at the consensus meeting voted to abandon the current pT2 substaging category. Given the favourable prognosis of organ-confined disease, it can also be questioned whether substaging is at all justified.[50]

Extraprostatic extension (pT3a)

The prostatic capsule is a poorly defined structure and not a true capsule, but is rather a transition between condensed prostatic stroma and the extraprostatic connective tissue. This structure is particularly poorly defined around the apex, the anterior prostate, and at the base of the gland. For these reasons, EPE is considered a more appropriate terminology than capsule penetration. Extraprostatic extension is most frequently encountered in the posterolateral region at the neurovascular bundle (Fig. 6.3.7). Tumour adjacent to or that invades the adipose tissue is a criterion for the diagnosis of extraprostatic extension. However, contrary to the situation with core biopsies, it was also agreed to diagnose prostatectomy specimens with EPE even when extraprostatic lesions are surrounded by desmoplastic connective tissue. Thus, tumour within a fibrous band, beyond the prostatic parenchyma, or the condensed smooth muscle, is sufficient to diagnose extraprostatic disease.

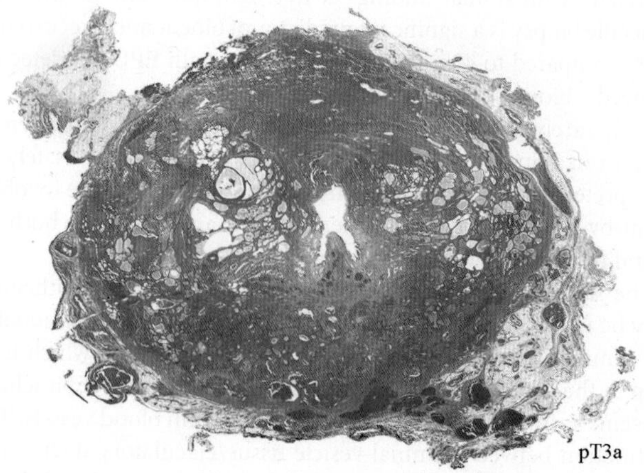

Fig. 6.3.7 Whole-mount section of the prostate with extraprostatic extension in the posterolateral region.

In areas where the so-called capsule is particularly poorly defined, such as at the anterior, the apex and at the bladder neck, growth into or at the level of adipose tissue is needed to identify extraprostatic extension. At the apex and anteriorly, there is a continuous transition between prostatic tissue and the striated muscle tissue of the pelvic floor. Hence, it was agreed that tumour growth around striated muscle does not indicate in any case EPE.

Extraprostatic extension can be classified as focal or established (or extensive or non-focal).[50] Patients with focal extraprostatic extension are characterized by a more favourable outcome after RP compared to patients with extensive EPE, thus recommending to describe the extent of EPE in the reports. There is, however, no consensus on the definition of these categories and measures such as 'a few glands outside the prostate' or 'less than one high-power field' have been used to define focal EPE.[50,56] Recently, Sung *et al.* suggested the employment of the radial distance of extraprostatic extension, with a cut-off at 0.75 mm having prognostic significance.[57] This method has some disadvantages; for instance, it is labour intensive and because the prostatic capsule is so poorly defined, it is very difficult to know from where this distance should be measured. It was recommended at the consensus conference that extraprostatic extension be stratified as focal or established, but no consensus was reached as to the definitions of these categories.[50,56]

Seminal vesicle invasion (pT3b)

Seminal vesicle invasion or SVI is defined as the invasion into the muscular coat of the seminal vesicle by cancer cells. SVI has been previously associated with the prognosis of patients with PCa[58,59] PCa can invade the seminal vesicles by three main mechanisms[60]:

(i) by extension to the ejaculatory duct complex;

(ii) by spread across the base of the prostate without other evidence of EPE or involvement from tumour affecting the seminal vesicles from the periprostatic and periseminal vesicle adipose tissue;

(iii) as an isolated tumour deposit without continuity with the primary PCa tumour focus.

While in most cases, seminal vesicle invasion occurs in glands with EPE, the latter cannot be reported in a minority of these cases. Many of these patients present only a minimal involvement of the seminal vesicles, or harbour tumours affecting only the portion of the seminal vesicles that is, at least in part, intraprostatic. Patients in this subgroup were associated with a favourable prognosis, similar to patients without SVI. Despite this, the prognostic value of these categories has not been confirmed by others.[61]

Locally advanced disease (pT4)

In previous editions of the TNM classification, bladder neck invasion was classified as pT4 disease, even when invasion was microscopic rather than macroscopic. It has, however, been shown that these patients have an outcome similar to those with ordinary extraprostatic extension, and it was agreed that the TNM classification should be revised accordingly. Indeed, in the latest edition, microscopic bladder neck invasion is now considered pT3a disease, while macroscopic bladder neck invasion is classified as pT4.[50,52]

Surgical margins and residual tumour (R)

In general, a prostatectomy specimen is surrounded by a thin layer of connective tissue and a wide surgical margin cannot be expected. Cancer must be seen extending to an inked margin for that margin to be considered positive.[51,62] A margin is reported as negative if cancer is separated from the inked surface by as little as a few collagen fibres. Tumour close to, but not extending to a margin, should be recorded as a margin negative as this does not influence prognosis. Positive margins are most common seen at the apex of the gland but may occur anywhere. Similar to extraprostatic extension, stratification of margin positivity into focal and more than focal may be useful, but the consensus conference failed to agree on methods for defining this. Among proposed definitions of focal margin positivity were: (i) only a few tumour cells in contact with the inked margin; (ii) margin positivity involving one gland in one section; (iii) 3 mm or less of positive margin in one section; and (iv) limited margin positivity in only one or two areas. Until a clinically relevant cut-off is decided upon, it was recommended to report the linear extent of margin positivity. As in the case of EPE, a consensus was reached about the necessity to report the location of any tumour positive margin, as this gives important feedback to the clinician.

Residual tumour after therapy with curative intent (e.g. surgical resection) is classified by the R classification, which may be employed by the surgeon to report the residual tumour status after surgical resection. For the pathologist, the R classification deals with the margins of surgical resection specimens; patients with positive resection margins on pathologic examination may be considered to have residual tumour. These patients may be classified based on the macroscopic or microscopic involvement.[51,62]

Lymphovascular invasion

The TNM system uses the category LVI to indicate the presence of lymphatic or venous invasion. Most of the time when vascular invasion is noted it is in tumours with fairly advanced pathology, such that it is unclear as to its independent prognostic significance. It has been shown that LVI correlates with risk of recurrence after RP, both in univariate and multivariate analysis.[42]

Perineural invasion

Perineural invasion is almost ubiquitously present in RP specimens, such that it is not useful as a prognostic parameter and we do not record it in the pathology reports of RP. Several studies investigated the prognostic role of (intraprostatic) perineural invasion. At this time, it is not entirely clear whether there are differences in terms of prognosis between intraprostatic and extraprostatic perineural invasion.[63]

Volume of cancer

There are several methods to estimate tumour volume, including planimetry, the grid method, assessment of the percentage of the specimen involved by cancer and measurement maximum tumour diameter.[42,50,55] Volume of PCa correlates with other prognostic factors, including grade, stage, and ploidy, and also with prognosis in patients who have undergone RP. Some authors have reported that tumour volume does not independently predict the prognosis when Gleason score, the presence of extraprostatic extension, positive surgical margins, and seminal vesicle involvement are included into the analysis. Other studies, based on series with larger tumours, have reported that tumour volume represents an independent prognostic factor. Because of these conflicting data, it was recommended that measurement of tumour volume should not be mandatory but that it was reasonable to give an objective assessment of tumour size, reporting the diameter of the largest tumour focus.

Conclusions

Substantial effort has been expended in the years in describing the morphologic features of cancer and determining its predictive value for staging, cancer recurrence, and patient survival in prostate carcinoma. Molecular knowledge of PCa can improve prediction of prognosis, but has not yet yielded information that is ready to be routinely incorporated into clinical practice.

Further reading

Berney DM, Wheeler TM, Grignon DJ, *et al.* and the ISUP Prostate Cancer Group International Society of Urological Pathology (ISUP) Consensus Conference on Handling and Staging of Radical Prostatectomy Specimens. Working group 4: seminal vesicles and lymph nodes. *Mod Pathol* 2011; **24**:39–47.

Bostwick DG, Cheng L. Precursors of prostate cancer. *Histopathology* 2012; **60**:4–27.

Egevad L, Mazzucchelli R, Montironi R. Implications of the International Society of Urological Pathology modified Gleason grading system. *Arch Pathol Lab Med* 2012; **136**:426–34.

Magi-Galluzzi C, Evans AJ, Delahunt B, *et al.* and the ISUP Prostate Cancer Group International Society of Urological Pathology (ISUP) Consensus Conference on Handling and Staging of Radical Prostatectomy Specimens. Working group 3: extraprostatic extension, lymphovascular invasion and locally advanced disease. *Mod Pathol* 2011; **24**:26–38.

Montironi R, Mazzucchelli R, Lopez-Beltran A, Scarpelli M, Cheng L. Prostatic intraepithelial neoplasia: its morphological and molecular diagnosis and clinical significance. *BJU Int* 2011; **108**:1394–401.

Samaratunga H, Montironi R, True L, *et al.* International Society of Urological Pathology (ISUP) Consensus Conference on Handling and Staging of Radical Prostatectomy Specimens. Working group 1: specimen handling. *Mod Pathol* 2011; **24**:6–15.

Tan PO, Cheng L, John R Srigley JR, *et al.* and the ISUP Prostate Cancer Group International Society of Urological Pathology (ISUP) Consensus Conference on Handling and Staging of Radical Prostatectomy Specimens. Working group 5: surgical margins. *Mod Pathol* 2011; **24**:48–57.

van der Kwast TH, Amin MB, Billis A, *et al.* and the ISUP Prostate Cancer Group International Society of Urological Pathology (ISUP) Consensus Conference on Handling and Staging of Radical Prostatectomy Specimens. Working group 2: T2 substaging and prostate cancer volume. *Mod Pathol* 2011; **24**:16–25.

References

1. Srigley JR, Amin MB, Boccon-Gibod L, *et al.* Prognostic and predictive factors in prostate cancer: historical perspectives and international consensus initiatives. *Scand J Urol Nephrol* 2005; **216**:8–19.
2. Nelson WG, De Marzo AM, Isaacs WB. Prostate cancer. *N Engl J Med* 2003; **349**:366–81.
3. Crawford ED. Epidemiology of prostate cancer. *Urology* 2003; **62**:3–12.
4. Bostwick DG, Cheng L. Precursors of prostate cancer. *Histopathology* 2012; **60**:4–27.
5. Montironi R, Mazzucchelli R, Lopez-Beltran A, Scarpelli M, Cheng L. Prostatic intraepithelial neoplasia: its morphological and molecular diagnosis and clinical significance. *BJU Int* 2011; **108**:1394–401.
6. Eskicorapci SY, Guliyev F, Islamoglu E, Ergen A, Ozen H. The effect of prior biopsy scheme on prostate cancer detection for repeat biopsy population: results of the 14-core prostate biopsy technique. *Int Urol Nephrol* 2007; **39**:189–95.
7. Kronz JD, Allan CH, Shaikh AA, Epstein JI. Predicting cancer following a diagnosis of high-grade prostatic intraepithelial neoplasia on needle biopsy: data on men with more than one follow-up biopsy. *Am J Surg Pathol* 2001; **25**:1079–85.
8. Hull D, Ma J, Singh H, Hossain D, Qian J, Bostwick DG. Precursor of prostate-specific antigen expression in prostatic intraepithelial neoplasia and adenocarcinoma: a study of 90 cases. *BJU Int* 2009; **104**:915–8.
9. Robinson B, Magi-Galluzzi C, Zhou M. Intraductal carcinoma of the prostate. *Arch Pathol Lab Med* 2012; **136**:418–25.
10. Cohen RJ, Shannon BA, Weinstein SL. Intraductal carcinoma of the prostate gland with transmucosal spread to the seminal vesicle: a lesion distinct from high-grade prostatic intraepithelial neoplasia. *Arch Pathol Lab Med* 2007; **131**:1122–5.
11. Tavora F, Epstein JI. High-grade prostatic intraepithelial neoplasia like ductal adenocarcinoma of the prostate: a clinicopathologic study of 28 cases. *Am J Surg Pathol* 2008; **32**:1060–67.
12. Montironi R, Scattoni V, Mazzucchelli R, Lopez-Beltran A, Bostwick DG, Montorsi F. Atypical foci suspicious but not diagnostic of malignancy in prostate needle biopsies (also referred to as "atypical small acinar proliferation suspicious for but not diagnostic of malignancy"). *Eur Urol* 2006; **50**:666–74.
13. Bostwick DG, Qian J, Frankel K. The incidence of high grade prostatic intraepithelial neoplasia in needle biopsies. *J Urol* 1995; **154**:1791–4.
14. Descazeaud A, Rubin MA, Allory Y, *et al.* What information are urologists extracting from prostate needle biopsy reports and what do they need for clinical management of prostate cancer? *Eur Urol* 2005; **48**:911–5.
15. Park S, Shinohara K, Grossfeld GD, Carroll PR. Prostate cancer detection in men with prior high grade prostatic intraepithelial neoplasia or atypical prostate biopsy. *J Urol* 2001; **165**:1409–14.
16. Leite KR, Mitteldorf CA, Camara-Lopes LH. Repeat prostate biopsies following diagnoses of prostate intraepithelial neoplasia and atypical small gland proliferation. *Int Braz J Urol* 2005; **31**:131–6.
17. Scattoni V, Roscigno M, Freschi M, *et al.* Predictors of prostate cancer after initial diagnosis of atypical small acinar proliferation at 10 to 12 core biopsies. *Urology* 2005; **66**:1043–7.
18. Schlesinger C, Bostwick DG, Iczkowski KA. High-grade prostatic intraepithelial neoplasia and atypical small acinar proliferation: predictive value for cancer in current practice. *Am J Surg Pathol* 2005; **29**:1201–7.
19. Humphrey PA. Focal glandular atypia. (pp. 219–25) In: Humphrey PA (ed). *Prostate Pathology*. Chigago, IL: ASCP Press, 2003.
20. Epstein JI. Diagnosis of limited adenocarcinoma of the prostate. *Histopathology* 2012; **60**:28–40.
21. Humphrey PA. Diagnosis of adenocarcinoma in prostate needle biopsy tissue. *J Clin Pathol* 2007; **60**:35–42.
22. Montironi R, Mazzucchelli R, Lopez-Beltran A, Cheng L. Prostate cancer origins, diagnosis, and prognosis in clinical practice. (pp. 92–155) In: Mikuz G (ed). *Clinical Pathology of Urologic Tumors*. London, UK: Informa Healtcare, 2007.
23. Del Rosario AD, Bui HX, Abdulla M, Ross JS. Sulfur-rich prostatic intraluminal crystalloids: A surgical pathologic and electron probe x-ray microanalytic study. *Hum Pathol* 1993; **24**:1159–67.
24. Molberg KH, Mikhail A, Vuitch F. Crystalloids in metastatic prostatic adenocarcinoma. *Am J Clin Pathol* 1994; **101**:266–8.
25. Goldstein NS, Qian J, Bostwick DG. Mucin expression in atypical adenomatous hyperplasia of the prostate. *Hum Pathol* 1995; **26**:887–91.

26. Hameed O, Humphrey PA. Pseudoneoplastic mimics of prostate and bladder carcinomas. *Arch Pathol Lab Med* 2010; **134**:427–43.
27. Shah RB, Zhou M, LeBlanc M, Snyder M, Rubin MA. Comparison of the basal cell specific markers, 34betaE12 and p 63 in the diagnosis of prostate cancer. *Am J Surg Pathol* 2002; **26**:1161–8.
28. Jiang Z, Wu CL, Woda BA, *et al.* P504S/Alpha-Methylacyl-CoA racemase: a useful marker for diagnosis of small foci of prostatic carcinoma on needle biopsy. *Am J Surg Pathol* 2002; **26**:1169–74.
29. Zhou M, Chinnaiyan AM, Kleer CG, Lucas PC, Rubin MA. Alpha-Methylacyl-CoA racemase: a novel tumor marker over-expressed in several human cancers and their precursor lesions. *Am J Surg Pathol* 2002; **26**:926–31.
30. Yang XJ, Wu CL, Woda BA, *et al.* Expression of Alpha-Methylacyl-CoA racemase (P504S) in atypical adenomatous hyperplasia of the prostate. *Am J Surg Pathol* 2002; **26**:921–5.
31. Egevad L, Mazzucchelli R, Montironi R. Implications of the International Society of Urological Pathology modified Gleason grading system. *Arch Pathol Lab Med* 2012; **136**:426–34.
32. Delahunt B, Miller RJ, Srigley JR, Evans AJ, Samaratunga H. Gleason grading: past, present and future. *Histopathology* 2012; **60**:75–86.
33. Montironi R, Cheng L, Lopez-Beltran A, *et al.* Original Gleason system versus 2005 ISUP modified Gleason system: the importance of indicating which system is used in the patient's pathology and clinical reports. *Eur Urol* 2010; **58**:369–73.
34. Uemura H, Hoshino K, Sasaki T, *et al.* Usefulness of the 2005 International Society of Urologic Pathology Gleason grading system in prostate biopsy and radical prostatectomy specimens. *BJU Int* 2009; **103**:1190–94.
35. Epstein JI. An update of the Gleason grading system. *J Urol* 2010; **183**:433–40.
36. Moch H, Humphrey PA, Ulbright TM, Reuter V. *WHO Classification of tumours of the urinary system and male genital organs*. Lyon, France: International Agency for Research on Cancer; 2016.
37. Pierorazio PM, Walsh PC, Partin AW, Epstein JI. Prognostic Gleason grade grouping: data based on the modified Gleason scoring system. *BJU Int* 2013; **111**:753–60.
38. Epstein JI, Algaba F, Allbrook WC Jr, *et al.* Tumours of the prostate. Acinar adenocarcinoma. (pp. 162–92) In: Eble JN, Sauter G, Epstein JI, Sesterhenn IA (eds). *Pathology and Genetics: Tumors of the Urinary System and Male Genital Organs*. Lyon, France: IARC Press, 2004.
39. Montironi R, Mazzucchelli R, Scarpelli M, Lopez-Beltran A, Fellegara G, Algaba F. Gleason grading of prostate cancer in needle biopsies or radical prostatectomy specimens: contemporary approach, current clinical significance and sources of pathology discrepancies. *BJU Int* 2005; **95**:1146–52.
40. Freedland SJ, Aronson WJ, Terris MK, *et al.* The percentage of prostate needle biopsy cores with carcinoma from the more involved side of the biopsy as a predictor of prostate specific antigen recurrence after radical prostatectomy: results from the Shared Equal Access Regional Cancer Hospital (SEARCH) database. *Cancer* 2003; **98**:2344–50.
41. Kattan MW, Eastham JA, Wheeler TM, *et al.* Counseling men with prostate cancer: a nomogram for predicting the presence of small, moderately differentiated, confined tumors. *J Urol* 2003; **170**:1792–7.
42. Fine SW, Amin MB, Berney DM, *et al.* A contemporary update on pathology reporting for prostate cancer: biopsy and radical prostatectomy specimens. *Eur Urol* 2012; **62**:20–39.
43. Montironi R, Scarpelli M, Mazzucchelli R, Cheng L, Lopez-Beltran A, Montorsi F. Extent of cancer of less than 50% in any prostate needle biopsy core: how many millimeters are there? *Eur Urol* 2012; **61**:751–6.
44. Cohen RJ, Stables S. Intra-prostatic fat. *Hum Pathol* 1998; **29**:424–5.
45. Epstein JI. Diagnosis and reporting of limited adenocarcinoma of the prostate on needle biopsy. *Mod Pathol* 2004; **17**:307–15.
46. Quinn DI, Henshall SM, Brenner PC, *et al.* Prognostic significance of preoperative factors in localized prostate carcinoma treated with radical prostatectomy: importance of percentage of biopsies that contain tumor and the presence of biopsy perineural invasion. *Cancer* 2003; **97**:1884–93.
47. Vargas SO, Jiroutek M, Welch WR, Nucci MR, D'Amico AV, Renshaw AA. Perineural invasion in prostate needle biopsy specimens. Correlation with extraprostatic extension at resection. *Am J Clin Pathol* 1999; **111**:223–8.
48. Holmes GF, Walsh PC, Pound CR, Epstein JI. Excision of the neurovascular bundle at radical prostatectomy in cases with perineural invasion on needle biopsy. *Urology* 1999; **53**:752–6.
49. Beard CJ, Chen MH, Cote K, *et al.* Perineural invasion is associated with increased relapse after external beam radiotherapy for men with low-risk prostate cancer and may be a marker for occult, high-grade cancer. *Int J Radiat Oncol Biol Phys* 2004; **58**:19–24.
50. Cheng L, Montironi R, Bostwick DG, Lopez-Beltran A, Berney DM. Staging of prostate cancer. *Histopathology* 2012; **60**:87–117.
51. Montironi R, Mazzucchelli R, Scarpelli M, Lopez-Beltran A, Mikuz G. Prostate carcinoma I: prognostic factors in radical prostatectomy specimens and pelvic lymph nodes. *BJU Int* 2006; **97**:485–91.
52. American Joint Committee on Cancer. Genitourinary sites. Prostate. (pp. 525–38) In: Edge SB, Byrd DR, Compton CC, Friz AG, Green FL, Trotti A (eds). *AJCC Cancer Staging Handbook*, 7th edition. New York, NY: Springer, 2009.
53. Sobin LH, Gospodarowicz MK, Wittekind CH (eds). Urological tumours: Prostate (pp. 243–8). In: *TNM Classification of Malignant Tumours*, 7th edition. Chichester, UK: Wiley-Blackwell, 2009.
54. Noguchi M, Stamey TA, McNeal JE, Nolley R. Prognostic factors for multifocal prostate cancer in radical prostatectomy specimens: lack of significance of secondary cancers. *J Urol* 2003; **170**:459–63.
55. van der Kwast TH, Amin MB, Billis A, *et al.* and the ISUP Prostate Cancer Group International Society of Urological Pathology (ISUP) Consensus Conference on Handling and Staging of Radical Prostatectomy Specimens. Working group 2: T2 substaging and prostate cancer volume. *Mod Pathol* 2011; **24**:16–25.
56. Magi-Galluzzi C, Evans AJ, Delahunt B, *et al.* and the ISUP Prostate Cancer Group International Society of Urological Pathology (ISUP) Consensus Conference on Handling and Staging of Radical Prostatectomy Specimens. Working group 3: extraprostatic extension, lymphovascular invasion and locally advanced disease. *Mod Pathol* 2011; **24**:26–38.
57. Sung MT, Lin H, Koch MO, Davidson DD, Cheng L. Radial distance of extraprostatic extension measured by ocular micrometer is an independent predictor of prostate-specific antigen recurrence: a new proposal for the substaging of pT3a prostate cancer. *Am J Surg Pathol* 2007; **31**:311–18.
58. Debras B, Guillonneau B, Bougaran J, Chambon E, Vallancien G. Prognostic significance of seminal vesicle invasion on the radical prostatectomy specimen. Rationale for seminal vesicle biopsies. *Eur Urol* 1998; **33**:271–7.
59. Tefilli MV, Gheiler EL, Tiguert R, *et al.* Prognostic indicators in patients with seminal vesicle involvement following radical prostatectomy for clinically localized prostate cancer. *J Urol* 1998; **160**:802–6.
60. Ohori M, Scardino PT, Lapin SL, Seale-Hawkins C, Link J, Wheeler TM. The mechanisms and prognostic significance of seminal vesicle involvement by prostate cancer. *Am J Surg Pathol* 1993; **17**:1252–61.
61. Berney DM, Wheeler TM, Grignon DJ, *et al.* and the ISUP Prostate Cancer Group International Society of Urological Pathology (ISUP) Consensus Conference on Handling and Staging of Radical Prostatectomy Specimens. Working group 4: seminal vesicles and lymph nodes. *Mod Pathol* 2011; **24**:39–47.
62. Tan PO, Cheng L, John R Srigley JR, *et al.* and the ISUP Prostate Cancer Group International Society of Urological Pathology(ISUP) Consensus Conference on Handling and Staging of Radical Prostatectomy Specimens. Working group 5: surgical margins. *Mod Pathol* 2011; **24**:48–57.
63. Bostwick DG, Grignon DJ, Hammond ME, *et al.* Prognostic factors in prostate cancer. College of American Pathologists Consensus Statement 1999. *Arch Pathol Lab Med* 2000; **124**:995–1000.

CHAPTER 6.4

Prostate-specific antigen and biomarkers for prostate cancer

Sven Wenske and Hans Lilja

Blood biomarkers

Introduction to human kallikreins

The human kallikrein family, located on chromosome 19q13,[1–3] has been identified to consist of 15 genes, encoding for serine proteases, several of which are mainly expressed in seminal fluid. To date, best described are the gene products encoded by *KLK2* (kallikrein-related peptidase 2 [hK2]) and *KLK3* (prostate-specific antigen [PSA]).[4] More expression, protein characteristics, and taxon-specific evolution of the *KLK* genes have been studied and described with distinct nomenclature.[2,5–7] Among these, *KLK2* and *KLK3* manifest the most extensive homology with ≈80% identity in amino acid sequence, relating to their ancestry and primate-specific duplication from a common predecessor, a non-functional pseudogene in rodents, and most other mammals except the canine species.[6]

Prostate-specific antigen and molecular isoforms

Prostate-specific antigen (PSA) is a ≈28-kD single chain kallikrein-related serine peptidase[6] expressed abundantly in normal human prostate epithelium, benign hyperplastic prostatic tissue (BPH), and prostate carcinoma.[8,9] Several studies have demonstrated very low level extra-prostatic production of PSA (≈10^{-4}-fold or lower compared to the levels found in human prostate epithelium) in human breast epithelium, endometrium, amniotic fluid, and periurethral glands.[10,11] The precursor of PSA is a 261 amino acid pre-pro-protein.[12] Subsequent processing by hK2 and other proteases leads to the conversion from the non-catalytic zymogen to catalytically active mature PSA comprising 237 amino acids.[13–15] Catalytically active PSA is a highly abundant single chain chymotrypsin-like serine-protease[16,17] that is critical to and responsible for the proteolysis of the gel-proteins semenogelin I (*SEMG1*) and II (*SEMG2*) and fibronectin in the seminal fluid, resulting in liquefaction of semen and release of motile spermatozoa.[18–20] In healthy men, PSA occurs in serum at concentrations corresponding to approximately 10^{-6} of those found in seminal fluid. In the seminal fluid, approximately 60–70% of PSA is found in catalytically active functional status,[16] forming complexes with different extracellular protease inhibitors, such as α_1-antichymotrypsin (ACT or *SERPINA3*), protein C inhibitor (*SERPINA5*), α_2-macroglobulin (*A2M*), and other *SERPIN*- or *A2M*-type inhibitors.[16,21–23]

About 30% of the PSA isolated from seminal fluid is catalytically inactive and unable to form complexes with ACT. Several different internal peptide bond cleavages render the catalytically active single chain form into non-catalytic multichain forms.[16,24] Subsequent studies implicate that that the proportion of free PSA with or without internal peptide cleavages at Lys145 and/or Lys146 is associated with risk of prostate cancer,[25,26] also among men at increased risk of unfavourable prostate cancer.[26] Other investigators have demonstrated that higher levels of pro-PSA are associated with prostate cancer,[14,27,28] especially in men with more aggressive disease and other adverse pathological features.[29,30]

Prostate-specific antigen and prostate cancer

As first reported in the early 1980s, PSA was detected in human serum and found to be significantly elevated in men with prostate cancer, and therefore suggested to be a novel and highly tissue-specific marker of this disease.[31–33] Subsequent reports by Stamey *et al.* in 1987 demonstrated the utility of PSA to detect and monitor treatment of prostate cancer, and that of Catalona *et al.* in 1991[43] found that also a modestly elevated PSA was associated with increased risk localized prostate cancer. Combined with many other largely consistent reports, the seminal studies by these authors led to rapid implementation and widespread use of the PSA test, particularly in the United States, with consequential dramatic increase in prostate cancer incidence during late 1980s and early 1990s, before the prostate cancer incidence started to stabilize from mid 1990s and onwards.[34] Since then, PSA has remained critical to early detection and screening, as well as disease monitoring in patients treated for prostate cancer, and still represents one of the most useful tumour markers in these settings.[4] However, it is also important to recognize that the current modalities of PSA testing has led to prostate cancer having one of the highest prevalence rates of all malignant diseases in men, with an overall lifetime risk of 18%, and approximately 3% risk of dying from this disease.[34–36] These numbers exemplify that the majority of prostate cancers may possibly be considered *insignificant*, that is, no life-threatening risk to the patient. However, distinguishing between *significant* and *insignificant* cancers remains one of the biggest challenges in the detection and treatment decision-making of prostate cancer, and controversy exists as to what degree PSA and other biomarkers may be able to help.[37] Due to the increasing use of PSA in the early detection and screening of prostate cancer, a migration of prostate cancer stages upon diagnosis has been observed towards earlier, lower stages (*stage migration*) during the past two decades since the implementation of PSA in clinical settings in the early 1980s.[37,38] However, with PSA being prostate-, but not cancer-specific, major challenges exist among men with significantly increased risk of prostate cancer as the conventional PSA test alone has low to modest specificity,[39,40] and therefore may quite poorly discriminate between a PSA elevated secondary to benign (BPH, prostatitis) compared to malignant prostate disease, particularly among previously screened men.[41] Consequently, constant research has led to the discovery and identification of additional biomarkers, such as different molecular forms of PSA in serum that may aid in increasing diagnostic accuracy for the early detection of prostate cancer. Additional biomarkers, such as free PSA and hK2, have been suggested to being incorporated into risk assessment armamentarium.

In the absence of data obtained from experimental animal models recapitulating the mechanisms required to enable PSA to enter the different extracellular compartments and subsequently disseminate into blood circulation, it has commonly been speculated that increased levels of PSA in blood associated with prostate cancer may be secondary to changes in the normal prostatic anatomy, such as disruption of the basal membrane, altered intercellular connections, and general tissue architecture changes during the development and progression of this disease. Both PSA and hK2 are potent catalytic peptidases that may contribute to modify extracellular matrix proteins and, possibly importantly, contribute to a dramatically elevated release.[42] Advanced cases of prostate cancer may therefore lead to a 1,000-fold increase of the physiologic release of PSA into circulation.

One of the first prospective analyses describing the utility of PSA as a screening test for men at risk for prostate cancer concluded that a serum concentration cut-off level of 4 ng/mL offered highest sensitivity and specificity to detect men with prostate cancer and to avoid unnecessary biopsies in men that do not harbour this disease.[43] However, the risk of finding evidence of prostate cancer at biopsy among the vast majority (85–90%) of men with PSA levels below commonly used cut-offs (e.g. 4 ng/mL) remains remarkably high and associated with risks of leaving an important proportion of prostate cancers undetected, with about 10% risk of finding prostate cancer at biopsy among 62–91-year-old men with PSA of about 1.0 ng/mL or less.[36,44] The use of lower PSA cut-offs have not been able to fully overcome this issue,[36,39,45] and were instead found to contribute to significant overdiagnosis and consequential overtreatment of men frequently harbouring prostate cancers of low grade and stage that are unlikely to lead to significant morbidity during the lifetime of the host and therefore likely may be considered as *insignificant* cancers. Hence, PSA is best interpreted in relationship to age, co-morbidity, and as a continuous variable representing a wide spectrum of disease and disease settings.[46] This is important as we also know that population-based levels of PSA in blood increase with advancing age,[4] likely due to higher prevalence of BPH and volume of BPH being associated with increasing age.[47]

Long-term prediction of prostate cancer risk using prostate-specific antigen

One of the first studies to predict long-term risk for prostate cancer reported on men with a PSA >2.5 ng/mL having an increased risk to being diagnosed with prostate cancer 10 years later, but was importantly limited due to significant sample degradation and a small sample size.[48] A subsequent report by Gann *et al.* also demonstrated that an elevated PSA preceded a prostate cancer diagnosis by several years.[49] PSA measured in blood provided at baseline between 1974 and 1986 by a highly representative group of men participating (72% participation) in the Malmö Preventive Project (MPP) in southern Sweden, to study cardiovascular and metabolic risk factors, demonstrated that also a modestly elevated PSA below age 50 is associated with an importantly increased risk of prostate cancer diagnosis many years later.[50] A update of this, including over 1,400 prostate cancer cases among 21,277 men aged 33–50 years at baseline who were followed for a median of 23 years, found that a single PSA measured at age 44–50 years predict a diagnosis of advanced prostate cancer (defined as clinical stage T3 or higher or evidence of metastasis at diagnosis) with an area under the receiver operating curve (AUR) of 0.75.[25] Using data and blood contributed in 1981 and 1982 from men invited to participate in the MPP at age 60 and followed for up to 25 years until death or age 85, demonstrated that a PSA level at age 60 was strongly associated with risk of metastasis (AUC of 0.86) and death (AUC of 0.90) many years later, with close to 90% of all subsequent events of metastasis or death from prostate cancer occurring among men with PSA levels in the top quartile at age 60 (i.e. ≥PSA of 2.0 ng/mL).[51] Also, a PSA blood level at or below median (i.e. ≤1 ng/mL) at age 60 confers insignificant lifetime risk of metastasis (≤0.5%) or death (≤0.2%) from prostate cancer, suggesting that about half of the men aged 60 or older (i.e. men aged ≥60 with a PSA of ≈≤1.0 ng/mL) may be exempt from any subsequent population-based PSA testing (Fig. 6.4.1).[51]

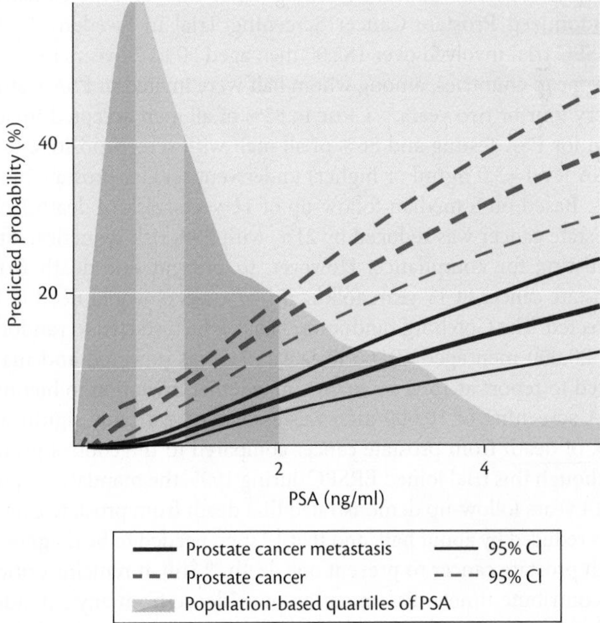

Fig. 6.4.1 Lifetime risk of clinically diagnosed prostate cancer or prostate cancer metastasis. Shaded region represents population-based distribution of prostate-specific antigen.

Reproduced from the *British Medical Journal*, Andrew J Vickers *et al.*, 'Prostate specific antigen concentration at age 60 and death or metastasis from prostate cancer: Case control study', Volume 341, c4521, DOI:10.1136/bmj.c4521, Copyright © 2010, British Medical Journal Publishing Group, with permission from BMJ Publishing Group Ltd.

These data suggest that the current intensely debated and troublesome ratio of benefits-to-harms associated with the current modality of PSA-based prostate cancer screening could possibly be improved by implementing risk stratifying approaches where men with little if any risk of significant cancer morbidity could be spared from frequent, elaborate testing, whereas men with; for example, PSA levels in the top decile or quartile at age 45 or later may benefit from more frequent and elaborate screening efforts.[53]

Randomized prostate cancer screening trials

In the United States, PSA-based prostate cancer screening became widely used already in early 1990s, which is long before any data from prospective randomized trials became available during the few years. This also resulted in significant problems in the interpretation of the data obtained by the randomized trial pursued by the Prostate, Lung, Colorectal, and Ovarian (PLCO) consortium at the National Cancer Institute in the United States, as about half of the men participating in this randomized trial had previously been subject to PSA screening, more than half of the control group continued to undergo PSA-based screening, and only a minority of the participants with a screen-positive test were subject to a prostate biopsy.[54] Undoubtedly, this may contribute to the fact that no significant differences in death from prostate cancer were found between the men invited to screening compared to the controls, as this trial rather may compare more systematic to less systematic screening regimens.[54] Therefore, the reported data from 11–14 years follow-up of the randomized trials in Europe contribute the most important and reliable data in reference to the theory that PSA-based screening among previously unscreened men in a highly significant statistical manner can reduce prostate cancer mortality after a follow-up of 10 years or longer (as reported by the European Randomized Study for Prostate Cancer Screening (ERSPC),[55] and the Göteborg randomized Prostate Cancer Screening Trial in Sweden).[56] The ERSPC trial involved over 182,00 men aged 50 to 74 years in seven European countries, among whom half were invited to PSA testing every four or two years.[57] Close to 83% of all men accepted invitation for PSA testing and 86% of all men with screen-positive tests (PSA level ≈3.0 ng/ml or higher) underwent sextant prostate biopsies. Based on a median follow-up of 11 years, risk of death from prostate cancer was reduced by 21%, with 29% risk reduction after adjusting for compliance. However, to prevent one death from prostate cancer at 11 years follow-up, 37 cancers would need to be detected. The Göteborg randomized trial, which started to randomize 20,000 men aged 50–66 in late 1994, was powered and mandated to report at 15 years follow-up whether invitation to biennial PSA screening of 10,000 men was associated with any significant risk of death from prostate cancer compared to the control group. Although this trial joined ERSPC during 1995, the mandated report at 14 years follow-up demonstrated that death from prostate cancer was reduced by about half, and that 12 men needed to be diagnosed with prostate cancer to prevent one death.[56] Still, it remains critical to contribute timely dissemination of evidence from any extended follow-up of these important trials to further our understanding of the ratio of benefits-to-harms associated with the current modality of population-based PSA screening.[58]

The largest randomized screening study in the United States, the PLCO Screening Study, involved more than 76,000 men that underwent either annual PSA screening, or usual medical care. There was no difference in the total numbers of cancers detected, nor in the overall mortality rates between the two groups. However, the biggest criticism of this study was the high contamination rate of men in the control group that did undergo PSA testing as part of their usual medical care; the other critique concerns PSA screening that had been performed in men before entering the study and randomization to one of the arms, which very likely altered the number of significant cancers in both arms, making it impossible to determine a difference, as reflected in the results.[59]

Prostate-specific antigen dynamics

PSA dynamics, and changes in PSA over time, have been studied extensively in the risk stratification of prostate cancer, and controversy exists as to whether they enhance the predictive accuracy of a single PSA measurement alone in various settings of this disease.

PSA velocity (PSAV) refers to changes of serum PSA levels over time, based on serial PSA measurements, and was shown to have a linear pattern in patients with BPH, whereas patients with prostate cancer seem to exhibit an exponential increase few years before diagnosis.[46,60] However, PSAV was not shown to add any significant diagnostic value for the detection of prostate cancer in addition to the use of a single total PSA level.[50] Especially in the setting of a low PSA, PSAV does not add any predictive accuracy, and should not be incorporated in this setting as it may raise the number of unnecessary biopsies with false-positive PSAV levels.[61] However, pretreatment PSAV may help in the identification of patients at risk for disease recurrence after prostate cancer treatment, as increasing PSAV was associated with poorer disease-specific survival,[46,62–64] but again, no added value beyond that of a single measured PSA value was gained.[65]

PSA doubling-time (PSA-DT) considers PSA levels at separate time points, and several publications have assessed the value of PSA-DT in the risk stratification of men with prostate cancer. A variety of different mathematical formulas to calculate PSA-DT have been used in the literature over the past two decades. The most comprehensive and only publication on the comparison of different definitions and on the assessment of PSA-DT in comparison to a single measured PSA value in the outcome prediction after prostate cancer treatment showed that no definition of PSA-DT enhanced the predictive accuracy of that of a single PSA value.[65]

A subset analysis of the ERSPC trial was able to show as well that PSA dynamics differed significantly between men with or without cancer on biopsy, but the predictive accuracy was of limited value for the practical application due to the high variability of those parameters.[66]

PSA density (PSAD), first described in 1992, reflects serum PSA level in relation to the patient's total prostate volume. Taking into consideration that PSA is prostate-specific, but not prostate cancer-specific, and therefore dependent on total prostate volume,[8] PSAD was shown to be higher in men that harbour prostatic malignancy due to significantly increased leakage of PSA into the bloodstream.[67] However, several limitations apply to the use of PSAD in clinical settings, as prostate volume assessment is provider-dependent; leakage of PSA into the blood may also be due to concomitant variable degree of prostatitis or physical activity, leading to false-positive results, or false-negative results in the setting where large BPH alone leads to significant leakage of PSA into the bloodstream and may mask PSA derived from a tumour within the prostate gland.

Overall, pretreatment PSAV, PSA-DT, and PSAD have been shown to be associated with oncological outcome of patients after treatment, but none of them were able to increase predictive accuracy of a single pretreatment PSA serum level.[65]

The various forms of prostate-specific antigen occurring in blood

Free prostate-specific antigen

The majority of total PSA is bound in complexes to α_1-antichymotrypsin (ACT; *SERPINA3*), protein C inhibitor (*SERPINA5*); and α_2-macroglobulin (*A2M*).[16,21,23,68]

Christensson *et al.* were first to demonstrate that a decrease in the relative proportion of PSA that is not bound in complexes; that is, a lower ratio-of-free-total PSA (or per cent-free PSA) is independent of total PSA associated with significantly increased risk of prostate cancer, particularly among men with modestly elevated levels of total PSA in blood (e.g. between 4 and 10 ng/mL).[69] Subsequently, this was found to both importantly enhance discrimination of men versus men without evidence of prostate cancer at biopsy and significantly increase the accuracy of total PSA alone in detecting prostate cancer at biopsy; for example, the lower the free-to-total PSA ratio, the higher the likelihood to harbour clinically significant prostate cancer, and free PSA increases the predictive accuracy of total PSA in men undergoing prostate biopsy.[46,70–72] Furthermore, lower preoperative free PSA seems to be associated also with biochemical recurrence and adverse pathological features in men undergoing radical prostatectomy for clinically localized prostate cancer.[73]

Intact and nicked prostate-specific antigen

Each of the different subforms of free PSA in serum is strongly implicated to be non-catalytic, as they appear to lack ability to react with any of the abundant protease inhibitors (e.g. ACT or A2M) present at 10,000-fold or higher excess in the blood. By contrast, the vast majority of PSA in semen occurs as free (unbound) forms of which about a third comprises inactive multichain forms.[16] The presence of latent, non-catalytic zymogen forms of single chain PSA (pro-PSA) has been demonstrated in androgen-dependent cell lines (e.g. LNCaP) and prostate cancer tissue but never been detected in seminal fluid.[74] Multichain forms, cleaved internally, for example at Lys_{145}, Lys_{146}, or between Lys_{182}-Ser_{183}, are predominantly contribute the non-catalytic forms of free PSA in seminal fluid,[16,24] while a very small fraction of non-catalytic PSA in seminal fluid comprises PSA covalently bound to the protein C inhibitor.[23]

In 2000, Nurmikko *et al.* reported on the development of a novel type of monoclonal antibodies that manifested high and very specific binding affinity to single chain forms of PSA, independent as to whether they were latent pro-PSA zymogen or catalytically active mature PSA forms capacity, whereas these '*intact*'-specific PSA-antibodies were completely unable to bind non-catalytic PSA containing internal cleavages at Lys_{145} and/or Lys_{146}.[75] The intact forms of free PSA seem to be more highly associated with prostate cancer,[25] and studies have described the development and validity of free PSA assays that are specific for intact PSA and do not recognize internally cleaved *nicked* PSA, and therefore may play a role in the discrimination and assessment of patients at risk for prostate cancer.[75–77] Several studies incorporated measurements of intact, free, and total PSA, combined with hK2 to predict the probability for prostate cancer on biopsy. Analysis of biopsy results and blood markers in samples from thousands of participants in the randomized screening trial (ERSPC) in Sweden, Netherlands, and France showed that a model based on intact PSA, total, free PSA, and hK2 levels contributed significantly to increased accuracy in predicting prostate cancer biopsy outcome compared to a base model using patient age and total PSA alone.[26,78–82] These studies incorporated men with distinct characteristics that importantly influences the discriminatory ability of the conventional PSA test, such as no prior PSA testing, a prior PSA test, or had a prior negative biopsy,[41] AUCs of the base model ranged from non-discriminatory up to close to 0.70 (Table 6.4.1).

Table 6.4.1 Four-kallikrein panel in the predictive accuracy of prostate biopsy outcome compared to a base model using patient age and total PSA alone, in different European trials

Cohert	Description	N	Increase in AUC: four-kallikrein model vs. PSA	Increase in AUC: panel plus DRE vs. PSA+DRE
Göteborg round 1[26]	Unscreened men	740	Any: 0.832 vs. 0.680 High grade: 0.870 vs. 0.816	Any: 0.836 vs. 0.724 High grade: 0.903 vs. 0.868
Göteborg subsequent rounds[80]	Men with a prior PSA test	1,241	Any: 0.674 vs. 0.564 High grade: 0.819 vs. 0.658	Any: 0.697 vs. 0.622 High grade: 0.828 vs. 0.717
Rotterdam round 1[78]	Unscreened men	2,186	Any: 0.764 vs. 0.637 High grade: 0.825 vs. 0.776	Any: 0.776 vs. 0.695 High grade: 0.837 vs. 0.806
Rotterdam subsequent rounds[79]	Men with a prior PSA test	1,501	Any: 0.713 vs. 0.557 High grade: 0.793 vs. 0.699	Any: 0.711 vs. 0.585 High grade: 0.798 vs. 0.709
Rotterdam prior neg biopsy[81]	Elevated PSA after negative biopsy	925	Not assessed	Any: 0.681 vs. 0.584 High grade: 0.873 vs. 0.764
ERSPC Tarn France[82]	Clinical work-up before biopsy	262	Not assessed	Any: 0.782 vs. 0.628 High grade: 0.870 vs. 0.767
Malmö, Sweden (MDC/EPIC)	Longitudinal follow-up without biopsy or screening	792	Any: 0.751 vs. 0.654 Advanced cancer*: 0.824 vs. 0.716	Not assessed

Source: data from Vickers AJ *et al.*, The relationship between prostate-specific antigen and prostate cancer risk: The Prostate Biopsy Collaborative Group, *Clinical Cancer Research*, Volume 16, Issue 17, pp. 4374–81, Copyright © 2010 American Association for Cancer Research.

However, importantly, the magnitude of enhanced accuracy was quite similar across all studies; for example, increase in AUC from 0.680 to 0.832 among previously unscreened ERSPC-participants in Sweden, also with importantly enhanced accuracy in predicting evidence of high-grade disease at biopsy (defined as presence of Gleason grade 4).[26] In addition, decision analytical methods were used to demonstrate that the clinical implication of these findings would be that the number of men recommended for a prostate biopsy could be reduced by about half, which would likely result in that up to 20% of the cancer diagnoses would be delayed, although the majority of these cases would be low-grade and stage cancer, and leaving only very few high-grade cancers undetected (Table 6.4.1).

Human kallikrein-related peptidase 2 (hk2) and other kallikrein-related peptidases

Human kallikrein-related peptidase 2 (hK2), another member of the kallikrein family encoded on chromosome 19q13, is also a secreted serine protease, and to 80% homologous in sequence to PSA. hK2 is primarily expressed in the prostate gland as well as in serum, but enzymatic activity of PSA and hK2 is different, and hK2 expression levels overall are 50-fold less than that of PSA.[2,83,84] hK2 has been shown to be overexpressed in men with prostate cancer as well, especially the ratio of hK2/PSA mRNA seems to increase with tumour grade.[85] However, this was contradicted by a analysis by Väänänen *et al.*[86] Several studies demonstrated that hK2 improves predictive accuracy of total and free PSA in the discrimination of men with vs. without prostate cancer in men with elevated total PSA.[26,87,88] Up to 15 human kallikrein gene loci have been identified to date in total, but hK2 and PSA (hK3) represent the best studied ones, and are the ones most significantly associated with prostate cancer.

Urine biomarkers

Prostate cancer gene 3

Prostate cancer gene 3 (*PCA3*) is a non-coding ribonucleic acid (RNA) that is expressed at low levels in normal prostate tissue, and highly overexpressed in prostate cancer tissue.[89,90] A quantitative reproducible assay for the detection of PCA3 in the urine has been developed,[91] and *PCA3* gained approval by the US Food and Drug Administration in 2010 for the use in men who show a persistently elevated PSA after having undergone a negative prostate biopsy.

Testing for the *PCA3* gene requires a sample of first-stream urine after a prostate massage with three strokes per lobe, and *PCA3* mRNA and PSA mRNA transcript copy numbers are consequently measured in the sample. This *PCA3* score is reported as a ratio of these two, with the PSA mRNA copy number accounting for and normalizing the variable number of prostate cancer cells in the sample.[91]

Several clinical studies have evaluated the use of the *PCA3* score in helping the decision-making of whether or not to biopsy patients at risk with elevated PSA serum levels. These studies included men undergoing a first prostate biopsy or men scheduled for a repeat biopsy.[92] In both settings, higher *PCA3* scores were shown to be associated with the presence of prostate cancer on biopsy,[91,92] while other trials have demonstrated the ability of *PCA3* to predict tumour burden on subsequent radical prostatectomy specimens.[94,95] Different cut-off levels for *PCA3* scores have been tested, and controversy still exists as to which threshold to use when decision is made on whether to perform a biopsy or not.[95] Initially a cut-off score of 35 was determined to be most appropriate in the early detection of prostate cancer on biopsy.[96,97] However, more studies confirmed that using this *PCA3* threshold, a large number of cancers are being left undetected, and that lowering the cut-off level would enhance the detection rate.[97,98]

Genetic markers and gene fusions

Single nucleotide polymorphisms and microseminoprotein-β

Genome-wide association studies identified several small nucleotide polymorphisms (SNP) that are associated with prostate cancer and advanced or aggressive disease.[99–101] SNPs are estimated to contribute significantly to the genetic inheritance of prostate cancer. One particular SNP, *rs10993994*, located on chromosome 10q11.1 in the promoter sequence of microseminoprotein-β (*MSMB*), was found to be prevalent and contribute an independently replicated, significant association of risk of prostate cancer.[102] The *MSMB*-gene product (MSP) is—similar to PSA—a highly abundantly expressed protein in the prostate epithelium that is present at very high levels in the seminal fluid,[103] that is also expressed at abundant in mucosal tissues.[104] Several studies were able to confirm that the *MSMB* SNP allele is very common (with a prevalence of 30–40% in Caucasians, and 70–80% in African-Americans), and significantly associated with an increased risk for the diagnosis of prostate cancer, whereas uncertainty remains regarding the association with adverse pathological features (higher stage and Gleason score). Using a nested case–control design with blood samples and data from the Multiethnic Cohort study, cancer risk was found to be associated with lower MSP across race, ethnicity, tumour stage or grade, and rs10993994-genotype. Therefore, regardless of race and ethnicity or rs10993994 genotype, men with low blood levels of MSP have increased risk of prostate cancer.[106] However, the predictive accuracy of SNPs alone is rather poor, and they do not seem to enhance the predictive accuracy of PSA.[102] Klein *et al.* evaluated previously identified SNPs for association with prostate cancer and accuracy in predicting prostate cancer in a large prospective population-based cohort of unscreened men. Few independent SNPs at four independent loci remained significant after multiple test correction ($p < 0.001$). However, prostate cancer risk prediction with SNPs alone was less accurate than with PSA measured at baseline (area under the curve of 0.57 vs. 0.79), with no benefit from combining SNPs with PSA.[102] Assessment of association between the six loci and prostate cancer risk in over 5,000 cases and 41,000 controls from Iceland, the Netherlands, Spain, Romania, and the United States showed that SNPs at 10q26 and 12q24 were exclusively associated with PSA levels, whereas four other loci also were associated with prostate cancer risk. We propose that a personalized PSA cut-off value, based on genotype, should be used when deciding to perform a prostate biopsy.[107]

Gene fusions

Gene fusions may occur during translocation or deletions of specific genome sequences. These genetic rearrangements may be oncogenetic trigger points in the development of malignant diseases.[108] The best studied gene fusion in prostate cancer involves the prostate-specific transmembrane protease serine 2 gene (*TMPRSS2*) and *ERG*, an *ETS* transcription factor gene, both located adjacent to each other on chromosome 21q22. *ERG* is a key oncogene in the development of prostate cancer, and the fusion with *TMPRSS2* occurs in about 50% of men with prostate cancer, which makes *TMPRSS2:ERG* the most prevalent gene fusion in human solid tumour development.[109,110] Similar to *PCA3, TMPRSS2:ERG* can be detected in the urine after prostatic massage, and has been described as an addition to PSA and other biomarkers in the prediction of prostate cancer.[96,111] As the fusion mechanism of *TMPRSS2:ERG* might be under the influence of androgens, publications studied the response of patients to hormonal therapy for advanced prostate cancer, and suggested that *ERG*-positive men showed a more favourable response, than patients that are *ERG*-negative.[112] However, data on the presence of *TMPRSS2:ERG* fusion and oncological outcomes remain controversial, as some studies suggest that it is associated with adverse pathological features and worse oncological outcome,[113,114] while others could not demonstrate such association.[115,116]

Acknowledgements

Funding: The work was supported in parts by grants from the National Cancer Institute [P50-CA92629, and P30-CA008748], the Sidney Kimmel Center for Prostate and Urologic Cancers, and David H. Koch through the Prostate Cancer Foundation, the National Institute for Health Research (NIHR) Oxford Biomedical Research Centre Program in UK, the Swedish Cancer Society (Cancerfonden project no. 14-0722), and the Swedish Research Council (VR-MH project no. 2016-02974).

Disclosures: Hans Lilja holds patents for free PSA, hK2, and intact PSA assays, and is named on a patent application for a statistical method to detect prostate cancer. The marker assay patents and the patent application for the statistical model has been licensed and commercialized as the 4K score by OPKO Diagnostics. Dr. Lilja receive royalties from sales of this test. Additionally, Dr. Lilja owns stock in OPKO.

Further reading

Becker C, Piironen T, Pettersson K, *et al.* Discrimination of men with prostate cancer from those with benign disease by measurements of human glandular kallikrein 2 (HK2) in serum. *J Urol* 2000; **163**(1):311–6.

Eeles RA, Kote-Jarai Z, Giles GG, *et al.* Multiple newly identified loci associated with prostate cancer susceptibility. *Nat Genet* 2008; **40**(3):316–21.

Etzioni R, Penson DF, Legler JM, *et al.* Overdiagnosis due to prostate-specific antigen screening: lessons from U.S. prostate cancer incidence trends. *J Natl Cancer Inst* 2002; **94**(13):981–90.

Lilja H, Ulmert D, Vickers AJ. Prostate-specific antigen and prostate cancer: prediction, detection and monitoring. *Nat Rev Cancer* 2008; **8**(4):268–78.

Lilja H. A kallikrein-like serine protease in prostatic fluid cleaves the predominant seminal vesicle protein. *J Clin Investig* 1985; **76**(5):1899–903.

Thompson IM, Pauler DK, Goodman PJ, *et al.* Prevalence of prostate cancer among men with a prostate-specific antigen level < or =4.0 ng per milliliter. *New Engl J Med* 2004; **350**(22):2239–46.

Vickers AJ, Cronin AM, Bjork T, Manjer J, Nilsson PM, Dahlin A, *et al.* Prostate specific antigen concentration at age 60 and death or metastasis from prostate cancer: case-control study. *BMJ* 2010; **341**:c4521.

References

1. Riegman PH, Vlietstra RJ, Suurmeijer L, Cleutjens CB, Trapman J. Characterization of the human kallikrein locus. *Genomics* 1992; **14**(1):6–11.
2. Yousef GM, Diamandis EP. The new human tissue kallikrein gene family: structure, function, and association to disease. *Endocr Rev* 2001; **22**(2):184–204.
3. Lawrence MG, Lai J, Clements JA. Kallikreins on steroids: structure, function, and hormonal regulation of prostate-specific antigen and the extended kallikrein locus. *Endocr Rev* 2010; **31**(4):407–46.
4. Lilja H, Ulmert D, Vickers AJ. Prostate-specific antigen and prostate cancer: prediction, detection and monitoring. *Nat Rev Cancer* 2008; **8**(4):268–78.
5. Diamandis EP. Prostate-specific antigen: a cancer fighter and a valuable messenger? *Clin Chem* 2000; **46**(7):896–900.
6. Olsson AY, Lilja H, Lundwall A. Taxon-specific evolution of glandular kallikrein genes and identification of a progenitor of prostate-specific antigen. *Genomics* 2004; **84**(1):147–56.
7. Lundwall A, Band V, Blaber M, *et al.* A comprehensive nomenclature for serine proteases with homology to tissue kallikreins. *Biol Chem* 2006; **387**(6):637–41.
8. Benson MC, Whang IS, Pantuck A, *et al.* Prostate specific antigen density: a means of distinguishing benign prostatic hypertrophy and prostate cancer. *J Urol* 1992; **147**(3 Pt 2):815–6.
9. Abrahamsson PA, Lilja H, Falkmer S, Wadstrom LB. Immunohistochemical distribution of the three predominant secretory proteins in the parenchyma of hyperplastic and neoplastic prostate glands. *Prostate* 1988; **12**(1):39–46.
10. Diamandis EP. Prostate-specific antigen: Its usefulness in clinical medicine. *Trends Endocrinol Metab* 1998; **9**(8):310–6.
11. Olsson AY, Bjartell A, Lilja H, Lundwall A. Expression of prostate-specific antigen (PSA) and human glandular kallikrein 2 (hK2) in ileum and other extraprostatic tissues. *Int J Cancer* 2005; **113**(2):290–7.
12. Lundwall A, Lilja H. Molecular cloning of human prostate specific antigen cDNA. *FEBS Lett* 1987; **214**(2):317–22.
13. Lovgren J, Rajakoski K, Karp M, Lundwall A, Lilja H. Activation of the zymogen form of prostate-specific antigen by human glandular kallikrein 2. *Biochem Biophys Res Commun* 1997; **238**(2):549–55.
14. Mikolajczyk SD, Marks LS, Partin AW, Rittenhouse HG. Free prostate-specific antigen in serum is becoming more complex. *Urology* 2002;**59**(6):797–802.
15. Kumar A, Mikolajczyk SD, Goel AS, Millar LS, Saedi MS. Expression of pro form of prostate-specific antigen by mammalian cells and its conversion to mature, active form by human kallikrein 2. *Cancer Res* 1997; **57**(15):3111–4.
16. Christensson A, Laurell CB, Lilja H. Enzymatic activity of prostate-specific antigen and its reactions with extracellular serine proteinase inhibitors. *Eur J Biochem* 1990; **194**(3):755–63.
17. Malm J, Hellman J, Hogg P, Lilja H. Enzymatic action of prostate-specific antigen (PSA or hK3): substrate specificity and regulation by Zn(2+), a tight-binding inhibitor. *Prostate* 2000; **45**(2):132–9.
18. Lilja H. A kallikrein-like serine protease in prostatic fluid cleaves the predominant seminal vesicle protein. *J Clin Investig* 1985; **76**(5):1899–903.
19. Lilja H, Oldbring J, Rannevik G, Laurell CB. Seminal vesicle-secreted proteins and their reactions during gelation and liquefaction of human semen. *J Clin Investig* 1987; **80**(2):281–5.
20. Lilja H, Abrahamsson PA, Lundwall A. Semenogelin, the predominant protein in human semen. Primary structure and identification of closely related proteins in the male accessory sex glands and on the spermatozoa. *J Biol Chem* 1989; **264**(3):1894–900.
21. Lilja H, Christensson A, Dahlen U, *et al.* Prostate-specific antigen in serum occurs predominantly in complex with alpha 1-antichymotrypsin. *Clin Chem* 1991; **37**(9):1618–25.
22. Koivunen E, Ristimaki A, Itkonen O, Osman S, Vuento M, Stenman UH. Tumor-associated trypsin participates in cancer

cell-mediated degradation of extracellular matrix. *Cancer Res* 1991; **51**(8):2107–12.
23. Christensson A, Lilja H. Complex formation between protein C inhibitor and prostate-specific antigen in vitro and in human semen. *Eur J Biochem* 1994; **220**(1):45–53.
24. Watt KW, Lee PJ, M'Timkulu T, Chan WP, Loor R. Human prostate-specific antigen: structural and functional similarity with serine proteases. *Proc Natl Acad Sci U S A* 1986; **83**(10):3166–70.
25. Nurmikko P, Pettersson K, Piironen T, Hugosson J, Lilja H. Discrimination of prostate cancer from benign disease by plasma measurement of intact, free prostate-specific antigen lacking an internal cleavage site at Lys145-Lys146. *Clin Chem* 2001; **47**(8):1415–23.
26. Vickers AJ, Cronin AM, Aus G, *et al.* A panel of kallikrein markers can reduce unnecessary biopsy for prostate cancer: data from the European Randomized Study of Prostate Cancer Screening in Göteborg, Sweden. *BMC Med* 2008;**6**:19.
27. Mikolajczyk SD, Marker KM, Millar LS, *et al.* A truncated precursor form of prostate-specific antigen is a more specific serum marker of prostate cancer. *Cancer Res* 2001; **61**(18):6958–63.
28. Sokoll LJ, Chan DW, Mikolajczyk SD, *et al.* Proenzyme psa for the early detection of prostate cancer in the 2.5-4.0 ng/ml total psa range: preliminary analysis. *Urology* 2003; **61**(2):274–6.
29. Catalona WJ, Bartsch G, Rittenhouse HG, Evans CL, Linton HJ, Horninger W, *et al.* Serum pro-prostate specific antigen preferentially detects aggressive prostate cancers in men with 2 to 4 ng/ml prostate specific antigen. *J Urol* 2004; **171**(6 Pt 1):2239–44.
30. Catalona WJ, Bartsch G, Rittenhouse HG, *et al.* Serum pro prostate specific antigen improves cancer detection compared to free and complexed prostate specific antigen in men with prostate specific antigen 2 to 4 ng/ml. *J Urol* 2003; **170**(6 Pt 1):2181–5.
31. Papsidero LD, Wang MC, Valenzuela LA, Murphy GP, Chu TM. A prostate antigen in sera of prostatic cancer patients. *Cancer Res*1980; **40**(7):2428–32.
32. Kuriyama M, Wang MC, Lee CI, *et al.* Use of human prostate-specific antigen in monitoring prostate cancer. *Cancer Res* 1981; **41**(10):3874–6.
33. Wang MC, Papsidero LD, Kuriyama M, Valenzuela LA, Murphy GP, Chu TM. Prostate antigen: a new potential marker for prostatic cancer. *Prostate* 1981; **2**(1):89–96.
34. Siegel R, Naishadham D, Jemal A. Cancer statistics, 2013. *CA Cancer J Clin* 2013; **63**(1):11–30.
35. Etzioni R, Penson DF, Legler JM, *et al.* Overdiagnosis due to prostate-specific antigen screening: lessons from U.S. prostate cancer incidence trends. *J Natl Cancer Inst* 2002; **94**(13):981–90.
36. Thompson IM, Pauler DK, Goodman PJ, *et al.* Prevalence of prostate cancer among men with a prostate-specific antigen level < or =4.0 ng per milliliter. *New Engl J Med* 2004; **350**(22):2239–46.
37. Albertsen PC. The unintended burden of increased prostate cancer detection associated with prostate cancer screening and diagnosis. *Urology* 2010; **75**(2):399–405.
38. Polascik TJ, Oesterling JE, Partin AW. Prostate specific antigen: a decade of discovery--what we have learned and where we are going. *J Urol* 1999; **162**(2):293–306.
39. Thompson IM, Chi C, Ankerst DP, *et al.* Effect of finasteride on the sensitivity of PSA for detecting prostate cancer. *J Natl Cancer Inst* 2006; **98**(16):1128–33.
40. Lilja H, Ulmert D, Bjork T, *et al.* Long-term prediction of prostate cancer up to 25 years before diagnosis of prostate cancer using prostate kallikreins measured at age 44 to 50 years. *J Clin Oncol* 2007; **25**(4):431–6.
41. Vickers AJ, Cronin AM, Roobol MJ, *et al.* The relationship between prostate-specific antigen and prostate cancer risk: the Prostate Biopsy Collaborative Group. *Clin Cancer Res* 2010; **16**(17):4374–81.
42. Lilja H. Biology of prostate-specific antigen. *Urology* 2003; **62**(5 Suppl 1):27–33.
43. Catalona WJ, Smith DS, Ratliff TL, *et al.* Measurement of prostate-specific antigen in serum as a screening test for prostate cancer. *New Engl J Med* 1991; **324**(17):1156–61.
44. Thompson IM, Pauler Ankerst D, Chi C, *et al.* Prediction of prostate cancer for patients receiving finasteride: results from the Prostate Cancer Prevention Trial. *J Clin Oncol* 2007; **25**(21):3076–81.
45. Krumholtz JS, Carvalhal GF, Ramos CG, *et al.* Prostate-specific antigen cutoff of 2.6 ng/mL for prostate cancer screening is associated with favorable pathologic tumor features. *Urology* 2002; **60**(3):469–73; discussion 73–4.
46. Shariat SF, Semjonow A, Lilja H, Savage C, Vickers AJ, Bjartell A. Tumor markers in prostate cancer I: blood-based markers. *Acta Oncol* 2011; **50**(Suppl 1):61–75.
47. Vickers AJ, Ulmert D, Serio AM, *et al.* The predictive value of prostate cancer biomarkers depends on age and time to diagnosis: towards a biologically-based screening strategy. *Int J Cancer* 2007; **121**(10):2212–7.
48. Stenman UH, Hakama M, Knekt P, Aromaa A, Teppo L, Leinonen J. Serum concentrations of prostate specific antigen and its complex with alpha 1-antichymotrypsin before diagnosis of prostate cancer. *Lancet* 1994; **344**(8937):1594–8.
49. Gann PH, Hennekens CH, Stampfer MJ. A prospective evaluation of plasma prostate-specific antigen for detection of prostatic cancer. *JAMA* 1995; **273**(4):289–94.
50. Ulmert D, Serio AM, O'Brien MF, *et al.* Long-term prediction of prostate cancer: prostate-specific antigen (PSA) velocity is predictive but does not improve the predictive accuracy of a single PSA measurement 15 years or more before cancer diagnosis in a large, representative, unscreened population. *J Clin Oncol* 2008; **26**(6):835–41.
51. Vickers AJ, Cronin AM, Bjork T, Manjer J, Nilsson PM, Dahlin A, *et al.* Prostate specific antigen concentration at age 60 and death or metastasis from prostate cancer: case-control study. *BMJ* 2010; **341**:c4521.
52. Moyer VA, Force USPST. Screening for prostate cancer: U.S. Preventive Services Task Force recommendation statement. *Ann Intern Med* 2012; **157**(2):120–34.
53. Vickers AJ, Roobol MJ, Lilja H. Screening for prostate cancer: early detection or overdetection? *Annu Rev Med* 2012; **63**:161–70.
54. Andriole GL, Crawford ED, Grubb RL 3rd, *et al.* Prostate cancer screening in the randomized Prostate, Lung, Colorectal, and Ovarian Cancer Screening Trial: mortality results after 13 years of follow-up. *J Natl Cancer Inst* 2012; **104**(2):125–32.
55. Schroder FH, Hugosson J, Roobol MJ, *et al.* Prostate-cancer mortality at 11 years of follow-up. *New Engl J Med* 2012; **366**(11):981–90.
56. Hugosson J, Carlsson S, Aus G, Bergdahl S, Khatami A, Lodding P, *et al.* Mortality results from the Göteborg randomised population-based prostate-cancer screening trial. *Lancet Oncol* 2010; **11**(8):725–32.
57. Schroder FH, Hugosson J, Roobol MJ, *et al.* Screening and prostate-cancer mortality in a randomized European study. *New Engl J Med* 2009; **360**(13):1320–8.
58. Carlsson S, Vickers AJ, Roobol M, *et al.* Prostate cancer screening: facts, statistics, and interpretation in response to the US Preventive Services Task Force Review. *J Clin Oncol* 2012; **30**(21):2581–4.
59. Andriole GL, Crawford ED, Grubb RL 3rd, *et al.* Mortality results from a randomized prostate-cancer screening trial. *New Engl J Med* 2009; **360**(13):1310–9.
60. Carter HB, Morrell CH, Pearson JD, *et al.* Estimation of prostatic growth using serial prostate-specific antigen measurements in men with and without prostate disease. *Cancer Res* 1992; **52**(12):3323–8.
61. Vickers AJ, Till C, Tangen CM, Lilja H, Thompson IM. An empirical evaluation of guidelines on prostate-specific antigen velocity in prostate cancer detection. *J Natl Cancer Inst* 2011; **103**(6):462–9.
62. D'Amico AV, Renshaw AA, Sussman B, Chen MH. Pretreatment PSA velocity and risk of death from prostate cancer following external beam radiation therapy. *JAMA* 2005; **294**(4):440–7.
63. D'Amico AV, Chen MH, Roehl KA, Catalona WJ. Preoperative PSA velocity and the risk of death from prostate cancer after radical prostatectomy. *New Engl J Med* 2004; **351**(2):125–35.
64. Carter HB, Ferrucci L, Kettermann A, *et al.* Detection of life-threatening prostate cancer with prostate-specific antigen velocity during a window of curability. *J Natl Cancer Inst* 2006; **98**(21):1521–7.

65. O'Brien MF, Cronin AM, Fearn PA, *et al.* Pretreatment prostate-specific antigen (PSA) velocity and doubling time are associated with outcome but neither improves prediction of outcome beyond pretreatment PSA alone in patients treated with radical prostatectomy. *J Clin Oncol* 2009; **27**(22):3591–7.
66. Raaijmakers R, Wildhagen MF, Ito K, *et al.* Prostate-specific antigen change in the European Randomized Study of Screening for Prostate Cancer, section Rotterdam. *Urology* 2004; **63**(2):316–20.
67. Stamey TA, Kabalin JN, McNeal JE, *et al.* Prostate specific antigen in the diagnosis and treatment of adenocarcinoma of the prostate. II. Radical prostatectomy treated patients. *J Urol* 1989; **141**(5):1076–83.
68. Stenman UH, Leinonen J, Alfthan H, Rannikko S, Tuhkanen K, Alfthan O. A complex between prostate-specific antigen and alpha 1-antichymotrypsin is the major form of prostate-specific antigen in serum of patients with prostatic cancer: assay of the complex improves clinical sensitivity for cancer. *Cancer Res* 1991; **51**(1):222–6.
69. Christensson A, Bjork T, Nilsson O, *et al.* Serum prostate specific antigen complexed to alpha 1-antichymotrypsin as an indicator of prostate cancer. *J Urol* 1993; **150**(1):100–5.
70. Catalona WJ, Partin AW, Slawin KM, *et al.* Use of the percentage of free prostate-specific antigen to enhance differentiation of prostate cancer from benign prostatic disease: a prospective multicenter clinical trial. *JAMA* 1998; **279**(19):1542–7.
71. Roddam AW, Duffy MJ, Hamdy FC, *et al.* Use of prostate-specific antigen (PSA) isoforms for the detection of prostate cancer in men with a PSA level of 2–10 ng/ml: systematic review and meta-analysis. *Eur Urol* 2005; **48**(3):386–99; discussion 98–9.
72. Wenske S, Korets R, Cronin AM, *et al.* Evaluation of molecular forms of prostate-specific antigen and human kallikrein 2 in predicting biochemical failure after radical prostatectomy. *Int J Cancer* 2009; **124**(3):659–63.
73. Shariat SF, Abdel-Aziz KF, Roehrborn CG, Lotan Y. Pre-operative percent free PSA predicts clinical outcomes in patients treated with radical prostatectomy with total PSA levels below 10 ng/ml. *Eur Urol* 2006; **49**(2):293–302.
74. Vaisanen V, Lovgren J, Hellman J, Piironen T, Lilja H, Pettersson K. Characterization and processing of prostate specific antigen (hK3) and human glandular kallikrein (hK2) secreted by LNCaP cells. *Prostate Cancer Prostatic Dis* 1999; **2**(2):91–7.
75. Nurmikko P, Vaisanen V, Piironen T, Lindgren S, Lilja H, Pettersson K. Production and characterization of novel anti-prostate-specific antigen (PSA) monoclonal antibodies that do not detect internally cleaved Lys145-Lys146 inactive PSA. *Clin Chem* 2000; **46**(10):1610–8.
76. Vaisanen V, Peltola MT, Lilja H, Nurmi M, Pettersson K. Intact free prostate-specific antigen and free and total human glandular kallikrein 2. Elimination of assay interference by enzymatic digestion of antibodies to F(ab')2 fragments. *Anal Chem* 2006; **78**(22):7809–15.
77. Peltola MT, Niemela P, Alanen K, Nurmi M, Lilja H, Pettersson K. Immunoassay for the discrimination of free prostate-specific antigen (fPSA) forms with internal cleavages at Lys((1)(4)(5)) or Lys((1)(4)(6)) from fPSA without internal cleavages at Lys((1)(4)(5)) or Lys((1)(4)(6)). *J Immunol Methods* 2011; **369**(1–2):74–80.
78. Vickers A, Cronin A, Roobol M, *et al.* Reducing unnecessary biopsy during prostate cancer screening using a four-kallikrein panel: an independent replication. *J Clin Oncol* 2010; **28**(15):2493–8.
79. Vickers AJ, Cronin AM, Roobol MJ, *et al.* A four-kallikrein panel predicts prostate cancer in men with screening: data from the European Randomized Study of Screening for Prostate Cancer, Rotterdam. *Clin Cancer Res* 2010; **16**(12):3232–9.
80. Vickers AJ, Cronin AM, Aus G, *et al.* Impact of screening on predicting the outcome of prostate cancer biopsy in men with elevated prostate-specific antigen: data from the European Randomized Study of Prostate Cancer Screening in Gothenburg, Sweden. *Cancer* 2010; **116**(11):2612–20.
81. Gupta A, Roobol MJ, Savage CJ, *et al.* A four-kallikrein panel for the prediction of repeat prostate biopsy: data from the European Randomized Study of Prostate Cancer screening in Rotterdam, Netherlands. *Br J Cancer* 2010; **103**(5):708–14.
82. Benchikh A, Savage C, Cronin A, *et al.* A panel of kallikrein markers can predict outcome of prostate biopsy following clinical work-up: an independent validation study from the European Randomized Study of Prostate Cancer screening, France. *BMC Cancer* 2010; **10**:635.
83. Schedlich LJ, Bennetts BH, Morris BJ. Primary structure of a human glandular kallikrein gene. *DNA* 1987; **6**(5):429–37.
84. Chapdelaine P, Paradis G, Tremblay RR, Dube JY. High level of expression in the prostate of a human glandular kallikrein mRNA related to prostate-specific antigen. *FEBS Lett* 1988; **236**(1):205–8.
85. Lintula S, Stenman J, Bjartell A, Nordling S, Stenman UH. Relative concentrations of hK2/PSA mRNA in benign and malignant prostatic tissue. *Prostate* 2005; **63**(4):324–9.
86. Väänänen R, Lilja H, Cronin A, *et al.* Association of transcript levels of 10 established or candidate-biomarker gene targets with cancerous versus non-cancerous prostate tissue from radical prostatectomy specimens. *Clin Biochem* 2013; **46**(0):670–4.
87. Becker C, Piironen T, Pettersson K, Hugosson J, Lilja H. Clinical value of human glandular kallikrein 2 and free and total prostate-specific antigen in serum from a population of men with prostate-specific antigen levels 3.0 ng/mL or greater. *Urology* 2000; **55**(5):694–9.
88. Becker C, Piironen T, Pettersson K, *et al.* Discrimination of men with prostate cancer from those with benign disease by measurements of human glandular kallikrein 2 (HK2) in serum. *J Urol* 2000; **163**(1):311–6.
89. Bussemakers MJ, van Bokhoven A, Verhaegh GW, *et al.* DD3: a new prostate-specific gene, highly overexpressed in prostate cancer. *Cancer Res* 1999; **59**(23):5975–9.
90. de Kok JB, Verhaegh GW, Roelofs RW, *et al.* DD3(PCA3), a very sensitive and specific marker to detect prostate tumors. *Cancer Res* 2002; **62**(9):2695–8.
91. Hessels D, Klein Gunnewiek JM, van Oort I, *et al.* DD3(PCA3)-based molecular urine analysis for the diagnosis of prostate cancer. *Eur Urol* 2003; **44**(1):8–15; discussion 15–16.
92. Haese A, de la Taille A, van Poppel H, *et al.* Clinical utility of the PCA3 urine assay in European men scheduled for repeat biopsy. *Eur Urol* 2008; **54**(5):1081–8.
93. Andriole G, Bostwick D, Brawley O, Gomella L, Marberger M, Tindall D, *et al.* Chemoprevention of prostate cancer in men at high risk: rationale and design of the reduction by dutasteride of prostate cancer events (REDUCE) trial. *J Urol* 2004; **172**(4 Pt 1):1314–7.
94. Whitman EJ, Groskopf J, Ali A, *et al.* PCA3 score before radical prostatectomy predicts extracapsular extension and tumor volume. *J Urol* 2008; **180**(5):1975–8; discussion 8–9.
95. van Poppel H, Haese A, Graefen M, *et al.* The relationship between Prostate Cancer gene 3 (PCA3) and prostate cancer significance. BJU Int 2012; **109**(3):360–6.
96. Salagierski M, Schalken JA. Molecular diagnosis of prostate cancer: PCA3 and TMPRSS2:ERG gene fusion. *J Urol* 2012; **187**(3):795–801.
97. Crawford ED, Rove KO, Trabulsi EJ, *et al.* Diagnostic performance of PCA3 to detect prostate cancer in men with increased prostate specific antigen: a prospective study of 1,962 cases. *J Urol* 2012; **188**(5):1726–31.
98. Roobol MJ, Schroder FH, van Leenders GL, *et al.* Performance of prostate cancer antigen 3 (PCA3) and prostate-specific antigen in Prescreened men: reproducibility and detection characteristics for prostate cancer patients with high PCA3 scores (>/= 100). *Eur Urol* 2010; **58**(6):893–9.
99. Eeles RA, Kote-Jarai Z, Giles GG, *et al.* Multiple newly identified loci associated with prostate cancer susceptibility. *Nat Genet* 2008; **40**(3):316–21.
100. Thomas G, Jacobs KB, Yeager M, *et al.* Multiple loci identified in a genome-wide association study of prostate cancer. *Nat Genet* 2008;**40**(3):310–5. Epub 2008/02/12.
101. Gudmundsson J, Sulem P, Rafnar T, *et al.* Common sequence variants on 2p15 and Xp11.22 confer susceptibility to prostate cancer. *Nat Genet* 2008; **40**(3):281–3.
102. Klein RJ, Hallden C, Gupta A, *et al.* Evaluation of multiple risk-associated single nucleotide polymorphisms versus prostate-specific antigen at baseline to predict prostate cancer in unscreened men. *Eur Urol* 2012; **61**(3):471–7.

103. Lilja H, Abrahamsson PA. Three predominant proteins secreted by the human prostate gland. *Prostate* 1988; **12**(1):29–38.
104. Weiber H, Andersson C, Murne A, *et al.* Beta microseminoprotein is not a prostate-specific protein. Its identification in mucous glands and secretions. *Am J Pathol* 1990; **137**(3):593–603.
105. Whitaker HC, Kote-Jarai Z, Ross-Adams H, *et al.* The rs10993994 risk allele for prostate cancer results in clinically relevant changes in microseminoprotein-beta expression in tissue and urine. *PloS One* 2010; **5**(10):e13363.
106. Haiman CA, Stram DO, Vickers AJ, *et al.* Levels of Beta-microseminoprotein in blood and risk of prostate cancer in multiple populations. *J Natl Cancer Inst* 2013; **105**(3):237–43.
107. Gudmundsson J, Besenbacher S, Sulem P, *et al.* Genetic correction of PSA values using sequence variants associated with PSA levels. *Sci Transl Med* 2010; **2**(62):62ra92.
108. Hoglund M, Frigyesi A, Mitelman F. A gene fusion network in human neoplasia. *Oncogene* 2006; **25**(18):2674–8.
109. Chinnaiyan AM, Palanisamy N. Chromosomal aberrations in solid tumors. *Prog Mol Biol Transl Sci* 2010; **95**:55–94.
110. Perner S, Mosquera JM, Demichelis F, al. TMPRSS2-ERG fusion prostate cancer: an early molecular event associated with invasion. *Am J Surg Pathol* 2007; **31**(6):882–8.
111. Hessels D, Smit FP, Verhaegh GW, Witjes JA, Cornel EB, Schalken JA. Detection of TMPRSS2-ERG fusion transcripts and prostate cancer antigen 3 in urinary sediments may improve diagnosis of prostate cancer. *Clin Cancer Res* 2007; **13**(17):5103–8.
112. Karnes RJ, Cheville JC, Ida CM, *et al.* The ability of biomarkers to predict systemic progression in men with high-risk prostate cancer treated surgically is dependent on ERG status. *Cancer Res* 2010; **70**(22):8994–9002.
113. Attard G, Clark J, Ambroisine L, *et al.* Duplication of the fusion of TMPRSS2 to ERG sequences identifies fatal human prostate cancer. *Oncogene* 2008; **27**(3):253–63.
114. Demichelis F, Fall K, Perner S, *et al.* TMPRSS2:ERG gene fusion associated with lethal prostate cancer in a watchful waiting cohort. *Oncogene* 2007; **26**(31):4596–9.
115. Rubio-Briones J, Fernandez-Serra A, Calatrava A, *et al.* Clinical implications of TMPRSS2-ERG gene fusion expression in patients with prostate cancer treated with radical prostatectomy. *J Urol* 2010; **183**(5):2054–61.
116. Hoogland AM, Jenster G, van Weerden WM, *et al.* ERG immunohistochemistry is not predictive for PSA recurrence, local recurrence or overall survival after radical prostatectomy for prostate cancer. *Mod Pathol* 2012; **25**(3):471–9.

CHAPTER 6.5

Screening for prostate cancer

Fritz H. Schröder

Introduction to screening for prostate cancer

The purpose of this introduction is to set the scene for the rest of this chapter by giving a summary of the most progress made in those randomized studies of screening for prostate cancer which contribute high quality data to level I evidence.

What is the proper level of evidence contributed by available data from randomized controlled trials?

To date, there have been five randomized controlled trials (RCTs) including a total of 341,342 participants aged 45 to 80 years that have tried to evaluate prostate-specific antigen (PSA)-based prostate cancer screening. Each has a different design, different criteria for the stratification of risk in the screening arm, and have suffered from either too little power (i.e. too small), contamination, or lack of methodological rigour. Considering this heterogeneity, producing level 1A evidence by combining the studies in meta-analysis is not easy or even impossible. Three such attempts have been published,[1–3] but contradict the outcome of the highest quality studies. In most experts' view, only two of the RCTs used in the first and second cited systematic review[1,2] qualify for consideration of the high level of evidence that allows inclusion in a systematic review. Meta-analyses are complicated and depend largely on what trials are available, how they were carried out (quality of the trials), and how the healthcare outcomes were measured.[4] While the statement in that 'all trials had one or more substantial methodological limitation' is correct, [1] all three attempted overview analyses in the views of the present authors do not adequately consider the differences in quality between the randomized trials included in the overview. This is also true for the paper on which the negative recommendations of the US Preventive Services Task Force are based.[3] The overview compares the large European and American study, which in the view of these authors should not be compared at the same level of evidence for reasons detailed.[5] The Prostate, Lung, Colorectal, and Ovarian (PLCO) study encountered pitfalls which are likely to significantly decrease the power of the study, and which preclude an outcome in line with the original purpose, that is, to show or exclude an effect of screening on prostate cancer mortality.[6] These include a very high level of 44% of screening prior to randomization, 53% of PSA use in the control group, and a compliance with biopsy indications of only about 40%.[7,8] In comparison to these facts, the methodological pitfalls of the European Randomized study of Screening for Prostate Cancer (ERSPC) study are relatively minor. The claim that treatment might have been more adequate and more aggressive in the screen arm is based on a brief statement in the summary of Wolters *et al.*[9] but is contradicted by a careful analysis of treatment in the screening and control arm of the Swedish study, which is claimed to be the main contributor to this contamination.[10] Another study included in the meta-analysis[11] can be criticized even more heavily on methodological grounds. During the first two rounds of screening, only rectal examination was applied. This leads to inadequate screening, which is also confirmed by the detection of 42 of 85 cancers diagnosed in the screening arm as interval cancers.[12]

For these and reasons detailed later, we will mainly focus on the studies presenting the highest level of evidence; namely the ERSPC study[13] and the Göteborg randomized screening trial,[10] which is also part of ERSPC.

Prostate cancer mortality reduction with screening—summary of the highest level of RCT evidence

As for all cancer screening trials, cancer mortality is the primary end point on which power calculations are based. Overall mortality is evaluated to assess the accuracy of randomization. Figures 6.5.1, 6.5.2, and 6.5.3, show the flow diagrams of the PLCO, ERSPC, and Göteborg screening trials. The PLCO trial showed no difference in PC mortality in the screen arm.[7] The ERSPC study, as a whole, shows at 11 years of follow-up that PSA screening produces a significant relative decrease in prostate cancer mortality of 21% and of 29% for screened men[13] (men who did not comply with randomization are excluded). The Swedish trial,[10] which started one year after the ERSPC study, but is part of ERSPC, reported in 2010 data based on 14 years of follow-up. This longer follow-up is due to the population-based character of the Swedish study where by law randomization to the control group was possible without informed consent allowing to randomize all participants at the same time. After 14 years, the trial reported a reduction of the relative risk of death from prostate cancer in the intention-to-screen analysis of 44% and for men in fact screened (attendees) of 56%.

Figures 6.5.4, 6.5.5, and 6.5.6, shows the Nelson–Aalen mortality curves of the PLCO (Fig. 6.5.4), the ERSPC, and Göteborg trials (Figs 6.5.5 and 6.5.6). The cumulative differences in mortality cited correspond to these curves. The authors of both studies acknowledge that prostate cancer screening is not yet ready for introduction at a population level, because of an imbalance in benefits and harms (the high rate of overdiagnosis and overtreatment is estimated in the range of 50%).[14] This issue and other aspects of quality of life have been used to calculate the net effect of screening in terms of quality of life adjusted life years.[15] As a result of modelling outcomes per 1,000 men of all ages within the ERSPC study, a lifelong

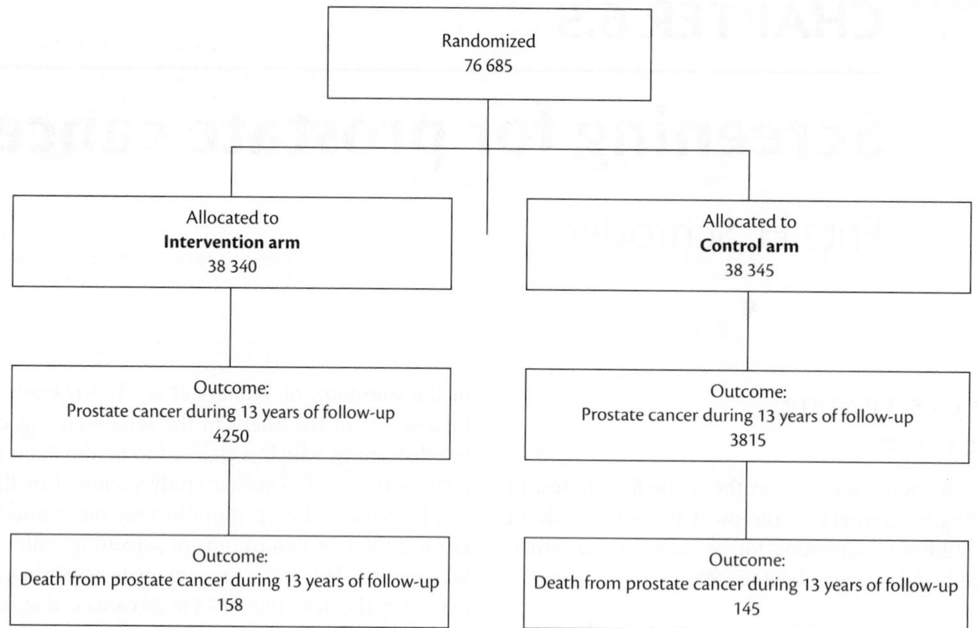

Fig. 6.5.1 Flow diagram for male participants in the Prostate, Lung, Colorectal, and Ovarian (PLCO) cancer screening trial.
Reproduced from Gerald L. Andriole *et al.*, 'Prostate Cancer Screening in the Randomized Prostate, Lung, Colorectal, and Ovarian Cancer Screening Trial: Mortality Results after 13 Years of Follow-up', *Journal of the National Cancer Institute*, Volume 104, Issue 2, pp. 125–32, Copyright © 2012, by permission of Oxford University Press.

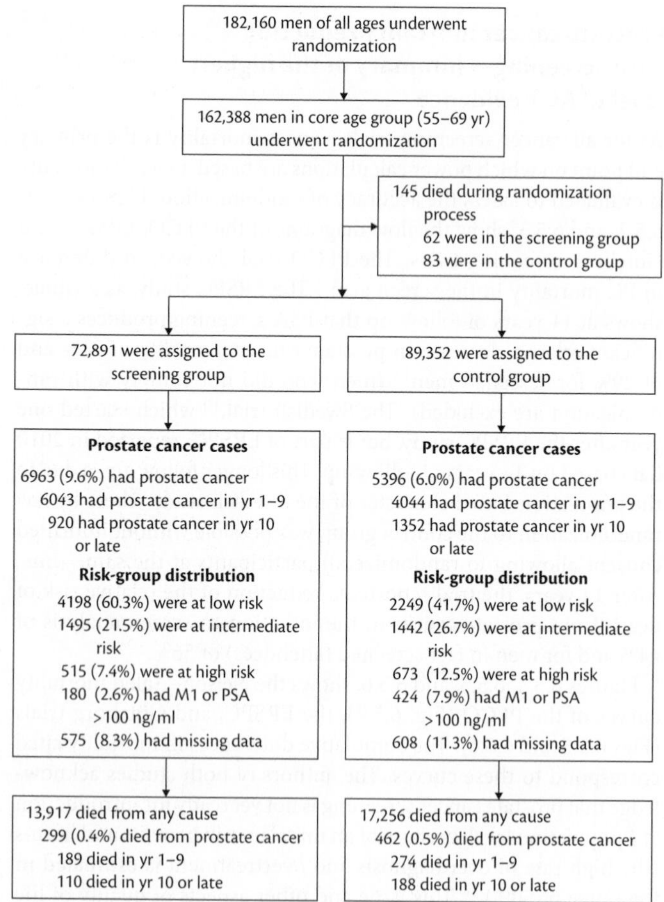

Fig. 6.5.2 Enrollment and outcomes in the ERSPC study.
From *The New England Journal of Medicine*, Fritz H. Schröder *et al*, 'Prostate-Cancer Mortality at 11 Years of Follow-up', Volume 366, Issue 11, pp. 981–90, Copyright © 2012 Massachusetts Medical Society. Reprinted with permission from Massachusetts Medical Society.

gain of 73 years or 8.4 years per prostate cancer death avoided was calculated. The number of quality of life adjusted life years gained was 56, a reduction of 23% from the 73 life years. This information will be important for healthcare providers and public health authorities in judging on the value of prostate cancer screening.

Definitions of screening

In this chapter, we follow the criteria of screening defined by Wilson and Jungner[16] in 1968. These criteria seem old but have survived and are still used in the critical assessment of cancer screening trials. These experts define screening as 'the presumptive identification of unrecognized disease or defect by the application of tests, examinations of other procedures which can be applied rapidly'. The authors then state that screening tests differentiate apparently well persons from those who probably have a disease. A screening test is not intended to be diagnostic. Furthermore, because all screening trials select for men at certain age groups, the definition of 'selective screening' applies. As the term is used for selection of high-risk populations, it may be applied to population-based screening. These procedures are strictly differentiated from 'case finding' of which the main object is 'to detect disease and bring patients to treatment, in contrast to epidemiological surveys'.

The criteria of Wilson and Jungner will be used to structure the present chapter. The criteria are given in Box 6.5.1.[16]

Quality requirements for screening trials, population screening, and case finding

This chapter will provide a step-by-step discussion of the ten prerequirements for population-based screening. In doing so, most information will be used to judge whether the requirements are presently met for prostate cancer screening trials and what the future perspectives may be.

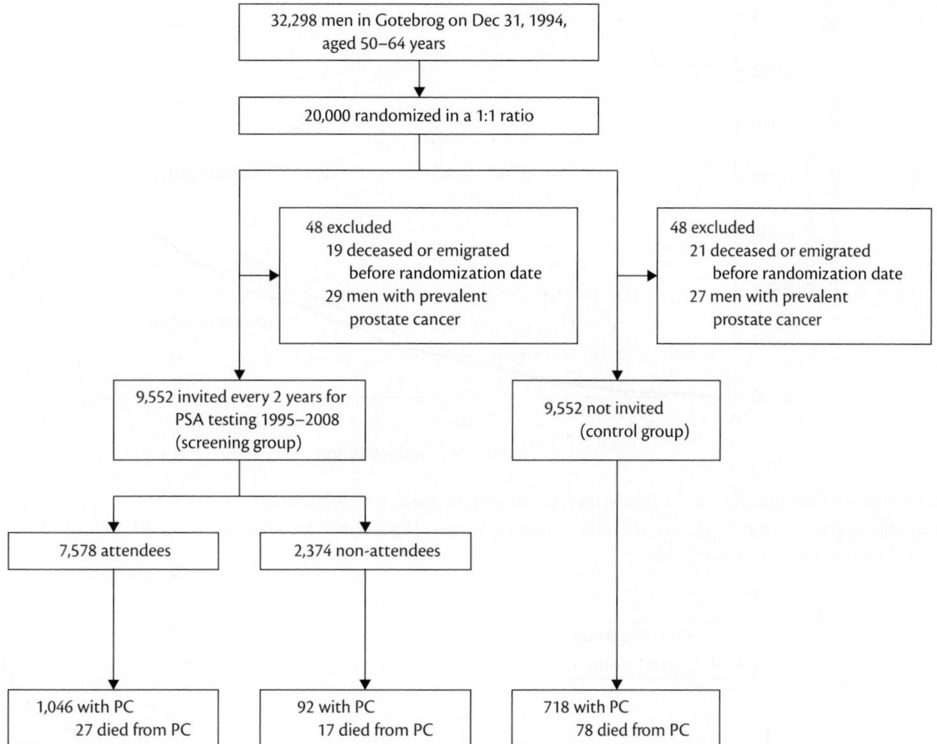

Fig. 6.5.3 Trial profile, ERSPC Göteborg.

Reprinted from *The Lancet Oncology*, Volume 11, Issue 8, Jonas Hugosson *et al.*, 'Mortality results from the Göteborg randomised population-based prostate-cancer screening trial', pp. 725–732, Copyright © 2010 Elsevier Ltd., with permission from Elsevier, http://www.sciencedirect.com/science/journal/14702045

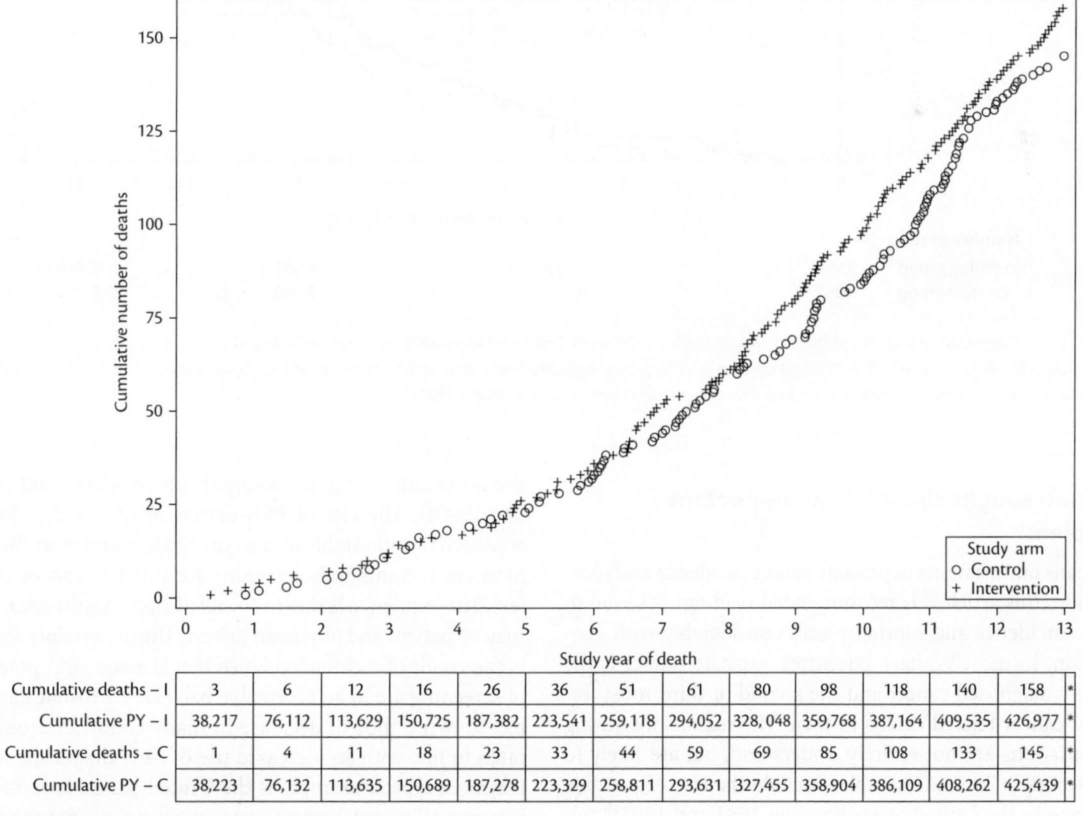

Cumulative deaths – I	3	6	12	16	26	36	51	61	80	98	118	140	158	*
Cumulative PY – I	38,217	76,112	113,629	150,725	187,382	223,541	259,118	294,052	328, 048	359,768	387,164	409,535	426,977	*
Cumulative deaths – C	1	4	11	18	23	33	44	59	69	85	108	133	145	*
Cumulative PY – C	38,223	76,132	113,635	150,689	187,278	223,329	258,811	293,631	327,455	358,904	386,109	408,262	425,439	*

Fig. 6.5.4 Nelson–Aalen curves of PLCO, ERSPC, and the Göteborg trial.

PLCO: Cumulative deaths from prostate cancer in the intervention and control arms from year 1 to 13; C: control arm; I: intervention arm; PY: person years.

Reproduced from Gerald L. Andriole *et al.*, 'Prostate Cancer Screening in the Randomized Prostate, Lung, Colorectal, and Ovarian Cancer Screening Trial: Mortality Results after 13 Years of Follow-up', *Journal of the National Cancer Institute*, Volume 104, Issue 2, pp. 125–32, Copyright © 2012, by permission of Oxford University Press.

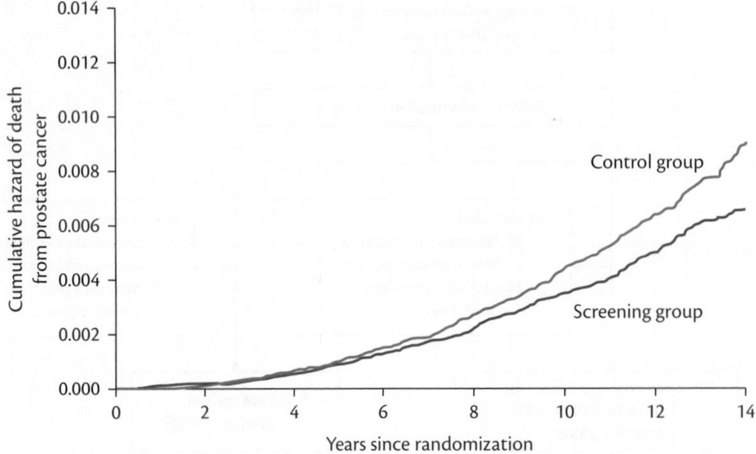

Fig. 6.5.5 Cumulative hazard of death from prostate cancer among men 55–69 years of age in the ERSPC study.
From *The New England Journal of Medicine*, Fritz H. Schröder *et al*, 'Prostate-Cancer Mortality at 11 Years of Follow-up', Volume 366, Issue 11, pp. 981–90, Copyright © 2012 Massachusetts Medical Society. Reprinted with permission from Massachusetts Medical Society.

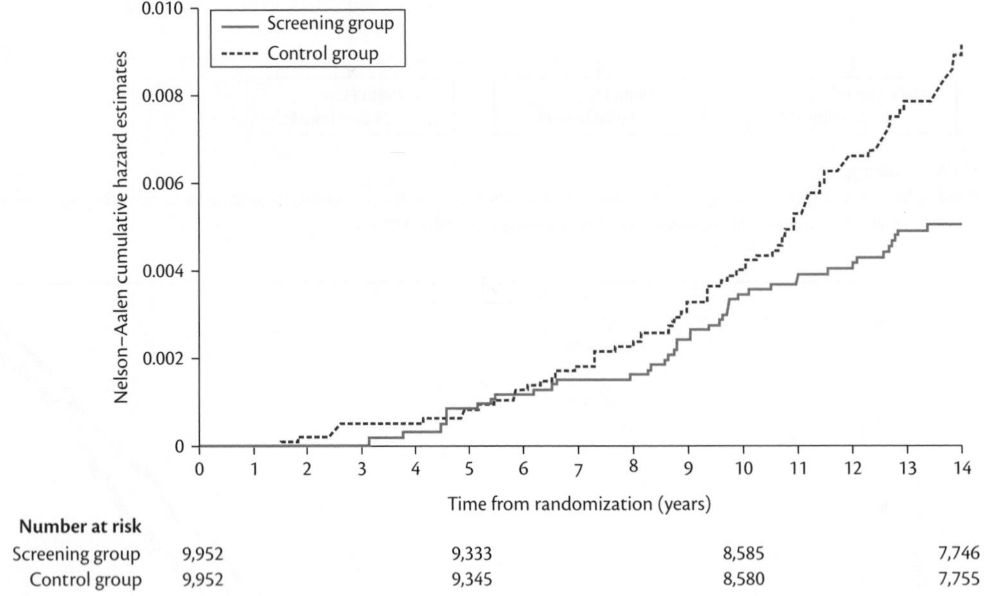

Fig. 6.5.6 ERSPC Göteborg—cumulative risk of death from prostate cancer using Nelson–Aalen cumulative hazard estimates.
Reprinted from *The Lancet Oncology*, Volume 11, Issue 8, Jonas Hugosson *et al.*, 'Mortality results from the Göteborg randomised population-based prostate-cancer screening trial', pp. 725–732, Copyright © 2010 Elsevier Ltd., with permission from Elsevier, http://www.sciencedirect.com/science/journal/14702045

'The condition sought should be an important health problem'

This section leans on variations in prostate cancer incidence and mortality worldwide (this article[17] is recommended reading). As seen in Figure 6.5.7,[17] incidence and mortality vary considerably with geographic location. In most Western countries, prostate cancer is the most frequently diagnosed cancer and the second or third most frequent cause of cancer related deaths in men. The reasons for strong geographic variations are not entirely understood, but are likely to involve PSA testing. Classical examples include the rise of prostate cancer incidence in the United States between 1983 and 1993[18] following PSA use advocacy, compared to a country where PSA use for early detection of prostate cancer has been strongly discouraged by the government (e.g. in Denmark the incidence did not rise in the late 1990s). The rise of PSA-driven incidence due to screening is considered undesirable and so no single country in the world at this moment recommends screening for prostate cancer using the PSA test. The incidence is due to so called 'opportunistic screening', which may be patient and physician driven. The uncertainty about screening is the result of lacking evidence that damage and potential benefits of screening are in an acceptable balance.[13] Prostate cancer mortality has shown trends to decrease in many countries around the world, often in line with an increased use of early diagnostic testing. Again, the most typical example is the United States. It is estimated[17] that between 1996 and 2005 prostate cancer mortality has decreased at an annual rate of 4.3%, a total decrease of 43%. Obviously, this mortality decrease, which in trend is seen in many other countries, can not be

Box 6.5.1 Pre-requirements for the application of screening

1. The condition sought should be an important health problem.
2. There should be an accepted treatment for patients with recognized disease.
3. Facilities for diagnosis and treatment should be available.
4. There should be a recognizable latent or early symptomatic stage.
5. The natural history of the condition, including development from latent to declared disease, should be adequately understood.
6. There should be an agreed policy on whom to treat as patients.
7. There should be a suitable test or examination.
8. The test should be acceptable to the population.
9. The cost of case finding (including diagnosis and treatment of patients diagnosed) should be economically balanced in relation to possible expenditure on medical care as a whole.
10. Case finding should be a continuing process and not a 'once and for all' project.

Reproduced with permission from Wilson JMG and Jungner G., *Principles and practice of screening for disease*, pp. 26–27, World Health Organization, Geneva, Switzerland, Copyright © World Health Organization 1968.

conclusively explained at this present time. In a two-centre modelling experiment, Etzioni *et al.*[19] suggest that 45–70% of the mortality decrease may be due to opportunistic screening. The remaining change in mortality is attributed to improvement in treatment, mainly by radical prostatectomy, radiotherapy, and maybe most importantly, radiotherapy combined with endocrine treatment in locally advanced disease.[20,21] An increase in incidence is also seen in some of the traditional low-risk countries of East Asia such as Japan. An unusual example is Korea, where incidence rise is accompanied with a rise in mortality. The best possible explanation for this may be the change of dietary habits in Korea, which in the past may have been the reason for the low incidence and mortality of this disease.

Considering the available data, there is little doubt that the first requirement is met and that prostate cancer can be considered an important health problem.

'There should be an accepted treatment for patients with recognized disease and facilities for diagnoses and treatment should be available'

Significant progress in treatment of locally confined, locally advanced, and metastatic prostate cancer has been made in years. Technical improvements of radical prostatectomy led to improvements of functional and oncological outcomes.[22,23] A large Scandinavian study compared radical prostatectomy to watchful waiting in 679 men randomized with a follow-up of 12.8 years.[24] The study recruited selected clinical participants and very few screen-detected cancers. The study group found an absolute risk

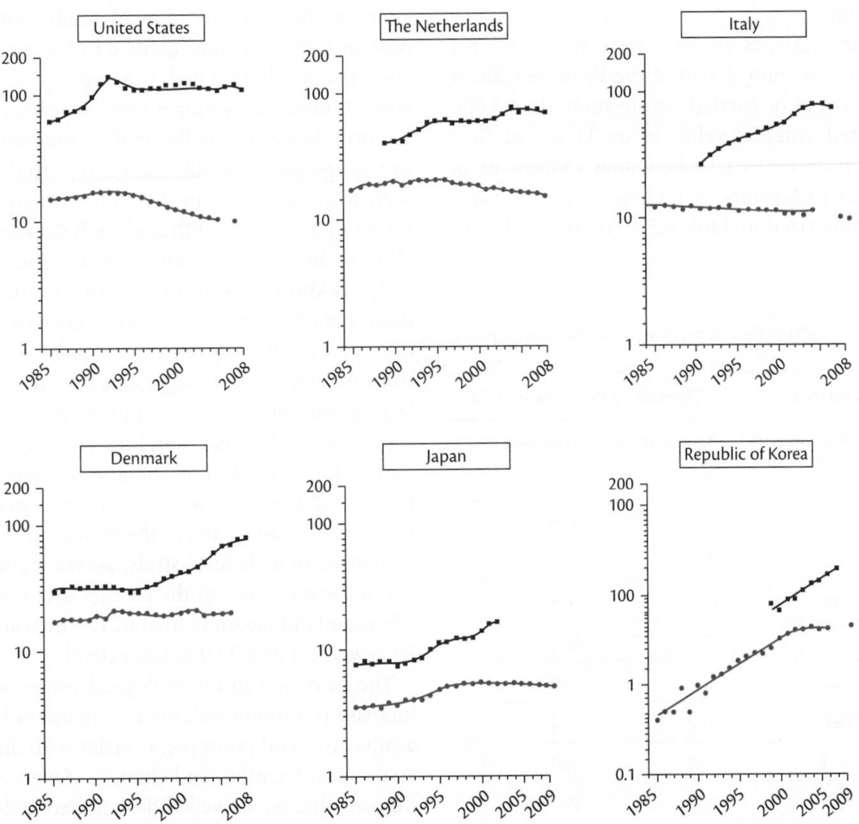

Fig. 6.5.7 Join point regression of incidence and mortality in six selected areas.

Reprinted from *European Urology*, Volume 61, Issue 6, Melissa M. Center *et al.*, 'International Variation in Prostate Cancer Incidence and Mortality Rates', pp. 1079–1092, Copyright © 2012 European Association of Urology, with permission from Elsevier, http://www.sciencedirect.com/science/journal/03022838

reduction of death from prostate cancer of 6.1% and a 38% relative reduction. Overall survival improved in a similar fashion. In a study of 415 patients with locally advanced disease treated by either radiotherapy alone or androgen suppression for a period of three years post-treatment, a study group of the European Organization for Research and Treatment of Cancer (EORTC) found with a 9.1-year follow-up significant improvements in prostate cancer specific and overall survival in the range of 25%.[20] After this keynote study, the question of whether hormone therapy might have the same effect remained open. This question was addressed by the Scandinavian Prostate Cancer Group in a study randomizing men with lymph node positive disease between endocrine treatment alone and endocrine treatment plus radiotherapy. The study found a significant advantage of the combination treatment. After this, for locally advanced disease radiotherapy plus endocrine treatment for a period of three years can be considered standard management. The period of post-radiotherapy treatment was subject to another EORTC study, which confirmed an advantage of the three-year treatment.[25] Metastatic disease is rarely diagnosed through screening. If so, standard forms of endocrine treatment are applied.

In most countries, facilities for diagnosis and treatment of prostate cancer are readily available. If anything, as indicated in the previous section, there may be an overutilization of the available diagnostic tests, including PSA and subsequent biopsies. The large differences between incidence and mortality seen in Figure 6.5.7 are also confirmed in the available randomized studies and overdiagnosis has been quantified to be in the range of 50%.[14] To curb opportunistic screening and the rates of overdiagnosis and overtreatment is one of the key issues to be dealt with in urological research in the nearby future.

The performance characteristics of PSA were unknown for many years, until the placebo control arm of the Prostate Cancer Prevention Trial (PCPT) could be carried out. In more than 5,000 men who initially presented with PSA values below 3.0 ng/mL (low risk), sextant prostate biopsies were carried out after a follow-up of seven years irrespective of PSA values or findings at rectal examination. The data are summarized in Table 6.5.1 and derived from Thompson *et al.*[26] In this setting where all men were biopsied positive and negative predictive values are identical to sensitivity and specificity. It is evident from the data shown that there is no cut-off where sensitivity and specificity would match in a reasonable way. Clearly, any of the usual cut-off values utilized such as a PSA value of ≥4.0 ng/mL or ≥3.0 ng/mL misses substantial numbers of cancers and also substantial numbers of aggressive cancers (characterized as having biopsy Gleason scores of ≥7). Unfortunately, no single more selective marker seems to become available in the nearby future. Some evidence from multiparametric MRI studies suggest selective detection of aggressive and non-aggressive prostate cancers when compared to ultrasound driven biopsies. These studies are very heterogeneous and require confirmation in prospective studies preferably in a multicentre and randomized setting.[27,28]

Table 6.5.1 Performance characteristics of prostate-specific antigen

	Any PCa vs. no PCa		Gleason ≥7 vs. <7 or no PCa	
PSA level	**True pos (%)**	**True neg (%)**	**True pos (%)**	**True neg (%)**
1.1	82.0	40.6	92.8	37.0
1.6	67.4	58.8	84.4	54.8
2.1	54.4	70.8	75.6	67.3
2.6	43.6	79.6	67.2	76.5
3.1	35.8	85.1	57.6	82.3
4.1	24.5	92.3	40.4	90.0
6.1	5.4	98.0	13.2	97.8
8.1	2.0	99.1	4.8	99.0
10.1	1.0	99.5	2.4	99.5

Reproduced from Ian M. Thompson *et al.*, 'Assessing Prostate Cancer Risk: Results from the Prostate Cancer Prevention Trial', *Journal of the National Cancer Institute*, Volume 98, Issue 8, pp. 529–34, Copyright © 2006, by permission of Oxford University Press.

In conclusion, on these two pre-requirements for screening, the answer could be: yes, adequate treatment is available. Unfortunately, while there is no doubt that PSA-driven diagnostic work-ups find prostate cancer at an early (often too early) stage, an optimal diagnostic regimen is still to be found.

There should be a recognizable latent or early symptomatic stage and the natural history of the condition, including development from latent to declared disease, should be adequately understood.

This issue cannot be discussed in detail without giving a description of the natural history of prostate cancer, including estimates of the time spent in each disease stage (Fig. 6.5.8; a schematic presentation of our understanding of initiation and progression of prostate cancer to clinical disease).

The best information on the pre-clinical prevalence of prostate cancer comes from autopsy studies. The classical paper by Franks[29] analysed the incidence of incidentally found prostate cancer at autopsy in 1,050 men subclassified in 10-year age groups. Remarkably, and in contradiction with the findings of Sakr,[30] no prostate cancer was found in men younger then 50 years. For the age groups 50–79, the prevalence of usually small lesions was 29–40%, rising to 67% in the age group 80–89. Sakr[30] reported autopsy findings on 249 men who died early in their life, usually of traffic accidents, and found in the fourth, fifth and sixth decade 'incidental invasive carcinoma' in 29%, 32%, and 55% of cases, respectively. Very little so far is known about mechanisms of disease initiation. The large discrepancies between the prevalence of autopsy detectable prostate cancer, clinically apparent disease, and the frequency of death from prostate cancer, suggests a selective progression process. The large geographic variation in prevalence of clinical disease,[17] is best explained by differences in lifestyle. A causal relationship between damaging or protective dietary substances has not conclusively been established. However, early evidence derived from Japanese migrants to Hawaii and to the mainland of the United States is confirmatory. In a classical study, Akazaki and Stemmermann[31] compared the incidence of the proliferative type of latent carcinoma in 239 mainland Japanese men to 158 migrants to Hawaii. The prevalence was 5.1 and 20.9%, respectively.

The next step in the biological progression of the disease is an increase in tumour volume that makes it biopsy detectable. This is a subjective end point (i.e. it varies with different biopsy schedules, anatomical location, and chance). An accepted definition of insignificant disease is well-differentiated (Gleason score ≤6), of low volume (below 0.5 mL or 0.2 mL), and with a low PSA value (e.g. <10 ng/mL). Considering the haphazard nature of blind ultrasound guided prostate biopsy, some of these cancers will inevitably be

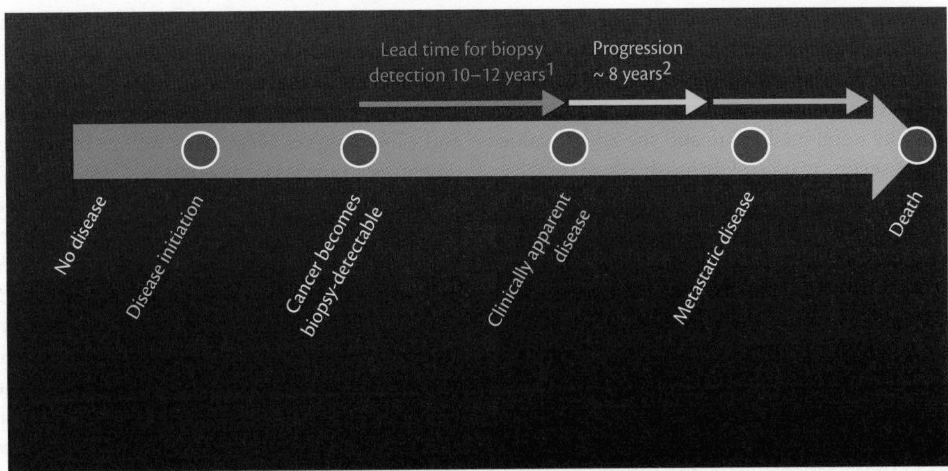

Fig. 6.5.8 Initiation and progression of prostate cancer.

detected. A comparison of biopsy detection rates with the proportion of cancer found incidentally at autopsy allows a limited quantification. One study found 42% of unsuspected prostate cancer in a systematic pathology evaluation of clinically unsuspicious prostates removed as part of cystoprostatectomy specimens in treating bladder cancer.[32] The data derived from the control arm of the PCPT study referred to above,[26] describes a detection rate of 21% in a setting where all men are biopsied. The cumulative incidence in the Dutch section of ERSPC, amounted to 11.6% with three to four screens conducted over 8 to 12 years.[13] This shows that even random sextant biopsies detect a large proportion of cancers otherwise only seen at autopsy.

The prevalence of clinically apparent disease varies strongly between geographical regions.[17] In the ERSPC control arm (non-screened), in Rotterdam, the cumulative incidence of clinically detected cases amounted to 5.6 in the age group 55–69 over an 11-year period. The difference between the screen and control group prevalence also gives an indication of the amount of overdiagnosis and potential overtreatment which occurs with screening. The time period by which the diagnosis of cancer is moved forward with respect to clinical detection is called lead time. The lead time was estimated to be in the range of 10–12 years.[14]

The remaining steps of the natural development of prostate cancer are indicated with time estimates in Figure 6.5.4. The progression period of eight years relates to men who have undergone radical prostatectomy and develop recurrence. The orange arrow indicates the time from development of metastatic disease to prostate cancer death. Overall, the known periods of natural history therefore add up to about 25 years. This long time of progressive development of prostate cancer needs to be taken into account when interpreting data coming from screening and treatment studies of this disease.

This section needs to be concluded by returning to statements by Wilson and Jungner. In answer, yes, there is a recognizable clinically latent stage. Its use in early detection however leads to significant amounts of overdiagnosis and overtreatment. Furthermore, there is a considerable knowledge about the natural history of prostate cancer. This knowledge, however, creates a complicated situation and considerable difficulty in interpreting the relevance of screen-detected cancers at a population level. For space reasons, this detailed discussion was limited to the diagnosis of prostate cancer in general and did not consider the progression from well-differentiated to more aggressive forms.

There should be an agreed policy on whom to treat (pre-requirement six)

At the first glance the answer to this question seems to be 'yes'. All major professional guidelines indicate all available treatment options for locally confined prostate cancer including active surveillance, radical prostatectomy, and radiotherapy (see latest EAU, AUA, and NCCN guidelines). Other options such as focal treatment are still under development. However, laymen and the medical advisors are confronted with difficult decision which require extensive discussion. Expected outcomes need to be predicted factoring in tumour characteristics, treatment options, potential side effects, expectations of quality of life, general health status, and life expectancy of the patient. While treatment options are clearly defined treatment choice remains difficult, and 'general agreement' while suggested by guidelines remains difficult to apply. Recent data from California show that even in the lowest risk group active, invasive treatments are still the preferred options with active surveillance only being applied in 6.8% of such cases.[33] Treatment options have already been dealt with under 2b.

There should be a suitable test or examination and the test should be acceptable to the population

The combination of digital rectal examination (DRE) and PSA can be considered as clinical standard for the diagnosis of non-metastatic prostate cancer, even in 2012. Both parameters are included in most current guidelines of professional organizations. Transrectal ultrasonography (TRUS) is usually only carried out if a biopsy of the prostate is indicated by either DRE, PSA, or both in conjunction. The value of TRUS as a screening test will be briefly discussed, but TRUS is no longer recommended as a primary screening tool.

Digital rectal examination as a screening test

The first suggestion that an induration in the prostate noticed by the palpating finger could indicate early prostate cancer came from a prospective non-comparative study carried out in the US army in the 1950s.[34] This study, which showed that DRE might be of value in diagnosing prostate cancer in a potentially curable state, had strong influence on the introduction of DRE based screening in Germany by law in 1971. Further discussion of the value of DRE in the context of this chapter is useful only in conjunction with PSA by addressing the combined value and the added value of DRE to this important serum marker. Obviously, the extensive international discussion of this issue during years could only take place after comprehensive studies of PSA as a marker for early prostate cancer. The first study presenting such evidence was.[35] Stamey and co-workers evaluated serum samples from 699 men presenting to their clinic of whom 378 had prostate cancer. Their study aimed at comparing prostate-specific antigen to prostatic acid phosphatase, the only marker available before the establishment of PSA. The authors found that PSA was elevated in 122 of 127 patients with newly diagnosed prostate cancer, prostatic acid phosphatase (PAP) was only elevated in 57 of those patients. Also, the authors describe for the first time that PSA was elevated in men with enlarged prostates as compared to PAP. Furthermore, they described a half-life of PSA after radical prostatectomy of 2.2 days, the effect of rectal examination on PSA levels, and they concluded that PSA is a more sensitive marker than PAP in the detection of prostate cancer. In 1991, another study showed that PSA was useful in early detection of prostate cancer and that it correlated with the extent of the disease.[36] During the following years the potential added value of DRE and TRUS became important issues in urological literature. This discussion will be limited to some of the most important studies. In an advertised screening setting Catalona *et al.* reported on 6,630 males above the age of 50 who underwent PSA testing and DRE. Quadrant biopsies were performed with PSA levels ≥4.0 ng/mL or with a suspicious rectal examination. Two-hundred and sixty-four cancers were detected with 1,167 biopsies, a detection rate of 4.5%. PSA detected significantly more tumours than DRE. However, the combined use of both predictors increased the positive predictive value (PPV) above that of PSA or DRE separately. The PPV of PSA in detecting locally confined disease was significantly higher. The authors concluded that both DRE and PSA should be used in conjunction. Their data, however, also showed a very low PPV of 10% of DRE for men with a PSA value of ≤4.0 ng/mL.[37]

The issue was again addressed within the ERSPC study. In total, 10,523 men age 54–76 who were randomly assigned to the screening arm were evaluated.[38] This study also correlated PSA levels to parameters of aggressiveness, particularly to the prevalence of potentially insignificant, overdiagnosed cancers. Four-hundred and seventy-three (473) cancers were found, a detection rate of 4.5%. The study confirmed a strong positive relation of PPV values to PSA ranges and a low PPV and detection rate of DRE alone of only about 10% in men with PSA values of ≤3.0 ng/mL, while the PPV of DRE above 3.0 ng/mL amounted to 46%. In addition, 42% of cancers identified with PSA values <4.0 ng/mL could be classified as 'minimal cancers'. These findings suggested that DRE might not be a useful test, at least in men with low PSA values.

The information described by Schröder *et al.*[38] eventually led to the omission of DRE from the screening algorithm of ERSPC all together. A validation of this step carried out during the year 2000 compared the test characteristics of PSA ≥3.0 ng/mL vs. PSA ≥4.0 ng/mL plus DRE in a comparative study of 7,943 vs. 8,612 participants, respectively. It turned out that the PPV of PSA ≥3.0 ng/mL amounted to 24.3% and was significantly higher than the 18.2% found with the combination of PSA and DRE as biopsy indications. These validation data confirmed the change of biopsy policies to PSA alone in ERSPC, but left open the question of the future fate of cancers that might have otherwise been detected by DRE. This issue was addressed later by evaluating the cancer detection rate and cancer aggressiveness, as well as interval cancers in men participating in the second round of screening four years after the initial screen. The findings in the second screening round were related to the results of DRE and TRUS during the first screening round. Somewhat surprisingly, the detection rate with or without an initially suspicious DRE was identical at 6% and obviously did not differ significantly. The proportion of clinically significant cancers by biopsy parameters was 2% and 1% for men with initially abnormal or normal DRE. Also, the proportion of interval cancers was low and amounted to 1.1% after four years in both groups. Logistic regression analysis also revealed no significant prediction of an initially abnormal rectal examination for the presence of prostate cancer in second and third screens. From this information, it was concluded that the omission of DRE as a screening test is acceptable and does not lead to missing more cancers and more significant cancers then using PSA alone as a biopsy indication.[39,40]

Prostate-specific antigen

As a result of using cut-off values in all clinical and screening studies reported, the true performance characteristics of PSA remained unknown, until data of a population of men who were all biopsied irrespective of their PSA value were published.[26] The results have been addressed above and showed that there is no level of sensitivity and specificity which matches to define a common cut-off value and that each cut-off value used will miss prostate cancers and aggressive prostate cancers. These findings, more than anything before, question the value of PSA as a marker for prostate cancer and stress the need for the development of markers which provide selectiveness for the identification of potentially insignificant or indolent versus aggressive disease. Preferentially, such markers should avoid the biopsy of prostates in men who are likely to harbour insignificant, potentially overdiagnosed lesions all together. At present, the identification of indolent cancer is possible, but only after the diagnosis has already been established.[41] Once prostate cancer is diagnosed, its carrier is burdened with lifelong worry and the need of follow-up, even if he harbours a tumour which will never progress during his lifetime and become life-threatening, and even if the choice of treatment is active surveillance.

Transrectal ultrasonography

TRUS is no longer utilized as a screening test but is essential for directing the biopsy needle when conducting prostatic biopsies. TRUS does not allow to identify details and even the claim that the prostate cancer presents as an hypoechogenic lesion is heavily debated. Because TRUS biopsy is non-targeted and random in character resulting in a very low specificity for detection of any PC and for the selective detection of aggressive PC, there is an urgent need to develop more targeted biopsy techniques. Multiparametric MRI offers a glimpse of hope in this respect.[27,28]

The authors have serious doubts about the 'suitability' of the presently available tests for all of the reasons outlined in this chapter, and feel that the answer to Wilson and Junger's prerequirement should be 'no' while available information suggests that present diagnostic procedures are well accepted by males in general. In the future, multiparametric MRI shows promise as a more specific (but expensive) tool for visualizing prostate cancer.

The cost of case finding (including diagnosis and treatment of patients diagnosed) should be economically balanced in relation to possible expenditure of medical care as a whole. Case finding should be a continuing process and not a 'once and for all' project.

A cost-effectiveness analysis combining early detection and treatment options of prostate cancer is at present not available. The fact is, however, that healthcare systems have accepted the expenses resulting from diagnoses made as a result of opportunistic screening. Once, if ever, screening for prostate cancer becomes a general healthcare policy, cost-effectiveness of early diagnosis and treatment has to be determined and put into perspective with the expenses of advanced prostate cancer, and also with accepted healthcare policies per country for affordable expenses per life-year saved.

Prerequirement 10 is easily met. The large randomized controlled trials of screening have all shown that repeated screening is feasible and acceptable.[42,43]

Conclusion

Screening for prostate cancer is common as 'opportunistic screening', but has not yet been established as a healthcare policy anywhere. While an effect on prostate cancer mortality has been shown by studies providing a high level of evidence, the harm caused by screening, mainly a high rate of overdiagnosis, prevents the formal introduction. This outlines the major need for progress of applied research which can be identified in 2013 in relation to screening for prostate cancer. The comparison of the present status of skills and knowledge with the prerequirements established by Wilson and Jungner identifies other areas where progress is needed in a potentially useful way.

Further reading

Andriole GL, Crawford ED, Grubb RL 3rd, *et al.* Prostate cancer screening in the randomized Prostate, Lung, Colorectal, and Ovarian Cancer Screening Trial: mortality results after 13 years of follow-up. *J Natl Cancer Inst* 2012; **104**(2):125–32.

Bolla M, de Reijke TM, van Tienhoven G, *et al.* for the EORTC Radiation Oncology Group and Genito-Urinary Tract Cancer Group. Duration of androgen suppression in the treatment of prostate cancer. *N Engl J Med* 2009; **360**:2516–27.

Bolla M, van Tienhoven G, Warde P, *et al.* External irradition with or without long-term androgen suppression for prostate cancer with high metastatic risk: 10-year results of an EORTC randomised study. *Lancet Oncol* 2010; **11**(11):1066–73.

Center MM, Jemal A, Lortet-Tieulent J, *et al.* International variation in prostate cancer incidence and mortality rates. *Eur Urol* 2012; **61**:1079–92.

Chou R, Croswell JM, Dana T, *et al.* Screening for prostate cancer: a review of the evidence for the US Preventive Services Task Force. *Ann Intern Med* 2011; **155**(11):762–71.

Draisma G, Boer R, Otto SJ, *et al.* Lead times and overdetection due to prostate-specific antigen screening: estimates from the European Randomized study of Screening for Prostate Cancer. *J Natl Cancer Inst* 2003; **95**(12):868–78.

Etzioni R, Tsodikov A, Mariotto A, *et al.* Quantifying the role of PSA screening in the US prostate cancer mortality decline. *Cancer Causes Control* 2008; **19**(2):175–81.

Heijnsdijk EAM, Wever EM, Auvinen A, *et al.* Quality-of-life effects of prostate-specific antigen screening. *N Engl J Med* 2012; **367**(7):595–605.

Hugosson J, Carlsson S, Aus G, *et al.* Mortality results from the Göteborg randomized population-based prostate-cancer screening trial. *Lancet Oncol* 2010; **11**(8):725–32.

Schröder FH, Hugosson J, Roobol MJ, *et al.* Prostate-cancer mortality at 11 years of follow-up. *N Engl J Med* 2012; **366**:981–90.

Schröder FH, Roobol MJ. ERSPC and PLCO prostate cancer screening studies: what are the differences? *Eur Urol* 2010; **58**(1):46–52.

Steyerberg EW, Roobol MJ, Kattan MW, van der Kwast TH, de Koning HJ, Schröder FH. Prediction of indolent prostate cancer: validation and updating of a prognostic nomogram. *J Urol* 2007; **177**(1):107–12.

Thompson IM, Ankerst DP, Chi C, *et al.* Assessing prostate cancer risk: results from the Prostate Cancer Prevention Trial. *J Natl Cancer Inst* 2006; **98**(8):529–34.

Ukimura O, Desai MM, Palmer S, *et al.* 3-Dimensional elastic registration system of prostate biopsy location by real-time 3-dimensional transrectal ultrasound guidance with magnetic resonance/transrectal ultrasound image fusion. *J Urol* 2012; **187**(3):1080–6.

Widmark A, Klepp O, Solberg A, *et al.* for the Scandinavian Prostate Cancer Group Study 7 and the Swedish Association for Urological Oncology 3. Endocrine treatment, with or without radiotherapy, in locally advanced prostate cancer (SPCG-7/SFUO-3): an open randomised phase III trial. *Lancet* 2009; **373**:301–8.

References

1. Djulbegovic M, Beyth RJ, Neuberger MM, Stoffs TL, Vieweg J, Djulbegovic B, Dahm P. Screening for prostate cancer: systematic review and meta-analysis of randomized controlled trials. *BMJ* 2010; **341**:c4543.
2. Ilic D, Neuberger MM, Djulbegovic M, Dahm P. Screening for prostate cancer. *Cochrane Database Syst Rev* 2013; **1**:CD004720.
3. Chou R, Croswell JM, Dana T, *et al.* Screening for prostate cancer: a review of the evidence for the US Preventive Services Task Force. *Ann Intern Med* 2011; **155**(11):762–71.
4. Cochrance Consumer Network—What is a systematic review? Available at: http://consumers.cochrane.org/[Accessed 18 August 2012] [Online].
5. Roobol MJ, Carlsson S, Hugosson J. Meta-analysis finds screening for prostate cancer with PSA does not reduce prostate cancer-related or all-cause mortality but results likely due to heterogeneity—the two highest quality studies identified do find prostate cancer-related mortality reduction. *Evid Based Med* 2011; **16**(1):20–1.
6. Schröder FH, Roobol MJ. ERSPC and PLCO prostate cancer screening studies: what are the differences? *Eur Urol* 2010; **58**(1):46–52.
7. Andriole GL, Crawford ED, Grubb RL 3rd, *et al.* Mortality results from a randomized prostate-cancer screening trial. *N Engl J Med* 2009; **360**(13):1310–9.
8. Andriole GL, Crawford ED, Grubb RL 3rd, *et al.* Prostate cancer screening in the randomized Prostate, Lung, Colorectal, and Ovarian Cancer Screening Trial: mortality results after 13 years of follow-up. *J Natl Cancer Inst* 2012; **104**(2):125–32.
9. Wolters T, Roobol MJ, Steyerberg EW, *et al.* The effect of study arm on prostate cancer treatment in the large screening trial ERSPC. *Int J Cancer* 2010; **126**(10):2387–93.
10. Hugosson J, Carlsson S, Aus G, *et al.* Mortality results from the Göteborg randomized population-based prostate-cancer screening trial. *Lancet Oncol* 2010; **11**(8):725–32.
11. Sandblom G, Varenhorst E, Rosell J, Löfman O, Carlsson P. Randomised prostate cancer screening trial: 20 year follow-up. *BMJ* 2011; **342**:d1539.
12. Schröder FH. Study has major shortcomings. *BMJ* 2011; **342**:d3704.
13. Schröder FH, Hugosson J, Roobol MJ, *et al.* Prostate-cancer mortality at 11 years of follow-up. *N Engl J Med* 2012; **366**:981–90.
14. Draisma G, Boer R, Otto SJ, *et al.* Lead times and overdetection due to prostate-specific antigen screening: estimates from the European Randomized study of Screening for Prostate Cancer. *J Natl Cancer Inst* 2003; **95**(12):868–78.
15. Heijnsdijk EAM, Wever EM, Auvinen A, *et al.* Quality-of-life effects of prostate-specific antigen screening. *N Engl J Med* 2012; **367**(7):595–605.

16. Wilson JMG, Jungner G. *Principles and practice of screening for disease.* WHO, Geneva, Switzerland, 1968. Available at: http://apps.who.int/iris/handle/10665/37650 [Online].
17. Center MM, Jemal A, Lortet-Tieulent J, *et al.* International variation in prostate cancer incidence and mortality rates. *Eur Urol* 2012; **61**:1079–92.
18. Siegel R, Naishadham D, Jemal A. Cancer statistics, 2012. *CA Cancer J Clin* 2012; **62**:10–29.
19. Etzioni R, Tsodikov A, Mariotto A, *et al.* Quantifying the role of PSA screening in the US prostate cancer mortality decline. *Cancer Causes Control* 2008; **19**(2):175–81.
20. Bolla M, van Tienhoven G, Warde P, *et al.* External irradition with or without long-term androgen suppression for prostate cancer with high metastatic risk: 10-year results of an EORTC randomised study. *Lancet Oncol* 2010; **11**(11):1066–73.
21. Widmark A, Klepp O, Solberg A, *et al.* for the Scandinavian Prostate Cancer Group Study 7 and the Swedish Association for Urological Oncology 3. Endocrine treatment, with or without radiotherapy, in locally advanced prostate cancer (SPCG-7/SFUO-3): an open randomised phase III trial. *Lancet* 2009; **373**:301–8.
22. Walsh PC, Donker PJ. Impotence following radical prostatectomy: insight into etiology and prevention. *J Urol* 1982; **128**(3):492–7.
23. Walsh PC. The discovery of the cavernous nerves and development of nerve sparing radical retropubic prostatectomy. *J Urol* 2007; **177**(5):1632–5.
24. Bill-Axelson A, Holmberg L, Ruutu M, *et al.* Radical prostatectomy versus watchful waiting in early prostate cancer. *N Engl J Med* 2011; **364**(18):1708–17.
25. Bolla M, de Reijke TM, van Tienhoven G, *et al.* for the EORTC Radiation Oncology Group and Genito-Urinary Tract Cancer Group. Duration of androgen suppression in the treatment of prostate cancer. *N Engl J Med* 2009; **360**:2516–27.
26. Thompson IM, Ankerst DP, Chi C, *et al.* Assessing prostate cancer risk: results from the Prostate Cancer Prevention Trial. *J Natl Cancer Inst* 2006; **98**(8):529–34.
27. Haffner J, Lemaitre L, Puech P, Haber GP, Leroy X, Jones JS, Villers A. Role of magnetic resonance imaging before initial biopsy: comparison of magnetic resonance imaging-targeted and systematic biopsy for significant prostate cancer detection. *BJU Int* 2011; **108**(8 Pt 2):E171–8.
28. Ukimura O, Desai MM, Palmer S, *et al.* 3-Dimensional elastic registration system of prostate biopsy location by real-time 3-dimensional transrectal ultrasound guidance with magnetic resonance/transrectal ultrasound image fusion. *J Urol* 2012; **187**(3):1080–6.
29. Franks LM. Latent carcinoma of the prostate. *J Pathol Bacteriol* 1954; **68**(2):603–16.
30. Sakr WA, Grignon DJ, Crissman JD, *et al.* High grade prostatic intraepithelial neoplasia (HGPIN) and prostatic adenocarcinoma between the ages of 20–69: an autopsy study of 249 cases. *In Vivo* 1994; **8**(3):439–43.
31. Akazaki K, Stemmermann GN. Comparative study of latent carcinoma of the prostate among Japanese in Japan and Hawaii. *J Natl Cancer Inst* 1973; **50**:1137–44.
32. Montironi R, Mazzucchelli R, Santinelli A, Scarpelli M, Beltran AL, Bostwick DG. Incidentally detected prostate cancer in cystoprostatectomies: pathological and morphometric comparison with clinically detected cancer in totally embedded specimens. *Hum Pathol* 2005; **36**(6):646–54.
33. Cooperberg MR, Broering JM, Carroll PR. Time trends and local variation in primary treatment of localized prostate cancer. *J Clin Oncol* 2010; **28**(7):1117–23.
34. Kimbrough JC. Carcinoma of the prostate: five-year follow-up of patients treated by radical surgery. *J Urol* 1956; **76**(3):287–91.
35. Stamey TA, Yang N, Hay AR, McNeal JE, Freiha FS, Redwine E. Prostate-specific antigen as a serum marker for adenocarcinoma of the prostate. *N Engl J Med* 1987; **317**(15):909–16.
36. Catalona WJ, Smith DS, Ratliff TL, *et al.* Measurement of prostate-specific antigen in serum as a screening test for prostate cancer. *N Engl J Med* 1991; **324**(17):1156–61.
37. Catalona WJ, Richie JP, Ahmann FR, *et al.* Comparison of digital rectal examination and serum prostate specific antigen in the early detection of prostate cancer: results of a multicenter clinical trial of 6,630 men. *J Urol* 1994; **151**:1283–90.
38. Schröder FH, van der Maas P, Beemsterboer P, *et al.* Evaluation of the digital rectal examination as a screening test for prostate cancer. *JNCI* 1998; **90**(23):1817–23.
39. Schröder FH, Roobol-Bouts M, Vis AN, van der Kwast TH, Kranse R. Prostate-specific antigen-based early detection of prostate cancer—validation of screening without rectal examination. *Urology* 2001; **57**:83–90.
40. Gosselaar C, Roobol MJ, van den Bergh RCN, Wolters T, Schröder FH. Digital rectal examination and the diagnosis of prostate cancer—a study based on eight years and three screenings within the European Randomized study of Screening for Prostate Cancer (ERSPC), Rotterdam. *Eur Urol* 2009; **55**(1):139–46.
41. Steyerberg EW, Roobol MJ, Kattan MW, van der Kwast TH, de Koning HJ, Schröder FH. Prediction of indolent prostate cancer: validation and updating of a prognostic nomogram. *J Urol* 2007; **177**(1):107–12.
42. Bentvelsen FM, Schröder FH. Modalities available for screening for prostate cancer. *Eur J Cancer* 1993; **29a**(6):804–11.
43. Essink-Bot ML, Korfage IJ, de Koning HJ. Include the quality-of-life effects in the evaluation of prostate cancer screening: expert opinions revisited? *BJU Int* 2003; **92**(Suppl 2):101–5.

CHAPTER 6.6

Clinical features, assessment, and imaging of prostate cancer

Anders Bjartell and David Ulmert

Introduction to clinical features of prostate cancer

Clinical features of prostate cancer have changed since the introduction of the prostate-specific antigen (PSA) blood test in the early nineties. The use of this test has produced a stage migration so that most cancers are now detected while locally confined to the prostate. Historically around one-third of cancers were detected with metatstases, one-third due to their advanced clinical stage (e.g. presenting with lower urinary tract symptoms), and only one-third were locally confined. Today, most patients are asymptomatic at the time of diagnosis and do not have any palpable tumour at digital rectal examination (DRE). Classification of newly diagnosed prostate cancer is now uniform worldwide and follows the tumour-node-metastases (TNM) system. An accurate assessment of disease extent is critical for predicting the outcome of curative treatment in men with clinically localized prostate cancer. For prognostication, the level of PSA in blood and tumour grade in prostate biopsies is also of major importance. Although the role of imaging has increased after technological improvements, there is still a need for pelvic lymph node dissection in many men for optimal staging of nodal status. Besides population-based screening for prostate cancer, men with symptoms from the urinary tract, skeletal pain, and general signs of malignacy need a DRE and PSA test. This is particularly true for men with first-degree relatives diagnosed with prostate cancer. In men with abberant DRE or PSA findings, a transrectal ultrasonography (TRUS)–guided prostate biopsy is then needed to clarify the diagnosis. The aim of clinical staging is to provide the urologist and the patient with correct information regarding whether the disease is localized, locally advanced, or metastatic, for optimized decision-making.

Clinical and pathological staging

Clinical staging is the assessment of disease extent based on clinical pretreatment parameters (DRE, PSA, prostate biopsy examination and imaging), whereas pathological staging utilizes the histopathological information obtained after surgical removal of the prostate and lymph node dissection. For prediction of outcome after prostatectomy, the following criteria are recognized to be important: tumour Gleason grade; surgical margin status (SMS); extraprostatic extension (EPE); seminal vesicle invasion (SVI); and pelvic lymph node involvement (LNI). For prediction of biochemical recurrence (BCR) after prostatectomy, nomograms have become popular.[1–3] Nomograms may be used pre- or postoperatively and allow prediction of prostate cancer recurrence for up to 15 years after radical prostatectomy.

The classification system used for clinical staging today is the TNM classification, which was introduced in 1975 by the American Joint Committee for Cancer Staging and End Results Reporting (AJCC).[4] It has since undergone several revisions, mainly concerning classification of palpable organ-confined tumours, or cT2. Although a non-palpable tumour detectable at TRUS is to be classified as T2, it is commonly considered as T1c today. The latest version of TNM staging for prostate cancer is available from the American Joint Committee on Cancer (AJCC) and the lastest version (7) was approved in 2016.[5,6]

Prediction of tumour extent

Digital rectal examination

Since the introduction of PSA testing, DRE is no longer the most important or common reason to diagnose prostate cancer. Nevertheless, the DRE is important to determine local disease extent (i.e. the primary clinical T-stage). The poor sensitivity, poor specificity, and the lack of reproducibility of DRE become obvious in populations screened using PSA. However, within such populations, an abnormal DRE is predictive of poorly differentiated prostate cancer (Gleason 8–10) or advanced tumour stage, and therefore abnormal DRE findings should be investigated with TRUS biopsy.[7,8] However, DRE has a poor accuracy for determining the extent of the disease. Many studies have described non-organ-confined prostate cancer at pathological examination (stage pT3) in patients whose tumour feels less advanced on DRE.[9] Taken together, DRE can both over and underestimate the local extent of prostate cancer, and it is best used in combination with PSA, Gleason grade, and other pretreatment parameters.

Prostate-specific antigen

The role of prostate-specific antigen (whether total or a subfraction) is described in more detail in Chapter 6.4. Despite the poor specificity of an elevated PSA, which may occur due to cancer, benign prostatic hyperplasia (BPH) or prostatitis at low or moderately elevated levels,[10] the usefulness of this parameter to predict disease extent can not be neglected. The level of PSA is a continous parameter. In general, increased values suggest an elevated risk of prostate cancer[11] and are reflective of increasing disease extent. Although it is rare, aggressive and poorly differentiated prostate cancer may not secrete PSA and therefore, it may be found in men with very low PSA levels.

Transrectal ultrasonography

The early detection of prostate cancer has not only benefited from PSA testing but also from systematic TRUS-guided prostate biopsy techniques. Transrectal ultrasonography was first described by Watanabe and colleagues,[12] and brought to routine clinical use after technical improvements and the introduction of the TRUS-guided systematic sextant biopsy protocols.[13,14] Today, it is the most commonly used imaging method for evaluation of the prostate, and usually performed in a greyscale mode. A transducer with a frequency range of 6–10 MHz is used in a side-fire endorectal probe. The examination usually starts by careful visualization of the gland from the base to the apex. The separation into different histological zones is not always easy to find, however the peripheral zone (PZ) and the transition zone (TZ) are sonographically visible in most glands. Measurement of the prostate total volume is performed in the transverse and sagittal plane and calculated by the formula of an ellipse (length × width × height × 0.52) (Fig. 6.6.1). The peripheral zone is then carefully examined for hypoechoic lesions, which may represent tumours. Unfortunately, other disease processes such as granulomatous prostatitis, prostatic infarct, and lymphoma may also give rise to hypoechoic areas. The TZ is enlarged, and the peripheral zone usually thin. Corpora amylacea are calcifications frequently observed along the surgical capsule in the border between TZ and PZ. Multiple small calcifications and cysts may be related to prior infection and not considered as signs of malignancy. The seminal vesicles and vasa deferentia should be fully visualized in the complete examination.

Typically, a tumour is identified as a hypoechoic area in the peripheral zone of the prostate gland. Most cancer lesions arise in this zone and therefore biopsies should be taken from all identified hypoechoic areas as well as throughout the PZ. The sensitivity and specificity of identifying tumour areas are not optimal, and TRUS is often considered as a less reliable method for identifying areas of malignant tissue at clinical stage T1c. Consequently, it is not possible to only rely on targeted biopsy, but instead it is necessary to systematically biopsy the whole gland. Early studies found that TRUS is unable to reliably localize low-volume prostate cancers with a detection rate of only 64% in patients undergoing prostatectomy.[15] In a study by Rifkin *et al.*[16] the overall accuracy of TRUS at detecting extracapsular extent was 46%, with sensitivity and specificity of 66% and 46%, respectively. A contemporary series of almost 4,000 patients, has confirmed that the value of TRUS for staging of pathologically confirmed prostate cancer is limited.[17] Colour Doppler function is available today and can show hypervascularized areas in the periperal zone representing tumours.[18] Although it may increase the accuracy in tumour detection, many urologists do not use it routinely and large prospective trials are not yet available. Taken together, greyscale TRUS is not reliable enough to detect tumours, and it is therefore not a candidate to replace systematic biopsies with additional targeted samples of suspect areas. The important roles of TRUS are to measure prostate size and as a guiding tool for biopsy.

Prostate biopsy

Guidelines for prostate biopsy, focusing on indications, techniques, and implications for patient care were reviewed by Ukimura *et al.*[19] The authors showed that the significance of prostate biopsy is not only pure cancer detection but also important for better characterization of clinically important cancer versus indolent cancers and to assist in clinical management of the individual patient. Local anaesthesia is generally recommended, and it is easily deposited as periprostatic infiltration with a fine needle in the biopsy channel of the transrectal probe.[20] Use of antibiotics prior to prostate biopsy is also strongly recommended. It can be administered intravenously, but it is most often given orally. Optimal dosing and length of treatment vary considerably. Ciprofloxacin is commonly used, although there may be an association between last year's increased resistance to quinilones and a rise in severe post-biopsy infections.[21] Severe infections with septicaemia and hospitalization may occur within a few days. Although the incidence was earlier considered as very low, this rate has increased as a consequence of antibiotic resistance strains.[22] A prospective multinational multicentre investigation (Global Prevalence Study of Infections in Urology, GPIU) was performed at 84 different centres over two weeks in 2010 to evaluate the incidence of infective complications after prostate biopsy and

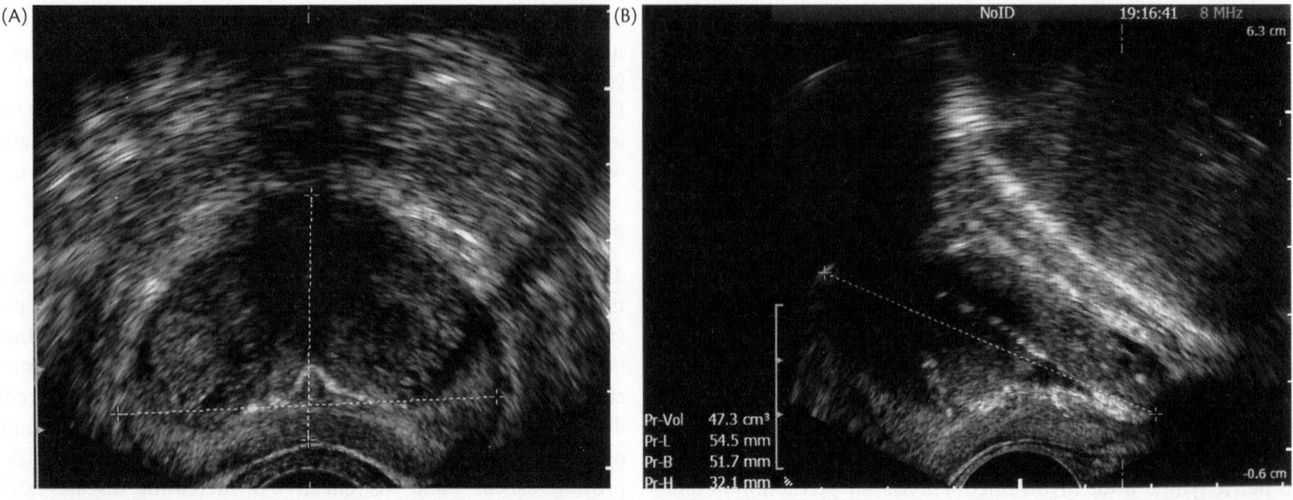

Fig. 6.6.1 (A) and (B) show transrectal ultrasonography measuring prostate size using an endorectal probe.

to identify risk factors.[23] Despite antibiotic prophylaxis, 5% of men (27/521) experienced an infective complication and required hospitalization in 3.1% (n = 16). A high incidence of fluoroquinolone resistance was confirmed. Complications after transrectal prostate biopy also include urinary retention, rectal bleeding, visible haematuria, and haematospermia. Warfarin and similar anticoagulantia are contraindicated, whereas aspirin is not.[24] Fine needle aspiration biopsy from the prostate is no longer considered good practice.

Initial biopsy

The most important indications for initial prostate biopsy are elevated PSA level and a suspicious DRE. Before deciding to biopsy, the patient's biological age, co-morbidities (Charlson co-morbidity index, CCI, or American Society of Anesthesiologists' identification system for a patient's medical status, ASA), and therapeutical options should be taken into consideration. If PSA is within the greyzone (3–10 ng/mL), then verification by a repeat PSA test after a few weeks may be recommended.[25] A search for confounding factors such as cystoscopy, catheterization, or urinary tract infection must be performed.[26] Risk stratification has become an important tool to reduce unnecessary prostate biopsies. Different risk calculators based on nomograms are available online for patients and doctors to support decision-making, and one of these is developed from the European Screening Study for Prostate Cancer (ERSPC).[27–29]

Recommendations of how many individual prostate biopsies should be obtained have changed. Sextant biopsy is no longer considered adequate. Recent data supports an extended protocol of 10–12 cores with additional cores where DRE or TRUS indicates a lesion[19] (Fig. 6.6.2, Fig. 6.6.2A). Haas *et al.*[30] performed a careful analysis with step-sections and revealed a detection rate of 80% with regard to clinically signficant tumours if a 12-core technique was used. This recommendation was empahsized in a study evaluating a 20-core prostate biopsy protocol.[31] Most studies underline the importance of lateral and apical sampling covering the peripheral zone.

As an alternative to transrectal biopsy, some urologists prefer to use an ultrasonography-guided perineal approach. This is also suitable in patients after rectal amputation. Improved cancer detection has been described by saturation biopsies, usually performed with a transperineal approach under anaesthesia in a hospital setting.[19] However, advantages with this technique have been questioned in subequent studies.[32] A contemporary study showed that the cancer detection rate is comparable between perineal and transrectal prostate biopsies.[33] A drawback with perineal saturation biopsy is an increased risk of urinary retention (10%),[34] and the risk of detecting indolent, less harmful cancers not requiring immediate treatment, which should also be taken into account.

Repeat biopsy

Around 20% of cancers are not detected on the first TRUS-guided biopsy. Indications for repeat biopsy are (i) a continous rising or a persistently elevated serum PSA; (ii) suspicious DRE or TRUS findings; (iii) the presence of atypical small acinar proliferation (ASAP) in previous biopsy samples; or (iv) multiple cores with prostatic intraepithelial neoplasia (PIN) in the previous biopsy.[25] The number of transrectal cores in repeat prostate biopsy should be at least 12 and should include samples from the TZ. Biopsies may be increased to 20 cores without an increased complication rate. When collecting adequate tissue for analysis, attention should be paid to include the PZ, the apical portion, as well as sampling from suspicious areas (Fig. 6.6.2B). Repeat biopsy is included in most protocols for active surveillance (AS) of men with clinically low-risk prostate cancer, but recommendations for the number and timing of rebiopsy vary.[19] The use of magnetic resonance imaging (MRI) to identify anterior tumours has become increasingly popular. MRI-guided prostate biopsy is available at many centres today, and MRI also have a role in AS protocols.[35] Diagnostic transurethral resection of the prostate (TURP) is considered of limited value for cancer detection and staging, and it is no longer recommended by the EAU Guidelines.[25] It can be concluded that the paradigm of initial and repeat prostate biopsy have changed, and it is expected to be further revised soon. This is not only due to rapid technical improvements, but is also a result of ongoing discussions of how to reduce overdiagnosis and overtreatment of low-risk prostate cancer.

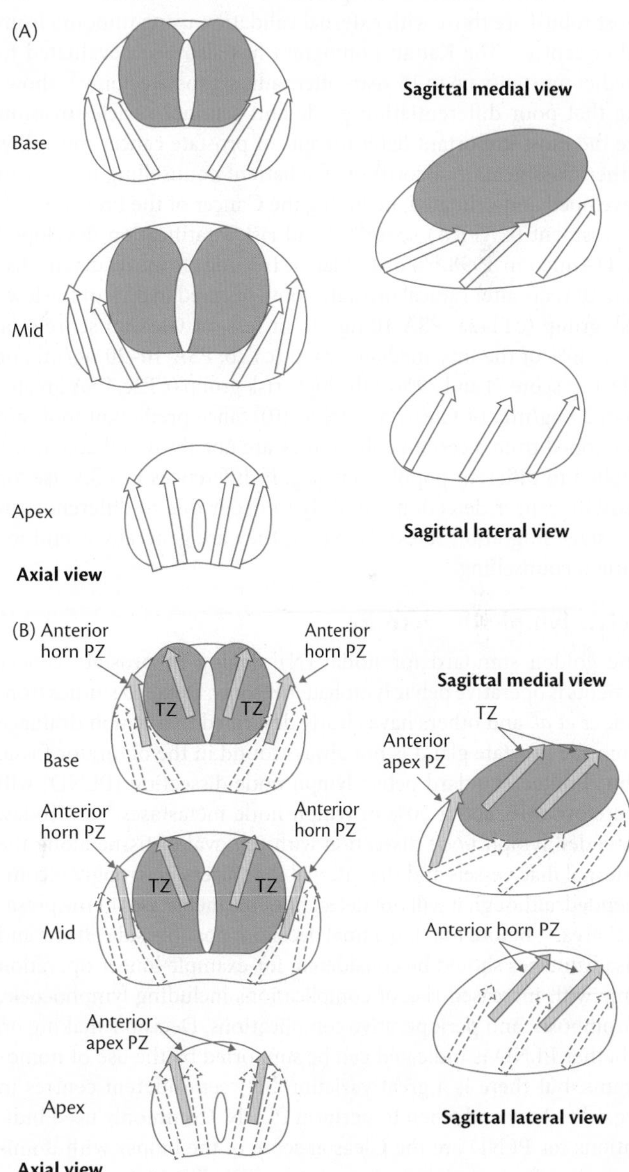

Fig. 6.6.2 Cartoons illustrate schemes for initial (A) and repeat prostate biopsy (B).

Reprinted from *European Urology*, Volume 63, Issue 2, Osamu Ukimura *et al.*, 'Contemporary Role of Systematic Prostate Biopsies: Indications, Techniques, and Implications for Patient Care', pp. 214–230, Copyright © 2012 European Association of Urology, with permission from Elsevier, http://www.sciencedirect.com/science/journal/03022838

Combination of multiple pretreatment parameters

Although several pretreatment parameters are used for prediction of tumour extent, none of these are good enough in isolation to predict the pathological stage accurately. The number of prediction tools using clinical parameters has increased markedly over the last few years.[3] Today, stage predictions are most precisely performed using nomograms or similar algorithms that integrate multiple clinical parameters. For example, age, DRE findings, clinical T-stage, serum PSA level, biopsy Gleason grade, and number of positive biopsies are usually combined to predict pathological T-stage, extracapsular extension, seminal vesicle invasion, lymph node involvement, and prostate cancer-specific survival 5–10 years after surgical treatment with curative intent. User-friendly prediction tools are available to the public on various websites.[1,2,36] The most robust are those with external validation using tumours from other centres. The Kattan nomogram has also been evaluated to predict mortality up to 15 years after radical prostatectomy[37] showing that poor differentiation grade and seminal vesicle invasion are the most important determinants of prostate cancer mortality. Other classification algorithms for patient counselling have been developed and validated, including the Cancer of the Prostate Risk Assessment (CAPRA) score[38,39] and risk stratification developed by D'Amico in 1998.[40] For the latter, freedom from recurrent disease 10 years after radical prostatectomy occured in 83% of the low-risk group (cT1-2a, PSA 10 ng/mL or less, or Gleason score 6 or less), 46% of the intermediate group (cT2b, PSA 10–20 ng/mL, or Gleason score 7) and 29% of the high-risk group (cT2c, PSA greater than 20 ng/mL, or Gleason score 8–10). Since prediction tools are developed from a certain cohort, they are not always reliable when applied to different populations (e.g. if differences in PSA use for prostate cancer detection are likely to occur due to differences in the stage migration rates). However, they are generally useful for patient counselling.

Pelvic lymphadenectomy

The golden standard for nodal (N) staging in prostate cancer patients is operative pelvic lymphadenectomy. Detailed studies from Studer *et al.* and others have clearly described that lymph drainage from the prostate gland is not always found in the obturator fossa. Thus limited/standard pelvic lymph node dissection (PLND) will therefore miss about 50% of lymph node metastases.[41–43] Today, extended lymph node dissection with removal of tissue along the external iliac vessels and the internal iliac artery is strongly recommended, although it will not detect possible metastases in the presacral area.[44] Before making a final decision, possible side effects and disadvantages should be considered, for example longer operation time with increased risk of complications including lymphocoele, thrombosis, and perioperative complications. Decision-making on whether PLND is indicated can be supported by the use of nomograms, but there is a great variation between different centres in regard to how and when to perform PLDN. Commonly used indications for PLND are the Gleason score of the biopsy with dominating grade 4 or higher, clinical stage T2b–T3, PSA greater than 10 ng/mL, or enlarged lymphnodes if radiographic evalaution has been performed. Recent improvements in imaging techniques to replace or to indicate PLDN to be performed are discussed below. CT scans have a poor accuracy for preoperative nodal-staging, as demonstrated by Briganti *et al.*[45] who evaluated a contemporary series of 1,541 patients undergoing radical prostatectomy and extended PLND between 2003 and 2010 at a single centre. Overall, sensitivity, specificity, and accuracy of CT scan were 13%, 96.0%, and 54.6%, respectively, and at multivariable analyses, inclusion of CT scan findings did not improve the accuracy of LNI prediction.

Molecular staging

Several attempts have been made to develop sensitive methods for the detection of metastatic spread by isolation of circulating tumour cells (CTCs) from peripheral blood. The semi-automated CellSearch® system (Janssen Diagnostics LLC, Raritan, NJ) is approved by the FDA in America for monitoring the treatment response in patients with metastatic breast and prostate cancer, but is not sensitive enough to be used for initial staging at diagnosis. This technology utilizes a combination of centrifugation and immunostainings to indirectly identify tumour cells with epithelial characteristics. A role of detecting CTCs in staging prostate cancer with limited tumour burden is still unclear, whereas the usefulness of measuring response to new treatments for metastastic prostate cancer is more proven.[46]

Imaging

Magnetic resonance imaging

One of the most promising developments in tumour detection and staging has been the use of multimodality MRI. Multiparametric MRI, which combines anatomic T2-weighted (T2W) imaging with MR spectroscopic imaging (MRSI), diffusion-weighted imaging (DWI), and/or dynamic contrast-enhanced MRI (DCE-MRI) appears relatively robust at detecting signficant prostate cancer (typically a lesion over 0.5 mL in volume), but is dependant upon the radiologist's experience and is only available at certain centres. The promise of a combination of anatomic, biologic, and functional dynamic information makes MRI likely to become the key tool in staging and monitoring prostate cancer patients. MRI has also been shown to add value in a nomogram setting.[47] One particular strength of MRI is its ability to detect tumours anteriorly in the prostate or in the transition zone. These are usually missed by TRUS biopsy (which preferentially samples the posterior prostate) and so MRI should be used in patients at risk of cancer (e.g. persistently high PSA level) but with a previous negative biopsy. Despite the proposed benefits of using MRI in localization of prostatic tumours, drawbacks are also well known. Lesions identified as possible tumour areas may represent post-biopsy haemorrhage or inflammation, and significant inter- and intraobserver variability also exist. Larger multicentre studies are needed to confirm the initial promising results and validate the use of multiparametric MRI for initial diagnosis of prostate cancer. Before such studies can be performed, there is a need to standardize imaging protocols and to determine reproducible quantitative parameters. A recent prospective study PROMIS (Prostate MRI Imaging Study) has evaluated the accuracy of multi-parametric MRI and TRUS biopsy in the diagnosis of prostate cancer. The study concluded that if used prior to prostate biopsy, mpMRI could prevent up to 27% of men from receiving biopsies while detecting 5% fewer clinically insignificant cancers, and improving the detection of clinically significant cancers. With further refinement of these findings, it is likely that mpMRI will play an important role in triaging men who would benefit from biopsy.[48]

CT and MRI have been evaluated in clinical staging of prostate cancer, but neither modality is sufficiently reliable to make their use mandatory in the assessment of local tumour invasion.[49,50] Combining endorectal MRI (e-MRI) with existing clinical variables may improve local staging,[51] particularly in the detection of extraprostatic extension (EPE) and SVI, although an experienced and dedicated genitourinary radiologist is required.[52,53] This was assessed when e-MRI was incorporated in a nomogram to predict organ-confined prostate cancer, and the greatest benefit was then seen in the intermediate and high-risk groups.[54] Using multimodality MRI, suspicious areas have been correlated with a pathological Gleason score, suggesting the potential for a MRI to distinguish between more or less aggressive forms of prostate cancer.[55]

MRI has also been evaluated for detection of lymph node metastases, but the interpretation of N-status rests solely on the presence of enlarged lymph nodes with a threshold of 1 cm in accordance with CT.[56] High-resolution MRI with lymphotrophic ultra-small super-paramagnetic iron oxide particles (USPIO) has shown promising results in detecting smaller lymph node metastases although the method is still considered as experimental.[57,58]

Positron emission tomography—computerized tomography

2-[^{18}F]-fluoro-2-deoxy-D-glucose (^{18}F-FDG)

The most widely used positron emission tomography (PET) tracer is the radiolabeled-glucose analogue ^{18}F-FDG. In its application for oncology, the tracer utilizes the Warburg effect; the observation that most cancer cells predominantly produce energy by a high rate of glycolysis.[59] The method has excelled as a clinical tool to assess metabolism for staging and monitoring of malignancies, providing invaluable diagnostic information. Unfortunately, prostate cancer is one malignancy where the clinical usefulness of ^{18}F-FDG is limited. The lack of success is due to both biological and technical factors; naturally low metabolic activity, multifocal distribution of cancer, interference with ^{18}F-FDG uptake at sites of inflammation, and the anatomical proximity to the high activity in the urinary bladder through which ^{18}F-FDG is excreted.

The biological explanation to the limited glycolytic uptake has not yet been fully resolved. In comparison to neoplasms in other organs, overexpression of glucose transporters is lower and only noted in some highly proliferative intraductal prostate cancers.[60] Several putative reasons for this have been suggested, such as an overall lower malignant metabolic activity,[61] or utilization of other hexoses such as fructose, which is highly abundant in prostatic fluid.

The multifocal distribution of neoplastic tissue further limit the tracer's role in primary diagnosis and in staging of prostate cancer because of the overlap of tracer accumulation in normal and abnormal prostate tissue. Studies evaluating ^{18}F-FDG-PET as an aid for detection of primary tumours have reported sensitivity and positive predictive values in the range of 60–80% for detecting tumours with a Gleason of 7 and greater in men with elevated PSA levels.[62,63] Also, studies evaluating ^{18}F-FDG as a method to detect disease recurrence after radical prostatectomy have been less than favourable. In one such example, comparing the performance of ^{18}F-FDG-PET/CT with PSA relapse following prostatectomy, PET was only true-positive in a third of the patients.[64]

Although limited as a tool for staging, ^{18}F-FDG-PET can be applied as a biomarker when monitoring therapy of advanced disease, especially skeletal metastasis.[65,66] While measuring direct tumour activity, rather than indirectly through bone turnover, ^{18}F-FDG complements bone scans (whether with ^{18}F-NaF PET or conventional single photon agents) by demarcating false-positive uptake in dormant or treated lesions, or false negative sites of lytic tumours (due to lack of bone turnover).

In summary, ^{18}F-FDG-PET is generally limited in the primary diagnosis, staging, and monitoring of prostate cancer. Although further investigation is still required, ^{18}F-FDG's use may be best as a complement to other biomarkers when evaluating treatment response in patients with generalized disease.

Choline PET-tracers (^{18}F-choline and ^{11}C-choline)

Choline is a precursor for biosynthesis of phospholipids. Choline kinase catalyses the phosphorylation of choline to form phosphorylcholine, followed by generation of phosphatidylcholine in the cell membrane in rapidly dividing cancer cells. Choline PET-tracers accumulate at a higher rate in malignant tissue due to increased cellular membrane synthesis.[67]

There are currently two clinical versions of choline-based radiotracers: ^{18}F-choline and ^{11}C-choline. The normal distribution of choline sees accumulation in several organs, including pancreas, liver, kidneys, and bowel.

Evaluation of choline as a diagnostic tool for primary prostate cancer is currently confounded by lack of protocol standardization.[68] Nonetheless, the most rigorous study to date does not support the use of choline PET as a sufficiently accurate tool for first-line diagnosis.[69] Comparison between tracer uptake and histopathology showed a limited correlation. Small and rind-like tumours were poorly detected, and standardized uptake values failed to distinguish between cancer, benign prostatic hypertrophy, and prostatitis.

Similar to ^{18}F-FDG, choline-based PET does not seem to be applicable as a method to detect biochemical recurrent or metastatic disease. The overall reported sensitivity for detection of recurrent or metastatic cancer ranges between 38% and 98%.[70] The wide range of sensitivity may relate to the heterogeneity of patient populations in terms of PSA level ranges, type of primary therapy, and the type and quality of validation criteria.

Tc99m-methylene diphosphonate

Scintigraphic techniques have long been the mainstay for assessing bone disease. Tc99m-methylene diphosphonate (MDP) is a metastable (^{99m}Tc) tagged phosphonate, which has a high affinity for adsorption and incorporation into the hydroxyapatite crystalline lattice of bone.[71] Uptake of MDP is a function of bone turnover (i.e. osteoblastic activity) and quantity of mineralized bone, but also blood supply, and local acid/base balance. Bone scintigraphy is very sensitive for osteogenic activity and allows for quick assessment of the entire skeleton. However, there are several limitations to the method. Bone scan findings depict indirect changes rather than the tumour itself. Evaluation of disease regression can be difficult to determine due to lingering radiotracer uptake in healing bone. Also, response assessment is confounded by the flare phenomenon, an increase in isotope uptake by metastatic lesions or the appearance of previously occult lesions after starting systemic therapy, a major obstacle that can occur up to 12 weeks post-effective treatment.[72]

Several methods to quantify the uptake of ^{99m}Tc-MDP have emerged over the years. One of the most successful techniques has been termed the bone scan index (BSI), which is a measure of the fractional volume of skeletal tumour burden.[73] Apart from being a valuable metric for estimating metastatic burden, BSI has also been shown to be a predictor of survival in patients with progressive prostate cancer (PCa).[74]

Fluorine-18–labelled sodium fluoride

Fluorine-18–labelled sodium fluoride (^{18}F-NaF) was one of the first tracers originally used for bone imaging with conventional gamma cameras. ^{18}F-NaF has re-emerged as a PET radiotracer.[75] The mechanism of ^{18}F-NaF uptake is similar to that of the phosphonates. Apart from the superior imaging characteristics provided by the PET technology itself (including the ability to quantify uptake in lesions), the advantages of ^{18}F-NaF over ^{99m}Tc-MDP include a higher affinity for bone, resulting in a more rapid blood clearance, a higher bone-to-background ratio, and a shorter time from tracer administration to imaging.[76] Although further validations are needed, studies show that ^{18}F-NaF outperforms ^{99m}Tc-MDP for the assessment of osteoblastic metastases, particularly when combined with the anatomic information derived from CT.[77]

Conclusions

Clinical staging is the assessment of disease extent based on pretreatment parameters (DRE, PSA, prostate biopsy examination, and imaging), which is of major importance both for prognostic evaluation and for decision-making regarding appropriate treatment. Lymph drainage from the prostate gland is not always found in the obturator fossa, and today, extended lymph node dissection with removal of tissue along the external iliac vessels and the internal iliac artery is strongly recommended when necessary. Before making a final decision, possible side effects, and disadvantages should be considered. The important roles of TRUS are to measure prostate size and to be used as a guiding tool for biopsy. Greyscale TRUS of the prostate gland is of limited use for visualization of tumour areas and is mainly used for biopsy guidance. It is therefore not a candidate to replace systematic biopsies. Multimodality MRI with a combination of anatomic, funtional and metabolic imaging modalities is the mainstay in evaluating the extent of local tumour, and it may also be used for guided prostate biopsy in the near future. Although several pretreatment parameters are used for prediction of tumour extent, none of these are good enough to alone predict the pathological stage accurately. The number of prediction tools has increased markedly the last few years and imaging modalities have also been incorporated. Today, this is most precisely performed using nomograms or similar algorithms that integrate multiple clinical parameters for improved staging.

The role of detecting CTCs in staging prostate cancer with limited tumour burden is still unclear, whereas it is more likely to be a successful tool when used to evaluate response to treatments in patients with metastastic disease.

Computed tomography and radionuclide bone scanning are mainly reserved for assessment of advanced disease. The total burden of skeletal metastases can be automatically estimated using bone scan index, which is of prognostic value but can also be useful in evaluation of treatment response. Several novel PET-tracers, which could be of importance in evaluating treatment response, are currently under evaluation.

Further reading

Briganti A, Blute ML, Eastham JH, *et al.* Pelvic lymph node dissection in prostate cancer. *Eur Urol* 2009; **55**(6):1251–65.

Danila DC, Fleisher M, Scher HI. Circulating tumor cells as biomarkers in prostate cancer. *Clin Cancer Res* 2011; **17**(12):3903–12.

Even-Sapir E, Metser U, Mishani E, Lievshitz G, Lerman H, Leibovitch I. The detection of bone metastases in patients with high-risk prostate cancer: 99mTc-MDP Planar bone scintigraphy, single- and multi-field-of-view SPECT, 18F-fluoride PET, and 18F-fluoride PET/CT. *J Nucl Med* 2006; **47**(2):287–97.

Heidenreich A, Bellmunt J, Bolla M, *et al.* EAU guidelines on prostate cancer. Part 1: screening, diagnosis, and treatment of clinically localised disease. *Eur Urol* 2011; **59**(1):61–71.

Jung AJ, Westphalen AC. Imaging prostate cancer. *Radiol Clin North Am* 2012; **50**(6):1043–59.

Lughezzani G, Briganti A, Karakiewicz PI, *et al.* Predictive and prognostic models in radical prostatectomy candidates: a critical analysis of the literature. *Eur Urol* 2010; **58**(5):687–700.

Preston MA1, Harisinghani MG, Mucci L, Witiuk K, Breau RH. Diagnostic tests in urology: magnetic resonance imaging (MRI) for the staging of prostate cancer. *BJU Int* 2013; **111**(3):514–7.

Sabbatini P, Larson SM, Kremer A, *et al.* Prognostic significance of extent of disease in bone in patients with androgen-independent prostate cancer. *J Clin Oncol* 1999; **17**(3):948–57.

Seitz M, Shukla-Dave A, Bjartell A, *et al.* Functional magnetic resonance imaging in prostate cancer. *Eur Urol* 2009; **55**(4):801–14.

Souvatzoglou M, Weirich G, Schwarzenboeck S, *et al.* The sensitivity of [11C]choline PET/CT to localize prostate cancer depends on the tumor configuration. *Clin Cancer Res* 2011; **17**(11):3751–9.

Ukimura O, Coleman JA, de la Taille A, *et al.* Contemporary role of systematic prostate biopsies: indications, techniques, and implications for patient care. *Eur Urol* 2013; **63**(2):214–30.

Ulmert D, O'Brien MF, Bjartell AS, Lilja H. Prostate kallikrein markers in diagnosis, risk stratification and prognosis. *Nat Rev Urol* 2009; **6**(7):384–91.

References

1. Stephenson AJ, Scardino PT, Eastham JA, *et al.* Preoperative nomogram predicting the 10-year probability of prostate cancer recurrence after radical prostatectomy. *J Natl Cancer Inst* 2006; **98**(10):715–7.
2. Center MS. *Prediction Tools – A Tool for Doctors and Patients.* [Cited 2013] Available at: http://www.nomograms.org [Online].
3. Lughezzani G, Briganti A, Karakiewicz PI, *et al.* Predictive and prognostic models in radical prostatectomy candidates: a critical analysis of the literature. *Eur Urol* 2010; **58**(5):687–700.
4. Wallace DM, Chisholm GD, Hendry WF. T.N.M. classification for urological tumours (U.I.C.C.) - 1974. *Br J Urol* 1975; **47**(1):1–12.
5. Sobin LH, Compton CC. TNM seventh edition: what's new, what's changed: communication from the International Union Against Cancer and the American Joint Committee on Cancer. *Cancer* 2010; **116**(22):5336–9.
6. Amin MB, Edge S, Greene F, *et al.* (eds). *AJCC Cancer Staging Manual.* Springer International Publishing AG. 2017.
7. Gosselaar C, Roobol MJ, van den Bergh RC, Wolters T, Schröder FH. Digital rectal examination and the diagnosis of prostate cancer-- a study based on 8 years and three screenings within the European Randomized Study of Screening for Prostate Cancer (ERSPC), Rotterdam. *Eur Urol* 2009; **55**(1):139–46.
8. Okotie OT, Roehl KA, Han M, Loeb S, Gashti SN, Catalona WJ. Characteristics of prostate cancer detected by digital rectal examination only. *Urology* 2007; **70**(6):1117–20.
9. Ohori M, Egawa S, Shinohara K, Wheeler TM, Scardino PT. Detection of microscopic extracapsular extension prior to radical prostatectomy for clinically localized prostate cancer. *Br J Urol* 1994; **74**(1):72–9.

10. Stamey TA, Caldwell M, McNeal JE, Nolley R, Hemenez M, Downs J. The prostate specific antigen era in the United States is over for prostate cancer: what happened in the last 20 years? *J Urol* 2004; **172**(4 Pt 1): 1297–301.
11. Ulmert D, O'Brien MF, Bjartell AS, Lilja H. Prostate kallikrein markers in diagnosis, risk stratification and prognosis. *Nat Rev Urol* 2009; **6**(7):384–91.
12. Watanabe H, Kato H, Kato T, Morita M, Tanaka M. *[Diagnostic application of ultrasonotomography to the prostate]*. Nihon Hinyokika Gakkai Zasshi 1968; **59**(4):273–9.
13. Hodge KK, McNeal JE, Stamey TA. Ultrasound guided transrectal core biopsies of the palpably abnormal prostate. *J Urol* 1989; **142**(1):66–70.
14. Hodge KK, McNeal JE, Terris MK, Stamey TA. Random systematic versus directed ultrasound guided transrectal core biopsies of the prostate. *J Urol* 1989; **142**(1):71–4; discussion 74–5.
15. Ellis WJ, Chetner MP, Preston SD, Brawer MK. Diagnosis of prostatic carcinoma: the yield of serum prostate specific antigen, digital rectal examination and transrectal ultrasonography. *J Urol* 1994; **152**(5 Pt 1): 1520–5.
16. Rifkin MD, Sudakoff GS, Alexander AA. Prostate: techniques, results, and potential applications of color Doppler US scanning. *Radiology* 1993; **186**(2):509–13.
17. Onur R, Littrup PJ, Pontes JE, Bianco FJ Jr. Contemporary impact of transrectal ultrasound lesions for prostate cancer detection. *J Urol* 2004; **172**(2):512–4.
18. Bree RL. The role of color Doppler and staging biopsies in prostate cancer detection. *Urology* 1997; **49**(3A Suppl):31–4.
19. Ukimura O, Coleman JA, de la Taille A, *et al.* Contemporary role of systematic prostate biopsies: indications, techniques, and implications for patient care. *Eur Urol* 2013; **63**(2):214–30.
20. Adamakis I, Mitropoulos D, Haritopoulos K, Alamanis C, Stravodimos K, Giannopoulos A. Pain during transrectal ultrasonography guided prostate biopsy: a randomized prospective trial comparing periprostatic infiltration with lidocaine with the intrarectal instillation of lidocaine-prilocain cream. *World J Urol* 2004; **22**(4):281–4.
21. Williamson DA, Roberts SA, Paterson DL, *et al.* Escherichia coli bloodstream infection after transrectal ultrasound-guided prostate biopsy: implications of fluoroquinolone-resistant sequence type 131 as a major causative pathogen. *Clin Infect Dis* 2012; **54**(10):1406–12.
22. Loeb S, Carter HB, Berndt SI, Ricker W, Schaeffer EM. Complications after prostate biopsy: data from SEER-Medicare. *J Urol* 2011; **186**(5):1830–4.
23. Wagenlehner FM, van Oostrum E, Tenke P, *et al.* Infective complications after prostate biopsy: outcome of the Global Prevalence Study of Infections in Urology (GPIU) 2010 and 2011, a prospective multinational multicentre prostate biopsy study. *Eur Urol* 2013; **63**(3):521–7.
24. Giannarini G, Mogorovich A, Valent F, *et al.* Continuing or discontinuing low-dose aspirin before transrectal prostate biopsy: results of a prospective randomized trial. *Urology* 2007; **70**(3):501–5.
25. Mottet N, Bellmunt J, Bolla M, *et al.* EAU-ESTRO-SIOG Guidelines on Prostate Cancer. Part 1: Screening, Diagnosis, and Local Treatment with Curative Intent. *Eur Urol* 2016 Aug 25; pii: S0302-2838(16)30470-5. doi: 10.1016/j.eururo.2016.08.003. [Epub ahead of print].
26. Stephan C, Lein M, Schnorr D, Loening SA, Jung K. Repeating the measurement of prostate-specific antigen in symptomatic men can avoid unnecessary prostatic biopsy. *BJU Int* 2004; **93**(9):1360–1.
27. Roobol MJ, Carlsson SV. Risk stratification in prostate cancer screening. *Nat Rev Urol* 2013; **10**(1):38–48.
28. Roobol MJ, Steyerberg EW, Kranse R, *et al.* A risk-based strategy improves prostate-specific antigen-driven detection of prostate cancer. *Eur Urol* 2010; **57**(1):79–85.
29. SWOP—The Prostate Cancer Research Foundation. *Calculate your prostate cancer risk*. Available at: http://www.prostatecancer-riskcalculator.com [Online].
30. Haas GP, Delongchamps NB, Jones RF, *et al.* Needle biopsies on autopsy prostates: sensitivity of cancer detection based on true prevalence. *J Natl Cancer Inst* 2007; **99**(19):1484–9.
31. Irani J, Blanchet P, Salomon L, *et al.* Is an extended 20-core prostate biopsy protocol more efficient than the the standard 12-core? A randomized multicenter trial. *J Urol* 2013; **190**(1):77–83.
32. Ashley RA, Inman BA, Routh JC, Mynderse LA, Gettman MT, Blute ML. Reassessing the diagnostic yield of saturation biopsy of the prostate. *Eur Urol* 2008; **53**(5):976–81.
33. Abdollah F, Novara G, Briganti A, *et al.* Trans-rectal versus trans-perineal saturation rebiopsy of the prostate: is there a difference in cancer detection rate? *Urology* 2011; **77**(4):921–5.
34. Moran BJ, Braccioforte MH, Conterato DJ. Re-biopsy of the prostate using a stereotactic transperineal technique. *J Urol* 2006; **176**(4 Pt 1): 1376–81; discussion 1381.
35. Lemaitre L, Puech P, Poncelet E, *et al.* Dynamic contrast-enhanced MRI of anterior prostate cancer: morphometric assessment and correlation with radical prostatectomy findings. *Eur Radiol* 2009; **19**(2):470–80.
36. Kattan MW, Eastham JA, Stapleton AM, Wheeler TM, Scardino PT. A preoperative nomogram for disease recurrence following radical prostatectomy for prostate cancer. *J Natl Cancer Inst* 1998; **90**(10):766–71.
37. Eggener SE, Scardino PT, Walsh PC, *et al.* Predicting 15-year prostate cancer specific mortality after radical prostatectomy. *J Urol* 2011; **185**(3):869–75.
38. Cooperberg MR, Freedland SJ, Pasta DJ, *et al.* Multiinstitutional validation of the UCSF cancer of the prostate risk assessment for prediction of recurrence after radical prostatectomy. *Cancer* 2006; **107**(10):2384–91.
39. Cooperberg MR, Pasta DJ, Elkin EP, *et al.* The University of California, San Francisco Cancer of the Prostate Risk Assessment score: a straightforward and reliable preoperative predictor of disease recurrence after radical prostatectomy. *J Urol* 2005; **173**(6):1938–42.
40. D'Amico AV, Whittington R, Malkowicz SB, *et al.* Clinical utility of percent-positive prostate biopsies in predicting biochemical outcome after radical prostatectomy or external-beam radiation therapy for patients with clinically localized prostate cancer. *Mol Urol* 2000; **4**(3):171–5; discussion 177.
41. Burkhard FC, Schumacher M, Studer UE. The role of lymphadenectomy in prostate cancer. *Nat Clin Pract Urol* 2005; **2**(7):336–42.
42. Janetschek G. Can sentinel pelvic lymph node dissection replace extended pelvic lymph node dissection in patients with prostate cancer? *Nat Clin Pract Urol* 2007; **4**(12):636–7.
43. Weckermann D, Dorn R, Trefz M, Wagner T, Wawroschek F, Harzmann R. Sentinel lymph node dissection for prostate cancer: experience with more than 1,000 patients. *J Urol* 2007; **177**(3):916–20.
44. Mattei A, Fuechsel FG, Bhatta Dhar N, *et al.* The template of the primary lymphatic landing sites of the prostate should be revisited: results of a multimodality mapping study. *Eur Urol* 2008; **53**(1):118–25.
45. Briganti A, Abdollah F, Nini A, *et al.* Performance characteristics of computed tomography in detecting lymph node metastases in contemporary patients with prostate cancer treated with extended pelvic lymph node dissection. *Eur Urol* 2012; **61**(6):1132–8.
46. Danila DC, Fleisher M, Scher HI. Circulating tumor cells as biomarkers in prostate cancer. *Clin Cancer Res* 2011; **17**(12):3903–12.
47. Shukla-Dave A, Hricak H, Akin O, *et al.* Preoperative nomograms incorporating magnetic resonance imaging and spectroscopy for prediction of insignificant prostate cancer. *BJU Int* 2012; **109**(9):1315–22.
48. Ahmed HU, El-Shater Bosaily A, Brown LC, et al. PROMIS study group. Diagnostic accuracy of multi-parametric MRI and TRUS biopsy in prostate cancer (PROMIS): a paired validating confirmatory study. *Lancet*. 2017 Feb 25; **389**(10071):815–822. doi: 10.1016/S0140-6736(16)32401-1.

49. Jager GJ, Severens JL, Thornbury JR, de La Rosette JJ, Ruijs SH, Barentsz JO. Prostate cancer staging: should MR imaging be used?—A decision analytic approach. *Radiology* 2000; **215**(2):445–51.
50. Lee N, Newhouse JH, Olsson CA, *et al.* Which patients with newly diagnosed prostate cancer need a computed tomography scan of the abdomen and pelvis? An analysis based on 588 patients. *Urology* 1999; **54**(3):490–4.
51. Masterson TA,Touijer K. The role of endorectal coil MRI in preoperative staging and decision-making for the treatment of clinically localized prostate cancer. *MAGMA* 2008; **21**(6):371–7.
52. Sala E, Akin O, Moskowitz CS, *et al.* Endorectal MR imaging in the evaluation of seminal vesicle invasion: diagnostic accuracy and multivariate feature analysis. *Radiology* 2006; **238**(3):929–37.
53. Wang L, Mullerad M, Chen HN, *et al.* Prostate cancer: incremental value of endorectal MR imaging findings for prediction of extracapsular extension. *Radiology* 2004; **232**(1):133–9.
54. Wang L, Hricak H, Kattan MW, Chen HN, Scardino PT, Kuroiwa K. Prediction of organ-confined prostate cancer: incremental value of MR imaging and MR spectroscopic imaging to staging nomograms. *Radiology* 2006; **238**(2):597–603.
55. Zakian KL, Sircar K, Hricak H, *et al.* Correlation of proton MR spectroscopic imaging with gleason score based on step-section pathologic analysis after radical prostatectomy. *Radiology* 2005; **234**(3):804–14.
56. Jager GJ, Barentsz JO, Oosterhof GO, Witjes JA, Ruijs SJ. Pelvic adenopathy in prostatic and urinary bladder carcinoma: MR imaging with a three-dimensional TI-weighted magnetization-prepared-rapid gradient-echo sequence. *AJR Am J Roentgenol* 1996; **167**(6):1503–7.
57. Harisinghani MG, Barentsz J, Hahn PF, *et al.* Noninvasive detection of clinically occult lymph-node metastases in prostate cancer. *N Engl J Med* 2003; **348**(25):2491–9.
58. Heesakkers RA, Fütterer JJ, Hövels AM, *et al.* Prostate cancer evaluated with ferumoxtran-10-enhanced T2*-weighted MR Imaging at 1.5 and 3.0 T: early experience. *Radiology* 2006; **239**(2):481–7.
59. Warburg O. On the origin of cancer cells. *Science* 1956; **123**(3191):309–14.
60. Reinicke K, Sotomayor P, Cisterna P, Delgado C, Nualart F, Godoy A. Cellular distribution of Glut-1 and Glut-5 in benign and malignant human prostate tissue. *J Cell Biochem* 2012; **113**(2):553–62.
61. Singh G, Lakkis CL, Laucirica R, Epner DE. Regulation of prostate cancer cell division by glucose. *J Cell Physiol* 1999; **180**(3):431–8.
62. Minamimoto R, Uemura H, Sano F, *et al.* The potential of FDG-PET/CT for detecting prostate cancer in patients with an elevated serum PSA level. *Ann Nucl Med* 2011; **25**(1):21–7.
63. Shiiba M, Ishihara K, Kimura G, *et al.* Evaluation of primary prostate cancer using 11C-methionine-PET/CT and 18F-FDG-PET/CT. *Ann Nucl Med* 2012; **26**(2):138–45.
64. Schöder H, Herrmann K, Gönen M, *et al.* 2-[18F]fluoro-2-deoxyglucose positron emission tomography for the detection of disease in patients with prostate-specific antigen relapse after radical prostatectomy. *Clin Cancer Res* 2005; **11**(13):4761–9.
65. Castellucci P, Jadvar H. PET/CT in prostate cancer: non-choline radiopharmaceuticals. *Q J Nucl Med Mol Imaging* 2012; **56**(4):367–74.
66. Morris MJ, Akhurst T, Larson SM, *et al.* Fluorodeoxyglucose positron emission tomography as an outcome measure for castrate metastatic prostate cancer treated with antimicrotubule chemotherapy. *Clin Cancer Res* 2005; **11**(9):3210–6.
67. Janardhan S, Srivani P, Sastry GN. Choline kinase: an important target for cancer. *Curr Med Chem* 2006; **13**(10):1169–86.
68. Bauman G, Belhocine T, Kovacs M, Ward A, Beheshti M, Rachinsky I. 18F-fluorocholine for prostate cancer imaging: a systematic review of the literature. *Prostate Cancer Prostatic Dis* 2012; **15**(1):45–55.
69. Souvatzoglou M, Weirich G, Schwarzenboeck S, *et al.* The sensitivity of [11C]choline PET/CT to localize prostate cancer depends on the tumor configuration. *Clin Cancer Res* 2011; **17**(11):3751–9.
70. Jadvar H. Molecular imaging of prostate cancer: PET radiotracers. *AJR Am J Roentgenol* 2012; **199**(2):278–91.
71. Subramanian G, McAfee JG. A new complex of 99mTc for skeletal imaging. *Radiology* 1971; **99**(1):192–6.
72. Pollen JJ, Witztum KF, Ashburn WL. The flare phenomenon on radionuclide bone scan in metastatic prostate cancer. *AJR Am J Roentgenol* 1984; **142**(4):773–6.
73. Imbriaco M, Larson SM, Yeung HW, *et al.* A new parameter for measuring metastatic bone involvement by prostate cancer: the Bone Scan Index. *Clin Cancer Res* 1998; **4**(7):1765–72.
74. Sabbatini P, Larson SM, Kremer A, *et al.* Prognostic significance of extent of disease in bone in patients with androgen-independent prostate cancer. *J Clin Oncol* 1999; **17**(3):948–57.
75. Grant FD, Fahey FH, Packard AB, Davis RT, Alavi A, Treves ST. Skeletal PET with 18F-fluoride: applying new technology to an old tracer. *J Nucl Med* 2008; **49**(1):68–78.
76. Segall G, Delbeke D, Stabin MG, *et al.* SNM practice guideline for sodium 18F-fluoride PET/CT bone scans 1.0. *J Nucl Med* 2010; **51**(11):1813–20.
77. Even-Sapir E, Metser U, Mishani E, Lievshitz G, Lerman H, Leibovitch I. The detection of bone metastases in patients with high-risk prostate cancer: 99mTc-MDP Planar bone scintigraphy, single- and multi-field-of-view SPECT, 18F-fluoride PET, and 18F-fluoride PET/CT. *J Nucl Med* 2006; **47**(2):287–97.

CHAPTER 6.7

Prostate cancer

Treatment of localized disease

Matthew Cooperberg and Peter Carroll

Introduction: the avoidable controversy of prostate cancer treatment

With a global incidence of over 900,000 cases per year and over 250,000 deaths annually, prostate cancer is among the most burdensome cancers facing men worldwide. Incidence varies up to 25-fold around the world, reflecting variation in genetics; diet, environmental, and lifestyle factors; access to healthcare overall; and, critically, intensity of prostate-specific antigen (PSA) screening.[1] Epidemiology trends in the United States reveal that since the advent of screening in the early 1990s, the age-adjusted population mortality rate has fallen nearly 50%, a success attributable in large part to screening and aggressive treatment of potentially lethal prostate cancer.[2] The cost of this progress, however, has been high: in the era of screening, prostate cancer has undergone a profound risk migration, such that most men are now diagnosed with low-risk prostate cancers,[3] which would in many cases cause no symptoms or threat to life had they never been detected.[4] Similar trends have been observed in other countries that have also adopted widespread screening.

Thus, many thousands of men have undergone surgery, radiation, and other treatments which likely did not benefit them in terms of quality or quantity of life, and too many of these men suffered long-term side effects of treatment.[5] Such men are said to have been overdiagnosed,[6] and then overtreated. The overdiagnosis and overtreatment of low-risk prostate cancer is felt by many to have reached epidemic proportions, to the point that prominent primary care organizations, including the influential US Preventive Services Task Force, are now recommending *against* PSA-based screening.[7] These recommendations are highly controversial, and if broadly adopted would have a substantial, adverse impact on prostate cancer morbidity and mortality. However, they highlight the shrinking patience on the part of primary care providers and policymakers for the avoidable morbidity and costs associated with overtreatment of low-risk prostate cancer.

Fortunately, this controversy can be largely solved, and the solution, while not necessarily *easy*, is relatively straightforward. Both screening and treatment can—and must—be done better. Screening efforts should focus on younger men with long life expectancy and those at higher risk for diagnosis.[8] Screening practices should reflect the desire to reduce prostate cancer mortality while minimizing the risks of overdiagnosis. Even more importantly, treatment must be focused on men at risk of prostate cancer mortality, and intensity of treatment should be matched appropriately to disease risk. Men with low-risk disease do not benefit from treatment, at least immediately after diagnosis,[9] and should be considered for active surveillance.[10] Conversely, those with higher-risk disease clearly benefit from local therapy,[9] even some who are older at time of diagnosis.[11,12] Treatments should be applied to minimize risks of adverse side effects, and in an era of constrained resources in many healthcare systems worldwide, must reflect consideration of costs. This chapter will describe approaches to patient risk stratification for initial management, and will introduce key aspects of the major primary treatment alternatives.

Prostate cancer presentation and risk stratification

Symptoms

In a screened population, the vast majority of prostate cancers are localized and asymptomatic at diagnosis.[3] However, prostate cancer which progresses, with or without prior treatment, can cause both local and distant symptoms. Local extension can produce both obstructive and irritative lower urinary tract symptoms (LUTS), due to growth of the tumour into the urethra, bladder neck, or trigone. It is important to note, however, that given the very high epidemiologic overlap between prostate cancer and benign prostatic hyperplasia (BPH), LUTS among men with clinically localized prostate cancer are much more likely attributable to BPH than to cancer. Local extension into both ureters can also produce symptoms of azotaemia. Metastatic prostate cancer spreads most commonly to the bones; bone metastases may cause pain and vulnerability to pathologic fracture. Metastases to the spinal column can also impinge on the spinal cord, causing symptoms of cord compression, including paraesthesia and weakness of the lower extremities, and urinary and/or faecal incontinence.

Signs

Digital rectal examination (DRE) may reveal induration or nodularity; in some cases gross extraprostatic extension may be detectable by DRE, particularly if there is effacement of the sulci lateral to the prostate on either side. Extensive regional lymphadenopathy, which is uncommon, may lead to lymphedema of the legs. Specific signs of cord compression depend on the level of the compression, potentially including weakness or spasticity of the legs, and a hyperreflexic bulbocavernosus reflex.

Laboratory and radiographic findings

The vast majority of prostate cancers are associated with an elevated PSA level, though some rare, poorly differentiated histologic subtypes produce little PSA. Some such tumours display neuroendocrine differentiation and may cause elevated serum levels of chromogranin A. Malignant obstruction of into one or both ureters may lead to elevated blood urea nitrogen and/or creatinine, and bone metastases may elevate alkaline phosphatase levels. Metastatic disease is also associated with anaemia and elevated lactate dehydrogenase.

Most prostate cancers in contemporary practice are diagnosed by transrectal ultrasound (TRUS)-guided biopsy. Though biopsies are usually performed on an 8- to 14-core mapped template intended to sample the whole gland, in some cases tumours are visible on TRUS as hypoechoic lesions; power Doppler examination may demonstrate hypervascularity. Extracapsular extension and/or seminal vesicle invasion can also be identified on TRUS, but accuracy of both diagnosis and staging are highly operator-dependent.

Men with low-risk tumour characteristics do not require further staging,[13] though unnecessary imaging tests are still very common in the United States[14–17]; indeed these cause so much avoidable ongoing cost and radiation exposure that *not* performing a bone scan for low-risk prostate cancer is now identified as a measure of high-quality care in the United States.[18] Higher-risk prostate cancer, on the other hand, does require an evaluation to rule out metastatic disease before local therapy is undertaken.

99-Technitium bone scintigraphy is the most common test to evaluate for skeletal metastases; some centres are now employing 18-fluoride-tagged sodium fluoride positron emission tomography together with computerized tomography (PET/CT) to improve sensitivity and detection of smaller metastases.[19] Full-body magnetic resonance imaging (MRI) has been studied as well with promising initial results, primarily in European countries where costs for this technology are lower.[20] Soft-tissue imaging, focusing in particular on lymphadenopathy, is typically performed via contrast-enhanced CT. Multiparametric pelvic MRI including diffusion-weighted and dynamic contrast sequences, together with spectroscopic imaging in some centres, can also evaluate lymph nodes, and provides better local staging of the prostate than CT.[21] Other PET tracers, including 13-carbon-tagged choline and acetate, also show promise for improved distant staging over conventional CT.[19]

Risk stratification

The suggestion that low-risk, indolent prostate cancers cannot be distinguished from high-risk, potentially lethal ones is an often-repeated calumny used to justify blanket recommendations against prostate cancer screening.[7] The simple truth is that prostate cancers can be risk-stratified with good accuracy using data available today in contemporary practice[22]—and that accuracy will improve further with emerging imaging tests and biomarkers. The problem is that while prostate cancer treatment *can* be targeted to tumour risk to minimize both over and undertreatment, in the reality of contemporary practice, treatment is *not* appropriately risk-adapted, but rather is inappropriately driven by age, financial, and legal incentives, and other non-clinical factors.[11,23]

Risk factors

Prostate-specific antigen

While the use of PSA as a screening test for prostate cancer is controversial, its use as a measure of cancer risk is not. With the exception of rare tumours that, as noted above, produce little PSA, PSA increases consistently with prostate cancer volume, stage, and aggressiveness. PSA is a key parameter in every multivariable risk stratification system, and is a key driver of decision-making for both staging and therapeutic intervention. PSA also forms the core of post-treatment monitoring protocols following virtually all treatments.

Grade

Prostate cancer is graded using the Gleason system, which assesses the histopathological architecture of the tumour glands under low-power microscopy. Historically, prostate cancer was graded on a 1 to 5 scale, with higher numbers indicating greater degrees of glandular fusion and abnormality. Under consensus guidelines adopted in 2005, however, patterns 1 and 2 are rarely assigned, especially for biopsy tissue. Thus, Gleason pattern 3 corresponds with low-grade disease (variable-sized glands that intercalate between normal-appearing glands); Gleason pattern 4 with intermediate grade (incompletely formed glands with variable amounts of fusion and a more infiltrative growth pattern), and Gleason pattern 5 with high grade (individually infiltrating cells with no gland formation) (Fig. 6.7.1).[24]

Pathologists assign a primary grade to the predominant pattern of cancer and a secondary grade to the second most commonly observed pattern in the specimen. If all the cancer is consistent with one pattern present, then both the primary and secondary grade are reported as the same (e.g. 3+3). The Gleason score or Gleason sum is obtained by adding the primary and secondary grades together. Thus, a Gleason score 6 (3+3) tumour is uniformly low grade. In risk stratifying intermediate- and high-grade tumours, the *primary* Gleason pattern is the more important driver of biologic risk: among Gleason score 7 tumours, Gleason 4+3 are more aggressive than Gleason 3+4 tumours. Many series do not distinguish between these two distinct grades (4+3 vs. 3+4); interpretation of such series must be guarded. A minor pattern may be noted as a tertiary score; when tertiary pattern 5 is noted (e.g. 3+4+5), the prognosis is worse. Recent analyses have suggested that improved information may be gained from the histology by *quantifying* the proportion of cancer that is high grade; tumours with 5% and 45% pattern 4 might both be assigned Gleason score 3+4, but the latter is more likely to demonstrate aggressive biology.[25]

Stage and other measures of tumour extent

Prostate cancer is staged using the American Joint Committee on Cancer (AJCC) TNM system (Box 6.7.1), with substages designated based on the local tumour extent (T-stage), lymph node involvement (N stage), and distant metastases (M stage). The staging system applies to both *clinical stage*, based on physical exam and imaging findings, and *pathologic stage*, determined after prostatectomy and/or lymphadenectomy—with the exception that T1 is only assigned in clinical staging; T2 is the lowest pathologic T-stage. It should be emphasized that assignment of clinical T-stage incorporates results of the DRE and TRUS, but not the results of the biopsy. Thus, if a patient has a palpable nodule on one side of the prostate and a biopsy demonstrating bilateral disease, his clinical

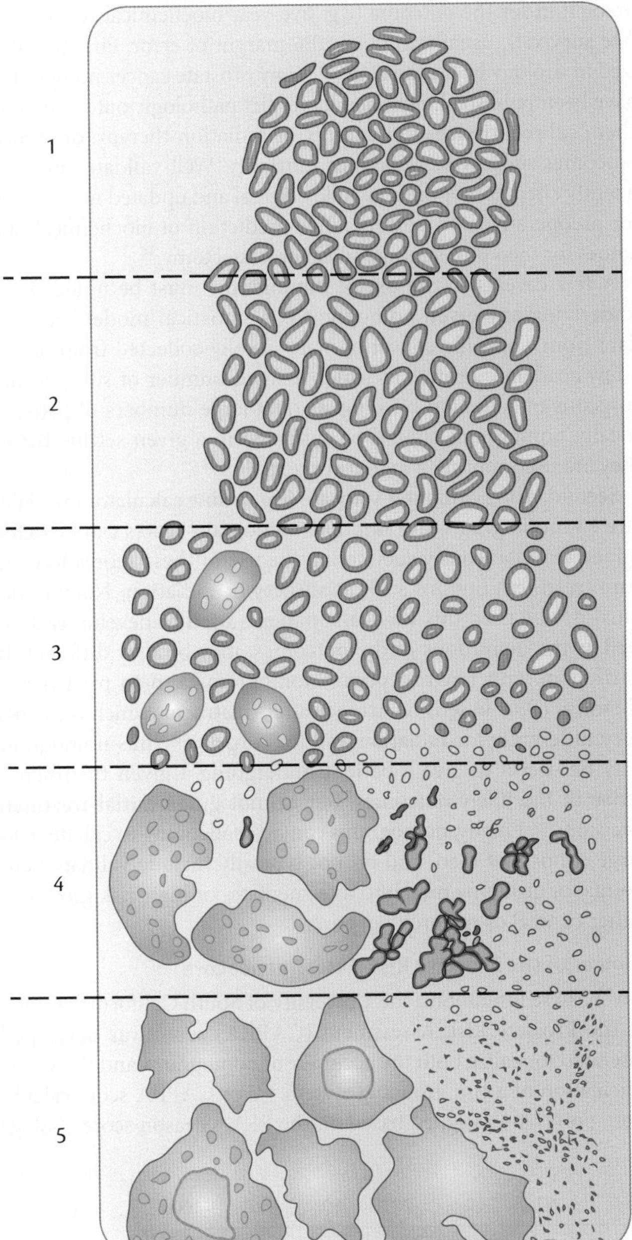

Fig. 6.7.1 Gleason grading system.
Reproduced with permission from Lippincott Williams and Wilkins/Wolters Kluwer Health: Epstein JI *et al.*, 'The 2005 International Society of Urological Pathology (ISUP) Consensus Conference on Gleason Grading of Prostatic Carcinoma', *The American Journal of Surgical Pathology*, Volume 29, Issue 9, pp. 1228–42, Copyright © 2005 Wolters Kluwer Health.

Box 6.7.1 TNM staging system for prostate cancer

TNM Staging System for Prostate Cancer
T Primary tumour
Tx Cannot be assessed
T0 No evidence of primary tumour
Tis Carcinoma *in situ* (PIN)
T1a ≤5% of tissue in resection for benign disease has cancer, normal DRE
T1b >5% of tissue in resection for benign disease has cancer, normal DRE
T1c Detected from elevated PSA alone, normal DRE, and imaging
T2a Tumour palpable by DRE or visible by imaging, involving less than half of one lobe of the prostate
T2b Tumour palpable by DRE or visible by imaging, involving more than half of one lobe of the prostate
T2c Tumour palpable by DRE or visible by imaging, involving both lobes of the prostate
T3a Extracapsular extension on one or both sides
T3b Seminal vesicle involvement on one or both sides
T4 Tumour directly extends into bladder neck, sphincter, rectum, levator muscles, or into pelvic sidewall
N—Regional lymph nodes (obturator, internal iliac, external iliac, presacral lymph nodes)
Nx Cannot be assessed
N0 No regional lymph node metastasis
N1 Metastasis in a regional lymph node or nodes
M—Distant metastasis
Mx Cannot be assessed
M0 No distant metastasis
M1a Distant metastasis in nonregional lymph nodes
M1b Distant metastasis to bone
M1c Distant metastasis to other sites
DRE, digital rectal examination; PIN, prostatic intraepithelial neoplasia; PSA, prostate-specific antigen; TRUS, transrectal ultrasound.

Used with the permission of the American Joint Committee on Cancer (AJCC), Chicago, Illinois. The original source for this material is the *AJCC Cancer Staging Manual, Seventh Edition* (2010) published by Springer Science and Business Media LLC, www.springer.com

stage remains T2a. If a patient has a normal DRE, with TRUS demonstrating a unilateral lesion and a biopsy positive for cancer, his clinical stage is also T2a (using results of DRE and TRUS). These rules are frequently misapplied in clinical practice as clinicians commonly assign stage based on biopsy.[26]

Compared to Gleason score and PSA levels, clinical T-stage in prostate cancer is a relatively weak prognostic factor, in part due to the subjectivity of both DRE and TRUS interpretation. A better estimation of tumour volume or extent can often be gained through assessment of biopsy core involvement, expressed alternatively as the number of biopsy cores positive, percent of cores positive, or percent of overall tissue positive for cancer. Given adjustment for these more objective measures of tumour volume, T-stage often drops out of multivariable models of prostate cancer prognosis, at least among clinically localized (T1-2) tumours.[27]

Multivariable risk assessment

No single parameter fully captures the risk of prostate cancer progression; rather, optimal risk stratification entails consideration of multiple parameters to generate an overall assessment of risk. Over 100 risk formulae, lookup tables, nomograms, and other instruments have been published toward this end; however, most have not been validated, and others suffer lack of discrimination, calibration, applicability, or other test characteristics.[22,28] Selected, widely described instruments are described below.

Risk groups

One of the first published approaches to risk stratification is a three-level risk group classification devised by D'Amico *et al.*[29] and formally endorsed by practice guidelines both in the US and in Europe.[30,31] In this classification, men are stratified across three groups as follows:

- *Low-risk*: PSA ≤10, Gleason ≤6, and clinical stage T1 or T2a
- *Intermediate-risk*: PSA 10–20, Gleason 7, or clinical stage T2b (sometimes modified to include T2c as well)
- *High-risk*: PSA >20, Gleason 8–10, or clinical stage T2c or T3a (sometimes modified to include T3a only)

The major advantage to this system is its simplicity, and it is used very commonly. However, it has significant drawbacks. First, it overweights T-stage which, as noted above, is not an accurate measure of tumour extent within the T1-2 category. Second, it does not differentiate Gleason 3+4 from 4+3 tumours which (also noted above) behave differently within the Gleason 7 category. Finally, the risk groups do not truly constitute a multivariable system in that they do not actually combine information from the various risk variables. A PSA 17, Gleason 4+3, stage T2b cancer and a PSA 3.4, Gleason 3+4, stage T1c cancer are both grouped in the 'intermediate risk' group, but would likely exhibit clearly divergent biological aggressiveness.[32]

Lookup tables and nomograms

Most multivariable risk instruments are derived multivariable logistic regression or Cox proportional hazards models, depending on the outcome of interest. For example, the well-validated tables first published by Partin *et al.* predict pathologic end points such as extracapsular extension and seminal vesicle invasion.[33] The term *nomogram* is frequently used synonymously to describe a risk model or predictive instrument. In fact, a nomogram is simply a graphical representation of a regression model, and is a visually accessible alternative to look up tables or computer software. To use a nomogram, a patient is assigned a number of points for each risk factor based on linear scales (Fig. 6.7.2); these are then summed to yield a prediction for the outcome (e.g. five-year biochemical recurrence-free survival), usually with a ±10% margin of error. First popularized in urology by Kattan *et al.*,[34] many prostate cancer nomograms have been published, intended to predict pathologic outcomes, biochemical recurrence after surgery or radiation therapy, or clinical outcomes such as metastasis or mortality. Well-validated and frequently cited nomograms include original and updated nomograms for preoperative and postoperative prediction of biochemical outcomes for men undergoing radical prostatectomy.[34–37]

A few caveats to the use of nomograms must be noted. First, underlying any given nomogram is a statistical model based on data from a specific cohort of men, usually collected from one or a few academic centres in which a small number of subspecialist surgeons or radiation oncologists treat large numbers of patients. Ideally nomograms should be validated in a given setting before they are used routinely in that context.[32,38,39]

Second, using computer software (e.g. online calculators available at www.nomograms.org) multiple nomogram scores can be determined simultaneously, facilitating the use of these scores to compare treatment options such as surgery or radiation. Nomograms must not be used this way—the patients used to develop each, as well as the definitions of the outcomes, may be very different. In particular, with few exceptions nomograms aim to predict biochemical (PSA-based) recurrence after treatment, which is defined very differently for radiation and for surgery.[40] Thus nomograms may be useful to give a patient undergoing a given treatment a sense of the likely outcomes, but cannot guide initial treatment decisions.[32] Finally, nomograms can be challenging to calculate for large cohorts of men, and do not typically include validated cut-points for grouping men into intermediate- or high-risk groups for either clinical or research purposes.

Cancer of the Prostate Risk Assessment score

Given these limitations, the University of South California's Cancer of the Prostate Risk Assessment (CAPRA) score was developed, intended to realize both the accuracy of nomograms and the simple calculation of a risk grouping system.[41] For CAPRA score calculation, points are assigned based on the PSA, Gleason score, T-stage,

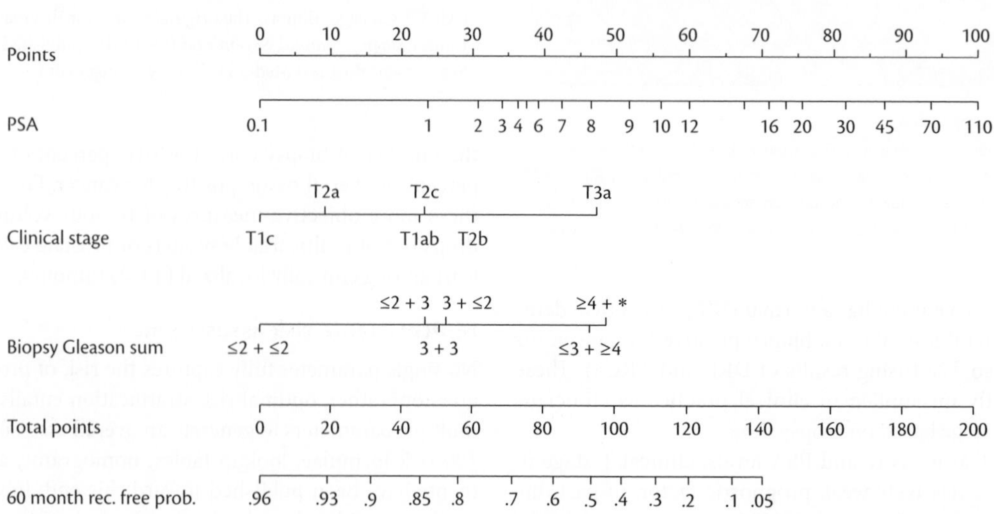

Fig. 6.7.2 Nomogram for prediction of biochemical recurrence after surgery.

Reproduced from Michael W. Kattan *et al.*, 'A Preoperative Nomogram for Disease Recurrence Following Radical Prostatectomy for Prostate Cancer', ***Journal of the National Cancer Institute***, Volume 90, Issue 10, pp. 766–71, Copyright © 2008 Oxford University Press, by permission of Oxford University Press.

Variable	Level	Points	Variable	Level	Points
PSA	≤6	0	T-stage	T1/T2	0
	6.1–10	1		T3a	1
	10.1–20	2			
	20.1–30	3	% of biopsy cores positive	<34%	0
	>30	4		≥34%	1
Gleason (primary/secondary)	1-3/1-3	0			
	1-3/4-5	1	Age	<50	0
	4-5/1-5	3		≥50	1

Fig. 6.7.3 Cancer of the Prostate Risk Assessment (CAPRA) score.
Adapted from *The Journal of Urology*, Volume 173, Issue 6, Cooperberg MR, *et al.*, The University of California, San Francisco Cancer of the Prostate Risk Assessment Score: A straightforward and reliable preoperative predictor of disease recurrence after radical prostatectomy, pp. 1938–42, Copyright © 2005 American Urological Association, with permission from Elsevier, http://www.sciencedirect.com/science/journal/00225347

per cent of biopsy cores positive, and age at diagnosis (Fig. 6.7.3). Points are added to generate a 0–10 score, with every two-point increase in score (e.g. from 1 to 3 or from 4 to 6) indicating roughly a doubling of risk. CAPRA scores in the 0–2 range correspond to relatively low-risk disease, CAPRA 3–5 tumours to intermediate risk, and CAPRA 6–10 tumours to high risk. The CAPRA score has been widely validated in multiple clinical settings on four continents, and in at least one study demonstrated superior accuracy compared to competing instruments in an independent head-to-head study.[42] The score has been shown to predict metastasis and mortality following surgery, radiation therapy, and hormonal therapy.[32,43]

Treatment options for localized prostate cancer

Treatment alternatives for localized prostate cancer endorsed by various international guidelines include active surveillance, radical prostatectomy, and radiation therapy.[30,31,44] As described above, intensity of treatment should be risk-adapted: most men with low-risk prostate cancer are candidates for at least a trial of active surveillance. Those with intermediate-risk disease are eligible for surgery or radiation monotherapy, and men with high-risk cancers often require multimodal therapy—either prostatectomy followed selectively by radiation depending on pathology and early biochemical outcomes, or combination radiation therapy with androgen deprivation therapy (ADT). Indeed, evolving evidence clearly supports a role for aggressive local therapy in the management of high-risk prostate cancer.[9,45–48] Western (as opposed to Asian) guidelines do not endorse ADT monotherapy as an alternative to surgery or radiation for localized disease because survival outcomes are inferior.[45] Likewise, cryotherapy, high-intensity focused ultrasound (HIFU), and other ablative treatments have not become standard options because they have not been shown clearly to yield better oncologic or quality of life (QoL) outcomes.

Active surveillance

As described above, a very substantial proportion of prostate cancers detected through screening efforts demonstrate indolent behaviour, and would never progress within the patient's lifetime without treatment. Studies on men with low-grade prostate cancer who never received surgery or radiation demonstrated that the vast majority die of other causes rather than prostate cancer.[12] The Prostate Intervention Versus Observation Trial (PIVOT) randomized men between surgery and conservative management, and found no benefit for surgery *for men with low-risk disease* within 10 years of diagnosis.[9] However, a subset of tumours which appeared to be low risk based on biopsy ultimately proved to be more aggressive, either due to undersampling on the original biopsy or to actual biological progression.

Therefore, men with apparently low-risk disease cannot be simply advised to ignore the diagnosis; rather, they are increasingly recognized to be good candidates for *active surveillance*, a protocol of observation under which men undergo periodic PSA tests and repeat biopsies, with intervention with intent to cure at first sign of progression.[10,49] Active surveillance is notably distinct from *watchful waiting*, a more passive strategy under which older men and/or those with significant co-morbidity are not followed regularly for prostate cancer, and are offered hormonal therapy for palliation if the cancer progresses to a symptomatic stage.

Eligibility criteria for active surveillance vary from one clinical centre to another, but generally include low PSA and/or PSA density (PSA divided by prostate volume in mL), low grade (Gleason 3+3, and in some cases Gleason 3+4), and low tumour volume as assessed by clinical stage and extent of biopsy core involvement. Progression is defined by rapid PSA rise, by increase in grade and/or tumour volume on repeat biopsy, or by treatment for any other reason. Between 20% and 46% of men on surveillance regimens may require treatment within five years of diagnosis. Thus in many cases active surveillance implies delayed rather than avoided treatment. Active surveillance is not without risks. Prostate biopsy is associated with a known risk of undersampling—that is, the likelihood that what looks like a low-grade, low-stage tumour on biopsy in fact is more aggressive. Aside from the risk of disease progression to an incurable stage during an internal of observation, serial biopsies are associated with low but rising risks of sepsis due to the spread of antibiotic resistant bacteria among community-dwelling men.[50]

Active surveillance is generally recognized to be underutilized as initial management for prostate cancer.[23,49] Aside from financial, legal, and other social pressures favouring treatment over surveillance, anxiety with respect to the possibility of disease progression tends to drive providers and patients to opt for early treatment.[51] Despite ongoing challenges in defining appropriate end points for research involving men on surveillance,[52–54] improved imaging tests such as multiparametric MRI and emerging biomarkers based on tissue, urine, and blood offer great hope for improved patient selection for both immediate and deferred treatment.[55]

Surgery

Radical prostatectomy includes removal of the prostate and seminal vesicles and anastomosis of the bladder neck to the membranous urethra. Pelvic lymphadenectomy may be performed concurrently with surgery for intermediate- and high-risk disease for improved staging. Open approaches to the procedure include retropubic (extraperitoneal) or perineal incisions. Laparoscopic radical prostatectomy can be accomplished via transperitoneal or extraperitoneal approaches, with or without the assistance of a surgical robot. The robot-assisted transperitoneal laparoscopic approach has become the most common approach to prostatectomy in the United States and is gaining in popularity in other countries.

Surgery is well-established by multiple randomized trials to offer a survival advantage over observation for men with intermediate- to high-risk prostate cancer, although not for low-risk disease.[9,56] Randomized trials comparing surgery to radiation have not been reported, but multiple carefully controlled cohort studies have suggested a survival benefit for surgery in favour of external beam radiation, especially for men with higher-risk disease.[23,47,57] Oncologic surveillance after surgery is relatively straightforward: in the absence of a prostate gland, the PSA should be undetectable within six to eight weeks after surgery, and detectable PSA indicates persistent benign or malignant prostate cells. Many labs now use ultrasensitive PSA assays with detection thresholds well under 0.1 ng/mL. Minimally detectable PSAs in the ultrasensitive range sometimes suggest persistence of benign prostate glands, and do not consistently predict further PSA rise.[58] On the other hand, rising PSAs in the setting of adverse pathology is highly suggestive of persistent disease, which may benefit from adjuvant or early salvage radiation therapy.[59,60] The natural history of recurrence after surgery is variable, and reflects factors such as the Gleason score and the PSA kinetics at time of recurrence.[61]

Aside from cancer cure, the principal goals of surgery are preservation of urinary and sexual function. The drivers of both urinary and sexual function outcomes are multifactorial, but are heavily influenced by technical factors during surgery—specifically, preservation of the external urinary sphincter and cavernous neurovascular bundles. The primary impact of surgery on urinary function is induction of at least temporary stress urinary incontinence (i.e. leakage with Valsalva manoeuvres). Continence tends to improve in the weeks and months after surgery up to at least one year, and can be improved with pelvic floor strengthening exercises (Kegel exercises). The likelihood of eventual recovery of continence varies greatly with surgeon skill and experience, and with patient factors such as age and co-morbidity—as well as with the specific definition of continence used. Of note, given high rates of concomitant BPH, many men with prostate cancer have baseline obstructive voiding symptoms (weak stream, hesitancy, and so on); these symptoms often improve after prostatectomy, whether or not continence is completely recovered.

Penile erections decline almost universally in the first months after surgery, then recover over a period lasting up to two years. Likelihood of erectile function recovery is driven by patient age, baseline sexual function, and extent and quality of neurovascular bundle preservation. Early use of phosphodiesterase-5 inhibitors (sildenafil, tadalafil, and so on) and other interventions to maximize penile blood flow (such as vacuum devices)—so-called 'penile rehabilitation'—may improve likelihood of eventual functional recovery. In terms of other aspects of sexual functioning after surgery, somatic sensory nerve function is not typically altered. Orgasm capacity may be preserved with or without erection recovery after surgery, but anejaculation is universal because the sources of seminal plasma (prostate and seminal vesicles) are removed.

Compared to open surgery, robot-assisted prostatectomy is associated with reduced blood loss and length of stay, fewer short-term complications, lower perioperative mortality, and comparable oncologic outcomes.[62–64] Perioperative mortality rates are 0.1% or less after both open and robot-assisted surgery in contemporary practice.[63] Differences in urinary and sexual outcomes are more controversial. Many papers from high-volume centres have shown improved outcomes for robot-assisted surgery over open surgery.[65,66] Population-based studies have not confirmed these results.[67] Possible explanations include low average surgical volumes and a long learning curve for prostatectomy,[68] as well as falsely high expectations (driven both by misleading advertising and by inherent cultural faith in technology) leading to decreased satisfaction and increased regret at any given level of objective functional recovery.[69–71]

Radiation therapy

The intent of radiation therapy for prostate cancer is irreversible damage to the cancer, and to the rest of the prostate gland. Most prostate radiation is delivered using photons administered either from sources external to the body (external beam radiotherapy, or EBRT), or from sources implanted, either permanently or temporarily, into the prostate gland (brachytherapy). Compared to surgery, radiation causes less stress urinary incontinence, but more irritative and/or obstructive urinary symptoms, and more gastrointestinal (GI) toxicity.[5,72,73] Radiation causes less early erectile dysfunction than surgery, but these differences attenuate with long-term follow-up.[74,75] Uncommon long-term complications include haemorrhagic cystitis, urethral stricture, rectourinary fistula, and secondary bladder or rectal cancer.[76] The rate of lethal complications is similar to the rate of perioperative mortality after surgery.[77]

Because the cytotoxic effects of radiation to prostate cancer cells may take years to accumulate, PSA levels fall more slowly than they do after surgery, and identifying persistent or recurrent disease can be difficult. Many definitions of recurrence after radiation have been proposed[78]; the most commonly accepted and cited ones are the 'ASTRO definition'—three consecutive rises in the PSA over the postradiation nadir, with the date of recurrence backdated to the midpoint of the first two rises—and more the 'Phoenix definition'—a rise in the PSA by 2 ng/mL over the nadir, with no backdating. The definition only allows reporting of outcomes at n-2 years if n is the median years of follow-up.[79]

The Phoenix definition, which has become the most commonly referenced standard, was chosen as the best surrogate for subsequent clinical progression and survival, not to identify all persistent cancer. This definition, like the older ASTRO definition, can be used to counsel patients and to compare outcomes across radiation series. However, given the different biologic effects of surgery and radiation on prostate cancer and the different intent of the definitions used to identify recurrence after surgery and radiation, biochemical (PSA-based) recurrence *cannot* be used as a valid surrogate end point for comparing of oncologic outcomes between surgery and radiation,[40] a very common error in comparative effectiveness research in prostate cancer.

External beam radiotherapy

Historically, EBRT was administered to a rectangular field based on bony landmarks using plain radiography or conventional tomography. More however, standard of care has involved three-dimensional pre-radiation planning using CT to reduce damage to surrounding tissues, allowing higher doses to be administered.[80] In the United States, the vast majority of EBRT is now administered as intensity-modulation radiation therapy (IMRT),[81] in which the intensity of the radiation beam can be varied as the radiation source is moved around the patient, allowing further increase in targeting precision. Compared to 3D conformal, non-intensity modulated EBRT, IMRT is associated with reduced GI toxicity but at the possible expense of greater urinary toxicity and/or more erectile dysfunction.[81,82]

IMRT is typically given to a dose of 72–80 Gy, and is administered over 40 or more treatment sessions spread over seven to nine weeks. Motion of the prostate can be substantial from day to day, depending on variables such as rectal fullness. Placement of radio-opaque fiducial markers or targeting beacons before starting treatment can help clinicians compensate for such variation. In general, higher-dose radiation is associated with lower rates of PSA recurrence, but has not been proven to improve long-term survival, and does come at the cost of greater GI toxicity.[83]

Radiation fields can also be planned to include the pelvic lymph nodes in cases of higher risk disease. Multiple randomized, controlled trials have also shown a clear mortality benefit for giving neoadjuvant ADT together with EBRT for intermediate- and high-risk disease.[77,84] The duration of neoadjuvant ADT varies from 4 to 36 months. ADT causes additional side effects—including hot flashes, fatigue, loss of muscle and bone mass, cognitive changes, and adverse effects on metabolism—and the optimal duration of therapy has not been well-established.

Many radiation oncologists now offer EBRT alternatives to typical IMRT, including stereotactic body radiation therapy (SBRT) and proton beam therapy. SBRT entails very frequent re-imaging of the prostate during each treatment session, with the radiation beam constantly adjusted to compensate for even minor target motion. SBRT thus allows higher doses to be given during each session, and therefore far fewer treatment sessions. As yet, there exist few long-term data comparing SBRT to IMRT or other radiation treatments.

Proton beam therapy has the theoretical advantage over other photon-based EBRT in that rather than passing through tissue, the protons stop at the target, thus minimizing the 'exit dose' to surrounding tissues. Proton beam therapy is extraordinarily expensive, extremely highly compensated, and aggressively marketed.[85] However, no clinical study to date has shown any clinical benefit, in terms of either cancer control or improved QoL. Indeed, a Medicare study found 25% *greater* rectal toxicity following proton beam therapy compared to IMRT,[81] and other analyses have questioned whether this approach could ever be cost-effective even when better clinical outcomes were theoretically demonstrable.[86]

Brachytherapy

Most brachytherapy is given via transperineal placement of radioactive iodine-125 or palladium-103 seeds, which remain indefinitely in the prostate even after they have expended their radiation. In *high dose rate* (HDR) brachytherapy, catheters are temporarily placed into the prostate, again using a transperineal approach, and a highly radioactive iridium-192 source is moved in and out of the catheters under robotic control, typically over a series of four treatments. Both types of brachytherapy generally require a regional or general anaesthetic. This is an outpatient procedure, though HDR sometimes entails an overnight stay to complete the set of treatments.

Relatively few studies have compared brachytherapy and EBRT directly. Both short- and long-term oncologic outcomes generally favour brachytherapy.[57,87,88] In terms of side effects, brachytherapy generally causes less GI toxicity but more urinary morbidity than IMRT.[89] Unlike EBRT, brachytherapy cannot be used to administer radiation to lymph nodes; therefore, for higher-risk cases brachytherapy is often combined with EBRT and/or ADT. Some studies have demonstrated improved oncologic outcomes for this combination over EBRT alone,[90] though at the cost of greater QoL impact.[91] Unlike the case with EBRT, ADT does not appear to improve the oncologic outcomes of men treated with brachytherapy. In some cases of BPH together with prostate cancer, however, ADT is used to shrink the prostate to facilitate the technical placement of the seeds. This combination does tend to cause more sexual dysfunction than brachytherapy alone.[91,92]

Ablative treatments

Cryosurgery—the ablation of tissue by local induction of extremely cold temperatures—is a relatively uncommon primary treatment for localized CaP,[23] although its use as a salvage option has increased as the technology has improved over the past several years.[93] Cryotherapy is performed under general or regional anaesthesia. Multiple probes are placed percutaneously under TRUS guidance, and using argon gas, an iceball is created covering the prostate, and two freeze-thaw cycles are typically used. Repeat freezing creates a larger tissue destruction area and theoretically brings the iceball edge and destruction zone edge closer together. The temperature at the edge of the iceball is 0°C to -2°C, while cell destruction requires -25°C to -50°C. Tissue destruction occurs a few millimetres inside the visible iceball edge and cannot be monitored precisely by ultrasound. Thermocouples therefore help monitor real-time temperatures. A urethral warming catheter is typically used to prevent urethral damage.

With contemporary cryotherapy technology, rates of incontinence, urethral sloughing, and rectal injury are low. Rates of biochemical control are comparable to those seen with other treatments (though similar controversies as those discussed above exist regarding optimal definitions of recurrence).[94,95] However, rates of erectile dysfunction are quite high, and generally compare unfavourably to rates achievable with contemporary radiation or nerve-sparing surgery.[95] This is a primary reason that cryotherapy remains a relatively uncommon treatment for newly diagnosed prostate cancer. Some centres are investigating focal or subtotal cryoablation of the prostate—initial studies reported promising findings, but this approach remains investigational.[96]

A wide variety of other energy-based ablative technologies has been applied to treatment of prostate cancer. Among these, the most widely used is HIFU, which is administered transrectally and induces coagulative necrosis of benign and malignant prostate tissue. The technology has some enthusiastic proponents, especially in continental Europe. However, outcomes in prospective series are mixed at best. The technology has never been approved in the United States. Two large centres in the United Kingdom ended their HIFU programmes due to poor outcomes,[97] and the UK health system does not recommend HIFU outside the context of a clinical trial. A Canadian systematic review likewise concluded that the data in support of HIFU are weak and the treatment should not be given outside of prospective trials.[98] Like cryotherapy, HIFU is being explored for focal therapy of prostate cancer,[99] but with short follow-up on small numbers of patients reported to date, this approach is very much experimental.

Comparative effectiveness

The comparative effectiveness of various treatment alternatives for localized prostate cancer remains the subject of significant on-going debate. No randomized, controlled trials including both primary surgery and primary radiation therapy patients have been completed, though one, the UK's ProtecT trial, has completed accrual.[100] This randomized clinical trial compared the treatment effectiveness of active monitoring (a surveillance programme), radical prostatectomy and external beam radiotherapy with neoadjuvant androgen deprivation therapy, and patient reported outcomes in a cohort of 1643 men with clinically localized prostate cancer detected by PSA testing in the United Kingdom. The results at 10-year median follow-up were published recently, showing a very low disease specific mortality with no differences between the three arms (around 1%). However, the study also demonstrated that radical treatments halved the rate of disease progression, while 80% of patients on active monitoring remained disease free and avoided treatment side effects. Patient reported outcomes showed different patterns of adverse event profiles for each treatment, with urinary and sexual function side-effects experienced mostly in men receiving surgery, and bowel symptoms after radiation, with some recovery over time. Similar side-effect profiles where demonstrated by two more recent large prospective observational studies from the US, consistent with findings of the ProtecT trial.[101–104] Cost-effectiveness studies, accounting for both oncologic and health-related quality of life (HRQoL) outcomes, generally have found that differences in effectiveness across treatments generally are not large, and that for low-risk disease active surveillance is often favoured over any local therapy.[105,106] However, costs vary substantially, particularly in the US system, with EBRT—IMRT in particular—accounting for substantially increased costs over surgery or brachytherapy.[106–108]

Varying financial and other incentives, limited high-quality comparative data, and resulting ambivalent guidelines all combine to yield very high regional and local variation in practice patterns.[23,109,110] Prostate cancer management is preference-sensitive—reflecting personal beliefs and preferences of clinicians and patients in the absence of clear data—and supply-sensitive—with utilization of some interventions correlating with extent of availability of those services.[110] Too much emphasis has been placed in years on technological innovation rather than appropriateness of care and universal outcomes assessment. Until this situation improves, overtreatment of low-risk prostate tumours and undertreatment of high-risk prostate cancer will continue to affect too many diagnosed with the disease, and to dilute the otherwise highly beneficial impact of well-intentioned screening and early detection protocols on the global burden of prostate cancer.

Further reading

Bill-Axelson A, Holmberg L, Ruutu M, *et al.* Radical prostatectomy versus watchful waiting in early prostate cancer. *N Engl J Med* 2011; **364**(18):1708–17.

Cooperberg MR, Broering JM, Carroll PR. Risk assessment for prostate cancer metastasis and mortality at the time of diagnosis. *J Natl Cancer Inst* 2009; **101**(12):878–87.

Cooperberg MR, Broering JM, Carroll PR. Time trends and local variation in primary treatment of localized prostate cancer. *J Clin Oncol* 2010; **28**:1117–23.

Cooperberg MR, Ramakrishna NR, Duff SB, *et al.* Primary treatments for clinically localized prostate cancer: a comprehensive lifetime cost-utility analysis. *BJU Int* 2013; **111**:437–50.

Freedland SJ, Humphreys EB, Mangold LA, *et al.* Risk of prostate cancer-specific mortality following biochemical recurrence after radical prostatectomy. *JAMA* 2005; **294**(4):433–9.

Ganz PA, Barry JM, Burke W, *et al.* National Institutes of Health State-of-the-Science Conference Statement: Role of active surveillance in the management of men with localized prostate cancer. *NIH Consens State Sci Statements* 2011; **28**(1):1–27.

Hayes JH, Ollendorf DA, Pearson SD, *et al.* Active surveillance compared with initial treatment for men with low-risk prostate cancer: a decision analysis. *JAMA* 2010; **304**(21):2373–80.

Heidenreich A, Bastian PJ, Bellmunt J, *et al.* EAU guidelines on prostate cancer. Part 1: screening, diagnosis, and local treatment with curative intent-update 2013. *Eur Urol* 2014; **65**(1):124–37.

Hummel S, Simpson EL, Hemingway P, Stevenson MD, Rees A. Intensity-modulated radiotherapy for the treatment of prostate cancer: a systematic review and economic evaluation. *Health Technol Assess* 2010; **14**(47):1–108, iii-iv.

Nguyen PL, Gu X, Lipsitz SR, *et al.* Cost implications of the rapid adoption of newer technologies for treating prostate cancer. *J Clin Oncol* 2011; **29**(12):1517–24.

Pardo Y, Guedea F, Aguilo F, *et al.* Quality-of-life impact of primary treatments for localized prostate cancer in patients without hormonal treatment. *J Clin Oncol* 2010; **28**(31):4687–96.

Sanda MG, Dunn RL, Michalski J, *et al.* Quality of life and satisfaction with outcome among prostate-cancer survivors. *N Engl J Med* 2008; **358**(12):1250–61.

Spencer BA, Miller DC, Litwin MS, *et al.* Variations in quality of care for men with early-stage prostate cancer. *J Clin Oncol* 2008; **26**(22):3735–42.

Tewari A, Sooriakumaran P, Bloch DA, Seshadri-Kreaden U, Hebert AE, Wiklund P. Positive surgical margin and perioperative complication rates of primary surgical treatments for prostate cancer: a systematic review and meta-analysis comparing retropubic, laparoscopic, and robotic prostatectomy. *Eur Urol* 2012; **62**(1):1–15.

Thompson I, Tangen C, Paradelo J, *et al.* Adjuvant radiotherapy for pathological T3N0M0 prostate cancer significantly reduces risk of metastases and improves survival: Long-term followup of a randomized clinical trial. *J Urol* 2009; **181**:956–62.

Thompson I, Thrasher JB, Aus G, *et al.* Guideline for the management of clinically localized prostate cancer: 2007 update. *J Urol* 2007; **177**(6):2106–31.

Wilt TJ, Brawer MK, Jones KM, *et al.* Radical prostatectomy versus observation for localized prostate cancer. *N Engl J Med* 2012; **367**(3):203–13.

Zelefsky MJ, Eastham JA, Cronin AM, *et al.* Metastasis after radical prostatectomy or external beam radiotherapy for patients with clinically localized prostate cancer: a comparison of clinical cohorts adjusted for case mix. *J Clin Oncol* 2010; **28**(9):1508–13.

References

1. Jemal A, Bray F, Center MM, Ferlay J, Ward E, Forman D. Global cancer statistics. *CA Cancer J Clin* 2011; **61**(2):69–90.
2. Etzioni R, Gulati R, Tsodikov A, *et al.* The prostate cancer conundrum revisited: treatment changes and prostate cancer mortality. *Cancer* 2012; **118**(23):5955–63.
3. Cooperberg MR, Broering JM, Kantoff PW, Carroll PR. Contemporary trends in low risk prostate cancer: risk assessment and treatment. *J Urol* 2007; **178**(3 Pt 2):S14–9.
4. Esserman L, Shieh Y, Thompson I. Rethinking screening for breast cancer and prostate cancer. *JAMA* 2009; **302**(15):1685–92.
5. Wei JT, Dunn RL, Sandler HM, *et al.* Comprehensive comparison of health-related quality of life after contemporary therapies for localized prostate cancer. *J Clin Oncol* 2002; **20**(2):557–66.
6. Draisma G, Etzioni R, Tsodikov A, *et al.* Lead time and overdiagnosis in prostate-specific antigen screening: importance of methods and context. *J Natl Cancer Inst* 2009; **101**(6):374–83.
7. Moyer VA. Screening for Prostate Cancer: U.S. Preventive Services Task Force Recommendation Statement. *Ann Intern Med* 2012; **157**(2):120–34.
8. Carroll PR, Albertsen PC, Greene K, *et al.* Prostate-Specific Antigen Best Practice Statement: 2009 Update. American Urological

Association, 2009. Available at: https://www.auanet.org/common/pdf/education/clinical-guidance/PSA-Archive.pdf [Online].
9. Wilt TJ, Brawer MK, Jones KM, *et al.* Radical prostatectomy versus observation for localized prostate cancer. *N Engl J Med* 2012; **367**(3):203–13.
10. Cooperberg MR, Carroll PR, Klotz L. Active surveillance for prostate cancer: progress and promise. *J Clin Oncol* 2011; **29**(27):3669–76.
11. Bechis SK, Carroll PR, Cooperberg MR. Impact of age at diagnosis on prostate cancer treatment and survival. *J Clin Oncol* 2011; **29**(2):235–41.
12. Lu-Yao GL, Albertsen PC, Moore DF, *et al.* Outcomes of localized prostate cancer following conservative management. *JAMA* 2009; **302**(11):1202–9.
13. O'Dowd GJ, Veltri RW, Orozco R, Miller MC, Oesterling JE. Update on the appropriate staging evaluation for newly diagnosed prostate cancer. *J Urol* 1997; **158**(3 Pt 1):687–98.
14. Cooperberg MR, Lubeck DP, Grossfeld GD, Mehta SS, Carroll PR. Contemporary trends in imaging test utilization for prostate cancer staging: data from the cancer of the prostate strategic urologic research endeavor. *J Urol* 2002; **168**(2):491–5.
15. Dinan MA, Curtis LH, Hammill BG, *et al.* Changes in the use and costs of diagnostic imaging among Medicare beneficiaries with cancer, 1999–2006. *JAMA* 2010; **303**(16):1625–31.
16. Lavery HJ, Brajtbord JS, Levinson AW, Nabizada-Pace F, Pollard ME, Samadi DB. Unnecessary imaging for the staging of low-risk prostate cancer is common. *Urology* 2011; **77**:274–79.
17. Palvolgyi R, Daskivich TJ, Chamie K, Kwan L, Litwin MS. Bone scan overuse in staging of prostate cancer: an analysis of a veterans affairs cohort. *Urology* 2011; **77**(6):1330–6.
18. Centers for Medicare & Medicaid Services. 2010 PQRI Measures List 2010 [20 January 2011]. Available at: https://http://www.cms.gov/PQRI/Downloads/2010_PQRI_MeasuresList_111309.pdf [Online].
19. Rioja J, Rodríguez-Fraile M, Lima-Favaretto R, *et al.* Role of positron emission tomography in urological oncology. *BJU Int* 2010; **106**(11):1578–93.
20. Lecouvet FE, Geukens D, Stainier A, *et al.* Magnetic resonance imaging of the axial skeleton for detecting bone metastases in patients with high-risk prostate cancer: diagnostic and cost-effectiveness and comparison with current detection strategies. *J Clin Oncol* 2007; **25**(22):3281–7.
21. Turkbey B, Mani H, Shah V, *et al.* Multiparametric 3T prostate magnetic resonance imaging to detect cancer: histopathological correlation using prostatectomy specimens processed in customized magnetic resonance imaging based molds. *J Urol* 2011; **186**(5):1818–24.
22. Cooperberg MR. Prostate cancer risk assessment: choosing the sharpest tool in the shed. *Cancer* 2008; **113**(11):3062–6.
23. Cooperberg MR, Broering JM, Carroll PR. Time trends and local variation in primary treatment of localized prostate cancer. *J Clin Oncol* 2010; **28**:1117–23.
24. Epstein JI, Allsbrook WC Jr, Amin MB, Egevad LL. The 2005 International Society of Urological Pathology (ISUP) Consensus Conference on Gleason Grading of Prostatic Carcinoma. *Am J Surg Pathol* 2005; **29**(9):1228–42.
25. Reese AC, Cowan JE, Brajtbord JS, Harris CR, Carroll PR, Cooperberg MR. The quantitative Gleason score improves prostate cancer risk assessment. *Cancer* 2012; **118**(24):6046–54.
26. Reese AC, Sadetsky N, Carroll PR, Cooperberg MR. Inaccuracies in assignment of clinical stage for localized prostate cancer. *Cancer* 2011; **117**(2):283–9.
27. Reese AC, Cooperberg MR, Carroll PR. Minimal impact of clinical stage on prostate cancer prognosis among contemporary patients with clinically localized disease. *J Urol* 2010; **184**(1):114–9.
28. Shariat S, Karakiewicz P, Margulis V, Kattan M. Inventory of prostate cancer predictive tools. *Curr Opin Urol* 2008; **18**(3):279–96.
29. D'Amico AV, Whittington R, Malkowicz SB, *et al.* Clinical utility of the percentage of positive prostate biopsies in defining biochemical outcome after radical prostatectomy for patients with clinically localized prostate cancer. *J Clin Oncol* 2000; **18**(6):1164–72.
30. Heidenreich A, Bellmunt J, Bolla M, *et al.* EAU guidelines on prostate cancer. Part 1: screening, diagnosis, and treatment of clinically localised disease. *Eur Urol* 2011; **59**(1):61–71.
31. Thompson I, Thrasher JB, Aus G, *et al.* Guideline for the management of clinically localized prostate cancer: 2007 update. *J Urol* 2007; **177**(6):2106–31.
32. Cooperberg M. Understanding and applying risk assessment for prostate cancer. PCRI Insights Patients and Physicians Co-Partnership, November 2010, Volume **13**, Number 4.
33. Makarov DV, Trock BJ, Humphreys EB, *et al.* Updated nomogram to predict pathologic stage of prostate cancer given prostate-specific antigen level, clinical stage, and biopsy Gleason score (Partin tables) based on cases from 2000 to 2005. *Urology* 2007; **69**(6):1095–101.
34. Kattan MW, Eastham JA, Stapleton AM, Wheeler TM, Scardino PT. A preoperative nomogram for disease recurrence following radical prostatectomy for prostate cancer. *J Natl Cancer Inst* 1998; **90**(10):766–71.
35. Kattan MW, Wheeler TM, Scardino PT. Postoperative nomogram for disease recurrence after radical prostatectomy for prostate cancer. *J Clin Oncol* 1999; **17**(5):1499–507.
36. Stephenson AJ, Scardino PT, Eastham JA, *et al.* Postoperative nomogram predicting the 10-year probability of prostate cancer recurrence after radical prostatectomy. *J Clin Oncol* 2005; **23**(28):7005–12.
37. Stephenson AJ, Scardino PT, Eastham JA, *et al.* Preoperative nomogram predicting the 10-year probability of prostate cancer recurrence after radical prostatectomy. *J Natl Cancer Inst* 2006; **98**(10):715–7.
38. Cooperberg MR, Hilton JF, Carroll PR. The CAPRA-S score: A straightforward tool for improved prediction of outcomes after radical prostatectomy. *Cancer* 2011; **117**(22):5039–46.
39. Greene KL, Meng MV, Elkin EP, *et al.* Validation of the Kattan preoperative nomogram for prostate cancer recurrence using a community based cohort: results from Cancer of the Prostate Strategic Urological Research Endeavor (CaPSURE). *J Urol* 2004; **171**(6, Part 1): 2255–9.
40. Nielsen ME, Makarov DV, Humphreys E, Mangold L, Partin AW, Walsh PC. Is it possible to compare PSA recurrence-free survival after surgery and radiotherapy using revised ASTRO criterion--"nadir + 2"? *Urology* 2008; **72**(2):389–93.
41. Cooperberg MR, Pasta DJ, Elkin EP, *et al.* The University of California, San Francisco Cancer of the Prostate Risk Assessment score: a straightforward and reliable preoperative predictor of disease recurrence after radical prostatectomy. *J Urol* 2005; **173**(6):1938–42.
42. Lughezzani G, Budaus L, Isbarn H, *et al.* Head-to-head comparison of the three most commonly used preoperative models for prediction of biochemical recurrence after radical prostatectomy. *Eur Urol* 2010; **57**(4):562–8.
43. Cooperberg MR, Broering JM, Carroll PR. Risk assessment for prostate cancer metastasis and mortality at the time of diagnosis. *J Natl Cancer Inst* 2009; **101**(12):878–87.
44. Kamidono S, Ohshima S, Hirao Y, *et al.* Evidence-based clinical practice Guidelines for Prostate Cancer (Summary—JUA 2006 Edition). *Int J Urol* 2008; **15**(1):1–18.
45. Cooperberg MR, Vickers AJ, Broering JM, Carroll PR. Comparative risk-adjusted mortality outcomes after primary surgery, radiotherapy, or androgen-deprivation therapy for localized prostate cancer. *Cancer* 2010; **116**(22):5226–34.
46. Warde P, Mason M, Ding K, *et al.* Combined androgen deprivation therapy and radiation therapy for locally advanced prostate cancer: a randomised, phase 3 trial. *Lancet* 2011; **378**(9809):2104–11.
47. Zelefsky MJ, Eastham JA, Cronin AM, *et al.* Metastasis after radical prostatectomy or external beam radiotherapy for patients with clinically localized prostate cancer: a comparison of clinical cohorts adjusted for case mix. *J Clin Oncol* 2010; **28**(9):1508–13.
48. Hoffman RM, Koyama T, Fan K-H, *et al.* Mortality after radical prostatectomy or external beam radiotherapy for localized prostate cancer. *J Natl Cancer Inst* 2013; **105**:711–18.
49. Ganz PA, Barry JM, Burke W, *et al.* National Institutes of Health State-of-the-Science Conference Statement: Role of active surveillance in the

management of men with localized prostate cancer. *NIH Consens State Sci Statements* 2011; **28**(1):1–27.
50. Nam RK, Saskin R, Lee Y, *et al.* Increasing hospital admission rates for urological complications after transrectal ultrasound guided prostate biopsy. *J Urol* 2010; **183**(3):963–8.
51. Latini DM, Hart SL, Knight SJ, *et al.* The relationship between anxiety and time to treatment for patients with prostate cancer on surveillance. *J Urol* 2007 Sep;**178**(3 Pt 1):826–31; discussion 31–2.
52. Porten SP, Whitson JM, Cowan JE, *et al.* Changes in prostate cancer grade on serial biopsy in men undergoing active surveillance. *J Clin Oncol* 2011; **29**(20):2795–800.
53. Ross AE, Loeb S, Landis P, *et al.* Prostate-specific antigen kinetics during follow-up are an unreliable trigger for intervention in a prostate cancer surveillance program. *J Clin Oncol* 2010; **28**(17):2810–6.
54. Whitson JM, Porten SP, Hilton JF, *et al.* The relationship between prostate specific antigen change and biopsy progression in patients on active surveillance for prostate cancer. *J Urol* 2011; **185**(5):1656–60.
55. Samaratunga H, Epstein J. What is the molecular pathology of low-risk prostate cancer? *World J Urol* 2008; **26**(5):431–6.
56. Bill-Axelson A, Holmberg L, Ruutu M, *et al.* Radical prostatectomy versus watchful waiting in early prostate cancer. *N Engl J Med* 2011; **364**(18):1708–17.
57. Kibel AS, Ciezki JP, Klein EA, *et al.* Survival among men with clinically localized prostate cancer treated with radical prostatectomy or radiation therapy in the prostate specific antigen era. *J Urol* 2012; **187**(4):1259–65.
58. Eisenberg ML, Davies BJ, Cooperberg MR, Cowan JE, Carroll PR. Prognostic implications of an undetectable ultrasensitive prostate-specific antigen level after radical prostatectomy. *Eur Urol* 2010; **57**(4):622–9.
59. Stephenson AJ, Scardino PT, Kattan MW, *et al.* Predicting the outcome of salvage radiation therapy for recurrent prostate cancer after radical prostatectomy. *J Clin Oncol* 2007; **25**(15):2035–41.
60. Thompson I, Tangen C, Paradelo J, *et al.* Adjuvant radiotherapy for pathological T3N0M0 prostate cancer significantly reduces risk of metastases and improves survival: Long-term followup of a randomized clinical trial. *J Urol* 2009; **181**: 956–62.
61. Freedland SJ, Humphreys EB, Mangold LA, *et al.* Risk of prostate cancer-specific mortality following biochemical recurrence after radical prostatectomy. *JAMA* 2005; **294**(4):433–9.
62. Barocas DA, Salem S, Kordan Y, *et al.* Robotic assisted laparoscopic prostatectomy versus radical retropubic prostatectomy for clinically localized prostate cancer: comparison of short-term biochemical recurrence-free survival. *J Urol* 2010; **183**(3):990–6.
63. Tewari A, Sooriakumaran P, Bloch DA, Seshadri-Kreaden U, Hebert AE, Wiklund P. Positive surgical margin and perioperative complication rates of primary surgical treatments for prostate cancer: a systematic review and meta-analysis comparing retropubic, laparoscopic, and robotic prostatectomy. *Eur Urol* 2012; **62**(1):1–15.
64. Hu JC, Gu X, Lipsitz SR, Barry MJ, *et al.* Comparative effectiveness of minimally invasive vs open radical prostatectomy. *JAMA* 2009; **302**(14):1557–64.
65. Ficarra V, Novara G, Ahlering TE, *et al.* Systematic review and meta-analysis of studies reporting potency rates after robot-assisted radical prostatectomy. *Eur Urol* 2012; **62**(3):418–30.
66. Ficarra V, Novara G, Rosen RC, *et al.* Systematic review and meta-analysis of studies reporting urinary continence recovery after robot-assisted radical prostatectomy. *Eur Urol* 2012; **62**(3):405–17.
67. Barry MJ, Gallagher PM, Skinner JS, Fowler FJ Jr. Adverse effects of robotic-assisted laparoscopic versus open retropubic radical prostatectomy among a nationwide random sample of medicare-age men. *J Clin Oncol* 2012; **30**(5):513–8.
68. Savage CJ, Vickers AJ. Low annual caseloads of United States surgeons conducting radical prostatectomy. *J Urol* 2009; **182**(6):2677–81.
69. Cooperberg MR. Urological cancer: For localized prostate cancer, does technology equal progress? *Nature Rev Clin Oncol* 2012; **9**(7):371–2.
70. Cooperberg MR, Odisho AY, Carroll PR. Outcomes for radical prostatectomy: Is it the singer, the song, or both? *J Clin Oncol* 2012; **30**(5):476–8.
71. Schroeck FR, Krupski TL, Sun L, *et al.* Satisfaction and regret after open retropubic or robot-assisted laparoscopic radical prostatectomy. *Eur Urol* 2008; **54**(4):785–93.
72. Sanda MG, Dunn RL, Michalski J, *et al.* Quality of life and satisfaction with outcome among prostate-cancer survivors. *N Engl J Med* 2008; **358**(12):1250–61.
73. Pardo Y, Guedea F, Aguilo F, *et al.* Quality-of-life impact of primary treatments for localized prostate cancer in patients without hormonal treatment. *J Clin Oncol* 2010; **28**(31):4687–96.
74. Alemozaffar M, Regan MM, Cooperberg MR, *et al.* Prediction of erectile function following treatment for prostate cancer. *JAMA* 2011; **306**(11):1205–14.
75. Litwin MS, Flanders SC, Pasta DJ, Stoddard ML, Lubeck DP, Henning JM. Sexual function and bother after radical prostatectomy or radiation for prostate cancer: multivariate quality-of-life analysis from CaPSURE. Cancer of the Prostate Strategic Urologic Research Endeavor. *Urology* 1999; **54**(3):503–8.
76. Abdel-Wahab M, Reis IM, Hamilton K. Second primary cancer after radiotherapy for prostate cancer--a SEER analysis of brachytherapy versus external beam radiotherapy. *Int J Radiat Oncol Biol Phys* 2008 Sep 1;**72**(1):58–68.
77. Jones CU, Hunt D, McGowan DG, *et al.* Radiotherapy and short-term androgen deprivation for localized prostate cancer. *N Engl J Med* 2011; **365**(2):107–18.
78. Cookson MS, Aus G, Burnett AL, *et al.* Variation in the definition of biochemical recurrence in patients treated for localized prostate cancer: the American Urological Association Prostate Guidelines for Localized Prostate Cancer Update Panel report and recommendations for a standard in the reporting of surgical outcomes. *J Urol* 2007; **177**(2):540–5.
79. Roach M 3rd, Hanks G, Thames H Jr, *et al.* Defining biochemical failure following radiotherapy with or without hormonal therapy in men with clinically localized prostate cancer: recommendations of the RTOG-ASTRO Phoenix Consensus Conference. *Int J Radiat Oncol Biol Phys* 2006; **65**(4):965–74.
80. Spencer BA, Miller DC, Litwin MS, *et al.* Variations in quality of care for men with early-stage prostate cancer. *J Clin Oncol* 2008; **26**(22):3735–42.
81. Sheets NC, Goldin GH, Meyer AM, *et al.* Intensity-modulated radiation therapy, proton therapy, or conformal radiation therapy and morbidity and disease control in localized prostate cancer. *JAMA* 2012; **307**(15):1611–20.
82. Hummel S, Simpson EL, Hemingway P, Stevenson MD, Rees A. Intensity-modulated radiotherapy for the treatment of prostate cancer: a systematic review and economic evaluation. *Health Technol Assess* 2010; **14**(47):1–108, iii-iv.
83. Viani GA, Stefano EJ, Afonso SL. Higher-than-conventional radiation doses in localized prostate cancer treatment: a meta-analysis of randomized, controlled trials. *Int J Radiat Oncol Biol Phys* 2009; **74**(5):1405–18.
84. Bolla M, de Reijke TM, Van Tienhoven G, *et al.* Duration of androgen suppression in the treatment of prostate cancer. *N Engl J Med* 2009; **360**(24):2516–27.
85. Aaronson DS, Odisho AY, Hills N, *et al.* Proton beam therapy and treatment for localized prostate cancer: if you build it, they will come. *Arch Int Med* 2012; **172**(3):280–3.
86. Konski A, Speier W, Hanlon A, Beck JR, Pollack A. Is proton beam therapy cost effective in the treatment of adenocarcinoma of the prostate? *J Clin Oncol* 2007; **25**(24):3603–8.
87. Pickles T, Keyes M, Morris WJ. Brachytherapy or conformal external radiotherapy for prostate cancer: a single-institution matched-pair analysis. *Int J Radiat Oncol Biol Phys* 2010; **76**(1):43–9.
88. Zelefsky MJ, Yamada Y, Pei X, *et al.* Comparison of tumor control and toxicity outcomes of high-dose intensity-modulated radiotherapy and brachytherapy for patients with favorable risk prostate cancer. *Urology* 2011; **77**(4):986–90.

89. Pinkawa M, Asadpour B, Piroth MD, *et al.* Health-related quality of life after permanent I-125 brachytherapy and conformal external beam radiotherapy for prostate cancer--a matched-pair comparison. *Radiother Oncol* 2009; **91**(2):225–31.
90. Pieters BR, de Back DZ, Koning CC, Zwinderman AH. Comparison of three radiotherapy modalities on biochemical control and overall survival for the treatment of prostate cancer: a systematic review. *Radiother Oncol* 2009; **93**(2):168–73.
91. Wu AK, Cooperberg MR, Sadetsky N, Carroll PR. Health related quality of life in patients treated with multimodal therapy for prostate cancer. *J Urol* 2008; **180**(6):2415–22; discussion 22.
92. Potters L, Torre T, Fearn PA, Leibel SA, Kattan MW. Potency after permanent prostate brachytherapy for localized prostate cancer. *Int J Radiat Oncol Biol Phys* 2001; **50**(5):1235–42.
93. Babaian RJ, Donnelly B, Bahn D, *et al.* Best practice statement on cryosurgery for the treatment of localized prostate cancer. *J Urol* 2008; **180**(5):1993–2004.
94. Jones JS, Rewcastle JC, Donnelly BJ, Lugnani FM, Pisters LL, Katz AE. Whole gland primary prostate cryoablation: initial results from the cryo on-line data registry. *J Urol* 2008; **180**(2):554–8.
95. Bahn DK, Lee F, Badalament R, Kumar A, Greski J, Chernick M. Targeted cryoablation of the prostate: 7-year outcomes in the primary treatment of prostate cancer. *Urology* 2002; **60**(2 Suppl 1):3–11.
96. Onik G, Vaughan D, Lotenfoe R, Dineen M, Brady J. The "male lumpectomy": focal therapy for prostate cancer using cryoablation results in 48 patients with at least 2-year follow-up. *Urol Oncol* 2008; **26**(5):500–5.
97. Challacombe BJ, Murphy DG, Zakri R, Cahill DJ. High-intensity focused ultrasound for localized prostate cancer: initial experience with a 2-year follow-up. *BJU Int* 2009; **104**(2):200–4.
98. Lukka H, Waldron T, Chin J, *et al.* High-intensity focused ultrasound for prostate cancer: a systematic review. *Clin Oncol (R Coll Radiol)* 2011; **23**(2):117–27.
99. Ahmed HU, Hindley RG, Dickinson L, *et al.* Focal therapy for localised unifocal and multifocal prostate cancer: a prospective development study. *Lancet Oncol* 2012; **13**(6):622–32.
100. Donovan JL, Peters TJ, Noble S, *et al.* Who can best recruit to randomized trials? Randomized trial comparing surgeons and nurses recruiting patients to a trial of treatments for localized prostate cancer (the ProtecT study). *J Clin Epidemiol* 2003; **56**(7):605–9.
101. Hamdy FC, Donovan JL, Lane JA, et al. ProtecT Study Group. 10-Year outcomes after monitoring, surgery, or radiotherapy for localised prostate cancer. *N Engl J Med.* 2016; **375**(15):1415–24.
102. Donovan JL, Hamdy FC, Lane JA, et al. ProtecT Study Group. Patient-reported outcomes after monitoring, surgery, or radiotherapy for prostate cancer. *N Engl J Med.* 2016; **375**(15):1425–37.
103. Barocas DA, Alvarez J, Resnick MJ, et al. Association between radiation therapy, surgery, or observation for localized prostate cancer and patient-reported outcomes after 3 years. *JAMA*. 2017 Mar 21; **317**(11):1126–40. doi: 10.1001/jama.2017.1704.
104. Chen RC, Basak R, Meyer AM, et al. Association between choice of radical prostatectomy, external beam radiotherapy, brachytherapy, or active surveillance and patient-reported quality of life among men with localized prostate cancer. *JAMA*. 2017 Mar 21; **317**(11):1141–50. doi: 10.1001/jama.2017.1652. PMID: 28324092.
105. Hayes JH, Ollendorf DA, Pearson SD, *et al.* Active surveillance compared with initial treatment for men with low-risk prostate cancer: a decision analysis. *JAMA* 2010; **304**(21):2373–80.
106. Cooperberg MR, Ramakrishna NR, Duff SB, *et al.* Primary treatments for clinically localized prostate cancer: systematic review and cost-utility analysis. *BJU Int* 2013; **111**:437–50.
107. Nguyen PL, Gu X, Lipsitz SR, *et al.* Cost implications of the rapid adoption of newer technologies for treating prostate cancer. *J Clin Oncol* 2011; **29**(12):1517–24.
108. Wilson LS, Tesoro R, Elkin EP, *et al.* Cumulative cost pattern comparison of prostate cancer treatments. *Cancer* 2007; **109**(3):518–27.
109. Shahinian VB, Kuo YF, Freeman JL, Goodwin JS. Determinants of androgen deprivation therapy use for prostate cancer: role of the urologist. *J Natl Cancer Inst* 2006; **98**(12):839–45.
110. Wennberg JE, Birkmeyer JD, Cooper MM, Wennberg DE. The Dartmouth Atlas of Health Care 1999: The Quality of Medical Care in the United States: A Report on the Medicare Program, 1999: pp. 1–333. Available at: http://www.dartmouthatlas.org/downloads/atlases/99Atlas.pdf [Online].

CHAPTER 6.8

Focal therapy for prostate cancer

Hashim Uddin Ahmed,
Louise Dickinson, and Mark Emberton

Introduction to focal therapy for prostate cancer

Men with localized prostate cancer have tough decisions to make. Their options straddle two ends of a spectrum, with active surveillance at one extreme and and radical treatment (surgery or radiotherapy) at the other. There seems to be a small absolute risk reduction in disease specific death—of approximately 5% over 10 years—between watchful waiting (a lesser form of active surveillance that is palliative in its intention) and radical surgery demonstrated in the Scandinavian Prostate Cancer Groups SPCG-4 randomized controlled trial.[1,2] The more Prostate Cancer Intervention versus Observation Trial (PIVOT) randomized controlled trial of watchful waiting versus radical prostatectomy in the era of prostate cancer screening showed no overall survival or prostate cancer specific survival advantage to survival over a 11-year period.[3] While further follow-up may demonstrate a survival advantage, this difference in mortality may be offset by a process of surveillance with intervention limited to those who exhibit signs of progression[4,5] as opposed to watchful waiting. As radical treatments carry significant periopertive morbidity (wound infection, haemorrhage, hospital stay), potentially lifelong side effects (such as incontinence, erectile dysfunction, rectal toxicity), and fail to cure many men, ablative therapies that reduce treatment burden while retaining acceptable cancer control have increasingly become areas of evaluation.

The overtreatment of low-risk prostate cancer and limited effect upon disease specific mortality is further brought into context by two randomized controlled trials assessing the efficacy of population prostate-specific antigen (PSA) screening. The North American Prostate Lung Colorectal and Ovarian (PLCO) screening trial showed no difference in prostate cancer specific mortality between the screened and non-screened arms with a mean follow-up of seven years, while the European Screening study (ERSPC) study showed that 1,400 men would need to be screened and 48 men treated to save one life within 10 years.[6] These numbers have dropped with further follow-up, but still remain relatively high. While arguments rage about the strengths and weaknesses of each study, what is very clear is that any advantage from screening and treatment is likely to be small if all cancers are treated uniformly. We are therefore left with abandoning the screening and diagnosis of prostate cancer or finding ways in which to identify those men that are likely to benefit from treatment—and in these men, offer tissue preserving therapy which is targeted to the cancer and not the whole organ, when it is morphometrically possible to do so (Fig. 6.8.1).

The conceptual basis for focal therapy

The problems associated with overtreatment are mitigated if both harms and costs are reduced. At the present time, most treatments for early prostate cancer are both expensive to administer and harmful to the patient (erectile function rates of 30–90%; pad requirement rates of 5–20%; and rectal symptoms occurring in 5–20% of men exposed to radiotherapy). Indeed, men may be willing to accept higher rates of genitourinary functional preservation with lower rates of survival. Trade-offs such as these are not unusual. In a published discrete choice experiment, men stated a need for an additional 26 months of life in order to compensate for lifelong urinary incontinence.[7]

There are two mitigation strategies that might be deployed. The first is a molecular/imaging phenotyping that would identify men who have clinically important cancer that might benefit from treatment.[8–11] Multiparametric MRI for instance has high rates of sensitivity and negative predictive value for Gleason 7 or greater and/or lesions with a volume of 0.5 cc or larger. This gives the test the optimal attributes for ruling out disease, which many (if not most) physicians would agree meets the threshold of what requires treatment rather than no treatment. The second strategy is to change the therapeutic target to the cancer (plus a margin) instead of the organ harbouring the cancer. In essence, little mitigation has occurred. Both surgery and radiotherapy have seen an escalation of complexity with minimal gains. Intensity-modulated radiotherapy on the one hand and robotic radical prostatectomy on the other have not resulted in the pathway transformation that was hoped for. For instance, a analysis has demonstrated few differences in quality-adjusted life years among the various surgical methods; surgical methods tended to be more effective than radiation, although combined external beam and brachytherapy radiation treatment for high-risk disease was the exception. Radiotherapy techniques were consistently more expensive than surgery although both were expensive,

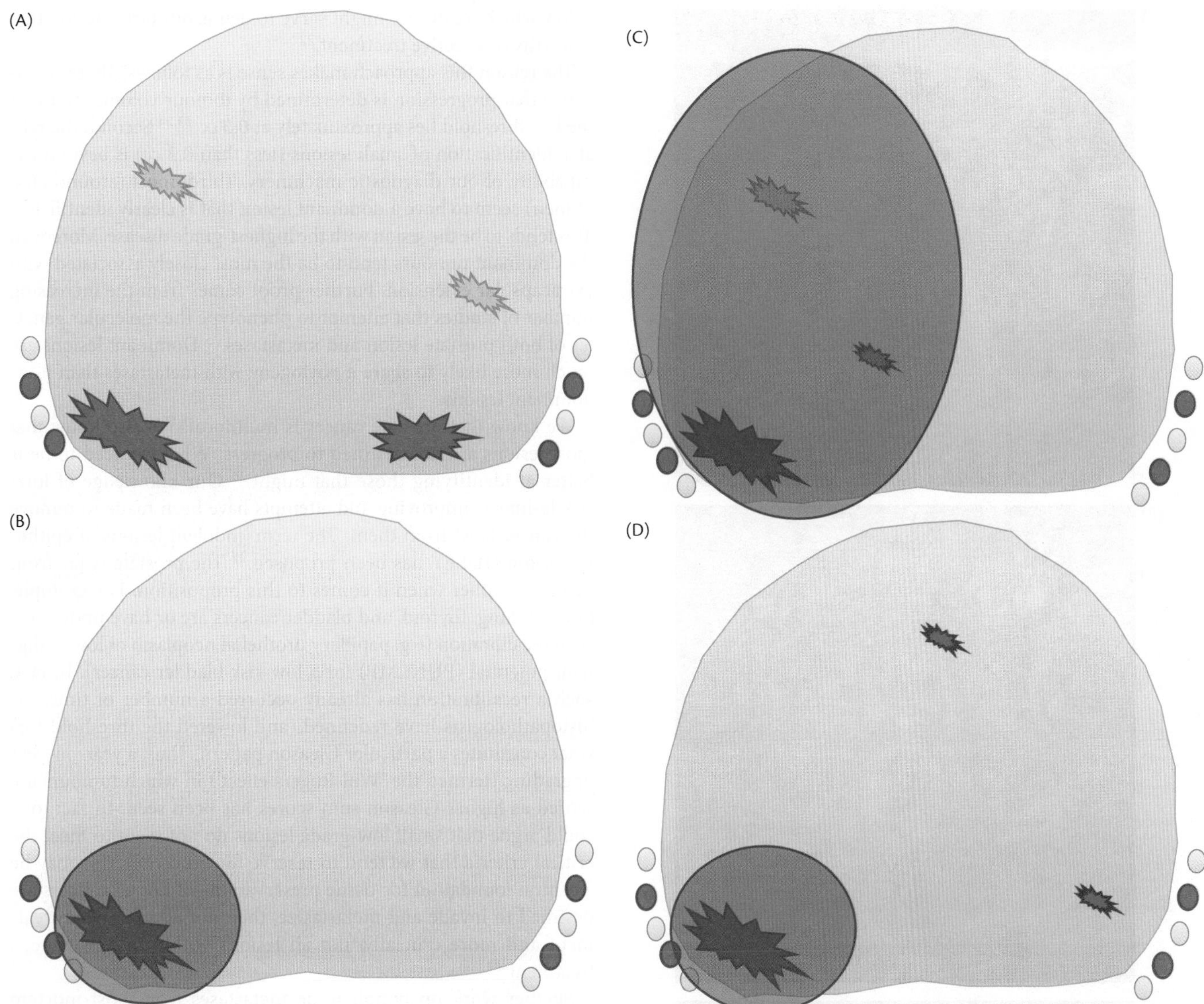

Fig. 6.8.1 (A) Multifocal clinically significant prostate cancer. Not suitable for focal therapy. (B) Unifocal clinically significant prostate cancer suitable for focal therapy. (C) Multifocal clinically significant and clinically insignificant prostate cancer. Suitable for focal therapy using hemiablation. (D) Multifocal clinically significant prostate cancer on one side and clinically insignificant lesions elsewhere. Suitable for focal therapy using index lesion ablation.

with costs ranging from \$19,901 (robot-assisted prostatectomy for low-risk disease) to \$50,276 (combined radiotherapy for high-risk disease).[12] Others have shown that cost savings are not realized, at in the first year and in the United States, between open and minimally invasive surgery.[13] Others have shown that proton beam therapy is significantly more expensive, even if it theoretically improved cancer outcomes, compared to photon beam standard radiotherapy.[14] In addition, there is little robust evidence that much has changed in relation to patient reported side effects.[15,16] It appears that an alternative strategy is going to be needed. One of the few on the table currently is to change our therapeutic target in the way that we have with renal and penile cancer.[17–21] In these two examples, we have witnessed a migration from an organ-based approach to one that attempts to treat the cancer plus a margin.

Prostate cancer biology—multifocality, the index lesion, and the idle lesion

The question then arises about the extent and nature of the margin. A hemiablation is easy to conceptualize and probably easy to standardize. However, for the smaller tumours it might also represent overtreatment. It has served as the entry point to focal therapy for many of the early phase studies. The alternative task of identifying the tumour in space and applying a volumetric margin is one that is much more exacting of both our risk stratification methods and our clinical competencies (Fig. 6.8.2).

This approach makes sense from the perspective of parsimony. It also makes sense from the perspective of biology. Small, low-risk cancer foci have very limited potential for harm. Generating a threshold (based on volume and grade) over which we treat and

(A)

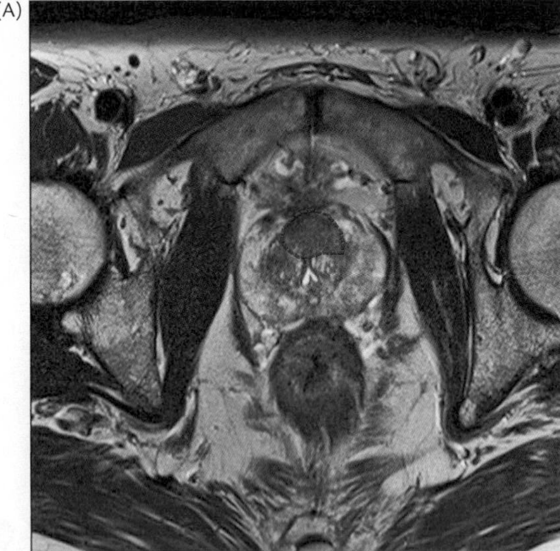

(B)

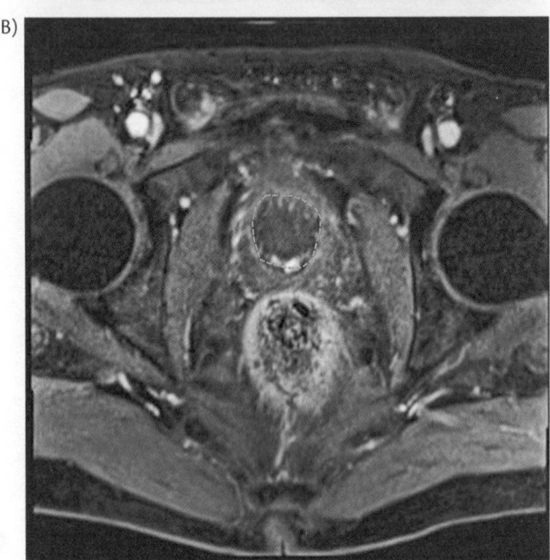

(C)

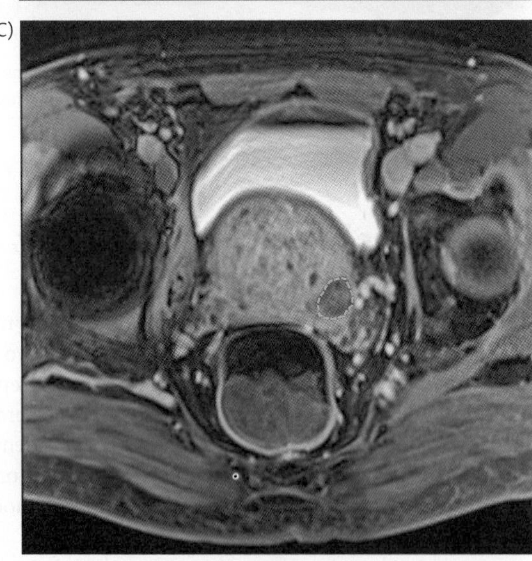

Fig. 6.8.2 (A) Pre-op axial T2W MRI showing anterior large lesion with Gleason 3+3 on template biopsies. PSA7.7. (B) Post-Focal HIFU 1 week contrast enhanced axial T1W MRI showing anterior area of poor perfusion corresponding to treatment area. PSA 1.1 at 3 months. (C) Another man with large >90 mL gland has left peripheral zone lesion Gleason 3+4, focally ablated with HIFU.

below which we do not might serve to define our target lesion that is worthy of selective treatment.[22]

The reason this approach makes sense is as follows. There is evidence that progression is determined by tumour volume, and that the key threshold lies approximately at 0.5 cc.[23,24] Second, the reliable identification of small lesions (less than 0.2 cc) is beyond the capability of our diagnostic machinery. Third, most (around 80% of men) seem to have a dominant lesion that is clearly identifiable. This tends to be the lesion with the highest-grade disease. Moreover, the dominant tumours tend to be the most closely associated with extracapsular extension. Further proof comes from the increasing number of studies that attempt to phenotype the molecular genetics of both prostate lesion and metastases.[25] Dominant lesions are much more likely to share a phylogeny with metastases than non-dominant lesions.

We know that prostate cancer is multifocal. We also know that most lesions are not destined to progress. What we need to be is better at identifying those that might.[26] Our knowledge of low-risk lesions is improving and attempts have been made to remove the cancer label from them. The term 'indolent lesions of epithelial origin (IDLE)' has been proposed.[27] The prostate is far from being an outlier when it comes to this proposition. For example, low-risk lung, thyroid, and bladder cancers are or have undergone such recalibration (e.g. papillary urothelial neoplasm of low malignant potential (PUNLMP) for a low-risk bladder cancer). In fact, such a recalibration has already occurred a number of times, as histopathologists have redefined (and lowered the threshold for) what constitutes a particular Gleason pattern. Thus, a year-on-year upgrading (termed the 'Will Rogers effect') in which tumours are scored as higher Gleason sum scores has been seen. In fact, one could argue that small low-grade lesions do not seem to meet the critical criteria that we tend to reserve for cancers.[28] This may be a central foundation for tissue preservation—if not all cancers are destined to invade and metastasize, then not all men need treatment and more crucially, not all lesions within one man need treatment.[29]

Further work on lymph node metastases from post-mortem studies has added to the knowledge. TMPRSS-ERG gene fusion has been seen in both index lesion and metastases, but have not been seen in lesser lesions.[30,31] Importantly, in those men who have metastases, these metastatic deposits share one common cell of origin.[32,33]

The low malignant potential of low-grade small lesions should not be surprising considering that one-third of the male population has a form of prostate cancer that will not manifest during their lives.[34] When prostates are removed for reasons other than prostate cancer, we see high levels of prevalence.[35] Furthermore, this low malignant potential for Gleason grade 6 disease is underlined by the finding in one study, which demonstrated that of 9,775 men who had pure Gleason 6 disease in radical whole-mount prostatectomy specimens, only three died of prostate cancer in a 15-year period.[36] Other groups have confirmed this, but in trials that used different end points.[37,38]

The assertion that there is a very low risk form of prostate cancer has been verified by the active surveillance series, where the rate of prostate cancer specific death is exceptionally low.[39] In the Toronto series, prostate cancer mortality occurred exclusively in men at higher risk.[40] Two reports from active surveillance cohorts derived from the ERSPC study add a further uncertainty in relation to intermediate-risk disease. The first from Rotterdam and Helsinki comprised 509 men; of these, 381 were low risk, and 128 were deemed to be intermediate risk. After a median 7.4 years follow-up, 221 men (43.4%) opted to defer their treatment. Just over a third in the low-risk group underwent treatment and just over half of the intermediate risk group crossed over to more radical therapy. Distant metastases were found in one low-risk and three intermediate-risk men. The Göteburg arm looked at 439 (45.7%) men who were managed with active surveillance from a total of just under 1,000 in the screening group[41]; half of these men were low risk (224; 51.0%), about one-quarter were very low risk (117; 27%), and most of the remaining were of intermediate risk (92; 21.0%). One or two were high risk (6; 1.4%). Two hundred and seventy-seven men remained on a surveillance strategy. However, by risk group, respectively, the following remained on surveillance: 133 (59%), 58 (50%), 46 (50%), and 3 (50%). Sixty men died during follow-up. Only one man—attributed and intermediate risk status—died from prostate cancer. This was over a decade after diagnosis. Despite these data indicating safety,[42] only 1 in 10 in the United States and 4 in 10 of men in the United Kingdom with low-risk disease are allocated to active surveillance.[43,44] This may be physician or patient-related, but likely a combination of both. With the uncertainty around longer follow-up, especially in the intermediate-risk group, this is hardly surprising, but does point to the need for improved therapeutic interventions that can minimize the harms of treatment if that is what men and their physicians choose.

Patient population

Any man with localized prostate cancer suitable for curative therapy should be regarded as potentially suitable for some form of focal therapeutic intervention. However, focal therapy has been seen by many, predominantly in the United States, as an alternative to active surveillance.[3] It is not. It should be part of a risk-stratified approach to care, in which the patient's disease status and his and his partner's wishes and preferences inform the therapeutic decision. It is complementary and not in competition to either surveillance or whole gland treatment (Fig. 6.8.3).[45]

Much argument has been proposed that cites focal therapy as an option for men who are unable to tolerate the idea of surveillance because or worry and or anxiety. This argument does not carry much weight, as the literature does not support widespread anxiety or decisional regret in this cohort of men. What is needed is risk stratification of high precision, clear communication of the risk stratification, and an openness to shared decision-making.[46–50]

The other side of this argument is that radical therapy should be reserved for clinically significant disease and that anything less would jeopardize oncological outcome. For this question to be truly resolved, we will need long-term data looking at metastases and or death from prostate cancer. This will require large cohorts monitored over one to two decades and adjusted for risk. Even this may not give us the answer if head-to-head randomized controlled trials (RCTs) comparing conservative strategies to radical therapy show no significant differences in overall survival.

Localization of disease

Even if focal therapy does not become the standard of care, it will have contributed towards overall health gain by making it an absolute requirement that precise risk stratification is obtained at

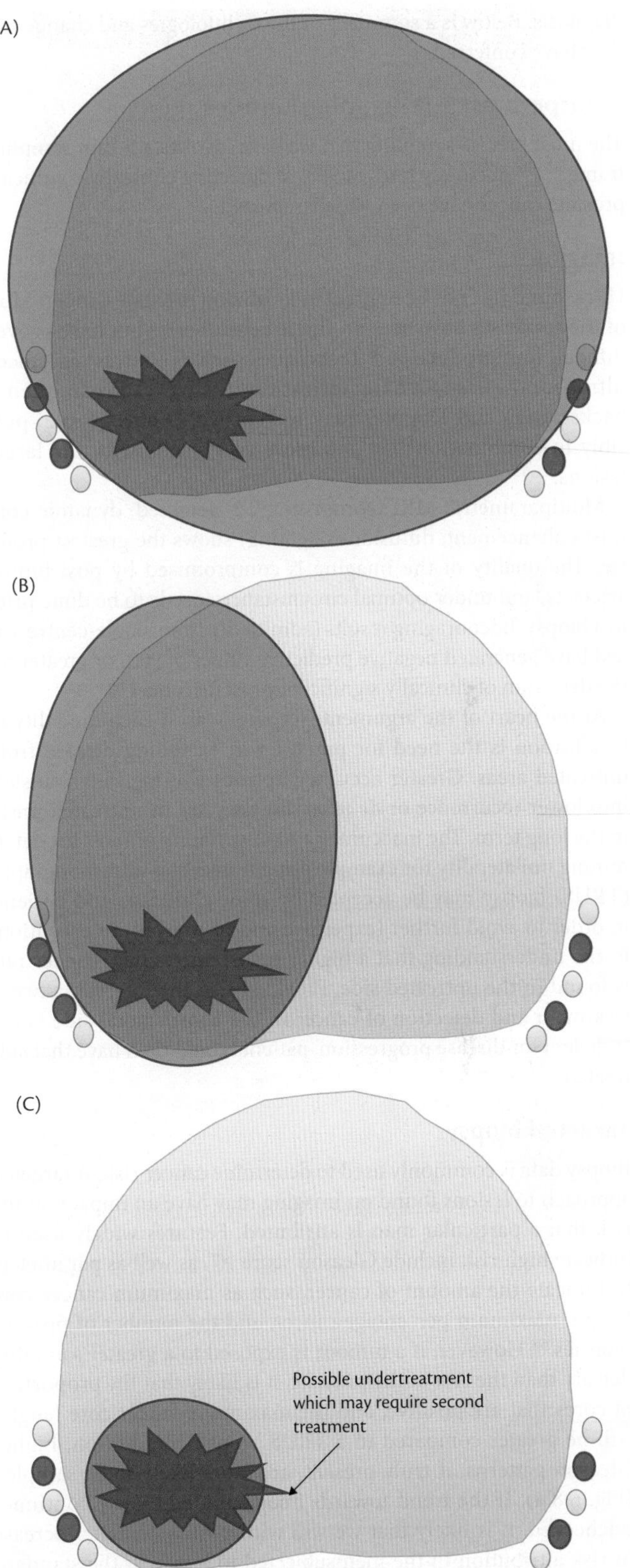

Fig. 6.8.3 (A) Large right peripheral zone lesion treated with wide margin—whole gland treatment. Higher likelihood of complete treatment but significant rates of genitourinary toxicity. (B) Large right peripheral zone lesion treated with wide margin but confined to lobe—hemiablation. Higher likelihood of complete ablation with fewer genitourinary toxicity compared to whole gland. (C) Large right peripheral zone lesion treated smaller margin—zonal or focal ablation. Lower likelihood of complete ablation but much fewer genitourinary toxicity.

diagnosis. Below is a summary of the technologies and change that they have conferred.

Transperineal 3-D mapping biopsies

The most precise sampling that we have invokes a 5-mm sampling frame.[51–56] Accuracy rates of 95% at detecting clinically significant prostate cancer have been widely reported.

Imaging

Ultrasound has not been great at localizing prostate cancer. Most of the successes have been in single centre series but have proved difficult to reproduce.[57,58] Techniques such as contrast enhanced ultrasound, tissue characterization (using radio-frequency backscatter) and Doppler may well prove to have a role, possibly in combination[59–63] and more specifically with the larger lesions.[64,65]

Multiparametric MRI (comprising T2-weighted, dynamic contrast enhancement, diffusion weighting) shows the greatest promise. The quality of the imaging is compromised by post-biopsy artefacts, and under optimal circumstances needs to be done prior to a biopsy. Encouraging results (admittedly from single-centre series) have generated negative predictive values of 90% or greater for the detection of clinically significant prostate cancer.[66,67]

At the heart of the arguments for and against each modality of localization is the need for precision in excluding disease from untreated areas. Greater accuracy upfront will logically translate into lower recurrence or *de novo* disease rates in untreated areas, in the long term. The inaccuracy and uncertainty of tools for determining unilaterality for example using transrectal ultrasonography (TRUS) biopsy may be accepted by some clinicians and patients in order to avoid further (expensive and/or morbid) interventions in the understanding that a higher recurrent/residual cancer rate is found in the untreated side. Provided that the interval between treatment and detection of cancer in the contralateral side is not sufficient for disease progression, patients could then have that side treated.

Targeted biopsy

Biopsy data is commonly used to determine cancer risk. A targeted approach to lesions found on imaging may have an impact on the risk that a particular man is attributed. Features widely used to indicate high risk include Gleason score ≥7, as well as parameters to indicate the amount of cancer, such as maximum cancer core length, maximum percentage cancer, and the number of positive biopsies.[68] However, if a tumour is exposed to a greater sampling density than the rest of the prostate, it is likely that the proportion of cores that are positive, and the maximum cancer core length, will be greater compared to a TRUS biopsy. In addition, higher Gleason patterns, if truly present, are more likely to be sampled (Fig. 6.8.4). If the trend towards image-guided biopsy continues unchecked, it is likely that we will witness a systematic increase in risk attribution in the men subjected to biopsy if the standard criteria for attributing risk are applied. It is therefore likely that new risk prediction models based on targeted biopsies will be required. As a start to correct what could be regarded as an artefactual increase in cancer risk derived from targeted biopsy, a risk stratification system that is independent of the number of positive cores could be considered.

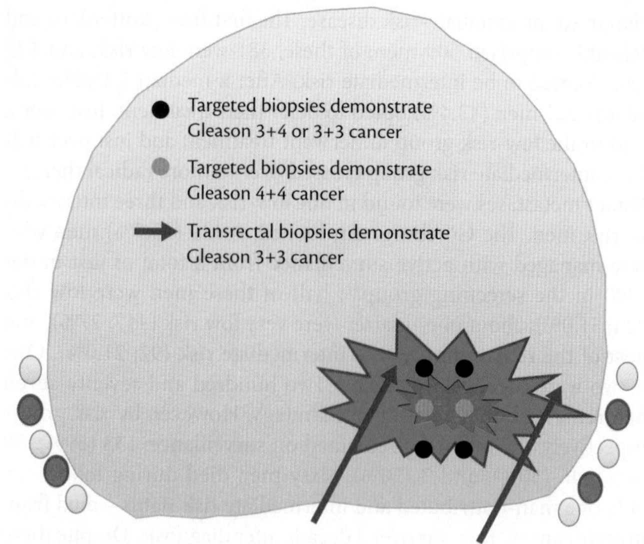
Targeted biopsies demonstrate Gleason 3+4 or 3+3 cancer
Targeted biopsies demonstrate Gleason 4+4 cancer
Transrectal biopsies demonstrate Gleason 3+3 cancer

Fig. 6.8.4 A Gleason 3+4 lesion in the left peripheral zone which through targeted biopsies may be miss-classified as very low risk on transrectal biopsies and very high risk 4+4 through a true-hit into the central pattern 4 using current risk stratification systems.

Ablative technology

There are numerous ways by which tissue can be selectively destroyed.[69] High-intensity focused ultrasound (HIFU) and cryosurgery—old technologies that have been adapted for use in focal therapy—are the only two modalities that benefit from retrospective and prospective published data. In summary, men can expect a 95% and 85% probability—for HIFU and Cryotherapy respectively—of preserving genitourinary function compared to baseline.[70,71] Other techniques such as brachytherapy, stereotactic radiotherapy, irreversible electroporation, radio-frequency ablation, magnetic resonance hyperthermia using magnetic nanoparticles, and toxin injections into the prostate are all under investigation.[72,73]

Clinical outcomes of focal therapy

So far, only single institution case series have reported as full publications, although prospective trial data is starting to emerge at the time of writing (Table 6.8.1 and Table 6.8.2). One of the first ever series reported was that by Onik.[74,75] He reported the fate of 55 men treated with cryotherapy hemiablation that had one year follow-up. Ninety-five per cent (52/55) exhibited PSA stability (as defined by ASTRO criteria) and of the 51 potent prior to the procedure, 44 (86%) remained potent after hemiablation. Four (7%) required retreatment due to infiled recurrence. This study was one of the first to highlight the imprecision of TRUS guided biopsy. In Onik's hands, when transperineal template biopsies (5 mm sampling frame) were applied as the reclassification tool over half the men that were deemed to have unilateral disease on TRUS criteria were verified as having this.[76–80] Bahn *et al.*[78] reported another cryotherapy with longer follow-up (70 months). In this report, biochemical disease-free status was seen in 93% of patients. This was associated with a 96% negative-biopsy rate. Potency (erections sufficient for penetration) was seen in the majority (89%). The series

Table 6.8.1 Focal therapy of prostate cancer using cryotherapy

Name and device	Onik *et al.* (2009) (Endocare)	Ellis *et al.* (2007) (Endocare)	Lambert *et al.* (2007) (Oncura)	Bahn *et al.* (2006) (Endocare)*	Crawford/ Barqawi (2009) (Endocare)	COLD Registry (2009) (Endocare)	Bahn *et al.* (2012) (Endocare)*
Type of study	Retrospective	Retrospective	Retrospective	Retrospective	Prospective	Retrospective	Retrospective
No.	112	60	25	31	100	795	73
Therapy	Hemi	Hemi	Hemi	Hemi	Focal	'Focal/Partial'	Hemiablation
Biopsy	Template	TRUS	TRUS	TRUS +Doppler	Template	TRUS	TRUS+Doppler
Mean PSA (ng/ml)	8.3	7.2 +/− 4.7	6 (range 1–13)	4.95	5.2 +/− 4.1	Not reported	5.4 (range 0.01–20)
Gleason Score	≤6	</=8	</=7	</=7	</=7	</=8	</=4+3
Potency	85%	70.6%	70.8%	89%	83%	65%	86%
Incontinence	0%	3.6%	0%	0%	NR	2.8%	0%
F/U (mean, months)	43.2	15.2	28	70	NR	12	Median 3.7yrs
Disease control	93% NED	76.7% (biopsy)	88% (>50% nadir reduction)	96% (biopsy) 92% (ASTRO)	97% (biopsy at 12/12)	4.5% (36/295) 25% (36/199) 83% (ASTRO)	70% reduction in PSA12/48 (25%) positive biopsies ◆ contralateral side: 11/12 ◆ ipsilateral: 1/12

*likely to be same but updated series.

Table 6.8.2 Focal therapy of prostate cancer using high-intensity focused ultrasound

Name and device	Muto *et al.* (2008) (Sonablate500)	Barret (2009) (Ablatherm)	Ahmed *et al.* (2009) (Sonablate500)	Ahmed *et al.* (2012)
Type of study	Retrospective	Retrospective	Prospective	Prospective
No.	29	12	20	41
Therapy	Hemiablation	Hemiablation	Hemiablation	Focal (unifocal and bilateral)
Biopsy	TRUS biopsy	TRUS Biopsy	MRI and template mapping biopsies	MRI and template mapping biopsies
Mean PSA (ng/ml)	5 (range 2–25)	<10	<15	<15
Gleason Score	</=8	</=7	</=4+3	</=4+3
Potency	Not reported	Not reported	19/20 (95%)	31/35 (89%)
Incontinence (pad-free)	Not reported	0%	1/20 (5%)	0/38 (0%)
Disease Control	76.5% (biopsy)	58% (10 years)	Biopsy positive ◆ 2/19 (10%) (any cancer) ◆ 0/19 (0%) (significant cancer)	Biopsy positive ◆ 9/39 (23%) (any cancer) ◆ 3/39 (8%) (significant cancer)

was subsequently updated in a more publication reporting on 73 men.[81] There is some evidence to show that penile rehabilitation may be more effective if tissue is preserved.[82] Some reports, particularly those that relied upon a TRUS based diagnostic strategy, have not fared so well and have required some men to undergo retreatment.[83] Ward and Jones reported on 1,160 men who underwent focal cryotherapy within the Cryo On-Line Database (COLD) registry sowing very encouraging rates of biochemical control and functional outcomes although the data was limited by lack of formal validated questionnaires and histological determination of treatment success or failure.[84]

HIFU, probably because it was less widely available than cryotherapy, has been evaluated more formally (Table 6.8.2). Muto and colleagues were the first to report. They did hemiablation using a Sonablate® 500 HIFU platform on a rather heterogeneous series.[82] Men with unilateral disease on TRUS biopsy (n = 29) had ablation directed to both peripheral zones and one-half of the transition zone. Despite the poor characterization only 10% (3/28) had positive biopsies when assessed at six months. However, a further 26% (4/17) had positive biopsies at the 12-month assessment. Urinary symptoms were stable prior to and following therapy. Sexual outcomes were not reported.

We now have a number of prospective studies that we can use to advise patients. The group at University College London (UCL) in the United Kingdom have reported on a hemiablation series that was both registered and prospective. In summary, 20 men (characterized by multiparametric MRI and template prostate mapping) exhibited an early return of baseline genitourinary function by three to six months. Ninety-five per cent (95%) reported having erections sufficient for penetration, 95% were pad-free. Oncological outcomes were favourable. Within field 90% were free of significant cancer (<1 core positive, Gleason 3+3, </=3 mm).[83]

In a further study (n = 41) by the UCL group, this time exploring the outcome of focal/zonal ablation using HIFU similar results were obtained.[84] The third study of the trilogy recruited 56 men and had treatment to the index lesion plus a margin. Currently the UK INDEX (a prospective and multicentre study) is both larger and longer term with three-year mapping biopsy as the primary outcome. This will inform the medium term oncological outcome

Conclusion

For men diagnosed with medium risk early prostate cancer, the therapeutic dilemma remains a stark one. It is not helped by the inherent inaccuracies of our current diagnostic pathway in which transrectal biopsies are used as the verification test. Tissue preserving therapy relies on the accurate diagnosis, characterization, and localization of disease within the prostate so that therapy can be targeted to the cancer—something we do all the time in other tumours. Early small series have shown that toxicity is very much lower. However, there is still much to determine. Reproducibility and longevity of cancer control are important for both physician and patient confidence. Indeed, with very little in the way of survival advantage for radical therapies against surveillance in the long term, reproducibility across centres with acceptable disease control rates in the medium term may well be the level of evidence required to change practice.

Further reading

Ahmed HU, Arya M, Freeman A, Emberton M. Do low-grade and low-volume prostate cancers bear the hallmarks of malignancy? *Lancet Oncol* 2012; **13**(11):e509–17.

Ahmed HU, Hindley RG, Dickinson L, *et al.* Focal therapy for localised unifocal and multifocal prostate cancer: a prospective development study. *Lancet Oncol* 2012; **13**(6):622–32.

Ahmed HU, Pendse D, Illing R, Allen C, van der Meulen JH, Emberton M. Will focal therapy become a standard of care for men with localized prostate cancer? *Nat Clin Pract Oncol* 2007; **4**(11):632–42.

Ahmed HU. The index lesion and the origin of prostate cancer. *N Engl J Med* 2009; **361**(17):1704–6.

Eggener S, Salomon G, Scardino PT, De la Rosette J, Polascik TJ, Brewster S. Focal therapy for prostate cancer: possibilities and limitations. *Eur Urol 2010; 58(1):57–64. Erratum in: Eur Urol* **2010; 58**(4):644.

Ganz PA, Barry JM, Burke W, *et al.* National Institutes of Health State-of-the-Science Conference: role of active surveillance in the management of men with localized prostate cancer. *Ann Intern Med* 2012; **156**(8):591–5.

Turkbey B, Pinto PA, Choyke PL; Medscape. Imaging techniques for prostate cancer: implications for focal therapy. *Nat Rev Urol* 2009; **6**(4):191–203.

Wilt TJ, Brawer MK, Jones KM, *et al.* Prostate Cancer Intervention versus Observation Trial (PIVOT) Study Group. Radical prostatectomy versus observation for localized prostate cancer. *N Engl J Med* 2012; **367**(3):203–13. *Erratum in: N Engl J Med* 2012; **367**(6):582.

References

1. Bill-Axelson A, Holmberg L, Filén F, *et al.*; Scandinavian Prostate Cancer Group Study Number 4. Radical prostatectomy versus watchful waiting in localized prostate cancer: the Scandinavian prostate cancer group-4 randomized trial. *J Natl Cancer Inst* 2008; **100**(16):1144–54.
2. Bill-Axelson A, Holmberg L, Ruutu M, *et al.* Scandinavian Prostate Cancer Group Study No. 4. Radical prostatectomy versus watchful waiting in early prostate cancer. *N Engl J Med* 2005; **352**(19):1977–84.
3. Wilt TJ, Brawer MK, Jones KM, *et al.* Prostate Cancer Intervention versus Observation Trial (PIVOT) Study Group. Radical prostatectomy versus observation for localized prostate cancer. *N Engl J Med* 2012; **367**(3):203–13. Erratum in: *N Engl J Med* 2012; **367**(6):582.
4. Dall'Era MA, Carroll PR. Outcomes and follow-up strategies for patients on active surveillance. *Curr Opin Urol* 2009; **19**(3):258–62.
5. van As NJ, Parker CC. Active surveillance with selective radical treatment for localized prostate cancer. *Cancer J* 2007; **13**(5):289–94.
6. Schröder FH, Hugosson J, Roobol MJ, *et al.*; ERSPC Investigators. Screening and prostate-cancer mortality in a randomized European study. *N Engl J Med* 2009; **360**(13):1320–8.
7. King MT, Viney R, Smith DP, *et al.* Survival gains needed to offset persistent adverse treatment effects in localised prostate cancer. *Br J Cancer* 2012; **106**(4):638–45.
8. Ahmed HU, Kirkham A, Arya M, *et al.* Is it time to consider a role for MRI before prostate biopsy? *Nat Rev Clin Oncol* 2009; **6**(4):197–206.
9. Macura KJ. Multiparametric magnetic resonance imaging of the prostate: current status in prostate cancer detection, localization, and staging. *Semin Roentgenol* 2008; **43**(4):303–13.
10. Kurhanewicz J, Vigneron D, Carroll P, Coakley F. Multiparametric magnetic resonance imaging in prostate cancer: present and future. *Curr Opin Urol* 2008; **18**(1):71–7.
11. Turkbey B, Pinto PA, Choyke PL; Medscape. Imaging techniques for prostate cancer: implications for focal therapy. *Nat Rev Urol* 2009; **6**(4):191–203.
12. Cooperberg MR, Ramakrishna NR, Duff SB, *et al.* Primary treatments for clinically localised prostate cancer: a comprehensive lifetime cost-utility analysis. *BJU Int* 2013; **111**(3):437–50.
13. Lowrance WT, Eastham JA, Yee DS, *et al.* Costs of medical care after open or minimally invasive prostate cancer surgery: a population-based analysis. *Cancer* 2012; **118**(12):3079–86.
14. Konski A, Speier W, Hanlon A, Beck JR, Pollack A. Is proton beam therapy cost effective in the treatment of adenocarcinoma of the prostate? *J Clin Oncol* 2007; **25**(24):3603–8.
15. Berryhill R Jr, Jhaveri J, Yadav R, *et al.* Robotic prostatectomy: a review of outcomes compared with laparoscopic and open approaches. *Urology* 2008; **72**(1):15–23.
16. Sanghani M, Mignano J. Intensity modulated radiation therapy: a review of current practice and future directions. *Technol Cancer Res Treat* 2006; **5**(5):447–50.
17. Karavitakis M, Ahmed HU, Abel PD, Hazell S, Winkler MH. Tumor focality in prostate cancer: implications for focal therapy. *Nat Rev Clin Oncol* 2011; **8**(1):48–55.
18. Lindner U, Trachtenberg J, Lawrentschuk N. Focal therapy in prostate cancer: modalities, findings and future considerations. *Nat Rev Urol* 2010; **7**(10):562–71.
19. de la Rosette J, Ahmed H, Barentsz J, *et al.* Focal therapy in prostate cancer-report from a consensus panel. *J Endourol* 2010; **24**(5):775–80.
20. Eggener S, Salomon G, Scardino PT, De la Rosette J, Polascik TJ, Brewster S. Focal therapy for prostate cancer: possibilities and limitations. *Eur Urol* 2010; **58**(1):57–64. Erratum in: *Eur Urol* 2010; **58**(4):644.

21. Ahmed HU, Pendse D, Illing R, Allen C, van der Meulen JH, Emberton M. Will focal therapy become a standard of care for men with localized prostate cancer? *Nat Clin Pract Oncol* 2007; **4**(11):632–42.
22. Scardino PT. Focal therapy for prostate cancer. *Nat Rev Urol* 2009; **6**(4):175.
23. Stamey TA, Freiha FS, McNeal JE, Redwine EA, Whittemore AS, Schmid HP. Localized prostate cancer. Relationship of tumor volume to clinical significance for treatment of prostate cancer. *Cancer* 1993; **71**(3 Suppl):933–8.
24. Epstein JI, Walsh PC, Carmichael M, Brendler CB. Pathologic and clinical findings to predict tumor extent of nonpalpable (stage T1c) prostate cancer. *JAMA* 1994; **271**(5):368–74.
25. Liu W, Laitinen S, Khan S, *et al.* Copy number analysis indicates monoclonal origin of lethal metastatic prostate cancer. *Nat Med* 2009; **15**(5):559–65. Erratum in: *Nat Med* 2009; **15**(7):819.
26. Ganz PA, Barry JM, Burke W, *et al.* National Institutes of Health State-of-the-Science Conference: role of active surveillance in the management of men with localized prostate cancer. *Ann Intern Med* 2012; **156**(8):591–5.
27. Esserman L, Shieh Y, Thompson I. Rethinking screening for breast cancer and prostate cancer. *JAMA* 2009; **302**(15):1685–92.
28. Hanahan D, Weinberg RA. The hallmarks of cancer. *Cell* 2000; **100**(1):57–70.
29. Ahmed HU, Arya M, Freeman A, Emberton M. Do low-grade and low-volume prostate cancers bear the hallmarks of malignancy? *Lancet Oncol* 2012; **13**(11):e509–17.
30. Guo CC, Wang Y, Xiao L, Troncoso P, Czerniak BA. The relationship of TMPRSS2-ERG gene fusion between primary and metastatic prostate cancers. *Hum Pathol* 2012; **43**(5):644–9.
31. Perner S, Svensson MA, Hossain RR, *et al.* ERG rearrangement metastasis patterns in locally advanced prostate cancer. *Urology* 2010; **75**(4):762–7.
32. Ahmed HU. The index lesion and the origin of prostate cancer. *N Engl J Med* 2009; **361**(17):1704–6.
33. Liu W, Laitinen S, Khan S, *et al.* Copy number analysis indicates monoclonal origin of lethal metastatic prostate cancer. *Nat Med* 2009; **15**(5):559–65.
34. Sakr WA, Grignon DJ, Haas GP, *et al.* Age and racial distribution of prostatic intraepithelial neoplasia. *Eur Urol* 1996; **30**:138–44.
35. Nevoux P, Ouzzane A, Ahmed HU, *et al.* Quantitative tissue analyses of prostate cancer foci in an unselected cystoprostatectomy series. *BJU Int* 2012; **110**(4):517–23.
36. Eggener SE, Scardino PT, Walsh PC, *et al.* Predicting 15-year prostate cancer specific mortality after radical prostatectomy. *J Urol* 2011; **185**(3):869–75.
37. Lee EW, Laze J, Lepor H. Outcomes of extremely low risk prostate cancer following radical prostatectomy. *Prostate Cancer Prostatic Dis* 2011; **14**(3):266–9.
38. Miyamoto H, Hernandez DJ, Epstein JI. A pathological reassessment of organ-confined, Gleason score 6 prostatic adenocarcinomas that progress after radical prostatectomy. *Hum Pathol* 2009; **40**(12):1693–8.
39. Dahabreh IJ, Chung M, Balk EM, *et al.* Active surveillance in men with localized prostate cancer: a systematic review. *Ann Intern Med* 2012; **156**(8):582–90.
40. Klotz L. Active surveillance for favorable-risk prostate cancer: background, patient selection, triggers for intervention, and outcomes. *Curr Urol Rep* 2012; **13**(2):153–9.
41. Klotz L, Zhang L, Lam A, Nam R, Mamedov A, Loblaw A. Clinical results of long-term follow-up of a large, active surveillance cohort with localized prostate cancer. *J Clin Oncol* 2010; **28**(1):126–31.
42. Bul M, van den Bergh RC, Zhu X, *et al.* Outcomes of initially expectantly managed patients with low or intermediate risk screen-detected localized prostate cancer. *BJU Int* 2012; **110**(11):1672–7.
43. Godtman RA, Holmberg E, Khatami A, Stranne J, Hugosson J. Outcome following active surveillance of men with screen-detected prostate cancer. results from the göteborg randomised population-based prostate cancer screening trial. *Eur Urol* 2013; **63**(1):101–7.
44. Dahabreh IJ, Chung M, Balk EM, *et al.* Active surveillance in men with localized prostate cancer: a systematic review. *Ann Intern Med* 2012; **156**(8):582–90.
45. McVey GP, McPhail S, Fowler S, McIntosh G, Gillatt D, Parker CC. Initial management of low-risk localized prostate cancer in the UK: analysis of the British Association of Urological Surgeons Cancer Registry. *BJU Int* 2010; **106**(8):1161–4.
46. Cooperberg MR, Lubeck DP, Meng MV, Mehta SS, Carroll PR. The changing face of low-risk prostate cancer: trends in clinical presentation and primary management. *J Clin Oncol* 2004; **22**(11):2141–9.
47. Ahmed HU, Emberton M. Re: Focal therapy for localized prostate cancer: a critical appraisal of rationale and modalities. *J Urol* 2008; **180**(2):780–1; author reply 781–3.
48. Bergman J, Litwin MS. Quality of life in men undergoing active surveillance for localized prostate cancer. *J Natl Cancer Inst Monogr* 2012; **2012**(45):242–9.
49. Loeb S, Carter HB, Berndt SI, Ricker W, Schaeffer EM. Is repeat prostate biopsy associated with a greater risk of hospitalization? Data from SEER-Medicare. *J Urol* 2013; **189**(3):867–70.
50. Fujita K, Landis P, McNeil BK, Pavlovich CP. Serial prostate biopsies are associated with an increased risk of erectile dysfunction in men with prostate cancer on active surveillance. *J Urol* 2009; **182**(6):2664–9.
51. Hilton JF, Blaschko SD, Whitson JM, Cowan JE, Carroll PR. The impact of serial prostate biopsies on sexual function in men on active surveillance for prostate cancer. *J Urol* 2012; **188**(4):1252–8.
52. Glaser AP, Novakovic K, Helfand BT. The impact of prostate biopsy on urinary symptoms, erectile function, and anxiety. *Curr Urol Rep* 2012; **13**(6):447–54.
53. Crawford ED, Wilson SS, Torkko KC, *et al.* Clinical staging of prostate cancer: a computer-simulated study of transperineal prostate biopsy. *BJU Int* 2005; **96**(7):999–1004.
54. Barzell WE, Melamed MR. Appropriate patient selection in the focal treatment of prostate cancer: the role of transperineal 3-dimensional pathologic mapping of the prostate--a 4-year experience. *Urology* 2007; **70**(6 Suppl):27–35.
55. Onik G, Miessau M, Bostwick DG. Three-dimensional prostate mapping biopsy has a potentially significant impact on prostate cancer management. *J Clin Oncol* 2009; **27**(26):4321–6.
56. Lecornet E, Ahmed HU, Hu Y, *et al.* The accuracy of different biopsy strategies for the detection of clinically important prostate cancer: a computer simulation. *J Urol* 2012; **188**(3):974–80.
57. Hu Y, Ahmed HU, Carter T, *et al.* A biopsy simulation study to assess the accuracy of several transrectal ultrasonography (TRUS)-biopsy strategies compared with template prostate mapping biopsies in patients who have undergone radical prostatectomy. *BJU Int* 2012; **110**(6):812–20.
58. Ahmed HU, Hu Y, Carter T, *et al.* Characterizing clinically significant prostate cancer using template prostate mapping biopsy. *J Urol* 2011; **186**(2):458–64.
59. Gravas S, Mamoulakis C, Rioja J, *et al.* Advances in ultrasound technology in oncologic urology. *Urol Clin North Am* 2009; **36**(2):133–45, vii.
60. Pallwein L, Mitterberger M, Pelzer A, *et al.* Ultrasound of prostate cancer: advances. *Eur Radiol* 2008; **18**(4):707–15.
61. Pallwein L, Aigner F, Faschingbauer R, *et al.* Prostate cancer diagnosis: value of real-time elastography. *Abdom Imaging* 2008; **33**(6):729–35.
62. Braeckman J, Autier P, Soviany C, *et al.* The accuracy of transrectal ultrasonography supplemented with computer-aided ultrasonography for detecting small prostate cancers. *BJU Int* 2008; **102**(11):1560–5.
63. Turkbey B, Choyke PL. Multiparametric MRI and prostate cancer diagnosis and risk stratification. *Curr Opin Urol* 2012; **22**(4):310–5.
64. Padhani AR. Integrating multiparametric prostate MRI into clinical practice. *Cancer Imaging* 2011; 11 Spec No A:S27–37.
65. Epstein JI. Prognostic significance of tumor volume in radical prostatectomy and needle biopsy specimens. *J Urol* 2011; **186**(3):790–7.

66. Ahmed HU, Moore C, Emberton M. Minimally-invasive technologies in uro-oncology: The role of cryotherapy, HIFU and photodynamic therapy in whole gland and focal therapy of localised prostate cancer. *Surg Oncol* 2009; **18**(3):219–32.
67. Moore CM, Pendse D, Emberton M; Medscape. Photodynamic therapy for prostate cancer—a review of current status and future promise. *Nat Clin Pract Urol* 2009; **6**(1):18–30.
68. Lindner U, Weersink RA, Haider MA, *et al.* Image guided photothermal focal therapy for localized prostate cancer: Phase I Trial. *J Urol* 2009; **182**(4):1371–7.
69. Salvador-Morales C, Gao W, Ghatalia P, *et al.* Multifunctional nanoparticles for prostate cancer therapy. *Expert Rev Anticancer Ther* 2009; **9**(2):211–21.
70. Rubinsky J, Onik G, Mikus P, Rubinsky B. Optimal parameters for the destruction of prostate cancer using irreversible electroporation. *J Urol* 2008; **180**(6):2668–74.
71. Hossack T, Patel MI, Huo A, *et al.* Location and pathological characteristics of cancers in radical prostatectomy specimens identified by transperineal biopsy compared to transrectal biopsy. *J Urol* 2012; **188**(3):781–5.
72. Huo AS, Hossack T, Symons JL, *et al.* Accuracy of primary systematic template guided transperineal biopsy of the prostate for locating prostate cancer: a comparison with radical prostatectomy specimens. *J Urol* 2012; **187**(6):2044–9.
73. Taira AV, Merrick GS, Bennett A, *et al.* Transperineal template-guided mapping biopsy as a staging procedure to select patients best suited for active surveillance. *Am J Clin Oncol* 2013; **36**(2):116–20.
74. Onik G, Narayan P, Vaughan D, Dineen M, Brunelle R. Focal "nerve-sparing" cryosurgery for treatment of primary prostate cancer: a new approach to preserving potency. *Urology* 2002; **60**:109–114.
75. Onik G, Vaughan D, Lotenfoe R, Dineen M, Brady J. "Male lumpectomy": focal therapy for prostate cancer using cryoablation. *Urology* 2007; **70**(6 Suppl):16–21.
76. Ayres BE, Montgomery BS, Barber NJ, *et al.* The role of transperineal template prostate biopsies in restaging men with prostate cancer managed by active surveillance. *BJU Int* 2012; **109**(8):1170–6.
77. Bahn DK, Silverman P, Lee F Sr, Badalament R, Bahn ED, Rewcastle JC. Focal prostate cryoablation: initial results show cancer control and potency preservation. *J Endourol* 2006; **20**(9):688–92.
78. Bahn D, de Castro Abreu AL, Gill IS, *et al.* Focal cryotherapy for clinically unilateral, low-intermediate risk prostate cancer in 73 men with a median follow-up of 3.7 years. *Eur Urol* 2012; **62**(1):55–63.
79. Ellis DS, Manny TB Jr, Rewcastle JC. Focal cryosurgery followed by penile rehabilitation as primary treatment for localized prostate cancer: initial results. *Urology* 2007; **70**(6 Suppl):9–15.
80. Lambert EH, Bolte K, Masson P, Katz AE. Focal cryosurgery: encouraging health outcomes for unifocal prostate cancer. *Urology* 2007; **69**(6):1117–20.
81. Ward JF, Jones JS. Focal cryotherapy for localized prostate cancer: a report from the national Cryo On-Line Database (COLD) Registry. *BJU Int* 2012; **109**(11):1648–54.
82. Muto S, Yoshii T, Saito K, Kamiyama Y, Ide H, Horie S. Focal therapy with high-intensity-focused ultrasound in the treatment of localized prostate cancer. *Jpn J Clin Oncol* 2008; **38**(3):192–9.
83. Ahmed HU, Freeman A, Kirkham A, *et al.* Focal therapy for localized prostate cancer: A Phase I/II Trial. *J Urol* 2011; **185**(4):1246–54.
84. Ahmed HU, Hindley RG, Dickinson L, *et al.* Focal therapy for localised unifocal and multifocal prostate cancer: a prospective development study. *Lancet Oncol* 2012; **13**(6):622–32.

CHAPTER 6.9

High-risk prostate cancer

Steven Joniau, Siska Van Bruwaene, R. Jeffrey Karnes, Gert De Meerleer, Paolo Gontero, Martin Spahn, and Alberto Briganti

Introduction to high-risk prostate cancer

An important tenant in prostate cancer (PCa) is to identify and treat men who are at risk of suffering or dying from their disease, without over treating men with indolent cancer, who are likely to die of another cause. Defining these PCa patients who are at risk and selecting an appropriate treatment for everyone is an important, multidisciplinary challenge.

Defining high-risk prostate cancer

Definition

The outcome of PCa is strongly related to its TNM (tumour node metastasis) clinical stage, biopsy Gleason score (GS) and pre-treatment serum prostate-specific antigen (PSA) levels. Since no single criterion is able to adequately identify all patients with localized PCa who have a high likelihood of progression after therapy, a combination of the parameters seems preferable. In 1998, D'Amico *et al.*[1] defined high-risk localized PCa (i.e. >50% probability of PSA failure at five years after curative treatment) as stage cT2c, or PSA >20 ng/mL, or GS 8–10. These criteria were adopted by the American Association of Urology (AUA). In contrast, the European Association of Urology (EAU) guidelines and the National Comprehensive Cancer Network (NCCN) guidelines define high-risk PCa as stage ≥cT3a or PSA >20 ng/mL or GS 8–10.[2,3] Both guidelines also define very high-risk PCa as cT3b-T4 N0 (i.e. invasion in the seminal vesicles or adjacent structures) or any T with N1. Indeed, Epstein and co-workers[4] found that 10 years after radical prostatectomy (RP) only 27% of T3b patients and none of the patients with T4 disease or lymph node (LN) metastases were progression-free. Results were significantly better for men with localized disease (pT2) and either focal or established capsular penetration (pT3a) (84.7 vs. 67.7 and 58.4%, respectively).

At this moment, there is still no definitive consensus on the definition of high-risk PCa (Table 6.9.1). Importantly, whatever definition used, not all patients diagnosed with high-risk PCa have an invariably poor prognosis. Several reports indicate heterogeneous outcomes for groups defined as high-risk PCa patients. For example, Yossepowitch *et al.*[5] compared eight different definitions of high-risk PCa and reported a 5-year biochemical relapse free survival (BRFS) after RP that ranged from 49% to 80%. This means that further risk stratification within this group is important in order to identify patients that can be cured with local therapy, versus those that might benefit from a multimodality approach.

Table 6.9.1 Definitions of high-risk prostate cancer (PCa)

D'Amico[1]	PSA ≥20 ng/mL or Gleason sum 8–10 or Clinical stage ≥T2c
American Urological Association (AUA)	PSA ≥20 ng/mL or Gleason sum 8–10 or Clinical stage ≥T2c
National Comprehensive Cancer Network (NCCN)	PSA ≥20 ng/mL or Gleason sum 8–10 or Clincal stage ≥T3 or Any two of the following: T2b/c, Gleason sum 7, PSA 10–20 ng/mL
European Association of Urology (EAU)	PSA ≥20 ng/mL or biopsy Gleason 8–10 or clinical stage T3a or higher
Radiation Therapy Oncology Group (RTOG)	PSA 20–100 ng/mL Biopsy Gleason 8–10 and any clinical stage or clinical stage ≥T2c or PSA <100 ng/mL and Gleason 8–10

Source: data from D'Amico AV *et al*, 'Biochemical outcome after radical prostatectomy, external beam radiation therapy, or interstitial radiation therapy for clinically localised prostate cancer', *Journal of American Medical Association*, Volume 280, Number 11, pp. 969–974, Copyright © 1998 American Medical Association; Mohler JL *et al.*, National Comprehensive Cancer Network, *Clinical Practice Guidelines in Oncology: Prostate Cancer*, Copyright © 2012 National Comprehensive Cancer Network, available from: http://www.nccn.org/professionals/physician_gls/f_guidelines.asp; American Urological Association, Ian Thompson *et al.*, *Prostate Cancer: Guideline for the Management of Clinically Localized Prostate* Cancer: 2007 Update, Copyright © 2007 American Urological Association Education and Research, Inc., available from https://www.auanet.org/education/clinical-practice-guidelines.cfm; Heidenreich A *et al.*, European Association of Urology, *Guidelines on Prostate Cancer*, Copyright © 2012 Uroweb, available from: https://uroweb.org/guideline/prostate-cancer/; and Radiation Therapy Oncology Group (RTOG), Publication Table, Copyright © RTOG, available from https://www.rtog.org/Publications/PublicationsTable.aspx

Prevalence

Despite PSA screening and early detection of PCa, a fair proportion of patients still present at diagnosis with high-risk PCa. Indeed,

Cooperberg *et al.* evaluated the trend in high-risk PCa in the US between 1990–2007. This revealed the percentage of patients presenting with high-risk PCa defined by the NCCN definition, went from 27.4% in 1990–1994 to 21.7% in 1995–1999, to 26.3% in 2000–2003 and to 13.7% between 2004–2007.[6] Furthermore, in the published European Randomized Study of Screening for PCa (ERSPC), 9.8% of the patients had T3/T4 tumours and 8.8% had GS >7 in the screening arm, while in the control arm, these figures were 15.8% and 19.5%, respectively.[7] Interestingly, in the Rotterdam arm of the ERSPC trial, 76.8% of the men who developed metastasis and/or died from PCa despite screening were patients with high-risk PCa.[8]

Natural history

In discussions of high-risk prostate cancer, the age and co-morbidities of the patient should always be taken into account. Albertsen *et al.* showed that a higher co-morbidity score is associated with higher overall mortality and lower prostate cancer-specific mortality.[9] Furthermore, cancer-specific survival data for PCa patients treated conservatively without curative intent improved over the years. This is probably due to stage migration, overdiagnosis related to PSA testing or advances in medical care in general.[10] Albertsen *et al.* reported in 2005 the outcome of patients with localized PCa managed by observation or androgen deprivation therapy (ADT) alone.[11] They concluded that patients with high-grade PCa (Gleason 8–10) have a high probability of dying from PCa within 10 years of diagnosis (50–61%). Lu-Yao *et al.* presented a similar study in 2009, representing patients in the post PSA era.[10] In this study the 10-year cancer-specific mortality was only 25%. A Swedish study by Akre *et al.* in 2011 evaluated the mortality in a large cohort of men (12,184 patients) with locally advanced PCa (cT3 or cT4 or cT2 with PSA between 50 and 99 ng/mL) managed with non-curative intent. They described a cumulative PCa-specific mortality at eight years of follow-up of 52% in patients with biopsy GS 8 and 64% in those with biopsy GS 9-10 PCa.[12]

Most in 2012 Rider *et al.*[13] presented the 15-year mortality estimates for PCa death in non-curatively treated men in a nationwide population-based cohort in Sweden. Patients with high-risk PCa (T3 or PSA 20–50 ng/mL or GS ≥8) had a cumulative risk of PCa death of 35.5% rising to 49.1% in patients with more adverse features (T4 or N1 or PSA 50–100 ng/mL). When comparing all-cause mortality data with a matched comparison cohort (randomly selected men free of PCa) the curves for low-risk PCa were superimposed during the entire 15-year follow-up, the curves for intermediate-risk PCa only diverged after five years, while for both high-risk PCa and metastatic disease the curves clearly diverge soon after diagnosis.

Staging in high-risk prostate cancer

T-staging

Downstaging of clinical T3 prostate cancer (on digital rectal examination or ultrasound) to a pathological T2 tumour is relatively frequent and occurs in +/– 30% of cases (Table 6.9.2). This has an obvious consequence for prognosis. Briganti *et al.*, showed that patients with specimen-confined disease after RP (i.e. pT2-T3aR0N0 patients), have significantly higher 10-year cancer-specific survival (CSS) rates (98%) than patients with non-specimen-confined disease (88%).[14] On the other hand, depending on PSA and Gleason score, 6–68% of cT3a tumours were shown to be understaged, either invading the seminal vesicles (SVs) (pT3b) or neighbouring organs (pT4).[15] Downgrading to lower Gleason scores occurred in 34-55% of patients with poorly differentiated prostate cancer (Table 6.9.2). The probability of downgrading increased with lower clinical stages.[16] Downgraded cases showed significantly better biochemical progression-free survival (56% vs. 27%).[16] Interestingly, biopsy Gleason score remained strongly associated with progression even when controlling for the pathological Gleason score, so it can be incorporated independently into post-operative nomograms.[17]

Increasing evidence shows the superiority of magnetic resonance imaging (MRI) in the prediction of extraprostatic extensions when compared to digital rectal examination (DRE) or ultrasound.[18] A study showed overstaging in only 6% of patients and a clear impact on surgical strategy. Patients with imaging findings suggesting >cT2 were less likely to undergo neurovascular bundle sparing.[19] Likewise, MRI guided biopsies are significantly more representative of true Gleason grade.[20] Therefore, in a high-risk PCa population, preoperative MRI might be a useful tool in risk stratification to identify patients in whom primary cancer control is possible and in whom nerve-sparing techniques are a safe option.

Several nomograms and tools have been developed to predict pathological stage. The Partin tables have been widely used to predict the final pathological stage after RP based on combinations of preoperative serum PSA, biopsy Gleason sum, and clinical stage.[21] However, these tables were mainly based on data from patients with T1c–T2c PCa. Therefore, several tools have been developed to predict the pathology at RP in patients with clinical T3–4 PCa. Briganti *et al.* designed a nomogram—including pretreatment PSA, age, clinical stage, and biopsy Gleason sum—that can predict the presence of specimen-confined disease at RP with 72% accuracy.[14] In addition, Joniau *et al.*, using data from the European Multi-centre Prostate Cancer Clinical and Translational research group (EMPaCT), created a look-up table using a combination of pretreatment PSA and biopsy Gleason sum to predict final histopathology.[15]

N-staging

Computed tomography (CT) is a commonly used non-invasive procedure for PCa LN staging. In a study by Briganti *et al.*, the sensitivity, specificity, and accuracy of CT scan for LN staging in high-risk prostate cancer were only 52.3%, 50.5%, and 56.1%, respectively. They estimated that in the presence of pathologically defined LN invasion, CT scan would show positive findings only in roughly 2 of 10 patients with high-risk prostate cancer, suggesting that CT scan for preoperative nodal staging is no better than tossing a coin.[22] Notwithstanding these limitations, preoperative CT scan in high-risk PCa remains a reliable imaging modality to detect bulky and/or nodal disease that may prevent successful ablative surgery.[23]

The question of whether we can overcome these problems by using modern imaging techniques has yet to be solved.[23] In years, many functional imaging modalities were introduced, reflecting metabolic changes such as [11C] choline positron emission tomography (PET)-CT and tissue characteristics such as diffusion-weighted MRI. Although these modern imaging techniques seem to have great potential, their current resolution is too low to accurately detect LN metastases that are not detected by a contrast-enhanced CT scan.[24,25] In a small study of Budiharto *et al.*[26] sensitivity of [11C] choline PET-CT and diffusion-weighted MRI were only 9.4% and 18.8%, respectively. Until now, only high-resolution MRI with magnetic nanoparticles has proven to succeed in accurately detecting small and otherwise undetectable LN metastases in PCa patients, with an increase in sensitivity to 100% on a patient-based analysis.[27] Unfortunately, no magnetic nanoparticle agent is currently approved for diagnostic use nor has any type of study validated these findings or replicated, so sufficiently accurate imaging techniques are still lacking.

An alternative, or better a parallel tool to imaging is the use of nomograms to predict LN metastasis. Several nomograms have been developed to predict the patient's risk of lymph node invasion (LNI) based on pretreatment parameters (mainly PSA, clinical stage, Gleason sum).[28] However, most of them are based on findings derived from limited pelvic lymph node dissection (PLND), which should no longer be performed, as it misses at least half of the LNs involved.[29] Briganti *et al.* proposed a nomogram based on findings from extended PLND (ePLND)[30] and suggested a cut-off risk to perform a lymphadenectomy of 5%. Nomograms could provide additional information, both for urologists—helping them to guide surgical practice—and for radiation oncologists, helping them to better define radiation fields during treatment planning.

It is generally accepted that until now, pelvic LN dissection (LND) has proved to be the most accurate and reliable nodal staging procedure.[28–30] Both NCCN and EAU guidelines[2,3] indicate that at the time a RP is performed in (very) high-risk patients, it must be combined with an ePLND because LN involvement is common in these patients (up to 46%).[29]

M—staging

Skeletal metastases (M staging) are currently assessed by bone scan. Promising results have been reported with preoperative use of PET/CT scans with ^{18}F-fluorocholine and ^{18}F-fluoride in patients with high-risk prostate cancer and a negative or inconclusive bone scan. For 20% of the patients the results of the PET/CT scans changed the treatment plan.[25,31] Another study similarly showed that MRI of the axial skeleton identified metastases in seven (30%) of 23 patients considered negative and eight (47%) of 17 patients considered equivocal by other strategies (bone scan, targeted X-rays, and MRI on request), which altered the initially planned therapy.[32]

Risk stratification

In addition, to improve counselling of high-risk patients regarding their prognosis, there is a need for substratification of high-risk patients into prognostic categories. Retrospective analysis of data from the EMPaCT research group showed that the cumulative number of risk factors at diagnosis (i.e. PSA >20 ng/mL, biopsy Gleason sum ≥ 8 and clinical stage ≥ cT3), was significantly associated with unfavourable histopathology, clinical progression, adjuvant treatment, salvage treatment and increased cancer-specific mortality (CSM).[33] Similar conclusions were reached in a retrospective study on high-risk patients treated with external beam radiotherapy (EBRT) ± ADT.[34] Based on this idea, several nomograms were developed to predict either a patient's risk of biochemical or clinical recurrence after RP, or his risk of CSM after RP, using a combination of the primary risk factors pretreatment PSA, biopsy Gleason sum, and clinical stage. Unfortunately, most of these predictive tools were developed based on data from patients with cT1–2 PCa. Therefore, new nomograms for high-risk PCa patients are needed.

Alternatively, high-risk patients might be substratified into three prognostic subgroups based on particular combinations of the primary risk factors: (i) a good-prognosis subgroup, comprising patients with only a single risk factor; (ii) an intermediate-prognosis subgroup, with patients having a PSA >20 ng/mL and cT3–4; and (iii) a poor prognosis subgroup, including patients with biopsy Gleason sum 8–10 in combination with at least one other high-risk factor. The 10-year CSS rates were 95.4%, 88.3%, and 79.7% for the good-, intermediate- and poor-risk subgroups, respectively.[35] Therefore, patients in the good-prognosis subgroup might be treated adequately with RP alone, while in patients in the poor prognosis subgroup adjuvant treatment should be tested prospectively. As such, this easy-to-use model might facilitate patient counselling and might help clinical trial investigators in selecting a patient population that could benefit from (neo) adjuvant treatments.

To improve risk stratification, it has been proposed to add secondary risk factors to the 'standard' prognostic models, such as extent of cancer in the needle biopsy, pre-diagnosis PSA velocity >2 ng/mL/year, PSA-DT, cancer volume at initial diagnosis (i.e. % of positive biopsy cores) or presence of a tertiary Gleason pattern 5. However, the additional clinical value of these secondary risk factors remains uncertain, as some of these parameters are not routinely collected in clinical practice.[36,37] In addition, the potential prognostic value of several biomarkers is currently being explored. For high-risk prostate cancer, it was found that progressive downregulation of micro-RNA (miR) 221 in the RP specimen was associated with a poor prognosis. miR-221 even had a higher prognostic value than the Gleason sum, which is known to be one of the strongest predictors of tumour recurrence. Most likely, in the future, not a single biomarker but a combination of a multiple biomarkers will be needed to accurately predict outcomes for each individual patient.[38]

Radical prostatectomy for high-risk prostate cancer

The management of locally advanced and/or high-risk PCa is one of the most compelling contemporary challenges. In the absence of a randomized trial comparing the true benefit of currently available treatment modalities (i.e. surgery, radiation therapy (RT), ADT) or a combination of these, it is very difficult to properly counsel patients on the optimal treatment. Cooperberg *et al.* published the local variation and time trends in primary treatment of localized PCa.[39] Data were analysed from the Cancer of the Prostate Strategic Urologic Research Endeavor (CaPSURE) registry. PCa risk was assessed using the D'Amico risk groups. Of the 11,892 patients, 1,790 patients (15.1%) had high-risk PCa. Of those, 3.2% opted for active surveillance, 7.5% for brachytherapy, 18.1% for external RT, 32.8% for hormonal therapy, 6.1% underwent cryotherapy and 32.2% underwent RP. This means 36% of them did not receive local treatment and over 50% were delivered hormonal therapy as exclusive or adjunctive treatment (combined therapy with radiation). Rider *et al.*[13] reported even lower rates with only 27% of high-risk PCa patients receiving curative intent treatment.

Surgery for high-risk prostate cancer (GS >7, PSA >20, >cT2)

Historically, RP was not considered an acceptable treatment option for patients with high-risk non-metastatic PCa, due to the high incidence of positive section margins, positive pelvic LNs, and poor long-term survival rate. Nowadays, RP combined with an ePLND is a valid strategy accepted by international guidelines.[2,3] The putative benefits of RP as first-line treatment are to achieve tumour volume reduction and optimal local control. Furthermore, pathologic examination of the resection specimen and postoperative PSA allows for better treatment individualization by carefully selecting patients that require adjuvant treatment. In a study Spahn *et al.*[40] found that patients with pT3b disease with positive surgical margins at the bladder neck had the highest risk of death (five-year CSS 60.0% and overall survival 52.3%), while pT3a disease (regardless of positive surgical margin location and lymph node invasion) and pT3b tumours with negative bladder neck margins had eight-year prostate cancer specific survival and overall survival rates of 92.0% and 84.9%, respectively.

Indeed, in high-risk PCa, RP can often be combined with adjuvant RT or ADT. For instance, in a large retrospective analysis conducted by the Mayo Clinic, approximately 75% of patients with cT3 PCa were not controlled by surgery alone.[41] On the other hand up to 30% of patients are overstaged and are potentially cured with surgery alone. Briganti published CSM data of high-risk PCa patients treated with RP. CSM ranged from 5.9% to 9.8% at 10 years depending on age category[42] while the CSM rate in a non-curatively treated population reaches 28.8%.[11]

Large retrospective series have analysed the oncological outcomes of surgery in men with high-risk non-metastatic PCa. These data are shown in Table 6.9.2. Ten-year CSS and ten-year overall survival (OS) rates were excellent, varying respectively between 83% and 92% and between 70% and 77%. Even though more than half of the patients received adjuvant hormonal therapy and/or RT in most of the presented studies, the high CSS suggests that local cancer control remains important in men with locally advanced disease.

Table 6.9.2 Outcome after radical prostatectomy in high-risk prostate cancer

Study	Time span	N	Pathological outcomes (% of pts)						OS (% of pts)			CSS (% of pts)			Adjuvant/ salvage Tx (%)
			pT2	pT3a	pT3b	pN1	SM+	GS 8-10	5 y	10 y	15 y	5 y	10 y	15 y	
cT3a															
Ward (2005)[43]	1987–1997	841	27	—	—	27	56	18	90	76	53	95	90	79	78
Carver (2006)[44]	1983–2003	176	30	—	—	19	27	15	—	—	—	94	85	76	47
Hsu (2007)[45]	1987–2004	200	24	57	16	9	34	41	96	77	—	99	92	—	56
Freedland (2007)[46]	1987–2003	58	9	—	—	31	22	41	—	—	—	98	91	84	26
Yossepowitch (2008)[47]	1985–2005	243	22	—	—	23	26	28	—	—	—	96	89	—	—
Xylinas (2009)[48]	1995–2005	100	21	53	26	17	61	9	—	—	—	90	—	—	31
Stephenson (2009)[49]	1987–2005	254	—	—	—	—	—	—	—	—	—	—	85	62	—
Walz (2010)[50]	1987–2005	293	—	—	—	12	37	30	—	—	—	—	—	—	—
GS 8–10 at biopsy															
Donohue (2006)[51]	1983–2004	238	34	—	—	18	32	55	—	—	—	—	—	—	—
Bastian (2006)[52]	1982–2004	220	—	—	—	17	29	66	—	—	—	—	—	—	—
Yossepowitch (2008)[47]	1985–2005	401	35	—	—	19	30	52	—	—	—	96	88	—	—
Stephenson (2009)[49]	1987–2005	702	—	—	—	—	—	—	—	—	—	—	84	66	—
Walz (2010)[50]	1987–2005	269	—	—	—	14	38	45	—	—	—	—	—	—	—
PSA >20 ng/mL															
Zwergel (2007)[53]	1986–2005	275	21	42	33	28		49	87	70	58	93	83	71	≥47%
Magheli (2007)[54]	1984–2005	265	—	—	—	24	41	30	—	—	—	—	—	—	—
Yossepowitch (2008)[47]	1985–2005	441	33	—	—	15	46	16	—	—	—	97	91	—	—
Stephenson (2009)[49]	1987–2005	726	—	—	—	—	—	—	—	—	—	—	90	78	—
Walz (2010)[50]	1987–2005	370	—	—	—	16	46	11	—	—	—	—	—	—	—
Gontero (2011)[55]	1987–2005	712	21	28	38	24	55	26	90	73	—	95	89	—	≥50

pts: patients, OS: overall survival, CSS: cancer-specific survival, Tx: treatment, N: number of patients, y: years, SM+: positive section margin.

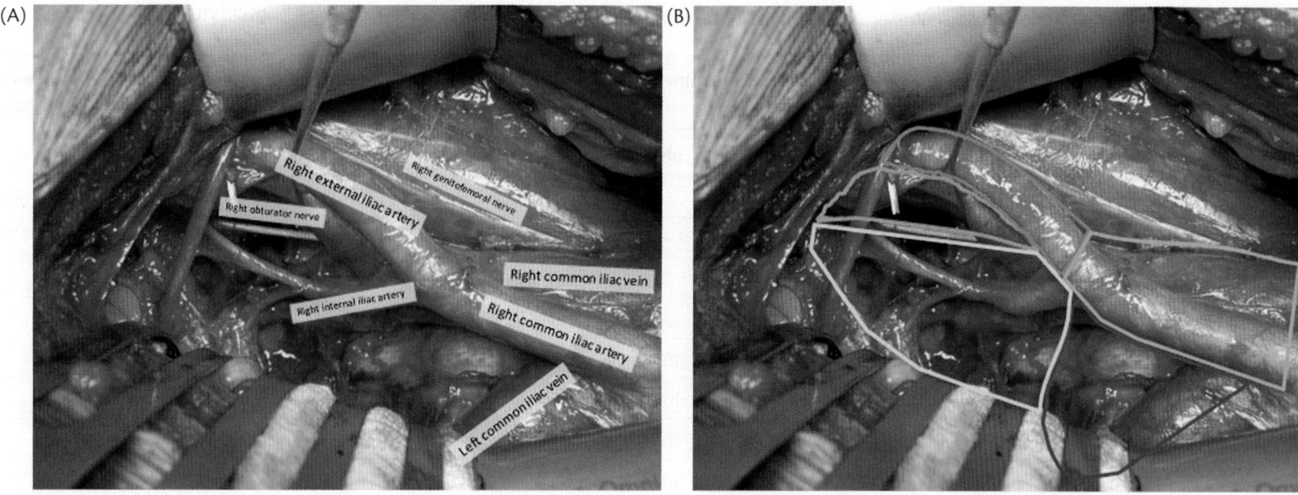

Fig. 6.9.1 Extended lymphadenectomy in prostate cancer. Lymph node dissection: external iliac region (blue); obturator fossa region (green); internal iliac region (yellow); common iliac region (orange); and presacral region (purple). (A) Denominates the different vessels. (B) Shows the different lymph node regions.

Reprinted from *European Urology*, Volume 63, Edition 3, Joniau S *et al.*, 'Mapping of Pelvic Lymph Node Metastases in Prostate Cancer', pp. 450–458, Copyright © 2015 European Association of Urology, with permission from Elsevier, http://www.sciencedirect.com/science/journal/03022838

Pelvic lymph node dissection

Both NCCN and EAU guidelines[2,3] indicate that when RP is performed in (very-) high-risk patients, it must be combined with an ePLND, because LN involvement is common in these patients (up to 45%).[29] The extent of PLND should be anatomically defined instead of counting the number of lymph nodes removed (see Fig. 6.9.1). Abdollah *et al.* promoted to use a cut-off number of 20 lymph nodes to obtain a 90% probability of correct staging.[56] However node density is variable between individuals. In the study of Joniau *et al.* a super-extended LND was performed in all patients but the number of lymph nodes retrieved ranged from 7 to 49.[29] For these reasons, the definition of adequate PLND in PCa should not be based on the number of lymph nodes removed but on the anatomical extent of dissection. The LND template should include at least bilateral removal of all lymphatic tissue in the obturator fossa and along the internal and the external iliac vessels.[2,57] The reason for this extensive approach resides in the anatomic complexity of lymphatic drainage of the prostatic gland. All urologists should be aware that limited PLND to the obturator fossa only is the equivalent of no PLND at all since half of patients with positive LN are missed (Table 6.9.3).[29] Therefore, this, would leave only two possible options: ePLND or no PLND.[58] Joniau *et al.* suggested including the presacral area in this ePLND template. This landing site was invaded by PCa in 9% of the cases (alone or in combination with other anatomic sites). Standard ePLND plus dissection of the presacral region would correctly stage 97% of patients and would remove all nodal metastases in 88% of them. This would improve staging without significantly increasing either complication rates or surgical time.[29] Dissection of the common iliac region did not improve the number of correctly staged N+ patients[29] and is probably a secondary landing site since no patients have been identified with positive common iliac nodes but negative lymph nodes in the lower pelvic areas.[29,59] Therefore, dissection of this area might be reserved for patients with more aggressive cancer features.

Table 6.9.3 Impact of the extent of lymphadenectomy on nodal staging and treatment

	Number of patients that were correctly staged	Number of patients in whom all positive LN were removed
Obturator fossa only	47%	15%
Extended LAD	94%	76%
Extended LAD + presacral	97%	88%
Extended LAD + presacral + common iliac	97%	97%

Source: data from *European Urology*, Volume 63, Issue 3, Steven Joniaua *et al.*, 'Mapping of Pelvic Lymph Node Metastases in Prostate Cancer', pp. 450–458, Copyright © 2012 European Association of Urology.

Surgery for very high-risk prostate cancer (T3b-T4 and N1)

Very high-risk PCa patients present two specific challenges: a need for local control as well as a need to treat any potential micrometastases. The optimal treatment approach usually necessitates multiple modalities. A population-based study used data from the Surveillance, Epidemiology and End Results (SEER) database and showed that clinical staging is highly accurate in predicting extraprostatic disease in this population. Only 4.7% and 15.8% of cT3b and T4 tumours, respectively, appeared to have organ-confined disease on pathology.[60]

Johnstone *et al.* also using the SEER database, showed that patients who underwent RP for cT4 PCa had a better survival than those who received ADT alone or RT alone and had a survival comparable with that of patients who received RT plus ADT.[61] The five-year CSS was 88% and the five-year OS was 73% (Table 6.9.4). Joniau *et al.* reported an excellent 10-year CSS of 91.9% in clinically T3b/T4 tumours with 25% of patients remaining free of additional therapies.[62] These results suggest that RP may be a reasonable step

Table 6.9.4 Outcome after radical prostatectomy in very high-risk prostate cancer

Study	Time span	N	Pathological outcomes (% of pts)							OS (% of pts)			CSS (% of pts)			Adjuvant Tx (%)
			pT2	pT3a	pT3b	pT4	pN1	SM+	GS 8–10	5 y	10 y	15 y	5 y	10 y	15 y	
cT3b-T4																
Johnstone (2006)[61]	1995–2001	72	33			43	—	—	—	73	—	—	88	—	—	31
Joniau (2012)[62]	1989–2004	51	8	29	45	18	22	63	—	88	71	—	92	92	—	65
Any T and N1																
Schumacher (2008)[63]	1989–2007	122	24	26	40	10	100	—	—	83	52	42	85	60	45	50
Da Pozzo (2009)[64]	1988–2002	250	8	15	61	16	100	62	33	—	—	—	89	80	—	100
Engel (2010)[65]	1988–2007	688	—	—	—	—	100	—	—	84	64	—	95	86	—	≥72
Steuber (2010)[66]	1992–2004	108	5	19	61	16	100	—	—	79	69	—	84	76	—	≥90
Briganti (2011)[67]	1988–2003	364	2	9	83	7	100	71	34	85	60	—	90	75	—	100

pts: patients; OS: overall survival; CSS: cancer-specific survival; Tx: treatment; N: number of patients; y: years; SM+: positive section margin.

in the context of a multimodality treatment approach in selected patients with cT3b-T4 PCa, provided that the tumour is not fixed to the pelvic wall or invaded into the urethral sphincter.

Although the incidence of LN metastasis has dramatically decreased in the PSA era, LN invasion is still diagnosed in up to 45% of patients submitted to extended PLND.[29] Historically, patients with LN invasion were considered to be affected by a systemic, non-curable disease and not considered suitable for a surgical approach. However, studies detail excellent survival outcomes after surgery for pathologically (but not clinically) positive LN, with 5-, 10- and 15-year CSS ranging from 84-95%, 51-86% and 45%, respectively. OS at 5, 10 and 15 years ranged from 79–85%, 36–69%, and 42%, respectively (Table 6.9.4).

Two retrospective studies have shown that, if patients show clinical evidence of LNI or if positive LNs are found during ePLND, patients still benefit from removal of the primary tumour.[65,66] Indeed, analysis of data from the Munich cancer registry showed significantly higher 5- and 10-year OS rates for the 688 N+ patients in whom RP was continued (84% and 64%, respectively), compared with the 250 N+ patients in whom RP was abandoned (60% and 28%, respectively).[65] Steuber *et al.* corroborated these observations in a single-centre study showing that 5- and 10-year CSS was significantly higher in the 108 N+ patients with completed RP (84% and 76%, respectively) than in the 50 N+ patients with aborted RP (81% and 46%, respectively). Thus, removing the primary tumour in patients who are N+ at the time of surgery (i.e. in very high-risk patients), can dramatically improve the patient prognosis.[66] Furthermore, both Schröder[68] and Messing[69] have investigated patients with surgically discovered nodal disease in EORTC and ECOG trials, respectively. Schröder investigated immediate or deferred hormonal therapy without treatment of the primary tumour. On the other hand, in the ECOG/Messing trial, immediate vs. deferred hormonal therapy was offered after radical prostatectomy and PLND. In the first study, overall five-year survival data were 63% and 69% respectively, which were worse than the five-year survival data of 90% and 74% in the Messing trial, respectively. Thus, this indirectly supports the concept of primary tumour treatment in high-risk disease.

The prognosis of node-positive patients is probably related to the number of lymph nodes involved supporting either the staging and/or therapeutic capabilities of an extended PLND over a limited one or none at all in high-risk disease. Schumacher[63] demonstrated that salvage ADT (at disease progression) was necessary in 36%, 41%, and 69% of patients with 1, 2, and >2 positive lymph nodes, respectively. When comparing patients with ≤2 or >2 positive nodes removed, median CSS at 10 years was 78.6% and 33.4%, respectively (p <0.001). Briganti *et al.*[70] confirmed these data showing a CSS at 15-year follow-up of 84% vs. 62%, for ≤2 or >2 positive nodes, respectively (p <0.001); thus, advocating more research to investigate a potential curative role of RP + PLND in this selected category of limited nodal disease patients.

Technical aspects/complications

Surgery for T3-4 patients clearly differs from RP for patients with low- or intermediate-risk PCa. It is a radical extirpation, including an ePLND, clean apical dissection, neurovascular bundle resection at the tumour-bearing side, complete resection of the SVs and resection of the bladder neck.[71] Gontero *et al.* compared the results of RP in very high-risk PCa with those having localized PCa. There were no significant differences in surgical morbidity except for blood transfusion, operative time, and lymphoceles.[72] Lerner[73] as well as Joniau[74] described complication rates that equal the results after RP for organ-confined disease. Joniau *et al.*[74] reported rectal injury and injury of the obturator nerve both in 0.7% of cases. Lymphatic leakage was noted in 2.2% of patients and 1.4% experienced prolonged drainage of urine. In 7.2%, wound-related problems occurred. Anastomotic stricture occurred in 2.9%. At 12 months, complete continence was 87.8% and erectile function had fully recovered in 6% and 10% of patients who underwent a non-nerve-sparing or unilateral nerve-sparing procedure, respectively. It is incumbent on the surgeon to be ready to perform such surgery which could involve wider margins of excision and a resultant more complex reconstruction depending on intraoperative findings to obtain the best local control of the primary.

Table 6.9.5 Characteristics of the randomized controlled trials comparing observation versus adjuvant RT after RP in pT3 or positive SM patients

Study	Study population	N (RT/obs)	% of pts with tPSA >0.2 ng/mL prior to randomization (RT/obs)	% of pts with SM+ (RT/obs)	Median FU (RT/obs)	Adjuvant EBRT regimen	Primary end point
SWOG 8,794 (Thompson *et al.* 2006,[78])	pT3N0M0	214/211	35%/32%	67%*/68%*	12.7 yr/ 12.5 yr	60–64 Gy to pelvis fossa	Metastasis-free survival
EORTC 22911 (Bolla *et al.* 2012,[79])	cT0-3pN0M0 + ≥ 1 pathological risk factor at RP (SVI, SM+, ECE)	502/503	10.7%	62.2%/63.0%	10.6 yr	50 Gy to prostate and SV + 10 Gy boost	BRFS
ARO 96-02/ AUO AP 09/ 95 (Wiegel *et al.* 2009,[80])	pT3-4pN0M0 + postoperative tPSA <0.1 ng/mL	114/154	0% (pts with tPSA ≥0.1 ng/mL excluded before randomization)	68%/61%	4.5 yr	60 Gy to prostate and SV	BRFS

*ECE or SM+.

ARO: Arbeitsgemeinschaft Radiologische Onkologie; AUO: Arbeitsgemeinschaft Urologische Onkologie; BRFS: biochemical recurrence-free survival; EBRT: external beam radiation therapy; ECE: extracapsular extension; EORTC: European Organisation for Research and Treatment of Cancer; ECE: extracapsular extension; FU: follow-up; obs: observation; pts: patients; RP: radical prostatectomy; RT: radiotherapy; SM+: positive surgical margins; SV(I): seminal vesicle (invasion); SWOG: Southwest Oncology Group; tPSA: total prostate-specific antigen; yr: year.

Adjuvant/salvage radiotherapy

Although some patients with high-risk PCa will benefit from RP alone, many patients with high-risk PCa will progress after surgery and require additional treatment with RT and/or ADT. The eradication of microscopic residual disease within the prostate bed after RP in high-risk prostate cancer can potentially be achieved with the use of RT by two distinct strategies: in the adjuvant setting shortly after surgery, but in the absence of any measurable PSA, or in the salvage setting at the time of biochemical recurrence (BCR) or later at clinical recurrence. The lack of randomized trials comparing adjuvant vs. salvage RT has created a longstanding dilemma: which one is best?

Three randomized controlled trials (RCT) have compared RP followed by immediate RT with RP alone in patients with pT3N0 PCa or with pT2 tumours and positive surgical margins (SM+) (Table 6.9.5). A meta-analysis, including these three RCTs, showed that adjuvant RT after RP improved OS, CSS, and metastasis-free survival only after 10 years compared with RP alone, but not after five years.[75] Local control and BRFS were improved both at 5 and at 10 years in the RP + RT group compared with the RP-alone group. An unpublished subgroup analysis also indicated that adjuvant RT provided a benefit in BRFS regardless of the presence of pathological risk factors at RP (SM+, extra capsular extension (ECE) and/or seminal vesicle invasion (SVI)).[76] In contrast, the benefit in OS was only seen in patients with SM+, ECE and/or SVI (data only for SWOG 8794 trial after median follow-up of 13.2 years). And even this survival advantage seems to disappear when correcting for concomitant disease.[77]

Important is the fact that the randomized population differed with respect to the postoperative PSA level prior to randomization for adjuvant RT between the three trials. In the German ARO 96-02 trial,[80] only men with a PSA <0.1 ng/mL were eligible for randomization, whereas in the EORTC trial[79] 11% had a PSA level >0.2 ng/mL prior to randomization. In the SWOG trial[78] this percentage was even higher (34%). This indicates that in the EORTC and SWOG trial a substantial number of patients received 'salvage' RT for a non-normalized PSA rather than adjuvant RT. In a subanalysis of the SWOG trial, Swanson *et al.*[81] showed that men in all categories of post-RP PSA level (<0.2, 0.2–1.0, >1.0 ng/mL) showed improvement of metastasis-free survival. But, a higher pre-radiation PSA resulted in a smaller advantage for radiotherapy compared to observation. This indicates that, although less effective in this study, also salvage RT may be beneficial to improve metastasis-free survival. Stephenson *et al.* created a nomogram and look-up table to assess the probability of six-year BPF survival after salvage RT.[82]

Three studies have attempted to compare adjuvant vs. salvage RT using a matched-controlled study design. Ost *et al.* matched 178 patients.[83] In the whole-group comparisons, the five-year BRFS of 84% favoured the adjuvant treatment group vs. 68% for salvage treatment group (p = 0.04). Subgroup analysis however, showed no difference between adjuvant and early salvage RT (eSRT) (PSA <0.5 ng/mL) with five-year BRFS of 92% versus 86%, respectively (p = 0.67). Trabulsi *et al.* compared 192 matched patients.[84] Again, the results favoured the adjuvant treatment group, with a five-year BRFS of 75% vs. 66% for salvage treatment group (p = 0.049). In this study the median PSA level before RT in the salvage cohort was 0.7 ng/mL, with a range of 0.2–2 ng/mL which represents a late salvage group. Therefore, Briganti *et al.*[85] published a match-controlled analysis of adjuvant versus eSRT (PSA pre-radiation ≤0.5 ng/mL). In contrast to the previous studies, these authors included in the eSRT arm also men without recurrence who therefore did not receive any salvage therapy. The proportion of these patients who were free from radiotherapy was comparable to what reported in the observational arm of the three previously mentioned prospective randomized studies testing the role of adjuvant RT.[75–77] The five-year BCR-free survival rates were 78.4% in aRT versus 81.8% in patients who underwent initial observation and eSRT in cases of relapse (p = 0.9). This suggests that timely administration of eSRT is comparable to aRT in improving BCR-free survival in the majority of pT3pN0 PCa patients. Therefore, eSRT may not compromise cancer control but significantly reduces overtreatment associated with aRT.

Four ongoing clinical trials which compare adjuvant RT with observation and early salvage RT (NCT00667069; Radiotherapy and Androgen Deprivation In Combination After Local Surgery (RADICALS) (ISRCTN40814031); RAVES (NCT00860652); EORTC 30041-22043, accessible at www.clinicaltrials.gov) will hopefully provide us with further answers to the lingering dilemma whether observation and early salvage RT is equally as good as adjuvant RT. Furthermore, these trials may clarify uncertainties related to differences in early and late toxicity between adjuvant versus early salvage RT.

Another relevant question concerns the dose that should be applied in the postoperative setting. It is beyond a doubt that in the primary setting a higher dose leads to better bRFS[86] and might reduce the risk of developing metastatic disease.[87,88] With modern technology, higher doses can be safely applied in the post-prostatectomy setting[89] as well and although not randomized, more evidence arises that also in the postoperative salvage setting,[90,91] a higher dose is beneficial. This is currently tested in the randomized SAKK 09/10 trial (accessible at http://sakk.ch/en/sakk-provides/our-trials/).

At present, the EAU guidelines stipulate that patients with pT3N0M0 should receive immediate postoperative EBRT to the surgical bed, upon recovery of urinary function, to improve OS and biochemical and clinical recurrence-free survival (RFS), with the highest impact for patients with SM+. It is only in the updated version of 2012 that early eSRT when PSA < 0.5 ng/mL is proposed as optional.[2] Similarly, the NCCN guidelines indicate that adjuvant/salvage RT after RP should be offered to all men with adverse pathological or laboratory features or detectable PSA and no evidence of disseminated disease.[3]

Adjuvant/salvage hormone therapy

There are currently no strong data available to suggest that the use of adjuvant ADT after surgery for locally advanced PCa is associated with a significant survival benefit. In the Early PCa (EPC) trial programme, the administration of oral bicalutamide 150 mg/day to surgically-treated patients with locally advanced disease (T3-T4) was not associated with an improvement in OS.[92] Similarly, Wirth *et al.* did not show a significant difference in OS in the ADT arm compared with the RP-only arm in 309 men with pT3-4N0 PCa after a median follow-up of 6.1 years.[93] On the other hand, Dorff *et al.* described the results of the SWOG-S9921 study[94] with two years of adjuvant ADT alone or in combination with mitoxantrone chemotherapy after RP for high-risk PCa (GS ≥ 8; preoperative PSA ≥ 15 ng/mL; pT3b, pT4, or pN1 or N1 disease; or GS of 7 with either preoperative PSA >10 ng/mL or a positive margin). They reported excellent OS of 96% at five years and 88% at eight years in the ADT-alone arm. The authors concluded that two years of ADT after RP resulted in an extremely low rate of disease recurrence and PCa-related death for high-risk PCa patients in SWOG-S9921. These data seem to support the consideration of adjuvant ADT in patients with high-risk PCa after RP and perhaps adjuvant ADT is best accomplished with LH-RH agonists rather than oral non-steroidal antiandrogens. Schubert *et al.*[95] performed a retrospective case matched analysis of 172 high-risk PCa patients from the EMPaCT database with positive section margins or non-organ-confined disease and negative lymph nodes to receive adjuvant ADT (group 1, n = 86) or no adjuvant ADT (group 2, n = 86). Estimated 5–10-year clinical progression-free survival was 96.9% (94.3%) for group 1 and 73.7% (67.0%) for group 2, respectively (p <0.01). Subgroup analysis showed that patients with T2/T3a tumours are at low-risk for metastatic disease and cancer-related death and do not need adjuvant ADT while they identified men with T3b margin positive disease at highest risk for clinical progression which therefore might benefit from immediate adjuvant ADT. This is concordant with the data of Spahn *et al.* who identified T3b patients with positive surgical margins at the bladder neck at highest risk of progression.[40]

Further, early ADT has been reported to provide a survival benefit in patients with nodal metastases in the Messing trial (ECOG 3886). In an assessment of 98 patients with nodal metastases who had undergone prostatectomy and lymphadenectomy, after a median follow-up of 11.9 years, immediate ADT was associated with a significant improvement in OS (HR 1.84, 95% CI: 1.01–3.35, p = 0.04), CSS (HR 4.09, 95% CI: 1.76–9.49, p = 0.0004) and CPFS (HR 3.42, 95% CI: 1.96-5.98, p <0.0001) compared with deferred ADT.[69] Nevertheless, this was a small study including patients before the PSA era with large cancer volumes, high proportion of seminal vesicle invasion, positive margins, and bulky nodal disease and were therefore at very high risk of recurrence, regardless of their LN status.[96] Patients were either given immediate adjuvant ADT or late ADT at the appearance of symptoms. Nowadays, patients usually present with lower stage/lower volume disease and mostly present with low-burden nodal disease. Furthermore, PSA is an extremely useful parameter during follow-up, allowing early salvage RT/ADT. Thus, it is unclear whether the conclusions drawn from this study are still valid at present. Notably, two retrospective studies in N+ patients failed to show a survival benefit with adjuvant ADT after RP.[97,98] Nevertheless, adjuvant ADT is still indicated in the EAU and NCCN guidelines for N+ patients after RP.[2,3]

The potential benefit of neoadjuvant ADT before RP in patients with high-risk non-metastatic PCa has been investigated in two systematic reviews.[99,100] These studies concluded that neoadjuvant ADT before RP reduces positive SM+ rates, organ confinement, and LNI, but does not significantly improve OS or CSS. Accordingly, neoadjuvant ADT before RP is not recommended in the EAU guidelines nor in the NCCN guidelines.[2,3] However, three abstracts have investigated whether more extensive androgen suppression prior to RP could improve pathological and biochemical outcomes in patients with high-risk localized PCa.[101–103] For that purpose, standard ADT—using luteinizing hormone-releasing hormone agonists, which inhibit androgen production by the testes—was combined with other agents targeting the androgen signalling pathway[104] like the 5α-reductase inhibitor dutasteride, the CYP17 inhibitors ketoconazole or abiraterone acetate and the androgen receptor inhibitor (antiandrogen) bicalutamide. All three studies demonstrated that neoadjuvant total androgen suppression can improve pathological and biochemical outcomes compared with standard ADT. However, the impact of this new neoadjuvant approach on survival remains to be investigated.

Adjuvant/salvage combination radiotherapy and hormone therapy

In a retrospective study done by Briganti *et al.*, 117 pT2-4pN1 patients treated with adjuvant ADT + RT (whole pelvis) were compared with 247 pT2-4pN1 patients treated with adjuvant ADT alone.[105] Patients in the RT + ADT group had significantly higher CSS and OS rates compared with patients in the ADT-alone group at 5, 8, and 10 years after RP, regardless of the extent of LNI. These results indicate that a multimodal approach might be optimal for node-positive patients after RP. But also in node-negative patients, the addition of ADT to high-dose radiotherapy in the adjuvant setting significantly improved bRFS and cRFS with a hazard ratio of 0.2.[106]

Regarding the node-negative group, several RCTs have been initiated to explore the potential benefits of combining adjuvant RT and ADT in patients with adverse pathological features after RP. These include the UK Medical Research Council RADICALS trial, the EORTC 30041-22043 trial, and the radiation therapy oncology group (RTOG) 96-01 trial (accessible at www.clinicaltrials.gov). Preliminary data from the RTOG 96-01 trial after a median follow-up of 7.1 years suggested that addition of two years of antiandrogens (bicalutamide) to RT can reduce the incidence of PSA progression and metastasis in patients with SM+, ECE and/or SVI and elevated PSA after RP.[99] The RTOG 96-01 trial is the first trial showing an overall survival benefit in favour of the combined treatment arm. Final data from the other trials are awaited to confirm this result.[107]

Thus, it is clear that several treatment options (RP, RT, ADT, CT) might be combined in (very) high-risk patients, either sequentially or simultaneously. The EAU guidelines emphasize that management decisions for patients with (very) high-risk PCa should be made after all treatments have been discussed by a multidisciplinary team (including urologists, radiation oncologists, medical oncologists, and radiologists). It is also of paramount importance to inform the patient about the likelihood of such a multimodality approach. In addition, the balance of the benefits and side effects of each treatment modality should been considered by the patients with regard to their own individual circumstances.[2]

Radiotherapy for high-risk prostate cancer

External beam radiation therapy

As monotherapy, external beam radiation therapy (EBRT) has only a modest success rate in patients with high-risk localized PCa. Indeed, in the EBRT alone arm of the RTOG 86-10[108] and RTOG 85-31 trials[109] only 10 and 21% of patients were free from biochemical recurrence five years after RT (44–46 Gy to the pelvic lymph nodes and 65–70 Gy to the prostatic bed), respectively. Therefore, EBRT as monotherapy should not be considered as a valid treatment option in HRPC.

High-dose, hypofractionated radiotherapy

To reduce the risk of biochemical failure, i.e. to achieve sufficient local control, dose escalation is essential, as shown in a meta-analysis by Viani *et al.*[110] Therefore, 74 Gy is currently recommended as a minimum dose (in combination with ADT) in the EAU guidelines.[2] Nowadays, several RT techniques are available that can deliver high radiation doses to the prostate without increasing the risk of morbidity, including intensity-modulated RT (IMRT) with or without image-guided RT (IGRT), stereotactic body RT, dose-escalated three-dimensional conformal RT (3D-CRT) and EBRT combined with low-dose-rate brachytherapy (LDR-BT; radioactive seed implantation) or high-dose-rate brachytherapy (HDR-BT). However, good quality data comparing these methods are scarce. In a systematic review of 182 publications,[111] EBRT combined with HDR-BT was associated with superior biochemical control and overall survival compared with EBRT alone (≥75 Gy). Although these results should be interpreted with caution—as the different treatment cohorts were not balanced for baseline variables, patients were not stratified according to their progression risk, and the definition of biochemical control differed among studies—the conclusion of this systematic review was confirmed in a RCT in 218 patients with localized PCa, with >50% of them being high-risk patients.[112] After a median follow-up of 7.1 years, EBRT (35.75 Gy in 13 fractions) followed by a HDR-BT boost (2 × 8.5 Gy in 24 h) resulted in a significant improvement in biochemical/clinical RFS and a 31% reduction in the risk of recurrence ($p = 0.01$) compared with EBRT alone (55 Gy in 20 daily fractions). However, there were no significant differences in OS, and the incidence of severe late urinary and rectal toxicity was similar between both treatment groups. Another RCT in 168 high-risk patients showed that hypofractionation (62 Gy in 20 fractions in five weeks (equivalent to a delivered dose of 75 Gy)) might improve biochemical RFS (BRFS) after three years compared with conventional fractionation (80 Gy in 40 fractions in eight weeks) 3D-CRT,[113] without increase in late toxicity. Together, these data indicate that high radiation doses to the prostate are key to achieve local control. However, more RCTs comparing the different techniques, doses, and dose fractionation schedules are urgently awaited before definite conclusions can be drawn.

Radiotherapy and (neo)adjuvant androgen deprivation therapy

As monotherapy with conventional-dose EBRT only yielded modest success rates in patients with high-risk PCa, it was investigated in many trials whether addition of neoadjuvant, concomitant and/or adjuvant ADT could increase efficacy. Indeed, as PCa is a hormone-dependent tumour, ADT was hypothesized (i) to reduce the tumour size before RT, enabling optimal targeting of the prostate while avoiding morbidity to the surrounding tissues; (ii) to induce apoptosis and to enhance radiosensitivity; and (iii) to reduce the risk of distant metastases by eliminating micrometastases that persist within the prostate after primary RT.[114]

The trials evaluating the potential benefit of adding ADT to RT in patients with high-risk non-metastatic PCa have been summarized in several systematic reviews and meta-analyses.[114–118] All of them concluded that addition of ADT to RT significantly improves OS and prostate CSS compared with RT alone. The results of the meta-analysis done by Bria *et al.*,[115] including seven trials and 4,387 patients (Table 6.9.5), confirm this.

Compared with RT alone, addition of neoadjuvant, concomitant and/or adjuvant ADT to RT decreased the risk of PCa-specific mortality (–24%), all-cause mortality (–14%), biochemical failure (–24%), clinical progression (–19%), local relapse (–36%), and distant metastases (–28%). Pooling of toxicity data did not show any significant differences in overall genitourinary or gastrointestinal toxicity, nor in cardiac deaths between both treatment arms. In contrast, some trials suggested that the toxicity associated with ADT might become more obvious—and even affect survival—in patients with co-morbidities such as cardiovascular disease.[119–120]

With regard to the optimal duration of adjuvant ADT in patients with high-risk PCa, two major trials demonstrated that long-term adjuvant ADT to RT significantly improves survival compared with short-term ADT. The EORTC 22961 non-inferiority trial reported five-year overall mortality rates of 19.0% in 483 men receiving adjuvant ADT for six months vs. 15.2% in 487 men receiving adjuvant ADT for three years.[121] Similarly, the RTOG 92-02 trial reported an improved 10-year OS and CSS in 166 patients with Gleason sum 8–10 receiving long-term (24 months) ADT + RT compared with 171 men receiving short-term (four months) ADT + RT.[122] Consequently, long-term ADT prior to and during EBRT is

Table 6.9.6 Overview of RCTs with neoadjuvant, concomitant or adjuvant ADT to RT, included in the meta-analysis done by Bria *et al.*[107]

Studies included in meta-analysis	Study population	# randomized pts	Treatment	Median follow-up
Neoadjuvant and concomitant ADT to RT				
TTROG 96-01 (Denham *et al.* 2005,[125]; Denham *et al.* 2012,[126])	T2b-4 N0 M0	818	RT alone (66 Gy to prostate and SV)vs RT + 2-mo neoadjuvant ADT + 1-mo concomitant ADT vs RT + 5-mo neoadjuvant ADT + 1-mo concomitant ADT	5.9 yr
RTOG 86-10 (Pilepich *et al.* 2002,[108]; Roach *et al.* 2008,[127])	T2-T4 N0-x M0	456	RT alone (44-46 Gy to WP + 21-24 Gy boost to prostate) vs RT + 2-mo neoadjuvant ADT + 2-mo concomitant ADT	12.6 yr
Concomitant and long-term adjuvant ADT to RT				
EORTC 22861 (Bolla *et al.* 2002,[128]) EORTC 22863[129]	T1-T2 grade 3 M0 or T3-T4 N0-1 M0	415	RT alone (50 Gy to WP; 20 Gy boost to prostate and SV) vs RT + 3-yr concomitant and adjuvant ADT	9.1 yr
Long-term adjuvant ADT to RT				
RTOG (Bolla *et al.* 2008,[109]; Pilepich *et al.* 2005,[130])	cT1-T2 N1 M0 or cT3-4 N0-1 M0 or pT3 after RP	977	RT alone (44-46 Gy to WP + 21-24 Gy boost to prostate) vs RT + adjuvant ADT until progression	7.6 yr
EPCP (See *et al.* 2006,[131])	T1-4 Nx-1 M0	1370	RT alone (64 Gy)vs RT + adjuvant ADT (median 1.8 yr)	7.2 yr
Neoadjuvant, concomitant, and adjuvant HT to RT				
L-101 (Laverdière *et al.* 2004,[132])	cT2-T3	161	RT alone (64 Gy) vs RT + 3-mo neoadjuvant ADT vs RT + 10-mo neoadjuvant, concomitant, and adjuvant ADT	5 yr
(D'Amico *et al.* 2008,[120])	cT1b-T2b N0 M0 and PSA > 10 ng/mL, Gleason sum 7–10, or radiographic evidence of extraprostatic disease	206	RT alone (3D-CRT) vs RT + 6-mo neoadjuvant, concomitant, and adjuvant ADT	7.6 yr

3D-CRT: 3-dimensional conformal radiation therapy; ADT: androgen-deprivation therapy; EORTC: European Organisation for Research and Treatment of Cancer; EPC: Early Prostate Cancer Programme; HT: hormone therapy; mo: month(s); PSA: prostate-specific antigen; RP: radical prostatectomy; RT: radiotherapy; RTOG: Radiation Therapy Oncology Group; SV: seminal vesicles; TTROG: Trans-Tasman Radiation Oncology Group; WP: whole pelvis; yr: year.

Reprinted from *International Journal of Radiation Oncology*Biology*Physics*, Volume 78, Issue 3, Supplement 1, W.U. Shipley, D. *et al.*, 'Initial Report of RTOG 9601: A Phase III Trial in Prostate Cancer: Anti-androgen Therapy (AAT) with Bicalutamide during and after Radiation Therapy (RT) Improves Freedom from Progression and Reduces the Incidence of Metastatic Disease in Patients following Radical Prostatectomy (RP) with pT2-3, N0 Disease, and Elevated PSA Levels', p. S27, Copyright © 2010, with permission from Elsevier, http://www.sciencedirect.com/science/journal/03603016

recommended both in the EAU guidelines (three years) and in the NCCN guidelines (two to three years).

However, it should be noted that in the majority of trials comparing ADT + RT with RT alone, the radiation doses were suboptimal (usually whole pelvic fields to 50 Gy, with a subsequent boost to the prostate; total dose ≤70 Gy) (Table 6.9.6). Hence, it might be possible that ADT was mainly required to compensate for the inadequate radiation doses that were used at that time.[123,124] As such, new RCTs are needed to reinvestigate the value of adding ADT to RT in contemporary RT settings (IMRT/IGRT, dose-escalated 3D-CRT, HDR-BT, and so on), using adequate doses for patients with high-risk PCa.

Whole-pelvic versus prostate-only (+ seminal vesicles) radiotherapy

In addition, it should be reinvestigated whether radiation to the whole pelvis is required in patients at high-risk of LN invasion or whether it can be restricted to the prostate and SVs. Indeed, the results of the RTOG 94-13[133,134] and the GETUG-1 trials[135] have evoked quite some debate,[136,137] both on the need for pelvic LN irradiation and on the selection of patients who would benefit from it. The Roach formula ([2/3 × PSA] + [Gleason score − 6] × 10) was shown to be still an accurate tool for predicting nodal involvement in contemporary PCa patients,[138] however the authors provoked a cut-off for pelvic irradiation of 6% instead of the conventional 15%. Hence, the formula is used for patient selection in the ongoing RTOG 09-24 trial, which compares whole-pelvic RT with RT to the prostate and SVs only—both in combination with neoadjuvant ADT and with a RT boost to the prostate and the SVs—in patients with unfavourable intermediate-risk and favourable high-risk PCa (www.clinicaltrials.com). IMRT will be used as radiation technique, as it appeared to be better than 3D-CRT for targeting the pelvic LNs while minimizing damage to other pelvic organs such as the rectum and the bladder.[139] Hopefully, the results of this ongoing trial, which is expected to be completed by the end of 2019, will answer the remaining questions.

Radiotherapy versus surgery

Unfortunately, there are no contemporary RCTs comparing RP with RT for patients with high-risk non-metastatic PCa.[140] To date, only data from observational studies are available.

A large retrospective study from the Memorial Sloan-Kettering Cancer Centre (MSKCC) compared metastasis-free survival rate in cT1-3 patients treated either with IMRT (≥81 Gy) or with RP + ePLND (done by experienced high-volume surgeons) between 1993 and 2002.[141] After adjustment for case mix, surgery was associated with a reduced risk of metastasis compared with RT. However, it should be noted that in the RT group, pelvic LNs were not irradiated. Moreover, high-risk patients did not receive long-term adjuvant ADT, although this has been shown to improve survival compared with RT alone (see above). In addition, salvage therapy was offered more quickly after recurrence to patients treated with primary RP (within a median time of 13 months) than to patients treated with primary RT (within a median time of 69 months). Therefore, it is likely that the RT results would not have been significantly different from the RP outcomes, if pelvic LNs had been irradiated and if long-term adjuvant ADT and/or (salvage) brachytherapy boosts had been given.[140] Similar data were obtained from the CaPSURE registry, including 7,538 men with localized PCa treated between 1987 and 2007. These results indicated that, compared with RP, and after adjusting for age, disease risk, and co-morbidity, the risk of dying of PCa was about twofold greater (HR = 2.21; 95% CI: 1.50–3.24) in patients who received EBRT, and about threefold greater (HR = 3.22; 95% CI: 2.16–4.81) in patients who received primary ADT monotherapy.[142] Interestingly, differences between treatment modalities were the largest in the high-risk group. However, this study had similar limitations as the above-mentioned study from the MSKCC: CaPSURE did not include consistent data on radiation dose and technique, only about two-thirds of the high-risk patients receiving EBRT also received neoadjuvant and/or adjuvant ADT, and there were insufficient events to control adequately for type and timing of salvage therapies.

Several retrospective studies focused specifically on high-risk patients. Arcangeli *et al.* compared 122 high-risk patients who underwent RP with 162 high-risk patients who underwent EBRT (80 Gy) ± ADT (nine months) between 2003 and 2007.[143] Patients with adverse pathological features at RP underwent adjuvant EBRT (66 Gy) ± adjuvant ADT. Both groups were balanced for clinical stage, biopsy Gleason sum, and initial PSA. After three years, biochemical failure was significantly more likely in the RP group (30.2%) than in the EBRT ± ADT group (13.2%) ($p = 0.001$). In contrast, in a competing-risks survival analysis in 132,706 high-risk patients with clinically localized PCa from 17 SEER registries (1988–2006), RP was associated with a lower CSM than RT in patients aged ≤69 years, but with a higher CSM in patients >70 years old.[144] Again, in this study, data on adjuvant or salvage ADT, and on RT doses and techniques were lacking. Boorjian *et al.* analysed data from high-risk patients treated between 1988 and 2004.[145] He did not find any significant differences in CSM between the RP group (N = 1,238) and the EBRT + ADT group (N = 344) (median RT dose: 72 Gy, including pelvic LNs; median duration of adjuvant ADT: 22.8 months) after adjustment for case mix. However, the risk of all-cause mortality was greater after EBRT + ADT than after RP. Thus, in the quest for the optimal treatment modality, impact of treatment on non-cancer-related mortality and on QoL should be considered as well. This was also emphasized in a decision analysis model, indicating that the choice of the optimal treatment modality for high-risk PCa patients is very sensitive to small increases in the risk of all-cause mortality.[146]

Although the data from these observational studies might give us some guidance, they should be interpreted with caution.[140,144] As indicated above, data on radiation dose and technique, and on adjuvant and salvage therapies were often lacking or inconsistent. Moreover, these studies were unable to account for the evolution in RP and RT techniques during the relatively long treatment periods, and for possible confounders such as PSA. Finally, and most importantly, these retrospective series suffered from selection bias due to a lack of randomization among treatment groups. This was clearly demonstrated by Giordano *et al.*, showing that patients who underwent RP for PCa actually had better survival outcomes than a control population of patients without cancer.[147] Therefore, we can conclude that, as long as there are no data from RCTs showing a clear benefit of one treatment option over another, no single treatment can be universally recommended. Very often, a multimodality approach is warranted to optimize patient outcomes,[140] and this treatment should be tailored to the patient's individual situation and preferences.

ADT for high-risk PCa

Ever since Huggins and Hodges demonstrated >70 years ago that PCa is an androgen-dependent cancer.[148,149] ADT has become the mainstay for (symptomatic) metastatic PCa management. It is used to palliate symptoms, delay progression and prevent potentially catastrophic complications (e.g. spinal cord compression, pathological fractures, ureteral obstruction). More ADT has also been increasingly used in patients with non-metastatic disease and in patients with PSA relapse after RP or RT, either as monotherapy, or as part of a multimodality approach.

The benefit of treating patients with high-risk prostate cancer locally over primary endocrine treatment is very clear for surgery (CSM in reference 11 versus 42) as well as for radiotherapy.[150] However, according to a French non-interventional study, 16.6% of all PCa patients had a contraindication to local therapy and therefore received ADT in a localized disease stage.[151] There is currently no conclusive evidence that ADT as monotherapy prolongs survival.[2] Indeed, a large population-based cohort study indicated that immediate primary ADT did not increase OS compared with conservative management (no RP, RT or ADT), not even in elderly men with poorly differentiated (i.e. high-grade) localized PCa.[152] Similarly, the Early Prostate Cancer Programme (EPCP)—comprising of three RCTs comparing ADT (150 mg bicalutamide once daily) with watchful waiting—showed a trend towards decreased OS in the ADT group in men with localized (T1-2N0-x) disease. However, in men with locally advanced/high-risk (T3-4, any N; any T, N+) PCa, ADT tended to improve OS.[153] Thus, it is clear that, if there is a survival benefit of primary ADT in patients with high-risk PCa, it is only modest. Moreover, it should be outweighed against the side effects of prolonged (or even lifelong) ADT, such as cardiovascular morbidity, peripheral artery disease, venous thromboembolism, metabolic syndrome, osteoporosis, fatigue, erectile dysfunction, and so on.[9,154,155] Probably initiation of ADT as monotherapy is best guided by baseline PSA and/or PSA doubling time

(PSA-DT). Indeed, a subanalysis of the EORTC 30891 trial showed that patients with a baseline PSA >50 ng/mL and/or PSA-DT <12 months had an increased risk of dying from PCa.[156] Therefore, these patients might benefit from immediate ADT.

Chemotherapy and future perspectives

It is likely that some patients with high-risk localized PCa have occult micrometastases at diagnosis, which would explain that they are unlikely to be cured by local therapy alone. In analogy with other types of carcinoma (e.g. breast, colon, lung), neoadjuvant or adjuvant chemotherapy are being explored in phase 2 and 3 trials with the hope to help improve the curative rate of definitive therapies.

It is currently investigated whether addition of chemotherapy to ADT after RP might improve outcomes in patients with high-risk non-metastatic PCa. Unfortunately, the SWOG 99-21 trial comparing two years of ADT alone with ADT plus six cycles of mitoxantrone and prednisone in 983 men with high-risk features at RP was halted prematurely due to three cases of acute myelogenous leukaemia in the chemotherapy arm.[157] Other trials exploring the potential benefit of (neo)adjuvant chemotherapy in patients with high-risk non-metastatic PCa—either in combination with RT, RP and/or ADT—are ongoing.[158]

Further reading

Bolla M, Collette L, Blank L, *et al.* Long-term results with immediate androgen suppression and external irradiation in patients with locally advanced prostate cancer (an EORTC study): a phase III randomised trial. *Lancet* 2002; **360**(9327):103–6.

Bolla M, Van Poppel H, Tombal B, *et al.* European Organisation for Research and Treatment of Cancer, Radiation Oncology and Genito-Urinary Groups. Postoperative radiotherapy after radical prostatectomy for high risk prostate cancer: long-term results of a randomized controlled trial (EORTC trial 22911). *Lancet* 2012; **380**(9858):2018–27.

Briganti A, Spahn M, Joniau S, *et al.* on behalf of the European Multicenter Prostate Cancer Clinical and Translational Research Group (EMPaCT). Impact of age and comorbidities on long-term survival of patients with high-risk prostate cancer treated with radical prostatectomy: A multi-institutional competing-risks analysis. *Eur Urol* 2013; **63**(4):693–701.

Briganti A, Wiegel T, Joniau S, *et al.* Early salvage radiation therapy does not compromise cancer control in patients with pT3N0 prostate cancer after radical prostatectomy: results of a match-controlled multi-institutional analysis. *Eur Urol* 2012; **62**(3):472–87.

Joniau S, Van den Bergh L, Lerut E, *et al.* Mapping of pelvic lymph node metastases in prostate cancer. *Eur Urol* 2013; **63**(3):450–8.

McLeod DG, Iversen P, See WA, Morris T, Armstrong J, Wirth MP. Casodex Early Prostate Cancer Trialists' Group. Bicalutamide 150 mg plus standard care vs standard care alone for early prostate cancer. *BJU Int* 2006; **97**(2):247–54.

Messing EM, Manola J, Yao J, *et al.* Eastern Cooperative Oncology Group study EST 3886. Immediate versus deferred androgen deprivation treatment in patients with node-positive prostate cancer after radical prostatectomy and pelvic lymphadenectomy. *Lancet Oncol* 2006; 7(6):472–9.

Partin AW, Mangold LA, Lamm DM, Walsh PC, Epstein JI, Pearson JD. Contemporary update of prostate cancer staging nomograms (Partin Tables) for the new millennium. *Urology* 2001; **58**(6):843–8.

Rider JR, Sandin F, Andrén O, Wiklund P, Hugosson J, Stattin P. Long-term outcomes among noncuratively treated men according to prostate cancer risk category in a nationwide, population-based study. *Eur Urol* 2013; **63**(1):88–96.

Schubert M, Joniau S, Gontero P, *et al.* The role of adjuvant hormonal treatment after surgery for localized high-risk prostate cancer: results of a matched multiinstitutional analysis. *Adv Urol* 2012; **2012**:612707.

Schumacher MC, Burkhard FC, Thalmann GN, Fleischmann A, Studer UE. Good outcome for patients with few lymph node metastases after radical retropubic prostatectomy. *Eur Urol* 2008; **54**(2):344–52.

Studer UE, Collette L, Whelan P, *et al.* Using PSA to guide timing of androgen deprivation in patients with T0-4 N0-2 M0 prostate cancer not suitable for local curative treatment (EORTC 30891). *Eur Urol* 2008; **53**(5):941–9.

Thompson IM Jr, Tangen CM, Paradelo J, *et al.* Adjuvant radiotherapy for pathologically advanced prostate cancer: a randomized clinical trial. *JAMA* 2006; **296**(19):2329–35.

Widmark A, Klepp O, Solberg A, *et al.* Endocrine treatment, with or without radiotherapy, in locally advanced prostate cancer (SPCG-7/SFUO-3): an open randomised phase III trial. *Lancet* 2009; **373**(9660):301–8.

Wiegel T, Bottke D, Steiner U, *et al.* Phase III postoperative adjuvant radiotherapy after radical prostatectomy compared with radical prostatectomy alone in pT3 prostate cancer with postoperative undetectable prostate-specific antigen: ARO 96–02/AUO AP 09/95. *J Clin Oncol* 2009; **27**(18):2924–30.

References

1. D'Amico AV, Whittington R, Malkowicz SB, *et al.* Biochemical outcome after radical prostatectomy, external beam radiation therapy, or interstitial radiation therapy for clinically localised prostate cancer. *JAMA* 1998; **280**(11):969–74.
2. Heidenreich A, Bastian PJ, Bellmunt J, *et al.* European Association of Urology guidelines on prostate cancer. [Updated 2012 Feb]. Available at: https://uroweb.org/guideline/prostate-cancer/ [Online].
3. Mohler JL, Armstrong AJ, Bahnson RR, *et al.* National Comprehensive Cancer Network clinical practice guidelines in oncology: Prostate cancer. 2012 [updated 2012 March]. Available at: http://www.nccn.org/professionals/physician_gls/f_guidelines.asp [Online].
4. Epstein JI, Partin AW, Sauvageot J, Walsh PC. Prediction of progression following radical prostatectomy. A multivariate analysis of 721 men with long-term follow-up. *Am J Surg Pathol* 1996; **20**(3):286–92.
5. Yossepowitch O, Eggener SE, Bianco FJ Jr, *et al.* Radical prostatectomy for clinically localized, high risk prostate cancer: critical analysis of risk assessment methods. *J Urol* 2007; **178**(2):493–99.
6. Cooperberg MR, Cowan J, Broering JM, Caroll PR. High-risk prostate cancer in the United States, 1990–2007. *World J Urol* 2008; **26**(3):211–18.
7. Schröder FH, Hugosson J, Roobol MJ, *et al.* Prostate-cancer mortality at 11 years of follow-up. *N Engl J Med* 2012; **366**(11):981–90.
8. Zhu X, van Leeuwen PJ, Bul M, Bangma CH, Roobol MJ, Schröder FH. Identifying and characterizing "escapes"-men who develop metastases or die from prostate cancer despite screening (ERSPC, section Rotterdam). *Int J Cancer* 2011; **129**(12):2847–54.
9. Albertsen PC, Moore DF, Shih W, Lin Y, Li H, Lu-Yao GL. Impact of comorbidity on survival among men with localized prostate cancer. *J Clin Oncol* 2011; **29**(10):1335–41.
10. Lu-Yao GL, Albertsen PC, Moore DF, *et al.* Outcomes of localized prostate cancer following conservative management. *JAMA* 2009; **302**(11):1202–9.
11. Albertsen PC, Hanley JA, Fine J. 20-year outcomes following conservative management of clinically localised prostate cancer. *JAMA* 2005; **293**(17):2095–101.
12. Akre O, Garmo H, Adolfsson J, Lambe M, Bratt O, Stattin P. Mortality among men with locally advanced prostate cancer managed with noncurative intent: a nationwide study in PCBaSe Sweden. *Eur Urol* 2011; **60**(3):554–63.
13. Rider JR, Sandin F, Andrén O, Wiklund P, Hugosson J, Stattin P. Long-term outcomes among noncuratively treated men according to prostate

cancer risk category in a nationwide, population-based study. *Eur Urol* 2013; **63**(1):88–96.

14. Briganti A, Joniau S, Gontero P, *et al.* Identifying the best candidate for radical prostatectomy among patients with high-risk prostate cancer. *Eur Urol* 2012; **61**(3):584–92.
15. Joniau S, Hsu C-Y, Lerut E, *et al.* A pretreatment table for the prediction of final histopathology after radical prostatectomy in clinical unilateral T3a prostate cancer. *Eur Urol* 2007; **51**(2):388–94.
16. Donohue JF, Bianco F J, Kuroiwa K, *et al.* Poorly differentiated prostate cancer treated with radical prostatectomy: long-term outcome and incidence of pathological downgrading. *J Urol* 2006; **176**(3):991–5.
17. Fitzsimons NJ, Presti JC Jr, Kane CJ, *et al.* Is biopsy Gleason score independently associated with biochemical progression following radical prostatectomy after adjusting for pathological Gleason score? *J Urol* 2006; **176**(6 Pt 1):2453–8.
18. Xylinas E, Yates DR, Renard-Penna R, *et al.* Role of pelvic phased array magnetic resonance imaging in staging of prostate cancer specifically in patients diagnosed with clinically locally advanced tumours by digital rectal examination. *World J Urol* 2013; **31**(4):881–6.
19. Roethke MC, Lichy MP, Kniess M, *et al.* Accuracy of preoperative endorectal MRI in predicting extracapsular extension and influence on neurovascular bundle sparing in radical prostatectomy. *World J Urol* 2013; **31**(5):1111–6.
20. Hambrock, T, Hoeks C, Hulsbergen-van de Kaa C, *et al.* Prospective assessment of prostate cancer aggressiveness using 3-T diffusion-weighted magnetic resonance imaging-guided biopsies versus a systematic 10-core transrectal ultrasound prostate biopsy cohort. *Eur Urol* **61**(1):177–84.
21. Partin AW, Mangold LA, Lamm DM, Walsh PC, Epstein JI, Pearson JD. Contemporary update of prostate cancer staging nomograms (Partin Tables) for the new millennium. *Urology* 2001; **58**(6):843–8.
22. Briganti A, Abdollah F, Nini A, *et al.* Performance characteristics of computed tomography in detecting lymph node metastases in contemporary patients with prostate cancer treated with extended pelvic lymph node dissection. *Eur Urol* 2012; **61**(6):1132–8.
23. Joniau S, Van den Bergh L, Peeters C, Haustermans K, Spahn M. Nodal staging in prostate cancer: still an unresolved issue. *Eur Urol* 2012; **61**(6):1139–41.
24. Hovels AM, Heesakkers RA, Adang EM, *et al.* The diagnostic accuracy of CT and MRI in the staging of pelvic lymph nodes in patients with prostate cancer: a meta-analysis. *Clin Radiol* 2008; **63**(4):387–95.
25. Poulsen MH, Bouchelouche K, Høilund-Carlsen PF, *et al.* [(18) F]fluoromethylcholine (FCH)positron emission tomography/ computed tomography (PET/CT) for lymph node staging of prostate cancer: a prospective study of 210 patients. *BJU Int* 2012; **110**(11):1666–71.
26. Budiharto T, Joniau S, Lerut E, *et al.* Prospective evaluation of 11-choline positron emission tomography/computed tomography and diffusion-weighted magnetic resonance imaging for the nodal staging of prostate cancer with a high risk of lymph node metastases. *Eur Urol* 2011; **60**(1):125–30.
27. Harisinghani MG, Barentsz J, Hahn PF, *et al.* Noninvasive detection of clinically occult lymph-node metastases in prostate cancer. *N Engl J Med* 2003; **348**(25):2491–9.
28. Briganti A, Blute ML, Eastham JH, Graefen M, Heidenreich A, Karnes JR, Montorsi F, Studer UE. Pelvic lymph node dissection in prostate cancer. *Eur Urol* 2009; **55**(6):1251–65.
29. Joniau S, Van den Bergh L, Lerut E, *et al.* Mapping of pelvic lymph node metastases in prostate cancer. *Eur Urol* 2013; **63**(3):450–8.
30. Briganti A, Larcher A, Abdollah F, *et al.* Updated nomogram predicting lymph node invasion in patients with prostate cancer undergoing extended pelvic lymph node dissection: the essential importance of percentage of positive cores. *Eur Urol* 2012; **61**(3):480–7.
31. Kjölhede H, Ahlgren G, Almquist H, *et al.* Combined (18) F-fluorocholine and (18) F-fluoride positron emission tomography/ computed tomography imaging for staging of high-risk prostate cancer. *BJU Int* 2012; **110**(10):1501–6.
32. Lecouvet FE, Geukens D, Stainier A, *et al.* Magnetic resonance imaging of the axial skeleton for detecting bone metastases in patients with high-risk prostate cancer: diagnostic and cost-effectiveness and comparison with current detection strategies. *J Clin Oncol* 2007; **25**(22):3281–7.
33. Spahn M, Joniau S, Gontero P, *et al.* Outcome predictors of radical prostatectomy in patients with prostate-specific antigen greater than 20 ng/ml: a European multi-institutional study of 712 patients. *Eur Urol* 2010; **58**(1):1–7.
34. Stenmark MH, Blas K, Halverson S, Sandler HM, Feng FY, Hamstra DA. Continued benefit to androgen deprivation therapy for prostate cancer patients treated with dose-escalated radiation therapy across multiple definitions of high-risk disease. *Int J Radiat Oncol Biol Phys* 2011; **81**(4):e335–44.
35. Joniau S, Spahn M, Briganti A, *et al.* Stratification of high-risk patients into prognostic categories; a European multi-institutional study. *Eur Urol* 2012; **11**(1):e158.
36. Bastian PJ, Boorjian SA, Bossi A, *et al.* High-risk prostate cancer: from definition to contemporary management. *Eur Urol* 2012; **61**(6):1096–106.
37. Rosenthal SA, Sandler HM. Treatment strategies for high-risk locally advanced prostate cancer. *Nat Rev Urol* 2010; **7**(1):31–8.
38. Spahn M, Kneitz S, Scholz CJ, *et al.* Expression of microRNA-221 is progressively reduced in aggressive prostate cancer and metastasis and predicts clinical recurrence. *Int J Cancer* 2010; **127**(2):394–403.
39. Cooperberg MR, Broering JM, Carroll PR. Time trends and local variation in primary treatment of localized prostate cancer. *J Clin Oncol* 2010; **28**(7):1117–23.
40. Spahn M, Briganti A, Capitanio U, *et al.* Outcome predictors of radical prostatectomy followed by adjuvant androgen deprivation deprivation in patients with clinical high risk prostate cancer and pT3 surgical margin positive disease. *J Urol* 2012; **188**(1):84–90.
41. Ward JF, Slezak JM, Blute ML, Bergstralh EJ, Zincke H. Radical prostatectomy for clinically advanced (cT3) prostate cancer since the advent of prostate-specific antigen testing: 15-year outcome. *BJU Int* 2005; **95**(6):751–6.
42. Briganti A, Spahn M, Joniau S, *et al.*; on behalf of the European Multicenter Prostate Cancer Clinical and Translational Research Group (EMPaCT). Impact of age and comorbidities on long-term survival of patients with high-risk prostate cancer treated with radical prostatectomy: A multi-institutional competing-risks analysis. *Eur Urol* 2013; **63**(4):693–701.
43. Ward JF, Slezak JM, Blute ML, Bergstralh EJ, Zincke H. Radical prostatectomy for clinically advanced (cT3) prostate cancer since the advent of prostate-specific antigen testing: 15-year outcome. *BJU Int* 2005; **95**(6):751–6.
44. Carver BS, Bianco FJ Jr, Scardino PT, Eastham JA. Long-term outcome following radical prostatectomy in men with clinical stage T3 prostate cancer. *J Urol* 2006; **176**(2):564–8.
45. Hsu CY, Joniau S, Oyen R, Roskams T, Van poppel H. Outcome of surgery for clinical unilateral T3a prostate cancer: a single-institution experience. *Eur Urol* 2007; **51**(1):121–128.
46. Freedland SJ, Partin AW, Humphreys EB, Mangold LA, Walsh PC. Radical prostatectomy for clinical stage T3a disease. *Cancer* 2007; **109**(7):1273–8.
47. Yossepowitch O, Eggener SE, Serio AM, *et al.* Secondary therapy, metastatic progression, and cancer-specific mortality in men with clinically high-risk prostate cancer treated with radical prostatectomy. *Eur Urol* 2008; **53**(5):950–9.
48. Xylinas E, Drouin SJ, Comperat E, *et al.* Oncological control after radical prostatectomy in men with clinical T3 prostate cancer: a single-centre experience. *BJU Int* 2009; **103**(9):1173–8.

49. Stephenson AJ, Kattan MW, Eastham JA, *et al.* Prostate cancer-specific mortality after radical prostatectomy for patients treated in the prostate-specific antigen era. *J Clin Oncol* 2009; **27**(26):4300–5.
50. Walz J, Joniau S, Chun FK, *et al.* Pathological results and rates of treatment failure in high-risk prostate cancer patients after radical prostatectomy. *BJU Int* 2011; **107**(5):765–70.
51. Donohue JF, Bianco FJ Jr, Kuroiwa K, *et al.* Poorly differentiated prostate cancer treated with radical prostatectomy: long-term outcome and incidence of pathological downgrading. *J Urol* 2006; **176**(3):991–5.
52. Bastian PJ, Gonzalgo ML, Aronson WJ, *et al.* Clinical and pathologic outcome after radical prostatectomy for prostate cancer patients with a preoperative Gleason sum of 8 to 10. *Cancer* 2006; **107**(6):1265–72.
53. Zwergel U, Suttmann H, Schroeder T, Siemer S, Wullich B, Kamradt J, Lehmann J, Stoeckle M. Outcome of prostate cancer patients with initial PSA > or = 20 ng/ml undergoing radical prostatectomy. *Eur Urol* 2007; **52**(4):1058–65.
54. Magheli A, Rais-Bahrami S, Peck HJ, *et al.* Importance of tumor location in patients with high preoperative prostate specific antigen levels (greater than 20 ng/ml) treated with radical prostatectomy. *J Urol* 2007; **178**(4 Pt 1):1311–15.
55. Gontero P, Spahn M, Tombal B, *et al.* Is there a prostate-specific antigen upper limit for radical prostatectomy? *BJU Int* 2011; **108**(7):1093–100.
56. Abdolah F, Sun M, Thuret R, *et al.* Lymph node count threshold for optimal pelvic lymph node staging in prostate cancer. *Int J Urol* 2012; **19**(7):645–51.
57. Briganti A, Blute ML, Eastham JH, *et al.* Pelvic lymph node dissection in prostate cancer. *Eur Urol* 2009; **55**(6):1251–65.
58. Briganti A, Suardi N, Gallina A, Abdollah F, Montorsi F. Pelvic lymph node dissection in prostate cancer: the mistery is taking shape. *Eur Urol* 2013; **63**(3):459–61.
59. Briganti A, Suardi N, Capgrosso P, *et al.* Lymphatic spread of nodal metastases in high-risk prostate cancer: The ascending pathway from the pelvis to the retroperitoneum. *Prostate* 2012; 72(2):186–92.
60. Schreiber D, Rineer J, Sura S, *et al.* Radical prostatectomy for cT3–4 disease: an evaluation of the pathological outcomes and patterns of care for adjuvant radiation in a national cohort. *BJU Int* 2011; **108**(3):360–5.
61. Johnstone PA, Ward KC, Goodman M, Assikis V, Petros JA. Radical prostatectomy for clinical T4 prostate cancer. *Cancer* 2006; **106**(12):2603–9.
62. Joniau S, Hsu CY, Gontero P, Spahn M, Van Poppel H. Radical prostatectomy in very high-risk localized prostate cancer: long-term outcomes and outcome predictors. *Scand J Urol Neprol* 2012; **46**(3):164–71.
63. Schumacher MC, Burkhard FC, Thalmann GN, Fleischmann A, Studer UE. Good outcome for patients with few lymph node metastases after radical retropubic prostatectomy. *Eur Urol* 2008; **54**(2):344–52.
64. Da Pozzo LF, Cozzarini C, Briganti A, *et al.* Long-term follow-up of patients with prostate cancer and nodal metastases treated by pelvic lymphadenectomy and radical prostatectomy: the positive impact of adjuvant radiotherapy. *Eur Urol* 2009; **55**(5):1003–11.
65. Engel J, Bastian PJ, Baur H, *et al.* Survival benefit of radical prostatectomy in lymph node-positive patients with prostate cancer. *Eur Urol* 2010; **57**(5):754–61.
66. Steuber T, Budäus L, Walz J, *et al.* Radical prostatectomy improves progression-free and cancer-specific survival in men with lymph node positive prostate cancer in the prostate-specific antigen era: a confirmatory study. *BJU Int* 2011; **107**(11):1755–61.
67. Briganti A, Karnes RJ, Da Pozzo LF, *et al.* Combination of adjuvant hormonal and radiation therapy significantly prolongs survival of patients with pT2–4 pN+ prostate cancer: results of a matched analysis. *Eur Urol* 2011; **59**(5):832–40.
68. Schröder FH, Kurth KH, Fosså SD, *et al.* Members of the European Organisation for the Research and Treatment of Cancer Genito-urinary Group. Early versus delayed endocrine treatment of pN1-3 M0 prostate cancer without local treatment of the primary tumor: results of European Organisation for the Research and Treatment of Cancer 30846--a phase III study. *J Urol* 2004; **172**(3):923–7.
69. Messing EM, Manola J, Yao J, *et al.* Eastern Cooperative Oncology Group study EST 3886. Immediate versus deferred androgen deprivation treatment in patients with node-positive prostate cancer after radical prostatectomy and pelvic lymphadenectomy. *Lancet Oncol* 2006; **7**(6):472–9.
70. Briganti A, Karnes JR, Da Pozzo LF, *et al.* Two positive nodes represent a significant cut-off value for cancer specific survival in patients with node positive prostate cancer. A new proposal based on a two-institution experience on 703 consecutive N+ patients treated with radical prostatectomy, extended pelvic lymph node dissection and adjuvant therapy. *Eur Urol* 2009; **55**(2):261–70.
71. Van Poppel H, Joniau S. An analysis of radical prostatectomy in advanced stage and high-grade prostate cancer. *Eur Urol* 2008; **53**(2):253–9.
72. Gontero P, Marchioro G, Pisani R, *et al.* Is radical prostatectomy feasible in all cases of locally advanced non-bone metastatic prostate cancer? Results of a single-institution study. *Eur Urol* 2007; **51**(4):922–9.
73. Lerner SE, Blute ML, Zincke H. Extended experience with radical prostatectomy for clinical stage T3 prostate cancer: outcome and contemporary morbidity. *J Urol* 1995; **154**(4),1447–52.
74. Joniau S, Van Baelen A, Hsu CY, Van Poppel H. Complications and functional results of surgery for locally advanced prostate cancer. *Adv Urol* 2012; **2012**:706309.
75. Daly T, Hickey BE, Lehman M, Francis DP, See AM. Adjuvant radiotherapy following radical prostatectomy for prostate cancer. *Cochrane Database Syst Rev* 2011; (12):CD007234.
76. Morgan SC, Walker-Dilks C, Goldman B, *et al.* Does the benefit of adjuvant radiotherapy following radical prostatectomy for pathologic T3 or margin-positive prostate cancer extend to all pathologic subgroups? A meta-analysis of the randomised trials. *Int J Radiat Oncol Biol Phys* 2010; **78**(3):S29–30.
77. Zakeri K, Rose BS, Gulaya S, D'Amico AV, Mell LK. Competing event risk stratification may improve the design and efficiency of clinical trials: Secondary analysis of SWOG 8794. *Contemp Clin Trials* 2013; **34**(1):74–9.
78. Thompson IM Jr, Tangen CM, Paradelo J, *et al.* Adjuvant radiotherapy for pathologically advanced prostate cancer: a randomized clinical trial. *JAMA* 2006; **296**(19):2329–35.
79. Bolla M, Van Poppel H, Tombal B, *et al.* European Organisation for Research and Treatment of Cancer, Radiation Oncology and Genito-Urinary Groups. Postoperative radiotherapy after radical prostatectomy for high risk prostate cancer: long-term results of a randomized controlled trial (EORTC trial 22911). *Lancet* 2012; **380**(9858):2018–27.
80. Wiegel T, Bottke D, Steiner U, *et al.* Phase III postoperative adjuvant radiotherapy after radical prostatectomy compared with radical prostatectomy alone in pT3 prostate cancer with postoperative undetectable prostate-specific antigen: ARO 96–02/AUO AP 09/95. *J Clin Oncol* 2009; **27**(18):2924–30.
81. Swanson GP, Hussey MA, Tangen CM, *et al.*; SWOG 8794. Predominant treatment failure in postprostatectomy patients is local: analysis of patterns of treatment failure in SWOG 8794. *J Clin Oncol* 2007; **25**(16):2225–9.
82. Stephenson AJ, Scardino PT, Kattan MW, *et al.* Predicting the outcome of salvage radiation therapy for recurrent prostate cancer after radical prostatectomy. *J Clin Oncol* 2007; **25**(15):2035–41.
83. Ost P, De Troyer B, Fonteyne V, Oosterlink W, De Meerleer G. A matched control analysis of adjuvant and salvage high-dose postoperative intensity-modulated radiotherapy for prostate cancer. *Int J Radiat Oncol Biol Phys* 2011; **80**(5):1316–22.
84. Trabulsi EJ, Valicenti RK, Hanlon AL, *et al.* A multi-institutional matched-control analysis of adjuvant and salvage postoperative radiation therapy for pT3–4N0 prostate cancer. *Urology* 2008; **72**(6):1298–302.

85. Briganti A, Wiegel T, Joniau S, *et al.* Early salvage radiation therapy does not compromise cancer control in patients with pT3N0 prostate cancer after radical prostatectomy: results of a match-controlled multi-institutional analysis. *Eur Urol* 2012; **62**(3):472–87.
86. Viani GA, Stefano EJ, Afonso SL. Higher-than-conventional radiation doses in localized prostate cancer treatment: a meta-analysis of randomized, controlled trials. *Int J Radiat Oncol Biol Phys* 2009; **74**(5):1405–18.
87. Coen JJ, Zietman AL, Thakral H, Shipley WU. Radical radiation for localized prostate cancer: local persistence of disease results in a late wave of metastases. *J Clin Oncol* 2002; **20**(15):3199–205.
88. Zelefsky MJ, Yamada Y, Fuks Z, *et al.* Long-term results of conformal radiotherapy for prostate cancer: impact of dose escalation on biochemical tumor control and distant metastases-free survival outcomes. *Int J Radiat Oncol Biol Phys* 2008; **71**(4):1028–33.
89. Ost P, Fonteyne V, Villeirs G, Lumen N, Oosterlinck W, De Meerleer G. Adjuvant high-dose intensity-modulated radiotherapy after radical prostatectomy for prostate cancer: clinical results in 104 patients. *Eur Urol* 2009; **56**(4):669–75.
90. King CR, Kapp DS. Radiotherapy after prostatectomy: is the evidence for dose escalation out there? *Int J Radiat Oncol Biol Phys* 2008; **71**(2):346–50.
91. Bernard JR Jr, Buskirk SJ, Heckman MG, *et al.* Salvage radiotherapy for rising prostate-specific antigen levels after radical prostatectomy for prostate cancer: dose-response analysis. *Int J Radiat Oncol Biol Phys* 2010; **76**(3):735–40.
92. McLeod DG, Iversen P, See WA, Morris T, Armstrong J, Wirth MP; Casodex Early Prostate Cancer Trialists' Group. Bicalutamide 150 mg plus standard care vs standard care alone for early prostate cancer. *BJU Int* 2006; **97**(2):247–54.
93. Wirth MP, Weissbach L, Marx FJ, *et al.* Prospective randomized trial comparing flutamide as adjuvant treatment versus observation after radical prostatectomy for locally advanced, lymph node-negative prostate cancer. *Eur Urol* 2004; **45**(3):267–70.
94. Dorff TB, Flaig TW, Tangen CM, *et al.* Adjuvant androgen deprivation for high-risk prostate cancer after radical prostatectomy: SWOG S9921 study. *J Clin Oncol* 2011; **29**(15):2040–5.
95. Schubert M, Joniau S, Gontero P, *et al.* The role of adjuvant hormonal treatment after surgery for localized high-risk prostate cancer: results of a matched multiinstitutional analysis. *Adv Urol* 2012; **2012**:612707.
96. Isbarn H, Boccon-Gibod L, Carroll PR, *et al.* Androgen deprivation therapy for the treatment of prostate cancer: consider both benefits and risks. *Eur Urol* 2009; **55**(1):62–75.
97. Wong YN, Freedland S, Egleston B, Hudes G, Schwartz JS, Armstrong K. Role of androgen deprivation therapy for node-positive prostate cancer. *J Clin Oncol* 2009; **27**(1):100–5.
98. Boorjian SA, Thompson RH, Siddiqui S, *et al.* Long-term outcome after radical prostatectomy for patients with lymph node positive prostate cancer in the prostate specific antigen era. *J Urol* 2007; **178**:864–70.
99. Shelley MD, Kumar S, Wilt T, Staffurth J, Coles B, Mason MD. A systematic review and meta-analysis of randomised trials of neo-adjuvant hormone therapy for localised and locally advanced prostate carcinoma. *Cancer Treat Rev* 2009; **35**(1):9–17.
100. Kumar S, Shelley M, Harrison C, Coles B, Wilt TJ, Mason MD. Neo-adjuvant and adjuvant hormone therapy for localised and locally advanced prostate cancer. *Cochrane Database Syst Rev* 2006; (4):CD006019.
101. Mostaghel EA, Nelson P, Lange PH, *et al.* Neoadjuvant androgen pathway suppression prior to prostatectomy. *J Clin Oncol* 2012; **30**(15 Suppl):282s (abs.4520).
102. Taplin ME, Montgomery RB, Logothetis C, *et al.* Effect of neoadjuvant abiraterone acetate (AA) plus leuprolide acetate (LHRHa) on PSA, pathological complete response (pCR), and near pCR in localized high-risk prostate cancer (LHRPC): Results of a randomized phase II study. *J Clin Oncol* 2012; **30**(15 Suppl):282s (abs.4521).
103. Efstathiou E, Davis JW, Troncoso P, *et al.* Cytoreduction and androgen signaling modulation by abiraterone acetate (AA) plus leuprolide acetate (LHRHa) versus LHRHa in localized high-risk prostate cancer (PCa): Preliminary results of a randomized preoperative study. *J Clin Oncol* 2012; **30**(15 Suppl):291s (abs.4556).
104. Ryan CJ, Tindall DJ. Androgen receptor rediscovered: the new biology and targeting the androgen receptor therapeutically. *J Clin Oncol* 2011; **29**(27):3651–8.
105. Briganti A, Karnes RJ, Da Pozzo LF, *et al.* Combination of adjuvant hormonal and radiation therapy significantly prolongs survival of patients with pT2–4 pN+ prostate cancer: results of a matched analysis. *Eur Urol* 2011; **59**(5):832–40.
106. Ost P, Cozzarini C, De Meerleer G, *et al.* High-dose adjuvant radiotherapy after radical prostatectomy with or without androgen deprivation therapy. *Int J Radiat Oncol Biol Phys* 2012; **83**(3):960–5.
107. Shipley WU, Hunt D, Lukka H, *et al.* Initial report of RTOG 9601: A phase III trial in prostate cancer: Anti-androgen therapy (AAT) with bicalutamide during and after radiation therapy (RT) improves freedom from progression and reduces the incidence of metastatic disease in patients following radical prostatectomy (RP) with pT2–3, N0 disease, and elevated PSA levels. *Int J Radiat Oncol Biol Phys* 2010; **78**:S27 (abs.58).
108. Pilepich MV, Winter K, John MJ, *et al.* Phase III radiation therapy oncology group (RTOG) trial 86–10 of androgen deprivation adjuvant to definitive radiotherapy in locally advanced carcinoma of the prostate. *Int J Radiat Oncol Biol Phys* 2001; **50**(5):1243–52.
109. Lawton CA, Winter K, Murray K, *et al.* Updated results of the phase III Radiation Therapy Oncology Group (RTOG) trial 85–31 evaluating the potential benefit of androgen suppression following standard radiation therapy for unfavorable prognosis carcinoma of the prostate. *Int J Radiat Oncol Biol Phys* 2001; **49**(4):937–46.
110. Viani GA, Stefano EJ, Afonso SL. Higher-than-conventional radiation doses in localized prostate cancer treatment: a meta-analysis of randomized, controlled trials. *Int J Radiat Oncol Biol Phys* 2009; **74**(5):1405–18.
111. Pieters BR, de Back DZ, Koning CCE, Zwinderman AH. Comparison of three radiotherapy modalities on biochemical control and overall survival for the treatment of prostate cancer: a systematic review. *Radiother Oncol* 2009; **93**(2):168–73.
112. Hoskin PJ, Rojas AM, Bownes PJ, Lowe GJ, Ostler PJ, Bryant L. Randomised trial of external beam radiotherapy alone or combined with high-dose-rate brachytherapy boost for localised prostate cancer. *Radiother Oncol* 2012; **103**(2):217–22.
113. Arcangeli G, Saracino B, Gomellini S, *et al.* A prospective phase III randomized trial of hypofractionation versus conventional fractionation in patients with high-risk prostate cancer. *Int J Radiat Oncol Biol Phys* 2010; **78**(1):11–18.
114. Shelley MD, Kumar S, Wilt T, Staffurth J, Coles B, Mason MD. A systematic review and meta-analysis of randomised trials of neo-adjuvant hormone therapy for localised and locally advanced prostate carcinoma. *Cancer Treat Rev* 2009; **35**(1):9–17.
115. Bria E, Cuppone F, Giannarelli D, *et al.* Does hormone treatment added to radiotherapy improve outcome in locally advanced prostate cancer?: meta-analysis of randomized trials. *Cancer* 2009; **115**(15):3446–56.
116. Shelley MD, Kumar S, Coles B, Wilt T, Staffurth J, Mason MD. Adjuvant hormone therapy for localised and locally advanced prostate carcinoma: a systematic review and meta-analysis of randomised trials. *Cancer Treat Rev* 2009; **35**(7):540–6.
117. Verhagen PC, Schröder FH, Collette L, Bangma CH. Does local treatment of the prostate in advanced and/or lymph node metastatic disease improve efficacy of androgen-deprivation therapy? A systematic review. *Eur Urol* 2010; **58**(2):261–9.
118. Kumar S, Shelley M, Harrison C, Coles B, Wilt TJ, Mason MD. Neo-adjuvant and adjuvant hormone therapy for localised and locally

advanced prostate cancer. *Cochrane Database Syst Rev* 2006 Oct 18;(4):CD006019.
119. Nanda A, Chen MH, Braccioforte MH, Moran BJ, D'Amico AV. Hormonal therapy use for prostate cancer and mortality in men with coronary artery disease-induced congestive heart failure or myocardial infarction. *JAMA* 2009; **302**(8):866–73.
120. D'Amico AV, Chen MH, Renshaw AA, Loffredo M, Kantoff PW. Androgen suppression and radiation vs radiation alone for prostate cancer: a randomized trial. *JAMA* 2008; **299**(3):289–95.
121. Bolla M, de Reijke TM, van Tienhoven G, *et al.* Duration of androgen suppression in the treatment of prostate cancer. *N Engl J Med* 2009; **360**(24):2516–27.
122. Horwitz EM, Bae K, Hanks GE, *et al.* Ten-year follow-up of radiation therapy oncology group protocol 92–02: a phase III trial of the duration of elective androgen deprivation in locally advanced prostate cancer. *J Clin Oncol* 2008; **26**(15):2497–504.
123. Harmenberg U, Hamdy FC, Widmark A, Lennernas B, Nilsson S. Curative radiation therapy in prostate cancer. *Acta Oncol* 2011; **50**(Suppl 1):98–103.
124. Zelefsky MJ, Pei X, Chou JF, *et al.* Dose escalation for prostate cancer radiotherapy: predictors of long-term biochemical tumor control and distant metastases-free survival outcomes. *Eur Urol* 2011; **60**(6):1133–9.
125. Denham JW, Steigler A, Lamb DS, *et al.* Short-term androgen deprivation and radiotherapy for locally advanced prostate cancer: results from the Trans-Tasman Radiation Oncology Group 96.01 randomised controlled trial. *Lancet Oncol* 2005; **6**(11):841–50.
126. Denham JW, Steigler A, Lamb DS, *et al.* Short-term neoadjuvant androgen deprivation and radiotherapy for locally advanced prostate cancer: 10-year data from the TROG 96.01 randomised trial. *Lancet Oncol* 2011; **12**(5):451–9.
127. Roach M, Bae K, Speight J, *et al.* Short-term neoadjuvant androgen deprivation therapy and external-beam radiotherapy for locally advanced prostate cancer: long-term results of RTOG 8610. *J Clin Oncol* 2008; **26**(4):585–91.
128. Bolla M, Collette L, Blank L, *et al.* Long-term results with immediate androgen suppression and external irradiation in patients with locally advanced prostate cancer (an EORTC study): a phase III randomised trial. *Lancet* 2002; **360**(9327):103–6.
129. Bolla M, Collette L, Van Tienhoven G, *et al.* Ten year results of long term adjuvant androgen deprivation with goserelin in patients with locally advanced prostate cancer treated with radiotherapy: a phase III EORTC study. *Int J Radiat Oncol Biol Phys* 2008; **72**:S30–1. (abs. 65).
130. Pilepich MV, Winter K, Lawton CA, *et al.* Androgen suppression adjuvant to definitive radiotherapy in prostate carcinoma--long-term results of phase III RTOG 85–31. *Int J Radiat Oncol Biol Phys* 2005; **61**(5):1285–90.
131. See WA, Tyrrell CJ. The addition of bicalutamide 150 mg to radiotherapy significantly improves overall survival in men with locally advanced prostate cancer. *J Cancer Res Clin Oncol* 2006; **132**(Suppl 1):S7–S16.
132. Laverdière J, Nabid A, De Bedoya LD, Ebacher A, Fortin A, Wang CS, Harel F. The efficacy and sequencing of a short course of androgen suppression on freedom from biochemical failure when administered with radiation therapy for T2-T3 prostate cancer. *J Urol* 2004; **171**(3):1137–40.
133. Roach M, DeSilvio M, Lawton C, *et al.* Phase III trial comparing whole-pelvic versus prostate-only radiotherapy and neoadjuvant versus adjuvant combined androgen suppression: Radiation Therapy Oncology Group 9413. *J Clin Oncol* 2003; **21**(10):1904–11.
134. Lawton CA, DeSilvio M, Roach M, *et al.* An update of the phase III trial comparing whole pelvic to prostate only radiotherapy and neoadjuvant to adjuvant total androgen suppression: updated analysis of RTOG 94–13, with emphasis on unexpected hormone/radiation interactions. *Int J Radiat Oncol Biol Phys* 2007; **69**(3):646–55.
135. Pommier P, Chabaud S, Lagrange JL, *et al.* Is there a role for pelvic irradiation in localized prostate adenocarcinoma? Preliminary results of GETUG-01. *J Clin Oncol* 2007; **25**(34):5366–73.
136. Nguyen PL, D'Amico AV. Targeting pelvic lymph nodes in men with intermediate- and high-risk prostate cancer despite two negative randomized trials. *J Clin Oncol* 2008; **26**(12):2055–6.
137. Roach M. Targeting pelvic lymph nodes in men with intermediate- and high-risk prostate cancer, and confusion about the results of the randomized trials. *J Clin Oncol* 2008; **26**(22):3816–17.
138. Abdollah F, Cozzarini C, Suardi N, *et al.* Indications for pelvic nodal treatment in prostate cancer should change. Validation of the Roach formula in a large extended nodal dissection series. *Int J Radiat Oncol Biol Phys* 2012; **83**(2):624–9.
139. Wang-Chesebro A, Xia P, Coleman J, Akazawa C, Roach M. Intensity-modulated radiotherapy improves lymph node coverage and dose to critical structures compared with three-dimensional conformal radiation therapy in clinically localized prostate cancer. *Int J Radiat Oncol Biol Phys* 2006; **66**(3):654–62.
140. Bastian PJ, Boorjian SA, Bossi A, *et al.* High-risk prostate cancer: from definition to contemporary management. *Eur Urol* 2012; **61**(6):1096–106.
141. Zelefsky MJ, Eastham JA, Cronin AM, *et al.* Metastasis after radical prostatectomy or external beam radiotherapy for patients with clinically localized prostate cancer: a comparison of clinical cohorts adjusted for case mix. *J Clin Oncol* 2010; **28**(9):1508–13.
142. Cooperberg MR, Vickers AJ, Broering JM, Carroll PR. Comparative risk-adjusted mortality outcomes after primary surgery, radiotherapy, or androgen-deprivation therapy for localized prostate cancer. *Cancer* 2010; **116**(22):5226–34.
143. Arcangeli G, Strigari L, Arcangeli S, *et al.* Retrospective comparison of external beam radiotherapy and radical prostatectomy in high-risk, clinically localized prostate cancer. *Int J Radiat Oncol Biol Phys* 2009; **75**(4):975–82.
144. Abdollah F, Sun M, Thuret R, *et al.* A competing-risks analysis of survival after alternative treatment modalities for prostate cancer patients: 1988–2006. *Eur Urol* 2011; **59**(1):88–95.
145. Boorjian SA, Karnes RJ, Viterbo R, Rangel LJ, Bergstralh, Horwitz EM. Long-term survival after radical prostatectomy versus external-beam radiotherapy for patients with high-risk prostate cancer. *Cancer* 2011; **117**(13):2883–91.
146. Parikh R, Sher DJ. Primary radiotherapy versus radical prostatectomy for high-risk prostate cancer: a decision analysis. *Cancer* 2012; **118**(1):258–67.
147. Giordano SH, Kuo YF, Duan Z, Hortobagyi GN, Freeman J, Goodwin JS. Limits of observational data in determining outcomes from cancer therapy. *Cancer* 2008; **112**(11):2456–66.
148. Huggins C, Stevens R, Hodges CV. Studies on prostatic cancer. II. The effects of castration on advanced carcinoma of the prostate gland. *Arch Surg* 1941; **43**(2):209–23.
149. Huggins C, Hodges CV. Studies on prostatic cancer. I. The effect of castration, of estrogen and of androgen injection on serum phosphatases in metastatic carcinoma of the prostate. *Cancer Res* 1941; **1**:293–7.
150. Widmark A, Klepp O, Solberg A, *et al.* Endocrine treatment, with or without radiotherapy, in locally advanced prostate cancer (SPCG-7/SFUO-3): an open randomised phase III trial. *Lancet* 2009; **373**(9660):301–8.
151. de la Taille A. Circumstances of prescription of hormone therapy for patients with prostate cancer. *Prog Urol* 2009; **19**(5):313–20.
152. Lu-Yao GL, Albertsen PC, Moore DF, *et al.* Survival following primary androgen deprivation therapy among men with localized prostate cancer. *JAMA* 2008; **300**(2):173–81.
153. McLeod DG, Iversen P, See WA, Morris T, Armstrong J, Wirth MP. Bicalutamide 150 mg plus standard care vs standard care alone for early prostate cancer. *BJU Int* 2006; **97**(2):247–54.

154. Schulman CC, Irani J, Morote J. Androgen-deprivation therapy in prostate cancer: a European expert panel review. *Eur Urol* 2010; **9**(7):675–91.
155. Hu JC, Williams SB, O'Malley AJ, Smith MR, Nguyen PL, Keating NL. Androgen-deprivation therapy for nonmetastatic prostate cancer is associated with an increased risk of peripheral arterial disease and venous thromboembolism. *Eur Urol* 2012; **61**(6):1119–28.
156. Studer UE, Collette L, Whelan P, *et al.* Using PSA to guide timing of androgen deprivation in patients with T0-4 N0-2 M0 prostate cancer not suitable for local curative treatment (EORTC 30891). *Eur Urol* 2008; **53**(5):941–9.
157. Flaig TW, Tangen CM, Hussain MHA, Stadler WM, Raghavan D, Crawford ED, Glodé LM. Randomization reveals unexpected acute leukemias in Southwest Oncology Group prostate cancer trial. *J Clin Oncol* 2008; **26**(9):1532–6.
158. Rosenthal SA, Sandler HM. Treatment strategies for high-risk locally advanced prostate cancer. *Nat Rev Urol* 2010; **7**(1):31–8.

CHAPTER 6.10

Technology and prostatectomy

Giacomo Novara, Alexander Mottrie, Filiberto Zattoni, and Vincenzo Ficarra

Introduction to technology and prostatectomy

Radical prostatectomy (RP) is the gold standard surgical treatment for patients with clinically localized prostate cancer (PCa) and life expectancy more than 10 years.[1] RP allows excellent local control of PCa and confers cancer-specific survival benefit over watchful waiting. Moreover, long-term oncological data after RP showed 25-year biochemical recurrence (BCR)-free survival and cancer-specific survival as high as and 55% and 80%, respectively.[2]

In the last decades, the desire to reduce the invasiveness of open retropubic RP (RRP) produced an increasing interest towards laparoscopic techniques. The shift from open to laparoscopic surgery represents a completely new experience for the surgeon, who must learn a new surgical anatomy, new operative procedures, and deal with new surgical tools. More specifically, the reduction of the range of motion (only 4 degrees of freedom (df)), two-dimensional vision (two-dimensional camera and display), the impaired eye–hand coordination (disorientation between real and visible movements), and the reduced haptic sense (minimal tactile feedback) are the main restrictions associated with a steep learning curve.[3] For surgeons with no experience with laparoscopy, the learning period could amount to hundreds of cases, extending over several years, which limited the application of laparoscopy to complex procedures such RP.

Robotic platforms have been introduced in an attempt to reduce the difficulty in performing complex laparoscopic procedures, particularly for non-laparoscopic surgeons. The first system, with a surgeon's console and remotely controlled telemanipulators, was developed with funding from the US Department of Defense in 1991 and came to be called the Stanford Research Institute Green Telepresence Surgery System after Phil Green, PhD.[3] That early system had only 4 df, similar to standard laparoscopic instruments. In 1995, Fredrick Moll licensed the commercial rights to the SRI Green Telepresence Surgery System and used this acquisition to found Intuitive Surgical Systems. After further development, a renovated master–slave clinical system was released in April 1997 in prototype form as the da Vinci surgical system, which received US Food and Drug Administration approval in July 2000. The da Vinci robot includes a true three-dimensional imaging system that provides magnification up to ×12. This system also incorporates the patented EndoWrist technology, which duplicates the dexterity of the surgeon's forearm and wrist at the operative site, thus providing 7 df.[3] Although the acceptance of traditional laparoscopic radical prostatectomy (LRP) was limited primarily by the steep learning curve of the procedure, robotic-assisted laparoscopic radical prostatectomy (RARP) had a rapid and wide diffusion in the world. Today, in the United States, more than 75% of the radical prostatectomy are performed using Intuitive Surgical's da Vinci platform and the procedure is largely adopted in several countries in the Western world.

Surgical technique

According to Pasadena recommendations, RARP has the same indications accepted for RRP and LRP procedures. Specifically, patients with low- and intermediate-risk localized prostate cancer and a life expectancy >10 yr are the best candidates for RARP.[4] Moreover, the procedure can be performed in patients with stage T1a disease and a life expectancy >15 yr or Gleason score 7; in selected patients with low volume high-risk localized PCa and in highly selected patients with very high-risk localized PCa (cT3b–T4 N0 or any T N1) in the context of multimodal treatment. According to the most important international guidelines, in patients with high or very high-risk disease the procedure must be anticipated from extended pelvic lymphadenectomy. This last category of patients together with those who are obese (BMI >30), with large prostate (prostate volume >70 gr), median lobe or receiving previous transurethral resection of prostate (TURP) or other procedure for benign prostatic hyperplasia (BPH) should be avoided in the learning curve step and reserved only for experienced surgeons. Similarly, patients requiring salvage RARP after radiation failure should be treated by very experienced surgeons.

The majority of robotic surgeons perform RARP using a transperitoneal, antegrade (from bladder neck to the apex) approach. The patient is placed in supine position with the legs in a semi-lithotomy position with compression stockings and sequential compression device for deep vein thrombosis prophylaxis, using well-padded Allen stirrups. The preferred primary access for pneumoperitoneum is represented by the Hasson technique, and only few surgeons still use the Verres needle. Usually, a longitudinal camera port incision is performed. However, Beck *et al.* proposed to use a transverse camera port incision to reduce the risk of camera port site hernia due to specimen extraction, particularly in obese patients and/or patients with large prostates.[5] After the insertion of the primary port, the abdomen is insufflated to a pressure of 15 mmHg. Then, the remaining ports are placed under direct camera supervision. Figure 6.10.1 shows the most used trocars placement. The definitive degree of Trendelenburg inclination is not standardized, and a wide range (between 10 and 40 degrees) is reported in the literature. The minimum possible degree of

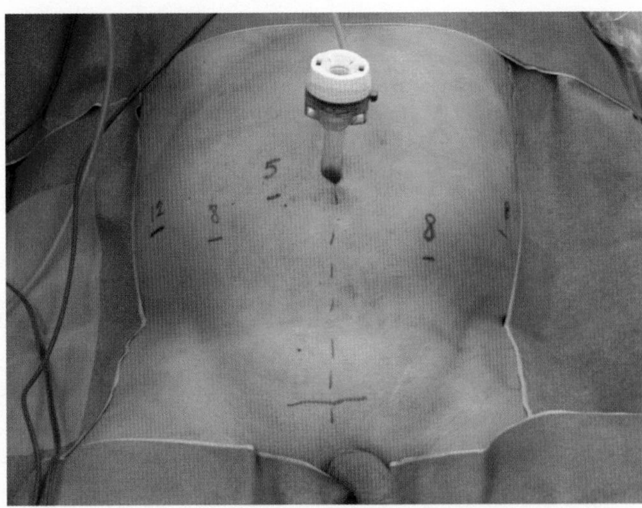

Fig. 6.10.1 Two 8 mm instrument trocars are placed approximately 7–10 cm (one hand breadth) lateral of the umbilicus in the direction of the anterior superior iliac spine. A third 8 mm robotic port (for the fourth arm) is placed 7–10 cm lateral to the left robotic port 2 cm above and anteriorly to the anterior superior iliac spine. Finally, a 5 mm assistant port is placed lateral to the camera port and superior to the right robotic port. A second 12 mm assistant port is placed 7–10 cm directly lateral to the right robotic port.

Trendelenburg inclination should be performed to minimize the potential anesthesiology issues and to reduce the traction during the urethrovesical anastomosis step.

After complete mobilization of the bladder, the periprostatic fat is removed from the endopelvic fascia and from the prostate. The majority of surgeons prefer opening the endopelvic fascia to gain access to the lateral surface of the prostate gland. Different techniques were described to show a clear outline of the prostatovesical junction. Then, the bladder neck is incised in the midline and deepened until the anterior muscular layer of the Denonvilliers' fascia is encountered. The majority of robotic surgeons perform a bladder neck preservation to increase the continence rate and to improve the quality of the urethrovesical anastomosis.

A transverse incision is made on anterior Denonvilliers' fascia close to the prostate. Most of the robotic surgeons suggest an athermal dissection or a minimal use of cautery in the area of the seminal vesicles, in order to avoid injury to cavernous nerves. Vas deferens are divided and the seminal vesicles are completely dissected using a sharp dissection. Some surgeons spare the seminal vesicle tip in low-risk patients in order to minimize the injury at level of cavernous nerves. Moreover, in low-risk patients where nerve preservation is feasible, the posterior layer of Denonvilliers fascia can be left on the rectum while in high-risk patients it should be included with the specimen. The Denonvillier's fascia incision is made few millimetres below the base of the prostate. Once incised, the perirectal fat is visible covering the fascia propria of rectum and the incision is continued on Denonvillier's fascia laterally along the entire width of prostate. The rectum can be separated from the prostate using scissors, under direct vision. The plane between rectum and prostate is defined by blunt and sharp dissection, continuing distally. The fascial space is dissected down all the way to the apex and laterally over the neurovascular bundles.

Anatomical studies showed multiple compartments, which could be developed from the levator fascia to the prostate capsule by entering different fascial planes during surgery. According to the wide variability and subjectivity among surgeons regarding these facets of the procedure, Pasadena Panel suggested using the newer concept of nerve-sparing procedures instead of old interfascial or intrafascial definitions. In detail, the first consensus conference on best practices in RARP proposed the following new definitions: (i) maximum preservation of cavernous nerves (full nerve-sparing), which is obtained by following the plane between the prostatic capsule and the multilayer tissue of the prostatic fascia; (ii) the less extended nerve-sparing technique (partial nerve-sparing) within the multilayer tissue of prostatic fascia; and (iii) the minimal nerve-sparing procedure preserving only the fibres running posterolaterally.

After the antegrade release of the lateral cavernous nerves, the prostatic vascular pedicles are dissected so that large Hem-o-lock clips can be placed to secure them. The cavernous nerves can be damaged by direct mechanical trauma, traction, or thermal energy. Most of robotic surgeons support the cautery-free dissection to avoid thermal injury of cavernous nerves. In high-risk patients, after ligation and division of prostatic pedicles, the prostatectomy is continued anteriorly with an extrafascial technique, with resection of the prostatic fascia and of the neurovascular bundles up to the apex. Then the puboprostatic ligaments and the dorsal vein complex are dissected to isolate the prostatic apex. Different surgical techniques can be used to realize this step of the procedure. The anterior urethral wall is opened just below the apical limit, exposing the Foley catheter. The posterior wall and the underlying rectourethralis muscle are then divided close to the prostate. The division of the rectourethralis muscle completely frees the specimen, which is placed in an Endobag sac.

During the reconstructive steps of the procedure, some robotic surgeons perform posterior muscolo-fascial plate reconstruction with the aim of shortening the time to the recovery of urinary continence recovery and to reduce the risk of bleeding and anastomosis leakage. Several techniques were proposed to perform this step of the procedure and no comparative studies showed what is the best one. Recent systematic reviews showed only a minimal advantage in favour of posterior musculofascial reconstruction in terms of urinary continence recovery within 1 month of RP. The urethrovesical anastomosis is the last step of the procedure. Most robotic surgeons prefer to use running sutures. Therefore, the use of interrupted stitches representing the gold standard in the era of open surgery has been abandoned. An 18 Ch catheter is placed into the bladder and usually removed after four to six days.

Perioperative outcomes and complication rates

RARP can be performed routinely in a reasonably short operative time, with low risk of blood loss and low transfusion rates. Specifically, a systematic review of the literature demonstrated overall mean operative time was 152 min (range: 90–291 min), mean blood loss of 166 ml (range: 69–534 mL), mean transfusion rate as low as 2% (range: 0.5–5%), mean catheterization time of 6.3 d (range: 5–8.6 d), and mean in-hospital stay as low as 1.9 d (range: 1–6 d)[6] (Table 6.10.1). Some patient characteristics such as high BMI, large prostate volume, prior abdominal surgery, prior BPH surgery, or presence of median lobe may make the surgical procedure more difficult, possibly increasing operative time,

Table 6.10.1 Perioperative outcomes in a robotic-assisted laparoscopic radical prostatectomy (RARP) series of studies

Author	Institution	Cases	Study design	Median/Mean operative time (min.)	Median/Mean blood loss (ml)	Transfusion rate (%)	Catheterization-duration (days)	In-hospital stay (days)
Patel (2008)[7]	Global robotic institute, Celebration, FL, US	1,500	Prospective case series	105 (55–300)	111 (50–500)	0.4%	6.3 (4–28)	1
Tewari (2008)[8]	Weill Cornell Medical College, NY, US	215	Prospective case series	120–240	150 ± 195	3%	7 (4–14)	—
Carlucci (2009)[9]	Mount Sinai Medical Center, NY, US	700	Prospective case series	124 (48–266)	69 (5—400)	0	7 (4–30)	1
Greco (2009)[10]	Northwesterm Univ, Chicago, IL, US	180	Prospective case series	291	359	—	—	1.8
Jaffe (2009)[11]	Montsuris, Paris, France	293	Prospective case series	158 ± 51	534 ± 416		8.6 ± 3.5	5 ± 2.6
Martin (2009)[12]	Mayo Clinic Arizona, Phoenix, AZ, US	509	Retrospective case series	190 ± 50	155 ± 212	1.2%	—	—
Murphy (2009)[13]	Melbourne, Australia	400	Prospective case series	186 ± 49	—	2.5%	8.2 ± 3.1	3.1 ± 1.4
Coelho (2010)[14]	Global robotic institute, Celebration, FL, US	2,500	Prospective case series	90 (75–100)	100 (100–150)	0.5%	5 (4–6)	1
Davis (2010)[15]	University of Texas MD Anderson Cancer Center, Houston, TX, US	178	Prospective case series	246 (126–378)	200 (35–850)	0.5%	—	1.8
Jeong (2010)[16]	Robert Wood Johnson Medical School, NJ, US	200	Retrospective case series	212 (110–540)	189 (50–800)	0		1.13
Lasser (2010)[17]	Warren Alpert Medical School at Brown University, Providence, RI, US	239	Prospective case series	231.9 (125–537)	—	4%	—	2.37 (1–23)
Lee (2010)[18]	Yonsei University College of Medicine, Seoul, South Korea	307	Unclear	210 ± 46	337 ± 287	2%	11.4 ± 4	5.1 ± 3
Novara (2010)[19]	Univ. of Padua, Italy	415	Prospective case series	184 ± 56	300 (150–400)	5%	5 (4–7)	6 (5–7)
Ploussard (2010)[20]	Creteil, Paris, France	206	Prospective case series	160	504	3%	8.2	4.3
Bolenz (2011)[21]	University of Texas Southwestern Medical Center, Dallas, TX, US	264	Retrospective case series	235 (209–270)	—	5%	—	1 (1–2)
Heldt (2011)[22]	Loma Linda University, US	418	Retrospective case series	291.1 ± 6.9	154.6 ± 10.3	—	—	1.7 ± 0.2
Jayram (2011)[23]	Univ. of Chicago, IL, US	148 D'amico high risk	Prospective case series	—	150 (25–1,000)	3%	6 (5–8)	—

Adapted from *European Urology*, Volume 62, Issue 3, Novara G *et al.*, 'Systematic review and meta-analysis of perioperative outcomes and complications after robot-assisted radical prostatectomy', pp. 431–52, Copyright © 2012, with permission from Elsevier, http://www.sciencedirect.com/science/journal/03022838

blood loss, or catheterization time. Similarly, surgeon experience (i.e. number of cases performed, achieving a fellowship training in RARP) are associated with better perioperative outcomes.

Postoperative complications are relatively uncommon, with overall mean rate around 10%. High-grade severe complications are very uncommon following RARP. Specifically, the mean complication rate is as low as 9% (range: 3–26%), with grade 1 complications being as prevalent as 4% (range: 2–11.5%); grade 2, 3% (range: 2–9%); grade 3, 2% (range: 0.5–7%); grade 4, 0.4% (range: 0–1.5%); grade 5, 0.02% (range: 0–0.5%) (6). Lymphocele or lymphorrea (mean 3.1%; range 1.2–29%), urinary leak (mean 1.8%; range 0.1–6.7%) and reoperation (mean 1.6%; range 0.5–7%) were the commonest surgical complications.[6]

Several studies have compared perioperative outcomes and complications in RRP, LRP, and RARP (Table 6.10.2). With regard to RARP and RRP, a systematic review and meta-analysis showed statistically significant differences in terms of rates for blood loss (weight mean difference [WMD]: 582.77; 95% CI, 435.25–730.29; p <0.00001) and transfusion (odds ratio [OR]: 4.85; 95% CI, 2.86–8.22; p <0.00001) in favour of RARP, whereas rates for operative time (WMD: −15.8; 95% CI, −68.65 to 37; p = 0.56) and overall complications (OR: 1.1; 95% CI, 0.59–2.04; p = 0.76) were similar for RARP and RRP. Conversely, rates for operative time (WMD: 34.78; 95% CI, −1.36–70.93; p = 0.06), blood loss (WMD: 54.21; 95% CI, −75.17–183.59; p = 0.41), and overall complications (OR: 1.24; 95% CI, 0.8–1.93; p = 0.34) were similar in LRP and RARP. Only the transfusion rate (OR: 2.56; 95% CI, 1.65–3.96; p <0.00001) was significantly lower in RARP patients.[6,24–26]

Urinary continence

According to a systematic review of the literature, 12-month urinary incontinence rates following RARP ranged from 4% to 31%, with a mean value of 16% in studies adopting the continence definition of 'no pad'. Considering studies using 'no pad or safety pad' as the continence definition, 12-month urinary incontinence rates ranged from 8% to 11%, with a mean value of 9%.[44] Some patient characteristics such as age, high BMI, large prostate volume, surgical experience can affect the probability to recover urinary continence after RARP. Similarly, several surgical aspects can influence continence rates, anterior and posterior anastomosis reconstruction techniques being the most relevant.[44]

Table 6.10.3 summarizes the data of studies comparing posterior reconstruction or anterior and posterior reconstruction (total reconstruction) versus the standard procedure. Specifically, a cumulative analysis of comparative studies demonstrated a small advantage in favour of posterior reconstruction (OR: 0.76; 95% CI, 0.59–0.98; p = 0.04) for continence recovery one month after RARP. Conversely, posterior reconstruction showed no advantage for continence at three months (OR: 1.11; 95% CI, 0.78–1.57; p = 0.57) and 6 months (OR: 0.95; 95% CI, 0.54–1.68; p = 0.86) after RARP over the standard approach.[44] Regardless of continence rates, posterior reconstruction is a quick and safe surgical detail which may ease subsequent steps of vesicourethral anastomosis. Similarly, total (anterior and posterior) reconstruction was evaluated in a few comparative studies and a cumulative analysis showed a small statistically significant difference in favour of total reconstruction at one-month continence rates (OR: 0.40; 95% CI, 0.16–0.96; p = 0.04) after the RARP.[44–54]

Recently, Srivastava *et al.* reported a large series on the association between extent of preservation of neurovascular bundles and continence rates, demonstrating that grade of preservation was strongly associated with continence. Specifically, patients receiving grade 1 preservation (i.e. the greatest extent of nerve preservation with incision of the Denonvilliers' fascia and the lateral pelvic fascia (LPF) just outside the prostatic capsule) had significantly higher early continence rates, as compared to those receiving partial/incremental nerve-sparing or non-nerve-sparing procedures.[67] Table 6.10.4 summarizes the comparative studies reporting continence rates in RRP, LRP, and RARP. With regard to RARP and RRP, a systematic review and meta-analysis showed that absolute risk of 12-month urinary incontinence was 11.3% after RRP and 7.5% after RARP. Therefore, the absolute risk reduction was 3.8% in favour of RARP (OR: 1.53; 95% CI, 1.04–2.25; p = 0.03). Similarly, with regard to RARP and LRP, the same systematic review demonstrated significant advantages in 12-month continence rates in favour of RARP (OR: 2.39; 95% CI, 1.29–4.45; p = 0.006).[44]

Erectile function

According to a systematic review, the mean values of the 3-, 6-, 12-, and 24-month potency recovery rates were 50% (32–68%), 65% (50–86%), 70% (54–90%), and 79% (63–94%), respectively. Notably, considering only the studies with high methodological quality (according to the Mulhall criteria), the mean 3-, 6-, 12-, and 24-month potency rates were 48% (32–68%), 68% (50–86%), 76% (62–90%), and 82% (69–94%), respectively. Conversely, studies with poorer quality showed values of 3-, 6-, 12-, and 24-month potency rates as high as 56%, 62% (53–70%), 66% (62–83%), and 63%, respectively.[74]

The adopted definition of potency can vary among studies, which, by itself, justifies major differences among the reported series. Moreover, several predictors can affect potency rates following RARP, including patient age, preoperative potency status, presence of co-morbidities, BMI, and extent of the nerve-sparing procedure. Series including both the unilateral and bilateral nerve-sparing procedure showed 3-, 6-, 12-, and 24-month potency rates of 32%, 53%, 69% (62–90%), and 63%, respectively, whereas the same rates in case of full bilateral nerve-sparing surgery were 56%, 69% (50–86%), 74% (62–90%), and 82% (69–94%), respectively.[74–79]

More controversial is the impact of thermal and athermal dissection of the neurovascular bundles during surgery. Ahlering *et al.* demonstrated significantly higher 24-month potency rates in patients younger than 65 and preoperatively fully potent receiving athermal dissection compared to patients receiving cautery in a prospective study.[80] Conversely, Samadi *et al.* demonstrated differences only in 3-month potency rates.[54] Similarly, the literature on the impact of extension of the nerve-sparing procedure on potency rate is sparse. Shikanov *et al.* evaluated 110 patients having 'extrafascial' dissection of the neurovascular bundles and 703 who underwent 'intrafascial' RARP, demonstrating significantly higher potency rates for those patients treated with an intrafascial technique.[81] Tewari *et al.* reported potency rates in a large series of patients stratifying data according to the extent of preservation defined with a novel grading system (grade 1: incision of the Denonvilliers' and LPF just outside the prostatic capsule; grade

Table 6.10.2 Perioperative parameters and complication rates in comparative studies evaluating robotic radical prostatectomy (RRP) and RARP, or laparoscopic radical prostatectomy (LRP) and RARP

Author	Cases	Median/Mean operative time (min.)	Median/Mean blood loss (ml)	Transfusion rate (%)	Catheterization duration (d)	In-hospital stay (d)	Overall complication rate (%)
RARP vs. RRP							
Caballero-Romeu (2008)[27]	62 RRP	210 (160–240)	1,500 (1,200–2,000)	81%	22 (19–26)	8 (7–9)	84%
	60 RARP	210 (158–240)	400 (213–500)	11%	12 (11–14)	5 (4–6)	42%
Drouin (2009)[28]	83 RRP	208 ± 76	821 ± 582	10%	14.7	7	16%
	71 RARP	199 ± 36	310 ± 205	6%	8.1	4.4	8%
Ficarra (2009)[29]	105 RRP	135	500	14%	6	7	13%
	103 RARP	185	300	2%	5	6	10%
Ou (2009)[30]	30 RRP	213 ± 37	912 ± 370	60%	9.2 ± 2.8	8.4 ± 2.2	10%
	30 RARP	205 ± 102	314 ± 284	13%	7.7 ± 2	7.3 ± 2.3	17%
Rocco (2009)[31]	240 RRP	160	800	—	7	6	—
	120 RARP	215	200		6	3	
Carlsson (2010)[32]	485 RRP	—	—	—	—	—	45%
	1,253 RARP						10%
Breyer (2010)[33]	695 RRP	—	—	8%	—	—	—
	293 RARP			1%			
Doumerc (2010)[34]	502 RRP	148 (75–330)	—	2%	7.9 (6–20)	5.5 (3–10)	1%
	212 RARP	192 (119–525)		1%	6.3 (6–21)	2.8 (2–7)	2%
Kordan (2010)[35]	414 RRP	—	450 (300–600)	3.4%	—	—	—
	830 RARP		100 (50–200)	0.8%			
Lo (2010)[36]	20 RRP	289 ± 64	—	65%	18 ± 7	17 ± 7	—
	20 RARP	306 ± 85		5%	12 ± 7	8 ± 6	
Truesdale (2010)[37]	217 RRP	204 ± 33	904 ± 615	—	—	—	—
	99 RARP	153 ± 51	160 ± 105				
Di Pierro (2011)[38]	75 RRP	253 ± 41	—	3%	—	—	37%
	75 RARP	330 ± 54		0			40%
RARP vs. LRP							
Caballero-Romeu (2008)[27]	70 LRP	345 (3,250–375)	1,270 (700–2,000)	49%	22 (17–28)	8 (5–10)	74%
	60 RARP	210 (158–240)	400 (213–500)	11%	12 (11–14)	5 (4–6)	42%
Cho (2009)[39]	60 LRP	321	289	—	14.2	16.4	25%
	60 RARP	224	208		8.4	12.3	7%
Drouin (2009)[28]	85 LRP	257 ± 94	558 ± 574	6%	8.9	6.1	7%
	71 RARP	199 ± 36	310 ± 205	6%	8.1	4.4	8%
Hakimi (2009)[40]	75 LRP	232	311	—	—	3.4	15%
	75 RARP	199	230			1.9	11%
Trabulsi (2010)[41]	45 LRP	300	299	4%	—	2.6	—
	205 RARP	190	259	2%		1.6	
Park (2011)[42]	62 LRP	308 (158–456)	214 (50–600)	0	9	7	11%
	44 RARP	371 (240–720)	220 (50–700)	2%	8	7	11%
Asimakopoulos (2011)[43]	64 LRP	—	—	5%	7.45 ± 2.3	—	8%
	52 RARP			0	7.25 ± 2.7		15%

Adapted from *European Urology*, Volume 62, Issue 3, Novara G *et al.*, 'Systematic review and meta-analysis of perioperative outcomes and complications after robot-assisted radical prostatectomy', pp. 431–52, Copyright © 2012, with permission from Elsevier, http://www.sciencedirect.com/science/journal/03022838

Table 6.10.3 Urinary continence rates reported in studies comparing RARP posterior or anterior and posterior reconstruction versus standard vesicourethral anastomosis

Authors	Cases (n)	Studydesign	Continence definition	Data collection	Urinary continence rates (%)			
					1-mo	3-mo	6-mo	12/24-mo
Posterior reconstruction versus standard vesicourethral anastomosis								
Krane (2009)[55]	PR (42) Standard (42)	Retrospective comparative	0–1 safety pad	Interview	85% 86%	—	—	—
Kim (2009)[56]	PR (30) Standard (30)	Retrospective comparative	Not reported	Not reported	49% 35%	89% 64%	96% 90%	—
Woo (2009)[57]	PR (69) Standard (63)	Prospective comparative	0–1 safety pad	Validated questionnaire	Mean time to continence 90 days Mean time to continence 150 days			
Joshi (2010)[58]	PR (53) Standard (54)	Prospective comparative	0 pad	Validated questionnaire	—	52% 63%	76% 84%	—
Kim (2010)[59]	PR (25) Standard (25)	Retrospective comparative	0 pad	Validated questionnaire	72% 68%	84% 76%	96% 96%	—
Coelho (2011)[60]	PR (473) Standard (330)	Prospective comparative	0 pad	Validated questionnaire	51% 42%	91% 92%	97% 96%	—
Sutherland (2011)[61]	PR (47) Standard (47)	RCT	0–1 safety pad	Validated questionnaire	—	63% 81%	—	—
Anterior and posterior reconstruction versus standard vesicourethral anastomosis								
Menon (2008)[62]	A+PR (59) Standard (57)	RCT	0–1 safety pad	Validated questionnaire	80% 75%	—	—	—
Sammon (2010)[63]	A+PR (46) Standard (50)	RCT	0 pad	Validated questionnaire	42% 47%	—	—	83%* 80%*
Koliakos (2010)[64]	A + PR (24) Standard (26)	RCT	0–1 safety pad	Validated questionnaire	65% 33%	—	—	—
Hurtes (2012)[65]	A + PR (39) Standard (33)	RCT	No leak, total control, no pad	Validated questionnaire	26.5% 7.1%	45.2% 15.4%	65.4% 57.9%	—
Tan (2010)[66]	A + PR (1,383) AR (303) Standard (214)	Prospective comparative	0–1 safety pad	Validated questionnaire	—	91% 77% 50%	95% 86% 62%	98% 92% 82%

*24 months.

Adapted from *European Urology*, Volume 62, Issue 3, Novara G *et al.*, 'Systematic review and meta-analysis of perioperative outcomes and complications after robot-assisted radical prostatectomy', pp. 431–52, Copyright © 2012, with permission from Elsevier, http://www.sciencedirect.com/science/journal/03022838

2: Incision through the Denonvilliers' fascia, leaving deeper layers on the rectum, and LPF just outside the layer of veins of the prostate capsule; grade 3: incision through the outer compartment of the LPF, leaving some yellow adipose and neural tissue on the specimen, and excising all layers of Denonvilliers' fascia; grade 4: wide excision of the LPF and Denonvilliers' fascia containing most of the periprostatic neurovascular tissue) (see Tewari *et al.* 2011).[82] Evaluating only patients with preoperative Sexual Health Inventory For Men (SHIM) scores >21 and with ≥1 year follow-up, the authors demonstrated that 90.9%, 81.4%, 73.5%, and 62% of grade 1 to 4 patients were able to achieve intercourse (p <0.001), respectively, and 81.7%, 74.3%, 66.1%, and 54.5% of grade 1 to 4 patients returned to baseline SHIM scores (p <0.001). Moreover, the strict selection criteria adopted to indicate patients for the different grades of preservation allowed authors to achieve similar positive surgical margin rates in all groups.[82] Table 6.10.5 summarizes potency rates in comparative studies evaluating RARP with RRP or LRP.

With regard to RARP and RRP, a systematic review and meta-analyses demonstrated that the prevalence of erectile dysfunction according to different definitions was 47.8% after RRP and 24.2% after RARP, with a statistically significant absolute risk reduction of 23.6% (OR: 2.84; 95% CI, 1.48–5.43; p = 0.002). Conversely, evaluating the comparative studies on RARP and LRP, the prevalence of erectile dysfunction was 55.6% after LRP and 39.8% after RARP, with an absolute risk reduction on 14.8% (OR: 1.89; 95% CI, 0.70–5.05; p = 0.21).[74]

Oncolgical outcome

As RARP is a relatively young procedure, data on cancer-specific survival following RARP are currently immature. However,

Table 6.10.4 Urinary continence in comparative studies evaluating RRP and RARP, or LRP and RARP

Authors	Cases (n)	Study design	Continence definition	Data collection	Urinary continence recovery (%)	
					6-mo	12-mo
RARP vs. RRP						
Tewari (2003)[68]	RRP (100) RARP (200)	Prospective comparison	0 pad	Interview	Median 160 days Median 44 days	
Caballero-Romeu (2008)[27]	RRP (62) RARP (60)	Historical control	0 pad	Unspecified	54% 40%	—
Krambeck (2009)[69]	RRP (564) RARP (286)	Retrospective series	0 pad	Institutional questionnaire	—	93.7% 91.8%
Ficarra (2009)[29]	RRP (105) RARP (103)	Prospective comparison	0 pad	Validated questionnaire	—	88% 97%
Rocco (2009)[31]	RRP (240) RARP (120)	Historical control	0–1 safety pad	Interview	84% 93%	88% 97%
Ou (2010)[70]	RRP (30) RARP (30)	Retrospective series	0 pad	Unspecified	83% 97%	97% 100%
Di Pierro (2011)[38]	RRP (75) RARP (75)	Prospective comparison	0 pad	Institutional questionnaire	—	80% 89%
Kim (2011)[71]	RRP (235) RARP (528)	Prospective comparison	0 pad	Validated questionnaire	Median 4.3 mo Median 3.7 mo	
RARP vs. LRP						
Joseph (2005)[72]	LRP (50) RARP (50)	Historical control	0 pad	Interview	92% 90%	—
Caballero-Romeu (2008)[27]	LRP (70) RARP (60)	Historical control	0 pad	Unspecified	64% 40%	—
Hakimi (2009)[40]	LRP (75) RARP (75)	Historical control	0 pad	Unspecified	—	90% 93%
Lee (2009)[73]	LRP (31) RARP (21)	Retrospective series	0–1 safety pad	Institutional questionnaire	81% 81%	—
Trabulsi (2010)[41]	LRP (45) RARP (205)	Historical control	0–1 safety pad	Unspecified	71% 91%	82% 94%
Asimakopoulos (2011)[43]	LRP (64) RARP (52)	RCT	0 pad	Interview		83% 94%
Park (2011)[42]	LRP (62) RARP (44)	Retrospective series	0–1 safety pad	Interview	76% 93%	95% 94%

Adapted from *European Urology*, Volume 62, Issue 3, Novara G *et al.*, 'Systematic review and meta-analysis of perioperative outcomes and complications after robot-assisted radical prostatectomy', pp. 431–52, Copyright © 2012, with permission from Elsevier, http://www.sciencedirect.com/science/journal/03022838

surrogate measures for prostate cancer mortality, such as lymph node yield, positive surgical margin (PSM) rates, and PSA (biochemical) free survival, are available. Few series have reported lymph node yield, adopting an extended template for lymph node dissection (involving the external iliac, internal iliac, and obturator lymph nodes).[78,83,84] Such study demonstrated lymph node yields and positive node rates ranging from 11% to 24%, according to the different patient characteristics. On the whole, these data suggest extended lymph node dissection is feasible during RARP, although, to be strict, most of the other reported series failed to adopt appropriate lymph node dissection templates.

A systematic review demonstrated the prevalence of PSMs ranged from 6.5% to 32%, with a mean value of 15%. The most prevalent site of PSM were prostate apex in 5% (range: 1–7%) of the cases, anterior prostate in 0.6% (range: 0.2–2%), at the bladder neck in 1.6% (range: 1–2%), and posterolaterally in 2.6% (range: 2–21%). Finally, the mean PSM rate was 9% (range: 4–23%) in pT2 cancers, 37% (range: 29–50%) in pT3 cancers, and 50% (range: 40–75%) in pT4 cancers.[85] With regards to predictors of PSMs, some cancer characteristics (including prostate volume, clinical T stage, and biopsy Gleason score, presence of perineural invasion), and surgeon experience (i.e. number of cases performed, presence of

Table 6.10.5 Potency rates in comparative studies evaluating RRP and RARP, or LRP and RARP

Authors	Cases (n)	Patient characteristics (RARP)	Surgical aspects (RARP)	Study design	Potency Definition	Data collection	12-mo	24-mo
RARP vs. RRP								
Tewari (2003)[68]	RRP (100) RARP (200)	—	—	Prospective comparison	Presence of erection	Interview	Median 440 days Median 180 days	
Ficarra (2009)[29]	RRP (41) RARP (64)	Mean age 61 Preop potent Bilateral NS	Intrafascial Clipless (monopolar dissection)	Prospective comparison	SHIM >17	Validated questionnaire	49% 81%	—
Krambeck (2009)[69]	RRP (417) RARP (203)	Mean age: 61 Preop potent Mono/Bilat NS	Interfascial Clipless (monopolar cautery)	Retrospective, contemporary series	ESI	Institutional questionnaire	63% 70%	—
Rocco (2009)[31]	RRP (214) RARP (78)	Mean age: 63 Preop Potent	Athermal dissection	Historical control	ESI	Interview	41% 61%	—
Ou (2010)[70]	RRP (2) RARP (16)	Mean age: 67 Preop potent Mono/Bilat NS	Athermal dissection	Retrospective contemporary series	ESI	Unspecified	50% 60%	—
Di Pierro (2011)[38]	RRP (47) RARP (22)	Mean age 62 Preop potent Bilateral NS	Interfascial Athermal	Prospective comparison	ESI	Institutional questionnaire	26% 55%	—
Kim (2011)[71]	RRP (122) RARP (373)	Mean age: 64 Preop potent Mono/Bilat NS	Athermal dissection	Prospective comparison	ESI	Validated questionnaire	28% 57%	47% 84%
RARP vs. LRP								
Cho (2009)[39]	LRP (41) RARP (53)	Mean age: 66 Preop potent Mono/Bilat NS	Unclear	Historical control	ESI	Interview	78% 81%	—
Hakimi (2009)[40]	LRP (45) RARP (51)	Mean age: 59 Preop potent Bilateral NS	Unclear	Historical control	ESI	Validated questionnaire	72% 76%	—
Asimakopoulos (2011)[43]	LRP (64) RARP (52)	Mean age: 59 Preop potent Bilateral NS	Athermal Intrafascial dissection	RCT	ESI	Validated questionnaire	32% 77%	—
Park (2011)[42]	LRP (62) RARP (44)	Mean age: 62.7 Preop potent Mono/Bilat NS	Unclear	Retrospective, contemporary series	ESI	Interview	48% 55%	—

Adapted from *European Urology*, Volume 62, Issue 3, Novara G *et al.*, 'Systematic review and meta-analysis of perioperative outcomes and complications after robot-assisted radical prostatectomy', pp. 431–52, Copyright © 2012, with permission from Elsevier, http://www.sciencedirect.com/science/journal/03022838

fellowship training in robotic surgery), are usually considered useful.[86–92] More controversial is the impact of the extent of preservation of neurovascular bundles dissection on PSM rates. Tewari *et al.* demonstrated similar prevalence of PSMs regardless of the adopted approach.[82] However, it must be kept in mind that the most aggressive grade 1 preservation is for reserved to patients with cT1c cancer, primary Gleason pattern 3, PSA <10 ng/mL, <5% of cancer in the biopsy, and negative MRI, whereas patients with more adverse clinical features (including Gleason pattern 4, Gleason score 8, PSA >10 ng/mL, more extended disease on biopsy, and/or positive MRI) were reserved grade 3 or 4 procedures.[82] Consequently, it might be hypothesized that a risk-stratified selection of patients for the different extent of nerve preservation might not jeopardize oncological outcome. Table 6.10.6 summarizes the comparative studies evaluating RARP to either RRP or LRP that report PSM rates. Systematic review reveals non-statistically significant differences in PSM rates following RRP and RARP (21% and 20%; OR: 1.21; 95% CI, 0.91–1.63; $p = 0.19$) and PSM rates in pT2 cancers (12% and

Table 6.10.6 Positive surgical margin in comparative studies evaluating RRP and RARP, or LRP and RARP

Author	Cases	Overall PSM	pT2 PSM	Author	Cases	Overall PSM	pT2 PSM
RARP vs. RRP				**RARP vs. LRP**			
Caballero-Romeu (2008)[27]	62 RRP 60 RARP	52% 31%	—	Caballero-Romeu (2008)[27]	70 LRP 60 RARP	46% 31%	—
Drouin (2009)[28]	83 RRP 71 RARP	18% 17%	7% 10%	Cho (2009)[39]	60 LRP 60 RARP	38% 23%	34% 22%
Ficarra (2009)[29]	105 RRP 103 RARP	21% 34%	12% 12%	Drouin (2009)[28]	85 LRP 71 RARP	19% 17%	11% 10%
Laurila (2009)[93]	84 RRP 88 RARP	14% 12%	15% 10%	Hakimi (2009)[40]	75 LRP 75 RARP	14% 12%	13% 11%
Ou (2009)[30]	30 RRP 30 RARP	20% 50%	0 3%	Trabulsi (2010)[41]	45 LRP 205 RARP	24% 16%	20% 10%
White (2009)[94]	50 RRP 50 RARP	36% 22%	34% 19%	Asimakopoulos (2011)[43]	64 LRP 52 RARP	10% 15%	8% 7%
Barocas (2010)[95]	491 RRP 1,413 RARP	30% 20%	—	Magheli (2011)[96]	522 LRP 522 RARP	13% 20%	7% 9%
Breyer (2010)[33]	695 RRP 293 RARP	16% 18%	—	Park (2011)[42]	62 LRP 44 RARP	21% 20%	—
Doumerc (2010)[34]	502 RRP 212 RARP	17% 21%	10% 12%				
Lo (2010)[36]	20 RRP 20 RARP	25% 20%	—				
Di Pierro (2011)[97]	75 RRP 75 RARP	32% 16%	24% 8%				
Kim (2011)[71]	235 RRP 528 RARP	25% 27%	9% 13%				
Magheli (2011)[96]	522 RRP 522 RARP	14% 20%	7% 9%				

Adapted from *European Urology*, Volume 62, Issue 3, Novara G *et al.*, 'Systematic review and meta-analysis of perioperative outcomes and complications after robot-assisted radical prostatectomy', pp. 431–52, Copyright © 2012, with permission from Elsevier, http://www.sciencedirect.com/science/journal/03022838

11%; OR: 1.25; 95% CI, 0.81–1.93; $p = 0.31$).[85] Similarly, overall PSM rates (18% and 18%; OR: 1.12; 95% CI, 0.81–1.55; $p = 0.47$) and PSM rates in pT2 cancers (11% and 12%; OR: 0.99; 95% CI, 0.73–1.35; $p = 0.97$) were similar in LRP and RARP.[85]

With regard to BCR, few series reported on BCR estimates following RARP with acceptably long follow-up duration. Menon *et al.* reported on 1,384 patients at a median follow-up duration of 60 months, demonstrating found 3-, 5-, and 7-year BCR rates of 90%, 87%, and 81%, respectively, with 95.5% cancer-specific survival.[98] Similar figures were reported by Suardi *et al.* in a smaller series of patients treated at the OLV Robotic Surgery Institute, Aalst, Belgium, and evaluated at a median follow-up of 67.5 months[99] and by Sooriakumaran *et al.* on about 1,000 patients from Karolinska University Hospital, Stockholm, Sweden evaluated at a median follow-up of 6.3 years.[100] A limited comparison of RRP, LRP, and RARP reveals no significant differences (HR: 0.9; 95% CI, 0.7–1.2; $p = 0.526$) or between LRP and RARP (HR: 0.5; 95% CI, 0.2–1.3; $p = 0.141$).[85]

Downsides of RARP

It is clear that RARP is not devoid of downsides. One of the claimed benefits of the robot-assisted approach is that it reduces the difficulty associated with conventional LRP, reducing the learning curve to as few as 12 cases.[101] Long operative times remain a definite downside of robotic-assisted laparoscopic prostatectomy (RALP) in the early experience of many centres. Moreover, the learning curve is clearly a much more complex than simply achieving acceptable operative times, and outcomes in terms of PSMs, continence, and potency must also be considered.[101] Surely, evaluating learning curve for functional outcomes is a very complex issue because of inconsistencies and subjectivity in outcome reporting for these variables across all approaches for RP. For oncological outcomes, Vickers *et al.* have clearly shown the impact of experience on BCR-free survival rates following RRP[102] and LRP.[103] Specifically, the authors demonstrated that cancer control after radical prostatectomy improves as a surgeon's experience increases (during the first 250 RRP or 750 LRP cases performed).[102,103] Unfortunately, a similar analysis of the learning curve for RARP is not available so far.

The most significant downside of RARP is clearly represented by the cost of the robotic platform. The installation cost is approximately US$1.8 million (US$ 2.0 million for the dual-console version), with maintenance costs of about $100,000 per annum. Robotic consumables cost around US$1,500 per case. The lack of a competitor in this area has contributed to costs remaining prohibitively high for many hospitals and indeed many countries, thereby preventing equitable availability of this technology across diverse healthcare systems.[101]

Proponents of RARP often claim that it leads to shorter hospitalization, faster return to work, and other benefits that justify the expense of the robot-assisted approach. However, these claims are usually unsubstantiated and are often limited by the great variation in health economies from one country to another.[101] Scales *et al.* demonstrated cost-equivalence of RARP with RRP based on 10 cases per week and cost superiority based on 14 cases per week in the United States.[104] Conversely, other health-economic analyses performed in UK demonstrated that excess cost related to purchase and maintenance can be reduced maintaining a case volume for each robotic system of at least 100–150 procedures per year.[105] A systematic review on the costs of RARP strongly suggested that it was not cost-effective in comparisons with RRP, with differences in costs ranging from $2,000 to $4,000.[106] However, the quality of the available literature in the field is quite limited.

There is little doubt that the fact that Intuitive Surgical retain a monopoly of the market does not help in limiting costs. For example, EndoWrist instruments have to be discarded after 10 or so uses, whereas EndoWrist training instruments often work very well for many sessions.[101] Although several companies are currently working on new platform, it is highly unlikely that new platforms with the high level of excellence currently achieved by da Vinci system will be available for clinical use in the short future.

Conclusions

RARP is a popular approach to perform RP in Western countries. Surgical technique is currently very well standardized and several studies are available in literature. According to the available data, RARP can be performed routinely with a relatively small risk of complications and with excellent functional outcomes. Clinical patient characteristics, surgical experience and surgical technique, and cancer characteristics may affect the risk of complications as well as continence and potency recovery. PSM rates are similar following RARP, RRP, and LRP. The few data available on BCR from high-volume centres are promising, but definitive comparisons with RRP or LRP are not currently possible. Moreover, significant data on cancer-specific survival are not available. Finally, high cost for purchasing and maintenance of the robotic platform is the most critical limitation of RARP.

Acknowledgement

Text extracts reproduced from Tewari AK *et al.*, 'Anatomical grades of nerve sparing: A risk-stratified approach to neural-hammock sparing during robot-assisted radical prostaectomy (RARP)', *BJU International*, Volume 108, Issue 6b, pp. 984–992, Copyright © 2011 The Authors and BJU International, with permission from 2011 John Wiley and Sons.

Further reading

Bolenz C, Freedland SJ, Hollenbeck BK, *et al.* Costs of radical prostatectomy for prostate cancer: a systematic review. *Eur Urol* 2014; **65**(2):316–24.

Ficarra V, Cavalleri S, Novara G, Aragona M, Artibani W. Evidence from robot-assisted laparoscopic radical prostatectomy: a systematic review. *Eur Urol* 2007; **51**(1):45–56.

Ficarra V, Novara G, Ahlering TE, *et al.* Systematic review and meta-analysis of studies reporting potency rates after robot-assisted radical prostatectomy. *Eur Urol* 2012; **62**(3):418–30.

Ficarra V, Novara G, Artibani W, *et al.* Retropubic, laparoscopic, and robot-assisted radical prostatectomy: a systematic review and cumulative analysis of comparative studies. *Eur Urol* 2009; **55**(5):1037–63.

Ficarra V, Novara G, Rosen RC, *et al.* Systematic review and meta-analysis of studies reporting urinary continence recovery after robot-assisted radical prostatectomy. *Eur Urol* 2012; **62**(3):405–17.

Ficarra V, Novara G, Secco S, *et al.* Predictors of Positive Surgical Margins After Laparoscopic Robot Assisted Radical Prostatectomy. *J Urol* 2009; **182**(6):2682–8.

Heidenreich A, Bellmunt J, Bolla M, *et al.* EAU guidelines on prostate cancer. Part 1: screening, diagnosis, and treatment of clinically localised disease. *Eur Urol* 2011; **59**(1):61–71.

Menon M, Bhandari M, Gupta N, *et al.* Biochemical recurrence following robot-assisted radical prostatectomy: Analysis of 1384 patients with a median 5-year follow-up. *Eur Urol* 2010; **58**(6):838–46.

Menon M, Shrivastava A, Bhandari M, Satyanarayana R, Siva S, Agarwal PK. Vattikuti Institute prostatectomy: technical modifications in 2009. *Eur Urol* 2009; **56**(1):89–96.

Murphy DG, Bjartell A, Ficarra V, *et al.* Downsides of robot-assisted laparoscopic radical prostatectomy: limitations and complications. *Eur Urol* 2010; **57**(5):735–46.

Novara G, Ficarra V, Mocellin S, *et al.* Systematic review and meta-analysis of studies reporting oncologic outcome after robot-assisted radical prostatectomy. *Eur Urol* 2012; **62**(3):382–404.

Novara G, Ficarra V, Rosen RC, *et al.* Systematic review and meta-analysis of perioperative outcomes and complications after robot-assisted radical prostatectomy. *Eur Urol* 2012; **62**(3):431–52.

Patel VR, Coelho RF, Rocco B, *et al.* Positive surgical margins after robotic assisted radical prostatectomy: A multi-institutional study. *Int Braz J Urol* 2011; **37**(4):540–1.

Ramsay C, Pickard R, Robertson C, *et al.* Systematic review and economic modelling of the relative clinical benefit and cost-effectiveness of laparoscopic surgery and robotic surgery for removal of the prostate in men with localised prostate cancer. *Health Technology Assessesment* 2012; **16**(41):1–313.

Sooriakumaran P, Haendler L, Nyberg T, *et al.* Biochemical recurrence after robot-assisted radical prostatectomy in a european single-centre cohort with a minimum follow-up time of 5 years. *Eur Urol* 2012; **62**(5):768–74.

Srivastava A, Chopra S, Pham A, *et al.* Effect of a risk-stratified grade of nerve-sparing technique on early return of continence after robot-assisted laparoscopic radical prostatectomy. *Eur Urol* 2013; **63**(3):438–44.

Suardi N, Ficarra V, Willemsen P, *et al.* Long-term biochemical recurrence rates after robot-assisted radical prostatectomy: analysis of a single-center series of patients with a minimum follow-up of 5 years. *Urology* 2012; **79**(1):133–8.

Tewari A, Sooriakumaran P, Bloch DA, Seshadri-Kreaden U, Hebert AE, Wiklund P. Positive surgical margin and perioperative complication rates of primary surgical treatments for prostate cancer: a systematic review and meta-analysis comparing retropubic, laparoscopic, and robotic prostatectomy. *Eur Urol* 2012; **62**(1):1–15.

Tewari AK, Srivastava A, Huang MW, *et al.* Anatomical grades of nerve sparing: A risk-stratified approach to neural-hammock sparing during robot-assisted radical prostatectomy (RARP). *BJU Int* 2011; **108**(6 B):984–92.

References

1. Heidenreich A, Bellmunt J, Bolla M, *et al.* EAU guidelines on prostate cancer. Part 1: screening, diagnosis, and treatment of clinically localised disease. *Eur Urol* 2011; **59**(1):61–71.
2. Ficarra V, Novara G, Artibani W, *et al.* Retropubic, laparoscopic, and robot-assisted radical prostatectomy: a systematic review and cumulative analysis of comparative studies. *Eur Urol* 2009; **55**(5):1037–63.
3. Ficarra V, Cavalleri S, Novara G, Aragona M, Artibani W. Evidence from robot-assisted laparoscopic radical prostatectomy: a systematic review. *Eur Urol* 2007; **51**(1):45–56.
4. Montorsi F, Wilson TG, Rosen RC, *et al.* Best practices in robot-assisted radical prostatectomy: Recommendations of the Pasadena consensus panel. *Eur Urol* 2012; **62**(3):368–81.
5. Beck S, Skarecky D, Osann K, Juarez R, Ahlering TE. Transverse versus vertical camera port incision in robotic radical prostatectomy: Effect on incisional hernias and cosmesis. *Urology* 2011; **78**(3):586–90.
6. Novara G, Ficarra V, Rosen RC, *et al.* Systematic review and meta-analysis of perioperative outcomes and complications after robot-assisted radical prostatectomy. *Eur Urol* 2012; **62**(3):431–52.
7. Patel VR, Palmer KJ, Coughlin G, Samavedi S. Robot-assisted laparoscopic radical prostatectomy: Perioperative outcomes of 1500 cases. *J Endourol* 2008; **22**(10):2299–305.
8. Tewari A, Rao S, Martinez-Salamanca JI, *et al.* Cancer control and the preservation of neurovascular tissue: How to meet competing goals during robotic radical prostatectomy. *BJU Int* 2008; **101**(8):1013–8.
9. Carlucci JR, Nabizada-Pace F, Samadi DB. Robot-assisted laparoscopic radical prostatectomy: Technique and outcomes of 700 cases. *Int J Biomed Sci* 2009; **5**(3):201–8.
10. Greco KA, Meeks JJ, Wu S, Nadler RB. Robot-assisted radical prostatectomy in men aged ≥70 years. *BJU Int* 2009; **104**(10):1492–5.
11. Jaffe J, Castellucci S, Cathelineau X, *et al.* Robot-assisted laparoscopic prostatectomy: a single-institutions learning curve. *Urology* 2009; **73**(1):127–33.
12. Martin GL, Nunez RN, Humphreys MD, *et al.* Interval from prostate biopsy to robot-assisted radical prostatectomy: Effects on perioperative outcomes. *BJU Int* 2009; **104**(11):1734–7.
13. Murphy DG, Kerger M, Crowe H, Peters JS, Costello AJ. Operative details and oncological and functional outcome of robotic-assisted laparoscopic radical prostatectomy: 400 cases with a minimum of 12 months follow-up. *Eur Urol* 2009; **55**(6):1358–67.
14. Coelho RF, Palmer KJ, Rocco B, *et al.* Early complication rates in a single-surgeon series of 2500 robotic-assisted radical prostatectomies: report applying a standardized grading system. *Eur Urol* 2010; **57**(6):945–52.
15. Davis JW, Kamat A, Munsell M, Pettaway C, Pisters L, Matin S. Initial experience of teaching robot-assisted radical prostatectomy to surgeons-in-training: Can training be evaluated and standardized? *BJU Int* 2010; **105**(8):1148–54.
16. Jeong J, Choi EY, Kim IY. Clavien classification of complications after the initial series of robot-assisted radical prostatectomy: The cancer institute of new Jersey/Robert wood Johnson medical school experience. *J Endourol* 2010; **24**(9):1457–61.
17. Lasser MS, Renzulli J Ii, Turini GA Iii, Haleblian G, Sax HC, Pareek G. An unbiased prospective report of perioperative complications of robot-assisted laparoscopic radical prostatectomy. *Urology* 2010; **75**(5):1083–9.
18. Lee JW, Jeong WJ, Park SY, Loreazo EIS, Oh CK, Rha KH. Learning curve for robot-assisted laparoscopic radical prostatectomy for pathologic T2 disease. *Korean J Urol* 2010; **51**(1):30–3.
19. Novara G, Ficarra V, D'Elia C, Secco S, Cavalleri S, Artibani W. Prospective evaluation with standardised criteria for postoperative complications after robotic-assisted laparoscopic radical prostatectomy. *Eur Urol* 2010; **57**(3):363–70.
20. Ploussard G, Xylinas E, Salomon L, *et al.* Robot-assisted extraperitoneal laparoscopic radical prostatectomy: Experience in a high-volume laparoscopy reference centre. *BJU Int* 2010; **105**(8):1155–60.
21. Bolenz C, Gupta A, Roehrborn CG, Lotan Y. Predictors of costs for robotic-assisted laparoscopic radical prostatectomy. *Urologic Oncology: Seminars and Original Investigations* 2011; **29**(3):325–9.
22. Heldt JP, Jellison FC, Yuen WD, *et al.* Patients with end-stage renal disease are candidates for robot-assisted laparoscopic radical prostatectomy. *J Endourol* 2011; **25**(7):1175–80.
23. Jayram G, Decastro GJ, Large MC, *et al.* Robotic radical prostatectomy in patients with high-risk disease: A review of short-term outcomes from a high-volume center. *J Endourol* 2011; **25**(3):455–7.
24. Fischer B, Engel N, Fehr JL, John H. Complications of robotic assisted radical prostatectomy. *World J Urol* 2008; **26**(6):595–602.
25. Agarwal PK, Sammon J, Bhandari A, *et al.* Safety profile of robot-assisted radical prostatectomy: A standardized report of complications in 3317 patients. *Eur Urol* 2011; **59**(5):684–98.
26. Lebeau T, Rouprêt M, Ferhi K, *et al.* Assessing the complications of laparoscopic robot-assisted surgery: The case of radical prostatectomy. *Surgical Endoscopy and Other Interventional Techniques* 2011; **25**(2):536–42.
27. Caballero-Romeu JP, Palacios Ramos J, Pereira Arias JG, Gamarra Quintanilla M, Astobieta Odriozola A, Ibarluzea González G. Radical prostatectomy: Evaluation of learning curve outcomes laparoscopic and robotic-assisted laparoscopic techniques with radical retropubic prostatectomy. *Prostatectomía radical: Comparación de los resultados obtenidos durantelas curvas de aprendizaje de la técnica laparoscópica pura y de la técnicaasistida por robot con la prostatectomía radical retropúbica* 2008; **32**(10):968–75.
28. Drouin SJ, Vaessen C, Hupertan V, *et al.* Comparison of mid-term carcinologic control obtained after open, laparoscopic, and robot-assisted radical prostatectomy for localized prostate cancer. *World J Urol* 2009; **27**(5):599–605.
29. Ficarra V, Novara G, Fracalanza S, *et al.* A prospective, non-randomized trial comparing robot-assisted laparoscopic and retropubic radical prostatectomy in one european institution. *BJU Int* 2009; **104**(4):534–9.
30. Ou YC, Yang CR, Wang J, Cheng CL, Patel VR. Comparison of robotic-assisted versus retropubic radical prostatectomy performed by a single surgeon. *Anticancer Res* 2009; **29**(5):1637–42.
31. Rocco B, Matei DV, Melegari S, *et al.* Robotic vs open prostatectomy in a laparoscopically naive centre: A matched-pair analysis. *BJU Int* 2009; **104**(7):991–5.
32. Carlsson S, Nilsson AE, Schumacher MC, *et al.* Surgery-related complications in 1253 robot-assisted and 485 open retropubic radical prostatectomies at the Karolinska University Hospital, Sweden. *Urology* 2010; **75**(5):1092–7.
33. Breyer BN, Davis CB, Cowan JE, Kane CJ, Carroll PR. Incidence of bladder neck contracture after robot-assisted laparoscopic and open radical prostatectomy. *BJU Int* 2010; **106**(11):1734–8.
34. Doumerc N, Yuen C, Savdie R, *et al.* Should experienced open prostatic surgeons convert to robotic surgery? the real learning curve for one surgeon over 3 years. *BJU Int* 2010; **106**(3):378–84.
35. Kordan Y, Barocas DA, Altamar HO, *et al.* Comparison of transfusion requirements between open and robotic-assisted laparoscopic radical prostatectomy. *BJU Int* 2010; **106**(7):1036–40.
36. Lo KL, Ng CF, Lam CNY, Hou SSM, To KF, Yip SKH. Short-term outcome of patients with robot-assisted versus open radical prostatectomy: For localised carcinoma of prostate. *Hong Kong Med J* 2010; **16**(1):31–5.
37. Truesdale MD, Lee DJ, Cheetham PJ, Hruby GW, Turk AT, Badani KK. Assessment of lymph node yield after pelvic lymph node dissection in men with prostate cancer: A comparison between robot-assisted radical prostatectomy and open radical prostatectomy in the modern era. *J Endourol* 2010; **24**(7):1055–60.
38. Di Pierro GB, Baumeister P, Stucki P, Beatrice J, Danuser H, Mattei A. A prospective trial comparing consecutive series of open retropubic and robot-assisted laparoscopic radical prostatectomy in a centre with a limited caseload. *Eur Urol* 2011; **59**(1):1–6.

39. Cho JW KT, Sung GT. Laparoscopic radical prostatectomy versus robot-assisted laparoscopic radical prostatectomy. *Korean J Urol* 2009; **50**(12):1198–202.
40. Hakimi AA, Blitstein J, Feder M, Shapiro E, Ghavamian R. Direct comparison of surgical and functional outcomes of robotic-assisted versus pure laparoscopic radical prostatectomy: single-surgeon experience. *Urology* 2009; **73**(1):119–23.
41. Trabulsi EJ, Zola JC, Gomella LG, Lallas CD. Transition from pure laparoscopic to robotic-assisted radical prostatectomy: A single surgeon institutional evolution. *Urologic Oncology: Seminars and Original Investigations* 2010; **28**(1):81–5.
42. Park JW, Won Lee H, Kim W, *et al.* Comparative assessment of a single surgeon's series of laparoscopic radical prostatectomy: Conventional versus robot-assisted. *J Endourol* 2011; **25**(4):597–602.
43. Asimakopoulos AD, Pereira Fraga CT, Annino F, Pasqualetti P, Calado AA, Mugnier C. Randomized comparison between laparoscopic and robot-assisted nerve-sparing radical prostatectomy. *J Sex Med* 2011; **8**(5):1503–12.
44. Ficarra V, Novara G, Rosen RC, *et al.* Systematic review and meta-analysis of studies reporting urinary continence recovery after robot-assisted radical prostatectomy. *Eur Urol* 2012; **62**(3):405–17.
45. Finley DS, Osann K, Chang A, Santos R, Skarecky D, Ahlering TE. Hypothermic robotic radical prostatectomy: Impact on continence. *J Endourol* 2009; **23**(9):1443–50.
46. Lee DJ CP, Badani KK. Predictors of early urinary continence after robotic prostatectomy. *Can J Urol* 2010; **17**(3):5200–5.
47. Novara G, Ficarra V, D'Elia C, *et al.* Evaluating urinary continence and preoperative predictors of urinary continence after robot assisted laparoscopic radical prostatectomy. *J Urol* 2010; **184**(3):1028–33.
48. Shikanov S, Desai V, Razmaria A, Zagaja GP, Shalhav AL. Robotic radical prostatectomy for elderly patients: probability of achieving continence and potency 1 year after surgery. *J Urol* 2010; **183**(5):1803–7.
49. Martin AD, Nakamura LY, Nunez RN, Wolter CE, Humphreys MR, Castle EP. Incontinence after radical prostatectomy: A patient centered analysis and implications for preoperative counseling. *J Urol* 2011; **186**(1):204–8.
50. Patel VR, Sivaraman A, Coelho RF, *et al.* Pentafecta: A new concept for reporting outcomes of robot-assisted laparoscopic radical prostatectomy. *Eur Urol* 2011; **59**(5):702–7.
51. Xylinas E, Durand X, Ploussard G, *et al.* Evaluation of combined oncologic and functional outcomes after robotic-assisted laparoscopic extraperitoneal radical prostatectomy: Trifecta rate of achieving continence, potency and cancer control. *Urol Oncol* 2013; **31**(1):99–103.
52. Park SY, Cho KS, Ham WS, Choi HM, Hong SJ, Rha KH. Robot-assisted laparoscopic radical cystoprostatectomy with ileal conduit urinary diversion: Initial experience in Korea. *J Laparoendosc Adv Surg Tech A* 2008; **18**(3):401–4.
53. Link BA, Nelson R, Josephson DY, *et al.* The impact of prostate gland weight in robot assisted laparoscopic radical prostatectomy. *J Urol* 2008; **180**(3):928–32.
54. Samadi DB, Muntner P, Nabizada-Pace F, Brajtbord JS, Carlucci J, Lavery HJ. Improvements in robot-assisted prostatectomy: the effect of surgeon experience and technical changes on oncologic and functional outcomes. *J Endourol* 2010; **24**(7):1105–10.
55. Krane LS, Wambi C, Bhandari A, Stricker HJ. Posterior support for urethrovesical anastomosis in robotic radical prostatectomy: single surgeon analysis. *Can J Urol* 2009; **16**(5):4836–40.
56. Kim SD KT, Cho JW, You YC, Sung GT. Effect of posterior urethral reconstruction (pur) in early recovery of urinary continence after robotic-assisted radical prostatectomy. *Korean J Urol* 2009; **50**(12):1203–7.
57. Woo JR, Shikanov S, Zorn KC, Shalhav AL, Zagaja GP. Impact of posterior rhabdosphincter reconstruction during robot-assisted radical prostatectomy: Retrospective analysis of time to continence. *J Endourol* 2009; **23**(12):1995–9.
58. Joshi N, de Blok W, van Muilekom E, van der Poel H. Impact of posterior musculofascial reconstruction on early continence after robot-assisted laparoscopic radical prostatectomy: results of a prospective parallel group trial. *Eur Urol* 2010; **58**(1):84–9.
59. Kim IY, Hwang EA, Mmeje C, Ercolani M, Lee DH. Impact of posterior urethral plate repair on continence following robot-assisted laparoscopic radical prostatectomy. *Yonsei Med J* 2010; **51**(3):427–31.
60. Coelho RF, Chauhan S, Orvieto MA, *et al.* Influence of modified posterior reconstruction of the rhabdosphincter on early recovery of continence and anastomotic leakage rates after robot-assisted radical prostatectomy. *Eur Urol* 2011; **59**(1):72–80.
61. Sutherland DE, Linder B, Guzman AM, *et al.* Posterior rhabdosphincter reconstruction during robotic assisted radical prostatectomy: Results from a phase II randomized clinical trial. *J Urol* 2011; **185**(4):1262–7.
62. Menon M, Muhletaler F, Campos M, Peabody JO. assessment of early continence after reconstruction of the periprostatic tissues in patients undergoing computer assisted (robotic) prostatectomy: results of a 2 group parallel randomized controlled trial. *J Urol* 2008; **180**(3):1018–23.
63. Sammon JD MF, Peabody JO, Diaz-Insua M, Satyanaryana R, Menon M. Long-term functional urinary outcomes comparing single- vs double-layer urethrovesical anastomosis: two-year follow-up of a two-group parallel randomized controlled trial. *Urology* 2010; **76**(5):1102–7.
64. Koliakos N, Mottrie A, Buffi N, De Naeyer G, Willemsen P, Fonteyne E. Posterior and anterior fixation of the urethra during robotic prostatectomy improves early continence rates. *Scand J Urol Nephrol* 2010; **44**(1):5–10.
65. Hurtes X RM, Vaessen C, Pereira H, Faivre d'Arcier B, Cormier L, Bruyère F. Anterior suspension combined with posterior reconstruction during robot-assisted laparoscopic prostatectomy improves early return of urinary continence: a prospective randomized multicentre trial. *BJU Int* 2012; **110**(6):875–83.
66. Tan G, Srivastava A, Grover S, *et al.* Optimizing vesicourethral anastomosis healing after robot-assisted laparoscopic radical prostatectomy: Lessons learned from three techniques in 1900 patients. *J Endourol* 2010; **24**(12):1975–83.
67. Srivastava A, Chopra S, Pham A, *et al.* Effect of a risk-stratified grade of nerve-sparing technique on early return of continence after robot-assisted laparoscopic radical prostatectomy. *Eur Urol* 2013; **63**(3):438–44.
68. Tewari A, Srivasatava A, Menon M. A prospective comparison of radical retropubic and robot-assisted prostatectomy: Experience in one institution. *BJU Int* 2003; **92**(3):205–10.
69. Krambeck AE, DiMarco DS, Rangel LJ, *et al.* Radical prostatectomy for prostatic adenocarcinoma: A matched comparison of open retropubic and robot-assisted techniques. *BJU Int* 2009; **103**(4):448–53.
70. Ou YC, Yang CR, Wang J, Cheng CL, Patel VR. Robotic-assisted laparoscopic radical prostatectomy: Learning curve of first 100 cases. *Int J Urol* 2010; **17**(7):635–40.
71. Kim SC, Song C, Kim W, *et al.* Factors determining functional outcomes after radical prostatectomy: Robot-assisted versus retropubic. *Eur Urol* 2011; **60**(3):413–9.
72. Joseph JV, Vicente I, Madeb R, Erturk E, Patel HRH. Robot-assisted vs pure laparoscopic radical prostatectomy: Are there any differences? *BJU Int* 2005; **96**(1):39–42.
73. Lee HW LH, Seo SI. Comparison of initial surgical outcomes between laparoscopic radical prostatectomy and robot-assisted laparoscopic radical prostatectomy performed by a single surgeon. *Korean J Urol* 2009; **50**(5):468–74.
74. Ficarra V, Novara G, Ahlering TE, *et al.* Systematic review and meta-analysis of studies reporting potency rates after robot-assisted radical prostatectomy. *Eur Urol* 2012; **62**(3):418–30.
75. Park SY, Ham WS, Choi YD, Rha KH. Robot-assisted laparoscopic radical prostatectomy: Clinical experience of 200 cases. *Korean J Urol* 2008; **49**(3):215–20.

76. Rodriguez E Jr, Finley DS, Skarecky D, Ahlering TE. single institution 2-year patient reported validated sexual function outcomes after nerve sparing robot assisted radical prostatectomy. *J Urol* 2009; **181**(1):259–63.
77. Shikanov SA, Zorn KC, Zagaja GP, Shalhav AL. Trifecta outcomes after robotic-assisted laparoscopic prostatectomy. *Urology* 2009; **74**(3):619–23.
78. Menon M, Shrivastava A, Bhandari M, Satyanarayana R, Siva S, Agarwal PK. Vattikuti Institute prostatectomy: technical modifications in 2009. *Eur Urol* 2009; **56**(1):89–96.
79. Novara G, Ficarra V, D'Elia C, *et al.* preoperative criteria to select patients for bilateral nerve-sparing robotic-assisted radical prostatectomy. *J Sex Med* 2010; **7**(2 PART 1):839–45.
80. Ahlering TE, Rodriguez E, Skarecky DW. Overcoming obstacles: Nerve-sparing issues in radical prostatectomy. *J Endourol* 2008; **22**(4):745–9.
81. Shikanov S, Woo J, Al-Ahmadie H, *et al.* Extrafascial versus interfascial nerve-sparing technique for robotic-assisted laparoscopic prostatectomy: comparison of functional outcomes and positive surgical margins characteristics. *Urology* 2009; **74**(3):611–6.
82. Tewari AK, Srivastava A, Huang MW, *et al.* Anatomical grades of nerve sparing: A risk-stratified approach to neural-hammock sparing during robot-assisted radical prostatectomy (RARP). *BJU Int* 2011; **108**(6 B):984–92.
83. Feicke A, Baumgartner M, Talimi S, *et al.* Robotic-assisted laparoscopic extended pelvic lymph node dissection for prostate cancer: surgical technique and experience with the first 99 cases. *Eur Urol* 2009; **55**(4):876–84.
84. Ham WS, Park SY, Rha KH, Kim WT, Choi YD. Robotic radical prostatectomy for patients with locally advanced prostate cancer is feasible: Results of a single-institution study. *J Laparoendosc Adv Surg Tech A* 2009; **19**(3):329–32.
85. Novara G, Ficarra V, Mocellin S, *et al.* Systematic review and meta-analysis of studies reporting oncologic outcome after robot-assisted radical prostatectomy. *Eur Urol* 2012; **62**(3):382–404.
86. Liss M, Osann K, Ornstein D. Positive surgical margins during robotic radical prostatectomy: A contemporary analysis of risk factors. *BJU Int* 2008; **102**(5):603–7.
87. Ficarra V, Novara G, Secco S, *et al.* Predictors of Positive Surgical Margins After Laparoscopic Robot Assisted Radical Prostatectomy. *J Urol* 2009; **182**(6):2682–8.
88. Ploussard G, Xylinas E, Paul A, *et al.* Is robot assistance affecting operating room time compared with pure retroperitoneal laparoscopic radical prostatectomy? *J Endourol* 2009; **23**(6):939–43.
89. Shikanov S, Song J, Royce C, *et al.* Length of positive surgical margin after radical prostatectomy as a predictor of biochemical recurrence. *J Urol* 2009; **182**(1):139–44.
90. Coelho RF, Chauhan S, Orvieto MA, Palmer KJ, Rocco B, Patel VR. Predictive factors for positive surgical margins and their locations after robot-assisted laparoscopic radical prostatectomy. *Eur Urol* 2010; **57**(6):1022–9.
91. Tewari AK PN, Leung RA, *et al.* Visual cues as a surrogate for tactile feedback during robotic-assisted laparoscopic prostatectomy: posterolateral margin rates in 1340 consecutive patients. *BJU Int* 2010; **106**(4):528–36.
92. Patel VR, Coelho RF, Rocco B, *et al.* Positive surgical margins after robotic assisted radical prostatectomy: A multi-institutional study. *Int Braz J Urol* 2011; **37**(4):540–1.
93. Laurila TAJ, Huang W, Jarrard DF. Robotic-assisted laparoscopic and radical retropubic prostatectomy generate similar positive margin rates in low and intermediate risk patients. *Urol Oncol* 2009; **27**(5):529–33.
94. White MA, De Haan AP, Stephens DD, Maatman TK, Maatman TJ. Comparative analysis of surgical margins between radical retropubic prostatectomy and RALP: are patients sacrificed during initiation of robotics program? *Urology* 2009; **73**(3):567–71.
95. Barocas DA, Salem S, Kordan Y, *et al.* Robotic assisted laparoscopic prostatectomy versus radical retropubic prostatectomy for clinically localized prostate cancer: Comparison of short-term biochemical recurrencefree survival. *J Endourol* 2010; **24**(6):893–4.
96. Magheli A, Gonzalgo ML, Su LM, *et al.* Impact of surgical technique (open vs laparoscopic vs robotic-assisted) on pathological and biochemical outcomes following radical prostatectomy: An analysis using propensity score matching. *BJU Int* 2011; **107**(12):1956–62.
97. Di Pierro GB, Besmer I, Hefermehl LJ, *et al.* Intra-abdominal fire due to insufflating oxygen instead of carbon dioxide during robot-assisted radical prostatectomy: Case report and literature review. *Eur Urol* 2010; **58**(4):626–8.
98. Menon M, Bhandari M, Gupta N, *et al.* Biochemical recurrence following robot-assisted radical prostatectomy: Analysis of 1384 patients with a median 5-year follow-up. *Eur Urol* 2010; **58**(6):838–46.
99. Suardi N, Ficarra V, Willemsen P, *et al.* Long-term biochemical recurrence rates after robot-assisted radical prostatectomy: Analysis of a single-center series of patients with a minimum follow-up of 5 years. *Urology* 2012; **79**(1):133–8.
100. Sooriakumaran P, Haendler L, Nyberg T, *et al.* Biochemical recurrence after robot-assisted radical prostatectomy in a european single-centre cohort with a minimum follow-up time of 5 years. *Eur Urol* 2012; **62**(5):768–74.
101. Murphy DG, Bjartell A, Ficarra V, *et al.* Downsides of robot-assisted laparoscopic radical prostatectomy: limitations and complications. *Eur Urol* 2010; **57**(5):735–46.
102. Vickers AJ, Bianco FJ, Serio AM, *et al.* The surgical learning curve for prostate cancer control after radical prostatectomy. *J Nat Cancer Inst* 2007; **99**(15):1171–7.
103. Vickers AJ, Savage CJ, Hruza M, *et al.* The surgical learning curve for laparoscopic radical prostatectomy: a retrospective cohort study. *Lancet Oncol* 2009; **10**(5):475–80.
104. Scales CD Jr, Jones PJ, Eisenstein EL, Preminger GM, Albala DM. Local cost structures and the economics of robot assisted radical prostatectomy. *J Urol* 2005; **174**(6):2323–9.
105. Ramsay C, Pickard R, Robertson C, *et al.* Systematic review and economic modelling of the relative clinical benefit and cost-effectiveness of laparoscopic surgery and robotic surgery for removal of the prostate in men with localised prostate cancer. *Health Technology Assessesment* 2012; **16**(41):1–313.
106. Bolenz C, Freedland SJ, Hollenbeck BK, *et al.* Costs of radical prostatectomy for prostate cancer: a systematic review. *Eur Urol* 2014; **65**(2):316–24.

CHAPTER 6.11

Metastatic disease in prostate cancer

Noel W. Clarke

Metastatic mechanisms in the primary tumour

The fundamental problem arising from of prostate cancer is its propensity to metastasize. Without this, the disease would not be the major public health problem it currently is. This tendency is predicated on specific molecular mechanisms and interactions resulting in the coordinated and inexorable process of local invasion, extravasation, and distal migration from the primary followed by the establishment of site specific metastases at secondary locations. Basic knowledge relating to this structured mechanism has improved in recent years but our understanding of the hows and whys of this process remains poor. Improved understanding of the molecular mechanisms underpinning metastases is essential and would potentially open the way for the application of novel therapies to treat this incurable condition.

Local invasion

Local invasion is the fundamental early step in the metastatic process and without it, tumour spread would not occur. For tumour invasion, epithelial cells must break free from adhesion to each other and to their connective tissue scaffold, they must become motile, and acquire the ability to break down the extracellular matrix using degradative enzymes. The means by which cells transformed by the malignant process, invade, and migrate has been described as the three-step invasion and metastasis theory:

- Step 1: Attachment to underlying extracellular matrix
- Step 2: Digestion of basement membrane
- Step 3: Migration to the interstitium

From the interstitium, cells must enter the vascular or lymphatic circulation by breaching the endothelial barrier.[1,2] The cell then migrates in the blood or lymphatic circulation and arrests at a secondary endothelial site, where the process of endothelial binding, extravasation, and endothelial transmigration occur once more. Only cancer cells have the ability to cross the endothelial barrier[1] and implant as a micrometastasis. They will only do this if the environment at the secondary site is favourable. In prostate cancer, these environmental properties are clearly present in lymph nodes and particularly, the red bone marrow.[3]

Clinical features

Bone metastases from prostate cancer are a major unresolved clinical problem. More than 80% of men with these will die from prostate cancer (PCa) within five years of first presentation[4] and they are present in most men dying from the disease.[5] Morbidity and death is usually the direct result of red bone marrow infiltration. Once established there, malignant cells grow prolifically, disturbing the integrated structure and function of the bone and bone marrow, producing the classical clinical picture of marrow failure, bone pain, pathological fracture, and spinal cord compression.

Prevalence

Bone metastases in prostate cancer occur in 35–85% of patients,[6,7] homing to the axial skeleton (lumbar spine: 60%, ribs: 50%, appendicular skeleton: 38%, skull: 14%).[8] Dissemination in the skeleton is haematogenous and metastasis distribution correlates closely with red marrow distribution.[9,10] Affinity for red marrow is the most likely factor determining this distribution pattern. Emphasis has been placed on the Batsons' theory of 'valveless' venous spread.[11] However, the high incidence of metastases in the lumbar spine and pelvis is likely to be a consequence of anatomical proximity and venous drainage, which dictates that this skeletal region has the highest exposure to cells released from the primary and therefore the highest number of epithelial 'hits' on the bone marrow endothelium. Prostate epithelial cell/bone marrow endothelial binding is a rapid process[12] and a critical number of cellular 'hits' are needed for metastatic development.[13] The environment for metastatic implantation and growth is therefore at its height in the red bone marrow of the pelvis and lumbar spine.

Pathophysiology

Circulating epithelial cells arrest in bone marrow by binding to the endothelium; this is site-selective[14,15] and despite significant numbers of cells measurable in circulation even in clinically localized disease, widespread multiorgan metastases are a relatively late event. Tumour cells bind to endothelial cell–cell junctional regions (Fig. 6.11.1) then migrate actively through by a complex process of chemoattraction, cell movement and homing/binding to bone marrow stroma (for detailed description of this, see [2,3,16]).

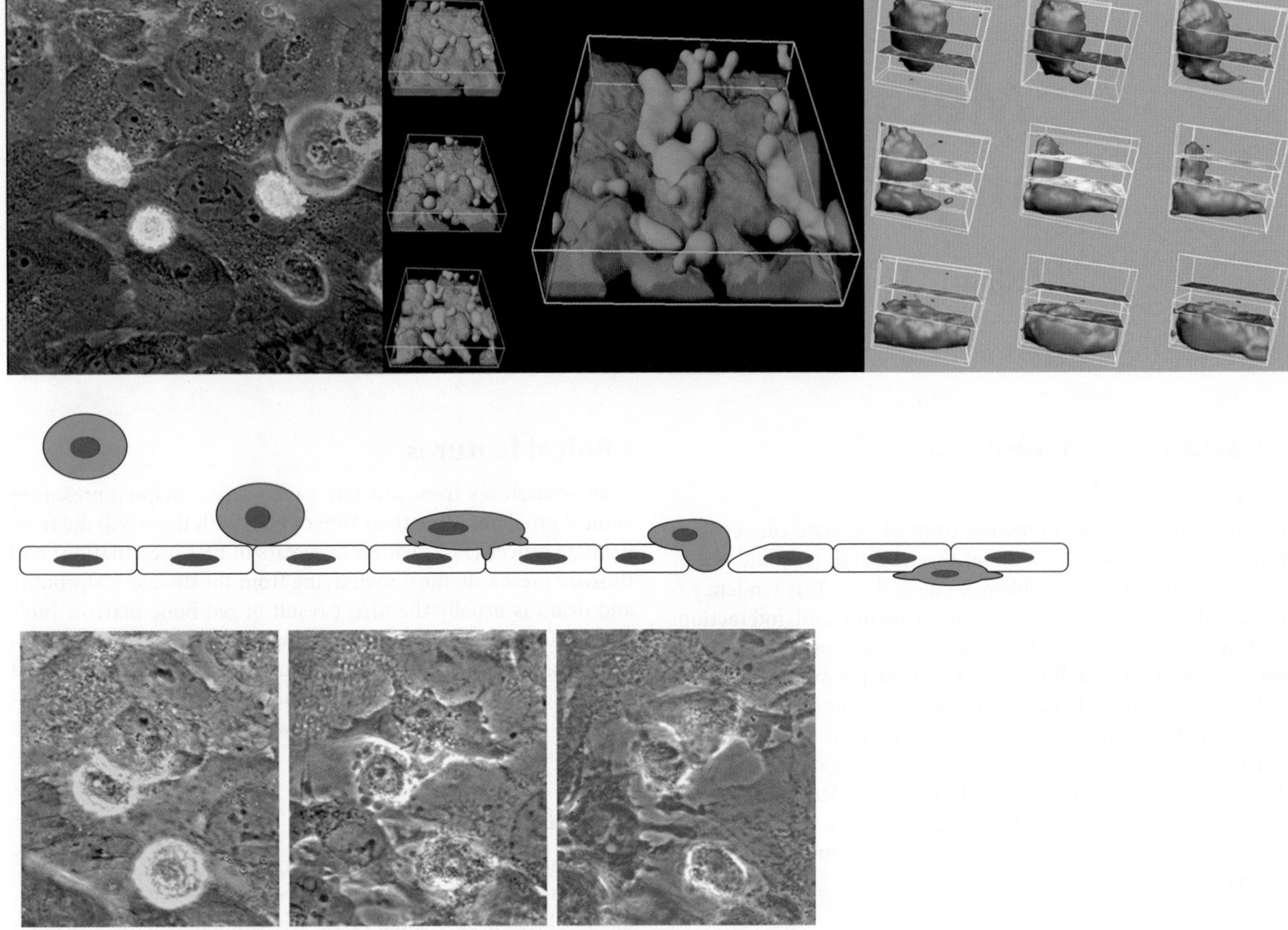

Fig. 6.11.1 Epithelial migration of prostate cancer cells across the bone marrow endothelium. The prostate cancer cells (green) bind to the endothelium (grey) at junctional areas. The prostate cancer cells then change shape (amoeboid to mesenchymal transition) and then move across the endothelial barrier. The binding process is completed within one hour and the migration within 24 hours.

Reprinted by permission from Macmillan Publishers Ltd on behalf of Cancer Research UK: *British Journal of Cancer*, Volume 92, Issue 3, C A Hart *et al.*, 'Invasive characteristics of human prostatic epithelial cells: understanding the metastatic process', pp. 503–512, Copyright © 2005 Rights Managed by Nature Publishing Group.

Within bone marrow cancer cells require several key elements to be present before an overt metastasis develops: there are many uncertainties about these and their interactions. Most migrating cancer cells die and some can remain dormant in bone marrow for considerable periods of time. However, once a cell colony propagates, the micrometastasis develops in the bone marrow space in close association with the bone surface disturbing the local microenvironment. It has been postulated that the first event in this process is osteoclast mediated resorption leading to release of stimulatory cytokines from the bone surface and culminating in a self-propagating cycle of bone resorption, cytokine release, tumour stimulation, and more resorption. This so-called 'vicious cycle' is almost certainly a later event and the first step in the early metastatic process is always a stimulation of fibroblastic elements in the bone marrow and osteoblasts on the bone surface. As metastases develop, the balance of bone resorption coupled to formation is disrupted, resulting in accelerated bone formation *and* destruction. This is caused by changes in local cytokine production and interaction. Several stimulating factors have been identified in relation to 'osteoblastic' metastases in prostate cancer. These selectively stimulate the mesodermal cell lineages thereby increasing osteoblast and fibroblast activity. They include fibroblast growth factors, TGFβ, bone morphorgenetic protein (BMP) and endothelin-1.[17] This overactivity is responsible for the measurable increase in bone volume[16,18,19] and for the measured acceleration in bone mineralization.[20] The tumour-generated bone deposited is abnormal 'woven' bone. This is characteristic of bone produced in high turnover states and is responsible for the well-described sclerotic appearance seen radiologically,[21] and measured histomorphometrically[19] and biochemically[22] in this disease.

In parallel with osteoblastic overactivity, PCa destroys bone by osteolysis driven by hyper-stimulated osteoclasts.[19,22–24] The paradox of increasing bone volume (sclerosis) accompanied by wholesale bone destruction is explained by histomorphometric measurement of bone metastases[19] showing that skeletal resorption is accompanied by synchronous replacement by abnormal woven bone, which, itself, undergoes further resorption. The lytic process is a consequence of abnormal levels of tumour-generated soluble growth factors. These overstimulate osteoclast recruitment, differentiation, and activation. One proven mechanism of this process is the stimulation of osteoblasts by macrophage colony stimulating factor (M-CSF), the receptor activator of the NFkb ligand (RANK-Ligand) and osteoprotegerin.[25,26] Osteoblasts then secrete the protein, RANK-Ligand which induces osteoclast differentiation by binding to the RANK surface receptor on the osteoclast precursor, stimulating osteoclastogenesis.[26] The protein osteoprotegerin plays a key regulatory role in this process by competing for the RANK binding site on osteoclast precursors. Knowledge of this process forms the basis for RANK-Ligand inhibition in clinical practice using the drug, denosumab.

Diagnosis

The basis of diagnostic imaging is Tc99 bone scanning, conventional radiology, and cross-sectional imaging with CT and/or MR scanning. None of these modalities is perfect and all have advantages and drawbacks.

Isotope bone scanning

The predilection of radionuclides for the bony skeleton has been known since 1929, when Martland and Humphries, in a classical paper, described the development of osteosarcomata in painters of luminous watch dials. It had also been known for some years that scintigraphic imaging was a better discriminator of metastatic disease in bone[27,28] and that bisphosphonate-labelled technetium was the most accurate and reliable isotope.[29] However, since that time there has been little evolution of any consequence in scintigraphic techniques for prostate cancer (PCa) in bone.[30] Most diagnostic pathways for metastatic staging in bone still rely heavily on Tc-99m bone scan, which is known to lack diagnostic specificity,[31,32] particularly at low levels of prostate-specific antigen (PSA), where it is a poor discriminator of microscopic disease. Indeed, its use at low PSA levels is of limited value: the positive detection rate of a bone scan in a patient with a PSA level <10 ng/mL is approximately 1%.

Thus, its use in an unstratified and routine manner is neither accurate nor cost effective. In cases where there is diagnostic uncertainty because of unspecific high uptake on scan (old fractures, Pagets disease, degenerative joint conditions, and so on) further characterization with supplementary targeted X-rays/scans is required to help discriminate benign from malignant lesions.[33]

MRI of the spine is routinely used for the imaging of suspected vertebral fractures or spinal cord compression in cancer patients and now, in the axial skeleton (AS-MRI) it is being used increasingly to detect metastases in the bone marrow/bone in prostate and other cancers.[34] AS-MRI has proved highly sensitive in detecting bone metastases in cancer patient.[34–38] Its superiority over BS in this regard is reported.[39–41] For example, in a well conducted single centre study, AS-MRI was able to identify bone metastases earlier than Tc-99m bone scan and its sensibility/specificity was superior to the standard imaging with Tc-99 BS and targeted X-rays.[42] However, skeletal MR needs to be better standardized: there is a lack of agreement regarding scan protocols (e.g. axial MR vs. whole body imaging, magnet power and sequences, and so on) and there is still a significant false negative and positive rate. Further work is ongoing in this area to refine and define the place of this technique in diagnosis and staging and it is likely that this imaging modality will ultimately supplant the isotopic bone scan.

Measurement of prostate cancer's treatment response and progression in bone is also a major problem. The conventional way to measure therapeutic response in soft tissue is to utilize RECIST criteria. These are based on the ability to measure the size of a solid tumour in two dimensions by clinical examination or cross sectional scanning.[43] With metastatic disease in bone this cannot be done, thereby confounding the application of RECIST in the skeleton.[43–46] This is particularly problematic for prostate cancer as metastases are mainly detected in bone (65–75%), with measurable lesions in lymph nodes or soft tissues being present in <40%, except in late-stage disease.[47,48] In the absence of robust imaging techniques for treatment response in bone, clinicians rely on techniques such as counting the number of scan hot spots, measuring their area and subjectively documenting scan intensity, interpreting this as regression or progression. However, these methods are notoriously unreliable for various reasons; for example, increased intensity can be the result regression of tumour (scan flare: occurring in up to 30%), healing in previously lytic areas can look like progression and methods involving counting of hotspots fail to account for the size of individual metastases (e.g. when the whole of the iliac blade is affected this counts as a single 'hotspot'). Other methods utilizing composite end points have been developed. These have mainly included radiological or clinical SREs (skeletal-related events). While these are useful, they are relatively crude instruments for measuring subtle changes in disease activity/regression in the skeleton. For future practice, it has become much more important, particularly for the development drugs targeted against bone metastasis to have better methods for measurement of response in bone.[49–51]

To this end, phase I studies to develop a single step MRI technique of the axial skeleton (AS-MRI) to quantify bone metastases have been undertaken to measure tumour response. Interestingly, tumour extension and response to therapy could be measured using CT scanner or AS-MRI.[52] This increased the proportion of RECIST measurable data from 29% to 65%.

Metastasis prevention

The most obvious way to prevent bone metastases is to remove the primary or kill off the cancer cells therein with radiation-based strategies. However, in a proportion of high-risk cases this strategy fails and where there is biochemical evidence of disease failure with the primary *in situ* (e.g. after 'curative' radiotherapy) or with an isolated PSA rise post prostatectomy then there then there is a significant chance of developing metastases in bone. A rapid PSA doubling time (PSADT) in M0 disease is a key prognostic factor for this.[53]

Strategies have been developed whereby systemic treatments are used to limit the development of bone metastases in high-risk clinical M0 patients. Examples include large scale trials using zoledronic acid, such as the ZEUSS or STAMPEDE trials,[54] which use zoledronic acid administered monthly over extended periods. Results of these studies have, however, been disappointing. The results using denosumab were positive.[55] This was effective for reducing the rate of M1 conversion, reducing the development of bone metastases by 15% by comparison with placebo. Subanalysis of this trial, studying groups with low PSADTs showed this reduction became more marked when the PSADT was <4 months, where the risk reduction here was 29%.[56] Although this level 1 evidence makes a case for the stratified use of this agent as a bone metastasis preventer in the high-risk setting, it awaits larger scale adoption by clinicians for this indication.

Clinical and metabolic effects

Morbidity and death from PCa is most commonly linked to skeletal metastatic spread. Disturbance in balanced bone and bone marrow function manifests as marrow failure, altered calcium metabolism, pathological fracture, and spinal cord compression.

Bone marrow failure

This is a direct consequence of red marrow infiltration by metastatic prostate cancer (Fig. 6.11.2). This displaces the erythroid and blast cell precursors, inducing dysfunction and depletion in leukoid and erythroid lineages. The commonest clinical consequence of this is anaemia, although immunological dysfunction, platelet malfunction, and overt DIC are known sequelae. Anaemia is common, especially in late stage disease.[57] inducing lethargy and shortness of breath, particularly when the haemoglobin falls below 8 g/dl. At this Hb level transfusion facilitates symptomatic improvement and is an effective palliative measure.[58,59]

Erythropoetin (EPO) has been used[60] and it also helps counteract the erythroid suppression produced by combined androgen blockade. A limited number of studies have used this agent in castrate-resistant prostate cancer (CRPC): a small study using EPO over 12 weeks showed a 2 g/dl increase in Hb.[61] A further report using EPO (5,000 units ×3/week) claimed significant benefit without major side effects, with 43% of patients experiencing improved quality of life (QoL) with Hb increases of >2 g/dl.[62] However, the short life expectancy of patients and cost of therapy have limited its use in this patient population.

Skeletal dysfunction

Metabolic effects

Derangement of skeletal function by prostatic infiltration disturbs calcium metabolism. Other cancers such as breast typically induce hypercalcaemia but this is uncommon in PCa occurring in only 1–5%.[63] Patients usually have low serum calcium because the excessive bone formation in metastases induces a 'calcium sink' effect,[64] utilizing the excess calcium released by osteolysis to meet the calcium demand from osteoblast overactivity. The increased calcium mobilization leads to mild hyperparathyroidism and a chronic increase in bone resorption in areas of the skeleton not involved by cancer which, in turn, potentiates the bone loss from androgen deprivation.[19]

Pathological fracture

Clinical pathological fracture has been perceived as a relatively uncommon event in prostate cancer with a proposed incidence of 3%,[65] contrasting with a rate of 9% in malignancies overall and 16% in breast cancer.[66,67] More recent analysis has shown that pathological fracture is a much more common problem than was previously thought. In CRPC the fracture rate has been reported to be as high as 33% when measured radiologically, with approximately

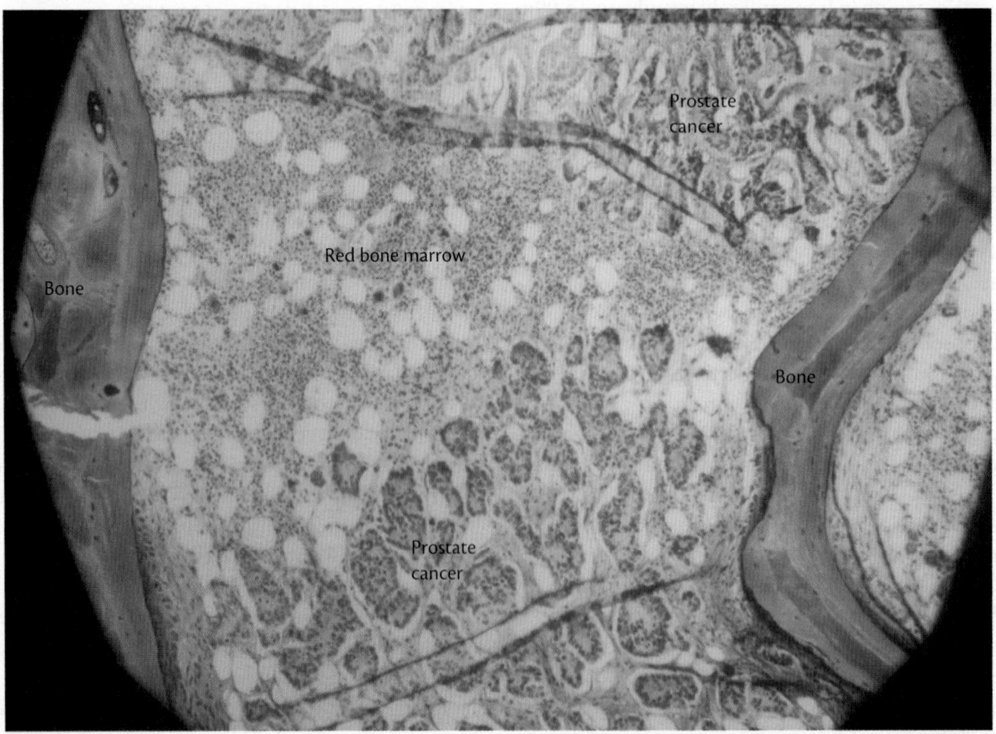

Fig. 6.11.2 Bone biopsy from a bone metastasis in hormone refractory prostate cancer. The trabeculae of the cancellous bone (solid blue) frame the marrow space containing normal red bone marrow (centre to upper left) and encroaching prostate cancer cells (lower central and upper right). The prostate cancer cells are displacing the red bone marrow progressively. The advancing front of malignant cells replaces the normal red marrow until the marrow space ultimately becomes populated completely by prostate cancer cells which in turn, induce osteoblast and osteoclast hyper-activity (as seen on the contiguous bone surfaces). It should be noted that the marrow replacement is not a compression phenomenon, as shown by the preservation of the architecture of the normal red marrow at the cancer/bone marrow interface. The marrow displacement is responsible for the anaemia and general haematological dysfunction seen commonly in hormone-refractory prostate cancer (HRPC).

two-thirds occurring in the vertebral column and one-third in the long bones.[68] This risk is exacerbated by the long-term use of androgen suppression.[69] However, there is controversy about the clinical importance of these 'skeletal-related events'—and it is important to discriminate between SRE's classified radiologically and those presenting clinically (the so-called 'clinical SRE', defined as a pathological fracture or a specific clinical intervention for a skeletal symptom such as local radiotherapy or intervention orthopaedic surgery).[70] When a clinical pathological fracture occurs, it is associated with a significant reduction in patient survival.[71] The incidence of these fractures can be reduced by the use of agents to reduce osteoclast overactivity. Other treatments include prophylactic local irradiation of lytic metastases in the shafts of long bones and in the neck of the femur. However, when a pathological fracture occurs in a long bone, it is important to treat this rapidly with orthopaedic fixation or joint replacement (Fig. 6.11.3). This is highly effective in reducing pain and restoring mobility. Fixation is usually supplemented by treatment with local radiotherapy two to four weeks after the surgery.

Spinal cord compression

This is a devastating complication of metastatic bone disease (Fig. 6.11.4). Prostate cancer is the commonest cause of malignant cord compression and its clinical manifestations occur in over 10% of patients.[65,72] Patients at risk can often be identified by simple clinical parameters: in a retrospective review of 68 patients[73] it was shown that heavy skeletal tumour load, long-standing duration of continuous androgen suppression and low Hb concentration effectively identified a population 'at risk'. Subsequent MRI scanning of such patients facilitated identification of men whose disease might be treated locally (e.g. with radiotherapy) before development of irreversible neurological deterioration. There is also good evidence to suggest that addition of a bisphosphonate or RANK-Ligand inhibition with denosumab to this group of patients will decrease the risk of cord compression still further.[65,74,75]

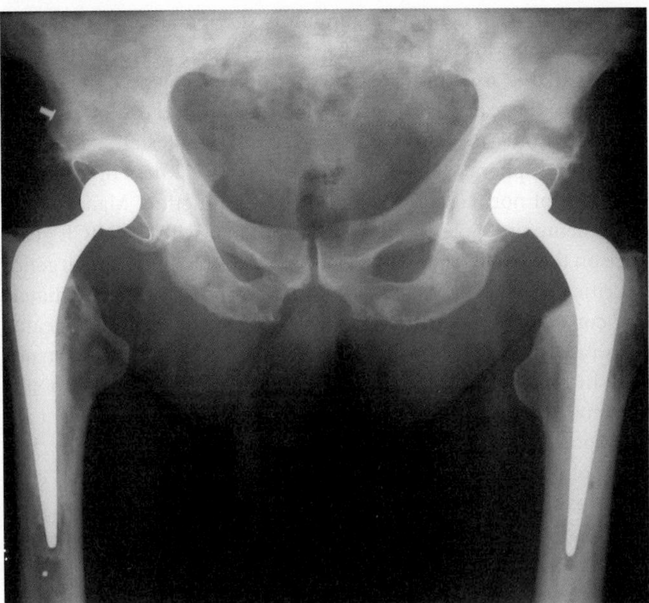

Fig. 6.11.3 Radiograph of a 63-year-old man with hormone refractory prostate cancer illustrating the problem of long bone fracture. Multiple sclerotic bone metastases are seen throughout the pelvis. Pathological fractures secondary to tumour mediated bone destruction have occurred separately in the necks of both femora over a 12-month period. These have been treated by prosthetic joint replacement and subsequent local radiotherapy.

Unfortunately, many patients present acutely, the underlying pathophysiological cause being a collapse of an affected vertebral

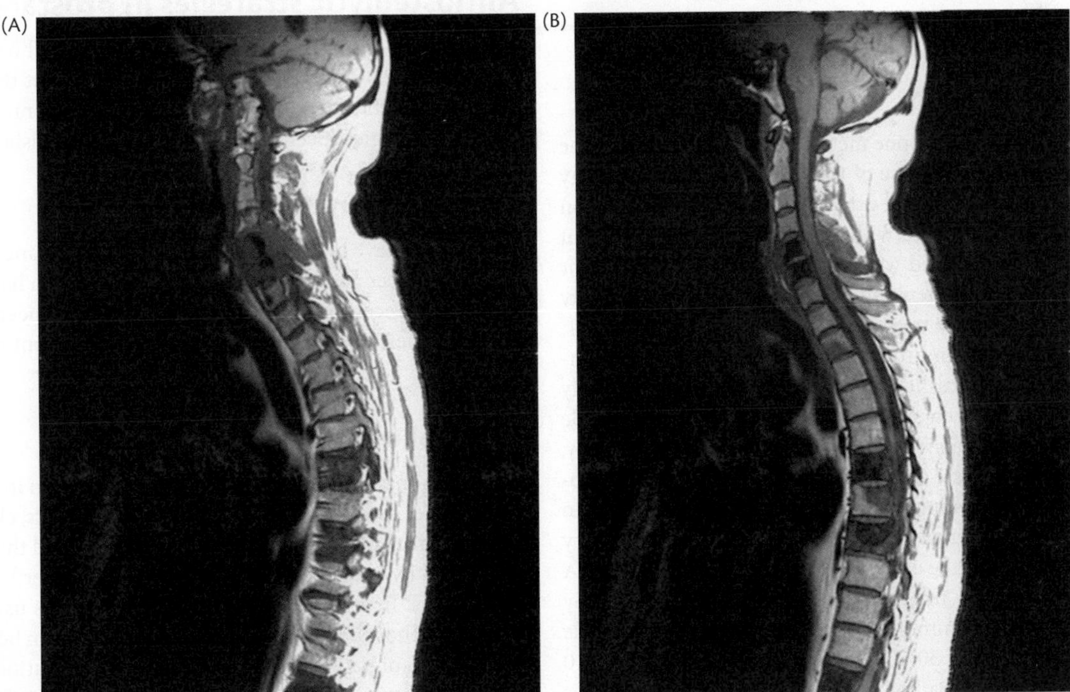

Fig. 6.11.4 MR scan of metastatic castrate resistant prostate cancer in the (A) cervical and (B) thoracic spine inducing spinal cord compression in HRPC. The serial scans from the same patient show destructive lesions in multiple vertebrae and illustrate that compression often occurs at multiple levels simultaneously. Early treatment is required for the best clinical outcome but paraplegia at presentation is usually an indicator of poor outcome.

body or encroachment of the tumour in the spinal canal itself. This tends to cause maximal trouble in the thoracic spine where the spinal canal is at its most narrow.[76] Prodromal symptoms tend to manifest as an excruciating 'band-like' pain around the lower abdomen (90% of cases) although more subtle manifestations include isolated peripheral neuropathy/lower limb weakness or spontaneous loss of normal bladder and/or bowel function. Management of the acute situation should be in accordance with the NICE guidance on the management of spinal cord compression[77] and urgency is critical. Dexamethasone should be administered immediately and consideration then given to whether the patient is best treated with radiotherapy or surgery. A reasoned balance must be struck here in relation to outcome and survival, as the response to surgery may be limited, especially if paraplegia has been present for >24 hours and if there is critical compression at multiple levels. In a study of 69 patients (52 with CRPC)[78] presenting with spinal cord compression, only 52% had a functional motor improvement after treatment, the majority seeing this within the first week of therapy. Many patients had multiple levels of compression (Fig. 6.11.4), a problem best categorized by MRI. Patients of younger age (<65) with single compression levels fared better: when these factors were excluded, there was no additional benefit arising from high irradiation dose (>30 Gy) or surgical decompression.[78] In a further study of spinal cord decompression only 8 of 19 men with CRPC had recovery of mobility postoperatively: perioperative mortality was 8% and a high proportion died within the year after surgery. Predictors of good outcome were the ability to walk preoperatively and rapid intervention after the onset of symptoms. Immobility, an onset of >24 hours and established paraplegia were particularly bad signs, the latter being a 'consistently accurate indication of poor long-term prognosis'.[79] This raises the question of whether or not laminectomy is justified in all CRPC patients with this particular problem: the answer is clearly 'no' but some will respond well and this needs carefully consideration by an expert team.

Management of bone pain and the use of ionizing radiation

Many patients with prostatic bone metastases will experience bone pain at some point in the course of their disease[8,80]: its aetiology is incompletely understood. The extent of disease in the skeleton does not necessarily correlate with the pain experienced,[81] but whether the pain is associated with a single isolated metastasis or a heavy skeletal load, it is often a source of considerable morbidity requiring multidisciplinary treatments by urologists, oncologists, and palliative care teams in order to bring symptoms under control. Many second and third-line therapies were developed recently and are now available when systemic therapy fails. These include the use of external beam or systemically administered radiotherapy, novel hormonal or cytotoxic chemotherapy, analgesics, and bisphosphonates. Focal radiotherapy is very effective for pain localized to specific metastases or defined areas of the skeleton. Regimens vary in different countries and the optimal treatment is still debated.[82] A typical European regimen might involve single dose 8 Gy or 4 Gy in six fractions while a commonly used North American schedule involves administration of 30 Gy given as 3 Gy fractions over 10 treatments.[83] 'Single shot' radiotherapy seems to be as efficacious as multifraction treatment in this situation. In a controlled study of single fraction 8 Gy versus 10 fractions of 3 Gy, there was no significant difference in outcome.[84] Whatever the regimen used, approximately 90% of patients will have a response and this will be complete in 40%.[85] Pain may recur at the same site of treatment but further local radiotherapy is then possible.[86]

When multiple sites are painful and other systemic therapies have failed, hemi-body irradiation (HBI) or administration of systemic radionuclides are effective. HBI will induce responses in 91% of patients (45% of these complete responses) within 3–8 days. Fractionated treatment is most effective[87] and two HBI doses of 3 Gy on consecutive days have shown to be as effective as 3 Gy over five days.[83] Toxicity, mainly nausea, vomiting, diarrhoea, and haematological suppression is usually transitory although the latter can be persistent.[88] Systemic radiotherapy using bone seeking isotopes can be very effective. Agents have previously focused on γ emitters like strontium[89] although phosphorus,[32] samarium, and rhenium[86] are also effective.[89] The half-life of Strontium is 50 days and a number of well-constructed randomized trials have confirmed its efficacy as a single dose administration. The response rate is in the region of 80%, with 33% experiencing a complete response.[90,91] Treatment is associated with mild haematological toxicity, inducing an average platelet count drop of 30%. This reaches its nadir at 6 weeks but it usually recovers by 12 weeks.[89] The treatment can be repeated if necessary. Its overall efficacy compares favourably with HBI[92] but it is less toxic. More recently evidence has emerged showing the utility of radium-223 (Alpharadin), an α emitter.[70] In a large scale randomized trial administering this agent to CRPC patients over six 'cycles' not only was quality of life improved, there was a reduction in pain, *clinical* SREs, and a prolongation of survival by four months. Furthermore, the toxicity of the drug was very low, with minimal suppression of the bone marrow. These striking results mean that this agent is likely to become a standard of care in bone related disease in PCa in the near future.

Antiosteolytic strategies in prostate cancer

The utility of antiresorptive agents in preventing bone loss arising from androgen deprivation is well established but this will not be discussed further herein. This section will concentrate on antiresorptive strategies specifically in relation to established metastases.

Bisphosphonates

These drugs have been used extensively in malignancy, particularly in breast cancer and myeloma. Their utility in PCa has been uncertain but in recent years their effects have now been established, although their clinical usage is variable in different countries and regions.

Control of bone pain

Bisphosphonates can alleviate refractory bone pain in CRPC. Open label studies using the earlier and less potent agents, clodronate[93,94] and pamidronate[95] reported a beneficial effect and these results are supported by positive findings using more powerful later generation drugs. In an open label study of 25 patients using the intravenous bisphosphonate 'Ibandronate', reductions in bone pain were seen in 92% of patients, with concomitant diminution in analgesic requirements and improvement in performance.[96] These findings have not, however, been replicated in larger controlled studies with clodronate[97,98] or pamidronate.[99] This may be a consequence of their lower potency by comparison with stronger drugs such as zoledronate and ibandronate. In a large scale randomized trial using zoledronate, currently the most potent bisphosphonate available, there was a significant decrease in pain requirement for those receiving the drug, although quality of life and performance were not affected significantly.[74] The reason for the variability of the results is unclear. Notwithstanding this, bisphosphonates do have a place in the management of refractory pain in CRPC. Patients most likely to benefit from bisphosphonates used as a pain relieving therapy are those with painful bone metastases which are difficult to control by other means.

Antiosteolytic effects on pathological fracture/cord compression

This class of drugs reduces bone resorption in CRPC[22] but their clinical benefit to the patient in reducing skeletal related morbid events has been open to question. Early controlled studies using less potent agents in small number studies (e.g.[100]) showed no effect from treatment by comparison with controls. Latterly, larger studies have shown differences even with less potent agents. A randomized UK MRC study assigned 311 patients with CRPC to receive the bisphosphonate clodronate or placebo with results showing a reduction in time to symptomatic bone progression.[101] In a second study using the same agent with chemotherapy (mitoxantrone and prednisone), subset analysis showed that moderate to severe bone pain was improved although the palliative effects were not different.[97] In a large randomized placebo-controlled study using zoledronic acid, serial use of the drug as monotherapy combined with standard palliative care reduced the incidence of skeletal related events by 11%.[74] This leads to the question of whether or not all patients with M1 CRPC should receive bisphosphonates. The view of some experts is that the cost/benefit from such a policy is insufficiently great[102] and added to this, there is the small but significant risk of osteonecrosis of the jaw (ONJ) with prolonged use, particularly in the presence of poor dental hygiene, and of renal toxicity. However, the same authors accept that there are patients who are likely to benefit from such a regimen. These patients include those with heavy skeletal tumour load, particularly in the thoracolumbar spine and femoral bones and those who have been on long-term LR/RH therapy or maximal androgen blockade. One future way of focusing this therapy may be to utilize serum and urinary markers to predict the 'at risk' population. Patients with high markers of bone turnover are known to represent a population with an increased risk of developing pathological fracture[103] and targeting this group may result in the most effective outcome.

Denosumab

Denosumab (XGEVA, Amgen) is a fully human monoclonal antibody that specifically targets the receptor activator of nuclear factor kappa B ligand (RANKL). This receptor/activator pathway plays a key role in bone destruction and tumour growth in metastatic cancers and denosumab inhibits it very effectively.[104] In a large scale randomized trial testing its efficacy against zoledronic acid in CRPC, where the latter drug was already known to reduce SREs by 11%, a further 18% reduction in first and subsequent SREs was demonstrated.[75] This agent is therefore the most effective antiosteolytic therapy currently available and it is of utility in advanced prostate cancer. It also has the added advantage that it is administered as a monthly subcutaneous injection and can be used when renal function is impaired.

Neither denosumab nor zoledronic acid have been shown to have a beneficial effect on overall or cancer specific survival and their use must be precautionary in relation to hypocalcaemia and ONJ. These agents can both induce clinical hypocalcaemia, and have to be given in conjunction with oral calcium and supplementary vitamin D. There is also a cumulative risk of osteonecrosis of the jaw; over two-year usage it was 13% with denosumab and 6% with zoledronic acid. Attention to treatment of dental hygiene is therefore necessary before and during use.

Conclusion

Bone metastases from prostate cancer are common and are a source of considerable morbidity. The understanding of their pathogenesis and natural history is improving but the overall knowledge and comprehension of the mechanisms of skeletal spread and subsequent marrow and skeletal dysfunction thereby induced is incomplete. A number of new drugs and approaches have been developed in recent years and there is evidence for their utility in prostate cancer in the palliative, end stages of metastatic PCa.

Further reading

Brown M, Roulson J, Hart C, Tawadros T, Clarke NW. Arachidonic acid induction of Rho-mediated transendothelial migration in prostate cancer. *Br J Canc* 2014; **110**(8):2099–108.

Brown MD, Hart C, Gazi E, Gardner P, Lockyer N, Clarke N. The influence of the omega 6 PUFA arachidonic acid and bone marrow adipocytes on metastatic spread from prostate cancer. *Brit J Canc* 2010; **102**(2):403–13.

Clarke NW, Brown MD. Molecular mechanisms of metastasis in prostate cancer. In: Partin A, Kirby R, Feneley M, Parsons J (eds). *Prostate Cancer*. New York, NY: Taylor & Francis, 2006.

Clarke NW, McClure J, George NJR. Morphometric evidence from bone resorption and replacement in prostate cancer. *Brit J Urol* 1991; **68**:74–80.

Coleman RE. Metastatic bone disease and the role of biochemical markers of bone metabolism in benign and malignant diseases. *Cancer Treat Rev* 2001; **27**:133–5.

Fizazi K, Carducci M, Smith M, *et al.* Denosumab versus zoledronic acid for treatment of bone metastases in men with castration-resistant prostate cancer: a randomised, double-blind study. *Lancet* 2011; **377**:813–22.

Hart CA, Brown M, Bagley S, Sharrard M, Clarke NW. Invasive characteristics of human prostatic epithelial cells: understanding the metastatic process. *Br J Canc* 2005; **92**:503–12.

Lang SH, Clarke NW, George NJR, Allen TD, Testa NG. Interaction of prostatic epithelial cells from benign and malignant tumour tissue with bone marrow stoma. *Prostate* 1998; **34**:203–13.

Lecouvet FE, Geukens D, Stainier A, *et al.* Magnetic resonance imaging of the axial skeleton for detecting bone metastases in patients with high-risk prostate cancer: diagnostic and cost-effectiveness and comparison with current detection strategies. *J Clin Oncol* 2007; **25**:3281–7.

Quilty PM, Kirk D, Bolger JJ, *et al.* Comparison of the palliative effects of Strontrium 89 and external beam radiotherapy in metastatic prostate cancer. *Radiother Oncol* 1994; **31**:33–40.

Saad F, Gleason DM, Murray R, *et al.* A randomised placebo-controlled trial of zoledronic acid in patients with hormone-refractory metastatic prostate carcinoma. *J Natl Canc Inst* 2002; **94**(19):1458–68.

Scott LJ, NW Clarke, JH Shanks, NG Testa, SH Lang. Interaction of human prostatic epithelial cells with bone marrow endothelium: banding and invasion. *Br J Cancer* 2001; **84**(10):1417–23.

White BD, Stirling AJ, Paterson E, Asquith-Coe K, Melder A. Guideline Development Group. Diagnosis and management of patients at risk of or with metastatic spinal cord compression: summary of NICE guidance. *BMJ* 2008; **337**:a2538.

References

1. Hart CA, Brown M, Bagley S, Sharrard M, Clarke NW. Invasive characteristics of human prostatic epithelial cells: understanding the metastatic process. *Br J Canc* 2005; **92**:503–12.
2. Brown M, Roulson J, Hart C, Tawadros T, Clarke NW. Arachidonic acid induction of Rho-mediated transendothelial migration in prostate cancer. *Br J Canc* 2014; **110**(8):2099–108.
3. Clarke NW, Brown MD. Molecular mechanisms of metastasis in prostate cancer. In: Partin A, Kirby R, Feneley M, Parsons J (eds). *Prostate Cancer*. New York, NY: Taylor & Francis, 2006.
4. Blackard CE, Byyar DP, Jordan WP. Orchiectomy for advanced prostatic carcinoma. A reevaluation. *Urology* 1973; **1**:553–60.
5. Abrams HL, Spiro R, Goldstein N. Metastases in Carcinoma. Analysis of 1000 Autopsied cases. *Cancer* 1950; **3**:74–85.
6. Galasko CSB. Development of skeletal metastases. (pp. 22–51) In: *Skeletal Metastases*. London, UK: Butterworth, 1986.
7. Carlin B, Andriole GL. The natural history of skeletal complications and management of bone metastases in patients with prostate cancer. *Cancer* 2000; **88**:2989–94.
8. Tofe J. Correlation of neoplasms with incidence and localisation of skeletal metastases: an analysis of 1355 Bisphosphonate scans. *J Nucl Med* 1975; **16**:986–9.
9. Willis RA. Secondary tumours in bone. (pp. 229–50) In: Willis RA (ed). *The Spread of Tumours in the Human Body*, 3rd edition. London, UK: Butterworth, 1973.
10. Dodds PR, Coride VJ, Lytton B. The role of the vertebral veins in the dissemination of prostate cancer. *J Urol* 1981; **126**:753–5.
11. Batson OV. The function of the vertebral veins and their role in the spread of metastases. *Ann Surg* 1940; **112**:138–49.
12. Scott LJ, NW Clarke, JH Shanks, NG Testa, SH Lang. Interaction of human prostatic epithelial cells with bone marrow endothelium: banding and invasion. *Br J Cancer* 2001; **84**(10):1417–23.
13. Lang SH, Clarke NW, George NJR, Allen TD, Testa NG. Interaction of prostatic epithelial cells from benign and malignant tumour tissue with bone marrow stoma. *Prostate* 1998; **34**:203–13.
14. Nicholson GL, Winkelhoake JL. Organ specification of blood borne tumour metastasis determined by cell adhesions? *Nature* 1975; **255**:230–2.
15. Auerbach R, Lu WC. Specification of adhesions between murine tumour cells and capillary endothelium: an in vitro correlate of preferential metastasis in vivo *Cancer Res* 1987; **47**:1492–96.
16. Brown MD, Hart C, Gazi E, Gardner P, Lockyer N, Clarke N. The influence of the omega 6 PUFA arachidonic acid and bone marrow adipocytes on metastatic spread from prostate cancer. *Brit J Canc* 2010; **102**(2):403–13.
17. Guise TA, Mundy GR. Cancer and bone. *Endocr Rev* 1998; **19**:18–54.
18. Charhon SA, Chapoy MC, Devlin, *et al.* Histomorphometric analysis of sclerotic bone metastasis from prostatic carcinoma from prostate cancer with special reference to osteomalacia. *Cancer* 1983; **51**:918–24.
19. Clarke NW, McClure J, George NJR. Morphometric evidence from bone resorption and replacement in prostate cancer. *Brit J Urol* 1991; **68**:74–80.
20. Clarke NW, McClure J, George NJR. Osteoblast function and osteomalacia in prostate cancer. *Eur Urol* 1993; **24**:286–90.
21. Cook GB, Watson FR. Events in the natural history of prostate cancer: rising salvage, mean age distribution and contingency co-efficient. *J Urol* 1968; **99**:87–96.
22. Clarke NW, McClure J, George NJR. Disodium Pamidronate identifies differential osteoclastic bone resorption in metastatic prostate cancer. *Br J Urol* 1992; **69**:64–70.
23. Galasko CSB. Mechanisms of one destruction in the development of skeletal metastases. *Nature* 1976; **263**:507–10
24. Urwin GH, Percival RC, Harvey WJ, *et al.* Generalised increase in bone resorption in carcinoma of the prostate. *Br J Urol* 1985; **57**:721–72.
25. Tietelbaum SL. Bone resorption by osteoclasts. *Science* 2000; **289**;1504–8.
26. Suda T, Takahashi N, Udagawa N, Jimi E, Gillespie MT, Martin TJ. Modulation of osteoclast differentiation and function modulation by new members of the tumour factor receptor by new members of the tumour necrosis factor receptor and ligand families. *Endocr Rev* 1999; **20**(3):345–57.
27. O'Donohue EPN, Constable AR, Sherwood T, Stephenson JJ, Chisholm GD. Bone scanning and plasma phosphatases in carcinoma of the prostate. *Br J Urol* 1978; **50**:172–7.
28. Fitzpatrick JM, Constable AR, Sherwood T, Stephenson JJ, Chisholm GD, O'Donohue EPN. Serial bone scanning: the assessment of treatment response in carcinoma of the prostate. *Br J Urol* 1978; **50**:555–61.
29. Subramanian G, McAfee SG. A new compound of 99m Tc for skeletal imaging. *Radiology* 1971; **99**:192–6.
30. Clarke NW. The origin of the bone scan as a tumour marker in prostate cancer. *Eur Urol* 2006; **50**:873–8.
31. Jacobson AF, Fogelman I. Bone scanning in clinical oncology: does it have a future? *Eur J Nucl Med* 1998; **25**:1219–23.
32. Schirrmeister H, Guhlmann A, Kotzerke J, *et al.* Early detection and accurate description of extent of metastatic bone disease in breast cancer with fluoride ion and positron emission tomography. *J Clin Oncol* 1999; **17**:2381–9.
33. Chybowski FM, Larson-Keller JJ, Bergstrahl EJ, Oesterling JE. Predicting radionuclide bone scan findings in patients with newly diagnosed, untreated prostate cancer: prostate specific antigen is superior to all other clinical parameters. *J Urol* 1992; **148**:313–8.
34. Daffner RH, Lupetin AR, Dash N, *et al.* MRI in the detection of malignant infiltration of bone marrow. *AJR Am J Roentgenol* 1986; **146**:353–8.
35. Gosfield E 3rd, Alavi A, Kneeland B. Comparison of radionuclide bone scans and magnetic resonance imaging in detecting spinal metastases. *J Nucl Med* 1993; **34**:2191.
36. Eustace S, Tello R, DeCarvalho V, *et al.* A comparison of whole-body turboSTIR MR imaging and planar 99mTc-methylene diphosphonate scintigraphy in the examination of patients with suspected skeletal metastases. *AJR Am J Roentgenol* 1997; **169**:1655–61.
37. Sanal SM, Flickinger FW, Caudell MJ, *et al.* Detection of bone marrow involvement in breast cancer with magnetic resonance imaging. *J Clin Oncol* 1994; **12**:1415–21.
38. Traill ZC, Talbot D, Golding S, Gleeson FV. Magnetic resonance imaging versus radionuclide scintigraphy in screening for bone metastases. *Clin Radiol* 1999; **54**:448–51.
39. Frank JA, Ling A, Patronas NJ, *et al.* Detection of malignant bone tumors: MR imaging vs scintigraphy. *AJR Am J Roentgenol* 1990; **155**:1043–8.
40. Haubold-Reuter BG, Duewell S, Schilcher BR, *et al.* The value of bone scintigraphy, bone marrow scintigraphy and fast spin-echo magnetic resonance imaging in staging of patients with malignant solid tumours: a prospective study. *Eur J Nucl Med* 1993; **20**:1063–9.
41. Kattapuram SV, Khurana JS, Scott JA, el-Khoury GY. Negative scintigraphy with positive magnetic resonance imaging in bone metastases. *Skeletal Radiol* 1990; **19**:113–16.
42. Lecouvet FE, Geukens D, Stainier A, *et al.* Magnetic resonance imaging of the axial skeleton for detecting bone metastases in patients with high-risk prostate cancer: diagnostic and cost-effectiveness and comparison with current detection strategies. *J Clin Oncol* 2007; **25**:3281–7.
43. Therasse P, Arbuck SG, Eisenhauer EA, *et al.* New guidelines to evaluate the response to treatment in solid tumors. European Organization for Research and Treatment of Cancer, National Cancer

Institute of the United States, National Cancer Institute of Canada. *J Natl Cancer Inst* 2000; **92**:205–16.
44. Dreicer R. Metastatic prostate cancer: assessment of response to systemic therapy. *Semin Urol Oncol* 1997; **15**:28–32.
45. Papac RJ. Bone marrow metastases. A review. *Cancer* 1994; **74**:2403–13.
46. Hanks C, Myers C, Scardino P. Cancer of the prostate. (pp. 1073–113) In: DeVita VT, Hellman S, Rosenberg SA. *Cancer: Principles and Practice of Oncology*, 5th edition. Philadelphia, PA: Lippincott Co., 1993.
47. Petrylak DP, Tangen CM, Hussain MH, *et al.* Docetaxel and estramustine compared with mitoxantrone and prednisone for advanced refractory prostate cancer. *N Engl J Med* 2004; **351**:1513–20.
48. Tannock IF, de Wit R, Berry WR, *et al.* Docetaxel plus prednisone or mitoxantrone plus prednisone for advanced prostate cancer. *N Engl J Med* 2004; **351**:1502–12.
49. Dearnaley DP, Sydes MR, Mason MD, *et al.* A double-blind, placebo-controlled, randomized trial of oral sodium clodronate for metastatic prostate cancer (MRC PR05 Trial). *J Natl Cancer Inst* 2003; **95**:1300–11.
50. Jimeno A, Carducci M. Atrasentan: targeting the endothelin axis in prostate cancer. *Expert Opin Investig Drugs* 2004; **13**:1631–40.
51. Saad F, Gleason DM, Murray R, *et al.* Long-term efficacy of zoledronic acid for the prevention of skeletal complications in patients with metastatic hormone-refractory prostate cancer. *J Natl Cancer Inst* 2004; **96**:879–82.
52. Tombal B, Rezazadeh A, Therasse P, *et al.* Magnetic resonance imaging of the axial skeleton enables objective measurement of tumor response on prostate cancer bone metastases. *Prostate* 2005; **65**:178–87.
53. Saylor PJ, Lee RJ, Smith MR. Emerging therapies to prevent skeletal complications in men with metastatic prostate cancer. *J Clin Oncol* 2011; **29** (27):3705–14.
54. Cancertrials.gov website, 2013. Available at: https://clinicaltrials.gov/ [Online].
55. Fizazi K1, Carducci M, Smith M, *et al.* Denosumab versus zoledronic acid for treatment of bone metastases in men with castration-resistant prostate cancer: a randomised, double-blind study. *Lancet* 2011; **377**(9768):813–22.
56. Smith MR, Saad F, Shore ND, *et al.* Effect of denosumab on prolonging bone-metastasis-free survival (BMFS) in men with nonmetastatic castrate-resistant prostate cancer (CRPC) presenting with aggressive PSA kinetics. J Clin Oncol 2012; **30**(15):4510.
57. Khafagy R, Shackley D, Samuel J, O'Flynn K, Betts C, Clarke NW. Complications arising in the final year of life in men dying from advanced prostate cancer. *J Pall Med* 2007; **10**(3):705–11.
58. Globel BH. Bleeding disorders. (pp. 575–607) In: Groenwald S, Frogge M, Goodman M, Yarbru C (eds). *Cancer Nursing—Principles and Practice,* 3rd edition. Boston MA: Jones Bartlett, 1993.
59. Esper P, Pienta KJ. Supportive core in the patient with hormone refractory prostate cancer. *Semin Urol Oncol* 1997; **15**(1):56–64.
60. Alpoers P, Chappell R, Schaibold H. Erythropoietin in Urology Oncology. *Eur Urol* 2001; **39**:1–8.
61. Beshara S, Letochka H, Linde T Anaemia associated with advanced prostatic adenocarcinoma effects of recombinant human Erythropoietin. *Prostate* 1997; **31**:153–60.
62. Johannsson JE, Wersall P, Brandberg Y, Andersson SO, Nordström L; EPO-Study Group. Efficiency of epoetin beta on hemoglobin, quality of life, and transfusion needs in patients with anemia due to hormone-refractory prostate cancer—a randomized study. *Scand J Urol Nephrol* 2001; **35**(4):288–94.
63. Mahadevia P, Ramaswamy A, Greenwald E, Wollner D, Markham D. Hypercalcaemia in prostate cancer. *Arch Intern Med* 1983; **143**:1339–42.
64. Spencer H, Lewin I. Derangements of calcium metabolism in patients with neoplastic bone involvement. *J Chronic Dis* 1963; **16**:713–26.
65. Soerdjbalie-Maikeov, Pelger RE, Lycklama à Nijeholt GA, *et al.* Strontium-89 (Metastron) and the bisphosphonate olpadronate reduce the incidence of spinal cord compression in patients with hormone-refractory prostate cancer metastatic to the skeleton. *Eur J Nucl Med Mol Imaging* 2002; **29**(4):494–508.
66. Coleman RE, Rubens RD. The clinical course of bone metastases from breast cancer. *Brit J Cancer* 1987; **55**:61–6.
67. Neville-Webb HC, Holden I, Coleman RE. The anti-tumour activity of Bisphosphonates. *Cancer Treatment Rev* 2002; **28**(2):305–19.
68. Berrutt A, Dogliotti L, Tucci M, Tarabuzzi R, Fontana D, Angeli A. Metabolic bone disease induced by prostate cancer: Rational for use of bisphosphonates. *J Urol* 2001; **166**:2023–31.
69. Townsend MF, Saunders WH, Northway RO, Graham SD Jr. Bone fractures associated with luteinizing hormone-releasing hormone agonists used in prostate carcinoma. *Can Urol* 1997; **79**:545–50.
70. Parker C, Nilsson S, Heinrich D, *et al.* Updated analysis of the phase III, double-blind, randomized, multinational study of radium-223 chloride in castration-resistant prostate cancer (CRPC) patients with bone metastases (ALSYMPCA). *J Clin Oncol* 2012; **30**(Suppl) [abstr LBA4512].
71. Oefefein MG, Ricchiutti, Conrand W, *et al.* Skeletal fractures negatively correlate with overall survival in men with prostate cancer. *J Urol* 2002; **168**:1005–7.
72. Osbourn J, Getzenberg RH, Trump DL. Spinal cord compression in prostate cancer. *J Neurooncol* 1995; **23**(2):135–47.
73. Bayley A, Milosevic M, Bland R, *et al.* A prospective study of factors predicting clinically occult spinal and compression in patients with metastatic prostate carcinoma. *Cancer* 2001; **92**(2):303–10.
74. Saad F, Gleason DM, Murray R, *et al.* A randomised placebo-controlled trial of zoledronic acid in patients with hormone-refractory metastatic prostate carcinoma. *J Natl Canc Inst* 2002; **94**(19):1458–68.
75. Fizazi K, Carducci M, Smith M, *et al.* Denosumab versus zoledronic acid for treatment of bone metastases in men with castration-resistant prostate cancer: a randomised, double-blind study. *Lancet* 2011; **377**:813–22.
76. Kuban DA, el-Mahid AM, Siegried SV, Schellhammer PF, Babb TJ. Characteristics of spinal cord compression in adenocarcinoma of the prostate. *Urology* 1986; **28**:364–9.
77. White BD, Stirling AJ, Paterson E, Asquith-Coe K, Melder A; Guideline Development Group. Diagnosis and management of patients at risk of or with metastatic spinal cord compression: summary of NICE guidance. *BMJ* 2008; **337**:a2538.
78. Huddart RA, Rajan B, Lau M, *et al.* Spinal cord decompression and carcinoma of the prostate: treatment outcome and prognostic factors. *Radiotherapy Oncol* 1997; **44**:229–36.
79. Iacovou J, Marks JC, Abrams PH, Gingell JC, Ball AJ. Cord compression and carcinoma of prostate: Is laminectomy justified? *Br J Urol* 1985; **57**:733–6.
80. Pollen JJ, Schmidt JD. Bone pain in metastatic cancer of the prostate. *Urology* 1979; **13**:129–34.
81. Shuttleworth ED, Blandy J. P Carcinoma of the prostate. (pp. 773–6) In: Blandy JP (ed). *Urology*. Oxford, UK: Blackwell Scientific Publications, 1976.
82. Rose MR, Kagan AR. The final report on the expert panel for the radiation oncology bone metastasis work group of the American College of Radiology. *Int J Radiat Oncol Biol Phys* 1998; **40**:1117–24.
83. Staniland E, Leir J, van Houwelingen H, *et al.* The effect of a single fraction compared to multiple fractions on painful bone metastases: a global analysis of the Dutch Bone Metastasis Study. *Radiotherapy Oncol* 1999; **52**(2):101–9.
84. Price P, Hosking RJ, Easton D, *et al.* Prospective randomised trial of single and multi fractional radiotherapy schedules in the treatment of painful bony metastases. *Radiother Oncol* 1986; **65**:247–55.
85. Hosking PJ. Scientific and clinical aspects of radiotherapy in the relief of bone pain. *Cancer Surv* 1988; **7**(1):69–86.
86. Tong D, Gillick L, Hendrickson FR. The palliation of symptomatic osseous metastases. Final results of the Radiation Therapy Oncology Group. *Cancer* 1982; **50**:893–9.
87. Zelefsky MJ, Scher H, Forman JD, *et al.* Palliative hemiskeletal irradiation for widespread metastatic prostate cancer: A comparison

of single and fractionated regimens. *Int J Rad Oncol Biophys* 1989; **17**(6):1281–5.

88. Friedland J. Local and systemic radiation for palliation of metastatic disease. *Urol Clin N America* 1999; **76** (2):391–402.
89. Jaeger PL, Kvoistia A, Piers DA. Treatment within 89 radioactive strontium for patients with bone metastases from prostate cancer. *Brit J Urol Int* 2000; **86**:929–34.
90. Lang AH, Ackerly DM, Bayly RJ, *et al.* Strontium-89 chloride for pain palliation in prostatic skeletal malignancy. *Brit J Radiol* 1991: **64**(765):816–22.
91. Lewington VJ, McEwan AJ, Ackery DM, *et al.* A prospective randomised double-blind cross-over study to examine the efficacy of Strontrium 89 in pain palliation in patients with advanced prostate cancer metastatic to bone. *Eur J Cancer* 1991; **27**:954–8.
92. Quilty PM, Kirk D, Bolger JJ, *et al.* Comparison of the palliative effects of Strontrium 89 and external beam radiotherapy in metastatic prostate cancer. *Radiother Oncol* 1994; **31**:33–40.
93. Kylmälä T, Tammela TL, Lincholm TS, Seppänen J. The effect of combined intravenous and oral Clodronate treatment on bone pain in patients with metastatic prostate cancer. *Ann Chir Gynaecol* 1994; **83**:316–9.
94. Cresswell SM, English PJ, Hall RR, *et al.* Pain relief and quality-of-life assessment following intravenous and oral Clodronate in hormone escape metastatic prostate cancer. *Brit J Urol* 1995; **76**:360–5.
95. Purhoit OP, Anthony C, Radstone CR, *et al.* High-dose intravenous pamidronate for metastatic bone pain. *Br J Cancer* 1994; **70**:554–8.
96. Heidenreich A, Elert A, Hoffmann R. Ibandronate in the treatment of prostate cancer associated with painful osseous metastases. *Prostate Cancer Prostatic Dis* 2002; **2**(5):231–5.
97. Ernst DS, Brasher P, Hagan N, Paterson AH, MacDonald RN, Bruera E. A randomised controlled trail of intravenous Clodronate in patients with metastatic bone disease and pain. *J Pain Symptom Manage* 1997; **13**:319–26.
98. Kylmälä T, Taube T, Tammela TL, Risteli L, Risteli J, Elomaa I. Concomitant i.v. and oral clodronate in the relief of bone pain—a double-blinded placebo-controlled study in patients with prostate cancer. *Br J Cancer* 1997; **76**:939–42.
99. Lipton A, Glover, Garvey H, *et al.* Pamidronate in the treatment of bone metastases: results of 2 dose ranging trials in patients with breast or prostate cancer. *Ann Oncol* 1994; **5**(Suppl 7):35–53.
100. Smith JA. Palliation of painful bone metastases from prostate cancer using sodium etidronate: results of a randomised, prospective placebo controlled study. *J Urol* 1989: **141**:85–7.
101. Dearnaley DP, Sydes MR. Preliminary evidence that oral clodronate delays symptomatic progression of bone metastases from prostate cancer. First results of the MRC PRO5 trial. ASCO 2001 # 1693.
102. Canil CM, Tannock IF. Should bisphosphonates be used routinely in patients with prostate cancer metastatic to bone. *J Natl Cancer Inst* 2002; **94**(19):1422–3.
103. Coleman RE. Metastatic bone disease and the role of biochemical markers of bone metabolism in benign and malignant diseases. *Cancer Treat Rev* 2001; **27**:133–5.
104. Fizazi K, Lipton A, Mariette X, *et al.* Randomized phase II trial of denosumab in patients with bone metastases from prostate cancer, breast cancer or other neoplasms after intravenous bisphsophonates. *J Clin Oncol* 2009; **27**:1564–71.

CHAPTER 6.12

Novel therapies and emerging strategies for the treatment of patients with castration-resistant prostate cancer

Deborah Mukherji, Aurelius Omlin, Carmel Pezaro, and Johann De Bono

Introduction

Suppression of gonadal androgens remains first-line treatment for patients with advanced prostate cancer. The response to androgen deprivation is not durable however, and progressive prostate cancer, despite castrate levels of testosterone (termed castration-resistant prostate cancer CRPC) is usually fatal.

Castration resistance typically develops two to three years after starting androgen deprivation therapy and may be detected by a rising prostate-specific antigen (PSA) or the development of new metastases. Prostate cancer typically metastasizes to the bone; however, nodal and visceral disease is commonly seen. Significant morbidity related to skeletal metastases such as bone pain, spinal cord compression, and pathological fracture is common in advanced disease. In 2004, docetaxel chemotherapy was shown to improve survival in advanced CRPC and became the standard of care for treatment of men with progressive, symptomatic disease. In the last six years, the immunotherapy sipuleucel-T, chemotherapy cabazitaxel, androgen biosynthesis inhibitor abiraterone acetate, alpha-emitting radioisotope radium-223, and the novel antiandrogen enzalutamide have all been shown to improve survival in randomized phase III studies.[1–5] The optimal use and sequencing of these new agents has yet to be determined and treatment paradigms for advanced prostate cancer are changing rapidly.

The success of abiraterone and enzalutamide confirmed the hypothesis that advanced prostate cancer remains driven by androgen receptor (AR) signalling and that targeting this pathway remains an effective strategy for disease control. There is also evidence that tubulin-binding taxane chemotherapies inhibit AR signalling and thereby block AR nuclear accumulation.[6] The term 'hormone-resistant prostate cancer' is incorrect and has been replaced by CRPC. Using 'maximal androgen blockade' to describe the combination of a luteinizing hormone releasing hormone (LHRH) agonist with an antiandrogen such as bicalutamide is also inaccurate, as intratumoral androgen synthesis and androgens derived from adrenal steroid precursors continue to drive tumour growth.

Targeting androgen receptor signalling

CYP17 inhibition: abiraterone acetate

A key enzyme in the androgen biosynthesis is CYP17, which has a dual function as a 17α-hydroxylase and 17,20-lyase. Non-specific CYP17 inhibitors, namely ketoconazole and aminoglutethimide, have modest activity in advanced prostate cancer but are not widely used due to their unfavourable side effect profiles.[7,8]

Abiraterone acetate (abiraterone; Zytiga, Janssen) is a novel 17α-hydroxylase and 17,20-lyase inhibitor.[9] Early clinical trials reported encouraging clinical activity with ≥50% PSA declines in 50–60% of patients.[10–13] Symptoms relating to mineralocorticoid excess (namely hypertension, hypokalaemia, and fluid retention) were the main side effects of abiraterone treatment and were successfully abrogated with the addition of low-dose glucocorticoids such as dexamethasone, prednisolone, or the mineralocorticoid receptor antagonist eplerenone. Two phase III trials in advanced prostate cancer have since been completed. In the post-docetaxel COU-301 trial, 1,195 patients with CRPC were randomized in a 2:1 ratio to treatment with abiraterone plus prednisone/prednisolone, or placebo plus prednisone/prednisolone. In this study, 30% of patients had received two lines of chemotherapy. The median overall survival (OS) on abiraterone was significantly longer than on placebo (interim analysis revealed a survival benefit of 3.9 months (14.8 months vs. 10.9 months, hazard ratio (HR) 0.65, 95% confidence interval (CI) 0.54–0.77) for abiraterone).[3] At final analysis the benefit had extended to 4.6 months.[14] The main drug-related side effects were mild to moderate. Symptoms of mineralocorticoid excess were more common in the abiraterone-treated patients, including fluid retention (31% vs. 22%, $p = 0.04$), hypokalaemia (17% vs. 8% $p < 0.001$) and hypertension (10% vs. 8%). Subgroup analysis confirmed the benefit of abiraterone in elderly patients aged ≥75 (14.9 months vs. 9.3 months, HR 0.52, 95% CI 0.38–0.71), in patients with visceral disease (12.6 months vs. 8.4 months HR 0.7, 95% CI 0.52–0.94), and in patients with significant baseline pain (worst pain ≥4 on brief pain inventory: 12.9 months vs. 8.9 months, HR 0.68, 95% CI 0.53–0.85). Abiraterone was licenced by the United States Food and Drug Administration (US FDA) in April 2011 and later that year in Europe for use in advanced prostate cancer following docetaxel-based chemotherapy.

Abiraterone has also been approved for use in the pre-docetaxel setting following the publication of the COU-302 phase III trial in chemotherapy-naive patients. A total of 1,088 patients were randomized 1:1 to abiraterone plus prednisone/prednisolone (n = 546) or prednisone/prednisolone and placebo (n = 542). The trial defined co-primary end points of radiographic progression-free survival (rPFS) and OS. The interim analysis, conducted after 311 deaths, showed a statistically significant improvement in rPFS with abiraterone compared to placebo (median rPFS not reached (NR) vs. 8.3; HR 0.43, 95% CI 0.35–0.52). A strong trend for improvement in median OS with abiraterone was also reported (median OS NR vs. 27.2 m; HR 0.75, 95% CI 0.61–0.93).[15] The trial was unblinded based on the recommendations of the independent data monitoring committee, although this decision was contentious due to the failure of the survival analysis to meet the pre-specified level of significance. On longer follow-up, median survival in the abiraterone group was 34.7 m versus 30.3 m on the prednisone arm, which was both clinically and statistically significant.[16]

Abiraterone is a well-tolerated oral therapy but requires regular review and active management of toxicities related to mineralocorticoid excess. Monitoring should include measurements of blood pressure, weight, potassium levels, and liver function tests. Abiraterone is a substrate of CYP3A4, therefore concomitant strong CYP3A4 inhibitors (such as clarithromycin) or inducers (such as phenytoin) should be avoided or used with caution. Early treatment discontinuation for rising PSA in the absence of clinical progression should be avoided. Additionally, early changes in bone scans may represent bone flares rather than disease progression.[17]

Orteronel (TAK-700, Takeda Phamarceuticals) is a novel inhibitor of androgen biosynthesis with greater selectivity for the 17,20-lyase, potentially allowing administration without concomitant corticosteroid medication. In a phase II trial of 97 chemotherapy-naive patients, orteronel was tested at different doses and ≥50% PSA declines were observed in 63%, 50%, 41%, and 60% in the 300 mg twice daily, 400 and 600 mg twice daily with prednisone, and 600 mg once daily groups, respectively.[18] The most frequently observed side effects of Common Terminology Criteria for Adverse Events (CTCAE) grade ≥3 were fatigue (12%) and hypokalaemia (8%). Phase III clinical trials with orteronel combined with prednisolone were conducted in similar populations to the abiraterone 301 and 302 trials. Both trials failed to meet the primary end point of improved OS and the further development of orteronel in CRPC was stopped.[19,20]

Next generation antiandrogen: enzalutamide and novel androgen receptor antagonists

Antiandrogens compete with endogenous androgen ligand for the ligand-binding pocket of the AR. Second-generation AR antagonists have been rationally designed and selected to avoid agonist activity even in models overexpressing AR.

Enzalutamide (MDV3100, XTANDI, Medivation) is a second-generation non-steroidal AR antagonist, approved for the treatment of advanced prostate cancer by the US Food and Drug Administration in August 2012. Enzalutamide was selected for development after demonstrating high affinity for the AR, inhibiting AR nuclear translocation and binding to DNA.[21] The Phase I-II clinical trial included 140 men with metastatic CRPC and reported encouraging antitumour activity such as ≥50% PSA declines in 56% of patients.[22] The pivotal double-blind phase III AFFIRM trial included 1,199 men pretreated with chemotherapy and randomized them in a 2:1 ratio to receive enzalutamide 160 mg/day or placebo. Enzalutamide treatment resulted in a 4.8-month improvement in survival (median OS 18.4 months vs. 13.6 months, HR 0.631, 95% CI 0.53–0.75).[4] The survival advantage was maintained in all subgroups, including patients with visceral disease (median OS of 13.4 months on enzalutmide vs. 9.5 months on placebo (HR 0.78, 95% CI 0.56–1.09)). PSA declines of ≥50% were documented in 54% patients on enzalutamide compared to 2% on placebo. Enzalutamide showed superiority in secondary end points including soft tissue responses (29% vs. 4%), time to first skeletal-related event (SRE, 16.7 months vs. 13.3 months) and quality of life measurements. A low frequency of grade ≥3 events were reported on both study arms, including fatigue (6% vs. 7%), diarrhoea (1% vs. <1%) and hot flushes (no grade 3 events). Five men (0.6%) on enzalutamide had seizures compared to none on the placebo arm, even though patients with a seizure history or known cerebral metastases were excluded. Alternative aetiologies for seizures were identified in several cases, including cerebral metastases (two patients) and concomitant centrally acting medications. Due to the possibility that enzalutamide may lower the threshold for seizures, it was recommended to avoid enzalutamide in men with a history of seizures, stroke, or unexplained loss of consciousness and to consider concomitant medications. Patients who remain well despite PSA progression should continue on enzalutamide until documentation of radiographic progression.

A second phase III trial in chemotherapy-naive men with CRPC (PREVAIL) randomized 1,717 patients to receive either enzalutamide 160 mg daily or placebo. The study was stopped after a planned interim analysis showed improved rPFS at 12 months of 65% in the enzalutamide arm compared with 14% in the placebo arm (HR 0.19, 95% CI 0.15–0.23). At the time of analysis, 72% of patients in the enzalutamide arm were alive compared with 63% of the patients in the placebo arm (HR 0.71, 95% CI 0.6–0.84).[23] Regulatory approval for the use of enzalutamide for CRPC in the pre-chemotherapy setting was granted in 2014.

ARN-509 (apalutamide, Aragon Pharmaceuticals, Inc.) is a second-generation AR antagonist that has structural similarity to enzalutamide. Preliminary data from a phase I trial showed durable PSA declines at doses between 30–300 mg/day.[22,24] It has been postulated that this agent has lower central nervous system penetration and may be associated with a lower risk of seizures. Clinical trials are ongoing, including a randomized phase III study in combination with abiraterone.

Androgen receptor splice variants

Mechanisms of resistance to AR-targeted therapies include AR gene amplification or overexpression, gain of function mutations involving the AR ligand-binding domain and AR splice variants, among others.[25] The presence of AR splice variants, particularly the AR-V7, has been correlated with both primary and acquired resistance to abiraterone and enzalutamide.[26,27] Ongoing studies are validating the AR-V7 variant as a treatment-selection biomarker and investigating the strategy of targeting the N-terminal domain of the AR in order to overcome this mechanism of resistance.[28]

Cytotoxic chemotherapy

Docetaxel

For more than a decade, chemotherapy has been regarded as a standard of care for men with CRPC. The pivotal trial establishing docetaxel as the first-line chemotherapy of choice was the phase III TAX-327 trial, which enrolled 1,006 men and tested docetaxel with prednisone, in either a weekly or three-weekly schedule, against the previous standard of mitoxantrone. Considering the primary survival analysis, the superior three-weekly schedule of docetaxel resulted in median OS of 18.9 months, compared to 16.5 months with mitoxantrone (HR 0.76, $p = 0.009$).[29] Docetaxel treatment was also associated with improvements in pain and quality of life.

Although docetaxel has been widely used since the publication of TAX-327 in 2004, a number of aspects regarding its use remain unclear. The schedule is usually continuous; intermittent dosing according to PSA response has also been proposed, but never formally compared to continuous treatment.[30,31] Likewise the optimal number of cycles remains unclear, with anecdotal reports of ongoing benefit for patients treated beyond 10 cycles.[32] Translational research focused on earlier assessment of response has included enumeration of circulating tumour cell (CTC) counts on chemotherapy. An exploratory analysis in a prospective study of 276 CRPC patients suggested that conversion from unfavourable (defined as ≥5 CTC/7.5 mL blood) to favourable counts (<5 CTC/7.5 mL blood) was associated with OS similar to that of patients with favourable counts throughout.[33] CTC counts on chemotherapy appeared superior to PSA in predicting OS.

A number of phase III trials have attempted to improve on the benefit achieved with docetaxel alone; however, none have shown positive results or impacted the standard schedule. Docetaxel retreatment may be considered an acceptable second-line therapy in men who had a good response to initial treatment. There is phase II trial evidence to support this strategy, demonstrating ≥50% PSA declines in 25–48% patients,[34,35] but as yet there is no level I evidence from a prospective randomized trial.

Cabazitaxel

Cabazitaxel (Jevtana, Sanofi-Aventis) is a semi-synthetic taxane compound that was selected for further development after preclinical studies suggested activity in docetaxel-resistant cell lines. Two phase I studies were performed in patients with solid tumours and showed that neutropenia was the primary dose limiting toxicity at 25–30 mg/m^2.[34–37] The formally published phase I trial included eight men with CRPC and two of these men achieved radiographic partial responses accompanied by >50% PSA declines.

Following this encouraging early-phase activity, the phase III TROPIC trial was performed. TROPIC was an open-label study in 755 men with progressive CRPC following docetaxel. More than 70% of participants had progressed on or within three months of completing docetaxel treatment. Men were randomized 1:1 to receive prednisone with either cabazitaxel or mitoxantrone.[2] Cabazitaxel treatment resulted in median OS of 15.1 months, a 2.4-month improvement compared to mitoxantrone (HR 0.70, $p < 0.0001$). Patients received a median of six cycles of cabazitaxel on trial, compared to four cycles of mitoxantrone. Planned analysis showed maintenance of cabazitaxel benefit across all subgroups, including patients who progressed on docetaxel. Secondary end points of pressure flow studies, time to progression, and response by PSA and imaging were significantly improved by cabazitaxel. Quality of life was not examined in the TROPIC study, but was explored in an early access programme within the United Kingdom, which suggested that cabazitaxel treatment led to improvement in pain control and preservation of quality of life.[38] Cabazitaxel received FDA approval in June 2011 as the second-line treatment in men with metastatic CRPC.

Cabazitaxel treatment in the TROPIC study appeared generally well tolerated, with a toxicity profile that included neutropenia (grade 3/4 in 303 patients; 82%) with febrile neutropenia in 28 patients (8%). Other grade 3/4 toxicities reported in at least 5% cabazitaxel recipients included anaemia (39 patients, 11%), diarrhoea (23 patients, 6%), fatigue (18 patients, 5%), and asthenia (17 patients, 5%). Neutropenia and diarrhoea were key contributors to treatment-related mortality of almost 5%, with additional risk factors of older age and prior radiotherapy. Neuropathy is rare with cabazitaxel. Geographic variation in treatment-related mortality was observed, likely reflecting differences in febrile neutropenia management and supportive care. The TROPIC study did not allow primary prophylaxis with granulocyte colony stimulating factor (G-CSF), but supplementary data recommended consideration of primary prophylaxis for high-risk patients, as well as therapeutic G-CSF and secondary prophylaxis for patients at increased risk of neutropenic complications.

The phase III PROSELICA trial compared cabazitaxel at 20mg/m^2 to 25mg/m^2 and demonstrated non-inferiority for OS with an improved safety profile for the lower dose.[39] Cabazitaxel was also tested in the first-line setting compared to docetaxel in the phase III FIRSTANA study however failed to demonstrate superior OS.[40]

The optimal number of cabazitaxel cycles has not been defined, with a maximum of 10 cycles mandated in the TROPIC study and no data regarding benefit from more prolonged treatment.

Immunotherapy

Sipuleucel-T

The approval of sipuleucel-T (Provenge®, Dendreon) by the US FDA for prostate cancer in April 2010 heralded the first antigen-specific immunotherapy to be approved for cancer treatment. Sipuleucel-T is individually manufactured for each patient in a process that involves harvesting peripheral-blood mononuclear cells (PBMCs), *ex vivo* incubation with a chimeric protein linking granulocyte-macrophage colony stimulating factor (GM-CSF) to prostatic acid phosphatase (PAP) and subsequent reinfusion to stimulate an immune response against cancer cells carrying the PAP antigen. Three intravenous infusions are given over a four-week period.

In a randomized phase III trial involving 512 patients with asymptomatic or minimally symptomatic CRPC, median OS was 25.8 months in the sipuleucel-T group, compared with 21.7 months in the placebo group (unadjusted HR 0.77; 95% CI 0.61–0.97, $p = 0.02$).[1] There was no difference in time to objective or clinical disease progression between the two study arms. There is ongoing controversy regarding the trial design and validity of the IMPACT trial results.[41] Adverse events occurring more frequently in the sipuleucel-T group included chills, fever, and headache; there were no reports of anaphylaxis following infusion of sipuleucel-T and no evidence of autoimmune adverse events. The high cost of $93,000 for a one-month course of treatment has impacted the uptake of sipuleucel-T.[42]

Other immuno-oncology agents

The modulation of immune checkpoints that cause cancer immune tolerance is an attractive therapeutic strategy. The targeting of cytotoxic T lymphocyte-associated receptor 4 (CTLA-4) and programmed death 1 (PD-1) are particularly attractive and have become standard of care agents in other solid tumours including melanoma, renal cell carcinoma, and lung cancer. CTLA-4 and PD-1 are both members of the CD28 family of co-receptors that negatively regulate T-cell responses.

Ipilimumab (Yervoy®, Bristol-Myers Squibb/Medarex) is a humanized anti-CTLA4 antibody that has been investigated for the treatment of prostate cancer.[43] Two phase III trials were conducted in CRPC. The first compared ipilimumab and placebo following radiotherapy in patients with mCRPC who progressed following docetaxel chemotherapy and a second trial was performed in chemotherapy-naive patients with metastatic CRPC.[44,45] Unfortunately, both trials with ipilimumab failed to meet the primary end point of improved overall survival.

PD-1 inhibition: A PD-1 antagonist nivolumab (MDX-1106,Bristol-Myers Squibb) has shown promising clinical activity in a phase 1 trial of 15 men with CRPC, with partial response in one patient (6.7%) and stable disease (>4 months) in three patients (20%).[46] Further studies of this agent and other PD-1 inhibitors are planned.

Bone-directed therapy

Bone metastases are a major cause of prostate cancer-specific morbidity and mortality. The treatment and prevention of SREs in prostate cancer is a priority and bone-targeted agents have the potential to impact both symptoms and survival in advanced disease. Bisphosphonates such as zoledronic acid[47] and bone-targeted radiopharmaceuticals such as samarium-153 and strontium-89 are used as monotherapy and in combination with chemotherapy (zoledronic acid).[48,49] Novel approaches to bone-targeted therapy include an alpha-emitting radiopharmaceutical radium-223 and receptor activation of nuclear factor kappa-B ligand (RANK-L) inhibitors.

Radium-223

Radium-223 chloride (Xofigo, Bayer) is a novel bone-targeting alpha-emitting agent that improved survival in patients with CRPC and symptomatic bone metastasis. The phase III ALSYMPCA study enrolled CRPC patients with symptomatic bone metastases, no evidence of visceral disease or significant lymphadenopathy and who had either received docetaxel or were deemed unfit for docetaxel chemotherapy. A planned interim analysis showed median OS of 14 months with radium-223 compared to 11.2 months with placebo (HR = 0.695, 95% CI 0.55–0.88, two-sided p = 0.00185), so the trial was halted and patients on the placebo arm offered radium-223. All of the secondary end points were improved with radium-223 treatment, including time to first symptomatic skeletal event (15.6m vs. 9.8m, HR 0.66, p <0.001) and improvement in bone turnover markers. Radium-223 appeared to be well tolerated with low frequencies of myelosupression (grade 3/4 neutropenia 2.2% vs. 0.7% and grade 3/4 thrombocytopenia 6.3% vs 2% in the radium-223 and placebo arms, respectively).[5] Studies combining radium-223 with chemotherapy and AR pathway targeted therapies are underway.

Denosumab

RANK signalling has been identified as a potent stimulus for osteoclast proliferation and bone resorption. Denosumab (Xgeva®, Amgen) is a fully humanized monoclonal antibody-targeting RANK-ligand that has recently been shown to be superior to zoledronic acid in preventing or delaying SREs in patients with bone metastases from CRPC.[50] A large double-blind phase III non-inferiority study randomized 1,904 patients to denosumab 120 mg subcutaneously monthly or zoledronic acid 4 mg intravenously monthly. The primary composite end point was time to SRE as defined by pathological fracture, radiotherapy to bone, surgery to bone, or spinal cord compression. The adverse event profile was similar in both arms. Denosumab was shown to be superior to zoledronic acid for prevention of SRE (median time to SRE 20.7 months vs. 17.1 months; HR 0.82, p = 0.008).[50] A separate phase III placebo-controlled study demonstrated that denosumab significantly improved bone metastasis-free survival in men with CRPC (29.5 vs. 25.2 months, HR 0.85 95% CI 0.73–0.98, p = 0.028), however there was no improvement in OS.[51]

Denosumab has advantages over zoledronic acid including ease of subcutaneous administration and reduced requirement for renal monitoring, however drug-related costs are significantly higher. Importantly the risk of osteonecrosis of the jaw, a well-known side effect of bisphosphonate treatment with significant impact on quality of live was reported to be 2.3% on denosumab compared to 1.3% on zoledronic acid. The cost per quality of life adjusted year (QALY) gained with denosumab has been estimated at $1.25 million.[52] Denosumab was approved by the US FDA in November 2010 for the prevention of SREs from solid tumours. Both denosumab and zoledronic acid are considered standard therapies for patients with symptomatic bone metastases.

Targeting intracellular signalling

Cabozantinib (XL184, Exelixis) is a small-molecule inhibitor of MET, VEGFR2, AXL, RON, and other molecular targets. Although cabozantinib appeared promising in preliminary CRPC trials, with striking pain palliation and bone scan responses observed, the post-docetaxel phase III COMET-1 study failed to demonstrate a survival advantage and development in CRPC was halted.[53]

In *AKT* inhibition, the phosphoinositide 3-kinase (PI3K)-AKT-mammalian target of rapamycin (mTOR) signalling pathway plays a central role in cell growth and survival. This intracellular signalling pathway is activated in most advanced prostate cancers, largely through loss of the negative regulator *PTEN*. Inhibition of either PI3K/AKT/mTOR or AR signalling can drive reciprocal activation of the other pathway providing the rationale for combining AKT and AR inhibitors in CRPC.[54] Data from a randomized phase II study of the oral AKT inhibitor ipatasertib plus abiraterone versus abiraterone alone in CRPC suggest that patients with tumours showing loss of PTEN may derive significant benefit from the combination strategy.[55] Further studies are planned using *PTEN* loss as a treatment-selection biomarker.

Response assessment in castration-resistant prostate cancer

The clinical spectrum of prostate cancer is such that only a minority of patients with metastatic disease will have measurable disease on cross-sectional imaging. The majority of patients with metastatic CRPC have only skeletal disease that can be challenging to objectively quantify. PSA can be an informative marker of disease progression, however PSA changes in response to systemic treatment cannot be reliably used as a surrogate for clinical benefit or survival.[56]

In 1999, the Prostate-Specific Antigen Working Group (PCWG1) produced the first consensus recommendations for the conduct of clinical trials in prostate cancer,[57] which were followed in 2000 by the introduction of the Response Evaluation Criteria in Solid Tumors (RECIST).[58] Since the publication of these guidelines, advances have been made in our understanding of the biology of prostate cancer and with the advent of both AR-directed and molecularly targeted therapies. Updated recommendations for these were published in 2008 (PCWG2).[59] PCWG2 recognized that cytotoxic agents typically produce PSA responses and regression of target lesions, whereas non-cytotoxic agents slowing tumour growth, inhibiting bone destruction, or targeting angiogenesis may not. The most recent recommendations (PCWG3) emphasize the need for biomarker-driven studies with serial biologic profiling of disease to better enable treatment selection based on disease biology.[60]

Despite the use of software designed to quantify changes in bone scan uptake, bone scintigraphy remains a relatively crude method for the assessment of treatment response in metastatic CRPC. New imaging techniques using diffusion-weighted magnetic resonance imaging (MRI)[61] and positron emission tomography/computed tomography (PET/CT) using choline and prostate-specific membrane antigen (PSMA) are being developed to improve the assessment of bone metastases in prostate cancer.[62] Guidance for response assessment in clinical practice have been incorporated in the recommendations of the St Gallen Advanced Prostate Cancer Consensus Conference (APCCC).[63]

The use of circulating biomarkers such as CTCs or circulating tumour-DNA for treatment selection and response assessment is an area of active research. Despite the use of software designed to quantify changes in bone scan uptake, bone scintigraphy remains a relatively crude method for the assessment of treatment response in metastatic CRPC.

CTC enumeration has been included as an efficacy-response question in a number of ongoing phase III trials and it is hoped that this will provide an early signal of treatment effect on which to inform clinical decisions. An early, validated surrogate end point could form the basis of regulatory approval in a time and cost-efficient manner, allowing faster access to active treatments for patients. Specific biomarkers associated with response to all treatment modalities are urgently required to guide treatment selection and sequencing.

Conclusion

With five novel therapies shown to improve survival in advanced CRPC in the last six years, the pace of drug development in this field is unprecedented (Table 6.12.1). The successes of abiraterone acetate and enzalutamide have conclusively shown that AR signalling remains a key driver of advanced prostate cancer. Median survival from a diagnosis of CRPC was 13–19 months in the pre-docetaxel era and is now exceeding 30 months with novel treatments.[64,65]

The clinical heterogeneity of prostate cancer has long been appreciated and we are now developing the tools to dissect the molecular heterogeneity of this disease. With so many therapeutic options now in the clinic and under investigation in clinical trials, strategies for treatment selection, combination, and sequencing are urgently required.

Table 6.12.1 Phase III clinical trials demonstrating improved overall survival in metastatic castration resistant prostate cancer (mCRPC)

Trial	Disease state	Trial design	HR	Median survival (m)	Reference
TAX327 N = 1,006	mCRPC	Docetaxel/prednisone vs. mitoxantrone/ prednisone	0.76	18.9 vs. 16.5	Tannock (2004)[29]
IMPACT N = 512	Pre-chemotherapy mCRPC	Sipuleucel-T vs. control	0.78	25.8 vs. 21.7	Kantoff (2010)[1]
TROPIC N = 755	mCRPC Post-docetaxel	Cabazitaxel/prednisone vs. mitoxantron/prednisone	0.70	15.1 vs. 12.7	de Bono (2010)[2]
COU-AA-301 N = 1,195	mCRPC Post-docetaxel	Abiraterone/prednisone vs. placbo/prednisone	0.65	15.8 vs. 11.2	de Bono (2011)[3]
ALSYMPCA N = 922	mCRPC Post-docetaxel or unfit for docetaxel	Radium-223 vs. placebo	0.70	14 vs. 11.2	Parker (2012)[5]
AFFIRM N = 1,199	mCRPC Post-docetaxel	Enzalutamide vs. placebo	0.63	18.4 vs. 13.6	Scher (2012)[4]

Acknowledgements

Abiraterone acetate was developed at The Institute of Cancer Research, which therefore has a commercial interest in the development of this agent. J.S.d.B. received consulting fees from Ortho Biotech Oncology Research and Development (a unit of Cougar Biotechnology); consulting fees and travel support from Amgen, Astellas, AstraZeneca, Boehringer Ingelheim, Bristol-Myers Squibb, Dendreon, Enzon, Exelixis, Genentech, GlaxoSmithKline, Medivation, Merck, Novartis, Pfizer, Roche, Sanofi-Aventis, Supergen, and Takeda; and grant support from AstraZeneca.

A.O.: travel support (Astellas, Bayer, Sanofi), advisory role (compensated, institutional: Astellas, Janssen, Bayer, Sanofi, Roche), research support (institutional): TEVA, Janssen.

C.P: advisory boards (compensated) including Novartis; honoraria including Janssen, Pfizer, Sanofi, Novartis, Astellas; travel support courtesy Pfizer and Sanofi.

DM: travel support (Astellas, Merck), advisory role (compensated, Janssen, Astellas, MSD, Roche, Sanofi).

Further reading

Darshan MS, Loftus MS, Thadani-Mulero M, *et al.* Taxane-induced blockade to nuclear accumulation of the androgen receptor predicts clinical responses in metastatic prostate cancer. *Cancer Res* 2011; **71**(18):6019–29.

de Bono JS, Logothetis CJ, Molina A, *et al.* Abiraterone and increased survival in metastatic prostate cancer. *N Engl J Med* 2011; **364**(21):1995–2005.

de Bono JS, Oudard S, Ozguroglu M, *et al.* Prednisone plus cabazitaxel or mitoxantrone for metastatic castration-resistant prostate cancer progressing after docetaxel treatment: a randomised open-label trial. *Lancet* 2010; **376**(9747):1147–54.

Fizazi K, Carducci M, Smith M, *et al.* Denosumab versus zoledronic acid for treatment of bone metastases in men with castration-resistant prostate cancer: a randomised, double-blind study. *Lancet* 2011; **377**(9768):813–22.

Kantoff PW, Higano CS, Shore ND, *et al.* Sipuleucel-T immunotherapy for castration-resistant prostate cancer. *N Engl J Med* 2010; **363**(5):411–22.

Olmos D, Arkenau HT, Ang JE, *et al.* Circulating tumour cell (CTC) counts as intermediate end points in castration-resistant prostate cancer (CRPC): a single-centre experience. *Ann Oncol* 2009; **20**(1):27–33.

Scher HI, Fizazi K, Saad F, *et al.* Increased survival with enzalutamide in prostate cancer after chemotherapy. *New Engl J Med* 2012; **367**(13):1187–97.

Scher HI, Halabi S, Tannock I, *et al.* Design and end points of clinical trials for patients with progressive prostate cancer and castrate levels of testosterone: recommendations of the Prostate Cancer Clinical Trials Working Group. *J Clin Oncol* 2008; **26**(7):1148–59.

Scher HI, Jia X, de Bono JS, *et al.* Circulating tumour cells as prognostic markers in progressive, castration-resistant prostate cancer: a reanalysis of IMMC38 trial data. *Lancet Oncol* 2009; **10**(3):233–9.

Tannock IF, de Wit R, Berry WR, *et al.* Docetaxel plus prednisone or mitoxantrone plus prednisone for advanced prostate cancer. *N Engl J Med* 2004; **351**(15):1502–12.

References

1. Kantoff PW, Higano CS, Shore ND, *et al.* Sipuleucel-T immunotherapy for castration-resistant prostate cancer. *N Engl J Med* 2010; **363**(5):411–22.
2. de Bono JS, Oudard S, Ozguroglu M, *et al.* Prednisone plus cabazitaxel or mitoxantrone for metastatic castration-resistant prostate cancer progressing after docetaxel treatment: a randomised open-label trial. *Lancet* 2010; **376**(9747):1147–54.
3. de Bono JS, Logothetis CJ, Molina A, *et al.* Abiraterone and increased survival in metastatic prostate cancer. *N Engl J Med* 2011; **364**(21):1995–2005.
4. Scher HI, Fizazi K, Saad F, *et al.* Increased survival with enzalutamide in prostate cancer after chemotherapy. *New Engl J Med* 2012; **367**(13):1187–97.
5. Parker C, Nilsson S, Heinrich D, *et al.* Alpha emitter radium-223 and survival in metastatic prostate cancer. *N Engl J Med* 2013; **369**(3):213–23.
6. Darshan MS, Loftus MS, Thadani-Mulero M, *et al.* Taxane-induced blockade to nuclear accumulation of the androgen receptor predicts clinical responses in metastatic prostate cancer. *Cancer Res* 2011; **71**(18):6019–29.
7. Small EJ, Baron AD, Fippin L, Apodaca D. Ketoconazole retains activity in advanced prostate cancer patients with progression despite flutamide withdrawal. *J Urol* 1997; **157**(4):1204–7.
8. Figg WD, Dawson N, Middleman MN, *et al.* Flutamide withdrawal and concomitant initiation of aminoglutethimide in patients with hormone refractory prostate cancer. *Acta Oncol* 1996; **35**(6):763–5.
9. Barrie SE, Potter GA, Goddard PM, Haynes BP, Dowsett M, Jarman M. Pharmacology of novel steroidal inhibitors of cytochrome P450(17) alpha (17 alpha-hydroxylase/C17-20 lyase). *J Steroid Biochem Mol Biol* 1994; **50**(5-6):267–73.
10. Attard G, Reid AH, Yap TA, *et al.* Phase I clinical trial of a selective inhibitor of CYP17, abiraterone acetate, confirms that castration-resistant prostate cancer commonly remains hormone driven. *J Clin Oncol* 2008; **26**(28):4563–71.
11. Ryan CJ, Smith MR, Fong L, *et al.* Phase I clinical trial of the CYP17 inhibitor abiraterone acetate demonstrating clinical activity in patients with castration-resistant prostate cancer who received prior ketoconazole therapy. *J Clin Oncol* 2010; **28**(9):1481–8.
12. Reid AH, Attard G, Danila DC, *et al.* Significant and sustained antitumor activity in post-docetaxel, castration-resistant prostate cancer with the CYP17 inhibitor abiraterone acetate. *J Clin Oncol* 2**010**; **28**(9):1489–95.
13. Danila DC, Morris MJ, de Bono JS, *et al.* Phase II multicenter study of abiraterone acetate plus prednisone therapy in patients with docetaxel-treated castration-resistant prostate cancer. *J Clin Oncol* 2010; **28**(9):1496–501.
14. Fizazi K, Scher HI, Molina A, *et al.* Abiraterone acetate for treatment of metastatic castration-resistant prostate cancer: final overall survival analysis of the COU-AA-301 randomised, double-blind, placebo-controlled phase 3 study. *Lancet Oncol* 2012; **13**(10):983–92.
15. Ryan CJ, Smith MR, de Bono JS, *et al.* Abiraterone in metastatic prostate cancer without previous chemotherapy. *N Engl J Med* 2013; **368**:138–48.
16. Ryan CJ, Smith MR, Fizazi K, *et al.* Abiraterone acetate plus prednisone versus placebo plus prednisone in chemotherapy-naive men with metastatic castration-resistant prostate cancer (COU-AA-302): final overall survival analysis of a randomised, double-blind, placebo-controlled phase 3 study. *Lancet Oncol* 2015; **16**(2):152–60.
17. Ryan CJ, Shah S, Efstathiou E, *et al.* Phase II study of abiraterone acetate in chemotherapy-naive metastatic castration-resistant prostate cancer displaying bone flare discordant with serologic response. *Clin Cancer Res* 2011; **17**(14):4854–61.
18. Hussain M, Corn PG, Michaelson MD, *et al.* Phase II study of single-agent orteronel (TAK-700) in patients with nonmetastatic castration-resistant prostate cancer and rising prostate-specific antigen. *Clin Cancer Res* 2014; **20**(16):4218–27.
19. Fizazi K, Jones R, Oudard S, *et al.* Phase III, randomized, double-blind, multicenter trial comparing orteronel (TAK-700) plus prednisone with placebo plus prednisone in patients with metastatic castration-resistant prostate cancer that has progressed during or after docetaxel-based therapy: ELM-PC 5. *J Clin Oncol* 2015; **33**(7):723–31.
20. Saad F, Fizazi K, Jinga V, *et al.* Orteronel plus prednisone in patients with chemotherapy-naive metastatic castration-resistant prostate

cancer (ELM-PC 4): a double-blind, multicentre, phase 3, randomised, placebo-controlled trial. *Lancet Oncol* 2015; **16**(3):338–48.

21. Tran C, Ouk S, Clegg NJ, *et al.* Development of a second-generation antiandrogen for treatment of advanced prostate cancer. *Science* 2009; **324**(5928):787–90.
22. Scher HI, Beer TM, Higano CS, *et al.* Antitumour activity of MDV3100 in castration-resistant prostate cancer: a phase 1-2 study. *Lancet* 2010; **375**(9724):1437–46.
23. Beer TM, Armstrong AJ, Rathkopf DE, *et al.* Enzalutamide in metastatic prostate cancer before chemotherapy. *N Engl J Med* 2014; **371**(5):424–33.
24. Rathkopf DE, Morris MJ, Danila DC, *et al.* A phase I study of the androgen signaling inhibitor ARN-509 in patients with metastatic castration-resistant prostate cancer (mCRPC). *J Clin Oncol* 2012; **30**(Suppl; abstr 4548).
25. Watson PA, Arora VK, Sawyers CL. Emerging mechanisms of resistance to androgen receptor inhibitors in prostate cancer. *Nat Rev Cancer* 2015; **15**(12):701–11.
26. Antonarakis ES, Lu C, Wang H, *et al.* AR-V7 and resistance to enzalutamide and abiraterone in prostate cancer. *N Engl J Med* 2014; **371**(11):1028–38.
27. Nakazawa M, Lu C, Chen Y, *et al.* Serial blood-based analysis of AR-V7 in men with advanced prostate cancer. *Ann Oncol* 2015; **26**(9):1859–65.
28. Antonarakis ES, Chandhasin C, Osbourne E, Luo J, Sadar MD, Perabo F. Targeting the N-terminal domain of the androgen receptor: A new approach for the treatment of advanced prostate cancer. *Oncologist* 2016; Sep 14: pii: theoncologist.2016-0161[Epub ahead of print].
29. Tannock IF, de Wit R, Berry WR, *et al.* Docetaxel plus prednisone or mitoxantrone plus prednisone for advanced prostate cancer. *N Engl J Med* 2004; **351**(15):1502–12.
30. Beer TM, Ryan CW, Venner PM, *et al.* Intermittent chemotherapy in patients with metastatic androgen-independent prostate cancer: results from ASCENT, a double-blinded, randomized comparison of high-dose calcitriol plus docetaxel with placebo plus docetaxel. *Cancer* 2008; **112**(2):326–30.
31. Mountzios I, Bournakis E, Efstathiou E, *et al.* Intermittent docetaxel chemotherapy in patients with castrate-resistant prostate cancer. *Urology* 2011; **77**(3):682–7.
32. Pond GR, Armstrong AJ, Wood BA, *et al.* Evaluating the value of number of cycles of docetaxel and prednisone in men with metastatic castration-resistant prostate cancer. *Eur Urol* 2012; **61**(2):363–9.
33. de Bono JS, Scher HI, Montgomery RB, *et al.* Circulating tumor cells predict survival benefit from treatment in metastatic castration-resistant prostate cancer. *Clin Cancer Res* 2008; **14**(19):6302–9.
34. Buonerba C, Palmieri G, Di Lorenzo G. Docetaxel rechallenge in castration-resistant prostate cancer: scientific legitimacy of common clinical practice. *Eur Urol* 2010; **58**(4):636–7.
35. Di Lorenzo G, Buonerba C, Faiella A, *et al.* Phase II study of docetaxel re-treatment in docetaxel-pretreated castration-resistant prostate cancer. *BJU Int* 2011; **107**(2):234–9.
36. Mita AC, Denis LJ, Rowinsky EK, *et al.* Phase I and pharmacokinetic study of XRP6258 (RPR 116258A), a novel taxane, administered as a 1-hour infusion every 3 weeks in patients with advanced solid tumors. *Clin Cancer Res* 2009; **15**(2):723–30.
37. Bissery M-C, Bouchard H, Riou JF, *et al.* Preclinical evaluation of TXD258, a new taxoid. *Proc Am Assoc Cancer Res* 2000; **41**:214 (abstr. 1364).
38. Bahl A, Masson S, Malik Z, *et al.* Cabazitaxel for metastatic castration-resistant prostate cancer (mCRPC): Interim safety and quality-of-life (QOL) data from the U.K. early access program (NCT01254279). *J Clin Oncol* 2012; **30**(Suppl 5):abstr 44.
39. De Bono JS, Hardy-Bessard AC, Kim CS, *et al.* Phase III non-inferiority study of cabazitaxel (C) 20mg/m^2 (C20) versus 25mg/m^2 (C25) in patients (pts) with metastatic castration-resistant prostate cancer (mCRPC) previously treated with docetaxel (D). *J Clin Oncol* 2016; **24**(Suppl):Abstr 5008.
40. Sartor AO OS, Sengelov L, Daugaad G, *et al.* Cabazitaxel vs docetaxel in chemotherapy-naive (CN) patients with metastatic castriation-resistant prostate cancer (mCRPC): A three-arm phase III study (FIRSTANA). *J Clin Oncol* 2016; **34**(Suppl):Abstr 5006.
41. Huber ML, Haynes L, Parker C, Iversen P. Interdisciplinary critique of sipuleucel-T as immunotherapy in castration-resistant prostate cancer. *J Natl Cancer Inst* 2012; **104**(4):273–9.
42. Longo DL. New therapies for castration-resistant prostate cancer. *N Engl J Med* 2010; **363**(5):479–81.
43. Slovin SF BT, Higano CS. Initial phase II experience of ipilimumab (IPI) alone and in combination with radiotherapy (XRT) in patients with metastatic castration resistant prostate cancer (mCRPC). *J Clin Oncol* 2009; **27**(15 Suppl):Abstract 5138.
44. Kwon ED, Drake CG, Scher HI, *et al.* Ipilimumab versus placebo after radiotherapy in patients with metastatic castration-resistant prostate cancer that had progressed after docetaxel chemotherapy (CA184-043): a multicentre, randomised, double-blind, phase 3 trial. *Lancet Oncol* 2014; **15**(7):700–12.
45. Beer TM, Kwon ED, Drake CG, *et al.* Randomized, double-blind, phase III trial of ipilimumab versus placebo in asymptomatic or minimally symptomatic patients with metastatic chemotherapy-naive castration-resistant prostate cancer. *J Clin Oncol* 2016; JCO691584.
46. Brahmer JR, Drake CG, Wollner I, *et al.* Phase I study of single-agent anti-programmed death-1 (MDX-1106) in refractory solid tumors: safety, clinical activity, pharmacodynamics, and immunologic correlates. *J Clin Oncol* 2010; **28**(19):3167–75.
47. Saad F, Gleason DM, Murray R, *et al.* Long-term efficacy of zoledronic acid for the prevention of skeletal complications in patients with metastatic hormone-refractory prostate cancer. *J Natl Cancer Inst* 2004; **96**(11):879–82.
48. Fizazi K, Beuzeboc P, Lumbroso J, *et al.* Phase II trial of consolidation docetaxel and samarium-153 in patients with bone metastases from castration-resistant prostate cancer. *J Clin Oncol* 2009; **27**(15):2429–35.
49. Tu SM, Millikan RE, Mengistu B, *et al.* Bone-targeted therapy for advanced androgen-independent carcinoma of the prostate: a randomised phase II trial. *Lancet* 2001; **357**(9253):336–41.
50. Fizazi K, Carducci M, Smith M, *et al.* Denosumab versus zoledronic acid for treatment of bone metastases in men with castration-resistant prostate cancer: a randomised, double-blind study. *Lancet* 2011; **377**(9768):813–22.
51. Saad F SM, Shore ND, Oudard S, *et al.* Effect of denosumab on prolonging bone-metastasis free survival (BMFS) in men with nonmetastatic castrate-resistant prostate cancer (CRPC) presenting with aggressive PSA kinetics. *J Clin Oncol* 2012; **30**(Suppl):Abstract 4510.
52. Snedecor SJ CJ, Kaura S, Botteman M. Cost-effectiveness of zoledronic acid (ZOL) versus denosumab (Dmab) in prevention of skeletal-related events (SREs) in castration-resistant prostate cancer metastatic to the bone (mCRPC). *J Clin Oncol* 2011; **29**(Suppl):Abstract 4581.
53. Smith M, De Bono J, Sternberg C, *et al.* Phase III study of cabozantinib in previously treated metastatic castration-resistant prostate cancer: COMET-1. *J Clin Oncol* 2016; **34**(25):3005–13.
54. Carver BS, Chapinski C, Wongvipat J, *et al.* Reciprocal feedback regulation of PI3K and androgen receptor signaling in PTEN-deficient prostate cancer. *Cancer Cell* 2011; **19**(5):575–86.
55. De Bono JS DGU, Massard C, Bracarda S, *et al.* PTEN loss as a predictive biomarker for the AKT inhibitor ipatasertib combined with aberaterone acetate in patients with metastatic castration-resistant prostate cancer (mCRPC). *Ann Oncol* 2016; **26**(Suppl 6):Abstract 1780.
56. Fleming MT, Morris MJ, Heller G, Scher HI. Post-therapy changes in PSA as an outcome measure in prostate cancer clinical trials. *Nat Clin Pract Oncol* 2006; **3**(12):658–67.
57. Bubley GJ, Carducci M, Dahut W, *et al.* Eligibility and response guidelines for phase II clinical trials in androgen-independent prostate cancer: recommendations from the Prostate-Specific Antigen Working Group. *J Clin Oncol* 1999; **17**(11):3461–7.
58. Therasse P, Arbuck SG, Eisenhauer EA, *et al.* New guidelines to evaluate the response to treatment in solid tumors. European

Organization for Research and Treatment of Cancer, National Cancer Institute of the United States, National Cancer Institute of Canada. *J Natl Cancer Inst* 2000; **92**(3):205–16.

59. Scher HI, Halabi S, Tannock I, *et al.* Design and end points of clinical trials for patients with progressive prostate cancer and castrate levels of testosterone: recommendations of the Prostate Cancer Clinical Trials Working Group. *J Clin Oncol* 2008; **26**(7):1148–59.
60. Scher HI, Morris MJ, Stadler WM, *et al.* Trial design and objectives for castration-resistant prostate cancer: Updated recommendations from the prostate cancer clinical trials working group 3. *J Clin Oncol* 2016; **34**(12):1402–18.
61. Messiou C, Collins DJ, Giles S, de Bono JS, Bianchini D, de Souza NM. Assessing response in bone metastases in prostate cancer with diffusion weighted MRI. *Eur Radiol* 2011; **21**(10):2169–77.
62. Ceci F, Castellucci P, Nanni C, Fanti S. PET/CT imaging for evaluating response to therapy in castration-resistant prostate cancer. *Eur J Nucl Med Mol Imaging* 2016; **43**(12):2103–4.
63. Gillessen S, Omlin A, Attard G, *et al.* Management of patients with advanced prostate cancer: recommendations of the St Gallen Advanced Prostate Cancer Consensus Conference (APCCC) 2015. *Ann Oncol* 2015; **26**(8):1589–604.
64. Armstrong A, Haggman M, Stadler WM, *et al.* Phase II study of tasquinimod in chemotherapy-naive patients with metastatic castrate-resistant prostate cancer (CRPC): Safety and efficacy analysis including subgroups. *J Clin Oncol* 2011; **29**(Suppl 7): Abstract 126.
65. Pezaro CJ, Omlin AG, Mukherji D, *et al.* Survival in metastatic castration resistant prostate cancer (mCRPC) trial participants. *J Clin Oncol* 2012; **30**(Suppl):Abstract e15136.

CHAPTER 6.13

Bladder and upper urinary tract cancer

Maria E. Goossens, Frank Buntinx, and Maurice P. Zeegers

Epidemiology, pathology, and demographics

Introduction to bladder cancer

Cancer of the bladder is estimated to be the ninth most common cause of cancer worldwide (382,660 cases in 2008)[1] and the thirteenth most frequent cause of death from cancer (145,000 deaths). It is relatively common in developed countries, where 63% of cases occur, and where it ranks sixth in frequency (225,000 cases), with high rates in North America and Europe, where 59% of all incident cases occur. The majority (77%) of the patients who suffer from bladder tumours are male. Population-based five-year survival rates range from 40% to 80% depending on whether non-invasive lesions are included in the computation.[2]

The most common histological type in Western countries is transitional cell carcinoma (TCC), which comprises some 95–97% of cancers in European populations. In Africa, the majority of bladder cancers are also TCCs. Substantial proportions of squamous cell carcinomas (SCC) are observed in Zimbabwe (37.8%) and Egypt (19,9%) related to the prevalence of infection with Schistosoma haematobium (Bilharziasis).[3] In South Africa, the national pathology-based registry shows marked differences in histology between blacks (36% SCC, 41% TCC) and whites (2% SCC, 94% TCC).[2]

In the United States and probably in most Western countries, urinary bladder cancer (UBC), has the greatest per-patient lifetime cost for cancer in terms of healthcare expenditure[4] compared to all other types of cancer. The annual cost of care for all patients with muscle-invasive bladder cancer (MIBC) is 70% more than for patients with non-muscle-invasive bladder cancer (non-MIBC). The mean, annual post-diagnosis continuing care costs per case is $4,975, $7,100, and $17,437 for those with CIS- Ta, T1, and MIBC. The major cost drivers, regardless of disease stage, are diagnostic/surveillance and complications, accounting for up to 43% and 37% of bladder cancer care costs, respectively.[5]

We reviewed the main established risk factors associated with bladder cancer aetiology. Data were extracted from previous reviews and meta-analyses and original articles identified from PubMed searches, reference lists, and book chapters dealing with the reviewed topics.

Pathology

Worldwide, UBC, formerly known as *transitional cell carcinoma*, is the most prevalent histological type of bladder tumour (80%) (Fig. 6.13.1). Bilharziasis is the leading cause of *squamous cell carcinoma* worldwide, with the highest incidence in Egypt (up to 59% of all bladder cancer cases). A lag period of approximately 30 years has been reported between bilharzial infection and subsequent development of the disease. The median age of SCC is 46 years. The male-to-female ratio is 5:1. Primary SCC in the non-bilharzial bladder is uncommon, accounting for 2% to 5%. Patients with spinal cord injury represent the largest group of patients affected by SCC in non-Bilharzia regions. SCC also is likely to occur in patients with chronic inflammatory disorders of the bladder, persistent calculi, chronic cystitis, and bladder diverticuli, and the overall five-year survival rate is poor (16%). *Adenocarcinoma* of the bladder is the third most common histologic type of bladder carcinoma. It accounts for 0.5% to 2.0% of all bladder tumours. It is the most common tumour arising in the bladder of patients with exstrophy. Adenocarcinoma of the bladder may also occur in association with schistosomiasis, endometriosis, bladder augmentation, and other irritative conditions of the urinary bladder. The mean patient age at diagnosis is around 66 years.[6] Adenocarcinoma is virtually always invasive and has a 5-year survival rate of 19%.[7] *Small-cell carcinoma of the bladder* (SCCB) is rare (incidence of 0.7%), highly aggressive, and diagnosed mainly at advanced stages. The majority of patients are male, with the mean sex ratio equal to 5:1. The mean age at time of first diagnosis is 67 years. Histological tests show a tumour, which is indistinguishable from small-cell lung carcinoma. Most patients are diagnosed with an advanced stage. Up to 70% of SCCB is associated with TCC. The overall five-year survival rate in all stages is 19% due to high metastatic potential and lack of symptoms in earlier stages of the disease.[8–10] *Keratinizing squamous metaplasia* is infrequently, and its clinical significance remains unclear, with studies linking it to the development of invasive SCC. Both synchronous diagnosis of urothelial tumour (up to 22%) and subsequent tumour development on follow-up has been identified.[11] *Inflammatory myofibroblastic tumour* of the genitourinary tract should be considered a neoplasm of uncertain malignant potential.[12] *Micropapillary urothelial carcinoma* of the urinary bladder is a rare anatomico-pathological variant of aggressive behaviour.[13]

The scope of this chapter is mainly on TCC, seen the great prevalence of TCC worldwide and since most studies examined risk factors on TCC.

Carcinogenesis

Superficial bladder cancer (non-MIBC) encompasses patients with stage Ta T1 tumours and patients with carcinoma *in situ* (CIS) (70%

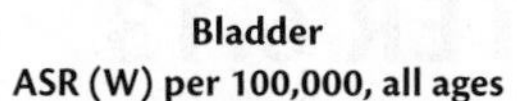

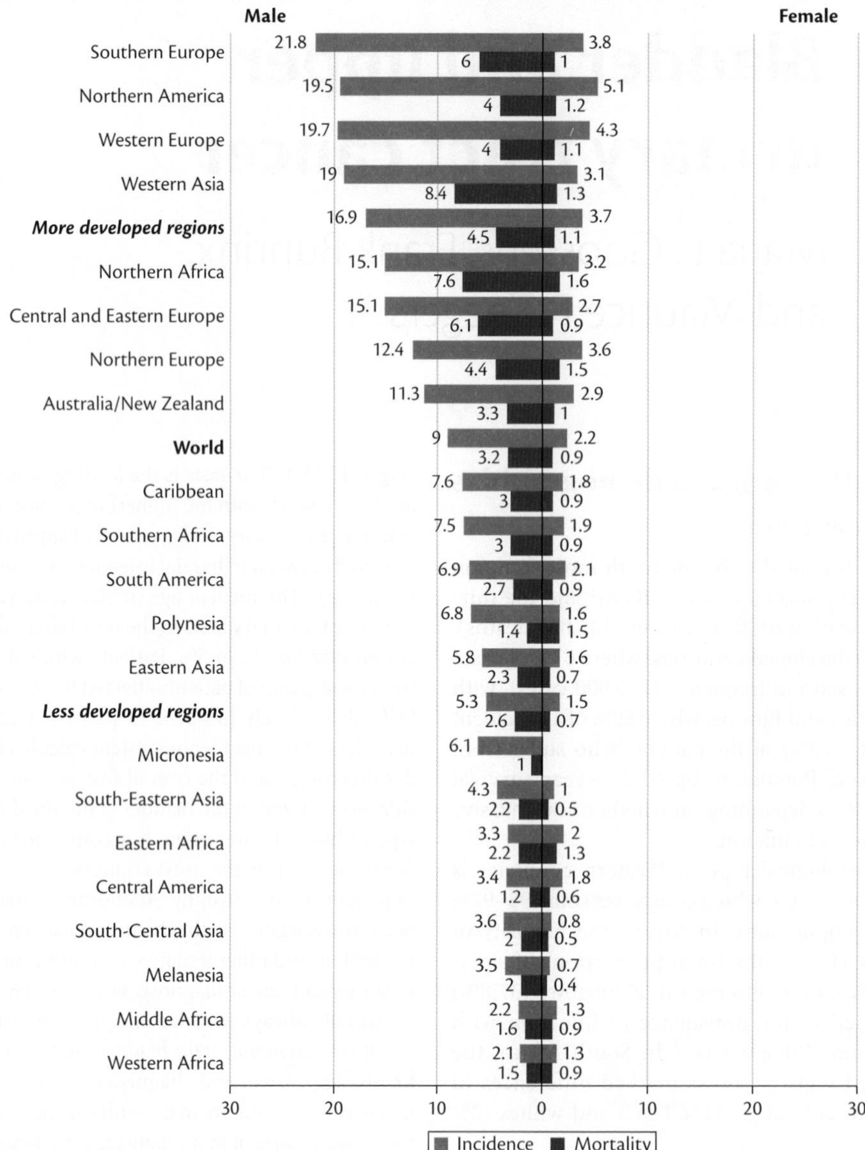

Fig. 6.13.1 Incidence of bladder cancer worldwide.

Reproduced with permission Ferlay J., Soerjomataram I., Ervik M., Dikshit R., Eser S., Mathers C., Rebelo M., Parkin D.M., Forman D., Bray, F. *GLOBOCAN 2012 v1.0, Cancer Incidence and Mortality Worldwide: IARC CancerBase No. 11* [Internet]. Lyon, France: International Agency for Research on Cancer; 2013. Available from: http://globocan.iarc.fr

at first diagnosis). The WHO grading of 1973[14] distinguishes well-differentiated tumours that have orderly arrangement of normal cell lining delicate papillae as grade 1 tumours, moderately differentiated tumours that have some focal variation in nuclear appearance as grade 2 tumours and poorly differentiated tumours that have the most extreme nuclear abnormalities as grade 3 tumours. Both grade 2 and 3 are high-grade tumours in the WHO grading of 2004.[15] Both grading systems are still in use.[16] The current TNM classification[17] of UBC describes Ta tumours as non-invasive and papillary, confined to the mucosa, CIS, as a flat tumour confined to the mucosa too, and T1 invasive tumours that invade the sub-epithelial connective tissue. Ta tumours account for approximately 70% of superficial TCC. Carcinoma *in situ* is a flat intraepithelial carcinoma and is characterized by flat disordered proliferation of cells with marked cytological abnormalities. CIS is a high-grade tumour and comprises approximately 10% of all cases of UBC. T2 and higher lesions are muscle-invasive tumours (MIBC). These patients are treated with radical cystectomy as they are at increased risk of lymph node, distant metastases, and death from UBC.[18]

The most important prognostic factors for recurrence are the prior recurrence rate, the number of tumours, and the tumour size; whereas for progression, the most important prognostic factors are staging, grade, and presence of CIS. Treatment with intravesical Bacillus Calmette-Guérin reduces both the risk of recurrence and the risk of progression, and is the treatment of choice for high-risk papillary tumours and for patients with CIS. Natural history of patients with superficial bladder cancer differs between patients with only stage Ta T1 TCC and patients with CIS. Without intravesical treatment after transurethral resection (TUR), 47% of the patients recurred and 9% progressed to muscle-invasive disease based on a median follow-up of about five years. Approximately one-third of the patients died and one-third of the deaths were due to malignant disease. On the other hand, CIS, which cannot be eradicated by TUR alone, has a much higher progression rate. Fifty-four per cent (54%) of these patients progressed to muscle-invasive disease. Intravesical chemotherapeutic agents such as thiotepa, doxorubicin, epirubicin, and mitomycin C prolong the time of the first recurrence and reduce the risk on recurrence by 20% and increase the eight-year disease-free rate to 45%. However, intravesical chemotherapy had no effect on delaying or preventing progression to muscle-invasive disease.[19]

Men have a 3,7% risk of developing UBC. They are at a three to four times higher risk than women for developing UBC, while women present more advanced diseases (71% versus 63% with non-MICB).[20] Women have more multifocal (50% vs. 29%, $p = 0.005$) and larger tumours (5.2 vs. 3.8 cm, $p = 0.03$). There is no uniform theory to explain the differential presentation and behaviour of UBC between genders.[21,22]

Age is now widely accepted as the greatest single risk factor for developing UBC. The median age at diagnosis is 70 years. The peak incidence of UBC occurs at 85 years old.[23] Mortality from UBC is also higher for the elderly. The ratio of cancer-specific mortality to incidence for men and women in the USA aged 65–69 years is 14% and 18%, respectively, whereas for men and women age 80–84 years it is 30% and 37%, respectively (SEER, 1973–97).[21] UBC rarely occurs below the age of 40 years. Below the age of 40 years UBC is more common in male patients. It starts mainly with gross painless haematuria, is more commonly located at bladder trigone/ureteral orifices and has a greater chance for unifocality, low-grade, and low-stage tumours.[24]

Risk factors

A rating system, adapted from the World Cancer Research Fund.[25] has been used to summarize the level of scientific evidence for each risk factor; it consists of five levels: convincing, probable, limited suggestive, limited-no conclusion, and substantial effect on risk unlikely. The rating has been based on the number of epidemiologic studies (cohort and/or case–control studies) showing consistent associations and whether or not supportive mechanistic evidence (biologically plausible and supportive laboratory evidence) is present (Table 6.13.1). The level of association is based on the previous results of published meta-and pooled analyses of case–control and cohort studies. The levels of association are categorized as substantially increased risk ($RR \geq 2.5$), moderately increased risk ($1.5 \leq RR < 2.5$), slightly (or small) increased risk ($1.2 \leq RR < 1.5$), no association ($0.8 \leq RR < 1.2$), slightly (or small) decreased risk ($0.7 \leq RR < 0.8$), moderately decreased risk ($0.4 \leq RR < 0.7$), and substantially decreased risk ($RR < 0.4$). We constructed a matrix in which the levels of evidence were combined with the levels of association (Table 6.13.2).

Occupational exposure

It is estimated that 20–27% of bladder cancers are attributable to occupational exposures.[26] There is convincing evidence for a slightly increased risk of UBC for *miners* (SRR= 1.31 (95% CI, 1.09–1.57)), *bus drivers* (SRR = 1.29 (95% CI, 1.08–1.53)), *rubber workers* (SRR = 1.29 (95% CI, 1.06–1.58)), *motor mechanics* (SRR = 1.27 (95% CI, 1.10–1.46)), *leather workers* (SRR = 1.27 (95% CI, 1.07–1.49)), *blacksmiths* (SRR = 1.27 (95% CI, 1.02–1.58)), *mechanics* (SRR = 1.21 (95% CI, 1.12–1.31)), *hairdressers* (SRR = 1.23 (95% CI, 1.11–1.37)), and a probable evidence for a slightly increased risk of UBC *machine setters* (SRR = 1.24 (95% CI, 1.09–1.42)).[27] For hairdressers, holding their job more than 10 years, there is a moderately increased risk (1.70 (95% CI, 1.01–2.88)).[28] There is convincing evidence, based on a meta-analysis, including more than 2,900 incident cases or deaths from bladder cancer among *painters* reported in 41 cohort and 30 case–control studies for a slightly increased risk of UBC (SRR = 1.25 (95% CI 1.16–1.34)). Furthermore, exposure-response analyses suggested that the risk increased with duration of employment.[29] For workers in the *petroleum industry*, there is probable evidence for a slightly increased risk based on the pooled risk of eight case–control studies (OR = 1.4 (95% CI, 1.27–1.54)).[30] There is probable evidence for a slightly increased risk of UBC for workers in *aluminium production* (pooled RR = 1.29, 95% CI 1.12–1.49; 8 cohort studies) and in the iron and steel foundries (pooled RR = 1.29, 95% CI 1.06–1.57; 7 cohort studies), a moderately increased risk for workers in the coal gasification (pooled RR = 2.39, 95% CI 1.36–4.21; 2 cohort studies).[31] There is convincing evidence for firefighters after 40 or more years of employment, that their risk of UBC mortality was significantly increased for bladder cancer, SRR = 5.7 (95% CI, 1.56–14.63). There is probable evidence for a slightly decreased risk of UBC for farmers based on meta-analyses of cancer mortality and incidence surveys with 29 studies reported (RR = 0.79).

The International Agency for Research on Cancer (IARC) has classified specific aromatic amines such as 4-aminobiphenyl, arsenic, benzo[a]pyrene, benzidine and N,N-bis(2-chloroethyl)-2-naphthylamine (chlornaphazine) as carcinogenic to humans and 4,4'-methylenebis(2-methylaniline) and ortho-toluidine as possible carcinogenic to humans. Rubber and aluminium industries and both magenta and auramine manufacturing expose to carcinogenic circumstances while petroleum refining and petrochemical

Table 6.13.1 Summary of levels of evidence for aetiological risk factors for disease adapted from the World Cancer Research Fund (2007)

Level of evidence	No. of studies	Supportive mechanistic evidence
Convincing	At least two independent cohort studies and case–control studies	Yes, and strong and plausible experimental evidence
Probable	At least two independent cohort studies, or at least five case–control studies	Yes
Limited—suggestive	At least two independent cohort studies, or at least five case–control studies (heterogeneity present)	Yes
Limited—no conclusion	No sufficient studies available, effect inconsistent	Yes/No
Substantial effect on risk unlikely	At least two independent cohort studies and case–control studies	No

Source: data from World Cancer Research Fund and American Institute for Cancer Research, *Food, Nutrition, Physical Activity, and the Prevention of Cancer: a Global Perspective*, American Institute for Cancer Research (AIRC), Washington, USA, Copyright © 2007.

Table 6.13.2 Levels of evidence and levels of association for risk factors (exposed vs. not exposed) for UBC

Evidence	Convincing	Probable	Limited suggestive	Limited—no conclusion	Substantial effect on risk unlikely
Substantially increased risk[a]	Men Smoking	Bilharziasis Renal cell cancer	Phenacetine	Organ transplantation UTI Human papilloma virus Users of menopause hormone replacement therapy Cyclophosphamide Salted meat Barbecued meat Soy products Spices	
Moderately increased risk[b]	Prostate cancer Arsenic Radiation	Coal gasification GSTP1	Dialysis	Hair dyes Gonorrhoea Urinary tract stones Personal hair dye use	
Slightly increased risk[c]	Coffee consumption men Uterus cancer Diabetesmellitus Painters Firefighters (>40 years of work) rs9642880[T] rs798766[T]	Tap water Machine setters Petroleum industry Aluminium production Iron and steel founderies NAT2 slow acetylation		Asthma Miners Bus drivers Rubber workers Motor mechanics Leather workers Blacksmiths Mechanics Hairdressers Disinfection by-products in drinking water rs2736100[C]	
No association[d]	Coffee consumption women Alcohol Fish Tea NSAIDs Physical activity	Paracetamol Fruit Vegetables ERCC2 D312N NBN E185Q XPC A499V	Waterpipe smoking Green tea Other tea Decaffeinated coffee	Syphilis Phenobarbital Isoniazid Chlonaphazine Asperin Total fluid Nickel	
Slightly decreased risk[e]		Farmers			
Moderately decreased risk[f]	Selenium			Dietary acrylamide Vitamines Citrus fruit Carrots	
Substantially decreased risk[g]					

[a] RR ≥2.5.

[b] 1.5 ≤ RR <2.5.

[c] 1.2 ≤ RR <1.5.

[d] 0.8 ≤ RR <1.2.

[e] 0.7 ≤ RR <0.8.

[f] 0.4 ≤ RR <0.7.

[g] RR <0.4.

manufacturing and exposure to diesel exhaust expose to probably carcinogenic circumstances. Occupational exposure as a barber or hairdresser is listed as probably carcinogenic exposure circumstances, while dry cleaning is listed as possible.[26,32]

Environmental factors

Contaminants in drinking water

Several contaminants in drinking water are associated with an increased risk of UBC. A WHO report[33] states that *arsenic* exposure via drinking water is related to UBC. There is sufficient evidence in humans that arsenic in drinking water causes cancers of the urinary bladder.[34] Although there is convincing evidence that exposure to high levels of arsenic in drinking water is associated with a moderately increased UBC risk,[35] lower exposures (e.g. <100–200 microg/L) generally are not. *Disinfection by-products in drinking water and swimming pools* are formed when disinfectants (chlorine, ozone, chlorine dioxide, or chloramines) react with naturally occurring organic matter, anthropogenic contaminants, bromide, and iodide during the production of drinking water. A recent epidemiologic study found that much of the risk for bladder cancer associated with drinking water was associated with three factors: Trihalomethane (THM) levels, showering/bathing/swimming (i.e. dermal/inhalation exposure), and genotype (having the GSTT1-1 gene). There is limited, non-conclusive evidence for a slightly increased risk between nitrate in drinking water and UBC. There were positive associations for bladder cancer with relative risks across nitrate quartiles = 1, 1.69, 1.10, and 2.83.[36]

Radiation

A UN report from 2000 reported that there is convincing evidence of a relation between radiation exposure and bladder cancer risk, based on the atomic bomb survivor data, especially for women (RR = 1.74 (95% CI, 0.71–3.22)). Several populations medically exposed to radiation for benign or malignant diseases also showed an increased risk of bladder cancer.[37]

Lifestyle factors

Tobacco

Tobacco smoking is the main known cause of UBC in humans (Fig. 6.13.2). An association has been observed in epidemiological studies conducted since the late 1950s, and its causal nature was established in the 1980s.[38] According to the meta-analysis of 35 case–control and eight cohort studies of Zeegers *et al.*[20] cigarette smoking was accounting for a more than threefold higher risk for men (OR = 3.18 (95% CI 2.35, 4.29) and nearly a threefold higher risk for women (OR = 2.90 (95% CI 2.01, 4.19). The IARC analysed the data of 42 case–control and 24 cohort studies reporting on cigarette smoking and cancer of the lower urinary tract. The 24 cohort studies consistently showed an excess of deaths from UBC among smokers (RR between 3.0 and 5.4 for smokers of 20 or more cigarettes/day). Also, the starting age of smoking has been found to be positively associated with risk; smokers who started smoking at an earlier age were at a higher risk for UBC.[39] The pooled analyses of Brennan *et al.*[40,41] showed an increasing risk of UBC with increasing duration of smoking, ranging from approximately a twofold increased risk for a duration less than 10 years (OR = 1.9, 95% CI 1.1, 3.1) to over a fourfold increased risk for a duration greater than 40 years (OR = 4.1, 95% CI 3.0, 5.5) for women and ranging from an odds ratio of 1.96 after

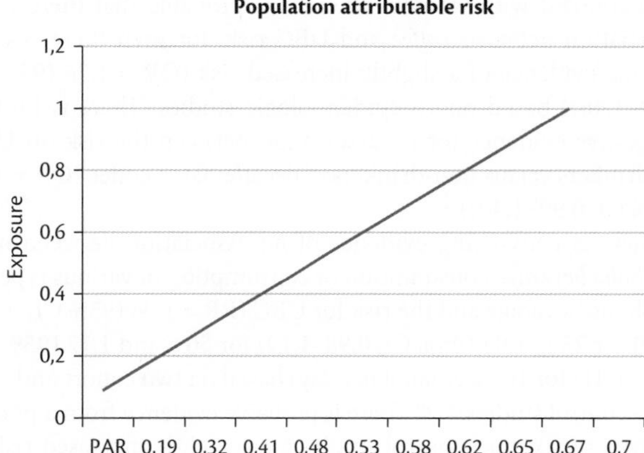

Fig. 6.13.2 Population attributable risk (PAR) of smoking for UBC (RR = 3.3). In a country where 40% of the people are smokers, smoking causes 50% of the bladder cancer incidence.

20 years of smoking (95% CI 1.48, 2.61) to 5.57 after 60 years (CI 4.18, 7.44) for men. A dose-response relationship was observed between number of cigarettes smoked per day and UBC up to a threshold limit of 15–20 cigarettes per day, OR = 3.8 (95% CI 2.7, 5.4) for women and OR = 4.50 (95% CI 3.81, 5.33) for men, after which no increased risk was observed. A lowering of risk after stopping cigarette smoking is seen in almost all the studies of the IARC and confirmed in the pooled analysis of Brennan *et al.*: the decrease is over 30% in the immediate 1-4 years after cessation. However, even after 25 years the decrease in risk did not reach the level of the never-smokers.[41] The relative risks for smokers of black tobacco were 1.5 to 2 times higher than those for smokers of blond tobacco.[39] Based on a pooled analysis of six case–control studies on men, the OR for pure pipe smoking was 1.9 (95% CI 1.2, 3.1) and that for pure cigar smoking 2.3 (95% CI 1.6, 3.5).[42] Studies conducted in populations with a high proportion of non-transitional cell carcinomas, such as Egypt and Zimbabwe, also reported a positive association with tobacco smoking.[38] Data on involuntary smoke and use of smokeless tobacco products are limited, but do not suggest an increased risk of UBC.[38] Waterpipe tobacco may not have an effect on UBC based on the result of one small Egyptian case–control study. There is convincing evidence for a substantially increased risk of UBC and smoking cigarettes, probable evidence for a moderately increased risk of UBC and smoking pipe and cigars. Fifteen studies investigated the influence of smoking on prognosis. All reported an increased risk of recurrence, but only one was statistically significant.[43]

Physical activity

Based on eight cohort and two case–control studies, there is convincing evidence for no association between physical activity and UBC risk.[44,45]

Personal hair dye use

There is limited non-conclusive evidence from two case–control studies of a moderately increased risk using hair dyes and UBC risk.[46]

Drinks

There is convincing evidence for no association between UBC risk and *tea* (both green and other) consumption based (OR = 1.0 (95% CI, 0.9–1.1)).[47]

In contrast with women, where it is probable that there is no association between *coffee* and UBC risk, for men there is convincing evidence of a slightly increased risk (OR = 1.26 (95% CI 1.09–1.46)) based on 16 epidemiologic studies. There is limited suggestive evidence for no association between the risk on UBC for drinkers versus non-drinkers of decaffeinated coffee (OR = 1.18 (95% CI, 0.99–1.40)).[47]

There is convincing evidence of no association between total *alcoholic beverage* consumption or consumption of various types of alcoholic beverage and the risk for UBC (RR = 1.04 (95% CI, 0.99–1.09) for 25 g, 1.08 (95% CI, 0.98–1.19) for 50 g and 1.17 (95% CI, 0.97–1.41) for 100 g ethanol per day) based on two cohort and nine case–control studies.[48,49] There is probable evidence from a pooled analysis of six case–control studies for a slightly increased risk of drinking >2 L/day of *tap water* vs. £0.5 L/day (OR=1.46 (95% CI, 1.20–1.78)).[50]

The available evidence on a possible relation between the *total fluid intake* and the risk of UBC is not conclusive seen the conflicting effect.[51]

Diet

There is convincing evidence that *fish* is not significantly associated with a decreased UBC risk (RR 0.86 (95% CI, 0.61–1.12)) in a meta-analysis of five cohort and nine case–control studies.[52] For *dietary acrylamide*, a probable human carcinogen, found in French fries and potato chips, there is limited, non-conclusive evidence for not-statistically a moderately decreased risk (RR highest versus lowest quintile: 0.60 (95% CI 0.39–0.94), *p*-trend: 0.13) for UBC only for women.[53] Trace elements, such as selenium, and nickel are found naturally in the environment, and human exposure derives from a variety of sources, including air, drinking water, and food. In contrast, with *nickel* exposure where there is limited, non-conclusive evidence for no association and UBC risk,[54] for *selenium*, there is convincing evidence for a moderately decreased risk (RR = 0.67 (95% CI, 0.46–0.97)) suggesting a protective effect of higher selenium concentrations in toenail, serum, or plasma against UBC.[55,56] The incidence of bladder cancer decreases by 25% if the plasma selenium increases by 10 ng/mL.[57] There is limited, non-conclusive evidence for association of *vitamins* and UBC risk: based on four case–control studies, of a moderately reduced risk associated with vitamin A including both retinol and carotenoids was found. A similar inverse association was also observed for the B group vitamins (two studies), vitamin C (two studies), vitamin E (one study), and isothiocyanates (one study). No associations were observed for vitamins D (one study), and K (one study).[51] There is convincing evidence of no bladder carcinogenicity for saccharin and other *sweeteners*.[51,58] There is probable evidence for no association between UBC risk and *fruit* (SRR for high versus low consumption of fruit was 0.87 (95% CI, 0.63–1.12). or *vegetables* consumption (SRR for high versus low consumption was 0.94 (95% CI, 0.72–1.16).[59] There is limited, non-conclusive evidence for a moderately decreased risk of UBC for citrus fruits, and yellow-orange vegetables, particularly carrots, and for a substantially increased risk of UBC for salted and barbecued meat, soy products, and spices.[51]

Medical history

For *asthma*, there is limited non-conclusive evidence (only two studies) for a slightly increase risk on UBC.[60]

For diabetes mellitus (DM), there is convincing evidence that diabetes provokes a slightly increased risk on UBC (RR = 1.24 (95% CI 1.08–1.42)).[61] In West European countries where the prevalence of diabetes is about 7%.[62] DM is responsible for 2% of the UBC cases (Fig. 6.13.3).

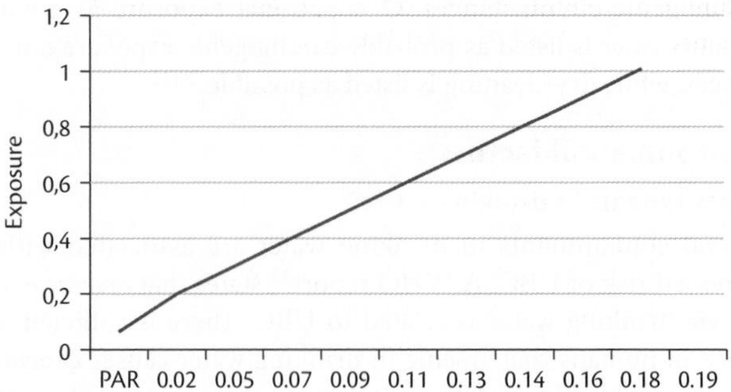

Fig. 6.13.3 PAR of UBC, according to prevalence of diabetes mellitus.
Source: data from *Diabetes Research and Clinical Practice*, Volume 87, Issue 1, Shaw JE *et al*, 'Global estimates of the prevalence of diabetes for 2010 and 2030', pp. 4–14, Copyright © 2009 Elsevier Ireland Ltd. Published by Elsevier Inc. All rights reserved.

There is limited non-conclusive evidence that *organ transplantation* may lead to a substantially increased risk of UBC (RR = 3.1) due to the immunosuppressed status after organ transplantation.[63]

There is limited non-conclusive evidence for a moderately increased risk for *urinary tract stones* and UBC.[58] and for a substantially increased risk between users of menopause *hormone replacement therapy* (OR = 3.29 (95% CI 1.49–7.25)) and UBC.[58]

Urinary tract infections

There is limited non-conclusive evidence for *bacterial infections* and the risk of UBC. Due to *Escherichia coli* and a *Proteus sp.* (RR respectively between 2 to 3.8, and 2.5 to 10) there is a substantially increased risk of TCC and SCC in neuropathic bladders after urinary tract infections (UTIs). Limited evidence is provided for gonorrhoea with a moderately increased risk (RR = 2.1 (95% CI, 1.0–4.5)) and no association for syphilis (RR = 1.1 (95% CI 0.2–7.0)).[64] There is limited non-conclusive evidence, based on case–control studies alone, that there is a substantially increased risk between *human papilloma virus* and UBC (RR = 3.2 (95% CI 1.19–8.60)).[64]

There is probable evidence, from case–control studies alone, that there is a substantially increased risk between infection with *Schitsosomiasis haematobium* (Bilharziasis) and UBC (OR of 2.0–14).[64] The overall prevalence of *S. haematobium* infection in Egypt is 37–48% and urinary bladder cancer accounts for about 31% of the total incidence of cancers in Egypt.[65] Until recent years, bladder cancer has been the most frequently diagnosed cancer and the most common cause of death in men aged 20–44 years in Egypt. In some countries with a high rate of schistosomal infections (such as Iraq, Malawi, Zambia, and Kuwait), bladder cancer was reported to be the leading malignant disease. Based on all these findings, the IARC has classified S. haematobium infection as carcinogenic.[66] The most recent study from Egypt, found that the OR for urinary schistosomiasis was higher in subjects who were younger at first diagnosis (OR of 3.3 for <15 years) and with a long time since the first diagnosis (OR of 3.0 for >35 years), suggesting a duration–risk relationship and a long-term effect of urinary schistosomiasis on bladder cancer.[67] Eradication of the parasitic menace results in a decrease of bladder cancer.[68]

Based on the information retrieved from cancer registries, there is convincing evidence of a substantially increased risk for UBC patients to develop subsequent cancers of the kidney and other urinary organs (SIR = 11,08 for males (p = 0.05) and 17.79 for females (p = 0.05)). There is a slightly increased risk for UBC after cancer of the uterus (SIR=1.41, p = 0.05),[69] a substantially increased risk for UBC after renal cell carcinoma (SIR = 4,7, p = 0.05)[69,70] and a moderately increased risk after prostate cancer.[71] Part of these excess risks can be result from indication bias.

Bladder cancer patients have a higher *co-morbidity* score and are more likely to have coexisting medical condition then patients without bladder cancer.[5] Men between 65 and 74 years are 10 times more likely to suffer from hypertension, cerebral ischaemic events, diabetes and asthma, 20 times more likely to suffer from depression, and 25 times more of cardial ischaemic events and chronic obstructive pulmonary disease (COPD). Men older than 75 year have 15 times more likely to suffer from depression, 20 times more likely to suffer from hypertension, cerebral ischaemic events and asthma, and 25 times more likely to suffer from cardial ischaemic events, diabetes, and COPD. Women between 65 and 74 years are 20 times more likely to suffer from hypertension, 30 times more likely to suffer from cerebral ischaemic events. Women older than 75 year are 10 times more likely to suffer from diabetes and COPD, 15 times more likely to suffer from depression, 20 times more likely to suffer from cerebral ischaemic events, 25 times more likely to suffer from asthma, and 40 times more likely to suffer from hypertension.[72]

Haematuria

Macroscopic haematuria has an overall predictive value of 0.83 (95% CI, 0.80–0.85) based on seven homogeneous studies. The predictive value is the highest in patients, aged 40 or more (0.41 (95% CI, 0.10–0.78)).[73]

Medication

There is no convincing association between regular use (>2 times/week) of non-aspirin *NSAIDs* compared and UBC (OR = 0.81 (95% CI, 0.63–1.05) for case–control studies and hazard ratio of 0.92 (95% CI, 0.81–1.04) for cohort studies),[74] as for *aspirin*, there is limited, non-conclusive evidence of no association with UBC.[75]

For *dialysis*, there is limited suggestive evidence of a moderately increased risk of UBC (RR = 2.2).[76] *Phenacetine* is responsible with limited suggestive evidence for a substantially increased risk of UBC (OR and RR, respectively, 5.4 and 5.3).[77] On the other hand, for acetaminophen (*paracetamol*), the major metabolite of phenacetine, probable evidence has been found of no association with UBC.[58] There is limited non-conclusive evidence of inconsistent effect of *phenobarbital*.[58] Non-conclusive evidence has been provided concerning bladder cancer and the risk associated with *isoniazid* therapy nor for *chlornaphazine*, a chloroethyl-derivative of 2-naphthyl-amine, used to treat polycythemia vera based on 61 patients of whom 13 developed UBC, of which eight invasive.[32] Also for *cyclophosphamide*, based on only two case–control studies and one cohort study, there is limited, non-conclusive evidence of a substantially increased risk of UBC.[58]

The IARC concluded that analgesic mixtures containing phenacetin and phenacetin are carcinogenic to humans,[78] just like cyclophosphamide.[32] Phenobarbital is possibly carcinogenic to humans.[79]

Genetics

Family history of UBC

Familial bladder cancer clusters with cancers of the stomach, larynx, kidney, endometrium and leukaemia due to both genetic and shared environmental factors (smoking habits). Family members also share prognosis of bladder cancer, either good or poor survival.[80–82] First degree relatives of patients with bladder cancer have a twofold increased risk of bladder cancer but high-risk bladder cancer families are extremely rare. There is no clear Mendelian inheritance pattern that can explain the increased familial risk. This makes classical linkage studies for the mapping of susceptibility genes impossible. The disease is probably caused by a combination of exposure to exogenous carcinogens and a large number of susceptibility genes with modest effects.[81] Candidate gene studies looked at susceptible genes and the occurrence of UBC. Genome-wide association studies make it possible to examin the existence of correlation between loci on a gene region and incidence of UBC.

Genes associated with UBC risk

Among the low-penetrant genes, the variants within the genes encoding metabolic enzymes have been consistently associated with susceptibility to bladder cancer and the evidence is compelling for NAT2 slow acetylator and GSTM1 null genotypes.[82] There is probable evidence from 30 case–control studies alone for a slightly increased risk of UBC for the NAT2 slow acetylation phenotype (defined by *NAT2* haplotypes) (SRR for *NAT2* slow acetylators), compared with rapid/intermediate acetylators was 1.4 (95% CI, 1.2–1.6; p <0.0001)) and *NAT2* and smoking interaction (SRR 1.2 (95% CI, 1.1–1.5; p = 0.009) for all populations combined.[80] There is probable evidence from case–control studies alone that GSTP1 Ile 105Val is associated with a moderately increased risk of UBC (unadjusted summary OR for GSTP1 Ile/Val and Val/Val compared with *GSTP1* Ile/Ile were 1.54 (95% CI, 1.21–1.99; p <0.001) and 2.17 (95% CI, 1.27–3.71; p = 0.005)).[81] There is probable evidence for no association between DNA repair genes: ERCC2 D312N (rs1799793; per-allele OR = 1.10 (95% CI, 1.01–1.19; p = 0.021)), NBN E185Q (rs1805794; per-allele OR = 1.09 (95% CI, 1.01–1.18; p = 0.028)), and XPC A499V (rs2228000; per-allele OR = 1.10 (95% CI, 1.00–1.21; p = 0.044)).[82] Only *NAT2* and *GSTM1* have consistently been demonstrated to be germline genetic susceptibility markers for UBC. The recent shift to an agnostic genome-wide association approach led to the identification of several UBC susceptibility loci, and provided valuable leads for new mechanistic insights into UBC carcinogenesis.[83]

Whole-exome sequencing of bladder tumours has identified mutations of chromatin remodelling genes such as *KDM6A* and *MLL3*, and of *STAG2*, which encodes a protein involved in sister chromatid cohesion. Moreover, four mutation signatures, principally comprising different combinations of C:G>T:A and G:C>C:G substitutions, have been detected in some bladder cancers, although their origins remain unclear.[84–89] Whole-genome sequence data at sufficiently high depth for variant calling have not been reported yet for bladder cancers.[90–94]

Genome-wide association studies

There is convincing evidence for a slightly increased risk of UBC and the SNP rs9642880[T] on the locus 8q24.21of the *MYC* gene region (OR =1.22 (95% CI, 1.15–1.29))[84] and the T allele of rs798766 on 4p16.3 of the TACC3/FGFR3 (OR = 1.24 (95% CI, 1.17–1.31)), which often harbours activating somatic mutations in low-grade, non-invasive UBC. Notably, rs798766[T] shows stronger association with low-grade and low-stage UBC than with more aggressive forms of the disease and is associated with higher risk of recurrence in low-grade stage Ta tumours. The frequency of rs798766[T] is higher in Ta tumours that carry an activating mutation in FGFR3 than in Ta tumours with wild-type *FGFR3*.[85] There is strong evidence for no association with UBC risk, but nonetheless of genome-wide significance, for rs710521[A] on 3q28 located near TP63 (OR = 1.19 (95% CI, 1.12–1.27)),[84] rs2736098[A] on 5p15.33 corresponds to A305A in the telomerase reverse transcriptase (TERT) protein (OR = 1.16 (95% CI, 1.08–1.23)), rs401681[C] on 5p15.33 of the gene region *CLPTM1L* (cisplatin resistance related protein CRR9p) (OR = 1.12 (95% CI, 1.06–1.18)),[86] for rs2294008 on chromosome 8q24.3 in the *PSCA* gene (OR = 1.15 (95% CI, 1.10–1.20)),[87] and for three new regions associated with UBC on chromosomes 22q13.1, 19q12 and 2q37.1: rs1014971, ($p = 8 \times 10–12$) maps to a non-genic region of chromosome 22q13.1, rs8102137 ($p = 2 \times 10–11$) on 19q12 maps to *CCNE1* and rs11892031 ($p = 1 \times 10–7$) maps to the *UGT1A* cluster on 2q37.1.[88] There is limited, non-conclusive evidence for a slightly increased risk of UBC for rs2736100 on 5p15, per C allele (OR = 1.23 (95% CI, 1.02–1.48).[89]

Several candidate gene studies looked for the association between germline genetic polymorphisms and the risk of recurrence and progression of mainly non-muscle-invasive bladder cancer (NMIBC) patients. These are small-size studies and the results of statistical significant findings of single studies should be tested for replication in larger, independent patient series.[83]

Conclusion

Seen the large effect of age, gender, and smoking habits on bladder cancer risk, the effect of all other risk factors tends to be modified by these three factors. It was not possible to go in that level of detail in this overview. Nevertheless, factors worth to be mentioned as increasing the risk of bladder cancer are: occupational exposures (dyes), prostate cancer, uterus cancer, diabetes mellitus, radiation, arsenic in drinking water, and coffee for men. NAT2 slow acetylator and GSTM1 null genotypes are also associated with an increased risk of this cancer. Potential factors that can decrease the risk of bladder cancer are high blood selenium levels and the intake of citrus fruit and carrots. The impact of diet will be further investigated in more detail by pooling data of case–control and cohort studies.

Regarding prognosis, there is little knowledge on the predictive role of environmental and occupational exposures and genetic polymorphisms on tumour recurrence and progression and survival. Although active tobacco smoking is the most commonly studied factor, no definitive conclusion can be drawn from the literature. Today, two ongoing studies examine the effect of the intake of high-selenium yeast on the recurrence of UBC. One study found a significantly decrease in time to recurrence with the intake of high doses of vitamins. This result has not yet been. The most important primary prevention measure for MIBC is to eliminate smoking and Bilharziasis.

Further reading

Abol-Enein H. Infection: is it a cause of bladder cancer? *Scand J Urol Nephrol Suppl* 2008; (218):79–84.

Abol-Enein H, Kava BR, Carmack AJ. Nonurothelial cancer of the bladder. *Urology* 2007; **69**(Suppl 1):93–104.

Brinkman M, Zeegers MP. Nutrition, total fluid and bladder cancer. *Scand J Urol Nephrol Suppl* 2008; (218):25–36.

Dennert G, Zwahlen M, Brinkman M, *et al.* Selenium for preventing cancer. Cochrane Database of Systematic Reviews [Internet] 2011; (5). Available at: http://www.mrw.interscience.wiley.com/cochrane/clsysrev/articles/CD005195/frame.html.[Online].

Ferlay J, Shin H, Bray F, Forman D, Mathers C, Parkin D. GLOBOCAN 2008, Cancer Incidence and Mortality Worldwide: IARC CancerBase No. 10 [Internet]. Lyon, France: International Agency for Research on Cancer, 2010. Available at: http://globocan.iarc.fr [Online].

Grotenhuis AJ, Vermeulen SH, Kiemeney LA. Germline genetic markers for urinary bladder cancer risk, prognosis and treatment response. *Future Oncol* 2010; **6**(9):1433–60.

IARC. Monographs on the Evaluation of Carcinogenic Risks to Humans Overall Evaluations of Carcinogenicity: An Updating of IARC Monographs. *IARC Monogr Eval Carcinog Risks Hum* 1987; (Suppl 7):1–42.

IARC. Occupational exposures in paint manufacture and painting. *IARC Monogr Eval Carcinog Risks Hum* 1989; **47**:329–442.

IARC. Coffee, tea, mate, methylxanthines and methylglyoxal. *IARC Monogr Eval Carcinog Risks Hum* 1997; **51**:41–272.

IARC. Tobacco smoke. International Agency for Research on Cancer, *IARC Monogr Eval Carcinog Risks Hum* 2004; **83**:53–1187.

IARC. Alcohol consumption and ethyl carbamate. *IARC Monogr Eval Carcinog Risks Hum* 2010; **96**:720–41.

Kiemeney LA, Sulem P, Besenbacher S, *et al.* A sequence variant at 4p16.3 confers susceptibility to urinary bladder cancer. *Nat Genet* 2010; **42**(5):415–9.

Kiemeney LA, Thorlacius S, Sulem P, *et al.* Sequence variant on 8q24 confers susceptibility to urinary bladder cancer. *Nat Genet* 2008; **40**(11):1307–12.

Murta-Nascimento C, Schmitz-Drager BJ, Zeegers MP, *et al.* Epidemiology of urinary bladder cancer: from tumor development to patient's death. *World J Urol* 2007; **25**(3):285–95.

Navarro Silvera SA, Rohan TE. Trace elements and cancer risk: a review of the epidemiologic evidence. *Cancer Causes Control* 2007; **18**(1):7–27.

Pelucchi C, La Vecchia C. Alcohol, coffee, and bladder cancer risk: a review of epidemiological studies. *Eur J Cancer Prev* 2009; **18**(1):62–8.

Research WCRFAIfC. Food, Nutrition, Physical Activity, and the Prevention of Cancer: a Global Perspective. Washington DC: AICR, 2007. Available at: http://www.aicr.org/assets/docs/pdf/reports/Second_Expert_Report.pdf [Online].

Reulen RC, Kellen E, Buntinx F, Brinkman M, Zeegers MP. A meta-analysis on the association between bladder cancer and occupation. *Scand J Urol Nephrol Suppl* 2008; (218):64–78.

Zeegers MP, Tan FE, Dorant E, van Den Brandt PA. The impact of characteristics of cigarette smoking on urinary tract cancer risk: a meta-analysis of epidemiologic studies. *Cancer* 2000; **89**(3):630–9.

Zeegers MP, Tan FE, Goldbohm RA, van den Brandt PA. Are coffee and tea consumption associated with urinary tract cancer risk? A systematic review and meta-analysis. *Int J Epidemiol* 2001; **30**(2):353–62.

References

1. Ferlay J, Shin H, Bray F, Forman D, Mathers C, Parkin D. GLOBOCAN 2008, Cancer Incidence and Mortality Worldwide: IARC CancerBase No. 10 [Internet]. Lyon, France: International Agency for Research on Cancer, 2010. Available at: http://globocan.iarc.fr [Online].
2. Parkin DM. The global burden of urinary bladder cancer. *Scand J Urol Nephrol Suppl* **2008**(218):12–20.
3. Sitas F, Parkin DM, Chirenje M, Stein L, Abratt R, Wabinga H. Part II: Cancer in Indigenous Africans—causes and control. *Lancet Oncol* 2008; **9**(8):786–95.
4. Botteman MF, Pashos CL, Redaelli A, Laskin B, Hauser R. The health economics of bladder cancer: a comprehensive review of the published literature. *Pharmacoeconomics* 2003; **21**(18):1315–30.

5. Cooksley CD, Avritscher EB, Grossman HB, *et al.* Clinical model of cost of bladder cancer in the elderly. *Urology* 2008; **71**(3):519–25.
6. Ploeg M, Aben KK, Hulsbergen-van de Kaa CA, Schoenberg MP, Witjes JA, Kiemeney LA. Clinical epidemiology of nonurothelial bladder cancer: analysis of the Netherlands Cancer Registry. *J Urol* 2010; **183**(3):915–20.
7. Abol-Enein H, Kava BR, Carmack AJ. Nonurothelial cancer of the bladder. *Urology* 2007;**69**(1 Suppl):93–104.
8. Ismaili N, Arifi S, Flechon A, *et al.* Small cell cancer of the bladder: pathology, diagnosis, treatment and prognosis. *Bull Cancer* 2009; **96**(6):E30–44.
9. Pant-Purohit M, Lopez-Beltran A, Montironi R, MacLennan GT, Cheng L. Small cell carcinoma of the urinary bladder. *Histol Histopathol* 2010; **25**(2):217–21.
10. Pan CX, Zhang H, Lara PN, Jr., Cheng L. Small-cell carcinoma of the urinary bladder: diagnosis and management. Expert review of anticancer therapy. 2006; **6**(12):1707–13.
11. Ahmad I, Barnetson RJ, Krishna NS. Keratinizing squamous metaplasia of the bladder: a review. *Urol Int* 2008; **81**(3):247–51.
12. Cheng L, Foster SR, MacLennan GT, Lopez-Beltran A, Zhang S, Montironi R. Inflammatory myofibroblastic tumors of the genitourinary tract—single entity or continuum? *J Urol* 2008;**180**(4):1235–40.
13. Astigueta Perez J, Abad Licham M, Morante Deza C, Pow-Sang Godoy M, Meza Montoya L, Destefano Urrutia V. [Micropapillary urothelial carcinoma of the bladder: case report and review of the literature]. Actas urologicas espanolas. 2008; **32**(5):552–5. Carcinoma urotelial micropapilar de vejiga: Aportacion de un caso y revision de la literatura.
14. Epstein JI, Amin MB, Reuter VR, Mostofi FK. The World Health Organization/International Society of Urological Pathology consensus classification of urothelial (transitional cell) neoplasms of the urinary bladder. Bladder Consensus Conference Committee. *Am J Surg Pathol* 1998; **22**(12):1435–48.
15. Sauter G, Algaba F, Amin MB, *et al.* Tumours of the urinary system: non-invasive urothelial neoplasias. (pp. 29–34) In: Eble JN, Sauter G, Epstein Jl, Sesterhenn I (eds). *WHO Classification of Tumours: Pathology and Genetics of Tumours of the Urinary System and Male Genital Organs*. Lyon, France: IARC Press, 2004.
16. Stenzl A, Cowan NC, De Santis M, *et al.* Update of the Clinical Guidelines of the European Association of Urology on muscle-invasive and metastatic bladder carcinoma. *Actas Urol Esp* 2010; **34**(1):51–62.
17. Sobin LH, Gospodariwicz M, Wittekind C (eds). *TNM Classification of Malignant Tumours. UICC International Union Against Cancer*, 7th edition. Chichester, UK: Wiley-Blackwell. 2009: pp. 262–5.
18. Josephson DY, Pasin E, Stein JP. Superficial bladder cancer: part 1. Update on etiology, classification and natural history. *Expert Rev Anticancer Ther* 2006; **6**(12):1723–34.
19. Sylvester RJ. Natural history, recurrence, and progression in superficial bladder cancer. *Scientific World Journal* 2006; **6**:2617–25.
20. Zeegers MP, Tan FE, Dorant E, van Den Brandt PA. The impact of characteristics of cigarette smoking on urinary tract cancer risk: a meta-analysis of epidemiologic studies. *Cancer* 2000; **89**(3):630–9.
21. Shariat SF, Sfakianos JP, Droller MJ, Karakiewicz PI, Meryn S, Bochner BH. The effect of age and gender on bladder cancer: a critical review of the literature. *BJU Int* 2010; **105**(3):300–8.
22. Scosyrev E, Trivedi D, Messing E. Female bladder cancer: incidence, treatment, and outcome. *Curr Opin Urol* 2010; **20**(5):404–8.
23. Schultzel M, Saltzstein SL, Downs TM, Shimasaki S, Sanders C, Sadler GR. Late age (85 years or older) peak incidence of bladder cancer. *J Urol* 2008; **179**(4):1302–5; discussion 5–6.
24. Paner GP, Zehnder P, Amin AM, Husain AN, Desai MM. Urothelial neoplasms of the urinary bladder occurring in young adult and pediatric patients: a comprehensive review of literature with implications for patient management. *Adv Anat Pathol* 2010; **18**(1):79–89.
25. Research WCRFAIfC. Food, Nutrition, Physical Activity, and the Prevention of Cancer: a Global Perspective. Washington DC: AICR, 2007. Available at: http://www.aicr.org/assets/docs/pdf/reports/Second_Expert_Report.pdf [Online].
26. Delclos GL, Lerner SP. Occupational risk factors. *Scand J Urol Nephrol Suppl* 2008; (218):58–63.
27. Reulen RC, Kellen E, Buntinx F, Brinkman M, Zeegers MP. A meta-analysis on the association between bladder cancer and occupation. *Scand J Urol Nephrol Suppl* 2008; (218):64–78.
28. Harling M, Schablon A, Schedlbauer G, Dulon M, Nienhaus A. Bladder cancer among hairdressers: a meta-analysis. *Occup Environ Med* 2010; **67**(5):351–8.
29. Guha N, Steenland NK, Merletti F, Altieri A, Cogliano V, Straif K. Bladder cancer risk in painters: a meta-analysis. *Occup Environ Med* 2010; **67**(8):568–73.
30. Baena AV, Allam MF, Diaz-Molina C, Del Castillo AS, Abdel-Rahman AG, Navajas RF. Urinary bladder cancer and the petroleum industry: a quantitative review. *Eur J Cancer Prev* 2006; **15**(6):493–7.
31. Bosetti C, Boffetta P, La Vecchia C. Occupational exposures to polycyclic aromatic hydrocarbons, and respiratory and urinary tract cancers: a quantitative review to 2005. *Ann Oncol* 2007;**18**(3):431–46.
32. IARC. Monographs on the Evaluation of Carcinogenic Risks to Humans Overall Evaluations of Carcinogenicity: An Updating of IARC Monographs. *IARC Monogr Eval Carcinog Risks Hum* 1987; (Suppl 7): 1–42.
33. WHO. IPCS environmental health criteria 224 Arsenic and arsenic compounds. Geneva: International Programme on Chemical Safety, World Health Organization, 2001. Available at: http://apps.who.int/iris/bitstream/10665/42366/1/WHO_EHC_224.pdf [Online].
34. IARC. Monographs. 2004; **84** (mono84–6). Available at: https://monographs.iarc.fr/ENG/Monographs/vol84/mono84.pdf [Online].
35. Rahman MM, Ng JC, Naidu R. Chronic exposure of arsenic via drinking water and its adverse health impacts on humans. *Environ Geochem Health* 2009; **31**(Suppl 1):189–200.
36. Weyer PJ, Cerhan JR, Kross BC, *et al.* Municipal drinking water nitrate level and cancer risk in older women: the Iowa Women's Health Study. *Epidemiology* 2001; **12**(3):327–38.
37. Hall P. Radiation-associated urinary bladder cancer. *Scand J Urol Nephrol Suppl* 2008; (218):85–8.
38. Boffetta P. Tobacco smoking and risk of bladder cancer. *Scand J Urol Nephrol Suppl* **2008**(218):45–54.
39. IARC. Tobacco smoke. International Agency for Research on Cancer, *IARC Monogr Eval Carcinog Risks Hum* 2004; **83**:53–1187.
40. Brennan P, Bogillot O, Cordier S, *et al.* Cigarette smoking and bladder cancer in men: a pooled analysis of 11 case-control studies. *Int J Cancer* 2000; **86**(2):289–94.
41. Brennan P, Bogillot O, Greiser E, *et al.* The contribution of cigarette smoking to bladder cancer in women (pooled European data). *Cancer Causes Control* 2001; **12**(5):411–7.
42. Pitard A, Brennan P, Clavel J, *et al.* Cigar, pipe, and cigarette smoking and bladder cancer risk in European men. *Cancer Causes Control* 2001;**12**(6):551–6.
43. Aveyard P, Adab P, Cheng KK, Wallace DM, Hey K, Murphy MF. Does smoking status influence the prognosis of bladder cancer? A systematic review. *BJU Int* 2002; **90**(3):228–39.
44. Leitzmann MF. Physical activity and genitourinary cancer prevention. *Recent Results Cancer Res* 2011; **186**:43–71.
45. Friedenreich CM, Neilson HK, Lynch BM. State of the epidemiological evidence on physical activity and cancer prevention. *Eur J Cancer* 2010; **46**(14):2593–604.
46. Rollison DE, Helzlsouer KJ, Pinney SM. Personal hair dye use and cancer: a systematic literature review and evaluation of exposure assessment in studies published since 1992. *J Toxicol Environ Health B Crit Rev* 2006;**9**(5):413–39.
47. Zeegers MP, Tan FE, Goldbohm RA, van den Brandt PA. Are coffee and tea consumption associated with urinary tract cancer risk? A systematic review and meta-analysis. *Int J Epidemiol* 2001; **30**(2):353–62.

48. IARC. Alcohol consumption and ethyl carbamate. *IARC Monogr Eval Carcinog Risks Hum* 2010; **96**:720–41.
49. Pelucchi C, La Vecchia C. Alcohol, coffee, and bladder cancer risk: a review of epidemiological studies. *Eur J Cancer Prev* 2009; **18**(1):62–8.
50. Villanueva CM, Cantor KP, King WD, *et al.* Total and specific fluid consumption as determinants of bladder cancer risk. *Int J Cancer* 2006; **118**(8):2040–7.
51. Brinkman M, Zeegers MP. Nutrition, total fluid and bladder cancer. *Scand J Urol Nephrol Suppl* 2008; (218):25–36.
52. Li Z, Yu J, Miao Q, *et al.* The association of fish consumption with bladder cancer risk: a meta-analysis. *World J Surg Oncol* 2011;**9**:107.
53. Hogervorst JG, Baars BJ, Schouten LJ, Konings EJ, Goldbohm RA, van den Brandt PA. The carcinogenicity of dietary acrylamide intake: a comparative discussion of epidemiological and experimental animal research. *Crit Rev Toxicol* 2010; **40**(6):485–512.
54. Navarro Silvera SA, Rohan TE. Trace elements and cancer risk: a review of the epidemiologic evidence. *Cancer Causes Control* 2007; **18**(1):7–27.
55. Dennert G, Zwahlen M, Brinkman M, *et al.* Selenium for preventing cancer. Cochrane Database of Systematic Reviews [Internet] 2011; (5). Available at: http://www.mrw.interscience.wiley.com/cochrane/clsysrev/articles/CD005195/frame.html.[Online].
56. Brinkman M, Buntinx F, Muls E, Zeegers MP. Use of selenium in chemoprevention of bladder cancer. *Lancet Oncol* 2006;**7**(9):766–74.
57. Kellen E, Zeegers M, Buntinx F. Selenium is inversely associated with bladder cancer risk: a report from the Belgian case-control study on bladder cancer. *Int J Urol* 2006; **13**(9):1180–4.
58. Murta-Nascimento C, Schmitz-Drager BJ, Zeegers MP, *et al.* Epidemiology of urinary bladder cancer: from tumor development to patient's death. *World J Urol* 2007; **25**(3):285–95.
59. Vainio H, Weiderpass E. Fruit and vegetables in cancer prevention. *Nutr Cancer* 2006; **54**(1):111–42.
60. Merrill RM, Isakson RT, Beck RE. The association between allergies and cancer: what is currently known? *Ann Allergy Asthma Immunol* 2007;**99**(2):102–16; quiz 17–9, 50.
61. Larsson SC, Orsini N, Brismar K, Wolk A. Diabetes mellitus and risk of bladder cancer: a meta-analysis. *Diabetologia* 2006; **49**(12):2819–23.
62. Shaw JE, Sicree RA, Zimmet PZ. Global estimates of the prevalence of diabetes for 2010 and 2030. *Diabetes Res Clin Pract* 2010; **87**(1):4–14.
63. Wallerand H, Ravaud A, Ferriere JM. Bladder cancer in patients after organ transplantation. *Curr Opin Urol* 2010; **20**(5):432–6.
64. Abol-Enein H. Infection: is it a cause of bladder cancer? *Scand J Urol Nephrol Suppl* 2008; (218):79–84.
65. Fried B, Reddy A, Mayer D. Helminths in human carcinogenesis. *Cancer Lett* 2010; **305**(2):239–49.
66. IARC. Schistosomes, Liver Flukes and Helicobacter pylori. *IARC Monogr Eval Carcinog Risks Hum* 1997; (volume 61).
67. Vennervald BJ, Polman K. Helminths and malignancy. *Parasite Immunol* 2009; **31**(11):686–96.
68. Salem S, Mitchell RE, El-Alim El-Dorey A, Smith JA, Barocas DA. Successful control of schistosomiasis and the changing epidemiology of bladder cancer in Egypt. *BJU Int* 2011; **107**(2):206–11.
69. Hayat MJ, Howlader N, Reichman ME, Edwards BK. Cancer statistics, trends, and multiple primary cancer analyses from the Surveillance, Epidemiology, and End Results (SEER) Program. *Oncologist* 2007; **12**(1):20–37.
70. Neuzillet Y, Lechevallier E, Coulange C. [Renal cancer and second cancer: critical review of the literature]. *Prog Urol* 2007; **17**(1):35–40.
71. Kellen E, Zeegers MP, Dirx M, *et al.* Occurrence of both bladder and prostate cancer in five cancer registries in Belgium, The Netherlands and the United Kingdom. *Eur J Cancer* 2007; **43**(11):1694–700.
72. [20 Years GP Practice in Flanders]. Available at: http://www.intego.be/ [Online].
73. Buntinx F, Wauters H. The diagnostic value of macroscopic haematuria in diagnosing urological cancers: a meta-analysis. *Family Practice* 1997; **14**(1):63–8.
74. Daugherty SE, Pfeiffer RM, Sigurdson AJ, Hayes RB, Leitzmann M, Schatzkin A, *et al.* Nonsteroidal antiinflammatory drugs and bladder cancer: a pooled analysis. *Am J Epidemiol* 2011; **173**(7):721–30.
75. Bosetti C, Gallus S, La Vecchia C. Aspirin and cancer risk: an updated quantitative review to 2005. *Cancer Causes Control* 2006; **17**(7):871–88.
76. Mandayam S, Shahinian VB. Are chronic dialysis patients at increased risk for cancer? *J Nephrol* 2008; **21**(2):166–74.
77. Colin P, Koenig P, Ouzzane A, *et al.* Environmental factors involved in carcinogenesis of urothelial cell carcinomas of the upper urinary tract. *BJU Int* 2009; **104**(10):1436–40.
78. IARC. Monograph Phenacetin. Monographs. 1987; **vol100A**(mono100A-25). Available at: http://monographs.iarc.fr/ENG/Monographs/vol100A/mono100A-25.pdf [Online].
79. IARC. Monograph Phenobarbital. Monographs. 1976, 1987; **vol79**(mono79-11). Available at: http://monographs.iarc.fr/ENG/Monographs/vol79/mono79-11.pdf [Online].
80. Garcia-Closas M, Malats N, Silverman D, *et al.* NAT2 slow acetylation, GSTM1 null genotype, and risk of bladder cancer: results from the Spanish Bladder Cancer Study and meta-analyses. *Lancet* 2005; **366**(9486):649–59.
81. Kellen E, Hemelt M, Broberg K, *et al.* Pooled analysis and meta-analysis of the glutathione S-transferase P1 Ile 105Val polymorphism and bladder cancer: a HuGE-GSEC review. *Am J Epidemiol* 2007; **165**(11):1221–30.
82. Stern MC, Lin J, Figueroa JD, *et al.* Polymorphisms in DNA repair genes, smoking, and bladder cancer risk: findings from the international consortium of bladder cancer. *Cancer Res* 2009; **69**(17):6857–64.
83. Grotenhuis AJ, Vermeulen SH, Kiemeney LA. Germline genetic markers for urinary bladder cancer risk, prognosis and treatment response. *Future Oncol* 2010; **6**(9):1433–60.
84. Kiemeney LA, Thorlacius S, Sulem P, *et al.* Sequence variant on 8q24 confers susceptibility to urinary bladder cancer. *Nat Genet* 2008; **40**(11):1307–12.
85. Kiemeney LA, Sulem P, Besenbacher S, *et al.* A sequence variant at 4p16.3 confers susceptibility to urinary bladder cancer. *Nat Genet* 2010; **42**(5):415–9.
86. Rafnar T, Sulem P, Stacey SN, *et al.* Sequence variants at the TERT-CLPTM1L locus associate with many cancer types. *Nat Genet* 2009; **41**(2):221–7.
87. Wu X, Ye Y, Kiemeney LA, *et al.* Genetic variation in the prostate stem cell antigen gene PSCA confers susceptibility to urinary bladder cancer. *Nat Genet* 2009; **41**(9):991–5.
88. Rothman N, Garcia-Closas M, Chatterjee N, *et al.* A multi-stage genome-wide association study of bladder cancer identifies multiple susceptibility loci. *Nat Genet* 2010; **42**(11):978–84.
89. Gago-Dominguez M, Jiang X, Conti DV, *et al.* Genetic variations on chromosomes 5p15 and 15q25 and bladder cancer risk: findings from the Los Angeles-Shanghai bladder case-control study. *Carcinogenesis* 2011; **32**(2):197–202.
90. Gui Y, Guo G, Huang Y, *et al.* Frequent mutations of chromatin remodeling genes in transitional cell carcinoma of the bladder. *Nat Genet* 2011; **43**:875–8.
91. Balbas-Martinez, C. *et al.* Recurrent inactivation of STAG2 in bladder cancer is not associated with aneuploidy. *Nat Genet* (2013).
92. Guo, G. *et al.* Whole-genome and whole-exome sequencing of bladder cancer identifies frequent alterations in genes involved in sister chromatid cohesion and segregation. *Nat Genet* 2013; **45**:1464–9.
93. Solomon DA, Kim JS, Bondarak J, *et al.* Frequent truncating mutations of *STAG2* in bladder cancer. *Nat Genet* 2013; **45**:1428–30.
94. Alexandrov LB, Nik-Zainal S, Wedge DC, *et al.* Signatures of mutational processes in human cancer. *Nature* 2013; **500**:415–21.

CHAPTER 6.14

Molecular biology of bladder cancer

Neveen Said and Dan Theodorescu

Introduction to molecular biology of bladder cancer

Bladder cancer is the most common malignancy involving the urinary system, caused primarily by tobacco use and exposure to industrial chemicals with an estimated 73,510 patients affected and 14,880 deaths in 2012.[1] Urothelial (transitional cell) carcinoma (UC) is the predominant histological type in the United States and Europe and accounts for ~90% of bladder cancers.[1]

UC arises from the mucosal lining of the bladder, and is frequently multifocal. Numerous factors, including chromosomal markers, genetic polymorphisms, and genetic and epigenetic alterations may be involved in tumorigenesis, progression, and metastasis (Figs 6.14.1 and 6.14.2). Initially 70% of patients with UC present with non-muscle-invasive (formerly known as 'superficial'), and 30% present with muscle-invasive disease.[2,3] Despite a good prognosis for patients with non-muscle-invasive UC, recurrence is common and is associated with development of muscle-invasive disease in up to 30%. Also, 50% of patients presenting with muscle-invasive UC have occult distant metastases and a poor five-year survival rate. Clinical data from human disease as well as experimental rodent models of carcinogenesis and metastasis revealed that, in addition to regional lymph node metastasis, muscle-invasive bladder cancer most commonly metastasizes to the lungs.[2,3] In this chapter, we will summarize the molecular events implicated in the multistep carcinogenesis and metastasis cascades of bladder cancer.

Molecular mechanisms of non-invasive bladder cancer

Gain-of-function mutations: *HRAS* and *FGFR3*

HRAS

The *HRAS* gene, which codes for p21Ras, a small GTPase, was the first identified human oncogene and was found in the T24/EJ urothelial cell line.[4–6] In the normal urothelium, normal *HRAS* protein diminishes with differentiation, with highest expression in the basal (progenitor) cells.[7] The role of *HRAS* in UC is supported by its ability to transform SV40-immortalized human urothelial cells into invasive transitional cell carcinomas.[8,9] In addition, in elegant transgenic studies, Ras overexpression has been shown to lead to non-muscle-invasive disease.[10] Ras interacts with Raf, a serine/threonine kinase, which is activated in tumour cells containing enhanced growth signalling pathways in both non-muscle invasive, muscle-invasive, and metastatic disease with subsequent activation of MAPK.[11,12] The activation of Ras depends on the addition of a lipid (farnesyl) moiety to its carboxy terminal, thus farnesyl transferase inhibitors and MAPK inhibitors may be of therapeutic potential.[11,12]

In UC, *HRAS* mutations were associated with both non-muscle-invasive (NMI),[13] and in muscle-invasive (MI) UC,[14–18] suggesting that hyperactive *HRAS* in UC can be due to activating mutations, or via either overexpression of the *HRAS* gene and/or increased signalling by upstream receptor tyrosine kinases (RTKs).[4,5] In a recent study,[19] primary bladder tumours from 257 patients and 184 recurrences from 54 patients were examined for mutations in a variety of genes. Of primary tumours 11% were mutant for RAS. Interestingly, FGFR3 mutations (discussed below) were mutually exclusive with RAS mutations and co-occurred with PIK3CA mutations. Mutations in the RAS genes were not predictors for recurrence-free, progression-free, and disease-specific survival. Taken together, Ras appears to be an important player in urothelial cancer and one most likely associated with non-muscle-invasive cancer.

FGFR3

Somatic activating mutations and/or overexpression of *FGFR3* were first described in UC over ten years ago and are common in UC with low malignant potential, low-stage and -grade, lower risk of progression, and better survival.[20,21] *FGFR3* mutations occur in around 50% of both lower and upper urinary tract tumours and these cluster in three distinct hotspots in exons 7, 10, and 15.[21] The most common mutations in exon 7 and 10 favour ligand-independent dimerization, transactivation, and signalling.[22–26] Mutations in exon 15 are rare, and induce a conformational change in the kinase domain resulting in ligand-independent receptor activation and signalling as well as FGFR3 cellular localization, with aberrant endoplasmic reticulum signalling.[27] *FGFR3* mutations are thought to occur early during urothelial transformation, as they are reported in over 80% preneoplastic lesions,[22,23] pointing to an overall 'benign' effect of *FGFR3* mutation in the bladder.[26,28] *FGFR3* mutant tumours were more chromosomally stable than their wild-type counterparts and a mutually exclusive relationship between *FGFR3* mutation and overrepresentation of 8q was observed in NMI tumours.[29] A recent study found that around 80% of NMIUC and 54% of MIUC have dysregulated *FGFR3* with discordant mutation and protein expression patterns, suggesting a key role of *FGFR3* in both NMI and MI disease either through mutation, overexpression, or both.[30] These discrepancies may reflect differential downstream signalling of wild-type and mutant receptors or the different molecular pathways instigating the development of these

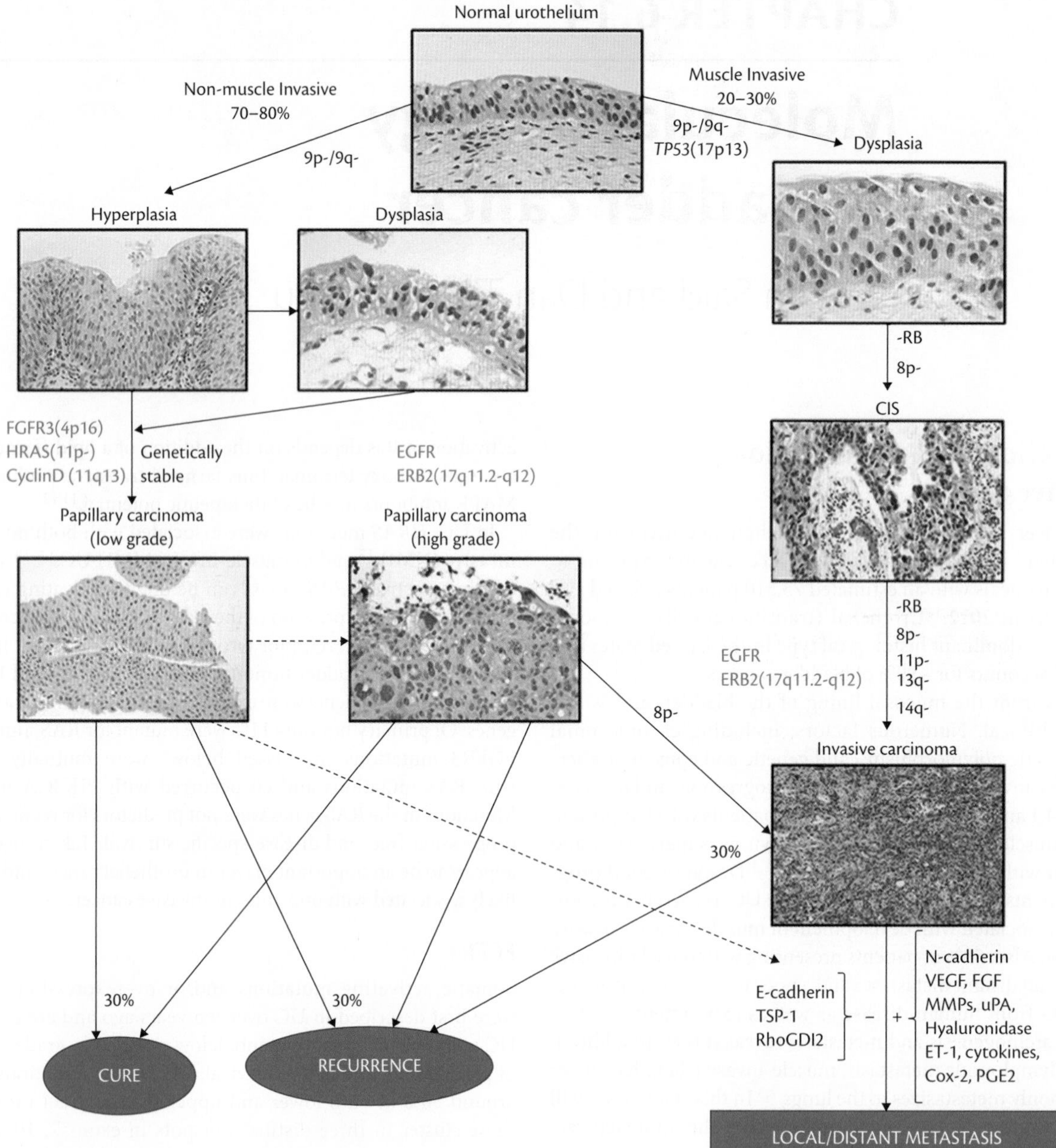

Fig. 6.14.1 Pathways of urothelial carcinoma (UC) development. At presentation, most tumours (70–80%) are diagnosed as non-muscle-invasive disease (superficial), and 20–30% as muscle-invasive disease. For the non-muscle-invasive disease, the preneoplastic lesions progress from hyperplasia/dysplasia, with stable genetic alterations and progress into non-invasive low or high malignant UC. The preneoplastic lesions of muscle-invasive UC are severe dysplasia/CIS, that accumulate unstable genetic alterations progress into invasive, high-grade UC.

Reproduced from Neveen Said and Dan Theodorescu, 'Bladder Cancer', in David Lyden, Danny R. Welece and Bethan Psaila (Eds.), *Cancer Metastasis: Biologic Basis and Therapeutics*, Cambridge University Press, Cambridge, UK, Copyright © 2011, with permission from Cambridge University Press.

tumours. The mechanisms driving FGFR3 overexpression in UC are largely unknown, although a recent study has shown the regulation of FGFR3 expression in urothelial cells by two microRNAs (miR-99a/100), that are often downregulated in UC, particularly in low-grade and low-stage tumours.[31]

Deletions of chromosome 9: allelic losses on the long arm (9q)

Events affecting chromosome 9 are common. Deletions of tumour suppressor genes at 9p21 (*CDKN2A*, *CDKN2B*), 9q22 (*PTCH*), 9q33 (DBC1), and 9q34 (TSC1) were reported in hyperplasia and throughout advanced grades and stages.[32] Homozygous deletions at 9p21.3 were associated with high stage and grade, while no associations between TSC1 copy number loss and stage, grade, or other copy number alterations were observed.[32] Loss of heterozygosity (LOH) analyses of UC have revealed a number of genomic regions of possible importance for UC development. LOH in 9p was seen in 70% and in 9q in 77% of the cases indicating chromosome 9 as the most frequently affected chromosome in UC[33] with LOH at 9p and 9q was equally distributed

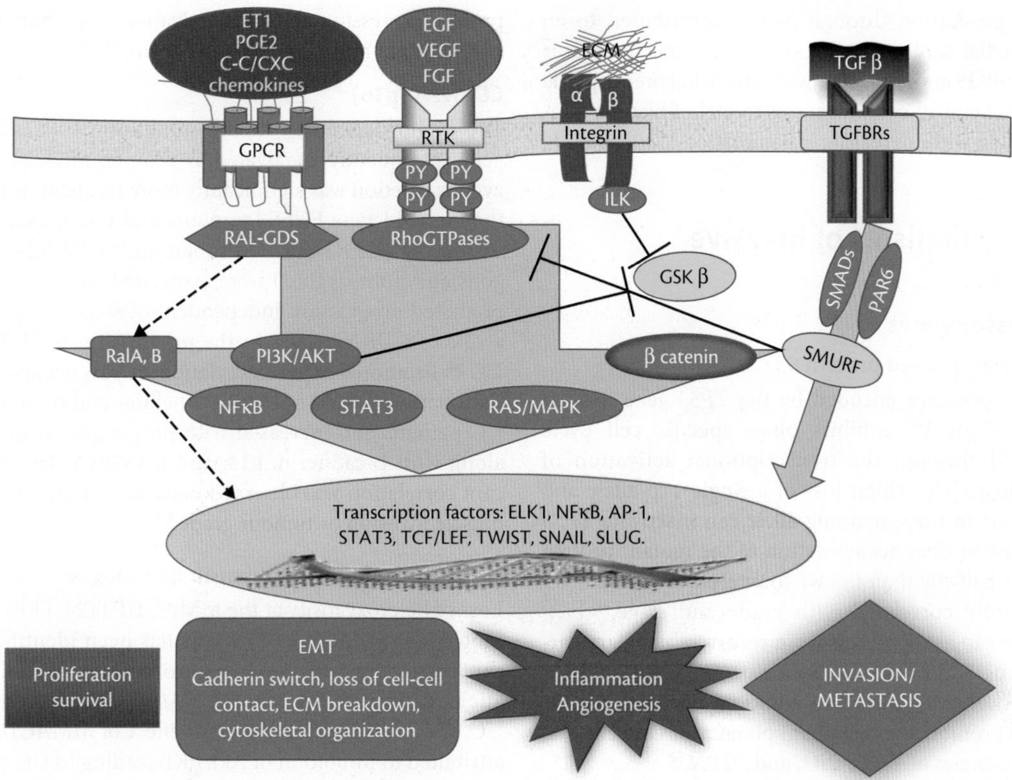

Fig. 6.14.2 Signalling pathways in UC. Receptor tyrosine kinases (EGFR, VEGFR, FGFR) contain a cytoplasmic tyrosine kinase domain, a single transmembrane domain, and an extracellular domain that upon binding to cognate ligands and activate downstream signalling through simultaneous activation of multiple pathways, which either lead to activation of Ras/MAPK, AKT/PI3K, with subsequent activation of multiple transcription factors resulting in cell proliferation/ survival, epithelial–mesenchymal transition (EMT) inflammation, angiogenesis, and lymphangiogenesis. Cross-talk between ECM-integrin-ILK, TGFβ, GSKβ/β-catenin directly affects cell adhesion and/or the cytoskeletal dynamics, through their effect on Rho GTPases. The convergence of these signalling pathways eventually leads to cancer cell invasion and metastasis.

Reproduced from Neveen Said and Dan Theodorescu, 'Bladder Cancer', in David Lyden, Danny R. Welece and Bethan Psaila (Eds.), *Cancer Metastasis: Biologic Basis and Therapeutics*, Cambridge University Press, Cambridge, UK, Copyright © 2011, with permission from Cambridge University Press.

among the tumour stages, whereas allelic losses at the remaining chromosomes correlated with higher stages. A similarly high frequency of allelic loss of chromosome 9 was reported by Koed *et al.*[34] with LOH at 9p amounting to 42% and in 9q to 67% affecting all chromosome arms. In both studies,[33,34] Ta tumours showed a significantly lower frequency of LOH than T1 tumours, whereas T1 and ≥T2 cases were similar in this respect. Also Chan *et al.*[35] demonstrated an association of LOH of high grade and high stage with a high incidence of LOH at 9p and 9q, 76% and 67%, respectively. Recently, homozygous deletions of other genes were reported[29] as HD of miR-31 and ELAVL2 (HuB; HelN1). The latter is a member of the Hu family of RNA-binding proteins which are implicated in post-transcriptional regulation and differentiation with several putative mRNA targets including the cyclin-dependent kinase inhibitor p21.[29] HD at 9p24 and 9p23 were detected in UC.[29,36]

Y chromosome loss

Y chromosome losses have been described in as an early event occurring in 10–40% of bladder cancers[37] and were suggested to be age-related. However, the clinical significance of chromosome Y losses is currently largely unknown.[37,38]

Polymorphisms in genes associated with detoxification of environmental carcinogens

Glutathione S-transferase M1 (GSTM1), N-acetyltransferase-1 and 2 (NAT1 and NAT2) and microsomal epoxide hydrolase, and the cytochrome P-450 enzymes 2D6, 1A1, 2A6, and 2E1 are phase II enzymes involved in xenobiotic metabolism. Polymorphisms of these enzymes have been long related to increased bladder cancer risk among different populations and racial backgrounds and are believed to influence the types of acquired mutations of oncogenes and tumour suppressors involved bladder cancer initiation and progression.[39–45]

Reactive oxygen and nitrogen species

Growing evidence suggests that genetic alterations result in higher levels of reactive oxygen species (ROS) in human cancer cells than in their normal counterparts.[46] ROS comprise a variety of reactive, oxygen-containing chemical metabolites, including hydrogen peroxide (H_2O_2) and superoxide (O_2^-).[46] ROS trigger genetic programmes associated with transformation such as those involving the cell cycle and mitogenic signalling.[47] NADPH oxidase (NOX) a major source of cellular ROS, exhibits high expression in UC and precancerous lesions such as dysplasia but not in normal urothelium. ROS generation through NOX4 contributed to an early step of urothelial carcinogenesis and cancer cell survival.[47] Increasing levels of ROS are associated with urothelial preneoplasia and neoplasia in a chemical carcinogenesis model of bladder cancer and are associated with increasing inflammation (*Said et al., In Press*).

Molecular mechanisms of invasive bladder cancer

Tumour suppressor genes

TP53 (transformation-related protein 53)

The p53 tumour suppressor encoded by the *TP53* gene located on chromosome 17p13.1[48] inhibits phase-specific cell cycle progression (G1-S) through the transcriptional activation of $p21^{WAF1/CIP1}$.[49] Most UCs exhibit loss of a single 17p allele and additional mutations in the remaining allele can inactivate *TP53* leading to increased nuclear accumulation of the mutant protein which has a longer half-life than the wt counterpart.[50] *TP53* deletion was significantly correlated with grade and stage.[46,51–55] Invasive carcinoma can also progress from recurrent papillary carcinoma by acquiring additional alterations in *TP53, RB1, PTEN, EGFRs, CCND1, MDM2*, or *E2F*.[56] In addition, oncogenic HRas has been shown to promote the malignant potency of UC cells that have acquired deficiencies of *TP53, RB1*, and *PTEN*.[56]

Mutations in the *TP53* gene that result in a truncated protein (or no protein), homozygous deletion of both alleles of the gene or gene silencing by methylation of the promoters of both alleles cannot be detected by nuclear accumulation of p53 protein,[57,58] thus limiting the sensitivity of immunohistochemistry (IHC) for p53 alterations. Nevertheless, even with this caveat, overexpression of nuclear p53 protein by IHC has been used as a surrogate marker for detection of mutant p53 in clinical specimens. p53 expression has been associated with increased risk of progression, or mortality in NMI and MI tumours respectively, independent of tumour grade, stage, and lymph node status.[48,49,59–70] Interestingly, this has not been borne out in patients treated with cystectomy in a recently reported randomized prospective trial.[71] This discordance in the identification of p53 as an independent prognostic marker for UC progression, recurrence, mortality and response to therapy in this latter and other studies may be due to genetic and epigenetic status of patients, cohort selection as well as technical and statistical variations.[46,72–74]

Rb1 (retinoblastoma 1)

Deletions of the long arm of chromosome 13, including the *Rb* locus on 13q14, were detected in MIUC.[75] Altered *Rb* expression in patients with MIUC, positively correlated with proliferative indices, and negatively correlated with patient survival.[64,76,77] Normal expression of Rb and p53 proteins favours good prognosis in patients with T1 tumours, whereas patients with abnormal expression of either or both proteins had a significant increase in progression.[78] Therefore, *P53* and *Rb* nuclear protein status could potentially be used in stratification of NMIUC patients (Ta, T1 and CIS) for conservative or aggressive treatment options.[79,80] In addition, analysis of multiple cell cycle regulatory proteins (pRb, p53, and $p21^{waf1/CIP1}$, with or without $p16^{ink4a}$) predicted disease outcome more accurately than any single marker, and independent of standard clinicopathologic prognostic factors.[74,81–84] Other than cell cycle deregulation, LOH of 13q14 and loss of Rb protein expression and/or inactivation contribute to UC progression through repression of E-cadherin.[2,81,85]

CDKN2A (p16)

The cyclin-dependent kinase inhibitor 2A (*CDKN2A*, $p16^{ink4a}$) gene is frequently inactivated by deletion in UC. *CDKN2A* homozygous deletion was significantly more frequent in *FGFR3*-mutated than in wild-type *FGFR3* tumours and was associated with MIUC within the *FGFR3*-mutated subgroup.[86] *CDKN2A* losses (hemizygous and homozygous) were associated with UC progression and predicted progression independent of stage and grade, suggesting a role of *CDKN2A* loss in the progression NMI FGFR3-mutated UC.[86] Promoter hypermethylation of p16 occurred frequently in both pathologically normal urothelium and tumour samples from UC patients and increased with progression from normal to UC along with E-cadherin, p14, and RASSF1A. However, no significant correlation was observed between p16 hypermethylation and muscle invasion or tumour grade.[87]

PTEN (phosphatase and tensin homologue)

Loss of heterozygosity at the MMAC1/PTEN/TEP1 locus is a common event in MIUC.[88,89] *PTEN* has been identified as a tumour suppressor gene mapped to chromosome 10q23,[90,91] and somatic mutations or deletions of *MMAC1/PTEN* have been found in UC.[90,91] The tumour suppressor effect of *MMAC1/PTEN* in UC is attributed to inhibition of Akt/PKB leading to UC growth suppression and enhancing chemosensitivity to doxorubicin.[89] In addition, *PTEN* synergizes with another tumour suppressor Lkb1 kinase is a tumour suppressor which regulates the TSC1/2 complex which has been found mutated in human UC.[92] Simultaneous deletion of *PTEN* and Lkb1 leads to upregulation of the mTOR pathway and the hypoxia marker GLUT1 in bladder epithelial cells, and increased their proliferation and tumourigenicity of UC.[92] In UC models, inhibitory effects of *PTEN* on cell motility were observed and these translate into suppression of *in vivo* invasion.[93] Surprisingly, this work revealed that *PTEN* can inhibit tumour invasion even in the absence of its lipid phosphatase activity.

Extracellular matrix (ECM) and adhesion molecules

Cadherins

E-cadherin, a calcium-dependent cell adhesion molecule mediates the homotypic interactions that maintain tight epithelial integrity and urine impermeability in the normal urothelium.[94,95] Reduced E-cadherin has been reported in experimental models and human tissues of UC[96] as part of the epithelial–mesenchymal transition (EMT) machinery involved in invasiveness and metastasis.[3,11,94–98] Methylation of the E-cadherin promoter, and subsequent gene silencing have been reported in early and late UC, and the frequency of methylation significantly correlated with progression and poor prognosis,[99–101] depth of muscle invasion, lymph node metastasis,[87,102–108] tumour recurrence,[101,109] and five-year survival.[87,110–113] Concomitant with loss of E-cadherin expression, N-cadherin, which is not expressed in normal urothelium, appeared in stage pT1 and increased in pT2-pT3 tumours. Progression-free survival and multivariate analyses revealed that N-cadherin expression is an independent prognostic marker for the progression of NMIUC to MIUC.[114] N-cadherin has a key role in determining the invasive capacity of UC cells via activation of PI3 kinase/Akt signalling.[114–116]

Integrins

The most commonly expressed integrin in the basal layer of the normal urothelium is $\alpha_6\beta_4$ whose expression is altered as an early event in the development of UC[117] suggesting its utility as a marker or driver of tumour formation.[89,118,119] Conversely, integrin α_v shows a grade and stage-dependent overexpression in UC, suggesting its importance in disease progression.[120] Recently the $\alpha_5\beta_1$ integrin (a fibronectin receptor) has been proposed as the initiating cellular signalling for intravesical immune and gene therapy.[120,121] The integrin-linked kinase (ILK) is a major signalling integrator from integrins cognate anchored to ECM ligands. In UC, ILK is overexpressed in MIUC and plays an important role in the EMT via the control of E-cadherin and MMP-9 expression.[122]

Versican

Versican is a highly conserved structural component of the ECM involved myriad physiological and pathological contexts and is associated with the invasive and metastatic signatures of many cancers including UC. Differential RNA splicing gives rise to four isoforms of versican (V0, V1, V2, and V3), which vary by the presence or absence of two glycosaminoglycan (GAG) binding domains named αGAG and βGAG.[123] Versican expression is regulated by cytokines, chemokines, and hypoxia. It functions not only as a scaffold or substrate to be consumed during tumour cell invasion, but represents a central component of cancer-related inflammation, as it can bind multiple types of cell adhesion receptors, growth factor receptors, and chemokines to provide a complex set of environmental cues to inflammatory and cancer cells in versican-rich sites.[123] Using common patterns of gene expression between UC models and cohorts of human UC tumours versican has been associated with tumour migration *in vitro* and advanced tumour stage in patients.[124] In addition, a recent mechanistic linkage between reduced expression of the metastasis suppressor Rho-GDI2 (discussed below) and high versican expression was found.[123] The expression of versican, was correlated with expression of inflammatory cytokines such as *CCL2* that *CCL2* leading to versican-driven metastasis through recruitment of inflammatory macrophages to the distant site.[123] Pharmacologic/immunologic targeting of *CCL2/CCR2* axis suppressed these inflammatory factors in the tumour microenvironment and ameliorated versican-induced lung metastasis.[123]

CD24

CD24, is a glycosyl phosphatidyl inositol–linked surface protein, that has been identified as a downstream target of the Ral family GTPases (discussed below)[125,126] and hypoxia-inducible factor 1α (HIF1α).[127] CD24 is highly expressed in bladder as well as other cancers. Loss of CD24 function in cancer cell lines was found to be associated with decreased cell proliferation and anchorage-independent growth, changes in the actin cytoskeleton, and induction of apoptosis.[125] Recent reports indicated the regulation of CD24 by HIF1α and their association with progression and metastasis in animal models of UC.[127] Overexpression of CD24 is also associated with poor outcome in UC patients. Furthermore, high levels of CD24 were found in primary bladder tumours and patient-matched nodal metastases[128] while targeting CD24 with monoclonal antibodies decreased metastatic burden.[128] In addition, CD24 expression was found to be androgen regulated in preclinical models of UC,[129] implying the important role for CD24 in urothelial tumorigenesis and metastasis in males and providing the foundation for UC therapy with antiandrogens.[129]

Hyaluronic acid/Hyaluronidase/Hyaluronic acid synthase

Hyaluronic acid (HA), a non-sulfated glycosaminoglycan, is an important component of the extracellular matrix (ECM).[130] In tumour tissues, elevated HA levels are contributed by both the tumour-associated stroma and tumour cells. HA is degraded by tumour cell-derived endoglycosidase hyaluronidase (HAase), specifically hyaluronidase 1 (HYAL1).[131–133] The secretion of HAase by tumour cells has been shown to induce angiogenesis, through cleavage of HA into angiogenic hyaluronic acid fragments that are detected in the urine of UC patients.[134] Urinary HA and HAase levels correlate with their levels in tissues, and are elevated the urine of UC patients and may serve as diagnostic markers.[131–133,135] HA synthesis occurs at the plasma membrane by a transmembrane HA synthase (HAS1, HAS2, or HAS3).[136–139] Tumour HAS1 expression has been shown to be a predictor of UC recurrence and treatment failure.[140–143] HA also regulates cell adhesion, migration, and proliferation by interacting with receptors such as CD44. Pericellular HA produced by tumour cells binds CD44, a transmembrane glycoprotein,[130] and induces a lipid raft-associated, signalling complex containing phosphorylated ErbB2 (p-ErbB2) and PI3-kinase,[95,144–148] signalling molecules shown to be important in UC biology.

Proteases and their regulators

High levels of matrix metalloproteinases (MMP) MMP-1, MMP-2 and MMP-9 mRNA were found in both NMIUC, and MIUC. Higher levels of MMP-2 and -9 associated with decreased survival,[149] and their urinary levels were associated to high tumour grade and stage, as well as with tissue polypeptide-specific antigen (TPS) and nuclear matrix protein 22 (NMP22).[150–155] Decreased expression of tissue inhibitor of metalloproteinases (TIMPs), TIMP-1 and TIMP-2 (inhibitors of MMP-9, and TIMP-2, respectively) is associated with advanced stage and grade.[149–151,156–161] High expression of tissue and urokinase plasminogen activator (tPA and uPA), urokinase plasminogen activator receptor (uPAR) and plasminogen activating inhibitor-1 (PAI-1) correlate with an unfavourable prognosis in invasive UC.[1,162]

Miscellaneous extracellular matrix and adhesion proteins

Aberrant glycosylation of tumours has been shown to drive tumour progression. Expression of specific carbohydrate epitopes such as the Sialosyl-Lewis^X (SLe^X) epitope in UC can affect invasive and metastatic ability in models and correlates with metastasis and poor survival in patients.[163] This aberrant glycosylation also increases adhesion of tumour cells to endothelial E-selectin possibly explaining one way that this change can affect metastatic ability.[163] Both laminin and type IV collagen, two major basement membrane (BM) components have been used as tumour markers, however their prognostic value is unclear.[95,164] The concentrations of tumour BM components such as laminin, elastase, and fibronectin were significantly higher in UC than in normal urothelium. Serum and urine laminin concentrations have been demonstrated to possess a high predictive value in the diagnosis of invasive UC, and together with interruption of the BM laminin staining pattern, suggest BM breakdown and loss consistent with aggressive disease.[95]

Growth factors and receptors

Epidermal growth factor family of ligands and receptors

Epidermal growth factor receptor (EGFR) expression levels in UC positively correlate with tumour progression, increasing grade and stage,[165,166] higher rates of recurrence[167] and phenotypic transition from NMIUC to MIUC.[168] EGFR overexpression in UC is not due to gene amplification and gene rearrangement[169] but rather correlated with the *HRAS* status suggesting a role of *HRAS* in transcriptional regulation of EGFR, in addition to its role in EGFR signal transduction.[15,170,171] Amplification and protein overexpression of the *ErbB2* gene located on 17q11.2-q12, has been suggested as a prognostic markers for patients with recurrent progressive UC.[172] Importantly, the ligand for EGFR, EGF, is found at 10-fold greater concentrations in urine than those found in blood, and likely potentiates the consequences of EGFR overexpression.[167,173,174] The uroplakin II gene promoter was used to drive the urothelial overexpression of EGFR in transgenic mice and this led to urothelial hyperplasia.[103] When coexpressed with the activated Ha-ras oncogene in double transgenic mice, EGFR had no tumour-enhancing effects over the urothelial hyperplastic phenotype induced by Ha-ras oncogene. However, when coexpressed with the SV40 large T antigen, EGFR accelerated tumour growth and converted the carcinoma *in situ* of the SV40T mice into high-grade bladder carcinomas, without triggering tumour invasion.

Vascular endothelial growth factor family

The vascular endothelial growth factor (VEGF) ligands and receptor family includes, VEGF-A, VEGF-B, VEGF-C, VEGF-D, and phosphatidylinositol glycan anchor biosynthesis class F (PlGF). In humans, VEGF-A exists in three isoforms 121,165, and 189-amino acid, and binds and activates VEGFR1 and VEGFR2 (two receptor tyrosine kinases), and is a potent inducer of angiogenesis.[175] PlGF and VEGF-B bind and activate only VEGFR1. VEGFR3 is mainly expressed in lymphatic endothelial cells and ligation by VEGF-C and -D regulates lymphangiogenesis.[175] VEGF-C or VEGF-D-overexpressing tumours are lymphangiogenic and highly metastatic to lymph nodes.[175] High levels of VEGF-A mRNA, and protein tumours expression and serum VEGF predicted earlier recurrence and increased risk of progression in patients with low or intermediate grade T1 UC,[176] correlated with increasing stage, grade, vascular invasion, and metastatic disease.[177,178] Mitogenic effects of the VEGF pathway includes the activation of PKC, sphingosine kinase (SPK), Ras (H-Ras and N-Ras activation, but not K-Ras activation) and mitogen-activated protein kinases (ERK1/2).[7,179–182] VEGF-D overexpression positively correlated with tumour stages and regional lymph node metastasis, and negatively correlated with disease-free survival.[183–185]

Fibroblast growth factors and receptors

Two isoforms of the potent angiogenic factor, fibroblast growth factor (FGF) are implicated in the pathogenesis of bladder cancer are the acidic FGF1 (aFGF) and the basic FGF2 (bFGF). Both are tightly bound to heparan-sulfates of the ECM and are thought to be released by proteases as a consequence of ECM degradation during cancer progression.[2,95] Both FGF1 and FGF2 contribute to a more aggressive phenotype in UC.[2,95] FGFs and their cognate receptors have been shown to play a role in reciprocal signalling from epithelial to mesenchymal compartments.[186] FGFR2IIIb mRNA is distributed throughout normal urothelium except for the umbrella cells, and low levels of FGFR2IIIc are detected in the stroma, whereas bladder carcinoma cell lines generally express no FGFR2IIIc isoform and very little FGFR2IIIb compared with normal urothelium.[187] In bladder carcinoma, low expression or complete loss of FGFR2IIIb expression is associated with poor prognosis.[22,187,188]

GTPase family molecules and regulators

The larger Ras superfamily in humans comprises over 100 small (20–30 kDa), related monomeric guanine nucleotide-binding proteins including six subfamilies: Ras, Rho, Arf, Rab, Ran, and Rad. H-Ras molecule stimulates the activation of other downstream signalling pathways which are associated with enhanced cell motility and invasion[189] including other GTPases such as Ral. Underlying the functional diversity of the Ras family is a common guanosine triphosphate (GTP)/guanosine diphosphate (GDP) cycle. Small G proteins cycle between inactive (GDP-bound) and active (GTP-bound) forms. Since only the latter can interact with downstream effectors, these proteins act as molecular switches coupling extracellular stimuli to intracellular effectors producing cellular responses. This cycling is regulated by guanine nucleotide exchange factors (GEFs), which promote GTP binding and GTPase activating proteins (GAPs), which promote GTP hydrolysis and GDP dissociation inhibitors (GDIs) that bind to Ras proteins in the cytoplasm, conferring aqueous solubility, and blocking activation. These proteins act as molecular switches coupling extracellular stimuli to intracellular effectors producing cellular responses.

Rho GTPases

The Rho subfamily has been implicated as a nexus for signal transduction pathways that affect the cell adhesion, migration, cell cycle progression, cell survival, membrane recycling, and gene expression. Cross-talk between Ras and Rho proteins was observed in several biological processes, including cell transformation, cell migration and epithelial–mesenchymal transition (EMT).[190,191] The role of Rho and ROCK in bladder cancer was investigated using Western blotting in paired tumour and non-tumour patient samples. RhoA, RhoC, and ROCK were more abundant in tumours and metastatic lymph nodes than in non-tumour bladder and uninvolved lymph nodes. Amounts of RhoA and RhoC protein, and ROCK protein expression correlated positively with one another and high RhoA, RhoC, and ROCK expression were related to poor tumour differentiation, muscle invasion, and patient outcome. By multivariate analysis, only RhoC was independently influenced in disease-free survival and RhoA and RhoC in overall survival. In contrast, RhoB expression was inversely related to the grade and stage, and its higher expression is associated with better overall survival.[190] More recently, biochemical studies indicated that the oncogene Src effects are mediated through phosphorylation of p190RhoGAP and these pathways converge to reduce activity of RhoA, RhoC, and Rho effector ROCK1. Treatment with a ROCK inhibitor reduced lung metastasis in experimental UC models *in vivo*, suggesting a pharmacologically tractable common downstream signalling pathway.[128]

Ral-GTPases

Ras-like (Ral) guanyl nucleotide-binding proteins, RalA and RalB are two members of Ras family of monomeric G proteins that share 85% amino acid identity.[192,193] Ral proteins are involved in endocytosis, exocytosis, actin cytoskeletal dynamics, and transcription. Ral activation has been reported as a mediator of EGF-stimulated migration in human UC cells.[194] Ral activation and expression in human UC and cell lines revealed that activated RalA and RalB are associated with the *G12V HRAS* oncogene and Ral effectors as RalBP1 and CD24 are overexpressed in MIUC.[126] Neither the activation of RalA nor RalB was significantly associated with mutation status for the seven bladder cancer genes (*KRAS, p53, RB, CDKN2a, PTEN, PIK3CA*, and *FGFR3*), suggesting independence of Ral activity from these common molecular lesions.[195] Using comparative gene expression and proteomic profiling of multiple independent data sets ($n = 522$) as well as 40 cell lines (BL-40) and genetically-engineered cells depleted of Ral A and/or B, Smith and colleagues[195] developed a Ral signature of 91 genes combining Ral A and Ral B effectors defined as 'Ral signature probes'. They found that NMIUC (stage pTa, pT1) had lower signature scores and clustered with the Ral-depleted cells, whereas MIUC (stage pT2+) had higher scores and clustered with control-treated cells. Signature scores that indicated high Ral activity were associated with poor patient prognosis.

RhoGDI2 (Rho GDP dissociation inhibitor beta)

Rho GDIs bind to Rho proteins in the cytoplasm, conferring aqueous solubility, and blocking activation or function through inhibiting the dissociation of bound nucleotides and their interactions with GEFs, GAPs, and effectors. RhoGDI2 (also known as D4-GDI or Ly-GDI) was initially believed to be exclusively expressed in haematopoietic cells[196] is highly expressed in the epithelium of genitourinary tract.[125] Reduced expression of RhoGDI2 correlated with increasing invasive and metastatic activity in human UC lines.[197,198] Expression analysis and follow-up mechanistic work on a novel animal model of UC metastasis identified RhoGDI2 as a metastasis suppressor gene.[194] In human bladder tumours, the RhoGDI2 level inversely correlated with development of metastatic disease, and multivariate analysis, identified RhoGDI2 as an independent prognostic marker of tumour recurrence following radical cystectomy.[197]

Tumour microenvironment

Hypoxia-inducible factor 1 and 2 (HIF1 and HIF2)

Hypoxia-inducible factor-1 (HIF-1) is a key transcription factor that regulates the cellular response to hypoxia. HIF-1 is a transactivator of a large number of genes that are related to regulation of angiogenesis, erythropoiesis, cell adhesion, and glucose transport in physiological and pathological conditions including cancer.[199] In UC, HIF1α is overexpression as a function of tumour grade and stage and correlated with tumour proliferation and vascular indices angiogenesis, inflammatory macrophage infiltration, and poor outcome.[200–203] HIF1α overexpression induced the prometastatic CD24 mRNA and protein with subsequent increased in cancer cell survival *in vitro* and *in vivo* at the levels of primary and metastatic tumour growth.[127] Analysis of clinical tumour specimens revealed a correlation between HIF-1α and CD24 levels and an association of their coexpression to decreased patient survival.[127] HIF2α along with HIF1α expression correlated with tumour grade, stage, markers of tumour angiogenesis, and recurrence or progression to MIUC.[202]

Endothelin axis

Endothelins (ETs) are a family of three 21-amino acid peptides ET-1, ET-2, and ET-3, which mediate their action by activating two G-protein-coupled receptor (GPCR) of $G\alpha_q$ and $G\alpha_s$ subtypes, ETA receptor (ET_AR) and ETB receptor (ET_BR). The endothelin axis is relevant role in various cancer and stromal cells interactions leading to autocrine/paracrine loops with subsequent aberrant proliferation, angiogenesis, immune modulation, invasion, and metastatic dissemination. The importance of endothelin axis in UC has been identified by virtue of ET-1 being regulated by RhoGDI2. The loss of RhoGDI2 expression in UC cell lines was correlated with upregulation of ET-1 expression.[189] ET-1 and ET_AR mRNA and protein expression in patient cohorts revealed that levels of ET-1 are higher in patients with MIUC, which are associated with higher incidence of metastasis, and that high ET-1 levels are associated with decreased patient survival. Consistent with its pro-inflammatory activity, we found that tumour-derived ET-1 acts through endothelin-1 receptor ET_AR to enhance migration and invasion of both tumour cells and macrophages and induces expression of inflammatory cytokines and proteases.[204] Preclinical models using cells depleted of ET-1 and pharmacologic blockade of ETRs indicated that tumour ET-1 expression and ET_AR activity are necessary for metastatic lung colonization in animal models of UC and that this process is preceded by and dependent on macrophage infiltration of the lung. In contrast, tumour ET-1 expression and ET_AR activity appeared less important in established primary or metastatic tumour growth. These findings strongly suggest that ET_AR inhibitors might be more effective as adjuvant therapeutic agents than as initial treatment for advanced primary or metastatic disease.[204,205]

Cytokines, chemokines, and their receptors

Interleukin-8 (IL-8) expression is increased in muscle-invasive tumours and carcinoma *in situ* when compared with non-invasive papillary tumours.[178,206] IL-6 and CCl2 were shown to be overexpressed in MIUC compared to NMIUC[123,204] and positively correlated with increased levels with the prometastatic molecules such as ET-1 and Versican while negatively correlated with RhoGDI2.[123,204,205] CCL2 and its receptor CCR2 were required for establishing pulmonary macrophage infiltration as prerequisite for bladder cancer lung metastases in preclinical models of UC cancer metastasis.[123] The expression levels of IL-5, IL-20, and IL-28A were increased in patients with MIUC and correlated with *in vitro* increase aggressiveness of UC cell lines with upregulation of MMP-2 and MMP-9 and activation of the transcription factors NF-kappaB and AP-1, activation of MAPK and Jak-Stat signalling pathways.[207]

Cycloxygenases, arachidonates, and prostaglandins receptors

Cyclooxygenase-2 (Cox-2) is not expressed in normal bladder urothelium,[82] but overexpressed at the molecular level in invasive UC. Cox-2 expression was associated with markers of aggressive disease, angiogenesis, lymph node metastasis, increased risk of disease recurrence and disease-specific mortality.[82,204,208–211]

Further reading

Chaffer CL, Dopheide B, Savagner P, Thompson EW, Williams ED. Aberrant fibroblast growth factor receptor signaling in bladder and other cancers. *Differentiation* 2007; **75**:831–42.

Chan MW, Hui AB, Yip SK, *et al.* Progressive increase of genetic alteration in urinary bladder cancer by combined allelotyping analysis and comparative genomic hybridization. *Int J Oncol* 2009; **34**:963–70.

Knowles MA. Molecular subtypes of bladder cancer: Jekyll and Hyde or chalk and cheese? *Carcinogenesis* 2006; **27**:361–73.

Kompier LC, van Tilborg AA, Zwarthoff EC. Bladder cancer: novel molecular characteristics, diagnostic, and therapeutic implications. *Urol Oncol* 2010; **28**:91–6.

Overdevest JB, Knubel KH, Duex JE, *et al.* CD24 expression is important in male urothelial tumorigenesis and metastasis in mice and is androgen regulated. *Proc Natl Acad Sci U S A* 2012; **109**(51):E3588–96.

Overdevest JB, Thomas S, Kristiansen G, Hansel DE, Smith SC, Theodorescu D. CD24 offers a therapeutic target for control of bladder cancer metastasis based on a requirement for lung colonization. *Cancer Res* 2011; **71**:3802–11.

Said N, Sanchez-Carbayo M, Smith SC, Theodorescu D. RhoGDI2 suppresses lung metastasis in mice by reducing tumor versican expression and macrophage infiltration. *J Clin Invest* 2012; **122**:1503–18.

Said N, Smith S, Sanchez-Carbayo M, Theodorescu D. Tumor endothelin-1 enhances metastatic colonization of the lung in mouse xenograft models of bladder cancer. *J Clin Invest* 2011; **121**:132–47.

Wallerand H, Reiter RR, Ravaud A. Molecular targeting in the treatment of either advanced or metastatic bladder cancer or both according to the signalling pathways. *Curr Opin Urol* 2008; **18**:524–32.

Wang HCR, Choudhary S. Reactive oxygen species-mediated therapeutic control of bladder cancer. *Nat Rev Urol* 2011; **8**:608–16.

References

1. Siegel R, Naishadham D, Jemal A. Cancer statistics. *CA: Cancer J Clin* 2012; **62**:10–29.
2. Knowles MA. Molecular subtypes of bladder cancer: Jekyll and Hyde or chalk and cheese? *Carcinogenesis* 2006; **27**:361–73.
3. Wasco MJ, Daignault S, Zhang Y, *et al.* Urothelial carcinoma with divergent histologic differentiation (mixed histologic features) predicts the presence of locally advanced bladder cancer when detected at transurethral resection. *Urology* 2007; **70**:69–74.
4. Taparowsky E, Suard Y, Fasano O, Shimizu K, Goldfarb M, Wigler M. Activation of the T24 bladder carcinoma transforming gene is linked to a single amino acid change. *Nature* 1982; **300**:762–5.
5. Parada LF, Tabin CJ, Shih C, Weinberg RA. Human EJ bladder carcinoma oncogene is homologue of Harvey sarcoma virus ras gene. *Nature* 1982; **297**:474–8.
6. Kawano H, Komaba S, Yamasaki T, *et al.* New potential therapy for orthotopic bladder carcinoma by combining HVJ envelope with doxorubicin. *Cancer Chemother Pharmacol* 2008; **61**:973–8.
7. Oxford G, Theodorescu D. The role of Ras superfamily proteins in bladder cancer progression. *J Urol* 2003; **170**:1987–93.
8. Christian BJ, Kao CH, Wu SQ, Meisner LF, Reznikoff CA. EJ/ras neoplastic transformation of simian virus 40-immortalized human uroepithelial cells: a rare event. *Cancer Res* 1990; **50**:4779–86.
9. Pratt CI, Kao CH, Wu SQ, Gilchrist KW, Oyasu R, Reznikoff CA. Neoplastic progression by EJ/ras at different steps of transformation in vitro of human uroepithelial cells. *Cancer Res* 1992; **52**:688–95.
10. Wu X, Pandolfi PP. Mouse models for multistep tumorigenesis. *Trends Cell Biol* 2001; **11**:S2–9.
11. Fondrevelle ME, Kantelip B, Reiter RE, *et al.* The expression of Twist has an impact on survival in human bladder cancer and is influenced by the smoking status. *Urol Oncol* 2008; **27**(3):268–76.
12. Wallerand H, Reiter RR, Ravaud A. Molecular targeting in the treatment of either advanced or metastatic bladder cancer or both according to the signalling pathways. *Curr Opin Urol* 2008; **18**:524–32.
13. Fitzgerald JM, Ramchurren N, Rieger K, *et al.* Identification of H-ras mutations in urine sediments complements cytology in the detection of bladder tumors. *J Natl Cancer Inst* 1995; **87**:129–33.
14. Theodorescu D, Cornil I, Fernandez BJ, Kerbel RS. Overexpression of normal and mutated forms of HRAS induces orthotopic bladder invasion in a human transitional cell carcinoma. *Proc Natl Acad Sci U S A* 1990; **87**:9047–51.
15. Theodorescu D, Cornil I, Sheehan C, Man MS, Kerbel RS. Ha-ras induction of the invasive phenotype results in up-regulation of epidermal growth factor receptors and altered responsiveness to epidermal growth factor in human papillary transitional cell carcinoma cells. *Cancer Res* 1991; **51**:4486–91.
16. Czerniak B, Cohen GL, Etkind P, *et al.* Concurrent mutations of coding and regulatory sequences of the Ha-ras gene in urinary bladder carcinomas. *Hum Pathol* 1992; **23**:1199–204.
17. Czerniak B, Deitch D, Simmons H, Etkind P, Herz F, Koss LG. Ha-ras gene codon 12 mutation and DNA ploidy in urinary bladder carcinoma. *Br J Cancer* 1990; **62**:762–3.
18. Fontana D, Bellina M, Scoffone C, *et al.* Evaluation of c-ras oncogene product (p21) in superficial bladder cancer. *Eur Urol* 1996; **29**:470–6.
19. Kompier LC, van Tilborg AA, Zwarthoff EC. Bladder cancer: novel molecular characteristics, diagnostic, and therapeutic implications. *Urol Oncol* 2010; **28**:91–6.
20. Billerey C, Chopin D, Aubriot-Lorton MH, *et al.* Frequent FGFR3 mutations in papillary non-invasive bladder (pTa) tumors. *Am J Pathol* 2001; **158**:1955–9.
21. di Martino E, Tomlinson DC, Knowles MA. A decade of FGF receptor research in bladder cancer: past, present, and future challenges. *Adv Urol* **2012**:429213.
22. Bernard-Pierrot I, Brams A, Dunois-Larde C, *et al.* Oncogenic properties of the mutated forms of fibroblast growth factor receptor 3b. *Carcinogenesis* 2006; **27**:740–7.
23. Chaffer CL, Dopheide B, Savagner P, Thompson EW, Williams ED. Aberrant fibroblast growth factor receptor signaling in bladder and other cancers. *Differentiation* 2007; **75**:831–42.
24. Hart KC, Robertson SC, Kanemitsu MY, Meyer AN, Tynan JA, Donoghue DJ. Transformation and Stat activation by derivatives of FGFR1, FGFR3, and FGFR4. *Oncogene* 2000; **19**:3309–20.
25. Knowles MA. Role of FGFR3 in urothelial cell carcinoma: biomarker and potential therapeutic target. *World J Urol* 2007; **25**:581–93.
26. van Rhijn BW, Montironi R, Zwarthoff EC, Jobsis AC, van der Kwast TH. Frequent FGFR3 mutations in urothelial papilloma. *J Pathol* 2002; **198**:245–51.
27. Lievens PMJ, Roncador A, Liboi E. K644E/M FGFR3 Mutants Activate Erk1/2 from the Endoplasmic Reticulum through FRS2α and PLCγ-independent Pathways. *J Molecular Biology* 2006; **357**:783–92.
28. van Rhijn BW, van der Kwast TH, Vis AN, *et al.* FGFR3 and P53 characterize alternative genetic pathways in the pathogenesis of urothelial cell carcinoma. *Cancer Res* 2004; **64**:1911–4.
29. Hurst CD, Platt FM, Taylor CF, Knowles MA. Novel tumor subgroups of urothelial carcinoma of the bladder defined by integrated genomic analysis. *Clin Cancer Res* 2012; **18**(21):5865–77.
30. Tomlinson DC, Baldo O, Harnden P, Knowles MA. FGFR3 protein expression and its relationship to mutation status and prognostic variables in bladder cancer. *J Pathol* 2007; **213**:91–8.
31. Catto JW, Miah S, Owen HC, *et al.* Distinct microRNA alterations characterize high- and low-grade bladder cancer. *Cancer Res* 2009; **69**:8472–81.
32. Höglund M. The bladder cancer genome; chromosomal changes as prognostic makers, opportunities, and obstacles. *Urol Oncol* 2012; **30**:533–40.
33. Hoque MO, Lee CC, Cairns P, Schoenberg M, Sidransky D. Genome-wide genetic characterization of bladder cancer: a comparison of high-density single-nucleotide polymorphism arrays and PCR-based microsatellite analysis. *Cancer Res* 2003; **63**:2216–22.
34. Koed K, Wiuf C, Christensen LL, *et al.* High-density single nucleotide polymorphism array defines novel stage and location-dependent allelic imbalances in human bladder tumors. *Cancer Res* 2005; **65**:34–45.
35. Chan MW, Hui AB, Yip SK, *et al.* Progressive increase of genetic alteration in urinary bladder cancer by combined allelotyping analysis and comparative genomic hybridization. *Int J Oncol* 2009; **34**:963–70.
36. Heidenblad M, Lindgren D, Jonson T, *et al.* Tiling resolution array CGH and high density expression profiling of urothelial carcinomas delineate genomic amplicons and candidate target genes specific for advanced tumors. *BMC Med Genomics* 2008; **1**:3.
37. Obermann EC, Junker K, Stoehr R, *et al.* Frequent genetic alterations in flat urothelial hyperplasias and concomitant papillary bladder cancer as detected by CGH, LOH, and FISH analyses. *J Pathol* 2003; **199**:50–57.

38. Minner S, Kilgue A, Stahl P, *et al.* Y chromosome loss is a frequent early event in urothelial bladder cancer. *Pathology* 2010; **42**:356–9.
39. Brockmoller J, Kaiser R, Kerb R, Cascorbi I, Jaeger V, Roots I. Polymorphic enzymes of xenobiotic metabolism as modulators of acquired P53 mutations in bladder cancer. *Pharmacogenetics* 1996; **6**:535–45.
40. Altayli E, Gunes S, Yilmaz AF, Goktas S, Bek Y. CYP1A2, CYP2D6, GSTM1, GSTP1, and GSTT1 gene polymorphisms in patients with bladder cancer in a Turkish population. *Int Urol Nephrol* 2009; **41**:259–66.
41. Lesseur C, Gilbert-Diamond D, Andrew AS, *et al.* A case-control study of polymorphisms in xenobiotic and arsenic metabolism genes and arsenic-related bladder cancer in New Hampshire. *Toxicol Lett* 2012; **210**:100–6.
42. Ouerhani S, Rouissi K, Marrakchi R, *et al.* Do smoking and polymorphisms in xenobiotic metabolizing enzymes affect the histological stage and grade of bladder tumors? *Bull Cancer* 2009; **96**:E23–29.
43. Rouissi K, Ouerhani S, Hamrita B, *et al.* Smoking and polymorphisms in xenobiotic metabolism and DNA repair genes are additive risk factors affecting bladder cancer in Northern Tunisia. *Pathology Oncol Res* 2011; **17**:879–86.
44. Zhang R, Xu G, Chen W, Zhang W. Genetic polymorphisms of glutathione S-transferase P1 and bladder cancer susceptibility in a Chinese population. *Genet Test Mol Biomarkers* 2011; **15**:85–88.
45. Sasaki T, Horikawa M, Orikasa K, *et al.* Possible relationship between the risk of Japanese bladder cancer cases and the CYP4B1 genotype. *Jpn J Clin Oncol* 2008; **38**:634–40.
46. Wang HCR, Choudhary S. Reactive oxygen species-mediated therapeutic control of bladder cancer. *Nat Rev Urol* 2011; **8**:608–16.
47. Shimada K, Fujii T, Anai S, Fujimoto K, Konishi N. ROS generation via NOX4 and its utility in the cytological diagnosis of urothelial carcinoma of the urinary bladder. *BMC Urol* 2011; **11**:22.
48. Mitra AP, Datar RH, Cote RJ. Molecular pathways in invasive bladder cancer: new insights into mechanisms, progression, and target identification. *J Clin Oncol* 2006; **24**:5552–64.
49. Mitra AP, Birkhahn M, Cote RJ. p53 and retinoblastoma pathways in bladder cancer. *World J Urol* 2007; **25**:563–71.
50. Iggo R, Gatter K, Bartek J, Lane D, Harris AL. Increased expression of mutant forms of p53 oncogene in primary lung cancer. *Lancet* 1990; **335**:675–9.
51. Fujimoto K, Yamada Y, Okajima E, *et al.* Frequent association of p53 gene mutation in invasive bladder cancer. *Cancer Res* 1992; **52**:1393–8.
52. Soini Y, Turpeenniemi-Hujanen T, Kamel D, *et al.* p53 immunohistochemistry in transitional cell carcinoma and dysplasia of the urinary bladder correlates with disease progression. *Br J Cancer* 1993; **68**:1029–35.
53. Moch H, Sauter G, Moore D, Mihatsch MJ, Gudat F, Waldman F. p53 and erbB-2 protein overexpression are associated with early invasion and metastasis in bladder cancer. *Virchows Arch A Pathol Anat Histopathol* 1993; **423**:329–34.
54. Matsuyama H, Pan Y, Mahdy EA, *et al.* p53 deletion as a genetic marker in urothelial tumor by fluorescence in situ hybridization. *Cancer Res* 1994; **54**:6057–60.
55. Yamamoto S, Masui T, Murai T, *et al.* Frequent mutations of the p53 gene and infrequent H- and K-ras mutations in urinary bladder carcinomas of NON/Shi mice treated with N-butyl-N-(4-hydroxybutyl) nitrosamine. *Carcinogenesis* 1995; **16**:2363–8.
56. Choudhary S, Wang HCR. Proapoptotic ability of oncogenic H-Ras to facilitate apoptosis induced by histone deacetylase inhibitors in human cancer cells. *Mol Cancer Ther* 2007; **6**:1099–111.
57. Chaffer CL, Thomas DM, Thompson EW, Williams ED. PPARgamma-independent induction of growth arrest and apoptosis in prostate and bladder carcinoma. *BMC Cancer* 2006; **6**:53.
58. Thomas CY, Theodorescu D. Molecular markers of prognosis and novel therapeutic strategies for urothelial cell carcinomas. *World J Urol* 2006; **24**:565–78.
59. Esrig D, Spruck CH 3rd, Nichols PW, *et al.* p53 nuclear protein accumulation correlates with mutations in the p53 gene, tumor grade, and stage in bladder cancer. *Am J Pathol* 1993; **143**:1389–97.
60. Esrig D, Elmajian D, Groshen S, *et al.* Accumulation of nuclear p53 and tumor progression in bladder cancer. *N Engl J Med* 1994; **331**:1259–64.
61. Spruck CH 3rd, Ohneseit PF, Gonzalez-Zulueta M, *et al.* Two molecular pathways to transitional cell carcinoma of the bladder. *Cancer Res* 1994; **54**:784–8.
62. Stavropoulos NE, Filliadis I, Ioachim E, *et al.* CD44 standard form expression as a predictor of progression in high risk superficial bladder tumors. *Int Urol Nephrol* 2001; **33**:479–83.
63. Stavropoulos NE, Ioachim E, Charchanti A, *et al.* Tumor markers in stage P1 bladder cancer. *Anticancer Res* 2001; **21**:1495–8.
64. Ioachim E, Charchanti A, Stavropoulos NE, Skopelitou A, Athanassiou ED, Agnantis NJ. Immunohistochemical expression of retinoblastoma gene product (Rb), p53 protein, MDM2, c-erbB-2, HLA-DR and proliferation indices in human urinary bladder carcinoma. *Histol Histopathol* 2000; **15**:721–7.
65. Lianes P, Orlow I, Zhang ZF, *et al.* Altered patterns of MDM2 and TP53 expression in human bladder cancer. *J Natl Cancer Inst* 1994; **86**:1325–30.
66. Sarkis AS, Dalbagni G, Cordon-Cardo C, *et al.* Nuclear overexpression of p53 protein in transitional cell bladder carcinoma: a marker for disease progression. *J Natl Cancer Inst* 1993; **85**:53–9.
67. Sarkis AS, Bajorin DF, Reuter VE, *et al.* Prognostic value of p53 nuclear overexpression in patients with invasive bladder cancer treated with neoadjuvant MVAC. *J Clin Oncol* 1995; **13**:1384–90.
68. Stavropoulos NE, Filiadis I, Ioachim E, *et al.* Prognostic significance of p53, bcl-2 and Ki-67 in high risk superficial bladder cancer. *Anticancer Res* 2002; **22**:3759–64.
69. Peyromaure M, Ravery V. Prognostic value of p53 overexpression in bladder tumors treated with Bacillus Calmette-Guerin. *Expert Rev Anticancer Ther* 2002; **2**:667–70.
70. Moonen PM, Witjes JA. Risk stratification of Ta, Tis, T1 cancer. (pp. 281–6) In: Lerner S, Schoenberg M, Sternberg C (eds). *Textbook of Bladder Cancer*. Oxford, UK: Taylor and Francis, 2006.
71. Stadler WM, Lerner SP, Groshen S, *et al.* Phase III study of molecularly targeted adjuvant therapy in locally advanced urothelial cancer of the bladder based on p53 status. *J Clin Oncol* 2011; **29**:3443–9.
72. Malats N, Bustos A, Nascimento CM, *et al.* P53 as a prognostic marker for bladder cancer: a meta-analysis and review. *Lancet Oncol* 2005; **6**:678–86.
73. Ecke TH, Sachs MD, Lenk SV, Loening SA, Schlechte HH. TP53 gene mutations as an independent marker for urinary bladder cancer progression. *Int J Mol Med* 2008; **21**:655–61.
74. Hutterer GC, Karakiewicz PI, Zippe C, *et al.* Urinary cytology and nuclear matrix protein 22 in the detection of bladder cancer recurrence other than transitional cell carcinoma. *BJU Int* 2008; **101**:561–5.
75. Cairns P, Proctor AJ, Knowles MA. Loss of heterozygosity at the RB locus is frequent and correlates with muscle invasion in bladder carcinoma. *Oncogene* 1991; **6**:2305–9.
76. Cordon-Cardo C, Sheinfeld J, Dalbagni G. Genetic studies and molecular markers of bladder cancer. *Semin Surg Oncol* 1997; **13**:319–27.
77. Cordon-Cardo C, Wartinger D, Petrylak D, *et al.* Altered expression of the retinoblastoma gene product: prognostic indicator in bladder cancer. *J Natl Cancer Inst* 1992; **84**:1251–6.
78. Grossman HB, Liebert M, Antelo M, *et al.* p53 and RB expression predict progression in T1 bladder cancer. *Clin Cancer Res* 1998; **4**:829–34.
79. Cordon-Cardo C. p53 and RB: simple interesting correlates or tumor markers of critical predictive nature? *J Clin Oncol* 2004; **22**:975–7.
80. Kikuchi E, Menendez S, Ohori M, Cordon-Cardo C, Kasahara N, Bochner BH. Inhibition of orthotopic human bladder tumor growth by lentiviral gene transfer of endostatin. *Clin Cancer Res* 2004; **10**:1835–42.

81. Shariat SF, Tokunaga H, Zhou J, *et al.* p53, p21, pRB, and p16 expression predict clinical outcome in cystectomy with bladder cancer. *J Clin Oncol* 2004; **22**:1014–24.
82. Margulis V, Shariat SF, Ashfaq R, *et al.* Expression of cyclooxygenase-2 in normal urothelium, and superficial and advanced transitional cell carcinoma of bladder. *J Urol* 2007; **177**:1163–8.
83. Shariat SF, Ashfaq R, Sagalowsky AI, Lotan Y. Predictive value of cell cycle biomarkers in nonmuscle invasive bladder transitional cell carcinoma. *J Urol* 2007; **177**:481–7; discussion 487.
84. Shariat SF, Zlotta AR, Ashfaq R, Sagalowsky AI, Lotan Y. Cooperative effect of cell-cycle regulators expression on bladder cancer development and biologic aggressiveness. *Mod Pathol* 2007; **20**:445–59.
85. Arima Y, Inoue Y, Shibata T, *et al.* Rb depletion results in deregulation of E-cadherin and induction of cellular phenotypic changes that are characteristic of the epithelial-to-mesenchymal transition. *Cancer Res* 2008; **68**:5104–12.
86. Schepeler T, Lamy P, Laurberg JR, *et al.* A high resolution genomic portrait of bladder cancer: correlation between genomic aberrations and the DNA damage response. *Oncogene* 2012; **32**(31):3577–86.
87. Lin HH, Ke HL, Wu WJ, Lee YH, Chang LL. Hypermethylation of E-cadherin, p16, p14, and RASSF1A genes in pathologically normal urothelium predict bladder recurrence of bladder cancer after transurethral resection. *Urol Oncol* 2012; **30**:177–81.
88. Ahmad I, Morton JP, Singh LB, *et al.* Beta-catenin activation synergizes with PTEN loss to cause bladder cancer formation. *Oncogene* 2011; **30**:178–89.
89. Tanaka M, Koul D, Davies MA, Liebert M, Steck PA, Grossman HB. MMAC1/PTEN inhibits cell growth and induces chemosensitivity to doxorubicin in human bladder cancer cells. *Oncogene* 2000; **19**:5406–12.
90. Liu J, Babaian DC, Liebert M, Steck PA, Kagan J. Inactivation of MMAC1 in bladder transitional-cell carcinoma cell lines and specimens. *Mol Carcinog* 2000; **29**:143–50.
91. Teng DH, Hu R, Lin H, *et al.* MMAC1/PTEN mutations in primary tumor specimens and tumor cell lines. *Cancer Res* 1997; **57**:5221–5.
92. Shorning BY, Griffiths D, Clarke AR. Lkb1 and Pten synergise to suppress mTOR-mediated tumorigenesis and epithelial-mesenchymal transition in the mouse bladder. *PLoS ONE* 2011; **6**:e16209.
93. Gildea JJ, Herlevsen M, Harding MA, *et al.* PTEN can inhibit in vitro organotypic and in vivo orthotopic invasion of human bladder cancer cells even in the absence of its lipid phosphatase activity. *Oncogene* 2004; **23**:6788–97.
94. Thiery JP. Epithelial-mesenchymal transitions in tumour progression. *Nat Rev Cancer* 2002; **2**:442–54.
95. Gontero P, Banisadr S, Frea B, Brausi M. Metastasis markers in bladder cancer: a review of the literature and clinical considerations. *Eur Urol* 2004; **46**:296–311.
96. Julien S, Puig I, Caretti E, *et al.* Activation of NF-kappaB by Akt upregulates Snail expression and induces epithelium mesenchyme transition. *Oncogene* 2007; **26**:7445–56.
97. Xie XY, Yang X, Zhang JH, Liu ZJ. Analysis of hTERT expression in exfoliated cells from patients with bladder transitional cell carcinomas using SYBR green real-time fluorescence quantitative PCR. *Ann Clin Biochem* 2007; **44**:523–8.
98. Zhang Z, Xie D, Li X, *et al.* Significance of TWIST expression and its association with E-cadherin in bladder cancer. *Hum Pathol* 2007; **38**:598–606.
99. Bornman DM, Mathew S, Alsruhe J, Herman JG, Gabrielson E. Methylation of the E-cadherin gene in bladder neoplasia and in normal urothelial epithelium from elderly individuals. *Am J Pathol* 2001; **159**:831–5.
100. Dhawan D, Hamdy FC, Rehman I, *et al.* Evidence for the early onset of aberrant promoter methylation in urothelial carcinoma. *J Pathol* 2006; **209**:336–43.
101. Muramaki M, Miyake H, Terakawa T, Kusuda Y, Fujisawa M. Expression profile of E-cadherin and N-cadherin in urothelial carcinoma of the upper urinary tract is associated with disease recurrence in patients undergoing nephroureterectomy. *Urology* 2011; **78**:1443.e1447–3.e1412.
102. Sanchez-Carbayo M, Socci ND, Charytonowicz E, *et al.* Molecular profiling of bladder cancer using cDNA microarrays: defining histogenesis and biological phenotypes. *Cancer Res* 2002; **62**:6973–80.
103. Cheng J, Huang H, Zhang ZT, *et al.* Overexpression of epidermal growth factor receptor in urothelium elicits urothelial hyperplasia and promotes bladder tumor growth. *Cancer Res* 2002; **62**:4157–63.
104. Sun W, Herrera GA. E-cadherin expression in urothelial carcinoma in situ, superficial papillary transitional cell carcinoma, and invasive transitional cell carcinoma. *Hum Pathol* 2002; **33**:996–1000.
105. Nakopoulou L, Zervas A, Gakiopoulou-Givalou H, *et al.* Prognostic value of E-cadherin, beta-catenin, P120ctn in patients with transitional cell bladder cancer. *Anticancer Res* 2000; **20**:4571–8.
106. Ashida S, Nakagawa H, Katagiri T, *et al.* Molecular features of the transition from prostatic intraepithelial neoplasia (PIN) to prostate cancer: genome-wide gene-expression profiles of prostate cancers and PINs. *Cancer Res* 2004; **64**:5963–72.
107. Gao J, Huang HY, Pak J, *et al.* p53 deficiency provokes urothelial proliferation and synergizes with activated Ha-ras in promoting urothelial tumorigenesis. *Oncogene* 2004; **23**:687–96.
108. Sun W, Herrera GA. E-cadherin expression in invasive urothelial carcinoma. *Ann Diagn Pathol* 2004; **8**:17–22.
109. Mahnken A, Kausch I, Feller AC, Kruger S. E-cadherin immunoreactivity correlates with recurrence and progression of minimally invasive transitional cell carcinomas of the urinary bladder. *Oncol Rep* 2005; **14**:1065–70.
110. Byrne RR, Shariat SF, Brown R, *et al.* E-cadherin immunostaining of bladder transitional cell carcinoma, carcinoma in situ and lymph node metastases with long-term followup. *J Urol* 2001; **165**:1473–9.
111. Kim JH, Shariat SF, Kim IY, *et al.* Predictive value of expression of transforming growth factor-beta(1) and its receptors in transitional cell carcinoma of the urinary bladder. *Cancer* 2001; **92**:1475–83.
112. Shariat SF, Pahlavan S, Baseman AG, *et al.* E-cadherin expression predicts clinical outcome in carcinoma in situ of the urinary bladder. *Urology* 2001; **57**:60–5.
113. Rao J, Seligson D, Visapaa H, *et al.* Tissue microarray analysis of cytoskeletal actin-associated biomarkers gelsolin and E-cadherin in urothelial carcinoma. *Cancer* 2002; **95**:1247–57.
114. Rieger-Christ KM, Lee P, Zagha R, *et al.* Novel expression of N-cadherin elicits in vitro bladder cell invasion via the Akt signaling pathway. *Oncogene* 2004; **23**:4745–53.
115. Clairotte A, Lascombe I, Fauconnet S, *et al.* Expression of E-cadherin and alpha-, beta-, gamma-catenins in patients with bladder cancer: identification of gamma-catenin as a new prognostic marker of neoplastic progression in T1 superficial urothelial tumors. *Am J Clin Pathol* 2006; **125**:119–26.
116. Lascombe I, Clairotte A, Fauconnet S, *et al.* N-cadherin as a novel prognostic marker of progression in superficial urothelial tumors. *Clin Cancer Res* 2006; **12**:2780–87.
117. Harabayashi T, Kanai Y, Yamada T, *et al.* Reduction of integrin beta4 and enhanced migration on laminin in association with intraepithelial spreading of urinary bladder carcinomas. *J Urol* 1999; **161**:1364–71.
118. Grossman HB, Lee C, Bromberg J, Liebert M. Expression of the alpha6beta4 integrin provides prognostic information in bladder cancer. *Oncol Rep* 2000; **7**:13–6.
119. Watanabe T, Shinohara N, Sazawa A, *et al.* An improved intravesical model using human bladder cancer cell lines to optimize gene and other therapies. *Cancer Gene Ther* 2000; **7**:1575–80.
120. Kausch I, Ardelt P, Bohle A, Ratliff TL. Immune gene therapy in urology. *Curr Urol Rep* 2002; **3**:82–9.
121. Chen F, Zhang G, Iwamoto Y, See WA. Bacillus Calmette-Guerin initiates intracellular signaling in a transitional carcinoma cell line by cross-linking alpha 5 beta 1 integrin. *J Urol* 2003; **170**:605–10.

122. Matsui Y, Assi K, Ogawa O, *et al.* The importance of integrin-linked kinase in the regulation of bladder cancer invasion. *Int J Cancer* 2012; **130**:521–31.
123. Said N, Sanchez-Carbayo M, Smith SC, Theodorescu D. RhoGDI2 suppresses lung metastasis in mice by reducing tumor versican expression and macrophage infiltration. *J Clin Invest* 2012; **122**:1503–18.
124. Kim WJ, Bae SC. Molecular biomarkers in urothelial bladder cancer. *Cancer Sci* 2008; **99**:646–52.
125. Smith SC, Oxford G, Wu Z, *et al.* The metastasis-associated gene CD24 is regulated by Ral GTPase and is a mediator of cell proliferation and survival in human cancer. *Cancer Res* 2006; **66**:1917–22.
126. Konety BC PR. Urothelial carcinoma: Cancers of the bladder, ureter, and renal pelvis. (pp. 308–27) In: Tanagho EA, McAninch JW (eds). *Smith's General Urology*. New York, NY: McGraw-Hill Company, Inc. 2007.
127. Thomas S, Harding MA, Smith SC, *et al.* CD24 Is an effector of HIF-1-driven primary tumor growth and metastasis. *Cancer Res* 2012; **72**(21):5600–12.
128. Overdevest JB, Thomas S, Kristiansen G, Hansel DE, Smith SC, Theodorescu D. CD24 offers a therapeutic target for control of bladder cancer metastasis based on a requirement for lung colonization. *Cancer Res* 2011; **71**:3802–11.
129. Overdevest JB, Knubel KH, Duex JE, *et al.* CD24 expression is important in male urothelial tumorigenesis and metastasis in mice and is androgen regulated. *Proc Natl Acad Sci U S A* 2012; **109**(51):E3588–96.
130. Naor D, Sionov RV, Ish-Shalom D. CD44: structure, function, and association with the malignant process. *Adv Cancer Res* 1997; **71**:241–319.
131. Lokeshwar VB, Block NL. HA-HAase urine test. A sensitive and specific method for detecting bladder cancer and evaluating its grade. *Urol Clin North Am* 2000; **27**:53–61.
132. Lokeshwar VB, Obek C, Pham HT, *et al.* Urinary hyaluronic acid and hyaluronidase: markers for bladder cancer detection and evaluation of grade. *J Urol* 2000; **163**:348–56.
133. Lokeshwar VB, Selzer MG. Differences in hyaluronic acid-mediated functions and signaling in arterial, microvessel, and vein-derived human endothelial cells. *J Biol Chem* 2000; **275**:27641–9.
134. Lokeshwar VB, Obek C, Soloway MS, Block NL. Tumor-associated hyaluronic acid: a new sensitive and specific urine marker for bladder cancer. *Cancer Res* 1997; **57**:773–7.
135. Habuchi T, Marberger M, Droller MJ, *et al.* Prognostic markers for bladder cancer: International Consensus Panel on bladder tumor markers. *Urology* 2005; **66**:64–74.
136. Hautmann SH, Lokeshwar VB, Schroeder GL, *et al.* Elevated tissue expression of hyaluronic acid and hyaluronidase validates the HA-HAase urine test for bladder cancer. *J Urol* 2001; **165**:2068–74.
137. Hautmann SH, Schroeder GL, Civantos F, *et al.* [Hyaluronic acid and hyaluronidase. 2 new bladder carcinoma markers]. *Urologe A* 2001; **40**:121–6.
138. Lokeshwar VB, Schroeder GL, Carey RI, Soloway MS, Iida N. Regulation of hyaluronidase activity by alternative mRNA splicing. *J Biol Chem* 2002; **277**:33654–63.
139. Golshani R, Lopez L, Estrella V, Kramer M, Iida N, Lokeshwar VB. Hyaluronic acid synthase-1 expression regulates bladder cancer growth, invasion, and angiogenesis through CD44. *Cancer Res* 2008; **68**:483–91.
140. Kuncova J, Kostrouch Z, Viale M, Revoltella R, Mandys V. Expression of CD44v6 correlates with cell proliferation and cellular atypia in urothelial carcinoma cell lines 5637 and HT1197. *Folia Biol (Praha)* 2005; **51**:3–11.
141. Kuncova J, Urban M, Mandys V. Expression of CD44s and CD44v6 in transitional cell carcinomas of the urinary bladder: comparison with tumour grade, proliferative activity and p53 immunoreactivity of tumour cells. *APMIS* 2007; **115**:1194–205.
142. Muramaki M, Miyake H, Kamidono S, Hara I. Over expression of CD44V8–10 in human bladder cancer cells decreases their interaction with hyaluronic acid and potentiates their malignant progression. *J Urol* 2004; **171**:426–30.
143. Muramaki M, Miyake H, Kurahashi T, Takenaka A, Inoue TA, Fujisawa M. Prognostic significance of adjuvant cisplatin-based combination chemotherapy following radical cystectomy in patients with invasive bladder cancer. *Int J Urol* 2008; **15**:314–8.
144. Sugino T, Gorham H, Yoshida K, *et al.* Progressive loss of CD44 gene expression in invasive bladder cancer. *Am J Pathol* 1996; **149**:873–82.
145. Garcia del Muro X, Torregrosa A, Munoz J, *et al.* Prognostic value of the expression of E-cadherin and beta-catenin in bladder cancer. *Eur J Cancer* 2000; **36**:357–62.
146. Lipponen P, Aaltoma S, Kosma VM, Ala-Opas M, Eskelinen M. Expression of CD44 standard and variant-v6 proteins in transitional cell bladder tumours and their relation to prognosis during a long-term follow-up. *J Pathol* 1998; **186**:157–64.
147. Hong RL, Pu YS, Chu JS, Lee WJ, Chen YC, Wu CW. Correlation of expression of CD44 isoforms and E-cadherin with differentiation in human urothelial cell lines and transitional cell carcinoma. *Cancer Lett* 1995; **89**:81–7.
148. Hong RL, Pu YS, Hsieh TS, Chu JS, Lee WJ. Expressions of E-cadherin and exon v6-containing isoforms of CD44 and their prognostic values in human transitional cell carcinoma. *J Urol* 1995; **153**:2025–8.
149. Kanayama H. Matrix metalloproteinases and bladder cancer. *J Med Invest* 2001; **48**:31–43.
150. Di Carlo A, Terracciano D, Mariano A, Macchia V. Urinary gelatinase activities (matrix metalloproteinases 2 and 9) in human bladder tumors. *Oncol Rep* 2006; **15**:1321–6.
151. Papathoma AS, Petraki C, Grigorakis A, *et al.* Prognostic significance of matrix metalloproteinases 2 and 9 in bladder cancer. *Anticancer Res* 2000; **20**:2009–2013.
152. Eissa S, Ali-Labib R, Swellam M, Bassiony M, Tash F, El-Zayat TM. Noninvasive diagnosis of bladder cancer by detection of matrix metalloproteinases (MMP-2 and MMP-9) and their inhibitor (TIMP-2) in urine. *Eur Urol* 2007; **52**:1388–96.
153. Monier F, Mollier S, Guillot M, Rambeaud JJ, Morel F, Zaoui P. Urinary release of 72 and 92 kDa gelatinases, TIMPs, N-GAL and conventional prognostic factors in urothelial carcinomas. *Eur Urol* 2002; **42**:356–63.
154. Monier F, Surla A, Guillot M, Morel F. Gelatinase isoforms in urine from bladder cancer patients. *Clin Chim Acta* 2000; **299**:11–23.
155. Grignon DJ, Sakr W, Toth M, *et al.* High levels of tissue inhibitor of metalloproteinase-2 (TIMP-2) expression are associated with poor outcome in invasive bladder cancer. *Cancer Res* 1996; **56**:1654–9.
156. Grossman HB, Tangen CM, Cordon-Cardo C, *et al.* Evaluation of Ki67, p53 and angiogenesis in patients enrolled in a randomized study of neoadjuvant chemotherapy with or without cystectomy: a Southwest Oncology Group Study. *Oncol Rep* 2006; **16**:807–10.
157. Sanchez-Carbayo M, Socci ND, Lozano J, Saint F, Cordon-Cardo C. Defining molecular profiles of poor outcome in patients with invasive bladder cancer using oligonucleotide microarrays. *J Clin Oncol* 2006; **24**:778–89.
158. Wallard MJ, Pennington CJ, Veerakumarasivam A, *et al.* Comprehensive profiling and localisation of the matrix metalloproteinases in urothelial carcinoma. *Br J Cancer* 2006; **94**:569–77.
159. Gakiopoulou H, Nakopoulou L, Siatelis A, *et al.* Tissue inhibitor of metalloproteinase-2 as a multifunctional molecule of which the expression is associated with adverse prognosis of patients with urothelial bladder carcinomas. *Clin Cancer Res* 2003; **9**:5573–81.
160. Reis ST, Leite KR, Piovesan LF, *et al.* Increased expression of MMP-9 and IL-8 are correlated with poor prognosis of bladder cancer. *BMC Urol* 2012;**12**:18.
161. Rodriguez Faba O, Palou-Redorta J, Fernandez-Gomez JM, *et al.* Matrix metalloproteinases and bladder cancer: what is new? *ISRN Urol* 2012; **2012**:581539.

162. Seddighzadeh M, Steineck G, Larsson P, *et al.* Expression of UPA and UPAR is associated with the clinical course of urinary bladder neoplasms. *Int J Cancer* 2002; **99**:721–6.
163. Numahata K, Satoh M, Handa K, *et al.* Sialosyl-Le(x) expression defines invasive and metastatic properties of bladder carcinoma. *Cancer* 2002; **94**:673–85.
164. Al-Sukhun S, Hussain M. Molecular biology of transitional cell carcinoma. *Crit Rev Oncol Hematol* 2003; **47**:181–93.
165. Lipponen P, Eskelinen M. Expression of epidermal growth factor receptor in bladder cancer as related to established prognostic factors, oncoprotein (c-erbB-2, p53) expression and long-term prognosis. *Br J Cancer* 1994; **69**:1120–5.
166. Gorgoulis VG, Barbatis C, Poulias I, Karameris AM. Molecular and immunohistochemical evaluation of epidermal growth factor receptor and c-erb-B-2 gene product in transitional cell carcinomas of the urinary bladder: a study in Greek patients. *Mod Pathol* 1995; **8**:758–64.
167. Chow NH, Liu HS, Lee EI, *et al.* Significance of urinary epidermal growth factor and its receptor expression in human bladder cancer. *Anticancer Res* 1997; **17**:1293–6.
168. Nguyen PL, Swanson PE, Jaszcz W, *et al.* Expression of epidermal growth factor receptor in invasive transitional cell carcinoma of the urinary bladder. A multivariate survival analysis. *Am J Clin Pathol* 1994; **101**:166–76.
169. Sauter G, Haley J, Chew K, *et al.* Epidermal-growth-factor-receptor expression is associated with rapid tumor proliferation in bladder cancer. *Int J Cancer* 1994; **57**:508–14.
170. Theodorescu D, Laderoute KR, Calaoagan JM, Guilding KM. Inhibition of human bladder cancer cell motility by genistein is dependent on epidermal growth factor receptor but not p21ras gene expression. *Int J Cancer* 1998; **78**:775–82.
171. Theodorescu D, Laderoute KR, Gulding KM. Epidermal growth factor receptor-regulated human bladder cancer motility is in part a phosphatidylinositol 3-kinase-mediated process. *Cell Growth Differ* 1998; **9**:919–28.
172. Ravery V, Grignon D, Angulo J, *et al.* Evaluation of epidermal growth factor receptor, transforming growth factor alpha, epidermal growth factor and c-erbB2 in the progression of invasive bladder cancer. *Urol Res* 1997; **25**:9–17.
173. Messing EM, Reznikoff CA. Normal and malignant human urothelium: in vitro effects of epidermal growth factor. *Cancer Res* 1987; **47**:2230–5.
174. Messing EM, Young TB, Hunt VB, Emoto SE, Wehbie JM. The significance of asymptomatic microhematuria in men 50 or more years old: findings of a home screening study using urinary dipsticks. *J Urol* 1987; **137**:919–22.
175. Shibuya M. Vascular endothelial growth factor-dependent and -independent regulation of angiogenesis. *BMB Rep* 2008; **41**:278–86.
176. Crew JP, O'Brien T, Bradburn M, *et al.* Vascular endothelial growth factor is a predictor of relapse and stage progression in superficial bladder cancer. *Cancer Res* 1997; **57**:5281–5.
177. Bouck N, Campbell S. Anti-cancer dividends from captopril and other inhibitors of angiogenesis. *J Nephrol* 1998; **11**:3–4.
178. Campbell CL, Savarese DM, Quesenberry PJ, Savarese TM. Expression of multiple angiogenic cytokines in cultured normal human prostate epithelial cells: predominance of vascular endothelial growth factor. *Int J Cancer* 1999; **80**:868–74.
179. Inoue K, Kamada M, Slaton JW, *et al.* The prognostic value of angiogenesis and metastasis-related genes for progression of transitional cell carcinoma of the renal pelvis and ureter. *Clin Cancer Res* 2002; **8**:1863–70.
180. Shu X, Wu W, Mosteller RD, Broek D. Sphingosine kinase mediates vascular endothelial growth factor-induced activation of ras and mitogen-activated protein kinases. *Mol Cell Biol* 2002; **22**:7758–68.
181. Wu W, Shu X, Hovsepyan H, Mosteller RD, Broek D. VEGF receptor expression and signaling in human bladder tumors. *Oncogene* 2003; **22**:3361–70.
182. Wu XX, Kakehi Y, Nishiyama H, Habuchi T, Ogawa O. elomerase activity in urine after transurethral resection is not a predictive marker for recurrence of superficial bladder cancer. *Int J Urol* 2003; **10**:117–8.
183. Herrmann E, Bogemann M, Bierer S, *et al.* The role of the endothelin axis and microvessel density in bladder cancer - correlation with tumor angiogenesis and clinical prognosis. *Oncol Rep* 2007; **18**:133–8.
184. Herrmann E, Eltze E, Bierer S, *et al.* VEGF-C, VEGF-D and Flt-4 in transitional bladder cancer: relationships to clinicopathological parameters and long-term survival. *Anticancer Res* 2007; **27**:3127–33.
185. Herrmann E, Eltze E, Kopke T, *et al.* [New markers for pharmacological targeting in bladder cancer with lymph node metastasis]. *Aktuelle Urol* 2007; **38**:392–7.
186. Ornitz DM, Itoh N. Fibroblast growth factors. *Genome Biol* 2001; **2**(3):REVIEWS3005.
187. Ricol D, Cappellen D, El Marjou A, *et al.* Tumour suppressive properties of fibroblast growth factor receptor 2-IIIb in human bladder cancer. *Oncogene* 1999; **18**:7234–43.
188. Bernard-Pierrot I, Ricol D, Cassidy A, *et al.* Inhibition of human bladder tumour cell growth by fibroblast growth factor receptor 2b is independent of its kinase activity. Involvement of the carboxy-terminal region of the receptor. *Oncogene* 2004; **23**:9201–11.
189. Oxford G, Owens CR, Titus BJ, *et al.* RalA and RalB: antagonistic relatives in cancer cell migration. *Cancer Res* 2005; **65**:7111–20.
190. Kamai T, Tsujii T, Arai K, *et al.* Significant association of Rho/ROCK pathway with invasion and metastasis of bladder cancer. *Clin Cancer Res* 2003; **9**:2632–41.
191. Ellenbroek SI, Collard JG. Rho GTPases: functions and association with cancer. *Clin Exp Metastasis* 2007; **24**:657–72.
192. Bos JL. Ras-like GTPases. *Biochim Biophys Acta* 1997; **1333**:M19–31.
193. Feig LA. Ral-GTPases: approaching their 15 minutes of fame. *Trends Cell Biol* 2003; **13**:419–25.
194. Gildea JJ, Harding MA, Seraj MJ, Gulding KM, Theodorescu D. The role of Ral A in epidermal growth factor receptor-regulated cell motility. *Cancer Res* 2002; **62**:982–5.
195. Smith SC, Baras AS, Owens CR, Dancik G, Theodorescu D. Transcriptional signatures of Ral GTPase are associated with aggressive clinicopathologic characteristics in human cancer. *Cancer Res* 2012; **72**:3480–91.
196. Scherle P, Behrens T, Staudt LM. Ly-GDI, a GDP-dissociation inhibitor of the RhoA GTP-binding protein, is expressed preferentially in lymphocytes. *Proc Natl Acad Sci U S A* 1993; **90**:7568–72.
197. Nicholson BE, Frierson HF, Conaway MR, *et al.* Profiling the evolution of human metastatic bladder cancer. *Cancer Res* 2004; **64**:7813–21.
198. Seraj MJ, Harding MA, Gildea JJ, Welch DR, Theodorescu D. The relationship of BRMS1 and RhoGDI2 gene expression to metastatic potential in lineage related human bladder cancer cell lines. *Clin Exp Metastasis* 2000; **18**:519–25.
199. Clifford SC, Astuti D, Hooper L, Maxwell PH, Ratcliffe PJ, Maher ER. The pVHL-associated SCF ubiquitin ligase complex: molecular genetic analysis of elongin B and C, Rbx1 and HIF-1alpha in renal cell carcinoma. *Oncogene* 2001; **20**:5067–74.
200. Chai CY, Chen WT, Hung WC, *et al.* Hypoxia-inducible factor-1alpha expression correlates with focal macrophage infiltration, angiogenesis and unfavourable prognosis in urothelial carcinoma. *J Clin Pathol* 2008; **61**:658–64.
201. Deniz H, Karakok M, Yagci F, Guldur ME. Evaluation of relationship between HIF-1alpha immunoreactivity and stage, grade, angiogenic profile and proliferative index in bladder urothelial carcinomas. *Int Urol Nephrol* 2010; **42**:103–7.
202. Ioachim E, Michael M, Salmas M, Michael MM, Stavropoulos NE, Malamou-Mitsi V. Hypoxia-inducible factors HIF-1alpha and HIF-2alpha expression in bladder cancer and their associations with other angiogenesis-related proteins. *Urol Int* 2006; **77**:255–63.
203. Chen WT, Hung WC, Kang WY, *et al.* Overexpression of cyclooxygenase-2 in urothelial carcinoma in conjunction with

tumor-associated-macrophage infiltration, hypoxia-inducible factor-1alpha expression, and tumor angiogenesis. *APMIS* 2009; **117**(3):176–84.

204. Said N, Smith S, Sanchez-Carbayo M, Theodorescu D. Tumor endothelin-1 enhances metastatic colonization of the lung in mouse xenograft models of bladder cancer. *J Clin Invest* 2011; **121**:132–47.
205. Said N, Theodorescu D. Permissive role of endothelin receptors in tumor metastasis. *Life Sci* 2012; **91**:522–7.
206. Black PC, Agarwal PK, Dinney CP. Targeted therapies in bladder cancer—an update. *Urol Oncol* 2007; **25**:433–8.
207. Lee SJ, Lee EJ, Kim SK, *et al.* Identification of pro-inflammatory cytokines associated with muscle invasive bladder cancer; the roles of IL-5, IL-20, and IL-28A. *PloS One* 2012; 7:e40267.
208. Hammam OA, Aziz AA, Roshdy MS, Abdel Hadi AM. Possible role of cyclooxygenase-2 in schistosomal and non-schistosomal-associated bladder cancer. *Medscape J Med* 2008; **10**:60.
209. Alvarez A, Lokeshwar VB. Bladder cancer biomarkers: current developments and future implementation. *Curr Opin Urol* 2007; **17**:341–6.
210. Kawakami K, Enokida H, Tachiwada T, *et al.* Identification of differentially expressed genes in human bladder cancer through genome-wide gene expression profiling. *Oncol Rep* 2006; **16**:521–31.
211. Czachorowski MJ, Amaral AF, Montes-Moreno S, *et al.* Cyclooxygenase-2 expression in bladder cancer and patient prognosis: results from a large clinical cohort and meta-analysis. *PloS One* 2012; 7:e45025.

CHAPTER 6.15

Pathology of bladder and upper urinary tract tumours

Simone Bertz and Arndt Hartmann

Urothelial tumours of the urinary tract

The epithelium of the urinary tract (termed urothelium) lines the renal calyses to the mid-urethra. Tumours arising from this epitehlium share similar etiologies, histopathological features, and prognosis, regardless of anatomical location. As such, they may be discussed together. While the majority of tumours are urothelial carcinoma in histological subtype, up to 10% are either squamous cell, adenocarcinoma or rare tumours (such as lymphoma, sarcoma, melanoma, and so on).[1,2]

Flat lesions of the urinary tract

Flat urothelial hyperplasia

According to the 2004 World Health Organization (WHO) classifcation, urothelial hyperplasia is defined as focal marked thickening of the otherwise mature urothelium due to an increase in the number of cell layers with few or no cytolgical atypia.[3] Flat urothelial hyperplasia may be found in the context of inflammatory and neoplastic changes of the bladder. The concept of urothelial hyperplasia as a premalignant lesion is based on molecular studies showing coincidental genetic alterations in urothelial hyperplasia and concomitant papillary bladder cancer.[4] However, if found separately there is no evidence for a malignant potential of this lesion.

Reactive urothelial atypia

Reactive (inflammatory) atypia is defined as a lesion associated with acute or chronic inflammatory conditions of the urothelium, for example previous therapy, surgery, or bladder stones. Significant changes in cytology and increased mitotic figures may occur. Differential diagnosis from neoplastic changes may be difficult in reactive atypia. Knowledge of the patient history may be helpful for a correct diagnosis.

Urothelial atypia of unknown significance

According to the WHO classifcation of 2004, urothelial atypia of unknown significance represents a descriptive term for cases with severe atypia disproportionate to the grade of inflammation. In these cases, true dysplasia cannot be reliably distinguished from reactive atypia as it is found in acute or chronic inflammation of the urothelium. Cases diagnosed as urothelial atypia of unknown significance would thus benefit from clinical follow-up. According to the literature there is no association with adverse outcomes and the clinical value of diagnosing urothelial atypia of unknown significance is very limited. Therefore, the diagnosis of urothelial atypia of unknown significance should be avoided.

Urothelial dysplasia/low-grade intraurothelial neoplasia

The 2004 WHO classification defines low-grade intraurothelial neoplasia as a flat urothelial lesion with appreciable cytologic and architectural changes which fall short of carcinoma *in situ* (CIS).[3] The importance of this preneoplastic lesion is based on molecuar studies, suggesting that low-grade intraurothelial neoplasia in association with non-invasive papillary urothelial neoplasms would indicate molecular instability and adverse patient outcome. According to the literature progression from *de novo* low-grade intraurothelial neoplasia to bladder neoplasia occurs in up to 19% of cases.[5,6]

Carcinoma *in situ*/high-grade intraurothelial neoplasia

CIS is defined as a non-papillary lesion with malignant cytological changes of the urothelium.[3] Histologically flat urothelium with marked cytological atypia and loss of stratification of the urothelium, without evidence of invasive tumour growth are diagnostic characteristics of CIS (Fig. 6.15.1). Primarily diagnosis of CIS required involvement of the full thickness of the urothelium. The extended definition includes lesions with a preserved umbrella cell layer undermined by otherwise definite CIS.[7] In the last few years immunohistochemistry has become important in diagnosis of CIS.

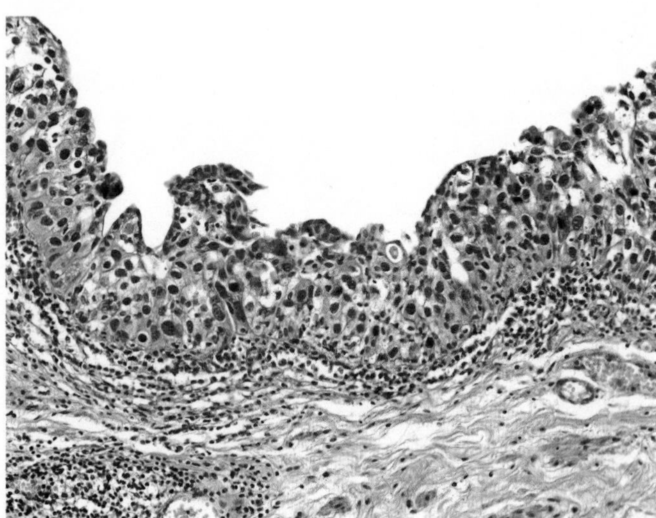

Fig. 6.15.1 Haematoxylin and eosin stain (H&E) of urothelial carcinoma *in situ*, objective ×20.

Especially CK20 has been established as a marker of differentiation of urothelium. In normal urothelium expression of CK20 is confined to umbrella cells. In contrast to this, in CIS there is an aberrant expression pattern of CK20 with usually strong expression in all urothelial cell layers. In some cases of dysplastic urothelium/CIS complete loss of CK20 expression or—in cases of pagetoid CIS—a patchy staining confined to neoplastic cells may be found. In reactive urothelium expression of CK20 may be increased, in equivocal cases additional markers such as CD44 may be used to differentiate between neoplastic and reactive urothelial changes.[8,9] Usually combinations of Ki-67, p53 and CK20 or p53, CD44 and CK20 are used to distinguish CIS and reactive changes of the urothelium.

According to the TNM classification, CIS is classified as pTis, in contrast to non-invasive papillary carcinomas of the urothelium which are classified as pTa (Table 6.15.1 and Table 6.15.2).[10] CIS has a considerable molecular instability and is associated with adverse patient outcome. CIS is frequently found in association with high-grade papillary urothelial tumours, but also rarely occurs as an isolated lesion as primary CIS. The term secondary CIS refers to CIS in patients with previously detected urothelial tumour and the term concurrent CIS refers to CIS concomitant with an exophytic urothelial tumour, whereas the term primary CIS is found in absence of previous or concomitant exophytic tumours.[11] Additionally, primary CIS is frequently associated with urothelial dysplasia.

Preneoplastic urothelial lesions are predominantly 'flat lesions', implicating that detection of those lesions during cystoscopy may be a particular problem. In CIS a patchy erythematous granular or velvety aspect with occasional erosion as well as cystoscopically undetectable lesions have been described. In some cases, additional cytological examination of urine/bladder irrigation may be helpful.

CIS is more frequent in men, where it presents at 60–70 years of age. While about 25% of patients are asymptomatic, other cases present with symptoms of interstitial cystitis (i.e. haematuria, dysuria, pain, nocturia, sterile pyuria).[12] CIS is detected most frequently at the trigone, lateral wall, and bladder dome, and multifocal growth sometimes with extent to the upper urinary tract is frequent.[13]

If untreated, progression of CIS to invasive carcinoma occurs in up to 80% and the mean interval between CIS diagnosis and progression is five years.[14] CIS is more frequent in tumours of higher stage and grade. There is higher risk of progression and cancer specific death in cases with invasive urothelial carcinoma with concomitant CIS compared to primary CIS.[15] In the case of CIS concomitant with non-invasive papillary urothelial carcinoma, outcome does not differ from isolated CIS.[13] In consequence CIS is proven to be the clinically relevant lesion. Furthermore, concomitant CIS has been shown to increase the risk of recurrence after cystectomy in patients with non-muscle-invasive tumour stages and stage pT2-tumours and decrease cancer specific survival in non-muscle-invasive tumour stages.[16] Whether multicentricity of CIS is of clinical importance is still under discussion. However, several studies have shown an association between CIS and a high risk of progression.[15,17] In patients with non-muscle-invasive bladder cancer, concomitant CIS is a risk factor for tumour recurrence in the upper urinary tract.[15] After cystectomy risk of upper urinary tract recurrence has been described to be higher in patients with CIS than in patients with muscle-invasive tumours.[18] An association between concomitant CIS in urothelial bladder cancer and involvement of the urethra has been described for patients who had radical cystectomy and pelvic lymphadenectomy.[16]

Table 6.15.1 2010 TNM classification of urinary bladder cancer[10]

T—Primary tumour	
TX	Primary tumour cannot be assessed
T0	No evidence of primary tumour
Ta	Non-invasive papillary carcinoma
Tis	Carcinoma *in situ*
T1	Tumour invades subepithelial connective tissue
T2	Tumour invades muscle
◆ T2a	◆ Tumour invades superficial muscle (inner half)
◆ T2b	◆ Tumour invades deep muscle (outer half)
T3	Tumour invades perivesical tissue
◆ T3a	◆ Microscopically
◆ T3b	◆ Macroscopically (extravesical mass)
T4	Tumour invades any of the following: prostate, uterus, vagina, pelvic wall, abominal wall
◆ T4a	◆ Tumour invades prostate, uterus, or vagina
◆ T4b	◆ Tumour invades pelvic wall or abdominal wall
N—Lymph nodes	
NX	Regional lymph nodes cannot be assessed
N0	No regional lymph node metastasis
N1	Metastasis in a single lymph node in the true pelvis (hypogastric, obturator, external iliac, or presacral)
N2	Metastasis in multiple lymph nodes in the true pelvis (hypogastric, obturator, external iliac, or presacral)
N3	Metastasis in common iliac lymph node(s)
M—Distant metastasis	
MX	Distant metastasis cannot be assessed
M0	No distant metastasis
M1	Distant metastasis

Used with the permission of the American Joint Committee on Cancer (AJCC), Chicago, Illinois. The original and primary source for this information is the *AJCC Cancer Staging Manual, Seventh Edition* (2010) published by Springer Science+Business Media, LLC (SBM). For complete information and data supporting the staging tables, visit www.springer.com. Any citation or quotation of this material must be credited to the AJCC as its primary source. The inclusion of this information herein does not authorize any reuse or further distribution without the expressed, written permission of Springer SBM, on behalf of the AJCC.

Prostatic involvement by urothelial CIS occurs significantly more frequent in bladder tumours located in the trigone and in cases with CIS of the bladder.[19] According to the TNM classification system of 2010 only direct infiltration of the prostatic stroma is classified T4a. Prostatic CIS even in the case of subepithelial invasion does not justify the classification pT4a.[10]

Histomorphological variants of urothelial CIS have been described, including large cell CIS, pagetoid CIS, denuding CIS, small cell CIS, micropapillary CIS, and CIS with glandular or squamous differentiation. Recognition of most of those variants is of low clinical importance. An association of glandular differentiated CIS with pure invasive adenocarcinoma or micropapillary CIS with micropapillary

Table 6.15.2 2010 TNM classification of the ureter and renal pelvis[10]

T—Primary tumour	
TX	Primary tumour cannot be assessed
T0	No evidence of primary tumour
Ta	Non-invasive papillary carcinoma
Tis	Carcinoma *in situ*
T1	Tumour invades subepithelial connective tissue
T2	Tumour invades muscularis
T3	*(Renal pelvis)* Tumour invades beyond muscularis into peripelvic fat or renal parenchyma*(Ureter)* Tumour invasdes beyond muscularis into periureteric fat
T4	Tumour invades adjacent organs or through the kidney into perinephric fat
N—Lymph nodes	
NX	Regional lymph nodes cannot be assessed
N0	No regional lymph node metastasis
N1	Metastasis in a single lymph node 2 cm or less in greatest dimension
N2	Metastasis in a single lymph node more than 2 cm but none more than 5 cm in greatest dimension, or multiple lymph nodes, none more than 5 cm in greatest dimension
N3	Metastasis in a lymph node more than 5 cm in greatest dimension
M—Distant metastasis	
MX	Distant metastasis cannot be assessed
M0	No distant metastasis
M1	Distant metastasis

Used with the permission of the American Joint Committee on Cancer (AJCC), Chicago, Illinois. The original and primary source for this information is the *AJCC Cancer Staging Manual, Seventh Edition* (2010) published by Springer Science+Business Media, LLC (SBM). For complete information and data supporting the staging tables, visit www.springer.com. Any citation or quotation of this material must be credited to the AJCC as its primary source. The inclusion of this information herein does not authorize any reuse or further distribution without the expressed, written permission of Springer SBM, on behalf of the AJCC.

variant of urothelial carcinoma has not yet been described.[20,21] Subsequent development of prognostically poor subtypes of invasive carcinoma may occur especially in patients with *in situ* adenocarcinoma of the bladder.[20] For therapeutic reasons it is of striking clinical importance to differentiate between pagetoid CIS and extramammary Paget disease extending into the urothelium.

Finally, reactive atypia of the urothelium, frequently following previous inflammation, but also following therapeutic (surgical) intervention or drug-related reactive atypia may mimic CIS. Cytologic atypia and architectural changes in this non-neoplastic urothelium can be marked and may persist for weeks to months after treatment. Information on previous treatment or operative manipulation or irritation is absolutely necessary for the pathologist in order to prevent a misdiagnosis of CIS.

Papillary lesions of the urinary tract

Papillary urothelial hyperplasia

According to the WHO classifcation of 2004 urothelial hyperplasia is defined as focal marked thickening of the otherwise mature urothelium due to an increase in the number of cell layers with few or no cytolgical atypia.[3] Morphological changes of papillary urothelial hyperplasia include undulating folds of normal urothelium with lack of fibrovascular cores and lack of cytolgic atypia.

As flat urothelial hyperplasia papillary hyperplasia may be found in the context of inflammatory and neoplastic changes of the bladder. Especially papillary urothelial hyperplasia is frequently accompanied by papillary bladder tumours. Few genetic studies suggest that papillary urothelial hyperplasia without atypia may be a precursor of low-grade papillary neoplasms.[22] Additionally a few studies suggest papillary urothelial hyperplasia with atypia as a preursor of lesions with molecular instability such as high-grade papillary neoplasms and carcinoma *in situ*.[23]

Urothelial papilloma

The current WHO classification of 2004 defines urothelial papilloma as an usually singular benign urothelial neoplasm with low incidence (1–4%) composed of a delicate fibrovascular core covered by normal urothelium with sometimes metaplastic changes.[3]

The most frequent locations are the posterior or lateral wall close to the ureteric orifices and the urethra. The mean age at diagnosis is 57 years (range 22–89 years), the male to female ratio is 1.9:1.[6] Usually urothelial papillomas occur as *de novo* neoplasms but there are occasional cases of secondary papilloma occurring in patients with history of bladder cancer. Due to their benign behaviour, recurrence rates are low in urothelial papilloma (about 8%).[24]

Diffuse papillomatosis is a rare lesion where most or all of a circumscribed region of the bladder mucosa is covered by multiple papillary processes with minimal or no architectural changes, little or mild nuclear atypia and absence of mitotic figures. There is a typical 'velvety' cystoscopic aspect of the mucosal surface.[25] This lesion may be found in patiens with a known history of papillary bladder tumours. Diffuse papillomatosis is a lesion is of uncertain malignant potential.[15,26]

Inverted urothelial papilloma

Inverted growth, i.e. invagination of sheets and strands of cytologically normal or minimally atypical urothelium into the lamina propria and complete absence of exophytic papillary tumour growth are histomorphologic features essential for the diagnosis of inverted papilloma. If diagnosed according to these strictly defined criteria, inverted papilloma is a benign lesion. Inverted papilloma is a usually singular lesion which occurs more frequently in men with a male to female ratio of 4–5:1. Inverted papillomas account for less than 1% of urothelial neoplasms, recurrence rates are below 1%. Progression to carcinoma is extremely rare if inverted papilloma is diagnosed properly.[3]

Papillary urothelial neoplasia of unknown malignant potential

Papillary urothelial neoplasia of unknown malignant potential (PUNLMP) is defined as a non-invasive papillary urothelial neoplasia with marked thickening of the urothelium similar to urothelial hyperplasia, with minimal or no cytological atypia. This entity has been defined in the WHO classification of 2004 in order to stratify the group of non-invasive papillary carcinoma according to clinical outcome and to prevent a psycosoccial stigmatization of patients who would be otherwise diagnosed with cancer. PUNLMP represents a group of tumours with favourable prognosis due to a mostly benign course of disease, which according to the 1973 WHO grading system would be at the least aggressive end of grade 1 urothelial carcinoma.

However, the concept of PUNLMP is controversial since there is still a risk of progression for this entity of up to 8% and for recurrence of up to 60%.[27,28] To reflect tumour biology some authors propose to replace this entity by low-grade urothelial carcinoma. Diagnosis of PUNLMP is rare and requires extensive histological examination. Prospective clinical trials and molecular studies will be essential to reliably differentiate between lesions which need to be diagnosed and treated as carcinoma.

Malignant epithelial lesions/tumours of the bladder

Grading and staging of bladder cancer

Until recently, urinary bladder cancer was categorized into 'superficial' (pTa, pT1, CIS) and 'invasive' (pT2-4) tumours. This categorization should be abandoned as multiple studies have revealed two genetic subtypes corresponding to high and low-grade categories and significant differences in outcome between stage pTa and pT1 tumours,[29,30] that is, genetically stable tumours including low-grade pTa tumours and genetically instable tumours including high-grade pTa tumours, CIS and invasive urothelial carcinoma (pT1-4) (please see Chapter 6.14, 'Molecular biology of bladder cancer'). Together with early reurrence, size of the tumour, multifocal tumour growth and CIS, histologic grade is an established risk factor associated with tumour recurrence and progression.[31–33] Grade of differentiation is reported according to the WHO classification system which is based on the degree of nuclear atypia and architectural changes of the dysplastic urothelium within the least differentiated area of the tumour.[26] Several grading systems have been introduced during the last years. All of them include papilloma as a separate category, whereas there is no complete correlation between the remaining categories.

The original 1973 WHO grading system was a three-tiered system with well differentiated (G1), moderately differentiated (G2), and poorly differentiated (G3/G4) tumours, based on cytologic and architectural changes of the urothelium as applied to most carcinoma in other anatomical sites. The latest WHO grading system of 2004 is a two-tiered system differentiating between low- and high-grade tumours and additionally introducing the new entity of PUNLMP,[3] which is composed of a part of the former grade 1 group. The group of low-grade tumours of the 2004 grading system consists of the residual grade 1 tumours not defined as PUNLMP and the better differentiated proportion of the grade 2 group. The former grade 3 group represents the new high-grade group together with the poorly differentiated proportion of the grade 2 group (Fig. 6.15.2).

Applying the two-tiered WHO 2004 pathologic grading system of urothelial carcinoma, low-grade cancer represents a relatively indolent tumour confined to the mucosa. Histomorphologically architecture of the urothelium is preserved but cytologic atypia is obvious. Variations in nuclear size, polarity, and shape and mostly basally located mitoses may occur. Long-term follow-up is needed in those patients due to recurrence rates of about 70% and risk of progression and cancer related death of about 5%.[15,34,35]

Papillary high-grade tumours show moderate to severe architectural and cytological changes. Risk of recurrence is about 73% and risk of progression has been documented in about 23% of non-invasive high-grade tumours.

Despite the improvement of interobserver variability for this two-tiered grading system of urothelial cancer, the former 1997 three-tiered WHO grading system has not lost its impact as an established risk factor for the majority of urologists (as it has been validated in most clinical trials and it has been proven as an important parameter contributing to risk tables and consequently therapeutic decisions).[36,37] This is why reporting of both grading systems is recommended by most authors.[15,38] As a result of a combination of both grading systems a 4-tiered grading system (grades 1–4) has been proposed recently with PUNLMP classified grade 1, low-grade tumours classified grade 2 and high-grade tumours classified grade 3 and grade 4, respectively.[15]

Depending on the depth of infiltration within the bladder wall invasive urothelial carcinoma is classified according to the TNM classification system of 2010 (for further information please see https://www.cancerstaging.org).[10] Pathologic stage is the most important predictor of outcome in bladder cancer and the most important factor for therapeutic decisions.[39] Transurethral resection of the bladder (TUR-B) allows accurate staging of bladder cancer up to stage pT2. Substaging into pT2a and pT2b is not possible in the majority of TUR-B specimens, due to the lack of orientation and tangential sectioning in tissue specimens obtained from transurethral resections. The transurethral resection of the bladder specimen should contain parts of the muscularis propria to minimize the risk of understaging of bladder cancer due to a sampling error.[40–42]

Assessment of higher tumour stages requires evaluation of the cystectomy and lymphadenectomy specimen.

Non-invasive papillary urothelial carcinoma—low grade and high grade

Non-invasive papillary urothelial carcinoma is defined as a neoplasm of urothelium lining papillary fronds, which shows low or

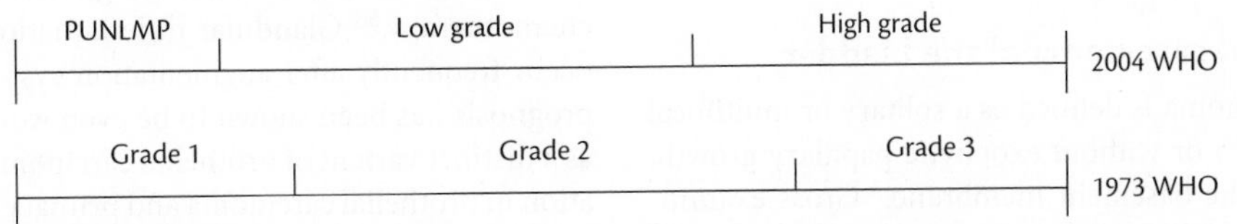

Fig. 6.15.2 Comparison of the 1973 and 2004 WHO grading systems.

Reprinted from *European Urology*, Volume 51, Issue 4, Gregory T. MacLennan *et al.*, Histologic Grading of Noninvasive Papillary Urothelial Neoplasms, pp. 889–898, Copyright © 2007 European Association of Urology, with permission from Elsevier, http://www.sciencedirect.com/science/journal/03022838

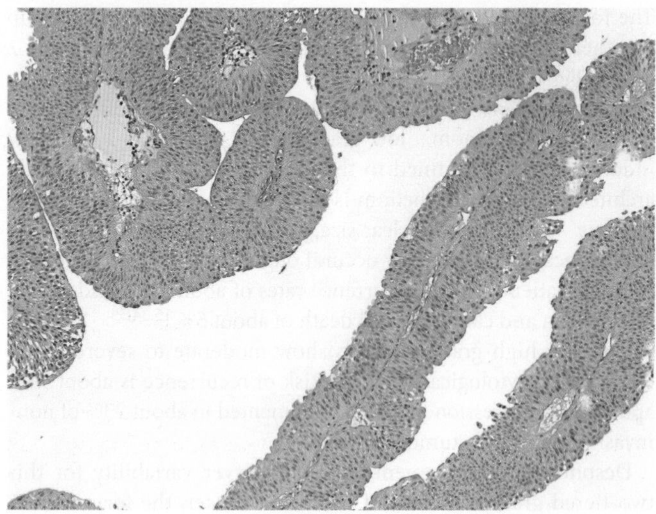

Fig. 6.15.3 H&E of non-invasive papillary urothelial carcinoma (pTa G1/low grade), objective ×5.

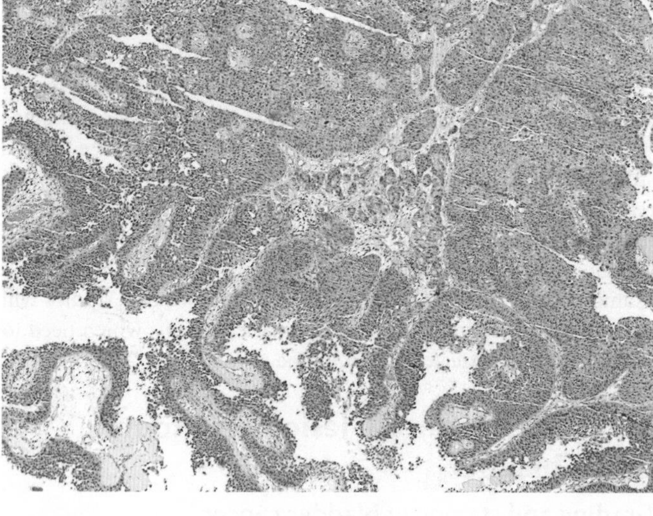

Fig. 6.15.4 H&E of invasive papillary urothelial carcinoma (pT1, G2/high grade), objective ×5.

high-grade architectural and cytological features as described above. Non-invasive papillary urothelial carcinoma comprises about 70% of primary urothelial neoplasms.

The neoplastic urothelium of low-grade non-invasive papillary urothelial carcinoma is characterized by minimal but easily recognizable changes in cytology and architecture. Mitotic figures are infrequent and mostly confined to the lower half of the urothelium (Fig. 6.15.3).

Histomorphological changes of the urothelium in high-grade non-invasive papillary urothelial carcinoma are severe, showing distortion in architecture and prominent cytological atypia. Mitotic figures are frequent and distributed over the whole thickness of the atypical urothelium and may be atypical.

About 70% of low-grade non-invasive papillary urothelial carcinomas will recur and up to 18% of will progress in stage whereas tumour progression in high-grade non-invasive papillary urothelial carcinomas occurs in up to 65%.[3,43] Risk of recurrence and progression has been shown to be higher in large, multifocal, and diffuse tumours.[44,45] Recurrent tumours and those with short disease-free intervals have an even higher risk of another recurrence whereas risk of recurrence has been described to decrease with each normal interval cystoscopy.[3,46] In the case of concurrent CIS, outcome was not influenced by the non-invasive papillary tumour component.[14]

As mentioned above histologic grade is an important prognostic factor regarding recurrence and progression in non-invasive urothelial neoplasia. Anyway there is a substantial difference in survival rates comparing papilloma and PUNLMP with non-invasive papillary urothelial carcinoma, as the former show survival rates comparable with the non-tumour population.[3]

Infiltrating urothelial carcinoma of the bladder

Invasive urothelial carcinoma is defined as a solitary or multifocal urothelial neoplasm, with or without exophytic papillary growth, that infiltrates beyond the basement membrane.[3] Gross examination shows solitary or multifocal tumours with a wide range of appearances including papillary, solid, nodular, polypoid, and ulcerated lesions. Low histologic grade is an exception in invasive urothelial carcinomas and occurs in only about 4% of tumours.[39,47]

Most pTa/pT1 cancers are papillary tumours (Fig. 6.15.4) whereas tumours of higher stages (pT2-4), that is, muscle-invasive tumours, are usually non-papillary tumours (Fig. 6.15.5). Muscle-invasive cancers represent a highly progressive, lethal disease requiring aggressive surgical treatment.[48] About one-third of bladder cancers are muscle-invasive at presentation. About 10–15% of muscle-invasive cancers are derived from preexisting non-muscle-invasive tumours. Some authorities separate these two groups of the invasive tumours (such as the first EAU guidelines).[49]

Subtypes of urothelial carcinoma

Apart from focal squamous and glandular differentiation of urothelial carcinoma, a number of subtypes of urothelial cancer have been described.[50]

These variants usually occur in variable proportions within otherwise urothelial differentiated tumours. Several subtypes may co-exist within one tumour and recognition of most of the subtypes is of clinical importance, due to significantly poorer outcomes in the majority of tumour subtypes.

Squamous differentiation is found in 21% of urothelial carcinoma of the bladder and needs to be distinguished from pure squamous cell carcinoma. Frequency of squamous differentiation increases with higher histologic grade and stage.[50] Poor response to radiotherapy and possibly chemotherapy have been described.[51,52] Low-grade tumours with a focal squamous component have higher recurrence rates.[15]

Glandular differentiation may occur in 6–18% of urothelial carcinomas.[3,53] As in tumours with squamous differentiation, there is an association with higher histologic grade and poor prognosis despite chemotherapy.[53] Glandular differentiation has been described to occur frequently after augmentation cystoplasty. In these tumours prognosis has been shown to be even worse and they are regarded as a distinct variant of urothelial carcinoma.[54] Glandular differentiation in urothelial carcinoma and primary adenocarcinoma are rare lesions. Metastasis from other localizations needs to be ruled out.

Only a few cases of urothelial carcinoma with villoglandular differentiation have been reported. This subtype will be diagnosed in the case of an additional tumour component with villous architecture.

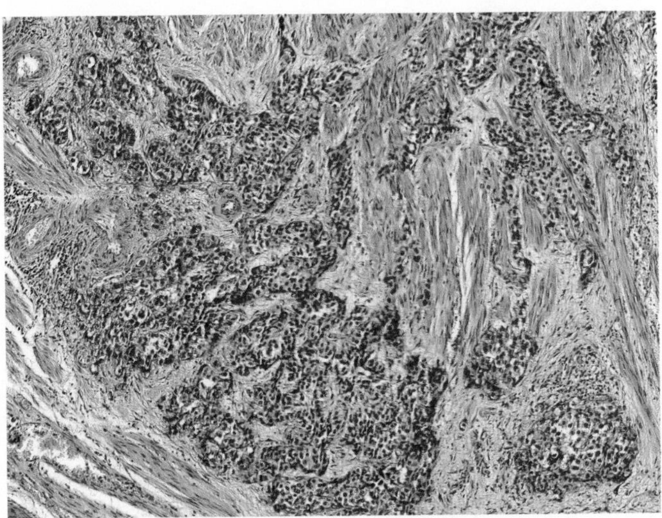

Fig. 6.15.5 H&E of muscle-invasive bladder cancer, objective ×10.

This probably aggressive variant has frequently been described together with cystitis cystica and glandularis. Furthermore, an association with adenocarcinoma of the bladder has been discussed.[55,56] In both glandular and villoglandular subtype recognition of invasive or non-inasive urothelial differentiated areas is essential.

Nested variant of urothelial carcinoma is a rare and highly aggressive variant of urothelial carcinoma associated with poor prognosis. Infiltration of the muscularis propria at the time of diagnosis is frequent and represents an important diagnostic feature of this subtype as typical nuclear and architectural features of malignancy may occur only focally.[57]

The micropapillary variant of bladder carcinoma is usually combined with conventional urothelial carcinoma and identifies an aggressive tumour. Muscle-invasive tumour stages, vascular and/or lymphatic invasion and consequently metastasis at the time of diagnosis are frequent. In the case of non-muscle-invasive micropapillary urothelial carcinoma, a repeat transurethral resection should be considered to exclude a sampling error and consideration to primary radical cystectomy given. Recognition of micropapillary histomorphology is especially important in carcinoma of unknown primary in women without gynecologic tumour.[58,59] Prognosis in micropapillary variant of urothelial carcinoma has been shown to be dependent on the percentage of micropapillary areas and the depth of infiltration (Fig. 6.15.6).[60,61]

Plasmacytoid urothelial carcinoma is another rare histological variant of bladder cancer, characterized by aggressive behaviour with frequent distant metastasis and early recurrence after chemotherapy. Reported frequency rates are about 2%. The nomenclature refers to histomorphological features of this variant as it imitates plasmacytoma cytologically and architecturally due to discoesive growth of the tumour cells. Immunohistochemistry for differential diagnosis especially of plasmacytoma and lobular-invasive breast cancer and diffuse cancers of other anatomic sites (e.g. gastric cancer may be required). Epithelial markers verify the epithelial origin of those tumours and loss of E-Cadherine expression is typical. Only few tumours with pure plasmacytoid histology have been reported.[62] Clinical diagnosis of this subtype is challenging as typical clinical symptoms may be absent.[63] Furthermore these tumours rarely appear as macroscopically identifiable masses. Plasmacytoid urothelial carcinoma usually presents with advanced tumour stages at the time of diagnosis and is frequently associatd with peritoneal dissemination.[64,65] Successful systemic therapy and radical cystectomy has been reported in a few cases only (Fig. 6.15.7).[66]

According to molecular studies primary small cell carcinoma of the bladder is derived from the same clonal population as conventional urothelial carcinoma.[67] Small cell differentiation even if only focally is associated with a dismal prognosis and requires different therapy schemes and therefore should be diagnosed as small cell carcinoma.[3] Metastatic small cell carcinoma from other sites and histomorphological mimics of small cell carcinoma (i.e. lymphoma and others), need to be excluded.

Only few cases of microcystic variant have been described in literature. Despite its glandular aspect, there is no relation to primary adenocarcinoma, but most notably to the nested type of urothelial carcinoma.[15] If there is an association to clinical outcome, it is not yet clear.[65,68]

(A)
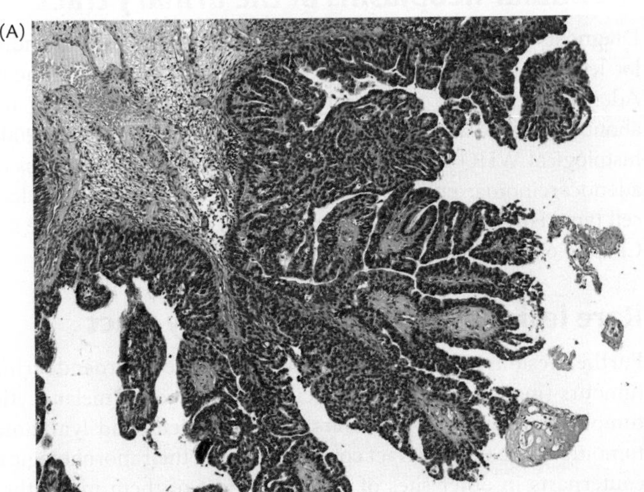

(B)
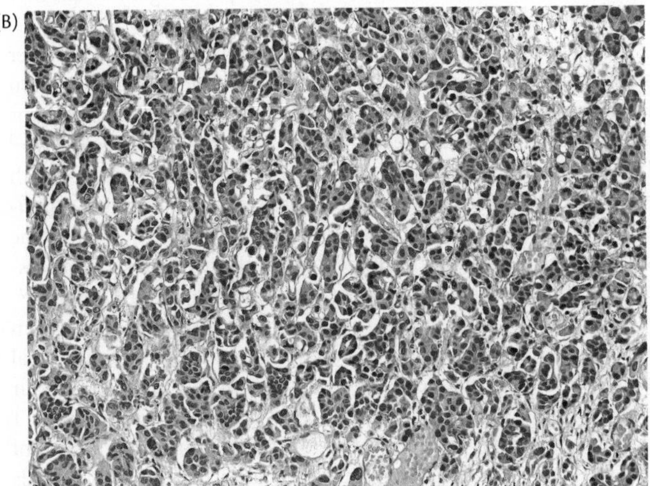

Fig. 6.15.6 H&E of (A) urothelial carcinoma, micropapillary variant, superficial component, objective ×10, H&E; and (B) urothelial carcinoma, micropapillary variant, invasive component, objective ×20.

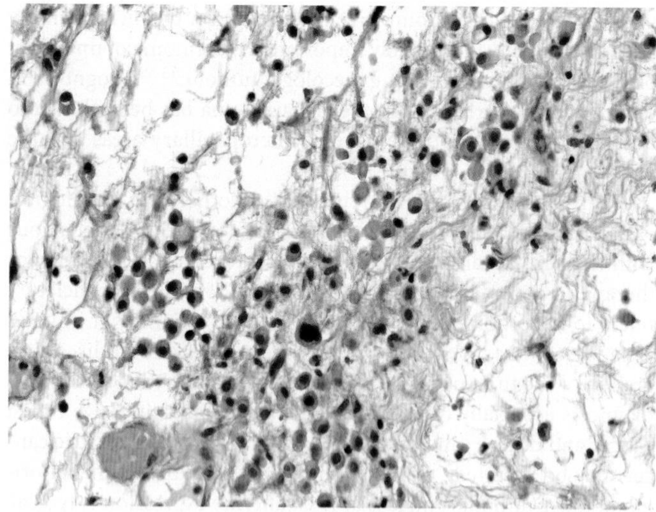

Fig. 6.15.7 H&E of urothelial carcinoma, plasmacytoid variant, objective ×40.

Further variants of urothelial carcinoma, named according to their predominant architectural and cytological features, are lymphoepithelioma-like carcinoma, lymphoma-like carcinoma, sarcomatoid carcinoma, clear cell variant, lipid cell variant, carcinoma with giant cells, carcinoma with trophoblastic differentiation, and undifferentiated carcinoma. Those variants are usually associated with poorly differentiated conventional urothelial carcinoma. Poor patient outcome is typical in most subtypes of bladder cancer.[3]

Risk factors in urothelial carcinoma of the bladder

The 5-year survival rate of muscle-invasive urothelial carcinoma is about 50%.[15] Apart from clinical prognostic factors (i.e.—among others—multifocality and tumour size >3 cm)[69] during previous years, morphological factors have been investigated with regard to their prognostic value, especially within the group of pT1 bladder cancers. Histologic grading according to the three-tiered WHO classification system of 1997 has been shown to have predictive value regarding cancer specific survival in pT1 urothelial bladder cancer. For muscle-invasive tumour stages the prognostic value of histologic grading is limited, as most of those tumours are high grade and G3 tumours, respectively. The pT category is another established prognostic factor.

Concurrent carcinoma *in situ* is associated with tumours of higher stage and grade. Furthermore, lymphatic and/or vascular invasion is associated with shorter survival in pT1 tumours. Margin status after cystectomy has also been shown to be a predictor of prognosis.[3] Lymphovascular invasion has also been shown to be associated with poor outcome independent of histologic grade. It is found significantly more frequently in large non-papillary tumours (>5 cm). One study revealed significantly different survival rates dependent of presence or absence of lymphovascular invasion in stage pT1 tumours.[70]

In pT1 tumours, several methods of substaging have been proposed. Apart from substaging systems based on anatomical structures of the bladder wall, the extent of the invasive tumour component has been investigated. First attempts to substage pT1 tumours based on the infiltration of the anatomical structure of the muscularis propria may in future be displaced by methods measuring the absolute extent of the tumour beyond the basement membrane. This is due to a number of retrospective studies during the last years which revealed significant differences in patient outcome discriminating between focally and extensively invasive pT1 tumours.[71–74]

An association of tumour growth pattern at the invasion front with tumour outcome has been postulated in several publications. Infiltrative growth patterns have been shown to be associated with adverse outcome in those tumours.[75,76] These recently published results need to be confirmed in prospective studies and may in future substantially contribute to the therapeutic decision.

Squamous neoplasms of the urinary tract

Squamous papilloma

This rare benign neoplasm is composed of papillary cores covered by squamous epithelium without cytological atypia. Squamous papilloma usually occurs in elderly women; recurrence is infrequent. Squamous papilloma needs to be distinguished from condyloma accuminatum as association with human papilomavirus (HPV) infection, nuclear accumulation of p53, and aggressive clinical behaviour have only been described for the latter.[77] Further helpful differential diagnostic features of condylomas are association with condyloma of external genitalia, immunosuppression, extensive growth, and multifocality.

Squamous cell carcinoma

Diagnosis of squamous cell carcinoma is defined by a pure squamous lesion (i.e. without any invasive or *in situ* urothelial component).[3] For details on squamous cell carcinoma of the bladder please refer to Chapter 6.23, 'Squamous cell bladder cancer'.

Verrucous carcinoma

Verrucous carcinoma is a rare variant of squamous cell carcinoma, usually, but not always associated with schistosoma-infection.[78,79] There is no evidence for a pathogenetic role of HPV in verrucous carcinoma.[77] Histomorphological features correspond to those of verrucous carcinoma localized at other sites of the body. Unlike conventional squamous cell carcinoma there is a minimal risk of progression despite high recurrence rates.[15]

Glandular neoplasms of the urinary tract

Diagnosis of adenocarcinoma is defined by a pure glandular lesion without any invasive or *in situ* urothelial component. Adenocarcinoma of the bladder is uncommon accounting for about 0.5–2% of all bladder malignancies. According to the 2004 histological WHO classification system there are four subtypes of adenocarcinoma: enteric, mucinous, signet-ring-cell, and clear cell type. For details on adenocarcinoma of the bladder, please see Chapter 6.24, 'Adenocarcinoma of the bladder'.

Rare lesions of the of the urinary tract

Further lesions of the urinary tract comprise neuroendocrine tumours (including small cell carcinoma; see above), melanocytic tumours, mesenchymal tumours, haematopoietic and lymphoid tumours of the urinary tract corresponding to their morphological couterparts in other sites of the body. Most of them may either occur as primary tumours or as secondary tumours in the context of systemic disease.

Metastatic tumours and secondary extension in urinary bladder

There is a broad range of tumours secondarily infiltrating the urinary bladder. Most commonly there is direct invasion from adjacent primary sites in decreasing frequency: colorectal carcinoma, prostatic carcinoma, and carcinoma of the cervix.[80] Metastatic spread is much less frequent and usually located in the bladder neck or trigone. Primary tumours are most frequently located in the stomach, skin, lung, and breast.[81] Most of those tumours are adenocarcinomas and only few secondary tumours have distinctive histomorphological and immunohistochemical features. Patient history and results of clinical examinations are therefore of utmost importance for sufficient diagnosis.

Upper urinary tract tumours

Upper tract tumours comprise tumours of the renal pelvis and ureter. They account for 5–10% of all urothelial carcinomas and occur in less than 10% of patients with bladder tumours.[2,3] The incidence of these tumours is about 0.7 to 1.1 per 100,000 inhabitants.[3] Upper urinary tract tumours are more common in older patients (mean 70 years)[15]; 90% of all upper tract carcinomas are urothelial carcinomas. Localization in the pyelocaliceal system occurs twice as frequent as in the ureter and multifocality is frequent.[3] Another interesting fact is that there are hereditary cases of upper urinary tract urothelial carcinoma occurring in association with hereditary non-polyposis colorectal cancer-syndrome (HNPCC/ Lynch-Syndrome), usually in patients <60 years of age and/or other HNPCC associated cancers in their own history or family history.[82] Benign epithelial tumours comprise urothelial and inverted papilloma, squamous papilloma, and villous adenoma with histomorphological features corresponding to the homonyous lesions in the bladder. For flat urothelial atypia the histomorphological categorization corresponds to that in the bladder.

According to the literature the risk or upper urinary tract recurrence increases in patients with multiple and high-risk tumours.[83] Furthermore, history of bladder cancer and multifocality of upper urinary tract tumours seem to be risk factors for bladder recurrences after surgery for upper urinary tract urothelial cell carcinoma.[84]

Regarding non-invasive and invasive urothelial carcinoma the basic histomorphological features of upper urinary tract tumours are identical to bladder tumours including the entire morphological range of histological subtypes. As in bladder carcinoma, squamous differentiation occurs quite frequently, comprising 44% of all tumours of the renal pelvis. An association between positive margins during cystectomy and upper urinary tract recurrence has been shown.[85]

About 60% of upper urinary tract urothelial carcinomas reveal invasive tumour stages at the time of diagnosis, which is much more frequent than in bladder cancer. Occurrence of tumours of higher histologic grade at the time of diagnosis is also higher compared to bladder tumours.[86,87] Compared to tumours of the bladder there is a different TNM classification and Union for International Cancer Control (UICC) staging system of upper urinary tract tumours mostly due to different anatomical conditions.[10]

As in bladder cancer histological grading is carried out according to the WHO classifications of 1973 and 2004.

The most important prognostic histopathological factors in upper urinary tract cancer are tumour stage, grade, and vascular invasion.[88,89] Muscle-invasive tumours and tumours of histological grade G3 go along with a very poor prognosis with five-year survival rates of less than 50%.[89,90] Further factors of adverse clinical outcome after radical nephroureterectomy are extensive tumour necrosis and solid tumour growth.[91,92] As in bladder cancer concomitant CIS and large size of the tumour are associated with adverse outcomes in organ-confined disease. Intravesical recurrence occurs with a frequency ranging from 15 to 50% after surgery for upper urinary tract tumours, necessitating strict follow-up, especially of patients with risk factors including low-tumour stage and multfocality.[84]

Conclusion

Bladder and urinary tract cancer comprise a wide range of histomorphologic appearances and clinical courses. Apart from histologic grading, staging, multifocality of tumours, and tumour size, histomorphological characteristics such as concomitant CIS, vascular invasion, infiltration patterns, and the extent of the invasive tumour component have become important features for prognostic stratification of tumours. Divergent differentiation is typical for urothelial carcinoma, especially of higher grade and stage. Recognition and correct diagnosis of histomorphological subtypes of bladder cancer is crucial for therapeutic implications and prognosis.

Further reading

Babjuk M, Oosterlinck W, Sylvester R, *et al.* EAU guidelines on non-muscle-invasive urothelial carcinoma of the bladder, the 2011 update. *Eur Urol* 2011; **59**(6):997–1008.

Bates AW, Baithun SI. The significance of secondary neoplasms of the urinary and male genital tract. *Virchows Arch* 2002; **440**(6):640–7.

Bertz S, Denzinger S, Otto W, *et al.* Substaging by estimating the size of invasive tumour can improve risk stratification in pT1 urothelial bladder cancer-evaluation of a large hospital-based single-centre series. *Histopathology* 2011; **59**(4):722–32.

Cheng L, Jones TD, McCarthy RP, *et al.* Molecular genetic evidence for a common clonal origin of urinary bladder small cell carcinoma and coexisting urothelial carcinoma. *Am J Pathol* 2005; **166**(5):1533–9.

Cheng L, López-Beltrán A, Bostwick DG. Bladder Pathology. Hoboken, NJ: Wiley-Blackwell, 2012.

Cheng L, Neumann RM, Bostwick DG. Papillary urothelial neoplasms of low malignant potential. Clinical and biologic implications. *Cancer* 1999; **86**(10):2102–8.

Eble JN, World HH, International AAO. *Pathology and Genetics of Tumours of the Urinary System and Male Genital Organs.* Lyon, France: IARC Press; Oxford University Press (distributor), 2004.

Epstein JI, Amin MB, Reuter VR, Mostofi FK. The World Health Organization/International Society of Urological Pathology consensus classification of urothelial (transitional cell) neoplasms of the urinary bladder. Bladder Consensus Conference Committee. *Am J Surg Pathol* 1998; **22**(12):1435–48.

Fritsche HM, Burger M, Denzinger S, Legal W, Goebell PJ, Hartmann A. Plasmacytoid urothelial carcinoma of the bladder: histological and clinical features of 5 cases. *J Urol* 200; **180**(5):1923–7.

Fujii Y, Kawakami S, Koga F, Nemoto T, Kihara K. Long-term outcome of bladder papillary urothelial neoplasms of low malignant potential. *BJU Int* 2003; **92**(6):559–62.

Holmäng S, Johansson SL. The nested variant of transitional cell carcinoma—a rare neoplasm with poor prognosis. *Scand J Urol Nephrol* 2001; **35**(2):102–5.

López-Beltrán A, Cheng L. Histologic variants of urothelial carcinoma: differential diagnosis and clinical implications. *Hum Pathol* 2006; **37**(11):1371–88.

Olgac S, Mazumdar M, Dalbagni G, Reuter VE. Urothelial carcinoma of the renal pelvis: a clinicopathologic study of 130 cases. *Am J Surg Pathol* 2004; **28**(12):1545–52.

Rhijn BWV, Kwast THVD, Alkhateeb SS, *et al.* A new and highly prognostic system to discern T1 bladder cancer substage. *Eur Urol* 2012; **61**(2):378–84.

Rouprêt M, Catto J, Coulet F, *et al.* Microsatellite instability as indicator of MSH2 gene mutation in patients with upper urinary tract transitional cell carcinoma. *J Med Genet* 2004; **41**(7):e91.

Rouprêt M, Zigeuner R, Palou J, *et al.* EAU Guidelines on Upper Urinary Tract Urothelial Cell Carcinomas [Internet]. 06_UUTUCC.pdf. 2012; Available at: http://www.uroweb.org/guidelines/online-guidelines/ [Online].

Sobin LH. *TNM Classification of Malignant Tumours*. Chichester, UK: Wiley-Blackwell, 2010.

References

1. Jemal A, Bray F, Center MM, Ferlay J, Ward E, Forman D. Global cancer statistics. *CA Cancer J Clin* 2011; **61**(2):69–90.
2. Green DA, Rink M, Xylinas E, *et al.* Urothelial carcinoma of the bladder and the upper tract: disparate twins. *J Urol* 2013; **189**(4):1214–21.
3. Eble JN, World HH, International AAO. *Pathology and Genetics of Tumours of the Urinary System and Male Genital Organs*. Lyon, France: IARC Press; Oxford University Press (distributor), 2004.
4. Obermann EC, Junker K, Stoehr R, *et al.* Frequent genetic alterations in flat urothelial hyperplasias and concomitant papillary bladder cancer as detected by CGH, LOH, and FISH analyses. *J Pathol* 2003; **199**(1):50–7.
5. Zuk RJ, Rogers HS, Martin JE, Baithun SI. Clinicopathological importance of primary dysplasia of bladder. *J Clin Pathol* 1988; **41**(12):1277–80.
6. Cheng L, Darson M, Cheville JC, *et al.* Urothelial papilloma of the bladder. Clinical and biologic implications. *Cancer* 1999; **86**(10):2098–101.
7. Williamson SR, Montironi R, López-Beltrán A, MacLennan GT, Davidson DD, Cheng L. Diagnosis, evaluation and treatment of carcinoma in situ of the urinary bladder: the state of the art. *Crit Rev Oncol Hematol* 2010; **76**(2):112–26.
8. Sobin LH. *TNM Classification of Malignant Tumours*. Chichester, UK: Wiley-Blackwell, 2010.
9. Sylvester RJ, van der Meijden A, Witjes JA, *et al.* High-grade Ta urothelial carcinoma and carcinoma in situ of the bladder. *Urology* 2005; **66**(6 Suppl 1):90–107.
10. Hodges KB, López-Beltrán A, Davidson DD, Montironi R, Cheng L. Urothelial dysplasia and other flat lesions of the urinary bladder: clinicopathologic and molecular features. *Hum Pathol* 2010; **41**(2):155–62.
11. Cheng L, Cheville JC, Neumann RM, Bostwick DG. Natural history of urothelial dysplasia of the bladder. *Am J Surg Pathol* 1999; **23**(4):443–7.
12. Cheng L, Cheville JC, Neumann RM, *et al.* Survival of patients with carcinoma in situ of the urinary bladder. *Cancer* 1999; **85**(11):2469–74.
13. Cheng L, López-Beltrán A, Bostwick DG. *Bladder Pathology*. Hoboken, NJ: Wiley-Blackwell, 2012.
14. Shariat SF, Palapattu GS, Karakiewicz PI, *et al.* Concomitant carcinoma in situ is a feature of aggressive disease in patients with organ-confined TCC at radical cystectomy. *Eur Urol* 2007; **51**(1):152–160.
15. Takenaka A, Yamada Y, Miyake H, Hara I, Fujisawa M. Clinical outcomes of bacillus Calmette-Guérin instillation therapy for carcinoma in situ of urinary bladder. *Int J Urol* 2008; **15**(4):309–13.
16. Solsona E, Iborra I, Ricós JV, Dumont R, Casanova JL, Calabuig C. Upper urinary tract involvement in patients with bladder carcinoma in situ (Tis): its impact on management. *Urology* 1997; **49**(3):347–52.
17. Patel SG, Cookson MS, Barocas DA, Clark PE, Smith JA, Chang SS. Risk factors for urothelial carcinoma of the prostate in patients undergoing radical cystoprostatectomy for bladder cancer. *BJU Int* 2009; **104**(7):934–7.
18. Chan TY, Epstein JI. In situ adenocarcinoma of the bladder. *Am J Surg Pathol* 2001; **25**(7):892–9.
19. Miller JS, Epstein JI. Noninvasive urothelial carcinoma of the bladder with glandular differentiation: report of 24 cases. *Am J Surg Pathol* 2009; **33**(8):1241–8.
20. Taylor DC, Bhagavan BS, Larsen MP, Cox JA, Epstein JI. Papillary urothelial hyperplasia. A precursor to papillary neoplasms. *Am J Surg Pathol* 1996; **20**(12):1481–8.
21. Swierczynski SL, Epstein JI. Prognostic significance of atypical papillary urothelial hyperplasia. *Hum Pathol* 2002; **33**(5):512–7.
22. Magi-Galluzzi C, Epstein JI. Urothelial papilloma of the bladder: a review of 34 de novo cases. *Am J Surg Pathol* 2004; **28**(12):1615–20.
23. Mostofi FK. Pathological aspects and spread of carcinoma of the bladder. *JAMA* 1968; **206**(8):1764–9 passim.
24. Bostwick DG, Mikuz G. Urothelial papillary (exophytic) neoplasms. *Virchows Arch* 2002; **441**(2):109–16.
25. Fujii Y, Kawakami S, Koga F, Nemoto T, Kihara K. Long-term outcome of bladder papillary urothelial neoplasms of low malignant potential. *BJU Int* 2003; **92**(6):559–62.
26. Cheng L, Neumann RM, Bostwick DG. Papillary urothelial neoplasms of low malignant potential. Clinical and biologic implications. *Cancer* 1999; **86**(10):2102–8.
27. Nieder AM, Soloway MS. Eliminate the term "superficial" bladder cancer. *J Urol* 2006; **175**(2):417–8.
28. Bryan RT, Wallace DM. 'Superficial' bladder cancer—time to uncouple pT1 tumours from pTa tumours. *BJU Int* 2002; **90**(9):846–52.
29. Epstein JI, Amin MB, Reuter VR, Mostofi FK. The World Health Organization/International Society of Urological Pathology consensus classification of urothelial (transitional cell) neoplasms of the urinary bladder. Bladder Consensus Conference Committee. *Am J Surg Pathol* 1998; **22**(12):1435–48.
30. Larsson P, Wijkström H, Thorstenson A, *et al.* A population-based study of 538 patients with newly detected urinary bladder neoplasms followed during 5 years. *Scand J Urol Nephrol* 2003; **37**(3):195–201.
31. Malmström PU, Busch C, Norlén BJ. Recurrence, progression and survival in bladder cancer. A retrospective analysis of 232 patients with greater than or equal to 5-year follow-up. *Scand J Urol Nephrol* 1987; **21**(3):185–95.
32. Holmäng S, Hedelin H, Anderström C, Holmberg E, Busch C, Johansson SL. Recurrence and progression in low grade papillary urothelial tumors. *J Urol* 1999; **162**(3 Pt 1):702–7.
33. Holmäng S, Andius P, Hedelin H, Wester K, Busch C, Johansson SL. Stage progression in Ta papillary urothelial tumors: relationship to grade, immunohistochemical expression of tumor markers, mitotic frequency and DNA ploidy. *J Urol* 2001; **165**(4):1124–8; discussion 1128–30.
34. May M, Brookman-Amissah S, Roigas J, *et al.* Prognostic accuracy of individual uropathologists in noninvasive urinary bladder carcinoma: a multicentre study comparing the 1973 and 2004 World Health Organisation classifications. *Eur Urol* 2010; **57**(5):850–8.
35. Sylvester RJ, van der Meijden AP, Oosterlinck W, *et al.* Predicting recurrence and progression in individual patients with stage Ta T1 bladder cancer using EORTC risk tables: a combined analysis of 2596 patients from seven EORTC trials. *Eur Urol* 2006; **49**(3):466–5; discussion 475–7.
36. Babjuk M, Oosterlinck W, Sylvester R, *et al.* EAU guidelines on non-muscle-invasive urothelial carcinoma of the bladder, the 2011 update. *Eur Urol* 2011; **59**(6):997–1008.
37. Cheng L, Montironi R, Davidson DD, López-Beltrán A. Staging and reporting of urothelial carcinoma of the urinary bladder. *Mod Pathol* 2009; **22**(Suppl 2):S70–95.
38. Cheng L, Neumann RM, Weaver AL, Spotts BE, Bostwick DG. Predicting cancer progression in patients with stage T1 bladder carcinoma. *J Clin Oncol* 1999; **17**(10):3182–7.

39. Herr HW. The value of a second transurethral resection in evaluating patients with bladder tumors. *J Urol* 1999; **162**(1):74–6.
40. Trias I, Orsola A, Español I, Vidal N, Raventós CX, Bucar S. [Bladder urothelial carcinoma stage T1: substaging, invasion morphological patterns and its prognosis significance]. *Actas Urol Esp* 2007; **31**(9):1002–8.
41. Cheng L, Neumann RM, Nehra A, Spotts BE, Weaver AL, Bostwick DG. Cancer heterogeneity and its biologic implications in the grading of urothelial carcinoma. *Cancer* 2000;**88**(7):1663–70.
42. Heney NM, Ahmed S, Flanagan MJ, *et al.* Superficial bladder cancer: progression and recurrence. *J Urol* 1983; **130**(6):1083–6.
43. Fitzpatrick JM, West AB, Butler MR, Lane V, O'Flynn JD. Superficial bladder tumors (stage pTa, grades 1 and 2): the importance of recurrence pattern following initial resection. *J Urol* 1986; **135**(5):920–2.
44. Holmäng S, Hedelin H, Anderström C, Johansson SL. The relationship among multiple recurrences, progression and prognosis of patients with stages Ta and T1 transitional cell cancer of the bladder followed for at least 20 years. *J Urol* 1995; **153**(6):1823–6; discussion 1826–7.
45. Messing EM, Vaillancourt A. Hematuria screening for bladder cancer. *J Occup Med* 1990; **32**(9):838–45.
46. López-Beltrán A, Cheng L. Stage pT1 bladder carcinoma: diagnostic criteria, pitfalls and prognostic significance. *Pathology* 2003; **35**(6):484–91.
47. López-Beltrán A, Martín J, García J, Toro M. Squamous and glandular differentiation in urothelial bladder carcinomas. Histopathology, histochemistry and immunohistochemical expression of carcinoembryonic antigen. *Histol Histopathol* 1988; **3**(1):63–8.
48. Martin JE, Jenkins BJ, Zuk RJ, Blandy JP, Baithun SI. Clinical importance of squamous metaplasia in invasive transitional cell carcinoma of the bladder. *J Clin Pathol* 1989; **42**(3):250–3.
49. Sakamoto N, Tsuneyoshi M, Enjoji M. Urinary bladder carcinoma with a neoplastic squamous component: a mapping study of 31 cases. *Histopathology* 1992; **21**(2):135–41.
50. López-Beltrán A, Cheng L. Histologic variants of urothelial carcinoma: differential diagnosis and clinical implications. *Hum Pathol* 2006; **37**(11):1371–88.
51. Sung MT, Zhang S, López-Beltrán A, *et al.* Urothelial carcinoma following augmentation cystoplasty: an aggressive variant with distinct clinicopathological characteristics and molecular genetic alterations. *Histopathology* 2009; **55**(2):161–73.
52. Cheng L, Montironi R, Bostwick DG. Villous adenoma of the urinary tract: a report of 23 cases, including 8 with coexistent adenocarcinoma. *Am J Surg Pathol* 1999; **23**(7):764–71.
53. Lim M, Adsay NV, Grignon D, Osunkoya AO. Urothelial carcinoma with villoglandular differentiation: a study of 14 cases. *Mod Pathol* 2009; **22**(10):1280–6.
54. Holmäng S, Johansson SL. The nested variant of transitional cell carcinoma—a rare neoplasm with poor prognosis. *Scand J Urol Nephrol* 2001; **35**(2):102–5.
55. Amin MB, Ro JY, el-Sharkawy T, *et al.* Micropapillary variant of transitional cell carcinoma of the urinary bladder. Histologic pattern resembling ovarian papillary serous carcinoma. *Am J Surg Pathol* 1994; **18**(12):1224–32.
56. Johansson SL, Borghede G, Holmäng S. Micropapillary bladder carcinoma: a clinicopathological study of 20 cases. *J Urol* 1999; **161**(6):1798–802.
57. Wang JK, Boorjian SA, Cheville JC, *et al.* Outcomes following radical cystectomy for micropapillary bladder cancer versus pure urothelial carcinoma: a matched cohort analysis. *World J Urol* 2012; **30**(6):801–6.
58. Samaratunga H, Khoo K. Micropapillary variant of urothelial carcinoma of the urinary bladder; a clinicopathological and immunohistochemical study. *Histopathology* 2004; **45**(1):55–64.
59. Gaafar A, Garmendia M, de Miguel E, *et al.* [Plasmacytoid urothelial carcinoma of the urinary bladder. A study of 7 cases]. *Actas Urol Esp* 200; **32**(8):806–10.
60. Ro JY, Shen SS, Lee HI, *et al.* Plasmacytoid transitional cell carcinoma of urinary bladder: a clinicopathologic study of 9 cases. *Am J Surg Pathol* 2008; **32**(5):752–7.
61. Dayyani F, Czerniak BA, Sircar K, *et al.* Plasmacytoid urothelial carcinomas—a chemo-sensitive cancer with poor prognosis, and peritoneal carcinomatosis. *J Urol* 2013; **189**(5):1656–61.
62. Fritsche HM, Burger M, Denzinger S, Legal W, Goebell PJ, Hartmann A. Plasmacytoid urothelial carcinoma of the bladder: histological and clinical features of 5 cases. *J Urol* 200; **180**(5):1923–7.
63. Hayashi T, Tanigawa G, Fujita K, *et al.* Two cases of plasmacytoid variant of urothelial carcinoma of urinary bladder: systemic chemotherapy might be of benefit. *Int J Clin Oncol* 2011; **16**(6):759–62.
64. Cheng L, Jones TD, McCarthy RP, *et al.* Molecular genetic evidence for a common clonal origin of urinary bladder small cell carcinoma and coexisting urothelial carcinoma. *Am J Pathol* 2005; **166**(5):1533–9.
65. Leroy X, Leteurtre E, De La Taille A, Augusto D, Biserte J, Gosselin B. Microcystic transitional cell carcinoma: a report of 2 cases arising in the renal pelvis. *Arch Pathol Lab Med* 2002; **126**(7):859–61.
66. Young RH, Eble JN. Unusual forms of carcinoma of the urinary bladder. *Hum Pathol* 1991; **22**(10):948–65.
67. Rodriguez-Alonso A, Pita-Fernandez S, Gonzalez-Carrera J, Nogueira-March JL. Multivariate analysis of survival, recurrence, progression and development of mestastasis in T1 and T2a transitional cell bladder carcinoma. *Cancer* 2002; **94**(6):1677–84.
68. Lopez JI, Angulo JC. The prognostic significance of vascular invasion in stage T1 bladder cancer. *Histopathology* 1995; **27**(1):27–33.
69. Cheng L, Weaver AL, Neumann RM, Scherer BG, Bostwick DG. Substaging of T1 bladder carcinoma based on the depth of invasion as measured by micrometer: A new proposal. *Cancer* 1999; **86**(6):1035–43.
70. Bertz S, Denzinger S, Otto W, *et al.* Substaging by estimating the size of invasive tumour can improve risk stratification in pT1 urothelial bladder cancer-evaluation of a large hospital-based single-centre series. *Histopathology* 2011; **59**(4):722–32.
71. Rhijn BWV, Kwast THVD, Alkhateeb SS, *et al.* A new and highly prognostic system to discern T1 bladder cancer substage. *Eur Urol* 2012; **61**(2):378–84.
72. Brimo F, Wu C, Zeizafoun N, *et al.* Prognostic factors in T1 bladder urothelial carcinoma: the value of recording millimetric depth of invasion, diameter of invasive carcinoma, and muscularis mucosa invasion. *Hum Pathol* 2013; **44**(1):95–102.
73. Denzinger S, Burger M, Fritsche HM, *et al.* Prognostic value of histopathological tumour growth patterns at the invasion front of T1G3 urothelial carcinoma of the bladder. *Scand J Urol Nephrol* 2009; **43**(4):282–7.
74. Jimenez RE, Gheiler E, Oskanian P, *et al.* Grading the invasive component of urothelial carcinoma of the bladder and its relationship with progression-free survival. *Am J Surg Pathol* 2000; **24**(7):980–7.
75. Cheng L, Leibovich BC, Cheville JC, *et al.* Squamous papilloma of the urinary tract is unrelated to condyloma acuminata. *Cancer* 2000; **88**(7):1679–86.
76. Oida Y, Yasuda M, Kajiwara H, Onda H, Kawamura N, Osamura RY. Double squamous cell carcinomas, verrucous type and poorly differentiated type, of the urinary bladder unassociated with bilharzial infection. *Pathol Int* 1997; **47**(9):651–4.
77. Holck S, Jørgensen L. Verrucous carcinoma of urinary bladder. *Urology* 1983; **22**(4):435–7.
78. Bates AW, Baithun SI. The significance of secondary neoplasms of the urinary and male genital tract. *Virchows Arch* 2002; **440**(6):640–7.
79. Bates AW, Baithun SI. Secondary neoplasms of the bladder are histological mimics of nontransitional cell primary tumours: clinicopathological and histological features of 282 cases. *Histopathology* 2000; **36**(1):32–40.
80. Rouprêt M, Catto J, Coulet F, *et al.* Microsatellite instability as indicator of MSH2 gene mutation in patients with upper urinary tract transitional cell carcinoma. *J Med Genet* 2004; **41**(7):e91.
81. Millán-Rodríguez F, Chéchile-Toniolo G, Salvador-Bayarri J, Huguet-Pérez J, Vicente-Rodríguez J. Upper urinary tract tumors after primary

superficial bladder tumours: prognostic factors and risk groups. *J Urol* 2000; **164**(4):1183–7.
82. Azémar MD, Comperat E, Richard F, Cussenot O, Rouprêt M. Bladder recurrence after surgery for upper urinary tract urothelial cell carcinoma: frequency, risk factors, and surveillance. *Urol Oncol* 2011; **29**(2):130–6.
83. Raj GV, Tal R, Vickers A, *et al.* Significance of intraoperative ureteral evaluation at radical cystectomy for urothelial cancer. *Cancer* 2006; **107**(9):2167–72.
84. Rouprêt M, Zigeuner R, Palou J, *et al.* EAU Guidelines on Upper Urinary Tract Urothelial Cell Carcinomas [Internet]. 06_UUTUCC. pdf. 2012; Available at: http://www.uroweb.org/guidelines/online-guidelines/ [Online].
85. Olgac S, Mazumdar M, Dalbagni G, Reuter VE. Urothelial carcinoma of the renal pelvis: a clinicopathologic study of 130 cases. *Am J Surg Pathol* 2004; **28**(12):1545–52.
86. Langner C, Hutterer G, Chromecki T, Winkelmayer I, Rehak P, Zigeuner R. pT classification, grade, and vascular invasion as prognostic indicators in urothelial carcinoma of the upper urinary tract. *Mod Pathol* 2006; **19**(2):272–9.
87. Lehmann J, Suttmann H, Kovac I, *et al.* Transitional cell carcinoma of the ureter: prognostic factors influencing progression and survival. *Eur Urol* 2007; **51**(5):1281–8.
88. Abouassaly R, Alibhai SM, Shah N, Timilshina N, Fleshner N, Finelli A. Troubling outcomes from population-level analysis of surgery for upper tract urothelial carcinoma. *Urology* 2010; **76**(4):895–901.
89. Remzi M, Haitel A, Margulis V, *et al.* Tumour architecture is an independent predictor of outcomes after nephroureterectomy: a multi-institutional analysis of 1363 patients. *BJU Int* 2009; **103**(3):307–11.
90. Zigeuner R, Shariat SF, Margulis V, *et al.* Tumour necrosis is an indicator of aggressive biology in patients with urothelial carcinoma of the upper urinary tract. *Eur Urol* 2010; **57**(4):575–81.
91. Pieras E, Frontera G, Ruiz X, Vicens A, Ozonas M, Pizá P. Concomitant carcinoma in situ and tumour size are prognostic factors for bladder recurrence after nephroureterectomy for upper tract transitional cell carcinoma. *BJU Int* 2010; **106**(9):1319–23.
92. Terakawa T, Miyake H, Muramaki M, Takenaka A, Hara I, Fujisawa M. Risk factors for intravesical recurrence after surgical management of transitional cell carcinoma of the upper urinary tract. *Urology* 2008; **71**(1):123–7.

CHAPTER 6.16

Screening for bladder cancer

Maree Brinkman and Maurice Zeegars

Introduction to screening for bladder cancer

In 1968, Wilson and Jungner proposed criteria for the successful implementation of disease screening programmes.[1] Specifically, effective screening required a cost-efficient, accurate safe test, which could be applied to a definable, compliant population, to detect a disease whose natural history may be altered by earlier detection and treatment. The goal of screening is to reduce disease-specific mortality, but screening may lead to over diagnosis of indolent disease, provide false reassurance to patients with false negative results, and may be harmful to the individual. Finally, screening is expensive to healthcare providers and only provides a public health benefit if high compliance rates are achieved in the target population. Consequently, in most countries, population screening is only recommended when benefits outweigh risks, such as for cervical, breast and colorectal cancers (see Table 6.16.1).

To date, there are no known screening programmes of asymptomatic individuals for bladder cancer (BC) anywhere in the world. This is despite the fact that BC ranks as the ninth most common malignancy worldwide, is one of the most expensive to treat and manage, has clearly identified aetiological associations (please see Chapter 6.13 for a bladder cancer overview and aetiology)[2,3] and at-risk populations, and that disease outcomes have not improved over the last 25 years.[4] suggesting the need to downstage tumours at diagnosis. Furthermore, the ease of access to representative biological fluids (urine) makes it a promising target of non-invasive screening. There are a range of urinary-based tests available for the detection and diagnosis of BC in those presenting with haematuria, irritative voiding symptoms, or who have a history of the disease. While BC screening may reduce mortality,[5–7] the United States Preventive Services Task Force recently concluded there was insufficient data to reach a conclusion regarding the benefit of this approach.[8] The main problem with BC screening is the identification of a sufficiently high-risk population to justify the cost. This is true given the prevalence of the main aetiological factors: namely cigarette smoking, pollution and occupational chemical exposure, and the highest risk groups, namely elderly males. This problem could be overcome if high-risk groups were defined using epidemiologic and genetic risk factors.[9] Here we will review screening for BC in the context of the Wilson and Jungers criteria.

Screening tests

An ideal screening test should be safe and acceptable to the patient, reliable and replicable technologically, economically affordable, and accurate (measured with sensitivity and specificity, and so on). For BC, most developed tests have assessed urinary contents for cancer-specific biomarkers. They are safe and acceptable to patients but may not be sufficiently robust or reliable in disease detection.

Haematuria

Urinalysis to test for haematuria, is one of the most common and least invasive of any initial screening test for bladder cancer. It has been reported that approximately 85% of BC cases present with visible haematuria.[10] Detection rates for BC are not as high for non-visible (microscopic or dipstick) haematuria, which requires the use of reagents/indicators or a microscope to test for blood in the urine. Non-visible haematuria can be identified from a positive dipstick test where the presence of haemoglobin causes the indicator to change colour, or the presence of more than three erythrocytes (red blood cells—RBCs) per high powered field from urine specimens.[11]

While the sensitivity of haematuria for BC is high, specificity is lower due to other factors producing haematuria, including urinary tract infection, nephrologic conditions (commonly IgA nephropathy), menstruation, and even dehydration.[11] Population-based screening studies report 16% to 24% of men <50 yrs have haematuria.[12] Dipsticks detect red blood cells using the peroxidase-like properties of haemoglobin to oxidize a chromogen, resulting in a colour change. Consequently, false positive results may be produced by other peroxidases (e.g. myoglobin or other oxidizing agents), and less commonly interfering agents (e.g. ascorbic acid) may cause false negative results. Haematuria does not automatically equate to a malignancy, neither does its absence necessarily exclude the possibility of BC. Haematuria may also be intermittent and require testing repeatedly across several time intervals before it is detected.[5] As weekly haematuria testing is impractical on a wide scale basis, it is suggested daily tests for 10-14 days every 6–12 months are a compromise for disease detection.[13]

A prospective analysis of urological patients from the United Kingdom, reported that 18.9% of the 948 patients with macroscopic haematuria were found to have BC on cystoscopy compared with only 4.8% confirmed BC cases of the 982 patients presenting with microscopic haematuria.[14] Furthermore, detection rates were typically higher for older individuals (>50 years) in both groups and for females (16%) compared with males (4%) among the patients with microscopic haematuria.

The effectiveness of a haematuria home screening program for healthy men 50 years and older using a chemical reagent strip (Ames Hemastix) was compared with a state-wide population-based sample of men the same age from a US tumour registry.[5] Similar proportions of low-grade superficial versus high-grade or invasive cases were found in both groups however, the proportion

Table 6.16.1 Screening recommendations and evidence for bladder, breast, cervix, and colorectal cancer screening, based on NCI's physician data query (PDQ) cancer information summary

Cancer type		Bladder cancer	Breast cancer	Cervix cancer	Colorectal cancer
European Union Recommendation		None	Mammography screening for breast cancer in women aged 50 to 69	Pap smear screening for cervical cancer precursors starting not before the age of 20 and not later than the age of 30	Faecal occult blood screening for colorectal cancer in men and women aged 50 to 74
Benefits		There is inadequate evidence to determine whether screening for bladder and other urothelial cancers has an impact on mortality	Based on fair evidence, screening mammography in women aged 40 to 70 years decreases breast cancer mortality. The benefit is higher for older women, in part because their breast cancer risk is higher	Based on solid evidence, regular screening of appropriate women for cervical cancer with the Pap test reduces mortality from cervical cancer. Screening is not beneficial in women older than 60 years if they have had a history of recent negative tests	Based on solid evidence, screening for colorectal cancer reduces colorectal cancer (CRC) mortality, but there is little evidence that it reduces all-cause mortality, possibly because of an observed increase in other causes of death
Description of the evidence	Study design	There are no studies that directly address this question	Meta-analysis of individual data from four randomized controlled trials and three additional RCTs	Population-based and cohort studies	Randomized controlled trials and case–control studies
	Internal validity	N/A	RCTs: varies from poor to goodMeta-analysis: good	Good	Good
	Consistency	N/A	Fair	Good	Good
	Magnitude of effects on health outcomes	N/A	Cancer-specific mortality is decreased by 15% for follow-up analysis and 20% for evaluation analysis. Absolute mortality benefit for women screened annually starting at age 40 years is 4 per 10,000 at 10.7 years. The comparable number for women screened annually starting at age 50 years is approximately 5 per 1,000. Absolute benefit is approximately 1% overall but depends on inherent breast cancer risk, which rises with age	Regular Pap screening decreases cervix cancer incidence and mortality by at least 80%	15–33% reduction in mortality for faecal occult blood testing (FOBT), 60–70% for left colon using colonoscopy
	External validity	N/A	Good	Good	Fair

Harms		Based on fair evidence, screening for bladder and other urothelial cancers would result in unnecessary diagnostic procedures with attendant morbidity	Treatment of insignificant cancers (overdiagnosis, true positives) can result in breast deformity, lymphedema, thromboembolic events, new cancers, or chemotherapy-induced toxicities	Regular screening with the Pap test leads to additional diagnostic procedures and treatment for low-grade squamous intraepithelial lesions (LSIL), with long-term consequences for fertility and pregnancy. These harms are greatest for younger women	Reguar screening with FOBT results in a high rate of false positive test that can lead to further invasiev diagnostic procedures (colonoscopy, flexible sigmoidoscopy)
Description of the Evidence	Study design	Opinions of respected authorities based on clinical experience, descriptive studies, or reports of expert committees	Descriptive population-based studies	Cohort or case–control studies	RCT and case–control studies
	Internal validity	N/A	Good	Good	Good
	Consistency	N/A	Good	Good	Good
	Magnitude of effects on health outcomes	Good evidence for rare harms	Overdiagnosis in 33% of cancer detected, 50% additional testing in 50% of women over 10 years, 25% of whom will have biopsy, 6–46% of invasive cancer will have false negative mammograms, radiation induced cancer estimated between 10–32/10,000 exposed to a cumulative dose of 1 Sv	Additional diagnostic procedures were performed in 50% of women undergoing regular Pap testing. Approximately 5% were treated for LSIL. The number with impaired fertility and pregnancy complications is unknown	Low PPV for the FOBT with 80% of false positives tests. Clinically significant complications can occur with colonosopy and sigmoidoscopy but are rare. They include perforations, bleeding, cardiovascular events, and other adverse events are rare
	External validity	N/A	Good	Good	Good

N/A: Not applicable; RCT: Randomized controlled trial.

Reprinted from *European Urology*, Volume 63, Issue 6, Stéphane Larré *et al.*, 'Screening for Bladder Cancer: Rationale, Limitations, Whom to Target, and Perspectives', pp. 104–58, Copyright © 2013, European Association of Urology, with permission from Elsevier, http://www.sciencedirect.com/science/journal/03022838

of late-stage disease was lower in the screened patients. At 14 years of follow-up, 20.4% of the tumour registry patients had died from BC compared with none of the participants with BC detected by screening.[5]

Urinalysis for haematuria is inexpensive and without adverse side effects, but a low positive predictive value (PPV) of around 8% limits its effectiveness as a routine screening tool, particularly as a one-off test.[5] Messing *et al.* showed it is an acceptable test to the population as most (97.7%) subjects completed ≥10 of 14 repeated tests.[15]

Urine cytology

Following haematuria analysis, the next simplest test is to examine the cellular appearance of urinary cells. These are usually obtained by spontaneous voiding, but can be retrieved by bladder washing (so-called barbotage).[16] Urinary samples are centrifuged to concentrate the cells, which are then fixed in alcohol and stained using the Papanicolaou technique.[11] Due to the potential for cytolysis, specimens that have been stored in the bladder overnight (first voided urine of the morning) or stored in a collection container for several hours should not be used for cytological analysis.[17]

Cytopathologists identify and classify exfoliated cells as either normal, atypical/indeterminate, suspicious, or malignant.[18] High-grade urothelial carcinoma cells (UCC) from exophytic tumours or carcinoma *in situ* (CIS) are more abnormal in appearance than low-grade cells, and so their presence is usually detected and often indicative of malignancy.[11] Compared with normal urothelial cells, tumour cells have a higher nuclear to cytoplasmic ratio, hyperchromatic and eccentrically located nuclei, and prominent nucleoli.[11] In high-grade UCC, cytology has a high specificity and sensitivity. Low-grade UCC more closely resembles normal urothelial cells[11] and so these tumours are often missed by cytology. This contributes to cytology's relatively low sensitivity rate (34%), combined with the different evaluation criteria used between cytopathologists.[16,19] Classification of cells may be complicated by previous treatments such as chemotherapy/radiotherapy, particularly within the past 12 months, cytotoxic drugs such as cyclophosamide, or other urological/nephrological conditions.[11] Generally, however, urinary cytology has a specificity reported to be very high (99%) and so a positive cytology result should be investigated as this can indicate a malignancy in a majority of patients, especially those with high-grade tumours.[17,19]

Cytology is widely used and considered to be the best available non-invasive screening test for BC.[16] It performs better at detecting high-grade tumours but has poorer detection rates, sensitivity, and specificity for well and moderately differentiated cells, which might make it an inappropriate test for screening the general population. Some authors suggest that the detection of low-grade UCC is not vital in screening programmes, as these rarely cause mortality (reviewed in[9]). The performance of cytology can be improved when used in conjunction with other biomarkers.[16]

New urine biomarkers

There are several novel or experimental soluble and cell-based urine biomarkers that have been reported and introduced for the clinician. These have been developed for potential use as either a replacement or to be used in conjunction with traditional screening tests.[20] Of these, the most mature are the NMP22 test and fluorescence *in situ* hybridization (FISH) for chromosomal alterations (UroVysion®).

Nuclear matrix protein 22 (NMP22)

Among the promising group of new urine biomarkers that have been approved by the United States Food and Drug Administration (FDA) for use in screening and monitoring of patients with a history of BC is Nuclear matrix protein 22 (NMP22).[16] This nuclear protein regulates cellular mitotic activity and is measured quantitatively using an enzyme-linked immunosorbent assay (ELISA) in the NMP22 BC Test®. Alternatively the qualitative NMP22 BladderChek Test® is a point of care test kit. There have been reports of NMP22 levels being five times higher in BC patients compared with those without a bladder tumour.[21] Elevated levels, however, can also be due to many other non-malignant conditions as well. A recent systematic review of the existing literature reported that NMP22 has a relatively high sensitivity of 68% for bladder cancer but the specificity was only 79%.[22] A study from a Veterans' Affairs urology practice compared the performance of NMP22 to cytology and office cystoscopy procedures over one year.[23] The authors reported a similar specificity for NMP22 (96%) compared with cytology (97%) both of which were higher than cystoscopy (88%). NMP22 also had a higher sensitivity (51% vs. 35%) and was cheaper than cytology ($8,750 vs. $52,500 for the same group).[23] This study suggests that NMP22 could be a useful test for the detection of lower grade tumours as an adjunct to cytology. Of note, NMP22 point of care testing is approved by the FDA only in combination with cystoscopy.

Bladder tumour antigen

The bladder tumour antigen (BTA) test can detect the human complement factor H-related protein which is produced and secreted by BC cells.[16] This biomarker can be measured in the BTA stat® point of care qualitative immunoassay and the quantitative BTA TRAK® ELISA.[16] These assays have both been approved by the FDA for surveillance of BC when used in conjunction with cystoscopy.[16] A clinical cohort of 126 subjects reported that BTA had a sensitivity of 72% and specificity of 53% for detecting BC.[24] These results vary from those reported from a follow-up study on BC (FinnBladder studies) which found that from 501 voided urine samples BTA had 56% and 85.7% sensitivity and specificity, respectively.[25] While BTA is more sensitive than urinary cytology, false positives can result from the presence of infection, inflammation, and haematuria.[25]

UroVysion®

UroVysion® is a cytogenetic biomarker for BC that uses fluorescence *in situ* hybridization to detect aneuploidy for chromosomes 3, 7, and loss of 9p21 locus of the P16 tumour suppressor gene.[26] UroVysion® was approved for use by the FDA in 2001 to monitor BC recurrence and as a screening test for patients with haematuria but with no history of BC in 2005.[27] Results from the UroScreen Study consisting of 1,609 subjects indicated that FISH with a specificity of 96.97% and a negative predictive value of 99.26% is comparable to cytology in terms of detecting BC.[26]

ImmunoCyt™

ImmunoCyt™ has been approved for BC surveillance. This test combines cytology with an immunofluorescence for two mucin-like antigens and high molecular weight glycosylated carcinoembryonic antigen.[16] A sensitivity of 82% (76–89%) and specificity of

85% (71–85%) for ImmunoCyt's have been reported in a pooled analysis.[22] The interpretation of ImmunoCyt requires specialized laboratory technicians, limiting this test's clinical application.[16]

Minichromosome maintenance proteins

The minichromosome maintenance (MCM) family of proteins (MCM proteins 2–7 collectively) are involved in DNA synthesis and are highly expressed in proliferating cells making them other potential biomarkers for detecting BC.[28] The levels of MCM proteins can be measured in urine sediments using an immunofluorometric assay.[28] A prospective blinded observational study of 1,677 patients undergoing investigation for urinary tract malignancy reported that BC was detected with 69% sensitivity and a 93% negative predictive value (NPV) using Mcm5.[28] This study compared Mcm5 with NMP22 and found both biomarkers shared similar strengths and limitations. Gender differences were also reported in the performances of both tests.[28] Furthermore, the combined use of the two tests increased detection rates of almost all advanced BC cases to around 95% of clinically significant disease.[28]

Another study reported using immunocytochemistry to test urine samples from 497 patients attending a urological clinic for MCM protein 2.[29] These patients presented with either gross haematuria or were undergoing cystoscopic surveillance. BC was detected with 81.3% sensitivity, 76% specificity, and a 92.7% NPV for the group presenting with gross haematuria. Sensitivity, specificity, and the NPV were 62.3%, 89.9% and 89.9% for the patients undergoing cystoscopy, respectively.[29]

Other novel urinary biomarkers that are also emerging but still under investigation are: additional nuclear matrix proteins BLCA-1 and BLCA-4, cytokeratins that are overexpressed in BC and can be detected by ELISA or RT-PCR; hyaluronic acid (promotes cell adhesion) and hyaluronidase (breaks down hyaluronic acid) both of which can be measured by ELISA-like assays; survivin which is an inhibitor of apoptosis and is measured by RT-PCR; telomerase, fibrin degradation products, DD23 monoclonal antibody, and Lewis X antigen.[30]

Cystoscopy and imaging studies

Cystoscopy is considered the gold standard diagnostic tool for detecting BC either alone or in conjunction with other tests.[16] Haematuria, positive urine cytology, or biomarker results should all be followed up with a detailed cystoscopic examination.[31] Patients who present with urgency, frequency, nocturia, and urge incontinence should also undergo cystoscopic investigation as these voiding symptoms can indicate an underlying malignancy, especially for CIS tumours.[31] Cystoscopy is used to detect the presence, location, and number of initial and recurrent tumours.[17] It also guides the urologist during transurethral resections of bladder tumours.

Flexible cystoscopy and rigid white light cystoscopy are widely used for the diagnosis and surveillance of BC.[28] Traditional white light cystoscopy, however, is thought to lack the sensitivity of hexaminolevulinate fluorescence cystoscopy to detect small flat lesions (e.g. CIS).[32] Cystoscopy is also invasive, uncomfortable, expensive and reportedly can cause infection in up to about 5% of cases.[33] According to best practice guidelines of the American Urological Association cystoscopy should be avoided in patients at low risk of UCC with imaging preferably preceding this procedure.[34]

Computerized tomography, magnetic resonance imaging, intravenous urography, and ultrasonography are the more commonly used imaging tests for diagnostic rather than for screening purposes.[34] These modalities are often conducted in conjunction with cystoscopy and are useful in assessing the presence of upper tract tumours that can be present in patients with a history of BC.[34] Some urologists recommend annual urography in high-risk BC patients.

Bladder cancer as a screening target

The outcome from BC has not improved for 20–30 years, suggesting the need to introduce attempts to down stage the disease at diagnosis (through screening) or to identify better treatments.[4] Diseases that make suitable targets for screening should be serious (either cause death or severe disability), have a known natural history (e.g. a non-invasive stage that progresses to invasion) and have an early, identifiable stage that can be treated to alter its natural history. Ideally, the disease should also be common. In 2008 there were an estimated 386,300 newly diagnosed cases and 150,200 deaths due to BC worldwide.[35] BC is a heterogeneous disease, with distinct molecular pathways.[36,37] Around two-thirds of tumours are low-grade and non-invasive (low risk) tumours. These may cause symptoms and bother, but only very rarely cause death (<5%). Therefore, early detection of these tumours is unnecessary. The remaining one-third of BCs are of high grade. These may present with or before the onset of muscle invasion. Early radical treatment of high-grade non-muscle-invasive (NMI) or invasive BC before the onset of metastasis, is known to prevent BC deaths and alter the natural history of this aggressive cancer. Therefore, detection of BC through screening should be targeted towards high-grade disease.[17,37]

One problem with asymptomatic population screening is the detection of incidental or latent cancers. These tumours are slow growing and would not have presented clinically within the owner's lifetime. The detection of incidental tumours (and their subsequent treatment) is an adverse outcome of a screening programme and should be avoided if possible. While breast and prostate cancers have a large proportion of incidental disease within the general population, this does not appear true of BC. Incidental BC is rarely found at autopsy.[38,39]

One of the key factors for health providers to consider with screening is a cost-benefit analysis. BC is currently ranked the ninth most common malignancy worldwide, but is one of the most expensive to manage.[40,41] The cost of BC was estimated in 2001 as being between $96,000 and $187,000 per patient (US dollars).[3] In 2002, the British government spent £55.4M on BC.[42] Much of this money is spent on managing patients with advanced disease. Hence the early detection of aggressive cancers, and the cheaper cost of treating localized BCs would favour screening.

Populations to screen

It is important to identify a population with sufficient background cases (prevalence) of a disease to make screening an economically viable proposal. For bladder cancer, one can consider the entire general population, a selection of the general population or focus upon persons exposed to known bladder carcinogens.[43]

Screening the general population for bladder cancer

There are two large reported studies of BC screening within the general population (reviewed in[9]). The first study screened 1,575

North American men for dipstick haematuria for 14 consecutive days, twice (nine months apart). Men (283 in total) with haematuria underwent cystoscopy. In total, 21 BCs were diagnosed (including one with muscle invasion).[44] The stage at diagnosis and BC specific survival was favourable in screened men when compared to a matched unscreened cohort of 509 men from the local cancer registry. Specifically, screened men were ten times less likely to be diagnosed with muscle-invasive cancer (4.8% vs. 45.5% (unscreened men)). Screened men also had a lower BC mortality (0% vs. 20.4% (unscreened men)) than the general population.[5]

In the second study, Britton *et al.*[45] tested 2,356 British men (aged 60–85) for haematuria using dipsticks (weekly for 10 weeks). Urine testing was positive in 20% of men (vs. 16% in[44]) and BC diagnosed in 17. No men with muscle-invasive BC were found, but more than half (9 out of 17) had high-grade non-muscle-invasive tumours. No comparisons with unscreened men were made. With follow-up, the impact on survival was not as favourable as in[44], as more than half of the high-risk patients (five out of nine) progressed to a muscle-invasive cancer and three died from BC.[46] This high BC mortality rate suggests that understaging or under-treatment within this population.

Hedelin *et al.*[47] screened 1,096 men (aged 60–70) through random mailing invitation for BC using dipstick haematuria testing and a bladder tumour biomarker (UBC). Non-visible haematuria was present in around a quarter of men and further investigation was restricted to men with either urinary bother (defined as an IPSS score >10) or a positive UBC test or more than 25 RBC/μl. In total, 7 BC were detected (0.6%) in current or ex-smokers.

As seen in these reports, the background rate of BC is low in the general, asymptomatic population (even when restricted to men over 60 years of age). Screening for BC in the general population is therefore not viable.[48]

Screening high-risk fractions within the general population

To alter the disease-specific survival within a population, screening needs to capture most high-grade non-metastatic BCs in a population. This population should be at high risk, to make screening economically viable, and could be defined using known aetiological factors for BC. These factors primarily include increasing age, male gender, cigarette smoking, and occupational carcinogen exposure.

Cigarette smoking is the most common acquired risk factor for BC. It is estimated that smoking accounts for approximately 50% of BC in men and 30% in women.[49] Cessation of smoking is reported to reduce the risk of BC and to lower subsequent recurrence and progression rates in BC patients.[50] With regards to age and gender, the highest incidence of BC occurs in ageing Caucasian males from Westernized countries.[35] BC rarely occurs before the age of 40 years,[51] and the male to female ratio is around 3:1.[51] There appears to be differences between different ethnic groups in the risk of developing bladder cancer. Caucasian American males typically have twice the risk of African American males but mortality rates are higher in the latter group of males while Asian populations have traditionally had the lowest rates of BC.[35]

A recent evaluation of the US Prostate, Lung, Colorectal, and Ovarian Screening Trial (PLCO) cohort used 149,619 individuals aged 55–75 years and decision-analytical methodology to incorporate these risk factors to determine BC risk.[43] Using patient age, gender, smoking history, and family history of BC, the authors created a risk scoring system that ranked individuals for screening. Screening the high-risk cohort (representing 25% of the entire population) would have detected 60% of all significant BCs (57 of 95). The highest risk scores were allocated to males, over 65 years old with a smoking history of ≥20 more pack-years. Van der Molen *et al.* suggested classifying populations into low (≤50 years old with invisible haematuria), medium (>50 years with invisible /≤50 years with visible haematuria) and high BC risk (>50 years with visible haematuria) using age, the extent of haematuria and exposure to known risk factors (such as analgesic use (e.g. phenacetin), environmental exposure to carcinogens (e.g. occupation and patient history of urological cancer, repeated infections, and irradiation).[52] They reported that for patients presenting with visible haematuria, malignancy was found in 10–28% of cases overall and up to 10% of patients under 40 years of age. The risk of urological cancer was lower for patients presenting with recurrent non-visible haematuria (8.9%) and even less for patients with non-visible haematuria and younger than 50 years (no cases of BC).

Screening workers with occupational carcinogen exposure

Occupational exposure to carcinogens is considered the second commonest acquired risk factor for BC. These chemical carcinogens include aromatic amines (beta-naphtylamine, aminobiphenyls, benzidine, and so on) and polycyclic aromatic hydrocarbons. Exposure occurs in a variety of occupations in industries including: hairdressing, automotive and petrochemical, plumbing, leather, clothing, rubber, aluminium, painting/dyes, printing, and dry cleaning.[50] Authors have reported screening workers exposed to the occupational carcinogens (reviewed in [9]) and find BC in 0–1.6% of screen attendees (see Table 6.16.2).

Lotan *et al.* screened 1,175 male and 327 female smokers or carcinogen exposed-workers using the NMP22 BladderCheck urine test.[53,54] Three per cent (3%) had never smoked and 34% worked for >15 years in high-risk occupations. The NMP22 test was positive in 5.7% of the population, 15% had microscopic haematuria and two non-invasive tumours were found in male heavy smokers (>40 pack-years of smoking).[53] The PPV of NMP22 was 2.4%. The authors suggested screening women and light smokers was not worthwhile.

Very high-risk populations

Certain very high-risk exposures for urothelial carcinoma are known. One such agent is aristolochic acid found in various Chinese herb medicinal products and contaminated wheat in the Balkans. Zlotta *et al.* followed 43 patients with high aristolochic acid exposures and the resultant nephropathy.[55] With 7.7 years of follow-up (median) a total of 22 BCs (51%) had been found. None were invasive at diagnosis and all treated. All similar patients (n = 3) who declined screening died from metastatic BC.

Family history and genetics

To date, the role of genetic predisposition has not been evaluated as a tool to aid BC screening. In the future it is likely this may be part of an assessment to stratify BC screening. With regards to genetics, a few case-series of families with high BC penetrance have been reported.[56] These may be due to general cancer syndromes, such as Li-Fraumeni (p53 mutation), retinoblastoma and lynch syndrome (DNA mismatch repair) kindreds.[57,58] However, currently there are no known familial cancer genes that predispose to only BC.

Table 6.16.2 Summary of bladder cancer cohort screening studies

Author	Reference*	Place	Year	Targeted population	Age	No.	Test	No. pos tests	% pos tests	Diagnostic procedure	No. cystoscopy	No. Bca	% Bca found	Estimated incidence per 100,000 per year
Messing	5,22, 31, 34	USA	1989–92	Men >50	63	1,575	Dipstick 14 days repeated 9 months later	258	16.4	Cystoscopy	258	21	1.33	1,333
Whelan	23 24, 33, 35	UK	1989, 92	Men 60–85	69	2,356	Weekly dipstick for 10 weeks	474	20.1	Cystoscopy	317	17	0.72	722
Roobol	25	The Netherlands	2008	Men 50-75	50–75	1,611	Dipstick 14 days. If positive NMP22, FGFR3, Microsatellite, methylations	378	3.6%[1]	Cystoscopy	58	1	0.06	62
Hedelin	26	Sweden	<2006	Men 60–70	60–70	1,096	Dipstick and UBC test	174	15.9	Cystoscopy (white and fluorescent)	174	7	0.64	639
Zlotta AR	27	Belgium	2011	Aristocholic acid	—	43	Cystoscopy ×2/y + systematic Bx	22	51.2	Cystoscopy + Bx	43	22	51.2	5,116
Steiner	28	Austria	2007	Smokers >= 40 pack-years	60	183	Dipstick, NMP22, cytology, and UroVysion	75	41	Cystoscopy	75	3	1.64	1,639
Lotan	29	USA	2006-07	Both sex >50 and smokers (>10y) +/- professional exposure (>15 years)	62.5	1,502	NMP22	85	5.7	Cystoscopy	69	2	0.13	133
Davies M	49	UK	1970	Workers	—	4,636	>2 cells/HPF or albumin>10 mg/100 mL on 2 repeat exams	84	1.8	Repeat urine test, if positive: intravenous urogram (IVU) and cystoscopy	—	3	0.06	65
Pesch B	50	Germany	2010	Exp AA	60	1,323	Dipstick, blood cell count, cytology, NMP22, urovysion	—	—	Cystoscopy	—	14	1.06	1,058
Crosby	51	USA	<1991	Exp AA (BN)		541	Cytology on a 33-month programme	64	11.8	Cystoscopy	24	7	1.29	470
Marsh	52	USA	1986–01	Exp AA (BN)		277	Urinanalysis, cytology, quantitative fluorescence analysis, annual, or semi-annual screens	51	18.4	Cystoscopy + Bx	40	3	1.08	1,080

(*continued*)

Table 6.16.2 (Continued)

Author	Reference*	Place	Year	Targeted population	Age	No.	Test	No. pos tests	% pos tests	Diagnostic procedure	No. cystoscopy	No. Bca	% Bca found	Estimated incidence per 100,000 per year
Hemstreet	19	China	1991–97	Exp benzidine	55	1,788	Dipstick, cytology, DNA ploïdy, p300	153	8.6	Cystoscopy	116	28	1.57	263
Hemstreet	19	China	1991–97	Non-exposed	58	373	Dipstick, cytology, DNA ploïdy, p300	26	7	Cystoscopy	20	2	0.54	87
Ward	45	USA	1968–79	Exp BD (MBOCA)		200	Cystoscopy	—	—	Cystoscopy	200	3	1.5	1,500
Ward	45	USA	1968-79	Exp BD (MBOCA)		385	Cytology	21	5.5	Cystoscopy	21	0	0	0
Ward	45	USA	1968-79	Exp BD (MBOCA)		385	Dipstick, cytology, NMP22 repeated 3 days + US	60	15.6	Cystoscopy	60	1	0.26	260
Chen	37	Taiwan	<2005	Exp BD (MBOCA)	38	70	Dipstick, cytology, NMP22	15	21.4	Cystoscopy	15	0	0	0
Chen	37	Taiwan	<2005	Non-exposed	37	92	Dipstick, cytology, NMP22	22	23.9	Cystoscopy	22	0	0	0
Thériaut	6	Quebec	1980–86	Exp PAH (AW)			Symptoms			Cystoscopy		30		
Thériaut	6	Quebec	1970–79	Exp PAH (AW)			Cytology			Cystoscopy		49		
Giberti	36	Itay	2006–08	Exp PAH (CW)	43	152	Dipstick, cytology, uCyt+	18	11.8	Cystoscopy	18	0	0	0

[1] 23.5% using dipstick only.

BCa: bladder cancer, N: number, exp: exposed to, AA: aromatic amines, PAH: polycyclic aromatic hydrocarbons, BN: beta-naphtylamine, BD: benzidine derivatives, AW: aluminium workers, CW: coke workers) pos: positive, HPF: high powered field, US ultra sound, Bx: biopsy.

* Please note that references in this table coincide with those provided in the paper by Larre *et al.*9

Reprinted from *European Urology*, Volume 63, Issue 6, Stéphane Larré *et al.*, 'Screening for Bladder Cancer: Rationale, Limitations, Whom to Target, and Perspectives', pp. 104–58, Copyright © 2013, European Association of Urology, with permission from Elsevier, http://www.sciencedirect.com/science/journal/03022838

A family history of BC among first-degree relatives is associated with a twofold increased likelihood of BC.[57] This risk may be due to shared acquired carcinogens (smoking habits and occupations are often shared in families) or genetic inheritance. For the latter, it is known that common polymorphisms of detoxification genes increase an individual's risk of BC. These genes include phase I metabolizing enzymes, for example cytochrome P450s (CYPs) involved in the first stage of metabolism (activation of carcinogens to reactive intermediate species).[59] This stage is followed by phase II metabolizing enzymes that detoxify carcinogenic metabolites to hydrophilic by-products, which can be readily excreted from the body.[59] Single nucleotide polymorphisms (SNPs) in genes coding for phase II enzymes, such as glutathione-S-transferases (GSTs), N-acetylation transferases (NATs), and sulfotransferases (SULTs), are common in Caucasian populations and associated with BC risk.[60] GSTs belong to a superfamily of enzymes that also detoxify environmental carcinogens (e.g. polycyclic aromatic hydrocarbons).[59] NATs are other enzymes involved in this pathway that work to remove other environmental carcinogens such as heterocyclic amines from the body. A slower metabolism of carcinogens enables them to react with DNA and form adducts leading to somatic mutations and cancer.[59] Polymorphisms in the methylenetetrahydrofolate reductase gene (MTHFR), which is involved in the one-carbon metabolism pathway, have also been associated with

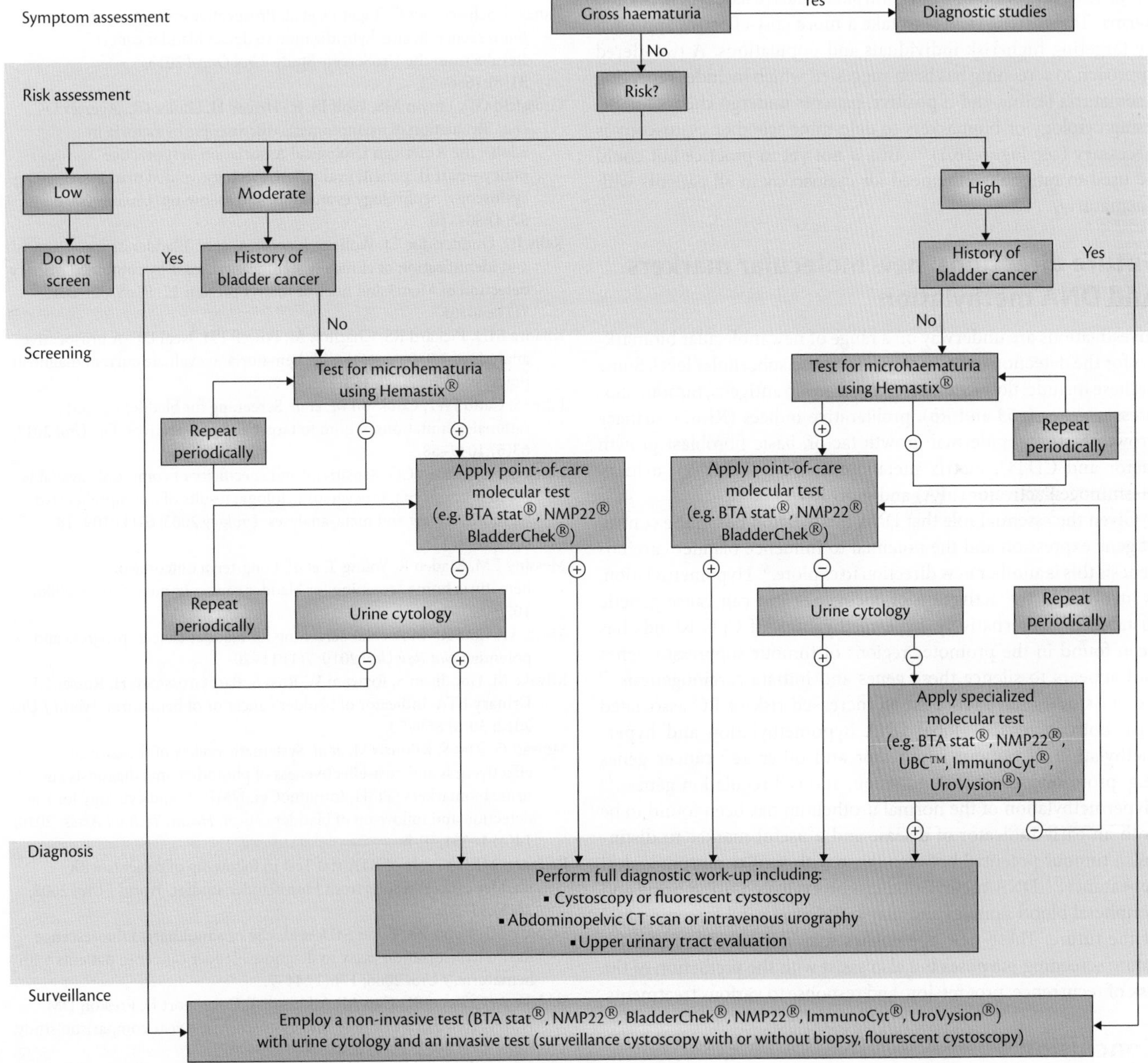

Fig. 6.16.1 Proposed protocol for screening for bladder cancer based on repeated haematuria testing.
Adapted with permission from Macmillan Publishers Ltd: *Nature Reviews Urology*, Volume 7, Issue 1, Anirban P. Mitra and Richard J. Cote, Molecular screening for bladder cancer: progress and potential, pp. 11–20, Copyright © 2010. Rights Managed by Nature Publishing Group.

risk of UCC.[61] Recent genome-wide association studies have identified additional SNPs involved in various cellular processes across the genome that may also have a role in bladder carcinogenesis.[62]

Recommendations for screening

According to US National Cancer Institute 'screening for bladder and other urothelial cancers would result in unnecessary diagnostic procedures with attendant mortality'.[63] The United States Preventive Services Task Force (USPSTF) also found 'inadequate evidence that screening for BC or treatment of screen-detected BC leads to improved disease-specific or overall morbidity or mortality'.[64] Similarly, the European Association of Urology (EAU) is unconvinced that any appropriate routine screening tests are currently available.[31] Before routine screening is considered, there needs to be large randomized controlled trials to assess benefits and harms. The current view is to take a more cost-effective approach by targeting high-risk individuals and populations. A two-tiered approach to screening has been suggested which includes repeating haematuria testing and if positive, patients undergo checks for BC using cytology or biomarkers to determine whether cystoscopy is necessary (see Fig. 6.16.1).[64] This is not yet in practice but could be used to rationalize the need for cystoscopy in all patients with haematuria.

Future directions: new molecular markers and DNA methylation

Investigations are underway on a range of new molecular biomarkers for the detection of BC at the cellular and subcellular level. Some of these include: flow cytometry, blood group antigens, tumour suppressor genes (*p53* and *Rb*), proliferative indices (Ki-67), urinary growth factors (epidermal growth factor, basic fibroblast growth factor and CD44), matrix metalloproteinase (MMP-9), urinary plasminogen activator (uPA) and short RNAs.[65,66]

Given the essential role that DNA methylation has in the control of gene expression and the potential to influence bladder carcinogenesis this is another new direction to explore.[67] Hypomethylation, is involved in the activation of oncogenes and can cause genetic instability.[68] Alternatively, hypermethylation of CpG islands has been found in the promoter regions of tumour suppressor genes and appears to silence these genes and initiate carcinogenesis.[69] Recent studies have reported an increased risk of BC associated with both increased global DNA hypomethylation and hypermethylation of tumour suppressor and other key cancer genes (e.g. proto-oncogenes, cell adhesion, and cell regulation genes).[70] Hypermethylation of the normal urothelium has been found to be both an early indicator of disease and a useful marker to distinguish tumour potential between those with similar morphological appearance.[71] DNA methylation can be evaluated using urine and peripheral blood samples and may serve as a useful screening tool of the future. These new approaches may not only be useful for future screening purposes but also assist with the prediction of the risk of recurrence, progression, and response to various treatments.

Conclusion

While there are many new and innovative tests at various stages of development for the detection of bladder cancer there are currently none that can meet all the criteria that would allow them to replace the existing best practice guidelines: testing for haematuria, urinary cytology with urological referral and subsequent cystoscopy and imaging. FDA approved biomarkers however, may be used as adjuncts to existing practices to improve the accuracy and rates of detection as well lower the frequency of the more invasive procedures. Furthermore, at this stage there is no evidence to suggest that routine screening can lower disease-specific mortality and morbidity rates and so screening should be restricted to individuals presenting with symptoms and deemed to be at higher risk of bladder cancer.

Further reading

Babjuk M, Oosterlinck W, Sylvester R, *et al.* EAU guidelines on non-muscle-invasive urothelial carcinoma of the bladder, the 2011 update. *Eur Urol* 2011; **59**(6):997–1008.

Banek S, Schwentner C, Tager D, et al. Prospective evaluation of fluorescence-in situ-hybridization to detect bladder cancer: Results from the UroScreen-Study. *Urol Oncol* 2013; **31**(8):1656–62.

Grossfeld GD, Litwin MS, Wolf JS, Jr., Hricak H, Shuler CL, Agerter DC, *et al.* Evaluation of asymptomatic microscopic hematuria in adults: the American Urological Association best practice policy—part II: patient evaluation, cytology, voided markers, imaging, cystoscopy, nephrology evaluation, and follow-up. *Urology* 2001; **57**(4):604–10.

Kelly JD, Dudderidge TJ, Wollenschlaeger A, *et al.* Bladder cancer diagnosis and identification of clinically significant disease by combined urinary detection of Mcm5 and nuclear matrix protein 22. *PLoS One* 2012; **7**(7):e40305.

Khadra MH, Pickard RS, Charlton M, Powell PH, Neal DE. A prospective analysis of 1,930 patients with hematuria to evaluate current diagnostic practice. *J Urol* 2000; **163**(2):524–7.

Larré S, Catto JWF, Cookson M, *et al.* Screening for bladder cancer: rationale, limitations, whom to target and perspectives. *Eur Urol* 2013; **63**(6):1049–58.

Lotan Y, Roehrborn CG. Sensitivity and specificity of commonly available bladder tumor markers versus cytology: results of a comprehensive literature review and meta-analyses. *Urology* 2003; **61**(1):109–18; discussion 118.

Messing EM, Madeb R, Young T, *et al.* Long-term outcome of hematuria home screening for bladder cancer in men. *Cancer* 2006; **107**(9):2173–9.

Mitra AP, Cote RJ. Molecular screening for bladder cancer: progress and potential. *Nat Rev Urol* 2010; 7(1):11–20.

Miyake M, Goodison S, Rizwani W, Ross S, Bart Grossman H, Rosser CJ. Urinary BTA: indicator of bladder cancer or of hematuria. *World J Urol* 2012; **30**(6):869–73.

Mowatt G, Zhu S, Kilonzo M, *et al.* Systematic review of the clinical effectiveness and cost-effectiveness of photodynamic diagnosis and urine biomarkers (FISH, ImmunoCyt, NMP22) and cytology for the detection and follow-up of bladder cancer. *Health Technol Assess* 2010; **14**(4):1–331, iii-iv.

Raitanen MP. The role of BTA stat Test in follow-up of patients with bladder cancer: results from FinnBladder studies. *World J Urol* 2008; **26**(1):45–50.

Sarosdy MF, Kahn PR, Ziffer MD, et al. Use of a multitarget fluorescence in situ hybridization assay to diagnose bladder cancer in patients with hematuria. *J Urol* 2006; **176**(1):44–7.

Schlake A, Crispen PL, Cap AP, Atkinson T, Davenport D, Preston DM. NMP-22, urinary cytology, and cystoscopy: a 1 year comparison study. *Can J Urol* 2012; **19**(4):6345–50.

Wadhwa N, Jatawa SK, Tiwari A. Non-invasive urine based tests for the detection of bladder cancer. *J Clin Pathol* 2012; **65**(11):970–5.

References

1. Wilson J, Jungners G (eds). *Principles and Practice of Screening for Disease*. Geneva, Switzerland: World Health Organization, 1968.
2. Parkin DM. The global burden of urinary bladder cancer. *Scand J Urol Nephrol Suppl* 2008; (218):12–20.
3. Botteman MF, Pashos CL, Redaelli A, Laskin B, Hauser R. The health economics of bladder cancer: a comprehensive review of the published literature. *Pharmacoeconomics* 2003; **21**(18):1315–30.
4. Howlader N, Noone AM, Krapcho M, *et al.* SEER Cancer Statistics Review, 1975–2009 (Vintage 2009 Populations). Bethesda, MA: National Cancer Institute, 2012. Available at: http://seer.cancer.gov/csr/1975_2009_pops09 [Online].
5. Messing EM, Madeb R, Young T, *et al.* Long-term outcome of hematuria home screening for bladder cancer in men. *Cancer* 2006; **107**(9):2173–9.
6. Theriault GP, Tremblay CG, Armstrong BG. Bladder cancer screening among primary aluminum production workers in Quebec. *J Occup Med* 1990; **32**(9):869–72.
7. Friedman GD, Hiatt RA, Quesenberry CP Jr, Selby JV, Weiss NS. Problems in assessing screening experience in observational studies of screening efficacy: example of urinalysis screening for bladder cancer. *J Med Screen* 1995; **2**(4):219–23.
8. Chou R, Dana T. Screening adults for bladder cancer: a review of the evidence for the U.S. preventive services task force. *Ann Intern Med* 2010; **153**(7):461–8.
9. Larré S, Catto JWF, Cookson M, *et al.* Screening for bladder cancer: rationale, limitations, whom to target and perspectives. *Eur Urol* 2013; **63**(6):1049–58.
10. Lokeshwar VB, Soloway MS. Current bladder tumor tests: does their projected utility fulfil clinical necessity? *J Urol* 2001; **165**(4):1067–77.
11. Reynard J, Brewster S, Biers S. *Oxford Handbook of Urology*. Oxford, UK: Oxford University Press, 2006.
12. Konety B, Lotan Y. Urothelial bladder cancer: biomarkers for detection and screening. *BJU Int* 2008; **102**(9 Pt B):1234–41.
13. Messing EM, Young TB, Hunt VB, Wehbie JM, Rust P. Urinary tract cancers found by home screening with hematuria dipsticks in healthy men over 50 years of age. *Cancer* 1989; **64**(11):2361–7.
14. Khadra MH, Pickard RS, Charlton M, Powell PH, Neal DE. A prospective analysis of 1,930 patients with hematuria to evaluate current diagnostic practice. *J Urol* 2000; **163**(2):524–7.
15. Messing EM, Young TB, Hunt VB, *et al.* Home screening for hematuria: results of a multiclinic study. *J Urol* 1992; **148**(2 Pt 1):289–92.
16. Mitra AP, Cote RJ. Molecular screening for bladder cancer: progress and potential. *Nat Rev Urol* 2010; **7**(1):11–20.
17. Babjuk M, Oosterlinck W, Sylvester R, *et al.* EAU guidelines on non-muscle-invasive urothelial carcinoma of the bladder, the 2011 update. *Eur Urol* 2011; **59**(6):997–1008.
18. Villicana P, Whiting B, Goodison S, Rosser CJ. Urine-based assays for the detection of bladder cancer. *Biomark Med* 2009; **3**(3):265.
19. Lotan Y, Roehrborn CG. Sensitivity and specificity of commonly available bladder tumor markers versus cytology: results of a comprehensive literature review and meta-analyses. *Urology* 2003; **61**(1):109–18; discussion 118.
20. Wadhwa N, Jatawa SK, Tiwari A. Non-invasive urine based tests for the detection of bladder cancer. *J Clin Pathol* 2012; **65**(11):970–5.
21. Jamshidian H, Kor K, Djalali M. Urine concentration of nuclear matrix protein 22 for diagnosis of transitional cell carcinoma of bladder. *Urol J* 2008; **5**(4):243–7.
22. Mowatt G, Zhu S, Kilonzo M, *et al.* Systematic review of the clinical effectiveness and cost-effectiveness of photodynamic diagnosis and urine biomarkers (FISH, ImmunoCyt, NMP22) and cytology for the detection and follow-up of bladder cancer. *Health Technol Assess* 2010; **14**(4):1–331, iii-iv.
23. Schlake A, Crispen PL, Cap AP, Atkinson T, Davenport D, Preston DM. NMP-22, urinary cytology, and cystoscopy: a 1 year comparison study. *Can J Urol* 2012; **19**(4):6345–50.
24. Miyake M, Goodison S, Rizwani W, Ross S, Bart Grossman H, Rosser CJ. Urinary BTA: indicator of bladder cancer or of hematuria. *World J Urol* 2012; **30**(6):869–73.
25. Raitanen MP. The role of BTA stat Test in follow-up of patients with bladder cancer: results from FinnBladder studies. *World J Urol* 2008; **26**(1):45–50.
26. Banek S, Schwentner C, Tager D, *et al.* Prospective evaluation of fluorescence-in situ-hybridization to detect bladder cancer: Results from the UroScreen-Study. *Urol Oncol* 2013; **31**(8):1656–62.
27. Sarosdy MF, Kahn PR, Ziffer MD, *et al.* Use of a multitarget fluorescence in situ hybridization assay to diagnose bladder cancer in patients with hematuria. *J Urol* 2006; **176**(1):44–7.
28. Kelly JD, Dudderidge TJ, Wollenschlaeger A, *et al.* Bladder cancer diagnosis and identification of clinically significant disease by combined urinary detection of Mcm5 and nuclear matrix protein 22. *PLoS One* 2012; **7**(7):e40305.
29. Saeb-Parsy K, Wilson A, Scarpini C, *et al.* Diagnosis of bladder cancer by immunocytochemical detection of minichromosome maintenance protein-2 in cells retrieved from urine. *Br J Cancer* 2012; **107**(8):1384–91.
30. Parker J, Spiess PE. Current and emerging bladder cancer urinary biomarkers. *Scientific World Journal* 2011; **11**:1103–12.
31. Babjuk M, Oosterlinck W, Sylvester R, *et al.* EAU Guidelines on Non-Muscle-Invasive Bladder Cancer (TaT1 & CIS), 2012 [25 September 2012]; Available at: http://www.uroweb.org [Online].
32. Fradet Y, Grossman HB, Gomella L, *et al.* A comparison of hexaminolevulinate fluorescence cystoscopy and white light cystoscopy for the detection of carcinoma in situ in patients with bladder cancer: a phase III, multicenter study. *J Urol* 2007; **178**(1):68–73; discussion 73.
33. Almallah YZ, Rennie CD, Stone J, Lancashire MJ. Urinary tract infection and patient satisfaction after flexible cystoscopy and urodynamic evaluation. *Urology* 2000; **56**(1):37–9.
34. Grossfeld GD, Litwin MS, Wolf JS, Jr., Hricak H, Shuler CL, Agerter DC, *et al.* Evaluation of asymptomatic microscopic hematuria in adults: the American Urological Association best practice policy—part II: patient evaluation, cytology, voided markers, imaging, cystoscopy, nephrology evaluation, and follow-up. *Urology* 2001; **57**(4):604–10.
35. Jemal A, Bray F, Center MM, Ferlay J, Ward E, Forman D. Global cancer statistics. *CA Cancer J Clin* 2011; **61**(2):69–90.
36. Dudziec E, Goepel JR, Catto JW. Global epigenetic profiling in bladder cancer. *Epigenomics* 2011; **3**(1):35–45.
37. Reynard J, Turner K, Mark S, Armenakas N, Feneley M, Sullivan MJ. *The Oxford Specialist Handbook of Urological Surgery*. Oxford, UK: Oxford University Press, 2008.
38. Resseguie LJ, Nobrega FT, Farrow GM, Timmons JW, Worobec TG. Epidemiology of renal and ureteral cancer in Rochester, Minnesota, 1950–1974, with special reference to clinical and pathologic features. *Mayo Clin Proc* 1978; **53**(8):503–10.
39. Kishi K, Hirota T, Matsumoto K, Kakizoe T, Murase T, Fujita J. Carcinoma of the bladder: a clinical and pathological analysis of 87 autopsy cases. *J Urol* 1981; **125**(1):36–9.
40. Sievert KD, Amend B, Nagele U, *et al.* Economic aspects of bladder cancer: what are the benefits and costs? *World J Urol* 2009; **27**(3):295–300.
41. Ploeg M, Aben KK, Kiemeney LA. The present and future burden of urinary bladder cancer in the world. *World J Urol* 2009; **27**(3):289–93.
42. Sangar VK, Ragavan N, Matanhelia SS, Watson MW, Blades RA. The economic consequences of prostate and bladder cancer in the UK. *BJU Int* 2005; **95**(1):59–63.
43. Vickers AJ, Bennette C, Kibel AS, *et al.* Who should be included in a clinical trial of screening for bladder cancer?: A decision analysis of data from the Prostate, Lung, Colorectal and Ovarian Cancer Screening Trial. *Cancer* 2012.

44. Messing EM, Young TB, Hunt VB, *et al.* Comparison of bladder cancer outcome in men undergoing hematuria home screening versus those with standard clinical presentations. *Urology* 1995; **45**(3):387–96; discussion 96–7.
45. Britton JP, Dowell AC, Whelan P, Harris CM. A community study of bladder cancer screening by the detection of occult urinary bleeding. *J Urol* 1992; **148**(3):788–90.
46. Mayfield MP, Whelan P. Bladder tumours detected on screening: results at 7 years. *Br J Urol* 1998; **82**(6):825–8.
47. Hedelin H, Jonsson K, Salomonsson K, Boman H. Screening for bladder tumours in men aged 60–70 years with a bladder tumour marker (UBC) and dipstick-detected haematuria using both white-light and fluorescence cystoscopy. *Scand J Urol Nephrol* 2006; **40**(1):26–30.
48. Kelly JD, Fawcett DP, Goldberg LC. Assessment and management of non-visible haematuria in primary care. *BMJ* 2009; **338**:a3021.
49. Zeegers MP, Tan FE, Dorant E, van Den Brandt PA. The impact of characteristics of cigarette smoking on urinary tract cancer risk: a meta-analysis of epidemiologic studies. *Cancer* 2000; **89**(3):630–9.
50. Kiriluk KJ, Prasad SM, Patel AR, Steinberg GD, Smith ND. Bladder cancer risk from occupational and environmental exposures. *Urol Oncol* 2012; **30**(2):199–211.
51. Shariat SF, Sfakianos JP, Droller MJ, Karakiewicz PI, Meryn S, Bochner BH. The effect of age and gender on bladder cancer: a critical review of the literature. *BJU Int* 2010; **105**(3):300–8.
52. van der Molen AJ, Hovius MC. Hematuria: a problem-based imaging algorithm illustrating the recent Dutch guidelines on hematuria. *AJR Am J Roentgenol* 2012; **198**(6):1256–65.
53. Lotan Y, Elias K, Svatek RS, Bagrodia A, Nuss G, Moran B, *et al.* Bladder cancer screening in a high risk asymptomatic population using a point of care urine based protein tumor marker. *J Urol* 2009; **182**(1):52–7; discussion 8.
54. Elias K, Svatek RS, Gupta S, Ho R, Lotan Y. High-risk patients with hematuria are not evaluated according to guideline recommendations. *Cancer* 2010; **116**(12):2954–9.
55. Zlotta AR, Roumeguere T, Kuk C, *et al.* Select screening in a specific high-risk population of patients suggests a stage migration toward detection of non-muscle-invasive bladder cancer. *Eur Urol* 2011; **59**(6):1026–31.
56. Wu X, Ros MM, Gu J, Kiemeney L. Epidemiology and genetic susceptibility to bladder cancer. *BJU Int* 2008; **102**(9 Pt B):1207–15.
57. Mueller CM, Caporaso N, Greene MH. Familial and genetic risk of transitional cell carcinoma of the urinary tract. *Urol Oncol* 2008; **26**(5):451–64.
58. Catto JW, Azzouzi AR, Amira N, *et al.* Distinct patterns of microsatellite instability are seen in tumours of the urinary tract. *Oncogene* 2003; **22**(54):8699–706.
59. Miller MC 3rd, Mohrenweiser HW, Bell DA. Genetic variability in susceptibility and response to toxicants. *Toxicol Lett* 2001; **120**(1–3):269–80.
60. Garcia-Closas M, Malats N, Silverman D, *et al.* NAT2 slow acetylation, GSTM1 null genotype, and risk of bladder cancer: results from the Spanish Bladder Cancer Study and meta-analyses. *Lancet* 2005; **366**(9486):649–59.
61. Kouidhi S, Rouissi K, Khedhiri S, Ouerhani S, Cherif M, Benammar-Elgaaied A. MTHFR gene polymorphisms and bladder cancer susceptibility: a meta-analysis including race, smoking status and tumour stage. *Asian Pac J Cancer Prev* 2011; **12**(9):2227–32.
62. Rothman N, Garcia-Closas M, Chatterjee N, *et al.* A multi-stage genome-wide association study of bladder cancer identifies multiple susceptibility loci. *Nat Genet* 2010; **42**(11):978–84.
63. National Cancer Institute. Bladder and Other Urothelial Cancers Screening 2012 [25 September 2012]. Available at: http://www.cancer.gov/cancertopics [Online].
64. Moyer VA. Screening for bladder cancer: U.S. Preventive Services Task Force recommendation statement. *Ann Intern Med* 2011; **155**(4):246–51.
65. Miah S, Dudziec E, Drayton RM, *et al.* An evaluation of urinary microRNA reveals a high sensitivity for bladder cancer. *Br J Cancer* 2012; **107**(1):123–8.
66. Netto GJ. Molecular biomarkers in urothelial carcinoma of the bladder: are we there yet? *Nat Rev Urol* 2012; **9**(1):41–51.
67. Reinert T. Methylation markers for urine-based detection of bladder cancer: the next generation of urinary markers for diagnosis and surveillance of bladder cancer. *Adv Urol* 2012; **2012**:503271.
68. Esteller M. Epigenetics in cancer. *N Engl J Med* 2008; **358**(11):1148–59.
69. Jones PA, Laird PW. Cancer epigenetics comes of age. *Nat Genet* 1999; **21**(2):163–7.
70. Moore LE, Pfeiffer RM, Poscablo C, *et al.* Genomic DNA hypomethylation as a biomarker for bladder cancer susceptibility in the Spanish Bladder Cancer Study: a case-control study. *Lancet Oncol* 2008; **9**(4):359–66.
71. van der Kwast TH, Bapat B. Predicting favourable prognosis of urothelial carcinoma: gene expression and genome profiling. *Curr Opin Urol* 2009; **19**(5):516–21.

CHAPTER 6.17

General overview of bladder cancer

Richard J. Bryant and James W.F. Catto

Demographics

BC is an important cause of cancer morbidity and mortality. It is the fourth commonest malignancy diagnosed in men in the United Kingdom and the ninth most common in women. In 2010 there were around 10,000 new cases per annum and around 3,000 disease-specific deaths in the United Kingdom alone (http://www.cancer-researchuk.org/cancer-info/cancerstats/types/bladder/incidence/uk-bladder-cancer-incidence-statistics).[1] The incidence is changing in both men and women reflecting falling rates of smoking in the former. The malignancy is more common with increasing age and the mean age at diagnosis is around 70 years. There is approximately a 3:1 male:female sex distribution of BC incidence but this is likely to alter in the future as smoking becomes more common in women. Caucasians have a greater propensity to develop BC compared with Afro-Caribbean or Hispanic patients. In the industrialized world the development of this malignancy is also associated with occupational carcinogen exposure. In the developing world squamous cell carcinoma of the bladder is associated with the parasitic infection *Schistosomiasis*.[2,3] BC is one of the most expensive malignancies in terms of lifetime costs per patient.[4,5] This cost is mainly due to the cost of prolonged bladder surveillance following endoscopic tumour resection, and partly due to the care necessary for patients with advanced BC.

Aetiology

A number of aetiological agents are implicated in the causation of BC and the two most important of these are tobacco smoking and occupational carcinogen exposure. Tobacco smoking confers an approximate fourfold relative risk of BC development and accounts for around half of all cancers.[6,7] Individuals who give up smoking reduce their risk of further bladder tumours in subsequent years. The risk of BC varies in smokers due the type of tobacco (blonde versus black), delivery (filtered versus non-filtered cigarettes), dose (pack years of smoking) and genetic variation in the enzymatic properties of detoxification enzymes.[8] Individuals with slow detoxification acetylators have an increased risk of developing BC compared against those with fast acetylators, due to a prolonged accumulation of carcinogenic toxins.[9] With regards to occupational exposure the most common carcinogens are aromatic amines and polycyclic aromatic hydrocarbons (PAHs).[10] Aromatic amines are used in the rubber, chemical, dye, and petroleum industries, while PAHs are found in the aluminium, coal, and roofing industries. Other factors known to increase urothelial cancer risk include the use of phenacetin analgesia, and intravesical chronic inflammatory processes such as pelvic irradiation and cyclophosphamide treatment.

Histological features

The predominant histological subtype of BC is urothelial cell carcinoma (UCC) which accounts for around 90% of all cases. Around 3–7% of BCs are squamous cell carcinoma (SCC), and around 1–2% of tumours are adenocarcinomas which may arise from the embryological remnant of the urachus. Rare types of bladder tumours include small cell carcinoma of the bladder, melanoma, lymphoma, and metastases from other sites.

Various grading systems are in use for BC. The commonest are the 1973 WHO and the more recent 2004 WHO grade definitions.[11] The 2004 WHO grading system uses two categories of grade (high and low-grade) for bladder carcinoma rather than the three used in 1973 (well, moderately, and poorly differentiated). The 2004 grading system also developed a new classification of PUNLMP (papillary urothelial neoplasm of low malignant potential) for well-differentiated non-invasive indolent lesions.

BCs are staged according to the TNM classification.[11] At the time of presentation around 75–80% of BC cases are non-muscle-invasive (NMI) BCs and these are manageable with endoscopic surgical resection.[12] Of the NMI BCs around 70% are non-invasive (pTa), 20% invade the lamina propria (pT1), and 10% are CIS.[13] Around 20–30% of NMIBCs will become muscle-invasive BC (MIBC) during follow-up.[14] This emphasizes the need for careful and regular bladder surveillance.[15] The remaining 20–25% of tumours are muscle-invasive (MIBC) (stage $\geq$ pT2) and approximately half of these patients will have occult metastases.[16] Overall 55–60% of all BCs are histologically of low grade at the time of clinical presentation whereas the remaining 40–45% are high-grade lesions, half of which will be found in MIBC.

Clinical presentation

Around 75% of BC cases present with painless visible haematuria. The remainder present with persistent irritative symptoms (such as dysuria, frequency, urgency, and suprapubic pain), symptoms of or proven recurrent or antibiotic-refractory urinary infections (UTIs), non-visible haematuria, or are found by chance during the investigation of other unrelated symptoms. Physical examination in affected patients is often unremarkable. Haematuria may be either visible or non-visible and may have associated symptoms or be non-symptomatic. The incidence of BC in patients presenting with visible haematuria is between 17 and 18.9%, while it is between 4.8 and 6% in patients with non-visible haematuria.[17–19]

In advanced BC, the patient may present with flank pain secondary to malignant ureteric obstruction and hydronephrosis, renal failure due to unilateral or bilateral ureteric obstruction, or with a pelvic mass. Lower limb lymphoedema may occur due to local compression of lymphatics by the primary tumour or secondary to lymph node metastases. Patients with metastatic BC may initially present with weight loss, constitutional symptoms, and metastases to liver, lung, bone, and adrenal glands, causing additional symptoms such as bone pain, respiratory symptoms, or jaundice.

SCC is more common in patients who have had bilharzia (infection with *Schistosomiasis haematobium*),[20] in patients with chronic bladder inflammation secondary to intravesical stones or a long-term indwelling catheter, and in patients with a neuropathic bladder (e.g. individuals with spinal cord injury or spina bifida). Clinicians should be concerned if such patients develop haematuria, urinary catheter blockages, recurrent UTIs, or new-onset irritative LUTS.

Primary adenocarcinoma of the bladder is rare but may be associated with a history of bladder extrophy, bladder tuberculosis infection, or in patients who have previously undergone a cystoplasty. Other tumours such as colorectal cancer, cervical cancer, or uterine cancer may also involve the bladder due to local invasion from these adjacent organs. Very occasionally other malignancies such as breast cancer or malignant melanoma can metastasize to the bladder.

Screening for bladder cancer

The aim of screening is to identify cases of a particular disease at an earlier stage when it is more amenable to treatment. The population to potentially be screened for BC is not currently known however it is likely that patients at high risk for developing this disease would benefit most from screening.[21] Most research to date regarding BC screening has focussed on the detection of haematuria using simple urinalysis, or the potential use of urinary cytology, however the optimum screening test has not yet been identified for this malignancy. Moreover, there have been no high quality randomized controlled trials or high quality observational studies comparing screening to non-screening for BC.[22] At the present time therefore screening for BC is not advocated.

Transurethral resection of a bladder tumour

After initial investigations have suggested the presence of a BC, the next step is to remove or sample the lesion. Transurethral resection of the bladder tumour (TURBT) is performed using a rigid cystoscope fitted with a resecting element and termed a resectoscope (Fig. 6.17.1). The aim of the TURBT is to fully remove the cancer (if NMI) and to fully stage the cancer and identify other pathologies.[23] The management of BC depends upon the distinctions between

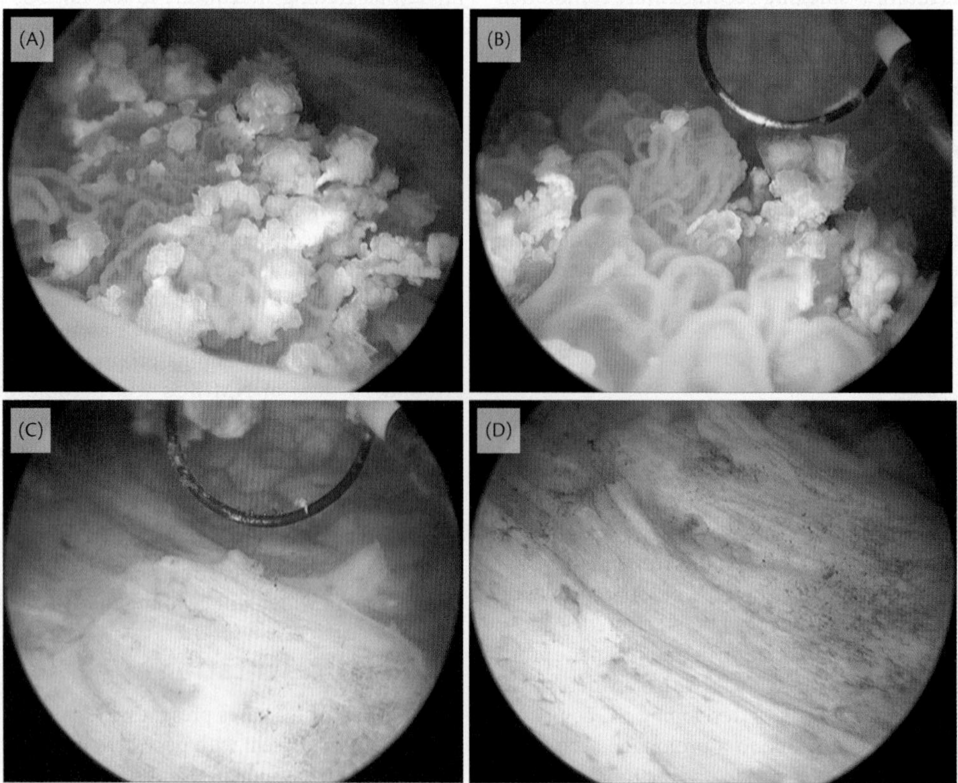

Fig. 6.17.1 Transurethral resection of a bladder tumour. (A) Exophytic partly calcified tumour within the bladder; (B) the resectoscope loop is visible prior to resection; (C) and (D) the tumour is resected flat into the detrusor muscle. Bleeding vessels and edges are cauterized.

Reproduced with permission from James Catto and Frank Gardiner, 'Fingertip Urology: Superficial bladder cancer', Primary slides, *BJU International*, Copyright © 2007, available from http://www.bjui.org/ftu/sup_bladder_prim/player.html

low and high-grade disease and between the presence of NMIBC and MIBC.

Prior to the patient undergoing a TURBT a urine sample should be cultured and any active urinary tract infection should be treated with antibiotics wherever possible. A full blood count should be performed to exclude anaemia and urea and electrolytes should be checked to exclude renal failure prior to the patient undergoing an anaesthetic. Many patients with BC are elderly or have significant co-morbidities therefore a thorough anaesthetic review is required prior to the surgical procedure which may be performed under general and/or regional anaesthetic.

The patient needs to be positioned in the lithotomy position therefore particular care needs to be taken if an individual has prosthetic knee or hip joints or arthritic conditions. Care should be taken to protect the patient's pressure points with pads particularly the common peroneal nerve to avoid neuropraxia and footdrop. A bimanual examination (per rectum in men and per vagina in women) is required to assess the size, mobility, and extent of the tumour both before and after resection. Under appropriate prophylactic antibiotic cover a 28 Ch resectoscope is passed per urethra and the bladder is inspected with a 30 degree (and if necessary a 70 degree) lens prior to resection of the tumour. Occasionally a 120 degree lens is required to adequately inspect the anterior bladder neck. The bladder must be adequately distended in order to be able to visualize and resect the tumour, and suprapubic pressure may be required to facilitate resection of tumours at the dome of the bladder, however care must be taken to avoid overdistension of the bladder as this increases the risk of bladder perforation. Continuous irrigation via the resectoscope is required during resection in order to maintain clear vision. As a TURBT aims to obtain tissue for diagnosis and to accurately stage the disease, it is important to first carefully resect the superficial aspect of the tumour down to the tumour base without causing excessive diathermy artefact, which would impede pathological evaluation. These initial resection chippings should then be collected for histology. Separate deep tumour resection biopsies should then be taken in order to obtain detrusor muscle without causing bladder perforation. These deeper specimens should be carefully labelled with adequate clinical information and macroscopic tumour characteristics to aid the pathologist, and then sent to the pathology laboratory in a pot separate from that containing the more superficial tumour samples.

In many cases the tumour is small and may be suitable for removal with the cold-cup biopsy forceps to avoid diathermy destruction. In these cases, subsequent resection biopsies of the tumour base including detrusor muscle should be obtained. Multifocal tumours require careful mapping within the bladder and multiple tumour samples should be sent to the pathologist in separate pots. If however the tumour is clearly muscle-invasive at the time of TURBT then the aim should be to adequately sample deep muscle for the purposes of staging, and to clear as much of the disease burden as is safely possible prior to future treatment with either radical cystectomy or radiotherapy. In patients who are unfit for radical treatment then the TURBT should be as thorough as safely possible in order to maximize local control for as long as possible.

Bladder tumours within diverticula require particular care during surgical resection, as diverticula lack muscularis propria. There is therefore a greater chance of bladder perforation than during resection in other areas. Given the difficulties of resecting tumours within a diverticulum it may be more appropriate in selected patients to proceed to a diverticulectomy or partial cystectomy rather than to rely on transurethral resection, particularly for high-grade bladder lesions as the lack of muscularis propria increases the risk of local extension of the tumour outside of the bladder.

If the patient has a general anaesthetic and has a tumour overlying the side wall of the bladder, then muscle paralysis may be indicated to reduce the chance that diathermy used during resection may induce an obturator reflex muscle jerk and a resultant bladder perforation. Other techniques to avoid bladder perforation include reducing the diathermy current, using a specially designed resection loop with an extension guard beyond the wire loop preventing deep wall penetration, or the use of cold-cup biopsy forceps followed by cauterization with coagulating diathermy.

If tumour is seen overlying or emerging from a ureteric orifice, then this should be resected with care. It is uncommon to see ureteric stenosis following the use of cutting diathermy however coagulating diathermy should be used as little as possible in these areas, and it may be advisable to place a ureteric stent to prevent short-term ureteric obstruction due to postoperative oedema. A retrograde ureteropyelogram and ureteroscopy may be needed to obtain tissue from within the ureter for further diagnosis and staging. It is often advisable to perform postoperative imaging with intravenous urography (IVU), CT urography (CTU), or dynamic renogram at four to six weeks after ureteric orifice resection in order to exclude upper urinary tract obstruction.

Any 'red patches' within the bladder either adjacent to the primary tumour or more remotely situated, or in the prostatic urethra, should be biopsied to identify concomitant CIS. It is important to sample flat urothelium around and distant to the tumour in cases of high-grade cancer, as the presence of CIS is one of the most predictive prognostic factors.[24,25] In low-grade tumours, the use of random bladder biopsies is unhelpful and may be harmful to patients as they may cause scarring and create sites of potential tumour cell implantation. While the histology of a tumour may be unknown at the time of resection, an experienced surgeon should be able to identify indolent versus aggressive looking BCs, and tailor the use of resection or biopsy accordingly. If the patient is potentially a suitable candidate for an orthotopic bladder reconstruction following future cystectomy, then it is helpful to perform bladder neck resection biopsies at the time of the initial TURBT in order to exclude disease at the bladder neck.

Once the resection aspect of the TURBT has been completed haemostasis should be ensured using coagulation diathermy. Care should be taken not to use excessive coagulation diathermy close to the ureteric orifices as this has the potential risk of inducing a ureteric stricture. At the end of the resection the bladder should be emptied and a further bimanual examination should be performed without a catheter *in situ* in order to accurately stage the disease and in particular to detect any residual bladder mass suggestive of pT3 disease. A large irrigating indwelling urethral catheter is then placed in the bladder in order to maintain drainage during the postoperative period while any further minor haematuria settles. Following the initial TURBT the patient should receive a single intravesical instillation of a chemotherapeutic agent such as mitomycin C which reduces the risk of NMIBC recurrence.[26,27]

Photodynamic diagnosis of bladder cancer

The use of photodynamic diagnosis (PDD) during TURBT has been reported to improve the detection rate of malignant epithelium during the resection procedure due to improved visualization of bladder tumours compared with standard white-light TURBT.[28] The underlying principle of PDD is that the presence of an endogenous or exogenous photosensitizer causes abnormal cells to fluoresce under a specific wavelength of light. PDD-assisted TURBT in current practice utilizes exogenous photosensitizers derived from the heme biosynthetic pathway. The starting point of the heme pathway is 5-aminolevulinic acid (5-ALA) which is instilled into the bladder two hours preoperatively. Under normal (i.e. benign) circumstances nucleated cells convert non-active molecules to the active fluorescent molecule protoporphyrin IX (PPIX) which is then rapidly converted to heme. Malignant urothelial cells have significant differences in heme metabolism compared with benign cells, resulting in the accumulation of PPIX in cancerous cells. PPIX absorbs light at 400nm (blue) and emits fluorescence at 635 nm (red), hence inspection of malignant urothelium with an excitation light source called a D-light through a yellow filter with a slow shutter speed results in the absorption of all blue light and amplification of red light, causing the malignant areas to appear bright red. Artefact fluorescence can sometimes occur due to folds of urothelium or at the trigone or ureteric orifices, however despite these slight limitations PDD-assisted TURBT has an overall sensitivity of 93% compared with 73% for white-light TURBT[29] and this difference is largely due to the improved detection of CIS. The use of PDD-assisted TURBT also improves the residual tumour rate following resection compared with white-light TURBT. PDD-assisted cystoscopy is useful in examining patients with positive urinary cytology but negative white-light cystoscopy, and it is also useful during the training of urological surgeons.

While cystoscopy with cytology are currently considered to be the gold-standard investigations for the detection and follow-up of BC a number of new optical imaging modalities are being developed in order to overcome the limitations of current techniques. Newer technologies include narrow band imaging, raman spectroscopy, and optical coherence tomography.[30] These newer techniques need further investigation before they can be advocated in the investigation of haematuria or in the diagnosis and treatment of BC, while the efficacy of urothelial inspection with these methods will also need to be carefully considered in terms of financial cost.

Radiological staging

Following TURBT, patients with high-grade or invasive disease who are considered for further treatment require full tumour staging. To complement the TURBT a number of radiological imaging options are available. These should examine the bladder in cross section, the regional lymph nodes for metastases, and common sites of metastases (such as the lungs and liver). In symptomatic patients further specific targeted imaging may be needed (such as a bone scan for patients with back pain). Furthermore, coexisting lung cancer may be present in many BC patients due to their shared aetiological agent (i.e. smoking).[31] It is important to wait for a minimum of seven days after the TURBT before performing cross-sectional imaging, as the initial resection may cause artefact in the surrounding tissues resulting in potential overstaging of the disease.[32]

If a CTU has been performed to investigate haematuria then this may be used to give provisional staging information for the bladder cancer, including possible pelvic or para-aortic lymphadenopathy, and visceral or bony metastases. A triple phase computed tomography scan (CT) (i.e. pre-contrast, and arterial and portal-venous post-contrast phases) of the abdomen and pelvis is necessary to fully stage the cancer. We also advocate CT of the thorax to look for pulmonary and mediastinal lesions. MRI is an alternative to CT and is thought to be slightly better for local bladder staging of a tumour and for detecting local lymphadenopathy. Both CT and MRI may understage the true disease burden by missing small nodal or visceral metastatic lesions in up to 30% of cases. In order to improve upon this several authors have examined the role of staging PET CT scans.[33,34] Currently this modality appears promising but it has a poor specificity due to the overdiagnosis of metastases.

Conclusions

In summary bladder cancer is a common malignancy that usually presents with visible painless haematuria. Rapid diagnosis and treatment is required to reduce mortality and morbidity from this cancer. Endoscopic resection is vital in the initial treatment and assessment of tumours.

Further reading

Babjuk M, Oosterlinck W, Sylvester R, *et al.* EAU guidelines on non-muscle-invasive urothelial carcinoma of the bladder, the 2011 update. *Eur Urol* 2011; **59**(6):997–1008.

Freedman ND, Silverman DT, Hollenbeck AR, Schatzkin A, Abnet CC. Association between smoking and risk of bladder cancer among men and women. *JAMA* 2011; **306**(7):737–45.

Jocham D, Stepp H, Waidelich R. Photodynamic diagnosis in urology: state-of-the-art. *Eur Urol* 2008; **53**(6):1138–48.

Kirkali Z, Chan T, Manoharan M, *et al.* Bladder cancer: epidemiology, staging and grading, and diagnosis. *Urology* 2005; **66**(6 Suppl 1):4–34.

References

1. Cancer Research UK: Bladder cancer incidence statistics. Available at: http://www.cancerresearchuk.org/cancer-info/cancerstats/types/bladder/incidence/uk-bladder-cancer-incidence-statistics [Online].
2. Kirkali Z, Chan T, Manoharan M, *et al.* Bladder cancer: epidemiology, staging and grading, and diagnosis. *Urology* 2005; **66**(6 Suppl 1):4–34.
3. Shokeir AA. Squamous cell carcinoma of the bladder: pathology, diagnosis and treatment. *BJU Int* 2004; **93**(2):216–20.
4. Botteman MF, Pashos CL, Redaelli A, Laskin B, Hauser R. The health economics of bladder cancer: a comprehensive review of the published literature. *Pharmacoeconomics* 2003; **21**(18):1315–30.
5. Sangar VK, Ragavan N, Matanhelia SS, Watson MW, Blades RA. The economic consequences of prostate and bladder cancer in the UK. *BJU Int* 2005; **95**(1):59–63.
6. Baris D, Karagas MR, Verrill C, *et al.* A case-control study of smoking and bladder cancer risk: emergent patterns over time. *J Natl Cancer Inst* 2009; **101**(22):1553–61.
7. Freedman ND, Silverman DT, Hollenbeck AR, Schatzkin A, Abnet CC. Association between smoking and risk of bladder cancer among men and women. *JAMA* 2011; **306**(7):737–45.
8. Gandini S, Botteri E, Iodice S, *et al.* Tobacco smoking and cancer: a meta-analysis. *Int J Cancer* 2008; **122**(1):155–64.
9. Risch A, Wallace DM, Bathers S, Sim E. Slow N-acetylation genotype is a susceptibility factor in occupational and smoking related bladder cancer. *Hum Mol Genet* 1995; **4**(2):231–6.
10. Reulen RC, Kellen E, Buntinx F, Brinkman M, Zeegers MP. A meta-analysis on the association between bladder cancer and occupation. *Scand J Urol Nephrol Suppl* 2008; (218):64–78.
11. Amin MB, McKenney JK, Paner GP, *et al.* ICUD-EAU International Consultation on Bladder Cancer 2012: Pathology. *Eur Urol* 2013; **63**(1):16–35.

12. Burger M, Oosterlinck W, Konety B, *et al.* ICUD-EAU International Consultation on Bladder Cancer 2012: Non-muscle-invasive urothelial carcinoma of the bladder. *Eur Urol* 2013; **63**(1):36–44.
13. Ro JY, Staerkel GA, Ayala AG. Cytologic and histologic features of superficial bladder cancer. *Urol Clin North Am* 1992; **19**(3):435–53.
14. Thomas F, Noon AP, Rubin N, Goepel J, Catto JW. Comparative outcomes of primary, recurrent and progressive high-risk non-muscle invasive bladder cancer. *Eur Urol* 2013; **63**(1):145–54.
15. Babjuk M, Oosterlinck W, Sylvester R, *et al.* EAU guidelines on non-muscle-invasive urothelial carcinoma of the bladder, the 2011 update. *Eur Urol* 2011; **59**(6):997–1008.
16. Stenzl A, Cowan NC, De Santis M, *et al.* Treatment of muscle-invasive and metastatic bladder cancer: update of the EAU guidelines. *Eur Urol* 2011; **59**(6):1009–18.
17. Edwards TJ, Dickinson AJ, Natale S, Gosling J, McGrath JS. A prospective analysis of the diagnostic yield resulting from the attendance of 4020 patients at a protocol-driven haematuria clinic. *BJU Int* 2006; **97**(2):301–5; discussion 305.
18. Datta SN, Allen GM, Evans R, Vaughton KC, Lucas MG. Urinary tract ultrasonography in the evaluation of haematuria—a report of over 1,000 cases. *Ann R Coll Surg Engl* 2002; **84**(3):203–5.
19. Mishriki SF, Nabi G, Cohen NP. Diagnosis of urologic malignancies in patients with asymptomatic dipstick hematuria: prospective study with 13 years' follow-up. *Urology* 2008; **71**(1):13–6.
20. Zheng YL, Amr S, Saleh DA, *et al.* Urinary bladder cancer risk factors in Egypt: a multicenter case-control study. *Cancer Epidemiol Biomarkers Prev* 2012; **21**(3):537–46.
21. Kamat AM, Hegarty PK, Gee JR, *et al.* ICUD-EAU International Consultation on Bladder Cancer 2012: Screening, diagnosis, and molecular markers. *Eur Urol* 2013; **63**(1):4–15.
22. Chou R, Dana T. Screening adults for bladder cancer: a review of the evidence for the U.S. preventive services task force. *Ann Intern Med* 2010; **153**(7):461–8.
23. Blandy JP, Notley RG, Reynard JM. *Transurethral Resection*, 5th edition. Oxford, UK: Taylor & Francis, 2004.
24. Thomas F, Rosario DJ, Rubin N, Goepel JR, Abbod MF, Catto JW. The long-term outcome of treated high-risk non-muscle invasive bladder cancer: Time to change treatment paradigm? *Cancer* 2012; **118**(22):5525–34.
25. Sylvester RJ, van der Meijden AP, Oosterlinck W, *et al.* Predicting recurrence and progression in individual patients with stage Ta T1 bladder cancer using EORTC risk tables: a combined analysis of 2596 patients from seven EORTC trials. *Eur Urol* 2006; **49**(3):466–75; discussion 475–7.
26. Sylvester RJ, Oosterlinck W, van der Meijden AP. A single immediate postoperative instillation of chemotherapy decreases the risk of recurrence in patients with stage Ta T1 bladder cancer: a meta-analysis of published results of randomized clinical trials. *J Urol* 2004; **171**(6 Pt 1):2186–90, quiz 2435.
27. Oddens JR, van der Meijden AP, Sylvester R. One immediate postoperative instillation of chemotherapy in low risk Ta, T1 bladder cancer patients. Is it always safe? *Eur Urol* 2004; **46**(3):336–8.
28. Grossman HB, Stenzl A, Fradet Y, *et al.* Long-term decrease in bladder cancer recurrence with hexaminolevulinate enabled fluorescence cystoscopy. *J Urol* 2012; **188**(1):58–62.
29. Jocham D, Stepp H, Waidelich R. Photodynamic diagnosis in urology: state-of-the-art. *Eur Urol* 2008; **53**(6):1138–48.
30. Patel P, Bryan RT, Wallace DM. Emerging endoscopic and photodynamic techniques for bladder cancer detection and surveillance. *TheScientificWorldJournal* 2011; **11**:2550–8.
31. Levi F, Randimbison L, Te VC, La Vecchia C. Second primary cancers in patients with lung carcinoma. *Cancer* 1999; **86**(1):186–90.
32. Kim JK, Park SY, Ahn HJ, Kim CS, Cho KS. Bladder cancer: analysis of multi-detector row helical CT enhancement pattern and accuracy in tumor detection and perivesical staging. *Radiology* 2004; **231**(3):725–31.
33. Vargas HA, Akin O, Schoder H, *et al.* Prospective evaluation of MRI, (11)C-acetate PET/CT and contrast-enhanced CT for staging of bladder cancer. *Eur J Radiol* 2012; **81**(12):4131–7.
34. Swinnen G, Maes A, Pottel H, *et al.* FDG-PET/CT for the preoperative lymph node staging of invasive bladder cancer. *Eur Urol* 2010; **57**(4):641–7.

CHAPTER 6.18

The investigation of haematuria

Richard J. Bryant and James W.F. Catto

Haematuria

Haematuria is defined as the presence of red blood cells in the urine. It may be visible or non-visible, and symptomatic or non-symptomatic.[1] Non-visible haematuria may be further classified as microscopic or dipstick, depending on the investigation used to detect it. Haematuria is an important clinical sign as approximately 40% of affected patients have significant underlying pathology. However, visible haematuria is a common symptom and is found in around 2.5% of the general population.[2] The investigation of haematuria is best performed in the setting of a one-stop haematuria clinic, unless in the presence of trauma in which case patients require careful radiological investigation for an underlying urological injury such as a renal laceration. The regional guidelines provide protocols regarding the optimal investigation of haematuria (such as that of Babjuk *et al.* 2011[3]).

The haematuria clinic

Many centres have dedicated 'haematuria clinics' which enable patients to be referred urgently by their primary care physician for thorough and prompt urological evaluation including urinalysis +/− urinary cytology, history-taking and physical examination, flexible cystoscopy, and upper tract radiological investigation. Some centres run these clinics on a 'one-stop' basis whereby the patient undergoes all of these procedures on the same day thereby reducing patient anxiety and diagnostic delay.

Causes of haematuria

Approximately 40% of patients with haematuria have significant underlying pathology (abbreviated list in Table 6.18.1). Individuals with visible haematuria have a greater risk of harbouring an underlying malignancy compared with those with non-visible haematuria, and this risk increases with advancing age, however the degree of haematuria does not always correlate with the risk of underlying malignancy. Probably the most important cause of haematuria is one of several urological malignancies and these are found in around 22–24.2% of cases (see Khadra *et al.* 2000).[2] The commonest cancer in patients presenting with haematuria is bladder cancer (BC), followed by renal cell carcinoma (RCC) or upper tract urothelial cell carcinoma (UTUCC). Less commonly haematuria may be due to prostate or urethral cancer. After cancer, the next commonest causes of haematuria are urinary tract infection (UTI), stones, and nephrological disorders. The latter are more common in younger patients and include focal glomerular disorders such as membranoproliferative glomerulonephritis, interstitial renal diseases including drug-induced nephropathy, and systemic conditions such as systemic lupus erythematosis. For these it is important to measure the blood pressure and serum creatinine levels, and to test the urine for proteinuria. If no urological cause of haematuria is identified then patients with hypertension, proteinuria (especially if the total protein excretion is greater than 1,000 mg/24 hours) or red cell casts within their urine, and/or renal impairment should be referred to a nephrologist. Patients with proteinuria on dipstick urinalysis should have urine sent for protein:creatinine or albumin:creatinine ratio measurement and they should have their glomerular filtration rate measured, for example using creatinine clearance. Serum immunological investigations may be required if an underlying immune-related renal disorder is suspected, and a renal biopsy may be indicated to establish the precise nature of any underlying renal parenchymal disease.

Anticoagulant medication such as warfarin, clopidogrel, or aspirin may precipitate haematuria, however it is important that patients taking these medications are still thoroughly investigated as tumours, stones, and infections may be present, which further increase the risk of bleeding in these patients. Other medications (such as phenytoin or rifampicin) and beetroot ingestion may colour the urine so that it appears red and bloody. 'Loin pain haematuria syndrome' refers to a syndrome in which patients present with a combination of flank pain and visible haematuria in the absence of demonstrable pathology, despite extensive investigations (including angiography and renal biopsy). The condition is commoner in women and may continue for many years with intermittent development of symptoms.

Investigation of haematuria

Given the broad range of potential diseases that can present with haematuria it is best to have a logical protocol to investigate such patients (e.g. Fig. 6.18.1).

Urinalysis

Non-visible haematuria describes the microscopic presence of red blood cells (RBCs) in a centrifuged urine sample and the use of a reagent strip to chemically detect the presence of RBCs in a freshly voided sample of urine. Asymptomatic non-visible haematuria is common with a reported population prevalence of 0.19–21% depending on the individuals being studied.[4–7] The precise definition of microscopic haematuria is contentious in terms of the required number of RBCs per high power field (HPF) for clinical significance. The AUA defined microscopic haematuria as ≥3 RBCs per HPF on evaluation of urinary sediment from two

Table 6.18.1 Common causes of haematuria

Aetiology	Disease	
Cancer	Bladder tumours	
	Upper tract tumours	
	Renal tumours	
	Prostate cancer	
	Metastasis	
Urinary stones		
Strictures	Urethral	
Inflammation	Bladder	Cystitis
	Kidney	Pyelonephritis
	Loin pain haematuria	
Trauma	Exercise	Joggers
	Injury	
Congenital	Upper tract	Pelviureteric junction obstruction
From adjacent viscera	Bowel	Divericulitis
		Appendicitis
	Uterine	Endometriosis
Nephrological	Glomerulonephirits	
	Nephritic syndrome	
	PCKD	
	Analgesic nephropathy	
Inflammatory	Bladder	Interstitial cystitis
	Prostate	Benign prostate hyperplasia
	Iatrogenic	Instrumentation
	Prostate	Post-TURP
	Bladder	Radiotherapy
Haematological	Haemolytic syndromes	
Medication	Anticoagulants	
	Colourants	Phenytoin, rifampicin, and beetroot

of three properly collected urinalysis specimens. Given the relatively limited specificity (65–99% for 2–5 RBCs per HPF) of the dipstick method the AUA recommend that the initial suggestion of microscopic haematuria based on dipstick urinalysis should be confirmed by microscopy of the urinary sediment.[8–11] Guidelines in the United Kingdom suggest that this is no longer necessary.[1] Patients with non-visible haematuria have a 10% chance of harbouring an underlying urological malignancy the most common of which is BC.[2,12]

Dipstick urinalysis is commonly performed as a rapid office based test for haematuria. The dipstick test is based on the ability of haemoglobin, released by lysed RBCs, to oxidize an adherent chromogen to produce a colour change. Most dipsticks detect <3 RBCs/HPF, but can also appear positive with other oxidizing agents such as free haemoglobin, myoglobin, and bleach. The presence of reducing agents such as vitamin C may give false negative results. Most commercially available dipsticks quantify non-visible haematuria as either a 'trace', +, ++ or +++, and recent British guidelines suggest that a 'trace' of haematuria does not require urological investigation per se.[1] It is good practice to confirm the microscopic presence of RBC in patients with dipstick haematuria.[13]

Several conditions may be confused with haematuria. Pseudohaematuria describes a reddish-brown discoloration of urine secondary to artificial colourings from certain foodstuffs or drugs. Patients with factitious disorders may deliberately contaminate their urine as an attention-seeking behaviour in order to undergo medical examination and investigation. Menstruation may also cause a false positive urine microscopy or dipstick test result.

Urine cytology

The primary advantage of performing urinary cytology is that this non-invasive test has a high specificity for poorly differentiated urothelial cell carcinoma (UCC). As such it is safe and relatively cost efficient and may support the diagnosis of BC from cystoscopy or raise the suspicion of a missed UCC in patients with normal investigations. Some authors suggest that the combination of cytology and cystoscopy is superior to cystoscopy alone. Urine cytology is better at detecting high-grade UCC cells, as are found in grade 3 cancers and carcinoma-*in-situ* (CIS), than in detecting low-grade UCC. As such cytology has a high specificity (around 96%) for UCC and outperforms other currently available bladder tumour markers. Cytology has a low sensitivity (44%) for UCC as it may miss grade 1/low-grade lesions.[14] Cytology has a high positive predictive value for UCC as it is only positive when malignant cells are identified by the pathologist. Disadvantages of a cytology test include the high level of specialist pathology support required and the associated expense of having the investigation available. Occasionally the urine cytology is positive in the presence of a normal cystoscopy and normal upper tract imaging and this diagnostic difficulty will require further investigations such as photodynamic diagnosis (PDD) cystoscopy and/or bilateral ureteroscopy and upper tract urinary cytology.

Urinary molecular markers

A number of urinary biomarkers have been described in the literature for use in the diagnosis and follow-up of BC including NMP22, BTA, BTA-Trak, BTA-Stat, telomerase and fluorescence in situ hybridization (FISH).[15,16] Despite a plethora of publications describing these and other various tests in the diagnosis of BC at the current time there have been very few randomized clinical trials conducted in this area. While the relative performance of each of these tests varies widely between studies none of them outperform cystoscopy, and therefore at present these tests are best used as an adjunct to cystoscopy rather than a replacement investigation. For example, NMP22 is approved by the US Food and Drug Administration (FDA) for the diagnosis of BC when used with cystoscopy, but not when used alone. No current biomarker has a better specificity than urinary cytology.[17] Combinations of these urinary biomarkers have been evaluated and demonstrate higher sensitivity and positive predictive values compared to the isolated use of each test.

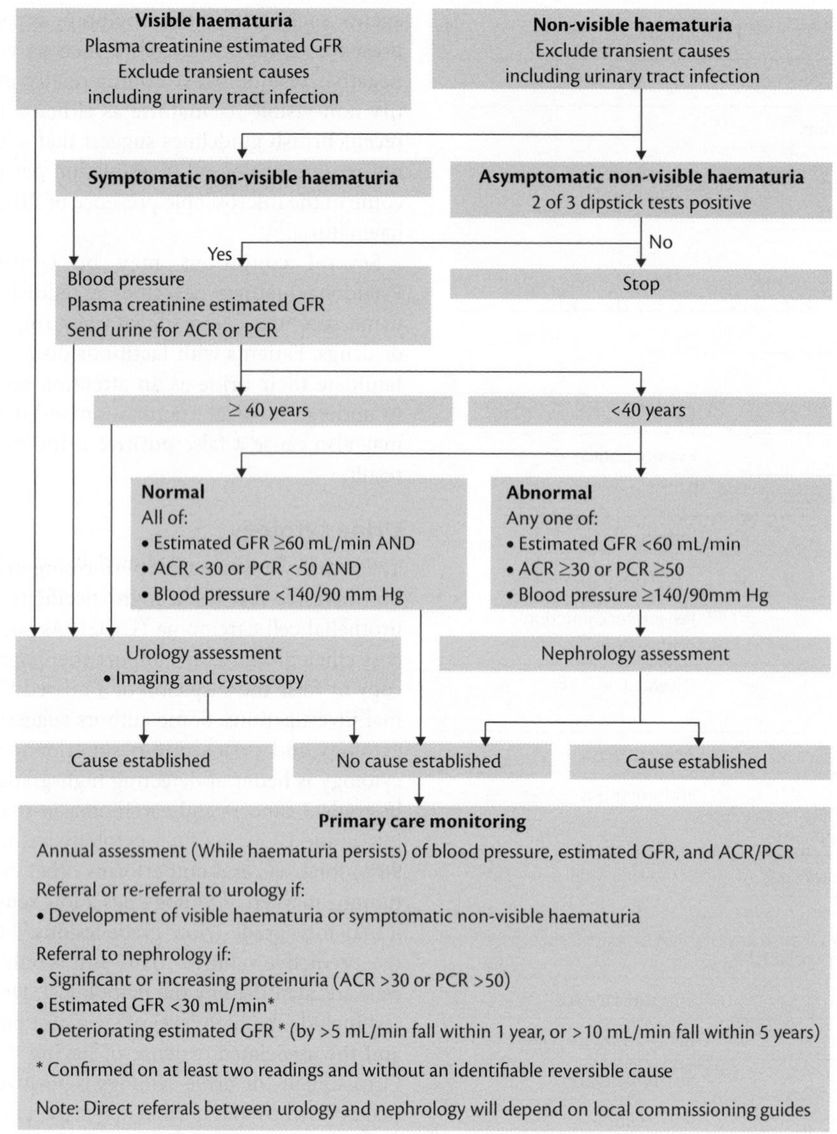

Fig. 6.18.1 Decision algorithm for the investigation of haematuria and the subsequent referral criteria adopted by the British Association of Urological Surgeons and the Renal Association.

GFR = glomerular filtration rate; PCR = protein:creatinine ratio; ACR = albumin:creatinine ratio.

Reproduced from *The British Medical Journal*, John D Kelly *et al.*, 'Assessment and management of non-visible haematuria in primary care', Volume 338, a3021, Copyright © 2009, British Medical Journal Publishing Group, with permission from BMJ Publishing Group Ltd.

Cystoscopy

The primary investigation for suspected BC is direct cystoscopic inspection of the lower urinary tract. White light cystoscopy (WLC) is an investigative procedure for BC and is recommended by both the AUA and the EAU.[3,18] WLC may be performed using either a flexible or rigid cystoscope. Flexible cystoscopy has the advantage that it can be performed under local anaesthetic in the clinic and this test can be incorporated into the diagnostic work-up of patients with haematuria and/or possible BC. It is however reasonable not to perform this invasive test in those patients with a bladder tumour seen on prior imaging and these patients may proceed directly to transurethral resection.

A fresh midstream specimen of urine (MSU) should be dipstick tested for blood, protein (renal disease), nitrates (infection) and glucose (diabetes) ahead of the flexible cystoscopy. Asymptomatic patients suspected of having a UTI on the dipstick test should undergo the flexible cystoscopy under antibiotic cover. Patients with a symptomatic UTI should have this treated first and have the flexible cystoscopy deferred until the infection has cleared. Many centres give a single dose of prophylactic antibiotic ahead of all flexible cystoscopies.

Flexible cystoscopes have narrow irrigation and instrumentation channels therefore it is difficult to simultaneously irrigate the bladder through the instrument and use a biopsy forceps or diathermy probe. Prior to the advent of flexible cystoscopies patients with suspected BC underwent rigid cystoscopy which facilitates excellent bladder irrigation and visualization however the larger size of the rigid cystoscope necessitates general or regional anaesthesia, especially in men. Nowadays patients with suspected BC undergo an initial flexible cystoscopy and thereafter proceed to formal transurethral resection. Some patients may undergo a rigid cystoscopy for some other reason, for example during an optical urethrotomy for urethral stricture disease, and be found to harbour a BC once the bladder is directly visualized.

Upper tract imaging

Imaging of the upper urinary tract (kidneys and ureters) is an essential part of the diagnostic evaluation of patients with haematuria.[19] Around 0.2–0.7% of patients investigated for haematuria have a RCC or UTUCC.[2,20] The upper urinary tract may be evaluated by several imaging modalities including ultrasound (USS), intravenous urography (IVU), CT urography (CTU) or magnetic resonance imaging (MRI). Each has strengths and weaknesses, and conflicting views of which is best are common. USS is relatively cheap and is safe as it does not use radiation, and can image the renal parenchyma and detect hydronephrosis. However, it is user dependent, the static images can be hard to interpret, and it may miss small ureteric or renal pelvis pathologies, and may miss the presence of upper tract calculi. IVU has traditionally been useful to investigate the urothelium for the presence of possible filling defects indicative of UTUCC. However, IVU involves radiation, is user dependant, may often be equivocal, and the necessary skills for this procedure are gradually being lost in radiology departments. CTU enables evaluation of both the renal parenchyma and the urothelium of the upper urinary tract and bladder, and this is becoming the gold standard investigation for visible haematuria. CTU has a high sensitivity for detecting other conditions in the urinary tract which might cause haematuria such as urinary calculi. An approach to imaging the upper tract that balances the risks and expense of investigations with diagnostic yield is best. USS may be used for patients with non-visible haematuria, especially in the case of younger patients, given the lower incidence of upper tract malignancy in these individuals (compared with those with visible haematuria) and its associated safety. USS should be combined with KUB X-ray (for stones) and flexible cystoscopy as initial investigations. These should be followed by an IVU or CTU if no abnormalities are detected and if there is persistent haematuria. Following normal investigations in an individual over 40 years of age over a follow-up period of 4 years there is a less than 1% chance of missing a urological tumour.[20] For patients with a higher risk of pathology (i.e. those with visible haematuria or those over 50 years of age) then it is sensible to replace USS/KUB/IVU with CTU along with a flexible cystoscopy. CTU has a reported sensitivity of 96% and a specificity of 99% in detecting upper urinary tract carcinomas.[21] In these patients the disadvantages of CTU (including the high cost of the procedure, high radiation dose and the need for contrast medium) are outweighed by its diagnostic performance. In many urological centres CTU has replaced a combination of USS and IVU in the diagnostic evaluation of patients with visible haematuria or recurrent non-visible haematuria, while USS continues to have a place in the evaluation of patients with non-visible haematuria.

Renal biopsy

Younger patients, particularly those under 40 years of age, often have a glomerular cause for their (non-visible) haematuria. These patients should have their blood pressure, urinary protein (by dipstick initially) and serum creatinine measured. Young adults with persistent haematuria have a 0.7% chance of developing end-stage renal failure (34-fold higher than in patients without persistent microscopic haematuria) over the next 20 years.[7] Thus, depending upon these findings it may be more appropriate for this group of patients to be referred to a renal physician for a nephrological evaluation. If nephrological consultation is not made, then the patients GP should follow these parameters over the next few years to ensure that any possible development of renal impairment is detected.

Treatment of intractable haematuria

A minority of patients with urological pathology present with constant and intractable haematuria. This can be very difficult to manage. Pathological examples include bleeding from advanced BC or prostate cancer and radiation cystitis following previous pelvic radiotherapy. The treatment of this bleeding is usually palliative and depends upon the cause. For BC and prostate cancer several options can be used including debridement of the intraluminal surface of the tumour by endoscopic resection or intravesical irrigation with pro-coagulant fluids such as alum or mitomycin-C. For all advanced cancers palliative radiotherapy (provided there has been no previous radiotherapy exposure) and/or radiological embolization of the feeding vessels may be used. These treatments are often unsuccessful and regular transfusion of blood may be needed. Occasionally bleeding from benign disease (e.g. radiotherapy cystitis) becomes such a problem that a cystectomy is warranted.

Further reading

Babjuk M, Oosterlinck W, Sylvester R, *et al.* EAU guidelines on non-muscle-invasive urothelial carcinoma of the bladder, the 2011 update. *Eur Urol* 2011; **59**(6):997–1008.

Kamat AM, Hegarty PK, Gee JR, *et al.* ICUD-EAU International Consultation on Bladder Cancer 2012: Screening, diagnosis, and molecular markers. *Eur Urol* 2013; **63**(1):4–15.

Kelly JD, Fawcett D, Goldberg LC. Assessment and management of non-visible haematuria in primary care. *BMJ* 2009; 338(a3021).

Khadra MH, Pickard RS, Charlton M, Powell PH, Neal DE. A prospective analysis of 1,930 patients with hematuria to evaluate current diagnostic practice. *J Urol* 2000; **163**(2):524–7.

Mowatt G, Zhu S, Kilonzo M, *et al.* Systematic review of the clinical effectiveness and cost-effectiveness of photodynamic diagnosis and urine biomarkers (FISH, ImmunoCyt, NMP22) and cytology for the detection and follow-up of bladder cancer. *Health Technol Assess* 2010; **14**(4): 1–331, iii-iv.

References

1. Kelly JD, Fawcett D, Goldberg LC. Assessment and management of non-visible haematuria in primary care. *BMJ* 2009; **338**(a3021).
2. Khadra MH, Pickard RS, Charlton M, Powell PH, Neal DE. A prospective analysis of 1,930 patients with hematuria to evaluate current diagnostic practice. *J Urol* 2000; **163**(2):524–7.
3. Babjuk M, Oosterlinck W, Sylvester R, *et al.* EAU guidelines on non-muscle-invasive urothelial carcinoma of the bladder, the 2011 update. *Eur Urol* 2011; **59**(6):997–1008.
4. Chou R, Dana T. Screening adults for bladder cancer: a review of the evidence for the U.S. preventive services task force. *Ann Int Med* 2010; **153**(7):461–8.
5. Brown RS. Has the time come to include urine dipstick testing in screening asymptomatic young adults? *JAMA* 2011; **306**(7):764–5.

6. Grossfeld GD, Litwin MS, Wolf JS, *et al.* Evaluation of asymptomatic microscopic hematuria in adults: the American Urological Association best practice policy—part I: definition, detection, prevalence, and etiology. *Urology* 2001; **57**(4):599–603.
7. Vivante A, Afek A, Frenkel-Nir Y, *et al.* Persistent asymptomatic isolated microscopic hematuria in Israeli adolescents and young adults and risk for end-stage renal disease. *JAMA* 2011; **306**(7):729–36.
8. Mariani AJ, Luangphinith S, Loo S, Scottolini A, Hodges CV. Dipstick chemical urinalysis: an accurate cost-effective screening test. *J Urol* 1984; **132**(1):64–6.
9. Sutton JM. Evaluation of hematuria in adults. *JAMA* 1990; **263**(18):2475–80.
10. Messing EM, Young TB, Hunt VB, Emoto SE, Wehbie JM. The significance of asymptomatic microhematuria in men 50 or more years old: findings of a home screening study using urinary dipsticks. *J Urol* 1987; **137**(5):919–22.
11. Woolhandler S, Pels RJ, Bor DH, Himmelstein DU, Lawrence RS. Dipstick urinalysis screening of asymptomatic adults for urinary tract disorders. I. Hematuria and proteinuria. *JAMA* 1989; **262**(9):1214–9.
12. Sultana SR, Goodman CM, Byrne DJ, Baxby K. Microscopic haematuria: urological investigation using a standard protocol. *Br J Urol* 1996; **78**(5):691–6; discussion 697–698.
13. Rao PK, Gao T, Pohl M, Jones JS. Dipstick pseudohematuria: unnecessary consultation and evaluation. *J Urol* 2010; **183**(2):560–4.
14. Mowatt G, Zhu S, Kilonzo M, *et al.* Systematic review of the clinical effectiveness and cost-effectiveness of photodynamic diagnosis and urine biomarkers (FISH, ImmunoCyt, NMP22) and cytology for the detection and follow-up of bladder cancer. *Health Technol Assess* 2010; **14**(4):1–331, iii-iv.
15. Kamat AM, Hegarty PK, Gee JR, *et al.* ICUD-EAU International Consultation on Bladder Cancer 2012: Screening, diagnosis, and molecular markers. *Eur Urol* 2013; **63**(1):4–15.
16. Robinson VL, Porter M, Messing E, Fradet Y, Kamat AM, Lotan Y. BCAN Think Tank session 2: Molecular detection of bladder cancer: the path to progress. *Urol Oncol* 2010; **28**(3):334–7.
17. Glas AS, Roos D, Deutekom M, Zwinderman AH, Bossuyt PM, Kurth KH. Tumor markers in the diagnosis of primary bladder cancer. A systematic review. *J Urol* 2003; **169**(6):1975–82.
18. Hall MC, Chang SS, Dalbagni G, *et al.* Guideline for the management of nonmuscle invasive bladder cancer (stages Ta, T1, and Tis): 2007 update. *J Urol* 2007; **178**(6):2314–30.
19. Feldstein MS, Hentz JG, Gillett MD, Novicki DE. Should the upper tracts be imaged for microscopic haematuria? *BJU Int* 2005; **96**(4):612–7.
20. Edwards TJ, Dickinson AJ, Natale S, Gosling J, McGrath JS. A prospective analysis of the diagnostic yield resulting from the attendance of 4020 patients at a protocol-driven haematuria clinic. *BJU Int* 2006; **97**(2):301–5; discussion 305.
21. Chlapoutakis K, Theocharopoulos N, Yarmenitis S, Damilakis J. Performance of computed tomographic urography in diagnosis of upper urinary tract urothelial carcinoma, in patients presenting with hematuria: Systematic review and meta-analysis. *Eur J Radiol* 2010; **73**(2):334–8.

CHAPTER 6.19

Low and intermediate risk non-muscle-invasive bladder cancer

Aditya Bagrodia and Yair Lotan

Epidemiology and presentation

Bladder cancer is the fourth most common cancer in men and the fifth most common malignancy overall.[1] In the United States in 2012, 73,510 new cases of bladder urothelial carcinoma and 14,880 deaths from bladder cancer are expected to occur.[2] Bladder cancer is four times more common in males than females, with an age standardized incidence rate of 10.1/100,000 for males and 2.5/100,000 for females.[1] Approximately 1 in 26 males and 1 in 87 females will develop urinary bladder cancer over the course of their life.[2]

The bladder is particularly susceptible to cancer, as it acts as a storage chamber for excreted carcinogens. Smoking is the most important risk factor for bladder cancer and is responsible for 50–75% of cases in men and 14–35% of cases in women.[3,4]

Carcinogens in tobacco include polyaromatic hydrocarbons such as 2-Naphthylamine, which are excreted by the kidneys and exert a carcinogenic effect on the entire urinary system. Following smoking, occupational exposure to carcinogens, namely aromatic amines (benzidine, 4-aminobiphenyl, b-naphthylamine, 4-chloro-o-toluidine), polycyclic aromatic hydrocarbons, and chlorinated hydrocarbons, is responsible for 20% of all bladder cancer cases. These occupational exposures are associated with chemical, oil, and dye-based industries.[3,5,6] While smoking and occupational exposures are associated with urothelial cell carcinoma (UCC, previously known as transitional cell carcinoma) which is the predominant histologic subtype of bladder cancer seen in the US and Europe, Schistosomiasis infection is associated with squamous cell carcinoma, and is the dominant subtype (75%) in areas of the world where bilharziasis is endemic.[7] UCC comprises the majority (90%) of bladder cancers in non-endemic regions, with squamous and adenocarcinoma constituting 5% and 1% of bladder tumours, respectively.[8,9]

Bladder cancer is broadly separated into two categories: non-muscle-invasive tumours and tumours that invade the muscularis propria. This dichotomy has significant implications, as patients with muscle-invasive tumours are generally treated with radical cystectomy while attempts are made to spare the bladder for non-muscle-invasive disease. Approximately 70–85% of bladder tumours are non-muscle-invasive at initial presentation (Ta, T1, Tis) and will be the focus of this chapter.

Diagnosis

Haematuria (blood in the urine) is the most common presenting symptom in patients with bladder cancer. Bladder cancer is found on initial evaluation in 13–34.5% of patients with gross (macroscopic) haematuria and in 0.5–10.5% of patients with microscopic haematuria.[10–14] Irritative voiding symptoms are also a symptom of bladder cancer, especially carcinoma *in situ* (CIS). These can manifest with primary symptoms, such as urgency, dysuria, frequency and nocturia, or be mis-diagnosed as recurrent bacterial cystitis. The latter is more common in females and may, in part, lead to the worse prognosis for females with bladder cancer, when compared to males. Approximately 80% of patients with CIS present with irritative voiding symptoms, and the presence of these symptoms doubles the risk of harbouring CIS (5% vs. 10.5%) among patients with haematuria.[11,15] However, both haematuria and voiding symptoms are seen commonly with other urologic conditions such as enlarged prostates, urinary tract infection, and urolithiasis and may result in diagnostic difficulties in many patients.

Patients suspected of having bladder cancer due to haematuria or symptoms should first undergo office cystoscopy. If imaging or cytology is highly suggestive of malignancy, initial cystoscopy may be performed under anaesthesia at the time of biopsy. Not all tumours are readily visible on conventional white light (WL) cystoscopy, and CIS is notorious for being indistinguishable from normal urothelium or inflamed mucosa.

Diagnostic difficulties with conventional WL cystoscopy have led investigators to explore more accurate technologies for detection of bladder cancer. Fluorescence based photodynamic diagnostic (PDD) techniques utilize the fact that photoactive compounds preferentially accumulate in hypermetabolic malignant tissue compared to normal tissue and fluoresce red under blue light illumination.[16] δ-aminolevulinic acid (5-ALA) was an initial compound used for PDD; however, it has largely been supplanted by hexyl aminolevulinate (HAL), a more lipophilic derivate that allows significantly shorter bladder instillation times and superior cystoscopic examination.[17,18] Clinical studies demonstrate that HAL may be superior to traditional WL cystoscopy at detection of bladder tumours. Over three hundred patients underwent WL cystoscopy followed by HAL in a multicentre study evaluating detection of non-invasive bladder cancer.[19] For Ta tumours, detection rates were significantly higher for HAL cystoscopy than WL cystoscopy (96% vs. 83% respectively, $p = 0.0001$). More T1 tumours were also detected with HAL cystoscopy than WL cystoscopy (95% vs. 86%, respectively, $p = 0.3$). A smaller prospective phase III study including 146 patients with known or suspected bladder cancer demonstrated that HAL cystoscopy improved overall tumour detection over WL cystoscopy with detection rates for dysplasia (93% vs. 48%), carcinoma *in situ* (95% vs. 68%) and superficial papillary tumours (96% vs. 85%) favouring HAL cystoscopy.[20]

The clinical relevance of increased tumour detections rates with HAL cystoscopy is also being investigated. A multinational, prospective study accrued 814 patients at high risk for bladder cancer recurrence and randomized them to HAL or WL cystoscopy. Patients were deemed to have an increased risk of recurrence based on more than one initial or recurrent bladder tumours or recurrence within 12 months of a previous bladder tumour.[21] In the PDD cohort, 286 patients had at least 1 Ta or T1 tumour (intent to treat) and in 47 patients (16%) at least one of the tumours was seen only with fluorescence ($p = 0.001$). During the nine-month follow-up, recurrence was assessed in 271 and 280 patients in the PDD and WL group, respectively. Tumours recurred in 128 of 271 patients (47%) in the PDD group and 157 of 280 (56%) in the WL group ($p = 0.026$). In the patients with high-grade Ta/T1 tumours the recurrence was 54.8% versus 56.6% in the fluorescence and WL groups, respectively ($p = 0.48$). More low-grade tumours recurred in the WL versus HAL group, (55.4% vs. 45.4%, respectively, $p = 0.02$). In this study that was restricted to high-risk patients, the benefit of PDD was limited to patients with low-grade non-invasive tumours. The benefit of HAL technology in patients with standard risk remains to be determined.

A metanalysis of prospective trials assessing the utility of PDD found that 20% more tumours and 23% more CIS were detected using PDD in comparison to traditional WL cystoscopy.[22] The improved detection rate using HAL technology translated into decreased recurrence rates at 12 months (15.8–27% better than WL) and 24 months (12–15% better than WL).[22] Conflicting data on the utility of PDD, practical issues related to instillation of the fluorescing agents and cost considerations have precluded it from widespread use.[23]

Initial management: tumour resection to establish histology

Once a bladder malignancy is suspected (based on imaging, cytology, or diagnostic cystoscopy), transurethral resection of the tumour is required to make a definitive diagnosis.[24] Complete tumour resection when safely possible is requisite. Non-conducting bladder irrigants such as sterile water, sorbitol, mannitol, or glycine solutions have traditionally been used; however, newer bipolar electrical resection allows for the use of normal saline, which may mitigate obturator reflexes during posteriolateral resection.[25] Under general or regional anaesthesia, cystoscopy is performed with both a 30° and 70° lens to visualize all aspects of the bladder. A flexible cystoscope may alternatively be employed. The size, number, location, and character (papillary versus nodular or sessile) of tumours and erythematous patches should be noted since these parameters have prognostic and management implications.[26–28] A bladder map is helpful for operative planning. Small tumours may be removed en bloc with a portion of the underlying detrusor muscle using cold-cup biopsy forceps followed by electrofulguration with Bugbee electrode. Representative samples of erythematous patches concerning for CIS are also amenable to cold-cup biopsy. Cold-cup biopsy has the advantage of removing cautery artefact on histological analysis.

Larger tumours are resected with a 30 degree resectoscope. Technical tenets of transurethral resection of a bladder tumour (TURBT) include ensuring that the resection loop is always visible, lifting the tumour off of the detrusor to minimize the risk of perforation, and safely obtaining detrusor muscle within the sample for accurate staging.[29] A complete and thorough transurethral resection of all visible tumours should be performed, as high quality tumour removal is associated with better prognosis.[30] Further, a sample of the detrusor muscle is necessary for accurate staging. A separate pass through the tumour bed after tumour resection may be taken to ensure adequate detrusor muscle sampling. Detrusor muscle in the specimen is important for decreasing early recurrences due to residual disease. The recurrence rate on first follow-up cystoscopy is significantly higher when detrusor muscle is absent (44.4%) than present (21.7%).[31]

If no lesions are visible in the bladder and cytology is positive or if there is a high suspicion for CIS, random bladder biopsies should be taken from the trigone, dome, posterior, lateral, and anterior walls. The theoretical reasons for taking random bladder biopsies are that CIS may exist in normal appearing urothelium and that certain small or endophytic tumours may not be visible. Multiple groups from the United States, Europe, and Asia have looked at the yield of random bladder biopsies. The rate of finding malignancy varies from 8–12.4%, with highest yield in patients with high-risk tumours.[32–35] Random bladder biopsies can be omitted in low-risk tumours (papillary appearance and negative cytology) as the incidence of concomitant CIS is less than 2% in this population.[34] The prostate may also be involved with tumour in patients with non-muscle-invasive bladder tumours. Risk factors for prostatic involvement include trigonal or bladder neck tumours, CIS, and multifocal malignancies.[36] Transurethral biopsies of the prostate should be taken when intraprostatic tumours are identified or when the aforementioned risk factors are present with positive cytology and no visible tumours.

Staging and classification

The American Joint Committee on Cancer classification, or Tumour-Node-Metastases (TNM) system, is the most widely used staging system for bladder cancer (for further information on staging please see www.cancerstaging.org).[37] Non-muscle-invasive tumours include Ta, T1, and carcinoma *in situ* (Tis). The bladder wall is generally divided into four layers (Fig. 6.19.1): the urothelial mucosal surface, subepithelial connective tissue (lamina propria), the detrusor muscle (or muscularis propria), and the surrounding fat.

Ta tumours are confined to the mucosa, Tis is a high-grade tumour that does not invade into the lamina propria, and T1 tumours invade into the subepithelial connective tissue. Some groups advocate a T1b subclassification for tumours that invade into the deep subepithelial connective tissue but the prognostic value of this schema has not been validated and it is not widely used.[38] Tumours invading the bladder muscular wall are stage T2 with tumour invading the superficial muscularis propria (inner

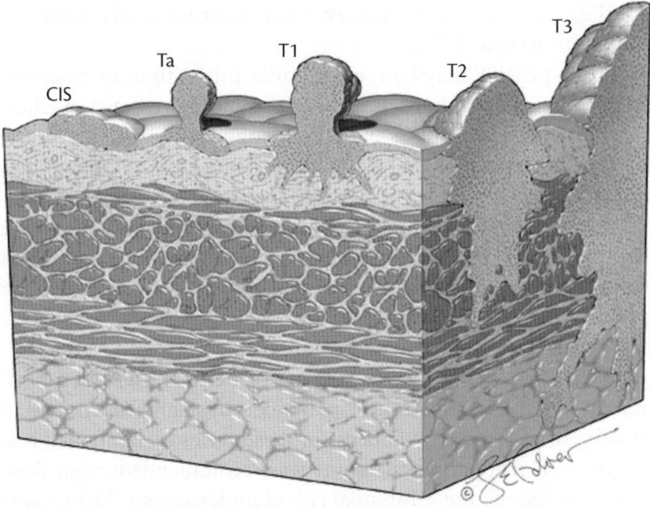

Fig. 6.19.1 Bladder wall divided into four layers.
Reproduced with courtesy of Lewis E. Calver.

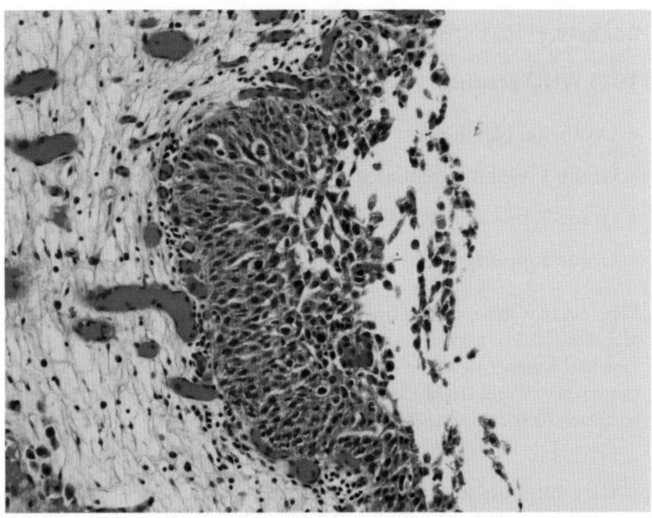

Fig. 6.19.3 Bladder CIS is a non-invasive, high-grade tumour by definition.
Reproduced with courtesy of Payal Kapur.

half) categorized as T2a and tumours invading the deep muscularis propria (outer half) as T2b. The bladder wall is surrounded by fat and tumours that invade the fat are classified as T3. Most non-muscle-invasive tumours on initial presentation are papillary tumours that do not invade the lamina propria.[39] Ta tumours are usually solitary, coral-like tumours that are generally low grade (Fig. 6.19.2). Low-grade Ta tumours are associated with a high rate of tumour recurrence (15–70% at one year) but low rate of progression to higher stage disease with less than 5% progressing to muscle-invasive disease.[27,40–43] The minority of tumours that are Ta with high grade have between a 13–40% chance of progressing to lamina propria invasion, and between 6–25% chance of becoming muscle-invasive.[44] T1 tumours comprise approximately one-quarter of all non-muscle-invasive tumours at initial presentation.[39] They may be papillary or nodular on gross appearance and have worse malignant potential than Ta tumours in terms of recurrence (80%) and

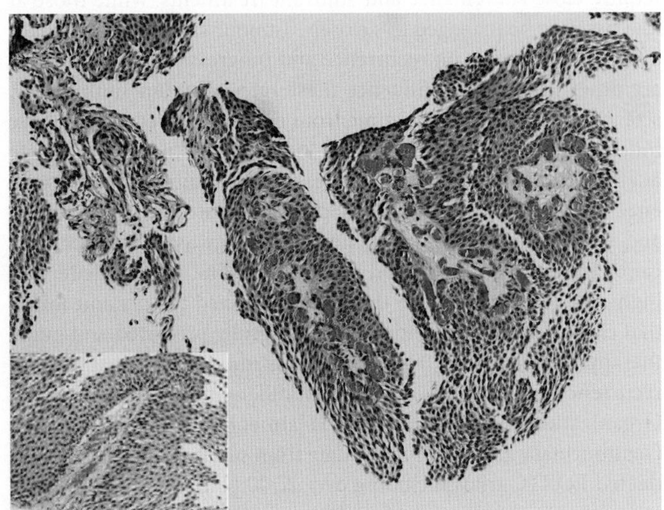

Fig. 6.19.2 Ta tumours are usually solitary, coral-like tumours that are generally low grade.
Reproduced with courtesy of Payal Kapur.

progression (50% within three years).[42,45,46] There is also a significant concern about understaging of T1 tumours, which is the reason for performing a repeat resection of the scar and the bladder (re-TUR) to confirm the absence of muscle invasion. Bladder CIS is a non-invasive, high-grade tumour by definition (Fig. 6.19.3). CIS in reference to bladder cancer does not denote a premalignant or precursor lesion. CIS is not always visualized on cystoscopic exam but often presents as erythematous, or velvety, patch that may diffusely occupy the bladder mucosa. This makes it difficult to identify and eradicate during transurethral resection. CIS most commonly occurs concurrently with other bladder tumours and is associated with high rates of recurrence (82%) and progression (42–83%) especially if not treated with adjuvant intravesical therapy.[44,47,48]

Tumour grade has a dramatic impact on progression and survival in patients with non-muscle-invasive bladder cancer. For non-muscle-invasive tumours, grade has a greater prognostic significance than tumour stage for predicting progression.[14,40–42,44,45] The World Health Organization (WHO) bladder cancer grading system of 1973 classified cancers as urothelial papilloma, grade 1 (well differentiated), grade 2 (moderately differentiated), and grade 3 (poorly differentiated) carcinoma (Box 6.19.1 and 6.19.2).[24,49] The WHO and International Society of Urological Pathologists amended the 1973 classification in 2004 with two substantial changes. First, a new category named papillary urothelial neoplasia of low malignant potential (PUNLMP) was created to describe lesions without cellular characteristics of malignancy but with papillary appearance and increased cell layers.[24,49] Secondly, tumours were to be categorized as either high grade or low grade, to avoid overclassification as WHO 1973 grade 2 lesions (moderately differentiated) that displayed more variable clinical behaviour.[24,49] The 2004 classification is demonstrated to have less interobserver variability than the previous version.[50] Neither system has been demonstrated to have prognostic superiority as of yet.[50,51]

Clinical staging incorporates the physical exam (including bimanual examination under anaesthesia before and after transurethral resection of bladder tumour—TURBT), radiographic imaging, and histological findings at TURBT. Urinary cytology and other urine-based markers may also be used. Clinically palpable

Box 6.19.1 1973 WHO grading of urothelial lesions[49]

1973 WHO grading

- Urothelial papilloma
- Grade 1: well differentiated
- Grade 2: moderately differentiated
- Grade 3: poorly differentiated

Reproduced with permission from Mostofi FK *et al.*, Histological typing of urinary bladder tumours, *International Histological Classification of Tumours*, Number 10, World Health Organization, Geneva, Switzerland, Copyright © World Health Organization 1973, http://apps.who.int/iris/bitstream/10665/41533/1/9241760109_eng.pdf

primary tumours and lymph nodes are not consistent with non-muscle-invasive bladder cancer. Along with cystoscopy, intravenous urography (IVU) or computed tomography urography (CTU) are often used as a part of the haematuria evaluation to identify concomitant filling defects in the upper tract collecting system, hydronephrosis suggesting bulky ureteral tumours or muscle-invasive bladder tumours near a ureteral orifice, and large tumours within the bladder. CTU has the advantage of assessing the kidneys, extent of local invasion, and potentially enlarged pelvic lymph nodes. Urine cytology from a voided or barbotaged specimen is helpful in the diagnosis and monitoring of patients with urothelial carcinoma. The sensitivity of urine cytology approaches 90% in patients with high-grade tumours and CIS but drops substantially for low-grade tumours.[52] A host of FDA-approved urine-based markers are commercially available with a promising role in the diagnosis and surveillance of bladder cancer, including nuclear matrix protein 22 (NMP22) and UroVysion®; however, none have replaced cytology or cystoscopy to date.[53,54]

Box 6.19.2 2004 WHO grading of urothelial lesions[49]

2004 WHO grading

- Flat lesions
- Hyperplasia (flat lesion without atypia or papillary aspects)
- Reactive atypia (flat lesion with atypia)
- Atypia of unknown significance
- Urothelial dysplasia
- Urothelial carcinoma in situ (CIS)
- Papillary lesions
- Urothelial papilloma (completely benign lesion)
- Papillary urothelial neoplasm of low malignant potential (PUNLMP)
- Low-grade papillary urothelial carcinoma
- High-grade papillary urothelial carcinoma

Text extracts reproduced with permission from Jonathan Epstein *et al.*, The World Health Organization/ International Society of Urological Pathology Consensus Classification of Urothelial (Transitional Cell) Neoplasms of the Urinary Bladder, *The American Journal of Surgical Pathology*, Volume 22, Issue 12, pp. 1435–1448, Copyright © 1998 Wolters Kluwer Health.

Repeat TURBT may be required after initial tumour resection if the initial tumour burden was not completely resected, medical instability of the patient or anaesthetic complication required early termination of the procedure, if all tumours were not anatomically accessible (i.e. large median lobe precluding resection of posterior tumours), or if visibility was excessively impaired. Restaging TURBT should also be considered in certain circumstances even if the aforementioned factors were not present, for instance when muscle is not identified in the initial specimen.

There is a significant risk of tumour understaging after initial TURBT. When cystectomy is performed for presumed non-muscle-invasive bladder cancer, pathologic upstaging is reported in 34–50% of patients.[55–58] Patients in these series certainly had risk factors such that early cystectomy was recommended; regardless, they demonstrate the substantial risk of understaging. T1 tumours should be restaged within two to six weeks of the initial resection. Residual disease after initial resection of T1 disease is identified in one-third to one-half of patients.[59–61] Approximately 20% of patients that undergo repeat tumour resection will have their tumour upstaged; this figure rises to 60% if no muscle was present on the initial specimen.[56,62] Repeat transurethral resection alters management strategy in 33% of patients and may improve survival as well.[63,64]

Prognostic indicators for future recurrence and progression: defining risk

While a bladder tumour can be removed by endoscopic resection (where possible), most patients develop further cancers within their lifetime. These subsequent tumours may arise from residual tissue at the site of the primary cancer (from an incomplete transurethral resection) or distant to this region from widespread molecular changes that have occurred following global carcinogen exposure (so-called 'field change'). The risk of further recurrences (a similar cancer to the previous) or progression (worse cancer to the previous) is key to the management of that patient. Those at high risk require close surveillance and adjuvant treatments, while those at low risk may be managed less closely. Tumour stage and grade have a significant impact on recurrence and progression rates but there are other factors that influence these rates. Tumour multiplicity, size, concomitant CIS, and time from resection to recurrence have independent prognostic value.[42,65] In a Spanish study, multivariate analysis demonstrated; stage, grade, tumour multiplicity and presence of CIS to be independent factors of recurrence, progression, and survival in patients with non-muscle-invasive bladder cancer.[65] These authors stratified patients into low, intermediate, and high-risk groups based on the aforementioned factors and found that clinical outcomes could be meaningfully predicted and guide therapy. Despite over 1,000 patients, this study was limited because recurrence and progression were not differentiated. The European Organization for Research and Treatment of Cancer (EORTC) Genitourinary group combined data from seven prospectively conducted EORTC trials including over 2,500 patients and found that recurrence and progression could be predicted based on; tumour multiplicity, diameter, primary recurrence rate (<1 year), tumour stage, presence of CIS, and grade. These six variables were given weighted values to calculate a final score and stratify patients into low, intermediate, and high-risk groups. Recurrence rates at one and five years were 15% and 31% for low-risk patients, between 24–38% at one year and 31–46% at five years for intermediate risk patients, and 61% and 78% for high-risk patients, respectively.[42] Progression rates at one and five years were substantially lower for low-risk patients (0.2 and 0.8%, respectively) than high-risk patients (4–24% progression at one year and 14–55% progression at five years).[42]

Pathologic features and molecular markers have also been evaluated for prognostic significance in non-muscle-invasive bladder cancer. Tumours that invade into the deep subepithelial connective tissue (proposed T1b classification) may be associated with higher progression rates.[38] Lymphovascular invasion (LVI) is an independent predictor of overall mortality, cancer-specific mortality, local, and distant recurrence in patients receiving cystectomy for bladder cancer.[66] It is an ominous finding if identified on TURBT specimen.[66] Recurrence rates (48% vs. 34%) and progression rates (30 vs. 10%) are found to be worse in patients with LVI than those without LVI, respectively.[67] The prognostic utility of regulatory biomarkers including pRb, p53, p21, and various growth factors is also studied in bladder cancer.[68–76] Altered expression of cell cycle regulators such as p53, p21, p27, cyclin E, and proliferative markers including Ki-67 are associated with increased recurrence and progression rates. Combining these markers allows for statistically significant risk stratification.[68] Tissue-based markers are still largely in the investigational stage and are not widely used for clinical decision making.

Surveillance

Due to the high recurrence rates of non-muscle-invasive bladder tumours, patients require close surveillance. Patients should be queried about voiding symptoms and gross haematuria at each follow-up appointment. Cystoscopy is also performed at regular intervals, as non-invasive methods utilizing urinary biomarkers for surveillance are still in the investigation phases.[77] Cystoscopy is usually performed in the outpatient setting, precluding the need for general anaesthesia. Intraurethral anaesthetic and use of a flexible cystoscope is commonly utilized.

The first cystoscopy following TURBT should take place at three months, since recurrence at this time is recognized as an important prognosticator for both recurrence and progression.[42,78,79] After urinalysis confirms the absence of infection, cystoscopy should be performed. This frequently includes a barbotaged urine specimen that is sent for cytology, however, the benefit of cytology in patients with low-grade tumours has been questioned due to low sensitivity. The National Comprehensive Cancer Network guidelines recommend cystoscopic evaluation every three to six months and then at increasing intervals as appropriate.[37] There is no consensus on optimal follow-up regimen, but conventionally patients are assessed cystoscopically at three-month intervals for the first two years, and then at six-month intervals for the next two to three years, and then annually thereafter.[80] For low-risk tumours, however, the EAU guidelines recommend cystoscopy at three months and if negative then another cystoscopy at 12 months and annually thereafter for the next five years.[81]

The surveillance cycle restarts every time a tumour is identified. If a tumour is identified on surveillance cystoscopy, the patient will require another TURBT to reassess the stage, grade, and pathological characteristics of the recurrent tumour for oncologic control of the tumour and proper patient counselling. In select patients that have a long history of only low-grade Ta tumours, small tumours may be laser or electrofulgurated in the ambulatory setting with the use of an intravesical anesthetic[43] or even managed without resection (so-called active surveillance) given their low propensity for progression and to avoid multiple operations and anaesthetics.[82,83]

Tumour markers

In an effort to eliminate or minimize the need for cystoscopy and also to decrease missed lesions due to operator error, difficult to diagnose CIS patches, and diagnostically challenging areas of acute inflammation or chronic catheter irritation, considerable effort has been spent on developing non-invasive, urine-based tumour markers. The development of adequate biomarkers could also potentially decrease the significant cost associated with bladder cancer surveillance.[39]

Urine-based tumour markers are usually compared to cytology in terms of ability to detect when cancer is present and reliably predict when there is no malignancy. Urine cytology has an acceptable sensitivity for detecting high-grade bladder cancer, yet lacks sensitivity for detect low-grade tumours, ranging from 4% to 31%. Cytology is also limited by the fact that results are not immediately available and a specialized cytopathologist is required for interpretation; results generally take one week to report, and possibly longer if no pathologist is readily available.[84] Unfortunately, the fact that cytology misses up to 20–30% of high-grade tumours means that it cannot replace or delay cystoscopy. Finally, frequently there are inconclusive results such as atypical cytology which make it difficult to interpret.

An ideal bladder tumour marker would accurately detect and monitor patients with a history of bladder cancer, identify recurrence early and prevent disease progression. Because of the relatively low prevalence of bladder cancer in general, screening the whole population would not be cost effective.[85] An accurate marker would also have the potential to replace, delay, or complement cystoscopy and/or cytology in the detection and monitoring of patients with bladder cancer. An ideal bladder cancer monitoring test would be non-invasive, objective, easy to perform and interpret, with high sensitivity and specificity, and would provide an immediate or rapid result. As noted above, the most commonly used adjunct for identification of bladder cancer is cytology which detects neoplastic cells in the urine.[86] Below the more commonly used and rigorously examined tumour markers will be discussed.

NMP22® (Alere Inc.) and BTA stat® are two extensively studied, urine-based protein-based tumour markers. The BTA stat® is a qualitative point-of-care test and the BTA TRAK is a quantitative test that detect human complement factor H-related protein (as well as complement factor H) which is present in the urine of patients with bladder cancer.[87] Nuclear matrix proteins have been attributed roles in DNA replication, in ribonucleic acid transcription and in the regulation of gene expression. One member of this family, nuclear mitotic apparatus protein 22 (NMP22), is much more prevalent in malignant urothelial cells than in their normal counterparts and is released in the urine during apoptosis.

ImmunoCyt™ (Diagnocure) is a test that combines cytology with an immunofluorescence assay.[88] ImmunoCyt™ detects cellular markers for bladder cancer in exfoliated urothelial cells using three fluorescent monoclonal antibodies to detect a high molecular weight form of carcinoembryonic antigen and two bladder tumour cell-associated mucins. At this time, the test requires the use of a fluorescence microscope by trained personnel and, as a consequence, is performed in a reference laboratory. Multiple chromosomes, such as 1, 3, 4, 7, 8, 9, 11, and 17 are altered in cancers of the urinary tract.

UroVysion™ (Abbott) is a genetic test with a multitarget fluorescence *in situ* hybridization (FISH) assay that detects increased numbers of chromosomes 3, 7, 17 as well as loss of the 9p21 locus. The FISH test combines assessment of the morphologic changes of conventional cytology with molecular DNA changes. The kit contains a mixture of unlabeled blocking DNA to suppress sequences contained within the target loci that are common to other chromosomes. A minimum of 25 morphologically abnormal cells are viewed. The case is considered positive for a tumour if four or more cells exhibit polysomy of chromosomes 3, 7 or 17, or if there is loss of chromosome 9 in nine cells.[89] However, no uniform criterion exists for a positive UroVysion assay at this time.

The main disadvantage of current markers is their lower specificity compared with cytology. For example, there is a substantially higher level of NMP22 in the urine of patients with bladder cancer. However, because this protein is released from dead and dying urothelial cells, many benign conditions of the urinary tract, such as stones, infection, inflammation, and haematuria carry these proteins as well and cystoscopy can cause a false-positive reading. At this time, it is difficult to make clear recommendations regarding the use of urine markers. The potential clinical scenarios for use of markers is in lieu of cystoscopy for either detection or surveillance, as an adjunct to cystoscopy for detection or surveillance or in combination with cystoscopy and cytology. The available markers are not sensitive enough to replace cystoscopy. Most studies have evaluated markers in combination with cystoscopy and cytology, with tumour markers improving sensitivity.[90,91] Unlike cytology which has a very high specificity, markers suffer from issues with lower specificity such that many patients with a positive marker do not have cancer. As a consequence, patients with a positive marker are usually monitored more closely but do not have recommendation to undergo bladder biopsies.

Upper urinary tract surveillance

There is a risk of developing metachronous tumours in the upper urinary tracts associated with bladder tumours. The overall percentage of patients with bladder tumours that synchronously or subsequently develop upper tract urothelial carcinomas is low (2%) but has been reported to be as high as 18% in high-risk patients.[92,93] The risk of upper tract malignancy increases with advanced tumour grade, location near the ureteral orifices, and in patients with haematuria.[94,95] Tumour multiplicity, frequent recurrences, presence of bladder CIS, and intravesical therapy failures are also identified as relatively higher risk characteristics.[96]

There is no consensus for who requires upper tract imaging and how often. Most patients receive imaging of their upper urinary tracts during initial evaluation if haematuria is the presenting symptom. Upper tract imaging may be postponed in patients with low risk (Ta/T1, low grade) unless haematuria develops or cytology is positive without identifiable lesions. In patients at higher risk, upper tract imaging should be considered annually. Intravenous urography was traditionally employed for upper tract surveillance but is limited in ability to evaluate the renal parenchyma.[94] Retrograde pyelography may be performed in a single setting in patients that are to undergo TURBT or may be required in patients with renal insufficiency or contrast allergy. CTU is increasingly being used for upper tract surveillance because of better sensitivity and specificity than IVU for detecting upper tract urothelial carcinomas.[97]

Prevention of recurrence and progression

TURBT is the cornerstone for initial diagnosis and management of non-muscle-invasive bladder tumours. Nearly one-half of patients will have a tumour recurrence within one year of initial TURBT. Of greater importance, approximately 0.4–24% will progress to muscle-invasive or metastatic disease.[42] Tumour recurrence is postulated to occur because of incomplete resection, occult tumours that were not visualized and resected at initial TURBT, floating tumour cells reimplanting after resection, and *de novo* tumour formation secondary to the known field effect of bladder cancer. Intravesical chemotherapy and immunotherapy are the two most extensively utilized and studied treatment modalities for the prevention of recurrence and progress.

Intravesical chemotherapy

Intravesical chemotherapy may be administered as a single perioperative dose within 24 hours of TURBT, as a six to eight week induction course following resection, or as a full course of induction + maintenance therapy. The perioperative dose decreases recurrence by preventing reimplantation of circulating tumour cells and by destroying non-resected tumour. Circulating tumour cells are covered by extracellular matrix within hours of reimplantation following TURBT, emphasizing the need for early postoperative chemotherapy.[98] While instillation of chemotherapeutic within 24 hours of TURBT is deemed acceptable, early instillation immediately following TURBT may be superior.[99,100] Suspected extra- or intraperitoneal bladder rupture or bleeding requiring continuous bladder irrigation precludes the safe use of postoperative chemotherapy and is an absolute contraindication. Sylvester and colleagues conducted a metanalysis of seven randomized trials comparing TURBT alone to TURBT with a single postoperative dose of intravesical chemotherapy (mitomycin C in two trials, epirubicin in three trials, thiotepa in one trial, and pirarubicin in one trial). Notably, no single cytotoxic chemotherapeutic drug was demonstrated to be superior to others with respect to efficacy and all show beneficial effect.[101] Over a 3.4 year median follow-up in 1,476 patients, 36.7% recurred in the cytotoxic chemotherapy arm versus 48.4% in the TURBT alone arm, for a reduction in the odds of recurrence of 39%.[101] The majority of patients in this metanalysis had solitary tumours (80%). More recent studies suggest that patients with low-risk tumours (EORTC recurrence scores 0–2) derive the greatest benefit from single dose perioperative chemotherapy while patients with higher risk tumours receive little or no benefit.[102] Of note, single dose intravesical chemotherapy has not demonstrated a reduction in progression-free survival rates. A clinically significant difference in progression rates are more difficult to demonstrate given the overall low rates of progression in the low-risk patients that are included in these particular trials. Furthermore, there has not been a direct comparison between a single postoperative dose of intravesical chemotherapy and induction chemotherapy, and these two adjuvant options are often combined in clinical trials and meta-analyses. In patients with low-risk non-invasive bladder cancer, a single dose of postoperative mitomycin is considered standard of care. An induction course may be considered as clinical scenario warrants.[101,103]

There are a host of intravesical chemotherapeutics that are available, including doxorubicin, mitomycin C, thiotepa, epirubicin, and valrubicin. As mentioned previously, none has definitively been shown to be superior to the others. Mitomycin C is the most commonly used intravesical agent used in the United States. Mitomycin C is prepared for intravesical instillation by combining 20–60 mg of mitomycin C in 20–40 mL of sterile water or normal saline. A concentration of 40 mg/40 mL is the most commonly used formulation. Confirming complete bladder drainage and restricting fluid prior to instillation allows for the highest concentration of solution to be exposed to the urothelium.[104]

Maintenance intravesical chemotherapy may be considered in patients that are at higher risk for recurrence. First and foremost, a decision must be made if the goal is to prevent recurrence (low-grade tumours) or progression (high-grade tumours) based on the histology from the TURBT specimen. Intravesical chemotherapy, including maintenance regimens, prevents recurrence but not progression in primary and recurrent tumours.[105–107] No trials directly compare a short course of postoperative intravesical chemotherapy (either as a single postoperative dose or as a postoperative course of <2 months duration) to an induction course and maintenance chemotherapy. Further, the schedule of maintenance instillations is not standardized. However, in metanalyses of patients with primary and recurrent non-invasive tumours without CIS, an induction course of chemotherapy alone had higher rates of recurrence than an induction course with one to two years of maintenance chemotherapy.[105,106] While metanalyses on induction-only versus induction plus maintenance chemotherapy for preventing recurrence of bladder tumour suggest a benefit of maintenance chemotherapy; the optimal length of treatment, frequency of instillations, and dose of chemotherapeutic agent remain to be elucidated.[107]

Intravesical immunotherapy

In 1976, Alvaro Morales described an antitumour effect of Bacillus Calmette–Guérin (BCG), an attenuated mycobacterium, for bladder cancer.[108] Since the initial reports, intravesical instillation of BCG has replaced percutaneous inoculation for the prevention of recurrence and progression in non-invasive urothelial carcinoma.[109] Instillation of BCG into the bladder triggers an extensive local immunologic and antiangiogenic response largely mediated by the release of cytokines that activate downstream cell-mediated cytotoxic pathways as well as both T-helper Type I and II responses.[110–112] Ultimately, this inflammatory reaction results in the anti-neoplastic activity of BCG.

Intravesical formulation of BCG is prepared by combining 50 mL of saline to a powdered form of the attenuated mycobacterium. The solution is instilled through a urethral catheter into the bladder for two hours. Some groups have reported similar efficacy with reduced concentrations of BCG to reduce treatment-related morbidity.[113] However, the incidence of severe systemic adverse events is comparable between the standard and reduced-dosed groups. Further, there may be an advantage to full dose BCG in multifocal tumours.[114,115] Anecdotally, the patient can be sequentially rotated 90 degrees every half an hour to bathe the entire surface of the bladder. Following instillation, the bladder is drained through the urethral catheter and the catheter may be removed. Systemic absorption of BCG may lead to significant complications; as such administration of intravesical BCG is usually delayed two to four weeks after TURBT, once the bladder mucosa has an opportunity to heal. Further, treatment after episodes of gross haematuria or traumatic catheterization should be delayed for one week to allow for re-epithelialization of the mucosa prior to instillation. Urinalysis prior to administration of BCG allows for diagnosis of cystitis, which potentially enhances systemic absorption and subsequent complications.

BCG is recognized to be superior to intravesical chemotherapy for the prevention of recurrence and progression of non-invasive bladder cancer and for the treatment of CIS. However, BCG has a substantially worse toxicity profile than intravesical chemotherapy, including infectious complications that do not exist with chemotherapy. The higher incidence and more severe nature of BCG adverse events limit its uniform use. Broadly, in patients with low-risk tumours (based on EORTC criteria), who are at a very low risk of progression, intravesical chemotherapy is favoured due to fewer adverse effects. On the opposite end of the spectrum, patients in the high risk category should receive BCG if early cystectomy is not planned. For patients at intermediate risk for recurrence and progression, BCG is more effective than intravesical chemotherapy for prevention yet carries a higher risk of adverse effects. For these patients, both intravesical chemotherapy and immunotherapy are reasonable options and should be tailored to the clinical scenario and patient preference. Serious systemic side effects of BCG are limited to <5% of patients and most of these can be effectively managed with prompt diagnosis and treatment.[116] Nevertheless, in a large multicentre study, 20% of patients stopped BCG due to untoward side effects, including BCG-induced cystitis, fever, and general malaise. Notably, the incidence of side effects decreased with increased length of BCG treatment.[116]

The Impact of Bacille Calmette–Guérin therapy on recurrence and progression

BCG is consistently demonstrated to be better than TURBT alone for the prevention of recurrent tumours. Early single and multicentre studies demonstrated that BCG reduced tumour recurrence rates compared to TURBT alone by 20–65%.[117–119] Subsequently, multiple metanalyses confirmed that adjuvant intravesical BCG after TURBT is superior to TURBT alone and TURBT plus intravesical chemotherapy.[120–123] In a prospective, randomized trial, Lamm *et al.* reported an improved first-recurrence-free survival interval for patients receiving BCG compared to mitomycin C.[124] A meta-analysis of 11 trials comparing BCG to intravesical chemotherapy demonstrated that overall 38.6% of the patients receiving BCG and 46.4% of those in the mitomycin C arm had tumour recurrence.[123] In the subgroup treated with maintenance BCG, six studies uniformly showed significant superiority of BCG over mitomycin C (OR 0.43, $p < 0.001$) for the prevention of recurrence.[123] Randomized clinical trials of patients with intermediate and high-risk tumours have also illustrated the superiority of BCG compared to combination therapy of epirubicin and interferon, mitomycin C, and epirubicin alone.[125–128] In one study comparing mitomycin C to BCG with nine-year follow-up, 80% in the MMC group experienced recurrence compared to 59% receiving BCG.[126] Similarly, when comparing combination of epirubicin/interferon to BCG, 62% were disease-free in the combination arm as opposed to 73% in the BCG cohort.[125] In summary, BCG is more effective than TURBT alone or TURBT plus intravesical chemotherapy for prophylaxis against tumour recurrence.

The prevention of tumour progression is a more clinically significant end point than preventing recurrence, and the role of BCG in achieving this outcome is inconclusive. Herr and colleagues presented long-term data of BCG versus control in 86 high-risk patients and reported that progression occurred in 95% of controls versus 53% of BCG-treated patients.[129] Furthermore, time to disease progression and cystectomy was significantly delayed by BCG treatment. Ultimately, radical cystectomy was performed in 42% of controls and 26% of patients receiving BCG. In a metanalysis of 24 trials on 4,863 patients and a median follow-up of 2.5 years, 9.8% of patients on BCG had progression compared to 13.8% in controls for a reduction of 27% in the odds of progression on BCG.[130] The progression rate for patients with papillary tumours was low (6.4%) compared to those with CIS (13.9%); the overall low progression rates were attributed to primarily relatively low-risk patients being enrolled in trials and the short duration of follow-up. Of note, only patients receiving maintenance BCG benefited and there was no statistically significant difference in either overall survival or cancer-specific survival for patients receiving BCG. The authors of the EORTC metanalysis concluded that BCG plus maintenance is the preferred treatment for patients with intermediate and high-risk papillary tumours and those with CIS.[130] Bohle and associated conducted a metanalysis that specifically compared BCG to intravesical chemotherapy.[131] This metanalysis included 1,277 patients treated with BCG and 1,133 with mitomycin C from nine trials with a median follow-up of 26 months. Tumour progression occurred in 7.7% of patients in the BCG group and 9.4% of patients in the mitomycin C group. In all nine individual studies and in the combined results, no statistically significant difference in the odds ratio for progression between the BCG and MMC-treated groups was found (combined OR = 0.77, p = 0.081). However, the combined result of the five individual studies where patients received maintenance BCG demonstrated a statistically significant superiority of BCG plus maintenance over MMC (OR = 0.66, p = 0.02). In summary, BCG is superior to TURBT alone, TURBT plus intravesical chemotherapy, and TURBT plus other intravesical immunotherapy, such as interferon, for the prevention of tumour progression but only if administered with maintenance regimens. Currently there exists conflicting data regarding potential benefit of BCG over controls for the clinical end points of metastasis-free survival, cancer-specific survival, and overall survival following a repeated meta-analysis using individual patient data.[127,132]

Bacille Calmette–Guérin for the management of CIS

Carcinoma is situ is by definition a high-grade tumour and is difficult to cure with TURBT alone. Furthermore, if CIS is found concomitantly with Ta/T1 tumours, there is an increased risk of recurrence and progression.[42] Management options for CIS include adjuvant BCG therapy + maintenance or early cystectomy. No clinical trials have specifically analysed outcomes in patients with exclusively CIS treated with intravesical instillations; however, in a subgroup of 403 patients with CIS in the EORTC-GU metanalysis, BCG reduced the risk of progression by 35% compared to controls. BCG has higher efficacy than intravesical chemotherapy in terms of both initial response (68% vs. 49%), durability of response (68% vs. 47% of initial responders), and overall disease-free survival (51% vs. 27%) for patients with CIS.[44,133] No trials compared BCG to early cystectomy in patients with CIS. Early cystectomy is associated with excellent cancer-specific survival rates yet up to half of patients would be overtreated since durable response rates have been reported in the 30–50% range.[118] In summary, BCG is superior to intravesical chemotherapy for CIS. A lack of randomized trials comparing BCG versus early cystectomy leave both of these as reasonable options that must be dictated based on individual clinical scenario.

The preferred Bacille Calmette–Guérin treatment schedule

As alluded to previously, individual studies and metanalyses consistently demonstrate that the benefits of BCG are improved when it is administered with a maintenance course. Morales initially described an arbitrary six-week induction course of BCG, and this is still the most commonly utilized induction regimen.[108] Han and Pan conducted a metanalysis assessing recurrence rates in patients with non-invasive bladder cancer.[120] They included 10 studies comparing patients who only received induction BCG (n = 2,072) to those that received BCG plus maintenance (n = 1,070) and found that maintenance decreased the risk of recurrence with an odds ratio of 0.47 (p = 0.004). In the metanalyses by Sylvester and Bohle that assess tumour progression rates, BCG was superior to controls if given with maintenance (37% reduction in odds or progression) and was statistically no different from controls if no maintenance was administered. The optimal dose, duration/type of induction course, and maintenance schedule are unknown. The Southwest Oncology Group (SWOG) utilized a six-week induction course of BCG followed by three weekly instillations at three months, six months, and then every six months thereafter for a total of three years.[134] The results were convincingly in favour of maintenance, with a median recurrence-free survival of 77 months in the maintenance arm compared to 36 months in the control group. However, only 16% of patients tolerated the full three-year schedule, and the majority of patients that stopped BCG did so in the first six months. As such, it is postulated that shorter course of maintenance may be adequate as this is what most patients actually receive. In their metanalsyes assessing recurrence and progression, Bohle and colleagues concluded that at least one year of maintenance BCG therapy is requisite to make BCG more effective than intravesical chemotherapy.[123,131]

Treatment of refractory disease

Non-muscle-invasive bladder cancer is considered refractory to intravescial treatment if (i) muscle-invasive disease develops; (ii) if tumour persists despite intravesical therapy; or (iii) worsening of the disease develops with either higher T stage, advanced grade, new CIS, or more frequent recurrences despite intravesical chemotherapy or immunotherapy. Failure of intravesical chemotherapy may be treated with BCG.[135] A second induction courses of BCG is effective in 25–30% of patients with persistent or recurrent disease after an initial induction course.[123,130,135–137] However, 20–50% of patients treated with BCG after a second induction course will progress.[138] Because of the high risk of progression, early cystectomy is advocated in intravesical treatment failures. If patients refuse cystectomy or are medically unfit, alternative experimental intravesical instillations may be considered.[139–143]

Conclusion

Non-muscle-invasive bladder cancer is a heterogeneous clinical entity, ranging from low-grade tumours with an indolent natural history to clinically aggressive, high-grade tumours. Accurate staging and risk stratification is paramount to identify which patients are at risk for recurrence and progression. This information is then used to thoughtfully integrate adjuvant treatment such that overtreatment is minimized in patients with indolent tumours and promptly incorporated for patients at higher risk. The goal in patients with aggressive tumours is to prevent or delay progression with the use of intravesical therapy and allow for preservation of the bladder as long as safely possible. Radical cystectomy is reserved for patients that are refractory to more conservative treatment or that progress to muscle invasion. Periodic surveillance with cystoscopy is required given the substantial recurrence rates for bladder tumours. The role of tumour markers to augment or replace cystoscopy is currently being investigated.

Acknowledgements

We would like to acknowledge Payal Kapur from the UT Southwestern Pathology Department for providing the histology slides and annotations. We also acknowledge Lewis Calver from the UT Southwestern Biomedical Arts Department for his drawing of the various bladder cancer stages.

Further reading

Babjuk M, Oosterlinck W, Sylvester R, *et al.* EAU Guidelines on Non-Muscle-Invasive Urothelial Carcinoma of the Bladder, the 2011 Update. *Eur Urol* 2011; **59**:997–1008.

Grossman HB, Gomella L, Fradet Y, *et al.* A phase III, multicenter comparison of hexaminolevulinate fluorescence cystoscopy and white light cystoscopy for the detection of superficial papillary lesions in patients with bladder cancer. *J Urol* 2007; **178**(1):62–7.

Lamm DL, Blumenstein BA, Crissman JD, *et al.* Maintenance bacillus Calmette-Guerin immunotherapy for recurrent TA, T1 and carcinoma in situ transitional cell carcinoma of the bladder: a randomized Southwest Oncology Group Study. *J Urol* 2000; **163**(4):1124–9.

Lotan Y, Roehrborn CG. Sensitivity and specificity of commonly available bladder tumor markers versus cytology: results of a comprehensive literature review and meta-analyses. *Urology* 2003; **61**(1):109–18; discussion 18.

Shariat SF, Ashfaq R, Sagalowsky AI, Lotan Y. Predictive value of cell cycle biomarkers in nonmuscle invasive bladder transitional cell carcinoma. *J Urol* 2007; **177**(2):481–7; discussion 487.

Sylvester RJ, Oosterlinck W, van der Meijden AP. A single immediate postoperative instillation of chemotherapy decreases the risk of recurrence in patients with stage Ta T1 bladder cancer: a meta-analysis of published results of randomized clinical trials. *J Urol* 2004; **171**(6 Pt 1):2186–90, quiz 435.

Sylvester RJ, van der MA, Lamm DL. Intravesical bacillus Calmette-Guerin reduces the risk of progression in patients with superficial bladder cancer: a meta-analysis of the published results of randomized clinical trials. *J Urol* 2002; **168**(5):1964–70.

Sylvester RJ, van der Meijden AP, Oosterlinck W, *et al.* Predicting recurrence and progression in individual patients with stage Ta T1 bladder cancer using EORTC risk tables: a combined analysis of 2596 patients from seven EORTC trials. *Eur Urol* 2006; **49**(3):466–5; discussion 75–7.

Wang LJ, Wong YC, Huang CC, Wu CH, Hung SC, Chen HW. Multidetector computerized tomography urography is more accurate than excretory urography for diagnosing transitional cell carcinoma of the upper urinary tract in adults with hematuria. *J Urol* 2009; **183**(1):48–55.

Zeegers MP, Tan FE, Dorant E, van Den Brandt PA. The impact of characteristics of cigarette smoking on urinary tract cancer risk: a meta-analysis of epidemiologic studies. *Cancer* 2000; **89**(3):630–9.

References

1. Ploeg M, Aben KK, Kiemeney LA. The present and future burden of urinary bladder cancer in the world. *World J Urol* 2009; **27**(3):289–93.
2. Siegel R, Naishadham D, Jemal A. Cancer statistics, 2012. *CA Cancer J Clin* 2012; **62**(1):10–29.
3. Zeegers MP, Tan FE, Dorant E, van Den Brandt PA. The impact of characteristics of cigarette smoking on urinary tract cancer risk: a meta-analysis of epidemiologic studies. *Cancer* 2000; **89**(3):630–9.
4. Samanic C, Kogevinas M, Dosemeci M, *et al.* Smoking and bladder cancer in Spain: effects of tobacco type, timing, environmental tobacco smoke, and gender. *Cancer Epidemiol Biomarkers Prev* 2006; **15**(7):1348–54.
5. Fernandez MI, Lopez JF, Vivaldi B, Coz F. Long-term impact of arsenic in drinking water on bladder cancer health care and mortality rates 20 years after end of exposure. *J Urol* 2012; **187**(3):856–61.
6. Zeegers MP, Swaen GM, Kant I, Goldbohm RA, van den Brandt PA. Occupational risk factors for male bladder cancer: results from a population based case cohort study in the Netherlands. Occupational and environmental medicine. 2001; **58**(9):590–6.
7. El-Bolkainy MN, Mokhtar NM, Ghoneim MA, Hussein MH. The impact of schistosomiasis on the pathology of bladder carcinoma. *Cancer* 1981; **48**(12):2643–8.
8. Fleshner NE, Herr HW, Stewart AK, Murphy GP, Mettlin C, Menck HR. The National Cancer Data Base report on bladder carcinoma. The American College of Surgeons Commission on Cancer and the American Cancer Society. *Cancer* 1996; **78**(7):1505–13.
9. Kantor AF, Hartge P, Hoover RN, Fraumeni JF, Jr. Epidemiological characteristics of squamous cell carcinoma and adenocarcinoma of the bladder. *Cancer Res* 1988; **48**(13):3853–5.
10. Golin AL, Howard RS. Asymptomatic microscopic hematuria. *J Urol* 1980; **124**(3):389–91.
11. Mohr DN, Offord KP, Owen RA, Melton LJ 3rd. Asymptomatic microhematuria and urologic disease. A population-based study. *JAMA* 1986; **256**(2):224–9.
12. Khadra MH, Pickard RS, Charlton M, Powell PH, Neal DE. A prospective analysis of 1,930 patients with hematuria to evaluate current diagnostic practice. *J Urol* 2000; **163**(2):524–7.
13. Lee LW, Davis E, Jr. Gross urinary hemorrhage: a symptom, not a disease. *J Am Med Assoc* 1953; **153**(9):782–4.
14. Varkarakis MJ, Gaeta J, Moore RH, Murphy GP. Superficial bladder tumor. Aspects of clinical progression. *Urology* 1974; **4**(4):414–20.
15. Zincke H, Utz DC, Farrow GM. Review of Mayo Clinic experience with carcinoma in situ. *Urology* 1985; **26**(4 Suppl):39–46.
16. Krieg RC, Messmann H, Rauch J, Seeger S, Knuechel R. Metabolic characterization of tumor cell-specific protoporphyrin IX accumulation after exposure to 5-aminolevulinic acid in human colonic cells. *Photochem Photobiol* 2002; **76**(5):518–25.
17. Witjes JA, Douglass J. The role of hexaminolevulinate fluorescence cystoscopy in bladder cancer. *Nat Clin Pract Urol* 2007; **4**(10):542–9.
18. Jichlinski P, Guillou L, Karlsen SJ, *et al.* Hexyl aminolevulinate fluorescence cystoscopy: new diagnostic tool for photodiagnosis

of superficial bladder cancer—a multicenter study. *J Urol* 2003; **170**(1):226–9.
19. Grossman HB, Gomella L, Fradet Y, *et al.* A phase III, multicenter comparison of hexaminolevulinate fluorescence cystoscopy and white light cystoscopy for the detection of superficial papillary lesions in patients with bladder cancer. *J Urol* 2007; **178**(1):62–7.
20. Jocham D, Witjes F, Wagner S, *et al.* Improved detection and treatment of bladder cancer using hexaminolevulinate imaging: a prospective, phase III multicenter study. *J Urol* 2005; **174**(3):862–6; discussion 6.
21. Stenzl A, Burger M, Fradet Y, *et al.* Hexaminolevulinate guided fluorescence cystoscopy reduces recurrence in patients with nonmuscle invasive bladder cancer. *J Urol* 2010; **184**(5):1907–13.
22. Kausch I, Sommerauer M, Montorsi F, *et al.* Photodynamic diagnosis in non-muscle-invasive bladder cancer: a systematic review and cumulative analysis of prospective studies. *Eur Urol* 2010; **57**(4):595–606.
23. Schumacher MC, Holmang S, Davidsson T, Friedrich B, Pedersen J, Wiklund NP. Transurethral resection of non-muscle-invasive bladder transitional cell cancers with or without 5-aminolevulinic Acid under visible and fluorescent light: results of a prospective, randomised, multicentre study. *Eur Urol* 2010; **57**(2):293–9.
24. Epstein JI, Amin MB, Reuter VR, Mostofi FK. The World Health Organization/International Society of Urological Pathology consensus classification of urothelial (transitional cell) neoplasms of the urinary bladder. Bladder Consensus Conference Committee. *Am J Surg Pathol* 1998; **22**(12):1435–48.
25. Shiozawa H, Aizawa T, Ito T, Miki M. A new transurethral resection system: operating in saline environment precludes obturator nerve reflexes. *J Urol* 2002; **168**(6):2665–7.
26. Lutzeyer W, Rubben H, Dahm H. Prognostic parameters in superficial bladder cancer: an analysis of 315 cases. *J Urol* 1982; **127**(2):250–2.
27. Heney NM, Ahmed S, Flanagan MJ, *et al.* Superficial bladder cancer: progression and recurrence. *J Urol* 1983; **130**(6):1083–6.
28. Kunju LP, You L, Zhang Y, Daignault S, Montie JE, Lee CT. Lymphovascular invasion of urothelial cancer in matched transurethral bladder tumor resection and radical cystectomy specimens. *J Urol* 2008; **180**(5):1928–32; discussion 32.
29. Holzbeierlein JM, Smith JA Jr. Surgical management of noninvasive bladder cancer (stages Ta/T1/CIS). *Urol Clin North Am* 2000; **27**(1):15–24, vii-viii.
30. Brausi M, Collette L, Kurth K, *et al.* Variability in the recurrence rate at first follow-up cystoscopy after TUR in stage Ta T1 transitional cell carcinoma of the bladder: a combined analysis of seven EORTC studies. *Eur Urol* 2002; **41**(5):523–31.
31. Mariappan P, Zachou A, Grigor KM. Detrusor muscle in the first, apparently complete transurethral resection of bladder tumour specimen is a surrogate marker of resection quality, predicts risk of early recurrence, and is dependent on operator experience. *Eur Urol* 2010; **57**(5):843–9.
32. May F, Treiber U, Hartung R, Schwaibold H. Significance of random bladder biopsies in superficial bladder cancer. *Eur Urol* 2003; **44**(1):47–50.
33. Swinn MJ, Walker MM, Harbin LJ, *et al.* Biopsy of the red patch at cystoscopy: is it worthwhile? *Eur Urol* 2004; **45**(4):471–4; discussion 4.
34. van der Meijden A, Oosterlinck W, Brausi M, Kurth KH, Sylvester R, de Balincourt C. Significance of bladder biopsies in Ta,T1 bladder tumors: a report from the EORTC Genito-Urinary Tract Cancer Cooperative Group. EORTC-GU Group Superficial Bladder Committee. *Eur Urol* 1999; **35**(4):267–71.
35. Fujimoto N, Harada S, Terado M, Sato H, Matsumoto T. Multiple biopsies of normal-looking urothelium in patients with superficial bladder cancer: Are they necessary? *Int J Urol* 2003; **10**(12):631–5.
36. Mungan MU, Canda AE, Tuzel E, Yorukoglu K, Kirkali Z. Risk factors for mucosal prostatic urethral involvement in superficial transitional cell carcinoma of the bladder. *Eur Urol* 2005; **48**(5):760–3.
37. Edge S, Byrd DR, Compton CC, Fritz AG, Greene FL, Trotti A (eds). *AJCC Cancer Staging Manual*, 7th edition. New York, NY: Springer; 2010.
38. Younes M, Sussman J, True LD. The usefulness of the level of the muscularis mucosae in the staging of invasive transitional cell carcinoma of the urinary bladder. *Cancer* 1990; **66**(3):543–8.
39. Donat SM. Evaluation and follow-up strategies for superficial bladder cancer. *Urol Clin North Am* 2003; **30**(4):765–76.
40. Kurth KH, Denis L, Bouffioux C, *et al.* Factors affecting recurrence and progression in superficial bladder tumours. *Eur J Cancer* 1995; **31A**(11):1840–6.
41. Allard P, Bernard P, Fradet Y, Tetu B. The early clinical course of primary Ta and T1 bladder cancer: a proposed prognostic index. *Br J Urol* 1998; **81**(5):692–8.
42. Sylvester RJ, van der Meijden AP, Oosterlinck W, *et al.* Predicting recurrence and progression in individual patients with stage Ta T1 bladder cancer using EORTC risk tables: a combined analysis of 2596 patients from seven EORTC trials. *Eur Urol* 2006; **49**(3):466–5; discussion 75–7.
43. Herr HW, Donat SM, Reuter VE. Management of low grade papillary bladder tumors. *J Urol* 2007; **178**(4 Pt 1):1201–5; discussion 5.
44. Sylvester RJ, van der Meijden A, Witjes JA, *et al.* High-grade Ta urothelial carcinoma and carcinoma in situ of the bladder. *Urology* 2005; **66**(6 Suppl 1):90–107.
45. Kiemeney LA, Witjes JA, Heijbroek RP, Verbeek AL, Debruyne FM. Predictability of recurrent and progressive disease in individual patients with primary superficial bladder cancer. *J Urol* 1993; **150**(1):60–4.
46. Herr HW. Tumour progression and survival in patients with T1G3 bladder tumours: 15-year outcome. *Br J Urol* 1997; **80**(5):762–5.
47. Hudson MA, Herr HW. Carcinoma in situ of the bladder. *J Urol* 1995; **153**(3 Pt 1):564–72.
48. Utz DC, Zincke H. The masquerade of bladder cancer in situ as interstitial cystitis. *J Urol* 1974; **111**(2):160–1.
49. Sauter G, Algaba F, Amin MB. Tumors of the urinary system: non-invasive urothelial neoplasias. In: Eble JN, Sauter G, Epstein JI, Sesterhenn I (eds). *Pathology and Genetics of Tumours of the Urinary System and Male Genital Organs*. Lyon, France: IARCC Press, 2004.
50. May M, Brookman-Amissah S, Roigas J, *et al.* Prognostic accuracy of individual uropathologists in noninvasive urinary bladder carcinoma: a multicentre study comparing the 1973 and 2004 World Health Organization classifications. *Eur Urol* 2010; **57**(5):850–8.
51. Burger M, van der Aa MN, van Oers JM, *et al.* Prediction of progression of non-muscle-invasive bladder cancer by WHO 1973 and 2004 grading and by FGFR3 mutation status: a prospective study. *Eur Urol* 2008; **54**(4):835–43.
52. Gaston KE, Pruthi RS. Value of urinary cytology in the diagnosis and management of urinary tract malignancies. *Urology* 2004; **63**(6):1009–16.
53. Lotan Y, Roehrborn CG. Sensitivity and specificity of commonly available bladder tumor markers versus cytology: results of a comprehensive literature review and meta-analyses. *Urology* 2003; **61**(1):109–18; discussion 18.
54. Lokeshwar VB, Habuchi T, Grossman HB, *et al.* Bladder tumor markers beyond cytology: International Consensus Panel on bladder tumor markers. *Urology* 2005; **66**(6 Suppl 1):35–63.
55. Freeman JA, Esrig D, Stein JP, *et al.* Radical cystectomy for high risk patients with superficial bladder cancer in the era of orthotopic urinary reconstruction. *Cancer* 1995;**76**(5):833–9.
56. Dutta SC, Smith JA Jr, Shappell SB, Coffey CS, Chang SS, Cookson MS. Clinical under staging of high risk nonmuscle invasive urothelial carcinoma treated with radical cystectomy. *J Urol* 2001; **166**(2):490–3.
57. Stein JP, Lieskovsky G, Cote R, *et al.* Radical cystectomy in the treatment of invasive bladder cancer: long-term results in 1,054 patients. *J Clin Oncol* 2001; **19**(3):666–75.
58. Ficarra V, Dalpiaz O, Alrabi N, Novara G, Galfano A, Artibani W. Correlation between clinical and pathological staging in a series

of radical cystectomies for bladder carcinoma. *BJU Int* 2005; **95**(6):786–90.

59. Brauers A, Buettner R, Jakse G. Second resection and prognosis of primary high risk superficial bladder cancer: is cystectomy often too early? *J Urol* 2001; **165**(3):808–10.
60. Chauvet V, Tian X, Husson H, *et al.* Mechanical stimuli induce cleavage and nuclear translocation of the polycystin-1 C terminus. *J Clin Invest* 2004; **114**(10):1433–43.
61. Miladi M, Peyromaure M, Zerbib M, Saighi D, Debre B. The value of a second transurethral resection in evaluating patients with bladder tumours. *Eur Urol* 2003; **43**(3):241–5.
62. Dalbagni G, Vora K, Kaag M, *et al.* Clinical outcome in a contemporary series of restaged patients with clinical T1 bladder cancer. *Eur Urol* 2009; **56**(6):903–10.
63. Herr HW. The value of a second transurethral resection in evaluating patients with bladder tumors. *J Urol* 1999; **162**(1):74–6.
64. Grimm MO, Steinhoff C, Simon X, Spiegelhalder P, Ackermann R, Vogeli TA. Effect of routine repeat transurethral resection for superficial bladder cancer: a long-term observational study. *J Urol* 2003; **170**(2 Pt 1):433–7.
65. Millan-Rodriguez F, Chechile-Toniolo G, Salvador-Bayarri J, Palou J, Algaba F, Vicente-Rodriguez J. Primary superficial bladder cancer risk groups according to progression, mortality and recurrence. *J Urol* 2000; **164**(3 Pt 1):680–4.
66. Lotan Y, Gupta A, Shariat SF, *et al.* Lymphovascular invasion is independently associated with overall survival, cause-specific survival, and local and distant recurrence in patients with negative lymph nodes at radical cystectomy. *J Clin Oncol* 2005; **23**(27):6533–9.
67. Cho KS, Seo HK, Joung JY, *et al.* Lymphovascular invasion in transurethral resection specimens as predictor of progression and metastasis in patients with newly diagnosed T1 bladder urothelial cancer. *J Urol* 2009; **182**(6):2625–30.
68. Shariat SF, Ashfaq R, Sagalowsky AI, Lotan Y. Predictive value of cell cycle biomarkers in nonmuscle invasive bladder transitional cell carcinoma. *J Urol* 2007; **177**(2):481–7; discussion 487.
69. Shariat SF, Bolenz C, Godoy G, *et al.* Predictive value of combined immunohistochemical markers in patients with pT1 urothelial carcinoma at radical cystectomy. *J Urol* 2009; **182**(1):78–84.
70. Shariat SF, Karakiewicz PI, Ashfaq R, *et al.* Multiple biomarkers improve prediction of bladder cancer recurrence and mortality in patients undergoing cystectomy. *Cancer* 2008; **112**(2):315–25.
71. Shariat SF, Tokunaga H, Zhou J, *et al.* p53, p21, pRB, and p16 expression predict clinical outcome in cystectomy with bladder cancer. *J Clin Oncol* 2004; **22**(6):1014–24.
72. Cote RJ, Esrig D, Groshen S, Jones PA, Skinner DG. p53 and treatment of bladder cancer. *Nature* 1997; **385**(6612):123–5.
73. Korkolopoulou P, Christodoulou P, Konstantinidou AE, Thomas-Tsagli E, Kapralos P, Davaris P. Cell cycle regulators in bladder cancer: a multivariate survival study with emphasis on p27Kip1. *Hum Pathol* 2000; **31**(6):751–60.
74. Sarkis AS, Bajorin DF, Reuter VE, *et al.* Prognostic value of p53 nuclear overexpression in patients with invasive bladder cancer treated with neoadjuvant MVAC. *J Clin Oncol* 1995; **13**(6):1384–90.
75. Sarkis AS, Dalbagni G, Cordon-Cardo C, *et al.* Nuclear overexpression of p53 protein in transitional cell bladder carcinoma: a marker for disease progression. *J Natl Cancer Inst* 1993; **85**(1):53–9.
76. Serth J, Kuczyk MA, Bokemeyer C, *et al.* p53 immunohistochemistry as an independent prognostic factor for superficial transitional cell carcinoma of the bladder. *Br J Cancer* 1995; **71**(1):201–5.
77. Shariat SF, Marberger MJ, Lotan Y, *et al.* Variability in the performance of nuclear matrix protein 22 for the detection of bladder cancer. *J Urol* 2006; **176**(3):919–26; discussion 26.
78. Solsona E, Iborra I, Dumont R, Rubio-Briones J, Casanova J, Almenar S. The 3-month clinical response to intravesical therapy as a predictive factor for progression in patients with high risk superficial bladder cancer. *J Urol* 2000; **164**(3 Pt 1):685–9.
79. Holmang S, Johansson SL. Stage Ta-T1 bladder cancer: the relationship between findings at first followup cystoscopy and subsequent recurrence and progression. *J Urol* 2002; **167**(4):1634–7.
80. Sengupta S, Blute ML. The management of superficial transitional cell carcinoma of the bladder. *Urology* 2006; **67**(3 Suppl 1):48–54; discussion 54–5.
81. Babjuk M, Oosterlinck W, Sylvester R, Kaasinen E, Bohle A, Palou-Redorta J. EAU guidelines on non-muscle-invasive urothelial carcinoma of the bladder. *Eur Urol* 2008; **54**(2):303–14.
82. Soloway MS, Bruck DS, Kim SS. Expectant management of small, recurrent, noninvasive papillary bladder tumors. *J Urol* 2003; **170**(2 Pt 1):438–41.
83. Pruthi RS, Baldwin N, Bhalani V, Wallen EM. Conservative management of low risk superficial bladder tumors. *J Urol* 2008; **179**(1):87–90; discussion 90.
84. Paez A, Coba JM, Murillo N, *et al.* Reliability of the routine cytological diagnosis in bladder cancer. *Eur Urol* 1999; **35**(3):228–32.
85. Lotan Y, Svatek RS, Sagalowsky AI. Should we screen for bladder cancer in a high-risk population?: A cost per life-year saved analysis. *Cancer* 2006; **107**(5):982–90.
86. Papanicolaou GN, Marshall VF. Urine Sediment Smears as a Diagnostic Procedure in Cancers of the Urinary Tract. *Science* 1945; **101**(2629):519–20.
87. Kinders R, Jones T, Root R, *et al.* Complement factor H or a related protein is a marker for transitional cell cancer of the bladder. *Clin Cancer Res* 1998; **4**(10):2511–20.
88. Tetu B, Tiguert R, Harel F, Fradet Y. ImmunoCyt/uCyt+ improves the sensitivity of urine cytology in patients followed for urothelial carcinoma. *Mod Pathol* 2005; **18**(1):83–9.
89. Sokolova IA, Halling KC, Jenkins RB, *et al.* The development of a multitarget, multicolor fluorescence in situ hybridization assay for the detection of urothelial carcinoma in urine. *J Mol Diagn* 2000; **2**(3):116–23.
90. Sarosdy MF, Schellhammer P, Bokinsky G, *et al.* Clinical evaluation of a multi-target fluorescent in situ hybridization assay for detection of bladder cancer. *J Urol* 2002; **168**(5):1950–4.
91. Mian C, Lodde M, Haitel A, Egarter Vigl E, Marberger M, Pycha A. Comparison of two qualitative assays, the UBC rapid test and the BTA stat test, in the diagnosis of urothelial cell carcinoma of the bladder. *Urology* 2000; **56**(2):228–31.
92. Herr HW, Cookson MS, Soloway SM. Upper tract tumors in patients with primary bladder cancer followed for 15 years. *J Urol* 1996; **156**(4):1286–7.
93. Oldbring J, Glifberg I, Mikulowski P, Hellsten S. Carcinoma of the renal pelvis and ureter following bladder carcinoma: frequency, risk factors and clinicopathological findings. *J Urol* 1989; **141**(6):1311–3.
94. Herranz-Amo F, Diez-Cordero JM, Verdu-Tartajo F, Bueno-Chomon G, Leal-Hernandez F, Bielsa-Carrillo A. Need for intravenous urography in patients with primary transitional carcinoma of the bladder? *Eur Urol* 1999; **36**(3):221–4.
95. Wright JL, Hotaling J, Porter MP. Predictors of upper tract urothelial cell carcinoma after primary bladder cancer: a population based analysis. *J Urol* 2009; **181**(3):1035–9; discussion 9.
96. Hurle R, Losa A, Manzetti A, Lembo A. Upper urinary tract tumors developing after treatment of superficial bladder cancer: 7-year follow-up of 591 consecutive patients. *Urology* 1999; **53**(6):1144–8.
97. Wang LJ, Wong YC, Huang CC, Wu CH, Hung SC, Chen HW. Multidetector computerized tomography urography is more accurate than excretory urography for diagnosing transitional cell carcinoma of the upper urinary tract in adults with hematuria. *J Urol* 2009; **183**(1):48–55.
98. Pode D, Alon Y, Horowitz AT, Vlodavsky I, Biran S. The mechanism of human bladder tumor implantation in an in vitro model. *J Urol* 1986; **136**(2):482–6.
99. Hendricksen K, Witjes WP, Idema JG, *et al.* Comparison of three schedules of intravesical epirubicin in patients with non-muscle-invasive bladder cancer. *Eur Urol* 2008; **53**(5):984–91.

100. Kaasinen E, Rintala E, Hellstrom P, *et al.* Factors explaining recurrence in patients undergoing chemoimmunotherapy regimens for frequently recurring superficial bladder carcinoma. *Eur Urol* 2002; **42**(2):167–74.
101. Sylvester RJ, Oosterlinck W, van der Meijden AP. A single immediate postoperative instillation of chemotherapy decreases the risk of recurrence in patients with stage Ta T1 bladder cancer: a meta-analysis of published results of randomized clinical trials. *J Urol* 2004; **171**(6 Pt 1):2186–90, quiz 435.
102. Gudjonsson S, Adell L, Merdasa F, *et al.* Should all patients with non-muscle-invasive bladder cancer receive early intravesical chemotherapy after transurethral resection? The results of a prospective randomised multicentre study. *Eur Urol* 2009; **55**(4):773–80.
103. Bouffioux C, Kurth KH, Bono A, *et al.* Intravesical adjuvant chemotherapy for superficial transitional cell bladder carcinoma: results of 2 European Organization for Research and Treatment of Cancer randomized trials with mitomycin C and doxorubicin comparing early versus delayed instillations and short-term versus long-term treatment. European Organization for Research and Treatment of Cancer Genitourinary Group. *J Urol* 1995; **153**(3 Pt 2):934–41.
104. Au JL, Badalament RA, Wientjes MG, *et al.* Methods to improve efficacy of intravesical mitomycin C: results of a randomized phase III trial. *J Natl Cancer Inst* 2001; **93**(8):597–604.
105. Huncharek M, Geschwind JF, Witherspoon B, McGarry R, Adcock D. Intravesical chemotherapy prophylaxis in primary superficial bladder cancer: a meta-analysis of 3703 patients from 11 randomized trials. *J Clin Epidemiol* 2000; **53**(7):676–80.
106. Huncharek M, McGarry R, Kupelnick B. Impact of intravesical chemotherapy on recurrence rate of recurrent superficial transitional cell carcinoma of the bladder: results of a meta-analysis. *Anticancer Res* 2001; **21**(1B):765–9.
107. Pawinski A, Sylvester R, Kurth KH, *et al.* A combined analysis of European Organization for Research and Treatment of Cancer, and Medical Research Council randomized clinical trials for the prophylactic treatment of stage TaT1 bladder cancer. European Organization for Research and Treatment of Cancer Genitourinary Tract Cancer Cooperative Group and the Medical Research Council Working Party on Superficial Bladder Cancer. *J Urol* 1996; **156**(6):1934–40, discussion 1940–1.
108. Morales A, Eidinger D, Bruce AW. Intracavitary Bacillus Calmette-Guerin in the treatment of superficial bladder tumors. *J Urol* 1976; **116**(2):180–3.
109. Brosman SA. Experience with bacillus Calmette-Guerin in patients with superficial bladder carcinoma. *J Urol* 1982; **128**(1):27–30.
110. Shen Z, Shen T, Wientjes MG, O'Donnell MA, Au JL. Intravesical treatments of bladder cancer: review. *Pharm Res* 2008; **25**(7):1500–10.
111. Luo Y, Chen X, O'Donnell MA. Role of Th1 and Th2 cytokines in BCG-induced IFN-gamma production: cytokine promotion and simulation of BCG effect. *Cytokine* 2003; **21**(1):17–26.
112. Bohle A, Brandau S. Immune mechanisms in bacillus Calmette-Guerin immunotherapy for superficial bladder cancer. *J Urol* 2003; **170**(3):964–9.
113. Oddens J, Brausi M, Sylvester R, *et al.* Final results of an EORTC-GU cancers group randomized study of maintenance bacillus Calmette-Guerin in intermediate- and high-risk Ta, T1 papillary carcinoma of the urinary bladder: one-third dose versus full dose and 1 year versus 3 years of maintenance. *Eur Urol* 2013; **63**(3):462–72.
114. Martinez-Pineiro JA, Flores N, Isorna S, *et al.* Long-term follow-up of a randomized prospective trial comparing a standard 81 mg dose of intravesical bacille Calmette-Guerin with a reduced dose of 27 mg in superficial bladder cancer. *BJU Int* 2002; **89**(7):671–80.
115. Martinez-Pineiro JA, Martinez-Pineiro L, Solsona E, *et al.* Has a 3-fold decreased dose of bacillus Calmette-Guerin the same efficacy against recurrences and progression of T1G3 and Tis bladder tumors than the standard dose? Results of a prospective randomized trial. *J Urol* 2005; **174**(4 Pt 1):1242–7.
116. van der Meijden AP, Sylvester RJ, Oosterlinck W, Hoeltl W, Bono AV. Maintenance Bacillus Calmette-Guerin for Ta T1 bladder tumors is not associated with increased toxicity: results from a European Organisation for Research and Treatment of Cancer Genito-Urinary Group Phase III Trial. *Eur Urol* 2003; **44**(4):429–34.
117. Krege S, Giani G, Meyer R, Otto T, Rubben H. A randomized multicenter trial of adjuvant therapy in superficial bladder cancer: transurethral resection only versus transurethral resection plus mitomycin C versus transurethral resection plus bacillus Calmette-Guerin. Participating Clinics. *J Urol* 1996; **156**(3):962–6.
118. Herr HW, Wartinger DD, Fair WR, Oettgen HF. Bacillus Calmette-Guerin therapy for superficial bladder cancer: a 10-year followup. *J Urol* 1992; **147**(4):1020–3.
119. Melekos MD, Chionis H, Pantazakos A, Fokaefs E, Paranychianakis G, Dauaher H. Intravesical bacillus Calmette-Guerin immunoprophylaxis of superficial bladder cancer: results of a controlled prospective trial with modified treatment schedule. *J Urol* 1993; **149**(4):744–8.
120. Han RF, Pan JG. Can intravesical bacillus Calmette-Guerin reduce recurrence in patients with superficial bladder cancer? A meta-analysis of randomized trials. *Urology* 2006; **67**(6):1216–23.
121. Shelley MD, Kynaston H, Court J, *et al.* A systematic review of intravesical bacillus Calmette-Guerin plus transurethral resection vs transurethral resection alone in Ta and T1 bladder cancer. *BJU Int* 2001; **88**(3):209–16.
122. Shelley MD, Wilt TJ, Court J, Coles B, Kynaston H, Mason MD. Intravesical bacillus Calmette-Guerin is superior to mitomycin C in reducing tumour recurrence in high-risk superficial bladder cancer: a meta-analysis of randomized trials. *BJU Int* 2004; **93**(4):485–90.
123. Bohle A, Jocham D, Bock PR. Intravesical bacillus Calmette-Guerin versus mitomycin C for superficial bladder cancer: a formal meta-analysis of comparative studies on recurrence and toxicity. *J Urol* 2003; **169**(1):90–5.
124. Lamm DL, Blumenstein BA, David Crawford E, Crissman JD, Lowe BA, Smith JA, Jr., *et al.* Randomized intergroup comparison of bacillus calmette-guerin immunotherapy and mitomycin C chemotherapy prophylaxis in superficial transitional cell carcinoma of the bladder a southwest oncology group study. *Urol Oncol* 1995; **1**(3):119–26.
125. Duchek M, Johansson R, Jahnson S, *et al.* Bacillus Calmette-Guerin is superior to a combination of epirubicin and interferon-alpha2b in the intravesical treatment of patients with stage T1 urinary bladder cancer. A prospective, randomized, Nordic study. *Eur Urol* 2010; **57**(1):25–31.
126. Jarvinen R, Kaasinen E, Sankila A, Rintala E. Long-term efficacy of maintenance bacillus Calmette-Guerin versus maintenance mitomycin C instillation therapy in frequently recurrent TaT1 tumours without carcinoma in situ: a subgroup analysis of the prospective, randomised FinnBladder I study with a 20-year follow-up. *Eur Urol* 2009; **56**(2):260–5.
127. Sylvester RJ, Brausi MA, Kirkels WJ, *et al.* Long-term efficacy results of EORTC genito-urinary group randomized phase 3 study 30911 comparing intravesical instillations of epirubicin, bacillus Calmette-Guerin, and bacillus Calmette-Guerin plus isoniazid in patients with intermediate- and high-risk stage Ta T1 urothelial carcinoma of the bladder. *Eur Urol* 2010; **57**(5):766–73.
128. Lundholm C, Norlen BJ, Ekman P, *et al.* A randomized prospective study comparing long-term intravesical instillations of mitomycin C and bacillus Calmette-Guerin in patients with superficial bladder carcinoma. *J Urol* 1996; **156**(2 Pt 1):372–6.
129. Herr HW, Laudone VP, Badalament RA, *et al.* Bacillus Calmette-Guerin therapy alters the progression of superficial bladder cancer. *J Clin Oncol* 1988; **6**(9):1450–5.

130. Sylvester RJ, van der MA, Lamm DL. Intravesical bacillus Calmette-Guerin reduces the risk of progression in patients with superficial bladder cancer: a meta-analysis of the published results of randomized clinical trials. *J Urol* 2002; **168**(5):1964–70.
131. Bohle A, Bock PR. Intravesical bacille Calmette-Guerin versus mitomycin C in superficial bladder cancer: formal meta-analysis of comparative studies on tumor progression. *Urology* 2004; **63**(4):682–6; discussion 6–7.
132. Malmstrom PU, Sylvester RJ, Crawford DE, *et al.* An individual patient data meta-analysis of the long-term outcome of randomised studies comparing intravesical mitomycin C versus bacillus Calmette-Guerin for non-muscle-invasive bladder cancer. *Eur Urol* 2009; **56**(2):247–56.
133. O'Donnell MA. Advances in the management of superficial bladder cancer. *Semin Oncol* 2007; **34**(2):85–97.
134. Lamm DL, Blumenstein BA, Crissman JD, *et al.* Maintenance bacillus Calmette-Guerin immunotherapy for recurrent TA, T1 and carcinoma in situ transitional cell carcinoma of the bladder: a randomized Southwest Oncology Group Study. *J Urol* 2000; **163**(4):1124–9.
135. Huncharek M, Kupelnick B. Impact of intravesical chemotherapy versus BCG immunotherapy on recurrence of superficial transitional cell carcinoma of the bladder: metaanalytic reevaluation. *Am J Clin Oncol* 2003; **26**(4):402–7.
136. Haaff EO, Dresner SM, Ratliff TL, Catalona WJ. Two courses of intravesical bacillus Calmette-Guerin for transitional cell carcinoma of the bladder. *J Urol* 1986; **136**(4):820–4.
137. Kavoussi LR, Torrence RJ, Gillen DP, *et al.* Results of 6 weekly intravesical bacillus Calmette-Guerin instillations on the treatment of superficial bladder tumors. *J Urol* 1988; **139**(5):935–40.
138. Nadler RB, Catalona WJ, Hudson MA, Ratliff TL. Durability of the tumor-free response for intravesical bacillus Calmette-Guerin therapy. *J Urol* 1994; **152**(2 Pt 1):367–73.
139. Dalbagni G, Russo P, Bochner B, *et al.* Phase II trial of intravesical gemcitabine in bacille Calmette-Guerin-refractory transitional cell carcinoma of the bladder. *J Clin Oncol* 2006; **24**(18):2729–34.
140. Barlow L, McKiernan J, Sawczuk I, Benson M. A single-institution experience with induction and maintenance intravesical docetaxel in the management of non-muscle-invasive bladder cancer refractory to bacille Calmette-Guerin therapy. *BJU Int* 2009; **104**(8):1098–102.
141. Steinberg G, Bahnson R, Brosman S, Middleton R, Wajsman Z, Wehle M. Efficacy and safety of valrubicin for the treatment of Bacillus Calmette-Guerin refractory carcinoma in situ of the bladder. The Valrubicin Study Group. *J Urol* 2000; **163**(3):761–7.
142. Joudi FN, Smith BJ, O'Donnell MA. Final results from a national multicenter phase II trial of combination bacillus Calmette-Guerin plus interferon alpha-2B for reducing recurrence of superficial bladder cancer. *Urol Oncol* 2006; **24**(4):344–8.
143. Yates DR, Roupret M. Failure of bacille Calmette-Guerin in patients with high risk non-muscle-invasive bladder cancer unsuitable for radical cystectomy: an update of available treatment options. *BJU Int* 2010; **106**(2):162–7.

CHAPTER 6.20

Bladder cancer
High-grade non-muscle-invasive disease

Richard P. Meijer, Alexandre R. Zlotta, and Bas W.G. van Rhijn

Introduction to bladder cancer

High-grade non-muscle-invasive bladder cancer (HG-NMIBC) represents the spectrum of NMI urothelial carcinoma (UC) with the highest risk for recurrence and progression to muscle-invasive bladder cancer (MIBC). This collective term includes all high-grade non-muscle-invasive (NMI) UC, such as those without invasion (pTa), those with lamina propria invasion (pT1) and those that are only/have concomitant *carcinoma in situ* (CIS; pTis). As such, HG-NMIBC represents a locally confined aggressive disease, and patients should be managed carefully and counselled about the potential outcomes. Disease progression, in this context is defined as the onset of MIBC or metastases from a NMI cancer. This event is associated with a dramatic deterioration in the prognosis for the patient (from around 80% to less than 50% five-year survival) and a change in treatment intent (perhaps from conservative to radical). As such, progression is the key clinical event in the management of patients with HG-NMIBC, and their care is directed towards its prevention or early detection. Of note, while these tumours are usually locally confined, around 5% of patients with HG-NMIBC have metastases at diagnosis.

To enable recurrence and progression risk assessment for patients with NMIBC, the European Organisation for Research and Treatment of Cancer (EORTC) has developed a risk calculator (www.eortc.be/tools/bladdercalculator) based on six variables (Table 6.20.1). High-grade pTa tumours have a 20–25% risk of progression to muscle-invasive disease, in contrast to pT1 tumours where the risk if between 25-75%.[1–3] Thus, the exact classification of high-risk lesions is of the utmost importance. Despite defined histopathological criteria, there is significant inter-observer variability among pathologists when classifying Ta versus T1 tumours and in grading UC. Concordance between pathologists ranges from 40–60% for staging (Ta versus T1) and from 70–78% for classifying CIS.[3–5] Therefore, central revision of histopathology by dedicated uro-pathologists has been advised for all high-grade and pT1 tumours (Ta versus T1).[6,7] Treatment for HG-NMIBC consists primarily of complete transurethral resection of the bladder tumour (TUR-BT), followed by adjuvant intravesical instillations of Bacillus Calmette–Guérin (BCG) or primary radical cystectomy.[6,8–10] The latter should be considered for primary high-risk HGNMI-BC (such as large tumours, those lesions with mutlifocality, those with CIS), HGNMI-BC that does not respond to BCG and in patients who are young, symptomatic and perhaps in females (who respond more poorly than men to BCG).[11] To further elucidate the risk profiles of T1 tumours, a system of substaging has recently been proposed, dividing these tumours in T1-microinvasive (T1m) and T1-extensive-invasive (T1e) tumours.[7] The aim of this staging system is to increase concordance between pathologist and better

Table 6.20.1 Weighting used to calculate recurrence and progression rates

Factor	Recurrence	Progression
Number of tumours		
Single	0	0
2–7	3	3
>8	6	3
Tumour diameter		
<3 cm	0	0
>3 cm	3	3
Prior recurrence rate		
Primary	0	0
<1 recurrence/year	2	2
>1 recurrence/year	4	2
Tumour stage		
pTa	0	0
pT1	1	4
Tumour grade (WHO 1973)		
G1	0	0
G2	1	0
G3	2	5
Concomitant CIS		
No	0	0
Yes	1	6
Total score	0–17	0–23

WHO = World Health Organization; CIS = carcinoma *in situ*.

Reprinted from *European Urology*, Volume 49, Issue 3, Richard J. Sylvester *et al.*, 'Predicting Recurrence and Progression in Individual Patients with Stage Ta T1 Bladder Cancer Using EORTC Risk Tables: A Combined Analysis of 2596 Patients from Seven EORTC Trials', pp. 466–477, Copyright © 2006 Elsevier B.V., with permission from Elsevier, http://www.sciencedirect.com/science/journal/03022838

stratify tumours with high and low progression risk. For patients with recurrence or persistence of HG-NMIBC during BCG treatment (BCG refractory disease), radical cystectomy is advised.[12] In those not fit or choosing to avoid radical surgery, alternate approaches such as repeated BCG, BCG with an immune-modulating agent (such as interferon), intravesical chemotherapy (such as gemcitabine) or device assisted chemotherapy (such as mitomycin-c delivered using hyperthermia or electromotive drug administration (EDMA)).[13]

Diagnosis

Symptoms

Visible haematuria is the most common presenting symptom for bladder cancer. However, in contrast to low risk papillary cancers, tumours with CIS (automatically defined as HGNMI-BC) may also commonly present with irritative lower urinary tract symptoms (such as urgency, frequency, pollakisuria, and dysuria). In females, these symptoms may be misdiagnosed as recurrent or antibiotic-refractory bacterial urinary infections. As with other UC, smoking and occupational carcinogen exposures are the most common causes of HGNMI-BC. However, smoking status does not predict bladder cancer stage or grade.

Investigations and initial treatment

Urinary cytology has a moderate sensitivity and high specificity for HG-NMIBC.[3,14] The performance of cytology is even better for CIS, in which the lesions lack of cellular cohesion and often shed cells into the urine. As such, urinary cytology can be an accurate test to accompany cystoscopy for bladder surveillance.[3] Urinary molecular markers have been extensively investigated, but (with respect to HG-NMIBC) they have not been proven to be of substantial value in daily clinical practice.

Cystoscopy is the most important tool in the diagnosis of bladder cancer, and the trained operator should usually be able to distinguish an indolent looking papillary low risk tumour from an aggressive HGNMI-BC. The latter appear more vascular, may have necrosis, may be multifocal, and may have solid elements. CIS appears as a flat red spreading lesion, and can be missed by white light cystoscopy (reports suggest up to 53% of specimens with CIS were missed).[15,16] For this reason, the combination of cystoscopy with urinary cytology is of importance. Furthermore, in recent years the introduction of photodynamic diagnostics (PDD) has proven to be of significant importance in the identification of CIS. Prior to fluorescence cystoscopy, the bladder is filled with a fluorescent substance (hexyl-aminovulinic acid), which accumulates primarily in tumour cells. During fluorescence cystoscopy blue ultraviolet light is used, causing the photosensitizing substance to emit a red fluorescence, thereby highlighting the suspect regions in the bladder (Fig. 6.20.1).[17] The application of PDD has shown to improve diagnostic accuracy for CIS with 39% versus white light cystoscopy.[18,19]

UC may originate anywhere in the urinary tract, although upper urinary tract tumours are relatively rare (comprising 5–10% of all UC).[20,21] Nevertheless, in selected cases of HG-NMIBC (especially tumours on the bladder trigone and adjacent to either ureteric orifice) it is important to exclude upper urinary tract tumours that may cause present as seedlings within the bladder.[22] Therefore, upper tract imaging should be performed (e.g. CT-urography). CIS may be found anywhere in the urinary tract. In cases of abnormal urinary cytology, and the absence of lesions on cystoscopy or CT-urography, selective urinary cytology of each upper urinary tract and sampling of the prostatic urethra should be considered.[6]

Transurethral resection of the bladder tumour (TUR-BT) is both a diagnostic and therapeutic procedure. Main goal of the procedure is to perform a complete resection of the bladder tumour. Furthermore, to obtain adequate material to (sub)stage the tumour. Thus adequate resection of detrusor muscle underneath the tumour is necessary. For staging purposes separate (cold-cup) biopsies can be taken from the tumour-bed.

Risk estimation

To estimate the risk of future recurrence or progression from a new NMIBC, EORTC developed a risk calculator (www.eortc.be/tools/bladdercalculator) based on six variables (Table 6.20.1). Of these, tumour grade is the strongest predictor, followed by stage and the presence of concomitant CIS. While CIS in many organs

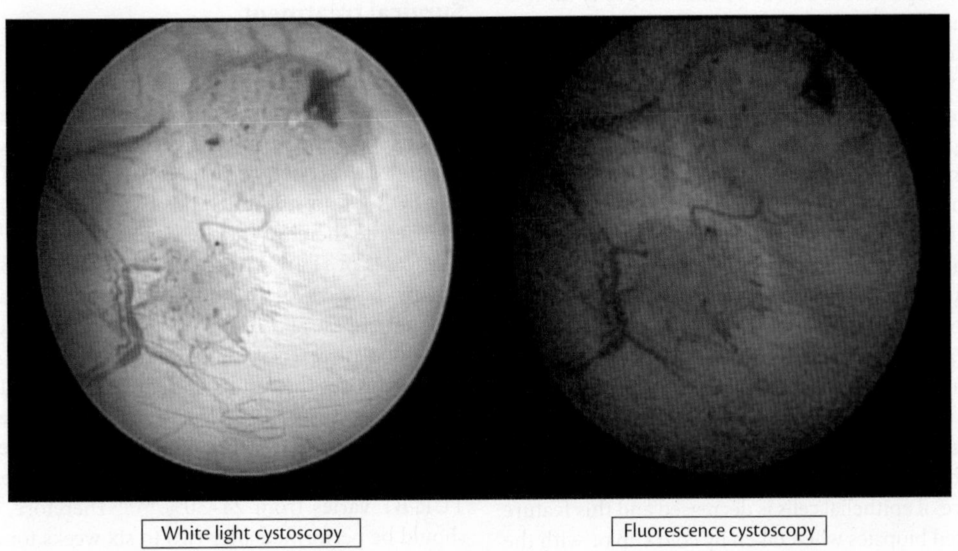

Fig. 6.20.1 White light cystoscopy (A) versus florescence cystoscopy (B).

is a premalignant (and often indolent) disease, CIS of the bladder is an aggressive cancer. If untreated (or does not respond to BCG), CIS in the bladder may progress to muscle-invasive disease in approximately 50% of patients, intravesical disease recurrence in up to 90% of patients,[23,24] and at diagnosis 5% or more already have nodal metastases. CIS can be found in isolation within the urinary tract (i.e. primary CIS) or in combination with UC either concomitantly (i.e. synchronous CIS with an exophytic UC) or subsequently (i.e. metachronously after previous UC).[3,25] Although, it has been reported that patients with primary CIS have a better prognosis than patients with concomitant or secondary CIS, the risk profiles of these three clinical types of CIS have not yet been fully clarified.[26–28] It should be noted that UC associated with concomitant CIS are usually HG-NMIBC (typically pT1 lesions). It is unusual for these UC to be low grade (grade 1 or grade 2 using 1973), but in this case the CIS is the most aggressive and important lesion. To provide a risk profile for CIS, a new subdivision has been proposed that identifyies patients with high-risk CIS (i.e. diffuse CIS, prostatic urethra involvement and/or overexpression of p53). These patients are at high risk of progression and metastatses and affected patients should be offered primary radical cystectomy without BCG. Lower risk CIS (i.e. focal CIS, lack of overexpression of p53, isolated lesion within the bladder) may be offered bladder-preserving therapy[29] (such as BCG) or primary radical cystectomy. CIS of the bladder is a recognized risk factor for the development of upper urinary tract tumours after radical cystectomy.[30]

For better assessment of NMIBC prognosis, a wide variety of molecular markers have been investigated. Some of these have been shown to be associated with aggressive disease and hold promise to predict progression if used in combination.[9,31,32] Conversely, the *FGFR3*-mutation has been found to be a selective marker for favourable disease in several reports.[32–34] Still the value of these molecular markers over traditional histo-pathology is not clear. Nevertheless, these markers may offer a better understanding of the biology of NMIBC and future research might lead to their use in clinical decision-making.

Pathology and staging

The histopathological report from a TUR-BT should specify tumour grade, depth of tumour invasion, and whether the lamina propria, sufficient muscle, and flat urothelial tissue are present in the specimen.[6] In addition, pathological variants and lymphovascular invasion should be reported. As stated, HG-NMIBC is a collective term including all high-grade NMI UC, such as those without invasion (pTa), those with lamina propria invasion (pT1), and those that are only or have concomitant CIS; pTis).

About 20% of all Ta tumours are high grade.[35,36] Given that most high-grade lesions are invasive (pT1 or pT2+), the pathologist and surgeon should ensure that lamina propria and muscularis propria are seen clearly, before agreeing upon the diagnosis of a high-grade pTa lesion. In case of doubt, an early re-resection of the UC scar is advised. CIS is often a multifocal disease and can involve regions beyond the bladder (such as the prostatic urethra or upper urinary tracts). CIS is frequently associated with invasive bladder cancer and is suspected to be the biological precursor of these lesions.[12,37] In CIS, the adherence of epithelial cells is decreased and this feature may result in denuded biopsies when taken by cold cup or with the resection loop.[16] Although CIS is defined as an overt high grade lesion, consensus on the diagnosis does not always exist when the specimen is reviewed by several pathologists. There is both intra-observer and inter-observer variability, even between severe dysplasia and CIS.[16,38] Most HG-NMIBC are pT1 lesions. These are invading the lamina proporia but stop short of the detrusor muscle. The risk of progression to invasion for a pT1 lesion varies considerably (25–75%) and can be predicted by the depth of invasion and the presence of CIS elsewhere in the bladder. As for other HG-NMIBCs, the surgeon and pathologist should ensure that detrusor muscle has been seen and sampled clearly, before exdluding muscle invasion (stage pT2). High-grade T1 disease represents a dilemma for the clinician, as conservative treatment may result in progression to life-threatening disease, whereas radical cystectomy may be overtreatment of non-progressive disease. Therefore, attempts have been made to develop a system of substaging that provides prognostic information to guide clinical decision-making in these patients. Some studies have proposed a system of substaging of T1 bladder cancer according to invasion above the muscularis mucosae-vascular plexus (MM-VP) (T1a), in the MM-VP (T1b), or beyond the MM-VP (T1c). Most studies found substage to be an important prognostic factor.[39,40] However, there was a high degree of inter-observer variability between pathologists regarding the identification of the MM-VP at the site of invasion of the tumour.[41] Finally, lack of consensus among pathologists led to the rejection of the T1a/b/c system by the WHO in 2004. A new system of T1 substaging was recently proposed, discerning T1-microinvasive (T1m) and T1-extensive invasive (T1e) tumours.[7] The definition of T1m was a single focus of lamina propria invasion with a diameter of ≤0.5 mm (within one high-power field objective ×40). The definition of T1e represents a larger area with invasion or multiple microinvasive areas. The latter system of substaging (T1m and T1e) appears to be user-friendly and highly predictive of T1 bladder cancer behaviour, although further validation of this system is required. To further reduce inter-observer variability, the WHO 2004 adopted a modified grading system for urothelial carcinomas. In this WHO 2004 grading system, high grade consists of a part of the WHO 1973 grade 2 and of the WHO 1973 grade 3.[42,43]

Treatment

Surgical treatment

The primary treatment for NMIBC is TUR-BT. During TUR-BT the tumour should be resected completely. A surprisingly high variability has been reported in recurrence rates after TUR-BT between various institutions, implying important differences in the quality of surgical resection of bladder tumours.[44] PDD may be used during TUR-BT to minimize positive surgical margins and residual disease and thereby reducing recurrence rates.[45]

In cases of HG-NMIBC, a re-staging TUR-BT is recommended within 6 weeks of the initial resection, because of the risk of residual disease and/or understaging. After initial TUR-BT the risk of residual disease varies between 36–63%.[46,47] Although the use of PDD improves the results of the initial TUR-BT, there is still a risk of residual disease of 12%, justifying a second resection. In samples without adequate detrusor muscle, a second resection is essential to adequately stage the patient. The risk of understaging at primary TUR-BT varies from 24–30%.[46,48] Therefore, a second TUR-BT should be performed after two to six weeks for all high-grade Ta-1 tumours, in patients opting for bladder sparing treatment.

The dilemma of bladder sparing treatment for patients with HG-NMIBC versus early cystectomy has been mentioned earlier.[49] Some reports have been published on the results of early cystectomy for patients with primary CIS. Although the disease-specific survival (DSS) rates in these series are generally excellent (ranging from 85-91%), the rate of overtreatment with early cystectomy is substantial (up to 50% of patients).[50,51] On the other hand, the window of opportunity to optimally treat these patients with high-risk NMIBC must be taken into account. In a retrospective analysis, the disease-specific survival proved to be significantly poorer for patients with progressive MIBC (five years DSS 28%) versus patients with primary MIBC (five years DSS 55%).[52] A possible explanation for this worse outcome of patients with progressive MIBC may be found that in high-risk NMIBC tumour biology consists of therapy-sensitive cells and therapy-insensitive cells. Intravesical instillations may lead to selection of resistant cell-lines and a more aggressive tumour biology that subsequently progresses to invasive disease.[52] For high-grade T1 disease, early radical cystectomy may be considered for selected high-risk patients (e.g. young patients with multifocal disease, concomitant CIS, and tumour in the prostatic urethra, micropapillary UC).[12]

Adjuvant treatment

In contrast to low-grade Ta bladder tumours, the instillation mitomycin-C (MMC) is insufficient for HG-NMIBC. For patients with HG-NMIBC, evidence suggests the best bladder sparing approach is intravesical BCG immunotherapy. This may be administered as a single course (Induction regimen: six weekly doses) or as a maintenance regimen over three years (with repeated intravesical inoculations).[6] The response to BCG treatment should be assessed three months after the first instillation. The classic BCG maintenance (so-called SWOG regimen) schedule consists of an induction period with six weekly instillations, followed by the maintenance period with three weekly instillations at months 3, 6, 12, 18, 24, 30, and 36 (i.e. 27 BCG instillations in three years). In cases of no response to BCG (persisting HG-NMIBC), another six weekly course of BCG induction may be considered or the patient may be eligible for cystectomy.

The choice between adjuvant intravesical treatment, namely, chemotherapy or BCG immunotherapy, depends on the risk that needs to be reduced: recurrence or progression. Several meta-analyses have shown that adjuvant intravesical treatment (chemotherapy or BCG) reduces NMIBC recurrence.[6,9] BCG is more effective but also more toxic. Furthermore, BCG in a maintenance schedule, but not intravesical chemotherapy, also reduces the risk of progression.[8] However, a meta-analysis restricted to BCG induction (6-weekly instillations) only versus maintenance BCG (1–3 years) treatment has not been done, and follow-up in the largest meta-analysis was short (2.5 years).[8] In the trials directly comparing maintenance BCG with induction BCG alone, progression was found in 30% of the patients who received maintenance as compared to 33% in the induction group.[53] In addition, a recent study has shown that T1 HG-NMIBC treated conservatively with BCG progressed to muscle invasion in 30% of cases and that one-third of progressive events occurred after three years of follow-up.[54] Treatment with BCG is currently considered to be the first-line approach for HG-NMIBC. It is a major concern that despite grade A recommendations in the guidelines, Surveillance Epidemiology and End Results data on 685 primary NMIBC patients indicated that such intravesical therapy was used in only 31% of patients in academic institutions.[6,55,56] In a subset of 350 high-risk NMIBC patients, only 42% received intravesical therapy, suggesting significant undertreatment.[56]

BCG failure is defined as the presence of HG-NMIBC after three to six months of BCG treatment, upstaging of disease (Ta to T1) under BCG treatment, appearance of CIS during BCG treatment and progression to MIBC despite BCG treatment.[13] BCG failure may be subdivided into *BCG intolerant disease* (i.e. recurrence of disease due to inadequate treatment because of symptomatic intolerance or adverse events), *BCG refractory disease* (i.e. failure to achieve disease-free status by six months after BCG induction and maintenance or after re-induction at three months; non-improving or worsening disease despite BCG) and *BCG resistant disease* (i.e. recurrence or persistent disease after initial induction and disease-free status six months after repeat TUR-BT and retreatment).[57,58] There have been reports on additional conservative treatment after BCG failure (e.g. hyperthermia and MMC; photodynamic therapy; BCG plus interferon alpha), but the results are still investigational. Therefore, a cystectomy is generally recommended for patients with BCG failure.[6]

Follow-up

Follow-up protocol

Follow-up of patients with HG-NMIBC consists primarily of regular cystoscopy and urinary cytology every three months for the first two years. In year three, these investigations should be performed every 4 months, the six monthly until year 5 and annually thereafter.[6] Most guidelines recommend lifelong follow-up of patients with HG-NMIBC. A recent study has shown that, despite a recurrence-free period of five years after BCG treatment, recurrence, and especially progression outside of the bladder still occur, thus concluding that the follow-up of HG-NMIBC should indeed continue for at least 10–15 years.[59] Furthermore, during follow-up imaging of the upper urinary tract is recommended every year.[6] At present, urinary markers other than cytology, are not incorporated into the standard follow-up schedule for HG-NMIBC.

Bacillus Calmette–Guérin toxicity

Intravesical BCG treatment is associated with more toxicity than intravesical chemotherapy. In a large trials, 75.2% of patients experience local side effects (cystitis, haematuria, frequency) and 39.4% of patients had systemic side effects (fever, general malaise), resulting in a discontinuation of treatment in 20.3% of patients. In most patients who discontinued BCG treatment because of toxicity, this was during the first six months of treatment. While local side effects (cystitis, haematuria, and frequency) were encountered during the entire treatment period, while the systemic side effects were seen more frequently in the first six months. Thus suggesting that systemic side effects depend more on the patient than on the number of instillations. Furthermore, the hypothesis that BCG induced side effects increase with time during maintenance treatment does not appear to be true.[60]

Severe complications (BCG sepsis, pneumonitis, osteomyelitis, tuberculosis) are rare. Nevertheless, such severe complications may occur after systemic absorption of BCG. For this reason, BCG treatment is contraindicated in patients with haematuria, after traumatic catheterization, and within two weeks after TUR-BT.[6]

Such systemic side effects may require treatment with prednisolone and tuberculostatic drugs.

Conclusions

The term HG-NMIBC includes NMI bladder cancers with a high risk of recurrence and progression to muscle-invasive disease (MIBC). These represent aggressive cancers that are typically locally confined to the bladder. As such, patients with these cancers require close surveillance and treatment to reduce the risk of progression to muscle invasion. Currently, intravesical BCG (maintenance regimen) is the most popular treatment for HG-NMIBC. Primary radical cystectomy should be offered to patients whose tumours are at high risk of progression or those who have a good performance status (such a young age or very fit) and so may subsequently fail BCG. However, cystectomy represents over treatment for many patients with HG-NMIBC. Follow-up of HG-NMIBC should continue for at least 10–15 years, consisting primarily of cystoscopy and urinary cytology, and intermittent imaging of the upper urinary tract.

Further reading

Babjuk M, Oosterlinck W, Sylvester R, *et al.* EAU guidelines on non-muscle-invasive urothelial carcinoma of the bladder, the 2011 update. *Eur Urol* 2011; **59**:997–1008.

Brausi M, Collette L, Kurth K, *et al.* Variability in the recurrence rate at first follow-up cystoscopy after TUR in stage Ta T1 transitional cell carcinoma of the bladder: a combined analysis of seven EORTC studies. *Eur Urol* 2002; **41**:523–31.

Herr HW. Is maintenance Bacillus Calmette-Guerin really necessary? *Eur Urol* 2008; **54**(5):971–3.

Kulkarni GS, Hakenberg OW, Gschwend JE, *et al.* An updated critical analysis of the treatment strategy for newly diagnosed high-grade T1 (previously T1G3) bladder cancer. *Eur Urol* 2010; **57**:60–70.

Malmström PU, Sylvester RJ, Crawford DE, *et al.* An individual patient data meta-analysis of the long-term outcome of randomised studies comparing intravesical mitomycin C versus bacillus Calmette-Guerin for non-muscle-invasive bladder cancer. *Eur Urol* 2009; **56**(2):247–56.

Meijer RP, van Onna IE, Kok ET, *et al.* The risk profiles of three clinical types of carcinoma in situ of the bladder. *BJU Int* 2011; **108**(6):839–43.

Schrier BP, Hollander MP, van Rhijn BW, Kiemeney LA, Witjes JA. Prognosis of muscle-invasive bladder cancer: difference between primary and progressive tumours and implications for therapy. *Eur Urol* 2004; **45**:292–6.

Sylvester RJ, van der Meijden AP, Oosterlinck W, *et al.* Predicting recurrence and progression in individual patients with stage Ta T1 bladder cancer using EORTC risk tables: a combined analysis of 2596 patients from seven EORTC trials. *Eur Urol* 2006; **49**:466–75; discussion 475–7.

Thomas F, Noon A, Rubin N, Goepel JR, Catto JWF. Comparative outcomes of primary, recurrent and progressive high-risk non-muscle invasive bladder cancer. *Eur Urol* 2013; **63**(1):145–54.

van der Meijden AP, Sylvester RJ, Oosterlinck W, *et al.* Maintenance Bacillus Calmette-Guerin for Ta T1 bladder tumors is not associated with increased toxicity: results from a European Organisation for Research and Treatment of Cancer Genito-Urinary Group Phase III Trial. *Eur Urol* 2003; **44**:429–34.

van Rhijn BW, Burger M, Lotan Y, *et al.* Recurrence and progression of disease in non-muscle-invasive bladder cancer: from epidemiology to treatment strategy. *Eur Urol* 2009; **56**:430–42.

van Rhijn BW, van der Kwast TH, Alkhateeb SS, *et al.* A new and highly prognostic system to discern T1 bladder cancer substage. *Eur Urol* 2012; **61**:378–84.

Witjes JA, Redorta JP, Jacqmin D, *et al.* Hexaminolevulinate-guided fluorescence cystoscopy in the diagnosis and follow-up of patients with non-muscle-invasive bladder cancer: review of the evidence and recommendations. *Eur Urol* 2010; **57**:607–14.

Yates DR, Brausi MA, Catto JW, *et al.* Treatment options available for bacillus Calmette-Guérin failure in non-muscle-invasive bladder cancer. *Eur Urol* 2012; **62**(6):1088–96.

References

1. Droller MJ. Urothelial cancer—mucosally confined disease can be aggressive. *J Urol* 2000; **163**:79–80.
2. Millan-Rodriguez F, Chechile-Toniolo G, Salvador-Bayarri J, *et al.* Primary superficial bladder cancer risk groups according to progression, mortality and recurrence. *J Urol* 2000; **164**:680–4.
3. Sylvester RJ, van der Meijden A, Witjes JA, *et al.* High-grade Ta urothelial carcinoma and carcinoma in situ of the bladder. *Urology* 2005; **66**(6 Suppl 1):90–107.
4. Bol MG, Baak JP, Buhr-Wildhagen S, *et al.* Reproducibility and prognostic variability of grade and lamina propria invasion in stages Ta, T1 urothelial carcinoma of the bladder. *J Urol* 2003; **169**:1291–4.
5. Witjes, JA, Moonen PM, van der Heijden AG. Review pathology in a diagnostic bladder cancer trial: effect of patient risk category. *Urology* 2006; **67**:751–5.
6. Babjuk M, Oosterlinck W, Sylvester R, *et al.* EAU guidelines on non-muscle-invasive urothelial carcinoma of the bladder, the 2011 update. *Eur Urol* 2011; **59**:997–1008.
7. van Rhijn BW, van der Kwast TH, Alkhateeb SS, *et al.* A new and highly prognostic system to discern T1 bladder cancer substage. *Eur Urol* 2012; **61**:378–84.
8. Sylvester RJ, van der Meijden, Lamm DL. Intravesical bacillus Calmette-Guerin reduces the risk of progression in patients with superficial bladder cancer: a meta-analysis of the published results of randomized clinical trials. *J Urol* 2002; **168**:1964–70.
9. van Rhijn BW, Burger M, Lotan Y, *et al.* Recurrence and progression of disease in non-muscle-invasive bladder cancer: from epidemiology to treatment strategy. *Eur Urol* 2009; **56**:430–42.
10. Thomas F, Rosario DJ, Rubin N, *et al.* The long-term outcome of treated high-risk nonmuscle-invasive bladder cancer: time to change treatment paradigm? *Cancer* 2012; **118**:5525–34.
11. Thomas F, Noon AP, Rubin N, Goepel JR, Catto JW. Comparative outcomes of primary, recurrent, and progressive high-risk non-muscle-invasive bladder cancer. *Eur Urol* 2013; **63**:145–54.
12. Burger M, Witjes JA, Babjuk M, *et al.* Second international consultation on bladder cancer. (pp. 249–68) In: Soloway MS, Khoury S (eds). *Bladder Cancer*, 2nd edition. Paris, France: Editions 21, 2012.
13. Yates DR, Brausi MA, Catto JW, *et al.* Treatment options available for bacillus Calmette-Guerin failure in non-muscle-invasive bladder cancer. *Eur Urol* 2012; **62**:1088–96.
14. Brown FM. Urine cytology. It is still the gold standard for screening? *Urol Clin North Am* 2000; **27**:25–37.
15. Zaak D, Hungerhuber E, Schneede P, *et al.* Role of 5-aminolevulinic acid in the detection of urothelial premalignant lesions. *Cancer* 2002; **95**:1234–8.
16. van der Meijden AP, Sylvester R, Oosterlinck W, *et al.* EAU guidelines on the diagnosis and treatment of urothelial carcinoma in situ. *Eur Urol* 2005; **48**:363–71.
17. Witjes JA, Redorta JP, Jacqmin D, *et al.* Hexaminolevulinate-guided fluorescence cystoscopy in the diagnosis and follow-up of patients with non-muscle-invasive bladder cancer: review of the evidence and recommendations. *Eur Urol* 2010; **57**:607–14.
18. Jocham D, Witjes F, Wagner S, *et al.* Improved detection and treatment of bladder cancer using hexaminolevulinate imaging: a prospective, phase III multicenter study. *J Urol* 2005; **174**:862–6; discussion 866.
19. Kausch I, Sommerauer M, Montorsi F, *et al.* Photodynamic diagnosis in non-muscle-invasive bladder cancer: a systematic review and cumulative analysis of prospective studies. *Eur Urol* 2010; **57**:595–606.
20. Munoz JJ, Ellison LM. Upper tract urothelial neoplasms: incidence and survival during the last 2 decades. *J Urol* 2000; **164**:1523–5.

21. Tawfiek ER, Bagley DH. Upper-tract transitional cell carcinoma. *Urology* 1997; **50**:321–9.
22. Palou J, Rodriguez-Rubio F, Huguet J, *et al.* Multivariate analysis of clinical parameters of synchronous primary superficial bladder cancer and upper urinary tract tumor. *J Urol* 2005; **174**:859–61.
23. Lamm DL. Carcinoma in situ. *Urol Clin North Am* 1992; **19**:499–508.
24. Wolf H, Melsen F, Pedersen SE, Nielsen KT. Natural history of carcinoma in situ of the urinary bladder. *Scand J Urol Nephrol Suppl* 1994; **157**:147–51.
25. Lamm DL, Herr H, Jakse G, *et al.* Updated concepts and treatment of carcinoma in situ. *Urol Oncol* 1908; **4**:130–8.
26. Griffiths TR, Charlton M, Neal DE, Powell PH. Treatment of carcinoma in situ with intravesical bacillus Calmette-Guerin without maintenance. *J Urol* 2002; **167**:2408–12.
27. Witjes JA. Bladder carcinoma in situ in 2003: state of the art. *Eur Urol* 2004; **45**:142–6.
28. Meijer RP, van Onna IE, Kok ET, *et al.* The risk profiles of three clinical types of carcinoma in situ of the bladder. *BJU Int* 2011; **108**(6):839–43.
29. Hudson MA, Herr HW. Carcinoma in situ of the bladder. *J Urol* 1995; **153**:564–72.
30. Volkmer BG, Schnoeller T, Kuefer R, *et al.* Upper urinary tract recurrence after radical cystectomy for bladder cancer—who is at risk? *J Urol* 2009; **182**:2632–7.
31. Stein JP, Grossfeld GD, Ginsberg DA, *et al.* Prognostic markers in bladder cancer: a contemporary review of the literature. *J Urol* 1998; **160**:645–59.
32. van Rhijn BW, Vis AN, van der Kwast TH, *et al.* Molecular grading of urothelial cell carcinoma with fibroblast growth factor receptor 3 and MIB-1 is superior to pathologic grade for the prediction of clinical outcome. *J Clin Oncol* 2003; **21**:1912–21.
33. Burger M, van der Aa MN, van Oers JM, *et al.* Prediction of progression of non-muscle-invasive bladder cancer by WHO 1973 and 2004 grading and by FGFR3 mutation status: a prospective study. *Eur Urol* 2008; **54**:835–43.
34. Hernandez S, Lopez-Knowles E, Lloreta J, *et al.* Prospective study of FGFR3 mutations as a prognostic factor in nonmuscle invasive urothelial bladder carcinomas. *J Clin Oncol* 2006; **24**(22):3664–71.
35. Sylvester RJ, van der Meijden AP, Oosterlinck W, *et al.* Predicting recurrence and progression in individual patients with stage Ta T1 bladder cancer using EORTC risk tables: a combined analysis of 2596 patients from seven EORTC trials. *Eur Urol* 2006; **49**:466–75; discussion 475–7.
36. Amling CL. Diagnosis and management of superficial bladder cancer. *Curr Probl Cancer* 2001; **25**:219–78.
37. Dyrskjot L, Zieger K, Kruhoffer M, *et al.* A molecular signature in superficial bladder carcinoma predicts clinical outcome. *Clin Cancer Res* 2005; **11**:4029–36.
38. Sharkey FE, Sarosdy MF. The significance of central pathology review in clinical studies of transitional cell carcinoma in situ. *J Urol* 1997; **157**(1):68–70; discussion 70–1.
39. Holmang S, Hedelin H, Anderstrom C, *et al.* The importance of the depth of invasion in stage T1 bladder carcinoma: a prospective cohort study. *J Urol* 1997; **157**:800–3; discussion 804.
40. Smits G, Schaafsma E, Kiemeney L, *et al.* Microstaging of pT1 transitional cell carcinoma of the bladder: identification of subgroups with distinct risks of progression. *Urology* 1998; **52**(6):1009–13; discussion 1013–4.
41. Nieder AM, Brausi M, Lamm D, *et al.* Management of stage T1 tumors of the bladder: International Consensus Panel. *Urology* 2005; **66**:108–25.
42. MacLennan GT, Kirkali Z, Cheng L. Histologic grading of noninvasive papillary urothelial neoplasms. *Eur Urol* 2007; **51**:889–97; discussion 897–8.
43. van Rhijn BW, van Leenders GJ, Ooms BC, *et al.* The pathologist's mean grade is constant and individualizes the prognostic value of bladder cancer grading. *Eur Urol* 2010; **57**:1052–7.
44. Brausi M, Collette L, Kurth K, *et al.* Variability in the recurrence rate at first follow-up cystoscopy after TUR in stage Ta T1 transitional cell carcinoma of the bladder: a combined analysis of seven EORTC studies. *Eur Urol* 2002; **41**:523–31.
45. Mowatt G, N'Dow J, Vale L, *et al.* Photodynamic diagnosis of bladder cancer compared with white light cystoscopy: Systematic review and meta-analysis. *Int J Technol Assess Health Care* 2011; **27**:3–10.
46. Miladi M, Peyromaure M, Zerbib M, *et al.* The value of a second transurethral resection in evaluating patients with bladder tumours. *Eur Urol* 2003; **43**:241–5.
47. Divrik T, Yildirim U, Eroğlu AS, Zorlu F, Ozen H. Is a second transurethral resection necessary for newly diagnosed pT1 bladder cancer? *J Urol* 2006; **175**:1258–61.
48. Dutta SC, Smith JA Jr, Shappell SB, Coffey CS, Chang SS, Cookson MS. Clinical under staging of high risk nonmuscle invasive urothelial carcinoma treated with radical cystectomy. *J Urol* 2001; **166**:490–3.
49. Kulkarni GS, Hakenberg OW, Gschwend JE, *et al.* An updated critical analysis of the treatment strategy for newly diagnosed high-grade T1 (previously T1G3) bladder cancer. *Eur Urol* 2010; **57**:60–70.
50. Tilki D, Reich O, Svatek RS, *et al.* Characteristics and outcomes of patients with clinical carcinoma in situ only treated with radical cystectomy: an international study of 243 patients. *J Urol* 2010; **183**:1757–63.
51. Shariat SF, Palapattu GS, Amiel GE, *et al.* Characteristics and outcomes of patients with carcinoma in situ only at radical cystectomy. *Urology* 2006; **68**:538.
52. Schrier BP, Hollander MP, van Rhijn BW, Kiemeney LA, Witjes JA. Prognosis of muscle-invasive bladder cancer: difference between primary and progressive tumours and implications for therapy. *Eur Urol* 2004; **45**:292–6.
53. Herr HW. Is maintenance Bacillus Calmette-Guerin really necessary? *Eur Urol* 2008; **54**(5):971–3.
54. Kakiashvili DM, van Rhijn BW, Trottier G, *et al.* Long-term follow-up of T1 high-grade bladder cancer after intravesical bacille Calmette-Guerin treatment. *BJU Int* 2011; **107**:540–6.
55. Brausi M, Witjes JA, Lamm D, *et al.* A review of current guidelines and best practice recommendations for the management of nonmuscle invasive bladder cancer by the International Bladder Cancer Group. *J Urol* 2011; **186**:2158–67.
56. Huang GJ, Hamilton AS, Lo M, *et al.* Predictors of intravesical therapy for nonmuscle invasive bladder cancer: results from the surveillance, epidemiology and end results program 2003 patterns of care project. *J Urol* 2008; **180**:520–4.
57. O'Donnell MA, Boehle A. Treatment options for BCG failures. *World J Urol* 2006; **24**:481–7.
58. Rosevear HM, Lightfoot AJ, Birusingh KK, *et al.* Factors affecting response to bacillus Calmette-Guerin plus interferon for urothelial carcinoma in situ. *J Urol* 2011; **186**:817–23.
59. Holmang S, Strock V. Should follow-up cystoscopy in bacillus Calmette-Guerin-treated patients continue after five tumour-free years? *Eur Urol* 2012; **61**:503–7.
60. van der Meijden AP, Sylvester RJ, Oosterlinck W, *et al.* Maintenance Bacillus Calmette-Guerin for Ta T1 bladder tumors is not associated with increased toxicity: results from a European Organisation for Research and Treatment of Cancer Genito-Urinary Group Phase III Trial. *Eur Urol* 2003; **44**:429–34.

CHAPTER 6.21

Muscle-invasive bladder cancer

Pascal Zehnder and George N. Thalmann

Introduction to muscle-invasive bladder cancer

In the United States, approximately 65,000 individuals (male to female ratio 3:1) are diagnosed with bladder cancer each year.[1] Of those, twenty to 40% have muscle-invasive disease requiring radical surgery. Overall, more than 13,000 patients in the USA die of the disease annually, making it the ninth most common cause of cancer deaths in males. Similarly, bladder cancer represented the eighth most common cause of cancer-specific death in Europe in 2008.[2] Focusing on the United Kingdom, more than 10,000 people are yearly diagnosed with bladder cancer and more than 4,000 die of it every year, accounting for 1 in 30 cancer deaths.[3] Bladder cancer typically affects individuals around their seventies. Although the disease potentially affects people at any age, the incidence progressively increases with age.

The high incidence and need for surveillance makes bladder cancer one of the most expensive to manage. While the initial diagnosis and staging work-up are performed by the majority of urologists, patients are usually referred to centres of expertise when it comes to radical surgery, the mainstay of therapy for patients with non-metastatic muscle-invasive bladder cancer. Evidence suggests better outcomes for patients undergoing radical cystectomy in high-volume units.

Pathologic subgroups

Urothelial cell cancer

The majority of bladder tumours are urothelial cell cancer (UCC: around 90%) in subtype. These can be classified according to tumour growth pattern (e.g. sessile, papillary, nodular, infiltrating, flat, and mixed). About one-fifth of UCC consist of mixed architectural elements. In this chapter we focus upon those that are invading the bladder wall (detrusor muscle/muscularis propria). Around one-third of new UCC are muscle-invasive at presentation. Of the remainder, up to half are high-grade and 25% of these may progress to invasion with time.[4]

Non-urothelial cell cancer

The remaining 5–10% of bladder tumours are non-UCC in cell type. Most of these are aggressive tumours that are invasive at presentation or have a very high risk of progression.[5] As such, most are treated as invasive tumours. Given the rarity of these cancers, there is a lack of evidence about their best treatment regimens. Most clinicians extrapolate care from UCC pathways and histologically similar tumours in other organs (e.g. squamous lung cancer, rectal adenocarcinoma). *Squamous cell carcinomas* reflect 2–3% of all bladder cancer worldwide and up to 75% in areas with endemic *Schistosoma haematobium* (e.g. Egypt). The peak of bilharzial cancers is 10 to 20 years earlier than the classic urothelial carcinoma and the rate of lymph node involvement or distant metastases is low. *Adenocarcinomas* represent less than 2% of bladder cancers. These are categorized into three groups: arising in the bladder urothelium (often around the trigone); in the urachus (at the dome: have a worse outcome than trigonal tumours); and secondary adenocarcinoma invading the bladder (often prostate or colorectal). Primary adenocarcinoma may occur in patients with former extrophic bladders, typically after a long latency and despite early surgical correction. Primary tumours of the stomach, intestinal tract, endometrium, breast, ovary, and prostate potentially metastasize to the urinary bladder. *Small cell carcinoma* is an aggressive tumour derived from neuroendocrine stem cells and requires cisplatin-based chemotherapy before radical surgery/radiotherapy. Despite a combined radical approach, prognosis remains poor. The majority of patients harbour lymph node metastases, although long-term disease-free survival is possible for patients with organ-confined tumours. *Carcinosarcoma* are very aggressive but rare tumours containing malignant mesenchymal and epithelial tissues.

Metastatic carcinoma

Basically any tumour can metastasize into the bladder with a certain predominance of primary tumours from prostate, uterus, ovaries, intestinal tract, lung, breast, kidney, and stomach.

TNM classification and tumour grading

Bladder cancer is classified according to 7th edition of the American Joint Cancer Committee (AJCC) staging manual applying the TNM criteria.[6] The clinical staging describes the extent of disease before any treatment and uses the prefix 'c', using clinical examination, cystoscopy, plus biopsy and imaging studies. Pathological staging describes the extent of disease through completion of definitive surgery and uses the prefix 'p'. It bases on the pathologic analysis of the cystectomy and lymphadenectomy specimens as well as imaging studies. Since tumour staging following transurethral bladder tumour biopsy and/or resection is heterogeneously reported either as cT- or pT-stage this is potentially misleading. Staging of surgical specimens following neoadjuvant treatments is further specified with the prefix 'yp'. Currently, both the 1973 and the 2004 World Health Organization (WHO) grading classifications are used, since many published studies were based on the old WHO grading system.

Staging requirements and modalities

The staging of bladder cancer requires a multimodal approach. The clinician should evaluate the primary lesion by inspection (at cystoscopy and transurethral resection of a bladder tumour (TURBT)) and palpation (under anaesthesia), and the pathologist evaluate the specimen for grade, histological subtype, and depth of invasion. High-grade and invasive lesions require staging for depth of invasion and metastatic spread to the abdominal/pelvic nodes, liver, and the chest. Uncommon site of metastases should be screened in symptomatic patients (e.g. brain and bone). Synchronous tumours in the upper urinary tract need excluding. Finally, shared etiologies exist with lung and other cancers (smoking). As such, imaging for these should be performed in patients undergoing major surgery.

Transurethral resection of bladder tumour (TURBT)

Every urologist should be aware that TURBT is a critical oncologic procedure. Immediately after visual tumour detection, the surgeon has to decide regarding the procedural strategy (Fig. 6.21.1). In case of a suspected non-muscle invasive tumour, the goal will be to entirely resect the lesion along with underlying bladder muscle and herewith cure the patient. If the macroscopic appearance suggests muscle-invasive growth the procedural objectives include the performance of a representative biopsy along with underlying bladder muscle to determine both tumour entity and muscle invasion (Fig. 6.21.2). Attempts to completely remove the tumour/

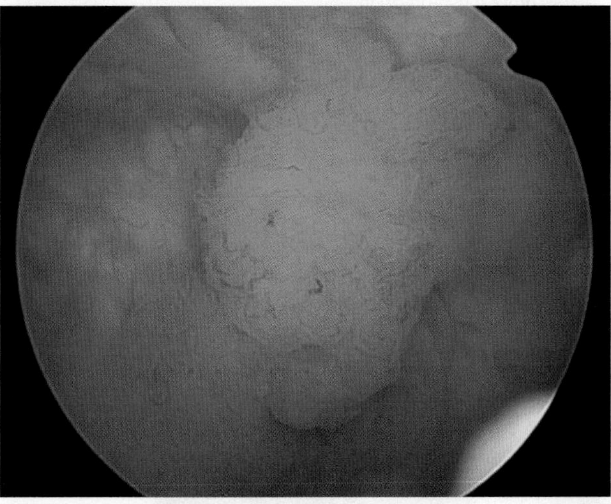

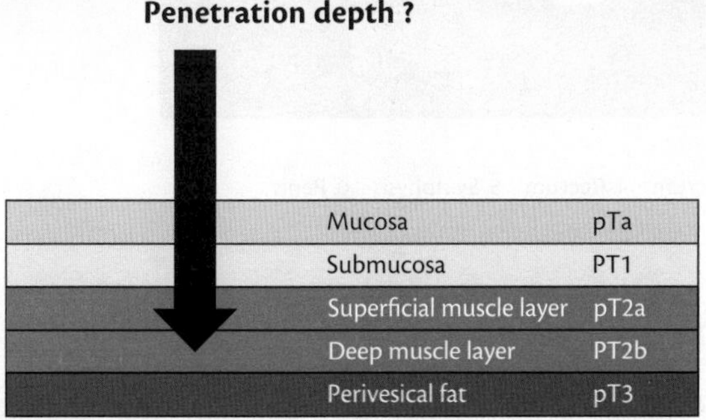

Fig. 6.21.1 Decision-making for transurethral resection of a bladder tumour (TURBT).

tumours in potential cystectomy candidates bear the unnecessary risk of bladder perforation and high-pressure resection with vascular tumour cell emboli/extravasation. Tumour localization in relation to the bladder neck and prostatic urethra is an important issue in view of performing nerve-sparing surgery and choice of urinary diversion. Hence, cold cup biopsies at the bladder neck (females) and within the prostatic urethra at the colliculus (males) are required in patients who may qualify for an orthotopic bladder substitute.

Invasive tumours surrounding or completely covering the ureteric orifices require an identical approach. In case of post interventional ureteric obstruction or the need for optimizing kidney function, the collecting system can be decompressed with the placement of a nephrostomy tube. Solid tumours within bladder diverticula are considered cT4 lesions. In these cases, the risk of bladder perforation in the frame of TURBT is substantially increased, and therefore these patients primarily undergo radical cystectomy.

Bimanual examination

Bimanual examination helps to judge whether locally advanced tumours with suspected extravesical growth are surgically removable or not. Optimally, the exam is performed under anaesthesia to allow a relaxed abdominal wall and pelvic floor, enabling a conclusive deep palpation.

Computed tomography scan

Ideally, any imaging study should be performed prior to TURBT, because it can be difficult to distinguish post-resection alterations from tumour infiltration. Urologists should consider cross sectional imaging for either all new tumours or those that appear invasive on flexible cystoscopy. Overall, staging accuracy by computed tomography (CT) scan ranges from 58% to 80%.[7] The limited accuracy originates from the CT technology that identifies pathology based on the size of a structure or process. Hence, only gross extravesical tumour manifestation and enlarged lymph nodes (>1 cm) are detectable. The fact that following radical cystectomy about 25% of clinically cN0M0 patients were found to have previously undetected lymph node metastases[8] clearly underlines the limitations of our current imaging armamentarium for staging. Many workers advocate CT chest as well, to fully stage the bladder tumour. This may detect metastases to the lung and primary bronchogenic tumours arising in smokers. Alternatives include a chest X-ray or PET scan (see below).

Magnetic resonance imaging

Magnetic resonance imaging (MRI) offers better soft tissue resolution than CT and is currently a modality often used for the evaluation of bladder cancers involving adjacent pelvic organs or for high-grade non-invasive lesions. Diffusion-weighted MRI seems to offer a better differentiation of non-muscle-invasive versus muscle-invasive bladder cancer.[9] The accuracy levels of MRI and CT in non-organ-confined bladder cancer staging are similar[7] (Fig. 6.21.3), although recent reports suggest metallic contrast agents may be used to improve the performance of MRI.[10]

Nuclear imaging

A bone scan is mandatory to accurately stage patients with boney symptoms and bladder cancer. The detection rate is low in

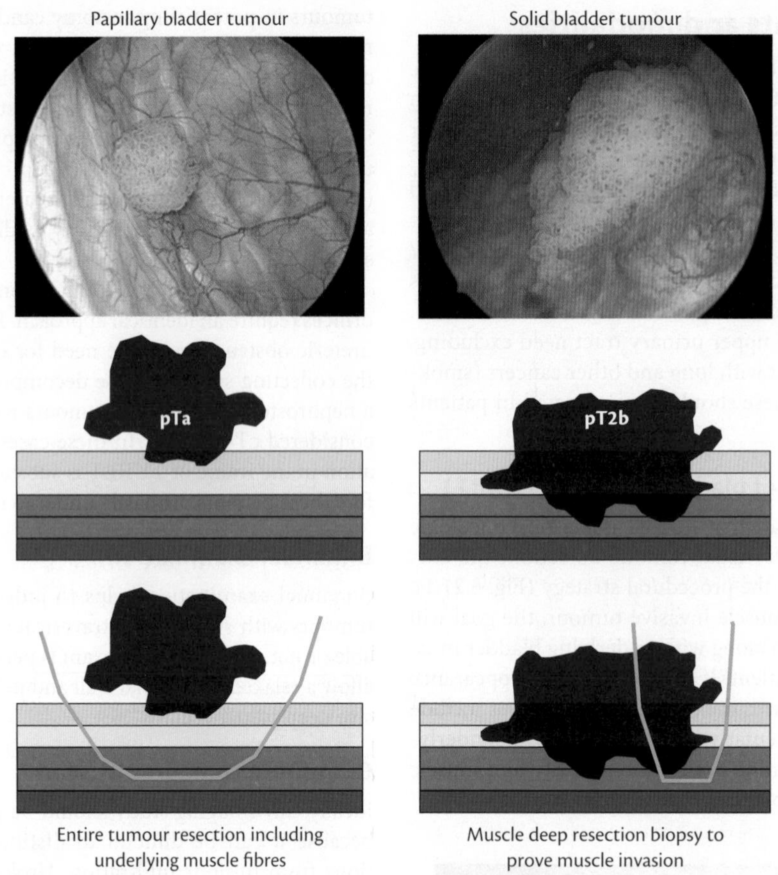

Fig. 6.21.2 TURBT resection strategies.

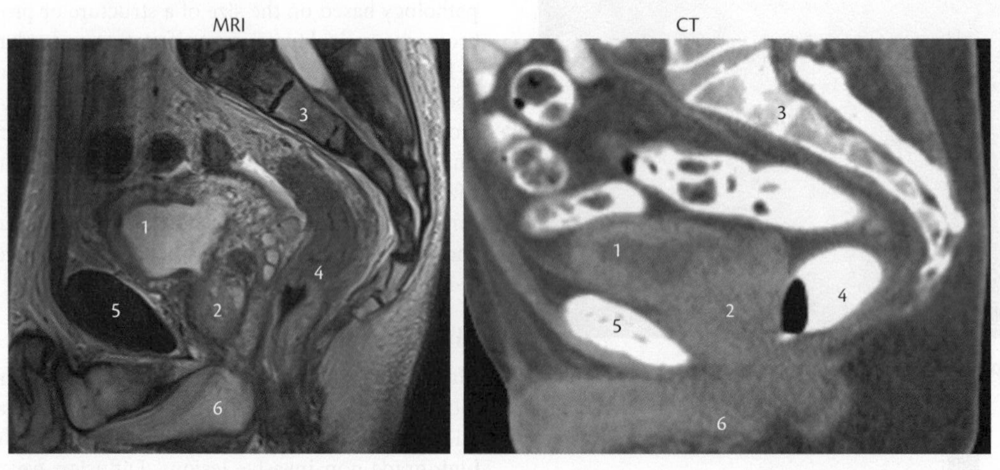

Fig. 6.21.3 Staging computed tomography (CT) and magnetic resonance imaging (MRI).

asymptomatic patients, and so usage should be by local protocols or agreements. Several workers are evaluating FDG-PET staging of bladder cancer prior to cystectomy.[11] This modality has a moderate specificity and sensitivity for metastases, and may detect lesions missed by cross sectional imaging. However, non-metastatic lesions may also appear active, leading to delays in definitive surgery, and most FDG-PET positive lesions are apparent on cross sectional imaging.

Treatment for muscle-invasive bladder cancer

Maximal transurethral resection of a bladder tumour

Attempts have been made to treat patients suffering from muscle-invasive bladder cancer with TURBT alone. It has been shown that radical TURBT can be a successful therapeutic strategy in selected patients with initially small (<2–3 cm) muscle-invasive bladder cancers who have no residual tumour on a second resection of the primary tumour site.[12] However, recurrence and progression rates in some consecutive series were substantial. Therefore, maximal and repeated TURBT eventually combined with intravesical Bacillus Calmette–Guérin instillation is limited to (solitary) pT1G3 tumours and patients refusing or unfit to undergo radical cystectomy.

Chemotherapy

Considering the underlying substantial staging error, chemotherapy as solitary treatment strategy does not achieve durable complete responses. On the other hand, chemotherapy may lead to down staging of the primary tumour. Therefore, and limited to very selected patients, an organ preserving strategy including TURBT and systemic cisplatin-based chemotherapy may allow for survival with the native bladder.[13] However, this is not standard treatment.

External beam radiotherapy

Similarly to chemotherapy, external beam radiotherapy (EBRT) and more recently intensity modulated radiotherapy[14] as monotherapies or combined with brachytherapy[15] consecutively to TURBT represent only an option in highly selected patients; for example, individuals unfit for radical surgery, those with unifocal disease and no carcinoma *in situ* (CIS), those with few urinary symptoms and good bladder function.[16] Besides the aim of local control, EBRT sometimes temporarily stops bleeding in patients where hemostasis cannot be achieved by transurethral intervention.

Multimodality approach

In contrast to the previously mentioned mono- or combined therapies, all three treatment modalities are combined in the multimodality bladder preserving approach. It is crucial to understand that a multimodality approach is only suitable for highly selected patients. This includes individuals with a solitary tumour <5 cm, a low organ-confined tumour stage, a complete TURBT with a negative second TURBT, no signs of ureteric obstruction, and no evidence of metastases to pelvic lymph nodes. Of all these variables, the completeness of TURBT was identified to be the most important prognostic factor for overall survival.[17] Patients with multifocal tumours and concomitant carcinoma *in situ*, which is not radio- nor chemosensitive, are at increased risk of recurrent or *de novo* tumour development despite primarily complete response.

Typically, the radiation dose to the bladder is 55 Gy to 70 Gy, with an additional 45 Gy to 50 Gy for the pelvic lymph nodes. Various fractionation regimes and doses such as hyper-fractionation, dose escalation, or accelerated radiation therapy are applied with the aim to overcome radio-resistance. Radiotherapy is combined with chemotherapy according to an induction/neoadjuvant, concurrent, or adjuvant concept. The cytotoxic agents are thought to sensitize tumour cells to radiation and to inhibit repopulation during radiotherapy. This combination aims at improving local control. In addition, systemic cytotoxic treatment is required to eradicate eventual occult distant micrometastases. Yet, the optimal cytotoxic regimen and combination with radiotherapy has to be established. Single chemotherapeutic agents used are cisplatin, gemcitabine, and taxanes. Alternatively, combinations such as methotrexate, cisplatin, and vinblastine are applied.[18,19] A typical trimodality treatment starts with a thorough, if possible complete TURBT, followed by an induction radio-chemotherapy. Four to six weeks after completion response to this treatment is evaluated by a restaging TURBT. While complete responders proceed to consolidation therapy, patients with residual muscle-invasive tumour will undergo salvage cystectomy. Approximately 20% to 30% of patients will present with residual tumour at restaging TURBT and another 20% to 30% with initial complete response will develop recurrent or *de novo* muscle-invasive or non-muscle-invasive tumours in the urinary bladder.[20]

With regard to radiation induced side effects, gastrointestinal or urogenital problems are frequent. About 1.5% of patients experience late gastrointestinal toxicity in terms of bowel obstruction requiring surgical therapy. At least 10% of patients complain of increased voiding frequency or urinary incontinence. Finally, about two percent of patients require a cystectomy in the course due to a low capacity shrunken bladder.[17] Therefore, multimodal organ preserving therapy of muscle-invasive bladder cancer should be considered only in select cases.

Radical cystectomy

For muscle-invasive bladder cancer, radical cystectomy with bilateral extended lymph node dissection represents the mainstay of therapy and offers cure to a substantial number of patients. The surgical principles were first described in 1950[21] and 1956.[22] While initially perioperative mortality was high (5–10%), radical cystectomy has become refined and is now the standard treatment for this disease (1–2% 90-day mortality rate in experienced centres).[23] While the default approach for this procedure is still through an open incision, advances in laparoscopy and namely in robotic surgery have made these routes a potential option in select cases.[24,25]

Pelvic lymph node dissection

Pelvic lymph node dissection is an integral part of the cystectomy procedure, as the critical axiom in oncologic surgery requires both the removal of the primary tumour and the primary echelon of lymphatic drainage. The urinary bladder has a complex lymphatic draining system recently demonstrated with a Technetium-based mapping study showing a median of 24 primary lymphatic landing sites per bladder.[26] Only 8–10% of primary lymphatic landing sites were found to be located above the mid-upper third of the common iliac vessels. In concordance with previous pathologic mapping studies, no so-called solitary extra pelvic radioactive lymph nodes (skip lesions) were detected.

Currently, there are two ongoing prospective randomized trials investigating the impact of the extent of lymph node dissection using different templates on oncologic outcome. At present, however, the evidence is based on observational studies such as the two consecutive retrospective interinstitutional template comparisons analysing patient outcome in relation to the extent of lymph node dissection at three high volume cystectomy centres.[27,28] Compared to the limited template, lymph node dissection up to the mid-upper

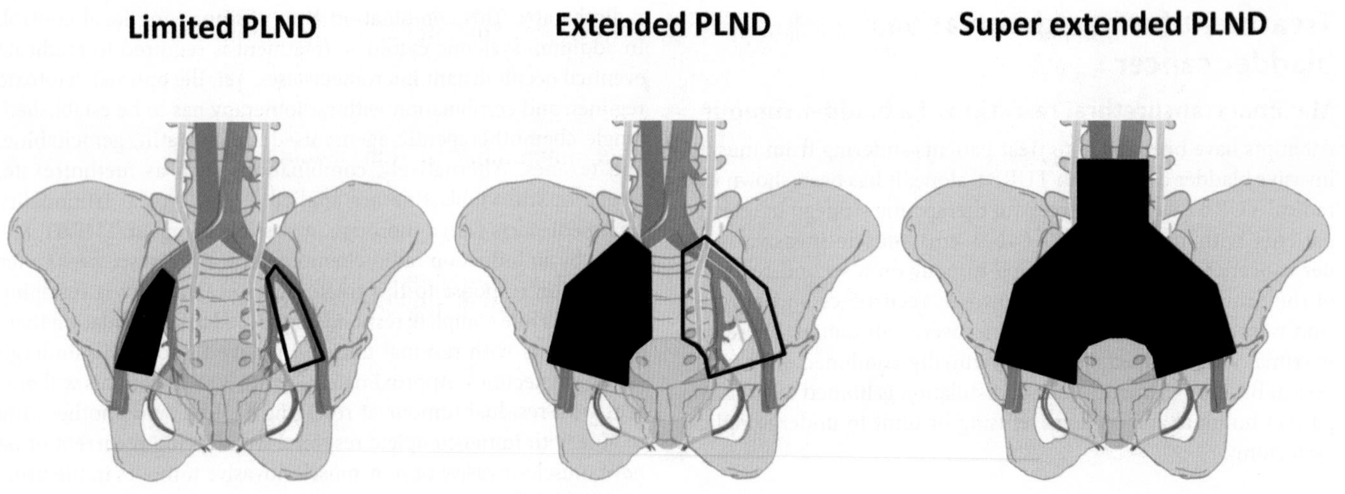

Limited PLND Extended PLND Super extended PLND

Fig. 6.21.4 Illustration of the three applied and debated pelvic lymph node dissection (PLND) templates. According to the currently available evidence, an extended PLND should respect the following boundaries of dissection and be regarded as the standard template: The genitofemoral nerve and the pelvic side wall laterally, the circumflex iliac vein and Cloquet's node distally, the obturator fossa with full exposure of the intrapelvic course of the obturator nerve (Triangle of Marcille) posterolaterally and the internal iliac vessels posteriorly including the tissue medial to these vessels. The template proximally ends at the mid-upper-third of the common iliac vessels.

Reprinted from *The Journal of Urology*, Volume 186, Issue 4, Pascal Zehnder *et al.*, Super Extended Versus Extended Pelvic Lymph Node Dissection in Patients Undergoing Radical Cystectomy for Bladder Cancer: A Comparative Study, pp. 1261–1268, Copyright © 2011 American Urological Association Education and Research, Inc. Published by Elsevier Inc. All rights reserved., with permission from Elsevier, http://www.sciencedirect.com/science/journal/00225347

third of the common iliac vessels removed significantly more positive lymph nodes and finally provided better outcomes. The further comparison with a super-extended template up to the inferior mesenteric artery did not confer an additional outcome benefit but bears the risk of harm to the autonomic nerves that may have a role in sexual and pelvic floor function postoperatively. Therefore, any radical cystectomy should be accompanied by a meticulous extended pelvic lymph node dissection up to the mid-upper third of the common iliac vessels (Fig. 6.21.4). From a practical stand point, performing pelvic lymph node dissection before cystectomy allows to have a better visualization with identification of the relevant structures, hence facilitating the transection of the vascular pedicles.

Male cystectomy

With the patient placed in the supine position including a Trendelenburg tilt, access to the peritoneal cavity is achieved via infraumbilical laparotomy. The urachal remnant/ ligaments are dissected off the umbilicus in such a way that a triangular peritoneal flap can be dissected towards the urinary bladder. Now, the space of Retzius is opened behind the pubic bone. Cranio-laterally, both vas deferens are identified and ligated near the internal inguinal ring. The dorsal peritoneum is bilaterally incised along the external iliac vessels and over the ureters. Cecum and sigmoid colon are detached from the lateral abdominal wall allowing for an increased working space. This is the moment where the extended meticulous pelvic lymph node dissection is performed. Consecutively, the skeletonized dorso-lateral bladder pedicles (superior/inferior vesical vessels and prostatic branches) are divided and ligated. At their entrance into the urinary bladder, the ureters are dissected, divided, and ligated. On both sides, a ureteral segment of 5 mm is sent for frozen section analysis. The peritoneum in the Douglas' space is incised at the level of the seminal vesicles and the virtual space between bladder/seminal vesicles/prostate and rectum is opened mainly by blunt dissection. This exposes the dorsomedial bladder pedicles which are divided step-wise between clamps. The procedure continues ventrally by opening the endopelvic fascia on either side of the prostate and sliding off the levator muscle fibres. With the help of a bent Babcock clamp Santorini's plexus is bunched, ligated, and transected. The prostate is dissected by sharp preparation along its ventral aspect towards the apex. Dissection from the side offers a better exposure of the usually donut-like organ curvature at the apex. Once the ventral urethral wall is transected, the Foley catheter is retracted followed by the transection of the posterior urethral wall distally to the verumontanum. The fused layers of Denovilliers fascia are dissected sharply and thus the entire passage between the rectum and the prostate from the former peritoneal reflection is opened. The remaining dorso-lateral prostatic pedicles are divided and ligated in a retrograde manner and the specimen sent for analysis. Hemostasis is achieved with an additional suture ligation at Santorini's plexus and if required along the remaining neurovascular structures.

Male nerve-sparing

This requires a modification at two stages, if the extent of cancer allows such an approach. First, transection of the dorsomedial pedicles has to be performed close to the posterior bladder wall and immediately on and lateral to the seminal vesicles. Using an Overholt clamp (bent) for this step facilitates direct dissection towards the bladder neck, along and not across the course of the pelvic plexus (Fig. 6.21.5). Electrocautery and other energy sources should be avoided at this stage. Second, following the bilateral opening of the endopelvic fascia, the periprostatic fascia is incised which allows to gently dissect the neurovascular bundles off the entire lateral aspect of the prostate. Importantly, too much exposure of the urethral stump, especially the lateral aspect has to be avoided.

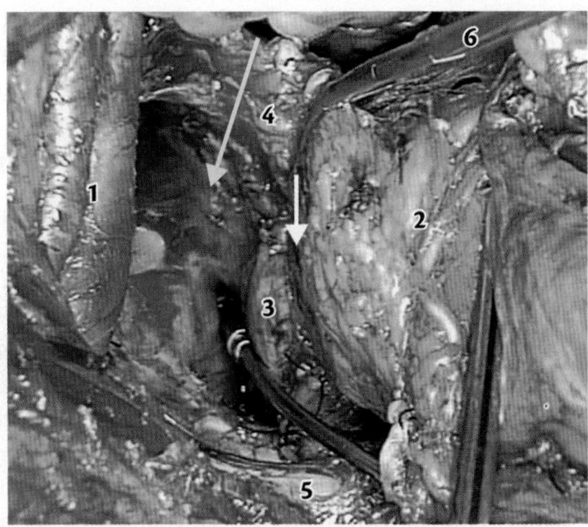

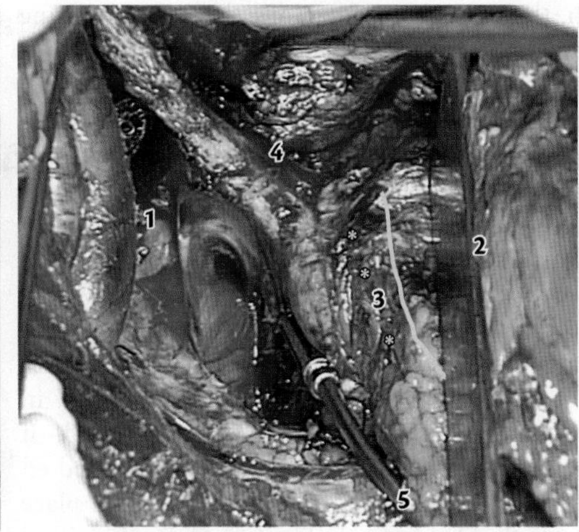

Fig. 6.21.5 Male nerve-sparing. Transection of the right dorsomedial bladder pedicle with the Kelly clamp close to the bladder wall towards the bladder neck (white arrow) instead of straight towards the pelvic floor (yellow arrow) allows for pelvic plexus preservation. Consecutively, the periprostatic fascia is incised allowing to dissect the neurovascular bundles* off the lateral aspect of the prostate (dotted yellow line):

1. Right external iliac vessels
2. Urinary bladder, right side wall
3. Right lateral aspect of the prostate
4. Right pelvic plexus
5. Pubic bone
6. Kelly clamp

Urethrectomy

Urethrectomy is indicated in patients with tumours involving the bladder neck in women or the prostatic urethra in men. In order to avoid a prolonged procedure, it may be safe to defer urethrectomy (e.g. by three months) rather than perform at the same time as cystectomy.[29] This requires the most distal transection of the proximal urethra during radical cystectomy. With the patient in a lithotomy position for the second stage, wide access to the perineum is gained with a U-shaped incision. Importantly, the cutaneous flap is mobilized with the entire subcutaneous tissue to avoid necrosis. Following a midline incision of the bulbocavernous muscle, the corpus spongiosum/urethra is now sharply dissected off the cavernosal bodies. Towards the glans penis, traction on the urethra inverts the penis, allowing urethral mobilization up to the coronal sulcus. The external urethral meatus is circumferentially incised deeply into the glans where the incision meets the previous dissection plane at the level of the coronal sulcus. With the entire penile urethra mobilized, the defect at the glans penis is closed with a few interrupted sutures. Once the bulbar arteries are ligated, the dissection is further deployed towards the symphysis and finally ends with the removal of the proximal urethra. While this approach is through a subscrotal incision, an alternative is through a prepubic approach through the same incision as the cystectomy.[30] This spares morbidity, is easier at the same time as the cystectomy, but has poor access to the urethrorectal junction.

Female cystectomy

The approach and pelvic exposure in females is similar to the previously described procedure in males. Anterior pelvic exenteration, to include the bladder, urethra, ovaries, uterus, fallopian tubes, and anterior vaginal wall, is considered the default procedure. This may be modified in carefully selected (e.g. younger) patients who wish to remain sexually active, to keep their ovaries, or who chose orthotopic bladder reconstruction. Extended pelvic lymph node dissection, division and transection of the dorso-lateral blood supply as well as dissection of both ureters is performed exactly the way it is done in males.

Cystohysterectomy

When the tumour is in the region of the bladder floor or dorsal wall then cysto-hysterectomy is warranted. Using a uterine clamp, gentle traction exposes the peritoneal reflection between the posterior wall of the uterus/vagina and the anterior rectal surface. Following the incision at the peritoneal reflection blunt dissection in the midline displays the vaginal vault. The dorsomedial bladder pedicles are dissected bilaterally to the pararectal region, at least 8 mm away from the bladder wall. With the uterus anteverted, full-thickness transverse incision of the vaginal dome, posterior to the cervix, and consecutive resection of the anterior vaginal wall is performed. Pulling on the Foley catheter back through the open vagina helps to identify the external urethral orifice, which then can be circumferentially excised. Bleeding from the clitoral plexus needs to be anticipated. The vaginal closure is obtained with an inverted running suture where the remaining most cranial posterior vaginal wall is brought to the remaining anterior vaginal wall and each side of the now V-shaped vaginal opening is sutured. Finally, a vascularized peritoneal flap is pulled over the suture line to prevent fistula formation.

Nerve-sparing female cystectomy

In case the bladder tumour is located anteriorly then nerve-sparing (+/− uterus preserving) cystectomy is feasible. To preserve the uterus and eventually the anterior vaginal wall, a transverse peritoneal incision is performed along the anterior surface of the uterus. Herewith, the avascular plane along the ventral uterine surface can be deployed until one identifies the vaginal wall as a white structure. In order to preserve laterally the paravaginal nerve fibres that innervate the urethra, the dissection runs close to the posterior bladder wall along the antero-lateral paravaginal plane, no further dorsal than the 2 or 10 o'clock position. The dorsomedial bladder pedicles are step-wise transected until finally the bladder neck is reached. Ideally, cold-cupping and ligatures are used to prevent potential thermal damage to the neurovascular structures. According to the oncologic principles, the anterior vaginal wall is in general resected during radical female cystectomy. However, it may be preserved partially or completely in patients with strict anterior tumour location. The vaginal wall—if necessary—is incised at the level of the cervix and resected en block with the bladder. Transection of the urethra takes place immediately distal to the bladder neck (Fig. 6.21.6). Further distal urethral mobilization and exposure must be avoided in order not to harm the nerves. The vaginal closure is obtained and a vascularized peritoneal flap pulled over the suture line to prevent fistula formation.

Individualized cystectomy

Nowadays, radical surgery has two goals to achieve: First, complete removal of the urinary bladder with the tumour and with negative surgical margins including the resection of all potential primary lymphatic landing sites; second to preserve as much pelvic functionality as possible in order to maintain postoperative quality of life and body image. This can be summarized as individualized cystectomy. As there is no place for compromise from an oncologic standpoint preoperative planning has to include the evaluation of the possibility of nerve-sparing and the form of urinary diversion as these are closely related and responsible for functional outcome.

Reconstruction—urinary diversions

Over time, urinary diversion has evolved from a simple diversion to protect the upper urinary tract to maximal functional and anatomic restoration with preservation of the patient's body image. Today, orthotopic reconstruction is the preferred choice of diversion at high volume cystectomy centres. Nevertheless, the most frequently performed urinary diversion worldwide remains the ileal conduit, first described in 1950 by Bricker.[31] According to a recent consensus conference our patient counselling on urinary diversion should be based on the following aspects: The safest method for cancer control with the fewest short and long-term complications, providing the easiest adjustment for patient's lifestyle and thereby supporting the best quality of life.[32]

Ileal conduit

Prior to surgery, the localization of the future cutaneous nipple requires careful assessment. Ideally, stoma position is tested in different positions in order to avoid loosening of the stoma plate or disturbance by skin folds. The impact of co-morbidities and manual dexterity needs to be taken into consideration as well. Intraoperatively, approximately 25 cm oral to the ileocecal valve a 15–20 cm long ileal segment is isolated and the proximal end closed with a seromuscular running suture. Usually, the stoma is situated below and to the right of the umbilicus. Therefore, the left ureter is passed over the aorta to the right paracaval area above the offspring

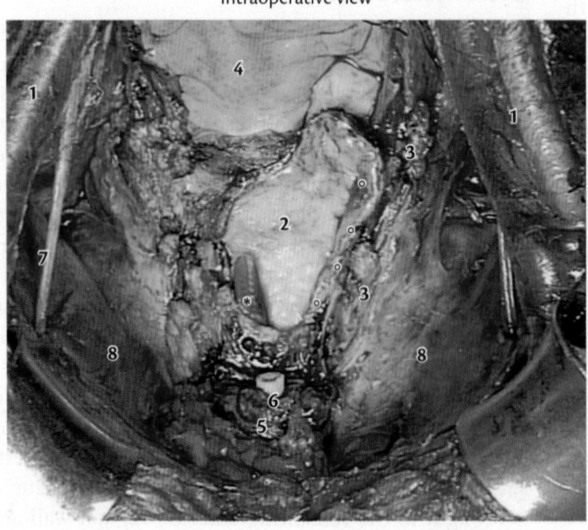

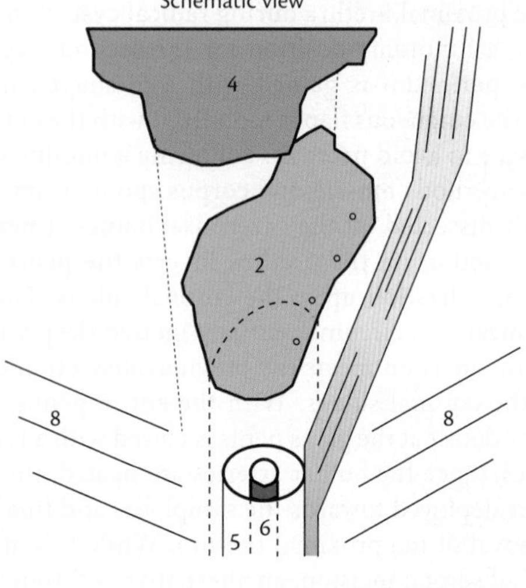

Fig. 6.21.6 Female nerve-sparing. Intraoperative situs following left-sided nerve-sparing. The anterior vaginal wall is resected including the majority of the right lateral vaginal wall and right pelvic plexus:

1. External iliac vessels
2. Posterior vaginal wall with intravaginal dressing forceps*
3. Preserved pelvic plexus right side with a more substantially remaining lateral vaginal wall
4. Anterior rectal wall, covered with peritoneum
5. Urethral stump
6. Transected Foley catheter
7. Right obturator nerve
8. Levator muscle fibres/pelvic floor

of the inferior mesenteric artery in order to avoid a nutcracker phenomenon. Following spatulation over 1.5 cm, both ureters are implanted into the proximal part of the ileal segment applying the Nesbit technique.[33] The anastomoses should be stented with ureteral catheters at least over five days. It is important that the tunnel for the ileum conduit passes through the rectus muscle to avoid herniation and stomal problems. Then the ileal conduit nipple is confected.

Complications

Peristomal skin lesions are common and can be managed with local treatment. Parastomal hernias occur in 10–15% and recurrence following repair is common. Alternatively, the cutaneous nipple can be repositioned to the contra lateral side or mesh material used to reinforce a weak fascia. Regarding the upper urinary tract, one-third of patients have radiographic or functional deterioration at five years increasing to 50% at 15 years.[34] Loss of glomerular filtration rate is mostly due to reflux, obstruction, or chronic infection. Stone development occurs in approximately 10% of patients.[34] Although the ileal conduit diversion is the most commonly performed urinary diversion, the rate of early and late complications is considerable.

Orthotopic bladder substitutes

The most common form of neobladder performed is the ileal reservoir. There exist differing techniques such as the W-shaped reservoir,[35] the Kock pouch,[36] or the ileal reservoir described by Studer using an afferent limb.[37] We describe the construction of an orthotopic bladder substitute according to Studer: approximately 25 cm oral to the ileocecal valve a 54-cm long ileal segment is isolated (Fig. 6.21.7). After restoration of bowel continuity, both ends of the isolated segment are closed with a seromuscular running suture. The distal 40 cm of the ileal segment are opened on the antimesenteric border leaving a 14 cm intact afferent ileal segment. Detubularization is important to decrease muscular contractions of the intestine. Both spatulated ureters are anastomosed to the proximal end of the afferent tubular limb applying the Nesbit technique. Now, the two medial ileal edges of the detubularized U-shaped ileal segment are approximated with a seromuscular running suture (Fig. 6.21.7B). The bottom of the U folded over results in a spherical reservoir (Fig. 6.21.7C). The neobladder is anastomosed at the most caudal part of the reservoir (Fig. 6.21.7D) to the urethral stump using six interrupted stitches. The reservoir is drained with both a Foley and suprapubic catheter and finally completely closed.

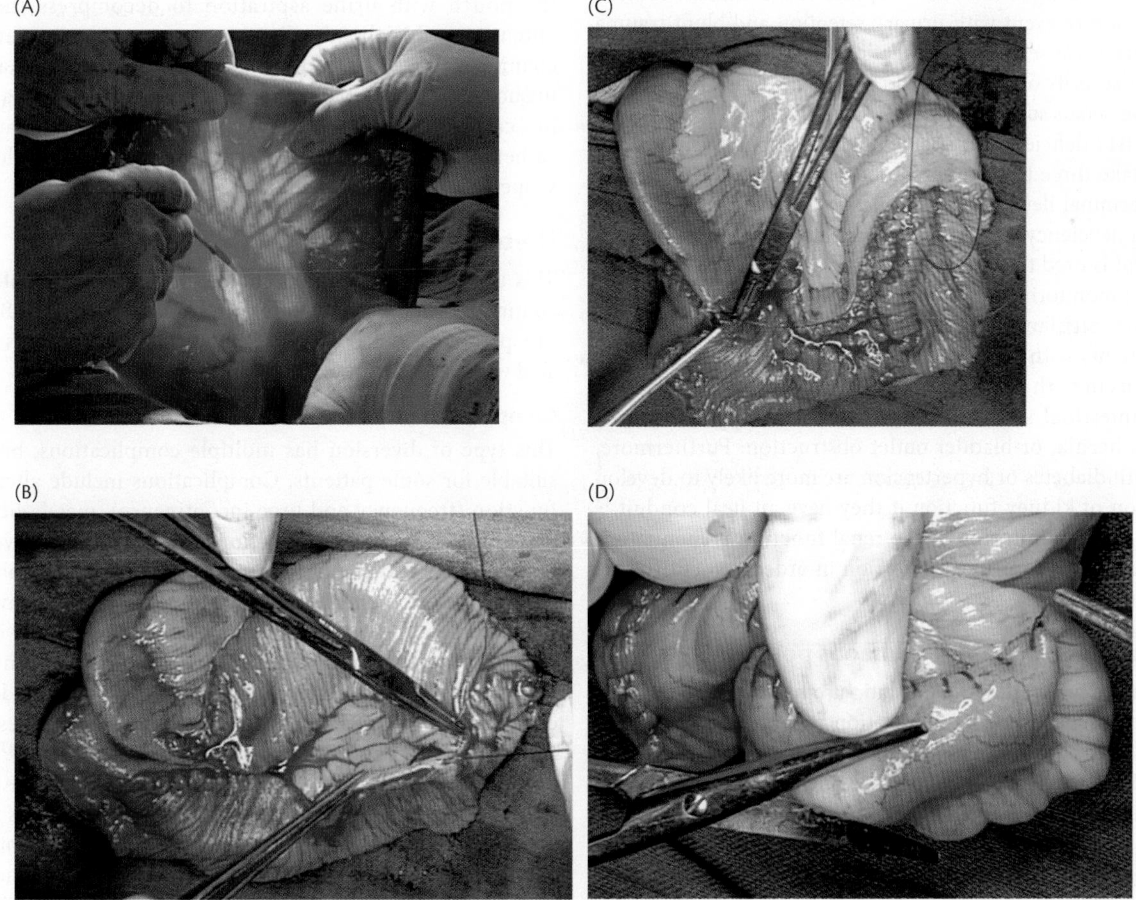

Fig. 6.21.7 Orthotopic bladder substitute. (A) Isolation of a 54 cm ileal segment with the help of the translumination technique; (B) U-shaped folding of the antimesenteric opened ileum. Running suture to close the posterior wall of the reservoir; (C) cross-folding with creation of the spherical reservoir; and (D) creation of the anastomotic opening at the most caudal part and not at the funnel shaped end of the suture line.

Complications

During the first months after Foley removal, patients are at increased risk of metabolic acidosis as the H+ ions in the urine are being reabsorbed by the ileal reservoir. Furthermore, patients lose salt with the urine. Besides the oral substitution with sodium bicarbonate, complete emptying of the bladder substitute is essential and requires regular controls. With high fluid intake and sodium rich alimentation sodium bicarbonate therapy can usually be abandoned with time.[38] Urinary tract infection may occur in the initial postoperative phase and later, but the urine in the bladder substitutes usually becomes sterile in the course. Any proven bacterial growth requires antibiotic treatment because infection negatively impacts both continence status and voiding function.[39] Few patients may even develop urinary retention in the frame of a urinary infection due to increased mucus production. The rate of uretero-intestinal strictures in patients with freely refluxing end-to-side anastomoses (Nesbit) is estimated around 3%. The stricture rate increases to 13.5% if an antirefluxing nipple valve is used.[40] Strictures are predominantly due to ischaemic scarring. Particularly the left ureter, usually left longer because it is passed under the left colonic mesentery to the right paracaval area, is at danger. Chronic infection may also play a role. Endoscopic balloon dilatation and stenting may only be successful in short (≤1.0 cm) strictures with recurrence rates around 50%. Open surgical reimplantation is by far more successful (>86%) and recommended as primarily therapeutic strategy in patients with long strictures.[41] Rupture of a continent urinary diversion is a rare event with urinary retention and blunt trauma being the major causes.[42] Catheterization with pouchogram allows to assess the severity of the defect and guides the decision regarding conservative versus surgical therapy.

Vitamin B12 deficiency in a patient with preoperatively normal levels can take three to five years to become manifest. Preserving 25 cm of terminal ileum before the ileocecal valve may even prevent such a deficiency. Nevertheless, patients in whom an isolated ileal segment is used to confect the urinary diversion need lifelong vitamin B12 monitoring.

Over time, median glomerular filtration rate values decrease in both patients with ileal conduits and bladder substitutes. The main reasons in both cohorts are due to urinary obstruction such as ureterointestinal stricture, stomal stenosis, nipple stricture, parastomal hernia, or bladder outlet obstruction. Furthermore, patients with diabetes or hypertension are more likely to develop deterioration of kidney function if they have an ileal conduit.[43] Therefore, close monitoring of the renal function is mandatory in all patients with an urinary diversion in order to identify correctable causes.

Continent catheterizable cutaneous pouch

Bladder cancer infiltrating the prostatic urethra in males or bladder neck in females is a contraindication for an orthotopic urinary diversion. In addition, patients with previous pelvic irradiation, major pelvic surgery, or severe underlying neurologic disorders are not optimal candidates either. In this case, a continent catheterizable pouch represents an attractive alternative for selected patients.

From a surgical stand point, a bladder substitute analogous to an orthotopic bladder can be used or another form of diversion. Usually, the umbilicus is the site for the catheterizable channel. Alternatively, one of the lower iliac fossae may be considered. Various tissues can be used to create the catheterizable channel.[44] If available, appendix is the preferable choice. Alternatively, a Yang-Monti nipple is constructed with the use of a detubularized 2 cm small bowel segment or even a fallopian tube can be utilized. The nipple/channel is then placed in the trough responsible for continence which is created on the anterior aspect of the pouch.[45] The spatulated tip of the channel is anastomosed to the mucosa according to Nesbit and the catheterizable channel wrapped within the trough by interrupted single stitches. The pouch is tacked to the anterior abdominal wall and the umbilicus incised in a V-shaped manner so that a skin flap is created. This decreases the risk of future cutaneous nipple strictures.

Complications

Channel-related complications such as stomal stenosis, false passage, and incontinence are most frequent.[46] Despite the fact that up to 25% of patients may experience some sort of problems requiring more or less invasive treatment, postoperative patient satisfaction, and quality of life in general is good. However, the majority of patients with stomal stenosis can be treated with incision and dilatation. False passages are mainly treated with temporarily catheter drainage alone. Reasons for channel revisions include recurrent scarring with inability to catheterize or persistent incontinence.

In the rare case a patient with continent catheterizable pouch presents with acute urinary retention in the emergency department treatment consists of ultrasound guided puncture of the pouch with urine aspiration to decompress the system. Oftentimes, this already allows to pass a guidewire through the channel followed by catheter placement. If such an attempt is unsuccessful, the pouch is permanently drained with a suprapubic catheter over a few days. Thereafter, another attempt to catheterize the channel—e.g. with the use of a flexible ureteroscope—can be undertaken.

Ureterosigmoidostomy

This used to be a common choice for younger patients needing continent urinary diversion (e.g. in bladder extrophy, TB bladder). Preoperatively, anal continence and rectal capacity status are evaluated with an enema ('porridge/slurry test').

Complications

This type of diversion has multiple complications, but may be suitable for some patients. Complications include altered bowel function (frequency and urge incontinence), metabolic acidosis, ascending urinary tract infections despite antirefluxive ureteral implantation and tumour formation (around the anastomosis). Acidosis and to some extent ascending infections may be positively influenced by regular rectal evacuation every two to three hours during daytime and once or twice at night. Patients with an ureterosigmoidostomy are at a 500 times higher risk of developing colonic tumours than the normal population. First described in 1929, this specific complication is diagnosed frequently.[47] Tumours occur with a mean lag of 21 years if surgery was before the age of 40. This mean lag substantially decreases to eight years if surgery took place after the age of 40. Interestingly, the risk of tumours persists even in patients converted to ileal conduits shortly after formation of the ureterosigmoidostomy. All patients with ureterosigmoidostomies require digital rectal examination, occult blood stool tests every 6–12 months, as well as regular colonoscopy starting five years postoperatively.

Cutaneous ureterostomy

Due to ureteral/stomal stenosis, this type of urinary diversion is warranted in patients requiring palliative urinary diversion or those with short bowel syndrome. Often, these individuals have a reduced general health status and benefit from the relatively low procedural morbidity of extra peritoneal preparation. Additionally, one regularly has to deal with patients, in whom locally advanced disease has completely deteriorated unilateral kidney function, making the intervention necessary on one side only.

Complications

Cutaneous stomal stenosis occurs in up to 50% of patients.[48] This may be reduced to 5% by using skin flap interposition or even avoided with a permanent postoperative stent placement and consecutive exchanges at six-week intervals.

Systemic chemotherapy

Approximately 25% of patients with clinically no nodal involvement are found postoperatively to harbour lymph node metastases,[49–51] reflecting the poor accuracy of staging tools. Despite radical surgery, the survival of patients with muscle-invasive bladder cancer is around 50% at five years.[52,53] Hence, invasive bladder cancer is often a systemic disease, requiring systemic chemotherapy. Interestingly, oncologic outcomes did not improve over the last three decades despite an increased use of systemic therapies.[54]

Neoadjuvant chemotherapy

Neoadjuvant chemotherapy is better tolerated than adjuvant therapy because patients do not have to recover from surgery. Therefore, it is easier to assess neoadjuvant regimens in randomized trials, for this reason (better compliance). The quality of evidence reflects this, showing a benefit for neoadjuvant chemotherapy that is greater than for adjuvant therapy. With neoadjuvant treatment, success (tumour regression and down staging) can be assessed prior to surgery using CT scans. Some authors advocate changing radical options (to radiotherapy) in the case of good response, although there is little evidence to support this approach. Although neoadjuvant cisplatin-containing combination chemotherapy is recommended by the European Association of Urology (EAU),[55] uptake varies between countries[56] reflecting clinical concerns about delaying radical treatment and healthcare design.

Pooled data from seven platinum-based combination chemotherapy studies demonstrate a significantly improved survival by 5–7%.[57] While classically methotrexate, vinblastine, doxorubicin, and cisplatin (MVAC) combination therapy was used prior to cystectomy, this regimen has been replaced by gemcitabine and cisplatin,[58] due to lower toxicity with comparable downstaging effects.[59] Usually, clinical restaging is performed after two induction courses. Patients with good response will continue with another two chemotherapy cycles. Non-responders or those with partial but insufficient treatment response are evaluated in terms of salvage cystectomy versus switch to a second line chemotherapy.

There have been recent developments in oncology substituting cisplatinum with carboplatin for its lesser side effects. As of now there exist only three phase II randomized studies that show a poorer response with carboplatin.[60,61] In patients with compromised kidney function due to neoplastic ureteric obstruction, the collecting system requires decompression previous to treatment initiation. Endourologic stent placement has to be avoided in order to prevent tumour spillage to the upper urinary tract. Therefore, nephrostomy tubes are preferred.

Adjuvant chemotherapy

Few studies are available regarding the adjuvant setting. A prospective randomized European Organisation for Research and Treatment of Cancer (EORTC) trial even had to be closed due to insufficient patient recruitment. Inherent to all retrospective studies is the substantial underlying patient selection bias. The advantage of an adjuvant strategy is that treatment administration is based on pathological staging, hence decreasing the rate of overtreatment. Furthermore, there is no delay in radical surgery particularly in patients with no or only limited tumour chemosensitivity. In contrast, even in the frame of randomized trials only 48–69% of participants finally receive the planed adjuvant treatment dose[62] (e.g. due to prolonged postoperative rehabilitation and impaired recovery).

Typically, it is the relatively young patient at risk with locally advanced disease and/or nodal involvement with extracapsular extension[63] who finally undergoes adjuvant chemotherapy. Again, gemcitabine and cisplatin combination therapy is the first choice. However, patients with compromised kidney function (<60 mL/min creatinin clearance) and those with inner ear hearing loss will not receive cisplatin. Instead, carboplatin is used which has been shown to be not as effective. Therefore, in patients ineligible for a cisplatin-based regimen the indication for adjuvant postoperative chemotherapy should be balanced against the limited effectivity and side effects. Finally, it remains unresolved whether immediate adjuvant chemotherapy or chemotherapy at the time of disease recurrence are preferable.

Radiotherapy

Neoadjuvant radiotherapy

In the frame of retrospective studies, neoadjuvant radiotherapy has been shown to downstage resectable cT3 tumours without increasing toxicity following radical cystectomy.[64] While results in the older literature even suggest a lower rate of local recurrences following neoadjuvant radiotherapy, this vague benefit clearly has to be balanced against the potential side effects. Of relevance here is the impact of radiotherapy on the neurovascular structures required in the setting of an orthotopic urinary diversion. A randomized clinical trial is ongoing in Germany.

Adjuvant radiotherapy

There exist only sparse and mainly outdated data in terms of adjuvant radiotherapy following radical cystectomy. Considering late gastrointestinal toxicity such as bowel obstruction requiring surgical therapy[17] and the moderate effectivity this approach has been mostly abandoned. The value of targeted radiotherapy in the management of limited positive surgical margins or patients with locally advanced and therefore only incomplete resectable tumours remains to be elucidated.

Follow-up

Patients who undergo radical cystectomy require lifelong follow up (for oncologic and functional reasons), adapted to tumour stage, nodal status, and patient performance. There is debate about the benefits of detection of asymptomatic postoperative recurrence, given that most treatments are aimed at symptom palliation. However, it is clear that further urothelial recurrences in the remaining urinary tract (urethra, upper tracts) occur in 5–10% of cases and can be cured at an early stage. Urethral barbotage cytology for early detection of urethral carcinoma *in situ* and cross sectional imaging studies to detect soft tissue metastases or upper tract disease are the most useful investigations in a follow-up protocol after any urinary diversion but certainly with an ileal orthotopic bladder substitute.[65]

Focusing on the functional aspects of urinary diversion, all patients with any form of urinary diversion require routine follow-up visits irrespective whether they had cancer or not. Continuous follow up with regular control examinations warrant excellent functional outcomes in terms of urinary continence, voiding pattern, upper urinary tract function preservation and metabolic alterations

Prognosis and prognostic factors

Overall, 20–40% of patients diagnosed with bladder cancer initially present with muscle-invasive disease. For those with no evidence of metastases, radical cystectomy with extended pelvic lymph node dissection is the mainstay of therapy. Postoperative tumour stage and nodal status are important predictors of outcome. Node negative patients with postoperative tumour stages pT0, pTa and pT1 have the best outcome with recurrence-free rates at 5 and 10 years of >90%.[66] Recurrence-free rates for patients with pT2 pNany (pN0-pN2) tumours can be expected around 75% and 70% at 5 and 10 years, respectively. The rates drop to 45–50% and 45% at 5 and 10 years respectively for patients with pT3 pNany tumours.[28] Patients with pT4 tumours represent a heterogeneous cohort with recurrence-free rates around 45% and 35% at 5 and 10 years, respectively (Fig. 6.21.8).[50,52,66] Overall, it is the patient with an organ-confined primary tumour and limited nodal involvement[67] following radical surgery that has the best chance for long-term cure. Nevertheless, even patients with intraoperatively grossly node positive disease have a 25% chance of long-term cure following radical surgery including a meticulous pelvic lymph node dissection.[68] Currently, postoperative tumour stage according to the TNM classification, specifically postoperative lymph node status as well as soft tissue margin status represent the factors that predominantly impact patient's outcome after radical cystectomy.[8,69,70] A variety of other factors such as BMI[71] and preoperative hydronephrosis[72,73] were individually reported but data are conflicting. In contrast, based on a meticulous extended pelvic lymph node dissection followed by a thorough pathologic work-up, the prognosis of a cystectomy patient can be determined quite reliably upon the underlying histological findings. Within this context, extracapsular extension of lymph node metastases was found to be an even stronger outcome predictor compared to tumour stage and number/percentage of metastatic nodes.[63] Similarly, lympho-vascular invasion was identified to be strongly associated with clinical outcome in lymph node negative patients.[74] Furthermore, attempts are undertaken to identify individual molecular risk profiles in order to stratify our patients and to guide them to neoadjuvant and/or adjuvant treatments.

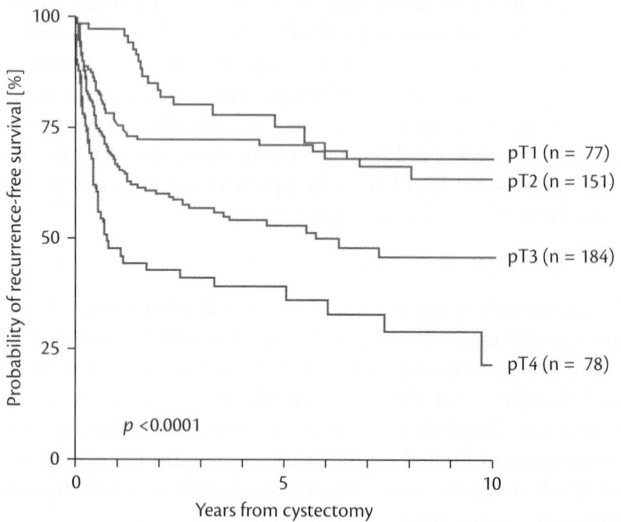

Fig. 6.21.8 Recurrence-free survival stratified according to primary tumour stage, irrespective of nodal status.

Reprinted with permission. Copyright © 2003 American Society of Clinical Oncology. All rights reserved. From Madersbacher S, et al: Radical Cystectomy for Bladder Cancer Today — A Homogeneous Series Without Neoadjuvant Therapy, *Journal of Clinical Oncology*, Volume 21, Issue 4, 2003, pp. 690–696.

Further reading

Bruins HM, Huang GJ, Cai J, Skinner DG, Stein JP, Penson DF. Clinical outcomes and recurrence predictors of lymph node positive urothelial cancer after cystectomy. *J Urol* 2009; **182**(5):2182–7.

Ghoneim MA, el-Mekresh MM, el-Baz MA, el-Attar IA, Ashamallah A. Radical cystectomy for carcinoma of the bladder: critical evaluation of the results in 1,026 cases. *J Urol* 1997; **158**(2):393–9.

Hautmann RE, de Petriconi RC, Pfeiffer C, Volkmer BG. Radical cystectomy for urothelial carcinoma of the bladder without neoadjuvant or adjuvant therapy: long-term results in 1100 patients. *Eur Urol* 2012; **61**(5):1039–47.

Herr HW. Transurethral resection of muscle-invasive bladder cancer: 10-year outcome. *J Clin Oncol* 2001; **19**(1):89–93.

Neoadjuvant chemotherapy in invasive bladder cancer: a systematic review and meta-analysis. *Lancet* 2003; **361**(9373):1927–34.

Roth B, Wissmeyer MP, Zehnder P, *et al.* A new multimodality technique accurately maps the primary lymphatic landing sites of the bladder. *Eur Urol* 2010; **57**(2):205–11.

Stein JP, Lieskovsky G, Cote R, *et al.* Radical cystectomy in the treatment of invasive bladder cancer: long-term results in 1,054 patients. *J Clin Oncol* 2001; **19**(3):666–75.

Stenzl A, Cowan NC, De Santis M, *et al.* Treatment of muscle-invasive and metastatic bladder cancer: update of the EAU guidelines. *European urology* 2011; **59**(6):1009–18.

Studer UE, Varol C, Danuser H. Orthotopic ileal neobladder. *BJU Int* 2004; **93**(1):183–93.

Zehnder P, Studer UE, Skinner EC, *et al.* Super extended versus extended pelvic lymph node dissection in patients undergoing radical cystectomy for bladder cancer: a comparative study. *J Urol* 2011; **186**(4):1261–8.

References

1. Chavan S BF, Lortet-Teulent J, Goodman MM, Jemal A. International variations in bladder cancer incidence and mortality. *Eur Urol* 2014; **66**(1):59–73.
2. Ferlay J, Parkin DM, Steliarova-Foucher E. Estimates of cancer incidence and mortality in Europe in 2008. *Eur J Cancer* 2010; **46**(4):765–81.
3. Cooper N, Cartwright R. Bladder. (pp. 39–50) In: Quinn M, Wood H, Cooper N, Rowan S (eds). *Cancer Atlas of the United Kingdom and Ireland 1991–2000*. London, UK: Office for National Statistics, 2005.

4. Thomas F, Noon AP, Rubin N, Goepel JR, Catto JW. Comparative outcomes of primary, recurrent, and progressive high-risk non-muscle-invasive bladder cancer. *Eur Urol* 2013; **63**(1):145–54.
5. Rogers CG, Palapattu GS, Shariat SF, *et al.* Clinical outcomes following radical cystectomy for primary nontransitional cell carcinoma of the bladder compared to transitional cell carcinoma of the bladder. *J Urol* 2006; **175**(6):2048–53; discussion 53.
6. Edge SB Byrd DR, Compton CC, Fritz AG, Greene FL, Trotti A (eds). *AJCC Cancer Staging Manual*, 7th edition. New York, NY: Springer; 2010.
7. Vargas HA, Akin O, Schoder H, *et al.* Prospective evaluation of MRI, (11)C-acetate PET/CT and contrast-enhanced CT for staging of bladder cancer. *Eur J Radiol* 2012; **81**(12):4131–7.
8. Stein JP, Lieskovsky G, Cote R, *et al.* Radical cystectomy in the treatment of invasive bladder cancer: long-term results in 1,054 patients. *J Clin Oncol* 2001; **19**(3):666–75.
9. El-Assmy A, Abou-El-Ghar ME, Mosbah A, *et al.* Bladder tumour staging: comparison of diffusion- and T2-weighted MR imaging. *Eur Radiol* 2009; **19**(7):1575–81.
10. Birkhauser FD, Studer UE, Froehlich JM, *et al.* Combined ultrasmall superparamagnetic particles of iron oxide-enhanced and diffusion-weighted magnetic resonance imaging facilitates detection of metastases in normal-sized pelvic lymph nodes of patients with bladder and prostate cancer. *Eur Urol* 2013; **64**(6):953–60.
11. Maurer T, Souvatzoglou M, Kubler H, *et al.* Diagnostic efficacy of [11C]choline positron emission tomography/computed tomography compared with conventional computed tomography in lymph node staging of patients with bladder cancer prior to radical cystectomy. *Eur Urol* 2012; **61**(5):1031–8.
12. Herr HW. Transurethral resection of muscle-invasive bladder cancer: 10-year outcome. *J Clin Oncol* 2001; **19**(1):89–93.
13. Sternberg CN, Pansadoro V, Calabro F, *et al.* Can patient selection for bladder preservation be based on response to chemotherapy? *Cancer* 2003; **97**(7):1644–52.
14. Meijer GJ, van der Toorn PP, Bal M, Schuring D, Weterings J, de Wildt M. High precision bladder cancer irradiation by integrating a library planning procedure of 6 prospectively generated SIB IMRT plans with image guidance using lipiodol markers. *Radiother Oncol* 2012; **105**(2):174–9.
15. Koning CC, Blank LE, Koedooder C, *et al.* Brachytherapy after external beam radiotherapy and limited surgery preserves bladders for patients with solitary pT1-pT3 bladder tumors. *Ann Oncol* 2012; **23**(11):2948–53.
16. Piet AH, Hulshof MC, Pieters BR, Pos FJ, de Reijke TM, Koning CC. Clinical results of a concomitant boost radiotherapy technique for muscle-invasive bladder cancer. *Strahlenther Onkol* 2008; **184**(6):313–8.
17. Rodel C, Grabenbauer GG, Kuhn R, *et al.* Combined-modality treatment and selective organ preservation in invasive bladder cancer: long-term results. *J Clin Oncol* 2002; **20**(14):3061–71.
18. James ND, Hussain SA, Hall E, *et al.* Radiotherapy with or without chemotherapy in muscle-invasive bladder cancer. *New Engl J Med* 2012; **366**(16):1477–88.
19. Kotwal S, Choudhury A, Johnston C, Paul AB, Whelan P, Kiltie AE. Similar treatment outcomes for radical cystectomy and radical radiotherapy in invasive bladder cancer treated at a United Kingdom specialist treatment center. *Int J Radiat Oncol Biol Phys* 2008; **70**(2):456–63.
20. Rodel C, Weiss C, Sauer R. Trimodality treatment and selective organ preservation for bladder cancer. *J Clin Oncol* 2006; **24**(35):5536–44.
21. Leadbetter WF, Cooper JF. Regional gland dissection for carcinoma of the bladder; a technique for one-stage cystectomy, gland dissection, and bilateral uretero-enterostomy. *J Urol* 1950; **63**(2):242–60.
22. Marshall VF, Whitmore WF Jr. The present position of radical cystectomy in the surgical management of carcinoma of the urinary bladder. *J Urol* 1956; **76**(4):387–91.
23. Quek ML, Stein JP, Daneshmand S, *et al.* A critical analysis of perioperative mortality from radical cystectomy. *J Urol* 2006; **175**(3 Pt 1):886–9; discussion 9–90.
24. Snow-Lisy DC, Campbell SC, Gill IS, *et al.* Robotic and laparoscopic radical cystectomy for bladder cancer: long-term oncologic outcomes. *Eur Urol* 2014; **65**(1):193–200.
25. Azzouni FS, Din R, Rehman S, *et al.* The first 100 consecutive, robot-assisted, intracorporeal ileal conduits: evolution of technique and 90-day outcomes. *Eur Urol* 2013; **63**(4):637–43.
26. Roth B, Wissmeyer MP, Zehnder P, *et al.* A new multimodality technique accurately maps the primary lymphatic landing sites of the bladder. *Eur Urol* 2010; **57**(2):205–11.
27. Dhar NB, Klein EA, Reuther AM, Thalmann GN, Madersbacher S, Studer UE. Outcome after radical cystectomy with limited or extended pelvic lymph node dissection. J Urol 2008; **179**(3):873–8; discussion 8.
28. Zehnder P, Studer UE, Skinner EC, *et al.* Super extended versus extended pelvic lymph node dissection in patients undergoing radical cystectomy for bladder cancer: a comparative study. *J Urol* 2011; **186**(4):1261–8.
29. Boorjian SA, Kim SP, Weight CJ, Cheville JC, Thapa P, Frank I. Risk factors and outcomes of urethral recurrence following radical cystectomy. *Eur Urol* 2011; **60**(6):1266–72.
30. Joniau S, Shabana W, Verlinde B, Van Poppel H. Prepubic urethrectomy during radical cystoprostatectomy. *Eur Urol* 2007; **51**(4):915–21.
31. Bricker EM. Bladder substitution after pelvic evisceration. *Surg Clin North Am* 1950; **30**(5):1511–21.
32. Hautmann RE, Abol-Enein H, Hafez K, *et al.* Urinary diversion. *Urology* 2007; **69**(1 Suppl):17–49.
33. Nesbit RM. Ureterosigmoid anastomosis by direct elliptical connection; a preliminary report. *J Urol* 1949; **61**(4):728–34.
34. Madersbacher S, Schmidt J, Eberle JM, *et al.* Long-term outcome of ileal conduit diversion. *J Urol* 2003; **169**(3):985–90.
35. Hautmann RE. Surgery illustrated—surgical atlas ileal neobladder. *BJU Int* 2010; **105**(7):1024–35.
36. Skinner DG, Boyd SD, Lieskovsky G, Bennett C, Hopwood B. Lower urinary tract reconstruction following cystectomy: experience and results in 126 patients using the Kock ileal reservoir with bilateral ureteroileal urethrostomy. *J Urol* 1991; **146**(3):756–60.
37. Studer UE, Varol C, Danuser H. Orthotopic ileal neobladder. *BJU Int* 2004; **93**(1):183–93.
38. Varol C, Studer UE. Managing patients after an ileal orthotopic bladder substitution. *BJU Int* 2004; **93**(3):266–70.
39. Zehnder P, Dhar N, Thurairaja R, Ochsner K, Studer UE. Effect of urinary tract infection on reservoir function in patients with ileal bladder substitute. *J Urol* 2009; **181**(6):2545–9.
40. Studer UE, Danuser H, Thalmann GN, Springer JP, Turner WH. Antireflux nipples or afferent tubular segments in 70 patients with ileal low pressure bladder substitutes: long-term results of a prospective randomized trial. *J Urol* 1996; **156**(6):1913–7.
41. Schondorf D, Meierhans-Ruf S, Kiss B, *et al.* Ureteroileal strictures after urinary diversion with an ileal segment—is there a place for endourological treatment at all? *J Urol* 2013; **190**(2):585–90.
42. Nippgen JB, Hakenberg OW, Manseck A, Wirth MP. Spontaneous late rupture of orthotopic detubularized ileal neobladders: report of five cases. *Urology* 2001; **58**(1):43–6.
43. Jin XD, Roethlisberger S, Burkhard FC, Birkhaeuser F, Thoeny HC, Studer UE. Long-term renal function after urinary diversion by ileal conduit or orthotopic ileal bladder substitution. *Eur Urol* 2012; **61**(3):491–7.
44. Castellan MA, Gosalbez R, Labbie A, Ibrahim E, Disandro M. Outcomes of continent catheterizable stomas for urinary and fecal incontinence: comparison among different tissue options. *BJU Int* 2005; **95**(7):1053–7.
45. Baradaran N, Stec AA, Gupta A, Keating MA, Gearhart JP. Using a serosal trough for fashioning a continent catheterizable stoma: technique and outcomes. *BJU Int* 2012; **111**(5):828–33.

46. Thomas JC, Dietrich MS, Trusler L, *et al.* Continent catheterizable channels and the timing of their complications. *J Urol* 2006; **176**(4 Pt 2):1816–20; discussion 20.
47. Leadbetter GW Jr, Zickerman P, Pierce E. Ureterosigmoidostomy and carcinoma of the colon. *J Urol* 1979; **121**(6):732–5.
48. MacGregor PS, Montie JE, Straffon RA. Cutaneous ureterostomy as palliative diversion in adults with malignancy. *Urology* 1987; **30**(1):31–4.
49. Vazina A, Dugi D, Shariat SF, Evans J, Link R, Lerner SP. Stage specific lymph node metastasis mapping in radical cystectomy specimens. *J Urol* 2004; **171**(5):1830–4.
50. Madersbacher S, Hochreiter W, Burkhard F, *et al.* Radical cystectomy for bladder cancer today—a homogeneous series without neoadjuvant therapy. *J Clin Oncol* 2003; **21**(4):690–6.
51. Herr HW, Bochner BH, Dalbagni G, Donat SM, Reuter VE, Bajorin DF. Impact of the number of lymph nodes retrieved on outcome in patients with muscle invasive bladder cancer. *J Urol* 2002;**167**(3):1295–8.
52. Stein JP, Skinner DG. Radical cystectomy for invasive bladder cancer: long-term results of a standard procedure. *World J Urol* 2006; **24**(3):296–304.
53. Ghoneim MA, el-Mekresh MM, el-Baz MA, el-Attar IA, Ashamallah A. Radical cystectomy for carcinoma of the bladder: critical evaluation of the results in 1,026 cases. *J Urol* 1997; **158**(2):393–9.
54. Zehnder P, Studer UE, Skinner EC, *et al.* Unaltered oncological outcomes of radical cystectomy with extended lymphadenectomy over three decades. *BJU Int* 2013; **112**(2):E51–8.
55. Stenzl A, Cowan NC, De Santis M, *et al.* Treatment of muscle-invasive and metastatic bladder cancer: update of the EAU guidelines. European urology. 2011; **59**(6):1009–18.
56. Fedeli U, Fedewa SA, Ward EM. Treatment of muscle invasive bladder cancer: evidence from the National Cancer Database, 2003 to 2007. *J Urol* 2011; **185**(1):72–8.
57. Neoadjuvant chemotherapy in invasive bladder cancer: a systematic review and meta-analysis. *Lancet* 2003; **361**(9373):1927–34.
58. Pal SK, Ruel NH, Wilson TG, Yuh BE. Retrospective analysis of clinical outcomes with neoadjuvant Cisplatin-based regimens for muscle-invasive bladder cancer. Clin genitourinary cancer. 2012; **10**(4):246–50.
59. Roberts JT, von der Maase H, Sengelov L, *et al.* Long-term survival results of a randomized trial comparing gemcitabine/cisplatin and methotrexate/vinblastine/doxorubicin/cisplatin in patients with locally advanced and metastatic bladder cancer. *Ann Oncol* 2006; **17**(Suppl 5):v118–22.
60. Dogliotti L, Carteni G, Siena S, *et al.* Gemcitabine plus cisplatin versus gemcitabine plus carboplatin as first-line chemotherapy in advanced transitional cell carcinoma of the urothelium: results of a randomized phase 2 trial. *Eur Urol* 2007; **52**(1):134–41.
61. Rexer H. [First line therapy for local advanced or metastasized urothelial carcinoma: randomized double-blind phase II study to compare gemcitabin and cisplatin in combination with OGX-427 or placebo for advanced transitional cell carcinoma of the bladder (OGX-427—AB 39/11 of the Working Group Urological Oncology)]. *Der Urologe Ausg A* 2011; **50**(12):1617–8.
62. Studer UE, Bacchi M, Biedermann C, *et al.* Adjuvant cisplatin chemotherapy following cystectomy for bladder cancer: results of a prospective randomized trial. *J Urol* 1994; **152**(1):81–4.
63. Fleischmann A, Thalmann GN, Markwalder R, Studer UE. Extracapsular extension of pelvic lymph node metastases from urothelial carcinoma of the bladder is an independent prognostic factor. *J Clin Oncol* 2005; **23**(10):2358–65.
64. Cole CJ, Pollack A, Zagars GK, Dinney CP, Swanson DA, von Eschenbach AC. Local control of muscle-invasive bladder cancer: preoperative radiotherapy and cystectomy versus cystectomy alone. *Int J Radiat Oncol Biol Phys* 1995; **32**(2):331–40.
65. Giannarini G, Kessler TM, Thoeny HC, Nguyen DP, Meissner C, Studer UE. Do patients benefit from routine follow-up to detect recurrences after radical cystectomy and ileal orthotopic bladder substitution? *Eur Urol* 2010; **58**(4):486–94.
66. Hautmann RE, de Petriconi RC, Pfeiffer C, Volkmer BG. Radical cystectomy for urothelial carcinoma of the bladder without neoadjuvant or adjuvant therapy: long-term results in 1100 patients. *Eur Urol* 2012; **61**(5):1039–47.
67. Bruins HM, Huang GJ, Cai J, Skinner DG, Stein JP, Penson DF. Clinical outcomes and recurrence predictors of lymph node positive urothelial cancer after cystectomy. *J Urol* 2009; **182**(5):2182–7.
68. Herr HW, Donat SM. Outcome of patients with grossly node positive bladder cancer after pelvic lymph node dissection and radical cystectomy. *J Urol* 2001; **165**(1):62–4; discussion 4.
69. Ghoneim MA, Abdel-Latif M, el-Mekresh M, *et al.* Radical cystectomy for carcinoma of the bladder: 2,720 consecutive cases 5 years later. *J Urol* 2008; **180**(1):121–7.
70. Rink M, Hansen J, Cha EK, *et al.* Outcomes and prognostic factors in patients with a single lymph node metastasis at time of radical cystectomy. *BJU Int* 2012; **111**(1):74–84.
71. Hafron J, Mitra N, Dalbagni G, Bochner B, Herr H, Donat SM. Does body mass index affect survival of patients undergoing radical or partial cystectomy for bladder cancer? *J Urol* 2005; **173**(5):1513–7.
72. Hofner T, Haferkamp A, Knapp L, *et al.* Preoperative hydronephrosis predicts advanced bladder cancer but is not an independent factor for cancer-specific survival after radical cystectomy. *Urol Int* 2011; **86**(1):25–30.
73. Stimson CJ, Cookson MS, Barocas DA, *et al.* Preoperative hydronephrosis predicts extravesical and node positive disease in patients undergoing cystectomy for bladder cancer. *J Urol* 2010; **183**(5):1732–7.
74. Shariat SF, Svatek RS, Tilki D, *et al.* International validation of the prognostic value of lymphovascular invasion in patients treated with radical cystectomy. *BJU Int* 2010; **105**(10):1402–12.

CHAPTER 6.22

Treatment of metastatic bladder cancer

Fabio Calabrò and Cora N. Sternberg

Introduction to treatment of metastatic bladder cancer

Urothelial bladder carcinoma is the fifth most common malignancy diagnosed in the United States with an estimated 73,510 new cases and 14,880 deaths in 2012.[1] In males, the global incidence is 297,300 per year with 112,300 deaths[2] and 5% have metastatic disease at presentation.[3] Despite adequate local control, most patients ultimately die due to distant disease. Systemic chemotherapy remains the standard of care for patients with metastatic urothelial carcinoma of the bladder. On the basis of the relatively high response rate obtained with combination chemotherapy, urothelial cancer can be considered a relatively chemosensitive disease. Nevertheless, long-term survival remains low and chemotherapy may provide the potential for cure in only selected patients. Despite partial understanding of the molecular aberrations driving urothelial carcinoma, this knowledge has yet to be translated into clinical success with targeted therapies.

Prognostic factors

Various prognostic features and factors predictive of response to chemotherapy have been identified. These can be divided into those reflecting the biology of the tumour and those reflecting the fitness of the patient. With the M-VAC (methotrexate, vinblastine, adriamycin, cisplatin) chemotherapy regimen[4] factors predicting lower response rates, increased toxicity and poor overall survival are: (i) the presence of visceral metastases; (ii) abnormal concentrations of serum alkaline phosphatase; and (iii) poor patient performance status.[5–7] Performance status is a strong predictive factor for survival in most malignancies. Various authors have reported survival stratified by these factors; the intergroup study found median survival varied from 4.4 to 18.2 months in patients treated with M-VAC depending upon the combination of these prognostic factors.[5] None of the patients with liver or bone metastases were alive at six years.[7] Physicians from Memorial Sloan Kettering Cancer Center (MSKCC) stratified 203 patients treated with M-VAC using Karnofsky performance status and the presence or absence of visceral metastases.[8] For patients with none, one, or two of these adverse features, the five-year survival rates were 33%, 11%, or 0% respectively. Similar results were obtained by the Spanish Oncology Genitourinary Group (SOGUG), in a phase I/II study of 56 patients with advanced urothelial tumours treated with paclitaxel, cisplatin, and gemcitabine. Factors associated with a poorer survival were performance status >0, presence of visceral metastasis, and more than one site of malignant disease. In a multivariate model, performance status ($p = 0.044$) and visceral disease ($p = 0.008$) were independent predictors for survival. Median survival times in patients with zero, one, or two of these risk factors were 32.8 months, 17 months, and 9.6 months, respectively.[9]

The proportion of patients in each prognostic group can help to put phase II trial results into perspective, can help compare results between studies and can be used to prospectively stratify patients in phase III trials.

Systemic chemotherapy

First-line chemotherapy in fit patients

Systemic chemotherapy remains the mainstay of treatment for fit patients with metastatic bladder carconoma. Multiagent cisplatin-based regimens, such as M-VAC, yield pathological complete remissions in some patients with metastatic disease and long-term survival in more than 60–70% of complete responders.[10] Patients with measurable lesions have an overall 72% response rate (RR) and 36% attain a complete response. Patients who achieved a complete response, with M-VAC and surgery, have twice the survival of patient's with only a partial response. Chemotherapy is more effective for nodal disease than in visceral metastases.[10,11] On the basis of these results, M-VAC is considered a standard of care in the treatment of metastatic bladder cancer (reproducible response rates in the range of 40–70% and median survival of approximately one year). In particular, prospective randomized trials have demonstrated the superiority of M-VAC (both in terms of response rate and survival) over cisplatin monotherapy[5,7] and CISCA (cisplatin, cyclofosfamide, adriamycin) combination therapy.[11] Of note, in one trial only 3.7% of the patients randomized to M-VAC were alive and continuously disease-free at six years, indicating cure in only a small fraction of patients.[7] However, M-VAC can be associated with significant toxicity; including myelosuppression, neutropenic fever, sepsis, mucositis, nausea, vomiting and a 3–4% toxic death rate[5,10] when growth factors are not used. The ideal candidate for M-VAC is a healthy patient with nodal and/or soft tissue disease. These patients have a 10% to 15% chance of prolonged progression-free survival with six cycles of chemotherapy. With the use of G-CSF (granulocyte-colony stimulating factor), toxic complications can be dramatically reduced and full M-VAC doses administered.

Various attempts have been made to improve response rates or reduce toxicity. Several phase II trials have evaluated dose-intense M-VAC with either GM-CSF (granulocyte macrophage-colony stimulating factor) or G-CSF. These trials report the possibility of increasing doses (by as much as 60%[12]), but with greater toxicity.[13–15] The EORTC 30924 phase III trial compared standard M-VAC to dose-intensified high dose M-VAC (with growth factor support: HD-M-VAC) in 263 patients. Patients receiving HD-M-VAC had significantly higher complete response rates (21% vs. 9%; p = 0.007), borderline higher progression-free survival rates (PFS; 9.1 vs. 8.2 months) but no difference in overall survival (OS). Importantly, there was less leukopenia, neutropenic fever, and mucositis with HD-M-VAC.[16] At seven-year follow-up, HD-M-VAC was associated with fewer cases of progression and death [Hazard Ratio (HR) = 0.73; p = 0.017].[17] Thus, a subset of fit patients could benefit from the intensified regimen.

Gemcitabine has been evaluated in a number of phase I/II trials.[18] Overall response (OR) rates range from 23–29% and CR rates from 4–13% in previously treated and untreated patients.[19–22] Toxicity, particularly myelosuppression, is mild and generally without grade 4 toxicities, as compared to M-VAC. Four phase II trials evaluated the combination of cisplatin and gemcitabine (GC) at different dosages and schedules. In patients with locally advanced and/or metastatic bladder cancer, the OR rates ranged from 41–57% with CR rates from 18–22%.[23–26] Toxicity was acceptable and median survival rates between 12.5 and 13.5 months. These preliminary results led to a large randomized trial of GC versus M-VAC,[27] powered to detect a four-month survival difference in favour of GC. A total of 405 patients were enrolled and overall survival found to be similar in both arms (HR = 1.04; 95% confidence interval, 0.82 to 1.32; p = 0.75). When first published, at a median follow-up of 19 months, overall survival in the GC group was 13.8 months similar to 14.8 months in the M-VAC group. of importance, this trial was not designed to detect equivalency (for this many more patients would have been needed). The toxicity profile was different in the two arms. Patients receiving GC had lower rates of grade 3–4 neutropenia (72% vs. 84%), neutropenic fever (2% vs. 14%) and grade 3–4 mucositis (1% vs. 22%), when compared to M-VAC. While there was a lower rate of thrombocytopenia and anaemia in the M-VAC arm, the toxic death rate was 3% with M-VAC and 1% with GC. The quality of life profile was similar for both arms. There was a non-significant trend to less fatigue with GC.

In a recent update,[28] overall survival was similar in both arms (HR = 1.09; 95% CI, 0.88 to 1.34; p = 0.66) with a median survival of 14.0 months for GC and 15.2 months for M-VAC. The five-year overall survival rates were 13.0% and 15.3%, respectively (p = 0.53). The median PFS was 7.7 months for GC and 8.3 months for M-VAC (HR = 1.09). The five-year PFS rates were 9.8% and 11.3%, respectively (p = 0.63). Significant prognostic factors favouring overall survival included performance score (>70), low/normal alkaline phosphatase level, number of disease sites (<or = three), and the absence of visceral metastases. By adjusting for these prognostic factors, the HR was 0.99 for overall survival and 1.01 for PFS. The five-year overall survival rates for patients with and without visceral metastases were 6.8% and 20.9%, respectively. On the basis of this conceived more favourable risk-benefit ratio, many have considered the GC regimen as a standard treatment in metastatic urothelial cancer. However, it is also possible that much of the toxicity in the M-VAC group could have been avoided with the prophylactic use of G-CSF, which was not administered in the M-VAC arm in this trial.

Attempts to improve upon GC have included adding a third drug. The combination of paclitaxel, gemcitabine, and cisplatin (PGC) has been studied in a phase I/II trial of 61 patients with advanced or metastatic urothelial carcinoma. Sixteen complete responders (27.6%) and 29 partial responders (50%) were observed (OR rate of 77.6% (95% CI: 60–98%). The median survival time available for the phase I part of the study was 24.0 months.[29] Subsequently, the EORTC 30987/Intergroup study randomized 627 patients to either PGC or GC, with the primary end point being survival. At a median follow-up of 4.6 years, the median OS was 15.8 months with PCG versus 12.7 months with GC (p = 0.075). OS in the subgroup of all eligible patients was somewhat longer on PCG, as was the case in patients with bladder primary tumours. The addition of paclitaxel to GC provided a 3.1-month survival benefit that did not reach statistical significance. PFS was not significantly longer on PCG (p = 0.11). Overall response rate was 55.5% on PCG and 43.6% on GC (p = 0.0031). Both treatments were well tolerated, with more thrombocytopenia and bleeding on GC than PCG (11.4% vs. 6.8%) and more febrile neutropenia on PCG than GC (13.2% vs. 4.3%).[30] The trial raised an issue of clinical importance. In a post hoc analysis, there was evidence of a greater and statistically significant survival benefit in patients with a bladder primary (median survival 15.9 months for PCG vs. 11.9 months for GC) in contrast to patients with non-bladder primary tumours, in whom there was no benefit. These results appear to confirm that despite morphologic similarities, there are genetic and epigenetic differences which separate urothelial carcinoma in the upper and lower urinary tracts.

Other regimens have been investigated in the first-line metastatic setting. A phase III randomized trial compared docetaxel and cisplatin (DC) with M-VAC and was reported by the Hellenic Cooperative Oncology Group.[31] Patients were randomly assigned to receive M-VAC (n = 109 patients) or DC (n = 111) (both treatment arms received G-CSF). The overall response rate (54.2% vs. 37.4%; p = 0.017), median time to progression (TTP; 9.4 vs. 6.1 months; p = 0.003) and median survival (14.2 vs. 9.3 months; p = 0.026) favoured the M-VAC regimen. After adjusting for prognostic factors, difference in TTP remained significant (HR = 1.61; p = 0.005), whereas the survival difference was non-significant at the 5% level (HR = 1.31; p = 0.089). M-VAC caused more frequent grade 3 or 4 neutropenia (35.4% vs. 19.2%; p = 0.006), thrombocytopenia (5.7% vs. 0.9%; p = 0.046), and neutropenic sepsis (11.6% vs. 3.8%; p = 0.001) but the toxicity with M-VAC was considerably lower than that previously reported for M-VAC administered without G-CSF. The authors concluded that M-VAC is more effective than DC in advanced urothelial cancer and that G-CSF-supported M-VAC is well tolerated and could be used instead of classic M-VAC as first-line treatment in advanced urothelial carcinoma. Of note, there was no prospective stratification for performance status in this trial and when analysed there was a higher proportion of patients with poor performance status in the DC arm (which may have partly contributed to the poor outcomes in this arm).

A randomized study of 130 patients compared a dose dense regimen with gemcitabine and cisplatin (DD-GC) with dose dense M-VAC (DD-M-VAC) in advanced urothelial cancer.[32] The median OS and PFS were 19 and 8.5 months for DD-M-VAC versus 18 and 7.8 months for DD-GC ($p = 0.98$ and 0.36, respectively). Neutropenic infections were less frequent for DD-GC than for DD-M-VAC (0% vs. 8%). More patients on DD-GC received at least six cycles of treatment (85% versus 63%, $p = 0.011$) and the discontinuation rate was lower for DD-GC (3% vs. 13%).[32]

Carboplatin-based regimens in fit patients

Several studies have compared carboplatin and cisplatin-containing regimens in patients with adequate renal function.[33–36] The former is less toxic than cisplatin. In general, these trials have demonstrated the superiority of cisplatin-based over carboplatin-based combinations. For example, phase II trials evaluated the combination of paclitaxel (dose between 150–225 mg/m^2) with carboplatin (administered at an area under the curve (AUC) of 5–6) and reported overall response rates of 14–65%, with CRs in 0–40%.[37–41] This regimen was well tolerated with mild haematologic and neurologic toxicities. A phase III trial conducted by the Eastern Cooperative Oncology Group (ECOG) compared M-VAC to paclitaxel-carboplatin.[35] Patients with previously untreated metastatic bladder carconoma were randomized to standard M-VAC or paclitaxel 225 mg/m^2 plus carboplatin AUC 6 every three weeks. After 2.5 years the study was closed due to poor accrual (only 85 of the planned 330 patients enrolled). Compared with carboplatin-paclitaxel, patients treated with M-VAC had more myelosuppression, mucositis, and renal toxicity. Interestingly a quality of life evaluation revealed non-significant differences between the two arms. Patients treated with carboplatin had an overall response rate of 28.2% compared to 35.9% for the M-VAC arm. At reporting (median follow-up of 32.5 months), the median survival for patients treated with M-VAC was 15.4 months versus 13.8 months for patients treated with carboplatin-paclitaxel ($p = 0.65$, log-rank test). These results are not significantly different. Due to the low number of patients enrolled definitive conclusions cannot be drawn.

A meta-analysis of 286 cisplatin-eligible patients from three randomized phase II studies and one randomized phase III study comparing cisplatin versus carboplatin-based regimens, in patients with metastatic urothelial carcinoma of the bladder, showed that cisplatin-based chemotherapy was associated with a significantly higher likelihood of achieving a complete response (risk ratio = 3.54; 95% CI = 1.48–8.49; $p = 0.005$) and overall response rate (risk ratio = 1.34; 95% CI = 1.04–1.71; $p = 0.02$). Survival end points could not be adequately assessed due to inconsistent reporting among trials.[42]

Based on this evidence, cisplatin remains the standard of care in fit patients with good performance status and adequate renal function.

Sequential regimens

Administration of non-cross-resistant agents in a sequential fashion may improve outcome by targeting tumour cells with different sensitivity profiles. Based on the effectiveness of this strategy in breast cancer, this option has been studied in metastatic bladder cancer. On the basis of the established activity of doxorubicin and gemcitabine (AG) as single agents, a phase I trial of sequential chemotherapy with these two drugs followed by ifosfamide, paclitaxel, and cisplatin (ITP), was conducted at MSKCC. After completion of a phase I trial,[43] a dose of doxorubucin 50 mg/m^2 and gemcitabine 2,000 mg/m^2 (at an infusion rate of 10 mg/m^2/min) every two weeks for six cycles with G-CSF was chosen. This was then followed by ITP in a phase II study. In a preliminary report of the phase II trial,[44] this sequenced therapy was associated with an 87% RR rate with a 43% CR rate in patients who completed the ITP portion of the study. The dose intensity (mg/m^2/week) for doxorubicin and cisplatin were significantly higher than that obtained with conventional M-VAC. In the final results of this study, myelosuppression was seen as 68% of patients who experienced grade 3 to 4 neutropenia and 25% had febrile neutropenia. The median PFS was 12.1 months (95% CI, 9.0 to 14.8 months), and median overall survival was 16.4 months (95% CI, 14.0 to 22.5 months). The authors concluded that this sequential regimen was associated with significant toxicity and that did not clearly offer a benefit compared to nonsequential, cisplatin-based regimens.[45] A similar regimen consisting of sequential adriamycin and gemcitabine followed by paclitaxel plus carboplatin has been explored in patients with impaired renal function.[46] Myelosuppression was the major toxicity reported in the 25 patients treated, with 28% of patients experiencing grade 3–4 neutropenia with only 2 (8%) episodes of febrile neutropenia. There were five complete responses and nine partial responses for an overall response rate of 56% (95% CI: 35–76%). The median survival was 15 months (95% CI: 11–30).

Docetaxel and methotrexate (DM) followed by gemcitabine and cisplatin (GC) has also been evaluated.[47] Patients received three cycles of DM (40 mg/m^2 methotrexate on days 1 and 8 and 100 mg/m^2 docetaxel on day 8 repeated every 21 days) followed by GC (1,000 mg/m^2 gemcitabine on days 1 and 8 and 75 mg/m^2 cisplatin on day 1 repeated every 21 days). The most common toxicities were haematologic, with grade 3/4 neutropenia and thrombocytopenia observed in 4 and 2 patients, respectively. A 33% response rate was observed after DM and a 67% response rate after GC for an overall response rate of 54%. Three patients who progressed on DM responded to GC and three responders to DM achieved a further response to GC. Median overall survival was 13.6 months.

Although sequential drug regimens cannot be recommended as standard treatment in patients with metastatic urothelial carcinoma, the provocative results in terms of median survival suggest that testing of novel agents in sequence is a feasible treatment strategy.

Platinum-free regimens in fit patients

In an additional effort to avoid cisplatin related toxicities, trials have been conducted using platinum-free combinations. After a phase I dose escalating trial of gemcitabine and paclitaxel in several solid tumours demonstrated these two drugs could be given simultaneously on an every two-week schedule,[48] a phase II trial in patients with urothelial cancer (who had failed prior cisplatin-based chemotherapy) was undertaken.[49] Forty-one patients were treated with an outpatient regimen of gemcitabine 2,500–3,000 mg/m^2 and paclitaxel 150 mg/m^2 every two weeks. The OR rate was 60% with a 28% CR rate. Median survival in these pretreated patients was 14.4 months. Median duration of response was six months (range 2–44+ months). There was no grade 3–4 anaemia or thrombocytopenia. Patients who had been treated with this combination after failing prior adjuvant or neoadjuvant cisplatin-based chemotherapy responded better than patients who had been previously treated for metastatic disease. This regimen every two weeks was found to be a well-tolerated outpatient regimen with minimal toxicity. In another study, 30 patients with progressive disease were treated with either six cycles of three-weekly gemcitabine (1,250 mg/m^2 day 1 and 8) and paclitaxel (175 mg/m^2 day 1) or with every two-week therapy with gemcitabine 1,000 mg/m^2 day 1 and paclitaxel 120 mg/m^2 day 2).[50] Responses were observed in pretreated patients.

Based on these data, an every two-week schema was developed primarily for chemonaive patients, but also for pretreated patients with up to two prior regimens. In a multicentre phase II study, paclitaxel 150 mg/m^2 and gemcitabine 3,000 mg/m^2 were given every two weeks. Fifty-six (chemonaive and six pretreated patients) were entered. Of 55 eligible patients, 17 had a partial and five had a complete response rate for an overall response rate of 40% (27–54%). One complete response and one partial response were observed in the six previously treated patients. Overall median survival was 11.8 months (11.9 months in the chemonaive cohort). Grade 3 or 4 myelosuppression occurred in 56%, but only four serious infections were observed. The investigators felt that this regimen was active and well tolerated, with perhaps compromised efficacy in comparison to cisplatin-containing regimens.[50]

In another American phase II trial, 54 patients[51] with advanced urothelial carcinoma received paclitaxel 200 mg/m^2 in a one-hour infusion on day 1 and gemcitabine 1,000 mg/m^2 on days 1, 8, and 15 every three weeks. Twenty-nine of 54 patients (54% CI: 40–67%) had objective responses, with 7% CR. At a median follow-up of 24 months, 16 patients (30%) were alive and 9 (17%) were progression-free. The median survival for the entire group was also 14.4 months, with 1 and 2-year actuarial survival rates of 57% and 25%, respectively. Of note, 7 of 15 (47%) patients previously treated with platinum-based chemotherapy responded to paclitaxel and gemcitabine. Grade 3/4 toxicity was primarily haematologic, including leukopenia (46%), thrombocytopenia (13%), and anaemia (28%). Ten patients (19%) required hospitalization for neutropenia and fever, and one patient had treatment-related septic death. The schedule of this regimen with only one week of rest may be responsible for the haematologic toxicity. In a multicenter Italian trial, 48 chemonaive patients with metastatic urothelial cancer were treated with gemcitabine 2,500 mg/m^2 in 30 min and paclitaxel 150 mg/ m^2 in three hours every 2 weeks.[52] The response rate in 33 evaluable patients was 37%, with 5 complete responses and 15 partial responses. Haematologic toxicity was predominant but manageable. The median survival was 13.2 months, and the median time to disease progression was 5.8 months. This regimen shows promise but may be most useful for patients unable to receive cisplatin. In another study from UCLA, the combination of gemcitabine plus docetaxel was studied in 27 patients with unresectable metastatic or locally advanced transitional cell carcinoma of the urothelial tract.[53] The first 10 patients received gemcitabine 800 mg/m^2 days 1, 8, and 15 of a 28-day treatment cycle plus docetaxel 80 mg/m^2. Due to dose-limiting toxicity (neutropenia), the initial dose of docetaxel was reduced to 60 mg/m^2 for the remaining 17 patients who entered the study. Neutropenia was the most common adverse event (grade 3 in 37% and grade 4 in 22.2%). The objective response rate was 33.3% with 2 of 27 patients (7.4%) achieving a complete response. The median duration of response was 20 weeks and median survival was 52 weeks.

The available data on the combination of gemcitabine and taxanes in advanced urothelial carcinoma demonstrate that the combination is active and tolerable and that complete responses can be attained. Mature phase II trials and data from randomized trials are needed to determine the future role of these combinations in the management of advanced urothelial carcinoma of the bladder. At the present time, patients who are eligible for cisplatin should be treated with cisplatin-based combination chemotherapy.

First-line regimens in patients unfit for cisplatin

In patients considered not eligible for cisplatin, carboplatin-based regimens have demonstrated activity.[41,46,54,55] The definition of 'unfitness for cisplatin' may be based on different factors: (a) age, although advanced age may not be associated with an increased likelihood of developing severe toxicities with cisplatin-based chemotherapy; (b) renal function, although the optimal threshold of renal function level that should preclude cisplatin is still unclear; (c) solitary kidney, usually applicable in patients with urothelial carcinoma of the upper urinary tract who undergo nephroureterectomy in whom adequate hydration and splitting cisplatin in two days is usually considered; (d) functional status and co-morbidities because poor functional status has been associated with increased toxicity and decreased efficacy in patients treated with cisplatin and because some co-morbidities can be exacerbated by cisplatin (e.g. neurotoxicity and ototoxicity).

Because of the significant variability in the definition of patients 'unfit' for cisplatin, a uniform definition of cisplatin ineligibility criteria for clinical trials has been suggested by a working group and includes: (i) ECOG performance status of 2; (ii) creatinine clearance <60 mL/min; (iii) Common Terminology Criteria for Adverse Events (CTCAE) Grade ≥2 hearing loss; (iv) CTCAE Grade ≥2 neuropathy.[56] According to this definition, patients should meet at least one of these criteria to be defined unfit for cisplatin.

For this 'unfit' group, gemcitabine has been combined with carboplatin to avoid the nephrotoxicity often associated with cisplatin. In four small trials[55,57] gemcitabine was given at 1,000 mg/m^2 on days 1 and 8 every 21 days and carboplatin at an AUC of 5 on day 1. This combination has shown activity with OR of 45% to 68%. The major toxicities encountered have been myelosuppression with grade 3–4 neutropenia and thrombocytopenia in 60–68% of patients.

Although several phase II trials have explored other chemotherapeutic regimens for this population, the first II/III randomized trial in this setting was conducted by the EORTC Genito-Urinary Group. In this trial, gemcitabine and carboplatin (GCa) was compared to methotrexate, carboplatin, and vinblastine (M-CAVI) in 238 unfit patients. Median OS was 9.3 months in the GCa arm and 8.1 months in the M-CAVI arm with a hazard ratio of 0.94 (95% CI, 0.72 to 1.22; p =.64). The hypothesized increase in OS from 9 months with M-CAVI regimen to 13.5 months with GCa was not reached. The primary end point of the study (OS) showed no statistically significant difference between the two treatment arms. Median PFS was 5.8 months in the GCa arm and 4.2 months in the M-CAVI arm in the intent-to-treat analysis, with a hazard ratio of 1.04 (95% CI, 0.80 to 1.35). Severe acute toxicity (death, grade 4 thrombocytopenia with bleeding, grade 3 or 4 renal toxicity, neutropenic fever, or mucositis) was observed in 9.3% of patients receiving GCa and in 21.2% of patients receiving M-CAVI.[58] This study has shown that M-CAVI is clearly more toxic than GCa in this patient population, particularly in patients with impaired renal function.

Dividing the cisplatin dose with hydration and administering it over two days is another viable option in patients with impaired renal function. In a Spanish trial, 38 patients with locally advanced or metastatic urothelial carcinoma with creatinine clearance between 35 and 59 mL/min received gemcitabine 2,500 mg/m^2 and cisplatin 35 mg/m^2 on day 1 and day 15 for a 28-day schedule. Fifteen partial responses (39%) were reported and 12 patients had stable disease (31%). Median PFS and overall survival were 3.5 and 8.5 months, respectively. Grade 3–4 haematological toxicities were: neutropenia 9%, anaemia 6% and thrombocytopenia 16%. No patient developed renal toxicity.[59]

Splitting the cisplatin dose in two days could be considered an option for unfit patients. However, as the results seem not to be superior to those obtained with carboplatin-based regimens in this population of patients, the combination of carboplatin and gemcitabine can be considered the standard of care in patients unfit for cisplatin. New agents with improved efficacy and tolerability may eliminate the need to evaluate patients with metastatic urothelial bladder cancer in separate cohorts in the future.

Second-line treatments

The outcome for patients with advanced transitional cell carcinoma who relapse or progress on first-line treatment is extremely poor. Poor prognostic factors including visceral metastasis and Karnofsky performance status of less than 80 have substantially been shown to affect outcomes in patients treated with first-line chemotherapy.[8] These recognized prognostic factors might continue to have an effect in the second-line setting. A recent retrospective analysis of patients who received second-line vinflunine identified ECOG performance status higher than 0, haemoglobin less than 100 g/L, and liver metastasis as poor prognostic factors.[60] Additionally, a shorter duration of TTP after first-line therapy, response to first-line chemotherapy, prior exposure to cisplatin and whether chemotherapy was administered in the perioperative or metastatic setting have an impact on sensitivity to second-line therapy.

Many chemotherapeutic agents have been tested in the second-line setting showing poor or no activity in phase II trials although a few yield modest response rates of 10–20%, median PFS of two to three months and median overall survival of six to nine months.[61–64] Multidrug combinations have been thoroughly investigated as second-line therapy for metastatic bladder cancer and have generally yielded better response rates, but not necessarily better survival outcomes, and often higher toxicities. Second-line combinations of gemcitabine and paclitaxel or gemcitabine and ifosfamide have been investigated and outcomes seem somewhat better than in monotherapy trials, although these trials have enrolled patients with favourable response characteristics.[49,65]

A case for non-cross-resistant combination second-line therapy could be made for patients with good performance and rapidly progressive or visceral disease. Re-administration of the first-line combination chemotherapy regimen might be considered if the previous quality of response was excellent (eg, complete response) or the TTP was long (e.g. >12 months); limited data supporting this strategy exist for M-VAC.[66]

Vinflunine ditartrate is a novel anti-tubulin agent obtained by a semisynthetic process from a vinca alkaloid base that has demonstrated higher antitumour activity compared with parent compounds. Single-agent vinflunine was studied in several phase I trials utilizing different schedules leading to the selection of the three-week schedule for phase II evaluation.[67–69] A multicenter phase II trial to determine the efficacy of vinflunine as second-line therapy in patients with advanced urothelial carcinoma of the bladder has been conducted in patients that failed or progressed after first-line platinum-containing regimens for advanced or metastatic disease, or had progressive disease after platinum-containing chemotherapy given with adjuvant or neoadjuvant intent.[70] Of 51 patients treated with 320 mg/m^2 of vinflunine, nine patients responded to the therapy yielding an OR rate of 18% (95% CI: 8.4–30.9%) and 67% (95% CI: 52.1–79.3%) achieved disease control (partial response plus stable disease). Of note, responses were seen in patients with relatively poor prognostic factors such as a short (<12 months) interval from prior platinum therapy (19%, including an 11% response rate in those progressing <3 months after platinum treatment), prior treatment for metastatic disease (24%), prior treatment with vinca alkaloids (14%) and visceral involvement (20%). The median duration of response was 9.1 months (95% CI: 4.2–15.0) and the median PFS was 3.0 months (95% CI: 2.4–3.8). The median OS was 6.6 months (95% CI: 4.8–7.6). The main haematological toxicity was grade 3–4 neutropenia, in 67% of patients (42% of cycles). Febrile neutropenia was observed in five patients (10%) and was fatal in two. Constipation was frequently observed and was grade 3-4 in 8% of patients. The incidence of grade 3 nausea and vomiting was very low, neither grade 3-4 sensory neuropathy nor severe venous irritation was observed. Moreover, and of importance in this particular study population, no grade 3-4 renal function impairment was observed.

In a subsequent phase III trial in the second-line setting of metastatic urothelial bladder cancer, 370 patients were randomized to vinflunine plus best supportive care (BSC) versus BSC alone.[71] In the intent-to-treat population, the difference in overall survival was not statistically significant (6.9 months for vinflunine plus BSC vs. 4.6 months for BSC) (HR = 0.88; 95% CI, 0.69 to 1.12; $p = 0.287$). In a subset of 357 eligible patients, the median OS was significantly longer for the vinflunine group (6.9 versus 4.3 months). Grade 3–4 toxicities included neutropenia (50%), febrile neutropenia (6%), anaemia (19%), fatigue (19%), and constipation (16%). There was one drug-related death on study. On the basis of these results, vinflunine has been approved for use in Europe but not in the United States.

Given the lack of definitive randomized data, there remains no well-defined standard of care for second-line chemotherapy for metastatic transitional cell carcinoma of the bladder cancer and participation in clinical trials should be encouraged.

New strategies

Overcoming platinum resistance

With platinum analogues being the most active drugs against urothelial cancer, the emergence of cisplatin resistance in the course of disease clearly limits treatment options and ultimately has an impact on survival. Many DNA repair pathways have been identified. The excision repair cross-complementation group 1 (ERCC1) is required to excise damaged nucleotides and has been shown to predict response to cisplatin-based chemotherapy. In 57 patients with advanced or metastatic bladder cancer treated with either GC or GCP, the ERCC1 mRNA expression levels correlated with survival, time to disease progression and chemotherapy response with median survival being significantly higher in patients with low ERCC1 levels (25.4 vs. 15.4 months; $p = 0.03$).[72] The same group reported that ERCC1 expression by immunohistochemistry can predict disease specific survival in patients treated with cisplatin-based chemotherapy.[73]

BRCA1 (Breast Cancer 1 gene) plays a central role in DNA repair pathways and low BRCA1 expression has been associated with sensitivity to cisplatin and longer survival in lung and ovarian cancer patients. In 57 patients with locally advanced bladder cancer treated with neoadjuvant cisplatin-based chemotherapy, both pathologic response (66% vs. 22%; $p = 0.01$) and median survival (168 vs. 34 months, $p = 0.002$) were better in patients with low/intermediate BRCA1 levels as compared with patients with high BRCA1 levels. BRCA1 expression may predict the efficacy of cisplatin-based neoadjuvant chemotherapy and may help to customize therapy in bladder cancer patients.[74]

The multidrug resistance gene 1 (MDR1) encodes P-glycoprotein (Pgp), a membrane protein that acts as an energy-dependent cellular efflux pump. Pgp can reduce intracellular concentrations of chemotherapy drugs such as anthracyclines and vinca alkaloids, resulting in decreased cytotoxicity. Furthermore, it appears that chemotherapy drugs induce MDR1 and lead to drug resistance.[75] In patients with locally advanced bladder cancer receiving adjuvant chemotherapy, high MDR1 expression is associated with inferior survival.[76] After two years, more than 65% of patients with high MDR1 expression had progressed compared to only 25% of patients with low MDR1 expression. After five years, only 23% of patients with high MDR1 expression were still alive versus 62% of patients with low MDR1 expression (HR 0.25, $p = 0.0006$).

The hope is that these emerging strategies will help pave the road towards personalized therapy in advanced bladder cancer.

Genetic markers

Several studies have been conducted using a combination of genetic markers to predict response to chemotherapy. Takata *et al.* analysed the gene expression profile of 27,648 genes from 27 invasive bladder cancers using a cDNA microarray.[77] Profiles of tumours from patients who responded to M-VAC neoadjuvant chemotherapy were compared to nonresponders to develop a scoring system of 14 predictive genes. This system was able to accurately predict drug response in eight out of nine patients. It was applied to 22 additional cases of bladder cancer and correctly predicted clinical response for 19 cases.[78] Another approach uses the co-expression extrapolation (COXEN) algorithm derived from expression microarray data of the National Cancer Institute (NCI)-60 cell line panel to predict drug sensitivity of bladder cancer cell lines.[79] The COXEN-based gene expression model was able to effectively stratify chemosensitivity and predict the three-year overall survival in patients treated with M-VAC.[80]

Genome sequencing

Recent successes with molecularly based targeted drugs, have made personalized medicine a reality. The success of these new drug strategies can be in part attributed to the identification of the genetic mechanisms responsible for the development and progression of metastatic cancers. Recently, the advances in sequencing technology have allowed for comprehensive mutation analysis of tumours and have led to the identification of a number of genes involved in the aetiology and progression of many types of cancer. The whole-genome sequencing has been used to to investigate the genetic basis of a durable remission of metastatic bladder cancer in a patient treated with everolimus, a drug that inhibits the mTOR (mammalian target of rapamycin) signalling pathway, in a phase II trial (NCI 00805129). Among the somatic mutations was a loss-of-function mutation in TSC1 (tuberous sclerosis complex 1), a regulator of mTOR pathway activation. Targeted sequencing revealed TSC1 mutations in about 8% of 109 additional bladder cancers examined, and TSC1 mutation correlated with everolimus sensitivity.[81] These results demonstrate the feasibility of using whole-genome sequencing in the clinical setting to identify previously occult biomarkers of drug sensitivity that can aid in the identification of patients most likely to respond to targeted anticancer drugs.

As the methodology and costs associated with next-generation sequencing continue to improve, this technology will be rapidly adopted into routine clinical oncology practices and will significantly impact on personalized therapy.

Targeted therapies

Targeting angiogenesis

Vascular endothelial growth factor (VEGF) receptors are another interesting target. The VEGF monoclonal antibody bevacizumab in combination with cisplatin and gemcitabine was tested in 43 chemotherapy-naive patients with metastatic or unrespectable urothelial carcinoma with an overall response rate of 72%. Median PFS was 8.2 months (95% CI, 6.8 to 10.3 months) with a median OS of 19.1 months (95% CI, 12.4 to 22.7 months). The study-defined goal of 50% improvement in PFS was not met. Three treatment-related deaths (central nervous system haemorrhage, sudden cardiac death, and aortic dissection) were observed.[82] On the basis of these preliminary results the Cancer and Leukemia Group B (CALGB) is conducting a phase III trial with the same regimen.

The oral multitargeted tyrosine kinase inhibitor (TKI) Sorafenib showed no objective responses in either the first or second-line treatment setting.[83,84] However, two other drugs in the same category produced different results. Sunitinib, used as second-line therapy for patients with metastatic bladder cancer led to a 43% partial response and stable disease[60,85] while when administered as first-line therapy to patients ineligible for cisplatin a partial response in 2 of 16 patients was obtained.[86] In order to evaluate the role of maintenance sunitinib after response to chemotherapy 54 patients were randomized to oral sunitinib or placebo. The six-month progression rate was 81%, median TTP five months for sunitinib and 75% and 2.7 months with placebo.[87]

The efficacy and safety of gemcitabine, cisplatin, and sunitinib in metastatic and muscle-infiltrating bladder cancer was tested in parallel phase II trials. Trial 1 enrolled 36 patients with metastatic bladder cancer who were chemotherapy naive; trial 2 enrolled 9 patients with muscle-infiltrating bladder cancer. Both trials were stopped early due to excessive toxicity. Grade 3 to 4 haematologic toxicities occurred in 70% (23/33) of patients in trial 1 and 22% (2/9) of patients in trial 2. In trial 1, the response rate was 49% (95% CI, 31–67%); in trial 2, the pathologic complete response was 22% (2/9).[88]

Pazopanib, a multitargeted TKI that targets vascular endothelial growth factor receptor (VEGFR)-1, -2, and -3; platelet derived growth factor receptor (PDGFR)-a and PDGFR-ß, and c-Kit, has been tested in 41 patients with urothelial carcinoma unresponsive or relapsing after at least one or more lines of cisplatin-based chemotherapy for metastatic disease; 21 (51%) of 41 patients were given pazopanib as third-line or further-line treatment.[89] Seven patients (17%) had a confirmed partial response, 14 patients had confirmed stable disease. Nineteen patients (46%) had a clear necrotic evolution of multiple metastases and/or a decreased standard uptake value on PET scan consistent with a partial response. The only grade 3 toxicity was hypertension in two patients. Median PFS was 2.6 months (95% CI 1.7–3.7) and median overall survival was 4.7 months (95% CI 4.2–7.3). Fatigue, hypertension, and anorexia were the most frequent grade 1 or 2 treatment-related side effects. Overall, there were 12 (29%) cases of grade 3 side effects. This study highlights the need for new criteria or modifications to existing criteria to assess response with cystostatic angiogenesis inhibitors.

Vandetanib is an oral once-daily selective TKI of key signalling pathways in cancer, including VEGFR-2 and epidermal growth factor receptor (EGFR). Early clinical trials showed that this agent alone or in combination with docetaxel had an acceptable adverse effect profile and produced tumour responses.[90] In a randomized double blinded trial, Vandetanib in combination with docetaxel was compared to docetaxel plus placebo in 142 patients with advanced urothelial cancer, who progressed on prior platinum-based chemotherapy. Median PFS was 2.56 months for the docetaxel plus vandetanib as compared to 1.58 months for docetaxel plus placebo (HR = 1.02;95% CI, 0.69–1.49; $p = .9$). Overall response rate and OS were not different between both arms. Grade 3 or higher toxicities were more commonly seen in the docetaxel plus vandetanib arm and included rash/photosensitivity (11% vs. 0%) and diarrhoea (7% vs. 0%). Among 37 patients who crossed over to single-agent vandetanib, overall response rate was 3% and OS was 5.2 months.[91]

Antiangiogenic agents are still in a very preliminary phase of clinical research in urothelial cancer and although the biological basis of angiogenesis in urothelial tumours is well known, their influence in the prognosis of these malignancies has yet to be demonstrated.

Targeting epidermal growth factor receptor

Many growth factor receptors and ligands have been shown to be overexpressed in urothelial cancer including human epidermal growth factor receptor 2 (HER2/neu), epidermal growth factor receptor (EGFR), and epidermal growth factor. Despite immunohistochemical confirmation of strong expression of EGFR on pre-treatment biopsies in a second-line trial with the EGFR inhibitor Gefitinib, the median PFS was only two months[92] and the same drug combined with GC in a phase II trial failed to improve response rate as compared to historical controls.[93] The absence of EGFR mutations at exons 19 to 21 in urothelial carcinoma may be responsible of the lack of activity of the EGFR inhibitors.[94]

Her2/neu is variably expressed on urothelial carcinomas and has been evaluated as a possible therapeutic target. One study screened 109 patients with advanced urothelial cancer and found that Her2-positive patients (52%) had more metastatic sites and higher rates of visceral disease than Her2-negative patients.[95] Forty-four patients were treated with trastuzumab, paclitaxel, carboplatin, and gemcitabine with an overall response rate of 70% with 57% confirmed responses. Median survival was 14.1 months. Toxicities included 93% grade 3–4 myelosuppression, 14% grade 3 sensory neuropathy, 22.7% grade 1–3 of cardiotoxicity (4.5% grade 3), and three therapy-related deaths.

Lapatinib, a dual EGFR and HER2 TKI, has been tested in 59 patients with advanced bladder cancer who progressed after cisplatin-based chemotherapy. This study was considered to be negative because it did not meet its primary end point (response rate) but demonstrated improved OS in a subset of patients with tumours overexpressing EGFR and/or HER-2 (30.3 weeks as compared to 10.6).[96] EGFR expression has been demonstrated on 50% of bladder tumours,[97] and trials are ongoing with cetuximab (NCT00645593).

New drugs

Eribulin, a halichondrin B derivative with microtubule inhibitory action, showed activity in the first-line treatment setting with a 34% response rate.[98] In a subsequent phase Ib/II study, eribulin was combined with cisplatin and gemcitabine. The recommended phase II dose of eribulin in combination with gemcitabine and cisplatin was established as 1.0 mg/m^2. Eribulin combined with standard GC chemotherapy is feasible and has encouraging clinical activity. Haematologic toxicity is the main limiting factor.[99]

Nab-paclitaxel (ABI-007), an albumin bound nanoparticle formulation of paclitaxel was tested as a single agent in 40 patients with platinum-refractory metastatic urothelial carcinoma. Single-agent nab-paclitaxel was well tolerated with a response rate (CR+PR) of 33% (12/36) and a clinical benefit rate (CR+PR+SD) of 58% (21/36), representing one of the highest reported response rates to date in the second-line setting.[100] Future trials are planned.

Immunotherapy

Immunotherapy continues to be one of the most rapidly evolving fields in oncology. In recent years, numerous immunotherapies have shown efficacy, safety, and durability across a variety of tumour types. Not since the days of M-VAC have we observed such important, long-lasting results. Bladder cancer is characterized by a high mutational load, a great deal of neo-antigens and is, therefore, highly immunogenic. Immunotherapy with checkpoint inhibitors has become increasingly important in the treatment of advanced bladder cancer.

PD-L1 checkpoint blockade has received FDA approval for metastatic urothelial cancer refractory to standard chemotherapy. In May 2016, the FDA approved the PD-L1 inhibitor atezolizumab for the second-line treatment of patients with advanced or metastatic recurrent urothelial cancer, based on a single-arm, phase II study. The FDA then granted Breakthrough Therapy Designation in June 2016 for nivolumab, an anti PD-1 monoclonal antibody based on the nivolumab CheckMate 032 study.

Rosenberg *et al.* published results on 310 patients in the IMvigor 210 trial (NCT021086529).[101] Cohort 2 was a phase II study of patients who had received >1 platinum-containing regimen. Patients were given 1200 mg intravenous atezolizumab every 21 days until progression. With a median follow-up of 11.7 months (95% CI 11.4–12.2), ongoing responses were recorded in 38 (84%) of 45 responders. The results led to FDA approval of atezolizumab in metastatic urothelial cancer refractory to standard chemotherapy. In further analysis of the results, PDL-1 expression, the Cancer Genome Atlas (TCGA) subtype (particularly the luminal subgroup) and mutational load were found to be independent predictors of response to atezolizumab. The luminal subgroup was associated with a more inflamed environment than the basal subtype. The luminal subtype was also found to have high Teffector cells and low stromal gene expression. Assessment of these characteristics may define drivers of immune responses. Further work on the biology of immune response to checkpoint inhibits is clearly a priority.

Meanwhile, Balar *et al.*[102] reported on atezolizumab as first-line treatment in cisplatin-ineligible patients from the same IMvigor 210 trial, in a single-arm, multicentre, phase 2 trial. There were 123 patients, of whom 119 received one or more doses of atezolizumab. At 17.2 months' median follow-up, the objective RR was 23% (95% CI 16–31), the CR rate was 9% (n = 11), and 19 of 27 responses were ongoing. Median response duration was not reached. From this portion of the trial, responses occurred across all PD-L1 and poor prognostic factor subgroups. Median PFS was 2.7 months (2.1–4.2). Median OS was 15.9 months (10.4 to not estimable). Tumour mutation load was associated with response. Atezolizumab showed encouraging durable response rates, survival, and tolerability, supporting its therapeutic use in untreated metastatic urothelial cancer.

Nivolumab monotherapy has also been evaluated in recurrent metastatic urothelial carcinoma in the CheckMate 032 trial (NCT01928394): a multicentre, open-label, two-stage, multiarm, phase 1/2 trial by Sharma *et al.*[103] This was part of a larger phase I/II open-label study of nivolumab monotherapy mg/kg administered intravenously every two weeks until disease progression or treatment discontinuation; or nivolumab combined with ipilimumab in subjects with advanced or metastatic solid tumours, in which 78 patients received single-agent nivolumab. The minimum follow-up was nine months (median 15.2 months, IQR 12.9–16.8). A confirmed investigator-assessed objective response was achieved in 19 (24.4%, 95% CI 15.3–35.4) of 78 patients.

At the European Society of Medical Oncology (ESMO) Meeting (7–11 October 2016; Copenhagen, Denmark 2016, LBA31), Galsky *et al.*[104] presented (Checkmate 275; NCT02387996) further results of of the PD-1 blocking antibody nivolumab in unresectable urothelial cancer patients who had progressed or recurred following treatment with a platinum agent.

Enrolment continued until approximately 70 patients with confirmed PD-L1 expression ≥5% were treated. The CheckMate 275 trial assessed the activity and safety of nivolumab in 270 patients and is the largest phase II study of a PD-1 inhibitor in bladder cancer reported. Patients were treated with nivolumab at 3 mg/kg until progression or unacceptable toxicity, and could be treated beyond progression under specific circumstances, but PFS was recorded at the time of first documented progression. The primary end point was objective RR in all treated patients and in patients with tumour PD-L1 expression ≥5%- and also ≥1% following a protocol amendment. ORR was defined as the proportion of patients with best overall response of confirmed complete (CR) or partial response (PR) assessed by a blinded independent review committee, using RECIST v1.1 criteria. Secondary end points included progression-free survival. Exploratory end points included investigator-assessed PFS (RECIST v1.1), safety, patient quality of life, and biomarker analyses of peripheral blood and tumour tissue. There was a minimum follow-up of six months at the time of the database lock.

Nivolumab resulted in a clinically meaningful objective RR of 19.6% in all treated patients, as assessed by blinded independent review, with 2% of patients achieving CR. Efficacy was observed, regardless of baseline tumour PD-L1 expression status, including patients with PD-L1 expression less than 1%. The median duration of response was not reached, with a minimum follow-up of six months. The median PFS was 2 months in all treated patients, 3.5 months in the PD-L1 greater than or equal to 1% cohort, and 1.8 months in both PD-L1 <1% and PD-L1 <5% cohorts. The median OS was 8.74 months in all treated patients, with medians ranging from 5.9 months in the PD-L1 less than 1% cohort, and 11.30 months (95% CI: 9.63, N.A.) in those patients with PD-L1 expression equal or greater than 1%. These findings, with only a median follow-up of 7 months, compare favourably to single-agent chemotherapy historical control medians for OS of approximately seven months.

This is the second study to evaluate nivolumab, a PD-1 checkpoint inhibitor as second-line therapy for urothelial cancer. In the 265 patients evaluated for efficacy, the primary end point of objective RR was 19.6%. In both patients with tumours expressing higher and lower levels of PD-L1 (including those with less than 1% PD-L1), the objective RR was above that achieved historically with chemotherapy. The results are consistent with the results from the nivolumab CheckMate 032 study. The strongest interferon gene signature expression occurred in the patients with the basal 1 subtype, with expression at least three times higher than other subtypes.

Based on these findings, the European Medicines Agency (EMA) has initiated an official review. Results suggesting that the strongest signature is associated with the basal 1 subtype differ from the results presented by Rosenberg *et al.*[101] with atezolizumab favouring the luminal subtype in terms of second-line therapy response (NCT02108652). This will have to be evaluated further as to which specific subtypes benefit most from immunotherapy.

A Phase III Randomized Clinical Trial of Pembrolizumab (MK-3475) Versus Paclitaxel, Docetaxel or Vinflunine in Subjects With Recurrent or Progressive Metastatic Urothelial Cancer (KEYNOTE-045; NCT02256436) is an open-label trial that was presented by Bellmunt *et al.* at the Society of Immunotherapy of Cancer (SITC 2016) meeting at National Harbor, MD, 9–13 November 2016.[105]

Some 542 patients with advanced urothelial carcinoma of the renal pelvis, ureter, bladder, or urethra, with predominantly transitional cell carcinoma, with progression after one to two lines of platinum-based chemotherapy or recurrence within 12 months of perioperative platinum-based therapy were randomized between pembrolizumab 200 mg IV Q3W for two years, or the physician's choice of either paclitaxel 175 mg/m^2 Q3W or docetaxel 75 mg/m^2 Q3W or vinflunine 320 mg/m^2 Q3W. The primary end point was OS and PFS in total and PD-L1 combined positive score (CPS) of tumour and immune cell PD-L1 expression ≥10% populations.

The median OS with pembrolizumab was 10.3 months (8.0–11.8 months) as compared to 7.4 months (6.1–8.3 months) with chemotherapy (HR = 0.73 (0.59–0.91; $p = 0.0022$). At 12 months, OS was 43.9% with pembrolizumab as compared to 30.7% with chemotherapy. OS for CPS, which included both tumour and inflammatory cells, ≥10% was 8.0 months (5.0–12.3 months) versus 5.2 months (4.0–7.4 months); HR = 0.57 (0.37–0.88, $p = 0.0048$). There was no significant difference in PFS between the two arms. ORR with pembrolizumab was 21.1%. A CR was seen in 7% and a PR in 14.1%. With chemotherapy, the ORR was 11.4%, with 3.3% CR and 8.1% PR. There was a difference of 9.6% ($p = 0.0011$). With pembrolizumab 68% had a response ≥12 months and with chemotherapy, 35% of patients had a response duration ≥12 months.

Pembrolizumab monotherapy reduced the risk of death by 27% compared with chemotherapy for patients with advanced urothelial carcinoma, whose disease progressed after prior treatment. The results set another new second-line standard for bladder cancer. The adverse event profile for pembrolizumab was consistent with previous experience with other similar agents.

Pembrolizumab was also presented in the phase 2 KEYNOTE-052; NCT02335424 study by Balar *et al.* at ESMO 2016; 7–11 October 2016; Copenhagen, Denmark.[106] This is a phase II study using pembrolizumab for first-line treatment in patients with advanced/unresectable (inoperable) or metastatic urothelial cancer who are ineligible for cisplatin-based therapy. The primary study objective was to determine the objective RR in all participants, in participants whose tumours rely on (PD-L1) protein (PD-L1-positive tumours), and in participants with strongly PD-L1-positive tumours.

Preliminary analysis of the first 100 patients enrolled in the trial were presented. The primary end point of ORR in PD-L1–unselected patients was 24%. The biomarker cut point to identify patients most likely to respond to the drug was determined to be 10% or greater total PD-L1 expression in immune cells or tumour cells. Thirty patients had this level of expression, of whom 11 (37%) responded to treatment. The median duration of response had not yet been reached and treatment was well tolerated.

Pembrolizumab has substantial activity with a favourable safety profile as first-line therapy in cisplatin-ineligible patients with metastatic bladder cancer. The biomarker cut point requires validation in the full study population, but appears to identify patients most likely to respond to pembrolizumab. Immunotherapy is rapidly redefining our treatment approach for patients that are ineligible for cisplatin-based chemotherapy.

Other agents such as durvalumab and tremelimumab are being evaluated in bladder cancer. The phase III Danube (NCT02516241) clinical trial is aiming to move immune single-agent and immune combination therapy into the frontline setting in bladder cancer. The trial has three arms: chemotherapy versus single-agent durvalumab, versus a combination of durvalumab and tremelimumab. The hope is that chemotherapy can be replaced. The estimated enrolment of 1005 patients has already been achieved.

Urothelial cancer is extremely sensitive to checkpoint inhibition with both anti PD-1 and anti PD-L1 antibodies. The future seems brighter with the advent of these new therapies.

Conclusions

Although important progress has been made in the management of advanced bladder cancer, 50% of the patients with invasive cancer still succumb to their disease. Chemotherapy remains the mainstay of treatment of metastatic urothelial carcinoma and cisplatin combination chemotherapy has to be considered the standard of care in patients with good performance status and adequate renal function.

In patients unfit for cisplatin, carboplatin-based regimens have demonstrated activity, but new agents with improved efficacy and tolerability may eliminate the need to evaluate patients with metastatic urothelial carcinoma in separate cohorts in the future.

Given the lack of definitive randomized data, there remains no well-defined standard of care for second-line chemotherapy for metastatic bladder cancer and participation in clinical trials should be encouraged. Development of less toxic, more effective agents is critical.

A better understanding of the molecular biology of bladder cancer will undoubtedly influence the selection of new therapeutic modalities. Several signalling pathways are activated in bladder urothelial carcinoma, but no targeted therapy, either alone or in combination with conventional cytotoxic chemotherapy, has been shown to significantly improve treatment outcomes. Whether or not this approach to therapy will lead to better results must still be determined. The future of metastatic urothelial carcinoma treatment lies in the ability to deliver personalized therapy. This area remains an active research field today and participation in clinical trial needs to be prioritized.

Further reading

Bajorin DF, Dodd PM, Mazumdar M, *et al.* Long-term survival in metastatic transitional-cell carcinoma and prognostic factors predicting outcome of therapy. *J Clin Oncol 1999*; **17**(10):3173–81.

Bellmunt J, Paz-Ares L, Cuello M, *et al.* Gene expression of ERCC1 as a novel prognostic marker in advanced bladder cancer patients receiving cisplatin-based chemotherapy. *Ann Oncol* 2007; **18**(3):522–8.

Bellmunt J, von der Maase H, Mead GM, *et al.* Randomized phase iii study comparing paclitaxel/cisplatin/ gemcitabine and gemcitabine/cisplatin in patients with locally advanced or metastatic urothelial cancer without prior systemic therapy: EORTC Intergroup Study 30987. *J Clin Oncol* 2012; **30**(10):1107–13.

Bellmunt Molins J, von der Maase H, Theodore C, *et al.* Phase III trial of vinflunine plus best supportive care compared with best supportive care alone after a platinum-containing regimen in patients with advanced transitional cell carcinoma of the urothelial tract. *J Clin Oncol* 2009; **27**(27):4454–61.

De Santis M, Bellmunt J, Mead G, *et al.* Randomized phase II/III trial assessing gemcitabine/carboplatin and methotrexate/carboplatin/vinblastine in patients with advanced urothelial cancer who are unfit for cisplatin-based chemotherapy: EORTC study 30986. *J Clin Oncol* 2012; **30**(2):191–9.

Galsky MD, Chen GJ, Oh WK, *et al.* Comparative effectiveness of cisplatin-based and carboplatin-based chemotherapy for treatment of advanced urothelial carcinoma. *Ann Oncol* 2012; **23**(2):406–10.

Galsky MD, Hahn NM, Rosenberg JE, *et al.* Treatment of patients with metastatic urothelial cancer "unfit" for cisplatin-based chemotherapy. *J Clin Oncol* 2011; **29**(17):2432–8.

Iyer G, Hanrahan AJ, MIlowsky MI, *et al.* Genome sequencing identifies a basis for everolimus sensitivity. *Science* 2012; **338**(6104):221.

Sternberg CN, de Mulder P, Schornagel JH, *et al.* Seven year update of an EORTC phase III trial of high dose intensity M-VAC chemotherapy and G-CSF versus classic M-VAC in advanced urothelial tract tumors (EORTC protocol 30924). *Eur J Cancer* 2006; **42**(1):50–4.

Sternberg CN, Yagoda A, Scher HI, *et al.* M-VAC (methotrexate, vinblastine, doxorubicin and cisplatin) for advanced transitional cell carcinoma of the bladder. *J Urol* 1988; **139**:461–9.

von der Maase H, Hansen SW, Roberts JT, *et al.* Gemcitabine and cisplatin versus methotrexate, vinblastine, doxorubicin, and cisplatin in advanced or metastatic bladder cancer: results of a large, randomized, multinational, multicenter, phase III study. *J Clin Oncol* 2000; **18**(17):3068–77.

Williams PD, Cheon S, Havaleshko DM, *et al.* Concordant gene expression signatures predict clinical outcomes of cancer patients undergoing systemic therapy. *Cancer Res* 2009; **69**(21):8302–9.

References

1. Siegel R, Naishadham D, Jemal A. Cancer statistics, 2012. *CA Cancer J Clin* 2012; **61**(1):10–29.
2. Chavan S, Bray F, Lortet-Teulent J, Goodman MM, Jemal A. International variations in bladder cancer incidence and mortality. *Eur Urol* 2014; **66**(1):59–73.

3. Rosenberg JE, Carroll PR, Small EJ. Update on chemotherapy for advanced bladder cancer. *J Urol* 2005; **174**(1):14–20.
4. Sternberg CN, Yagoda A, Scher HI, *et al.* M-VAC (methotrexate, vinblastine, doxorubicin and cisplatin) for advanced transitional cell carcinoma of the bladder. *J Urol* 1988; **139**:461–9.
5. Loehrer PJ Sr, Einhorn LH, Elson PJ, *et al.* A randomized comparison of cisplatin alone or in combination with methotrexate, vinblastine, and doxorubicin in patients with metastatic urothelial carcinoma: a cooperative group study. *J Clin Oncol* 1992; **10**(7):1066–73.
6. Geller NL, Sternberg CN, Penenberg D, Scher H, Yagoda A. Prognostic factors for survival of patients with advanced urothelial tumors treated with methotrexate, vinblastine, doxorubicin, and cisplatin chemotherapy. *Cancer* 1991; **67**:1525–31.
7. Saxman SB, Propert KJ, Einhorn LH, *et al.* Long-term follow-up of a phase III intergroup study of cisplatin alone or in combination with methotrexate, vinblastine, and doxorubicin in patients with metastatic urothelial carcinoma: a cooperative group study. *J Clin Oncol* 1997; **15**(7):2564–9.
8. Bajorin DF, Dodd PM, Mazumdar M, *et al.* Long-term survival in metastatic transitional-cell carcinoma and prognostic factors predicting outcome of therapy. *J Clin Oncol* 1999; **17**(10):3173–81.
9. Bellmunt J, Albanell J, Paz-Ares L, *et al.* pretreatment prognostic factors for survival in patients with advanced urothelial tumors treated in a phase i/ii trial with paclitaxel, cisplatin, and gemcitabine. *Cancer* 2002; **95**(4):751–7.
10. Sternberg CN, Yagoda A, Scher HI, *et al.* M-VAC for advanced transitional cell carcinoma of the urothelium: Efficacy, and patterns of response and relapse. *Cancer* 1989; **64**:2448–58.
11. Logothetis CJ, Dexeus F, Finn L, *et al.* A prospective randomized trial comparing CISCA to MVAC chemotherapy in advanced metastastic urothelial tumors. *J Clin Oncol* 1990; **8**:1050–5.
12. Sternberg C, de Mulder P, van Oosterom AT, *et al.* Escalated M-VAC chemotherapy and recombinant human granulocyte macrophage colony stimulating factor (GM-CSF) in patients with advanced urothelial tract tumors. *Ann Oncol* 1993; **4**(5):403–7.
13. Loehrer PJ, Elson P, Dreicer R, *et al.* A phase I-II study: escalated dosages of methotrexate (M), vinblastine (V), doxorubicin (A), and cisplatin (C) plus rhG-CSF in advanced urothelial carcinoma: An ECOG trial. *Proc Amer Soc Clin Onc* 1992; **11**:201.
14. Logothetis C, Finn L, Amato R, Hossan E, Sella A. Escalated (ESC) MVAC +/- rhGM-CSF (Schering-Plough) in metastatic transitional cell carcinoma (TCC): Preliminary results of a randomized trial. *Proc Amer Soc Clin Onc* 1992; **11**:202.
15. Seidman AD, Scher HI, Gabrilove JL, *et al.* Dose-intensification of methotrexate, vinblastine, doxorubicin, and cisplatin with recombinant granulocyte-colony stimulating factor as initial therapy in advanced urothelial cancer. *J Clin Oncol* 1992; **11**:414–20.
16. Sternberg CN, de Mulder PHM, Schornagel JH, *et al.* Randomized phase iii trial of high dose intensity methotrexate, vinblastine, doxorubicin, and cisplatin (MVAC) chemotherapy and recombinant human granulocyte colony-stimulating factor versus classic MVAC in advanced urothelial tract tumors: European Organization for Research and Treatment of Cancer. Protocol No. 30924. *J Clin Oncol* 2001; **19**(10):2638–46.
17. Sternberg CN, de Mulder P, Schornagel JH, *et al.* Seven year update of an EORTC phase III trial of high dose intensity M-VAC chemotherapy and G-CSF versus classic M-VAC in advanced urothelial tract tumors (EORTC protocol 30924). *Eur J Cancer* 2006; **42**(1):50–4.
18. Sternberg CN. Gemcitabine in bladder cancer. *Sem Oncol* 2000; **27**(1) (Suppl 2):31–9.
19. Lorusso V, Pollera CF, Antimi M, *et al.* A phase II study of gemcitabine in patients with transitional cell carcinoma of the urinary tract previously treated with platinum. *Eur J Cancer* 1998; **34**(8):1208–12.
20. Moore MJ, Tannock IF, Ernst DS, Huan S, Murray N. Gemcitabine: a promising new agent in the treatment of advanced urothelial cancer. *J Clin Oncol* 1997; **15** (12):3441–5.
21. Stadler WM, Kuzel T, Roth B, Raghavan D, Dorr FA. Phase II study of single-agent gemcitabine in previously untreated patients with metastatic urothelial cancer. *J Clin Oncol* 1997; **15**(11):3394–8.
22. Gebbia V, Testa A, Borsellino N, *et al.* Single agent 2',2'-difluorodeoxycytidine in the treatment of metastatic urothelial carcinoma: a phase II study. *Clin Ter* 1999; **150**(1):11–5.
23. von der Maase H. Gemcitabine and cisplatin in locally advanced and/or metastatic blaccer cancer. *Eur J Cancer* 2000; **36**(Suppl 2):13–6.
24. Kaufman D, Raghavan D, Carducci M, *et al.* Phase II trial of gemcitabine (G) and paclitaxel (P) in patients with metastatic urothelial cancer. *J Clin Oncol* 2000; **18**(9):1921–7.
25. Lorusso V, Manzione L, De Vita F, Antimi M, Selvaggi FP, De Lena M. gemcitabine plus cisplatin for advanced transitional cell carcinoma of the urinary tract: a phase ii multicenter trial. *J Urol* 2000; **164**(1):53–6.
26. Moore MJ, Winquist EW, Murray N, *et al.* Gemcitabine plus cisplatin, an active regimen in advanced urothelial cancer: a phase ii trial of the national cancer institute of canada trials group. *J Clin Oncol* 1999; **17**(9):2876–81.
27. von der Maase H, Hansen SW, Roberts JT, *et al.* Gemcitabine and cisplatin versus methotrexate, vinblastine, doxorubicin, and cisplatin in advanced or metastatic bladder cancer: results of a large, randomized, multinational, multicenter, phase III study. *J Clin Oncol* 2000; **18**(17):3068–77.
28. von der Maase H, Sengelov L, Roberts JT, *et al.* Long-term survival results of a randomized trial comparing gemcitabine plus cisplatin, with methotrexate, vinblastine, doxorubicin, plus cisplatin in patients with bladder cancer. *J Clin Oncol* 2005; **23**(21):4602–8.
29. Bellmunt J, Guillem V, Paz-Ares L, *et al.* Phase I-II study of paclitaxel, cisplatin, and gemcitabine in advanced transitional-cell carcinoma of the urothelium. *J Clin Oncol* 2000; **18**(18):3247–55.
30. Bellmunt J, von der Maase H, Mead GM, *et al.* Randomized phase iii study comparing paclitaxel/cisplatin/ gemcitabine and gemcitabine/ cisplatin in patients with locally advanced or metastatic urothelial cancer without prior systemic therapy: EORTC Intergroup Study 30987. *J Clin Oncol* 2012; **30**(10):1107–13.
31. Bamias A, Aravantinos G, Deliveliotis C. Docetaxel and cisplatin with granulocyte colony-stimulating factor (G-CSF) versus M-VAC with G-CSF in advanced urothelial carcinoma: a multicenter, randomized, phase III study from the Hellenic Cooperative Oncology Group. *J Clin Oncol* 2004; **22**:220–8.
32. Bamias A, Dafni U, Karadimou A, *et al.* Prospective, open-label, randomized, phase III study of two dose-dense regimens MVAC versus gemcitabine/cisplatin in patients with inoperable, metastatic or relapsed urothelial cancer: a Hellenic Cooperative Oncology Group study (HE 16/03). *Ann Oncol* 2013; **24**(4):1011–7.
33. Petrioli R, Frediani B, Manganelli A, *et al.* Comparison between a cisplatin-containing regimen and a carboplatin-containing regimen for recurrent or metastatic cancer patients: A randomized phase II study. *Cancer* 1996; **77**:344–51.
34. Bellmunt J, Ribas A, Eres N, *et al.* Carboplatin-based versus cisplatin-based chemotherapy in the treatment of surgically incurable advanced bladder carcinoma. *Cancer* 1997; **80**:1966–72.
35. Dreicer R, Manola J, Roth BJ, *et al.* Phase III trial of methotrexate, vinblastine, doxorubicin, and cisplatin versus carboplatin and paclitaxel in patients with advanced carcinoma of the urothelium. *Cancer* 2004; **100**(8):1639–45.
36. Dogliotti L, Cartenì G, Siena S, *et al.* Gemcitabine plus cisplatin versus gemcitabine plus carboplatin as first-line chemotherapy in advanced transitional cell carcinoma of the urothelium: results of a randomized phase 2 trial. *Eur Urol* 2007; **52**(1):134–41.
37. Small EJ, Lew D, Redman BG, *et al.* Southwest oncology group study of paclitaxel and carboplatin for advanced transitional cell carcinoma: the importance of survival as a clinical trial end point. *J Clin Oncol* 2000; **18**(13):2537–44.

38. Redman BG, Smith DC, Flaherty L, Du W, Hussain M. Phase II trial of paclitaxel and carboplatin in the treatment of advanced urothelial carcinoma. *J Clin Oncol* 1998; **16**(5):1844–8.
39. Vaughn DJ, Malkowicz SB, Zoltick B, *et al.* Paclitaxel plus carboplatin in advanced carcinoma of the urothelium: an active and tolerable outpatient regiment. *J Clin Oncol* 1998; **16**(1):255–60.
40. Pycha A, Grbovic M, Posch B, *et al.* Paclitaxel and carboplatin in patients with metastatic transitional cell cancer of the urinary tract. *Urology* 1999; **53**(3):510–5.
41. Vaughn DJ, Manola J, Dreicer R, See W, Levitt R, Wilding G. Phase II study of paclitaxel plus carboplatin in patients with advanced carcinoma of the urothelium and renal dysfunction (E2896): a trial of the Eastern Cooperative Oncology Group. *Cancer* 2002; **95**(5):1022–7.
42. Galsky MD, Chen GJ, Oh WK, *et al.* Comparative effectiveness of cisplatin-based and carboplatin-based chemotherapy for treatment of advanced urothelial carcinoma. *Ann Oncol* 2012; **23**(2):406–10.
43. Dodd PM, McCaffrey JA, Hilton S, *et al.* Phase I evaluation of sequential doxorubicin gemcitabine then ifosfamide paclitaxel cisplatin for patients with unresectable or metastatic transitional cell carcinoma of the urothelial tract. *J Clin Oncol* 2000; **18**(4):840–6.
44. Maluf FC, Hilton S, Nanus DM, *et al.* Sequential doxorubicin/gemcitabine (AG) and ifosfamide, paclitaxel and cisplatin (ITP) chemotherapy (AG-ITP) in patients (Pts) with metastatic or locally advanced transitional cell carcinoma of the urothelium (TCC). *Proc Am Soc Clin Oncol* 2000;**19**:342a.
45. MIlowsky MI, Nanus DM, Maluf FC, *et al.* Final results of sequential doxorubicin plus gemcitabine and ifosfamide, paclitaxel and cisplatin chemotherapy in patients with metastatic or locally advanced transitional cell carcinoma of the urothelium. *J Clin Oncol* 2009; **27**(25):4062–7.
46. Galsky MD, Iasonos A, Mironov S, Scattergood J, Boyle MG, Bajorin DF. Phase II trial of dose-dense doxorubicin plus gemcitabine followed by paclitaxel plus carboplatin in patients with advanced urothelial carcinoma and impaired renal function. *Cancer* 2007; **109**(3):549–55.
47. Artz A, Stadler WM, Vogelzang NJ, Zimmerman T, Ryan C. A phase II trial of sequential chemotherapy with docetaxel and methotrexate followed by gemcitabine and cisplatin for metastatic urothelial cancer. *Am J Clin Oncol* 2005; **28**(2):109–13.
48. Rothenberg ML, Sharma A, Weiss GR, *et al.* Phase I trial of paclitaxel and gemcitabine administered every two weeks in patients with refractory solid tumors. *Ann Oncol* 1998; **9**(7):733–8.
49. Sternberg CN, Calabrò F, Pizzocaro G, Marini L, Schnetzer S, Sella A. Chemotherapy with every-2-week gemcitabine and paclitaxel in patients with transitional cell carcinoma who have received prior cisplatin-based therapy. *Cancer* 2001; **92**(12):2993–8.
50. Fechner GH, Siener R, Reimann M, *et al.* Randomized phase II trial of gemcitabine and paclitaxel with or without maintenance treatment in patients with cisplatin refractory transitional cell carcinoma. *J Urol* 2002; **167**(4 Suppl):284.
51. Meluch AA, Greco FA, Burris HA, *et al.* Paclitaxel and gemcitabine chemotherapy for adanced transitional-cell carcinoma of the urothelial tract: a Phase II trial of the Minnie Pearl Cancer Research Network. *J Clin Oncol* 2001; **19**(12):3018–24.
52. Calabrò F, Lorusso V, Rosati G, *et al.* Gemcitabine and paclitaxel every 2 weeks in patients with previously untreated urothelial carcinoma. *Cancer* 2009; **115**(12):2652–9.
53. Gitlitz BJ, Baker C, Chapman Y, *et al.* A phase II study of gemcitabine and docetaxel therapy in patients with advanced urothelial carcinoma. *Cancer* 2003; **98**(9):1863–9.
54. Linardou H, Aravantinos G, Efstathiou E, *et al.* Gemcitabine and carboplatin combination as first-line treatment in elderly patients and those unfit for cisplatin-based chemotherapy with advanced bladder carcinoma: Phase II study of the Hellenic Co-operative Oncology Group. *Urology* 2004; **64**(3):479–84.
55. Bellmunt J, de Wit R, Albanell J, Baselga J. A feasibility study of carboplatin with fixed dose of gemcitabine in 'unfit' patients with advanced bladder cancer. *Eur J Cancer* 2001; **37**(17):2212–5.
56. Galsky MD, Hahn NM, Rosenberg JE, *et al.* Treatment of patients with metastatic urothelial cancer "unfit" for cisplatin-based chemotherapy. *J Clin Oncol* 2011; **29**(17):2432–8.
57. Carles J, Nogue M, Domenech M, *et al.* Carboplatin-gemcitabine treatment of patients with transitional cell carcinoma of the bladder and impaired renal function. *Oncology* 2000; **59**(1):24–7.
58. De Santis M, Bellmunt J, Mead G, *et al.* Randomized phase II/III trial assessing gemcitabine/carboplatin and methotrexate/carboplatin/vinblastine in patients with advanced urothelial cancer who are unfit for cisplatin-based chemotherapy: EORTC study 30986. *J Clin Oncol* 2012; **30**(2):191–9.
59. Morales-Barrera R, Bellmunt J, Suarez C, Valverde C, Guix M, Serrano C. Cisplatin and gemcitabine administered every two weeks in patients with locally advanced or metastatic urothelial carcinoma and impaired renal function. *Eur J Cancer* 2012; **48**(12):1816–21.
60. Bellmunt J, Chow WH, Fougeray R, *et al.* Prognostic factors in patients with advanced transitional cell carcinoma of the urothelial tract experiencing treatment failure with platinum-containing regimens. *J Clin Oncol* 2010; **28**(11):1850–5.
61. Vaughn DJ, Broome CM, Hussain M, Gutheil JC, Markowitz AB. Phase II trial of weekly paclitaxel in patients with previously treated advanced urothelial cancer. *J Clin Oncol* 2002; **20**(4):937–40.
62. Sweeney CJ, Roth BJ, Kabbinavar FF, *et al.* Phase II study of pemetrexed for second-line treatment of transitional cell cancer of the urothelium. *J Clin Oncol* 2006; **24**(21):3451–7.
63. Witte RS, Elson P, Bono B, *et al.* Eastern Cooperative Group phase II trial of ifosfamide in the treatment of previously treated advanced urothelial carcinoma. *J Clin Oncol* 1997; **15**(2):589–93.
64. Galsky MD, Mironov S, Iasonos A, Scattergood J, Boyle MG, Bajorin DF. Phase II trial of pemetrexed as second-line therapy in patients with metastatic urothelial carcinoma. *Invest New Drugs* 2007; **25**(3):265–70.
65. Pectasides D, Aravantinos G, Kalofonos H, *et al.* Combination chemotherapy with gemcitabine and ifosfamide as second-line treatment in metastatic urothelial cancer. A phase II trial conducted by the Hellenic Cooperative Oncology Group. *Ann Oncol* 2001; **12**(10):1417–22.
66. Kattan J, Culine S, Theodore C, Droz JP. Second-line M-VAC therapy in patients previously treated with the M-VAC regimen for metastatic urothelial cancer. *Ann Oncol* 1993; **4**(9):793–4.
67. Bennouna J, Fumoleau P, Armand JP, *et al.* Phase I and pharmacokinetic study of the new vinca alkaloid vinflunine administered as a 10-min infusion every 3 weeks in patients with advanced solid tumours. *Ann Oncol* 2003; **14**(4):630–7.
68. Delord JP, Stupp R, Pinel M, Nguyen L, Vermorken J. Phase I study of Vinflunine given as a 10 minute intravenous infusion on a weekly schedule in patients with advanced solid tumours. *Proc Annu Meet Am Soc Clin Oncol* 2001; **20**:111a.
69. Johnson P, Geldart T, Fumoleau P, Pinel MC, Nguyen L, Judson I. Phase I study of vinflunine administered as a 10-minute infusion on days 1 and 8 every 3 weeks. I*nvest New Drugs* 2006; **24**(3):223–31.
70. Culine S, Theodore C, De Santis M, *et al.* A phase II study of vinflunine in bladder cancer patients progressing after first-line platinum-containing regimen. *Br J Cancer* 2006; **94**(10):1395–401.
71. Bellmunt Molins J, von der Maase H, Theodore C, *et al.* Phase III trial of vinflunine plus best supportive care compared with best supportive care alone after a platinum-containing regimen in patients with advanced transitional cell carcinoma of the urothelial tract. *J Clin Oncol* 2009; **27**(27):4454–61.
72. Bellmunt J, Paz-Ares L, Cuello M, *et al.* Gene expression of ERCC1 as a novel prognostic marker in advanced bladder cancer patients receiving cisplatin-based chemotherapy. *Ann Oncol* 2007; **18**(3):522–8.
73. Guix M, Lema L, Lloreta J, *et al.* Excision repair cross-complementing 1 (ERCC1) and survival in advanced bladder cancer: Confirmatory results using immunohistochemistry. *Proc Annu Meet Am Soc Clin Oncol* 2009; **27**(15s).

74. Font A, Taron M, Gago JL, *et al.* BRCA1 mRNA expression and outcome to neoadjuvant cisplatin-based chemotherapy in bladder cancer. *Ann Oncol* 2011; **22**(1):139–44.
75. Tada Y, Wada M, Kuroiwa K, *et al.* MDR1 gene overexpression and altered degree of methylation at the promoter region in bladder cancer during chemotherapeutic treatment. *Clin Cancer Res* 2000; **6**(12):4618–27.
76. Hoffmann AC, Wild P, Leicht C, *et al.* MDR1 and ERCC1 expression predict outcome of patients with locally advanced bladder cancer receiving adjuvant chemotherapy. *Neoplasia* 2010; **12**:628–36.
77. Takata R, Katagiri T, Kanehira M, *et al.* Predicting response to methotrexate, vinblastine, doxorubicin, and cisplatin neoadjuvant chemotherapy for bladder cancers through genome-wide gene expression profiling. *Clin Cancer Res* 2005; **11**:2625–36.
78. Takata R, Katagiri T, Kanehira M, *et al.* Validation study of the prediction system for clinical response of M-VAC neoadjuvant chemotherapy. *Cancer Sci* 2007; **98**(1):113–7.
79. Lee JK, Havaleshko DM, Cho H, *et al.* A strategy for predicting the chemosensitivity of human cancers and its application to drug discovery. *Proc Natl Acad Sci U S A* 2007; **104**:13086–91.
80. Williams PD, Cheon S, Havaleshko DM, *et al.* Concordant gene expression signatures predict clinical outcomes of cancer patients undergoing systemic therapy. *Cancer Res* 2009; **69**(21):8302–9.
81. Iyer G, Hanrahan AJ, MIlowsky MI, *et al.* Genome sequencing identifies a basis for everolimus sensitivity. *Science* 2012; **338**(6104):221.
82. Hahn NM, Stadler WM, Zon RT, *et al.* Phase II trial of cisplatin, gemcitabine, and bevacizumab as first-line therapy for metastatic urothelial carcinoma: Hoosier Oncology Group GU 04–75. *J Clin Oncol* 2011; **29**(12):1525–30.
83. Sridhar SS, Winquist E, Eisen A, *et al.* A phase II trial of sorafenib in first-line metastatic urothelial cancer: a study of the PMH Phase II Consortium. *Invest New Drugs* 2011; **29**(5):1045–9.
84. Dreicer R, Li H, Stein M, *et al.* Phase II trial of sorafenib in patients with advanced urothelium cancer: A trial of the Eastern Cooperative Oncology Group. *Cancer* 2009; **115**(18):4090–5.
85. Gallagher DJ, MIlowsky MI, Gerst SR, *et al.* Phase II study of sunitinib in patients with metastatic urothelial cancer. *J Clin Oncol* 2010; **28**(8):1373–9.
86. Bellmunt J, Maroto P, Mellado B, *et al.* Phase II study of sunitinib as first line treatment in patients with advanced urothelial cancer ineligible for cisplatin-based chemotherapy. Genitourinary Cancer Symposium, 2008.
87. Grivas P, Nanus DM, Stadler WM, *et al.* Randomized phase II trial of maintenance sunitinib versus placebo following response to chemotherapy (CT) for patients (pts) with advanced urothelial carcinoma (UC). Genitourinary Cancer Symposium. *J Clin Oncol* 2012; **30**(Suppl 5; abstr 265).
88. Galsky MD, Hahn NM, Powles T, Hellerstedt BA, Lerner SP, Gardner TA. Gemcitabine, cisplatin and sunitinib for metastatic urothelial carcinoma and as preoperative therapy for muscle-invasive bladder cancer. *Clin Genitourin Cancer* 2013; **11**(2):175–81.
89. Necchi A, Mariani L, Zaffaroni N, *et al.* Pazopanib in advanced and platinum-resistant urothelial cancer: an open-label, single group, phase 2 trial. *Lancet Oncol* 2012; **13**(8):810–6.
90. Morabito A, Piccirillo MC, Falasconi F, *et al.* Vandetanib (ZD6474), a dual inhibitor of vascular endothelial growth factor receptor (VEGFR) and epidermal growth factor receptor (EGFR) tyrosine kinases: current status and future directions. *Oncologist* 2009; **14**(4):378–90.
91. Choueiri TK, Ross RW, Jacobus S, *et al.* Double-blind, randomized trial of docetaxel plus vandetanib versus docetaxel plus placebo in platinum-pretreated metastatic urothelial cancer. *J Clin Oncol* 2012; **30**(5):507–12.
92. Petrylak DP, Tangen CM, Van Veldhuizen PJ Jr, *et al.* Results of the Southwest Oncology Group phase II evaluation (study S0031) of ZD1839 for advanced transitional cell carcinoma of the urothelium. *BJU Int* 2010; **105**(3):317–21.
93. Philips G, Halabi S, Sanford BL, Bajorin D, Small EJ, Cancer and Leukemia Group B. A Phase II trial of cisplatin (C), gemcitabine (G) and gefitinib for advanced urothelial carcinoma: Results of Cancer and Luekemia Group B (CALGB) 90102. *Ann Oncol* 2009; **10**(6):1074–9.
94. Chaux A, Cohen JS, Schultz L, *et al.* High epidermal growth factor receptor immunohistochemical expression in urothelial carcinoma of the bladder is not associated with EGFR mutations in exons 19 and 21: a study using formalin-fixed, paraffin-embedded archival tissues. *Hum Pathol* 2012; **43**(10):1590–5.
95. Hussain MH, MacVicar GR, Petrylak DP, *et al.* Trastuzumab, paclitaxel, carboplatin, and gemcitabine in advanced human epidermal growth factor receptor-2/neu-positive urothelial carcinoma: results of a multicenter phase II National Cancer Institute trial. *J Clin Oncol* 2007; **25**(16):2118–24.
96. Wuelfing C, Machiels J, Richel D, *et al.* A single arm, multicenter, open label, phase II study of lapatinib as second-line treatment of pts with locally advanced or metastatic transitional cell carcinoma. *Cancer* 2009; **115**(13):2881–90.
97. Neal DE, Sharples L, Smith K, Fennelly J, Hall RR, Harris AL. The epidermal growth factor receptor and the prognosis of bladder cancer. *Cancer* 1990; **65**(7):1619–25.
98. Quinn DI, Aparicio A, Tsao-Wei DD, *et al.* Phase II study of eribulin (E7389) in patients (pts) with advanced urothelial cancer (UC)-Final report: A California Cancer Consortium-led NCI/CTEP-sponsored trial. *J Clin Oncol* 2010; **28**(15s) (Suppl; abstr 4539).
99. Vogelzang NJ, Conkling P, Duran I, *et al.* Phase Ib/II study of eribulin mesylate administered in combination with gemcitabine/cisplatin as first-line therapy for locally advanced or metastatic bladder cancer: Phase Ib results. *J Clin Oncol* 2012; **30**(Suppl 5; abstr 273).
100. Sridhar SS, Canil CM, Mukherjee SD, *et al.* A phase II study of single-agent nab-paclitaxel as second-line therapy in patients with metastatic urothelial carcinoma. Genitourinary Cancer Symposium, 2010. *J Clin Oncol* 2010; **28**(15):TPS231.
101. Rosenberg JE, Hoffman-Censits J, Powles T, *et al.* Atezolizumab in patients with locally advanced and metastatic urothelial carcinoma who have progressed following treatment with platinum-based chemotherapy: a single-arm, multicentre, phase 2 trial. *Lancet* 2016; **387**(10031):1909–20.
102. Balar AV, Galsky MD, Rosenberg JE, *et al.* Atezolizumab as first-line treatment in cisplatin-ineligible patients with locally advanced and metastatic urothelial carcinoma: a single-arm, multicentre, phase 2 trial. *Lancet* 2016; **387**(10031):1909–20.
103. Sharma P, Callahan MK, Bono P, *et al.* Nivolumab monotherapy in recurrent metastatic urothelial carcinoma (CheckMate 032): a multicentre, open-label, two-stage, multi-arm, phase 1/2 trial. *Lancet Oncol* 2017; **17**(11):1590–8.
104. Galsky MD, Retz M, Siefker-Radtke AO, *et al.* Efficacy and safety of nivolumab monotherapy in patients with metastatic urothelial cancer (mUC) who have received prior treatment: Results from the phase II CheckMate 275 study. *Ann Oncol* 2016; **27**(Suppl 6) (LBA31):vi552–87.
105. Bellmunt J, de Wit R, Vaughn DJ, *et al.* A Phase III Randomized Clinical Trial of Pembrolizumab (MK-3475) Versus Paclitaxel, Docetaxel or Vinflunine in Subjects With Recurrent or Progressive Metastatic Urothelial Cancer (KEYNOTE-045; NCT02256436). Society of Immunotherapy of Cancer (SITC 2016) meeting at National Harbor, MD. 9–13 November 2016.
106. Balar A, Bellmunt J, O'Donnell PH, *et al.* Pembrolizumab (pembro) as first-line therapy for advanced/unresectable or metastatic urothelial cancer: Preliminary results from the phase 2 KEYNOTE-052 study. *Ann Oncol* 2016; **27**(Suppl 6)(LBA32):vi552–87.

CHAPTER 6.23

Squamous cell bladder cancer

Roman Mayr and Maximilian Burger

Introduction to squamous cell bladder cancer

In the developed countries, over 90% of all bladder cancer cases are urothelial carcinomas, with squamous cell carcinoma (SCC), adenocarcinomas, and rare types of bladder cancer comprising the remaining 10% of bladder cancer cases.[1] In Western regions pure SCC of the bladder constitutes 1.2–4.5% of all bladder tumours.[2–5] SCC can occur in both non-bilharzial and bilharzial bladders; the two subtypes differ in epidemiology, pathogenesis, and clinical outcome. SCC in the bilharzial bladder is an endemic disease in many regions of the Middle East, Africa, Southeast Asia, and South America. The highest incidence of schistosomiasis-associated bladder cancer in men is observed in Egypt (19/100.000).[6] In an Egyptian radical cystectomy series, SCC represented 59% of all specimens.[7] The non-bilharzial type occurs in the developed countries and represents less than 5% of all bladder tumours; it occurs most often in the seventh decade of life, where patients usually present with painless haematuria, with no previous history of bladder cancer. The knowledge of SCC of the bladder is nevertheless important due to different aetiology, clinical pathways, and clinical outcome.

Histophathology

Keratinization and/or intercellular bridges are classical morphological features found in squamous differentiation. SCC of the bladder is defined as a malignant neoplasm derived from the urothelium that shows a pure squamous cell phenotype[8–10] (see Fig. 6.23.1). When urothelial elements (including urothelial carcinoma *in situ*) are present, the tumour should be classified as urothelial carcinoma with squamous differentiation. The diagnosis of SCC is reserved for bladder cancers that are composed of entirely keratin-forming carcinoma cells.[11] Keratinizing squamous metaplasia may be present in the adjacent epithelium in cases of SCC of the bladder and frequently shows the full spectrum of dysplastic lesion and/or carcinoma *in situ*.[8] Invasive SCC of the bladder displays a range of differentiation, from well differentiated to poorly differentiated, with a histologic spectrum that can vary from well-defined islands of squamous cells with keratinization, prominent intercellular bridges, and minimal nuclear pleomorphism, to tumours exhibiting marked nuclear pleomorphism and only focal evidence of squamous differentiation. The histological grading is based on the amount of keratinization and the degree of nuclear pleomorphism using a

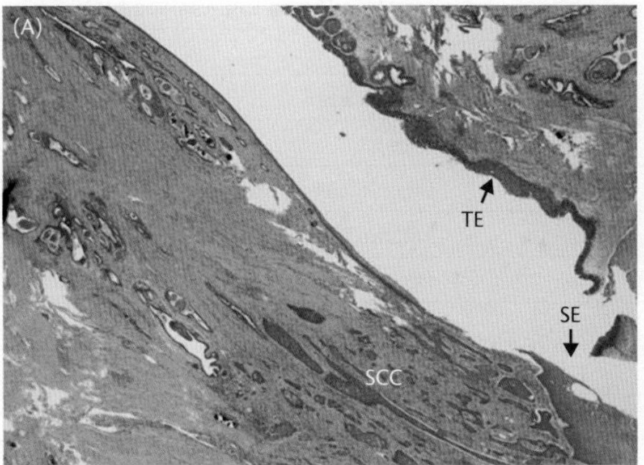

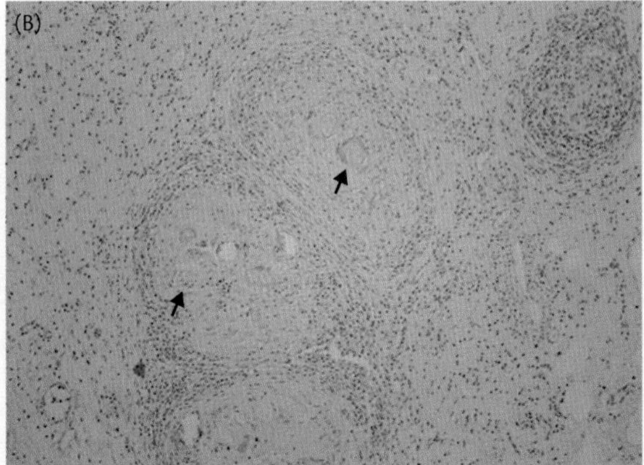

Fig. 6.23.1 Histological slides of non-bilharzial squamous cell carcinom (A) and bilharziosis of the bladder (B). Non-bilharzial squamous cell carcinoma of the bladder (A): squamous epithelial (SE) and transition epithelial (TE) are visualized with black arrows. Invasive squamous cell carcinoma (SCC) infiltrating the subconective tissue. Bladder bilharziasis (B): histological photographs of a bladder with S. hematobium infection, showing calcified parasite eggs (arrow) sorrounded by granulomas.

Reproduced with kind permission of Dr Reinhard Kluge and Dr Esther Hanspeter, Department of Pathology, and Chairman, Dr Guido Mazzoleni, Central Hospital of Bolzano, Italy.

three-tiered system (Grade 1–3).[9,12] About 20% of urothelial carcinomas contain areas of squamous or glandular differentiation. Its frequency depends on stage and grade. Tumours with any identifiable urothelial element are classified as urothelial carcinoma with squamous differentiation, and an estimate of the percentage of squamous component should be provided. However, recognition of squamous differentiation in a non-keratinizing or poorly differentiated invasive carcinoma is often difficult. Immunohistochemistry using CK14, Mac 387, and CK20 may help. Urothelial carcinoma is typically CK20 positive and is negative for CK 14 and Mac 387.[13–15] Areas showing squamous differentiation, both keratinizing and non-keratinizing, are typically CK14 positive, Mac387 positive, and negative for CK20.

Aetiology

SCC can occur in both non-bilharzial and bilharzial bladders. These two subtypes differ in epidemiology, pathogenesis, and clinicopathological features. Differences of the characteristics associated with non-bilharzial and bilharzial SCC are listed in Table 6.23.1.[16]

Bilharzial squamous cell bladder cancer

Bilharziasis is an endemic disease in many regions of the Middle East, Africa, Southeast Asia, and South America, secondary to schistosomiasis. Schistosomes have a typical trematode vertebrate-invertebrate lifecycle, with humans being the definitive host (see Fig. 6.23.2). Globally, an estimated 207 million people are currently infected, and more than 90% of them live in Africa. The highest incidence of the bilharzial bladder is in Egypt. Moreover, an estimated 700 million people are at risk with an annual death of about 20,000 people.[17,18] The mean age of patients affected from bilharzial cancer is 10–20 years lower than in non-bilharzial cancer.[19] The latency period between initial infestation with bilharziasis and the subsequent development of bladder cancer is about 30 years. A male predominance is observed, probably due to the increased exposure of males to schistosome infestation from work within infested fields.[20]

The aetiology of bladder carcinogenesis is probably related to bacterial and viral infections, commonly associated with bilharzial infestation, rather than the parasite itself.[21] Urinary bacteria have a double action: (a) the secretion of ß-glucoronidase enzyme which may clear conjugated carcinogens, yielding free carcinogenic product; and (b) the production of carcinogenic nitrosamines from their precursors in urine.[22] HPV may play a role in the carcinogenesis as it was detected in nearly a quarter of cases of bilharzial bladder SCC.[22] The possibility of carcinogenic product of parasite origin is not supported.[22] However, local mechanical irritation by schistosome eggs appears to be an important promoting factor.[22]

Non-bilharzial squamous cell bladder cancer

In Western regions pure SCC of the bladder constitutes of 1.2–4.5% of all vescical tumours.[2–5,23] The tumour is usually diagnosed in the seventh decade of live with a slight male predominance. Whites show a lower incidence compared to black patients, even in the presence of the same environmental factors. In Western countries SCC is usually diagnosed in patients with prolonged indwelling catheters.[24,25] An incidence of nearly 10% for SCC of the bladder in patients with a catheter indwelling for ≥10 years has been described.[26] Inflammation from chronic urinary tract irritation, either from bacterial infections, foreign bodies, bladder calculi, or chronic bladder outlet obstruction have been implicated in the pathogenesis of SCC.[27] Many of these factors are

Table 6.23.1 Comparison between non-bilharzial and bilharzial SCC of the bladder

Feature	Non-bilharzial	Bilharzial
Geographical distribution	Western countries	East, Africa, South-East Asia, South America
% of all bladder tumours	1.2–4.5%	59%
Age	Seventh decade	Fifth decade
Gender predominance	Slightly more male	Male 5:1
Risk factors	Prolonged catheterization, chronic UTI	Chronic infections associated with bilharzial infestation
Principal symptom	Haematuria	Irritative bladder
Cystoscopic findings	Lower vescical hemisphere	Upper vescical hemisphere
Tumour shape	Ulcerative	Nodular
Pathology		
Stage	Mostly advanced	Mostly advanced
Grade	High grade	Low to moderate
Lymphnode-disease	8–10%	18.7%
Treatment of choice	Radical cystectomy	Radical cystectomy
General prognosis	Poor	Good
Prevention	Avoid prolonged indwelling catheterization, early detection	Eliminate and treat bilharzias, early detection

Adapted with permission from A.A. Shokeir, 'Squamous cell carcinoma of the bladder: pathology, diagnosis and treatment', *BJU International*, Volume 96, Issue 2, pp. 216–20, Copyright © 2003 John Wiley and Sons.

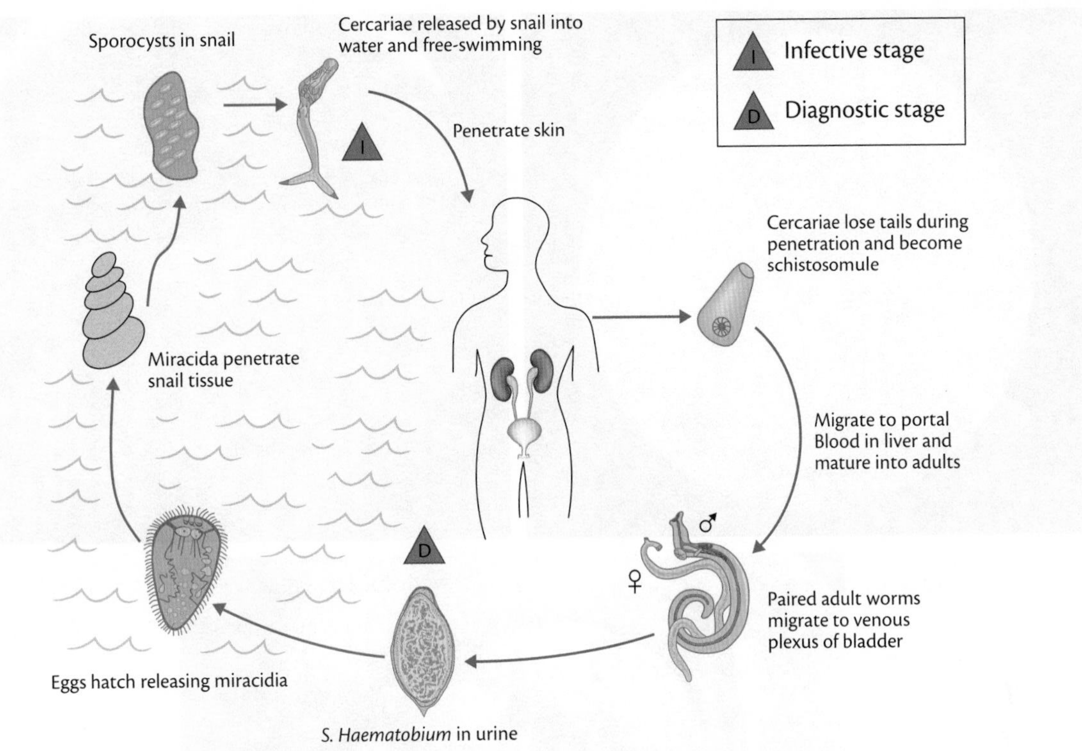

Fig. 6.23.2 Lifecycle of *S. Haematobium.*
Reproduced from Centers for Disease Control and Prevention, *Parasites – Schistosomiasis*, DPDx, November 2012, available from http://www.cdc.gov/parasites/schistosomiasis/biology.html

present in patients with spinal cord injury and long-term indwelling catheters.

Diagnosis and prognostic factors

SCC in the bilharzial bladder is a distinct clinical and pathological entity and different from the entity in the Western world.[16] The classic presentation of bilharzial bladder cancer is characterized by symptoms of cystitis, painful micturition, frequency, and haematuria. Urographic examinations reveal an extensive irregular filling defect in the cystographic phase.[28] The diagnostic work up depends on cystoscopy (see Fig. 6.23.3), transurethral bladder biopsies, and carful bimanual examination under anaesthesia.[29] Eighty per cent of patients affected from bilharzial bladder cancer present with at least pT3 tumour stage.[30] In non-bilharzial SCC of the bladder haematuria is the principal symptom in 63–100% of patients, irritative bladder symptoms occur in 33–67% and in 35% there is weight loss, back, or pelvic pain or frank obstructive symptoms, all of which are suggestive of advanced disease.[3,4,8] A concomitant urinary tract infection is present in 93% of patients at diagnosis.[3] In non-bilharzial bladder cancer a toumor stage ≥pT3 is found in 90% of patients at presentation.[31] At cystoscopy most of the tumours are solitary, extensive and associated with leukoplakia (see Fig. 6.23.3B). The localization of the tumour in the bladder is variable but there is a predilection for the trigone and lateral walls. Macroscopically tumours are ulcerating and infiltrating but rarely papillary (see Fig. 6.23.3C). The tumour may occupy a diverticulum and may also associate with bladder stones.[3,4] For urine cytology a low sensitivity of 44% and a specificity of 91.3% for the detection of bladder cancer in a group with a significant proportion of patients with SCC have been described.[32] However, in the same study, NMP22 had a superior sensitivity (85%) and a high specificity (100%). SCC of the non-bilharzial bladder has a low incidence (8–10%) of distant metastasis.[33] However, the prognosis of SCC of the bladder is discouraging because most of the patients present with advanced disease and die from locoregional recurrence.[31] About 90% of deaths from SCC are cause by locoregional recurrence within three years. In contrast, in urothelial carcinoma the cause of death is much more often caused by metastasis. Because urothelial carcinoma of the bladder frequently develops focal squamous differentiation, it is important to differentiate SCC from urothelial carcinoma with squamous differentiation. Because the findings on a small biopsy sometimes may not represent the entire pathological spectrum of the tumour, SCC should not be diagnosed solely on a small bladder biopsy. Extensive transurethral resection of the bladder is needed for a decent diagnostic workup. Lymphovascular invasion has been shown to be an independent predictor of cancer-specific mortality, but not for disease recurrence in SCC of the bladder after radical cystectomy.[34] Lymphonadal disease at radical cystectomy was not independently associated with disease recurrence, nor cancer-specific survival. However, a prognostic marker score (COX-2, p53, Caspase, and BAX) has been shown to predict disease-free survival and cancer-specific survival. These patients could benefit from a multimodal therapy.[34]

Therapy and follow-up

The majority of patients with non-bilharzial SCC typically present with a poorly differentiated, muscle-invasive tumour with no previous

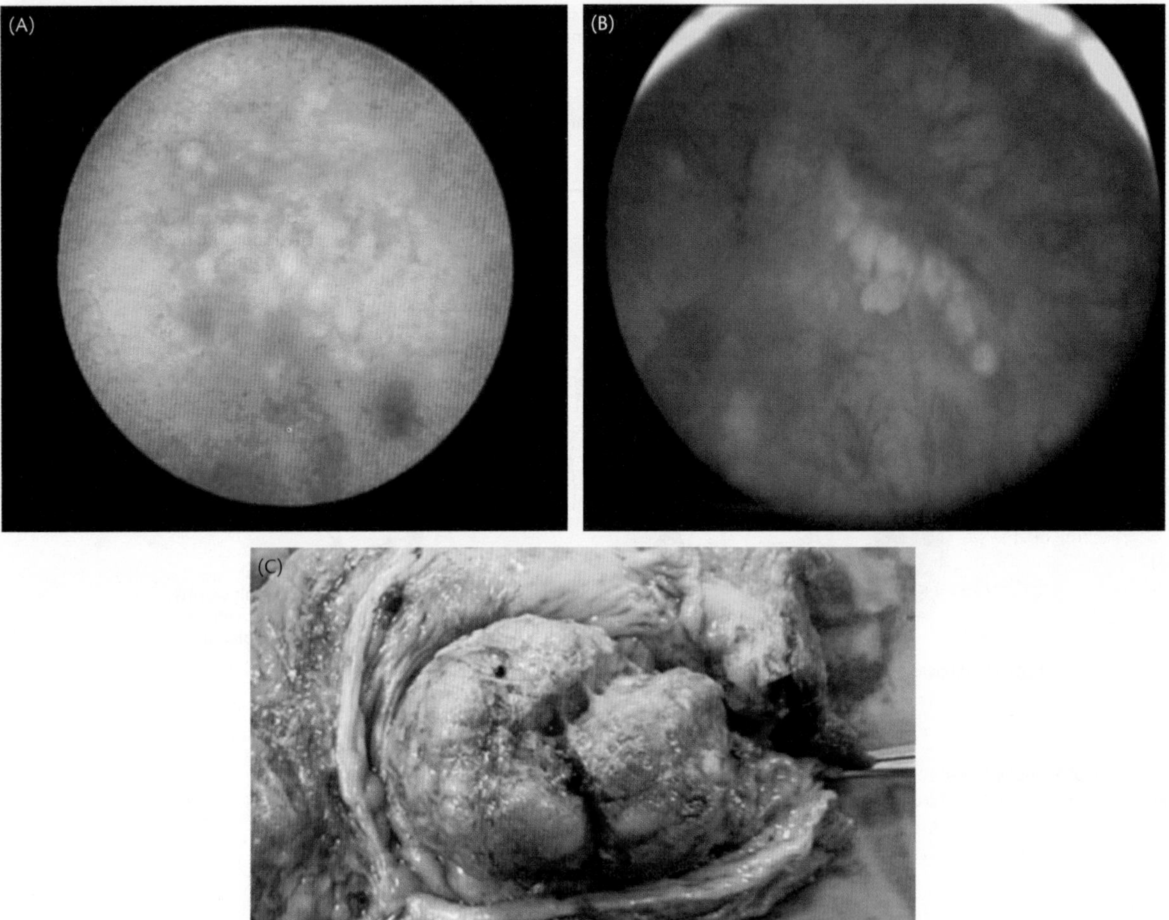

Fig. 6.23.3 Bilharziasis of the bladder. (A) Cystoscopy: active bilharziosis of the bladder; (B) cystoscopic view of leukoplakia patches, these lesions are precancerous to SCC; and (C) operative specimen of bulky squamous cell carcinoma of the bladder.

(A) Reproduced form Springer, *Endoskopische Urologie Atlas und Lehrbuch*, R. Hofmann (Hrsg.), Copyright © Springer Medizin Verlag Heidelberg 2009. With kind permission of Springer Science+Business Media; (B) and (C) Reproduced from Springer, *World Journal of Urology*, Volume 30, Issue 1, 2012, pp. 31–8, Khalaf I., Urologic complications of genitourinary schistosomiasis. With kind permission from Springer Science and Business Media.

history of urothelial carcinoma.[4] The gold standard therapy for muscle-invasive bladder cancer remains radical cystectomy with pelvic lymph node dissection and consecutive urinary diversion.[35,36] At the time of radical cystectomy the rate of non-organ confined disease was higher in SCC patients compared to their urothelial carcinoma counterparts, who underwent radical cystectomy.[37] In a single centre report of 27 cases nearly a quarter of the patients were not eligible for immediate surgery, however a downstaging with consecutive radical cystectomy with neoadjuvant therapies had no success.[31] A recent retrospective study involving 12.311 patients from the SEER database showed that patients with non-bilharzial SCC harbour a more advanced disease at radical cystectomy than patients with urothelial carcinoma.[37] However, cancer-specific mortality rates did not differ in these two subgroups after adjusting for tumour stage.[37] Another retrospective study showed that SCC was more aggressive than urothelial carcinoma in patients with non-organ confined disease.[38] There is no evidence of different cancer-specific survival or overall survival in patients with SCC and those with squamous diffentiation treated with radical cystectomy.[39] However, surgical resection is critical to achive local tumour control and improves survival in patients with SCC.

The standard treatment for metastatic urothelial cancer of the bladder is the gemcitabine/cisplatin chemotherapeutic regimen.[40] Urothelial carcinoma with squamous differentiation and pure SCC of the bladder are treated with the same regimen as the pure urothelial carcinoma of the bladder. The response rates of pure SCC of the bladder are less favourable to platinum-based chemotherapy when compared to urothelial carcinoma with squamous differentiation and urothelial carcinoma of the bladder (27%, 34%, and 44%).[41] Advanced or metastatic pure SCC may also respond less favourably to platinum-based chemotherapy, but overall survival of these patients is similar to patients with urothelial carcinoma of the bladder.[41]

The two-year overall survival rate of non-bilharzial SCC was reported to be 48% and recurrence-free survival rate 33% in a single centre report of 27 patients.[31] Patients who survived underwent radical cystectomy.[3,5,31,33,42,43] Survival depends on local disease expansion, which is in contrast to the urothelial carcinoma of the bladder where the main cause of death is systemic recurrence.[31]

Follow-up strategies in patients affected from SCC of the bladder do not much differ from strategies applied in patients suffering from urothelial carcinoma. Important in SCC patients is the locoregional control of the disease, which is the main cause of death in these patients.

Further reading

Bichler KH, Savatovsky I; Members of the Urinary Tract Infection (UTI) Working Group of the Guidelines Office of the European Association of Urology (EAU), *et al.* EAU guidelines for the management of urogenital schistosomiasis. *Eur Urol* 2006; **49**(6):998–1003.

Ehdaie B, Maschino A, Shariat SF, *et al.* Comparative outcomes of pure squamous cell carcinoma and urothelial carcinoma with squamous differentiation in patients treated with radical cystectomy. *J Urol* 2012; **187**(1):74–9.

Kassouf W, Spiess PE, Siefker-Radtke A, *et al.* Outcome and patterns of recurrence of nonbilharzial pure squamous cell carcinoma of the bladder: a contemporary review of The University of Texas M D Anderson Cancer Center experience. *Cancer* 2007; **110**(4):764–9.

Khalaf I, Shokeir A, Shalaby M. Urologic complications of genitourinary schistosomiasis. *World J Urol* 2012; **30**(1):31–8.

Lagwinski N, Thomas A, Stephenson AJ, *et al.* Squamous cell carcinoma of the bladder: a clinicopathologic analysis of 45 cases. *Am J Surg Pathol* 2007; **31**(12):1777–87.

Michaud DS. Chronic inflammation and bladder cancer. *Urol Oncol* 2007; **25**(3):260–8.

Rogers CG, Palapattu GS, Shariat SF, *et al.* Clinical outcomes following radical cystectomy for primary nontransitional cell carcinoma of the bladder compared to transitional cell carcinoma of the bladder. *J Urol* 2006; **175**(6):2048–53; discussion 2053.

Salem HK, Mahfouz S. Changing patterns (age, incidence, and pathologic types) of schistosoma-associated bladder cancer in egypt in the past decade. *Urology* 2012; **79**(2):379–83.

Shanks JH, Iczkowski KA. Divergent differentiation in urothelial carcinoma and other bladder cancer subtypes with selected mimics, *Histopathology* 2009; **54**(7):885–900.

Shokeir AA. Squamous cell carcinoma of the bladder: pathology, diagnosis and treatment. *BJU Int* 2004; **93**(2):216–20.

Youssef R, Kapur P, Shariat SF, *et al.* Prognostic value of apoptotic markers in squamous cell carcinoma of the urinary bladder. *BJU Int* 2012; **110**(7):961–6.

References

1. Lynch CF, Cohen MB. Urinary system. *Cancer* 1995; **75**(1 Suppl):316–29.
2. Miller A, Mitchell JP, Brown NJ. The Bristol bladder tumour registry. *Br J Urol* 1969; **41**(Suppl):1–64.
3. Johnson DE, Schoenwald MB, Ayala AG, Miller LS. Squamous cell carcinoma of the bladder. *J Urol* 1976; **115**(5):542–4.
4. Rundle JS, Hart AJ, McGeorge A, Smith JS, Malcolm AJ, Smith PM. Squamous cell carcinoma of bladder. A review of 114 patients. *Br J Urol* 1982; **54**(5):522–6.
5. Serretta V, Pomara G, Piazza F, Gange E. Pure squamous cell carcinoma of the bladder in western countries. Report on 19 consecutive cases. *Eur Urol* 2000; **37**(1):85–9.
6. Ferlay J, Bray F, Forman D, Mathers C, Parkin DM. *GLOBOCAN 2008 v2.0, Cancer Incidence and Mortality Worldwide: IARC CancerBase No. 10.* Lyon, France: International Agency for Research on Cancer; 2010. [Accessed 11 October 2012] Available at: http://globocan.iarc.fr [Online].
7. Ghoneim MA, el-Mekresh MM, el-Baz MA, el-Attar IA, Ashamallah A. Radical cystectomy for carcinoma of the bladder: critical evaluation of the results in 1,026 cases. *J Urol* 1997; **158**(2):393–9.
8. Bessette PL, Abell MR, Herwig KR. A clinicopathologic study of squamous cell carcinoma of the bladder. *J Urol* 1974; **112**(1):66–7.
9. Faysal MH. Squamous cell carcinoma of the bladder. *J Urol* 1981; **126**(5):598–9.
10. Lagwinski N, Thomas A, Stephenson AJ, *et al.* Squamous cell carcinoma of the bladder: a clinicopathologic analysis of 45 cases. *Am J Surg Pathol* 2007; **31**(12):1777–87.
11. Grignon DJ, El-Bolkainy MN, Schmitz-Dräger BJ, Simon R, Tyczynski JE. Squamous cell carcinoma. (pp. 124–7) In: Eble JN, Sauter G, Epstein JI, Sesterhenn IA (eds). *World Health Organization Classification of Tumours: Tumours of the Urinary System and Male Genital Organs.* Lyon, France: IARC Press, 2004.
12. Newman DM, Brown JR, Jay AC, Pontius EE. Squamous cell carcinoma of the bladder. *J Urol* 1968; **100**(4):470–3.
13. Harnden P, Southgate J. Cytokeratin 14 as a marker of squamous differentiation in transitional cell carcinomas. *J Clin Pathol* 1997; **50**(12):1032–3.
14. Tungekar MF, Heryet A, Gatter KC. The L1 antigen and squamous metaplasia in the bladder. *Histopathology* 1991; **19**(3):245–50.
15. Lopez-Beltran A, Requena MJ, Alvarez-Kindelan J, Quintero A, Blanca A, Montironi R. Squamous differentiation in primary urothelial carcinoma of the urinary tract as seen by MAC387 immunohistochemistry. *J Clin Pathol* 2007; **60**(3):332–5.
16. Shokeir AA. Squamous cell carcinoma of the bladder: pathology, diagnosis and treatment. *BJU Int* 2004; **93**(2):216–20.
17. World Health Organization. Schistosomiasis: burden and trends. 2008; Available at: http://www.who.int/bulletin/volumes/86/10/08-058669/en/ [Online].
18. World Health Organization. Schistosomiasis. 2012; Available at: http://www.who.int/mediacentre/factsheets/fs115/en/index.html [Online].
19. el-Boulkany MN, Ghoneim MA, Mansour MA. Carcinoma of the bilharzial bladder in Egypt. Clinical and pathological features. *Br J Urol* 1972; **44**(5):561–70.
20. el-Sebai I, Sherif M, el-Bolkainy MN, Mansour MA, Ghoneim MA.Verrucose squamous carcinoma of bladder. *Urology* 1974; **4**(4):407–10.
21. El-Bolkainy MN. *Topographical Pathology of Cancer.* Cairo University, Egypt: The National Cancer Institute, 1998: pp. 59–63.
22. El-Merzabani MM, El-Aaser AA, Zakhary NI. A study on the aetiological factors of bilharzial bladder cancer in Egypt--1. Nitrosamines and their precursors in urine. *Eur J Cancer* 1979; **15**(3):287–91.
23. Rogers CG, Palapattu GS, Shariat SF, *et al.* Clinical outcomes following radical cystectomy for primary nontransitional cell carcinoma of the bladder compared to transitional cell carcinoma of the bladder. *J Urol* 2006; **175**(6):2048–53; discussion 2053.
24. Navon JD, Soliman H, Khonsari F, Ahlering T. Screening cystoscopy and survival of spinal cord injured patients with squamous cell cancer of the bladder. *J Urol* 1997; **157**(6):2109–11.
25. Stonehill WH, Goldman HB, Dmochowski RR. The use of urine cytology for diagnosing bladder cancer in spinal cord injured patients. *J Urol* 1997; **157**(6):2112–4.
26. Locke JR, Hill DE, Walzer Y. Incidence of squamous cell carcinoma in patients with long-term catheter drainage. *J Urol* 1985; **133**(6):1034–5.
27. Michaud DS. Chronic inflammation and bladder cancer. *Urol Oncol* 2007; **25**(3):260–8.
28. Khalaf I, Shokeir A, Shalaby M. Urologic complications of genitourinary schistosomiasis. *World J Urol* 2012; **30**(1):31–8.
29. Ghoneim MA. Non-transitional cell bladder cancer. (pp. 679–870) In: Krane RJ, Siroky MB, Fitzpatrick JM (eds). *Clinical Urology.* Philadelphia, PA: Lippincott Co. 1994.
30. El-Sebaie M, Zaghloul MS, Howard G, Mokhtar A. Squamous cell carcinoma of the bilharzial and non-bilharzial urinary bladder: a review of etiological features, natural history, and management. *Int J Clin Oncol* 2005; **10**(1):20–5.
31. Kassouf W, Spiess PE, Siefker-Radtke A, *et al.* Outcome and patterns of recurrence of nonbilharzial pure squamous cell carcinoma of the bladder: a contemporary review of The University of Texas M D Anderson Cancer Center experience. *Cancer* 2007; **110**(4):764–9.
32. Eissa S, Swellam M, Sadek M, Mourad MS, El Ahmady O, Khalifa A. Comparative evaluation of the nuclear matrix protein, fibronectin, urinary bladder cancer antigen and voided urine cytology in the detection of bladder tumors. *J Urol* 2002; **168**(2):465–9.

33. Swanson DA, Liles A, Zagars GK. Preoperative irradiation and radical cystectomy for stages T2 and T3 squamous cell carcinoma of the bladder. *J Urol* 1990; **143**(1):37–40.
34. Youssef R, Kapur P, Shariat SF, *et al.* Prognostic value of apoptotic markers in squamous cell carcinoma of the urinary bladder. *BJU Int* 2012; **110**(7):961–6.
35. Stein JP, Lieskovsky G, Cote R, *et al.* Radical cystectomy in the treatment of invasive bladder cancer: long-term results in 1,054 patients. *J Clin Oncol* 2001; **19**(3):666–75.
36. Madersbacher S, Hochreiter W, Burkhard F, *et al.* Radical cystectomy for bladder cancer today--a homogeneous series without neoadjuvant therapy. *J Clin Oncol* 2003; **21**(4):690–6.
37. Abdollah F, Sun M, Jeldres C, *et al.* Survival after radical cystectomy of non-bilharzial squamous cell carcinoma vs urothelial carcinoma: a competing-risks analysis. *BJU Int* 2012; **109**(4):564–9.
38. Scosyrev E, Yao J, Messing E. Urothelial carcinoma versus squamous cell carcinoma of bladder: is survival different with stage adjustment? *Urology* 2009; **73**(4):822–7.
39. Ehdaie B, Maschino A, Shariat SF, *et al.* Comparative outcomes of pure squamous cell carcinoma and urothelial carcinoma with squamous differentiation in patients treated with radical cystectomy. *J Urol* 2012; **187**(1):74–9.
40. von der Maase H, Sengelov L, Roberts JT, *et al.* Long-term survival results of a randomized trial comparing gemcitabine plus cisplatin, with methotrexate, vinblastine, doxorubicin, plus cisplatin in patients with bladder cancer. *J Clin Oncol* 2005; **23**(21):4602–8.
41. Kastritis E, Dimopoulos MA, Antoniou N, *et al.* The outcome of patients with advanced pure squamous or mixed squamous and transitional urothelial carcinomas following platinum-based chemotherapy. *Anticancer Res* 2006; **26**(5B):3865–9.
42. Richie JP, Waisman J, Skinner DG, Dretler SP. Squamous carcinoma of the bladder: treatment by radical cystectomy. *J Urol* 1976; **115**(6):670–2.
43. Jones MA, Bloom HJ, Williams G, Trott PA, Wallace DM. The management of squamous cell carcinoma of the bladder. *Br J Urol* 1980; **52**(6):511–4.

CHAPTER 6.24

Adenocarcinoma of the bladder

Roy Mano and Ofer Yossepowitch

Introduction to adenocarcinoma of the bladder

Adenocarcinoma of the bladder constitutes the third most common histologic subtype of bladder malignancies. These tumours are typically classified as primary (arising from the bladder), urachal (arising from the remnant of the urachus) and secondary (metastatic from another primary tumour). While adenocarcinoma present in a similar clinical fashion to urothelial cell carcinoma of the bladder (UCC), these tumours differ in epidemiological, aetiological, and pathological factors. In general, adenocarcinoma carry an unfavourable prognosis, mostly due to their aggressive biological nature and advanced stage at diagnosis.

Demographics

Adenocarcinoma of the bladder is the third most common histologic subtype of bladder tumour. These tumours represent around 0.5–2.0% of all bladder cancers.[1–3] For example, in two large epidemiologic series derived from a population-based registry in the United States and the Netherlands, adenocarcinoma comprised 1–1.5% of newly diagnosed bladder cancers.[4,5] Similar to most common malignancies, the incidence of this disease increases steadily with age.[4] Typically the age at diagnosis is around 64 years, and is an average of 3–4.5 years younger than that of bladder UCC.[5,6] Although adenocarcinoma of the bladder has a male predominance (male to female ratio 1.7–2.2:1.[4–7]), it is more common in females than UCC (where ratio is 2.5:1). Primary adenocarcinoma of the bladder is also relatively more frequent in non-Caucasians than UCC.[4–6]

Adenocarcinoma of the urachus is less common than primary adenocarcinoma of the bladder. Urachal tumours account for 0.17–0.34% of all bladder neoplasms. Based on several small single institution studies, urachal carcinoma was initially believed to represent approximately one-third of primary bladder adenocarcinomas.[8–27] Recently, two large population-based studies found that urachal adenocarcinoma comprises only 10–20% of bladder adenocarcinoma.[7,28] Patients with urachal carcinoma were younger (median age of 56 years compared to 69 years in patients with non-urachal adenocarcinoma), and a higher proportion of female patients was observed (45%).[7]

Aetiology

Traditionally, metaplastic changes in potentially unstable urothelium were considered the primary causative factor for development of urinary bladder adenocarcinoma. Chronic irritation and infection of the bladder may predispose to these changes.[29,30] More recently, however, several studies have refuted this theory, showing that although cystitis cystica and glandularis or intestinal metaplasia (representing the histological correlate of chronic inflammation) may coexist with bladder adenocarcinoma, they do not increase the risk of its development.[31,32]

To date, bladder adenocarcinoma is the most common tumour observed in bladder exstrophy patients and is more frequently diagnosed in geographic regions where schistosomiasis is endemic.[1–3] In addition, endometriosis, bladder augmentation, and other irritative conditions of the urinary tract may predispose the bladder to development of adenocarcinoma.[3]

Schistosomiasis

In three large series from Egypt, where bilharzia is endemic, the incidence of primary adenocarcinoma of the bladder ranged from 5.2–9.9%.[19,23,33] This is higher than reported in regions without endemic bilharzia, and supports a causative association. Indeed, bilharzial eggs were found in up to 82% of patients.[19] Chronic vesical irritation and associated bacterial or viral infections in patients with bilharzial cystitis may explain the higher incidence of adenocarcinoma in this population. Of note, squamous cell carcinoma of the bladder is more common than adenocarcinoma in patients with bilharzia.

Bladder exstrophy

Adenocarcinoma of the bladder remnant is the second largest category of neoplasia in treated and non-treated exstrophy patients. It arises in 4% of patients, at an almost 700-fold greater incidence compared to the age-matched general population.[34,35] This neoplasia occurs most commonly in men, at a mean age of 44 years.[34–37] In non-treated patients, exposure of the exstrophied bladder to an *ex vivo* environment results in constant irritation and infections culminating in glandular metaplasia and the potential for malignant transformation.[34] In treated patients, bladder augmentation may play a role in promoting carcinoma in the repaired bladder.[37]

Enteric bladder augmentation

In patients whose bladder has been augmented, adenocarcinoma appears the most common histologic subtype of tumour (around 63% of tumours in ileocystoplasties, 53% of all tumours in colocystoplasties and 3.4% of patients undergoing gastrocystoplasty). Typically, the lesions develop at the junction between the intestinal mucosa and urothelium. The median latency period between augmentation and cancer evolvement is generally prolonged (17–22 years) and depends predominantly on the bowel segment used for augmentation (colonic segments tend to develop cancers more rapidly) and the reason for the augmentation.[38–40] It is unclear whether the augmentation process by itself leads to malignancy or whether the underlying bladder pathology is, in fact, the primary oncogenic determinant. While most reported adenocarcinoma are found in patients whose bladders were augmented following tuberculosis infection, postradiotherapy, postextsrophy, or following neuropathic problems. No increased risk of adenocarcinoma was reported in patients whose bladders were augmented for detrusor overactivty.

Pathology

Adenocarcinoma of the urinary bladder is best classified according to its site of origin: primary tumours arising from the bladder or urachal remnant, and secondary (metastatic) adenocarcinoma. The latter usually represent local extension of primary colon, prostate, or ovarian malignancy.[29] As a rule, metastatic carcinoma to the bladder is more common than primary adenocarcinoma. As such, a second tumour must be excluded before establishing the diagnosis of primary bladder adenocarcinoma.[1,41]

With regards to primary adenocarcinoma, the distinction between urachal and non-urachal origin is often challenging as both share similar morphologic features and immunohistochemical profiles.[42] Bladder location is usually the best guide to tissue of origin; urachal lesions at the dome and non-urachal lesions at the base or side walls. The urachus contains three distinct tissue layers: a luminal layer composed of cuboidal or transitional epithelium, an intermediate submucosal connective tissue layer, and an outer smooth muscle layer.[21] The majority of urachal tumours are high-grade adenocarcinomas (84–100% of cases),[12,21,24,25] arising either from the luminal layer or from residual enteric rests during embryological development.[20,26]

Mostofi *et al.* proposed the initial diagnostic criteria for urachal adenocarcinoma which included: (i) tumour location in the bladder dome; (ii) absence of cystitis cystica and cystitis glandularis in the bladder; (iii) predominant invasion of the muscularis propria or deeper tissues with a sharp demarcation between the tumour and surface bladder urothelium that is free of glandular or polypoid proliferation; (iv) urachal remnants within the tumour; (v) involvement of the space of Retzius, anterior abdominal wall, or umbilicus; (vi) no evidence of a primary neoplasm elsewhere.[43] Johnson *et al.* deemed these criteria too restrictive and suggested that location of the tumour in the bladder dome, sharp demarcation between the tumour and the surface epithelium, and exclusion of primary adenocarcinoma elsewhere should be the delineating features of urachal carcinomas.[44] A more practical approach was proposed by several other investigators who indicated that all enteric type adenocarcinoma located at the bladder dome should be considered of urachal origin until proven otherwise.[12,16,29]

Pathology

Macroscopically, adenocarcinomas can have a papillary, nodular, flat, or ulcerated architecture. Some variants tend to present with prominent bladder wall thickening ('linitis plastica') without apparent growth due to diffuse infiltration of the bladder wall with tumour cells.[42] Microscopically, these tumours show pure glandular morphology with varying histological growth patterns.[42,45] Based on their morphologic appearance, Grignon *et al.* divided the tumours into five distinct histologic subtypes: enteric, when the architectural and cytological features resemble those of typical colonic adenocarcinomas (Fig. 6.24.1, Fig. 6.24.1AB); mucinous, when the tumour is characterized by single cells or nests of cells floating in lakes of extracellular mucin; signet ring, when the tumour is composed of single signet-ring cells diffusely permeating the tissues (Fig. 6.24.1C and D); adenocarcinoma not-otherwise-specified (NOS), when the pattern does not fit into any of the aforementioned categories; and mixed, when the tumour shows two or more of the patterns with no dominant pattern accounting for more than 75% of the material. Urachal and non-urachal tumours share similar morphologic features, although urachal tumours are more frequently categorized as mucinous type.[14]

Two additional rare categories exist: clear cell and hepatoid subtypes. Clear cell adenocarcinoma resembles tumours of the female genital tract. It mostly affects women and is usually located in the posterior, lateral walls, or trigone of the bladder and immunostains for CA-125.[46] The hepatoid type of adenocarcinoma has the morphological characteristics of hepatocellular carcinoma, may appear with hyaline globules and bile production, and stains for α-fetoprotein.[42]

Grading and staging

Non-urachal tumours are staged and graded in a similar fashion to UCC, endorsing the TNM and WHO classification systems.[19] For urachal tumours, three distinct staging systems have been formulated: the Sheldon,[12] Ontario,[22] and Mayo[21] classifications (Table 6.24.1). While the Sheldon staging system is the most commonly utilized, it is relatively complex. The more recently published Mayo system offers simplicity and an improved ability to predict survival.[21]

Most primary adenocarcinomas (47–100%) are classified as moderately to poorly differentiated at initial diagnosis. The majority of tumours, both urachal (25–64%) and non-urachal (29–92%), are locally advanced at presentation. Metastatic disease at presentation is found in 4–31% of urachal tumours and 4–44% of non-urachal tumours.[6,7,10,11,14,16,18–26,28] Compared to UCC, bladder adenocarcinoma has a higher propensity for muscle invasion, extravesical spread, and metastases.[5,6] Urachal tumours are more likely to be diagnosed at advanced stage involving distant organs,[7] particularly in patients younger than 45 years.[28]

The most common location of metastases in non-urachal tumours were lungs (40%), liver (37%) and skeleton (37%).[10] Urachal tumours tend to spread by local extension to adjacent pelvic structures followed by hematogenous dissemination to distant organs. Distant metastases are most commonly seen in the lungs (50%), lymph nodes (46%), bone (30%), bowel (30%), brain (20%), and liver (16%). Metastases to multiple organs are a common feature of advanced stage.[25]

Primary adenocarcinoma of non-urachal and urachal origin

Clinical presentation

Painless visible haematuria is the most frequent symptom in patients with bladder adenocarcinoma. It is reported in 48–92% of urachal and non-urachal tumours. Irritative or obstructive urinary voiding symptoms are also common, but are generally seen in patients with non-urachal tumours (48% vs. 13% in urachal tumours). Lack

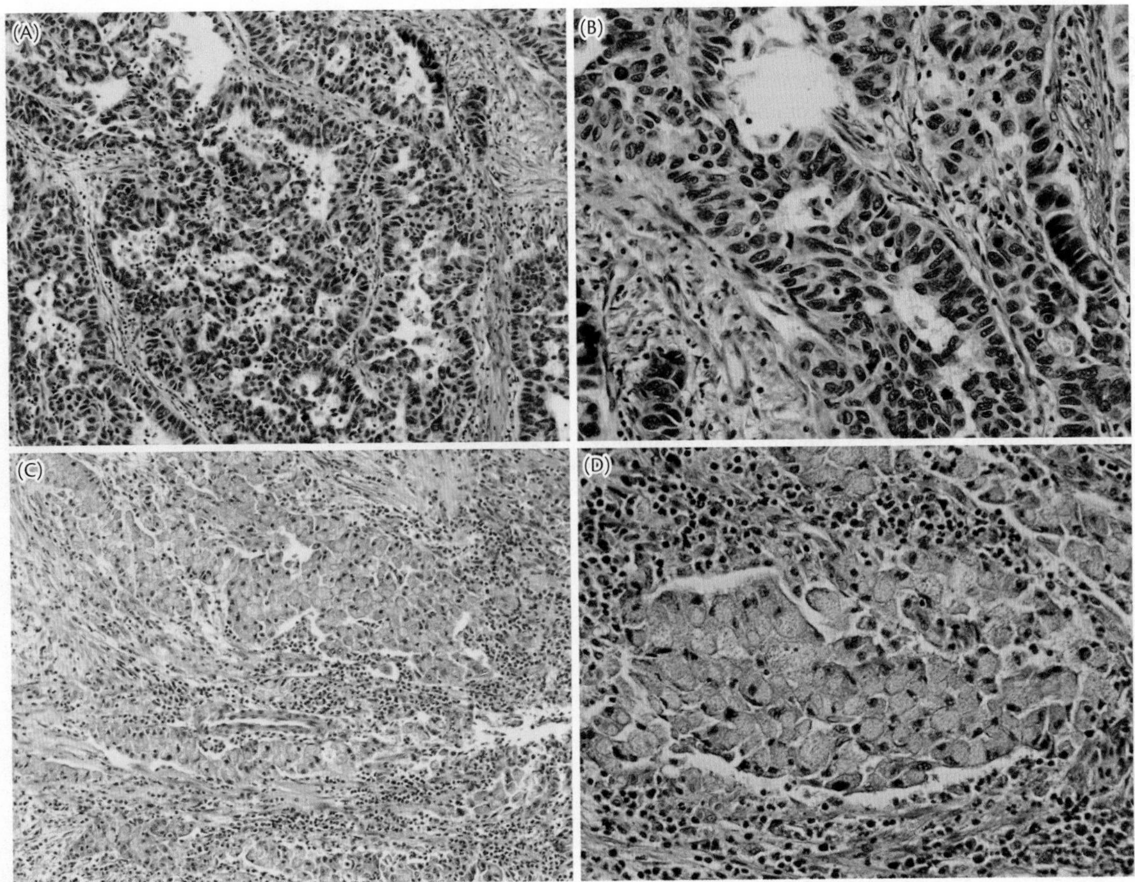

Fig. 6.24.1 Primary non-urachal adenocarcinoma of the bladder, enteric type (haematoxylin-eosin, original magnification ×100 (A) and ×200 (B)). Urachal adenocarcinoma of the bladder, signet-ring cell type (haematoxylin-eosin, original magnification ×100 (C) and ×200 (D)).

Table 6.24.1 Staging systems for urachal cancer

Stage	Sheldon[12]	Mayo[21]	Stage	Ontario[22]*
I	Tumour confined to the urachal mucosa	Tumours confined to the urachus and/or bladder	T1	Tumour confined to submucosa
II	Invasion confined to the urachus	Tumours extending beyond the muscular layer of the urachus and/or the bladder	T2	Tumour confined to muscular wall of bladder
III	Local extension	Tumours infiltrating the regional lymph nodes	T3	Tumour extended into the periurachal or vesical soft tissue
IIIA	◆ to the bladder			
IIIB	◆ to the abdominal wall		T4	Tumour invaded adjacent organs, including the abdominal wall
IIIC	◆ to the peritoneum			
IIID	◆ to viscera other than the bladder			
IV	Metastatic disease	Tumours infiltrating non-regional lymph nodes or other distant sites		
IVA	◆ to regional lymph nodes			
IVB	◆ to distant sites			

*Staging system for primary tumours, regional nodes, and distant metastases are considered separately.

Reprinted from *The Journal of Urology*, Volume 131, Issue 1, Sheldon CA, *et al.*, Malignant urachal lesions, pp. 1–8, Copyright © 1984, with permission from Elsevier, http://www.sciencedirect.com/science/article/pii/S0022534711041437; Richard A. *et al.*, Urachal carcinoma: Clinicopathologic features and long-term outcomes of an aggressive malignancy, *Cancer*, Volume 107, Issue 4, pp. 712–20, Copyright © 2006 John Wiley and Sons; and *The Journal of Urology*, Volume 175, Issue 6, Jehonathan H. Pinthus *et al.*, Population Based Survival Data on Urachal Tumors, pp. 2042–2047, Copyright © 2006, with permission from Elsevier, http://www.sciencedirect.com/science/article/pii/S0022534711041437

of symptoms allows urachal adenocarcinoma to escape clinical detection for a long time and leads to the advanced stage typically found at diagnosis.[21] While all adenocarcinomas secret mucin to a certain extent, mucosuria is a relatively uncommon finding and is mostly associated with urachal tumours. Mucosuria is reported in up to 17% of patients with urachal and only in 2% of patients with non-urachal adenocarcinomas.[10,11,14–18,21,25–27] Additional infrequent findings in patients with urachal adenocarcinoma include a draining mucoid sinus to the skin, recurrent urinary tract infections, palpable abdominal mass, and abdominal or suprapubic pain.[16,17,21,25,26]

Positive urinary cytology can be found in approximately 40% of patients with urachal adenocarcinoma, largely associated with high tumour grade. Cystoscopy is diagnostic in virtually all patients, demonstrating a protruding mass at the dome or anterior bladder wall.[14,16,21,25,26] Serum tumour markers may be elevated in some patients with urachal tumours, providing means of monitoring the response to therapy, and early diagnosis of disease recurrence or progression during follow-up. In one series elevated CEA, CA 19-9 and CA-125 were found in 59%, 60%, and 44% of patients respectively.[20]

Adenocarcinoma of the bladder can exhibit distinctive findings on imaging studies. In non-urachal tumours, particularly of the signet-ring cell subtype, markedly increased bladder wall thickness combined with diffused perivesical stranding are common.[47] Urachal adenocarcinoma often manifests as a mixed cystic and solid mass, arising from the midline of the bladder dome (Fig. 6.24.2 and Fig. 6.24.3). Associated calcifications, varying from fine punctate deposits to extensive areas of calcification, are visible in 33–72% of the patients, most often in the periphery of the mass.[12,21,48] An additional unique feature of adenocarcinomas includes focal areas of high signal intensity on sagittal T2-weighted MR images, secondary to mucin production.[49]

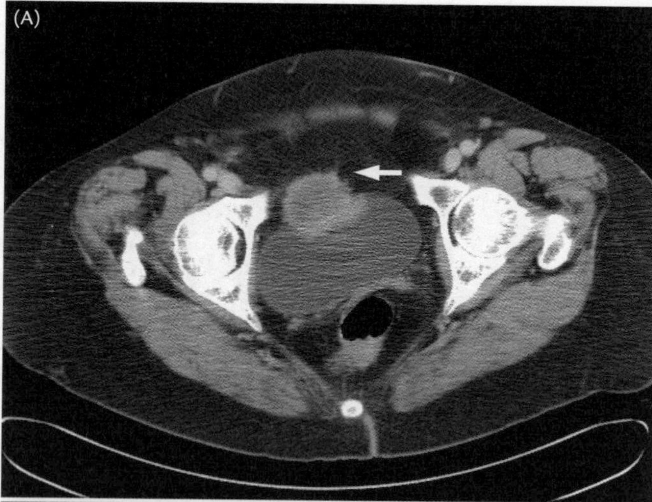

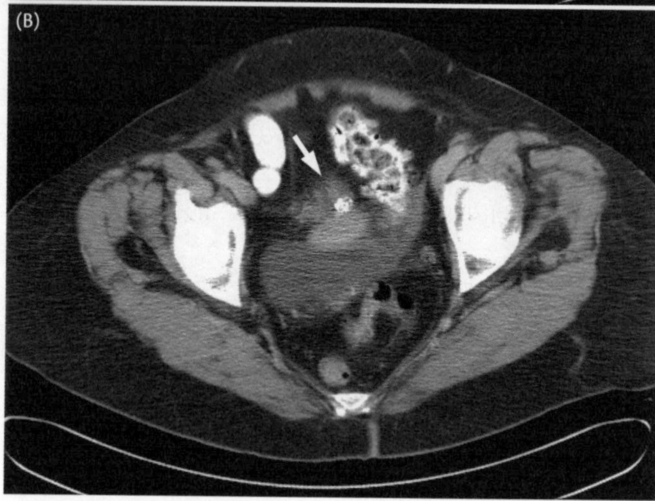

Fig. 6.24.2 A 64-year-old female with urachal adenocarcinoma of the bladder. Axial computed tomography images showing (A) a midline mass involving the dome of the bladder (arrow), with (B) a thick peripheral calcification in its superior aspect (arrow).

Treatment of localized non-urachal adenocarcinoma

Most studies addressing the management of primary bladder adenocarcinoma are small, retrospective, and include several treatment modalities. Therefore, the optimal therapeutic strategy for these patients has yet to be defined.[19]

Bladder-sparing surgery

Transurethral resection of the tumour has a poor success as monotherapy for non-urachal adenocarcinoma of the bladder. The reported five-year survival rates are around 19–33% and are not improved by the addition of adjuvant radiotherapy.[9,10,50] Partial cystectomy can be used for localized disease when feasible. Feasibility, means that the tumour is in a mobile component of the bladder and is small enough to allow resection with a margin of normal bladder that will leave sufficient bladder volume for quality of life. The oncologic outcomes are generally dismal for partial cystectomy,[19] except for one series reporting a five-year survival rate of 54% after partial bladder resection alone.[10] This report may be due to most careful patient selection.

Radical cystectomy and pelvic lymphadenectomy

Radical cystectomy and pelvic lymphadenectomy are the mainstay of treatment for non-urachal adenocarcinoma of the bladder. In relatively large series, the five-year survival rates of patients treated by radical cystectomy were 21–55%.[10,19,23] The most important predictor of survival was tumour stage. Reported five-year overall

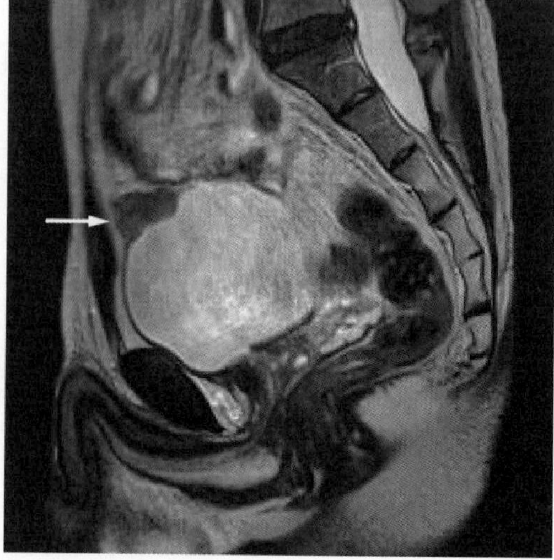

Fig. 6.24.3 A T2-weighted sagittal pelvic magnetic resonance imaging scan demonstrating a mass arising from the dome of the urinary bladder (arrow), consistent with adenocarcinoma of the bladder.

survival rates are around 100%, 54%, 50%, and 35% for stage I, II, III, and IV, respectively.[23]

Radiotherapy

Traditionally, adenocarcinoma of the bladder was considered radio-resistant.[19] The reported five-year survival rate among patients treated with external radiation therapy alone was less than 20%.[8,10,13] However, postoperative adjuvant radiation therapy to target the entire pelvis may offer a clinical benefit. In one series, a significantly improved disease free survival was observed in patients with pathologically advanced disease treated with adjuvant radiation therapy (61%) compared to cystectomy alone (37%).[23] The radiation was not associated with delayed morbidity and resulted in a substantially improved local failure rate.

Treatment of localized urachal adenocarcinoma

Partial and radical cystectomy

The standard of care for localized urachal carcinoma entails extended partial cystectomy with en bloc resection of the entire urachus (including the umbilicus), the posterior rectus fascia, a generous portion of the overlying peritoneum and perivesical soft tissue extending out to the lateral pelvic sidewalls. Removal of the bladder dome must leave sufficient bladder volume for a functional quality of life. Resection of involved adjacent organs (bowel) is carried out when necessary to remove all macroscopic disease. Bilateral pelvic lymph node dissection is considered a mandatory adjunct, including common iliac, external iliac, obturator, and hypogastric lymph nodes.[24] Wide excision with negative soft tissue and bladder margins is critical to minimize the risk of local recurrence.[22] In univariate analysis, complete urachectomy and umbilectomy were significant predictors of survival.[21] In fact, radical cystectomy did not show any survival advantage over properly performed extended partial cystectomy.[14,16,20–22,24,28] Minimally invasive surgical techniques including laparoscopic and robot-assisted laparoscopic partial cystectomy with urachal resection have been reported as a reasonable alternative to the traditional open approach.[51,52]

In a review of surgically treated urachal cancer series, Herr *et al.* noted that the long-term disease specific survival rates ranged from 33% to 88%, with nearly half of the patients dead of disease at a median follow-up time of five years.[24] However, restricting the data to patients who, in addition to partial cystectomy, had concomitant wide resection of the urachus, a significantly improved five-year survival rate was observed, reaching as high as 70%.[24,25]

Treatment failure manifested as local relapse in the pelvis or bladder occurs in 15–18% of patients, and generally within the first two years after treatment.[21,24] Surgical resection of local tumour recurrence resulted in long-term cure (median follow-up of 15 years) in more than 50% of the patients.[21] It is important to note that while local recurrence in the bladder is amenable to salvage therapy, pelvic recurrence outside the bladder portends an ominous prognosis. In one study, two-thirds of the patients with disease relapse in the bladder were cured with salvage surgery alone, whereas only 17% of the patients with pelvic relapse had responded to combined chemotherapy and surgical resection.[24] None of the patients were salvaged successfully with radiation therapy.[21]

Distant metastases developed in 32–54% of the patients who presented with localized disease. Most patients (92%) with metastatic urachal carcinoma died of their disease at a median time of 12 to 24 months. Survival was not related to the particular site of metastases.[20,21]

Multimodality treatment

Siefker-Radtke *et al.* described the use of 5-fluorouracil and cisplatin-based neoadjuvant chemotherapy in two patients with locally advanced disease prior to surgical treatment. At a median follow-up time of 17 months, no evidence of disease was observed.[20] In contrast, adjuvant therapy (chemotherapy, radiation, or a combination thereof) in patients with positive lymph nodes or involved surgical margins did not prove to be of any therapeutic benefit.[20,21]

Radiotherapy

Ashely *et al.* described six patients treated by primary external beam radiation therapy using a median radiation dose of 50 Gy. These patients had a worse outcome when compared with surgically treated patients, but were older, had higher grade tumours, and a more advanced disease.[21]

Treatment of metastatic disease

Relying on treatment paradigms used in patients with gastrointestinal adenocarcinoma, 5-fluorouracil (5-FU) based chemotherapy was initially attempted by several investigators in small groups of patients with bladder adenocarcinoma. Response rates were generally inconsistent suggesting that 5-FU may provide some therapeutic benefit in these patients.[53–55] In one study, Logothetis *et al.* reported on the use of 5-FU, doxorubicin, and mitomycin in urachal adenocarcinoma with an initial response rate of 65% but no durable response.[54] Cisplatin-based chemotherapy regimens were assessed in several small studies. Galsky *et al.* reported on 11 patients with unresectable or metastatic bladder adenocarcinoma treated with ifosfamide, paclitaxel and cisplatin (ITP). Overall response rate was 36%, most of which was partial response. In two patients the response to systemic chemotherapy downsized the tumour allowing performance of radical cystectomy for previously unresectable disease. Median survival was 24.8 months.[56] Siefker-Radtke *et al.* showed that chemotherapy administered to patients with metastatic urachal adenocarcinoma, most of whom developed distant relapse after failure of surgical treatment for locally advanced disease, resulted in a median overall survival of 20 months. Objective initial response was achieved in 20% of patients (mostly partial). Most clinical responses were observed with 5-fluorouracil/cisplatin-based regimens, implying that chemotherapy generally used for colon adenocarcinomas may be more beneficial to patients with urachal adenocarcinoma than traditional chemotherapy regimens used in urothelial tumours. Only 5% of the patients had long-term disease-free survival.[20] Molina *et al.* reported the clinical outcome of 10 patients with either disease relapse after surgical treatment for locally advanced disease or metastatic urachal adenocarcinoma treated with 5-FU based regimens, MVAC, VP-16/platinum and Taxol/platinum. The median survival after chemotherapy was 20.4 months. Progression of disease was usually seen when single agent 5-FU was used. Conversely, platinum-containing regimens resulted in stable disease or partial response in 71% of cases.[25] Tatokoro *et al.* analysed the clinical efficacy of combination chemotherapy consisting of ifosfamide, 5-FU, etoposide and cisplatin (IFEP) in metastatic adenocarcinoma of the urachus after definitive surgery. Objective initial responses were observed in three of four patients (75%). One patient required salvage surgery and two were treated with consolidative radiotherapy. The median survival was 26 months.[57]

A study summarizing the chemotherapy regimens for metastatic urachal carcinoma showed that the highest response rates and progression-free survival were noticed with the use of 5-FU- and CPT-11-based regimens.[58]

Prognosis

Overall 5 and 10-year survival rates are reported to be around 18–57% and 28% in non-urachal adenocarcinoma and 34–70% and 31–46% in urachal adenocarcinoma, respectively.[5–7,9,10,14–18,20–26,28,59] Three large population-based studies showed that patients with urachal tumours had a lower risk of all cause and disease specific mortality compared to patients with non-urachal tumours,[7] and that stage and grade-adjusted cancer-specific mortality rates are similar in patients diagnosed with adenocarcinoma and urothelial carcinoma. Thus, the worse overall survival seen in adenocarcinoma is likely attributed to the more advanced stage distribution at presentation.[5,6]

Tumour stage is a significant predictive factor for prognosis in most series.[5,7,10,14,17,19,20,22–25,28] In one population-based series, the five-year survival rates decreased as the stage of the disease increased, with survival rates of 57%, 29%, and 11% in patients with disease stage II, III, and IV, respectively.[5] Additional prognostic factors included—tumour grade,[7,10,19,21,22] lymph node involvement,[19,20,23,28] surgical margin status,[20,21,24,27] macroscopic residual tumour,[28] histologic type (mucinous and signet-ring histological subtypes predicted lower survival rates),[17,23,27] tumour size,[10] and age.[7] In addition, a study assessing the prognostic value of the cell-cycle specific biomarkers—p53, p21, p27, Ki-67, and cyclin E in adenocarcinoma of the bladder showed that the combined alterations of p27 and Ki-67 and of all five biomarkers were associated with increased probability of disease recurrence and cancer-specific mortality.[60]

Secondary adenocarcinoma

The bladder can be affected by the direct extension of cancer from adjacent viscera, or spread from distant foci via blood or lymphatic channels. In a comprehensive literature review, Velcheti and Govindan indicated the most common source of metastases to the bladder to be the genitourinary tract (35%) followed by the colon and rectum (28%), melanoma (9%), breast (8%) and gastric carcinoma (8%).[41] Metastatic involvement of the bladder does not manifest with typical urinary symptoms and might be overlooked on cystoscopy as it generally infiltrates the bladder wall rather than cause ulceration of the mucosal lining.[41] On imaging, the tumour usually presents as thickening of the bladder wall, frequently involving the bladder neck and trigone. Colonic tumours involve the fundus more commonly.[61,62]

Differentiating primary and secondary bladder adenocarcinoma

It can be challenging to distinguish primary and metastatic adenocarcinoma of the bladder using only histological appearance. The presence of intestinal type metaplasia and cystitis glandularis along with *in situ* adenocarcinoma within the tumour or elsewhere in the bladder can be indicative of primary adenocarcinoma. Unfortunately, these features appear in only a small percentage of patients.[41] An overlying intact urothelium may suggest a secondary source, although a metastatic tumour may also cause ulceration of the epithelium without emanating from it.[61]

Immunohistochemical staining may assist in distinguishing metastatic colon adenocarcinoma from enteric type primary bladder adenocarcinoma but specific monoclonal antibodies have proven useful only in some patients.[62] Cytokeratin (CK) 7 and CK20 are both positive in more than half of the patients with primary bladder adenocarcinoma, whereas in the typical colonic adenocarcinoma CK7 staining is negative and CK20 is positive.[63,64] Thrombomodulin, an endothelial thrombin receptor, is positive in 59% of bladder adenocarcinomas and in none of the colonic adenocarcinomas.[64] β-catenin is typically accumulated in the nucleus of colorectal adenocarcinoma tumour cells, and β-catenin nuclear staining was found in 81% of colorectal metastases to the bladder. Conversely, a membranous β-catenin staining pattern was observed in 88% of primary bladder adenocarcinoma, 93% of urachal adenocarcinoma, and all cases of metastatic adenocarcinoma. Thus, the nuclear versus membranous staining pattern of β-catenin may be of diagnostic value.[26,64] Positive expression of 34βE12, a high-molecular-weight cytokeratin, occurs in 66% of urachal adenocarcinomas and 11% of colonic adenocarcinomas; therefore a strong diffuse positivity would favour urachal over colonic origin.[26] Villin, an actin-binding protein, is expressed in 98% of colorectal adenocarcinomas, and 65% of primary bladder adenocarcinomas. Lack of villin immunoreactivity suggests a bladder origin.[65] Nuclear CDX-2 transcription factor expression was initially thought to be restricted to colonic adenocarcinoma.[65] However, recent studies showed similar expression in bladder adenocarcinoma eliminating CDX-2 as a tool for differentiating between the two.[42] In a study of patients diagnosed with adenocarcinoma of the urinary tract and a previously resected colorectal carcinoma, deleted-in-colon-cancer (DCC) immunoreactivity, a prognostic marker for colorectal cancer, was observed consistently in the bladder lesion when the primary colorectal mass expressed DCC. In addition, positive DCC protein expression was related to a more favourable prognosis.[66]

Differentiating bladder adenocarcinoma from prostate adenocarcinoma is possible with the use of prostate-specific antigen (PSA) staining, which is negative in bladder adenocarcinomas.[42] PAP positivity may also imply a prostatic origin, although it may be positive in some bladder adenocarcinomas as well.[61]

In practice, knowledge of a history of tumour elsewhere and comparison with the original histology will establish the secondary nature of a bladder tumour in many cases, particularly as tumours that had spread to the bladder tend to be at an advanced stage.[61]

Treatment of secondary adenocarcinoma of the bladder

Differentiating primary urothelial adenocarcinoma from secondary tumour involving the urinary tract is important when deciding on the appropriate treatment strategy. While primary muscle-invasive adenocarcinoma of the urinary bladder may prompt removal of the bladder, treatment of metastatic adenocarcinoma to the bladder is often only a secondary consideration depending on the stage and prognosis of the primary cancer, as well as its chemosensitivity and radiosensitivity.[41]

Although wide surgical excision followed by the administration of adjuvant therapy would yield the longest survival, the decision of treating the patient with partial cystectomy, radical cystectomy or pelvic exenteration should rely not only on the anatomical location of the tumour, but primarily on the patients' performance status and life expectancy.[66]

Conclusions

Adenocarcinomas of the bladder are classified into three categories according to their origin, namely non-urachal, urachal, and metastatic. While all share similar clinical and histological characteristics, differentiating between the tumours is important as treatment of the disease varies substantially. Since most studies are of small size and retrospective, the optimal treatment regimen for metastatic cancer has yet to be defined. In general, primary adenocarcinoma of the bladder has a poor prognosis.

Further reading

Abol-Enein H, Kava BR, Carmack AJ. Nonurothelial cancer of the bladder. *Urology* 2007; **69**(Suppl 1):93–104.

Dahm P, Gschwend JE. Malignant non-urothelial neoplasms of the urinary bladder: a review. *Eur Urol* 2003; **44**(6):672–81.

Lughezzani G, Sun M, Jeldres C, *et al.* Adenocarcinoma versus urothelial carcinoma of the urinary bladder: comparison between pathologic stage at radical cystectomy and cancer-specific mortality. *Urology* 2010; **75**(2):376–81.

Roy S, Parwani AV. Adenocarcinoma of the urinary bladder. *Arch Pathol Lab Med* 2011; **135**(12):1601–5.

Wang HL, Lu DW, Yerian LM, *et al.* Immunohistochemical distinction between primary adenocarcinoma of the bladder and secondary colorectal adenocarcinoma. *Am J Surg Pathol* 2001; **25**(11):1380–7.

Wright JL, Porter MP, Li CI, Lange PH, Lin DW. Differences in survival among patients with urachal and nonurachal adenocarcinomas of the bladder. *Cancer* 2006; **107**(4):721–8.

References

1. Dahm P, Gschwend JE. Malignant non-urothelial neoplasms of the urinary bladder: a review. *Eur Urol* 2003; **44**(6):672–81.
2. Manunta A, Vincendeau S, Kiriakou G, Lobel B, Guille F. Non-transitional cell bladder carcinomas. *BJU Int* 2005; **95**(4):497–502.
3. Abol-Enein H, Kava BR, Carmack AJ. Nonurothelial cancer of the bladder. *Urology* 2007; **69**(Suppl 1):93–104.
4. Kantor AF, Hartge P, Hoover RN, Fraumeni JF Jr. Epidemiological characteristics of squamous cell carcinoma and adenocarcinoma of the bladder. *Cancer Res* 1988; **48**(13):3853–5.
5. Ploeg M, Aben KK, Hulsbergen-van de Kaa CA, Schoenberg MP, Witjes JA, Kiemeney LA. Clinical epidemiology of nonurothelial bladder cancer: analysis of the Netherlands Cancer Registry. *J Urol* 2010; **183**(3):915–20.
6. Lughezzani G, Sun M, Jeldres C, *et al.* Adenocarcinoma versus urothelial carcinoma of the urinary bladder: comparison between pathologic stage at radical cystectomy and cancer-specific mortality. *Urology* 2010; **75**(2):376–81.
7. Wright JL, Porter MP, Li CI, Lange PH, Lin DW. Differences in survival among patients with urachal and nonurachal adenocarcinomas of the bladder. *Cancer* 2006; **107**(4):721–8.
8. Thomas DG, Ward AM, Williams JL. A study of 52 cases of adenocarcinoma of the bladder. *Br J Urol* 1971; **43**(1):4–15.
9. Kramer SA, Bredael J, Croker BP, Paulson DF, Glenn JF. Primary non-urachal adenocarcinoma of the bladder. *J Urol* 1979; **121**(3):278–81.
10. Anderstrom C, Johansson SL, von Schultz L. Primary adenocarcinoma of the urinary bladder. A clinicopathologic and prognostic study. *Cancer* 1983; **52**(7):1273–80.
11. Bennett JK, Wheatley JK, Walton KN. 10-year experience with adenocarcinoma of the bladder. *J Urol* 1984; **131**(2):262–3.
12. Sheldon CA, Clayman RV, Gonzalez R, Williams RD, Fraley EE. Malignant urachal lesions. *J Urol* 1984; **131**(1):1–8.
13. Gill HS, Dhillon HK, Woodhouse CR. Adenocarcinoma of the urinary bladder. *Br J Urol* 1989; **64**(2):138–42.
14. Grignon DJ, Ro JY, Ayala AG, Johnson DE, Ordonez NG. Primary adenocarcinoma of the urinary bladder. A clinicopathologic analysis of 72 cases. *Cancer* 1991; **67**(8):2165–72.
15. Wilson TG, Pritchett TR, Lieskovsky G, Warner NE, Skinner DG. Primary adenocarcinoma of bladder. *Urology* 1991; **38**(3):223–6.
16. Henly DR, Farrow GM, Zincke H. Urachal cancer: role of conservative surgery. *Urology* 1993; **42**(6):635–9.
17. Nakanishi K, Kawai T, Suzuki M, Torikata C. Prognostic factors in urachal adenocarcinoma. A study in 41 specimens of DNA status, proliferating cell-nuclear antigen immunostaining, and argyrophilic nucleolar-organizer region counts. *Hum Pathol* 1996; **27**(3):240–7.
18. Dandekar NP, Dalal AV, Tongaonkar HB, Kamat MR. Adenocarcinoma of bladder. *Eur J Surg Oncol* 1997; **23**(2):157–60.
19. el-Mekresh MM, el-Baz MA, Abol-Enein H, Ghoneim MA. Primary adenocarcinoma of the urinary bladder: a report of 185 cases. *Br J Urol* 1998; **82**(2):206–12.
20. Siefker-Radtke AO, Gee J, Shen Y, *et al.* Multimodality management of urachal carcinoma: the M. D. Anderson Cancer Center experience. *J Urol* 2003; **169**(4):1295–8.
21. Ashley RA, Inman BA, Sebo TJ, *et al.* Urachal carcinoma: clinicopathologic features and long-term outcomes of an aggressive malignancy. *Cancer* 2006; **107**(4):712–20.
22. Pinthus JH, Haddad R, Trachtenberg J, *et al.* Population based survival data on urachal tumors. *J Urol* 2006; **175**(6):2042–7; discussion 7.
23. Zaghloul MS, Nouh A, Nazmy M, *et al.* Long-term results of primary adenocarcinoma of the urinary bladder: a report on 192 patients. *Urol Oncol* 2006; **24**(1):13–20.
24. Herr HW, Bochner BH, Sharp D, Dalbagni G, Reuter VE. Urachal carcinoma: contemporary surgical outcomes. *J Urol* 2007; **178**(1):74–8; discussion 8.
25. Molina JR, Quevedo JF, Furth AF, Richardson RL, Zincke H, Burch PA. Predictors of survival from urachal cancer: a Mayo Clinic study of 49 cases. *Cancer* 2007; **110**(11):2434–40.
26. Gopalan A, Sharp DS, Fine SW, *et al.* Urachal carcinoma: a clinicopathologic analysis of 24 cases with outcome correlation. *Am J Surg Pathol* 2009; **33**(5):659–68.
27. Thomas AA, Stephenson AJ, Campbell SC, Jones JS, Hansel DE. Clinicopathologic features and utility of immunohistochemical markers in signet-ring cell adenocarcinoma of the bladder. *Hum Pathol* 2009; **40**(1):108–16.
28. Bruins HM, Visser O, Ploeg M, Hulsbergen-van de Kaa CA, Kiemeney LA, Witjes JA. The clinical epidemiology of urachal carcinoma: results of a large, population based study. *J Urol* 2012; **188**(4):1102–7.
29. Wheeler JD, Hill WT. Adenocarcinoma involving the urinary bladder. *Cancer* 1954; **7**(1):119–35.
30. Allen TD, Henderson BW. Adenocarcinoma of the Bladder. *J Urol* 1965; **93**:50–6.
31. Corica FA, Husmann DA, Churchill BM, *et al.* Intestinal metaplasia is not a strong risk factor for bladder cancer: study of 53 cases with long-term follow-up. *Urology* 1997; **50**(3):427–31.
32. Smith AK, Hansel DE, Jones JS. Role of cystitis cystica et glandularis and intestinal metaplasia in development of bladder carcinoma. *Urology* 2008; **71**(5):915–8.
33. el-Boulkany MN, Ghoneim MA, Mansour MA. Carcinoma of the bilharzial bladder in Egypt. Clinical and pathological features. *Br J Urol* 1972; **44**(5):561–70.
34. Smeulders N, Woodhouse CR. Neoplasia in adult exstrophy patients. *BJU Int* 2001; **87**(7):623–8.
35. Beare JB, Tormey AR Jr, Wattenberg CA. Exstrophy of the urinary bladder complicated by adenocarcinoma. *J Urol* 1956; **76**(5):583–94.
36. Mc IJ, Worley G Jr. Adenocarcinoma arising in exstrophy of the bladder: report of two cases and review of the literature. *J Urol* 1955; **73**(5):820–9.

37. Woodhouse CR, North AC, Gearhart JP. Standing the test of time: long-term outcome of reconstruction of the exstrophy bladder. *World J Urol* 2006; **24**(3):244–9.
38. Austen M, Kalble T. Secondary malignancies in different forms of urinary diversion using isolated gut. *J Urol* 2004; **172**(3):831–8.
39. Soergel TM, Cain MP, Misseri R, Gardner TA, Koch MO, Rink RC. Transitional cell carcinoma of the bladder following augmentation cystoplasty for the neuropathic bladder. *J Urol* 2004; **172**(4 Pt 2):1649–51; discussion 51–2.
40. Castellan M, Gosalbez R, Perez-Brayfield M, *et al.* Tumor in bladder reservoir after gastrocystoplasty. *J Urol* 2007 Oct; **178**(4 Pt 2):1771–4; discussion 4.
41. Velcheti V, Govindan R. Metastatic cancer involving bladder: a review. *Can J Urol* 2007; **14**(1):3443–8.
42. Roy S, Parwani AV. Adenocarcinoma of the urinary bladder. *Arch Pathol Lab Med* 2011; **135**(12):1601–5.
43. Mostofi FK, Thomson RV, Dean AL Jr. Mucous adenocarcinoma of the urinary bladder. *Cancer* 1955; **8**(4):741–58.
44. Johnson DE, Hodge GB, Abdul-Karim FW, Ayala AG. Urachal carcinoma. *Urology* 1985; **26**(3):218–21.
45. Williamson SR, Lopez-Beltran A, Montironi R, Cheng L. Glandular lesions of the urinary bladder:clinical significance and differential diagnosis. *Histopathology* 2011; **58**(6):811–34.
46. Adeniran AJ, Tamboli P. Clear cell adenocarcinoma of the urinary bladder: a short review. *Arch Pathol Lab Med* 2009; **133**(6):987–91.
47. Hughes MJ, Fisher C, Sohaib SA. Imaging features of primary nonurachal adenocarcinoma of the bladder. *AJR Am J Roentgenol* 2004; **183**(5):1397–401.
48. Thali-Schwab CM, Woodward PJ, Wagner BJ. Computed tomographic appearance of urachal adenocarcinomas: review of 25 cases. *Eur Radiol* 2005; **15**(1):79–84.
49. Rafal RB, Markisz JA. Urachal carcinoma: the role of magnetic resonance imaging. *Urol Radiol* 1991; **12**(4):184–7.
50. Malek RS, Rosen JS, O'Dea MJ. Adenocarcinoma of bladder. *Urology* 1983; **21**(4):357–9.
51. Colombo JR Jr, Desai M, Canes D, *et al.* Laparoscopic partial cystectomy for urachal and bladder cancer. *Clinics (Sao Paulo)* 2008; **63**(6):731–4.
52. Spiess PE, Correa JJ. Robotic assisted laparoscopic partial cystectomy and urachal resection for urachal adenocarcinoma. *Int Braz J Urol* 2009; **35**(5):609.
53. Nevin JE 3rd, Melnick I, Baggerly JT, Easley CA Jr, Landes R. Advanced carcinoma of bladder: treatment using hypogastric artery infusion with 5-fluorouracil, either as a single agent or in combination with bleomycin or adriamycin and supervoltage radiation. *J Urol* 1974; **112**(6):752–8.
54. Logothetis CJ, Samuels ML, Ogden S. Chemotherapy for adenocarcinomas of bladder and urachal origin: 5-fluorouracil, doxorubicin, and mitomycin-C. *Urology* 1985; **26**(3):252–5.
55. Hatch TR, Fuchs EF. Intra-arterial infusion of 5-fluorouracil for recurrent adenocarcinoma of bladder. *Urology* 1989; **33**(4):311–2.
56. Galsky MD, Iasonos A, Mironov S, *et al.* Prospective trial of ifosfamide, paclitaxel, and cisplatin in patients with advanced non-transitional cell carcinoma of the urothelial tract. *Urology* 2007; **69**(2):255–9.
57. Tatokoro M, Kawakami S, Yonese J, *et al.* Preliminary report of multimodal treatment with ifosfamide, 5-fluorouracil, etoposide and cisplatin (IFEP chemotherapy) against metastatic adenocarcinoma of the urachus. *Int J Urol* 2008; **15**(9):851–3.
58. Yazawa S, Kikuchi E, Takeda T, *et al.* Surgical and chemotherapeutic options for urachal carcinoma: report of ten cases and literature review. *Urol Int* 2012; **88**(2):209–14.
59. Xiaoxu L, Jianhong L, Jinfeng W, Klotz LH. Bladder adenocarcinoma: 31 reported cases. *Can J Urol* 2001; **8**(5):1380–3.
60. Kapur P, Lotan Y, King E, *et al.* Primary adenocarcinoma of the urinary bladder: value of cell cycle biomarkers. *Am J Clin Pathol* 2011; **135**(6):822–30.
61. Bates AW, Baithun SI. Secondary neoplasms of the bladder are histological mimics of nontransitional cell primary tumours: clinicopathological and histological features of 282 cases. *Histopathology* 2000; **36**(1):32–40.
62. Morichetti D, Mazzucchelli R, Lopez-Beltran A, *et al.* Secondary neoplasms of the urinary system and male genital organs. *BJU Int* 2009; **104**(6):770–6.
63. Torenbeek R, Lagendijk JH, Van Diest PJ, Bril H, van de Molengraft FJ, Meijer CJ. Value of a panel of antibodies to identify the primary origin of adenocarcinomas presenting as bladder carcinoma. *Histopathology* 1998; **32**(1):20–7.
64. Wang HL, Lu DW, Yerian LM, *et al.* Immunohistochemical distinction between primary adenocarcinoma of the bladder and secondary colorectal adenocarcinoma. *Am J Surg Pathol* 2001; **25**(11):1380–7.
65. Suh N, Yang XJ, Tretiakova MS, Humphrey PA, Wang HL. Value of CDX2, villin, and alpha-methylacyl coenzyme A racemase immunostains in the distinction between primary adenocarcinoma of the bladder and secondary colorectal adenocarcinoma. *Mod Pathol* 2005; **18**(9):1217–22.
66. Yossepowitch O, Koren R, Konichezki M, Livne PM, Baniel J. Deleted-in-colon-cancer protein expression in patients with adenocarcinoma of the urinary tract and a history of colorectal cancer. *Urology* 2004; **64**(6):1133–8.

CHAPTER 6.25

Urothelial carcinomas of the upper urinary tract

Tarek P. Ghoneim, Pierre Colin, and Morgan Rouprêt

Epidemiology

Incidence

Upper urinary tract urothelial carcinomas (UTUCs) are relatively rare tumours. They account for 5–10% of urothelial carcinomas. It is estimated that about 7,200 new cases of tumour of the renal pelvis or ureter occur each year in the European Union.[1,2] In the United States, Munoz and Ellison estimated the incidence at 0.73 of 100,000 person-years for ureteral transitional cell carcinoma and at 1.0 of 100,000 person-years for renal pelvis transitional cell carcinoma, between 1985 and 1995.[3] However, worldwide incidence of renal pelvis tumours is inaccurate since these tumours can be included in kidney tumours according to studies.[2,4]

Age

Most recent series report an average age of occurrence of 70 years; with incidence increasing with age.[5]

Sex-ratio

As with bladder cancer, men are more likely than women to suffer from UTUCs. In fact, occurrence is up to two times higher for male patients, but this discrepancy can probably be attributed to the greater likelihood of men being exposed to the effects of major carcinogens for many years.[1,5]

Risk factors

Environmental factors

Exposure to tobacco increases the relative risk (RR) of developing a UTUC to 2.5–7. Number of cigarettes a day, and number of years of exposure appear to influence that risk. Multiple substances (aromatic amine, benzopyrene, dimethylbenzathracene) inhaled in the cigarette smoke play a role in the upper urinary tract carcinogenesis.

Occupational exposure is another important environmental risk factor. Indeed, employees of many industries (dyes, textiles, rubber, chemicals, petrochemicals, coal, coke, tar) are exposed to several chemical carcinogens (aromatic amines, polycyclic aromatic hydrocarbons, chlorinated solvents). An average exposure of about seven years is needed for developing UTUC and the interval of occurrence after exposure can be up to 20 years.[1,6,7]

It has been noticed that in the Balkans in South Eastern Europe, incidence is multiplied by 60 to 100 times the incidence of the rest of the world. However, since first described in the 1950s the difference of incidence has decreased dramatically. UTUC of the Balkans is associated with Balkan Endemic Nephropathy, a degenerative interstitial nephropathy.[8,9] But the exact aetiology is yet to be determined. Many hypotheses have been put forth. Exposure to professional carcinogens, infectious exposure has been suggested.

More recently, Chinese herb nephropathy has been described in patients exposed to a Chinese herbal product containing *Aristolochia fangchi*.[10] Half of these patients then develop UTUC. *Aristolochia fangchi*, as well as *Aristolochia clematis* (a plant endemic to the Balkans) contains aristolochic acid, which is described as a carcinogen responsible of a genetic mutation.[11]

Southwestern and northeastern Taiwan are other regions of endemic UTUC. It has been suggested a link between UTUC and the Blackfoot disease (BFD), which is a vasculitis caused by chronic exposure to arsenic in the water of artesian wells. However, arsenic pollution is not an issue in the northeastern part of the country and patients suffering from UTUC in the southwest often do not present BFD. The role of arsenic in the carcinogenesis is probably not sufficient to explain the higher incidence on this Asian island.

Phenacetin was widely used as an analgesic for 40 years but has been abandoned since the 1980s when its role as a carcinogen for the upper urinary tract was demonstrated.[12,13] As the average latency for appearance of UTUC is 22 years, the number of cases described today is decreasing. Carcinogenesis appears to be related to papillary necrosis caused by phenacetin.

Chronic exposure to alkylating chemotherapy (cyclophosphamide, ifosfamide) and laxatives seems to be implicated in the appearance of UTUC, though only small studies have reported those.

Chronic inflammation and other endogenous factors

Chronic urinary tract infections may be implicated in the carcinogenesis of UTUC with an OR of 1.5–2. Through chronic irritation, presence of lithiasis in the urinary tract may promote cancer proliferation. The risk increases with female gender, renal pelvis calcifications, history of concomitant infections, and number of hospital-related disease lithiasis. Arterial hypertension may harbour a risk for UTUC though mechanism remains unclear; with a RR of 1.3.

Heredity and genetic polymorphism

HNPCC (hereditary non-polyposis colorectal cancer) syndrome also known as Lynch syndrome is the commonest monogenetic predisposition for colorectal cancer. The lifetime risk of malignancies is 80%. Apart from colorectal cancer, patients with this syndrome also have a risk of developing other malignant tumours, such as endometrial, ovarian, small bowel, stomach, hepato-biliary, skin, brain, or urogenital cancers, mostly UTUCs.[14] Typically, these patients are younger than sporadic cases. In case of suspicion for a hereditary carcinoma, several tests are recommended: microsatellite instability analysis, immunochemistry, and DNA sequencing. It has recently been stated that a significant proportion of patients with newly diagnosed UTUC were misclassified as sporadic and may have HNPCC as a cause. A prediction tool to attempt indentifying patients who may have HNPCC was proposed based on clinical criterias: age at diagnosis, sex, personal, and family history of other cancers associated to HNPCC.

In addition the evidence suggesting an individual genetic susceptibility (i.e. polymorphism) to known risk factors has grown recently. The carcinogenesis due to toxic exposure is probably in most cases, related to genetic variants of the detoxification enzymatic system.

Natural history

Carcinogenesis biology—molecular pathways

Aside from constitutional mutations, from a germline mutation, present in almost all cells of the body; genetic (mutation, deletion) and epigenetic (DNA methylation) alterations occur. An unstable balance is represented by two type of genes: proto-oncogenes and tumour suppressor genes. When one of these type of genes is altered; the cell may follow the pathological path of oncogenesis.

Proto-oncogenes code for several types of proteins such as growth factors, receptors, or nuclear proteins helping regulate cell growth and differentiation. Either spontaneously or after exposure to an exogenous carcinogen, the promoter of the proto-oncogene may be altered. This transforms the proto-oncogene into an oncogene and the protein is overexpressed. The two main proto-oncogenes assessed for UTUC are:

- FGFR3 (fibroblast growth factor receptor 3): it is a tyrosine kinase receptor. Its inactivation may be associated to better survival and lower grade. Also present for bladder cancer, there appears that incidence of mutation is similar in UTUC or bladder carcinomas.
- EGF (epidermal growth factor) receptor and ligand: it is a transmembrane protein complex, with a tyrosine kinase activity. Ten to 55% of UTUC have EGF overexpression and it might be correlated to advanced stage and grade. Also, mutation of epidermal growth factor receptor might be linked to histopathological characteristics such as metaplastic squamous and/or glandular differentiation.

Tumour suppressor genes code for proteins implied in the control of cell growth with a repressive effect on cell cycle regulation or promoting apoptosis; for proteins protecting genomic integrity (DNA repair proteins) or intercellular interaction (metastasis suppressors). The main tumour suppressor genes studied for UTUC are the following:

- *p53*: it is encoded by the *TP53* gene located on the short arm of chromosome 17 (17p13.1). p53 is a protein helping to lead the cell towards apoptosis when DNA damage is impossible. If damage on DNA is limited it can actually activate DNA repair. A mutant p53 allows cellular replication with DNA damage that might lead to cancerous proliferation. Mutations of *TP53* generally occur (90% of cases) on exon 5 to 8 and the type of mutation is probably different according to the type of exogenous carcinogen exposition.
- *RB1*: located on chromosome 13; it codes for a protein playing a role in cell cycle regulation.
- *CDH1*: located on chromosome 16, it codes for Cadherin-E protein (epithelial cadherin), which plays a role in the cell–cell adhesion system. Loss of function allows increasing proliferation, invasion, and metastasis.

Epigenetic mutations play also a role in oncogenesis. CpG islands are regions of the DNA with higher concentrations of CpG sites. Methylation of CpG islands is probably responsible for inactivation of tumour suppressor genes. This mechanism has been suggested as a possible cause for inactivation of several tumour suppressor genes such as *CDH1, hMLH1, hMSH2, GSTP1, MGMT, p16*, and *p14*.

Genomic instability is indicated by microsatellite instability (MSI). MSI is defined by the expansion or deletion of one or two repeat units. It correlated with the mutation of a mismatch repair gene and is detected with polymerase chain reaction (PCR) on DNA from normal and tumour tissue. MSI are detected in nearly all HNPCC, UTUC, and in 25% of sporadic tumours.[14]

Tumour location and multifocality

Renal pelvis tumours are more common than ureteral ones. And within the ureter, distal localization is more frequent than proximal ones. However, UTUC is a pan-urothelial disease and multifocal, synchronous lesions are not rare: ipsilateral multifocality occurs in about 20% of cases. Bilateral tumours are extremely rare either they be synchronous or metachronous (1.6 to 3.1%, respectfully). Chronic exposure to phenacetin, black foot disease, or Balkan nephropathy might be a risk factor to bilateral tumours. Multiple recurrences of bladder tumours might also be a risk factor.

Theories for multifocal tumours are either the 'field effect' of carcinogens on urothelial cells that can be separate in location resulting in oligoclonality; or the 'seed theory' with intraluminal or intraepithelial spread of a single mutated cell.[15,16,17]

Association of UTUC and bladder carcinoma is well described. In 17% of cases, concurrent bladder cancer is present. Recurrence of disease in the bladder occurs in 22–47% of UTUC patients.[18,19,20] The most frequent site of recurrence is the ipsilateral ureteral meatus. Recurrence occurs in the majority of cases in the two years following UTUC management but no real risk factor have been identified yet; only multifocality of UTUC lesions.[21]

Upper urinary tract recurrence after an invasive bladder tumour is rare (rate of 2 to 5%).[22] They occur mostly in the 3 years following radical cystectomy. Several risk factors have been identified such as a history of carcinoma *in situ* in the bladder, a history of bladder cancer recurrence, of cystectomy for non-muscle-invasive bladder cancer and tumour involvement of the ureter on the cystectomy specimen.[22]

Local, regional, lymphatic, and metastatic spread

Epithelial spread, either through the 'field theory' or the 'seed theory', is antegrade or retrograde.

The muscle layer surrounding the urothelium of the renal pelvis and the ureter constitutes a barrier to the spread of the tumour.

However, this layer is very thin. Invasive tumours will easily spread to the muscle and the adventitia and surrounding tissues.

Higher grade and localization may be directly linked to local spread. Muscle layer is thinner for the ureter than for the renal pelvic making local spread easier and thus regional and metastatic dissemination easier.[23,24] Ureteral location seems to be associated to higher stage tumours. Renal parenchyma may constitute a thicker and more protective barrier for calyceal localization of tumours.

Lymphatic system of the upper urinary tract is as following:

- renal pelvis is drained first in to hilar nodes and then to para and retrocaval nodes on the right and para-aortic nodes on the left;
- proximal ureter is either drained directly to para and retrocaval nodes on the right and para-aortic nodes on the left or through the hilar nodes;
- distal ureter is drained towards pelvic lymph nodes.

Lymphatic spread depends on localization of the tumour and on its grade and stage.

Once these nodes are affected, extension progresses towards the thoracic duct, mediastinum, and supraclavicular nodes.

Metastases are rarely inaugural. Most common sites are bone (32%), lung (25%) and liver (24%).[25,26] Tumour grade, stage, and presence of lymphovascular invasion appear to be most important predictors of metastatic dissemination.

Pathology

Normal urothelium is the epithelium that covers the entire urinary tract including the bladder and the urethra. The aspect that matters the most for pathology classification and management decisions, is the thickness of the underlying tissues: a muscular mucosa in the renal pelvis, laying on the renal hilum fat; a thin subepithelial connective tissue for the ureter.

Histological types

Urothelial carcinomas constitute the vast majority of upper urinary tract tumours (95%). Of these, transitional origin is the most common; followed by squamous cell carcinomas and adenocarcinomas. They are very similar to bladder urothelial carcinomas.

Urothelial carcinomas are of several types:

- papillary tumours are the most common (85%). They are more or less differentiated. The pelvic location is the most frequent (Figs 6.25.1 and 6.25.2). There, they can be bulky and infiltrate the renal parenchyma. In the ureter, they may be revealed by an obstructive symptom (Figs 6.25.3).

Non-invasive tumours are characterized by an exophytic papillary proliferation of the urothelium. The layers of urothelium are multiplied but the lamina propria is preserved. Depending on the cellular and architectural deterioration, the grade of the tumour changes. These lesions are classified as pTa.

Infiltrating tumours are defined as a crossing of the lamina propria. When only the subepithelial connective tissue is invaded, the tumour is classified as pT1. pT2 tumours are defined as those invading the muscle layer. At this point, all tumours are considered as high grade. If periureteric or peripelvic fat or renal parenchyma is invaded, then the tumour is considered pT3 and pT4 if adjacent organs or perinephric fat are invaded.

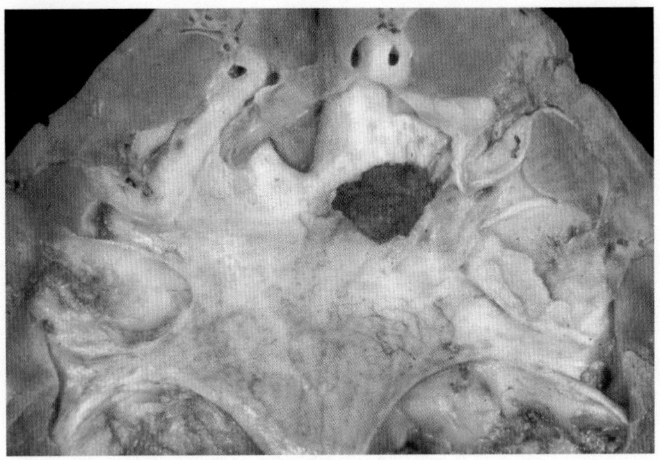

Fig. 6.25.1 Non-invasive tumour of the renal pelvis.

- Carcinoma *in situ* is frequently associated to high-grade infiltrating papillary tumours. It is actually considered by some to be a precursor of infiltrating tumours. Though lamina propria is preserved, cyto-nuclear atypias, mitosis, and architectural disorders are seen. It may be single or multifocal.[28,29]
- Sessile tumours are rare. They are often infiltrating and of high grade.

Other subtypes of carcinomas are rare:

- squamous cell carcinoma constitutes 0.7 to 7% of the UTUC. Usually single, localization is often pelvic. They are often of high grade and have a poor prognosis. Association to chronic infection, or calculi is common.
- Adenocarcinoma may occur. It represents less than 1% of upper tract tumours. Association to chronic infection and calculi is common. Three types are described: tubulovillous, and mucinous, more common and more aggressive, and papillary nonintestinal type, rare but with a better prognosis.

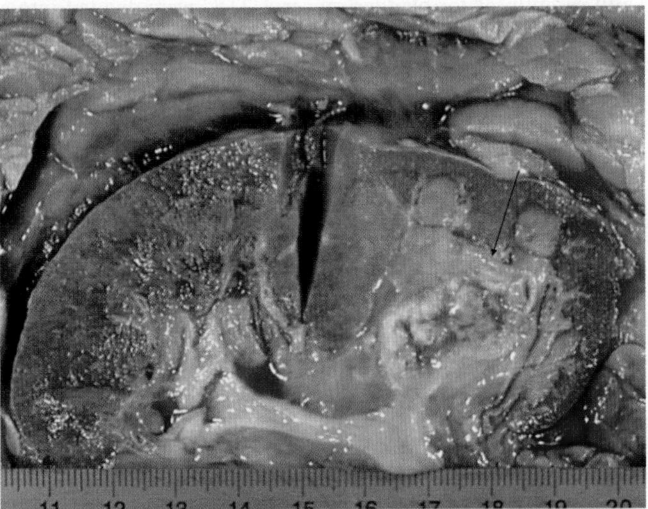

Fig. 6.25.2 Tumour of the renal pelvis which starts to invade the renal parenchyma.

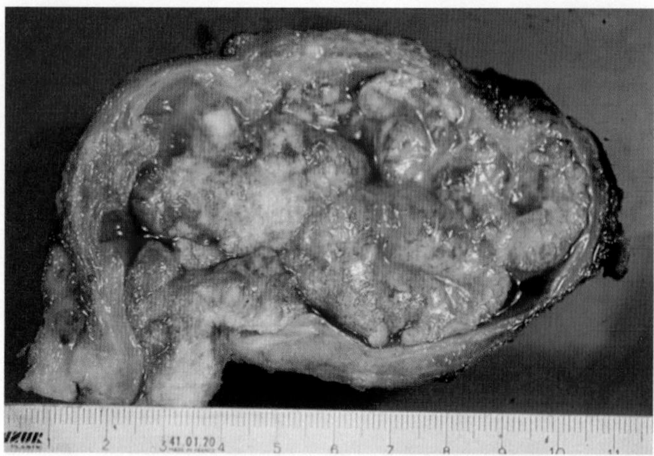

Fig. 6.25.3 Obstructive and bulky tumour of the ureter.

- Neuroendocrine carcinomas represent less than 0.5% of urinary tract tumours and include: small cell carcinomas (40 cases described), large cell carcinomas, and carcinoid tumours. They are usually associated with an urothelial contingent.

Tumour classification

Classifications mimic those of the bladder. The actual Tumour Node Metastasis staging system is the Union Internationale Contre le Cancer (UICC) 2009 TNM classification. It allows a prognostic classification of tumours.

It has been suggested that for pelvic tumours pT3 tumours should be divided into pT3a for a microscopic invasion of the renal parenchyma (<5 mm) and pT3b for a macroscopic invasion invasion of the renal parenchyma or invasion of peripelvic fat. Langner and al showed that pT3a and pT3b tumours have similar prognosis to pT2 and pT4 tumours respectfully.

Papillary lesions are more often of higher stage than sessile ones.

A correlation between stage and grade has been proven, with both characteristics evolving the same way.

Grading system

Until recently, as for bladder cancer, UTUC were divided into a grade 1 to 3 classification.[28,29] That was the 1973 World Health Organization (WHO) classification. But advances in molecular biology allow distinguishing three groups of non-invasive tumours: papillary urothelial neoplasia of low malignant potential (extremely rare), low-grade carcinomas and high-grade carcinomas (WHO 2004 classification).

However, this new classification is limited by the conversion from the 1973 classification:

- 1973 grade 1 includes the low malignant potential papillary urothelial neoplasia and part of the low-grade carcinomas;
- 1973 grade 2 includes the rest of the low-grade and some of the high-grade carcinomas;
- 1973 grade 3 includes the rest of the high-grade carcinomas.

Prognostic factors

The most important prognostic factors appear to be tumour stage and lymph node status.

Patient-related factors

Age of occurrence of UTUC is high and the older the patient is, the worse the prognosis is. Several studies have concluded that worse prognosis is associated with chronological age.

Historically female sex was considered a pejorative prognostic factor. However, after several recent large multi-institutional studies have established that female or male patients have the same survival rates, gender is not considered to be a prognostic factor any longer.

Health status is increasingly being assessed as a potential prognostic factor.

This characteristic is important since the population affected by UTUC is often old and presents important co-morbidities. Two health status scores have been assessed:

The American Society of Anaesthesiologist score (taking into account several co morbidities) in a recent retrospective multi-institutional study (including 554 patients) was correlated to oncological outcome after radical treatment.

However, the Eastern Cooperative Oncology Group Performance Status score (ECOG PS) was assessed in another recent retrospective collaborative study including 427 patients and was not associated to recurrence-free survival or specific survival after radical treatment.

Lastly, current smokers at diagnosis have a higher risk for poor oncologic outcomes; obesity and higher BMI adversely impact cancer outcomes in UTUCs

Tumour stage and grade

Tumour stage is probably certainly the most significant prognostic factor for UTUC. There is clear cut-off for survival between non-invasive and invasive tumours. Five year cancer-specific survival rates are 90%, 85–90%, 70–80%, 30–50%, and 0–30% for Ta tumours, pT1, pT2, pT3, and pT4 tumours, respectively.[31] A recent retrospective study, from Shariat *et al.* suggests that pT3 pelvicalyceal tumours should be subclassified as pT3a (microscopic invasion of the renal parenchyma) and pT3b (macroscopic infiltration of the renal parenchyma); as the latter stage had worse recurrence-free and cancer-specific survival and was identified as an independent prognostic factor.

Tumour grade as a prognostic factor is debated.[32–38] High grade is strongly associated to tumour stage; invasive lesions being very often of grade 3. Whether tumour grade influences survival was a matter of debate at the time of single institution small retrospective studies. But more recent collaborative group studies show that higher grade is associated with worse oncological outcome.

Clinical grade (biopsy tumour grade) allows a prediction of final grade though sensitivity is not perfect, as we will see in the diagnostic paragraph. Clinical stage is much more unreliable than clinical grade; either through biopsy (difficulty to obtain underlying muscle) or through imaging (poor predictive value).[39–50]

Tumour location

Intuitively one would think that ureteral location confers worse prognosis to UTUC because of the thin wall surrounding the ureter compared to the thickness of the renal parenchyma.

However, according to recent findings, there is a prognostic impact of tumour location when adjusted for tumour stage: ureteral and multifocal tumours have a worse prognosis than renal pelvis tumours.[51,52,53]

Others pathologic factors

Whether a sessile or papillary tumour is more aggressive has been the subject of several reports. Most conclude that a sessile lesion has a worse prognosis. A sessile architecture appears to be correlated to invasive, higher grade, lymph node involvement, and lymphovascular invasion.

Lymphovascular invasion (LVI) is an important step of the metastatic spread and it is present in nearly 20% of UTUCs.[54,55] First, the lymphovascular space of the peritumoral space is invaded before extension to the first lymph node involved. LVI is associated to tumour stage, grade, sessile architecture, positive lymph nodes, concomitant carcinoma *in situ* (CIS) and tumour necrosis; all of pejorative prognosis and is also an independent predictor of poor prognosis for cancer-specific survival and recurrence-free survival.[56]

Lymph node involvement is a predictor of aggressiveness. It is correlated to tumour stage and grade. Cancer-specific survival is around 30% at 5 years in case of positive lymph nodes.[57]

Lymph node density is defined as the rate of positive lymph nodes on the overall number of lymph nodes retrieved from the lymph node dissection. Bolenz and al stratified patients according to their lymph node density: over 30% of lymph node density; cancer-specific and recurrence-free survival worsens.[59] However, the templates of lymph node dissection are not precisely defined yet as we will see later in this chapter.

Concomitant CIS in the final nephroureterectomy specimen is probably a risk factor for worse recurrence-free and cancer-specific survival according to several studies.[59,60,61]

On the other hand, CIS alone on the specimen has a fairly good prognosis (90%) cancer-specific survival at three years if radical treatment is applied.

Tumour necrosis is observed in several types of cancers. It is usually a reflection of tumour aggressiveness from intense proliferation.[62] Neovascularisation is necessary but if growth is to rapid; hypoxia induces necrosis. Two large multi-institutional studies have assessed tumour necrosis as a potential prognostic factor. However most single studies state that tumor necrosis (especially if extensive, accounting for more than 10% of total tumour mass) is a pejorative prognostic factor for recurrence-free and cancer-specific survival.

Other factors

It appears from several studies that preoperative hydronephrosis at imaging is correlated to advanced stage and to worse prognosis.[63,64,65] Symptoms at diagnosis are probably not related to cancer-specific survival though advanced lesions seem more symptomatic than non-invasive tumours.

Molecular markers

Several molecular markers have been assessed for UTUC but due to the rarity of this disease and the limited number of patients of the studies, none of the markers has fulfilled the clinical criteria necessary to support their introduction in clinical decision-making.[66]

Multiple tissue-based markers have been assessed. p53 is probably correlated with tumour aggressiveness. Overexpression of Ki-67, EGFR, Bcl2, and survivin have been studied and either correlate to tumour aggressiveness or were proven to be independently correlated to survival.[66,67] For blood-based markers, such as C-reactive protein (CRP) elevation or elevated blood cells counts were assessed in small retrospective studies and were correlated to survival. However, the data is to scarce to allow definite conclusions. Microsatellite instability may be a predictor of overall survival (conclusion from a single institutional study) but has to be assessed in further studies.[68–71]

Prediction tools in UTUC

Few prediction tools have been developed to help clinicians in their management decision-making.

Two preoperative models for prediction of tumour stage have been developed:

- Margulis and al developed their nomogram using preoperative data such as tumour grade, architecture, and location; achieving 76.6% of accuracy for predicting non-organ confined tumours.[72]
- Favaretto and al combined preoperative imaging and endoscopic data (local invasion and hydronephrosis on imaging; high-grade tumour at ureteroscopy and tumour location at ureteroscopy) to creat a predicting tool with around 70% prediction accuracy for muscle-invasive and non-organ confined lesions.[73]

There are two nomograms that can predict survival rates in a post-operative setting based on standard pathologic features: one coming from an international group and the other one built from a european population only (available at http://labs.fccc.edu/nomograms/nomogram.php?id=66&audience=1). Both are based on age, pT and pN stage, and tumour grade.[74,75]

Diagnostic

Symptoms

Gross haematuria is the most common symptom at diagnosis of UTUC. It can be gross or microscopic; total or terminal if the tumour affects the very distal part of the ureter. Depending on the series, haematuria occurs in 70 to 80% of cases. Flank pain can occur in 20 to 30% of cases. Renal colic is possible due to a blood clot in the upper tract or to the migration of a fragment of tumour. However, often, the pain is dull, with a slow and chronic obstruction of the upper urinary tract. A flank or abdominal mass can be palpable in some advanced cases. Locally or metastatic disease might be revealed by asthenia, anorexia, weight loss.In some rare cases (10%), diagnosis is fortuitous.[76]

Imaging

Historically, intravenous pyelography was the gold standard for UTUC diagnosis. However, it is now superseded by computed tomographic urography (CT urography).[77,78,79]

Intravenous pyelography has a sensitivity of about 55 to 90% according to the series.

Radiocontrast agent must be of low osmolarity to avoid dilution by diuresis.

The description of the lesions is well established:

- Filling defects are classical. They may be single or multiple; smooth, irregular, or stippled.
- Obstructing tumours may present with stricture like images and with ureteric dilatation. At the most, renal function might be poor and contrast excretion delayed or non-existent.
- Calcifications occur in 2 to 7% of tumours and may mimic standard renal or ureteral calculi.

Retrograde pyelography is usually performed during cystocopy under general anaesthesia. Description of the lesions is very similar to intravenous pyelography. Selective cytology being possible during the same procedure, retrograde pyelography is very sensitive and specific (96 and 97%).

CT urography is nowadays the imaging technique with the highest accuracy for UTUC.[80,81,82] It allows a vision of the entire urinary tract in a single breath-hold, assessment of the urinary tract lumen and wall and a loco regional evaluation.

Acquisition protocol is rigorously set. It is multiphasic:

- First phase is performed pre-enhancement to exclude a lithiasis.
- An early corticomedullary, late arterial phase follows (40 seconds after infusion), ruling out a possible vascular abnormality. This phase is not mandatory.
- A nephrographic phase (90 to 120 seconds after infusion) allows assessment of the renal parenchyma and tumour vascularization.
- Finally an excretory phase of the entire urinary tract is necessary (6 to 8 minutes after infusion) is necessary for the assessment of the urothelium.

A hyperdiuresis is often performed by furosemid infusion or hyperhydration allowing a complete opacification of the entire urinary tract in a single acquisition, which is particularly useful for the distal ureter considering ureteral peristaltsis.

Post-processing with MIP (maximum intensity projection) and MPR (multiplanar reformatted images) allows three-dimensional reformations. Coronal reformation is particularly useful allowing an equivalent of intravenous pyelography.

Urothelial tumours have a tissue density (40–50 UH) within the urinary tract, isodense to renal parenchyma, with moderate enhancement after contract infusion (60-70 UH) and appear as filling defects at the excretory phase (Figs 6.25.4 and 6.25.5).

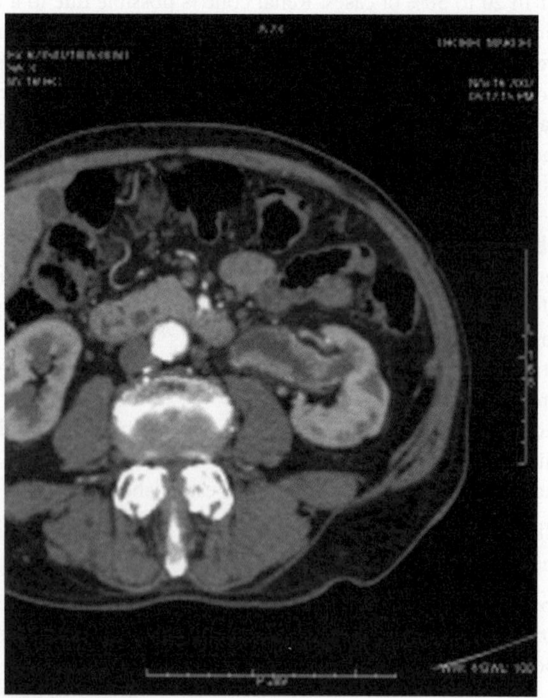

Fig. 6.25.4 Computed tomographic (CT) urography: multifocal upper urinary tract urothelial carcinoma (UTUC) of the left renal pelvis (thickness of upper tract wall).

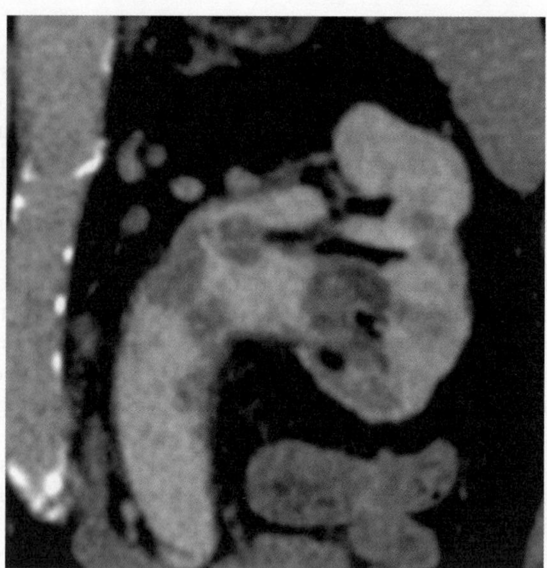

Fig. 6.25.5 CT urography: multifocal UTUC of the ureter and renal pelvis.

Differential diagnoses of filling defects are calculi, blood clots, fungus ball, or ureteritis cystica.

CT urography may be useful for staging: in pelvicaliceal lesions are separated from the renal parenchyma by a fat plane or of contrast medium, the tumour is considered T1 or T2. Infiltrating renal pelvis tumours usually preserve the shape of the kidney, unlike renal cell carcinoma an infiltrating ureteral lesion will appear as an irregular wall thickening with or without upstream dilatation.[83,84]

On a recent meta-analysis CT urography was proven to have a pooled sensitivity and specificity of 96% and 99%, respectfully.[77,79]

MR urography may be useful in cases of contraindication of CT urography only.[85] UTUC being isointense to renal parenchyma in T1 and T2 weighted phases, gadolinium use is recommended to obtain a certain enhancement, which will however not be as intense as for renal parenchyma allowing a differentiation between both tissues. However, MR urography with gadolinium-based contrast media is also contraindicated in patients with severe renal impairment (<30 mL/min creatinine clearance) due to the risk of nephrogenic systemic fibrosis.

Ureteroscopy

Flexible ureteroscopy is a precious diagnostic tool for UTUC (Fig. 6.25.6). It is superior to rigid ureterosopy in that it allows an exploration of the calyceal cavities. Examination of the ureter is possible and must be performed from the pelvis to the bladder otherwise vision is mediocre.

The exploration of the renal tract allows direct vision of the lesions, biopsies, selective cytology.[86,87,88] However, it can happen that inferior calyx cannot be biopsied as the introduction of the biopsy forceps limits the deflection capacities of the ureterosope. Diagnostic sensitivity of biopsies reaches 89 to 95%.

The biopsy is better in predicting grade than stage. However, grade prediction sensitivity varies greatly according to studies, from 58% to 92%, of accuracy in prediction of high-grade tumours and upgrading from after radical treatment is not uncommon. The limits of the biopsy are mainly the quality of the material sent to

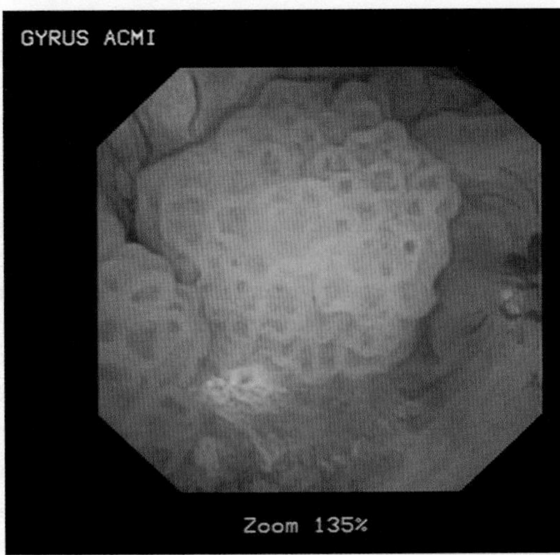

Fig. 6.25.6 Flexible ureteroscopy: digital magnified vision of a tumour at the bottom of the lower cayx (zoom 135%).

pathology: sample sizes, no papillary fronds, crush artefacts, and distorted architecture. The size of the sample (avoiding urinary tract perforation) limits the ability of predicting stage.

Flexible ureteroscopy is a rapidly evolving technology: endoscopes are smaller, more flexible allowing exploration of over 95% of the urinary tract. Vision is better with digital endoscopes.[1,89]

The recent digital endoscopes allow narrow band imaging (NBI). This optical technique of imaging enhancement uses the capacity of tissue to more or less absorb narrow band light: several interference filters are used limiting the wavelength of white light to a narrow band (415–540 nm). At such a wavelight, blood vessels, tumours absorb the light being immediately emphasized by NBI. Initial studies report increased detection rates for NBI versus conventional white light (about 22%).[90]

Photodynamic diagnosis is starting to be assessed for upper tract lesions. It has been proven to be efficient for tumour detection in bladder. Fluorochromes are instilled and are absorbed by the urothelium. After excitation at a certain wavelength, fluorescence contrast between normal and pathological urothelium theoretically allows distinction. However, only few small studies have assessed this technology for the upper tract.

Cystoscopy will be performed to exclude a concomitant bladder tumour. It also performed when a retrographe pyelography is planned.

Cytology

It is the analysis of cells obtained from desquamation of the urothelium. The sample is taken either from voiding or from endoscopy.

Specificity is relatively high (>90%)but sensitivity is limited, especially for low-grade tumours (35–65%).[1] A mean of improving sensitivity is to perform a selective cytology directly in the concerned tract. If cystoscopy is normal, with bladder CIS excluded, a positive cytology is highly indicative of a probable UTUC.

Often, cytology is obtained directly *in situ* after retrograde pyelography. However, it has been suggested that contrast agents, affect directly the quality of the sampling by falsely worsening it.

Pathologists use Papanicolaou's classification. Though sensitivity is not high, combining cytology, to imaging with a filling defect for example is very significant. Cytology may also benefit from fluroscence *in situ* hybridization (FISH) (Urovysion kit from Abbot): it allows detecting molecular abnormalities in cells during the interphase. Sensitivity varies between 81 and 85% with a specificity of 97%, though sensitivity decreases for low-grade tumours in preliminary reports.

Markers

Several biological tests (NMP22, BTA test, Immunocyt) have been developed for diagnosis of urothelial carcinomas. Initially intended for bladder tumours, they have been studied in the upper tract context but no one has entered daily practice so far.

To date, the following investigations are recommended for the diagnosis of UTUC: urinary, cytology, cystoscopy, CT urography, retrograde ureteropyelopgraphy and diagnosis ureteroscopy and biopsy (if suspicion of small volume tumour).

Treatment

Localized disease

Radical treatment: nephroureterectomy

Radical nephroureterectomy (RNU) has remained to date the gold standard treatment for UTUC for 75 years. The rule is to remove the entire upper urinary tract, kidney (perinephric fat included), and ureter, as well as a 2 cm bladder cuff which is essential. Another imperative is to preserve the urinary tract to avoid tumour cell dissemination. Open RNU was the gold standard of radical treatment but laparoscopic surgery is increasingly popular.[84–88] It seems that laparoscopic oncological results are equivalent to open surgery as long as experimented laparoscopic surgeons perform it. However, locally advanced tumours might benefit more from open surgery than laparoscopy, as in a prospective randomized trial comparing both approach, pT3 tumours had worse survival after laparoscopy.

The delay between diagnosis and radical treatment is important as a delay longer than three months for invasive tumours was associated with cancer-specific survival.

Open surgery

Two modalities of access are available and have equivalent oncological results:

- A single midline incision allowing access to both the kidney and the distal ureter.
- Two separate incision: a lumbotomy for the kidney and a second incision (Gibson incision, Pfannenstiel, or a short subumbilical midline incision) for the distal ureter and bladder cuff.

Laparoscopic surgery

Allowing less perioperative morbidity and earlier hospital discharge, laparoscopic approach must be performed respecting all the oncologic rules that apply to open surgery.

A transperitoneal or retroperitoneal approach is possible, depending on the surgeon's experience; neither has been proven to be superior to the other. The only matter of discussion concerns the management of the distal ureter as we will learn later.

Robotic surgery is being assessed as well; but only small reports exist and no definite conclusion can be made. According to the most recent data, open and laparoscopic access are equivalent in terms of efficacy.

Distal ureter management

Bladder cuff resection is a priority in the radical management of UTUC. Several techniques have been described. The classical gold standard is open management. The lower ureter is clipped and removed with the bladder cuff in the en-bloc specimen.

Pure laparoscopic management of the distal ureter is possible. Two main techniques of securing the ureter are described:

- Extravesical stapling of the ureter. This technique is combined with the unroofing technique described further in this paragraph. The ureter is dissected, gently pulled, and a stapler is place near the ureterovesical junction. Disadvantages are that there is not precise control on the intramural ureter; there is a theoretical risk of lithiasis formation on the metallic staples.
- The transvesical approach: transvesical laparoscopic ports are placed, allowing intramural dissection of the ureter orifice after placement of a PDS Endoloop at the ureter tip preventing urine leakage.

Several endoscopic techniques have been described, allowing shorter operative time and are especially useful for patients with poor health status.[77,79] Though comparative studies versus open bladder are small and retrospective, it seems that most techniques have higher recurrence or positive margins rate.

- The stripping of the ureter is performed by introducing an uretheral catheter in the ureter and at the end of the nephrectomy; the ureter is sectioned above the catheter which is attached to the ureter. By pulling on the catheter, the ureter is then stripped. The introverted ureter is freed from the bladder with an endoscopic section.
- In the pluck technique, the ureteral orifice is disarticulated from the bladder wall in performing an endoscopic resection of the entire intramural ureter with a theoretical risk of cancerous cell dissemination. To minimize that risk, a PDS Endoloop or clip can be placed endoscopically on the ureteral orifice.
- The unroofing technique is performed by sectioning the intramural ureter on its anterior part; electrocautering the posterior intramural ureter. To avoid urine leakage an uretheral dilatation balloon is placed in the renal pelvis and the ureter is dissected laparoscopically and detached.

In conclusion, a bladder cuff must always be performed when possible; with open technique still being the gold standard.

Lymphadenectomy

Allowing a better staging of the disease, lymphadenectomy gives a chance to reduce tumour mass and eventually giving a chance of systemic adjuvant treatment. However, the template of lymph node dissection still has to be defined. For Kondo *et al.* the site of lymphadenectomy should depend on initial tumour location. For a pelvic or upper ureter, tumour lymph node dissection should include para cava, retro cava, and interaortico cava nodes for the right side and para-aortic nodes on the left side. For a lower ureter location, a pelvic lymph node dissection should be performed.

Therapeutic benefice of lymph node dissection remains a moot point. For Roscigno and al lymphadenectomy should be performed for patients suspicious of invasive tumours since pNx patients had worse survival rates than pN0 for pT2-4 patients. However, another study from Lughezzani and al concluded in contradictory results with no benefit observed from lymph node dissection. The lack of standardized template or indications for lymph node dissection is an explanation of discrepancies in the results. Some teams have suggested that the number of lymph nodes removed plays a prognostic role: 8 nodes being the threshold for better survival. Still, lymphadenectomy remains recommended in all cases of invasive UTUC.

Nephron-sparing procedures

Initially reserved for imperative indications (solitary kidney, bilateral lesions, major co-morbidities) conservative management has become an option along with radical treatment for selected patients: imperative indications, or low-stage, low-grade, and single lesions. The choice of the technique depends on surgeon's experience, location of the tumour. Close follow-up is necessary after these techniques.

Segmental ureterectomy

In case of a distal ureter tumour, segmental ureterectomy can be proposed. A bladder cuff remains mandatory. The resection is followed by an ureterovesical anastomosis, with or without antireflux mechanism or on a psoic bladder. Laparoscopic and robotic cases have been described. If the tumour is located in the mid-ureter, a segmental ureterectomy is possible with a direct ureteroureteral anastomosis.

In case of pyelocalyceal location, the nephrectomy, or a subtotal nephro-ureterectomy may be performed. Partial renal pelvis resections have been described but are technically difficult and have poor oncological outcomes.

Oncological outcomes after segmental ureterectomy are acceptable when indications are respected.[94,95,96]

Endoscopic management

Endoscopic management has flourished with the coming of smaller, digital ureteroscopes, and laser allows direct management of the tumours during endoscopy. With advances in fiberoptic technology and ever smaller calibre instruments, open surgery is being superseded progressively by less invasive endoscopic procedures. Consequently, first-line nephron-sparing strategies (NSS) are being increasingly performed; not only for imperative cases (i.e. solitary kidney, bilateral disease, or renal insufficiency) but also for patients with a normal contralateral kidney.[90–93]

Ureteroscopic management

This is, by far, the most promising technique to treat UTUC and its use in on constant expansion worldwide. Small lesions may be removed directly with the biopsy pliers. Otherwise laser vaporization will help treat the tumours. A ureteral catheter will be placed and keeped for 24/48 hours after resection. Inferior calyces locations may be a limit to this treatment and voluminous lesions may require several sessions of treatment. In all cases, complete resection is mandatory as well as cauterization of the implantation zone of the tumour. Rare cases of ureter perforation or postoperative stenosis occur but do not seem to impact overall prognosis. When it comes to ureteroscopy, most teams deal exclusively with pure flexibles endoscopes nowadays rather than than rigid ureteroscopes.[90–93]

Percutaneous management

Reserved for pyelocalyceal or proximal ureter lesions, this approach is progressively being abandoned with technological progresses for ureteroscopes. A theoretical risk of tumour seeding exists but has actually very rarely been described.[97,98]

According to the last guidelines, nephron-sparing procedures in UTUCs should be advocated in: unifocal tumour, small tumour, low-grade tumour (cytology or biopsies) without evidence of an infiltrative lesion on CT urography.

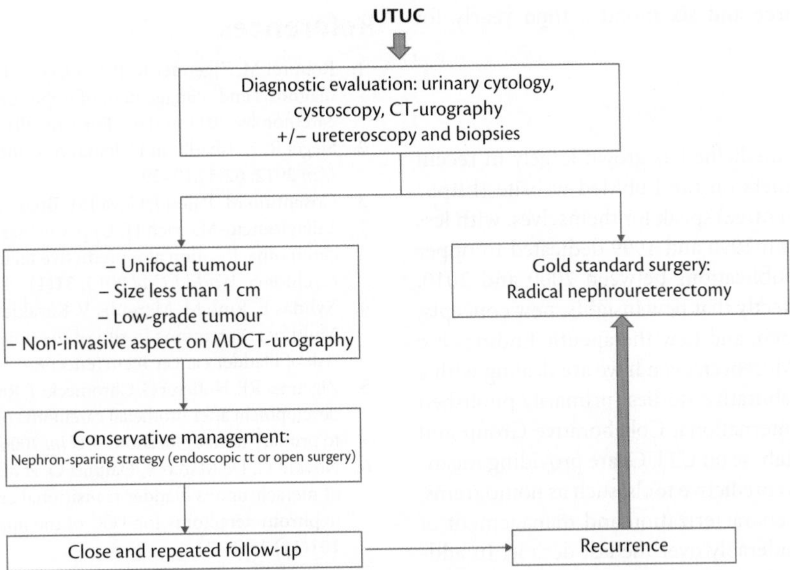

Fig. 6.25.7 Flow chart for the management of UTUC.

To summarize UTUC management, we propose the flow chart in Figure 6.25.7.

Adjuvant topical therapy

Adjuvant therapies instilled percutaneously or through a ureteral stent have been assessed after conservative management. Bacille Calmette-Guérin (BCG) or mitomycin C have been used.[99,100,101]

The major drawback for instillation in the upper tract relies on whether or not treatment would remain at the tumour site for a sufficient period to cause a satisfactory antitumour effect, with a relative short duration of exposure. The most reliable access to the upper urinary tract remains via a nephrostomy tube large enough (e.g. 10F) left in place after percutaneous resection or fulguration, or placed under local anaesthesia and in the prone position, under ultrasound control. This procedure allows for reliable and iterative exposure of the urothelium to the topical agent. The topical agent can be delivered by retrograde reflux from the bladder with an indwelling double-J stent in the Trendelenbourg position.

One major drawback with ureteric stents[3] 4F is the possible ureteric obstruction and subsequent pyelovenous influx during instillation. Furthermore, a ureteric catheter can theoretically lead to an increased risk of injury of the pyelocaliceal mucosae. In addition, it is often difficult to complete filling of the pyelocaliceal system and often the superior calyx remains unfilled. A role for BCG in the management of UT CIS has been demonstrated in retrospective studies, although a definitive efficacy of adjuvant topical therapy after endoscopic resection of Ta/T1 tumours has not yet been proven. No individual study has shown a statistical improvement in survival and recurrence rates.

Advanced disease

Radical nephroureterectomy

RNU is not recommended in the setting of metastatic tumours. However, it may be performed for symptomatic patients in a palliative situation to ease pain and local symptoms.[1,102,103,104,105]

Chemotherapy

Chemotherapy regimens are the same as for bladder cancer. They are platinum based. Contrary to what has been demonstrated for bladder cancer, there have been no reported effects of neoadjuvant chemotherapy for UTUCs in the only study published so far. Results of adjuvant chemotherapy come from small studies and conclusions are difficult to make. There is probably a gain in recurrence-free survival but no gain of cancer-specific survival in particular for advanced stage (<pT3) or metastatic patients. In addition, not all the patients receive this treatment because of co-morbidities and impaired renal function after radical surgery. Adjuvant chemotherapy can somehow achieve a recurrence-free rate of up to 50% but has clearly no impact on survival. Further data are awaited from the ongoing prospective randomized POUT trial (PeriOperative chemotherapy or sUrveillance in upper Tract urothelial cancer) with was launched in 2012 in the United Kingdom.[1,104,105,106,107]

Radiotherapy

Adjuvant radiotherapy has a very limited role in UTUC. Local control, or survival does not seem influenced by radiation therapy. Combination to chemotherapy is advised but benefice is very limited.

Follow-up

Most recurrences occur in the two years following radical treatment. Radical treatment allows minimizing the risk of local recurrence and the risk is mainly a regional or distant recurrence, with risk factors described earlier. However, regular cystoscopy is mandatory because bladder recurrence is always possible.[1]

After RNU, cystoscopy and urinary cytology must be performed at 3 month after treatment than yearly for 5 years according to european guidelines. A CT Urography has to be performed every year for five years for non-invasive tumours but every 6 months for two years than yearly for three years for invasive tumours.

In case of a conservative management, follow-up is extremely important and stringent. Cystoscopy, ipsilateral ureteroscopy and *in situ* cytology are required at three, six months, than every six months for two years and than yearly for three years. CT Urography should be performed at three and six months, then yearly for five years.

Conclusion

The field of evidence-based medicine has grown largely in recent years for UTUCs. The numbers on the PubMed website (http://www.ncbi.nlm.nih.gov/sites/entrez) speak for themselves, with less than 306 publications between 1990 and 1999 dedicated to upper tract tumours versus 778 publications between 2000 and 2010. This trend demonstrates perfectly that new insights, new concepts, new clinical and basic research, and new therapeutic findings are becoming readily available. Moreover, even if we are dealing with a rare tumour type, more collaborative studies (primarily published by two groups, the UTUC International Collaborative Group and the French Collaborative Database on UTUC) are providing meaningful scientific data and even predictive tools, such as nomograms. To conclude, the molecular characterization and management of UTUCs has progressed considerably over the last decade. In addition, surgery is moving towards minimally invasive techniques that spare the kidney's functional unity as much as possible. However, it has taken a century to move from the era of treating the 'urinary apparatus' to tumour detection and identification by molecular biology techniques.

Further reading

Colin P, Koenig P, Ouzzane A, *et al.* Environmental factors involved in carcinogenesis of urothelial cell carcinomas of the upper urinary tract. *BJU Int* 2009; **104**(10):1436–40.

Herrmann TR, Liatsikos EN, Nagele U, Traxer O, Merseburger AS. EAU guidelines on laser technologies. *Eur Urol* 2012; **61**(4):783–95.

Kondo T, Hashimoto Y, Kobayashi H, *et al.* Template-based lymphadenectomy in urothelial carcinoma of the upper urinary tract: impact on patient survival. *Int J Urol* 2010 Oct; **17**(10):848–54.

Lughezzani G, Burger M, Margulis V, *et al.* Prognostic factors in upper urinary tract urothelial carcinomas: a comprehensive review of the current literature. *Eur Urol* 2012; **62**(1):100–14.

Margulis V, Shariat SF, Matin SF, *et al.* Outcomes of radical nephroureterectomy: a series from the Upper Tract Urothelial Carcinoma Collaboration. *Cancer* 2009; **115**(6):1224–33.

Roscigno M, Brausi M, Heidenreich A, *et al.* Lymphadenectomy at the time of nephroureterectomy for upper tract urothelial cancer. *Eur Urol* 2011; **60**(4):776–83.

Rouprêt M, Yates DR, Comperat E, Cussenot O. Upper urinary tract urothelial cell carcinomas and other urological malignancies involved in the hereditary nonpolyposis colorectal cancer (lynch syndrome) tumor spectrum. *Eur Urol* 2008; **54**(6):1226–36.

Rouprêt M, Zigeuner R, Palou J, *et al.* European guidelines for the diagnosis and management of upper urinary tract urothelial cell carcinomas: 2011 update. *Eur Urol* 2011; **59**(4):584–94.

Vassilakopoulou M, de la Motte Rouge T, Colin P, *et al.* Outcomes after adjuvant chemotherapy in the treatment of high-risk urothelial carcinoma of the upper urinary tract (UUT-UC): results from a large multicenter collaborative study. *Cancer* 2011; **117**(24):5500–8.

Wang LJ, Wong YC, Huang CC, Wu CH, Hung SC, Chen HW. Multidetector computerized tomography urography is more accurate than excretory urography for diagnosing transitional cell carcinoma of the upper urinary tract in adults with hematuria. *J Urol* 2010; **183**(1):48–55.

Yates DR, Hupertan V, Colin P, *et al.* Cancer-specific survival after radical nephroureterectomy for upper urinary tract urothelial carcinoma: proposal and multi-institutional validation of a post-operative nomogram. *Br J Cancer* 2012; **106**(6):1083–8.

References

1. Rouprêt M, Zigeuner R, Palou J, *et al.* European guidelines for the diagnosis and management of upper urinary tract urothelial cell carcinomas: 2011 update. *Eur Urol* 2011; **59**(4):584–94.
2. Siegel R, Naishadham D, Jemal A. Cancer statistics, 2012. *CA Cancer J Clin* 2012; **62**(1):10–29.
3. Cosentino M, Palou J, Gaya JM, Breda A, Rodriguez-Faba O, Villavicencio-Mavrich H. Upper urinary tract urothelial cell carcinoma: location as a predictive factor for concomitant bladder carcinoma. *World J Urol* 2013; **31**(1):141–5.
4. Xylinas E, Rink M, Margulis V, Karakiewicz P, Novara G, Shariat SF. Multifocal carcinoma in situ of the upper tract is associated with high risk of bladder cancer recurrence. *Eur Urol* 2012; **61**(5):1069–70.
5. Zigeuner RE, Hutterer G, Chromecki T, Rehak P, Langner C. Bladder tumour development after urothelial carcinoma of the upper urinary tract is related to primary tumour location. *BJU Int* 2006; **98**(6):1181–6.
6. Novara G, De Marco V, Dalpiaz O, *et al.* Independent predictors of metachronous bladder transitional cell carcinoma (TCC) after nephroureterectomy for TCC of the upper urinary tract. *BJU Int* 2008; **101**(11):1368–74.
7. Li WM, Shen JT, Li CC, *et al.* Oncologic outcomes following three different approaches to the distal ureter and bladder cuff in nephroureterectomy for primary upper urinary tract urothelial carcinoma. *Eur Urol* 2010; **57**(6):963–9.
8. Novara G, De Marco V, Dalpiaz O, *et al.* Independent predictors of contralateral metachronous upper urinary tract transitional cell carcinoma after nephroureterectomy: multi-institutional dataset from three European centers. *Int J Urol* 2009; **16**(2):187–91.
9. Babjuk M, Oosterlinck W, Sylvester R, *et al.* EAU guidelines on non-muscle-invasive urothelial carcinoma of the bladder, the 2011 update. *Eur Urol* 2011; **59**(6):997–1008.
10. Margulis V, Shariat SF, Matin SF, *et al.* Outcomes of radical nephroureterectomy: a series from the Upper Tract Urothelial Carcinoma Collaboration. *Cancer* 2009; **115**(6):1224–33.
11. Shariat SF, Favaretto RL, Gupta A, *et al.* Gender differences in radical nephroureterectomy for upper tract urothelial carcinoma. *World J Urol* 2011; **29**(4):481–6.
12. Rouprêt M, Yates DR, Comperat E, Cussenot O. Upper urinary tract urothelial cell carcinomas and other urological malignancies involved in the hereditary nonpolyposis colorectal cancer (lynch syndrome) tumor spectrum. *Eur Urol* 2008; **54**(6):1226–36.
13. Audenet F, Colin P, Yates DR, *et al.* A proportion of hereditary upper urinary tract urothelial carcinomas are misclassified as sporadic according to a multi-institutional database analysis: proposal of patient-specific risk identification tool. *BJU Int* 2012; **110**(11 Pt B):E583–9.
14. McLaughlin JK, Silverman DT, Hsing AW, *et al.* Cigarette smoking and cancers of the renal pelvis and ureter. *Cancer Res* 1992; **52**(2):254–7.
15. Colin P, Koenig P, Ouzzane A, *et al.* Environmental factors involved in carcinogenesis of urothelial cell carcinomas of the upper urinary tract. *BJU Int* 2009; **104**(10):1436–40.
16. Chen CH, Dickman KG, Moriya M, *et al.* Aristolochic acid-associated urothelial cancer in Taiwan. *Proc Natl Acad Sci U S A* 2012; **109**(21):8241–6.
17. Laing C, Hamour S, Sheaff M, Miller R, Woolfson R. Chinese herbal uropathy and nephropathy. *Lancet* 2006; **368**(9532):338.
18. Rouprêt M, Drouin SJ, Cancel-Tassin G, Comperat E, Larre S, Cussenot O. Genetic variability in 8q24 confers susceptibility to urothelial carcinoma of the upper urinary tract and is linked with patterns of disease aggressiveness at diagnosis. *J Urol* 2012; **187**(2):424–8.
19. Rouprêt M, Cancel-Tassin G, Comperat E, *et al.* Phenol sulfotransferase SULT1A1*2 allele and enhanced risk of upper urinary tract urothelial cell carcinoma. *Cancer Epidemiol Biomarkers Prev* 2007;**16**(11):2500–3.
20. Orsola A, Trias I, Raventos CX, Espanol I, Cecchini L, Orsola I. Renal collecting (Bellini) duct carcinoma displays similar characteristics to upper tract urothelial cell carcinoma. *Urology* 2005; **65**(1):49–54.

21. Rink M, Robinson BD, Green DA, *et al.* Impact of histological variants on clinical outcomes of patients with upper urinary tract urothelial carcinoma. *J Urol* 2012; **188**(2):398–404.
22. Sobin L, Gospodarowicz M, Wittekind C. Urological tumours. renal pelvis and ureter. In: *TNM Classification of Malignant Tumours*, 7th edition. Chichester, UK: Wiley-Blackwell, 2009: pp. 258–261.
23. Roscigno M, Cha EK, Rink M, *et al.* International validation of the prognostic value of subclassification for AJCC stage pT3 upper tract urothelial carcinoma of the renal pelvis. *BJU Int* 2012; **110**(5):674–81.
24. Lopez-Beltran A, Bassi P, Pavone-Macaluso M, Montironi R. Handling and pathology reporting of specimens with carcinoma of the urinary bladder, ureter, and renal pelvis. *Eur Urol* 2004; **45**(3):257–66.
25. Sauter G, Algaba F, Amin M. Tumors of the urinary system. (pp. 110–23) In: *World Health Organization Classification of Tumors: Pathology and Genetics of Tumors of the Urinary System and Male Genital Organs*. Lyon, France: IARC Press, 2004.
26. Raman JD, Shariat SF, Karakiewicz PI, *et al.* Does preoperative symptom classification impact prognosis in patients with clinically localized upper-tract urothelial carcinoma managed by radical nephroureterectomy? *Urol Oncol* 2011; **29**(6):716–23.
27. Cowan NC, Turney BW, Taylor NJ, McCarthy CL, Crew JP. Multidetector computed tomography urography for diagnosing upper urinary tract urothelial tumour. *BJU Int* 2007; **99**(6):1363–70.
28. Fritz GA, Schoellnast H, Deutschmann HA, Quehenberger F, Tillich M. Multiphasic multidetector-row CT (MDCT) in detection and staging of transitional cell carcinomas of the upper urinary tract. *Eur Radiol* 2006; **16**(6):1244–52.
29. Maheshwari E, O'Malley ME, Ghai S, Staunton M, Massey C. Split-bolus MDCT urography: Upper tract opacification and performance for upper tract tumors in patients with hematuria. *AJR Am J Roentgenol* 2010; **194**(2):453–8.
30. Wang LJ, Wong YC, Chuang CK, Huang CC, Pang ST. Diagnostic accuracy of transitional cell carcinoma on multidetector computerized tomography urography in patients with gross hematuria. *J Urol* 2009; **181**(2):524–31; discussion 31.
31. Wang LJ, Wong YC, Huang CC, Wu CH, Hung SC, Chen HW. Multidetector computerized tomography urography is more accurate than excretory urography for diagnosing transitional cell carcinoma of the upper urinary tract in adults with hematuria. *J Urol* 2010; **183**(1):48–55.
32. Van Der Molen AJ, Cowan NC, Mueller-Lisse UG, Nolte-Ernsting CC, Takahashi S, Cohan RH. CT urography: definition, indications and techniques. A guideline for clinical practice. *Eur Radiol* 2008; **18**(1):4–17.
33. Dillman JR, Caoili EM, Cohan RH, Ellis JH, Francis IR, Schipper MJ. Detection of upper tract urothelial neoplasms: sensitivity of axial, coronal reformatted, and curved-planar reformatted image-types utilizing 16-row multi-detector CT urography. *Abdom Imaging* 2008; **33**(6):707–16.
34. Xu AD, Ng CS, Kamat A, Grossman HB, Dinney C, Sandler CM. Significance of upper urinary tract urothelial thickening and filling defect seen on MDCT urography in patients with a history of urothelial neoplasms. *AJR Am J Roentgenol* 2010; **195**(4):959–65.
35. Messer JC, Terrell JD, Herman MP, *et al.* Multi-institutional validation of the ability of preoperative hydronephrosis to predict advanced pathologic tumor stage in upper-tract urothelial carcinoma. *Urol Oncol* 2013 Aug;**31**(6):904–8.
36. Messer J, Shariat SF, Brien JC, *et al.* Urinary cytology has a poor performance for predicting invasive or high-grade upper-tract urothelial carcinoma. *BJU Int* 2011; **108**(5):701–5.
37. Lee KS, Zeikus E, DeWolf WC, Rofsky NM, Pedrosa I. MR urography versus retrograde pyelography/ureteroscopy for the exclusion of upper urinary tract malignancy. *Clin Radiol* 2010; **65**(3):185–92.
38. Rojas CP, Castle SM, Llanos CA, *et al.* Low biopsy volume in ureteroscopy does not affect tumor biopsy grading in upper tract urothelial carcinoma. *Urol Oncol* 2013; **31**(8):1696–700.
39. Clements T, Messer JC, Terrell JD, *et al.* High-grade ureteroscopic biopsy is associated with advanced pathology of upper-tract urothelial carcinoma tumors at definitive surgical resection. *J Endourol* 2012; **26**(4):398–402.
40. Ishikawa S, Abe T, Shinohara N, *et al.* Impact of diagnostic ureteroscopy on intravesical recurrence and survival in patients with urothelial carcinoma of the upper urinary tract. *J Urol* 2010; **184**(3):883–7.
41. Brien JC, Shariat SF, Herman MP, *et al.* Preoperative hydronephrosis, ureteroscopic biopsy grade and urinary cytology can improve prediction of advanced upper tract urothelial carcinoma. *J Urol* 2010; **184**(1):69–73.
42. Traxer O, Geavlete B, de Medina SG, Sibony M, Al-Qahtani SM. Narrow-band imaging digital flexible ureteroscopy in detection of upper urinary tract transitional-cell carcinoma: initial experience. *J Endourol* 2011; **25**(1):19–23.
43. Jeldres C, Sun M, Isbarn H, *et al.* A population-based assessment of perioperative mortality after nephroureterectomy for upper-tract urothelial carcinoma. *Urology* 2010; **75**(2):315–20.
44. Lughezzani G, Burger M, Margulis V, *et al.* Prognostic factors in upper urinary tract urothelial carcinomas: a comprehensive review of the current literature. *Eur Urol* 2012; **62**(1):100–14.
45. Li CC, Chang TH, Wu WJ, *et al.* Significant predictive factors for prognosis of primary upper urinary tract cancer after radical nephroureterectomy in Taiwanese patients. *Eur Urol* 2008; **54**(5):1127–34.
46. Fajkovic H, Cha EK, Jeldres C, *et al.* Prognostic value of extranodal extension and other lymph node parameters in patients with upper tract urothelial carcinoma. *J Urol* 2012; **187**(3):845–51.
47. Fernandez MI, Shariat SF, Margulis V, *et al.* Evidence-based sex-related outcomes after radical nephroureterectomy for upper tract urothelial carcinoma: results of large multicenter study. *Urology* 2009; **73**(1):142–6.
48. Shariat SF, Godoy G, Lotan Y, *et al.* Advanced patient age is associated with inferior cancer-specific survival after radical nephroureterectomy. *BJU Int* 2010; **105**(12):1672–7.
49. Chromecki TF, Ehdaie B, Novara G, *et al.* Chronological age is not an independent predictor of clinical outcomes after radical nephroureterectomy. *World J Urol* 2011; **29**(4):473–80.
50. Matsumoto K, Novara G, Gupta A, *et al.* Racial differences in the outcome of patients with urothelial carcinoma of the upper urinary tract: an international study. *BJU Int* 2011; **108**(8 Pt 2):E304–9.
51. Isbarn H, Jeldres C, Shariat SF, *et al.* Location of the primary tumor is not an independent predictor of cancer specific mortality in patients with upper urinary tract urothelial carcinoma. *J Urol* 2009; **182**(5):2177–81.
52. Yafi FA, Novara G, Shariat SF, *et al.* Impact of tumour location versus multifocality in patients with upper tract urothelial carcinoma treated with nephroureterectomy and bladder cuff excision: a homogeneous series without perioperative chemotherapy. *BJU Int* 2012; **110**(2b):E7–E13.
53. Ouzzane A, Colin P, Xylinas E, *et al.* Ureteral and multifocal tumours have worse prognosis than renal pelvic tumours in urothelial carcinoma of the upper urinary tract treated by nephroureterectomy. *Eur Urol* 2011; **60**(6):1258–65.
54. Chromecki TF, Cha EK, Fajkovic H, *et al.* The impact of tumor multifocality on outcomes in patients treated with radical nephroureterectomy. *Eur Urol* 2012; **61**(2):245–53.
55. Ehdaie B, Furberg H, Zabor EC, *et al.* Impact of smoking status at diagnosis on disease recurrence and death in upper tract urothelial carcinoma. *BJU Int* 2013; **111**(4):589–95.
56. Rink M, Xylinas E, Margulis V, *et al.* Impact of smoking on oncologic outcomes of upper tract urothelial carcinoma after radical nephroureterectomy. *Eur Urol* 2013; **63**(6):1082–90.
57. Simsir A, Sarsik B, Cureklibatir I, Sen S, Gunaydin G, Cal C. Prognostic factors for upper urinary tract urothelial carcinomas: stage, grade, and smoking status. *Int Urol Nephrol* 2011; **43**(4):1039–45.
58. Kikuchi E, Margulis V, Karakiewicz PI, *et al.* Lymphovascular invasion predicts clinical outcomes in patients with node-negative upper tract urothelial carcinoma. *J Clin Oncol* 2009; **27**(4):612–8.

59. Bolenz C, Shariat SF, Fernandez MI, Margulis V, Lotan Y, Karakiewicz P, *et al.* Risk stratification of patients with nodal involvement in upper tract urothelial carcinoma: value of lymph-node density. *BJU Int* 2009; 103(3):302-6. Epub 2008/11/08
60. Colin P, Ouzzane A, Yates DR, *et al.* Influence of positive surgical margin status after radical nephroureterectomy on upper urinary tract urothelial carcinoma survival. *Ann Surg Oncol* 2012; **19**(11):3613–20.
61. Zigeuner R, Shariat SF, Margulis V, *et al.* Tumour necrosis is an indicator of aggressive biology in patients with urothelial carcinoma of the upper urinary tract. *Eur Urol* 2010; **57**(4):575–81.
62. Remzi M, Haitel A, Margulis V, *et al.* Tumour architecture is an independent predictor of outcomes after nephroureterectomy: a multi-institutional analysis of 1363 patients. *BJU Int* 2009; **103**(3):307–11.
63. Fritsche HM, Novara G, Burger M, *et al.* Macroscopic sessile tumor architecture is a pathologic feature of biologically aggressive upper tract urothelial carcinoma. *Urol Oncol* 2012; **30**(5):666–72.
64. Otto W, Shariat SF, Fritsche HM, *et al.* Concomitant carcinoma in situ as an independent prognostic parameter for recurrence and survival in upper tract urothelial carcinoma: a multicenter analysis of 772 patients. *World J Urol* 2011; **29**(4):487–94.
65. Wheat JC, Weizer AZ, Wolf JS Jr, *et al.* Concomitant carcinoma in situ is a feature of aggressive disease in patients with organ confined urothelial carcinoma following radical nephroureterectomy. *Urol Oncol* 2012; **30**(3):252–8.
66. Pieras E, Frontera G, Ruiz X, Vicens A, Ozonas M, Piza P. Concomitant carcinoma in situ and tumour size are prognostic factors for bladder recurrence after nephroureterectomy for upper tract transitional cell carcinoma. *BJU Int* 2010; **106**(9):1319–23.
67. Youssef RF, Shariat SF, Lotan Y, *et al.* Prognostic effect of urinary bladder carcinoma in situ on clinical outcome of subsequent upper tract urothelial carcinoma. *Urology* 2011; **77**(4):861–6.
68. Berod AA, Colin P, Yates DR, *et al.* The role of American Society of Anesthesiologists scores in predicting urothelial carcinoma of the upper urinary tract outcome after radical nephroureterectomy: results from a national multi-institutional collaborative study. *BJU Int* 2012; **110**(11 Pt C):E1035–40.
69. Martinez-Salamanca JI, Shariat SF, Rodriguez JC, *et al.* Prognostic role of ECOG performance status in patients with urothelial carcinoma of the upper urinary tract: an international study. *BJU Int* 2012; **109**(8):1155–61.
70. Ehdaie B, Chromecki TF, Lee RK, *et al.* Obesity adversely impacts disease specific outcomes in patients with upper tract urothelial carcinoma. *J Urol* 2011; **186**(1):66–72.
71. Eltz S, Comperat E, Cussenot O, Rouprêt M. Molecular and histological markers in urothelial carcinomas of the upper urinary tract. *BJU Int* 2008; **102**(5):532–5.
72. Margulis V, Youssef RF, Karakiewicz PI, *et al.* Preoperative multivariable prognostic model for prediction of nonorgan confined urothelial carcinoma of the upper urinary tract. *J Urol* 2010; **184**(2):453–8.
73. Favaretto RL, Shariat SF, Savage C, *et al.* Combining imaging and ureteroscopy variables in a preoperative multivariable model for prediction of muscle-invasive and non-organ confined disease in patients with upper tract urothelial carcinoma. *BJU Int* 2012; **109**(1):77–82.
74. Cha EK, Shariat SF, Kormaksson M, *et al.* Predicting clinical outcomes after radical nephroureterectomy for upper tract urothelial carcinoma. *Eur Urol* 2012; **61**(4):818–25.
75. Yates DR, Hupertan V, Colin P, *et al.* Cancer-specific survival after radical nephroureterectomy for upper urinary tract urothelial carcinoma: proposal and multi-institutional validation of a post-operative nomogram. *Br J Cancer* 2012; **106**(6):1083–8.
76. Lughezzani G, Sun M, Perrotte P, *et al.* Should bladder cuff excision remain the standard of care at nephroureterectomy in patients with urothelial carcinoma of the renal pelvis? A population-based study. *Eur Urol* 2010; **57**(6):956–62.
77. Phe V, Cussenot O, Bitker MO, Rouprêt M. Does the surgical technique for management of the distal ureter influence the outcome after nephroureterectomy? *BJU Int* 2011; **108**(1):130–8.
78. Zigeuner R, Pummer K. Urothelial carcinoma of the upper urinary tract: surgical approach and prognostic factors. *Eur Urol* 2008; **53**(4):720–31.
79. Xylinas E, Rink M, Cha EK, *et al.* Impact of distal ureter management on oncologic outcomes following radical nephroureterectomy for upper tract urothelial carcinoma. *Eur Urol* 2014; **65**(1):210–7.
80. Sundi D, Svatek RS, Margulis V, *et al.* Upper tract urothelial carcinoma: impact of time to surgery. *Urol Oncol* 2012; **30**(3):266–72.
81. Waldert M, Karakiewicz PI, Raman JD, *et al.* A delay in radical nephroureterectomy can lead to upstaging. *BJU Int* 2010; **105**(6):812–7.
82. Roscigno M, Brausi M, Heidenreich A, *et al.* Lymphadenectomy at the time of nephroureterectomy for upper tract urothelial cancer. *Eur Urol* 2011; **60**(4):776–83.
83. Lughezzani G, Jeldres C, Isbarn H, *et al.* A critical appraisal of the value of lymph node dissection at nephroureterectomy for upper tract urothelial carcinoma. *Urology* 2010; **75**(1):118–24.
84. Capitanio U, Shariat SF, Isbarn H, *et al.* Comparison of oncologic outcomes for open and laparoscopic nephroureterectomy: a multi-institutional analysis of 1249 cases. *Eur Urol* 2009; **56**(1):1–9.
85. Favaretto RL, Shariat SF, Chade DC, *et al.* Comparison between laparoscopic and open radical nephroureterectomy in a contemporary group of patients: are recurrence and disease-specific survival associated with surgical technique? *Eur Urol* 2010; **58**(5):645–51.
86. Walton TJ, Novara G, Matsumoto K, *et al.* Oncological outcomes after laparoscopic and open radical nephroureterectomy: results from an international cohort. *BJU Int* 2011; **108**(3):406–12.
87. Ariane MM, Colin P, Ouzzane A, *et al.* Assessment of oncologic control obtained after open versus laparoscopic nephroureterectomy for upper urinary tract urothelial carcinomas (UUT-UCs): results from a large French multicenter collaborative study. *Ann Surg Oncol* 2012; **19**(1):301–8.
88. Simone G, Papalia R, Guaglianone S, *et al.* Laparoscopic versus open nephroureterectomy: perioperative and oncologic outcomes from a randomised prospective study. *Eur Urol* 2009; **56**(3):520–6.
89. Adibi M, Youssef R, Shariat SF, *et al.* Oncological outcomes after radical nephroureterectomy for upper tract urothelial carcinoma: Comparison over the three decades. *Int J Urol* 2012; **19**(12):1060–6.
90. Daneshmand S, Quek ML, Huffman JL. Endoscopic management of upper urinary tract transitional cell carcinoma: long-term experience. *Cancer* 2003; **98**(1):55–60.
91. Cutress ML, Stewart GD, Zakikhani P, Phipps S, Thomas BG, Tolley DA. Ureteroscopic and percutaneous management of upper tract urothelial carcinoma (UTUC): systematic review. *BJU Int* 2012; **110**(5):614–28.
92. Bagley DH, Grasso M 3rd. Ureteroscopic laser treatment of upper urinary tract neoplasms. *World J Urol* 2010; **28**(2):143–9.
93. Herrmann TR, Liatsikos EN, Nagele U, Traxer O, Merseburger AS. EAU guidelines on laser technologies. *Eur Urol* 2012; **61**(4):783–95.
94. Jeldres C, Lughezzani G, Sun M, *et al.* Segmental ureterectomy can safely be performed in patients with transitional cell carcinoma of the ureter. *J Urol* 2010; **183**(4):1324–9.
95. Lughezzani G, Jeldres C, Isbarn H, *et al.* Nephroureterectomy and segmental ureterectomy in the treatment of invasive upper tract urothelial carcinoma: a population-based study of 2299 patients. *Eur J Cancer* 2009; **45**(18):3291–7.
96. Colin P, Ouzzane A, Pignot G, *et al.* Comparison of oncological outcomes after segmental ureterectomy or radical nephroureterectomy in urothelial carcinomas of the upper urinary tract: results from a large French multicentre study. *BJU Int* 2012; **110**(8):1134–41.
97. Rouprêt M, Traxer O, Tligui M, *et al.* Upper urinary tract transitional cell carcinoma: recurrence rate after percutaneous endoscopic resection. *Eur Urol* 2007; **51**(3):709–13; discussion 14.
98. Palou J, Piovesan LF, Huguet J, Salvador J, Vicente J, Villavicencio H. Percutaneous nephroscopic management of upper urinary tract

transitional cell carcinoma: recurrence and long-term followup. *J Urol* 2004; **172**(1):66–9.

99. Giannarini G, Kessler TM, Birkhauser FD, Thalmann GN, Studer UE. Antegrade perfusion with bacillus Calmette-Guerin in patients with non-muscle-invasive urothelial carcinoma of the upper urinary tract: who may benefit? *Eur Urol* 2011; **60**(5):955–60.
100. Irie A, Iwamura M, Kadowaki K, Ohkawa A, Uchida T, Baba S. Intravesical instillation of bacille Calmette-Guerin for carcinoma in situ of the urothelium involving the upper urinary tract using vesicoureteral reflux created by a double-pigtail catheter. *Urology* 2002; **59**(1):53–7.
101. O'Brien T, Ray E, Singh R, Coker B, Beard R. Prevention of bladder tumours after nephroureterectomy for primary upper urinary tract urothelial carcinoma: a prospective, multicentre, randomised clinical trial of a single postoperative intravesical dose of mitomycin C (the ODMIT-C Trial). *Eur Urol* 2011; **60**(4):703–10.
102. Kaag MG, O'Malley RL, O'Malley P, *et al.* Changes in renal function following nephroureterectomy may affect the use of perioperative chemotherapy. *Eur Urol* 2010; **58**(4):581–7.
103. Lane BR, Smith AK, Larson BT, *et al.* Chronic kidney disease after nephroureterectomy for upper tract urothelial carcinoma and implications for the administration of perioperative chemotherapy. *Cancer* 2010; **116**(12):2967–73.
104. Matin SF, Margulis V, Kamat A, *et al.* Incidence of downstaging and complete remission after neoadjuvant chemotherapy for high-risk upper tract transitional cell carcinoma. *Cancer* 2010; **116**(13):3127–34.
105. Hellenthal NJ, Shariat SF, Margulis V, *et al.* Adjuvant chemotherapy for high risk upper tract urothelial carcinoma: results from the Upper Tract Urothelial Carcinoma Collaboration. *J Urol* 2009; **182**(3):900–6.
106. Vassilakopoulou M, de la Motte Rouge T, Colin P, *et al.* Outcomes after adjuvant chemotherapy in the treatment of high-risk urothelial carcinoma of the upper urinary tract (UUT-UC): results from a large multicenter collaborative study. *Cancer* 2011; **117**(24):5500–8.
107. Czito B, Zietman A, Kaufman D, Skowronski U, Shipley W. Adjuvant radiotherapy with and without concurrent chemotherapy for locally advanced transitional cell carcinoma of the renal pelvis and ureter. *J Urol* 2004; **172**(4 Pt 1):1271–5.

CHAPTER 6.26

The aetiology, epidemiology, clinical features, and investigation of kidney cancer

Nilay Patel†, David Cranston, and Mark Sullivan

Introduction to renal cancer

Renal cancer is the most lethal malignancy, with 33–44% of patients dying as a result of the disease.[1,2] While 50% of patients present with organ-confined disease, 25% of present with metastases and another 25% of patients with go on to develop recurrent or metastatic disease during follow-up. Surgery is the mainstay of treatment for organ-confined and locally advanced disease. A plethora of novel targeted therapies are now available for the treatment of metastatic disease, some with promising results.

Renal cancers arise most commonly from the renal parenchyma. More than 90% of kidney tumours are renal cell carcinoma, which has several distinct subtypes—clear cell, papillary, chromophobe, and collecting duct. The remaining 10% are comprised of upper tract urothelial carcinoma, lymphoma, sarcoma, and benign solid tumours such as oncocytoma and angiomyolipoma. Around, 96% of cases of renal cancers are sporadic with 4% occurring in patients with known hereditary renal cancer syndrome.

Incidence

Worldwide, 271,000 new cases of kidney cancer were diagnosed in 2008 making it the thirteenth most common malignancy in the world.[3] The incidence of kidney cancer varies across and within continents, with the highest incidence rates recorded in Europe and North America, and the lowest rates in Asia and Africa. In the European Union approximately 88,400 new cases of kidney cancer were diagnosed in 2008,[4] making it the tenth most common cancer. Malignant tumours of the kidney accounted for about 4% of cancers in the United States, with over 54,000 new diagnoses in 2008.[1] In the United Kingdom, kidney cancer is the eighth most common cancer, accounting for approximately 3% of all new cases. Statistics from Cancer Research UK showed that in 2009, there were 9,286 new cases of kidney cancer in the United Kingdom; 5,706 (61%) in men and 3,580 (39%) in women. The male to female ratio for renal cancer incidence rates vary from 1.6–2:1.[5]

Age-adjusted incidence rates are considered the best way of evaluating incidence rates and patterns of disease. In Europe the estimated age standardized kidney cancer incidences per 100,000 (ASR) for males is 15.8 and 7.1 for females,[4] while worldwide the ASR for males is 5.2 and 2.8 for females.[3] The incidence of renal cancer has been by increasing worldwide since the early 1970s by approximately 2% per year. In European, the ASR incidence rates have more than doubled between 1975–1977 and 2007–2009. This trend has started to change in recent years, with the incidence of renal cancer in Sweden, Finland, and the Netherlands starting to decrease. In the United Kingdom the incidence of renal cancer has increased for all age groups since the mid-1970s with the largest increase observed in people over 75 years of age (Fig. 6.26.1). Similar increases have been observed in the United States, where the incidence of kidney cancers diagnosed between 1975 and 2006 has risen consistently over time, with the most rapidly increasing kidney cancer incidence seen in patients younger than 40 or those aged 60 to 79.[1] A relative decrease in incidence has been observed above the age of 80, though this may be a consequence of lower investigation rates in this population group. Contemporary data from the United States has shown that the age-adjusted incidence rate of renal cancer rose from 7.6 in 1988 to 11.7 in 2006 which equates to a estimated annual percentage increase of 2.4%.[6]

The introduction of computed tomography (CT), into everyday medical practice for evaluation of abdominal symptoms or follow-up of other unrelated malignancies has contributed to the increased detection of incidental renal tumours over the past three decades. Historically renal tumours were diagnosed on the basis of excretory urograpy or renal ultrasound. The use of computed tomography (CT) scanning has increased exponentially during the 1990s, and the improved sensitivity of CT imaging for identifying renal masses has resulted in a downward stage migration at presentation with an increasing proportion of patients presenting with incidental localized renal tumours. The increased incidence of renal cancer is not however, confined just to localized disease. A historical study conducted in the United States using a SEER data set from 1975–1995 found that kidney cancer incidence increased for localized and more advanced tumours.[7] This observation suggests that the increase in incidence is the result of increased detection and additional unidentified environmental influences. Subsequent data from the SEER database showed that this pattern had changed with increases confined to localized tumours, with the greatest rise in incidence seen in patients with tumours <2 cm in size.[1] The most recent update using stage-specific age-adjusted incidence rates showed that the incidence of localized disease has continued

† Deceased

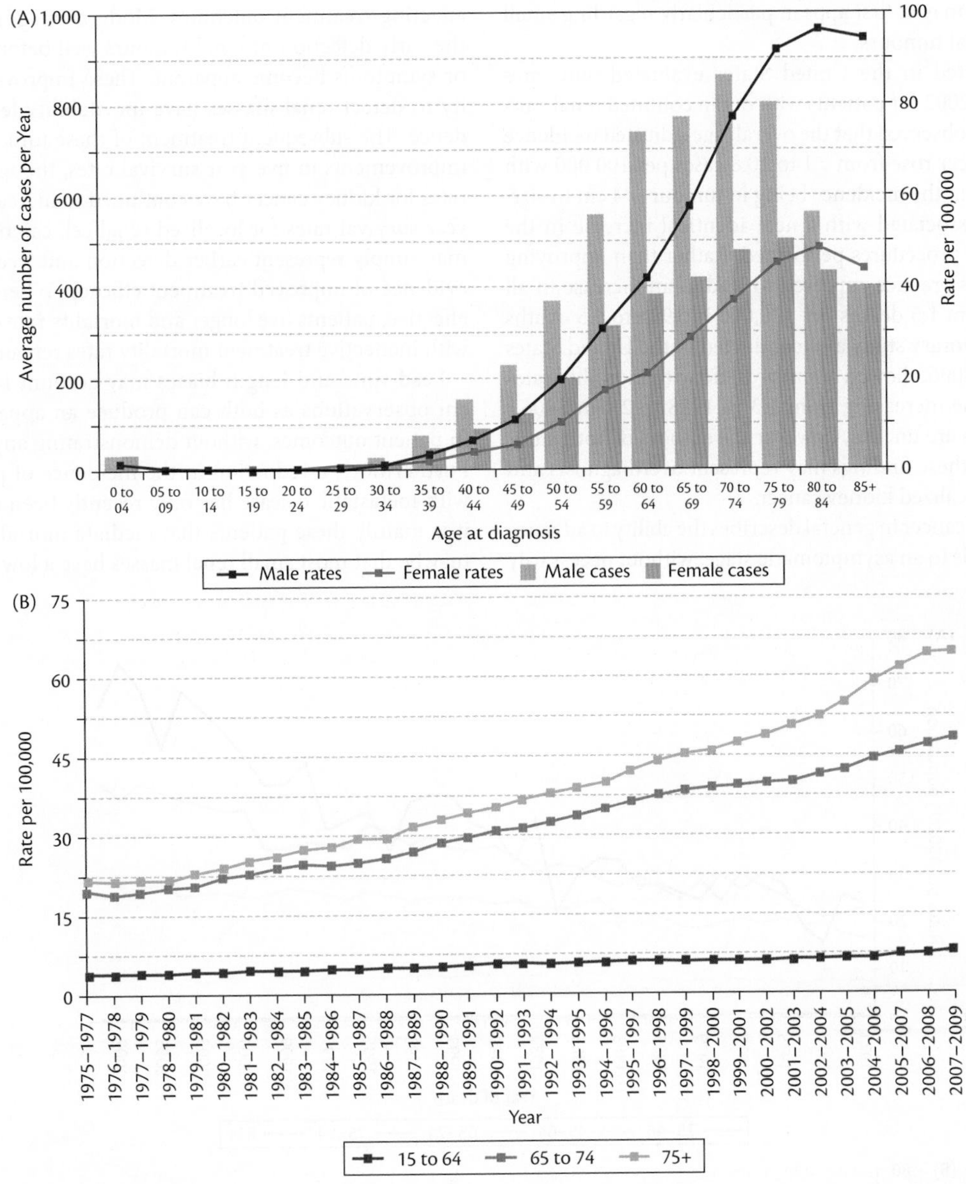

Fig. 6.26.1 (A) Kidney cancer: average number of new cases per year and age-specific incidence rates, UK, 2007–2009; (B) kidney cancer European age-standardized incidence rates, by age in Great Britain, 1975–2009.

Reproduced with permission from Cancer Research UK, *Kidney cancer incidence statistics*, Copyright © Cancer Research UK, http://www.cancerresearchuk.org/cancer-info/cancerstats/types/kidney/incidence, accessed July 2013.

to increase from 3.8 in 1988 to 8.2 in 2006 while metastatic disease rates decreased during the same period from 2.1 to 1.6.[6] The observed stage migration has as expected been accompanied by a reduction in average tumour size at presentation: tumours of less than 4 cm account for 48–66% of new kidney cancers.[8,9]

Mortality

In 2008, kidney cancer resulted in 116,000 deaths worldwide, with mortality rates twice as high in males compared to females.[3] Global mortality rates mirror incidence rates with the highest mortality rates in Europe, North America, and Australia and the lowest rates in Africa and Asia. In 2008, approximately 2–3% of cancer deaths were attributed to renal cancer; 39,300 in Europe, 3,800 in the United Kingdom, and 13,000 in the Unites States.[1,4]

Kidney cancer mortality rates in the United Kingdom for both men and women have increased steadily over the past 30 years. Male age standardized mortality rates have gone from 4.3 per 100,000 in 1971 to around 6.0 per 100,000 in 2008 and female rates have increased over the same period from 2.1 to 3.1 per 100,000. Over the course of the past decade, death rates in the United Kingdom have started to stabilize. In Europe, mortality rates increased consistently up until the early 1990s, where after they plateaued. Mortality rates in parts of Scandinavia, France, Germany, and the Netherlands, have actually decreased in the past decade.[4]

It is possible that the downward stage migration of newly diagnosed renal cancers has started to affect mortality rates. Historically there has been an assumption that early treatment of low-stage disease will result in better survival outcomes. This notion may not be as clear cut as it may at first appear, particularly regarding small organ confined renal tumours.

A study conducted in the United States evaluated outcomes between 1983 and 2002 for patients with organ confined renal cancers.[10] The authors observed that the overall age-adjusted incidence rate for kidney cancer rose from 7.1 to 10.8 cases per 100 000 with the most rapid rise in the incidence being in tumours <4 cm in size. This in turn was associated with a near identical increase in the number of surgical procedures performed. Rather than improving mortality rates, this practice appeared to lead to an increase in all cause mortality from 1.5 deaths per 100,000 in 1983 to 6.5 deaths in 2002. A contemporary study also conducted in the United States between 1988 and 2006, showed a similar trend with mortality rates for localized disease increasing from 1.3 in 1988 to 2.4 in 2006.[6] The reasons for this are unclear, however the authors of both studies speculated that these findings may represent overdiagnosis and overtreatment of localized kidney cancer.

Overdiagnosis of cancer in general describes the ability to advance the time of diagnosis to an asymptomatic stage, without necessarily affecting treatment outcomes. Modern imaging modalities allow the early detection of renal tumours well before any clinical signs or symptoms become apparent. These improvements in the ability to detect renal masses have inevitability led to a rise in incidence. The subsequent treatment of these tumours has resulted in improvements in five-year survival rates, though overall mortality rates for kidney cancer have continued to increase. The rise in five-year survival rates for localized renal cell carconoma (RCC) cases may simply represent earlier detection and treatment, rather than evidence of improved treatment efficacy. When early treatment is effective, patients live longer and mortality rate decreases, however with ineffective treatment mortality rates remain unchanged.

Lead-time and length biases may account for these inconsistent observations as both can produce an apparent improvement in patient outcomes, without demonstrating any mortality benefit. Furthermore, a reduction in the incidence of patients presenting with metastatic disease has only recently been demonstrated, and it is mainly these patients that mediate mortality (Fig. 6.26.2). It may be that most small renal masses have a low intrinsic mortality

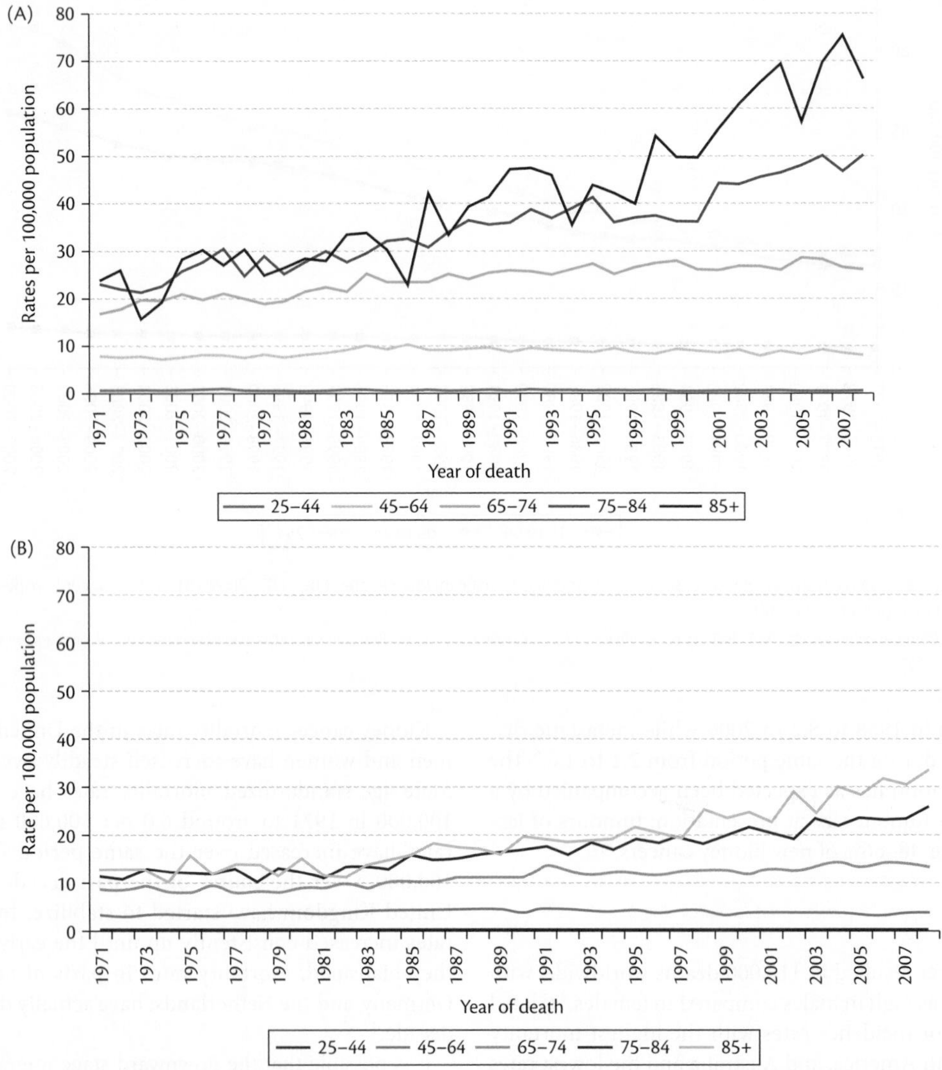

Fig. 6.26.2 (A) Age-specific mortality rates for kidney cancer, UK males, 1971–2008; (B) age-specific mortality rates for kidney cancer, UK females, 1971–2008.
Reproduced with permission from Cancer Research UK, *Kidney cancer incidence statistics*, Copyright © Cancer Research UK, http://www.cancerresearchuk.org/cancer-info/cancerstats/types/kidney/mortality/, accessed July 2013.

rates,[11] which is only altered fractionally by early treatment, thus overall mortality remains unaffected.

There is emerging evidence that overdiagnosis and overtreatment of small renal masses may actually be causing harm instead of improving outcomes. Numerous papers have demonstrated excessive cancer-specific or other-cause mortality in patients with small localized cancers treated with radical nephrectomy as compared to partial nephrectomy.[12–15] It has been shown that a significant proportion of these patients develop mild chronic kidney disease following surgery,[16] the development of which is an established independent risk factor for cardiovascular disease and death.[17,18] This may in part explain the observation from the UK that the largest increases in mortality rates are in older patients (Fig. 6.26.2). These data suggest that at least a proportion of these small detectable lesions represent an indolent form of kidney cancer that may not merit surgical intervention.[19,20]

Risk factors

Race

Incidence of RCC varies considerably among different ethnic populations.[1,5,21] In the USA the age-adjusted incidence rates of renal cell cancer are nearly twice as high in black men and woman compared to the white population.[22] Interestingly the higher incidence of renal cell cancer among blacks is almost entirely in patients with localized disease. This observation is in direct contrast to the low incidence of renal cancer in African countries.[3] The incidence of renal cancer in Asians is low both in their countries of origin and in the Unites States. Immigrants to the USA from Latin America have a much higher incidence of renal cancer than countries in South America. These ethnic differences in incidence may be attributable to various environmental factors.

Obesity

Obesity is believed to have played a causal role in the development of approximately one-third of renal cancers in Europe and the Unites States.[1,5,21] Obesity has been identified as a risk factor for RCC in a number of studies. Individuals who are overweight or obese have an increased risk of developing renal cancer in a dose-response manner. A meta-analysis,[23] demonstrated that the risk of renal cancer increased with elevated body mass index (BMI), with summary risk estimates (per 5 kg/m^2 increase in BMI) of 1.24 in men and 1.34 in women. The increased risk in obese patients has been attributed to numerous factors including increased exposure to oestrogens and androgens, chronic tissue hypoxia, insulin resistance, and compensatory hyperinsulinemia, obesity-induced inflammatory response, and lipid peroxidation and oxidative stress.[1,5,21] The global rise in obesity is likely to have contributed to the increase in incidence of renal cancer over the three decades. The prevalence of obesity has started to stabilize in parts of the Western world, which may in turn impact on the incidence of renal cancer in the future.

Cigarette smoking

Cigarette smoking is a well-established risk factor for renal cancer.[1,5,21] A meta-analysis of 24 studies showed that a history of smoking increases the risk of renal cancer compared to never smoking.[24] Compared with people who have never smoked, the risk of developing renal cancer is increased by approximately 50% in male and 20% in female smokers. The association between smoking and RCC demonstrates a clear dose-response relationship with higher risk estimates associated with heavier smoking. There is only limited evidence to suggest that smoking cessation may reduce the risk of RCC in ever-smoking men after 10 years of non-smoking.[25]

Cigarette smoking is hypothesized to increase the risk of renal cancer through chronic tissue hypoxia resulting from carbon monoxide exposure.[1,5,21] Experimental studies have suggested that increased sensitivity to nicotine-derived nitrosamine ketone in cigarette smoke may predispose susceptible individuals to an elevated risk of developing renal cancer. Mutations within chromosome 3p are frequently found in renal cancers. Benzo-α-pyrene diolepoxide is a metabolic product of the cigarette smoke constituent benzo-α-pyrene that increases the risk of developing renal cancer in susceptible individuals. The prevalence of cigarette smoking has declined in Europe and the USA over the last 30 years, which suggests that the relative importance of cigarette smoking in the development of kidney cancer might fall in developed regions.

Hypertension

Hypertension and the use of antihypertensive medications are associated with an increased risk of renal cancer.[1,5,21] Studies have shown a clear dose-response relationship between elevated blood pressure and an increased risk of RCC. The independent contributions of hypertension and the use of antihypertensive medications have been difficult to separate, as most studies are based on a diagnosis of hypertension which is inevitably associated with treatment with antihypertensive drugs. Limited prospective data indicate that it is high blood pressure, rather than the use of antihypertensive medication that increases renal cancer risk.[26] Better control of blood pressure may lower renal cancer risk, whereas the use of antihypertensive medications, is probably not a risk factor. A cohort study with sequential blood pressure measurements, observed that the risk of developing renal cancer increased with elevation of blood pressure and decreased with reduction in blood pressure, suggesting that effective control of blood pressure might reduce renal cancer risk.[27] The biological mechanisms behind the causal relationship between hypertension and renal cancer are unclear.

Acquired renal cystic disease

Acquired renal cystic disease (ARCD) arises predominantly in patients with end-stage renal disease receiving haemodialysis.[1,5,21] The incidence of RCC in ARCD is up to six times higher than in the general population. The risk of developing RCC does not appear to decrease after renal transplantation. The pattern of renal cancer in those with end-stage renal disease (ESRD) differs from renal cancer in the general population, with patients being younger and having a higher male preponderance.

Diabetes

Diabetes mellitus has been shown to be associated with an increased risk of several cancers. A history of diabetes has been linked to an increased risk of developing renal cancer in several cohort studies, however it has not been possible to demonstrate that diabetes is a risk factor independent from obesity and hypertension.[1,5,21]

Nutritional factors and diet

High daily intakes of fat and protein are associated with increased incidence of kidney cancer in both men and women. A weak association has been observed between with a high intake of processed meat and the development of renal cancer (≥27 g/day), even after adjustment for known risk factors.[1,5,21] A pooled analysis of 13 cohort studies found that fruit and vegetable consumption was associated with a lower risk of renal cancer.[28] Recent studies showed a 28% risk reduction in individuals who consumed at least 15 g of alcohol, regardless of type of alcoholic beverage.[1,5,21]

Occupation

Though not generally considered an occupational disease, some weak associations have been observed between renal cancer and a number of known carcinogens.[1,5,21] Trichloroethylene is a solvent that has been widely used as metal degreaser and chemical additive. There is increasing evidence linking trichloroethylene to the development of renal cancer with a large number of studies reporting an increase in risk with increasing levels of exposure. Occupational exposure to carcinogenic metals and products has been evaluated in parts of Europe. A statistically significant association has been found for lead, glass fibres, mineral wool fibres, and brick dust.

Hereditary renal cancer syndromes

Numerous hereditary renal cancer syndromes have been described all of which have an autosomal dominant inheritance pathway. The application of molecular techniques has identified a number of defective genes that share common metabolic pathways.[29,30]

Von Hippel-Lindau (VHL) disease arises as a result of silencing mutations in the *VHL* gene (3p25). The VHL protein regulates intracellular levels of hypoxia inducible factor (HIF). Dysfunctional VHL occurs in VHL disease and results in the constitutive over expression of HIF and its downstream targets. VHL disease is associated with development of clear cell renal cell carcinoma, phaechromocytoma, retainal/CNS haemangiobalstomas and pancreatic cysts.

Hereditary papillary renal cell carcinoma (HPRCC) has been linked to mutations in the *MET* gene (7q31), a cell surface receptor for hepatocyte growth factor. Activating mutations of *MET* leads to increased intracellular signalling, which in turn promotes proliferation, transformation, and invasion. HPRCC is associated with the development of multifocal, bilateral type 1 papillary renal cell carcinoma. No extra renal manifestations have been described.

Hereditary leiomatosis RCC (HLRCC) arises as a result of mutations in the fumarate hydratase gene (1q42) a key component of the Kreb's cycle. Inactivating mutations in fumarate hydratase result in the accumulation of fumarate which in turn results in decreased degradation of HIF. HLRCC is characterized by the development of aggressive type 2 papillary RCCs, uterine leiomyoma/lyomyosarcoma and cutaneous leiomyoma/lyomyosarcomas.

Birt-Hogg-Dubé (BHD) syndrome is associated with mutations in the folliculin gene (17p11). Folliculin is a tumour suppressor gene that plays a role in signalling through the AMPK-mTOR pathways. Features of BHD include the development of multiple and bilateral renal cancers (chromophobe, oncocytoma, hybrid oncocytic, clear cell), cutaneous fibro-folliculoma, lung cysts/spontaneous pneumothoraces, colonic polyps, and cancer.

Initial assessment

In contemporary practice, more than 50% of renal cancers are diagnosed incidentally as a consequence investigations for unrelated abdominal symptoms or conditions.[9,31,32] This increased use of cross-sectional imaging has led to a downward stage migration at presentation. Approximately 60% of newly diagnosed tumours are localized, 19% have regional lymph node involvement and 21% have metastatic disease.[1]

Table 6.26.1 Paraneoplastic syndromes associated with renal cancer

Syndrome	% of cases	Pathophysiology
Non-metastatic Hypercalcaemia	13–20	Parathyroid hormone-related peptide
Hypertension	40	Renin
Polycythemia	1–8	Erthythropoetin
Anaemia	—	Erthythropoetin, poor nutrition, chronic disease state
Liver dysfunction (Stauffer Syndrome)	3–20	IL-6
Fever, weight loss, malaise	20–30	Cytokines–TNFa, IL1, IL6, PGE, INF
Amyloidosis	3–8	AA protein

Source: data from Ganesh S. Palapattu *et al.*, 'Paraneoplastic syndromes in urologic malignancy: the many faces of renal cell carcinoma', *Reviews in Urology*, Volume 4, Number 4, Copyright. © 2002 MedReviews, LLC.

A careful medical history and thorough physical examination are essential components in the assessment of patients with newly diagnosed renal cancers. Most patients with renal tumours are asymptomatic, with the classic triad of symptoms associated with renal malignancies; palpable mass, haematuria, and flank pain present in less than 15% of patients with renal cell cancer. These symptoms occur more commonly in isolation; haematuria (60%), loin pain (40%), abdominal mass (25%). It is estimated, that 10–40% of patients with renal cancer present with a paraneoplastic syndrome (Table 6.26.1).[33] A few patients present with metastatic disease present with symptoms such as bone pain, persistent cough, or focal neurological disorders.

In the vast majority of cases physical examination is normal. Abnormal physical signs associated with renal cancers include; palpable abdominal mass; palpable cervical lymphadenopathy; non-reducing left sided varicocele arising as a consequence of an obstructing tumour thrombus in the left renal vein and bilateral lower extremity oedema suggestive of vena caval involvement and obstruction.

Baseline blood tests should include a full blood count, urea and electrolytes, liver function tests, and calcium. Some groups have additionally advocated the use of inflammatory markers such as the erythrocyte sedimentation rate (ESR) and C-reactive protein (CRP).[34,35]

Radiological assessment

A significant proportion of renal cancers are diagnosed as incidental renal masses during the course of abdominal imaging focused on the evaluation of other organs (e.g. colon CT). Incidental renal masses have been reported in up to 40% of patients who undergo abdominal imaging, though not all of these are malignant.[36] Renal masses comprise a spectrum of pathologies ranging from simple benign cysts to advanced renal carcinomas. It is essential that the correct imaging be performed during the evaluation and staging of a renal mass, as these images are the basis upon which treatments plans are made.

Computed tomography and magnetic resonance imaging (MRI) are considered the imaging modalities of choice for the evaluation and staging of renal masses.[32] For patients with allergies to iodinated contrast medium gadolinium-enhanced MRI or contrast-enhanced US can be helpful instead. A chest CT should be performed routinely to stage the thorax, though a plain chest radiograph may be sufficient for patients with tumours felt to have a low metastatic potential. MRI scans of the brain and Technetium-99m-methylene diphosphonate bone scans are indicated only in patients with signs and symptoms suggestive of metastatic disease at these sites.

Computed tomography

Most renal masses can be diagnosed accurately using imaging alone. Guidelines written by the European Association of Urology recommend the use of CT or MRI in the diagnostic assessment of renal masses.[32] The most important criterion for the diagnosis of malignant lesions is the presence of enhancement, as such imaging must be performed both before and after administration of intravenous contrast medium. Typical multidetector CT (MDCT) protocols comprise an unenhanced phase where the abdominal viscera are imaged with 3–5 mm slices.[37,38] The unenhanced images of the kidneys permit detection of calcification or fat in the kidney and provide a baseline to enable assessment of enhancement following the administration of contrast. After the administration of 100–150 mL of iodinated intravenous contrast (given at a flow rate of 2–3 mL/s), contrast-enhanced images focused on the kidneys are taken at a number of different phases; arterial (15–30s), corticomedullary/portal venous (45–60s), nephrographic (80–90s), and excretory phases (minimum of 180s). With CT, enhancement is determined by comparing Hounsfield unit (HU) readings before and after contrast administration. An increase of 20 HU is indicative of enhancement and thus malignancy (Fig. 6.26.3). An increase of 10–20 HU should be regarded as indeterminate and further imaging performed. The nephrographic phase, is considered the optimal phase for the assessment of renal tumours, with malignant lesions appearing as areas of reduced enhancement compared to the normal surrounding renal parenchymal. Also, parenchymal phase imaging avoids the potential pitfall of small intrarenal lesions not being recognized because they are considered to be normal renal medulla, (which enhances later than the cortex), as can happen with cortico-medullary phase imaging. The combination of excretory and nephrographic phases has been shown to improve lesion detection and staging. The late arterial phase provides a useful angiographic image of arterial and venous supply to the kidney but has limited additional usefulness for lesion detection and characterization when a nephrographic phase is used. Abdominal contrast-enhanced CT angiography is a useful tool in selected cases to obtain detailed information about the kidney vascular supply. Multiplanar reformatted reconstructions of images are enormously helpful in allowing visualization of the relationships of structures during surgical planning.

In addition to identifying the primary tumour, cross-sectional imaging also provides information on the function of the contralateral kidney; primary tumour extension with extrarenal spread; venous involvement; enlargement of locoregional lymph nodes; condition of adrenal glands and the liver (Box 6.26.1).[39]

CT imaging is able to provide an accurate assessment of both cystic or solid renal mass lesions. Cystic renal masses are common, with approximately 40% of patients having at least one renal cyst incidentally discovered on abdominal CT. The prevalence of renal cysts increases with age from <10% in patients under 40 years to >60% in those over 80 years of age.[36] Use of the Bosniak classification allows stratification of cystic lesions into those that can be ignored, those that need to be followed up, and those that require urological referral for consideration of removal.[40] The Bosniak classification was originally developed for CT but can also be applied to MRI or contrast-enhanced ultrasound. It is based on the identification of a number of cyst characteristics: fluid density, wall and septal thickness, enhancement, and calcification (Table 6.26.2). The main area of difficulty is in differentiating between a Bosniak II and III cyst. This is of considerable importance as surgical excision is the standard of care for Bosniak III cysts, whereas category II cysts do not require intervention or follow-up. This difficulty led to the introduction of category IIF; which represents cysts that are more complex than a Bosniak II cyst, for example with more thin septa or with minimal enhancement of the septa that warrant follow-up imaging rather than surgery.

All enhancing solid renal mass without a macroscopic fat content should be regarded as potentially malignant renal lesions. Solid

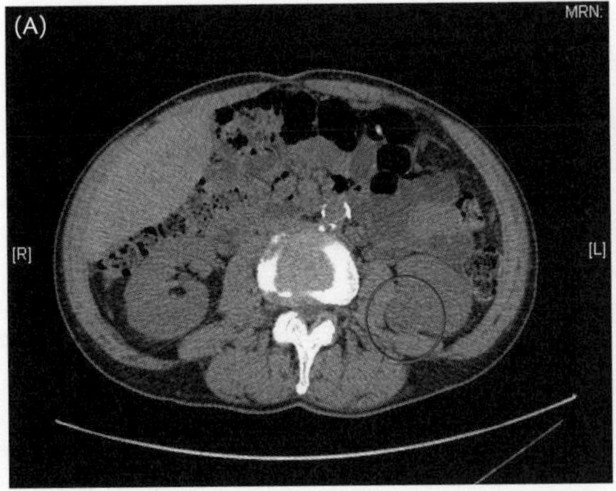

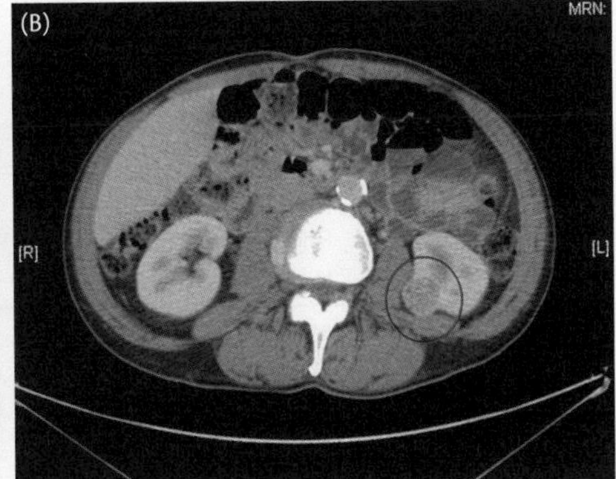

Fig. 6.26.3 A computer tomography scan of a small renal mass seen pre- and postcontrast. The renal tumour in the left kidney is seen as an area of reduced enhancement in comparison with the surrounding renal parenchyma. The lesion enhances by >20 HU postcontrast indicating a likely renal cancer.

Box 6.26.1 Important renal tumour characteristics evaluated with cross-sectional imaging

- Maximal tumour size
- Presence of enhancement (>20 HU)
- Fat invasion (perinephric/renal sinus)
- Venous involvement and extent (renal vein/IVC)
- Adjacent organ involvement (adrenal/liver/pancreas/bowel)
- Position (upper/lower pole, hilar, anterior/posterior location)
- Percentage exophytic or endophytic
- Proximity to collecting system and hilar vessels
- Number of vessels (arteries and veins)
- Number of ureters
- Collateral neovascularity
- Presence and nature of contralateral kidney
- Formal TNM staging

Source: data from Chapin BF *et al.*, 'Renal Cell Carcinoma: What the Surgeon and Treating Physician Need to Know', *American Journal of Roentgenology*, Volume 196, Number 6, pp. 1255–62, Copyright © 2011 American Roentgen Ray Society.

masses do demonstrate considerable variability in their appearance on CT.[37,38] Clear cell RCC have a more heterogeneous in appearance than other histologic subtypes and tend to demonstrate greater enhancement postcontrast particularly in the cortico-mudullary phase. Papillary tumours on the other hand appear more homogeneous and have a much lower degree of enhancement than in non-papillary tumours. The presence of macroscopic fat within a renal lesion at CT is diagnostic of an angiomyolipoma (AML) and these lesions warrant treatment (excision or embolization) once they are larger than 4 cm as beyond this they are at significant risk of spontaneous haemorrhage.

Oncocytoma is the most common solid benign renal tumour and accounts for approximately 5% of all renal masses. The classical histo-pathological appearance of an oncocytoma is a central stellate scar, which can sometimes be seen on CT. Unfortunately, areas of necrosis can mimic these scars, and as such oncocytomas cannot reliably distinguished from renal cancers on imaging alone. Upper tract urothelial carcinomas account for between 5–10% of renal malignancies, and usually present with haematuria. These tumours are best seen in the excretory phase as a filling defects within the collecting system. Large, advanced upper tract urothelial cell carcinoma may extend into the renal parenchyma in an infiltrating pattern and should always be considered as a possible diagnosis in central renal masses.

Magnetic resonance imaging

MRI has similar overall staging accuracy to CT and is generally reserved for cases of a severe allergy to iodinated contrast, pregnancy, or when CT imaging has been indeterminate.[32,37,38] It is important to consider the risks of nephrogenic systemic fibrosis in patients with significantly impaired renal function, which is thought to be associated with the administration of gadolinium contrast.

MRI sequences should include axial dual echo in phase and opposed-phase T1W, gradient echo (GRE); fat-saturated, coronal T2W; and fat-saturated, three-dimensional (3D) T1W pre and post-gadolinium imaging.[38] The corticomedullary phase will occur approximately 30s after contrast injection, and the nephrographic phase at around two min.

MRI has been shown to have similar diagnostic accuracy to CT in the characterization of renal cysts.[41] The superior contrast resolution offered by gadolinium enhanced MRI is helpful in further characterizing lesions that have indeterminate enhancement (10–20 HU) with CT or in patients unable to have iodinated contrast medium. Enhancement can be assessed on MRI, by evaluating signal intensity pre and post-gadolinium in the same manner as at CT. An increase of >15% on the contrast-enhanced images can be taken to signify enhancement. MRI is unable to detect calcification, which is a key component of the Bosniak classification system. However, the importance of calcification as a prognostic feature within the Bosniak classification is now questionable, as calcification within a lesion does not appear to be associated with an increased risk of malignancy.

Table 6.26.2 Bosniak classification of renal cysts

Bosniak category	Risk of malignancy (%)	Typical feature	Management
I	0	Simple benign cyst Hairline thin wall No other features Water dense No enhancement	Discharge—no follow-up
II	<10	Few hairline septa Fine calcification in wall/septa Hyperdense cyst <3 cm	Discharge—no follow-up
IIF	<10	Multiple hairline septa Minimal enhancement or thickening of wall/septa Thick/nodular calcification Hyperdense cyst >3 cm	Radiological surveillance
III	50	Thickened irregular wall/septa with enhancement	Surgical excision
IV	80–90	Malignant cystic lesion with enhancing soft tissue elements	Surgical excision

Adapted with permission from Israel GM and Bosniak MA, 'Follow-up CT of moderately complex cystic lesions of the kidney (Bosniak category IIF)', *American Journal of Roentgenology*, Volume 181, Number 3, pp. 627–33, Copyright ©2003 American Roentgen Ray Society.

Fat-suppressed MRI sequences are able to identify the fat within an AML, with similar diagnostic accuracy as CT. Much like CT, MRI is unable to differentiate oncocytomas from renal cancer. Clear cell renal cancers can appear hyperintense on T2-weighted imaging, and show strong heterogeneous enhancement postcontrast.[42] Papillary renal cancers on the other hand can appear hypointense on T2-weighted imaging, and have low-level homogeneous enhancement postcontrast.

Ultrasound

Ultrasonography is often the modality through which incidental renal masses are picked up. Ultrasound is good at differentiating between cystic and solid lesions; as cystic lesions typically are anechoic structures, which have strong posterior acoustic enhancement. Sharply marginated cysts without any internal contents can safely be catagorized as Bosniak I simple cysts using ultrasound alone. The finding of more complex features on ultrasound, such as nodularity, calcification, multiple septa, septal, or wall thickening, warrants a CT or MRI examination for a more accurate assessment. Contrast-enhanced ultrasonography is showing promise as an alternative means of evaluating complex cystic renal masses, though at present is not the standard of care.[43]

Ultrasound can have problems visualizing the retroperitoneum and perinephric tissues clearly. Solid renal masses will only be accurately identified on ultrasound if they are of different echogenicity to the normal renal cortex or have altered the normal contours of the kidney anatomy. As such ultrasound has reported accuracies for T staging of only 77–85%.[37] Fat-containing AMLs can readily be seen on ultrasound as echo bright masses, however other solid masses have appearances similar to normal renal cortex, making them difficult to characterize under 2 cm in size. All solid renal masses detected at ultrasound need further evaluation with CT or MRI. Intraoperative ultrasound can be extremely useful for the identification of endophytic hilar tumours in patients undergoing nephron-sparing surgery.

Positron emission tomography

In contrast to CT and MRI, positron emission tomography (PET) scans provide functional, rather than structural, information on physiologic activity. Combining this functional information with anatomical imaging is now feasible with 'combined' PET-CT machines that utilize PET and CT images obtained contemporaneously during the same study. There is some evidence to suggest that ^{18}F-FDG-PET-CT may have a role in staging and disease relapse or metastasis in renal cancer.[44] Diagnostic PET-CT has its limitations, but its utility might be enhanced by using immuno-PET with 124I-cG250 which uses radiolabelled monoclonal antibodies against carbonic anhydrase IX. In the future, functional imaging may play a role in monitoring responses to targeted therapies and personalized treatment planning. At present the true value of PET in the diagnosis and follow-up of renal cancer remains to be determined.

Evaluation of tumour thrombus

Tumour thrombus within the lumen of the renal vein and inferior vena cava (IVC) has been observed in 4–23% of cases of renal carcinoma. MRI has historically been the investigation of choice for evaluating the presence of tumour thrombus and determining the cephalad extent of an IVC thrombus. More recently contrast-enhanced MDCT has been shown to have equivalent diagnostic accuracy as MRI.[45] Doppler ultrasound can also be useful for assessing the presence and extent of venous thrombus, with detection rates of 87%.[46] Accurate preoperative identification of a tumour thrombus, its level and any evidence of luminal infiltration are of great importance in making decisions regarding surgical approach for caval and cardiac tumours.

Radiological scoring systems

The past decade has seen a drive towards treating T1 renal masses with nephron-sparing surgery. This has led to the introduction of a number of standardized scoring systems (RENAL nephrometry score, PADUA score, and C index) that have developed to characterize renal tumour anatomy and complexity in a reproducible, quantifiable manner (Table 6.26.3).[47–49] The aim of these scoring systems is to allow meaningful comparison of renal masses in clinical practice and help to identify predictors of complications and surgical outcomes. By recognizing a number of key anatomic considerations these scoring systems can assist surgeons in determining the feasibility and safety of the different approaches to partial nephrectomy. All three anatomic classification systems have been shown to predict surgical outcome, though at present none is superior to the other.[50,51]

Table 6.26.3 Comparison of radiological scoring systems for organ-confined renal masses

(A) RENAL nephrometry	(B) PADUA	(C) C INDEX
Radius of tumour	Polar location (superior, inferior, medial)	Distance between kidney centre and tumour centre
Eexophytic, endophytic nature Nearness to collecting system or sinus	Exophytic or endophytic nature Renal rim (lateral or medial) Renal sinus involvement	Radius of tumour
Anterior or posterior location Location relative to polar lines	Collecting system involvement Tumour size (radius) Anterior or posterior location	

(A) Reprinted from *The Journal of Urology*, Volume 182, Issue 3, Alexander Kutikov and Robert G. Uzzo, 'The R.E.N.A.L. Nephrometry Score: A Comprehensive Standardized System for Quantitating Renal Tumor Size, Location and Depth', pp. 844–853, Copyright © 2009 American Urological Association, with permission from Elsevier, http://www.sciencedirect.com/science/journal/00225347; (B) Reprinted from *European Urology*, Volume 56, Issue 5, Ficarra V *et al.*, 'Preoperative Aspects and Dimensions Used for an Anatomical (PADUA) Classification of Renal Tumours in Patients who are Candidates for Nephron-Sparing Surgery', pp. 786–793, Copyright © 2009 European Association of Urology, with permission from Elsevier, http://www.sciencedirect.com/science/journal/03022838; and (C) Reprinted from *The Journal of Urology*, Volume 183, Issue 5, Matthew N. Simmons *et al.*, 'Kidney Tumor Location Measurement Using the C Index Method', pp. 1708–1713, Copyright © 2010 American Urological Association, with permission from Elsevier, http://www.sciencedirect.com/science/journal/00225347

Renal imaging in patients with renal dysfunction

The use of intravenous contrast greatly increases sensitivity and specificity for the detection and evaluation of renal masses. The use of intravenous contrast is safe in patients with normal renal function, with acute adverse events reported in 0.2–0.7% of patients receiving low-osmolality iodinated contrast media and 0.07–0.16% in patients receiving gadolinium-based contrast media (GBCA). Acute adverse effects of contrast media are most commonly allergic-like ('anaphylactoid') reactions.

The administration of intravenous contrast medium has been linked to the development of contrast-induced nephropathy (CIN) and acute kidney injury. A retrospective study compared the incidence of CIN in 11,588 patients who underwent either contrast-enhanced and unenhanced CT scans. No significant difference was observed in the overall incidence of CIN between the group that received the contrast medium and the control group (8.2% vs. 5.9%)[52] below a baseline creatinine of 159 μmol/L. Only patients with a baseline serum creatinine greater than 159.1 μmol/L had an increased risk of CIN.

Much of the literature investigating the incidence of CIN has failed to include a control group of patients not receiving contrast medium. A number of prospective studies have evaluated the risk of CIN and renal failure following the administration of CT contrast. In total seven studies monitored up 1,175 patients with known renal impairment following the use of low and iso-osmolar contrast-enhanced CT scans. The overall incidence of CIN was 5.4% with 0% of patients going on to need dialysis for acute renal failure.[53] Guidelines issued by the Royal College of Radiologists and the American College of Radiology (ACR) do not set an standardized creatinine or eGFR threshold beyond which iodinated contrast medium should not be given. The ACR state that there is insufficient good data to prescribe a specific recommended threshold. They go on to state that the risk of CIN from intravenous contrast media is sufficiently low up to a threshold of 177 μmol/L.

The most serious potential adverse effect of Gadolinium based contrast agents (GBCA) is nephrogenic system fibrosis (NSF). NSF is a rare adverse reaction to GBCA that occurs almost exclusively in patients with severe chronic kidney disease or acute renal failure for which there is no proven curative therapy.[54,55] The overall incidence of NSF in stages 4 and 5 chronic kidney disease (eGFR <30 mL/min/1.73 m^2) is estimated at between 1% and 7%. The Royal College of Radiologists guidelines state that the used of GBCA are contraindicated below an eGFR of 30 mL/min/1.73 m^2.

Renal mass biopsy

The accuracy and reliability of cross-sectional imaging in the diagnosis of renal cancers have been sufficiently high, that most patients with renal masses proceed directly to definitive treatment without first having a tissue diagnosis.[32] Concerns regarding the risk of bleeding and tumour seeding have meant that percutaneous renal biopsies have historically only been performed for a limited number of indications; a renal mass in patients with a history of a second malignancy, suspected renal lymphoma, a differential diagnosis of a renal tumour/abscess/inflammatory mass. Renal biopsy is now also indicated in patients with metastatic renal cancer who are being considered for treatment with targeted therapies such as Sunitinib.

Changes in the pattern of presentation and the management of renal cancer have led to a re-evaluation on the role of image guided biopsy in the assessment of small renal masses.[56] The increasing incidence of small renal masses and the associated rise in number of surgical treatments performed has resulted in many patients having surgery for benign renal masses. Histological confirmation of benign histology has been demonstrated in 20% of masses under 4 cm in size and 30% of masses under 2 cm in size.[57] Percunateous renal biopsy is increasingly being advocated in the assessment of these small renal masses as unnecessary surgery can be avoided for benign renal tumours, such as oncocytomas and angiomyolipomas.[20] This is of particular importance in elderly patients with multiple medical co-morbidities. The results of a renal biopsy can also be a useful aid for treatment planning histologically proven malignant small renal masses. For example, the presence of high-grade disease may be seen as a contraindication to managing patients with active surveillance. Percutaneous biopsy should be considered before ablative therapy and can be performed following treatment to ensure successful ablation.

Percutaneous renal biopsies aim to identify the presence of malignancy, tumour type, and grade. Historical case series of renal tumour biopsies have overall reported diagnostic rates between 70–97.5% and diagnostic accuracy of 86–100%.[20,56] An analysis of biopsies performed since 2001, found that an accurate diagnosis could be made in 95% of cases with an adequate biopsy.[58] Historically up to 30% of biopsies have been non-diagnostic and these patients offered either a re-biopsy or excision. Analysis of outcomes following re-biopsy show a diagnostic rate of 80–86% which is similar to the initial biopsy rate, and a cancer detection rate approaching 80%.[59] These data suggests that a non-diagnostic biopsy should not be regarded as a benign diagnosis and patients can safely be offered a repeat diagnostic biopsy.

The diagnosis of histological subtype is possible in most renal tumour biopsies, with low interobserver variability in pathologic subtyping. The main diagnostic challenge can be in differentiating between oncocytomas and chromophobe renal carcinomas.[60] The application of immuno-histochemistry panels and other molecular techniques may improve diagnostic accuracy in the future. Accurate Fuhrman grading can be challenging on renal core biopsies with reported accuracy rates of 70–83%.[61] In many ways categorizing tumours as low (Fuhrman I–II) or high (Fuhrman III–IV) grade on core biopsy may be more clinically relevant.

The previously noted concerns regarding the safety of contemporary renal biopsy seem unfounded. Most centres now perform core biopsies through a coaxial needle. An 18-gauge automated biopsy gun will produce cores of 15–22 mm in maximal length and two passes can produce a reliable specimen in 97% of cases. With this technique significant bleeding is reported in <1% of cases, and no cases of renal tumour seeding after biopsy have been reported in the literature.[20,56,62] All cases of renal tumour seeding occurred before the use a coaxial cannula which minimizes the risk of tumour spill into the tissues between the skin and tumour surface.

Screening

Routine screening for renal cancer is currently not recommended by the UK National Screening Committee or the European Association of Urology.[32] The criteria for screening proposed by Wilson and Jungner apply as much today as they did in 1968.[63] An assessment of the merits of screening for kidney cancer can be made by taking each criterion in turn.

(i) *The condition should be an important health problem*—As discussed earlier in the chapter, renal cancer is a significant health problem worldwide with an increasing incidence and mortality rate in some parts of the world. Of all urological malignancies it has the highest mortality rate.

(ii) *There should be a treatment for the condition*—Surgery is the mainstay of treatment for organ confined disease.[32] Oncological outcomes are better for early stage disease compared to locally advanced or metastatic disease–5-year survival rates for T1 tumours = 85–95%, T2 tumours = 65–75%, T3 tumours = 40–65%.[64,65] Survival rates are significantly lower for metastatic disease, however the introduction of novel targeted therapies may lead to significant improvements in oncological outcomes.[66]

(iii) *Facilities for diagnosis and treatment should be available*—Renal/abdominal ultrasound would be the screening investigation of choice. This is a simple, safe, and well-established investigation for identifying solid renal masses and readily available to most patients. A proportion of patients with a renal mass will go on to have further imaging with CT/MRI. Most patients would have easy access to treatment as renal cancer surgery is a routine part of urological practice.

(iv) *There should be a latent stage of the disease*—More than 50% of newly diagnosed renal cancers are small organ confined renal masses. These masses are believed 17.008 ptto be the precursors to more advanced and metastatic disease.

(v) *There should be a test or examination for the condition*—Screen detected renal masses would require further characterization with dedicated cross-sectional imaging (CT/MRI) and in some circumstances a percutaneous renal biopsy. CT/MRI are readily available in most hospitals and have a high sensitivity and specificity for the detection of renal cancer. In contemporary practice percuanteous renal biopsy is a safe and accurate procedure with a high diagnostic rate, which would reduce the rate of unnecessary surgery for benign disease.[56,59,62]

(vi) *The test should be acceptable to the population*—Abdominal ultrasonography is a quick and non-invasive investigation that would be acceptable to the general population, as shown by screening programmes for abdominal aortic aneurysms.

(vii) *The natural history of the disease should be adequately understood*—Renal cancers are extremely heterogenous in their biology and behaviour with a spectrum of presentation from the asymptomatic small renal mass to large tumours with aortocaval involvement. A greater understanding of the natural history of renal masses is changing attitudes towards treatment as all small renal masses do not inevitably progress to large symptomatic tumours with a propensity to metastasize. Tumours under 4 cm in size grow on average at between 2–3 mm per year and have a metastatic rate of less than 1% per year.[11,67] Over a three-year period between 30–50% of tumour do not grow at all.[19,68] Aggressive treatment of all screen detected small renal tumours may in some cases represent overtreatment of indolent disease. Increased detection of small renal masses over the past three decades has resulted in an increase in the number of surgical procedures for renal cancer. There is little evidence to show that this has led to a reduction in mortality rate from renal cancer.[6,10] In fact a significant

Box 6.26.2 2010 TNM classification for renal cancer developed by the International Union Against Cancer (UICC) and the American Joint Committee on Cancer (AJCC)

T Primary tumour

Tx Primary tumour cannot be assessed No evidence of primary tumour

T1 Tumour ≤7 cm in greatest dimension, limited to the kidney

T1a Tumour ≤4 cm in greatest dimension, limited to the kidney

T1b Tumour >4 cm but ≤7 cm in greatest dimension

T2 Tumour >7 cm in greatest dimension, limited to the kidney

T2a Tumour >7 cm but ≤10 cm in greatest dimension

T2b Tumours >10 cm limited to the kidney

T3 Tumour extends into major veins or directly invades adrenal gland or perinephric tissues but not into the ipsilateral adrenal gland and not beyond Gerota's fascia

T3a Tumour grossly extends into the renal vein or its segmental (muscle-containing) branches or tumour invades perirenal and/or renal sinus (peripelvic) fat but not beyond Gerota's fascia

T3b Tumour grossly extends into the vena cava below the diaphragm

T3c Tumour grossly extends into vena cava above the diaphragm or invades the wall of the vena cava

T4 Tumour invades beyond Gerota's fascia (including contiguous extension into the ipsilateral adrenal gland)

N Regional lymph nodes

NX Regional lymph nodes cannot be assessed

N0 No regional lymph node metastasis

N1 Metastasis in a single regional lymph node

N2 Metastasis in more than one regional lymph node

M Distant metastasis

M0 No distant metastasis

M1 Distant metastasis

TNM stage grouping

Stage I T1N0M0

Stage II T2N0M0

Stage III T3N0M0 or T1/2/3N1M0

Stage IV T4N0/1/2M0 or AnyTN2M0 or anyTanyNM1

Used with the permission of the American Joint Committee on Cancer (AJCC), Chicago, Illinois. The original and primary source for this information is the *AJCC Cancer Staging Manual, Seventh Edition (2010)* published by Springer Science+Business Media, LLC (SBM). For complete information and data supporting the staging tables, visit www.springer.com. Any citation or quotation of this material must be credited to the AJCC as its primary source. The inclusion of this information herein does not authorize any reuse or further distribution without the expressed, written permission of Springer SBM, on behalf of the AJCC.

proportion of patients with small renal masses who are treated with surgery go on to develop chronic kidney disease, which may in turn result in reduced overall survival.[16]

(viii) *There should be an agreed policy on whom to treat*—The pick up rate for screen detected renal masses in general population is 0.1–0.3%.[69,70] This low pick up rate may not justify screening the general population. Screening high risk population groups may however be justified—patients with ESRF/ARCD are at a high risk of developing renal cancer. Screening projects for renal cancer in patients on dialysis have reduced the risk of death from all causes by 35%, compared with that in the group with detection by symptoms. Other high-risk groups include kidney transplant recipients, hereditary renal cancer syndromes, and a previous history of renal cancer. These criteria may even be extended to smokers with hypertension and a high BMI.

(ix) *The total cost of finding a case should be economically balanced in relation to medical expenditure as a whole*—The cost of screening the entire population would be high and perhaps unjustified. If screening led to a reduction in the incidence of metastatic disease these costs could be offset by a reduction in the costs of targeted therapies which at present are £25,000 per patient per year. The cost effectiveness of such a screening programme could be improved by combining the US for AAA with renal cancer screening which is currently offered to males aged 65.

(x) *Case-finding should be a continuous process, not just a 'once and for all' project*—This would require serial scans over the lifetime of a patient e.g. every five years.

National screening programmes for renal cancer at present are unjustified as the natural history of the disease is still poorly understood, the benefits of treatment of early stage disease are still unproved, the detection rate in the general population is very low and the costs of screening and treatment high. Focused screening programmes identifying high risk populations groups may prove to be beneficial in the future.

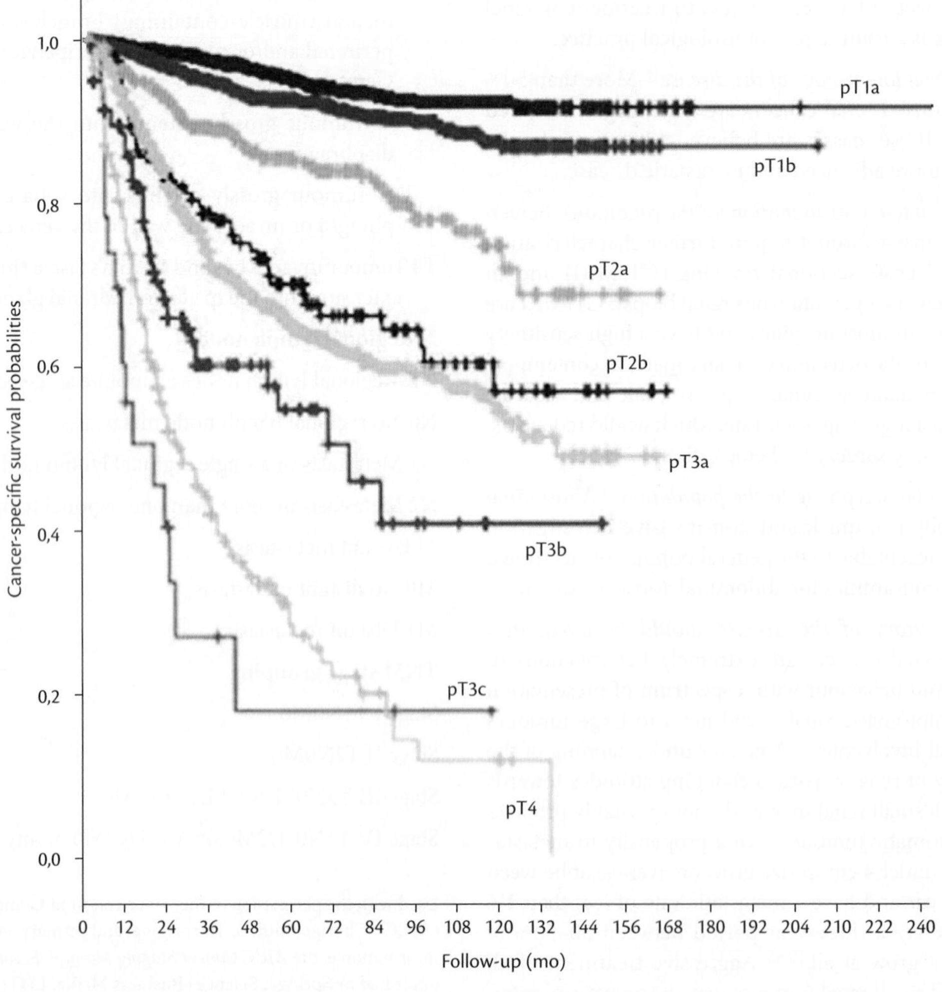

Fig. 6.26.4 Cancer-specific survival (CSS) probability according to the 2009 TNM staging system (log-rank pooled over strata $p < 0.0001$). Five-year CSS was 94.9% in pT1a (blue curve), 92.6% in pT1b (green curve), 85.4% in pT2a (grey curve), 70% in pT2b (violet curve), 64.7% in pT3a (yellow curve), 54.7 in pT3b (red curve), 17.9 in pT3c (light blue curve), and 27.1% in pT4 (light grey curve). All the pairwise survival differences among the different pT stages were statistically significant with the exception of those observed between pT2b and pT3a cancers (log-rank pairwise $p = 0.34$) and between pT3c and pT4 cancers (log-rank pairwise $p = 0.26$).[64]

Reprinted from *European Urology*, Volume 58, Issue 4, Novara G *et al.*, 'Validation of the 2009 TNM version in a large multi-institutional cohort of patients treated for renal cell carcinoma: are further improvements needed?', pp. 588–95, Copyright © 2010 European Association of Urology, with permission from Elsevier, http://www.sciencedirect.com/science/journal/03022838

Staging

Accurate clinical staging is an essential component of the assessment and evaluation of patients with renal cancer. Tumour size, presence of venous involvement, evidence of local organ invasion, presence of lymphadenopathy, or distant metastatic disease are all key factors in determining the most appropriate therapeutic approach. The TNM classification developed by the International Union Against Cancer (UICC) and the American Joint Committee on Cancer (AJCC) is recognized as the standard method of staging urological malignancies (Box 6.26.2).[71] The aim of the TNM staging system is to allow effective communication of tumour characteristics, permit the evaluation of different treatment strategies, determine the selection criteria for clinical trials and ultimately aid the selection process for treating an individual patient. The classification system was revised in 2010 in response to a significant shift towards managing T1/2 renal masses with partial nephrectomy and new prognostic data on tumour size and local invasion. In comparison with the 2002 staging system the 2010 revisions included (i) T2 cancers were subclassified into two subgroups based on a tumour size cut-off point of 10 cm (T2a 7–10 cm vs T2b >10 cm); (ii) tumours with renal vein involvement or perinephric fat involvement were classified as T3a (iii) tumours with adrenal involvement were classified as T4 cancers. External validation of the revised 2009 classification was performed and showed the following five-year cancer-specific survival (CSS) rates; T1a = 94.9%. T1b = 92.6%, T2a = 85.4%, T2b = 70%, T3a = 64.7%, T3b = 54.7%, T3c = 17.9% and T4 = 27.1% (Fig. 6.26.4).[64]

Conclusion

Renal cancer is an increasing healthcare burden across the world, with evidence of rising incidence rates, mortality rates, and healthcare costs. Significant strides have been made in our understanding of the genetic basis and natural history of the disease. The continued identification and modification of risk factors for the development of renal cancer may in time lead to a reduction in incidence. Future work will need to focus on reducing mortality rates by determining how best to treat patients with localized tumours and those with advanced metastatic disease.

Further reading

American College of Radiology. Manual on Contrast Media. Version 10.2. Available at: http://www.acr.org/Quality-Safety/Resources/Contrast-Manual [Online].

Chawla SN, Crispen PL, Hanlon AL, Greenberg RE, Chen DYT, Uzzo RG. The natural history of observed enhancing renal masses: meta-analysis and review of the world literature. *J Urol* 2006; **175**(2):425–31.

Chow WH, Devesa SS. Contemporary epidemiology of renal cell cancer. *Cancer J* 2008; **14**(5):288–301.

Ferlay J, Shin H-R, Bray F, Forman D, Mathers C, Parkin DM. Estimates of worldwide burden of cancer in 2008: GLOBOCAN 2008. *Int J Cancer* 2010; **127**(12):2893–917.

Filipas D, Spix C, Schulz-Lampel D, *et al.* Screening for renal cell carcinoma using ultrasonography: a feasibility study. *BJU Int* 2003; **91**(7):595–9.

Go AS, Chertow GM, Fan D, McCulloch CE, Hsu C-Y. Chronic kidney disease and the risks of death, cardiovascular events, and hospitalization. *N Engl J Med* 2004; **351**(13):1296–305.

Hollingsworth JM, Miller DC, Daignault S, Hollenbeck BK. Rising incidence of small renal masses: a need to reassess treatment effect. *J Natl Cancer Inst* 2006; **98**(18):1331–4.

Israel GM, Bosniak MA. Follow-up CT of moderately complex cystic lesions of the kidney (Bosniak category IIF). *AJR Am J Roentgenol* 2003; **181**(3):627–33.

Jewett MAS, Mattar K, Basiuk J, *et al.* Active surveillance of small renal masses: progression patterns of early stage kidney cancer. *Eur Urol* 2011; **60**(1):39–44.

Linehan WM, Srinivasan R, Schmidt LS. The genetic basis of kidney cancer: a metabolic disease. *Nat Rev Urol* 2010; **7**(5):277–85.

Ljungberg B, Campbell SC, Cho HY, *et al.* The epidemiology of renal cell carcinoma. *Eur Urol* 2011; **60**(4):615–21.

Ljungberg B, Cowan NC, Hanbury DC, *et al.* EAU guidelines on renal cell carcinoma: the 2010 update. *Eur Urol* 2010; **58**(3):398–406.

Ng CS, Wood CG, Silverman PM, Tannir NM, Tamboli P, Sandler CM. Renal Cell carcinoma: Diagnosis, staging, and surveillance. *AJR Am J Roentgenol* 2008; **191**(4):1220–32.

Novara G, Ficarra V, Antonelli A, *et al.* Validation of the 2009 TNM version in a large multi-institutional cohort of patients treated for renal cell carcinoma: are further improvements needed? *Eur Urol* 2010; **58**(4):588–95.

Patel N, Cranston D, Akhtar MZ, *et al.* Active surveillance of small renal masses offers short-term oncological efficacy equivalent to radical and partial nephrectomy. *BJU Int* 2012; **110**(9):1270–5.

Phé V, Yates DR, Renard-Penna R, Cussenot O, Roupret M. Is there a contemporary role for percutaneous needle biopsy in the era of small renal masses? *BJU Int* 2011 Sep 2; [Epub ahead of print].

Smaldone MC, Kutikov A, Egleston BL, *et al.* Small renal masses progressing to metastases under active surveillance: A systematic review and pooled analysis. *Cancer*; **118**(4):997–1006.

Sun M, Thuret R, Abdollah F, *et al.* Age-adjusted incidence, mortality, and survival rates of stage-specific renal cell carcinoma in North America: A trend analysis. *Eur Urol* 2011; **59**(1):135–41.

Volpe A, Cadeddu JA, Cestari A, *et al.* Contemporary management of small renal masses. *Eur Urol* 2011; **60**(3):501–15.

Wilson JM, Jungner YG. [Principles and practice of mass screening for disease]. *Bol Oficina Sanit Panam* 1968; **65**(4):281–393.

References

1. Chow WH, Devesa SS. Contemporary epidemiology of renal cell cancer. *Cancer J* 2008; **14**(5):288–301.
2. Ferlay J, Parkin DM, Steliarova-Foucher E. Estimates of cancer incidence and mortality in Europe in 2008. *Eur J Cancer* 2010; **46**(4):765–81.
3. Ferlay J, Shin H-R, Bray F, Forman D, Mathers C, Parkin DM. Estimates of worldwide burden of cancer in 2008: GLOBOCAN 2008. *Int J Cancer* 2010; **127**(12):2893–917.
4. Levi F, Ferlay J, Galeone C, *et al.* The changing pattern of kidney cancer incidence and mortality in Europe. *BJU Int* 2008; **101**(8):949–58.
5. Ljungberg B, Campbell SC, Cho HY, *et al.* The epidemiology of renal cell carcinoma. *Eur Urol* 2011; **60**(4):615–21.
6. Sun M, Thuret R, Abdollah F, *et al.* Age-adjusted incidence, mortality, and survival rates of stage-specific renal cell carcinoma in North America: A trend analysis. *Eur Urol* 2011; **59**(1):135–41.
7. Hock LM, Lynch J, Balaji KC. Increasing incidence of all stages of kidney cancer in the last 2 decades in the United States: an analysis of surveillance, epidemiology and end results program data. *J Urol* 2002; **167**(1):57–60.
8. Nguyen MM, Gill IS, Ellison LM. The evolving presentation of renal carcinoma in the United States: Trends from the surveillance, epidemiology, and end results program. *J Urol* 2006; **176**(6):2397–400.
9. Gill IS, Aron M, Gervais DA, Jewett MAS. Clinical practice. Small renal mass. *N Engl J Med* 2010; **362**(7):624–34.
10. Hollingsworth JM, Miller DC, Daignault S, Hollenbeck BK. Rising incidence of small renal masses: a need to reassess treatment effect. *J Natl Cancer Inst* 2006; **98**(18):1331–4.
11. Smaldone MC, Kutikov A, Egleston BL, *et al.* Small renal masses progressing to metastases under active surveillance: A systematic review and pooled analysis. *Cancer*; **118**(4):997–1006.

12. Kates M, Badalato GM, Pitman M, McKiernan JM. Increased Risk of Overall and Cardiovascular Mortality After Radical Nephrectomy for Renal Cell Carcinoma 2 cm or Less. *J Urol* 2011; **186**(4):1247–53.
13. Weight CJ, Larson BT, Fergany AF, *et al.* Nephrectomy induced chronic renal insufficiency is associated with increased risk of cardiovascular death and death from any cause in patients with localized cT1b renal masses. *J Urol* 2010; **183**(4):1317–23.
14. Thompson RH, Boorjian SA, Lohse CM, *et al.* Radical nephrectomy for pT1a renal masses may be associated with decreased overall survival compared with partial nephrectomy. *J Urol* 2008; **179**(2):468–71; discussion 472–3.
15. Weight CJ, Larson BT, Gao T, *et al.* Elective partial nephrectomy in patients with clinical t1b renal tumors is associated with improved overall survival. *Urology* 2010; **76**(3):631–7.
16. Huang WC, Levey AS, Serio AM, *et al.* Chronic kidney disease after nephrectomy in patients with renal cortical tumours: a retrospective cohort study. *Lancet Oncol* 2006; **7**(9):735–40.
17. Hemmelgarn BR, Manns BJ, Lloyd A, *et al.* Relation between kidney function, proteinuria, and adverse outcomes. *JAMA* 2010; **303**(5):423–9.
18. Go AS, Chertow GM, Fan D, McCulloch CE, Hsu C-Y. Chronic kidney disease and the risks of death, cardiovascular events, and hospitalization. *N Engl J Med* 2004; **351**(13):1296–305.
19. Patel N, Cranston D, Akhtar MZ, *et al.* Active surveillance of small renal masses offers short-term oncological efficacy equivalent to radical and partial nephrectomy. *BJU Int* 2012; **110**(9):1270–5.
20. Volpe A, Cadeddu JA, Cestari A, *et al.* Contemporary management of small renal masses. *Eur Urol* 2011; **60**(3):501–15.
21. Chow W-H, Dong LM, Devesa SS. Epidemiology and risk factors for kidney cancer. *Nat Rev Urol* 2010; **7**(5):245–57.
22. Lipworth L, McLaughlin JK, Tarone RE, Blot WJ. Renal cancer paradox. *Eur J Cancer Prev* 2011; **20**(4):331–3.
23. Renehan AG, Tyson M, Egger M, Heller RF, Zwahlen M. Body-mass index and incidence of cancer: a systematic review and meta-analysis of prospective observational studies. *Lancet* 2008; **371**(9612):569–78.
24. Hunt JD, van der Hel OL, McMillan GP, Boffetta P, Brennan P. Renal cell carcinoma in relation to cigarette smoking: meta-analysis of 24 studies. *Int J Cancer* 2005; **114**(1):101–8.
25. Parker AS, Cerhan JR, Janney CA, Lynch CF, Cantor KP. Smoking cessation and renal cell carcinoma. *Ann Epidemiol* 2003; **13**(4):245–51.
26. Weikert S, Boeing H, Pischon T, *et al.* Blood pressure and risk of renal cell carcinoma in the European prospective investigation into cancer and nutrition. *Am J Epidemiol* 2008; **167**(4):438–46.
27. Chow W-H, Gridley G, Fraumeni JF, Järvholm B. Obesity, hypertension, and the risk of kidney cancer in men. *N Engl J Med* 2000; **343**(18):1305–11.
28. Lee JE, Männistö S, Spiegelman D, *et al.* Intakes of fruit, vegetables, and carotenoids and renal cell cancer risk: a pooled analysis of 13 prospective studies. *Cancer Epidemiol Biomarkers Prev* 2009; **18**(6):1730–9.
29. Verine J, Pluvinage A, Bousquet G, *et al.* Hereditary renal cancer syndromes: An update of a systematic review. *Eur Urol* 2010; **58**(5):701–10.
30. Linehan WM, Srinivasan R, Schmidt LS. The genetic basis of kidney cancer: a metabolic disease. *Nat Rev Urol* 2010; **7**(5):277–85.
31. Luciani LG, Cestari R, Tallarigo C. Incidental renal cell carcinoma-age and stage characterization and clinical implications: study of 1092 patients (1982-1997). *Urology* 2000; **56**(1):58–62.
32. Ljungberg B, Cowan NC, Hanbury DC, *et al.* EAU guidelines on renal cell carcinoma: the 2010 update. *Eur Urol* 2010; **58**(3):398–406.
33. Palapattu GS, Kristo B, Rajfer J. Paraneoplastic syndromes in urologic malignancy: the many faces of renal cell carcinoma. *Rev Urol* 2002; **4**(4):163–70.
34. Wu Y, Fu X, Zhu X, *et al.* Prognostic role of systemic inflammatory response in renal cell carcinoma: a systematic review and meta-analysis. *J Cancer Res Clin Oncol* 2011; **137**(5):887–96.
35. Steffens S, Köhler A, Rudolph R, *et al.* Validation of CRP as prognostic marker for renal cell carcinoma in a large series of patients. *BMC Cancer* 2012; **12**(1):399.
36. Carrim ZI, Murchison JT. The prevalence of simple renal and hepatic cysts detected by spiral computed tomography. *Clin Radiol* 2003; **58**(8):626–9.
37. Ng CS, Wood CG, Silverman PM, Tannir NM, Tamboli P, Sandler CM. Renal Cell carcinoma: Diagnosis, staging, and surveillance. *AJR Am J Roentgenol* 2008; **191**(4):1220–32.
38. Bradley AJ, Lim YY, Singh FM. Imaging features, follow-up, and management of incidentally detected renal lesions. *Clin Radiol* 2011; **66**(12):1129–39.
39. Chapin BF, Delacroix SE, Wood CG. Renal cell carcinoma: What the surgeon and treating physician need to know. *AJR Am J Roentgenol* 2011; **196**(6):1255–62.
40. Israel GM, Bosniak MA. Follow-up CT of moderately complex cystic lesions of the kidney (Bosniak category IIF). *AJR Am J Roentgenol* 2003; **181**(3):627–33.
41. Israel GM, Hindman N, Bosniak MA. Evaluation of cystic renal masses: comparison of CT and MR imaging by using the Bosniak classification system. *Radiology* 2004; **231**(2):365–71.
42. Sun MRM, Ngo L, Genega EM, *et al.* Renal cell carcinoma: dynamic contrast-enhanced MR imaging for differentiation of tumor subtypes--correlation with pathologic findings. *Radiology* 2009; **250**(3):793–802.
43. Quaia E, Bertolotto M, Cioffi V, *et al.* Comparison of contrast-enhanced sonography with unenhanced sonography and contrast-enhanced CT in the diagnosis of malignancy in complex cystic renal masses. *AJR Am J Roentgenol* 2008; **191**(4):1239–49.
44. Lawrentschuk N, Davis ID, Bolton DM, Scott AM. Functional imaging of renal cell carcinoma. *Nat Rev Urol* 2010; **7**(5):258–66.
45. Guzzo TJ, Pierorazio PM, Schaeffer EM, Fishman EK, Allaf ME. The accuracy of multidetector computerized tomography for evaluating tumor thrombus in patients with renal cell carcinoma. *J Urol* 2009; **181**(2):486–90; discussion 491.
46. Habboub HK, Abu-Yousef MM, Williams RD, See WA, Schweiger GD. Accuracy of color Doppler sonography in assessing venous thrombus extension in renal cell carcinoma. *AJR Am J Roentgenol* 1997; **168**(1):267–71.
47. Kutikov A, Uzzo RG. The R.E.N.A.L. Nephrometry score: A comprehensive standardized system for quantitating renal tumor size, location and depth. *J Urol* 2009; **182**(3):844–53.
48. Ficarra V, Novara G, Secco S, *et al.* Preoperative aspects and dimensions used for an anatomical (PADUA) classification of renal tumours in patients who are candidates for nephron-sparing surgery. *Eur Urol* 2009; **56**(5):786–93.
49. Simmons MN, Ching CB, Samplaski MK, Park CH, Gill IS. Kidney tumor location measurement using the C index method. *J Urol* 2010; **183**(5):1708–13.
50. Hew MN, Baseskioglu B, Barwari K, *et al.* Critical appraisal of the PADUA classification and assessment of the R.E.N.A.L. nephrometry score in patients undergoing partial nephrectomy. *J Urol* 2011; **186**(1):42–6.
51. Okhunov Z, Rais-Bahrami S, George AK, *et al.* The comparison of three renal tumor scoring systems: C-Index, P.A.D.U.A., and R.E.N.A.L. nephrometry scores. *J Endourol* 2011; **25**(12):1921–4.
52. Bruce RJ, Djamali A, Shinki K, Michel SJ, Fine JP, Pozniak MA. Background fluctuation of kidney function versus contrast-induced nephrotoxicity. *Am J Roentgenol* 2009; **192**(3):711–8.
53. Katzberg RW, Newhouse JH. Intravenous contrast medium-induced nephrotoxicity: Is the medical risk really as great as we have come to believe? *Radiology* 2010; **256**(1):21–8.
54. Natalin RA, Prince MR, Grossman ME, Silvers D, Landman J. Contemporary applications and limitations of magnetic resonance imaging contrast materials. *J Urol* 2010; **183**(1):27–33.
55. Poff JA, Hecht EM, Ramchandani P. Renal imaging in patients with renal impairment. *Curr Urol Rep* 2010; **12**(1):24–33.

56. Phé V, Yates DR, Renard-Penna R, Cussenot O, Rouupret M. Is there a contemporary role for percutaneous needle biopsy in the era of small renal masses? *BJU Int* 2011 Sep 2; [Epub ahead of print].
57. Frank I, Blute ML, Cheville JC, Lohse CM, Weaver AL, Zincke H. An outcome prediction model for patients with clear cell renal cell carcinoma treated with radical nephrectomy based on tumor stage, size, grade and necrosis: the SSIGN score. *J Urol* 2002; **168**(6):2395–400.
58. Lane BR, Samplaski MK, Herts BR, Zhou M, Novick AC, Campbell SC. Renal mass biopsy--a renaissance? *J Urol* 2008; **179**(1):20–7.
59. Leveridge MJ, Finelli A, Kachura JR, *et al.* Outcomes of small renal mass needle core biopsy, nondiagnostic percutaneous biopsy, and the role of repeat biopsy. *Eur Urol* 2011; **60**(3):578–84.
60. Kümmerlin I, Kate ten F, Smedts F, *et al.* Core biopsies of renal tumors: a study on diagnostic accuracy, interobserver, and intraobserver variability. *Eur Urol* 2008; **53**(6):1219–25.
61. Neuzillet Y, Lechevallier E, Andre M, Daniel L, Coulange C. Accuracy and clinical role of fine needle percutaneous biopsy with computerized tomography guidance of small (less than 4.0 cm) renal masses. *J Urol* 2004; **171**(5):1802–5.
62. Volpe A, Mattar K, Finelli A, *et al.* contemporary results of percutaneous biopsy of 100 small renal masses: A single center experience. *J Urol* 2008; **180**(6):2333–7.
63. Wilson JM, Jungner YG. [Principles and practice of mass screening for disease]. *Bol Oficina Sanit Panam* 1968; **65**(4):281–393.
64. Novara G, Ficarra V, Antonelli A, *et al.* Validation of the 2009 TNM version in a large multi-institutional cohort of patients treated for renal cell carcinoma: are further improvements needed? *Eur Urol* 2010; **58**(4):588–95.
65. Tsui KH, Shvarts O, Smith RB, Figlin RA, deKernion JB, Belldegrun A. Prognostic indicators for renal cell carcinoma: a multivariate analysis of 643 patients using the revised 1997 TNM staging criteria. *J Urol* 2000; **163**(4):1090–5; quiz 1295.
66. Patard JJ, Pignot G, Escudier B, *et al.* ICUD-EAU International Consultation on Kidney Cancer 2010: Treatment of metastatic disease. *Eur Urol* 2011; **60**(4):684–90.
67. Chawla SN, Crispen PL, Hanlon AL, Greenberg RE, Chen DYT, Uzzo RG. The natural history of observed enhancing renal masses: meta-analysis and review of the world literature. *J Urol* 2006;**175**(2):425–31.
68. Jewett MAS, Mattar K, Basiuk J, *et al.* Active surveillance of small renal masses: progression patterns of early stage kidney cancer. *Eur Urol* 2011; **60**(1):39–44.
69. Turney BW, Reynard JM, Cranston DW. A case for screening for renal cancer. *BJU Int* 2006; **97**(2):220–1.
70. Filipas D, Spix C, Schulz-Lampel D, *et al.* Screening for renal cell carcinoma using ultrasonography: a feasibility study. BJU Int 2003; **91**(7):595–9.
71. Edge S, Byrd D, Compton C, Fritz A. *AJCC Cancer Staging Manual*, 7th edition. American Joint Committee on Cancer. New York, NY: Springer-Verlag, 2010.

CHAPTER 6.27

Genetics and molecular biology of renal cancer

Mariam Jafri and Eamonn R. Maher

Introduction to genetics and molecular biology of renal cancer

Though familial kidney cancers represent around 3% of kidney cancers,[1] studies of the molecular pathology of inherited kidney cancer syndromes have provided important insights into the pathophysiology of sporadic renal cell carcinoma (RCC). In the last two decades, knowledge of the molecular pathology of RCC led to the use of novel targeted therapies which have revolutionized the clinical management of individuals with RCC. Furthermore, these agents developed in kidney cancer are now being successfully used in the management of other cancers both common e.g. breast cancer and less common (i.e. neuroendocrine cancers).

In this chapter, we will discuss the clinical and pathophysiological features of the common familial kidney cancer syndromes and the molecular pathology of sporadic renal cell carcinoma.

A brief overview of molecular genetics of cancers

Cancer is most simply described as a 'disease involving dynamic changes in the genome'.[2] Cancers thrive and cause tissue destruction because of their ability to adapt to differing milieu's such as inadequate blood supply and therapeutic agents by gaining new genetic alterations allowing them to evolve with time. The key genetic changes driving cancer cell proliferation occur in two sets of genes (i) oncogenes and (ii) tumour suppressors. Mutations in oncogenes lead to a dominant gain in function and mutations in tumour suppressor genes (TSGs) cause a loss of function. The mechanism of TSG inactivation and oncogene activation are shown in Figure 6.27.1. In addition, alterations in DNA repair pathways act to promote the acquisition of mutations in oncogenes and TSGs.

Oncogenes

The archetypical oncogene is RAS, which was demonstrated to have transforming function in the late 1970s.[3] Work on RAS has not only demonstrated that gain of function mutations can lead to cell transformation but also led to the discovery of other oncogenes. As more genes were found to be altered in cancer, it became apparent that the progression from the normal to malignant phenotype occurred due to the gain of alterations that enabled cells to evade the normal homeostatic mechanisms.[3] Oncogenes usually promote cancer growth by dysregulating finely controlled intracellular signalling pathways leading to increased production of pro-growth factors. The *MET* oncogene is commonly mutated in papillary carcinoma and its oncogenic function is described below.

Tumour suppressor genes

The normal function of a tumour suppressor gene is to negatively regulate cell growth and promote differentiation. TSG inactivation is a major feature of cancer cells, though some TSGs such as *TP53* are inactivated in many types of cancer, other TSGs (e.g. *VHL*) are involved in specific tumour types. For most TSGs (including *VHL*) it is necessary to inactivate both alleles ('copies of the gene') for tumour initiation (see Fig. 6.27.1). The *VHL* gene product pVHL promotes ubiquitinization and inactivation of hypoxia-inducible factors (HIF). Biallelic *VHL* inactivation and loss of functional pVHL leads to accumulation of HIF which consequently increases cell growth by production of growth factors such as vascular endothelial growth factor (VEGF) and transforming growth factor (TGF).[4] In individuals with inherited mutations in a TSG, inactivation of the one normal (wild type) allele is required for tumour initiation (i.e. a single mutational event) whereas in sporadic cancers two independent mutational events ('two hits') are required to produce biallelic TSG inactivation. The earlier age at diagnosis of RCC in VHL disease compared to sporadic RCC is consistent with this model. Inactivation of the *VHL* TSG occurs in >80% of sporadic clear cell RCC. TSGs can be inactivated by a number of mechanisms, including intragenic alterations in DNA sequence (mutations), larger scale events that lead to loss of multiple genes and epigenetic changes (e.g. DNA methylation) that cause gene silencing. Multiple mechanisms may result in oncogene activation (e.g. mutations, genomic rearrangements, increased gene copy) but the mutation spectrum is much more restricted than for TSGs (many different mutations can inactivate a TSG but activation of an oncogene requires more specific effects on function). Though inactivation of the *VHL* TSG is an early and critical event in the pathogenesis of most clear cell RCC, it is insufficient for tumourigenesis and additional changes occur. Thus, cancers develop in a process analogous to Darwinian evolution where successive genetic changes allow cells to gain growth advantages. This leads to the progressive conversion of normal cells into cancer cells.[5] With the clonal evolution of cancers, an accumulation of genetic changes occurs, resulting in the presence of numerous mutations some of which are thought to drive the process of oncogenesis whereas other mutations are so-called 'passenger' mutations (promoted by

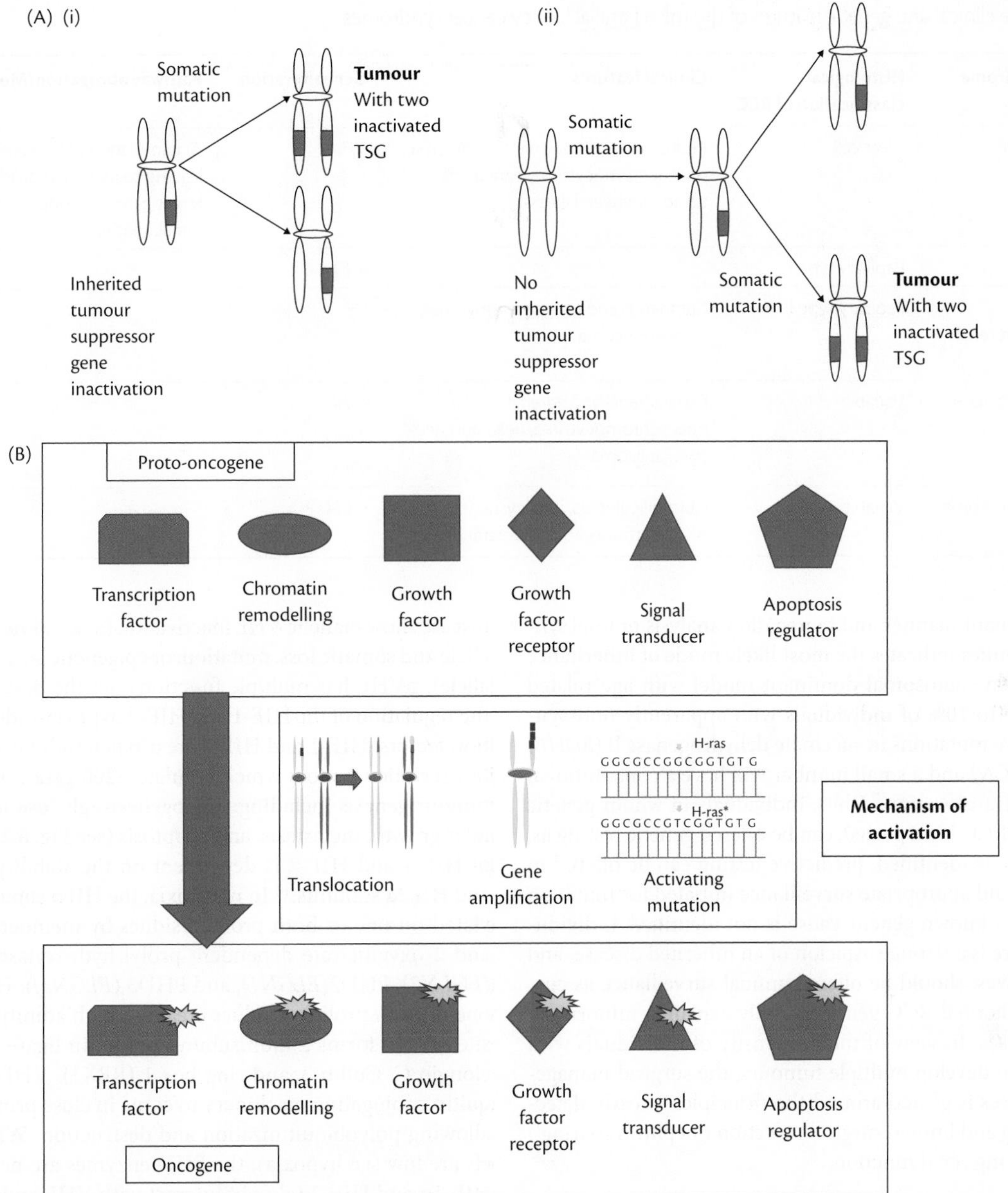

Fig. 6.27.1 Tumour suppressor and oncogenes. (A) Tumour suppressor genes (TSGs) are typically autosomal dominantly inherited. (i) Individuals with an inherited cancer predisposition (familial cancer predisposition syndrome); for example. von Hippel-Lindau disease individuals have only one functioning 'wild-type' TSG (*VHL*). This is subsequently inactivated by mutation, translocation, or deletion allowing tumour formation. (ii) In sporadic disease (e.g. in clear cell renal carcinoma) both alleles need to be inactivated—'a double hit' in order for oncogenesis to occur; and (B) oncogenes exist in all cells as proto-oncogenes, they tend to be genes with one of the following functions: transcription factors, chromatin remodelling, growth factors, growth factor receptors, signal transducers, and apoptosis regulation. In the normal cell, their expression and function is closely controlled by finely controlled mechanisms such as phosphorylation via signalling cascades. In cancers, they are constitutively activated by a number of different mechanisms including translocation, activating mutations, and gene amplification. Thus, mutations in these genes are associated with the initiation of tumour formation and tumour growth.

abnormal DNA repair mechanisms). The study of familial cancer syndromes represents an approach to identifying which genes are likely to harbour driver mutations.

Inherited kidney cancers

Inherited kidney cancer disorders may be divided into syndromic and non-syndromic. The clinical and molecular features of the main kidney cancer syndromes are described in Table 6.27.1. Many cases (but not all) of inherited kidney cancer will have a family history of RCC or extrarenal features of one of the specific syndromes listed and multicentric/bilateral tumours are frequent. Familial kidney cancers typically present at an earlier age at diagnosis than sporadic RCC. A specific disorder may be suggested by the presence of extra-renal features and RCC histopathology. Thus, hereditary papillary carcinoma is associated with a *MET* mutation and type I papillary cancer and RCC associated with VHL disease are always clear cell. The known syndromic causes of familial RCC are inherited in an

Table 6.27.1 The clinical and genetic features of the main familial kidney cancer syndromes

Familial RCC syndrome	Histological classification of RCC	Clinical features	Genealteration	Pathway abrogation/Molecular pathology
Von Hippel-Lindau	Clear cell	Retinal and CNS haemangioblastoma, phaeochromocytoma, pancreatic tumours, visceral cysts	*VHL*	Accumulation of hypoxia-inducible factor leading to increased production of HIF-target genes, causing angiogenesis and oncogenesiss
HRPC1	Papillary type I		*MET*	
Heriditary leiomyomatosisand renal cancer	Papillary type II	Cutaneous and uterine leiomyomas, leiomyosarcoma	*FH*	
Succinate dehydrogenase subunitmutations	Variable	Extra adrenal and adrenal phaeochromocytoma, head and neck paraganglioma	*SDHB* *SDHD* *SDHC*	
Birt-Hogg-Dubé syndrome	Variable	Fibrofolliculomas, lung cysts, pneumothorax and colorectal polyps	*FLCN*	

autosomal dominant manner and segregation analysis of non-syndromic RCC families indicates the most likely mode of inheritance to be a single gene autosomal dominant model with age related penetrance.[6] Up to 10% of individuals with apparently non-syndromic RCC have mutations in succinate dehydrogenase B (*SDHB)* or folliculin (*FLCN)* and a small number will have a constitutional chromosome 3 translocation.[7] Thus, individuals in whom genetic susceptibility to RCC is suspected, can be offered genetic testing as, if a genetic cause is identified, predictive testing can be offered to at-risk relatives and appropriate surveillance initiated for mutation carriers. Even if a known genetic cause is not identified, individuals in whom there is a strong suspicion of an inherited disease, and their close relatives, should be offered annual surveillance as currently known inherited RCC genes can only explain a minority of familial RCC cases. In view of the propensity of individuals with inherited RCC to develop multiple tumours, the surgical management of such cases is geared around the principles of early detection by screening and limited surgical resection ('nephron sparing') aimed at preserving renal function.

Von Hippel-Lindau disease

Von Hippel-Lindau disease (VHL) is the commonest cause of inherited RCC with an incidence of about 1 in 35,000 live births. Lifetime risk of developing a clear cell RCC is >70% in many cases.[1] Other clinical features include: retinal and cerebellar haemangioblastomas, phaeochromocytoma, renal, pancreatic, and epididymal cysts. About 20% of *VHL* mutations occur *de novo* and such individuals do not have a family history.[8] Molecular genetic testing has been available since 1993[9] and is indicated in all suspected cases. Once a mutation has been detected in an individual, family members can be tested and those testing negative for the gene mutation do not require surveillance. In contrast, individuals testing positive are offered regular screening for retinal and central nervous system haemangioblastomas, RCC, pancreatic tumours, and phaeochromocytomas.[8] The precise *VHL* mutation detected may predict risk for some tumours (e.g. phaeochromocytoma, RCC) and allow more personalized screening protocols.

VHL disease is caused by germline mutations in the *VHL* TSG. RCC and other VHL-related tumours from individuals with VHL disease show biallelic *VHL* inactivation (a germline mutation in one allele and somatic loss, mutation, or epigenetic silencing of the other allele). pVHL has multiple functions but the best characterized is the regulation of the HIF-1 and HIF-2 hypoxia-inducible transcription factors. HIF-1 and HIF-2 are α/β heterodimeric DNA-binding transcription factors which regulate >200 genes with key roles in tumourigenesis including: angiogenesis, glucose metabolism, cellular growth, metastasis, and apoptosis (see Fig. 6.27.2). Expression of HIF-1 and HIF-2 is dependent on the stability of the HIF 1α and HIF2α subunits.[10] In normoxia, the HIFα subunits are hydroxylated on one or both prolyl residues by members of the oxygen and 2-oxyglutarate dependent prolyl hydroxylase family (PHD1 *(EGLN2)*, PHD2*(ELGN1)*, and PHD3 (*ELGN3)*). Hydroxylation of one or both proline residues creates a high affinity pVHL binding site. pVHL forms a multisubunit ubiquitin ligase with elongin B, elongin C, Cullin 2, and ring-box 1 (RBX1). VHL allows the ubiquitin conjugating machinery to come in close proximity with HIF allowing polyubiquitinization and destruction. When oxygen levels are low (i.e hypoxia), the PHD enzymes are not activated, and HIF-1α and HIF-2α do not interact with VHL and are thus able to accumulate and heterodimerize with HIF-β subunit activating their target genes. If *VHL* is inactivated, lack of pVHL has a similar effect to that of hypoxia with HIF-1α and HIF-2α stabilization allowing transactivation of HIF-target genes.[11]

Both HIF-1 and HIF-2 degradation is regulated by pVHL, but there is evidence that HIF-2 overexpression is more important for RCC development. Over two hundred direct HIF responsive genes have been described; these include genes responsible for cell proliferation such as transforming growth factor and epidermal growth factor receptor; angiogenesis (vascular endothelial growth factor, platelet-derived growth factor B, interleukin-8), glucose uptake and metabolism (e.g. glucose transporter 1), chemotaxis (e.g stromal cell derived factor), and cell cycle control (e.g. cyclin D1 is an important target of HIF-2 and is upregulated in VHL null cancer models).[12]

VHL inactivation can also contribute to tumourigenesis in a HIF independent manner. Thus, VHL can regulate p53 function in a HIF independent manner by suppressing p53 ubiquitinization and so enhancing its transcriptional activity.

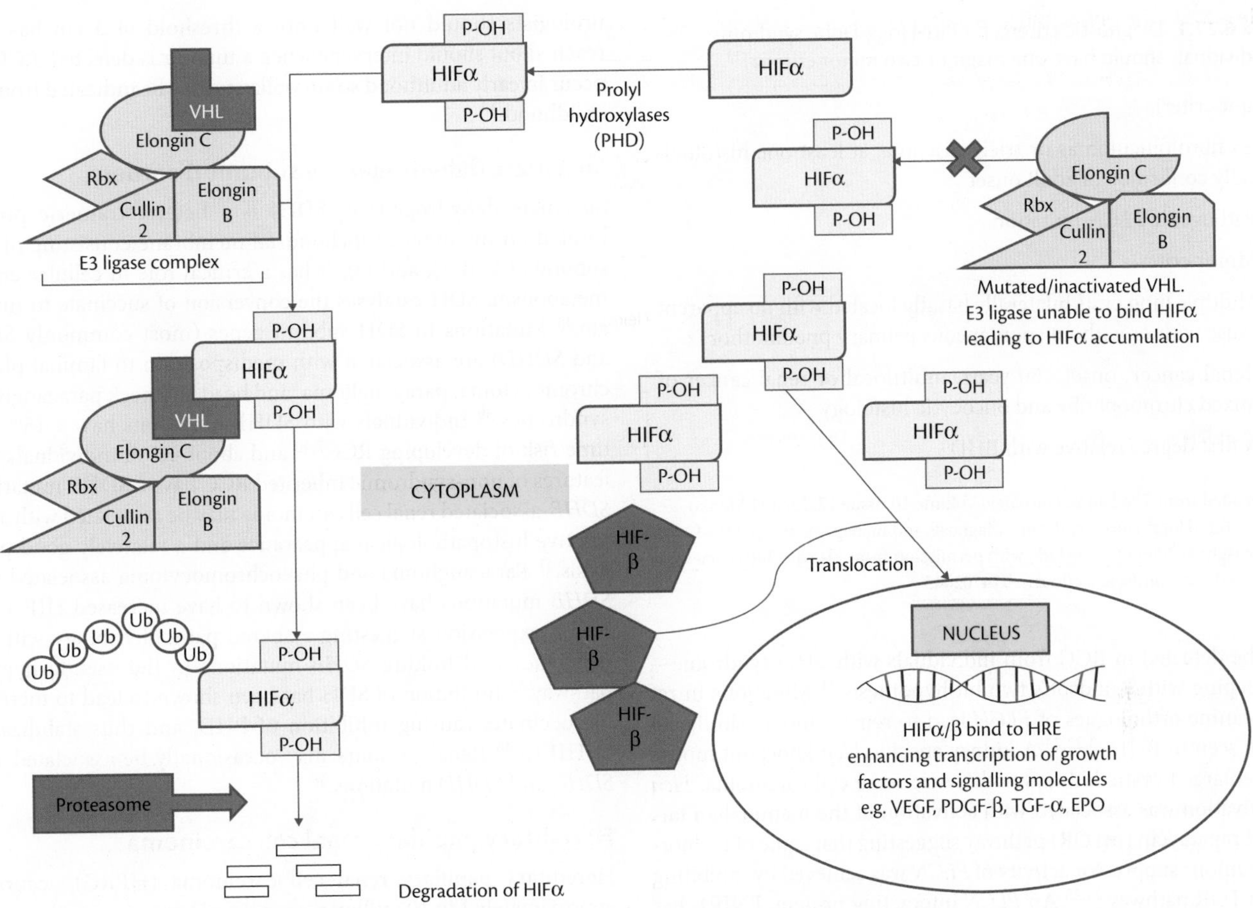

Fig. 6.27.2 The role of VHL in the hypoxic response. The role of the product of *VHL* (pVHL) in the hypoxic response. HIF is hydroxylated on one of two preserved prolyl residues by one of three prolyl hydroxylase (PHD). These enzymes are sensitive to oxygen concentration changes over a physiological range.[4] When oxygen levels are low, HIFα is stable. When oxygen is available HIFα is hydroxylated on one or both proline residues generating a binding site for VHL. Recruitment of the VHL E3 ligase complex containing elongin C, elongin B, cullin 2, RING-box protein 1 (RBX1), leads to the polyubiquitylation and proteasomal degradation of HIFα. If *VHL* is inactivated, HIFα cannot be ubiquinated and thus accumulates in the cytoplasm. It dimerizes with HIFβ and translocates to the nucleus. The HIFα/β heterodimer enhances transcription of >200 genes. These include proteins regulating: (i) glucose uptake and metabolism (e.g. GLUT-1); (ii) angiogenesis (e.g. VEGF); (iii) extracellular matrix formation and turnover (e.g. matrix metalloproteinase 1); (iv) chemotaxis (e.g. C-X-C chemokine receptor 4); (v) survival and proliferation (e.g. transforming growth factor α); and (vi) the epithelial to mesenchymal transition.

Birt-Hogg-Dubé syndrome

Birt-Hogg-Dubé (BHD) syndrome is an autosomal dominant condition characterized by skin lesions, multiple lung cysts, spontaneous pneumothorax, and kidney cancer.[13] A classical triad of skin lesions can occur in BHD syndrome, these consist of fibrofolliculinomas (the most common lesions), trichodiscomas, and achrocordomas.[14] This syndrome was first described in 1977 and 25 years later was found to be caused by mutations in a gene called folliculin (*FLCN*).[15] Clinical diagnostic criteria for BHD are available for diagnosis (Box 6.27.1) but a *FLCN* mutation can be detected in most cases.

The first clinical presentation of BHD syndrome may be to the urologist as a renal tumour, or to the acute physician with a spontaneous pneumothorax.[13] BHD is likely under-diagnosed as the dermatological features (typically facial fibrofolliculomas) appear after age 20 years but may be absent or, if sparse, overlooked.[14,16] Individuals with BHD are estimated to be at a seven fold increased risk of renal cell carcinoma.[17] In contrast to VHL disease, BHD is associated with a variety of histological subtypes of RCC including; clear cell carcinoma, chromophobe renal cell carcinoma, and a hybrid of oncocytoma and chromophobe RCC.[6] In a large UK study of individuals with familial kidney cancer without known mutations in *VHL*, *MET*, and *FH*, BHD was found in 4.3% of cases. Though there are no universally agreed guidelines for surveillance, annual renal MRI (or ultrasound) is recommended from age 20 years.[6] If a renal tumour is detected the management is generally similar to that in VHL disease—removal when 3 cm in diameter by nephron sparing surgery. Often there is considerable phenotypic variation within families (e.g. some individuals with only cutaneous lesions, others with pneumothorax, and others with renal cell carcinoma).[14] In addition to the three major features of BHD syndrome, there is also a reported association with colorectal cancer—though this is not universally accepted.[17] It has been suggested that only some *FLCN* mutations may predispose to colorectal cancer.[18]

FLCN encodes a 579 amino acid protein which is evolutionarily well conserved.[14,15,19] The vast majority of *FLCN* pathogenic mutations lead to truncated proteins.[20,21] *FLCN* is believed to function act as a tumour suppressor and somatic *FLCN* mutations

Box 6.27.1 Diagnostic criteria for Birt-Hogg-Dubé syndrome (individuals should have one major or two minor criteria)[13]

Major criteria

- ≥5 fibrofolliculomas or trichodiscoma, at least one histologically confirmed of adult onset
- Pathogenic *FLCN* mutation

Minor criteria

- Multiple lung cysts bilaterally basally located with no apparent cause with or without spontaneous primary pneumothorax
- Renal cancer: onset <50 years, multifocal or renal cancer of mixed chromophobe and oncocytic histology
- A first degree relative with BHD

Reprinted from *The Lancet Oncology*, Volume 10, Issue 12, Fred H Menko *et al.*, 'Birt-Hogg-Dubé syndrome: diagnosis and management', pp. 119–1206, Copyright © 2009 Elsevier Ltd., with permission from Elsevier, http://www.sciencedirect.com/science/journal/14702045

can be detected in RCC from individuals with BHD syndrome—in keeping with Knudson's two hit hypothesis.[21] Mutations in rat and canine orthologues of *FLCN* lead to renal tumours similar to those seen in BHD.[13,22,23] A kidney specific *Flcn* knockout mouse had enlarged cystic kidneys with cystic renal cell carcinoma. *Flcn* inactivation was associated with activation of the mammalian target of rapamycin (mTOR) pathway suggesting that some of the normal tumour suppressor activity of *FLCN* was achieved by inhibiting the mTOR pathway.[24,25] An *FLCN* interacting protein, FNIP1, has been identified, this interacts with 5′-AMP–activated protein kinase (AMPK), an important energy sensor in cells that negatively regulates the mTOR.[26–28] Treatment of *Flcn* knockout mice with mTOR inhibitors lead to decreased tumour growth and increased survival[29] but in other models the effect of folliculin deficiency on mTOR activity has been inconsistent and folliculin regulation of mTOR may be context dependent. Folliculin may also have a role in regulating TGF-β pathway signalling,[30] mitochondrial function[31] and HIF transcription activity.[32]

Hereditary leiomyomatosis and renal cell carcinoma

Heriditary leiomyomatosis (HLRCC) is a dominantly inherited disorder associated with cutaneous leiomyoma, uterine leiomyomas, and in some individuals an aggressive type II papillary renal cell carcinoma.[33] RCC is seen in 20% of HLRCC families.[34] HLRCC is caused by mutations in the fumarate hydratase (*FH*) gene. Biallelic inactivation of *FH* occurs in HLRCC-associated renal tumours.[34] Fumarate hydatase is an enzyme of the Kreb cycle that catalyses the conversion of fumarate to malate. FH inactivation increases cellular fumarate which inhibits the hypoxia-inducible factor prolyl hydroxylase enzymes (HIF-PHDs). Proline hydroxylation of HIF1 and HIF2 are critical for pVHL regulation of HIF transcription factor levels. FH inactivation causes stabilization of HIF and the upregulation of HIF-target genes (mimicking the effect of VHL inactivation).[35,36]

HLRCC associated RCC are typically solitary and unilateral, have a high nuclear grade and are aggressive. Most patients will die of metastatic disease within five years after diagnosis—even with small T1 tumours. Thus, unlike in other familial cancer syndromes, urologists should not wait until a threshold of 3 cm has been reached but should intervene when a tumour is detected. RCC can occur in early adulthood so surveillance may be indicated from late childhood.[37]

Succinate dehydrogenase subunit disorders

Succinate dehydrogenase (SDH) is a heterotetrameric protein located on the inner mitochondrial membrane consisting of four subunits (A, B, C, and D). It has a critical role in cellular energy metabolism. SDH catalyses the conversion of succinate to fumarate.[38] Mutations in SDH subunit genes (most commonly *SDHB* and *SDHD*) are associated with predisposition to familial phaeochromocytoma, paraganglioma, and head and neck paraganglioma syndromes.[39] Individuals with SDHB mutations have ~15% lifetime risk of developing RCC[7,40] and about 4% of individuals with features of non-syndromic inherited RCC have a SDHB mutation.[7] *SDHB*-associated renal cell carcinoma may be associated with a distinctive histopathological appearance and a relatively good prognosis.[41] Paraganglioma and phaeochromocytoma associated with *SDHB* mutations have been shown to have increased HIF-1 and VEGF expression suggesting a shared pathophysiology with FH deficiency and linking *SDHB* mutations to the pseudo-hypoxic pathway.[42] Inhibition of SDH has been shown to lead to increases in succinate, causing inhibition of PHD, and thus stabilization of HIF1α.[43] Renal tumours may occasionally be associated with *SDHC* and *SDHD* mutations.[38]

Hereditary papillary renal cell carcinoma

Hereditary papillary renal cell carcinoma (HPRC) occurs in approximately 1 in 10 million persons[1] and has an incomplete penetrance (90% likelihood of developing RCC at 80 years of age).[44] It is caused by activating mutations in the *MET* proto-oncogene. HPRC is inherited in an autosomal dominant manner and is associated with the development of multiple bilateral type I PRCC.[45] 13% of sporadic papillary renal cell carcinoma also contain a *MET* mutation.[46,47] Identification of the *MET* mutation was facilitated by the fact that type I papillary renal cell carcinomas are associated with trisomy 7, and thus linkage analysis was performed and the proto-oncogene identified on 7q34.[47,48] Breast, pancreas, and stomach cancers have been associated with HPRC in some families.[37] By age 50, only around 30% of *MET* mutation carriers have developed renal cancer. Individuals with inherited papillary renal cell carcinoma can have over 1,000 microscopic papillary carcinoma in resected specimens,[49] though HRPC tumours have a better prognosis than those associated with HLRCC. Met is the tyrosine kinase receptor for hepatocyte growth factor.[50] Point mutations occur in both sporadic and inherited papillary renal cell carcinoma leading to constitutive activation of the receptor pathway. Interestingly, *MET* expression has also been found to be upregulated in some clear cell renal carcinoma models,[50,51] suggesting that the MET/HGF pathway maybe have more general relevance in the pathogenesis of RCC.[52]

Translocation

Inherited renal cell carcinoma may be associated with a constitutional translocation, most commonly involving the short arm of chromosome 3 (3p) and thus karyotyping is a standard investigation for patients suspected of inherited RCC. Initially autosomal dominantly inherited familial RCC was reported in association with a constitutional t(3:8)(p12;q24) and since then eleven further RCC-associated translocations have been identified.[53] Investigation of these translocations has led to the identification of candidate TSGs, for example *FHIT, TRC8, LSAMP*, and *NORE1*. In some cases it has been suggested that the genes disrupted by the translocation function, like *VHL*, act as TSGs with a 'two hit model of tumourigenesis', but in others predisposition to renal tumorigenesis appears to result from instability of the translocated chromosome such that 3p is lost from the cell and then a somatic *VHL* mutation occurs on the remaining chromosome 3. In a recent population-based study, RCC individuals with translocations were at a similar age to individuals with *FLCN* or *VHL* mutations, and often had multiple tumours.[53]

Low penetrance RCC susceptibility genes: Polymorphic variation in the *MITF* gene was reported to predispose to RCC and melanoma and variants associated with HIF-2 and Cyclin D1 regulation have been linked to RCC.[54,55]

The molecular genetics of sporadic kidney cancer

Chromosomal changes in sporadic kidney cancer

As mentioned previously, the role of VHL in sporadic kidney cancers is pivotal with >80% of clear cell RCC demonstrating *VHL* inactivation.[56] *VHL* resides on chromosome 3p and early cytogenetic studies indicated 3p allele loss in over 60% of sporadic kidney cancers.[57] Detailed mapping of the 3p area did not demonstrate a single area of critical allele loss, and 3p was found to contain a number of TSGs.[58] Important TSGs on 3p include *RASSF1A*, which was silenced by methylation in about a half of kidney cancers[59,60] and *PBRM1* which is mutated in about 40% of RCC.[61] Microarray-based studies have revealed areas of increased copy number (1q, 2q, 5q, 7q, 8q, 12p and 20q) and decreased number (1p, 3p, 4q, 6q, 8p, 9p, and 14q).[62] These differences in copy number can help identify possible genes of interest in the pathogenesis of kidney cancer.

A specific somatic cytogenetic abnormality, Xp11.2 translocation, occurs in a rare subset of papillary RCC. Xp11.2 translocation positive tumours account for up to a third of paediatric or young adult RCC cases but are rare in older cases. Xp11.2 translocation positive cancers have an aggressive course. The translocations results in a fusion between the transcription factor on chromosome Xp11 with one of a number of other genes (at least six).[63] The tumour tends to be a mixture of papillary and alveolar type. In adults, Xp11 translocations are relatively rare with one study suggesting an incidence of only 1.6%[64] The type of translocation may also be associated with disease severity. Interestingly, there is interplay between this pathway and the MET pathway, as TFE translocations are associated with upregulation of c-met and then increased intracellular signalling.[65] TFE has also been shown to be upregulated in *FLCN* null cells, indicating that TFE may have a more prevalent role in kidney cancer than previously identified.[66]

Somatic mutations in sporadic kidney cancer

Following the identification of frequent *VHL* gene mutations in sporadic clear cell RCC it was more than 15 years before a second frequently mutated gene was identified. Thus exome sequencing revealed truncating mutations in the *PBRM1* gene on chromosome 3p21 in 41% of clear cell RCC.[61] *PBRM1* encodes the chromatin targeting subunit of the PBAF SWI/SNF chromatin remodelling complex. Prior to this finding resequencing of 3,500 candidate cancer genes in RCC identified three genes were each mutated in ~3% of sporadic RCC and which were each implicated in histone modification.[66] These were the histone 3 lysine demethylases UTX/KDM6A and JARID1C/KDM5C and the H3 lysine methylase SETD2. These finding suggested that disruption of normal patterns of chromatin modification play a key role in RCC development. Interestingly, neurofibromatosis 2 gene (*NF2*) mutations were detected in a small subset of tumours without *VHL* mutations.[67]

Epigenetic changes in sporadic kidney cancer

Epigenetic modifications have been implicated in the pathogenesis of many cancers. The best studied feature of cancer epigenetics is epigenetic silencing of TSGs by *de novo* promoter region hypermethylation.[68] *VHL* was one of the first human TSGs in which epigenetic inactivation was demonstrated. Though genetic changes (mutation or allele loss) are more common sources of *VHL* inactivation than *de novo* DNA methylation, the *RASSF1A* TSG is inactivated much more frequently by promoter region hypermethylation than by intragenic mutations. More than 40 candidate TSGs genes are reported to be methylated in more than 20% of kidney cancers[58] and this number will expand as the results of large scale cancer genome projects are released. More detailed knowledge of the patterns of epigenetic inactivation of TSGs in RCC will offer opportunities for therapeutic intervention. Thus, a key feature of epigenetic TSG inactivation is that it is potentially reversible (promoter hypermethylation may be reversed by demethylating agents). In addition, delineation of the key signalling pathways that are dysregulated by epigenetic TSG inactivation will offer new possibilities for targeted therapies.

The clinical impact of understanding key kidney cancer pathways

As described above the two major pathways implicated in renal cell oncogenesis are the hypoxia-inducible pathway and the mTOR pathway. There is some interaction between the two pathways and other genes found to be important in familial or sporadic renal cancer influence these pathways (see Fig. 6.27.3). Novel targeted agents are described elsewhere in this book, and thus will be mentioned only briefly here. However, before 2005 the only systemic treatment available for RCC was immunotherapy. Since then, the first drugs developed were orally available tyrosine kinase inhibitors. One such drug, sunitinib targets VEGF, PDGFRα, FLT3, and c-kit pathways. This is now the UK standard of care for advanced renal cell carcinoma and in clinical trials more than doubled progression-free survival from five to eleven months.[69] In the second line setting and in the first line in those with poor prognostic features (on clinical evaluation), mTOR inhibitors have been used effectively. Temsirolimus is used in individuals with high risk renal cell carcinoma and is the only targeted agent shown to improve overall survival (HR = 0.75) in advanced disease.[70] Everolimus is an oral preparation used in the second line setting and has also improved progression-free survival from two months to five months.[71] Furthermore, new agents are being evaluated and licenced in the management of RCC with the tyrosine kinase inhibitors pazopanib[72] and axitinib[73] entering clinical practice. These drugs have also been utilized in so-called orphan cancers where historically there has been less investment in drug development for example sunitinib and everolimus are now used in neuroendocrine cancers,[74,75] and sorafenib

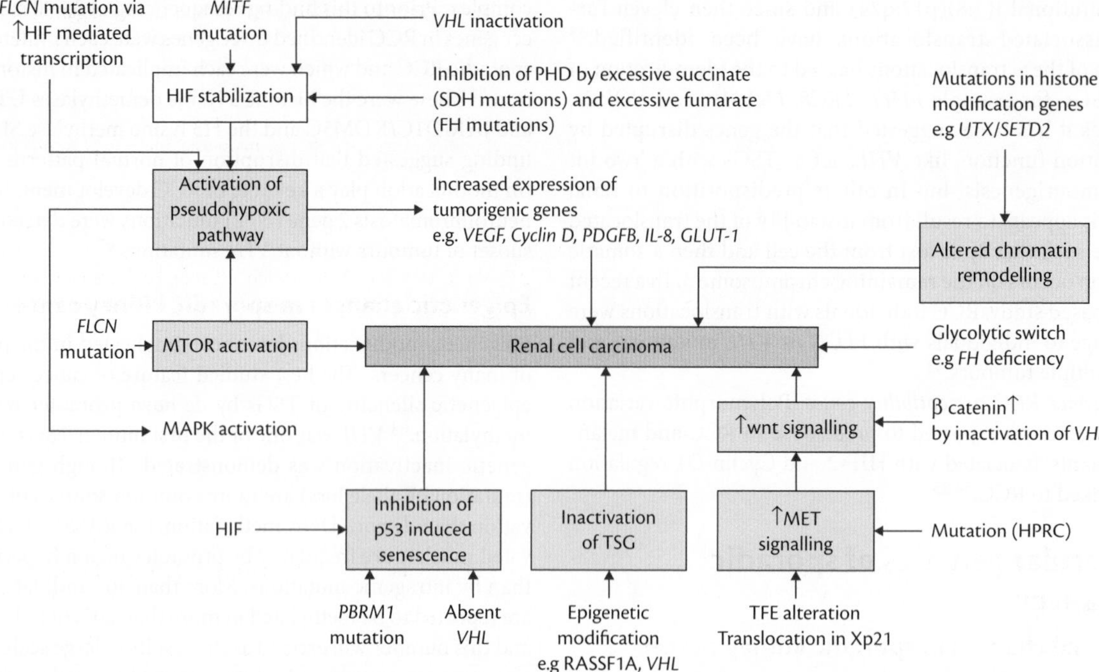

Fig. 6.27.3 An interaction between the key pathways involved in the development of renal cell carcinoma. Within an individual tumour there is likely to abrogation of a number of signalling pathways, which have already been exploited therapeutically. However, with a better understanding of the mutation spectrum in individual patients, in the future patients may receive personalized care on the basis of the mutations found in their cancer.

in hepatocellular carcinoma.[76] These targeted agents are also being used in common cancers, everolimus has recently been shown to be efficacious in hormone-receptor-positive breast cancer.[77] Thus, understanding the molecular biology of RCC has helped improve the care for individuals with other cancers. Over the next few years, there will be further improvements in the understanding of the genetic basis of familial and sporadic renal cancers. This will provide increased opportunities for personalized medicine, where the individual is treated on the basis of the genetic alterations seen in their tumour. Furthermore, with the development of more novel therapies, chemo-preventative treatments for those with inherited susceptibilities may become a possibility.

Conclusions

Familial kidney cancers represent a diagnostic and clinical challenge to those involved in the management of individuals with inherited susceptibilities. The cornerstones of effective clinical care are: (i) recognition of potential inherited RCC syndromes; (ii) characterization of responsible gene mutation (if detectable); (iii) regular renal imaging for affected individuals and at-risk relatives (unless shown not to be mutation carriers); and (iv) excellent interdisciplinary working. The studies of individuals with these conditions have revealed the key pathways in kidney cancer oncogenesis. The two most important pathways are those of the hypoxia-inducible pathway and the mTOR pathway. These pathways have been found to play important roles in the development of sporadic as well as inherited RCC. Over the last decade, treatments based on the abnormalities in the hypoxia-inducible pathway and mTOR pathway have revolutionized patient management and improved survival in patients with advanced disease.

Further reading

Adams J, Ratcliffe PJ, Pollard PJ. Novel insights into FH-associated disease are KEAPing the lid on oncogenic HIF signalling. *Oncotarget* 2011; **2**(11):820–1.

Hanahan D, Weinberg RA. Hallmarks of cancer: the next generation. *Cell* 2011; **144**(5):646–74.

Kaelin Jr WG. The von Hippel-Lindau tumour suppressor protein: O2 sensing and cancer. *Nat Rev Cancer* 2008; **8**(11):865–73.

Keefe SM, Nathanson KL, Rathmell WK. The molecular biology of renal cell carcinoma. *Semin Oncol* 2013; **40**(4):421–8.

Latif FTK, Gnarra J, Yao M, *et al.* Identification of the von Hippel-Lindau disease tumor suppressor gene. *Science* 1993; **260**(5112):1317–20.

Linehan WM, Rathmell WK. Kidney cancer. *Urol Oncol* 2012; **30**(6):948–51.

Linehan WM, Srinivasan R, Schmidt LS. The genetic basis of kidney cancer: a metabolic disease. *Nat Rev Urol* 2010; 7(5):277–85.

Maher ER. Genetics of familial renal cancers. *Nephron Exp Nephrol* 2011; **118**(1):e21–6.

Maher ER. Genomics and epigenomics of renal cell carcinoma. *Semin Cancer Biol* 2013; **23**(1):10–7.

Menko FH, van Steensel MAM, Giraud S, *et al.* Birt-Hogg-Dubé syndrome: diagnosis and management. *Lancet Oncol* 2009; **10**(12):1199–206.

Moch H. An overview of renal cell cancer: pathology and genetics. *Semin Cancer Biol* 2013; **23**(1):3–9.

Morris MR ME. Epigenetics of renal cell carcinoma: the path towards new diagnostics and therapeutics. *Genome* Med 2010; **2**(9):59.

Morrison PJ, Donnelly DE, Atkinson AB, *et al.* Advances in the genetics of familial renal cancer. *Oncologist* 2010; **15**(6):532–8.

Ricketts C, Woodward ER, Killick P, *et al.* Germline SDHB mutations and familial renal cell carcinoma. *J Nat Cancer Inst* 2008; **100**(17):1260–2.

Schimdt L, Duh FM, Chen F, Kishida T, *et al.* Germline and somatic mutations in the tyrosine kinase domain of the MET proto-oncogene in papillary renal carcinomas. *Nat Genet* 1997; **16**(1):68–73.

Selak MA, Armour SM, MacKenzie ED, *et al.* Succinate links TCA cycle dysfunction to oncogenesis by inhibiting HIF-α prolyl hydroxylase. *Cancer Cell* 2005; **7**(1):77–85.

Shen C, Kaelin WG Jr. The VHL/HIF axis in clear cell renal carcinoma. *Semin Cancer Biol* 2013; **23**(1):18–25.

Singer EA, Gupta GN, Marchalik D, Srinivasan R. Evolving therapeutic targets in renal cell carcinoma. *Curr Opin Oncol* 2013 May;**25**(3):273–80.

Sudarshan S, Karam JA, Brugarolas J, *et al.* Metabolism of kidney cancer: from the lab to clinical practice. *Eur Urol* 2013; **63**(2):244–51.

Varela I, Tarpey P, Raine K, *et al.* Exome sequencing identifies frequent mutation of the SWI/SNF complex gene PBRM1 in renal carcinoma. *Nature* 2011; **469**(7331):539–42.

References

1. Maher ER. Genetics of familial renal cancers. *Nephron Exp Nephrol* 2011; **118**(1):e21–6.
2. Hanahan D, Weinberg RA. Hallmarks of cancer: the next generation. *Cell* 2011; **144**(5):646–74.
3. Pylayeva-Gupta Y, Grabocka E, Bar-Sagi D. RAS oncogenes: weaving a tumorigenic web. *Nat Rev Cancer* 2011; **11**(11):761–74.
4. Kaelin WG Jr. The von Hippel-Lindau tumour suppressor protein: O2 sensing and cancer. *Nat Rev Cancer* 2008; **8**(11):865–73.
5. Hanahan D, Weinberg RA. The hallmarks of cancer. *Cell* 2000; **100**(1):57–70.
6. Woodward ER, Ricketts C, Killick P, *et al.* Familial non-VHL clear cell (conventional) renal cell carcinoma: clinical features, segregation analysis, and mutation analysis of FLCN. *Clin Cancer Res* 2008; **14**(18):5925–30.
7. Ricketts C, Woodward ER, Killick P, *et al.* Germline SDHB mutations and familial renal cell carcinoma. *J Nat Cancer Inst* 2008; **100**(17):1260–2.
8. Maher ER, Neumann HP, Richard S. von Hippel-Lindau disease: a clinical and scientific review. *Eur J Hum Genet* 2011; **19**(6):617–23.
9. Latif FTK, Gnarra J, Yao M, *et al.* Identification of the von Hippel-Lindau disease tumor suppressor gene. *Science* 1993; **260**(5112):1317–20.
10. Raval RR, Lau KW, Tran MGB, *et al.* Contrasting properties of hypoxia-inducible factor 1 (HIF-1) and HIF-2 in von Hippel-Lindau-associated renal cell carcinoma. *Mol Cell Biol* 2005; **25**(13):5675–86.
11. Li M, Kim WY. Two sides to every story: the HIF-dependent and HIF-independent functions of pVHL. *J Cell Mol Med* 2011; **15**(2):187–95.
12. Zatyka M, da Silva NF, Clifford SC, *et al.* Identification of cyclin D1 and other novel targets for the von Hippel-Lindau tumor suppressor gene by expression array analysis and investigation of cyclin d1 genotype as a modifier in von Hippel-Lindau Disease. *Cancer Res* 2002; **62**(13):3803–11.
13. Menko FH, van Steensel MAM, Giraud S, *et al.* Birt-Hogg-Dubé syndrome: diagnosis and management. *Lancet Oncol* 2009; **10**(12):1199–206.
14. Schmidt LS, Nickerson ML, Warren MB, *et al.* Germline BHD-mutation spectrum and phenotype analysis of a large cohort of families with Birt-Hogg-Dube syndrome. *Am J Hum Genet* 2005; **76**(6):1023–33.
15. Nickerson ML, Warren MB, Toro JR, *et al.* Mutations in a novel gene lead to kidney tumors, lung wall defects, and benign tumors of the hair follicle in patients with the Birt-Hogg-Dube syndrome. *Cancer Cell* 2002; **2**(2):157–64.
16. Toro JR, Wei MH, Glenn GM, *et al.* BHD mutations, clinical and molecular genetic investigations of Birt–Hogg–Dubé syndrome: a new series of 50 families and a review of published reports. *J Med Genet* 2008; **45**(6):321–31.
17. Zbar B, Alvord WG, Glenn G, *et al.* Risk of renal and colonic neoplasms and spontaneous pneumothorax in the Birt-Hogg-Dubé Syndrome. *Cancer Epidemiol Biomarkers Prev* 2002; **11**(4):393–400.
18. Nahorski MS, Lim DHK, Martin L, *et al.* Investigation of the Birt–Hogg–Dubé tumour suppressor gene (FLCN) in familial and sporadic colorectal cancer. *J Med Genet* 2010; **47**(6):385–90.
19. Schmidt LS, Warren MB, Nickerson ML, *et al.* Birt-Hogg-Dubé Syndrome, a genodermatosis associated with spontaneous pneumothorax and kidney neoplasia, maps to chromosome 17p11.2. *Am J Hum Genet* 2001; **69**(4):876–82.
20. Lim DHK, Rehal PK, Nahorski MS, *et al.* A new locus-specific database (LSDB) for mutations in the folliculin (FLCN) gene. *Hum Mutat* 2010; **31**(1):E1043–E51.
21. Vocke CD, Yang Y, Pavlovich CP, *et al.* High frequency of somatic frameshift BHD gene mutations in Birt-Hogg-Dubé–associated renal tumors. *J Natl Cancer Inst* 2005; **97**(12):931–5.
22. Okimoto K, Sakurai J, Kobayashi T, *et al.* A germ-line insertion in the Birt-Hogg-Dube (BHD) gene gives rise to the Nihon rat model of inherited renal cancer. *Proc Natl Acad Sci U S A* 2004; **101**(7):2023–7.
23. Lingaas F, Comstock KE, Kirkness EF, *et al.* A mutation in the canine BHD gene is associated with hereditary multifocal renal cystadenocarcinoma and nodular dermatofibrosis in the German Shepherd dog. *Hum Mol Genet* 2003; **12**(23):3043–53.
24. Chen J, Futami K, Petillo D, *et al.* Deficiency of FLCN in mouse kidney led to development of polycystic kidneys and renal neoplasia. *PloS One* 2008; **3**(10):e3581.
25. Hasumi Y, Baba M, Ajima R, *et al.* Homozygous loss of BHD causes early embryonic lethality and kidney tumor development with activation of mTORC1 and mTORC2. *Proc Natl Acad Sci* 2009; **106**(44):18722–7.
26. Baba M, Hong S-B, Sharma N, *et al.* Folliculin encoded by the BHD gene interacts with a binding protein, FNIP1, and AMPK, and is involved in AMPK and mTOR signaling. *Proc Natl Acad Sci* 2006; **103**(42):15552–7.
27. Hasumi H, Baba M, Hong SB, *et al.* Identification and characterization of a novel folliculin-interacting protein FNIP2. *Gene* 2008; **415**(1–2):60–7.
28. Takagi Y, Kobayashi T, Shiono M, *et al.* Interaction of folliculin (Birt-Hogg-Dube gene product) with a novel Fnip1-like (FnipL/Fnip2) protein. *Oncogene* 2008; **27**(40):5339–47.
29. Hartman TR, Nicolas E, Klein-Szanto A, *et al.* The role of the Birt-Hogg-Dube protein in mTOR activation and renal tumorigenesis. *Oncogene* 2009; **28**(13):1594–604.
30. Hong S-B, Oh H, Valera V, *et al.* Tumor suppressor FLCN inhibits tumorigenesis of a FLCN-null renal cancer cell line and regulates expression of key molecules in TGF-beta signaling. *Mol Cancer* 2010; **9**(1):160.
31. Klomp J, Petillo D, Niemi N, *et al.* Birt-Hogg-Dube renal tumors are genetically distinct from other renal neoplasias and are associated with up-regulation of mitochondrial gene expression. *BMC Med Genomics* 2010; **3**(1):59.
32. Preston RS, Philp A, Claessens T, *et al.* Absence of the Birt-Hogg-Dube gene product is associated with increased hypoxia-inducible factor transcriptional activity and a loss of metabolic flexibility. *Oncogene* 2011; **30**(10):1159–73.
33. Kiuru M, Lehtonen R, Arola J, *et al.* Few FH mutations in sporadic counterparts of tumor types observed in hereditary leiomyomatosis and renal cell cancer families. *Cancer Res* 2002; **62**(16):4554–7.
34. Verine J, Pluvinage A, Bousquet G, *et al.* Hereditary renal cancer syndromes: An update of a systematic review. *Eur Urol* 2010; **58**(5):701–10.
35. Lehtonen HJ, Makinen MJ, Kiuru M, *et al.* Increased HIF1 alpha in SDH and FH deficient tumors does not cause microsatellite instability. *Int J Cancer* 2007; **121**(6):1386–9.
36. Adams J, Ratcliffe PJ, Pollard PJ. Novel insights into FH-associated disease are KEAPing the lid on oncogenic HIF signalling. *Oncotarget* 2011; **2**(11):820–1.
37. Morrison PJ, Donnelly DE, Atkinson AB, *et al.* Advances in the genetics of familial renal cancer. *Oncologist* 2010; **15**(6):532–8.

38. Malinoc A, Sullivan M, Wiech T, *et al.* Biallelic inactivation of the SDHC gene in renal carcinoma associated with paraganglioma syndrome type 3. *Endocr Relat Cancer* 2012; **19**(3):283–90.
39. Jafri M, Maher ER. Genetics in endocrinology: The genetics of phaeochromocytoma: using clinical features to guide genetic testing. *Eur J Endocrinol* 2012; **166**(2):151–8.
40. Vanharanta S, Buchta M, McWhinney SR, *et al.* Early-onset renal cell carcinoma as a novel extraparaganglial component of SDHB-associated heritable paraganglioma. *Am J Hum Genet* 2004;**74**(1):153–9.
41. Gill AJ, Pachter NS, Chou A, *et al.* Renal tumors associated with germline SDHB mutation show distinctive morphology. *Am J Surg Pathol* 2011; **35**(10):1578–85.
42. Pollard PJ, Brière JJ, Alam NA, *et al.* Accumulation of Krebs cycle intermediates and over-expression of HIF1α in tumours which result from germline FH and SDH mutations. *Hum Mol Genet* 2005; **14**(15):2231–9.
43. Selak MA, Armour SM, MacKenzie ED, *et al.* Succinate links TCA cycle dysfunction to oncogenesis by inhibiting HIF-α prolyl hydroxylase. *Cancer Cell* 2005; **7**(1):77–85.
44. Linehan WM, Srinivasan R, Schmidt LS. The genetic basis of kidney cancer: a metabolic disease. *Nat Rev Urol* 2010;7(5):277–85.
45. Schimdt L, Duh FM, Chen F, Kishida T, *et al.* Germline and somatic mutations in the tyrosine kinase domain of the MET proto-oncogene in papillary renal carcinomas. *Nat Genet* 1997; **16**(1):68–73.
46. Sweeney P, El-Naggar AK, Lin S-H, Pisters LL. Biological significance of C-met over expression in papillary renal cell carcinoma. *J Urol* 2002; **168**(1):51–5.
47. Schmidt L, Junker K, Nakaigawa N, *et al.* Novel mutations of the MET proto-oncogene in papillary renal carcinomas. *Oncogene* 1999; **18**(14):2343–50.
48. Zhuang Z, Park WS, Pack S, *et al.* Trisomy 7-harbouring non-random duplication of the mutant MET allele in hereditary papillary renal carcinomas. *Nat Genet* 1998; **20**(1):66–9.
49. Ornstein DK, Lubensky IA, Venzon D, Zbar B, Linehan WM, Walther MM. Prevalence of microscopic tumors in normal appearing renal parenchyma of patients with hereditary papillary renal cancer. *J Urol* 2000; **163**(2):431–3.
50. Nakaigawa N, Yao M, Baba M, *et al.* Inactivation of von Hippel-Lindau gene induces constitutive phosphorylation of MET protein in clear cell renal carcinoma. *Cancer Res* 2006; **66**(7):3699–705.
51. Oh RR, Park JY, Lee JH, *et al.* Expression of HGF/SF and Met protein is associated with genetic alterations of VHL gene in primary renal cell carcinomas. *APMIS* 2002; **110**(3):229–38.
52. Horie S, Aruga S, Kawamata H, Okui N, Kakizoe T, Kitamura T. Biological role of hgf/met pathway in renal cell carcinoma. *J Urol* 1999; **161**(3):990–7.
53. Woodward ER, Skytte A-B, Cruger DG, Maher ER. Population-based survey of cancer risks in chromosome 3 translocation carriers. *Genes Chromosomes Cancer* 2010; **49**(1):52–8.
54. Schodel J, Bardella C, Sciesielski LK, *et al.* Common genetic variants at the 11q13.3 renal cancer susceptibility locus influence binding of HIF to an enhancer of cyclin D1 expression. *Nat Genet* 2012; **44**(4):420–5.
55. Yu J, Habuchi T, Tsuchiya N, *et al.* Association of the cyclin D1 gene G870A polymorphism with susceptibility to sporadic renal cell carcinoma. *J Urol* 2004; **172**:2410–3.
56. Nickerson ML, Jaeger E, Shi Y, *et al.* Improved identification of von Hippel-Lindau gene alterations in clear cell renal tumors. *Clin Cancer Res* 2008; **14**(15):4726–34.
57. Zbar B, Branch H, Talmadge C, Linehan M. Loss of alleles of loci on the short arm of chromosome 3 in renal cell carcinoma. *Nature* 1987; **327**(6124):721–4.
58. Maher ER. Genomics and epigenomics of renal cell carcinoma. *Semin Cancer Biol* 2013; **23**(1):10–7.
59. Dreijerink K, Braga E, Kuzmin I, *et al.* The candidate tumor suppressor gene, RASSF1A, from human chromosome 3p21.3 is involved in kidney tumorigenesis. *Proc Nat Acad Sci U S A* 2001; **98**(13):7504–9.
60. Morrissey C, Martinez A, Zatyka M, *et al.* Epigenetic inactivation of the RASSF1A 3p21.3 tumor suppressor gene in both clear cell and papillary renal cell carcinoma. *Cancer Res* 2001; **61**(19):7277–81.
61. Varela I, Tarpey P, Raine K, *et al.* Exome sequencing identifies frequent mutation of the SWI/SNF complex gene PBRM1 in renal carcinoma. *Nature* 2011; **469**(7331):539–42.
62. Beroukhim R, Brunet J-P, Di Napoli A, *et al.* Patterns of gene expression and copy-number alterations in von-Hippel Lindau disease-associated and sporadic clear cell carcinoma of the kidney. *Cancer Res* 2009; **69**(11):4674–81.
63. Armah HB, Parwani AV. Xp11.2 Translocation renal cell carcinoma. *Arch Pathol Lab Med* 2010; **134**(1):124–9.
64. Komai Y, Fujiwara M, Fujii Y, *et al.* Adult Xp11 Translocation renal cell carcinoma diagnosed by cytogenetics and immunohistochemistry. *Clin Cancer Res* 2009; **15**(4):1170–6.
65. Tsuda M, Davis IJ, Argani P, *et al.* TFE3 fusions activate MET signaling by transcriptional up-regulation, defining another class of tumors as candidates for therapeutic MET inhibition. *Cancer Res* 2007; **67**(3):919–29.
66. Hong S-B, Oh H, Valera VA, Baba M, Schmidt LS, Linehan WM. Inactivation of the FLCN Tumor suppressor gene induces TFE3 transcriptional activity by increasing its nuclear localization. *PloS One* 2010; **5**(12):e15793.
67. Dalgliesh GL, Furge K, Greenman C, *et al.* Systematic sequencing of renal carcinoma reveals inactivation of histone modifying genes. *Nature* 2010; **463**(7279):360–3.
68. Morris MR ME. Epigenetics of renal cell carcinoma: the path towards new diagnostics and therapeutics. *Genome Med* 2010;**2**(9):59.
69. Motzer RJ, Hutson TE, Tomczak P, *et al.* Overall survival and updated results for sunitinib compared with interferon alfa in patients with metastatic renal cell carcinoma. *J Clin Oncol* 2009; **27**(22):3584–90.
70. Hudes G, Carducci M, Tomczak P, *et al.* Temsirolimus, interferon alfa, or both for advanced renal-cell carcinoma. *New Engl J Med* 2007; **356**(22):2271–81.
71. Motzer RJ, Escudier B, Oudard S, *et al.* Phase 3 trial of everolimus for metastatic renal cell carcinoma. *Cancer* 2010; **116**(18):4256–65.
72. Sternberg CN, Davis ID, Mardiak J, *et al.* Pazopanib in locally advanced or metastatic renal cell carcinoma: Results of a randomized phase III trial. *J Clin Oncol* 2010; **28**(6):1061–8.
73. Rini BI, Escudier B, Tomczak P, *et al.* Comparative effectiveness of axitinib versus sorafenib in advanced renal cell carcinoma (AXIS): a randomised phase 3 trial. *Lancet* 2011; **378**(9807):1931–9.
74. Yao JC, Shah MH, Ito T, *et al.* Everolimus for advanced pancreatic neuroendocrine tumors. *New Engl J Med* 2011; **364**(6):514–23.
75. Raymond E, Dahan L, Raoul J-L, *et al.* Sunitinib malate for the treatment of pancreatic neuroendocrine tumors. *New Engl J Med* 2011; **364**(6):501–13.
76. Llovet JM, Ricci S, Mazzaferro V, *et al.* Sorafenib in Advanced Hepatocellular Carcinoma. *New Engl J Med* 2008; **359**(4):378–90.
77. Baselga J, Campone M, Piccart M, *et al.* Everolimus in postmenopausal hormone-receptor–positive advanced breast cancer. *New Engl J Med* 2012; **366**(6):520–9.

CHAPTER 6.28

Pathology of renal cancer and other tumours affecting the kidney

Antonio Lopez-Beltran, Rodolfo Montironi, and Liang Cheng

Introduction to pathology of renal cancer and other tumours affecting the kidney

The current classification of renal cell tumours was proposed in 2004 by the World Health Organization (WHO).[1,2] It describes categories and entities based on pathological and genetic analyses, and previous classifications, in particular the Mainz and Heidelberg classifications.[2–4] Since this is a rapidly expanding field of research, new entities and morphologic variants of common categories have recently been described.[1–3,5–135] This chapter gives an overview on recent developments in the classification of kidney tumours in chidren and adults.

Familial renal cancer

Hereditary renal cancers show a tendency to be multiple and bilateral, may have a family history, and present at an earlier age.[10,12,20,27,36,37,39,41,58] Table 6.28.1 lists known inherited syndromes that predispose to renal tumours.[1,2]

Von Hippel-Lindau clear cell renal cell carcinoma

Like its sporadic counterpart, von Hippel-Lindau (VHL) clear cell renal cell carcinoma (RCC) harbours defective VHL tumour suppressor genes. Genetic alteration in the *VHL* gene in the tumour can include deletion, nonsense, or frame-shift mutations or missense mutations.[10]

Hereditary papillary renal cell carcinoma

Hereditary papillary RCC are typically bilateral, multifocal type 1 papillary RCC. Genetic alterations involve a proto-oncogene, c-MET, located at 7q31.1. Similar to what is found in sporadic papillary renal cell carcinoma, trisomy 7 and 17 are identified.[27]

Hereditary leiomatosis renal cell carcinoma

Hereditary leiomyomatosis-associated RCC patients develop cutaneous and uterine leiomyomas and type 2 papillary RCC. The pathologic findings in this disease are caused by mutations in the fumarate hydratase gene located at 1q42.[36] Architectural patterns

Table 6.28.1 Familial renal tumours

Syndrome	Gene	Tumour
Von Hippel-Lindau (VHL)	*VHL* (3p25)	Clear cell
Tuberous sclerosis	*TSC1, TSC2*	Angiomyolipoma, clear cell, other
Familial renal carcinoma	Gene not identified	Clear cell
Constitutional chromosome 3 translocation	Responsible gene not found*	Clear cell
Hereditary PRCC	*c-MET*	Papillary type 1
Birt-Hogg-Dubé (BHD)	*BHD*	Chromophobe**
Familial oncocytoma	Loss of multiple chromosomes	Oncocytoma
Hereditary leiomyomatosis RCC	*FH*	Papillary type 2

**VHL* gene mutated in some families.

**Renal oncocytomas, hybrid oncocytic, and clear cell carcinomas may occur.

Reproduced from Springer, *Rare Tumors* and *Tumor-like Conditions in Urological Pathology*, 'Renal Tumors and Tumor-Like Conditions', 2015, pp.1–61, Antonio Lopez-Beltran *et al.*, Springer International Publishing, Copyright © 2015 Springer International Publishing Switzerland. With permission of Springer Science+Business Media.

are papillary, tubulopapillary, tubular, solid, or mixed. The hallmark of the hereditary leiomyomatosis RCC, is the presence of large nucleus with a very prominent eosinophilic nucleolus, surrounded by a clear halo.[15] These tumours are associated with poor prognosis.[15,36]

Birt-Hogg-Dubé syndrome

Birt-Hogg-Dubé is an autosomal dominant cancer syndrome characterized by benign skin and renal tumours, and spontaneous pneumothorax.[37] The disease-related gene has been mapped to chromosome 17p11.2. Birt-Hogg-Dubé is characterized by a spectrum of mutations, and clinical heterogeneity among and within families. Renal epithelial tumours with hybrid features are seen in this syndrome.[37,45]

Renal cell carcinoma

Clear cell renal cell carcinoma

Most clear cell RCC are variably sized solitary cortical neoplasms, rarely bilateral (<5%) or multicentric (4%),[84] typically golden yellow. Necrosis, cystic degeneration, haemorrhage, calcification, ossification, and extension into the renal vein may occur. Clear cell tumours of any size are considered malignant (Table 6.28.2).[1,2,48,84]

Microvascular invasion and microscopic tumour coagulative necrosis may be relevant predictors in low stage RCC.[2,4,17,18,84] Clear cell RCC has a worse prognosis when compared with chromophobe or papillary subtypes, and may progress into a sarcomatoid carcinoma which is an ominous prognostic sign.

The international Society of Urological Pathologists (ISUP) suggested that clear cell RCC grading should be based upon nucleolar features and not Fuhrman grading for grade 1 to 3 tumours.[48,110] Sporadic clear cell RCC displays frequent chromosome 3p losses (Table 6.28.2, Fig. 6.28.1).[4,63]

Clear cell RCC may have acidophilic cytoplasm, angioleiomyoma-like stroma or pseudopapillary architecture but retains the characteristic 3p loss (Table 6.28.3).[9,14,81,104,108,111,135]

Multilocular cystic renal cell carcinoma

The 2004 WHO classification of kidney tumours recognizes multilocular cystic RCC (MCRCC) as a variant of clear cell RCC with

Table 6.28.2 Main histotypes of renal cell tumours seen in adults with associated genetic alterations

Malignant renal cell tumours	**Main genetic alterations**
◆ Clear cell renal cell carcinoma	−3p, +5q22, −6q, −8p, −9p, −14q
◆ Multilocular cystic renal cell neoplasm of low malignant potential (multilocular clear cell renal cell carcinoma)	*VHL* gene mutation
◆ Papillary renal cell carcinoma	+3q, +7,+8, +12, +16, +17, +20, −Y
◆ Chromophobe renal cell carcinoma	−1, −2,−6,−10, −17, −21, hypodiploidy
◆ Carcinoma of the collecting ducts of Bellini	−1q, −6p, −8p, −13q, −21q, −3p (rare)
◆ Tubulocystic carcinoma	Variable trisomy of chromosome 17
◆ Renal medulary carcinoma	Rare loss of chromosome 22
◆ MiT family translocation RCC (renal carcinoma associated with Xp11.2 translocations/TFE3 gene fusions (MiTF/TFE family translocation carcinomas)	t(X;1)(p11.2;q21), t(X;17)(p11.2;q25), t(X;1)(p11.2;p34), t(X;17)(p11.2;q23), others
◆ Renal cell carcinoma in long-term survivors after neuroblastoma	Allelic imbalance at 20q13
◆ Mucinous tubular and spindle cell carcinoma	−1, −4, −6, −8, −13, −14, +7, +11, +16, +17
◆ Renal cell carcinoma unclassified	Unknown
Renal cell neoplasms in end-stage renal disease	
◆ Acquired cystic disease-related RCC	Variable gains chromosomes 7 and 17, no *VHL* gene deletions, rare gains 1, 2, 6, 10
◆ Clear cell papillary RCC	Lacked the gains of chromosome 7, no loss of Y chromosome, lack 3p deletions
Benign renal cell tumours	
◆ Papillary adenoma	Similar to papillary RCC but less extensive
◆ Oncocytoma	Chromosomes 1 and/or 14 loss and frequent alterations of mitochondrial DNA, 11q13 translocation, no chromosome 3p loss
◆ Metanephric tumours: adenoma, adenofibroma, stromal metanephric	Normal karyotypes, 2p deletion, others
Mixed stromal and epithelial tumours	
◆ *Renal epithelial and stromal tumour (REST)	Nonrandom X-chromosomeInactivation, others

*Include categories listed in other classifications as cystic nephroma or mixed epithelial and stromal tumour.

Adapted from *European Urology*, Volume 49, Issue 5, Antonio Lopez-Beltran *et al.*, '2004 WHO Classification of the Renal Tumors of the Adults', pp. 798–805, Copyright © 2006 European Association of Urology, with permission from Elsevier, http://www.sciencedirect.com/science/journal/03022838

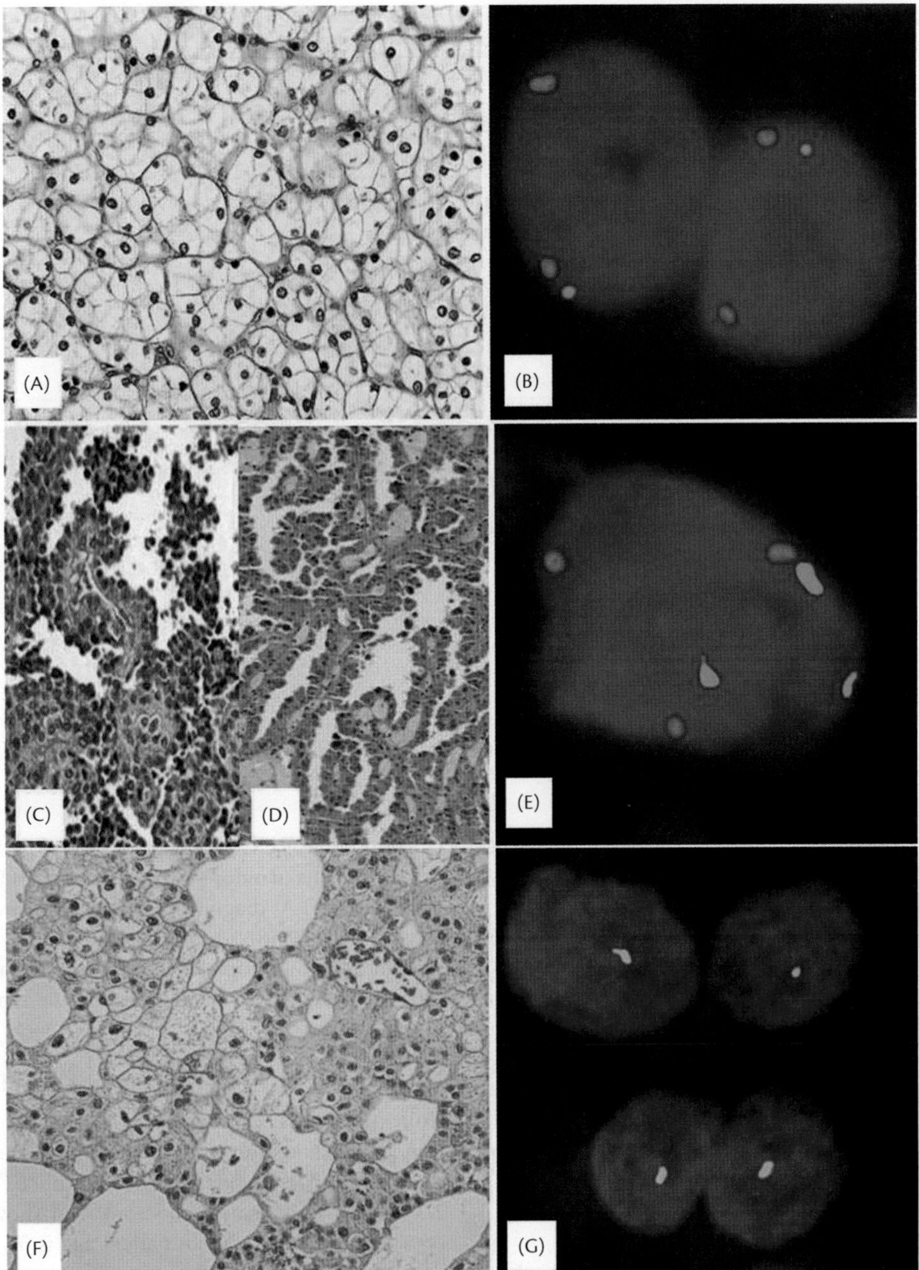

Fig. 6.28.1 Main histologic types of renal cell carcinoma. Clear cell type (A) showing chromosome 3p deletion (one single green signal) (B); papillary type 1 (C) and type 2 (D) showing trisomy 7 and 17 (three signals green and three signals red) (E); chromophobe type (F) showing chromosome 10 monosomy (one single blue signal) (G). (B, E, G: fluorescent *in situ* hybridization analysis).

a good prognosis.[2] This is a tumour entirely composed of cysts of variable size separated from the kidney by a fibrous capsule. The cyst are lined by a single layer of clear to pale cells but occasionally shows a few small papillae.[2] The septa are composed of fibrous tissue that may have epithelial cells with clear cytoplasm that resemble those lining the cysts (Table 6.28.2). Cases with expansive nodules are excluded. *VHL* gene mutations in MCRCC supports its classification as a type of clear cell RCC.[32] No progression of MCRCC has been reported. It has been suggested to rename MCRCC as multilocular cystic renal cell neoplasm of low malignant potential.[32]

Papillary renal cell carcinoma

Papillary RCC has a less aggressive clinical course than clear cell RCC.[1,2] Papillary RCC has variable proportions of papillae and may be bilateral or multifocal with haemorrhage, necrosis or cystic degeneration (Table 6.28.2, Fig. 6.28.1).[2] The papillae contain a fibrovascular core with aggregates of foamy macrophages, calcified concretions, and frequent hemosiderin granules.[85] Cellular type 1 and type 2 tumours have papillae covered by small cells with scanty cytoplasm arranged in a single layer in type1, and tumour cells of higher nuclear grade, eosinophilic cytoplasm, and

Table 6.28.3 Immunohistochemical profile of common renal neoplasms

Tumour histotype	
Clear cell RCC	**Positive for:** vimentin, AE1/AE3, CD10, RCCm, CD15, PAX2, PAX8, and carbonic anhydrase IX **Negative for:** HMWCK, CK7, CK20, CD117, Ksp-cadherin, parvalbumin
Papillary RCC and mucinous tubular and spindle cell carcinoma	**Positive for:** vimentin, AE1/AE3, CK7, AMACR, RCC Marker, PAX2, and PAX8 **Negative for:** CD117, Ksp-cadherin, and parvalbumin
Chromophobe RCC/oncocytoma	**Positive for:** E-cadherin, Ksp-cadherin, parvalbumin, CD117, AE1/AE3 **Negative for:** vimentin, CK7 (or weak), carbonic anhydrase IX, and AMACR
Collecting duct carcinoma	**Positive for**: p63 and HMWCK, Some positive for PAX2 and PAX8 When p63 and uroplakin III positive more likely urothelial carcinoma
Papillary clear cell RCC	**Positive for:** CK7, PAX2, and PAX8 **Negative for:** AMACR
Xp11.2 translocation carcinoma	**Positive for:** CD10, RCC Marker, TFE3, PAX2, and PAX8 **Usually negative** or focally positive for AE1/AE3
Urothelial carcinoma (renal pelvis)	**Positive for:** CK7 and p63 (70%), CK5/6 and CK20, uroplakin III, HMWCK, and thrombomodulin **Negative for:** RCC Marker, CD10, PAX2, and PAX8
Epithelioid angiomyolipoma	**Positive for**: HMB-45, Mart-1, or Melan-A, micropthalmia transcription factor, tyrosinase, and muscle-specific actin **Negative for**: AE1/AE3, EMA, CD10, RCC Marker, PAX2, and PAX

RCC: Renal cell carcinoma.

Adapted with permission from Shen SS *et al.*, 'Role of Immunohistochemistry in Diagnosing Renal Neoplasms: When Is It Really Useful?', *Archives of Pathology and Laboratory Medicine*, Volume 136, pp.410–417, Copyright © 2012 College of American Pathologists.

pseudostratified nuclei in type 2.[2,3,49,75,76] Type 1 tumours have longer survival.[25,74,75] Trisomy or tetrasomy 7, trisomy 17 and loss of chromosome Y are the cytogenetic signature (Fig. 6.28.1).[26,61] Stage, tumour proliferation, and sarcomatoid change being correlated with outcome. It has been suggested that papillary RCC grading should be based upon nucleolar features and not Fuhrman grading for grade 1 to 3 tumours.[28] Age and sex distribution of papillary RCC is similar to clear cell RCC. Recent molecular genetic studies provide evidences for the independent origin of multifocal papillary tumours in patients with papillary RCC.[90] An oncoytic variant of papillary RCC has been reported.[11,86] One patient died of metastases on follow-up (Table 6.28.3).[11]

Chromophobe renal cell carcinoma

Less aggressive than other RCC, the chromophobe type is characterized by huge pale cells with reticulated cytoplasm and prominent cell membrane (Table 6.28.2, Fig. 6.28.1).[1,78] It accounts for 5% of renal epithelial tumours.[3,33,47,59,76] Chromophobe RCC is solid and appears orange turning grey or sandy after fixation. The eosinophilic variant needs to be differentiated from oncocytoma.[62] Sarcomatoid transformation is associated to aggressive disease.[47,64,67] Diffuse cytoplasmic Hale's iron colloid stain is characteristic. The relationship between oncocytoma and chromophobe RCC is still unclear. Both seems to derive from the intercalated cell of the collecting duct, both have rearrangement of mitochondrial DNA, increased mitochondria in oncocytoma[19] and numerous mitochondria-derived microvesicles in chromophobe RCC, and both are frequently observed in oncocytosis with or without Birt-Hogg-Dubé syndrome.[59] There are reports of hybrid tumour composed of oncocytic and chromophobe elements.[13] Therefore, oncocytoma might be the benign counterpart of chromophobe RCC.[14,62] Loss of several chromosomes characterizes chromophobe RCC (Table 6.28.2, Fig. 6.28.1).[7,29] Recognizing occassional occurrence of metastases and 10% mortality is of clinical relevance. At diagnosis most patients are in the sixth decade, stage T1 or T2 (86%) and similar gender incidence. Fuhrman grading is not appropiated to grade chromophome RCC with an international consensus on that chromophobe RCC should not be graded at present (Table 6.28.3).[76]

Carcinoma of the collecting ducts of Bellini

Collecting duct carcinoma (CDC), also known as Bellini's tumour, accounts for <1% of renal malignancies and derives from the 'principal cells' of the collecting duct (Table 6.28.2); ranges 2.5 to 12 cm, is centrally located, and shows a firm grey-white appearance.[6,30,66,106] Mean patient age is 55 years with male predominance. When small, origin within a medullary pyramid may be seen. At diagnosis, most tumours are in advanced stage with metastasis and morphologic criteria for diagnosis are the presence of an infiltrative tubular or tubulopapillary pattern, associated with desmoplastic stromal reaction, necrosis, and cells displaying high Fuhrman grade. CDC is positive for low and high molecular weight keratins, c-KIT, and vimentin, but molecular alterations of CDC are poorly understood (Table 6.28.2).[6,30,66,106,114] The main differential diagnoses of CDC include type 2 PRCC, renal pelvic adenocarcinoma, or urothelial carcinoma with glandular differentiation.[6,66,106]

Renal medullary carcinoma

It is a rapidly growing rare tumour of the renal medulla regarded as an aggressive variant of collecting duct carcinoma[106] that was initially considered of renal pelvis origin. Some may have solid or rhabdoid phenotype.[73] With few exceptions this tumour is seen in young male blacks with sickle cell trait (mean age 22 years), presenting with haematuria, flank pain, weight loss, and palpable mass. Metastatic disease may be the initial clinical evidence and the reported prognosis is poor.[73,106]

Tubulocystic carcinoma

Is a rare renal tumour composed of tubular and cystic structures (Table 6.28.2).[42] The genomic alterations of tubulocystic carcinoma are alike but not identical to those of papillary RCC. Like papillary RCC, it often exhibits trisomy of chromosome 17, but it does not show trisomy 7.[42] It does not exhibit monosomy of chromosomes 1, 6, 14, 15, and 22 and frequent allelic loss on chromosomal arms 1q, 6p, 8p, 13q, and 21q, which are frequently seen in collecting duct cancer.[42] Immunohistochemistry showed variable expression of CD10, AMACR, parvalbumin, 34βE12, PAX-2, and CK19.[114] A recent report on 13 cases showed one case with lymph node metastasis.[42] Some may coexist with papillary RCC.[42] It is considered a poorly defined entity.

MiTF/TFE family translocation carcinomas

This type of RCC is defined by different translocations involving chromosome Xp11.2, all resulting in gene fusions involving the TFE3 gene (Table 6.28.2, Fig. 6.28.2).[51–57] This carcinoma predominantly affects children and young adults, but may be seen in adults. The ASPL-TFE3 translocation carcinomas characteristically present at an advanced stage associated with lymph node metastases.[51–57] RCC associated with Xp11.2 translocations resemble clear cell RCC on gross examination and seems to have an indolent evolution, even with metastasis.[65] The histopathologic appearance is that of a papillary carcinoma with clear cells and cells with granular eosinophilic cytoplasm with foci of calcifications regardless of the type of translocation. TFE3 immunostainings were positive in only 82% of TFE3 translocation carcinomas.[65] Both TFE3 and TFEB renal translocation carcinomas expressed CD10 and alpha-methylacyl-coenzyme-A racemase[65] (Table 6.28.3). Another subset of renal tumours are associated with a translocation t(6;11)(p21;q12) involving the transcription factor EB (TFEB).[107] Argani and Ladanyi have[51–57] recently proposed to regroup these neoplasms under the category of 'MiTF/TFE family translocation carcinomas'. Translocation involving TFE3 and TFEB can be specifically identified by immunohistochemistry, but diagnosis may also be performed by FISH analysis.[51–57,107]

Mucinous, tubular, and spindle cell carcinoma

This entity,[2] is a low-grade carcinoma composed of tightly packed tubules separated by pale mucinous stroma and a spindle cell component.[68,78,80] It seems to derive from the distal nephron. This tumour has a combination of losses involving chromosomes 1, 4, 6, 8, 13 and 14 and gains of chromosome 7, 11, 16, and 17.[24,80] A recent immunohistochemical analysis found a significant overlap with papillary RCC,[21] and some authors believe this is a variant of papillary RCC with spindle cell differentiation (Table 6.28.3).[21] There is a female predominance and the mean age is 53 years at diagnosis. One patient developed metastases on follow-up. It is a poorly defined entity.[68,78,80]

Renal cell carcinoma in long-term survivors after neuroblastoma

A few cases of RCC arise in long-term survivors of childhood neuroblastoma.[8] This group is heterogeneous that shows oncocytoid features. Allelic imbalances occur at the 20q13 locus.[8,78] The prognosis is similar to other RCC. Uni- or bilateral lesions develop at mean age of 13.5 years.[78]

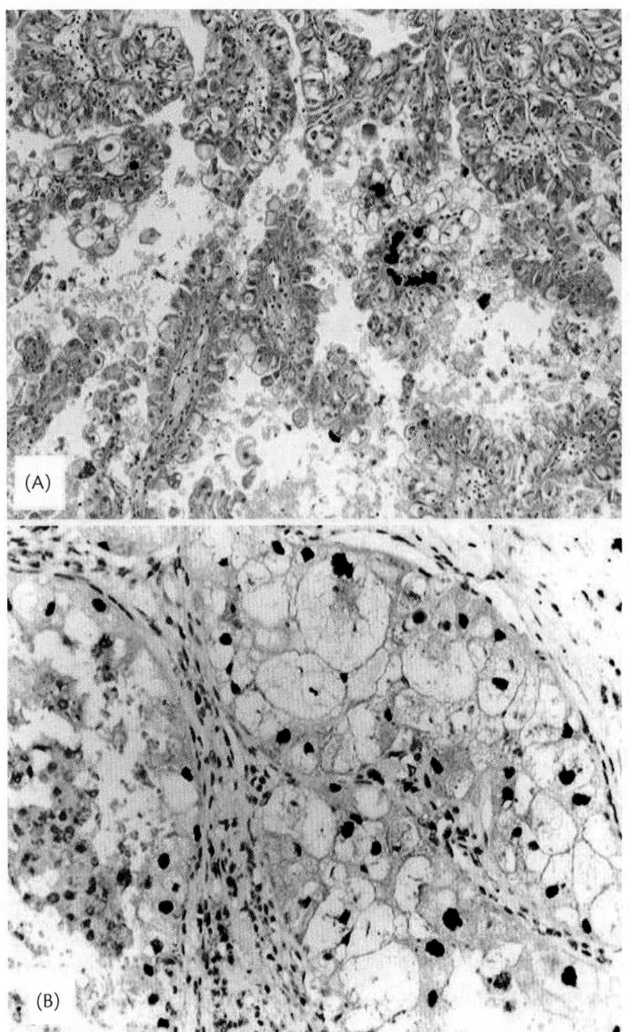

Fig. 6.28.2 Renal cell carcinoma in a case of Xp.11 translocation showing papillary arechitecture, eosinophilic and clear cells, and focal calcification (A); nuclear immunoreactivity for TFE-3 protein (B).

RCC with sarcomatoid or rhabdoid differentiation

Current WHO classification does not consider sarcomatoid RCC as an entity but rather as a progression of any RCC main type.[2,25,67,74] Pure sarcomatoid morphology without recognizable epithelial elements falls into the unclassified RCC category.[2,25,47] RCC with sarcomatoid elements show higher proliferative activity than other renal cell carcinoma types and usually exhibit highly malignant behaviour with a predilection for increased local invasiveness and a higher likelihood of distant metastasis.[67,74]

Sarcomatoid components may be seen in clear cell, papillary, chromophobe, and collecting duct carcinomas.[2,64,67] It is speculated that the sarcomatoid components of RCC represent areas of dedifferentiation or epithelial-mesenchyma transition.[25,67,74]

Jones *et al.*[91] examined the patterns of allelic loss and of nonrandom X-chromosome inactivation in clear cell and sarcomatoid components of RCC from 22 patients and concluded that both clear cell and sarcomatoid components of RCC are derived from the same progenitor cell.[91] The specific molecular mechanisms responsible for sarcomatoid transformation of a renal tumour are unknown, although some studies suggest a link with mutations of the *TP53* tumour suppressor gene.[64,67,71,91,111]

RCC with rhabdoid differentiation is a rare and aggressive neoplasm with poor prognosis. Most patients are at high stage at diagnosis, develop metastases soon after, and died of the disease withing a year of diagnosis.[112–114] Rhabdoid cells are large with eccentric atypical nucleus and eosinophilic intracytoplasmic inclusion that is positive for vimentin, EMA, and cytokeratin. Ocassionally sarcomatoid change and rhabdoid features may coexist.

Renal cell carcinoma, unclassified

This represents 4–6% of renal tumours. At diagnosis, most are of high grade and stage with poor survival.[2,109,111] The WHO criteria include: (i) composites of recognized types; (ii) pure sarcomatoid morphology; (iii) mucin production; (iv) rare mixtures of epithelial and stromal elements; and (v) unrecognizable cell types.[2,115] Reported data suggest that it is an aggressive form of RCC (Table 6.28.1), as confirmed in a recent study based on 56 cases. The prognosis of these patients is mainly related to pT stage, tumour size, microvascular invasion, tumour necrosis, or recurrence after surgery.[43,115]

Renal cell neoplasms in end-stage renal disease

The spectrum of renal tumours associated with end-stage renal disease is quite varied with examples of clear cell, papillary, or chromophobe RCC, CDC, tubulocystic carcinoma, angiomyolipoma, oncocytoma, and mixed epithelial and stromal tumour. Two new histologic subtypes of RCC have been reported to occur in patients with end-stage renal disease.[34,70,93,94]

Acquired cystic disease-associated renal cell carcinoma

These are composed of cells with abundant eosinophilic cytoplasm and variably solid, cribriform, tubulocystic, and papillary architecture.[70] Tickoo *et al.*[34] analysed the status of the *VHL* gene and chromosomes 7 and 17 with FISH in 43 tumours and found no *VHL* gene deletions, although gains of chromosomes 7 and 17 were observed in some cases. Cossu-Rocca *et al.*[70] studied three additional cases and found[70] deposits of calcium oxalate crystals in each tumour. FISH analysis showed no losses or gains of chromosomes 1, 2, 6, 10, or 17 in one tumour; gains of chromosomes 1, 2, and 6 were noted in two tumours, one of these also showed gains of chromosome 10.[70,93,94]

Clear cell papillary (tubulopapillary) renal cell carcinoma

These are renal carcinomas composed mainly of papillary structures proliferating within cystic spaces, lined by cells with clear cytoplasm.[93,94] Gobbo *et al.* investigated a group of seven tumours from five patients with FISH and immunohistochemistry.[82] All tumours lacked the gains of chromosome 7 and loss of Y that are typical for papillary renal cell carcinoma and furthermore lack the 3p deletion which is typical of clear cell RCC (Table 6.28.3). These tumours also occur in patients unrelated to end-stage renal disease. It remains poorly defined.

Recently described entities not included in the current WHO classification of urologic tumours

Various studies relating to leiomyomatous (RCC with angioleiomyoma-like stroma) RCC,[9] oncocytic papillary RCC, follicular (thyroid-like) RCC,[31,101] succinate dehydrogenase B-associated RCC, *ALK*-translocation RCC, and hybrid oncocytic tumours in Birt-Hogg-Dubé syndrome had been reported, the overerall opinion is that clinical and histological features are not sufficiently understood to permit classification of these as distinctive tumour histotypes at present.[109–113]

Benign tumours

Papillary adenoma

Papillary adenoma is usually solitary, 0.5 cm or smaller, well-circumscribed, greyish or white lesion in the renal cortex that shows a tubulopapillary architecture similar to cellular types 1 and 2 in papillary RCC (Fig. 6.28.3).[85] Papillary adenoma is the most common neoplasm of the epithelium of the renal tubules.[61] It is found in 10% to 40% of specimens and shows genetic alterations similar to papillary RCC but less extensive. 'Renal adenomatosis' refers to the occasional occurrence of multiple and/or bilateral papillary adenomas.[61,85]

Metanephric tumours: adenoma, adenofibroma, and metanephric stromal tumour

This group includes metanephric adenoma, metanephric adenofibroma, and metanephric stromal tumour.[2,72]

Metanephric adenoma is an epithelial neoplasm that occurs in children and adults with female preponderance;[51,89] half are incidental. An exceptional case with metastasis has been reported, and therefore, appropriated follow-up is adviced.[77] May coexist with Wilms' tumour or RCC.[72,85] A case of high-grade sarcoma arising in association with metanephric adenoma (metanephric adenosarcoma) has been described. Metanephric adenomas are 3 to 6 cm, usually solitary and not encapsulated (Fig. 6.28.3).[89,121,122] Metanephric adenofibroma shows an epithelial component similar to metanephric adenoma which is embedded in a fibroblast-like stroma. Metanephric adenoma has a normal karyotype.[60,61,72,83] Rare cases of metanephric stromal tumour, entirely composed of stromal elements have been described.[120–122]

Renal oncocytoma

Oncocytoma is a benign renal epithelial neoplasm that derives from the intercalated cells.[50] It is well-circumscribed, non-encapsulated, mahogany-brown, or pale yellow with a central stellate scar. The 'oncocyte' has densely granular eosinophilic cytoplasm and round and regular nuclei (Fig. 6.28.3). Mitotic activity and necrosis are uncommon. Chromosomes 1 and/or 14 loss and alterations of mitochondrial DNA are frequent. Oncocytoma comprises 3% to 9% of all primary renal neoplasms.[50] Most are incidental and sporadic but few are symptomatic.

The eosinophilic variants of chromophobe RCC are difficult to distinguish from renal oncocytomas on haematoxylin and eosin stained sections.[50] The distinction is important, as chromophobe renal cell carcinoma is a malignant tumour while oncocytoma is benign. Reports of 'malignant' or 'metastatic' oncocytomas are

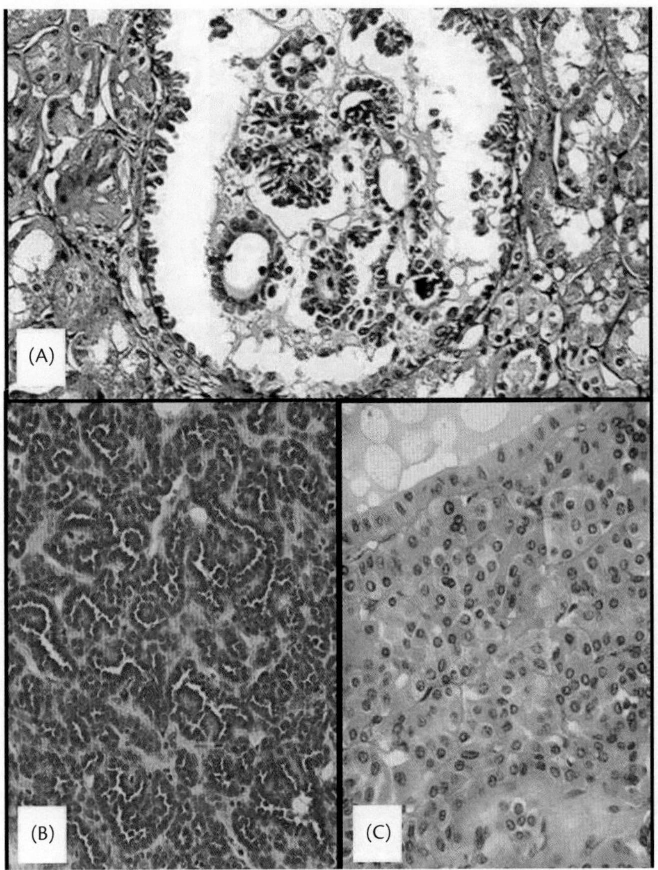

Fig. 6.28.3 Histologic features in benign epithelial tumours of the kidney including papillary adenoma (A), metanephric adenoma (B), and oncocytoma (C).

postulated to actually represent misdiagnosed chromophobe renal cell carcinomas.[88] The Hale's colloidal iron stain shows a diffuse and strong reticular pattern in almost 100% of chromophobe RCC, and it is frequently patchy and focal in oncocytoma (Table 6.28.3).[23,50]

The term oncocytosis (oncocytomatosis) refers to a small subset of oncocytic tumours removed surgically because of a dominant mass that microscopically has the features of oncocytoma, although some may have either chromophobe RCC or hybrid features.[35,69]

Cystic nephroma and mixed epithelial and stromal tumours

Cystic nephroma is a benign mixed epithelial and stromal neoplasm frequently unilateral, encapsulated, solitary, and multilocular with no solid areas or necrosis.[16,46,78]

Adult cases present after age of 30 with female predominance. Some are associated with pleuropulmonary blastoma.[87] Clonal analysis supports its neoplastic nature.[16,46,78]

Mixed epithelial and stromal tumour of kidney is a rare renal neoplasm composed of a mixture of stromal solid areas and epithelial (mostly cystic) elements previously reported as cystic hamartoma of renal pelvis or adult mesoblastic nephroma.[46] Some stromal cells react with antibodies to oestrogen and progesterone. There is a female predominance with history of oestrogen therapy. All cases have been seen in adults. Some may experience malignant sarcomatous transformation. A recent report suggests that cystic nephroma and mixed epithelial and stromal tumours are part of the same spectrum of lesions, and therefore, they should be named as 'renal epithelial and stromal tumour'.[16,38]

Mesenchymal neoplasms

Medullary fibroma (renomedullary interstitial cell tumour)

These tumours are frequently multiple and found incidentally at autopsy or surgery for another condition. Tumours are unencapsulated, circumscribed, white or grey, and paucicellular, measuring 0.1–0.5 cm. The cells are small stellate, spindle or polygonal in a loose basophilic stroma and seems to originate from prostaglandin-producing interstitial cells in renal medulla. Amyloid deposits may be present.[1,2]

Juxtaglomerular cell tumour

A benign renin-secreting tumour derived from modified smooth muscle cells of the juxtaglomerular apparatus in patients with refractory hypertension and high plasma rennin activity. Most tumours are <4 cm unilateral, encapsulated, solitary, cortical and occur in females (mean age of 27 years).[134] Histologically, sheets of uniform round, polygonal, or spindled cells are present with uniform, round to oval nuclei with scattered mitotic figures.[134] Thin and thick-walled blood vessels are often prominent. Immunoreactivity for renin, actin, vimentin, and CD34 is characteristic. Ultrastructurally, cells contain rhomboid renin-specific crystals.[134]

Angiomyolipoma

Angiomyolipoma (AML) is a benign tumour associated with several hereditary disorders including von Recklinghausen disease, von Hippel-Lindau syndrome, Autosomal dominant (adult) polycystic kidney disease or tuberous sclerosis.

It occurs in 80% of patients with tuberous sclerosis. The mean age of patients with 'sporadic' AML ranges 45–55 years but drops to 25–35 years of age in patients with tuberous sclerosis. AML is thought to be derived from perivascular epithelioid cell. AML frequently exhibits loss of heterozygosity in portions of the *TSC2* gene locus on chromosome 16p13 (in both sporadic and tuberous sclerosis cases), and less often in the *TSC1* gene on chromosome 9q34. May occur in renal cortex, medulla or in perirenal soft tissues and may coexist with other renal neoplasms (RCC, oncocytoma) or being associated with lymphangioleiomyomatosis of lung. AML is typically unencapsulated, yellow to tan-pink, range from 3 to 20 cm and is composed of variable admixtures of mature adipose tissue, smooth muscle, and abnormally formed blood vessels. Smooth muscle proliferations often appear to spin off perpendicularly from the outer layers of blood vessel walls. Smooth muscle cells may be spindled with mild degrees of nuclear atypia. Involvement of intrarenal veins, renal vein, vena cava, and regional lymph nodes are indicative of multifocal growth, rather than invasion or metastasis. AML is characterized by coexpression of melanocytic markers (HMB-45, HMB50, CD63, MART-1/Melan-A, microphthalmia transcription factor) (Fig. 6.28.4) and smooth muscle markers (muscle-specific actin, smoothmuscle actin, desmin) (Table 6.28.3).

Epithelioid angiomyolipoma

A potentially malignant mesenchymal neoplasm closely related to classic AML. Half of recorded cases have a history of tuberous

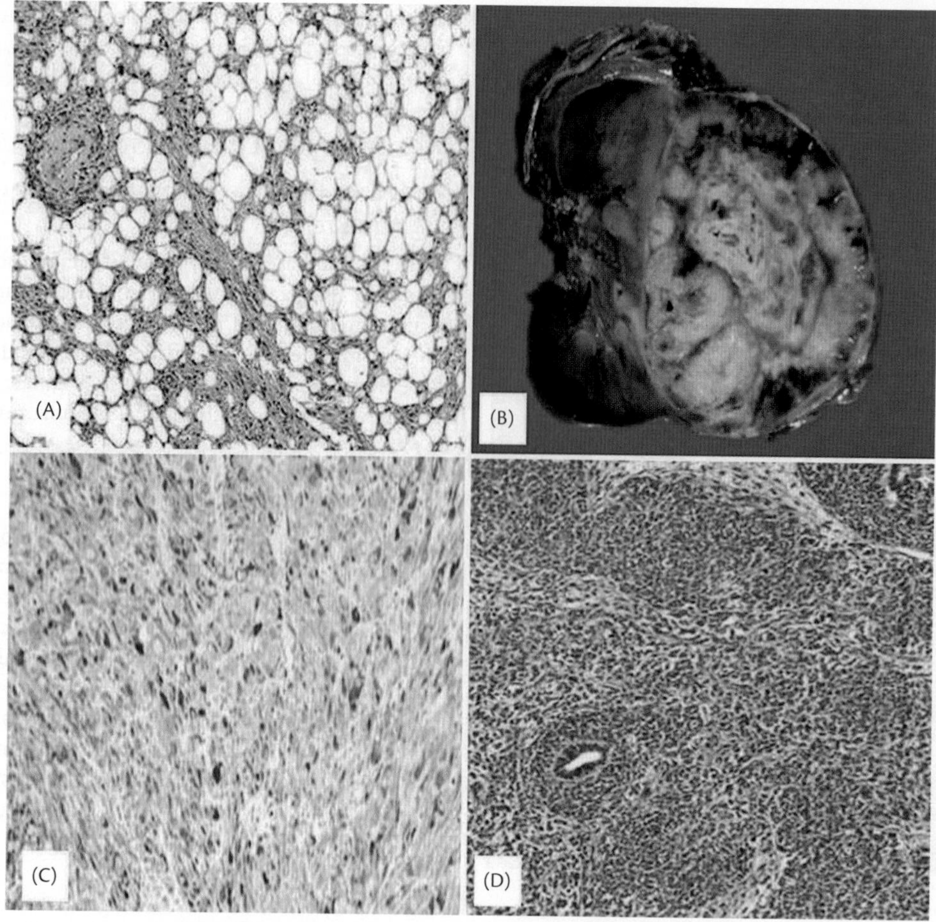

Fig. 6.28.4 Histologic features of angiomyolipoma including mature adipose tissue, smooth muscle, and blood vessels (A), and immunorreactivity for HMB-45 in a case of epithelioid angiomyolipoma (B). Gross features (C) and classic triphasic histology (blastema, epithelium, stroma) (D) in Wilms' tumour.

sclerosis.[2,75] Tumours exhibit allelic loss of the *TS2*-containing region. Most are large, haemorrhagic, and locally infiltrative with sheets of cytologically malignant epithelioid cells, and is easy to misdiagnose as high-grade carcinoma.[75] The immunohistochemical profile is similar to that of classic AML. Some patients sufered metastasis and/or death.

Wilms' tumour and other renal neoplasms in children

Nephrogenic rests and nephroblastomatosis

Nephrogenic rests are abnormally persistent foci of embryonal cells identifiable in 1% of post-mortem kidneys in infants and considered capable of developing into nephroblastoma. May be present in 25–40% of kidneys harbouring nephroblastoma.[123–128] If diffuse and multifocal, the term 'nephroblastomatosis' is applicable. Nephrogenic rests are subclassified into perilobar (more common and multifocal) and intralobar (unifocal) types. The later is at higher risk of development of nephroblastoma.[123–128]

Nephroblastoma (Wilms' tumour)

Usually occurs between six months and three years of age; rare after three years of age. It comprises 85% of paediatric renal neoplasms and 5% of childhood cancers.[123–133]

Five per cent (5%) are multicentric, 5% are bilateral, and 5% are anaplastic. Lung metastasis is common and is frequently associated with cryptorchidism, hypospadias, hemihypertrophy, aniridia, renal ectopia, and horseshoe kidney. Known risk factors include Beckwith–Wiedemann (hemihypertrophy) associated with the WT2 gene, Wilms–aniridia–genital anomaly–retardation syndrome: associated with the WT1 gene, Denys–Drash syndrome (glomerulonephritis, pseudohermaphroditism, and nephroblastoma) associated with the WT1 gene, Trisomy 18, and multicystic dysplastic kidney.[123–133] Putative tumour suppressor genes are WT1 (chromosome 11p13), WT2 (chromosome 11p15.5), and WT3 (chromosome 16q).

Most are circumscribed large tumours (>5 cm) (Fig. 6.28.4) that may be cystic or multicentric. Typical histology is triphasic tumour including blastema, epithelial component (abortive tubules and glomeruli) and stroma (skeletal muscle (most common), spindle cells, or cartilage). Positive WT1, vimentin, neuron-specific enolase (focal), (focal), and desmin (focal) is the diagnostic signature.[123–133]

Anaplasia is one of the criteria for placing Wilms' tumour under unfavourable histology category[123–133]—the other is the development of a high-grade sarcoma or carcinoma within nephroblastoma. Anaplasia indicates increased resistance to therapy rather than increased aggressiveness. Definiton of anaplasia incude multipolar polyploid mitotic figures and each component of the

Table 6.28.4 Staging nephroblastoma (fifth protocol, National Wilms' Tumor Study Group)

Stage I	Limited to kidney and completely resected. Renal capsule is intact. Renal sinus soft tissue may be minimally infiltrated
Stage II	Tumour infiltrates beyond kidney, but is completely resected. Tumour extends beyond renal capsule. Tumour infiltrates vessels within the renal sinus. Tumour with prior open or large core needle biopsies. Tumour with local spillage confined to flank
Stage III	Residual non-hematogenous tumour confined to abdomen. Tumour in abdominal lymph nodes. Diffuse peritoneal contamination: direct tumour growth, tumour implants, and spillage into peritoneum before or during surgery. Gross or microscopic involvement of specimen margins. Residual tumour in abdomen. Tumour removed noncontiguously (piece-meal resection)
Stage IV	Haematogenous metastases
Stage V	Bilateral renal involvement at diagnosis (tumour in each kidney should be separately substaged)

Reproduced from Springer, *Rare Tumors and Tumor-like Conditions in Urological Pathology*, 'Renal Tumors and Tumor-Like Conditions', 2015, pp. 1–61, Antonio Lopez-Beltran *et al.*, Springer International Publishing, Copyright © 2015 Springer International Publishing Switzerland. With permission of Springer Science+Business Media.

abnormal metaphase must be as large as or larger than a normal metaphase, markedly enlarged and hyperchromatic nuclei (at least three times larger than adjacent non-neoplastic nuclei). Anaplasia is confined to renal parenchyma.[123–133] Table 6.28.4 shows current staging.

Main differential diagnosis includes clear cell sarcoma, rhabdoid tumour, neuroblastoma, synovial sarcoma, and primitive neuroectodermal tumour (PNET) of the kidney.[133]

Cystic partially differentiated nephroblastoma

Most are detected as palpable masses in children <4 years old with benign clinical course.[123–133] Usually are 5–10 cm in diameter with fibrous pseudocapsule. Tumour is entirely composed of variably sized cysts, some of those may have papillary excrescences. Cysts are separated by septa of variable thickness and lined by flat, cuboidal, or hobnail epithelium. Septa contain blastema, nephroblastomatous epithelial elements, and differentiated and/or undifferentiated mesenchymal elements (skeletal muscle, cartilage, fat, or myxoid mesenchyme). Solid expansile nodules warrant a diagnosis of cystic nephroblastoma. If no nephroblastomatous elements are seen in the fibrous septa, some apply the diagnostic term 'cystic nephroma'[132]; however, these lesions are viewed as being different from similar lesions in in adults.

Congenital mesoblastic nephroma

Most common congenital renal neoplasm and 90% of patients are <1-year-old. It accounts for 2% of all paediatric renal tumours and presents as a palpable mass.[123–133] Metastasis and tumour-related death is rare; recurrences are attributable to incomplete initial resection. Two morphologic patterns: 'classic congenital mesoblastic nephroma' and 'cellular congenital mesoblastic nephroma (translocation t)'[12,15] which confirms that it is an infantile fibrosarcoma of the kidney. Classic congenital mesoblastic nephroma (CMN) is viewed as infantile fibromatosis (no translocation identified).

Usually are unilateral (mean diameter is 6 cm), solitary tumours that may have cysts, haemorrhage, and necrosis. The classic form shows intersecting bundles of spindle cells resembling fibroblasts and prominent irregular vascular spaces.[123–133] Cellular form shows plump spindle cells, arranged in poorly formed fascicles. Mitotic figures are present. Mixed congenital mesoblastic nephroma shows features of both types. On immunohistochemistry, positive vimentin, actin, desmin (rare), and negative CD34, cytokeratins, and S100 protein are the signature.[123–133]

Clear cell sarcoma of the kidney

This accounts for about 3% of all malignant paediatric renal neoplasms, it is twice as common in males ranging from 2 months to 54 years).[123–133] It is typically large (mean diameter 11 cm), has propensity for bone metastasis, unilateral, unicentric, soft to firm, homogeneous, light brown or grey and encapsulated; 5% involve the renal vein.

The classic pattern includes epithelioid or spindled cells arranged in nests or cords separated by fibrovascular septa of variable thickness. Cells are separated by myxoid extracellular matrix material that mimics clear cytoplasm. Cell nuclei are round to oval, with dispersed chromatin and inconspicuous, or no nucleoli mitotic activity is low. Many pattern variations have been described: myxoid, sclerosing, cellular, epithelioid, spindle cell, and palisading. Differential diagnosis from nephroblastoma may be difficult, likwise, pale H&E staining and negative immunostaining for all markers except vimentin and BCL2 suggests clear cell sacoma.[123–133]

Rhabdoid tumour of the kidney

Accounts for about 2% of all paediatric renal tumours and 80% of patients have metastases at the time of diagnosis.[123–133] Most patients die within one year. Almost all patients are <3 years old. Identical tumours involve other sites; especially central nervous system.[131] The typical case is unilateral, large, unencapsulated, with haemorrhage and necrosis, sometimes with satellite intrarenal metastases. Histologically, rhabdoid tumour is composed of sheets of monotonous discohesive large cells with vesicular nuclei, prominent nucleoli, and hyaline eosinophilic cytoplasmic inclusions of intermediate filaments. Usually there is extensive vascular invasion. Rhabdoid tumours in all sites are characterized by mutation or deletion of the INI1 tumour suppressor gene on the long arm of chromosome 22q11.[131]

Neuroblastoma

Tumours are unencapsulated, haemorrhagic and poorly circumscribed with tipical organoid arrangement of cells, 'salt and pepper' nuclear chromatin, and Homer-Wright rosettes.[129] Cell are usually positive for neuron-specific enolase, synaptophysin, S100 protein, and chromogranin supportive of neuronal differentiation.

Primitive neuroectodermal tumour

Most patients are adolescent or young adults (range 1 month–72 years) showing poorly circumscribed tumours composed of primitive round cells with varying degrees of rosette formation.[133] The nuclei shows coarse nuclear chromatin and nuclei do not overlap. Typically, cells are CD99 and FLI1positive and WT1 negative. Characteristic translocations include especially t (11;22)(q24;q12).

Synovial sarcoma

Large variably cystic tumours (mean diameter 11 cm) composed of primitive spindle cells with overlapping ovoid nuclei and scant cytoplasm admixed with variably sized cystic spaces that represent trapped dilated native renal tubules and ducts. Proliferating cells are typically WT1 negative but show t(X;18) translocation.[125]

Other rare tumours

Other uncommon tumours seen in the kidney may virtually include the whole spectrum of neoplastic diseases.[1,2] Examples are lymphoma (frequently in post-transplant patients), leukaemia, plasmacytoma, ossifying renal tumour of infancy, hemangiopericytoma, leiomyosarcoma, primary osteosarcoma, angiosarcoma, leiomyoma, hemangioma, lymphangioma, schwannoma, paraganglioma, solitary fibrous tumour, or germ cell tumours.[1,2]

Secondary tumours

Secondary tumours to the kidney usually occur as part of a widespread dissemination.[119] Renal involvement is frequently bilateral and in a multinodular fashion. Primary sources include lung, thyroid, skin (melanoma), contralateral kidney, and gastrointestinal tract.[97–99,119]

Renal cell carcinoma immunohistochemical markers, such as RCC marker and CD10, and urothelial carcinoma markers, such as uroplakin and thrombomodulin, can be of some utility when combined with other specific markers, including thyroid transcription factor-1 (lung and thyroid) and melanoma markers (HMB45 and Melan-A). (Table 6.28.3) There are some primary tumours from the thyroid that very closely mimic primary kidney tumours (i.e. follicular thyroid-like RCC), a poorly defined primary RCC negative with thyroglobulin and thyroid transcription factor 1 (both positive in thyroid carcinoma).[31,97–99,101,102,119] PAX2 and/or PAX8 are considered most useful for the diagnosis of primary renal tumour metastasis in other organs.[119]

Percutaneous biopsy of renal tumours

Renal tumour biopsy today has limited morbidity and allows histologic diagnosis in the majority of cases.[103,104,117] The increasing incidence of small renal masses, the development of conservative and minimally invasive treatments for low-risk RCC and benign renal tumours, and the discovery of targeted treatments for metastatic disease have provided the rationale for indications of percutaneous renal tumour biopsy. Renal tumour biopsy can avoid unnecessary surgeries, can confirm success after thermal ablation of small renal mases and support the selection of the appropriate systemic therapy for metastatic RCC.[103,104,117] Current diagnostic yield of biopsies ranges from 78% to 100%, with sensitivity and specificity for the diagnosis of 86–100% and 100%, respectively. Diagnostic accuracy for tumour subtyping ranges from 86% to 98%. An immunohistochemical panel, including parvalbumin, CD10, a-methylacyl-coenzyme A racemase, cathepsin K, S100A1, cytokeratin 7, and carbonic anhydrase IX, seems to be the most promising.[117]

Conclusion

Pathologists and urologists are aware that RCC it is not a single disease and that their molecular and clinical properties define a number of pathologic entities whose recognition is important in clinical practice. The classification of epithelial tumours of the kidney has been expanded in recent years and a modified working classification is now in use. In the era of targeted therapy, the fact that different histotypes have different outcome and different response to therapy represents a major adavance. Introduction of modern percutaneous biopsy protocols in clinical practice allows quality histologic diagnosis in the majority of cases. This methodology is also suitable for molecular diagnostic purpose and represents a changing paradigm in renal cancer.

Further reading

Algaba F, Akaza H, Lopez-Beltran A, *et al.* Current pathology keys of renal cell carcinoma. *Eur Urol* 2011; **60**:634–43.

Cheng L, Williamson SR, Zhang S, MacLennan GT, Montironi R, Lopez-Beltran A. Understanding the molecular genetics of renal cell neoplasia: implications for diagnosis, prognosis and therapy. *Expert Rev Anticancer Ther* 2010; **10**:843–64.

Delahunt B, Sika-Paotonu D, Bethwaite PB, *et al.* Grading of clear cell renal cell carcinoma should be based on nucleolar prominence. *Am J Surg Pathol* 2011; **35**(8):1134–9.

Ficarra V, Brunelli M, Cheng L, *et al.* Prognostic and therapeutic impact of the histopathologic definition of parenchymal epithelial renal tumors. *Eur Urol* 2010; **58**:655–68.

Lopez-Beltran A, Kirkali Z, Montironi R, *et al.* Unclassified renal cell carcinoma: a report of 56 cases. *BJU Int* 2012; **110**:786–793.

Lopez-Beltran A, Montironi R, Egevad L, *et al.* Genetic profiles in renal tumors. *Int J Urol* 2010; **17**:6–19.

Morichetti D, Mazzucchelli R, Lopez-Beltran A, *et al.* Secondary neoplasms of the urinary system and male genital organs. *BJU Int* 2009; **104**:770–6.

Shen SS, Truong LD, Scarpelli M, Lopez-Beltran A. Role of immunohistochemistry in diagnosing renal neoplasms: when is it really useful?. *Arch Pathol Lab Med* 2012; **136**:410–17.

Srigley JR, Delahunt B. Uncommon and recently described renal carcinomas. *Mod Pathol* 2009; **22**:S2–23.

Suzigan S, Lopez-Beltran A, Montironi R, *et al.* Multilocular cystic renal cell carcinoma: a report of 45 cases of a kidney tumor of low malignant potential. *Am J Clin Pathol* 2006; **125**:217–22.

Tickoo SK, dePeralta-Venturina MN, Harik LR, *et al.* Spectrum of epithelial neoplasms in end-stage renal disease: an experience from 66 tumor-bearing kidneys with emphasis on histologic patterns distinct from those in sporadic adult renal neoplasia. *Am J Surg Pathol* 2006; **30**:141–53.

Volpe A, Finelli A, Gill IS, *et al.* Rationale for percutaneous biopsy and histologic characterisation of renal tumours. *Eur Urol* 2012; **62**:491–504.

References

1. Lopez-Beltran A, Scarpelli M, Montironi R, Kirkali Z. 2004 WHO classification of the renal tumors of the adults. *Eur Urol* 2006; **49**:798–805.
2. Eble JN, Sauter G, Epstein JI, Sesterhenn IA. *Pathology and Genetics: Tumors of the Urinary System and Male Genital Organs.* Lyon, France: IARC Press, 2004.
3. Thoenes W, Storkel S, Rumpelt HJ, Moll R. Cytomorphological typing of renal cell carcinoma—a new approach. *Eur Urol* 1990; **18**(Suppl 2):6–9.
4. Kovacs G, Akhtar M, Beckwith BJ, *et al.* The Heidelberg classification of renal cell tumours. *J Pathol* 1997; **183**:131–3.
5. Jung SJ, Chung JI, Park SH, Ayala AG, Ro JY. Thyroid follicular carcinoma-like tumor of kidney: a case report with morphologic, immunohistochemical, and genetic analysis. *Am J Surg Pathol* 2006; **30**:411–15.
6. Filosa A, Fabiani A. Angiogenesis and molecular markers as specific therapeutic targets in renal cell carcinomas. *Anal Quant Cytol Histol* 2008; **30**:185–6.

7. Kovacs A, Kovacs G. Low chromosome number in chromophobe renal cell carcinomas. *Genes Chromosomes Cancer* 1992; **4**:267–8.
8. Koyle MA, Hatch DA, Furness PD 3rd, Lovell MA, Odom LF, Kurzrock EA. Long-term urological complications in survivors younger than 15 months of advanced stage abdominal neuroblastoma. *J Urol* 2001; **166**:1455–8.
9. Kuhn E, De Anda J, Manoni S, Netto G, Rosai J. Renal cell carcinoma associated with prominent angioleiomyoma-like proliferation: Report of 5 cases and review of the literature. *Am J Surg Pathol* 2006, **30**:1372–81.
10. Latif F, Duh FM, Gnarra J, *et al.* von Hippel-Lindau syndrome: cloning and identification of the plasma membrane Ca(++)-transporting ATPase isoform 2 gene that resides in the von Hippel-Lindau gene region. *Cancer Res* 1993; **53**:861–7.
11. Lefevre M, Couturier J, Sibony M, *et al.* Adult papillary renal tumor with oncocytic cells: clinicopathologic, immunohistochemical, and cytogenetic features of 10 cases. *Am J Surg Pathol* 2005; **29**:1576–81.
12. Lendvay TS, Marshall FF. The tuberous sclerosis complex and its highly variable manifestations. *J Urol* 2003; **169**:1635–42.
13. Mancini V, Battaglia M, Ditonno P, *et al.* Current insights in renal cell cancer pathology. *Urol Oncol* 2008; **26**:225–38.
14. Martignoni G, Brunelli M, Gobbo S, *et al.* Role of molecular markers in diagnosis and prognosis of renal cell carcinoma. *Anal Quant Cytol Histol* 2007; **29**:41–9.
15. Merino MJ, Torres-Cabala C, Pinto P, Linehan WM. The morphologic spectrum of kidney tumors in hereditary leiomyomatosis and renal cell carcinoma (HLRCC) syndrome. *Am J Surg Pathol* 2007; **31**:1578–85.
16. Montironi R, Mazzucchelli R, Lopez-Beltran A, *et al.* Cystic nephroma and mixed epithelial and stromal tumour of the kidney: opposite ends of the spectrum of the same entity? *Eur Urol* 2008; **54**:1237–46.
17. Montironi R, Mikuz G, Algaba F, *et al.* Epithelial tumours of the adult kidney. *Virchows Arch* 1999; **434**:281–90.
18. Montironi R, Scarpelli M, Martignoni G, Cheng L, Lopez-Beltran A. Splitting and lumping adult renal epithelial tumours: is that what the urologists want? *Eur Urol* 2008; **53**:673–675; discussion 676–80.
19. Nagy A, Wilhelm M, Sukosd F, Ljungberg B, Kovacs G. Somatic mitochondrial DNA mutations in human chromophobe renal cell carcinomas. *Genes Chromosomes Cancer* 2002; **35**:256–60.
20. Nickerson ML, Warren MB, Toro JR, *et al.* Mutations in a novel gene lead to kidney tumors, lung wall defects, and benign tumors of the hair follicle in patients with the Birt-Hogg-Dube syndrome. *Cancer Cell* 2002, **2**:157–64.
21. Paner GP, Srigley JR, Radhakrishnan A, *et al.* Immunohistochemical analysis of mucinous tubular and spindle cell carcinoma and papillary renal cell carcinoma of the kidney: significant immunophenotypic overlap warrants diagnostic caution. *Am J Surg Pathol* 2006; **30**:13–19.
22. Patard JJ, Pouessel D, Bensalah K, Culine S. Targeted therapy in renal cell carcinoma. *World J Urol* 2008; **26**:135–40.
23. Presti JC Jr, Moch H, Reuter VE, Huynh D, Waldman FM. Comparative genomic hybridization for genetic analysis of renal oncocytomas. *Genes Chromosomes Cancer* 1996; **17**:199–204.
24. Rakozy C, Schmahl GE, Bogner S, Storkel S. Low-grade tubular-mucinous renal neoplasms: morphologic, immunohistochemical, and genetic features. *Mod Pathol* 2002; **15**:1162–71.
25. Ro JY, Ayala AG, Sella A, Samuels ML, Swanson DA. Sarcomatoid renal cell carcinoma: clinicopathologic. A study of 42 cases. *Cancer* 1987; **59**:516–26.
26. Sanders ME, Mick R, Tomaszewski JE, Barr FG. Unique patterns of allelic imbalance distinguish type 1 from type 2 sporadic papillary renal cell carcinoma. *Am J Pathol* 2002; **161**:997–1005.
27. Schmidt L, Duh FM, Chen F, *et al.* Germline and somatic mutations in the tyrosine kinase domain of the MET proto-oncogene in papillary renal carcinomas. *Nat Genet* 1997; **16**:68–73.
28. Sika-Paotonu D, Bethwaite PB, McCredie MR, William Jordan T, Delahunt B. Nucleolar grade but not Fuhrman grade is applicable to papillary renal cell carcinoma. *Am J Surg Pathol* 2006; **30**:1091–6.
29. Speicher MR, Schoell B, du Manoir S, *et al.* Specific loss of chromosomes 1, 2, 6, 10, 13, 17, and 21 in chromophobe renal cell carcinomas revealed by comparative genomic hybridization. *Am J Pathol* 1994; **145**:356–64.
30. Srigley JR, Eble JN. Collecting duct carcinoma of kidney. *Semin Diagn Pathol* 1998; **15**:54–67.
31. Sterlacci W, Verdorfer I, Gabriel M, Mikuz G. Thyroid follicular carcinoma-like renal tumor: a case report with morphologic, immunophenotypic, cytogenetic, and scintigraphic studies. *Virchows Arch* 2008; **452**:91–5.
32. Suzigan S, Lopez-Beltran A, Montironi R, *et al.* Multilocular cystic renal cell carcinoma: a report of 45 cases of a kidney tumor of low malignant potential. *Am J Clin Pathol* 2006; **125**:217–22.
33. Thoenes W, Storkel S, Rumpelt HJ, *et al.* Chromophobe cell renal carcinoma and its variants--a report on 32 cases. *J Pathol* 1988; **155**:277–87.
34. Tickoo SK, dePeralta-Venturina MN, Harik LR, *et al.* Spectrum of epithelial neoplasms in end-stage renal disease: an experience from 66 tumor-bearing kidneys with emphasis on histologic patterns distinct from those in sporadic adult renal neoplasia. *Am J Surg Pathol* 2006; **30**:141–53.
35. Tickoo SK, Reuter VE, Amin MB, *et al.* Renal oncocytosis: a morphologic study of fourteen cases. *Am J Surg Pathol* 1999; **23**:1094–101.
36. Tomlinson IP, Alam NA, Rowan AJ, *et al.* Germline mutations in FH predispose to dominantly inherited uterine fibroids, skin leiomyomata and papillary renal cell cancer. *Nat Genet* 2002; **30**:406–10.
37. Toro JR, Wei MH, Glenn GM, *et al.* BHD mutations, clinical and molecular genetic investigations of Birt-Hogg-Dube syndrome: a new series of 50 families and a review of published reports. *J Med Genet* 2008; **45**:321–331.
38. Turbiner J, Amin MB, Humphrey PA, *et al.* Cystic nephroma and mixed epithelial and stromal tumor of kidney: a detailed clinicopathologic analysis of 34 cases and proposal for renal epithelial and stromal tumor (REST) as a unifying term. *Am J Surg Pathol* 2007; **31**:489–500.
39. Weirich G, Glenn G, Junker K, *et al.* Familial renal oncocytoma: clinicopathological study of 5 families. *J Urol* 1998; **160**:335–40.
40. Went P, Dirnhofer S, Salvisberg T, *et al.* Expression of epithelial cell adhesion molecule (EpCam) in renal epithelial tumors. *Am J Surg Pathol* 2005; **29**:83–88.
41. Woodward ER. Familial non-syndromic clear cell renal cell carcinoma. *Curr Mol Med* 2004; **4**:843–8.
42. Yang XJ, Zhou M, Hes O, *et al.* Tubulocystic carcinoma of the kidney: clinicopathologic and molecular characterization. *Am J Surg Pathol* 2008; **32**:177–87.
43. Zisman A, Chao DH, Pantuck AJ, *et al.* Unclassified renal cell carcinoma: clinical features and prognostic impact of a new histological subtype. *J Urol* 2002; **168**:950–5.
44. Adley BP, Papavero V, Sugimura J, Teh BT, Yang XJ. Diagnostic value of cytokeratin 7 and parvalbumin in differentiating chromophobe renal cell carcinoma from renal oncocytoma. *Anal Quant Cytol Histol* 2006; **28**:228–36.
45. Adley BP, Smith ND, Nayar R, Yang XJ. Birt-Hogg-Dube syndrome: clinicopathologic findings and genetic alterations. *Arch Pathol Lab Med* 2006; **130**:1865–70.
46. Adsay NV, Eble JN, Srigley JR, Jones EC, Grignon DJ. Mixed epithelial and stromal tumor of the kidney. *Am J Surg Pathol* 2000; **24**:958–70.
47. Akhtar M, Tulbah A, Kardar AH, Ali MA. Sarcomatoid renal cell carcinoma: the chromophobe connection. *Am J Surg Pathol* 1997; **21**:1188–95.
48. Algaba F, Trias I, Scarpelli M, Boccon-Gibod L, Kirkali Z, Van Poppel H. Handling and pathology reporting of renal tumor specimens. *Eur Urol* 2004; **45**:437–43.
49. Amin MB, Corless CL, Renshaw AA, Tickoo SK, Kubus J, Schultz DS. Papillary (chromophil) renal cell carcinoma: histomorphologic

characteristics and evaluation of conventional pathologic prognostic parameters in 62 cases. *Am J Surg Pathol* 1997; **21**:621–35.

50. Amin MB, Crotty TB, Tickoo SK, Farrow GM. Renal oncocytoma: a reappraisal of morphologic features with clinicopathologic findings in 80 cases. *Am J Surg Pathol* 1997; **21**:1–12.
51. Argani P. Metanephric neoplasms: the hyperdifferentiated, benign end of the Wilms tumor spectrum? *Clin Lab Med* 2005; **25**:379–92.
52. Argani P, Antonescu CR, Couturier J, *et al.* PRCC-TFE3 renal carcinomas: morphologic, immunohistochemical, ultrastructural, and molecular analysis of an entity associated with the t(X;1)(p11.2;q21). *Am J Surg Pathol* 2002; **26**:1553–66.
53. Argani P, Antonescu CR, Illei PB, *et al.* Primary renal neoplasms with the ASPL-TFE3 gene fusion of alveolar soft part sarcoma: a distinctive tumor entity previously included among renal cell carcinomas of children and adolescents. *Am J Pathol* 2001; **159**:179–92.
54. Argani P, Ladanyi M. Translocation carcinomas of the kidney. *Clin Lab Med* 2005; **25**:363–78.
55. Argani P, Lae M, Hutchinson B, *et al.* Renal carcinomas with the t(6;11)(p21;q12): clinicopathologic features and demonstration of the specific alpha-TFEB gene fusion by immunohistochemistry, RT-PCR, and DNA PCR. *Am J Surg Pathol* 2005; **29**:230–40.
56. Argani P, Lal P, Hutchinson B, Lui MY, Reuter VE, Ladanyi M. Aberrant nuclear immunoreactivity for TFE3 in neoplasms with TFE3 gene fusions: a sensitive and specific immunohistochemical assay. *Am J Surg Pathol* 2003; **27**:750–61.
57. Argani P, Olgac S, Tickoo SK, *et al.* Xp11 translocation renal cell carcinoma in adults: expanded clinical, pathologic, and genetic spectrum. *Am J Surg Pathol* 2007; **31**:1149–60.
58. Bonne AC, Bodmer D, Schoenmakers EF, van Ravenswaaij CM, Hoogerbrugge N, van Kessel AG. Chromosome 3 translocations and familial renal cell cancer. *Curr Mol Med* 2004; **4**:849–54.
59. Bruder E, Passera O, Harms D, *et al.* Morphologic and molecular characterization of renal cell carcinoma in children and young adults. *Am J Surg Pathol* 2004; **28**:1117–32.
60. Brunelli M, Eble JN, Zhang S, Martignoni G, Cheng L. Metanephric adenoma lacks the gains of chromosomes 7 and 17 and loss of Y that are typical of papillary renal cell carcinoma and papillary adenoma. *Mod Pathol* 2003; **16**:1060–3.
61. Brunelli M, Eble JN, Zhang S, Martignoni G, Cheng L. Gains of chromosomes 7, 17, 12, 16, and 20 and loss of Y occur early in the evolution of papillary renal cell neoplasia: a fluorescent in situ hybridization study. *Mod Pathol* 2003; **16**:1053–9.
62. Brunelli M, Eble JN, Zhang S, Martignoni G, Delahunt B, Cheng L. Eosinophilic and classic chromophobe renal cell carcinomas have similar frequent losses of multiple chromosomes from among chromosomes 1, 2, 6, 10, and 17, and this pattern of genetic abnormality is not present in renal oncocytoma. *Mod Pathol* 2005; **18**:161–9.
63. Brunelli M, Eccher A, Gobbo S, *et al.* Loss of chromosome 9p is an independent prognostic factor in patients with clear cell renal cell carcinoma. *Mod Pathol* 2008; **21**:1–6.
64. Brunelli M, Gobbo S, Cossu-Rocca P, *et al.* Chromosomal gains in the sarcomatoid transformation of chromophobe renal cell carcinoma. *Mod Pathol* 2007; **20**:303–9.
65. Camparo P, Vasiliu V, Molinie V, *et al.* Renal translocation carcinomas: clinicopathologic, immunohistochemical, and gene expression profiling analysis of 31 cases with a review of the literature. *Am J Surg Pathol* 2008; **32**:656–70.
66. Chao D, Zisman A, Pantuck AJ, *et al.* Collecting duct renal cell carcinoma: clinical study of a rare tumor. *J Urol* 2002; **167**:71–4.
67. Cheville JC, Lohse CM, Zincke H, *et al.* Sarcomatoid renal cell carcinoma: an examination of underlying histologic subtype and an analysis of associations with patient outcome. *Am J Surg Pathol* 2004; **28**:435–41.
68. Cossu-Rocca P, Eble JN, Delahunt B, *et al.* Renal mucinous tubular and spindle carcinoma lacks the gains of chromosomes 7 and 17 and losses of chromosome Y that are prevalent in papillary renal cell carcinoma. *Mod Pathol* 2006; **19**:488–93.
69. Cossu-Rocca P, Eble JN, Zhang S, *et al.* Interphase cytogenetic analysis with centromeric probes for chromosomes 1, 2, 6, 10, and 17 in 11 tumors from a patient with bilateral renal oncocytosis. *Mod Pathol* 2008; **21**:498–504.
70. Cossu-Rocca P, Eble JN, Zhang S, Martignoni G, Brunelli M, Cheng L. Acquired cystic disease-associated renal tumors: an immunohistochemical and fluorescence in situ hybridization study. *Mod Pathol* 2006; **19**:780–7.
71. Dal Cin P, Sciot R, Van Poppel H, Balzarini P, Roskams T, Van den Berghe H. Chromosome changes in sarcomatoid renal carcinomas are different from those in renal cell carcinomas. *Cancer Genet Cytogenet* 2002; **134**:38–40.
72. Davis CJ Jr, Barton JH, Sesterhenn IA, Mostofi FK. Metanephric adenoma. Clinicopathological study of fifty patients. *Am J Surg Pathol* 1995; **19**:1101–14.
73. Davis CJ Jr, Mostofi FK, Sesterhenn IA. Renal medullary carcinoma. The seventh sickle cell nephropathy. *Am J Surg Pathol* 1995; **19**:1–11.
74. de Peralta-Venturina M, Moch H, Amin M, *et al.* Sarcomatoid differentiation in renal cell carcinoma: a study of 101 cases. *Am J Surg Pathol* 2001; **25**:275–84.
75. Delahunt B, Eble JN. Papillary renal cell carcinoma: a clinicopathologic and immunohistochemical study of 105 tumors. *Mod Pathol* 1997; **10**:537–44.
76. Delahunt B, Sika-Paotonu D, Bethwaite PB, *et al.* Fuhrman grading is not appropriate for chromophobe renal cell carcinoma. *Am J Surg Pathol* 2007; **31**:957–60.
77. Drut R, Drut RM, Ortolani C. Metastatic metanephric adenoma with foci of papillary carcinoma in a child: a combined histologic, immunohistochemical, and FISH study. *Int J Surg Pathol* 2001; **9**:241–7.
78. Eble JN. Mucinous tubular and spindle cell carcinoma and post-neuroblastoma carcinoma: newly recognised entities in the renal cell carcinoma family. *Pathology* 2003; **35**:499–504.
79. Eble JN, Amin MB, Young RH. Epithelioid angiomyolipoma of the kidney: a report of five cases with a prominent and diagnostically confusing epithelioid smooth muscle component. *Am J Surg Pathol* 1997; **21**:1123–30.
80. Fine SW, Argani P, DeMarzo AM, *et al.* Expanding the histologic spectrum of mucinous tubular and spindle cell carcinoma of the kidney. *Am J Surg Pathol* 2006; **30**:1554–60.
81. Fuzesi L, Gunawan B, Bergmann F, Tack S, Braun S, Jakse G. Papillary renal cell carcinoma with clear cell cytomorphology and chromosomal loss of 3p. *Histopathology* 1999; **35**:157–61.
82. Gobbo S, Eble JN, Grignon DJ, *et al.* Clear cell papillary renal cell carcinoma: a distinct histopathologic and molecular genetic entity. *Am J Surg Pathol* 2008; **32**(8):1239–45.
83. Granter SR, Fletcher JA, Renshaw AA. Cytologic and cytogenetic analysis of metanephric adenoma of the kidney: a report of two cases. *Am J Clin Pathol* 1997; **108**:544–9.
84. Grignon DJ, Che M. Clear cell renal cell carcinoma. *Clin Lab Med* 2005; **25**:305–16.
85. Grignon DJ, Eble JN. Papillary and metanephric adenomas of the kidney. *Semin Diagn Pathol* 1998; **15**:41–53.
86. Hes O, Brunelli M, Michal M, *et al.* Oncocytic papillary renal cell carcinoma: a clinicopathologic, immunohistochemical, ultrastructural, and interphase cytogenetic study of 12 cases. *Ann Diagn Pathol* 2006; **10**:133–9.
87. Ishida Y, Kato K, Kigasawa H, Ohama Y, Ijiri R, Tanaka Y. Synchronous occurrence of pleuropulmonary blastoma and cystic nephroma: possible genetic link in cystic lesions of the lung and the kidney. *Med Pediatr Oncol* 2000; **35**:85–7.
88. Jockle GA, Toker C, Shamsuddin AM. Metastatic renal oncocytic neoplasm with benign histologic appearance. *Urology* 1987; **30**:79–81.
89. Jones EC, Pins M, Dickersin GR, Young RH. Metanephric adenoma of the kidney. A clinicopathological, immunohistochemical, flow cytometric, cytogenetic, and electron microscopic study of seven cases. *Am J Surg Pathol* 1995; **19**:615–26.

90. Jones TD, Eble JN, Wang M, *et al.* Molecular genetic evidence for the independent origin of multifocal papillary tumors in patients with papillary renal cell carcinomas. *Clin Cancer Res* 2005; **11**:7226–33.
91. Jones TD, Eble JN, Wang M, Maclennan GT, Jain S, Cheng L. Clonal divergence and genetic heterogeneity in clear cell renal cell carcinomas with sarcomatoid transformation. *Cancer* 2005; **104**:1195–203.
92. Mostofi FK, Davis CJ Jr. *Histological Typing of Kidney Tumors.* New York, NY: Springer-Verlag, 1998.
93. Tickoo SK, de Peralta-Venturina MN, Salama M, Wang Y, Moch H, Amin MB. Spectrum of epithelial tumors in end stage renal disease (ESRD): emphasis on histologic patterns distinct from those in sporadic adult renal neoplasia. *Lab Invest* 2003; **83**:173A.
94. Gobbo S, Eble JN, Martignoni G, *et al.* Clear-cell papillary renal cell carcinoma: a distinct histopathological and molecular genetic entity. *Am J Surg Pathol* 2008; **32**:1239–45.
95. Lopez-Beltran A, Kirkali Z, Cheng L, *et al.* Targeted therapies and biological modifiers in urologic tumors: pathobiology and clinical implications. *Semin Diagn Pathol* 2008; **25**:232–44.
96. Lopez-Beltran A, Carrasco JC, Cheng L, Scarpelli M, Kirkali Z, Montironi R. 2009 update on the classification of renal epithelial tumors in adults. *Int J Urol* 2009; **16**:432–43.
97. Honda H, Coffman CE, Berbaum KS, Barloon TJ, Masuda K. CT analysis of metastatic neoplasms of the kidney. Comparison with primary renal cell carcinoma. *Acta Radiol* 1992; **33**:39–44.
98. Mazzucchelli R, Morichetti D, Giorgini S, Barbisan F. Classification and reclassification of adult renal epithelial tumors. *Anal Quant Cytol Histol* 2008; **30**:247–8.
99. Requena MJ, Carrasco JC, Alvarez-Kindelan J. Role of molecular markers in diagnosis and prognosis of renal cell carcinoma. *Anal Quant Cytol Histol* 2008; **30**:336–7.
100. Martignoni G, Brunelli M, Gobbo S, *et al.* Role of molecular markers in diagnosis and prognosis of renal cell carcinoma. *Anal Quant Cytol Histol* 2007; **29**:41–9.
101. Jung SJ, Chung JI, Park SH, Ayala AG, Ro JY. Thyroid follicular carcinoma-like tumor of kidney: a case report with morphologic, immunohistochemical, and genetic analysis. *Am J Surg Pathol* 2006; **30**:411–15.
102. Gupta R, Viswanathan S, D'Cruz A, Kane SV. Metastatic papillary carcinoma of thyroid masquerading as a renal tumour. *J Clin Pathol* 2008; **61**:143.
103. Lhermitte B, Leval L. Interpretation of needle biopsies of the kidney for investigation of renal masses. *Virchows Arch* 2012; **461**:13–26.
104. Filosa A, Fabiani A. From biopsy to active surveillance in small renal masses: Is it feasible? *Anal Quant Cyt Hist* 2012; **34**:109–10.
105. Volpe A, Finelli A, Gill IS, *et al.* Rationale for percutaneous biopsy and histologic characterisation of renal tumours. *Eur Urol* 2012; **62**:491–504.
106. Gupta R, Billis A, Shah RB, *et al.* Carcinoma of the collecting ducts of bellini and renal medullary carcinoma clinicopathologic analysis of 52 cases of rare aggressive subtypes of renal cell carcinoma with a focus on their interrelationship. *Am J Surg Pathol* 2012; **36**:1265–78.
107. Rao Q, Liu B, Cheng L, *et al.* A clinicopathologic study emphasizing unusual morphology, novel alpha-TFEB gene fusion point, immunobiomarkers, and ultrastructural features, as well as detection of the gene fusion by fluorescence in situ hybridization. *Am J Surg Pathol* 2012; **36**:1327–8.
108. Bianconi M, Scartozzi M, Faloppi L, *et al.* Angiogenetic pathway as a therapeutic target in renal cell carcinoma. *Anal Quant Cyt Hist* 2012; **34**:15–22.
108. Brunelli M, Delahunt B, Ficarra V, *et al.* Utility of tissue microarrays for assessment of chromosomal abnormalities in chromophobe renal cell carcinoma. *Anal Quant Cytol Histol* 2009; **31**:401–9.
109. Lopez-Beltran A, Montironi R, Egevad L, *et al.* Genetic profiles in renal tumors. *Int J Urol* 2010; **17**:6–19.
110. Delahunt B, Sika-Paotonu D, Bethwaite PB, *et al.* Grading of clear cell renal cell carcinoma should be based on nucleolar prominence. *Am J Surg Pathol* 2011; **35**(8):1134–9.
111. Cheng L, Williamson SR, Zhang S, MacLennan GT, Montironi R, Lopez-Beltran A. Understanding the molecular genetics of renal cell neoplasia: implications for diagnosis, prognosis and therapy. *Expert Rev Anticancer Ther* 2010; **10**:843–64.
112. Algaba F, Akaza H, Lopez-Beltran A, *et al.* Current pathology keys of renal cell carcinoma. *Eur Urol* 2011; **60**:634–43.
113. Srigley JR, Delahunt B. Uncommon and recently described renal carcinomas. *Mod Pathol* 2009; **22**:S2–S23.
114. Shen SS, Truong LD, Scarpelli M, Lopez-Beltran A. Role of immunohistochemistry in diagnosing renal neoplasms: when is it really useful?. *Arch Pathol Lab Med* 2012; **136**:410–17.
115. Lopez-Beltran A, Kirkali Z, Montironi R, *et al.* Unclassified renal cell carcinoma: a report of 56 cases. *BJU Int* 2012; **110**:786–793.
116. *Ibid.* **34**.
117. *Ibid.* **105**.
118. Ficarra V, Brunelli M, Cheng L, *et al.* Prognostic and therapeutic impact of the histopathologic definition of parenchymal epithelial renal tumors. *Eur Urol* 2010; **58**:655–68.
119. Morichetti D, Mazzucchelli R, Lopez-Beltran A, *et al.* Secondary neoplasms of the urinary system and male genital organs. *BJU Int* 2009; **104**:770–6.
120. Argani P, Beckwith JB. Metanephric stromal tumor: report of 31 cases of a distinctive pediatric renal; neoplasm. *Am J Surg Pathol* 2000; **24**:917–26.
121. Arroyo MR, Green DM, Perlman EJ, *et al.* The spectrum of metanephric adenofibroma and related lesions. *Am J Surg Pathol* 2001; **25**:433–44.
122. Brunelli M, Eble JN, Zhang S, *et al.* Metanephric adenoma lacks the gain of chromosomes 7 and 17 and loss of Y which are typical of papillary renal cell carcinoma and adenoma. *Mod Pathol* 2003; **16**:1060–3.
123. Davidoff AM. Wilms's tumor. *Curr Opin Pediatr* 2009; **21**:357–64.
124. Vujanić GM, Sandstedt B. The pathology of Wilms' tumour (nephroblastoma): the International Society of Paediatric Oncology approach. *J Clin Pathol* 2010; **63**(2):102–9.
125. Sebire NJ, Vujanić GM. Paediatric renal tumours: recent developments, new entities and pathological features. *Histopathology* 2009; **54**(5):516–28.
126. Muir TE, Cheville JC, Lager DJ. Metanephric adenoma, nephrogenic rests, and Wilms' tumor. *Am J Surg Pathol* 2001; **25**:1290–6.
127. Weeks DA, Beckwith JB, Mierau GW. Benign nodal lesions mimicking metastases from pediatric renal neoplasms: a report of the National Wilms' Tumor Study Pathology Center. *Hum Pathol* 1990; **21**(12):1239–44.
128. Beckwith JB, Kiviat NB, Bonadio JF. Nephrogenic rests, nephroblastomatosis, and the pathogenesis of Wilms' tumor. *Pediatr Pathol* 1990; **10**(1–2):1–36.
129. Davenport KP, Blanco FC, Sandler AD. Pediatric malignancies: neuroblastoma, Wilm's tumor, hepatoblastoma, rhabdomyosarcoma, and sacroccygeal teratoma. *Surg Clin North Am* 2012; **92**(3):745–67.
130. Fan R. Primary renal neuroblastoma--a clinical pathologic study of 8 cases. *Am J Surg Pathol* 2012; **36**(1):94–100.
131. Venneti S, Le P, Martinez D, *et al.* Malignant rhabdoid tumors express stem cell factors, which relate to the expression of EZH2 and Id proteins. *Am J Surg Pathol* 2011; **35**(10):1463–72.
132. Van den Hoek J. Cystic nephroma, cystic partially differentiated nephrobastoma and cystic Wilm's tumor in children: a spectrum with therapeutic dilemmas. *Urol Int* 2009; **82**:65–70.
133. Angel JR, Alfred A, Sakhuja A, Sells RE, Zechlinski JJ. Ewing's sarcoma of the kidney. *Int J Clin Oncol* 2010; **15**(3):314–8.
134. Martin SA, Mynderse LA, Lager DJ, *et al.* Juxtaglomerular cell tumor: a clinicopathologic study of four cases and review of the literature. *Am J Clin Pathol* 2001; **116**:854–63.
135. Filosa A, Fabiani A. Renal cell carcinoma: molecular and genetic markers as new prognostic and therapeutic tools. *Anal Quant Cytol Histol* 2008; **30**:341–3.

CHAPTER 6.29

Treatment of localized renal cell cancer

Ashraf Almatar and Michael A.S. Jewett

Introduction to treatment of localized renal cell cancer

Surgery remains the mainstay of curative treatment for renal cell cancer (RCC). Historically, radical nephrectomy (RN) with or without adrenalectomy or lymphadenectomy has been the gold standard treatment for localized kidney cancer, which we define as stage T1-2N0M0.[1] Laparoscopic radical nephrectomy (LRN) and robot-assisted laparoscopic radical nephrectomy (RARN) are increasingly being performed because of decreased morbidity and comparable survival.[2–6]

The incidence of RCC has increased in the last three decades. This appears to be mainly related to the increase in the detection rate of early stage carcinoma as small renal masses (SRMs), due to widespread use of cross-sectional imaging for unrelated conditions.[7] RN for these SRMs is now usually considered overtreatment, as we increasingly understand the long-term deleterious impact of nephrectomy on renal function, the correlation with chronic kidney disease (CKD), and increased risk of morbid cardiac events and death, plus the equivalent therapeutic efficacy of partial nephrectomy (PN).[8,9] As a result, surgical options for localized RCC have expanded in the last two decades to include nephron-sparing partial nephrectomy (with open or laparoscopic/robotic approaches) or probe ablation by cryotherapy or radiofrequency ablation (RFA).[10] Active surveillance (AS) with delayed treatment for progression has become a reasonable option, especially in the elderly with co-morbidities and shorter life expectancy where the risk from intervention outweighs the risk of dying from the cancer.[11,12]

In the personalized medicine era, the goal of treatment for localized RCC is to individualize the treatment plan after histologically and morphologically characterizing the tumour, assessing renal function, and considering the patient's age and co-morbidity. This should be done while maintaining the very high rate of cancer control that we have achieved in the past with nephrectomy and by using as minimally invasive technology as possible.[13]

Diagnosis and staging

More than 50% of RCCs are discovered incidentally by imaging for unrelated indications and these tumours are more likely to be localized to the kidney.[14,15] The goal of diagnosis and staging of a new RCC is to plan optimal treatment, which begins with taking a history, conducting a physical examination, and performing selected laboratory tests. Symptomatic presentation could be due to local tumour effects including pain, bleeding, venous involvement and paraneoplastic syndromes, or metastasis.[16] Paraneoplastic syndromes are found in 20% of all patients with RCC and include: elevated erythrocyte sedimentation rate, hypertension, anaemia, cachexia and weight loss, pyrexia, abnormal liver function, hypercalcaemia, polycythaemia, neuromyopathy, and amyloidosis.[17] The classical triad of flank pain, haematuria, and abdominal mass is now found in only 10% of RCC patients and virtually never in early stage disease.[18] The triad is of historical interest only in the developed world with early diagnosis. Flank pain is caused by intrarenal haemorrhage, tumour invasion of surrounding structures, or the collecting system with haematuria and blood clots causing obstruction.[16] Palpable lymph nodes (especially cervical) suggest lymphatic involvement and the presence of constitutional symptoms suggests advanced disease, as do varicocele or lower limb oedema with venous involvement. Persistent cough and bone pain may result from metastases.[16]

Standard imaging includes a chest X-ray or computed tomography (CT), and a contrast study of the abdomen and pelvis. The most commonly used is tri-phasic computerized tomography.[19] CT scanning is a familiar imaging modality for urologists and will provide information about tumour size, location, renal vessels, anomalous vessels, possible adjacent tissue involvement, venous and lymph node involvement, the condition of both adrenal glands, and metastasis to other organs.[16] A solid mass or a tumour containing a complex renal cyst (Bosniak 3 or 4) that is an RCC enhances by more than 15 Hounsfield units (HU). The presence and function of the other kidney should also be assessed and recorded. MRI, pre- and post-gadolinium, is usually reserved for patients with suspected venous involvement, those who are allergic to iodine contrast, and those with renal insufficiency. A bone scan should be done in patients with skeletal symptoms or elevated alkaline phosphatase. Brain imaging for central nervous system (CNS) symptoms and a CT scan of the chest when the chest X-ray is abnormal, are indicated.[16] While positron emission tomography (PET) scans are not usually of use for staging RCC, they can discriminate the biology of lung lesions.

Renal tumour biopsy

Renal needle core tumour biopsy is indicated if there is any suspicion that a renal mass is a metastasis, lymphoma, abscess, or when there is a need to establish a pathological diagnosis in patients who are candidates for systemic therapy with disseminated disease or when the tumour is unresectable.[19] The role for biopsy in suspected early stage RCC is more controversial, but is being increasingly used when the result will change management. With an expanding range of management options, biopsy is increasingly used to investigate enhancing SRMs ≤3–4 cm in axial diameter before recommending surgery or thermal ablation therapy (with cryotherapy or radiofrequency (RFA)). Initial AS may be indicated, especially in some tumour types, and the follow-up strategy may change if the biopsy is benign.[13,20] Twenty to thirty per cent (20–30%) of SRMs (≤4 cm) are benign and immediate intervention may be avoided. The accuracy and safety of renal tumour biopsy has improved with experience, and the diagnostic rate is well over 90%, especially if a repeat biopsy is done following a non-diagnostic first biopsy.[21,22] Serious complications occur in less than 2% of biopsies, and tumour spillage or seeding is extremely rare. We now know that there is heterogeneity in the biological aggressiveness of T1a tumours and biopsy may aid the informed decision-making process to select appropriate treatment.[22,23] However, the American Society of Clinical Oncology (ASCO) clinical practice guidelines in the management of small renal masses recently recommended that all patients with SRMs should be considered for a renal biopsy if the results may alter the management.[24]

Surgical anatomy of the kidney

The retroperitoneal kidneys have an adherent parenchymal capsule, which is surrounded by perinephric fat within the perinephric or Gerota's fascia, which in turn is covered by paranephric fat. Anatomic knowledge of the structures adjacent to the kidneys is important to avoid injury to these structures. Posteriorly, there are the psoas and quadratus lumborum muscles and the eleventh and twelfth ribs (Fig. 6.29.1) for anterior relations. The renal arteries originate from the lateral side of the aorta, just inferior of the superior mesenteric artery. The renal veins lie anterior to the renal arteries. The right renal artery origins below the left renal vein and posterior to the inferior vena cava. The renal arteries divide into two main branches, posterior and anterior, and the anterior branch in turn usually divides into four segmental arteries (Fig. 6.29.2). The kidney can be considered to have four segments (superior, anterior, posterior, and inferior) that are supplied by the segmental arteries (which are end arteries). Ligation or injury of a segmental artery will devitalize parenchymal tissue. Venous tributaries correspond to the renal segmental arteries and drain into a single renal vein that in turn drains into the inferior vena cava (IVC). The left renal vein is longer than the right and passes anterior to the aorta. The left renal vein receives the gonadal, adrenal, and lumbar veins, while the right vein does not usually receive any vein. There is a rich network anastomosis between the segmental tributaries, so that if a tributary is ligated or injured, it will not affect the drainage of that segment. Multiple renal arteries are a common vascular anomalous variation that occur in one-third of patients and this can have surgical implications.[25–27] Preoperative image review is imperative.

Radical nephrectomy

The basic principles of RN for RCC include the sequential ligation of the renal artery and then vein, removal of the kidney within an intact perinephric (Gerota's) fascia with the ipsilateral adrenal gland, and lymph node dissection from the crus of the diaphragm to the aortic bifurcation.[1] Routine removal of the ipsilateral adrenal gland is no longer standard with localized RCC if preoperative imaging does not show involvement. The procedure can be done open, laparoscopically, or with robotic assistance.

Indications

RN is indicated for T1 tumours not amenable to PN (see indications of PN) and is the standard of care for localized ≥T2 disease.[13,28–30]

Role of lymphadenectomy in localized RCC

The role of lymph node dissection (LND) with RN for RCC was originally codified by Charles Robson and included the ipsilateral

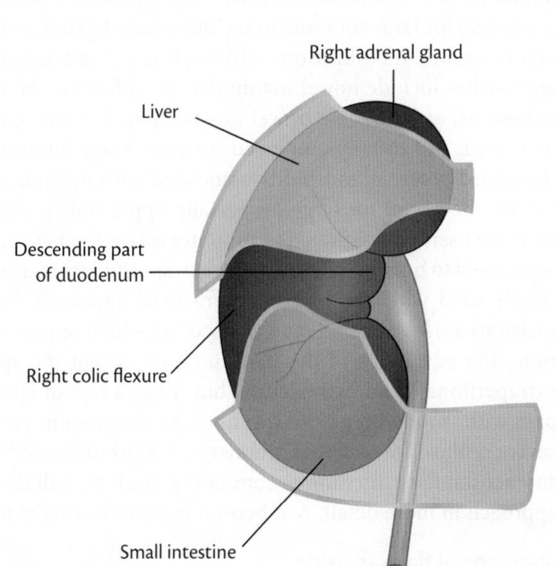

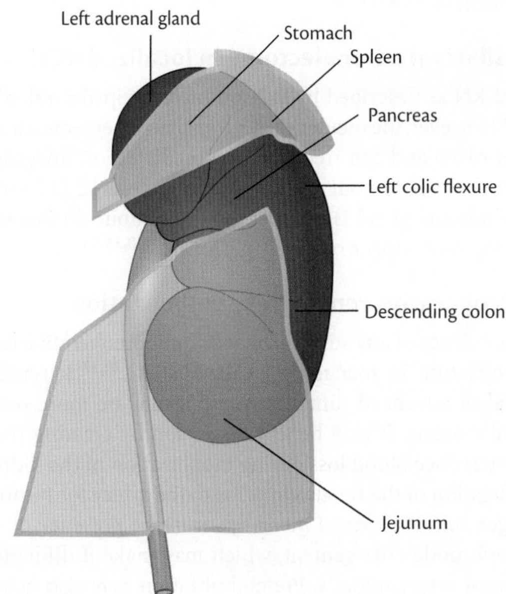

Fig. 6.29.1 Anterior relations to the kidneys.
Reprinted from Alan J. Wein *et al.*, *Campbell-Walsh Urology*, Tenth Edition, Saunders an imprint of Elsevier Inc., Copyright © 2012, by permission of Elsevier.

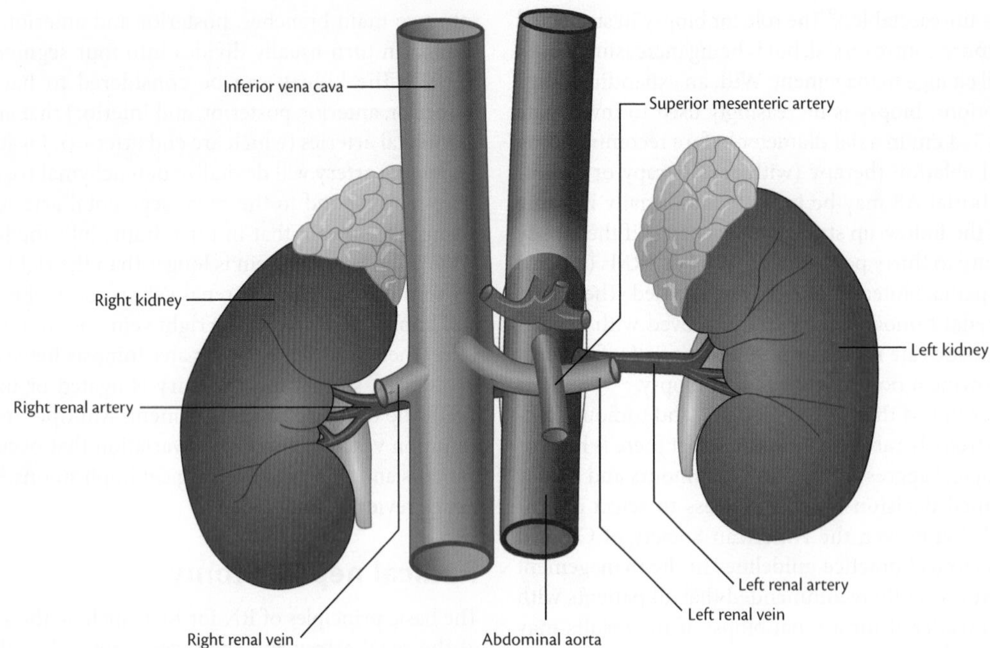

Fig. 6.29.2 Relationship of the kidneys to great vessels.
Reprinted from Alan J. Wein *et al.*, *Campbell-Walsh Urology*, Tenth Edition, Saunders an imprint of Elsevier Inc., Copyright © 2012, by permission of Elsevier.

paracaval or para-aortic nodes from the crus of the diaphragm to the aortic bifurcation.[1] The therapeutic benefit of LND in localized RCC was studied in a recent European Organization for Research and Treatment of Cancer (EORTC) multicentre prospective randomized trial of LND in localized RCC.[31] While there are limitations of this trial, it did not show any benefit in overall survival (OS) or progression-free survival with LND.[20,31–34] In the absence of high-level evidence, the US National Comprehensive Cancer Network (NCCN) and European Association of Urology (EAU) guidelines recommended LND for palpable or radiologically enlarged nodes for staging purposes, but acknowledge that this has uncertain therapeutic benefit.[20,32–34]

Role of ipsilateral adrenalectomy in localized RCC

The classical RN as described by Robson includes ipsilateral adrenalectomy.[1] However, the incidence of adrenal involvement in localized RCC is <10% and can frequently be predicted on imaging.[35] Therefore, unless the tumour is in the upper pole, ≥T2 (≥7 cm in size), or the adrenal gland is involved by the tumour on imaging, adrenalectomy is no longer routinely performed.[20,34,36]

Role of preoperative renal artery embolization

There is no evidence of any survival benefit from preoperative renal artery embolization in managing localized RCC.[20,37] It remains controversial in advanced tumours where it may be more useful for technical reasons. It may benefit dissection by creating tissue oedema, may reduce blood loss during mobilization of the kidney; allow early ligation of the renal vein prior to the artery for tumours that are larger, hilar, or extend medially; or in the presence of significant lymph node enlargement, which may make it difficult to locate the renal artery initially. Pre-embolization may also help to shrink arterialized thrombus to facilitate thrombectomy.[16,38] The procedure is generally safe. The most common complication is postinfarction syndrome characterized by nausea, vomiting, fever, and flank pain.[39]

Surgical approaches

Open radical nephrectomy

The choice of surgical incision is determined by surgeon preference, tumour location and size, body habitus, prior surgical history, and the planned extent of lymphadenectomy. The aims are to have comfortable exposure, decreased risk of injury to other structures, and to minimize the risk of complications. Three types of incisions are commonly employed: anterior abdominal midline or subcostal, flank, and thoracoabdominal. The approach is usually transperitoneal for large tumours to facilitate early ligation of the vessels before kidney mobilization—although the disadvantages of this approaches include bowel manipulation with potential ileus, later adhesions, and possible bowel obstruction. A thoracoabdominal incision is not usually employed for early stage tumours and has the added potential morbidity associated with opening the pleura but can be useful for larger, especially upper pole masses. It may be more useful for right-sided tumours where the IVC and hepatic veins need to be controlled. A flank extraperitoneal incision is commonly used with an eleventh supracostal approach. Supracostal incisions are less morbid than transcostal, which requires rib resection. The advantage of the flank incision is that the approach is extraperitoneal and extrapleural, but it has a risk of chronic flank pain with wound bulge and it is not a good option in patients with severe scoliosis or severe pulmonary co-morbidities.[25,26] Since the supracostal flank incision is commonly used, we will describe this approach in more detail. A subcostal incision is usually too low.

Supracostal flank incision

After induction of anaesthesia sustained with endotracheal intubation and with a urethral catheter connected to a urine bag, the patient is placed in the lateral position with the tip of the twelfth rib over the point of table flexion with the kidney lift. The dependent leg is flexed at the knee and hip with the upper leg kept straight. A pillow is placed between the knees. Other pressure points are padded. The kidney lift is elevated until the flank muscles become tense and the table is adjusted to bring the flank into a horizontal orientation. The patient is secured to the table with wide adhesive tapes or another device. After skin preparation and draping, the incision over the eleventh rib can be made as long as from the posterior axillary line and extended medially to the rectus sheath, although a much reduced incision is usually made centred on the rib tip. The incision is carried down through the subcutaneous tissue to expose the latissimus dorsi and serratus posterior inferior muscles, which in turn are incised to expose the intercostal muscles. The external and internal oblique muscles are incised anteriorly to expose the transverse abdominal muscle. The retroperitoneum is entered by incising the lumbodorsal fascia at the tip of the rib. With the index finger, the peritoneum is swept medially and inferiorly and the transverse abdominal muscle is incised or split medially. Inadvertent opening of the peritoneum can be closed primarily. The intercostal muscle is cut along the upper margin of the rib while displacing the extrapleural facia and pleura with the diaphragmatic leaves. The diaphragm is identified and divided close to its origin to displace the pleura superiorly. If the pleura is opened inadvertently, it can be closed primarily, aspirating air and any pooled blood.

The Robson principle of RN is early, individual ligation of the renal artery and vein by dissecting the hilum and isolating them separately. The renal artery is posterior to the vein. The artery is doubly ligated or clipped and divided, followed by the vein. The kidney is mobilized outside Gerota's fascia with sharp and blunt dissection. The ureter is identified and ligated or clipped as distal as possible. A metallic clip is useful for localization in the future if needed. Indications for removal of the adrenal gland and for lymphadenectomy have been discussed. An abdominal drain is not necessary and a chest tube is usually unnecessary even if the pleura is opened, unless there is concern about inadequate closure or pulmonary disease. A chest X-ray is indicated immediately postoperatively if there is a concern. The wound is closed in layers with the surgical table partially deflexed.[25,26]

Laparoscopic/robotic radical nephrectomy

The first laparoscopic nephrectomy was performed by Clayman and colleagues in 1991.[40] Since then, this procedure has been adopted and performed widely. It is now indicated for T1 and many T2 tumours.[41,42] It is generally contraindicated in locally advanced disease or with tumour involvement of the inferior vena cava. Multiple studies have shown the feasibility of laparoscopic nephrectomy despite renal vein involvement, significant prior surgeries, and even in morbidly obese patients in experienced hands.[16,42] It has gained popularity because of the similar oncological outcomes and shorter convalescence than the open approach. Four approaches can be used: transperitoneal, retroperitoneal, hand-assisted, and robotically assisted.[43] There is no significant difference in efficacy and safety between the transperitoneal and the retroperitoneal approach.[44,45] The robotic approach appears to have similar oncological and operative outcomes as laparoscopic surgery, but with higher cost and longer operative time, at least initially.[4] The technique is well described and it follows the same principles of open radical nephrectomy.[46]

Results

The risk of postoperative recurrence increases with clinical and pathological tumour stage.[16,47–49] Overall, reported recurrence with metastasis after RN is 24% and is stage dependent (pT1 7%, pT2 27%, and pT3 39%). Local recurrence in the renal fossa, ipsilateral adrenal gland, or ipsilateral retroperitoneal lymph node appears to be rare and is detected in 2–4% of cases.[16] Forty per cent (40%) of local recurrence are isolated, while 60% are associated with distant metastasis.[16,48] The most common site of metastasis is the lung followed in decreasing order by bone, liver, and brain.[48] Most but not all relapses are detected within the first three years after surgery and some may occur years later.[48] The risk is increased with unfavourable pathology such as collecting duct, medullary, or sarcomatoid variant tumours. The finding of positive lymph nodes also increase the risk. There appears to be no difference in recurrence rates between open and laparoscopic radical nephrectomy.[3,5]

Partial nephrectomy

Czerny was the first to describe PN for malignant kidney disease in 1890.[50] Revived in the 1990s, it has become the standard treatment for small, localized RCC. The widespread use of imaging with the increased incidence of SRMs, experience with renal vascular surgery, improvement in the strategies to prevent renal ischaemic injury, and outcomes for imperative PN with solitary kidneys and multiple tumours have led to the adoption in PN where feasible despite a normal contralateral kidney.[16] PN is defined as removal of the kidney tumour while preserving as much normal parenchyma as possible. Decreased risk of CKD, and overtreatment of benign kidney tumours by radical nephrectomy are the advantages of PN.[16]

Indications

Traditionally, indications of PN are divided into three categories: imperative or absolute, relative, and elective.[51] Indications that are imperative include a tumour in a solitary kidney or bilateral renal tumours; relative include tumours with an impaired contralateral kidney or with conditions that may cause CKD in the future such as diabetes mellitus, hypertension, glomerulopathy, obstruction, stone disease, and chronic pyelonephritis[51]; or elective for a tumour with two anatomically and functionally normal kidneys. Generally T1a tumours (<4 cm in diameter) are managed by PN but there is increasing experience with T1b and even T2 tumours.[28] It is generally believed that oncological outcomes with PN and RN for T1 tumours are equivalent, although the report from the EORTC randomized trial controversially raised some questions about the validity of this opinion.[13,28,29,52,53–58]

Surgical approaches

Open partial nephrectomy

The supra eleventh rib extrapleural, extraperitoneal flank incision is commonly used for this procedure, which provides good exposure. A thoracoabdominal incision can be used, especially for large upper pole tumours.[25] Some surgeons use a transabdominal midline approach. The preparation, position, and skin incision is the same as of the RN described earlier.

The basic principles of PN are full mobilization of the kidney, early vascular control, tumour excision with negative margins,

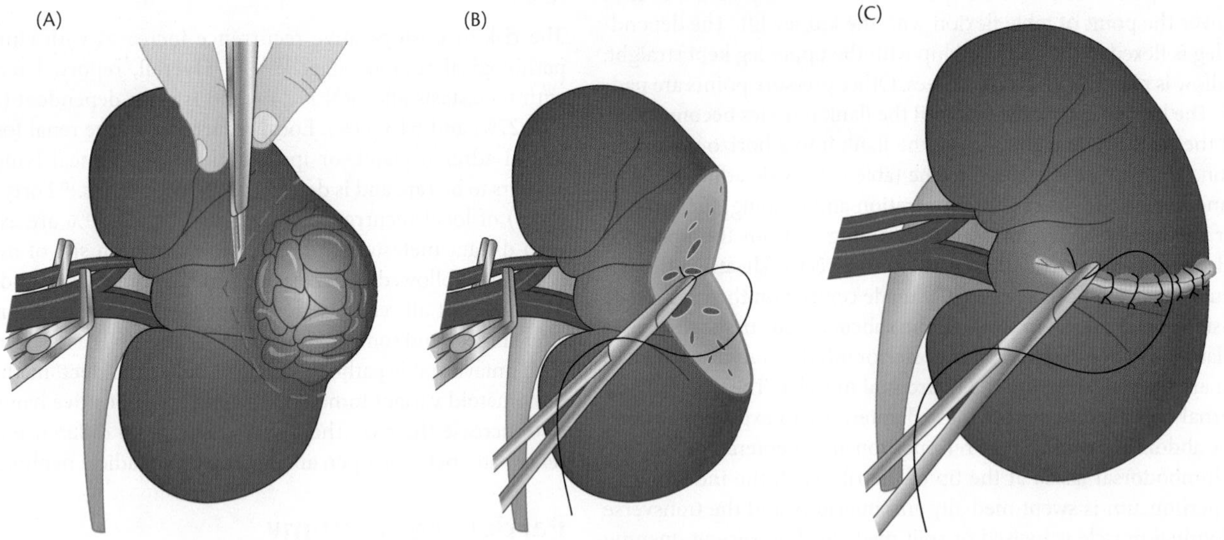

Fig. 6.29.3 Main principles of partial nephrectomy. (A) Early vascular control, tumour excision with negative margins; (B and C) renorrhaphy with ligation of the bleeding vessels and closure of the collecting system and then approximation of the capsule.

Reprinted from Alan J. Wein *et al., Campbell-Walsh Urology*, Tenth Edition, Saunders an imprint of Elsevier Inc., Copyright © 2012, by permission of Elsevier.

minimization of ischaemic injury, and repair of the renal defect or renorrhaphy (Fig. 6.29.3).[25]

After entering the retroperitoneum, the kidney is mobilized within Gerota's fascia attempting to leave the perinephric fat overlying the tumour intact, as up to 25% of localized RCC extend into the fat.[16] The vessels in the renal pedicle are then dissected free to prepare for vascular control. Vessel loops can be used. The ureter is identified and can also be encircled with a vessel loop. The renal artery or the branch supplying the tumour is then clamped; the renal vein and/the whole hilum are usually clamped as well. Decreased intraoperative blood loss, better visualization, and reduction in kidney tissue turgor are the main advantages of clamping the renal artery. *In situ* hypothermia, administration of intravenous mannitol 5–10 min prior to arterial clamping, and maintaining patency of the renal vein appear to minimize renal ischaemic injury.[25,59] Inducing hypothermia is difficult with the laparoscopic approach but with open PN, it is achieved with ice slush around the entire kidney for 10 minutes immediately after the artery occlusion and before starting the excision of the tumour. The objective is to keep the core temperature of the kidney at 20°C. Maintaining a low temperature permits up to three hours ischaemia time without permanent injury to the kidney.[25,60] Keeping the vein patent not only minimizes ischaemia, but it also permits identification of venous bleeding during tumour excision. The evidence for these manoeuvres is not strong but is being studied (please refer to the clinical trials.gov website for the ongoing Ottawa trial on hypothermia). Intraoperative ultrasonography may be useful to delineate tumours not visible or palpable on the surface of the kidney. The tumour is excised using sharp and blunt dissection to achieve a negative surgical margin while preserving as much as parenchyma as possible. Many techniques are described to remove the tumour including enucleation, wedge resection, polar segmental nephrectomy, transverse resection, and extracorporeal PN with autotransplantation. The renal capsule should be excised with the tumour. Arterial and venous branches identified during the resection and that are bleeding should be ligated or clipped. After tumour excision, any bleeding source should be ligated with small 4-0 figure of eight absorbable ligatures to secure haemostasis. At least 20% of the renal tissue is required for a functioning kidney without the need for dialysis.[16,51] A ureteral stent could be inserted prior to the procedure if collecting system entry is anticipated. Collecting system defects can be better identified with the aid of methylene blue instilled through a ureteral catheter. The collecting system is then closed with 4-0 monocryl suture. A haemostatic bolster of rolled Surgicel® is then applied at the defect and a haemostatic can be added to the bolster. The renorrhaphy is performed by mattress suturing the cortical edges with 2-0 or 3-0 interrupted sutures over the bolster. The sutures should be free of tension. The renal artery or hilum is then unclamped. A retroperitoneal drain is usually left in place and double J stent can be inserted when there is a major reconstruction of the collecting system.[25,51,61]

Laparoscopic/robotic partial nephrectomy

Open partial nephrectomy (OPN) remains the standard treatment for SRMs and RN should not be done when PN is feasible. Patient and physician preference for decreased morbidity with minimal invasive surgery led to the dissemination of laparoscopic techniques and laparoscopic partial nephrectomy (LPN) replaced the open approach in experienced laparoscopic centres. Winfield was the first to report this procedure in 1993.[39] It has the advantage of decreased operative time (with surgeon experience), decreased blood loss, and shorter hospital stay with the same oncological and renal functional outcomes.[6,62] The indications are the same as OPN.[63] The same principles of OPN are followed. It can be done through a transperitoneal or extraperitoneal approach. The transperitoneal approach has longer warm ischaemia time, longer operative time, and longer hospital stay, but the perioperative complications and analgesia requirements remain the same between the two approaches.[64] The transperitoneal approach has the advantage of a bigger working space, familiarity with anatomic landmarks, and technical ease of suturing. The choice of approach depends on the surgeon's experience and the location of the tumour.

Robot-assisted laparoscopic partial nephrectomy (RALPN) is safe and has similar oncological and morbidity outcomes with a primary benefit of easy intracorporeal suturing.[65,66] The advantage of 3D visualization that replicates the open experience makes the procedure more comfortable for most surgeons. The additional cost of these procedures is a significant issue, but RALPN appears to be replacing LPN when a robot is available.

Results

Local recurrence after PN is seen in up to 10% of cases, but is as low as 1–3% for T1a tumours.[28,29,50,51] Recurrence can be due to incomplete resection or a new primary. Disease specific survival is >90%, which is comparable to RN.[28,51,67,68] The rate of recurrence or metastasis is stage dependent. In pT1, the rate of local recurrence and metastasis are 0% and 4.4%, respectively, 2% and 5.3% in pT2, 8.2%, 11.5% in pT3a, and 10.6% and 15% in pT3b.[59] Approximately 80% of recurrence is detected in the first three years. The prevalence of positive surgical margin after partial nephrectomy is 0–7% with no difference in open, laparoscopic, or robotic approach. There is no difference in metastasis and cancer-specific survival in comparison to patients who have had negative surgical margins.[69,70]

Complications of open surgery

The proximity of the kidneys to major vessels and vital visceral structures may result in damage to these structures with complications. Understanding the anatomy of the kidneys and their relation to the nearby structures is essential.

The overall complication rates for RN and PN are approximately16% and 19%, respectively, with a mortality rate of 0.3% mainly due to myocardial infarction and pulmonary embolism.[71] There is no difference in the overall complication rates between open and laparoscopic RN, but the vascular complications are more common with the laparoscopic group.[3] LPN has higher complication rates than OPN; especially bleeding and reoperation rate of urological procedures. It is associated with longer ischaemic time, but this did not reflect on the renal function since the functional outcomes are the same in the two groups.[6,29] RAPN appears to have lower complication rates.[66]

Intraoperative complications

Vascular injury

This occurs in about 10.7% and the rate of significant bleeding (>1 L blood loss) is 1.2% with RN and 3.1% with PN.[72] To decrease the risk of bleeding, anticoagulants should be stopped before surgery and the anatomy of the renal vasculature should be carefully defined on the preoperative imaging. Predictable sites for bleeding include the renal hilum, collateral tumour vessels, the anterior or lateral IVC, lumber veins, and the right adrenal vein. Vascular injury can be controlled with standard vascular repair techniques. Control of a lumbar vein injury may be complicated by the end retracting towards the spine. A small Allis clamp may be useful to gain control.[25] The superior mesenteric artery can be mistaken for the left renal artery when large left tumours are approached and ligated in error.

Injury to the pleura

This is reported to occur in 9.3% of RNs and 11.5% of PNs.[73] Incision at or above the eleventh rib carries a greater risk.[26] If a pleural tear is recognized intraoperatively, the defect closure is begun and then a red rubber catheter is inserted into the defect, before hyperinflating the lungs. With this manoeuvre, the air and fluid are drained out the catheter and the defect can be closed with the preplaced purse-string suture. A chest X-ray should be performed in the recovery room to rule out pneumothorax. A chest tube is inserted if there is 15–20% pneumothorax or in case of tension pneumothorax.[25]

Injury to colon, small intestine, duodenum, spleen, liver, and pancreas

These complications can be associated with both transperitoneal and retroperitoneal approaches. The biggest risk is to the duodenum during right renal surgery. Awareness and immediate repair are critical. Injury to or limited resection of the liver may occur during right RN. Superficial laceration can be managed with electrocoagulation on 'spray' setting or argon beam laser, or with application of one of the haemostatic materials to the defect. The spleen and pancreas can be injured during the attempt to divide the splenorenal ligament during left RN and by excessive mobilization or traction during exposure. Splenectomy and/or pancreatic resection may be necessary.[25,26]

Postoperative complications

Pulmonary

Pneumothorax after a pleural incision or lung parenchymal injury can occur when the chest is opened and a chest tube is not left in place. A chest tube should be inserted postoperatively if there is >15–20% pneumothorax, or if there is tension and a chest X-ray should be done immediately postoperatively if the pleura is opened intraoperatively. There is an increased risk of atelectasis and pneumonia after surgery in the flank position. Fever in the first postoperative day is the hallmark of atelectasis. It should be managed appropriately. Diaphragmatic palsy is a rare occurrence after extended thoracoabdominal approach or with diaphragmatic resection.

Intrabdominal

Prolonged ileus and intestinal obstruction can occur after a transperitoneal approach with bowel manipulation. Pancreatitis, pancreatic pseudocyst, or abscess formation is rare but can occur if pancreatic injury was not recognized and managed during the procedure. Pancreatitis can present with persistent abdominal pain and prolonged ileus, but can be managed conservatively. Drainage is rarely necessary.[25]

Renal

Chronic kidney disease is a significant risk after RN or PN due to loss of nephrons. About half of RN patients, despite normal preoperative renal function, develop new onset CKD and this is reduced by 50% to one-quarter after PN.[8,74] The renal injury with PN may also be attributed to the ischaemic injury from vascular clamping. In solitary kidneys where the creatinine level reflects the function of the operated kidney, risk factors for the development of acute kidney injury are large tumour size (>7 cm), resection of more than 50% of the normal parenchyma, long ischaemia time (>60 minutes), and *ex vivo* surgery.[75] Measures to minimize injury include intraoperative administration of mannitol, hypothermia, and minimization of the ischaemic time. The risk of temporary dialysis is 8% and permanent dialysis 4% after PN in a solitary kidney.

Patients who undergo PN, especially those with a small amount of parenchymal may develop hyperfiltration renal injury with a risk for proteinuria, focal segmental glomerulosclerosis, and progressive renal failure. This may occur when more than 50% of the renal parenchyma is removed from a solitary kidney.[16] Long-term monitoring of renal function is mandatory.

Incisional

Abdominal incisional hernia after open surgery and flank wound bulge due to injury to the intercostal nerves can occur.[25,26,61,76]

Bleeding

Pain, flank, or abdominal swelling, signs of hypovolemia or drainage of blood through the wound site can all occur with bleeding from a major vessel, injury to the liver, spleen, or a mesenteric vessel, or even from the kidney itself after PN. It can be self-limited in the retroperitoneum and be managed by bed rest, serial haemoglobin and haematocrit measurement with frequent vital signs monitoring, and blood transfusion as needed. Renal angiogram with embolization may be required or even re-exploration to control the bleeding points. Reoperation for complications is higher with the PN compared to RN (4.4 vs. 2.4%).[73] Delayed bleeding may occur with arteriovenous malformation, which may be managed percutaneously.[25]

Urinary fistula

This is the most common complication after PN with an occurrence rate of 4.4%.[77] Central, large tumours, and surgery that requires major reconstruction of the pelvicalyceal system are risk factors.[61] Fistula is diagnosed when there is persistent drainage of fluid and the fluid creatinine level is more than twice the serum creatinine.[77] Most fistulas will close spontaneously with watchful waiting if there is no distal ureteric obstruction. The surgical drain should be left in place until drainage has decreased to a small daily volume of <50–100 cc. Persistent fistula is managed by bladder drainage with a catheter to reduce upper tract pressure followed by imaging with US or CT to rule out a urinoma that may require percutaneous drainage. If there is hydronephrosis or any evidence of obstruction, a ureteral catheter for drainage may be helpful.

Follow-up after surgery

The only consensus regarding the follow-up strategy after RN or PN surgery for RCC is that it should be intensified with increased pathological stage. Follow-up should monitor for postoperative complications and recurrence, kidney function, as well as local and distant recurrence. There are many proposed guidelines in the literature.[20,34,48,49,78–81] Patients can be followed up in six weeks for postoperative complications with history, physical examination, creatinine, and haemoglobin. The Canadian Urological Association (CUA) has proposed guidelines for follow-up depending on the initial pathological stage.[49] For T1 disease the patient could be followed with clinical assessment, biochemistry, and chest X-ray at one year from surgery and then every year for five years, and CT or ultrasound abdomen at two and five years from surgery. For PT2 disease, follow-up will include clinical assessment, biochemistry, and chest X-ray at six months from surgery, then every six months for three years, then yearly thereafter. CT or ultrasound scans of the abdomen could be done one year from surgery then every two years for 10 years.[49] Several nomograms have been designed to quantify the risk of recurrence and metastasis after surgery for localized RCC and these have been classified as low, intermediate, and high risk.[78,81–84] The EAU guidelines adopted these nomograms for follow-up, which intensify as the risk increases.[20] The total length of follow-up is not usually specified in the guidelines but late recurrence is seen in RCC. Most recurrence is diagnosed in the first three years.

Active surveillance

The incidence of RCC has increased and although the number of surgical procedures has increased accordingly, mortality due to RCC has not decreased significantly.[7,14] This and other observations have led to the reassessment of immediate treatment of SRMs and the necessity of treating all cases. About half of the patients with SRMs are more than 65 years old and a significant number of these patients have co-morbidities.[7,85] A recent study showed that treatment of localized renal tumours with surgery does not increase the overall survival in patients more than 75 years old.[74] Surgical morbidity is higher in these groups of patients and the surgical risk may outweigh the progression of the SRM.[72] Twenty per cent (20%) of SRMs are benign and up to two-thirds of RCCs appear to have low growth potential so that initial excision of these tumours may be considered as overtreatment.[29,86,87] Although SRMs grow slowly (0.28 cm/year) and one-third do not grow, the rate does not differentiate between benign and malignant tumours and it does not correlate with the aggressiveness of RCC.[85,88] Renal cell cancer <4 cm have lower rate of progression and metastasis (1%) than those >4 cm in three-year follow-up.[85,89] So far there are no radiographic characteristics that can predict the aggressiveness and progression of SRMs.[29,90] For these reasons, AS for SRMs with delayed intervention until the diameter reaches 3–4 cm is a reasonable initial option that should be discussed. The patient should be counselled about the growth rate that it does not predict malignancy or clearly the aggressive potential of the mass. This approach does not appear to result in a loss of the window for nephron-sparing surgery (NSS) upon progression in the short term. The patient should also be counselled for the low but real risk for progression and metastasis and the lack of salvage treatment in this situation.[13] The mass should be imaged every three to six months initially until the growth rate is determined and may extend the follow-up after that. Renal biopsy may help.[21,29]

Thermal ablation therapy

Thermal ablation therapy with either heating by cryoblation or heating with radiofrequency (RFA) are acceptable minimally invasive treatments for SRMs. Ablation can be done with a laparoscopic approach or percutaneously. Elderly patients with significant co-morbidities who are not fit for surgery are good candidates. It can be used for local recurrence after NSS and in patients with hereditary RCC with multifocal tumours where multiple PNs are not possible.[10,16,29]

The best results are achieved with tumours ≤3 cm that are exophytic, peripheral, and away from major vessels or the renal collecting system.[54] Decreased morbidity, shorter or no hospital stay, shorter convalescence, and the ability to treat high-risk patients for surgery are potential advantages for this treatment.[29] There are a few concerns with the ablation therapies. First, they have a recurrence rate of 5–12%, which is higher than with surgical treatment.[91] Second, the follow-up reported in most studies is short. Third, complete ablation of all tumours is difficult at the time of treatment. Finally, salvage surgical treatment, if required, is difficult because of the perinephric fibrosis.[29,54]

Special situations

Bilateral renal tumours

Bilateral synchronous sporadic RCC occurs in up to 5% of cases. Most centres prefer a staged surgical approach, using PN for the tumours more amenable for NSS (smaller or in a more accessible location), followed by PN or RN for the contralateral kidney with the larger tumour. This allows the ipsilateral kidney to recover and establish its function before surgery to the other kidney, reducing the risk of dialysis postoperatively.[16,54,92]

Tumour associated with hereditary kidney diseases

Tumours in patients with hereditary kidney tumour diseases including Von Hippel-Lindau disease, familial papillary RCC, hereditary leiomyomatosis and RCC syndrome, and the Birt-Hogg-Dubé syndrome, differ from sporadic renal cell cancer in presentation and natural history. They occur in a younger age group, are bilateral, multifocal, and have higher rate of recurrence (2–51%).[54,93,94] The five-year free survival rate for local recurrence is 71% but it is only 15% at 10 years and 23% end up with end-stage renal disease requiring dialysis.[94] Options of treatment include PN with subsequent resections for recurrences; or AS for new or existing tumours until they reach 3 cm in maximal axial diameter since the rate of metastasis is very low, but it increases to 27.4% when it is >3 cm which warrant treatment.[95] This approach is not recommended for hereditary leiomyomatosis because of its aggressive nature and should be treated even if it is <3 cm.[95] Partial nephrectomy in this situation may carry an increased risk of local recurrence. Thermal ablation is an attractive treatment modality especially if there was previous ipsilateral surgery, impaired renal function, and clamping the hilum may worsen the condition, and in significant multifocal disease.[16,54,96] The final option is bilateral radical nephrectomy with renal replacement therapy.

Tumour in a solitary kidney

Tumour in a solitary kidney is an absolute indication for a NSS attempt. However, there are several concerns. Twenty per cent (20%) of the renal parenchyma needs to be preserved to avoid end-stage renal disease and dialysis.[16] Even if more than this amount remained, there is an 8% risk for postoperative dialysis and 4% may require permanent dialysis.[54,97] The other concern is the effect of pronged ischaemia time on renal function. Vascular clamping with cold or warm ischaemia are associated with acute and chronic renal failure and warm ischaemia >20 minutes is associated with increased incidence of permanent dialysis (10% vs. 4%).[54,98] This has a clinical implication in selecting the appropriate modality of treatment with the aim to adequately control the hilum and minimize the ischaemic time. Open PN may be a better option than LPN because it may be associated with a shorter ischaemia time and a lower rate of dialysis (10% vs. 0.6%).[54,99]

Conclusion

There has been evolution in the management of localized RCC in the last few years. The management options range from surgery (PN or RN), either open or minimally invasive (laparoscopic or robotic), to thermal ablation therapy and active surveillance. Partial nephrectomy is now the standard of care for T1a and some T1b tumours even with a normal contralateral kidney. RN is reserved for larger tumours or when PN is not feasible. RN should be done laparoscopically unless this approach is contraindicated.

There is no proven therapeutic role for LND, and it should be reserved for cases with radiological or palpable lymph node enlargement for staging purposes. Ipsilateral adrenalectomy is indicated only if the adrenal gland appears to be involved, or at risk of involvement depending on the size and location of the renal tumour.

Follow-up after surgery should be individualized according to pathological stage. Thermal ablation therapy is an acceptable option for elderly patients with significant co-morbidities who are not fit for surgery. Ablation can be used for local recurrences and in patients with hereditary RCC with multifocal tumours. Active surveillance is an attractive option for SRMs, especially for elderly patients with co-morbidities and short life expectancy. Renal mass biopsy is safe and can help in patient counselling and decision-making regarding the treatment option.

Further reading

Campbell SC, Lane BR. Malignant renal tumor. (pp.1413–74) In: Kavoussi L, Novick A, Partin A, Peters C (eds). *Campbell's-Walsh Urology*, Vol 2, 10th edition. Philadelphia, PA: Saunders, 2012.

Campbell SC, Novick AC, Belldegrun A, et al. Guideline for management of the clinical stage 1 renal mass. American Urological Association Education and Research, Inc., ©2009. Available at: http://www.auanet.org/content/guidelines-and-quality-care/clinical-guidelines/main-reports/renalmass09.pdf [Online].

Chawla SN, Crispen PL, Hanlon AL, Greenberg RE, Chen DY, Uzzo RG. The natural history of observed enhancing renal masses: meta-analysis and review of the world literature. *J Urol* 2006; **175**(2):425–31.

Gill IS, Kavoussi LR, Lane BR, *et al.* Comparison of 1,800 laparoscopic and open partial nephrectomies for single renal tumors. *J Urol 2007*; **178**(1):41–6.

Kassouf W, Siemens R, Morash C, *et al.* Follow-up guidelines after radical or partial nephrectomy for localized and locally advanced renal cell carcinoma. *Can Urol Assoc* 2009; **3**(1):73–6.

Kavoussi LR SM, Gill IS. Laparoscopic surgery of the kidney. (pp. 1628–69) In: Kavoussi L (ed). *Campbell's Walsh Urology*. Philadelphia, PA: Saunders, 2012.

Kenney PWC. Contemporary open surgery of the kidney. (pp. 1554–627) In: Kavoussi L (ed). *Campbell's Walsh Urology*. Philadelphia, PA: Saunders, 2012.

Kunkle DA, Egleston BL, Uzzo RG. Excise, ablate or observe: the small renal mass dilemma--a meta-analysis and review. *J Urol* 2008; **179**(4):1227–33; discussion 33–4.

Ljungberg B, Bensalah K, Bex A, *et al.* EAU Guidelines on Renal Cell Carcinoma. Uroweb 2016. Available at: http://uroweb.org/wp-content/uploads/EAU-Guidelines-Renal-Cell-Carcinoma-2016.pdf [Online].

National Comprehensive Cancer Network. Kidney Cancer (version 2.2017). Accessed date 10 November 2016. Available at: http://www.nccn.org/professionals/physician_gls/pdf/kidney.pdf [Online].

Nguyen CT, Campbell SC, Novick AC. Choice of operation for clinically localized renal tumor. *Urol Clin North Am* 2008; **35**(4):645–55; vii.

Pouliot F LJ, Pantuck AJ. Treatment of localized kidney cancer. (pp. 329–42) In: Dahm P DR, (ed). *Evidence-Based Urology.* West Sussex, UK: Wiley-Blackwell, 2010.

Smith JA, Howards SS, Preminger GM. *Hinman's Atlas of Urologic Surgery*. Philadelphia, PA: WB Saunders, 2012.

Uzzo RG, Novick AC. Nephron sparing surgery for renal tumors: indications, techniques and outcomes. *J Urol* 2001; **166**(1):6–18.

Van Poppel H, Becker F, Cadeddu JA, *et al.* Treatment of localised renal cell carcinoma. *Eur Urol* 2011; **60**(4):662–72.

Van Poppel H, Da Pozzo L, Albrecht W, *et al.* A prospective, randomised EORTC intergroup phase 3 study comparing the oncologic outcome of elective nephron-sparing surgery and radical nephrectomy for low-stage renal cell carcinoma. *Eur Urol* 2011; **59**(4):543–52.

References

1. Robson CJ, Churchill BM, Anderson W. The results of radical nephrectomy for renal cell carcinoma. *J Urol* 1969; **101**(3):297–301.
2. Borin JF. Laparoscopic radical nephrectomy: long-term outcomes. *Curr Opin Urol* 2008; **18**(2):139–44.
3. Hemal AK, Kumar A, Kumar R, Wadhwa P, Seth A, Gupta NP. Laparoscopic versus open radical nephrectomy for large renal tumors: a long-term prospective comparison. *J Urol* 2007; **177**(3):862–6.
4. Hemal AK, Kumar A. A prospective comparison of laparoscopic and robotic radical nephrectomy for T1-2N0M0 renal cell carcinoma. *World J Urol* 2009; **27**(1):89–94.
5. Dunn MD, Portis AJ, Shalhav AL, *et al.* Laparoscopic versus open radical nephrectomy: a 9-year experience. *J Urol* 2000; **164**(4):1153–9.
6. Gill IS, Kavoussi LR, Lane BR, *et al.* Comparison of 1,800 laparoscopic and open partial nephrectomies for single renal tumors. *J Urol* 2007; **178**(1):41–6.
7. Hollingsworth JM, Miller DC, Daignault S, Hollenbeck BK. Rising incidence of small renal masses: a need to reassess treatment effect. *J Natl Cancer Inst* 2006; **98**(18):1331–4.
8. Lucas SM, Stern JM, Adibi M, Zeltser IS, Cadeddu JA, Raj GV. Renal function outcomes in patients treated for renal masses smaller than 4 cm by ablative and extirpative techniques. *J Urol* 2008; **179**(1):75–9; discussion 9–80.
9. Go AS, Chertow GM, Fan D, McCulloch CE, Hsu CY. Chronic kidney disease and the risks of death, cardiovascular events, and hospitalization. *New Engl J Med* 2004; **351**(13):1296–305.
10. Kunkle DA, Egleston BL, Uzzo RG. Excise, ablate or observe: the small renal mass dilemma--a meta-analysis and review. *J Urol* 2008; **179**(4):1227–33; discussion 33–4.
11. Jewett MA, Zuniga A. Renal tumor natural history: the rationale and role for active surveillance. *Urol Clin North Am* 2008; **35**(4):627–34; vii.
12. Van Poppel H, Joniau S. Is surveillance an option for the treatment of small renal masses? *Eur Urol* 2007; **52**(5):1323–30.
13. Campbell SC, Novick AC, Belldegrun A, *et al.* Guideline for management of the clinical T1 renal mass. *J Urol* 2009; **182**(4):1271–9.
14. Chow WH, Devesa SS, Warren JL, Fraumeni JF Jr. Rising incidence of renal cell cancer in the United States. *JAMA* 1999; **281**(17):1628–31.
15. Pantuck AJ, Zisman A, Rauch MK, Belldegrun A. Incidental renal tumors. *Urology* 2000; **56**(2):190–6.
16. Campbell SC, Lane BR. Malignant renal tumor. (pp.1413–74) In: Kavoussi L, Novick A, Partin A, Peters C (eds). *Campbell's-Walsh Urology*, Vol **2**, 10th edition. Philadelphia, PA: Saunders, 2012.
17. Gold PJ, Fefer A, Thompson JA. Paraneoplastic manifestations of renal cell carcinoma. *Semin Urol Oncol* 1996; **14**(4):216–22.
18. Jayson M, Sanders H. Increased incidence of serendipitously discovered renal cell carcinoma. *Urology* 1998; **51**(2):203–5.
19. Herts BR, Baker ME. The current role of percutaneous biopsy in the evaluation of renal masses. *Semin Urol Oncol* 1995; **13**(4):254–61.
20. Ljungberg B, Bensalah K, Bex A, *et al.* EAU Guidelines on Renal Cell Carcinoma. Uroweb 2016. Available at: http://uroweb.org/wp-content/uploads/EAU-Guidelines-Renal-Cell-Carcinoma-2016.pdf [Online].
21. Leveridge MJ, Finelli A, Kachura JR, *et al.* Outcomes of small renal mass needle core biopsy, nondiagnostic percutaneous biopsy, and the role of repeat biopsy. *Eur Urol* 2011; **60**(3):578–84.
22. Richard PO, Jewett MA, Bhatt JR, *et al.* Renal tumor biopsy for small renal masses: a single-center 13-year experience. *Eur Urol* 2015; **68**(6):1007–13.
23. Shannon BA, Cohen RJ, de Bruto H, Davies RJ. The value of preoperative needle core biopsy for diagnosing benign lesions among small, incidentally detected renal masses. *J Urol* 2008; **180**(4):1257–61; discussion 61.
24. Finelli A, Ismaila N, Bro B, *et al.* Management of small renal masses: American Society of Clinical Oncology Clinical Practice Guideline. *J Clin Oncol* 2017 Jan 17; Jco2016699645.
25. Kenney PWC. Contemporary open surgery of the kidney. (pp. 1554–627) In: Kavoussi L (ed). *Campbell's Walsh Urology*. Philadelphia, PA: Saunders, 2012.
26. Wotkowicz C, Libertino JA. Renal cell cancer: radical nephrectomy. *BJU Int* 2007; **99**(5 Pt B):1231–8.
27. el-Galley RE, Keane TE. Embryology, anatomy, and surgical applications of the kidney and ureter. *Surg Clin North Am* 2000; **80**(1):381–401, xiv.
28. Leibovich BC, Blute M, Cheville JC, Lohse CM, Weaver AL, Zincke H. Nephron sparing surgery for appropriately selected renal cell carcinoma between 4 and 7 cm results in outcome similar to radical nephrectomy. *J Urol* 2004; **171**(3):1066–70.
29. Van Poppel H, Becker F, Cadeddu JA, *et al.* Treatment of localised renal cell carcinoma. *Eur Urol* 2011; **60**(4):662–72.
30. Dash A, Vickers AJ, Schachter LR, Bach AM, Snyder ME, Russo P. Comparison of outcomes in elective partial vs radical nephrectomy for clear cell renal cell carcinoma of 4-7 cm. *BJU Int* 2006; **97**(5):939–45.
31. Blom JH, van Poppel H, Marechal JM, *et al.* Radical nephrectomy with and without lymph-node dissection: final results of European Organization for Research and Treatment of Cancer (EORTC) randomized phase 3 trial 30881. *Eur Urol* 2009; **55**(1):28–34.
32. Pantuck AJ, Zisman A, Dorey F, *et al.* Renal cell carcinoma with retroperitoneal lymph nodes. Impact on survival and benefits of immunotherapy. *Cancer* 2003; **97**(12):2995–3002.
33. Pouliot F LJ, Pantuck AJ. Treatment of localized kidney cancer. (pp. 329–42) In: Dahm PDR, (ed). *Evidence-Based Urology*. West Sussex, UK: Wiley-Blackwell, 2010.
34. National Comprehensive Cancer Network. Kidney Cancer (version 2.2017). Accessed date 10 November 2016. Available at: http://www.nccn.org/professionals/physician_gls/pdf/kidney.pdf [Online].
35. Antonelli A, Cozzoli A, Simeone C, *et al.* Surgical treatment of adrenal metastasis from renal cell carcinoma: a single-centre experience of 45 patients. *BJU Int* 2006; **97**(3):505–8.
36. O'Malley RL, Godoy G, Kanofsky JA, Taneja SS. The necessity of adrenalectomy at the time of radical nephrectomy: a systematic review. *J Urol* 2009; **181**(5):2009–17.
37. May M, Brookman-Amissah S, Pflanz S, Roigas J, Hoschke B, Kendel F. Pre-operative renal arterial embolisation does not provide survival benefit in patients with radical nephrectomy for renal cell carcinoma. *Br J Radiol* 2009; **82**(981):724–31.
38. Wszolek MF, Wotkowicz C, Libertino JA. Surgical management of large renal tumors. *Nat Clin Pract Urol* 2008; **5**(1):35–46.
39. Schwartz MJ, Smith EB, Trost DW, Vaughan ED, Jr. Renal artery embolization: clinical indications and experience from over 100 cases. *BJU Int* 2007; **99**(4):881–6.
40. Clayman RV, Kavoussi LR, Soper NJ, *et al.* Laparoscopic nephrectomy: initial case report. *J Urol* 1991; **146**(2):278–82.
41. Berger AD, Kanofsky JA, O'Malley RL, *et al.* Transperitoneal laparoscopic radical nephrectomy for large (more than 7 cm) renal masses. *Urology* 2008; **71**(3):421–4.
42. Mattar K, Finelli A. Expanding the indications for laparoscopic radical nephrectomy. *Curr Opin Urol* 2007; **17**(2):88–92.
43. Kavoussi LR SM, Gill IS. Laparoscopic surgery of the kidney. (pp. 1628–69) In: Kavoussi L (ed). *Campbell's Walsh Urology*. Philadelphia, PA: Saunders, 2012.
44. Desai MM, Strzempkowski B, Matin SF, *et al.* Prospective randomized comparison of transperitoneal versus retroperitoneal laparoscopic radical nephrectomy. *J Urol* 2005; **173**(1):38–41.
45. Nambirajan T, Jeschke S, Al-Zahrani H, Vrabec G, Leeb K, Janetschek G. Prospective, randomized controlled study: transperitoneal

laparoscopic versus retroperitoneoscopic radical nephrectomy. *Urology* 2004; **64**(5):919–24.

46. Schwartz MJ, Kavoussi LR. Laparoscopic and robotic surgery of the kidney. (pp. 1446–83) In: Wein AJ (ed). *Campbell-Walsh Urology*. Philadelphia, PA: Elsevier, Inc, 2016.
47. Stephenson AJ, Chetner MP, Rourke K, *et al.* Guidelines for the surveillance of localized renal cell carcinoma based on the patterns of relapse after nephrectomy. *J Urol* 2004; **172**(1):58–62.
48. Levy DA, Slaton JW, Swanson DA, Dinney CP. Stage specific guidelines for surveillance after radical nephrectomy for local renal cell carcinoma. *J Urol* 1998; **159**(4):1163–7.
49. Kassouf W, Siemens R, Morash C, *et al.* Follow-up guidelines after radical or partial nephrectomy for localized and locally advanced renal cell carcinoma. *Can Urol Assoc* 2009; **3**(1):73–6.
50. Herr HW. A history of partial nephrectomy for renal tumors. *J Urol* 2005; **173**(3):705–8.
51. Uzzo RG, Novick AC. Nephron sparing surgery for renal tumors: indications, techniques and outcomes. *J Urol* 2001; **166**(1):6–18.
52. Long CJ, Canter DJ, Kutikov A, *et al.* Partial nephrectomy for renal masses >/= 7 cm: technical, oncological and functional outcomes. *BJU Int* 2012; **109**(10):1450–6.
53. Ganesamoni R, Mavuduru R, Agarwal MM. Re: Hendrik van Poppel, Luigi da Pozzo, Walter Albrecht, *et al.* A prospective, randomised EORTC intergroup phase 3 study comparing the oncologic outcome of elective nephron-sparing surgery and radical nephrectomy for low-stage renal cell carcinoma. *Eur Urol* 2011; **59**:543–52.
54. Nguyen CT, Campbell SC, Novick AC. Choice of operation for clinically localized renal tumor. *Urol Clin North Am* 2008; **35**(4):645–55; vii.
55. Lee CT, Katz J, Shi W, Thaler HT, Reuter VE, Russo P. Surgical management of renal tumors 4 cm. or less in a contemporary cohort. *J Urol* 2000; **163**(3):730–6.
56. Van Poppel H, Da Pozzo L, Albrecht W, *et al.* A prospective, randomised EORTC intergroup phase 3 study comparing the oncologic outcome of elective nephron-sparing surgery and radical nephrectomy for low-stage renal cell carcinoma. *Eur Urol* 2011; **59**(4):543–52.
57. Kluth LA, Xylinas E, Shariat SF. Words of wisdom: re: a prospective, randomised EORTC intergroup phase 3 study comparing the oncologic outcome of elective nephron-sparing surgery and radical nephrectomy for low-stage renal cell carcinoma. *Eur Urol* 2013; **63**(2):399–400.
58. Taneja SS. Re.: A prospective, randomised EORTC intergroup phase 3 study comparing the oncologic outcome of elective nephron-sparing surgery and radical nephrectomy for low-stage renal cell carcinoma. *J Urol* 2011; **185**(5):1637–8.
59. Hafez KS, Novick AC, Campbell SC. Patterns of tumor recurrence and guidelines for followup after nephron sparing surgery for sporadic renal cell carcinoma. *J Urol* 1997; **157**(6):2067–70.
60. Luttrop W, Nelson CE, Nilsson T, Olin T. Study of glomerular and tubular function after in situ cooling of the kidney. *J Urol* 1976; **115**(2):133–5.
61. Smith JA, Howards SS, Preminger GM. *Hinman's Atlas of Urologic Surgery*. Philadelphia, PA: WB Saunders, 2012.
62. Lane BR, Gill IS. 7-year oncological outcomes after laparoscopic and open partial nephrectomy. *J Urol* 2010; **183**(2):473–9.
63. Turna B, Aron M, Gill IS. Expanding indications for laparoscopic partial nephrectomy. *Urology* 2008; **72**(3):481–7.
64. Ng CS, Gill IS, Ramani AP, *et al.* Transperitoneal versus retroperitoneal laparoscopic partial nephrectomy: patient selection and perioperative outcomes. *J Urol* 2005; **174**(3):846–9.
65. Scoll BJ, Uzzo RG, Chen DY, *et al.* Robot-assisted partial nephrectomy: a large single-institutional experience. *Urology* 2010; **75**(6):1328–34.
66. Choi JE, You JH, Kim DK, Rha KH, Lee SH. Comparison of perioperative outcomes between robotic and laparoscopic partial nephrectomy: a systematic review and meta-analysis. *Eur Urol* 2015; **67**(5):891–901.
67. Patard JJ, Shvarts O, Lam JS, *et al.* Safety and efficacy of partial nephrectomy for all T1 tumors based on an international multicenter experience. *J Urol* 2004; **171**(6 Pt 1):2181–5, quiz 435.
68. Mitchell RE, Gilbert SM, Murphy AM, Olsson CA, Benson MC, McKiernan JM. Partial nephrectomy and radical nephrectomy offer similar cancer outcomes in renal cortical tumors 4 cm or larger. *Urology* 2006; **67**(2):260–4.
69. Borghesi M, Brunocilla E, Schiavina R, Martorana G. Positive surgical margins after nephron-sparing surgery for renal cell carcinoma: incidence, clinical impact, and management. *Clin Genitourin Cancer* 2013; **11**(1):5–9.
70. Ani I, Finelli A, Alibhai SM, Timilshina N, Fleshner N, Abouassaly R. Prevalence and impact on survival of positive surgical margins in partial nephrectomy for renal cell carcinoma: a population-based study. *BJU Int* 2013; **111**(8):E300–5.
71. Stephenson AJ, Hakimi AA, Snyder ME, Russo P. Complications of radical and partial nephrectomy in a large contemporary cohort. *J Urol* 2004; **171**(1):130–4.
72. Abouassaly R, Alibhai SM, Tomlinson GA, Urbach DR, Finelli A. The effect of age on the morbidity of kidney surgery. *J Urol* 2011; **186**(3):811–6.
73. Van Poppel H, Da Pozzo L, Albrecht W, *et al.* A prospective randomized EORTC intergroup phase 3 study comparing the complications of elective nephron-sparing surgery and radical nephrectomy for low-stage renal cell carcinoma. *Eur Urol* 2007; **51**(6):1606–15.
74. Lane BR, Abouassaly R, Gao T, *et al.* Active treatment of localized renal tumors may not impact overall survival in patients aged 75 years or older. *Cancer* 2010; **116**(13):3119–26.
75. Partial Nephrectomy. Urology Surgery—urologysurgery.wordpress.com. [cited 10 November 2016]. Available at: http://urologysurgery.wordpress.com/2008/09/21/partial-nephrectomy/1 [Online].
76. Chatterjee S, Nam R, Fleshner N, Klotz L. Permanent flank bulge is a consequence of flank incision for radical nephrectomy in one half of patients. *Urol Oncol* 2004; **22**(1):36–9.
77. Kundu SD, Thompson RH, Kallingal GJ, Cambareri G, Russo P. Urinary fistulae after partial nephrectomy. *BJU Int* 2010; **106**(7):1042–4.
78. Chin AI, Lam JS, Figlin RA, Belldegrun AS. Surveillance strategies for renal cell carcinoma patients following nephrectomy. *Rev Urol* 2006; **8**(1):1–7.
79. Ljungberg B, Alamdari FI, Rasmuson T, Roos G. Follow-up guidelines for nonmetastatic renal cell carcinoma based on the occurrence of metastases after radical nephrectomy. *BJU Int* 1999; **84**(4):405–11.
80. Sandock DS, Seftel AD, Resnick MI. A new protocol for the followup of renal cell carcinoma based on pathological stage. *J Urol* 1995; **154**(1):28–31.
81. Lam JS, Shvarts O, Leppert JT, Pantuck AJ, Figlin RA, Belldegrun AS. Postoperative surveillance protocol for patients with localized and locally advanced renal cell carcinoma based on a validated prognostic nomogram and risk group stratification system. *J Urol* 2005; **174**(2):466–72; discussion 72; quiz 801.
82. Kattan MW, Reuter V, Motzer RJ, Katz J, Russo P. A postoperative prognostic nomogram for renal cell carcinoma. *J Urol* 2001; **166**(1):63–7.
83. Leibovich BC, Blute ML, Cheville JC, *et al.* Prediction of progression after radical nephrectomy for patients with clear cell renal cell carcinoma: a stratification tool for prospective clinical trials. *Cancer* 2003; **97**(7):1663–71.
84. Karakiewicz PI, Briganti A, Chun FK, *et al.* Multi-institutional validation of a new renal cancer-specific survival nomogram. *J Clin Oncol* 2007; **25**(11):1316–22.
85. Jewett MA, Mattar K, Basiuk J, *et al.* Active surveillance of small renal masses: progression patterns of early stage kidney cancer. *Eur Urol* 2011; **60**(1):39–44.

86. Frank I, Blute ML, Cheville JC, Lohse CM, Weaver AL, Zincke H. Solid renal tumors: an analysis of pathological features related to tumor size. *J Urol* 2003; **170**(6 Pt 1):2217–20.
87. Remzi M, Ozsoy M, Klingler HC, *et al.* Are small renal tumors harmless? Analysis of histopathological features according to tumors 4 cm or less in diameter. *J Urol* 2006; **176**(3):896–9.
88. Kunkle DA, Crispen PL, Chen DY, Greenberg RE, Uzzo RG. Enhancing renal masses with zero net growth during active surveillance. *J Urol* 2007; **177**(3):849–53; discussion 53-4.
89. Chawla SN, Crispen PL, Hanlon AL, Greenberg RE, Chen DY, Uzzo RG. The natural history of observed enhancing renal masses: meta-analysis and review of the world literature. *J Urol* 2006; **175**(2):425–31.
90. Remzi M, Katzenbeisser D, Waldert M, *et al.* Renal tumour size measured radiologically before surgery is an unreliable variable for predicting histopathological features: benign tumours are not necessarily small. *BJU Int* 2007; **99**(5):1002–6.
91. Matin SF, Ahrar K, Cadeddu JA, *et al.* Residual and recurrent disease following renal energy ablative therapy: a multi-institutional study. *J Urol* 2006; **176**(5):1973–7.
92. Booth J, Matin SF, Ahrar K, Tamboli P, Wood CG. Contemporary strategies for treating nonhereditary synchronous bilateral renal tumors and the impact of minimally invasive, nephron-sparing techniques. *Urol Oncol* 2008; **26**(1):37–42.
93. Roupret M, Hopirtean V, Mejean A, *et al.* Nephron sparing surgery for renal cell carcinoma and von Hippel-Lindau's disease: a single center experience. *J Urol* 2003; **170**(5):1752–5.
94. Steinbach F, Novick AC, Zincke H, *et al.* Treatment of renal cell carcinoma in von Hippel-Lindau disease: a multicenter study. *J Urol* 1995; **153**(6):1812–6.
95. Duffey BG, Choyke PL, Glenn G, *et al.* The relationship between renal tumor size and metastases in patients with von Hippel-Lindau disease. *J Urol* 2004; **172**(1):63–5.
96. Shingleton WB, Sewell PE Jr. Percutaneous renal cryoablation of renal tumors in patients with von Hippel-Lindau disease. *J Urol* 2002; **167**(3):1268–70.
97. Campbell SC, Novick AC, Streem SB, Klein E, Licht M. Complications of nephron sparing surgery for renal tumors. *J Urol* 1994; **151**(5):1177–80.
98. Thompson RH, Frank I, Lohse CM, *et al.* The impact of ischemia time during open nephron sparing surgery on solitary kidneys: a multi-institutional study. *J Urol* 2007; **177**(2):471–6.
99. Lane BR, Novick AC, Babineau D, Fergany AF, Kaouk JH, Gill IS. Comparison of laparoscopic and open partial nephrectomy for tumor in a solitary kidney. *J Urol* 2008; **179**(3):847–51; discussion 52.

CHAPTER 6.30

Ablative technologies for renal cancer

Stephen Faddegon, Ephrem O. Olweny, and Jeffrey A. Cadeddu

Introduction to ablative technologies for renal cancer

Background and indications for renal ablation

The term 'renal ablation' (RA) encompasses numerous technologies and energy sources used for the destruction of renal neoplasms *in situ*. Radiofrequency ablation (RFA) and cryoablation (CA) are the most widely studied RA modalities and will represent the focus of this chapter. Various changes in the demographics of renal tumours and renal failure in the general population have lead to the need for less aggressive treatments, such as RA. These demographic changes include the rising prevalence of small asymptomatic lesions detected through abdominal scanning and that tumours are now commonly found in patients with poor renal function.

The outcomes of RA can be difficult to interpret from the literature. Definitions of treatment failure may differ between reports, and treated masses are not always biopsied to confirm malignancy. Furthermore, there are no randomized trials comparing ablation modalities, or comparing ablation to extirpative surgery, the gold standard for treatment of renal masses. Well-recognized indications for RA include patients with small renal masses who are either poor surgical candidates or at risk of renal insufficiency. This includes patients with solitary kidneys, bilateral renal masses, hereditary syndromes such as von Hippel-Lindau's disease (VHL), and those with renal insufficiency. The optimal tumour size for RA appears to be equal to or less than less than three cm, although there is no established cutoff. A recent series of 159 tumours treated by RFA reported significantly higher 5-year disease-free survival for tumours <3 cm compared to those >3 cm (91% vs. 79%, p = 0.001).[1] Complication rates may also increase with tumours >3 cm, particular when treated by CA.[2] Although the American Urological Association (AUA) guidelines suggest that tumours greater than 4 cm may be treated by RA,[3] many centres avoid ablation of T1b tumours, regardless of co-morbidity status, for these reasons.[4,5] When RA is reserved for smaller tumours, several studies report of achievement of oncologic efficacy similar to that for partial nephrectomy.[5–8] Relative contraindications to RA include short life expectancy that would preclude any survival benefit to ablation, and patients who may not tolerate sedation or anaesthesia (such as an acute illness or unstable cardiovascular status). Central or hilar tumours may be poorly suited to thermal ablation due to increased risk for complications and 'heat sink' phenomena, which impairs ablation efficacy. Additionally, underlying coagulopathy must be corrected prior to treatment.[9]

The rationale for renal ablation

The increased prevalence of small renal masses (SRMs), due to the widespread use of abdominal imaging for other reasons, has fuelled interest in active surveillance and minimally invasive treatment options.[6,10] Only 20-25% of SRMs have highly aggressive histological features, while 55–60% are malignant but display indolent behaviour.[11–13] Surgical therapy for indolent and benign tumours, which represent the majority of SRMs, might be considered overtreatment, but preoperative distinction from malignant tumours with aggressive histology is unreliable. Although surgery is traditionally recommended for younger patients, active surveillance is an option, given low associated rates of metastasis.[14] Elderly patients are more often counselled towards active surveillance, although those who live long enough may experience tumour growth and eventually require treatment. For all patient age groups with SRMs, RA could be considered a treatment compromise, offering the opportunity for treatment while minimizing patient morbidity. Indeed, RA is associated with shorter convalescence and fewer complications than surgery,[15] with minimal impact on post-treatment renal function.[16,17]

Radiofrequency ablation

Background

Radiofrequency (RF) waves are defined as the portion of the electromagnetic spectrum with frequencies between 3Hz and 300GHz. Their interaction with biological tissues was described as early as 1891, when D'Arsonval demonstrated that RF waves passed though biological tissues raised tissue temperatures.[18] In 1926, Bovie and Cushing described the use of a Bovie knife to resect a brain tumour, a device that used RF current for alternate cutting and cauterization.[19] However, it was not until 1990 that the use of RF energy to produce focal areas of tissue ablation was first reported. That year, two independent investigators described the use of an insulated RF needle designed for percutaneous insertion that created a zone of ablation centred around the un-insulated needle tip.[20,21] Use of this device for solid organ (liver tumour) ablation was first reported in 1993[22] while use in kidney ablation was first reported in 1997.[23]

Mechanism of action

During ablation, alternating current applied to the probe (cathode) causes water molecules closest to the probe to vibrate at high frequency so as to align with the current. Some of the resulting kinetic energy is displaced as heat due to friction between adjacent vibrating molecules. The tissue temperature is raised, being highest closest to the probe and dropping off exponentially with increasing distance from the probe. The probe itself is not heated by the current.[24] Tissue death and vaporization respectively occur at 55ºC and 100ºC. Ablation efficacy is primarily determined efficiency of energy deposition and tissue conductivity. If the tissue temperature is raised too rapidly, tissue vaporization results in carbonization and charring around the probe, raising the tissue impedance and limiting transmission of further electrical and thermal energy. Conversely, proximity to blood vessels that are greater than three mm in diameter results in a 'heat sink' effect, whereby heat is absorbed by circulating blood, limiting the success of achieving target temperatures within the tissue.[24]

Several techniques are employed by current RF systems to optimize efficiency of energy delivery. The maximum amount of RF current that can be delivered is dependent on both the generator output and electrode surface area. Modern RF generators are capable of outputs of up from 200 to 250 W.[24] During treatment delivery, the two most commonly used generators utilize either temperature monitoring (whereby power is modulated to maintain target temperature and minimize tissue impedance; Angiodynamics, Queensbury, NY, USA) or impedance monitoring (whereby power is cycled and increased to drive impedance high without monitoring of temperature or time; Radionics, Burlington, MA, USA). Commonly used electrode designs include use of multi-tined probes to increase tissue contact surface area thereby increasing ablation zones,[25] and use of cooled tip electrodes which minimize charring around the RF probe.[26]

Surgical technique

Percutaneous RFA

Depending on treating physician preference, either conscious sedation or general anaesthesia is employed, and the procedure is performed on an outpatient basis. In the authors' experience, general anaesthesia is safe for the majority of patients, enables control of respirations during probe positioning and lesion biopsy, and generally does not preclude same-day patient discharge. Intravenous prophylactic antibiotics are administered, a Foley catheter is placed, and the patient is positioned in either a prone or modified flank position on the computed tomography (CT) gantry, generally with the torso supported on bolsters. The choice of position is largely dictated by the tumour location. A non-contrast CT is first obtained to confirm tumour size and position in the prone or lateral position, and a contrast-enhanced CT is then obtained to better delineate the tumour. A 20-gauge finder needle is inserted under CT-guidance to guide the desired trajectory of the RF probe. At the authors' institution, a 14-gauge Starburst XL (RITA Medical Systems, Mountain View, CA) probe is then deployed and its position is adjusted to ensure complete lesion coverage plus a peritumoural margin of at least 5 mm. This is done using serial limited CT scans through the kidney employing 3 mm cuts. Use of fine cuts ensures that individual ablation probe tines are within three mm of each other, which represents the maximum heat dispersion distance from each tine. After probe positioning, an 18-gauge CT-guided TruCut biopsy is obtained by inserting the biopsy needle parallel to the ablation probe. Probe and biopsy needle positioning and adjustments are performed with breath holding at end-expiration. Ablation cycles of 5, 7, and 8 minutes at a target temperature of 105°C are then delivered for tine deployments of <2 cm, 2–4 cm, and ≥4 cm respectively, with two cycles delivered per treatment. During the brief intervening period between treatment cycles, the passive tissue temperature in each quadrant should be at least 70°C. A contrast-enhanced CT is repeated post-treatment to assess completeness of ablation and to rule out complications. If inadequately treated areas are identified, the RF probe is repositioned and the treatment is repeated. Occasionally, for more anteriorly located tumours, a 5% dextrose solution in water is infused into the perinephric space to increase the distance between the renal lesion and closely neighbouring structures. Heat sinks due to small vessels can often be overcome by ablation of the vessels. The Foley catheter is monitored for haematuria at all times, and the probe depth is readjusted as needed if haematuria is noted. The probe tract is ablated during probe withdrawal. For ablation of larger lesions, some authors have described the use of non-conducting temperature probes placed at the peripheral and deep margins of the tumour for active temperature monitoring.[27] Rather than multi-tined probes, multiple individual probes can also be used in overlapping ablations.[6]

Laparoscopic RFA

Laparoscopic RFA may be used for ablation anterior or centrally located tumours. A transperitoneal approach is generally used. The kidney is mobilized, Gerota's fascia is entered, and the lesion is exposed. The radiofrequency probe is inserted percutaneously through a separate stab incision and is deployed under laparoscopic ultrasound guidance, ensuring that the treatment tines extend beyond the tumour edge and the deep margin. At conclusion of the treatment cycles, a 5 mm toothed forceps is used to obtain a biopsy of the mass, following which Gerota's fascia is re-approximated prior to port removal and closure.

Cryoablation

Background

The earliest applications of extreme cold temperatures in the clinical setting were described as far back as the early 1900s, when the use of liquid air and liquid carbon dioxide were employed for the treatment of skin lesions.[28,29] The clinical application of liquid nitrogen as a cryogen was first introduced in 1950,[30] with the earliest use for urological application (prostate ablation) described in 1966,[31] and the first use for renal tumour ablation reported in 1995.[32] Liquid nitrogen is capable of achieving cooling temperatures nearing −200°C. Despite limited early applications, CA did not become mainstream until the development of intraoperative ultrasound monitoring and the introduction of argon gas cryoprobes. Intraoperative ultrasound guidance improved effectiveness by facilitating accurate probe placement within the tumour and real-time verification of ice ball propagation beyond the tumour margins.[33,34] The use of argon gas improved the efficiency of CA by enabling shorter treatment times due to its rapid cooling property.[35]

There have been several recent advancements in cryotherapy technology. These include ultra-thin 17-gauge needle probes which allow precise positioning within the tumour and may minimize the risk of bleeding following probe removal.[36] In a multi-institutional study of 144 patients, the ultra-thin probes resulted in a 15% complication rate of which half were minor and did not require secondary intervention.[37] Additional research is being conducted in CT-guided stereotactic probe positioning to increase the accuracy of probe placement.[36]

Mechanism of action

Cooling during CA is achieved through the Joule-Thomson effect in which pressurized liquid gas cools as it expands to a gaseous state at the tip of the cryoprobe, achieving temperatures as low as -195°C (range –80°C to –195°C). The thaw phase is usually achieved with helium gas, which warms rather than cools as it is depressurized. Depending on the size and shape of the tumour, multiple ablation probes can be used to ensure adequate tumour coverage.[8]

The mechanism of cell death involves intracellular dehydration, direct injury to proteins and cell membranes, and local ischaemia. During freezing, extracellular ice formation establishes as osmotic gradient that causes a fluid shift from the intracellular space to extracellular space, resulting in intracellular dehydration and changes in pH. Intracellular and extracellular ice formation also result in direct damage to cell membranes[8] and protein denaturation that impairs vital enzyme pathways.[38,39] Local ischaemia results from disruption of the microvasculature.[8] Finally, reperfusion injury during the thaw phase results in thrombosis, coagulative necrosis, apoptosis.[40,41]

Surgical technique

Treatment approach

CA can be performed via laparoscopic, percutaneous, or open approaches, although the open approach is rarely performed in favour of the more minimally invasive options. The majority of published series describe a laparoscopic approach[5] although there is an increasing number of percutaneous CA series.[6]

Laparoscopic CA is favoured for anterior, anteromedial and hilar masses, and is typically performed through a transperitoneal approach. The kidney is mobilized and the fat overlying the tumour is cleared to allow for complete visualization and intraoperative ultrasound monitoring. Some practitioners choose to expose the hilum in the event of haemorrhage. Core biopsies are obtained after which cryoprobes are inserted under direct vision with ultrasound assistance.[5,8] Selection of probe size and number is dependent upon tumour size. Animal studies suggest that for 17-gauge mm elliptical ice ball cryoprobes (1.47-mm diameter; Galil Medical, Arden Hill, MN, USA), a single probe is inadequate for complete ablation of most renal tumours, while use of three probes in a triangular template with 1.5 cm spacing achieved the largest zones of necrosis, sufficient for lesions <4 cm in size.[42] However, based on isotherm studies in gel and in *ex vivo* and *in vivo* porcine kidneys, Young and Clayman found that *ex vivo* isotherm data are inadequate for predicting *in vivo* tissue temperatures during CA, and recommended cryoprobe deployment several millimetres beyond the targeted lesion along with tissue temperature monitoring using thermosensors.[43] Intraoperative ultrasonography is essential for probe placement and monitoring of ice ball propagation.[6]

Posterior tumours can be accessed percutaneously with the patient supine under general or conscious sedation. Probes positioning and ice ball monitoring are done under CT or magnetic resonance imaging (MRI) guidance.[8] Advantages of the percutaneous approach include decreased pain, shorter hospital stay, and superior cost-effectiveness.[44] Disadvantages compared to the laparoscopic approach include the inability to assess for acute haemorrhage.[8] Unlike percutaneous RFA, the percutaneous puncture tract cannot be treated during probe removal.

Imaging

Renal imaging is central to the evaluation, treatment, and postoperative assessment of cryoablated tumours. A high-quality preoperative contrast-enhanced CT or MRI provides information about tumour size, location, and proximity to surrounding organs, the renal hilum, or the collecting system. As previously mentioned, intraoperative imaging guides probe placement and monitoring of ice ball propagation; ultrasound is utilized for laparoscopic approaches while CT or MRI is employed during percutaneous ablation.[6] For percutaneous CA, a post-ablative contrast-enhanced CT or MRI scan is also essential to confirm treatment success and evaluate for acute haemorrhage.[8]

Treatment monitoring

Monitoring of treatment efficacy during CA employs imaging of the ablation zone and monitoring of thermocouples. Tumour cell death is reliably achieved at target temperatures of –40°C.[45] Although the cryoprobe tip reaches temperatures of –140°C to –190°C, there is a steep temperature gradient which falls to 0°C at the edge of the ice ball.[46] Temperatures of less than –20°C are achieved at a distance of 3.1 mm inside the edge of the ice ball.[47] For these reasons, the ice ball should propagate 1 cm beyond the tumour margin to ensure temperatures of –40°C at the tumour margin.[45] The ice ball appears as a hypoechoic area with a hyperechoic rim on ultrasound.[8] Although it is easily visualized, posterior acoustic shadowing can impair accurate assessment of the ice ball depth, emphasizing the importance of accurate probe placement before the initiation of treatment.[5] Thermosensors may also be placed at the peripheral tumour margin to ensure that target temperatures are achieved.[48]

Treatment cycles

Two freeze/thaw cycles are standard, which stems from a prospective study in female dogs that demonstrated a larger and more complete area of necrosis following two cycles as compared to a single cycle.[49] The second ice ball is usually propagated beyond the initial border of ablation to ensure complete ablation.[5] There is no standard duration for a freeze cycle because, unlike RFA, the freeze time itself is not considered clinically significant as long as target temperatures are reached.[8] Ten minutes is commonly used during the initial cycle while the second cycle is generally shorter, lasting 6–8 minutes.[31,50] Such practice is supported by a study of female pigs in which freeze cycles of five minutes resulted in inadequate necrosis, while 15 minutes was associated with higher rates of tissue fracture. Ten minute freeze cycles represented an optimal compromise with adequate tumour necrosis and few complications.[51]

While the thaw cycle can be done passively, helium gas is generally employed to reduce the thaw time. Few studies have compared these two approaches and there is no present standard of care. At least one animal study found no difference in necrosis between active and passive thawing,[49] but prospective human studies have not been performed to date.[31] Following the second cycle thaw, the probe is gently twisted and if there is no resistance, it can be removed atraumatically.[5]

Post-ablation follow-up

Routine post-ablation follow-up includes a periodic history and physical, chest X-ray, abdominal CT, and laboratory tests including a complete metabolic profile. There is considerable variability in the follow-up routine used at individual treatment centres, and an optimal follow-up regimen has not been defined. At most centres, the first post-ablation CT or MRI is obtained at 4–12 weeks. If persistent enhancement is identified in any portion of the treated lesion on this study, it is classified as incompletely ablated and repeat ablation is scheduled. Radiographic success is defined as loss of enhancement accompanied by involution of the treated lesion on follow-up scans.[52] However, radiographic findings can be variable, for example loss of enhancement without accompanying involution or enhancement that is due to inflammatory changes without tumour recurrence.[52] The role of a routine post-ablation biopsy is controversial and studies have yielded conflicting data on its utility.[23,53–59] Taking the dual limitations of imaging studies and biopsy findings into consideration, a recent multi-institutional study on the incidence and patterns of recurrence following energy ablative therapy concluded that radiographic detection of residual or recurrent disease was the current state of the art when performed correctly.[60] However, when enhancement and involution are incongruent, or whenever recurrence is suspected, multisite-directed core biopsies should be considered.[52]

Outcomes of radiofrequency and cryoablation

Oncologic outcomes

To date, outcome reporting for oncologic efficacy of thermal ablative therapy is limited by small cohort sizes, short follow-up, inclusion of patients with benign masses, lack of pre-ablation biopsy, inclusion of patients with confounding features for renal cell carcinoma (RCC) recurrence such as hereditary cancer syndromes, variable definitions of recurrence, and other limitations.[4] However, recent studies with reasonable numbers of patients (≥30) have emphasized reporting of long-term oncologic outcomes in patients with biopsy-proven RCC, either primarily or within subset analyses, and these studies form the basis for the oncologic outcomes of ablative therapies discussed in this chapter.[61–69] Some of these studies however, are confounded by inclusion of patients with hereditary cancer syndromes and/or prior RCC treatment. Tables 6.30.1 and 6.30.2 summarize RCC-specific outcomes for RFA and CA respectively in select series with intermediate to long-term follow-up. For RFA, local recurrence-free outcomes range between 88% and 95% while rates for CA are 80% to approximately 87%. Metastasis-free survival and cancer-specific survival exceed 90% in virtually all series. Although studies drawing comparisons with partial nephrectomy are limited by unmatched tumour sizes and inconsistent definitions of post-ablation recurrence, data to date suggest that progression-free survival and disease-specific survival are similar for energy ablative therapy and extirpative therapy in the intermediate term (five years), exceeding 90% in each case. In a head-to-head comparison of RFA and PN in patients with sporadic unilateral T1a RCC, five-year actual local recurrence-free survival, overall disease-free survival, and progression-free survival were statistically similar between the cohorts.[63] In this series, persistent enhancement on the initial post-ablation imaging study was classified as incomplete ablation and was treated by repeat ablation in the majority of cases. Oncologic outcomes were then assessed after complete treatment (i.e. after complete loss of enhancement) was achieved.[63] Similar studies to date comparing oncologic outcomes for CA and partial nephrectomy in matched cohorts are limited by

Table 6.30.1 RCC-specific outcomes following RFA of renal tumours

Author, year	No. patients (no. tumours)	Follow-up (yr)	Tumour size, cm	Approach	Local recurrence	Metastatic recurrence	Overall disease-free survival	Cancer-specific survival	Overall survival
Psutka *et al.* (2012)[62]	185 (185)	Median 6.43 (range 0.5–13.4)	Median 3 (range 1–6.5)	Perc	5-yr RFS 95.2%	5-yr MFS 99.4%	5-yr DFS 87.6%	5-yr CSS 99.4%	5-yr OS 73.3%
Tracy *et al.* (2010)[63] (subgroup analysis)	160 (179)	Mean 2.25 (range 0.13–7.5)	Mean 2.4* (range 1.0–5.4)	Perc and Lap	5-yr RFS 90%	5-yr MFS 95%	—	5-yr CSS99%	5-yr OS 85%*
Zagoria *et al.* (2011)[64]	41 (48)	Median 4.67 (IQR 3–5.3)	Median 2.6 (range 0.7–8.2)	Perc	5-yr RFS 88%	3/41 (7%) developed metastases	5-yr DFS 83%**	1/41 (2.4%) died of RCC	5-yr OS 66%
Olweny *et al.* (2012)[61]	37 (37)	Median 6.5 (IQR 5.8–7.1)	Median 2.1 (IQR 1.8–2.8)	Perc and Lap	5-yr RFS 91.7%	5-yr MFS 97.2%	5-yr DFS 89%	5-yr CSS 97.2%	5-yr OS 97.2%
Levinson *et al.* (2008)[59] (subgroup analysis)	18 (18)	Mean 4.8 (range 3.4–6.7)	Mean 2.1 (range 1–4)	Perc	5-yr RFS 79.9%	5-yr MFS 100%	5-yr DFS 79.9%	5-yr CSS 100%	5-yr OS 58.3%
McDougal *et al.* (2005)[60]	16 (20)	Mean 4.6 (4–6)	Mean 3.2 (range 1.1–7.1)	Perc	4-yr RFS 91%	4-yr MFS 100%	—	4-yr CSS 100%	4-yr OS 68.7%

*Overall survival for entire cohort, including 22% with non-diagnostic or benign histology.

**No recurrences observed in patients with tumours <4 cm in size.

Table 6.30.2 RCC-specific outcomes following CA of renal tumours

Author, year	No. patients (no. tumours)	Follow-up (yr)	Tumour size, cm	Approach	Local recurrence	Metastatic recurrence	Overall disease-free survival	Cancer-specific survival	Overall survival
Aron *et al.* (2010)[65] (subgroup analysis)	55 (55)	Median 7.8 (range 5–11)	Mean 2.3 (range 0.9–5.0)	Lap	7/55 (12.7%) had local/ loco-regional recurrence	6/55 (11%) developed metastases	5-yr DFS 81%	5-yr CSS 92%	5-yr OS84%
Guazzzoni *et al.* (2010)[66] (subgroup analysis)	44	Mean 5.1	Median 2.14(range 0.5–4)	Lap	3 patients had loco-regional recurrence*	2 patients had metachronous recurrence*	—	5-yr CSS100%	5-yr OS 93.2%
Tanagho *et al.* (2012)[67] (subgroup analysis)	35	Mean 6.3 (SD 3.3)	Mean 2.5 (SD 0.98)	Lap	6-yr RFS 80%	6-yr MFS 100%	6-yr DFS 80%	6-yr CSS100%	6-yr OS 76.2%

*Although these patients received salvage therapy by RFA or radical nephrectomy, the authors did not include them in their analysis of recurrences.

inclusion of patients with benign histologies, rendering interpretation of recurrence outcomes inconclusive.[15, 70,71]

As is evident from Tables 6.30.1 and 6.30.2, recent series including at least 30 patients and greater than 5 years of follow-up have reported outcomes for RFA[63–66] and cryoablation[67–69] at individual institutions. A meta-analysis of these data could be of value in informing future recommendations for the role of these therapies in the primary management of Stage 1 RCC. Furthermore, recent studies with intermediate to long-term follow-up have helped to better inform patient selection criteria for energy ablative therapy. In the study by Best *et al.*, following RFA of 108 biopsy-proven RCC tumours the, five-year overall disease-free survival for those with tumours <3 cm was 95%, significantly dropping to 78% for those with tumours ≥3 cm (p = 0.002).[1] Similarly, in the study by Psutka *et al.*, five-year recurrence-free survival and overall disease-free survival after RFA in 143 patients with T1a RCC were 96.1% and 91.5%, respectively, compared with 91.9% and 74.5% in a comparative group of 42 patients with T1b tumours.[64] In the study by Tanagho *et al.*, a subset of 35 patients with biopsy-proven RCC who underwent laparoscopic cryoablation with a mean (SD) follow-up of 76[39] months had a six-year overall disease-free survival of 80%. On a multivariate analysis, only tumour size ≥2.6 cm was a significant predictor of oncological failure (hazard ratio 28.9; 95% CI = 1.1–794; p = 0.046).[69]

Surgical approach may be an important consideration influencing oncologic outcomes for RFA and cryoablation. For RFA, only one study to date has specifically investigated comparative oncologic outcomes for percutaneous vs. laparoscopic approaches. Young *et al.* reported that three-year RCC-specific radiographic recurrence-free probability for percutaneous vs. laparoscopic RFA was 92% vs. 91.5%, respectively (p = 0.84).[72] Oncologic success (absence of viable tumour on post-ablation biopsy) in these groups was 94% vs. 100% (p = 0.16) for percutaneous *vs.* laparoscopic RFA respectively. Tumours treated by laparoscopic RFA were on average 0.1 cm larger (p <0.05) and more likely anteriorly located.[72] In contrast, in a comparative multi-institutional study involving 145 patients with a mean follow-up of about 38 months, Strom *et al.* reported a significantly increased risk of local recurrence in patients who underwent percutaneous *vs.* laparoscopic cryoablation (16.4% vs. 5.9%; p = 0.042).[73] However, in this study, there was a significantly greater proportion of patients with biopsy-proven RCC in the percutaneous cryoablation group (76.4% vs. 58.3%; p = 0.035). Similar studies with shorter follow-up have reported statistically similar oncologic outcomes for percutaneous and laparoscopic cryoablation.[74,75] Additional studies with longer follow-up and with reporting of RCC-specific outcomes are needed to address the importance of surgical approach on treatment outcomes for thermal ablation.

Treatment complications

A recent meta-analysis classified postoperative complications into major urologic, major non-urologic, and minor complications. While partial nephrectomy had the highest rate of major urologic complications, there was no significant difference in the rate of major urologic complications between CA and RFA, which was 4.9% and 6%, respectively. These complications included postoperative haemorrhage requiring transfusion or intervention, ureteral obstruction, urine leak, abscess, or unexpected loss of renal function.[3] Haemorrhage occurs in less than 2% of patients following RFA, as the probe tract is ablated during probe withdrawal.[6] On the other hand, haemorrhage is the most commonly reported complication following CA, and often accompanies renal or tumour fracture.[3] Risk factors for fracture appear to be large tumours and utilization of multiple probes,[2,6] and may lead to significant haemorrhage requiring transfusion in up to 17–38% of cases.[2,50] If encountered during a laparoscopic CA, intraoperative bleeding can normally be controlled with hemostatic agents and pressure, although partial nephrectomy may be necessary in some cases.[5] Postoperative haemorrhage may present as flank pain, prolonged ileus, and dropping haematocrit and can be confirmed by a non-contrast abdominal CT scan.[5] Management includes bed rest and serial hematocrits, with angioembolization rarely being necessary.[6]

Complications involving the collecting system are rare. Ablation of tumours abutting the intrarenal collecting system rarely leads to urinary leakage.[76–78] However the renal pelvis and ureter should be clear of the ablation zone to avoid stricture formation and obstruction.[6]

In the meta-analysis by Campbell *et al.*,[3] major non-urologic complications were found to be more common following CA than RFA (4.9% vs. 4.4%). Bowel injuries are rare, particularly when ablation is restricted to tumours separated from bowel by >1 cm.[6,79] Percutaneous hydrodistension, in which water is injected between the tumour and visceral structures, may be considered to increase separation distance from neighbouring vital structures.

Minor complications from ablation include pain or paraesthesia at the cutaneous puncture site, mild haematuria, and urinary tract infections.[3]

Renal function outcomes

Several series report preservation of renal function after CA and RFA.[9,80–84] Patients that may be at risk for renal functional decline are those with significant preoperative renal insufficiency or solitary kidneys, although even these patients generally have favourable post-ablation renal function preservation.[8,85,86]

Some studies have compared renal function outcomes of ablation and partial nephrectomy. Unlike partial nephrectomy, RFA and CA do not require hilar occlusion and warm ischaemia. On the other hand, ablation may result in greater loss of normal nephron mass as the zone of ablation typically extends 1 cm beyond the tumour. A recent study comparing renal function outcomes of patients undergoing RFA, partial nephrectomy, or radical nephrectomy found radical nephrectomy to result in the greatest glomerular filtration rate (GFR) decline, while GFR loss after RFA and partial nephrectomy were not statistically different. The three-year freedom from Stage 3 chronic kidney disease progression for RFA, PN, and RN was 95.2%, 70.7%, and 39.9%, respectively (p <0.001).[87] In a multicentre study, patients with solitary kidneys undergoing RFA had a lower one-year GFR decline than for open partial nephrectomy under cold ischaemia (24.5% vs. 10.4%, p <0.001).[86] These data suggest that RFA and CA have minimal impact on renal function, and are at least equivalent to nephron-sparing surgery.

Novel ablative technologies

RFA and CA for the treatment of small renal tumours have been a part of the clinical landscape for at least a decade and preliminary data confirming their long-term efficacy has recently emerged and continues to mature. In recent years, several groups have additionally reported on a wide range of alternative ablative modalities, many of which have undergone preliminary evaluation in the clinical setting. Olweny and Cadeddu recently reviewed the literature on novel methods for renal tissue ablation.[88] Modalities such as microwave ablation, laser ablation, irreversible electroporation, high-intensity focused ultrasound, and MR-guided radiotherapy have undergone phase I or phase II evaluation at select centres, while promising techniques such as RCC electrovaporazation, and histotripsy have thus far only been evaluated in the experimental setting.[88] Additionally, techniques aimed at improving the efficacy, ablation size and safety of RFA, including bipolar and multipolar ablation, have yielded preliminary promising results.[89,90] A selection of promising novel ablation technologies are reviewed below.

Microwave ablation

Although its use for renal tumour ablation is relatively recent, microwave energy has been used effectively for liver tumour ablation for several years. Microwaves oscillate at two to five times higher frequencies than RF waves resulting in more rapid tissue heating, higher tissue temperatures, and creation of larger lesions.[91] Theoretical advantages of microwave energy over RF include a better convection profile given a broader power density field (up to 2 cm surrounding the antenna), thereby eliminating the need for reliance on efficient thermal conduction for heat dispersion beyond a few millimetres from the ablation probe, as is characteristic of RFA. Furthermore, the larger heating zone and higher temperatures theoretically translate towards less susceptibility to heat sink effects.[91] In initial small series, the use of microwave ablation (MWA) for primarily exophytic, biopsy-proven T1a RCC yielded 100% recurrence-free outcomes in the short term (median 6–11 months).[92,93] However, in 10 patients unselected for tumour size or location, with tumours ranging in size between 2.0 and 5.5 cm, Castle *et al.* reported a local recurrence rate of 38% after MWA at a mean follow-up of 17.9 months (range 14–24).[94] Furthermore MWA was associated with a 40% postoperative complication rate, including three Clavien IIIb complications in two patients.[94] These findings suggest that before the broader advantages of MWA over RFA can be realized, additional technological improvements are needed, and its current use should be considered investigational.

Irreversible electroporation

Irreversible electroporation (IRE) is a novel technique in which tissue ablation is created by the application of pulsatile, direct current high electrical voltages across cell membranes, resulting in membrane permeabilization by generation of 'nanopores'. Under certain electrical field conditions, the membrane permeabilization is reversible, a property exploited by several researchers over the past two decades for intracellular gene transfer and drug delivery.[95] Davalos *et al.* first described the ablative potential of IRE in 2005, which was previously regarded only as an undesirable side effect of reversible electroporation.[96] In animal experiments of renal ablation with IRE, it was found to create discrete ablation lesions with NADH-confirmed cellular non-viability, with sparing of blood vessels and the collecting system.[97,98] An interesting feature of IRE ablation is lesion resolution over time, thought to be related to absence of secondary ischaemia-related cell death in tissues within the ablation zone that results from small vessel destruction (e.g. as for the thermal modalities).[97,98] The potential clinical significance of this finding is presently unknown, and requires further investigation. In a recent phase I proof-of-concept clinical study, IRE was found to be safe in humans when performed with full muscle paralysis and electrocardiographic gating.[99]

Laser ablation

Although laser ablation has been successfully used for the ablation of malignant liver neoplasms for several years, only two studies to date have reported its use in renal tumour ablation.[100,101] The study by Dick *et al.* demonstrated only reduction in, but not loss of enhancing tumour volume during a mean follow-up of 16.9 (3–32) months following MR-guided Nd-YAG laser ablation; however no disease progression was observed.[100] More recently, Kariniemi *et al.* reported 100% recurrence-free outcomes during a mean follow-up of 20 (12–30) months in eight patients with 10 T1a RCC tumours who underwent laser ablation using an Nd-YAG laser.[101] Further evaluation in additional patients is warranted given these promising initial findings.

Conclusions

As the incidence of RCC continues to rise, with a preponderance of newly detected Stage 1 renal tumours, ablative therapies will play an increasingly important role among the management options for small renal masses. Emerging long-term data for RFA and CA suggest that treatment efficacy for these modalities is similar to that for extirpative surgical therapy. Pending further maturation of outcomes data, technological enhancements to improve efficacy for ablation of larger tumours, evaluation in diverse patient populations, better elucidation of patient selection criteria, improvements in techniques for detection and monitoring of recurrences and other considerations, their use presently remains restricted to elderly patients and/or patients with advanced co-morbidities who are poor surgical candidates. Emerging novel technologies demonstrate early potential to expand the renal ablative capabilities of energy-based ablative devices pending additional evaluation in experimental and clinical settings. Energy-based ablation carries a number of advantages over traditional surgical approaches, including lower morbidity, decreased technical demands, excellent preservation of post-treatment renal function and decreased cost. Future prospective randomized trials would be invaluable in better defining the clinical role of renal ablation in comparison to established alternative strategies.

Further reading

Altunrende F, Autorino R, Hillyer S, *et al.* Image guided percutaneous probe ablation for renal tumors in 65 solitary kidneys: functional and oncological outcomes. *J Urol* 2011; **186**(1):35–41.

Aron M, Kamoi K, Remer E, Berger A, Desai M, Gill I. Laparoscopic renal cryoablation: 8-year, single surgeon outcomes. *J Urol* 2010; **183**(3):889–95.

Best SL, Park SK, Yaacoub RF, *et al.* Long-term outcomes of renal tumor radio frequency ablation stratified by tumor diameter: size matters. *J Urol* 2012; **187**(4):1183–9.

Campbell SC, Novick AC, Belldegrun A, *et al.* Guideline for management of the clinical T1 renal mass. *J Urol* 2009; **182**(4):1271–9.

Hong K, Georgiades C. Radiofrequency ablation: mechanism of action and devices. *J Vasc Interv Radiol* 2010; **21**(Suppl 8):S179–86.

Lucas SM, Stern JM, Adibi M, Zeltser IS, Cadeddu JA, Raj GV. Renal function outcomes in patients treated for renal masses smaller than 4 cm by ablative and extirpative techniques. *J Urol* 2008; **179**(1):75–9; discussion 9–80.

Matin SF, Ahrar K, Cadeddu JA, *et al.* Residual and recurrent disease following renal energy ablative therapy: a multi-institutional study. *J Urol* 2006; **176**(5):1973–7.

Matin SF. Determining failure after renal ablative therapy for renal cell carcinoma: false-negative and false-positive imaging findings. *Urology* 2010; **75**(6):1254–7.

Olweny EO, Cadeddu JA. Novel methods for renal tissue ablation. *Curr Opin Urol* 2012; **22**(5):379–84.

Olweny EO, Park SK, Tan YK, Best SL, Trimmer C, Cadeddu JA. Radiofrequency ablation versus partial nephrectomy in patients with solitary clinical T1a renal cell carcinoma: Comparable oncologic outcomes at a minimum of 5 years of follow-up. *Eur Urol* 2012; **61**(6):1156–61.

Psutka SP, Feldman AS, McDougal WS, McGovern FJ, Mueller P, Gervais DA. Long-term oncologic outcomes after radiofrequency ablation for t1 renal cell carcinoma. *Eur Urol* 2013; **63**(3):486–92.

Strom KH, Derweesh I, Stroup SP, *et al.* Second prize: Recurrence rates after percutaneous and laparoscopic renal cryoablation of small renal masses: does the approach make a difference? *J Endourol* 2011; **25**(3):371–5.

Tanagho YS, Roytman TM, Bhayani SB, *et al.* Laparoscopic cryoablation of renal masses: single-center long-term experience. *Urology* 2012; **80**(2):307–15.

Tracy CR, Raman JD, Donnally C, Trimmer CK, Cadeddu JA. Durable oncologic outcomes after radiofrequency ablation: experience from treating 243 small renal masses over 7.5 years. *Cancer* 2010; **116**(13):3135–42.

Young EE, Castle SM, Gorbatiy V, Leveillee RJ. Comparison of safety, renal function outcomes and efficacy of laparoscopic and percutaneous radio frequency ablation of renal masses. *J Urol* 2012; **187**(4):1177–82.

Young JL, Clayman RV. Cryoprobe isotherms: a caveat and review. *J Endourol* 2010; **24**(5):673–6.

Zagoria RJ, Pettus JA, Rogers M, Werle DM, Childs D, Leyendecker JR. Long-term outcomes after percutaneous radiofrequency ablation for renal cell carcinoma. *Urology* 2011; **77**(6):1393–7.

References

1. Best SL, Park SK, Yaacoub RF, *et al.* Long-term outcomes of renal tumor radio frequency ablation stratified by tumor diameter: size matters. *J Urol* 2012; **187**(4):1183–9.
2. Lehman DS, Hruby GW, Phillips CK, McKiernan JM, Benson MC, Landman J. First Prize (tie): Laparoscopic renal cryoablation: efficacy and complications for larger renal masses. *J Endourol* 2008; **22**(6):1123–7.
3. Campbell SC, Novick AC, Belldegrun A, *et al.* Guideline for management of the clinical T1 renal mass. *J Urol* 2009; **182**(4):1271–9.
4. Faddegon S, Cadeddu JA. Does renal mass ablation provide adequate long-term oncologic control? *Urol Clin North Am* 2012; **39**(2):181–90.
5. Graversen JA, Mues AC, Landman J. Laparoscopic ablation of renal neoplasms. *J Endourol* 2011; **25**(2):187–94.
6. Karam JA, Ahrar K, Matin SF. Ablation of kidney tumors. *Surg Oncol Clin N Am* 2011; **20**(2):341–53, viii.
7. Stern JM, Svatek R, Park S, *et al.* Intermediate comparison of partial nephrectomy and radiofrequency ablation for clinical T1a renal tumours. *BJU Int* 2007; **100**(2):287–90.
8. Mues AC, Landman J. Results of kidney tumor cryoablation: renal function preservation and oncologic efficacy. *World J Urol* 2010; **28**(5):565–70.
9. Raman JD, Hall DW, Cadeddu JA. Renal ablative therapy: radiofrequency ablation and cryoablation. *J Surg Oncol* 2009; **100**(8):639–44.
10. Jayson M, Sanders H. Increased incidence of serendipitously discovered renal cell carcinoma. *Urology* 1998; **51**(2):203–5.
11. Russo P. Should elective partial nephrectomy be performed for renal cell carcinoma >4 cm in size? *Nat Clin Pract Urol* 2008; **5**(9):482–3.
12. Thompson RH, Kurta JM, Kaag M, *et al.* Tumor size is associated with malignant potential in renal cell carcinoma cases. *J Urol* 2009; **181**(5):2033–6.
13. Frank I, Blute ML, Cheville JC, Lohse CM, Weaver AL, Zincke H. Solid renal tumors: an analysis of pathological features related to tumor size. *J Urol* 2003; **170**(6 Pt 1):2217–20.
14. Cutress ML, Ratan HL, Williams ST, O'Brien MF. Update on the management of T1 renal cortical tumours. *BJU Int* 2010; **106**(8):1130–6.
15. Desai MM, Aron M, Gill IS. Laparoscopic partial nephrectomy versus laparoscopic cryoablation for the small renal tumor. *Urology* 2005; **66**(Suppl 5):23–8.
16. Shingleton WB, Sewell PE Jr. Cryoablation of renal tumours in patients with solitary kidneys. *BJU Int* 2003; **92**(3):237–9.
17. Raman JD, Thomas J, Lucas SM, *et al.* Radiofrequency ablation for T1a tumors in a solitary kidney: promising intermediate oncologic and renal function outcomes. *Can J Urol* 2008; **15**(2):3980–5.
18. D'Arsonval MA. Action physiologique des courants alternatifs. *C R Soc Biol* 1891; **43**:283–6.

19. Bovie WT, Cushing H. Electrosurgery as an aid to the removal of intracranial tumors with a preliminary note on a new surgical-current generator. *Surg Gynecol Obstet* 1928; **47**:751–84.
20. McGahan JP, Browning PD, Brock JM, Tesluk H. Hepatic ablation using radiofrequency electrocautery. *Invest Radiol* 1990; **25**(3):267–70.
21. Rossi S, Fornari F, Pathies C, Buscarini L. Thermal lesions induced by 480 KHz localized current field in guinea pig and pig liver. *Tumori* 1990; **76**(1):54–7.
22. McGahan JP, Scheider P, Brock JM, Teslik H. Treatment of liver tumors by percutaneous radiofrequency electrocautery. *Semin Intervent Radiol* 1993; **10**(2):143–9.
23. Zlotta AR, Wildschutz T, Raviv G, *et al.* Radiofrequency interstitial tumor ablation (RITA) is a possible new modality for treatment of renal cancer: ex vivo and in vivo experience. *J Endourol* 1997; **11**(4):251–8.
24. Hong K, Georgiades C. Radiofrequency ablation: mechanism of action and devices. *J Vasc Interv Radiol* 2010; **21**(Suppl 8):S179–86.
25. Rossi S, Buscarini E, Garbagnati F, *et al.* Percutaneous treatment of small hepatic tumors by an expandable RF needle electrode. *AJR Am J Roentgenol* 1998; **170**(4):1015–22.
26. Goldberg SN, Gazelle GS, Solbiati L, Rittman WJ, Mueller PR. Radiofrequency tissue ablation: increased lesion diameter with a perfusion electrode. *Acad Radiol* 1996; **3**(8):636–44.
27. Carey RI, Leveillee RJ. First prize: direct real-time temperature monitoring for laparoscopic and CT-guided radiofrequency ablation of renal tumors between 3 and 5 cm. *J Endourol* 2007; **21**(8):807–13.
28. Pusey WA. The use of carbon dioxide snow in the treatment of nevi and other lesions of the skin. *J Am Med Assoc* 1907; **49**:1354–6.
29. White AC. Possibilities of liquid air to the physician. *JAMA* 1901; **198**:426–8.
30. Allington HV. Liquid nitrogen in the treatment of skin diseases. *Calif Med* 1950; **72**:153–5.
31. Levy D, Avallone A, Jones JS. Current state of urological cryosurgery: prostate and kidney. *BJU Int* 2010; **105**(5):590–600.
32. Uchida M, Imaide Y, Sugimoto K, Uehara H, Watanabe H. Percutaneous cryosurgery for renal tumours. *Br J Urol* 1995 Feb;75(2):132–6; discussion 6–7.
33. Onik G, Cooper C, Goldberg HI, Moss AA, Rubinsky B, Christianson M. Ultrasonic characteristics of frozen liver. *Cryobiology* 1984; **21**(3):321–8.
34. Onik G, Gilbert J, Hoddick W, *et al.* Sonographic monitoring of hepatic cryosurgery in an experimental animal model. *AJR Am J Roentgenol* 1985 May;**144**(5):1043–7.
35. Rewcastle JC, Sandison GA, Saliken JC, Donnelly BJ, McKinnon JG. Considerations during clinical operation of two commercially available cryomachines. *J Surg Oncol* 1999; **71**(2):106–11.
36. Autorino R, Haber GP, White MA, Stein RJ, Kaouk JH. New developments in renal focal therapy. *J Endourol* 2010; **24**(5):665–72.
37. Laguna MP, Beemster P, Kumar V, *et al.* Perioperative morbidity of laparoscopic cryoablation of small renal masses with ultrathin probes: a European multicentre experience. *Eur Urol* 2009; **56**(2):355–61.
38. Hoffmann NE, Bischof JC. The cryobiology of cryosurgical injury. *Urology* 2002; **60**(2 Suppl 1):40–9.
39. Lovelock JE. The haemolysis of human red blood-cells by freezing and thawing. *Biochim Biophys Acta* 1953; **10**(3):414–26.
40. Kahlenberg MS, Volpe C, Klippenstein DL, Penetrante RB, Petrelli NJ, Rodriguez-Bigas MA. Clinicopathologic effects of cryotherapy on hepatic vessels and bile ducts in a porcine model. *Ann Surg Oncol* 1998; **5**(8):713–8.
41. Weber SM, Lee FT Jr, Chinn DO, Warner T, Chosy SG, Mahvi DM. Perivascular and intralesional tissue necrosis after hepatic cryoablation: results in a porcine model. *Surgery* 1997; **122**(4):742–7.
42. Breda A, Lam JS, Riggs S, *et al.* In vivo efficacy of laparoscopic assisted percutaneous renal cryotherapy: evidence based guidelines for the practicing urologist. *J Urol* 2008; **179**(1):333–7.
43. Young JL, Clayman RV. Cryoprobe isotherms: a caveat and review. *J Endourol* 2010; **24**(5):673–6.
44. Badwan K, Maxwell K, Venkatesh R, *et al.* Comparison of laparoscopic and percutaneous cryoablation of renal tumors: a cost analysis. *J Endourol* 2008; **22**(6):1275–7.
45. Gill IS, Novick AC. Renal cryosurgery. *Urology* 1999; **54**(2):215–9.
46. Gill W, Fraser J, Carter DC. Repeated freeze-thaw cycles in cryosurgery. *Nature* 1968; **219**(5152):410–3.
47. Campbell SC, Krishnamurthi V, Chow G, Hale J, Myles J, Novick AC. Renal cryosurgery: experimental evaluation of treatment parameters. *Urology* 1998; **52**(1):29–33; discussion 33–4.
48. Rukstalis DB, Khorsandi M, Garcia FU, Hoenig DM, Cohen JK. Clinical experience with open renal cryoablation. *Urology* 2001; **57**(1):34–9.
49. Woolley ML, Schulsinger DA, Durand DB, Zeltser IS, Waltzer WC. Effect of freezing parameters (freeze cycle and thaw process) on tissue destruction following renal cryoablation. *J Endourol* 2002; **16**(7):519–22.
50. White WM, Kaouk JH. Ablative therapy for renal tumors: In: Walsh PC, Retik AB, Stamey TA, Vaughan ED (eds). *Campbell's Urology*, 10th edition. Philadelphia, PA: WB Saunders Co, 2012.
51. Auge BK, Santa-Cruz RW, Polascik TJ. Effect of freeze time during renal cryoablation: a swine model. *J Endourol* 2006; **20**(12):1101–5.
52. Matin SF. Determining failure after renal ablative therapy for renal cell carcinoma: false-negative and false-positive imaging findings. *Urology* 2010; **75**(6):1254–7.
53. Klingler HC, Marberger M, Mauermann J, Remzi M, Susani M. 'Skipping' is still a problem with radiofrequency ablation of small renal tumours. *BJU Int* 2007; **99**(5):998–1001.
54. Lin CH, Moinzadeh A, Ramani AP, Gill IS. Histopathologic confirmation of complete cancer-cell kill in excised specimens after renal cryotherapy. *Urology* 2004; **64**(3):590.
55. Matlaga BR, Zagoria RJ, Woodruff RD, Torti FM, Hall MC. Phase II trial of radio frequency ablation of renal cancer: evaluation of the kill zone. *J Urol* 2002; **168**(6):2401–5.
56. Michaels MJ, Rhee HK, Mourtzinos AP, Summerhayes IC, Silverman ML, Libertino JA. Incomplete renal tumor destruction using radio frequency interstitial ablation. *J Urol* 2002; **168**(6):2406–9; discussion 9–10.
57. Raman JD, Stern JM, Zeltser I, Kabbani W, Cadeddu JA. Absence of viable renal carcinoma in biopsies performed more than 1 year following radio frequency ablation confirms reliability of axial imaging. *J Urol* 2008; **179**(6):2142–5.
58. Rendon RA, Kachura JR, Sweet JM, *et al.* The uncertainty of radio frequency treatment of renal cell carcinoma: findings at immediate and delayed nephrectomy. *J Urol* 2002; **167**(4):1587–92.
59. Weight CJ, Kaouk JH, Hegarty NJ, *et al.* Correlation of radiographic imaging and histopathology following cryoablation and radio frequency ablation for renal tumors. *J Urol* 2008; **179**(4):1277–81; discussion 81–3.
60. Matin SF, Ahrar K, Cadeddu JA, *et al.* Residual and recurrent disease following renal energy ablative therapy: a multi-institutional study. *J Urol* 2006; **176**(5):1973–7.
61. Levinson AW, Su LM, Agarwal D, *et al.* Long-term oncological and overall outcomes of percutaneous radio frequency ablation in high risk surgical patients with a solitary small renal mass. *J Urol* 2008 Aug;**180**(2):499–504; discussion
62. McDougal WS, Gervais DA, McGovern FJ, Mueller PR. Long-term followup of patients with renal cell carcinoma treated with radio frequency ablation with curative intent. *J Urol* 2005; **174**(1):61–3.
63. Olweny EO, Park SK, Tan YK, Best SL, Trimmer C, Cadeddu JA. Radiofrequency ablation versus partial nephrectomy in patients with solitary clinical T1a renal cell carcinoma: Comparable oncologic outcomes at a minimum of 5 years of follow-up. *Eur Urol* 2012; **61**(6):1156–61.
64. Psutka SP, Feldman AS, McDougal WS, McGovern FJ, Mueller P, Gervais DA. Long-term oncologic outcomes after radiofrequency ablation for t1 renal cell carcinoma. *Eur Urol* 2013; **63**(3):486–92.
65. Tracy CR, Raman JD, Donnally C, Trimmer CK, Cadeddu JA. Durable oncologic outcomes after radiofrequency ablation: experience

from treating 243 small renal masses over 7.5 years. *Cancer* 2010; **116**(13):3135–42.

66. Zagoria RJ, Pettus JA, Rogers M, Werle DM, Childs D, Leyendecker JR. Long-term outcomes after percutaneous radiofrequency ablation for renal cell carcinoma. *Urology* 2011; **77**(6):1393–7.
67. Aron M, Kamoi K, Remer E, Berger A, Desai M, Gill I. Laparoscopic renal cryoablation: 8-year, single surgeon outcomes. *J Urol* 2010; **183**(3):889–95.
68. Guazzoni G, Cestari A, Buffi N, *et al.* Oncologic results of laparoscopic renal cryoablation for clinical T1a tumors: 8 years of experience in a single institution. *Urology* 2010; **76**(3):624–9.
69. Tanagho YS, Roytman TM, Bhayani SB, *et al.* Laparoscopic cryoablation of renal masses: single-center long-term experience. *Urology* 2012; **80**(2):307–15.
70. Guillotreau J, Haber GP, Autorino R, *et al.* Robotic partial nephrectomy versus laparoscopic cryoablation for the small renal mass. *Eur Urol* 2012; **61**(5):899–904.
71. Klatte T, Grubmuller B, Waldert M, Weibl P, Remzi M. Laparoscopic cryoablation versus partial nephrectomy for the treatment of small renal masses: systematic review and cumulative analysis of observational studies. *Eur Urol* 2011; **60**(3):435–43.
72. Young EE, Castle SM, Gorbatiy V, Leveillee RJ. Comparison of safety, renal function outcomes and efficacy of laparoscopic and percutaneous radio frequency ablation of renal masses. *J Urol* 2012; **187**(4):1177–82.
73. Strom KH, Derweesh I, Stroup SP, *et al.* Second prize: Recurrence rates after percutaneous and laparoscopic renal cryoablation of small renal masses: does the approach make a difference? *J Endourol* 2011; **25**(3):371–5.
74. Finley DS, Beck S, Box G, *et al.* Percutaneous and laparoscopic cryoablation of small renal masses. *J Urol* 2008; **180**(2):492–8; discussion 8.
75. Hui GC, Tuncali K, Tatli S, Morrison PR, Silverman SG. Comparison of percutaneous and surgical approaches to renal tumor ablation: metaanalysis of effectiveness and complication rates. *J Vasc Interv Radiol* 2008; **19**(9):1311–20.
76. Warlick CA, Lima GC, Allaf ME, *et al.* Clinical sequelae of radiographic iceball involvement of collecting system during computed tomography-guided percutaneous renal tumor cryoablation. *Urology* 2006; **67**(5):918–22.
77. Janzen NK, Perry KT, Han KR, *et al.* The effects of intentional cryoablation and radio frequency ablation of renal tissue involving the collecting system in a porcine model. *J Urol* 2005; **173**(4):1368–74.
78. Brashears JH 3rd, Raj GV, Crisci A, *et al.* Renal cryoablation and radio frequency ablation: an evaluation of worst case scenarios in a porcine model. *J Urol* 2005; **173**(6):2160–5.
79. Weizer AZ, Raj GV, O'Connell M, Robertson CN, Nelson RC, Polascik TJ. Complications after percutaneous radiofrequency ablation of renal tumors. *Urology* 2005; **66**(6):1176–80.
80. Bourne AE, Kramer BA, Steiner HL, Schwartz BF. Renal insufficiency is not a contraindication for cryoablation of small renal masses. *J Endourol* 2009; **23**(7):1195–8.
81. Gill IS, Remer EM, Hasan WA, *et al.* Renal cryoablation: outcome at 3 years. *J Urol* 2005; **173**(6):1903–7.
82. Altunrende F, Autorino R, Hillyer S, *et al.* Image guided percutaneous probe ablation for renal tumors in 65 solitary kidneys: functional and oncological outcomes. *J Urol* 2011; **186**(1):35–41.
83. Pettus JA, Werle DM, Saunders W, *et al.* Percutaneous radiofrequency ablation does not affect glomerular filtration rate. *J Endourol* 2010; **24**(10):1687–91.
84. Johnson DB, Taylor GD, Lotan Y, Sagalowsky AI, Koenemann KS, Cadeddu JA. The effects of radio frequency ablation on renal function and blood pressure. *J Urol* 2003; **170**(6 Pt 1):2234–6.
85. Malcolm JB, Logan JE, Given RW, *et al.* Renal functional outcomes after cryoablation of small renal masses. *J Endourol* 2010; **24**(3):479–82.
86. Raman JD, Raj GV, Lucas SM, *et al.* Renal functional outcomes for tumours in a solitary kidney managed by ablative or extirpative techniques. *BJU Int* 2010; **105**(4):496–500.
87. Lucas SM, Stern JM, Adibi M, Zeltser IS, Cadeddu JA, Raj GV. Renal function outcomes in patients treated for renal masses smaller than 4 cm by ablative and extirpative techniques. *J Urol* 2008; **179**(1):75–9; discussion 9–80.
88. Olweny EO, Cadeddu JA. Novel methods for renal tissue ablation. *Curr Opin Urol* 2012; **22**(5):379–84.
89. Neuhaus J, Blachut L, Rabenalt R, *et al.* Efficiency analysis of bipolar and multipolar radiofrequency ablation in an in vivo porcine kidney model using three-dimensional reconstruction of histologic section series. *J Endourol* 2011; **25**(5):859–67.
90. Okhunov Z, Roy O, Duty B, *et al.* Clinical evaluation of a novel bipolar radiofrequency ablation system for renal masses. *BJU Int* 2012; **110**(5):688–91.
91. Simon CJ, Dupuy DE, Mayo-Smith WW. Microwave ablation: principles and applications. *Radiographics* 2005; **25**(Suppl 1):S69–83.
92. Carrafiello G, Mangini M, Fontana F, *et al.* Single-antenna microwave ablation under contrast-enhanced ultrasound guidance for treatment of small renal cell carcinoma: preliminary experience. *Cardiovasc Intervent Radiol* 2010; **33**(2):367–74.
93. Liang P, Wang Y, Zhang D, Yu X, Gao Y, Ni X. Ultrasound guided percutaneous microwave ablation for small renal cancer: initial experience. *J Urol* 2008; **180**(3):844–8; discussion 8.
94. Castle SM, Salas N, Leveillee RJ. Initial experience using microwave ablation therapy for renal tumor treatment: 18-month follow-up. *Urology* 2011; **77**(4):792–7.
95. Rubinsky B. Irreversible electroporation in medicine. *Technol Cancer Res Treat* 2007; **6**(4):255–60.
96. Davalos RV, Mir IL, Rubinsky B. Tissue ablation with irreversible electroporation. *Ann Biomed Eng* 2005; **33**(2):223–31.
97. Deodhar A, Monette S, Single GW Jr, *et al.* Renal tissue ablation with irreversible electroporation: preliminary results in a porcine model. *Urology* 2011; **77**(3):754–60.
98. Tracy CR, Kabbani W, Cadeddu JA. Irreversible electroporation (IRE): a novel method for renal tissue ablation. *BJU Int* 2011; **107**(12):1982–7.
99. Pech M, Janitzky A, Wendler JJ, *et al.* Irreversible electroporation of renal cell carcinoma: a first-in-man phase I clinical study. *Cardiovasc Intervent Radiol* 2011; **34**(1):132–8.
100. Dick EA, Joarder R, De Jode MG, Wragg P, Vale JA, Gedroyc WM. Magnetic resonance imaging-guided laser thermal ablation of renal tumours. *BJU Int* 2002; **90**(9):814–22.
101. Kariniemi J, Ojala R, Hellstrom P, Sequeiros RB. MRI-guided percutaneous laser ablation of small renal cell carcinoma: Initial clinical experience. *Acta Radiol* 2010; **51**(4):467–72.

CHAPTER 6.31

Kidney cancer
Treatment of locally advanced and low volume metastatic disease

Tim O'Brien and Amit Patel

Locally advanced renal cell cancer

Venous involvement

Macroscopic invasion of the renal vein or inferior vena cava is seen in approximately 5–10% of patients undergoing nephrectomy.[1,2] Suspicion should be raised in patients with clinical signs of venous obstruction (e.g. varicocoele, lower limb swelling, or dilated abdominal veins). Shortness of breath is usually seen if extension into the right atrium has occurred.

The cephalad extension of venous thrombus is now classified into three stages (TNM 2010)[3]: stage 3a, into renal vein; 3b, extension into the inferior vena cava (IVC) below the diaphragm; 3c, extension above the diaphragm. Many authorities advocate MRI as the best technique both for assessing tumour extent and for assessing the risk of venous wall invasion.[4,5] Modern multiplanar computed tomography (CT) imaging is also very accurate. MRI and CT have replaced the need for invasive venocavography. Preoperative emobolization on the renal artery can be performed however Subramanian *et al.* found that this did not significantly reduce blood loss or complications from nephrectomy.[6]

A number of different incisions can be employed dependent on the cephalad extent of the thrombus and the size of the primary tumour (see Fig. 6.31.1 for thrombus level). Level 1 or 2 thrombus is usually best approached through an abdominal incision (i.e. Subcostal, Mercedes, Chevron). Traditional nephrectomy techniques suffice for level 1 as long as ligation of the renal vein is confirmed to be clear of the tumour thrombus. A Satinsky clamp 'side-swiping' the IVC allows division of the renal vein at its ostium. Level 2 thrombus often requires clamping of the IVC above and below the thrombus and control of the contralateral renal vein. Mobilization of the right lobe of the liver aids access as does division of small branches to the caudate lobe. If the thrombus is free floating the renal ostium is opened and thrombus removed. If the thrombus is adherent en bloc excision of part of or all of the IVC may be required with patching or grafting of the IVC (see Fig. 6.31.2.). Veno-veno bypass may be utilized to maintain the circulation when grafting is required.[7]

Level 3 thrombus requires extensive dissection and mobilization of adjacent organs. Access is often best achieved with a chevron and/or sternotomy incision. If thrombus can be milked back into the subdiaphragmatic IVC then the techniques employed in high level 2 thrombus may suffice but usually cardiopulmonary bypass and hypothermic circulatory arrest is the preferred option to allow extraction of the tumour in a contolled fashion from the IVC and right atrium. Twenty minutes of circulatory arrest at a temperature of 22°C seems to be associated with a very low chance of neurological sequelae. Bypass techniques require anticoagulation and post surgical coagulopathy is a real risk.

Around 40% of tumours with venous extension can be cured with aggressive surgical management alone.[8–9] If lymph nodes are involved or if the vein wall is directly invaded then the prognosis is worse.[10] Most authors agree that the higher the thrombus in the IVC the worse the prognosis.[9–14]

Regional lymph nodes

The role of lymphadenectomy in renal cell cancer (RCC) remains controversial. In a classic study Robson *et al.* showing 22.7% of lymph nodes to be positive in nephrectomy specimens but the lymphadenectomy appeared to add no survival benefit.[15] A European Organisation for Research and Treatment of Cancer (EORTC) randomized trial showed little added morbidity from lymphadenectomy for clinical N0 patients but no benefit was seen in oncological outcome.[16]

When nodes are obviously involved more distant metastases are often present and this may explain why lymphadenectomy in this scenario is thought to be rarely beneficial. Conversely, Canfield *et al.* performed lymphadenectomy in 54 patients with clinical node positive, non-metastatic disease with a median survival of 20.3 months.[17] In the absence of a randomized trial in this particular scenario, the true benefits in oncological outcome cannot be confirmed. The advantages may lie in targeting these patients for trials of adjuvant treatment and for better estimates of prognosis.

Adjacent organ infiltration

Pathological infiltration of adjacent organs represents 2% of surgical cases.[18] On the left this may be spleen, colon, adrenal, pancreas, or duodenum; and on the right, adrenal, colon, liver, or duodenum. These patients often present with pain from infiltration of the posterior abdominal wall and paraspinous muscles. Direct infiltration of the liver is often suspected from preoperative imaging but rarely confirmed at surgery. In the absence of metastasis, en bloc resection of the kidney and adjacent infiltrated organs is usually indicated but outcomes remain poor: Karellas *et al.* demonstrated that 90%

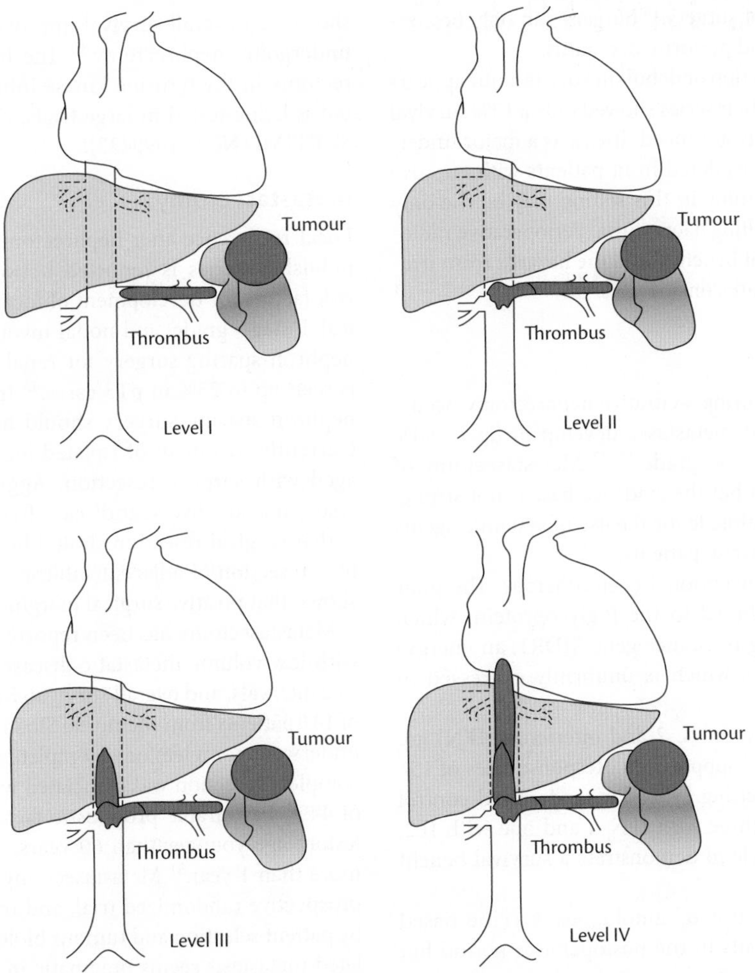

Fig. 6.31.1 The Mayo classification of macroscopic venous invasion in renal cell carcinoma. Level I: tumour thrombus is either at the entry of the renal vein or within the inferior vena cava (IVC). Level II: thrombus extends within the IVC >2 cm above the confluence of the renal vein and IVC but still remains below the hepatic veins. Level III: thrombus involves the intrahepatic IVC. The size of the thrombus ranges from a narrow tail that extends into the IVC to one that fills the lumen and enlarges the IVC. Level IV: thrombus extends above the diaphragm or into the right atrium.

Reprinted from *European Urology*, Volume 52, Issue 3, Ziya Kirkali and Hein Van Poppel, 'A Critical Analysis of Surgery for Kidney Cancer with Vena Cava Invasion', pp. 658–662, Copyright © 2007 European Association of Urology, with permission from Elsevier, http://www.sciencedirect.com/science/journal/03022838

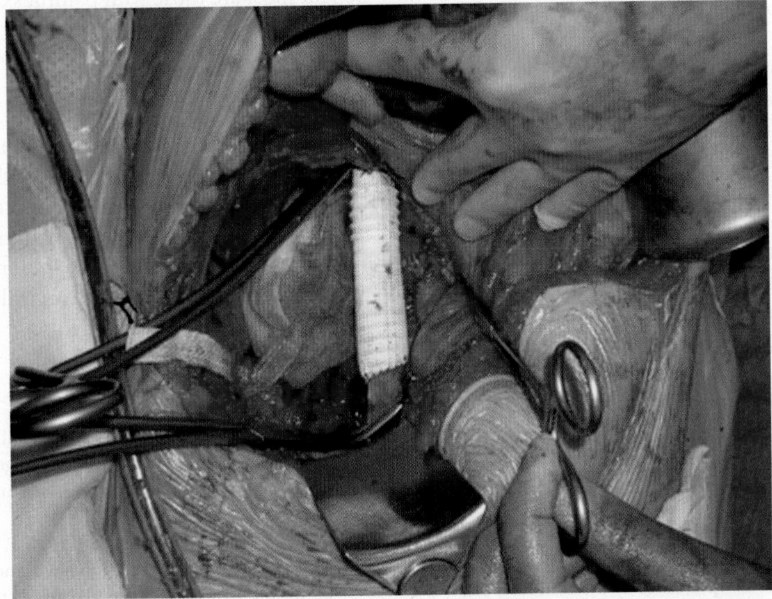

Fig. 6.31.2 En bloc resection and grafting of the inferior vena cava.

recurred within 12 months of surgery.[18] Surgery can only be considered in patients with a good performance status.

The role of incomplete resection or debulking of a tumour appears limited. De Kernion *et al.* in their series showed only a 12% survival at 1 year.[19] Resection of locally advanced disease is a major undertaking and should only be considered in fit patients with curative intent. Occasionally nephrectomy in this setting may be the only satisfactory method of controlling haematuria. Perioperative radiotherapy is not thought to be of benefit[20] and the hazards from irradiating adjacent small bowel are considerable.

Adjuvant therapy

Isolated local recurrence following a curative nephrectomy occurs in only 2–5% of patients but metastases develop in up to 50% depending on primary stage and grade.[21–22] Metastasectomy of single metastases is an option but the evidence base is not strong. Thus, there is a convincing rationale for the use of systemic agents in the adjuvant setting in high-risk patients.

RCC is not sensitive to conventional chemotherapy. The poor response rate has been attributed to the P-glycoprotein, which is a product of the multidrug resistance gene MDR1, an energy-dependant drug efflux pump, which is uniformly expressed in RCCs.[23]

Immunotherapy in the form of IL-2 and interferon (IFN) are thought to be active in tumour suppression. Response rates of 15–20% have been seen in this setting.[24,25] Four randomized control trials have been performed, three with IFN-α and one with IL2. None of these studies were able to demonstrate a survival benefit from immunotherapy.[26–29]

There has been work in use of autologous vaccine-based approaches to vaccinate patients in the postoperative period but with no success. The Oncophage trial reported no benefit.[30]

Currently trials investigating the use of targeted molegular agents such as the tyrosine kinase inhibitors and m-TOR inihibitors are under investigation in the adjuvant setting.

Cytoreduction

In the era of multimodal therapy, the role of cytoreductive nephrectomy continues to be explored. It is thought that a bulky primary tumour might inhibit the immune system which is critical for innate mechanisms to combat tumours. There have been rare, well described instances of disease regression of metastatic deposits after nephrectomy[31–34] and pre-clinical data suggests large primary tumours may inhibit T-cell function.[35,36] Systemic agents such as cytokines may also be less effective in the presence of a large primary tumour.[37]

The potential immune benefits of a cytoreductive nephrectomy have to be set against the morbidity and occasional mortality from the procedure and the potential delay to the delivery of systemic therapy. Nephrectomy alone in the context of metastatic disease is not thought to improve outcomes. A further concern about patients managed with cytoreductive intent is that many patients may never receive the planned systemic treatment: a review of patients who underwent nephrectomy and proposed IL-2 therapy showed only 55% of patients received the adjuvant treatment. Surgical morbidity and rapid disease progression were common factors for failure of delivery.[38] The SWOG 8949 trial, examining interferon-α-2b alone versus cytoreductive nephrectomy and interferon-α-2b showed an overall survival improvement of 3 months in the arm undergoing nephrectomy.[39] The benefit of cytoreductive nephrectomy in the tyrosine kinase inhibitor (TKI) era is not known, but is being tested in large trials, CARMENA (NCT00930033) & SURTIME(NCT01099423).

Metastasectomy

Local recurrence after nephrectomy remains a rare event and in published series is reported between 2–4%.[40–44] The strongest risk factors for development of local recurrence appear to be clinical T-stage, grade, and nodal involvement. Recurrence following nephron-sparing surgery for renal cancer is more common and is seen up to 25% in pT3 cases.[45] Intrarenal recurrence following nephron-sparing surgery should be treated as *de novo* tumour. Currently treatment of isolated local recurrence should be managed with surgical resection. Aggressive surgical resection can result in a 30% five-year disease-free survival.[42–43,46–49] The caveat is that surgical resection should be radical and complete with en bloc resection of adjacent/infiltrated organs as these studies have shown that positive surgical margins lead to poorer outcomes.[46,50.]

Metastasectomy has been reported by several groups in patients with low volume metastatic disease, showing favourable disease-free intervals, and overall survival. Kavolius *et al.* published a series of 141 patients from Memorial Sloan Kettering Cancer Center, who underwent complete or incomplete metastasectomy. In this series complete resection was associated with a five-year overall survival of 44%. Favourable prognostic factors were a solitary metastatic lesion, age younger than 60 years, and a disease-free interval of more than 1 year.[51] Metastasectomy has not been considered in a prospective randomized trial, and reported series could be biased by patient selection and tumour biology. However, resection of isolated metastasis seems pragmatic in patients with reasonable performance status.

Palliative surgery

In some patients who are heavily symptomatic, palliative nephrectomy can be performed. Disappointingly not all paraneoplastic manifestations will improve post operatively. Patients who seem to benefit most are those with painful skeletal metastases managed by excision and prosthetics.

Conclusions

Surgery remains the main therapeutic option for patients with locally advanced disease and those with symptomatic renal tumours with low volume metastases. Clinical trials are currently evaluating the efficacy of surgery in combination with modern systemic therapy (such as the tyrosine kinase inhibitors and m-TOR inihibitors). Careful patient selection and surgical team experience are vital to obtain the best results for patients.

Further reading

Blute ML, Leibovich BC, Lohse CM, Cheville JC, Zincke H. The Mayo Clinic experience with surgical management, complications and outcome for patients with renal cell carcinoma and venous tumour thrombus. *BJU Int* 2004; **94**:33–41.

Canfield SE, Kamat AM, Sánchez-Ortiz RF, Detry M, Swanson DA, Wood CG. Wood renal cell carcinoma with nodal metastases in the absence of distant metastatic disease (clinical stage TxN1–2M0): The impact of aggressive surgical resection on patient outcome. *J Urol* 2006; **175**(3):864–9.

Hatcher PA, Anderson EE, Paulson DF, Carson CC, Robertson JE. Surgical management and prognosis of renal cell carcinoma invading the vena cava. *J Urol* 1991; **145**(1):20–3; discussion 23–4.

Kavolius JP, Mastorakos DP, Pavlovich C, *et al.* Resection of metastatic renal cell carcinoma. *J Clin Oncol* 1998; **16**:2261–6.

Kirkali Z, Van Poppel H. A critical analysis of surgery for kidney cancer with vena cava invasion. *Eur Urol* 2007; **52**(3):658–62.

Leibovich BC, Cheville JC, Lohse CM, *et al.* A scoring algorithm to predict survival for patients with metastatic clear cell renal cell carcinoma: A stratification tool for prospective clinical trials. *J Urol* 2005; **174**:1759–63.

Leibovich BC, Cheville JC, Lohse CM, *et al.* Cancer specific survival for patients with pT3 renal cell carcinoma-can the 2002 primary tumor classification be improved? *J Urol* 2005; **173**:716–9.

Marcus SG, Choyke PL, Reiter R, *et al.* Regression of metastatic renal cell carcinoma after cytoreductive nephrectomy. *J Urol* 1993; **150**:463–6.

Marshall FF. Renal cell carcinoma: surgical management or regional lymph nodes and inferior vena cava tumour thrombus. *Semina Surg Oncol* 1988; **4**:129–32.

Middleton Jr AW. Indications for and results of nephrectomy for metastatic renal cell carcinoma. *Urol Clin North Am* 1980; **7**:711–17.

Schrodter S, Hakenberg OW, Manseck A, Leike S, Wirth MP. Outcome of surgical treatment of isolated local recurrence after radical nephrectomy for renal cell carcinoma. *J Urol* 2002; **167**(4):1630–3.

Wagner B, Patard JJ, Méjean A, *et al.* Prognostic value of renal vein and inferior vena cava involvement in renal cell carcinoma. *Eur Urol* 2009; **55**:452–60.

Wiesner C, Jakse G, Rohde D. Therapy of local recurrence of renal cell carcinoma. *Oncol Rep* 2002; **9**:189–92.

References

1. Leibovich BC, Cheville JC, Lohse CM, *et al.* A scoring algorithm to predict survival for patients with metastatic clear cell renal cell carcinoma: A stratification tool for prospective clinical trials. *J Urol* 2005; **174**:1759–63.
2. Marshall FF. Renal cell carcinoma: surgical management or regional lymph nodes and inferior vena cava tumour thrombus. *Semina Surg Oncol* 1988; **4**:129–32.
3. Sobin LH, Gospodarowicz MK, Wittekind C, International Union against Cancer. *TNM Classification of Malignant Tumours*. Chichester, UK: Wiley-Blackwell, 2010.
4. Kallman DA, King BF, Hattery RR, *et al.* Renal vein and inferior vena cava tumor thrombus in renal cell carcinoma: CT, US, MRI and venacavography. *J Comput Assist Tomogr* 1992; **16**:240–7.
5. Oto A, Herts BR, Remer EM, Novick AC. Inferior vena cava tumor thrombus in renal cell carcinoma: staging by MR imaging and impact on surgical treatment. *AJR Am J Roentgenol* 1998; **171**:1619–24.
6. Subramanian VS, Stephenson AJ, Goldfarb DA, Fergany AF, Novick AC, Krishnamurthi V. Utility of preoperative renal artery embolization for management of renal tumors with inferior vena caval thrombi. *Urology* 2009; **74**(1):154–9.
7. Kirkali Z, Van Poppel H. A critical analysis of surgery for kidney cancer with vena cava invasion. *Eur Urol* 2007; **52**(3):658–62.
8. Blute ML, Leibovich BC, Lohse CM, Cheville JC, Zincke H. The Mayo Clinic experience with surgical management, complications and outcome for patients with renal cell carcinoma and venous tumour thrombus. *BJU Int* 2004; **94**:33–41.
9. Zisman A, Wieder JA, Pantuck AJ, *et al.* Renal cell carcinoma with tumor thrombus extension: biology, role of nephrectomy and response to immunotherapy. *J Urol* 2003; **169**(3):909–16.
10. Hatcher PA, Anderson EE, Paulson DF, Carson CC, Robertson JE. Surgical management and prognosis of renal cell carcinoma invading the vena cava. *J Urol* 1991; **145**(1):20–3; discussion 23–4.
11. Pantuck AJ, Zisman A, Dorey F, *et al.* Renal cell carcinoma with retroperitoneal lymph nodes. *Cancer* 2003; **97**:2995–3002.
12. Leibovich BC, Cheville JC, Lohse CM, *et al.* Cancer specific survival for patients with pT3 renal cell carcinoma-can the 2002 primary tumor classification be improved? *J Urol* 2005; **173**:716–9.
13. Kim HL, Zisman A, Han KR, *et al.* Prognostic significance of venous thrombus in renal cell carcinoma. Are renal vein and inferior vena cava involvement different? *J Urol* 2004; **171**: 588–91.
14. Wagner B, Patard JJ, Méjean A, *et al.* Prognostic value of renal vein and inferior vena cava involvement in renal cell carcinoma. *Eur Urol* 2009; **55**:452–60.
15. Robson CJ, Churchill BM, Anderson W. The results of radical nephrectomy for renal cell carcinoma. *J Urol* 1969; **101**:297–301.
16. Blom JH, van Poppel H, Marechal JM, *et al.* Radical nephrectomy with and without lymph node dissection: preliminary results of the EORTC randomized phase III protocol 30881. *Eur Urol* 1999; **36**:570–5.
17. Canfield SE, Kamat AM, Sánchez-Ortiz RF, Detry M, Swanson DA, Wood CG. Wood renal cell carcinoma with nodal metastases in the absence of distant metastatic disease (clinical stage TxN1–2M0): The impact of aggressive surgical resection on patient outcome. *J Urol* 2006; **175**(3):864–9.
18. Karellas ME, Jang TL, Kagiwada MA, Kinnaman MD, Jarnagin WR, Russo P. Advanced-stage renal cell carcinoma treated by radical nephrectomy and adjacent organ or structure resection. *BJU Int* 2009; **103**:160–4.
19. DeKernion JB, Ramming KP, Smith RB. The natural history of metastatic renal cell carcinoma: A computer analysis. *J Urol* 1978; **120**:148–52.
20. Kjaer M, Frederiksen PL, Engelholm SA. Postoperative radiotherapy in stage II and III renal adenocarcinoma. A randomized trial by the Copenhagen Renal Cancer Study Group. *Int J Radiat Oncol Biol Phys* 1987; **13**(5):665–72.
21. Itano NB, Blute ML, Spotts B, Zincke H. Outcome of isolated renal cell carcinoma fossa recurrence after nephrectomy. *J Urol* 2000; **164**(2):322–5.
22. Schrodter S, Hakenberg OW, Manseck A, Leike S, Wirth MP. Outcome of surgical treatment of isolated local recurrence after radical nephrectomy for renal cell carcinoma. *J Urol* 2002; **167**(4):1630–3.
23. Chapman AE, Goldstein LJ. Multiple drug resistance: biologic basis and clinical significance in renal-cell carcinoma. *Semin Oncol* 1995; **22**(1):17–28.
24. Motzer R, Russo P. Systemic therapy for renal cell carcinoma. *J Urol* 2000; **163**:408–17.
25. Margolin K, Gordon MS, Holmgren E, *et al.* Phase Ib trial of intravenous recombinant humanized monoclonal antibody to vascular endothelial growth factor in combination with chemotherapy in patients with advanced cancer: pharmacologic and long-term safety data. *J Clin Oncol* 2001; **19**(3):851–6.
26. Porzolt F, on behalf of the Delta-P Study Group. Adjuvant therapy of renal cell cancer (RCC) with interferon alfa. *Proc Am Soc Clin Oncol* 1992; **11**:202.
27. Messing EM, Manola J, Wilding G, *et al.* Eastern Cooperative Oncology Group/Intergroup trial. Phase III study of interferon alfa-NL as adjuvant treatment for resectable renal cell carcinoma: an Eastern Cooperative Oncology Group/Intergroup trial. *J Clin Oncol* 2003; **21**:1214–22.
28. Pizzocaro G, Piva L, Colavita M, *et al.* Interferon adjuvant to radical nephrectomy in Robson stages II and III renal cell carcinoma: a multicentric randomized study. *J Clin Oncol* 2001; **19**:425–31.
29. Clark JI, Atkins MB, Urba WJ, *et al.* Adjuvant high-dose bolus interleukin-2 for patients with high-risk renal cell carcinoma: a cytokine working group randomized trial. *J Clin Oncol* 2003; **21**:3133–40.
30. Wood C, Srivastava P, Bukowski R, *et al.* An adjuvant autologous therapeutic vaccine (HSPPC-96; vitespen) versus observation alone for patients at high risk of recurrence after nephrectomy for renal cell carcinoma: a multicentre, open-label randomized phase III trial. *Lancet* 2008; **372**:145–54.
31. Bloom HJ. Proceedings: Hormone-induced and spontaneous regression of metastatic renal cancer. *Cancer* 1973; **32**:1066–71.

32. Middleton AW Jr. Indications for and results of nephrectomy for metastatic renal cell carcinoma. *Urol Clin North Am* 1980; 7:711–17.
33. Snow RM, Schellhammer PF. Spontaneous regression of metastatic renal cell carcinoma. *Urology* 1982; **20**:177–181.
34. Marcus SG, Choyke PL, Reiter R, *et al.* Regression of metastatic renal cell carcinoma after cytoreductive nephrectomy. *J Urol* 1993; **150**:463–6.
35. Bukowski RM, Rayman P, Uzzo R, *et al.* Signal transduction abnormalities in T lymphocytes from patients with advanced renal carcinoma: clinical relevance and effects of cytokine therapy. *Clin Cancer Res* 1998; **4**:2337–47.
36. Uzzo RG, Rayman P, Kolenko V, *et al.* Mechanisms of apoptosis in T cells from patients with renal cell carcinoma. *Clin Cancer Res* 1999; **5**:1219–29.
37. Wagner JR, Walther MM, Linehan WM, *et al.* Interleukin-2 based immunotherapy for metastatic renal cell carcinoma with the kidney in place. *J Urol* 1999; **162**:43–5.
38. Walther MM, Yang JC, Pass HI, *et al.* Cytoreductive surgery before high dose interleukin-2 based therapy in patients with metastatic renal cell carcinoma. *J Urol* 1997; **158**:1675–8.
39. Flanigan RC, Salmon SE, Blumenstein BA, *et al.* Nephrectomy followed by interferon alfa-2b compared with interferon alfa-2b alone for metastatic renal-cell cancer. *N Engl J Med* 2001; **345**:1655–9.
40. Sandock DS, Seftel AD, Resnick MI. A new protocol for the followup of renal cell carcinoma based on pathological stage. *J Urol* 1995; **154**:28–31.
41. Levy DA, Slaton JW, Swanson DA, *et al.* Stage specific guidelines for surveillance after radical nephrectomy for local renal cell carcinoma. *J Urol* 1998; **159**:1163–7.
42. Itano NB, Blute ML, Spotts B, *et al.* Outcome of isolated renal cell carcinoma fossa recurrence after nephrectomy. *J Urol* 2000; **164**:322–5.
43. Schrodter S, Hakenberg OW, Manseck A, *et al.* Outcome of surgical treatment of isolated local recurrence after radical nephrectomy for renal cell carcinoma. *J Urol* 2002; **167**:1630–3.
44. Dimarco DS, Lohse CM, Zincke H, *et al.* Long-term survival of patients with unilateral sporadic multifocal renal cell carcinoma according to histologic subtype compared with patients with solitary tumors after radical nephrectomy. *Urology* 2004; **64**:4627.
45. Stephenson AJ, Chetner MP, Rourke K, *et al.* Guidelines for the surveillance of localized renal cell carcinoma based on the patterns of relapse after nephrectomy. *J Urol* 2004; **172**:58–62.
46. Tanguay S, Pisters LL, Lawrence DD, *et al.* Therapy of locally recurrent renal cell carcinoma after nephrectomy. *J Urol* 1996; **155**:26–9.
47. Wiesner C, Jakse G, Rohde D. Therapy of local recurrence of renal cell carcinoma. *Oncol Rep* 2002; **9**:189–92.
48. Gogus C, Baltaci S, Beduk Y, *et al.* Isolated local recurrence of renal cell carcinoma after radical nephrectomy: experience with 10 cases. *Urology* 2003; **61**:926–9.
49. Bruno JJ II, Snyder ME, Motzer RJ, *et al.* Renal cell carcinoma local recurrences: impact of surgical treatment and concomitant metastasis on survival. *BJU Int* 2006; **97**:9338.
50. Sandhu SS, Symes A, A'Hern R, *et al.* Surgical excision of isolated renal-bed recurrence after radical nephrectomy for renal cell carcinoma. *BJU Int* 2005; **95**:522–5.
51. Kavolius JP, Mastorakos DP, Pavlovich C, *et al.* Resection of metastatic renal cell carcinoma. *J Clin Oncol* 1998; **16**:2261–6.

CHAPTER 6.32

Treatment of metastatic renal cancer

Han Hsi Wong, Basma Greef, and Tim Eisen

Introduction to treating metastatic renal cancer

Historically, 30% of patients with renal cell carcinoma (RCC) present with metastatic disease at the time of diagnosis. Recent data suggested that this figure is changing, with a rising incidence of overall RCC cases and a decline in the incidence of metastatic disease at diagnosis to approximately 14%.[1] This is largely attributed to the increased use of radiological imaging. The commonest site of metastasis is the lungs (75%), but involvements of the bone (30%), liver (25%), brain (7%), and lymph nodes (30–70%) are also common.[2–8] The management of renal cancer is challenging as it is relatively insensitive to conventional chemotherapy and radiotherapy. Although outcome of those with metastatic disease is still poor, improved diagnostic and surgical procedures, coupled with the increased understanding of the molecular biology of RCC and the development of targeted agents, have doubled median survival (MS) from 10 to 22 months for patients with intermediate risk.[9]

The major histological subtypes of RCC are the clear cell (75%) and non-clear cell tumours (types I and II papillary—12%; chromophobe—4%; collecting duct—<1%; oncocytoma, a benign variant—4%, and unclassified histology -3–5%).[10] The biology of renal cancer is highly variable and some patients with relatively indolent disease can be safely monitored for years. As such, several factors should be considered when deciding on the appropriateness and timing of treatment, including the patient's performance status, co-morbidities, site, and volume of disease, rate of disease progression, and prognostic scores.

Prognostic score in metastatic disease

Prediction of a patient's outcome by means of a reliable, validated prognostic system is important to help select patients for specific treatment options, including surgery, systemic therapy, or to enter into clinical trials. One of the earliest prognostic models is the Memorial Sloan-Kettering Cancer Center (MSKCC) or Motzer score.[11] In a study of 670 patients, patients were scored, based on the following risk factors:

- Karnofsky performance status <80%
- Haemoglobin <lower limit of normal
- Corrected calcium >10 mg/dL (2.5 mmol/L)
- Lactate dehydrogenase (LDH) >1.5× upper limit of normal
- Absence of prior nephrectomy

A score of 0, 1 to 2 and >=3 were found to be associated with MS of 20, 10, and 4 months, respectively. This system was later modified after the benefit of interferon (IFN)-α was shown after nephrectomy.[12] Instead of 'absence of prior nephrectomy', the 'interval from disease diagnosis to therapy of <1 year' was used in the scoring system. A score of 0, 1 to 2, and >=3 were associated with MS of 30, 14, and 5 months, respectively. An MSKCC score of patients previously treated with systemic therapy for metastatic disease has also been developed, for which low Karnofsky performance status, low haemoglobin, and high corrected calcium were identified as adverse features—a score of 0, 1, and 2 to 3 predicted MS of 22.1, 11.9, and 5.4 months, respectively.[13]

The MSKCC system was subsequently validated and elaborated by investigators at the Cleveland Clinic Foundation (CCF), which studied 353 patients entered into clinical trials involving immunotherapy. This consists of four prognostic factors from the modified MSKCC score (Karnofsky performance status was excluded) and four additional factors of prior radiotherapy, presence of hepatic, pulmonary, or retroperitoneal lymph node metastases (Table 6.32.1).[14]

Table 6.32.1 CCF-extended MSKCC prognostic system for patients with metastatic renal cell carcinoma

Score	Risk	1-year survival	Median survival (months)
0–1	Favourable	81%	26
2	Intermediate	58%	14.4
≥3	Poor	23%	7.3
Score one for each of:			
Haemoglobin <lower limit of normal			
Corrected calcium >10 mg/dL (2.5 mmol/L)			
Lactate dehydrogenase >1.5x upper limit of normal			
Interval from diagnosis to study entry of <1 year			
Prior radiotherapy*			
Hepatic metastasis*			
Pulmonary metastasis*			
Retroperitoneal lymph node metastasis*			

*Additional prognostic markers added to the MSKCC score

Source: data from Mekhail, T. M. *et al.*, 'Validation and extension of the Memorial Sloan-Kettering prognostic factors model for survival in patients with previously untreated metastatic renal cell carcinoma', *Journal of Clinical Oncology*, Volume 23, Number 4, pp. 832–41, Copyright © 2005 American Society of Clinical Oncology.

Table 6.32.2 Prognostic factors in patients with metastatic renal cell carcinoma treated with VEGF-targeted agents

Score	Risk	2-year survival	Median survival (months)
0	Favourable	75%	>48
1–2	Intermediate	53%	27
3–6	Poor	7%	8.8

Score one for each of:
Karnofsky performance status <80%
Haemoglobin <lower limit of normal
Calcium >upper limit of normal
Neutrophil count >upper limit of normal
Platelet count >upper limit of normal
Time of diagnosis to systemic therapy of <1 year

Source: data from Heng, D. Y. C. *et al.*, 'Prognostic factors for overall survival in patients with metastatic renal cell carcinoma treated with vascular endothelial growth factor-targeted agents: results from a large, multicenter study', *Journal of Clinical Oncology*, Volume 27, Number 34, pp. 5794–9, Copyright © 2009 American Society of Clinical Oncology.

Since the development of agents targeting the vascular endothelial growth factor (VEGF) pathway, a new prognostic scoring system was developed by Heng *et al.* to reflect the current treatment paradigm for patients with metastatic RCC.[15] The Database Consortium Model was based on the outcome of 645 patients treated with sunitinib (61%), sorafenib (31%), and bevacizumab (8%). This is summarized in Table 6.32.2, where neutrophil and platelet counts were also considered as prognostic factors. This model was subsequently validated in an independent multinational data set including 849 patients treated with antiangiogenic targeted therapies, with a MS of 43, 22.5, and 7.8 months in good, intermediate, or poor prognosis groups.[16]

In a crowded field in which there were a number of different prognostic scoring systems in use, the International Kidney Cancer Working Group sought to develop a unified prognostic model using an international database of 3,748 patients with metastatic RCC.[17] Nine clinical factors were used: days from diagnosis to start of treatment; Eastern Cooperative Oncology Group (ECOG) performance status; number of metastatic sites; prior immunotherapy; haemoglobin, LDH, and white blood count; alkaline phosphatase and serum calcium. MS for the favourable, intermediate, and poor-risk groups are 26.9, 11.5, and 4.2 months, respectively. The formula for risk calculation is more complex than the other models. Moreover, cross-model comparison has shown that it yields patient classification similar to simpler models, such as the Database Consortium Model.[16]

It is important to note that a patient's prognosis is dynamic and it changes with time, such that someone who remains alive after a period of time on treatment will have a better prognosis than someone who is newly diagnosed—this concept is known as conditional survival. Harshman *et al.* have demonstrated that for patients with metastatic RCC commenced on targeted therapy, the two-year conditional survival probability increased from 44% at 0 months to 51% at 18 months since the beginning of treatment.[18] After extensive investigation in large data sets, prognostic models based on clinical parameters have most likely reached the limit of their accuracy. Further improvements in the accuracy of prognostic models will most likely depend on the identification of prognostic biomarkers.[16]

Surgery in metastatic disease

Patients who presented with metastatic RCC or who developed recurrent/metastatic disease after initial treatment are usually treated with systemic therapy. However, surgery may be beneficial in selected patients in one of the following:

- Palliative nephrectomy for symptom control
- Cytoreductive surgery to reduce the tumour burden
- Metastasectomy for solitary or limited number of metastases

Nephrectomy

Nephrectomy is indicated in good or intermediate performance status patients with uncontrolled haematuria and/or pain from the primary tumour. Angioinfarction is a less invasive alternative for inoperable patients. Significant systemic symptoms such as fatigue, hypercalcaemia, and fever may sometimes be improved by nephrectomy. However, these are often best treated with systemic therapy as the surgical outcome is likely to be poor in patients with these problems and the symptoms often remain due to the presence of residual metastatic disease. While the regression of metastases has been reported after nephrectomy in ≤1% of cases (mainly in the lungs), the surgical morbidity and 2% mortality rate means that this must not be the sole indication for debulking surgery.[19]

For patients with good performance status, cytoreductive nephrectomy prior to cytokine treatment has been shown to confer survival benefit. Nevertheless, these trial data are mainly of historical interest, since cytokine immunotherapy has now largely been superseded by the molecularly targeted agents. Two trials had randomized patients with metastatic RCC to undergo radical nephrectomy, followed by therapy with IFN-α, or to receive IFN-α alone—the Southwest Oncology Group (SWOG)-8949 trial of 241 patients[20] and the smaller European Organization for Research and Treatment of Cancer (EORTC)-30947 trial of 83 patients.[21] Combined analysis of these two trials demonstrated an MS of 13.6 months with nephrectomy, compared to 7.8 months without, representing a 31% decrease in the risk of death ($p = 0.002$).[22] Metastatic non-clear cell carcinoma has a worse prognosis than clear cell carcinoma in patients who underwent cytoreductive surgery.[23]

In contrast to the lack of response of the primary tumour with cytokine-based immunotherapy, significant tumour shrinkage has been observed with antiangiogenic tyrosine kinase inhibitors (TKIs).[24,25] The improved efficacy and tolerability of these treatments has prompted the re-evaluation of the need and timing nephrectomy in patients with advanced and metastatic RCC. In a retrospective study of 314 patients treated with targeted therapy, those who underwent cytoreductive nephrectomy had a much longer survival compared to those who did not (19.8 vs. 9.4 months).[26] Two phase III trials were designed to define the roles of nephrectomy and molecularly targeted agents. Both trials faced recruitment challenges. The CARMENA (Clinical Trial to Assess the Importance of Nephrectomy) study continues to recruit and aims to compare nephrectomy and the tyrosine kinase inhibitor sunitinib versus sunitinib alone in patients with metastatic disease. The EORTC SURTIME 30073 trial stopped recruitment and aimed to compare immediate nephrectomy followed by sunitinib versus pre-surgical sunitinib followed by nephrectomy and sunitinib. Until evidence from randomized trials is available, there is no current consensus as to whether cytoreductive nephrectomy should be performed prior to the initiation of systemic therapy. Careful patient selection is essential, as patients may run the risk of not being able to receive targeted agents due to rapid disease progression or post-surgical complications. If the novel immunotherapeutic therapies discussed below become established first-line treatments, then debulking surgery prior to immunotherapy is likely to return as a frequent indication.

The retroperitoneal lymph nodes are the commonest regional site of metastasis. The presence of nodal involvement in patients with metastatic RCC undergoing cytoreductive nephrectomy has an adverse effect on survival and response to subsequent immunotherapy.[27,28] One retrospective analysis reported an improvement in survival in patients with radiological evidence of nodal involvement, who had lymph node dissection (LND) but no benefit found for patients undergoing prophylactic dissection.[29] This finding was not reproduced by another retrospective series which showed no benefit for LND.[30] This remains an area of controversy in the surgical management of metastatic renal cancer, in the absence of prospective, randomized trial data.

Metastasectomy

There is an important role for metastasectomy in a highly selected population of patients. In one series, resection of solitary metastasis could lead to survival of five years or more in about a third of patients.[31] For most patients the realistic benefit of surgery is to remain free of disease and to spare systemic therapy and its side effects for a significant period of time.

In a retrospective study, 278 patients either underwent resection of all metastases with curative intent, partial resection of metastatic disease, or were treated non-surgically.[31] The respective five-year survival rates were 44%, 14%, and 11%. Predictors of prolonged survival include disease-free interval from nephrectomy to the detection of metastasis of >1 year, solitary rather than multiple sites of metastases, and age of <60 years. Survival rates after complete resection of second and third metastases were not different compared with initial metastasectomy. Resection of isolated metastases to soft tissue sites gave the best result (five-year survival of 75%), followed by glandular sites (thyroid, salivary, pancreas, adrenal, and ovary—63%), pulmonary (54%), bone (40%), and brain (18%) metastases.

Surgical excision of metastatic RCC in the bone could be performed for local tumour control, pain relief, and improving function.[32] In a retrospective series, 295 patients with RCC and bone metastases underwent surgical procedures that include curettage with cementing and/or internal fixation, *en bloc* resection, closed nailing, and amputation.[33] The overall one- and five-year survival rates were 47% and 11%, respectively. The best results were seen in patients with clear cell histology and with solitary bone metastasis, or multiple but bone-only metastases.

Surgery for brain metastasis may provide symptom relief from the mass effect of the tumour. It could also result in long-term survival. In a series of 138 patients, removal of solitary brain metastasis was found to be associated with a recurrence-free survival of 13 months compared to four months for those who had >1 lesions.[34]

Lee *et al.* described 31 patients with metastatic RCC who relapsed after an initial response to IL-2.[35] These patients underwent metastasectomy on disease relapse, resulting in a two-year progression-free survival (PFS) of 37%. The evidence for metastasectomy in patients who had received targeted therapy is lacking, arising from small retrospective case series. In a small study of 22 patients, 11 patients were disease-free at a median of 43 weeks after surgery.[36] Metastatic sites include the retroperitoneum, lungs, adrenal glands, bowels, mediastinum, bone, brain, and inferior vena cava. Overall, 21 patients were still alive at a median follow-up of just over two years. Orlova *et al.* recently reported a larger cohort of 147 patients, 47 of whom underwent incomplete metastasectomy followed by targeted therapies, while the remainder were treated with targeted therapies alone.[37] There was improved PFS to first-line treatment in the metastasectomy patients (p = 0.018) but no significant difference in overall survival between the groups, in this albeit small sample. Retrospective data of this type are open to selection bias and should be interpreted with caution, but in the absence of randomized evidence serve to aid the discussion between clinician and patient.

There is a balance to be drawn between offering surgery immediately once a solitary metastasis is noted and waiting for a period of observation to ascertain that the behaviour of the disease is truly oligometastatic. Immediate surgery runs a significant risk of proving futile since many patients will quickly develop further metastases. Too long a period of observation runs the risk of missing the opportunity of removing all macroscopic disease. Our practice is to monitor patients with a single or limited number of resectable metastases at presentation for three to six months before metastasectomy is considered. This is especially so for patients who are at risk of surgical complications (e.g. poor performance status, significant co-morbidities) or whose disease is expected to progress rapidly. Systemic treatment with molecularly targeted agents is more suitable for these patients. However, one must also take into account the risk of a resectable lesion becoming unresectable due to local disease progression, such as central thoracic lesions.

General non-surgical management of metastatic disease

Interventional radiology

Interventional radiological procedures provide an alternative to surgery in local tumour control and symptom palliation. These include arterial embolization or angioinfarction, cryoablation, and radiofrequency ablation (RFA). So far, no randomized trial has compared these techniques with surgery in metastatic RCC.

Several case series have consistently shown the effectiveness of renal artery embolization in improving pain and controlling intractable haematuria from the primary tumour, with no survival benefit.[38–43] Embolization agents used include metallic microcoils, acrylic gelatine microspheres, polyvinyl alcohol particles, absolute ethanol, and gelatine sponge. A common complication of this procedure is postinfarction syndrome, characterized by flank pain, fever, nausea, and vomiting, which is usually self-limiting.[39] Selective arterial embolization can also be used for local tumour control or haemostasis in cases such as disease infiltration into the gastrointestinal tract, bone, and pulmonary metastases.[44–47]

Cryoablation is the destruction of tissue by freezing to sub-zero temperatures. In a small study of 27 patients, multisite cryoablation of oligometastatic RCC was associated with low complication and local tumour recurrence rates.[48] RFA destroys tissue by using heat generated from high-frequency alternating electric current on the RFA probe, and has been used in the palliative setting for the destruction of lung metastases and in the control of painful bone lesions in combination with oesteoplasty.[49–52]

Radiotherapy

Radiotherapy can be given in the palliative setting for pain associated with bone metastasis, spinal cord compression, and brain metastasis. For patients with multiple brain metastases, whole-brain radiotherapy offers symptom control but no survival benefit.[53–55] Patients with up to three brain metastases of up to 2 cm in size may be treated with stereotactic radiosurgery. Although disappearance of the tumour is unusual, a tumour control rate as high as 96% has been reported.[56–58] An early 'good' response to radiosurgery—defined as 75% radiological tumour shrinkage one month after treatment—has been reported to be associated with prolonged MS (18.0 months vs. 9.0 months, $p = 0.025$).[59]

Bisphosphonates for bone metastasis

Intravenous bisphosphonates can be useful in pain from metastatic disease. A randomized phase III trial of 773 patients with bone metastases secondary to solid tumours other than breast or prostate cancer has demonstrated the efficacy of zoledronic acid in reducing skeletal-related events (SREs) (i.e. pathological fracture, spinal cord compression, bone pain requiring radiotherapy, and orthopaedic surgery).[60,61] In a subset analysis of 74 patients with RCC, zoledronic acid was found to significantly reduce the proportion of patients with SREs, skeletal morbidity rate, and time to progression of bone lesions.[62] The risk of developing an SRE was reduced by 61% compared to placebo. There was a non-statistically significant trend towards improved survival in the group that received zoledronic acid ($p = 0.179$).

Pre-clinical and early clinical studies have shown that zoledronic acid has antitumour properties that might improve the survival of patients with metastatic RCC.[63,64] A retrospective study of 76 patients suggested that the use of bisphosphonates in addition to sunitinib in patients with bone metastases from RCC might improve disease response and survival, compared to those who were not on bisphosphonates.[65] A possible survival benefit of zoledronic acid has also been suggested in trial of 45 patients (one-year survival of 80.8% compared to 59.1% for those who did not receive zoledronic acid, respectively; $p = 0.0034$).[66] The phase II RAZOR trial of RAD001 (everolimus) and zoledronic acid in 30 RCC patients with bone metastases demonstrated a longer survival for those who received combination treatment (7.5 months), compared to the everolimus-only group (5.4 months), although this was not statistically significant ($p = 0.11$).[67]

Denosumab, a human monoclonal anti-receptor activator of nuclear factor κ-B ligand antibody given subcutaneously, has been found to be at least as effective as zoledronic acid in preventing SREs in patients with metastatic cancer to the bone or myeloma.[68] In this randomized trial of 1,776 patients, 9% had RCC.

Systemic treatment of metastatic clear cell carcinoma

Systemic treatment of metastatic clear cell RCC has come full circle. An initial era of cytokine-based immunotherapy was followed by the widespread adoption of molecularly targeted agents in the mid-2000s. In recent years, there has been a resurgence of the role of immunotherapy, this time based on T-cell checkpoint modifiers. The treatment algorithm based on current evidence is summarized in Table 6.32.3.

Table 6.32.3 Treatment algorithm for metastatic renal cell carcinoma (RCC) based on current evidence. Risk categories refer to MSKCC metastatic RCC prognostic groupings

	Good risk	Intermediate risk	Poor risk
1st line	*Preferred:* Pazopanib Sunitinib *Selected patients:* HD-Il2 Bevacizumab + IFN-α	*Preferred:* Pazopanib Sunitinib *Selected patients:* Bevacizumab + IFN-α	Temsirolimus
2nd Line	Nivolumab Axitinib Lenvatinib and everolimus Cabozantinib Sorafenib	Nivolumab Axitinib Lenvatinib and everolimus Cabozantinib Sorafenib	Nivolumab

The immune system: Cytokine therapy and T-cell checkpoint inhibitors

The immune system plays an important role in cancer development and progression, particularly the T-lymphocytes.[69] The terms 'cancer immunosurveillance' and 'cancer immunoediting' are often used to describe how precancerous or cancerous cells are being detected and eliminated by the immune system.[70] Normally, the activation and proliferation of lymphocytes are regulated by interaction of the peptide-antigen-major histocompatibility complex with the T-cell receptor. The resulting immunological response will also depend on the balance between the binding of co-stimulatory and co-inhibitory molecules to other receptors found on T-cells. Binding of CD80 and CD86 to CD28 on T-cells will result in activation, whereas binding of these ligands to cytotoxic T-lymphocyte-associated antigen-4 (CTLA-4) can downregulate T-cell responses. Similarly, the programme death-ligand 1 (PD-L1 or B7-H1) can also bind to its receptor PD-1 on activated T-cells and immune cells to dampen the immunological response.[71] Within these complex interactions, when tumours progress they often develop ways to escape immune recognition and to downregulate the immune system.[72] For example, overexpression of PD-L1 by tumour cells has been found to promote T-cell apoptosis.[73].

The immune system is also tightly regulated by small proteins called cytokines, which are secreted by a variety of cells and mediate their effects by binding to cellular receptors. The rationale behind their use in cancer treatment is to stimulate an adequate and sustained T-cell and natural killer-cell-mediated antitumour immunity. IFN-α also has an antiangiogenic effect.[74]

Interferon-α

The activity of IFN-α monotherapy has previously been evaluated in a number of large randomized clinical trials.[20,75–78] A Cochrane meta-analysis by Coppin *et al.* that included four studies involving 644 patients showed that IFN-α improved the survival of patients with advanced RCC by a median of 3.8 months, with a reduction of one-year mortality by 44% and a 26% risk reduction of death during the first two years compared to controls.[79] The dose range was between 5 to 18 MIU subcutaneously, three times weekly.

Combination treatment of IFN-α with IL-2, cis-retinoic acid or chemotherapy has not been shown to improve overall survival compared to IFN-α monotherapy.[80–85] IFN-α therapy is characterized by slow partial response (about four months for objective response) and this seldom persists for more than a year. Common side effects include fatigue and flu-like symptoms, but treatment is generally well-tolerated. Its role in the monotherapy of advanced RCC has now been largely replaced by the more effective molecularly targeted therapies. However, it is still used in combination with bevacizumab in the first-line treatment of metastatic RCC.

Interleukin-2

A multicentre French study randomized 425 patients with metastatic RCC to receive either IL-2 (five-day continuous intravenous infusion at 18 MIU/m^2/day), IFN-α (18 MIU subcutaneously three times a week), or both (with IFN-α dose at 6 MIU three times a week).[75] Although response rate was much higher in the combination therapy group at 10 weeks (18.6% compared to 6.5% with IL-2 and 7.5% with IFN-α, respectively), there were no statistically differences in MS (Table 6.32.4). Toxicities were more frequent with high-dose IL-2, including moderate-to-severe hypotension (secondary to vascular leak syndrome), fever, nausea/vomiting, diarrhoea, as well as a range of respiratory (e.g. dyspnoea), renal/electrolyte (e.g. oliguria), and neurological (e.g. confusion, agitation) abnormalities.

In another study, Yang *et al.* randomized patients to receive either intravenous high-dose IL-2 (720,000 IU/kg/8 hourly), intravenous low-dose IL-2 (72,000 IU/kg/8 hourly), or low-dose subcutaneous IL-2 daily (Table 6.32.4).[86] Response rate was significantly higher in the high-dose group, that is, 21% compared to 13% in the low-dose intravenous group (p = 0.048), and 10% in the subcutaneous group (p = 0.033). Although there was no difference in OS, the duration of response and survival was superior in the high-dose group, which achieved a complete response (p = 0.04), but at the expense of more toxicities. A subsequent randomized study by the Cytokine Working Group compared high-dose IL-2 (600,000 IU/kg/8 hourly) intravenously with subcutaneous IL-2 and IFN-α in 192 patients with metastatic RCC.[87] This trial showed that high-dose treatment has a higher response rate (23.2% vs. 9.9%) and longer OS (17.5 vs. 13 months), although the latter was not statistically significant (Table 6.32.4). However, patients with bone or liver metastases, or a primary tumour still in place achieved a significantly higher response rate and survival with high-dose IL-2 compared to subcutaneous IL-2 and IFN-α. In addition, seven out of eight patients who initially achieved a complete response to high-dose IL-2 were able to sustain this after three years. The prospective cohort SELECT trial failed to validate other histological features that might predict patient's response to IL-2.[88]

In summary, high-dose IL-2 is an option for carefully selected patients who are expected to tolerate the toxicities associated with the treatment, due to its ability to induce a long-lasting response in a small subset of patients. Treatment with IL-2 requires hospital admission to a ward with close monitoring equipment and staff, and which can provide inotrope support when necessary. Patient selection criteria may include age of <60 years, good performance status, lack of significant co-morbidities, clear cell histology, lack of sarcomatoid features, >1 year since nephrectomy, a limited number of sites of metastasis, the absence of bone or liver metastases, and psychological motivation for intensive therapy.[75,89,90]

Nivolumab

The last few years has seen the introduction of T-cell check point inhibitors (TCCIs—a new class of treatments targeting the interaction between T-cells and tumour cells), to enhance the immune antitumour response. A number of drugs of this class have shown promise in clinical development (see 'Therapies in development'), but nivolumab is the first to have attained regulatory approval and be adopted into clinical practice in RCC. Nivolumab (Opdivo®, Bristol Myers-Squibb) is a fully human IgG4 programmed death 1 (PD-1) inhibitor. The Checkmate 025 trial randomized 821 patients with advanced clear cell RCC, who had received one or two previous lines of TKI treatment to nivolumab (3 mg/kg intravenously every two weeks) or everolimus.[91] Median OS was significantly prolonged in the nivolumab group (25.0 months vs. 19.6 months, p = 0.0018) (Table 6.32.4). In subgroup analyses, benefit from nivolumab was found to be independent of MSKCC prognostic group and of PD-L1 expression in the tumour. Nivolumab was relatively well-tolerated with a grade 3 or 4 toxicity rate of 19%, versus 35% for everolimus. Gastrointestinal, skin, and pulmonary toxicities predominate, but as the toxicities of this class of drug are largely autoimmune in origin due to the loss of self-tolerance, any organ can be affected. Therefore, vigilance for a wide range of rare and unusual toxicities is important. Other TCCI-based regimens are in clinical development. These include ongoing trials of dual TCCI-blockade and combinations with TKIs and with bevacizumab (see 'Therapies in development', below).

Tyrosine kinase inhibitors

The von Hippel-Lindau (*VHL*) gene product forms part of a protein complex with ubiquitin ligase activity that 'marks' a specific target protein for degradation. One of its targets is the hypoxia-inducible factor-α (HIF-α). In normoxic conditions, HIF-α is hydroxylated at its proline residues via an oxygen-dependent enzymatic reaction. This is recognized by the VHL complex, resulting in its proteosomal degradation. During hypoxia, HIF-α is not hydroxylated due to the lack of oxygen, and thus it does not bind to *VHL* and is not degraded. Moreover, inactivating mutations or gene silencing of *VHL* is found in up to 91% of sporadic clear cell RCC.[92–97] This causes HIF-α to accumulate and form a complex with HIF-β. The resulting transcription factor complex enters the nucleus and binds to the HIF-responsive element enhancer sequence, leading to the transcription of hypoxia-induced genes (Fig. 6.32.1). Of the two main HIF-α isoforms, HIF-1α and HIF-2α, the latter is predominantly expressed in RCC.[98] HIF-2α drives the expression of tumourigenic and angiogenic factors such as VEGF, transforming growth factor-α (TGF-α), platelet-derived growth factor (PDGF), and cyclin D1.[99]

These secreted growth factors bind to the extracellular domain of specific receptor tyrosine kinases located on endothelial, stromal, and tumour cells. Tyrosine kinases are enzymes which transfer a phosphate group from adenosine triphosphate to a protein at its tyrosine residue—this phosphorylation event could turn an inactive protein from its 'off' to its active 'on' state. Binding of ligand causes conformational changes to the receptor, activating its intracellular kinase activity (Fig. 6.32.1). This subsequently activates a cascade of events through phosphorylation of intracellular proteins.

Table 6.32.4 Phase III trials of therapies in metastatic RCC

Trial	Line of treatment	No. of patients	Patient group	Treatment	Objective response rate	Median PFS (months)	Median OS (months)
Groupe Français d'Immunothérapie (Négrier *et al.* 1998)[75]	1st	425	Treatment-naive metastatic RCC	IL-2 IFN-α IL-2 + IFN-α	6.5% 7.5% 18.6%	(PFS at 1 year of 15%, 12% and 20%, respectively for IL-2, IFN-α and combination)	12* 13* 17*
Yang *et al.* (2003)[86]	1st	400	Metastatic clear cell RCC with no previous IL-2 treatment	High-dose intravenous IL-2 Low-dose intravenous IL-2 Low-dose subcutaneous IL-2	21% 11% 10%	No difference in overall survival between the groups Survival of patients who had a complete response was longer with high-dose compared to low-dose IL-2 ($p = 0.04$)	
Cytokine Working Group (McDermott *et al.* 2005)[87]	1st	192	Metastatic RCC with no previous IL-2 or IFN-α treatment	High-dose IL-2 Subcutaneous IL-2 + IFN-α	23.2% 9.9%	3.1 3.1	17.5*[a] 13*
CheckMate025 (Motzer *et al.* 2015)[91]	2nd/3rd	821	Advanced clear cell RCC One or two previous antiangiogenic treatments—no previous mTOR inhibitor	Nivolumab Everolimus	25% 5%	4.6 4.4	25.0 19.6
NCT00083889 (Motzer *et al.* 2007)[7,103]	1st	750	Treatment-naive metastatic clear cell RCC	Sunitinib IFN-α	47% 12%	11 5	26.4 20.0[b]
VEG105192 (Sternberg *et al.* 2010)[6]	1st/2nd	435	Locally advanced or metastatic clear cell/ predominantly clear cell RCC(treatment-naive or cytokine-pretreated)	Pazopanib Placebo (2:1)	30% 3%	9.2 (11.1 for treatment-naive; 7.4 for cytokine-pretreated) 4.2 (2.8 for treatment-naive; 4.2 for cytokine-pretreated)	22.9 20.5 (23.5 for treatment-naive)[c]
TARGET (Escudier *et al.* 2007)[5,110]	2nd	903	Metastatic clear cell RCC which progressed after 1st-line cytokine therapy	Sorafenib Placebo	10% 2%	5.5 2.8	17.8 14.3[d]
AXIS (Rini *et al.* 2011)[116,117]	2nd	723	Metastatic clear cell RCC which progressed after 1st-line therapy with sunitinib, bevacizumab plus IFN-α, temsirolimus, or cytokines	Axitinib Sorafenib	19% 9%	6.7 4.7	20.1 19.2

METEOR Choueiri *et al.* (2016)[121]	2nd or higher	658	Advanced or metastatic clear cell RCC. One or more previous TKI	Cabozantinib	17%	7.4		21.4
				Everolimus	3%	3.9		16.5
AVOREN	1st	649	Treatment-naive metastatic clear cell RCC	Bevacizumab + IFN-α	31%	10.2		23.3*
(Escudier *et al.* 2007)[124,125]				Placebo + IFN-α	13%	5.4		21.3*
CALGB 90206	1st	732	Treatment-naive metastatic clear cell RCC	Bevacizumab + IFN-α	25.5%	8.5		18.3*
(Rini *et al.* 2008)[8,126]				IFN-α	13.1%	5.2		17.4*
Global ARCC (Hudes *et al.* 2007)[127]	1st	626	Previously untreated, poor prognosis metastatic RCC	Temsirolimus	8.6%	5.5		10.9
				IFN-α	4.8%	3.1		7.3
			(80% clear cell)	Temsirolimus + IFNα	8.1%	4.7		8.4
RECORD-1	2nd	416	Metastatic clear cell RCC which progressed on or within 6 months of stopping sunitinib, sorafenib, or both	Everolimus	1.8%	4.9		14.8
(Motzer *et al.* 2008)[4,128]				Placebo	0%	1.9		10.0[e]
				(2:1)				

[a]Survival was significantly better with high-dose IL-2 in patients with bone or liver metastases or a primary tumour in place.

[b]After censoring 25 patients who crossed over from the IFN-α group to the sunitinib group.

[c]Confounded by cross-over of more than half of the placebo patients to the pazopanib arm. Analysis using the rank-preserving structural failure time method (RPSFT) suggested a 50% reduction in the risk of death compared to placebo in treatment-naive patients.

[d]After censoring of patients who crossed over to the sorafenib arm.

[e]Estimated using the RPSFT method due to high rate of cross-over.

*not statistically significant.

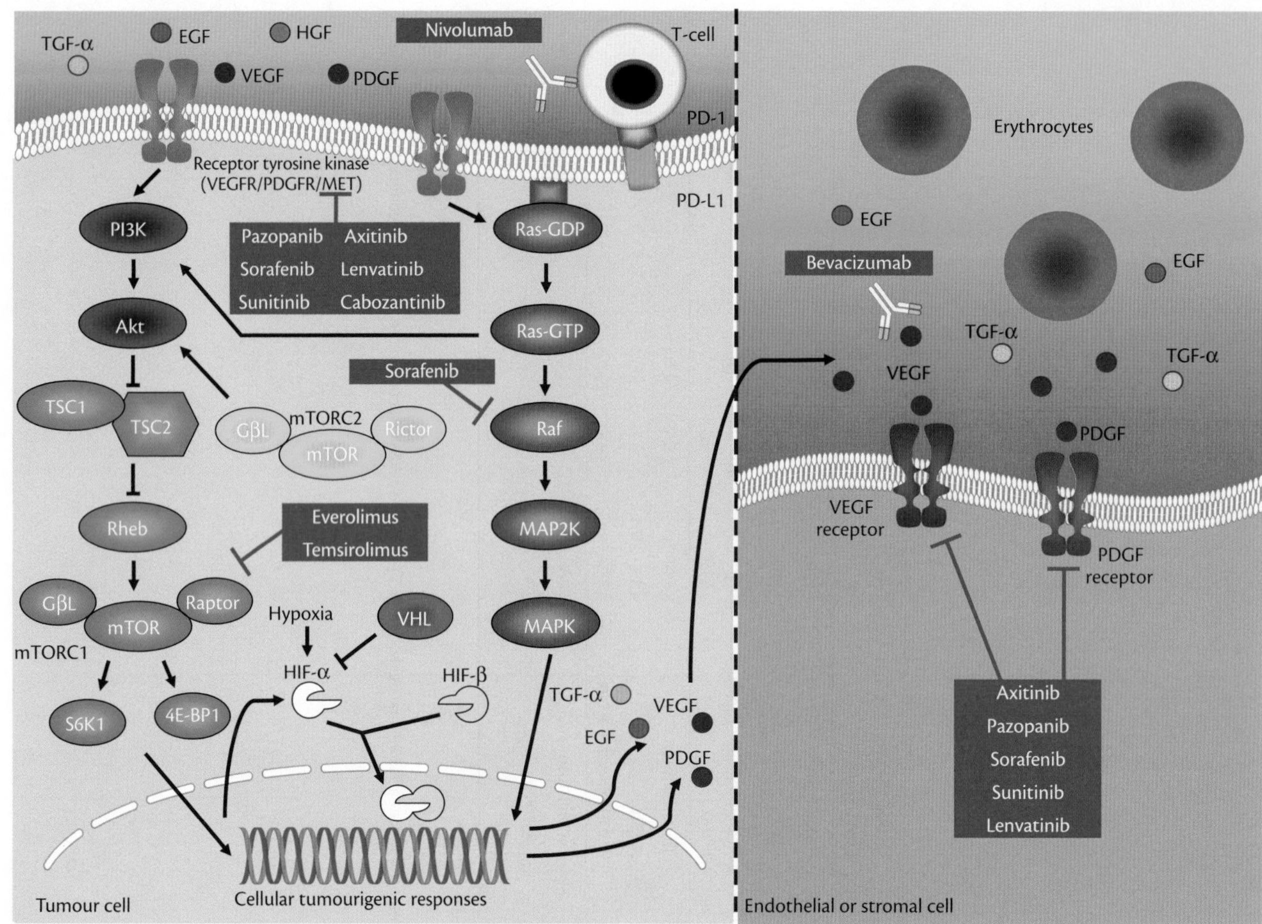

Fig. 6.32.1 Simplified schematic of signalling pathways and therapeutic targets in renal cell carcinoma. Binding of ligand to the growth factor receptor results in the activation of its intracellular tyrosine kinase. This phosphorylates and activates PI3K, which in turn activates Akt (PI3K can also be phosphorylated by activated Ras protein, which itself could lead to downstream tumourigenic cellular responses via the Raf-MAP2K-MAPK pathway). Akt in turn inhibits TSC2, which releases the inhibition of TSC2 on Rheb, leading to the activation of mTORC1. mTORC1 phosphorylates S6K1 and 4E-BP1, which control the translation of specific mRNAs and the synthesis of proteins involved in cell growth, proliferation, and angiogenesis, including HIF-α. In normoxic conditions, HIF-α is hydroxylated and subsequently recognized by the *VHL* complex which targets HIF-α for proteosomal degradation. However, during hypoxia or in the absence of VHL protein (secondary to gene mutation or silencing), HIF-α accumulates and forms a complex with HIF-β, resulting in the transcription of genes that encode for proteins such as EGF, TGF-α, VEGF, and PDGF. These secreted growth factors can act on surrounding stromal or endothelial cells, leading to their proliferation and angiogenesis. They can also exert their effect via an autocrine fashion by binding to receptors on cancer cells. Axitinib, pazopanib, sorafenib sunitinib, cabozantinib, and lenvatinib are TKIs that act primarily on the inhibition of endothelial cells (via the inhibition of the receptor tyrosine kinases VEGFR, PDGFR, and MET, among others), although direct antitumour effects independent of angiogenesis have been observed.[184,185] The mTOR inhibitors everolimus and temsirolimus form a complex with FKBP12, which then inhibits mTORC1. Bevacizumab is a humanized monoclonal antibody that binds circulating VEGF-A to inhibit angiogenesis. Nivolumab is a monoclonal antibody that binds to PD-1 on T-cells to prevent its binding with PD-L1 on tumour cells.

4E-BP1—eukaryotic translation initiation factor 4E-binding protein 1; EGF—epidermal growth factor; FKBP12 —FK506-binding protein 12; GDP—guanosine diphosphate; GTP—guanosine triphosphate; HGF—hepatocyte growth factor; HIF—hypoxia-inducible factor; MAP2K—mitogen-activated protein kinase; MAPK—mitogen-activated protein kinase; mRNA—messenger ribonucleic acid; mTOR—mammalian target of rapamycin; mTORC—mTOR complex; PD-1—programmed death 1; PD-L1—programmed death ligand 1; PDGF—platelet-derived growth factor; PI3K —phosphatidylinositol 3-kinase; S6K1—S6 kinase 1; TGF-α—transforming growth factor-α; TKI—tyrosine kinase inhibitor; TSC—tuberous sclerosis complex; VEGF—vascular endothelial growth factor; VHL—von Hippel-Lindau.

These pathways allow extracellular signals to be transmitted to the nucleus, and if dysregulated (e.g. overexpression of ligands, activating mutation of receptors), could result in changes to the cell's phenotype. TKIs are molecules that inhibit the intracellular kinase of these receptors, thereby blocking downstream signalling events such as cell proliferation, resistance to apoptosis, migration, metastasis, and tumour angiogenesis.

A number of TKIs including sunitinib, pazopanib, axitinib, and cabozantinib have demonstrated significant activity against metastatic RCC in randomized phase III trials. A common theme in most of these trials is the cross-over of patients in the placebo group to the treatment group on documented disease progression. Although this is ethically desirable and attractive to patients, a high rate of cross-over often masks the real impact of the investigational drug on OS. Furthermore, OS analysis normally requires long-term follow-up and a larger number of patients. Given these reasons, PFS is often used as a surrogate primary end point for OS.[100] Secondary end points of these trials normally include objective response rate (i.e. partial or complete response on radiological imaging), OS, safety, and quality of life measures.

In the clinical setting, objective assessment for patients on systemic therapy is usually undertaken by computed tomography scans (CT) every three months. The aim is to achieve the absence of progressive disease (i.e. response or stable disease).

Sunitinib

Sunitinib (Pfizer) is an orally active inhibitor of a number protein tyrosine kinases, including the receptors of VEGF (VEGFR-1 to -3), PDGF (PDGFR-α and -β), CD117 (c-Kit), Fms-like tyrosine kinase-3 (FLT-3), colony stimulating factor 1 receptor (CSF1R) and the receptor encoded by the proto-oncogene *RET*. Sunitinib has demonstrated efficacy in phase II trials in the second-line setting of metastatic RCC following progression with cytokine therapy.[101,102] Its role as a first-line treatment was studied in a landmark multinational phase III trial, where 750 treatment-naive patients with metastatic clear cell RCC were randomly assigned to receive either sunitinib or IFN-α 9 MIU subcutaneously thrice weekly.[7,103] Sunitinib demonstrated a survival benefit compared to IFN-α in the first-line setting—median PFS of 11 versus 5 months ($p < 0.001$) and OS of 26.4 versus 21.8 months (HR 0.818; $p = 0.049$), respectively (Table 6.32.4). When 25 patients who crossed over from the IFN-α arm to the sunitinib arm were censored, a clear OS benefit was noted (26.4 vs. 20 months; $p = 0.036$).[103]

After sunitinib became widely available, subsequent studies showed that sunitinib also has activity in patients with non-clear cell histology, poor performance status, age of >65 years, and brain metastases.[3,104]

Sunitinib is normally given at 50 mg daily on a four weeks on, two weeks off schedule, and thus the cycle repeated every 42 days. Dose reductions to 37.5 mg or 25 mg daily can be made to improve tolerability, although there is some concern that reduced drug exposure could impair efficacy.[105] Alternate dosing schedules have been explored to tread the balance between drug exposure and toxicity. Bjarmason *et al.* reported a phase II study of individualized toxicity-driven dosing of sunitnib.[106] The protocol included dose escalation for patients with minimal toxicity on 50 mg, and dose reduction and individualized treatment duration for those not tolerating treatment. In this small study, flexible dosing appeared safe and did not appear to compromise drug response.

Pazopanib

Pazopanib (Votrient®, GlaxoSmithKline) is an oral TKI targeting VEGFRs, PDGFRs, CSF1R, and CD117. In a phase III trial, 435 patients with locally advanced or metastatic RCC (treatment-naive or previous cytokine therapy) were randomized 2:1 to receive pazopanib 800 mg daily or placebo.[6] All patients had clear cell or predominantly clear cell histology. In the treatment-naive population, a median PFS of 11.1 months was noted in the pazopanib group compared to 2.8 months in the placebo group ($p < 0.0001$) (Table 6.32.4). An OS advantage was masked by a large number of patients (51%) in the placebo group who crossed over to receive pazopanib (22.9 months with pazopanib vs. 23.5 months with placebo). A post-hoc analysis designed to adjust for this cross-over showed that pazopanib reduced the risk of death by 50% compared to placebo in the treatment-naive patients. Analysis using data from sunitinib, pazopanib, IFN-α, and placebo showed that the estimated median OS were 27.8, 26.8, 15.8, and 12.1 months, respectively.[107] Pazopanib was subsequently compared to sunitinib in the first-line setting, in the phase III non-inferiority COMPARZ (Comparing the Efficacy, Safety and Tolerability of Pazopanib vs. Sunitinib) trial.[108] This trial randomized 1,100 treatment-naive patients with clear cell RCC to either continuous pazopanib 800 mg once daily or sunitinib. Pazopanib was non-inferior to sunitinib in terms of OS and PFS (Table 6.32.4). The efficacy of pazopanib is thus comparable to that of sunitinib, and it has been approved by UK's National Institute for Health and Clinical Excellence for the first-line treatment of advanced RCC who have not received prior cytokine therapy. Results from the PISCES (Patient Preference Study of Pazopanib versus Sunitinib in Advanced or Metastatic Kidney Cancer) cross-over trial of 168 patients showed that the majority of patients preferred pazopanib over sunitinib (70% vs. 22%), due to better quality of life and less fatigue.[109]

Sorafenib

Sorafenib (Nexavar®, Bayer) is a small molecule inhibitor against several tyrosine kinases, including VEGFRs, PDGFRs, FLT-3, CD117, RET, and Raf. Its role as a second-line agent in metastatic RCC has been tested in the large Treatment Approaches in Renal Cancer Global Evaluation Trial (TARGET), where 903 patients were randomized to receive sorafenib 400 mg twice daily or placebo.[5,110] The selected patients had metastatic clear cell RCC which had progressed after one systemic treatment within the previous eight months, had good performance status and were in the low-to-intermediate risk groups according to the MSKCC prognostic score. After correcting for the high rate of cross-over between the two treatment groups, median OS were found to be 17.8 and 14.3 months for sorafenib and placebo, respectively (HR = 0.78; $p = 0.029$) (Table 6.32.4). Subgroup analysis revealed that the clinical benefit and quality of life of those treated with sorafenib were similar among the older (≥70 years) and younger patients.[111]

The benefit of sorafenib as a first-line agent in metastatic RCC was shown to be similar to that of IFN-α in a phase II trial of 189 patients.[112] Other randomized trials showed no difference in PFS with first-line sorafenib monotherapy compared to sorafenib in combination with IFN-α, IL-2, trabaninib (AMG 386, a selective angiopoietin 1/2-neutralizing peptibody).[113–115] Sorafenib remains licensed for metastatic RCC, although higher level evidence exists for other TKIs, and subsequently this agent is less frequently used.

Axitinib

Axitinib (Inlyta®, Pfizer) is an orally active potent inhibitor of VEGFR-1 to -3 that can block these receptors at subnanomolar drug concentrations. It has weaker activity against PDGFRs and CD117. Axitinib is a second-generation TKI that is a highly potent and specific inhibitor of VEGF-signalling. These properties maximize on-target effects while minimizing off-target toxicities. In the AXIS (axitinib vs. sorafenib) trial, 723 patients with metastatic clear cell RCC who had progressed after first-line treatment with sunitinib, bevacizumab plus IFN-α, temsirolimus, or cytokines were randomized to receive axitinib (starting dose of 5 mg twice daily) or sorafenib.[116] The median PFS was longer in the axitinib group compared to the sorafenib group (6.7 vs. 4.7 months; HR = 0.665; $p < 0.0001$) (Table 6.32.4). The benefit was higher in patients previously treated with cytokines (12.1 vs. 6.5 months) compared to those treated previously with sunitinib (4.8 vs. 3.4 months). Final OS data—a secondary outcome measure—showed no significant difference between axitinib and sorafenib (20.1 vs. 19.2 months, HR 0.969, $p = 0.37$).[117] A phase 3 trial in the first-line setting randomized 288 previously untreated patients in a 2:1 ratio to axitinib or sorafenib.[118] There was no statistically significant difference in PFS, which was 10.1 months with axitinib, and 6.5 months for sorafenib (HR 0.77, $p = 0.038$).

Cabozantinib

Cabozantinib (Cabometyx®, Exelixis) is an oral small molecule inhibitor of a range of tyrosine kinases including VEGFRs, MET, and AXL. c-MET is has been found to be overexpressed in sporadic ccRCC, and is an independent predictor of poor prognosis.[119]

The phase III METEOR study randomized 658 patients with clear cell RCC who had progressed on at least one line of anti-VEGF TKI treatment to either cabozantinib 60 mg or everolimus.[120] Patients receiving cabozantinib had a significantly prolonged median OS of 21.4 months versus 16.5 months for everolimus (HR 0.66, $p = 0.00026$). Cabozantinib treatment also led to an improved PFS of 7.4 months versus 3.9 months for everolimus. Based on these results, cabozantinib has now become an established treatment in the second line. The phase II CABOSUN study recently reported results for cabozantinib in the first line in patients with poor or intermediate risk metastatic RCC.[121] Some 157 patients with untreated metastatic clear cell RCC were randomized to cabozantinib or sunitinib. The results were significantly in favour of cabozantinib with a PFS of 8.2 versus 5.6 months ($p = 0.012$) and an impressive ORR of 46% (vs. 18%).

Lenvatinib

Lenvatinib (Kisplyx®/Lenvima®, Eisai) is a oral multitarget tyrosine kinase inhibitor with targets including the VEGFRs 1-3, FGFRs 1-4, PDGFRα, RET, and KIT. Lenvatinib has been approved in combination with everolimus in the second line based on the results of an open-label phase 2 study. Some 153 patients were randomized to receive lenvatinib, everolimus, or both drugs combined.[122] The doses used in the combination arm were lenvatinib 18 mg and everolimus 5 mg, both once daily. The primary outcomes of investigator-assessed PFS were 14.6 months, 7.4 months, and 5.5 months in combination, lenvatinib, and everolimus arms, respectively. The difference in PFS between lenvatinib/everolimus combination and everolimus was significant (HR 0.40, $p = 0.0005$). There was also a statistically significant difference in PFS when comparing monotherapy with lenvatinib with that of everolimus (HR 0.61, $p = 0.048$). However there was no significant difference in PFS when comparing combination treatment with lenvatinib monotherapy (HR 0.66, $p = 0.12$).

Fatigue, reduced appetite, and diarrhoea were the most common adverse events in the combination arm, which had a slightly higher rate of grade 3 or 4 events compared to everolimus (45% vs. 38%). A post-hoc retrospective independent radiological review requested by regulatory authorities confirmed the PFS advantage of the lenvatinib/everolimus combination over single-agent everolimus with a PFS of 12.8 months vs. 5.6 months (HR 0.45, $p = 0.0029$).[123] In the independently reviewed analysis, there was no significant difference between lenvatinib monotherapy and everolimus monotherapy.

Antiangiogenic antibody

Bevacizumab (Avastin®, Roche) is a humanized mouse monoclonal IgG1 antibody that inhibits angiogenesis via its interaction with VEGF-A. In the phase III European AVOREN (Avastin® and Roferon® in RCC) trial, 649 patients with previously untreated metastatic RCC were randomized to receive IFN-α (9 MIU subcutaneously three times weekly) and bevacizumab (10 mg/kg intravenously every two weeks), or placebo and IFN-α111,112 (Table 6.32.4).[124,125] Median PFS was longer in the bevacizumab and IFN-α group compared to control (10.2 vs. 5.4 months; HR = 0.63; $p = 0.0001$). However, there was no significant difference in OS (23.3 vs. 21.3 months). Another trial performed by the Cancer and Leukemia Group B (CALGB) in the United States involved 732 previously untreated patients with metastatic clear cell RCC, randomized to receive either bevacizumab and IFN-α or IFN-α alone.[8,126] Again, there was an improvement in median PFS with combination treatment compared to IFN-α alone (8.5 vs. 5.2 months; HR = 0.72; $p < 0.001$), but no OS benefit was noted (18.3 vs. 17.4 months). The failure of translating improvement in PFS to better OS was likely to be the result of a large number of patients receiving subsequent treatments when they progressed during or after the trials, therefore masking the true benefit of adding bevacizumab.

mTOR inhibitors

The mTOR (mammalian target of rapamycin) signalling pathway plays an important role in cancer growth and progression. Upon activation by upstream growth factor receptor or Ras, the protein phosphatidylinositol 3-kinase (PI3K) phosphorylates Akt (Fig. 6.32.1). This releases the inhibition of tuberous sclerosis complex 2 (TSC2) on Rheb, resulting in the activation of mTOR. mTOR forms multimolecular complexes with either Raptor to form mTORC1, or Rictor to form mTORC2. mTORC1 phosphorylates S6 kinase 1 (S6K1, also known as $p70^{S6K}$) and eukaryotic translation initiation factor 4E-binding protein 1 (4E-BP1), both of which control the translation of specific mRNAs and the synthesis of proteins involved in a variety of cellular events, including cell proliferation, survival, resistance to apoptosis, angiogenesis, and invasion. Importantly, mTOR signalling also controls the synthesis of HIF-α. This pathway could be targeted by an mTOR inhibitor.

The first mTOR inhibitor, sirolimus (or rapamycin, so named as it was first isolated from *Streptomyces hygroscopicus* in the soil sample from Rapa Nui), was initially discovered as part of a screening programme for new antifungal agents. Rapamycin and its analogues were later found to have immunosuppressive and more importantly, antitumour properties. The mTOR inhibitors currently in clinical use for RCC are temsirolimus and everolimus. The main differences between these drugs lie in their chemical properties in terms of drug solubility and metabolism. Temsirolimus, a prodrug of sirolimus, is water soluble and is given intravenously, whereas everolimus has low solubility and therefore has to be administered orally.

Temsirolimus

The efficacy of temsirolimus (Torisel®, Pfizer) was evaluated in the Global Advanced RCC (ARCC) trial of 626 patients with previously untreated metastatic RCC with poor prognosis (defined as ≥3 of the following six factors: Karnofsky performance status of 60 or 70; haemoglobin <lower limit of normal; corrected calcium >10 mg/dL; LDH >1.5× upper limit of normal; time from initial diagnosis to randomization of <1 year; and metastases in multiple organs).[127] Patients (80% of whom had clear cell carcinoma) were randomized to receive either intravenous temsirolimus 25 mg weekly alone, IFN-α alone, or combination treatment. Patients who received temsirolimus alone had a longer median OS compared to IFN-α alone (10.9 vs. 7.3 months; HR = 0.73; $p = 0.008$). The combination of temsirolimus and IFN not only failed to improve PFS and OS but was associated with more serious adverse events. Subgroup analyses suggest that benefit may be limited to patients under the age of 65 and those with a KPS over 70%. The evidence from this trial supports the use of temsirolimus as a first-line treatment option for patients with poor-risk RCC who are able to tolerate treatment. Antihistamine is routinely given prior to temsirolimus to prevent hypersensitivity reactions.

Everolimus

Everolimus (Afinitor®, Novartis) is an orally administered mTOR inhibitor. In the RECORD-1 (Renal Cell Cancer Treatment with Oral RAD001 Given Daily) trial, 416 patients with metastatic RCC who had progressed on, or within six months of stopping sunitinib, sorafenib, or both were randomized 2:1 to receive everolimus 10 mg daily or placebo.[4,128] Median PFS was in favour of everolimus (4.9 vs. 1.9 months; p <0.001), although there was no difference in median OS (14.8 months with everolimus vs. 14.4 months with placebo). As 80% of patients in the placebo arm crossed over to everolimus, a recalculation estimated the MS of patients in the placebo group to be 10 months (i.e. 4.8 months less than that of the everolimus group). Shorter survival was associated with low performance status, hypercalcaemia, low haemoglobin, and prior sunitinib treatment.

Side effects of targeted treatment and their management

Side effects are common with the use of targeted therapies.[129] For multitargeted TKIs such as sunitinib and pazopanib, the intended antitumour targets are primarily those of the VEGF-angiogenesis signalling pathway. These 'on-target' toxicities are largely similar to those of the anti-VEGF antibody bevacizumab and include hypertension and dysphonia (Table 6.32.5). A number of 'off-target' toxicities are also common and are partly related to inhibitory effects on other kinases.

Symptoms such as fatigue, alopecia, anorexia, nausea, stomatitis, and dermatological toxicities are managed by patient education and prophylactic or early interventions. Hand-foot syndrome, or palmar-plantar erythrodysaesthesia, is a spectrum of skin reaction ranging from erythema to desquamation, and is thought to be due to the direct toxic effect and impaired vascular repair mechanism secondary to TKI exposure.[130] Avoidance of excessive trauma and application of emollients are effective preventative measures.[129]

Hypothyroidism occurred in 14% of patients on sunitinib.[103] This could be the result of a number of mechanisms, including impaired blood flow leading to thyroiditis, and the inhibition of RET resulting in thyroid follicular cell apoptosis.[131] Routine monitoring of thyroid function is required and replacement therapy needs to be started when necessary. Moderate-to-severe derangement in liver enzymes, usually asymptomatic and occurring within the first four months of treatment, have been reported in up to 12% of patients on pazopanib.[6] As such, close monitoring is essential and treatment interruptions may be needed.

TKIs can cause hypertension and cardiotoxicity.[132] Blood pressure is closely monitored and can be treated with antihypertensives. Echocardiogram and electrocardiogram (ECG) assessment are normally advised in elderly patients, in patients with a history of cardiovascular disease, or cardiovascular risk factors such as diabetes, both before and, if clinically indicated, during treatment. A left ventricular ejection fraction of ≥50% is normally considered safe to commence treatment, whereas significant ischaemic changes, arrhythmias, or prolonged QT interval on ECG must be taken with caution and referral to a cardiologist may be indicated. TKIs can also result in QT prolongation and may lead to ventricular arrhythmias including torsades de pointes. Other concomitant drugs that may cause QT prolongation should be used with caution, including ciprofloxacin, clarithromycin, erythromycin, domperidone, ondansetron, and the selective serotonin reuptake inhibitor (SSRI) antidepressants.

The mTOR inhibitors could also result in metabolic abnormalities such as hyperglycaemia, hypokalaemia, and hyperlipidaemia, which require careful monitoring. A non-infectious pneumonitis has been reported in about 10% of patients and this is best managed by early recognition and prompt intervention, usually by dose reduction or treatment interruption.[4,127,128] Corticosteroids may be needed in severe cases.

TKIs and mTOR inhibitors are primarily metabolized by the liver enzyme cytochrome $P_{450}3A4$ (CYP3A4). As a result, CYP3A4 inhibitors could increase plasma drug levels and toxicities, and should therefore be avoided (Table 6.32.6). Potent CYP3A4 inducers, on the other hand, could reduce drug concentrations and potentially treatment efficacy.

Table 6.32.5 On- and off-target toxicities of VEGF inhibition

On-target	Off-target
Hypertension	Anorexia
Proteinuria	Diarrhoea
Bleeding	Nausea and vomiting
Thrombosis	Fatigue
Poor wound healing	Hypothyroidism
Gastrointestinal perforation	Stomatitis
Hypothyroidism	Cardiotoxicity
Hand-foot syndrome	Alopecia
Dysphonia	Rash or skin discoloration
	Hand-foot syndrome
	Myelosuppression
	Hepatotoxicity

Table 6.32.6 Drugs that affect liver CYP3A4

CYP3A4 inhibitors (may increase levels of TKI or mTOR inhibitor)	
Strong inhibitors:	Moderate inhibitors:
Clarithromycin	Aprepitant
Indinavir	Ciclosporin
Itraconazole	Diltiazem
Ketoconazole	Erythromycin
Nelfinavir	Fluconazole
Ritonavir	Grapefruit juice
Voriconazole	Verapamil
CYP3A4 inducers (may decrease levels of TKI or mTOR inhibitor)	
Carbamazapine	
Dexamethasone	
Efavirenz	
Nevirapine	
Phenytoin	
Prednisolone	
Rifampicin	
St. John's Wort	

The introduction of TCCIs has brought with it a new range of toxicities, which the medical community has had to rapidly assimilate into its practice and learn to manage effectively. In the phase III trial of nivolumab in RCC, treatment was relatively well-tolerated overall with a grade 3/4 toxicitiy rate of 19%.[91] Treatment was discontinued due to adverse events in 8% of patients in the nivolumab arm. The commonest (all-grade) adverse events were fatigue (33%), nausea (14%), pruritis (14%), diarrhoea (12%), and decreased appetite (12%). Nivolumab, in common with other TCCIs, is associated with immune-related adverse events (irAEs), a group of autoimmune side effects resulting from activation of the immune system. Pneumonitis, endocrinopathies, colitis, and hepatitis have all been observed with nivolumab, although any system can be affected.[91,133,134] Management algorithms vary slightly depending on the system affected, but the general principle is to withhold treatment until symptoms resolve, with the addition of corticosteroids and other immunosuppressants, if required.

Patients with diarrhoea should be monitored for signs and symptoms of colitis, which include passing blood or mucus per rectum and abdominal pain.[133] Mild (grade 1) diarrhoea can be managed with supportive measures including loperamide and increasing oral fluid. If there are more than four bowel motions per day over baseline, then treatment should be withheld, with the introduction of steroids if there is no improvement.[133] Grade 3 diarrhoea mandates admission for steroids, with the addition of infliximab (5 mg/kg) if there is no improvement after three days. Asymptomatic pneumonitis should be managed by withholding treatment and giving corticosteroids (e.g. prednisolone 1 mg/kg/day PO). Treatment can be reintroduced once the radiological appearances have resolved.[133,134] For more severe pneumonitis, the patient should be admitted for intravenous corticosteroids, consideration should be given to the administration of empirical antibiotics and infliximab. Bronchoscopy with biopsy may also be appropriate.[133] Treatment should be permanently discontinued after a single episode of grade 3 pneumonitis.

Systemic treatment of metastatic non-clear cell carcinoma

Malignant non-clear cell RCCs are a clinically and histologically diverse group of cancers, They include chromophobe, collecting duct, and papillary (types I and II) tumours, as well as other rarer types that remain histologically unclassified. The chromophobe subtype is found in 4% of cases, and is often organ-confined and has a low risk of tumour progression, metastasis, and death.[10,135,136] In contrast, collecting duct RCC, although extremely rare (<1%), is aggressive and associated with a worse prognosis.[10,135] Papillary tumours are the second commonest histological subtype after clear cell, and account for 10–15% of all renal cancer. Localized disease has a favourable prognosis, but metastatic papillary carcinoma has a worse outcome in terms of survival and resistance to systemic therapy than clear cell carcinoma—this is particularly the case for the more aggressive, high-grade type II tumour.[135,137,138] In the pre-TKI era, MS were estimated to be 29, 11, and 5.5 months for chromophobe, collecting duct, and papillary tumours, respectively.[135]

Non-clear cell RCCs are far less common than their clear cell counterpart, and the majority of clinical trials have excluded these histological subtypes. With the exception of temsirolimus (subgroup analysis), phase III evidence for the systemic therapy of patients with metastatic non-clear cell RCC is lacking. A subgroup analysis of the Global ARCC trial (for which 124 patients (20%) had non-clear cell tumours, mainly papillary) demonstrated that temsirolimus was as effective in improving PFS and OS for patients with non-clear cell compared to clear cell carcinomas.[127,139] Most benefit was seen in patients with poor prognostic features.

Evidence for the use of TKIs and mTOR inhibitors and their relative efficacy in non-clear cell RCC has consisted of retrospective analyses, cohort studies, and a small number of phase 2 trials. In the expanded-access trial for sunitinib, Gore *et al.* showed that this agent conferred a response rate of 11% for patients with non-clear cell RCC.[3] Choueiri *et al.* performed a retrospective multicentre review of 53 patients with metastatic papillary and chromophobe RCCs who were treated with sunitinib or sorafenib.[140] The overall PFS for patients with chromophobe RCC was 10.6 months and 7.6 months for papillary RCC. Patients with papillary RCC treated with sunitinib had a much longer PFS (11.9 months) compared to those treated with sorafenib (5.1 months; p <0.001). A single-arm phase II trial of 57 patients treated with sunitinib suggested a much more limited benefit for sunitinib in papillary RCC with a PFS of only 1.6 months.[141] Patients with chromophobe histology had a much longer PFS of 12.7 months.

There are two recent phase II trials randomizing patients with non-clear cell RCC to everolimus and sunitinib, which have reported conflicting results. The ASPEN (Afinitor® versus Sutent® in Patients with Metastatic Non-Clear Cell RCC) trial compared sunitinib and everolimus in the previously untreated patients with non-clear cell RCC.[142] The study included 108 patients with papillary (65%), chromophobe (15%), and unclassified (19%) histology. Overall, sunitinib resulted in an improved PFS compared to everolimus (8.3 months vs. 5.6 months). Subgroup analyses showed interesting differential responses according to histological subtypes. Everolimus appeared superior for MSKCC poor-risk and chromophobe histology, while patients with good and intermediate-risk disease and non-chromophobe histology appeared to benefit most from sunitinib.

In contrast, the recently reported phase II ESPN study, which also randomized patients with non-clear cell histology (n = 68) to everolimus or sunitinib found no significant difference in PFS.[143]

Erlotinib, an oral epidermal growth factor receptor (EGFR) TKI, has been studied in a phase II trial of patients with advanced papillary RCC.[144] Of the 45 evaluable patients, the overall response rate was 11% and the median OS was 27 months. Although this was a single-arm study, the OS observed was higher than that reported previously.[135,140] There have been some phase II trials that have also shown some promising results for non-clear cell RCC with chemotherapy, alone, or in combination with TKIs (see 'Chemotherapy in metastatic renal cell carcinoma', below).

In summary, due to the lack of strong evidence for the systemic treatment of metastatic non-clear cell RCC, enrolment of patients into clinical trials is currently the preferred strategy.

Chemotherapy in metastatic renal cell carcinoma

Chemotherapy does not have an established role in the treatment of metastatic RCC. RCC is invariably insensitive to chemotherapy and data were normally obtained from small trials or case reports. Phase II studies of single-agent gemcitabine, or in combination with intravenous or oral fluoropyrimidines (5-fluorouracil, capecitabine or S-1) and cisplatin have reported response rates of 5 to 24.4% in metastatic RCC.[145–154] The addition of sorafenib to gemcitabine and metronomic capecitabine appeared to be more effective, resulting in partial response in 20 out of 40 patients studied and a median PFS of 11 months.[155] Michaelson *et al.* reported the results of a phase II study in which patients with poor-risk or sarcomatoid clear cell RCC were given a combination of sunitinib and gemcitabine.[156] The response rates were a promising 26% and 24% in the sarcomatoid and poor-risk patients, respectively, and the combination is being evaluated further.

A multicentre phase II trial of 23 patients with metastatic collecting duct tumour reported a response rate of 26%, PFS of 7.1 months, and OS of 10.5 months using gemcitabine with a platinum agent.[157] In RCC with sarcomatoid differentiation, which is associated with rapid progression and poor prognosis, the combination of doxorubicin and gemcitabine has shown moderate activity in small studies.[158–160]

Therapies in development

Many novel therapeutic agents are currently in development, and patients should be encouraged to enter clinical trials.

After the success of the TKIs and the improved understanding of the molecular biology of RCC, a substantial effort has been put into extracting maximum benefit from this treatment modality. This includes the optimization of dosing and scheduling with the currently approved drugs and the use of sequential or combination therapy. The development of predictive biomarkers of response to treatment would greatly aid treatment choice. For example, low plasma levels cytokine and angiogenic factors such as IL-6, IL-8, VEGF, osteopontin, and hepatocyte growth factor (HGF) were found to be associated with response and PFS from pazopanib treatment.[161]

In addition, a number of factors need to be considered during the development of new TKIs, such as the drug's pharmacokinetics and bioavailability, interaction with other drugs, target specificity, and toxicities. The ideal drug would be one that provides multiple tumour only-specific target inhibition at low concentration. It may also possible to re-engineer drugs to avoid off-target pathways if the underlying mechanism is known.[162]

Foretinib (GSK1363089, GlaxoSmithKline), inhibits the *MET*-encoded HGF receptor and VEGFR-2. Mutations of *MET* can be found in sporadic or hereditary papillary RCC, conditions with a poor prognosis that represent an area of unmet need.[163,164] Foretinib has shown promising activity in RCC in early phase trials, while another MET-inhibitor (savolitinib), is also currently undergoing evaluation in a phase II trial.[165,166] Cediranib (Recentin® or AZD2171, AstraZeneca) is a potent TKI against VEGFR-1 to -3. In a phase II trial, it has shown a response rate of 34% in patients with advanced clear cell RCC, resulting in a median PFS of 12.1 months compared to 2.8 months in the placebo group.[167]

One of the biggest advances in the management of metastatic RCC in the last decade has been the emergence of immunotherapy targeting T-cell checkpoints, aimed at stimulating the cytotoxic T-cell response. A number of other agents and combinations of agents targeting these pathways have shown promise and are undergoing further investigation. The phase III CheckMate214 study is combining nivolumab with the anti-CTLA4 antibody ipilimumab in the first-line treatment of metastatic RCC.[168] The comparator arm in this trial is sunitinib. Dudek *et al.* recently reported a phase I study in which the anti-PD-1 antibody pembrolizumab was safely combined with bevacizumab.[169] A number of other early phase trials are investigating combining the monoclonal anti-VEGF antibodies bevacizumab and aflibercept, with a number of other T-cell modulating agents including nivolumab, pembrolizumab, and atezolizumab.

Active immunotherapy in the form of vaccination has also been studied. AGS-003 (Arcelis®, Argos Therapeutics) is a form of personalized immunotherapy whereby a patient's own dendritic cells (DCs) are collected by leukapheresis, then co-electroporated with his/her own tumour mRNA and synthetic CD40 ligand RNA. The resulting cells are delivered back to the patient by intradermal injection. The rationale is that by combining DCs (the most important antigen-presenting cells) with tumour antigens and the immunostimulating CD40 ligand would result in a T-cell-mediated antitumour immunity. Phase II data showed that the combination of AGS-003 with sunitinib in patients with poor and intermediate-risk patients with RCC produced promising results.[170] The ongoing phase III ADAPT (Autologous Dendritic Cell Immunotherapy (AGS-003) Plus Standard Treatment of Advanced RCC) trial is expected to report in 2017.

Many other potential therapeutic targets and drugs are constantly being discovered in RCC. As mentioned earlier, the HIF pathway plays an important role in RCC progression, and inhibition of HIF has been shown to suppress tumour growth in the laboratory.[171,172] Inhibitors of HIF are currently in development.[173–176] In addition, the increased expression of tumour necrosis factor receptor-2 (which promotes VEGFR-2 signalling) and the activation of the Notch signalling pathway have also been found to be important in RCC development.[177–179] It is now known that some of the mutated genes found in RCC (i.e. *VHL, MET, TSC1, TSC2, FLCN* (folliculin), *FH* (fumarate hydratase), and *SDH* (succinate dehydrogenase)), can result in the dysregulation of a number of metabolic pathways involving oxygen, iron, nutrient and/or energy sensing.[180] These pathways could provide an opportunity for therapeutic targeting. *PBRM1* has been found to be mutated in 41% of clear cell RCC.[181] This gene encodes for the tumour suppressor protein polybromo-1 (Pb1) which is involved in chromatin remodelling.[182] This in turn controls the accessibility of DNA and regulates gene transcription. Inactivation of Pb1 could therefore result in abnormal transcriptional activity and subsequently tumourigenesis and disease progression.[183] It will be take some time before agents targeting these aberrations could be used clinically; nonetheless, the outcome of patients with metastatic RCC certainly looks promising in the coming years.

Conclusion

Currently about 14% of patients with RCC have metastatic disease at the time of diagnosis.[1] While this used to carry a dire prognosis, the MS of these patients have doubled over the last 10 years; this could be as high as 44 months for low-risk patients.[9] There are several reasons to be optimistic, not least because of improvement in diagnostic imaging and surgical techniques, but significant progress has also been made in understanding the molecular biology and clinical behaviour of RCC, as well as the emergence of new treatment modalities.

Prognostic scoring systems are invaluable for identifying patients that may be suitable for either conservative or more aggressive interventions. These include nephrectomy or other surgical and non-surgical procedures to prolong survival and for symptom control. Most patients do require and benefit from systemic treatment, and IFN-α and IL-2 used to be the main form of therapy before the arrival of targeted agents. IL-2 is effective and still being used, although this comes at the expense of inpatient treatment and severe toxicities. Over the last decade TKIs, mTOR inhibitors, and the anti-VEGF antibody bevacizumab completely revolutionized the treatment of metastatic RCC, resulting in improved survival with acceptable toxicities. In the last year, yet another paradigm shift has taken place in the treatment of metastatic renal cancer with the advent of the T-cell checkpoint inhibitors. The treatment algorithm based on currently available evidence is summarized in Table 6.32.3. It is expected this will change again in the coming years as more novel therapeutic approaches are being developed.

Further reading

Choueiri TK, Escudier B, Powles T, *et al.* Cabozantinib versus everolimus in advanced renal cell carcinoma. *Lancet Oncol* 2016; **17**:917–27.

Cohen HT, McGovern FJ. Renal-cell carcinoma. *N Engl J Med* 2005; **353**:2477–90.

Eisen T, Sternberg CN, Robert C, *et al.* Targeted therapies for renal cell carcinoma: review of adverse event management strategies. *J Natl Cancer Inst* 2012; **104**:93–113.

Escudier B, Eisen T, Stadler WM, *et al.* Sorafenib in advanced clear-cell renal-cell carcinoma. *N Engl J Med* 2007; **356**:125–34.

Escudier B, Pluzanska A, Koralewski P, *et al.* Bevacizumab plus interferon alfa-2a for treatment of metastatic renal cell carcinoma: a randomised, double-blind phase III trial. *Lancet* 2007; **370**:2103–11.

Flanigan RC, Salmon SE, Blumenstein BA, *et al.* Nephrectomy followed by interferon alfa-2b compared with interferon alfa-2b alone for metastatic renal-cell cancer. *N Engl J Med* 2001; **345**:1655–9.

Heng DY, Xie W, Regan MM, *et al.* Prognostic factors for overall survival in patients with metastatic renal cell carcinoma treated with vascular endothelial growth factor-targeted agents: results from a large, multicenter study. *J Clin Oncol* 2009; **27**:5794–9.

Hudes G, Carducci M, Tomczak P, *et al.* Temsirolimus, interferon alfa, or both for advanced renal-cell carcinoma. *N Engl J Med* 2007; **356**:2271–81.

Kavolius JP, Mastorakos DP, Pavlovich C, Russo P, Burt ME, Brady MS. *Resection of metastatic renal cell carcinoma. J Clin Oncol* 1998; **16**:2261–6.

McDermott DF, Regan MM, Clark JI, *et al.* Randomized phase III trial of high-dose interleukin-2 versus subcutaneous interleukin-2 and interferon in patients with metastatic renal cell carcinoma. *J Clin Oncol* 2005; **23**:133–41.

Mekhail TM, Abou-Jawde RM, Boumerhi G, *et al.* Validation and extension of the Memorial Sloan-Kettering prognostic factors model for survival in patients with previously untreated metastatic renl cell carcinoma. *J Clin Oncol* 2005; **23**:832–41.

Mickisch GH, Garin A, van Poppel H, de Prijck L, Sylvester R. Radical nephrectomy plus interferon-alfa-based immunotherapy compared with interferon alfa alone in metastatic renal-cell carcinoma: a randomised trial. *Lancet* 2001; **358**:966–70.

Motzer RJ, Bacik J, Schwartz LH, *et al.* Prognostic factors for survival in previously treated patients with metastatic renal cell carcinoma. *J Clin Oncol* 2004; **22**:454–63.

Motzer RJ, Escudier B, McDermott DF, *et al.* Nivolumab versus everolimus in advanced renal-cell carcinoma. *N Engl J Med* 2015; **373**:1803–13.

Motzer RJ, Escudier B, Oudard S, *et al.* Efficacy of everolimus in advanced renal cell carcinoma: a double-blind, randomised, placebo-controlled phase III trial. *Lancet* 2008; **372**:449–56.

Motzer RJ, Hutson TE, Cella D, *et al.* Pazopanib versus sunitinib in the metastatic renal-cell carcinoma. *N Engl J Med* 2013; **369**:722–31.

Motzer RJ, Hutson TE, Tomczak P, *et al.* Sunitinib versus interferon alfa in metastatic renal-cell carcinoma. *N Engl J Med* 2007; **356**:115–24.

Motzer RJ, Mazumdar M, Bacik J, Berg W, Amsterdam A, Ferrara J. Survival and prognostic stratification of 670 patients with advanced renal cell carcinoma. *J Clin Oncol* 1999; **17**:2530–40.

Négrier S, Escudier B, Lasset C, *et al.* Recombinant human interleukin-2, recombinant human interferon alfa-2a, or both in metastatic renal-cell carcinoma. Groupe Français d'Immunothérapie. *N Engl J Med* 1998; **338**:1272–8.

Rini BI, Escudier B, Tomczak P, *et al.* Comparative effectiveness of axitinib versus sorafenib in advanced renal cell carcinoma (AXIS): a randomised phase 3 trial. *Lancet* 2011; **378**:1931–9.

Rini BI, Halabi S, Rosenberg JE, *et al.* Bevacizumab plus interferon alfa compared with interferon alfa monotherapy in patients with metastatic renal cell carcinoma: CALGB 90206. *J Clin Oncol* 2008; **26**:5422–8.

Sternberg CN, Davis ID, Mardiak J, *et al.* Pazopanib in locally advanced or metastatic renal cell carcinoma: results of a randomized phase III trial. *J Clin Oncol* 2010; **28**:1061–8.

Weinstock M, McDermott D. Targeting PD-1/PD-L1 in the treatment of metastatic renal cell carcinoma. *Ther Adv Urol* 2015; **7**:365–77.

Yang JC, Sherry RM, Steinberg SM, *et al.* Randomized study of high-dose and low-dose interleukin-2 in patients with metastatic renal cancer. *J Clin Oncol* 2003; **21**:3127–32.

References

1. Sun M, Thuret R, Abdollah F, *et al.* Age-adjusted incidence, mortality, and survival rates of stage-specific renal cell carcinoma in North America: a trend analysis. *Eur Urol* 2011; **59**:135–41.
2. Barnholtz-Sloan JS, Sloan AE, Davis FG, Vigneau FD, Lai P, Sawaya RE. Incidence proportions of brain metastases in patients diagnosed (1973 to 2001) in the Metropolitan Detroit Cancer Surveillance System. *J Clin Oncol* 2004; **22**:2865–72.
3. Gore ME, Szczylik C, Porta C, *et al.* Safety and efficacy of sunitinib for metastatic renal-cell carcinoma: an expanded-access trial. *Lancet Oncol* 2009; **10**:757–63.
4. Motzer RJ, Escudier B, Oudard S, *et al.* Efficacy of everolimus in advanced renal cell carcinoma: a double-blind, randomised, placebo-controlled phase III trial. *Lancet* 2008; **372**:449–56.
5. Escudier B, Eisen T, Stadler WM, *et al.* Sorafenib in advanced clear-cell renal-cell carcinoma. *N Engl J Med* 2007; **356**:125–34.
6. Sternberg CN, Davis ID, Mardiak J, *et al.* Pazopanib in locally advanced or metastatic renal cell carcinoma: results of a randomized phase III trial. *J Clin Oncol* 2010; **28**:1061–8.
7. Motzer RJ, Hutson TE, Tomczak P, *et al.* Sunitinib versus interferon alfa in metastatic renal-cell carcinoma. *N Engl J Med* 2007; **356**:115–24.
8. Rini BI, Halabi S, Rosenberg JE, *et al.* Bevacizumab plus interferon alfa compared with interferon alfa monotherapy in patients with metastatic renal cell carcinoma: CALGB 90206. *J Clin Oncol* 2008; **26**:5422–8.
9. Procopio G, Verzoni E, Iacovelli R, *et al.* Prognostic factors for survival in patients with metastatic renal cell carcinoma treated with targeted therapies. *Br J Cancer* 2012; **107**:1227–32.
10. Cohen HT, McGovern FJ. Renal-cell carcinoma. *N Engl J Med* 2005; **353**:2477–90.
11. Motzer RJ, Mazumdar M, Bacik J, Berg W, Amsterdam A, Ferrara J. Survival and prognostic stratification of 670 patients with advanced renal cell carcinoma. *J Clin Oncol* 1999; **17**:2530–40.
12. Motzer RJ, Bacik J, Murphy BA, Russo P, Mazumdar M. Interferon-alfa as a comparative treatment for clinical trials of new therapies against advanced renal cell carcinoma. *J Clin Oncol* 2002; **20**:289–96.
13. Motzer RJ, Bacik J, Schwartz LH, *et al.* Prognostic factors for survival in previously treated patients with metastatic renal cell carcinoma. *J Clin Oncol* 2004; **22**:454–63.
14. Mekhail TM, Abou-Jawde RM, Boumerhi G, *et al.* Validation and extension of the Memorial Sloan-Kettering prognostic factors model

for survival in patients with previously untreated metastatic renl cell carcinoma. *J Clin Oncol* 2005; **23**:832–41.

15. Heng DY, Xie W, Regan MM, *et al.* Prognostic factors for overall survival in patients with metastatic renal cell carcinoma treated with vascular endothelial growth factor-targeted agents: results from a large, multicenter study. *J Clin Oncol* 2009; **27**:5794–9.
16. Heng DYC, Xie W, Regan MM, *et al.* External validation and comparison with other models of the International Metastatic Renal-Cell Carcinoma Database Consortium prognostic model: A population-based study. *Lancet Oncol* 2013; **14**:141–8.
17. Manola, J, Royston P, Elson P, *et al.* Prognostic model for survival in patients with metastatic renal cell carcinoma: results from the international kidney cancer working group. *Clin Cancer Res* 2011; **17**:5443–50.
18. Harshman LC, Xie W, Bjarnason GA, *et al.* Conditional survival of patients with metastatic renal-cell carcinoma treated with VEGF-targeted therapy: a population-based study. *Lancet Oncol* 2012; **13**:927–35.
19. Elhilali MM, Gleave M, Fradet Y, *et al.* Placebo-associated remissions in a multicentre, randomized, double-blind trial of interferon gamma-1b for the treatment of metastatic renal cell carcinoma. The Canadian Urologic Oncology Group. *BJU Int* 2000; **86**:613–8.
20. Flanigan RC, Salmon SE, Blumenstein BA, *et al.* Nephrectomy followed by interferon alfa-2b compared with interferon alfa-2b alone for metastatic renal-cell cancer. *N Engl J Med* 2001; **345**:1655–9.
21. Mickisch GH, Garin A, van Poppel H, de Prijck L, Sylvester R. Radical nephrectomy plus interferon-alfa-based immunotherapy compared with interferon alfa alone in metastatic renal-cell carcinoma: a randomised trial. *Lancet* 2001; **358**:966–70.
22. Flanigan RC, Mickisch G, Sylvester R, Tangen C, Van Poppel H, Crawford ED. Cytoreductive nephrectomy in patients with metastatic renal cancer: a combined analysis. *J Urol* 2004; **171**:1071–6.
23. Kassouf W, Sanchez-Ortiz R, Tamboli P, *et al.* Cytoreductive nephrectomy for metastatic renal cell carcinoma with nonclear cell histology. *J Urol* 2007; **178**:1896–900.
24. Rini BI, Campbell SC. The evolving role of surgery for advanced renal cell carcinoma in the era of molecular targeted therapy. *J Urol* 2007; **177**:1978–84.
25. van der Veldt AA, Meijerink MR, van den Eertwegh AJ, *et al.* Sunitinib for treatment of advanced renal cell cancer: primary tumor response. *Clin Cancer Res* 2008; **14**:2431–6.
26. Choueiri TK, Xie W, Kollmannsberger C, *et al.* The impact of cytoreductive nephrectomy on survival of patients with metastatic renal cell carcinoma receiving vascular endothelial growth factor targeted therapy. *J Urol* 2011; **185**:60–6.
27. Vasselli JR, Yang JC, Linehan WM, White DE, Rosenberg SA, Walther MM. Lack of retroperitoneal lymphadenopathy predicts survival of patients with metastatic renal cell carcinoma. *J Urol* 2001; **166**:68–72.
28. Pantuck AJ, Zisman A, Dorey F, *et al.* Renal cell carcinoma with retroperitoneal lymph nodes. Impact on survival and benefits of immunotherapy. *Cancer* 2003; **97**:2995–3002.
29. Pantuck AJ, Zisman A, Dorey F, *et al.* Renal cell carcinoma with retroperitoneal lymph nodes: role of lymph node dissection. *J Urol* 2003;**169**:2076–83.
30. Gershman B, Thompson RH, Moreira DM, *et al.* Lymph node dissection is not associated with improved survival among patients undergoing cytoreductive nephrectomy for metastatic renal cell carcinoma: A propensity-score based analysis. J Urol 2016, doi: 10.1016/j.juro.2016.09.074. [Epub ahead of print].
31. Kavolius JP, Mastorakos DP, Pavlovich C, Russo P, Burt ME, Brady MS. Resection of metastatic renal cell carcinoma. *J Clin Oncol* 1998; **16**:2261–6.
32. Kollender Y, Bickels J, Price WM, *et al.* Metastatic renal cell carcinoma of bone: indications and technique of surgical intervention. *J Urol* 2000; **164**:1505–8.
33. Lin PP, Mirza AN, Lewis VO, *et al.* Patient survival after surgery for osseous metastases from renal cell carcinoma. *J Bone Joint Surg Am* 2007; **89**:1794–801.
34. Shuch B, La Rochelle JC, Klatte T, *et al.* Brain metastasis from renal cell carcinoma: presentation, recurrence, and survival. *Cancer* 2008; **113**:1641–8.
35. Lee DS, White DE, Hurst R, Rosenberg SA, Yang J. Patterns of relapse and response to retreatment in patients with metastatic melanoma or renal cell carcinoma who responded to interleukin-2-based immunotherapy. *Cancer J Sci Am* 1998; **4**:86–93.
36. Karam JA, Rini BI, Varella L, *et al.* Metastasectomy after targeted therapy in patients with advanced renal cell carcinoma. *J Urol* 2011; **185**:439–44.
37. Orlova R, Borisov P, Karlov PA, *et al.* Efficacy of incomplete metastasectomy with targeted therapy in patients with metastatic renal cell carcinoma. *J Clin Oncol* 2016; **34**(Suppl); Abstract e16117.
38. Munro NP, Woodhams S, Nawrocki JD, Fletcher MS, Thomas PJ. The role of transarterial embolization in the treatment of renal cell carcinoma. *BJU Int* 2003; **92**:240–4.
39. Schwartz MJ, Smith EB, Trost DW, Vaughan ED. Renal artery embolization: clinical indications and experience from over 100 cases. *BJU Int* 2007; **99**:881–6.
40. Mukund A, Gamanagatti S. Ethanol ablation of renal cell carcinoma for palliation of symptoms in advanced disease. *J Palliat Med* 2010; **13**:117–20.
41. Nurmi M, Satokari K, Puntala P. Renal artery embolization in the palliative treatment of renal adenocarcinoma. *Scand J Urol Nephrol* 1987; **21**:93–6.
42. Maxwell NJ, Saleem Amer N, Rogers E, Kiely D, Sweeney P, Brady AP. Renal artery embolisation in the palliative treatment of renal carcinoma. *Br J Radiol* 2007; **80**:96–102.
43. Kalman D, Varenhorst E. The role of arterial embolization in renal cell carcinoma. *Scand J Urol Nephrol* 1999; **33**:162–70.
44. Koike Y, Takizawa K, Ogawa Y, *et al.* Transcatheter arterial chemoembolization (TACE) or embolization (TAE) for symptomatic bone metastases as a palliative treatment. *Cardiovasc Intervent Radiol* 2011; **34**:793–801.
45. Vogl TJ, Lehnert T, Zangos S, *et al.* Transpulmonary chemoembolization (TPCE) as a treatment for unresectable lung metastases. *Eur Radiol* 2008; **18**:2449–55.
46. Forauer AR, Kent E, Cwikiel W, Esper P, Redman B. Selective palliative transcatheter embolization of bony metastases from renal cell carcinoma. *Acta Oncol* 2007; **46**:1012–8.
47. Kobak J, Gandras EJ, Fleury L, Macura J, Shams J. Embolization for treatment of gastrointestinal hemorrhage secondary to recurrent renal cell carcinoma. *Cardiovasc Intervent Radiol* 2006; **29**:1117–20.
48. Bang HJ, Littrup PJ, Goodrich DJ, *et al.* Percutaneous cryoablation of metastatic renal cell carcinoma for local tumor control: feasibility, outcomes, and estimated cost-effectiveness for palliation. *J Vasc Interv Radiol* 2012; **23**:770–7.
49. Hoffmann RT, Jakobs TF, Trumm C, Weber C, Helmberger TK, Reiser MF. Radiofrequency ablation in combination with osteoplasty in the treatment of painful metastatic bone disease. *J Vasc Interv Radiol* 2008; **19**:419–25.
50. Soga N, Yamakado K, Gohara H, *et al.* Percutaneous radiofrequency ablation for unresectable pulmonary metastases from renal cell carcinoma. *BJU Int* 2009; **104**:790–4.
51. Lane MD, Le HB, Lee S, *et al.* Combination radiofrequency ablation and cementoplasty for palliative treatment of painful neoplastic bone metastasis: experience with 53 treated lesions in 36 patients. *Skeletal Radiol* 2011; **40**:25–32.
52. Shu Yan Huo A, Lawson Morris D, King J, Glenn D. Use of percutaneous radiofrequency ablation in pulmonary metastases from renal cell carcinoma. *Ann Surg Oncol* 2009; **16**:3169–75.
53. Meyners T, Heisterkamp C, Kueter JD, *et al.* Prognostic factors for outcomes after whole-brain irradiation of brain metastases from relatively radioresistant tumors: a retrospective analysis. *BMC Cancer* 2010; **10**:582.
54. Maor MH, Frias AE, Oswald MJ. Palliative radiotherapy for brain metastases in renal carcinoma. *Cancer* 1988; **62**:1912–7.

55. Wrónski M, Maor MH, Davis BJ, Sawaya R, Levin VA. External radiation of brain metastases from renal carcinoma: a retrospective study of 119 patients from the M. D. Anderson Cancer Center. *Int J Radiat Oncol Biol Phys* 1997; **37**:753–9.
56. Sheehan JP, Sun MH, Kondziolka D, Flickinger J, Lunsford LD. Radiosurgery in patients with renal cell carcinoma metastasis to the brain: long-term outcomes and prognostic factors influencing survival and local tumor control. *J Neurosurg* 2003; **98**:342–9.
57. Kim YH, Kim JW, Chung HT, *et al.* Brain metastasis from renal cell carcinoma. *Prog Neurol Surg* 2012; **25**:163–75.
58. Shuto T, Inomori S, Fujino H, Nagano H. Gamma knife surgery for metastatic brain tumors from renal cell carcinoma. *J Neurosurg* 2006; **105**:555–60.
59. Kim WH, Kim DG, Han JH, *et al.* Early significant tumor volume reduction after radiosurgery in brain metastases from renal cell carcinoma results in long-term survival. *Int J Rad Onc Biol Phys* 2012; **82**:1749–55.
60. Rosen LS, Gordon D, Tchekmedyian NS, *et al.* Long-term efficacy and safety of zoledronic acid in the treatment of skeletal metastases in patients with nonsmall cell lung carcinoma and other solid tumors: a randomized, Phase III, double-blind, placebo-controlled trial. *Cancer* 2004; **100**:2613–21.
61. Rosen LS, Gordon D, Tchekmedyian S, *et al.* Zoledronic acid versus placebo in the treatment of skeletal metastases in patients with lung cancer and other solid tumors: a phase III, double-blind, randomized trial--the Zoledronic Acid Lung Cancer and Other Solid Tumors Study Group. *J Clin Oncol* 2003; **21**:3150–7.
62. Lipton A, Zheng M, Seaman J. Zoledronic acid delays the onset of skeletal-related events and progression of skeletal disease in patients with advanced renal cell carcinoma. *Cancer* 2003; **98**:962–9.
63. Lang JM, Kaikobad MR, Wallace M, *et al.* Pilot trial of interleukin-2 and zoledronic acid to augment γδ T cells as treatment for patients with refractory renal cell carcinoma. *Cancer Immunol Immunother* 2011; **60**:1447–60.
64. Pandha H, Birchall L, Meyer B, *et al.* Antitumor effects of aminobisphosphonates on renal cell carcinoma cell lines. *J Urol* 2006; **176**:2255–61.
65. Keizman D, Ish-Shalom M, Pili R, *et al.* Bisphosphonates combined with sunitinib may improve the response rate, progression free survival and overall survival of patients with bone metastases from renal cell carcinoma. *Eur J Cancer* 2012; **48**:1031–7.
66. Yasuda Y, Fujii Y, Yuasa T, *et al.* Possible improvement of survival with use of zoledronic acid in patients with bone metastases from renal cell carcinoma. *Int J Clin Oncol* 2013; **18**(5):877–83.
67. Broom RJ, Hinder V, Sharples K, *et al.* RAD001 and zoledronic acid in renal cell carcinoma patients with bone metastases : a randomized first line phase II trial. *Clin Genitourin Cancer* 2015; **13**:50–8.
68. Henry DH, Costa L, Goldwasser F, *et al.* Randomized, double-blind study of denosumab versus zoledronic acid in the treatment of bone metastases in patients with advanced cancer (excluding breast and prostate cancer) or multiple myeloma. *J Clin Oncol* 2011; **29**:1125–32.
69. Shankaran V, Ikeda H, Bruce AT, *et al.* IFNgamma and lymphocytes prevent primary tumour development and shape tumour immunogenicity. *Nature* 2001; **410**:1107–11.
70. Dunn GP, Bruce AT, Ikeda H, Old LJ, Schreiber RD. Cancer immunoediting: from immunosurveillance to tumor escape. *Nat Immunol* 2002; **3**:991–8.
71. Weinstock M, McDermott D. Targeting PD-1/PD-L1 in the treatment of metastatic renal cell carcinoma. *Ther Adv Urol* 2015; **7**:365–77.
72. Bhardwaj N. Harnessing the immune system to treat cancer. *J Clin Invest* 2007; **117**:1130–6.
73. Dong H, Strome SE, Salomao DR, *et al.* Tumor-associated B7-H1 promotes T-cell apoptosis: a potential mechanism of immune evasion. *Nat Med* 2002; **8**:793–800.
74. Albini A, Marchisone C, Del Grosso F, *et al.* Inhibition of angiogenesis and vascular tumor growth by interferon-producing cells: A gene therapy approach. *Am J Pathol* 2000; **156**:1381–93.
75. Négrier S, Escudier B, Lasset C, *et al.* Recombinant human interleukin-2, recombinant human interferon alfa-2a, or both in metastatic renal-cell carcinoma. Groupe Français d'Immunothérapie. *N Engl J Med* 1998; **338**:1272–8.
76. [No authors listed]. Interferon-alpha and survival in metastatic renal carcinoma: early results of a randomised controlled trial. Medical Research Council Renal Cancer Collaborators. *Lancet* 1999; **353**:14–7.
77. Minasian LM, Motzer RJ, Gluck L, Mazumdar M, Vlamis V, Krown SE. Interferon alfa-2a in advanced renal cell carcinoma: treatment results and survival in 159 patients with long-term follow-up. *J Clin Oncol* 1993; **11**:1368–75.
78. Motzer RJ, Bacik J, Murphy BA, Russo P, Mazumdar M. Interferon-alfa as a comparative treatment for clinical trials of new therapies against advanced renal cell carcinoma. *J Clin Oncol* 2002; **20**:289–96.
79. Coppin C, Porzsolt F, Awa A, Kumpf J, Coldman A, Wilt T. Immunotherapy for advanced renal cell cancer. *Cochrane Database Syst Rev* 2005; **25**:CD001425.
80. Aass N, De Mulder PH, Mickisch GH, *et al.* Randomized phase II/III trial of interferon Alfa-2a with and without 13-cis-retinoic acid in patients with progressive metastatic renal cell Carcinoma: the European Organisation for Research and Treatment of Cancer Genito-Urinary Tract Cancer Group (EORTC). *J Clin Oncol* 2005; **23**:4172–8.
81. Motzer RJ, Murphy BA, Bacik J, *et al.* Phase III trial of interferon alfa-2a with or without 13-cis-retinoic acid for patients with advanced renal cell carcinoma. *J Clin Oncol* 2000; **18**:2972–80.
82. Atzpodien J, Kirchner H, Jonas U, *et al.* Interleukin-2- and interferon alfa-2a-based immunochemotherapy in advanced renal cell carcinoma: a Prospectively Randomized Trial of the German Cooperative Renal Carcinoma Chemoimmunotherapy Group (DGCIN). *J Clin Oncol* 2004; **22**:1188–94.
83. Fosså SD, Martinelli G, Otto U, *et al.* Recombinant interferon alfa-2a with or without vinblastine in metastatic renal cell carcinoma: results of a European multi-center phase III study. *Ann Oncol* 1992; **3**:301–5.
84. Neidhart JA, Anderson SA, Harris JE, *et al.* Vinblastine fails to improve response of renal cancer to interferon alfa-n1: high response rate in patients with pulmonary metastases. *J Clin Oncol* 1991; **9**:832–6.
85. Gore ME, Griffin CL, Hancock B, *et al.* Interferon alfa-2a versus combination therapy with interferon alfa-2a, interleukin-2, and fluorouracil in patients with untreated metastatic renal cell carcinoma (MRC RE04/EORTC GU 30012): an open-label randomised trial. *Lancet* 2010; **375**:641–8.
86. Yang JC, Sherry RM, Steinberg SM, *et al.* Randomized study of high-dose and low-dose interleukin-2 in patients with metastatic renal cancer. *J Clin Oncol* 2003; **21**:3127–32.
87. McDermott DF, Regan MM, Clark JI, *et al.* Randomized phase III trial of high-dose interleukin-2 versus subcutaneous interleukin-2 and interferon in patients with metastatic renal cell carcinoma. *J Clin Oncol* 2005; **23**:133–41.
88. McDermott DF, Cheng SC, Signoretti S, *et al.* The High-dose aldesleukin 'select' trial: a trial to prospectively validate predictive models of response to treatment in patients with metastatic renal cell carcinoma. *Clin Cancer Res* 2015; **21**:561–8.
89. Atkins MB, Sparano J, Fisher RI, *et al.* Randomized phase II trial of high-dose interleukin-2 either alone or in combination with interferon alfa-2b in advanced renal cell carcinoma. *J Clin Oncol* 1993; **11**:661–70.
90. Figlin R, Gitlitz B, Franklin J, *et al.* Interleukin-2-based immunotherapy for the treatment of metastatic renal cell carcinoma: an analysis of 203 consecutively treated patients. *Cancer J Sci Am* 1997; **3**(Suppl 1):S92–7.
91. Motzer RJ, Escudier B, McDermott DF, *et al.* Nivolumab versus everolimus in advanced renal-cell carcinoma. *N Engl J Med* 2015; **373**:1803–13.
92. Duan DR, Pause A, Burgess WH, *et al.* Inhibition of transcription elongation by the VHL tumor suppressor protein. *Science* 1995; **269**:1402–6.
93. Kibel A, Iliopoulos O, DeCaprio JA, Kaelin WG. Binding of the von Hippel-Lindau tumor suppressor protein to Elongin B and C. *Science* 1995; **269**:1444–6.

94. Pause A, Lee S, Worrell RA, *et al.* The von Hippel-Lindau tumor-suppressor gene product forms a stable complex with human CUL-2, a member of the Cdc53 family of proteins. *Proc Natl Acad Sci U S A* 1997; **94**:2156–61.
95. Shuin T, Kondo K, Torigoe S, *et al.* Frequent somatic mutations and loss of heterozygosity of the von Hippel-Lindau tumor suppressor gene in primary human renal cell carcinomas. *Cancer Res* 1994; **54**:2852–5.
96. Nickerson ML, Jaeger E, Shi Y, *et al.* Improved identification of von Hippel-Lindau gene alterations in clear cell renal tumors. *Clin Cancer Res* 2008; **14**:4726–34.
97. Gnarra JR, Tory K, Weng Y, *et al.* Mutations of the VHL tumour suppressor gene in renal carcinoma. *Nat Genet* 1994; **7**:85–90.
98. Turner, KJ, Moore JW, Jones A, *et al.* Expression of hypoxia-inducible factors in human renal cancer: relationship to angiogenesis and to the von Hippel-Lindau gene mutation. *Cancer Res* 2002; **62**:2957–61.
99. Raval RR, Lau KW, Tran MG, *et al.* Contrasting properties of hypoxia-inducible factor 1 (HIF-1) and HIF-2 in von Hippel-Lindau-associated renal cell carcinoma. *Mol Cell Biol* 2005; **25**:5675–86.
100. Hotte SJ, Bjarnason GA, Heng DY, *et al.* Progression-free survival as a clinical trial endpoint in advanced renal cell carcinoma. *Curr Oncol* 2011; **18** (Suppl 2):S11–9.
101. Motzer RJ, Rini BI, Bukowski RM, *et al.* Sunitinib in patients with metastatic renal cell carcinoma. *JAMA* 2006; **295**:2516–24.
102. Motzer RJ, Rini BI, Bukowski RM, *et al.* Activity of SU11248, a multitargeted inhibitor of vascular endothelial growth factor receptor and platelet-derived growth factor receptor, in patients with metastatic renal cell carcinoma. *J Clin Oncol* 2006; **24**:16–24.
103. Motzer RJ, Hutson TE, Tomczak P, *et al.* Overall survival and updated results for sunitinib compared with interferon alfa in patients with metastatic renal cell carcinoma. *J Clin Oncol* 2009; **27**:3584–90.
104. Gore ME, Hariharan S, Porta C, *et al.* Sunitinib in metastatic renal cell carcinoma patients with brain metastases. *Cancer* 2011; **117**:501–9.
105. Ravaud A, Bello CL. Exposure-response relationships in patients with metastatic renal cell carcinoma receiving sunitinib: maintaining optimum efficacy in clinical practice. *Anticancer Drugs* 2011; **22**:377–83.
106. Bjarnason GA, Knox JJ, Kollmannsberger CK, *et al.* Phase II study of individualized sunitnib as first line therapy for metastatic renal cancer. *J Clin Oncol* 2005; **33**(Suppl; abstr 4555).
107. NICE. Pazopanib for the first-line treatment of advanced renal cell carcinoma. Technology appraisal guidance [TA215] 2011. Available at: https://www.nice.org.uk/Guidance/ta215 [Online].
108. Motzer RJ, Hutson TE, Cella D, *et al.* Pazopanib versus sunitinib in the metastatic renal-cell carcinoma. *N Engl J Med* 2013; **369**:722–31.
109. Escudier B, Porta C, Bono P, *et al.* Randomized, controlled, double-blind, cross-over trial assessing treatment preference for pazopanib versus sunitinib in patients with metastatic renal cell carcinoma: PISCES Study. *J Clin Oncol* 2014; **32**:1412–18.
110. Escudier B, Eisen T, Stadler WM, *et al.* Sorafenib for treatment of renal cell carcinoma: Final efficacy and safety results of the phase III treatment approaches in renal cancer global evaluation trial. *J Clin Oncol* 2009; **27**:3312–8.
111. Eisen T, Oudard S, Szczylik C, *et al.* Sorafenib for older patients with renal cell carcinoma: subset analysis from a randomized trial. *J Natl Cancer Inst* 2008; **100**:1454–63.
112. Escudier B, Eisen T, Stadler WM, *et al.* Randomized phase II trial of first-line treatment with sorafenib versus interferon Alfa-2a in patients with metastatic renal cell carcinoma. *J Clin Oncol* 2009; **27**:1280–9.
113. Rini B, Szczylik C, Tannir NM, *et al.* AMG 386 in combination with sorafenib in patients with metastatic clear cell carcinoma of the kidney: A randomized, double-blind, placebo-controlled, phase 2 study. *Cancer* 2012; **118**(24):6152–61.
114. Procopio G, Verzoni E, Bracarda S, *et al.* Sorafenib with interleukin-2 vs sorafenib alone in metastatic renal cell carcinoma: the ROSORC trial. *Br J Cancer* 2011; **104**:1256–61.
115. Jonasch E, Corn P, Pagliaro LC, *et al.* Upfront, randomized, phase 2 trial of sorafenib versus sorafenib and low-dose interferon alfa in patients with advanced renal cell carcinoma: clinical and biomarker analysis. *Cancer* 2010; **116**:57–65.
116. Rini BI, Escudier B, Tomczak P, *et al.* Comparative effectiveness of axitinib versus sorafenib in advanced renal cell carcinoma (AXIS): a randomised phase 3 trial. *Lancet* 2011; **378**:1931–9.
117. Motzer RJ, Escudier B, Tomczak P, *et al.* Axitinib versus Sorafenib as second-line treatment for advanced renal cell carcinoma: overall survival analysis and updated results from a randomised phase 3 trial. *Lancet Oncol* 2013; **14**:552–62.
118. Hutson TE, Lesovoy V, Al-Shukri S, *et al.* Axitinib versus sorafenib as first-line therapy in patients with metastatic renal cell carcinoma: a randomised open-label phase 3 trial. *Lancet Oncol* 2013; **14**:1287–94.
119. Gibney GT, Aziz SA, Camp RL, *et al.* C-Met is a prognostic marker and potential therapeutic target in clear cell renal cell carcinoma. *Ann Oncol* 2013; **24**:343–9.
120. Choueiri TK, Escudier B, Powles T, *et al.* Cabozantinib versus everolimus in advanced renal cell carcinoma. *Lancet Oncol* 2016; **17**:917–27.
121. Choueiri TK, Halabi S, Sanford BL, *et al.* Cabozantinib versus sunitinib as initial targeted therapy for patients with metastatic renal cell carcinoma of poor or intermediate risk. *J Clin Oncol* 2016, DOI:10.1200/JCO.2016.70.7398. [Epub before print].
122. Motzer RJ, Hutson TE, Glen H, *et al.* Lenvatinib, everolimus and the combination in patients with metastatic renal cell carcinoma: a randomised, phase 2, open-label, multicentre trial. *Lancet Oncol* 2015; **16**:1473–82.
123. Motzer RJ, *et al.* Independent assessment of lenvatinib plus everolimus in patients with metastatic renal cell carcinoma. *Lancet Oncol* 2016; **17**(1):e4–5.
124. Escudier B, Escudier B, Bellmunt J, Négrier S, *et al.* Phase III trial of bevacizumab plus interferon alfa-2a in patients with metastatic renal cell carcinoma (AVOREN): final analysis of overall survival. *J Clin Oncol* 2010; **28**:2144–50.
125. Escudier B, Pluzanska A, Koralewski P, *et al.* Bevacizumab plus interferon alfa-2a for treatment of metastatic renal cell carcinoma: a randomised, double-blind phase III trial. *Lancet* 2007; **370**:2103–11.
126. Rini BI, Halabi S, Rosenberg JE, *et al.* Phase III trial of bevacizumab plus interferon alfa versus interferon alfa monotherapy in patients with metastatic renal cell carcinoma: final results of CALGB 90206. *J Clin Oncol* 2010; **28**:2137–43.
127. Hudes G, Carducci M, Tomczak P, *et al.* Temsirolimus, interferon alfa, or both for advanced renal-cell carcinoma. *N Engl J Med* 2007; **356**:2271–81.
128. Motzer, R. J. *et al.* Phase 3 trial of everolimus for metastatic renal cell carcinoma: final results and analysis of prognostic factors. *Cancer* 2010; **116**:4256–65.
129. Eisen T, Sternberg CN, Robert C, *et al.* Targeted therapies for renal cell carcinoma: review of adverse event management strategies. *J Natl Cancer Inst* 2012; **104**:93–113.
130. Lacouture ME, Wu S, Robert C, *et al.* Evolving strategies for the management of hand-foot skin reaction associated with the multitargeted kinase inhibitors sorafenib and sunitinib. *Oncologist* 2008; **13**:1001–11.
131. Torino F, Corsello SM, Longo R, Barnabei A, Gasparini G. Hypothyroidism related to tyrosine kinase inhibitors: an emerging toxic effect of targeted therapy. *Nat Rev Clin Oncol* 2009; **6**:219–28.
132. Force T, Krause DS, Van Etten RA. Molecular mechanisms of cardiotoxicity of tyrosine kinase inhibition. *Nat Rev Cancer* 2007; **7**:332–44.
133. Spain L, Diem S, Larkin J. Management of toxicities of immune checkpoint inhibitors. *Cancer Treat Rev* 2016; **44**:51–60.

134. European Medicines Agency (2016) (EMA), Nivolumab BMS EU Summary of Product Characteristics. Available at: http://ema.europa.eu. [Accessed November 2016] [Online].
135. Motzer RJ, Bacik J, Mariani T, Russo P, Mazumdar M, Reuter V. Treatment outcome and survival associated with metastatic renal cell carcinoma of non-clear-cell histology. *J Clin Oncol* 2002; **20**:2376–81.
136. Volpe A, Novara G, Antonelli A, *et al.* Chromophobe renal cell carcinoma (RCC): oncological outcomes and prognostic factors in a large multicentre series. *BJU Int* 2012; **110**:76–83.
137. Beck SD, Patel MI, Snyder ME, *et al.* Effect of papillary and chromophobe cell type on disease-free survival after nephrectomy for renal cell carcinoma. *Ann Surg Oncol* 2004; **11**:71–7.
138. Mejean A, Hopirtean V, Bazin JP, *et al.* Prognostic factors for the survival of patients with papillary renal cell carcinoma: meaning of histological typing and multifocality. *J Urol* 2003; **170**:764–7.
139. Dutcher JP, de Souza P, McDermott D, *et al.* Effect of temsirolimus versus interferon-alpha on outcome of patients with advanced renal cell carcinoma of different tumor histologies. *Med Oncol* 2009; **26**:202–9.
140. Choueiri TK, Plantade A, Elson P, *et al.* Efficacy of sunitinib and sorafenib in metastatic papillary and chromophobe renal cell carcinoma. *J Clin Oncol* 2008; **26**:127–31.
141. Tannir NM, Plimack E, Ng C, *et al.* A Phase 2 trial of sunitinib in patients with advanced non-clear cell renal cell carcinoma. *Eur Urol* 2012; **62**(6):1013–19.
142. Armstrong AJ, Halabi S, Eisen T, *et al.* Everolimus versus sunitinib for patients with metastatic non-clear cell renal cell carcinoma (ASPEN) a multicentre, open-label, randomised phase 2 trial. *Lancet Oncol* 2016; **17**:378–88.
143. Tannir N, Jonasch E, Albiges L, *et al.* Everolimus versus sunitinib prospective evaluation in metastatic non-clear cell renal cell carcinoma (ESPN): A randomized multicenter phase 2 trial. *Eur Urol* 2016; **69**(5):866–74.
144. Gordon MS, Hussey M, Nagle RB, *et al.* Phase II study of erlotinib in patients with locally advanced or metastatic papillary histology renal cell cancer: SWOG S0317. *J Clin Oncol* 2009; **27**:5788–93.
145. George CM, Vogelzang NJ, Rini BI, *et al.* A phase II trial of weekly intravenous gemcitabine and cisplatin with continuous infusion fluorouracil in patients with metastatic renal cell carcinoma. *Ann Oncol* 2002; **13**:116–20.
146. Van Veldhuizen PJ, Hussey M, Lara PN Jr, *et al.* A phase ii study of gemcitabine and capecitabine in patients with advanced renal cell cancer: southwest oncology group study S0312. *Am J Clin Oncol* 2009; **32**:453–9.
147. Stadler WM, Halabi S, Rini B, *et al.* A phase II study of gemcitabine and capecitabine in metastatic renal cancer: a report of Cancer and Leukemia Group B protocol 90008. *Cancer* 2006; **107**:1273–9.
148. Waters JS, Moss C, Pyle L, *et al.* Phase II clinical trial of capecitabine and gemcitabine chemotherapy in patients with metastatic renal carcinoma. *Br J Cancer* 2004; **91**:1763–8.
149. Tannir NM, Thall PF, Ng CS, *et al.* A phase II trial of gemcitabine plus capecitabine for metastatic renal cell cancer previously treated with immunotherapy and targeted agents. *J Urol* 2008; **180**:867–72; discussion 872.
150. Chung EK, Posadas EM, Kasza K, *et al.* A phase II trial of gemcitabine, capecitabine, and bevacizumab in metastatic renal carcinoma. *Am J Clin Oncol* 2011; **34**:150–4.
151. De Mulder PH, Weissbach L, Jakse G, Osieka R, Blatter J. Gemcitabine: a phase II study in patients with advanced renal cancer. *Cancer Chemother Pharmacol* 1996; **37**:491–5.
152. Mertens WC, Eisenhauer EA, Moore M, *et al.* Gemcitabine in advanced renal cell carcinoma. A phase II study of the National Cancer Institute of Canada Clinical Trials Group. *Ann Oncol* 1993; **4**: 331–2.
153. Naito, S. Eto M, Shinohara N, *et al.* Multicenter phase II trial of S-1 in patients with cytokine-refractory metastatic renal cell carcinoma. *J Clin Oncol* 2010; **28**:5022–9.
154. Rini BI, Vogelzang NJ, Dumas MC, Wade JL 3rd, Taber DA, Stadler WM. Phase II trial of weekly intravenous gemcitabine with continuous infusion fluorouracil in patients with metastatic renal cell cancer. *J Clin Oncol* 2000; **18**:2419–26.
155. Bellmunt J, Trigo JM, Calvo E, *et al.* Activity of a multitargeted chemo-switch regimen (sorafenib, gemcitabine, and metronomic capecitabine) in metastatic renal-cell carcinoma: a phase 2 study (SOGUG-02-06). *Lancet Oncol* 2010; **11**:350–7.
156. Michaelson MD, McKay RR, Werner L, *et al.* Phase 2 trial of sunitinib and gemcitabine in patients with sarcomatoid and/or poor risk metastatic renal cell carcinoma. *Cancer* 2015; **121**:3435–43.
157. Oudard S, Banu E, Vieillefond A, *et al.* Prospective multicenter phase II study of gemcitabine plus platinum salt for metastatic collecting duct carcinoma: results of a GETUG (Groupe d'Etudes des Tumeurs Uro-Génitales) study. *J Urol* 2007; **177**:1698–702.
158. Haas NB, Lin X, Manola J, *et al.* A phase II trial of doxorubicin and gemcitabine in renal cell carcinoma with sarcomatoid features: ECOG 8802. *Med Oncol* 2012; **29**:761–7.
159. Nanus DM, Garino A, Milowsky MI, Larkin M, Dutcher JP. Active chemotherapy for sarcomatoid and rapidly progressing renal cell carcinoma. *Cancer* 2004; **101**:1545–51.
160. Dutcher JP, Nanus, D. Long-term survival of patients with sarcomatoid renal cell cancer treated with chemotherapy. *Med Oncol* 2011; **28**:1530–3.
161. Tran HT, Liu Y, Zurita AJ, *et al.* Prognostic or predictive plasma cytokines and angiogenic factors for patients treated with pazopanib for metastatic renal-cell cancer: a retrospective analysis of phase 2 and phase 3 trials. *Lancet Oncol* 2012; **13**:827–37.
162. Fernández A, Sanguino A, Peng Z, *et al.* An anticancer C-Kit kinase inhibitor is reengineered to make it more active and less cardiotoxic. *J Clin Invest* 2007; **117**:4044–54.
163. Choi JS, Kim MK, Seo JW, *et al.* MET expression in sporadic renal cell carcinomas. *J Korean Med Sci* 2006; **21**:672–7.
164. Migliore C, Giordano S. Molecular cancer therapy: can our expectation be MET? *Eur J Cancer* 2008; **44**:641–51.
165. Eder JP. Shapiro GI, Appleman LJ, *et al.* A phase I study of foretinib, a multi-targeted inhibitor of c-Met and vascular endothelial growth factor receptor 2. *Clin Cancer Res* 2010; **16**:3507–16.
166. Choueiri TK, Vaishampayan U, Rosenberg JE, *et al.* Phase II and biomarker study of the dual MET/VEGFR2 inhibitor foretinib in patients with papillary renal cell carcinoma. *J Clin Oncol* 2013; **31**(2):181–6.
167. Mulders P, Hawkins R, Nathan P, *et al.* Cediranib monotherapy in patients with advanced renal cell carcinoma: results of a randomised phase II study. *Eur J Cancer* 2012; **48**:527–37.
168. Hammers HJ, Plimack ER, Sternberg C, *et al.* CheckMate214: A phase III, randomized, open-label study of nivolumab combined with ipilimumab versus suntinib monotherapy in patients with previously untreated metastatic renal cell carcinoma. *J Clin Oncol* 2015; **33**(Suppl; abstr TPS4578).
169. Dudek AZ, Sica A, Sidani A, *et al.* Phase Ib study of pembrolizumab in combination with bevacizumab for the treatment of renal cell carcinoma: Big Ten Cancer Research Consortium BTCRC-GU13-003. *J Clin Oncol* 2016; **34**(Suppl 2S; abstr 559).
170. Amin A, Dudek AZ, Logan TF, *et al.* Survival with AGS-003, an autologous dendritic cell-based immunotherapy, in combination with sunitinib in unfavourable risk patients with advanced renal cell carcinoma (RCC): Phase 2 study results. *J Immunother Cancer* 2015; **3**:14.
171. Zimmer M, Doucette D, Siddiqui N, Iliopoulos O. Inhibition of hypoxia-inducible factor is sufficient for growth suppression of VHL-/- tumors. *Mol Cancer Res* 2004; **2**:89–95.
172. Kondo K, Kim WY, Lechpammer M, Kaelin WG. Inhibition of HIF2alpha is sufficient to suppress pVHL-defective tumor growth. *PLoS Biol* 2003; **1**:E83.
173. Yeo EJ, Chun YS, Cho YS, *et al.* YC-1: a potential anticancer drug targeting hypoxia-inducible factor 1. *J Natl Cancer Inst* 2003; **95**:516–25.

174. Welsh SJ, Williams RR, Birmingham A, Newman DJ, Kirkpatrick DL, Powis G. The thioredoxin redox inhibitors 1-methylpropyl 2-imidazolyl disulfide and pleurotin inhibit hypoxia-induced factor 1alpha and vascular endothelial growth factor formation. *Mol Cancer Ther* 2003; **2**:235–43.
175. Welsh S, Williams R, Kirkpatrick L, Paine-Murrieta G, Powis G. Antitumor activity and pharmacodynamic properties of PX-478, an inhibitor of hypoxia-inducible factor-1alpha. *Mol Cancer Ther* 2004; **3**:233–44.
176. Carew JS, Esquivel JA 2nd, Espitia CM, *et al.* ELR510444 inhibits tumor growth and angiogenesis by abrogating HIF activity and disrupting microtubules in renal cell carcinoma. *PLoS One* 2012; **7**:e31120.
177. Al-Lamki RS, Sadler TJ, Wang J, *et al.* Tumor necrosis factor receptor expression and signaling in renal cell carcinoma. *Am J Pathol* 2010; **177**:943–54.
178. Sjölund J, Johansson M, Manna S, *et al.* Suppression of renal cell carcinoma growth by inhibition of Notch signaling in vitro and in vivo. *J Clin Invest* 2008; **118**:217–28.
179. Sjölund J, Boström AK, Lindgren D, *et al.* The notch and TGF-β signaling pathways contribute to the aggressiveness of clear cell renal cell carcinoma. *PLoS One* 2011; **6**:e23057.
180. Linehan WM, Srinivasan R, Schmidt LS. The genetic basis of kidney cancer: a metabolic disease. *Nat Rev Urol* 2010; **7**:277–85.
181. Varela I, Tarpey P, Raine K, *et al.* Exome sequencing identifies frequent mutation of the SWI/SNF complex gene PBRM1 in renal carcinoma. *Nature* 2011; **469**:539–42.
182. Thompson M. Polybromo-1: the chromatin targeting subunit of the PBAF complex. *Biochimie* 2009; **91**:309–19.
183. Pawłowski R, Mühl SM, Sulser T, Krek W, Moch H, Schraml P. Loss of PBRM1 expression is associated with renal cell carcinoma progression. *Int J Cancer* 2013; **132**(2):E11–7.
184. Flaherty KT. Sorafenib in renal cell carcinoma. *Clin Cancer Res* 2007; **13**:747s–752s.
185. Canter D, Kuitikov A, Glovine K, *et al.* Are all multi-targeted tyrosine kinase inhibitors created equal? An in vitro study of sunitinib and pazopanib in renal cell carcinoma cell lines. *Can J Urol* 2011; **18**:5819–25.

CHAPTER 6.33

Testicular cancer

Christian Winter and Peter Albers

Introduction to testicular cancer

While malignant tumours of the testis are rare, testicular cancer is the most common cancer among men between the ages of 15 to 40 years. These cancers represent the leading cause of cancer-related mortality and morbidity in this age group,[1,2] but generally have an excellent prognosis. The main factors contributing to the survival from affected patients are knowledge about the pathogenesis of testicular cancer, accurate staging at the time of diagnosis, early multimodal treatment (combination chemotherapy, radiotherapy and surgery) for appropriate cases and strict follow-up regimens and salvage therapies.

During the past decades major progress has been made in the efficacy of testicular cancer treatment. Perhaps the major factor for this has been the introduction of cisplatin-based combination chemotherapy. In the early 1970s Larry Einhorn and John Donohue conducted the first studies with cisplatin-based chemotherapy in patients with testicular cancer.[3] They showed cure rates for advanced testicular cancer improved from 5% to 60% by using combination chemotherapy with cisplatin, vinblastine and bleomycin (PVB).[4] In 1978 the combination chemotherapy cisplatin and etoposide was first evaluated as salvage chemotherapy, representing the first time that patients with solid tumour had been cured with second-line chemotherapy. In the early 1980s, the PVB regimen was replaced by the BEP regime (bleomycin/etoposide/cisplatin) which was proven to have higher cure rates with less toxicity.[4] The BEP regimen is now established as standard chemotherapy in primary treatment of testicular cancer. The surgical treatment remains an important part in therapy of testicular cancer. For most patients with low-stage disease, surgical resection of the affected testis by a radical orchiectomy is the only recommended treatment option. With the use of a risk-adapted treatment management, about 50% of patients with early stage germ cell tumours (GCTs) will choose close surveillance instead of immediate adjuvant treatment (e.g. chemotherapy) following orchiectomy. Surveillance is an effective means of managing early stage testicular germ cell tumour patients despite variability in protocols and patient compliance.[5] The overall disease-free survival in these patients is around 100%.

The treatment of advanced testicular GCTs is based on risk stratification according to clinical features and International Germ Cell Cancer Collaborative Group (IGCCCG) classification. Cisplatin-based chemotherapy is proven to be the optimal treatment regimen for good-risk patients: cure rates using chemotherapy with or without surgery approximate 90%.[6] For patients with advanced disease and intermediate/poor prognosis, intensification of treatment is being investigated to increase long-term cure rates. These patients can achieve long-term freedom from disease (five-year overall progression-free survival up to 70%) when chemotherapy is combined with surgical treatment by a complete resection of residual post-chemotherapy masses.[7]

Pathology, pathogenesis, and risk factors

Pathology

The majority of patients with testicular cancer presents with primary tumour in the testis. In the minority (around 5%), the primary tumour is extragonadal in the retroperitoneum or in the mediastinum. Most (95%) primary testicular tumours are GCT, and the remainder include non-germinal neoplasms such as Leydig cell and Sertoli cell tumours, or lymphomas. Histopathologically, GCTs divide into two major groups: seminoma and non-seminoma. Major groups and subtypes of testicular germ cell tumour are histologically classified in the World Health Organization (WHO) System (Table 6.33.1).[8]

Seminomas, which are not pluripotent, appear as sheets of undifferentiated cells that resemble primitive germ cell.[9] Non-seminomatous tumours display a variety of histological forms and differentiate along an embryonic lineage (embryonal carcinoma, teratoma, teratocarcinoma) or extra-embryonic tissue components (yolk sac tumour, choriocarcinoma). Teratoma as a special subgroup of germ cell tumours show tremendous histologic diversity, containing a variety of tissue elements derived from all three embryonic germ cell layers. WHO classification recognizes three histological subtypes: mature, immature, and teratomas with malignant transformation. In addition, the finding of any of these histological germ cell tumour types within a seminoma defines the tumour as a non-seminomatous germ cell tumour (NSGCT), primarily because the natural history of these tumours is less favourable than that of pure seminoma.[10]

Pathogenesis and risk factors

Testicular maldescent

While parts of the pathogenesis of testicular cancer remain unknown, several risk factors are identified. The strongest risk factor of testicular cancer is cryptorchidism or testis maldescent. This link was suggested as early as in the beginning of the nineteenth century. A recent meta-analysis has estimated the relative risk of germ cell tumour among men with prior cryptorchidism to be 4.8 fold (95% CI = 4.0-5.7),[11] but reported ranges varying between 5-10-fold.[12] Only 10% of testicular cancer develops in men with prior cryptorchidism. The risk of testicular malignancy is higher with bilateral than with unilateral cryptorchidism. In men with unilateral cryptorchidism, most tumours occur in the affected side, although malignant degeneration is found on the contralateral side in about 20% of cases.[13] Several reports

Table 6.33.1 WHO classification of tumours of the testis

Germ cell tumours derived from germ cell neoplasia in situ	
Non-invasive germ cell neoplasia	
Germ cell neoplasia in situ	9064/2
Specific forms of intratubular germ cell neoplasia	
Tumours of a single histological type (pure forms)	
Seminoma	9061/3
Seminoma with syncytiotrophoblast cells	
Non-seminomatous germ cell tumours	
Embryonal carcinoma	9070/3
Yolk sac tumour, postpubertal-type	9071/3
Trophoblastic tumours	
Choriocarcinoma	9100/3
Non-choriocarcinomatous trophoblastic tumours	
Placental site trophoblastic tumour	9104/1
Epitheloid trophoblastic tumour	9105/3
Cystic trophoblastic tumour	
Teratoma, postpubertal-type	9080/3
Teratoma with somatic-type malignancy	9084/3
Non-seminomatous germ cell tumours of more than one histological type	
Mixed germ cell tumours	9085/3
Germ cell tumours of unknown type	
Regressed germ cell tumours	9080/1
Germ cell tumours unrelated to germ cell neoplasia in situ	
Spermatocytic tumour	9063/3
Teratoma, prepubertal-type	9084/0
Dermoid cyst	
Epidermoid cyst	
Well-differentiated neuroendocrine tumour (monodermal teratoma)	8240/3
Mixed teratoma and yolk sac tumour, prepubertal-type	9085/3
Yolk sac tumour, prepubertal-type	9071/3
Sex cord–stromal tumours	
Pure tumours	
Leydig cell tumour	8650/1
Malignant Leydig cell tumour	8650/3
Sertoli cell tumour	8640/1
Malignant Sertoli cell tumour	8640/3
Large cell calcifying Sertoli cell tumour	8642/1
Intratubular large cell hyalinizing Sertoli cell neoplasia	8643/1*
Granulosa cell tumour	
Adult granulose cell tumour	8620/1
Juvenile granulose cell tumour	8322/1*
Tumours in the fiborna–thecoma group	8600/0
Mixed and unclassified sex cord–stromal tumours	
Mixed sex cord–stromal tumour	8592/1
Unclassified sex cord–stromal tumour	8591/1
Tumour containing both germ cell and sex cord–stromal elements	
Gonadoblastoma	9073/1
Miscellaneous tumours of the testis	
Ovarian epithelial–type tumours	
Serous cystadenoma	8441/0
Serous tumour of borderline malignancy	8442/1
Serous cystadenocarcinoma	8441/3
Mucinous cystadenoma	8470/0
Mucinous borderline tumour	8472/1
Mucinous cystadenocarcinoma	8470/3
Endometrioid adenocarcinoma	8380/3
Clear cell adenocarcinoma	8310/3
Brenner tumour	9000/0
Juvenile xanthogranuloma	
Haemangioma	9120/0
Haematolymphoid tumours	
Diffuse large B-cell lymphoma	9680/3
Follicular lymphoma, NOS	9690/3
Extranodal NK/T-cell lymphoma, nasal-type	9719/3
Plasmacytoma	9734/3
Myeloid sarcoma	9930/3
Rosai–Dorfman disease	
Tumours of collecting duct and rete testis	
Adenoma	8140/0
Adenocarcinoma	8140/3

The morphology codes are from the International Classification of Diseases for Oncology (ICD-O) {917A}. Behaviour is coded /0 for benign tumours; /1 for unspecified, borderline, or uncertain behaviour; /2 for carcinoma in situ and grade III intraepithelial neoplasia; and /3 for malignant tumours. The classification is modified from the previous WHO classification {756A}, taking into account changes in our understanding of these lesions.

*New code approved by the IARC/WHO Committee for ICD-O.

Reproduced with permission from Eble, JN, Sauter, G, Epstein JI, Sesterhenn IA. World Health Organization Classification of Tumours. *Pathology and Genetics of Tumours of the Urinary System and Male Genital Organ*. Volume 7. IARC, Lyon, 2004.

showed no ethnic discrepancy in the incidence of cryptorchidism.[14] Despite the pronounced discrepancy in incidence of testicular cancer.[15] In addition, Kallmann Syndrome, a condition of congenital hypogonadotropic hypogonadism, is characterized by cryptorchidism, but not by increased risk for testis cancer.[16] Furthermore the prevalence of cryptorchidism has been reported by some studies to have increased between the 1950s and the 1980s, but the proportion of testicular cancer patients with cryptorchidism appears to have remained constant at approximately 10%.[17] So it is not clear whether cryptorchidism predisposes to testis cancer or whether the GCT and maldescent share common risk factors. The complex genetical disruption is clinically summarized as the so-called 'testicular dysgenesis syndrome' including maldescent, atrophy, and infertiliy.

Contralateral testicular tumour

A previous history of testicular GCT is a well-established risk factor for developing contralateral testicular cancer. For example, studies from Denmark and New Zealand showed relative risks of a contralateral germ cell tumour are 24.5–27.5-fold for GCT patients.[18,19] Fosså *et al.*[20] reported a cohort study involving 29,515 men in the United States, in which GCT patients had a 12.4-fold risk of a metachronous contralateral testicular cancer when compared to the general population.

While the primary tumour histology does not affect the incidence of metachronous contralateral tumours, the incidence is markedly influenced by the patient's age at the time of presentation.[21] For example, younger patients (<30 years of age at initial diagnosis) have a higher incidence of bilateral metachronous seminoma compared with older men (3.9% (<30 years) vs. 1.9% (>30 years), $p \leq 0.01$).

Perinatal risk factors

The hypothesis that the development of testicular cancer is initiated in very early life has focused research onto possible perinatal factors, such as birth weight, gestational age, maternal age, maternal smoking, maternal parity, and birth order.[22] For example, low birth weight was reported to be associated with GCT development risk in several studies.[23,24] However, a recent meta-analysis found only modest support for this relationship (estimated odds ratio of 1.28 (95% CI = 0.99–1.65)).[25] In contrast, it does appear that a decreased gestational age is associated with an increased risk of testicular cancer.[26] In summary, these studies suggest tentative evidence that birth weight and gestational age are associated with the risk of testicular cancer.

With regards to maternal factors, researchers have examined age, smoking, and various perinatal factors. Reports suggest that maternal age is linked to the risk of developing GCTs.[27–29] However, the exact relationship is unclear, as tumour risk appears increased in sons of both younger (<20 years) and older (≥30 years) mothers. Several conflicting reports have detailed an association between maternal smoking and the risk of testicular cancer.[30,31] However, a recently published case–control study from Scandinavia and meta-analysis suggest no association between maternal smoking during pregnancy and the risk of testicular cancer in male offspring.[32] A number of other perinatal factors, such as maternal body weight, maternal socioeconomic, hyperemesis gravidarum, or breech presentation, have been associated with risk for testicular cancer. However, findings of these parameters do not concur and so currently there is no definitive evidence to support any association of these factors and testicular tumour risk.

Indirect evidence suggests that the intrauterine hormonal milieu may increase the risk of testicular cancer. An increased risk to developed GCT reported among first born sons and dizygotic twins may be related to higher maternal oestrogen levels.[33] Furthermore, maternal obesity, a condition consistent with increased serum free estradiol levels, has also been associated with GCT risk.[34] Because of these associations, the 'oestrogen hypothesis' was formally introduced in the 1990s.[35] The effect of exogenous, as well as endogenous, estrogene exposure has also been examined in several studies. Multiple case reports have noted the occurrence of testicular cancer in sons of estrogen-exposed mothers.[36] Other researchers have reported conflicting results and reviews of the literature have concluded, in general, that the supporting data are equivocal.[37] Endocrine disrupting chemical (EDC) exposure could potentially alter the hormonal intrauterine environment.[38] EDCs have been defined as exogenous agents that interfere with the production, release, transport, metabolism, binding, action, or elimination of the natural hormones in the body.[39] Persistent organochlorine pesticides (e.g. dichlorodiphenyltrichloroethane (DDT), dichlorodiphenyldichloroethylene (DDE)) are important representative of EDCs. Several epidemiologic studies of EDCs and testicular cancer have been reported. For example, McGlynn *et al.* investigated the role of pesticides early life exposure in GCT development.[40] In a case–control study they showed that high serum levels of the pesticide DDE were significantly associated with an increased risk of development of testicular cancer. An exposure to these persistent organic pesticides during fetal life or via breastfeeding may increase the risk of GCT in young men. Another US study, however, did not find any associations between testis cancer and organochlorine pesticides.[41] Differences in the dates of sample collection may explain some of the discrepancy in results.

Postnatal risk factors

A number of studies have examined associations between postnatal factors and testicular cancer. It was shown that several factors such as body mass index, puberty age, and body size are not associated with risk of testicular cancer. But height, in contrast, has been positively associated with a risk of germ cell cancer in most studies, although further confirmation is needed.[42] An association between diet and the risk of testicular cancer has been proposed and studied in several contexts. High fat intake and dairy products, largely in childhood, lead to an increased risk of testicular cancer.[43–45] Garner *et al.* examined the association between 17 food groups and the risk of testicular cancer, and found that luncheon meats and cheese were significantly associated with an increased risk of testicular cancer.[46] A protective effect of childhood physical activity has been reported by several studies[47,48], but not by others.[49,50] In addition, one study found a direct association between physical activity and testis cancer risk.[51] Overall, however, the evidence suggests that decreased childhood physical activity and GCT risk may be associated.

Occupational studies of testicular cancer have not confirmed any single profession as a risk factor. Some studies have found an increased risk of testicular tumours among firefighters,[52] metal workers,[53] leather workers,[54] aircraft technicians,[55] and agricultural workers.[56] In general, white collar workers have been found to be at higher risk of testicular germ cell tumour (TGCT) than blue collar workers, thus observed occupational associations could be confounded by socioeconomic status.[57] Early studies indicated that higher socioeconomic status was associated with an increased risk[58] while more current studies have found little association.[59]

An infectious aetiology of testicular cancer was suggested based on epidemiologic parallels with Hodgkin disease.[60] In several reports an increased risk of testicular cancer was found among men infected with human immunodeficiency virus (HIV).[61,62] Two members of the herpes virus family, Epstein-Barr virus and cytomegalovirus (CMV) have been suggested to have oncogenic potential.[63] Both viruses have been implicated in the aetiology of testicular cancer.[64,65]

There have been several reports linking trauma to the testicle or scrotum with testicular cancer, but epidemiological evidence is inconclusive because of the difficulty in assessing trauma retrospectively.[66,67]

Sperm abnormalities are frequently found in patients with testis tumours. As the incidence of testicular cancer has increased over the past 30 years, there has been a corresponding decrease in fertility and semen quality among men in Western countries.[68] Subsequently, several studies have shown an association between male infertility or subfertility and testicular cancer.[69,70] So Raman *et al.* reported that infertile men with abnormal semen analyses had a 20 times greater incidence of testicular cancer than the general population.[71] While studies support the existence of common aetiological factors between subfertility and testicular cancer, the exact causative factors have yet to be thoroughly defined.

Genetic factors

Familial studies have provided the strongest evidence supporting a role for inherited susceptibility for testicular cancer. In comparison with the general population, the risk of testicular cancer has been reported to be eightfold higher in brothers and fourfold higher in sons of affected men.[72,73] Migration studies, especially from Finland, Sweden, and Denmark, where the incidence of testicular cancer is low, medium and high, respectively, support the hypothesis of shared genes rather than shared environmental exposures. The risk of testicular cancer in Finnish men migrating to Sweden remained low regardless of age of migration,[74] and the risk of testicular cancer in Danish men migrating to Sweden remained high.[75]

Testicular cancer has been also associated with genetic alterations. Rapley *et al.*[76] first reported evidence for a testicular cancer susceptibility gene, TGCT1, located on chromosome Xq27. Data suggest that several loci must contribute to GCT susceptibility and that no one locus explains a large fraction of the familial risk. Several studies showed that GCTs are also characterized by gain of the short arm of chromosome 12 in almost all cases.[77,78] Genome-wide association studies in cohorts of patients with testicular cancer identified a specific single nucleotide polymorphisms relating to genes involved in early gonadal development, including DMRT1[79] and KITLG.[80,81] This observation is of significant relevance in the context of the origin of the cancer, and might be a putative target for identification of high-risk individuals in specific populations.

Epidemiology

Testicular cancer is the most common cancer among men between the ages of 15 to 45 years. It has been shown that 84% of testis cancers occurs among men at ages of 15 and 44 years, whereas only 15% of the GCT occur in men aged 45 years and older. The incidence of non-seminoma peaks at approximately age 25 years, while the incidence of seminoma peaks at age 35 years.

In 2008, the global age-standardized incidence rate of testicular cancer was 1.5 per 100,000 men per year.[82] The incidence of GCTs shows marked variations among different countries. The highest incidence rates in the world occur in populations of Scandinavia (15.2 per 100,000 per year). Men from northern Europe, in particular Norwegian and Danish men, have incidence rates five to ten times higher than African and Asian men (e.g. Japan: 0.8 per 100,000 per year). In the United States, it is estimated that 8,400 men diagnosed with and 380 men died of testicular cancer in the year 2009.

Testicular cancer incidence varies considerably among racial and ethnic groups. For example, in the United States, the incidence of testicular cancer between 1973 and 2004 among white men was 5.46 per 100,000, while the incidence among black men was 0.95 per 100,000.[83]

The incidence of testicular cancer has doubled in the past 30 years and is still increasing.[15] A large geographic difference exists hypothesizing a combination of genetic factors and environmental influences, but the reason for this development is still unexplained.

Diagnostic procedures in testicular cancer

Clinical presentation and first diagnostic steps

Most testicular cancer patients present with a primary tumour in the testis. Delay in diagnosing germ cell cancer may be caused either by patients who ignore symptoms too long or by physicians who fail to make the correct diagnosis: for example, misclassifying a testicular mass as epididymitis or back pain from retroperitoneal disease resulting from vertebral disc problems. Therefore, a high level of suspicion should be maintained in young men with any of these clinical features. In a minority of patients, the primary tumour manifestation is located extragonadally, that is, in the retroperitoneum or the mediastinum.

When assessing the patient's history, the following risk factors for the development of testicular tumours should be addressed: contralateral testicular tumour, undescended testis/cryptorchidism, history of infertility and testicular tumour among first-degree relatives, particularly in the father and/or brothers.

In patients suspicious of a testicular tumour diagnostic examinations including testis palpation, ultrasound of the testes (7.5 MHz transducer) and the determination of serum tumour markers alpha-fetoprotein (AFP), ß-human chorionic gonadotropin, and lactic dehydrogenase (LDH) are mandatory.

Tumour markers

Serum tumour markers play a crucial role in the management of patients with testicular cancer, contributing to diagnosis, staging, and risk assessment, evaluation of response to treatment and detection of relapse. Alpha-fetoprotein (AFP), HCG and lactate dehydrogenase (LDH) are established serum markers. Other serum tumour markers like placental alkaline phosphatase (PLAP) have been evaluated but provide limited additional clinical information.

Alpha-fetoprotein

Alpha-fetoprotein (AFP) is a homolog of albumin and is thought to act as a carrier protein in the foetus. During pregnancy, AFP is initially produced by the yolk sac and later by the fetal liver.[84] After birth, circulating concentrations decrease with a half-life of 5 days, falling to adult levels (less 10–15 μg/L). In adults with testicular cancer AFP is a sensitive marker for non-seminomatous tumours especially in yolk sac tumours and increases in 50–70% of NSGCT patients. Rising levels of serum AFP indicate persistent germ cell tumour, even in the absence of radiographic evidence of disease. Elevated serum concentrations of AFP occur in most hepatocellular carcinomas and 10-30% of other gastrointestinal cancers, but these diseases are rare in patients with testicular cancer. Also benign liver disease, in particular hepatitis, and liver damage induced by chemotherapy are often associated with moderately elevated serum AFP levels, and may result in misinterpretation especially if levels are rising.[85,86]

Human chorionic gonadotropin

Human chorionic gonadotropin (HCG) is a member of the glycoprotein hormone family, which includes luteinizing hormone (LH), follicle stimulating hormone (FSH), and thyroid stimulating hormone. HCG is secreted at low levels by the pituitary, producing plasma levels that are measurable by sensitive methods. The serum concentrations may increase with age, the upper reference limit for men below 50 years of age is 0.7 U/L and for men above this age 2.1 U/L.[87] The β-subunit of HCG (HCGß) is secreted by germ cell tumours especially seminoma and choriocarcinoma. An increased hCG is seen in 40–60% of NSGCT patients and up to 30% of seminomas can present or develop an elevated HCG level.

It is important to note that chemotherapy often causes gonadal suppression that increases the HCG levels. Therefore, levels increasing from below 2 up to 5–8 U/L during chemotherapy are often iatrogenic and do not necessarily indicate relapse. Moderately elevated levels of HCG may be of pituitary origin, especially if accompanying with higher serum levels of LH and FSH and are attributed to interrupted feedback inhibition from the gonads.[88,89]

Lactate dehydrogenase

The enzyme lactate dehydrogenase (LDH) exists as a tetramer that may contain various combinations of two subunits, LDH-A, LDH-B. The various subunits can combine in five isoenzymes (LDH1, LDH-2, LDH-3, LDH-4, LDH-5). LDH is expressed in many tissues and elevated levels may be caused by a wide variety of diseases like hemolysis, meningitis, encephalitis, acute pancreatitis, and HIV. Despite its lack of specificity, LDH is a useful marker in germ cell tumours.[90] Its level may be elevated in 80% of patients with advanced testicular cancer and LDH concentration is proportional to tumour volume.

Other serum tumour markers

A tumour-associated isoenzyme of alkaline phosphatase was first described in a patient with lung cancer and later detected in serum of patients with other cancers and identified as PLAP. PLAP is elevated most frequently in patients with seminoma (60–70%), and less frequently in those with other GCTs. Serum concentrations of PLAP are increased up to 10-fold in smokers,[91] and so this limits its clinical application. PLAP detection is not routinely included in the diagnostic work up of testicular cancer patients.

Neuron-specific enolase (NSE) is elevated in about 30–50% of patients with seminomas and less often in NSGCT patients.[92,93] However, in spite of these promising results, the use of NSE is limited and apart from the possible diagnosis of primitive neuroectodermal differentiated tumours (PNET) after chemotherapy, not routinely recommended.

Inguinal exploration, orchiectomy, and partial orchiectomy

Surgical exploration is obligatory for suspected tumours. If the patient has life-threatening metastatic disease or massive elevation of markers in conjunction with large metastatic masses, an orchiectomy should not delay chemotherapy and may be deferred until clinical stabilization (usually end of chemotherapy). If the histological origin of the metastatic disease in this scenario is unclear a biopsy of the tumour mass could be performed. A combined elevation of hCG and AFP is extremely suspicious of germ cell cancer even without a testicular mass. In cases with extragonadal origin a computed tomography (CT) scan of the abdomen is indicated followed by guided biopsy of any retroperitoneal mass. An open surgical exploration of the abdomen in the presence of a dual marker rise should be avoided.

Radical orchiectomy should be performed through an inguinal incision and a division of the spermatic cord at the internal inguinal ring if a tumour is found. If the testicular cancer diagnosis is not clear, a biopsy is taken for frozen section histological examination. In cases of small testicular masses, histology by frozen section should be performed in order to avoid orchiectomy for benign tumours. Organ-sparing surgery can be attempted in special cases (e.g. bilateral testicular tumours, metachronous contralateral tumours, tumour in a solitary testis with normal preoperative testosterone levels).[94] These options must be carefully discussed with the patient and surgery performed in a centre with experience.[95]

Contralateral biopsy

Contralateral biopsy has been advocated to rule out the presence of GCNIS (germ cell neoplasia *in situ*), a malignant pre-invasive testicular germ cell lesion. Without treatment 70% of GCNIS progresses to a definitive germ cell tumour within 7 years. Up to 9% (approximately 2.5%) of the patients with testicular cancer have a GCNIS in contralateral testis.[96,97]

According to current guidelines, a biopsy of the contralateral testis is recommended for high-risk patients to look for germ cell neoplasia *in situ*. High risk is defined as a patient with a testicular volume of less than 12 mL, an age less then 40 years, a history of cryptorchidism or poor spermatogenesis (less than 15 million sperms per millilitre of semen).[98] The benefit of biopsy (i.e. diagnosis and treatment of GCNIS) must be weighed against its risk (trauma to/reduction in volume of a solitary testicle) and the risks of GCNIS treatment (infertility following radiotherapy to the solitary testicle) and the low mortality rates from contralateral tumours. A recent prospectively randomized study from SWENOTECA showed in 988 patients with early stage non-seminoma that the proportion of bilateral cancers was similar in biopsy-negative patients (3.6%) and patients without a biopsy (3.0%).[99] They documented a high proportion of false negative biopsies, which might explain why patients with negative biopsy had the same risk of contralateral tumour as patients not undergoing biopsy. These results may lead to change current guidelines and not to recommend contralateral biopsy in GCT patients.

Imaging procedures

After histopathological classification of the tumour, further staging is necessary. This comprises radiological (usually CT) scanning of the thorax, abdomen, and pelvis, and measuring the kinetics of serum tumour markers. A chest X-ray could be considered as the only thoracic examination in seminoma patients in whom abdominal and pelvic CT scans are negative. Magnetic resonance imaging can be helpful when CT scan is inconclusive, when CT scan is contraindicated or in cases of concern about radiation exposure. Other examinations, such as brain or spinal CT, bone scan, or liver ultrasound, should be performed in presence of symptoms or a suspicion of metastases to these organs (Table 6.33.2). A fluorodeoxyglucose-PET (FDG-PET) scan in the initial staging

Table 6.33.2 Diagnostic procedures

	Diagnostic procedure
Laboratory findings	Tumour markers: ◆ α-fetoprotein (AFP) ◆ β-human chorionic gonadotropin (β-HCG) ◆ Lactate dehydrogenase (LDH)
Imaging	Testicular ultrasound (7.5-MHz transducer)Chest X-ray (seminoma CS I) CT scan of abdomen and pelvis Chest CT scan (not mandatory for seminoma CS I) MRT of chest and abdomen (only if contraindication for CT scan) CT of central nervous system (in advanced disease or in presence of symptoms) Ultrasound of liver (only in presence of symptoms) Bone scan (only in presence of symptoms) PET scan: identification viable tissue in residual lesion in seminoma (follow-up)
Fertility investigations	Total testosterone, LH, FSHSemen analysis Sperm banking / cryopreservation

examination of testicular cancer is not recommended, but seems to be useful in the follow-up of patients with seminoma to detect residual tumours after chemotherapy.[100]

Further diagnostic procedures

In patients with testicular cancer a pretreatment fertility assessment with determination of testosterone, LH, and FSH serum levels should be performed (baseline examination to follow-up possible hormonal long-term toxicity), and semen analysis and cryopreservation should be offered to the patients.

Classification

After completing histological analysis and staging investigations, the clinical stage (CS) based on UICC/TNM classification and serum tumour markers should be defined (Tables 6.33.3 and 6.33.4). Metastatic disease is classified according to the IGCCCG criteria including the histological features, location of primary and metastatic lesions and tumour marker levels (after orchiectomy) (Table 6.33.5). The optimal individual treatment strategy is predicated on the CS and the IGCCCG classification.[101,102]

Summary and conclusion

Testicular cancer is the most common malignancy in men 15 to 45 years of age. The global age-standardized incidence rate of testicular cancer is 1.5 per 100,000 men per year but increases up to 10 per 100,000 men per year in Northern Europe. Despite the increasing rates of testicular germ cell tumours seen during the last decades, the aetiology of testicular cancer remains in some parts poorly understood. Geographic and ethnic discrepancies suggest both environmental and genetic factors contribute to the development of germ cell tumours. The association with perinatal risk factors and congenital anomalies, as well as young age of onset, suggest that the tumour may originate in utero. Risk factors

Table 6.33.3 TNM classification

TNM staging	Unit	Value
Primary tumour (T)	pTX	Primary tumour cannot be assessed. (If no radical orchiectomy has been performed, Tx is used)
	pT0	No evidence of primary tumour (e.g. histologic scar in testis)
	pTis	Intratubular germ cell neoplasia (germ cell neoplasia *in situ*)
	pT1	Tumour limited to the testis and epididymis without vascular/ lymphatic invasion. Tumour may invade into the tunica albuginea but not the tunica vaginalis
	pT2	Tumour limited to the testis and epididymis with vascular/lymphatic invasion, or tumour extending through the tunica albuginea with involvement of the tunica vaginalis
	pT3	Tumour invades the spermatic cord with or without vascular/lymphatic invasion
	pT4	Tumour invades the scrotum with or without vascular/lymphatic invasion
Regional lymph nodes (N)	NX N0 N1	Regional lymph nodes cannot be assessedNo regional lymph node metastasis Metastasis with a lymph node mass 2 cm or less in greatest dimension; or multiple lymph nodes, none more than 2 cm in greatest dimension
	N2	Metastasis with a lymph node mass, more than 2 cm but not more than 5 cm in greatest dimension; or multiple lymph nodes, any one mass greater than 2 cm but not more than 5 cm in greatest dimension
	N3	Metastasis with a lymph node mass more than 5 cm in greatest dimension
Metastasis (M)	MX	Distant metastasis cannot be assessed
	M0	No distant metastasis
	M1	Distant metastasis
	M1a	Non-regional nodal or pulmonary metastasis
	M1b	Other metastasis (non-pulmonary visceral metastasis)
Serum tumour markers (S) (after orchiectomy)	SX S0 S1	Marker studies not available or not performed Marker study levels within normal limits LDH <1.5 × normal and HCG (mIU/mL) <5,000 and AFP (ng/mL) <1,000
	S2	LDH 1.5-10 × normal or HCG (mIU/mL) 5,000–50,000 or AFP (ng/mL) 1,000–10,000
	S3	LDH >10 × normal or HCG (mIU/mL) >50,000 or AFP (ng/mL) >10,000

From Sobin LH, Gospodariwicz M, Wittekind C (Eds), *TNM classification of malignant tumors, UICC International Union Against Cancer, Seventh Edition*, pp. 249–254, Copyright © Wiley-Blackwell 2009. Reproduced with permission of Blackwell Publishing Ltd.

Table 6.33.4 Clinical stages (CSs)

Clinical stage	CS	TNM classification
Stage I (CS I)	IA	pT1 N0 M0 S0
(no metastasis (M0) and	IB	pT2 N0 M0 S0
negative regional lymph nodes (N0))		pT3 N0 M0 S0
		pT4 N0 M0 S0
	IS	pT1-4 N0 M0 S1-3
Stage II (CS II)	II A	pT1-4 N1 M0 S0
		pT1-4 N1 M0 S1
(positive regional lymph nodes (N+))	II B	pT1-4 N2 M0 S0
		pT1-4 N2 M0 S1
	II C	pT1-4 N3 M0 S0
		pT1-4 N3 M0 S1
Stage III (CS III)	III A	pT1-4 N1-3 M1A S0
		pT1-4 N1-3 M1A S1
(metastasis (M+))	III B	pT1-4 N1-3 M0 S2
		pT1-4 N1-3 M1A S2
	III C	pT1-4 N1-3 M0 S3
		pT1-4 N1-3 M1A S3
		pT1-4 N1-3 M1B S0-1

Adapted with permission from P. Albers (Chair), W. Albrecht, F. Algaba *et al.*, Guidelines on Testicular Cancer, p.11, European Association of Urology, Copyright © European Association of Urology 2015, available from http://uroweb.org/wp-content/uploads/11-Testicular-Cancer_LR1.pdf. Source: data from Sobin LH, Gospodariwicz M, Wittekind C (Eds), *TNM classification of malignant tumors*, UICC International Union Against Cancer, Seventh Edition, pp. 249–254, Copyright © Wiley-Blackwell 2009.

for testicular cancer include cryptorchidism (maldescensus testis), family history, and white race. If testicular cancer is diagnosed early, the cure rate is nearly 99%. Patients presenting with a painless testicular mass, scrotal heaviness, a dull ache, or acute pain should receive a thorough examination. Testicular masses should be examined with scrotal ultrasonography. In every case of suspicion of testicular cancer tumour marker detection (AFP, hCG, LDH) is mandatory and a surgical exploration of the intratesticular mass is obligatory. Radical orchiectomy should be performed through an inguinal incision if a tumour is found to be malignant. Furthermore, radiological examinations including abdominopelvic CT scan and chest CT scan are required as initial staging investigations. In addition to imaging, the patient has to be classified with a CS based on UICC/TNM classification. For this purpose, serum tumour markers should be determined after orchiectomy. Patients with advanced disease are classified according to the IGCCCG classification. The correct individual classification of patients with testicular cancer according to diagnostic results followed by risk-adapted treatment plan is crucial for the success of the treatment.

In early stage patients the recent aim of testicular cancer treatment is to avoid overtreatment and decrease short- and long-term toxicity. With the use of a risk-adapted treatment management, about a half of patients with early stage GCT will favour close surveillance instead of adjuvant treatment. Surveillance develops to be the preferred and most effective treatment option in managing early stage testicular germ cell tumour patients. In spite of compliance problems, the overall disease-free survival in these patients is approaching 100%.

The therapy of advanced testicular germ cell tumours is based on risk stratification according to clinical features and IGCCCG classification. In patients with 'good prognosis' features chemotherapy

Table 6.33.5 IGCCCG classification

IGCCCG	NSGCT	Seminoma
Good prognosis	◆ Testis or primary extragonadal retroperitoneal tumour ◆ No non-pulmonary visceral metastases ◆ AFP <1, 000 ng/mL ◆ ß-HCG <1,000 ng/mL (<5,000 IU/l) ◆ LDH <1.5 × normal level	◆ Any primary localization ◆ No non-pulmonary visceral metastases ◆ Any marker level
Intermediate prognosis	◆ Testis or primary extragonadal retroperitonealtumour ◆ No presence of non-pulmonary visceral metastases ◆ AFP 1,000–10,000 ng/mL and/or ◆ ß-HCG 1,000–10,000 ng/mL (5,000–50,000 IU/l) and/or ◆ LDH 1.5–10 × normal	◆ Any primary localization ◆ Presence of non-pulmonary visceral metastases (liver, CNS,bone, intestinum) ◆ Any tumour marker level
Poor prognosis	◆ Primary mediastinal germ cell tumour with or without testis or primary retroperitoneal tumour ◆ Presence of non-pulmonary visceral metastases (liver, CNS, bone, intestinum) and/or ◆ AFP >10,000 ng/mL and/or ◆ ß-HCG >10,000 ng/mL (50.000 IU/l) and/or ◆ LDH >10 × normal level	Does not exist

Adapted with permission from P. Albers (Chair), W. Albrecht, F. Algaba *et al.*, *Guidelines on Testicular Cancer*, p. 12, European Association of Urology, Copyright © European Association of Urology 2015, available from http://uroweb.org/wp-content/uploads/11-Testicular-Cancer_LR1.pdf

with three cycles BEP or four cycles EP is the optimal treatment regimen and cure rates with either regimen with or without surgery approximate 90%. For patients with advanced disease and 'intermediate/poor prognosis' features, intensification of the standard treatment (four cycles BEP) is being investigated to increase long-term cure rates. These patients can have long-term freedom from disease progression when chemotherapy is combined with complete resection of residual masses. Future investigations should focus on further improving diagnostic procedures and treatment strategies to reduce the risk of late toxicities and improve cure rates.

Further reading

Bosl GJ, Motzer RJ. Testicular germ-cell cancer. *N Engl J Med* 1997; **337**:242–53.

Dieckmann KP, Pichlmeier U. Clinical epidemiology of testicular germ cell tumors. *World J Urol* 2004; **22**:2–14.

Kanetsky PA, Mitra N, Vardhanabhuti S, *et al.* Common variation in kitlg and at 5q31.3 predisposes to testicular germ cell cancer. *Nat Genet* 2009; **41**:811–5.

Krege S, Beyer J, Souchon R, *et al.* European consensus conference on diagnosis and treatment of germ cell cancer: a report of the second meeting of the european germ cell cancer consensus group (egcccg): Part I. *Eur Urol* 2008; **53**:478–96.

Krege S, Beyer J, Souchon R, *et al.* European consensus conference on diagnosis and treatment of germ cell cancer: a report of the second meeting of the european germ cell cancer consensus group (egcccg): Part II. *Eur Urol* 2008; **53**:497–513.

McGlynn KA, Cook MB. Etiologic factors in testicular germ-cell tumors. *Future Oncol* 2009; **5**:1389–402.

McGlynn KA, Quraishi SM, Graubard BI, Weber JP, Rubertone MV, Erickson RL. Persistent organochlorine pesticides and risk of testicular germ cell tumors. *J Natl Cancer Inst* 2008; **100**:663–71.

Rapley EA, Turnbull C, Al Olama AA, *et al.* A genome-wide association study of testicular germ cell tumor. *Nat Genet* 2009; **41**:807–10.

Ulbright TM. Germ cell tumors of the gonads: A selective review emphasizing problems in differential diagnosis, newly appreciated, and controversial issues. *Mod Pathol* 2005; **18**(Suppl 2):S61–79.

Winter C, Albers P. Testicular germ cell tumors: Pathogenesis, diagnosis and treatment. *Nat Rev Endocrinol* 2011; 7:43–53.

References

1. Bosl GJ, Motzer RJ. Testicular germ-cell cancer. *N Engl J Med* 1997; **337**:242–53.
2. Winter C, Albers P. Testicular germ cell tumors: Pathogenesis, diagnosis and treatment. *Nat Rev Endocrinol* 2011; 7:43–53.
3. Einhorn LH, Donohue JP. Improved chemotherapy in disseminated testicular cancer. *J Urol* 1977; **117**:65–9.
4. Einhorn LH. Treatment of testicular cancer: A new and improved model. *J Clin Oncol* 1990; **8**:1777–81.
5. Ernst DS, Brasher P, Venner PM, *et al.* Compliance and outcome of patients with stage 1 non-seminomatous germ cell tumors (nsgct) managed with surveillance programs in seven canadian centres. *Can J Urol* 2005; **12**:2575–80.
6. Feldman DR, Motzer RJ. Good-risk-advanced germ cell tumors: Historical perspective and current standards of care. *World J Urol* 2009; **27**:463–70.
7. Shayegan B, Carver BS, Stasi J, Motzer RJ, Bosl GJ, Sheinfeld J. Clinical outcome following post-chemotherapy retroperitoneal lymph node dissection in men with intermediate- and poor-risk nonseminomatous germ cell tumour. *BJU Int* 2007; **99**:993–7.
8. Eble JN, Sauter G, Epstein JI, Sesterhenn IA. *World Health Organization Classification of Tumours: Pathology and Genetics of Tumours of the Urinary System and Male Genital Organs*. Lyon, France: IARC Press 2004: pp. 250–62.
9. Ulbright TM, Roth LM. Recent developments in the pathology of germ cell tumors. *Semin Diagn Pathol* 1987; **4**:304–19.
10. Ulbright TM. Germ cell tumors of the gonads: A selective review emphasizing problems in differential diagnosis, newly appreciated, and controversial issues. *Mod Pathol* 2005; **18**(Suppl 2):S61–79.
11. Dieckmann KP, Pichlmeier U. Clinical epidemiology of testicular germ cell tumors. *World J Urol* 2004; **22**:2–14.
12. Garner MJ, Turner MC, Ghadirian P, Krewski D. Epidemiology of testicular cancer: An overview. *Int J Cancer* 2005; **116**:331–9.
13. Batata MA, Chu FC, Hilaris BS, Whitmore WF, Golbey RB. Testicular cancer in cryptorchids. *Cancer* 1982; **49**:1023–30.
14. Berkowitz GS, Lapinski RH, Godbold JH, Dolgin SE, Holzman IR. Maternal and neonatal risk factors for cryptorchidism. *Epidemiology* 1995; **6**:127–31.
15. McGlynn KA, Devesa SS, Sigurdson AJ, Brown LM, Tsao L, Tarone RE. Trends in the incidence of testicular germ cell tumors in the united states. *Cancer* 2003; **97**:63–70.
16. Ginsburg J. Unanswered questions in carcinoma of the testis. *Lancet* 1997; **349**:1785–6.
17. Petersen PM, Skakkebaek NE, Vistisen K, Rorth M, Giwercman A. Semen quality and reproductive hormones before orchiectomy in men with testicular cancer. *J Clin Oncol* 1999; **17**:941–7.
18. Osterlind A, Berthelsen JG, Abildgaard N, *et al.* Risk of bilateral testicular germ cell cancer in denmark: 1960-1984. *J Natl Cancer Inst* 1991; **83**:1391–5.
19. Colls BM, Harvey VJ, Skelton L, Thompson PI, Frampton CM. Bilateral germ cell testicular tumors in new zealand: Experience in auckland and christchurch 1978-1994. *J Clin Oncol* 1996; **14**:2061–5.
20. Fossa SD, Chen J, Schonfeld SJ, *et al.* Risk of contralateral testicular cancer: A population-based study of 29,515 U.S. men. *J Natl Cancer Inst* 2005; **97**:1056–66.
21. Theodore C, Terrier-Lacombe MJ, Laplanche A, *et al.* Bilateral germ-cell tumours: 22-year experience at the institut gustave roussy. *Br J Cancer* 2004; **90**:55–9.
22. McGlynn KA, Cook MB. Etiologic factors in testicular germ-cell tumors. *Future Oncol* 2009; **5**:1389–402.
23. Brown LM, Pottern LM, Hoover RN. Prenatal and perinatal risk factors for testicular cancer. *Cancer Res* 1986; **46**:4812–6.
24. Akre O, Ekbom A, Hsieh CC, Trichopoulos D, Adami HO. Testicular nonseminoma and seminoma in relation to perinatal characteristics. *J Natl Cancer Inst* 1996; **88**:883–9.
25. Richiardi L, Pettersson A, Akre O. Genetic and environmental risk factors for testicular cancer. *Int J Androl* 2007; **30**:230–40; discussion 240–31.
26. Richiardi L, Akre O, Bellocco R, Ekbom A. Perinatal determinants of germ-cell testicular cancer in relation to histological subtypes. *Br J Cancer* 2002; **87**:545–50.
27. Cook MB, Graubard BI, Rubertone MV, Erickson RL, McGlynn KA. Perinatal factors and the risk of testicular germ cell tumors. *Int J Cancer* 2008; **122**:2600–6.
28. Sabroe S, Olsen J. Perinatal correlates of specific histological types of testicular cancer in patients below 35 years of age: A case-cohort study based on midwives' records in denmark. *Int J Cancer* 1998; **78**:140–3.
29. Wanderas EH, Grotmol T, Fossa SD, Tretli S. Maternal health and pre- and perinatal characteristics in the etiology of testicular cancer: A prospective population- and register-based study on norwegian males born between 1967 and 1995. *Cancer Causes Control* 1998; **9**:475–86.
30. Pettersson A, Kaijser M, Richiardi L, Askling J, Ekbom A, Akre O. Women smoking and testicular cancer: One epidemic causing another? *Int J Cancer* 2004; **109**:941–4.
31. Pettersson A, Akre O, Richiardi L, Ekbom A, Kaijser M. Maternal smoking and the epidemic of testicular cancer--a nested case-control study. *Int J Cancer* 2007; **120**:2044–6.

32. Tuomisto J, Holl K, Rantakokko P, *et al.* Maternal smoking during pregnancy and testicular cancer in the sons: A nested case-control study and a meta-analysis. *Eur J Cancer* 2009; **45**:1640–8.
33. Bernstein L, Depue RH, Ross RK, Judd HL, Pike MC, Henderson BE. Higher maternal levels of free estradiol in first compared to second pregnancy: Early gestational differences. *J Natl Cancer Inst* 1986; **76**:1035–9.
34. Henderson BE, Ross R, Bernstein L. Estrogens as a cause of human cancer: The Richard and Hinda Rosenthal Foundation award lecture. *Cancer Res* 1988; **48**:246–53.
35. Sharpe RM, Skakkebaek NE. Are oestrogens involved in falling sperm counts and disorders of the male reproductive tract? *Lancet* 1993; **341**:1392–5.
36. Strohsnitter WC, Noller KL, Hoover RN, *et al.* Cancer risk in men exposed in utero to diethylstilbestrol. *J Natl Cancer Inst* 2001; **93**:545–51.
37. Newbold RR. Lessons learned from perinatal exposure to diethylstilbestrol. *Toxicol Appl Pharmacol* 2004; **199**:142–50.
38. Goldenberg RC, Fortes FS, Cristancho JM, *et al.* Modulation of gap junction mediated intercellular communication in tm3 leydig cells. *J Endocrinol* 2003; **177**:327–35.
39. Kavlock RJ, Daston GP, DeRosa C, *et al.* Research needs for the risk assessment of health and environmental effects of endocrine disruptors: A report of the u.S. Epa-sponsored workshop. *Environ Health Perspect* 1996; **104**(Suppl 4):715–40.
40. McGlynn KA, Quraishi SM, Graubard BI, Weber JP, Rubertone MV, Erickson RL. Persistent organochlorine pesticides and risk of testicular germ cell tumors. *J Natl Cancer Inst* 2008; **100**:663–71.
41. Biggs ML, Davis MD, Eaton DL, *et al.* Serum organochlorine pesticide residues and risk of testicular germ cell carcinoma: A population-based case-control study. *Cancer Epidemiol Biomarkers Prev* 2008; **17**:2012–8.
42. Dieckmann KP, Hartmann JT, Classen J, Ludde R, Diederichs M, Pichlmeier U. Tallness is associated with risk of testicular cancer: Evidence for the nutrition hypothesis. *Br J Cancer* 2008; **99**:1517–21.
43. Davies TW, Palmer CR, Ruja E, Lipscombe JM. Adolescent milk, dairy product and fruit consumption and testicular cancer. *Br J Cancer* 1996; **74**:657–60.
44. Sigurdson AJ, Chang S, Annegers JF, *et al.* A case-control study of diet and testicular carcinoma. *Nutr Cancer* 1999; **34**:20–6.
45. Ganmaa D, Li XM, Wang J, Qin LQ, Wang PY, Sato A. Incidence and mortality of testicular and prostatic cancers in relation to world dietary practices. *Int J Cancer* 2002; **98**:262–7.
46. Garner MJ, Birkett NJ, Johnson KC, Shatenstein B, Ghadirian P, Krewski D. Dietary risk factors for testicular carcinoma. *Int J Cancer* 2003; **106**:934–41.
47. Cook MB, Zhang Y, Graubard BI, Rubertone MV, Erickson RL, McGlynn KA. Risk of testicular germ-cell tumours in relation to childhood physical activity. *Br J Cancer* 2008; **98**:174–8.
48. [No authors listed]. Social, behavioural and medical factors in the aetiology of testicular cancer: results from the UK study. UK Testicular Cancer Study Group. *Br J Cancer* 1994; **70**:513–20.
49. Dosemeci M, Hayes RB, Vetter R, *et al.* Occupational physical activity, socioeconomic status, and risks of 15 cancer sites in turkey. *Cancer Causes Control* 1993; **4**:313–21.
50. Paffenbarger RS Jr, Hyde RT, Wing AL. Physical activity and incidence of cancer in diverse populations: A preliminary report. *Am J Clin Nutr* 1987; **45**:312–7.
51. Srivastava A, Kreiger N. Relation of physical activity to risk of testicular cancer. *Am J Epidemiol* 2000; **151**:78–87.
52. Stang A, Jockel KH, Baumgardt-Elms C, Ahrens W. Firefighting and risk of testicular cancer: Results from a german population-based case-control study. *Am J Ind Med* 2003; **43**:291–4.
53. Rhomberg W, Schmoll HJ, Schneider B. High frequency of metalworkers among patients with seminomatous tumors of the testis: A case-control study. *Am J Ind Med* 1995; **28**:79–87.
54. Marshall EG, Melius JM, London MA, Nasca PC, Burnett WS. Investigation of a testicular cancer cluster using a case-control approach. *Int J Epidemiol* 1990; **19**:269–73.
55. Foley S, Middleton S, Stitson D, Mahoney M. The incidence of testicular cancer in royal air force personnel. *Br J Urol* 1995; **76**:495–6.
56. Moller H. Work in agriculture, childhood residence, nitrate exposure, and testicular cancer risk: A case-control study in denmark. *Cancer Epidemiol Biomarkers Prev* 1997; **6**:141–4.
57. Van den Eeden SK, Weiss NS, Strader CH, Daling JR. Occupation and the occurrence of testicular cancer. *Am J Ind Med* 1991; **19**:327–37.
58. Ross RK, McCurtis JW, Henderson BE, Menck HR, Mack TM, Martin SP. Descriptive epidemiology of testicular and prostatic cancer in los angeles. *Br J Cancer* 1979; **39**:284–92.
59. Coupland CA, Forman D, Chilvers CE, Davey G, Pike MC, Oliver RT. Maternal risk factors for testicular cancer: A population-based case-control study (UK). *Cancer Causes Control* 2004; **15**:277–83.
60. Newell GR, Mills PK, Johnson DE. Epidemiologic comparison of cancer of the testis and hodgkin's disease among young males. *Cancer* 1984; **54**:1117–23.
61. Logothetis CJ, Newell GR, Samuels ML. Testicular cancer in homosexual men with cellular immune deficiency: Report of 2 cases. *J Urol* 1985; **133**:484–6.
62. Frisch M, Biggar RJ, Engels EA, Goedert JJ. Association of cancer with aids-related immunosuppression in adults. *JAMA* 2001; **285**:1736–45.
63. Morris JD, Eddleston AL, Crook T. Viral infection and cancer. *Lancet* 1995; **346**:754–8.
64. Akre O, Lipworth L, Tretli S, *et al.* Epstein-Barr virus and cytomegalovirus in relation to testicular-cancer risk: A nested case-control study. *Int J Cancer* 1999; **82**:1–5.
65. Lyter DW, Bryant J, Thackeray R, Rinaldo CR, Kingsley LA. Incidence of human immunodeficiency virus-related and nonrelated malignancies in a large cohort of homosexual men. *J Clin Oncol* 1995; **13**:2540–6.
66. Brown LM, Pottern LM, Hoover RN. Testicular cancer in young men: The search for causes of the epidemic increase in the United States. *J Epidemiol Community Health* 1987; **41**:349–54.
67. Haughey BP, Graham S, Brasure J, Zielezny M, Sufrin G, Burnett WS. The epidemiology of testicular cancer in upstate new york. *Am J Epidemiol* 1989; **130**:25–36.
68. Carlsen E, Giwercman A, Keiding N, Skakkebaek NE. Evidence for decreasing quality of semen during past 50 years. *BMJ* 1992; **305**:609–13.
69. Skakkebaek NE, Jorgensen N. Testicular dysgenesis and fertility. *Andrologia* 2005; **37**:217–8.
70. Mancini M, Carmignani L, Gazzano G, *et al.* High prevalence of testicular cancer in azoospermic men without spermatogenesis. *Hum Reprod* 2007; **22**:1042–6.
71. Raman JD, Nobert CF, Goldstein M. Increased incidence of testicular cancer in men presenting with infertility and abnormal semen analysis. *J Urol* 2005; **174**:1819–22; discussion 1822.
72. Westergaard T, Olsen JH, Frisch M, Kroman N, Nielsen JW, Melbye M. Cancer risk in fathers and brothers of testicular cancer patients in denmark. A population-based study. *Int J Cancer* 1996; **66**:627–31.
73. Sonneveld DJ, Sleijfer DT, Schrafford Koops H, *et al.* Familial testicular cancer in a single-centre population. *Eur J Cancer* 1999; **35**:1368–73.
74. Ekbom A, Richiardi L, Akre O, Montgomery SM, Sparen P. Age at immigration and duration of stay in relation to risk for testicular cancer among finnish immigrants in sweden. *J Natl Cancer Inst* 2003; **95**:1238–40.
75. Hemminki K, Li X. Cancer risks in nordic immigrants and their offspring in sweden. *Eur J Cancer* 2002; **38**:2428–34.
76. Rapley EA, Crockford GP, Teare D, *et al.* Localization to xq27 of a susceptibility gene for testicular germ-cell tumours. *Nat Genet* 2000; **24**:197–200.
77. Korkola JE, Houldsworth J, Bosl GJ, Chaganti RS. Molecular events in germ cell tumours: Linking chromosome-12 gain, acquisition of pluripotency and response to cisplatin. *BJU Int* 2009; **104**:1334–8.

78. Korkola JE, Houldsworth J, Feldman DR, *et al.* Identification and validation of a gene expression signature that predicts outcome in adult men with germ cell tumors. *J Clin Oncol* 2009; **27**:5240–7.
79. Kanetsky PA, Mitra N, Vardhanabhuti S, *et al.* A second independent locus within dmrt1 is associated with testicular germ cell tumor susceptibility. *Hum Mol Genet* 2011; **20**:3109–17.
80. Kanetsky PA, Mitra N, Vardhanabhuti S, *et al.* Common variation in kitlg and at 5q31.3 predisposes to testicular germ cell cancer. *Nat Genet* 2009; **41**:811–5.
81. Rapley EA, Turnbull C, Al Olama AA, *et al.* A genome-wide association study of testicular germ cell tumor. *Nat Genet* 2009; **41**:807–10.
82. Ferlay J, Shin HR, Bray F, Forman D, Mathers C, Parkin DM. Estimates of worldwide burden of cancer in 2008: Globocan 2008. *Int J Cancer* 2010; **127**:2893–917.
83. Shah MN, Devesa SS, Zhu K, McGlynn KA. Trends in testicular germ cell tumours by ethnic group in the united states. *Int J Androl* 2007; **30**:206–13; discussion 213–14.
84. Abelev GI. Alpha-fetoprotein as a marker of embryo-specific differentiations in normal and tumor tissues. *Transplant Rev* 1974; **20**:3–37.
85. Germa JR, Llanos M, Tabernero JM, Mora J. False elevations of alpha-fetoprotein associated with liver dysfunction in germ cell tumors. *Cancer* 1993; **72**:2491–4.
86. Morris MJ, Bosl GJ. Recognizing abnormal marker results that do not reflect disease in patients with germ cell tumors. *J Urol* 2000; **163**:796–801.
87. Alfthan H, Haglund C, Dabek J, Stenman UH. Concentrations of human choriogonadotropin, its beta-subunit, and the core fragment of the beta-subunit in serum and urine of men and nonpregnant women. *Clin Chem* 1992; **38**:1981–7.
88. Catalona WJ, Vaitukaitis JL, Fair WR. Falsely positive specific human chorionic gonadotropin assays in patients with testicular tumors: Conversion to negative with testosterone administration. *J Urol* 1979; **122**:126–8.
89. Stenman UH, Alfthan H, Hotakainen K. Human chorionic gonadotropin in cancer. *Clin Biochem* 2004; **37**:549–61.
90. Sturgeon CM, Duffy MJ, Stenman UH, *et al.* National academy of clinical biochemistry laboratory medicine practice guidelines for use of tumor markers in testicular, prostate, colorectal, breast, and ovarian cancers. *Clin Chem* 2008; **54**:e11–79.
91. De Broe ME, Pollet DE. Multicenter evaluation of human placental alkaline phosphatase as a possible tumor-associated antigen in serum. *Clin Chem* 1988; **34**:1995–9.
92. Kuzmits R, Schernthaner G, Krisch K. Serum neuron-specific enolase. A marker for responses to therapy in seminoma. *Cancer* 1987; **60**:1017–21.
93. Fossa SD, Klepp O, Paus E. Neuron-specific enolase--a serum tumour marker in seminoma? *Br J Cancer* 1992; **65**:297–9.
94. Heidenreich A, Weissbach L, Höltl W, *et al.* Organ sparing surgery for malignant germ cell tumor of the testis. *J Urol* 2001; **166**:2161–5.
95. Heidenreich A, Höltl W, Albrecht W, Pont J, Engelmann UH. Testis-preserving surgery in bilateral testicular germ cell tumours. *Br J Urol* 1997; **79**:253–7.
96. von der Maase H, Rorth M, Walbom-Jorgensen S, *et al.* Carcinoma in situ of contralateral testis in patients with testicular germ cell cancer: Study of 27 cases in 500 patients. *Br Med J* 1986; **293**:1398–401.
97. Harland SJ, Cook PA, Fossa SD, *et al.* Intratubular germ cell neoplasia of the contralateral testis in testicular cancer: Defining a high risk group. *J Urol* 1998; **160**:1353–7.
98. Dieckmann KP, Loy V. Prevalence of contralateral testicular intraepithelial neoplasia in patients with testicular germ cell neoplasms. *J Clin Oncol* 1996; **14**:3126–32.
99. Tandstad TS, Solberg A, Hakansson U, *et al.* Bilateral testicular cancer within two prospective, population-based swenoteca protocols in clinical stage i nonseminoma. *J Clin Oncol* 2012; **30**(15):Abstract 4508.
100. De Santis M, Becherer A, Bokemeyer C, *et al.* 2-18fluoro-deoxy-d-glucose positron emission tomography is a reliable predictor for viable tumor in postchemotherapy seminoma: An update of the prospective multicentric sempet trial. *J Clin Oncol* 2004; **22**:1034–9.
101. Krege S, Beyer J, Souchon R, *et al.* European consensus conference on diagnosis and treatment of germ cell cancer: A report of the second meeting of the european germ cell cancer consensus group (egcccg): Part I. *Eur Urol* 2008; **53**:478–96.
102. Krege S, Beyer J, Souchon R, *et al.* European consensus conference on diagnosis and treatment of germ cell cancer: A report of the second meeting of the european germ cell cancer consensus group (egcccg): Part II. *Eur Urol* 2008; **53**:497–513.

CHAPTER 6.34

Pathology of testicular tumours

John Goepel

Introduction to pathology of testicular tumours

Though testis tumours are rare, they are the most frequent malignant tumour of young adults comprising 27% of cancers in males 15 to 24 years, and have the highest cure rates of all male malignancies with 96% five-year survival.[1] So a correct prompt diagnosis and management has potential huge benefits. The contribution of urological surgeons may involve initial diagnosis, orchidectomy to remove the primary tumour, and sometimes the resection of residual nodal masses after chemotherapy. These comments apply to germ cell tumours (seminoma and teratoma), which constitute the great majority of testis tumours, but there are several other tumours that can occur.

Germ cell tumours

Germ cell tumours comprise 95% of all testis tumours. They arise from spermatogonia within the seminiferous tubules, and may mimic their normal counterparts in differentiating into a wide variety of embryonic or extra-embryonic tissues. This results in a bewildering variety of histological patterns and descriptive categories that may be helpful to pathologists in their diagnosis, but can be confusing for clinical staff particularly when there are no differences in therapy or outcome. The matter is further confused by the use of the same word 'teratoma' to have a somewhat different meaning in the British and WHO classifications, as will be explained later. The term germ cell tumour will be used to cover the two broad categories of seminoma and non-seminoma.

Incidence of germ cell tumours and risk factors

The incidence varies considerably between countries, being highest in Western Europe (7.8 per 100,000) and lowest in Western Africa (0.2). In Western Europe it has doubled over the last three decades, though may have stopped rising, and is currently 7 per 100,000 males in the United Kingdom.[2,3] Testicular maldescent is a recognized risk factor, though there is still debate as to whether, or to what extent, it is causative, or a reflection of a common risk pathway, as corrective surgery does not abrogate the risk completely. In subjects with unilateral cryporchidism undergoing orchidopexy before the age of about 10 to 12 years there is a continuing relative risk of about 2 to 3 for a germ cell tumour. Delaying orchidopexy until after this age or not operating confers a relative risk of about 6.[4,5] Hypospadias similarly confers an increased risk of a tumour, slightly less than cryptorchidism, but these risk factors do not seem to be familial traits.[6] The other established risk factors are a contralateral testis tumour, relative risk 25, and a family history, relative risk 3 to 10.[7,8]

Men with infertility have the precursor lesion intratubular germ cell neoplasia, unclassified (IGCNU) in up to 1% of cases,[9] but incidental abnormalities on ultrasound are generally benign, such as scars or Leydig cell lesions.[10]

Germ cell tumours are predominantly diseases of young adult males, with a peak incidence for non-seminoma in the third decade and for seminoma in the fourth decade, with relatively fewer in later life. Germ cell tumours in infancy are discussed later: there are no germ cell tumours in the rest of childhood.

Pathogenesis

The neoplastic changes arise *in utero* in primordial germ cells before migration into the testis (or aberrant migration to thymus or pineal) where they occupy the germ cell niche. The tumour cells abnormally retain transcription factors for totipotent development, with aberrant expression of OCT3/4 (POU5F1) and NANOG as well as expressing placental alkaline phosphatase (PLAP) similar to primordial germ cells. After puberty there is expansion of this clone of abnormal germ cells, initially basally situated but later filling the seminiferous tubule with cells with abundant clear cytoplasm and an enlarged nucleus, referred to as carcinoma *in situ* or IGCNU, with expression of OCT3/4, NANOG, PLAP, and c-Kit (CD117). This situation can persist for many years, but the acquisition of extra copies of chromosome 12p, typically paired as isochromosomes i12p, confers an invasive phenotype and the establishment of the germ cell tumour.[11–13] Seminomas continue to express this phenotype, whereas embryonal carcinoma additionally expresses SOX2 as seen in their embryonal stem cell counterparts. Embryonal carcinoma expresses CD30, and this can be demonstrated in some morphological IGCNU, suggesting differentiation to intratubular embryonal carcinoma.[14] The other patterns of germ cell tumour described below reflect the pluripotent precursors, with embryonic and extra-embryonic differentiation options.

The risk of progression from IGCNU to cancer is approximately 50% in five years, rising to 70% at seven years.[11] The contralateral testis to the one with a tumour has a 5% risk of harbouring IGCNU, but the morbidity for treating it is such that it may not be advisable to undertake a biopsy.[15]

Clinical presentation

A scrotal swelling, generally but not always painless, will be the presentation in 90% of patients with testicular germ cell tumours[16]; though often large enough to be confidently recognized as a mass in the testis, there are also many patients who benefit from ultrasound examination of the testis to identify the location and character of a more subtle mass. However, with incidental testicular ultrasound alterations 80% are benign, so a conservative approach is appropriate in this scenario.[17] Biopsy of testis lesions is regarded as scrotal violation, and alleged to lead to a poorer outcome, but this has been challenged and may be preferable to intraoperative frozen section.[18]

The remainder of patients present with metastatic spread. Para-aortic node deposits may cause backache, while a supraclavicular node may be visible. Pulmonary metastases may be so extensive as to cause dyspnoea, and with choriocarcinoma (malignant teratoma trophoblastic) they may cause haemoptysis; this particularly aggressive variant also is more likely to result in brain or visceral deposits liable to haemorrhage and rupture. Sometimes the testis primary will be tiny or regressed, though IGCNU may still be detectable.[19]

Germ cell tumours may also be primary at extragonadal sites in 2 to 10% of cases,[19,20] particularly the retroperitoneum and mediastinum, but also the brain. This is said to be a consequence of incomplete or aberrant migration of primordial germ cells from the yolk sac to the genital ridge during embryonic development. However, before accepting an extragonadal origin a testis primary tumour must be carefully excluded. In general, extragonadal germ cell tumours carry a poorer prognosis, particularly non-seminomas.[21]

Sometimes ultrasound examination of the testis shows microlithiasis. It is common to observe rounded calcified bodies within seminiferous tubules in the vicinity of germ cell tumours or IGCNU, so finding microlithiasis should prompt a careful evaluation of the testis. But if no tumour is found there is no proven benefit in an extended period of repeated examinations in anticipation of early detection of a tumour.[22]

Classification of germ cell tumours

Taken as a whole, germ cell tumours have been divided into five groups,[11] three of which arise in the testis. Type I is tumours in neonates and infants, and type III is spermatocytic seminoma: these are discussed later. Type II is the tumours of adults which fall into two broad categories of seminoma and non-seminoma. Categorization of non-seminomas has been contentious, with the British Testicular Tumour Panel (BTTP)[20] describing them all as malignant teratomas and then subdividing them according to the patterns of differentiation observed. In contrast, the WHO[23] restricts the term teratoma to those tumours that have somatic differentiation such as resemblance to neural tissue, adipose tissue, or intestine. In other words, a teratoma shows the capacity to differentiate along the three lineages of ectoderm, mesoderm, and endoderm. The WHO then applies other terms to the other patterns of differentiation described below, and describes tumours as mixed when there is more than one pattern. Despite the inelegance of grouping tumours by what they are not, the BTTP system has not been kept up to date, so the WHO system is to be preferred. Comparison between BTTP and WHO designations is shown in Table 6.34.1.

Seminoma

Approximately half of all testis germ cell tumours are seminoma without other patterns of tumour.[19] They do not occur before puberty, and are uncommon before the third decade, reaching a peak in the fourth decade with further cases throughout adult life. The macroscopic appearance is of a uniform pale mass, which may have necrosis in larger tumours, and there may be multiple

Table 6.34.1 Types of germ cell tumour arising is testis, adapted from Oosterhuis and Looijenga

Type	Phenotype	Age	Genotype
I	Teratoma Yolk sac tumour	Neonates and children	Diploid (teratoma) Aneuploid (yolk sac tumour) Gain of 1q, 12(p13) and 20q Loss of 1p, 4, 6q
II	Seminoma Non-seminoma	>15 years	Aneuploid (+/- triploid) Gain of X, 7, 8, 12p, 21 Loss of Y, 1p, 11, 13, 18
III	Spermatocytic seminoma	>50 years	Aneuploid Gain of 9

Adapted by permission from Macmillan Publishers Ltd: *Nature Reviews Cancer*, Volume 5, Issue 3, J. Wolter Oosterhuis and Leendert H. J. Looijenga, 'Testicular germ-cell tumours in a broader perspective', pp. 210–22, Copyright © 2005.

separate nodules corresponding to multiple foci of invasion from the precursor IGCNU. Spread within the testis results in invasion of the rete testis, the network of tubules connecting the seminiferous tubules to the epididymis. This interstitial rete invasion seems to correlate with an increased risk of dissemination.[24]

Microscopy shows a relatively uniform cell type with moderately abundant clear cytoplasm containing glycogen, and an open nucleus with readily visible nucleolus. The cells are generally not arranged in any particular pattern and lack cohesion though some variants are described.[23] The stroma usually contains lymphocytes, which can be very abundant (Fig. 6.34.1). There may also be epithelioid histiocytes, and some cases are so floridly granulomatous that the seminoma can be obscured, giving a challenging differential diagnosis between a granulomatous seminoma and granulomatous orchitis. Seminoma cells are positive for the same markers as their intratubular precusor, OCT3/4, CD117 and PLAP, and are generally negative for cytokeratins though focal staining can be seen. Immunohistochemistry is rarely required to make the diagnosis in a testis tumour, but can be valuable if the sample comes from a distant lymph node or extragonadal tumour. About 7% of seminomas have recognizable syncytiotrophoblast cells scattered singly within them (in occasional tumours they are quite numerous) and these tumours have elevated serum human chorionic gonadotrophin (hCG). This variant, seminoma with syncytiotrophoblast cells, does not differ in clinical behaviour from classical seminoma.

Following growth within the testis, seminoma will typically give rise to lymph node metastasis in para-aortic nodes. Sometimes lympho-vascular invasion can be seen in peritumoural or more distant vessels, and this correlates with increased risk of nodal disease.[24] Nodal disease can extend to supraclavicular fossa, but vascular dissemination to the lungs or elsewhere is very uncommon. With the exception of those cases secreting hCG, there is no available tumour marker for seminoma.

Teratoma

Used in the narrower WHO sense, this is a tumour with somatic differentiated elements.[23] The macroscopic appearance is mixed solid and cystic. There are often cysts resembling gut or bronchus with a range of squamous or glandular epithelial patterns of differentiation. Smooth muscle may encircle these structures, and there may

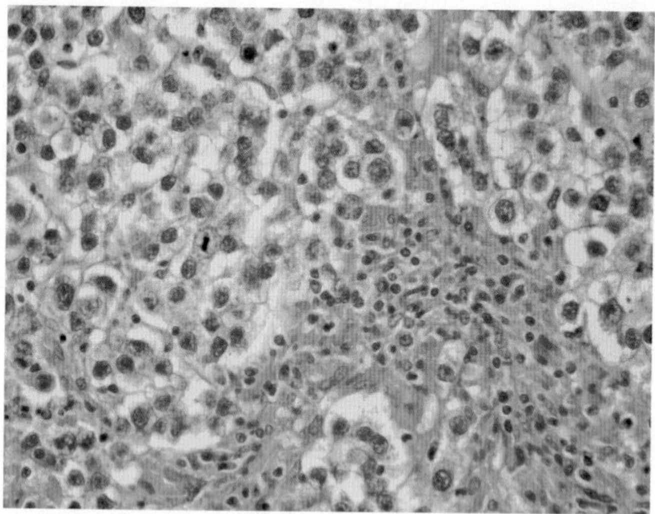

Fig. 6.34.1 Seminoma histology.

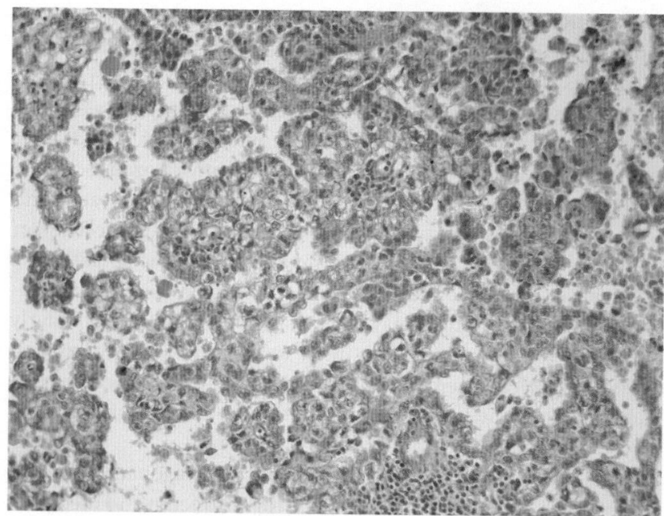

Fig. 6.34.3 Embryonal carcinoma histology.

be islands of cartilage, adipose tissue, or neural tissue (Fig. 6.34.2). Although representation of all three germ cell layers is usual, some teratomas are more restricted in their range of differentiation. Pure teratoma is only 2–4% of adult testis tumours.[16,19]

In up to 6% of teratomas there is development of a somatic malignancy, carcinoma or more often sarcoma, and these tumours have a more aggressive course.[25]

Embryonal carcinoma

Embryonal carcinoma (EC) tumour resembles a poorly differentiated adenocarcinoma. There are different possible architectural patterns, with a tubulo-papillary configuration often seen (Fig. 6.34.3). Necrosis is common. The cells are more cohesive than seminoma, and more dysplastic, but confusion is possible. Immunohistochemistry shows a positive reaction for OCT3/4 and sometimes PLAP, but unlike seminoma SOX2 expression signifies the next step of differentiation with resemblance to embryonal stem cells,[13] and cytokeratins and CD30 are also positive. Scattered syncytiotrophoblast cells may be present.

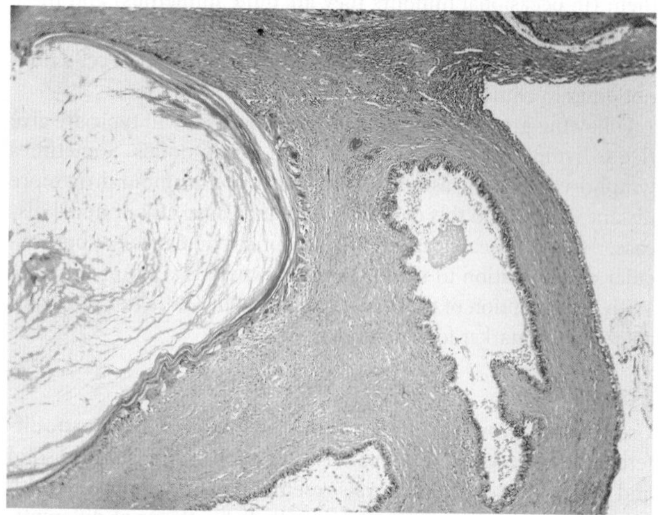

Fig. 6.34.2 Teratoma histology.

Yolk sac tumour

Many different histological patterns are possible within this designation, and there is ongoing debate about the suitability of the term. The patterns seen most often are cystic formations with a lining of attenuated or cuboidal epithelium, sometimes arranged around a central vascular core (a Schiller-Duval body), or loose blastema. The epithelial cells secrete, and stain positive for alpha fetoprotein (AFP), which is valuable as a tumour marker as well as histological diagnosis, particularly as yolk sack tumour (YST) is negative for OCT3/4 staining.

As regards invasion and dissemination, EC and YST behave in the same way. There is local invasion in the testis with eventual spread into adjacent tissues; invasion of peritumoural vessels is an important indicator of increased risk of dissemination, and features in the TNM staging system, as well as frequently influencing decisions about adjuvant treatment. Lymphatic spread is to the para-aortic nodes, and vascular metastasis is common to the lungs.

Choriocarcinoma

This variant of germ cell tumour is histologically similar to the gestational tumour though clearly has a very different origin. Aggregates of atypical cytotrophoblast cells lie juxtaposed with atypical syncytiotrophoblast cells lying over their free border in a bilaminar manner reminiscent of chorionic villi. Vascular invasion is usual, and the tumours are generally haemorrhagic, sometimes to the extent that it appears to be a haematoma and a careful search is needed to find viable tumour cells. Vascular invasion also often results in extensive metastatic spread not only to the lungs but also the brain, liver, or other sites, where it may present with haemorrhage, and serum hCG levels may be extremely elevated.

Very rarely there are other primary testicular trophoblastic tumours such as placental site trophoblastic tumour, which is composed of extra-villous trophoblast cells.[26]

Mixed germ cell tumour

Non-seminomatous tumours of one histological type are rare, and between one-third and one-half of all germ cell tumours of the testis have more than one histological pattern; all combinations

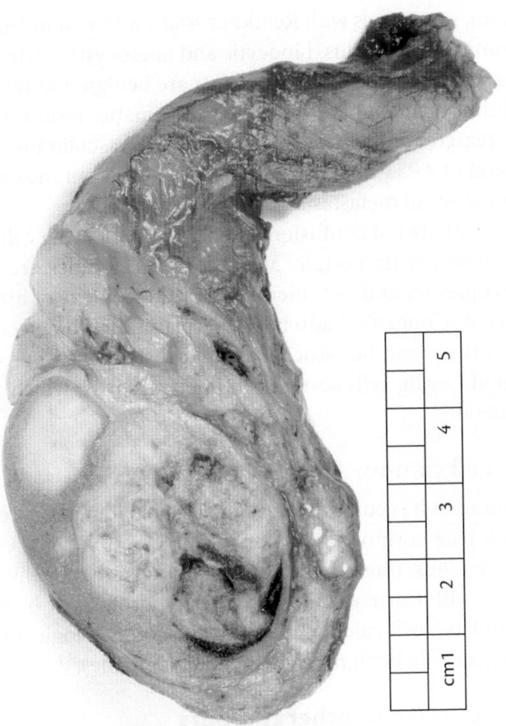

Fig. 6.34.4 Mixed germ cell tumour. The pale nodule in the upper pole is typical of seminoma, while the variegated larger mass is non-seminoma.

are possible (Fig. 6.34.4). The descriptor mixed germ cell tumour should then be followed by a listing of the components present. In the BTTP classification the presence of a separate mass of seminoma along with any variety of non-seminoma is referred to as a combined tumour, followed by an indication as to what components are present; microscopic foci of seminoma do not affect the category (Table 6.34.2).

Table 6.34.2 Comparison of WHO and BTTP systems for classifying germ cell tumours

WHO term	BTTP term
Seminoma (S)	Seminoma (S)
Teratoma (T)	Teratoma differentiated (TD)
Embryonal carcinoma (EC)	Malignant teratoma undifferentiated (MTU)
Yolk sac tumour (YST)	Malignant teratoma undifferentiated (MTU)
Choriocarcinoma (chorio)	Malignant teratoma trophoblastic (MTT)
Mixed germ cell tumour T and any EC or YST	Malignant teratoma intermediate (MTI)
Mixed germ cell tumour Chorio in any combination	Malignant teratoma trophoblastic (MTT)

BTTP reproduced with permission from Collins DH and Pugh RCB, 'Classification and frequency of testicular cancer', *British Journal of Urology*, Volume 36, Supplement 1, pp. 1-11, Copyright © 1964 John Wiley and Sons. Source: WHO data in table compiled from Eble, JN, Sauter, G, Epstein JI and Sesterhenn IA, *World Health Organization Classification of Tumours: Pathology and Genetics of Tumours of the Urinary System and Male Genital Organ*, Volume 7, IARC, Lyon, Copyright © 2004.

Germ cell tumours in the infant testis

Neonates and infants have germ cell tumours type I, rather than the adult Type II.[11] These are not confined to the testis, indeed the sacral region is the most frequent. Their molecular pathology is quite different with different chromosomal abnormalities. Morphologically they are either teratomas or yolk sac tumours, with a benign or malignant behaviour, respectively.

Staging testicular tumours

The TNM system for testis tumours,[27] has the usual subdivisions to indicate the extent of tumour locally, node involvement, and metastatic spread, with the difference that peritumoural lymphovascular invasion defines the difference between pT1 and pT2. There is an additional S category, to indicate the degree of elevation of serum tumour markers. This is taken into account when deriving the TNM stage group from the T, N, M, and S information.

The Royal Marsden Hospital (RMH) staging system[28] (Table 6.34.3) is widely used by oncologists. This recognizes four stages according to the extent of spread and volume of disease, and also takes account of tumour marker elevation.

Another clinical staging and prognostic system for guiding treatment options is that of the International Germ Cell Cancer Collaborative Group (IGCCCG).[29]

Outline of clinical management

Orchidectomy is the usual initial treatment and for RMH stage 1 is often followed by surveillance. Tumours with a high risk of metastatic spread or proven metastasis are offered chemotherapy. Management is greatly aided by the availability of tumour markers. Lactate dehydrogenase (LDH) is a generic tumour marker, while AFP and hCG are sufficiently specific to be invaluable in monitoring tumour burden

Table 6.34.3 Royal Marsden Hospital staging system for testicular tumours—the full system also includes designation of the sites of metastatic disease

Royal Marsden Hospital staging system, extract	
Stage 1 1 M	No evidence of metastasis No evidence of metastasis, but rising serum marker
Stage 2 A 2 B 2 C	Abdominal nodes up to 2 cm diameter From 2 to 5 cm Over 5 cm
Stage 3	Supradiaphragmatic node metastasis
Stage 4	Extranodal metastasis (lung, liver brain, etc)
Lung metastasis	
L1	Fewer than three metastases
L2	3 or more metastases, up to 2 cm
L3	3 or more metastases, one over 2 cm

Reprinted from *The Lancet*, Volume 325, Issue 8419, 'Prognostic factors in advanced non-seminomatous germ-cell testicular tumours: Results of multicentre study. Report from the Medical Research Council Working Party on Testicular Tumours', pp. 8–11, Copyright © 1985, with permission from Elsevier, http://www.sciencedirect.com/science/journal/01406736

Cure rates are very high, even for presentation with metastatic disease, and range from 90% down to 50% depending on the amount of tumour. Overall cures exceed 90% for seminoma and is 99% for RMH stage 1.[19] The marked sensitivity to chemotherapy is a consequence of its unusual molecular biology.[13]

Residual masses after chemotherapy

If there is a residual mass after chemotherapy, for example retroperitoneal, with no raised tumour marker then there are several possible explanations, and it is usual to proceed to surgical resection. There are four common outcomes: necrotic tumour with none viable, fibrosis only, differentiated teratoma only, or viable other tumour types (EC or YST usually).[19] Much less often there is a new somatic tumour arisen from the teratoma, such as sarcoma or adenocarcinoma.

Spermatocytic seminoma

This is an uncommon testicular tumour, generally in older men, and is a germ cell tumour type III.[11] It has a distinctive molecular biology, with chromosome 9 changes seen most often. The histology is characterized by spermatocyte-like cells, hyperchromatic small cells, and scattered giant cells, often mononuclear; the stroma may be oedematous and lacks a lymphocytic infiltrate. IGCNU is not seen. The differential diagnosis is from seminoma and lymphoma; spermatocytic seminoma is positive for SSX, XPA and MAGE-A4, and lacks expression of OCT3/4 and PLAP.[11,30] The usual spermatocytic seminoma is benign, so orchidectomy is curative. A rare malignant variant has a sarcoma developing from within the tumour.

Lymphoma

Lymphoma of the testis is about 4% of tumours, and tends to arise in older men. Diffuse large B-cell lymphoma is the particular variety seen most often, characterized by large lymphoid cells positive for CD20. Diffuse infiltration of the testis gives a destructive mass, though frequently some seminiferous tubules remain surrounded by tumour. This is an aggressive lymphoma, and though some cases are confined to the testis, it is common for the tumour to have spread locally or widely. The usual treatment is to offer multidrug chemotherapy. As the disease runs its course, testis lymphoma seems to have a particular predilection for recurrence in the central nervous system, even if CNS prophylactic treatment has been attempted.[31]

The testis is also a potential site of recurrence of lymphoblastic leukaemias.

Sex cord stromal tumours

Less frequent than germ cell tumours, these arise from other specialized tissue within the testis; similar tumours are seen in the ovary.

Leydig cell tumour

These tumours comprise 1% of all testis tumours and may occur at any age including children. Children may have isosexual precocious puberty, and adults may have gynaecomastia. The tumour forms a rounded mass within the body of the testis, characteristically yellow or tan, and the cells have moderately abundant eosinophilic cytoplasm, sometimes with Reinke crystals, with a rounded nucleus and prominent nucleolus. Lipocytic and microcystic variants occur

At least 90% of Leydig cell tumours are benign, but histological recognition of malignancy can be problematic. Features such as size, increased mitotic activity, Ki67 fraction, vascular invasion and expression of *TP53* correlate with malignancy,[32] but the only proof is the presence of metastasis.

A different area of confusion is separation of Leydig cell tumour from a hyperplastic nodule. Multiple small nodules are unlikely to be neoplastic, and are often seen in the context of atrophy in maldescent. Congenital adrenal hyperplasia due to defective hormone synthesis can be associated with substantial and progressive nodules of Leydig cells several centimetres across; which are usually bilateral.[33]

Sertoli cell tumour

A rare tumour, it is composed of tubules or solid nests of columnar cells with pale eosinophilic cytoplasm like Sertoli cells. Usually a tumour of adults, those presenting in children are more likely to be associated with Carney or Peutz-Jegher syndromes, or be bilateral. There are large cell calcifying and sclerosing histological variants. Though generally benign, there are malignant ones.[34]

Granulosa cell and other tumours

Other types of sex cord stromal tumours such as granulosa cell tumour are occasionally recorded in the testis.[35] Juvenile granulosa cell tumours may be congenital or in neonates.[36]

Other tumours, benign and malignant

There are several other uncommon tumours particularly seen in or around the testis, as well as tumours that can be found at any location, such as sarcoma.

Epidermoid cyst

This is a firm round mass with a wall lined by keratinizing squamous epithelium without dysplasia or adnexa, and lamellated keratin filling the cavity. Ultrasound typically has regular concentric echoes in a unilocular cyst, but neither this nor MRI are completely sensitive and specific.[37] This is a benign lesion that can be managed by local resection. It is quite distinct from teratoma, and there is no associated IGCNU.

Adenomatoid tumour

Most often arising in relation to the head of the epididymis, this is a pale somewhat ill defined and slightly infiltrative mass. It is composed of anastomosing tubules and cysts of mesothelial cells.[38] Despite the capacity to infiltrate into the testis, this is a benign neoplasm and simple excision is curative.

Carcinoid tumour

Carcinoid tumours may arise in children or adults, only sometimes with a teratoma component too. Most are benign but some progress to carcinoid syndrome.[39,40]

Malignant mesothelioma of tunica vaginalis

This tumour gives a hydrocele and mass lesion around the testis, but is rarely diagnosed preoperatively. Asbestos exposure may have occurred, but some patients are young. Survival is poor, particularly after local recurrence.[41,42]

Müllerian tumour of borderline malignancy

The appendix of the testis is a Müllerian remnant, and so these rare tumours may be derived from it. They present with persistent or recurrent hydrocele, and progress to a mass surrounding and subsequently invading the testis.[43]

Papillary cystadenoma of epididymis

An uncommon tumour, it has a strong association with von Hipple-Lindau disease, and in this context may be bilateral.[44]

Paratesticular rhabdomyosarcoma

This is a distinctive neoplasm of children and young adults, presenting as a mass adjacent to or surrounding the testis. The spindle cell variant embryonal rhabdomyosarcoma is the most frequent type. Metastasis may occur to para-aortic lymph nodes. Localized disease has a very good outcome.[45,46]

Liposarcoma of spermatic cord

Adipocytic tumours of the cord need to be viewed with some caution. The tissue derives from the retroperitoneum, and the tumours reflect this. Many of tumours will be well differentiated liposarcoma, sometimes with only minimal or focal cytological atypia. There is then the risk of evolution to a dedifferentiated liposarcoma.[47] One of the surgical problems is defining the limits of the well differentiated component, due to its resemblance to normal adipose tissue.

Further reading

Cancer Registration Statistics England, 2010. Available at: http://www.ons.gov.uk/ons/rel/vsob1/cancer-statistics-registrations—england—series-mb1-/no—41—2010/rft-cancer-registrations-2010.xls [Online].

Horwich A, Shipley J, Huddart R. Testicular germ-cell cancer. *Lancet* 2006; **367**(9512):754–65.

Oosterhuis J, Looijenga L. Testicular germ-cell tmours in a broader perspective. *Nat Rev Cancer* 2005; **5**:210–22.

Wood HM, Elder JS. Cryptorchidism and testicular cancer: separating fact from fiction. *J Urol* 2009; **181**:452–61.

Woodward PJ, Heidenreich A, Looijenga LHJ, Oosterhuis JW, McLeod DG, Møller H. Testicular germ cell tumors. (pp. 217–78) In: Eble JN, Sauter G, Epstein JI, Sesterhann IA (eds). *World Health Organization Classification of Tumours: Pathology and Genetics of the Urinary System and Male Genital Organs*. Lyon, France: IARC Press, 2004.

References

1. ONS Cancer Statistics, 2010. Available at: http://www.ons.gov.uk/ons/rel/vsob1/cancer-statistics-registrations--england--series-mb1-/no--41--2010/rft-cancer-registrations-2010.xls [Online].
2. The Globocan project, 2012. Available at: http://globocan.iarc.fr/ [Online].
3. Bray F, Richiardi L, Ekbom A, Pukkala E, Cuninkova M, Møller H. Trends in testicular cancer incidence and mortality in 22 European countries: continuing increases in incidence and declines in mortality. *Int J Cancer* 2006; **118**:3099–111.
4. Walsh TJ, Dall'Era MA, Croughan MS, Carroll PR, Turek PJ. Prepubertal orchiopexy for cryptorchidism may be associated with lower risk of testicular cancer. *J Urol* 2007; **178**:1440–6.
5. Wood HM, Elder JS. Cryptorchidism and testicular cancer: separating fact from fiction. *J Urol* 2009; **181**:452–61.
6. Schnack TH, Poulsen G, Myrup C, Wohlfahrt J, Melbye M. Familial coaggregation of cryptorchidism, hypospadias, and testicular germ cell cancer: a nationwide cohort study. *J Natl Cancer Inst* 2010; **102**:187–92.
7. Dieckmann KP, Pichlmeier U. Clinical epidemiology of testicular germ cell tumors. *World J Urol* 2004; **22**:2–14.
8. Nicholson PW, Harland SJ. Inheritance and testicular cancer. *Br J Cancer* 1995; **71**:421–6.
9. Dieckmann KP, Skakkebaek NE. Carcinoma in situ of the testis: review of biological and clinical features. *Int J Cancer* 1999; **83**:815–22.
10. Eifler JB Jr, King P, Schlegel PN. Incidental testicular lesions found during infertility evaluation are usually benign and may be managed conservatively. *J Urol* 2008; **180**:261–4.
11. Oosterhuis J, Looijenga L. Testicular germ-cell tmours in a broader perspective. *Nat Rev Cancer* 2005; **5**:210–22.
12. Looijenga LH, Gillis AJ, Stoop HJ, Hersmus R, Oosterhuis JW. Chromosomes and expression in human testicular germ-cell tumors: insight into their cell of origin and pathogenesis. *Ann N Y Acad Sci* 2007; **1120**:187–214.
13. Looijenga LHJ, Gillis AJM, Stoop H, Biermann K, Oosterhuis JW. Dissecting the molecular pathways of (testicular) germ cell tumour pathogenesis; from initiation to treatment- resistance. *Int J Androl* 2011; **34**:e2–e6.
14. Berney DM, Lee A, Randle SJ, Jordan S, Shamash J, Oliver RT. The frequency of intratubular embryonal carcinoma: implications for the pathogenesis of germ cell tumours. *Histopathology* 2004; **45**:155–61.
15. Heidenreich A. Contralateral testicular biopsy in testis cancer: current concepts and controversies. *BJU Int* 2009; **104**:1346–50.
16. Germa-Lluch JR, Garcia del Muro X, Maroto P, *et al.* Clinical pattern and therapeutic results achieved in 1490 patients with germ-cell tumours of the testis: the experience of the Spanish Germ-Cell Cancer Group (GG). *Eur Urol* 2002; **42**:553–62.
17. Carmignani L, Gadda F, Gazzano G, *et al.* High incidence of benign testicular neoplasms diagnosed by ultrasound. *J Urol* 2003; **170**:1783–6.
18. Soh E, Berman LH, Grant JW, Bullock N, Williams MV. Ultrasound-guided core-needle biopsy of the testis for focal indeterminate intratesticular lesions. *Eur Radiol* 2008; **18**:2990–6.
19. Horwich A, Shipley J, Huddart R. Testicular germ-cell cancer. *Lancet* 2006; **367**(9512):754–65.
20. Collins DH, Pugh RCB. Classification and frequency of testicular cancer. *Br J Urol* 1964; **36**:Suppl 1–11.
21. Bokemeyer C, Nichols C, Droz JP. Extragonadal germ cell tumors of the mediastinum and the retroperitoneum: results from an international analysis. *J Clin Oncol* 2002; **20**:1864–73.
22. Shanmugasundaram R, Singh JC, Kekre NS. Testicular microlithiasis: Is there an agreed protocol? *Indian J Urol* 2007; **23**:234–9.
23. Woodward PJ, Heidenreich A, Looijenga LHJ, Oosterhuis JW, McLeod DG, Møller H. Testicular germ cell tumors. (pp. 217–78) In: Eble JN, Sauter G, Epstein JI, Sesterhann IA (eds). *World Health Organization Classification of Tumours: Pathology and Genetics of the Urinary System and Male Genital Organs*. Lyon, France: IARC Press, 2004.
24. Valdevenito JP, Gallegos I, Fernandez C, Acevedo C, Palma R. Correlation between primary tumor pathologic features and presence of clinical metastasis at diagnosis of testicular seminoma. *Urology* 2007; **70**:777–80.
25. Comiter CV, Kibel AS, Richie JP, Nucci MR, Renshaw AA. Prognostic features of teratomas with malignant transformation: a clinicopathological study of 21 cases. *J Urol* 1998; **159**:859–63.
26. Ulbright TM, Young RH, Scully RE. Trophoblastic tumors of the testis other than classic choriocarcinoma: "monophasic" choriocarcinoma and placental site trophoblastic tumor: a report of two cases. *Am J Surg Pathol* 1997; **21**:282–8.
27. Sobin LH, Gospodarowicz MK, Wittekind CH. *TNM Classification of Malignant Tumours*, 7th edition. Oxford, UK: Wiley-Blackwell, 2009.
28. [No authors listed]. Prognostic factors in advanced non-seminomatous germ-cell testicular tumours: results of multicentre study. Report from the Medical Research Council Working Party on Testicular Tumours. *Lancet* 1985; **1**:8–11.

29. {No authors listed]. International Germ-Cell Cancer Collaborative Group (IGCCCG). A prognostic factor-based staging system for metastatic germ cell cancers. *J Clin Oncol* 1997; **87**:293–8.
30. Rajpert-De Meyts E, Jacobsen GK, Bartkova J, *et al.* The immunohistochemical expression pattern of Chk2, p53, p19INK4d, MAGE-A4 and other selected antigens provides new evidence for the premeiotic origin of spermatocytic seminoma. *Histopathology* 2003; **42**:217–26.
31. Guirguis HR, Cheung MC, Mahrous M, *et al.* Impact of central nervous system (CNS) prophylaxis on the incidence and risk factors for CNS relapse in patients with diffuse large B-cell lymphoma treated in the rituximab era: a single centre experience and review of the literature. *Br J Haematol* 2012; **159**:39–49.
32. McCluggage WG, Shanks JH, Arthur K, Banerjee SS. Cellular proliferation and nuclear ploidy assessments augment established prognostic factors in predicting malignancy in testicular Leydig cell tumours. *Histopathology* 1998; **33**:361–8.
33. Rutgers JL, Young RH, Scully RE. The testicular "tumor" of the adrenogenital syndrome. A report of six cases and review of the literature on testicular masses in patients with adrenocortical disorders. *Am J Surg Pathol* 1988; **12**:503–13.
34. Plata C, Algaba F, Andujar M, *et al.* Large cell calcifying Sertoli cell tumour of the testis. *Histopathology* 1995; **26**:255–9.
35. Hanson JA, Ambaye AB. Adult testicular granulosa cell tumor: a review of the literature for clinicopathologic predictors of malignancy. *Arch Pathol Lab Med* 2011; **135**:143–6.
36. Harms D, Kock LR. Testicular juvenile granulosa cell and Sertoli cell tumours: a clinicopathological study of 29 cases from the Kiel Paediatric Tumour Registry. *Virchows Archiv* 1997; **430**:301–9.
37. Ozturk M, Mavili E, Erdogan N, Demirci D. Epidermoid cyst of the testicle: unusual magnetic resonance imaging findings. *Acta Radiologica* 2004; **45**:882–4.
38. Delahunt B, Eble JN, King D, Bethwaite PB, Nacey JN, Thornton A. Immunohistochemical evidence for mesothelial origin of paratesticular adenomatoid tumour. *Histopathology* 2000; **36**:109–15.
39. Abbosh PH, Zhang S, Maclennan GT, *et al.* Germ cell origin of testicular carcinoid tumors. *Clin Cancer Res* 2008; **14**:1393–6.
40. Wang WP, Guo C, Berney DM, *et al.* Primary carcinoid tumors of the testis: a clinicopathologic study of 29 cases. *Am J Surg Pathol* 2010; **34**:519–24.
41. Chekol SS, Sun CC. Malignant mesothelioma of the tunica vaginalis testis: diagnostic studies and differential diagnosis. *Arch Pathol Lab Med* 2012; **136**:113–7.
42. Plas E, Riedl CR, Pfluger H. Malignant mesothelioma of the tunica vaginalis testis: review of the literature and assessment of prognostic parameters. *Cancer* 1998; **83**:2437–46.
43. De Nictolis M, Tommasoni S, Fabris G, Prat J. Intratesticular serous cystadenoma of borderline malignancy. A pathological, histochemical and DNA content study of a case with long-term follow-up. *Virchows Arch A Pathol Anat Histopathol* 1993; **423**:221–5.
44. Odrzywolski KJ, Mukhopadhyay S. Papillary cystadenoma of the epididymis. *Arch Pathol Lab Med* 2010; **134**:630–3.
45. Keskin S, Ekenel M, Basaran M, Kilicaslan I, Tunc M, Bavbek S. Clinicopathological characteristics and treatment outcomes of adult patients with paratesticular rhabdomyosarcoma (PRMS): A 10-year single-centre experience. *Can Urol Assoc J* 2012; **6**:42–5.
46. Reeves HM, MacLennan GT. Paratesticular Rhabdomyosarcoma. *J Urol* 2009; **182**:1578–9.
47. Schwartz SL, Swierzewski SJ 3rd, Sondak VK, Grossman HB. Liposarcoma of the spermatic cord: report of 6 cases and review of the literature. J Urol 1995; **153**:154–7.

CHAPTER 6.35

Testis cancer

Treatment

Axel Heidenreich

Therapeutic concept

Inguinal orchiectomy remains the initial step in treatment prior to any other systemic cytotoxic or radio-oncological therapy. Only in cases where chemotherapy needs to be initiated due to life threatening symptoms of extensive metastatic disease *and* in whom the diagnosis of a germ cell tumour is without doubt can inguinal orchiectomy be delayed.[1–3]

Inguinal orchiectomy is not an emergency procedure and can be safely performed as an elective operation. Patients should be given time for semen cryopreservation (especially those with a solitary testicle, bilateral tumours, or even if they wish to in the presence of an apparently normal contralateral testis). A treatment delay of 2 to 3 weeks does not result in an impairment of the prognosis.[1–3] Treatment, however, should be initiated as early as possible.

Surgical treatment: inguinal orchiectomy

Inguinal exploration and orchiectomy with early clamping of the spermatic cord is the treatment of choice for testicular cancer. The specimen reveals accurate histopathology and pathological stage classification.[4,5] A properly performed radical orchiectomy is associated with minimal morbidity and provides excellent local control of the primary tumour in the vast majority of patients. However, any testicular mass of uncertain ranking must be explored by the inguinal approach to verify or exclude malignancy. Since benign testicular lesions are recognized with increasing frequency, frozen section analysis should be considered intraoperatively, which accurately differentiates malignant from benign testicular lesions with high sensitivity and specificity.[6,7] The procedure may be performed using general, spinal, or local anaesthesia on an outpatient basis as described previously.[4,5] Surgical complications occur in less than 5% of patients with postoperative bleeding representing the most common complication, which may occasionally result in a scrotal or retroperitoneal haematoma.[8] Wound infection and paraesthesia of the scrotum are less common postoperative complications.

Prior inguinal or scrotal surgery may alter the normal lymphatic drainage of the testis so that specific measures have to be taken in cases of scrotal violation (such as an emergency scrotal exploration identifies a tumour rather than torsion), which is reported in a frequency of 4–17%.[9,10] A meta-analysis of patients with a history of scrotal violation at initial therapy demonstrated the local recurrence rate was 2.9% compared to 0.4% for patients undergoing an inguinal radical orchiectomy.[9] The current recommendations for the management of scrotal violation are: (i) in patients with low-stage seminoma, the radiation portals should be extended to include the ipsilateral inguinal region and scrotum; (ii) in patients with low-stage non-seminomatous germ cell tumour, the scrotal scar should be widely excised with the spermatic cord at the time of retroperitoneal lymph node dissection (RPLND); (iii) patients receiving induction chemotherapy for metastatic disease should have the cord stump excised at the time of PC-RPLND; however, given the relative absence of local relapse after systemic chemotherapy, an extensive inguinal dissection or hemiscrotectomy should not be performed.

Surgical treatment: testis-sparing surgery

Considering the growing attention to functional issues of cancer survivorship, surgical management of primary testicular tumours has to reflect potential long-term effects of orchidectomy, quality-of-life issues, and the potential impact on the endocrine and the exocrine function of the testis.

Organ preserving surgery of testicular tumours is indicated under the following conditions:[1–3,11,12]

- benign testicular tumour such as epidermoid cysts, Leydig cell tumour, Sertoli cell tumour, and so on;
- benign epididymal masses such as adenomatoid tumours;
- synchronous bilateral testicular germ cell tumours;
- metachronous testicular germ cell tumours;
- unilateral testicular germ cell tumours in a solitary testicle.

The aim of organ preserving testicular surgery is (i) to maintain endocrine function with physiological levels of testosterone, (ii) to preserve fertility with the option to father a child, and (iii) to maintain quality of life.

In patients with synchronous or metachronous bilateral testicular germ cell tumours or a germ cell tumours arising in a solitary testicle, organ preservation can be attempted if the tumour is smaller than 2 cm in diameter (or at least smaller than 50% of the testicular volume). Furthermore, the serum levels of both testosterone and luteinizing hormone (LH) should be in the normal range. An elevated LH in the presence of physiological testosterone levels indicates compensated Leydig cell insufficiency, which might decompensate after local surgery and adjuvant radiation therapy. Another key aspect of patient selection is the compliance

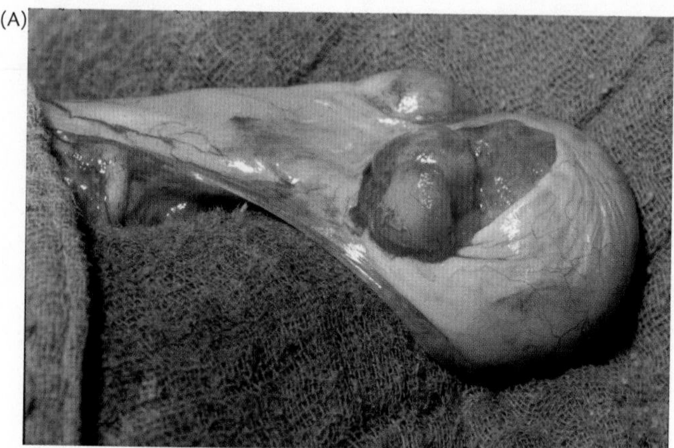

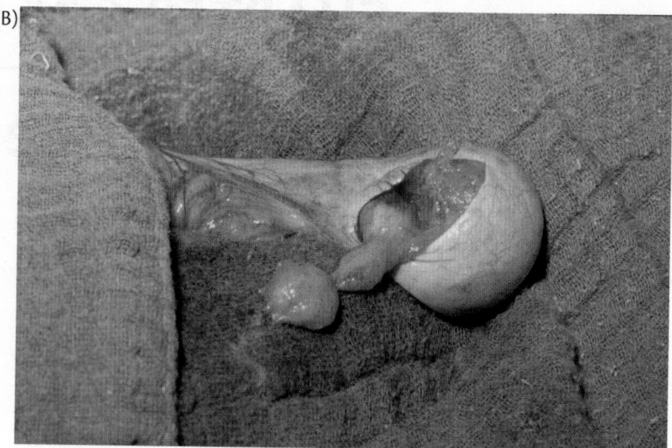

Fig. 6.35.1 Tumour enucleation in testicular germ cell tumours. (A) Identification of small intratesticular tumours after incision of the tunica albuginea just above the palpable tumour nodules. (B) Enucleation of multiple intratesticular tumours.

of both patient and physician. In addition, a semen analysis should be obtained in order to assess fertility and to discuss the option of cryopreservation. Also testicular ultrasonography must be performed preoperatively with a 7.5–10 MHz scanner in order to assess intratesticular location and diameter of the tumour.

The initial steps of the organ-sparing procedure are identical to the inguinal orchiectomy outlined above with all manipulations being performed under cold ischaemia. Warm ischaemia can result in damage of the Sertoli and the Leydig cells with consecutive impairment of the endocrine and the exocrine function of the testis. If the tumour is palpable the tunica albuginea is incised immediately above the testicular mass. Once the tumour is exposed the adjacent testicular parenchyma can be scraped away with a small swab or the blade of a scalpel due to the pseudocapsule surrounding most of the small lesions (see Fig. 6.35.1). The testicular tumour is to be completely enucleated and send for frozen section examination to identify the histology (benign versus malignant) and to assess the surgical margins. Once the tumour is completely removed, four biopsies are taken from the tumour bed and send for frozen section examination.

The current studies demonstrate a five-year survival rate of 98% and maintenance of physiological testosterone serum levels in about 90% of the patients without the need for testosterone substitution. The disease-free survival rate was 99%, local recurrence developed in 5.5%, and normal testosterone serum levels were maintained in 85% of the patients.

The use of testicular sparing surgery in testicular cancer requires a close follow-up for the early detection of possible local recurrences. The best modality for local follow-up is scrotal ultrasonography. We recommend the first ultrasound to be done four to six weeks postoperatively, a time when scar tissue has replaced the intraparenchymatous traumatic oedema. Thereafter, scrotal images should be taken every two months for the first year to adequately document the developing scar tissue for further follow-up studies. Afterwards, six-month intervals seem to be adequate for early identification of local recurrences. In patients having undergone local adjuvant radiation therapy, scrotal ultrasonography can be safely omitted and the patient should be educated to self palpate the remaining testicle. In patients developing a local recurrence, radical orchiectomy has to be performed and androgen substitution has to be initiated.

Surgical treatment: contralateral testis biopsy

About 5% of all patients with a unilateral testicular germ cell tumour will harbour testicular intraepithelial neoplasia (TIN) in their contralateral testicle, which will be detected by an immunohistochemical evaluation of a randomly taken testis biopsy at the time of orchiectomy.[13] In a recent prospective trial it has been shown that a systematic two-site biopsy of the testis improves sensitivity to detect TIN and the diagnostic extra yield imparted was 18%.[14] Currently, there exists controversy about the clinical utility of the contralateral biopsy, which is supposedly unnecessary for 95% of patients.[1–3,15] An evidence-based meta-analysis of all studies concerned with the detection of TIN suggests that it is justified to recommend contralateral biopsy for men with a testis volume <12 mL and age <30 years at the time of diagnosis, since their risk for contralateral TIN is >34% (Table 6.35.1).[1–3] It must be emphasized that the biopsy specimen should be fixed in Bouin's or in Stieve's solution to preserve TIN cells for diagnosis.

Table 6.35.1 Clinical risk factors for contralateral TIN in patients with unilateral testicular germ cell tumors

Risk factor	Relative risk	95% confidence intervel
Testicular atrophy (<12 mL)	4.3	2.83–6.44
History of cryptorchidism	2.1	1.21–3.63
Age <30 years	1.7	1.17–2.6
Family history of testis cancer	2.2	1.25–12.3
Infertility	1.6	1.10–10

Source: data from Krege S *et al.*, 'European consensus conference on diagnosis and treatment of germ cell cancer: a report of the second meeting of the European Germ Cell Cancer Consensus group (EGCCCG): Part I', *European Urology*, Volume 53, Issue 3, pp. 478–96, Copyright © 2008 European Association of Urology; Albers *et al.*, 'EAU guidelines on testicular cancer: 2011 update', *European Urology*, Volume 60, Issue 2, pp. 304–19, Copyright © 2011 European Association of Urology; and Beyer J *et al.*, 'Maintaining success, reducing treatment burden, focusing on survivorship: Highlights from the third European consensus conference on diagnosis and treatment of germ-cell cancer', *Annals of Oncology*, Volume 24, Issue 4, pp. 878–888, Copyright © 2013, Oxford University Press.

About one-third of patients with extragonadal germ cell cancer harbour TIN within one or both testicles which otherwise appear normal. The cumulative risk of developing a metachronous testicular cancer 10 years after diagnosis and treatment of extragonadal germ cell tumours is only 10%, and higher among patients with non-seminomatous histology or retroperitoneal location than among patients with pure seminomatous histology (1.4%) or primary mediastinal location (6.2%).[16,17] However, since all patients with extragonadal germ cell cancer will receive platinum-based chemotherapy which will eliminate a substantial percentage of TIN, a routinely performed bilateral testicular biopsy is not recommended. Nevertheless, if biopsy is planned in patients with a higher risk for TIN following an extragonadal germ cell tumour, this should be preferably performed prior to chemotherapy. If performed thereafter, testicular biopsy may be considered not earlier than two years after the completion of chemotherapy.

There are three possible therapeutic options for TIN: orchiectomy, radiotherapy with 20 Gy, or a surveillance strategy, which should be discussed with the patient.[1–3] Both orchiectomy or radiotherapy offer definitive treatment of TIN, but will destroy any potential residual fertility. Since the interval between diagnosis of TIN and the development of a testicular tumour is usually long, a surveillance strategy is justified for patients who want to father children and have residual spermatogenesis at least sufficient for assisted fertilization. In the case of a surveillance strategy regularly performed evaluation of the TIN bearing testicle by ultrasound is mandatory.

If radiation treatment is chosen a total dose of 20 Gy (single doses of 2 Gy, 5 fractions per week) seems to be the most appropriate treatment, which is able to safely eliminate all TIN loci.

Treatment of seminomatous testicular germ cell tumours

Clinical stage I seminoma

Despite negative computerized tomography (CT) scans, there is a risk of 12% to 32% of occult retroperitoneal lymph node metastases depending on the absence or presence negative prognostic markers. The cure rate of clinical stage I seminomatous germ cell cancer is close to 100% and can be achieved by the three different therapeutic options: active surveillance, radiation therapy, and carboplatin mono-chemotherapy.

No prognostic classification system has been prospectively validated, and there is controversial evidence from Canadian surveillance studies that the size of the primary tumour (≤4 cm versus >4 cm) and infiltration of the rete testis might represent independent prognostic indicators for occult metastases.[18] In contrast to the initial analyses from the Canadian group, however, these risk factors could not be validated in subsequent series for the identification of seminoma patients with a high-risk of occult metastases.[19–24] Patients with both factors represent a high-risk population with a relapse rate of around 35%, so that these histopathological parameters still should be documented. Patient age (<34 versus ≥34 years) and the presence of vascular invasion (VI) are of equivocal prognostic relevance but they are of non-significant.

Adjuvant radiotherapy

Adjuvant retroperitoneal radiation therapy to the para-aortic or paracaval region was the most frequently used approach resulting in a relapse-free long-term survival of 97%.[1–3] Adjuvant radiotherapy results in a relapse rate of 3–4%. Almost all of these recurrences are located outside the irradiated area, mostly in the pelvis, or close to the border of the radiation fields especially in the area of the renal hilum. The target volume of irradiation includes the infradiaphragmal paraaortal/paracaval lymphatics. The upper and lower field margins are defined by the upper edge of the thoracic vertebra 11 and the lower edge of the lumbar vertebra 5. Ipsilateral to the primary tumour the lateral field margin should be extended to the renal hilum; the contralateral margin has to include the processus transversus of the lumbar vertebrae. The total dose is 20 Gy (single doses of 2.0 Gy each, five fractions per week) based on the results of the prospective randomized trial of the Medical Research Council (MRC) which compared 30 Gy with 20 Gy.[24] A recent follow-up analysis of the TE10, TE 18, and TE 19 trial including a total 2,466 clincal stage I seminoma patients confirmed the non-inferiority of 20 Gy versus 30 Gy with a relapse rate of only 0.2% after three years.[25,26] Adjuvant radiation therapy with limited target volume and doses may be associated with mild acute side effects (usually WHO grade I–II), predominantly in the form of gastrointestinal symptoms. Compared to no adjuvant treatment there is a small risk of secondary malignancies after radiation therapy.[27,28] Statistically significantly increased risks of solid cancers were observed among patients treated with radiotherapy alone (RR = 2.0, 95% CI = 1.9– 2.2), chemotherapy alone (RR = 1.8, 95% CI = 1.3–2.5), and both (RR = 2.9, 95% CI = 1.9–4.2). For patients diagnosed with seminomas or non-seminomatous tumours at age 35 years, cumulative risks of solid cancer 40 years later (i.e. to age 75 years) were 36% and 31%, respectively, compared with 23% for the general population. Cancers of the lung (RR = 1.5, 95% CI = 1.2–1.7), colon (RR = 2.0, 95% CI = 1.7–2.5), bladder (RR = 2.7, 95% CI = 2.2–3.1), pancreas (RR = 3.6, 95% CI = 2.8–4.6), and stomach (RR = 4.0, 95% CI = 3.2–4.8) accounted for almost 60% of the total excess. Similar results were reported for a group of 2,707 long-term survivors with a mean follow-up of 17 years.[29] The risk of secondary malignancies was 2.6-fold (95% CI, 1.7–4.0-fold) increased after subdiaphragmatic radiotherapy. Based on these data of long-term toxicities adjuvant radiation therapy is no longer recommended by the major European guidelines on the management of testicular cancer.[2]

Active surveillance

A surveillance strategy should be used as the preferred treatment option in patients in whom this approach is considered feasible. This recommendation is based on the results of numerous prospective non-randomized studies of surveillance.[30–36] The data in these series are now mature and relapse rates have consistently been reported to be approximately 15% in unselected populations of patients with stage I disease. The predominant site of relapse in all studies was in the para-aortic lymph nodes in about 85% of all cases with relapses. The median time to relapse ranged from 12 to 18 months, but late relapses (>5 years) have been reported in some series. Disease-specific survival is 99% overall and thus comparable to other options.

An optimal follow-up strategy for patients on surveillance has not yet been determined. Most relapses occur within two years of diagnosis and less than 10% of recurrences are diagnosed beyond the third year of follow-up.[1–3] About 35% of relapses are detected by cross-sectional imaging techniques beyond the third year so that these examinations might be limited to the first years of follow-up. Furthermore, surveillance programmes with a high volume of imaging apparently do not lead to earlier detection or less advanced stage at the time of relapse as compared to protocols with low-volume imaging.[34] Routine chest X-ray and serum marker estimation are likely of no value in follow-up protocols.[35,36]

Adjuvant chemotherapy

The MRC in the United Kingdom has conducted a randomized phase III study of 1,447 patients comparing adjuvant radiotherapy and a single course of carboplatin.[37] Carboplatin was dosed based on an area under the curve (AUC) of 7 which is typically around 15% greater than using a m^2 dosing regimen. A recent update of the study with 6.5 years median follow-up the five-year relapse rates were 4% and 5.3%, respectively, for radiotherapy and chemotherapy, HR 1.25 (90% C.I. 0.83–1.89).[38] Sixty-seven per cent (67%) of those who relapsed in the carboplatin arm did so in the retroperitoneum alone. An unexpected finding in this study was a reduction in the observed number of second primary germ cell tumours in patients treated with adjuvant chemotherapy with a five-year event rate of 1.96% with radiotherapy versus 0.54% with chemotherapy.

This dosing schedule was also used in the Spanish Germ Cell Cancer Cooperative Group trials[32] which reported on the prospective treatment of patients with risk factors for recurrence (tumours >4 cm and/or Rete testis invasion) with two cycles of AUC7 carboplatin and the five-year relapse rate was 3.8%. As observed in the MRC TE19 study most relapses were retroperitoneal, hence necessitating ongoing abdomino-pelvic CT imaging. When giving a single dose of carboplatin at an AUC of 7, it is important to calculate the dose based on an accurate measurement of the glomerular filtration rate and not to rely on a calculation of the creatine clearance based on the serum creatinine level.

One major unanswered question about carboplatin chemotherapy in this setting is whether there are late effects of treatment. Like radiation, platinum-based chemotherapy has been associated with an increased risk of cancer and heart disease. Although the total dose of the chemotherapy used in the treatment of stage I seminoma is low compared to the chemotherapy given for more advanced stage disease, only long-term follow-up studies will inform us whether there are long-term health issues associated with one or two doses of carboplatin.

The relapse pattern after adjuvant single-agent carboplatin mandates that continued cross-sectional imaging of the retroperitoneal lymph nodes is required (similar to surveillance). The vast majority of relapses occur within the first three years and follow-up efforts should thus concentrate on this time period with less frequent visits thereafter.[39]

Stage II seminoma

At work-up after orchidectomy, about 15–20% of patients have radiologically involved para-aortic lymph nodes. Until now the standard treatment in CS IIA/B seminoma has been radiotherapy. Total doses in the range of 30–36 Gy seems reasonable: In CS IIA 30 Gy and in CS IIB 36 Gy, respectively, are administered homogeneously with single doses of 2Gy at five fractions per week.[40–43] With modern radiation techniques this treatment results in a relapse-free survival at six years of 95% for stage IIA and 89% for stage IIB. Overall survival is close to 100%.[1–3] The target volume includes the para-aortic and ipsilateral iliac lymphatics. The upper field margin is the upper border of the thoracic vertebra 11, the lower field margin is the upper border of the acetabulum. In CS IIA, the lateral field margins for the para-aortic fields are identical to those for CS I. In CS IIB the lateral field margins are individually modified according to the extension of the lymph nodes with a safety margin of 1.0 to 1.5 cm. To reduce the risk of impairment of fertility due to scatter radiation dose shielding of the remaining testicle during irradiation is mandatory. Three months post radiation therapy, abdominal and pelvic CT scans should be performed to document the treatment effect and as a basis for follow-up.

In stage IIB chemotherapy with three cycles of standard dose cisplatin, etoposide and bleomycin (BEP), or four cycles of cisplatin and etoposide (EP) represents a treatment alternative to radiotherapy, particularly in patients with larger multinodal retroperitoneal disease, but may be associated with a higher risk of acute toxicity as compared to radiotherapy.[44] Single-agent carboplatin has not shown to safely eradicate retroperitoneal metastases in patients with stage II seminoma despite a dosage of AUC 7.[45]

Seminoma, stage ≥IIC

For patients with 'good' prognosis disease, according to International Germ Cell Cancer Collaboration Group (IGCCCG) criteria,[46] standard treatment is three cycles of BEP. In cases of contraindications against bleomycin four cycles of cisplatin and etoposide can be given. The original five-day BEP regimen (etoposide 100 mg/m^2 and cisplatin 20 mg/m^2 each day, bleomycin 30 mg on days 1, 8, and 15) remains standard treatment for four cycles required in 'intermediate' prognosis patients. In seminomas, there is no poor prognosis group. Chemotherapy should be given without dose reductions at 22-day intervals. Postponing treatment (i.e. maximum of three days for each decision) should rarely be considered in cases of existing fever, neutrophils <500 /μl, or platelets <100,000 /μl at day 1 of a subsequent cycle.

With the introduction of an 'intermediate' prognosis group by the IGCCCG classification a group of patients has been defined who may reach a five-year survival of 80%. Available data support four cycles BEP as standard treatment in these patients.

PC-RPLND in advanced seminomas

Following primary cisplatin-based chemotherapy, viable cancer can be demonstrated in about 12–30% of men with residual masses >3 cm and in less than 10% in those with residual masses <3 cm in diameter. Following guideline-adapted cytotoxic protocols, however, the incidence of viable cancer in residual seminomatous masses has decreased to 20% irrespective of their size.[47–56] Adhering to the former recommendation to resect all residual masses >3 cm diameter would result in an overtreatment rate of 80% without any therapeutic benefit for the patient reducing PC-RPLND to a mere invasive staging procedure. Furthermore, surgical resection of residual seminomatous elements is technically challenging due to the severe desmoplastic reaction between the regressing mass and the adjacent vascular and visceral structures resulting in a higher frequency of additional intraoperative procedures and an increased rate of postoperative complications.[54]

In order to better select patients who might benefit from PC-RPLND, the role of FDG—PET to predict the presence of viable tumour in residual masses of advanced seminomas was prospectively evaluated. After initial positive results, studies were expanded to 54 patients with 74 documented residual masses on computed tomography ranging from 1 cm to 11 cm.[47] After PET scanning the patients either underwent surgery or were followed clinically; any growing lesion was assumed to be malignant whereas regressing lesions or residual masses remaining stable for ≥24 months were considered to contain non-viable elements only. The sensitivity and specificity to detect viability with FDG-PET was 80% and 100%, respectively; there was no false—positive scan and there were three false negative PET scans. In accordance with the current recommendation of the European Germ Cell Cancer Consensus Group (EGCCCG), post chemotherapy as well as post-radiotherapy residual masses in seminoma patients should not necessarily be resected, irrespective of their size, but should be closely followed by imaging investigations and tumour marker determinations.[1–3] In patients with residual lesions of < 3 cm in size, the use FDG-PET scanning is optional. No resection or any other treatment modality besides further active surveillance is necessary in patients with a negative PET scan, while a positive PET scan, if performed more than six weeks after day 21 of the last chemo-/radiotherapy, is a strong and reliable predictor of viable tumour tissue in patients with residual lesions.[46] In FDG-PET positive patients, histology should be obtained by biopsy or resection. Further treatment should be based on the results of histology and may include observation, surgery, radiation, or further chemotherapy. In patients with progressive disease after first-line chemotherapy histology should be obtained and salvage chemotherapy given after confirmation of seminoma.[1–3]

Treatment of patients with non-seminoma CS I

If treatment is performed correctly, the cure rate of patients with CS I non-seminomatous germ-cell tumors (NSGCT) should be 99%, regardless of the management chosen. Basically, three treatment options with the same high cure rate but significantly differences in frequency and type of treatment-associated toxicities might be offered to the patient: active surveillance, primary chemotherapy with one to two cycles of cisplatin, etoposide, and bleomycin (PEB) and nerve-sparing RPLND (Fig. 6.35.2). When choosing a risk-adapted approach in clinical stage I NSGCT one has to reflect that all of the patients will be long-term survivors so that long-term side effects of treatment should be minimal or non-existent. According

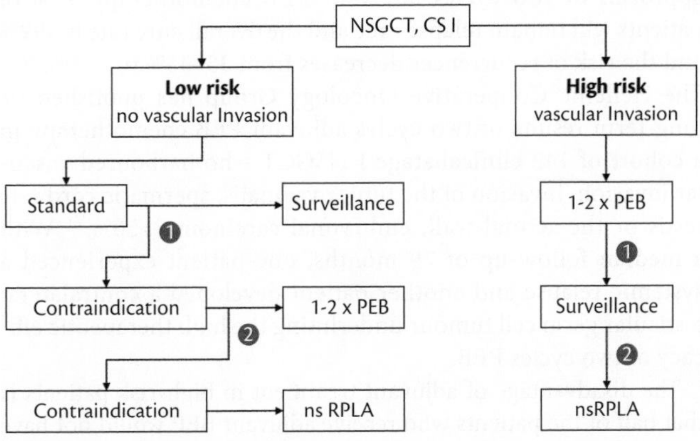

Fig. 6.35.2 Treatment options in clinical stage I NSGCT.
Source: data from Albers P *et al*, European Association of Urology, 'EAU guidelines on testicular cancer: 2011 update', *European Urolology*, Volume 60, Issue 2, pp. 304–19, Copyright © 2011 European Association of Urology.

to the most recommendations of the European Germ Cell Cancer Consensus Group Conference (EGCCCG) low-risk patients should be primarily offered active surveillance,[1–3] whereas systemic chemotherapy with two cycles of PEB represents the treatment of choice for high-risk patients.

Active surveillance

Active surveillance represents a treatment strategy with the aim to detect retroperitoneal or systemic relapses and to treat only those patients with documented metastatic disease thereby decreasing the risk of unnecessary overtreatment.

When recommending active surveillance for low risk or in certain scenarios also for stage I high-risk NSGCT, two major important aspects have to be considered: (i) risk of secondary malignancies due to the repetitive radiation exposure of the imaging studies and (ii) more intensive treatment in case of relapse (three cycles PEB ± post-chemotherapy RPLND) as compared to primary active therapy (one cycle PEB).

In the case of active surveillance for CS I, low-risk NSGCT, the relapse rate is 27–30% when considering a long-term follow-up of ≤20 years.[1–3] Relapses occur in the retroperitoneum in 54–78% of patients, in the lung in 13–31%, but are very rarely found in more than one visceral organ. With this approach 78–86% of patients do not need any further treatment after orchiectomy. If a patient under surveillance relapses, the administration of chemotherapy will result in a cure rate close to 100%.

Patients with a low risk of relapse (no VI) should be managed by surveillance according to the EGCCCG recommendations for follow-up, which require at least five CT scans performed at 0, 3, 12, 18, and 24 months.[1–3] This follow-up protocol with extensive imaging studies, however, might lead to a high radiation exposure with significant long-term consequences for the patients.

In a recent study Tarin *et al.*[57] estimated the risk of secondary cancer associated with imaging related radiation during surveillance of stage I NSGCT using CT. In their analysis they evaluated surveillance protocols recommending about 16 CT scans over a five-year period and they took into consideration a 64-slice CT scanner obtaining images of the abdomen and pelvis with and without the chest. For calculation of organ specific radiation dose, a standardized, phantom male patient was used using the Monte Carlo simulation techniques. Lifetime attributable risks of cancer were estimated using the approach outlined in the Biological Effects of Ionizing Radiation VII Phase 2 report.[58] With a five-year surveillance protocol the lifetime cancer risk ranged from 1 in 52 (1.9%) for an 18-year old to 1 in 63 (1.2%) for a 40-year old patient. If chest CTs were also obtained the risk increases to 1 in 39 (2.6%) and 1 in 58 (1.6%), respectively. The relative risk of a secondary malignancy with surveillance compared to a single scan after RPLND is approximately 15.2.

Various studies have been designed to reduce the number of CT scans during the surveillance strategy.[59,60] In order to reduce the number of CT scans during follow-up, the prospective randomized Medical Research Council Trial TE08 was initiated which compared the diagnostic efficacy of two versus five CT scans during the first two years of follow-up to detect the number of patients who relapse with intermediate and poor prognosis disease at relapse.[60] Some 247 patients and 167 patients were randomized to the two-scan and the five-scan group, respectively. Besides CT scans, all patients underwent follow-up assessments at various time intervals: clinical examination, evaluation of serum tumour markers AFP, ß-hCG, and lactate dehydrogenase (LDH), as well as chest X-ray. With a median follow-up of 40 months, 37 (15%) relapses have developed in the two-scan and 33 (20%) relapses have occurred in the five-scan group. None of the patients had poor prognosis disease at time of relapse, but two (0.8%) patients and one (0.6%) patient had intermediate prognosis disease. There were, however, some other statistically significant differences between the two groups with regard to the indicators of relapse. The proportion of patients in whom elevated tumour markers were the first indicators of relapsing disease was 21.6% and 6.1% in the two-scan and the five-scan group, respectively. Interestingly, 16 patients had normal markers at time of orchiectomy but elevated markers at time of relapse underlining the importance of serum tumour markers measurements in every patient with CS I NSGCT who undergoes active surveillance. In the two arms combined a total of 11 patients developed lung metastases, of whom 7 were tumour marker negative. The following conclusions can be drawn from this large prospective randomized trial: (i) fewer CT scans reduce the radiation exposure and costs without harming the patient; (ii) regular measurements of ß-hCG, AFP, and LDH together with chest X-rays and two abdominal CT scans are necessary for a surveillance programme, and (iii) it is unclear if this approach of reduced imaging studies can be applied for high-risk patients since only 10% of the recruited NSGCT demonstrated vascular invasion with a relapse rate of 32%.

Non-risk-adapted active surveillance

Vascular invasion (VI) of the primary tumour is the most important prognostic indicator for relapse. Patients with VI have a 48% risk of developing metastatic disease whereas only 14–22% of patients without VI will relapse.[61–64] A risk-adapted strategy based on the presence of VI with the application of two cycles PEB chemotherapy is the recommended standard procedure according to the EGCCCG and the EAU guidelines although.[2]

Kakiashvili *et al.*[65] reported on the largest experience of nonrisk adapted surveillance in 371 patients with clinical stage I NSGCT. With regard to outcome measurements, patients were stratified into two cohorts based on the time of diagnosis with group 1 being diagnosed between 1981 and 1992 and group 2 being diagnosed between 1993–2005. The median follow-up is 6.3 years and the median time to relapse is 7.1 months. Presence of vascular invasion and pure embryonal carcinoma were identified as independent predictors of relapse in both cohorts. Some 42% and 27.6% of both cohorts were high-risk patients and 54.5% and 49.2% of those patients relapsed as compared to only 18.7% and 14.2% in the low-risk group. Interestingly, the number of high-risk patients decreased over time which might be a result of improved diagnostic modalities and a more precise definition of high-risk disease. This nonrisk adapted surveillance strategy resulted in a five-year disease-specific and overall survival rate of 99.2% and 98.2%, respectively. This approach will spare unnecessary treatment in 50% of high-risk patients and it will thereby reduce the overall treatment burden in these young men. The retroperitoneum was the relapsing site in 75% of the patients, in another 10% of the patients, relapse was only diagnosed by a tumour marker rise.

In another retrospective study, 223 clinical stage I NSGCT underwent surveillance independent on their prognostic risk profile.[66] Vascular invasion was present, absent or unknown in 66%, 27%, and 7%, respectively. After a median follow-up, 59 (26%) patients relapsed with good prognosis disease and all were salvaged by systemic chemotherapy, 8% of the patients needed to undergo post-chemotherapy RPLND. Only half of the relapsing patients demonstrated vascular invasion in their orchiectomy specimen.

Furthermore, recent studies have questioned the high recurrence rate of close to 50%. In the retrospective study from Divrik *et al.*[67] the relapse rate was only 35.9% in CS I NSGCT with only one risk factor which was defined as either presence of vascular invasion or percentage of embryonal carcinoma >50%. Rustin *et al.*[60] reported a 32% two-year relapse rate among patients with vascular invasion. Also, Stephenson *et al.*[68] described a progression rate of only 33% in patients with CS I NSGCT who would undergo surveillance. Based on these findings some authors offered surveillance even to patients with high-risk CS I NSGCT with excellent outcome. Al-Thourah *et al.*[69] retrospectively evaluated 107 CS I patients with predominant embryonal carcinoma who underwent active surveillance or nerve-sparing RPLND. With a median follow-up of four years 33% in the surveillance group experienced relapse and were salvaged with chemotherapy and post-chemotherapy RPLND. In the RPLND group 18 (56%) patients had pathological stage I and 14 (44%) had pathological stage II disease. Four patients experienced a systemic relapse outside the boundaries of resection and all were cured by chemotherapy. Comparing both therapeutic approaches, 33% of patients in the surveillance group and 46% of patients in the RPLND group needed systemic chemotherapy. Patients with both embryonal carcinoma and VI experienced systemic relapse in 59% and 57% of the cases in the surveillance arm and the RPLND arm, respectively whereas patients with none of the risk factors were cured in 65% by either treatment.

Active surveillance might be used in both low and high-risk clinical stage I NSGCTs. Whereas it represents the standard approach in low-risk patients with an expected relapse rate of 12–15%, high-risk patients and physicians who follow the surveillance strategy have to be informed about the high relapse risk and the urgent need to adhere to strict follow-up schedules in order to maintain the high cure rate.

Primary chemotherapy

According to the EGCCCG and the EAU guidelines, patients with a high risk of relapse (VI present) should receive adjuvant chemotherapy with two cycles of BEP.[1–3] By the recommended approach of two cycles adjuvant PEB chemotherapy 97% of patients will remain relapse-free and the overall cure rate is >99% and the risk of recurrences decreases from 35–45% to 2–3%.[70,71] The Hellenic Cooperative Oncology Group has published its long-term results of two cycles adjuvant PEB chemotherapy in a cohort of 142 clinical stage I NSGCT who harboured vascular invasion, invasion of the tunica vaginalis, spermatic cord rete testis or the scrotal wall, embryonal carcinoma >50%.[71] With a median follow-up of 79 months, one patient experienced a systemic relapse and another patient developed a contralateral testicular germ cell tumour underlining the high therapeutic efficacy of two cycles PEB.

The disadvantage of adjuvant treatment in high-risk patients is that half of the patients who receive adjuvant BEP would not have required chemotherapy at all and may be unnecessarily exposed to the side effects of chemotherapy, a possible transient decrease in fertility[39] and possibly a small risk of secondary malignancies, as reported from patients receiving higher doses of chemotherapy.

In order to decrease the potential long-term side effects associated with adjuvant chemotherapy, various groups have applied only one cycle of PEB chemotherapy in high-risk CSI NSGCT.[72–75] In a prospective randomized clinical phase III trial the German Testicular Cancer Study Group (GTCSG) randomized 382 patients with CS I NSGCT to either receive one cycle of PEB chemotherapy or RPLND.[74] After a median follow-up of 4.7 years, 2 (1.04%) and 15 (7.8%) recurrences were detected in the chemotherapy and in the RPLND arm, respectively, resulting in a two-year recurrence-free survival rate of 99.46% versus 91.87% ($p = 0.001$). Although RPLND was associated with a significantly higher relapse rate, one has to consider that RPLND was performed in numerous centres with variable surgical experience which might have contributed to the relatively high frequency of intraabdominal relapses as compared to other studies. Quality of surgery, which could not be compared in all of the 61 participating centres (two-thirds of patients were recruited by only 12 institutions), is currently recognized as one of the main limitations of RPLND in a national setting.

In another large prospective community-based multicenter management programme the Swedish and Norwegian Testicular Cancer Project (SWENTOCA) evaluated the therapeutic outcome of one cycle adjuvant chemotherapy according to the PEB regime in 745 CS I NSGCT patients.[75] Treatment strategy was based on the presence or absence of vascular invasion. At a median follow-up of 4.7 years a total of 51 relapses were observed. 41.7% and 13.2% of patients with or without vascular invasion experienced relapse whereas only 3.2% and 1.3% of the patients developed recurrences following one cycle of chemotherapy. After a follow-up of more than four years, the data seem to be mature and one cycle of PEB chemotherapy might become the standard of therapy reducing both the total burden of chemotherapy for high-risk clinical stage I NSGCT compared to surveillance or adjuvant therapy with two cycles of PEB.

Retroperitoneal lymph node dissection

According to the EGCCCG and the EAU guidelines, patients unwilling to undergo a surveillance strategy or adjuvant chemotherapy, nerve-sparing lymphadenectomy (NS-RPLND, see Fig. 6.35.3) may be performed.[1–3]

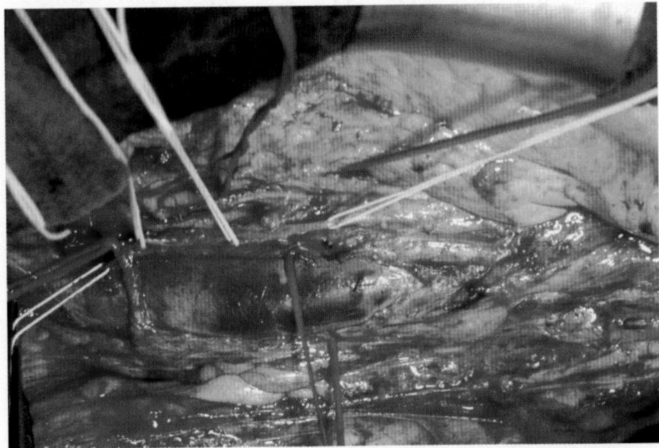

Fig. 6.35.3 Intraoperative situs of a nerve-sparing bilateral RPLND for clinical stage I nonseminatous germ cell tumour demonstrating the sympathetic chain and ganglia and the sympathetic nerves running into the hypogastric plexus.

Primary RPLND is still widely practice in the United States for high-risk patients although less so in Canada and Europe. RPLND provides accurate staging information regarding RP lymph node status. With proper selection of patients for RPLND, two-thirds have low burden pathologic stage (pS) II disease, and almost 90% will be cured by surgery only.[68] The rationale for primary nerve-sparing RPLND for patients with CS I NSGCT is based on the evidence that the RP represents the primary metastatic site in more than 80% of patients and that it is also the most frequently involved site of chemoresistant mature teratoma.[76,77] Virtually all patients who relapse after primary RPLND are chemotherapy naïve and eventually cured by usually three cycles of cisplatin-based chemotherapy. Only a minority of CS I NSGCT harbours occult systemic metastatic disease and might be better managed by inductive systemic chemotherapy. RPLND simplifies follow-up and makes it more liberal. Subsequent RP relapse is rare, and abdominal imaging can be restricted to one baseline CT a few months after surgery. With the introduction of nerve-spearing technique along with various modified templates, antegrade ejaculation rates 90–100% have been reported, with significantly reduced morbidity and virtually unknown mortality.[78–81] Patients selection factors on outcome after primary RPLND have been reported and the application of these parameters might allow a risk-adapted indication RPLND.[76] The authors analysed a cohort of 453 patients with CS I to IIB NSGCT who underwent RPLND between 1989 and 2002. Of those, 308 (68%) and 122 (27%) presented with CS I and CS IIA disease, respectively. Whereas the frequency of mature teratoma remained fairly constant in the two time periods (22% vs. 21%) the number of patients with low-volume disease (pN1) increased significantly from 40–64% ($p = 0.01$). Some 217 (70%) patients of the 308 CS I NSGCTs demonstrated true pathological stage I disease after RPLND. The four-year progression-free probability in this cohort was 97%; the risk of systemic progression decreased from 14% before 1999 to 1.3% after 1999 suggesting an improved risk stratification for systemic disease based on the selection criteria developed after critical analysis of the first patient cohort being treated between 1989 and 1999.

For CS, I NSGCT-elevated postorchiectomy tumour markers appear to be associated with a significantly increased risk of progression which was as high as 72%. Stephenson *et al.*[82] analysed the outcome of 267 patients with CS I and CS IIA NSGCTs with one or two of the aforementioned risk factors who underwent nsR-PLND. ECA and VI were present in 31% of the patients and ECA without VI was identified in 10% whereas 58% demonstrated VI without ECA. The presence of both risk factors was associate with a significantly higher risk of retroperitoneal metastases (54% vs. 37%, $p = 0.009$). Patients with pathological stage I were followed actively and did not receive adjuvant chemotherapy whereas 22% and 83% of patients with pN1 and pN2 disease received two cycles PEB, respectively. All patients remained disease-free during the complete follow-up period. 16% of pathological stage II patients had teratoma in the retroperitoneum which would not have been eliminated by primary chemotherapy. 211 patients did not receive adjuvant chemotherapy. All relapsing patients could be salvage by four cycles EP chemotherapy. Summarizing the data of the total cohort of 267 patients, 80 (29.9%) CS I/IIA high-risk patients received either adjuvant or salvage chemotherapy. If only high-risk CS I NSGCT are considered an estimated 89% would have been free of progression five years after chemotherapy.

In a similar approach, Nicolai *et al.*[83] reviewed their experience of primary RPLND with no adjuvant chemotherapy in a cohort of 322 consecutive CS I NSGCT who were followed for a median time of 17 years. Some 262 (81.4%) patients were staged as pathological stage I, whereas 41 (12.7%) and 19 (5.9%) patients demonstrated pathological stage IIA and IIB, respectively. However, 50 patients (15.5%) developed a recurrence with 96% occurring the first two years of follow-up. The majority of relapses (n = 44) were located outside the retroperitoneum, whereas six and four relapses developed in the retroperitoneum and in the contralateral testis. Some 271 (84.1%) patients of the total cohort did not experience relapsing disease including 68.3% of the patients with pathological stage IIA/B. Based on multivariate analysis, presence of vascular invasion, percentage of embryonal carcinoma >50%, presence of lymph node metastases increased the probability of relapses by the factor 2.7, 3.5, and 2.9, respectively.[84]

Although rare with an incidence of only 2–5%, clinical stage I mature teratoma of the testis harbour a risk of about 16%[85,86] for retroperitoneal lymph node metastases. The majority of these patients will demonstrate teratomatous elements in the retroperitoneal lymph node metastases, so that nerve-sparing RPLND represents the treatment of choice.

When discussing nerve-sparing RPLND as primary treatment option in patients with CS I NSGCT, potential surgery-related complications have to be considered. The German Testicular Cancer Study Group evaluated the outcome of 239 CS I NSGCT who underwent nerve-sparing RPLND.[87] Minor complications and major complications were observed in 14.2% and in 5.4%, respectively. Antegrade ejaculation could be preserved in 93.3% of the patients and the frequency of ejaculation correlated significantly with the experience of the single surgeon. 14 (.8%) patients developed relapses with the majority (n = 11) being located in the extraperitoneal areas.

In summary, nerve-sparing RPLND seems to cure about 85% to 90% of patients with high-risk CS I NSGCT. Whereas, 67% of low-risk NSGCT are overtreated due to true pathological stage I in 70% of the patients and a low systemic recurrence rate of 3%, high-risk patients might benefit from surgery.

Stage IIA/B non-seminomatous germ cell tumours

Low-stage testicular disease comprises clinical stages IIA and IIB associated with a cure rate of approximately 98%.[1–3] Patients with low-volume disease and abnormal tumour marker levels of AFP, ß-hCG, or LDH are treated according to the algorithm of the IGCCCG and the EGCCCG recommendations (Fig. 6.35.4). Patients with marker negative retroperitoneal lymph nodes suspected to be clinical stage IIA might be offered two treatment options: nerve-sparing RPLND or surveillance. Primary RPLND is a viable approach in clinical stage IIA, since an overstaging is faced in about 20% of patients who would have been subjected to unnecessary chemotherapy otherwise; additional advantages of nerve-sparing RPLND are preservation of sympathetic nerves in 80% of patients and accurate staging in all patients. Furthermore, adjuvant chemotherapy will only be necessary in patients with positive lymph node disease and unfavourable prognostic markers.[88,89] Risk of relapse is only about 15% if fewer than three lymph nodes are involved; the maximum lymph node diameter is <2 cm and there is no extranodal extension, so not all patients must undergo adjuvant chemotherapy and a subgroup of patients might be followed by surveillance. If primary surveillance without nsRPLND is chosen, follow-up at six-week intervals is indicated to document any growth or regression of the lesion. A growing mass indicates vital cancer and therapy can be initiated. A lesion decreasing in size usually does not harbour malignant disease and can be followed. As in clinical stage I disease, both therapeutic options should be intensively discussed with the patient, and parameters such as the wish to father a child, compliance of both patient and physician, and the need for safety must be integrated into the decision. The only exceptions are patients with elevated markers following radical orchiectomy but no visible metastases on CT scans, who should undergo primary chemotherapy with three cycles of PEB.[90]

Patients with clinical stage IIB testicular cancer, however, will undergo primary chemotherapy depending on the serum concentrations of the markers AFP, ß-hCG and LDH with three or four cycles of PEB followed by secondary RPLND in about 30% of cases, although basically the same three therapeutic options are available as for clinical stage IIA.

Treatment of patients with advanced NSGCT

For patients with 'good' prognosis disease, according to IGCCCG criteria (Tables 6.35.2, Table 6.35.3, and Table 6.35.4),[46] standard treatment is three cycles of BEP. In cases of contraindications against bleomycin four cycles of cisplatin and etoposide (EP) can be given.[1–3] Chemotherapy should be given without dose reductions

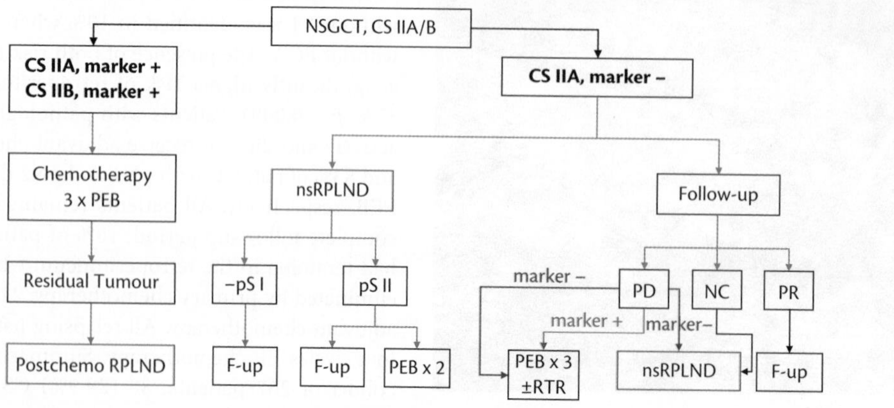

Fig. 6.35.4 Treatment options in CS IIA NSGCT.
Source: data from Albers P *et al*, European Association of Urology, 'EAU guidelines on testicular cancer: 2011 update', *European Urolology*, Volume 60, Issue 2, pp. 304–19, Copyright © 2011 European Association of Urology.

Table 6.35.2 IGCCCG risk classification for advanced non-seminomatous germ cell tumours

Prognosis	5-OS	Nonseminoma
Good	90%	Testis or primary extragonadal retroperitoneal tumour and low markers AFP <1,000 ng/mL, β-HCG <1,000 ng/mL (<5,000 IU/l) and LDH <1.5 × normal level and no non-pulmonary visceral metastases
intermediate	75%	Testis or primary extragonadal retroperitoneal tumour and intermediate markers AFP 1,000–10,000 ng/mL β-HCG 1,000–10,000 ng/mL, LDH 1.5–10 × normal level and presence of non-pulmonary visceral metastases
poor	50%	Primary mediastinal germ cell tumour or presence of non-pulmonary visceral metastases and/or 'high markers' AFP >10,000 ng/mL, -HCG >10,000 ng/mL LDH >10 × UNL

Source: data from International Germ Cell Cancer Collaborative Group (IGCCCG), 'The International Germ Cell Consensus Classification: a prognostic factor based staging system for metastatic germ cell cancer', *Journal of Clinical Oncology*, Volume 15, Number 2, pp. 594–603, Copyright © 1997 American Society of Clinical Oncology.

at 22-day intervals. Postponing treatment (i.e. maximal of three days for each decision) should rarely be considered in cases of existing fever, neutrophils <500 /µl, or platelets <100,000 /µl at day 1 of a subsequent cycle.

There is no indication for routine prophylactic application of haematopoietic growth factors, such as granulocyte-colony stimulating factor (G-CSF). However, if serious infectious complications have occurred during one preceding chemotherapy cycle, prophylactic administration of G-CSF is recommended in subsequent cycles.[1–3] Since dose reductions due to neutropenia should be avoided, prophylactic G-CSF should also be used if prolonged neutropenia occurs for maintenance of the required dose intensity.

With the introduction of an 'intermediate' prognosis group by the IGCCCG classification, a group of patients has been defined who may reach a five-year survival of 80%. Available data support four cycles BEP as standard treatment in these patients.[1–3] For patients with 'poor' prognosis standard treatment consists of four cycles of BEP. Four cycles of etoposide, ifosfamide, and cisplatin

Table 6.35.3 IGCCCG risk classification for advanced seminomatous germ cell tumours

Prognosis	5-OS	Seminoma
Good	90%	Any primary localizationany marker level and no non-pulmonary visceral metastases
Intermediate	75%	Any primary localization and presebce of non-pulmonary visceral metastases (liver, CNS, bone, intestinum) any marker level
Poor		Non-existant in seminomas

Source: data from International Germ Cell Cancer Collaborative Group (IGCCCG), 'The International Germ Cell Consensus Classification: a prognostic factor based staging system for metastatic germ cell cancer', *Journal of Clinical Oncology*, Volume 15, Number 2, pp. 594–603, Copyright © 1997 American Society of Clinical Oncology.

Table 6.35.4 Treatment recommendations according to IGCCCG risk group classification

Prognosis	5-OS	Treatment Recomendation
Good	90%	3 × PEB oder 4 × EP
Intermediate	75%	4 × PEB
Poor	50%	4 × PEB

Source: data from International Germ Cell Cancer Collaborative Group (IGCCCG), 'The International Germ Cell Consensus Classification: a prognostic factor based staging system for metastatic germ cell cancer', *Journal of Clinical Oncology*, Volume 15, Number 2, pp. 594–603, Copyright © 1997 American Society of Clinical Oncology.

(VIP) are equally effective, but cause more acute myelotoxicity and are not recommended as standard. In the IGCCCG analysis, five-year progression-free and overall survival were 41% and 48%, respectively. In individual patients, VIP may be preferred to BEP in order to avoid possible bleomycin-induced lung injury in already pulmonary compromised patients. Patients with extensive liver-, pulmonary- or CNS-involvement may benefit from an immediate brief course of reduced-dose chemotherapy before full-dose chemotherapy cycles are started.

Three randomized trials have shown no advantage in high-dose chemotherapy for the overall group of 'poor prognosis' patients.[91–93] Only patients with a slow marker decline after the first or second cycle may represent a subgroup with inferior prognosis in whom dose-intensified chemotherapy might be indicated.

Since a matched-pair analysis resulted in a better survival rate,[1–3] poor prognosis patients should still be treated in ongoing prospective trials, investigating the value of dose-intensified or high-dose chemotherapy. Patients with 'poor prognosis' should be treated in a reference centre because a better outcome was reported for intermediate and poor prognosis patients who had been treated within a clinical trial in a high volume centre.

PC-RPLND in advanced NSGCT

In patients who achieve complete remission, that is, normalized tumour markers and no residual lesions after chemotherapy, post-chemotherapy surgery is not required. In patients with any residual mass irrespective of size and normalization of tumour markers the residual masses should be resected. Histology of residual masses after first-line chemotherapy will be necrosis, mature teratoma and vital cancer in about 50%, 35% and 15% of patients, respectively.[94–97]

In patients with residual lesions <1 cm, PC-RPLND also should be strongly considered since it has been shown in various retrospective single-centre analysis that up to 20% and 8% of the patients will harbour mature teratoma and vital cancer, despite the small sized lesions. There is an even increased risk of residual teratoma, if teratoma was present in the initial histology. In persistent retroperitoneal disease, retroperitoneal surgery should include all areas of initial metastatic sites. However, this approach has been challenged by recent retrospective studies from three groups.[98–100] Kollmannsberger *et al.*[98] analysed 276 patients who underwent systemic chemotherapy for metastatic NSGCT. Some 161 patients (58.3%) achieved a complete remission which was defined by the presence of residual lesions <1 cm and all patients were followed without surgical resection. After a mean follow-up of 40 (2–128) months relapses were observed in 6% of the patients and none of them died after appropriate salvage therapy. However, 94% of the patients belonged to the IGCCCG good prognosis group and only 3% belonged to the intermediate and the poor-risk group. In a similar approach, Ehrlich *et al.*[99] evaluated 141 patients who were observed after systemic chemotherapy and residual lesions <1 cm. After a mean follow-up of up to 15 years, 9% of the patients relapsed and 3% of the patients died due to testis cancer. IGCCCG risk group classification predicted the outcome best: recurrence-free survival and cancer-specific survival were 95% and 99%, respectively, in men who belonged to the good-risk group, whereas it dropped to 91% and 73% if the patients belonged to the intermediate and poor-risk group. However, only six out of 12 relapses developed in the retroperitoneum, so that only 50% of the patients would have had a potential benefit from PC-RPLND. Quite recently, the GTCSG analysed the outcome of 392 patients who underwent PC-RPLND for residual lesions of any size and they correlated the final pathohistological findings with the size of the residual masses and the IGCCCG risk profile[100] 9.4% and 21.8% of the men with residual lesions smaller than 1 cm harboured vital cancer and mature teratoma in the resected specimens, respectively. These numbers increased to 21% and 25% in patients with residual lesions of 1–1.5 cm and to 36% and 42% in men with lesions larger than 1.5cm. The IGCCCG risk profile was not identified as an independent risk to predict the final pathohistology of small residual lesions. The GTCSG draw the conclusion that all patients with any visible residual masses should be resected in a tertiary referral centre.

Considerations for the most appropriate surgical strategy

PC-RPLND is a challenging surgical procedure which requires detailed knowledge of the retroperitoneal anatomy, familiarity with surgical techniques of the vascular and intestinal structures as well as profound experience in the management of patients with testicular cancer. Depending on the size and the extent of the residual lesions, the surgeon has to modify his surgical approach to the retroperitoneal space. An abdominal midline incision from the xyphoid to the symphysis can be used in most patients with unilateral and infrahilar disease, whereas a Chevron incision might be more suitable in those men with bilateral and suprahilar disease. About 10% of the patients demonstrate persistent retrocrural disease so that a thoracoabdominal approach will be best to easily and safely explore this anatomical region.[101–103] Although the morbidity of PC-RPLND exceeds that of primary nerve-sparing RPLND, modifications of cytotoxic regimes, the surgical approach, and perioperative care have resulted in a decreased incidence of acute and long-term complications. Due to the high treatment-related acute morbidity, however, surgery of residual masses should be performed at specialized centres only.[1–3]

In patients with residual masses at multiples sites, an individual decision should be made regarding the number and extension of resections. Decisions on the extent of surgery should be based on the risk of relapse of an individual patient and on quality-of-life issues. Resection of residual tumours outside the abdomen or lung should also be considered on an individual basis, since discordant histology is found in 35–50% of patients.[104] Pulmonary or mediastinal residual masses harbour necrosis/fibrosis only in 90% if the retroperitoneal masses did not contain mature teratoma or viable cancer. Therefore, these lesions might be managed by surveillance and elective surgery at time of progression. If, however, pulmonary or mediastinal nodules were found to contain necrosis/fibrosis at primary resection, about 45% of retroperitoneal residual masses will demonstrate a discordant histology so that PC-RPLND is indicated.

Preoperative imaging studies

Prior to PC-RPLND, a complete metastatic and physical evaluation including: (i) computed tomography of the chest, the abdomen and the small pelvis about six to eight weeks following the last cycle of chemotherapy; (ii) measurement of the serum tumour markers; and (iii) pulmonary function testing in men with an increased risk of pulmonary toxicity (four cycles PEB, >40 years, smoking history, renal insufficiency) should be performed prior to PC-RPLND.

Especially in patients with large residual masses, imaging studies should allow an adequate assessment of the large retroperitoneal vascular structures since involvement of the inferior vena cava (IVC) and the abdominal aorta can be expected in about 6–10% and 2%, respectively (Fig. 6.35.5).[105–109] Magnetic resonance imaging represents the most appropriate imaging technique to predict infiltrations of the vessel wall and the presence of an intracaval tumour thrombus. Infiltrations of the IVC wall or IVC thrombi should be completely resected since about two-thirds of the patients harbour vital cancer or mature teratoma in the infiltrating masses. Usually intraoperative reconstruction or replacement of the IVC is not necessary since chronic venous sequalae are to be expected in less than 5% of all patients.[107]

The necessity for aortic replacement is rare and usually accompanied by large residual masses involving additional adjacent structures and making additional surgical procedures necessary such as nephrectomy, IVC resection, small bowel resection, and hepatic resection. In the majority of cases mature teratoma or vital carcinoma was identified in the aortic wall.[109]

Timing of PC—RPLND

Once residual masses have been diagnosed PC-RPLND should be initiated as soon as possible with a complete resection of all retroperitoneal and intraperitoneal masses. Complete resection of residual masses is of very important prognostic significance. Sonneveld *et al.*[110] demonstrated that about 50% of all patients with locoregional recurrences after PC-RPLND had an incomplete resection at time of first surgery. Hendry *et al.*[111] retrospectively analysed the outcome of 443 patients undergoing either immediate or elective PC-RPLND once progression of the residual masses was demonstrated. A significant benefit with regard to progression-free survival (83% vs. 62%, $p = 0.001$) and cancer-specific survival (89% vs. 56%, $p = 0.001$) was identified for the immediate surgical approach. Incomplete resection and large size of the residual mass were identified as prognostic risk factors predicting poor outcome. Both parameters were observed more frequently in the group of patients who underwent elective PC-RPLND.

PC—RPLND: extent of surgery

The anatomical extent of PC-RPLND has been discussed controversially for many years. It has been common practice to perform a full bilateral template dissection deriving from experiences of the 1980s when most patients presented with high-volume residual disease when undergoing retroperitoneal surgery. The boundaries of a full bilateral template include the crura of the diaphragm, the bifurcation of the common iliac arteries and the ureters thereby including the primary and secondary landing zones of the right

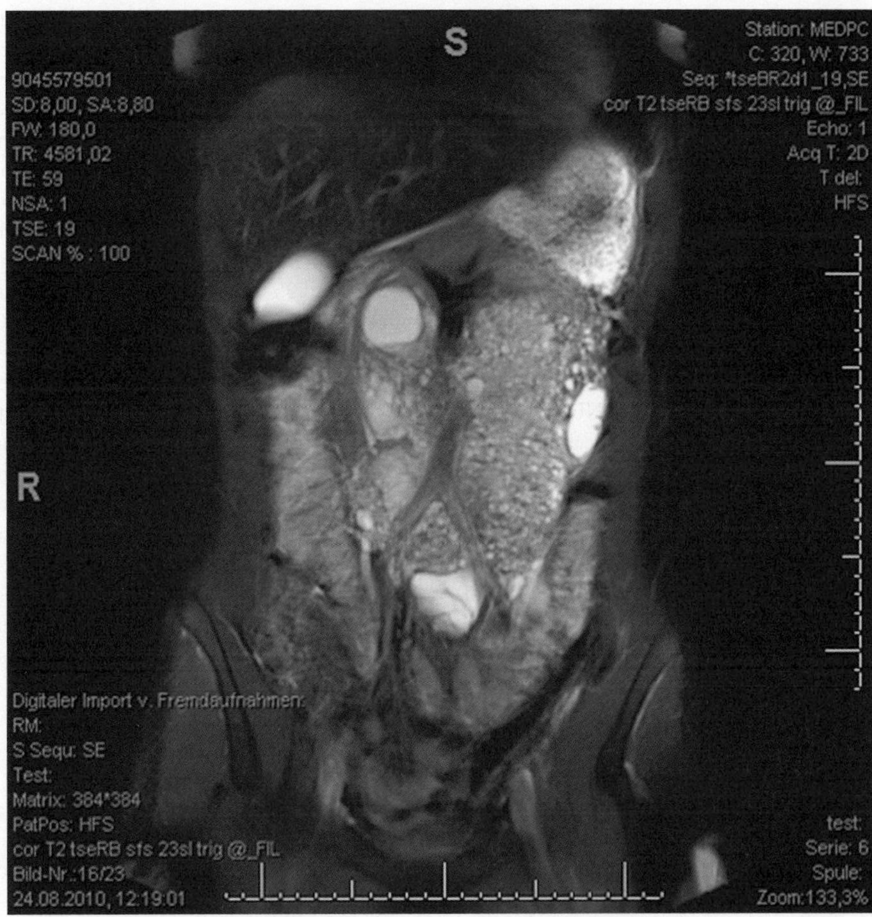

Fig. 6.35.5 Encasement of the infrarenal aorta by mature teratoma.

(paracaval, interaortocaval) and the left (para-aortic, preaortic) testicles. Wood *et al.*[112] demonstrated an 8% incidence of contralateral spread among 113 patients with bulky disease undergoing full bilateral PC-RPLND after cisplatin- or carboplatin-based chemotherapy. Similarly, Qvist *et al.*[113] and Rabbani *et al.*[114] reported a 5.7% and a 2.6% incidence of teratomatous residues outside the boundaries of a modified template dissection. Nowadays, however, systemic chemotherapy is delivered for relatively low-volume retroperitoneal disease (clinical stages IIB) with most metastases being restricted to the primary landing zone of the tumour-bearing testicle. Although the potential of contralateral spread does exist especially from right to left, it is usually not common in low-volume residues questioning the appropriateness of full bilateral dissection for any residual disease. In a retrospective analysis, Aprikian *et al.*[115] analysed the outcome of 40 patients undergoing limited or bilateral radical PC-RPLND. A limited approach was chosen if intraoperative frozen section analysis (FSA) of the resected mass demonstrated necrosis or fibrosis, whereas a radical RPLND was used in the presence of mature teratoma or viable cancer. Some 20% of the patients experienced recurrences (14% and 26% in the limited and radical RPLND, respectively) with none of the recurrences located in the retroperitoneum. The authors suggested to use intraoperative FSA to trigger the most appropriate surgical approach in the clinical scenario of PC-RPLND. Herr[116] analysed the therapeutic outcome of limited versus full bilateral PC-RPLND based on the results of FSA of the resected mass. If FSA demonstrated necrosis a limited RPLND was performed, in all other cases patients underwent bilateral RPLND. After a median follow-up of 6 years, 14 relapses were observed with only two developing in the retroperitoneum; furthermore, six major surgical complications were observed with five after bilateral RPLND. Modified PC-RPLND was considered to be a safe surgical procedure in a well selected group of patients with advanced testicular cancer. These early retrospective and single-centre studies indicate that a modified PC-RPLND might be a safe approach in men with limited retroperitoneal disease and right/left primary tumours with no evidence of teratoma or viable cancer on FSA of the residual mass. However, application of the modified unilateral template to PC-RPLND still is discussed controversially among tertiary referral centres based on the 3–8% incidence of mature teratoma or viable cancer in the contralateral landing zone.[117,118] Quite recently, two experienced groups—the Indiana group and the German Testicular Cancer Study Group—reported their experience of patients undergoing modified unilateral template PC-RPLND.[119,120] The group at Indiana University has performed a limited PC-RPLND in 100 men with low-volume retroperitoneal disease (<5 cm) confined to the primary landing zone of the primary tumour.[76] After a mean follow-up of 32 months. only four patients relapsed, all outside the boundaries of the modified and even of the bilateral template. The two-year and five-year disease-free survival was 95%.

It was the purpose of the GTCSG to assess the oncological necessity of full bilateral retroperitoneal PC-RPLND in 152 patients with normalized or plateauing serum tumour markers.[120] Depending on the size of the residual mass or the location of the primary testicular tumour a full bilateral template resection (n = 54) or a modified template resection (n = 98) was performed. If patients exhibited a well-defined lesion ≤2 cm modified PC-RPLND was performed, lesions >5 cm were always treated by a full bilateral PC-RPLND. Lesions 2–5 cm in diameter were approached dependent on the site of the primary and the location of the mass: interaortacaval residuals were always approached with a full bilateral PC-RPLND, whereas as para-aortic and paracaval lesions were treated by a modified PC-RPLND if the metastatic site corresponded to site of the primary; otherwise, a full bilateral PC-RPLND was initiated. There were no significant intraoperative complications; there was, however, a significant difference with regard to postoperative morbidity between bilateral and modified PC-RPLND with more complications in patients undergoing extended surgery (p <0.001). Antegrade ejaculation was preserved in 85% of patients undergoing modified PC-RPLND whereas it could not preserved in 75% of the cases undergoing full bilateral PC-RPLND (p = 0.02), respectively. Eight (5.2%) recurrences were observed after a mean follow-up of 39 (6–105) months: one in-field relapse following modified PC-RPLND and seven recurrences outside the boundaries of full bilateral PC-RPLND. Two-year disease-free survival was 78.6% and 92.8% for bilateral and modified PC-RPLND, respectively. Limitations are a still short follow-up, limited number of patients; and retrospective nature. There was no significant correlation with extent of surgery and frequency and location of relapses.

Based on the data presented, full bilateral PC-RPLND is not always required and it should be considered as surgical approach of choice in patients with extensive residual masses, interaortacaval location, or a location of the residual mass not corresponding to the site of the primary testis tumour. In well-defined small masses <5 cm, a modified template residual tumour resection (RTR) does not interfere with oncological outcome but decreases treatment-associated morbidity.

PC-RPLND after salvage chemotherapy or previous retroperitoneal surgery

Patients who have undergone salvage chemotherapy, prior primary or PC-RPLND, those judged to be unresectable and those with disease progression prior to retroperitoneal surgery are at high risk for both a poor therapeutic outcome and an increased frequency of surgery—associated complications. The presence of anyone of these poor prognostic parameters increases the risk of relapse from 12% to 45%.[121–126]

The presence of residual tumour masses after salvage chemotherapy is associated with a higher frequency of viable cancer, a higher likelihood of incomplete surgical resection and a higher risk of postoperative relapse as compared to those patients undergoing PC-RPLND after first-line chemotherapy. Recently, Eggener *et al.*[118] demonstrated that modern chemotherapeutic salvage regimes containing taxanes significantly reduced the presence of viable cancer from 42% to 14% (p = 0.01) when compared to earlier cisplatin-based cytotoxic regimes; the rates of teratoma in the residual tumours was similar with 31% and 33%. They found a 10-year disease-specific survival of 70% so that PC-RPLND even after multiple chemotherapy regimes is indicated if the masses appear to be completely resectable.

Although rare, a subset of patients needs repeat RPLND due to metastatic tumour recurrence after primary RPLND or PC-RPLND because of incomplete tumour resection during initial surgery.[121–126] Repeat RPLND itself represents a poor risk factor associated with a significantly lower five-year survival rate of only 55% as compared to 86% in the group of patients undergoing adequate PC-RPLND. The long-term outcome after repeat RPLND relies on the complete resection of all residual retroperitoneal masses which will harbour viable cancer and mature teratoma in 20–25% and 35–40%, respectively. Whereas the cure rate for those with mature teratoma only approaches 100%, it decreases significantly to 44% and 20% in the presence of viable cancer and teratoma with malignant transformation, respectively. Repeat RPLND is a challenging surgical procedure associated with higher rates of adjunctive surgical procedures with ipsilateral nephrectomy and vascular procedures being the most frequent adjunctive surgeries.

Repeat RPLND often represents the last chance of cure for patients with in-field recurrences and it usually can be performed with an acceptable morbidity. Repeat RPLND will result in a long-term survival of 67% to 75%; if patients present with in-field recurrences and elevated markers, systemic chemotherapy followed by PC-RPLND should be initiated. In patients with negative markers immediate RPLND should be performed since most masses will harbour mature teratoma only.

Desperation PC-RPLND

The term 'desperation RPLND' applies to patients with persistently elevated or increasing serum tumour markers after primary inductive chemotherapy or after salvage chemotherapy due to either intrinsic or extrinsic chemoresistance. PC-RPLND in this cohort of patients is associated with a higher frequency of adjunctive surgeries and a poorer outcome. Usually, surgery alone is felt to result in a low likelihood of cure due to widespread systemic disease. However, according to the data of various groups, the five-year overall survival is 54% to 67% so that surgery might be indicated in well selected subset cohort of patients.[126,127] In recent series, increasing preoperative ß-hCG, elevated AFP, redo RPLND, and incomplete resection had been identified as negative risk factors associated with a poor survival. Despite elevated serum tumour markers about 45% to 50% of all patients harbour mature teratoma or necrosis/fibrosis in the surgical specimen resulting in a high cure rate. Patients with elevated but declining serum tumour markers and patients who had received first-line chemotherapy only had the highest likelihood to demonstrate teratoma or necrosis in the resected specimen. On the other hand, patients with incomplete resection demonstrate a poor prognosis and most likely do not benefit from extensive surgery. It is of utmost importance to identify those patients with potentially complete resection of residual masses who might benefit most from immediate surgery.

Adjunctive surgery in patients undergoing PC-RPLND

Additional surgical procedures of adjacent vascular or visceral structures might be necessary in up to 25% of the patients undergoing PC-RPLND in order to achieve complete resection of the residual masses: En bloc nephrectomy represents the most common type of adjunctive surgery for complete tumour clearance. Additional vascular procedures such as aortic replacement and resection of the inferior vena cava due to tumour infiltration will be necessary in about 1.5% and 10%, respectively.[128–130]

Complications after PC-RPLND

Whereas the frequency of complications is low in patients undergoing primary nerve-sparing RPLND for clinical stage I NSGCT,[87] it increases significantly in PC-RPLND for large-volume residual disease. Although the frequency of associated complications has been decreased in recent series as compared to series of the 1990s, it still approaches 10%.[131] The most common complications include minor complications such as wound infections, paralytic ileus, transient hyperamylasemia, pneumonitis/atelectasis, whereas significant complications such as acute renal failure, chylous ascites, or obstructive ileus develop in less than 2% of the patients.[132]

Consolidation chemotherapy after secondary surgery

After resection of necrosis or teratoma no further treatment is required. When viable undifferentiated tumour is found, the role of further consolidation chemotherapy is uncertain. A retrospective analysis demonstrated an improved progression-free survival with adjuvant chemotherapy, but failed to show an improvement in overall survival. Therefore, a 'wait-and-watch' strategy may also be justified.[133,134] Patients in the 'good' prognosis group, according to the IGCCCG classification, with complete resection of residual masses and with <10% vital tumour cells in the resected specimens have a favourable outcome even without adjuvant chemotherapy. If completely resected tumour presents >10% of viable cancer, or if completeness of the resection is in doubt, consolidation chemotherapy might be justified.

Management of brain metastases

Approximately 10% of all patients with advanced germ cell cancer present with brain metastases (i.e. 1–2% of all patients with testicular cancer). At relapse, metastases in the central nervous system (CNS) usually occur as part of a systemic relapse and rarely as an isolated sanctuary site relapse after previously successful treatment. Patients who present with brain metastases at initial diagnosis have a long-term survival probability of 30–40%, whereas patients who develop metastases during first-line treatment or in the context of recurrent disease outside of the brain have a five-year survival rate of only 2–5%.[135–137] The best prognostic group consists of patients with a solitary brain lesion discovered by initial staging investigations. The presence of metastatic choriocarcinoma indicates a poor prognosis independent from any form of treatment.[137]

The optimal sequence of treatment modalities (chemotherapy, radiotherapy, operation) has not yet been finally defined. Curative intent chemotherapy is necessary in all patients with brain metastases (EBM III: 217). In a multivariate analysis cranial irradiation added to systemic chemotherapy improved the overall prognosis of patients who present with brain metastasis (EBM III: 218). It has not yet been defined whether post-chemotherapy irradiation of the CNS is required after complete remission has been achieved by chemotherapy alone. It also remains unclear, whether or not secondary resection of a solitary residual mass is required after chemotherapy (MRI scans are mandatory for detection of micrometastases).

References

1. Krege S, Beyer J, Souchon R, *et al.* European consensus conference on diagnosis and treatment of germ cell cancer: a report of the second meeting of the European Germ Cell Cancer Consensus group (EGCCCG): part I. *Eur Urol* 2008; **53**(3):478–96.
2. Albers P, Albrecht W, Algaba F, *et al.* EAU guidelines on testicular cancer: 2011 update. *Eur Urol* 2011; **60**(2):304–19.
3. Beyer J, Albers P, Altena R, *et al.* Maintaining success, reducing treatment burden, focusing on survivorship: highlights from the third European consensus conference on diagnosis and treatment of germ-cell cancer. *Ann Oncol* 2013; **24**(4):878–88.
4. Daneshmand S, Skinner EC. Surgery for testicular cancer: radical orchiectomy. (pp. 93–7) In: Raghavan D (ed). *American Cancer Society Atlas of Clinical Oncology—Germ Cell Tumors.* Decker, Hamilton, 2003.
5. Carver BS, Heidenreich A, Sogani P. Radical orchiectomy and testis sparing procedures for the management of germ cell tumors. (pp. 125–30) In: Laguna MP, Bokemeyer C, Richie JP (eds). *Cancer of the Testis.* London, UK: Springer, 2010.
6. Tokuc R, Sakr W, Pontes JE, Haas GP. Accuracy of frozen section examination of testicular tumors. *Urology* 1992; **40**:512–16.
7. Elert A, Olbert P, Hegele A, Barth P, Hofmann R, Heidenreich A. Accuracy of frozen section examination of testicular tumors of uncertain dignity. *Eur Urol* 2002; **41**:290–3.
8. Bochner BH, Lerner SP, Kawachi M, Williams RD, Scardino PT, Skinner DG. Postradical orchiectomy hemorrhage: should an alteration in staging strategy for testicular cancer be considered? *Urology* 1995; **46**:408–11.
9. Capelouto C, Clark P, Ransil B, Loughlin K. A review of scrotal violation in testicular cancer: Is adjuvant local therapy necessary? *J Urol* 1995; **153**:1397–401.
10. Leibovitch I, Baniel J, Foster RS, Donohue JP. The clinical implications of procedural deviations during orchiectomy for nonseminomatous germ cell cancer. *J Urol* 1995; **154**:935–9.
11. Heidenreich A, Weißbach L, Höltl W, *et al.* Organ sparing surgery for malignant germ cell tumor of the testis. *J Urol* 2001; **166**:2161–5.
12. Heidenreich A, Bonfig R, Derschum W, von Vietsch H, Wilbert DM. A conservative approach to bilateral testicular germ cell tumors. *J Urol* 1995; **153**:1147–50.
13. Dieckmann KP, Loy V. Prevalence of contralateral intraepithelial neoplasia in patients with testicular germ cell neoplasms. *J Clin Oncol* 1996; **14**:3126–32.
14. Dieckmann KP, Kulejewski M, Pichlmeyer U, Loy V. Diagnosis of contralateral testicular intraepithelial neoplasia (TIN) in patients with testicular germ cell cancer: systematic two-site biopsies are more sensitive than a single random biopsy. *Eur Urol* 2007; **51**:175–83.
15. Heidenreich A. Contralateral testicular biopsy in testis cancer: current concepts and controversies. *BJU Int* 2009; **104**(9 Pt B):1346–50.
16. Hartmann JT, Fosså SD, Nichols CR, *et al.* Incidence of metachronous testicular cancer in patients with extragonadal germ cell tumors. *J Natl Cancer Inst* 2001; **93**:1733–8.
17. Daugaard G, Rørth M, von der Maase H, Skakkebæk NE. Management of extragonadal germ cell tumors and the significance of bilateral testicular biopsies. *Ann Oncol* 1992; **3**:283–9.
18. Warde P, Specht L, Horwich A, *et al.* Prognostic factors for relapse in stage I seminoma managed by surveillance. *J Clin Oncol* 2002; **20**:4448–52.
19. Tandstad T, Smaaland R, Solberg A, *et al.* Management of seminomatous testicular cancer: a binational prospective population-based study from the Swedish norwegian testicular cancer study group. *J Clin Oncol* 2011; **29**(6):719–25.
20. Chung P, Mayhew LA, Warde P, Winquist E, Lukka H. Genitourinary Cancer Disease Site Group of Cancer Care Ontario's Program in Evidence-based Care. Management of stage I seminomatous testicular cancer: a systematic review. *Clin Oncol (R Coll Radiol)* 2010; **22**(1):6–16
21. Fosså SD, Aass N, Heilo A, *et al.* Testicular carcinoma in situ in patients with extragonadal germ-cell tumours: the clinical role of pre-treatment biopsy. *Ann Oncol* 2003; **14**:1412–18.
22. Bamberg M, Shmidberger H, Meisner C, *et al.* Radiotherapy for stage I, IIA/B testicular seminoma. *Int J Cancer* 1999; **83**:823–7.
23. Fosså SD, Horwich A, Russel JM, *et al.* Optimal planning target volume for stage I testicular seminoma: a Medical Research Council randomized trial. *J Clin Oncol* 1999; **17**:1146–54.

24. Jones WG, Fosså SD, Mead GM, *et al.* Randomized trial of 30 versus 20 Gy in the adjuvant treatment of stage I testicular seminoma: a report on Medical Research Council Trial TE 18, European Organisation for the research and Treatment of Cancer Trial 30942. *J Clin Oncol* 2005; **23**:1200–8.
25. Mead GM, Fosså SD, Oliver RT, *et al.* Randomized trials in 2466 patients with stage I seminoma: patterns of relapse and follow-up. *J Natl Cancer Inst* 2011; **103**(3):241–9.
26. Power RE, Kennedy J, Crown J, *et al.* Pelvic recurrence in stage I seminoma: a new phenomenon that questions modern protocols for radiotherapy and follow-up. *Int J Urol* 2005; **12**:378–82.
27. Taylor MB, Carrington BM, Livsey JE, Logue JP. The effects of radiotherapy treatment changes on sites of relapse in stage I testicular seminoma. *Clin Radiol* 2001; **56**:116–19.
28. Travis LB, Fosså SD, Schonfeld SJ, *et al.* Second cancers among 40,576 testicular cancer patients: focus on long-term survivors. *J Natl Cancer Inst* 2005; **97**(18):1354–6.
29. van den Belt-Dusebout AW, de Wit R, Gietema JA, *et al.* Treatment-specific risks of second malignancies and cardiovascular disease in 5-year survivors of testicular cancer. *J Clin Oncol* 2007; **25**(28):4370–8.
30. Warde P, Huddart R, Bolton D, Heidenreich A, Gilligan T, Fosså S. Management of localized seminoma, stage I-II: SIU/ICUD Consensus Meeting on Germ Cell Tumors (GCT), Shanghai 2009. *Urology* 2011; **78**(4 Suppl):S435–43.
31. Cummins S, Yau T, Huddart R, Dearnaley D, Horwich A. Surveillance in stage I seminoma patients: a long-term assessment. *Eur Urol* 2010; **57**(4):673–8.
32. Aparicio J, Germà JR, García del Muro X, *et al.* Risk-adapted management for patients with clinical stage I seminoma: the Second Spanish Germ Cell Cancer Cooperative Group study. *J Clin Oncol* 2005; **23**(34):8717–23.
33. Germà-Lluch JR, García del Muro X, Maroto P, *et al.* Clinical pattern and therapeutic results achieved in 1490 patients with germ-cell tumours of the testis: the experience of the Spanish Germ-Cell Cancer Group (GG). *Eur Urol* 2002; **42**(6):553–62.
34. Classen J, Souchon R, Hehr T, Hartmann M, Hartmann JT, Bamberg M. Posttreatment surveillance after paraaortic radiotherapy for stage I seminoma: a systematic analysis. *J Cancer Res Clin Oncol* 2010; **136**(2):227–32.
35. Tolan S, Vesprini D, Jewett MA, *et al.* No role for routine chest radiography in stage I seminoma surveillance. *Eur Urol* 2010; **57**(3):474–9.
36. Vesprini D, Chung P, Tolan S, *et al.* Utility of serum tumor markers during surveillance for stage I seminoma. *Cancer* 2012; **118**(21):5245–50.
37. Oliver RT, Mason MD, Mead GM, *et al.* Radiotherapy versus single-agent arboplatin in adjuvant treatment of stage I seminoma: a randomised trial. *Lancet* 2005; **366**:293–300.
38. Oliver RT, Mead GM, Rustin GJ, *et al.* Randomized trial of carboplatin versus radiotherapy for stage I seminoma: mature results on relapse and contralateral testis cancer rates in MRC TE19/EORTC 30982 study (ISRCTN27163214). *J Clin Oncol* 2011; **29**(8):957–62.
39. Classen J, Schmidberger H, Meisner C, *et al.* Radiotherapy for stages IIA/B testicular seminoma: final report of a prospective multicenter clinical trial. *J Clin Oncol* 2003; **21**:1101–6.
40. Schmidberger H, Bamberg M, Meisner C, *et al.* Radiotherapy in stage IIA and IIB testicular seminoma with reduced portals: a prospective multicenter study. *Int J Radiol Oncol Biol Phys* 1997; **39**:321–6.
41. Patterson H, Norman AR, Mitra SS, *et al.* Combination carboplatin and radiotherapy in the management of stage II testicular seminoma: comparison with radiotherapy treatment alone. *Radiother Oncol* 2001; **59**:5–11.
42. Zagars GK, Pollack A. Radiotherapy for stage II testicular seminoma. *Int J Radiat Oncol Biol Phys* 2001; **51**:643–9.
43. von der Maase H. Do we have a new standard of treatment for patients with seminoma stage IIA and stage IIB? *Radiother Oncol* 2001; **59**:1–3.
44. Arranz JA, García del Muro X, Germà J, *et al.* E 400P in advanced seminoma of good prognosis according to the International Germ Cell Cancer Collaboration Group (IGCCCG) classification: The Spanish Germ Cell Cancer Group experience. *Ann Oncol* 2001; **12**:487–91.
45. Krege S, Boergermann C, Baschek R, *et al.* Single-agent carboplatin for CS II-A/B testicular seminoma. A phase II study of the German Testicular Cancer Study Group (GTCSG). *Ann Oncol* 2006; **17**:276–80.
46. International Germ Cell Cancer Collaborative Group (IGCCCG). The International Germ Cell Consensus Classification: a prognostic factor based staging system for metastatic germ cell cancer. *J Clin Oncol* 1997; **15**:594–603.
47. Bachner M, Loriot Y, Gross-Goupil M, *et al.* 2–18fluoro-deoxy-D-glucose positron emission tomography (FDG-PET) for postchemotherapy seminoma residual lesions: a retrospective validation of the SEMPET trial. *Ann Oncol* 2012; **23**(1):59–64.
48. Flechon A, Bompas E, Biron P, Droz JP. Management of post-chemotherapy residual masses in advanced seminoma. *J Urol* 1979; **168**:1975–9.
49. Friedman EL, Garnick MB, Stomper PC, Mauch PM, Harrington DP, Richie JP. Therapeutic guidelines and results in advanced seminoma. *J Clin Oncol* 1985; **3**:1325–32.
50. Schultz SM, Einhorn LH, Conces DJ, Williams SD, Loehrer PJ. Management of postchemotherapy residual mass in patients with advanced seminoma: Indiana University experience. *J Clin Oncol* 1989; **7**:1497–503.
51. Fosså SD, Borge L, Aass N, Johannessen NB, Stenwig AE, Kaalhus O. The treatment of advanced metastatic seminoma: experience in 55 cases. *J Clin Oncol* 1987; **5**(7):1071–7.
52. Ravi R, Rao RR, Shanta V. Integrated approach to the management of patients with advanced germ cell tumors of the testis. *J Surg Oncol* 1994; **55**(1):47–51.
53. Puc HS, Heelan R. Mazumdar M, *et al.* Management of residual mass in advanced seminoma: results and recommendations from the Memorial Sloan Kettering Cancer Center. *J Clin Oncol* 1996; **14**:454–60.
54. Mosharafa AA, Foster RS, Leibovich CC, Bihrle R, Johnson C, Donohue JP. Is post chemotherapy resection of seminomatous elements associated with higher acute morbidity? *J Urol* 2003; **169**:2126–8.
55. Kamat MR, Kulkarni JN, Tongoankar HB, Ravi R. Value of retroperitoneal lymph node dissection in advanced testicular seminoma. *J Surg Oncol* 1992; **51**:65–7.
56. Herr HW, Sheinfeld J, Puc HS, *et al.* Surgery for a post-chemotherapy residual mass in seminoma. *J Urol* 1997; **157**:860–2.
57. Tarin TV, Sonn G, Shinghal R. Estimating the risk of cancer associated with imaging related radiation during surveillance for stage I testicular cancer using computerized tomography. *J Urol* 2009; **181**(2):627–32.
58. Tubiana M, Aurengo A, Averbeck D, Masse R. Recent reports on the effect of low doses of ionizing radiation and its dose-effect relationship. *Radiat Environ Biophys* 2006; **44**(4):245–51.
59. Atsü N, Eskiçorapçi S, Uner A, *et al.* A novel surveillance protocol for stage I nonseminomatous germ cell testicular tumours. *BJU Int* 2003; **92**(1):32–5.
60. Rustin GJ, Mead GM, Stenning SP, *et al.* Randomized trial of two or five computed tomography scans in the surveillance of patients with stage I nonseminomatous germ cell tumors of the testis: Medical Research Council Trial TE08, ISRCTN56475197--the National Cancer Research Institute Testis Cancer Clinical Studies Group. *J Clin Oncol* 2007; **25**(11):1310–5.
61. Read G, Stenning SP, Cullen MH, *et al.* Medical Research Council prospective study of surveillance for stage I testicular teratoma. Medical Research Council Testicular Tumors Working Party. *J Clin Oncol* 1992; **10**:1762–8.
62. Heidenreich A, Sesterhenn IA, Mostofi FK, *et al.* Prognostic factors that identify patients with clinical stage I nonseminomatous germ cell tumors at low risk and high risk for metastasis. *Cancer* 1998; **83**:1002–11.

63. Albers P, Siener R, Kliesch S, *et al.* Risk factors for relapse in clinical stage I nonseminomatous testicular germ cell tumors: results of the German Testicular Cancer Study Group Trial. *J Clin Oncol* 2003; **21**(8):1505–12.
64. Perrotti M, Ankem M, Bancilla A, deCarvalho V, Amenta P, Weiss R. Prospective metastatic risk assignment in clinical stage I nonseminomatous germ cell testis cancer: a single institution pilot study. *Urol Oncol* 2004; **22**(3):174–7.
65. Kakiashvili DM, Zuniga A, Jewett MA. High risk NSGCT: case for surveillance. *World J Urol* 2009; **27**(4):441–7.
66. Kollmannsberger C, Moore C, Chi KN, *et al.* Non-risk-adapted surveillance for patients with stage I nonseminomatous testicular germ-cell tumors: diminishing treatment-related morbidity while maintaining efficacy. *Ann Oncol* 2010; **21**(6):1296–301.
67. Divrik RT, Akdogan B, Özen H, Zorlu F. Outcomes of surveillance protocol of clinical stage I nonseminomatous germ cell tumors—is shift to risk adapted policy justified? *J Urol* 2006; **176**:1424–30.
68. Stephenson AJ, Bosl GJ, Motzer RJ, *et al.* Retroperitoneal lymph node dissection for nonseminomatous germ cell testicular cancer: impact of patient selection factors on outcome. *J Clin Oncol* 2005; **23**:2781–8.
69. Al-Tourah AJ, Murray N, Coppin C, Kollmansberger C, Man A, Chi KN. Minimizing treatment without compromising cure with primary surveillance for clinical stage I embryonal predominant carcinoma noneminomatous testicular cancer: a population based analysis from British Columbia. *J Urol* 2005; **174**:2209–13.
70. Tandstad T, Cohn-Cedermark G, Dahl O, *et al.* Long-term follow-up after risk-adapted treatment in clinical stage 1 (CS1) nonseminomatous germ-cell testicular cancer (NSGCT) implementing adjuvant CVB chemotherapy. A SWENOTECA study. *Ann Oncol* 2010; **21**(9):1858–63.
71. Bamias A, Aravantinos G, Kastriotis I, *et al.* Report of the long-term efficacy of two cycles of adjuvant bleomycin/etoposide/cisplatin in patients with stage I testicular nonseminomatous germ-cell tumors (NSGCT): A risk adapted protocol of the Hellenic Cooperative Oncology Group. *Urol Oncol* 2011; **29**(2):189–93.
72. Gilbert DC, Norman AR, Nicholl J, Dearnaley DP, Horwich A, Huddart RA. Treating stage I nonseminomatous germ cell tumours with a single cycle of chemotherapy. *BJU Int* 2006; **98**(1):67–9.
73. Westermann DH, Schefer H, Thalmann GN, Karamitopoulou-Diamantis E, Fey MF, Studer UE. Long-term followup results of 1 cycle of adjuvant bleomycin, etoposide and cisplatin chemotherapy for high risk clinical stage I nonseminomatous germ cell tumors of the testis. *J Urol* 2008; **179**(1):163–6.
74. Albers P, Siener R, Krege S, *et al.* Randomized phase III trial comparing retroperitoneal lymph node dissection with one course of bleomycin and etoposide plus cisplatin chemotherapy in the adjuvant treatment of clinical stage I Nonseminomatous testicular germ cell tumors: AUO trial AH 01/94 by the German Testicular Cancer Study Group. *J Clin Oncol* 2008; **26**(18):2966–72.
75. Tandstad T, Dahl O, Cohn-Cedermark G, *et al.* Risk-adapted treatment in clinical stage I nonseminomatous germ cell testicular cancer: the SWENOTECA management program. *J Clin Oncol* 2009; **27**(13):2122–8.
76. Stephenson AJ, Bosl GJ, Motzer RJ, Kattan MW, Stasi J, Bajorin DF, Sheinfeld J. Retroperitoneal lymph node dissection for nonseminomatous germ cell testicular cancer: impact of patient selection factors on outcome. *J Clin Oncol* 2005; **23**:2781–8.
77. Baniel J, Foster RS, Einhorn LH, *et al.* Late relapse of clinical stage I testicular cancer. *J Urol* 1995; **154**:1370–2.
78. Yoon GH, Stein JP, Skinner DG. Retroperitoneal lymph node dissection in the treatment of low-stage nonseminomatous germ cell tumors of the testicle: an update. *Urol Oncol* 2005; **23**:168–77.
79. Jewett MA, Kong YS, Goldberg SD, *et al.* Retroperitoneal lymphadenectomy for testis tumor with nerve sparing for ejaculation. *J Urol* 1988; **139**:1220–4.
80. Donohue JP, Thornhill JA, Foster RS, *et al.* Primary retroperitoneal lymph node dissection in clinical stage A nonseminomatous germ cell testis cancer. Review of the Indiana University experience 1965–1989. *Br J Urol* 1993; **71**:326–35.
81. Donohue JP, Foster RS, Rowland RG, *et al.* Nerve-sparing retroperitoneal lymphadenectomy with preservation of ejaculation. *J Urol* 1990; **144**:287–91; discussion 291–2.
82. Stephenson AJ, Bosl GJ, Bajorin DF, Stasi J, Motzer RJ, Sheinfeld J. Retroperitoneal lymph node dissection in patients with low stage testicular cancer with embryonalcarcinoma predominance and/or lymphovascular invasion. *J Urol* 2005; **174**:557–60.
83. Nicolai N, Miceli R, Necchi A, *et al.* Retroperitoneal lymph node dissection with no adjuvant chemotherapy in clinical stage I nonseminomatous germ cell tumours: Long-term outcome and analysis of risk factors of recurrence. *Eur Urol* 2010; **58**(6):912–8.
84. Rassweiler JJ, Scheitlin W, Heidenreich A, Laguna MP, Janetschek G. Laparoscopicretroperitoneal lymph node dissection: does it still have a role in the management of clinical stage I nonseminomatous testis cancer? A European perspective. *Eur Urol* 2008; **54**(5):1004–15.
85. Leibovitch I, Foster RS, Ulbright TM, Donohue JP. Adult primary pure teratoma of the testis. The Indiana experience. *Cancer* 1995; **75**(9):2244–50.
86. Heidenreich A, Moul JW, McLeod DG, Mostofi FK, Engelmann UH. The role of retroperitoneal lymphadenectomy in mature teratoma of the testis. *J Urol* 1997; **157**(1):160–3.
87. Heidenreich A, Albers P, Hartmann M, *et al.* Complications of primary nerve sparing retroperitoneal lymph node dissection for clinical stage I nonseminomatous germ cell tumors of the testis: experience of the German Testicular Cancer Study Group. *J Urol* 2003; **169**(5):1710–4.
88. Pizzocaro G, Monfardini S. No adjuvant chemotherapy in selected patients with pathological stage II nonseminomatous germ cell tumors of the testis. *J Urol* 1994; **131**:677–80.
89. Weißbach L, Bussar-Maatz R, Flechtner H, *et al.* RPLND or primary chemotherapy in clinical stage IIA/B nonseminomatous germ cell tumors? Results of a prospective multicenter trial including quality of life assessment. *Eur Urol* 2000; **37**:582–94.
90. Motzer RJ, Nichols CJ, Margolin KA, *et al.* Phase III randomized trial of conventional-dose chemotherapy with or without high-dose chemotherapy and autologous hematopoietic stem-cell rescue as first-line treatment for patients with poor-prognosis metastatic germ cell tumors. *J Clin Oncol* 2007; **25**(3):247–56.
91. Droz JP, Kramar A, Biron P, *et al.* Genito-Urinary Group of the French Federation of Cancer Centers (GETUG). Failure of high-dose cyclophosphamide and etoposide combined with double-dose cisplatin and bone marrow support in patients with high-volume metastatic nonseminomatous germ-cell tumours: mature results of a randomised trial. *Eur Urol* 2007; **51**(3):739–46; discussion 747–8.
92. Daugaard G, Skoneczna I, Aass N, *et al.* A randomized phase III study comparing standard dose BEP with sequential high-dose cisplatin, etoposide, and ifosfamide (VIP) plus stem-cell support in males with poor-prognosis germ-cell cancer. An intergroup study of EORTC, GTCSG, and Grupo Germinal (EORTC 30974). *Ann Oncol* 2011; **22**(5):1054–61.
93. Motzer RJ, Mazumdar M, Bajorin DF, *et al.* High-dose carboplatin, etoposide, and cyclophosphamide with autologous bone marrow transplantation in first-line therapy for patients with poor-risk germ cell tumors. *J Clin Oncol* 1997; **15**(7):2546–52.
94. Fosså SD, Ous S, Lien HH, Stenwig AE. Post-chemotherapy lymph node histology in radiologically normal patients with metastatic nonseminomatous testicular cancer. *J Urol* 1989; **141**:557–9.
95. Toner GC, Panicek DM, Heelan RT, *et al.* Adjunctive surgery after chemotherapy for nonseminomatous germ cell tumors: recommendations for patient selection. *J Clin Oncol* 1990; **8**:1683–94.
96. Aprikian AG, Herr HW, Bajorin DF, Bosl GJ. Resection of postchemotherapy residual masses and limited retroperitoneal lymphadenectomy in patients with metastatic testicular nonseminomatous germ cell tumors. *Cancer* 1994; **74**:1329–34.

97. Herr HW. Does necrosis on frozen-section analysis of a mass after chemotherapy justify a limited retroperitoneal resection in patients with advanced testis cancer? *Br J Urol* 1997; **80**:653–7.
98. Kollmannsberger C, Daneshmand S, So A, *et al.* Management of disseminated nonseminomatous germ cell tumors with risk-based chemotherapy followed by response-guided postchemotherapy surgery. *J Clin Oncol* 2010; **28**(4):537–42.
99. Ehrlich Y, Brames MJ, Beck SD, Foster RS, Einhorn LH. Long-term follow-up of Cisplatin combination chemotherapy in patients with disseminated nonseminomatous germ cell tumors: is a postchemotherapy retroperitoneal lymph node dissection needed after complete remission? *J Clin Oncol* 2010; **28**(4):531–6.
100. Pfister D, Busch J, Winter C, *et al.* Pathohistological findings in patients with nonseminomatous germ cell tumours who undergo postchemotherapy retroperitoneal lymph node dissection for small tumours. *J Urol* 2011; AUA Abstract #830.
101. Albers P, Höltl W, Heidenreich A, Aharinejad S. Thoracoabdominal resection of retrocrural residual tumors. *Aktuelle Urol* 2004; **35**:141–50.
102. Fujioka T, Nomura K, Okamoto T, Aoki H, Ohhori T, Kubo T. Retroperitoneal lymph node dissection for testicular tumors using the thoracoabdominal approach. *Int Surg* 1993; **78**:154–8.
103. Skinner DG, Melamud A, Lieskovsky G. Complications of thoracoabdominal retroperitoneal lymph node dissection. *J Urol* 1982; **127**:1107–10.
104. Hartmann JT, Candelaria M, Kuczyk MA, Schmoll HJ, Bokemeyer C. Comparison of histological results from the resection of residual masses at different sites after chemotherapy for metastatic non-seminomatous germ cell tumours. *Eur J Cancer* 1997; **33**:843–7.
105. Beck SD, Foster RS, Bihrle R, Koch MO, Wahle GR, Donohue JP. Aortic replacement during post-chemotherapy retroperitoneal lymph node dissection. *J Urol* 2001; **165**:1517–20.
106. Christmas TJ, Smith GL, Kooner R. Vascular interventions during post-chemotherapy retroperitoneal lymph node dissection for metastatic testis cancer. *Eur J Surg Oncol* 1998; **24**(4):292–7.
107. Beck SD, Lalka SG. Long-term results after inferior vena cava resection during retroperitoneal lymphadenectomy for metastatic germ cell cancer. *J Vasc Surg* 1998; **28**:808–14.
108. Heidenreich A, Derakhshani P, Krug B, Engelmann UH. Evaluation of the inferior vena cava by magnetic resonance imaging in advanced testicular germ cell tumors. *Eur Urol* 1998; **49**:196.
109. Winter C, Pfister D, Busch J, *et al.* Residual tumor size and IGCCCG risk classification predict additional vascular procedures in patients with germ cell tumors and residual tumor resection: a multicenter analysis of the German Testicular Cancer Study Group. *Eur Urol* 2012; **61**(2):403–9.
110. Sonneveld DJ, Sleijfer DT, Koops HS, Keemers-Gels ME, Molenaar WM, Hoekstra HJ. Mature teratoma identified after postchemotherapy surgery in patients with disseminated nonseminomatous testicular germ cell tumors: a plea for an aggressive surgical approach. *Cancer* 1998; **82**:1343–51.
111. Hendry WF, Norman AR, Dearnaley DP, *et al.* Metastatic nonseminomatous germ cell tumors of the testis: results of elective and salvage surgery for patients with residual retroperitoneal masses. *Cancer* 2002; **94**:1668–76.
112. Wood DP, Herr HW, Heller G, *et al.* Distribution of retroperitoneal metastases after chemotherapy in patients with nonseminomatous germ cell tumors. *J Urol* 1992; **148**:1812–16.
113. Qvist HL, Fosså SD, Ous S, Hoie J, Stenwig AE, Giercksky KE. Post-chemotherapy tumor residuals in patients with advanced nonseminomatous testicular cancer. Is it necessary to resect all residual masses? *J Urol* 1991; **145**:300–2.
114. Rabbani F, Goldenberg SL, Gleave ME, Paterson RF, Murray N, Sullivan LD. Retroperitoneal lymphadenectomy for post-chemotherapy residual masses: is a modified dissection and resection of the residual mass sufficient? *Br J Urol* 1998; **81**:295–300.
115. Aprikian AG, Herr HW, Bajorin DF, Bosl GJ. Resection of postchemotherapy residual masses and limited retroperitoneal lymphadenectomy in patients with metastatic testicular nonseminomatous germ cell tumors. *Cancer* 1994; **74**:1329–34.
116. Herr HW. Does necrosis on frozen-section analysis of a mass after chemotherapy justify a limited retroperitoneal resection in patients with advanced testis cancer? *Br J Urol* 1997; **80**:653–7.
117. Ehrlich Y, Yossepovitch O, Kedar D, Baniel J. Distribution of nodal metastases after chemotherapy in nonseminomatous testis cancer: a possible indication for limited dissection. *BJU Int* 2006; **97**:1221–4.
118. Eggener SE, Carver BS, Loeb S, Kondagunta GV, Bosl GJ, Sheinfeld J. Pathologic findings and clinical outcome of patients undergoing retroperitoneal lymph node dissection after multiple chemotherapy regimes for metastatic testicular germ cell tumors. *Cancer* 2007; **109**:528–35.
119. Beck SD, Foster RS, Bihrle R, Donohue JP, Einhorn LH. Is full bilateral retroperitoneal lymph node dissection always necessary for postchemotherapy residual tumor? *Cancer* 2007; **110**:1235–40.
120. Heidenreich A, Pfister D, Witthuhn R, Thüer D, Albers P. Postchemotherapy retroperitoneal lymph node dissection in advanced testicular cancer: radical or modified template resection. *Eur Urol* 2009; **55**(1):217–24.
121. Waples MJ, Messing EM. Redo retroperitoneal lymphadenectomy for germ cell tumor. *Urology* 1993; **42**:1–4.
122. Cespedes RD, Peretsman SJ. Retroperitoneal recurrences after retroperitoneal lymph node dissection for low-stage nonseminomatous germ cell tumors. *Urology* 1999; **54**:548–52.
123. Sexton WJ, Wood CG, Kim R, Pisters LL. Repeat retroperitoneal lymph node dissection for metastatic testis cancer. *J Urol* 2003; **169**:1353–6.
124. McKiernan JM, Motzer RJ, Bajorin DF, Bacik J, Bosl GJ, Sheinfeld J. Reoperative retroperitoneal surgery for nonseminomatous germ cell tumor: clinical presentation, patterns of recurrence and outcome. *Urology* 2003; **62**:732–6.
125. Heidenreich A, Ohlmann C, Hegele A, Beyer J. Repeat retroperitoneal lymphadenectomy in advanced testicular cancer. *Eur Urol* 2005; **47**:64–71.
126. Albers P, Ganz A, Hannig E, Miersch WD, Müller SC. Salvage surgery of chemorefractory germ cell tumors with elevated markers. *J Urol* 2000; **164**:381–4.
127. Beck SD, Foster RS, Bihrle R, Einhorn LH, Donohue JP. Outcome analysis for patients with elevated serum tumor markers at postchemotherapy retroperitoneal lymph node dissection. *J Clin Oncol* 2005; **23**:6149–56.
128. Nash PA, Leibovitch I, Foster RS, Bihrle R. Rowland RG, Donohue JP. En bloc nephrectomy in patients undergoing post-chemotherapy retroperitoneal lymph node dissection for nonseminomatous testis cancer: indications, implications and outcomes. *J Urol* 1998; **159**:707–10.
129. Stephenson AJ, Tal R, Sheinfeld J. Adjunctive nephrectomy at post-chemotherapy retroperitoneal lymph node dissection for nonseminomatous germ cell testicular cancer. *J Urol* 2006; **176**:1996–9.
130. Heidenreich A, Seger M, Schrader AJ, Hofmann R, Engelmann UH. Surgical considerations in residual tumor resection following inductive chemotherapy for advanced testicular cancer. *Eur Urol* 2004; (Suppl 3):162.
131. Heidenreich A. Residual tumor resection following inductive chemotherapy in advanced testicular cancer. *Eur Urol* 2007; **51**:299–301
132. Leibovitch I, Mor Y, Golomb J, Ramon J. The diagnosis and management of postoperative chylous ascites. *J Urol* 2002; **167**:449–57.
133. Fizazi K, Tjulandin S, Salvioni R, *et al.* Viable malignant cells after primary chemotherapy for disseminated nonseminatous germ cell tumors: prognostic factors and role of postsurgery chemotherapy results from an international study. *J Clin Oncol* 2001; **19**:2647–57.

134. Fizazi K, Oldenburg J, Dunant A, *et al.* Assessing prognosis and optimizing treatment in patients with postchemotherapy viable nonseminomatous germ-cell tumors (NSGCT): results of the sCR2 international study. *Ann Oncol* 2008; **19**(2):259–64.
135. Spears WT, Morphis JG, Lester SG, *et al.* Brain metastases and testicular tumors: long-term survival. *Int J Radiat Oncol Biol Phys* 1991; **22**:17–22.
136. Kollmannsberger C, Nichols C, Bamberg M, *et al.* First-line high dose chemotherapy ± radiation in patients with metastatic germ-cell cancer and brain metastases. *Ann Oncol* 2000; **11**:553–9.
137. Oechsle K, Bokemeyer C. Treatment of brain metastases from germ cell tumors. *Hematol Oncol Clin North Am* 2011; **25**(3):605–13.

CHAPTER 6.36

Penile cancer

Rosa Djajadiningrat and Simon Horenblas

Introduction to penile cancer

Penile cancer is a rare malignancy, which is often associated with a long delay before diagnosis.[1,2] Reasons for this delay include perception of shame, fear, and ignorance. Squamous cell carcinoma accounts for more than 95% of penile malignancies. The pattern of dissemination is predominantly lymphogenic to the inguinal nodes. Localized squamous cell carcinoma can be cured in the most patients. But even with lymph node metastases cure is possible in a majority of patients. Prevention should be focussed on early management of phimosis, prevention of high-risk human papilloma virus (HPV) infection and on health education for laymen and physicians. The low incidence poses a challenge for clinicians as many aspects in the management are based on a limited amount of scientific evidence.

Epidemiology and aetiology

Penile cancer is rare in Western countries, accounting for less than 1% of male cancers. This number can be as high as 10% in Asia, Africa, and South America.[3] The substantial worldwide variation in penile cancer incidences is most likely due to the differences in socio-economic conditions and religious practices like neonatal circumcision.[4] Penile cancer occurs predominantly in elderly men, although the disease may also occasionally present in young men. The mean age at diagnosis of patients is 60 years.[5,6]

Risk factors

The aetiology of penile cancer is multifactorial and several risk factors are identified with an association with its development. Established risk factors include phimosis, HPV infection, smoking, age, chronic inflammatory conditions such as lichen sclerosis, psoralen-UV-A photochemotherapy, penile injury, genital warts, and HIV infection.

Circumcision

The most important risk factor for penile cancer is non-circumcision of the penis. Current estimates have suggested that over 25% of all men worldwide are circumcised.[7] Penile cancer is rarely seen in populations who routinely practice circumcision during the neonatal or childhood period.[7–10] The positive effect of circumcision is mainly explained by preventing conditions such as poor hygiene, smegma retention, and phimosis, which have been reported as risk factors for penile cancer.[8,10,11] Phimosis, or narrowness of the opening of the foreskin, leads invariably to the retention of normally desquamated epidermal cells and urinary products (smegma) resulting in conditions of chronic irritation with of without bacterial inflammation of the prepuce and the glans.[12–14] The main causes of acquired phimosis are chronic inflammation, balanoposthitis, forceful foreskin retraction, lichen sclerosis, and diabetes mellitus.

Human papillomavirus

A major risk factor for penile carcinoma is infection with human papillomavirus (HPV). Risk of infection with HPV is increased by number of sexual partners, history of genital warts, or other sexually transmitted diseases.[11] Interestingly, the HPV prevalence is lower in circumcised men compared to those who have not been circumcised.[15,16] Some studies have shown an association between HPV and penile cancer comparable to that of cervical cancer, where HPV has been considered responsible for almost all cases. For penile cancer, the role of high-risk HPV infection seems to vary between 30–100%.[8,17,18] HPV 16, HPV 18, and HPV 45 are the most common oncogenic subtypes. Of all HPV subtypes in penile cancer, HPV-16 is the predominant subtype, found in 60–63% of the cases. The prognostic value of HPV expression and penile cancer remains unclear with conflicting data in several studies.[11,19–22]

Smoking

Smoking shows a dose-dependent association with penile cancer. The use of any form of tobacco is a risk factor for the development of penile cancer.[10,11,23] The risk of penile cancer among men who smoke at diagnosis is 2.8 times higher than among men who have never smoked.[8] The exact mechanism is not understood.

Chronic inflammatory conditions

Inflammation may represent a critical component in tumour development or progression as many penile cancers arise at sites of infection, chronic irritation, or injury. A chronic inflammatory skin disorder that is restricted to the glans and foreskin is lichen sclerosis et atrophicus (LS) or synonymous, balanitis xerotica obliterans (BXO). It occurs almost exclusively in uncircumcised men and has been associated with phimosis.[24] It presents most commonly in men between 30–40 years. Initially, Lichen sclerosis et atrophicus (LS) was considered a benign condition, however, histological progression from chronic inflammation to dysplasia and eventually to malignant transformation has been reported.[25–27] Although LS is considered to be a premalignant condition in the European guidelines, the precancerous nature is not well established.[26–28] In vulvar cancer, lichen sclerosis has shown more definitively to progress to invasive cancer in 4-5% of cases.[29]

Psoralen ultraviolet photochemotherapy

Patients with psoriasis undergoing psoralen ultraviolet photochemotherapy (PUVA) have an increased risk for the development of penile cancer.[30] Here also there is a strong dose-dependent relation.

Genital warts and HIV infection

Men with a history of genital warts have an almost six times higher risk of developing penile cancer than men who have no risk of warts.[8] Likewise, there is an eightfold increased risk of penile cancer in patients with HIV, although this might be related to the higher incidence of HPV among men with HIV.[31]

Clinical features

Penile cancer has been associated with significant delay in presentation. Presentation varies from an area of induration to an ulcer or a papillary exophytic growth (see Fig. 6.36.1). With continued neglect, the lesion advances until a purulent discharge is seen exuding from beneath a frequently phimotic, non-retractive prepuce. Phimosis can obscure a lesion and allow a tumour to progress silently. Finally, the disease penetrates Buck's fascia and the tunica albuginea and extends along the penile shaft to involve the corpora cavernosa. Penile squamous cell carcinoma (SCC) has a strong tendency for lymphatic dissemination, with hematogenic spread predominately in cases with advanced lymphatic invasion.[32] Without treatment, patients with penile SCC will develop metastases and usually die within two years after diagnosis of the primary lesion. In general, patients die because of the locoregional uncontrollable process rather than from distant metastases.

Invasive penile carcinoma initially occurs on the glans (48%), prepuce (25%), glans and prepuce (9%), coronal sulcus (6%), and shaft (2%). Squamous cell carcinoma of the penis subsequently invades local structures, corpora cavernosa, and the urethra.[33] The most reliable way of diagnosis is a biopsy.

The inguinal lymph nodes are the first site of metastasis followed by the pelvic nodes and sometimes the retroperitoneal nodes. Metastatic sites that are rarely involved are liver, lungs, and bones (1–10%).[33,34]

Patients with advanced disease can present with symptoms associated with metastatic disease such as generalized weakness, weight loss, pain, or hypercalcaemia.[35]

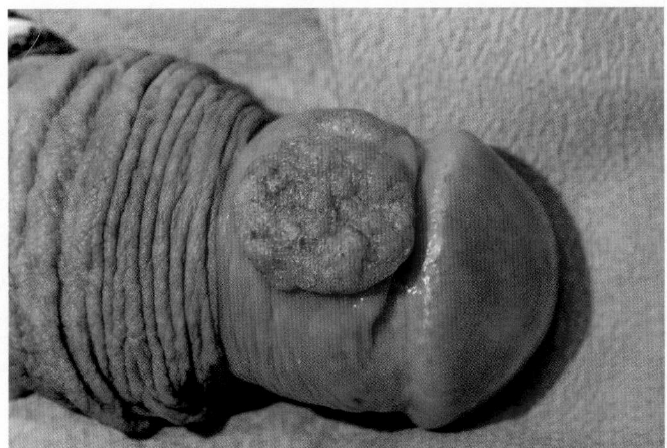

Fig. 6.36.1 Primary papillary tumour of the penile shaft.

Pathology and staging

The most commonly used staging system in penile carcinoma is the 2009 TNM classification (Table 6.36.1). Virtually all penile carcinomas are of squamous cell origin and include the following subtypes: verrucous carcinoma, warty carcinoma (verruciform) and, basaloid carcinoma, papillary, and sarcomatoid carcinomas.[36–38] Although they are less common subtypes, warty carcinoma, and basaloid carcinoma appear to be more highly associated with HPV, than typical squamous cell carcinoma or verrucous carcinoma of the penis. Histopathologic grading is based on the amount of cellular anaplasia seen within the tumour on histopatholical examination according to Broders.[39] Grade 1 is well differentiated, grade 2 is moderately differentiated and grade 3 is poorly differentiated.

Recently, the TNM classification system for penile cancer was updated. The important changes in the new system are subcategorization of T1 into T1a and T1b based on grade and presence of lymphovascular invasion (LVI). This identifies patients with a high- and low-risk for lymph node involvement.

The classification needs a further update for the definition of T2 category, as recent publications have shown prognostic differences for corpus spongiosum invasion and corpus cavernosum invasion, being worse in the latter.[40,41] Furthermore, the N-category is revised with extracapsular nodal extension as a poor prognosticator.[42–44]

Physical examination

Physical examination of the primary penile lesion should evaluate and document the number of lesions, tumour dimensions, sites involved (foreskin, glans, shaft), morphology (flat, papillary, nodular, ulcerating, fungating), relationship with other structures (corpus spongiosum, corpora cavernosa, urethra), boundaries, and penile length.[45,46] The groins should be palpated and in case of lymphadenopathy the following points have to be assessed: node consistency, node location, diameter of nodes or masses, unilateral, or bilateral location, number of nodes identified in each inguinal area, mobile or fixed node or masses, relationship (infiltration or perforation) to other structures, such as the skin, vascular structures and oedema of leg and/or scrotum.

The accuracy of palpation alone is not sufficient to select patients in whom inguinal lymphadenectomy is necessary. Palpable inguinal lymphadenopathy is present at diagnosis in 30–60% of patients.[47] In about 70% of these patients, this is caused by metastatic invasion and in the other 30% by inflammatory reactions. The easiest way to confirm lymph node metastases in patients with palpable nodes is by fine needle aspiration cytology. Note that the result is only reliable if positive, false-negative rates are reported up to 29%.[48,49] If negative, another fine needle aspiration is recommended as soon as possible. If negative again and in the presence of clinical suspicion, an excisional biopsy is advised. Occult nodal metastasis is present in approximately 20% of patients presenting with impalpable nodes.[50,51]

Management of primary tumour

Surgical resection has been the mainstay of treatment in penile carcinoma. The goals of treatment are cure, organ preservation, and avoidance of disease, and treatment related morbidity. Traditionally, amputation or radiotherapy has been the cornerstone of treatment of penile cancer. Amputation definitely provides excellent locoregional control, but unfortunately it is associated with urinary and

Table 6.36.1 2009 TNM classification of penile cancer

Clinical classification			
T-	**Primary tumour**		
	TX	Primary tumour cannot be assessed	
	T0	No evidence of primary tumour	
	Tis	Carcinoma *in situ*	
	Ta	Non-invasive verrucous carcinoma, not associated with destructive invasion	
	T1	Tumour invades subepithelial connective tissue	
		T1a	Tumour invades subepithelial connective tissue without lymphovascular invasion and is not poorly differentiated or undifferentiated (T1G1-2)
		T1b	Tumour invades subepithelial connective tissue with lymphovascular invasion or is poorly differentiated or undifferentiated (T1G3-4)
	T2*	Tumour invades corpus spongiosum/corpora cavernosa	
	T3	Tumour invades urethra	
	T4	Tumour invades adjacent structures	
N-	**Regional lymph nodes**		
	NX	Regional lymph nodes cannot be assessed	
	N0	No palpable or visibly enlarged inguinal lymph node	
	N1	Palpable mobile unilateral inguinal lymph node	
	N2	Palpable mobile multiple or bilateral inguinal lymph nodes	
	N3	Fixed inguinal nodal mass or pelvic lymphadenopathy, unilateral or bilateral	
M-	**Distant metastasis**		
	M0	No distant metastasis	
	M1	Distant metastasis	
Pathological classification			
The pT categories correspond to the T categories. The pN categories are based upon biopsy or surgical excision			
pN-	**Regional lymph nodes**		
	pNx	Regional lymph nodes cannot be assessed	
	pN0	No regional lymph nodes metastasis	
	pN1	Intranodal metastasis	
	pN2	Metastasis in multiple or bilateral inguinal lymph nodes	
	pN3	Metastasis in pelvic lymph node(s), unilateral or bilateral of extranodal extension of regional lymph node metastasis	
pM-	**Distant metastasis**		
	pM0	No distant metastasis	
	pM1	Distant metastasis	
G	**Histopathological grading**		
	Gx	Grade of differentiation cannot be assessed	
	G1	Well differentiated	
	G2	Moderately differentiated	
	G3-4	Poorly differentiated or undifferentiated	

**The definition of the T2 category needs a further update. Two recent publications have shown that the prognosis for corpus spongiosum invasion is much better than for corpora cavernosum invasion.*

Reproduced with permission from TNM Online: Leslie H. Sobin, Mary K. Gospodarowicz, and Christian Wittekind (Eds.), *TNM Classification of Malignant* Tumours, Seventh Edition; Christian Wittekind, *TNM Supplement: A Commentary on Uniform Use, Fourth Edition*; and Mary K. Gospodarowicz, Brian O'Sullivan, and Leslie H. Sobin (Eds.), *Prognostic Factors in Cancer, Third Edition*, Copyright © 1999-2014 by John Wiley and Sons,available from http://onlinelibrary.wiley.com/book/10.1002/9780471420194

sexual dysfunction, just as a significant psychological morbidity.[52] Penile-preserving techniques have been developed without jeopardizing oncological results combined with minimal loss of anatomy and function, minimizing the devastating psychosexual effect in patients.

Non-surgical management

Non-surgical approaches are mainly reserved for superficial lesions like premalignant lesions, carcinoma *in situ*, and Ta lesions. Non-surgical therapies include the use of topical chemotherapy, immunotherapy, and photodynamic therapy. Topical options are 5-fluorouracil cream and imiquimod. 5-fluorouracil is a chemotherapeutical cream, which can be applied directly on the penis for four to six weeks. Imiquimod 5% is a locally applied immune modulator. Small series showed moderately effectiveness with little toxicity.[53]

Laser therapy

Laser therapy is an elegant organ-preserving option with excellent cosmetic and functional results for superficial lesions. Either a CO_2-laser or a neodymium:YAG (Nd:YAG) laser can be used. The greatest difference between these two lasers is their tissue penetration. The Nd:YAG laser tends to penetrate deeper than the CO_2-laser in human tissue with a 4–6 mm cutting depth. It is a very well-tolerated procedure, but this treatment shows high overall local recurrence rates, which makes retreatment necessary. A wide variety of recurrence rates have been described, ranging from 6.3% to 42%[54–59] Complications occur in 1–7% and include bleeding, moderate pain, and preputial lymphedema.[54,56,60] Laser therapy is mainly used for carcinoma *in situ*, but is also used to treat invasive disease (smaller than half of the glans).[61]

Local excision

The most common treatment for superficial penile carcinoma is local excision with of without circumcision.[61,62] Primary closure of the defect is possible if the lesion is small. Local excision of T1 tumours located at the midshaft is also possible.

Circumcision

Circumcision alone is very effective for the treatment of lesions that affect the foreskin only (T1G1-3) and spare the glans.[35] Recurrence rates are as high as 30–50% for circumcision alone.[63]

Moh's micrographic surgery

Moh's microsurgery is a minimally invasive option for superficial tumours initially performed in 1930 and now used in multiple malignancies. Tissue is consecutive sliced in thin layers and immediately reviewed under microscopy to secure microscopic tumour-negative margins.[64] However, also in this procedure relatively high recurrence rates have been described.[65]

Total glans resurfacing

Total glans resurfacing is a technique where the epithelium is removed and replaced with a skin graft.[66] This approach allows preservation of maximal penile length, form, and function with excellent oncological control. Graft take is good, and the cosmetic appearance six weeks after surgery is excellent. The most relevant complication is graft necrosis.

Glans amputation

Patients with T2 lesions of the glans are eligible total glansectomy, as opposed to the traditional partial amputation. An alternative treatment for very carefully selected patients is partial glansectomy of tumours encompassing less than half of the glans.

Traditionally, a 20 mm macroscopic clear margin proximal to the lesion was required, but there was no evidence to support this conception. Two studies regarding margins showed that oncological control could also be achieved with a margin of only a few millimetres.[67,68]

Glans amputation aims at removing only the glans, leaving the corpora cavernosa intact.[69] The exposed corporal heads can be covered with a skin graft that has been quilted to the corpora to prevent hematoma formation.[70,71]

Also the urethra can be used by everting the urethral mucosa to cover the corpora tips, the shaft skin is sutured closely to it, and no split-thickness graft is necessary.[72]

Partial penectomy

Patients with tumours involving the glans penis or distal penile shaft, not suitable for penile-preserving therapies should be treated with a partial penectomy. These are mostly patients presenting with palpable penile lesions extended from to glans penis to the distal tunica albuginea and corpus cavernosum. The aim is to ensure tumour removal with adequate tumour-free margins, while preserving enough length for the patient to void in standing position and to continue sexual activity.

A circumcoronal incision of the penile shaft skin is made with partial degloving of the penis. Once the skin and the superficial fascial layers are dissected, Bucks fascia is identified. The area where the corpus cavernosum is going to be transacted is marked. The neurovascular bundle is mobilized, ligated, and divided prior to the transaction of the penis. A tourniquet placed at the base of the penis will minimize the bleeding when transecting the corpus cavernosum. If transacted, the corpora are mobilized off the non-involved urethra and the urethra will then be divided ensuring that it is approximately two centimetres longer than the corporal margins in order to unable adequate spatulation of the urethra. The corpora are over sewn and the tourniquet can be released. The urethra is spatulated dorsally and sutured to the corporal margins. The penile skin is brought forward and used to cover the corporal tips. A skin graft can be used if there is paucity of penile skin. The most common complication of partial penectomy is meatal stenosis (3.5–9%).[61,73]

Total penectomy

Total penectomy is the therapy for patients where tumour involvement is so extensive that the penile shaft necessitates complete excision of penis and crura to achieve tumour-free margins. The urethra is redirected to the perineum (perineal urethrostomy). The skin and the superficial fascia are divided. The penis is mobilized and the deep dorsal vein and neurovascular bundle are ligated and divided. The suspensory ligament is divided and the dissection continues proximately. For the creation of a perineal urethrostomy a separate inverted U-incision is made in the perineum. The urethra is identified and mobilized. Ensuring that there is an adequate urethral length, the urethra is transected and spatulated ventrally in order to allow the tip of the U to be incorporated ventrally. The crura are followed until de pubic bone and completely separated off the pubic bone. The dorsal artery has to be identified and ligated. The remnants of the crura are oversewn and the skin is the sutured to the urethra. Similar to partial amputation the most common complication is meatal stenosis.[61,73]

Local recurrence

The definition of local recurrence differs between authors and can be defined as follows: the same cancer was left behind, consequently residual disease occurs after primary surgery, or a synchronous recurrence; that is secondary tumour was already present, or a metachronous recurrence (i.e. a new cancer developed simultaneously).

The local recurrence rate after partial or total penectomy is 4%.[61,73–76] Recurrences after penis preserving therapies vary from 9-50%.[65,70–72,77] In surgical penile-preserving therapies, positive surgical margins are the most predictive factor for local recurrence.[54,57,61] In addition, in penile-preserving techniques glans skin can be left behind that has potential for developing cancer. Most local recurrences develop during the first two to three years after treatment. Often local recurrences are treated with another penile-sparing therapy with partial penectomy preserved for more extensive recurrences.[70,71,77] Local recurrence does not seem to have an effect on survival.[57,61]

Management of lymph nodes

The presence of nodal involvement is the single most important prognostic factor in penile SCC.[2,42–44,51,78,79] The first draining lymph nodes (the 'first-echelon' or 'sentinel' nodes) are invariably within the inguinal lymphatic region. Thereafter, dissemination is to the pelvic nodes and/or distant sites. At initial presentation, distant metastases are present in only 1–2% of patients. Generally, patients with distant metastasis have also clinical evidence of (at least) inguinal nodal involvement.[32] Primary haematogenic spread has only been seen in sarcomatoid subtypes only.[80] Therefore, preoperative staging focuses primarily on the locoregional situation.

There is no controversy about the need for lymphadenectomy in patients with clinical evident nodal involvement. However, the optimal management of clinically node-negative (cN0) patients is subject of debate, since non-invasive staging techniques are limited in detecting small metastatic deposits. Approximately 20–25% of these cN0 patients have occult metastasis.[50] Current imaging techniques such as ultrasound, computed tomography (CT) and positron emission tomography (PET), as well as risk prediction based on primary tumour characteristics, have so far been unable to identify cN0 patients with occult metastases within reasonable limits.[48,81,82]

Removal of nodal metastases at the earliest possible time, preferably in patients with impalpable lymph nodes and microscopic invasion only, improves survival considerably compared with surgical removal at the time when metastases become clinically apparent.[80] Some clinicians manage these cN0 patients with close surveillance, while others treat them with an elective inguinal node dissection based upon 'risk-adapted approaches'.[83] While the former may lead to unintentional delay because of outgrowth of occult metastases in 20–25% of cN0 patients, the latter results in unnecessary lymph node dissection in 75–80% of cases, because of absence of metastasis.[84] Moreover, inguinal lymphadenectomy is associated with a high morbidity rate. Up to 35–70% of patients have short- or long-term complications.[85–88]

Lymphatic drainage of the penis

The primary drainage of penile SCC is to the lymph nodes in the groin, and secondary drainage is to the lymph nodes in the pelvis. Bilateral inguinal drainage is considered the normal lymphatic anatomy of the penis. The anatomy of the inguinal nodes has been described by various authors.[89–91] It is customary to divide inguinal nodes into two groups: superficial and deep. The superficial nodes are located beneath Scarpa's fascia and above the fascia lata covering the muscles of the thigh; around 8 to 25 nodes are present. There are three to five deep inguinal lymph nodes and these are situated around the fossa ovalis, the opening in the fascia lata where the saphenous vein drains into the femoral vein. The deep inguinal nodes connect the superficial nodes to the pelvic nodes. The deep inguinal nodes receive their afferents from the superficial nodes and directly from the deeper structures of the penis. The distinction of superficial and deep inguinal lymph nodes is clinically irrelevant since physical examination (palpation) cannot discern these anatomical entities from each other.[47]

The so-called 'node of Cloquet' or 'Rosenmüller' is the most constant and usually largest inguinal node, located just underneath the inguinal ligament and medially to the femoral vein. Daseler *et al.* divided the inguinal region into five sections by drawing a horizontal and vertical line through the point where the saphenous vein drains into the femoral vein with one central zone directly overlying the junction.[92] With some individual variation, the nodes that are most frequently involved in penile SCC are typically located in Daseler's superiomedial section.[93] Skip metastases, circumventing the inguinal lymphatic region, to the pelvic lymph nodes are extremely rare and probably anecdotal.[94,95] The pelvic nodes are located around the iliac vessels and in the obturator fossa, approximately 12–20.

Dynamic sentinel node biopsy

Sentinel lymph node biopsy is a fairly new technique in medical practice that is becoming the standard of care for regional lymph node staging of many solid tumours. This technique is based on the hypothesis of step-wise distribution of malignant cells in the lymphatic system. The absence of tumour cells in the first lymph node(s) in the lymphatic drainage of the tumour indicates the absence of further spread in regional lymph node basin(s). Sentinel lymph node biopsy is the preferred method of lymph node staging in melanoma and breast cancer.[96] This procedure has been included in the 2009 European Association of Urology guidelines on penile cancer.[40]

Since 1994, dynamic sentinel node biopsy (DSNB) has been performed at the authors' institution to stage cN0-patients.[97]

The best definition of a sentinel node is probably that of Morton: '... the first lymph node that receives afferent drainage from a primary tumor'.[98] It is important to realize, that there is individual variation in the location of the sentinel node. Moreover, although the location is usually in the area traditionally known as the regional lymph node basin, aberrant locations can be seen in a minority of patients. Also more than one sentinel node can be present. All these variations can only be found if one combines all the preoperative information from the lymphoscintigraphy with the findings during surgery.

Lymphoscintigraphy

To localize the sentinel node preoperatively, lymphoscintigraphy is usually performed after intradermal peritumoral injection of colloid particles labelled with technetium-99m. The tracer is transported through the lymphatic channels to the first draining nodes in the groin and made visible on the lymphoscintigram as a 'hot spot'. Lymph node uptake is based on the ingestion of the colloid particles by the macrophages. Lymphoscintigraphy is usually performed the day or morning before surgery.

Guided by the imaging, the location of the sentinel node is marked on the skin to enable peroperative localization using the handheld gamma ray detection probe, usually the following day.[99] Lymphoscintigraphy has been shown to be a very reproducible mode of imaging. In a study of 20 patients, 2 separate lymphoscintigrams were made and compared. There was virtually 100% concordance between the two studies.[100] Recently, hybrid SPECT-CT scanners have become available, allowing for the mapping of lymphatic drainage, after injection with a radioactive tracer, with unprecedented detail and in relation to anatomical landmarks obtained from the CT images (see Fig. 6.36.2).

Perioperatively, patent blue dye can visualize lymphatic vessels and helps to differentiate sentinel nodes from second-echelon nodes (see Fig. 6.36.3). However, the use of blue dye alone is insufficient to reliably detect sentinel nodes. Differences between lymphatic mapping with radio-labelled colloid and blue dye occur fairly often.[101–103] The two lymphatic mapping techniques are complementary. If only blue dye was used, almost 30% of the sentinel nodes would have been missed, because almost all harvested sentinel nodes were hot, whereas only about 70% were blue as well.

Lymphadenectomy: indication

Surgery remains the treatment of choice in patients with metastatic disease in the groins. Cure can be attained in approximately 80% of patients who have one or two involved inguinal nodes without extranodal extension. Ipsilateral inguinal lymphadenectomy

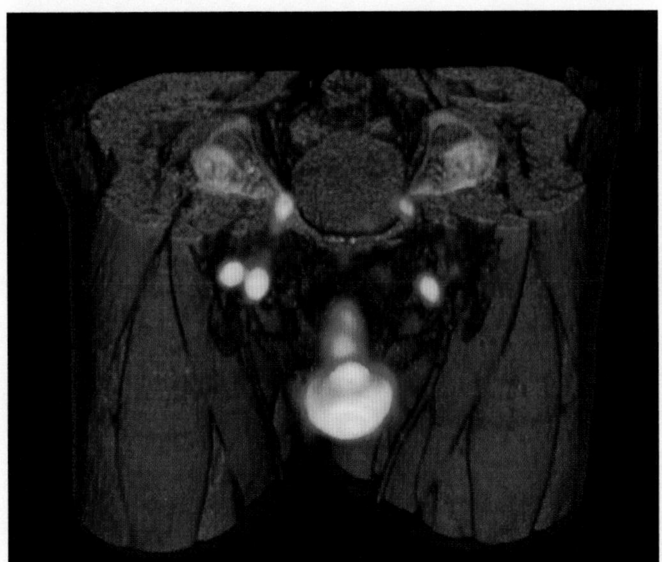

Fig. 6.36.2 SPECT/CT after administration of radioactive tracer showing two sentinel nodes in the right groin and one in the left groin.

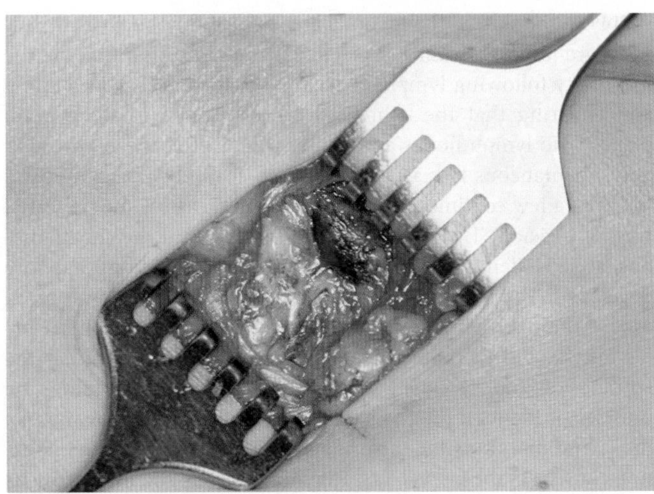

Fig. 6.36.3 Perioperative illustration of a blue sentinel node in the groin with a blue lymphatic duct.

is indicated when tumour-bearing lymph nodes are found with DSNB, fine needle aspiration cytology (FNAC), or excision biopsy. Previous studies have suggested that the likelihood of bilateral inguinal involvement is related to the number of involved nodes in the unilateral resected inguinal specimen.[44,51] With two or more metastases the probability of occult lateral involvement is 30% and this may warrant an early contralateral inguinal lymphadenectomy. Currently, ultrasound-guided FNAC and DSNB are used to solve this problem in the authors' institute in those patients presenting with unilateral positive nodes. Patients with contralateral groins with tumour-negative sentinel nodes are kept under close surveillance.

Approximately 20–30% of all patients with positive inguinal nodes harbour tumour-positive pelvic nodes.[44,79,104] Although patients with pelvic lymph node involvement are considered to have a poor outcome, pelvic lymphadenectomy can be curative in some patients. Particularly patients with occult pelvic metastases benefit. Several studies have shown that the likelihood of pelvic nodal involvement is related to the number of positive nodes in the inguinal specimen and presence of nodal extension.[25,37–42] At the authors' institute a pelvic dissection is considered unnecessary in patients with one intranodal inguinal metastasis. In all other patients with two or more inguinal nodes involved or extranodal extension, an ipsilateral pelvic lymphadenectomy is performed. Contralateral pelvic lymphadenectomy is not recommended, since there is no evidence that cross-over from groin to the contralateral pelvic area does occur.[51,79,104] Therefore, contralateral pelvic lymphadenectomy is not recommended in patients with unilateral nodal involvement. Patients with preoperative evidence of pelvic metastases are unlikely to be cured by surgery alone and are candidates for neoadjuvant chemotherapy before undergoing surgery (see later in this chapter).[105]

Inguinal lymphadenectomy

Several surgical approaches have been described in order to minimize the complications associated with the procedure. The patient is placed supine with the legs abducted and externally rotated. A variety of incisions can be used. For inguinal node dissection the incisions can be divided into horizontal and vertical. The vascular supply to the skin of the inguinal area is such that horizontal incisions are preferred over vertical ones. The key to minimizing the morbidity following lymphadenectomy is correct tissue handling and ensuring that the skin flaps are developed in the correct plane.[51] No lymph nodes are found in the layer between the skin and subcutaneous fascia. At the authors' institute a para-inguinal incision, a few centimetres below the groin crease, is the preferred type of incision. The skin should be incised until the subcutaneous fascia is identified. Then the proximal and distal skin flaps are developed. The boundaries of the dissection are as follows: proximally, the inguinal ligament; distally, the crossing of the sartorius muscle and the adductor longus muscle (also referred as the entrance of Hunter's canal, where the femoral vessels go under the muscles of the leg); the medial boundary is the adductor muscle; the lateral margin is the sartorius muscle. The floor of the dissection consists of the fascia lata, the femoral vessels and the pectineus muscle (see Fig. 6.36.4). As the femoral nerve is located beneath the fascia lata, it is not seen during standard lymphadenectomy. Since inguinal lymphadenectomy can be a curative procedure, it is important to meticulously remove all of the lymphatic tissue. After performing the dissection, the skin edges are carefully inspected; any area with doubtful viability should be excised. There are no comparative studies on the use of antibiotics but it seems reasonable to give prophylactic antibiotics at the time of surgery, as this type of surgery should be considered a contaminated procedure, because of coexisting inflammatory reactions within the lymph nodes. Prior to closing the wound, suction drains are inserted in order to prevent lymphocele formation. Postoperative antibiotic use is variable among surgeons performing the procedure. Some centres continue antibiotics until the drain is removed. After one week the vacuum is removed and spontaneous drainage observed. Drains are removed if the drainage is <50 mL/day although some centres wait until it is <30mL/day. Immediately after surgery ambulation is strongly advised and supported with individually fitted elastic stockings. Skin closure following lymphadenectomy can be difficult in patients with extensive metastatic disease with overlying skin involvement. The skin involved should be excised, although inevitably, this leaves a large defect. Various methods can be used to manage this surgical problem. After a sartorius transposition the wound can heal by secondary intention. Healing can be improved and hastened by a split skin graft on the granulation tissue. Another method is the so-called 'skin-stretch' method[106]; by gradually increasing the pressure on the skin edges in a cyclic fashion, large skin defects are closed with no tension. Island flaps that can be useful for closure are the rectus abdominis pedicle, gracilis pedicle, and the tensor fascia lata pedicle.[107,108] In cases of en-bloc removal, scrotal skin and mobilized abdominal wall can be used to assist in the closure of the defect. The femoral vessels can be protected by transposition of the scrotal content and suturing the scrotal content to the inguinal ligament.

Pelvic lymphadenectomy

Pelvic lymphadenectomy can be undertaken simultaneously at the time of inguinal node dissection or as a separate procedure. In the first scenario, removal of the lymph nodes using one or two incisions has been described; most authors prefer two separate incisions. A comparison of the various types of incisions has shown that the lowest complication rate occurs when two separate incisions are used.[86,87] The pelvic node dissection is undertaken either through a lower abdominal midline incision or a unilateral muscle splitting incision. The boundaries of the pelvic node dissection are proximally, the common iliac vessels; distally, the passage of lymphatic vessels to the groin; laterally, the ilioinguinal nerve; medially, the bladder and prostate; and the base is the deepest part of the obturator fossa. Care must be taken to completely remove the obturator fossa, especially the space behind the external iliac vessels, all the way to the sacrum. A large node can usually be found there and if left is prone to recurrence with intractable pain, because of neural in growth. After the dissection suction drains are left in place.

Complications of lymph node dissection

The morbidity (complication rate) from lymphadenectomy limits its applicability to all patients. The reported complication rate varies from 35% to 88%[85–88] and is increased by pelvic node dissection

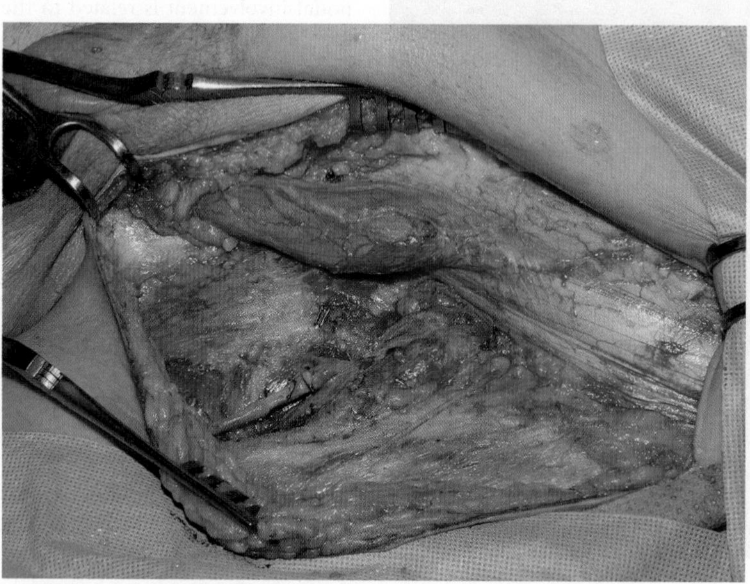

Fig. 6.36.4 Anatomical boundaries of an inguinal lymph node dissection.

and radiotherapy.[79,87] The most commonly cited complications are wound infection (15 ± 10%), skin necrosis with or without wound dehiscence (14 ± 50%), lymphocele/seroma formation (10 ± 10%), lymphoedema (27 ± 30%), and other complications including haemorrhage, thrombosis, and even death. Although a recent series has shown that the complications rate of lymphadenectomy has decreased, the incidence and magnitude of complications appears to remain significant with a complication rate of 58% per patient.[88]

Minimizing the morbidity of lymphadenectomy

Standard lymphadenectomy consists of the removal of all lymph nodes in the inguinal region. Recent lymphoscintigraphical and anatomical data indicate that limiting the dissection field to the central and craniomedial part may provide sufficient oncological control.[93,104] Further mapping studies are necessary to test the safety of this modified lymphadenectomy template. Moreover, to be of real clinical value, there should be evidence of a reduction in the complication rate. An alternative option which could minimize the morbidity associated with the procedure involves minimal invasive techniques like video endoscopic inguinal lymphadenectomy (VEIL). Some small series have now shown promising results with lower complication rates compared with an open procedure. Tobias-Machado *et al.* have reported their initial results of 10 patients without palpable lymph nodes who underwent VEIL on one side and the standard open approach on the contralateral side. Although operative times were longer with the endoscopic approach compared with the open method, the mean numbers of retrieved and tumour-positive lymph nodes were similar. Moreover, there was a trend towards decreased postoperative morbidity. In another study reporting on their expanding experience, the VEIL approach led also to a significant decreased hospital stay (mean of 1 day vs. 6.4 days in patients who had undergone standard lymphadenectomy on one limb).[109] The robot assisted procedures have also recently been published in a case report.[110]

Management of complications

After removing the suction drains a lymphocele can develop in 10–20% of patients. This can usually be managed by outpatient aspiration with a large needle and a large syringe. After natural resolution of the space in which the lymphocele develops, the accumulation of lymphatic fluid stops. Large wound defects can be closed using a so-called vacuum assisted closure (VAC) system. A sponge is inserted in the wound and sealed with plastic and a draining tube is attached to a low vacuum pump. Excellent results have been obtained, decreasing the time to secondary healing. If the defect remains large a split skin graft can be laid on top of the granulation tissue.

Despite the use of elastic stockings, lymphedema can still develop in approximately 10% of patients, especially those in whom extensive surgery together with radiation therapy was necessary because of the burden of disease. Supporting therapy includes lymph massage and compression therapy. Surgical therapy using lymphatic-venous anastomies have not been entirely successful. Legs with lymphedema are infection prone, especially with streptococcus A bacteria, leading to erisypelas. At the author's institution antibiotic prophylaxis with monthly penicillin depots is strongly advised after two bouts of erisypelas-like infections.

Adjuvant radiotherapy

Although no randomized studies comparing different treatment options are available, radiation therapy has been offered as an adjuvant therapy to inguinal nodes patients after lymphadenectomy to improve locoregional tumour control. This is in compliance with adjuvant radiotherapy in head and neck squamous cell carcinomas showing improvement of regional control.[111] Patients eligible for this, are patients with extensive metastases and/or extranodal spread, but control is achieved at the cost of severe side effects as severe oedema and pain.

Advanced disease

Locally advanced disease

Some patients delay treatment and seek care only when disease is far advanced with extensive local and/or regionally involvement. Sometimes these lesions have led to bulky fungating masses that have eroded the epidermis and destructed large amounts of surrounding tissues.

The only option for direct palliation is often surgical removal of all diseased tissue. Such surgery often leads to large wound defects with sometimes exposure of femoral artery and veins which can be

(A)
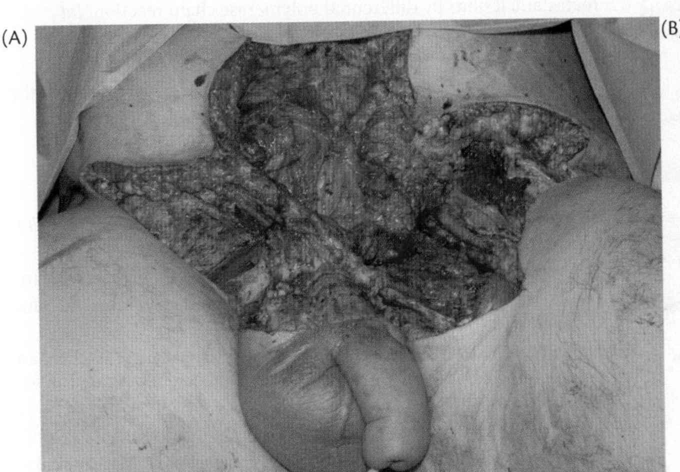

(B)
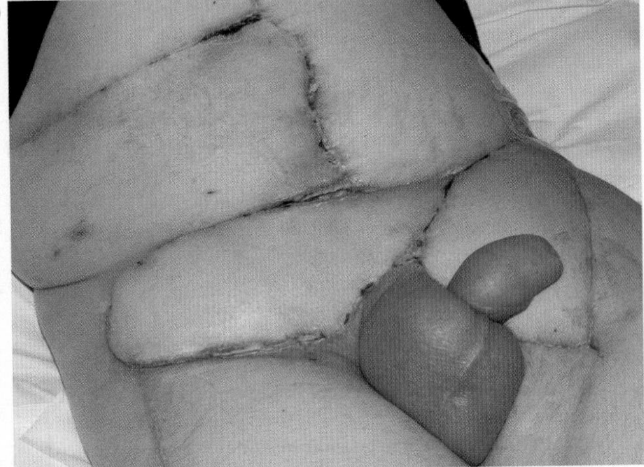

Fig. 6.36.5 (A) Large defect after surgical removal of bulky metastasis; and (B) Vertical rectus abdominis myocutaneous flap covering the defect.

covered using pedicled skin flaps. Primary closure may be obtained by scrotal skin flaps,[112] abdominal wall advancement flap,[113] or a myocutaneous flap based on the tensior fascia lata,[108] or the rectus abdominis for more extensive defects.[107,114] The latter is most used in the authors' institute (see Fig. 6.36.5). Results regarding cure are disappointing, however.

Role of neoadjuvant chemotherapy

In locally advanced cases, induction chemotherapy followed by surgery is an option. Due to rarity of disease, no randomized controlled trials are available. Small studies have demonstrated modest efficacy of bleomycin, methotrexate, cisplatin, and 5-FU, either as single agents or as combination therapy.[32] Recently, taxanes have been introduced as chemotherapeutic agent, after showing good results in advanced head and neck squamous cell carcinomas.[115] Promising therapeutic results have been obtained with taxane-based (T) therapy in combination with cisplatin-fluorouracil (PF)[116] for salvage of primarily unresectable or relapsed nodal metastases. Taxanes in combination with ifosfamide and cisplatin demonstrated clinically meaningful responses in patients with bulky regional lymph nodes.[117,118]

Further reading

Bleeker MC, Heideman DA, Snijders PJ, Horenblas S, Dillner J, Meijer CJ. Penile cancer: epidemiology, pathogenesis and prevention. *World J Urol* 2009; **27**(2):141–50.

Cubilla AL. The role of pathologic prognostic factors in squamous cell carcinoma of the penis. *World J Urol* 2009 Apr; **27**(2):169–77.

Culkin DJ, Beer TM. Advanced penile carcinoma. *J Urol* 2003; **170**(2 Pt 1): 359–65.

Daling JR, Madeleine MM, Johnson LG, *et al.* Penile cancer: importance of circumcision, human papillomavirus and smoking in in situ and invasive disease. *Int J Cancer* 2005; **116**(4):606–16.

Deem S, Keane T, Bhavsar R, El-Zawahary A, Savage S. Contemporary diagnosis and management of squamous cell carcinoma (SCC) of the penis. *BJU Int* 2011; **108**(9):1378–92.

Hegarty PK, Shabbir M, Hughes B, *et al.* Penile preserving surgery and surgical strategies to maximize penile form and function in penile cancer: recommendations from the United Kingdom experience. *World J Urol* 2009; **27**(2):179–87.

Heideman DA, Waterboer T, Pawlita M, *et al.* Human papillomavirus-16 is the predominant type etiologically involved in penile squamous cell carcinoma. *J Clin Oncol* 2007; **25**(29):4550–6.

Horenblas S. Lymphadenectomy in penile cancer. *Urol Clin North Am* 2011; **38**(4): 459–69, vi–vii.

Horenblas S. Sentinel lymph node biopsy in penile carcinoma. *Semin Diagn Pathol* 2012; **29**(2):90–5.

Ornellas AA, Kinchin EW, Nóbrega BLB, Wisnescky A, Koifman N, Quirino R. Surgical treatment of invasive squamous cell carcinoma of the penis: Brazilian National Cancer Institute long-term experience. *J Surg Oncol* 2008; **97**(6):487–95.

Pizzocaro G, Algaba F, Horenblas S, Solsona E, Van der Poel H, Watkin N. EAU penile cancer guidelines 2009. *Eur Urol* 2010; **57**(6):1002–12.

References

1. Kroon BK, Horenblas S, Nieweg OE. Contemporary management of penile squamous cell carcinoma. *J Surg Oncol* 2005; **89**(1):43–50.
2. Ornellas AA, Kinchin EW, Nóbrega BLB, Wisnescky A, Koifman N, Quirino R. Surgical treatment of invasive squamous cell carcinoma of the penis: Brazilian National Cancer Institute long-term experience. *J Surg Oncol* 2008; **97**(6):487–95.
3. Misra S, Chaturvedi A, Misra NC. Penile carcinoma: a challenge for the developing world. *Lancet Oncol* 2004; **5**(4):240–7.
4. Barnholtz-Sloan JS, Maldonado JL, Pow-sang J, Giuliano AR, Guiliano AR. Incidence trends in primary malignant penile cancer. *Urol Oncol* 2007; **25**(5):361–7.
5. Guimarães GC, Cunha IW, Soares FA, *et al.* Penile squamous cell carcinoma clinicopathological features, nodal metastasis and outcome in 333 cases. *J Urol* 2009; **182**(2):528–34; discussion 534.
6. Goodman MT, Hernandez BY, Shvetsov YB. Demographic and pathologic differences in the incidence of invasive penile cancer in the United States, 1995-2003. *Cancer Epidemiol Biomarkers Prev* 2007; **16**(9):1833–9.
7. Moses S, Bailey RC, Ronald AR. Male circumcision: assessment of health benefits and risks. *Sex Transm Infect* 1998; **74**(5):368–73.
8. Maden C, Sherman KJ, Beckmann AM, *et al.* History of circumcision, medical conditions, and sexual activity and risk of penile cancer. *J Nat Cancer Instit* 1993; **85**(1):19–24.
9. Schoen E, Oehrli M, Colby C, Machin G. The highly protective effect of newborn circumcision against invasive penile cancer. *Pediatrics* 2000; **105**(3):E36.
10. Dillner J, von Krogh G, Horenblas S, Meijer CJ. Etiology of squamous cell carcinoma of the penis. *Scand J Urol Nephrol Suppl* 2000; (205):189–93.
11. Daling JR, Madeleine MM, Johnson LG, *et al.* Penile cancer: importance of circumcision, human papillomavirus and smoking in in situ and invasive disease. *Int J Cancer* 2005; **116**(4):606–16.
12. Bromage SJ, Crump A, Pearce I. Phimosis as a presenting feature of diabetes. *BJU Int* 2008; **101**(3):338–40.
13. Hayashi Y, Kojima Y, Mizuno K, Kohri K. Prepuce: phimosis, paraphimosis, and circumcision. *ScientificWorld Journal* 2011; **11**:289–301.
14. Mcgregor TB, Pike JG, Leonard MP. Pathologic and physiologic phimosis. *Can Fam Physician* 2007; **53**:445–8.
15. Castellsagué X, Bosch F, Munoz N, Meijer CJLM, Shah K, de Sanjosé P. *N Engl J Med* 2002; **346**(15):1105–12.
16. Nielson CM, Harris RB, Dunne EF, *et al.* Risk factors for anogenital human papillomavirus infection in men. *J Infect Dis* 2007; **196**(8):1137–45.
17. Rubin MA, Kleter B, Zhou M, *et al.* Detection and typing of human papillomavirus DNA in penile carcinoma: evidence for multiple independent pathways of penile carcinogenesis. *Am J Pathol* 2001; **159**(4):1211–8.
18. McCance DJ, Kalache A, Ashdown K, *et al.* Human papillomavirus types 16 and 18 in carcinomas of the penis from Brazil. *Int J Cancer* 1986; **37**(1):55–9.
19. Wiener JS, Effert PJ, Humphrey PA, Yu L, Liu ET, Walther PJ. Prevalence of human papillomavirus types 16 and 18 in squamous-cell carcinoma of the penis: a retrospective analysis of primary and metastatic lesions by differential polymerase chain reaction. *Int J Cancer* 1992; **50**(5):694–701.
20. Bezerra AL, Lopes A, Santiago GH, Ribeiro KC, Latorre MR, Villa LL. Human papillomavirus as a prognostic factor in carcinoma of the penis: analysis of 82 patients treated with amputation and bilateral lymphadenectomy. *Cancer* 2001; **91**(12):2315–21.
21. Gregoire L, Cubilla AL, Reuter VE, Haas GP, Lancaster WD. Preferential association of human papillomavirus with high-grade histologic variants of penile-invasive squamous cell carcinoma. *J Nat Cancer Inst* 1995; **87**(22):1705–9.
22. Lont AP, Kroon BK, Horenblas S, *et al.* Presence of high-risk human papillomavirus DNA in penile carcinoma predicts favorable outcome in survival. *Int J Cancer* 2006; **119**(5):1078–81.
23. Hellberg D, Valentin J, Eklund T, Nilsson S. Penile cancer: is there an epidemiological role for smoking and sexual behaviour? *BMJ* 1987; **295**(6609):1306–8.
24. Kiss A, Király L, Kutasy B, Merksz M. High incidence of balanitis xerotica obliterans in boys with phimosis: prospective 10-year study. *Pediatr Dermatol* 2005; **22**(4):305–8.

25. Das S, Tunuguntla HS. Balanitis xerotica obliterans--a review. *World J Urol* 2000; **18**(6):382–7.
26. Nasca MR, Innocenzi D, Micali G. Penile cancer among patients with genital lichen sclerosus. *J Am Acad Dermatol* 1999; **41**(6):911–4.
27. Barbagli G, Palminteri E, Mirri F, Guazzoni G, Turini D, Lazzeri M. Penile carcinoma in patients with genital lichen sclerosus: a multicenter survey. *J Urol* 2006; **175**(4):1359–63.
28. Velazquez EF, Cubilla AL. Lichen sclerosus in 68 patients with squamous cell carcinoma of the penis: frequent atypias and correlation with special carcinoma variants suggests a precancerous role. *Am J Surg Pathol* 2003; **27**(11):1448–53.
29. Carli P, Cattaneo A, De Magnis A, Biggeri A, Taddei G, Giannotti B. Squamous cell carcinoma arising in vulval lichen sclerosus: a longitudinal cohort study. *Eur J Cancer Prev* 1995; **4**(6):491–5.
30. Stern RS, Bagheri S, Nichols K. The persistent risk of genital tumors among men treated with psoralen plus ultraviolet A (PUVA) for psoriasis. *J Am Acad Dermatol* 2002; **47**(1):33–9.
31. Engels EA, Pfeiffer RM, Goedert JJ, *et al.* Trends in cancer risk among people with AIDS in the United States 1980-2002. *AIDS* 2006; **20**(12):1645–54.
32. Culkin DJ, Beer TM. Advanced penile carcinoma. *J Urol* 2003; **170**(2 Pt 1):359–65.
33. Burgers JK, Badalament RA, Drago JR. Penile cancer. Clinical presentation, diagnosis, and staging. *Urol Clin North Am* 1992; **19**(2):247–56.
34. Heinlen JE, Buethe DD, Culkin DJ. Advanced penile cancer. *Int Urol Nephrol* 2012; **44**(1):139–48.
35. Deem S, Keane T, Bhavsar R, El-Zawahary A, Savage S. Contemporary diagnosis and management of squamous cell carcinoma (SCC) of the penis. *BJU Int* 2011; **108**(9):1378–92.
36. Schwartz RA. Verrucous carcinoma of the skin and mucosa. *J Am Acad Dermatol* 1995; **32**(1):1–21; quiz 22–4.
37. Bezerra AL, Lopes A, Landman G, Alencar GN, Torloni H, Villa LL. Clinicopathologic features and human papillomavirus dna prevalence of warty and squamous cell carcinoma of the penis. *Am J Surg Pathol* 2001; **25**(5):673–8.
38. Cubilla AL, Reuter VE, Gregoire L, *et al.* Basaloid squamous cell carcinoma: a distinctive human papilloma virus-related penile neoplasm: a report of 20 cases. *Am J Surg Pathol* 1998; **22**(6):755–61.
39. Broders A. Squamous cell-epithelioma of the skin. *Ann Surg* 1921; **43**(2):141–59.
40. Pizzocaro G, Algaba F, Horenblas S, Solsona E, Van der Poel H, Watkin N. EAU penile cancer guidelines 2009. *Eur Urol* 2010; **57**(6):1002–12.
41. Leijte J a P, Gallee M, Antonini N, Horenblas S. Evaluation of current TNM classification of penile carcinoma. *J Urol* 2008; **180**(3):933–8; discussion 938.
42. Pandey D, Mahajan V, Kannan RR. Prognostic factors in node-positive carcinoma of the penis. *J Surg Oncol* 2006; **93**(2):133–8.
43. Ravi R. Correlation between the extent of nodal involvement and survival following groin dissection for carcinoma of the penis. *Br J Urol* 1993; **72**(5 Pt 2):817–9.
44. Srinivas V, Morse MJ, Herr HW, Sogani PC, Whitmore WF. Penile cancer: relation of extent of nodal metastasis to survival. *J Urol* 1987; **137**(5):880–2.
45. Heyns CF, Mendoza-Valdés A, Pompeo ACL. Diagnosis and staging of penile cancer. *Urology* 2010; **76**(2 Suppl 1):S15–23.
46. *Ibid.* 40.
47. Horenblas S. Lymphadenectomy for squamous cell carcinoma of the penis. Part 1: diagnosis of lymph node metastasis. *BJU Int* 2001; **88**(5):467–72.
48. Horenblas S, Van Tinteren H, Delemarre JF, Moonen LM, Lustig V, Kröger R. Squamous cell carcinoma of the penis: accuracy of tumor, nodes and metastasis classification system, and role of lymphangiography, computerized tomography scan and fine needle aspiration cytology. *J Urol* 1991; **146**(5):1279–83.
49. Senthil Kumar MP, Ananthakrishnan N, Prema V. Predicting regional lymph node metastasis in carcinoma of the penis: a comparison between fine-needle aspiration cytology, sentinel lymph node biopsy and medial inguinal lymph node biopsy. *Br J Urol* 1998; **81**(3):453–7.
50. Abi-Aad AS, deKernion JB. Controversies in ilioinguinal lymphadenectomy for cancer of the penis. *Urol Clin North Am* 1992; **19**(2):319–24.
51. Horenblas S, Van Tinteren H. Squamous cell carcinoma of the penis. III Treatment of regional lymph nodes. *J Urol* 1993; **149**(3):492–7.
52. Opjordsmoen S, Fosså SD. Quality of life in patients treated for penile cancer. A follow-up study. *Br J Urol* 1994; **74**(5):652–7.
53. Alnajjar HM, Lam W, Bolgeri M, Rees RW, Perry MJ, Watkin NA. Treatment of carcinoma in situ of the glans penis with topical chemotherapy agents. *Eur Urol* 2012; **62**(5):923.
54. Tietjen DN, Malek RS. Laser therapy of squamous cell dysplasia and carcinoma of the penis. *Urology* 1998; **52**(4):559–65.
55. Frimberger D, Hungerhuber E, Zaak D, Waidelich R, Hofstetter A, Schneede P. Penile carcinoma. Is Nd:YAG laser therapy radical enough? *J Urol* 2002; **168**(6):2418–21; discussion 2421.
56. Windahl T, Andersson S-O. Combined laser treatment for penile carcinoma: results after long-term followup. *J Urol* 2003; **169**(6):2118–21.
57. Meijer RP, Boon TA, van Venrooij GEPM, Wijburg CJ. Long-term follow-up after laser therapy for penile carcinoma. *Urology* 2007; **69**(4):759–62.
58. Schlenker B, Tilki D, Seitz M, Bader MJ, Reich O, Schneede P, *et al.* Organ-preserving neodymium-yttrium-aluminium-garnet laser therapy for penile carcinoma: a long-term follow-up. *BJU Int* 2010; **106**(6):786–90.
59. Tewari M, Rai P, Kumar M, Shukla HS. Long-term outcome of treatment of early carcinoma of the lip with Nd:YAG laser. *World J Surg* 2008; **32**(4):543–7.
60. Bandieramonte G, Colecchia M, Mariani L, *et al.* Peniscopically controlled CO_2 laser excision for conservative treatment of in situ and T1 penile carcinoma: report on 224 patients. *Eur Urol* 2008; **54**(4):875–82.
61. Lont a P, Gallee MPW, Meinhardt W, van Tinteren H, Horenblas S. Penis conserving treatment for T1 and T2 penile carcinoma: clinical implications of a local recurrence. *J Urol* 2006; **176**(2):575–80; discussion 580.
62. Wells MJ, Taylor RS. Mohs micrographic surgery for penoscrotal malignancy. *Urol Clin North Am* 2010; **37**(3):403–9.
63. Davis J, Schellhammer P, Schlossberg SM. Conservative surgical therapy for penile and urethral carcinoma. *Urology* 1999; **53**(203):386–92.
64. Mohs FE, Snow SN, Messing EM, Kuglitsch ME. Microscopically controlled surgery in the treatment of carcinoma of the penis. *J Urol* 1985; **133**(6):961–6.
65. Shindel AW, Mann MW, Lev RY, *et al.* Mohs micrographic surgery for penile cancer: management and long-term followup. *J Urol* 2007; **178**(5):1980–5.
66. Hegarty PK, Shabbir M, Hughes B, *et al.* Penile preserving surgery and surgical strategies to maximize penile form and function in penile cancer: recommendations from the United Kingdom experience. *World J Urol* 2009; **27**(2):179–87.
67. Minhas S, Kayes O, Hegarty P, Kumar P, Freeman A, Ralph D. What surgical resection margins are required to achieve oncological control in men with primary penile cancer? *BJU Int* 2005; **96**(7):1040–3.
68. Agrawal A, Pai D, Ananthakrishnan N, Smile SR, Ratnakar C. The histological extent of the local spread of carcinoma of the penis and its therapeutic implications. *BJU Int* 2000; **85**(3):299–301.
69. Veeratterapillay R, Sahadevan K, Aluru P, Asterling S, Rao GS, Greene D. Organ-preserving surgery for penile cancer: description of techniques and surgical outcomes. *BJU Int* 2012; **110**(11):1792–5.
70. Pietrzak P, Corbishley C, Watkin N. Organ-sparing surgery for invasive penile cancer: early follow-up data. *BJU Int* 2004; **94**(9):1253–7.

71. Palminteri E, Berdondini E, Lazzeri M, Mirri F, Barbagli G. Resurfacing and reconstruction of the glans penis. *Eur Urol* 2007; **52**(3):893–8.
72. Brown CT, Minhas S, Ralph DJ. Conservative surgery for penile cancer: subtotal glans excision without grafting. *BJU Int* 2005; **96**(6):911–2.
73. Korets R, Koppie TM, Snyder ME, Russo P. Partial penectomy for patients with squamous cell carcinoma of the penis: the Memorial Sloan-Kettering experience. *Ann Surg Oncol* 2007; **14**(12):3614–9.
74. Leijte JP, Kirrander P, Antonini N, Windahl T, Horenblas S. Recurrence patterns of squamous cell carcinoma of the penis: recommendations for follow-up based on a two-centre analysis of 700 patients. *Eur Urol* 2008; **54**(1):161–8.
75. *Ibid.* **2**.
76. Ficarra V, Maffei N, Piacentini I, Rabi NA, Cerruto MA. Local treatment of penile squamous. *Urol Int* 2002;169–73.
77. Bissada NK, Yakout HH, Fahmy WE, *et al.* Multi-institutional long-term experience with conservative surgery for invasive penile carcinoma. *J Urol* 2003; **169**(2):500–2.
78. Sánchez-Ortiz RF, Pettaway CA. The role of lymphadenectomy in penile cancer. *Urol Oncol* 2004; **22**(3):236–44; discussion 244–5.
79. Lont AP, Kroon BK, Gallee MPW, van Tinteren H, Moonen LMF, Horenblas S. Pelvic lymph node dissection for penile carcinoma: extent of inguinal lymph node involvement as an indicator for pelvic lymph node involvement and survival. *J Urol* 2007; **177**(3):947–52; discussion 952.
80. Kroon BK, Horenblas S, Lont AP, Tanis PJ, Gallee MPW, Nieweg OE. Patients with penile carcinoma benefit from immediate resection of clinically occult lymph node metastases. *J Urol* 2005; **173**(3):816–9.
81. Hegarty PK, Kayes O, Freeman A, Christopher N, Ralph DJ, Minhas S. A prospective study of 100 cases of penile cancer managed according to European Association of Urology guidelines. *BJU Int* 2006; **98**(3):526–31.
82. Sadeghi R, Gholami H, Zakavi SR, Kakhki VRD, Horenblas S. Accuracy of 18 F-FDG PET/CT for diagnosing inguinal lymph node involvement in penile squamous cell carcinoma. *Clin Nucl Med* 2012; **37**:436–41.
83. Solsona E, Algaba F, Horenblas S, Pizzocaro G, Windahl T. EAU Guidelines on Penile Cancer. *Eur Urol* 2004; **46**(1):1–8.
84. Ficarra V, Zattoni F, Cunico SC, *et al.* Lymphatic and vascular embolizations are independent predictive variables of inguinal lymph node involvement in patients with squamous cell carcinoma of the penis: Gruppo Uro-Oncologico del Nord Est (Northeast Uro-Oncological Group) Penile Cancer data bas. *Cancer* 2005; **103**(12):2507–16.
85. Johnson DE, Lo RK. Complications of groin dissection in penile cancer. Experience with 101 lymphadenectomies. *Urology* 1984; **24**(4):312–4.
86. Ornellas AA, Seixas AL, de Moraes JR. Analyses of 200 lymphadenectomies in patients with penile carcinoma. *J Urol* 1991; **146**(2):330–2.
87. Ravi R. Morbidity following groin dissection for penile carcinoma. *Br J Urol* 1993; **72**(6):941–5.
88. Bevan-Thomas R, Slaton JW, Pettaway CA. Contemporary morbidity from lymphadenectomy for penile squamous cell carcinoma: the M.D. Anderson Cancer Center Experience. *J Urol* 2002; **167**(4):1638–42.
89. Cabanas R. Anatomy and biopsy of sentinel nodes. *Urol Clin North Am* 1992; **19**(2):267–76.
90. Crawford ED, Daneshgari F. Management of regional lymphatic drainage in carcinoma of the penis. *Urol Clin North Am* 1992; **19**(2):305–17.
91. Dewire D, Lepor H. Anatomic considerations of the penis and its lymphatic drainage. *Urol Clin North Am* 1992; **19**:211–9.
92. Daseler EH, Anson BJ, Reimann AF. Radical excision of the inguinal and iliac lymph glands; a study based upon 450 anatomical dissections and upon supportive clinical observations. *Surg Gynecol Obstet* 1948; **87**(6):679–94.
93. Leijte JP, Valdés Olmos RA, Nieweg OE, Horenblas S. Anatomical mapping of lymphatic drainage in penile carcinoma with SPECT-CT: implications for the extent of inguinal lymph node dissection. *Eur Urol* 2008; **54**(4):885–90.
94. Lopes A, Bezerra L, Serrano SV, Hidalgo GS. Iliac nodal metastases from carcinoma of the penis treated surgically. *BJU Int* 2000; **86**(6):690–3.
95. Wood HM, Angermeier KW. Anatomic considerations of the penis, lymphatic drainage, and biopsy of the sentinel node. *Urol Clin North Am* 2010; **37**(3):327–34.
96. Berveiller P, Mir O, Veyrie N, Barranger E. The sentinel-node concept: a dramatic improvement in breast-cancer surgery. *Lancet Oncol* 2010; **11**(9):906.
97. Leijte JAP, Kroon BK, Valdés Olmos RA, Nieweg OE, Horenblas S. Reliability and safety of current dynamic sentinel node biopsy for penile carcinoma. *Eur Urol* 2007; **52**(1):170–7.
98. Morton DL, Bostick PJ. Will the true sentinel node please stand? *Ann Surg Oncol* 1999; **6**(1):12–4.
99. Valdés Olmos RA, Tanis PJ, Hoefnagel CA, *et al.* Penile lymphoscintigraphy for sentinel node identification. *Eur J Nucl Med Mol Imag* 2001; **28**(5):581–5.
100. Kroon BK, Valdés Olmos RA, van Tinteren H, Nieweg OE, Horenblas S. Reproducibility of lymphoscintigraphy for lymphatic mapping in patients with penile carcinoma. *J Urol* 2005; **174**(6):2214–7.
101. Horenblas S, Jansen L, Meinhardt W, Hoefnagel CA, de Jong D, Nieweg OE. Detection of occult metastasis in squamous cell carcinoma of the penis using a dynamic sentinel node procedure. *J Urol* 2000; **163**(1):100–4.
102. Kroon BK, Horenblas S, Estourgie SH, Lont AP, Valdés Olmos RA, Nieweg OE. How to avoid false-negative dynamic sentinel node procedures in penile carcinoma. *J Urol* 2004; **171**(2):2191–4.
103. Kroon BK, Horenblas S, Meinhardt W, *et al.* Dynamic sentinel node biopsy in penile carcinoma: evaluation of 10 years experience. *Eur Urol* 2005; **47**(5):601–6; discussion 606.
104. Zhu Y, Zhang S-L, Ye D-W, *et al.* Prospectively packaged ilioinguinal lymphadenectomy for penile cancer: the disseminative pattern of lymph node metastasis. *J Urol* 2009; **181**(5):2103–8.
105. Horenblas S, Van Tinteren H. Squamous cell carcinoma of the penis. IV. Prognostic factors of survival: analysis of tumor, nodes and metastasis classification system. *J Urol* 1994; **151**:1239–43.
106. Melis P, Bos KE, Horenblas S. Primary skin closure of a large groin defect after inguinal lymphadenectomy for penile cancer using a skin stretching device. *J Urol* 1998; **159**(1):185–7.
107. Kayes OJ, Durrant CA, Ralph D, Floyd D, Withey S, Minhas S. Vertical rectus abdominis flap reconstruction in patients with advanced penile squamous cell carcinoma. *BJU Int* 2007; **99**(1):37–40.
108. Airhart RA, deKernion JB, Guillermo EO. Tensor fascia lata myocutaneous flap for coverage of skin defect after radical groin dissection for metastatic penile carcinoma. *J Urol* 1982; **128**(3):599–601.
109. Tobias-Machado M, Tavares A, Silva MNR, *et al.* Can video endoscopic inguinal lymphadenectomy achieve a lower morbidity than open lymph node dissection in penile cancer patients? *J Endourology* 2008; **22**(8):1687–91.
110. Sotelo R, Sanchez-Salas R, Clavijo R. Endoscopic inguinal lymph node dissection for penile carcinoma: the developing of a novel technique. *World J Urol* 2009; **27**(2):213–9.

111. Bartelink H, Breur K, Hart G, Annyas B, van Slooten E, Snow G. The value of postoperative radiotherapy as an adjuvant to radical neck dissection. *Cancer* 1983; **52**(6):1008–13.
112. Skinner DG. Management of extensive, localized neoplasms of lower abdominal wall. Pubectomy and scrotal skin transfer technique. *Urology* 1974; **3**(1):34–7.
113. Tabatabaei S, McDougal WS. Primary skin closure of large groin defects after inguinal lymphadenectomy for penile cancer using an abdominal cutaneous advancement flap. *J Urol* 2003; **169**(1):118–20.
114. Bare RL, Assimos DG, McCullough DL, Smith DP, DeFranzo AJ, Marks MW. Inguinal lymphadenectomy and primary groin reconstruction using rectus abdominis muscle flaps in patients with penile cancer. *Urology* 1994; **44**(4):557–61.
115. Shin DM, Glisson BS, Khuri FR, *et al.* Phase II study of induction chemotherapy with paclitaxel, ifosfamide, and carboplatin (TIC) for patients with locally advanced squamous cell carcinoma of the head and neck. *Cancer* 2002; **95**(2):322–30.
116. Pizzocaro G, Nicolai N, Milani A. Taxanes in combination with cisplatin and fluorouracil for advanced penile cancer: preliminary results. *Eur Urol* 2009; **55**(3):546–51.
117. Pagliaro LC, Williams DL, Daliani D, *et al.* Neoadjuvant paclitaxel, ifosfamide, and cisplatin chemotherapy for metastatic penile cancer: a phase II study. *J Clin Oncol* 2010; **28**(24):3851–7.
118. Bermejo C, Busby JE, Spiess PE, Heller L, Pagliaro LC, Pettaway CA. Neoadjuvant chemotherapy followed by aggressive surgical consolidation for metastatic penile squamous cell carcinoma. *J Urol* 2007; **177**(4):1335–8.

CHAPTER 6.37

Adrenocortical cancer

Steve Ball and Sajid Kalathil

Adrenal gland: anatomy, embryology, and physiology

The adrenal glands are paired retroperitoneal structures that lie at the anterosuperior and medial aspect of kidneys. They are pyramidal; weigh approximately 5 gm each in healthy adults; and measure approximately 5 cm × 2 cm× 1 cm. The right adrenal lies above the kidney, posterolateral to inferior vena cava while the left adrenal lies above left kidney behind the pancreas and splenic artery.

The adrenal gland is composed of an outer cortex and an inner medulla. While closely related anatomically, these two layers are developmentally and functionally discrete. Foetal adrenal gland is evident from six to eight weeks of gestation and rapidly increases in size. The adrenal cortex derives from mesenchymal cells attached to the coelomic cavity lining adjacent to the urogenital ridge. Two distinct zones are evident within the developing cortex: an inner prominent foetal zone which later regresses; and an outer definitive zone that goes on to form the adult cortex. In contrast, the adrenal medulla is derived from cells of the neural crest that migrate at the seventh week of life and enter the foetal cortex. Primitive adrenal medulla is formed by week 20 but a distinct medulla is not apparent until atrophy of the foetal zone of the cortex.

The adrenals have a rich blood supply, estimated at 6–7 mL/g per minute. The inferior phrenic artery is the main arterial supply with additional branches from aorta and renal artery. Venous drainage is into the posterior surface of inferior vena cava on the right and into the left renal vein on the left

The adrenal cortex is made of three layers. These have functional as well as morphological differences. The zona gomerulosa (ZG) is the outermost layer, comprised of closely packed small cells. The middle zona fasciculata (ZF) is made of larger cells and constitutes up to three-quarters of the cortex. The innermost layer is the Zona reticularis (ZR). The adrenal cortex synthesizes and secretes steroid hormones. However, there are key differences in the pattern of mineralocorticoid, glucocorticoid, and androgens produced by the three layers. The ZG alone secretes the mineralocorticoid aldosterone and is the only cortical layer to express the enzyme aldosterone synthase. The ZF secretes mainly cortisol with some androgen precursors. The ZR secretes androgens in addition to DHEA and androstenedione, as well as cortisol (Fig. 6.37.1). The secretion of cortisol and sex steroid precursors by the ZF and ZR are regulated by pituitary adrenocorticotropic hormone (ACTH). In contrast, aldosterone production by the ZG is controlled mainly by the renin-angiotensin system and circulating electrolyte concentration.

The adrenal medulla is effectively a large sympathetic nerve terminal, made of chromaffin cells which secrete noradrenaline and adrenaline in response to neuro-humeral activation by the autonomic nervous system and other endocrine mediators.

Adrenocortical cancer

Introduction

Adrenocortical cancer (ACC) is a rare malignancy and has a poor prognosis. The incidence is estimated at 0.7–2 cases per 1 million. While it is most common in those aged between 40–50 years, it can present at any age. ACC in children suggests an inherited predisposition (Li-Fraumeni syndrome and Beckwith-Wiederman syndrome)[(1)]. The unusually high incidence of ACC seen in a subset of children in southern Brazil (3.4–4.2 versus 0.3 per 1 million children under the age of 15 across the world) reflects a high background prevalence of germ line loss of function mutations in the *TP53* tumour-suppression gene (responsible for Li-Fraumeni syndrome) in this population.[1,2] ACC is more common in males than females.

Clinical presentation can be with symptoms and signs of steroid hormone excess (functional tumours); mass effects; or as an incidental radiological finding. Presentation in the young person is more commonly with functional disease. Non-functional ACC tends to present later in the natural history and with more advanced disease.

Aetiology and pathophysiology

While the aetiology of ACC is still not clearly understood, there has been progress in understanding some of the molecular mechanisms of tumour development. Comparative genomic hybridization has identified chromosome losses at 1p,17p,22p,22q,2q and 11q in 62% of people with sporadic ACC.[3] Microsatellite marker analysis has revealed a high prevalence of loss of heterozygosity or allelic imbalance at 11q13 (≥90%), 17p13 (≥85%) and 2p16 (92%).[4,5] Many of these loci correspond to known oncogenes and/or tumour suppressor genes, supporting a causative role in pathogenesis (Table 6.37.1). Some of these molecular characteristics have been shown to have prognostic significance.

ACC is associated with two inherited tumour predisposition syndromes: Li-Fraumeni and Beckwith-Weidemann syndromes. Li-Fraumeni syndrome (LFS) is a rare, autosomal dominant disorder linked to germ line loss of function mutations of the p53 tumour suppressor gene. P53 mutations can be inherited or can arise *de novo* early in embryogenesis. LFS is associated with a range of other malignancies including sarcoma, breast cancer, and leukaemia.

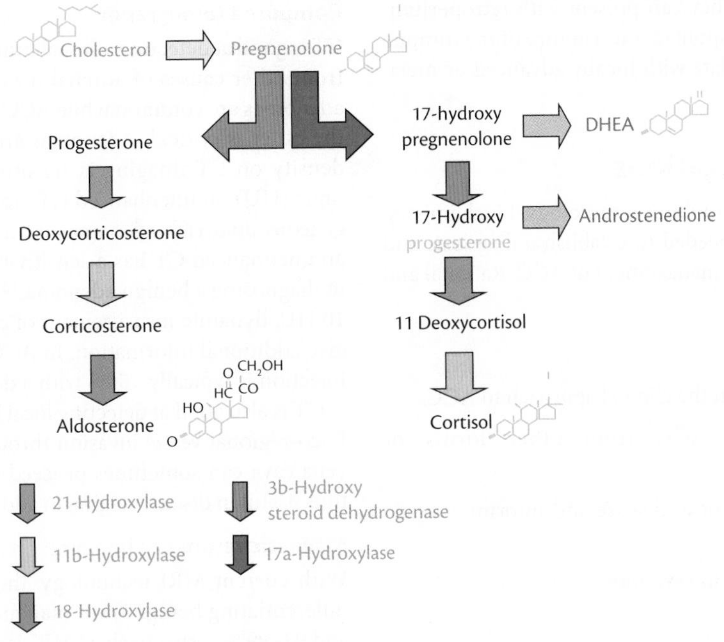

Fig. 6.37.1 Adrenal steroidogenesis: outline of metabolic pathways generating glucocorticoids, mineralocorticoids, and androgens in the adrenal cortex. DHEA: dihydroepiadrosterone.

Clinical presentation

The most common presentation of ACC (50–60%) is with clinical evidence of adrenal steroid hormone excess,[6–10] most often with Cushing's syndrome. Androgen production can lead to presentation with symptoms and signs of androgen excess in women. Conversely, oestrogen production can lead to presentation with symptoms and signs of feminization in the male. Aldosterone and other mineralocorticoid production can result in hypertension and hypokalaemia.

Cushing's syndrome

Less than 5% of all presentations with Cushing's syndrome are attributable to ACC. Classical features of Cushing's syndrome may dominate: centripetal obesity, hirsutism, plethora, proximal myopathy, and abdominal striae. Hypokalaemia is a feature of severe hypercortisolaemia. Rapid onset of symptoms from cortisol excess is a feature of ACC. If tumour growth is rapid, presentation with glucocorticoid excess may be atypical. There may be little or no weight gain; while muscle atrophy, severe hypertension, and diabetes mellitus may be dominant features.

Table 6.37.1 Oncogenes and tumour suppressor genes associated with adrenocortical cancer (ACC)

Oncogenes and associated signalling pathways	Tumour suppressor genes
IGF-2: IGF signalling pathway	P53
β catenin: Wnt signalling pathway	Melanocortin 2 suppressor gene (MC2R)
Steroidogenic factor 1: developmental transcription factor	
Fibroblast growth factor 2 (FGF2),	
Transforming growth factor (TGFα, TGFβ),	
Vascular endothelial growth factor (VEGF)	

Testosterone secreting tumours

Virilization is the hallmark of testosterone secreting ACCs. They are rare and most of them are found in women. Testosterone secretion is autonomous. Signs and symptoms of androgen excess include acne, hirsutism, androgenetic affluvium, oligomenorrhoea. Virilization may manifest with or without concomitant Cushing's syndrome.

Oestrogen secreting adrenocortical cancer

Most feminizing ACCs occur in men. They are usually larger and behave more aggressively than other forms of ACC. Presenting symptoms include gynaecomastia. Impotence or decreased libido with associated testicular atrophy may occur. Some clinical features may be due to peripheral aromatization of co-secreted weak adrenal androgens. Only 7% of cases with ACC in the German Adrenocortical cancer registry showed evidence of feminization.[11]

Aldosterone secreting adrenocortical cancer

While primary hyperaldosteronism or Conn's syndrome can be caused by ACC, it is usually in combination with excess glucocorticoid or androgen secretion. Hypertension and profound hypokalaemia are the dominant clinical features. It is unusual for benign adrenal adenomas producing Conn's syndrome to be larger than 3 cm. Conn's syndrome presenting with larger adrenal lesions should therefore raise the suspicion of ACC.

Non-functioning adrenocortical cancer

Patients with non-functioning ACC usually present with symptoms of abdominal discomfort, nausea, vomiting, or back pain caused by the local mass effects. Rarely, they can present with retroperitoneal haemorrhage secondary to spontaneous rupture of the tumour. Presentation may be relatively late with locally advanced or metastatic disease.

Diagnosis and investigations

A multidisciplinary approach combining radiology, biochemistry, and tissue-based pathology is needed to establish a diagnosis and patient-centred approach to the management of ACC. Rational and thorough investigation is key.

The role of imaging

Imaging plays important roles in the clinical approach to ACC.

- Diagnosis: differentiating ACC from other forms of adrenal tumour
- Staging: establishing the extent of disease and informing a tailored approach to treatment
- Assessing disease response to intervention
- Monitoring for recurrence
- Computed tomography (CT) and MRI are effective in all these roles, while there are emerging data on positron emission tomography (PET) (Table 6.37.2)

Computed tomography

CT is good at detecting adrenal tumours and in differentiating ACC from other causes of adrenal mass. This is important, as adrenal adenomas are common while ACC is rare. Differentiating one from the other is critical. Adenomas are generally lipid-rich. As tissue density on CT imaging is sensitive to lipid content, Hounsfield units (HU) on unenhanced CT are useful in differentiating homogeneous lipid-rich adenomas from ACC. A threshold of 10HU on an unenhanced CT has a sensitivity of 71% and specificity of 98% in diagnosing a benign adenoma.[12] When baseline density is above 10 HU, dynamic measurement of contrast-enhanced densities can give additional information. In ACC, washout after contrast media injection is typically <50% with a delayed attenuation of >35 HU.[13]

CT is also good at detecting local invasion and distant metastases. Loco-regional vessel invasion through the renal veins and inferior vena cava can sometimes proceed up to the right atrium.[14] CT is thus useful in disease staging in addition to establishing a diagnosis.

Magnetic resonance imaging

With current MRI technology, the sensitivity and specificity for differentiating benign from malignant lesions range from 81–89% and 92–99%, respectively.[15] MRI is good for differentiating adrenal masses from surrounding soft-tissue structures and thus very useful in guiding an approach to surgery. ACC has the same signal intensity as liver on T1 weighted and increased intensity on T2

Table 6.37.2 Radiological features of ACC relative to adrenal adenoma

Feature	ACC	Adrenal adenoma
General	Irregular Heterogeneous >4 cm	
CT	>10 HU non-enhanced CT Enhancement washout <50% Delayed attenuation >35%	<10 HU non-enhanced CT Absolute enhancement washout >60% Relative enhancement washout >40%
MRI	Hypo-intense T1 Hyper-intense T2 Chemical shift properties	

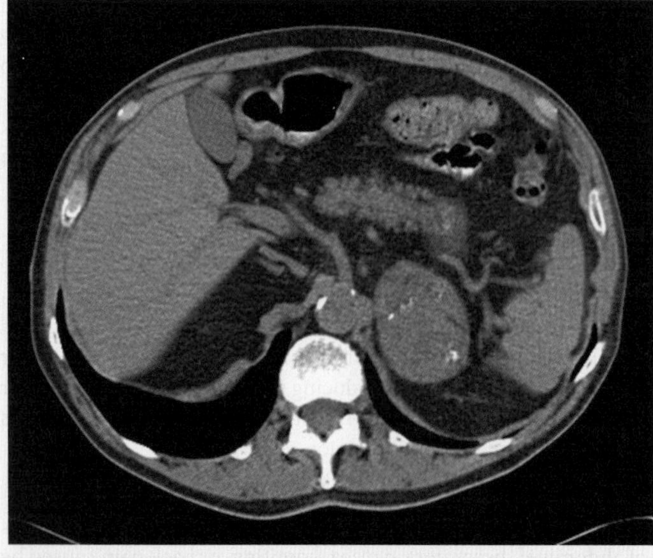

weighted sequences. Given concerns over cumulative radiation exposure, MRI has a clear role in long-term surveillance for local recurrence after surgery in young patients.

^{18}F-flurodeoxyglucose—positron emission tomography

PET is emerging as a new tool in the study of adrenal tumours. Because of its high metabolic activity, ACC demonstrates high uptake of ^{18}F-flurodeoxyglucose (FDG) relative to other adrenal lesions. Sensitivity has been reported to be as high as 100% with a specificity of 88% in differentiating ACC from adrenal adenomas.[16] PET may therefore have a role in the differential diagnosis of those lesions with indeterminate features on CT/MRI.

Emerging approaches to lesions with indeterminate imaging characteristics

CT, MRI, and FDG-PET cannot always differentiate ACC from other adrenal lesions reliably. Metomidate is emerging as an imaging agent that may help in this area. Metomidate binds specifically to 11 B-hydroxylase and aldosterone synthase. Coupling with a radio-tracer thus produces a radio-ligand with high specificity for adrenocortical cells, suitable for use in PET and CT-SPECT imaging.[17,18]

Image-guided biopsy

Needle biopsy is not usually advised as a tool in the differential diagnosis of ACC. Adrenal haemorrhage and tumour rupture are significant concerns. It can be considered in specific circumstances.

- Confirmation of metastatic disease where surgery is not intended
- Exclusion of metastatic disease to the adrenal in those with additional extra-adrenal malignancy

Biochemical investigation: establishing function and identifying biomarkers

As with radiology, clinical biochemistry has multiple roles in the diagnosis and management of ACC.

- Characterizing any clinical syndrome of increased adrenal steroid hormone production: to aid patient management
- Excluding phaeochromocytoma in the differential diagnosis of an adrenal mass
- Identifying an endocrine or other circulating biomarker for use in identifying ACC and in disease monitoring/surveillance

Standardized approaches to establishing endocrine function of a potential or established ACC can be helpful in balancing the need for speed and accuracy in progressing the differential diagnosis. A rational approach is outlined in Table 6.37.3.

Differentiating ACC from adrenal adenoma simply on imaging can be challenging. A metabolomics approach using biomarkers for ACC would be a great asset. One such approach, using mass spectrometry based steroid profiling has shown promising initial results. This study looked at 32 distinct adrenal-derived steroids in 24 hour urine samples from patients with ACC and adrenal adenoma. Results revealed a pattern of predominantly immature, early stage steroidogenesis in ACC. Generalized Matrix Learning Vector Quantization (GMLVQ) analysis identified a subset of nine steroids that performed best in differentiating ACC from adrenocortical adenoma (ACA) with a sensitivity and specificity of 88%.[19]

Table 6.37.3 Biochemical investigation of ACC

Purpose	Test
Exclude glucocorticoid excess	24-hour urine free cortisol 0900 plasma cortisol and ACTH Overnight dexamethasone suppression test
Exclude phaeochromocytoma	Timed overnight urine metanephrines Plasma metanephrines
Exclude mineralocorticoid excess	Serum K^+ Plasma aldosterone/renin ratio
Exclude sex steroid excess	Plasma DHEA-S Plasma testosterone Plasma oestrodiol (men and postmenopausal women)

ACTH: Adrenocorticotropic hormone; DHEA-S: Dehydroepiandrosterone-sulphate.

Tissue-based pathology

Perhaps surprisingly, tissue-based pathology diagnoses of ACC can be difficult in the absence of local spread or distant metastasis. Standard criteria are based on macroscopic and microscopic morphology criteria. Assessment should be by an experienced pathologist who is accustomed to dealing with adrenal tumours. Reliability and reproducibility of assessment is key, and can be improved through standardized training packages.[20] Importantly, evolving proteomic and genomic approaches are likely to support new classification systems that take into account molecular and functional data.[21]

Macroscopic features indicative of ACC are tumour size, haemorrhage, and breached tumour capsule. The most popular microscopic diagnostic tool is the Weiss scoring system. This incorporates nine parameters relating to tumour structure, cytology and evidence of local invasion (Table 6.37.4).[22] In experienced hands and using specific cut-offs (scores of 2 or less classed as benign; a score of 3 or more considered indicative of ACC) the system has a reported sensitivity and specificity of 100% and 96%, respectively.[23]

Table 6.37.4 Weiss Scoring system for classification/diagnosis of ACC

Cytology	1	High mitotic rate (>5 of 50 hpf)
	2	Atypical Mitosis
	3	High nuclear grade
Structure	4	Diffuse architecture
	5	Necrosis
	6	Low percentage of clear cells
Invasion	7	Capsular invasion
	8	Sinusoidal invasion
	9	Vein invasion

Reproduced with permission from Lippincott Williams and Wilkins/Wolters Kluwer Health: Weiss LM, 'Comparative histologic study of 43 metastasizing and nonmetastasizing adrenocortical tumors', *American Journal of Surgical Pathology*, Volume 8, Issue 3, pp. 163–169, Copyright © 1984 Wolters Kluwer Health, Inc.

Table 6.37.5 Staging in ACC

WHO Stage	TMN Stage	ENSAT Stage (2008)
Stage I	T1, N0, M0	T1, N0, M0
Stage II	T2, N0, M0	T2, N0, M0
Stage III	T1-2, N1, M0 T3, N0, M0	T1-2, N1, M0 T3-4, N0-1, M0
Stage IV	T3, N1, M0 T4, N0, M0 T4, N0, M0 T4, N1, M0 Tx, Nx, M1	T1-4, N0-1, M0-1

A number of staging classifications have been developed over time, combining features of primary tumour, local-regional, and distant disease.

T1, tumour size ≤5 cm; T2, tumour size >5 cm; T3, tumour infiltration in surrounding tissue; T4, tumour invasion in adjacent organs or venous tumour thrombus in vena cava or renal vein. N0, no positive lymph nodes; N1, positive lymph node(s); M0, no distant metastases; M1, presence of distant metastasis. Abbreviations: M, metastasis; N, lymph node; T, tumour; ENSAT, European Network for the Study of Adrenal Tumors.

Source: data from De Lellis RA *et al.*, *Pathology and genetics of tumors of endocrine organs, International Agency for Research on Cancer*, Lyon, France, Copyright © 2004 IARC; American Joint Committee on Cancer (AJCC), *AJCC Cancer Staging Manual, Seventh Edition*, Science+Business Media, LLC, Copyright © 2010 AJCC; and Fassnacht M *et al.*, 'Limited prognostic value of the 2004 International Union Against Cancer staging classification for adrenocortical carcinoma: proposal for a Revised TNM Classification', *Cancer*, Volume 1215, Issue 2, pp. 243–50, Copyright © 2008 American Cancer Society.

Tumour staining with Ki-67 can help to differentiate carcinomas from adenomas. High Ki-67 index is shown to have shortened disease free interval and overall survival.[24]

Staging in adrenocortical cancer

Tumour staging has important roles in the management of patients with ACC.

- Tailoring therapy
- Establishing prognosis and guiding patient and clinician expectation
- Monitoring response to intervention and guiding escalation of therapy
- Guiding patient and clinician adaptation to disease progression

A range of staging systems have been published (Table 6.37.5).

Approaches to the treatment of adrenocortical cancer

Management of patients with ACC requires a multidisciplinary approach. To date, the absence of a strong evidence base supported by large, randomized controlled trials remains problematic. The development and recruitment to such trials is to be recommended.

Surgery

Surgery remains the mainstay of treatment offering the prospect of cure. While there remains some debate as to the relative merits of a laparoscopic versus an open approach, the former can be considered appropriate at least for stage I and II disease. Local lymph nodes should be excised/sampled.[25] In patients with infiltrating disease, lymph node or vessel involvement (stage III), open surgery may be required.

Complete resection and volume of residual disease are important outcome predictors.[26] For this reason, surgery should be limited to centres with significant experience in surgery for ACC.

Adjuvant therapy

Most published data indicate high recurrence rate of ACC even after complete resection. Against this background, adjuvant therapy has been considered. Figure 6.37.2 outlines an approach to treatment of ACC amenable to surgery.

Mitotane or O,p'DDD (Ortho, para', Dichloro, Diphenyl-, Dichloroethane) is an adrenolytic agent used for the adjuvant therapy in ACC. Many centres currently recommend mitotane adjuvant therapy after complete resection. Mitotane can induce partial tumour regression and prolong recurrence-free survival. An impact on overall survival has not been demonstrated. Tolerability can be limited by systemic toxicity.[27,28,29] In addition to its adrenolytic properties, mitotane inhibits adrenocortical steroid synthesis by inhibiting cholesterol side chain cleavage and 11 Beta-hydroxylation. Mitotane also affects extra-adrenal cortisol metabolism by inducing hepatic clearance. Mitotane dose titration and supportive therapies require close clinical supervision.

In patients with localized tumour and apparent complete (R0) resection, adjuvant radiotherapy to the tumour bed is not routinely recommended. It should be considered if the primary tumour measures >8 cm in greatest dimension; there is evidence of microscopic tumour invasion in blood vessels; or if there is a Ki-67 index of >10%. Adjuvant radiotherapy to the tumour bed can be considered in patients at high risk for local recurrence (e.g. incomplete/R1resection).[30]

Recurrent disease

Further surgery should be offered for recurrent disease if complete resection is feasible.[31] Adjuvant chemotherapy with mitotane should be considered after surgery for recurrent disease. For recurrence despite mitotane adjuvant therapy, second-line chemotherapy such as that used for advanced disease should be considered after further surgery or if surgery is not appropriate.[32]

Advanced disease

The rarity of ACC has limited clinical studies of cytotoxic chemotherapeutic agents. In advanced disease, surgery has limited advantage but debulking surgery is considered for patients with severe hormone excess that cannot be controlled otherwise. Medical therapy should be initiated as soon as possible.[32,33] Treatment decisions should be based on clinical judgement, tumour progression, and local policies. All drugs exhibit clinical toxicity and therefore treatment should be administered by experienced physicians. Adrenal insufficiency and gastrointestinal side effects are common with mitotane and the majority of patients will require higher than standard-dose hydrocortisone replacment therapy. Additional treatment options with metronomic Capecitabine and Gemcitabine as additional-line therapy have been published.[34] Newer targeted therapy like IGF-1 receptor inhibitor showed promising initial results but they are still under investigation.

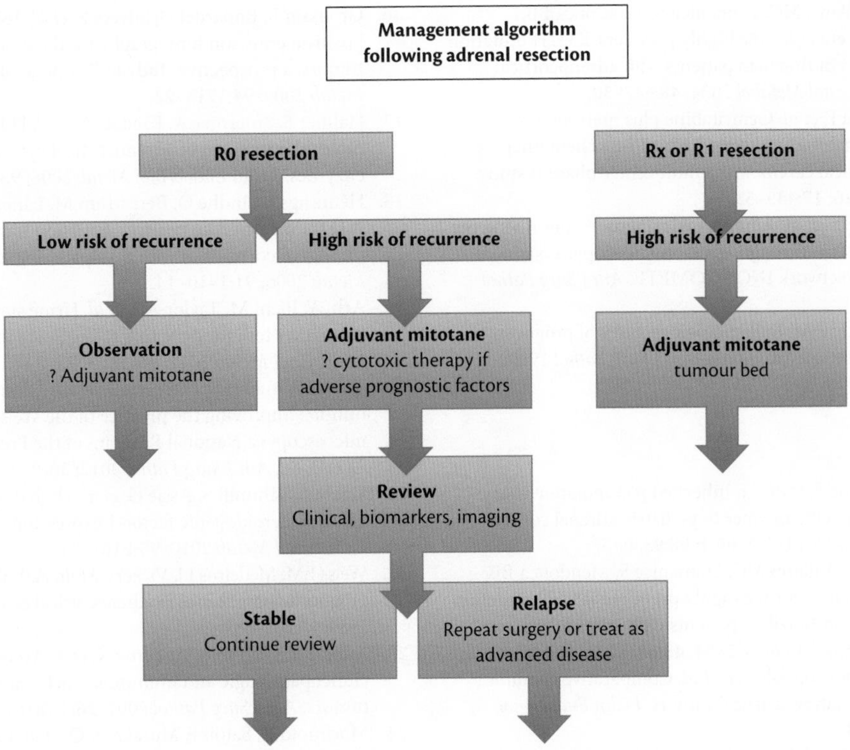

Management algorithm following adrenal resection

R0 resection

Low risk of recurrence

Observation
? Adjuvant mitotane

High risk of recurrence

Adjuvant mitotane
? cytotoxic therapy if adverse prognostic factors

Review
Clinical, biomarkers, imaging

Stable
Continue review

Relapse
Repeat surgery or treat as advanced disease

Rx or R1 resection

High risk of recurrence

Adjuvant mitotane
tumour bed

Fig. 6.37.2 An outline approach to the treatment of adrenocortical cancer amenable to complete resection.
Abbreviations: R0 = complete resection; R1 = incomplete resection; Rx = unsure resection status; EBRT = external beam radiotherapy.

Radiotherapy can play an important role in the care of patients with advanced ACC. In a palliative setting, radiotherapy may be used for symptomatic metastasis to bone, brain, or for vena caval obstruction.[30]

Follow-up of patients with adrenocortical cancer

Recurrence is not uncommon even in patients with localized ACC. Early detection of recurrence can influence the outcome. For this reason, close follow-up is advised after initial treatment. Follow-up with cross sectional imaging using CT or MRI chest and abdomen should be carried out every three months in the initial stage. Endocrine biomarkers should also be monitored if they have been identified. Monitoring interval can be gradually increased after a stable period of two years. Follow-up in patients without recurrence is recommended for a minimum period of 10 years.

Prognosis

ACC carries poor prognosis. Five-year overall survival rate is 37–47%.[35] The most consistently cited factors associated with poor outcome are advanced stage and incomplete surgical resection. High-grade tumour, older age and hormone hyper-secretion have also been found to be associated with poorer prognosis in some studies.[14,29,36]

Further reading

Abiven G, Coste J, Groussin L, *et al.* Clinical and biological features in the prognosis of adrenocortical cancer: poor outcome of cortisol-secreting tumors in a series of 202 consecutive patients. *J Clin Endocrinol Metab* 2006; **91**:2650–5.

Arlt W, Biehl M, Taylor AE, *et al.* Urine steroid metabolomics as a biomarker tool for detecting malignancy in adrenal tumors. *J Clin Endocrinol Metab* 2011; **96**(12):3775–84.

Berruti A, Terzolo M, Sperone P, *et al.* Etoposide, doxorubicin and cisplatin plus mitotane in the treatment of advanced adrenocortical carcinoma: a large prospective phase II trial. *Endoc Relat Cancer* 2005; **12**:657–66.

Crucitti F, Bellantone R, Ferrante A, Boscherini M, Crucitti P. The Italian Registry for Adrenal Cortical Carcinoma: analysis of a multiinstitutional series of 129 patients. The ACC Italian Registry Study Group. *Surgery* 1996; **119**:161–70.

Fassnacht M. Allolio, B. Clinical management of adrenocortical carcinoma. *Best Pract Res Clin Endocrinol Metab* 2009; **23**:273–89.

Groussin L, Bonardel G, Silvéra S, *et al.* 18F-Fluorodeoxyglucose positron emission tomography for the diagnosis of adrenocortical tumors: a prospective study in 77 operated patients. *J Clin Endocrinol Metab* 2009; **94**:1713–22.

Hennings J, Lindhe O, Bergström M, Långström B, Sundin A, Hellman P. [11C]metomidate positron emission tomography of adrenocortical tumors in correlation with histopathological findings. *J Clin Endocrinol Metab* 2006; **91**:1410–14.

Khan TS, Imam H, Juhlin C, *et al.* Streptozocin and o,p'DDD in the treatment of adrenocortical cancer patients: long-term survival in its adjuvant use. *Ann Oncol* 2000; **11**:1281–7.

Luton JP, Cerdas S, Billaud L, *et al.* Clinical features of adrenocortical carcinoma, prognostic factors, and the effect of mitotane therapy. *N Engl J Med* 1990; **322**:1195–201.

Morimoto R, Satoh F, Murakami O, *et al.* Immunohistochemistry of a proliferation marker Ki67/MIB1 in adrenocortical carcinomas: Ki67/MIB1 labeling index is a predictor for recurrence of adrenocortical carcinomas. *Endocr J* 2008; **55**:49–55.

Park BK, Kim CK, Kim B, Lee JH. Comparison of delayed enhanced CT and chemical shift MR for evaluating hyper-attenuating incidental adrenal masses. *Radiology* 2007; **243**:760–5.

Pinto EM, Billerbeck AE, Villares MC, Domenice S, Mendonça BB, Latronico AC. Founder effect for the highly prevalent R337H mutation of tumor suppressor p53 in Brazilian patients with adrenocortical tumors. *Arq Bras Endocrinol Metabol* 2004; **48**:647–50.

Sperone P, Ferrero A, Daffara F, *et al.* Gemcitabine plus metronomic 5-fluorouracil or capecitabine as a second-/third-line chemotherapy in advanced adrenocortical carcinoma: a multicenter phase II study. *Endocr Relat Cancer* 2010; **17**:445–53.

Tissier F, Aubert S, Leteurtre E, *et al.* Adrenocortical tumors: improving the practice of the Weiss system through virtual microscopy: a National Program of the French Network INCa-COMETE. *Am J Surg Pathol* 2012; **36**(8):1194–201.

Weiss LM, Medeiros LJ, Vickery AL Jr. Pathologic features of prognostic significance in adrenocortical carcinoma. *Am J Surg Pathol* 1989; **13**:202–6.

References

1. Raul C. Ribeiro, Sandrinie F, *et al.* An inherited p53 mutation that contributes in a tissue-specific manner to pediatric adrenal cortical carcinoma. *Proc Natl Acad Sci U S A* 2001; **98**:9330–5.
2. Pinto EM, Billerbeck AE, Villares MC, Domenice S, Mendonça BB, Latronico AC. Founder effect for the highly prevalent R337H mutation of tumor suppressor p53 in Brazilian patients with adrenocortical tumors. *Arq Bras Endocrinol Metabol* 2004; **48**:647–50.
3. Sidhu S, Marsh DJ, Theodosopoulos G, *et al.* Comparative genomic hybridization analysis of adrenocortical tumors. *J Clin Endocrinol Metab* 2002; **87**:3467–74.
4. Kjellman M, Roshani L, Teh BT, *et al.* Genotyping of adrenocortical tumors: very frequent deletions of the MEN1 locus in 11q13 and of a 1-centimorgan region in 2p16. *J Clin Endocrinol Metab* 1999; **84**:730–5.
5. Gicquel C, Bertagna X, Gaston V, *et al.* Molecular markers and long-term recurrences in a large cohort of patients with sporadic adrenocortical ENSAT tumors. *Cancer Res* 2001; **61**, 6762–7.
6. Crucitti F, Bellantone R, Ferrante A, Boscherini M, Crucitti P. The Italian Registry for Adrenal Cortical Carcinoma: analysis of a multiinstitutional series of 129 patients. The ACC Italian Registry Study Group. *Surgery* 1996; **119**:161–70.
7. Schulick RD, Brennan MF. Adrenocortical carcinoma. *World J Urol* 1999; **17**:26–34.
8. Dackiw AP, Lee JE, Gagel RF, Evans DB. Adrenal cortical carcinoma. *World J Surg* 2001; **25**:914–26.
9. Abiven G, Coste J, Groussin L, *et al.* Clinical and biological features in the prognosis of adrenocortical cancer: poor outcome of cortisol-secreting tumors in a series of 202 consecutive patients. *J Clin Endocrinol Metab* 2006; **91**:2650–5.
10. Samuels MH, Loriaux DL. Cushing's syndrome and the nodular adrenal gland. *Endocrinol Metab Clin North Am* 1994; **23**(3):555–69.
11. Universität Würzburg Offizielle Homepage des Deutsche Nebennierenkarzinom-Registers, 2010. Available at: http://www.nebennierenkarzinom.de/ [Online].
12. Fassnacht M. Allolio, B. Clinical management of adrenocortical carcinoma. *Best Pract Res Clin Endocrinol Metab 2009;* **23**:273–89.
13. Peña CS, Boland GW, Hahn PF, Lee MJ, Mueller PR. Characterization of Indeterminate (Lipid-poor) Adrenal Masses: Use of Washout Characteristics at Contrast-enhanced CT. *Radiology* 2000; **217**:798–802.
14. Icard P, Goudet P, Charpenay C, *et al.* Adrenocortical carcinomas: surgical trends and results of a 253-patient series from the French Association of Endocrine Surgeons study group. *World J Surg* 2001; **25**:891–7.
15. Park BK, Kim CK, Kim B, Lee JH. Comparison of delayed enhanced CT and chemical shift MR for evaluating hyper-attenuating incidental adrenal masses. *Radiology* 2007; **243**:760–5.
16. Groussin L, Bonardel G, Silvéra S, *et al.* 18F-Fluorodeoxyglucose positron emission tomography for the diagnosis of adrenocortical tumors: a prospective study in 77 operated patients. *J Clin Endocrinol Metab* 2009; **94**:1713–22.
17. Hahner S, Stuermer A, Kreissl M, *et al.* [123 I]Iodometomidate for molecular imaging of adrenocortical cytochrome P450 family 11B enzymes. *J Clin Endocrinol Metab* 2008; **93**:2358–65.
18. Hennings J, Lindhe O, Bergström M, Långström B, Sundin A, Hellman P. [11C]metomidate positron emission tomography of adrenocortical tumors in correlation with histopathological findings. *J Clin Endocrinol Metab* 2006; **91**:1410–14.
19. Arlt W, Biehl M, Taylor AE, *et al.* Urine steroid metabolomics as a biomarker tool for detecting malignancy in adrenal tumors. *J Clin Endocrinol Metab* 2011; **96**(12):3775–84.
20. Tissier F, Aubert S, Leteurtre E, *et al.* Adrenocortical tumors: improving the practice of the Weiss system through virtual microscopy: a National Program of the French Network INCa-COMETE. *Am J Surg Pathol* 2012; **36**(8):1194–201.
21. Sbiera S, Schmull S, Assie G, *et al.* High diagnostic and prognostic value of steroidogenic factor-1 expression in adrenal tumors. *J Clin Endocrinol Metab* 2010; **95**:E161–71.
22. Weiss LM, Medeiros LJ, Vickery AL Jr. Pathologic features of prognostic significance in adrenocortical carcinoma. *Am J Surg Pathol* 1989; **13**:202–6.
23. Aubert S, Wacrenier A, Leroy X, *et al.* Weiss system revisited: a clinicopathologic and immunohistochemical study of 49 adrenocortical tumors. *Am J Surg Pathol* 2002; **26**(12):1612–9.
24. Morimoto R, Satoh F, Murakami O, *et al.* Immunohistochemistry of a proliferation marker Ki67/MIB1 in adrenocortical carcinomas: Ki67/MIB1 labeling index is a predictor for recurrence of adrenocortical carcinomas. *Endocr J* 2008; **55**:49–55.
25. Brix D, Allolio B, Fenske W, *et al.* Laparoscopic versus open adrenalectomy for adrenocortical carcinoma: surgical and oncologic outcome in 152 patients. *Eur Urol* 2010; **58**:609–15.
26. Murphy MM, Witkowski ER, Ng SC, *et al.* Trends in adrenalectomy: a recent national review. *Surg Endosc* 2010; **24**:2518–26.
27. Terzolo, M. *et al.* Adjuvant mitotane treatment for adrenocortical carcinoma. *N Engl J Med* 2007; **356**:2372–80.
28. Hahner S, Fassnacht M. Mitotane for adrenocortical carcinoma treatment. *Curr Opin Investig Drugs* 2005; **6**:386–94.
29. Luton JP, Cerdas S, Billaud L, *et al.* Clinical features of adrenocortical carcinoma, prognostic factors, and the effect of mitotane therapy. *N Engl J Med* 1990; **322**:1195–201.
30. Polat B, Fassnacht M, Pfreundner L, *et al.* Radiotherapy in adrenocortical carcinoma. *Cancer* 2009; **115**:2816–23.
31. Erdogan I, Hahner S, Johanssen S, *et al.* Impact of surgery on clinical outcome in patients with recurrence of adrenocortical carcinoma. *Endocrine Abstracts* 2009; **20**:194.
32. Khan TS, Imam H, Juhlin C, *et al.* Streptozocin and o,p'DDD in the treatment of adrenocortical cancer patients: long-term survival in its adjuvant use. *Ann Oncol* 2000; **11**:1281–7.
33. Berruti A, Terzolo M, Sperone P, *et al.* Etoposide, doxorubicin and cisplatin plus mitotane in the treatment of advanced adrenocortical carcinoma: a large prospective phase II trial. *Endoc Relat Cancer* 2005; **12**:657–66.
34. Sperone P, Ferrero A, Daffara F, *et al.* Gemcitabine plus metronomic 5-fluorouracil or capecitabine as a second-/third-line chemotherapy in advanced adrenocortical carcinoma: a multicenter phase II study. *Endocr Relat Cancer* 2010; **17**:445–53.
35. *Ibid.* **9**.
36. Kebebew E, Reiff E, Duh QY, *et al.* Extent of disease at presentation and outcome for adrenocortical carcinoma: have we made progress? *World J Surg* 2006; **30**:872–8.

CHAPTER 6.38

Treatment of adrenal tumours

Atul Bagul and Saba Balasubramanian

Introduction to the treatment of adrenal tumours

Bartholomaeus Eustachius, the Roman anatomist was the first to describe the adrenal gland in 1552; the *'Glandulae renibus incumbentes'* (gland lying on the kidney). It was only in the latter half of the nineteenth century that the gland's association with disease was described by Thomas Addison and others. A link with hormonal secretion was then made leading to the discovery of the first hormone 'adrenaline' in 1897.[1] The early reports of adrenalectomy procedures in the late nineteenth and early twentieth century were for large tumours irrespective of function; and the elaborate description of the operations clearly emphasized the problems with surgical exposure and access to the adrenals.

In the twentieth century, the focus of adrenal pathology changed significantly—from hypoadrenalism due to predominantly infective causes (i.e. tuberculosis) to hyperfunction due to neoplastic processes. The variety of hormonal syndromes relating to adrenal glands underlies the spectrum of clinical manifestations with which patients with adrenal disease present. More recently, the management of incidentally detected adrenal lesions (incidentalomas) have been the focus of attention; although the vast majority are non-functional and benign, a significant proportion may be associated with subtle hormonal abnormalities and a small minority may represent adrenocortical cancer.

This chapter will focus on adrenal tumours and its management as it relates to the surgeon. For more detailed understanding of endocrine pathophysiology, the reader is referred to other sources. Non-neoplastic pathology such as autoimmune conditions and infective processes in the adrenal glands are beyond the scope of this chapter.

Anatomy and physiology

The two adrenal glands are retroperitoneal structures, golden yellow in colour, each weighing approximately 5 g. They lie within the renal fascia, in relation to the upper-pole of the kidneys (T11-12 vertebrae). The right gland is like an irregular tetrahedron and is located behind the inferior vena cava (IVC) and the right hepatic lobe. The left is semilunar in shape and anteromedial to the kidney. The superior, middle, and inferior arteries arise from the phrenic, abdominal aorta, and renal arteries, respectively. The main adrenal vein drains into the IVC on the right and renal vein on the left.[2]

The adrenal gland is divided into an embryologically, structurally and functionally different outer cortex (from the mesoderm) and an inner medulla (from the neuroectoderm). The adrenal cortex has three layers and produce hormones which are cholesterol derivatives:

- Zona Glomerulosa (outer layer)—mineralocorticoids (aldosterone)
- Zona Fasciculata (middle layer)—glucocorticoids (cortisol)
- Zona Reticularis (inner layer)—sex hormones (DHEA: dehydroepiandrosterone and androstenedione)

Cortisol secretion is controlled by a negative feedback involving the hypothalamo-pituitary-adrenal axis [Corticotrophin releasing factor (CRF)—adrenocorticotropic hormone (ACTH)—cortisol]. Cortisol plays a role in stress response, carbohydrate, lipid, and protein metabolism, and has some mineralocorticoid effects promoting salt and water retention. Aldosterone is secreted under the control of renin-angiotensin system and leads to renal re-absorption of sodium and excretion of potassium and hydrogen. The adrenal sex hormones are under control of ACTH and are weakly androgenic and when in excess, can cause virilization in women.

The adrenal medulla secretes catecholomines—adrenaline (epinephrine), noradrenaline (norepinephrine), and dopamine. Their actions are mediated via adrenergic and dopaminergic receptors. The physiological effect (also called 'flight or fight response') is characterized by increase in heart rate, blood pressure, and cardiac output, excitation of the central nervous system, increased blood flow to muscles, reduced splanchnic circulation, and breakdown of lipids and glycogen.

Classification of adrenal tumours

Adrenal tumours may be classified depending on the site of origin, pathology, and function. A pragmatic approach is shown in Table 6.38.1. Other adrenal lesions that may not be classified as 'adrenal tumours' include amyloidosis, cysts, granulomas, haematomas, hamartomas, and xanthomas. The commonly used eponymous names Cushing's and Conn's refer to adrenal lesions associated with hypercortisolism and hyperaldosteronism respectively.

Investigation for adrenal tumours

Biochemical tests

The exact nature and extent of biochemical investigations depend on the presentation and the nature of the suspected diagnosis. Patients may be referred to the endocrinologist or physician with clinical features of hypercortisolism, hyperaldosteronism or phaeochromocytoma where adrenal hyperfunction (hormonal excess) is suspected. Very occasionally, adrenal tumours may produce

Table 6.38.1 Classification of adrenal tumours

Site of origin	Benign	Malignant
Cortex	Adenoma (functioning and non-functioning) Hyperplasia (functioning and non-functioning) ◆ Micronodular ◆ Macronodular	Adrenocortical cancer
Medulla	Phaeochromocytoma	Malignant phaeochromocytoma
Miscellaneous	Myelolipoma Neurofibroma Teratoma Ganglioneuroma	Metastases (from breast, lung, melanoma, leukaemia) Lymphoma Neuroblastoma Ganglioneuroblastoma Sarcomas

excessive sex-steroid hormones resulting in virilizing or feminizing features. If adrenal hyperfunction is suspected, a biochemical diagnosis should be made before the use of imaging. This is to avoid the detection of small incidental findings of no significance.

An increasing number of patients now present with incidentally detected adrenal lesions (incidentalomas) during abdominal and/or thoracic imaging for non-adrenal indications. The detection of an incidentaloma should lead to a biochemical screen even in the absence of any symptoms or signs of hormonal excess. This is to minimize the risk of overlooking biochemical syndromes that will influence the management of these lesions.

A summary of commonly used investigations is as follows.[3]

(i) An overnight 1 mg dexamethasone suppression test is often done as a first test to rule out hypercortisolism. Alternative tests include urinary free cortisol, late night salivary cortisol, and midnight plasma cortisol levels.

(ii) In patients with hypertension, serum potassium, aldosterone, and plasma renin activity will help in establishing the diagnosis of primary hyperaldosteronism. The lack of hypokalaemia alone does not rule out this condition. Testing is not necessary in patients who are not hypertensive.

(iii) DHEAS (dehydroepiandrosterone) levels are done to rule out sex hormone excess.

(iv) 24 hour urinary catecholamines and metanephrines have been used as a standard test for several years now for the diagnosis of a phaeochromocytoma. Recent evidence points to plasma free metanephrines as being more accurate with the added advantage being the avoidance of a 24-hour collection. However, this may not be available in all centres.

These tests are best done in accordance to locally determined endocrinology protocols. Surgeons should be aware that several medications can influence the results of endocrine biochemical tests and tests often need repeating after appropriate changes in interfering medications. There may be other factors at play; for example, in urine biochemistry, the 24-hour urine collection may not have been complete. Also, a number of these tests do not have a clear cut-off value; rather a normal range, borderline range, and an abnormal range. Test results that are borderline or equivocal need to be repeated. A detailed knowledge of endocrinology and biochemistry is required for the correct interpretation of results and a comprehensive discussion of these issues is beyond the scope of this chapter.

Cross-sectional imaging

Cross-sectional imaging such as computed tomography (CT) scan or MRI is the standard form of radiological assessment for adrenal tumours. They also account for the vast majority of incidentally detected adrenal lesions. The aims of these tests include localization of a suspected biochemical syndrome, determination of the nature of an adrenal lesion and exclusion of other coexistent pathology. General features of malignancy lesions on CT/MRI include heterogeneity, irregular borders, local invasion, lymphadenopathy, and rapid growth on sequential scans. The density of an adrenal lesion (measured by Housnfield units—HU) on a non-contrast CT scan is helpful to determine the likelihood of malignancy. Benign cortical lesions are generally 'fat rich' and appear as low density, while phaeochromocytomas and malignant lesions are high density. A level of less than 10 HU (Hounsfield Units) is generally regarded as a good indicator of a benign lesion. Lesions with Hounsfield units of between 10 and 30 can be further characterized by studying washout on delayed images in a three phase CT scan or by MR imaging. The use of chemical shift imaging on MRI provides information that is a good discriminant between lipid-rich and lipid poor lesions; the latter being more likely to be malignant or phaeochromocytomas.[4]

Functional imaging

Functional imaging is performed in certain specific situations to corroborate a suspected pathological or biochemical diagnosis. In patients with an indeterminate adrenal lesion, FDG-PET (Fluro-deoxyglucose positron emission tomography) scan may be useful; increased uptake in adrenal cancer, phaeochromocytoma, metastases, and lymphoma may help differentiate from benign adrenal tumours.[5] In patients with a biochemical diagnosis of phaeochromocytoma where bilateral, metastatic or extra-adrenal pathology is suspected; ^{123}I MIBG (metaiodobenzylguanidine) scanning may identify extent of disease and may influence the management approach.

Selective venous sampling is occasionally used in patients with proven biochemical adrenal hyperfunction to enable lateralization (the side) of the pathology. It has a specific indication in Conn's syndrome (primary hyperaldosteronism); this will be discussed later.

Biopsy

Biopsy of adrenal gland lesions is rarely performed as they do not help to diagnose malignancy in either cortical or medullary lesions. In addition, there are concerns relating to dissemination of cancer along the biopsy tract if the lesions are malignant. Occasionally, a fine needle imaging guided biopsy may be required to confirm uncommon pathology such as tuberculosis, lymphoma, or metastases from another primary source. If this is required, biochemical tests should be performed first to rule out phaeochromocytoma to avoid the problems associated with catecholamine release.[6]

Clinical syndromes of surgical interest

Adrenal incidentaloma

Adrenal incidentaloma is characterized by the incidental discovery of an adrenal mass larger than 1cm in diameter on cross-sectional imaging performed for non-adrenal pathology. The prevalence of such adrenal incidentalomas on cross-sectional imaging is thought to be up to 5% but increases with age, resolution of the imaging modality used and the presence of background medical problems. The prevalence is higher in patients with a history of malignancy.[7]

The pathology could be any of the ones listed in Table 6.38.1. Less than 5% are due to primary adrenal cancer.[8]

Management

The detection of an adrenal incidentaloma should be followed by a biochemical assessment of adrenal function as outlined earlier. This may not be appropriate in all patients such as those with terminal illness and metastatic disease. Tumours that are functional in nature should be considered for excision. The management of non-functional lesions is controversial, but guidelines suggest that surgery be considered in lesions of over 4 cm, as increasing size correlates with malignancy.[3] Other relative indications include equivocal findings on radiology such as heterogeneity or delayed washout of contrast. Increasingly, uptake on a PET scan is considered to be an indication for surgery in lesions around 4 cm. In smaller, non-functioning, benign appearing lesions, recommended follow up protocols vary; although most authors would advise further evaluation of size and function at six to nine months before patients are reassured and discharged.[8]

Cushing's syndrome

Cushing's syndrome is a rare disorder characterized by increased levels of circulating glucocorticoids, mostly adults in second to fifth decade of life. The prevalence is 10 cases per million per year. The aetiology is either ACTH dependent disease (80%), where the primary pathology is outside the adrenal gland or ACTH independent disease, where the primary pathology is in the adrenal (20%). The former may be due to ACTH excess from pituitary disease or other ectopic sources. ACTH independent (or adrenal) hypercortisolism may be commonly due to an adrenal adenoma or carcinoma and rarely due to bilateral adrenal hyperplasia, primary pigmented nodular adrenal disease or McCune Albright syndrome.[9]

Clinical features

The clinical features along with their frequency are listed in Table 6.38.2.

Table 6.38.2 Clinical features of Cushing's syndrome

Clinical feature	Occurrence rate (%)
Obesity	95
Facial plethora	90
Decreased libido	90
Thin skin	85
Decreased linear growth in children	75
Menstrual irregularity	80
Hypertension	75
Hirsutism	75
Depression/emotional lability	70
Easy bruising	65
Glucose intolerance	60
Weakness	60
Acne	50
Osteopenia or fracture	50
Nephrolithiasis	50

Reproduced from John A. H. Wass and Paul M. Stewart, *Oxford Textbook of Endocrinology and Diabetes, Second Edition*, Table 5.7.2, p. 826, Oxford University Press, Oxford, UK, Copyright © 2011, by permission of Oxford University Press.

Investigations

This involves a confirmation of the diagnosis based on demonstration of high cortisol levels and loss of negative feedback control of hypothalamic-pituitary-adrenal (HPA) axis. A low dose dexamethasone suppression test to demonstrate failure of cortisol suppression by the HPA axis and low plasma ACTH levels are usually sufficient in patients with hypercortisolism secondary to adrenal pathology; although in some of these cases and in hypercortisolism not due to adrenal pathology, additional biochemical testing is required. Patients with suspected adrenal source of hypercortisolism are further investigated by a CT or MRI scan, as discussed earlier.

Management

Adrenalectomy is the definitive treatment of choice for benign and malignant adrenal tumours with hypercortisolism. Bilateral adrenalectomy is also considered to address the problem of hypercortisolism in patients with ACTH dependent Cushing's in certain scenarios such as failed pituitary surgery and hypercortisolism due to ectopic ACTH secretion where the ectopic source cannot be treated adequately.

Medical treatment of hypercortisolism with drugs that inhibit steroid synthesis such as metapyrone (11-β hydroxylase inhibitor) and ketaconazole (P-450 enzyme inhibitor) are sometimes used in patients with significant hypercortisolism for adequate optimization before surgery.

Phaeochromocytoma

Phaeochromoctoma is a functioning tumour of chromaffin cells which is characterized by excessive synthesis and release of catecholamines and their metabolites (such as metanephrines). Chromaffin cell tumours occur mostly in the adrenal medulla (80-85%) and occasionally (15–20%) in extra-adrenal tissue—paragangliomas.[10] Phaeochromocytoma was first described by Frankel in 1886 and has an incidence of 1–2 per 100,000 population. They are termed as the 10% tumour as approximately 10% are extra-adrenal, 10% bilateral, 10% malignant, 10% occur in children, and 10% are familial. The '10% familial' rule is no longer valid as more recent studies show that up to one-third of patients have a genetic predisposition. The familial lesions are usually seen in patients under the age of 40 years and are associated with multiple endocrine neoplasia type II (MEN 2A & 2B: chromosome 10), von Hippel-Lindau disease (chromosome 3), Neurofibromatosis Type 1 (NF 1 gene: chromosome 17) and paraganglioma syndromes (SDH B and D mutations in chromosome 8 and 4, respectively). A number of other genes have recently been described with mutations that predispose to phaeochromocytomas and paragangliomas.

Clinical features

Although a number of phaeochromocytomas are detected following investigations for severe hypertension or the occurrence of an unexplained cardiovascular event, some may be detected

Box 6.38.1 Clinical features in phaeochromocytoma

- Sustained or paroxysmal hypertension
- Headache
- Palpitations
- Sweating
- Pallor
- Nausea
- Flushing
- Weight loss
- Tiredness
- Psychological symptoms (anxiety, panic)
- Orthostatic hypotension
- Hyperglycaemia

during biochemical investigation of an adrenal incidentaloma. Box 6.38.1 lists the features most commonly associated with phaeochromocytomas.

Investigations

Biochemical investigations and imaging for phaeochromocytoma have been explained earlier. It is important to note that while adrenal lesions may produce a variety of catecholamines and metanephrines; extra-adrenal lesions do not release adrenaline or metanephrines—this is due to the absence of phenylethanolamine-N-methyl transferase (PNMT) in extra-adrenal chromaffin tissue. This enzyme catalyses the conversion of noradrenaline to adrenaline in the adrenal medulla. Repeat biochemical testing is often necessary; especially in patients with borderline levels. Several drugs that interfere with the synthesis, release, uptake, and degradation of catecholamines may be associated with spurious biochemical results.[11] These include sympathomimetic agents (such as amphetamine), monoamine oxidase (MAO) inhibitors (such as tranylcypromine), adrenaline and noradrenaline reuptake inhibitors (such as venlafaxine), adrenergic receptor blockers, and drugs that interfere with catecholamine hormone assays (such as paracetamol). These may have to be stopped or replaced by other agents before repeat testing.

Management

Adrenalectomy is recommended for all patients with phaeochromocytoma.[12–15] Earlier concerns regarding the feasibility and safety of laparoscopic surgery have now been satisfactorily addressed by several studies. Careful preoperative workup and management is however mandatory. Simple procedures like an anaesthetic induction or a percutaneous intervention may precipitate a hypertensive crisis in patients who have not been given adequate alpha blockade. The aim of preoperative medical treatment should be maximum tolerated alpha blockade. Phenoxybenzamine is commenced at 10 mg bd and gradually increased until symptoms become troublesome. Selective α_1 blocker like doxazosine is a good alternative.[16] Beta-blockers can precipitate a hypertensive crisis and must only be used to control tachycardia after effective alpha blockade is achieved.[17] In the preoperative period, patients should be encouraged to take fluids liberally and 1–2 L normal saline may be infused overnight prior to surgery to expand the intravascular volume. These preoperative measures will help reduce the risk of postoperative hypotension.

During surgery, close monitoring of cardiovascular parameters by an experienced anaesthetist; appropriate and judicious use of inotropes and vasodilatory agents; and good communication between the surgeon and anaesthetist during tumour handling and vein ligation are all essential to ensure a good outcome. Postoperatively, hypotension and hypoglycaemia should be anticipated and treated. We currently offer annual, lifelong biochemical screening to detect and treat recurrent or metachronous phaeochromocytoma.

Malignant phaeochromocytoma is rare and often only suspected when the disease recurs in local or distant sites. Recurrent disease should be resected if possible. Patients with unresectable disease may be treated with alpha blockade and therapeutic ^{131}I-MIBG. Response rates of 57% have been reported with chemotherapy (cyclophosphamide, vincristine, and dacarbazine). The five-year survival is around 20%.[12]

Primary aldosteronism (Conn's syndrome)

Primary aldosteronism is a syndrome characterized by excessive production of aldosterone in the adrenal cortex. It was first described by Jerome Conn in 1955. It is now thought to be prevalent in around 10% of all hypertensive patients. It may be caused by idiopathic bilateral (or occasionally unilateral) hyperplasia in up to 75% of patients and an adrenal adenoma in the remainder.[13] Rarer causes include adrenal carcinoma and glucocorticoid-suppressible hyperaldosteronism. Only adrenal adenoma causing primary aldosteronism will be discussed further as those are the patients referred for surgical treatment.

Clinical features

The clinical features of primary hyperaldosteronism mimic that of severe essential hypertension. Patients may present with renal failure or the cardiovascular consequences of hypertension and chronic salt and water load. Although the pathogenesis of hypertension involves volume expansion, oedema is typically absent. Hypokalaemia (if present) may lead to muscle weakness, cramps, fatigue, polyuria, polydipsia, and cardiac arrhythmias.[14]

Investigations

Patients that need to be investigated for the presence of primary hyperaldosteronism include those with hypertension and any one of the following:

(i) Hypokalaemia

(ii) Hypertension resistant to drug therapy

(iii) Adrenal incidentalomas

(iv) Any reason to suspect secondary hypertension such as young age, strong family history of hypertension or stroke in young age

Routine blood tests are often normal and hypokalaemia only occurs in approximately 25% of patients. A high plasma aldosterone concentration to plasma renin activity ratio (high aldosterone and low renin) is usually sufficient to diagnose primary hyperaldosteronism. Occasionally additional tests such as (oral or intravenous) salt loading to demonstrate lack of aldosterone suppression may be required. Imaging typically shows a small (usually less than 2 cm) adrenal lesion with features of benign cortical origin. Due to the frequent occurrence of some nodularity in both adrenal glands and the small size of lesions causing Conn's syndrome, most experts recommend adrenal venous sampling of aldosterone levels prior to unilateral adrenalectomy. This will ensure that the correct side is operated upon and that patients with bilateral disease do not undergo unnecessary surgery.

Management

Medical therapy using aldosterone antagonists such as spironolactone and eplerenone, in combination with other antihypertensives are often effective in controlling hypertension. This is the treatment of choice in patients with bilateral disease and in the initial stages of management of those with unilateral pathology (Conn's adenoma). Surgery (unilateral laparoscopic adrenalectomy) is an excellent definitive treatment option for those with Conn's adenoma with the objective of reducing dependence on lifelong medical treatment and its attendant costs and side effects. Hypertension improves in all patients and may be cured in 30-60% of them.[13]

Adrenocortical carcinoma

Adrenocortical carcinoma is rare; but one of the most lethal of endocrine tumours. It has an incidence of one to two cases per million per year.[15] It presents with two peak incidences, the first and fifth decade of life and is more common in females. Around 60% of tumours are functioning and produce a combination of steroid hormones and their precursors.[16]

Clinical features

Patients presenting with hormonal excess often present with severe hypercortisolism. Features of other hormone excess such as virilizing or feminizing symptoms (due to sex hormones) and hyperaldosteronism may coexist or occasionally present in isolation.[15] Patients with non-functioning tumours present either as an incidentalomas or with local symptoms such as abdominal pain.

Investigations

Briefly, biochemical investigations (described earlier) will help confirm hyperfunction. Tumours secreting multiple hormones are more likely to be malignant. Cross-sectional imaging such as CT or MRI of the adrenal and functional imaging such as PET scan provide valuable clues as to the possibility of cancer and help alert the surgeon and ensure that a complete resection is performed. The differentiation between benign and malignant tumours can be difficult even on histological examination. Weiss proposed criteria[17] based on the presence of at least three of nine histological features to diagnose malignancy. These include high nuclear grade (III or IV), high mitotic rate (>5/50 high-power fields), atypical mitoses, clear cells comprising 25% or less of the tumour, diffuse architecture, microscopic necrosis, and invasion of venous, sinusoidal, and capsular structures. This is widely used, although other indices such as Ki67 (cell proliferation marker) and molecular markers have recently been proposed.[18]

Tumour staging

Several staging systems have been proposed to enable optimum prognostication in adrenal cancer. An overall scheme incorporating the different systems is presented in Table 6.38.3. As illustrated, the more recent system proposed by the European Network for the Study of Adrenal Tumours (ENSAT) restricts stage IV to patients with distant metastases. More than 50% of patients present with stage III or stage IV tumours. Five-year disease specific survival rates for stage I, II, III, and IV disease are reported to be 82%, 61%, 50%, and 13%, respectively.[19]

Management

Surgical resection offers the only prospect for cure. A radical resection of the tumour along with any enlarged lymph nodes is potentially curative in patients without distant metastases. For large tumours invading adjacent structures such as the kidney and the liver, en bloc resection should be performed whenever possible. For cancers with tumour emboli into the vena cava, macroscopic clearance should still be attempted. Tumour embolectomy and/or resection of a segment of the vena cava may occasionally be necessary. Debulking procedures may have a role for palliation; especially in those with functioning tumours or local symptoms.

As preoperative diagnosis for patients with local disease can be difficult, the index of suspicion for adrenal cancer should be

Table 6.38.3 Staging of adrenocortical cancer

Stage	Macfarlane (1958)/Sullivan (1978)	UICC/TNM (2004)	ENSAT (2009)
I	Tumour ≤5 cm, with no local invasion, nodal or distant metastasis	T1, N0, M0	T1, N0, M0
II	Tumour >5 cm, with no local invasion, nodal or distant metastasis	T2, N0, M0	T2, N0, M0
III	Tumour with local invasion *or* nodal disease; but without distant metastasis	T1-2, N1, M0 T3, N0, M0	Any T, N1, M0 T3-4, N0, M0
IV	Tumour with local invasion *and* nodal disease; or tumours with distant metastasis	T4, N0, M0 T3-4, N1, M0 Any T, Any N, M1	Any T, Any N, M1

TNM classification: T1 = ≤5 cm; T2 = >5 cm; T3 = infiltration into surrounding tissue; T4 = invasion into adjacent organs; N0 = no positive lymph node metastasis; N1 = positive lymph nodes present; M0 = no distant metastasis; M1 = distant metastasis present.

Adapted from *European Journal of Cancer*, Volume 46, Issue 4, Lughezzani G *et al.*, 'The European Network for the study of adrenal tumours staging system is prognostically superior to the international union against cancer - staging system: A North American validation', pp. 713–9, Crown Copyright © 2009 Published by Elsevier Ltd, with permission from Elsevier, http://www.sciencedirect.com/science/journal/09598049 Source: data from Guthrie T and Jasani N, 'Contemporary management of adrenocortical carcinoma', *Cancer Therapy*, Volume 6, pp. 597–602, Copyright © 2008; De Lellis RA *et al.*, *Pathology and genetics of tumors of endocrine organs*, International Agency for Research on Cancer, Lyon, France, Copyright © 2004 IARC; McFarlane DA, 'Cancer of the adrenal cortex: The natural history, prognosis and treatment in the study of fifty cases. Hunterian Lecture Delivered at the Royal College of Surgeons of England on 6th March 1958', *Annals of The Royal College of Surgeons of England*, Volume 23, Issue 3, pp. 155–186, Copyright © 1958; Sullivan M *et al.*, Adrenal cortical carcinoma, *Journal of Urology*, Volume 120, Issue 6, pp. 660–5, Copyright © 1968; and Fassnacht M *et al.*, 'Limited prognostic value of the 2004 International Union Against Cancer staging classification for adrenocortical carcinoma: proposal for a Revised TNM Classification', *Cancer*, Volume 1215, Issue 2, pp. 243–50, Copyright © 2008 American Cancer Society.

low. Although laparoscopic resection may be performed and has equivalent outcomes to open resection in experienced hands,[20] most authors advocate open surgery in large lesions likely to be malignant. This is to reduce the risk of capsule rupture, tumour seeding, and peritoneal and port site recurrences.

The role of adjuvant therapy such as mitotane for resected tumours is controversial, but may be considered for high risk patients (stage III disease, incomplete resection, Ki67 >10%).[21] Postoperative surveillance includes a combination of physical examination, imaging, and biochemical assessment (for functional tumours).

For resectable recurrences and metastases, surgery should still be considered in addition to mitotane and cytotoxic chemotherapy. Symptoms relating to hormonal excess may require additional adrenostatic drugs such as metyrapone and ketoconazole.[15]

Secondary adrenal tumours

Metastasis could arise from tumours such as breast, bronchus, and melanoma. A large metastasis could destroy adrenal tissue and lead to adrenal insufficiency; which may present as an acute (Addisonian) crisis. These are however often identified on cross-sectional imaging done for staging or surveillance as part of the management of the primary tumour. Investigations should be done as previously discussed. In addition, a CT guided biopsy may occasionally help confirm the diagnosis. Isolated adrenal metastasis may be considered for resection if the primary tumour has been adequately treated, the patient's general condition is appropriate and if there is no obvious evidence of disease elsewhere.[22]

Adrenalectomy: the surgical procedures

Thornton performed the first reported adrenalectomy in 1889 for a 9 kg tumour. Although several approaches have been described for an open operation, adrenal surgery has always been considered a major challenge due to its anatomy. Laparoscopic adrenalectomy was described first by Gagner in 1992 and has now become the standard approach for most adrenal lesions. Key advantages with the laparoscopic approach include the reduction in access related complications (wound dehiscence, hernias, acute and chronic pain), adhesions, ileus, and respiratory morbidity; leading to shorter hospital stay and earlier recovery. The disadvantages are a steep learning curve and longer operative times, especially in the early phase of learning. For large tumours (>7 cm), a hand-assist approach serves as a useful technique and largely preserves the advantages of laparoscopy. Both open and laparoscopic procedures can be performed by anterior, lateral, and posterior routes; the ideal approach needs to be tailored to the patient and dependent upon tumour pathology, tumour size, patient habitus, previous surgery, surgeon's experience, and whether a bilateral procedure is being planned. Table 6.38.4 illustrates the advantages and disadvantages of various approaches. Robotic techniques are now being introduced to facilitate laparoscopic resection, but the precise nature of the advantages is unclear and is not thought to outweigh the significant costs involved.

Informed consent

A detailed discussion of indications for adrenalectomy, risks of complications, and the implications of surgery including the need for postoperative steroid replacement is mandatory. General complications include venous thromboembolism, respiratory, and cardiac problems. Specific complications that should be discussed include

- Complications related to surgical access and exposure: wound infection, delayed healing, wound dehiscence & hernia formation (increased with hypercortisolism) and damage to adjacent viscera (bowel, kidneys, great vessels, diaphragm, liver on the right, and spleen and pancreas on left side).
- Pathology specific complications:
  (a) Cushing's syndrome: contralateral adrenal suppression (after unilateral adrenalectomy) and need for steroid replacement; need for lifelong steroids after bilateral adrenalectomy.
  (b) Phaeochromocytoma: perioperative hypertensive crisis with consequent cardiovascular and cerebrovascular morbidity, postoperative hypotension, and hypoglycaemia.
  (c) Conn's syndrome: persistent hypertension.
  (d) Adrenocortical cancer: tumour rupture, persistent, and recurrent disease.

Key principles in adrenal surgery

Correct positioning of the patient, appropriate port sites, and incisions, identification of anatomical landmarks, and careful dissection are all important to successful adrenal surgery. 'Surrounding structures and organs are dissected off the adrenal gland'. When malignancy is suspected, resection should include the entire gland including the surrounding fat and any lymph nodes. Adjacent viscera may need to be excised *en bloc* if there is evidence of local invasion.

In some patients (such as those with bilateral phaeochromocytomas and Conn's syndrome), partial or cortical sparing adrenalectomy has been advocated to avoid steroid dependence. This is however often unsuccessful as patients have a higher risk of recurrent disease and may still need steroid supplementation. Good perioperative care is vital especially in patients with functioning tumours and requires close collaboration with an experienced anaesthetist and medical endocrinology team.

Postoperative adrenal insufficiency

This is a medical emergency and can occur in patients who undergo bilateral adrenalectomy (for example for bilateral phaeochromocytoma or for ACTH dependent hypercortisolism) or unilateral adrenalectomy (for cortisol producing adrenal tumours where they may be contralateral adrenal suppression). This may occur despite compliance with steroid medication and could be precipitated by infection, surgery, trauma, or sepsis; conditions where steroid requirements increase significantly.

Patients may present with malaise, tiredness, weakness, anorexia, and abdominal pain. Findings at presentation include hypovolaemia, hypotension refractory to fluid loading, hyponatraemia, hypoglycaemia, hyperkalaemia, and hypercalcaemia. A short synacthen test confirms adrenal insufficiency.

These patients should be hydrated with normal saline and supraphysiological doses of hydrocortisone in the acute phase. After treatment of the acute phase, long term steroid replacement with glucocorticoids (hydrocortisone) and mineralocorticoids (fludrocortisone) is necessary.

Table 6.38.4 Approaches for an adrenalectomy

Approach		Advantages	Disadvantages
Laparoscopic	Anterior/ transperitoneal	Short learning curve for established laparoscopic surgeons	Problems inherent in transperitoneal access
	Retroperitoneal	Ideal for small lesions and patients with history of abdominal surgery Avoids disadvantages of entering peritoneal cavity	Not suitable for large lesions Difficult orientation for low volume surgeons
Open	Anterior	Better suited to large (>7 cm) lesions suspicious for cancer	Increased morbidity in comparison to laparoscopic approach (ileus, adhesions, hernia, respiratory complications)
	Retroperitoneal	Direct route (but very rarely performed nowadays)	Significant pain/morbidity associated with rib excision
Open thoracoabdominal		Very wide exposure; optimal for very large tumours with diaphragmatic or vena cava involvement	Wound problems, pain, hernias, and respiratory complications

Prevention of this complication after discharge from hospital involves patient education on the importance of compliance to medication, use of a 'Medic-alert' bracelet or steroid card, and awareness of the need to increase steroid dose including use of a pre-dosed syringe (100 mg hydrocortisone) for self-administration when acutely unwell.

Summary

The management of adrenal tumours is associated with numerous potential pitfalls for the inexperienced. A clear understanding of anatomy, pathophysiology, and the natural course of different adrenal diseases is fundamental to securing the best possible patient outcomes. In addition, a multidisciplinary approach that involves surgeons, endocrinologists, diagnostic and interventional radiologists, and oncologists in determining appropriate treatment strategies is important in ensuring optimal outcomes.

References

1. Welbourn RB. The adrenal glands. (p. 382) In: Welbourn RB (ed). *The History of Endocrine Surgery*. New York, NY: Praeger, 1990.
2. Dyson M. Endocrine system. (pp. 1900–5) In: Williams PL (ed). *Gray's Anatomy: The Anatomical Basis of Medicine and Surgery*, 38th edition. New York, NY: Churchill Livingstone, 1995.
3. Nieman LK. Approach to the patient with an adrenal incidentaloma. *J Clin Endocrinol Metab* 2010; **95**(9):4106–13.
4. Goenka AH, Shah SN, Remer EM, Berber E. Adrenal imaging: a primer for oncosurgeons. *J Surg Oncol* 2012; **106**(5):543–8.
5. Blake MA, Prakash P, Cronin CG. PET/CT for adrenal assessment. *AJR Am J Roentgenol* 2010; **195**(2):W91–5.
6. Sood SK, Balasubramanian SP, Harrison BJ. Percutaneous biopsy of adrenal and extra-adrenal retroperitoneal lesions: beware of catecholamine secreting tumours! *Surgeon* 2007; **5**(5):279–81.
7. Grumbach MM, Biller BM, Braunstein GD, *et al.* Management of the clinically inapparent adrenal mass ("incidentaloma"). *Ann Intern Med* 2003; **138**(5):424–9.
8. Arnaldi G, Boscaro M. Adrenal incidentaloma. *Best Pract Res Clin Endocrinol Metab* 2012; **26**(4):405–19.
9. Newell-Price J. Diagnosis/differential diagnosis of Cushing's syndrome: a review of best practice. *Best Pract Res Clin Endocrinol Metab* 2009; **23**(Suppl 1):S5–14.
10. Lenders JW, Eisenhofer G, Mannelli M, Pacak K. Phaeochromocytoma. *Lancet* 2005; **366**(9486):665–75.
11. Neary NM, King KS, Pacak K. Drugs and pheochromocytoma--don't be fooled by every elevated metanephrine. *N Engl J Med* 2011; **364**(23):2268–70.
12. John H, Ziegler WH, Hauri D, Jaeger P. Pheochromocytomas: can malignant potential be predicted? *Urology* 1999; **53**(4):679–83.
13. Young WF Jr. Minireview: primary aldosteronism--changing concepts in diagnosis and treatment. *Endocrinology* 2003; **144**(6):2208–13.
14. Carey RM. Primary aldosteronism. *J Surg Oncol* 2012; **106**(5):575–9.
15. Allolio B, Fassnacht M. Clinical review: Adrenocortical carcinoma: clinical update. *J Clin Endocrinol Metab* 2006; **91**(6):2027–37.
16. Lafemina J, Brennan MF. Adrenocortical carcinoma: past, present, and future. *J Surg Oncol* 2012; **106**(5):586–94.
17. Weiss LM. Comparative histologic study of 43 metastasizing and nonmetastasizing adrenocortical tumors. *Am J Surg Pathol* 1984; **8**(3):163–9.
18. Papotti M, Libe R, Duregon E, Volante M, Bertherat J, Tissier F. The Weiss score and beyond--histopathology for adrenocortical carcinoma. *Horm Cancer* 2011; **2**(6):333–40.
19. Fassnacht M, Johanssen S, Quinkler M, *et al.* Limited prognostic value of the 2004 International Union Against Cancer staging classification for adrenocortical carcinoma: proposal for a Revised TNM Classification. *Cancer* 2009; **115**(2):243–50.
20. Brix D, Allolio B, Fenske W, *et al.* Laparoscopic versus open adrenalectomy for adrenocortical carcinoma: surgical and oncologic outcome in 152 patients. *Eur Urol* 2010; **58**(4):609–15.
21. Berruti A, Fassnacht M, Baudin E, *et al.* Adjuvant therapy in patients with adrenocortical carcinoma: a position of an international panel. *J Clin Oncol* 2010; **28**(23):e401–2; author reply e3.
22. Sancho JJ, Triponez F, Montet X, Sitges-Serra A. Surgical management of adrenal metastases. *Langenbecks Arch Surg* 2012; **397**(2):179–94.

SECTION 7

Andrology

Section editor: David John Ralph

CHAPTER 7.1

Infertility

Assessment

Gert R. Dohle

Introduction: aetiology and prevalence

Male infertility is defined as the absence of spontaneous pregnancy after one year of unprotected intercourse. About 15% of couples with an active wish for children do not achieve a pregnancy within one year. Half of these couples will have a spontaneous pregnancy in the next year; eventually 4% of couples will remain unwillingly childless.[1]

The main cause and associated factors of male infertility are listed in Box 7.1.1.

Predictive factors for spontaneous pregnancy are female age and ovarian function, duration of infertility, and semen quality. The cumulative pregnancy rate in infertile couples with two years of follow-up and oligozoospermia as the primary cause of infertility is 27%.[2] In Western societies, female age has become the most important single variable influencing spontaneous pregnancy and outcome in assisted reproduction.[3]

History and physical examination

Assessment of couples with infertility is extensively described in the *WHO Manual for the Standardized Investigation and Diagnosis of the Infertile Couple*.[4] History taking should focus on the main causes and associated factors of male infertility (Boxes 7.1.1 and 7.1.2). Physical examination includes body composition, signs of male hypogonadism, a close examination of the inguinal region and evaluation of the scrotal contents (Box 7.1.3). Rectal examination is only indicated in case of micturition disturbances or genital infections.

Laboratory examinations

Semen analysis

Andrological evaluation is indicated if semen analysis shows abnormalities compared with reference values (WHO Manual) (Table 7.1.1). Important treatment decisions are based on the results of semen analysis and standardization of the complete laboratory work-up is essential. Ejaculate analysis has been standardized by the WHO and disseminated by continuing work and publications in the *WHO Laboratory Manual for Human Semen and Sperm-Cervical Mucus Interaction* (fifth edition).[5] The diagnosis of male infertility relies to a great extent on semen analysis. In spite of detailed technical guidelines and external quality control programmes for sperm laboratories, a large degree of inter- and intralaboratory variability

Box 7.1.1 Main causes and associated factors of male infertility

- Testicular insufficiency
  - Congenital: testicular dysgenesis syndrome (TDS)
  - (Viral) orchitis
  - Testicular torsion
  - Cytotoxic therapy (chemotherapy)
  - Radiation therapy
- Genetic abnormalities
  - Klinefelter's syndrome, Y-chromosomal deletions, *CFTR* gene mutations,
- Hypogonadotrophic hypogonadism (low LH and FSH)
  - Primary forms: Kallmann's syndrome, idiopathic congenital hypogonadotrophic hypogonadism
  - Secondary forms: pituitary dysfunction (adenoma, infection, haemochromatosis, drugs)
  - Anabolic steroids
  - Morbid obesity
- Obstructions of the seminal pathway
  - Congenital bilateral absence of the vas deferens (CBAVD)
  - Midline prostatic cysts
  - Epididymal obstruction
  - Obstruction caused by previous scrotal and inguinal surgery
- Urogenital infections/male accessory gland infection
- Other causes
  - Sperm antibodies
  - Drugs
  - Chronic disease
  - Varicocele
  - Sexual problems
  - Ejaculatory dysfunction
- Idiopathic male infertility (30–40%)

Box 7.1.2 History taking in male infertility patients

Duration of the infertility (months)
Primary or secondary form; children in a previous relationship
Cryptorchidism
Inguinal and scrotal surgery
Urogenital infections, sexually transmitted diseases, tuberculosis
Urogenital trauma and testicular torsion
Previous malignancy
Lifestyle factors: smoking, alcohol abuse, anabolic steroids
Puberty (age)
Chronic diseases
Family history (infertility, congenital abnormalities, genetic abnormalities)
Occupational exposure to chemicals and irradiation
Sexual problems

in WHO sperm parameters exists. In addition to the technical variation, semen analyses in consecutive samples of an individual are known to be subject to individual biological variation.[6] Although sperm parameters like concentration, motility, and morphology are used to classify men as infertile, subfertile, or fertile, none of these parameters are diagnostic of infertility.[7]

If the results of semen analysis are normal according to WHO criteria, one test should be sufficient. If the results are abnormal in at least two tests, further andrological investigation is recommended. It is important to distinguish between the following:

- oligozoospermia: <15 million spermatozoa/mL;
- asthenozoospermia: <32% motile spermatozoa;
- teratozoospermia: <4% normal forms.

Quite often, these three abnormalities occur simultaneously, referred to as the *OAT-syndrome*.

Reproductive hormones

Increased levels of lutenizing hormone (LH) and follicle-stimulating hormone (FSH) occur frequently in men with infertility due to testicular insufficiency with disturbed spermatogenesis, together with decreased testicular volume and low testosterone.

Men with low levels of gonadotrophins (hypogonadotrophic hypogonadism) usually have extreme oligozoospermia or azoospermia. The prevalence of low reproductive hormone levels in infertile men ranges from 0.6–8.9%.[8] Box 7.1.4 highlights the two main types of hypogonadism and the aetiology.

Determination of reproductive hormones can also help differentiate between obstructive and non-obstructive forms of azoospermia: an elevated FSH indicates a non-obstructive form of azoospermia.

Box 7.1.3 Physical examination in an infertile man

Gynaecomastia, male body composition, length/weight/body mass index
Investigation of the inguinal region (hernia, scars, lymphadenopathy)
Penile abnormalities (hypospadias, meatal stenosis, deformity)
Testes: volume, consistency (firm, soft), scrotal position, palpable abnormalities
Epididymis: dilatation, defects, induration, cysts
Vas deferens abnormalities
Spermatic cord: varicocele (upright position), Valsalva manoeuvre

Table 7.1.1 Lower reference limits (fifth centiles and their 95% confidence intervals) for semen characteristics

Parameter	Lower reference limit
Semen volume (mL)	1.5 (1.4–1.7)
Total sperm number (mill. per ejaculate)	39 (33–46)
Sperm concentration (mill. per mL)	15 (12–16)
Total motility (progressive, non-progressive, %)	40 (38–42)
Progressive motility (PR, %)	32 (31–34)
Vitality (live spermatozoa, %)	58 (55–63)
Sperm morphology (normal forms, %)	4 (3.0–4.0)
Other consensus threshold values	
pH	≥7.2
Peroxidase-positive leukocytes (mill. per mL)	<1.0
MAR test (motile spermatozoa with bound particles, %)	<50
Immunobead test (motile spermatozoa with bound beads, %)	<50
Seminal zinc (μmol/ejaculate)	≥2.4
Seminal fructose (μmol/ejaculate)	≥13
Seminal neutral glucosidase (mU/ejaculate)	≥20

Source: data from World Health Organization, *WHO Laboratory Manual for the Examination of Human Semen and Sperm-Cervical Mucus Interaction, Fifth Edition*, Cambridge University Press, Cambridge, UK, Copyright © 2010.

Microbiology

Infections of the male urogenital tract are potentially correctable causes of male infertility. There is however no strong evidence that links male accessory gland infections to male infertility.[9,10] In contrast to the situation in women, not much is known about the consequences of sexual transmitted diseases (e.g. chlamydial infections) in men and their impact on semen quality. Studies suggest that genital tract infections in young men, including epididymitis, are often attributable to chlamydia. Epididymitis is thought to be important because fertility might be affected due to inflammation, obstruction, and functional impairment, especially where both epididymi are affected. There are, however, no conclusive studies showing that men infected with chlamydia trachomatis are less fertile than uninfected men. Male genital chlamydial infection is mainly a threat to the female genital organs. Some bacteria may cause a chronic infection of the prostate and the epididymis, resulting in (partial) obstruction of the ejaculatory ducts with low seminal volume and oligozoospermia.[11] Treatment can eradicate bacteria in the accessory glands, but leucocytes and reactive oxygen species (ROS) production may continue to be produced and infertility will persist.[12]

Box 7.1.4 Hypogonadism classified according to the level of lutenizing hormone and follicle-stimulating hormone and its main causes

Hypergonadotrophic hypogonadism (high FSH/LH)

- Causes: testicular insufficiency, disturbed or absent spermatogenesis
- Congenital forms: Klinefelter's syndrome, cryptorchidism, anorchia, testicular dysgenesis
- Acquired forms: orchitis, testicular torsion, castration, chemotherapy, irradiation, testicular tumour

Hypogonadotrophic hypogonadism (low FSH/LH)

- Causes: insufficient production of gonadotrophins (hypothalamic-pituitary dysfunction)
- Congenital forms: Kallmann's syndrome, idiophatic hypogonadotrophic hypogonadism (IHH)
- Acuired forms: pituitary tumour (prolactinoma), anabolic steroids, morbid obesity
- In case of hypogonadotrophic hypogonadism a CT scan or MRI scan of the pituitary gland is indicated

Leucocytospermia

According to WHO classification, >1 × 10^6 WBC per mL is defined as leukocytospermia. Leucocytospermia is often found in men without obvious signs of urogenital infection and with negative cultures. Leucocytes, especially neutrophilic granulocytes can produce large amounts of ROS and cytokines, which may influence sperm function.[13]

Reactive oxygen species

Impairment of sperm function can be caused by the formation of an excess of reactive oxygen species.[13] Spermatozoa are more vulnerable to ROS than other cells due to the structure of the sperm membrane and a poor defence system against free oxygen radicals. Mitochondria are particularly vulnerable to oxidative stress, thus influencing sperm motility. Especially within the epididymis exposure time to ROS is quite long and the amount of scavengers is limited.[14] Oxidative stress is known to cause sperm DNA damage (see 'Sperm DNA damage').

Sperm DNA damage

Determination of sperm DNA fragmentation, as assessed by the COMET and TUNEL assays and the sperm chromatin structure assay (SCSA), may be an important tool for the evaluation of semen quality and male fertility. The biological variation of the sperm DNA fragmentation is much less compared to the variation of classical sperm parameters.[15] Sperm DNA fragmentation tests can be applied as an additional sperm quality tool to be used in both clinical and research settings.[16] Interestingly, even semen samples with normal concentration, motility, and morphology can harbour abnormalities in sperm chromatin structure that are possibly related to reduced male fertility.[17] In addition, high levels of sperm DNA fragmentation are associated with a low chance of spontaneous conception and conception after intrauterine insemination.[16,18] Several studies have documented that conditions like fever, increased scrotal temperature (varicoceles), smoking, and urogenital infections can alter sperm DNA integrity.[19] Sperm DNA fragmentation can be the result of a defective spermatogenesis and of post-testicular events, such as the effect of excessive ROS.

Genetic evaluation

Genetic abnormalities are more common in men with unexplained oligozoospermia and azoospermia, including numerical and structural chromosomal abnormalities, deletions of the Azoospermia factor region of the Y chromosome and mutations in the cystic fibrosis transmembrane conductance regulator gene, commonly associated with congenital vas deferens abnormalities.[20] The frequency of cytogenetic abnormalities was found to be as high as 13.7% in men with non-obstructive azoospermia and 4.6% in men with oligozoospermia.[21] The more severe is the testicular deficiency, the higher is the frequency of cytogenetic abnormalities and Y chromosome deletions. The most frequent chromosomal aneuploidy found in azoospermic men is the Klinefelter syndrome.[22] Numeric and structural chromosomal aberrations may result in spontaneous abortions and in an unbalanced karyotype in the offspring and multiple congenital abnormalities. Y chromosome deletions will cause infertility in the male offspring. *CFTR* gene mutations can result in a child with a mild or severe form of cystic fibrosis.[23]

Scrotal ultrasound

Scrotal ultrasound is widely used for the diagnosis of male infertility. Benign and (pre)malignant scrotal abnormalities are often found in infertile men. Scrotal ultrasound can detect substantially more abnormalities compared with physical examination. The sensitivity of scrotal ultrasound to detect abnormalities is almost 100%. It can help to establish a diagnosis in male infertility and initiate causal treatment. Combined with colour Doppler, it can detect vascular pathology (varicocele) and inflammatory processes (epididymo-orchitis). We found a 38% prevalence of scrotal abnormalities in a series of 1,372 infertile men, including varicocele (29.7%), testicular tumours (0.5%), testicular cysts (0.7%), and testicular microlithiasis (0.9%). Only 33% of the sonographic findings were also discovered by palpation.[24]

Varicoceles

Palpation of the spermatic cord has a low detection rate of grade 1 and 2 varicoceles and a substantial interobserver variability as compared with colour Doppler ultrasound. Scrotal ultrasounds allows a more objective and precise assessment of varicoceles, including flow characteristics. Based on our experience with scrotal ultrasound, we propose a new classification system for varicoceles that should include the following three observations:

- Diameter of the veins >3 mm at rest/supine position;
- Increase in diameter in upright position;
- Reflux/retrograde flow >2 sec spontaneous or with a Valsalva manoeuvre.

Testicular tumours and microcalcifications

Malignant testicular tumours and potentially premalignant conditions like microlithiasis are incidental findings during ultrasound screening of infertile men. Testicular tumours represent only 1% to

2% of malignant tumours in men, but are a common malignancy in young men.[1] In infertile men, testicular malignancies are found in 0.5–1%. Ultrasound has a near 100% sensitivity for detecting testicular tumours.[25]

Testicular microlithiasis are calcifications in the lumina of the seminiferous tubules. Microlithiasis has an incidence of 3% in the general population. In men investigated for scrotal abnormalities, microlithiasis is often found next to malignant disorders. In men with a history of cryptorchidism microlithiasis is found in 11.7%; in male infertility in 0.8–15%. Microlithiasis is associated with an increased risk for carcinoma *in situ* of the testis.[25]

Testicular biopsy

Testicular biopsy was considered the cornerstone of male infertility diagnosis for many years in men with unexplained infertility and men with azoospermia. Recent guidelines for male infertility have limited the indications for a diagnostic testicular biopsy to the confirmation of obstructive azoospermia in men with normal size testes and normal reproductive hormones. Testicular biopsy is also performed in men with risk factors for testicular malignancy (see 'Testicular tumours and microcalcifications'). For an accurate histological classification, proper tissue handling, fixation, preparation of the specimen, and evaluation are needed. A standardized approach to testicular biopsy is recommended.[26] In addition, for the detection of carcinoma *in situ* of the testis, immunohistochemistry is mandatory. Testicular biopsies, performed for sperm harvesting as well as those for assessing spermatogenic status, should be evaluated for the presence of CIS.

Nowadays, testicular biopsies are mainly performed for sperm harvesting in men with non-obstructive azoospermia, to be used for intracytoplasmic sperm injection (ICSI). Spermatozoa can be harvested from the testes of men with non-obstructive azoospermia in 40–60% of patients. Since testicular spermatozoa can successfully be used for ICSI it is strongly recommended to perform cryopreservation of (part of the) testicular tissue for future ICSI, if spermatozoa are available.

Further reading

Assche van E, Bonduelle M, Tournaye H, *et al.* Cytogenetics of infertile men. *Hum Reprod* 1996; **11**(Suppl 4):1–24.

De Braekeleer M, Ferec C. Mutations in the cystic fibrosis gene in men with congenital bilateral absence of the vas deferens. *Mol Hum Reprod* 1996; **2**(9):669–77.

Dohle GR, Elzanaty S, van Casteren NJ. Testicular biopsy: clinical practice and interpretation. *Asian J Androl* 2012; **14**(1):88–93.

Guzick DS, Overstreet JW, Factor-Litvak P, *et al.* Sperm morphology, motility, and concentration in fertile and infertile men. *N Engl J Med* 2001; **345**(19):1388–93.

Krausz C. Genetic aspects of male infertility. *Eur Urol Rev* 2009; **3**(2):93–6.

La Vignera S, Vicari E, Condorelli RA, D'Agata R, Calogero AE. Male accessory gland infection and sperm parameters (review). *Int J Androl* 2011; **34**:e330–47.

Lanfranco F, Kamischke A, Zitzmann M, *et al.* Klinefelter's syndrome. *Lancet* 2004; **364**(9430):273–83.

Nieschlag E, Behre HM. *Andrology: Male Reproductive Health and Dysfunction*, 2nd edition. Berlin, Germany: Springer-Verlag: pp. 83–87.

Pierik FH, Dohle GR, van Muiswinkel JM, Vreeburg JTM, Weber RFA. Is routine scrotal ultrasound in infertile men advantageous? *J Urol* 1999; **162**:1618–20.

Smit M, Dohle GR, Hop WC, Wildhagen MF, Weber RF, Romijn JC. Clinical correlates of the biological variation of sperm DNA fragmentation in infertile men attending an andrology outpatient clinic. *Int J Androl* 2007; **30**(1):48–55.

van Casteren NJ, Looijenga LH, Dohle GR. Testicular microlithiasis and carcinoma in situ overview and proposed clinical guideline. *Int J Androl* 2009; **32**(4):279–87.

World Health Organization. *WHO Laboratory Manual for the Examination of Human Semen and Sperm-Cervical Mucus Interaction*, 5th edition. Cambridge, UK: Cambridge University Press, 2010.

World Health Organization. *WHO Manual for the Standardized Investigation and Diagnosis of the Infertile Couple.* Cambridge, UK: Cambridge University Press, 2000.

References

1. Nieschlag E, Behre HM. *Andrology: Male Reproductive Health and Dysfunction*, 2nd edition. Berlin, Germany: Springer-Verlag: pp. 83–87.
2. Snick HK, Snick TS, Evers JL, Collins JA. The spontaneous pregnancy prognosis in untreated subfertile couples: the Walcheren primary care study. *Hum Reprod* 1997; **12**(7):1582–8.
3. Rowe T. Fertility and a woman's age. *J Reprod Med* 2006; **51**(3); 157–63.
4. World Health Organization. *WHO Manual for the Standardized Investigation and Diagnosis of the Infertile Couple.* Cambridge, UK: Cambridge University Press, 2000.
5. World Health Organization. *WHO Laboratory Manual for the Examination of Human Semen and Sperm-Cervical Mucus Interaction*, 5th edition. Cambridge, UK: Cambridge University Press, 2010.
6. Alvarez C, Castilla JA, Martinez L, Ramirez JP, Vergara F, Gaforio JJ. Biological variation of seminal parameters in healthy subjects. *Hum Reprod* 2003; **18**(10):2082–8.
7. Guzick DS, Overstreet JW, Factor-Litvak P, *et al.* Sperm morphology, motility, and concentration in fertile and infertile men. *N Engl J Med* 2001; **345**(19):1388–93.
8. Behre HM, Nieschlag E, Partsch CJ, *et al.* Diseases of the hypothalamus and the pituitary gland. (pp. 169–92) In: Nieschlag E, Behre HM, Nieschlag S (eds). *Andrology: Male Reproductive Health and Dysfunction*, 3rd edition. Berlin, Germany: Springer-Verlag, 2010.
9. Purvis K, Christiansen E. Infection of the male reproductive tract. Impact, diagnosis and treatment in relation to male infertility. *Int J Androl* 1993; **16**:1–13.
10. Weidner W, Krause W, Ludwig M. Relevance of male accessory gland infection for subsequent fertility with special focus on prostatitis. *Hum Reprod Update* 1999; **5**:421–32.
11. Dohle GR. Inflammatory-associated obstructions of the male reproductive tract. *Andrologia* 2003; **35**(5):321–4.
12. Vicari E Effectiveness and limits of antimicrobal treatments on seminal leucocyte concentration and related reactive oxygen species production in patients with male accessory gland infection. *Hum Reprod* 2000; **12**:2536–44.
13. Depuydt CE, Bosmans E, Zalata A, Schoonjans F, Comhaire FH. The relation between reactive oxygen species and cytokines in andrological patients with or without male accessory gland infection. *J Androl* 1996; **17**:699–707.
14. La Vignera S, Vicari E, Condorelli RA, D'Agata R, Calogero AE. Male accessory gland infection and sperm parameters (review). *Int J Androl* 2011; **34**:e330–47.
15. Smit M, Dohle GR, Hop WC, Wildhagen MF, Weber RF, Romijn JC. Clinical correlates of the biological variation of sperm DNA fragmentation in infertile men attending an andrology outpatient clinic. *Int J Androl* 2007; **30**(1):48–55.
16. Evenson DP, Wixon R. Clinical aspects of sperm DNA fragmentation detection and male infertility. *Theriogenology* 2006; **65**(5):979–91.

17. Saleh RA, Agarwal A, Nelson DR, *et al.* Increased sperm nuclear DNA damage in normozoospermic infertile men: a prospective study. *Fertil Steril* 2002; **78**(2):313–8.
18. Bungum M, Humaidan P, Spano M, *et al.* The predictive value of sperm chromatin structure assay (SCSA) parameters for the outcome of intrauterine insemination, IVF and ICSI. *Hum Reprod* 2004; **19**:1401.
19. Zini A, Dohle G. Are varicoceles associated with increased deoxyribonucleic acid fragmentation? *Fertil Steril* 2011; **96**(6):1283–7.
20. Krausz C. Genetic aspects of male infertility. *Eur Urol Rev* 2009; **3**(2):93–6.
21. Assche van E, Bonduelle M, Tournaye H, *et al.* Cytogenetics of infertile men. *Hum Reprod* 1996; **11**(Suppl 4):1–24.
22. Lanfranco F, Kamischke A, Zitzmann M, *et al.* Klinefelter's syndrome. *Lancet* 2004; **364**(9430):273–83.
23. De Braekeleer M, Ferec C. Mutations in the cystic fibrosis gene in men with congenital bilateral absence of the vas deferens. *Mol Hum Reprod* 1996; **2**(9):669–77.
24. Pierik FH, Dohle GR, van Muiswinkel JM, Vreeburg JTM, Weber RFA. Is routine scrotal ultrasound in infertile men advantageous? *J Urol* 1999; **162**:1618–20.
25. van Casteren NJ, Looijenga LH, Dohle GR. Testicular microlithiasis and carcinoma in situ overview and proposed clinical guideline. *Int J Androl* 2009; **32**(4):279–87.
26. Dohle GR, Elzanaty S, van Casteren NJ. Testicular biopsy: clinical practice and interpretation. *Asian J Androl* 2012; **14**(1):88–93.

CHAPTER 7.2

Surgical treatment of male infertility

Gert R. Dohle

Introduction to surgical treatment of male infertility

Surgical treatment of male infertility involves diagnostic procedures (i.e. testis biopsy), (micro)surgical correction of obstructive azoospermia, varicocele repair, and sperm aspiration from the epididymis (MESA) and testes (TESE).

Testis biopsy can be performed for diagnostic purposes, for instance to differentiate obstructive azoospermia from non-obstructive forms.[1] This applies to men with normal testicular volume and normal reproductive hormones. In men with azoospermia and elevated follicle-stimulating hormone (FSH), a non-obstructive form is present and a testis biopsy is not indicated for diagnostic purposes. A testis biopsy can also be used to harvest spermatozoa to be used for intracytoplasmic sperm injection (TESE and ICSI).

Primary obstructions of the male genital tract are found in 10–20% of men with infertility. The patients present with azoospermia, normal testicular volume, and normal reproductive hormones. The site of the obstruction is commonly at the epididymal level or in the vas deferens, resulting is dilation of the epididymis. The aetiology of the epididymal obstruction is either congenital (idiopathic) or due to an epididymal infection or surgery.[2] About 10% of the men with obstructive azoospermia have a structural abnormality of the genital tract, such as congenital bilateral absence of the vas deferens (CBAVD), a mild form of cystic fibrosis. In these men, part of the epididymis and the scrotal vas deferens are absent, due to a regression of the wolffian duct during early pregnancy.[3]

Obstructions of the ejaculatory ducts are found in men with recurrent prostatitis and in men with prostatic cysts in the midline of the prostate. Signs of distal obstructions of the genital tract can be found on transrectal ultrasound in the prostate and the seminal vesicles. Dilations of the ejaculatory ducts and the seminal vesicles can be observed as well as calcifications in this region.[4]

Varicoceles are found in about 10% of all men and in 25% of men with abnormal semen analysis.[5] Correction of a varicocele often results in an improvement of semen parameters. Spontaneous pregnancies occur in 25–30% of couples within one year after varicocele repair.[6]

Sperm retrieval for ICSI can be performed by open surgery of the epididymis (MESA) in case of obstructive azoospermia and of the testis (TESE), but also by percutaneous fine needle aspiration of spermatozoa from the epididymis (PESA) or the testis (TEFNA).[7,8]

Diagnostic procedures

Obstructive azoospermia is likely to be present in men with normal size testes and normal gonadotrophins. An exception is men with a late block in spermatogensis (maturation arrest) who may also present with the same clinical features. Scrotal and transrectal ultrasound can be helpful in confirming the presence of an obstruction of the male genital tract. Ultrasonographic signs of obstruction are dilatation of the rete testis, the epididymis, and the seminal vesicles in the case of ejaculatory duct obstruction.[9] In selective cases, an MRI-scan of the genital region may help in the diagnostic process. Scrotal ultrasound can also detect the presence of a varicocele and potential (pre)malignant abnormalities of the testes.[10] Transrectal ultrasound is indicated in men with low seminal volume, a normal FSH, an azoospermia or severe oligospermia: in these men an obstruction of the ejaculatory ducts may be present. Dilatation of the seminal vesicles and the presence of cystic lesion in the prostatic midline can be found in these cases.[11]

The diagnosis CBAVD can be made on careful examination of the patient and on basis of the results of semen analysis: azoospermia, a low seminal volume, low pH, and low or absent fructose in the ejaculate indicates CBAVD. Additional genetic testing for cystic fibrosis gene mutations in both the patient and his partner should be performed before a sperm aspiration (MESA) and intracytoplasmic sperm injection (ICSI) is performed.[3]

Testis biopsy

Before scrotal exploration is performed in men with azoospermia, a testis biopsy can be done to confirm the diagnosis of obstruction. In men with low volume testes and elevated levels of FSH, an impairment of spermatogenesis is likely to be present and a diagnostic testicular biopsy is not indicated. Instead, in men with non-obstructive azoospermia (NOA) sperm aspiration from the testes can be performed for future ICSI. It is advised to cryopreserve testicular tissue from a diagnostic biopsy for future artificial reproductive techniques (ART) in case spermatozoa are present. Also, the pathologist should perform additional immunostaining of the histological specimen to detect carcinoma *in situ* of the testis, which has a higher incidence in men with NOA.[1] Testicular biopsy can be performed under local and general anaesthesia. Usually, the procedure is performed as day-care surgery in an outpatient clinic setting. For a diagnostic testicular biopsy, a scrotal incision of 2–3 cm should allow enough exposure of the tunica albuginea of the testicular. A small incision in the capsule of the testicle of about 0.5 cm is made for obtaining a biopsy of about 3 × 3 × 3 mm. For adequate classification of spermatogenesis, the removed tissue should contain at least 100 seminiferous tubules. The tissue should not be squeezed with a forceps since this may disrupt testicular tissue architecture and hamper proper evaluation of the seminiferous tubules. The wound is closed with absorbable sutures.

An alternative to an open diagnostic testicular biopsy could be a transcutaneous puncture of the testis with either a true-cut needle or a testicular fine needle aspiration (TEFNA). The advantage of fine needle aspiration of the testis is that is does not require surgical equipment and experience and can be performed in an outpatient setting under local anaesthesia.[8]

Microsurgery

Microsurgery in urology mainly involves procedures for obstructive male infertility. Since the results of microsurgical procedures are grossly dependent on the skills of the surgeon, adequate microsurgical training and clinical experience are the keys to success. Practical teaching courses can be very helpful, but a learning curve should be taken into account. As in other surgical procedures, patience, good microsurgical instruments, and gentle tissue handling are important prerequisites for good results. Successful microsurgical correction of an obstruction of the male genital tract has clear benefits over ART in terms of healthcare costs and lower associated obstetric and neonatal problems in case of spontaneous pregnancy.[12]

Vasovasostomy

Microsurgical vasectomy reversal is a challenge for the physician but successful treatment depends on many pre- and intraoperative factors (Box 7.2.1). The main prognostic factors determining the outcome of surgery are the duration of the obstructve interval and the age of the female partner. After an interval of more than 10 years, patency decreases to <75% and pregnancy results are less than 30%.[13] Epididymal dysfunction with poor motility score and secondary epididymal obstruction appeares to be common after a long interval. Furthermore, in men with partners older than 35 years of age, pregnancy is limited due to a decline in ovarian reserve in older woman.[14]

A microsurgical repair after vasectomy can be a very successful and rewarding procedure, since both patency and pregnancy results are high under good surgical conditions.[15] The advantage of microsurgery is that it enables the surgeon to adequately observe the tissue conditions at the level of the planned anastomosis and to perform a delicate and exact alignment between the proximal and distal part of the dissected vas deferens.

Box 7.2.1 Preoperative and intraoperative factors influencing the outcome of vasectomy reversal

- Age and fertility status of the female partner
- Interval between vasectomy and vasectomy reversal
- Microsurgical skills and experience
- The use of optical magnification
- The presence of spermatozoa in the proximal vas deferens
- Gentle tissue handling, with meticulous care for the blood supply
- Tension free and leak-proof anastomosis
- A modified one-layer or a two-layer microsurgical anastomosis
- Bipolar cautery and the use of non-absorbable 9/0 or 10/0 sutures

In men with a long obstructive interval between vasectomy and reversal, an obstruction of the epididymis can be found due to a blow-out of the epididymal tubule with subsequent leakage of semen in the organ and fibrosis. A vasoepididymostomy procedure is needed to treat the obstruction. The results of vasectomy reversal procedures can be improved substantially if the surgeon is able to perform a vasoepididymostomy in cases of a secondary epididymal obstruction, occurring in about 25% of men with an interval of more than 10 years.[16]

Secondary stenosis of the anastomosis appears in about 12–18% of the patients within one year. Failure after a first vasovasostomy is usually caused by stricture and fibrosis at the anastomosis site. Only in a minority of men is an epididymal dysfunction or a testicular insufficiency the cause of the failure.

Vasoepididymostomy

A vasoepididymostomy is indicated in men with an obstructive azoospermia due to an epididymal blockage. Common causes for this type of obstruction are epididymitis and vasal obstruction with secondary blow-out of the epididymal tubule. A vasoepididymostomy is a difficult operation to perform, even for experienced microsurgons. Recent refinements of the technique, such as invagination of a single epididymal loop into the lumen of the vas deferens have facilitated the operation and improved surgical outcome.[17]

After exposure of the scrotum, the epididymis is inspected under the operating microscope. Tubule fluid is aspirated for examination in the laboratory and cryopreservation, starting in the tail of the epididymis. The vas is then pulled through the tunica vaginalis and the serosa of the vas is fixated to the tunica vaginalis of the epididymis. A dilated part of the epididymal tubule is dissected under the microscope and 11/0 nylon sutures are used for the anastomsis between the opened tubule and the lumen of the vas deferens.

After the operation, it may take several months before spermatozoa appear in the ejaculate. Cryopreservation of motile spermatozoa is advised, because in about 20% the anastomosis may be secondarily blocked due to fibrosis, resulting in azoospermia after initial patency.

The patency rate of the procedure is 60–70% and spontaneous pregnancies occur in 20–30%.[18] Factors determing the success rate of the procedure are epididymal function, the presence of antisperm antibodies, and the duration of the obstruction. Passage through a substantial portion of the epididymis seems essential for the fertilizing capacity of the spermatozoa and anastomisis between the vas deferens and the head of the epididymis may not result in spontaneous pregnancies. IVF/ICSI procedures are still required for these couples.[19]

Varicocele repair

The role of varicocoele repair in improving spontaneous pregnancy has not yet been shown in a meta-analysis of randomized controlled trials.[20] Sperm improvement is usually observed after varicocoele repair but it seems difficult to show that varicocelctomy also improves fertility outcome.[21] However, there seems to be a benefit

Table 7.2.1 Advantages, disadvantages, and complications of different treatment modalities for varicocele repair

Treatment	Advantage	Recurrence/ persistence (reference)	Complication and disadvantages
Antegrade sclerotherapy (Tauber)	Minimal invasive, can be performed under local anaesthesia	9%	Complication rate 0.3–2.2%; testicular atrophy; scrotal haematoma; epididymitis
Retrograde embolization	Minimal invasive, under local aneathesia	10–15%	Bleeding/haematoma; radiological complication (e.g. reaction to contrast media); misplacement or migration of coils; retroperitoneal haemorrhage; high dosis of irradiation
Open operation			
Scrotal operation	Easy accessible, local anaesthesia may be possible	13–30%	Testicular atrophy; arterial damage with risk of devascularization and gangrene of testicle; potentially high risk of recurrence; vasal damage
Inguinal approach (Ivanisevich)		13%	Possibility of missing out a branch of testicular vein; arterial damage; bleeding en infection; vassal damage
High inguinal ligation (Palomo)		16–29%	5–10% incidence of hydrocele; retroperitoneal bleeding and haematoma
Microsurgery	Minimal invasive; fast recovery	1–4%	Arterial injury; potential loss of the testis due to necrosis; haematoma
Laparoscopy	Bilateral correction possible in one session	7–15%	Injury to testicular artery and lymph vessels; intestinal, vascular and nerve damage; peritonitis; bleeding; postoperative pain (due to diaphragmatic stretching during pneumoperitoneum); pneumoscrotum; wound infection

for young couples with an infertility duration of at least two years, a clinical varicocele, oligozoospermia, and otherwise unexplained infertility.[22] Recently, several studies have shown an improvement of DNA fragmentation of spermatozoa observed after surgical varicocoele repair indicating a real effect of varicocelectomy on semen parameters.[21,23]

The size of the varicocoele may be important in the decision for repair or observation: in three randomized controlled trials of the effect of subclinical varicocele repair on spontaneous pregnancy, treatment appeared to be as good as no treatment.[24–26] Also in normospermic men varicocoelectomy showed no benefit as compared to controls.[27,28] In fact, varicocoeles are frequently observed in men with normal semen analysis and routine treatment of all varicocoeles would be overtreatment if the fertility status of the patient and his partner is not considered.[29] In many infertile couples female factors, such as ovulatory disorders, coincide with the presence of the varicocoele and successful correction of these factors could also account for the increase in spontaneous pregnancies.[30,31]

Varicocele repair results in spontaneous pregnancy in about 25–30% of couples within one year of observation after treatment.[6,31] There are different ways to correct a varicocele and all of these treatments have advantages and drawbacks, such as recurrences and complications.[32] Table 7.2.1 highlights the main treatment modalities for varicocele repair.

Microsurgical correction of a varicocele seems to be to most efficient treatment in terms of recurrences and complications, but randomized studies comparing different treatment modalities are still lacking.[33]

Surgical sperm aspiration

Men with azoospermia may be offered surgical or percutaneous sperm retrieval for the use of ICSI. In men with obstructive azoospermia there is a high chance of finding viable spermatozoa in the epididymis. Percutaneous puncture and sperm aspiration of the epididymis (PESA) under local anaesthesia is usually successful in these men. As an alternative, an open scrotal exploration can be performed and spermatozoa are aspirated from dilated tubles of the epididymis usisng microscopical magnification (MESA). The potential advantage of this procedure is that a substantial number of spermatozoa can be harvested, thus allowing multiple ICSI cycles. Also, if no spermatozoa are found in the epididymis, a testis biopsy can be performed for sperm retrieval (TESE) in the same procedure.[7]

Testis biopsy can be part of an ICSI treatment in patients with clinical evidence of NOA. Spermatogenesis may be focal: in about 50–60% of men with NOA spermatozoa can be found that can be used for ICSI. Most authors recommend taking several testicular samples.[34] A good correlation is seen between diagnostic biopsy histology and the likelihood of finding mature sperm cells during testicular sperm retrieval and ICSI.[35] No clear relationship has been found between successful sperm harvesting and FSH, inhibin B, or testicular volume. In case of complete AZFa and AZFb microdeletions, no spermatozoa can be retrieved. Testicular sperm extraction is the technique of choice and shows excellent repeatability.[34] Microsurgical testicular sperm extraction may increase retrieval rates, although comparative studies are not available yet.[36] After opening the testis, fluid from large calibre tubules is aspirated with the aid of the operating microscope; complications appear to be lower than with classical TESE. Positive retrievals are reported even in conditions such as Sertoli cell only syndrome.[37]

Testicular fine needle aspiration may be a good alternative for TESE, especially in men with normal size testis and normal gonadotrophins.[8] Disadvantage of this technique of sperm harvesting is that does not allow histological examination to detect (for instance) carcinoma *in situ* (CIS) and testicular malignancies.

Further reading

Ammar T, Sidhu PS, Wilkins CJ. Male infertility: the role of imaging in diagnosis and management. *Br J Radiol* 2012; **85**(Spec No 1):S59–68.

Baazeem A, Belzile E, Ciampi A, *et al.* Varicocele and male factor infertility treatment: a new meta-analysis and review of the role of varicocele repair. *Eur Urol* 2011; **60**(4):796–808.

Beliveau ME, Turek PJ. The value of testicular 'mapping' in men with non-obstructive azoospermia. *Asian J Androl* 2011; **13**(2):225–30.

Belker AM, Thomas AJ, Fuchs EF, Konnak JW, Sharlip ID. Results of 1469 microsurgical vasectomy reversals by the vasovasostomy group. *J Urol* 1991; **145**:505–11.

Cayan S, Shavakhabov S, Kadioğlu A.Treatment of palpable varicocele in infertile men: a meta-analysis to define the best technique. *J Androl* 2009; **30**(1):33–40.

Dabaja AA, Schlegel PN. Microdissection testicular sperm extraction: an update. *Asian J Androl* 2013; **15**(1):35–9.

Dohle GR, Elzanaty S, van Casteren N. Testicular biopsy: clinical practice and interpretation. *Asian J Androl* 2012; **14**(1):88–93.

Dubin L, Amelar RD. Varicocoelectomy: 986 cases in a twelve-year study. *Urology* 1977; **10**(5):446–9.

Esteves SC, Miyaoka R, Agarwal A. Sperm retrieval techniques for assisted reproduction. *Int Braz J Urol* 2011; **37**(5):570–83.

Goldstein M, Tanrikut C. Microsurgical management of male infertility. *Nat Clin Pract Urol* 2006; **3**(7):381–91.

Jungwirth A, Giwercman A, Tournaye H, *et al.* European Association of Urology Working Group on Male Infertility. European Association of Urology guidelines on Male Infertility: the 2012 update. *Eur Urol* 2012; **62**(2):324–32.

Lee R, Li PS, Goldstein M, Tanrikut C, Schattman G, Schlegel PN. A decision analysis of treatments for obstructive azoospermia. *Hum Reprod* 2008; **23**(9):2043–9.

Marmar JL. Modified vasoepididymostomy with simultaneous double needle placement, tubulotomy and tubular invagination. *J Urol* 2000; **163**:483–6.

Silber SJ, Grotjan HE. Microscopic vasectomy reversal 30 years later: a summary of 4010 cases by the same surgeon. *J Androl* 2004; **25**(6):845–59.

Vernaeve V, Verheyen G, Goossens A, Van Steirteghem A, Devroey P, Tournaye H. How successful is repeat testicular sperm extraction in patients with azoospermia? *Hum Reprod* 2006; **21**(6):1551–4.

References

1. Dohle GR, Elzanaty S, van Casteren N. Testicular biopsy: clinical practice and interpretation. *Asian J Androl* 2012; **14**(1):88–93.
2. Jungwirth A, Giwercman A, Tournaye H, *et al.* European Association of Urology Working Group on Male Infertility. European Association of Urology guidelines on Male Infertility: the 2012 update. *Eur Urol* 2012; **62**(2):324–32.
3. Oates RD. The genetic basis of male reproductive failure. *Urol Clin North Am* 2008; **35**(2):257–70.
4. Jarrow JP. Transrectal ultrasonography in infertile men. *Fert Steril* 1993; **60**:1035–9.
5. The influence of varicocele on parameters of fertility in a large group of men presenting to infertility clinics. World Health Organization. *Fertil Steril* 1992; **57**:1289–93.
6. Dubin L, Amelar RD. Varicocoelectomy: 986 cases in a twelve-year study. *Urology* 1977; **10**(5):446–9.
7. Esteves SC, Miyaoka R, Agarwal A. Sperm retrieval techniques for assisted reproduction. *Int Braz J Urol* 2011; **37**(5):570–83.
8. Beliveau ME, Turek PJ. The value of testicular 'mapping' in men with non-obstructive azoospermia. *Asian J Androl* 2011; **13**(2):225–30.
9. Ammar T, Sidhu PS, Wilkins CJ. Male infertility: the role of imaging in diagnosis and management. *Br J Radiol* 2012; **85**(Spec No 1):S59–68.
10. Pierik FH, Dohle GR, van Muiswinkel JM, Vreeburg JT, Weber RF. Is routine scrotal ultrasound advantageous in infertile men? *J Urol* 1999; **162**(5):1618–20.
11. Engin G, Celtik M, Sanli O, Aytac O, Muradov Z, Kadioğlu A. Comparison of transrectal ultrasonography and transrectal ultrasonography-guided seminal vesicle aspiration in the diagnosis of the ejaculatory duct obstruction. *Fertil Steril* 2009; **92**(3):964–70.
12. Lee R, Li PS, Goldstein M, Tanrikut C, Schattman G, Schlegel PN. A decision analysis of treatments for obstructive azoospermia. *Hum Reprod* 2008; **23**(9):2043–9.
13. Belker AM, Thomas AJ, Fuchs EF, Konnak JW, Sharlip ID. Results of 1469 microsurgical vasectomy reversals by the vasovasostomy group. *J Urol* 1991; **145**:505–11.
14. Kolettis PN, Sabanegh ES, Nalesnik JG, D'Amico AM, Box LC, Burns JR. Pregnancy outcomes after vasectomy reversal for female partners 35 years old or older. *J Urol* 2003; **169**(6):2250–2.
15. Silber SJ, Grotjan HE. Microscopic vasectomy reversal 30 years later: a summary of 4010 cases by the same surgeon. *J Androl* 2004; **25**(6):845–59.
16. Elzanaty S, Dohle GR. Vasovasostomy and predictors of vasal patency: a systematic review. *Scand J Urol Nephrol* 2012; **46**(4):241–6.
17. Marmar JL. Modified vasoepididymostomy with simultaneous double needle placement, tubulotomy and tubular invagination. *J Urol* 2000; **163**:483–6.
18. Chan PT, Brandell RA, Goldstein M. Prospective analysis of outcomes after microsurgical intussusception vasoepididymostomy. *BJU Int* 2005; **96**(4):598–601.
19. Berardinucci D, Zini A, Jarvi K. Microsurgical reconstruction for epididymal obstruction. *J Urol* 1998; **159**:831–4.
20. Baazeem A, Belzile E, Ciampi A, *et al.* Varicocele and male factor infertility treatment: a new meta-analysis and review of the role of varicocele repair. *Eur Urol* 2011; **60**(4):796–808.
21. Argawal A, Deepinder F, Cocuzza M, *et al.* Efficacy of varicocoelectomy in improving semen parqameters: new meta-analytical approach. *Urology* 2007; **70**:532–8.
22. Dohle GR. Varicocoele repair: the role of the duration of infertility. *Int J Androl* 2011; **34**(3):193–4.
23. Smit M, Romijn JC, Wildhagen MF, Veldhoven JL, Weber RF, Dohle GR. Decreased sperm DNA fragmentation after surgical varicocoelectomy is associated with increased pregnancy rate. *J Urol* 2010; **183**(1):270–4.
24. Grasso M, Lania M, Castelli M, Galli L, Franzoso F, Rigatti P. Low-grade left varicocoele in patients over 30 years old: the effect of spermatic vein ligation on fertility. *BJU Int* 2000; **85**(3):305–7.
25. Unal D, Yeni E, Verit A, Karatas OF. Clomiphene citrate versus varicocoelectomy in treatment of subclinical varicocoele: a prospective randomized study. *Int J Urol* 2001; **8**(5):227–30.
26. Yamamoto M, Hibi H, Hirata Y, Miyake K, Ishigaki T. Effect of varicocoelectomy on sperm parameters and pregnancy rates in patients with subclinical varicocele: a randomized prospective controlled study. *J Urol* 1996; **155**(5):1636–8.
27. Nilsson S, Edvinsson A, Nilsson B. Improvement of semen and pregnancy rate after ligation and division of the internal spermatic vein: fact or fiction? *Br J Urol* 1979; **51**(6):591–6.
28. Breznik R, Vlaisavljevic V, Borko E. Treatment of varicocoele and male fertility. *Arch Androl* 1993; **30**(3):157–60.
29. Zargooshi J. Sperm count and sperm motility in incidental high-grade varicocoele. *Fertil Steril* 2007; **88**(5):1470–3.
30. Baker HW, Burger HG, de Kretser DM, Hudson B, Rennie GC, Straffon WG. Testicular vein ligation and fertility in men with varicocoeles. *Br Med J* 1985; **291**(6510):1678–80.
31. Nieschlag E, Hertle L, Fischedick A, Abshagen K, Behre HM. Update on treatment of varicocoele: counselling as effective as occlusion of the vena spermatica. *Hum Reprod* 1998; **13**:2147–50.

32. Cayan S, Shavakhabov S, Kadioğlu A.Treatment of palpable varicocele in infertile men: a meta-analysis to define the best technique. *J Androl* 2009; **30**(1):33–40.
33. Goldstein M, Tanrikut C. Microsurgical management of male infertility. *Nat Clin Pract Urol* 2006; **3**(7):381–91.
34. Vernaeve V, Verheyen G, Goossens A, Van Steirteghem A, Devroey P, Tournaye H. How successful is repeat testicular sperm extraction in patients with azoospermia? *Hum Reprod* 2006; **21**(6):1551–4.
35. Shulze W, Thoms F, Knuth UA. Testicular sperm extraction: comprehensive analysis with simultaneously performed histology in 1418 biopsies from 766 subfertile men. *Hum Reprod* 1999; **14**(1):82–96.
36. Dabaja AA, Schlegel PN. Microdissection testicular sperm extraction: an update. *Asian J Androl* 2013; **15**(1):35–9.
37. Colpi GM, Piediferro G, Nerva F, Giacchetta D, Colpi EM, Piatti E. Sperm retrieval for intra-cytoplasmic sperm injection in non-obstructive azoospermia. *Minerva Urol Nefrol* 2005; **57**(2):99–107.

CHAPTER 7.3

Infertility
Sperm retrieval

Oliver Kayes and Akwasi Amoako

Introduction to sperm retrieval

Azoospermia, defined as the complete absence of sperm in the ejaculate, affects 1–3% of the male population and accounts for 10–15% of infertile males. It is usually classified into two distinct subgroups, obstructive and non-obstructive. Obstructive azoospermia (OA) constitutes 40% of cases. Spermatogenesis is normal as evidenced by normal testicular volume and normal serum follicle-stimulating hormone (FSH) and testosterone levels, but a mechanical obstruction of the ductile system prevents expulsion of spermatozoa in semen. Acquired causes of OA include vasectomy, genital tract infections, surgery (scrotal, inguinal, pelvic, or abdominal) and trauma. Congenital causes include cystic fibrosis, congenital absence of the vas deferens, ejaculatory duct, and prostatic cysts. The remaining 60% of azoospermic men have a defect in sperm production due to hypospermatogenesis or maturation arrest at the spermatid stage and these are classed as non-obstructive azoospermia (NOA).[1–3]

NOA can result from exposure to environmental toxins, medications, cryptorchidism, genetic, and congenital abnormalities, varicocele, trauma, viral orchitis, endocrine disorders, or it may be idiopathic. Historically, these men were considered sterile and the only chance of their partner becoming pregnant was through the use of donor sperm.

Several sperm retrieval techniques have been developed to obtain sperm from the vas deferens, the epididymis, or the testicular parenchyma in men with OA and NOA or ejaculatory problems. Surgical sperm retrieval combined with recent advances in *in vitro* fertilization (IVF) and the advent of intracytoplasmic sperm injection (ICSI) permit excellent prospects for pregnancy and allow infertile men without ejaculated sperm the opportunity to father their own genetic offspring.[1,2,4]

Sperm retrieval techniques

Techniques currently employed for sperm extraction can be broadly divided into aspiration techniques and open biopsy techniques and includes: vasal sperm aspiration; percutaneous epididymal sperm aspiration (PESA); microsurgical epididymal sperm aspiration (MESA); fine-needle testicular sperm aspiration (TESA); multibiopsy testicular sperm extraction (TESE); and microdissection testicular sperm extraction (micro-TESE). In men with OA, sperm retrieval can be successfully harvested from the vas deferens, epididymis, or the testicular parenchyma using either an aspiration or open biopsy technique. Testicular sperm extraction remains the only way to harvest sperm in men with NOA and yields clinically usable sperm in approximately 50% of these men.[5] The ideal surgical sperm retrieval technique should be able to retrieve high quality and adequate numbers of sperm for treatment and/or cryopreservation with minimal damage to the testicles. Sperm retrieval techniques may be performed using local, regional, or general anaesthesia. Our usual practice is to perform aspiration techniques under local anaesthesia while the open microsurgical techniques are completed under regional or general anaesthesia.

Vasal sperm aspiration

Vasal sperm aspiration involves extraction of sperm from the vas deferens in patients with congenital or acquired obstruction of the ductile system, vasectomized men, or men with ejaculatory problems. A small scrotal incision is made to identify the vas deferens and the lumen is entered via a small incision or puncture through its muscular wall. A fined-tipped syringe containing sperm culture medium is used to aspirate leaking vasal fluid. The incision made into the lumen of the vas is closed once adequate spermatozoa have been retrieved.[6] Vasal sperm aspiration yields more mature, highly motile, and fertilizable sperm than any of the other sperm retrieval techniques because sperm aspirated from the vas have undergone the extensive maturation process in the epididymis required to attain motility potential.[7] Vasal sperm has been used successfully in intrauterine insemination cycles, although is more commonly utilized in IVF/ICSI.[8] Short stay outpatient or day case surgery care is standard practice with associated rapid recovery within 24 hours. Although uncommon, complications include bleeding (1%), infection (1%), and scarring in the lumen of the vas deferens (5%).[3]

Epididymal sperm aspiration

Percutaneous epididymal sperm aspiration and microsurgical epididymal sperm aspiration are the two techniques currently used to obtain sperm from the epididymis of men with obstructive azoospermia. Men with OA have good prospects of successful sperm retrieval from their epididymis. PESA is normally undertaken as an outpatient procedure with local anaesthesia (+/− sedation) but can also be done under regional or general anaesthesia. The procedure involves stabilization of the epididymis between the index finger, thumb, and forefinger while cupping the testis in the palm. A 19 G needle attached to a tuberculin (1 mL) syringe containing gamete culture medium is directly inserted through the stretched scrotal skin into the epididymis. The plunger of the syringe is fully drawn back to create a negative pressure and the tip of the needle is gently moved in and out of the epididymis until slightly opalescent fluid is aspirated into the syringe. The needle is gently withdrawn from the epididymis and the aspirate flushed into sperm medium in a tube that is passed on to the laboratory personnel for microscopic examination.

The main advantages of PESA are reproducibility, the possibility of repeat procedures, reduced cost, reduced pain, and no requirement for intensive microsurgical training.[9]

MESA involves opening of the scrotal skin to expose the epididymis and allows direct visualization of the seminiferous tubules. A small incision is made in the selected epididymal tubule and fluid exuding from the tubule is aspirated using a silicone tube or blunted needle attached to a 1 mL tuberculin syringe. The aspirate is flushed into 0.5–1.0 mL of sperm medium at 37°C and the tube containing the epididymal aspirate is transferred to the laboratory for microscopic examination. The main advantage of MESA over PESA is the retrieval of higher numbers and better quality sperm. MESA however, is associated with more complications such as bleeding, haematoma, postoperative pain, infection, and fibrosis.[3] There are associated training and equipment restrictions that only permit MESA to be offered in limited centres.

During PESA or MESA, sufficient spermatozoa for ICSI or cryopreservation may be obtained in a single puncture and aspirate. The procedure can however be repeated with fresh materials at different sites of the same epididymis and/or from the contralateral epididymis until an adequate number of viable motile sperm have been recovered.[10] Successful sperm retrieval using either technique has been reported for 90–100% of men with OA. Motile sperm isolated with PESA and MESA has similar fertilization, cleavage, and clinical pregnancy rates to ejaculated sperm when used in ICSI cycles.[9] It is important to warn patients that potential microsurgical reconstructive techniques (i.e. epididymo-tubulo-vasostomy) may be impeded and compromised following epididymal breach and aspiration.

Testicular sperm aspiration

TESA is a blind procedure whereby a large gauge needle attached to a syringe is inserted through the stretched anterior scrotal skin into the anteromedial or anterolateral portion of the superior testicular pole in an oblique angle towards the middle and lower zones of the testis. A small piece of testicular tissue is aspirated and the needle is gently withdrawn from the testis while the negative pressure is maintained. The specimen is flushed into a tube containing 0.5–1.0 mL warm sperm medium and transferred to the laboratory for microscopic examination. TESA (or TESE) may be performed at the contralateral testis if insufficient or no sperm are obtained. Different areas of the testicles can be sampled.[6]

Testicular sperm extraction

Testicular sperm extraction (TESE) involves the use of single or multiple open biopsies to retrieve sperm from the testicular parenchyma. TESE is primarily used in cases of NOA but may be used where PESA and MESA have failed and in men with OA. This technique has been used historically as the method of choice to obtain sperm from the testicular parenchyma, although in recent years microsurgical TESE has become the preferred method with several perceived advantages over conventional TESE. Standard testicular sperm extraction (TESE) involves opening of the scrotal skin and tunica vaginalis to expose the tunica albuginea. Incisions are made through the tunica albuginea in different regions of each testis, usually three incisions per testicle, and the testicular tissues extruding from the incisions are excised. Gentle pressure is applied to the testis to extrude testicular parenchyma out of the small incision and assist in its removal. Some fragments (at least one per testis) are embedded within Bouin's solution for histological examination. The remaining testicular biopsies are passed on to the laboratory personnel for sperm retrieval. TESE can be repeated in a different testicular pole if a multiple biopsy approach is used.[3,11] Sperm retrieval rates using conventional TESE vary from 25% to 60%.[12]

Microdissection testicular sperm extraction (micro-TESE) is done similarly to the conventional TESE (see Fig. 7.3.1) by opening the scrotal skin and tunica vaginalis but instead of using multiple incisions, a single equatorial incision is made in the tunica albuginea to bi-valve the testis and expose the testicular parenchyma. Micro-TESE incorporates the use of an operating microscope with ×16–25 magnification to dissect the testicular parenchyma and search for dilated seminiferous tubules[12] that indicate potential areas of active spermatogenesis. Biopsies can be performed by removing these individual tubules. In the absence of dilated tubules, multiple random biopsies are taken from at least three regions of each testicle. Specimens are sent to the laboratory for processing and to search for sperm. The albuginea and scrotal layers are closed using absorbable sutures.

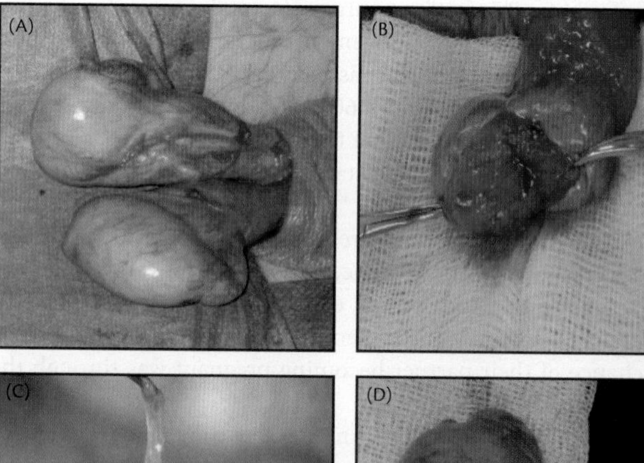

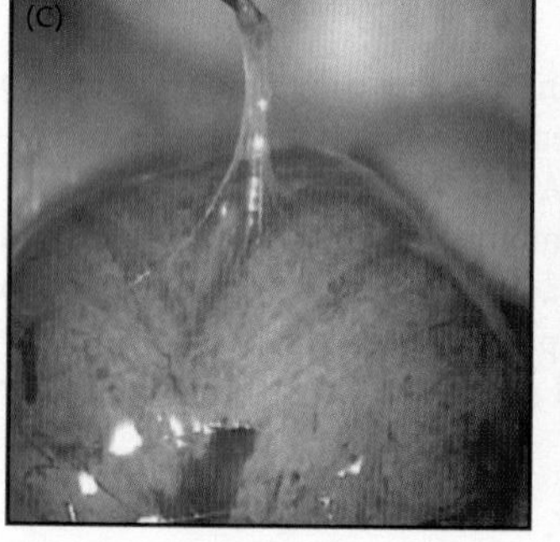

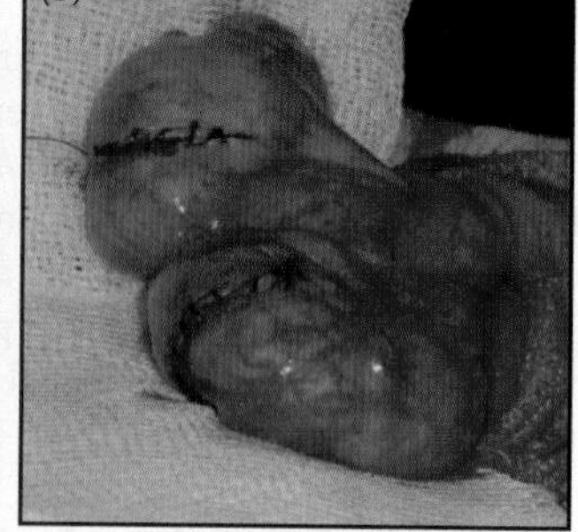

Fig. 7.3.1 Microdissection testicular sperm extraction (micro-TESE). (A) The testis are delivered through a midline skin incision and inspected for evidence of reduced function (size), obstruction (distended epididymis), infections (scarring, hydrocele), and general normal anatomy. (B) An equatorial incision is made, sparing the relevant blood supply and the testis is bivalved gently to expose the underlying parenchyma. (C) Using an operating microscope, the testicular parenchyma is inspected to identify potential areas of active spermatogenesis (i.e. dilated seminiferous tubules). Individual tubules are excised and placed in culture medium for inspection by the embryologist. (D) The tunica albuginea is closed with either interrupted on running sutures (4/0 vircyl™). Before closure of the dartos and skin, careful inspection for bleeding is completed, and delivery of a bilateral cord block is undertaken.

Table 7.3.1 Success rates of micro-TESE in non-obstructive azoospermic (NOA) men with known associated negative fertility factors

Condition	Success rate (%)
Clinical	
History of undescended testis	52–74%
Varicocele	63%
Infection (e.g. epididymitis, mumps)	67%
Torsion	>50%
Post chemotherapy	55–75%
Genetic	
Any AZF a +/or b microdeletion	0%
Isolated AZF c microdeletion	75%
Idiopathic	50–60%
Klinefelter's	30–50%
Biological	
High FSH; small testis	50%
Sertoli cell-only syndrome (SCOS)	40%
Maturation arrest (MA)	40%
Hypospermatogenesis	75%

Source: data from Ashraf CM *et al.*, 'Microdissection Testicular sperm extraction (Micro-TESE): Results of a large series from India', *Andrology*, Volume 3, Issue 1, 1000113, Copyright © 2014 Ashraf CM, *et al.* and Schlegel PN, 'Testicular sperm extraction: microdissection improves sperm yield with minimal tissue excision', *Human Reproduction*, Volume 14, Issue 1, pp. 131–5, Copyright © 1999 European Society of Human Reproduction and Embryology.

The success of micro-TESE at obtaining testicular sperm for ICSI has been reported in the region of 50–54% in all cases of NOA and in patients where dilated seminiferous tubules were clearly identified, the success rate was 73.6% (Table 7.3.1). Furthermore, sperm retrieved using micro-TESE techniques results in fertilization and embryo cleavage rates of 61% and 75% respectively, with a cumulative clinical pregnancy rate of 29.78% per ICSI cycle.[12] Additionally, micro-TESE offers the advantage of removing only a small amount of parenchymal tissue; thereby helping to preserve testicular androgen production in men with NOA who may already have compromised testicular size and function. Comparative studies have shown improved retrieval rates for micro-TESE against multiple biopsies (63% vs. 43%) and reduced average sampling volumes (9.4 mg vs. 720 mg).[4]

Conventional TESE or micro-TESE may be performed on the contralateral testis if insufficient or no sperm are obtained. Different areas of the testicles can be sampled. Patients are discharged on the same day and can return to normal activities one and three days after percutaneous and open techniques, respectively. Analgesics, scrotal ice packing, and support is recommended to control oedema and to alleviate pain. Patients should refrain from ejaculation and strenuous physical activity for approximately 14 days.[3]

Following TESE or micro-TESE, testicular tissue is placed in 2 mL of sperm medium and minced mechanically with sterile slides. The presence of spermatozoa is checked with an inverted microscope at ×3,400 magnification. Any motile sperm that are found are immediately frozen. If the initial microscopic evaluation did not show motile spermatozoa, the sperm suspension is transferred into a Falcon tube and centrifuged at 600 g for five minutes. The pellet is resuspended in 0.5 mL of sperm medium and incubated at 37°C and 5% CO_2 for one hour and the presence of motile sperm is checked again. After two hours of extensive search, if no sperm is found, the sample is discarded.

Current evidence in the literature regarding the ideal choice of sperm retrieval technique is restricted to non-comparative, descriptive, observational, and uncontrolled studies. Current evidence, however, suggests that micro-TESE performs better than conventional TESE, particularly in cases of sertoli cell-only syndrome (SCOS) where tubules containing active foci of spermatogenesis can be identified and in men with high FSH and smaller testes (see Table 7.3.1). Conventional TESE can yield better sperm retrieval rate than FNA.[13]

Fresh motile testicular sperm retrieved from NOA patients may have the same potential to achieve fertilization and pregnancy as sperm retrieved from OA patients. Sperm retrieval rates using micro-TESE have been evaluated in both OA and NOA men. In one study, sperm were retrieved from 17 of 40 (43%) patients with NOA and 18 of 18 (100%) with OA. Motile sperm retrieved in cases of NOA and OA using micro-TESE had similar fertilization and pregnancy rates.[14] Several variable such as age, serum FSH, and inhibin B levels, testicular size, genetic analysis, history of Klinefelter syndrome, history of cryptorchidism or varicocele have been used to preoperatively identify non-obstructive azoospermic men with a potentially high yield at the time of sperm extraction. To date, none of these factors absolutely predict the chance of successful sperm retrieval in men with NOA.

Histological examination of percutaneous or open testicular biopsy cannot absolutely predict future sperm retrieval success rates due to sampling errors and the phenomenon of sporadic spermatogenesis observed in the testes of some infertile men with NOA.[15] In recent years, fine-needle aspiration has been proposed as a means of systematically localizing areas of active spermatogenesis in the testis to aid biopsy and improve chance of successful sperm retrieval. This technique has not been scrutinized and the available evidence is currently restricted to data from only one centre.[6]

Role of adjuvant therapies prior to surgical sperm retrieval

Hormonal therapies have been empirically used prior to surgical sperm retrieval in patients with NOA to potentiate spermatogenic function and hopefully improve output and sperm quality. Although none of these treatments have been subjected to randomized controlled trials, the available evidence from various studies suggests a possible role.[16] Clomiphene citrate, human chorionic gonadotropin (hCG), and human menopausal gonadotropin (hMG) have been shown to increase endogenous FSH secretion and intratesticular testosterone levels, which are essential for spermatogenesis. A multicentre study involving 612 men with NOA reported that administration of clomiphene citrate, hCG, and hMG prior to micro-TESE resulted in the presence of sperm in the ejaculate which obviates the need for surgical sperm retrieval and a greater likelihood of successful sperm retrieval in those who remain azoospermic (57% vs. 33.6%) compared to the control group.[17,18] Pure FSH treatment prior to TESE in 108 men with NOA and normal FSH levels has also shown a higher sperm retrieval rate in the treated group (64% vs. 33%) compared to the control group.[19]

Aromatase inhibitors such as letrozole and anastrozole have also been used to correct the abnormal testosterone to oestradiol ratio that is commonly found in men with NOA. This imbalance is purported to result from an increase in aromatase activity from the hyperplastic Leydig cells which results in increased oestrogen production. Some investigators have reported a dramatic improvement in sperm concentration and motility in men with severe oligozoospermia.[20,21] The anti-oestrogen tamoxifen has also been used to correct the abnormal testosterone/oestrogen ratio in men with NOA and improve the results of testicular sperm recovery, as well as increasing the chance of pregnancy by ICSI.[22]

Varicocele has a substantial impact on sperm production and quality and varicocelectomy in patients with abnormal semen parameters, which leads to an improvement in sperm count and motility. However, the impact of varicocelectomy in improving sperm production in men with NOA and the chance of successful sperm recovery is currently not well established. Some studies have reported a positive effect on sperm retrieval rates following varicocelectomy. A retrospective review of 138 patients with clinical varicoceles who either had varicocelectomy or not prior to TESE shows similar sperm retrieval rate of 60% and 60%, respectively.[23] Further data is pending in this area.

Cryopreservation

Sperm that are retrieved surgically can be used for treatment in a fresh IVF cycle by timing oocyte retrieval day with surgical sperm retrieval; however, the logistics involved may not allow this and the absence of any retrieved sperm on the day of the of oocyte retrieval may result in cycle cancellation. Cryopreservation of human spermatozoa was introduced in the 1960s and provides an alternative by storing surgically retrieved spermatozoa before assisted reproduction treatments. Cryopreservation is known to have some deleterious effects on spermatozoa by altering important structures such as the sperm membrane, chromatin integrity, and DNA fragmentation, thereby decreasing overall viability and ability to survive the freeze-thaw process. These effects are even more marked in sperm retrieved from the testes.

However, emerging evidence suggests that cryopreservation has no significant effect on sperm viability. A retrospective cohort study involving a total of 337 IVF/ICSI cycles using sperm surgically retrieved on the day of oocyte retrieval (group A), the day before oocyte retrieval (group B), and frozen-thawed testicular spermatozoa (group C) from men with OA and NOA found similar fertilization rates of 70.7%, 68.7%, and 67.3%, clinical pregnancy rates of 31.3%, 30.9%, and 25.5%, and delivery rates of 28.9%, 28.5%, and 23.2% for groups A, B, and C, respectively. Neither the timing of TESE (on the day of or the day before oocyte retrieval) nor the use of frozen-thawed testicular sperm affected the outcome of ICSI-ET cycle when motile spermatozoa were obtained in azoospermic men. In addition, the aetiology of azoospermia does not have any influence on the outcome with different timings of microdissection TESE procedures for ICSI.[24]

Conclusion

Surgical sperm retrieval in combination with IVF/ICSI represents new therapeutic avenues in the fertility management of couples where the male partner has azoospermia which is not correctable. The current techniques have variable success rates but have not been subjected to randomized control trials—hence the paucity of good evidence to inform the choice of one technique over the others. In experienced hands, sufficient and good quality sperm can usually be harvested for treatment and/or cryopreservation.

Further reading

Donoso P, Tournaye H, Devroey P. Which is the best sperm retrieval technique for non-obstructive azoospermia? A systematic review. *Hum Reprod Update* 2007; **13**(6):539–49.

Kalsi J, Thum MY, Muneer A, Abdullah H, Minhas S. In the era of micro-dissection sperm retrieval (m-TESE) is an isolated testicular biopsy necessary in the management of men with non-obstructive azoospermia? *BJU Int* 2012; **109**(3):418–24.

Shin DH, Turek PJ. Sperm retrieval techniques. *Nat Rev Urol* 2013; **10**(12):723–30.

References

1. Silber SJ, Nagy ZP, Liu J, Godoy H, Devroey P, Van Steirteghem AC. Conventional in-vitro fertilization versus intracytoplasmic sperm injection for patients requiring microsurgical sperm aspiration. *Hum Reprod* 1994; **9**:1705–9.
2. Devroey P, Liu J, Nagy Z, *et al.* Pregnancies after testicular extraction (TESE) and intracytoplasmic sperm injection (ICSI) in non-obstructive azoospermia. *Hum Reprod* 1995; **10**:1457–60.
3. Esteves SC, Miyaoka R, Agarwal A. Surgical treatment of male infertility in the era of intracytoplasmic sperm injection—new insights. *Clinics* 2011; **66**(8):1463–77.
4. Schlegel PN. Testicular sperm extraction: microdissection improves sperm yield with minimal tissue excision. *Hum Reprod* 1999; **14**:131–5.
5. Shin DH, Turek PJ. Sperm retrieval techniques. *Nat Rev Urol* 2013; **10**(12):723–30.
6. Turek PJ. Sperm retrieval techniques. (pp. 453–65) In: Carrell DT, Peterson CM (eds). *Reproductive Endocrinology and Infertility*. New York, NY: Springer, 2010.
7. Qiu Y, Wang LG, Zhang LH, Zhang AD, Wang ZY. Quality of sperm obtained by penile vibratory stimulation and percutaneous vasal sperm aspiration in men with spinal cord injury. *J Androl* 2012; **33**(5):1036–46.
8. Saito K, Kinoshita Y, Suzuki K, Kawakami Y, Sato K, Matsuura K. Successful pregnancy with intrauterine insemination using vasal sperm retrieved by electric stimulation. *Fertil Steril* 2002; **77**(3):621–3.
9. Meniru GI, Gorgy A, Batha S, Clarke RJ, Podsiadly BT, Craft IL. Studies of percutaneous epididymal sperm aspiration (PESA) and intracytoplasmic sperm injection. *Hum Reprod Update* 1998; **4**(1):57–71.
10. Dohle, GR, Ramos, L, Pieters, MHEC, Braat, DDM, Weber RFA. Surgical sperm retrieval and intracytoplasmic sperm injection as treatment of obstructive azoospermia. *Hum Reprod* 1998: **13**(3):620–3.
11. Meseguer, M, Garrido, N, Remohi J, *et al.* Testicular sperm extraction (TESE) and ICSI in patients with permanent azoospermia after chemotherapy. *Hum Reprod* 2003; **18**(6):1281–5.
12. Ashraf CM, Dharmaraj P, Sankalp S, *et al.* Microdissection testicular sperm extraction (Micro-TESE): Results of a large series from india. *Andrology* 2014; **3**:113.
13. Donoso P, Tournaye H, Devroey P. Which is the best sperm retrieval technique for non-obstructive azoospermia? A systematic review. *Hum Reprod Update* 2007; **13**(6):539–49.
14. Kanto S, Sugawara J, Masuda H, Sasano H, Arai Y, Kyono K. Fresh motile testicular sperm retrieved from nonobstructive azoospermic patients has the same potential to achieve fertilization and pregnancy via ICSI as sperm retrieved from obstructive azoospermic patients. *Fertil Steril* 2008; **90**(5):2010.e5–7.

15. Carpi A, Sabanegh E, Mechanick J. Controversies in the management of nonobstructive azoospermia. *Fertil Steril* 2009; **91**(4):963–70.
16. Shiraishi K, Ohmi C, Shimabukuro T, Matsuyama H. Human chorionic gonadotrophin treatment prior to microdissection testicular sperm extraction in non-obstructive azoospermia. *Hum Reprod* 2012; **27**(2):331–9.
17. Hussein A, Ozgok Y, Ross L, Rao P, Niederberger C. Optimization of spermatogenesis-regulating hormones in patients with non-obstructive azoospermia and its impact on sperm retrieval: a multicentre study. *BJU Int* 2013; **111**(3 Pt B):E110–4.
18. Hussein A, Ozgok Y, Ross L, Niederberger C. Clomiphene administration for cases of nonobstructive azoospermia: a multicenter study. *J Androl* 2005; **26**(6):787–91.
19. Aydos K, Unlü C, Demirel LC, Evirgen O, Tolunay O. The effect of pure FSH administration in non-obstructive azoospermic men on testicular sperm retrieval. *Eur J Obstet Gynecol Reprod Biol* 2003; **108**(1):54–8.
20. Schlegel PN. Aromatase inhibitors for male infertility. *Fertil Steril* 2012; **98**(6):1359–62.
21. Gregoriou O, Bakas P, Grigoriadis C, Creatsa M, Hassiakos D, Creatsas G. Changes in hormonal profile and seminal parameters with use of aromatase inhibitors in management of infertile men with low testosterone to oestradiol ratios. *Fertil Steril* 2012; **98**(1):48–51.
22. Moein MR, Tabibnejad N, Ghasemzadeh J. Beneficial effect of tamoxifen on sperm recovery in infertile men with nonobstructive azoospermia. *Andrologia* 2012; **44**(Suppl 1):194–8.
23. Schlegel PN, Kaufmann J. Role of varicocelectomy in men with nonobstructive azoospermia. *Fertil Steril* 2004; **81**(6):1585–8.
24. Karacan M, Alwaeely F, Erkan S, *et al.* Outcome of intracytoplasmic sperm injection cycles with fresh testicular spermatozoa obtained on the day of or the day before oocyte collection and with cryopreserved testicular sperm in patients with azoospermia. *Fertil Steril* 2013; **100**(4):975–80.

CHAPTER 7.4

Infertility

Vasectomy

Yacov Reisman

Introduction to vasectomy

The purpose of the vasectomy is to provide reliable contraception.[1] In 2002, data collected in the United States show that vasectomy was used by 5.7% of men aged 15–44, which represents the fourth most commonly used contraceptive method. Another study from the United States estimates that about one out of every six men over the age of 35 has had a vasectomy.[2] Meanwhile, a UK study shows that 18% of men aged <70 years have had a vasectomy. Higher vasectomy rates are associated with higher levels of education and income.[3]

Research indicates that the level of effectiveness is 99.6%.[4] Compared to tubal sterilization, vasectomy is equally effective in preventing pregnancy; however, vasectomy is simpler, faster, safer, and less expensive.[5,6]

Counselling and relative contraindications

It is not a legal requirement to involve both partners in the decision-making and consent process. Nevertheless, it is good practice to involve both partners if the male agrees.

The history should include information about the patient's marital status, number of children, and motives for the procedure. His medical and surgical history should be reviewed as well and past history of surgical or anaesthetic complications should be noted.

The procedure should be described. Vasectomy is intended to be a permanent form of contraception; its benefits and potential complications should be explained as well. It should be emphasized that vasectomy does not produce immediate sterility and another form of contraception is required until vas occlusion is confirmed by post-vasectomy semen analysis.[1]

As pregnancy after vasectomy may have serious consequences, men should be always informed about the small possibility of vasectomy failure. The risk of pregnancy after vasectomy is approximately 1 in 2,000 for men who have post-vasectomy azoospermia.[7] Genital examination can be performed. Both vasa should be palpated, with particular attention paid to the mobility and the number of vasa.[4]

Over 10 years, about 2% of vasectomized men have a reversal operation, and sometimes additional artificial reproductive techniques are needed to achieve conception.[1]

There are no absolute contraindications. Relative contraindications may be the absence of children, young age (<30 years) (as the chance of a reversal request is increased in men who had a vasectomy at a young age and in those without children), severe illness, no current relationship, and scrotal pain.[1,4]

Surgical techniques

Vasectomy can performed in an outpatient setting under local anaesthesia. Prophylactic antimicrobials are not indicated routinely. The patient should be instructed to cleanse the genital area on the day of surgery. Aspirin should not be taken for one week before the procedure, while other platelet inhibitors and anticoagulants should be withheld for three to four days beforehand. If an anxiolytic has been prescribed, it should be taken 30 minutes before surgery.

The proper surgical environment includes a warm room to facilitate scrotal relaxation. The procedure is performed with the patient in the supine or dorsolithotomy position. Intravenous access is generally not required. Some surgeons shave the surgical area, and warmed povidone-iodine solution applied. The penis may then be retracted by taping it to the abdomen.

For anaesthesia, a 1–2 cm wheal should be made at the desired incision site, bilaterally. The needle is advanced parallel and adjacent to the vas and toward the external inguinal ring. After gentle aspiration, 2–5 mL of 1% lidocaine without adrenaline is injected.[1,4]

Although various vasectomy techniques have been described, all share three essential steps: isolation of the vas deferens, delivery and interruption of the vas, and management of the vasal ends.

Isolation of the vas can occasionally be challenging. The technique used to position the vas is the key to a successful procedure. A 'three-finger technique' for positioning the vas has been described, in which the non-dominant hand is used to manipulate the vas into a subcutaneous position.

After the vas is manoeuvred to the desired location, a 1–2 cm horizontal or vertical incision is made. Next, the soft tissue is bluntly dissected. A clamp is then advanced through the incision to grasp the vas and surrounding tissue. After, the fibrous layer surrounding the vas is incised longitudinally. Controversy exists regarding the length of the vas segment to be removed. In one study, removal of segments that were less than 14–16 mm in length was associated with increased rates of recanalization. Therefore, removal of at least 15 mm is recommended. There is no need for routine pathologic examination of the vas. A variety of surgical techniques for occluding the vas are used, but no single method has been shown to be superior to others. Options include ligation, clipping, cautery, proximal fascial interposition, and open-ended techniques. Combinations of these methods are usually performed. Ligation of the vasal ends is a common practice. Proximal fascial interposition involves the closure of the fascial sheath over the prostatic cut end of the vas in a purse-string fashion. This technique was shown to be effective and to cause few postoperative complications.[8–10] Following management of the vasal ends, the wound is then inspected and the incision is closed with absorbable suture.

The no-scalpel technique was developed in China in 1974 in the hope of improving the acceptance of vasectomy in that country. A ringed extracutaneous vas clamp is used to fixate the vas to the overlying skin, and a single midline incision is made by means of a sharpened clamp. The benefits of no-scalpel vasectomy include a shorter operating time, less pain and swelling, and faster recovery. Failure rates are similar to those associated with conventional techniques.[11]

Postoperative care and clearance

After the procedure is completed, postoperative instructions should be reviewed with the patient. Appropriate recommendations include intermittent ice applications to the scrotum, bed rest, scrotal support for 48 hours, and avoidance of heavy exertion for one week. Appropriate analgesia should be offered. Sexual activity should be avoided for one week. Another method of contraception should be used until semen analysis has confirmed azoospermia.

Many patients are not compliant with the protocol after vasectomy. There is general consensus that men can be given clearance if no spermatozoa are found in the ejaculate. At least 80% of men have no spermatozoa found in their ejaculate three months after vasectomy. In some men, low numbers of non-motile spermatozoa are present and can persist for a longer period of time. These men can be given clearance if <100,000 non-motile spermatozoa per millilitre are present three months after vasectomy. In case of persistent motile spermatozoa after six months of follow-up, it is advised that the vasectomy be redone. An adequate number of ejaculations, at least 20, should have occurred in those three months.[12–14]

Effectiveness

The World Health Organization (WHO) states that, 'vasectomy is highly effective when the procedure is properly performed and when the man waits for 3 months after the vasectomy before having unprotected intercourse'. Pregnancy rates associated with vasectomy are reported in the range of 0–2 per 100 operations, with most studies reporting failure rates of less than 1%.[15]

Vasectomy failure may be due to user failure or to failure of the technique itself. User failure occurs when alternate contraception is not used during the period after vasectomy but before all sperm are cleared from the reproductive tract. The most common cause of failure of the vasectomy technique itself is spontaneous recanalization of the vas, which can occur at any time after vasectomy. Early recanalization occurs before azoospermia is achieved, when sperm counts begin to rise before they have even fallen to zero. Late recanalization occurs after azoospermia has been demonstrated, when motile sperm reappear in the ejaculate. The pregnancy rate due to late recanalization is approximately 1 in 2,000.[1]

In a large review of randomized trials concerning different vasectomy methods, none of the trials found a difference between the groups for time to azoospermia. Fascial interposition was less likely to end in vasectomy failure at 34 weeks.[11]

Complications and late consequences

A low frequency of complications is associated with vasectomy. Different definitions of complications in the literature have resulted in different reported frequencies.

Postoperative bleeding and haematoma (4–22%) rarely, may require incision and drainage. If the haematoma is stable, allow it to resolve on its own. Some advocate the use of prophylactic antibiotics.[16] Infections (0.2–1.5%) are generally mild and limited to the wound site, but Fournier's disease has been reported.[17] Chronic scrotal pain (1–14%) is usually mild but sometimes is associated with negative impact on quality of life. Few of these men require additional surgery.

A sperm granuloma is the result of an inflammatory reaction to the leakage of sperm from the vas. Sperm granuloma develops in 15–40% of patients undergoing vasectomy and may cause pain in up to 3% of patients in whom it develops.[16] Sexual problems are no more prevalent among vasectomized men than they are among non-vasectomized men.[18]

Antisperm antibodies are found in between 8–21% of men in the general population and in 9–36% of infertility patients. In contrast, circulating sperm agglutinating antibodies are found in 50–80% of men in the first year after following vasectomy. Development of antisperm antibodies is thought to be related to breakdown of the blood-testis barrier and leakage of sperm antigens from the epididymis. Sperm antigens have been found in the serum of men as early as two weeks after vasectomy.

All available data indicate that vasectomy is safe and is not associated with increasing risk of serious, long-term side effects or disease, such as testicular or prostate cancer or heart disease.[19]

Further reading

Cook LA, Van Vliet H, Lopez LM, Pun A, Gallo MF. Vasectomy occlusion techniques for male sterilization. *Cochrane Database Syst Rev* 2007; **18**(2):CD003991.

Dohle GR, Diemer T, Kopa Z, *et al.* European Association of Urology guidelines on vasectomy. *Eur Urol* 2012; **61**:159–63.

Royal College of Obstetricians and Gynaecologists. *Male and Female Sterilization: Evidence-based Guideline no. 4.* London, UK: RCOG Press, 2004.

World Health Organization. *Selected Practice Recommendations for Contraceptive Use*, 2nd edition. Geneva, Switzerland: World Health Organization, 2004.

References

1. Dohle GR, Diemer T, Kopa Z, *et al.* European Association of Urology guidelines on vasectomy. *Eur Urol* 2012; **61**:159–63.
2. Labrecque M, Dufresne C, Barone MA, St-Hilaire K. Vasectomy surgical techniques: a systematic review. *BMC Med* 2004; **2**:21.
3. Rowlands S, Hannaford P. The incidence of sterilisation in the UK. *BJOG* 2003; **110**:819–24.
4. Sharlip ID, Belker AM, Honig S, *et al.* Vasectomy: AUA guidelines. *J Urol* 2012; **188**(6 Suppl):2482–91.

5. Royal College of Obstetricians and Gynaecologists. *Male and Female Sterilization: Evidence-based Guideline no. 4*. London, UK: RCOG Press, 2004.
6. Anderson JE, Jamieson DJ, Warner L, *et al.* Contraceptive sterilization among married adults: national data on who chooses vasectomy and tubal sterilization. *Contraception* 2012; **85**:552–7.
7. Alderman PM. The lurking sperm. A review of failures in 8879 vasectomies performed by one physician. *JAMA* 1988; **259**:3142–4.
8. Sokal D, Irsula B, Hays M, Chen-Mok M, Barone MA. Vasectomy by ligation and excision, with or without fascial interposition: a randomized controlled trial. *BMC Med* 2004; **2**:6.
9. Xiaozhang L. Vasectomy occlusion techniques for male sterilization: RHL commentary 2008. The WHO Reproductive Health Library. Geneva, Switzerland: World Health Organization, 2008. Available at: http://apps.who.int/rhl/fertility/contraception/CD003391_xiaozhangl_guide/en/ [Online].
10. Cook LA, Van Vliet H, Lopez LM, Pun A, Gallo MF. Vasectomy occlusion techniques for male sterilization. *Cochrane Database Syst Rev* 2007; **18**(2):CD003991.
11. Barone M (ed). *No-scalpel Vasectomy: A Training Curriculum for Surgeons*, 3rd edition. New York, NY: Engender Health, 2003.
12. Chawla A, Bowles B, Zini A. Vasectomy follow-up: clinical significance of rare nonmotile sperm in postoperative semen analysis. *Urology* 2004; **64**:1212–5.
13. Hancock P, McLaughlin E. British Andrology Society guidelines for the assessment of post vasectomy semen samples. *J Clin Pathol* 2002; **55**:812–6.
14. Korthorst RA, Consten D, van Roijen JH. Clearance after vasectomy with a single semen sample containing < than 100 000 immotile sperm/mL: analysis of 1073 patients. *BJU Int* 2010; **105**:1572–5.
15. World Health Organization. *Selected Practice Recommendations for Contraceptive Use*, 2nd edition. Geneva, Switzerland: World Health Organization, 2004.
16. Adams CE, Wald M. Risks and complications of vasectomy. *Urol Clin North Am* 2009; **36**:331–6.
17. Hartanto, Victor, Eric Chenven, David Di Piazza, *et al.* Fournier gangrene following vasectomy. *Infect Urol* 2001; **14**(3):80–2.
18. Smith A, Lyons A, Ferris J, Richters J, Pitts M, Shelley J. Are sexual problems more common in men who have had a vasectomy? A population-based study of Australian men. *J Sex Med* 2010; **7**:736–42.
19. Köhler TS, Fazili AA, Brannigan RE. Putative health risks associated with vasectomy. *Urol Clin North Am* 2009; **36**:337–45.

CHAPTER 7.5

The management of fertility in spinal cord injury

Mikkel Fode and Jens Sønksen

Causes of infertility in spinal cord injury

As normal ejaculation is mediated by sympathetic and parasympathetic fibres from segments T10–12 and S2–4, respectively, only about 10% of men with spinal cord injury (SCI) can ejaculate normally by sexual stimulation.[1–14] In addition, SCI can reduce semen quality. The reason for this is not entirely clear but factors in sperm transportation/storage, the seminal plasma, and the immune system are likely to be acountable. Meanwhile SCI does not significantly affect female fertility.

Treatments

Treatment of SCI induced infertility is dependent on obtaining viable sperm. The first choice is penile vibratory stimulation (PVS) (Fig. 7.5.1). This is performed by stimulating the glans penis for repeated periods of two to three minutes or until ejaculation. The penile skin should be inspected for bruises during breaks. PVS is most effective in men with an intact reflex arc, as men with injuries at T10 or above have an 88% success rate, while men with lower injuries have a 15% success rate. If a patient is unable to ejaculate initially, two vibrators can be applied at each side of the glans simultaneously. Although rare, the most serious side effect of PVS is an uninhibited sympathetic reflex response termed autonomic dysreflexia. This can occur in patients with an injury at or above T6. Patients at risk, can be given prophylactic nifedipine. If pre-symptoms (including hypertension, bradycardia, sweating, chills, headache, anxiety, and flushing) occur during stimulation, the procedure should be discontinued and the patient should be returned to an upright position.

If PVS is unsuccessful, electroejaculation (EEJ) can be attempted.[15–22] With this method, an electric current is delivered through a rectal probe (Fig. 7.5.2). First 5V of electricity is

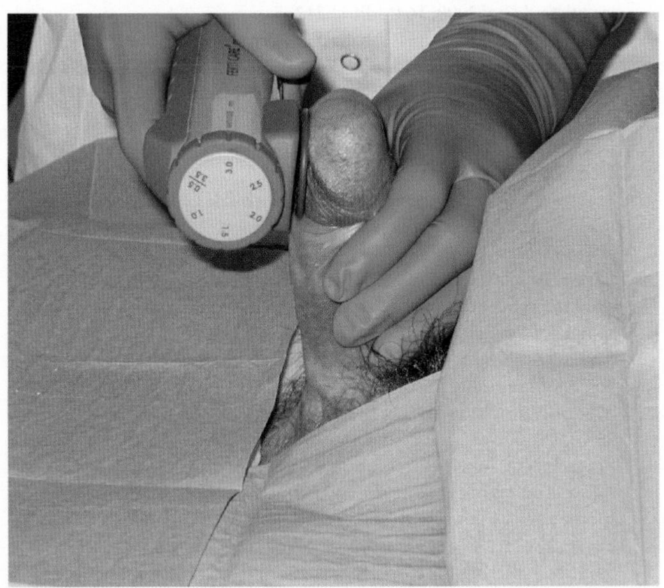

Fig. 7.5.1 Penile vibratory stimulation (PVS). PVS is performed by stimulating either the ventral or the dorsal side of the glans penis for repeated periods of two to three minutes until ejaculation. The optimal stimulation parameters have been shown to be an amplitude of 2.5 mm and a frequency of 100 Hz. If PVS is initially unsuccessful, dual stimulation of both sides of the glans with two vibrators can be attempted. The illustration depicts the FERTI CARE® vibrator (Multicept A/S, Frederiksberg, Denmark).

Reproduced courtesy of Jens Sonksen, MD, PhD, DMSci.

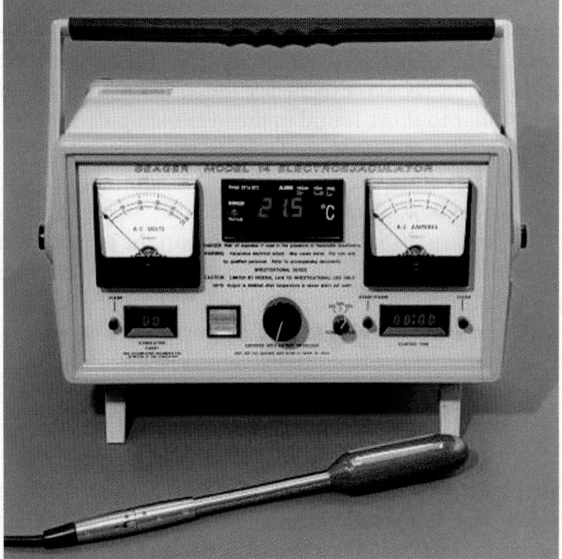

Fig. 7.5.2 Electroejaculation (EEJ). EEJ is performed with the patient placed in the lateral decubitus position. The probe is inserted into the rectum with the electrodes facing toward the seminal vesicles and the prostate. An electric current is then delivered in a wave-like pattern with a progressivly increasing voltage up to 30 V. A dribbling ejaculation takes place during breaks between stimulation waves and the ejaculate is collected by milking the urethra. The illustration depicts the Seager Model 14 Electroejaculator (Dalzell Medical Systems, USA).

Reproduced courtesy of Jens Sonksen, MD, PhD, DMSci.

delivered for five seconds, after which the current is abruptly discontinued. This causes pelvic muscle contractions during which ejaculation can occur. When the contractions have ended, subsequent waves of stimulation and pauses are initiated. The electricity is progressively increased to a maximum of 20–30 V. Waves are continued until no more ejaculate is obtained. As EEJ often results in a partly retrograde ejaculation the bladder can be emptied and a sperm-friendly medium instilled prior to EEJ. This allows sperm to be collected by catheterization following the procedure. In patients with preserved pelvic sensation, general anaesthesia is necessary. EEJ typically results in a lower total motile sperm count compared to PVS, but the procedure results in an ejaculate in almost all cases. The risk of autonomic dysreflexia is higher with EEJ than with PVS but the same considerations apply. In patients under general anaesthesia, blood pressure must be monitored as any abrupt increase should lead to discontinuation of the procedure.

Surgical sperm retrieval should only be considered as a last option, as these methods are both expensive and invasive and yield lower total motile sperm counts than PVS and EEJ.

Methods of insemination

Home insemination can be attempted in patients who are able to ejaculate with PVS and who have good semen quality. No cut-off point has been established but a reasonable estimate is a minimum of four million motile sperm. After instruction, the couple performs PVS around the time of ovulation. The ejaculate is collected in a cup and injected into the vagina by a needleless syringe. The largest study of its kind (n = 140) has recently shown a pregnancy rate of 43% and a median time to pregnancy of 22.8 months (range 6.0–98.4) with this method.

If the couple is unable to or does not wish to perform home insemination, assisted reproductive techniques (ART) can be performed at a fertility clinic. ART include intrauterine insemination (IUI), *in vitro* fertilization (IVF), and intracytoplasmic sperm injection (ICSI). Pregnancy outcomes with these methods are similar to those found in the overall population of infertile couples. The choice of method depends on the total motile sperm count. IUI may be attempted with counts above four million, while IVF or ICSI are recommended in case of lower sperm counts or in case of IUI failure. It is important to bear in mind that the number of motile sperm depends partly on the method of sperm retrieval as PVS yields the highest count while surgical sperm retrieval automatically commits the couple to IVF or ICSI.

Conclusion

The first choice for inducing ejaculation in SCI patients is PVS. If this is unsuccessful, EEJ should be employed. Depending on the total motile sperm count, couples can choose between performing home insemination or receiving a form of ART. The advantages of home insemination include low cost, a strong sense of patient control, and the possibility of multiple pregnancies without further treatment, while the disadvantages are a lower overall pregnancy rate than with ART and a relatively long median time to pregnancy. With the right treatment, it is possible for most SCI men to have children.

Further reading

Brackett NL, Ibrahim E, Iremashvili V, Aballa TC, Lynne CM. Treatment for ejaculatory dysfunction in men with spinal cord injury: an 18-year single center experience. *J Urol* 2010; **183**(6):2304–8.

Fode M, Krogh-Jespersen S, Brackett NL, *et al.* Ejaculatory disorder in men with spinal cord injury. *Eur Urol Rev* 2011; **6**(1):49–55.

Kafetsoulis A, Brackett NL, Ibrahim E, Attia GR, Lynne CM. Current trends in the treatment of infertility in men with spinal cord injury. *Fertil Steril* 2006; **86**(4):781–9.

National Spinal Cord Injury Statistical Center. Spinal cord injury facts and figures at a glance. *J Spinal Cord Med* 2010; **33**:439–440.

Sønksen J. Assisted ejaculation and semen characteristics in spinal cord injured males. *Scand J Urol Nephrol Suppl* 2003; (213):1–31.

Sønksen J, Biering-Sorensen F, Kristensen JK. Ejaculation induced by penile vibratory stimulation in men with spinal cord injuries. The importance of the vibratory amplitude. *Paraplegia* 1994; **32**(10):651–60.

Sønksen J, Fode M, Lochner-Ernst D, Ohl DA. Vibratory ejaculation in 140 spinal cord injured men and home insemination of their partners. *Spinal Cord* 2012; **50**(1):63–6.

Sønksen J, Ohl DA, Wedemeyer G. Sphincteric effects during penile vibratory ejaculation and electroejaculation in men with spinal cord injuries. *J Urol* 2001; **165**:426–9.

References

1. Brackett NL, Ibrahim E, Iremashvili V, Aballa TC, Lynne CM. Treatment for ejaculatory dysfunction in men with spinal cord injury: an 18-year single center experience. *J Urol* 2010; **183**(6):2304–8.
2. Ohl DA, Menge AC, Jarow JP. Seminal vesicle aspiration in spinal cord injured men: insight into poor sperm quality. *J Urol* 1999; **162**(6):2048–51.
3. Brackett NL, Davi RC, Padron OF, Lynne CM. Seminal plasma of spinal cord injured men inhibits sperm motility of normal men. *J Urol* 1996; **155**(5):1632–5.
4. Brackett NL, Lynne CM, Aballa TC, Ferrell SM. Sperm motility from the vas deferens of spinal cord injured men is higher than from the ejaculate. *J Urol* 2000; **164**(3 Pt 1):712–5.
5. Basu S, Lynne CM, Ruiz P, Aballa TC, Ferrell SM, Brackett NL. Cytofluorographic identification of activated T-cell subpopulations in the semen of men with spinal cord injuries. *J Androl* 2002; **23**(4):551–6.
6. Aird IA, Vince GS, Bates MD, Johnson PM, Lewis-Jones ID. Leukocytes in semen from men with spinal cord injuries. *Fertil Steril* 1999; **72**(1):97–103.
7. Trabulsi EJ, Shupp-Byrne D, Sedor J, Hirsch IH. Leukocyte subtypes in electroejaculates of spinal cord injured men. *Arch Phys Med Rehabil* 2002; **83**(1):31–4.
8. Basu S, Aballa TC, Ferrell SM, Lynne CM, Brackett NL. Inflammatory cytokine concentrations are elevated in seminal plasma of men with spinal cord injuries. *J Androl* 2004; **25**(2):250–4.
9. Cohen DR, Basu S, Randall JM, Aballa TC, Lynne CM, Brackett NL. Sperm motility in men with spinal cord injuries is enhanced by inactivating cytokines in the seminal plasma. *J Androl* 2004; **25**(6):922–5.
10. Brackett NL, Cohen DR, Ibrahim E, Aballa TC, Lynne CM. Neutralization of cytokine activity at the receptor level improves sperm otility in men with spinal cord injuries. *J Androl* 2007; **28**(5):717–21.
11. Sønksen J, Biering-Sorensen F, Kristensen JK. Ejaculation induced by penile vibratory stimulation in men with spinal cord injuries. The importance of the vibratory amplitude. *Paraplegia* 1994; **32**(10):651–60.
12. Kafetsoulis A, Brackett NL, Ibrahim E, Attia GR, Lynne CM. Current trends in the treatment of infertility in men with spinal cord injury. *Fertil Steril* 2006; **86**(4):781–9.
13. Sønksen J. Assisted ejaculation and semen characteristics in spinal cord injured males. *Scand J Urol Nephrol Suppl* 2003; (213):1–31.

14. Brackett NL, Kafetsoulis A, Ibrahim E, Aballa TC, Lynne CM. Application of 2 vibrators salvages ejaculatory failures to 1 vibrator during penile vibratory stimulation in men with spinal cord injuries. *J Urol* 2007; **177**(2):660–3.
15. Ekland MB, Krassioukov AV, McBride KE, Elliott SL. Incidence of autonomic dysreflexia and silent autonomic dysreflexia in men with spinal cord injury undergoing sperm retrieval: implications for clinical practice. *J Spinal Cord Med* 2008; **31**(1):33–9.
16. Steinberger RE, Ohl DA, Bennett CJ, McCabe M, Wang SC. Nifedipine pretreatment for autonomic dysreflexia during electroejaculation. *Urology* 1990; **36**(3):228–31.
17. Brindley GS. Electroejaculation: its technique, neurological implications and uses. *J Neurol Neurosurg Psychiatry* 1981; **44**(1):9–18.
18. Brackett NL, Ead DN, Aballa TC, Ferrell SM, Lynne CM. Semen retrieval in men with spinal cord injury is improved by interrupting current delivery during electroejaculation. *J Urol* 2002; **167**(1):201–3.
19. Perkash I, Martin DE, Warner H, Blank MS, Collins DC. Reproductive biology of paraplegics: results of semen collection, testicular biopsy and serum hormone evaluation. *J Urol* 1985; **134**(2):284–8.
20. Sarkarati M, Rossier AB, Fam BA. Experience in vibratory and electro-ejaculation techniques in spinal cord injury patients: a preliminary report. *J Urol* 1987; **138**(1):59–62.
21. Ohl DA, Sønksen J, Menge AC, McCabe M, Keller LM. Electroejaculation versus vibratory stimulation in spinal cord injured men: sperm quality and patient preference. *J Urol* 1997; **157**(6):2147–9.
22. Sønksen J, Fode M, Lochner-Ernst D, Ohl DA. Vibratory ejaculation in 140 spinal cord injured men and home insemination of their partners. *Spinal Cord* 2012; **50**(1):63–6.

CHAPTER 7.6

Mechanism of penile erection

Selim Cellek

Anatomy of the penis

The penis is composed of three cylindrical masses of cavernous tissue bound together by fibrous tissue (Buck's fascia) and covered with skin. The lateral two masses are known as the corpus cavernosum; the third is median and is termed the corpus spongiosum (Fig. 7.6.1). The corpus cavernosum is surrounded by a thick fibrous envelope called the tunica albuginea. The urethra is located within the corpus spongiosum, which is surrounded by a thinner and more elastic fibrous layer than the tunica albuginea of the corpus cavernosum (Fig. 7.6.1). The blood supply to the penile skin and corpus cavernosum is via external and internal pudendal arteries respectively. The internal pudendal artery exits Alcock's canal, and after giving off branches to the scrotum and the bulb becomes the common penile artery. This divides into the dorsal artery which supplies the glans, and the cavernosal artery which goes through the tunica albuginea at the hilum of the penis; then runs distally in the centre of each corpus while giving off numerous helicine branches. These corkscrew-shaped muscular vessels open directly into the lacunar spaces in the corpus cavernosum (Fig. 7.6.1). The venous drainage is via the superficial, intermediate, and deep venous systems. The superficial system, which lies above Buck's fascia, allows blood from multiple superficial veins primarily of the skin to drain into the superficial dorsal vein, which itself drains into the external branch of the internal saphenous vein. The intermediate venous system lies beneath Buck's fascia and comprises the deep dorsal vein and the multiple circumflex veins. This system drains blood from the glans, corpus spongiosum, and the distal two-thirds of the corpora. The deep dorsal vein runs in the groove dorsally between the corpus cavernosum (Fig. 7.6.1) and drains into the dorsal venous complex at the urethroprostatic junction. The deep drainage system consists of the cavernosal and crural veins. Emissary veins in the proximal third of the penis join to form one or two cavernosal veins, which pass between the bulb and crus of the penis to drain into the internal pudendal vein.[1]

Human sexual cycle

The classic human sexual cycle consists of four phases: desire, arousal, orgasm, and resolution.[2–4] Erection in man occurs during the arousal phase and continues through the orgasm phase until the

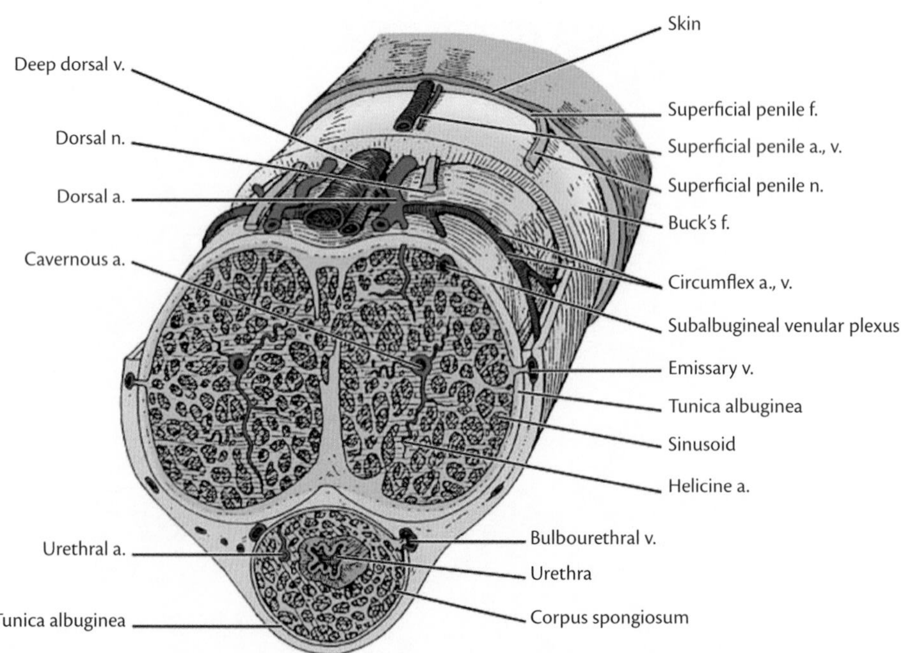

Fig. 7.6.1 Cross-section anatomy of penis. The penis is composed of three cylindrical masses of cavernous tissue bound together by fibrous tissue and covered with skin. Two of the masses are lateral, and are known as the corpus cavernosum; the third is median, and is termed the corpus spongiosum. The location of arteries, veins, and urethra are depicted.
Reprinted from Greg T MacLennan, *Hinman's Atlas of UroSurgical Anatomy, Second Edition*, Saunders an imprint of Elsevier, Philadelphia, USA, Copyright © 2012, with permission from Elsevier.

resolution phase. During the desire and arousal phases, the central nervous system receives, processes, and integrates tactile, visual, olfactory, and imaginative sexual stimuli. This leads to the activation of autonomic and somatic pathways which descend through the spinal cord to the peripheral tissues. Activation of the erectogenic autonomic pathways causes the relaxation of penile arterial and cavernosal smooth muscle, causing an increase in blood flow into the penis (Fig. 7.6.2). The rise in the blood flow triggers further activation of the endothelial cells lining the blood vessels and cavernosal sinusoidal spaces, which leads to further relaxation of the underlying smooth muscle (Fig. 7.6.2). Increased inflow due to arterial and cavernosal smooth muscle relaxation, decreased outflow due to physical compression of subtunical venules, and contraction of striated muscles lead to a further increase in intracavernosal pressure which reaches above the systemic blood pressure (Fig. 7.6.2); a hallmark of rigid erection.[5] In this chapter, the factors involved in this central-peripheral-smooth muscle axis will be introduced and the current knowledge around these mechanisms will be summarized.

Central mechanisms

Sexual stimuli are received by the brain from all parts of man's body. This information is then processed and integrated in the occipital lobe (visual), rhinencephalon (olfactory), thalamus (tactile), and limbic system (imaginative), leading to activation of two nuclei in the hypothalamus: the paraventricular nucleus (PVN) and medial preoptic area (MPOA).[6] These two nuclei send projections to autonomic and spinal centres regulating the peripheral events leading to erection. Within the PVN and MPOA, several neurotransmitters/neuropeptides such as dopamine, oxytocin, serotonin, adrenocorticotrophic hormone (ACTH), alpha-melanocyte stimulating hormone (α-MSH), gamma-aminobutyric acid (GABA), noradrenaline (NA), excitatory amino acids, opioid peptides, acetylcholine, and nitric oxide (NO) have been localized and most have been suggested to be involved in the central regulation of penile erection.[6]

Descending pathways from the brain through the spinal cord are both excitatory and inhibitory in nature. It is thought that without any sexual stimuli there is a continuous inhibitory tone on the descending pathways, while the excitatory component is silent. This tonic inhibition is lifted, which is called disinhibition, when the sexual stimuli increase above a threshold level. This leads to increased pro-erectile excitatory descending activity with activation of the peripheral autonomic and somatic pathways. The nucleus para gigantocellularis (nPGC) of the brain stem is thought to be the relay point where this tonic inhibition takes place.[7]

Below the brain stem, the descending excitatory path reaches two further critical relay points in the spinal cord: the thoracic centre at the level of T11-L2 and the sacral centre at the level of S2-S4. These two relay points are important in integrating the ascending and descending stimuli from and to the periphery and higher central

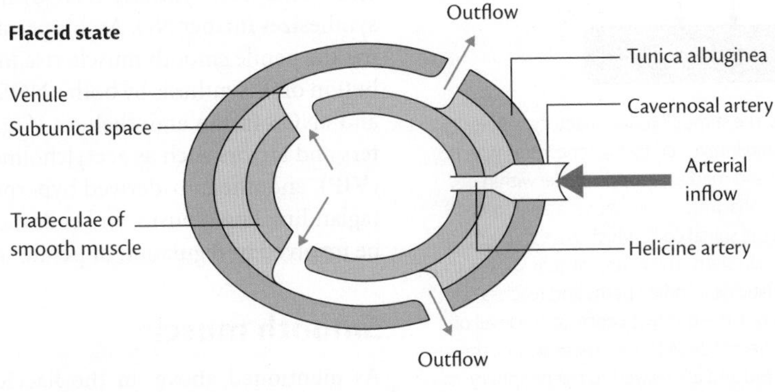

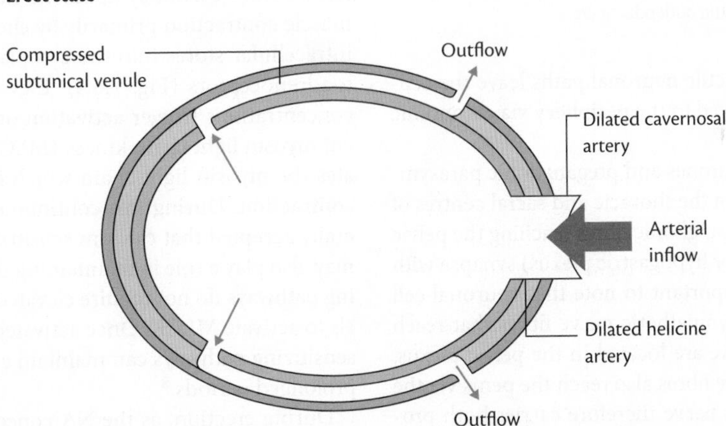

Fig. 7.6.2 Schematic representation of haemodynamic events during erection. During the flaccid state, the cavernosal and arterial smooth is contracted and subtunical venules are open. This causes outflow to exceed the inflow. During erection, cavernosal and arterial smooth muscle relaxes, which increases the inflow. Expansion of the cavernosal space leads to elongation and obstruction of subtunical venules; this decreases the outflow.

Reproduced with permission from Carson C, McMahon CJ. *Fast Facts: Erectile Dysfunction*, 4th edn. Oxford: Health Press Limited, 2008, fastfacts.com

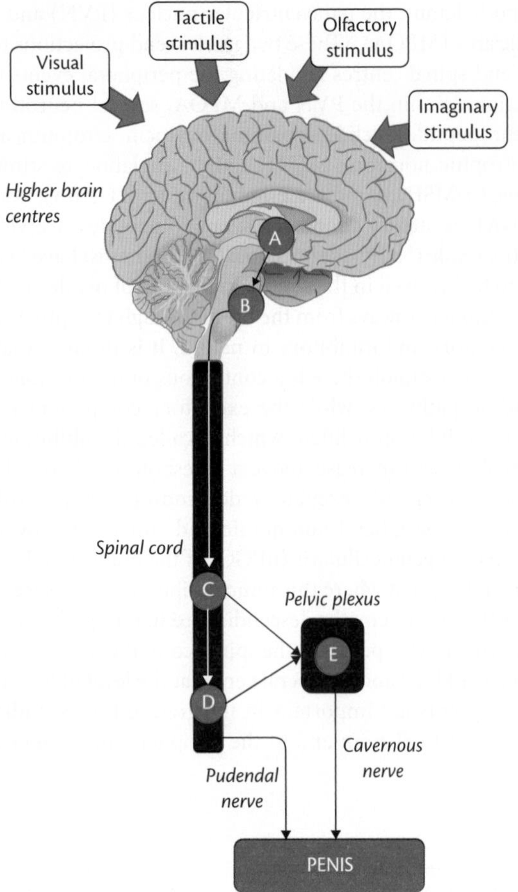

Fig. 7.6.3 Central-peripheral-penile axis: the stimuli (visual, olfactory, tactile, and imaginary) are received, processed, and integrated by higher centres which leads to activation of the paraventricular and medial preoptic nuclei within the hypothalamus (A). Activation of hypothalamic nuclei causes activation of descending excitatory pathway through the spinal cord, which goes through the nucleus paragigantocellularis (B) in the brain stem. The neuronal activation is then relayed through the autonomic and somatic descending paths and reaches two further critical relay points in the spinal cord: the thoracic centre at the level of T11-L2 (C) and the sacral centre at the level of S2–S4 (D). At these points, the erectile neuronal paths leave the spinal cord and are relayed to the periphery via autonomic and somatic nerves. The autonomic nerves are relayed further at the pelvic plexus (E) before reaching the penis via the cavernous nerve. The somatic nerve fibres reach the penis directly via the pudendal nerve.

regions. At these points, the erectile neuronal paths leave the central nervous system and are relayed to the periphery via autonomic and somatic nerves (Fig. 7.6.3).[6,7]

Preganglionic sympathetic neurones and preganglionic parasympathetic neurones are localized in the thoracic and sacral centres of the spinal cord, respectively. Preganglionic fibres reaching the pelvic plexus (also known as the inferior hypogastric plexus) synapse with postganglionic neurons. It is important to note that neuronal cell bodies of the pro-erectile parasympathetic nerve fibres that reach the penis via the cavernous nerve are located in the pelvic plexus. Postganglionic sympathetic nerve fibres also reach the penis via the cavernous nerve. The cavernous nerve therefore carries both pro-erectile parasympathetic and anti-erectile sympathetic nerve fibres to the penile vasculature and the cavernous body. Sacral motor neurones send direct projections to the striated ischiocavernosus and bulbospongiosus muscles via the pudendal nerve (Fig. 7.6.3).[6]

Sympathetic nerve fibres in the penis release low concentrations of the neurotransmitter NA continuously. NA causes contraction of vascular and cavernosal smooth muscle by activating α1-adrenoceptors. The tonic release of NA therefore causes a heightened smooth muscle tone under normal conditions (i.e. without sexual stimuli) keeping the penis flaccid. It should also be noted that parasympathetic nerve fibres release small amounts of NO during the flaccid phase; it is generally accepted that the heightened tone of the penile smooth muscle is the net result of a balance between contractile NA and relaxant NO (Fig. 7.6.4).[5] When the autonomic nerves are activated by higher centres as a result of sexual stimuli, two key events take place simultaneously:

(i) NO released from postganglionic parasympathetic nerve fibres increases significantly which causes relaxation of vascular and cavernosal smooth muscle. These nerve fibres are also known as nitrergic (Fig. 7.6.4) because of their expression of neuronal NO synthase (nNOS), which synthesizes NO.[8]

(ii) Acetylcholine released from parasympathetic nerve fibres simultaneously with NO inhibits the release of NA from sympathetic nerve fibres.[9,10]

This initial relaxation as a result of increased vasorelaxant NO and decreased vasoconstrictor NA leads to an increase in blood inflow into the cavernosal space. Increased blood flow generates increased shear stress on the endothelial cells lining the blood vessels and cavernosal sinusoids. Shear stress causes activation of endothelial NO synthase (eNOS) in the endothelial cells[11] which synthesizes further NO. At this point the NO concentrations reaching the penile smooth muscle rise to a peak level due to the contribution of its synthesis by both nNOS in the parasympathetic nerves and eNOS in the endothelium (Fig. 7.6.4). Other neurotransmitters and factors such as acetylcholine, vasoactive intestinal peptide (VIP), endothelium-derived hyperpolarizing factor (EDHF), prostaglandins, angiotensin, and endothelin have also been suggested to be involved in regulation of penile smooth muscle tone.[5]

Smooth muscle

As mentioned above, in the flaccid state, vascular, and cavernosal smooth muscle tone in the penis is elevated by continuous release of NA from sympathetic nerve fibres. NA causes smooth muscle contraction primarily by eliciting a release of calcium from intracellular stores into the cytoplasm secondary to activation of α-adrenoceptors (Fig. 7.6.4). Elevated intracellular free calcium concentrations trigger activation of calcium-calmodulin dependent myosin light chain kinase (MLCK), which in turn phosphorylates the myosin light chain which is essential for smooth muscle contraction. During this continuous contractile period, it is generally accepted that calcium sensitizing pathways such Rho-kinase may also play a role in maintaining the high tone. Calcium sensitizing pathways do not require elevated intracellular free calcium levels to activate MLCK. Once activated via α-adrenoceptors, calcium sensitizing pathways can maintain a high, smooth muscle tone for prolonged periods.[8]

During erection, as the NA concentration reaching the smooth muscle decreases, the concentration of NO increases. This causes a shift in the smooth muscle from contractile phase to relaxant phase. This shift is a result of the combination of decreased activation of contractile pathways (i.e. direct activation of MLCK by increased

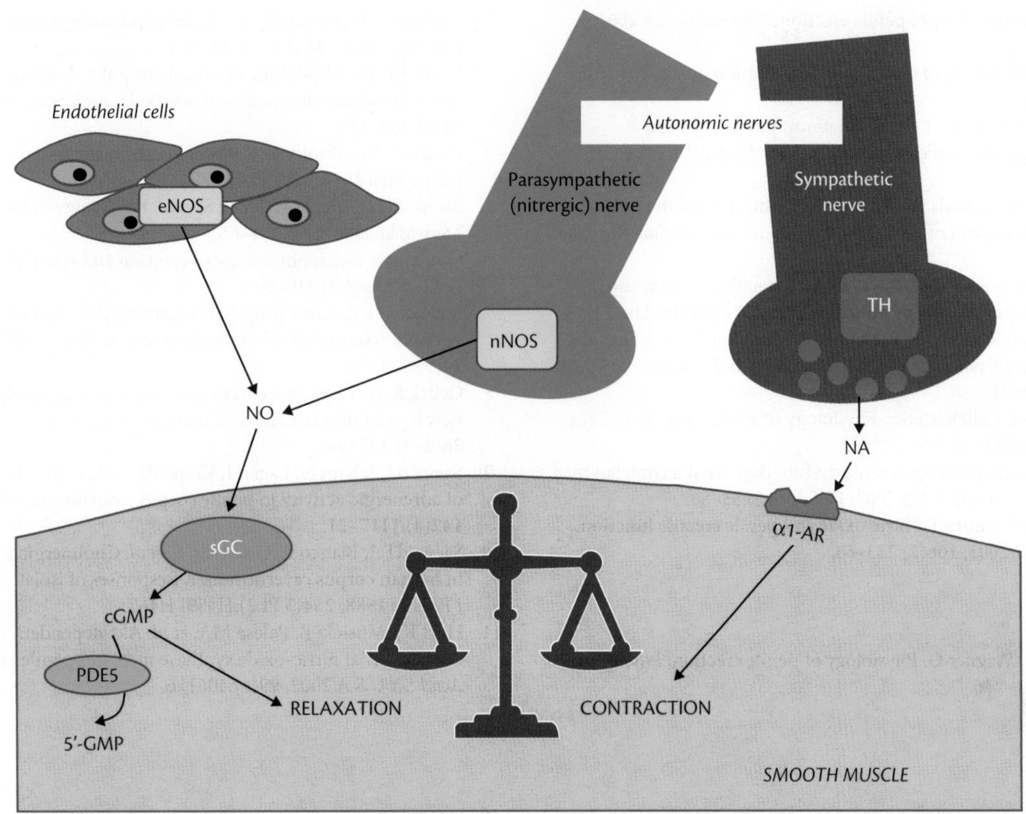

Fig. 7.6.4 Penile erection is governed by a balance between relaxant and contractile mechanisms in the smooth muscle: the cavernosal and vascular smooth muscle of the penis receive two opposing signals from endothelial cells and autonomic nerve fibres. The main relaxant mediator nitric oxide (NO) is synthesized by endothelial NO synthase (eNOS) in the endothelial cells and by neuronal NO synthase (nNOS) in the parasympathetic nerve fibres. The main contractile mediator noradrenaline (NA) is synthesized by tyrosine hydroxylase (TH) and stored in vesicles until its release (depicted as red circles) in the sympathetic nerve fibres. NO diffuses into the nearby smooth muscle cell and activates intracellular cytoplasmic soluble guanylate cyclase (sGC). Activation of sGC leads to an increased level of cyclic guanosine monophosphate (cGMP) concentrations in the smooth muscle cells. cGMP acts then on several pathways leading to relaxation. cGMP is quickly metabolized to inactive 5′-GMP by phosphodiesterase type 5 (PDE5). NA activates the α1-adrenoceptor (α1-AR) on the membrane of the smooth muscle cell, which leads to the contraction. For clarity, other relaxant or contractile factors such as vasoactive intestinal peptide, endothelial derived hyperpolarizing factor, and endothelin are not depicted.

calcium and calcium sensitizing pathways) and increased activation of relaxant pathways, which in turn has an inhibitory effect on the contractile pathways via different mechanisms.

The main relaxant mechanism is the activation of soluble guanylate cyclase (sGC) enzyme by NO. Activation of sGC leads to an increased level of cyclic guanosine monophosphate (cGMP) concentrations in the smooth muscle cells (Fig. 7.6.4). cGMP acts then on several pathways leading to relaxation. cGMP is quickly metabolized to inactive 5′-GMP by an enzyme called phosphodiesterase type 5 (PDE5) in the penile smooth muscle (Fig. 7.6.4).[5] Inhibition of PDE5 therefore causes an increase in cGMP concentrations in the penile smooth muscle, leading to potentiation of NO-driven erectile process.

Relaxation of vascular and cavernosal smooth muscle causes an increase in blood flow into the cavernosal space. This leads to engorgement of sinusoidal spaces with blood which results in reduced outflow due to compression of the subtunical venules. This is commonly called the veno-occlusive mechanism. Such an increased inflow and decreased outflow causes the intracavernosal pressure to reach the level of systemic arterial pressure. The pressure is further increased when striated muscles such as ischiocavernosus muscle contract as a results of activation of pudendal nerve fibres.

Conclusions

A brief summary of the current understanding of mechanisms involved in the regulation of penile erection is given. Although the main players in this important physiological function such as NO and noradrenaline have been identified and characterized, there remain several unanswered questions: what are the contribution of other factors (e.g. EDHF, VIP) to penile erection in men? Which central neurotransmitters are involved in regulation of erectile response in men and how are they linked to psychological aspects of sexual function? What are the relative contribution of eNOS and nNOS? What are the characteristics of a human nitrergic neurone (i.e. how does a nitrergic neurone transport nNOS enzyme through its axon)? It is hoped that with the help of technological breakthroughs these questions will be answered in the near future, which will eventually lead to better and newer treatment modalities for erectile dysfunction.

Further reading

Andersson KE, Wagner G. Physiology of penile erection. *Physiol Rev* 1995; **75**(1):191–236.

Andersson KE. Mechanisms of penile erection and basis for pharmacological treatment of erectile dysfunction. *Pharmacol Rev* 2011; **63**(4):811–59.

Andersson KE. Pharmacology of penile erection. *Pharmacol Rev* 2001; **53**(3):417–50.

Giuliano F. Neurophysiology of erection and ejaculation. *J Sex Med* 2011; **8**(Suppl 4):310–5.

Gratzke C, Angulo J, Chitaley K, *et al.* Anatomy, physiology, and pathophysiology of erectile dysfunction. *J Sex Med* 2010; **7**(1 Pt 2): 445–75.

McKenna KE. Some proposals regarding the organization of the central nervous system control of penile erection. *Neurosci Biobehav Rev* 2000; **24**(5):535–40.

Saenz de Tejada I, Angulo J, *et al.* Physiology of erectile function and pathophysiology of erectile dysfunction. (pp. 287–343) In: Lue TF, Basson R, Rosen R, Giuliano F, Khoury S, Montorsi F (eds). *Sexual Medicine: Sexual Dysfunction in Men and Women*. Paris, France: Health Publications, 2004.

Saenz dT, I, Angulo J, Cellek S, *et al.* Physiology of erectile function. *J Sex Med* 2004; **1**(3):254–65.

Stief CG. Central mechanisms of erectile dysfunction: what a clinician may want to know. *Int J Impot Res* 2003; **15**(Suppl 2):S3–S6.

Toda N, Ayajiki K, Okamura T. Nitric oxide and penile erectile function. *Pharmacol Ther* 2005; **106**(2):233–66.

References

1. Andersson KE, Wagner G. Physiology of penile erection. *Physiol Rev* 1995; **75**(1):191–236.
2. Masters WH, Johnson VE. The human female: anatomy of sexual response. *Minn Med* 1960; **43**:31–6.
3. Levin RJ. The physiology of sexual arousal in the human female: a recreational and procreational synthesis. *Arch Sex Behav* 2002; **31**(5):405–11.
4. deGroat WC, Booth AM. Physiology of male sexual function. *Ann Intern Med* 1980; **92**(2 Pt 2):329–31.
5. Saenz dT, I, Angulo J, Cellek S, *et al.* Physiology of erectile function. *J Sex Med* 2004; **1**(3):254–65.
6. Giuliano F. Neurophysiology of erection and ejaculation. *J Sex Med* 2011; **8**(Suppl 4):310–5.
7. McKenna KE. Some proposals regarding the organization of the central nervous system control of penile erection. *Neurosci Biobehav Rev* 2000; **24**(5):535–40.
8. Cellek S. Nitrergic-noradrenergic interaction in penile erection: a new insight into erectile dysfunction. *Drugs Today (Barc)* 2000; **36**(2–3):135–46.
9. Saenz dT, I, Kim N, Lagan I, Krane RJ, Goldstein I. Regulation of adrenergic activity in penile corpus cavernosum. *J Urol* 1989; **142**(4):1117–21.
10. Saenz dT, I, Blanco R, Goldstein I, *et al.* Cholinergic neurotransmission in human corpus cavernosum. I. Responses of isolated tissue. *Am J Physiol* 1988; **254**(3 Pt 2):H459–H467.
11. Hurt KJ, Musicki B, Palese MA, *et al.* Akt-dependent phosphorylation of endothelial nitric-oxide synthase mediates penile erection. *Proc Natl Acad Sci U S A* 2002; **99**(6):4061–6.

CHAPTER 7.7

Erectile dysfunction
Pathophysiology and assessment

Antonino Saccà and Andrea Salonia

Introduction to erectile dysfunction

Erection is a complex neurovascular phenomenon under hormonal and psychological control; this includes arterial dilation, trabecular smooth muscle relaxation, and activation of the corporeal veno-occlusive mechanism. Erectile dysfunction (ED)—defined as the persistent inability to attain and maintain an erection sufficient to permit satisfactory sexual performance—may occur from multifaceted, complex mechanisms including disruptions in neural, vascular, and hormonal signalling.

Penile erections are under psychological control and represent the result of subsequent complex vascular and neurological phenomena. Penile erections are normally classified as *central, reflexogenic,* and *nocturnal* erections (see Chapter 7.6).

Abnormalities of erectile function have been traditionally classified as *neurogenic* (failure to initiate), *arteriogenic* (failure to fill), and *venogenic* (failure to store).[1] However, the term *venogenic ED* reflects changes in the anatomy and histology of the corpus cavernosum, with alteration of the cavernous veno-occlusive mechanism. In addition, abnormalities of the sex hormone milieu may significantly affect the quality of penile erections, and this aspect has attracted much interest with regard to its role in the ageing population.[2]

This chapter will focus on one area of pathophysiology which leads to the development of ED: the ageing process. In addition the chapter will describe on the assessment of the patient seeking medical help for ED.

Ageing and erectile function impairment

Data from the European Male Ageing Study (EMAS) in European men aged 40–79 years old showed that around 30% of individuals reported ED and 6% reported severe orgasmic impairment, both of which were closely associated with age and concomitant morbidities.[3] Interestingly, concern about ED increased with age, peaking in the 50–59 years age band, but decreased thereafter.[3]

The process of ageing may affect all the components of the erectile process, including nerves, arteries, veins, cavernous tissue, and hormones. However, evidence in the literature of ageing-induced damage to these structures has certainly been influenced by the availability of techniques for identifying certain types of damage, and this is the reason for a leading role played by vascular and endocrine abnormalities affecting the male erectile system.[1,4–6] The process of ageing is multifactorial and depends on several factors, including metabolic rate, genetics, lifestyle, and environmental conditions.[7]

Irrespective of the initiating factor, the ultimate common pathologic process is smooth muscle cell (SMC) damage along with an increased penile fibrosis, which may ultimately decrease the vasodilator response. Age-related smooth muscle dysfunction has long been recognized in the respiratory,[8] gastrointestinal,[9] and cardiovascular[10] systems.

Likewise, ageing may also significantly affect the genitourinary tract; in this context, a frequent and co-causal association between lower urinary tract symptoms (LUTS) and sexual dysfunction (i.e. ED and ejaculatory disorders) has been widely observed.[11–14]

The exact mechanism that links ageing to SMC dysfunction within the CC is certainly not unique, and it is not completely understood. Normal erectile function is a delicate balance between vasoconstrictor and vasorelaxant mediators on corporal smooth muscle tone.[1,15] Endothelium-derived NO and endothelin-1 (ET-1) have been identified as modulators of erectile function. NO is a key regulator of cavernosal smooth muscle relaxation, whereas ET-1, being a potent vasoconstrictor agent, is believed to maintain penile flaccidity.[1,15,16] For instance, evidence suggests that there are age-related changes in the levels of these modulators when ED occurs.[17–20] Among others, Garbán *et al.*[17] showed a decreased NO synthase (NOS) activity and a reduction in NOS-containing nerve fibres within the corpus cavernosum in the penis of ageing male rats. Rajasekaran *et al.* reported age-related impairments in the expression of NO and ET-1 as well as in the production of growth factors, such as transforming growth factor-β1 (TGF-β1).[21] Published reports suggest that elevated RhoA/Rho-kinase signalling plays may role in the development of ED, and in other disorders of the urogenital tract such as benign prostatic hyperplasia, kidney failure, ejaculation disorders, prostate and bladder cancer initiation, and eventual metastasis.[22,23] Data would suggest that increased RhoA/Rho-kinase signalling is a major factor in the pathogenesis of age-associated ED and the mechanism involves increased penile smooth muscle contractility through inhibition of myosin light chain phosphatase.[12,24] This pathway involves RhoA, a small monomeric G-protein that activates Rho-kinase. Activated Rho-kinase phosphorylates the regulatory subunit of smooth muscle myosin phosphatase (SMPP-IM). Inhibitory phosphorylation of SMPP-IM leads to the sensitization of myofilaments to Ca++,[25] which translates into smooth muscle contraction. An age-related increase in RhoA expression has been documented in rat vascular tissues, and this overexpression has been suggested as being responsible for age-associated vascular disorders.[24,26]

Moreover, hypertension, which has been recognized as a well-known vascular risk factor for ED,[27–30] is also associated with elevated penile RhoA levels.[31] Conversely, inhibition of Rho-kinase activity has been found to be beneficial in attenuating the decline in erectile function in hypertensive rats.[32] In summary, the net result of the impairment of erection regulators, such as NO, ET-1, and Rho-kinase, is an increased penile smooth muscle tone, which may be responsible for the impaired erectile response seen throughout the ageing process in animal models. Overall, age-related morphological and functional changes in terms of smooth muscle and collagen content are observed in human corpus cavernosum as a possible contributing factor to the development of ED.[33,34]

A further major mechanism suggested as a potential cause of ED is pelvic atherosclerosis.[1] Atherosclerosis-induced arterial insufficiency is a common clinical problem in the elderly and remains the leading cause of death in the adult population.[35] In this context, ED has progressively emerged as an important sentinel marker of men's overall health, assuming major relevance exactly in the cardiovascular field.[36–41] This is particularly important in individuals with diabetes mellitus.[42–47] Overall, ED may be associated with a significantly increased risk of cardiovascular disease (CVD), coronary heart disease (CAD), stroke, overall atherosclerotic cardiovascular events,[48] and all-cause mortality,[36–41] and the increase is probably independent of conventional cardiovascular risk factors,[37,42] glyco-metabolic control, and ED severity.[43,44]

In pathophysiological terms, using animal models mimicking pelvic ischaemia and hypercholesterolemia, Azadzoi *et al.* demonstrated similar alterations in the smooth muscle cells of the detrusor and of the corpora, as result of pelvic atherosclerosis. Chronic ischaemia resulted in fibrosis, smooth muscle atrophy, and non-compliance of the bladder.[49] Chronic ischaemia is also involved in the deterioration of cavernosal smooth muscle and in the development of corporeal fibrosis, which in turn may lead to ED.[50,51] Moreover, pelvic atherosclerosis may damage the pudendal–cavernous–helicine arterial tree.[52] In the early stages of atherosclerosis this process results in decreased arterial blood flow to the corpus cavernosum and, as a consequence, leads to ED, while in more advanced stages, the erectile tissue loses its capability to produce the quantity of NO needed for smooth muscle relaxation, because of the down-regulation of the expression of the constitutive NOS.[53]

Chronic ischaemia is also responsible of the overexpression of TGF-β1. This protein is a pleotropic cytokine demonstrated to be an essential mediator of tissue fibrosis.[1,54,55] Overproduction of TGF-β1 decreases the smooth muscle–connective tissue ratio by inducing the expression of collagen, fibronectin, and proteoglycans while inhibiting the growth of smooth muscle cells and the activity of collagenase.[56–58]

Oxidative stress is another potential factor in the pathogenesis of ED in the elderly. Oxidative damage to the vasculature caused by reactive oxygen species (ROS) plays a fundamental role in the natural ageing process.[59] The interaction between ROS and NO has been indicated as crucial to the development of ED.[60,61] Specifically, NO would seem to interact with superoxide to form peroxynitrite, which has been reported to play a central role in atherogenesis.[62,63] In the presence of peroxynitrite, the enzyme responsible for inactivating superoxide is inhibited, which in turn results in a further increase of peroxynitrite and may drive a reduction in the concentration of the available NO.[62,63] Moreover, peroxynitrite and superoxide increase the incidence of apoptosis in the endothelium, leading to a further decrease in available NO. Finally, the reduction in NO concentration increases the adhesion of platelets and leukocytes to the endothelial cells, which react with a vasoconstriction stimulus mediated by thromboxane A2 and leukotrienes.[63] Because the reduced availability of NO and long-term endothelial damage are the two most important causes of ED, the role of oxidative stress in the corpora cavernosa is a critical determinant in the pathophysiology of ED. Endothelial dysfunction represents the first step in the pathophysiology of ED and can anticipate a major peripheral vascular problem.[64–66] Overall, endothelial dysfunction can be defined as an abnormal endothelial response that reduces the bioavailability of NO and impairs vasodilation.

Late-onset hypogonadism in the general male population can be defined by the presence of at least three sexual symptoms (i.e. decreased frequency of morning erections, ED, decreased frequency of sexual thoughts) associated with a total testosterone level of less than 11 nmol per litre (320 ng per dL) and a free testosterone (T) level of less than 220 pmol per litre (64 pg per mL).[67] The importance of an age-related reduction in the circulating testosterone in men remains clinically controversial.[67] In this context, hypogonadism is certainly a common condition which occurs more frequently in older men. It is characterized by low testosterone and is associated with symptoms which are often non-specific. A key symptom is low libido, but it can also be associated with ED, reduced muscle mass and strength, increased body fat, reduced bone mineral density and osteoporosis, reduced vitality, and depressed mood. Moreover, hypogonadism is linked with a variety of co-morbid conditions including the metabolic syndrome, diabetes, obesity, and osteoporosis.[2,5,68–70]

Erectile dysfunction assessment

An accurate diagnosis of ED represents a significant opportunity not only to diagnose the dysfunction per se, and the associated aetiological factors, but also to identify co-morbid and potentially life-threatening conditions.[71,72] Therefore, while maintaining the standards of simplicity, diagnosis of ED has to be as detailed as possible. This requires a careful medical and sexual history, a comprehensive physical examination, and laboratory testing. Conversely any assessment must be tailored to both patient complaints and individual risk factors.

Basic diagnostic assessment of erectile dysfunction

Medical history

The work-up for ED diagnosis should start by considering that ED shares several common risk factors with CVD.[73] In this context a comprehensive medical history regarding both modifiable (e.g. physical exercise, obesity, dyslipidemia, smoking and recreational drugs, excessive alcohol intake) and unmodifiable risk factors must be taken.[74–76] The latter include diabetes mellitus, hypertension, sleep disturbances (e.g. obstructive sleep apnoea syndrome), metabolic syndrome, late-onset hypogonadism/testosterone deficiency syndrome and other hormonal causes of male sexual dysfunctions.[77–84] The work-up should also consider symptoms and signs of either depression[85] or anxiety disorders.[86–88] Impairment of erectile functioning is also frequently co-morbid with either neurological disorders (i.e. multiple sclerosis, Parkinson's disease, and cerebrovascular disease)[89] or psychiatric disorder.[71] The history should also consider all major pelvic and retroperitoneal surgeries, which may also impact on male sexuality.[1,90]

ED is strongly related with ageing, with a steep incline in prevalence rates in men older than 40 years.[86,91] This increase of ED with age is also associated with a progressive increase in the prevalence LUTS.[12,92] whose presence and severity should also be assessed.

An evaluation of current treatments taken by the patient for any reason must complete the medical history. Indeed, a detailed knowledge of concurrent therapy including antidepressants, antipsychotics, and antihypertensives (e.g. thiazides, β-blockers,[93] nitrates, and nitrate donors, antiandrogens, and so on), not only has a role in helping the physician gain a better understanding of the possible pathophysiological pathways of ED, but it may also identify potential drug interaction, such as the potential interaction between PDE5 inhibitors and nitrate medication. Likewise, due to the highly prevalent co-presence of ED and LUTS, a comprehensive collection of information regarding the potential use of any α-blockers and 5α-reductase inhibitors should complete the medical history.[13]

Sexual history

Sexual history taking is mandatory in each patient complaining of any sexual dysfunction/disorder.[71,94] In this context, age, sexual orientation, marital status, sexual experience should be always considered in order to better understanding individual sexual ecology. After having inquired whether or not the patient is sexually active and either naive or not for seeking medical help, the basic work-up in men with ED should consider onset and duration of the erectile problem, along with a detailed investigation about the rigidity and duration of nocturnal/morning erections, erogenous erections, and erections obtained by self-masturbation, as well.[71,94]

Diagnosis of congenital or acquired penile curvature (e.g. secondary due to Peyronie's disease) is mainly based on medical and sexual histories.[95]

Physical examination

Physical examination in patients with ED usually does not reveal the diagnosis. In this context, according to the Recommendations of the International Consultation in Sexual Medicine (ICSM), for the Clinical Evaluation of Men and Women with Sexual Dysfunction,[96] physical examination is highly recommended, but not always necessary (grade C). Therefore, the aim of physical examination in men with ED is to assess genitourinary anatomy, as well as endocrine, vascular, and neurological systems.[71,97] Moreover, physical examination may reveal important information in patients with Peyronie's plaques or atrophic testicles. Local examination thus includes inspection of the penile shaft for size, position of the meatus, scars and skin abnormalities, and palpation for fibrous plaques. Testicular size and consistency are assessed. Digital rectal examination is advisable in patients above 45 years[97] of age (above 50 years according to European Association of Urology (EAU) guidelines)[71] and in men who might be possible candidates for testosterone replacement therapy.[71,97]

Moreover, a general examination ideally should include evaluation of male secondary sex characters, gynaecomastia, pulses, peripheral sensations, and scars from previous surgeries or trauma. Blood pressure and heart rate should be measured, especially if they have not been assessed throughout the previous three to six months.[71] Waist circumference measurement is helpful in counselling the patient about the risks related to obesity and the possibility of the metabolic syndrome.[81]

Laboratory assessment

According to the EAU guidelines on male sexual dysfunction, laboratory testing must be tailored to the patient's complaints and risk factors.[71] Moreover, according to the recommendations of the ICSM for the Clinical Evaluation of Men and Women with Sexual Dysfunction, it is once again highly recommended, but not always necessary (grade C).[96] Recommended laboratory tests include fasting glucose[71] and lipids profile.[71] if not assessed throughout the previous 12 months. Hormonal tests must include a morning sample of total testosterone.[71,83,84,97] Additional laboratory tests (e.g. thyroid function, prolactin, luteinizing hormone) may be performed at the discretion of the physician, based on the medical history and clinician's judgement.[71,97]

Specialized diagnostic tests

The vast majority of patients with ED can be adequately managed without further diagnostic assessments; conversely, some patients may actually benefit from specific diagnostic tests.[71] Among them, men with primary erectile disorders (neither associated with acquired organic disease nor with psychogenic disorder), young patients with arteriogenic ED coupled with a history of either pelvic or perineal trauma, patients with complex endocrine, psychiatric, or psychosexual disorders. Even more important, specific tests should be used in men with congenital or acquired penile deformities, who may eventually benefit from surgical correction.[97]

Rigiscan® assessment of nocturnal penile tumescence and rigidity

The Rigiscan® device allows assessment of nocturnal penile tumescence and rigidity. At least two consecutive nights of recording are necessary to evaluate nocturnal penile tumescence and rigidity recordings.[98] Nocturnal penile tumescence and rigidity with at least one erectile episode of tip penile rigidity greater than 60% and 10 minutes in duration may be associated with normal erectile function.[15,98]

Dynamic duplex ultrasound penile blood flow evaluation

In-office evaluation of ED by colour duplex Doppler ultrasound (CDDU) can help the decision-making process related to choosing the most appropriate therapy.[71,99] Standardized operating procedures (SOPs) for CDDU have been recently published.[99] Usually, CDDU is a dynamic test requiring intracavernosal injection of a vasoactive agent performed by an experienced sonographer in a physician's office or by a radiologist in a hospital setting. CDDU will assess arterial inflow, venous outflow and may help to understand the cause of the patients symptoms.

Dynamic infusion cavernosometry or cavernosography

The standard method of diagnosing venous leakage is by dynamic infusion cavernosometry and cavernosography (DICC).[71,99] Venous-occlusion dysfunction (VOD) is an organic cause of ED and it occurs when an abnormal venous drainage prevents a rigid erection in the presence of a normal penile arterial flow. VOD can be diagnosed by an abnormal cavernosometry and the site of the 'leakage' can be assessed through cavernosography.[99] DICC is not routinely performed; indeed, it should be performed only in patients failing to respond to oral/local therapy and who may be considered for vascular reconstructive surgery.[71]

Internal pudendal arteriography

Arteriography is the most invasive diagnostic test for vasculogenic ED. It should be only considered in highly selected cases of young men with decreased cavernosal arterial inflow by CDDU and a history of pelvic or perineal trauma,[71,98] where arteriography may highlight a discrete focus of arterial occlusion which may be corrected with microvascular surgery. Conversely, pudendal angiography, in conjunction with microembolization, is first-line therapy for high-flow/traumatic priapism.[100]

Conclusions

Overall, ED is age-linked and may be considered a reliable proxy of male general health status. In this context, it seems reasonable to suppose that, throughout the ageing process, erectile function impairment may be mostly considered as the result of athero-sclerosis-induced cavernosal ischaemia, which ultimately leads to both cavernosal fibrosis and to veno-occlusive dysfunction. Abnormalities in circulating levels of hormones controlling sexual organs—mainly testosterone—most probably play a significant role in some patients. In practical terms, these findings prompt us to further outline the importance of taking a comprehensive medical and sexual history and performing a focussed physical examination in all men with ED. Laboratory tests should be also considered in the minimal work-up for ED, whereas specialised diagnostic tests should be only dedicated to selected patients.

Further reading

Althof SE, Rosen RC, Perelman MA, Rubio-Aurioles E. Standard operating procedures for taking a sexual history. *J Sex Med* 2012; 10(1):26–35.

Buvat J, Maggi M, Gooren L, *et al.* Endocrine aspects of male sexual dysfunctions. *J Sex Med* 2010; 7:1627–56.

Buvat J, Maggi M, Guay A, Torres LO. Testosterone deficiency in men: systematic review and standard operating procedures for diagnosis and treatment. *J Sex Med* 2013; 10(1):245–84.

Corona G, Lee DM, Forti G, *et al.* Age-related changes in general and sexual health in middle-aged and older men: results from the European Male Ageing Study (EMAS). *J Sex Med* 2010; 7:1362–80.

Dong JY, Zhang YH, Qin LQ. Erectile dysfunction and risk of cardiovascular disease: meta-analysis of prospective cohort studies. *J Am Coll Cardiol* 2011; 58:1378–85.

Gacci M, Eardley I, Giuliano F, *et al.* Critical analysis of the relationship between sexual dysfunctions and lower urinary tract symptoms due to benign prostatic hyperplasia. *Eur Urol* 2011; 60:809–25.

Gratzke C, Angulo J, Chitaley K, *et al.* Anatomy, physiology, and pathophysiology of erectile dysfunction. *J Sex Med* 2010; **7**:445–75.

Gupta BP, Murad MH, Clifton MM, Prokop L, Nehra A, Kopecky SL. The effect of lifestyle modification and cardiovascular risk factor reduction on erectile dysfunction: a systematic review and meta-analysis. *Arch Intern Med* 2011; **171**:1797–803.

Hatzichristou D, Rosen RC, Derogatis LR, *et al.* Recommendations for the clinical evaluation of men and women with sexual dysfunction. *J Sex Med* 2010; 7:337–48.

Hatzimouratidis K, Amar E, Eardley I, *et al.* Guidelines on male sexual dysfunction: erectile dysfunction and premature ejaculation. *Eur Urol* 2010; **57**:804–14.

Hatzimouratidis K, Eardley I, Giuliano F, *et al.* EAU guidelines on penile curvature. *Eur Urol* 2012; **62**:543–52.

Jackson G, Montorsi P, Adams MA, *et al.* Cardiovascular aspects of sexual medicine. *J Sex Med* 2010; **7**:1608–26.

Maggi M, Buvat J, Corona G, Guay A, Torres LO. Hormonal causes of male sexual dysfunctions and their management (hyperprolactinemia, thyroid disorders, GH disorders, and DHEA). *J Sex Med* 2013; **10**(3):661–77.

Montorsi F, Briganti A, Salonia A, *et al.* Erectile dysfunction prevalence, time of onset and association with risk factors in 300 consecutive patients with acute chest pain and angiographically documented coronary artery disease. *Eur Urol* 2003; **44**:360–4.

Nunes KP, Labazi H, Webb RC. New insights into hypertension-associated erectile dysfunction. *Curr Opin Nephrol Hypertens* 2012; **21**:163–70.

Rosen R, Altwein J, Boyle P, *et al.* Lower urinary tract symptoms and male sexual dysfunction: the multinational survey of the aging male (MSAM-7). *Eur Urol* 2003; **44**:637–49.

Salonia A, Burnett AL, Graefen M, *et al.* Prevention and management of postprostatectomy sexual dysfunctions. Part 1: choosing the right patient at the right time for the right surgery. *Eur Urol* 2012; **62**:261–72.

Shoskes DA. The challenge of erectile dysfunction in the man with chronic prostatitis/chronic pelvic pain syndrome. *Curr Urol Rep* 2012; **13**:263–7.

Tajar A, Huhtaniemi IT, O'Neill TW, *et al.* Characteristics of androgen deficiency in late-onset hypogonadism: results from the European Male Ageing Study (EMAS). *J Clin Endocrinol Metab* 2012; **97**:1508–16.

Wu FC, Tajar A, Beynon JM, *et al.* Identification of late-onset hypogonadism in middle-aged and elderly men. *N Engl J Med* 2010; 363:123–35.

References

1. Gratzke C, Angulo J, Chitaley K, *et al.* Anatomy, physiology, and pathophysiology of erectile dysfunction. *J Sex Med* 2010; **7**:445–75.
2. Corona G, Mannucci E, Forti G, Maggi M. Hypogonadism, ED, metabolic syndrome and obesity: a pathological link supporting cardiovascular diseases. *Int J Androl* 2009; **32**:587–98.
3. Corona G, Lee DM, Forti G, *et al.* Age-related changes in general and sexual health in middle-aged and older men: results from the European Male Ageing Study *(EMAS)*. *J Sex Med* 2010; **7**:1362–80.
4. Shelton JB, Rajfer J. Androgen deficiency in aging and metabolically challenged men. *Urol Clin North Am* 2012; **39**:63–75.
5. Maggi M, Buvat J, Corona G, Guay A, Torres LO. Hormonal causes of male sexual dysfunctions and their management (hyperprolactinemia, thyroid disorders, GH disorders, and DHEA). *J Sex Med* 2013; **10**(3):661–77.
6. Wagle KC, Carrejo MH, Tan RS. The implications of increasing age on erectile dysfunction. *Am J Mens Health* 2012; **6**:273–9.
7. Schöneich C. Reactive oxygen species and biological aging: a mechanistic approach. *Exp Gerontol* 1999; **34**:19–34.
8. Rossi A, Ganassini A, Tantucci C, Grassi V. Aging and the respiratory system. *Aging (Milano)* 1996; **8**:143–61.
9. Bitar KN. Aging and neural control of the GI tract: V. Aging and gastrointestinal smooth muscle: from signal transduction to contractile proteins. *Am J Physiol Gastrointest Liver Physiol* 2003; **284**:G1–7.
10. Al-Shaer M, Choueiri NE, Correia ML, Sinkey CA, Barenz TA, Haynes WG. Effects of aging and atherosclerosis on endothelial and vascular smooth muscle function in humans. *Int J Cardiol* 2006; **109**:201–6.
11. Gacci M, Eardley I, Giuliano F, *et al.* Critical analysis of the relationship between sexual dysfunctions and lower urinary tract symptoms due to benign prostatic hyperplasia. *Eur Urol* 2011; **60**:809–25.
12. Mazur DJ, Helfand BT, McVary KT. Influences of neuroregulatory factors on the development of lower urinary tract symptoms/benign prostatic hyperplasia and erectile dysfunction in aging men. *Urol Clin North Am* 2012; **39**:77–88.
13. Seftel AD, de la Rosette J, Birt J, Porter V, Zarotsky V, Viktrup L. Coexisting lower urinary tract symptoms and erectile dysfunction: a systematic review of epidemiological data. *Int J Clin Pract* 2013; **67**:32–45.

14. Shoskes DA. The challenge of erectile dysfunction in the man with chronic prostatitis/chronic pelvic pain syndrome. *Curr Urol Rep* 2012; **13**:263–7.
15. Andersson KE. Mechanisms of penile erection and basis for pharmacological treatment of erectile dysfunction. *Pharmacol Rev* 2011; **63**(4):811–59.
16. Saenz de Tejada I, Carson MP, de las Morenas A, Goldstein I, Traish AM. Endothelin: localization, synthesis, activity, and receptor types in human penile corpus cavernosum. *Am J Physiol* 1991; **261**:H1078–85.
17. Garbán H, Vernet D, Freedman A, Rajfer J, González-Cadavid N. Effect of aging on nitric oxide-mediated penile erection in rats. *Am J Physiol* 1995; **268**:H467–75.
18. Carrier S1, Nagaraju P, Morgan DM, Baba K, Nunes L, Lue TF. Age decreases nitric oxide synthase-containing nerve fibers in the rat penis. *J Urol* 1997; **157**:1088–92.
19. Dahiya R, Chui R, Perinchery G, Nakajima K, Oh BR, Lue TF. Differential gene expression of growth factors in young and old rat penile tissues is associated with erectile dysfunction. *Int J Impot Res* 1999; **11**:201–6.
20. Toda N. Age-related changes in endothelial function and blood flow regulation. *Pharmacol Ther* 2012; **133**:159–76.
21. Rajasekaran M, Kasyan A, Jain A, Kim SW, Monga M. Altered growth factor expression in the aging penis: the Brown–Norway rat model. *J Androl* 2002; **23**:393–9.
22. Gur S, Kadowitz PJ, Hellstrom WJ. RhoA/Rho-kinase as a therapeutic target for the male urogenital tract. *J Sex Med* 2011; **8**:675–87.
23. Jiang X, Chitaley K. The promise of inhibition of smooth muscle tone as a treatment for erectile dysfunction: where are we now? *Int J Impot Res* 2012; **24**:49–60.
24. Jin L, Liu T, Lagoda GA, Champion HC, Bivalacqua TJ, Burnett AL. Elevated RhoA/Rho-kinase activity in the aged rat penis: mechanism for age-associated erectile dysfunction. *FASEB J* 2006; **20**:536–8.
25. Somlyo AP, Somlyo AV. Signal transduction by Gproteins, rho-kinase and protein phosphatase to smooth muscle and non-muscle myosin II. *J Physiol* 2000; **522**:177–85.
26. Miao L, Calvert JW, Tang J, Parent AD, Zhang JH. Age-related RhoA expression in blood vessels of rats. *Mech Ageing Dev* 2001; **122**:1757–70.
27. Johannes CB, Araujo AB, Feldman HA, Derby CA, Kleinman KP, McKinlay JB. Incidence of erectile dysfunction in men 40 to 69 years old: longitudinal results from the Massachusetts male aging study. *J Urol* 2000; **163**:460–3.
28. Nunes KP, Labazi H, Webb RC. New insights into hypertension-associated erectile dysfunction. *Curr Opin Nephrol Hypertens* 2012; **21**:163–70.
29. Scranton RE, Goldstein I, Stecher VJ. Erectile dysfunction diagnosis and treatment as a means to improve medication adherence and optimize comorbidity management. *J Sex Med* 2013; **10**(2):551–61.
30. Hannan JL, Blaser MC, Pang JJ, Adams SM, Pang SC, Adams MA. Impact of hypertension, aging, and antihypertensive treatment on the morphology of the pudendal artery. *J Sex Med* 2011; **8**:1027–38.
31. Lee DL, Webb RC, Jin L. Hypertension and RhoA/Rho-kinase signaling in the vasculature: highlights from the recent literature. *Hypertension* 2004; **44**:796–9.
32. Wilkes N, White S, Stein P, Bernie J, Rajasekaran M. Phosphodiesterase-5 inhibition synergizes rhokinase antagonism and enhances erectile response in male hypertensive rats. *Int J Impot Res* 2004; **16**:187–94.
33. González-Cadavid NF. Mechanisms of penile fibrosis. *J Sex Med* 2009; **6**(Suppl 3):353–62.
34. Ferrer JE, Velez JD, Herrera AM, *et al.* Age-related morphological changes in smooth muscle and collagen content in human corpus cavernosum. *J Sex Med* 2010; **7**:2723–8.
35. Feinstein M, Ning H, Kang J, Bertoni A, Carnethon M, Lloyd-Jones DM. Racial differences in risks for first cardiovascular events and noncardiovascular death: the Atherosclerosis Risk in Communities study, the Cardiovascular Health Study, and the Multi-Ethnic Study of Atherosclerosis. *Circulation* 2012; **126**:50–9.
36. Vlachopoulos C, Rokkas K, Ioakeimidis N, Stefanadis C. Inflammation, metabolic syndrome, erectile dysfunction, and coronary artery disease: common links. *Eur Urol* 2007; **52**:1590–600.
37. Dong JY, Zhang YH, Qin LQ. Erectile dysfunction and risk of cardiovascular disease: meta-analysis of prospective cohort studies. *J Am Coll Cardiol* 2011; **58**:1378–85.
38. Gupta BP, Murad MH, Clifton MM, Prokop L, Nehra A, Kopecky SL. The effect of lifestyle modification and cardiovascular risk factor reduction on erectile dysfunction: a systematic review and meta-analysis. *Arch Intern Med* 2011; **171**:1797–803.
39. Guo W1, Liao C, Zou Y, *et al.* Erectile dysfunction and risk of clinical cardiovascular events: a meta-analysis of seven cohort studies. *J Sex Med* 2010; **7**:2805–16.
40. Batty GD, Li Q, Czernichow S, *et al.* Erectile dysfunction and later cardiovascular disease in men with type 2 diabetes: prospective cohort study based on the ADVANCE (Action in Diabetes and Vascular Disease: Preterax and Diamicron Modified-Release Controlled Evaluation) trial. *J Am Coll Cardiol* 2010; **56**:1908–13.
41. Vlachopoulos C, Rokkas K, Ioakeimidis N, *et al.* Prevalence of asymptomatic coronary artery disease in men with vasculogenic erectile dysfunction: a prospective angiographic study. *Eur Urol* 2005; **48**:996–1002.
42. Montorsi F, Briganti A, Salonia A, *et al.* Erectile dysfunction prevalence, time of onset and association with risk factors in 300 consecutive patients with acute chest pain and angiographically documented coronary artery disease. *Eur Urol* 2003; **44**:360–4.
43. Rastrelli G, Corona G, Monami M, *et al.* Poor response to alprostadil ICI test is associated with arteriogenic erectile dysfunction and higher risk of major adverse cardiovascular events. *J Sex Med* 2011; **8**:3433–45.
44. Hermans MP, Ahn SA, Rousseau MF, *et al.* Erectile dysfunction, microangiopathy and UKPDS risk in type 2 diabetes. *Diabetes Metab* 2009; **35**:484–9.
45. Chang ST, Chu CM, Hsiao JF, *et al.* Coronary phenotypes in patients with erectile dysfunction and silent ischemic heart disease: a pilot study. *J Sex Med* 2010; **7**:2798–804.
46. García-Malpartida K, Mármol R, Jover A, *et al.* Relationship between erectile dysfunction and silent myocardial ischemia in type 2 diabetic patients with no known macrovascular complications. *J Sex Med* 2011; **8**:2606–16.
47. Araña Rosaínz Mde J, Ojeda MO, Acosta JR, *et al.* Imbalanced low-grade inflammation and endothelial activation in patients with type 2 diabetes mellitus and erectile dysfunction. *J Sex Med* 2011; **8**:2017–30.
48. Chew KK, Finn J, Stuckey B, *et al.* Erectile dysfunction as a predictor for subsequent atherosclerotic cardiovascular events: findings from a linked-data study. *J Sex Med* 2010; **7**:192–202.
49. Azadzoi KM, Tarcan T, Siroky MB, Krane RJ. Atherosclerosis-induced chronic ischemia causes bladder fibrosis and non-compliance in the rabbit. *J Urol* 1999; **161**:1626–35.
50. Montorsi F, Briganti A, Salonia A, *et al.* The ageing male and erectile dysfunction. *BJU Int* 2003; **92**:516–20.
51. Azadzoi KM, Master TA, Siroky MB. Effect of chronic ischemia on constitutive and inducible nitric oxide synthase expression in erectile tissue. *J Androl* 2004; **25**:382–8.
52. Sarteschi LM, Montorsi F, Menchini Fabris F, Guazzoni G, Lencioni R, Rigatti P. Cavernous arterial and arteriolar circulation in patients with erectile dysfunction: a power Doppler study. *J Urol* 1998; **159**:428–32.
53. Grein U, Schubert GE. Arteriosclerosis of penile arteries: histological findings and their significance in the treatment of erectile dysfunction. *Urol Int* 2002; **68**:261–4.
54. Nehra A, Azadzoi KM, Moreland RB, *et al.* Cavernosal expandability is an erectile tissue mechanical property which predicts trabecular histology in an animal model of vasculogenic erectile dysfunction. *J Urol* 1998; **159**:2229–36.

55. Nehra A, Gettman MT, Nugent M, *et al.* Transforming growth factor-beta1 (TGF-beta1) is sufficient to induce fibrosis of rabbit corpus cavernosum in vivo. *J Urol* 1999; **162**:910–5.
56. Border WA, Noble NA. Transforming growth factor beta in tissue fibrosis. *N Engl J Med* 1994; **331**:1286–92.
57. Bowen T, Jenkins RH, Fraser DJ, *et al.* MicroRNAs, transforming growth factor beta-1, and tissue fibrosis. *J Pathol* 2013; **229**:274–85.
58. Hubmacher D, Apte SS. The biology of the extracellular matrix: novel insights. *Curr Opin Rheumatol* 2013; **25**:65–70.
59. Angelopoulou R, Lavranos G, Manolakou P, *et al.* ROS in the aging male: model diseases with ROS-related pathophysiology. *Reprod Toxicol* 2009; **28**:167–71.
60. Rodríguez-Mañas L, El-Assar M, Vallejo S, *et al.* Endothelial dysfunction in aged humans is related with oxidative stress and vascular inflammation. *Aging Cell* 2009; **8**:226–38.
61. Jones RW, Rees RW, Minhas S, Ralph D, Persad RA, Jeremy JY. Oxygen free radicals and the penis. *Expert Opin Pharmacother* 2002; **3**:889–97.
62. Beckman JS, Koppenol WH. Nitric oxide, superoxide, and peroxynitrite: the good, the bad, and ugly. *Am J Physiol* 1996; **271**:C1424–37.
63. Agarwal A, Nandipati KC, Sharma RK, Zippe CD, Raina R. Role of oxidative stress in the pathophysiological mechanism of erectile dysfunction. *J Androl* 2006; **27**:335–47.
64. Vardi Y, Dayan L, Apple B, Gruenwald I, Ofer Y, Jacob G. Penile and systemic endothelial function in men with and without erectile dysfunction. *Eur Urol* 2009; **55**:979–85.
65. Vlachopoulos C1, Ioakeimidis N, Terentes-Printzios D, Stefanadis C. The triad: erectile dysfunction—endothelial dysfunction—cardiovascular disease. *Curr Pharm Des* 2008; **14**:3700–14.
66. Jackson G, Montorsi P, Adams MA, *et al.* Cardiovascular aspects of sexual medicine. *J Sex Med* 2010; **7**:1608–26.
67. Wu FC, Tajar A, Beynon JM, *et al.* Identification of late-onset hypogonadism in middle-aged and elderly men. *N Engl J Med* 2010; **363**:123–35.
68. Tajar A, Huhtaniemi IT, O'Neill TW, *et al.* Characteristics of androgen deficiency in late-onset hypogonadism: results from the European Male Ageing Study (EMAS). *J Clin Endocrinol Metab* 2012; **97**:1508–16.
69. Corona G, Rastrelli G, Vignozzi L, Mannucci E, Maggi M. How to recognize late-onset hypogonadism in men with sexual dysfunction. *Asian J Androl* 2012; **14**:251–9.
70. Isidori AM, Giannetta E, Gianfrilli D, *et al.* Effects of testosterone on sexual function in men: results of a meta-analysis. *Clin Endocrinol (Oxf)* 2005; **63**:381–94.
71. Hatzimouratidis K, Amar E, Eardley I, *et al.* Guidelines on male sexual dysfunction: erectile dysfunction and premature ejaculation. *Eur Urol* 2010; **57**:804–14.
72. Salonia A, Castagna G, Saccà A, *et al.* Is erectile dysfunction a reliable proxy of general male health status? The case for the international index of erectile function-erectile function domain. *J Sex Med* 2012; **9**:2708–15.
73. *Ibid.* **66.**
74. Derby CA, Mohr BA, Goldstein I, *et al.* Modifiable risk factors and erectile dysfunction: can lifestyle changes modify risk?. *Urology* 2000; **56**:302–6.
75. Glina S, Sharlip ID, Hellstrom WJ. Modifying risk factors to prevent and treat erectile dysfunction. *J Sex Med* 2013; **10**(1):115–9.
76. Mulhall J, Teloken P, Brock G, Kim E. Obesity, dyslipidemias and erectile dysfunction: a report of a subcommittee of the sexual medicine society of North America. *J Sex Med* 2006; **3**:778–86.
77. Malavige LS, Levy JC. Erectile dysfunction in diabetes mellitus. *J Sex Med* 2009; **6**:1232–47.
78. Hidalgo-Tamola J, Chitaley K. Review type 2 diabetes mellitus and erectile dysfunction. *J Sex Med* 2009; **6**:916–26.
79. *Ibid.* **28.**
80. Zias N, Bezwada V, Gilman S, Chroneou A. Obstructive sleep apnea and erectile dysfunction: still a neglected risk factor?. *Sleep Breath* 2009; **13**:3–10.
81. Lee RK, Chughtai B, Te AE, Kaplan SA. Sexual function in men with metabolic syndrome. *Urol Clin North Am* 2012; **39**:53–62.
82. Hammarsten J, Peeker R. Urological aspects of the metabolic syndrome. *Nat Rev Urol* 2011; **8**:483–94.
83. Buvat J, Maggi M, Gooren L, *et al.* Endocrine aspects of male sexual dysfunctions. *J Sex Med* 2010; **7**:1627–56.
84. Buvat J, Maggi M, Guay A, Torres LO. Testosterone deficiency in men: systematic review and standard operating procedures for diagnosis and treatment. *J Sex Med* 2013; **10**(1):245–84.
85. Perelman MA. Erectile dysfunction and depression: screening and treatment. *Urol Clin North Am* 2011; **38**:125–39.
86. Feldman HA, Goldstein I, Hatzichristou DG, Krane RJ, McKinlay JB. Impotence and its medical and psychosocial correlates: results of the Massachusetts Male Aging Study. *J Urol* 1994; **151**:54–61.
87. Hunt N, McHale S. Psychosocial aspects of andrologic disease. *Endocrinol Metab Clin North Am* 2007; **36**:521–31.
88. Zemishlany Z, Weizman A. The impact of mental illness on sexual dysfunction. *Adv Psychosom Med* 2008; **29**:89–106.
89. Fode M, Krogh-Jespersen S, Brackett NL, Ohl DA, Lynne CM, Sønksen J. Male sexual dysfunction and infertility associated with neurological disorders. *Asian J Androl* 2012; **14**:61–8.
90. Salonia A, Burnett AL, Graefen M, *et al.* Prevention and management of postprostatectomy sexual dysfunctions. Part 1: choosing the right patient at the right time for the right surgery. *Eur Urol* 2012; **62**:261–72.
91. Saigal CS, Wessells H, Pace J, Schonlau M, Wilt TJ; Urologic Diseases in America Project. Predictors and prevalence of erectile dysfunction in a racially diverse population. *Arch Intern Med* 2006; **166**:207–12.
92. Rosen R, Altwein J, Boyle P, *et al.* Lower urinary tract symptoms and male sexual dysfunction: the multinational survey of the aging male (MSAM-7). *Eur Urol* 2003; **44**:637–49.
93. Karavitakis M, Komninos C, Theodorakis PN, *et al.* Evaluation of sexual function in hypertensive men receiving treatment: a review of current guidelines recommendation. *J Sex Med* 2011; **8**:2405–14.
94. Althof SE, Rosen RC, Perelman MA, Rubio-Aurioles E. Standard operating procedures for taking a sexual history. *J Sex Med* 2012; **10**(1):26–35.
95. Hatzimouratidis K, Eardley I, Giuliano F, *et al.* EAU guidelines on penile curvature. *Eur Urol* 2012; **62**:543–52.
96. Hatzichristou D, Rosen RC, Derogatis LR, *et al.* Recommendations for the clinical evaluation of men and women with sexual dysfunction. *J Sex Med* 2010; **7**:337–48.
97. Ghanem HM, Salonia A, Martin-Morales A. SOP: Physical examination and laboratory testing for men with erectile dysfunction. *J Sex Med* 2013; **10**(1):108–10.
98. Hatzichristou DG, Hatzimouratidis K, Ioannides E, Yannakoyorgos K, Dimitriadis G, Kalinderis A. Nocturnal penile tumescence and rigidity monitoring in young potent volunteers: reproducibility, evaluation criteria and the effect of sexual intercourse. *J Urol* 1998; **159**:1921–6.
99. Sikka SC, Hellstrom WJ, Brock G, Morales AM. Standardization of vascular assessment of erectile dysfunction: standard operating procedures for Duplex Ultrasound. *J Sex Med* 2013; **10**(1):120–9.
100. Burnett AL, Sharlip ID. Standard operating procedures for priapism. *J Sex Med* 2013; **10**(1):180–94.

CHAPTER 7.8

Erectile dysfunction

Medical therapy

Hartmut Porst

Introduction to medical therapy

Many studies are witnessing that male sexual health is not maintained in many elderly men, a process which usually starts in the fifth decade and progressively increases in the aged population. This statement applies for all male sexual functions but especially for erectile function as has been shown in a Norwegian epidemiologic study.[1] Together with premature ejaculation (PE), erectile dysfunction is the most frequently reported male sexual disorder but shows in contrast to PE a clear age dependency, with a steep increase beyond the fifth decade. Whereas in age groups <50 years the prevalence rates for erectile dysfunction (ED) range between 9% and 39% and are <20% in most series, they increase to between 40–80% in the elderly population >70 years of age depending on the populations investigated.[2]

Management of risk factors to improve erectile dysfunction

In patients >40 years of age, ED is significantly associated with cardiovascular risk factors such as diabetes, hypertension, coronary artery disease (CAD), dyslipidemia, atherosclerosis, and metabolic syndrome. There is a strong correlation between ED and coronary artery disease.[3] In a recently published meta-analysis reviewing 12 prospective cohort studies with a total of 36,744 participants, the overall combined relative risks for men with ED compared with the reference group were 1.48 (95% confidence interval [CI]: 1.25–1.74) for CVD, 1.46 (95% CI: 1.31–1.63) for coronary heart disease, 1.35 (95% CI: 1.19–1.54) for stroke, and 1.19 (95% CI: 1.05–1.34) for all-cause mortality.[4] In addition, many epidemiological studies have provided evidence that ED is also closely linked to benign prostate hyperplasia (BPH) and that men suffering from lower urinary tract symptoms (LUTS) due to BPH have a 60–80% likelihood of suffering from simultaneous ED.[5] It has been shown by several studies that changes in lifestyle with giving up sedentary lifestyle and resuming regular physical activities, good control of diabetes with glycosylated haemoglobin values <7%, and changes of certain medications in the treatment of BPH, hypertension, and depression are able to improve erectile function per se or can add, respectively, to the efficacy of ED specific medications.[4–6] Last, but not least, several studies provided evidence that untreated hypogonadism may cause per se sexual dysfunctions such as ED, loss of libido and ejaculatory problems, or can contribute to poor or non-responsiveness to ED-specific medications, especially to PDE 5 inhibitors.[6]

The respective threshold levels below which sexual symptoms become evident are about 15 nmol/l (432 ng/dl) for libido and 8–10.4 nmol/l (230–300 ng/dl) for ED. In any case, T-replacement therapy in hypogonadal men with sexual disorders should be started first, followed by specific ED medications such as PDE5 inhibitors if T-replacement alone fails.

Medical treatment of erectile dysfunction

Oral drug therapy of erectile dysfunction

Phosphodiesterase (PDE)-5 inhibitors

PDE5 inhibitors are recommended in the guidelines of the world leading medical societies as first line therapy of ED.[7,8] PDE5 inhibitors inhibit the enzyme PDE5 competitively, thereby preventing the breakdown of its physiological target substance 3′5′-cGMP (cycloguanosine monophosphate).This mechanism of action results in an increase of the intracellular cGMP concentrations finally reaching the threshold level above which erection is triggered by a complex cascade of physiological actions (Fig. 7.8.1).The phosphodiesterase 5 enzyme is found in high concentrations in the entire urogenital system and especially in the cavernous bodies, as well as in lower concentrations in the vascular and gastrointestinal system.

Erection is initated in the cerebral sex centres by erotic stimuli, resulting in the release of erection stimulatory neurotransmitters such as dopamine, oxytocin and melanocortins (alpha-MSH). The erectile stimuli travel along oxytocinergic nerve fibres in the spinal cord to the spinal cord erection centres, which they leave at the level of S2–4 (called nervi erigentes) to join the inferior hypogastric plexus, before passing in the cavernous nerves that enter the cavernous bodies below the pelvic floor. The parasympathetic nerve fibres of the cavernous bodies finally lead into either cholinergic nerve terminals releasing ACH or in non-adrenergic, non-cholinergic (NANC) also called peptidergic nerve terminals, releasing either nitric oxide (NO) or vasoactive intestinal polypeptide (VIP). The NO release results in an activation of the enzyme guanylate cyclase which converts GTP to 3′5′-cGMP, the most important neurotransmitter for erection in the cavernous bodies.

A further natural pathway for triggering an erection is the release of VIP from NANC nerve terminals resulting in the activation of the adenylate cyclase and production of 3′5′-cAMP. Both cGMP and cAMP induce relaxation of the cavernosal smooth muscle cells, resulting in an increase of arterial inflow and decrease in venous outflow thereby causing penile tumescence and erection.

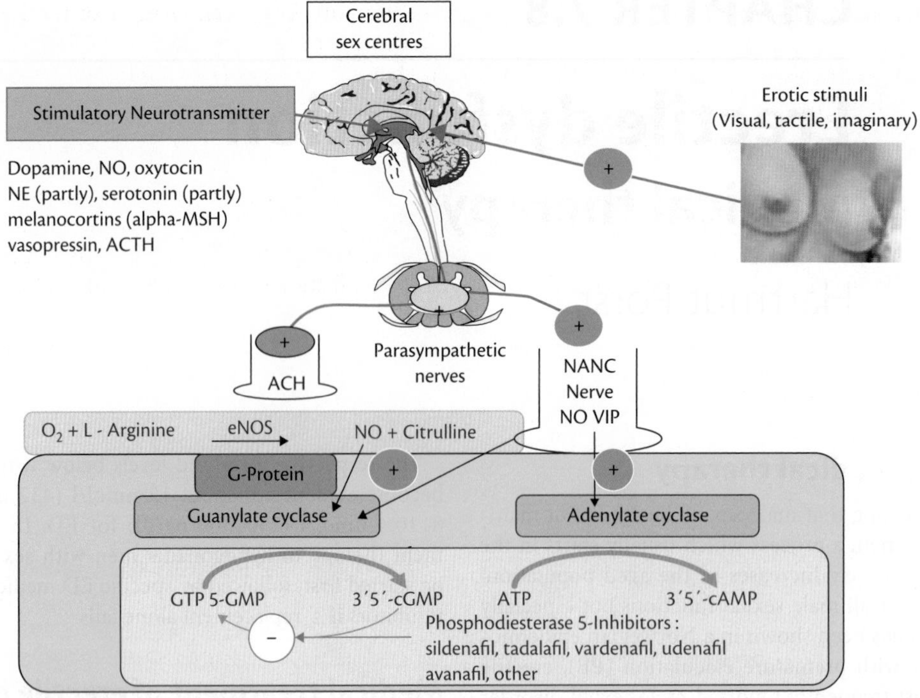

Fig. 7.8.1 Erectile circle and the mechanism of PDE5 inhibitors.
Whereas PDE5 inhibitors act through the cGMP pathway, prostaglandin E1 (alpostradil) and VIP act through the cAMP pathway.
ACH = acetylcholine; ACTH = adrenocorticotropic hormone; ATP = adenosine triphosphate; 3′5′-cAMP = cyclic adenosine monophosphate; 3′5′-cGMP = cyclic guanosine monophosphate; eNOS = endothelial nitric oxide synthase; GTP = guanosine triphphosphate; MSH = melanocyte-stimulating hormone; NANC = non-adrenergic, non-cholinergic; NE = noradrenaline; NO = nitric oxide; VIP = vasoactive intestinal polypeptide
Reproduced from Porst H, 'Oral pharmacotherapy of erectile dysfunction' pp. 75–93, in Porst H, and Buvat J (Eds.), *Standard Practice in Sexual Medicine*, Blackwell Publishing, Malden, MA, USA, Copyright © 2006, with permission from John Wiley & Sons, Inc.

Because both psychogenic ED, characterized by an increase of the sympathetic tone, and organic ED, characterized by a variety of negative mechanisms on erection, always result in a decrese of cGMP, PDE5 inhibitors show impressive efficacy rates (60–80%) in both aetiologic scenarios.

Usually PDE5 inhibitors are taken as needed (i.e. about one hour prior to sexual engagement). In general, all marketed PDE 5 inhibitors show a comparable efficacy with succesfully completed intercourse rates of between 60% and 75% depending on the underlying ED aetiology but discriminate themselves in terms of their pharmacokinetic profile with avanafil (Stendra®/Spedra®) showing the shortest T_{Max} and therefore the fastest onset of action and tadalafil (Cialis®) showing the longest $T_{1/2}$ with about 17 hours resulting in the longest period of efficacy among all PDE5 inhibitors. Several onset and duration of action studies have generated the following pharmacokinetic data as illustrated in Tables 7.8.1 and 7.8.2.

The efficacy of all PDE5 inhibitors can substantially be impaired by the following factors:

(i) Inadequate sexual stimulation
(ii) Inadequate timing between drug intake and sexual activities (see pharmacokinetics)
(iii) Intake of a fatty meal (impacts both efficacy and onset of action of avanafil, sidenafil, and vardenafil)
(iv) Neuropathy/damage of the autonomic parasympathetic penile nerve supply (i.e. in diabetes, alcohol abuse, pelvic surgery with injury of the cavernous nerves)

Table 7.8.1 Pharmacokinetics of the three PDE5 inhibitors sildenafil, tadalafil, and vardenafil (Cialis®, Levitra®, and Viagra® labels)

Drug	T_{Max} (min)	Onset of action (min) earliest	>50% pt. response	$T_{1/2}$ (h)	Duration of efficacy h (% successful coitus)	C_{Max} ng/mL
Sildenafil 100 mg	70 (30–120)	14	20	3.82 ± 0,84	8 (85%)	327 ± 236
Tadalafil 20 mg	120 (30–720)	16	30	17.5	36 (59% and 62%)	378
Vardenafil 20 mg	40 (15–180)	11	25	3.94 ± 1.31	8 ± 2 (69%)	20.9 ± 1.83

Reproduced from Porst H *et al.*, 'SOP conservative (medical and mechanical) treatment of erectile dysfunction', *Journal of Sexual Medicine*, Volume 10, Issue 1, pp. 130–171, Copyright © 2013 International Society for Sexual Medicine, with permission from John Wiley and Sons.

Table 7.8.2 Pharmacokinetics of the new PDE5 inhibitors

	Avanafil[16] 100 mg	Mirodenafil[17] 10 mg	Lodenafil[18] 160 mg	Udenafil[19] 100 mg
T_{Max} (h)	0.5–1.5	1.25	1.2	1–1.5
$T_{1/2}$ (h)	<1.5	2.5	2.4	11–13

Reproduced from Porst H *et al.*, 'SOP conservative (medical and mechanical) treatment of erectile dysfunction', *Journal of Sexual Medicine*, Volume 10, Issue 1, pp. 130–171, Copyright © 2013 International Society for Sexual Medicine, with permission from John Wiley and Sons.

(v) Untreated hypogonadism if T-values are <10.4 nmol/L (300 ng/dl)

Frequent drug-related side effects of PDE5 include headache in between 10% and 15%, flushing in between 5% and 15%, dypepsia in between 4% and 10%, rhinitis (stuffy nose) in between 4% and 10%. With sildenafil, temporary colour vision disturbances and increased brightness sensitivity was observed in up to 5% and with tadalafil back and muscle pain in up to 6%.[6]

Daily dosing of tadlafil/udenafil

Both tadalafil and udenafil show considerably longer half-lives of about 17 hours and 13 hours respectively than the other short acting PDE5 inhibitors and are therefore suitable for once a day dosing. With daily application of low doses efficacy rates comparable to p.r.n dosing of the maximum dose of either drug were reported (see relevant literature[6]). Tadalafil once a day in the dosages of 2.5 mg and 5 mg is approved worldwide for the treatment of ED and represents an attractive alternative regimen to p.r.n.dosing, especially for those patients who are suffering from both, ED and LUTS/BPH.[7–9]

Yohimbine

Yohimbine is the main alkaloid from the bark of the tree called *Coryanthe johimbe K. Schum* (yohimbehe tree), particularly growing in Central Africa. The main site of action of yohimbine are alpha2-adrenoceptors. Doses range from 5 mg to 15 mg three times a day.[10] Because of its weak efficacy, especially in patients with an organic ED aetiology, yohimbine is not recommended.[7,8]

L-Arginine

L-Arginine, a natural amino acid, is the basic compound for the synthesis of NO (see Fig. 7.8.1). Daily doses of beween 3–7 grammes have shown some efficacy in randomized trials—but the drug has never reached a broader market acceptance. In difficult to treat patients, L-Arginine may enhance the efficacy of PDE5 inhibitors.

Topical alprostadil (syn.PGE$_1$)

PGE$_1$ (Alprostadil) stimulates adenylate cyclase and increases the intracellular cAMP concentration thereby facilitating the relaxation of the cavernous smooth musculature. With a special topical PGE$_1$ gel preparation two large randomized placebo-controlled double-blind trials with doses of 100, 200 and 300 μg alprostadil were conducted in total of 1,732 patients (21% diabetes, 44% hypertension, 12% RRP, 21% CAD, 16% nitrate or alpha blocker medication). The mean changes of the IIEF-EF domain scores from baseline to end point were −0.7, 1.6, 2.5, and 2.4 points for each group, respectively (p <0.001).[11] Adverse events were mainly temporary and limited locally to the application site with penile oedema (1.4%), genital pain (17.5%), penile burning (23%), penile erythema (11.3%). Partners complained in 4.4% of vaginal burning and in 2.1% of vaginitis. Because of its limited efficacy as compared to PDE5 inhibitors, topical alprostadil is not suited as monotherapy for organic ED patients but might be considered for combination therapy with PDE5 inhibitors in difficult to treat patient groups.

Transurethral alprostadil (PGE$_1$) with MUSE® (medicated urethral system for erection)

An alprostadil preparation using a transurethral application with a small applicator for single use was introduced in 1994 and later marketed as MUSE® (medicated urethral system for erection).[6,7] Although the transurethral application route is preferable to intracavernosal self-injection therapy, the inferior efficacy data in direct comparative trials with intracavernously injected alprostadil limits its use as monotherapy for those patients who are non-responsive to PDE5 inhibitors. MUSE® is applied into the moistened urethra through the external orifice directly after emptying the bladder (Fig. 7.8.2). Typical frequent side effects are penile/urethral pain between 25% and 43% and urethral bleeding (around 5%). Infrequent adverse events include dizziness because of blood pressure fall (1–5%) and even the occurrence of syncope between 0.4% and 3%.

The efficacy of MUSE® may be enhanced by simultaneous application of a constriction bandage on the penis base to avoid fast venous drainage.

Intracavernosal self-injection therapy

The following vasoactive drugs have been used both for diagnostic and therapeutic purposes in the management of ED[6,7]:

PGE1 (prostaglandin E1, syn. alprostadil) (trade names: Caverject®, Edex®, Viridal®);

Papaverine (several generics available worldwide);

Combination papaverine/phentolamine-bimix (trade name: Androskat®: only available in some European countries);

Trimix (syn. triple drug): mixture of PGE$_1$/papaverine/phentolamine (no commercial product available);

Combination of vasoactive intestinal polypeptide and phentolamine (trade name Invicorp®, only available in Europe on a prescription basis).

Intracorporeal injection therapy is a second-line therapy in ED for those patients who are non- or poorly reponsive to PDE5 inhibitors, which is frequently the case in patients with long-term diabetes or patients after pelvic surgery with injury of the cavernous nerves. The overwhelming majority of patients conducting self-injection therapy uses alprostadil (PGE$_1$) usually in doses between 5 and 20 μg, which are available in user-friendly dual-chamber injection syringes for single use and marketed as Caverject® or Edex®/Viridal® in many countries worldwide. Patients have to be

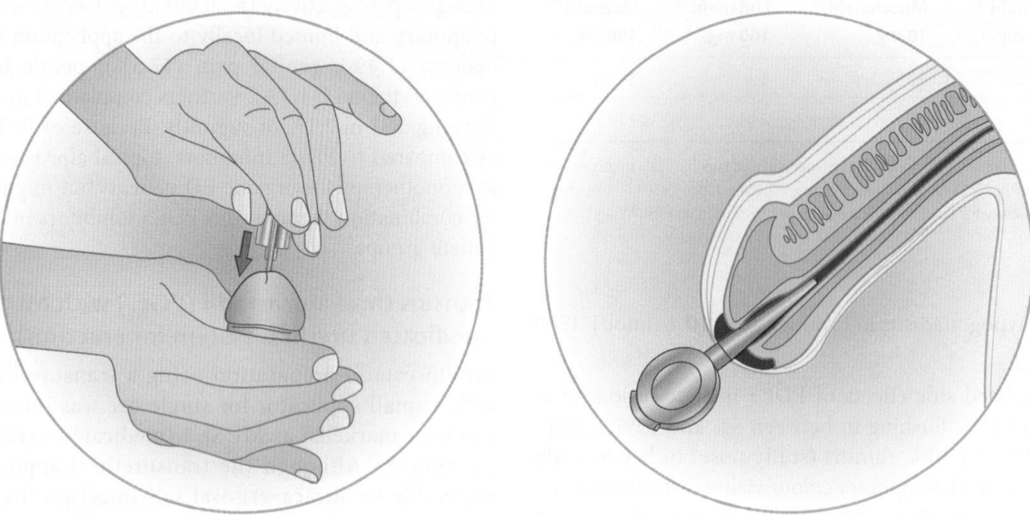

MUSE (**M**edical **U**rethral **S**ystem for **E**rection)
Single use system for application of Alprostadil into the urethra.

Fig. 7.8.2 Correct technique of transurethral application of MUSE (medicated urethral system for erection).

Reproduced from Porst H *et al.*, 'SOP conservative (medical and mechanical) treatment of erectile dysfunction', *Journal of Sexual Medicine*, Volume 10, Issue 1, pp. 130–171, Copyright © 2013 International Society for Sexual Medicine, with permission from John Wiley and Sons.

instructed in the correct self-injection technique which usually takes about two to three sessions.

Side effects are either attributed to the mode of application or the drug itself. Haematoma/bruising of the penile skin and scarring of the cavernous tissue with manifestation of Peyronie-like indurations with/without penile deviation are relatively frequent (see Table 7.8.3). Prolonged erections/priapism mostly occurs in the initation phase and are significantly more common with papaverine and phentolamine containing preparations (3–10%) than with PGE_1 mono-preparations (<1%). Priapism episodes lasting longer than six hours should be treated by intracavernosal injection of a sympathomimetically acting antidote (etilefrine, phenylephrine, or adrenaline) alone or by evacuation of the entrapped blood through a butterfly cannula depending on the duration of priapism.

Combination therapies

Combination therapies should considered in those ED patients not satisfactorily be served with either monotherapy. This is often observed in patients with severe organic ED and especially in patients with diabetes or after pelvic surgery.

In the literature, only two smaller studies were published using a combination of sildenafil and MUSE® in non-responders to either monotherapy.[14,15]According to the author's personal experience, combination therapy of daily dosing tadalafil 5 mg with either MUSE® or intracavernous alprostadil (Caverject®,Viridal®) is able to rescue a reasonable number of non-responders to PDE5 inhibitor monotherapy.[16–19]

Further readings

Corona G, Maggi M. The role of testosterone in erectile dysfunction. *Nat Rev Urol* 2010; 7:46–56.

Table 7.8.3 Penile fibroses in prospective long-term intracavernosal self-injection trials with alprostadil (PGE_1)

	No. pts.	Follow-up (months)	Fibrosis total	Nodules plaques	Deviations	Severe fibros.
Alprostadil st. powder (Caverject®-USA)	683	18	7.5% (51)	22	8	21
Alprostadil st. powder (Caverject®-Europe)	848 511	6 18	4% (34) 5.1% (26)	Not	published	
Alprostadil Alfadex (Viridal®-Europe)	162	48	11.7% (19)	10	6	3

Reproduced from Porst H *et al.*, 'SOP conservative (medical and mechanical) treatment of erectile dysfunction', Journal of Sexual Medicine, Volume 10, Issue 1, pp. 130–171, Copyright © 2013 International Society for Sexual Medicine, with permission from John Wiley and Sons.

Gacci M, Eardley I, Giuliano F, *et al.* Critical analysis of the relationship between sexual dysfunctions and lower urinary tract symptoms due to benign prostatic hyperplasia. *Eur Urol* 2011; **60**:809–25.

Hatzimouratidis K, Amar E, Eardley I, *et al.* Guidelines on male sexual dysfunction: erectile dysfunction and premature ejaculation. *Eur Urol* 2010; **57**:804–14.

Porst H. The rationale for prostaglandin E1 in erectile failure: A survey of world-wide experience. *J Urol* 1996; **155**:802–15.

Porst H, Burnett A, Brock G, *et al.*; and the ISSM Standards Committee for Sexual Medicine. SOP conservative (medical and mechanical) treatment of erectile dys-function. *J Sex Med* 2013; **10**:130–71.

Porst H, Kim ED, Casabé AR, *et al.*; for the LVHJ study team. Efficacy and safety of tadalafil once daily in the treatment of men with lower urinary tract symptoms suggestive of benign prostatic hyperplasia: Results of an international randomized, double-blind, placebo-controlled trial. *Eur Urol* 2011; **60**:1105–13.

Porst H, Rajfer J, Casabé A, *et al.* Long-term safety and efficacy of tadalafil 5 mg dosed once daily in men with erectile dysfunction. *J Sex Med* 2008; **5**:2160–9.

References

1. Mykletun A, Dahl AA, O'Leary MP, Fosså SD. Assessment of male sexual function by the Brief Sexual Function Inventory. *BJU Int* 2006; **97**(2):316–23.
2. Porst H, Sharlip I. History and epidemiology of male sexual dysfunction. (pp. 43–8) In: Porst H, Buvat J (eds). *Standard Practice in Sexual Medicine*. Chichester, UK: Blackwell Publishing, 2006.
3. Dong J-Y, Zhang Y-H, Li-Qiang Q. Erectile dysfunction and risk of cardiovascular disease: Meta-Analysis of prospective cohort studies. *J Am Coll Cardiol* 2011; **58**:1378–85.
4. Glina S, Sharlip ID, Hellstrom WJG. Modifying risk factors to prevent and treat erectile dysfunction. *J Sex Med* 2013; **10**:115–119.
5. Gacci M, Eardley I, Giuliano F, *et al.* Critical analysis of the relationship between sexual dysfunctions and lower urinary tract symptoms due to benign prostatic hyperplasia. *Eur Urol* 2011; **60**:809–25.
6. Porst H, Burnett A, Brock G, *et al.*; and the ISSM Standards Committee for Sexual Medicine. SOP conservative (medical and mechanical) treatment of erectile dysfunction. *J Sex Med* 2013; **10**:130–71.
7. Eardley I, Donatucci C, Corbin J, *et al.* Pharmacotherapy for erectile dysfunction. *J Sex Med* 2010; **7**:524–40.
8. Hatzimouratidis K, Amar E, Eardley I, *et al.* Guidelines on male sexual dysfunction: erectile dysfunction and premature ejaculation. *Eur Urol* 2010; **57**:804–14.
9. Porst H, McVary KT, Montorsi F, *et al.* Effects of once-daily tadalafil on erectile function in men with erectile dysfunction and signs and symptoms of benign prostatic hyperplasia. *Eur Urol* 2009; **56**:727–36.
10. Ernst E, Pittler MH. Yohimbin for erectile dysfunction: A systematic review and meta-analysis of randomized clinical trials. *J Urol* 1998; **159**:433–6.
11. Padma-Nathan H, Yeager JL. An integrated analysis of alprostadil topical cream for the treatment of erectile dysfunction in 1732 patients. *Urology* 2006; **68**(2): 386–91.
12. Porst H, Buvat J, Meuleman E, *et al.* Intracavernous Alprostadil Alfadex—an effective and well tolerated treatment for erectile dysfunction. Results of a long term European study. *Int J Impotence Res* 1998; **10**:225–31.
13. Linet OI, Ogrinc FG. Efficacy and safety of intracavernosal alprostadil in men with erectile dysfunction. The Alprostadil Study Group. *N Engl J Med* 1996; **334**(14):873–7.
14. Mydlo JH,Volpe MA, Maccia RJ. Inital results utilizing combination therapy for patients with a suboptimal response to either Alprostadil or Sildenafil monotherapy. *Eur Urol* 2000; **38**:30–4.
15. Nehra A, Jones WR, Hakim L, *et al.* Effectiveness of combination therapy of MUSE and Viagra in the salvage of erectile dysfunction patients desiring noninvasive therapy. *J Urol* 1999; **161**(Suppl 4):213.
16. Limin M, Johnsen N, Hellstrom WJ. Avanafil, a new rapidonset phosphodiesterase 5 inhibitor for the treatment of erectile dysfunction. *Expert Opin Investig Drugs* 2010; **19**:1427–37.
17. Paick JS, Ahn TY, Choi HK, *et al.* Efficacy and safety of mirodenafil, a new oral phosphodiesterase type 5 inhibitor, for treatment of erectile dysfunction. *J Sex Med* 2008; **5**:2672–80.
18. Glina S, Toscano I, Gomatzky C, *et al.* Efficacy and tolerability of lodenafil carbonate for oral therapy in erectile dysfunction: A phase II clinical trial. *J Sex Med* 2009; **6**:553–7.
19. Kim B, Lim H, Chung J, *et al.* Safety, tolerability, and phamacokinetics of udenafil, a novel PDE-5 inhibitor in healthy young Korean subjects. *Br J Clin Pharmacol* 2008; **65**:848–54.

CHAPTER 7.9

Erectile dysfunction
Surgical therapy

Carlo Bettocchi and Marco Spilotros

Introduction to surgery for erectile dysfunction

Since the introduction of PDE5 inhibitors and PGE_1 (prostaglandine E1) the treatment options for erectile dysfunction (ED) have radically changed. Furthermore, vacuum device therapy can also provide satisfactory results in selected patients. Despite that, a significant patient group does not achieve satisfactory erections and the sole available option to treat their condition is represented by surgery. In addition, this approach is advocated in those cases in which medical treatment is contraindicated, or when ED and severe corporal fibrosis with significant curvature of the penis coexist. Penile prosthetic surgery is the most common solution to restore erectile function in the abovementioned conditions, but venous ligation and penile arterial revascularization have some value in selected patients.

Penile prosthesis

Penile prosthesis implantation is recommended in patients with organ failure who do not respond to medical therapy, in case of severe corporal fibrosis due to priapism or when both ED and Peyronie's disease are diagnosed. There are several devices available with different features for the needs of each patient: adequate counselling before the procedure is mandatory in order to select the best option and reduce the postoperative dissatisfaction rate.[1]

Hydraulic and malleable penile implants are the most common devices used: the former can be three-piece (3P) or two-piece (2P) inflatable (Table 7.9.1).[2] Three-piece prostheses are characterized by two cylinders implanted into the corporas, a pump positioned in the scrotum, and a reservoir generally placed in the Retzius space. The system is filled with saline or contrast medium and its passage between the reservoir and the cylinder activates the pump, which produces an artificial erection while detumescence is achieved by deflating the cylinders. Two-piece prostheses do not have a separate reservoir and the fluid is contained in the bottom of the two cylinders and the pump provides the activation and deactivation of the device. With malleable prostheses, patients cannot reach penile detumescence and the hard rods placed into the corpora can be manually positioned upwards or downwards in order to allow sexual intercourse or conceal the device, respectively. The main difference between inflatable and malleable prostheses lies in the aesthetic outcome and ease of use: with the former, the result is excellent both during erection and detumescence but requires

Table 7.9.1 Principle penile prostheses available on the market

	AMS®	Coloplast®	Other companies
Malleable	Spectra™	Genesis™	Promedon Tube® Silimed® Jonas® Virilis I™ Virilis II™ Apollo™
Soft silicone			Subrini
Two-piece	Ambicor®		
Three-piece	AMS 700 CX™ AMS 700 CXR™ AMS LGX™	Alpha 1™ Titan™ Titan narrow base™	

reasonable manual dexterity, while the latter are extremely easy to use, but the aesthetic appearance is less natural. A third type of implant is the Subrini prosthesis, manufactured in soft silicone: these devices have been used in the past to restore erectile function and in more recent series to prevent penile shortening after Peyronie's disease surgical treatment.[3,4]

Several surgical approaches are described for penile prosthesis implantation and are related to the personal experience of the surgeon and to device itself. The incision can be performed at the tip of the penile shaft or along it (for a malleable implant) while it can be infrapubic or penoscrotal for both malleable and inflatable devices. Patient history and examination are mandatory to choose the better option: in case of obesity, the easiest approach is the penoscrotal option; while in the case of previous pelvic surgery, the infrapubic incision or a combined penoscrotal and abdominal one can be helpful and safer for the reservoir positioning.[1]

Penile prosthetic surgery has several critical steps.[5] In the penoscrotal approach, the isolation of both corpora and the indentification of the urethra represent the first one: the insertion of a Foley catheter at the beginning of the procedure and the use of a Scott retractor make the process easier. The site of the bilateral corporotomies is fundamental in order to bury the tubing: staying sutures, generally 2/0 or 0 Vicryl, are positioned in each corpora and the incision is performed between them followed by their dilation.

A preliminary blunt dissection of the erectile tissue with curved scissors both distally and proximally is useful prior to dilatation. Hegar and Brooks dilators are generally chosen in virgin cases, while Rosellos are suggested in case of several corporal fibrosis. At the end of this procedure, the simultaneous insertion of dilators in both corpora proximally and then distally confirms that both corpora have the same length and that cross-over between them has not occurred. Their exact length is then measured and after careful washing of the corpora with antibiotic solution, the cylinders are positioned and the staying sutures are tightened. For inflatable devices, the operation proceeds with the insertion of the pump and the reservoir. The pump should not be placed relatively superficial position to facilitate easy manipulation. The reservoir can be inserted through an infrapubic, abdominal, or penoscrotal incision, with the first two approaches recommended in cases of previous pelvic and abdominal surgery. Following a penoscrotal incision, a hole in the external inguinal ring is performed and the reservoir is placed in the Retzius space with the bladder empty. Since the introduction of the flatter reservoir, both by AMS (American Medical Systems, Minnetonka, MN) and Coloplast (Minneapolis, MN), there is an increasing trend in positioning them under the rectus muscle or even in the subcutaneous tissue in case of patients with a plentiful fat pad. The components are then connected and a careful haemostasis is performed: a drain can be left *in situ* for 24 hours and then removed with the catheter, with an alternative being a compressive bandage around the penile shaft and scrotum.

As mentioned above, this kind of operation although relatively simple can present several complications. Urethral perforation can be recognized by bleeding throughout the external meatus. Corporal perforation is occasionally seen in fibrotic corporas: in cases of proximal perforation, the rear tip extender of the prosthesis can be sutured to the corpora to fix the cylinder and thus prevent its migration, while distal lesions should be repaired to avoid the erosion of the prosthesis. Bladder injuries, can occur but are generally rare during the reservoir positioning, but if it occurs prolonged catheterization is recommended.[6]

Postoperative complications in penile prosthetic surgery can occur; however, their rate is low and surgical outcomes are improving, thanks to a progressively better experience regarding the technique and the enhancements in the prosthesis itself. Infection of the device represents the most serious complication of all, and for this reason meticulous attention to sterility during the operation and an adequate prophylactic antibiotic coverage is important. In order to reduce the bacterial colonization of the genital area showers with antibacterial soap for few days before surgery are recommended, followed by a prolonged washing with iodine-based soap in the operative room prior to surgery.[1] Furthermore, during the procedure it is recommended to irrigate the operative field and particularly both corpora before the insertion of the device with antibiotic solution. Antibiotic-soaked swabs should be used to prevent the contact between prosthesis and skin. In their 3P implants, AMS and Coloplast have introduced an antibiotic coating with minocycline and rifampicine, and a hydrophilic coating in polyvinylpyrrolidone (PVP), respectively, to further reduce this risk. The AMS device does not need to be soaked in an antibiotic solution before its insertion, while this is necessary for the Colopast prosthesis. These improvements have resulted in a significant decrease in the infection rate for virgin implants to 0.68% and 1.06%, respectively, for AMS and Coloplast implants.[7,8] In case of infection, the removal of the device is mandatory and at the same stage a new one can be placed after a salvage washing with antiseptic solutions (iodine, peroxide, and antibiotic); excellent results are reported in up to 84% of cases.[9–11] After infection, another common postoperative risk is mechanical malfunction such as leakage of liquid from the cylinders, cylinder aneurysm, or pump malfunction. Autoinflation of the prosthesis can occur following formation of a capsule around the pump—but thanks to the introduction of the lock-out valve, this event is now observed only in about 1% of cases.[12,13]

The low complication rate, the reliability of the devices, and the high satisfaction rate in patients and partners make penile prosthesis a safe and successful option to restore erectile function in patients who cannot be treated successfully with medical therapy.[14–16]

Penile arterial revascularization and venous ligation

Penile arterial revascularization is a feasible and satisfactory procedure in selected patients with arterial insufficiency secondary to trauma. Doppler ultrasound and arteriography are mandatory to document an arterial insufficiency, a stenosis in the internal pudendal artery, and to exclude a venous leakage. This kind of surgery is only suitable for those patients are relatively young, and do not suffer from vascular disease or diabetes.[17,18] To restore a satisfactory arterial flow in both corpora, the inferior epigastric artery can be anastomosed to the dorsal artery or to the deep dorsal vein, with or without venous ligation.[19,20] This approach, which requires experience in microsurgery, can provide excellent results if performed in the indicated patients although complications such as thrombosis of the anastomosis and glans hyperaemia can occur.[1,18,21] Outcomes of penile arterial revascularization have been gathered from several studies, but randomized controlled trials are not available. Babei *et al.*,[22] in a meta-analysis of the relevant publications about this topic up to 2008, concluded that this surgery can be successful in the long term, particularly for men younger than 30 years, non-smokers, and without venous leakage.

A further surgical approach to treat ED in men with congenital venous leakage due to large deep and dorsal veins and large crural veins is represented by venous ligation.[23,24] The same procedure is not recommended in older patients where the venous leakage occurs as a consequence of smooth muscle dysfunction.[23,25] To achieve successful results, the patency of the penile arterial supply is mandatory. Cayan *et al.*[26] reported their experience in 26 men with primary venous leakage treated with resection of the superficial and deep dorsal veins, ligation of the cavernous vein, and cruras proximal to the entrance of the cavernous artery. After one-year follow-up, they reported excellent results and patient satisfaction, especially in young patients with normal penile arterial system and no risk factors. Rahman *et al.*[27] showed similar results in 11 young patients with primary ED for congenital venous leakage. They performed in these patients a ligation of the two cruras proximally to the entrance of the cavernous artery and reported satisfactory and durable results after a median follow-up of 34 months. Venous ligation in young patients without systemic pathological conditions in which a congenital venous leakage is documented can provide satisfactory results even if data based on larger series are necessary.

Further reading

Anderson PGB, Jain S, Summerton DJ, Terry TR. Insertion of an inflatable penile prosthesis. *BJU Int* 2007; **99**:467–82.

Babaei AR, Safarinejad MR, Kolahi AA. Penile revascularization for erectile dysfunction: A systematic review and meta-analysis of effectiveness and complications. *J Urol* 2009; **6**:1–7.

Brant MD, Ludlow JK, Mulcahy JJ. The prosthesis salvage operation: Immediate replacement of the infected penile prosthesis. *J Urol* 1996; **155**:155–7.

Cayan S. Primary penile venous leakage surgery with crural ligation in men with erectile dysfunction. *J Urol* 2008; **180**:1056–9.

Hellstrome W, Montague D, Moncada I, *et al.* Implants, mechanical devices, and vascular surgery for erectile dysfunction. *J Sex Med* 2010; 7:501–23.

Kaygil O, Okulu E, Aldemir E, *et al.* Penile revascularization in vasculogenic erectile dysfunction (ED): long term follow-up. *BJU Int* 2011; **109**:109–15.

Mulcahy JJ, Austoni E, Barada JH, *et al.* The penile implant for erectile dysfunction. *J Sex Med* 2004; **1**:98–109.

Mulhall JP, Ahmed A, Branch J, Parker M. Serial assessment of efficacy and satisfaction profiles following penile prosthesis surgery. *J Urol* 2003; **169**:1429–33.

Natali A, Olianas R, Fisch M. Penile implantation in Europe: Successes and complications with 253 implants in Italy and Germany. *J Sex Med* 2008; 5:1503–12.

References

1. Hellstrome W, Montague D, Moncada I, *et al.* Implants, mechanical devices, and vascular surgery for erectile dysfunction. *J Sex Med* 2010; 7:501–23.
2. Mulcahy JJ, Austoni E, Barada JH, *et al.* The penile implant for erectile dysfunction. *J Sex Med* 2004; **1**:98–109.
3. Subrini L. Subrini penile implants: Surgical, sexual and psychological results. *Eur Urol* 1982; **8**:222–6.
4. Austoni E, Colombo F, Romanò AL, *et al.* Soft prosthesis implant and relaxing albugineal incision with saphenous grafting for surgical therapy of Peyronie's disease: a 5-year experience and long-term follow-up on 145 operated patients. *Eur Urol* 2005; **47**(2):223–9.
5. Anderson PGB, Jain S, Summerton DJ, Terry TR. Insertion of an inflatable penile prosthesis. *BJU Int* 2007; **99**:467–82.
6. Bettocchi C, Ditonno P, Palumbo F, *et al.* Penile prosthesis: what should we do about complications? *Adv Urol* 2008:573560.
7. Carson CC 3rd. Efficacy of antibiotic impregnation of inflatable penile prostheses in decreasing infection in original implants. *J Urol* 2004; **171**:1611–4.
8. Wolter CE, Hellstrom WJ. The hydrophiliccoated inflatable penile prosthesis: 1-year experience. *J Sex Med* 2004; **1**:221–4.
9. Brant MD, Ludlow JK, Mulcahy JJ. The prosthesis salvage operation: Immediate replacement of the infected penile prosthesis. *J Urol* 1996; **155**:155–7.
10. Mulcahy JJ. Treatment alternatives for the infected penile implant. *Int J Impot Res* 2003; **15**(Suppl 5):S147–9.
11. Mulcahy JJ. Long-term experience with salvage of infected penile implants. *J Urol* 2000; **163**:481–2.
12. Wilson SK, Henry GD, Delk JR Jr, Cleves MA. The mentor Alpha 1 penile prosthesis with reservoir lock-out valve: Effective prevention of autoinflation with improved capability for ectopic reservoir placement. *J Urol* 2002; **168**:1475–8.
13. Hollenbeck BK, Miller DC, Ohl DA. The utility of lockout valve reservoirs in preventing autoinflation in penile prostheses. *Int Urol Nephrol* 2002; **34**:379–83.
14. Mulhall JP, Ahmed A, Branch J, Parker M. Serial assessment of efficacy and satisfaction profiles following penile prosthesis surgery. *J Urol* 2003; **169**:1429–33.
15. Natali A, Olianas R, Fisch M. Penile implantation in Europe: Successes and complications with 253 implants in Italy and Germany. *J Sex Med* 2008; **5**:1503–12.
16. *Ibid.* **14**.
17. Zumbe J, Drawz G, Wiedemann A, Grozinger K, Engelmann U. Indications for penile revascularization and long-term results. *Andrologia* 1999; **31**(Suppl 1):83–7.
18. Kaygil O, Okulu E, Aldemir E, *et al.* Penile revascularization in vasculogenic erectile dysfunction (ED): long term follow-up. *BJU Int* 2011; **109**:109–15.
19. Sohn M, Martín-Morales A. Surgical treatment of erectile dysfunction. (pp. 126–48) In: Porst JB, Buvat J (eds). *Standard Practice in Sexual Medicine*. Hoboken, NJ: Wiley, 2006.
20. Virag R. Vasculogenic impotence: A review of 92 cases with 54 surgical operations. *Vas Surg* 1981; **15**:9–17.
21. Manning M, Junemann KP, Scheepe JR, *et al.* Long-term follow up and selection criteria for penile revascularization in erectile failure. *J Urol* 1998; **160**:1680–4.
22. Babaei AR, Safarinejad MR, Kolahi AA. Penile revascularization for erectile dysfunction: A systematic review and meta-analysis of effectiveness and complications. *J Urol* 2009; **6**:1–7.
23. Lue TF. Surgery for crural venous leakage. *Urology* 1999; **54**:739–41.
24. Ebbehoj J, Wagner G. Insufficient penile erection due to abnormal drainage of cavernous bodies. *Urology* 1979; **13**:507–10.
25. Montague DK, Barada JH, Belker AM, *et al.* Clinical guidelines panel on erectile dysfunction: summary report on the treatment of organic erectile dysfunction. *J Urol* 1996; **156**:2007–11.
26. Cayan S. Primary penile venous leakage surgery with crural ligation in men with erectile dysfunction. *J Urol* 2008; **180**:1056–9.
27. Rahman N, Dean R, Carrion R, *et al.* Crural ligation for primary erectile dysfunction: a case series. *J Urol* 2005; **173**:2064–6.

CHAPTER 7.10

Ejaculatory disorders

Chris G. McMahon

Introduction to ejaculatory disorders

Ejaculatory dysfunction is one of the most common male sexual disorders. The spectrum of ejaculatory dysfunction extends from premature ejaculation, through delayed ejaculation to a complete inability to ejaculate, anejaculation, and also includes retrograde ejaculation.

The anatomy and physiology of the ejaculatory response

The ejaculatory reflex comprises sensory receptors and areas, afferent pathways, cerebral sensory areas, cerebral motor centres, spinal motor centres, and efferent pathways. Neurochemically, this reflex involves a complex interplay between central serotonergic and dopaminergic neurons, with secondary involvement of cholinergic, adrenergic, oxytocinergic, and gamma aminobutyric acid (GABA) neurons. Serotonin, which inhibits emission/ejaculation, and dopamine, which promotes seminal emission/ejaculation, have emerged as key neurochemical factors.[1]

Premature ejaculation

Premature ejaculation (PE) has been estimated to occur in 4–39% of men in the general community[2–8] and is often reported as the most common male sexual disorder. There is, however, a substantial disparity between the incidence of PE in epidemiological studies which rely upon either patient self-report of PE or inconsistent and poorly validated definitions of PE,[7,9,10] and that suggested by community-based stopwatch studies of the intravaginal ejaculation latency time (IELT), the time interval between penetration and ejaculation.[11] The latter demonstrates that the distribution of the IELT was positively skewed, with a median IELT of 5.4 minutes (range 0.55–44.1 min), decreased with age and varied between countries, and supports the notion that IELTs of less than one minute are statistically abnormal compared to men in the general Western population (Fig. 7.10.1).[11]

Classification of premature ejaculation

The population of men with PE is not homogenous and comprises lifelong (primary) and acquired (secondary) PE[12] and has been recently expanded to include natural variable PE and premature-like ejaculatory dysfunction.[13]

- *Lifelong PE* is characterized by early ejaculation at every or nearly every intercourse within 30–60 seconds in the majority of cases (80%) or between one to two minutes (20%), with every or nearly every sexual partner and from the first sexual encounters onwards.

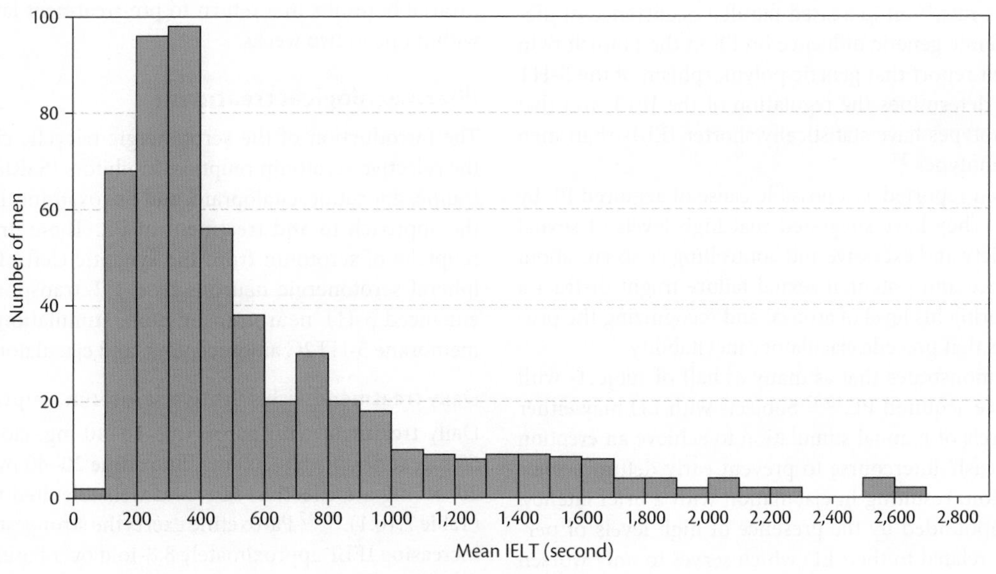

Fig. 7.10.1 Distribution of intravaginal ejaculatory latency times (IELT) values in a random cohort of 491 men.

Reproduced from Waldinger MD *et al*, 'Original Research—Ejaculation Disorders: A Multinational Population Survey of Intravaginal Ejaculation Latency Time', *Journal of Sexual Medicine*, Volume 2, Issue 2, pp. 492–7, Copyright © 2005 John Wiley and Sons, with permission from John Wiley and Sons.

- *Acquired PE* differs from lifelong PE, in that sufferers develop early ejaculation at some point in their life having previously had normal ejaculation experiences. Acquired PE may be due to sexual performance anxiety,[14] psychological or relationship problems,[14] erectile dysfunction (ED),[15] prostatitis,[16] hyperthyroidism,[17] or during withdrawal/detoxification from prescribed[18] or recreational drugs.[19]
- *Natural variable PE* should be regarded as a normal variation in sexual performance, as the IELT is never consistently rapid but merely coincidental and situational.[20]
- *Premature-like ejaculatory dysfunction* is characterized by a preoccupation with a subjective but false perception of PE by men who ejaculate with a normal IELT of three to six minutes.

Defining premature ejaculation

The first contemporary multivariate evidence-based definition of lifelong PE was developed in 2008 by a panel of international experts, convened by the International Society for Sexual Medicine (ISSM), who agreed that the diagnostic criteria necessary to define PE are: time from penetration to ejaculation; inability to delay ejaculation; and negative personal consequences from PE such as distress, bother, frustration and/or the development of sexual avoidance. This panel defined lifelong PE as a male sexual dysfunction characterized by '… ejaculation which always or nearly always occurs prior to or within about one minute of vaginal penetration, the inability to delay ejaculation on all or nearly all vaginal penetrations, and the presence of negative personal consequences, such as distress, bother, frustration and/or the avoidance of sexual intimacy'.[21]

The aetiology of premature ejaculation

Ejaculatory latency time is probably a biological variable, which is genetically determined and may differ between populations and cultures, ranging from extremely rapid through to average or slow ejaculation. The notion that lifelong PE has a genetic basis is supported by animal studies showing a subgroup of persistent rapidly ejaculating Wistar rats,[22] an increased familial occurrence of lifelong PE,[23] a moderate genetic influence on PE in the Finnish twin study,[24] and recent report that genetic polymorphism of the 5-HT transporter gene determines the regulation of the IELT and that men with LL genotypes have statistically shorter IELTs than men with SS and SL genotypes.[25]

Anxiety has been reported as a possible cause of acquired PE by multiple authors. They have suggested that high levels of sexual performance anxiety and excessive and controlling concerns about sexual performance and potential sexual failure might distract a man from monitoring his level of arousal and recognizing the prodromal sensations that precede ejaculatory inevitability.[26–31]

Recent data demonstrates that as many as half of subjects with ED also experience acquired PE.[15,32] Subjects with ED may either require higher levels of manual stimulation to achieve an erection or intentionally 'rush' intercourse to prevent early detumescence of a partial erection, resulting in ejaculation with a brief latency. This may be compounded by the presence of high levels of performance anxiety related to their ED which serves to only worsen their prematurity.

The majority of patients with thyroid hormone disorders experience sexual dysfunction.[17,32] Studies report a significant correlation between acquired PE and suppressed thyroid stimulating hormone (TSH) values[32] with an acquired PE prevalence of 50% in men with hyperthyroidism which fell to 15% after thyroid hormone normalization.[17]

Acute and chronic lower urogenital infection, prostatodynia, or chronic pelvic pain syndrome (CPPS) is associated with ED, PE, and painful ejaculation. Although physical and microbiological examination of the prostate in men with painful ejaculation or lower urinary tract symptoms (LUTS) is mandatory, there is insufficient evidence to support routine screening of men with PE for chronic prostatitis.

Treatment of premature ejaculation

Premature ejaculation treatment strategies include psychosexual counselling, daily or on-demand pharmacotherapy, either alone or in combination as part of an integrated treatment programme. Figure 7.10.2 is a flow chart for the management of PE.

Psychosexual counselling

The cornerstones of behavioural treatment are the Seman's 'stop-start' manoeuvre and its modification proposed by Masters and Johnson, the squeeze technique. Both are based on the theory that PE occurs because the man fails to pay sufficient attention to pre-orgasmic levels of sexual tension.[33,34] As most men with PE are aware of their anxiety and the sources of that anxiety tend to be relatively superficial, treatment success with these behavioural approaches is relatively good in the short term, but convincing long-term treatment outcome data are lacking.[35–38]

Cognitive behavioural therapy (CBT), especially when combined with pharmacotherapy, is an effective intervention for acquired PE related to sexual performance anxiety; a substantial proportion of men report sustained improvements on ejaculatory latency and control following cessation of pharmacotherapy.[39–41] However, men with lifelong PE rarely achieve symptomatic improvement with CBT alone and are best managed with either pharmacotherapy alone or in combination with CBT if there is a significant secondary psychogenic contribution, where cessation of pharmacotherapy invariably results in a return to pre-treatment latency and control within one to two weeks.

Pharmacological treatment

The introduction of the serotonergic tricyclic clomipramine and the selective serotonin reuptake inhibitors (SSRIs) paroxetine, sertraline, fluoxetine, citalopram, and fluvoxamine, has revolutionized the approach to and treatment of PE. These drugs block axonal reuptake of serotonin from the synaptic cleft of central and peripheral serotonergic neurons by 5-HT transporters, resulting in enhanced 5-HT neurotransmission, stimulation of post-synaptic membrane 5-HT2C autoreceptors, and ejaculatory delay.

Daily treatment with selective serotonin reuptake inhibitors

Daily treatment with paroxetine 10–40 mg, clomipramine 12.5–50 mg, sertraline 50–200 mg, fluoxetine 20–40 mg, and citalopram 20–40 mg are effective, safe, and well-tolerated treatments for PE (Table 7.10.1).[42–47] Paroxetine exerts the strongest ejaculation delay, increasing IELT approximately 8.8-fold over baseline.[42] Ejaculation delay usually occurs within 5–10 days of starting treatment, but the full therapeutic effect may require two to three weeks of treatment and is usually sustained during long-term use.[41] Patient should be

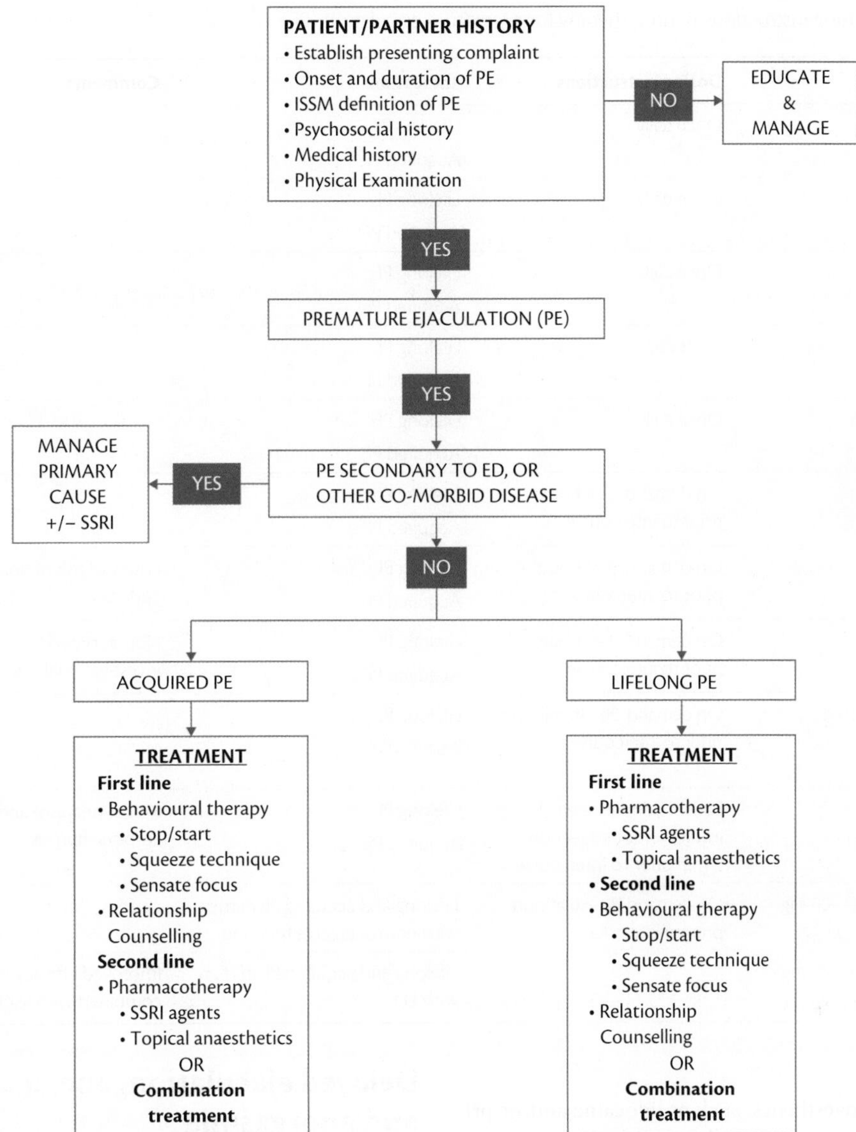

Fig. 7.10.2 Management algorithm for the office treatment of premature ejaculation.
Reproduced from David Rowland *et al.*, 'Disorders of Orgasm and Ejaculation in Men', *Journal of Sexual Medicine*, Volume 7, Issue 4, Part 2, pp. 1668–86, Copyright © International Society for Sexual Medicine 2010, with permission from John Wiley and Sons.

reviewed after four weeks of treatment and dose titrated according to response and tolerability. Although tachyphylaxis is uncommon, some patients report a reduced response after 6–12 months of treatment.

On-demand treatment with selective serotonin reuptake inhibitors

Administration of clomipramine and to a lesser extent, paroxetine, sertraline and fluoxetine four to six hours before intercourse is modestly efficacious and well tolerated but is associated with substantially less ejaculatory delay than daily treatment (Table 7.10.1).[48–51] On-demand treatment may be used following an initial four to eight week trial of daily treatment or combined with concomitant low dose daily treatment.[48–50]

On-demand treatment with dapoxetine

Dapoxetine (30 mg, 60 mg) is an SSRI, specifically developed for the treatment of PE. It is rapidly absorbed and has a brief plasma half-life of 0.5–0.8 hours with minimal plasma accumulation, suggesting a role as an on-demand treatment for PE.

The dapoxetine clinical trial programme includes more than 7,400 men and demonstrates superiority to placebo, with a dose-dependent fold increase in mean IELT of 2.5–3.0 over baseline, substantial improvements in ejaculatory control, patient and partner sexual satisfaction, and reductions in personal, partner, and relationship distress.[52]

On-demand treatment with tramadol

Tramadol is a centrally acting synthetic opioid analgesic with an unclear mode of action. The only double-blind well-designed study demonstrates a superiority to placebo, but a mediocre fold increase in IELT of 2.49, consistent with the weak serotonin reuptake inhibitor activity of tramadol.[53] The unclear safety profile and the potential for addiction discourages use of tramadol in PE clinical practice.

Table 7.10.1 Doses and dosing instructions of drug therapy for premature ejaculation (PE)

Drug	Dose	Dosing instructions	Indication	Comments	Level of evidence
Paroxetine	10–40 mg	Once daily	Lifelong PE Acquired PE		High
Sertraline	50–200 mg	Once daily	Lifelong PE Acquired PE		High
Fluoxetine	20–40 mg	Once daily	Lifelong PE Acquired PE		High
Citalopram	20–40 mg	Once daily	Lifelong PE Acquired PE		High
Clomipramine	12.5–50 mg	Once daily	Lifelong PE Acquired PE		High
	12.5–50 mg	On demand, 3–4 hours prior to intercourse	Lifelong PE Acquired PE		High
Tramadol	25–50 mg	On demand, 3–4 hours prior to intercourse	Lifelong PE Acquired PE	Potential risk of opiate addiction	Low
Dapoxetine	30–60 mg	On demand, 1–3 hours prior to intercourse	Lifelong PE Acquired PE	Non-approved investigational drug	High
Topical lignocaine/ priliocaine	Patient titrated	On demand, 20–30 minutes prior to intercourse	Lifelong PE Acquired PE		High
Alprostadil	5–20 mcg	Patient administered intracavernous injection 5 min prior to intercourse	Lifelong PE Acquired PE	Risk of priapism and corporal fibrosis	Very low
PDE5 inhibitors	Sildenafil 25–100 mg Tadalafil 10–20 mg Vardenafil 10–20 mg	On demand, 30–50 minutes prior to intercourse	Lifelong and acquired PE in men with normal erectile function		Very low
			Lifelong and acquired PE in men with ED	Improved efficacy if combined with SSRI	Moderate

Topical anaesthetics

The use of topical local anaesthetics, such as lidocaine and/or prilocaine as a cream, gel, or spray is well-established and is moderately effective in retarding ejaculation. A recent study reported that a metered-dose aerosol spray containing a eutectic mixture of lidocaine and prilocaine (TEMPE®) produced a 2.4-fold increase in baseline IELT and significant improvements in ejaculatory control and both patient and partner sexual quality-of-life.[54,55] The use of topical anaesthetics may be associated with significant penile hypoanaesthesia and possible transvaginal absorption, resulting in vaginal numbness and consequent female anorgasmia, unless a condom is used.

Phosphodiesterase inhibitors

Off-label on-demand or daily dosing of PDE5 inhibitors is not recommended for the treatment of lifelong PE in men with normal erectile function. ED pharmacotherapy alone or in combination with PE pharmacotherapy is recommended for the treatment of lifelong or acquired PE in men with co-morbid ED.

Surgery

Selective dorsal nerve neurotomy or hyaluronic acid gel glans penis augmentation is not recommended for the treatment of PE. Surgery may be associated with permanent loss of sexual function and is contraindicated in the management of PE.

Delayed ejaculation, anejaculation, and anorgasmia

Any psychological or medical disease or surgical procedure which interferes with either central control of ejaculation or the peripheral sympathetic nerve supply to the vas and bladder neck, the somatic efferent nerve supply to the pelvic floor, or the somatic afferent nerve supply to the penis can result in delayed ejaculation, anejaculation, and anorgasmia. As such, the causes of delayed ejaculation and anejaculation are manifold (Table 7.10.2).

Defining delayed ejaculation/anejaculation

Delayed ejaculation (DE) (inhibited ejaculation, retarded ejaculation) and anejaculation are probably the least common, least studied, and least understood of the male sexual dysfunctions. Again, there are a number of definitions for DE, but the DSM-IV definition again uses requirement for a recurrent symptom (delayed or absent ejaculation) combined with some degree of personal distress.[56]

Pathophysiology of delayed ejaculation/anejaculation

A number of pathophysiologies have been associated with ejaculatory problems. These include congenital disorders, as well as ones caused by trauma, infection, disease, and treatment for other disorders (Table 7.10.2). When a medical history or symptomatology

Table 7.10.2 Causes of delayed ejaculation, anejaculation, and anorgasmia

Ageing male psychogenic	Degeneration of penile afferent nerves causing inhibited ejaculation
Congenital	Müllerian duct cyst
	Wolfian duct abnormaility
	Prune belly syndrome
Anatomic causes	Transurethral resection of prostate
	Bladder neck incision
Neurogenic causes	Diabetic autonomic neuropathy
	Multiple sclerosis
	Spinal cord injury
	Radical prostatectomy
	Proctocolectomy
	Bilateral sympathectomy
	Abdominal aortic aneurysmectomy
	Para-aortic lympthadenectomy
Infective	Urethritis
	Genitourinary tuberculosis
	Schistosomiasis
Endocrine	Hypogonadism
	Hypothyroidism
Medication	Alpha-methyl dopa
	Thiazide diuretics
	Tricyclic and SSRI antidepressants
	Phenothiazine
	Alcohol abuse

so indicates, investigation of such possible aetiologies may be necessary.

Delayed ejaculation due to degeneration of psychogenic factors, penile afferent nerves, and pacinian corpuscles in the ageing male, diabetic autonomic neuropathy, SSRI antidepressants and major tranquillizers, radical prostatectomy, or other pelvic surgery are the most common causes of DE seen in clinical practice.

Psychogenic DE is usually related to sexual performance anxiety, which may draw the man's attention away from erotic cues that normally serve to enhance arousal. Other psychodynamic explanations emphasize psychosexual development issues and have attributed lifelong DE to a wide range of conditions, including fear, anxiety, hostility, orthodoxy of religious belief, and relationship difficulties.[57,58] Idiosyncratic and vigorous masturbation styles that cannot be replicated during intercourse with a partner, or an 'autosexual' orientation where men derive greater arousal and enjoyment from masturbation than from intercourse, are risk factors for DE.[59] Disparity between the reality of sex with the partner and the sexual fantasy used during masturbation may inhibit sexual arousal and thus represent another contributor to DE.

Delayed ejaculation and anejaculation is commonly seen in men with hypothyroidism and occasionally in hypogonadal men. The ability to ejaculate may be severely impaired in multiple sclerosis, diabetic autonomic neuropathy, and by spinal cord injury (SCI).[60]

Evaluation of men with delayed ejaculation/anejaculation

Assessment begins by determining whether DE is lifelong or acquired, global or situational. Its evaluation includes establishment of how often a man can ejaculate during intercourse and the time elapsed between penetration and ejaculation, the IELT. If ejaculation fails to occur, the duration of thrusting before suspension of intercourse, and the reasons for suspension of intercourse (e.g. fatigue, loss of erection, a sense of ejaculatory futility or partner request, and whether ejaculation can occur during post-coital self or partner-assisted masturbation must be determined) should be clarified.

In men with acquired DE, previous illness, surgery, medications, or life events/circumstances should be reviewed. The events may include a variety of life stressors and other psychological factors (e.g. following his wife's mastectomy where the man is afraid of hurting her and therefore is only partially aroused). Societal and religious attitudes that may interfere with excitement are noted, such as the 'spilling of seed as a sin'.

A focused physical and genital examination to determine whether the testes and epididymes are normal and whether the vasa are present or absent on each side, supported by a screening morning total testosterone level and any other hormonal or imaging investigations indicated by either history or physical examination will identify or exclude organic disease. The presence of a neuropathy may require electrophysiological evaluation of neural pathways controlling ejaculation, pudendal somatosensory and motor evoked potentials, sacral reflex arc testing, and sympathetic skin responses.

The occurrence of orgasm in the absence of prograde ejaculation suggests retrograde ejaculation and can be confirmed by the presence of spermatozoa in post-masturbation first-void urine. If the aetiology of DE is unclear, culture of expressed prostatic secretion and urine, urine cytology, and serum prostate specific antigen will exclude prostatitis, bladder, and prostatic cancer. Ultrasound scan of the testicles and epididymes may define any local disease.

Figure 7.10.3 is a flow chart for the management of DE.[61]

Treatment of men with delayed ejaculation/anejaculation

Treatment should be aetiology-specific, address the issue of infertility in men of a reproductive age, and may include patient/couple psychoeducation and/or psychosexual therapy, pharmacotherapy, or integrated treatment. Men/partners of reproductive age undergoing pelvic surgery should be informed of the risk of infertility due to anejaculation and the availability of sperm harvesting and assisted reproductive techniques.

Psychological strategies in the treatment of delayed ejaculation

Numerous psychotherapeutic processes are described for the management of delayed or inhibited ejaculation.[62,63] Among these strategies are: (i) sex education; (ii) reduction of goal-focused anxiety; (iii) increased, more genitally focused stimulation; (iv) patient role-playing an exaggerated ejaculatory response on his own and in

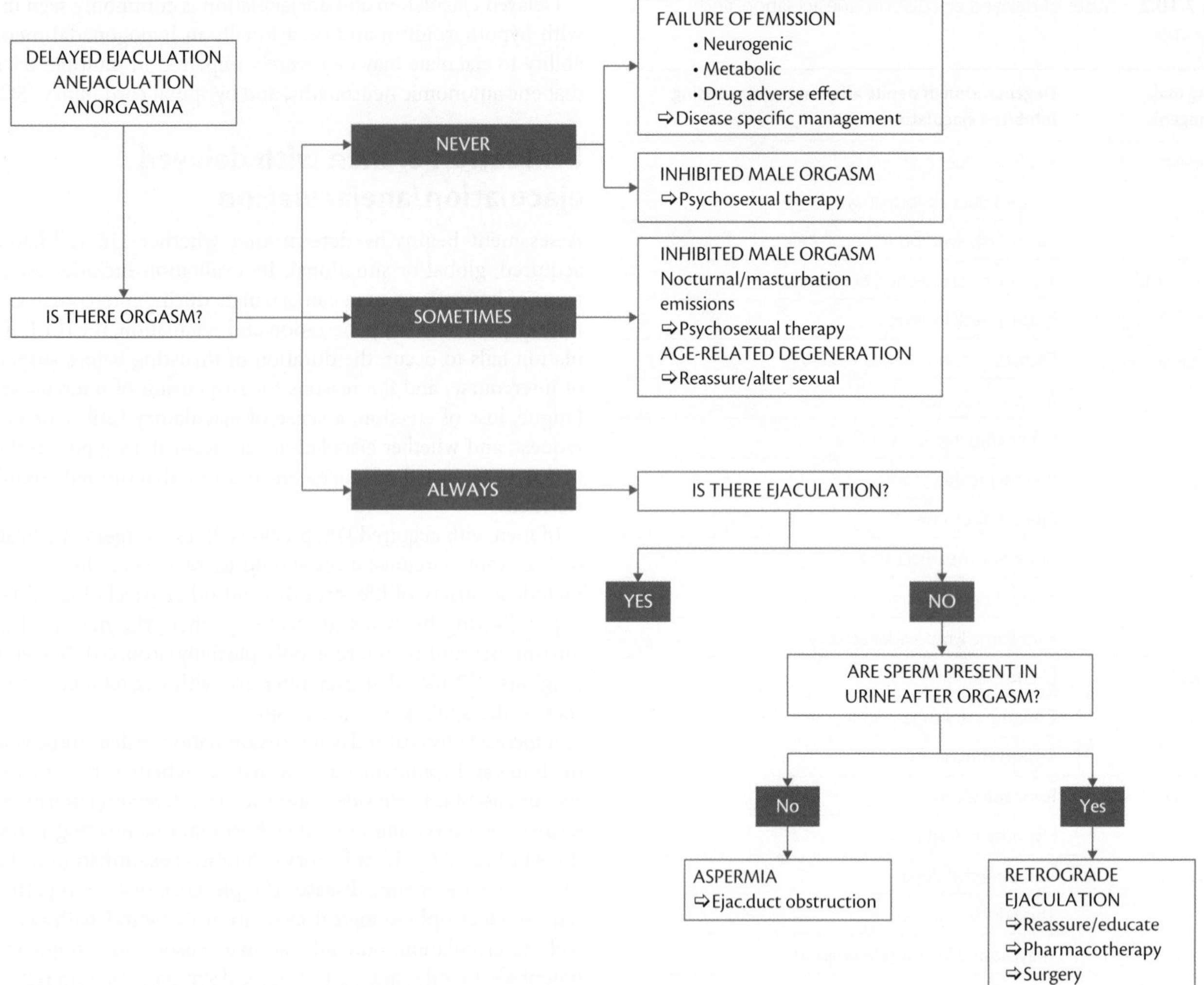

Fig. 7.10.3 Management algorithm for the office treatment of delayed ejaculation.

Reproduced from David Rowland *et al.*, 'Disorders of Orgasm and Ejaculation in Men', *Journal of Sexual Medicine*, Volume 7, Issue 4, Part 2, pp. 1668–86, Copyright © International Society for Sexual Medicine 2010, with permission from John Wiley and Sons.

front of his partner; (v) masturbatory retraining; and (vi) realignment of sexual fantasies and arousal strategies.

Most current sex therapy approaches to DE emphasize the importance of masturbation in the treatment of DE, with most of the focus on 'masturbatory retraining' integrated into sex therapy.[64]

An important component in the treatment of any type of DE is the removal of the 'demand' (and thus anxiety-producing) characteristics of the situation.[62] To reduce anxiety, treatment may include recognition of DE men's overeagerness to please their partners, validation of (though not necessarily encouragement of) the man's autosexual orientation, removal of stigmas suggesting hostility or withholding towards their partner, and general anxiety reduction techniques such as relaxation and desensitization.

Pharmacotherapy in the treatment of delayed ejaculation

Drug treatment of delayed or inhibited ejaculation has met with limited success (Table 7.10.3). These drugs facilitate ejaculation by either a central dopaminergic, anti-serotonergic, or oxytocinergic mechanism of action or a peripheral adrenergic mechanism of action. However, no drugs have been approved by regulatory agencies for this purpose, and most drugs that have been identified for potential use have limited efficacy, impart significant side effects, or are yet considered experimental in nature. Results are relatively poor in men with psychogenic DE and neuropathic DE.

Alpha-1 adrenergic receptor agonists such as on-demand precoital pseudoephedrine (120 mg one to two hours prior to intercourse) or the serotonin-noradrenaline reuptake inhibitors (SNRI) antidepressant reboxetine (4–8 mg daily) which inhibits synaptic noradrenaline reuptake have limited efficacy. The antihistamine cyproheptadine, a central serotonin antagonist, is anecdotally associated with the reversal of anorgasmia induced by the SSRI antidepressants, but no controlled studies have been reported.[65,66] These studies suggest an effective dose range of 2–16 mg, with administration on a chronic or 'on demand' basis. However, significant dose-related sedative effects are likely to diminish its overall efficacy.

Amantadine, an indirect stimulant of dopaminergic nerves both centrally and peripherally, has been reported to stimulate sexual behaviour and ejaculation in SSRI antidepressant induced anorgasmia when administered on demand (100–200 mg, five to six hours before coitus) or chronically (100–200 mg BID).[67]

Table 7.10.3 Adjunctive drug therapy for SSRI-induced sexual dysfunction

Drug	Dosage	
	As needed	**Daily**
Amantadine	100–400 mg (for two days prior to coitus)	100–200 mg bid
Cabergoline		0.25–0.5 mg every 3 days
Pseudoephedrine	60–120 mg (1–2 hrs prior to coitus)	
Reboxetine		4–8 mg
Oxytocin	24I U intranasal during coitus	
Bupropion		150 mg daily or bid
Buspirone		5–15 mg bid
Cyproheptadine	4–12 mg (3–4 hrs prior to coitus)	

A variety of other pharmacological agents including bromocriptine, cabergoline, bupropion, and buspirone have been anecdotally reported as potential DE pharmacotherapy, despite an absence of large population randomized controlled trials (RCTs). Of interest is the recent single case report of the intracoital administration of intranasal oxytocin in a case of treatment-resistant anorgasmia.[68] However, in the absence of robust RCT data, oxytocin cannot be recommended as a treatment for DE.

Retrograde ejaculation

Antegrade (normal) ejaculation requires a closed bladder neck (and proximal urethra). Surgical procedures that compromise the bladder neck closure mechanism and diabetes mellitus are the most common causes of retrograde ejaculation. Transurethral incision of the prostate (TUIP) results in retrograde ejaculation in 5%[69] to 45%[70] of patients and is probably related to whether one or two incisions are made and whether or not the incision includes primarily the bladder neck or extends to the level of the verumontanum. Transurethral resection of the prostate (TURP) carries a higher incidence of retrograde ejaculation than does TUIP. The reported incidence of retrograde ejaculation following TURP ranges from 42%[71] to 100%.[72] Retrograde ejaculation and failure of emission can be distinguished by examination of a post-masturbatory specimen of urine for the presence of spermatozoa and fructose.

Results of surgical treatment of retrograde ejaculation with bladder neck reconstruction remain consistently poor.[73] Drug treatment is the most promising approach. Several sympathomimetic agents, including pseudoephedrine, ephedrine, and phenylpropanolomine have been described as useful with mixed results.[74] The most useful is pseudoephedrine, which is administered at a dose of 120 mg 2–2.5 hours precoitally. The tricyclic antidepressant, imipramine, which blocks the reuptake of noradrenaline by the axon from the synaptic cleft, is also occasionally useful.[75] The usual dose is 25 mg twice daily and long-term treatment is likely to be more effective. In patients who do not achieve antegrade ejaculation with surgery or medication, sperm retrieval and artificial insemination is an alternative approach.

Painful ejaculation

Painful ejaculation or odynorgasmia is a poorly characterized syndrome. It may be associated with urethritis, benign prostatic hypertrophy (BPH), acute or chronic prostatitis, chronic pelvic pain syndrome, seminal vesiculitis, seminal vesicular calculi, or ejaculatory duct obstruction.[76–79] Often, no obvious aetiologic factor can be found. Painful ejaculation occurs in 17–23% of men with LUTS/BPH.[80–83] Men with BPH and painful ejaculation have more severe LUTS and report greater bother. In addition, they report a higher incidence of ED and a reduced ejaculation volume, compared to neb with LUTS only.[84] Treatment of men with LUTS with alpha-blocking drugs may be associated with painful ejaculation. A lower incidence of pain has been reported with the uroselective alpha-1 blocking drug, alfuzosin.[85] Management should focus on treatment of the underlying cause of symptoms.

Further reading

Althof S. The psychology of premature ejaculation: therapies and consequences. *J Sex Med* 2006; **3**(Suppl 4):324– 31.

Althof SE, Abdo CH, Dean J, *et al.* International Society for Sexual Medicine's guidelines for the diagnosis and treatment of premature ejaculation. *J Sex Med* 2010; 7(9):2947– 69.

McMahon CG, Althof SE, Waldinger MD, *et al.* An evidence-based definition of lifelong premature ejaculation: report of the International Society for Sexual Medicine (ISSM) ad hoc committee for the definition of premature ejaculation. *J Sex Med* 2008; **5**(7):1590–606.

McMahon CG, McMahon CN, Leow LJ, Winestock CG. Efficacy of type-5 phosphodiesterase inhibitors in the drug treatment of premature ejaculation: a systematic review. *BJU Int* 2006; **98**(2):259– 72.

Patrick DL, Althof SE, Pryor JL, *et al.* Premature ejaculation: an observational study of men and their partners. *J Sex Med* 2005; **2**(3):58–367.

Porst H, Montorsi F, Rosen RC, Gaynor L, Grupe S, Alexander J. The Premature Ejaculation Prevalence and Attitudes (PEPA) survey: prevalence, comorbidities, and professional help-seeking. *Eur Urol* 2007; **51**(3):816–23; discussion 24.

Rowland D, McMahon CG, Abdo C, *et al.* Disorders of orgasm and ejaculation in men. *J Sex Med* 2010; 7(4 Pt 2):1668–86.

Waldinger MD, Quinn P, Dilleen M, Mundayat R, Schweitzer DH, Boolell M. A multinational population survey of intravaginal ejaculation latency time. *J Sex Med* 2005; **2**:492–7.

References

1. McMahon CG, Abdo C, Incrocci L, *et al.* Disorders of orgasm and ejaculation in men. *J Sex Med* 2004; **1**(1):58–65.
2. Reading A, Wiest W. An analysis of self-reported sexual behavior in a sample of normal males. *Arch Sex Behav* 1984; **13**:69–83.
3. Nathan SG. The epidemiology of the DSM-III psychosexual dysfunctions. *J Sex Marital Ther* 1986; **12**(4):267–81.
4. Spector KR, Boyle M. The prevalence and perceived aetiology of male sexual problems in a non-clinical sample. *Br J Med Psychol* 1986; **59**(Pt 4):351–8.
5. Spector IP, Carey M. Incidence and prevalence of the sexual dysfunctions: a critical review of the empirical literature. *Arch Sex Behav* 1990; **19**:389.
6. Grenier G, Byers ES. The relationships among ejaculatory control, ejaculatory latency, and attempts to prolong heterosexual intercourse. *Arch Sex Behav* 1997; **26**(1):27–47.
7. Laumann EO, Paik A, Rosen RC. Sexual dysfunction in the United States: prevalence and predictors. *JAMA* 1999; **281**(6):537–44.
8. Porst H, Montorsi F, Rosen RC, Gaynor L, Grupe S, Alexander J. The Premature Ejaculation Prevalence and Attitudes (PEPA)

survey: prevalence, comorbidities, and professional help-seeking. *Eur Urol* 2007; **51**(3):816–23; discussion 24.
9. Patrick DL, Althof SE, Pryor JL, *et al.* Premature ejaculation: an observational study of men and their partners. *J Sex Med* 2005; **2**(3):58–367.
10. Giuliano F, Patrick DL, Porst H, *et al.* Premature ejaculation: results from a five-country European observational study. *Eur Urol* 2008; **53**(5):1048–57.
11. Waldinger MD, Quinn P, Dilleen M, Mundayat R, Schweitzer DH, Boolell M. A multinational population survey of intravaginal ejaculation latency time. *J Sex Med* 2005; **2**:492–7.
12. Schapiro B. Premature ejaculation, a review of 1130 cases. *J Urol* 1943; **50**: 374–9.
13. Waldinger MD. Premature ejaculation: definition and drug treatment. Drugs. 2007; **67**(4):547–68.
14. Hartmann U, Schedlowski M, Kruger TH. Cognitive and partner-related factors in rapid ejaculation: Differences between dysfunctional and functional men. *World J Urol* 2005; **10**:10.
15. Laumann EO, Nicolosi A, Glasser DB, *et al.* Sexual problems among women and men aged 40–80 y: prevalence and correlates identified in the Global Study of Sexual Attitudes and Behaviors. *Int J Impot Res* 2005; **17**(1):39–57.
16. Screponi E, Carosa E, Di Stasi SM, Pepe M, Carruba G, Jannini EA. Prevalence of chronic prostatitis in men with premature ejaculation. *Urology* 2001; **58**(2):198–202.
17. Carani C, Isidori AM, Granata A, *et al.* Multicenter study on the prevalence of sexual symptoms in male hypo- and hyperthyroid patients. *J Clin Endocrinol Metab* 2005; **90**(12):6472–9.
18. Adson DE, Kotlyar M. Premature ejaculation associated with citalopram withdrawal. *Ann Pharmacother* 2003; **37**(12):1804–6.
19. Peugh J, Belenko S. Alcohol, drugs and sexual function: a review. *J Psychoactive Drugs* 2001; **33**(3):223–32.
20. Waldinger MD, Schweitzer DH. Changing paradigms from a historical DSM-III and DSM-IV view toward an evidence-based definition of premature ejaculation. Part II—proposals for DSM-V and ICD-11. *J Sex Med* 2006; **3**(4):693–705.
21. McMahon CG, Althof SE, Waldinger MD, *et al.* An evidence-based definition of lifelong premature ejaculation: report of the International Society for Sexual Medicine (ISSM) ad hoc committee for the definition of premature ejaculation. *J Sex Med* 2008; **5**(7):1590–606.
22. Pattij T, Olivier B, Waldinger MD. Animal models of ejaculatory behavior. *Curr Pharma Des* 2005; **11**(31):4069–77.
23. Waldinger MD, Rietschel M, Nothen MM, Hengeveld MW, Olivier B. Familial occurrence of primary premature ejaculation. *Psychiatr Genet* 1998; **8**(1):37–40.
24. Jern P, Santtila P, Witting K, *et al.* Premature and delayed ejaculation: Genetic and environmental effects in a population-based sample of Finnish twins. *J Sex Med* 2007; **4**(6):1739–49.
25. Janssen PK, Bakker SC, Rethelyi J, *et al.* Serotonin transporter promoter region (5-HTTLPR) polymorphism is associated with the intravaginal ejaculation latency time in Dutch men with lifelong premature ejaculation. *J Sex Med* 2009; **6**(1):276–84.
26. Vandereycken W. Towards a better delineation of ejaculatory disorders. *Acta Psychiatr Belg* 1986; **86**(1):57–63.
27. Zilbergeld B. *Male Sexuality*. Toronto, ON: Bantam, 1978.
28. Zilbergeld B. *The New Male Sexuality*. New York, NY: Bantam, 1992.
29. Kaplan HS. *PE: How to Overcome Premature Ejaculation*. New York, NY: Brunner/Mazel, 1989.
30. Kockott G, Feil W, Revenstorf D, Aldenhoff J, Besinger U. Symptomatology and psychological aspects of male sexual inadequacy: results of an experimental study. *Arch Sex Behav* 1980; **9**(6):457–75.
31. Kaplan H. *The Evaluation of Sexual Disorders: The Urologic Evaluation of Ejaculatory Disorders*. New York, NY: Brunner/Mazel, 1983.
32. Corona G, Petrone L, Mannucci E, *et al.* Psycho-biological correlates of rapid ejaculation in patients attending an andrologic unit for sexual dysfunctions. *Eur Urol* 2004; **46**(5):615–22.
33. Masters WH, Johnson VE. *Human Sexual Inadequacy*. Boston, MA: Little Brown, 1970: pp. 92–115.
34. Semans JH. Premature ejaculation: a new approach. *South Med J* 1956; **49**(4):353–8.
35. McCarthy B. Cognitive-behavioural strategies and techniques in the treatment of early ejaculation. (pp. 141–67) In: Leiblum SR, Rosen R (eds). *Principles and Practices of Sex Therapy: Update for the 1990's*. New York, NY: Guilford Press, 1988.
36. de Carufel F, Trudel G. Effects of a new functional-sexological treatment for premature ejaculation. *J Sex Marital Ther* 2006; **32**(2):97–114.
37. De Amicis LA, Goldberg DC, LoPiccolo J, Friedman J, Davies L. Clinical follow-up of couples treated for sexual dysfunction. *Arch Sex Behav* 1985; **14**(6):467–89.
38. Hawton K, Catalan J, Martin P, Fagg J. Long-term outcome of sex therapy. *Behav Res Ther* 1986; **24**(6):665–75.
39. McMahon CG, Abdo C, Incrocci I, *et al.* Disorders of orgasm and ejaculation in men. (pp. 409–68) In: Lue TF, Basson R, Rosen R, Giuliano F, Khoury S, Montorsi F (eds). *Sexual Medicine: Sexual Dysfunctions in Men and Women* (2nd International Consultation on Sexual Dysfunctions-Paris). Paris, France: Health Publications, 2004.
40. Perelman MA. A new combination treatment for premature ejaculation: a sex therapist's perspective. *J Sex Med* 2006; **3**(6):1004–12.
41. McMahon CG. Long term results of treatment of premature ejaculation with selective serotonin re-uptake inhibitors. *Int J Imp Res* 2002; **14**(Suppl 3):S19.
42. Waldinger M. Towards evidenced based drug treatment research on premature ejaculation: a critical evaluation of methodology. *J Impot Res* 2003; **15**(5):309–13.
43. Atmaca M, Kuloglu M, Tezcan E, Semercioz A. The efficacy of citalopram in the treatment of premature ejaculation: a placebo-controlled study. *Int J Imp Res* 2002; **14**(6):502–5.
44. McMahon CG. Treatment of premature ejaculation with sertraline hydrochloride: a single-blind placebo controlled crossover study. *J Urol* 1998; **159**(6):1935–8.
45. Kara H, Aydin S, Yucel M, Agargun MY, Odabas O, Yilmaz Y. The efficacy of fluoxetine in the treatment of premature ejaculation: a double-blind placebo controlled study. *J Urol* 1996; **156**(5):1631–2.
46. Waldinger MD, Hengeveld MW, Zwinderman AH. Paroxetine treatment of premature ejaculation: a double-blind, randomized, placebo-controlled study. *Am J Psychiat* 1994; **151**(9):1377–9.
47. Goodman RE. An assessment of clomipramine (Anafranil) in the treatment of premature ejaculation. *J Int Med Res* 1980; **8**(Suppl 3):53–9.
48. McMahon CG, Touma K. Treatment of premature ejaculation with paroxetine hydrochloride as needed: 2 single-blind placebo controlled crossover studies. *J Urol* 1999; **161**(6):1826–30.
49. Strassberg DS, de Gouveia Brazao CA, Rowland DL, Tan P, Slob AK. Clomipramine in the treatment of rapid (premature) ejaculation. *J Sex Marital Ther* 1999; **25**(2):89–101.
50. Kim SW, Paick JS. Short-term analysis of the effects of as needed use of sertraline at 5 PM for the treatment of premature ejaculation. *Urology* 1999; **54**(3):544–7.
51. Waldinger MD, Zwinderman AH, Olivier B. On-demand treatment of premature ejaculation with clomipramine and paroxetine: a randomized, double-blind fixed-dose study with stopwatch assessment. *Eur Urol* 2004; **46**(4):510–5; discussion 6.
52. McMahon CG, Althof SE, Kaufman JM, *et al.* Efficacy and safety of dapoxetine for the treatment of premature ejaculation: integrated analysis of results from five phase 3 trials. *J Sex Med* 2010; **8**(2):524–39.
53. Bar-Or D, Salottolo KM, Orlando A, Winkler JV. A randomized double-blind, placebo-controlled multicenter study to evaluate the efficacy and safety of two doses of the tramadol orally disintegrating tablet for the treatment of premature ejaculation within less than 2 minutes. *Eur Urol* 2011; **61**(4):736–43.
54. Dinsmore WW, Hackett G, Goldmeier D, *et al.* Topical eutectic mixture for premature ejaculation (TEMPE): a novel aerosol-delivery form of

lidocaine-prilocaine for treating premature ejaculation. *BJU Int* 2007; **99**(2):369–75.

55. Henry R, Morales A, Wyllie MG. TEMPE: Topical Eutectic-Like Mixture for Premature Ejaculation. *Expert Opin Drug Deliv* 2008; **5**(2):251–61.
56. American Psychiatric Association. *Diagnostic and Statistical Manual of Medical Disorders*, 5th edition. Washington DC, WA: American Psychiatry Publishing, 2013.
57. Waldinger MD, Schweitzer DH. Retarded ejaculation in men: an overview of psychological and neurobiological insights. *World J Urol* 2005; **23**(2):76–81.
58. Munjack DJ, Kanno PH. Retarded ejaculation: a review. *Arch Sex Behav* 1979; **8**(2):139–50.
59. Perelman M. Idiosyncratic masturbation patterns: a key unexplored variable in the treatment of retarded ejaculation by the practicing urologist. *J Urol* 2005; **173**(Suppl 3):S340.
60. Comarr AE. Sexual function among patients with spinal cord injury. *Urol Int* 1970; **25**(2):134–68.
61. Rowland D, McMahon CG, Abdo C, *et al.* Disorders of orgasm and ejaculation in men. *J Sex Med* 2010; **7**(4 Pt 2):1668–86.
62. Apfelbaum B. Retarded ejaculation: A much-misunderstood syndrome. (pp, 168–206) In: Lieblum SR, Rosen RC (eds). *Principles and Practice of Sex Therapy: Update for the 1990's*, 2nd edition. New York, NY: Guilford Press. 1989.
63. McCarthy B. Strategies and techniques for the treatment of ejaculatory inhibition. *J Sex Ed Ther* 1981; **7**(2):20–3.
64. Kaplan H. *The Evaluation of Sexual Disorders: Psychological and medical Aspects*. New York, NY: Brunner/Mazel, 1995.
65. McCormick S, Olin J, Brotman AW. Reversal of fluoxetine-induced anorgasmia by cyproheptadine in two patients. *J Clin Psychiatry* 1990; **51**(9):383–4.
66. Ashton K, Hamer R, Rosen R. Serotonin reuptake inhibitor-induced sexual dysfunction and its treatment: a large-scale retrospective study of 596 psychiatric outpatients. *J Sex Marital Ther* 1997; **23**(3):165–75.
67. Balogh S, Hendricks S, Kang J. Treatment of fluoxetine-induced anorgasmia with amantadine. *J Clin Psychiatry* 1992; **53**(6):212–3.
68. Ishak WW, Berman DS, Peters A. Male anorgasmia treated with oxytocin. *J Sex Med* 2007; **5**(4):1022–4.
69. Hedlund H, Ek A. Ejaculation and sexual function after endoscopic bladder neck incision. *Br J Urol* 1985; **57**(2):164–7.
70. Kelly MJ, Roskamp D, Leach GE. Transurethral incision of the prostate: a preoperative and postoperative analysis of symptoms and urodynamic findings. *J Urol* 1989; **142**(6):1507–9.
71. Edwards L, Powell C. An objective comparison of transurethral resection and bladder neck incision in the treatment of prostatic hypertrophy. *J Urol* 1982; **128**:325–7.
72. Quinlan DM, Epstein JI, Carter BS, Walsh PC. Sexual function following radical prostatectomy: influence of preservation of neurovascular bundles. *J Urol* 1991; **145**:998–1002.
73. Abrahams JI, Solish GI, Boorjian P, Waterhouse RK. The surgical correction of retrograde ejaculation. *J Urol* 1975; **114**(6):888–90.
74. Kedia K, Markland C. The effect of pharmacological agents on ejaculation. *J Urol* 1975; **114**(4):569–73.
75. Nijman JM, Jager S, Boer PW, Kremer J, Oldhoff J, Koops HS. The treatment of ejaculation disorders after retroperitoneal lymph node dissection. *Cancer* 1982; **50**(12):2967–71.
76. Kochakarn W, Leenanupunth C, Muangman V, Ratana-Olarn K, Viseshsindh V. Ejaculatory duct obstruction in the infertile male: experience of 7 cases at Ramathibodi Hospital. *J Med Assoc Thai* 2001; **84**(8):1148–52.
77. Nickel JC, Elhilali M, Vallancien G, Group A-OS. Benign prostatic hyperplasia (BPH) and prostatitis: prevalence of painful ejaculation in men with clinical BPH. *BJU Int* 2005; **95**(4):571–4.
78. Corriere JN, Jr. Painful ejaculation due to seminal vesicle calculi. *J Urol* 1997; **157**(2):626.
79. Weintraub MP, De Mouy E, Hellstrom WJ. Newer modalities in the diagnosis and treatment of ejaculatory duct obstruction. *J Urol* 1993; **150**(4):1150–4.
80. Tubaro A, Polito M, Giambroni L, Famulari C, Gange E, Ostardo E. Sexual function in patients with LUTS suggestive of BPH. *Eur Urol* 2001; **40**(Suppl 1):19–22.
81. Vallancien G, Emberton M, Harving N, van Moorselaar RJ, Alf-One Study G. Sexual dysfunction in 1,274 European men suffering from lower urinary tract symptoms. *J Urol* 2003; **169**(6):2257–61.
82. Frankel SJ, Donovan JL, Peters TI, *et al.* Sexual dysfunction in men with lower urinary tract symptoms. *J Clin Epidemiol* 1998; **51**(8):677–85.
83. Brookes ST, Donovan JL, Peters TJ, Abrams P, Neal DE. Sexual dysfunction in men after treatment for lower urinary tract symptoms: evidence from randomised controlled trial. *BMJ* 2002; **324**(7345):1059–61.
84. Rosen R, Altwein J, Boyle P, *et al.* Lower urinary tract symptoms and male sexual dysfunction: the multinational survey of the aging male (MSAM-7). *Eur Urol* 2003; **44**(6):637–49.
85. van Moorselaar RJ, Hartung R, Emberton M, *et al.* Alfuzosin 10 mg once daily improves sexual function in men with lower urinary tract symptoms and concomitant sexual dysfunction. *BJU Int* 2005; **95**(4):603–8.

CHAPTER 7.11

Priapism

Asif Muneer and David Ralph

Priapism—historical background and classification

The ancient Greek god Priapus was thought to be the son of Aphrodite and through the jealousy of Hera who cast a spell, Priapus was born with an enormous phallus, large hands, and tongue. It is from Priapus, the ancient god of fertility and gardening that the term priapism has been derived. Priapism is defined as a prolonged penile erection which persists in the absence of sexual stimulation and despite orgasm. The condition is a rare urological emergency with an incidence of 1.5 cases per 100,000 person-years.[1] The earliest documented account of this disorder is the citation *'Gonorrhoea, Satyriasi et Priapisme'* by Petraeus.[2]

Although a complete understanding of the underlying pathophysiology of this condition is still far from complete, a renewed interest in priapism has emerged over the last two decades. Both clinical studies and *in vitro* work has helped to formulate novel theories in order to explain the pathophysiology of the condition and develop novel management strategies. There are three main subtypes which are differentiated by the development of ischaemia within the corpus cavernosum. Ischaemic (low-flow) priapism is the commonest subtype, followed by non-ischaemic (high-flow) priapism, and then the rarer stuttering (recurrent) priapism. Differentiation between these three subtypes depends on the clinical characteristics and the presence or absence of an ischaemic milieu in the corpus cavernosum.

Pathophysiology of priapism

Ischaemic (low-flow priapism)

Ischaemic priapism is the most common and extensively investigated subtype. The majority of clinical cases are idiopathic; however, several aetiological factors have been identified from case reports, case series, and anecdotal evidence. The commonest risk factors include hypercellular haematological disorders (including sickle cell disease), malignancy, neurological conditions, and pharmacological agents such as antipsychotics or intracavernosal injections used for erectile dysfunction (see Table 7.11.1). In ischaemic priapism, the underlying factor which results in the development of the characteristic clinical picture and its long-term sequelae is stasis of deoxygenated blood in a closed compartment, akin to a compartment syndrome. As the duration of the priapism increases, the blood within the corpus cavernosum becomes increasingly hypoxic and acidotic,[3] and eventually develops glucopoenia.[4] The development and maintenance of this ischaemic extracellular milieu results in corpus cavernosum smooth muscle dysfunction, which can become irreversible if the ischaemia is not promptly reversed and normal cavernosal blood flow resumed.[4]

Using electron microscopy, the early histological changes within the cavernosal smooth muscle include an increase in size of the perinuclear cytoplasm, endoplasmic reticulum, ribosomes, and Golgi apparatus after approximately 12 hours. Between 24 and 48 hours, widespread endothelial destruction and exposure of the basement membrane occurs with subsequent thrombocyte adherence. The smooth muscle cells also undergo a transformation as described above, as well as necrosis, which culminates in a phenotypic change into fibroblast-like cells.[5] Clinically, priapism lasting for more than 24 hours is associated with the development of some degree of erectile dysfunction. In cases lasting longer than 72 hours, it is unlikely that any long-term erectile function will be maintained.

The complex regulatory mechanisms involved in achieving a penile erection provide several areas in the pathway where dysregulation may occur and lead to a persistent penile erection. The precise nature of the initiating mechanism in this condition is still unclear; however, it is undoubtedly multifactorial, involving central neuronal pathways, alterations in the corpus cavernosum microenvironment, modulation of the smooth muscle contractile machinery and aberrant neurotransmitter regulation in the corpus cavernosum. During the maintenance phase, there is an imbalance between the regulatory factors mediating vasorelaxation and vasoconstriction pathways in the penis. Although earlier studies suggested that nitric oxide (NO)-mediated smooth muscle relaxation is unlikely to have a role in priapism,[6] *in vivo* work utilizing endothelial NO synthase (eNOS)-negative mutant mice as a model for stuttering priapism have proposed that reduced endothelial NO/cyclic guanosine monophosphate (cGMP) production results in phosphodiesterase-5 (PDE5) dysregulation with a lowering of the PDE5 functional set point. Therefore, when neuronally derived NO mediates smooth muscle relaxation, there is insufficient PDE5 available to degrade it. Combined with the impaired procontractile effects of Rho-kinase in the corpus cavernosum, the overall balance is towards unregulated smooth muscle relaxation, and hence a persistent erection.[7]

Non-ischaemic (high-flow) priapism

High-flow priapism is relatively uncommon, and follows blunt trauma to the perineum or genitalia (typically after straddle-type injuries) where the cavernosal artery is compressed against the pubic bone. Patients commonly present after a delay following the initial injury with a non-painful persistent erection and this may occur several weeks following the initial injury. Analysis of the aspirated blood from the corpus cavernosum characteristically shows normoxia with a normal blood pH. Provided that the intracavernosal blood remains normoxic, the corpus cavernosum is unlikely to develop irreversible smooth muscle dysfunction. It is therefore important to accurately differentiate between the priapism subtypes so that the correct management can be instituted.[8,9]

Stuttering (recurrent) priapism

An estimated 20–25 million individuals are thought to suffer from stuttering priapism. Although the exact aetiology is poorly understood, this condition is common in patients with sickle cell disease, although idiopathic stuttering priapism as an entity is now also increasingly recognized. Clinically, stuttering priapism characteristically occurs nocturnally with intermittent painful erections. Erections become painful if the duration of the erection exceeds one hour. However, in some individuals the erections become painful after a shorter period. In patients with sickle cell disease, the erections are associated with the development of ischaemia and hence smooth muscle dysfunction may result after several short-lived episodes. Very rarely, stuttering priapism may also be a manifestation of short-lived high-flow episodes as a fistula may intermittently open and spontaneously close.[10,11] It is possible that stuttering priapism may represent the early phase of a disease continuum that culminates in a case of ischaemic priapism which is refractory to medical or surgical intervention.

Management of priapism

Priapism is an emergency and therefore patients require an urgent assessment and treatment, as a diagnostic delay may result in irreversible smooth muscle dysfunction. Provided that the diagnosis is established promptly, ischaemic priapism requires urgent intervention, whereas non-ischaemic priapism can initially be treated conservatively. Diagnostic uncertainty can result if there have been attempted interventions prior to presentation, such as corporal blood aspirations or inexperienced radiological evaluation, which can incorrectly diagnose a non-ischaemic priapism when the actual underlying condition is an ischaemic priapism. However, provided that the clinical history, corporal blood aspiration, and radiological assessment is all interpreted correctly, there should be no doubt with the underlying diagnosis.

Table 7.11.1 Common aetiological factors for priapism

Idiopathic		30% risk
Haematological	Sickle cell disease	
	Leukaemia	
	Polycythaemia	
	Thalassemia	
	Fabry's disease	
Antipsychotics	Chlorpromazine	
	Clozapine	
	Hydralazine	
	Prazosin	
	Guanethidine	
Intracavernosal injections	Papaverine	5% risk
	Prostaglandin E_1	1% risk
Malignancy	Metastatic prostate cancer	
	Bladder caner	
Neurological	Cauda equina	
	Spinal stenosis	

Radiological assessment of patients presenting with priapism

Penile ultrasound with colour Doppler studies provides a convenient and relatively easy assessment of the patient presenting with priapism. Ischaemic priapism characteristically will show poor perfusion of the cavernosal tissue and in more prolonged cases, distal fibrosis is evident. In contrast, non-ischaemic priapism will demonstrate perfusion throughout the corpus cavernosum, as well as the site of the arteriosinusoidal fistula. Where the facility is available, penile MRI is useful in imaging cases where there is diagnostic uncertainty, or in prolonged ischaemic priapism to establish the viability of the cavernosal smooth muscle.

Management of ischaemic priapism

The initial management of patients with ischaemic priapism involves the administration of analgaesia. As the duration of the penile erection increases, the corpus cavernosum becomes increasingly hypoxic and acidotic. This results in painful stimuli via nociceptors in the penis, and opioid analgaesia is often required.[12] Once adequate pain relief has been administered to the patient a clinical history should establish whether there are any predisposing medical conditions or risk factors which have resulted in the development of the priapism. However, aspiration of stagnant blood from the corpus cavernosum normally aids in establishing a correct diagnosis. Following a local anaesthetic dorsal penile nerve block, a large-gauge needle can be inserted directly into the corpus cavernosum laterally to avoid the dorsal neurovascular bundle and urethra. Alternatively, the needle can be inserted directly through the glans penis and into the distal corpus cavernosum. Aspiration of deoxygenated and viscous blood is characteristic of ischaemic priapism. In some instances where the duration of priapism is short, this diagnostic procedure in itself may resolve the problem if veno-occlusion is successfully reversed and reperfusion with oxygenated blood allows penile detumescence.[13,14] The aspirated blood should undergo biochemical analysis in order to calculate the pO_2, pH, and glucose levels. This helps to verify that this is indeed an ischaemic priapism.[13–15] Unsuccessful detumescence following aspiration of blood from the corpus cavernosum requires additional pharmacological and surgical steps.

The next step involves the instillation of α-adrenergic agonists to induce smooth muscle contraction in the corpus cavernosum and the helicine arteries. This reduces the volume of stagnated blood within the penis and relieves the pressure on the subtunical venules and promotes successful detumescence. However, the cavernosal smooth muscle may still fail to contract due to the metabolic alterations in the immediate microenvironment of the cavernosal smooth muscle.

The most common agent utilized is the α-adrenergic agonist phenylephrine which is injected intracavernosally in aliquots of

200–500 µg.[15] Careful monitoring of the patient's blood pressure is required, as the adrenergic effects of the drug on the systemic circulation can lead to systemic hypertension particularly with repeated doses.[15] Alpha agonists attach to the α1 receptor on smooth muscle, resulting in an increase in the intracellular IP_3 levels. The IP_3 attaches to the sarcoplasmic reticulum, which releases Ca^{2+} into the sarcoplasm and stimulates myosin light chain kinase resulting in smooth muscle contraction (Fig. 7.11.1). Alternative α-adrenergic agents that have successfully been utilized include adrenaline, noradrenaline, and metaraminol.[15] Oral terbutaline has also been reported to be successful,[16,17] although it does have β_2 agonist effects and minor β_1 activity.[14] Alternative medical treatments such as methylene blue and etilefrine have been utilized in patients who fail to respond to these measures.

Methylene blue is a compound with several biological effects. It is a well-known inhibitor of soluble guanylate cyclase (sGC).[18] By inhibiting intracellular sGC and thereby reducing cGMP levels, cavernosal smooth muscle tone is increased. The use of methylene blue has been limited to anecdotal reports and small case series.[19–21] Etilefrine is an α-adrenergic agonist that has the advantage of oral administration as well as intracavernous use. It is successfully utilized in sickle cell patients.[22–24]

Surgical management of ischaemic priapism

The underlying physiological basis for surgical interventions is to divert ischaemic blood from the corpus cavernosum into the venous system by developing a new channel of blood flow. The main surgical procedures that have been utilized are listed in Table 7.11.2.[25,26]

The Winter shunt and the Ebbehoj procedure both allow a simple way of creating a shunt between the corpus spongiosum and the corpus cavernosum. A narrow-blade scalpel is inserted into the glans, dorsal to the urethral meatus and into the corpus cavernosum. Multiple incisions are made through the same entry site by rotating the scalpel blade by 90 degrees. The overlying glans is then closed using sutures. In contrast, Winter's procedure uses a Tru-cut biopsy needle to remove a core of tunica albuginea and therefore create fistulous communications. Several attempts may be required before detumescence occurs.

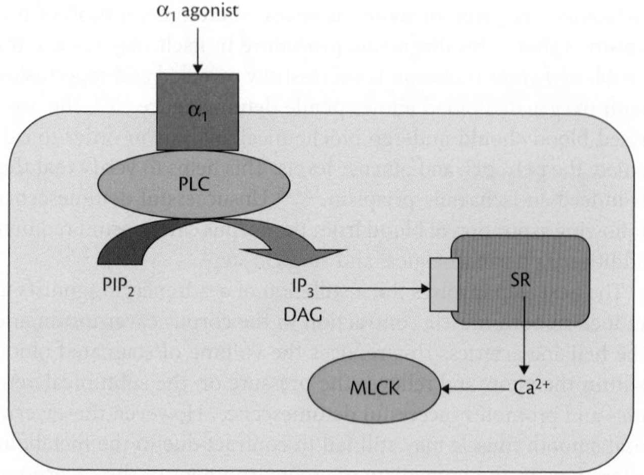

Fig. 7.11.1 Intracellular mechanism of alpha agonists to induce smooth muscle contraction.
SR: sarcoplasmic reticulum; MLCK: myosin light chain kinase; PLC: phospholipase C.

Table 7.11.2 Surgical interventions for ischaemic priapism

Year	Technique
1964	Quackels procedure
1964	Grayhack procedure
1975	Ebbehoj procedure
1976	Winter shunt
1976	Barry procedure
1981	Al Ghorab procedure
2008	Lue T shunt and tunnelling

Despite these surgical procedures, over 50% of patients still develop erectile dysfunction following successful detumescence with the erectile dysfunction rate being even higher when the duration of the priapism is longer.[12]

More complex shunt surgery has been attempted with limited success. Proximal shunts can be created between the proximal corpus spongiosum and corpus cavernosum by making a small corporotomy (called a Grayhack procedure) (Fig. 7.11.2), or between the saphenous vein and corpus spongiosum (termed a Quakels procedure) (Fig. 7.11.3). The success of these procedures is limited in prolonged cases, as the blood flow out of the ischaemic compartment is impaired.

Recently, further modifications of the shunt procedures have been described. The T shunt (Fig. 7.11.4) involves inserting a scalpel through the glans penis and into the tip of the corpus cavernosum followed by a 90-degree rotation of the scalpel. If there is still a failure of detumescence then the procedure is repeated on the opposite side. Failure of this manoeuvre is followed by inserting a small dilator through the glans penis and into the corpus cavernosum (known as tunnelling).

The high incidence of erectile dysfunction following prolonged ischaemic priapism episodes is due to the development of fibrosis in the corpus cavernosum. Depending on the amount of viable smooth muscle, treatment with PDE5 inhibitors may be successful but failure of pharmacological treatment ultimately requires insertion of a penile prosthesis. This surgical option provides girth and rigidity to allow penetrative intercourse, but the insertion of an

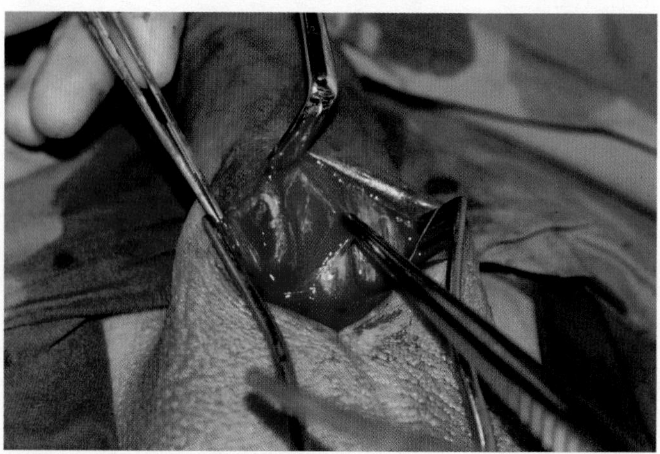

Fig. 7.11.2 Grayhack procedure.

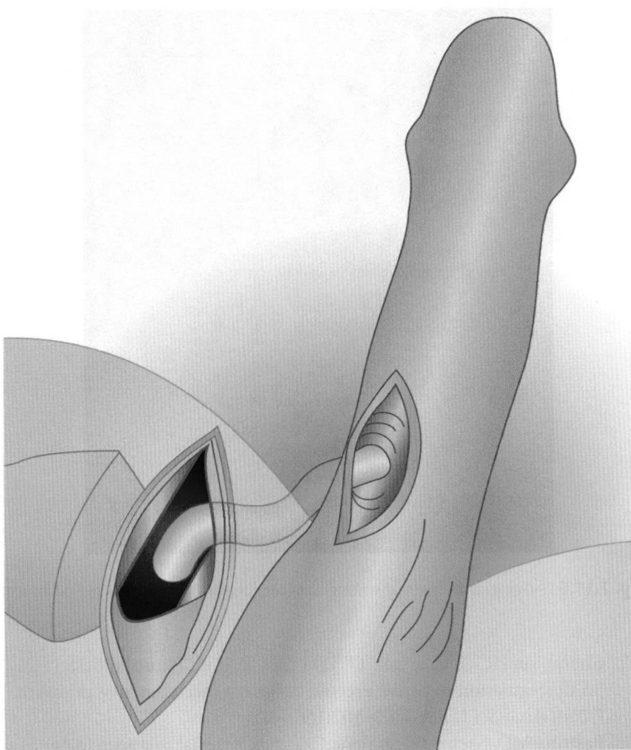

Fig. 7.11.3 Quakels procedure.

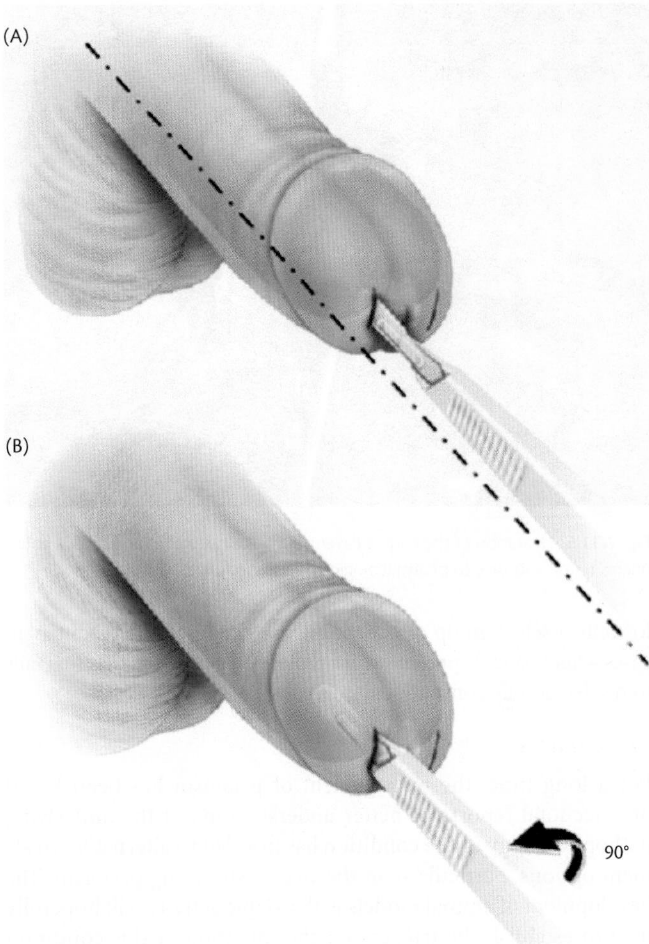

Fig. 7.11.4 T shunt. A scalpel is inserted through the glans penis (A) and into the corpus cavernosum followed by rotation in a direction away from the urethral meatus (B).

Reprinted by permission from Macmillan Publishers Ltd: *Nature Reviews Urology*, Yun-Ching Huang *et al.*, 'Evaluation and management of priapism: 2009 update', Volume 6, pp. 262–271, Copyright © 2009, Rights Managed by Nature Publishing Group, DOI:10.1038/nrurol.2009.50

implant in a heavily fibrosed corpora is notoriously difficult and is associated with complications such as urethral injury, crural perforation, failure to dilate, and prosthetic infection. Although additional surgical manouvres and special cavernotomes can aid in the delayed placement of a penile prosthesis, an alternative option is to insert a prosthesis at an earlier stage.[27] Ischaemic priapism with a prolonged duration and which is refractory to pharmacological or surgical intervention is suitable for immediate penile implant placement, provided that there is evidence of smooth muscle necrosis within the corpus cavernosum (see Fig. 7.11.5).[28] The advantage of this early placement is that the penile length is maintained and the space in the corpus cavernosum can be created without facing extensive fibrosis. Although malleable implants are easily inserted, exchange to an inflatable implant can be performed at a later date.

Management of non-ischaemic priapism

Although patients present with less pain due to the presence of normoxic blood within the corpus cavernosum, the persisting erection can still remain troublesome. Differentiating this condition from ischaemic priapism is a priority, and is aided by taking an accurate and thorough clinical history combined with Doppler studies that show an increased arterial blood flow to the penis. The blood is well oxygenated and the risk of ischaemic damage with eventual corporal fibrosis and impotence is low. Potency is reported to be preserved in 77–86% of patients with long-term follow-up.[8] Arteriography combined with superselective embolization using absorbable material (e.g. gelfoam), is the treatment of choice in this condition (see Fig. 7.11.6).[9,10] In the presence of fistulae at the base of the corpora, duplex ultrasound-guided compression can also be successful in reversing the high-flow priapism. Open arterial ligation using intraoperative ultrasound techniques has also been described.[11]

Management of stuttering priapism

Patients with problematic stuttering priapism can be offered oral medication, with refractory cases requiring surgical intervention. Several oral agents have been used in the past based solely on anecdotal evidence, including digoxin, procyclidine, pseudoephedrine, and terbutaline. More recently, 5-alpha reductase inhibitors and ketoconazole have also been used in small case series. However, the most efficacious treatments involve antiandrogens (cyproterone acetate) or lutenizing hormone-releasing hormone (LH-RH) analogues. Recent studies have also found that there is a paradoxical effect following the long-term administration of a PDE5 inhibitor, in that it can reduce the frequency of erections in these patients[29] based on studies using eNOS knockout mice.[7] Treatment failures have prompted surgical interventions in the form of phenylephrine drug delivery systems, which have been successful only in the short term. Ultimately, the insertion of a penile prosthesis can overcome problematic erections

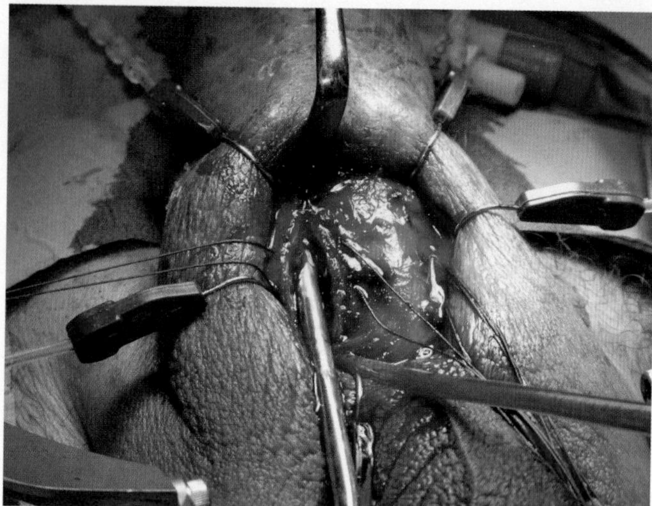

Fig. 7.11.5 Dilatation of the corpus cavernosum in a case of refractory low-flow priapism unresponsive to pharmacological treatment for 72 hours.

for only a select group of patients. These can be inserted acutely in cases where patients present with a prolonged penile erection that fails to resolve despite conventional medical treatment.[28]

Conclusion

For a long time, the management of priapism has been based on anecdotal reports. A better understanding of the underlying pathophysiology of the condition has now led to alternative treatment options, particularly in the area of stuttering priapism. The development of animal models with priapic activity will hopefully help to establish the triggers for the initiation of this condition and allow for better targeted therapies in the erectogenic pathway.

Acknowledgement

Chapter adapted with permission from Asif Muneer, *The Investigation of Corpus Cavernosum Smooth Muscle Dysfunction in Ischaemic Priapism*, A thesis submitted in fulfilment of the requirements for the degree of Doctor of Medicine, University College London, UK, Copyright © Asif Muneer 2007; and Asif Muneer et al, 'Management of Priapism', *Touch Urology*, Copyright © 2012, http://www.touchurology.com/articles/management-priapism

References

1. Earle CM, Stuckey BGA, Ching HL, Wisniewski ZS. The incidence and management of priapism in western Australia: a 16 year audit. *Int J Impot Res* 2003; **15**:272–6.
2. Hinman F. Priapism: report of cases in a clinical study of the literature with reference to its pathogenesis and surgical treatments. *Ann Surg* 1914; **60**:689.
3. Broderick GA, Harkaway R. Pharmacologic erection: time-dependent changes in the corporal environment. *Int J Impot Res* 1994; **6**(1):9–16.
4. Muneer A, Cellek S, Dogan A, *et al.* Investigation of cavernosal smooth muscle dysfunction in low-flow priapism using an in vitro model. *Int J Impot Res* 2005; **17**(1):10–18.
5. Spycher MA, Hauri D. The ultrastructure of the erectile tissue in priapism, *J Urol* 1986; **135**(1):142–7.
6. Kim JJ, Moon DG, Koh SK. The role of nitric oxide in vivo feline erection under hypoxia. *Int J Impot Res* 1998; **10**(3):145–50.

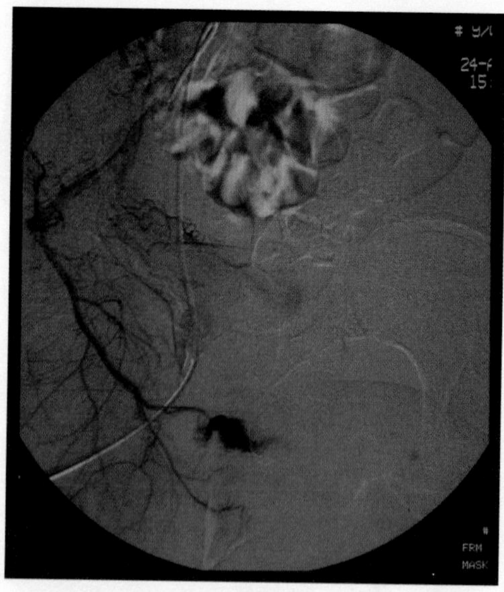

Fig. 7.11.6 Angiography demonstating a fistula causing non-ischaemic priapism.

7. Champion HC, Bivalacqua TJ, Takimoto E, *et al.* Phosphodiesterase-5A dysregulation in penile erectile tissue is a mechanism of priapism. *P Natl Acad Sci U S A* 2005; **102**:1661–6.
8. Bastuba MD, Saenz dT, Dinlenc CZ, *et al.* Arterial priapism: diagnosis, treatment and long-term follow-up. *J Urol* 1994; **151**(5):1231–7.
9. Hatzichristou D, Salpiggidis G, Hatzimouratidis K, *et al.* Management strategy for arterial priapism: therapeutic dilemmas. *J Urol* 2002; **168**(5):2074–7.
10. Volkmer BG, Nesslauer T, Kuefer R, *et al.* High-flow priapism: a combined interventional approach with angiography and colour Doppler. *Ultrasound Med Biol* 2002; **28**(2):165–9.
11. Brock G, Breza J, Lue TF, Tanagho EA. High-flow priapism: a spectrum of disease. *J Urol* 1993; **150**(3):968–71.
12. Pohl J, Pott B, Kleinhans G. Priapism: a three-phase concept of management according to aetiology and prognosis. *Br J Urol* 1986; **58**(2):113–18.
13. Lue TF, Hellstrom WJ, McAninch JW, Tanagho EA. Priapism: a refined approach to diagnosis and treatment. *J Urol* 1986; **136**(1):104–8.
14. Pautler SE, Brock GB. Priapism. From Priapus to the present time. *Urol Clin North Am* 2001; **28**(2):391–403.
15. Bochinski DJ, Deng DY, Lue TF. The treatment of priapism—when and how?. *Int J Impot Res* 2003; **15**(Suppl 5):S86–90.
16. Shantha TR, Finnerty DP, Rodriquez AP. Treatment of persistent penile erection and priapism using terbutaline. *J Urol* 1989; **141**(6):1427–9.
17. Ahmed I, Shaikh NA. Treatment of intermittent idiopathic priapism with oral terbutaline. *Br J Urol* 1997; **80**(2):341.
18. Trigo-Rocha F, Hsu GL, Donatucci CF, Lue TF. The role of cyclic adenosine monophosphate, cyclic guanosine monophosphate, endothelium and non-adrenergic, non-cholinergic neurotransmission in canine penile erection. *J Urol* 1993; **149**(4):872–7.
19. de Holl JD, Shin PA, Angle JF, Steers WD. Alternative approaches to the management of priapism. *Int J Impot Res* 1998; **10**(1):11–14.
20. Martinez PF, Hoang-Boehm J, Weiss J, *et al.* Methylene blue as a successful treatment alternative for pharmacologically-induced priapism. *Eur Urol* 2001; **39**(1):20–23.
21. Martinez Portillo FJ, Fernandez Arancibia MI, Bach S, *et al.* Methylene blue: an effective therapeutic alternative for priapism induced by intracavernous injection of vasoactive agents. *Arch Esp Urol* 2002; **55**(3):303–8.
22. Okpala I, Westerdale N, Jegede T, Cheung B. Etilefrine for the prevention of priapism in adult sickle cell disease. *Br J Haematol* 2002; **118**(3):918–21.

23. Gbadoe AD, Atakouma Y, Kusiaku K, Assimadi JK. Management of sickle cell priapism with etilefrine. *Arch Dis Child* 2001; **85**(1):52–3.
24. Albrecht W, Stackl W. Treatment of partial priapism with an intracavernous injection of etilefrine. *JAMA* 1997; **277**(5):378.
25. Ebbehoj J. A new operation for priapism. *Scand J Plast Reconstr Surg* 1974; **8**(3):241–2.
26. Winter CC. Cure of idiopathic priapism: new procedure for creating fistula between glans penis and corpora cavernosa. *Urology* 1976; **8**(4):389–91.
27. Bertram RA, Carson CC III, Webster GD. Implantation of penile prostheses in patients impotent after priapism. *Urology* 1985; **26**(4):325–7.
28. Rees RW, Kalsi J, Minhas S, *et al.* The management of lowflow priapism with the immediate insertion of a penile prosthesis. *BJU Int* 2002; **90**(9):893–7.
29. Burnett AL, Bivalacqua TJ, Champion HC, Musicki B. Feasibility of the use of Phosphodiesterase-5 Inhibitors in a pharmacological prevention programme for recurrent priapism. *J Sex Med* 2006; **3**:1077–84.

CHAPTER 7.12

The ageing male

Geoffrey I. Hackett

Introduction to the ageing male

As much of primary care management involves the prevention of cardiovascular events, the life expectancy of men has improved considerably over the last 30 years but life expectancy still lags an average of six years behind women in most European countries (Fig. 7.12.1).[1]

Patients would ideally like to enjoy a higher quality of life in these additional years, essentially extending the years of middle life rather than senility. Issues such as the prevention of osteoporosis or dementia in ageing men become more important as longevity is enhanced. These are issues that we rarely discuss with ageing men. Under the heading of 'the ageing male', somewhat different symptoms and complaints are listed by multiple authors.[2] These include:

(i) Physical changes, increased visceral and abdominal fat, decreased muscle strength, insulin resistance, type 2 diabetes, increasing severity of cardiovascular disease

(ii) Vegetative or somatoform complaints

(iii) Cognitative complaints; reduced concentration and forgetfulness

(iv) Affective and mood changes: depression, anxiety, tearfulness, irritability, and reduced sexual interest

(v) Behavioural changes, such as reduction in sexual activity or reduced time spent on hobbies once enjoyed

The contributions of biological and psychosocial determinants of age-related complaints remains controversial: similar complaints motivating middle-aged men to seek medical or psychological help have been interpreted by clinical and developmental psychologists as a 'mid-life crisis'. Psychosocial changes and transitions in middle-aged men, such as grown-up children leaving home ('empty nest'), unfulfilled life and career aspirations, ill elderly relatives, an increase vulnerability to economic changes in the workforce,

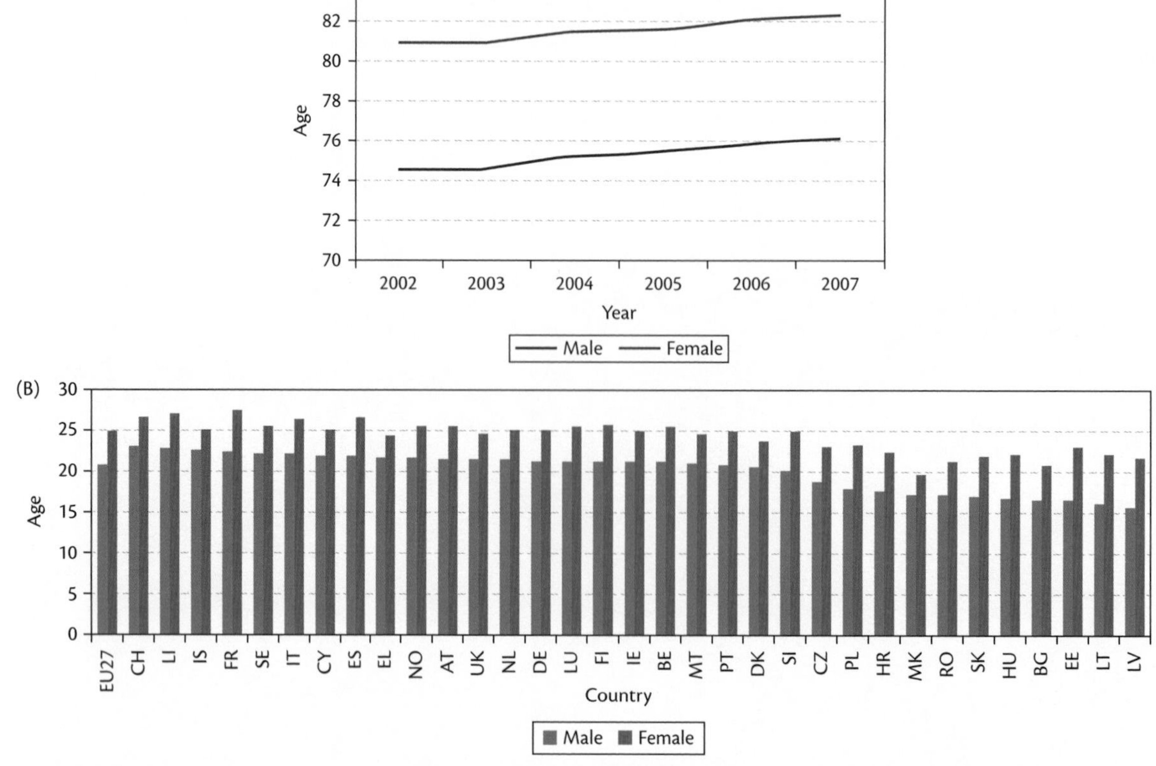

Fig. 7.12.1 (A) Time trends in life expectancy, by sex, EU27, 2002–2007; and (B) life expectancy from age 60 years, sex and country, latest year.

Reproduced with permission from European Commission, *The State of Men's Health in Europe*, Copyright © European Union, 1995–2015, available from http://ec.europa.eu/health/population_groups/docs/men_health_report_en.pdf. Source: data from Eurostat demo_mlexpec 1 2008 except EU27, BE, FR, IT, UK (2007).

and so on may culminate in significant distress in the age span 40–60. From this perspective, negative, age-related stereotypes of physical and mental stress contribute significantly to distress in middle-aged men along with dissatisfaction with their relationship and work. Age-related resources (experience, reflectiveness, caution) are seen as undervalued components of 'healthy ageing'.[2] A major research problem resides in the fact that the definitions of the ageing male are based on clinical samples with a lack of systematic studies in the ageing community. The MMAS[3] focused on the associations and impact of erectile dysfunction in an ageing population. Beutel *et al.* reviewed[2] stratified samples of 2,182 men in age groups (18–75) and found a continuous increase of physical, mental, and general fatigue and a reduction of activity and motivation with age. Exhaustion, cardiovascular, and musculoskeletal complaints increased, along with reduced health satisfaction and increased depression scores. Marked increase of certain complaints were more specific to certain age groups, dissatisfaction with sexuality increased markedly above 60, anxiety was greatest at ages 60–70 and then improved. Household income and employment were strong associations with anxiety and depression at all ages. The lack of a partner was consistently associated with poor satisfaction with health, particularly over 60.

The European report on men's health (2010)[1] focused on men's treatment-seeking behaviour at different ages across Europe. Men are low attenders at primary and secondary care services below the age of 45, but over the age of 75 account for significantly greater occupancy of acute hospital beds than women.[1] Such reports have led to greater interest in preventative strategies for men over 40 to reduce the huge secondary care burden created by the ageing male population.

Hormones and ageing

For over 30 years, physicians have been aware of the importance of multiple hormonal changes with ageing, including growth hormone, IGF-1, DHEa-sulphate, thyroxine, and melatonin. Leptin and sex hormone-binding globulin (SHBG) levels increase with age and oestrogen changes little with age.[4]

Testosterone levels fall progressively in men from the age of 30 by 1% per annum[5] but few primary care physicians consider measurement of testosterone in men presenting with symptoms, such as tiredness, sweating, poor concentration, altered mood, depression, or erectile dysfunction.[4] This is despite evidence-based guidelines from urology[6–8] and endocrine societies recommending testosterone measurement as best practice in cases of ED and type 2 diabetes. Androgen therapy has been viewed with suspicion by urologists, often perceived as quackery. Others have felt that it is inappropriate to interfere with normal ageing processes or that we must heed warnings from our enthusiasm for hormone replacement therapy (HRT) in females.

Several terms have been used for the condition of androgen deficiency in ageing males, but late-onset hypogonadism or testosterone deficiency syndrome (TDS) are currently preferred.[7] The term 'andropause' is not currently fashionable, as it suggests that there is a male equivalent to the female menopause. Other terms include androgen deficiency of the ageing male (ADAM), partial androgen deficiency of the ageing male, or partial androgen deficiency.

The current BSSM (British Society for Sexual Medicine), ISSAM (International Society for Study of the Aging Male), EAU (European Urology Association) definition of late onset hypogonadism[7] is: 'A biochemical syndrome associated with advancing age and characterised by a deficiency in serum androgen levels with or without a decreased genomic sensitivity to androgens. It may result in significant alterations in the quality of life and adversely affect the function of multiple organ systems.'

This state of hypogonadism causes a global decrease in energy and a decrease in the feeling of well-being. It also causes a change in sexual function and has other endocrine and metabolic repercussions. These can affect bones, muscles, and lipids, as well as cognitive function TDS or late-onset hypogonadism as defined on the basis of clinical symptoms associated with abnormal testosterone levels. The European Male Ageing Study[9] (EMAS) studied 3,369 men aged 40–79 at eight European centres and concluded that the three following cardinal symptoms were most likely to be related to low levels of testosterone:

- Erectile dysfunction
- Reduced sexual desire
- Loss of morning erections

Other symptoms such as hot flushes, sweats, tiredness, loss of vitality, reduced shaving frequency, gynaecomastia, depressed mood, poor concentration, and sleep disturbance were regarded as less specific.

Recent guidelines suggest that a level of total testosterone of <8 nmol/L or free testosterone of less than 180 pmol/L require testosterone replacement therapy and total testosterone of >12 nmol/L or free testosterone of >225 pmol/L do not. Between these levels, a trial of therapy for a minimum of six months should be considered based on symptoms (Fig. 7.12.2).[7]

Biochemical assessment of hypogonadism

Total testosterone should be measured between the hours of 7–11 am on two occasions at least one month apart and ideally be assessed by mass spectrometry (ID-GCMS). Equilibrium dialysis is currently the gold standard for free testosterone, as immunoassays based on analogue displacement are currently inaccurate.[7,8] The EAU/ISSM/BSSM management algorithm is shown in Figure 7.12.2.

Assessing symptoms of low testosterone

As many of the symptoms of hypogonadism are vague in nature, initial assessment and subsequent response may be best undertaken with the aid of one of the following validated questionnaires[8]:

- The Ageing Males' Symptoms (AMS) scale is a 17-item questionnaire and is useful in the diagnosis of hypogonadism and in monitoring changes in response to treatment with testosterone;
- The Androgen Deficiency in Ageing Men (ADAM) scale is a 10-item questionnaire that is useful for screening and within clinical consultations;
- The International Index of Erectile Function (IIEF); or
- The Sexual Health Inventory for Men (SHIM);
- The Hospital Anxiety and Depression Scale (HADS) or PHQ9 are currently used in primary care to assess depression in chronic medical conditions in primary care. Symptoms of depression and hypogonadism often overlap and antidepressants may exacerbate the symptoms of hypogonadism.

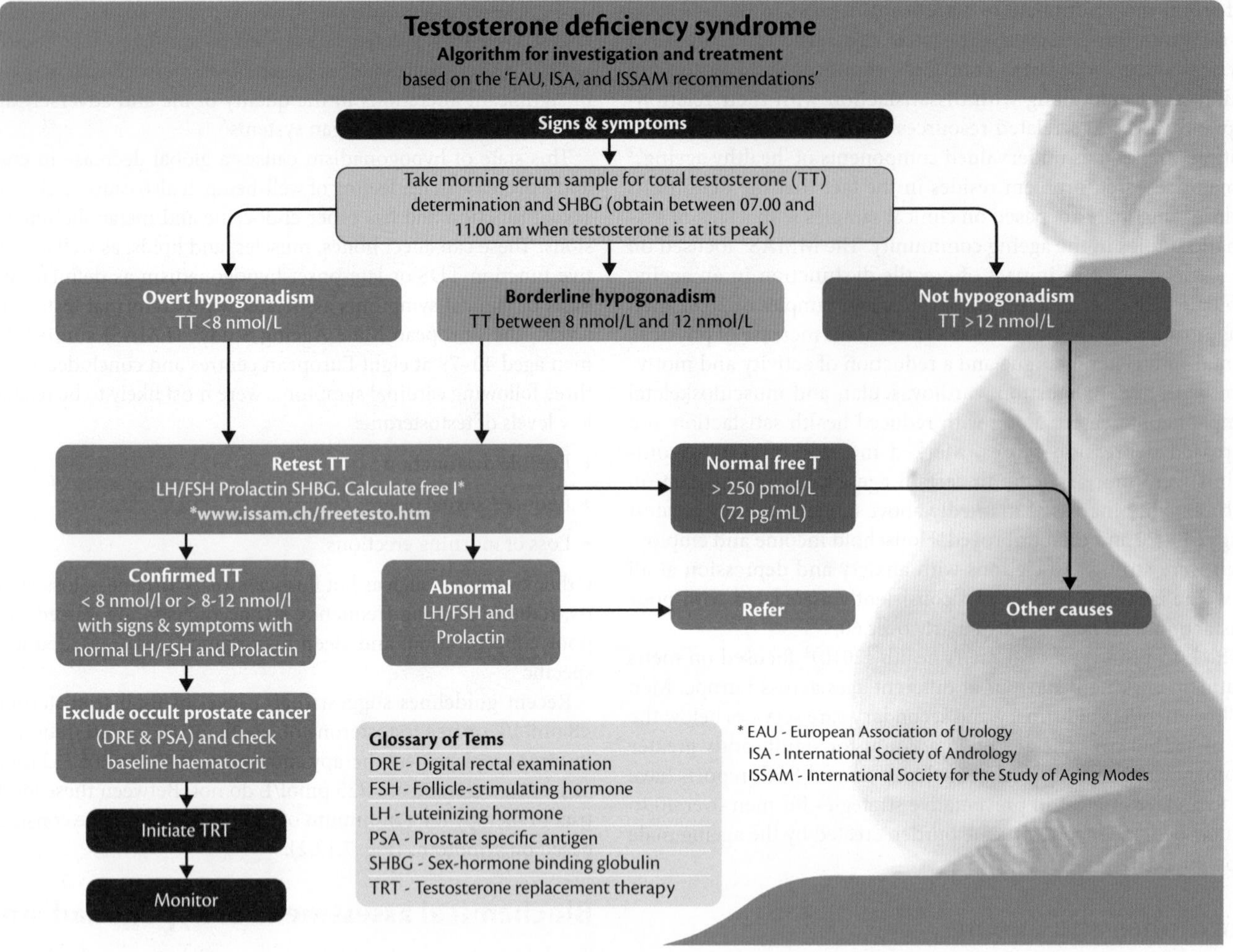

Fig. 7.12.2 Testosterone deficiency syndrome.

Reproduced with permission from E. Nieschlag *et al.*, Investigation, treatment and monitoring of late-onset hypogonadism in males: ISA, ISSAM, and EAU recommendations, *International Journal of Andrology*, Volume 28, Issue 3, pp. 125–127, Copyright © 2005 John Wiley and Sons.

Low testosterone and increased mortality

There is increasing evidence that TDS is associated with increased cardiovascular and all-cause mortality.[9–16] Two recent meta-analyses have looked at a large number of long-term studies linking low testosterone to increased cardiovascular and all-cause mortality. Araujo[19] concluded that the evidence for a link between low testosterone was strong but concluded that the differences in cohort selection and choice baseline testosterone measurement were important particularly as SHBG rises with age and falls with obesity and insulin resistance. Haring *et al.*[20] looked at the data in terms of several models and found that even after strict adjustment for co-morbidities there seems to be a link between mortality risk and testosterone level throughout the studies (Table 7.12.1).

A recent study of 3,637 community-dwelling men aged 70–88 in Western Australia[17] showed that low free testosterone, raised SHBG, and lutenizing hormone (LH) were associated with all-cause and cardiovascular deaths (HR 1.62 95% CI 18.2–24.8). An earlier study from the same authors studied 3,443 men[18] over 70 and showed an increased risk of stroke and transient ischaemic attack (TIA) associated with minor reductions in total and free testosterone <11.7 nmol/L (HR 1.99). Another recent study suggested that the combination of low free testosterone and low vitamin D were associated with increased all-cause mortality.

Mortality studies from high-risk groups

Malkin *et al.* (Fig. 7.12.3)[21] followed up to 930 men referred with coronary artery disease for 6.9 years. The prevalence of hypogonadism was 24%, mortality rates were 21% versus 12% ($p = 0.002$) for hypogonadal men versus eugonadal, and the study was halted early at 6.9 years. Only beta-blocker therapy and left ventricular failure were found to have a greater influence on survival.

Muraleedaran *et al.*[22] screened a primary care diabetic population of 587 patients and followed them up for 5.8 years. They found 475 of men had normal TT levels, 22% were overtly hypogonadal (<8 nmol/L) and 31% were in the borderline range. These percentages were in close agreement with earlier publications by Kapoor *et al.*[23] and Hackett *et al.*[24]

Effect of low testosterone on surrogate markers for cardiovascular risk

Decreases in serum total cholesterol have been noted as early as after four weeks[25] but most studies have reported a decrease after

Table 7.12.1 Association of low testosterone levels with all-cause mortality by difference cut-offs from recent studies

Cut-off for the definition of low total testosterone (TT)	MMAS; 8 TT <6.94 nmol/L (200 ng/dL)	Wang; 34 TT <8.0 nmol/L (230 ng/dL)	Rancho Bernardo 7 TT <8.36 nmol/L (241 ng/dL)	Male veterans Study; 35 TT <8.7 nmol/L (250 ng/dL)	HIM; 36 TT <10.41 nmol/L (300 ng/dL)	EPIC; 6 TT <12.5 nmol/L (360 ng/dL)	Age-specific cut-off <10th percentile
Low TT (n)	34	69	82	98	241	474	
Model 1	1.59 (0.83; 4.02)	1.96 (0.93; 3.63)	2.21 (1.26; 3.89)**	2.24 (1.41; 3.57)**	1.33 (0.93; 1.90)	1.28 (0.95; 1.72)	2.21 (1.40; 3.49)**
Model 2	2.12 (1.01; 4.46)*	2.08 (1.12; 3.86)*	2.33 (1.33; 4.12)**	2.10 (1.34; 3.29)**	1.28 (0.89; 1.84)	1.20 (0.88; 1.62)	2.26 (1.43; 3.59)**
Model 3	2.50 (1.18; 5.27)*	2.24 (1.21; 4.17)*	2.53 (1.43; 4.47)**	2.32 (1.38; 3.89)**	1.37 (0.95; 1.99)	1.28 (1.93; 1.75)	2.35 (1.47; 3.74)***
Model 4	2.68 (1.19; 6.04)*	2.13 (1.06; 4.26)*	2.56 (1.38; 4.76)**	1.92 (1.18; 3.14)**	1.11 (0.72; 1.69)	1.10 (0.78; 1.56)	2.25 (1.35; 3.75)**

Model 1: adjusted for age. Model 2: adjusted for age, and WC. Model 3: adjusted for model 2, smoking (3 categories), high-risk alcohol use, and physical activity. Model 4: adjusted for model 3, renal insufficiency, and DHEAS. HR, hazard ratio; CI, 95% confidence interval; CVD, cardiovascular disease; WC, waist circumference; DHEAS, dehydroepiandrosterone sulfate.

*p, 0.05.

**p, 0.01.

***p, 0.001.

Reproduced from Robin Haring *et al.*, 'Low serum testosterone levels are associated with increased risk of mortality in a population-based cohort of men aged 20–79', *European Heart Journal*, Volume 31, Issue 12, pp. 1494–1501, Copyright © 2010. Published on behalf of the European Society of Cardiology. All rights reserved. & The Author 2010, by permission of Oxford University Press.

three months.[25] Greater reductions were seen in obese men[25] with metabolic syndrome. The MRFIT[26] study showed that hypogonadal men had slightly increased triglycerides and high-density lipoproteins (HDL), leading to the suggestion that testosterone replacement therapy (TRT) might be expected to lower triglycerides and HDL.

The decrease in serum triglycerides follows a similar pattern: after four weeks with decrease over nine months[25] and maximum effect at 12 months.[25] The decrease in low-density lipoprotein cholesterol seems somewhat slower: after three months, after 40–44 weeks, or after 12 months.[25]

Studies have found both an increase and decrease in HDL cholesterol[25] dependent on the presence of diabetes or the use of statins. TRT has also been shown to reduce fibrinogen to levels similar to fibrates. Low androgen levels are associated with inflammation.[25] A decline was noted in IL6 and TNF-alpha within 16 weeks[25] and in another study after 16 weeks.[25] In the Moscow study, C-reactive protein was reduced by TRT at 30 weeks versus a placebo.[27]

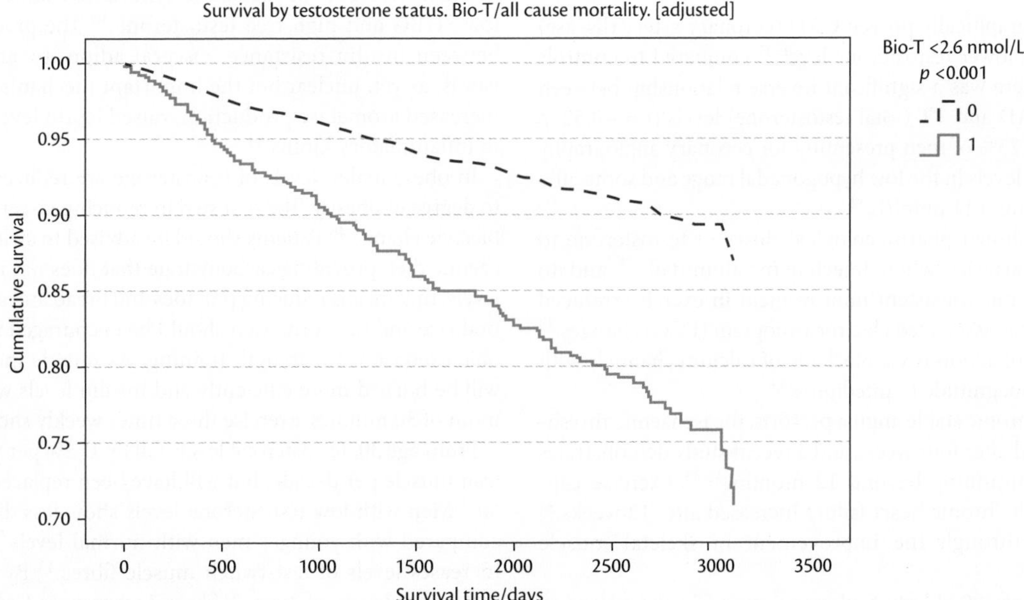

Fig. 7.12.3 Effect of baseline bioavailable testosterone on all-cause mortality in men with proven coronary heart disease (n = 930 mean follow-up of 6.9 years).

Reproduced from *Heart*, Chris J Malkin *et al.*, Low serum testosterone and increased mortality in men with coronary heart disease, Volume 96, Issue 22, pp. 1821–1825, 2010, with permission from BMJ Publishing Group Ltd.

Several studies have shown reduction in waist circumference, visceral fat, and BMI.[25] Preliminary longer term studies suggest considerable weight loss can be seen for up to four years. Placebo-controlled studies in untreated hypertension are difficult to conduct for ethical reasons. In some studies a decline in diastolic blood pressure has been observed, after 3–9 months,[25] and in systolic blood pressure.[25] Maximum effects were observed after 12 months.[25] A decrease in arterial stiffness measured as pulse wave velocity was measurable after 48 weeks,[25] and in large artery compliance after three months[25] a reduction on carotid artery intimal thickness was observed at 12 months in one study but this did not reach significance due to the small cohort size.[25]

The effects of testosterone replacement therapy on cardiovascular mortality

A prospective recent study of 587 men with type 2 diabetes[28] involved 5.8 years follow-up. Low testosterone was defined as TT <10.4 nmol/L. Fifty-eight men were treated with testosterone for two years or more. The mortality rate was 20% in the untreated group, 9.1% in the normal group independent of co-morbidities and therapies. Mortality was 8.6% in the treated group ($p = 0.049$).

A similar retrospective US study involved 1,031 men with 372 on TRT. The cumulative mortality was 21% in the untreated group versus 10% ($p = 0.001$) in the treated group, with greatest effect in younger men and those with type 2 diabetes.[29] In a recent paper of 145 patients with first ischaemic stroke and diabetes, 66% were found to be hypogonadal. In the testosterone-treated group, 7% had a recurrence of stroke in two years versus 16.6% in the control group with 28% of the treated men returning to work versus 6% of the control group. There were significant improvements in lipid profile and HbA1c.[30]

Effects on angina threshold and heart failure

Men with angiographically proven CAD (coronary artery disease) had significantly lower testosterone levels[31] compared to controls ($p < 0.01$) and there was a significant inverse relationship between the degree of CAD and TT (total testosterone) levels ($r = -0.52$, $p < 0.01$).[25] Nearly 25% of men presenting for coronary angiography had testosterone levels in the low hypogonadal range and some 50% had a TT of less than 11 nmol/L.[32]

Studies have shown pharmacological doses of testosterone to relax coronary arteries when injected intraluminally[33] and to produce modest but consistent improvement in exercise-induced angina and reverse-associated electrocardiogram (ECG) changes.[33] The mechanism of action is via blockade of calcium channels with effect of similar magnitude to nifedipine.[33]

In men with chronic stable angina pectoris, the ischaemic threshold had increased after four weeks and a recent study demonstrates improvement continuing beyond 12 months.[32,33] Exercise capacity in men with chronic heart failure increased after 12 weeks,[34] predominantly through the improvement in skeletal muscle performance.

A recent trial of 209 elderly frail men[35] over 65 randomized to receive either placebo or 100 g of topical testosterone gel was terminated early as there were 23 cardiac events (two deaths) in the 106 men in the testosterone group versus five in the placebo group, despite positive results in study end points. These events included myocardial infarction and dysrhythmias and hypertension. The authors conceded that there were more cardiovascular co-morbidities in the active treatment group and that the starting dose and escalation was outside the product licence. The active treatment group had more severe CAD. The study involved rapid escalation up to 150 mg per day, above the manufacturer's recommended dose, and many of the events were reported with inadequate validation.

Insulin resistance and type 2 diabetes

Studies have shown an inverse relationship between serum testosterone and fasting blood glucose and insulin levels.[3,26,36] Both hyperinsulinaemia and low testosterone have been shown to predict the development of type 2 diabetes (T2D).[3,26,37–43] Medications such as chronic analgesics, anticonvulsants, 5-ARIs, and androgen ablation therapy are associated with increased risk of testosterone deficiency and insulin resistance.[7,8]

Hypogonadism is a common feature of the metabolic syndrome.[6] Intra-abdominal adiposity (IAA) drives the progression of multiple risk factors directly, through the secretion of excess free fatty acids and inflammatory adipokines, and decreased secretion of adiponectin.[44] The important contributions of IAA to dyslipidaemia and insulin resistance provide an indirect, though clinically important, link to the genesis and progression of atherosclerosis and cardiovascular disease.[44] The presence of excess IAA is an important determinant of cardiometabolic risk. IAA is accompanied by elevated C-reactive protein and is associated with an inflammatory cascade, with the expression of a number of atherogenic inflammatory kinins leading to cardiovascular plaque and type 2 diabetes. The INTERHEART Study[45] involving 29,972 participants examined the contributory factors involved in a first acute myocardial infarction and found IAA to be an important predictive factor. It recommended waist circumference or hip–waist ratio as a standard measurement of cardiovascular risk. Women with T2D or metabolic syndrome characteristically have low SHBG and high free testosterone.[10] The precise interaction between insulin resistance, visceral adiposity, and hypogonadism is, as yet, unclear but the important mechanisms are through increased aromatase production, raised leptin levels, and increase in inflammatory kinins.[44]

In obese males, levels of testosterone are reduced in proportion to degree of obesity. The first step in reducing visceral fat is diet and lifestyle change.[46] Patients should be advised to switch to a low glycaemic diet, providing carbohydrate that does not increase glucose levels; that means reducing potatoes and bread and substituting natural rice and full corn. Men should be encouraged to combine aerobic exercise with strength training. As muscle increases, glucose will be burned more efficiently and insulin levels will fall. A minimum of 30 minutes' exercise three times weekly should be advised.

From age 30, testosterone levels fall by 1–2% per year and 3 kg of lean muscle per decade, but will have been replaced by even more fat.[3] Men with low testosterone levels show less diurnal variation compared with younger men with normal levels.[7,8] Testosterone increases levels of fast-twitch muscle fibres.[43] By increasing testosterone, levels of type 2 fibres increase and glucose burning improves. Weight loss will increase levels of testosterone and augment the effects of lifestyle and exercise advice.[46]

Table 7.12.2 Outcome of therapy in a population of men with type 2 diabetes and hypogonadism (BLAST)

	HbA1c (%) >7.5	Weight (kg)	BMI (kg/m²)	WC (cm)	TC (mml/l)	EF (IIEF)	AMS (pts)	HADS-D	GEQ (% imp)
30 weeks	−0.41	−0.7	−0.3	−2.5	−0.25	+3.0	−5.3	−1.01	46
p value	0.007	0.13	0.01	0.012	0.025	0.006	0.095	0.64	<0.001
82 weeks	−0.87	−2.7	−1.00	−4.2	−0.19	+4.31 +9.57 PDE5I	−8.1	−2.18	68–70
p value	0.009	0.016	0.019	<0.001	0.035	0.003	0.001	0.001	0.0001

Reproduced with permission from G. Hackett *et al.*, 'The response to testosterone undecanoate in men with type 2 diabetes is dependent on achieving threshold serum levels (the BLAST study)', International *Journal of Clinical Practice*, Volume 68, Issue 2, pp. 203–215, Copyright © 2014 John Wiley & Sons Ltd.

Diabetologists have traditionally considered the fall in testosterone level as being a consequence of obesity but studies now clearly show that low testosterone leads to visceral obesity and metabolic syndrome, and is also a consequence of obesity.[4] Four large long-term studies have shown that baseline levels of testosterone predict the later development of type 2 diabetes.[3,10,26,37] In the case of MMAS, a baseline total testosterone of less than 10.4 nmol/L was associated with a greater than fourfold incidence of type 2 diabetes over the next nine years and NHANES-III followed up men from as young as 20 and found a similar fourfold greater prevalence independent of obesity or ethnicity.[37] UK diabetes data from 2010[47] showed the prevalence of type 2 diabetes in men aged 35–44 to be doubled that of women, despite men in that age group having lower levels of obesity and taking more exercise. This effect was even more marked in southern Asian men.[47] A study has recently commenced in Australia to establish whether treating young obese men with low testosterone will reduce the incidence of type 2 diabetes. There is high-level evidence that TRT improves insulin resistance, as measured by HOMA-IR, reduces HbA1c[39] (by approximately 0.7% by 18 months),[42] and inflammatory markers (CRP, IL6, and TNF-alpha) in men with type 2 diabetes and metabolic syndrome.[27,38–43] There is high level of evidence for reduction in total cholesterol,weight, BMI and visceral fat (a significant marker for CV risk) and improvement of lean muscle mass. Improvements in sexual function were seen in men with baseline TT levels below 8 nmol/L with metabolic parameters requiring sustained levels above 14 nmol/L for 12–18 months. The BLAST study[27] suggested that men with depression (23% of the cohort with diabetes) were markedly less responsive (Table 7.12.2).

Osteoporosis, recurrent falls, and muscle strength

The prevalence of osteoporosis in men over 50 is 4–6%, and hypogonadism, particularly with onset in younger men, is an acknowledged risk factor (in around 20% of all male cases) with white men at greater risk (7%) than black (5%), or Hispanic American men (3%).[47,48,49] This becomes more important when population data show that by age 75 there are around 60 living men for every 100 living women.[1] The morbidity and mortality of osteoporotic fractures are significantly higher in men than women (Fig. 7.12.4).[50]

In terms of both primary and secondary prevention of osteoporosis, men are largely ignored, with the perception being that osteoporotic fracture is almost exclusively a problem in postmenopausal women.[49] Current NICE (National Institute of Health and Clinical Excellence) guidance[49] on osteoporosis concentrates exclusively on women and there is currently no guidance for men, although hypogonadism is frequently quoted as a major risk factor. NICE guidance on prostate cancer[50] does stress the importance of osteoporosis treatment in men on androgen ablation therapy.

The importance of androgen deficiency in relation to osteoporosis is more significant, as hypogonadism has been associated with cognitive impairment[51] and risk of falls in the elderly,[51] increasing fracture risk. The MINOS study looked at 1,040 French men aged 51–54 and the MrOS[52,53] study in the United States studied 2,587 community based men aged 65 to 99 and concluded that men with a bioavailable testosterone in the lower quartile had a 40% additional risk of fall. The effect was most apparent in the 65 to 69 age group, and in men aged over 80 testosterone levels were not associated with falls. The authors concluded that 'these results provide additional justification for trials of testosterone in older men and should aid in the design of those studies'.

Despite these findings, Kiebzak *et al.*[54] in a review of 363 patients admitted for osteoporotic fracture (110 men and 253 women) only 4.5% of men versus 27% of women had prior treatment. The 12-month mortality for men of 32% for osteoporosis is less clear but 30% of all hip fractures over 75 occur in men compared with 17% for women. At 12-month follow-up of survivors, 27% of men versus 71% of women were taking treatment (usually only calcium and vitamin D). Eleven per cent (11%) of men versus 27% of women received follow-up bone density assessment.

A long-term study on the effects of testosterone treatment showed that bone mineral density continues to increase in the lumbar spine after 18 to 30 months of treatment. Meta-regression analysis performed at the lumbar spine and femoral neck revealed a significant effect of TRT, and pooled results from eight randomized clinical trials (RCTs)[55] found that testosterone had a moderate effect on bone resorption markers. To date, no adequately powered trial has yet explored the impact of therapy on hip and vertebral fracture.

Recurrent falls in the elderly are associated with considerable mortality and economic burden. Risk of falling has been shown to be clearly associated with loss of lean muscle especially in the lower limbs of ageing men. Srinivas-Shanker *et al.*[56] studied 274 intermediate-frail and frail elderly hypogonadal (mean T 11.1 nmol/L) men, aged 65–90 years treated with 25–75 mg testosterone gel or placebo daily for six months and followed up for another six months after cessation of therapy. Mean T increased to 18.4 nmol/L at six months, and declined to 10.5 nmol/L at 12 months. Isometric knee extension peak torque, lean body mass (plus decreased body fat) and somatic and sexual symptoms improved significantly in the T-arm compared to placebo but

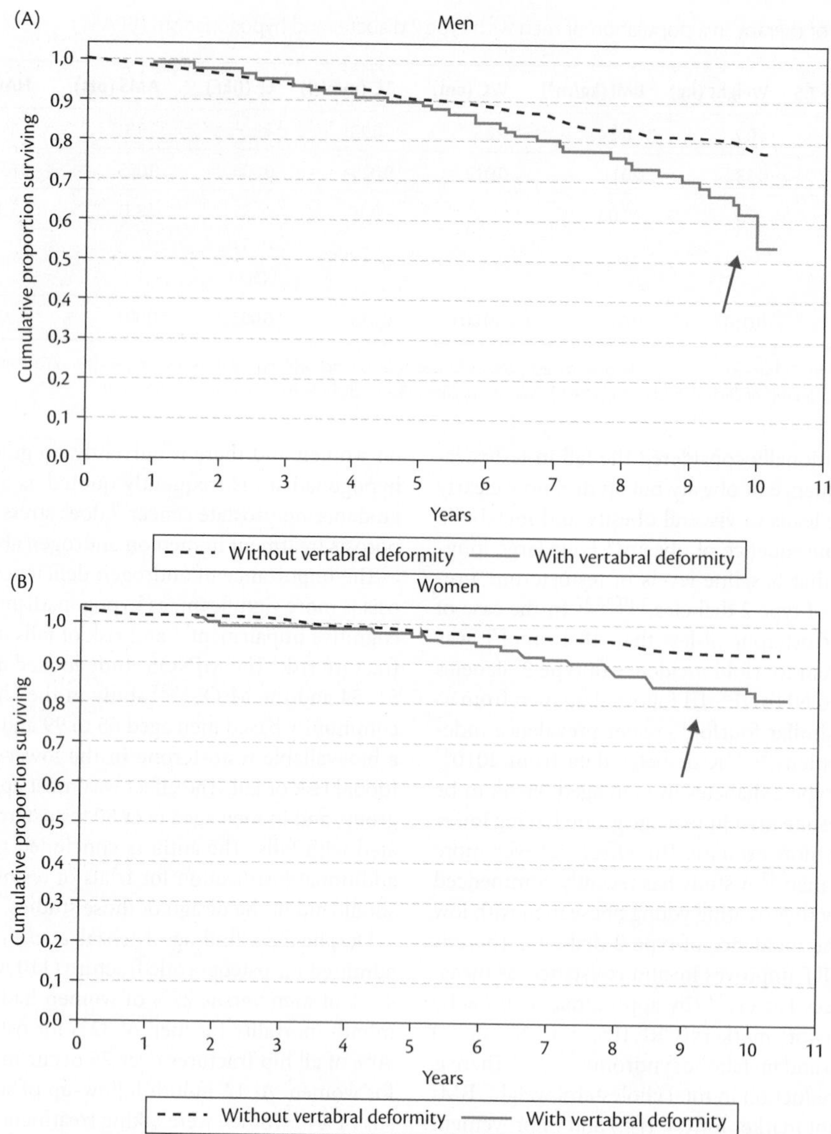

Fig. 7.12.4 Vertebral fractures and mortality. (A) Cumulative survival rate, adjusted to age 65 years, in men with a prevalent vertebral deformity, using deformity criterion—3 SD, at baseline compared with men without a vertebral deformity, during a 10-year follow-up period. (B) Cumulative survival rate, adjusted to age 65 years, in women with a prevalent vertebral deformity, using deformity criterion 3 SD, at baseline compared with women without a vertebral deformity, during a 10-year follow-up period.

Springer, *Osteoporosis International*, Volume 14, 2003, pp. 61–68, 'Prevalent vertebral deformities predict increased mortality and increased fracture rate in both men and women: A 10-year population-based study of 598 individuals from the Swedish cohort in the European Vertebral Osteoporosis Study', R. Hasserius, Figure 1 and 2, Copyright © International Osteoporosis Foundation and National Osteoporosis Foundation 2003. With kind permission from Springer Science and Business Media.

improvements were seen no more after six-month T-withdrawal. The message is that benefits occur relatively early but treatment must be considered for the long term.

Cognitive function

There is evidence that hypogonadism is associated with decreased cognitive function and that testosterone administration enhances performance on spatial cognition and mathematical reasoning.[51] In the MMAS,[3] there was no evidence that older age was associated with testosterone in terms of spatial ability, working memory and speed/attention when adjusted for age and covariants. However, in the 10-year longitudinal assessment of multiple cognitive domains, higher free testosterone predicted better scores on visual and verbal memory, visual-spatial functioning, visual motor scanning, and a reduced rate of longitudinal decline in visual memory.[57] Studies consistently show that T therapy improves mood, energy, and well-being in younger men, but the effects tend to be less clear in ageing men.[57] Nevertheless, benefits are consistently clear in a subset of ageing men with manifest low testosterone.[58]

Mood and depression

Symptoms associated with low testosterone are diminished energy, reduced vitality or well-being, increased fatigue, depressed mood, impaired cognition, decreased muscle mass, and strength, diminished bone density, and anaemia. The lifetime prevalence of depression, at 24%, is known to be three times higher in type 2 diabetics than the general population and the most commonly cited reason is the burden of co-morbidities in diabetes.[59] None of the papers reviewed in meta-analysis of 42 studies in 200,145 subjects considered androgen status, despite the obvious overlap in symptoms between hypogonadism and depression. Diabetes was found to be a greater risk factor for depression in male than in female type 2 diabetics and sexual problems were the complication most associated with depression.[60,61]

A randomized placebo-controlled study[62] of long-acting testosterone undecanoate for 30 weeks on 184 men with metabolic syndrome or type 2 diabetes (mean age 52 and mean baseline testosterone of 8 nmol/L) showed significant improvements in Beck Inventory scores (BDI) for testosterone versus placebo of 2.5 points and 7.4 points on the ageing male score, as well as three-point improvements on the IIEF. The recently published BLAST study in type 2 diabetes showed significant improvement in depression and anxiety scores along with all domains of sexual function, most marked after 12–18 months with long-acting testosterone undecanoate.[42] Presence of depression reduced the metabolic response to testosterone.

Although low testosterone has been shown to predict incident depression in ageing men, only two of nine RCTs (randomized clinical trials) have shown a significant improvement on depression scores in a general population of ageing men compared with placebo.[63] Combined therapy with antidepressants has been shown to be superior to antidepressant plus placebo in a group of younger men with refractory depression.[64]

Testosterone and Alzheimer's disease

Men are relatively protected from Alzheimer's disease compared with women. There is evidence that androgens confer protection from Alzheimer's disease in their own right and a recent study found a link between cognitive functioning and bioavailable testosterone.[65,66] Testosterone therapy has been shown to improve mood and quality of life in men with Alzheimer's disease despite cognitive improvement failing to reach clinical significance. The conclusion from these studies would be that free testosterone should be monitored in cases of Alzheimer's disease and a therapeutic trial may be appropriate in many cases.[67]

Testosterone and quality of life

Several studies have shown improvement in AMS scores with testosterone therapy but the validity of these finding have been questioned in patients with chronic illness. Validated quality of life (QoL) tools such as SF12 and SF36 have shown significant improvements in physical and mental health scores in general populations of ageing men both with and without diabetes.[68] In the BLAST diabetes study, at 12–18 months nearly 70% of mean (men age 62) stated that testosterone therapy had improved their health and in 38% that improvement was definite.[42]

Treatments

Long-term safety of testosterone therapy

A meta-analysis of 1,000 patient-years[69] versus placebo suggests a slight reduction in myocardial infarction and cerebrovascular accident (CVA) but a marked reduction in coronary interventions (Fig. 7.12.5). There was a 6% incidence of raised haematocrit (>50%) without significant consequences and no deaths in the active treatment group versus five in the placebo cohort.

Two recent publications in the United States based on healthcare databases[70,71] suggested a possible increase in cardiovascular events with TRT but both have been heavily criticised due to flawed methodology and statistics. Two retrospective studies, one on diabetes,[28,29] suggest lower mortality (Fig. 7.12.6).

Anderson *et al.*[73] reported 5,695 men followed up over three years and based on therapeutic levels of testosterone, showed a marked reduction in mortality and major coronary events (MACE) but non-significant reduction in absolute numbers of myocardial events. This suggests that testosterone in a marker of frailty and associated with the likelihood of surviving incident cardiac and non-cardiac events (see Fig. 7.12.7).

A 2015 paper based on four-year follow-up of 859 patients from the BLAST[74] study showed an independent reduction in mortality with both TRT and PDE5i therapy (Fig. 7.12.8), most marked in older men (Fig. 7.12.9). A further study evaluated 7,860 men with type 2 diabetes (mean age 70) and reported a 28% reduction in all-cause mortality in men prescribed PDE5 inhibitors for ED.[75] These findings are of significant importance as prescribing has been discouraged in older men due to a perception of increased risk.

At least seven observational studies have reported no association of lower urinary tract symptoms (LUTS) with serum testosterone level and five have shown an inverse relationship.[76] No studies to date show an increase in LUTS/BPH symptoms with higher serum testosterone levels.[77] The balance of studies of TRT suggest an *improvement* in LUTS. As TRT has been shown to up-regulate PDE5, increase pelvic blood flow and enhance the effect of PDE5is (now an accepted therapy for both ED and LUTS), it is no longer logical to advice avoidance of TRT in men with mild to moderate BPH.

Calof[69] also found that patients on testosterone were 12 times more likely to get a prostate biopsy but no more likely to have a positive finding.

Several studies and meta-analyses have failed to show a link between TRT and development of prostate cancer[76,78,79] but several have shown a tendency for more aggressive prostate cancer in men with low testosterone (Fig.7.12.10). One recent study of 279 consecutive patients referred for biopsy on the basis of abnormal digital rectal examination (DRE) or raised prostate-specific antigen (PSA) found that low bioavailable testosterone and high SHBG were associated with a 4.9 and 3.2-fold risk of positive biopsy.[80]

Current EAU, ISSAM, and BSSM guidance[7,8] is that there is 'no evidence TRT is associated with increased risk of prostate cancer or activation of subclinical cancer'.

Despite these conclusions, many patients are deprived clinical and metabolic benefit because of slight normal physiological increases in PSA and concerns that no long-term study has conclusively proved absolute safety. Because of logistic and ethical reasons, the ideal long-term study is unlikely to be done and until then physicians will have to practice on using the best available evidence.

Dehydroepiandrogen

This weak androgen precursor is available as a food supplement in the United States, with little convincing evidence for cardiovascular benefit. A recent 12-month double-blind placebo-controlled study

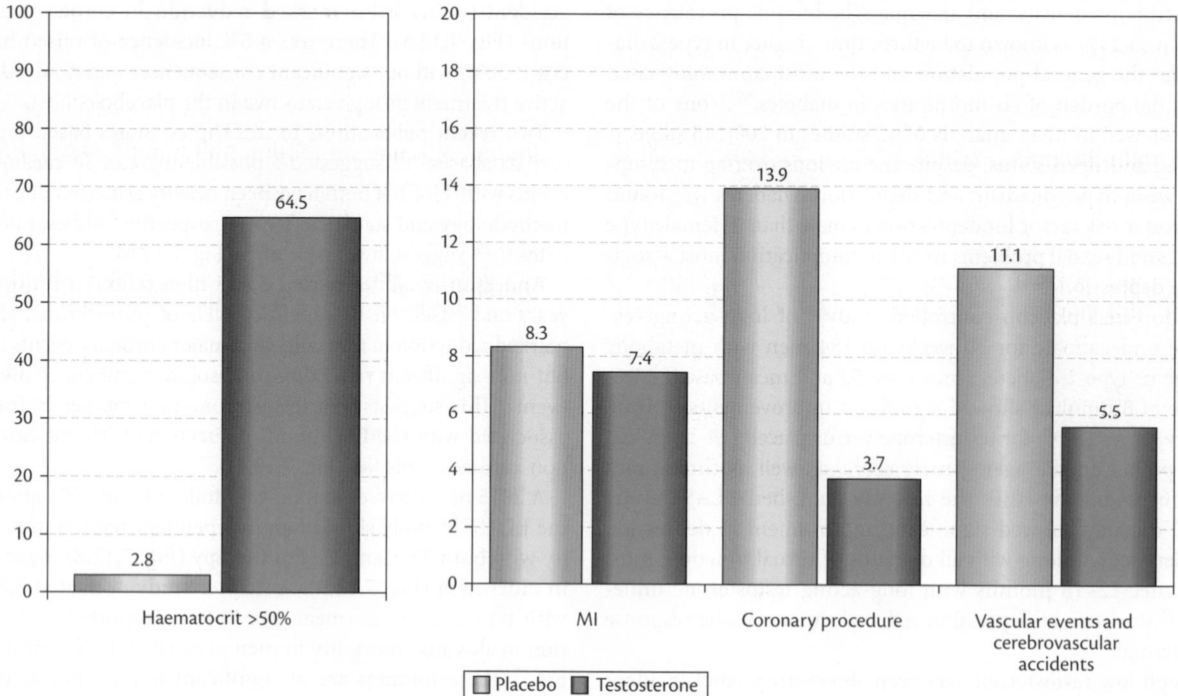

Fig. 7.12.5 Meta-analysis of placebo-controlled testosterone trials in middle-aged and older men: cardiovascular adverse event rates per 1,000 patient-years.

Notes: A meta-analysis of randomized clinical trials to determine the risks of adverse events associated with testosterone replacement in older men. The MEDLINE database was searched from 1966 to April 2004, using testosterone as the indexing term; limits included human, male, > or = 45 years old, and randomized controlled trial. Of the 417 studies thus identified, 19 met the inclusion criteria: testosterone replacement for at least 90 days, men > or = 45 years old with low or low-normal testosterone level, randomized controlled trial, and medically stable men. Odds ratios (ORs) were pooled using a random effects model, assuming heterogeneous results across studies, and were weighted for sample size. In the 19 studies that met eligibility criteria, 651 men were treated with testosterone and 433 with placebo. Testosterone-treated men were nearly four times as likely to have haematocrit >50% as placebo-treated men (OR = 3.69, 95% CI, 1.82–7.51). The frequency of cardiovascular events, or death was not significantly different between the two groups.

Source: data from Calof OM *et al.*, 'Adverse events associated with testosterone replacement in middle-aged and older men: a meta-analysis of randomized, placebo-controlled trials', *The Journals of Gerontology: Series A*, Volume 60, Issue 11, pp. 1451–7, Copyright © 2005, Oxford University Press.

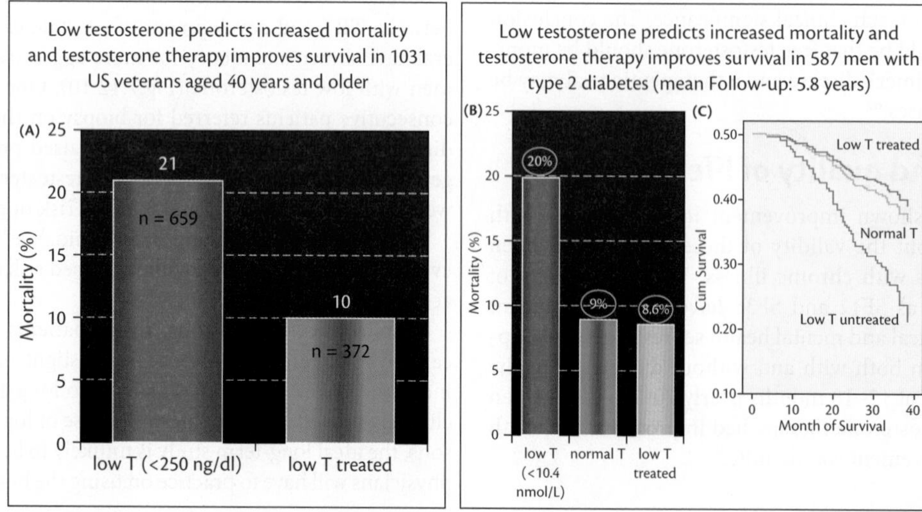

Fig. 7.12.6 Long-term mortality studies on testosterone replacement therapy (TRT).

(A) Source: data from Shores M *et al.*, 'Testosterone treatment and mortality in men with low testosterone', *The Journal of Clinical Endocrinology and Metabolism*, Volume 96, Issue 6, pp. 2011–2591, Copyright © 2015 Endocrine Society; (B) Source: data from Muraleedharan V. *et al.*, 'Testosterone deficiency is associated with increased risk of mortality and testosterone replacement improves survival in men with type 2 diabetes', *European Journal of Endocrinology*, Volume 169, Issue 6, pp. 725–733, Copyright © 2013 European Society of Endocrinology; and (C) Reproduced with permission from Muraleedharan V *et al.*, 'Testosterone deficiency is associated with increased risk of mortality and testosterone replacement improves survival in men with type 2 diabetes', *European Journal of Endocrinology*, Volume 169, Issue 6, pp. 725–733, Copyright © 2013 European Society of Endocrinology.

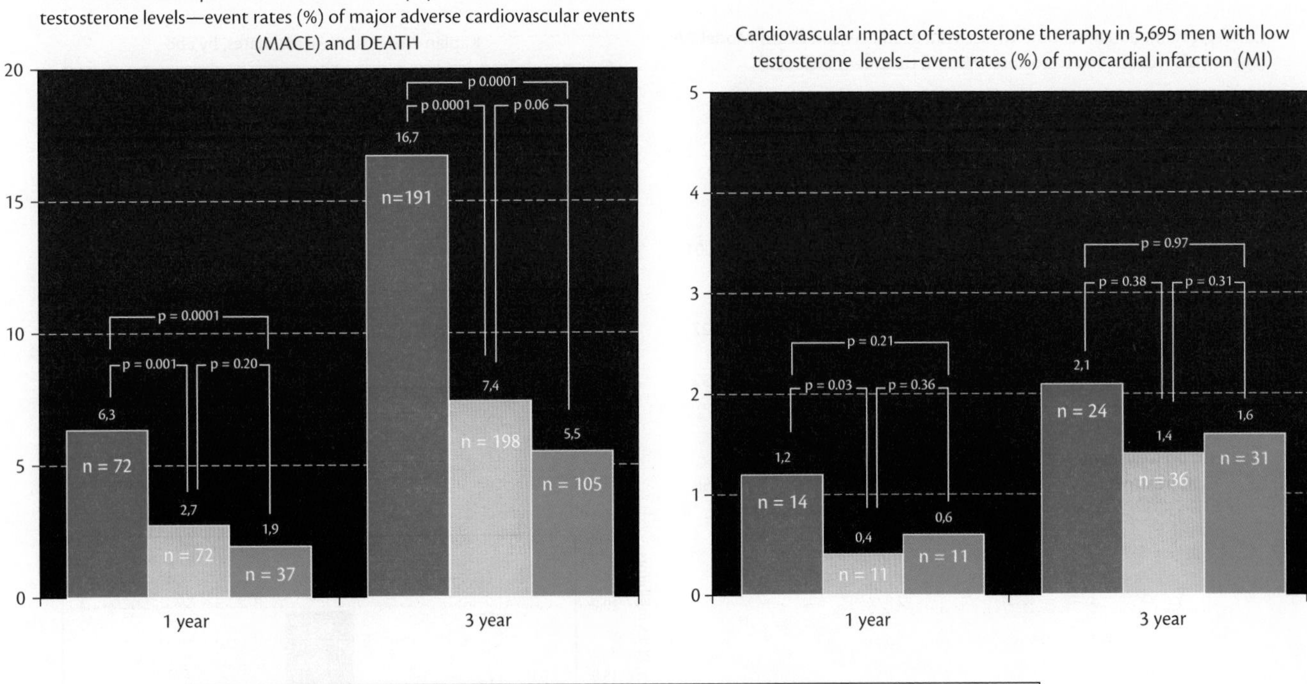

Fig. 7.12.7 TRT reduces mortality and major coronary events (MACE) and death but not absolute rate of mild cognitive impairment and cerebrovascular accident (CVA).

Source: data from Anderson JL *et al.*, 'Abstract 13220: Cardiovascular Impact of Testosterone Therapy in Men with Low Testosterone Levels', *Circulation*, Volume 130: Abstract 13220, Copyright © 2014, Wolters Kluwer Health.

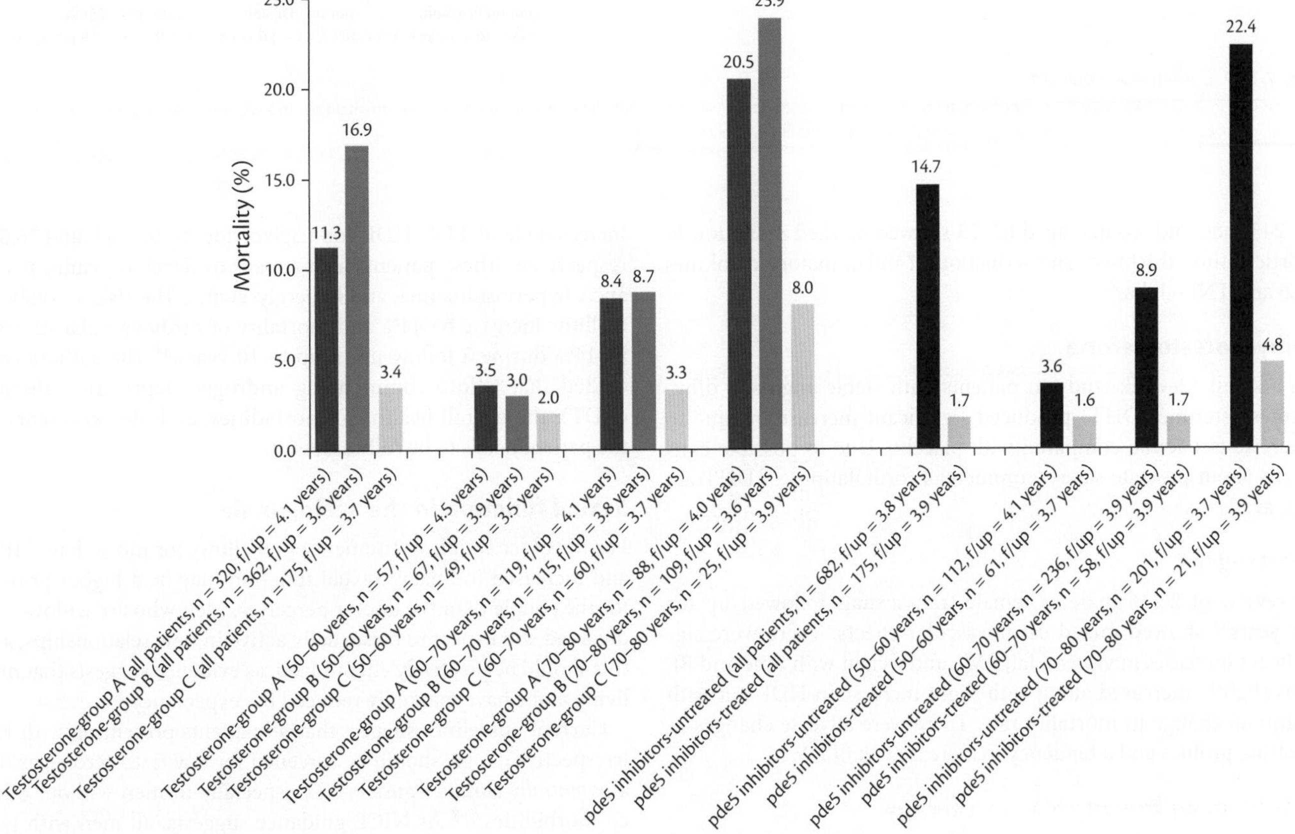

Fig. 7.12.8 Long-term mortality data in diabetes.

Source: data from G. Hackett *et al.*, 'The response to testosterone undecanoate in men with type 2 diabetes is dependent on achieving threshold serum levels (the BLAST study)', *International Journal of Clinical Practice*, Volume 68, Issue 2, pp. 203–215, Copyright © 2014 John Wiley & Sons Ltd.

Cox regression, outcome: time to last visit/death, censor: death Model 2A (age at visit 1/death and testosterone/statin treatment included)

n = 682 (patients not on PDE5 inhibitors)

Variables	HR (95 confidence intervals)	*p*
Age at last visit/death (continuous variable: years)	1.10 (1.07–1.12)	<0.001
Testosterone treatment		
Group A	0.62 (0.41–0.95)	0.027
Group B	Reference	
Group C	0.33 (0.12–0.92)	0.033
Statins		
Not on treatment	Reference	
On treatment	0.66 (0.44–1.01)	0.058

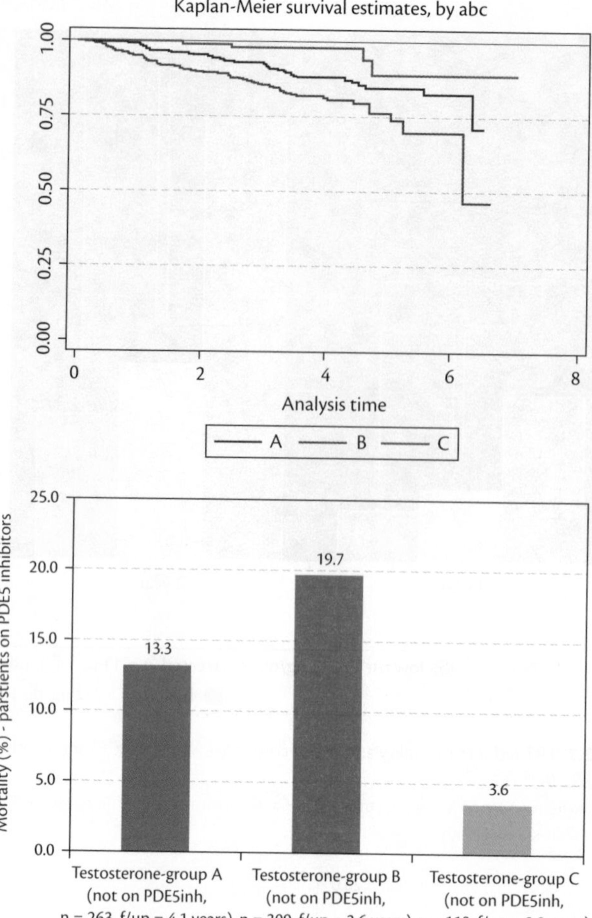

Fig. 7.12.9 Cox regression outcome.

Source: data from G. Hackett *et al.*, 'The response to testosterone undecanoate in men with type 2 diabetes is dependent on achieving threshold serum levels (the BLAST study)', *International Journal of Clinical Practice*, Volume 68, Issue 2, pp. 203–215, Copyright © 2014 John Wiley & Sons Ltd.

of 243 men and women aged 65–75 showed marked reduction in aortic intima thickness and reduction of inflammatory cytokines IL6 and TNF-alpha.[81]

Dihydrotestosterone

In a small 12-week study in patients with stable angina,[82] dihydrotestosterone (DHT) produced significant increase in time to exercise ischaemia compared with placebo. Due to possible concerns about prostate safety, commercial formulations of DHT are not available.

Oestrogens

A review of 2,236 male to female transsexuals followed up for 31 years[83] showed mixed cardiovascular effects. There were significant increases in visceral fat, BMI, and weight with time and BP was slightly increased along with slight increase in HDL but with minimal change in mortality rate. There were adverse changes in clotting profiles and a tendency to increase risk of DVT.

Effects of androgen ablation therapy

Men with prostate cancer, treated with androgen deprivation, develop an increase of fat mass with an altered lipid profile, increasing total, LDL, HDL and triglycerides by 9, 7, 11, and 26.5%, respectively. These patients also appear to develop insulin resistance, hyperinsulinemia, and hyperglycaemia. The risks of diabetes mellitus increase by 44% and mortality of cardiovascular diseases by 16% during a follow-up of up to 10 years.[84] The authors concluded that before commencing androgen deprivation therapy (ADT), the overall health, co-morbidities, and life expectancy of the patient needs to be fully assessed.

Sexual function in the ageing male

For the older couple, retirement often allows for more shared time and increased intimacy. Sexual function may be a higher priority for the couple than the doctor perceives. Men who are widowed or divorced still expect to be sexually active in new relationships, and this should be positively encouraged, as evidence suggests that men living alone have markedly reduced life expectancy.[1]

Current guidelines suggest that *all* patients presenting with ED, irrespective of age, should be screened for low testosterone, as it is a *potentially curable cause of ED,* especially in men without other co-morbidities.[6–8] As NICE guidance suggests, all men with type 2 diabetes should be assessed *annually* and the GP contract now includes routine assessment for ED in coronary heart disease

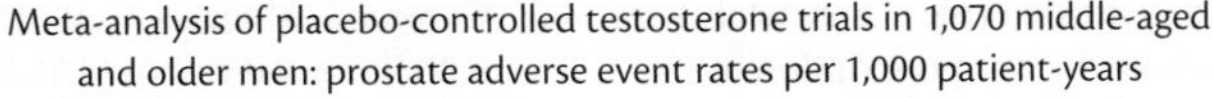

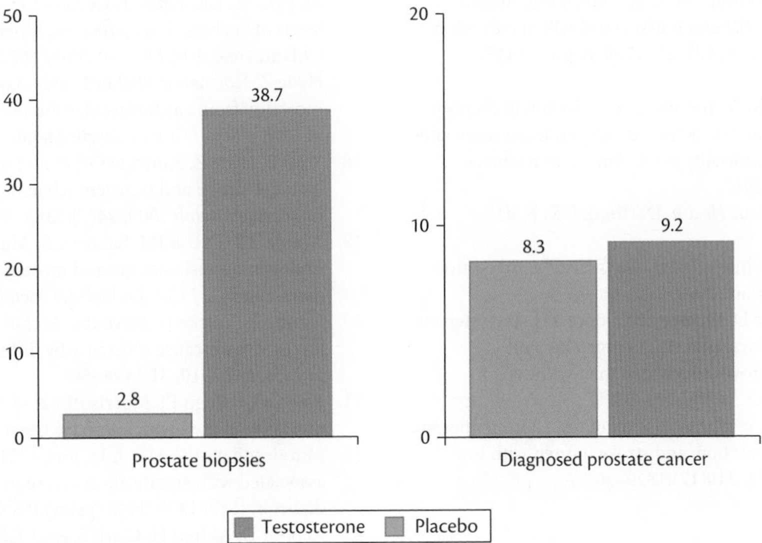

Fig. 7.12.10 Effects on the prostate of normalizing testosterone levels in hypogonadal men. Notes: A meta-analysis of randomized clinical trials to determine the risks of adverse events associated with testosterone replacement in older men.

METHODS: The MEDLINE database was searched from 1966 to April 2004, using testosterone as the indexing term; limits included human, male, ≥45 years old, and randomized controlled trial. Of the 417 studies thus identified, 19 met the inclusion criteria: testosterone replacement for at least 90 days, men ≥45 years old with low or low-normal testosterone level, randomized controlled trial, and medically stable men. RESULTS: In the 19 studies that met eligibility criteria, 651 men were treated with testosterone and 433 with placebo. The combined rate of all prostate events was significantly greater in testosterone-treated men than in placebo-treated men (OR = 1.78, 95% confidence interval [CI], 1.07–2.95). Rates of prostate cancer, prostate-specific antigen (PSA) >4 ng/mL, and prostate biopsies were numerically higher in the testosterone group than in the placebo group, although differences between the groups were not individually statistically significant. Testosterone replacement in older men was associated with a significantly higher risk of detection of prostate events and of haematocrit >50% than was placebo. These data reaffirm the need to monitor PSA, and digital examination of the prostate during testosterone replacement in older men.

Source: data from Calof OM *et al.*, 'Adverse events associated with testosterone replacement in middle-aged and older men: a meta-analysis of randomized, placebo-controlled trials', *Journal of Gerontology: Medical Sciences*, Volume 60A, Number 11, pp. 1451–7, Copyright © 2005 by The Gerontological Society of America.

(CHD) patients. Increased demand for testosterone supplementation will be a natural consequence of this correction of previous underdiagnosis and undertreatment.[85] Testosterone is involved at several sites in the erectile process up-regulates PDE5 in the corpora cavernosum, enhancing the effect of PDE5 inhibitors.[86] Oral ED drugs were shown to be effective in around 70% of men (55% in diabetes) during clinical trials with *unrestricted free medication*, such that responses are likely to be much low with restricted access.[6] Correcting low testosterone levels salvages 30–50% of men who would otherwise fail with oral therapy.[87–89]

When a low testosterone is detected, the anticipation of the patient would be that this abnormality will be corrected, irrespective of age. The patient will not be expecting the abnormality to be dismissed and for potentially lifelong, expensive, on-demand, self-funded ED therapy to be prescribed. TRT may provide a number of possible additional benefits beyond improving erections: namely

(i) Improving sexual desire (often diminished in ageing men with ED)
(ii) Improved morning erections
(iii) Improving ejaculatory and orgasmic function
(iv) Possible improvement in well-being, metabolic risk, cognitive function, depression, and quality of life[6–8]

Several studies have clearly shown that TRT can be effective as mono-therapy for ED,[87,88] generally in men without other multiple-co-morbidities, but also as a salvage procedure for patients who fail to respond to PDE5 inhibitors.[89] It is logical to restore testosterone levels to the normal range before re-introducing oral therapy. This process introduces some complex management and financial (for the patient and the physician) issues as both medications may be required long term for an effective outcome.

Conclusions

The benefits of conventional cardiovascular risk reduction by exercise and weight loss are fundamental to healthy ageing. There is considerable evidence of modest cardiac and metabolic benefits plus sexual, mood, and quality of life changes associated with testosterone replacement therapy and possibly PDE5 inhibitors that together may add up to substantial benefit to many patients. These may potentially denied to patients by fears over prostate and cardiovascular risk that are not currently supported by evidence. Ideally, we need large long-term studies to resolve these issues with certainty but such studies will be challenging for logistic and financial reasons. Until then, patients require advice and treatment based on current best evidence.

Further reading

Anderson JL, May HT, Lappe DL, *et al.* Impact of Testosterone Replacement Therapy on Myocardial Infarction, Stroke, and Death in Men With Low Testosterone Concentrations in an Integrated Health Care System. *Am J Cardiol* 2016; **117**(5):794–9.

Finkle WD, Greenland S, Ridgeway GK, *et al.* Increased risk of non-fatal myocardial infarction following testosterone therapy prescription in men. *PLoS One* 2014; **9**(1):e85805.

Anderson SG, Hutchings DC, Woodward M, et al. Phosphodiesterase type-5 inhibitor use in type 2 diabetes is associated with a reduction in all-cause mortality. *Heart* 2016; **102**(21):1750–6. doi:10.1136/heartjnl-2015-309223.

Hackett G, Ramachandran S, Heald A. Testosterone replacement therapy and pde5 inhibitor use in Type 2 diabetes are independently associated with a reduction in all-cause mortality 9-LB. American Diabetes Association (2015) 5–9 June 2015.

Hackett G. *Role of Androgens in Men's Health.* Dartford, UK: NSHI Publishing, 2011.

Kirby R, Carson CC, Kirby MG, White A (eds). *Men's Health*, 3rd edition. London, UK: Informa Healthcare, 2009.

Muraleedaran V, Marsh H, Kapoor D, Channer KS, Jones TH. Testosterone deficiency is associated with increased risk of mortality and testosterone replacement improves survival in men with type 2 diabetes. *Eur J Endocrinol* 2013; **169**(6):725–33.

Vigen R, O'Donnell CI, Baron AE, *et al.* Association of testosterone therapy with mortality, myocardial infarction, and stroke in men with low testosterone levels. *JAMA* 2013; **310**(17):1829–36.

References

1. The European Commision. The State of Men's Health in Europe. Available at: http://ec.europa.eu/health/population_groups/docs/men_health_report_en.pdf [Online].
2. Beutel M, Wiltink J, Schwarz R, Weidner W, Brahler E. Complaints of the Aging male based on a representative community study. *Eur Urol* 2002; **41**:85–93.
3. Stellato RK, Feldman HA, Hamdy O, Horton ES, McKinlay JB. Testosterone, sex hormone-binding globulin, and the development of type 2 diabetes in middle-aged men: prospective results from the Massachusetts male aging study. *Diabetes Care* 2000; **23**(4):490–4.
4. Hackett G. *Role of Androgens in Men's Health.* Dartford, UK: NSHI Publishing, 2011.
5. Rhoden EL Teloken C, Sogari PR, Souto CA. The relationship of serum testosterone to erectile function in normal ageing men. *J Urol* 2002; **167**(4):1745–8.
6. Hackett G, Kell P, Ralph D, *et al.* British Society for Sexual Medicine Guidelines on the management of erectile dysfunction. *J Sex Med* 2008; **5**(8):1841–6.
7. Wang C, Nieschlag E, Swerdloff RS, *et al.* Investigation, treatment, and monitoring of late-onset hypogonadism in males; ISA, ISSAM, EAU, EAA, and ASA recommendations. *Eur Urol* 2009; **55**:21–130.
8. Wylie K. Ress M, Hackett G, *et al.* Androgens, health and sexuality in men and women. *Maturitas* 2010; **67**(3):275–89.
9. Khaw KT, Dowsett M, Folkerd E, *et al.* Endogenous testosterone and mortality due to all causes, cardiovascular disease, and cancer in men: European Prospective Investigation into Cancer in Norfolk (EPIC-Norfolk) prospective population study. *Circulation* 2007: **116** (23);2694–701.
10. Oh JY, Barrett-Connor E, Wedick NM, Wingard DL; Rancho Bernardo Study. Endogenous sex hormones and the development of type 2 diabetes in older men and women; the Rancho Bernardo study. *Diabetes Care* 2002; **25**:55–60
11. Shores MM, Matsumoto AM, Sloan KL, *et al.* Low serum testosterone and mortality in male veterans. *Arch Intern Med* 2006; **166**:1660–65.
12. Hak AE, Witteman JCM, De Jong FH, *et al.* Low levels of endogenous androgens increase the risk of atherosclerosis in elderly men: the Rotterdam Study. *J Clin Endocrinol Metab* 2002; **87**:3632–9.
13. Tivesten A, Vandenput L, Labrie F, Karlsson M, *et al.* Low serum testosterone and estradiol predict mortality in elderly men. *J Clin Endocrinol Metab* 2009; **94**(7):2482–8.
14. Vikan T, Schirmer H, Njølstad I, Svartberg J. Endogenous sex hormones and the prospective association with cardiovascular disease and mortality in men: the Tromsø Study. *Eur J Endocrinol* 2009; **161**:435–42.
15. Corona G, Monami M, Boddi V, *et al.* Low testosterone is associated with increased risk of MACE lethality in subjects with erectile dysfunction. *J Sex Med* 2010; **7**:1557–63.
16. Maggio M, Laurentini F, Ceda GP, *et al.* Relationship between low levels of anabolic hormones and 6 year mortality in older men in the Chianti area. *Arch Int Med* 2007; **167**:2249–54.
17. Hyde Z, Norman P, Flicker L, *et al.* Low free testosterone predicts mortality from cardiovascular disease but not other causes: The Health in Men Study. *J Clin Endocrin Metab* 2012; (97)**1**:179–189.
18. Yeap B, Hyde Z, Almeida OP, *et al.* Low testosterone levels predict incident stroke and transient ichaemic attack in older men. *J Clin Endocrinol Metab* 2009; **94**(7):2353–9.
19. Araujo AB, Dixon JM, Suarez EA, Murad MH, Guey LT, Wittert GA. Endogenous testosterone and mortality in men:a systemic review and meta-analysis. *J Clin Endocrinol Metab* 2011; **96**(10):3007–19.
20. Haring R, Völzke H, Steveling A, *et al.* Association of low testosterone levels with all-cause mortality by different cut-offs from recent studies. *Eur Heary J* 2010; **31**:1494–501.
21. Malkin CJ, Pugh PJ, Morris PD, *et al.* Serum testosterone and increased mortality in men with coronary heart disease. *Heart* 2010; **96**:1821–5.
22. Muraleedharan V, Marsh H, Jones TH. Low testosterone level is associated with significant increase in mortality in patients with type 2 diabetes. ISSN 1470-3947 (print) ISSN 1479-6848 [Online].
23. Kapoor D, Aldred H, Clark S, *et al.* Clinical and biochemical assessment of hypogonadism in men with type 2 diabetes, Correlations with bioavailable testosterone and visceral adiposity. *Diabetes Care* 2007; **30**:911–17.
24. Hackett G, Cole N, Deshpande A, *et al.* Biochemical hypogonadism in men with type 2 diabetes. *Primary Care Practice* 2009; **9**: 5:226–31.
25. Saad F, Aversa A, Isidori A, *et al.* Onset of effects of testosterone replacement and time span until maximal effect is achieved. *Eur J Endocrinol* 2011; **165**:675–85.
26. Haffner SM, Shaten J, Stern MP, Smith GD, Kuller L. Low levels of sex hormone-binding globulin and testosterone predict the development of non-insulin-dependent diabetes mellitus in men. MRFIT Research Group. Multiple Risk Factor Intervention Trial. *Am J Epidemiol* 1996; **143**:889–97.
27. Kalinchenko S, Tishova Y, Mskhalaya G, Gooren L Giltay E, Saad F. Effects of testosterone supplementation on markers of the metabolic syndrome and inflammation in hypogonadal men with the metabolic syndrome: the double-blinded placebo-controlled Moscow study. *Clin Endocrinol* 2010; **73**(5):602–12.
28. Muraleedaran V, Marsh H, Kapoor D, Channer KS, Jones TH. Testosterone deficiency is associated with increased risk of mortality and testosterone replacement improves survival in men with type 2 diabetes. *Eur J Endocrinol* 2013; **169**(6):725–33.
29. Shores M, Smith NL, Forsberg CW, Anawalt BD, Marsumoto AM. Testosterone treatment and mortality in men with low testosterone. *J Clin Endocrin Metab* 2012; **97**(6):2050–8.
30. Morganuv L, Denisola I, Rohzkova T, *et al.* Androgen deficet and its treatment in stroke male patients with type II diabetes. *Zh Nevrol Pskihiatr Im S S Korsakova* 2011; **111**(8Pt2):21–4.
31. English KM, Mandour O, Steeds RP, Diver MJ, Jones TH, Channer KS. Men with coronary artery disease have lower levels of androgens than men with normal coronary angiograms. *Eur Heart J* 2000; **21**: 890–4.
32. Mathur A, Malkin C, Saleem B, Muthusammy R, Jones CH, Channer K. The long term benefits of testosterone on angina threshold and atheroma in men. *Eur J Endocrinol* 2009; **161**(3):443–9.
33. English KM, Steeds RP, Jones TH, Diver MJ, Channer KS. Low-dose transdermal testosterone therapy improves angina threshold in men with chronic stable angina: a randomized, double-blind, placebo-controlled study. *Circulation* 2000; **102**:1906–11.
34. Caminiti G, Volterrani M, Iellamo F, *et al.* Effect of long-acting testosterone treatment on functional exercise capacity, skeletal muscle performance, insulin resistance, and baroreflex sensitivity in elderly patients with chronic heart failure a double-blind, placebo-controlled, randomized study. *J Am Coll Cardiol* 2009; **54**:919–27.

35. Basaria S, Coviello AD, Travison TG, Storer TW Farwell WR, Jette AM. Adverse events associated with testosterone administration. *New Eng J Med* 2012; **363**(2):109–22.
36. Kapoor D, Aldred H, Clark S, *et al.* Clinical and biochemical assessment of hypogonadism in men with type 2 diabetes: correlations with bioavailable testosterone and visceral adiposity. *Diabetes Care* 2007; **30**:911–17.
37. Selvin E, Feinleib M, Zhang L, *et al.* Androgens and diabetes in men: results from the third National Health and Nutrition Survey (NHANES-III). *Diabetes Care* 2007; **30**:234–8.
38. Jones T. A placebo controlled study on the effects of transdermal testosterone gel in hypogonadal men with type ii diabetes or metabolic syndrome in diabetic control and insulin sensitivity: The TIMES 2 Study. *Diabetes Care* 2011; **34**:828–37.
39. Kapoor D, Goodwin E, Channer KS, *et al.* Testosterone replacement therapy improves insulin resistance, glycaemic control, visceral adiposity and hypercholesterolemia in hypogonadal men with Type 2 diabetes. *Eur J Endocrinol* 2006; **154**:899–906.
40. Naharci MI, Pinar M, Bolu E, Olgun A. Effect of testosterone on insulin sensitivity in men with idiopathic hypogonadotropic hypogonadism. *Endocr Pract* 2007; **13**:629–35.
41. Boyanov MA, Boneva Z, Christov VG. Testosterone supplementation in men with type 2 diabetes, visceral obesity and partial androgen deficiency. *Aging Male* 2003; **6**:1–7.
42. Hackett G, Cole N. Long acting testosterone undecanoate improves diabetes control v placebo in a hypogonadal population with type 2 diabetes PO-05-12. *J Sex Med* 2011; **8**(5):430.
43. Wang C Swerdloff RS, Iranmanesh R, *et al.* Testosterone gel improves sexual function, mood, muscle strength and body composition in hypogonadal men. J endocrinol. *Metab* 2000; **85**(8):2839–53.
44. Maggio M, Basaria S, Ble A, *et al.* Correlation between testosterone and the inflammatory marker soluble interleukin-6 receptor inolder men. *J Clin Endocrinol Metab* 2006; **91**:345–7.
45. MacLeod, Davey Smith G, Metcalfe C, Hart C. INTERHEART. *Lancet* 2005; **365**(9454):118–19.
46. Dwyer AA, Caronia LM, Lee H. Lifestyle modification can reverse hypogonadism in men impaired glucose tolerance. OR28-3 Endocrine Society 23–26 June 2012. Available at: https://www.diabetes.org.uk/Documents/Reports/Diabetes_in_the_UK_2010.pdf [Accessed 28 August 2012] [Online].
47. Murphy S, Kham ST, Cassidy A. Compston JE. Sex hormones and bone mineral density in elderly men. *Bone Miner* 1993; **20**:133–40.
48. Rudman D, Drinka PJ, Wilson CR, Mattson DE, Scherman F, Cuisinier MC. Relations of endogenous anabolic hormones and physical activity to bone mineral density and lean body mass in elderly men. *Clin Endocrinol* 1994; **40**:653–61.
49. NICE Guidance on Osteoporosis. Available at: www.nice.org.uk [Online].
50. NICE Guidance on Prostate Cancer. Available at: www.nice.org.uk [Online].
51. Fonda S, Bertrand R, O'Donnell A, Longcope C, Mc Kincley JB. Age, hormones and cognitive function among middle-aged and elderly men: cross sectional evidence from the Massachusetts Male Ageing study. *J Gerontology* 2005; **60A**:385–90.
52. Orwoll E, Lambert LC, Marshall LM, *et al.* For the osteoporotic fractures in men study group. Endogenous testosterone levels, physical performance and falls risk in older men. *Arch Int Med* 2006; **166**:2124–31.
53. Szulc P, Munoz F, Claustrat B, Garnero P, Marchand F. Bioavailable oestradiol may be an important determinant of osteoporosis in men; the MINOS study. *J Clin Endocrinol Metab* 2001; **86**:192–9.
54. Kiebzak GM. Beinart GA, Perzer K, Ambrose CG. Undertreatment of osteoporosis in men with hip fracture. *Arch Int Med* 2002; **162**:2217–22.
55. Wang BC, Cunningham G, Dobs A, *et al.* Long term testosterone gel treatment maintains beneficial effects on sexual function, lean and fat mass, and bone mineral density in hypogonadal men. *J Clin Endocrinol Metab* 2004; **89**:2085–98.
56. Srinivas-Shankar U, Roberts SA, Conolly MJ, *et al.* Effects of testosterone on muscle strength, physical function, body composition, and quality of life in intermediate-frail and frail elderly men: a randomized, double-blind, placebo-controlled study. *J Clin Endocrinol Metab* 2010; **95**:639–50.
57. Moffat SD, Zonderman AB, Metter EJ, Blackman MR, Harman SM. Resnick SM. Longitudinal assessment of serum free testosterone concentration predicts memory performance and cognitive status in elderly men. *J Clin Endocrinol Metab* 2002; **87**:5001–7.
58. Kaufman JM, Vermeulen A. The decline in androgen levels in elderly men and its clinical and therapeutic implications. *Endocrine Rev* 2005; **26**;833–76.
59. Goldney R, Phillips PJ, Fisher LJ, Wilson DH. Diabetes, depression and quality of life: A population study. *Diabetes Care* 2004; **27**(5):1066–70.
60. Anderson RJ, Freedland KE, Clouse RE, Lustman PJ. The prevalence of co-morbid depression in adults with diabetes: a meta-analysis. *Diabetes Care* 2001; **24**(6):1069–78.
61. De Groot M Anderson R, Freedland K, Clourse R, Lustman P. Association of Diabetes Complications and Depression; a meta-analysis. *Psychosom Med* 2001; **63**(4):619–30.
62. Giltay EJ, Tishova YA, Mskhalaya GJ, *et al.* Effects of testosterone supplementation on depressive symptoms and sexual dysfunction in hypogonadal men with the metabolic syndrome. *J Sex Med* 2010; **7**(7):2572–82.
63. Buvat J, Boujadoue G. Testosterone replacement in the ageing male. *J Men's Health Gender* 2005; **2**:396–9.
64. Pope HG, Cohane GH, Kanayama G, Siegel AJ, Hudson JL. Testosterone gel supplementation for men with refractory depression. A randomised placebo controlled study. *Am J Psychiatry* 2003; **160**:105–11.
65. Moffat SD, Zonderman AB, Metter EJ, *et al.* Free testosterone and risk for Alzheimer disease in older men. *Neurology* 2004; **62**(2):188–93.
66. Hogervorst E, Bandelow S, Combrinck M, Smith AD. Low free testosterone is an independent risk factor for Alzheimer's disease. *Exp Gerontol* 2004; **39**(11–12):1633.
67. Po H, Lu P, Masterman D, *et al.* Effects of testosterone on cognition and mood in male patients with Alzheimer disease and healthy male men. *Arch Neurol* 2006; **63**(2):177–85.
68. Tong SF, Ng CJ, Lee BC, *et al.* Effect of long lasting testosterone undecanoate treatment on quality of life in men with testosterone deficiency syndrome: a double blind randomised controlled trial. *Asian J Androl* 2012; **14**(4):604–11.
69. Calof OM, Singh AB, Lee ML, *et al.* Adverse events associated with testosterone replacement in middle aged and older men; A meta-analysis of randomised placebo controlled trials. *J Gerontol* 2005: **60**(11):1451–7.
70. Vigen R, O'Donnell CI, Baron AE, *et al.* Association of testosterone therapy with mortality, myocardial infarction, and stroke in men with low testosterone levels. *JAMA* 2013; **310**(17):1829–36.
71. Finkle WD, Greenland S, Ridgeway GK, *et al.* Increased risk of non-fatal myocardial infarction following testosterone therapy prescription in men. *PLoS One* 2014; **9**(1):e85805.
72. Sharma R, Oni OA, Gupta K, *et al.* Normalization of testosterone level is associated with reduced incidence of myocardial infarction and mortality in men. *Eur Heart J* 2015; **36**(40):2706–15.
73. Anderson JL, May HT, Lappe DL, *et al.* Impact of Testosterone Replacement Therapy on Myocardial Infarction, Stroke, and Death in Men With Low Testosterone Concentrations in an Integrated Health Care System. *Am J Cardiol* 2016; **117**(5):794–9.
74. Hackett G, Ramachandran S, Heald A. testosterone replacement therapy and pde5 inhibitor use in type 2 diabetes are independently associated with a reduction in all-cause mortality 9-LB. American Diabetes Association (2015) 5–9 June 2015.
75. Anderson SG, Hutchings DC, Woodward M, et al. Phosphodiesterase type-5 inhibitor use in type 2 diabetes is associated with a reduction in all-cause mortality. *Heart* 2016; **102**(21):1750–6. doi:10.1136/heartjnl-2015-309223.

76. Roddam AW, Allen NE, Appleby P, Key JJ. Endogenous sex hormones and prostate cancer: A collaborative analysis of 18 prospective studies. *J Nat Cancer Inst* 2008; **100**(3):170–83.
77. Parsons JK. Benign prostatic hypertrophy and lower urinary tract symptoms, epidemiology and risk factors. *Curr Bladder Dysfunct Rep* 2010; **5**:212–18.
78. Marks LS, Mazer NA, Mostaghel E, Hess DL, Dorey FJ Epstein JL. Effect of testosterone replacement therapy on prostate tissue in men with late onset hypogonadism; a randomised controlled trial. *JAMA* 2009; **296**(19):2351–61.
79. Shabsigh R, Crawford ED, Nehra, Slawin KM. Testosterone therapy in hypogonadal men and potential prostate cancer risk: a systematic review. *Int J Impot Res* 2009; **21**(1):9–23.
80. Garcia-Cruz E, Carrion A, Garcia-Larrosa A, *et al.* Higher sex hormone-binding globulin and lower bioavailable testosterone are linked to positive prostate cancer biopsy. *Scand J Urol* 2013; **47**(4):282–9.
81. Weiss E, Villareal D, Ehsani A, Fontana L, O'Holloszy J. DHEA replacement therapy in older adults improves indices of arterial stiffness. *Aging Cell* 2012; **11**(5):876–84.
82. Palusiński R, Barud W, Biłan A, Witczak A, Myśliński W, Hanzlik J. Effect of dihydrotestosterone treatment on exercise induced ischemia in men with stable ischemic heart disease. *Pol Merkur Lekarski* 2000; **9**(50):533–4.
83. Gooren L, Giltay EJ, Bunck M. Long-term treatment of transsexuals with cross-sex hormones: extensive clinical experience. *JCEM* 2008; **93**(1):19–25.
84. Keating NL, O'Malley AJ, Freedland SJ, Smith MR. Diabetes and cardiovascular disease during androgen deprivation therapy: observational study of veterans with prostate cancer. *J Natl Cancer Inst* 2010; **102**(1):39–46.
85. Home P, Mant J, Diaz J, Turner C, on behalf of the Guideline Development Group Management of type 2 diabetes: summary of updated NICE guidance. *BMJ* 2008; **336**:1306–8.
86. Isidori AM, Giannetta, Gianfrilli D, Greco EA, Bonifacio V, Aversa A. Effects of testosterone on sexual function in men: results of a meta-analysis. *Clin Endocrinol* 2005; **63**(4):381–94.
87. Saad F, Aversa A, Isidori A, Zafalon L, Zitzmann M, Gooren L. Onset of effects of testosterone replacement and time span until maximal effect is achieved. *Eur J Endocrinol* 2011; **165**(5):165–85.
88. Yassin AA, Saad F, Traish A. Testosterone undecanoate restores erectile function in a subset of patients with venous leakage: a series of case reports. *J Sex Med* 2006; **3**:727–35.
89. Eardley I. Optimising response to PDE5 inhibitors: converting non-responders to responders. *Eur Urol* 2006; **50**:31–3.

CHAPTER 7.13

Peyronie's disease, congenital curvature, and chordee

Epidemiology, pathophysiology, evaluation, and treatment

Laurence A. Levine, William Brant, and Stephen M. Larsen

Peyronie's disease

Introduction to Peyronie's disease

Peyronie's disease (PD) is a fibrotic wound healing disorder of the tunica albuginea. This physically and often psychologically devastating disorder causes penile deformities including curvature, hinging, narrowing, and shortening as well as painful erections. Penile pain is a common feature that resolves in most patients 6–18 months after onset. Pain and deformity progression occur during the acute phase, whereas pain resolution with either deformity regression or stabilization identifies its stable phase. PD data outcomes have been difficult to interpret without a validated questionnaire, and this is further complicated by a reported spontaneous improvement rate of 13–39%.[1,2] This chapter reviews the diagnosis and management of PD.

Epidemiology

PD is estimated to occur in 3–9% of adult men.[3,4] Although commonly diagnosed in the fourth and fifth decades of life, PD occurring before the age of 20 has been described.[5] Patients with diabetes and those who have received a radical prostatectomy are significantly more affected by this condition with incidence rates reaching 20% and 15.9%, respectively.[6,7] Approximately 30% of PD patients have diabetes. Other co-morbid conditions are reported to occur in association with PD including hypertension, dyslipidemia, and hypogonadism.[8] Low levels of androgens (DHEA and testosterone) when compared to age-matched non-PD controls, and these low plasma androgen concentrations possibly contribute to the pathogenesis and onset of PD.[9] Studies demonstrate serious psychological sequelae on both the PD patient and partner with a rate of clinical depression of 48%.[10] PD is associated with other collagen diseases such as Dupuytren's and Ledderhose disease.

Pathophysiology

PD is thought to occur in genetically susceptible individuals following penile trauma.[11] In the acute phase an inflammatory component is accompanied by subjective pain. A localized response to endogenous factors such as TGF-β released in response to repeated microtrauma leads to unregulated extracellular matrix deposition and ultimately to plaque formation.[12–15] PD tissue samples have reduced or absent levels of matrix metalloproteinases (MMPs) and elevated tissue inhibitors of matrix metalloproteinases (TIMPs). These findings suggest that PD fibroblasts may be manipulated to encourage scar remodelling in the final phase of wound healing and may be an avenue for future research and treatment.[16]

Evaluation and diagnosis

A standardized evaluation includes history, physical examination, diagnostic imaging, and questionnaires.[17] These questionnaires should address deformity, sexual function, impact of disease, as well as treatment satisfaction. The PD questionnaire (PDQ) was recently validated and includes assessment of psychological symptoms, penile pain, and PD symptom bother.[18]

The history should address onset, pain, deformity, palpable lump, trauma, and previous treatments. One may ask the patient to estimate the degree and direction of erect penile curvature, although only 20% of patients accurately report the degree of curvature with 56% overestimating and 26% underestimating curvature with an average difference of 20 degrees. Therefore, preoperative objective measures of erect deformity are necessary in order to accurately counsel patients, recommend appropriate treatment, and objectively evaluate outcomes.[19] The history should also address the presence of indentation, hinging/buckling with axial pressure, and the amount of shortening. Shortening may be the most psychologically devastating symptom, occurring in 70% of patients and ranging from 1–10 cm.[10,20,21] Questions regarding pre-Peyronie's erectile status are important and guide surgical planning. Diminished rigidity, which is commonly seen, may be psychogenic in nature and/or due to underlying medical conditions. Clinical depression and loss of self-esteem can also be seen, as well as devastating effects on the patient's sexual and social relationships.[10,21] Questions regarding sexual dysfunction should include ejaculation, orgasm, and change in sensation.

Physical examination of the penis is critical. A stretched penile length must be obtained because of the concern for further shortening. With the patient in the supine position, the glans is grasped, and pulled to full stretch perpendicular to the plane of the body.[22] A rigid ruler presses down on the suprapubic fat pad to the pubic bone, and the penis is measured to the corona or meatus depending on physician preference. Preoperative penile sensitivity can be assessed with light touch and biothesiometry, though no standard evaluation of this parameter has been established.

Deformity assessment of an erect penis is the most important part of the clinical diagnosis. Pharmacologically induced erection via injection of vasoactive agent is the most reliable method when compared to vacuum-induced or photograph.[23] If a full erection does not occur, administration of a second dose is recommended. Pressure can also be applied to the base of the penis if needed. Curvature is then measured in the erect state while a simple string can be used to measure girth at the base, subcoronal, and any area of indentation or hourglass narrowing.

Doppler ultrasound can be helpful if the diagnosis is in doubt. In the flaccid condition, corporal fibrosis and plaque calcification can be seen.[24] Up to 32% will have plaque calcification which can occur early after initial onset of the plaque formation and is therefore not an indicator of mature disease as was previously thought.[25]

Treatment

Non-surgical therapy

PD remains a therapeutic dilemma due to an incomplete understanding of its aetiopathophysiology and the relative paucity of randomized, placebo-controlled trials. Conservative management is commonly applied for early presentations of PD.[26] Indications for non-surgical therapy include men with early phase disease (i.e. less than 12 months' duration) who have unstable or progressive deformity and painful erections, as well as those not psychologically ready or interested in surgery.[26]

A recent report by the PD committee during the 2009 International Consultation on Sexual Medicine (ICSM) stated there is no evidence of benefit with respect to deformity with any oral or topical therapy or with shock wave treatment.[8] Preliminary reports demonstrate benefit with respect to curvature and length correction with external penile traction and/or vacuum therapy.[27,28] Intralesional injection of verapamil and interferon have also shown evidence of curvature reduction but large scale multicenter studies are needed.[29,30] Most recently, clostridial collagenase has been shown in randomized double-blind placebo-controlled studies to reduce curvature and deformity.[31] At the time of writing, the treatment has been licensed in the United States and in Europe.

The authors support the use of combination therapy using oral and injectable agents (for their biological effects) together with external traction therapy (for its mechanical effects) to create a synergy to reduce deformity and improve sexual function. Please see Table 7.13.1 for a depiction of the proposed mechanism of action, side effects, and effectiveness of non-surgical treatments.

Surgery for Peyronie's disease

The main indication for surgery for men with PD is stable disease, defined as at least one year from onset and at least six months of stable deformity with compromised ability to engage in coital activity due to deformity and/or inadequate rigidity. Extensive plaque calcification can also be an indication, as can significant PD accompanied by concurrent erectile dysfunction. Penile pain is a relative contraindication except when it may be due to a strong erection imparting torque-like pressure on the penis.[8]

It is important to have a frank discussion regarding the possibility of persistent or recurrent curvature, change in penile erect length, diminished rigidity, and decreased sexual sensation in order to set appropriate expectations regarding the outcome of surgery.[8] Persistent or recurrent curvature is unusual but has been shown in up to 16% of men.[32] Up to 30% of men may have some degree of postoperative loss of rigidity. Consideration for penile prosthesis should be discussed if the patient already has significant erectile dysfunction (ED) preoperatively.[8,32] Decreased sensation occurs in 20% of men acutely, but tends to resolve over the ensuing months.[33] Several surgical algorithms have been published and are summarized in Box 7.13.1.[34,35]

Tunical shortening procedures

All plication procedures shorten the long side of the penis and therefore can result in loss of length on that aspect. Men who have a ventral curvature of greater than 60 degrees tend to have the greatest potential loss of penile length.[33] Other drawbacks of any plication procedure are that it does not correct shortening, does not address hinge or hourglass effect, and indeed may exacerbate it. Several other side effects have been reported including narrowing (0–17%), pain associated with sutures, and tactile and sexual sensitivity changes (0–21%).[8,33]

The ICSM report stated that there was 'no evidence that one surgical approach provides better outcomes over another, but curvature correction can be expected with less risk of new ED' compared to grafting procedures.[8] See Table 7.13.2 for a summary of the outcomes of surgical straightening with tunica albuginea plication.

Tunical lengthening procedures (incision or partial excision and grafting)

Indications for incision or partial excision and grafting for surgical correction of PD include greater complexity of disease with several or all of the following: curvature greater than 60–70 degrees, shaft narrowing, hinging, and extensive plaque calcification. Good preoperative erections are of utmost importance.[36]

Predictors of postoperative ED include preoperative ED, age >55, evidence of corporal veno-occlusive dysfunction on duplex ultrasound (resistance index <0.80), ventral curvature, and possibly the severity of the curvature.[36,37]

Surgical grafting techniques include plaque incision, where an H or double-Y incision is made in the area of maximum curvature.[38] This allows the tunic to be expanded in this area, thereby correcting the curvature and shaft calibre. Partial plaque excision has also been suggested, where the area of maximum deformity is excised particularly if it is associated with severe indentation.[37–40] The key to these operations is to limit the trauma to the underlying cavernosal tissue to maintain the veno-occlusive relationship between the cavernosal tissue and the overlying tunic and graft.

Successful straightening has been reported in 63–100% with patient satisfaction ranging from 41–96%, partner satisfaction 77%, and successful coitus in 79–100%.[33,41–46] ED is reported in 0% to 35% of men with increased risk of ED when grafting is performed to correct ventral curvature.[33,43] Recurrence of greater than 30-degree curvature can be seen from 0% to 16%.[43–48] See Table 7.13.2 for a summary of the outcomes for penile straightening with plaque incision/excision and grafting.

Table 7.13.1 Conservative treatments for Peyronie's disease

Oral agents	Mechanism	Efficacy	Side effects	ICSM guidelines
Vitamin E 400 IU daily or BD	Antioxidant limits oxidative stress of reactive oxygen species shown to be increased in PD	No benefit with respect to pain, curvature, or plaque size	Possible cerebrovascular events, nausea, vomiting, diarrhoea, headache, dizziness	No benefit with respect to deformity
Colchicine 2.5 mg daily	Inhibits fibrosis and collagen deposition primarily by inhibiting neutrophil microtubules	No benefit with respect to pain, curvature, or plaque size	Myelosuppression, diarrhoea, nausea, vomiting	No benefit with respect to deformity
Potassium amino-benzoate 3 g six-hourly	Stabilizes tissue serotonin monoamine oxidase activity; antifibrotic effect due to a direct inhibitory effect on fibroblast glycosamineglycan secretion	Mean decrease in plaque size in 74.3%, no improvement in curvature	Anorexia, nausea, fever, skin rash, hypoglycaemia	No benefit with respect to deformity
Tamoxifen 40 mg daily	Affects the release of TGF from fibroblasts, and blocks TGF-receptors, reducing fibrogenesis	No demonstrable improvement in pain, curvature, or plaque size	Alopecia, retinopathy, thromboembolism, pancytopenia	No benefit with respect to deformity
Carnitine 1 g twice daily	Attenuates both collagen fibre deposition and elastogenesis	No significant improvement in pain, curvature, or plaque size	Seizure, diarrhoea, nausea, stomach cramps, vomiting	No benefit with respect to deformity
Procarbazine (100 mg/m^2)	Oral alkylating agent	91% failure or worsening	Hepatotoxicity, myelosuppression, central nervous system effects, and GI disturbances	Not addressed by ICSM guideline
Pentoxifylline400 mg twice daily	Nonspecific phosphodiesterase inhibitor, attenuates both collagen fibre deposition and elastogenesis	36.9% with mean decrease in curvature of 23 degrees	Indigestion, nausea, vomiting, dizziness, headache, angina, aplastic anaemia, leucopenia, thrombocytopenia	Further studies required to confirm findings
Injectable agents	**Mechanism**	**Efficacy**	**Side effects**	**ICSM guidelines**
Collagenase (10,000 units × injections at 0 and 3 months)	Lyses collagen, the primary component of PD plaques	57% had 25% reduced Curvature. IMPRESS trial demonstrates mean 34% decrease in curvature (17 degrees) with improvement in subjective symptoms as well	Penile pain, swelling, contusions, ecchymoses	Several small non-controlled trials showed limited benefit. (The ICSM process predated the publication of the large RCTs that demonstrated the efficacy of collagenase)
Verapamil (10 mg bi-weekly ×12 injections)	Inhibits local extracellular matrix production, reduces fibroblast proliferation, increases local collagenase activity	60% with mean decrease of 30 degrees, 57% with decreased plaque volume, and trend towards decreased curvature	Nausea, lightheadedness, penile pain, ecchymoses, no cardiovascular events	Appears to make scientific sense but no large scale placebo-controlled trials
Nicardipine (10 mg bi-weekly × 6 injections)	Ca2þ channel blocker, mechanism likely similar to verapamil	Improvement in IIEF scores, and plaque size, no specific values given	Headache, no hypotension or cardiovascular events	No guidelines
Corticosteroids (25 mg per week) (50 mg every 4–6 weeks)	Anti-inflammatory	100% resolution of pain, no significant difference in curvature, or plaque size	Tissue atrophy, thinning of skin, and immunosuppression	No objective measures of therapeutic benefit

(continued)

Table 7.13.1 Continued

Injectable agents	Mechanism	Efficacy	Side effects	ICSM guidelines
Orgotein (4 mg every 2 weeks)	Anti-inflammatory with pronounced superoxide dismutase activity	No benefit with regard to pain, deformity, or plaque size	Pain, swelling, stiffness, dysesthesias, and skin rashes	Not addressed by ICSM guidelines
Interferons (1–10,000 U per week)	Decrease fibroblast proliferation *in vitro*, reduce extracellular matrix production, and increase collagenase	Decreased curvature of 27%, resolution of pain in 67%,decreased plaque size by 54.6%	Myalgias, flu-like symptoms, fever	One placebo-controlled Trial showed an outcome benefit with interferon over saline
External energy agents	**Mechanism**	**Efficacy**	**Side effects**	**ICSM guidelines**
Penile ESWT (2,000 shocks weekly × 4)	Local inflammatory reaction leading to plaque lysis, improved vascularity, plaque resorption and contralateral scarring	Pain resolved in 53%, no benefit with regard to curvature or deformity	Bruising, skin haemorrhage, haematoma, urethral bleeding	Evidence that ESWT does not improve PD-related deformity
Electromotive drug administration (EMDA)-Iontophoresis (5–10 mg verapamil ± 8 mg dexamethasone at 2.4 mA for 20 min)	Decreased expression of bFGF mRNA and bFGF protein expression in excised Peyronie's plaques, verapamil same mechanism as intralesional	45% had at least 50% reduction of curvature, 88% with complete resolution of pain	Mild erythema	Several controlled trials had evidence of reduced deformity following iontophoresis treatment using verapamil and dexamethasone
Penile traction (2–9 hr per day)	Tension-induced cellular proliferation, reorientation collagen fibrils, upregulation of 'antifibrotic' genes	Decreased curvature of 33%	Local irritation	Early evidence from two small non-controlled prospective trials have reported a reduction of deformity and increased penile length

ESWT = extracorporeal shock wave therapy; GI = gastrointestinal; ICSM = International Consultation on Sexual Medicine; IIEF = International Index of Erectile Function; PD = Peyronie's disease; TGF = tumour growth factor.

Box 7.13.1 Peyronie's disease surgical algorithm

I. When rigidity adequate preoperatively with or without oral pharmacotherapy:
   A. Tunica plication when:
      (i) curvature <60–70 degrees
      (ii) no destabilizing hourglass or hinge
      (iii) predicted loss of length <20% erect length
   B. Plaque incision/partial excision and grafting when:
      (i) curvature >60–70 degrees
      (ii) destabilizing hinge
II. When rigidity suboptimal: penile prosthesis implantation
   A. Penis straight after implantation: no further straightening techniques necessary
   B. Manual modelling: if persistent curvature after implant
   C. Tunica incision
      (i) without grafting: defect created by incision <2 cm
      (ii) with graft: defect created by incision >2 cm

(I) Text extracts reprinted from *The Journal of Urology*, Volume 158, Issue 6, Laurence A. Levine and Eric L. Lenting, 'A surgical algorithm for the treatment of Peyronie's disease', pp. 2149–2152, Copyright © 1997 European Association of Urology, with permission from Elsevier, http://www.sciencedirect.com/science/journal/00225347; (II) Text extracts reproduced from John Mulhall *et al.*, 'Original Research—Surgery: A Surgical Algorithm for Men with Combined Peyronie's Disease and Erectile Dysfunction: Functional and Satisfaction Outcomes', *Journal of Sexual Medicine*, Volume 2, Issue 2, pp. 132–8, Copyright © 2005 John Wiley and Sons.

Penile prosthesis for men with Peyronie's disease

Insertion of a penile prosthesis in men with PD is indicated when there is concurrent ED refractory to PDE5 inhibitors.[34,35] An algorithm for penile straightening with insertion of penile prosthesis with additional straightening manoeuvres is provided in Box 7.13.1.

Techniques for straightening when placing penile prosthesis for Peyronie's disease

An inflatable penile prosthesis appears to be the preferred surgical implant, as the pressure within the cylinders allows for superior correction of curvature with manual modelling, as well as improved girth enhancement.[49] Manual modelling is recommended with a high-pressure inflatable cylinder, but all available three-piece and two-piece devices have been used successfully to correct deformity. The penis is then bent in the contralateral direction to the curvature for 60–90 seconds.[50] The modelling technique should be done gradually with no direct pressure on the glans as this will reduce the likelihood of injury to the tunic or urethra by distal extrusion of the prosthetic cylinders.[32,50] Sensory deficits after manual modelling are rare, but are a potential complication.[51] An alternative to modelling would be to perform a tunic plication contralateral to the curvature before placement of the prosthesis.[52]

When there is residual curve of greater than 30 degrees or residual indentation causing the inflated cylinder to buckle, tunical incision with or without grafting is recommended. The tunical incision is made with the cylinders deflated, using the cautery to release the tunic with an effort to preserve the cavernosal tissue over the implant.[53] Once the incision is made, the cylinders are re-inflated, and further modelling can be performed to optimize deformity correction. Grafting over the defect is recommended when the defect measures greater than 2 cm in any dimension.

A novel approach has recently been described where a long-nose nasal speculum is placed into the intracorporal space and expanded, thus disrupting the scar in a radial fashion and then longitudinal incisions with scissors or curved scalpel further disrupt the plaque. Sensory side effects are possible but not reported in over 230 cases.[54] Additional manoeuvres do not appear to increase the rate of mechanical failure or infection.[51]

Preoperative discussion is also focused on the goal of obtaining 'functional straightness', in which a residual curvature of 20 degrees or less in any direction would likely not compromise sexual activity.[55]

The most common postoperative complaint is length loss, which has been confirmed objectively by Wang *et al.*[56] Traction therapy used before penile prosthesis placement in men with PD may prevent further loss of length after prosthesis placement.[57] See Table 7.13.2 for a summary on the outcomes of penile straightening with penile prosthesis placement.

Congenital curvature and chordee

Introduction to congenital curvature and chordee

Congenital curvature and chordee may exist in isolation or in conjunction with hypospadias. Congenital curvature and chordee have historically been considered separate entities, although, as discussed below, they may have a common aetiology.

Epidemiology

The exact prevalence of congenital curvature is not known because firstly, mild curvatures cause no difficulty with intromission and, secondly, sexually naive subjects have no comparison, thus even painful intromission may be considered 'normal'. Those who present clinically are likely to represent a small fraction overall, as they are ones who have either noted the problem or who have had difficulty in coitus. A common presentation is that of unconsummated marriage.[58] Reported prevalence ranges from 0.6–10% of live births and is more commonly associated with hypospadias.[59,60]

Aetiology

The aetiology of congenital curvature is discrepant growth between the relatively longer, elastic dorsal tunica compared to the ventrum, while chordee can be due to skin tethering, fibrous dartos tissue, corporal disproportion, and urethral tethering.[61,62] In true congenital curvature, relative overelasticity results in a long phallus.[63,64] An ultra-structural study[65] using tissue from the convex side as the study site and the concave side as a control, found that the convex side had a more irregular collagen pattern, with widening, fragmentation, and more heterogeneous fibre size. Though most commonly ventral, chordee may manifest as a curvature in any direction.

Table 7.13.2 Summary of the outcomes of surgical straightening for Peyronie's disease with tunica albuginea plication, grafting, and insertion of penile prosthesis

Procedure type	Reference number	No. of patients	Mean duration of follow-up (mo.)	Straight at latest follow-up (%)	Erectile dysfunction (%)	Satisfaction rates (%)
Nesbit	94	218	89	86	12	84
	95	359	21	82	2	NA
	96	28	22	79	4	79
	97	9	31	NA	NA	67
Yachia	96	30	12	100	NA	83
	97	8	31	NA	NA	63
Tunica albuginea plication	98	124	31	85	6	96
	99	44	49	29	36	NA
	100	28	34	57	3.5	82
	101	29	34	79	38	81
	102	28	34	82	35	68
	33	22	20	91	9	NA
Dermal graft	103	15	17	73	12	70
	33	50	45	94	NA	NA
Saphenous vein grafts	45	113	12	86	15	96
	104	112	<18	96	12	92
	105	50	32	80	6	88
Buccal mucosa	43	15	12	100	0	100
	106	26	38.4	92.3	7.7	NA
Proximal crura	107	7	6	85.7	0	85.7
	108	31	NA	83.8	19.3	93.5
	109	27	NA	96.2	3.7	70.4
Tunica vaginalis	110	15	4–16	87.5	0	100
	111	25	42.2	88	68	NA
Dura mater	112	40	12–72	95	15	NA
	113	40	12–24	100	25	NA
Temporalis fascia	114	12	NA	100	0	100
Fascia lata	115	14	31	79	7	93
Pericardial graft	40	33	19	87.9	0	NA
Stratasis graft	103	13	7.8	76.9	NA	84.6
Small intestinal submucosa (SIS)	42	19	15	63	53	NA
	116	162	38	91	9	NA
Tutoplast pericardial graft	33	81	58	79	20	78
	46	19	22	84	16	74
	116	11	14	91	NA	NA
	103	11	19	91	0	NA

Insertion of inflatable penile prosthesis	Reference number	Prosthesis type	No. of patients	Mean follow-up (months)	Additional straightening manoeuvres (%)	Satisfaction rates (%)
	51	Inflatable	90	49	96	84
	50	Inflatable	138	NA	8	NA
	55	Inflatable	72	NA	8	67
	37	Inflatable	5	22	100	100

Non-surgical approaches

There is a paucity of studies addressing the non-surgical management of chordee. Androgen administration has been suggested as a potential treatment. The tunica albuginea of children with chordee has cytoplasmic androgen receptors and these receptors are not found in adults. In an effort to both understand aetiology and to treat congenital curvature, Catuogno and Romano administered either local androgens (to the convex side of the penis) or performed plication surgery in a non-randomized fashion to 70 subjects with ages ranging from four years to early twenties. They reported that younger subjects had 80–100% improvement of curvature, but this improvement was not seen in older patients (those over 15 years). On biopsies done at the time of surgery (in those who failed medical treatment or did not elect to undergo it), they found a relative reduction in androgen receptors on the concave aspect of the penis and that overall androgen receptor numbers decreased with increasing age.[66,67] Despite the success of this medical treatment, at least in children, there are no similar reports in the peer-reviewed literature.

Surgical techniques

Plication approaches

Many of the techniques that are currently used in the treatment of PD were originally developed for the correction of congenital curvatures (Table 7.13.3).[68–76] The classic, and possibly first, description of the issue is from the 1965 report by Nesbit on three patients. Essed and Schoeder described a modification of the Nesbit technique in 1985.[68] Another evolution in surgical treatment was described by Yachia in 10 patients, 9 of whom had congenital curvature.[69] Another alternative was described by Baskin and Duckett in 1994[70] for over 180 cases of paediatric chordee, with or without hypospadias. Later, after more careful study of the penile structural anatomy and recognition that the adult penis generates much higher intracorporal pressures than the paediatric erection,[71–74] the authors described a new technique for congenital curvature.[75] Another variation on this combined the location of the Baskin approach with the Yachia Heineke-Mikulicz principle.[76]

Rotational approaches

A different approach primarily used in the paediatric population involves a rotation of the corpora.[77–79] This approach is rarely employed in the treatment of adult congenital curvature because of the risk of urethral injury. Studies report good cosmetic results with few subjects requiring additional straightening manoeuvres and preservation of corporal length.[80,81]

Grafting approaches

It is intuitive to prefer an approach that preserves phallic size, particularly in children with chordee who already may have a short phallus. Grafting approaches are particularly appealing when there is severe curvature, in which shortening the longer side of the corpora would further shorten the phallus. As discussed earlier in this chapter, the result of surgery have demonstrated a greater risk of compromised erectile rigidity, mainly due to venous leak while the gain in length is more theoretical than actual. A variety of graft materials have been used (see Table 7.13.4).[81–84] Practice patterns vary widely.[85] In one survey, 20 degrees of ventral curvature was considered 'significant', with 75% recommending surgery, while 99% recommend surgery at 30 degrees. Most recommend plication if curvature is less than 40 degrees. At 40 degrees, there was an increased trend towards taking a 'ventral' (i.e. manipulation of the urethral plate or grafting) approach.

Results of surgery

One-hundred per cent (100%) of patients undergoing the Nesbit procedure had a subjective report of penile shortening versus 73.5% undergoing multiple parallel plications (MPP).[86]

Seventy-four per cent (74%) of patients complained of subjective loss of length with the Essed-Schröder plication technique, although 78% described overall satisfaction with the procedure.[87] A greater degree of penile curvature, as well as ventral curvature was associated with an increased per cent of mean length lost.

Baskin and Lue[75] reported a 10% recurrence rate, with at least one year of follow-up using the MPP technique with 80% satisfaction. Two patients (20%) requested reoperation for residual curvature of 15 degrees, which highlights the need for adequate preoperative counselling with regards to surgical outcomes.

Leonardo *et al.*[86] reported no recurrences following a Nesbit procedure at a mean follow-up of 141 months; 50% of patients had no curvature and 50% had minimal curvature of less than 30 degrees. The same study reported a 15.8% recurrence rate requiring revision) following the MPP technique. All of these recurrent cases were performed with use of absorbable suture and there were no recurrences when non-absorbable suture was used. Overall, with

Table 7.13.3 Surgical techniques for correcting congenital curvature

Year	Author	Technique	No. of subjects	Follow-up (months)	Complications	Suture
1965	Nesbit[61]	Nesbit	3	6–12	One early pull through suture with need for revision	Silk
1985	Essed and Schroeder[68]	Plication (for PD, not chordee)	5	Not reported	One patient complained of penile shortening	Non-absorbable
1990	Yachia[69]	Heineke-Mikulicz	10	Not reported	None reported	Absorbable
1994	Baskin and Duckett[70]	Buried tunica albuginea	182	Not reported	One repeat operation;six mild residual curvature;	Absorbable
1998	Baskin and Lue[75]	Midline pure plication	10	More than 12 months	One early recurrence	Braided non-absorbable
2004	Giammusso[76]	Midline Yachia	12	20 months	One ED; one penile shortening	

Table 7.13.4 Grafting techniques for congenital curvature

Citation	Technique	Long-term follow-up?	Complications/issues
117, 118	Dermal grafts	10-year average (52)	Only three sexually active (of 16 total): one using intracavernous injections.[2] Short-terms study revealed no erectile dysfunction or loss of subjective penile length
119	Buccal mucosa	No	Two incomplete corrections (12 patients total)
120–122	Tunica vaginalis graft	No	Up to 60% complications[9]
123–4	Small intestinal submucosa (SIS)	No	Higher rates of complications using 4-ply[14]

the MPP technique, 68.4% of patients had optimal correction, while 31.6% had minimal deviation at the end of follow-up. Notably, there was no significant difference between the two techniques with respect to rates of severe or mild recurrence of curvature.

Reoperation for recurrent curvature when using the Essed-Schröder tunical plication are required in approximately 12% of patients.[87] In this study, 24% of patients had improved erectile function after correction of curvature and 24% had persistent ED; no patients had worsening of their ED.

Suture choice

The original description of the Nesbit technique used silk sutures, but there has been an interest in using absorbable suture to avoid palpable knots. Traditionally, permanent sutures are utilized for penile plication because of the theoretical risk of recurrent curvature with suture failure or absorption. Patients were able to feel suture knots following the Essed-Schröder plication technique 50% of the time when using polytetrafluoroethylene suture, and as high as 88% with use of polypropylene suture.[87] Sutures were palpable in 75% and 100% following plication corporoplasty and the Nesbit technique, respectively. Following the MPP technique, 100% of patients could palpate suture where braided non-absorbable suture was used.[75]

Recently, a randomized trial compared absorbable and non-absorbable sutures for corporal plication. Both sutures resulted in acceptable correction of the curvature in most patients.[88] There was a trend favouring absorbable vicryl suture over non-absorbable nylon with regards to patient satisfaction. A significantly higher number of patients were able to palpate the suture material in the nylon group (39%) versus the vicryl group (6%).

Non-excisional plication has been shown to have an 86% success rate with 15 degrees of residual curvature or less at six months postoperatively.[89] About 28% of patients had suture failure but only half of these patients developed recurrent curvature and only a few felt it necessary to have a repeat operation.

The rates of the palpable sutures being bothersome ranges from 0–40%, regardless of suture material.[75,90] Very rarely does the discomfort of the suture interfere with sexual intercourse, with reported rates of 10%.[75]

Psychosocial aspects

Improvements in sexual relationships, overall relationships, confidence, libido, and satisfaction have been demonstrated with curvature correction.[91,92] Predictors of improvement included perceived straightness of the penis as well as preservation of penile length. In contrast, Cavallini and Caracciolo[93] found that despite vast improvements in the ability to achieve vaginal intromission and subjective correction of curvature, patients' interpersonal relationships, and rates of psychogenic ED did not improve. The authors cautioned that cosmetic surgery of the penis for the improvement of social relationships is of dubious value.

Conclusions

Peyronie's disease, congenital curvature, and chordee are often physically and psychologically devastating to patients and can pose quite a challenge, even for an experienced urologist. Given the myriad of treatment options available from non-surgical to surgical, patient counselling and education are of paramount importance. Surgical correction appears to be the gold standard with a variety of approaches being used with reasonable success and a relatively low rate of severe complications.[94–124] Managing patient expectations is important to achieve maximum patient satisfaction. With this in mind, the overall goal of the urologist and patient should be to restore adequate sexual function with functional straightness.

Further reading

Baskin LS, Lue TF. The correction of congenital penile curvature in young men. *BJU Int* 1998; **81**(6):895–9.

Bologna RA, Noah TA, Nasrallah PF, McMahon DR. Chordee: varied opinions and treatments as documented in a survey of the American Academy of Pediatrics, Section of Urology. *Urology* 1999; **53**(3):608–12.

Deveci S, Hopps CV, O'Brien K, *et al.* A retrospective review of 307 men with Peyronie's disease. *J Urol* 2002; **168**:1075–9.

Devine CJ Jr, Horton CE. Use of dermal graft to correct chordee. *J Urol* 1975; **113**(1):56–8.

Kaplan GW, Lamm DL. Embryogenesis of chordee. *J Urol* 1975; **114**(5):769–72.

Larsen SM, Levine LA. Peyronie's disease: Review of nonsurgical treatment options. *Urol Clin North Am* 2011; **38**:195–205.

Leonardo C, De Nunzio C, Michetti P, *et al.* Plication corporoplasty versus Nesbit operation for the correction of congenital penile curvature. A long-term follow-up. *Int Urol Nephrol* 2012; **44**(1):55–60.

Levine LA, Greenfield JM. Establishing a standardized evaluation of the man with Peyronie's disease. *Int J Impot Res* 2003; **15**(Suppl 5):S103–12.

Mulhall J, Anderson M, Parker M. A surgical algorithm for men with combined Peyronie's disease and erectile dysfunction. Functional and satisfaction outcomes. *J Sex Med* 2005; **2**:132–8.

Nesbit RM. Congenital curvature of the phallus: report of three cases with description of corrective operation. *J Urol* 1965; **93**:230–2.

Rahman NU, Carrion RE, Bochinski D, Lue TF. Combined penile plication surgery and insertion of penile prosthesis for severe penile curvature and erectile dysfunction. *J Urol* 2004; **171**:2346–9.

Ralph D, Gonzalez-Cadavid N, Mirone V, Perovic S, Sohn M, Usta M, Levine L. The management of Peyronie's disease: evidence-based 2010 guidelines. *J Sex Med* 2010; **7**(7):1259–74.

Schwarzer U, Sommer F, Klotz T, *et al.* The prevalence of Peyronie's disease: results of a large survey. *BJU Int* 2001; **88**:727–30.

Tal R, Nabulsi O, Nelson CJ, Mulhall JP. The psychosocial impact of penile reconstructive surgery for congenital penile deviation. *J Sex Med* 2010; **7**(1 Pt 1):121–8.

Taylor FL, Levine LA. Surgical correction of Peyronie's disease via tunica albuginea plication or partial plaque excision with pericardial graft: long-term follow up. *J Sex Med* 2008: **5**(9):2221–8.

Wessells H, Lue T, McAninch J. Penile length in the flaccid and erect states: guidelines for penile augmentation. *J Urol* 1996; **156**:995–7.

Wilson SK, Cleves MA, Delk JR 2nd. Long-term follow-up of treatment for Peyronie's disease: modeling the penis over an inflatable penile prosthesis. *J Urol* 2001; **165**(3):825–9.

References

1. Deveci S, Hopps CV, O'Brien K, *et al.* Defining the clinical characteristics of Peyronie's disease in young men. *J Sex Med* 2007; **4**:485–90.
2. Deveci S, Hopps CV, O'Brien K, *et al.* A retrospective review of 307 men with Peyronie's disease. *J Urol* 2002; **168**:1075–9.
3. Schwarzer U, Sommer F, Klotz T, *et al.* The prevalence of Peyronie's disease: results of a large survey. *BJU Int* 2001; **88**:727–30.
4. Mulhall JP, Creech SD, Boorjian SA, *et al.* Subjective and objective analysis of the prevalence of Peyronie's disease in a population of men presenting for prostate cancer screening. *J Urol* 2004; **171**:2350–3
5. Pryor JP, Ralph DJ. Clinical presentations of Peyronie's. *Int J Imp Res* 2002; **14**:414–17.
6. El-Sakka AI, Tayeb KA. Peyronie's disease in diabetic patients being screened for erectile dysfunction. *J Urol* 2005; **174**:1026–30.
7. Tal R, Heck M, Teloken P, *et al.* Peyronie's disease following radical prostatectomy: Incidence and predictors. *J Sex Med* 2010; **7**:1254–61.
8. Ralph D, Gonzalez-Cadavid N, Mirone V, *et al.* The management of Peyronie's disease: Evidence-based 2010 guidelines. *J Sex Med* 2010; **7**(7):1259–74.
9. Cavallini G, Biagiotti G, Lo Giudice C. Association between peyronie's disease and low serum testosterone levels: detection and therapeutic considerations. *J Androl* 2012; **33**(3):381–8.
10. Nelson CJ, Diblasio C, Kendirci M, *et al.* The chronology depression and distress in men with Peyronie's Disease. *J Sex Med* 2008; **5**:1985–90
11. Van de Water L. Mechanisms by which fibrin and fibronectin appear in healing wounds: implications for Peyronie's disease. *J Urol* 1997; **157**:306–10.
12. El-Sakka AI, Hassoba HM, Pillarisetty RJ, *et al.* Peyronie's disease is associated with an increase in transforming growth factor-beta protein expression. *J Urol* 1997; **158**:1391–4.
13. Mulhall JP, Anderson MS, Lubrano T, Shankey TV. Peyronie's disease cell culture models: phenotypic, genotypic and functional analyses. *Int J Impot Res* 2002; **14**:397–405.
14. Cantini LP, Ferrini MG, Vernet D, *et al.* Profibrotic role of myostatin in Peyronie's disease. *J Sex Med* 2008; **5**:1607–22.
15. Ryu JK, Piao S, Shin HY, *et al.* IN-1130, a novel transforming growth factor-beta type I receptor kinase (activin receptor-like kinase inhibitor, promotes regression of fibrotic plaque and corrects penile curvature in a rat model of Peyronie's disease. *J Sex Med* 2009; **6**:1284–96.
16. Del Carlo M, Cole AA, Levine LA. Differential calcium independent regulation of matrix metalloproteinases and tissue inhibitors of matrix metalloproteinases by interleukin-1beta and transforming growth factor-beta in Peyronie's plaque fibroblasts. *J Urol* 2008; **179**:2447–55.
17. Levine LA, Greenfield JM. Establishing a standardized evaluation of the man with Peyronie's disease. *Int J Impot Res* 2003; **15**(suppl 5):S103–12.
18. Hellstrom WJ, Feldman R, Rosen RC, *et al.* Bother and distress associated with Peyronie's disease: validation of the Peyronie's disease questionnaire. *J Urol* 2013; **190**(2):627–34.
19. Bacal V, Rumohr J, Sturm R, Lipshultz LI, Schumacher M, Grober ED. Correlation of degree of penile curvature between patient estimates and objective measures among men with Peyronie's disease. *J Sex Med* 2009; **6**(3):862–5.
20. Benson JS, Abern MR, Levine LA. Penile shortening after radical prostatectomy and Peyronie's surgery. *Curr Urol Rep* 2009; **10**:468–74.
21. Smith JF, Walsh TJ, Conti SL, *et al.* Risk factors for emotional and relationship problems in Peyronie's disease. *J Sex Med* 2008; **5**(9):2179–84.
22. Wessells H, Lue T, McAninch J. Penile length in the flaccid and erect states: guidelines for penile augmentation. *J Urol* 1996; **156**:995–7.
23. Ohebshalom M, Mulhall J, Guhring P, Parker M. Measurement of penile curvature in Peyronie's disease patients: comparison of three methods. *J Sex Med* 2007; **4**:199–203.
24. Montorsi F, Guazzoni G, Bergamaschi F, *et al.* Vascular abnormalities in Peyronie's disease: the role of color Doppler sonography. *J Urol* 1994; **15**:373–5.
25. Levine L, Rybak J, Corder C, Farrel MR. Peyronie's disease plaque calcification—prevalence, time to identification, and development of a new grading classification. *J Sex Med* 2013; **10**(12):3121–8.
26. Larsen SM, Levine LA. Peyronie's disease: Review of nonsurgical treatment options. *Urol Clin North Am* 2011; **38**:195–205.
27. Raheem AA, Garaffa G, Raheem TA, *et al.* The role of vacuum pump therapy to mechanically straighten the penis in Peyronie's disease. *BJU Int* 2010; **106**(8):1178–80.
28. Levine LA, Newell M, Taylor FL. Penile traction therapy for treatment of Peyronie's disease: a single-center pilot study. *J Sex Med* 2008; **5**(6):1468–73.
29. Rehman J, Benet A, Melman A. Use of intralesional verapamil to dissolve Peyronie's disease plaque: a long-term single-blind study. *Urology* 1998; **51**:620–6.
30. Hellstrom WJ, Kendirci M, Matern R, *et al.* Single-blind, multicenter placebo-controlled parallel study to assess the safety and efficacy of intralesional interferon alpha-2B for minimally invasive treatment for Peyronie's disease. *J Urol* 2006; **176**:394–8.
31. Gelbard M, Goldstein I, Hellstrom WJ, *et al.* Clinical efficacy, safety and tolerability of collagenase clostridium histolyticum for the treatment of peyronie disease in 2 large double-blind, randomized, placebo controlled phase 3 studies. *J Urol* 2013; **190**:199–207.
32. Taylor FL, Levine LA. Peyronie's disease. *Urol Clin North Am* 2007; **34**(4):517–34.
33. Taylor FL, Levine LA. Surgical correction of Peyronie's disease via tunica albuginea plication or partial plaque excision with pericardial graft: long-term follow up. *J Sex Med* 2008: **5**(9):2221–8.
34. Levine LA, Lenting EL. A surgical algorithm for the treatment of Peyronie's disease. *J Urol* 1997; **158**:2149–52.
35. Mulhall J, Anderson M, Parker M. A surgical algorithm for men with combined Peyronie's disease and erectile dysfunction. Functional and satisfaction outcomes. *J Sex Med* 2005; **2**:132–8.
36. Taylor F, Abern M, Levine LA. Predicting erectile dysfunction following surgical correction of peyronie's disease without inflatable penile prosthesis placement: vascular assessment and preoperative risk factors. *J Sex Med* 2012; **9**(1):296–301.
37. Flores S, Choi J, Alex B, Mulhall JP. Erectile dysfunction after plaque incision and grafting: short-term assessment of incidence and predictors. *J Sex Med* 2011; **8**(7):2031–7.
38. Gelbard MK. Relaxing incisions in the correction of penile deformity due to Peyronie's disease. *J Urol* 1995; **154**:1457–60.
39. Levine LA. Partial plaque excision and grafting for Peyronie's disease. *J Sex Med* 2011; **8**:1842–5.
40. Egydio PH, Lucon AM, Arap S. A single relaxing incision to correct different types of penile curvature: surgical technique based on geometrical principles. *BJU Int* 2004; **94**(7):1147–57.
41. Gur S, Limin M, Hellstrom WJ. Current status and new developments in Peyronie's disease: medical, minimally invasive and surgical treatment options. *Expert Opin Pharmacother* 2011; **12**(6):931–44.
42. Breyer BN, Brant WO, Garcia MM, *et al.* Complications of porcine small intestine submucosa graft for Peyronie's disease. *J Urol* 2007; **177**(2):589–91.

43. Cormio L, Zucchi A, Lorusso F, *et al.* Surgical treatment of Peyronie's disease by plaque incision and grafting with buccal mucosa. *Eur Urol* 2009; **55**(6):1469–75.
44. Simonato A, Gregori A, Varca V, *et al.* Penile dermal flap in patients with Peyronie's disease: long-term results. *J Urol* 2010; **183**(3):1065–8.
45. Kalsi J, Minhas S, Christopher N, Ralph D. The results of plaque incision and venous grafting (Lue procedure) to correct the penile deformity of Peyronie's disease. *BJU Int* 2005; **95**(7):1029–33.
46. Usta MF, Bivalacqua TJ, Sanabria J, *et al.* Patient and partner satisfaction and long-term results after surgical treatment for Peyronie's disease. *Urology* 2003; **62**(1):105–9.
47. Chung E, Clendinning E, Lessard L, Brock G. Five-year follow-up of Peyronie's graft surgery: Outcomes and patient satisfaction. *J Sex Med* 2011; **8**:594–600.
48. Montorsi F, Salonia A, Briganti A. Five year follow-up of plaque incision and vein grafting for Peyronie's disease. *J Urol* 2004; **171**:331.
49. Montorsi F, Guazzoni G, Bergamaschi F, Rigatti P. Patient-partner satisfaction with semirigid penile prosthesis for Peyronie's disease: A 5-year follow-up study. *J Urol* 1993; **150**:1819–21.
50. Wilson SK, Cleves MA, Delk JR 2nd. Long-term follow-up of treatment for Peyronie's disease: modeling the penis over an inflatable penile prosthesis. *J Urol* 2001; **165**(3):825–9.
51. Levine LA, Benson JS, Hoover C. Inflatable penile prosthesis placement in men with Peyronie's disease and drug-resistant erectile dysfunction: A single-center study. *J Sex Med* 2010; **7**:3775–83.
52. Rahman NU, Carrion RE, Bochinski D, Lue TF. Combined penile plication surgery and insertion of penile prosthesis for severe penile curvature and erectile dysfunction. *J Urol* 2004; **171**:2346–9.
53. Hakim LS, Kulaksizoglu H, Hamill BK, *et al.* Guide to safe corporotomy incisions in the presence of underlying inflatable penile cylinders: Results of in vitro and in vivo studies. *J Urol* 1996; **155**:918–23.
54. Perito P, Wilson S. The Peyronie's plaque "scratch": an adjunct to modeling. *J Sex Med* 2013; **10**(5):1194–7.
55. Akin-Olugbade O, Parker M, Guhring P, Mulhall J. Determinants of patients satisfaction following penile prosthesis surgery. *J Sex Med* 2006; **3**:743–8.
56. Wang R, Howard GE, Hoang A, *et al.* Prospective and long-term evaluation of erect penile length obtained with inflatable penile prosthesis to that induced by intracavernosal injection. *Asian J Androl* 2009; **11**(4):411–5.
57. Levine LA, Rybak J. Traction therapy for men with shortened penis prior to penile prosthesis implantation: a pilot study. *J Sex Med* 2011; **8**:2112–2117
58. Brant WO, Taylor M, Mobley E, Myers JB. "Emergent" repair of congenital penile curvature for unconsummated marriage. *J Sex Med* 2012; **9**(1):1.
59. Montag S, Palmer LS. Abnormalities of penile curvature: chordee and penile torsion. *ScientificWorldJournal* 2011; **11**:1470–8.
60. Stojanovic B, Bizic M, Majstorovic M, *et al.* Penile curvature incidence in hypospadias: can it be determined? *Adv Urol* 2011: **813205**.
61. Nesbit RM. Congenital curvature of the phallus: Report of three cases with description of corrective operation. *J Urol* 1965; **93**: 230–2.
62. Donnahoo KK, Cain MP, Pope JC, *et al.* Etiology, management and surgical complications of congenital chordee without hypospadias. *J Urol* 1998; **160**(3 Pt 2):1120–2.
63. Adams MC, Chalian VS, Rink RC. Congenital dorsal penile curvature: a potential problem of the long phallus. *J Urol* 1999; **161**(4):1304–7.
64. Kelami A. Classification of congenital and acquired penile deviation. *Urol Int* 1983; **38**(4):229–33.
65. Darewicz B, Kudelski J, Szynaka B, Nowak HF, Darewicz J. Ultrastructure of the tunica albuginea in congenital penile curvature. *J Urol* 2001; **166**(5):1766–8.
66. Gearhart JP, Linhard HR, Berkovitz GD, Jeffs RD, Brown TR. Androgen receptor levels and 5 alpha-reductase activities in preputial skin and chordee tissue of boys with isolated hypospadias. *J Urol* 1988; **140**(5 Pt 2):1243–6.
67. Tietjen DN, Uramoto GY, Tindall DJ, Husmann DA. Micropenis in hypogonadotropic hypogonadism: response of the penile androgen receptor to testosterone treatment. *J Urol* 1998; **160**(3 Pt 2):1054–7.
68. Essed E, Schroeder FH. New surgical treatment for Peyronie disease. *Urology* 1985; **25**(6):582–7.
69. Yachia D. Modified corporoplasty for the treatment of penile curvature. *J Urol* 1990; **143**(1):80–2.
70. Baskin LS, Duckett JW. Dorsal tunica albuginea plication for hypospadias curvature. *J Urol* 1994; **151**(6):1668–71.
71. Baskin LS, Lee YT, Cunha GR. Neuroanatomical ontogeny of the human fetal penis. *BJU Int* 1997; **79**(4):628–40.
72. Breza, Aboseif, Orvis, *et al.* Detailed anatomy of penile neurovascular structures: surgical significance. *J Urol* 1989; **141**(2):437–43.
73. Lue, Zeineh, Schmidt, Tanagho. Neuroanatomy of penile erection: its relevance to iatrogenic impotence. *J Urol* 1984; **131**(2):273–80.
74. Paick JS, Donatucci CF, Lue TF. Anatomy of cavernous nerves distal to prostate: microdissection study in adult male cadavers. *Urology* 1993; **42**(2):145–9.
75. Baskin LS, Lue TF. The correction of congenital penile curvature in young men. *BJU Int* 1998; **81**(6):895–9.
76. Giammusso B, Burrello M, Branchina A, *et al.* Modified corporoplasty for ventral penile curvature: description of the technique and initial results. *J Urol* 2004; **171**(3):1209–11.
77. Kass EJ. Dorsal corporeal rotation: an alternative technique for the management of severe chordee. *J Urol* 1993; **150**(2 Pt 2):635–6.
78. Kaplan GW, Lamm DL. Embryogenesis of chordee. *J Urol* 1975; **114**(5):769–72.
79. Glenister TW. The origin and fate of the urethral plate in man. *J Anat* 1954; **88**(3):413–25.
80. Dessanti A, Iannuccelli M, Falchetti D, *et al.* Correction of congenital chordee penis by 'ventral separation and outward rotation of corpora'. *J Pediatr Surg* 2002; **37**(9):1347–50.
81. Shaeer O. Shaeer's corporal rotation for length-preserving correction of penile curvature: modifications and 3-year experience. *J Sex Med* 2008; **5**(11):2716–24.
82. Kogan SJ, Reda EF, Smey PL, Levitt SB. Dermal graft correction of extraordinary chordee. *J Urol* 1983; **130**(5):952–4.
83. Lindgren BW, Reda EF, Levitt SB, Brock WA. Single and multiple dermal grafts for the management of severe penile curvature. *J Urol* 1998; **160**(3 Pt 2):1128–30.
84. Devine CJ Jr, Horton CE. Use of dermal graft to correct chordee. *J Urol* 1975; **113**(1):56–8.
85. Bologna RA, Noah TA, Nasrallah PF, McMahon DR. Chordee: varied opinions and treatments as documented in a survey of the American Academy of Pediatrics, Section of Urology. *Urology* 1999; **53**(3):608–12.
86. Leonardo C, De Nunzio C, Michetti P, *et al.* Plication corporoplasty versus Nesbit operation for the correction of congenital penile curvature. A long-term follow-up. *Int Urol Nephrol* 2012; **44**(1):55–60.
87. Van Der Horst C, Martinez-Portillo FJ, Seif C, *et al.* Treatment of penile curvature with Essed-Schröder tunical plication: aspects of quality of life from the patients' perspective. *BJU Int* 2004; **93**(1):105–8.
88. Basiri A, Sarhangnejad R, Ghahestani SM, Radfar MH. Comparing absorbable and nonabsorbable sutures in corporeal plication for treatment of congenital penile curvature. *J Urol* 2011; **8**(4):302–6.
89. Hsieh JT, Liu SP, Chen Y, *et al.* Correction of congenital penile curvature using modified tunical plication with absorbable sutures: the long-term outcome and patient satisfaction. *Eur Urol* 2007; **52**(1):261–6.
90. Van der Horst C, Martinez-Portillo FJ, Melchior D, *et al.* Polytetrafluoroethylene versus polypropylene sutures for Essed-Schroeder tunical plication. *J Urol* 2003; **170**(2 Pt 1):472–5.
91. Van der Drift DG, Vroege JA, Groenendijk PM, *et al.* The plication procedure for penile curvature: surgical outcome and postoperative sexual functioning. *Urol Int* 2002; **69**(2):120–4.

92. Tal R, Nabulsi O, Nelson CJ, Mulhall JP. The psychosocial impact of penile reconstructive surgery for congenital penile deviation. *J Sex Med* 2010; **7**(1 Pt 1):121–8.
93. Cavallini G, Caracciolo S. Pilot study to determine improvements in subjective penile morphology and personal relationships following a Nesbit plication procedure for men with congenital penile curvature. *Asian J Androl* 2008; **10**(3):512–9.
94. Savoca F, Scieri F, Pietropaolo F, *et al.* Straightening corporoplasty for Peyronie's disease: a review of 218 patients with median follow-up of 89 months. *Eur Urol* 2004; **46**(5):610–4.
95. Ralph DJ, al-Akraa M, Pryor JP. The Nesbit operation for Peyronie's disease: 16-year experience. *J Urol* 1995; **4**:1362–3.
96. Licht MR, Lewis RW. Modified Nesbit procedure for the treatment of Peyronie's disease: a comparative outcome analysis. *J Urol* 1997; **15**;460–3.
97. Mufti GR, Aitchison M, Bramwell SP, *et al.* Corporeal plication for surgical correction of Peyronie's disease. *J Urol* 1990; **144**:281–2.
98. Gholami SS, Lue TF. Correction of penile curvature using the 16-dot plication technique: A review of 132 patients. *J Urol* 2002; **167**:2066–9.
99. Chahal R, Gogoi NK, Sundaram SK, Weston PM. Corporal plication for penile curvature caused by Peyronie's disease: the patients' perspective. *BJU Int* 2001; **87**:352–6.
100. Geertsen UA, Brok KE, Andersen B, Nielsen HV. Peyronie's curvature treated by plication of the penile fasciae. *BJU Int* 1996; **77**:733–5.
101. Thiounn N, Missirliu A, Zerbib M, *et al.* Corporeal plication for surgical correction of penile curvature: Experience with 60 patients. *Eur Urol* 1998; **33**:401–8.
102. Van Der Horst C, Martinez-Portillo FJ, Seif C, *et al.* Treatment of penile curvature with Essed-Schröder tunical plication: aspects of quality of life from the patients' perspective. *BJU Int* 2004; **93**:105–8.
103. Kovac JR, Brock GB. Surgical outcomes and patient satisfaction after dermal, pericardial, and small intestinal submucosal grafting for Peyronie's disease. *J Sex Med* 2007; **4**:1500–8.
104. El-Sakka AI, Rashwan HM, Lue TF. Venous patch graft for Peyronie's disease. Part II: outcome analysis. *J Urol* 1998; **160**(6Pt1):2050–3.
105. Akkus E, Ozkara H, Alici B, *et al.* Incision and venous patch graft in the surgical treatment of penile curvature in Peyronie's disease. *Eur Urol* 2001; **40**:531–6.
106. Shioshvili TJ, Kakonahvili AP. The surgical treatment of Peyronie's disease: Replacement of plaque by free autograft of buccal mucosa. *Eur Urol* 2005; **48**:129–35.
107. Teloken C, Grazziotin T, Rhoden E, *et al.* Penile straightening with crural graft of the corpus cavernosum. *J Urol* 2000; **164**:107–8.
108. Schwarzer JU, Muhlen B, Schukai O. Penile corporoplasty using tunica albuginea free graft from proximal corpus cavernosum: a new technique for treatment of penile curvature in Peyronie's disease. *Eur Urol* 2003; **44**(6):720–3.
109. Da Ros CT, Graziottin TM, Ribeiro E, Averbeck MA. Long-term follow-up of penile curvature correction utilizing autologous albugineal crural graft. *Int Braz J Urol* 2012; **38**(2):242–7.
110. Das S. Peyronie's disease: Excision and autografting with tunica vaginalis. *J Urol* 1980; **124**:818–9.
111. O'Donnell PD. Results of surgical management of Peyronie's disease. *J Urol* 1992; **148**(4):1184–7.
112. Sampaio JS, Passarinho FA, Mendes CJ. Peyronie's disease. Surgical correction of 40 patients with relaxing incision and duramater graft. *Eur Urol* 2002; **41**:551–5.
113. Fallon B. Cadaveric dura mater graft for correction of penile curvature in Peyronie disease. *Urology* 1990; **35**(2):127–9.
114. Gelbard MK, Hayden B. Expanding contractures of the tunica albuginea due to Peyronie's disease with temporalis fascia free grafts. *J Urol* 1991; **145**(4):772–6.
115. Kalsi JS, Christopher N, Ralph DJ, Minhas S. Plaque incision and fascia lata grafting in the surgical management of Peyronie's disease. *BJU Int* 2006; **98**(1):110–4
116. Hellstrom WJ, Reddy S. Application of pericardial graft in the surgical management of Peyronie's disease. *J Urol* 2000; **163**(5):1445–7.
117. Simonato A, Gregori A, Ambruosi C, Ruggiero G, Traverso P, Carmignani G. Congenital penile curvature: dermal grafting procedure to prevent penile shortening in adults. *Eur Urol* 2007; **51**(5):1420–7.
118. Badawy H, Morsi H. Long-term followup of dermal grafts for repair of severe penile curvature. *J Urol* 2008; **180**(4 Suppl):1842–5.
119. Mokhless IA, Youssif ME, Orabi SS, Ehnaish MM. Corporeal body grafting using buccal mucosa for posterior hypospadias with severe curvature. J Urol 2009; **182**(4 Suppl):1726–9.
120. Braga LH, Pippi Salle JL, Dave S, Bagli DJ, Lorenzo AJ, Khoury AE. Outcome analysis of severe chordee correction using tunica vaginalis as a flap in boys with proximal hypospadias. *J Urol* 2007; **178**(4 Pt 2):1693–7; discussion 7.
121. Hayashi Y, Kojima Y, Mizuno K, *et al.* Demonstration of postoperative effectiveness in ventral lengthening using a tunica vaginalis flap for severe penile curvature with hypospadias. *Urology* 2010; **76**(1):101–6.
122. Ritchey ML, Ribbeck M. Successful use of tunica vaginalis grafts for treatment of severe penile chordee in children. *J Urol* 2003; **170**:1574–6.
123. Kropp BP, Cheng EY, Pope JC 4th, *et al.* Use of small intestinal submucosa for corporal body grafting in cases of severe penile curvature. *J Urol* 2002; **168**(4 Pt 2):1742–5; discussion 5.
124. Elmore JM, Kirsch AJ, Scherz HC, Smith EA. Small intestinal submucosa for corporeal body grafting in severe hypospadias requiring division of the urethral plate. *J Urol* 2007; **178**(4 Pt 2):1698–701; discussion 701.

CHAPTER 7.14

Male genital injury

Giulio Garaffa, Salvatore Sansalone, and David J. Ralph

Introduction to male genital injury

Genital injuries in civilian centres are relatively rare and in this setting penile fracture represents the most common cause of trauma. The scenario is completely different in the battlefield where the use of protective torso armour, which guarantees a relative protection to the abdominal viscera, has led to the survival of patients with extremely severe injuries to pelvis, genitals, and lower limbs caused by fragmentation weapons.

Surgical repair of genital injuries is critical as preservation of sexual and urinary function and cosmesis have a major impact on patient's satisfaction, self-esteem, and ultimately, quality of life.

Effects of trauma and protective mechanisms

The pendulous portions of the penis and the scrotum have an incredible capacity to resist injury, as their flaccidity limits the effect of the kinetic energy. The proximal, fixed part of the penis is more prone to blunt trauma, which can occur as a consequence of pelvic fracture or straddle injury. However, there is a limit above which the kinetic energy and speed of the weapon cannot be absorbed adequately by the elasticity of the tissues and this is why blunt traumas, which usually occur in road traffic accidents, cause much less damage to the pendulous portion of penis and scrotum than firearm and stab injuries. Pelvic fractures with symphyseal or pubic ramus displacement instead can cause severe injury to the deep structures of the penis, including avulsion of the crura of the corpora cavernosa from its vascular and neural supply.

While flaccidity represents a protective mechanism, rigidity renders the penis more susceptible to trauma; this is because the tunica albuginea becomes thinner and more fragile as it is stretched during the erection. Furthermore, forcibly bending an erect penis leads to an exponential increase in intracavernosal pressures, which can lead to a fracture of the already stretched tunica albuginea.

While on one hand the laxity of the genital skin plays a protective role, as it allows absorbtion of the kinetic energy during trauma, on the other hand rotating and suction devices can easily grab hold of a portion of the loose skin, which can be completely avulsed from the genitalia.

The type of vascular supply to a particular region of the genitalia also plays an important role in defining the type of damage that will occur following an insult. In particular, ischaemic loss of the penis or testicles is rare and is usually seen only in cases of complete amputation or prolonged constriction injury, as these structures receive blood supply from multiple sources, which need to be all compromised for ischaemia to occur. On the contrary, the skin receives its vascular supply only from the deep fascial layers and when these are affected total skin necrosis occurs.

When managing genital trauma, it is paramount to identify possible associated bony, vascular, bowel, and urinary tract injuries, which are present in up to 83% of cases, and which require immediate treatment as they may be potentially life-threatening. The management of the genital trauma should be deferred to a later stage, when associated injuries have been successfully dealt with and the patient's condition is stable.

Usually urethral injuries can be suspected by the presence of blood at the level of the urethral meatus and by the inability to void. These should be confirmed with a retrograde urethrogram.

The presence of haematuria indicates possible insult to the bladder or upper urinary tract, especially in patients who have sustained blunt abdominal trauma or penetrating stabbing and firearm injuries.

Types of injury

Classification of genital injuries is extremely complex, as an offending mechanism can lead to a broad spectrum of lesions and the same type of lesion can be produced by different causes.

According to the offending mechanism, genital injury can be subdivided in the following six categories:

Bites

Although bites are quite common, with almost 50% of the Western world's citizens treated at least once in their lifetime, genital injuries resulting from human or animal bites are rare and mostly presented in individual case reports.

The main problem in patients who have suffered a bite is the risk of infection, which occurs in up to 30% of cases, usually in the first 48 hours after the injury. Therefore accurate surgical debridement of all non-viable tissue and removal of any foreign body, irrigation of the wound with antiseptic solution and administration of broad-spectrum antibiotics is mandatory, even when there is no evidence of infection. Vaccination against tetanus or rabies might be also indicated. Human bites also carry the risk of transmission of sexually transmitted diseases such as HIV, herpes, and hepatitis.

With regards to surgical management, injuries should be initially treated conservatively with suturing and dressing. With the exception of complete amputation of the penis, which warrants immediate microsurgical anastomosis, reconstruction should not be attempted until the risk of infection has been ruled out and when the extent of necrosis has become obvious.

Penetrating injuries to the genitalia due to gunshot wounds and stabbing

During wartime, penetrating gunshot wounds account for two-thirds of all urologic injuries, while in civilian centres this type of injury is relatively rare. Up to 80% of patients with penile stabbing and gunshot wounds have associated injuries, usually involving scrotum, thighs, pelvis, and buttocks, which usually must be dealt with before addressing the genital injuries.

Important differences exist between military and civilian gunshot wounds; in particular, military injuries are typically caused by high velocity projectiles, which inflict much greater damage and cause more tissue loss than that seen in civilian centres, where bullets have a relatively low velocity. Due to the significant tissue loss observed in military injuries, immediate repair is frequently not feasible and patients may require urinary diversion followed by delayed repair.

In case of penetrating genital injuries, the penile shaft is the most commonly affected structure followed by the scrotum and the urethra. A retrograde urethrogram should be always performed to rule out urethral injury, which is present in up to 50% of cases and prompts urinary diversion with a suprapubic cystostomy and urethral repair.

Penetrating wounds due to stabbing and bullets require immediate exploration, removal of any residual foreign material and surgical reconstruction in order to guarantee adequate cosmetic and functional results. In general, the type of surgical repair is tailored to the type and extent of injury and should take account of the blood supply to the area.

In distal penile trauma, a circumcising subcoronal incision guarantees adequate exposure of the corpora cavernosa, allows identification of the exact site of injury and identifies urethral involvement where present. In patients who have experienced a proximal penile injury instead, a penoscrotal approach should be performed. Ideally, small corporeal defects should be repaired primarily with the use of interrupted absorbable sutures while larger defects, such as those produced by high velocity projectiles, may require the interposition of a graft. Urethral injuries should be repaired primarily with interrupted absorbable sutures over a silicone catheter, which should be left *in situ* for three weeks.

Testicular ruptures are not uncommon and require immediate repair of the tunica albuginea, a manoeuvre that preserves the testicles in up to 80% of cases if performed within 48 to 72 hours of the injury. After 72 hours, or if the reconstruction is not possible due to the presence of diffuse necrosis, simple orchiectomy is the only option.

Burns and necrotizing infections

Although genital burns in isolation are very rare, genitals are involved in up to 5–13% of cases in the presence of extensive body burns. Automobile and industrial accidents are the most frequent causes of burns in the genital area. The severity of the burns dictates the type of management required. First- and second-degree burns usually can be managed conservatively, while debridement of necrotic tissue and reconstruction with the use of local flaps and skin grafts is necessary in case of third-degree burns (Fig. 7.14.1). Meshed split-thickness skin grafts are ideal for scrotal reconstruction as they take well and heal mimicking the rugae present on the scrotum, although they play little if no role in the thermoregulation of the testicles. The penile shaft instead should be repaired with full-thickness skin grafts harvested from non-hair bearing areas of the body; this is because full-thickness grafts tend to heal with less contracture than their split-thickness counterpart and therefore allow the physiological girth and length expansion during the erections.

Necrotizing fasciitis, also known as Fournier's gangrene, is the most common cause of genital skin loss, accounting for up to 75% of cases. This condition usually occurs in the immunocompromized patient and the sources of infection are perirectal abscesses and urethral strictures and fistulas.

Early recognition and aggressive surgical debridement of all infected and necrotic tissues are mandatory in these patients in order to guarantee the best outcome. Reconstruction should be delayed until the wounds appear clean and granulating and requires the use of flaps and skin grafts to repair the tissue defects, as previously described.

Blunt trauma

The vast majority of blunt trauma results from sporting and traffic accidents and can be managed conservatively. Injury occurs when the testis is pushed violently against a bony structure, leading to testicular contusion or rupture, or when the erect penis is forcibly bent, causing a penile fracture.

In scrotal blunt trauma, testicular rupture should be excluded with an ultrasound scan, as immediate surgical repair allows testicular preservation in up to 80% of cases. If not treated promptly, testicular rupture leads invariably to testicular atrophy (Fig. 7.14.2).

Penile fracture is the most common type of penile trauma and can be defined as rupture of the tunica albuginea of the corpora cavernosa following blunt trauma to the erect penis. Hitting the female pelvis during enthusiastic sex or vigorous masturbation are the most common causes of penile fracture. It usually occurs in the erect state, when elongation and thinning of the tunica albuginea occurs and the most common location is the ventrolateral aspect of the penis, where the tunica is weakest, being unilayer in this area.

The clinical features of penile fracture are a snapping sound followed by immediate detumescence, swelling, and shaft contusion. If Buck's fascia has been breached, the haematoma tracks to the base of the shaft and spreads to the perineum, scrotum and lower abdomen (butterfly sign) (Fig. 7.14.3).

Isolated rupture of the urethra or of the deep dorsal vein of the penis can give a similar picture and therefore must be excluded with accurate history taking, examination, and imaging.

A concomitant urethral injury is present in up to 30% of cases and should be ruled out with a retrograde urethrography; blood at the urethral meatus, difficulty to pass urine, or inability to introduce a catheter are obvious signs, but they may not be apparent even when the urethra has been completely transected.

Conservative management of penile fractures has now become obsolete, as it is associated with formation of chordee, pseudoaneurysms of the corpora, penile deviation, and erectile dysfunction.

Therefore the modern management involves early surgery, which can be carried out either through a circumcising subcoronal or a penoscrotal approach and allows identification and repair with absorbable sutures of the corporal tear and any associated urethral injuries.

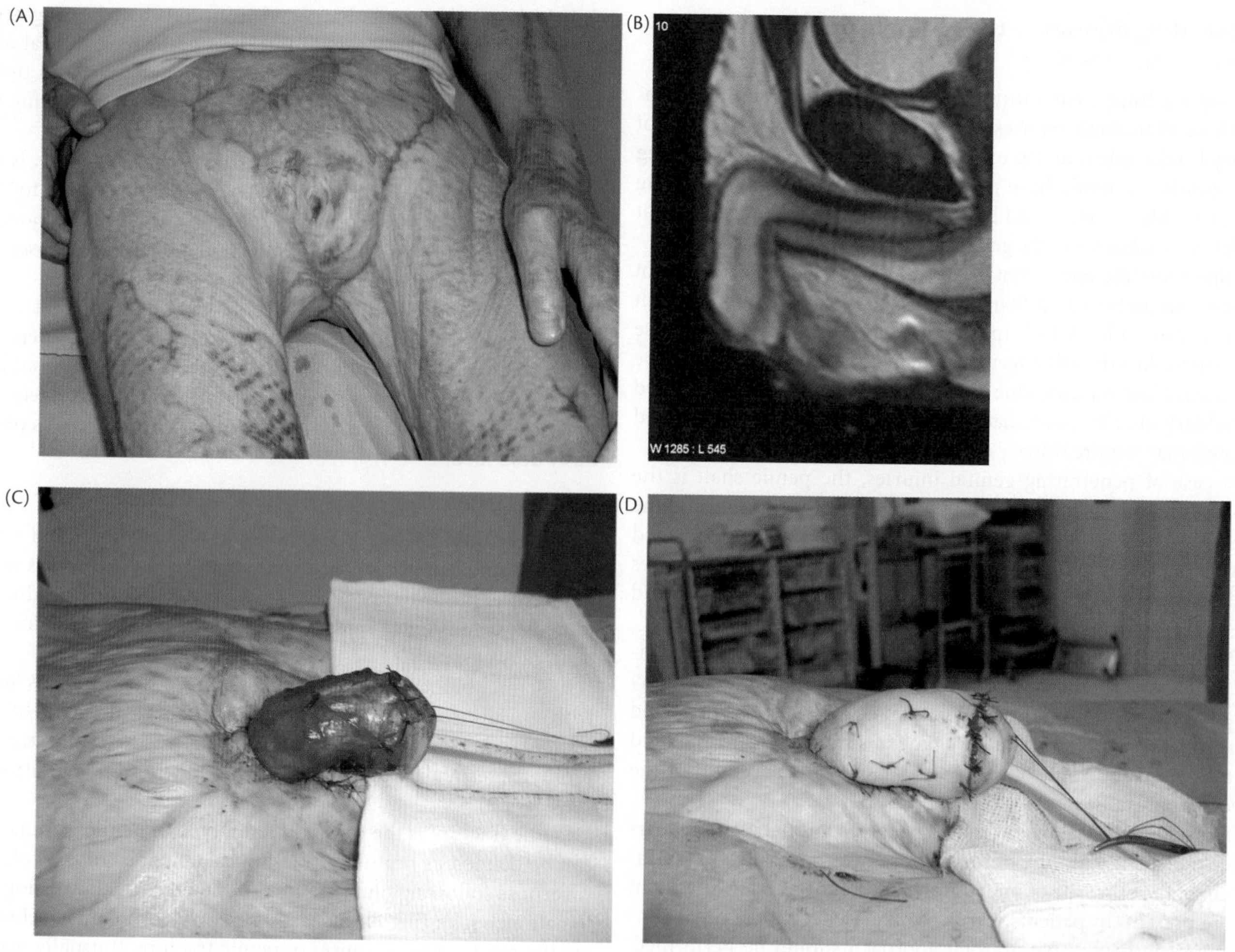

Fig. 7.14.1 Third-degree electrical burn involving the genitalia, previously repaired with a split-thickness skin graft. (A) Initial presentation of the patient after skin grafting. (B) Magnetic resonance imaging showing intact corpora cavernosa trapped underneath the skin graft. (C) The corpora are released and prepared for grafting; and (D) final result after penile reconstruction with the use of a full-thickness skin graft.

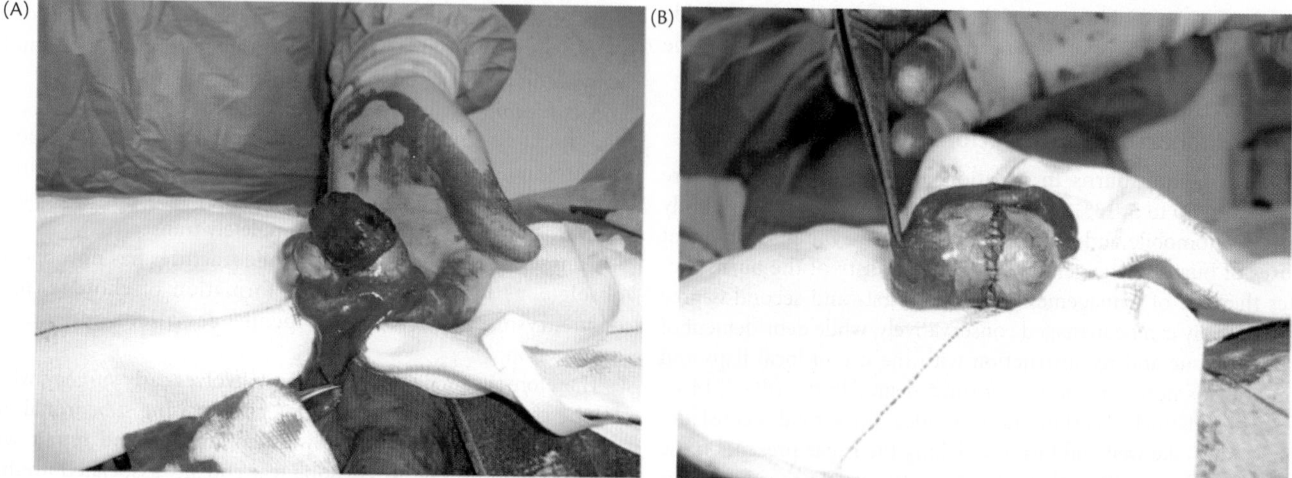

Fig. 7.14.2 Blunt scrotal trauma with testicular rupture. (A) The exposed testis presents a transversal breach of the tunica albuginea and the parenchyma is visible. (B) The tunica albuginea is repaired with a desorbable suture.

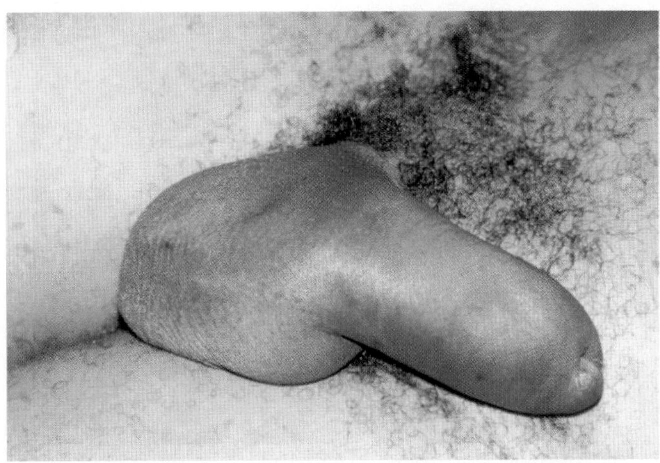

Fig. 7.14.3 Penile fracture with breach of Buck's fascia. The haematoma extends under the skin of the shaft and the scrotum.

Since subocoronal incisions and degloving are associated with significant complications such as haematoma formation, skin necrosis, and postoperative oedema, the procedure should be carried out through a small skin incision placed above the fracture site, which should have been precisely located with an ultrasound scan or magnetic resonance imaging. As more than two-thirds of all fractures occur at the base of the shaft, a penoscrotal incision represents the access of choice in the majority of patients (Figs 7.14.4 and 7.14.5).

(A)

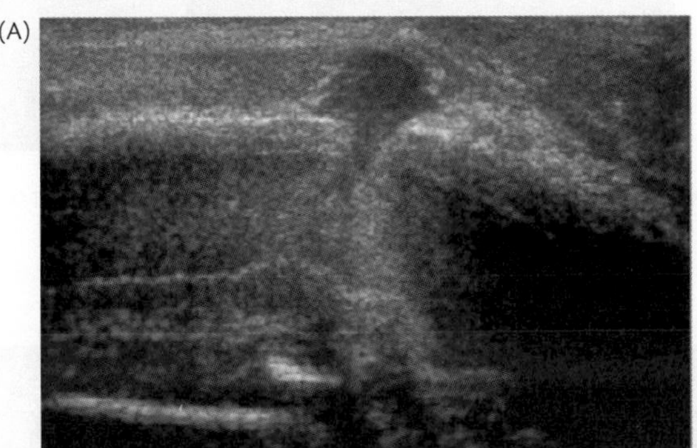

(B)

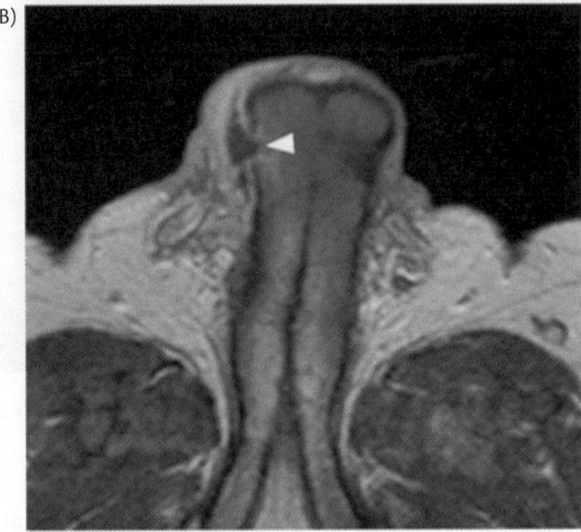

Fig. 7.14.4 Identification of the location of the rupture of the tunica albuginea. (A) Ultrasound scan of the corpora cavernosa identifying the rupture of the tunica albuginea and the associated haematoma. (B) Magnetic resonance imaging documenting the site of rupture of the corpora cavernosa.

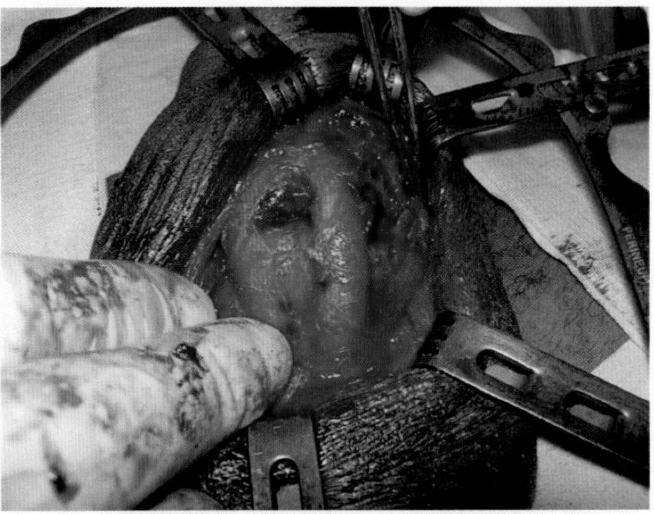

Fig. 7.14.5 A penoscrotal approach guarantees an excellent exposure of all proximal ruptures. The urethra can be easily assessed and has not been breached.

Long-term outcomes after early surgical repair are very encouraging with penile curvature and erectile dysfunction reported by only 5% and 1% of patients, respectively.

Another relatively common form of genital trauma is suspensory ligament rupture, which occurs when the erect penis is forcibly bent downwards during enthusiastic sex. Patients typically feel a 'snapping' sound and notice a degree of instability of the penis, which is directly related to the degree of damage occurred to the suspensory ligament. A noticeable gap between the base of the penis and the pubic bone is a common finding. This condition can be easily differentiated from rupture of the corpora cavernosa, as detumescence, swelling, and shaft contusion usually do not occur.

Suspensory ligament rupture does not require immediate surgical intervention, as the suspensory ligament does not play a key role in the male genitalia. Suspensory ligament repair is usually offered electively only in patients who complain of instability of the penis or have developed secondary erectile dysfunction.

Traumatic genital skin avulsion

Avulsion injuries usually result from a rapid deceleration in which the loose, elastic skin of the genitalia is caught in clothing or is trapped in rotating and suction devices and traumatically ripped. Due to the inherent elasticity of the genital skin, typically only the skin and Dartos fascia are avulsed.

Minor avulsions injuries, such as rupture of the frenulum during vigorous masturbation or enthusiastic sex, can be managed as simple lacerations, with immediate primary closure in layers after the administration of broad-spectrum antibiotics (Fig. 7.14.6).

In cases of complex avulsion, debridement should be limited to the obviously non-viable tissue and the skin edges should be reapproximated. Delayed debridement and reconstruction with the use of local flaps or skin grafts is often necessary in these cases. Due to its intrinsic elasticity, scrotal skin reconstruction can be almost

(A) (B) (C)

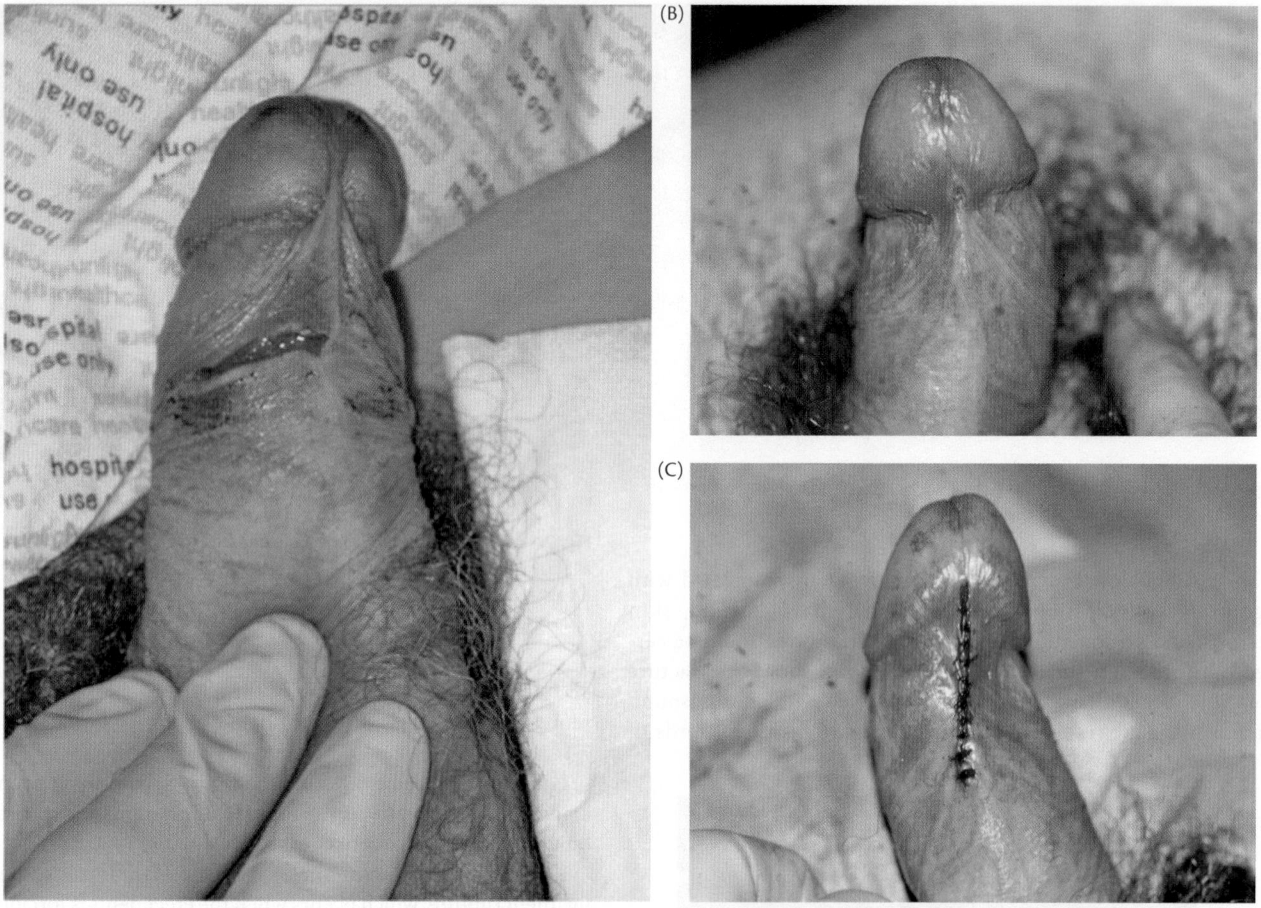

Fig. 7.14.6 Minor traumatic genital skin avulsions. (A) A preputial laceration; (B) chronic traumatic tears due to a relatively short frenom; and (C) acute frenular tear requiring immediate surgical repair.

always accomplished with primary closure, while full-thickness skin grafts are frequently necessary for penile skin repair.

Traumatic amputation and genital self-mutilation

The spectrum of genital amputation spans from mild forms, such as circumcision and dorsal preputial incisions, to the total amputation of the genitalia.

Penile and testicular amputation are rare injuries, which usually occurs as a result of assault or is self-inflicted by patients with psychosis or unresolved transsexual and religious issues (Fig. 7.14.7).

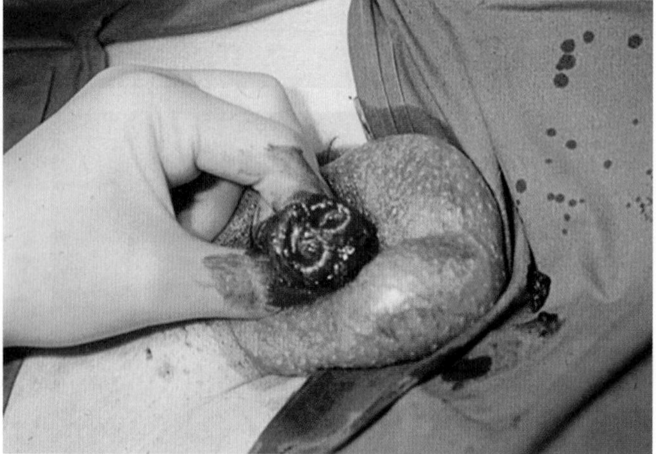

Fig. 7.14.7 Complete amputation of the penis. The transected corpora cavernosa and spongiosum are visible.

Once the patient has been resuscitated, conservative surgery should always be attempted; preservation of the genitals for up to 24 hours is possible if they are wrapped in a saline-soaked gauze in a sterile bag and maintained refrigerated in an ice-slush bath.

With regards to the penis, microscopical reconstruction of the dorsal penile nerves, arteries, and veins is required after replantation of the corporeal bodies and of the urethra. Anastomosis of the cavernosal arteries is technically difficult and should be avoided, as it leads to further cavernosal scarring, as the vessels have to be dissected to be prepared for the anastomosis, and is not associated with improved outcomes, in terms of postoperative erectile function. If reconstruction is not feasible, the distal corpora are sutured in around fashion and the urethra spatulated on the tip of the stump. Stump advancement with division of the suspensory ligament or total phallic reconstruction can be offered at a later stage in highly motivated patients (Figs 7.14.8 and 7.14.9).

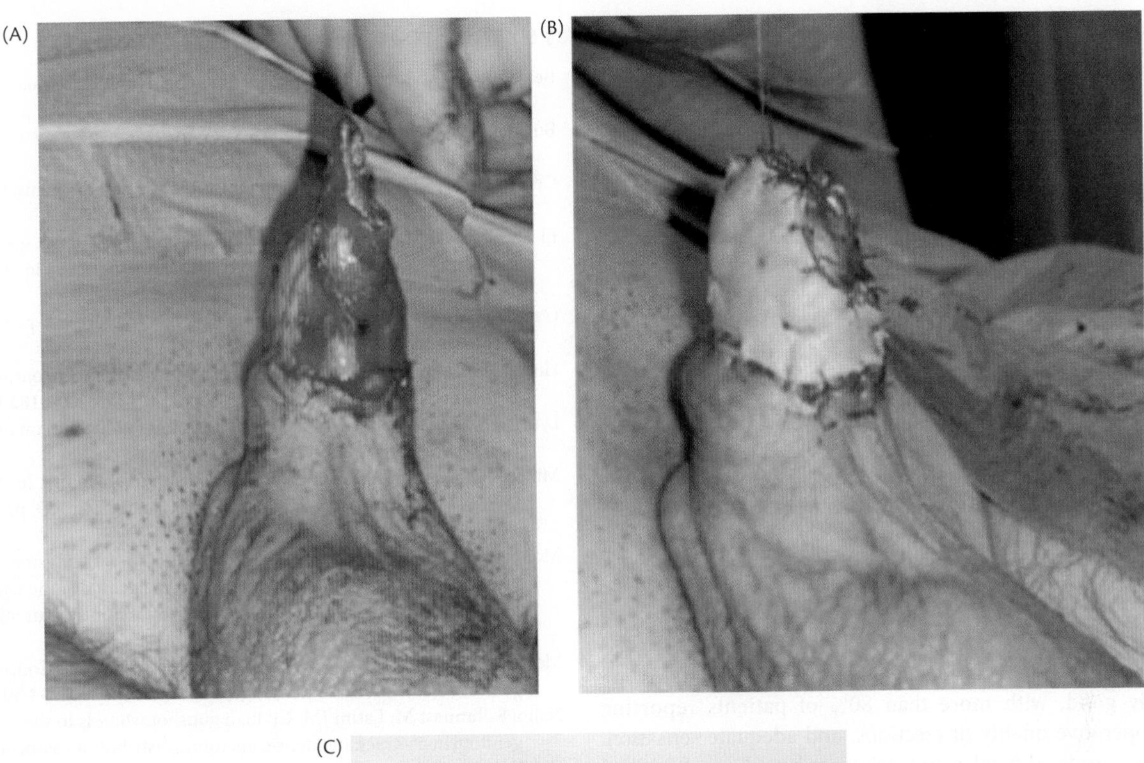

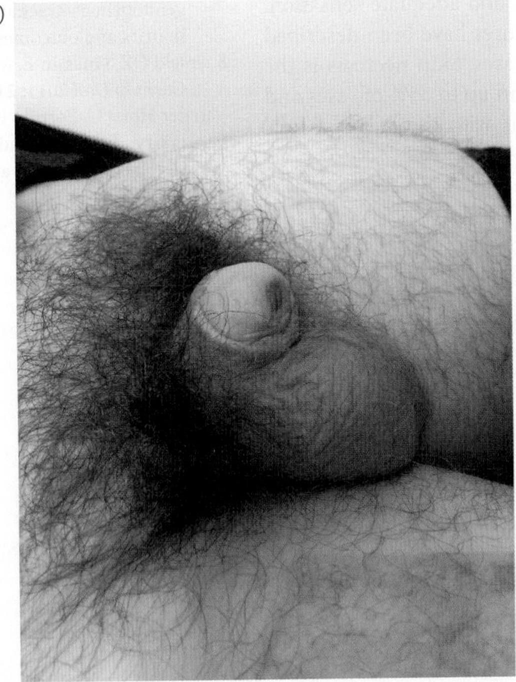

Fig. 7.14.8 Delayed penile reconstruction with the use of skin graft following partial traumatic amputation. (A) The distal corpora cavernosa are exposed and prepared for grafting. (B) A pseudo-glans is fashioned with the use of a split-thickness skin graft, which is placed on the tip of the corpora, after adequate spatulation of the urethral distal end. Extra penile length can be achieved with the division of the suspensory ligament. (C) The final result.

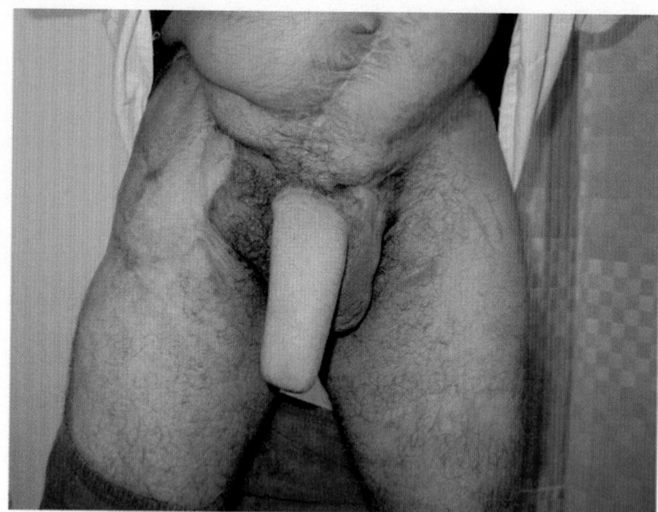

Fig. 7.14.9 Total phallic reconstruction with the use of a sensate forearm free flap based on the radial artery gives superior cosmetic and functional results.

Outcomes after microsurgical reattachment of the penis are surprisingly good, with more than 80% of patients reporting good postoperative quality of erections, and adequate sensation. Postoperative urethral fistulas and strictures have been described respectively in up to 10% and 20% of cases. Skin necrosis is the most common complication and occurs in up to 55% of cases and requires debridement followed by repair with the use of a full-thickness skin graft.

Further reading

Bertolotto M, Calderan L, Cova MA. Imaging in penile traumas-therapeutic implications. *Eur Radiol* 2005; **15**:2475–82.

Buckley JC, McAninch JW. Diagnosis and management of testicular ruptures. *Urol Clin N Am* 2006; **33**:111–16.

Cervinka WH, Block NL. Civilian gunshot injuries of the penis: the Miami experience. *J Urol* 2009; **73**(4):877–80.

El Atat R, Sfaxi M, Benslama MR, *et al.* Fracture of the penis: management and long term results of surgical treatment. Experience in 300 cases. *J Trauma* 2008; **64**:121–5.

Garaffa G, Abdel Raheem AM, Ralph DJ. Penile fracture and penile reconstruction. *Curr Urol Rep* 2011; **12**(6):427–31.

Hudak SJ, Hakim S. Operative management of the wartime genitourinary injuries at Balad air force theater hospital, 2005 to 2008. *J Urol* 2009; **182**:180–3.

Lynch TH, Martinez-Pineiro L, Plas E, *et al.* EAU guidelines on urological trauma. *Eur Urol* 2005; **47**:1–15.

Miller S, McAninch JW. Penile fracture and soft tissue injury. In: McAninch JW (ed). Traumatic and Reconstructive Urology. (Ch. 59; pp. 693–698) Philadelphia, PA; WB Saunders, 1996.

Mohr AM, Pham AM, Lavery RF, Sifri Z, Bargman V, Livingston DH. Management of trauma to the male external genitalia: the usefulness of American Association for the Surgery of Trauma organ injury scales. *J Urol* 2003; **170**:2311–15.

Morey AF, Metro MJ, Carney KJ, Miller KS, McAninch JW. Consensus on genitourinary trauma: external genitalia. *BJU Int* 2004; **94**:507–15.

Najibi S, Tannast M, Latini JM. Civilian gunshot wounds to the genitourinary tract: incidence, anatomic distribution, associated injuries and outcomes. *J Urol* 2010; **76**(4):977–81.

Shenfeld OZ, Gnessin E. Management of urogenital trauma: state of the art. *Curr Op Urol* 2011; **21**:449–54.

Van der Horst C, Portillo FJ, Seif C, Groth W, Junemann KP. Male genital injury: diagnostic and treatment. *BJU Int* 2004; **93**:927–30.

Wessells H, Long L. Penile and genital injuries. *Urol Clin N Am* 2006; **33**:117–26.

CHAPTER 7.15

Scrotal swelling

Ates Kadioglu and Emre Salabaş

Introduction to scrotal swelling

Scrotal swelling is a common condition encountered in urology and includes a variety of different diseases. (Table 7.15.1) The swelling may originate from testicles, epididymis, tunical layers, or the scrotum wall itself. Emergencies usually present with pain and short onset time while malignant lesions are usually smooth, solid, and painless. All should be regarded as malignant lesions until proven otherwise. Differential diagnosis and surgical treatment of the scrotal swelling will be described with a focus on benign pathologies.

Embrology

The descent of the testicle from the abdomen to the scrotum happens via the external and internal inguinal rings at gestational week 28. The peritoneum is extended in the process forming a vaginal conduit, the processus vaginalis, which usually closes in the first year of life. This conduit separates the peritoneal and vaginal cavities and the tunica vaginalis has both parietal and visceral layers, facing the inner scrotal wall and the tunica albuginea respectively (Fig. 7.15.1).[1]

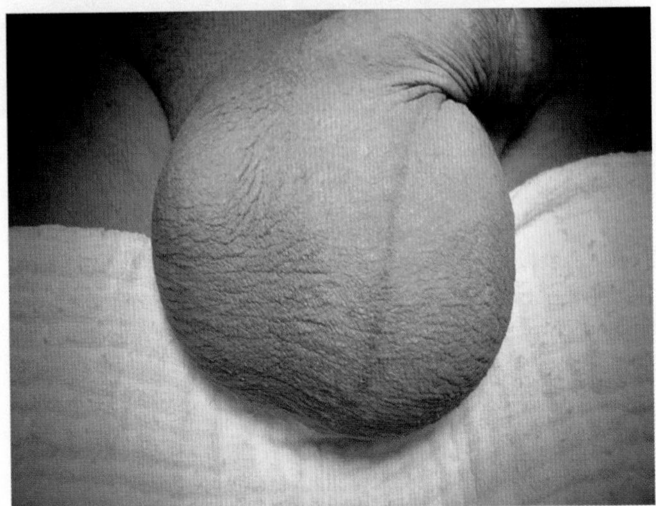

Fig. 7.15.1 Inspection of scrotal swelling (left hydrocele).

Hydrocele

Aetiology and diagnosis

A Hydrocele is an abnormal collection of serous fluid around the tunica albuginea of the testis and within the tunica vaginalis. The etymological roots of the word are based on hydros (water) and kele (mass). The cause in adult patients is the excessive fluid secretion of the tunica vaginalis accompanied by inadequate reabsorbtion. In children a communicating hydrocele may be present as a result of a patent processus vaginalis in the first 18 months of life and its treatment method should be similar to herniorrhaphy. While primary hydrocele is the most common variant, it may also occur secondary to trauma, infection, non-specific/tuberculous epididymitis, or tumours. Dissection of the spermatic vessels in renal transplantation, obstruction of the lymphatic system in inguinal or pelvic surgery, or a thickened tunical wall infested with filariasis are also less common causes of a secondary hydrocele.[2–4]

Table 7.15.1 Differential diagnosis for scrotal swellings

Scrotal swelling—differential diagnostics		
Benign	Malignant	Emergencies
Sebaceous cyst	Testicular tumours	Epididymitis
Epididymal cyst	Seminoma	Orchitis
Sperm granuloma	Embryonal cell	Testicular torsion
Hydrocele	Yolk sac	Trauma
Varicocele	Teratoma	Necrotizing fasciitis
Genital lymphoedema	Lymphoma	

Source: data from Chapter 16: 'Urological Surgery and Equipment', in Albala DM *et al.* (Eds), *Oxford American Handbook of Urology*, Oxford University Press, New York, USA, Copyright © 2011 Oxford University Press Inc.

Physical examination of a standing patient should be performed to exclude an inguinoscrotal hernia and to palpate the tense, painless, hemiscrotal swelling. Differential diagnoses include epididymal cyst and testis tumour, which may require scrotal ultrasound to differentiate them. Radiologic confirmation of the absence of the tumour is required because a secondary hydrocele accompanies 10% of testicular malignancies. Transillumination of a hydrocele or spermatocele under light illumination is a characteristic sign and is absent in tumours.[3]

Indication of surgery

Surgery is indicated in the presence of symptoms such as discomfort, pain, disability due to the size and cosmetic problems. Patients should be informed about possible complications. Surgical treatment is the gold standard for young healthy patients with its high success and low complication rate (Fig. 7.15.2).

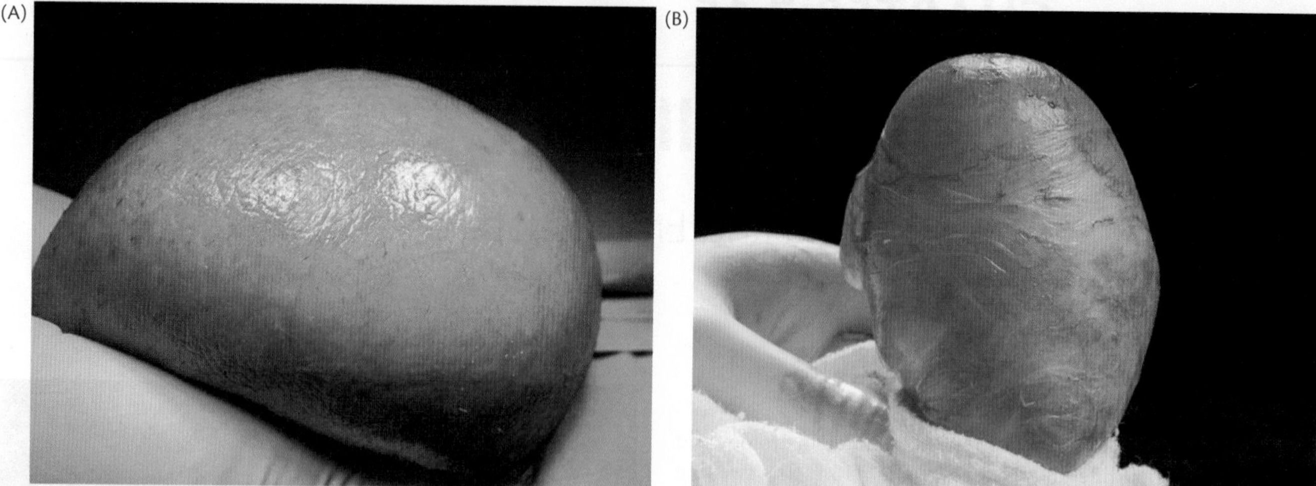

Fig. 7.15.2 Preoperative and intraoperative image of hydrocele. (A) Physical examination of tense, hemiscrotal swelling indicating hydrocele. (B) Intraoperative image of hydrocele sac containing entrapped fluid.

Preoperative preparation

The penoscrotal area should be shaved and draped after disinfection with antiseptics. General or regional anaesthesia can be used, as well as local anaesthesia with additional pre-medication. The genital branch of the genitofemoral nerve is located through the cord and local anaesthesia such as 1% lidocaine (7–10 mL) solution injected into the stretched cord and the intradermal area of the incision. No antibiotic prophylaxis is required. Bipolar forceps may be necessary for coagulation with minimal testicular trauma.[1,4]

Surgical techniques

A small transverse or midline scrotal incision facilitates delivery of the testis. In patients under local anaesthesia, pain in the flanks may be seen following traction of the cord. The hydrocele sac should be opened and completely dissected free from the testis after aspiration of the fluid.

Andrews/Jaboulay technique

In this technique, delivery of the testis is made through a 3 cm incision from the vaginal tunica prior to eversion of the hydrocele sac around it. The edges of the sac can be wrapped around the cord or left open. The scrotal closure should be done with two layer sutures, one for dartos and one for the skin.

Winkleman technique

The difference here is the greater resection of the sac leaving only a cuff around the testis. The free edges of the sac should be closed by a running suture around the cord for haemostasis with the help of electrocautery of the edges. The closure is again done with two layers.

Lord technique

In this technique, the incision length should be short enough for the delivery of testis. Prior to the placement of an Allis forceps around the edges sac, the tunical vagina should be opened without further dissection. Then circumferential (radial)plication of the tunica vaginalis is performed with multiple 2–0 or 3–0 absorbable sutures with 1 cm intervals between them and the bites. After the sutures are tied, the sac will resemble a collar around the testis and epididymis. The Lord technique should not be used for thick, multiloculated, and infected hydrocele sacs as the plicated bundle remains in the scrotum. The scrotum is closed, in two layers.[1,4]

Success and complications

Haematoma is the most common complication of the surgery followed by infection, persistent swelling, recurrence, spermatic vessel injury, and chronic pain. The excision technique has the highest complication and lowest recurrence rate. The overall complication rate is 19%. In large hydroceles, meticulous dissection should be applied to prevent possible trauma to the epididymis, vas or testis, and cause infertility as a result.[5]

Postoperative care

Although no drainage is required for these techniques, a Penrose drain may be inserted through a separate incision cases where there is hemostasis difficulties. The scrotum should be supported by a standard scrotal support. The scrotal swelling and pain may be decreased with the intermittent application of an icepack for 24 hours and oral analgesics.

Alternative treatments

In congenital hydroceles without concomitant hernia, the initial treatment is observation as it will resolve in most the patients after the first year. For the patients with an acquired symptomatic hydrocele but who are inappropriate for the surgery, an alternative treatment may be considered. Tetracycline (500 mg) insertion to the cavity as a sclerosant following aspiration of the fluid is possible although pain is common as is recurrence.[6] Ethanolamine oleate, polidocanol, sodium tetradecyl sulphate, phenol solutions (2.5%), and alcohol solutions (95%) have all been used sclerosant agents. Testicular loss, infection, pain, infertility, chemical epididymo-orchitis are reported side effects of this treatment and it is not recommended for healthy young males.

Recently 2–4 ml polidocanol (30 mg/mL) was administered to the 224 patients up to four times with a 94% satisfaction rate and only mild compliations.[7] Three per cent (3%) polidcanol was used in 190 patients with an overall cure rate of 83%, and a recurrence rate of 41% without any pain.[8] In a randomized controlled prospective trial in 90 patients, hydrocelectomy had a significantly higher postoperative fever (26.7% vs. 6.7%, p <0.05), infection (p <0.05), and satisfaction rate (95% vs. 62%, p <0.05) in comparision with sclerotherapy.[9]

Epididymitis

The epididymis may be palpated posterior to the testis. Increased size, induration, and pain imply epididymitis. In the acute phase of the disease, the testis and epididymis are palpated as an en bloc corpus and they may also adhere to a red, tender scrotum. Chlamydia trachomatis, Neisseria gonorrhoeae, *Escherichia coli* are the most common bacterial causes of the disease. Tuberculosis, schistosomiasis, and non-specific chronic epididymitis may cause chronic painless induration while pyuria, thick seminal vesicles, nodules in the prostate, and beads in the vas deferens are additional signs of tuberculosis.[10]

Spermatocele

Aetiology and diagnosis

The origins of the word 'spermatocele' come from the words 'spermatos' and 'kele', sperm, and cyst in Greek. It is a smooth, painless cystic structure originating from an efferent duct of rete testis and is filled with a milky fluid containing spermatozoa. Although it transiluminates in the same way as a hydrocele, the cysts are present outside of the vaginal tunica and may be incidentally diagnosed with ultrasonography in 30% of the patients.[11] Although clinical signs are adequate for diagnosis, ultrasonography may be necessary in case of impalpable testis with a huge or multiple epididymal cysts. Differential diagnosis is similar to hydrocele and other scrotal swellings.

The likely aetiology of the spermatocele is obstruction of epididymal ducts as a result of blockage by the shredded immature germ cells originating from seminiferous epithelial cells, leading to proximal dilation. Although trauma, infection, and inflammation are possible causes most cases are idiopathic. A spermatocele may originate from any point along the epididymis but the cephalo-posterior part of the testis is its most common location. Most of the time a spermatocele is palpated as scrotal swelling separate from the testis.[3–4]

Management

Pain, discomfort, and disability due to large size (>4 cm) and suspicion of malignancy are primary indications for surgery. In case of pain, patient should be informed the possible persistence of pain and high recurrence rate.[11]

Surgical treatment

The preoperative preparation and postoperative care is same as for hydrocele and are described above. General anaesthesia should be preferred for microscopic spermatoselectomy.

A scrotal transverse or midline incision is preferred for the initial approach. The surgical objective is removal of the intact cystic structure following sharp dissection and ligation of the epididymal duct without harming the testis or epididymis. The defect is be closed by approximation of the edges or placing fascia or tunica in the area. Hydrocelectomy may be necessary in some cases. A partial or total epididymectomy may be necessary in cases of severely adhesive spermatocele.[1,4]

Microsurgical spermatoselectomy

The technique uses up to 25× magnification. The efferent duct is ligated with a 5–0 or 6–0 absorbable suture prior to spermatocele removal. The epididymis is inspected for possible tubule trauma, leakage, or cauterization. Cystic fluid is examined under 400× magnification to differentiate a spermatocele from an epididymal cyst. Epididymal tunica is reapproximated with 9–0 interrupted monofilament sutures and the tunica vaginalis and scrotal skin is closed in the conventional fashion. Preservation of epididymis is confirmed by the absence of epidiymal tissue in cystic pathology specimen.[11]

Results of surgery

Haematoma of the scrotum is the most common complication. Infections of the wound, scrotal abscess, haematocele, testicular atrophy, reduced fertility, recurrent hydrocele or spermatocele are the other possible complications (10–30%).[4] A high epididymal injury rate (17–50%) has been reported in patients and it may cause an obstruction to sperm transit.[12] Success rates are high with a low incidence of recurrence (5–10%). In a study of 23 patients who underwent microsurgical spermatoselectomy, a single scrotal haematoma was the only reported complication (5%) with neither a reduction in sperm quality nor testicular atrophy or any other complications. Other scrotal pathologies accompanying spermatocele in this study were grade 2–3 varicocele (35%), hydrocele (26%) and congenital vasal aplasia (9%). None of the cases reoccurred after the surgery.[12]

Alternative treatment

Percutaneous aspiration and the sclerotherapy of the cyst are not recommended because of the risk of epididymal obstruction, chemical epididymitis, and recurrence. In a study of 28 patients with spermatocele, aspiration with sodium tetradecyl sulphate injection provided 85% patient satisfaction and may be considered for older patients.[13–14]

Sperm granuloma

Sperm granuloma is a complication of vasectomy seen in 1–10% of the patients. They are located at the ligation site of the vas deferens as small, hard, and tender swellings. A pea-shaped swelling superior and distinctly separate from the testis is palpated in a standing patient and inguinal hernia should be excluded in this examination. Sperm granuloma may be confused with epididymal cyst and the transillumination test should not be depended on. Although history of casectomy may help diagnosis, in some cases diagnosis can be made only at the time of the surgery.

Surgery is indicated for a discomforting, painful granuloma. The surgical excision principles are similar to epididymal cyst removal but the patient should be forewarned about recurrence risk and scrotal pain.[3]

Varicocele

A varicocele is the abnormal dilation of internal spermatic veins within the pampiniform plexus. It is found in 15–20% of healthy males and 40–70% of infertile patients.[15] Patients present with either infertility or inguinal pain. Almost all of the cases are left-sided but bilateral varicoceles are seen in 15–50% of the patients. Varicoceles cause progressive testicular damage, testicular development disorder (in adolescents), and reduction in spermatogenesis as a result of the elevated testicular temperature free radical formation and, venous reflux.

The diagnosis of varicocele is by physical examination with the findings on scrotal examination of the 'bag of worms' appearance. Venous blood flow reversal with the Valsalva manoeuvre or spermatic vein diameters of 3 mm or greater on Doppler ultrasound supports the diagnosis of varicocele but is not necessary (see Fig. 7.15.3).[16] A clinical grading system is outlined below:

Subclinic (only shown with Doppler ultrasound):

Grade 1: palpable during Valsalva manoeuvre, but not otherwise

Grade 2: palpable at rest, but not visible

Grade 3: visible and palpable at rest

Classification of varicocele reproduced with permission from Patrick J. Rowe *et al.*, *WHO Manual: For the standardized investigation, diagnosis and management of the infertile male*, Cambridge University Press, Cambridge, UK, Copyright © World Health Organization 2000.

Varicocelectomy is indicated in males with clinical varicocele (grade 1–3), subnormal semen parameters, fertile partners, who are infertile for two years. In adolescent patients the indication is progressive failure of testicular development documented by serial physical examinations or ultrasound assessment of testicular volume. Pain is a subjective indication for surgery and is not recommended in guidelines.

The main principle of the surgery is the ligation of internal and external spermatic veins while preserving arterial and lymphatic vessels. Microscopic inguinal or subinguinal varicocelectomy is the recommended technique with minimal recurrence and complication rate and substantial increase in semen parameters and spontaneous pregnancy (see also Chapter 7.2).[17]

Testicular tumours (see also Chapter 6.33)

The incidence of testicular tumours is 3–10/100,000/year and they constitute 5% of urological tumours.[18] Epidemiologic risk factors are undescended testis, Klinefelter's syndrome, familial history of testicular tumours among first-grade relatives, the presence of a contralateral tumour or intraepithelial tumour and infertility. Although initial surgical intervention may be performed in any urology clinic, improved relapse and overall survival rates has been reported for patients who received all the treatment in a reference centre.[19]

Most cases present with a unilateral painless testicular mass or with incidental ultrasound findings in their third decade.[20] Physical examination of scrotum, abdomen and lymph nodes should be performed in conjunction with scrotal ultrasound. Serum markers of AFP, B HCG, LDH should be determined.

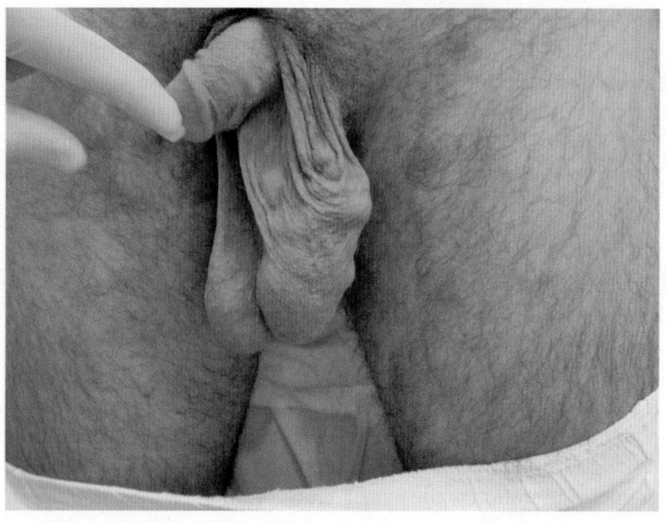

Fig. 7.15.3 Varicocele (Grade 3).

Surgical treatment is by radical orchidectomy with division of the spermatic cord at the internal inguinal ring. Further treatment is dealt with in Chapters 6.33–6.35.

Scrotal lymphedema

Scrotal lymphedema is an uncommon condition consisting of scrotal wall oedema, thickening, enlargement, and inflammation as a result of the obstruction of lymphatic ducts connected to the scrotum. The obstruction can be primary (congenital malformation of lymphatic system) or secondary (parasitic infestation, iatrogenic trauma after surgery, malignant lesions, post radiotherapy, lymphadenectomy) and it can result in a significant reduction in quality of life as a result of difficulties in voiding, mobilization, sexual intercourse, and local hygiene. Wuchereria bancrofti is the most common parasite leading to filiriazis and secondary giant recurrent lymphedema (Fig. 7.15.4).[21]

Surgery is indicated in all cases of moderate to severe genital lympedema.[22]

The preoperative preparation and postoperative care is same as for hydrocele.[4,22] Broad spectrum antibiotics are used for surgical prophylaxis.

Surgical treatment can be ablative with excision of excess skin and soft tissue or physiologic with creation of new channels for lymphatic fluid transportation.

In ablative surgery, skin grafting or primary closure is recommended for moderate/severe cases. Local flaps harvested from the thigh area or remnant skin are preferred for closure. Recently split thickness skin grafts harvested from radial and femoral regions have also been.

Lymphaplasty is performed by creating a lymphatic shunt between obstructed ducts and the superficial or deep inguinal lymphatics to increase the drainage. The technique can be performed in mild/moderate cases but the patient should be forewarned of possible recurrence.

(A) 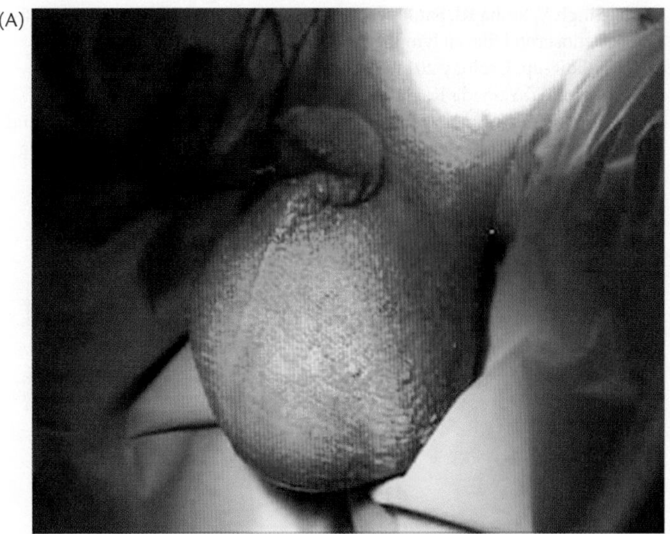

(B) 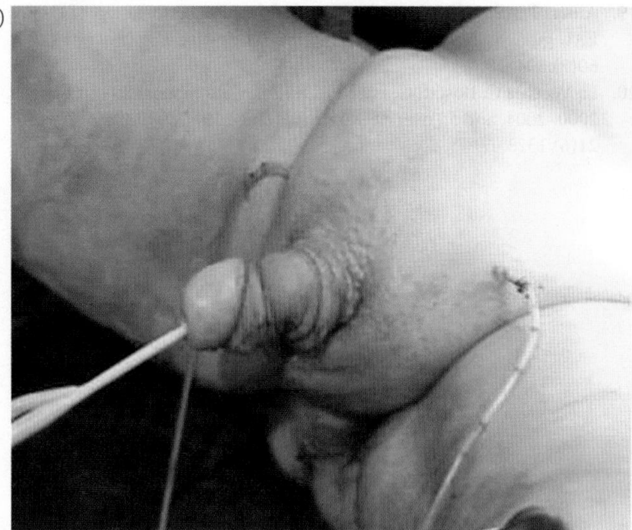

Fig. 7.15.4 Preoperative and postoperative lymphedema. (A) Scrotal lymphedema with thickened, enlarged and edematous scrotal wall. (B) Early postoperative photo of scrotal lymphedema.

In a recent study investigating patients who underwent ablative surgery and grafting, 100% cosmetic and satisfaction rate has been achieved with a 25% scrotal infection rate.[21]

Further reading

Albers P, Albrecht W, Algaba F, *et al.* European Association of Urology. EAU guidelines on testicular cancer: 2011 update. *Eur Urol* 2011; **60**(2):304–19.

Jungwirth A, Giwercman A, Tournaye H, *et al.* EAU Working Group on Male Infertility. European Association of Urology Guidelines on Male Infertility: the 2012 update. *Eur Urol* 2012; **62**(2):324–32.

Kauffman EC, Kim HH, Tanrikut C, Goldstein M. Microsurgical spermatocelectomy: technique and outcomes of a novel surgical approach. *J Urol* 2011; **185**(1):238–42.

Ku JH, Kim MH, Lee NK, Park YH. The excisional, plication and internal drainage techniques: a comparision of the results for idiopathic hydrocele. *BJU Int* 2001; **87**(1):82–4.

Nesbit JA. Hydrocele and spermatocele. In: Graham SD, Keane TE, Glenn JF (eds). *Glenn's Urologic Surgery*, 6th edition. Philadelphia: Lippincott Williams & Wilkins, 2004.

Rioja J, Sánchez-Margallo FM, Usón J, Rioja LA. Adult hydrocele and spermatocele. *BJU Int* 2011; **107**(11):1852–64.

Smith JA, Howards SS, Preminger GM. *Hinman's Atlas of Urologic Surgery*, 3rd edition. Philadelphia, PA: Elsevier Saunders, 2012.

Wein AJ, Kavoussi LR. *Campbell- Walsh Urology*, 10th edition. Philadelphia, PA: Elsevier Saunders, 2012.

References

1. Nesbit JA. Hydrocele and spermatocele. In: Graham SD, Keane TE, Glenn JF (eds). *Glenn's Urologic Surgery*, 6th edition. Philadelphia: Lippincott Williams & Wilkins, 2004.
2. Albala DM *et al.* Urological surgery and equipment. (Ch. 17) In: Reynard J, Brewster S, Biers S (eds). *Oxford American Handbook of Urology*. Oxford, UK: Oxford University Press, 2011.
3. Vissamsetti B, O'Flynn KJ. Diagnosis and treatment of benign scrotal swellings. *Trends in Urology & Men's Health* 2011; **3**:27–30.
4. Rioja J, Sánchez-Margallo FM, Usón J, Rioja LA. Adult hydrocele and spermatocele. *BJU Int* 2011; **107**(11):1852–64.
5. Ku JH, Kim MH, Lee NK, Park YH. The excisional, plication and internal drainage techniques: a comparision of the results for idiopathic hydrocele. *BJU Int* 2001; **87**(1):82–4.
6. Ali J, Anwar W, Akbar M, Akbar SA, Zafar A. Aspiration and tetracycline sclerotherapy of primary vaginal hydrocoele of testis in adults. *J Ayub Med Coll Abbottabad* 2008; **20**(2):93–5.
7. Jahnson S, Sandblom D, Holmäng S. A randomized trial comparing 2 doses of polidocanol sclerotherapy for hydrocele or spermatocele. *J Urol* 2011; **186**(4):1319–23.
8. Sallami S, Binous MY, Ben Rhouma S, *et al.* Sclerotherapy of idiopatic hydrocele with polidocanol: a study about 190 cases: *Tunis Med* 2011; **89**(5):440–4.
9. Khaniya S, Agrawal CS, Koirala R, Regmi R, Adhikary S. Comparison of aspiration-sclerotherapy with hydrocelectomy in the management of hydrocele: a prospective randomized study. *Int J Surg* 2009; **7**(4):392–5.
10. Tanagho EA, McAninch JW (eds). Physical examination of the genitourinary tract. In: *Smith's General Urology*. 17th edition. New York NY: McGraw-Hill Professional, 2008.
11. Walsh TJ, Seeger KT, Turek PJ. Spermatoceles in adults: when does size matter? *Arch Androl* 2007; **53**(6):345–8.
12. Kauffman EC, Kim HH, Tanrikut C, Goldstein M. Microsurgical spermatocelectomy: technique and outcomes of a novel surgical approach. *J Urol* 2011; **185**(1):238–42.
13. Beiko DT, Morales A. Percutaneous aspiration and sclerotherapy for treatment of spermatoceles. *J Urol* 2001; **166**(1):137–9.
14. Beiko DT, Kim D, Morales A. Aspiration and sclerotherapy versus hydrocelectomy for treatment of hydroceles. *Urology* 2003; **61**(4):708–12.
15. Witt MA, Lipshultz LI. Varicocele: a progressive or static lesion? *Urology* 1993; **42**:541–3.
16. Meacham RB, Townsend RR, Rademacher D, Drose JA. The incidence of varicoceles in the general population when evaluated by physical examination, gray scale sonography and color Doppler sonography. *J Urol* 1994; **151**(6):1535–8.
17. Jungwirth A, Giwercman A, Tournaye H, *et al.*; EAU Working Group on Male Infertility. European Association of Urology Guidelines on Male Infertility: the 2012 update. *Eur Urol* 2012; **62**(2):324–32.
18. Curado MP, Edwards B, Shin R, *et al. Cancer Incidence in Five Continents*, Vol **IX**. IARC Scientific Publications, 2007, No. 160.

19. Albers P, Albrecht W, Algaba F, *et al.*; European Association of Urology. EAU guidelines on testicular cancer: 2011 update. *Eur Urol* 2011; **60**(2):304–19.
20. La Vecchia C, Bosetti C, Lucchini F, *et al.* Cancer mortality in Europe, 2000–2004, and an overview of trends since 1975. *Ann Oncol* 2010; **21**(6):1323–60.
21. Singh V, Sinha RJ, Sankhwar SN, Kumar V. Reconstructive surgery for penoscrotal filarial lymphedema: A decade of experience and follow-up. Urology 2011; **77**(5):1228–31.
22. Otsuki Y, Yamada K, Hasegawa K, Kimata Y, Suami H. Overview of treatments for male genital lymphedema: critical literature review and anatomical considerations. *Plast Reconstr Surg* 2012; **129**(4):767e–9e.

CHAPTER 7.16

Penile reconstruction

Giulio Garaffa and David John Ralph

Introduction to penile reconstruction

Although the last decades have been characterized by the continuous evolution of reconstructive surgery and in particular of free tissue transfer techniques, repairing and reconstructing the penis remains anatomically, functionally, and aesthetically a great challenge. This is due to the unique architecture of the penis and to the absence in the whole human body of an alternative tissue that could adequately replace the corpora cavernosa in terms of colour, texture, structure, and ultimately, function.

In the patient who wishes to be sexually active, the primary goal of penile reconstruction is the creation of a cosmetically acceptable result that adequately resembles the natural features of a penis, including the capacity to void and ejaculate from the tip of the phallus and to engage in penetrative sexual intercourse with appropriate tactile and erogenous sensation.

This chapter will give an update in penile reconstruction, spanning from glans resurfacing to total phallic reconstruction in the case of amputation, aphallia, or micropenis.

Principles in penile reconstruction

Due to the unique characteristics of penile tissues, in cases of penile trauma, avulsion, partial, or complete excision, surgical repair should be immediate with preservation of as much viable tissue as possible. In particular, unless diffusely affected by chronic benign or malignant conditions such as lichen sclerosus (LS), carcinoma *in situ* (CIS) or squamous cell carcinoma (SCC) of the penis, genital skin should be used for primary repair, either in the form of a flap or of a skin graft (SG). This will guarantee a more realistic result in terms of texture and colour.

Even in cases of traumatic amputation with complete transection of the corpora cavernosa and spongiosum, microsurgical replantation can be successful if the penis is maintained in cold ischaemia for periods of up to 16 hours.

If primary repair with genital tissue is not feasible, either as a consequence of the lack of viable tissue or because the reconstruction is performed electively as a delayed procedure rather than in the acute setting, non-genital SGs, and a variety of local and free flaps are available for genital reconstruction.

Principles of skin grafting

Genital and non-genital skin grafts have been widely used for the reconstruction of the external male genitalia. Grafting consists of transferring tissue without bringing its own blood supply with it and therefore grafts initially rely on plasmatic imbibition from the recipient bed to survive until new vessels begin to grow into the transplanted skin. This process, called capillary inosculation, usually occurs within 36 hours.

In order to guarantee adequate plasmatic imbibition and capillary inosculation and ultimately a full graft take, the graft needs to be adequately secured to the recipient bed to prevent its movement and steps taken to prevent the formation of collections of blood and exudate, which would separate the bed from the graft and ultimately lead to graft failure. Usually the graft is quilted to the recipient bed and a compressive dressing applied to prevent movement. Grafts can be meshed to allow the exudate to be drained from the fenestrations without forming collections between the recipient bed and the graft, thus guaranteeing a higher chance of graft take. Meshing allows expansion of the graft and this proves particularly useful when the recipient area is relatively large, typically in patients with extensive burns. On the other hand, meshed grafts tend to heal with significant contracture and ultimately lead to poor cosmetic results. Therefore, meshed grafts should never be used when cosmesis is an issue.

Skin grafts can be subdivided into split thickness (STSG) and full thickness (FTSG). Split-thickness skin grafts, which include the epidermis and part of the dermis, are usually harvested with a dermatome, and the donor site is usually left to heal by re-epithelialization from the dermis and the surrounding skin. The thickness of the graft depends on the donor and recipient sites and on the needs of the patients. As a general role, as the thickness of the graft increases, the cosmetic result of the recipient site improves as contracture, discromia and induration become more less likely while healing of the donor site is associated with more severe scarring.

Full-thickness skin grafts instead include the epidermis and the entire thickness of the dermis and therefore contain hair follicula. As the dermis is completely removed with the graft, the donor site cannot heal by re-epithelialization and needs to be primarily closed. On the other hand, the cosmetic results at the recipient site tend to be superior to the one achieved with STSG as the presence of a full dermis guarantees less contracture and less discromia. As shaft, glans, and coronal skin are naturally hairless, FTSG should be preferably harvested from a non-hair bearing area of the body, in order to guarantee adequate cosmetic results.

Reconstruction of glans and corona

Reconstruction of the glans and corona in isolation is usually required following traumatic amputation or surgical excision for benign and malignant conditions. The procedures most commonly performed to remove benign and malignant lesions of the glans penis are partial/complete glans resurfacing, partial/complete glansectomy, and distal corporectomy.

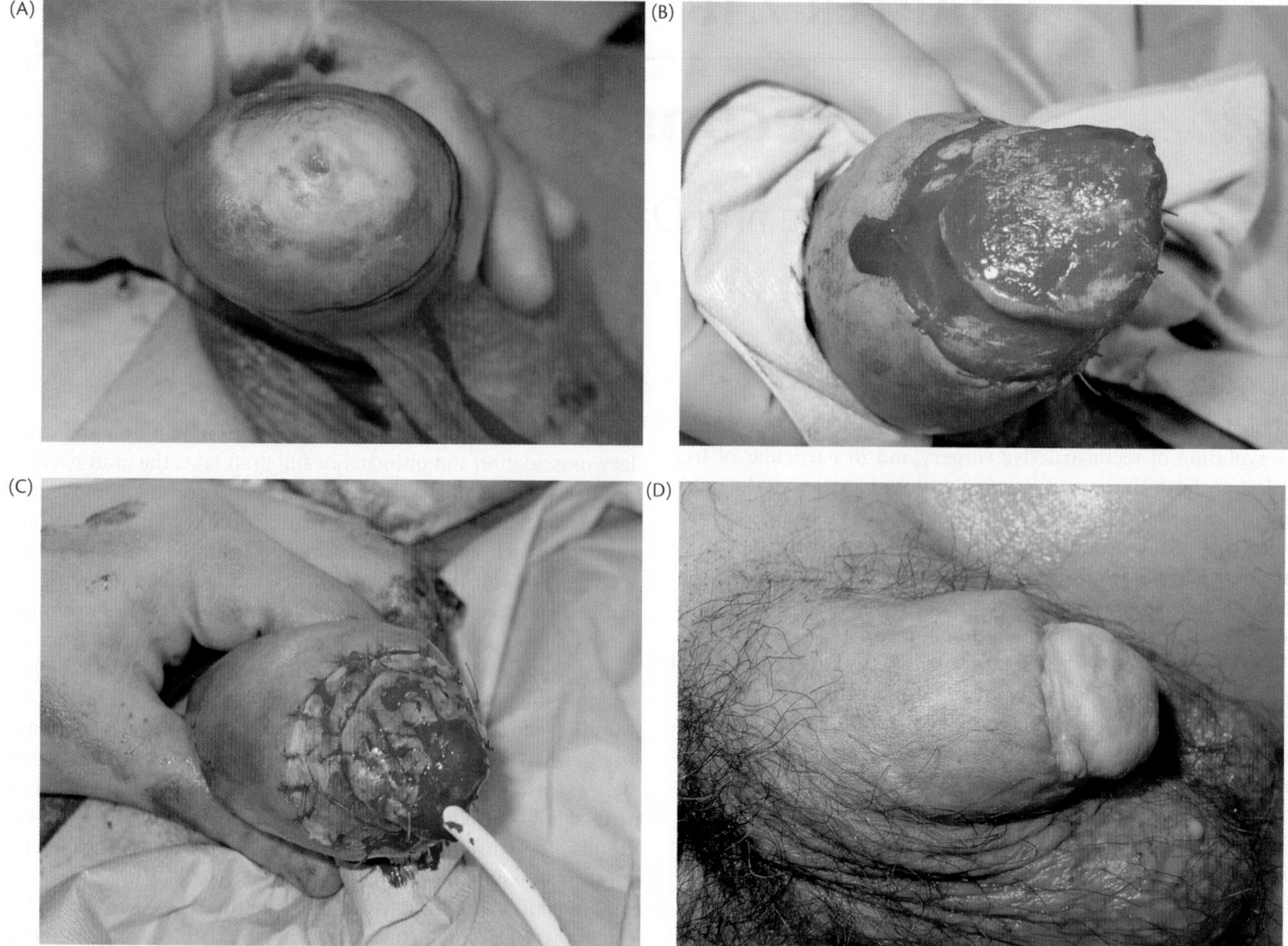

Fig. 7.16.1 Glans resurfacing for lichen sclerosus (LS) of the glans penis. (A) The glans is diffusely affected by LS. (B) The affected mucosa is dissected off the underlying spongiosum. (C) A split-thickness skin graft is quilted on the denuded spongiosum; and (D) the final result.

Glans resurfacing, which is indicated in patients with lichen sclerosus or carcinoma *in situ* of the glans penis, involves the partial or complete excision of the glans epithelium and subepithelial tissue off the underlying spongiosum followed by repair with the use of a STSG of non-genital skin, which is quilted to refashion the coronal ridge and groove and recreate a realistic cosmetic effect (Fig. 7.16.1).

Glansectomy is indicated for pT1 and pT2 squamous cell carcinoma of the glans penis and involves the complete excision of the glans penis, which is dissected off the tip of the corpora cavernosa. Distal corporectomy is required if the SCC invades the tip of the corpora cavernosa and involves the excision of the glans penis and of the corporeal heads in order to guarantee clearance of the malignancy. Although reconstruction is traditionally achieved with the use of a STSG, which is quilted to the corporeal heads to recreate the appearance of a pseudo-glans, excellent cosmetic results have been reported also using an inverted, spatulated distal urethral flap, which is used to cover the denuded distal corporeal heads. The main advantage of the use of an inverted urethral flap for glans reconstruction is the presence of a spongy component that might engorge during sexual activity, thus increasing sensation. On the other hand, this technique requires an extensive proximal urethral dissection and may cause a bowstring effect leading to ventral curvature if the urethra is relatively too short.

Glans reconstruction with the use of STSG or of inverted spatulated distal urethral flaps following glansectomy and distal corporectomy are simple and reproducible procedures that yield adequate cosmetic and functional results in more than 94% of cases. Almost all patients are able to retain sexual and urinary function using this method, although there is typically some loss of sensation.

Frenular grafting

Frenuloplasty, which can be offered to patients with a short or scarred frenulum, is based on the Heineke-Mikulicz principle. A transverse incision in the frenulum is sutured longitudinally, lengthening the frenulum at the expense of narrowing the prepuce.

Occasionally this leads to an unretractable foreskin in patients with a pre-existent degree of phimosis. Traditionally, to prevent this complication, circumcision has been the treatment of choice in patients with a degree of phimosis and associated short frenulum. Alternatively, frenular grafting can be offered to such patients who wish to preserve their foreskin. Frenular grafting initially involves a transverse incision of the frenulum, which leads to the creation of a diamond shaped defect. As a longitudinal primary closure would lead to narrowing of the prepuce, a FTSG or a thick STSG is applied to cover the defect. Full-thickness skin grafts are usually harvested from non-hair bearing areas such as the dorsal aspect of the prepuce or the retroauricular region (Wolfe's graft), while the inner thigh is the usual donor site for STSG. As a compressive dressing cannot be applied on the corona, adequate quilting of the graft to the recipient bed is necessary to guarantee an adequate take and satisfactory cosmetic and functional results. This technique, initially described by Ralph *et al.* in 2007, represents a simple and reproducible technique, and yields excellent cosmetic and functional results in virtually all patients.

Penile shaft skin loss

A variety of benign and malignant conditions can cause significant penile skin loss. Benign conditions include buried penis, genital lymphoedema, trauma, and necrotizing fasciitis while the most common malignant cause is SCC of the penis.

Traditionally, scrotal skin has been used for repair as scrotal tissue is redundant, generally well vascularized, and scrotal defects can be easily repaired primarily. Furthermore, scrotal flaps can be easily harvested and rotated on the penile shaft without disconnecting their vascular pedicle. Although scrotal flaps represent an easy solution for penile reconstruction, they usually lead to suboptimal cosmetic results, as scrotal skin presents rugae and hair follicles and has a very different texture from the one of the penis. Therefore, the use of scrotal flaps should be limited to older patients where cosmesis is of less importance.

As previously described for glans reconstruction, skin grafts harvested from a non-genital area represent the ideal solution for penile shaft skin defect repair. Non-hair bearing full-thickness skin grafts seem to guarantee superior cosmetic and functional results, as they heal with less contracture than STSG and therefore allow the physiological girth and length expansion during erections to occur.

Among the conditions that may cause significant penile loss, genital lymphoedema, and buried penis are discussed in detail, while genital trauma is discussed in Chapters 4.7 and 7.14.

Genital lymphoedema

Lymphoedema, which arises from the abnormal retention of lymphatic fluid in the subcutaneous tissues as a result of lymphatic obstruction can occur in isolation affecting either the scrotum, penis, or can involve both or it may be combined with generalized lower limb oedema. It may be classified as primary (idiopathic) due to an abnormal development of the subcutaneous lymphatic system or, more commonly, due to a secondary disorder. As the lymphatic drainage of the penis and scrotum is predominately to the inguinal lymph nodes bilaterally, it usually presents only when both lymph nodes chains have been affected either by surgery, trauma, radiation therapy, malignant infiltration, or venereal diseases. Recurrent episodes of cellulitis are common and are responsible for the loss of elastic fibres, hyperplasia of the collagenous connective tissue, and the formation of fibrosis that renders the swelling permanent with progressive loss of function and progressively deteriorating cosmesis.

The management of penile and scrotal lymphoedema is directed at preserving sexual and voiding functions and providing an acceptable cosmetic result. Underlying pathologies should be also actively treated. Conservative management consisting in elevation, compression, and lymph-draining massage may be effective in the early stages of the disease, when the elastic fibres have not yet been replaced by scar tissues. Compressive cycling shorts are often helpful.

In advanced cases or when repeated bouts of cellulitis have already led to the formation of fibrosis and to irreversible skin changes, surgical management becomes the only viable option. Surgery involves the excision of all the lymphoedematous tissue and overlying skin followed by repair with full-thickness skin grafts and/or local flaps.

When dealing with patients with genital lymphoedema, the following rules should be followed in order to achieve adequate cosmetic and functional results:

(i) Care must be paid not to undermine excessively the skin edges when excising the lymphoedematous tissue. As the blood supply to the skin derives from the underlying dartos, which is swollen by the lymphoedematous process, an aggressive excision can lead to skin necrosis.

(ii) In patients with combined penoscrotal lymphoedema, the scrotal lymphoedema should be addressed first, as this sometimes leads to spontaneous resolution of the penile swelling.

(iii) In patients with penile lymphoedema, the inner layer of the prepuce is usually not involved by the lymphoedema and is relatively intact, as it does not share the same lymphatic drainage pathways with the rest of the genitalia. Therefore, the inner prepuce should be always preserved and used as a flap for penile shaft cover. When further cover is necessary, non-hair bearing FTSG are the solution of choice in sexually active patients to minimize contracture and guarantee superior cosmetic and functional results.

Acquired buried penis

Acquired buried penis is a condition that can lead to urinary tract obstruction, poor hygiene, urinary and soft tissue infection, and severe impairment of sexual and urinary function. It can be the consequence of excessive circumcision, of excessive suprapubic adiposity, or of a combination of the two. It is relatively frequent in morbidly obese patients and the maceration of skin secondary to pooling of urine can lead to infection and skin changes such as LS. It is not uncommon that these patients develop phimosis secondary to LS and are managed with repeated circumcisions, which do not solve the problem, as the penis remains in a moist environment and the skin changes progressively spread to the proximal penile skin. Ultimately, the penile skin is completely removed with the repeated circumcisions and patients remain with a penile shaft completely buried into the abdominal skin, which gets then affected by LS and contracts around the glans penis.

Management of the buried penis therefore becomes imperative in these patients mainly to prevent urine pooling and chronic infection, which is frequently exacerbated by diabetes mellitus, and to reduce therefore the chance of developing SCC of the penis or urethral carcinoma. Usually these patients have multiple co-morbidities and pose a significant challenge from a surgical and anaesthetic perspective. Ideally, patients with excessive adiposity should be actively invited to lose weight first, or offered bariatric surgery, as this will improve the outcome of genital reconstruction.

Although liposuction represents a viable option to tackle localized suprapubic adiposity, apronectomy with suprapubic fat pad excision often represents the only solution in these patients as it also allows removal of the excess skin from the lower abdominal area. Usually the suprapubic adiposity is so extensive that the incision of the apronectomy has to be extended laterally well beyond the superior external iliac spine.

Once the penis shaft is exposed, reconstruction is achieved with FTSG in patients who wish to recover sexual function and with STSG in the remainder. Although postoperative recovery is almost always complicated by wound infection and partial dehiscence, the long-term outcome is usually good and patients are able to recover reasonable urinary and sexual function (see Fig. 7.16.2).

Buried penis secondary to lack of skin alone is instead a condition typical of the young male. It is usually the consequence of excessive neonatal circumcision or of widespread LS and it is rarely associated with pooling of urine, or with urinary tract and soft tissue infections. As these patients are young and their main concern is sexual dysfunction, achieving an adequate cosmetic and functional result is paramount. Meshed and STSG should therefore never be used and FTSG should be harvested from non-hair bearing areas where the skin matches the genital one in terms of thickness, texture, and colour. Ideally, the inner arm, the axilla, the iliac fossa, and the retroauricular regions represent the ideal donor sites. Usually the graft is quilted to the shaft penis and a compressive dressing is applied for seven days to improve the chance of take. The urine is diverted with a urethral catheter and the erections are inhibited with antiandrogens while the dressing is in place. Once the graft has taken, the dressing and the catheter are removed and nocturnal erections are encouraged with the administration of phosphodiesterase type 5 inhibitors (PDE5i) in order to promote an early stretch of the graft and minimize the risk of contracture.

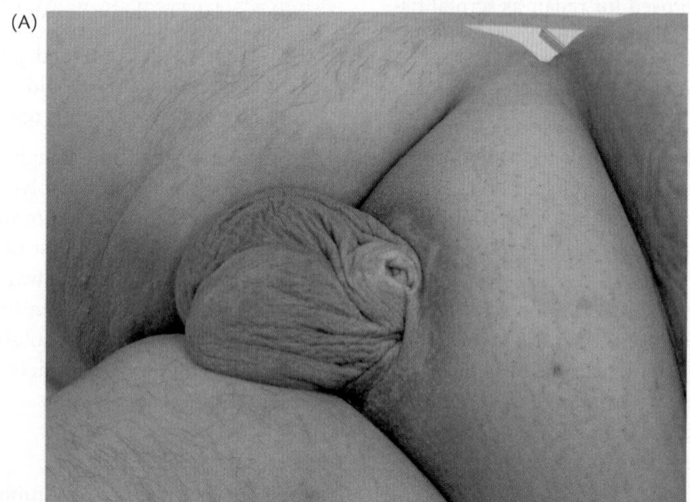

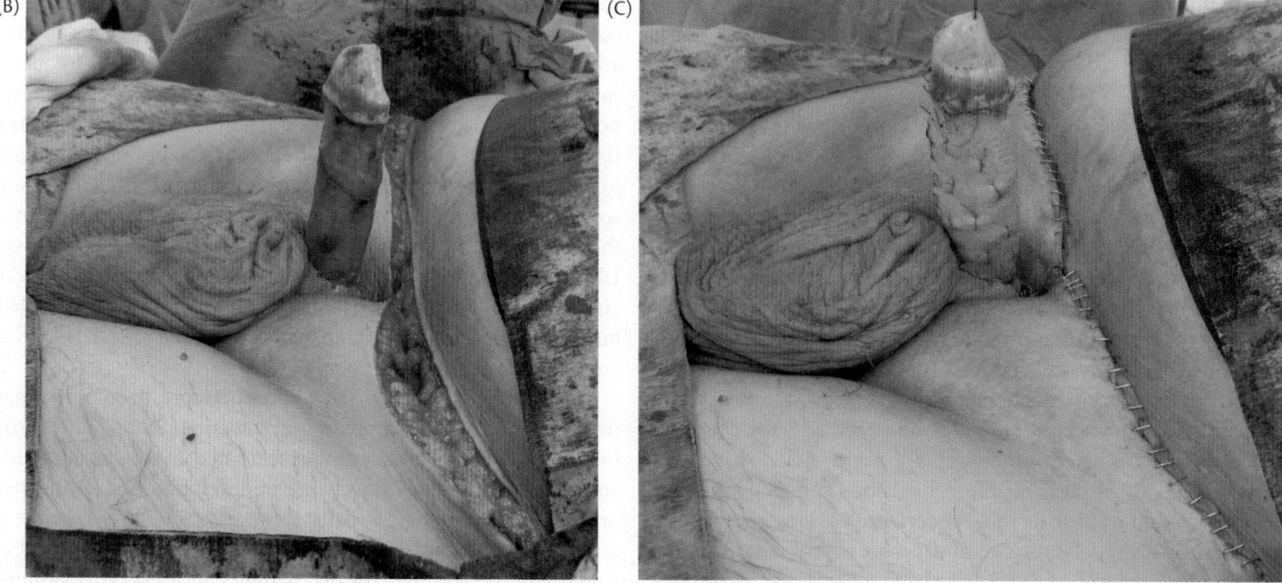

Fig. 7.16.2 Management of buried penis. (A) Buried penis secondary to excessive adiposity and LS. (B) An extensive apronectomy is performed and the penile shaft is released and prepared for grafting; and (C) a full-thickness skin graft harvested from the abdomen is applied to the penile shaft.

Total penile reconstruction

Indications for total penile shaft reconstruction are partial or subtotal penectomy, traumatic amputation of the penis, micropenis, aphallia, or penile agenesis and female to male transsexualism.

In cases of traumatic amputation with complete transection of the corpora cavernosa and spongiosum, the penis should be preserved in ice slush, as microsurgical replantation can be successfully attempted within 16 hours of cold ischaemia.

Following partial amputation for carcinoma, conservative management such as division of the suspensory ligament of the penis or excision of the suprapubic adiposity may allow a better 'exposure' of the penis, thereby maximizing the apparent length of the residual penile stump.

If these procedures result in an insufficient length gain, with the consequent inability of the patient to engage in penetrative sexual intercourse and void while standing, or if there is severe psychological distress as a consequence of the loss of penile length, patients should be offered total penile reconstruction.

Ideally, total phallic reconstruction should allow the creation of a cosmetically acceptable sensate phallus with an incorporated neourethra and enough bulk to house the cylinders of an inflatable penile prosthesis that allows the patient to resume sexual and urinary function with confidence. The procedure should be performed in as few surgical stages as possible and should be associated with minor donor site morbidity.

Despite a variety of surgical solutions that have been attempted over the last century, none of the techniques available to date can fulfil all of the above criteria.

Evolution of phalloplasty techniques

Although a variety of techniques of total phallic reconstruction have been described following Bogoras' pioneering attempt in 1936, when he used a random pedicled oblique abdominal singular tubularized flap to create a rudimental neophallus, the main breakthrough has been the advent of microsurgical techniques.

Song and Chang described the use of a radial artery-based free flap (RAFF) for phallic reconstruction in patients that had previously suffered penile amputation. This technique involved the creation of a 'tube within a tube' with the urethra fashioned from the relatively non-hair bearing ulnar aspect of the forearm flap. This technique allowed the creation of a cosmetically acceptable phallus; sensation was maintained with the coadaptation of the antebrachial nerves to the dorsal nerve of the penis or to the iliohypogastric and ilioinguinalis nerves. Following their success, many teams adopted this technique and applied some modifications in flap design in order to improve the cosmesis of the neophallus and to minimize the overall complication rate.

In further attempts to minimize donor site morbidity, free osteocutaneous fibular flaps, anterolateral thigh flaps, and upper arm flaps have all been described. However due to the nature of the flaps, the neourethra cannot be fashioned reliably according to the 'tube within a tube' technique and is instead prelaminated by tunnelling a skin graft or bladder mucosa graft, which in turn results in poor functional results.

Although minimal, donor site morbidity still represents the main drawback of the RAFF technique, as the forearm scar represents a 'stigma', which some patients are not ready to accept. Patients who wish to achieve cosmetic and functional results similar to the one provide by the RAFF phalloplasty but want to minimize the donor site morbidity at the level of the forearm, can be offered the incorporation of a 4-cm wide tubularized free flap based on the radial artery in a prefashioned infraumbilical flap phalloplasty. This technique, also known as radial artery urethroplasty, allows the formation of a patent neourethra and leads to a significantly smaller scar on the donor forearm.

Patients who wish to engage in penetrative sexual intercourse need either to wear an external baculum or have a stiffener incorporated into the phallus. Traditionally, incorporation of cartilage or bone grafts into the phallus has led to unsatisfactory cosmetic and functional results as the grafts were inevitably resorbed and were prone to fracture. For these reasons and for the difficulty of concealment, cartilage and bone grafts have been progressively abandoned. Implantation of a hydraulic inflatable penile prosthesis represents the only solution in these patients. Malleable devices can lead to pressure ulceration and ultimately are prone to erosion. Ideally, implantation of an inflatable penile prosthesis should be offered at least one year after the construction of the phallus to give

(A)
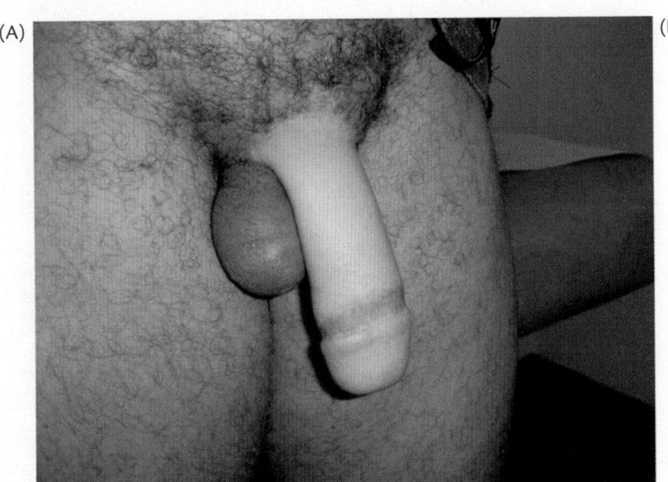

(B)
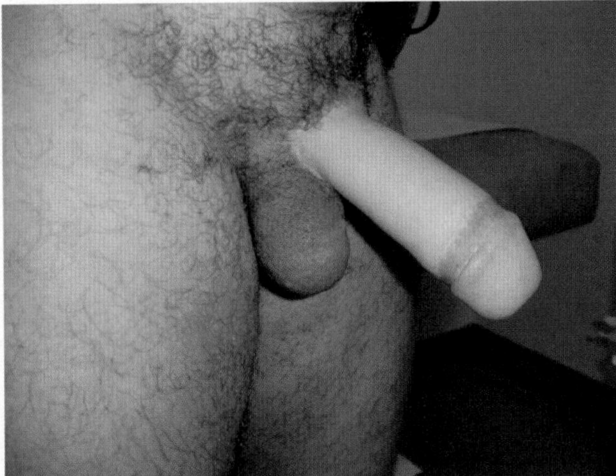

Fig. 7.16.3 The deflated (A) and inflated (B) state of a three-piece inflatable penile prosthesis in a patient who has undergone total phallic reconstruction with the use of RAFF.

enough time for cutaneous sensation to have developed and indeed are only indicated if there is reasonable phallic sensation. As phalluses lack tunica albuginea, the cylinders of the implant need to be housed in a Dacron or Goretex envelope, which allows anchoring to the pubic bone and minimizes the risk of distal extrusion.

Complication rates following penile prosthesis implantation in phalloplasty can be 20 times higher than in a normal penis, with up to 50% of patients requiring revision surgery within four years (Fig. 7.16.3).

Conclusion

A variety of surgical techniques can be used in the reconstruction of the penis. Skin grafts are most commonly used when some or all of the penile skin is lost, with split-thickness grafts being best suited to reconstruction of the glans penis, and full thickness grafts best suited for the shaft of the penis. With the increasing prevalence of obesity, there is an increasing demand for surgical treatment and reconstruction of the buried penis, which is often associated with coexisting lichen sclerosis, and which present a significant surgical (and anaesthetic) challenge.

Further reading

Chang TS, Hwang WY. Forearm flap in one-stage reconstruction of the penis. *Plast Reconstr Surg* 1984; **74**:251–8.

Garaffa G, Christopher AN, Ralph DJ. The management of genital lymphoedema. *BJU Int* 2008; **102**(4):480–4.

Garaffa G, Christopher NA, Ralph DJ. Total phallic reconstruction in female to male transsexuals. *Eur Urol* 2010; **57**(4):715–22.

Garaffa G, Raheem AA, Christopher NA, Ralph DJ. Total phallic reconstruction after penile amputation for carcinoma. *BJU Int* 2009; **104**(6):852–6.

Garaffa G, Ralph DJ, Christopher N. Total urethral construction with the radial artery based forearm free flap in the transsexual. *BJU Int* 2010; **106**(8):1206–10.

Hadway P, Corbishley CM, Watkin N. Total glans resurfacing for premalignant lesions of the penis: initial outcome data. *BJU Int* 2006; **98** (3):532–6.

Hoebeke PB, Decaesteker K, Beysens M, Opdenakker Y, Lumen N, Monstrey SM. Erectile implants in female-to-male-transsexuals: our experience in 129 patients. *Eur Urol* 2010; **57**(2):334–40.

Keyes O, Li CY, Spillings A, Ralph DJ. Frenular grafting: an alternative to circumcision in men with a combination of tight frenulum and phimosis. *J Sex Med* 2007; **4**(4):1070–3.

Morelli G, Pagni R, Mariani C, *et al.* Glansectomy with split-thickness skin graft for the treatment of penile carcinoma. *Int J Imp Res* 2009; **21**(5):311–4.

Morey AF, Rozansky TA. Genital and lower urinary tract trauma. (pp. 993–1022) In: Wein AJ, Kavoussi LR, Novick AC (eds). *Campbell-Walsh Urology*. Philadelphia, PA: Saunders Elsevier, 2007.

Pestana IA, Greenfield JM, Walsh M, Donatucci CF, Erdmann D. Management of "buried penis" in adulthood: an overview. *Plast Reconstr Surg* 2009; **124**(4):1186–95.

Pietrzak P, Corbishley, Watkin N. Organ-sparing surgery for invasive penile cancer: early follow-up data. *BJU Int* 2004; **94**(9):1253–7.

Selvaggi G, Monstrey S, Hoebeke P, *et al.* Donor-site morbidity of the radial forearm free flap after 125 phalloplasties in gender identity disorder. *Plast Reconstr Surg* 2006; **118**(5):1171–7.

Song R, Gao Y, Song Y, Yu Y, Song Y. The forearm flap. *Clin Plast Surg* 1982: **9**(1):21–6.

CHAPTER 7.17

Penile augmentation

Salvatore Sansalone, Giulio Garaffa, Ian Eardley, and David Ralph

Introduction to penile augmentation

Most patients who seek penile enhancement have a normally sized and functioning penis. Any man seeking penile augmentation benefits from a careful clinical assessment, together with counselling regarding the treatment options available and the results and complications of surgery. Indeed, for those with normal penile size, careful psychological assessment is essential before any physical treatment should be considered. If a man perceives his penis to be too small, when actually it is of normal size, the condition is termed penile dysmorphophobia.

In the history there should be an assessment of the patient's concerns and aspirations. Some are concerned about the penile length while others are concerned about the girth of their penis and for many it is a combination of both these features. Indeed, it is not always the erect length that concerns them, but more commonly the flaccid appearance which they may feel is embarrassing if seen by other men, for example in a sports changing room. This is the so-called 'locker room' syndrome. The scope of the appropriate psychological assessment is beyond the scope of this chapter, but can be found elsewhere.[1]

The man should be examined in a warm room and the penile dimensions should be measured. There are three potential measures of length that can be obtained: the flaccid length, the stretched length, and the erect length. The former varies with the ambient temperature and the degree of anxiety of the patient, and the last would involve an intracavernosal injection in the clinic. The stretched penile length appears to be the most reliable and reproducible measure, with measurement taken from the pubic bone to the tip of the glans penis following gentle stretching of the penis. There are several reported studies of what is 'normal' and a length of around 12–14 cm appears to be an average length in Caucasian men. The normal penile girth is around 9–10 cm. These epidemiological studies allow a normative 'range' to be calculated, with a true micropenis generally considered to be a stretched length of less than 7–8 cm. Another factor that is relevant is the patient's age and degree of masculinization. Penile size increases considerably during adolescence under the influence of androgens, and if there is doubt about the androgenic status of the patient, this should also be assessed.

One further issue that is increasingly relevant is the degree to which the penis is buried within the suprapubic fat pad. With central obesity becoming so prevalent, there is an increasing tendency for the penis to become buried, such that simple approaches to 'uncover' the penis can often be valuable.

For men with a normal penile size, psychotherapy is the first port of call and a variety of techniques are valuable.[1] Most importantly a discussion about what is actually normal is important, since the patient may have developed unrealistic perceptions of normality from the pornography that is now so freely available. A further issue is that of perspective. When a man looks at his own penis, he looks down and sees a foreshortened phallus. However, when he looks at another man, he sees the penis side-on, and this inevitably looks larger than his own. Simply viewing himself in a mirror can be helpful in restoring the perspective of himself.

There is preliminary evidence that stretching devices can be helpful in some men[2] and it is only when these options have been exhausted and the patient is fully aware of the lack of real evidence regarding the outcomes of surgery, that augmentation should be considered.[3,4] Even here, there are many who feel that such surgery is not justified in this group of men, given the lack of robust data regarding outcomes.[5] For patients with a true micropenis, the situation is more straightforward. Psychological therapy is not the way here, and the role of stretching devices is unproven. Surgery is the only option, even if the outcomes are less than ideal, and this chapter describes current augmentation techniques.

Penile lengthening

Abdominal and pelvic liposuction and lipectomy (apronectomy)

Removing the excess adipose tissue partially covering the proximal aspect of the penis provides merely visual shaft lengthening and is therefore indicated in patients with abundant pubic adiposity or a protruding abdomen such that the penis is buried. Since the technique does not affect the corpora cavernosa, neurovascular bundle or urethra, it is safe, practical, and entails no complications such as deformity or loss of sensation. However, its poor cosmetic and functional outcomes mean that only occasionally is it enough to resolve the 'problem' alone, and it is therefore commonly combined with other augmentation procedures (e.g. suspensory ligament division and girth enhancement).

Suspensory ligament division

Detachment of the suspensory ligament from the pubic symphysis brings forward the corpora cavernosa. The ligament is divided close to its attachment to the pubic bone to avoid vascular and nerve damage. Reattachment of the divided ligament with postoperative penile shortening is prevented by filling the space created by the dissection with a vascularized flap of lipomatous tissue or with biocompatible material (e.g. a testicular prosthesis). A suprapubic skin manoeuvre such as a Z plasty or V-Y plasty is required to advance suprapubic skin onto the penis. Postoperatively, penile traction with vacuum devices, traction appliances, or special weights attached to the coronal margin of the penis are applied to pull the penis away from the pubic bone and stretch the corpora cavernosa. The procedure only results in an 'apparent' lengthening of the flaccid penis without any significant change in the erect length; it is therefore indicated in patients with 'locker room syndrome'.

Studies of penile length increase by this procedure are few and result comparison is hampered by diverse length measurement methods and surgical techniques. Satisfaction with an average length increase of 1.3 cm was very low in 42 patients undergoing ligament division and silicone buffer insertion.[9]

Skin flaps and grafts

Skin flaps are indicated when the penopubic skin 'traps' the penis preventing elongation during erection, as in the case of skin loss due to excessive circumcision, lichen sclerosus, genital lymphoedema, trauma, and burns.[6,7] Other penopubic skin flaps and grafts are performed within more complex elongation procedures requiring full skin covering of the extended penis.[8–15]

A variety of techniques have been described, the commonest being the inverted V-Y advancement flap (or V-Y plasty) modified by Roos and co-workers (1994),[13] who combined it with suspensory ligament division. Other types include lower abdominal Z plasty and W flap reconstruction.

However, flaps bring unattractive hair-bearing skin onto the shaft and may cause pubic deformation. Moreover, in cases of suboptimal healing, especially due to poor surgical technique or surgeon experience, flap contracture may result in a buried penis or in a bowstring effect with penile curvature. Skin grafts are useful alternatives. Full-thickness skin grafts heal with less contracture than split-thickness grafts, preserving penis elasticity, and ensuring adequate erections. All areas with redundant non-hairy skin can be donor sites (groin crease, axilla, inner arm). Careful recipient site and graft preparation are critical, in particular quilting to the recipient site and application of a compressive dressing. Erections must be inhibited pharmacologically to optimize take.

Penile girth enhancement

Penile girth augmentation is even more controversial, since there are no indications for this procedure and no guidelines in the literature. None of the available techniques achieve the ideal outcome of a girth increase with appropriate symmetry, maintenance of physiological erection and micturition, and a reasonable complication rate.

Injectable materials

Initially considered to be very promising, injection of autologous abdominal fat harvested by liposuction into the dartos layer of the penis has progressively been abandoned because of high complication rates, in particular deformities such as penile curvature or asymmetry and formation of nodules of liquefied, necrotic, or calcified adipose tissue due to resorption or migration. Despite the unpredictable results, due to lack of an adequate blood supply to the injected material and to the risk of adipocyte necrosis, Panfilov[11] reported an average girth increase of 2.6 cm.

Injection of liquid injectable silicon (LIS) into the dartos fascia also carries a high rate of complications including swelling, penile distortion, granuloma formation, LIS migration, idiosyncratic reactions, and the risk of neurovascular bundle damage with loss of sensation and ultimately sexual dysfunction. Better known for its role in facial soft tissue augmentation, hyaluronic acid gel has also been used as a tissue filler for glans penis augmentation. Kim and co-workers[8] reported an average 1.5 cm increase in glans circumference without serious complications and high overall satisfaction in 187 men.

Graft procedures

Dermal fat grafts consisting of all skin layers and subcutaneous tissue are usually harvested from the abdomen and gluteal folds and placed around the shaft between dartos and Buck's fascia after removing the epidermis from the graft itself. Although complications such as donor site scarring and deformity, persistent penile oedema, and induration, venous congestion, and fibrosis leading to penile deformity are common, their success rate appears to be superior to fat injection.

Pedicled skin flaps are another option. Shaeer[15] reported excellent girth increase and cosmetic outcomes in patients with a malleable penile prosthesis. Although easily reproducible and safe, the procedure involves the risk of flap ischaemia and contracture with consequent penile curvature and shortening, especially in patients without a penile prosthesis.[16]

Allografts and xenografts offer an alternative to all the procedures discussed above. Advantages include shorter operating time, since the graft or flap does not need to be harvested; no donor site morbidity, high take, and low complication rates. Alloderm®, the commonest allograft used in penile girth enhancement, is an acellular, inert dermal matrix derived from donated human skin.[17] Porcine small intestinal submucosa (SIS®) and bovine pericardium (Peri-Guard®) are xenografts. Though rare, erosion, resorption, fibrosis and contracture, and skin loss are the most frequent complications of allografts.

A revolutionary approach uses scaffolds as grafts for girth augmentation by an *ex vivo* tissue engineering process where fibroblasts previously harvested from the patient's scrotal dermal tissue are seeded onto a pretreated tube-shaped biodegradable scaffold that is incubated for 24 hours before implantation around the shaft, between Buck's and dartos fascia. Postoperatively, the scaffold undergoes remodelling through infiltration by inflammatory cells and substitution with a collagen-rich hypervascularized tissue resembling the normal dartos layer. Perovic and colleagues[12] achieved girth augmentation with biodegradable scaffolds in 84 patients with penile dysmorphophobia and failed girth enhancement surgery, reporting an average girth increase of 3.1 cm, high satisfaction, and a complication rate of 8%.

Austoni's technique, involving real enlargement of the corpora cavernosa by bilateral venous graft implantation, is the only procedure providing increased girth in the erect state. It consists of a longitudinal incision of the tunica albuginea from the coronal sulcus to the proximal aspect of the shaft on each side of the urethra; the resulting defect is grafted with a saphenous vein patch to widen the corpora cavernosa. None of his 39 patients experienced postoperative complications or erectile dysfunction; girth increase was up to 2.1 cm, with all patients engaging in penetrative sexual intercourse and expressing satisfaction with the cosmetic and functional outcome. Its main limitation is that its reproducibility is strongly affected by technical factors and by preoperative erectile function, since corpora incision and grafting is associated with postoperative worsening of erectile function and long-term results tend to be poor.

Conclusion

Men with penile dysmorphophobia require careful assessment including psychological assessment. Guidelines agree that augmentation surgery should be confined to men with a true micropenis. This reflects the limited evidence of efficacy, together with the risk of complications which are often severe, and can include permanent disfigurement and impaired urinary and sexual function.

Further reading

Austoni E. *Atlas of Reconstructive Penile Surgery*. Pisa, Italy: Pacini Editore, 2010.

Perovic SV, Sansalone S, Djinovic R, Ferlosio A, Vespasiani G, Orlandi A. Penile enhancement using autologous tissue engineering with biodegradable scaffold: a clinical and hystomorphometric study. *J Sex Med* 2010; 7(9):3206–15.

Vardi Y, Harshai Y, Gil T, Gruenwald I. A critical analysis of penile enhancement procedures for patients with normal penile size: surgical techniques, success and complications. *Eur Urol* 2008; **54**:1042–50.

Wylie KR, Eardley I. Penile size and the 'small penis syndrome'. *BJU Int* 2007; **99**:1449–55.

References

1. Alter GJ, Jordan GH. Penile elongation and girth enhancement. *AUA Update Series* 2007; **26**:229–37.
2. Alter GJ. Penile enlargement surgery. *Tech Urol* 1998; **4**:70–6.
3. Alter GJ. Augmentation phalloplasty. *Urol Clin North Am* 1995; **22**:887–902.
4. Austoni E, Guarneri A, Cazzaniga A. A new technique for augmentation phalloplasty: albugineal surgery with bilateral saphenous grafts-three years of experience. *Eur Urol* 2002; **42**:245–53.
5. Bruno JJ 2nd. Senderoff DM, Fracchia JA, Armenakas NA. Reconstruction of penile wounds following complications of AlloDerm-based augmentation phalloplasty. *Plast Reconstr Surg* 2007; **119**:1e–4e.
6. Chung E, Clendinning E, Lessard L, Brock G. Five-year follow-up of Peyronie's graft surgery: outcomes and patient satisfaction. *J Sex Med* 2011; **8**(2): 594–600
7. Garaffa G, Christopher AN, Ralph DJ. The management of genital lymphoedema. *BJU Int* 2008; **102**(4):408–14.
8. Kim JJ, Kwak TI, Jeon BG, Cheon J, Moon DG. Human glans penis augmentation using Injectable hyaluronic acid gel. *Int J Imp Res* 2003; **15**:439–443.
9. Li C-Y, Kayes O, Kell PD, Christopher AN, Minhas S, Ralph DJ. Penile suspensory ligament division for penile augmentation: indications and results. *Eur Urol* 2006; **49**:729–33.
10. Moon DG, Yoo JW, Bae JH, Han CS, Kim YM, Kim JJ. Sexual function and psychological characteristics of penile paraffinoma. *Asian J Andro* 2003; **5**:191–4.
11. Panfilov DE. Augmentative phalloplasty. *Aesth Plast Surg* 2006; **30**:183–97.
12. Perovic SV, Byunb J, Scheplevic P, Djordjevica M, Kimd J, Bubanja T. New perspectives of penile enhancement surgery: tissue engineering with biodegradable scaffolds. *Eur Urol* 2006; **49**:139–47.
13. Roos H, Lissoos I. Penis lengthening. *Int J Aesth Restor Surg* 1994; **2**:89–96.
14. Sansalone S, Garaffa G, Djinovic R, *et al.* Simultaneous penile lengthening and penile prosthesis implantation in patient with Peyronie's disease, refractory erectile dysfunction and severe penile shortening. *J Sex Med* 2012; **9**(1):316–21.
15. Shaeer O. Supersizing the penis following penile prosthesis implantation. *J Sex Med* 2010; 7(7):2608–16.
16. Spyropoulos E, Christoforidis C, Borousas D, Mavrikos S, Bourounis M, Athanasiadis S. Augmentation phalloplasty surgery for penile dysmorphophobia in young adults: considerations regarding patient selection, outcome evaluation and techniques applied. *Eur Urol* 2005; **48**:121–8.
17. Whitehead ED. Allografts dermal matrix graft (Alloderm®) for pericavernosal penile widening in normal men. Abstract presented at: First World Congress of Aesthetic Medicine; March 15–17, 2004; Rio de Janeiro, Brazil.

SECTION 8

Paediatrics

Section editor: David F.M. Thomas

CHAPTER 8.1

Prenatal diagnosis and perinatal urology

David F.M. Thomas

Anatomical and functional development of the upper urinary tract

The kidney is formed by the interaction of the ureteric bud and the metanephric tissue during the fifth week of gestation. Nephron formation (nephrogenisis) is dependent on a process of reciprocal induction whereby the glomeruli, convoluted tubules, and loop of Henle are derived from the metanephric tissue while the renal pelvis, calyces, and collecting ducts originate from the ureteric bud. In man, nephrogenesis extends from the sixth to the thirty-sixth weeks of gestation, with the sequential formation of zones or 'generations' of nephrons within the developing renal cortex. Nephrogenisis ceases after 36 weeks, with the number of nephrons remaining fixed thereafter at approximately one million per kidney. During the sixth to tenth weeks of gestation, the kidneys undergo relative ascent on the posterior abdominal wall, acquiring segmental blood supply during this process.[1]

Urine production commences from around the ninth week of gestation and as gestation proceeds, the foetal kidneys excrete an increasingly large volume of urine. By the thirty-sixth week, foetal urine output is approximately 30–40 mL per hour and constitutes around 90% of the amniotic fluid volume.[2] In addition to its protective role of 'cushioning' the foetus within the uterus, amniotic fluid helps to promote normal lung development.[3] For this reason, abnormalities which cause significantly decreased urine output such as bilateral renal agenesis or foetal bladder outlet obstruction[4] result in a marked reduction in amniotic fluid (oligohydramnios) accompanied by congenital pulmonary hypoplasia.

Although the foetal kidneys play an active role in fluid excretion, glomerular function is minimal throughout gestation[5] and this component of excretory function is fulfilled by the placenta. Although circulatory changes at the time of birth are accompanied by a dramatic increase in renal blood flow, the corrected values for glomerular filtration rate nevertheless remain greatly reduced by comparison with older children and adults.[6,7] Glomerular filtration rate increases steadily in the early months of life but it is not until two years of age that corrected values reach the comparable adult range.

Immature tubular function in newborns and young infants is reflected in reduced concentrating capacity and relative inability to excrete a water load. As a consequence, newborn infants are at particular risk of fluid overload and dilutional hyponatraemia.

Abnormalities of the upper urinary tract

A number of different mechanisms can result in the complete absence of a kidney (renal agenesis) including failed induction of nephrogenesis and the intrauterine or postnatal involution of a multicystic dysplastic kidney. Although the term 'hypoplasia' is used to describe a small, but architecturally normal kidney, in practice most small kidneys also exhibit evidence of dysplasia. This is characterized by histological evidence of immature nephrons and abnormal mesenchymal tissue including fibromuscular tissue and cartilage.[8]

Renal dysplasia can result from defective interaction between the ureteric bud and metanephric mesenchyme (for example, in the dysplastic upper pole of a duplex kidney) or an insult to the developing kidney such as severe outflow obstruction caused by posterior urethral valves. Multicystic dysplastic kidney (MCDK) is usually associated with segemental atresia of the proximal ureter but can occasionally occur in conjunction with distal ureteric obstruction.

Renal anomalies such as horseshoe kidney, crossed-fused renal ectopia, and ectopic pelvic kidney are abnormalities of renal ascent and fusion dating from the sixth to tenth week of gestation.

Prenatal diagnosis

The widespread introduction of antenatal ultrasonography in the 1980s had a profound impact on the specialty of paediatric urology, when urological conditions which had previously presented with symptoms during the course of childhood were increasingly identified in newborns who were entirely healthy and asymptomatic at birth.

Currently, routine antenatal scanning for foetal anomalies is performed between 15–20 weeks gestation, but scans at 10–12 weeks are also being increasingly adopted in high-risk pregnancies—for example, for the early prenatal diagnosis of Down's syndrome.

The sensitivity of antenatal ultrasonography is highest for the detection of abnormalities which cause urinary tract dilatation and for renal cystic disease (Fig. 8.1.1). By contrast, renal agenesis and renal ectopia are less readily detectable in the second trimester.

It is also important to note that conditions such as pelviureteric junction obstruction, vesicoureteric reflux, upper tract duplication, and even posteriorurethral valves may not be visualized at 17–20 weeks because they have not yet given rise to detectable dilatation at that stage in gestation.[9,10]

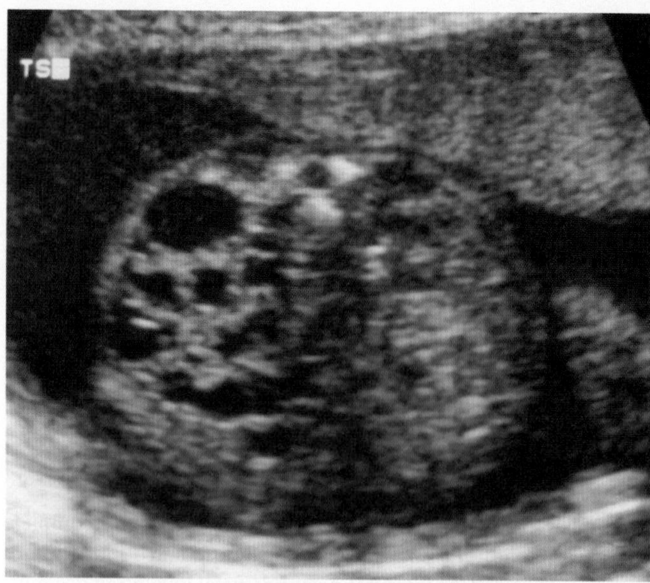

Fig. 8.1.1 Antenatal scan: transverse view of foetal abdomen demonstrating multiple fluid-containing spaces. Typical appearances of a large multicystic dysplastic kidney (MCDK).

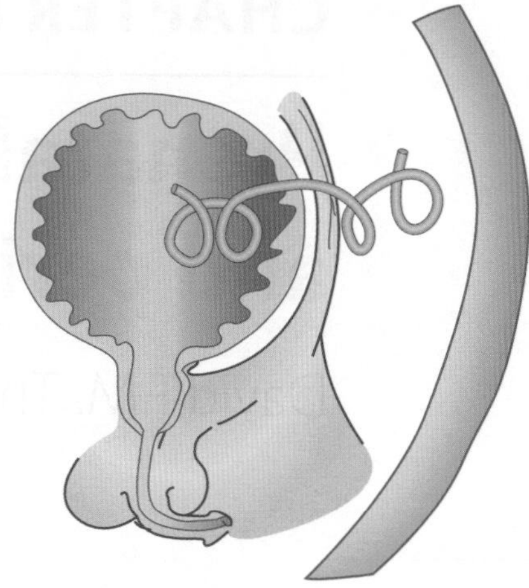

Fig. 8.1.2 Vesicoamniotic shunt. The shunt catheter is introduced percutaneously under ultrasound guidance with the intention of draining urine from the obstructed foetal bladder into the amniotic cavity.

Republished with permission of Taylor and Francis Group, LLC from *Essentials of Paediatric Urology*, David F. M. Thomas, Patrick G. Duffy, and Anthony M. K. Rickwood, (Eds.), CRC Press, Taylor and Francis Group, Florida, USA, Copyright © 2002; permission conveyed through Copyright Clearance Center, Inc.

Clinically significant abnormalities of the urinary tract are detected in approximately 1:500 pregnancies,[11] whereas 'pyelectasis' (mild dilatation of little clinical significance) is observed in as many in 1:100 pregnancies.[12]

Foetal intervention

Termination of pregnancy is the most widely practised form of foetal intervention—particularly for abnormalities such as bilateral renal agenesis or bilateral multicystic dysplastic kidney which are incompatible with survival.

Decisions surrounding the management of severe outflow obstruction are more problematic. The majority of severely affected foetuses are males with posterior urethral valves in whom the findings of oligohydramnios, gross dilatation, and echogenic cortex (denoting dysplasia) on a second trimester ultrasound denote a high risk of early onset renal failure.

In the presence of these unfavourable prognostic indicators, the options open to parents and their medical advisors comprise: continuing with the pregnancy, termination of the pregnancy, or foetal intervention, usually in the form of vesicoamniotic shunting.

The rationale for foetal intervention centres on the premise that the prognosis for renal function can be improved by decompression of the obstructed urinary tract *in utero*.[13] Open foetal surgery was first introduced in the 1980s[14] but was then rapidly superseded by 'vesicoamniotic shunting' in which an ultrasound-guided pigtail catheter is inserted percutaneously between the foetal bladder and amniotic cavity (Fig. 8.1.2).[15] Vesicoamniotic shunting has been widely practised on an unreported basis and the results have proved difficult to assess. Nevertheless, a critical analysis of the available evidence indicates that irreversible renal damage (in the form of dysplasia) is usually present by the time the abnormality has been detected and vesicoamniotic shunting is performed. Advocates of vesicoamniotic shunting have argued, however, that the technique has usually been reserved for the most severe end of the obstructive spectrum and that intrauterine decompression might genuinely improve the prognosis for renal function for those foetuses with less severe outflow obstruction.[16] Hopes that a multicentre-controlled trial in the United Kingdom might resolve these issues have been unfulfilled since the trial was abandoned because of difficulty in recruiting cases in adequate numbers.

Postnatal investigation and management

Many healthy, asymptomatic children with prenatally detected anomalies of the urinary tract were undoubtedly overinvestigated in the past—often with unnecessarily invasive tests.

In recent years, however, a more selective approach to postnatal investigation has evolved with the initial aim of identifying newborn infants who are at greatest risk of urinary tract infection or systemic sepsis in the early months of life (Fig. 8.1.3).

By contrast, the common antenatal finding of unilateral dilatation confined to the kidney rarely requires urgent investigation, since it is associated with a far lower risk of early morbidity.

An approach to investigation based on the findings of antenatal ultrasonography and the initial postnatal scan[17] can be summarized as follows:

Bilateral upper tract dilatation (collecting systems and/or ureters)

Impaired bladder emptying or a thick-walled bladder

These appearances point to lower urinary tract obstruction and/or high grade reflux.

Antibiotic prophylaxis is commenced and a postnatal ultrasound performed in the first 48 hours of life. If the findings confirm those seen prenatally a micturating cystourethrogram (MCUG) is performed to investigate outflow obstruction or vesicoureteric reflux.

Unilateral upper tract dilatation confined to the kidney (pelvis and/or calyces)

Pelviureteric junction (PUJ) obstruction is the commonest cause for this finding. A repeat ultrasound scan is performed at four to six

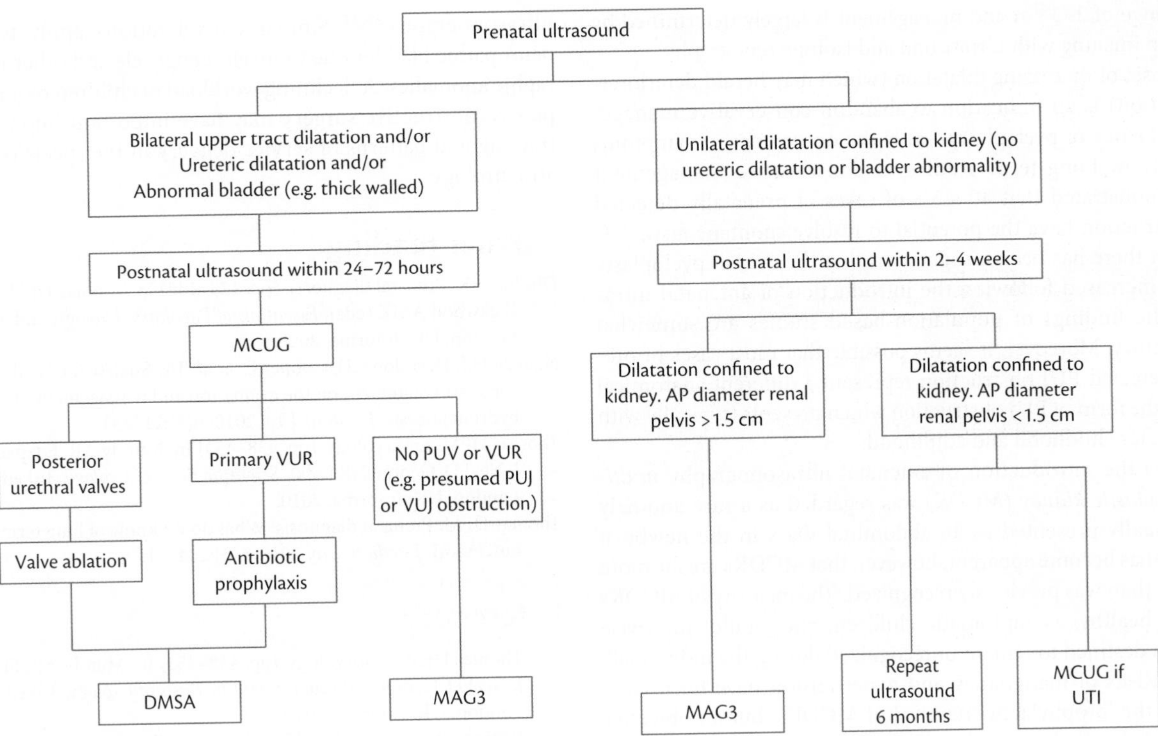

Fig. 8.1.3 Algorithm summarizing a selective approach to postnatal investigation.

weeks followed by ^{99m}TcMAG3 dynamic renography. However, this is best deferred for eight weeks or longer in view of the difficulty in interpreting drainage curve data in young infants with immature tubular function.

MCUG is no longer routinely performed for unilateral dilatation confined to the kidney. While this approach carries some risk of missing some infants with vesicoureteric reflux (VUR) it is offset by the far larger number of healthy infants who are no longer being submitted to unnecessary and invasive investigation.

Nevertheless, the parents of infants with upper tract dilatation should be advised of the importance of having the urine checked if their child develops any features of urinary infection or an unexplained febrile illness.

Mild dilatation confined to the kidney (anteroposterior diameter of the renal pelvis <1 cm)

An ultrasound scan is repeated within two to four weeks. Practice varies considerably with regard to further ultrasound follow-up, but the weight of evidence[18–20] indicates that the risk of morbidity associated with this common antenatal finding is extremely low and the majority of children can be safely discharged after a final scan at 6–12 months.

Cystic kidney

Multicystic dysplastic kidney (MCDK) is by far the commonest prenatally detected cystic malformation. The kidney is entirely replaced by non-communicating cysts and there is complete absence of solid renal tissue. If the diagnostic criteria for MCDK are fulfilled and the contralateral kidney appears normal, the only additional investigation needed to confirm the diagnosis (by demonstrating total absence of function) is a ^{99m}TcDMSA scan at six to eight weeks. ^{99m}TcDMSA is also the modality of choice for demonstrating the presence of ectopic kidneys.

Upper tract duplication (duplex kidney)

Antibiotic prophylaxis is commenced pending further investigation. Anatomical and functional assessment usually requires a combination of ultrasound, MCUG, and isotope renography in the first 8–12 weeks. Magnetic resonance urography can be very informative in the investigation of complex duplex anatomy and ectopic ureters but is rarely indicated in the first six months of life.

Impact of prenatal diagnosis

The results of some longer-term studies are now providing valuable information on the natural history of prenatally detected uropathies and, in turn, are contributing to a more evidence-based approach to investigation and management. A detailed account is beyond the scope of this chapter, but some of the key findings regarding the long-term outcome of common urological conditions can be briefly summarized as follows.

Pelviureteric junction obstruction accounts for 35–50% of clinically significant prenatally detected urinary tract abnormalities. Numerous studies have demonstrated a correlation between the natural history and outcome of prenatally detected PUJ and initial differential renal function and the severity of dilatation—as defined by the anteroposterior diameter of the renal pelvis or the grading system devised by the Society for Fetal Urology.[21,22]

The postnatal investigation and management of PUJ obstruction is detailed elsewhere but the findings of long-term studies[23] have endorsed a conservative approach for prenatally detected PUJ obstruction in cases where the AP (anteroposterior) diameter of the renal pelvis is <2 cm and differential function on isotope renography is >40%. Pyeloplasty is indicated when differential function is reduced below 40% or the AP diameter of the renal pelvis exceeds 3 cm. In many cases, the renal pelvic AP diameter is in the range of 2–3 cm and management is largely determined by follow-up imaging with ultrasound and isotope renography.

The onset of increasing dilatation (which may herald deteriorating function) is an indication to abandon conservative management in favour of pyeloplasty—as is the occurrence of symptoms or infection. Long-term studies of conservative management have demonstrated that 40–45% of cases of prenatally detected PUJ obstruction have the potential to resolve spontaneously.[23–27] Although there has been a suggestion that the overall pyeloplasty rate has increased following the introduction of antenatal ultrasound, the findings of population-based studies are somewhat contradictory. Moreover, it seems possible that most cases of prenatally detected PUJ obstruction represent a different anatomical entity to the form of PUJ obstruction which presents (typically with pain) in later childhood and adulthood.

Prior to the introduction of antenatal ultrasonography *multicystic dysplastic kidney (MCDK)* was regarded as a rare anomaly which usually presented as an abdominal mass in the newborn period. It has become apparent, however, that MCDKs are far more prevalent than was previously recognized. The majority of MCDKs occur in healthy, asymptomatic children, and would otherwise have been destined to remain unrecognized during the individual's lifetime. Risks of malignancy and hypertension have been cited to justify the 'prophylactic' removal of MCDKs, but an objective analysis of the evidence indicates that the risk of malignancy is exceedingly small[23,28–30] and the risk of developing hypertension is below 1%.[23,30,31]

With the advent of prenatal diagnosis, it had been anticipated that it would lead to an improved prognosis for renal function in boys with posterior urethral valves by facilitating early intervention and minimizing the risk of infection.

However, this proved not to be the case and it was found that the short- to medium-term prognosis for boys with prenatally detected posterior urethral valves (PUV) was inferior to that of boys in whom PUV presented clinically.[32,33] This apparent paradox can almost certainly be explained by the tendency of second trimester antenatal screening to selectively identify cases at the more severe end of the spectrum. Studies designed to assess the longer-term functional outcome have reported differing results. While one long-term study found no difference in the incidence of end-stage renal failure in patients with prenatally PUV when compared with those who had presented clinically,[34] another study did identify a probable benefit when outcomes were assessed in the second and third decades of life.[35]

Conclusion

Prenatal diagnosis has been beneficial for children with significant urological abnormalities by providing an opportunity to reduce their risk of morbidity and renal damage due to infection and high grade obstruction. By contrast, the detection of mild dilatation of little or no clinical significance has undoubtedly generated an unnecessary burden of parental anxiety and unwarranted investigation. However, there is now widespread recognition of the need to adopt a selective approach to postnatal investigation.

Paediatric urologists in many Western countries have encountered a declining number of referrals of newborns with bladder exstrophy, prune belly syndrome, and cloacal anomalies as a consequence of termination of pregnancies prompted by antenatal ultrasonography.[36,37] Similar considerations apply to cases of neuropathic bladder due to myelomengocele and other major dysraphic anomalies. A declining workload of children requiring complex reconstructive surgery may have important implications for training and patterns of service delivery in the specialty of paediatric urology.

Further reading

Dhillon HK. Prenatal diagnosis. (pp. 133–142) In: Thomas DFM, Duffy PG, Rickwood AMK (eds). *Essentials of Paediatric Urology,* 2nd edition. London, UK: Informa, 2008.

Nguyen HT, Herndon CD, Cooper C, *et al.* The Society for Fetal Urology consensus statement on the evaluation and management of antenatal hydronephrosis. *J Pediatr Urol* 2010; **6**(3):212–31.

Thomas DFM. Embryology. (pp. 438–453) In: Mundy AR, Fitzpatrick J, Neal D, George NR (eds). *Scientific Basis of Urology,* 3rd edition. London, UK: Informa, 2010.

Thomas DFM. Prenatal diagnosis: What do we know of long term outcomes?. *J Pediatr Urol* 2010; **6**(3):204–11.

References

1. Thomas DFM. Embryology. (pp. 438–453) In: Mundy AR, Fitzpatrick J, Neal D, George NR (eds). *Scientific Basis of Urology,* 3rd edition. London, UK: Informa, 2010.
2. Rabinowitz R, Peters MT, Vyas S, Campbell S, Nicolaides KH. Measurement of fetal urine production in normal pregnancy by real-time ultrasonography. *Am J Obstet Gynecol* 1989; **161**(5):1264–6.
3. De Mello D, Reid LM The kidney/lung loop. (pp. 62–77) In: Thomas DFM (ed). *Urological Disease in the Fetus and Infant.* Oxford, UK: Butterworth-Heinemann, 1997.
4. Glick PL, Harrison MR, Golbus MS *et al.* Management of the fetus with congenital hydronephrosis II. Prognostic criteria and selection for treatment. *J Pediatr Surg* 1985; **20**:376–87.
5. Haycock GB. Development of glomerular filtration and tubular sodium reabsorption in the human fetus and newborn. *Br J Urol* 1998; **81**:33–8.
6. Heilbron DC, Holliday MA, al-Dahwi A, Kogan BA. Expressing glomerular filtration rate in children. *Pediatr Nephrol* 1991; **5**(1):5–11
7. Trompetor R, Renal physiology and renal failure. (pp. 14–24) In: Thomas DFM, Duffy PG, Rickwood AMK (eds). *Essentials of Paediatric Urology,* 2nd edition. London, UK: Informa, 2008.
8. Risdon RA. Renal dysplasia. I. A clinico-pathological study of 76 cases. *J Clin Pathol* 1971; **24**(1):57–71.
9. Barker AP, Cave MM, Thomas DFM, Lilford RJ, Irving HC, Arthur RJ, Smith SEW. Fetal PUJ obstruction: predictors of outcome. *Br J Urol* 1995; **76**:649–52.
10. Hutton KAR, Thomas DFM, Arthur RJ, Irving HC, Smith SEW. Prenatally detected posterior urethral valves: is gestational age at detection a predictor of outcome? *J Urol* 1994; **152**:698–701.
11. Arthur RJ, Irving HC, Thomas DFM, Watters JK. Bilateral fetal uropathy: what is the outlook? *BMJ* 1989; **298**(6685):1419–20.
12. Chitty LS, Chudleigh P, Pembrey M, Campbell S. Renal pathology in fetuses with mild pyelectasis: prediction of outcome. *Ultrasound Obstet Gynaecol* 1999; **14**(Suppl 1):12.
13. Glick PL, Harrison MR, Adzick NS, Noall RA, Villa RL. Correction of congenital hydronephrosis in utero IV: in utero decompression prevents renal dysplasia. *J Pediatr Surg* 1984; **19**(6):649–57.
14. Crombleholme TM, Harrison MR, Langer JC, *et al.* Early experience with open fetal surgery for congenital hydronephrosis. *J Pediatr Surg* 1988; **23**(12):1114–21.
15. Rodeck CH, Nicolaides KH. Ultrasound guided invasive procedures in obstetrics. *Clin Obstet Gynaecol* 1983; **10**(3):515–39.
16. Clark TJ, Martin WL, Divakaran TG, Whittle MJ, Kilby MD, Khan KS. Prenatal bladder drainage in the management of fetal lower urinary

tract obstruction: a systematic review and meta-analysis. *Obstet Gynaecol* 2003; **102**(2):367–82.

17. Dhillon HK. Prenatal diagnosis. (pp. 133–142) In: Thomas DFM, Duffy PG, Rickwood AMK (eds). *Essentials of Paediatric Urology,* 2nd edition. London, UK: Informa, 2008.
18. Ismaili K, Hall M, Donner C, Thomas D, Vermeylen D, Avni F. Results of systematic screening for minor degrees of fetal renal pelvis in an unselected population. *Am J Obstet Gynaecol* 2003; **188**(1):242–6.
19. Thomas DFM, Madden NP, Irving HC, Arthur RJ, Smith SEW. Mild dilatation of the kidney: a follow up study. *Brit Journal Urol* 1994; **74**:236–9.
20. Damon-Elias HA, Luijnenburg SE, Visser GH, Stoutenbeek PH, de Jong TP. Mild pyelectesis diagnosed by prenatal ultrasound is not a predictor of urinary tract morbidity in childhood. *Prenat Diagn* 2005; **25**(13):1239–47.
21. Nguyen HT, Herndon CD, Cooper C, *et al.* The Society for Fetal Urology consensus statement on the evaluation and management of antenatal hydronephrosis. *J Pediatr Urol* 2010; **6**(3):212–31.
22. Maizels M, Reisman EM, Flom LS, Nelson J, Fernbach S, Firth CF. Grading nephroureteral dilatation detected in the first year of life—correlation with obstruction. *J Urol* 1992; **148**:609.
23. Thomas DFM. Prenatal diagnosis: What do we know of long term outcomes?. *J Pediatr Urol* 2010; **6**(3):204–11.
24. Ismail A, Elkholy A, Zaghmout O, *et al.* Postnatal management of antenatally diagnosed ureteroplevic junction obstruction. *J Urol* 2006; **2**:163–8.
25. Tombesi MM, Alconcher LF. Natural history of bilateral mild isolated antenatal hydronephrosis conservatively managed. *Pediatr Nephrol* 2012; **27**(7):1119–23.
26. Tombesi MM, Alconcher LF. Short-term outcome of mild isolated antenatal hydronephrosis conservatively managed. *J Pediatr Urol* 2012; **8**(2):129–33.
27. Longpre M, Nguan A, Macneily AE, Afshar K. Prediction of the outcome of antenatally diagnosed hydronephrosis: a multivariable analysis. *J Pediatr Urol* 2012; **8**(2):135–9.
28. Cambio A J, Evans CP, Kurzrock EA. Non surgical management of multicystic dysplastic kidney. *BJU Int* 2008; **101**:804–8
29. Narchi H. Risk of Wilms' tumour with multicystic kidney disease: a systematic review. *Arch Dis Child* 2005; **90**(2):147–9.
30. Aslam M, Watson AR; Trent and Anglia MCDK Study Group. Unilateral multicystic dysplastic kidney: long term outcomes. *Arch Dis Child* 2006; **91**(10):820–3.
31. Narchi H. Risk of hypertension with multicystic kidney disease: a systematic review. *Arch Dis Child* 2005; **90**(9):921–4.
32. Reinberg Y, De Castano I, Gonzalez R. Prognosis for patients with prenatally detected posterior urethral valves. *J Urol* 1992; **148**:125–6.
33. Cuckow P. Posterior urethral valves. (pp. 540–54) In: Stringer MD, Oldham KT, Mouriquand PDE (eds). *Paediatric Surgery and Urology: Long-term Outcomes.* Cambridge, UK: Cambridge University Press, 2006.
34. Ylinen E, Ala-Houhala M, Wikström S. Prognostic factors of posterior urethral valves and the role of antenatal detection. *Paedtr Nephrol* 2004; **19**:874–9.
35. Kousidis G, Thomas DFM, Morgan H, Haider N, Subramaniam R, Feather S. The long term outcome of prenatally detected posterior urethral valves: a 10 to 22 year follow up study. *BJUI* 2008; **102**(8):1020–4.
36. Cromie WJ, Lee K, Houde K, Holmes L. Implications of prenatal ultrasound screening in the incidence of major genitourinary malformations. *J Urol* 2001; **165**:1677–80.
37. Hsieh MH, Lai J, Saigal CS; Urologic Diseases in America Project. Trends in porenatal sonography use and subsequent urological diagnoses and abortions in the United States. *J Pediatr Urol* 2009; **5**:490–4.

CHAPTER 8.2

Urinary tract infection in children

David F.M. Thomas

Introduction to urinary tract infection in children

Urinary tract infection is one of the most important disorders of childhood because of its prevalence, its association with underlying abnormalities of the urinary tract and the threat of infective renal scarring leading to long-term morbidity.

Although urinary infection is now a rare cause of mortality, it remains a cause of severe systemic illness which may be accompanied by septicaemic complications. Even when confined to the lower tract (cystitis), recurrent urinary tract infections (UTIs) may have a significant impact on quality of life by interfering with schooling and requiring repeated GP and hospital attendances.

During the last two decades, a growing awareness of urinary tract infection among general practitioners coupled with the availability of sensitive reagent sticks for early diagnosis has led to many more children with normal urinary tracts being referred for investigation than in the past. Reliance on outdated diagnostic protocols resulted in large numbers of children with normal urinary tracts being over-investigated with unnecessarily invasive tests.[1] For this reason, the National Institute of Clinical Excellence (NICE) commissioned a group of experts to draw up new guidelines, which were published in 2007.[2] While the reasoning behind the guidelines has been broadly accepted, critics have raised concerns that implementation of some of the recommendations might carry a risk of underlying pathology being missed in some children.

Aetiology

Over the last decade it has become apparent that the concept of UTIs as the replication of bacteria within urine is oversimplistic. Proliferation of uropathogenic *Escherichia coli* is now thought to occur predominantly at an intracellular level within the urothelium—particularly in the bladder. The persistence of intracellular bacterial communities in vacuoles within urothelial cells forms a latent reservoir of organisms with the potential to cause further UTIs.[3,4]

Anatomical factors

Vesicouretericreflux (VUR) is the condition most commonly identified during the course of investigation. Stasis due to dysfunctional voiding is frequently implicated as a predisposing factor—particularly in girls with an acquired pattern of deferred voiding and incomplete bladder emptying. Abnormalities such as posterior urethral valves and pelviureteric junction obstruction which previously presented with UTI are often detected prenatally.

Although UTIs are 10 to 20 times less common in circumcised boys, the overall risk of UTI in the non-circumcised is low and does not represent a medical indication for routine newborn circumcision. By contrast, there is evidence to justify circumcision in boys with significant urological abnormalities which put them a considerably increased risk of infection.[5]

Bacterial pathogenicity

The organisms responsible for UTIs in children are similar to those in other age groups, namely *Escherichia coli*, *Klebsiella*, *Enterobacter*, and *Strep faecalis*. Fimbriated forms of *E. coli* are of particular virulence because of their ability to adhere to urothelial receptor sites and colonize the urinary tract. *Proteus mirabilis* is a urea-splitting organism which is implicated in the formation of infective calculi, particularly in uncircumcised male infants. Infection with *Pseudomonas aeruginosa* and other opportunistic pathogens is often associated with underlying anatomical abnormalities and may prove difficult to eradicate until the underlying stasis and/or reflux has been corrected.

Clinical aspects

Specimen collection

Although cooperative potty-trained children are capable of providing a clean catch midstream sample, other methods are needed for younger children and for those who are unable to provide a midstream specimen. The use of adhesive collection bags applied to the region of the genitalia remains the most common method for collecting urine samples in infants. Alternatively, pads or cotton wool balls placed inside the nappy can be used to collect a specimen of urine which is then aspirated from the material with a syringe.

Suprapubic puncture and aspiration of bladder urine is rarely indicated except to facilitate urgent diagnosis in a sick child. Once collected, the urine specimen should be sent promptly to the laboratory for microscopy and culture but a urine specimen may store in a refrigerator for up to 24 hours before being transported to the laboratory.

Laboratory diagnosis

The principle diagnostic criterion of infection is $>10^5$ colony forming units per mL of organisms in pure growth on culture. In a sample obtained by suprapubic puncture, any bacterial growth is regarded as significant. Criteria for the diagnosis of significant pyuria vary in different laboratories, but a leukocyte count corresponding >10 WBC/mm^3 is generally considered to be significant.

The early detection of UTIs has been greatly facilitated in recent years by the introduction of reagent dipsticks with nitrite and leukocyte esterase reagents.[6] Reagent sticks also test for haematuria and proteinuria—although neither are diagnostic for infection. A strongly positive result for proteinuria should, however, prompt further investigation of possible renal disease.

Clinical presentation

In newborns and infants, the clinical features of urinary tract infection are usually non-specific and may be difficult to differentiate from any other cause of febrile illness in this age group. For this reason, it is essential that urine microscopy and culture are always included in the 'septic work-up' of every child with unexplained fever. Dipstick testing will generally provide initial evidence of urinary infection, but whenever possible, a sample should be sent to the laboratory before antibiotic treatment is commenced. Recurrent or chronic infection in infants is characterized by failure to thrive and poor weight gain. Infective stone disease due to proteus infection may present with an insidious clinical picture and the presence of this organism in the urine should always prompt further investigations.

In children aged two years and upwards, the clinical picture is largely determined by whether infection is confined to the lower tract (cystitis) or whether the upper tract is involved (pyelonephritis). In practice, this distinction is not always clear cut, since children with pyelonephritis may also have lower tract symptoms.

Lower tract infection is characterized by dysuria, frequency, urgency, and suprapubic discomfort or pain. In addition, a recent onset of daytime and/or night-time enuresis is a relatively common feature of UTI in young children who were previously dry.

Asymptomatic bacteruria is relatively common in girls aged over four years and is almost invariably due to stasis and post-void residual urine in the bladder. Low-grade VUR may also be present. Despite the term, 'asymptomatic' chronic bacteruria is usually associated with malodorous urine and mild dysuria.

Upper tract infection (pyelonephritis) is characterized by fever >38°C, systemic ill health, loin pain, and tenderness. However not all these features are present in every child with pyelonephritis. Prompt diagnosis and effective antibiotic treatment are essential to minimize the risk of infective renal scarring.

History and examination

Parents should be asked about any known family history of reflux or other urological conditions and also whether any abnormality was detected on antenatal scanning. In older children, it is crucially important to enquire about voiding history—with an emphasis on any tendency to deferred voiding (particularly at school). Information should also be sought on fluid intake and any history of constipation.

Physical examination should include abdominal palpation combined with palpation and visual examination of the lower spine to look for possible stigmata of occult spinal dysraphism.

Treatment of urinary tract infection

Newborns and infants with suspected UTI and older children with pyelonephritis are usually admitted to hospital under the care of paediatricians. Treatment with intravenous antibiotics is commenced as soon as a urine specimen has been obtained for laboratory analysis and culture.

Children with symptomatic lower UTIs are treated with an appropriate oral antibiotic. From one authoritative review of the published evidence, it was concluded that a two- to four-day course of oral antibiotics appeared to be as effective as a seven- to fourteen-day course when treating lower tract UTI in children.[7] The 2007 NICE guidelines recommend a three-day course of antibiotic treatment for most cases.[2]

Long-term antibiotic prophylaxis forms the mainstay of the conservative management of vesicoureteric reflux (VUR) but in the absence of VUR, long-term antibiotic prophylaxis is not indicated—except perhaps as an adjunct to bladder retraining in children whose UTIs are related to dysfunctional voiding.

Investigation

Diagnostic imaging is aimed at identifying underlying anatomical abnormalities of the urinary tract which pose a risk of further UTIs, serious illness, or renal scarring.[8]

Historically, urological abnormalities (notably VUR) were identified in up to 30% of children referred for investigation. While this may still be true of young infants, the yield of positive findings in older children is now probably of the order of 10% or less. The benefits of investigation must therefore be balanced against the risk of overinvestigating children with normal urinary tracts.[2]

The benefits and drawback of imaging modalities used for this purpose in children are summarized in Table 8.2.1.

Ultrasound

Ultrasonography is widely used as an initial screening test to detect dilatation (regardless of cause) and for the assessment of renal size, renal outline, cortical scarring,[9] and the presence of calculi. Ultrasound also provides valuable information on bladder wall thickness, bladder emptying, and assessment of post-voiding residual urine.

It is not, however, a reliable modality for the detection of VUR. Blane and associates[10] found that ultrasound appearances were normal in 74% of refluxing units. Moreover, in 28% of cases the VUR 'missed' on ultrasound was grade III or higher. Similar results have been reported from other studies.

DMSA scintigraphy

Tc 99^m DMSA is the most sensitive modality for visualizing renal scarring and also provides an accurate measure of differential renal function.

Micturating cystourethrography

Although this invasive investigation is now used far more selectively than in the past, it retains an important role because it provides anatomical information on the lower urinary tract and permits grading of the severity of VUR. The study is performed under prophylactic antibiotic cover with contrast being introduced into the bladder using a 4–6 Fr feeding tube or via an indwelling catheter which has been left *in situ* at the time of cystoscopy. The radiation dosage has been greatly reduced by modern radiology techniques

Indirect MAG3 renocystography

Although this has been promoted as a non-invasive alternative to micturating cystourethrogram (MCUG), it nevertheless requires

Table 8.2.1 Summary of imaging modalities used in children following urinary tract infection

Imaging modality	Strengths	Weaknesses
Ultrasound	Non-invasive, readily available, and inexpensive Imaging not dependent upon functioning kidney(s) 'Real time' visualization of the bladder, with measurement of post-void residual	Unreliable for the detection of mild/moderate degrees of reflux Poor sensitivity for the detection of minor scarring Operator dependent
DMSA	Provides reliable, reproducible information on renal scarring and differential functionUseful for visualizing poorly functioning ectopic kidneys	Invasive (requires IV cannulation) Radiation dosage (small) Limited availability
Micturating cystourethrogram (MCUG)	Remains the 'gold standard' investigation for vesicoureteric reflux Visualization of lower tract anatomy (e.g. posterior urethral valves)	Invasive, requiring urethral catheterization Radiation exposure (although this is greatly reduced with modern techniques)
Indirect cystography (MAG3)	Less invasive than MCUG (but requires IV cannulation) More physiological for detection of VUR during normal voiding Provides additional information on renal function	Limited to children who are potty-trained and cooperative Requires IV cannulation Poor sensitivity for the detection of low grade VUR Does not provide the anatomical information yielded by MCUG
Intravenous urogram (IVU)	Potential to demonstrate detail of upper tract abnormalities not always evident on other modalities	Now rarely used in children because functional and anatomical information can be obtained using less invasive modalities

the intravenous injection of the tracer. Indirect nuclear cystography can only be used in toilet-trained children and does not yield the anatomical information provided by a conventional MCUG. Its use is therefore largely limited to follow up rather than initial investigation.

Intravenous urography

Intravenous urography (IVU) no longer plays any meaningful role in the investigation of UTI in children.

National Institute of Clinical Excellence guidelines

The diagnostic protocols advocated in the 2007 NICE guidelines can be applied across a range of primary, secondary, and tertiary practice.[2] Although many aspects of the guidelines have been widely accepted, concern has been expressed regarding the potential for significant underlying urological abnormalities to remain undetected if an ultrasound scan is no longer performed routinely in every child with a proven UTI. Of additional concern is the possible risk that the highly selective use of micturating cystourethrography advocated in the guidelines will result in clinically significant VUR remaining undiagnosed. From their experience, Lytzen and associates[11] concluded that use of the guidelines was not appropriate for children experiencing their first episode of pyelonephritis. By contrast, Deader and associates[12] analysed a series of 346 children with UTI and concluded that significant abnormalities would not have been missed if they had been investigated in accordance with the NICE guidelines.

A practical approach to investigation

This is largely determined by the age of the child and the severity and nature of the urinary tract infection.

Infants aged 0–6 months

For those who respond well to antibiotic treatment within 48 hours, an ultrasound scan should be performed within six weeks. If this is normal, no further investigations are required. The occurrence of further UTIs is, however, a strong indication for additional investigations, including DMSA and MCUG.

A DMSA scan is indicated when a UTI does not respond within 48 hours or is categorized as 'atypical'* according to the NICE guidelines. Where possible, this investigation should be deferred for four to six months in order to distinguish between acute, reversible changes and established renal scarring. Antibiotic prophylaxis should be maintained until the results of the DMSA (and MCUG) are known.

* An atypical UTI is defined by one or more of the following features:

- Systemic symptoms
- Fever >38.5°C
- Impaired urine flow
- Abdominal or bladder mass
- Elevated plasma creatinine
- Infecting organisms other than *E. coli*
- Positive family history (e.g. of VUR)

If the initial ultrasound scan reveals abnormal findings, further investigation is guided by the nature of the findings. For example a MAG3 scan would be more appropriate rather than a DMSA renogram if the appearances are indicative of obstruction and an MCUG would be indicated by the finding of a distended, thick-walled bladder.

Children aged six months to three years

The NICE guidelines do not advocate a routine ultrasound scan for children in this age range whose UTI responds well to antibiotic treatment within 48 hours. Nevertheless, many paediatric clinicians remain uncomfortable with this particular recommendation and continue to routinely screen young children with an ultrasound scan—even after a 'typical' UTI.

Children whose UTI does not respond promptly to antibiotic treatment or falls within the 'atypical' criteria (set out above) should be investigated by ultrasonography and, in most cases, a DMSA scan after four to six months.

Recurrent UTIs require investigation with a DMSA scan to look for scarring (denoting probable VUR)—even if the ultrasound findings are normal. MCUG is performed on a more selective basis in this age group, for example when there is a family history of VUR, any suggestion of poor urinary stream, ureteric or bladder dilatation on ultrasound, or cortical scarring on DMSA.

Children aged three years and upwards

No diagnostic imaging is required following a first UTI which responds well to treatment within 48 hours. Ultrasound is, however, indicated when a UTI does not respond promptly to antibiotic treatment or is accompanied by systemic symptoms or the 'atypical' features—as defined above.

In this age group, the NICE guidelines advocate a highly selective approach to the use of DMSA. Nevertheless, many clinicians continue to advise a DMSA scan if the clinical picture has been suggestive of upper tract infection (pyelonephritis).

When an abnormality is visualized on ultrasound, this should be investigated appropriately—for example, by MCUG if there is evidence of ureteric dilatation or a lower tract anomaly.

Conclusion

The greater risk of renal damage in infants and young children coupled with the higher yield of abnormal findings in this age group justifies a more intensive approach to investigation. By contrast, asymptomatic or low-grade UTIs in older children pose little or no threat of renal scarring or long-term morbidity. Any benefit in identifying the small percentage with underlying urological abnormalities must be balanced by the importance of minimizing the burden of unnecessary, invasive investigations in healthy children.[13] Nevertheless, every child should be assessed on an individual basis and in the final analysis; published guidelines should always be applied within the overall context of clinical judgement.

Further reading

Hiorns MP. Diagnostic imaging. (pp. 25–42) In: Thomas DFM, Duffy PG, Rickwood AMK (eds). *Essentials of Paediatric Urology,* 2nd edition. London, UK: Informa Healthcare, 2008.

National Institute for Health and Clinical Excellence. Guidelines on urinary tract infection in children, 2007. Available at: www.nice.org.uk/cgCG054 [Online].

O'Toole S J. Urinary tract infection. (pp. 43–55) In: Thomas DFM, Duffy PG, Rickwood AMK (eds). *Essentials of Paediatric Urology*, 2nd edition. London, UK: Informa Healthcare, 2008.

References

1. Verrier Jones K. Time to review the value of imaging after urinary tract infection in infants. *Arch Dis Child* 2005; **90**(7):663–4.
2. National Institute for Health and Clinical Excellence. Guidelines on urinary tract infection in children, 2007. Available at: www.nice.org.uk/cgCG054 [Online].
3. Anderson GG, Palermo JJ, Schilling JD, Roth R, Hueser J, Hultgren SJ. Intracellular bacterial biofilm—like pods in urinary tract infections. *Science* 2003; **301**(5629):105–7.
4. Mysorekar IU, Hultgren SJ. Mechanismms of uropathogenic Escherichia coli persistence and eradication from the urinary tract. *Proc Natl Acad Sci U S A* 2006; **103**(38):14170–5.
5. Singh-Grewal D, Macdessi J, Craig J. Circumcision for the prevention of urinary tract infection in boys: A systematic review of clinical trials and observation studies. *Arch Dis Child* 2005; **90**(8):853–8.
6. O'Toole S J. Urinary tract infection. (pp. 43–55) In: Thomas DFM, Duffy PG, Rickwood AMK (eds). *Essentials of Paediatric Urology*, 2nd edition. London, UK: Informa Healthcare, 2008.
7. Michael M, Hodson EM, Craig JC, Martin S, Moyer VA. Short compared with standard duration of antibiotic treatment for urinary tract infection: a systematic review of randomised controlled trials. *Arch Dis Child* 2002; **87**(2):118–23.
8. Hiorns MP. Diagnostic imaging. (pp. 25–42) In: Thomas DFM, Duffy PG, Rickwood AMK (eds). *Essentials of Paediatric Urology,* 2nd edition. London, UK: Informa Healthcare, 2008.
9. Christian MT, McColl JH, MacKenzie JR, Beattie TJ. Risk assessment of renal cortical scarring with urinary tract infection by clinical features and ultrasonography. *Arch Dis Child* 2000; **82**(5):376–80.
10. Blane CE, DiPietro MA, Zerin JM, Sedman AB, Bloom DA. Renal sonography is not a reliable screening examination for vesicoureteral reflux. *J Urol* 1993; **150**(2 Pt 2):752–5.
11. Lytzen R, Thorup J, Cortes D. Experience with the NICE guidelines for imaging studies in children with first pyelonephritis. *Eur J Pediatr Surg* 2011; **21**(5):283–6.
12. Deader R, Tiboni SG, Malone PS, Fairhurst J. Will the implementation of the 2007 National Institute for Health and Clinical Excellence (NICE) guidelines on childhood urinary tract infection (UTI) in the UK miss significant urinary tract pathology? *BJU Int* 2012; **110**(3):454–8.
13. Schroeder AR, Abidari JM, Kirpekar R, *et al.* Impact of a more restrictive approach to urinary tract imaging after febrile urinary tract infection. *Arch Pediatr Adolesc Med* 2011; **165**(11):1027–32.

CHAPTER 8.3

Vesicoureteric reflux

David F.M. Thomas

Aetiology

The anatomy of the normal ureterovesical junction creates a valve mechanism preventing the retrograde flow of urine at physiological bladder pressures. Factors contributing to the competence of the antireflux mechanism include: the passive 'flap valve' effect of the intramural and submucosal course of the ureter; concentric contraction of the distal ureteric wall; and elongation of the intramural ureter within Waldeyer's sheath at the time of voiding.

Primary vesicoureteric reflux (VUR) is congenital in origin and is believed to result from an abnormality of the ureteric bud. Congenital renal damage (dysplasia) is most commonly seen in association with high-grade VUR and is thought to reflect faulty reciprocal interaction between an aberrant ureteric bud and the metanephric mesenchyme.

VUR has a strong genetic basis with a reported incidence in excess of 30% in siblings.[1] The risk of VUR in the offspring of affected of parents may be as high 50%.[2] Although a considerable number of putative genes have been studied, attempts to identify a single 'reflux gene' have so far yielded consistently negative results.

Gender differences

The major differences between the characteristics of primary VUR in males and females[3] probably owe more to anatomical and functional differences in the lower urinary tract than any specific sex-linked genetic factors. VUR in girls typically presents with urinary infection between the age of 2 and 7 years, is of mild to moderate severity and is associated with detrusor instability or other features of acquired bladder dysfunction in upwards of 50% of cases. By contrast, primary VUR in boys is more often of higher grade and may be detected on antenatal ultrasonography by virtue of upper tract dilatation and poor bladder emptying. Intrauterine bladder dysfunction has been implicated in the aetiology of high-grade VUR in male infants[4] with some authors postulating impaired maturation of the sphincter complex as a cause of transient functional outflow obstruction in the foetus.[5] When primary VUR presents clinically with urinary tract infection, in boys it is generally in the first two years of life.[6]

Classification and grading of vesicoureteric reflux

VUR has been historically subdivided as being either primary or secondary in aetiology. Primary VUR is congenital in origin, has a strong genetic basis and is characterized by weakness or incompetence of the valve mechanism at the vesicoureteric junction.

Secondary VUR results from incompetence of the valve mechanism secondary to chronically elevated intravesical pressure, for example in cases of outflow obstruction due to posterior urethral valves (PUV) or cases of neuropathic bladder. Secondary VUR has the potential to resolve spontaneously once more normal, physiological bladder pressures have been restored, for example by ablation of PUV or by bladder augmentation for neuropathic bladder.

In practice, the distinction between primary (anatomical) and secondary (functional) VUR is often less precise and acquired patterns of dysfunctional voiding play an important role in causing or exacerbating low to moderate grade VUR in mid to later childhood.

The system devised by the international Reflux Study Committee[7] is the one most widely used for grading the VUR (Fig. 8.3.1).

Reflux-related renal damage (reflux nephropathy)

Experimental studies have demonstrated the importance of intrarenal reflux in promoting the transmission of organisms from the collecting system into the renal parenchyma. Abnormal papillae are located mainly in the upper and lower poles of the kidney, which are the areas at greatest risk of developing focal pyelonephritic scarring.[8,9]

The overwhelming weight of evidence indicates that focal renal scarring occurs as a consequence of pyelonephritis and that the reflux of sterile urine at normal voiding pressures does not cause ongoing renal damage.

The presence of congenital renal damage (dysplasia) is, however, relatively common, particularly in association with higher grades of VUR. Typically, a dysplastic kidney is small, has reduced function on DMSA, and has abnormally textured renal parenchyma on ultrasound. Although renal dysplasia can be diagnosed with some confidence on imaging in the newborn period it can prove difficult, if not impossible to accurately differentiate between infective and congenital mechanisms of renal damage once a kidney has been exposed to severe or recurrent pyelonephritis.

The risk of infective renal scarring is greatest in infancy and experimental evidence suggests that this risk is maximal after first major episode of pyelonephritis.

Clinical aspects

Although VUR is most commonly diagnosed during the investigation of UTI, it may occasionally come to light for the first time in children presenting with renal insufficiency or hypertension. High-grade VUR in male infants is increasingly diagnosed by antenatal ultrasound and asymptomatic VUR may be identified during screening of siblings of children with known VUR.

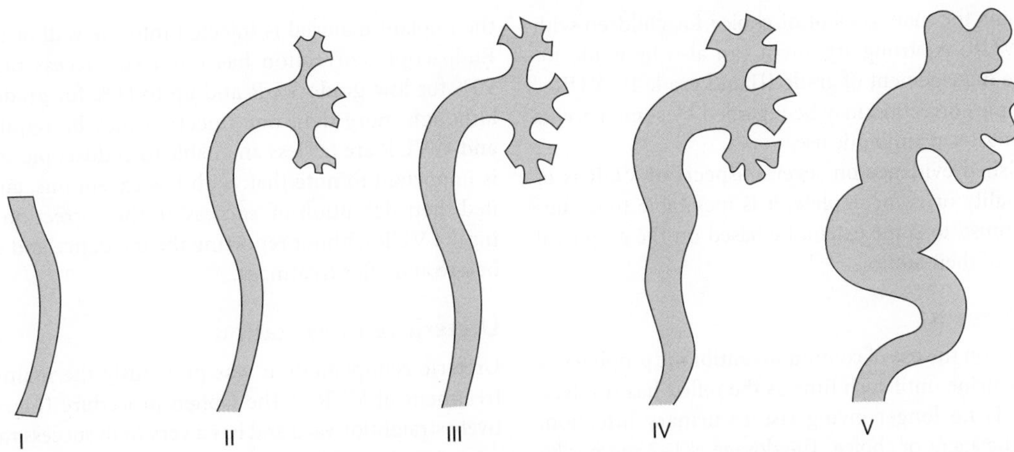

Fig. 8.3.1 Grading of Reflux. Grade I: Reflux into non-dilated ureter, reflux does not extend up to the kidney. Grade II: Non- dilating reflux extending up to the renal pelvis and calyces. Grade III: Mild to moderate dilatation of the ureter and collecting systems but with preservation of the papillary indentation of the calyces. Grade IV: Dilatation of moderate severity with some "blunting" of the calyces. V: Severe reflux into tortuous and grossly dilated ureter. Extensive "blunting" of the calyces and loss of papillary indentation.

Investigation

Ultrasound

Although a valuable screening tool in the investigation of urinary tract infection ultrasound has the major drawback of an unacceptably high 'false negative' rate for the detection of low to moderate grades of VUR. Even higher grades of VUR may be 'missed' on ultrasound in upwards of 25% of cases.[10]

Normal appearances on a 99^m DMSA scan do not exclude the presence of VUR but, conversely, evidence of scarring is strongly suggestive of underlying VUR and merits further investigation by micturating cystourethrography.[11]

Micturating cystourethrography

Reliance on this invasive investigation has declined considerably over the last two decades. Nevertheless, it remains the most accurate investigation for the diagnosis and grading of VUR and, unlike other imaging modalities, MCUG also permits detailed visualization of the anatomy of the bladder outflow and urethra. This is particularly important in males in view of the possible presence of outflow obstruction.

Natural history of vesicoureteric reflux

Numerous follow-up studies in sizeable cohorts of children have consistently documented the tendency for VUR to resolve spontaneously during the course of childhood.[12] The spontaneous resolution rate for grade I VUR is of the order of 85% and for grade II VUR 60%. Even grade III VUR has a spontaneous resolution rate of 45% to 50%. By contrast, the spontaneous resolution rate for higher grades of VUR is much lower, being of the order of 5–10% for grade IV VUR and less than 5% for grade V VUR. The spontaneous resolution of VUR probably results largely from an increase in the absolute and relative length of the intramural and submucosal ureter leading to strengthening of the 'flap valve' component of the antireflux valve mechanism.

Management

Historically, the management of VUR consisted of either 'medical' management—relying mainly on continuous antibiotic prophylaxis or open ureteric reimplantation. Over the last two decades, however, the surgical management of VUR has been revolutionized by the introduction of endoscopic treatment[13,14] with the result that open surgery now plays a far more limited role. Moreover, the efficacy of long-term antibiotic prophylaxis for the prevention of UTI has been called into question. One large, systematic literature review found no difference in the incidence of UTIs in children with VUR who were maintained on antibiotic prophylaxis compared with those who were not. However, the study populations were heterogeneous and the methodology employed in most published studies was not of high quality.[15] By contrast the Swedish randomized, controlled trial found that antibiotic prophylaxis was effective in reducing the incidence of UTIs in girls—but not in boys.[16] The published evidence is, however, more conclusive in demonstrating a reduced risk of new renal scarring in children receiving antibiotic prophylaxis.

Medical or surgical management?

Over the last three decades, a number of controlled studies have been undertaken in an attempt to determine which is more effective: medical or surgical treatment. The results of these trials have mostly been inconclusive with neither form of treatment being shown to be significantly superior to the other.[17–19]

Unlike earlier studies, the treatment arms of the recent Swedish reflux trial included endoscopic correction and 'surveillance' (in which children did not receive regular antibiotic prophylaxis, but were treated only if they developed a urinary tract infection). A total of 203 children with grades III or IV VUR were recruited to this prospective study and their outcomes were assessed after a minimum of two years.[20] Endoscopic treatment had the highest rate of resolution or downgrading (71%) of VUR, the corresponding figures for surveillance and antibiotic prophylaxis being 47% and 39%, respectively.[21] However, antibiotic prophylaxis had the lowest incidence of breakthrough UTIs (19% vs. 23% for endoscopic treatment and 57% in the surveillance arm of the study.[16] The incidence of new scarring (6%) was also lowest in those children receiving antibiotic prophylaxis.[22]

In summary, the weight of available evidence indicates that conservative management centred on the use of regular antibiotic prophylaxis remains the management of choice for children with grades I and II VUR. A strong argument can also be made for prophylaxis in the management of grade III and grade IV VUR—although endoscopic correction may be regarded by some parents as preferable to long-term antibiotic use.

Since the published evidence on several aspects of VUR is of poor scientific quality or is incomplete, it is inevitable that published guidelines must, to some extent, be based on the empirical recommendations of their authors.[23,24]

Medical management

This approach relies on the use of continuous antibiotic prophylaxis to maintain sterile urine until such time as the reflux has resolved spontaneously or is no longer giving rise to urinary infection. Trimethoprim is the agent of choice. The dosage is 1–2 mg per kg per day administered as single night-time dose. Nitrofurantoin is an alternative agent, but since this is often poorly tolerated, an oral cephalosporin may be a more palatable alternative. Active treatment of any underlying dysfunctional voiding is a key element of successful medical management, with particular emphasis on regular voiding and elimination of post-void residual urine.[25–27]

When there is evidence of detrusor instability, anticholinergic medication should also be considered. Antibiotic prophylaxis is maintained in younger children until they are fully potty-trained and have acquired a reliable voiding pattern. For those presenting later in childhood (usually girls), prophylaxis is maintained until any underlying dysfunctional voiding has been effectively treated and the urine has remained clear of infection for a year. It is not usually necessary to repeat the contrast MCUG before discontinuing prophylaxis in a child who is well and remaining infection-free.

Endoscopic correction

Developed and popularized by O'Donnell and Puri,[13,14] endoscopic treatment gained widespread acceptance following the introduction of dextranomer-hyaluronic acid copolymer as the injectable implant material. In the standard technique, the needle enters the submucosal plane below the ureteric orifice at a '6o'clock' position and the implant material is injected to create a mound, creating a crescent-shaped configuration at the ureteric orifice (Fig. 8.3.2A). In cases of high-grade VUR, the tip of the cystoscope can be advanced through the ureteric orifice and the implant material is injected into the wall of the distal ureter. Endoscopic correction has reported success rates in excess of 90% for low-grade VUR and up to 80% for grades II/III VUR—although more than one injection may be required. Grades IV and V VUR are far less amenable to endoscopic correction.[28,29] It is important to note that, with few exceptions, authors have limited their definition of 'success' to the correction (or downgrading) of VUR without reporting the incidence and severity of UTIs before and after treatment.

Ureteric reimplantation

Ureteric reimplantation was previously the mainstay of surgical treatment of VUR.[30] The Cohen procedure (Fig. 8.3.2B) is relatively straightforward and has a very high success rate coupled with a low incidence of complications. For grossly dilated ureters, the Politano-Leadbetter reimplantation may be preferable, particularly when combined with a psoas hitch procedure to obviate the risk of kinking at the entry site into the bladder (Fig. 8.3.2C). Extravesical antireflux procedures such as the Lich and Gregoir operations have gained increasing acceptance in recent years, since they are claimed to cause less postoperative discomfort than intravesical reimplantation techniques (Fig. 8.3.2D).

Other surgical options

Circumcision is a simple measure which can sometimes prove highly effective in preventing UTIs in infants with high-grade VUR for whom vesicostomy or ureteric reimplantation might otherwise be considered.

Correcting high-grade VUR in small infants is technically challenging, has a lower success rate, and is more prone to complications. For these reasons cutaneous vesicostomy is a valuable temporizing manoeuvre in this age group and is usually very effective in preventing symptomatic febrile UTIs and promoting drainage of the refluxing upper tracts. Ureteric reimplantation can be combined with closure of the vesicostomy towards the end of the second year of life. Refluxing loop ureterostomy has also been advocated for this purpose. Finally, nephroureterectomy may be considered when differential function is less than 10% and the contralateral kidney is healthy. With the advent of laparoscopic urology, this is a considerably less invasive procedure than the open approach employed in the past.

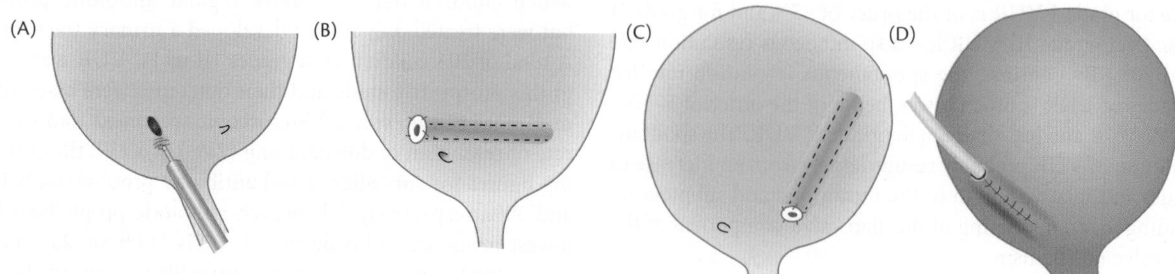

Fig. 8.3.2 Surgical options for correction of VUR. (A) Endoscopic. Submucoslal injection of implant material beneath refluxing ureteric orifice. (B) Cohen ureteric reimplantation; (C) Leadbetter ureteric reimplantion; and (D) Lich Gregoir ureteric reimplantation.

Republished with permission of Taylor and Francis Group, LLC from *Essentials of Paediatric Urology*, David F. M. Thomas, Patrick G. Duffy, and Anthony M. K. Rickwood, (Eds.), CRC Press, Taylor and Francis Group, Florida, USA, Copyright © 2002; permission conveyed through Copyright Clearance Center, Inc.

Conclusions

Vesicoureteric reflux is not a disease entity in the conventional sense but, rather, a variable manifestation of abnormal anatomy, disordered lower tract function, or the interaction of both factors. The principal aims of treatment are to prevent urinary tract infection and protect the kidneys against the risk of acquired renal scarring. Medical management remains the preferred option for children with mild to moderate VUR. In addition to long-term antibiotic prophylaxis, it is important to recognize and actively treat any underlying pattern of dysfunctional voiding. When surgical intervention is indicated, endoscopic correction is now the preferred technique for correcting mild to moderate grades of VUR. Ureteric reimplantation and other surgical options retain an important role in the management severe or complicated VUR.

Further reading

Tekgül S, Riedmiller H, Hoebeke P, *et al.* EAU Guidelines on vesicoureteral reflux in children. *Eur Urol* 2012; **62**(3):534–42.

Thomas DFM, Subramaniam R. Vesico ureteric reflux. (pp. 57–72) In: Thomas DFM, Duffy PG, Rickwood AMK (eds). *Essentials of Paediatric Urology*, 2nd edition. London, UK: Informa, 2008.

van der Voort JH, Verrier Jones K. Vesicoureteric reflux; definition and conservative management. (pp. 555–70) In: Stringer MD, Oldham KT, Mouriquand PDE (eds). *Paediatric Surgery and Urology: Long-term Outcomes*. Cambridge, UK: Cambridge University Press, 2006.

References

1. Jerkins GR, Noe HN. Familial vesicoureteral reflux: a prospective study. *J Urol* 1982; **128**(4):774–8.
2. Noe HN, Wyatt RJ, Peeden JN Jr, Rivas ML. The transmission of vesicoureteral reflux from parent to child. *J Urol* 1992; **148**(6):1869–71.
3. Yeung CK, Godley ML, Dhillion HK, *et al.* The characteristics of primary veisco-ureteric reflux in male and female infants with prenatal hydronephrosis. *Br J Urol* 1997; **80**:319–27.
4. Chandra M, Maddix H, McVicar M. Transient urodynamic dysfunction of infancy: relationship to urinary tract infections and vesicoureteral reflux. *J Urol* 1996; **155**(2):673–7.
5. Kokoua A, Homsy Y, Lavigne JF, *et al.* Maturation of the external urinary sphincter: a comparative histotopographic study in humans. *J Urol* 1993; **150**(2 Pt 2):617–22.
6. Caoine P, Villa M, Capozza N, De Gennaro M, Rizzoni G. Predictive risk factors for chronic renal failure in primary high-grade vesico ureteric reflux. *BJU Int* 2004; **93**:1309–12.
7. Lebowitz RL, Olbing H, Parkkulainen KV, Smellie JM, Tamminen-Möbius TE. International system of radiographic grading of vesicoureteric reflux. International Reflux Study in Children. *Pediatr Radiol* 1985; **15**(2):105–9.
8. Hodson CJ, Maling TM, McManamon PJ, Lewis MG. The pathogenesis of reflux nephropathy (chronic atrophic pyelonephritis). *Br J Radiol* 1975; Suppl **13**:1–26.
9. Ransley PG, Risdon RA. Renal papillary morphology and intrarenal reflux in the young pig. *Urol Res* 1975; **3**(3):105–9.
10. Blane CE, DiPietro MA, Zerin JM, Sedman AB, Bloom DA. Renal sonography is not a reliable screening examination for vesicoureteral reflux. *J Urol* 1993; **150**(2 Pt 2):752–5.
11. Sciagrà R, Materassi M, Rossi V, Ienuso R, Danti A, La Cava G. Alternative approaches to the prognostic stratification of mild to moderate primary vesicoureteral reflux in children. *J Urol* 1996; **155**(6):2052–5.
12. Skoog SJ, Belman AB, Majd M. A nonsurgical approach to the management of primary vesicoureteral reflux. *J Urol* 1987; **138**(4 Pt 2):941–6.
13. Puri P, O'Donnell B. Correction of experimentally produced vesicoureteric reflux in the piglet by intravesical injection of Teflon. *Br Med J (Clin Res Ed)* 1984; **289**(6436):5–7.
14. O'Donnell B, Puri P. Endoscopic correction of primary vesicoureteric reflux: results in 94 ureters. *Br Med J (Clin Res Ed)* 1986; **293**(6559):1404–6.
15. Williams G, Craig JC. Long-term antibiotics for preventing recurrent urinary tract infection in children. *Cochrane Database Syst Rev* 2011; **16**;(3):CD001534.
16. Brandström P, Esbjörner E, Herthelius M, Swerkersson S, Jodal U, Hansson S. The Swedish reflux trial in children: III. Urinary tract infection pattern. *J Urol* 2010; **184**(1):286–91.
17. Birmingham Reflux Study Group. Prospective trial of operative versus non-operative treatment of severe vesicoureteric reflux in children: five years' observation. *Br Med J (Clin Res Ed)* 1987; **295**(6592):237–41.
18. Olbing H, Smellie JM, Jodal U, Lax H. New renal scars in children with severe VUR: a 10-year study of randomized treatment. *Pediatr Nephrol* 2003; **18**(11):1128–31.
19. Medical versus surgical treatment of primary vesicoureteral reflux: report of the International Reflux Study Committee. *Pediatrics* 1981; **67**(3):392–400.
20. Brandström P, Esbjörner E, Herthelius M, *et al.* The Swedish reflux trial in children: I. Study design and study population characteristics. *J Urol* 2010; **184**(1):274–9.
21. Holmdahl G, Brandström P, Läckgren G, *et al.* The Swedish reflux trial in children: II. Vesicoureteral reflux outcome. *J Urol* 2010; **184**(1):280–5.
22. Brandström P, Nevéus T, Sixt R, Stokland E, Jodal U, Hansson S. The Swedish reflux trial in children: IV. Renal damage. *J Urol* 2010; **184**(1):292–7.
23. Tekgül S, Riedmiller H, Hoebeke P, *et al.* EAU Guidelines on vesicoureteral reflux in children. *Eur Urol* 2012; **62**(3):534–42.
24. Urinary tract infection: clinical practice guideline for the diagnosis and management of the initial UTI in febrile infants and children 2 to 24 months. Subcommittee on Urinary Tract Infection, Steering Committee on Quality Improvement and Management, Roberts KB. *Pediatrics* 2011; **128**(3):595–610.
25. van der Voort J H, Verrier Jones K. Vesicoureteric reflux: Definition and conservative management. (pp. 555–70) In: Stringer MD, Oldham KT, Mouriquand PDE (eds). *Paediatric Surgery and Urology: Long-term Outcomes*. Cambridge, UK: Cambridge University Press, 2006.
26. Koff SA, Wagner TT, Jayanthi VR. The relationship among dysfunctional elimination syndromes, primary vesicoureteral reflux and urinary tract infections in children. *J Urol* 1998; **160**(3 Pt 2):1019–22.
27. Sillén U, Brandström P, Jodal U, Holmdahl G, Sandin A, Sjöberg I, Hansson S. The Swedish reflux trial in children: v. Bladder dysfunction. *J Urol* 2010; **184**(1):298–304.
28. Läckgren G, Wåhlin N, Sköldenberg E, Stenberg A. Long-term followup of children treated with dextranomer/hyaluronic acid copolymer for vesicoureteral reflux. *J Urol* 2001; **166**(5):1887–92.
29. Puri P, Ninan GK, Surana R. Subureteric Teflon injection (STING). Results of a European survey. *Eur Urol* 1995; **27**(1):71–5.
30. Sung J, Skoog S.Surgical management of vesicoureteral reflux in children. *Pediatr Nephrol* 2012; **27**(4):551–61.

CHAPTER 8.4

Disorders of the kidney and upper urinary tract in children

Kim Hutton

Pelviureteric junction obstruction

The term 'hydronephrosis' is often loosely applied to this condition. Pelviureteric junction obstruction (PUJO) is characterized by defective transport of urine across the pelviureteric junction (PUJ) leading to elevated pressure within the renal collecting system and dilatation of the pelvis and calyces.

Aetiology

PUJO is caused by either intrinsic,[1–4] extrinsic or intraluminal abnormalities[5,6] in the vicinity of the PUJ. Horseshoe kidneys are prone to PUJO, as are duplex or pelvic kidneys. PUJO is also occasionally secondary to severe vesicoureteric reflux.[7]

Presentation

The majority of cases of PUJO are detected prenatally and most affected infants are completely asymptomatic at birth. Mild renal dilatation is present in 1% of foetuses whereas significant foetal uropathy occurs in 1 in 600 pregnancies. PUJO accounts for approximately 35% of significant foetal uropathies[8] and the overall incidence is in the region of 1 in 1,000–2,000 live births. Clinical presentation in older children typically consists of loin or abdominal pain, urinary tract infection (UTI), haematuria (often after relatively mild trauma), stone formation or, (rarely) hypertension. PUJO complicated by infection may present acutely as pyonephrosis, with swinging pyrexia and a tender flank/abdominal mass. PUJO occurs twice as commonly in males than females, the left kidney is involved in two-thirds of cases and in 10–20% of cases the condition is bilateral.

Diagnosis of obstruction

Obstruction can be defined as any restriction to urinary outflow, which, if left untreated, will lead to progressive deterioration of function in the affected kidney.[9] To clinicians, however, it seems illogical to wait until functional deterioration has occurred before intervening. One of the prime aims of investigation, therefore, is to differentiate between those hydronephrotic kidneys whose function is destined to deteriorate and those whose function is likely to be maintained and remain stable over time. Unfortunately there is no single 'gold standard' test for obstruction and for this reason, clinical decision-making often has to be guided by a pragmatic interpretation of the results of different diagnostic tests—notably renal ultrasound (Fig. 8.4.1) and technetium 99m mercaptoacetyltriglycine (MAG3) renography. Parameters taken into account include morphology of the kidney, severity of hydronephrosis, and whether it is stable or increasing. Functional assessment is based on differential function and the characteristics of the renogram curve, as classified by O'Reilly.[10] Magnetic resonance urography (MRU) is used increasingly as a means of obtaining anatomical and functional information from a single test. However it is relatively expensive and requires the use of sedation or general anaesthesia in children.[11] Although the interpretation of results is relatively straightforward in symptomatic children, this is more difficult in asymptomatic children—particularly infants with prenatally detected hydronephrosis.

The intravenous urogram is obsolete and the antegrade pressure-flow test devised by Whitaker is rarely used nowadays. However there is still a limited role for retrograde/antegrade contrast studies to delineate unusual anatomy or prior to 're do' pyeloplasty.

Management of prenatally detected PUJO

In cases of unilateral hydronephrosis the initial postnatal ultrasound scan can be deferred until 7–10 days of life. Indeed, scanning in the first 24–48 hours may underestimate the true severity of dilatation since urinary output is reduced in the early newborn period. However, an early postnatal scan is indicated for hydronephrosis affecting a solitary kidney or significant bilateral hydronephrosis. Evaluation of such cases should also include a micturating cystourethrogram (MCUG). By contrast, the MCUG can usually be omitted in cases with unilateral hydronephrosis since any coexisting vesicoureteric reflux (VUR) is likely to be low grade and self limiting. Diuretic renography is performed at 4–12 weeks of age depending of the severity of dilatation. A decision must then be taken on whether to proceed to early pyeloplasty or to adopt a conservative approach comprising regular ultrasound scans and MAG3 renography. Initially, conservative management is generally appropriate if the renal anterior-posterior (AP) pelvic diameter in the transverse plane is <30 mm and differential function 40% or greater. Of those infants who fulfil the criteria for conservative management the majority will experience resolution of their hydronephrosis over time. Twenty-five per cent (25%) of conservatively managed infants will, however, come to pyeloplasty—although very few of these experience irreversible loss of function.[12–15] A conservative approach can also be adopted for prenatally detected bilateral hydronephrosis providing that careful follow-up is maintained and strict indications for surgical intervention are observed.[16]

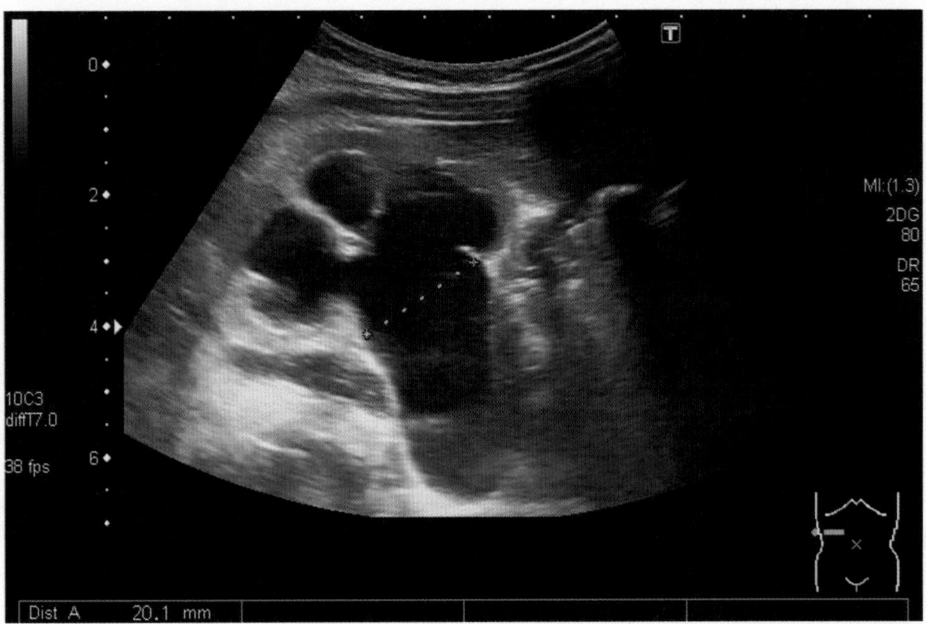

Fig. 8.4.1 Renal ultrasound of a four-month old infant with prenatally detected right hydronephrosis showing dilatation with an anterioposterior (AP) pelvic diameter of 20 mm and cortical thinning. The MAG3 renogram (not shown) revealed an obstructed curve with 20% differential function. This infant proceeded to pyeloplasty.

Surgical management of pelviureteric junction obstruction

Acute presentation with infection within the obstructed system (pyonephrosis) requires treatment with broad spectrum intravenous antibiotics and prompt percutaneous nephrostomy drainage under general anaesthesia. A subsequent antegrade study will confirm the presence of obstruction at the level of the PUJ and a technetium 99m dimercaptosuccinic acid (DMSA) scan after three to four weeks of temporary urinary diversion will then permit an informed decision on whether to proceed to pyeloplasty or nephrectomy (if residual differential function is less than 10–15%).

The majority of cases of PUJO do not present acutely and surgery can therefore be planned on an elective basis. Although a number of surgical options are available, the procedure of choice is almost invariably a dismembered pyeloplasty performed by either an open or laparoscopic approach.

Endourological procedures

Balloon dilatation or endopyelotomy can be performed by the antegrade or retrograde route. Success rates of between 65–100% have been reported in the 4–17 year age group.[17–19] But since the majority of children with PUJO undergo surgery in first year or two of life, even centres with sufficient expertise rarely perform these procedures because of technical limitations related to patient size. However, published results for secondary endopyelotomy after failed pyeloplasty of 94% success rate at 61 months' follow-up suggests this approach may be a reasonable alternative to re-do pyeloplasty.[19]

Open surgery

The 'gold standard' operation is still the Anderson and Hynes pyeloplasty[20] which can be performed via an open anterior, loin, or posterior lumbotomy approach. The duration of hospital admission has been dramatically reduced in recent years, with one centre reporting its experience of one day hospitalisation[21] and another reporting a median hospital stay of 11.5 hours for pyeloplasty performed though a small flank incision.[22] A minimally invasive open pyeloplasty using short incisions in children under one year of age has been described—with all patients being discharged from hospital in less than 23 hours.[23]

Laparoscopic pyeloplasty

Increasing experience with conventional and robotic-assisted laparoscopic pyeloplasty has confirmed the safety and efficacy of this procedure in children.[24–26] Laparoscopic pyeloplasty can be performed via a retroperitoneal or transperitoneal approach. The advantages claimed for laparoscopic pyeloplasty include shorter hospital stay, reduced analgesic requirement, and improved cosmesis.[27] However, operating times are longer and the benefits claimed by the proponents of laparoscopic pyeloplasty have yet to be adequately evaluated by randomized controlled trails.[28,29]

Laparoscopic transposition lower pole vessels

This technique is used in cases where the obstruction is thought to be caused by extrinsic vascular compression of the PUJ by lower polar crossing vessels (rather than intrinsic pathology of the PUJ). The renal vessels are mobilized, transposed superiorly, and fixed ('pexed') at a short distance from the PUJ by creating a sutured 'hammock' of anterior pelvis.[30,31] When used selectively the short term results appear encouraging.

Protection of the anastomosis/drainage

There is no consensus on the use of indwelling JJ stents to provide postoperative internal drainage across the anastomosis. A one-year multicentre audit of 220 pyeloplasties under the auspices of The British Association of Paediatric Urologists did not identify any difference in complications and outcomes between stented and unstented groups (K. Hutton, unpublished data). Unlike indwelling

JJ stents, nephrostent devices drain externally, and do not require cystoscopic removal under general anaesthesia.

Complications of surgery

The major complications are prolonged postoperative urinary leakage and persistent or recurrent obstruction. Less serious complications include haematoma, wound infection, UTI, and stent-related problems. Providing a wound drain has been placed in the perirenal space at the time of surgery, any urinary leakage usually settles within a few days. If leakage is significant and a non-stented anastomosis was performed consideration should be given to the endoscopic placement of a JJ stent. Leakage, if properly managed, does not appear to affect success rates of surgery.[32] Early post operative obstruction is rare and is managed with either a JJ stent or nephrostomy.

Results of surgery and long-term follow-up

The success rate of pyeloplasty is in excess of 95%, which is maintained thereafter, with a late recurrence risk of 1–2% after 5–10 years.[33] Re-do pyeloplasty or ureterocalycostomy for failed pyeloplasty have a similarly high success rate.

Vesicoureteric junction obstruction

Vesicoureteric junction obstruction (VUJO) is invariably associated with the ultrasound finding of megaureter (Fig. 8.4.2.). However, it is important to note that VUJO is only one cause of ureteric dilatation, the others being gross VUR ('refluxing' megaureter), non-obstructive dilatation, and a combination of reflux and obstruction—as described in King's classification of megaureter.[34] Primary VUJO is usually associated with the presence of an adynamic segment of distal ureter leading to inefficient urine transport. Anatomical narrowing (stenosis) of a distal ureteric segment is less common. Secondary obstruction can occur in cases of neuropathic bladder and bladder outflow obstruction.

Aetiology

A number of histological abnormalities have been identified in the distal portion of obstructed megaureters notably; increased collagen deposition, hypertrophy of circular muscle fibres and an additional circumferential layer of intramural smooth muscle.[35] Other reported abnormalities include increased myocyte apoptosis in the obstructed ureteric segment[36] and absent or reduced numbers of interstitial cells of Cajal.[37]

Clinical presentation

Most cases of primary nonrefluxing megaureter are now detected prenatally and affected infants are usually asymptomatic. Primary obstructive megaureter is more common in males, is more frequent on the left side and is bilateral in 25% of cases.[38] The features of clinical presentation are variable and include: urinary tract infection, haematuria, abdominal pain, urolithiasis, failure to thrive, and abdominal mass. VUJO may sometimes occur intermittently.[39]

Investigation

Ultrasound cannot reliably distinguish between obstruction and reflux and for this reason investigation of a megaureter should always include an MCUG. When VUR has been excluded, further investigation consists of a MAG3 renogram to evaluate function and drainage.

Bilateral dilatation of ureters and renal collecting systems (hydroureteronephrosis) demands urgent investigation by ultrasound and MCUG to exclude bladder outlet obstruction or high grade VUR. The administration of frusemide during the MAG3 is essential because drainage curves can be difficult to assess in the presence of marked ureteric dilatation. Imaging with the child in an upright position and obtaining post micturition views permits more reliable interpretation of the drainage curve. Contrast studies may be required where a coexisting PUJO and VUJO are suspected. Retrograde ureteric catheterization can be technically difficult in

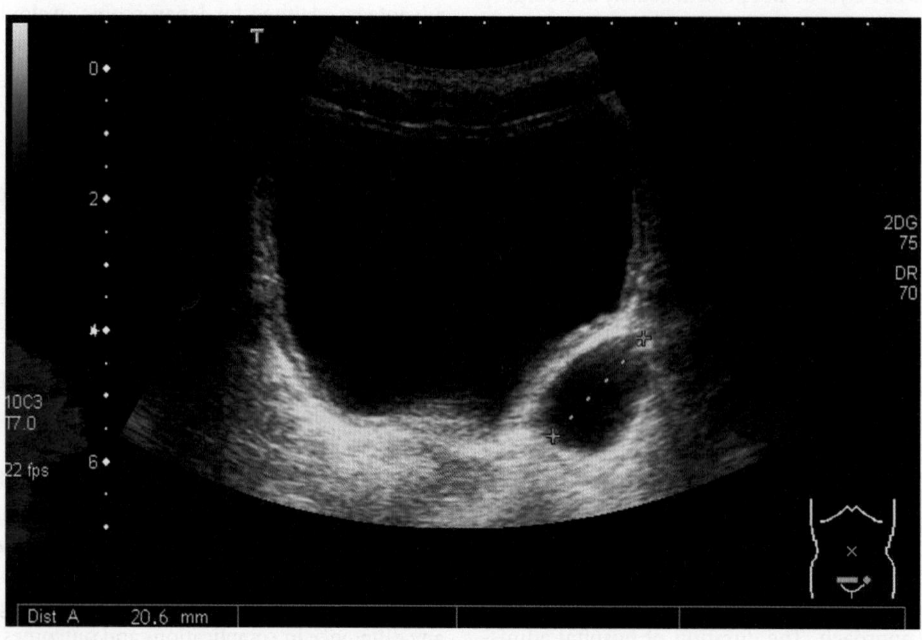

Fig. 8.4.2 Postnatal ultrasound showing hydroureter behind the bladder in a case of prenatally detected vesicoureteric junction obstruction (VUJO).

cases of VUJO and percutaneous renal puncture and antegrade pyelography may therefore be needed to accurately define the level of obstruction. Although not widely used at present, a MRU provides both anatomical and functional assessment in a single study.[40]

Management of prenatally detected vesicoureteric junction obstruction

The outcome of conservative management and the natural history of VUJO have been reported from a number of centres. For example, Liu *et al.* reported on 67 megaureters in 53 newborns with a median follow-up of 3.1 years. Dilatation resolved spontaneously in 23 megaureters (34%) but persisted in 33 (49%). Surgery was performed on 11 megaureters (17%) for breakthrough infection or deteriorating function.[41] Spontaneous resolution proceeds more slowly and is less likely to resolve completely when the anterior-posterior diameter of the dilated ureter exceeds 1 cm. The rate of surgical intervention is also higher.[42] Although congenital obstructed megaureter generally behaves as a benign condition,[43,44] the natural history is not entirely predictable and the occurrence of increasing dilatation and/or deteriorating function is well documented. Although rare, stone formation is another late complication. For these reasons it is probably prudent to maintain regular ultrasound surveillance until the individual reaches maturity—at least in those cases with persisting hydroureteronephrosis.[45] Most paediatric urologists prescribe prophylactic antibiotics in the first year or two of life but in the absence of any randomized controlled trials it is unclear whether prophylaxis is effective—and, if so, its optimal duration.

Surgical management

The principal indications comprise: reduced function (differential function <40%) on initial evaluation; deteriorating function on follow-up; increasing hydroureteronephrosis; and the development of symptoms such as pain or UTI. The decision to operate in clinically presenting cases is usually straightforward. Children presenting with minor UTI can be managed by antibiotic prophylaxis pending spontaneous resolution of the megaureter but surgery is indicated in cases of primary megaureter complicated by more severe or recurrent UTIs.

Temporary JJ stent insertion

The use of JJ stents as a temporizing manoeuvre in neonates and infants with VUJO has gained popularity since it was first described by Shenoy and Rance in 1999.[46] This approach avoids the difficulty of reimplanting a grossly dilated ureter into a small infant bladder and provides time for possible spontaneous resolution of obstruction. Complications include stent migration, stone formation and urinary infection (in 32–70% of patients). Endoscopic insertion is often not feasible in small infants and open transvesical stent placement is therefore required in 50–68% of cases. Although initially described as a temporizing manoeuvre it has been reported that a period of indwelling stent drainage may constitute definitive treatment in approximately 50% of cases, thus avoiding the need for open surgery following stent removal.[47,48] However, JJ stent drainage is not guaranteed to prevent further functional deterioration and one study reported a 13% nephrectomy rate despite JJ stenting.[48]

Other endourological procedures

Although rarely used, endoureterotomy combined with JJ stenting has been described, with a reported success rate of 90%.[49] High pressure balloon dilation and temporary JJ stenting has also been described as an alternative to open surgery, with a success rate of 77–100%.[50–52]

Temporary internal or external diversion in children under one year of age

Many surgeons prefer to avoid performing definitive surgery for megaureters in the first 6–12 months of life because of technical difficulties and anecdotal evidence of a subsequent risk of iatrogenic neuropathic bladder/sphincter dysfunction. Previously, a loop or end ureterostomy was employed as a temporary diversion to decompress the obstructed system pending reconstruction at a later date. More recently, a novel method of internal diversion has been described using a refluxing ureteral reimplant, with a proximal end to side anastomosis between the dilated ureter and bladder. This promising approach is preferable to an exteriorized ureterostomy and represents a reasonable alternative to temporary JJ stenting.[53,54]

Open surgery

The standard open surgical approach consists of excising the vesicoureteric junction and reimplanting the megaureter using either a Cohen cross-trigonal tunnel or, alternatively a Politano-Leadbetter reimplantation combined with psoas hitch. A grossly dilated ureter can be remodelled using an excisional tapering,[55] ureteric folding,[56] or imbrication[57] technique prior to reimplantation. More recently, an extravesical approach has been successfully employed for treating megaureters.[58]

Laparoscopic surgery

Although the feasibility of laparoscopic and robotic-assisted procedures has been documented, medium and long-term results are awaited.[59,60]

Complications of surgery

The major complications are; persisting obstruction or iatrogenic VUR due to a failure to create an adequate anti reflux mechanism at the time of reimplantation. Some degree of residual upper tract dilatation is not unusual but significantly impaired drainage requires careful re-evaluation and possible further intervention. Postoperative VUR often improves spontaneously or can be managed by endoscopic injection.

Results of surgery and long-term follow-up

Surgical correction of VUJO is highly effective with a success rate of 90–94%.[61–63] A successful surgical outcome almost invariably results in stabilization of renal function.[62]

Renal duplication anomalies

Post-mortem data put the incidence of duplication anomalies in the general population at 0.8%.[64] There is no predominant laterality but the anomaly is found bilaterally in 20–40% of cases. Girls are affected twice as frequently as boys and a there is strong genetic predisposition, with an 8% incidence in siblings of index cases. The mode of inheritance is believed to be autosomal dominant transmission with incomplete penetrance.[65,66]

Classification

The majority of duplication anomalies are 'incomplete' and consist of either a bifid pelvis or bifid ureters. Affected individuals are often asymptomatic. Duplication is defined as 'complete' when both ureters remain separate throughout their course and drain into the bladder via two distinct orifices. The Weigert-Meyer rule describes the usual anatomical pattern whereby the upper pole orifice lies in a more medial and caudal position than the lower pole orifice. This is a consequence of repositioning of the ureters during incorporation of the mesonephric duct into the trigone in early embryological development.

Additional abnormalities can affect either upper or lower pole ureters. In the case of the upper pole these are related to ureteric ectopia or a duplex system ureterocele. An intravesical ureterocele is located entirely within the bladder whereas all or part of an ectopic ureterocele is sited at the bladder neck or within the urethra.[67] Ureteroceles can be further classified as stenotic, sphincteric, sphincterostenotic, cecoureteroceles, blind, and non-obstructive.[68] They can also be defined by reference to the number of renal units in jeopardy.[69] The commonest associated abnormality of the lower pole is VUR.

Presentation

Duplex kidneys are being increasingly identified prenatally and it is usually possible to make a reasonably accurate anatomical diagnosis from the ultrasound findings.[70] Ultrasonographic features commonly comprise two separate renal pelvises and/or dilatation of a single moiety with a dilated ipsilateral ureter or ureterocele.[71] Affected newborns are mostly asymptomatic and their initial management consists of an ultrasound at three to seven days of life and commencement of a prophylactic antibiotic. More urgent imaging is indicated when antenatal ultrasonography has demonstrated bilateral upper tract dilatation associated with an ureterocele since this finding is suggestive of bladder outflow obstruction. In most cases, however, further imaging (MCUG and isotope renography) can be deferred until 6–12 weeks of age. When not detected prenatally, duplication anomalies present clinically with; severe systemic illness associated with septicaemia, acute or chronic retention, epididymo-orchitis, and in a girl a discoloured introital mass representing a prolapsed ureterocele, or dribbling incontinence. The latter is associated with an ectopic ureter and is almost exclusively restricted to girls.[72] MRU is a valuable means of demonstrating a cryptic duplex system and ectopic ureter causing incontinence (Fig. 8.4.3).

Vesicoureteric reflux

Urinary tract infection in association with children with duplication anomalies is most commonly linked to VUR.[73] This usually affects the lower pole moeity but both moeities are occasionally involved and ectopic ureters which drain into the urethra or bladder neck are also prone to reflux during voiding. Ultrasound typically shows a dysplastic or scarred lower moiety with a dilated lower pole collecting system and ureter. DMSA is used to assess parenchymal defects and estimate the differential function in the upper and lower poles of the affected kidney.

Conservative management of low grade (1 and 2) VUR is successful with resolution rates comparable for those in single system

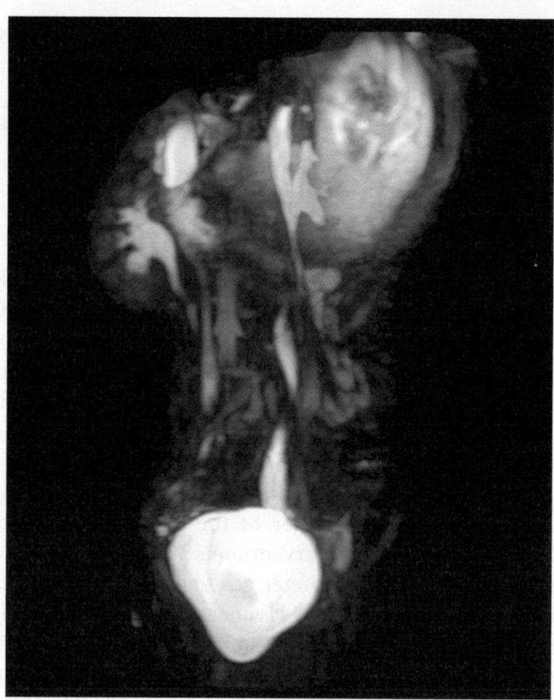

Fig. 8.4.3 Magnetic resonance urography (MRU) in a girl with dribbling incontinence. This demonstrates bilateral duplication. Interestingly, two ureteric orifices were seen on both sides of the bladder on cystoscopy. Retrograde studies showed an uncomplicated complete duplication on the right. On the left side, the medial and more caudal orifice was associated with a normal lower pole moiety, while the lateral and more cranial orifice was associated with a markedly dilated tubular structure accompanying the lower pole ureter but ending blindly in the iliac fossa. A left ureteric triplication with upper pole ectopic ureter was diagnosed. Left upper pole heminephrectomy was performed and her wetting ceased.

VUR. High grade VUR is more likely to require intervention due to breakthrough infections or new renal scarring.[74] Minimally invasive endoscopic correction has a reported success rate of 63–85% in treating VUR in duplex systems[75,76] while open surgery (either by intravesical reimplantation of both ureters within their common sheath[77] or an extravesical technique[78,79]) has a success rate of 98%. A relatively simple, effective but underused alternative consists of performing a low ureteroureterostomy between the refluxing ureter and non-refluxing upper pole ureter.[80,81] If the relevant expertise is available the procedure can be performed laparoscopically.[82] When function in the lower pole is poor (<10%) heminephroureterectomy is usually indicated,via an open or laparoscopic approach.

Ureteroceles

Non-operative management is possible in selected patients who do not have bladder outflow obstruction.[83–86] Endoscopic puncture can be performed to decompress and drain an acutely infected system or as a definitive treatment for intravesical ureteroceles.[87–90] However, endoscopic puncture is less suited to ectopic ureteroceles because of a significant failure rate and subsequent requirement for more extensive intervention (e.g. because of recurrent urinary infections). More definitive surgical management may include: ureterocele excision and reimplantation of upper and lower pole ureters; ipsilateral ureteroureterostomy or extensive reconstruction involving the ipsilateral upper and lower tracts. In cases without lower pole VUR, upper pole heminephrectomy is often curative.[91–93] Conversely, it may occasionally be reasonable to consider limiting surgery to correction of lower pole VUR while leaving a poorly functioning upper pole moiety *in situ*.[94]

Small, single system (orthotopic) ureteroceles may not require any form of intervention if they are not giving rise to obstruction. When accompanied by upper tract dilatation and evidence of obstruction on dynamic renography, treatment of an orthotopic, single system ureterocele is generally advisable in view of the risks of infection and stone formation. Endoscopic deroofing is preferable to simple puncture but definitive treatment consists of excision of the ureterocele combined with ureteric reimplantation.

Ectopic ureter in duplex kidneys

On prenatal ultrasonography ectopic ureters may be apparent as dilatation of the upper pole moeity and absence of a demonstrable ureterocele in the bladder. Ectopic ureters which enter the lower urinary tract above the sphincter mechanism (suprasphincteric) usually present with UTI whereas infrasphincteric ectopic ureters typically present in girls with dribbling incontinence superimposed on a background of normal voiding. Upper pole function is usually grossly impaired and treatment therefore consists of upper pole heminephrouretectomy. In the rare cases with salvageable upper pole function, ureteric reimplantation, or ipsilateral ureteroureterostomy may be considered. Upper to lower pole ureteroureterostomy has been described as a means of avoiding ablative upper pole surgery while also minimizing the risk of damage to the remaining moeity and reducing visible scarring. Although this necessarily entails leaving poorly functioning upper pole renal tissue *in situ*, reported results have been encouraging.[95,96]

Multicystic dysplastic kidney

Multicystic dysplastic kidney (MCDK) is the most common cystic kidney disorder of childhood. The kidney is replaced by tense non-communicating cysts of variable size with an absence of parenchymal tissue. The anomaly is usually associated with proximal ureteric atresia. MCDKs are non-functioning and when they occur bilaterally are invariably lethal.

Aetiology and embryology

MCDKs are thought to represent the outcome of an insult to the embryonic kidney caused by complete ureteric obstruction or, alternatively, defective interaction between the ureteric bud and metanephric mesenchyme. At a molecular level altered expression of specific genes has been documented.[97–99] Some cases of MCDK have been linked to prenatal exposure to antiepileptic drugs such as sodium valporate, carbamazepine, and phenobarbital.[100,101]

Incidence

The reported incidence varies between 1 in 3,000—1 in 5,000,[102] with one population-based study citing a figure of 1 in 4,300. Most cases are sporadic but familial occurrence with autosomal dominant inheritance with variable expressivity and reduced penetrance has been reported.[103]

Presentation

Unilateral MCDKs are more prevalent in boys (59%) and the left side is more commonly affected than the right.[102] The overwhelming majority of MCDKs are detected prenatally. Affected infants are usually entirely asymptomatic and the majority of prenatally detected MCDKs are impalpable on examination. Prior to the introduction of routine antenatal ultrasound screening MCDK was regarded as a rare anomaly which presented as an abdominal mass in the newborn. Although there are historic case reports of MCDK presenting with pain, haematuria, UTI, or hypertension in later life the accuracy of the diagnosis of MCDK in these cases is doubtful. A large palpable MCDK in a newborn infant can cause respiratory compromise, vomiting, or failure to thrive due to the mass effect of the lesion. In these cases early nephrectomy is advisable—although temporary management with ultrasound guided cyst aspiration has been described in sick, premature neonates.[104] Segmental MCDK is rare and usually affects the upper pole of a duplex kidney.[105] Some cases of unilateral renal agenesis diagnosed in adult life may represent the outcome of spontaneous involution of a MCDK.[106]

Associated anomalies

Coexisting renal tract anomalies are common, with a 20% incidence of VUR and 5% incidence of PUJO in the contralateral kidney. Other associated anomalies include; ureteroceles (1.3%), horseshoe kidney (0.6%) and posterior urethral valves (0.4%).[102] Progressive infundibular stenosis of the contralateral kidney has been reported.[107] Ipsilateral genital tract abnormalities are present in up to 15% of patients, including seminal vesical cyst in boys and Gartner duct cyst, blind ending hemivagina,[108] and cystic accessory uterine cavity in girls.[109]

Investigation

The typical ultrasound appearances of a MCDK are characterized by loss of normal renal outline, cysts of variable size, a lack of central renal sinus echo, and absence of renal parenchyma (Fig. 8.4.4).[110] DMSA imaging shows complete absence of function. Opinion is divided on the need for a routine MCUG to detect coexisting VUR but if the contralateral kidney appears normal on ultrasound any VUR is likely to be low grade and destined to resolve spontaneously. Several studies have confirmed the safety of omitting a routine MCUG in these circumstances.[111–113] More recently MRU has been recommended for evaluation of the contralateral kidney[114] but costs and risks have been questioned particularly when general anaesthesia is required.[115]

Potential risks and complications

Several large, systematic reviews have documented that MCDKs are associated with a very low risk of hypertension and malignant change.[116,117] A North American MCDK Registry documented minimal hypertension in 4 out of 441 children—which, in all cases was believed to be unrelated to the MCDK.[118] Hypertension is more likely to be due to pathology in the contralateral kidney than the MCDK itself. Using extrapolated data Beckwith calculated an incidence of 1 in 2,000 for Wilms tumour in MCDK.[119] More recent data suggest that the risk is even lower. Most patients with a MCDK exhibit a benign clinical course with spontaneous involution in the majority of cases. Complete involution occurs in 62% of MCDKs by 10 years of age, although those larger than 5 cm at birth are statistically less likely to regress.[120]

Controversies in management

There is no universal agreement on the management of MCDKs. A non-operative approach has been adopted by most paediatric

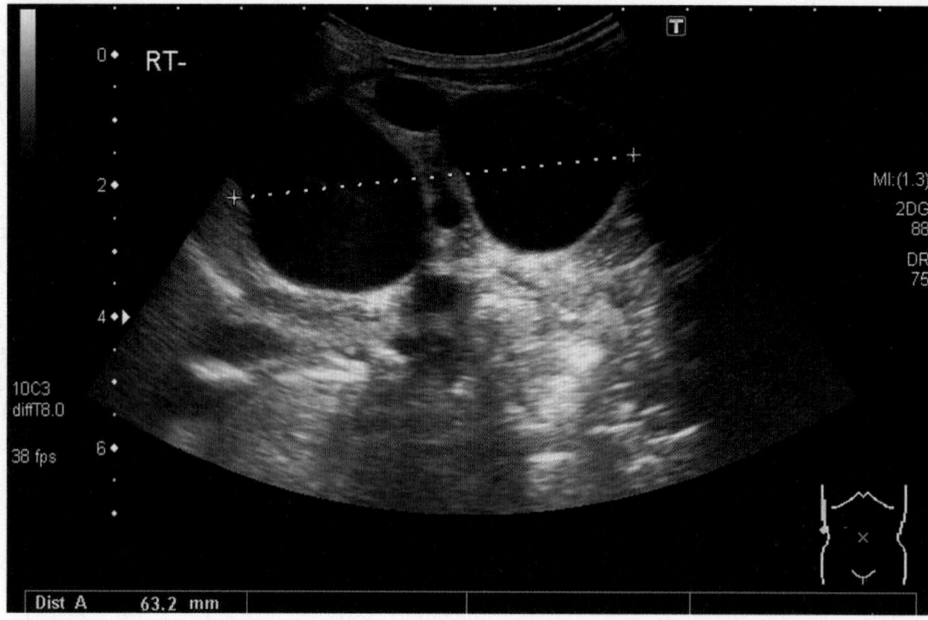

Fig. 8.4.4 Renal ultrasound of a MCDK showing cysts of varying size.

urologists because of the low risk of complications and knowledge that the majority of MCDKs involute spontaneously.[103,113,121,122] Nevertheless, some paediatric urologists continue to favour elective 'prophylactic' nephrectomy because of perceived risks of hypertension and malignant change.[123,124] However, it has been estimated that it would be necessary to remove 20,000 MCDKs in order to prevent one child dying from Wilms tumour.[118] The weight of published evidence indicates that the risk of hypertension associated with a genuine MCDK is very low—probably in the range 0.5% or less. The benefits of regular follow-up ultrasound has been questioned.[115] Onal and Kogan have suggested that children with MCDKs can be safely discharged from urological follow-up, with their primary care provider being responsible for further monitoring.[122]

Indications for surgery

Surgery should be reserved for symptomatic patients, cases of diagnostic difficulty and (very rarely) where the MCDK increases in size. Nephrectomy can be performed via an open or laparoscopic approach with minimal morbidity.[125,126]

Other cystic renal diseases in childhood

Bilateral cystic disease is almost invariably inherited in aetiology. The most common forms are autosomal recessive polycystic kidney disease (ARPKD), autosomal dominant polycystic disease (ADPKD), tuberous sclerosis complex (TSC1 and TSC2), and von Hipple-Lindau disease.[127]

ARPKD is due to a mutation of the *PKHD1* gene located on chromosome 6p21 and presents with bilateral renal enlargement and liver involvement with hepatic fibrosis. The diagnosis is often suspected prenatally and clinical features in the neonatal period include respiratory compromise due to pulmonary hypoplasia or size of the kidneys, hypertension, and renal insufficiency. Atypical presentation in later childhood is with hypertension or features of liver failure including portal hypertension and bleeding oesophageal varices. ADPKD is a more common, slowly progressive condition associated with two genetic defects—PKD1 on chromosome 16p13.3 and PKD2 on chromosome 4q21–23. Most children are asymptomatic and remain undiagnosed until adulthood. When ADPKD is detected prenatally or in the newborn period it carries a very poor prognosis.

Multilocular renal cysts are benign lesions that present with pain, haematuria, or an abdominal mass. Management is by nephrectomy or, when feasible, partial nephrectomy.[128] Simple renal cysts are rare in children and managed conservatively unless symptomatic. When indicated (usually because of pain) treatment consists of either aspiration or injection with ethanol or, alternatively laparoscopic de-roofing depending on the size and site of the cyst. Acquired cystic kidney disease is encountered in patients receiving renal replacement therapy.[129]

Horseshoe kidney and other anomalies of migration/fusion

Horseshoe kidney

Horseshoe kidney is the most common fusion anomaly, occurring in 1 in 400 to 1 in 1,800 individuals. It is twice as common in males. In 95% of cases, fusion involves the lower poles. Horseshoe kidney is associated with trisomy 18 (Edwards syndrome), Turner syndrome,[130] tuberous sclerosis complex,[131] and thrombocytopenia, absent radii (TAR) syndrome.[132] The most frequent associated urological anomaly is VUR (usually low grade) which is present in up to 80% of cases. Other associated conditions include: PUJO, renal calculi, unilateral multicystic dysplasia.[133] partial and complete ureteral duplication,[134,135] ureteric triplication.[136] supernumerary kidney,[137] pyelic fusion with single ureter,[138] and ectopic ureter in association with horseshoe kidney.[139] The risk of Wilms' tumour is slightly increased.[140–144] Most horseshoe kidneys are asymptomatic and the requirement for urological intervention centres on PUJO or stone disease. PUJO can be managed with conventional open surgery or with laparoscopic techniques.[145,146] Ureterocalicostomy can play a useful role—for both primary and re-do cases. Stones are

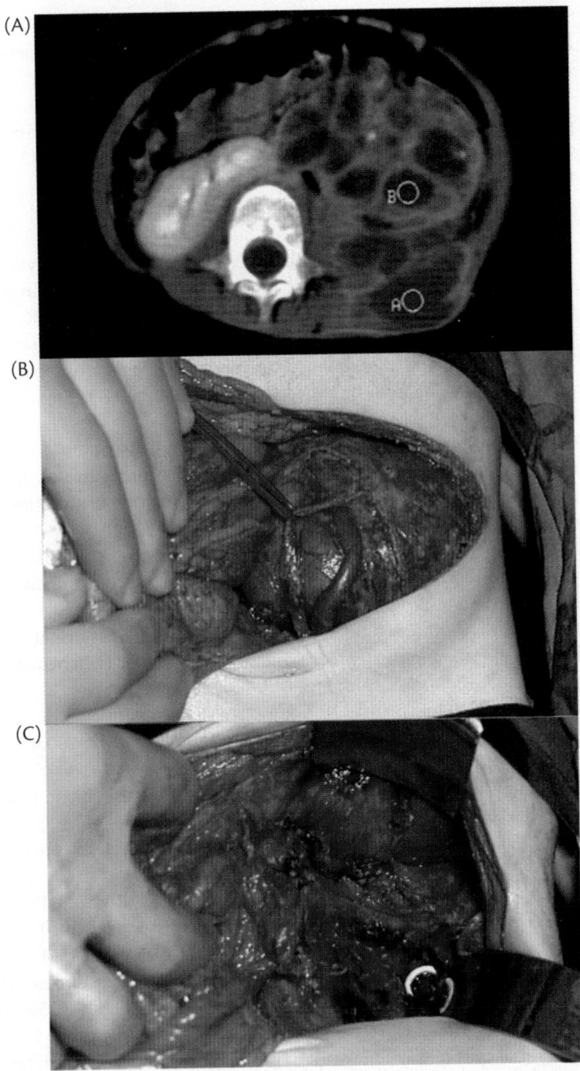

Fig. 8.4.5 (A) Computed tomography scan of a patient with a left paranephric abscess and xanthogranulomatous pyelonephritis within a horseshoe kidney. (B) Operative view of the large left renal mass. (C) Renal bed following resection of left half of the horseshoe kidney. Note the white pigtail drain that had been inserted into the paranephric abscess preoperatively.

often amenable to external shock wave lithotripsy or percutaneous nephrolithotomy.[147,148] Complicated pathology, for example xanthogranulomatous pyelonephritis in one-half of a horseshoe kidney, is probably best treated by an open surgical approach (Fig. 8.4.5).

Simple renal ectopia

Abnormal ascent of the kidney during early development most commonly results in a pelvic kidney. Rarer forms of ectopia include iliac and thoracic kidneys. The left side is affected more commonly[149] and there is an increased risk of urological abnormalities including VUR, simple ectopia, contralateral renal dysplasia, cryptorchidism, and hypospadias.[150] Coexisting defects in other systems may include; cardiac anomalies, scoliosis, hemivertibrae, and female genital tract anomalies (bicornuate, unicornuate, absent uterus, duplicate vagina, rudimentary vagina).[151] Ectopic kidney also features in the Mayer-Rokitansky-Küster-Hauser complex[152] and intrathoracic kidney has been described in association with congenital diaphragmatic hernia.[153] Eighty per cent (80%) of affected individuals are asymptomatic and the anomaly is identified either on routine antenatal ultrasound or as an incidental finding during ultrasound scanning in childhood.[150] Although differential function in ectopic kidneys is reduced (average 38%) this does not appear to affect overall function or blood pressure long term.[154]

Crossed renal ectopia

The different anatomical patterns of this condition include; cross-fused ectopia, cross-unfused ectopia, or (very rarely) solitary crossed ectopia or bilateral crossed ectopia. It is three times more common for the left kidney to cross to the right side than vice versa. The incidence is approximately 1in 7,000, with a male predominance. Occasional familial inheritance has been reported.[155] The majority of individuals are asymptomatic and the anomaly is either detected prenatally[150] or, postnatally as an incidental ultrasound finding. Occasionally it comes to light as an incidental clinical finding when the lower pole of the fused kidney is palpated during the course of abdominal examination. Associated VUR occurs in 20–40% of patients.[150,156] Although there is some evidence of functional impairment in 93% of crossed fused ectopic kidneys[156] longitudinal analysis has generally shown stable glomerular filtration rate and blood pressure through childhood.[154] Intervention is only required for cases complicated by obstruction, problematic VUR, or stone disease.

Conclusions

Upper tract abnormalities constitute a large part of paediatric urological practice. Whereas these conditions previously presented clinically many are now detected prenatally and the majority of affected infants are healthy and asymptomatic. The importance of protecting upper tract function must be balanced against the need to avoid submitting large numbers of asymptomatic children to unnecessary surgery. Long-term data are now emerging which will enable urologists to distinguish more reliably between those children who are likely to benefit from early surgery from those who can safely be managed conservatively.

Further reading

Aslam M, Watson AR; Trent & Anglia MCDK Study Group. Unilateral multicystic dysplastic kidney: long term outcomes. *Arch Dis Child* 2006; **91**:820–3.

Cuckow P. Management of ureteric duplication in childhood. *Eur Urol* 1998; 7:20–7.

Dhillon HK. Prenatally diagnosed hydronephrosis: the Great Ormond Street experience. *Br J Urol* 1998; **81**(Suppl 2):39–44.

Gearhart JP, Rink RC, Mouriquand PDE (eds). *Pediatric Urology*, 2nd edition. Philadelphia, PA: Saunders Elsevier, 2010.

Godbole P, Gearhart J, Wilcox D (eds). *Clinical Problems in Pediatric Urology*. Chichester, UK: Blackwell Publishing, 2006.

Hutton KAR, Shrestha R. Surgical management of renal tract problems. *Paediatr Child Health* 2008; **18**:259–63.

Pohl HG. Recent advances in the management of ureteroceles in infants and children: why less may be more. *Curr Opin Urol* 2011; **21**:322–7.

Shokeir AA, Nijman RJ. Primary megaureter: current trends in diagnosis and treatment. *BJU Int* 2000; **86**:861–8.

Thomas DFM, Duffy PG, Rickwood AMK (eds). *Essentials of Paediatric Urology*, 2nd edition. London, UK: Healthcare, 2008.

References

1. Hosgor M, Karaca I, Ulukus C, *et al.* Structural changes of smooth muscle in congenital ureteropelvic junction obstruction. *J Pediatr Surg* 2005; **40**:1632–6.
2. Kaya C, Bogaert G, de Ridder D, *et al.* Extracellular matrix degradation and reduced neural density in children with intrinsic ureteropelvic junction obstruction. *Urology* 2010; **76**:185–9.
3. Özel SK, Emir H, Dervişoğlu S, *et al.* The roles of extracellular matrix proteins, apoptosis and c-kit positive cells in the pathogenesis of ureteropelvic junction obstruction. *J Pediatr Urol* 2010; **6**:125–9.
4. Solari V, Piotrowska AP, Puri P. Altered expression of interstitial cells of Cajal in congenital ureteropelvic junction obstruction. *J Urol* 2003; **170**:2420–2.
5. Hutton KAR, Shrestha R. Surgical management of renal tract problems. *Paediatr Child Health* 2008; **18**:259–63.
6. Babu R, Hutton KA. Renal fungal balls and pelvi-ureteric junction obstruction in a very low birth weight infant: treatment with streptokinase. *Pediatr Surg Int* 2004; **20**:804–5.
7. Hollowell JG, Altman HG, Snyder HM 3rd, Duckett JW. Coexisting ureteropelvic junction obstruction and vesicoureteral reflux: diagnostic and therapeutic implications. *J Urol* 1989; **142**:490–3.
8. Thomas DF. Prenatally detected uropathy: epidemiological considerations. *Br J Urol* 1998; **81**(Suppl 2):8–12.
9. Koff SA. Problematic ureteropelvic junction obstruction. *J Urol* 1987; **138**:390.
10. O'Reilly PH, Lawson RS, Shields RA, Testa HJ. Idiopathic hydronephrosis—the diuresis renogram: a new non-invasive method of assessing equivocal pelvioureteral junction obstruction. *J Urol* 1979; **121**:153–5.
11. Kirsch AJ, McMann LP, Jones RA, Smith EA, Scherz HC, Grattan-Smith JD. Magnetic resonance urography for evaluating outcomes after pediatric pyeloplasty. *J Urol* 2006; **176**:1755–61.
12. Ransley PG, Dhillon HK, Gordon I, Duffy PG, Dillon MJ, Barratt TM. The postnatal management of hydronephrosis diagnosed by prenatal ultrasound. *J Urol* 1990; **144**:584–7.
13. Arnold AJ, Rickwood AM. Natural history of pelviureteric obstruction detected by prenatal sonography. *Br J Urol* 1990; **65**:91–6.
14. Madden NP, Thomas DF, Gordon AC, Arthur RJ, Irving HC, Smith SE. Antenatally detected pelviureteric junction obstruction. Is non-operation safe? *Br J Urol* 1991; **68**:305–10.
15. Dhillon HK. Prenatally diagnosed hydronephrosis: the Great Ormond Street experience. *Br J Urol* 1998; **81**(Suppl 2):39–44.
16. Onen A, Jayanthi VR, Koff SA. Long-term followup of prenatally detected severe bilateral newborn hydronephrosis initially managed nonoperatively. *J Urol* 2002; **168**:1118–20.
17. Doraiswamy NV. Retrograde ureteroplasty using balloon dilatation in children with pelviureteric obstruction. *J Pediatr Surg* 1994; **29**:937–40.
18. Tállai B, Salah MA, Flaskó T, Tóth C, Varga A. Endopyelotomy in childhood: our experience with 37 patients. *J Endourol* 2004; **18**:952–8.
19. Kim EH, Tanagho YS, Traxel EJ, Austin PF, Figenshau RS, Coplen DE. Endopyelotomy for pediatric ureteropelvic junction obstruction: A review of our 25-year experience. *J Urol* 2012; **188**:1628–33.
20. Anderson JC, Hynes W. Retrocaval ureter; a case diagnosed pre-operatively and treated successfully by a plastic operation. *Br J Urol* 1949; **21**:209–14.
21. Piedrahita YK, Palmer JS. Is one-day hospitalization after open pyeloplasty possible and safe? *Urology* 2006; **67**:181–4.
22. Ruiz E, Soria R, Ormaechea E, Lino MM, Moldes JM, de Badiola FI. Simplified open approach to surgical treatment of ureteropelvic junction obstruction in young children and infants. *J Urol* 2011; **185**:2512–6.
23. Chacko JK, Koyle MA, Mingin GC, Furness PD 3rd. The minimally invasive open pyeloplasty. *J Pediatr Urol* 2006; **2**:368–72.
24. Metzelder ML, Schier F, Petersen C, Truss M, Ure BM. Laparoscopic transabdominal pyeloplasty in children is feasible irrespective of age. *J Urol* 2006; **175**:688–91.
25. Lee RS, Retik AB, Borer JG, Peters CA. Pediatric robot assisted laparoscopic dismembered pyeloplasty: comparison with a cohort of open surgery. *J Urol* 2006; **175**:683–7.
26. Blanc T, Muller C, Abdoul H, *et al.* Retroperitoneal laparoscopic pyeloplasty in children: long-term outcome and critical analysis of 10-year experience in a teaching center. *Eur Urol* 2013; **63**(3):565–72.
27. Peters CA. Pediatric robot-assisted pyeloplasty. *J Endourol* 2011; **25**:179–85.
28. Mei H, Pu J, Yang C, Zhang H, Zheng L, Tong Q. Laparoscopic versus open pyeloplasty for ureteropelvic junction obstruction in children: a systematic review and meta-analysis. *J Endourol* 2011; **25**:727–36.
29. Freilich DA, Penna FJ, Nelson CP, Retik AB, Nguyen HT. Parental satisfaction after open versus robot assisted laparoscopic pyeloplasty: results from modified Glasgow Children's Benefit Inventory Survey. *J Urol* 2010; **183**:704–8.
30. Godbole P, Mushtaq I, Wilcox DT, Duffy PG. Laparoscopic transposition of lower pole vessels—the 'vascular hitch': an alternative to dismembered pyeloplasty for pelvi-ureteric junction obstruction in children. *J Pediatr Urol* 2006; **2**:285–9.
31. Singh RR, Govindarajan KK, Chandran H. Laparoscopic vascular relocation: alternative treatment for renovascular hydronephrosis in children. *Pediatr Surg Int* 2010; **26**:717–20.
32. Liss ZJ, Olsen TM, Roelof BA, Steinhardt GF. Duration of urinary leakage after open non-stented dismembered pyeloplasty in pediatric patients. *J Pediatr Urol* 2013; **9**(5):613–6.
33. Psooy K, Pike JG, Leonard MP. Long-term followup of pediatric dismembered pyeloplasty: how long is long enough? *J Urol* 2003; **169**:1809–12.
34. King LR. Megaloureter: definition, diagnosis and management. *J Urol* 1980; **123**:222–3.
35. Joseph DB. Ureterovesical junction anomalies: megaureters. (pp. 272–82
[Chapter 21]) In: Gearhart JP, Rink RC, Mouriquand PDE (eds). *Pediatric Urology*, 2nd edition. Philadelphia, PA: Saunders, 2010.
36. Payabvash S, Kajbafzadeh AM, Tavangar SM, Monajemzadeh M, Sadeghi Z. Myocyte apoptosis in primary obstructive megaureters: the role of decreased vascular and neural supply. *J Urol* 2007; **178**:259–64.
37. Arena E, Nicòtina PA, Arena S, Romeo C, Zuccarello B, Romeo G. Interstitial cells of Cajal network in primary obstructive megaureter. *Pediatr Med Chir* 2007; **29**:28–31.
38. Shokeir AA, Nijman RJ. Primary megaureter: current trends in diagnosis and treatment. *BJU Int* 2000; **86**:861–8.
39. Botelho L, Rincon JA, Nguyen HT, Bauer SB, Rust D, Estrada CR. Intermittent ureterovesical junction obstruction in children. *J Pediatr Urol* 2011; 7:579–81.
40. Jones RA, Grattan-Smith JD, Little S. Pediatric magnetic resonance urography. *J Magn Reson Imaging* 2011; **33**:510–26.
41. Liu HY, Dhillon HK, Yeung CK, Diamond DA, Duffy PG, Ransley PG. Clinical outcome and management of prenatally diagnosed primary megaureters. *J Urol* 1994; **152**:614–7.
42. McLellan DL, Retik AB, Bauer SB, *et al.* Rate and predictors of spontaneous resolution of prenatally diagnosed primary nonrefluxing megaureter. *J Urol* 2002; **168**:2177–80.
43. Arena S, Magno C, Montalto AS, *et al.* Long-term follow-up of neonatally diagnosed primary megaureter: rate and predictors of spontaneous resolution. *Scand J Urol Nephrol* 2012; **46**:201–7.
44. Baskin LS, Zderic SA, Snyder HM, Duckett JW. Primary dilated megaureter: long-term followup. *J Urol* 1994; **152**:618–21.
45. Shukla AR, Cooper J, Patel RP, *et al.* Prenatally detected primary megaureter: a role for extended followup. *J Urol* 2005; **173**:1353–6.
46. Shenoy MU, Rance CH. Is there a place for the insertion of a JJ stent as a temporizing procedure for symptomatic partial congenital vesico-ureteric junction obstruction in infancy? *BJU Int* 1999; **84**:524–5.
47. Castagnetti M, Cimador M, Sergio M, De Grazia E. Double-J stent insertion across vesicoureteral junction—is it a valuable initial approach in neonates and infants with severe primary nonrefluxing megaureter? *Urology* 2006; **68**:870–5.

48. Farrugia MK, Steinbrecher HA, Malone PS. The utilization of stents in the management of primary obstructive megaureters requiring intervention before 1 year of age. *J Pediatr Urol* 2011; **7**:198–202.
49. Kajbafzadeh AM, Payabvash S, Salmasi AH, Arshadi H, Hashemi SM, Arabian S, Najjaran-Tousi V. Endoureterotomy for treatment of primary obstructive megaureter in children. *J Endourol* 2007; **21**:743–9.
50. García-Aparicio L, Rodo J, Krauel L, Palazon P, Martin O, Ribó JM. High pressure balloon dilation of the ureterovesical junction—first line approach to treat primary obstructive megaureter? *J Urol* 2012; **187**:1834–8.
51. Torino G, Collura G, Mele E, Garganese MC, Capozza N. Severe primary obstructive megaureter in the first year of life: preliminary experience with endoscopic balloon dilation. *J Endourol* 2012; **26**:325–9.
52. Christman MS, Kasturi S, Lambert SM, Kovell RC, Casale P. Endoscopic management and the role of double stenting for primary obstructive megaureters. *J Urol* 2012; **187**:1018–22.
53. Lee SD, Akbal C, Kaefer M. Refluxing ureteral reimplant as temporary treatment of obstructive megaureter in neonate and infant. *J Urol* 2005; **173**:1357–60.
54. Kaefer M, Franke E, Rhee A, Rink R, Misser R. The reluxing ureteral reimplant for initial treatment of the obstructed megaureter. Presentation at the European Society for Paediatric Urology, Zurich, Switzerland May 09–12, 2012.
55. Hendren WH. Operative repair of megaureter in children. *J Urol* 1969; **101**:491–507.
56. Kaliciński ZH, Kansy J, Kotarbińska B, Joszt W. Surgery of megaureters—modification of Hendren's operation. *J Pediatr Surg* 1977; **12**:183–8.
57. Starr A. Ureteral plication. A new concept in ureteral tailoring for megaureter. *Invest Urol* 1979; **17**:153–8.
58. McLorie GA, Jayanthi VR, Kinahan TJ, Khoury AE, Churchill BM. A modified extravesical technique for megaureter repair. *Br J Urol* 1994; **74**:715–9.
59. Ansari MS, Mandhani A, Khurana N, Kumar A. Laparoscopic ureteral reimplantation with extracorporeal tailoring for megaureter: a simple technical nuance. *J Urol* 2006; **176**:2640–2.
60. Hemal AK, Nayyar R, Rao R. Robotic repair of primary symptomatic obstructive megaureter with intracorporeal or extracorporeal ureteric tapering and ureteroneocystostomy. *J Endourol* 2009; **23**:2041–6.
61. DeFoor W, Minevich E, Reddy P, *et al.* Results of tapered ureteral reimplantation for primary megaureter: extravesical versus intravesical approach. *J Urol* 2004; **172**:1640–3.
62. Fretz PC, Austin JC, Cooper CS, Hawtrey CE. Long-term outcome analysis of Starr plication for primary obstructive megaureters. *J Urol* 2004; **172**:703–5.
63. Ben-Meir D, McMullin N, Kimber C, Gibikote S, Kongola K, Hutson JM. Reimplantation of obstructive megaureters with and without tailoring. *J Pediatr Urol* 2006; **2**:178–81.
64. Nation EF. Duplication of the kidney and ureter: a statistical study of 230 new cases. *J Urol* 1944; **51**:456–465.
65. Nepple KG, Cooper CS, Snyder HM 3rd. Ureteral duplication, ectopy, and ureteroceles. (pp. 337–52 [Chapter 26]) In: Gearhart JP, Rink RC, Mouriquand PDE (eds). *Pediatric Urology*, 2nd edition. Philadelphia, PA: Saunders, 2010.
66. Rickwood AMK, Madden NP, Boddy SA. Duplication anomalies, ureteroceles and ectopic ureters. (pp. 93–108 [Chapter 7]) In: Thomas DFM, Duffy PG, Rickwood AMK (eds). *Essentials of Paediatric Urology*, 2nd edition. London, UK: Informa Healthcare, 2008.
67. Glassberg KI, Braren V, Duckett JW, *et al.* Suggested terminology for duplex systems, ectopic ureters and ureteroceles. *J Urol* 1984; **132**:1153–4.
68. Stephens D. Caecoureterocele and concepts on the embryology and aetiology of ureteroceles. *Aust N Z J Surg* 1971; **40**:239–48.
69. Churchill BM, Sheldon CA, McLorie GA. The ectopic ureterocele: a proposed practical classification based on renal unit jeopardy. *J Pediatr Surg* 1992; **27**:497–500.
70. Whitten SM, McHoney M, Wilcox DT, New S, Chitty LS. Accuracy of antenatal fetal ultrasound in the diagnosis of duplex kidneys. *Ultrasound Obstet Gynecol* 2003; **21**:342–6.
71. Adiego B, Martinez-Ten P, Perez-Pedregosa J, *et al.* Antenatally diagnosed renal duplex anomalies: sonographic features and long-term postnatal outcome. *J Ultrasound Med* 2011; **30**:809–15.
72. Ejaz T, Malone PS. Male duplex urinary incontinence. *J Urol* 1995; **153**:470–1.
73. Siomou E, Papadopoulou F, Kollios KD, *et al.* Duplex collecting system diagnosed during the first 6 years of life after a first urinary tract infection: a study of 63 children. *J Urol* 2006; **175**:678–81.
74. Afshar K, Papanikolaou F, Malek R, Bagli D, Pippi-Salle JL, Khoury A. Vesicoureteral reflux and complete ureteral duplication. Conservative or surgical management? *J Urol* 2005; **173**:1725–7.
75. Läckgren G, Wåhlin N, Sköldenberg E, Nevéus T, Stenberg A. Endoscopic treatment of vesicoureteral reflux with dextranomer/hyaluronic acid copolymer is effective in either double ureters or a small kidney. *J Urol* 2003; **170**:1551–5.
76. Molitierno JA Jr, Scherz HC, Kirsch AJ. Endoscopic injection of dextranomer hyaluronic acid copolymer for the treatment of vesicoureteral reflux in duplex ureters. *J Pediatr Urol* 2008; **4**:372–6.
77. Ellsworth PI, Lim DJ, Walker RD, Stevens PS, Barraza MA, Mesrobian HG. Common sheath reimplantation yields excellent results in the treatment of vesicoureteral reflux in duplicated collecting systems. *J Urol* 1996; **155**:1407–9.
78. Minevich E, Tackett L, Wacksman J, Sheldon CA. Extravesical common sheath detrusorrhaphy (ureteroneocystotomy) and reflux in duplicated collecting systems. *J Urol* 2002; **167**:288–90.
79. Barrieras D, Lapointe S, Houle H. Is common sheath extravesical reimplantation an effective technique to correct reflux in duplicated collecting systems? *J Urol* 2003; **170**:1545–7.
80. Amar AD. Ipsilateral ureteroureterostomy for single ureteral disease in patients with ureteral duplication: a review of 8 years of experience with 16 patients. *J Urol* 1978; **119**:472–5.
81. Chacko JK, Koyle MA, Mingin GC, Furness PD 3rd. Ipsilateral ureteroureterostomy in the surgical management of the severely dilated ureter in ureteral duplication. *J Urol* 2007; **178**:1689–92.
82. González R, Piaggio L. Initial experience with laparoscopic ipsilateral ureteroureterostomy in infants and children for duplication anomalies of the urinary tract. *J Urol* 2007; **177**:2315–8.
83. Shankar KR, Vishwanath N, Rickwood AM. Outcome of patients with prenatally detected duplex system ureterocele; natural history of those managed expectantly. *J Urol* 2001; **165**:1226–8.
84. Coplen DE, Austin PF. Outcome analysis of prenatally detected ureteroceles associated with multicystic dysplasia. *J Urol* 2004; **172**:1637–9.
85. Han MY, Gibbons MD, Belman AB, Pohl HG, Majd M, Rushton HG. Indications for nonoperative management of ureteroceles. *J Urol* 2005; **174**:1652–5.
86. Direnna T, Leonard MP. Watchful waiting for prenatally detected ureteroceles. *J Urol* 2006; **175**:1493–5.
87. Cooper CS, Passerini-Glazel G, Hutcheson JC, *et al.* Long-term followup of endoscopic incision of ureteroceles: intravesical versus extravesical. *J Urol* 2000; **164**:1097–9.
88. Byun E, Merguerian PA. A meta-analysis of surgical practice patterns in the endoscopic management of ureteroceles. *J Urol* 2006; **176**:1871–7.
89. Di Renzo D, Ellsworth PI, Caldamone AA, Chiesa PL. Transurethral puncture for ureterocele-which factors dictate outcomes? *J Urol* 2010; **184**:1620–4.
90. Merguerian PA, Taenzer A, Knoerlein K, McQuiston L, Herz D. Variation in management of duplex system intravesical ureteroceles: a survey of pediatric urologists. *J Urol* 2010; **184**:1625–30.
91. Husmann DA, Ewalt DH, Glenski WJ, Bernier PA. Ureterocele associated with ureteral duplication and a nonfunctioning upper pole segment: management by partial nephroureterectomy alone. *J Urol* 1995; **154**:723–6.

92. Decter RM, Sprunger JK, Holland RJ. Can a single individualized procedure predictably resolve all the problematic aspects of the pediatric ureterocele? *J Urol* 2001; **165**:2308–10.
93. Gomes J, Mendes M, Castro R, Reis A. Current role of simplified upper tract approach in the surgical treatment of ectopic ureteroceles: a single centre's experience. *Eur Urol* 2002; **41**:323–7.
94. Gran CD, Kropp BP, Cheng EY, Kropp KA. Primary lower urinary tract reconstruction for nonfunctioning renal moieties associated with obstructing ureteroceles. *J Urol* 2005; **173**:198–201.
95. Storm DW, Modi A, Jayanthi VR. Laparoscopic ipsilateral ureteroureterostomy in the management of ureteral ectopia in infants and children. *J Pediatr Urol* 2011; 7:529–33.
96. Prieto J, Ziada A, Baker L, Snodgrass W. Ureteroureterostomy via inguinal incision for ectopic ureters and ureteroceles without ipsilateral lower pole reflux. *J Urol* 2009; **181**:1844–8.
97. Winyard PJ, Risdon RA, Sams VR, Dressler GR, Woolf AS. The PAX2 tanscription factor is expressed in cystic and hyperproliferative dysplastic epithelia in human kidney malformations. *J Clin Invest* 1996; **98**:451–9.
98. Arena S, Fazzari C, Scuderi MG, Implatini A, Villari D, Torre S, Arena F, Di Benedetto V. Molecular events involved in the morphogenesis of multicystic dysplastic kidney. *Urol Int* 2010; **85**:106–11.
99. Guertl B, Senanayake U, Nusshold E, *et al.* Lim1, an embryonal transcription factor, is absent in multicystic renal dysplasia, but reactivated in nephroblastomas. *Pathobiology* 2011;**78**:210–9.
100. Carta M, Cimador M, Giuffrè M, *et al.* Unilateral multicystic dysplastic kidney in infants exposed to antiepileptic drugs during pregnancy. *Pediatr Nephrol* 2007; **22**:1054–7.
101. Ozkan H, Cetinkaya M, Köksal N, Yapici S. Severe fetal valproate syndrome: combination of complex cardiac defect, multicystic dysplastic kidney, and trigonocephaly. *J Matern Fetal Neonatal Med* 2011; **24**:521–4.
102. Schreuder MF, Westland R, van Wijk JA. Unilateral multicystic dysplastic kidney: a meta-analysis of observational studies on the incidence, associated urinary tract malformations and the contralateral kidney. *Nephrol Dial Transplant* 2009; **24**:1810–8.
103. Belk RA, Thomas DF, Mueller RF, Godbole P, Markham AF, Weston MJ. A family study and the natural history of prenatally detected unilateral multicystic dysplastic kidney. *J Urol* 2002; **167**:666–9.
104. Triest JA, Bukowski TP. Multicystic dysplastic kidney as cause of gastric outlet obstruction and respiratory compromise. *J Urol* 1999; **161**:1918–9.
105. Lin CC, Tsai JD, Sheu JC, Lu HJ, Chang BP. Segmental multicystic dysplastic kidney in children: clinical presentation, imaging finding, management, and outcome. *J Pediatr Surg* 2010; **45**:1856–62.
106. Hitchcock R, Burge DM. Renal agenesis: an acquired condition? *J Pediatr Surg* 1994; **29**:454–5.
107. Dally EA, Raman A, Webb NR, Farnsworth RH. Unilateral multicystic dysplastic kidney with progressive infundibular stenosis in the contralateral kidney: experience at 1 center and review of literature. *J Urol* 2011; **186**:1053–8.
108. Merrot T, Lumenta DB, Tercier S, Morisson-Lacombes G, Guys JM, Alessandrini P. Multicystic dysplastic kidney with ipsilateral abnormalities of genitourinary tract: experience in children. *Urology* 2006; **67**:603–7.
109. Farrugia MK, Hiorns MP, Mushtaq I. Multicystic dysplastic kidney and cystic accessory uterine cavity: a new prenatally diagnosed association. *Pediatr Surg Int* 2011; **27**:891–3.
110. Stuck KJ, Koff SA, Silver TM. Ultrasonic features of multicystic dysplastic kidney: expanded diagnostic criteria. *Radiology* 1982; **143**:217–21.
111. Ismaili K, Avni FE, Alexander M, Schulman C, Collier F, Hall M. Routine voiding cystourethrography is of no value in neonates with unilateral multicystic dysplastic kidney. *J Pediatr* 2005; **146**:759–63.
112. Feldenberg LR, Siegel NJ. Clinical course and outcome for children with multicystic dysplastic kidneys. *Pediatr Nephrol* 2000; **14**:1098–101.
113. Aslam M, Watson AR; Trent & Anglia MCDK Study Group. Unilateral multicystic dysplastic kidney: long term outcomes. *Arch Dis Child* 2006; **91**:820–3.
114. Kalisvaart J, Bootwala Y, Poonawala H, *et al.* Comparison of ultrasound and magnetic resonance urography for evaluation of contralateral kidney in patients with multicystic dysplastic kidney disease. *J Urol* 2011; **186**:1059–64.
115. Hollowell JG, Kogan BA. How much imaging is necessary in patients with multicystic dysplastic kidneys? *J Urol* 2011; **186**:785–6.
116. Narchi H. Risk of hypertension with multicystic kidney disease: a systematic review. *Arch Dis Child* 2005; **90**:921–4.
117. Narchi H. Risk of Wilms' tumour with multicystic kidney disease: a systematic review. *Arch Dis Child* 2005; **90**:147–9.
118. Wacksman J, Phipps L. Report of the Multicystic Kidney Registry: preliminary findings. *J Urol* 1993; **150**:1870–2.
119. Beckwith JB. Wilms tumor and multicystic dysplastic kidney disease. Editorial comment. *J Urol* 1997; **158**:2259–60.
120. Hayes WN, Watson AR; Trent & Anglia MCDK Study Group. Unilateral multicystic dysplastic kidney: does initial size matter? *Pediatr Nephrol* 2012; **27**:1335–40.
121. Chiappinelli A, Savanelli A, Farina A, Settimi A. Multicystic dysplastic kidney: our experience in non-surgical management. *Pediatr Surg Int* 2011; **27**:775–9.
122. Onal B, Kogan BA. Natural history of patients with multicystic dysplastic kidney what followup is needed? *J Urol* 2006; **176**:1607–11.
123. Webb NJ, Lewis MA, Bruce J, *et al.* Unilateral multicystic dysplastic kidney: the case for nephrectomy. *Arch Dis Child* 1997; **76**:31–4.
124. Homsy YL, Anderson JH, Oudjhane K, Russo P. Wilms tumor and multicystic dysplastic kidney disease. *J Urol* 1997; **158**:2256–9.
125. Borer JG, Cisek LJ, Atala A, Diamond DA, Retik AB, Peters CA. Pediatric retroperitoneoscopic nephrectomy using 2 mm. instrumentation. *J Urol* 1999; **162**:1725–9.
126. Liem NT, Dung LA, Viet ND. Single trocar retroperitoneoscopic nephrectomy for unilateral multicystic dysplastic kidney in children. *Pediatr Surg Int* 2012; **28**:641–3.
127. Sessa A, Righetti M, Battini G. Autosomal recessive and dominant polycystic kidney diseases. *Minerva Urol Nefrol* 2004; **56**:329–38.
128. Patel G, Choudhry M, Lakhoo K. The diagnostic dilemma of a multilocular renal cyst: a case report. *J Med Case Rep* 2009; **3**:**79**.
129. Acquired cystic kidney disease in children undergoing continuous ambulatory peritoneal dialysis. Kyushu Pediatric Nephrology Study Group. *Am J Kidney Dis* 1999; **34**:242–6.
130. Lippe B, Geffner ME, Dietrich RB, Boechat MI, Kangarloo H. Renal malformations in patients with Turner syndrome: imaging in 141 patients. *Pediatrics* 1988; **82**:852–6.
131. Niemi AK, Northrup H, Hudgins L, Bernstein JA. Horseshoe kidney and a rare TSC2 variant in two unrelated individuals with tuberous sclerosis complex. *Am J Med Genet A* 2011; **155A**:2534–7.
132. Bradshaw A, Donnelly LF, Foreman JW. Thrombocytopenia and absent radii (TAR) syndrome associated with horseshoe kidney. *Pediatr Nephrol* 2000; **14**:29–31.
133. Borer JG, Glassberg KI, Kassner EG, Schulsinger DA, Mooppan UM. Unilateral multicystic dysplasia in 1 component of a horseshoe kidney: case reports and review of the literature. *J Urol* 1994; **152**:1568–71.
134. Keskin S, Erdoğan N, Kurt A, Tan S, Ipek A. Bilateral partial ureteral duplication with double collecting system in horseshoe kidney. *Adv Med Sci* 2009; **54**:302–4.
135. Mirzazadeh M, Richards KA. Complete duplication of collecting system in a horseshoe kidney presenting with recurrent urinary tract infections: report of an exceedingly rare congenital anomaly and review of literature. *ScientificWorldJournal* 2011; **11**:1591–6.
136. Pode D, Shapiro A, Lebensart P. Unilateral triplication of the collecting system in a horseshoe kidney. *J Urol* 1983; **130**:533–4.

137. Ramasamy S, Paramasivam J, Janardhanam K. Supernumerary kidney presenting as pyonephrosis. *Indian J Urol* 2009; **25**:389–91.
138. Yesilli C, Erdem O, Akduman B, Erdem Z, Gundogdu S, Mungan NA. Horseshoe kidney with pyelic fusion and crossed single ureter. *J Urol* 2003; **170**:175–6.
139. Khong PL, Peh WC, Mya GH, Chan KL, Saing H. Horseshoe kidney with bilateral single system ectopic ureters. *Aust N Z J Surg* 1996; **66**:773–6.
140. Mesrobian HG, Kelalis PP, Hrabovsky E, Othersen HB Jr, deLorimier A, Nesmith B. Wilms tumor in horseshoe kidneys: a report from the National Wilms Tumor Study. *J Urol* 1985; **133**:1002–3.
141. Neville H, Ritchey ML, Shamberger RC, Haase G, Perlman S, Yoshioka T. The occurrence of Wilms tumor in horseshoe kidneys: a report from the National Wilms Tumor Study Group (NWTSG). *J Pediatr Surg* 2002; **37**:1134–7.
142. Huang EY, Mascarenhas L, Mahour GH. Wilms' tumor and horseshoe kidneys: a case report and review of the literature. *J Pediatr Surg* 2004; **39**:207–12.
143. Lee SH, Bae MH, Choi SH, *et al.* Wilms' tumor in a horseshoe kidney. *Korean J Urol* 2012; **53**:577–80.
144. Kapur VK, Sakalkale RP, Samuel KV, *et al.* Association of extrarenal Wilms' tumor with a horseshoe kidney. *J Pediatr Surg* 1998; **33**:935–7.
145. Kawauchi A, Fujito A, Yoneda K, *et al.* Laparoscopic pyeloplasty and isthmectomy for hydronephrosis of horseshoe kidney: a pediatric case. *J Endourol* 2005; **19**:984–6.
146. Talug C, Perlmutter AE, Kumar T, Zaslau S, Tarry WF. Laparoscopic pyeloplasty for ureteropelvic junction obstruction in a horseshoe kidney. *Can J Urol* 2007; **14**:3773–5.
147. Symons SJ, Ramachandran A, Kurien A, Baiysha R, Desai MR. Urolithiasis in the horseshoe kidney: a single-centre experience. *BJU Int* 2008; **102**:1676–80.
148. Abdeldaeim HM, Hamdy SA, Mokhless IA. Percutaneous nephrolithotomy for the management of stones in anomalous kidneys in children. *J Pediatr Urol* 2011; 7:239–43.
149. Schreuder MF. Unilateral anomalies of kidney development: why is left not right? *Kidney Int* 2011; **80**:740–5.
150. Guarino N, Tadini B, Camardi P, Silvestro L, Lace R, Bianchi M. The incidence of associated urological abnormalities in children with renal ectopia. *J Urol* 2004; **172**:1757–9.
151. Woodward M, Frank JD. Abnormal migration and fusion of the kidneys. (pp. 213–17 [Chapter 16]) In: Gearhart JP, Rink RC, Mouriquand PDE (eds). *Pediatric Urology*, 2nd edition. Philadelphia, PA: Saunders, 2010.
152. Pittock ST, Babovic-Vuksanovic D, Lteif A. Mayer-Rokitansky-Küster-Hauser anomaly and its associated malformations. *Am J Med Genet A* 2005; **135**:314–6.
153. Sesia SB, Haecker FM. Late-presenting diaphragmatic hernia associated with intrathoracic kidney: tachypnoea as unique clinical sign. *BMJ Case Rep* 2012; **23**;2012.
154. van den Bosch CM, van Wijk JA, Beckers GM, van der Horst HJ, Schreuder MF, Bökenkamp A. Urological and nephrological findings of renal ectopia. *J Urol* 2010; **183**:1574–8.
155. Rinat C, Farkas A, Frishberg Y. Familial inheritance of crossed fused renal ectopia. *Pediatr Nephrol* 2001; **16**:269–70.
156. Arena F, Arena S, Paolata A, Campenni A, Zuccarello B, Romeo G. Is a complete urological evaluation necessary in all newborns with asymptomatic renal ectopia? *Int J Urol* 2007; **14**:491–5.

CHAPTER 8.5

Disorders of the urethra

Kim Hutton and Ashok Daya Ram

Introduction to disorders of the urethra

Disorders of the urethra are mostly congenital in origin and occur predominantly in males. Posterior urethral valves is an exclusively male disorder with a reported incidence varying widely between 1 in 5,000 to 25,000 live births.[1,2] It commonly causes secondary changes in the upper urinary tract which exacerbate the effects of associated primary renal dysplasia. Posterior urethral valve disorder (PUV) remains the most common obstructive cause of end-stage renal disease in children.[3] Anterior urethral valves, urethral diverticulum, syringocele, urethral atresia, urethral stricture, and urethral polyp are far less common causes of obstructive uropathy. Urethral duplication can present as a double urinary stream or urinary incontinence. A urethral web can cause dysfunctional voiding with incontinence in female patients. Bulbar urethritis presents with terminal haematuria and is usually managed conservatively.

Posterior urethral valves

Hugh Hampton Young is credited with the first classification of PUV in 1919,[4] although earlier reports date from 1717.[5] Type I valves are the most common (95%) pattern, being likened to two 'sails of a ship' which fuse anteriorly and attach obliquely to the verumontanum posteriorly and the anterior urethral wall distally. Type II valves are mucosal folds arising from the proximal verumontanum which extend toward the bladder neck. They are not thought to be of clinical significance. Type III valves lie transversely across the urethra with a central aperture, are not attached to the verumontanum and lie distal to it. It has been suggested that PUV exists as a single entity—a congenital obstructive posterior urethral membrane—and that iatrogenic disruption from catheterization or instrumentation accounts for the features described in the original Young classification.[6]

Aetiology and associated conditions

The exact cause of PUV is not known. Although there are rare reports of familial occurrence the condition most commonly occurs on a sporadic basis. Stephens hypothesized that overdevelopment and abnormal anterior fusion of the mesonephric ducts lead to the formation of obstructing membranes.[7] PUV are more common in patients with prune belly syndrome and Down's syndrome. Sixteen per cent (16%) of PUV patients have associated undescended testes.[8]

Pathophysiology

The bladder fulfils storage and emptying functions from early foetal life. Abnormally elevated voiding pressures caused by urethral obstruction lead to pathological changes in the bladder, prostatic urethra, upper tracts, and renal parenchyma characterized by dilatation, distortion, and further damage to developing renal parenchyma.[9] Outflow obstruction in the early stages of gestation is a potent cause of renal dysplasia. The overall severity of congenital damage depends on the timing and degree of urethral obstruction, secondary pressure changes in the upper tract and the degree of irreversible primary renal dysplasia. Pressure 'pop off' mechanisms that may protect the upper tracts include the unilateral vesicoureteric reflux and renal dysplasia syndrome (VURD phenomenon), perinephric urinoma, bladder rupture with urinary ascites, patent urachus, and large bladder diverticula.[10–12]

Prenatal diagnosis

In the healthcare systems of Western countries, virtually all cases of severe foetal obstructive uropathy are picked up on routine antenatal ultrasound and followed up by serial sonographic examination. The differential diagnosis for presumed prenatally detected PUV includes gross primary vesicoureteric reflux (VUR); prune belly syndrome, ureteral duplication, megacystis-microcolon-intestinal hypoperistalsis syndrome, and urethral atresia. The classical ultrasound finding in PUV is a keyhole appearance of the dilated posterior urethra and bladder.[13]

Ultrasound predictors of impaired postnatal renal function include oligohydramnios, renal cortical echogenicity, and cortical cysts. By contrast, the severity of bladder distension is not, in itself, a reliable predictor.[14] Although foetal urinary electrolytes, osmolality, protein, and beta(2)-microglobulin levels have been studied as markers of foetal renal function, the authors of a large,systematic review concluded that they are of little or no value in predicting postnatal functional outcome.[15,16] It is important to note, however, that milder forms of PUV may not give rise to detectable abnormalities in the first two trimesters of pregnancy and will not be picked up if antenatal scanning is limited to a single, routine anomaly scan performed at 17–20 weeks.

Prenatal management

Antenatal counselling is a crucial part of prenatal management. Many parents opt for termination of pregnancy but in foetuses of less than 32 weeks gestation vesicoamniotic shunting is a therapeutic option.[2] Foetal intervention is considered in more detail in Chapter 8.1, 'Prenatal diagnosis and perinatal urology'. Although preliminary results from the PLUTO (percutaneous shunting for lower urinary tract obstruction) multicentre randomized controlled trial suggested a possible improvement in survival following shunting[17] the trial was subsequently abandoned because of recruitment problems. The weight of available evidence indicates that the effects of severe foetal obstructive uropathy on postnatal renal function are not ameliorated by intrauterine shunting.[18] Fetoscopic valve ablation has also been described.[19]

Postnatal presentation

In severe forms of PUV, the affected infant suffers from respiratory failure secondary to pulmonary hypoplasia which, in combination with renal failure can lead to neonatal death. PUV can give rise to varying degrees of urethral obstruction and the observation that a male infant is apparently voiding normally does not necessarily exclude this diagnosis. Similarly, upper tract changes are very variable in severity—as is the impact on renal function. The best outcome is achieved by early investigation and timely intervention with a multidisciplinary approach, involving paediatric urology, nephrology, and radiology and neonatology specialists. When the condition has not been detected prenatally it may present clinically in infancy or later childhood with urinary tract infection, voiding dysfunction, or incontinence.[20] The endoscopic appearance of non-obstructing mucosal folds in the posterior urethra is sometimes misinterpreted as playing a role in the aetiology of voiding dysfunction in older boys. Unless there is evidence of upper tract dilatation or markedly increased bladder wall thickness this relatively common endoscopic finding can be disregarded and no attempt should be made at resection. Management should concentrate, instead, on identifying and treating the causes of dysfunctional voiding. Very occasionally PUV remains undiagnosed until adolescence or adult life.[21–23]

Postnatal management

In prenatally detected cases or those presenting clinically in infancy, initial management consists of prompt relief of obstruction by passage of a 5 or 6 Fr feeding tube into the bladder, prophylactic antibiotics, and correction of any fluid, electrolyte, and acid-base disturbance. Decompression of the obstructed urinary tract can sometimes result in a significant post obstructive diuresis requiring regular measurement of plasma electrolyte and creatinine and judicious fluid management. It is important to note that plasma creatinine values at birth mirror those in the maternal circulation and during the early days of life do not provide a reliable indication of the true severity of renal impairment.

Micturating cystourethrography (MCUG) is the investigation of choice once the infant's condition has been stabilized (Fig. 8.5.1). The availability of dedicated paediatric endoscopes has made it possible to confirm the diagnosis and proceed to primary valve ablation in the majority of infants (Fig. 8.5.2).[24] Computer enhanced visual learning methods have recently been developed as an aid to endoscopic management and these are likely to play an increasingly valuable role for surgical trainees.[25] The surgical options for relieving the obstruction under direct vision include cold knife incision, diathermy ablation, or laser energy to disrupt the valve tissue. One study has suggested that cold knife incision is associated with a lower risk of stricture formation than diathermy ablation.[26] However, the senior author has encountered only one case of stricture in 65 PUV patients resected with diathermy—and this resolved with a single urethral dilatation. Bleeding is seldom a problem. A postoperative MCUG or endoscopy is performed some weeks later to confirm successful relief of obstruction. If necessary, further valve ablation is performed to remove any residual tissue.

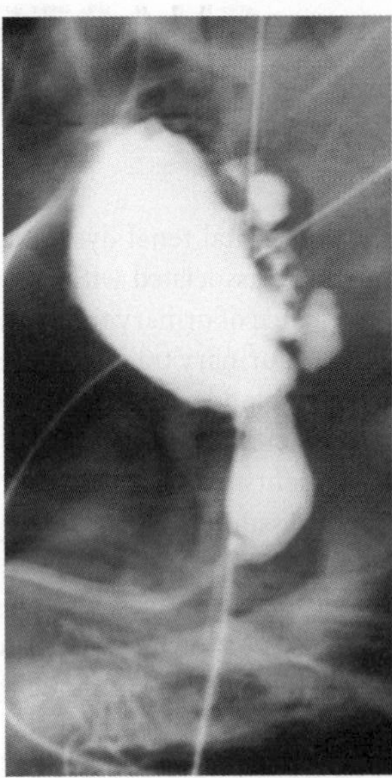

Fig. 8.5.1 Micturating cystourethrography (MCUG) showing trabeculated bladder with diverticula formation, dilated posterior urethra and abrupt calibre change at the level of the verumontanum consistent with a diagnosis of posterior urethral valves.

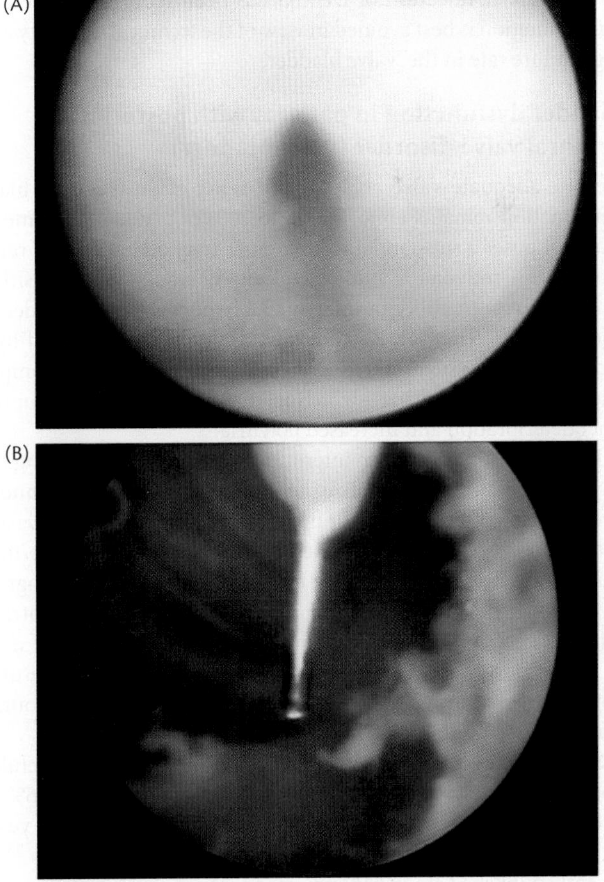

Fig. 8.5.2 (A) Endoscopic view of type 1 posterior urethral valves. (B) View after complete valve resection revealing capacious posterior urethra.

If primary valve ablation is not feasible, urinary diversion using vesicostomy or ureterostomy are alternatives, although their use has dramatically decreased in recent years.

Further management

Although irreversible congenital renal dysplasia is the most common cause of renal damage associated with PUV, damage can also be acquired as a consequence of urinary tract infection and bladder dysfunction. Prevention of urinary tract infection (UTI) and active management of the 'valve bladder' are therefore essential to minimize further functional deterioration and delay the onset of renal failure. Follow-up of patients with PUV should routinely include measurement of blood pressure, height and weight, urine dipstick analysis, renal tract ultrasound, and serum creatinine measurements. When indicated, follow-up may also entail isotope renography, videourodynamics, uroflowmetry and formal glomerular filtration rate (GFR) measurement. Antibiotic prophylaxis is usually administered for the first 6–12 months of life and is maintained for longer periods in boys with persisting VUR or renal scarring. There is growing evidence that circumcision can be beneficial in those boys who experience recurrent UTIs[27] but it is not used routinely as a prophylactic measure in most centres.

Unilateral or bilateral VUR occurs in 30–70% of cases of PUV but resolves spontaneously in more than half of these cases following valve resection. Persistent reflux is best managed conservatively with antibiotic prophylaxis combined with active treatment of any associated bladder dysfunction. Successful endoscopic correction by subureteric injection of Deflux® has been reported.[28] Ureteric reimplantation is best avoided in view of the technical difficulty and high failure rate in the 'valve bladder'.

Bladder dysfunction in patients with posterior urethral valve disorder (valve bladder)

Despite adequate valve ablation and relief of obstruction, bladder function remains abnormal in to 70% of patients, in some of whom it poses a substantial risk of upper tract dilatation and renal damage.[29] Urodynamic studies typically demonstrate a transition from hypercontractility in infancy to a hypocontractile bladder in adolescence.[30] The 'valve bladder' syndrome is characterized by a vicious cycle of polyuria, reduced bladder sensation, hypocompliance, and residual urine—which in turn provokes further upper tract deterioration and increased polyuria.

Double voiding and clean intermittent catheterization during the daytime may suffice to stabilize the situation but, if not, continuous overnight bladder catheter drainage may be required.[31] Invasive urodynamics (videourodynamics, cystometry, and pressure/flow studies) are usually reserved for boys with this pattern of progressive bladder dysfunction and/or renal impairment.[32] By contrast, safe and effective long-term follow-up for boys with PUV of mild to moderate severity can usually be limited to non-invasive uroflowmetry, measurement of post-void residual urine on ultrasound, bladder diary, and monitoring of plasma creatinine.

Symptoms of bladder dysfunction tend to resolve during childhood and adolescence—with one study finding that while 46% of patients had some residual impairment of continence at 10 years of age, this figure had fallen to 1% by the age of 20 years.[33] A recently published study has suggested that anticholinergic therapy in infants with high voiding pressures and/or small bladder capacity may have the potential to improve the prognosis for bladder function.[34] Alpha adrenergic blockers may enhance bladder emptying.[35] Clean intermittent catheterization is often poorly tolerated in boys with PUV because of their sensate urethra and to overcome this problem it may be necessary to create a continent catheterizable (Mitrofanoff) channel. Bladder augmentation is rarely required but can be performed using either ileum or, when available, redundant megaureter.

End-stage renal failure

An authoritative review of 34 studies involving 1,474 patients[36] documented an overall incidence of chronic renal failure and end-stage renal disease of 22% and 11%, respectively. For renal transplantation, graft survival rate is 81% at 5 years and 57% at 10 years. These rates are comparable to those for paediatric renal transplantation into normal bladders.[37]

Fertility

Contrary to many published reports, one recent, extensive long-term study found that long-term outcomes for fertility and sexual function in men with a history of PUV were similar to those of a healthy control population. Even men in chronic renal failure had satisfactory erectile function and paternity rates.[38]

Prognosis

This is determined largely by the degree of primary renal dysplasia. Other contributory factors include ongoing obstructive damage (before and after birth), persistent bladder dysfunction after valve ablation and acquired renal scarring due to UTIs and VUR. Favourable prognostic factors include presentation in later childhood and upper tract protection by 'pop off' mechanisms. Poor prognostic factors include maternal oligohydramnios, early postnatal presentation, proteinuria, bilateral VUR, incontinence persisting beyond five years of age,[39] elevated nadir creatinine levels and bladder wall thickness more than 1.3 mm on ultrasound.[40] In adult males with a history of PUV the incidence of troublesome lower urinary tract symptoms (e.g. hesitancy, weak stream, incomplete emptying, and straining, urge and stress incontinence) is two- to threefolds higher than the general population.[41]

Anterior urethral valve, Cowper's syringocele, and urethral diverticulum

These rare anomalies derive from cystic dilatation of a Cowper's gland duct (syringocele). Rupture of a cyst creates a diverticulum—with the anterior lip acting as an obstructive 'valve' in the anterior urethra.[42–45] Typically these conditions present with obstructed voiding, post micturition dribble, haematuria, or UTI. Their treatment consists of endoscopic resection, and outcomes are generally good.[46]

Urethral atresia, prune belly syndrome, megalourethra, urethral stricture, and urethral web

Urethral atresia is lethal unless it is accompanied by the presence of a patent urachus (or antenatal intervention is performed). Most affected pregnancies are terminated but in those that go to term the affected newborns either succumb to pulmonary hypoplasia and renal failure or, alternatively, progress rapidly to end-stage renal disease despite early intervention.[47] Urethral atresia is a feature of severe forms of prune belly syndrome. Although almost invariably lethal, this anomaly has been reportedly treated by progressive dilatation of the anterior urethra (PADUA procedure)[48] in conjunction with extensive surgical reconstruction of the urinary tract. Prune belly syndrome comprises extensive urinary tract dilatation, bilateral cryptorchidism, and absence of abdominal wall musculature. Skeletal abnormalities, notably kyphoscoliosis, may also be present. Although it has been suggested that the condition represents the outcome of self-limiting intra uterine urethral obstruction the aetiology remains uncertain. There is a broad spectrum of severity and some affected individuals progress into adulthood with well-preserved renal function. The birth incidence of prune belly syndrome has declined substantially in recent years as a consequence of prenatal diagnosis and termination of pregnancy.

Megalourethra is characterized by deficiency of the corpus spongiosum with or without deficiency of the corpora cavernosa. Two forms are recognized depending upon whether the dilatation of the urethra is saccular or fusiform in configuration. Megalourethra is often associated with other severe anomalies including prune belly syndrome or the VACTERL (**v**ertebral anomalies, **a**nal atresia, **c**ardiac defects, **t**racheoesophageal fistula, and **e**sophageal atresia, **r**enal anomalies, and **l**imb defects). Depending on its severity megalourethra is either managed conservatively or by surgical reconstruction.

Congenital bulbar strictures are rare and are usually amenable to endoscopic cold knife incision or urethroplasty. A posterior meatal web in girls causes deflection of the urinary stream anteriorly onto the clitoris, stimulating the bulbocavernosus reflex and causing sphincter activity, dysfunctional voiding, and subsequent daytime incontinence.[49] Treatment of this rare anomaly consists of simple incision—which is curative and leads to a much improved quality of life.

Urethral duplication

The duplicate urethra usually runs parallel to the native urethra in a sagittal plane—although occasionally a coronal plane. Duplication may be complete or incomplete—in which case the urethras may fuse proximally to create a Y type anomaly or distally to form a single channel.[50–52] The most widely used classification was developed by Effmann.[53] Surgical treatment is tailored to individual anatomy.

Urethral polyp

These benign lesions present with obstructive symptoms, UTI, or haematuria. The diagnosis is usually made on MCUG (Fig. 8.5.3, Fig. 8.5.3A).[54–56] Urethral polyps occur mainly in boys, in whom they arise from the verumontanum in the posterior urethra. Endoscopic resection is curative (Fig. 8.5.3B). Occasionally, the size of the polyp precludes its removal via the urethra following resection of the pedicle and in these situations percutaneous transvesical retrieval of the specimen is required. Urethral polyps are occasionally seen in girls.[57]

Bulbar urethritis

Also known as idiopathic urethrorrhagia, this benign self-limiting condition affects teenage boys and presents with dysuria, terminal haematuria, or blood spotting on the underwear.[58] The aetiology is unknown and although endoscopy is not routinely performed appearances are of roughened, inflamed urethral mucosa with fibrinous exudate.[59] Management is usually conservative although the use of urethral instillation of triamcinolone or a period of indwelling catheter drainage have been described for intractable cases. The progression to urethral stricture formation has been reported.[60]

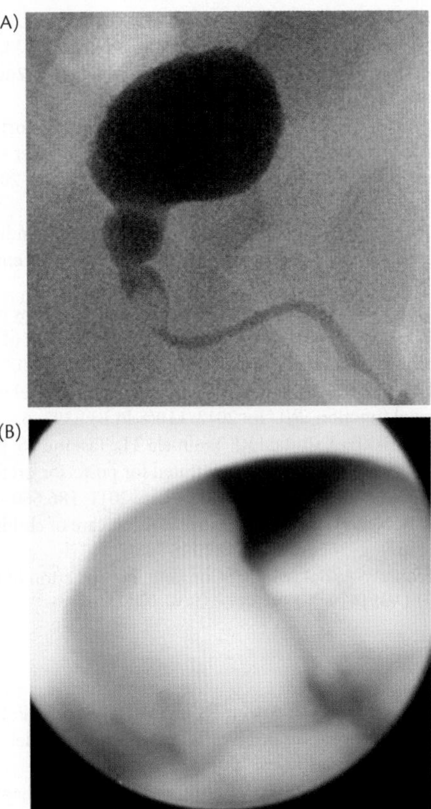

Fig. 8.5.3 This five-week-old male infant presented with a urinary tract infection (UTI) and a left perinephric abscess that required percutaneous ultrasound guided drainage. (A) MCUG showing filling defect in posterior urethra that altered position during voiding; and (B) endoscopic view of urethral polyp arising from the proximal limit of the verumontanum. Transurethral resection was performed and histology showed a benign fibroepithelial polyp. He has remained entirely asymptomatic in the five years since surgery.

Conclusions

Posterior urethral valves is the commonest cause of congenital outflow obstruction and its multidisciplinary management often commences from the time of first diagnosis on an antenatal ultrasound scan. Prompt decompression of the obstructed urinary tract is the initial priority but subsequent management of bladder dysfunction is of crucial importance to the preservation of renal function, overall prognosis, and long-term outcome. PUV may have lifelong consequences so it is important that adult urologists have a good understanding of this condition. The overall aim of management is to enable affected individuals to lead normal lives into adolescence and beyond.[61]

Further reading

Casale AJ. Posterior urethral valves. (pp. 3389–3410 [Chapter 126]) In: Wein AJ, Kavoussi LR (eds). *Campbell-Walsh Urology*, 10th edition. Philadelphia, PA: WB Saunders, 2011.

Desai DY, Duffy PG. Posterior urethral valves and other urethral abnormalities. (pp. 109–20 [Chapter 8]) In: Thomas DFM, Duffy PG, Rickwood AMK (eds). *Essentials of Paediatric Urology*, 2nd edition. London, UK: Informa Healthcare, 2008.

Hennus PM, van der Heijden GJ, Bosch JL, de Jong TP, de Kort LM. A systematic review on renal and bladder dysfunction after endoscopic treatment of infravesical obstruction in boys. *PLoS One* 2012; 7(9):e44663.

Koff SA, Mutabagani KH, Jayanthi VR. The valve bladder syndrome: pathophysiology and treatment with nocturnal bladder emptying. *J Urol* 2002; **167**:291–7.

Morris RK, Malin GL, Khan KS, Kilby MD. Systematic review of the effectiveness of antenatal intervention for the treatment of congenital lower urinary tract obstruction. *BJOG* 2010; **117**:382–90.

Taskinen S, Heikkilä J, Santtila P, Rintala R. Posterior urethral valves and adult sexual function. *BJU Int* 2012; **110**(8 Pt B):E392–6.

Tikkinen KA, Heikkilä J, Rintala RJ, Tammela TL, Taskinen S. Lower urinary tract symptoms in adults treated for posterior urethral valves in childhood: matched cohort study. *J Urol* 2011; **186**:660–6.

Woodhouse CR, Neild GH, Yu RN, Bauer S. Adult care of children from pediatric urology. *J Urol* 2012; **187**:1164–71.

Young HH, Frontz WA, Baldwin JC. Congenital obstruction of the posterior urethra. *J Urol* 1919; **3**:289–365.

References

1. Hutton KA, Thomas DF, Arthur RJ, Irving HC, Smith SE. Prenatally detected posterior urethral valves: is gestational age at detection a predictor of outcome? *J Urol* 1994; **152**(2 Pt 2):698–701
2. Casale AJ. Posterior urethral valves. (pp. 3389–3410 [Chapter 126]) In: Wein AJ, Kavoussi LR (eds). *Campbell-Walsh Urology*, 10th edition. Philadelphia, PA: WB Saunders, 2011.
3. Elder JS, Shapiro E. Posterior urethral valves. (pp. 781–92 [Chapter 56]) In: Ashcraft KW, Holcomb GW, Murphy JP (eds). *Pediatric Surgery*, 4th edition. Philadelphia, PA: Elsevier Saunders, 2005.
4. Young HH, Frontz WA, Baldwin JC. Congenital obstruction of the posterior urethra. *J Urol* 1919; **3**:289–365.
5. Levin TL, Han B, Little BP. Congenital anomalies of the male urethra. *Pediatr Radiol* 2007; **37**:851–62.
6. Dewan PA, Zappala SM, Ransley PG, Duffy PG. Endoscopic reappraisal of the morphology of congenital obstruction of the posterior urethra. *Br J Urol* 1992; **70**:439–44.
7. Stephens FD, Smith ED, Hutson JM. *Congenital Abnormalities of the Urinary and Genital Tracts*. Oxford, UK: Isis Medical Media, 1996.
8. Heikkilä J, Taskinen S, Toppari J, Rintala R. Posterior urethral valves are often associated with cryptorchidism and inguinal hernias. *J Urol* 2008; **180**:715–7.
9. Henneberry MO, Stephens FD. Renal hypoplasia and dysplasia in infants with posterior urethral valves. *J Urol* 1980; **123**:912–5.
10. Close CE, Mitchell ME. Posterior urethral valves. (pp. 437–45 [Chapter 33]) In: Gearhart JP, Rink RC, Mouriquand PDE (eds). *Pediatric Urology*, 2nd edition. Philadelphia, PA: Saunders Elsevier, 2010.
11. Rittenberg MH, Hulbert WC, Snyder HM 3rd, Duckett JW. Protective factors in posterior urethral valves. *J Urol* 1988; **140**:993–6.
12. Kaefer M, Keating MA, Adams MC, Rink RC. Posterior urethral valves, pressure pop-offs and bladder function. *J Urol* 1995; **154**:708–11.
13. Elder JS. Management of antenatally-diagnosed hydronephrosis. (pp. 793–808) In: Puri P (ed). *Newborn Surgery*, 2nd edition. London, UK: Hodder Arnold, 2003.
14. Morris RK, Malin GL, Khan KS, Kilby MD. Antenatal ultrasound to predict postnatal renal function in congenital lower urinary tract obstruction: systematic review of test accuracy. *BJOG* 2009; **116**:1290–9.
15. Lee J, Kimber C, Shekleton P, Cheng W. Prognostic factors of severe foetal megacystis. *ANZ J Surg* 2011; **81**:552–5.
16. Morris RK, Quinlan-Jones E, Kilby MD, Khan KS. Systematic review of accuracy of fetal urine analysis to predict poor postnatal renal function in cases of congenital urinary tract obstruction. *Prenat Diagn* 2007; **27**:900–11.
17. Morris R, Kilby M. The PLUTO trial: percutaneous shunting in lower urinary tract obstruction. Abstract 18. *Am J Obstet Gynecol* 2012; **206**(1):S14.
18. Morris RK, Malin GL, Khan KS, Kilby MD. Systematic review of the effectiveness of antenatal intervention for the treatment of congenital lower urinary tract obstruction. *BJOG* 2010; **117**:382–90.
19. Quintero RA, Hume R, Smith C,*et al.* Percutaneous fetal cystoscopy and endoscopic fulguration of posterior urethral valves. *Am J Obstet Gynecol* 1995; **172**:206–9.
20. Hendren WH. Posterior urethral valves in boys. A broad clinical spectrum. *J Urol* 1971; **106**:298–307.
21. Mahony DT, Laferte RO. Congenital posterior urethral valves in adult males. *Urology* 1974; **3**:724–34.
22. Schober JM, Dulabon LM, Woodhouse CR. Outcome of valve ablation in late-presenting posterior urethral valves. *BJU Int* 2004; **94**:616–9.
23. Mahadik P, Vaddi SP, Godala CM, Sambar V, Kulkarni S, Gundala R. Posterior urethral valve: delayed presentation in adolescence. *Int Neurourol J* 2012; **16**:149–52.
24. Desai DY, Duffy PG. Posterior urethral valves and other urethral abnormalities. (pp. 109–20 [Chapter 8]) In: Thomas DFM, Duffy PG, Rickwood AMK (eds). *Essentials of Paediatric Urology*, 2nd edition. London, UK: Informa Healthcare, 2008.
25. Matoka DJ, Marks AJ, Stoltz RS, Maizels M. Utilization of computer enhanced visual learning (CEVL) method improves endoscopic diagnosis of posterior urethral valves (PUV). *J Pediatr Urol* 2013; **9**(4):498–502
26. Babu R, Kumar R. Early outcome following diathermy versus cold knife ablation of posterior urethral valves. *J Pediatr Urol* 2013; **9**(1):7–10
27. Mukherjee S, Joshi A, Carroll D, Chandran H, Parashar K, McCarthy L. What is the effect of circumcision on risk of urinary tract infection in boys with posterior urethral valves? *J Pediatr Surg* 2009; **44**:417–21.
28. Oktar T, Acar O, Sancaktutar A, Sanlı O, Tefik T, Ziylan O. Endoscopic treatment of vesicoureteral reflux in children with posterior urethral valves. *Int Urol Nephrol* 2012; **44**:1305–9.
29. De Gennaro M, Capitanucci ML, Mosiello G, Caione P, Silveri M. The changing urodynamic pattern from infancy to adolescence in boys with posterior urethral valves. *BJU Int* 2000; **85**:1104–8.
30. Holmdahl G, Sillén U, Hanson E, Hermansson G, Hjälmås K. Bladder dysfunction in boys with posterior urethral valves before and after puberty. *J Urol* 1996; **155**:694–8.
31. Koff SA, Mutabagani KH, Jayanthi VR. The valve bladder syndrome: pathophysiology and treatment with nocturnal bladder emptying. *J Urol* 2002; **167**:291–7.
32. Capitanucci ML, Marciano A, Zaccara A, La Sala E, Mosiello G, De Gennaro M. Long-term bladder function followup in boys with posterior urethral valves: comparison of noninvasive vs invasive urodynamic studies. *J Urol* 2012; **188**:953–7.
33. Smith GH, Canning DA, Schulman SL, Snyder HM 3rd, Duckett JW. The long-term outcome of posterior urethral valves treated with primary valve ablation and observation. *J Urol* 1996; **155**:1730–4.
34. Casey JT, Hagerty JA, Maizels M, *et al.* Early administration of oxybutynin improves bladder function and clinical outcomes in newborns with posterior urethral valves. *J Urol* 2012; **188**:1516–20.
35. Abraham MK, Nasir AR, Sudarsanan B, *et al.* Role of alpha adrenergic blocker in the management of posterior urethral valves. *Pediatr Surg Int* 2009; **25**:1113–5.
36. Hennus PM, van der Heijden GJ, Bosch JL, de Jong TP, de Kort LM. A systematic review on renal and bladder dysfunction after endoscopic treatment of infravesical obstruction in boys. *PLoS One* 2012; 7(9):e44663.
37. Kamal MM, El-Hefnawy AS, Soliman S, Shokeir AA, Ghoneim MA. Impact of posterior urethral valves on pediatric renal transplantation: a single-center comparative study of 297 cases. *Pediatr Transplant* 2011; **15**:482–7.

38. Taskinen S, Heikkilä J, Santtila P, Rintala R. Posterior urethral valves and adult sexual function. *BJU Int* 2012; **110**(8 Pt B):E392–6.
39. Parkhouse HF, Barratt TM, Dillon MJ, Duffy PG, Fay J, Ransley PG, Woodhouse CR, Williams DI. Long-term outcome of boys with posterior urethral valves. *Br J Urol* 1988; **62**:59–62.
40. Lee YS, Jung HJ, Im YJ, Hong CH, Han SW. The significance of detrusor wall thickness as a prognostic factor in pediatric bladder outlet obstruction. *J Pediatr Surg* 2012; **47**:1682–7.
41. Tikkinen KA, Heikkilä J, Rintala RJ, Tammela TL, Taskinen S. Lower urinary tract symptoms in adults treated for posterior urethral valves in childhood: matched cohort study. *J Urol* 2011; **186**:660–6.
42. Campobasso P, Schieven E, Fernandes EC. Cowper's syringocele: an analysis of 15 consecutive cases. *Arch Dis Child* 1996; **75**:71–3.
43. Shintaku I, Ono Y, Katoh N, Takeda A, Ohshima S. Anterior urethral diverticulum produced by Cowper's gland duct cyst. *Int J Urol* 1996; **3**:412–3.
44. McLellan DL, Gaston MV, Diamond DA, Lebowitz RL, Mandell J, Atala A, Bauer SB. Anterior urethral valves and diverticula in children: a result of ruptured Cowper's duct cyst? *BJU Int* 2004; **94**:375–8.
45. Kajiwara M, Inoue K, Kato M, Usui A, Matsubara A, Usui T. Anterior urethral valves in children: a possible association between anterior urethral valves and Cowper's duct cyst. *Int J Urol* 2007; **14**:156–60.
46. Routh JC, McGee SM, Ashley RA, Reinberg Y, Vandersteen DR. Predicting renal outcomes in children with anterior urethral valves: a systematic review. *J Urol* 2010; **184**:1615–9.
47. González R, De Filippo R, Jednak R, Barthold JS. Urethral atresia: long-term outcome in 6 children who survived the neonatal period. *J Urol* 2001; **165**:2241–4.
48. Stalberg K, González R. Urethral atresia and anhydramnios at 18 weeks of gestation can result in normal development. *J Pediatr Urol* 2012; **8**:e33–5.
49. Hoebeke P, Van Laecke E, Raes A, Van Gool JD, Vande Walle J. Anomalies of the external urethral meatus in girls with non-neurogenic bladder sphincter dysfunction. *BJU Int* 1999; **83**:294–8.
50. Mane SB, Obaidah A, Dhende NP, Arlikar J, Acharya H, Thakur A, Reddy S. Urethral duplication in children: our experience of eight cases. *J Pediatr Urol* 2009; **5**:363–7.
51. Coleman RA, Winkle DC, Borzi PA. Urethral duplication: cases of ventral and dorsal complete duplication and review of the literature. *J Pediatr Urol* 2010; **6**:188–91.
52. Macedo A Jr, Rondon A, Bacelar H, Ottoni S, Liguori R, Garrone G, Ortiz V. Urethral duplication II-A Y type with rectal urethra: ASTRA approach and tunica vaginalis flap for first stage repair. *Int Braz J Urol* 2012; **38**:707–8.
53. Effmann EL, Lebowitz RL, Colodny AH. Duplication of the urethra. *Radiology* 1976; **119**:179–85.
54. Kearney GP, Lebowitz RL, Retik AB. Obstructing polyps of the posterior urethra in boys: embryology and management. *J Urol* 1979; **122**:802–4.
55. Raviv G, Leibovitch I, Hanani J, Hertz M, Goldwasser B, Jonas P. Hematuria and voiding disorders in children caused by congenital urethral polyps. Principles of diagnosis and management. *Eur Urol* 1993; **23**:382–5.
56. Eziyi AK, Helmy TE, Sarhan OM, Eissa WM, Ghaly MA. Management of male urethral polyps in children: experience with four cases. *Afr J Paediatr Surg* 2009; **6**:49–51.
57. Ben-Meir D, Yin M, Chow CW, Hutson JM. Urethral polyps in prepubertal girls. *J Urol* 2005; **174**:1443–4.
58. Kaplan GW, Brock WA. Idiopathic urethrorrhagia in boys. *J Urol* 1982; **128**:1001–3.
59. Walker BR, Ellison ED, Snow BW, Cartwright PC. The natural history of idiopathic urethrorrhagia in boys. *J Urol* 2001; **166**:231–2.
60. Docimo SG, Silver RI, González R, Müller SC, Jeffs RD. Idiopathic anterior urethritis in prepubertal and pubertal boys: pathology and clues to etiology. *Urology* 1998; **51**:99–102.
61. Woodhouse CR, Neild GH, Yu RN, Bauer S. Adult care of children from pediatric urology. *J Urol* 2012; **187**:1164–71.

CHAPTER 8.6

Neuropathic bladder and anorectal anomalies

Henrik Steinbrecher

Introduction to neuropathic bladder and anorectal anomalies

Successful management of the urinary tract in children with neuropathic bladder presents both a technical and intellectual challenge to the paediatric urologist. Although urological management must be adapted to individual differences in physical, social, and educational needs, it is guided by the same underlying basic principles.

In the past, some children with neuropathic bladder were not diagnosed until relatively late, were inadequately investigated or treated, and often denied the benefits of integrated care. During the last 20 to 30 years, however, a far better understanding of the physiology of neuropathic bladder dysfunction has emerged, leading, in turn, to a wider range of treatment options than was available in the past.

This chapter provides an overview of the urological management of the neuropathic bladder with an emphasis on myelomeningocoele. The urological aspects of anorectal malformations are also described.

Definition, classification, and pathophysiology

A neuropathic bladder is one in which function is abnormal as a consequence of an identifiable neurological lesion or disorder. Although the term 'neuropathic' usually refers to the bladder, it is important to recognize that the sphincter mechanism is also invariably involved.

There have been many attempts to classify and define the combination of clinical and physiological features of neuropathic bladder/sphincter dysfunction. These have ranged from purely neuroanatomical classifications to others based predominantly on clinical features. The latter are of more practical value to clinicians.

From a clinical perspective, a neuropathic bladder may be classified as being either overactive or underactive, and similarly the sphincter may also be considered as being overactive or underactive. However, many cases of neuropathic dysfunction demonstrate intermediate degrees of bladder overactivity and reduced compliance coupled with varying degrees of sphincter incompetence. The degree of preservation of urethral sensation also varies considerably between individuals.

Broadly speaking, an overactive bladder and overactive sphincter are manifestations of an upper motor neuron (suprasacral, spinal cord) lesion whereas an underactive bladder and underactive sphincter are associated with a lower motor neuron (sacral cord) lesion.

In an upper motor neuron lesion, the spinal reflexes (detrusor muscle reflex, anocutaneous reflex) are intact but this reflex activity is not modulated by higher centres. Consequently, there is loss of normal coordination between detrusor contraction and sphincter relaxation (detrusor/sphincter dyssynergia).

In a lower motor neuron lesion, the spinal reflexes are lost and the bladder fails to contract normally. In addition this pattern is almost invariably accompanied by variable degrees of sphincter weakness.

In practice, over 60% of children with myelomeningocoele or other structural spinal cord and vertebral defects, demonstrate a mixed upper and lower motor neuron picture and an intermediate pattern of bladder dysfunction. Clinical features in an individual case tend to be determined by the level of the lowest spinal nerve segment involved by the spinal cord lesion.

In cases of neuropathic bladder associated with closed or occult spinal dysraphism, the level of the vertebral abnormality is not a reliable predictor of the level of the spinal cord lesion, especially in the presence of a spinal cord syrinx or tethered cord.

A mixed picture can arise from four combinations of bladder–sphincter dysfunction.

(a) Hyperreflexic bladder with hyperreflexic sphincter (= dyssynergia)

(b) Hyperreflexic bladder with hyporeflexic sphincter

(c) Hyporeflexic bladder with hyperreflexic sphincter (= dyssynergia)

(d) Hyporeflexic bladder with hyporeflexic sphincter.

To understand the significance of these four patterns of dysfunction it is necessary to consider the basic functions of the bladder–sphincter mechanism during filling and emptying.

On filling, the normal bladder is capable of storing a reasonably high volume of urine at low pressure. The relationship between volume and pressure is described as compliance. A poorly compliant bladder is characterized by an inappropriate level of detrusor activity leading to an abnormal rise in intravesical pressure at small volumes of filling.

In the normal bladder, voiding proceeds to completion, and is under voluntary control once the child is potty trained.

An overactive (hyperreflexic) neuropathic bladder is unable to store normal, physiological volumes of urine, and generates abnormally elevated storage pressures (i.e. is poorly compliant). Involuntary voiding or leakage of urine leads to incontinence.

An underactive (hyporeflexic) bladder is characterized by high volume, low pressure storage of urine with incomplete emptying, and varying degrees of overflow incontinence.

An overactive (hyperreflexic) sphincter causes increased outlet resistance. Abnormally elevated bladder pressures must be generated to overcome this resistance during emptying. However, there is little, if any leakage on filling.

By contrast, an underactive (hyporeflexic) sphincter is associated with reduced outlet resistance. Bladder emptying occurs at low pressure and urinary leakage can occur during the filling phase without any detrusor contraction.

A 'safe' bladder is one in which urine is stored at low pressure storage compliance is adequate and there is no secondary vesicoureteric reflux. However, urinary leakage (incontinence) almost invariably occurs to a greater or lesser degree.

An 'unsafe' bladder is one where the upper tracts are at risk; this may be because of high-pressure storage (overactivity during storage or poor compliance) or emptying (caused by increased outlet resistance.) The presence of secondary vesicoureteric reflux may render the bladder 'unsafe'—as may incomplete voiding posing an increased risk of urinary infection.

Aetiology

Congenital causes of neuropathic bladder include:

- Myelomeningocoele
- Sacral agenesis
- Sacrospinal dysraphisms
- Congenital tumours (e.g. sacrococcygeal teratoma or neuroblastoma)
- Anorectal malformations associated with abnormalities of the vertebrae, sacrum, and spinal cord

Myelomeningocoele

Myelomeningocoele results from failure of fusion of the neural crest between days 23–27 after fertilization. Predisposing factors include maternal anticonvulsants, diabetes, and a positive family history. Folic acid supplements administered before and during pregnancy have been shown to reduce the incidence by up to 70%.

Sacral agenesis occurs in 1:25,000 live births and may be a component of the Currarino syndrome (an autosomal dominant condition characterized by sacral agenesis, anterior meningocele, or anorectal malformation).

Sacral agenesis

Sacral agenesis ranges in severity from complete absence of the sacrum to minor defects of sacral vertebral elements. The severity of the associated neurological deficit is usually proportional to the extent of the bony defect.

Sacral ageneisis often remains undetected in early childhood since there are no external physical signs and urinary and faecal incontinence may not be recognized as being abnormal until after the age of potty training.

Sacrospinal dysraphisms

Sacrospinal dysraphism encompasses a range of abnormalities including: lipomyelomeningocoele, lumbosacral lipoma, tight filum terminale, dorsal dermal sinus, and other causes of a tethered spinal cord. Although often termed 'occult dysraphism' these abnormalities are usually associated with some external evidence ('stigmata') of the underlying lesion. Unfortunately, these cutaneous lesions are sometimes overlooked or their significance not recognized. As a consequence, serious upper tract damage may have occurred by the time the neurological abnormality is diagnosed.

Cord tethering causing traction on the filum terminale poses a threat of progressive neurological deterioration during somatic growth, particularly in later childhood.

Congenital tumours

Sacrococcygeal teratoma is germ cell tumour occurring in 1:35,000 live births.[1] Treatment consists of early and complete excision of the lesion. Neuropathic bladder and bowel can arise either as a primary consequence of nerve compression or involvement by the tumour or, alternatively, following surgical excision (which invariably requires resection of part of the sacrum).

Neuroblastoma is a tumour arising from sympathetic neuroblasts derived from the neural crest. Most tumours involve the adrenal gland. However they can also arise from paravertebral sympathetic or pelvic plexuses—with resultant disturbance of bladder and bowel function.

Acquired causes are rarer in children but include:

- Spinal cord injury (typically road traffic or horse riding accidents)
- Iatrogenic injury to the pelvic nerves (e.g. following anorectal pull—through procedures)
- Transverse myelitis (viral, bacterial, or unknown aetiology)
- Spinal cord ischaemia (occurring as birth injury or a complication of thoracic or spinal surgery)
- Spinal tumours

Clinical assessment

History and examination

A multidisciplinary assessment of the relevant history is mandatory and should encompass the urological, gastrointestinal, orthopaedic, and neurological systems. In the urological history it is important to inquire about the urinary stream since, for example, sphincter incompetence is accompanied by continuous dribbling or incontinence on crying, straining, or upright posture. However, the voiding pattern in infants should be interpreted with caution since some degree of detrusor sphincter discoordination is common prior potty training.

A history of urinary infections suggests upper tract problems such as vesicoureteric reflux or (rarely) vesicoureteric junction obstruction.

Examination should include abdominal palpation to identify the presence of a full bladder. If urine can be readily expressed with minimal suprapubic pressure this is indicates probable sphincter weakness.

The genitalia should be examined to assess sensation. Examination of the spine is mandatory to look for external evidence of 'occult' dysraphism such as a hairy tuft, haemangioma, abnormal dimple, or asymmetry of buttock muscle mass. Neurological examination of the lower limbs is performed to assess tone, power, reflexes, and sensation.

As the child grows and develops it is essential to assess their level of cognitive and social abilities since these will have an important bearing on the individual's potential ability to manage their neuropathic bladder independently. Detailed information on family and social factors is important, since having a neuropathic bladder has lifelong implications for the family as well as the affected child.

Investigations

The priorities are to identify the pattern of neuropathic dysfunction and assess the threat posed to the kidneys. The risk of urinary infection should also be assessed since vesicoureteric reflux (particularly in conjunction with high storage pressures) poses a serious risk of renal damage.

Urinary tract ultrasound is used to evaluate renal size, shape, consistency, cortical thickness, scarring, corticomedullary differentiation, and dilatation of the pelvis calyceal systems and ureters.

Ultrasound also provides a measure of bladder wall thickness (although only when the bladder is filled to at least 50% of expected capacity).

Although a DMSA scan may not be performed routinely as part of the initial work up, it is indicated when there is a history of urinary infection or evidence of renal scarring or ureteric dilatation on ultrasound.

Videourodynamics (VUD) will establish the type of neuropathic bladder dysfunction (e.g. overactive, underactive, or intermediate patterns of bladder dysfunction and hypocompliance). Imaging during the study is helpful in assessing the continence mechanism and looking for VUR.

The VUD findings should make it possible to determine whether the bladder is 'safe' or 'unsafe'. In cases of congenital neuropathic bladder VUD studies are probably best carried out within the first three to four months to establish a baseline and to inform the decision on whether to commence clean intermittent catheterization (CIC) (plus anticholinergic medication when indicated).

However, in some cases of occult dysraphism where the extent (if any) of bladder involvement is initially unclear, it may be reasonable to defer VUD—with the proviso that that the infant is reviewed regularly and the upper tracts monitored closely with ultrasound.

It must also be emphasized, that even if the neuropathic bladder appears to be 'safe' in infancy there is a strong likelihood that it will change as the child grows and further VUD will be required to reassess bladder function in the future.

Videourodynamics is an invasive investigation and the insertion of urinary and rectal catheters can cause considerable distress in children. To minimize distress the use of suprapubic catheters is preferable to the urethral route when the urethra is sensate or anatomically abnormal.

Electromyographic (EMG) recordings are rarely performed in children.

Figure 8.6.1 shows two examples of urodynamic tracings in children with myelomeningocoele.

Testing for latex allergy should be considered in view of the likelihood of multiple investigations and procedures involving exposure to latex.[2,3]

Treatment strategies for the kidneys and bladder

The threat to renal function is greatest when one or more of the following are present; neurogenic detrusor overactivity, high storage pressure, poor compliance, detrusor sphincter dyssynergia, high leak point pressure, vesicoureteric reflux, and recurrent urinary infections.

Reducing bladder overactivity and storage pressure and improving compliance

All the various measures designed to reduce bladder pressure have the potential drawback of impeding bladder emptying. Before embarking on treatment it is therefore important to ensure that effective bladder emptying can be achieved by CIC.

A nurse specialist plays an invaluable role in teaching the technique to the child and parents and providing ongoing support and advice. In cases when CIC is not possible, for example because of inability on the part of the child or parents or sensate urethra, the alternatives comprise an indwelling suprapubic catheter or a suprapubic cystostomy button device. This incorporates a valve mechanism which can be closed and opened intermittently to drain the bladder (e.g. two to three hourly intervals).[4,5]

Even when regular bladder emptying has been established with CIC, anticholinergic medication is commonly required to reduce bladder pressure and detrusor overactivity and to increase compliance. Many oral preparations are available (tolteridine, oxybutynin, solifenacin)—with varying dosages. Intravesical instillation of oxybutynin is not used routinely in children but may be used on a selective basis once effective CIC has been established.[6]

Intravesical injection of botulinum toxin A (BOTOX A) is being increasingly used in this age group.[7] Typically, diluted aliquots of 0.5–1 mL are injected endoscopically into 20–30 sites in the bladder wall under general anaesthesia. The duration of therapeutic benefit (reduction in detrusor overactivity and improved compliance) extends over three to nine months. Ideally, videourodynamics should be repeated after 6–12 weeks to verify the effectiveness of the treatment.

Although repeated injections will be required to maintain the benefit[8] this may still represent an acceptable approach if continence is improved during the period when the child is maturing and becoming more self-sufficient prior to undergoing major bladder surgery. The extent to which the therapeutic effect of Botox A on detrusor activity and compliance is reproduced after repeated injections is still unclear.[9]

Secondary vesicoureteric reflux often resolves or decreases following reduction in bladder pressure—for example following augmentation. However, specific intervention may be required in children who experience symptomatic UTIs. Endoscopic correction ('STING' procedure) has been used in neuropathic bladders[10] but success rates are lower than those for endoscopic correction of primary VUR in non-neuropathic bladders.[11] Antibiotic prophylaxis is advisable while VUR persists.

Increasing bladder capacity

Bladder capacity may be reduced as a consequence of physical contraction, functional overactivity—or a combination of both factors.

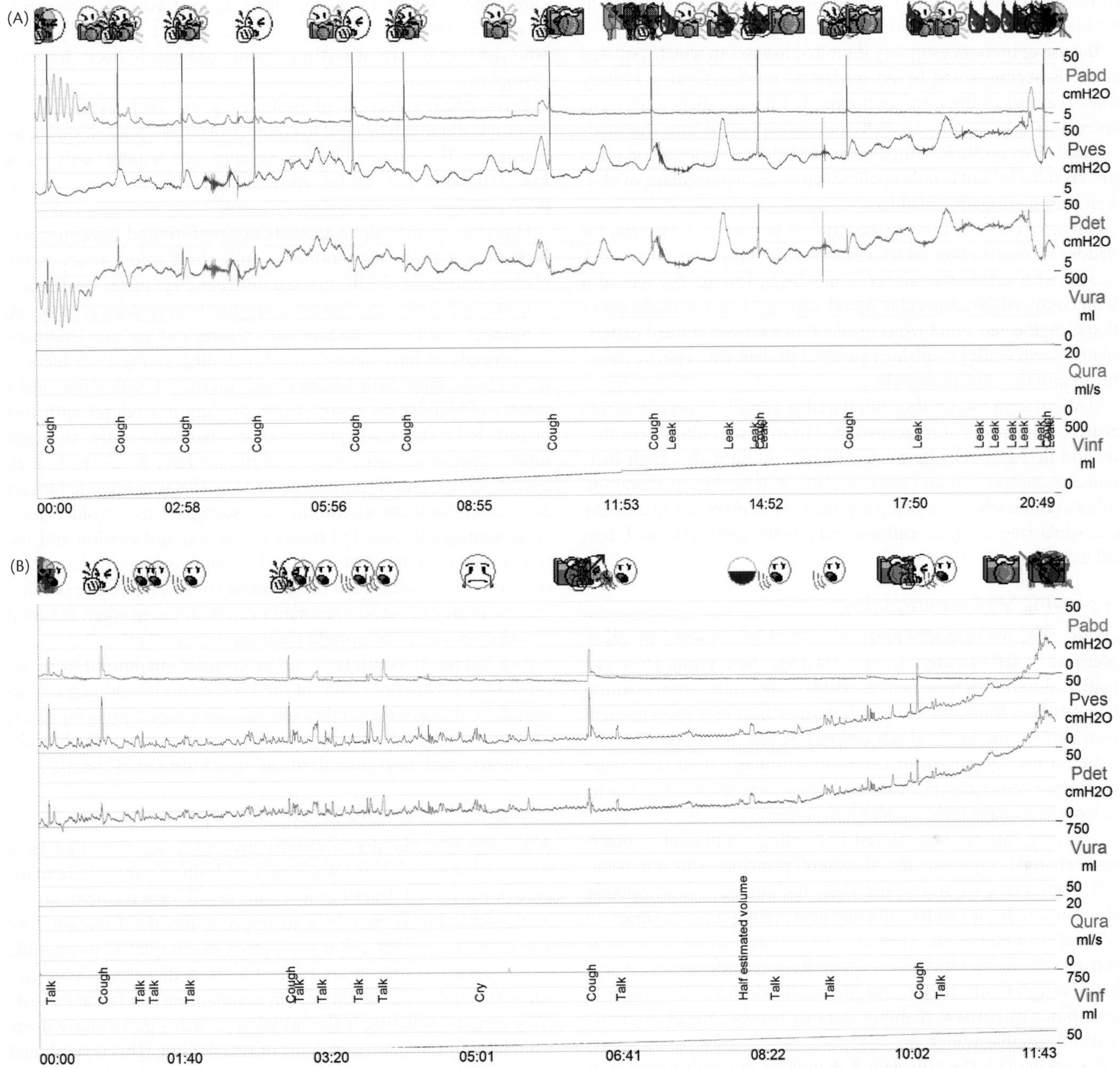

Fig. 8.6.1 (A) Urodynamic tracing demonstrating overactive bladder, leaking with contractions and compliance drift in a 13-year-old boy with myelomeningocoele. (B) Urodynamic tracing of 6.5 year old girl with thoracolumbar myelomeningocoele, wheelchair bound on four-hourly clean intermittent self-catheterization (CISC).

The use of intestinal segments to augment the neuropathic bladder (enterocystoplasty) has been widely practised in children for three decades. The most commonly performed procedure is 'clam ileocystoplasty' in which a 20–30 cm segment of distal ileum is isolated on its blood supply approximately 15 cm from the ileo caecal valve. The bowel is opened on its anti mesenteric aspect and then incorporated into the bladder after it has been widely opened ('bi-valved') in either the coronal or sagital plane. Ileum has the advantage of secreting less mucus than colon. Leaving the final 15 cm of terminal ileum *in situ* minimizes the risk of vitamin B12 malabsorption—which is a documented long-term complication of enterocystoplasty in children.[12] The use of stomach (gastrocystoplasty) has been largely abandoned because of dysuria and haematuria caused by acid secretion into the urine.

Other approaches have been explored to try and overcome the problems resulting from prolonged contact between urine and intestinal epithelium. In detrusorraphy or detrusorectomy the bladder wall muscle layer is incised or excised but the urothelial bladder lining is left *in situ*. Bladder capacity is thus increased by creating in effect, a large bladder diverticulum.[13]

Although both techniques have the advantage of retaining an urothelial-lined bladder they are unsuited for use in irregular, contracted bladders, and have a high long-term failure rate due to fibrosis and shrinkage. In the technique of seromuscular enterocystoplasty a 'demucosalized' bowel segment is attached to the bladder at the site of detrusorectomy.

The use of ureterocystoplasy is limited to cases in which a dilated ureter is accompanied by an ipsilateral nonfunctioning kidney. After removal of the nonfunctioning kidney the dilated ureter is opened, refashioned as a patch, and incorporated into the bladder wall. This urothelial-lined form of bladder augmentation gives good results[14,15] but is only applicable to a small percentage of children with neuropathic bladder.

Extensive research is being undertaken to develop a material for bladder reconstruction which combines the properties of smooth muscle with a tissue engineered urothelial lining. The use of a demucosalized seromuscular bowel segment lined with sheets of 'tissue engineered' autologous urothelium has been studied experimentally and while promising in animal studies, has yet to be introduced into the clinical domain.

Medium term results of a clinical trial in a small cohort of patients treated with a neobladder constructed from tissue cultured urothelial and detrusor cells have been disappointing with a high incidence of contraction and some instances of bladder perforation. Other avenues which are being explored experimentally include the use cellularized collagen scaffolds and possible applications of stem cell technology.[16–20]

Improving bladder emptying

Ideally, effective bladder emptying should be achieved by clean intermittent self catheterization (CISC) via the urethra. However, many children with neuropathic bladder often suffer from postural deformities or impaired manual dexterity which may prevent them from performing urethral self catheterization. Although CIC can be performed by parents or carers on an interim basis the longer term aim should always be to find some way of enabling young patients to manage their bladder independently.

For many, this can be achieved by creating a continent catheterizable channel employing the Mitofanoff principle. This is particularly helpful in girls and young women confined to a wheelchair who commonly encounter difficulty in accessing their urethra.

Many catheterizable conduits have been devised for the Mitrofanoff channel including; appendix, a reconfigured ileal segment (Yang/Monti), ureter, and prepucial skin tube. The choice is determined by tissue availability, distance between the bladder and skin and vascularity.[21,22]

The appendix is the Mitrofanoff channel of choice by virtue of its availability, reliability, ease of catheterization, and lower incidence of complications. Nevertheless, stenosis at the junction between the appendix and skin is common—although revision is a relatively simple procedure. Complications following the Mitrofanoff procedure tend to occur in the first year after surgery.[23]

Continence

Although achieving a socially acceptable degree of urinary continence is a secondary goal compared with the overriding priority of protecting upper tract function there seems little justification in subjecting a child or young person to major surgery unless they can also be offered the prospect of becoming dry.

If outflow resistance is sufficient, continence may sometimes be achieved simply by reducing intravesical pressure to below the 'leak point' pressure—for example, by bladder augmentation. However, additional measures are often needed to achieve complete continence (with CISC). An alpha agonist such as ephedrine 15 mg 3× /day may be effective and may also be useful in patients who develop recurrent wetting having previously been dry after cystoplasty.

Periurethral injection of bulking agents such as Deflux or Macroplastique can be used to enhance bladder neck and sphincter resistance. This minimally invasive approach requires only a day case admission and can be repeated on a number of occasions if necessary.

However, neither alpha agonists nor periurethral injections will be sufficient to create continence in a child whose neuropathic bladder is associated with marked outlet and sphincter weakness.

In this situation more invasive surgical intervention is required. A number of different bladder neck repairs and urethral lengthening procedures have been devised including Young Dees bladder neck repair, Pippi Salle bladder neck urethral lengthening, and a variety of bladder neck suspension or sling procedures with free or pedicled rectus fascia grafts and prosthetic materials. Although more effective in girls, these techniques have a relatively high overall failure rate in both sexes. The artificial urinary sphincter and periurethral constrictor are best suited for use in older boys. Disadvantages include the risks of infection and erosion and the requirement for the reservoir to be pumped to provide a fixed resistance. By contrast, the periurethral constrictor device is softer and the degree of outflow resistance can be adjusted when the child is conscious and in an upright position (Fig. 8.6.2).[24]

As a last resort, continence can be virtually guaranteed by surgical closure or disconnection of the bladder neck—although occasionally a fistula to the urethra necessitates a repeat procedure. It is self-evident that this approach can only be adopted if the bladder can be accessed for regular drainage via a Mitrofanoff channel.

Treatment strategies for the neuropathic bowel

A neuropathic bladder is almost invariably accompanied by a neuropathic bowel. It is important that both conditions are managed jointly—not least because successful management of the neuropathic bowel may help to improve bladder function. The aim is to ensure that colon is emptied as completely as possible on a regular and socially convenient basis. A diet rich in fibre and adequate fluid intake are helpful in maintaining soft faecal consistency. Regular toileting is the initial approach—particularly if the child has any sensation of colonic or rectal filling. This is combined with medical therapy comprising stool softeners (lactulose), stimulants (Sennakot or Movicol), suppositories (glycerine or dulcolax) or enemas such as phosphate enemas.

For many children, more intensive management is required to prevent constipation and minimize faecal soiling. In the first instance this is likely to consist of retrograde rectal or colonic washouts. While this approach provides predictability it is cumbersome, relatively messy, and unsuited for use in older children seeking to be less dependent on parents or carers. Moreover, some leakage of fluid and faecal material often occurs for a while after the enema. A containable form of washout using a closed system of irrigation and drainage (Peristeen) has been introduced recently and is being increasingly adopted (Fig. 8.6.3).[25]

Unlike conventional enemas administered via the rectal route antegrade colonic washouts empty the large bowel by administration of irrigating fluid through a tube positioned in the caecum. The child must be able to sit on a toilet for up to one hour and be

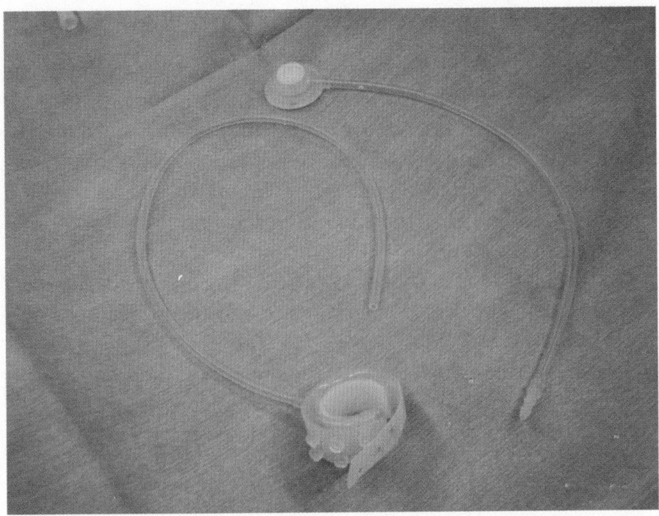

Fig. 8.6.2 Lima (SILIMED) urethral constrictor.

prepared to tolerate either a caecostomy tube or a caecostomy button device on the abdominal wall.

The MACE procedure (Malone antegrade continent enema) (Fig. 8.6.4), utilizes the Mitrofanoff principle and consists of a continent catheterizable conduit (usually appendix) connected to the large bowel. A catheter is passed via the conduit into the bowel for the administration of an antegrade colonic washout. The catheter is then removed, leaving only a small, discreet stoma flush with the abdominal wall which is often hidden within the umbilical cicatrix).[26]

Recent modifications of the MACE procedure include the use of a laparoscopic rather than open approach and placement of the conduit in the left side of the colon.[27,28] The acceptability and success of the MACE procedure is reflected in high satisfaction scores from patients and parents.[29,30]

Long-term follow-up and outcomes

Augmentation cystoplasty

Despite the need for major surgery and the risk of complications, bladder augmentation and continent urinary diversion receive high patient acceptability/satisfaction scores. Up to 90–95% of patients achieve acceptable continence rates while over 80% maintain stable long-term renal function. Among the commoner complications are stone formation (15–20%) and adhesive intestinal obstruction (5%).[31] The long-term risk of malignancy in augmented bladders remains unclear but is probably of the order 1–2%.

Mitrofanoff procedure

The incidence of stomal stenosis is of the order of 40%[31] and this complication occurs most frequently in the first postoperative year.

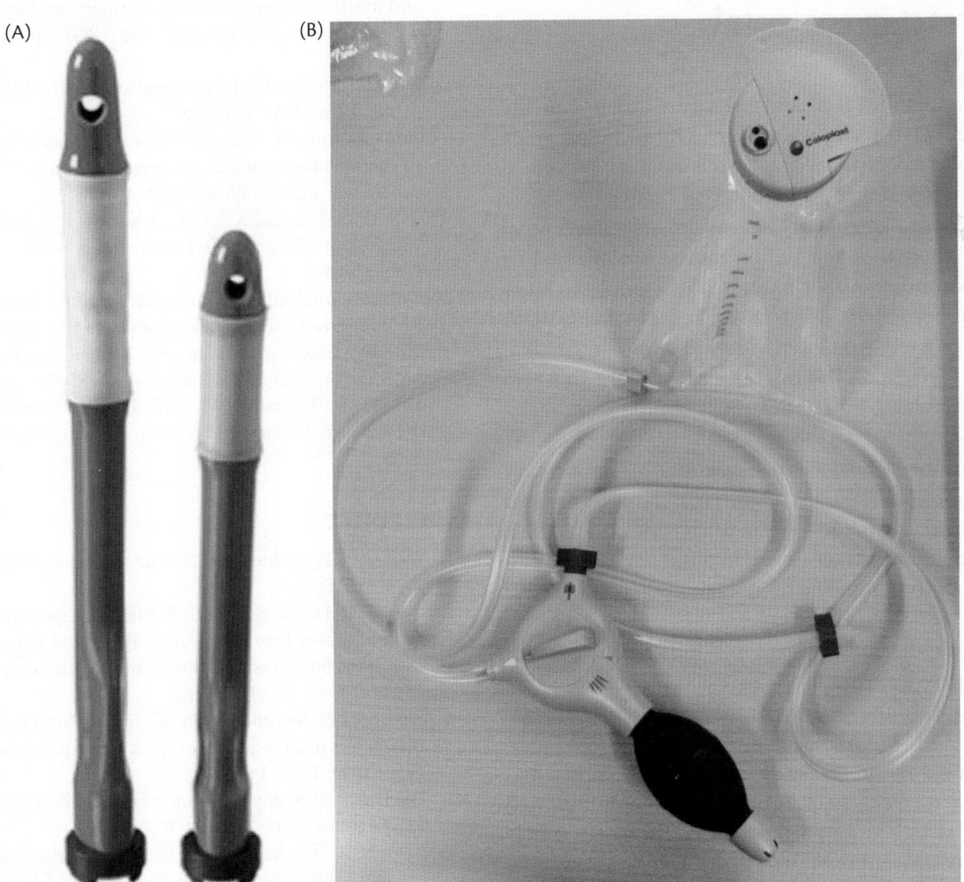

Fig. 8.6.3 (A) Peristeen washout tubing and irrigation set; and (B) peristeen rectal catheters.

(A) Reproduced with permission from COLOPLAST.

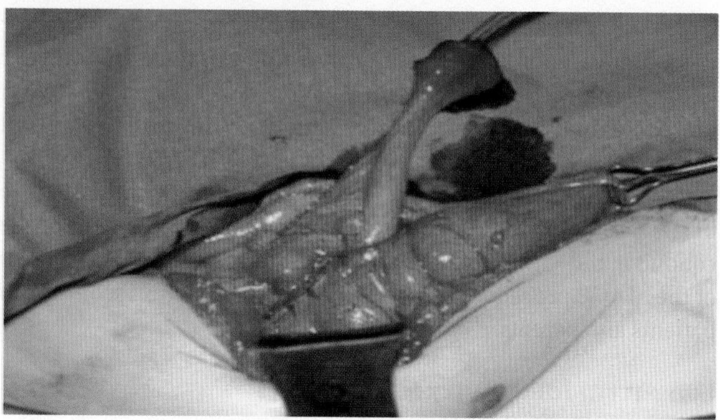

Fig. 8.6.4 Operative photograph of use of appendix for *in situ* MACE (Malone antegrade continence enema) procedure.

The use of a 'stopper' inserted into the stoma between catheterization has been reported to reduce the risk of this complication.[32]

Malone antegrade continent enema

The long-term success of the MACE procedure has been well established although it has become apparent that not all children will continue to use it into adulthood for various reasons. The technique of *in situ* appendicocaecostomy is preferred by many surgeons.[33]

The urinary tract in anorectal malformations

This spectrum of anomalies is characterized by absence of the anus on the perineum. In males with a high ano rectal anomaly the lower bowel joins the urinary tract via a congenital recto—urethral fistula. The incidence is 1:5,000 live births and many cases are now diagnosed antenatally because of associated renal or sacral vertebral anomalies—including those encompassed by the VACTERL association. Abnormalities of the upper urinary tract are present in more than 50% of cases. These include: VUR, PUJ obstruction, crossed fused renal ectopia, and renal dysplasia or agenesis. Vertebral abnormalities are present in up to 40% of cases—particularly those with more complex anorectal malformations.

Of the various protocols devised for evaluation of the urinary tract, the ARGUS protocol[34] is the author's preference. Infants with a low anorectal anomaly, a normal sacrum and normal appearances of the urinary tract on ultrasound are unlikely to experience bladder dysfunction and do not require more intensive investigation.

Conversely, videourodynamic evaluation is indicated in cases of high anorectal anomaly. Depending on the results of spinal imaging and urinary tract ultrasound further investigations may include spinal MRI scan, DMSA, and MCUG.

Surgical correction of anorectal malformations is complex and is often undertaken in stages, with an initial colostomy followed later by an anorectal pull through procedure. The most widely performed definitive procedure is the PSARP (posterior saggital anorectoplasty). Because up to 10% of children develop bladder dysfunction postoperatively, clinical and ultrasonographic follow-up is advisable until the child is fully potty trained.

Long-term outcomes

These are very variable and are determined to a large extent by the severity of the anorectal malformation, the extent of any associated sacral abnormality, presence of a neuropathic bladder and any associated other congenital problems. Bowel problems including constipation and soiling are often intractable and chronic constipation can compromise the outcome of bladder reconstruction by posing an increased risk of urinary infection and stone formation.

On rare occasions the only way of achieving independence and a socially acceptable degree of continence may be by creating a permanent colostomy.

The long-term outlook for renal function in children whose urinary tract abnormalities are associated with cloacal anaomalies is generally favourable although lifelong follow-up is essential.[35]

Conclusion

There have been very significant advances in the management of neuropathic bladder and bowel in children during the last 20 to 30 years. It is now possible to conserve renal function while offering the prospect of a socially acceptable degree of urinary continence in the majority of affected children. Increasing understanding of long-term outcomes is likely to lead to further advances in management.

Further reading

Boemers TML, Beek FJA, Bax NM. Guidelines for the urological screening and initial management of lower urinary tract dysfunction in children with anorectal malformations—the ARGUS protocol. *BJU Int* 1999; **83**:662–71.

Farrugia MK, Malone PS. Educational article: The Mitrofanoff procedure. *J Pediatr Urol* 2010; **6**(4):330–7.

Herndon CD, Rink RC, Cain MP, Lerner M, Kaefer M, Yerkes E, Casale AJ. In situ Malone antegrade continence enema in 127 patients: a 6-year experience. *J Urol* 2004; **172**(4 Pt 2):1689–91.

Johal NS, Hamid R, Aslam Z, Carr B, Vuckiw PM, Duffy PG. Ureterocystoplasty: long term functional results. *J Urol* 2008; **179**:2373–4.

López Pereira P, Salvador OP, Arcas JA, Martínez Urrutia MA, Romera RL, Monereo EJ. Transanal irrigation for the treatment of neuropathic bowel dysfunction. *J Pediatr Urol* 2010; **6**(2):134–8.

Steinbrecher HA, Malone PS, Ricjwood AMK. Neuropathic bladder. (pp. 171–87) In: Thomas DFM, Duffy PG, Rickwood AMK (eds). *Essentials of Paediatric Urology*, 2nd edition. London, UK: Informa Healthcare, 2008.

References

1. Ashcraft KW, Holder TM. Hereditary presacral teratoma. *J Pediatr Surg* 1974; **9**(5):691–7.
2. Cremer R, Hoppe A, Korsch E, Kleine-Diepenbruck U, Bläker F. Natural rubber latex allergy: prevalence and risk factors in patients with spina bifida compared with atopic children and controls. *Eur J Pediatr* 1998; **157**(1):13–16.
3. Ellsworth PI, Merguerian PA, Klein RB, Rozycki AA. Evaluation and risk factors of latex allergy in spina bifida patients: is it preventable? *J Urol* 1993; **150**(2 Pt 2):691–3.
4. Hitchcock RJ, Sadiq M. Button vesicostomy: a continent urinary stoma. *J Pediatr Urol* 2007; **3**(2):104–8.
5. Bennett SG, Bennett S, Bell TE. The gastrostomy button as a catheterizable urinary stoma: A pilot study. *J Urol* 2003; **170**(3):832–4.
6. Guerra LA, Moher D, Sampson M, Barrowman N, Pike J, Leonard M. Intravesical oxybutynin for children with poorly compliant neurogenic bladder: a systematic review. *J Urol* 2008; **180**:1091–7.

7. Schulte-Baukloh H, Michael T, Schobert J, Stolze T, Knispel H. Efficacy of botulinum-A toxin in children with detrusor hyperreflexia due to myelomeningocele: preliminary results. *Urology* 2002; **59**:325.
8 Schulte-Baukloh H, Knispel H, Stolze T, Weiss C, Michael T, Miller K. Repeated botulinum-A toxin injections in treatment of children with neurogenic detrusor overactivity. *Urology* 2005; **66**:865.
9. Gamé X, Mouracade P, Chartier-Kastler E, *et al.* Botulinum toxin-A (Botox®) intradetrusor injections in children with neurogenic detrusor overactivity/neurogenic overactive bladder: A systematic literature review. *J Pediatr Urol* 2009; **5**(3):156–64.
10. Quinn FM, Diamond T, Boston VE. Endoscopic management of vesico-ureteric reflux in children with neuropathic bladder secondary to myelomeningocoele. *Z Kinderchir* 1988; **43**(Suppl 2):43–45.
11. Granata C, Buffa P, Di Rovasenda E, *et al.* Treatment of vesico-ureteric reflux in children with neuropathic bladder: a comparison of surgical and endoscopic correction. *J Pediatr Surg* 1999; **34**(12):1836–8.
12. Blackburn SC, Parkar S, Prime M, *et al.* Ileal bladder augmentation and vitamin B12: levels decrease with time after surgery. *J Pediatr Urol* 2012; **8**(1):47–50.
13. Cartwright PC and Snow BW. Bladder auto-augmentation: partial detrusor excision to augment the bladder without the use of bowel. *J Urol* 1989; **142**:1050–3.
14. Churchill BM, Aliabadi H, Landau EH, *et al.* Ureteral bladder augmentation. *J Urol* 1993; **150**:716–20.
15. Johal NS, Hamid R, Aslam Z, Carr B, Vuckiw PM, Duffy PG. Ureterocystoplasty: long term functional results. *J Urol* 2008; **179**:2373–4.
16. Falke G, Caffaratti J, Atala A. Tissue engineering of the bladder. *World J Urol* 2000; **18**(1):36–43.
17. Fraser M, Thomas DF, Pitt E, Harnden P, Trejdosiewicz LK, Southgate J. A surgical model of composite cystoplasty with cultured urothelial cells: a controlled study of gross outcome and urothelial phenotype. *BJU Int* 2004; **93**(4):609–16.
18. Atala, A, Bauer SB, Soker S, *et al.* Tissue engineered autolagous bladder for patients needing cystoplasty. *Lancet* 2006; **367**:1241–6.
19. Stanasel I, Mirzazadeh M, Smith JJ 3rd. Bladder tissue engineering. *Urol Clin North Am* 2010; **37**(4):593–9.
20. Turner A, Subramanian R, Thomas DFM, *et al.* Transplantation of autologous differential urothelium in an experimental model of composite cystoplasty. *Eur Urol* 2011; **59**:447–54.
21. Cain MP, Casale AJ, King SJ, Rink RC. Appendicovesicostomy and newer alternatives for the Mitrofanoff procedure: results in the last 100 patients at Riley Children's Hospital. *J Urol* 1999; **162**(5):1749–52.
22. Farrugia MK, Malone PS. Educational article: The Mitrofanoff procedure. *J Pediatr Urol* 2010; **6**(4):330–7.
23. Thomas JC, Dietrich MS, Trusler L, *et al.* Continent catheterizable channels and the timing of their complications. *J Urol* 2006; **176**(4 Pt 2):1816–20; discussion 1820.
24. Farrugia MK, Lottmann HB, Neilson A, Nicholls G, Woodward M, Malone PS. Outcome of the lima periurethral constrictor in children and adolescents: a European perspective. *J Urol* 2012; **188**(4 Suppl):1555–60.
25. López Pereira P, Salvador OP, Arcas JA, Martínez Urrutia MA, Romera RL, Monereo EJ. Transanal irrigation for the treatment of neuropathic bowel dysfunction. *J Pediatr Urol* 2010; **6**(2):134–8.
26. Curry JI, Osborne A, Malone PS. The MACE procedure: experience in the United Kingdom. *J Pediatr Surg* 1999; **34**(2):338–40.
27. Sinha CK, Butler C, Haddad M. Eur Antegrade Continent Enema (LACE): review of the literature. *J Pediatr Surg* 2008; **18**(4):215–8.
28. Herndon CD, Rink RC, Cain MP, Lerner M, Kaefer M, Yerkes E, Casale AJ. In situ Malone antegrade continence enema in 127 patients: a 6-year experience. *J Urol* 2004; **172**(4 Pt 2):1689–91.
29. Ok JH, Kurzrock EA. Objective measurement of quality of life changes after ACE Malone using the FICQOL survey. *J Pediatr Urol* 2011; **7**(3):389–93.
30. Tiryaki S, Ergun O, Celik A, Ulman I, Avanoglu A. Success of Malone's antegrade continence enema (MACE) from the patients' perspective. *Eur J Pediatr Surg* 2010; **20**(6):405–7.
31. Bani-Hani AH, Cain MP, Kaefer M, Meldrum KK, King S, Johnson CS, Rink RC. The Malone antegrade continence enema: single institutional review. *J Urol* 2008; **180**(3):1106–10.
32. Peter Rubenwolf, Antje beissert, Elmar Gerharz, H Riedmiller. 15 years of continent urinary diversion and enterocystoplasty in children and adolescents: the Wuerzburg experience. *BJU Int* 2009; **105**:698–705.
33. Ardelt PU, Wodhouse CRJ, Riedmiller H, Gerhar EW. The efferent segment in continent cutaneous urinary diversion: a comprehensive review of the literature. *BJU Int* 2011; **109**:288–97.
34. Boemers TML, Beek FJA, Bax NM. Guidelines for the urological screening and initial management of lower urinary tract dysfunction in children with anorectal malformations—the ARGUS protocol. *BJU Int* 1999; **83**:662–71.
35. Braga LH, Lorenzo AJ, Dave S, Del-Valle MH, Khoury AE, Pippi-Salle JL. Long-term renal function and continence status in patients with cloacal malformation. *Can Urol Assoc J* 2007; **1**(4):371–6.

CHAPTER 8.7

Urinary incontinence and bladder dysfunction

Henrik Steinbrecher

Introduction to urinary incontinence and bladder dysfunction

Daytime (diurnal) and night-time (nocturnal) wetting are among the commonest symptoms of childhood. Successful management requires an understanding of normal maturation of the bladder cycle and the functional abnormalities which cause incontinence.

Terminology and definitions (ICCS classification)

The most widely used classification of bladder dysfunction is the one published International Children's Continence Society (ICCS).[1] Urinary incontinence is defined as the 'uncontrollable leakage of urine, which may be either continuous or intermittent'. However, intermittent incontinence is only regarded as being abnormal in children aged over five years.

Nocturnal enuresis is defined as 'the symptom of involuntary wetting during sleep without any inherent suggestion of frequency or pathophysiology'.[2]

Many common symptoms such as urgency, hesitancy, or delay before initiating the urinary stream cannot be reliably assessed until the age at which normal bladder control has been achieved. Moreover, an intermittent stream is not abnormal under the age of three years (unless it is accompanied by straining).

Children normally void between three and seven times per day. Normal bladder capacity in children over the age of 2 years can be estimated as follows; 30+ (age in years ×30) mL.

Prevalance, incidence, and epidemiology

Daytime wetting is common in children, with a prevalence of 15% in four year olds, declining to 5% in nine year olds. Mild nocturnal enuresis (occurring less than twice a week) affects >20% of children aged four to five years. By nine years of age, 8% of children are occasional bed wetters while 1–2% of this age group continues to experience more severe and regular nocturnal enuresis.[3] Nocturnal enuresis has a strong familial tendency and boys are affected more commonly than girls. Although the problem usually resolves over the course of childhood, a small percentage of adolescents continue to suffer from intractable nocturnal enuresis. Detrusor instability is a normal phenomenon in infancy and early childhood but resolves in 90% of children by the age of 5.[4,5]

Development and physiological maturation of the micturition cycle

The lower urinary tract is innervated by autonomic and somatic neural pathways. Parasympathetic pathways are represented by pre and postganglionic fibres from S2, S3, and S4 whereas the sympathetic innervation originates in the spinal cord at T10-L2. Somatic nerves originating in S2-S4 coalesce to form the pudendal nerves supplying the pelvic floor muscles and external urethral sphincter.

Newborns and small infants void approximately once an hour. Voiding is a reflex function at this age but neurological regulation of lower urinary tract function matures during the early years of childhood. During toilet training (and for a short time afterwards) voiding is associated with a transitional pattern of voluntary inhibition of the voiding reflex by supraspinal centres. The normal voiding cycle is usually established by seven years of age—by which time children normally void between three to seven times a days.

The key elements of the normal micturition cycle and bladder–sphincter interaction are illustrated in Figure 8.7.1.

Clinical assessment

History

A detailed history should be obtained from the child and parents with the aim of answering three key questions;

(i) *Is the urinary leakage continuous or intermittent?* Continuous leakage suggests an underlying structural abnormality (ectopic duplex ureter, congenitally short female urethra, female epispadias) or sphincter weakness whereas intermittent leakage is more suggestive of a functional aetiology.

(ii) *Does the incontinence occur both during the daytime and night or is it confined either to the day (diurnal enuresis) or night (nocturnal enuresis)?* Incontinence confined to the day in a child who is dry at night almost invariably has a functional basis. However, some forms of ectopic ureter may give rise to minimal leakage at night.

(iii) *Is the urinary incontinence primary or secondary?* Incontinence is defined as being primary if the child has never been reliably dry. This history points towards a structural or neurogenic cause. By contrast, if there has ever been a period when the child was consistently dry (even if only for a few months) this

NORMAL BLADDER (Storage - voiding) CYCLE

1. Bladder fills and urethra contracts (via T10–12 lumber sympathetics and S2-4 Voluntary somatic)

There is RECEPTIVE RELAXATION of the bladder giving HIGH COMPILANCE (dv/dp) = mL/cm water

2. Urethra relaxes (via S2–4 Voluntary somatic)

3. Pelvic floor relaxes (via S2–4 Voluntary somatic)

4. Bladder detrusor contracts (via parasympathetic S2–4)

5. Urinary flow to completion

6. Urethra contracts (via S2–4 Voluntary somatic)

NORMAL BLADDER/URETHRAL FUNCTION

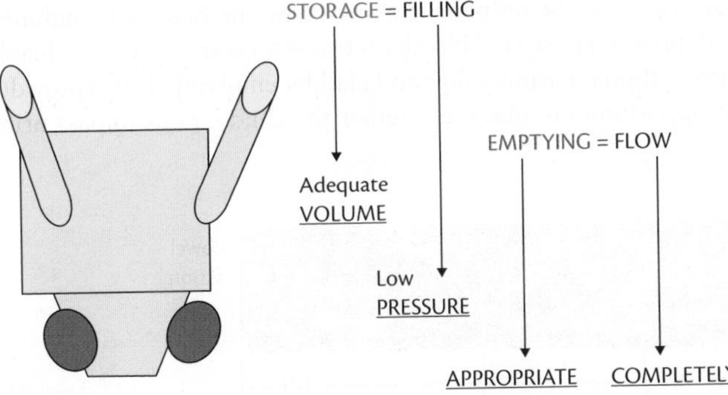

Fig. 8.7.1 The normal micturition cycle.

constitutes secondary incontinence—for which a functional cause is far more likely.The following aspects of the history may help guide the clinician towards a diagnosis.

Voiding frequency

Children normally void between three to seven times per day. More frequent voiding is suggestive of bladder instability or a hypersensitive bladder. Conversely children who void less frequently than normal may have an underactive bladder and an overflow pattern of incontinence.

Urgency and urge incontinence

Using simple language it is important to try and establish from the child and parent(s) whether the incontinence is accompanied by urgency.

Stress incontinence

Evidence of stress leakage is most apparent during coughing, sneezing, or sporting activity. It is important to note, however, that wetting provoked by laughter may be caused by the specific condition of giggle incontinence rather than stress leakage.

Urinary stream

Although the characteristics of the stream can be difficult to assess from the history in young children, it is nevertheless important to enquire about the strength of the stream and whether urine is passed with a continuous or intermittent flow. These observations may provide valuable clues to the presence of bladder–sphincter dyssynergia or outflow obstruction.

Urinary infection

Is there a history of isolated or recurrent urinary tract infections (UTIs)? Certain patterns of bladder dysfunction strongly predispose to urinary tract infection. In turn urinary tract infection can provoke bladder dysfunction.

Bowel function

The association between lower urinary tract symptoms and disordered bowel function (notably constipation) is well recognized and relatively common. The combination of urinary incontinence and faecal soiling (encopresis) is termed 'elimination disorder'.

Fluid input/output

The child and parents should be specifically questioned about fluid intake (type, amount) and urine output (amount and regularity). It is helpful to have a mug or cup available in the clinic to indicate the volumes involved since children and parents almost invariably overestimate daily fluid intake.

Family history and associated conditions

It is important to inquire about predisposing factors such as a family history of nocturnal enuresis, asthma (higher risk of stress incontinence), or associated behavioural and cognitive disorders. For example, attention deficit hyperactivity syndrome, autistic spectrum disorder, and trisomy 21 (Down's syndrome) all carry an increased risk of dysfunctional voiding and urinary incontinence. Children with these disorders are less likely to experience spontaneous resolution of their symptoms and have a lower response rate to treatment.

Social history

This includes information on size of the family, number of siblings, sleeping arrangements (e.g. bunk beds) and ease of access to a toilet at night. It is also important to enquire about the child's sleeping habits (e.g. depth of sleep and whether they can be aroused from sleep.)

Vaginal 'reflux'

Vaginal 'reflux' (retrograde filling of the vagina during voiding) is characterized by intermittent urinary incontinence immediately or shortly after voiding. Typically it occurs around the time of puberty when the body's habitus changes, but may also occur in girls who tend to sit on the toilet with their legs close together. Labial adhesions can also cause dribbling incontinence after voiding due to retrograde accumulation of urine within the partly occluded vagina, which then drains out involuntarily when the girl stands up to leave the toilet.

In its purest form, giggle incontinence only occurs during laughter and not at other times. This distressing condition has a neurological basis which is believed to be related to dissociation of upper neuronal control and relaxation of the pelvic floor and sphincter mechanism. *Giggle incontinence* is often exacerbated by coexistent bladder instability.

Examination

Every child with urinary incontinence should undergo a careful clinical examination including;

Abdominal examination/palpation. This may reveal, for example, evidence of constipation, faecal loading, or a palpably distended bladder.

Genital examination may reveal relevant abnormalities of the external genitalia—notably epispadias (both male and female) and labial adhesions.

Inspection and palpation of the spine is mandatory to look for external evidence of underlying spinal dysraphism (hairy tufts, haemangiomas, absent sacrum). Limited neurological examination of the lower limbs (sensation, tone, power, and reflexes) will determine if the lower lumbar and sacral spinal segments are functioning normally. However this is often difficult in small children.

Investigations

Perhaps the simplest aid to clinical assessment is a *frequency/volume chart* (Fig. 8.7.2). Despite some variation in design all such charts include a 24 hour time column, a column recording fluid intake and a column recording urinary output. The chart should also record when urinary leakage occurs and when the child has a bowel action. It is also useful to record the time when the child arises and goes to bed.

'Child friendly' features such as cartoons can be helpful in enlisting the child's compliance to improve the accuracy of the recorded information. A chart which has been accurately completed over 48 hours is usually sufficient to provide an informative picture of the child's fluid input, urinary output, and voiding habits. Moreover, in practice, it is difficult for families to maintain an accurate record for much longer than 48 hours. The commitment shown by the child and parents to the completion of an input/output chart can provide a helpful insight into the impact of the incontinence on the lives of the child and family and their commitment to comply with treatment.

Inevitably, charts tend to be compiled over a weekend and may not provide an accurate reflection of the normal school day when fluid intake and voiding habits tend to be disrupted by school routines, peer pressure, and phobia of school toilets.

Urinalysis is essential to test for infection or glycosuria. The onset of diabetes melitus (or, very rarely, diabetes insipidus) may be accompanied by polyuria, frequency, and incontinence.

A simple non–invasive *flow rate* measurement (which can be performed in the outpatient clinic or by the bedside) combined with pre- and post-void bladder ultrasound scan will yield valuable information on urinary flow and bladder emptying. It also provides an opportunity to observe whether the child strains to pass urine

Date			Degree of urgency				Wet episodes		Comments
Time	Volume in	Volume out	None	Mild	Moderate	Severe	Yes	No	
01:00									
02:00									
03:00									
04:00									
05:00									
06:00									
07:00									
08:00									
09:00									
10:00									
11:00									
12:00									
13:00									
14:00									
15:00									
16:00									
17:00									
18:00									
19:00									
20:00									
21:00									
22:00									
23:00									
00:00									

Bowel action

Return charts to your nurse/doctor at next visit.

Please complete this frequency volume chart everytime you have a drink or go to the toilet.

Please tick if wet or dry each time you go to the toilet and record level of wetting in comments column.
Please record on comments chart when you go for a poo.

Fig. 8.7.2 A typical frequency volume chart.

or, (in an older child) whether they are capable of voluntary midstream interruption of voiding.

An *ultrasound scan* of the urinary tract will provide information on the kidneys including their position, size, shape, and morphology (e.g. simplex or duplex). Imaging of the bladder should assess; pre-void bladder volume, post void bladder residual, bladder size, shape, and wall thickness.

Depending upon the results of initial investigations and the differential diagnosis further imaging may be indicated as follows;

Lumbo-sacral spinal X-ray and/or magnetic resonance imaging (MRI) of the spine and spinal cord

MRI is the investigation of choice if there is any suggestion of neurological deficit or external cutaneous abnormality denoting possible 'occult' dysraphism. Imaging in such cases may reveal cord tethering, syrinxes, or cord lipomas.

Magnetic resonance urography or laparoscopy can be very helpful in visualizing ectopic duplex ureters in the pelvis and occult dysplastic kidneys with ectopic drainage.

Cystourethroscopy is of particular value in assessing urethral size and length and bladder neck anatomy in girls with urogenital sinus anomalies.

Videourodynamic assessment rarely forms part of the routine investigation of children with non-neuropathic incontinence. This invasive investigation can be very distressing in this age group and information obtained in these circumstances may be potentially misleading and less informative than a carefully taken history.

Nevertheless videourodynamics can play a selective role in the investigation of older children and adolescents with intractable incontinence. Intervention such as bladder augmentation or botulinum toxin injection should never be contemplated without prior videourodynamic evaluation.

Treatment

Structural abnormalities

Surgery is invariably required for incontinence caused by anatomical abnormalities because there is no prospect of spontaneous resolution. An ectopic ureter can sometimes be managed by reimplantation or ureteroureterostomy, but since function in the upper moiety of a duplex kidney associated with an ectopic ureter is usually very poor, heminephrectomy is generally the preferred option.

Congenital short urethra is a poorly defined entity. Surgical intervention may be indicated if there is no response to simple measures for stress incontinence such as ephedrine 5 mg three times a day or pelvic floor exercises (which are not usually feasible in prepubertal children). The surgical options are similar to those for stress leakage in adult women and include bladder neck sling procedures and periurethral injection of bulking agents.

Female epispadias requires more extensive reconstructive surgery. This comprises open bladder neck repair and possible bladder augmentation and/or Mitrofanoff procedure, depending on the severity of the anomaly and urodynamic findings.

Labial adhesions causing post void dribbling can often be managed conservatively by the application of topical oestrogen cream (oestradiol 0.01% topical) twice daily for six weeks. Alternatively, separation can be performed under brief general anaesthesia.

Dribbling caused by retrograde filling of the vagina ('vaginal reflux' is managed by advice on positioning. The girl is encouraged to sit on the toilet with her legs further apart (or even astride the toilet) to facilitate more effective opening of the introitus. A gentle cough or Valsalva manoevre after voiding will help to expel any urine that has tracked up the vagina.

Simple strategies for functional urinary incontinence

One of the simplest and most effective forms of treatment consists of explaining the nature of the normal micturition cycle to the child and parents. This is accompanied by advice on simple measures intended to establish a more normal voiding pattern. These include emphasizing the importance of regular voiding (typically 5–6 times a day at two or three hourly intervals) and staying at the toilet long enough to ensure complete bladder emptying. The child should maintain a regular fluid intake with a total volume appropriate to her/his age. As an estimate this is 500 mL per day at five years of age, 750 mL at age seven, 1,000 mL at age 10, 1,250 mL at age 10, and 1,500—2,000 mL from 15 years upwards.

Guidelines on bedwetting published by the National Institute of Clinical Excellence[2] recommend slightly higher fluid intake than cited above.

Drinks to be avoided (especially in children with overactive bladders) include tea, coffee, hot chocolate, cola type drinks, and blackcurrent drinks. Apart from their diuretic properties some constituents of these drinks may also exert a direct stimulant effect on the detrusor.

Intake/output charts in children with nocturnal enuresis frequently reveal evidence of a high fluid intake in the afternoon and evening with a low fluid intake during the morning and early afternoon at school.

Initial advice should be reinforced by regular and frequent follow-up—either in the outpatient clinic or by telephone. A urology nurse specialist often plays a key role in this process.

When dysfunctional voiding is complicated by UTI, appropriate additional measures include; increasing fluid intake and voiding frequency (to promote more effective diuresis and bladder emptying), avoiding exposure to bubble baths which may change perineal bacterial flora and introducing bio-yoghurt into the diet.

The use of prophylactic antibiotics may be occasionally justified until the underlying bladder dysfunction has resolved.

Constipation is commonly implicated as a cause of urinary infection and bladder dysfunction. Regular administration of laxatives (e.g. sennakot 2.5–5 mL/day) or softening agents (e.g. Movicol Paediatric, half—one sachet/day or lactulose 2.5–5 mL day) can help to maintain an empty rectum and, in turn, promote more effective bladder function.

Advanced strategies for functional incontinence

If the simple measure outlined above do not result in any improvement more invasive measures must be considered, depending on symptoms and the pattern of bladder dysfunction.

Overactive bladder

Incontinence due to severe detrusor overactivity is characterized by frequency and urgency. Anticholinergic agents should be considered for those children whose symptoms do not respond to conservative measures. Typically, the first line of treatment is oxybutynin in an initial dose of 2.5 mg twice daily, increasing to 2.5 mg three times a day if necessary. The main alternative is tolteridine (1–2 mg twice a day). Slow release preparations are available (slow release oxybutynin 5–10 mg, once a day, slow release tolteridine 2–4 mg, once a day).

Because of their M1 antimuscarinic mode of pharmacological action these anticholinergics carry a risk of side effects including; dry eyes, dry mouth, constipation and, occasional, personality/behavioural changes. Solifenacin (an M3 anticholinergic agent with minimal systemic effects) is being increasingly used in older children in a dosage of 5–10 mg daily but is not yet licensed for use in children.

The use of *transcutaneous electrical nerve stimulation* has been reported with a typical treatment regimen comprising 20 minutes of use three times a week over a six week period. A success rate in selected cases of up to 60% has been claimed but the duration of symptomatic improvement is variable.

Intravesical injection of Botulinum A toxin is an option for young people with severe and intractable bladder overactivity which has failed to respond to other measures. It is essential that clean intermittent self-catheterization (CISC) is discussed and even taught prior to the procedure in view of the significant risk (5%) of incomplete bladder emptying or frank urinary retention following Botulinum toxin injection. The duration of action is between 3–9 months and repeated injections are often required.

Other, more invasive forms of treatment of a severely overactive bladder include

Posterior tibial nerve neurostimulation

This treatment has been used predominantly in adults in whom it appears to be more effective in treating overactive than underactive bladders.[6–8] Similar considerations apply to *sacral nerve stimulation*.[9,10] As a last resort, *bladder augmentation* is effective treatment of severe bladder over activity. However the balance between the potential benefits and drawbacks (including the probable need for intermittent catheterization) should be carefully considered before advising major reconstructive surgery in children and young people with non-neuropathic bladder dysfunction.

Bladder–sphincter dyssynergia/ dysfunctional voiding

This is characterized by a variable, intermittent urinary stream. However, this condition can only be reliably diagnosed by vieourodynamics—which typically demonstrate alternating detrusor contraction and relaxation in conjunction with incomplete sphincter relaxation. Bladder (detrusor)—spincter dyssynergia may be an acquired pattern of bladder behaviour which develops in response to incontinence caused by detrusor overactivity. Girls are affected more commonly than boys and the condition is often associated with urinary infections and secondary vesico-ureteric reflux. Management is based on a sustained programme of 're-education of the voiding mechanism' by utilizing cognitive bladder training with or without intermittent catheterization. This is a time-consuming and demanding process which may require one-to-one input from a trained urotherapist. Non-invasive biofeedback techniques using visual and sensory clues may be effective in teaching children to recognize their own bladder sensation and modify their bladder activity accordingly.

At its most extreme, bladder–sphincter dyssynergia can progress to mimic the features of neuropathic bladder. Termed 'non-neuropathic neuropathic bladder' or 'Hinman's syndrome' this serious condition shares the same radiological features as a genuine neuropathic bladder namely; trabeculation and 'fir tree' or 'cottage loaf' appearance on micturating cystourethrogram (MCUG) and videourodynamics. By the time the diagnosis has been established, secondary upper tract changes have often supervened. There may be a history of significant psychological or physical turmoil dating from the time of potty training. Because of the significant risk posed to the upper urinary tract, aggressive management must be instituted using similar measures to those employed in treating a genuine neuropathic bladder (see chapter 'Neuropathic bladder and anorectal anomalies').

Functional sensory urgency

This condition is poorly understood and while the onset may occasionally be traced to a minor urinary infection no aetiological factor can be identified in the majority of cases. Sensory urgency is commoner in girls and is generally unresponsive to anticholinergics. The mainstay of treatment is bladder training whereby children are instructed to defer voiding when they first experience the urge to void. Initially voiding is deferred by a 5–10 minute period but the duration is gradually increased depending on what the child can tolerate comfortably.

Functional underactivity of the bladder

This is characterized by a large capacity bladder with loss of normal detrusor activity which may be accompanied by 'overflow' leakage. It may occur as a late outcome of posterior urethral valves ('myogenic failure') or other forms of chronic outflow obstruction. It is also a feature of prune belly syndrome (triad syndrome). Clean intermittent catheterization (including via a Mitrofanoff catheterizable abdominal stoma) is the treatment of choice if the bladder is of good capacity and compliance is adequate.

Giggle incontinence

This distressing condition causes incontinence when the individual is giggling or laughing but not usually at other times. Giggle incontinence can have a debilitating impact on school and social life, especially since it often affects older children and teenagers. Although the precise mechanism is unknown it is thought to be allied to cataplexy in which a sudden, transient loss of muscular tone is triggered by strong emotions. Higher neural centres are clearly implicated in the pathophysiology.

Methylphenidate (ritalin) is probably the most effective form of treatment and its mode of action is thought to be mediated by its effect on reuptake inhibition of the monoamine transporters in the brain. Nevertheless, this agent is often unacceptable to parents because of its connotations with attention deficit hyperactivity disorder and the relatively high incidence of side effects. Moreover, it is necessary for the young patient to take the medication on a regular daily or twice daily basis to prevent symptoms which might occur only once a month.[11,12] Although ineffective for the treatment of pure giggle incontinence, anticholinergic therapy may be helpful in treating any coexistent detrusor overactivity.

Nighttime urinary incontinence (nocturnal enuresis)

Nocturnal enuresis has a strong familial basis with a positive family history in over 50% of affected children.

The 'Three Systems Model' described by Butler and Holland[13] identifies three main causative factors (Table 8.7.1).

Table 8.7.1 Three systems model for nocturnal enuresis

Cause	Signs and symptoms	Common treatments
Low release of AVP	Wetting soon after going to sleep and large wet patches	Enuresis alarm Medication (desmopressin)
Bladder overactivity	Frequent passing of urine, a sense of urgency, small amounts passed each time (during the day) and variable size of wet patch, and waking during or after wetting (at night)	Anticholinergic medication (relaxes bladder muscle) Bladder training
Lack of arousal from sleep	Wet patches but the child does not always wake, combined with signs listed above	A full waking assessment is required. This may involve asking the child what factors normally wake them. Individuals usually waken by stimulus that is important to the individual, not necessarily by loud noise, so alarms will not always work if the assessment shows that they are hard to wake. A combination or the treatments above may work, along with addressing needs such as anxiety of going to toilet in dark or other factors preventing he child from getting out of bed at night

Reproduced with permission from Butler R and Swinthinbank, L, *Nocturnal Enuresis and Daytime Wetting: A Handbook for Professionals*, ERIC, The Children's Bowel and Bladder Charity, Bristol, UK, Copyright © ERIC 2007.

(i) Impaired nocturnal secretion of arginine vasopressin (AVP) resulting in overproduction of urine at night

(ii) Bladder overactivity and associated daytime symptoms

(iii) Lack of arousal from sleep (usually combined with one or both of the causes above)

Treatment is aimed at correcting one or more of these three causative factors. Simple measures to reduce overnight urine production include: ensuring that the child does not drink after 6 pm and maintaining a regular, moderate fluid intake throughout the day (rather than drinking large volumes in the afternoon and early evening.)

If this proves ineffective a vasopressin analogue such as desmopressin can be prescribed to decrease obligatory urine production overnight. Nasal formulations of desmopressin are no longer recommended because of adverse reactions including hyponatraemia, seizures, and water intoxication. By contrast, oral formulations have a far more favourable safety profile.

Formulations in current use comprise Desmotabs (200–400 micrograms) or Desmomelt (120–240 micrograms) taken one hour prior to bedtime.

Imipramine is no longer recommended for the treatment of nocturnal enuresis in children.

Bed wetting alarms are designed to modify arousal mechanisms in children whose enuresis is related to a deep sleeping pattern. The equipment usually consists of a pad placed on the mattress, which triggers either an audible or vibratory signal when activated by the initial drops of urine. Over time, the child's level of awareness during sleep changes and he/she acquires the ability to wake before any urinary leakage has occurred. Bed wetting alarms are most effective when used in the context of a dedicated enuresis clinic providing support and practical advice. Nocturnal hypoxia has been implicated as a rare cause of nocturnal enuresis and tonsillectomy has been advocated as a treatment for primary nocturnal enuresis when this is supported by evidence of sleep studies. However this has not been endorsed by the findings of recent prospective controlled trials.[14–16]

If nocturnal enuresis is also accompanied by daytime wetting little progress will be made in treating it until the factors responsible for daytime wetting have been adequately treated and the child has become dry during the day.

Long-term outcomes

Parents seeking a 'quick fix' often express disappointment on learning that that treatment may have to be maintained for a number of years. Children with bedwetting may also have behavioural problems requiring specific attention.[17] Long-term treatment with desmopressin has been shown to be effective and is generally well-tolerated in children aged five years and above.[18]

For children with an overactive bladder it is often necessary to continue anticholinergic medication (in conjunction with bladder retraining) for a number of years. It is important to persist with this approach since up to 80% will become dry over the course of five years.[19]

More sophisticated treatments including biofeedback and behavioural therapy have a reported success rates of 60–80%[20,21] in the treatment of daytime incontinence but a lower success rate (50–60%) for the treatment of severe nocturnal enuresis.[22]

With the onset of puberty, physiological and anatomical changes are usually accompanied by greater awareness and increased motivation to comply with treatment. As a consequence, even children with persisting symptoms will mostly become dry by their mid-teens at the latest. Only a very small percentage of affected individuals are destined to experience a disabling degree of incontinence in adult life.

Conclusion

The treatment of urinary incontinence in children is rewarding but can be challenging and requires commitment on the part of the child, parents, and clinician. Children with daytime incontinence persisting to five years of age merit formal assessment and investigation.

Further reading

Butler R, Holland P. The three systems: a conceptual way of understanding nocturnal enuresis. *Scan J Urol Nephrol* 2000; **34**:270–7.

Butler RJ, Heron J. The prevalence of infrequent bedwetting and nocturnal enuresis in childhood: A large British cohort. *Scand J Urol Nephrol* 2008; **42**:257–64.

ERIC—The Children's Bowel and Bladder Charity. Available at: www.eric.org.uk [Online].

Haddad M, Besson R, Aubert D, *et al.* Sacral neuromodulation in children with urinary and fecal incontinence: a multicenter, open label, randomized, crossover study. *J Urol* 2010; **184**(2):696–701.

International Children's Incontinence Society. Available at: www.i-c-c-s.org [Online].

Nevéus T, von Gontard A, Hoebeke P, *et al.* The standardization of terminology of lower urinary tract function in children and adolescents: Report from the Standardisation Committee of the International Children's Continence Society. *J Urol* 2006; **176**:314–24.

NICE clinical guideline 111. Available at: www.nice.org.uk [Online].

References

1. Nevéus T, von Gontard A, Hoebeke P, *et al.* The standardization of terminology of lower urinary tract function in children and adolescents: Report from the Standardisation Committee of the International Children's Continence Society. *J Urol* 2006; **176**:314–24.
2. NICE clinical guideline 111. Available at: www.nice.org.uk [Online].
3. Butler RJ, Heron J. The prevalence of infrequent bedwetting and nocturnal enuresis in childhood: A large British cohort. *Scand J Urol Nephrol* 2008; **42**:257–64.
4. Linderholm BE. The cystometric findings in enuresis. *J Urol* 1966; **96**:718–22.
5. Mackeith R, Meadow R, Turner RK. How children become dry. (pp. 3–21) In: Colvin I, MacKeith RC, Meadows SR (eds). *Bladder Control and Enuresis.* Philadelphia, PA: Lippincott, 1973.
6. Van Balken M, Vandoninck V, Gisholf K, *et al.* Posterior tibial nerve stimulation as a neuromodulative treatment of lower urinary tract dysfunction. *J Urol* 2001; **166**(3):914–18.
7. De Genarro M, Capitanucci M, Mastracci P, Silveri M, Gatti C, Mosiello G. Percutaneous tibial nerve neuromodulation is well tolerated in children and effective for treating refractory vesical dysfunction. *J Urol* 2004; **171**(5):1911–13.
8. Capitanucci ML, Camannu D, Demelas F, Mosiello G, Zaccara A, De Gennaro M. Long-term efficacy of percutaneous tibial nerve stimulation for different types of lower urinary tract dysfunction in children. *J Urol* 2009; **182**(4):2056–61.
9. Roth T, Vandersteen D, Hollatz P, Inman B, Reinberg Y. Sacral neuromodulation for the dysfunctional elimination syndrome: A single center experience with 20 children. *J Urol* 2008; **180**(1):306–11.
10. Haddad M, Besson R, Aubert D, *et al.* Sacral neuromodulation in children with urinary and fecal incontinence: a multicenter, open label, randomized, crossover study. *J Urol* 2010; **184**(2):696–701.
11. Berry AK, Zderic S, Carr M. Methylphenidate for giggle incontinence. *J Urol* 2009; **182**(4):2028–32.
12. Glahn BE. Giggle incontinence (enuresis risoria). A study and an aetiological hypothesis. *Br J Urol* 1979; **51**(5):363–6.
13. Butler R, Holland P. The three systems: a conceptual way of understanding nocturnal enuresis. *Scan J Urol Nephrol* 2000; **34**:270–7.
14. Weider D, Hauri P. Nocturnal enuresis in children with upper airway obstruction. *Int J Pediatr Otorhinolaryngol* 1985; **9**(2):173–82.
15. Basha S, Bialowas C, Ende K, Szeremeta W. Effectiveness of adenotonsillectomy in the resolution of nocturnal enuresis secondary to obstructive sleep apnea. *Laryngoscope* 2005; **115**(6):1101–3.
16. Kalorin CM, Mouzakes JG, Gavin JP, Davis TD, Feustel P, Kogan BA. Tonsillectomy does not improve bedwetting: results of a prospective controlled trial. *J Urol* 2010; **184**(6):2527–31.
17. Joinson C, Heron J, Edmond A, Butler R. Psychological problems in children with bedwetting and combined (day and night) wetting: A UK population based study. *J Paediatr Psychol* 2007; **32**(5):605–16.
18. Lottmann H, Baydala L, Eggert P, Klein BM, Evans J, Norgaard JP. Long-term desmopressin response in primary nocturnal enuresis: open-label, multinational study. *Int J Clin Pract* 2009; **63**(1):35–45.
19. Vurran M J, Kaefer M, Peteres C, Logigian E, Bauer S. The overactive bladder in childhood: long term results with conservative management. *J Urol* 2000; **162**(2): 574–7.
20. Bachmann CJ, Heilenkötter K, Janhsen E, *et al.* Long-term effects of a urotherapy training program in children with functional urinary incontinence: a 2-year follow-up. *Scand J Urol Nephrol* 2008; **42**(4):337–43.
21. Heilenkötter K, Bachmann C, Janhsen E, *et al.* Prospective evaluation of inpatient and outpatient bladder training in children with functional urinary incontinence. *Urology* 2006; **67**(1):176–80.
22. Butler R, Swinthinbank L. *Nocturnal Enuresis and Daytime Wetting: A Handbook for Professionals.* Bristol, UK: ERIC, 2007.

CHAPTER 8.8

Abnormalities of the bladder

Peter Cuckow

Introduction to abnormalities of the bladder

This chapter provides an overview of the current management of the exstrophy–epispadias complex and other congenital abnormalities of the bladder. Neuropathic bladder is considered in Chapter 8.6.

Exstrophy, epispadias, and cloacal exstrophy

These anomalies are grouped together as the 'exstrophy–epispadias complex'. In the United Kingdom the treatment of children with exstrophy–epispadias anomalies is now concentrated in two supra-regional centres.

Classic bladder exstrophy

The incidence is approximately 1 in 30,000, with a male:female ratio of 3:1. Bladder exstrophy usually occurs as an isolated abnormality which is believed to have its origins in failure of mesodermal ingrowth between the layers of the cloacal membrane. Subsequent rupture of the cloacal membrane results in exposure of the bladder, which occupies the defect as an open plate. Bladder exstrophy is accompanied by separation of the pubic rami ('pubic diastasis'), division of the inferior rectus sheath and a low-set insertion of the umbilical cord (Fig. 8.8.1).

In boys, the exposed bladder is continuous with the exteriorized epispadiac urethra on the dorsal aspect of the penis. Because of their attachment to the widely separated inferior pubic rami, the origins of the corpora are also separated—leading to considerable reduction in the length of the penile shaft. In girls the urethral plate is shorter and ends in the midline at the introitus between the two halves of a separated (bifid) clitoris.

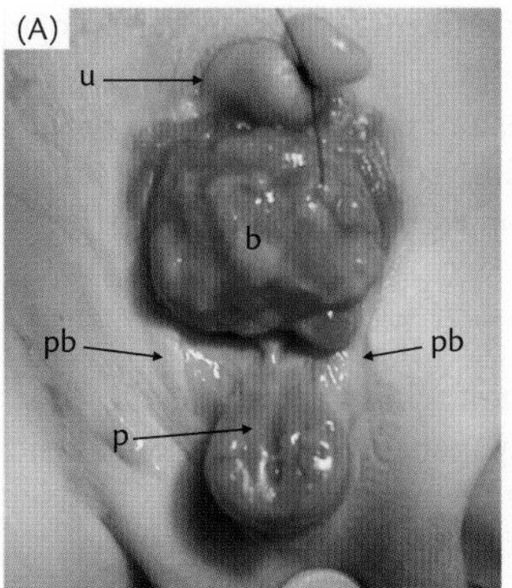

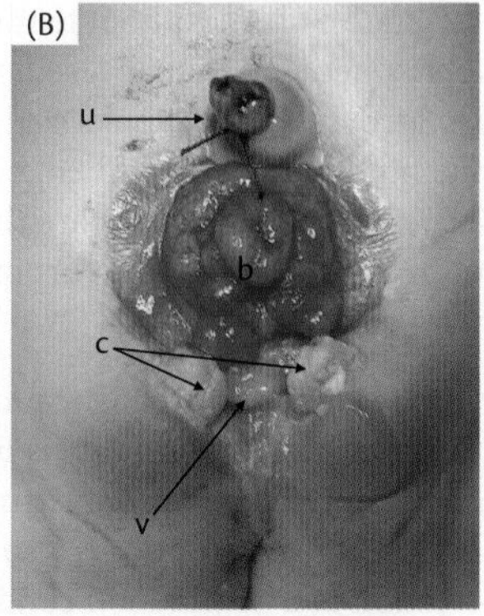

Fig. 8.8.1 Classic bladder exstrophy. (A) In the male, the bladder is continuous with the dorsal urethral plate on the penis (p). Above the umbilical cord (u) the rectus muscles separate to insert onto the split pubic bones on either side (pb). (B) In the female, the clitoris (c) and attached labia minora are divided on either side of the vaginal opening (v), which marks the lower limit of the urethral plate.

Approximately 50% of cases of classic bladder exstrophy are now diagnosed on antenatal ultrasound. Diagnostic findings include a low-lying umbilical cord, non-visualization of the bladder, and a shortened, thickened penis. Those countries where termination of pregnancy is practised have witnessed a marked decline in the birth incidence of bladder exstrophy. Prenatal counselling in a specialist centre enables parents to gain an informed perspective of the long-term outlook and permits planning of peri and postnatal care.

Primary bladder closure

Ideally this is performed in the first few days of life[1] but can be safely delayed if circumstances dictate. The use of bilateral iliac osteotomies to relieve tension on the bladder closure and reduce the risk of dehiscence is now usually limited to delayed primary closure or secondary closure after previous dehiscence. Osteotomies are still used, however, when there is a large defect[2] and in cloacal exstrophy. In surgery, the bladder plate is separated from the abdominal wall and the medial aspect of the rectus muscles, with the dissection continuing down to the level of the veru montanum in boys or the vaginal opening in girls. Once it has been fully mobilized, the bladder is then closed in the midline. Pelvic and abdominal wall tissues are then reconstituted, leaving the urethral opening sited at the base of the penis in boys and above the vaginal orifice in girls.

Complete primary reconstruction

This radical alternative entails a far more extensive primary procedure aimed at simultaneous anatomical reconstruction of the bladder, urethra, and penis.[3] It is usually delayed for several months and routinely includes osteotomies. While it carries a significant risk of complications, this approach offers a worthwhile prospect of normal voiding continence.[4]

Secondary procedures

Following successful primary closure, further surgery is required to create continence and to reconstruct the genitalia. In the 'modern staged repair' (as described by Jeffs)[2] correction of the penile abnormality is usually performed in the first year of life. The urethral plate is separated from the penile corpora, tubularized to the tip of the glans, and then relocated inferior to the corporal bodies. External rotation of the corpora corrects the dorsal chordee. When the bladder capacity has increased sufficiently a further operation is undertaken to reconstruct the bladder neck. In some children this combination of procedures may be sufficient to create an obstructed pattern of continence.

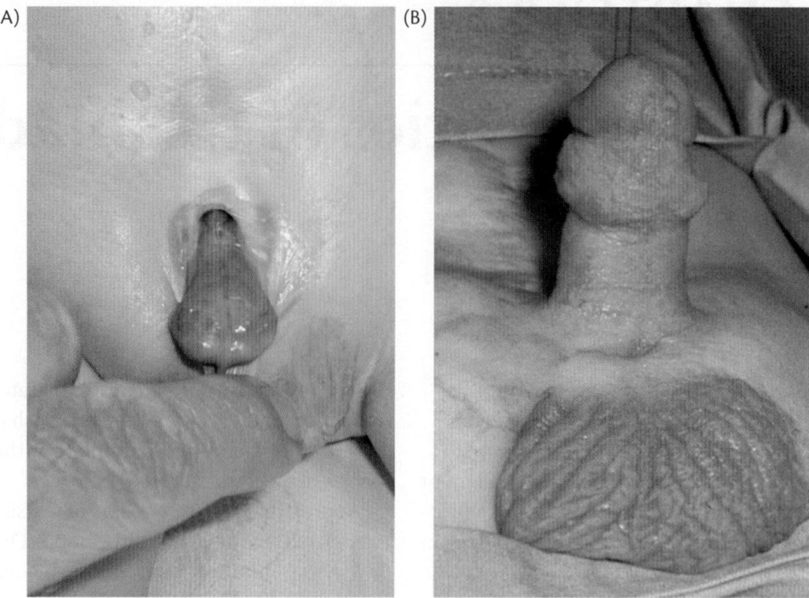

Fig. 8.8.2 Bladder exstrophy. (A) Appearances after primary bladder closure demonstrating epispadiac urethra; and (B) the emergent penis after a Kelly operation. The urethra opens in a hypospadiac position and the patient will subsequently undergo a staged urethroplasty. He is continent.

The Kelly operation[5] involves a radical reconstruction of the soft-tissues to restore normal anatomical relations of the bladder outlet, pelvic floor, urethra, and penis. It is performed at around one year and entails extensive mobilization of the corpora from the pubic rami and release of the pelvic floor, with careful preservation of the pudendal nerves and vessels. The ureters are reimplanted and the bladder neck is redefined and loosely reconstructed. The urethra is tubularized and the corpora approximated in the midline, thus enhancing penile length (Fig. 8.8.2).

In girls, complete mobilization of the clitoral corpora enables them to be joined in the midline. The urethra and vagina are both wrapped in muscle to form a notional sphincter.

Daytime continence develops in up to 70% of patients over the following three to four years with night-time continence ensuing as bladder capacity increases.

Continent diversion

This was the mainstay of treatment until the late 1990s and continues to play a role in children who do not achieve continence despite one of the procedures described above. A tight bladder neck reconstruction is performed to create high outlet resistance. Bladder capacity is increased by ileocystoplasty and emptying is achieved by a continent catheterizable channel (Mitrofanoff procedure).

Cloacal exstrophy

The incidence is approximately 1 in 300,000, with a male preponderance. Clocal exstrophy is thought to originate from failure of septation of the cloaca accompanied by a lack of mesodermal ingrowth into the cloacal membrane. The exposed bladder is usually divided into two halves lying on each side of a central section of exstrophic bowel. The intestinal component typically consists of an open caecum with the ileum entering it, one or two appendices, a blind-ending distal hindgut segment and an imperforate anus. The pelvic diastasis is far wider than in classic exstrophy and consequently the penis is even shorter or may be separated into two halves. In girls the vagina may be absent but is more often duplicated. The abdominal wall defect is usually accompanied by a large exomphalos above the exstrophy plate (Fig. 8.8.3).

Cloacal exstrophy is commonly complicated by prematurity and intrauterine growth retardation. There is also a high incidence of congenital anomalies affecting other systems.

Most cases are now detected antenatally and many parents opt for termination. When the pregnancy proceeds, neonatal mortality rate remains high—particularly in cases with an associated major cardiac or small bowel anomaly.

Initial management is aimed at stabilizing the infant's general condition and managing any complications of prematurity. This is followed by a detailed radiological assessment including urinary and spinal ultrasound and cardiac echo.

Abdominal closure

Surgery is often delayed to allow conservative management of the exomphalos and to treat complications of prematurity or other life-threatening conditions. Iliac osteotomies are invariably required to facilitate closure without tension, and the use of a temporary silo or a prosthetic mesh may also be necessary. The central bowel plate is isolated and then tubularized to restore intestinal continuity, with the hindgut distal to it being exteriorized as a terminal colostomy. The two bladder halves are then joined together with a narrowed outlet at the base of the corpora.

Continence

Since there is little realistic prospect of achieving faecal continence, the intestinal abnormality is usually managed by a permanent end colostomy. Further reconstruction of the bladder entails bladder neck reconstruction (or closure) combined with cystoplasty and a creation of a Mitrofanoff conduit.

Although the majority of affected individuals now have the potential to survive into adulthood, they are nevertheless likely to experience significant physical[6] and psychological morbidity. For this reason, the ongoing support provided by nurse specialists and psychologists is of paramount importance.

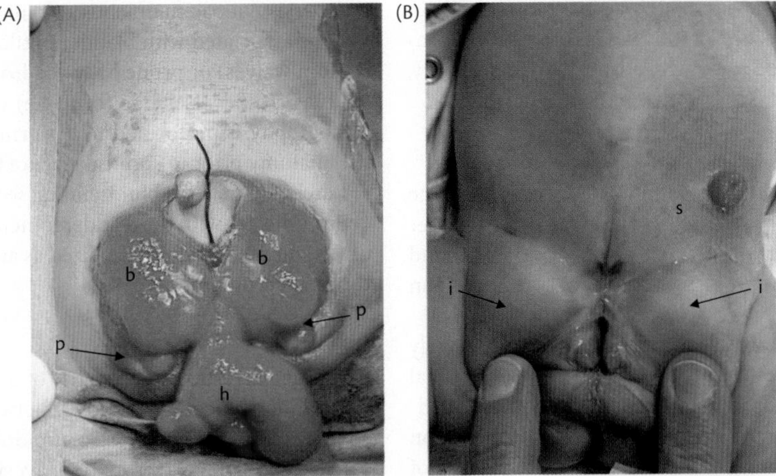

Fig. 8.8.3 Cloacal exstrophy. (A) Preoperative view showing two hemi-bladders (b) with a prolapsing hindgut segment (h) between them. The penis (p) is in two halves, attached to the widely separated pubic bones. There is no exomphalos. (B) Following midline closure with osteotomies, the two penile halves are joined together but require further reconstruction (Kelly operation). There is an L-sided end colostomy (s). Bilateral inguinal hernias (i) have developed.

Primary epispadias

This is more common in boys, in whom the estimated incidence is 1 in 150,000. The anomaly is characterized by an exposed urethral plate lying on the dorsum of the penis. Primary epispadias varies in severity from a localized deficiency of the glanular urethra (with preservation of normal continence) to extensive exteriorization of the penile and proximal urethra with an associated bladder neck abnormality (which is usually accompanied by urinary incontinence). The degree of bladder neck incompetence and reduction in bladder capacity generally correlates with the severity of the epispadiac anomaly. In girls, primary epispadias is characterized by a divided (bifid) clitoris, wide urethra, and bladder neck deficiency. Incontinence is inevitable (Fig. 8.8.4). Although some visible abnormality is invariably present from birth it may, nevertheless, remain undetected in girls until they are investigated for incontinence in later childhood. Likewise, distal epispadias in boys may be concealed by an intact foreskin and may not become apparent until the foreskin becomes retractile—or at the time of circumcision.

In severe cases, cystoscopy reveals marked deficiency of the bladder neck muscle with the veru montanum located within the bladder and abnormal appearances of the trigone. However, the cystoscopic findings do not reliably predict the eventual prognosis for continence.

Surgical repair

In boys who are continent, the Cantwell-Ransley epispadias repair[7] yields good results—although the penis may still appear relatively short. When epispadias is associated with incontinence, the Kelly operation is now the preferred option. Despite optimal reconstruction, however, it may be difficult to create continence and normal spontaneous voiding because of the dysplastic nature of the bladder neck and sphincter musculature.

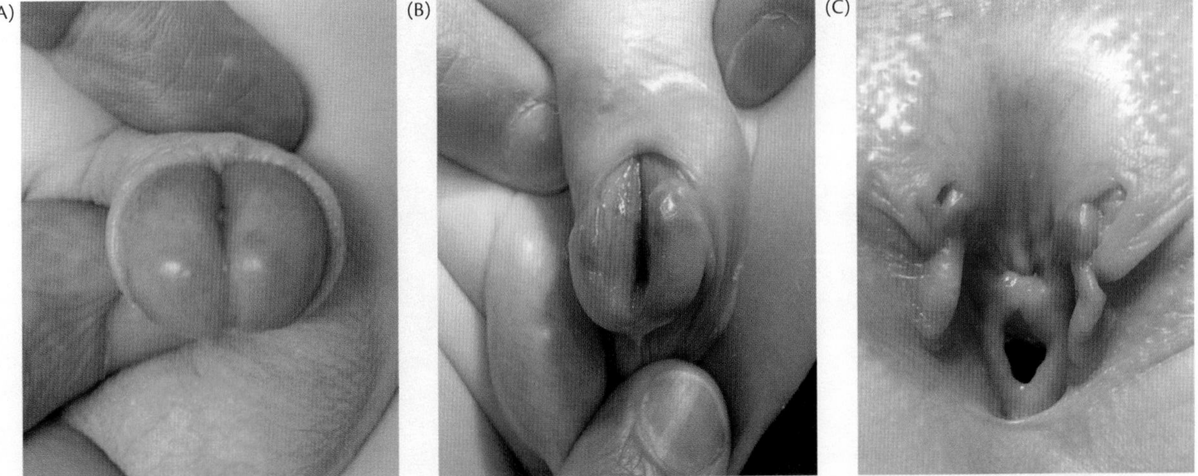

Fig. 8.8.4 Primary epispadias. (A) Glanular epispadias with dorsal cleft glans but a normal bladder neck is seen at cystoscopy. (B) A more severe case associated with an open bladder neck at cystoscopy. (C) A typical female case, showing the divided clitoris and dorsally deficient urethra. Late presentation during investigation for incontinence.

In girls, the Kelly operation has a high success rate—both in terms of continence and correction of the bifid clitoris. The alternative approach consists of bladder neck reconstruction, cystoplasty, and a Mitrofanoff procedure.

Urachal anomalies

In early gestation the urinary tract communicates freely with the amniotic cavity via the urachus, which extends from the bladder to the umbilicus. The lumen of the urachus normally closes around the twelfth week leaving a non-patent fibrous cord—the median umbilical ligament.

The commonest urachal anomaly (accounting for approximately 50% of cases) is a sinus in which a patent section of the residual urachus communicates with the umbilicus—but not with the bladder. Presentation is with umbilical discharge, persistent granulation tissue or pain, and localized tenderness. Investigation consists of ultrasound[8] and contrast sinography (to determine the proximal extent of the sinus). The standard treatment is surgical excision.

Urachal cysts account for approximately one-third of cases and usually present with infection, the commonest organism being *Staphylococcus aureus*. The diagnosis is confirmed by ultrasound. Asymptomatic urachal cysts are sometimes identified incidentally during ultrasound imaging for unrelated indications.

When infection is present, this is managed with antibiotics, combined with surgical drainage if necessary. Surgical excision[9] is best deferred until any infection has been eliminated. Asymptomatic cysts should also be excised in view of the reported long-term risk of adenocarcinoma.[10,11]

A persistent patent urachus accounts for around 10% of cases and may be associated with bladder outflow obstruction (e.g. posterior urethral valves) or prune belly syndrome. It is usually evident from birth as a fluid discharge (of urine) from the umbilicus. Contrast cystography is performed to confirm the diagnosis and delineate the anatomy prior to surgical closure (Fig. 8.8.5).

Rarely, a persistent blind-ending section of patent urachus which communicates with the bladder lumen can create a non-obstructive diverticulum, which is visualized as an incidental finding on a micturating cryptogram.

Bladder diverticula

A bladder diverticulum consists of a thin-walled out-pouching of the bladder mucosa protruding between bands of detrusor muscle. Diverticula occur more commonly in boys in whom they are often secondary to elevated intravesical pressure caused by outflow obstruction due to posterior urethral valves, syringocele, and urethral strictures. Other causes include neuropathic bladder, detrusor-sphincter dyssynergia, and prune belly syndrome.[12,13] Small secondary diverticula tend to resolve spontaneously after normal bladder dynamics have been restored, for example following ablation of posterior urethral valves.

Diverticula occur most commonly above and lateral to the ureteric orifice, from where they may extend outwards through the ureteric hiatus. Diverticula may also develop in this site as an iatrogenic complication of ureteric reimplantation. Other sites include the dome of the bladder, particularly in cases of severe outlet obstruction. Large diverticula in the region of the bladder neck or

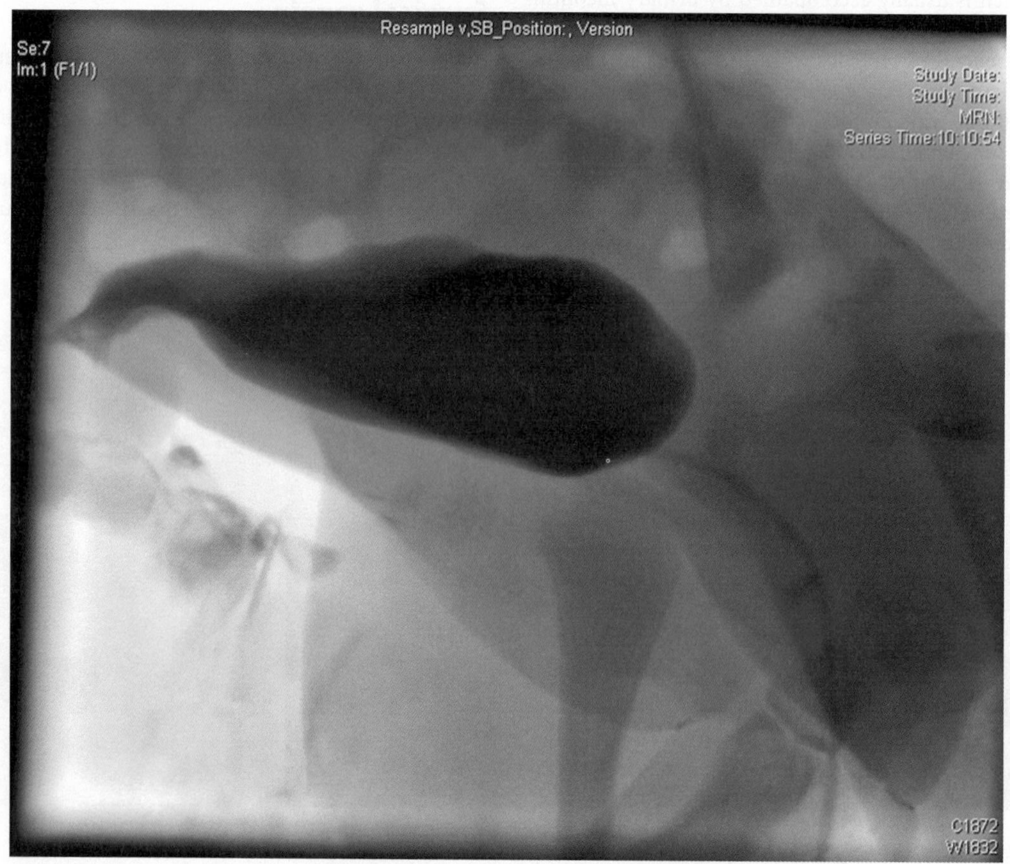

Fig. 8.8.5 Micturating cystourethrogram showing a patent urachus in a baby girl, presenting after birth as a discharge of urine from the umbilicus.

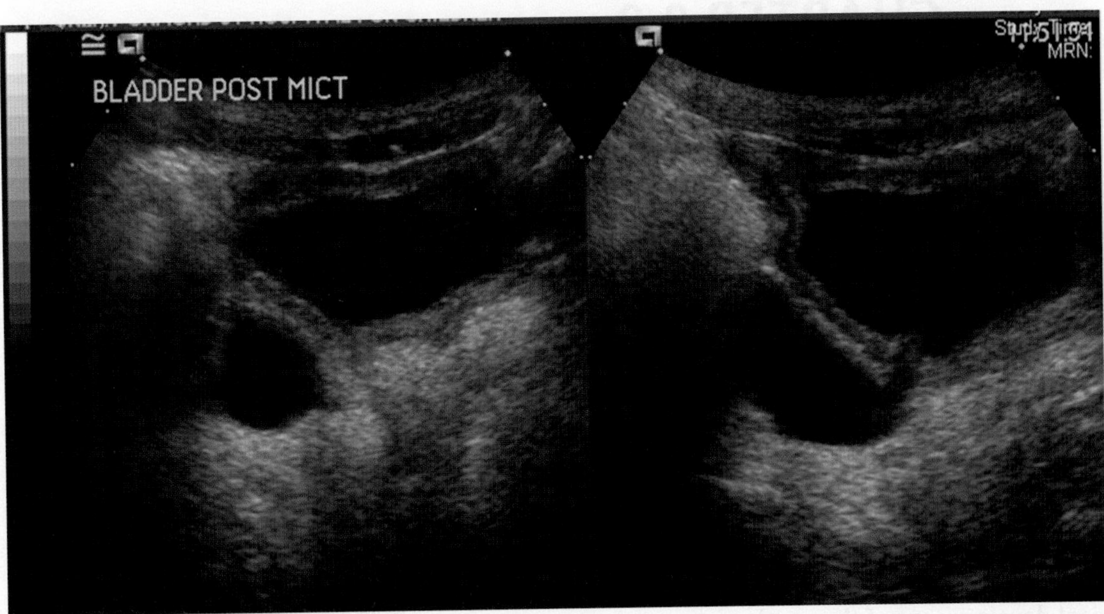

Fig. 8.8.6 Two ultrasound images of a large bladder diverticulum in a boy with posterior urethral valves. This persisted following valve resection and resulted in poor bladder emptying. The diverticulum was therefore excised.

proximal urethra can cause distortion or compression of the bladder outlet, thus exacerbating any outflow obstruction.

Bladder diverticula also occur in children with connective tissue disorders such as Menke's syndrome, Ehlers Danlos syndrome, cutis laxa, and Williams syndrome. In these conditions, there is a high incidence of recurrence following surgical excision. Primary diverticula of unknown aetiology can also occur in children (predominantly boys) with no identifiable underlying pathology. Excision is usually curative in such cases. The investigation of bladder diverticula is by pre- and post-void ultrasound (Fig. 8.8.6) and micturating cystourethrography.

Small asymptomatic diverticula can usually be managed conservatively, whereas surgical excision is indicated for larger diverticula giving rise to symptoms or complications.

Conclusions

The spectrum of congenital anomalies of the bladder includes some of the most severe abnormalities of the urinary tract compatible with survival. While the surgical management of urachal anomalies and bladder diverticula lie within the remit of every paediatric urologist, there are compelling arguments for concentrating the management of the exstrophy–epispadias complex in the hands of a small number of specialists. This model of service provision, which has already been adopted in the United Kingdom, offers the best prospect of improving the long-term outcome for children born with these rare conditions.

Further reading

Cendron M. Unusual conditions of the bladder, including bladder trauma, urachal anomalies and bladder diverticula. (pp. 1047–58) In: Docimo SG, Canning D, Khoury A (eds). *Textbook of Clinical Pediatric Urology*, 5th edition. London, UK: Taylor and Francis, 2007.

Cuckow P. Bladder exstrophy and epispadias. (pp. 199–211) In: Thomas DFM, Duffy PG, Rickwood AMK (eds). *Essentials of Paediatric Urology*, 2nd edition. London, UK: Informa Healthcare, 2008.

Gearhart JP. Exstrophy epispadias and other bladder anomalies. (p. 2189) In: Walsh PC, Retik AB, Vaughan D, Wein AJ (eds). *Campbell's Urology*, 8th edition. Philadelphia, PA: WB Saunders, 2002.

References

1. Mushtaq I, Garriboli M, Smeulders N, *et al.* Primary neonatal bladderexstrophy closure challenging the traditions. *J Urol* 2014; **191**(1):193–7.
2. Baird AD, Nelson CP, Gearhart JP. Modern staged repair of bladder exstrophy: a contemporary series. *J Pediatr Urol* 2007; **3**(4):311–5.
3. Grady RW, Mitchell ME. Complete primary repair of exstrophy. *J Urol* 1999; **162**(4):1415–20.
4. Shnorhavorian M, Grady RW, Andersen A, Joyner BD, Mitchell ME. Long-term followup of complete primary repair of exstrophy: the Seattle experience. *J Urol* 2008; **180**(4 Suppl):1615–9.
5. Kelly JH, Eraklis AJ. A procedure for lengthening the phallus in boys with exstrophy of the bladder. *J Pediatric Surgery* 1971; **6**(5):645–9.
6. McHoney M, Ransley PG, Duffy P, Wilcox DT, Spitz L. Cloacal exstrophy: morbidity associated with abnormalities of the gastrointestinal tract and spine. *J Pediatr Surg* 2004; **39**(8):1209–13.
7. Kajbafzadeh AM, Duffy PG, Ransley PG. The evolution of penile reconstruction in epispadias repair: a report of 180 cases. *J Urol* 1995; **154**(2 Pt 2):858–61.
8. Widni EE, Höllwarth ME, Haxhija EQ. The impact of preoperative ultrasound on correct diagnosis of urachal remnants in children. *J Pediatr Surg* 2010; **45**(7):1433–7.
9. Mesrobian HGO, Zacharias A, Balcom AH, Cohen RD. Ten years of experience with isolated urachal anomalies in children. *J Urol* 1997; **158**(3):1316–18.
10. Copp HL, Wong IY, Krishnan C, Malhotra S, Kennedy WA. Clinical presentation and urachal remnant pathology: implications for treatment. *J Urol* 2009; **182**(4 Suppl):1921–4.
11. Ashley RA, Inman BA, Routh JC, Rohlinger AL, Husmann DA, Kramer SA. Urachal anomalies: a longitudinal study of urachal remnants in children and adults. *J Urol* 2007; **178**(4 Pt 2):1615–8.
12. Blane CE, Zerin JM, Bloom DA. Bladder diverticula in children. *Radiology* 1994; **190**(3):695–7.
13. Psutka SP, Cendron M. Bladder diverticula in children. *J Pediatr Urol* 2013; **9**(2):129–38.

CHAPTER 8.9

Hypospadias

Peter Cuckow

Introduction to hypospadias

This chapter summarizes the aetiology and clinical features of hypospadias and describes the current surgical approach to the correction of this common urological anomaly.

Aetiology

Embryological development of the urethra

The penile urethra is formed when the urethral folds fuse in a proximal to distal direction on the genital tubercle and merge with an invagination or 'ingrowth' from the tip of the glans which gives rise to the glanular urethra. This process is testosterone-dependant and is completed by the fifteenth week of gestation. Abnormalities of the normal pattern of development give rise to hypospadias.[1,2]

Aetiological factors and epidemiology

Hypospadias has an incidence of approximately 1 in 250 to 1 in 300.[3] The aetiology is multifactorial and includes genetic, endocrine, developmental, and environmental factors. Approximately 8% of fathers and 14% of male siblings of infants with hypospadias also have the condition. Factors thought to interfere with normal virilization include; maternal progestogen treatment in early pregnancy, infertility treatment, and intrauterine growth retardation.[4] Intrauterine exposure to environmental pollutants with antiandrogenic or oestrogenic properties has also been suggested as a possible aetiological factor.[3] More severe forms of hypospadias merge with the spectrum of disorders of sexual development (DSD) and karyotyping and endocrine screening are therefore essential in such cases—particularly if the gonads are impalpable or asymmetric.

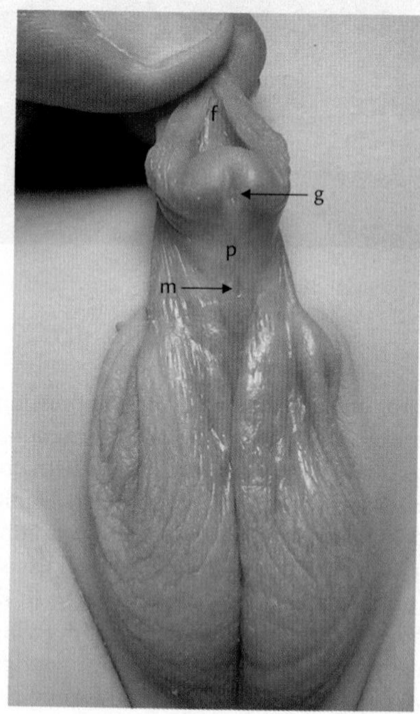

Fig. 8.9.1 Ventral urethral meatus located on the penile shaft (m). Urethral plate distal to the meatus (p) and dorsal hooded foreskin (f). Shallow glans groove and distal glanular pit (g).

Classification

Anatomical features

In hypospadias the urethral opening is located in an abnormal position, which may be sited at any point from the anterior anal margin to just below the tip of the glans. An exteriorized urethral plate extends from the urinary meatus to the glans, often terminating in a groove of varying depth. In some cases a blind ending urethral 'pit' is also present on the glans tip.

The foreskin is typically incomplete on its ventral aspect—giving rise to a characteristic dorsal 'hood'. Downward (ventral) curvature of the penile shaft ('chordee') is relatively common. In milder cases this may simply be due to tightness of the ventral skin (Fig. 8.9.1) but more severe chordee is either due to tethering of the penile corpora by abnormal dysgenetic tissue or intrinsic curvature of the corpora.

Broadly speaking, hypospadias is classified as: glanular, distal penile, proximal penile, or penoscrotal. In 80% of cases, the urethral meatus is located on the penile shaft or glans, whereas in the remaining 20% of cases it is sited more proximally at the base of the penile shaft or in the region of the penoscrotal junction. The more distally the urinary meatus is located, the straighter and better developed is the penis (and the greater the likelihood that the hypospadias will be amenable to single-stage surgical correction). Severe cases are characterized by a proximal meatus, more severe chordee, and relative hypoplasia of the shaft and glans. The more extensive reconstruction required in such cases typically comprises a two-stage repair (Fig. 8.9.2). A distally sited meatus may sometimes be deceptive since, in some cases, the spongiosum tissue is deficient and the urethra is thin walled and dysplastic. In the 'mega meatus intact prepuce' variant the prepuce is entirely normal but the urethra opens into a wide cleft in the glans. This anomaly may only become apparent at an age when the foreskin becomes fully retractile—or, alternatively, during the initial stage of circumcision.

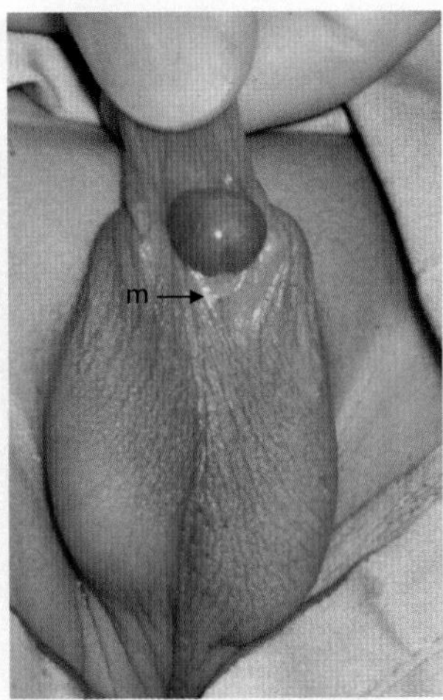

Fig. 8.9.2 More severe case than illustrated in Fig 8.9.1. Meatus located at the penoscrotal junction (m). The proximity of the meatus to the glans is indicative of severe chordee.

Presentation and assessment

Hypospadias is usually diagnosed at birth or during routine neonatal examination. In severe cases, the possibility of an underlying DSD should be considered and multidisciplinary assessment undertaken. Although the precise position of the urethral meatus may sometimes be difficult to identify on initial examination, impairment of urinary flow is very unusual and, indeed, if untreated hypospadias rarely has any impact on health in infancy.

Surgical management

Timing of surgery

Surgical correction is best deferred until at least nine months of age and in most UK centres, the preferred age is shortly after the first birthday. An initial urological consultation is advisable at around three months of age to determine the likely plan of management based on factors such as meatal position, the presence and severity of chordee, and overall development of the shaft and glans.

In a minority of cases the final decision regarding the choice of surgical procedure can only be made once the full extent of the chordee has been assessed intraoperatively by an artificial erection test.

General considerations

The priorities of surgical management are:

- Correction of chordee to create a straight penile shaft
- Reconstruction of the urethra to the penile tip
- Reconstruction of the glans and the urinary meatus

Reconfiguration of the penile shaft skin. This usually entails removing excess skin to create the appearances of a normal circumcised penis. Although reconstruction of the foreskin is also feasible in many cases this has been reported to carry an increased risk of complications.

Ultimately, the aims are to enable the affected individual to pass urine normally in a standing position like his peers, to ensure normal erectile function and to achieve a cosmetic appearance that is as normal as possible.

More than 200 named operations have been described since the 1800s and over 1,000 articles on hypospadias were published in major journals between 1990–2000.

Many of the historic techniques attributed to Ombredanne, Duplay, Byers, Dennis Browne and others have been incorporated into the procedures employed in current practice. The use of magnification, antibiotic prophylaxis, fine, absorbable sutures, urethral stents, and dressings have all contributed to greatly improved surgical success rates in recent years. However, the most important determinants of a successful outcome are the experience and commitment of the surgeon and regular peer-reviewed audit of results.

Single-stage repair

There is broad consensus that cases of distal hypospadias where the penis is straight following release of penile shaft skin can be repaired with a single-stage procedure. If the urethral plate is of sufficient width and is accompanied by a well-defined glans groove, it can be tubularized from the urethral opening to the tip of the glans using a technique based on the principle first described by Thiersch and Duplay. The MAGPI procedure (meatal advancement and glanuloplasty) devised by Duckett[5] for the correction of subcoronal hypospadias is also still widely used. The technique of incising the urethral plate in the midline prior to closure around a stent was first described by Orkiszewski in 1986 and forms the basis of the TIP (tubularized incised plate). Popularized by Snodgrass, this technique has been adopted by the majority of surgeons in the United Kingdom for the correction of distal hypospadias (Fig. 8.9.3).[6–8]

More severe forms of hypospadias with a proximal meatus and chordee can also be corrected with a single-stage operation using a variety of techniques. In the 1980s Asopa and Duckett devised urethroplasty techniques employing a tube or onlay flap derived from preputial skin mobilized on a vascular pedicle and then incorporated into the urethral plate to create the neo urethra.[9] Newer techniques (such as that described by Koyanagi) also employ a single-stage repair. However, the high complication rates of complex single-stage procedures have prompted many surgeons to switch to a staged approach.

Staged repair

Originally proposed by Dennis Browne, the two-stage approach is now favoured by most UK Paediatric Urologists for the repair of severe hypospadias or 'salvage' or 're do' cases.[10,11] During the first stage, the penile skin is mobilized from the shaft and dysplastic urethral plate tissue is dissected off the ventral surface of the corpora. An artificial erection test is then performed to accurately assess the severity of any residual chordee. When this is present it is corrected by mobilizing the neurovascular bundles off the dorso-lateral surface of the corporal bodies and then performing strategically placed plications ('tucks') on their convex surface. The effect is similar to that achieved by Nesbitt's procedure. A free graft of inner preputial skin is harvested and laid into the ventral surface of the shaft and glans—which has first been split open on its ventral aspect to create a wide, rectangular raw surface. The graft is secured with multiple circumferential and quilting sutures and a temporary pressure dressing is applied for a week during initial graft healing (Fig. 8.9.4). The remaining skin is then used to cover the penile shaft.

The second stage is performed once the graft has healed—usually a minimum of six months after the first stage procedure. Using a

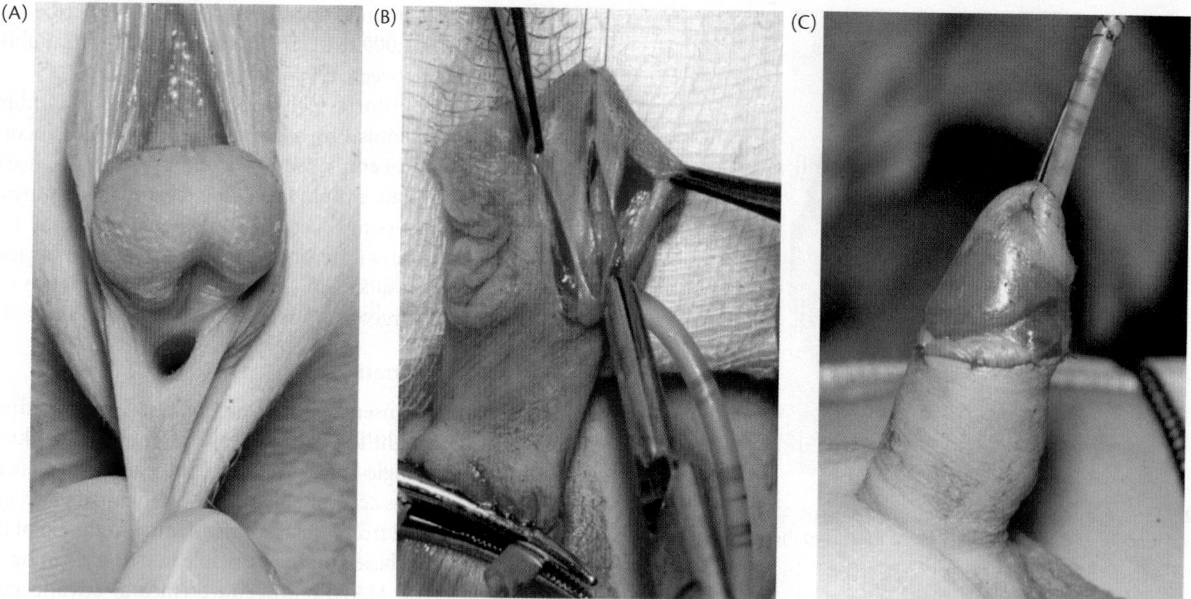

Fig. 8.9.3 (A) Distal hypospadias with a deep glans groove. No chordee. (B) Surgical correction by tubularization of the incised urethral plate, (C) leaving a circumcised appearance.

U-shaped incision, the graft is tubularized and the urethra reconstructed in at least three layers around a stent (Fig. 8.9.5).

Most hypospadias surgeons routinely use some form of postoperative dressing and a period of bladder drainage with an indwelling stent or catheter. A prophylactic antibiotic and an anticholinergic agent (to reduce bladder spasm) are prescribed if a stent has been left *in situ*.

Complications

Hypospadias surgery carries a wide range of complications.[12,13] Complete breakdown of the repair may be caused by infection, ischaemia, tension on the tissues used for urethroplasty or a combination of these factors. A tight urethral closure or swelling and inflammation of the penis may result in partially obstructed voiding and extravasation of urine through the suture line after removal of the stent and dressing. Treatment usually consists of a further period of catheter drainage—via a supra pubic route if necessary. The occurrence of severe complications in the early postoperative period carries a high risk of longer-term problems and the need for revision surgery.

Urethro cutaneous fistula is the commonest complication requiring further surgery. Typically, fistulas are caused by localized tissue breakdown in the vicinity of the suture line or poor urethral closure technique.

Scarring of the reconstructed urethra causes narrowing—either at the meatus (meatal stenosis) or in the neo urethra (urethral stricture). In turn this leads to partially obstructed voiding with impaired flow, secondary bladder dysfunction, and upper tract changes in severe cases. Flowmetry has been used for clinical research studies of voiding function following hypospadias repair[14,15] and is being increasingly incorporated into routine follow-up protocols in many centres.

Although dilatation may be effective, surgical revision is often necessary for the definitive treatment of more severe strictures or stenosis.

Widely varying complication rates have been reported following surgical repair of distal hypospadias. In the hands of experienced surgeons, however, the overall complication rate should probably be no higher than 10%. By contrast, the single-stage approach for the correction of proximal hypospadias entails lengthy, complex

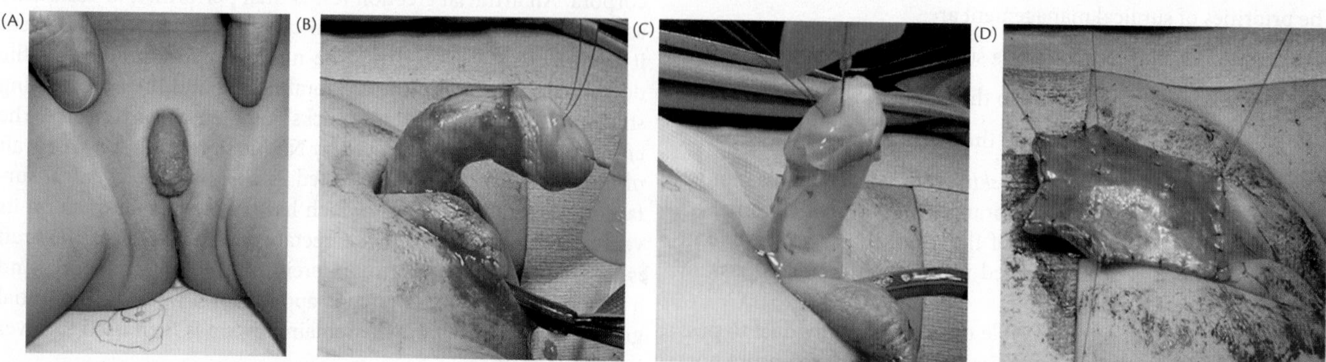

Fig. 8.9.4 (A) First stage of two-stage repair in a severe case. (B) Chordee, due to corporal curvature is shown by artificial erection. (C) This is corrected with dorsal tucks. (D) Excess prepuce is applied to the ventral shaft and split glans as a free graft.

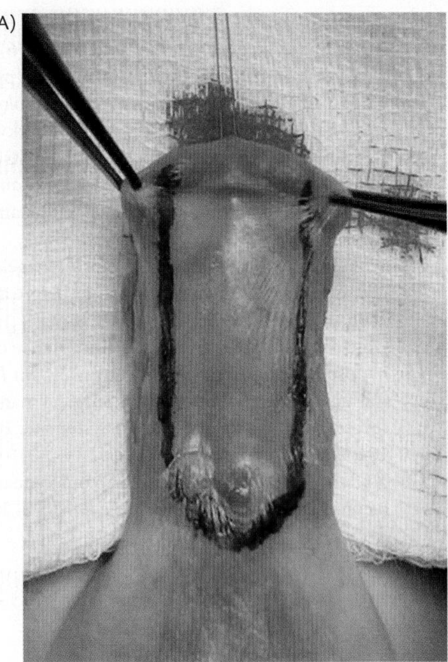

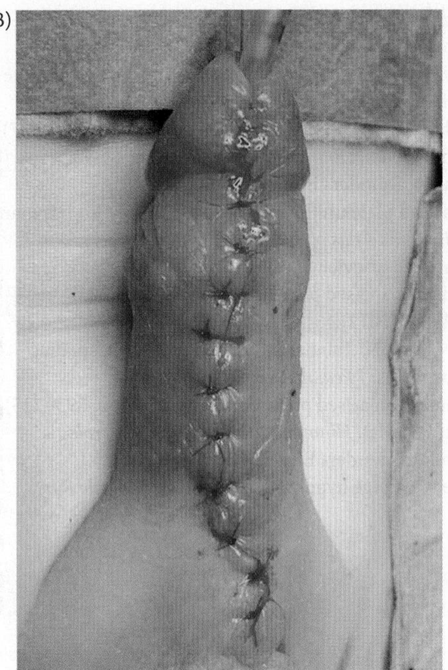

Fig. 8.9.5 Second stage repair. (A) The graft is incised with a U-shaped incision (B) The urethra is reconstructed in three layers.

surgical procedures. It not surprising, therefore, that re-operation rates of up to 50% have been reported—with fistulas and meatal stenosis occurring in up to 30% of cases.[16] Although the complication rate has been considerably reduced following the introduction of two-stage repairs, 20% of patients may nevertheless require an additional procedure.

The benefits of correcting minor forms of glanular hypospadias are questionable since they rarely impact on function and surgical correction introduces the potential risk of complications. Such cases can be managed by a modified circumcision to remove the preputial hood and, if necessary, a meatoplasty to improve the direction of the urinary stream. While the appearance of the penis may not be not entirely normal the cosmetic deficit is usually minimal.

Revision surgery

Dehiscence can often be corrected by simple re-closure of the urethra in accordance with a TIP repair—incorporating a buccal mucosa inlay graft if necessary.

Simple closure of urethro cutaneous fistulas is usually effective if there is no distal stenosis and if adequate tissue is available to achieve closure in three layers.

Persistent chordee is best managed by excision of ventral scar tissue and grafting of the penile shaft during the first stage of a two-stage revision procedure. Healthy inner preputial skin is the graft of choice but buccal mucosa and posterior auricular skin can be used if this is not available. For some patients, it may be preferable to accept a meatus of adequate calibre sited on the distal shaft rather than undergo repeated unsuccessful attempts to reconstruct the meatus on the tip of the glans.

Long-term results

Although the available evidence is limited[17] it clearly indicates that a proportion of patients experience unsatisfactory long-term outcomes. Balanitis Xerotica et Obliterans is a relatively common indication for late surgical revision in adults following hypospadias surgery in childhood.

While successful surgical repair can help to minimize any long-term psychological morbidity, a minority of patients will nevertheless experience significant psychological problems related to their condition. Long-term follow-up and support may therefore be beneficial for patients with severe forms of hypospadias.

Conclusion

Hypospadias is one of the commonest congenital abnormalities of the genitourinary tract. Approximately 80% of cases are of mild to moderate severity and can be successfully corrected with a single-stage procedure. A two-stage approach is being increasingly adopted for more complex cases. The experience and commitment of the surgeon, coupled with regular audit of results are the most important determinants of a successful surgical outcome.

Further reading

Hadidi A, Azmy AF. *Hypospadias Surgery: An Illustrated Guide*, 2nd edition. Berlin, Germany: Springer Verlag, 2013.

Snodgrass WT, Shukla AR, Canning DA. Hypospadias. (pp. 1204–38) In: Docimo SG, Canning D, Khoury A (eds). *Textbook of Clinical Pediatric Urology*, 5th edition. London, UK: Taylor and Francis, 2007.

Wilcox DT, Mouriquand PDE. Hypospadias. (pp. 213–31) In: Thomas DFM, Duffy PG, Rickwood AMK (eds). *Essentials of Paediatric Urology*, 2nd edition. London, UK: Informa Healthcare, 2008.

References

1. Baskin LS. Hypospadias and urethral development. *J Urol* 2000; **163**:951–6.
2. Thomas DFM. Embryology. (pp. 438–53) In: Mundy AR, Fitzpatrick J, Neal D, George NR (eds). *Scientific Basis of Urology*, 3rd edn. London, UK: Informa Healthcare, 2010.

3. Thomas DFM. Hypospadiology: Science and surgery. *BJU Int* 2004; **93**:470–3.
4. Fredell L, Kockum I, Hansson E, *et al.* Heredity of hypospadias and the significance of low birth weight. *J Urol* 2002; **167**(3):1423–7.
5. Duckett JW. Meatoplasty and glanuloplasy (MAGPI repair). (pp. 693–7) In: Hinman F, Baskin LS (eds). *Hinman's Atlas of Pediatric Urologic Surgery.* Philadelphia PA: Saunders Elsevier, 2009.
6. Snodgrass W. Tubularised plate urethroplasty. (pp. 716–25) In: Hinman F, Baskin LS (eds). *Hinman's Atlas of Pediatric Urologic Surgery.* Philadelphia PA: Saunders Elsevier, 2009.
7. Snodgrass W. Tubularized, incised plate urethroplasty for distal hypospadias. *J Urol* 1994; **151**(2):464–5.
8. Snodgrass W, Bush N, Cost N. Tubularisd incised plate hypospadias repair for distal hypospadias. *J Pediatr Urol* 2010; **6**:408–13.
9. Duckett JW. Transverse tubularised preputial island flap. (pp. 693–725) In: Hinman F, Baskin LS (eds). *Hinman's Atlas of Pediatric Urologic Surgery.* Philadelphia PA: Saunders Elsevier, 2009.
10. Bracka A. A versatile two-stage hypospadias repair. *Br J Plastic Surg* 1995; **48**:345–52.
11. Nitkunan T, Johal N, O'Malley K, Cuckow P. Secondary hypospadias repair in two stages. *J Pediatr Urol* 2006; **2**(6):559–63.
12. Snodgrass W. Hypospadias urethroplasty. (pp. 201–11) In: Wilcox DT, Godbole PP, Koyle MA (eds). *Pediatric Urology: Surgical Complications and Management.* Oxford, UK: Wiley-Blackwell, 2008.
13. Baskin LS. Hypospadias. (pp. 611–20) In Stringer MD, Oldham KT, Mouriquand PDE (eds). *Pediatric Surgery and Urology: Long-term Outcomes,* 2nd edition. Cambridge, UK: Cambridge University Press, 2006.
14. Wolffenbuttel KP, Wondergem N, Hoefnagels JJ, *et al.* Abnormal urine flow in boys with distal hypospadias before and after correction. *J Urol* 2006; **176**(4 Pt 2):1733–6.
15. González R, Ludwikowski BM. Importance of urinary flow studies after hypospadias repair: a systematic review. *Int J Urol* 2011; **18**(11):757–61.
16. Castagnetti M, El Ghoneimi A. Surgical management of primary severe hypospadias in children: Systematic 20 year review. *J Urol* 2010; **184**:1469–75.
17. Tourchi A, Hoebeke P. Long-term outcome of male genital reconstruction in childhood. *J Pediatr Urol* 2013; **9**(6):980–9.

CHAPTER 8.10

Disorders of the prepuce

Ahmed A. Darwish and Kim A.R. Hutton

Introduction to disorders of the prepuce

The prepuce (or foreskin) is the portion of penile skin covering and protecting the underlying surface of the glans. At birth, the foreskin is normally adherent to the glans, with the result that it is non-retractile. The term 'physiological phimosis' is applied to a healthy but non-retractile foreskin. During the first few years of life, spontaneous lysis of the adhesions between the foreskin and glans occurs, with the result that the foreskin gradually becomes retractile. However the rate at which this process occurs varies very considerably between different individuals.

The normal foreskin can be partly or completely retracted in 20% of boys at 6 months of age, in 50% at one year, 80% at two years, and in 90% by the age of three years.[1–5] In many boys, however, complete retraction of a healthy foreskin may not be possible until much later in childhood. Significant pathology affecting the foreskin generally presents with symptoms or cosmetic concerns.

Pathological phimosis

This term is largely synonymous with balanitis xerotica obliterans (BXO), a progressive inflammatory process of unknown aetiology affecting the male genitalia. First described in adults by Stuhmer in 1928,[6] the first published report of BXO in a child is credited to Catterall and Oates in 1962.[7] The disease is histologically identical to lichen sclerosis et atrophicus of the vulva. Balanitis xerotica obliterans typically presents with local irritation, dysuria, and bleeding, secondary (i.e. acquired) non-retraction of the foreskin or deteriorating urinary stream. Rarely, it presents with acute urinary retention or incontinence secondary to chronic outflow obstruction. In extreme cases there may be renal impairment.[8] Areas of greyish white discoloration and thickening of the skin develop at the preputial opening and on the inner layer of the foreskin and the glans penis. As the disease progresses, the skin becomes inelastic with whitish plaques coalescing to produce a fibrotic preputial ring (Fig. 8.10.1). When the disease is more extensive it may be accompanied by ulceration and involvement of the external urethral meatus and urethra. Although it was previously taught that BXO does not affect boys under the age of 5 years, recently published evidence has shown this to be incorrect. One published series of affected boys included five with histologically proven BXO who were under 4 years of age and one who was under two years of age.[9] Glanular involvement occurs in around half of paediatric cases of BXO, with meatal involvement in 20–30%. Depending upon the severity of meatal stenosis treatment consists of topical steroid therapy, meatal dilatation or meatotomy/meatoplasty.[10,11] Balanitis xerotica obliterans is widely regarded as an absolute indication for circumcision. The excised foreskin should be sent for histological examination to confirm the diagnosis.[12] Follow-up is indicated to monitor for the development of meatal stenosis.[10] In adult patients there is an association between BXO and squamous cell carcinoma (SCC) of the penis[13] but whether childhood BXO predisposes to the later development of SCC is entirely unclear.

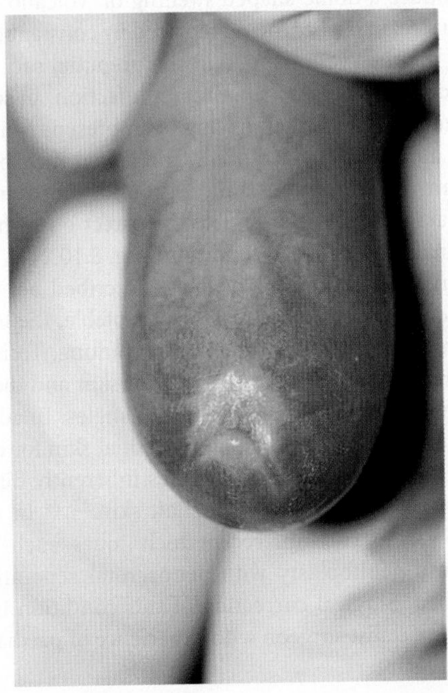

Fig. 8.10.1 Pathological phimosis in a 13-year-old boy due to balanitis xerotica obliterans. Note the whitish scarred appearance to the narrowed preputial orifice.

Paraphimosis

Paraphimosis is rare in childhood but can arise following retraction of a physiological phimosis by a boy (or parent) who is unaware of the importance of returning the foreskin to its original position over the glans. Circumferential constriction caused by physiological phimosis restricts venous return from the foreskin and glans leading to discoloration, oedema, and localized discomfort. Paraphimosis is a urological emergency which, if untreated can progress to tissue necrosis.[14,15] Several non-invasive techniques have been described for its reduction which involve manual compression in combination with; an 'iced glove' method,[16] osmotic agents such as sugar,[17] or mannitol,[18] and flexible, self-adhering bandages.[15] The Dundee technique of multiple needle puncture with expression of oedema fluid usually requires general anaesthesia in childhood.[19] A dorsal slit can be performed as a last resort. Since data from clinical trials are lacking the treatment of paraphimosis is usually based on local practice or local guidelines.[20] Paraphimosis is normally an isolated event and is not an indication for circumcision—except in boys experiencing recurrent episodes.

Congenital megaprepuce

First described in a case report in 1994,[21] this condition appears to be becoming more common. Typically, the preputial sac is significantly enlarged, surrounds the whole penile shaft and distends with urine to produce a dome-shaped swelling or 'volcano'-type penis. The urinary stream is poor, being replaced by constant dribbling of urine from the reservoir trapped in the preputial sac. Congenital megaprepuce rarely causes urinary tract infection. In some boys it may be genuinely congenital, having been present from birth but in others it appears to be acquired. Congenital megaprepuce can be confidently diagnosed on clinical grounds alone and imaging is unnecessary. Surgery is advisable to correct both the cosmetic and functional aspects of the condition (Fig. 8.10.2). A number of different surgical techniques have been described but while their short-term cosmetic outcome may be acceptable, the longer-term results are more variable and often disappointing. Technical difficulties centre on the paucity of penile shaft skin and the poor definition of the penopubic and penoscrotal angles. In addition it is invariably necessary to rely on inner preputial skin for coverage of at least part of the penile shaft. This has inherently different aesthetic properties to normal penile shaft skin.[22–24] In an attempt to simplify reconstruction, recent techniques such as ventral V-plasty[25] and genitoplasty with penoscrotal separation[26] have been described. Surgical correction of this condition is best performed by a specialist surgeon with experience of paediatric penile reconstructive surgery.

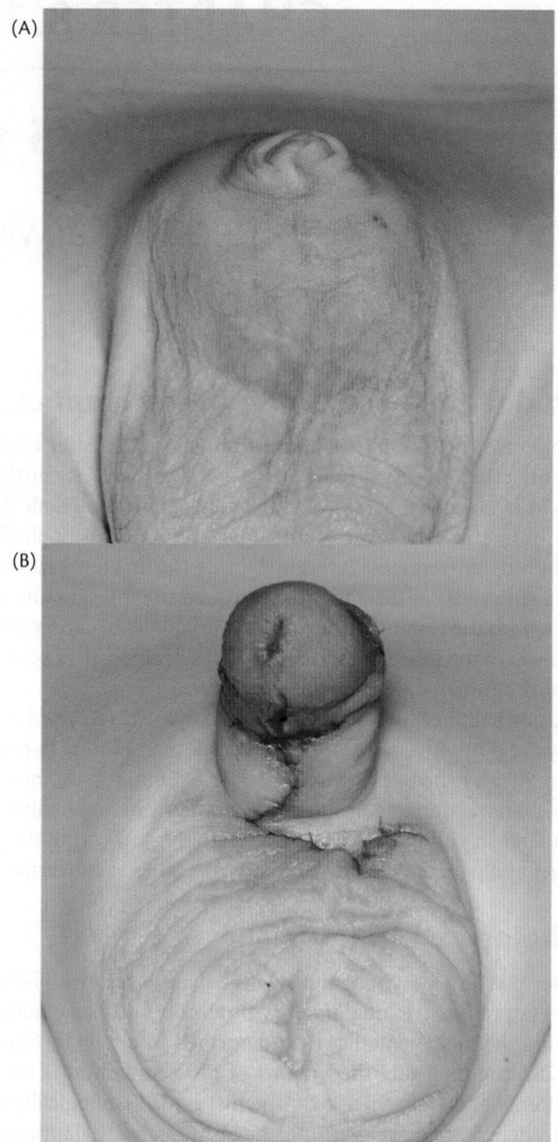

Fig. 8.10.2 (A) Congenital megaprepuce in an infant with a concealed penis from birth; and (B) postoperative appearance following a modified circumcision.

Other disorders of the prepuce

Preputial adhesions to the glans resolve spontaneously[3] and do not require any form of intervention. Smegma which accumulates behind an adherent prepuce can create the appearance of a yellowish 'cyst', also called a preputial 'pearl'.[27] This may also resemble the appearance of a mobile subcutaneous lipoma of the distal penile shaft. Such 'cysts' always resolve spontaneously. True mucous retention cysts of the foreskin are rare and are treated by surgical enucleation. Acute balanoposthitis (infection of the prepuce and glans) is a common condition resulting in localized erythema and oedema.[28] Although the infection is often self-limiting, a culture swab should be taken and oral antibiotics prescribed for more severe cases in which there is discharge of pus from the preputial opening. Balanoposthitis is not an indication for circumcision except when it occurs repeatedly. Many boys with mild infection or minor irritation are referred inappropriately for surgical assessment.[29] Rarely, genital involvement in cases of Henoch-Schönlein purpura can be mistaken for balanoposthitis.[30]

Circumcision and alternatives to circumcision

In the United Kingdom, medical indications for paediatric circumcision are restricted to boys with BXO, recurrent balanoposthitis, or repeated episodes of paraphimosis. Circumcision may also be justified as a prophylactic measure against urinary tract infection (UTI) in boys with significant urinary tract abnormalities such as posterior urethral valves or vesicoureteric reflux.[31,32] The American Academy of Pediatrics Task Force on Circumcision[33] has recently updated its guidance on circumcision, with a recommendation that the health benefits of newborn male circumcision outweigh the risks. The benefits claimed for routine neonatal circumcision include; prevention of urinary tract infections, reduced risks of acquiring some sexually transmitted infections (including HIV) and prevention of penile cancer. However, the authors of the American Academy of Pediatrics (AAP) recommendations have been strongly criticized on the grounds of cultural bias and flawed interpretation of the published evidence.[34] In most Western countries, routine neonatal circumcision is not considered to be a legitimate public health measure. Ritual circumcision of male infants and children is, however, widely performed in accordance with certain religious and cultural beliefs. In the United Kingdom this is usually undertaken in a community setting by individuals who may or may not be medically qualified. A range of techniques are employed, of which the use of a Plastibell disposable device is probably the commonest. Circumcision services are provided under the auspices of the National Health Service in some cities in the United Kingdom.

Clinical trials in countries with a high prevalence of HIV infection have demonstrated that transmission of HIV infection is significantly reduced by circumcision.[35,36]

The successful treatment of 'physiological' phimosis and non-retractile foreskins by the use of topical steroids has been reported in a number of studies.[37–39] This approach has also been reported to be effective in some cases of BXO.[40] Preputioplasty is a useful alternative to circumcision but is unsuited to use in younger boys who are less willing to comply with the requirement for regular retraction of the prepuce postoperatively.[41,42] Although most surgeons prefer circumcision to preputioplasty for the treatment of BXO, promising initial results have been reported for preputioplasty combined with intralesional steroid injection.[43]

Conclusion

Physiological phimosis (a non-retractile but otherwise healthy foreskin) is one of the commonest reasons for surgical referral in childhood. In most cases, all that is required is parental reassurance and an explanation that the foreskin will gradually become fully retractile. Balanitis xerotica obliterans is the main medical indication for circumcision and can be readily diagnosed from the clinical findings.

Further reading

Babu R, Harrison SK, Hutton KA. Ballooning of the foreskin and physiological phimosis: is there any objective evidence of obstructed voiding? *BJU Int* 2004; **94**:384–7.

Becker K. Lichen sclerosus in boys. *Dtsch Arztebl Int* 2011; **108**(4):53–8.

Cuckow PM. Circumcision. (pp. 664– 74 [Chapter 52]) In: Stringer MD, Oldham KT, Mouriquand PDE (eds). *Pediatric Surgery and Urology: Long- term Outcomes*, 2nd edition. Cambridge, UK: Cambridge University Press, 2006.

Gairdner D. The fate of the foreskin, a study of circumcision. *Br Med J* 1949; **2**(4642):1433–7.

Hutton AR. The prepuce. (pp. 233– 45 [Chapter 17]) In: Thomas DFM, Duffy PG, Rickwood AMK (eds). *Essentials of Paediatric Urology*, 2nd edition. London, UK: Informa Healthcare, 2008.

Malone P, Steinbrecher H. Medical aspects of male circumcision. *BMJ* 2007; **335**(7631):1206–9.

Oster J. Further fate of the foreskin. Incidence of preputial adhesions, phimosis, and smegma among Danish schoolboys. *Arch Dis Child* 1968; **43**:200–3.

References

1. Deibert GA. The separation of the prepuce in the human penis. *Anat Rec* 1933; **57**:387–99.
2. Hayashi Y, Kojima Y, Mizuno K, *et al.* A Japanese view on circumcision: nonoperative management of normal and abnormal prepuce. *Urology* 2010; **76**:21–4.
3. Gairdner D. The fate of the foreskin, a study of circumcision. *Br Med J* 1949; **2**(4642):1433–7.
4. Oster J. Further fate of the foreskin. Incidence of preputial adhesions, phimosis, and smegma among Danish schoolboys. *Arch Dis Child* 1968; **43**:200–3.
5. Weiss C. Routine non-ritual circumcision in infancy. A new look at an old operation. *Clin Pediatr (Phila)* 1964; **3**:560–3.
6. Stuhmer A. Balanitis xerotica obliterans (post-operationem) und ihre Beziehungen zur "Kraurosis glandis et praeputii penis". *Arch Derm Syph* 1928; **156**:613.
7. Catterall RD, Oates JK. Treatment of balanitis xerotica obliterans with hydrocortisone injections. *Br J Vener Dis* 1962; **38**:75–7.
8. Sandler G, Patrick E, Cass D. Long standing balanitis xerotica obliterans resulting in renal impairment in a child. *Pediatr Surg Int* 2008; **24**:961–4.
9. Jayakumar S, Antao B, Bevington O, Furness P, Ninan GK. Balanitis xerotica obliterans in children and its incidence under the age of 5 years. *J Pediatr Urol* 2012; **8**:272–5.
10. Holbrook C, Tsang T. Management of boys with abnormal appearance of meatus at circumcision for balanitis xerotica obliterans. *Ann R Coll Surg Engl* 2011; **93**:482–4.
11. Gargollo PC, Kozakewich HP, Bauer SB, *et al.* Balanitis xerotica obliterans in boys. *J Urol* 2005; **174**:1409–12.
12. Bochove-Overgaauw DM, Gelders W, De Vylder AM. Routine biopsies in pediatric circumcision: (non) sense? *J Pediatr Urol* 2009; **5**:178–80.
13. Barbagli G, Palminteri E, Mirri F, Guazzoni G, Turini D, Lazzeri M. Penile carcinoma in patients with genital lichen sclerosus: a multicenter survey. *J Urol* 2006; **175**:1359–63.
14. Hollowood AD, Sibley GN. Non-painful paraphimosis causing partial amputation. *Br J Urol* 1997; **80**:958.
15. Pohlman GD, Phillips JM, Wilcox DT. Simple method of paraphimosis reduction revisited: Point of technique and review of the literature. *J Pediatr Urol* 2013; **9**:104–7.
16. Houghton GR. The "iced-glove" method of treatment of paraphimosis. *Br J Surg* 1973; **60**:876–7.
17. González Fernández M, Sousa Escandón MA, Parra Muntaner L, López Pacios JC. [Sugar: treatment of choice in irreducible paraphimosis]. *Actas Urol Esp* 2001; **25**:393–5.
18. Anand A, Kapoor S. Mannitol for paraphimosis reduction. *Urol Int* 2013; **90**:106–8.
19. Reynard JM, Barua JM. Reduction of paraphimosis the simple way—the Dundee technique. *BJU Int* 1999; **83**:859–60.
20. Mackway-Jones K, Teece S. Best evidence topic reports. Ice, pins, or sugar to reduce paraphimosis. *Emerg Med J* 2004; **21**:77–8.
21. O'Brien A, Shapiro AM, Frank JD. Phimosis or congenital megaprepuce? *Br J Urol* 1994; **73**:719–20.
22. Summerton DJ, McNally J, Denny AJ, Malone PS. Congenital megaprepuce: an emerging condition—how to recognize and treat it. *BJU Int* 2000; **86**:519–22.
23. Ruiz E, Vagni R, Apostolo C, *et al.* Simplified surgical approach to congenital megaprepuce: fixing, unfurling and tailoring revisited. *J Urol* 2011; **185**(6 Suppl):2487–90.
24. Rod J, Desmonts A, Petit T, Ravasse P. Congenital megaprepuce: A 12-year experience (52 cases) of this specific form of buried penis. *J Pediatr Urol* 2013; **9**(6 Pt A):784–8.
25. Alexander A, Lorenzo AJ, Salle JL, Rode H. The Ventral V-plasty: a simple procedure for the reconstruction of a congenital megaprepuce. *J Pediatr Surg* 2010; **45**:1741–7.
26. Buluggiu A, Panait N, Anastasescu R, Merrot T, Alessandrini P. Congenital megaprepuce: surgical approach. *Urology* 2013; **81**(3):649–52.
27. Malone P, Steinbrecher H. Medical aspects of male circumcision. *BMJ* 2007; **335**(7631):1206–9.
28. Schwartz RH, Rushton HG. Acute balanoposthitis in young boys. *Pediatr Infect Dis J* 1996; **15**:176–7.
29. Griffiths D, Frank JD. Inappropriate circumcision referrals by GPs. *J R Soc Med* 1992; **85**:324–5.
30. Caliskan B, Guven A, Atabek C, Gok F, Demirbag S, Surer I. Henoch-Schönlein purpura presenting with symptoms mimicking balanoposthitis. *Pediatr Rep* 2009; **1**(1):e5.
31. Singh-Grewal D, Macdessi J, Craig J. Circumcision for the prevention of urinary tract infection in boys: a systematic review of randomised trials and observational studies. *Arch Dis Child* 2005; **90**:853–8.

32. Bader M, McCarthy L. What is the efficacy of circumcision in boys with complex urinary tract abnormalities? *Pediatr Nephrol* 2013; **28**(12):2267–72.
33. American academy of pediatrics task force on circumcision. Male circumcision. *Pediatrics* 2012; **130**(3):e756–85.
34. Frisch M, Aigrain Y, Barauskas V, *et al.* Cultural bias in the AAP's 2012 technical report and policy statement on male circumcision. *Pediatrics* 2013; **131**(4):796–800.
35. Bailey RC, Moses S, Parker CB, *et al.* Male circumcision for HIV prevention in young men in Kisumu, Kenya: a randomised controlled trial. *Lancet* 2007; **369**(9562):643–56.
36. Chang LW, Serwadda D, Quinn TC, Wawer MJ, Gray RH, Reynolds SJ. Combination implementation for HIV prevention: moving from clinical trial evidence to population-level effects. *Lancet Infect Dis* 2013; **13**:65–76.
37. Lund L, Wai KH, Mui LM, Yeung CK. Effect of topical steroid on non-retractile prepubertal foreskin by a prospective, randomized, double-blind study. *Scand J Urol Nephrol* 2000; **34**:267–9.
38. Orsola A, Caffaratti J, Garat JM. Conservative treatment of phimosis in children using a topical steroid. *Urology* 2000; **56**:307–10.
39. Elmore JM, Baker LA, Snodgrass WT. Topical steroid therapy as an alternative to circumcision for phimosis in boys younger than 3 years. *J Urol* 2002; **168**:1746–7.
40. Kiss A, Csontai A, Pirót L, Nyirády P, Merksz M, Király L. The response of balanitis xerotica obliterans to local steroid application compared with placebo in children. *J Urol* 2001; **165**:219–20.
41. Cuckow PM, Rix G, Mouriquand PD. Preputial plasty: a good alternative to circumcision. *J Pediatr Surg* 1994; **29**:561–3.
42. Fischer-Klein Ch, Rauchenwald M. Triple incision to treat phimosis in children: an alternative to circumcision? *BJU Int* 2003; **92**:459–62.
43. Wilkinson DJ, Lansdale N, Everitt LH, *et al.* Foreskin preputioplasty and intralesional triamcinolone: a valid alternative to circumcision for balanitis xerotica obliterans. *J Pediatr Surg* 2012; **47**:756–9.

CHAPTER 8.11

Undescended testis and inguinoscrotal conditions in children

David F.M. Thomas

Undescended testis (cryptorchidism)

Normal development and descent of the testis

The testis develops within the genital ridge from the sixth week of gestation onwards. Endocrine regulation of testicular descent is complex but Müllerian inhibitory substance plays a role in the first phase of testicular descent whereas the second phase occurs in response to testosterone stimulation between the twenty-eighth and thirty-fifth week of gestation. Descent is mediated by contraction of the gubernaculum, which guides the descending testis into the scrotum.[1] The testis has normally descended fully by the time of birth in a term infant. During descent the testis is accompanied by the processus vaginalis, a pouch-like protrusion extending downwards from the peritoneal cavity into the scrotum (Fig. 8.11.1, Fig. 8.11.1A).[1,2] Although the processus vaginalis normally undergoes spontaneous closure in the later stages of gestation (Fig. 8.11.1B)[2] it remains open in around 3–5% of term infants, thus creating a potential inguinal hernia or communicating hydrocele.

Although it was previously thought that the testis remains biologically quiescent until the onset of puberty it is now known that this is not the case.[3,4] Active maturation of germ cells commences from around six months of age with transformation from fetal gonocytes to primary spermatocytes continuing until the age of three to four years. However, the process of germ cell maturation only proceeds normally when the testis is located within the scrotum, where the temperature is 2–3°C lower than in the abdomen or groin. Germ cell maturation is impaired at higher temperatures and progressive temperature—related degenerative changes continue

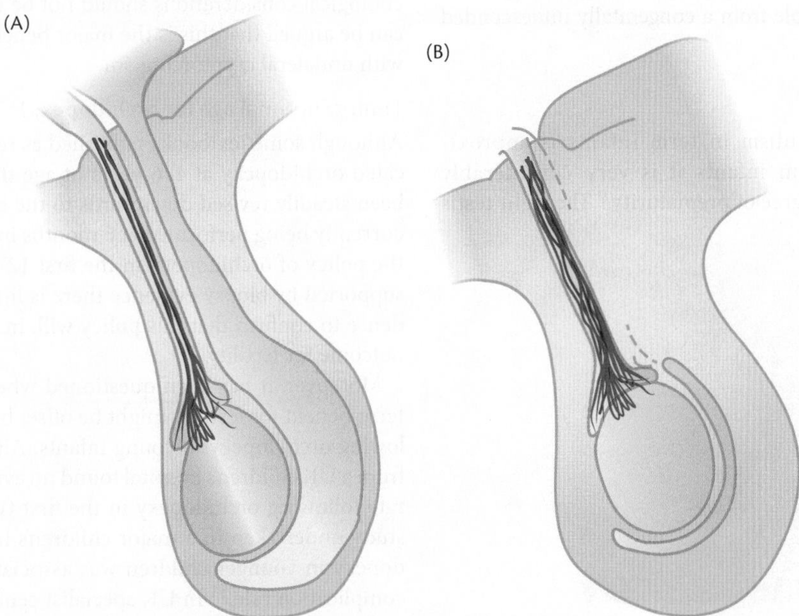

Fig. 8.11.1 Anatomy of processus vaginalis. (A) The processus vaginalis accompanies the testis during its descent into the scrotum; and (B) spontaneous closure of the processus vaginalis is normally complete by the time of birth in a term infant.

Republished with permission of Taylor and Francis Group, LLC from *Essentials of Paediatric Urology*, David F. M. Thomas, Patrick G. Duffy, and Anthony M. K. Rickwood, (Eds.), CRC Press, Taylor and Francis Group, Florida, USA, Copyright © 2002; permission conveyed through Copyright Clearance Center, Inc.

throughout childhood eventually culminating in total absence of germ cells after puberty.

Aetiology

Recognized factors[5] include:

- Impaired virilization due to defective androgen synthesis or partial and complete androgen sensitivity
- Mechanical factors (e.g. prune belly syndrome and abdominal wall defects)
- Genetically—determined syndromes (e.g. Prader-Willi syndrome)[6]
- Neurological disorders including spina bifida and cerebral palsy[7,8]

In the majority of cases, however, particularly of unilateral undescended testis (UDT), no specific aetiological factor can be identified.

Classification

It its simplest, the classification consists of *palpable* or *impalpable UDTs*. However, with patient and careful examination a testis which was initially thought to be impalpable can often be identified in the inguinal canal. *Intracanalicular testes* may be difficult to identify on clinical examination since they are often mobile and tend to move between the inguinal canal and abdominal cavity through a wide-mouthed patent processus vaginalis. *Inguinal undescended testes* are usually located just outside and above the external inguinal ring in the 'superficial inguinal pouch'. *Retractile testes* occur most commonly between three and seven years of age. So-called 'high retractile' testes also exhibit cremasteric overactivity but unlike normal retractile testes cannot be brought easily to the bottom of scrotum without tension on the spermatic cord. *Ascending testes* are those which have descended fully at birth but subsequently undergo secondary ascent during childhood to adopt an inguinal position which may be indistinguishable from a congenitally undescended testis (Fig. 8.11.2).

Incidence

The incidence of cryptorchidism in term infants is approximately 1.5% and in preterm infants it is very considerably higher, depending on the degree of prematurity.[9] The right testis is affected more commonly than the left and 25% of cases are bilateral.

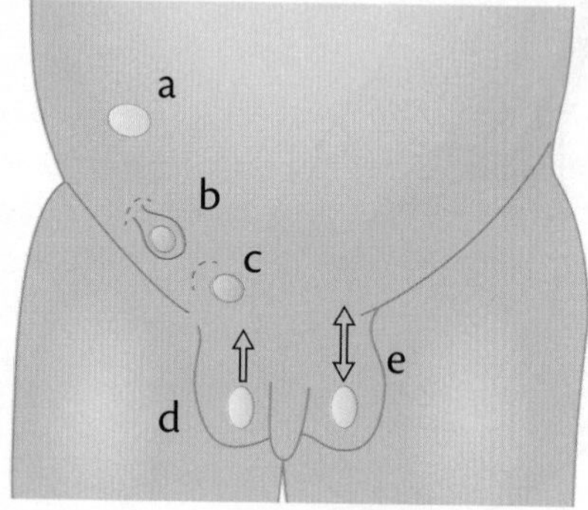

Fig. 8.11.2 Anatomical classification of cryptorchidism. (a) Intra-abdominal testis; (b) intracanalicular testis; (c) inguinal testis (lying outside inguinal canal); (d) ascending testis; and (e) retractile testis.

Clinical features

Most undescended testes are either identified during the course of neonatal examination or routine checks by health professionals in the first year of life. Occasionally a congenitally undescended testis undergoes spontaneous descent in the first six months of life but since this is rare, every infant with an undescended testis should be referred for a surgical opinion with a view to orchidopexy. *Examination* is best undertaken in a warm environment and should include inspection of the scrotum to assess the position of the testes prior to palpation. This should be performed gently and with warm hands to avoid evoking a cremasteric reflex.[10]

Orchidopexy

Indications

Recent evidence of germ cell transformation occurring in early childhood adds further weight to the arguments for performing orchidopexy at a young age to maximize potential fertility.[3,4] This applies particularly in cases of bilateral cryptorchidism. Testes which have been retained in the groin or abdomen into adult life undoubtedly carry an increased risk of malignancy. In one study, premalignant changes (intratubular germ cell neoplasia or 'carcinoma *in situ*') were documented in 25% of testes which had been retained within the abdomen into adulthood.[11] However, there is now a growing body of evidence that orchidopexy performed in early to mid-childhood can reduce the long-term risk of testicular cancer to a level closer to that in the normal population.[12,13] Orchidopexy probably protects the testis from trauma (although this is a largely intuitive rather than evidence-based indication) and also confers protection against the risk of torsion—particularly in intracanalicular UDTs. Finally, the importance of cosmetic/psychological considerations should not be underestimated. Indeed it can be argued that this is the major benefit of orchidopexy in boys with unilateral cryptorchidism.

Timing: optimal age for orchidopexy?

Although some textbooks published as recently as the 1980s advocated orchidopexy at 4–6 years of age the recommended age has been steadily revised downwards to the extent that orchidopexy is currently being performed at 6 months in some centres.[3] But while the policy of orchidopexy in the first 12 months of life is strongly supported by biopsy evidence there is little long-term clinical evidence to confirm that this policy will, in fact, lead to an improved outcome for fertility.

Moreover, it has been questioned whether the perceived long-term benefit for fertility might be offset by a higher failure rate following orchidopexy in young infants. Although a study published from a UK children's hospital found no evidence of a higher atrophy rate following orchidopexy in the first two years of life[14] another study undertaken in a major children's hospital found that orchidopexy in younger children was associated with a higher overall complication rate.[15] In UK specialist centres, orchidopexy appears to be most widely performed as a day case shortly after the first birthday.

Technical aspects of orchidopexy

For a detailed account of surgical technique the reader is referred to a textbook of operative paediatric surgery.[16,17]

Some of the key technical points can be summarized as follows:

- Examination under anaesthesia to establish the position of the testis prior to surgery;
- Skin crease incision;
- Opening the inguinal canal to facilitate mobilization of the cord structures to the level of the internal inguinal ring;
- Identifying, mobilizing, and transfixing any processus vaginalis from the cord structures. This can require a difficult dissection, particularly in cases of intracanalicular testis when the flimsy peritoneal sac is often closely adherent to the vas and vessels;
- Gentle tissue handling to avoid damage to the delicate vas and vessels.

Although it is standard practice to secure the testis within the scrotum by use of a 'dartos' pouch technique many experienced surgeons also take the added precaution of suture fixation to the scrotal pouch to minimize the risk of re-ascent. A scrotal approach is increasingly favoured for ascending or 'high retractile' testes.[18]

Orchidopexy: results and complications

Complications include; ischaemic atrophy of the testis, reascent (requiring re-do orchidopexy), iatrogenic injury to the vas deferens and dehiscence of the scrotal incision.

From his analysis of 64 publications (8,425 orchidopexies) Docimo identified a 92% overall success rate for orchidopexy for inguinal undescended testes, with corresponding figures for intracanalicular testes and abdominal testes of 87% and 74%, respectively.[19] A literature review undertaken by Hutton and Sau[20] found that published complication rates varied between 1.9% and 6%.[20]

Although a higher failure rate is reported following orchidopexy for intra-abdominal testes Docimo's analysis nevertheless identified an overall 67% success rate for the single stage Fowler-Stephens procedure and 77% for the two-stage procedure. More recently, success rates (defined by viability and scrotal position) in excess of 90% have been reported for the Fowler-Stephens orchidopexy.[21,22]

Fertility

Fertility can be assessed by measuring laboratory parameters of semen quality or by paternity. Both methods have potential weaknesses and do not always correlate closely.

The published evidence consistently demonstrates that bilateral cryptorchidism is associated with a significantly poorer outcome than unilateral cryptorchidism.[23,24] Indeed, for men with a history of unilateral cryptorchidism, paternity rates appear to be normal or only marginally reduced.[24] Studies of semen quality in men with a history of unilateral cryptorchidism nevertheless report widely differing results with the percentage of those with normal semen analysis ranging from 17% to 95%. Hutson concluded from his detailed examination of the evidence that more than 50% of men with a history of unilateral cryptorchidism have normal parameters of semen quality.[3] By contrast, men with a history of bilateral cryptorchidism experience a marked impairment of semen quality with the percentage of normal values ranging from 0% to 40% in 10 published series. Impairment of semen quality is mirrored in reduced prospects of achieving paternity—with reported paternity rates for men with a history of bilateral cryptorchidism ranging from 33% to 65%.[3]

Malignancy

Whereas studies in the 1940s and 1950s indicated that the risk of malignancy in undescended testes was increased by fifty fold, more recent studies have suggested that the actual figure is very considerably lower[12,13,25]—corresponding to only a five to ten fold increase in relative risk. The absolute lifetime risk of a man with a history of cryptorchidism developing testicular cancer is approximately 1:100 as opposed to a 1:500 in the normal population.

Does orchidopexy reduce the risk of developing malignancy? Although the evidence remains somewhat contradictory there is a growing body of evidence to indicate that this is indeed the case. In summary, the risk of malignancy was probably overstated in the past and the individual lifetime risk is probably of the order of 1%.

Follow-up consists of postoperative review at 6–12 months to assess the position and viability of the testis. Ideally, patients should be reviewed again in their mid-teens to confirm that pubertal testicular growth has occurred and to explain the rationale for testicular self-examination. Unfortunately this ideal is difficult to achieve in many healthcare systems.

Impalpable testis: Investigation

Ultrasound is an unreliable modality for determining whether an impalpable testis is genuinely absent (anorchia) or is present but located within the abdomen. However, ultrasound may occasionally be helpful in identifying an impalpable inguinal testis—for example, in boys with Prader-Willi syndrome. Computed tomography (CT) and MRI are reasonably sensitive for visualizing intra-abdominal testes in older boys but laparoscopy is unquestionably the investigation of choice in all age groups[26] (Fig. 8.11.3). Although there is some variation in published laparoscopic findings an abdominal testis is identified in around 40% of cases. In approximately 30% the testis is absent—as confirmed by the finding of blind ending vas and vessels and in approximately 20% the vas and vessels are seen to the enter inguinal canal, terminating in a 'nubbin' of atrophic tissue. In approximately 10% of cases the testis is present, but is either intracanalicular (moving between the inguinal canal and abdominal cavity) or is small and concealed within the inguinal canal, for example in boys with Prader-Willi syndrome.

Management of intra-abdominal testes

The implications of different laparoscopic findings and the relevant treatment options should be discussed with the parents prior to surgery. A small or morphologically abnormal testis is probably best excised at the time of laparoscopy. By contrast, it may be appropriate to consider orchidopexy if the testis appears normal. Currently, the favoured approach is the two stages Fowler-Stephens's technique.[26–29] The first stage consists of clipping the testicular vessels at the time of diagnostic laparoscopy. Over the ensuing 6–12 months the testis acquires an enhanced collateral blood supply via the vessels accompanying the vas. During the second stage (which can be performed as an open or laparoscopically assisted procedure) the testis is carefully mobilized with the vas and an adjacent strip of vascularized peritoneum and then relocated to the scrotum.

The laparoscopic two-stage Fowler-Stephens operation has largely superseded microvascular transfer—in which the testicular vessels are divided before the testis is repositioned the scrotum and revascularization achieved by microvascular anastomosis of testicular vessels to branches of the inferior epigastric vessels in the groin.[30]

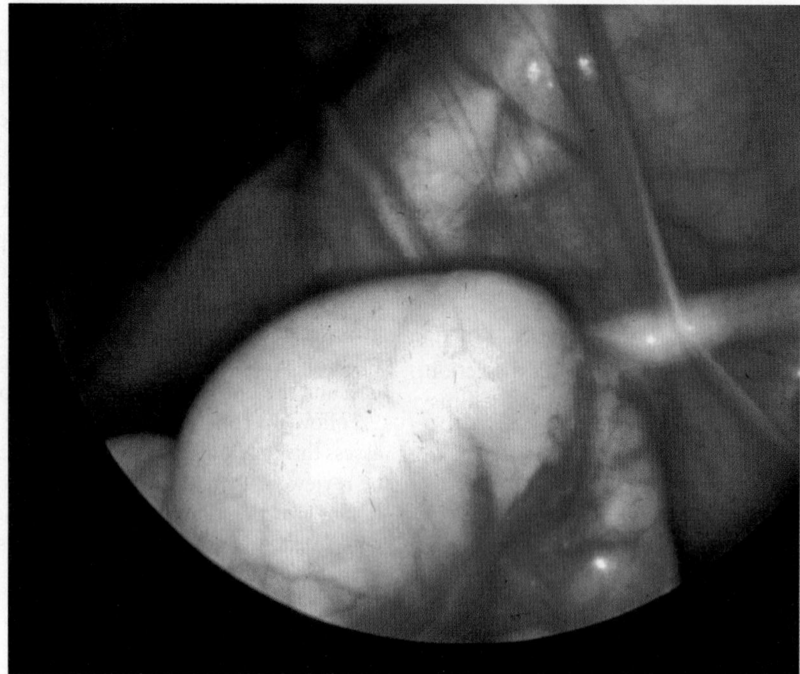

Fig. 8.11.3 Laparoscopic appearances of an intra-abdominal testis.

Newborns or infants with bilateral impalpable testes require specialist assessment to investigate possible chromosomal abnormalities or disorders of sex differentiation.

Retractile testis

Excessive activity of the cremasteric muscle fibres encircling the spermatic cord has the effect of elevating the testis from its normal scrotal position to a higher position in the scrotum or above.[31] Retractile testes are common, the peak incidence being between three and seven years of age. The diagnosis of 'retractile testis' should be viewed with caution in infants age under 12 months since this is more likely to represent mobility in an incompletely descended testis rather than cremasteric overactivity in a fully descended testis.

On examination, a genuine 'retractile' testis can be brought easily to the floor of the scrotum, where it remains without tension on the spermatic cord. Testes which fulfil these criteria can be managed conservatively since in the majority of cases the cremasteric overactivity gradually resolves, allowing the testis to revert permanently to a scrotal position. Nevertheless it is prudent to review boys with retractile testes on an annual or biannual basis since this outcome is not always predictable and a proportion of retractile testes progress to secondary ascent.

Although hormonal treatment with human chorionic gonadotrophin or luteinizing releasing hormone has a limited role in the treatment of 'high retractile' or ascending testes the majority of paediatric urologists favour the greater certainty afforded by orchidopexy.[32]

Ascending testis

The phenomenon of secondary testicular ascent has been convincingly documented in a sizeable number of published reports.[33] Hack and associates[34] found a bimodal distribution in the age at presentation of 221 boys with 258 undescended testes. Of those presenting in later childhood (at a mean age of 8.4 years) 73% of 'undescended' testes had nevertheless been previously recorded as lying in a normal scrotal position on at least one occasion in earlier childhood. Indeed, 48% of these testes had been recorded in a scrotal position on three previous examinations. Further evidence of the phenomenon of secondary ascent can be inferred from population—based data in which cumulative orchidopexy rates exceed the birth incidence of cryptorchidism.[35]

Although the mechanism is poorly understood, it has been reported that 25–40% of ascending testes have passed through a retractile phase.[36] The natural history of untreated ascending testes is poorly documented since the majority of urologists favour surgical intervention. However, Hack and associates followed 44 boys with 50 ascended testes through puberty and reported that 84% of these testes reverted to a scrotal position, while 16% required orchidopexy.[37]

The limited evidence of biopsy studies of ascending testes is difficult to assess but Hutson concluded that, 'even later in childhood, 5–10 years of non-scrotal position does cause secondary degeneration of the testes'.[3]

Orchidopexy for ascending testes is generally straightforward since extensive mobilization is rarely required. A scrotal approach can be used if the testis can be brought to the upper scrotum under anaesthesia.

Acute scrotal conditions

Testicular torsion accounts for approximately 90% of cases of acute scrotal pathology in adolescents.[38,39] By contrast the differential diagnosis is more varied in prepubertal boys, in whom torsion of a testicular appendage (hydatid of morgagni) accounts for 40–50% of cases. It is important to note, nevertheless, that even in prepubertal boys testicular torsion accounts for over 30% of cases of acute scrotal pathology. Other conditions include: idiopathic scrotal oedema, epididymo-orchitis, and Henoch-Schönlien purpuric vasculitis.

Testicular torsion

With the exception of 'neonatal torsion' the testis and cord structures almost invariably twist within the coverings of the tunica vaginalis (intravaginal torsion). This is a consequence of excessive mobility and an abnormally high attachment of the tunica vaginalis. This anatomical pattern ('bell clapper testis') probably represents one end of the normal anatomical spectrum, rather than a discrete pathological entity.[40] In cases of extravaginal torsion, the testis, and its coverings twist in their entirety. This pattern is virtually confined to the early newborn period.

The incidence of testicular torsion is approximately 1:4,000. Possible precipitating factors include trauma, cold weather, recent exercise, and sexual activity.[41]

Pathophysiology

Experimental studies in rat, porcine, and canine models have shown that 720-degree torsion consistently results in complete cessation of blood flow. Histological evidence of irreversible ischaemic damage is detectable after as little as two hours, with complete loss of seminiferous tissue after six hours.[42–44] There is more variability in the severity and timescale of ischaemic injury caused by less severe degrees of experimentally induced torsion. Evaluating the clinical evidence is more problematic—not least because of the poor scientific standard of most published studies. The progression from ischaemia to atrophy extends over many months. For this reason, published 'salvage' or 'viability' rates based on an assessment of potential viability at the time of exploration are highly misleading—unless the 'salvaged' testes have been reassessed after a minimum of six months. Few published studies meet these basic scientific criteria and the majority consist of retrospective case note reviews with little or no outcome data. One follow-up study found that 68% of 'saved' testes had atrophied when reassessed at four years.[45] In a study looking specifically at long-term atrophy rates in 'saved' or 'salvaged' testes in prepubertal boys it was found that in boys with symptoms of 7–12 hours duration, 83% of testes which had been judged to be viable at the time of exploration were nevertheless found to have atrophied on long-term follow-up. Even in boys operated upon within six hours of the onset of symptoms 33% of seemingly viable testes underwent atrophy.[46] When viability is retained, testicular volume may nevertheless be greatly reduced since atrophy is not an 'all or none' phenomenon.[47,48] The eight-hour viability 'watershed' identified in one widely cited study is misleading since closer scrutiny of the study data reveals that all the normal-sized viable testes had, in fact, been operated on within four to six hours while those operated upon between six to eight hours were abnormal on follow-up.[49] Reviewing a series of 104 boys with a median age of 13 years Saxena and associates reported an orchidectomy rate of 9% in boys presenting in less than six hours compared with 56% in those presenting after 6 hours. However, as in the majority of published studies, the authors provide no follow-up data and no information on the long-term atrophy rates in the 44% of testes left *in situ* in boys with a history exceeding six hours.[50] The assertion by the authors of one review article[51] that that it is 'commonly accepted' that viability declines sharply when symptoms exceed six hours is probably overoptimistic. Many clinicians appear to hold a misguided view of the timescale of potential viability based on uncritical acceptance of the flawed methodology and conclusions of the majority of retrospective clinical studies. This is particularly prevalent in the context of litigation.

A critical analysis of the more reliable published evidence indicates that the best prospect of retaining a viable, normal-sized testis lies in restoring its blood supply within four to six hours of the onset of torsion. Partial or complete atrophy is increasingly likely after six to eight hours. The experimental evidence suggests that beyond 6 hours the outcome is largely determined by the severity of torsion. There is probably little realistic prospect of conserving any viable testicular tissue after six to eight hours in cases of 720-degree torsion but preservation of a viable full sized testis may occasionally occur after 8–10 hours (or longer) in cases where vascular occlusion is incomplete because the torsion is mild in severity, intermittent, or resolves spontaneously.

The presence of circulating auto antibodies in some men with a history of torsion has been attributed to ischaemic damage to the blood/testis barrier. However the reported incidence of detectable anti sperm antibodies varies considerably in different published series and the clinical significance (if any) is uncertain.[52]

Clinical presentation, diagnosis, and management

Torsion classically presents with a sudden onset of severe pain accompanied by acute tenderness of the testis. Testicular pain is often referred to the groin and lower abdominal quadrant and, indeed, this may be the predominant symptom—leading to a misdiagnosis of appendicitis or enteritis. Confusingly, pain may sometimes be remarkably absent in the early stages of torsion—particularly in the prepubertal age group. The clinical assessment of any adolescent or child presenting with a sudden onset of inguinal or lower abdominal pain should always include examination of the testes. Palpation usually (but not invariably) reveals acute tenderness of the testis, which may be lying in an elevated position within the scrotum due to cremasteric contraction. Oedema and erythema of the overlying scrotal skin ensue as the timescale progresses.

Since testicular torsion accounts for around 90% of all cases of acute scrotal pathology in adolescents, urgent surgical exploration is mandatory in this age group unless there is compelling evidence of an alternative diagnosis.

Investigations such as ultrasound are rarely contributory and risk reducing the chances of conserving a viable testis by delaying surgical exploration. By contrast, the use of Doppler ultrasound may be justified in prepubertal boys since the differential diagnosis is wider in this age group. Nevertheless, surgical exploration should be performed as a matter of urgency if there is any doubt regarding the diagnosis.

Surgical exploration

Once the testis has been delivered through a scrotal incision the cord is untwisted and potential viability assessed. Favourable signs include a prompt change in colour signifying reperfusion and arterial bleeding when the tunica albuginea is incised. If the testis is judged to be potentially viable, it is fixed to the scrotal wall with a non-absorbable sutures at three sites.

Unfortunately, surgical optimism is often misplaced and, as already indicated, an appreciable proportion of testes which have been judged to be potentially viable at the time of exploration nevertheless proceed to undergo atrophy.[45,46,49]

Unless there is clear evidence of reperfusion to indicate potential viability it is therefore advisable to remove a 'doubtful' testis rather than leave it *in situ*. Because of the bilateral nature of the 'bell clapper' anomaly and the documented occurrence of asynchronous contralateral torsion, prophylactic suture fixation of the contralateral testis is a mandatory, regardless of the outcome on the affected side. Implantation of a testicular prosthesis should not be performed at the time of exploration because it is important that the young patient is adequately counselled and his scrotum has developed sufficiently to accommodate an adult-sized prosthesis (usually from the age of 15–16 years onwards).

Outcome

Studies in men with a history of testicular torsion in adolescence or early adulthood have consistently reported evidence of impaired semen quality, with the proportion of those affected exceeding 50% in some studies.[53] By contrast, the impact (if any) of reduced semen quality on paternity is not known since paternity rates in men with a history of testicular torsion have not been formally studied. Extrapolation from fertility data in men with unilateral testicular pathology or anorchia suggests despite some reduction in semen quality, paternity rates in men with a history of testicular torsion are likely to be normal or only marginally reduced.[54] Normal androgen levels are maintained regardless of whether the affected testis was conserved or removed[55] and the majority of studies have also reported normal levels of gonadotrophic hormones.

Neonatal torsion

So-called 'neonatal' torsion typically presents as a firm scrotal swelling with overlying skin discoloration which is identified shortly after delivery or in the first 48 hours of life. In the overwhelming majority of cases the torsion has occurred *in utero* rather than the newborn period.[56,57] Doppler ultrasound confirms the long-stranding nature of the changes in the testicular tissue and the absence of perfusion. A conservative approach to 'neonatal' torsion has been widely adopted on the rationale that the testis is invariably non-viable and (unlike torsion in other age groups) the extra-vaginal pattern of 'neonatal' torsion is not associated with an increased risk in the contralateral testis. However, the wisdom of this approach has been called into doubt by the authors of a growing number of case reports of synchronous and asynchronous contralateral torsion.[58] For this reason some surgeons have advocated a return to the previous practice of orchidectomy and fixation of the contralateral testis.

Other causes of acute scrotal pathology

Pain arising from torsion of a testicular appendage (hydatid of morgagni) is usually more insidious in onset and more localized than torsion of the testis. The peak incidence is around 10 years of age. Although infarction of the testicular appendage may be visible under the scrotal skin as the pathogmonic 'blue dot sign' this is often obscured by oedema and erythema of the overlying scrotal tissues. While an experienced clinician should be able to differentiate between torsion of a testicular appendage and testicular torsion on clinical grounds (with ultrasound confirmation if necessary) urgent surgical exploration is indicated if the diagnosis is in any doubt. Excision of the infarcted appendage may also be indicated if the pain is slow to resolve on conservative management.[59]

Epididymo-orchitis

This is a rare condition in children and young people and should not be diagnosed unless there is strong supportive evidence of urinary infection and/or a predisposing anatomical abnormality of the urogenital tract. Clinical features include marked tenderness of the testis, florid scrotal erythema, fever, dysuria, and systemic symptoms. Ultrasonography demonstrates perfusion within the testis and hyperaemia of the surrounding tissues. Treatment consists of antibiotics and analgesia. Appropriate imaging of the urinary tract is required in all cases to investigate the possibility of an underlying abnormality such as vesico ureteric reflux or a Müllerian remnant (pseudo vagina). Cases of testicular torsion associated with scrotal erythema and oedema are sometimes mistaken for epididymis orchitis but the presence of these features is almost always associated with a non-viable testis.

Ideopathic scrotal oedema

Ideopathic scrotal oedema is a distinctive disorder of early to mid-childhood which is characterized by painless scrotal swelling and erythema. The aetiology is unknown and the condition is sometimes recurrent. For a clinician familiar with this condition, the diagnosis is usually straightforward, but can be confirmed by the use of scrotal ultrasonography. Management is conservative and the condition usually resolves spontaneously within 48 to 72 hours.

Inguinal hernia

Inguinal hernias and hydroceles in children originate from failure of the normal closure of the processus vaginalis. When the mouth of the processus vaginalis remains widely patent it creates the potential for an indirect inguinal hernia whereas the persistence of a narrower processus gives rise to a communicating hydrocele (Fig. 8.11.4).[10]

The incidence of inguinal hernias in term infants is approximately 3–5%, rising to 30% in preterm infants.[60] Males outnumber females by approximately 10:1. The right side is more commonly affected than the left and 5–10% of hernias are bilateral.

In addition to prematurity, other predisposing factors include cryptorchidism, connective tissue disorders, chronic respiratory disease, and increased abdominal pressure.

Although inguinal hernias in infants and children typically present as a reducible inguinal swelling this may only appear intermittently and may be difficult to demonstrate during the course of a visit to the outpatient clinic. It may therefore be necessary to repeat the examination on more than one occasion or, rarely, to proceed to surgical exploration on the basis of a convincing description by the parents.

Hernias in infants under six months sometimes present acutely with a tense, irreducible swelling. In these circumstances every attempt should be made to reduce the hernia using analgesia or sedation, while deferring surgery for 24 or 48 hours to allow sufficient time for oedema and friability of the tissues to resolve. Regardless of age and pattern of presentation, all inguinal hernias in children should be managed surgically since they do not resolve spontaneously and carry a risk of incarceration and strangulation—predominantly in infants and younger children.

Surgical management

Uncomplicated inguinal hernias in older children can be treated by adult urologists with appropriate paediatric training. By

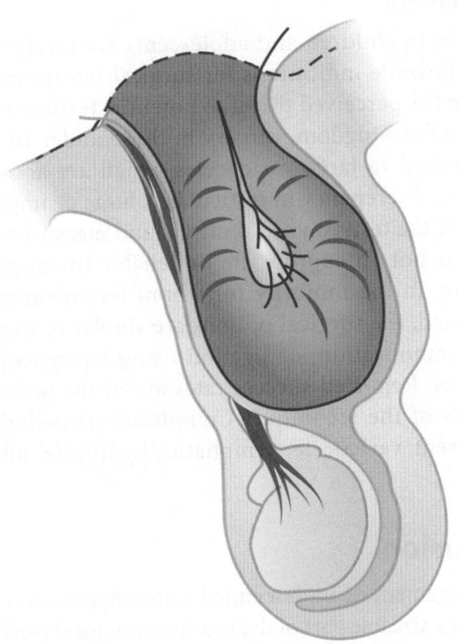

Fig. 8.11.4 Indirect inguinal hernia.
Republished with permission of Taylor and Francis Group, LLC from *Essentials of Paediatric Urology*, David F. M. Thomas, Patrick G. Duffy, and Anthony M. K. Rickwood, (Eds.), CRC Press, Taylor and Francis Group, Florida, USA, Copyright © 2002; permission conveyed through Copyright Clearance Center, Inc.

contrast, the surgical management of hernias in infancy requires specialist paediatric surgical expertise. Particular care is needed during the dissection of a flimsy sac to ensure that it is not torn and that its entire circumference is included in the transfixion suture. Since hernias in children are almost invariably indirect, simple herniotomy is usually sufficient—although it may be also advisable to insert some sutures to narrow the internal inguinal ring if it has been stretched by a particularly large hernia. Regardless of age it is important to check that the testis has been returned to the scrotum before closing the incision. Sizeable series of laparoscopic herniotomies have been published, with low complication rates.[61] Although the laparoscopic approach offers an advantage in simplifying the treatment of bilateral hernias it offers little, if any, cosmetic advantage over an open procedure performed through a small inguinal skin crease incision.

Surgical complications are unusual in older children but recurrence rates of 5% to 10% have been reported in small infants.[60,62] Other complications include ischaemic testicular atrophy and iatrogenic injury to the vas deferens.[63] It should be noted, however, that testicular atrophy following surgery for incarcerated hernia may have resulted from compression of the testicular vessels by the tense, obstructed hernia rather than a iatrogenic vascular injury.

Although the majority of girls with an inguinal hernia have a normal female karyoype, complete androgen insensitivity syndrome (46XY DSD) sometimes comes to light during a hernia operation in a child with a female external genital phenotype. Opinion is divided on the advisability of routine karyotyping of a girl with an inguinal hernia but in the author's opinion this option should be discussed with the parents at the initial consultation.

Hydrocele

Communicating hydroceles are present in up to 5% of newborn infants but mostly resolve when the processus vaginalis closes spontaneously during the first 12 months of life. An encysted hydrocele forms when the processus vaginalis closes to leave an isolated collection of fluid in the upper scrotum or groin. In most cases a hydrocele can be diagnosed on purely clinical grounds if the collection of fluid is confined to the scrotum. However, a large hydrocele extending between the inguinal canal and scrotum can be difficult to differentiate from an inguinoscrotal hernia on examination alone (Fig. 8.11.5).[64]

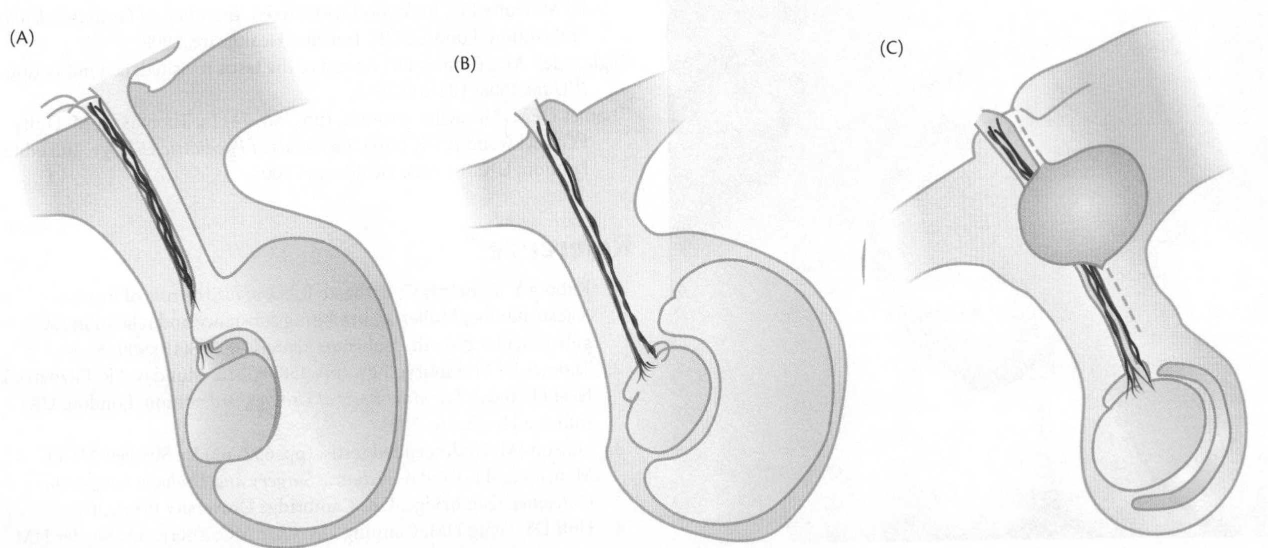

Fig. 8.11.5 (A) Persistent patent processus vaginalis resulting in a communicating hydrocele; (B) non-communicating hydrocele; and (C) encysted hydrocele.
Republished with permission of Taylor and Francis Group, LLC from *Essentials of Paediatric Urology*, David F. M. Thomas, Patrick G. Duffy, and Anthony M. K. Rickwood, (Eds.), CRC Press, Taylor and Francis Group, Florida, USA, Copyright © 2002; permission conveyed through Copyright Clearance Center, Inc.

Transillumination may not always reliably distinguish between a hydrocele and scrotal hernia in infancy—although it is a reliable physical sign in older children. Any suggestion of an abnormality of the testis on clinical examination or transillumination merits urgent investigation by ultrasound in view of the small but serious risk of underlying malignancy.

Hydroceles which are present from birth or appear in the first few weeks of life can usually be managed conservatively in the high expectation of spontaneous resolution following closure of the processus vaginalis. Indications for surgical intervention include persistence a hydrocele beyond one year of age or the appearance of a hydrocele in later childhood. The operation is similar to that for inguinal hernia. Once the communicating processus has been transfixed and divided, the distal portion is incised for a short length and a probe or a haemostat passed down into the hydrocele sac. Gentle pressure is applied to the scrotum to expel fluid retrogradely from the hydrocele sac prior to completion of the procedure. Occasionally, the processus vaginalis is found to be non- patent and the hydrocele is found to be of the non-communicating variety (Fig. 8.11.6). In this situation the sac is opened via a scrotal incision and is then everted or plicated using one of the techniques employed for adult non-communicating hydroceles.

Varicocele

Varicoceles in the paediatric age group share the same aetiology as young adults and the majority (90%) are left-sided. Asymptomatic varicoceles are occasionally identified incidentally during the course of examination performed for some other reason, but most referrals arise because the individual has become aware of a discrepancy between the two sides of his scrotum. The diagnosis is usually readily apparent on clinical examination but scrotal and abdominal ultrasonography should be performed to confirm the diagnosis, to assess testicular volume, and to exclude the remote possibility of a renal tumour.

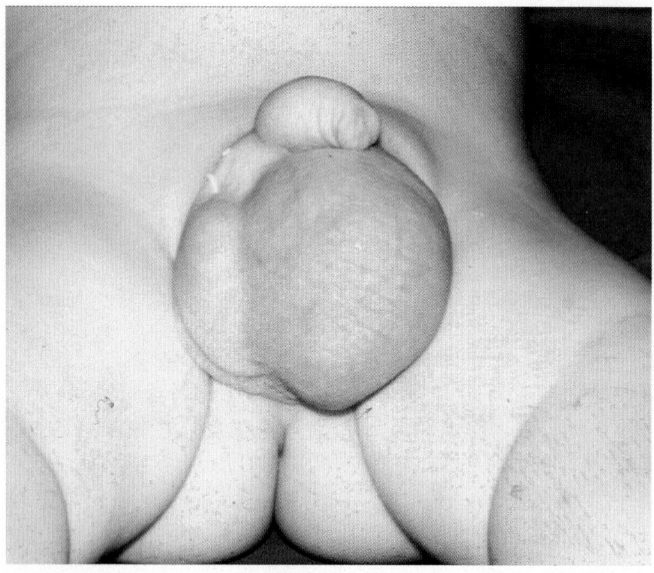

Fig. 8.11.6 Left-sided hydrocele. Although the majority of hydroceles in children are associated with the presence of a patent processus vaginalis some large, tense hydroceles are of the non-communicating variety—as in this child's case.

Management

Vricoceles in children and adolescents are rarely symptomatic and the possible indications for surgical intervention therefore centre on the perceived threat to potential fertility in adulthood. In the United Kingdom, surgery in those under 16 years is generally limited to large varicoceles which are accompanied by significant discrepancy in testicular volume or impaired growth velocity of the testis on serial ultrasound measurements. Semen analysis is not an appropriate or reliable investigation in this age group. In the minority for whom treatment is thought to be indicated, the surgical options are similar to those in adults, notably embolization, or ligation using laparoscopic, or open techniques. Reported success rates are of the order of 80–85% regardless of the technique. Complications include persistent or recurrent varicocele, lymphatic 'hydrocele' and testicular atrophy.

Conclusion

The management of undescended testes, hydroceles, and hernias comprises a sizeable part of the routine urological workload in children and young people. Testicular torsion is one of the few genuine surgical emergencies in this age group. Adult urologists who have received appropriate paediatric training can make an important contribution to the care of children with the common surgical disorders of the inguinoscrotal region.

Further reading

Hutson JM. Undescended testes. (pp. 652–3) In: Stringer MD, Oldham KT, Mouriquand PDE (eds). *Pediatric Surgery and Urology: Long-term Outcomes,* 2nd edition. Cambridge, UK: Cambridge University Press, 2006.

Hutton KAR, Sau I, Orchidopexy and orchidectomy. (pp. 170–81) In: Godbole PP, Wilcox DT, Koyle MA, (eds). *Pediatric Urology: Surgical Complications and Management.* Oxford, UK: Wiley-Blackwell, 2008.

Keys C, Heloury Y. Retractile testes: a review of the current literature. *J Pediatr Urol* 2012; **8**(1):2–6.

Madden NP. Testis hydrocoele and varicocoele. (pp. 248–63) In: Thomas DFM, Duffy PG, Rickwood AMK (eds). *Essentials of Paediatric Urology,* 2nd edition. London, UK: Informa Healthcare, 2008.

Taghizadeh AK, Thomas DF. Ascent of the testis revisited: fact not fiction. *BJU Int* 2008; **102**(6):676–8.

Thomas DFM. The acute scrotum. (pp. 266–74) In: Thomas DFM, Duffy PG, Rickwood AMK (eds). *Essentials of Paediatric Urology,* 2nd edition. London, UK: Informa Healthcare, 2008.

References

1. Kubota Y, Temelcos C, Bathgate RAD, *et al.* The role of insulin 3, testosterone, Mullerian inhibiting substance and relaxin in rat gubernacular growth. *Mol Hum Reprod* 2002; **8**(10):900–5.
2. Thomas DFM. Embryology. (pp. 438–53) In: Munday AR, Fitzpatrick J, Neal DE (eds). *Scientific Basis of Urology,* 3rd edition. London, UK: Informa Heathcare, 2003.
3. Hutson JM. Undescended testis. (pp. 652–63) In: Stringer MDO, Mouriquand KT (eds). *Pediatric Surgery and Urology: Long-term Outcomes.* Cambridge, UK: Cambridge University Press, 2006.
4. Huff DS, Fenig DM, Canning DA, Carr MG, Zderic SA, Snyder HM 3rd. Abnormal germ cell development in cryptorchidism. *Horm Res* 2001; **55**(1):11–7.
5. Chacko JK, Barthold JS. Genetic and environmental contributors to cryptorchidism. *Pediatr Endocrinol Rev* 2009; **6**(4):476–80.

6. Vogels A, Moerman P, Frijns JP, Bogaert GA. Testicular histology in boys with Prader-Willi syndrome: fertile or infertile? *J Urol* 2008; **180**(4 Suppl):1800–4.
7. Smith JA, Hutson JM, Beasley SW, Reddihough DS. The relationship between cerebral palsy and cryptorchidism. *J Pediatr Surg* 1989; **24**(12):1303–5.
8. Rundle JS, Primrose DA, Carachi R. Cryptorchism in cerebral palsy. *Br J Urol* 1982; **54**(2):170–1.
9. [No authors listed]. Cryptorchidism: a prospective study of 7500 consecutive male births, 1984–8. John Radcliffe Hospital Cryptorchidism Study Group. *Arch Dis Child* 1992; **67**(7):892–9.
10. Madden NP. Testis hydrocoele and varicocoele. (pp. 248–63) In: Thomas DFM, Duffy PG, Rickwood AMK (eds). *Essentials of Paediatric Urology,* 2nd edition. London, UK: Informa Healthcare, 2008.
11. Ford TF, Parkinson MC, Pryor JP. The undescended testis in adult life. *Br J Urol* 1985; **57**(2):181–4.
12. Pettersson A, Richiardi L, Nordenskjold A, Kaijser M, Akre O. Age at surgery for undescended testis and risk of testicular cancer. *N Engl J Med* 2007; **356**(18):1835–41.
13. Walsh TJ, Dall'Era MA, Croughan MS, Carroll PR, Turek PJ. Prepubertal orchiopexy for cryptorchidism may be associated with lower risk of testicular cancer. *J Urol* 2007; **178**(4 Pt 1):1440–6; discussion 1446.
14. Wilson-Storey D, McGenity K, Dickson JA. Orchidopexy: the younger the better? *J R Coll Surg Edinb* 1990; **35**(6):362–4.
15. Thorup J, Jensen CL, Langballe O, Petersen BL, Cortes D. The challenge of early surgery for cryptorchidism. *Scand J Urol Nephrol* 2011; **45**(3):184–9.
16. Hutson JM. Orchidopexy. (pp. 861–9) In: Spitz L, Coran A C (eds). *Operative Pediatric Surgery*, 6th edition. London, UK: Hodder Arnold, 2006.
17. Hutson JM. Inguinal orchiopexy (open technique). (pp. 597–606) In: Hinman F, Baskin LS (eds). *Hinman's Atlas of Pediatric Urologic Surgery.* Philadelphia PA: Saunders Elsevier, 2009.
18. Gordon M, Cervellione RM, Morabito A, Bianchi A. 20 years of transcrotal orchidopexy for undescended testis: results and outcomes. *J Pediatr Urol* 2010; **6**(5):506–12.
19. Docimo SG. The results of surgical therapy for cryptorchidism: a literature review and analysis. *J Urol* 1995; **154**(3):1148–52.
20. Hutton KAR, Sau I. Orchidopexy and orchidectomy. (pp. 170–81) In: Godbole PP, Wilcox DT, Koyle MA, (eds). *Pediatric Urology: Surgical Complications and Management.* Oxford, UK: Wiley-Blackwell, 2008.
21. Dhanani NN, Cornelius D, Gunes A, Ritchey ML. Successful outpatient management of the nonpalpable intra-abdominal testis with staged Fowler-Stephens orchiopexy. *J Urol* 2004; **172**(6 Pt 1):2399–401.
22. Elyas R, Guerra LA, Pike J, *et al.* Is staging beneficial for Fowler-Stephens orchiopexy? A systematic review. *J Urol* 2010; **183**(5):2012–8.
23. Miller KD, Coughlin MT, Lee PA. Fertility after unilateral cryptorchidism. Paternity, time to conception, pretreatment testicular location and size, hormone and sperm parameters. *Horm Res* 2001; **55**(5):249–53.
24. Lee PA, Coughlin MT. Fertility after bilateral cryptorchidism. Evaluation by paternity, hormone, and semen data. *Horm Res* 2001; **55**(1):28–32.
25. Wood HM, Elder JS. Cryptorchidism and testicular cancer: separating fact from fiction. *J Urol* 2009; **181**(2):452–61.
26. Moursy EE, Gamal W, Hussein MM. Laparoscopic orchiopexy for non-palpable testes: outcome of two techniques. *J Pediatr Urol* 2011; **7**(2):178–81.
27. Esposito C, Vallone G, Savanelli A, Settimi A. Long-term outcome of laparoscopic Fowler-Stephens orchiopexy in boys with intra-abdominal testis. *J Urol* 2009; **181**(4):1851–6.
28. Hvistendahl GM, Poulsen EU. Laparoscopy for the impalpable testes: experience with 80 intra-abdominal testes. *J Pediatr Urol* 2009; **5**(5):389–92.
29. Bogaert GA. Laparoscopic orchiopexy techniques. (pp. 597–606) In: Hinman F, Baskin L (eds). *Hinman's Atlas of Pediatric Urologic Surgery.* Philadelphia, PA: Saunders Elsevier, 2009.
30. Bianchi AM. Microvascular orchiopexy. (pp. 592–6) In: Hinman F, Baskin LS (eds). *Hinman's Atlas of Pediatric Urologic Surgery.* Philadelphia PA: Saunders Elsevier, 2009.
31. Keys C, Heloury Y. Retractile testes: a review of the current literature. *J Pediatr Urol* 2012; **8**(1):2–6.
32. Hazebroek, F.W., *et al.*, Why luteinizing-hormone-releasing-hormone nasal spray will not replace orchiopexy in the treatment of boys with undescended testes. *J Pediatr Surg* 1987; **22**(12):1177–82.
33. Taghizadeh AK, Thomas DF. Ascent of the testis revisited: fact not fiction. *BJU Int* 2008; **102**(6):676–8.
34. Hack WW, Meijer RW, Van Der Voort-Doedens LM, Bos SD, De Kok ME. Previous testicular position in boys referred for an undescended testis: further explanation of the late orchidopexy enigma? *BJU Int* 2003; **92**(3):293–6.
35. Fenton EJM, Woodward AA, Hudson IL, Marschner I. The ascending testis. *Pediatr Surg Int* 1990; **5**(1):6–9.
36. Lamah M, McCaughey ES, Finlay FO, Burge DM. The ascending testis: is late orchidopexy due to failure of screening or late ascent? *Pediatr Surg Int* 2001; **17**(5–6):421–3.
37. Hack WW, Meijer RW, van der Voort-Doedens LM, Bos SD, Haasnoot K. Natural course of acquired undescended testis in boys. *Br J Surg* 2003; **90**(6):728–31.
38. Nour S, MacKinnon AE. Acute scrotal swelling in children. *J R Coll Surg Edinb* 1991; **36**(6):392–4.
39. Ben-Chaim J, Leibovitch I, Ramon J, Winberg D, Goldwasser B. Etiology of acute scrotum at surgical exploration in children, adolescents and adults. *Eur Urol* 1992; **21**(1):45–7.
40. Caesar RE, Kaplan GW. Incidence of the bell-clapper deformity in an autopsy series. *Urology* 1994; **44**(1):114–6.
41. Williamson RC. Torsion of the testis and allied conditions. *Br J Surg* 1976; **63**(6):465–76.
42. Bergh A, Collin O, Lissbrant E. Effects of acute graded reductions in testicular blood flow on testicular morphology in the adult rat. *Biol Reprod* 2001; **64**(1):13–20.
43. Smith GI. Cellular changes from graded testicular ischemia. *J Urol* 1955; **73**(2):355–62.
44. Turner TT. Acute experimental testicular torsion. No effect on the contralateral testis. *J Androl* 1985; **6**(1):65–72.
45. Krarup T. The testes after torsion. *Br J Urol* 1978; **50**(1):43–6.
46. Macnicol MF. Torsion of the testis in childhood. *Br J Surg* 1974; **61**(11):905–8.
47. Anderson JB, Williamson RC. The fate of the human testes following unilateral torsion of the spermatic cord. *Br J Urol* 1986; **58**(6):698–704.
48. Thomas WE, Cooper MJ, Crane GA, Lee G, Williamson RC. Testicular exocrine malfunction after torsion. *Lancet* 1984; **2**(8416):1357–60.
49. Bartsch G, Frank S, Marberger H, Mikuz G. Testicular torsion: late results with special regard to fertility and endocrine function. *J Urol* 1980; **124**(3):375–8.
50. Saxena AK, Castellani C, Ruttenstock EM, Höllwarth ME. Testicular torsion: a 15-year single-centre clinical and histological analysis. *Acta Paediatr* 2012; **101**(7):e282–6.
51. Drlik M, Kocvara R. Torsion of spermatic cord in children: A review. *J Pediatr Urol* 2013; **9**(3):259–66.
52. Mastrogiacomo I, Zanchetta R, Graziotti P, Betterle C, Scrufari P, Lembo A. Immunological and clinical study of patients after spermatic cord torsion. *Andrologia* 1982; **14**(1):25–30.
53. Visser AJ, Heyns CF. Testicular function after torsion of the spermatic cord. *BJU Int* 2003; **92**(3):200–3.
54. Ferreira U, Netto Júnior NR, Esteves SC, Rivero MA, Schirren C. Comparative study of the fertility potential of men with only one testis. *Scand J Urol Nephrol* 1991; **25**(4):255–9.

55. Arap MA, Vicentini FC, Cocuzza M, *et al.* Late hormonal levels, semen parameters, and presence of antisperm antibodies in patients treated for testicular torsion. *J Androl* 2007; **28**(4):528–32.
56. Burge DM. Neonatal testicular torsion and infarction: aetiology and management. *Br J Urol* 1987; **59**(1):70–3.
57. John CM, Kooner G, Mathew DE, Ahmed S, Kenny SE. Neonatal testicular torsion—a lost cause? *Acta Paediatr* 2008; **97**(4):502–4.
58. Baglaj M, Carachi R. Neonatal bilateral testicular torsion: a plea for emergency exploration. *J Urol* 2007; **177**(6):2296–9.
59. Thomas DFM. The acute scrotum. (pp. 266–74) In: Thomas DFM, Duffy PG, Rickwood AMK (eds). *Essentials of Paediatric Urology,* 2nd edition. London, UK: Informa Healthcare, 2008.
60. Parkinson EJ. Inguinal and umbilical hernias. (pp. 286–95) In: Stringer MD, Oldham KT, Mouriquand PDE (eds). *Pediatric Surgery and Urology: Long-term Outcomes*, 2nd edition. Cambridge, UK: Cambridge University Press, 2006.
61. Schier F, Montupet P, Esposito C. Laparoscopic inguinal herniorrhaphy in children: a three-center experience with 933 repairs. *J Pediatr Surg* 2002; **37**(3):395–7.
62. Grosfeld JL, Minnick K, Shedd F, West KW, Rescorla FJ, Vane DW. Inguinal hernia in children: factors affecting recurrence in 62 cases. *J Pediatr Surg* 1991; **26**(3):283–7.
63. Parkhouse H, Hendry WF. Vasal injuries during childhood and their effect on subsequent fertility. *Br J Urol* 1991; **67**(1):91–5.
64. Squire R, Gough DC. Abdominoscrotal hydrocele in infancy. *Br J Urol* 1988; **61**(4):347–9.

CHAPTER 8.12

Disorders of sex development

David F.M. Thomas

Introduction to disorders of sex development

A revised classification of disorders of sex development (DSD) using less pejorative descriptive terminology has been widely adopted in recent years Table 8.12.1.[1] In the Western World the commonest patterns of DSD are masculinization of the external genitalia in female infants due to congenital adrenal hyperplasia (46XXDSD) and androgen receptor defects leading to undervirilization of infants with a 46XY karyotype.

The gender of individuals with DSD may be difficult to define in simple terms because of discordance between their karyoptype and gonadal and/or genital phenotype.

Aetiology and embryology

Normal development of the genital tracts

Male and female internal and external genitalia share identical precursors until the sixth week of gestation.[2] Subsequent sex differentiation in the female is mainly a passive process which is not dependent upon a single sex-determining gene. By contrast, normal sex differentiation in the male is ultimately dependent on the presence of a single testis-determining gene (SRY) located on the Y chromosome.

Male differentiation

The testis is formed by interaction of primordial germ cells and the primitive sex cords within the embryonic gonad. Müllerian inhibiting substance (MIS)—also termed anti-Müllerian hormone (AMH) is a glycoprotein hormone secreted by the pre-Sertoli cells of the testis from around the seventh week onwards. It is responsible for involution of the paramesonephric ducts and also stimulates testosterone production by the Leydig cells of the embryonic testis. MIS is also thought to play an important role in the first phase of testicular descent.[3]

In the male, the mesonephric ducts persist as the vas deferens and ejaculatory ducts. Although this process is testosterone-dependant the mechanism is incompletely understood. The external genitalia of male and female embryos initially share the same undifferentiated anatomical phenotype. Virilization of male external genitalia is dependent on the presence of circulating testosterone, 5α-reductase (for conversion to dihydrotestosterone) and functioning receptors in the target tissues. Differentiation of the male external genitalia occurs principally from the tenth week of gestation onwards, with formation of the urethra being completed by closure of the urogenital groove around the fifteenth week. The scrotum is derived from the labioscrotal folds.

Female differentiation

Unlike the male, differentiation of the internal and external genitalia in the female occurs as a passive process which is not dependent upon exposure to sex hormones at different stages in the differentiation pathway. In the absence of MIS the para mesonephric ducts persist as the Fallopian tubes, which fuse distally to form the uterus and upper two-thirds of the vagina. The lower third of the vagina is derived from the urogenital sinus. The mesonephric ducts undergo spontaneous involution and are represented only by vestigal remnants. In the female, the external genital phenotype retains a closer affinity to the original undifferentiated external genitalia of the six week embryo than the male.

Clinical aspects of disorders of sex development

Any infant born with ambiguous genitalia requires prompt and expert multidisciplinary assessment.[4] Congenital adrenal hyperplasia is the commonest DSD in the Western world—accounting for approximately 80% of cases. Early diagnosis and commencement of steroid replacement therapy are essential to minimize the risk of potentially life-threatening hyponatraemia in the salt losing forms of this condition. Other DSDs include virilization defects (notably due to complete or partial androgen insensitivity) mixed gonadal dysgenesis and ovotesticular DSD (true hermaphroditism).

While these conditions do not pose the same imminent threat to the health of the affected infant as congenital adrenal hyperplasia (CAH), prompt investigation and assessment is nevertheless essential to permit an informed decision on gender assignment.

Examination and investigation

A detailed clinical examination of the external genitalia is performed to evaluate the degree of virilization and to determine whether palpable gonads are present. The possible diagnosis of 46XXDSD due to CAH should always be considered in any infant with hypospadias and impalpable gonads.[4]

Initial investigations include:

- karyotype
- plasma biochemistry
- 17 hydroxyprogesterone (which is elevated in CAH).

A range of further endocrine investigations may then be indicated, depending upon the results of the initial tests. Further investigations may include: plasma testosterone (both before and after stimulation with human chorionic gonadotrophin); steroid assays; MIS assay; and evaluation of receptor activity in genital skin biopsies.

Table 8.12.1 Revised terminology and classification of disorders of sex development (DSD)

Previous terminology	Current terminology	Causes
Intersex states	Disorders of sex development (DSD)	
Female pseudohermaphroditism	44 XX DSD	Abnormal virilization of external genitalia +/− urogenital sinus ◆ Congenital adrenal hyperplasia ◆ Aromatase deficiency ◆ Maternal androgen-secreting tumour
Male pseudohermaphroditism	46XYDSD	Inadequate virilization ◆ Receptor defect. Complete androgen insensitivity defect (CAIS) previously 'testicular feminization syndrome' *or* partial androgen insensitivity syndrome ◆ Defective testosterone synthesis ◆ Bilateral anorchia
True hermaphroditism	Ovotesticular DSD	Differing patterns of gonadal dysgenesis associated with differing abnormal (or normal) karyoptypes
Mixed gonadal dysgenesis	Unchanged (i.e. mixed gonadal dysgenesis)	Gonadal dysgenesis. Varying genital phenotypes. Karyotype most commonly 45X/46XY mosaicism

Source: data from Christopher P. Houk *et al.*, 'Summary of Consensus Statement on Intersex Disorders and Their Management', *Pediatrics*, Volume 118, Issue 2, pp. 753–7, Copyright © 2006 by the American Academy of Pediatrics.

Diagnostic imaging

Ultrasound examination of the pelvic structures is performed to visualize pelvic or intra-abdominal gonads and the uterus. The presence of a fluid-filled persistent Müllerian remnant or 'pseudo vagina' may also be seen on ultrasound in some undervirilized male infants.

Magnetic resonance imaging is an excellent modality for the detailed assessment of pelvic anatomy but it is not usually employed for the initial work-up in newborns.

Although a contrast sinogram/urethrogram can be used to delineate the anatomy of the urethra, vagina and/or persistent urogenital sinus, information of greater direct relevance to surgical planning is usually provided by cystourethroscopy and vaginoscopy.[5] Laparoscopy has the advantage of combining diagnostic examination of the pelvic structures with biopsy of any internal gonads but since gonadal biopsy is only required in a minority of cases, laparoscopy is not usually undertaken in infancy.

Classification and patterns of disorders of sex development

46XX DSD (previously termed female pseudo hermaphroditism) is the commonest disorder of sex development and is usually due to virilization of the external genitalia in girls with CAH. Other, rarer causes of 46XX DSD include; aromatase deficiency and intrauterine virilization by androgens of maternal origin (e.g. androgen-secreting tumours).

Congenital adrenal hyperplasia

CAH is a genetically determined enzyme defect, which is most commonly inherited as an autosomal recessive trait.

Three distinct enzyme defects have been identified of which 21 hydroxylase deficiency is the commonest, with an estimated incidence 1:15,000.

An enzymatic block in the bio synthetic pathway of the adrenal hormones cortisol and aldosterone results in accumulation of steroid precursors which are then converted via 4-androstenedione to testosterone.[4] Exposure of the external genitalia to the high levels of circulating androgens produced by the adrenal glands leads to varying degrees of virilization—which, at its most extreme, may be characterized by a normal male genital phenotype (with the exception of palpable gonads) (Figs 8.12.1 and 8.12.2). By contrast, the internal genitalia are anatomically normal. Depending on the severity of virilization the vagina either opens on the perineum or, more commonly, fuses with the distal urethra to form a common urogenital sinus with a single perineal opening.

Early diagnosis is essential to ensure prompt correction of electrolyte disturbance associated with the 'salt losing state' which is present in more than 50% of cases. Once effective adrenal hormone

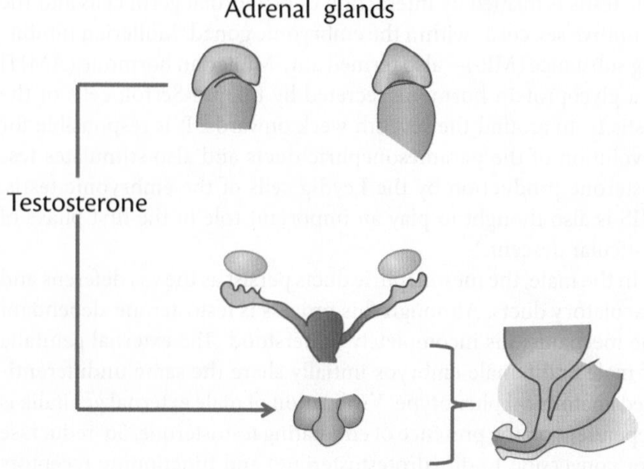

Fig. 8.12.1 Features of congenital adrenal hyperplasia. The external genitalia are virilized by intrauterine exposure to high levels of circulating androgens produced by the adrenal glands. Normal ovaries, uterus, and fallopian tubes. Fusion of vagina and urethra to form urogenital sinus with level of confluence depending on severity of virilization.

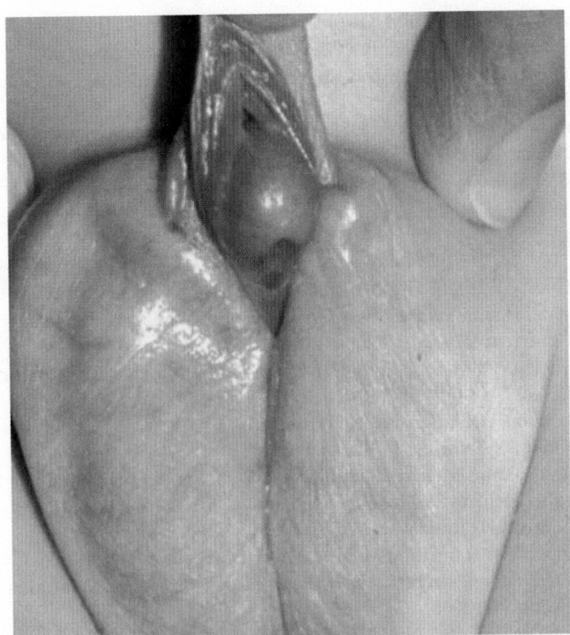

Fig. 8.12.2 Virilized external genitalia in a female infant with congenital adrenal hyperplasia comprising clitoral hypertrophy, urogenital sinus (not visible) and 'scrotalization' of labia majora.

replacement therapy has been instituted, testosterone levels fall, and the degree of virilization may gradually decrease in severity. In girls with milder degrees of virilization clitoral reduction surgery is not required. However, when more severe virilization is present at birth, any spontaneous improvement is unlikely to be sufficient to obviate the need to consider cosmetic genital reconstruction (feminizing genitoplasty).

The role of feminizing genitoplasty in the management of CAH has become the subject of heated controversy. Some advocacy groups and 'intersex rights' activists argue strongly that all forms of 'genital normalizing surgery' in childhood should be proscribed on the grounds that DSD phenotypes should not be regarded as abnormal but, rather 'part of the larger picture of sex variance'. It is unclear to what extent (if any) these pressure groups (some of which may include individuals with other forms of gender dysphoria) genuinely represent the views of the majority of DSD patients and their parents. Specialists caring for children with 46XXDSD are well aware of the long-term studies reporting evidence of sensory impairment and (rarely) clitoral atrophy in a proportion of women treated by early surgery.[6,7] Clitoral reduction is already being performed on a far more selective basis than in the past and it is reasonable to anticipate that improved long-term surgical outcomes will be achieved by current techniques in the hands of specialist surgeons. By contrast, withholding treatment from all girls with 46 XX DSD (as advocated by the more strident pressure groups) would effectively consign those with severely virilized genitalia to the prospect of spending their childhood and early adolescence as a girl with male external genitalia. The consequences of adopting this course of action in girls growing up in Western society are largely unknown and few parents are likely to volunteer their own daughter to participate in an uncontrolled experiment of this nature. In practice, most parents are unwilling to adopt a timescale which would leave their daughter with virilized genitalia and prominent phallic enlargement throughout her childhood. Specialist opinion therefore continues to favour cosmetic feminizing genitoplasty (including clitoral reduction) on a selective basis when this is judged by doctors and parents to be in the best interests of the child.

Surgery is usually performed between 6 and 18 months of age. Great care is needed to preserve and protect the neurovascular bundles during resection and debulking of erectile tissue in the corporeal bodies.[8,9] Where there is a low confluence of the urethra and vagina and short urogenital sinus, feminizing genitoplasty can reasonably be combined with a simple flap vaginoplasty.

In an alternative technique the urogenital sinus, distal urethra, and vagina are mobilized en bloc to permit exteriorization of the urethra and vagina on the perineum.[10]

When the vagina is small and is inserted high into the urethra/urogenital sinus, more extensive mobilization is required and vaginoplasty in these cases is probably best deferred until the midteens (or prior to the onset of sexual activity). At that age the individual herself can be actively involved in decision-making[11] and is more likely to be motivated to undertake postoperative dilatation following vaginoplasty.

46XY disorders of sex development (previously termed male pseudohermaphroditism)

This varied group of conditions is characterized by inadequate or absent virilization of the external genitalia. Causes include defective androgen synthesis, enzyme defects, and receptor defects in the target genital tissues.

Impairment of testosterone production may result from enzyme defects in the biosynthetic pathway, morphological abnormalities within the testis (Leydig cell aplasia) or bilateral anorchia.

Absent or impaired virilization despite exposure to normal or elevated levels of circulating androgens is usually caused by androgen receptor defects in the tissues of the external genitalia. At its most extreme, this is exemplified by complete androgen insensitivity syndrome (CAIS)—previously termed testicular feminization syndrome. Affected individuals have a female external genital phenotype combined with male internal genital structures—abdominal (or inguinal) testes, vas deferens, and ejaculatory ducts. This combination of features is explained by failure of the external genitalia to virilize despite exposure to testosterone, coupled with normal regression of Müllerian structures in response to MIS produced by the fetal testis. The explanation for the persistence and differentiation of mesonephric duct structures is less clear.

Complete androgen insensitivity syndrome usually remains unrecognized in childhood, with the diagnosis being made during the investigation of primary amenorrhoea. Occasionally, however, CAIS comes to light when a testis is unexpectedly identified during the course of a hernia operation in a child being reared as a normal female.

Individuals with CAIS have invariably been raised as females prior to the diagnosis being made and retain this gender throughout their lives. Although it has been standard practice to advise bilateral orchidectomy at some stage (in view of the high long-term risk of testicular malignancy)[12] this policy is currently being questioned.

Partial androgen insensitivity is characterized by varying degrees of impaired virilization. A number of different aetiologies (notably peripheral receptor defects) can give rise to this genital phenotype. However, even after extensive endocrine investigation the underlying cause can only be established in approximately 50% of cases.

Decisions on gender of rearing and surgical management are taken on an individual basis, taking into account the genital anatomy, the feasibility (or otherwise) of reconstructing a functioning penis of reasonable size and social/cultural factors.

Penile reconstruction is undertaken in accordance with the principles of the correction of proximal hypospadias with many paediatric urologists favouring preoperative treatment with testosterone. Scrotal transposition is often performed to create more normal appearances of the scrotum in childhood and orchidopexy is also required in many cases.

Mixed gonadal dysgenesis and ovotesticular disorders of sex development

These forms of DSD exhibit a range of different genital and gonadal phenotypes and are often associated with mosaicism of sex chromosomes (e.g. 45X/46XY karyotype). Although the gonads in affected individuals are often dysgenetic, a gonad containing Y chromosomal material may be capable of producing sufficient testosterone to maintain some degree of virilization of the external genitalia. Decision-making is taken on a case-by-case basis according to the findings of endocrine investigations and, where appropriate, gonadal biopsy. Female gender assignment is more appropriate in most cases but male gender assignment may be considered if the phallic size is adequate for reconstruction.[13]

Dysgenetic and/or discordant gonads are excised in view of the high risk of malignancy, whereas gonadal tissue which is consistent with the assigned gender may be conserved, for example, by orchidopexy. Nevertheless, the risk of malignancy in retained gonadal tissue remains significantly increased and lifelong surveillance is required.

Ovo testicular DSD (previously termed 'true hermaphroditism') is very rare in the Western World but is considerably less rare in Southern Africa. Genital ambiguity is accompanied by the presence of both testicular and ovarian tissue—which may either be present in separate gonads or located in the same gonad. Ovotesticular DSD is associated with a range of different karyotypes. Management and gender of rearing are determined on an individual basis according to the genital and gonadal phenotype and social and cultural factors.

Conclusion

Disorders of sex development are rare. The best overall long-term outcomes are achieved by specialized multidisciplinary teams consisting of paediatric endocrinologists, paediatric urologists, and psychologists and others with particular expertise in the management of DSD.[14] Patient and parent support groups can also play a valuable role. Despite optimal management, however, many children born with DSD face the prospect of impaired sexual and reproductive function coupled with potential psychological morbidity in later life.[15] Continuity of follow-up and coordination of care through adolescence and into adult life are of vital importance to their future wellbeing.[16]

Further reading

Balen AH, Creighton SM, Davies MC, MacDougall J, Stanhope R. *Paediatric and Adolescent Gynaecology: A Multidisciplinary Approach*. Cambridge, UK: Cambridge University Press, 2004.

Lottman H, Thomas DFM. Disorders of sex development. (pp. 275–93) In: Thomas DFM, Duffy PG, Rickwood AMK (eds). *Essentials of Paediatric Urology*, 2nd edition. London, UK: Informa Healthcare, 2008.

Report of Working Party on DSD Evaluation. Fondation Mérieux, Annecy, France, March 14–17 2012. (Multiple authors) *J Pediatr Urol* 2012; **8**(6):571–632.

References

1. Houk CP, Hughes IA, Ahmed SF, Lee PA. Summary of consensus statement on intersex disorders. International Intersex Consensus Conference. *Pediatrics* 2006; **118**(2):753–7.
2. Thomas DFM. Embryology. (pp. 438–53) In: Mundy AR, Fitzpatrick J, Neal D, George NR (eds). *Scientific Basis of Urology*, 3rd edition. London, UK: Informa Healthcare, 2010.
3. Kubota Y, Temelcos C, Bathgate RA, *et al.* The role of insulin 3, testosterone, Müllerian inhibiting substance and relaxin in rat gubernacular growth. *Mol Hum Reprod* 2002; **8**(10):900–5.
4. Lottman H, Thomas DFM. Disorders of sex development. (pp. 275–93) In: Thomas DFM, Duffy PG, Rickwood AMK (eds). *Essentials of Paediatric Urology*, 2nd edition, London, UK: Informa Healthcare, 2008.
5. Vanderbrink BA, Rink RC, Cain MP, *et al.* Does preoperative genitography in congenital adrenal hyperplasia cases affect surgical approach to feminizing genitoplasty? *J Urol* 2010 Oct; **184**(4 Suppl):1793–8.
6. Creighton SM, Minto CL, Steele SJ. Objective cosmetic and anatomical outcomes at adolescence of feminizing surgery for ambiguous genitalia done in childhood. *Lancet* 2001; **358**(9276):124–5.
7. Minto CL, Liao LM, Woodhouse CR, Ransley PG, Creighton SM. The effect of clitoral surgery on sexual outcome in individuals who have intersex conditions with ambiguous genitalia: a cross-sectional study. *Lancet* 2003; **361**:1252–7.
8. Donahoe PK, Pieretti RV, Schnitzer JJ. Surgical reconstruction of intersex abnormalities. (pp. 915–28) In: Spitz L, Coran AC (eds). *Operative Pediatric Surgery*, 6th edition. London, UK: Hodder Arnold, 2006.
9. Creighton S, Chernausek SD, Romao R, Ransley P, Salle JP. Timing and nature of reconstructive surgery for disorders of sex development—introduction. *J Pediatr Urol* 2012; **8**(6):602–10.
10. Rink RC, Metcalfe PD, Kaefer MA, Casale AJ, Meldrum KK, Cain MP. Partial urogenital mobilization: a limited proximal dissection. *J Pediatr Urol* 2006; **2**(4):351–6.
11. Creighton S. Long-term sequelae of genital surgery. (pp. 327–33) In: Balen AH, Creighton SM, Davies MC, MacDougall J, Stanhope R (eds). *Paediatric and Adolescent Gynaecology: A Multidisciplinary Approach*. Cambridge, UK: Cambridge University Press, 2004.
12. Deans R, Creighton SM, Liao LM, Conway GS. Timing of gonadectomy in adult women with complete androgen insensitivity syndrome (CAIS): patient preferences and clinical evidence. *Clin Endocrinol (Oxf)* 2012; **76**(6):894–8.
13. Baka-Ostrowska M, Gastol P Smigielski M, *et al.* Surgical dilemmas in mixed gonadal dysgenesis. *BJU Int* 2003; **91**(Suppl 1):40–1.
14. Houk CP, Hughes IA, Ahmed SF, Lee PA. Summary of consensus statement on intersex disorders. International Intersex Consensus Conference. *Pediatrics* 2006; **118**(2):753–7.
15. Auchus RJ, Witchel SF, Leight KR, *et al.* Guidelines for the development of comprehensive care centers for congenital adrenal hyperplasia: Guidance from the CARES Foundation Initiative. *Int J Pediatr Endocrinol* 2010; **2010**:275213.
16. Schober J, Nordenström A, Hoebeke P, *et al.* Disorders of sex development: Summaries of long-term outcome studies. *J Pediatr Urol* 2012; **8**(6):616–23.

CHAPTER 8.13

Urological malignancies in children

Roly Squire

Childhood renal tumours

Wilms tumour (nephroblastoma)

Following the publication in 1899 of his classical review of childhood kidney tumours,[1–4] Max Wilms remains eponymously linked to the commonest paediatric urological malignancy of childhood, nephroblastoma.

The peak incidence of Wilms tumour (WT) is at three years and nearly all cases present under five years of age. Wilms tumour most commonly presents as an asymptomatic abdominal or flank mass, but can also present with; haematuria, abdominal pain, symptomatic hypertension, or symptoms from lung metastases. In addition, a small number of Wilms tumours are identified by screening of children with a known genetic predisposition.

Almost 10% of Wilms tumours occur in children with a defined genetic risk.[5,6] These include; aniridia (WAGR: **W**ilms, **A**niridia, **G**enitourinary anomalies, mental **R**etardation),[7] Beckwith Weidemann syndrome (EMG: **E**xomphalos, **M**acroglossia, **G**igantism),[8–10] or Denys Drash (congenital nephropathy, Wilms tumour, intersex disorder).[11,12]

It is recommended that children who are at >5% risk of developing Wilms tumour should undergo ultrasound screening at three-monthly intervals until they reach five to seven years of age. Screening should be undertaken under the guidance of a clinical geneticist.[13] The genetic basis of WT is of particular scientific interest because, like retinoblastoma, the statistical comparison between unilateral and bilateral cases led to a step change in our understanding of cancer genetics.[14]

At the time of presentation the main differential diagnosis lies between Wilms tumour and the other major abdominal tumour of childhood, neuroblastoma. But whereas children with Wilms tumour generally appear healthy, those with neuroblastoma are often overtly unwell as a result of metastatic spread. Examination of a child with an abdominal mass must always include blood pressure measurement since both these tumours can cause hypertension. In cases of Wilms tumour hypertension is generally caused by renin secretion,[15,16] while in neuroblastoma it is due to catecholamine secretion.

The initial investigation of an abdominal mass in a child is by ultrasound. If the ultrasound appearances are suggestive of a renal tumour the following further investigations are then recommended:

- Urinary catecholamine metabolites (raised in neuroblastoma)
- Serum alpha-fetoprotein (AFP) measurement (raised in hepatoblastoma and teratoma)
- Computed tomography (CT) or MR scan of the abdomen and pelvis (to characterize the primary tumour, identify bilateral tumours, look for intravascular spread and intra-abdominal metastases) (Figs 8.13.1)
- CT scan of the chest (screen for lung metastases)

The standard staging for Wilms tumour [Table 8.13.1] is informed by the initial investigations, but also requires information derived from surgical resection. In the United Kingdom children are treated in accordance with international protocols published by SIOP (International Society of Paediatric Oncology), which currently include pre-surgical (neoadjuvant) chemotherapy in all cases presenting in children over six months of age.[17] In localized (stage I–III) tumours, neoadjuvant chemotherapy was initially given to shrink the tumour with the aim of reducing surgical morbidity.[18,19] This has been the subject of an important UK study (UKW3)with randomization between immediate and delayed resection. The results of this study confirmed that neoadjuvant chemotherapy reduces surgical complications and also downgrades some stage III tumours—thus allowing the subsequent burden of chemotherapy to be reduced.[20,21] However, the routine use of neoadjuvant chemotherapy for all children with localized tumours may result in some low risk tumours being overtreated. For this reason the protocols from the Children's Oncology Group in the USA continue to recommend immediate primary resection of localized tumours.[22] Protocols from the USA only recommend pre-resection chemotherapy for children with metastases, intravascular extension, or tumour in the contralateral kidney.

In the UK, histological confirmation of diagnosis is recommended before treatment is started. This entails an ultrasound-guided needle-core biopsy via a retroperitoneal approach.[23] The advantages of tumour biopsy lie in excluding rare non-malignant renal masses and in identifying histological subgroups that may require alternative chemotherapy regimens. This biopsy technique does not alter the tumour stage whereas a transperitoneal or incisional biopsy automatically upgrades the tumour to stage III.

Wilms tumour is a very chemo- and radio-sensitive malignancy, and multimodal therapy regimes have been refined over many clinical trials, initiated by the National Wilms Tumor Study (NWTS) in the United States.[24–29] Outcomes are now very good, with overall long-term survival of >70% for all tumours and a survival rate of >90% for low risk localized tumours with favourable histology.[30]

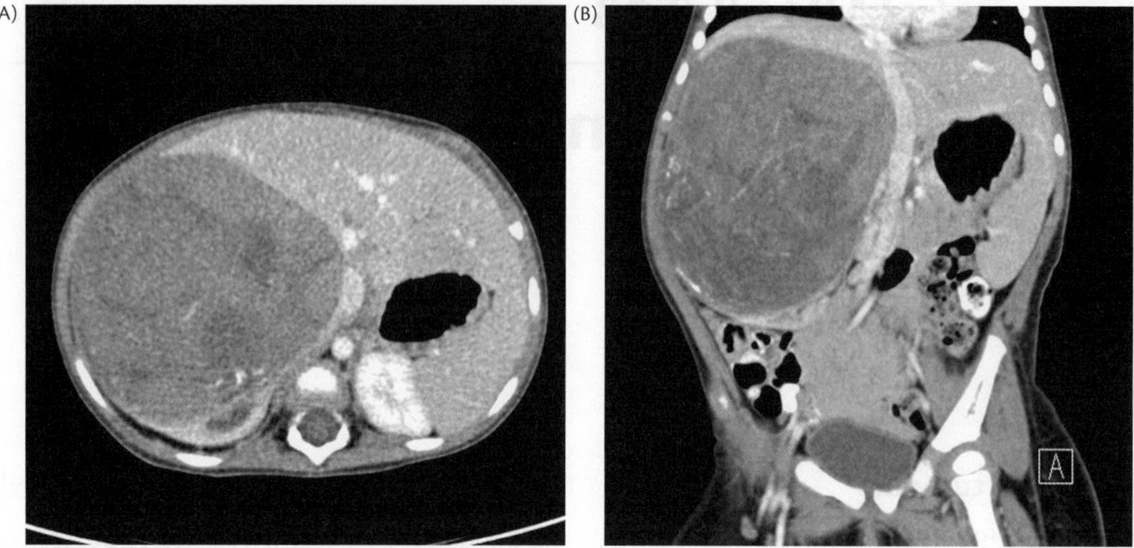

Fig. 8.13.1 (A) Axial image from a contrast computed tomography (CT) scan of a three-year-old boy who presented with an asymptomatic abdominal mass. The scan shows a very large Wilms tumour replacing most of the right kidney. Note the crescent of renal parenchyma splayed around the posterior margin of the tumour, showing that the tumour arises from the kidney. (B) A coronal reconstruction from the same CT scan, showing displacement of the inferior vena cava, but no evidence of intravascular spread. The CT scan is also important to exclude tumour in the contralateral kidney, to look for enlarged (and possibly involved) para-aortic lymph nodes, and to visualize other sites of potential intra-abdominal metastases.

Risk stratification is based upon histological classification, and is used to guide intensity of adjuvant therapy.[31]

Protocols are being developed which are aimed at intensifying treatment for high risk tumours, while decreasing therapy for low risk tumours and thus reducing adverse effects at the same time as maintaining the excellent outcomes.

Bilateral tumours and tumours with intracaval or intra-atrial extension present a particular surgical challenge. Following neoadjuvant chemotherapy it is usually possible to carry out nephron-sparing surgery on in stage V tumours, occasionally using bench surgery.[32,33] Although the use of neoadjuvant chemotherapy has reduced the number of cases with intravascular tumour extension, there are still occasions when cardiopulmonary bypass is required to achieve complete tumour resection.[34] In stage IV disease, metastases usually respond well to chemotherapy but there can be a role for metastatectomy to treat residual lesions.

Table 8.13.1 Staging system for Wilms tumour

Stage	Definition
I	Tumour confined to kidney and completely excised
II	Tumour extending beyond kidney into perinephric fat, adjacent organs, vena cava; completely excised
III	Incomplete excision of tumour; or complete excision with abdominal lymph node involvement; or preoperative/intraoperative tumour rupture; or peritoneal tumour deposits; or tumour thrombi present at resection margins of vessels or ureter
IV	Haematogenous metastases; or lymph node metastases outside abdomen/pelvis
V	Bilateral renal tumours

Reproduced with permission from National Wilms Tumor Study (NTWS), Copyright © NWTS, http://www.nwtsg.org

Mesoblastic nephroma

In infants under six months of age the differential diagnosis of renal tumours includes mesoblastic nephroma. Although it can be locally infiltrative, this renal tumour is usually benign.[35] Mesoblastic nephroma commonly presents as an incidental flank mass in early infancy, but can also present perinatally with associated features including; polyhydramnios, hydrops foetalis, and hypercalcaemia.[36,37] Treatment consists of total nephrectomy. The kidney is removed en bloc with surrounding perinephric fat to prevent recurrence.[38] No adjuvant treatment is required. Because of the difficulty in distinguishing mesoblastic nephroma from Wilms tumour on diagnostic imaging, immediate nephrectomy is recommended for renal tumours in this age group.

Nephroblastomatosis

The presence of foci of embryonal nephrogenic tissue may be observed in association with Wilms tumour, and these are considered to be potential precursors of nephroblastoma.[39] Some children present with benign aggregations or 'rests' of nephrogenic tissue and the appearances of these lesions on MR imaging may be sufficiently distinctive to permit observation rather than surgical intervention.[40]

Other renal tumours

Two rare malignancies, clear cell sarcoma and rhabdoid tumours, were previously classified as forms of Wilms tumour. However, their histological features and poorer outcomes distinguish them from other forms of Wilms tumour and their management entails more intensified adjuvant treatment.[41] Surgical management, however, is the same as for Wilms tumour.

Renal cell carcinoma occurs rarely in older children, and is treated as in adults.

Malignant tumours of the bladder

Rhabdomyosarcoma

The dominant bladder/prostate malignancy in children is rhabdomyosarcoma (RMS). This highly malignant tumour arises from primitive mesenchymal cells which are committed to differentiation into striated muscle.

The incidence of bladder/prostate RMS is bimodal with most cases presenting between two and five years of age, and a second, smaller group presenting in adolescence.[42]

Bladder/prostate RMS typically presents with either with haematuria or bladder outlet obstruction. The tumour mass is usually readily visualized on ultrasound examination.

A full histological and cytogenetic diagnosis is mandatory to distinguish embryonal and alveolar rhabdomyosarcoma since these two sub types require different therapeutic approaches and have markedly different outcomes.[43–45] Alveolar RMS is characterized by the cytogenetic translocation t[2,13] and is associated with a worse prognosis.[46]

Treatment usually starts with chemotherapy, preceded by tumour biopsy. Primary tumour resection should only be considered in those cases where it seems feasible to completely excise a tumour in the bladder dome without risk to bladder function. Bladder tumours are easily biopsied endoscopically, whereas biopsying a prostatic RMS may need a perineal or transrectal needle-core approach.

Treatment of RMS is risk-stratified, based upon pathological grading, site of disease, ease of resection, age at presentation, size of primary tumour, and lymph node involvement.[47,48] The aim of treatment is to achieve cure with the minimal amount of morbidity, particularly with regard to bladder function.[49,50] Unfavourable alveolar histology tends to be associated with other parameters of higher risk.[51]

The bladder outlet and prostatic region are unfavourable sites and for this reason bladder/prostate tumours are classified as high risk. Such tumours are likely to require aggressive neoadjuvant chemotherapy, attempted surgical resection, and adjuvant radiotherapy. A recently reported approach which combines resection of the tumour with prostatic brachytherapy is encouraging, since it may offer a higher chance of conserving the bladder.[52] Younger children with embryonal tumours are at intermediate risk, but still require multimodal therapy, albeit with a lower intensity. Even seemingly localized RMS is presumed to be micrometastatic, and so all children with RMS receive some chemotherapy.

Urothelial tumours

Urothelial tumours are exceedingly rare in childhood. Transitional cell carcinoma can very occasionally occur in older adolescents, and its treatment is the same as in adults. Outcomes in children are reported to be better than in adults. Urothelial neoplasms of low malignant potential (PUNLMP) can also occur in older adolescents,[53] and are treated according to adult guidelines.

Testicular tumours

Although the management of testicular masses in childhood generally mirrors their management in adults there are some important distinctions. Most malignant tumours of the testis in children present with an enlarging mass but, importantly, some present with a hydrocele.[54] Examination of a child with a hydrocele should therefore include careful palpation of the scrotal contents to ensure that the underlying testis is normal. If this is in any doubt ultrasound should be performed.[55] Blood tests for tumour markers (AFP and βHCG) are then performed prior to surgical exploration and orchidectomy via an inguinal approach. In order of frequency, the testicular tumours encountered in children are; mature teratoma, malignant germ cell tumour (yolk sac tumour) and paratesticular rhabdomyosarcoma.[56]

In principle, testicular sparing surgery can be considered for a mature teratoma, but in reality these tumours usually exceed the volume of the small prepubertal testis, and so there is no alternative to orchidectomy.

For a discreet lump within an otherwise normal testis preoperative ultrasound can be very valuable,in identifying benign masses such as an epidermoid cyst which can be enucleated. Nevertheless intraoperative frozen section is a recommended precaution in such cases.

Subsequent management, including imaging for metastases, is guided by the histological diagnosis—with adjuvant treatment depending on the stage and grade of tumour.[57] Lymph node involvement is generally identified on imaging rather than on biopsy.[58] Malignant germ cell tumours and paratesticular RMS both respond very well to treatment and have excellent outcomes.[59,60]

In the perinatal period an enlarged testis is most likely to be a consequence of intrauterine ('neonatal') testicular torsion, and is invariably beyond salvage. Since atrophy is the inevitable outcome, conservative management has been widely adopted in preference to surgical exploration.[61]

Poorly controlled congenital adrenal hyperplasia in adolescents may be associated with the development of hyperplastic nodules on both testes—with histological features resembling Leydig Cell tumours.[62] Surgical intervention is not required.

Conclusions

Urological malignancies are rare in childhood. Survival rates for Wilms tumour have improved dramatically over recent decades and the challenge is now to devise protocols which offer comparable outcomes with lower treatment-related morbidity. Rhabdomyosarcoma remains a challenging tumour to treat—both because of the tumour biology and the unfavourable anatomical location in many cases. Multimodal treatment is necessary to provide a reasonable prospect of cure with preservation of bladder function. The presentation and management of testicular tumours in children broadly mirrors that in adults. Management consists of radical orchidectomy with chemotherapy when this is indicated by tumour histology and staging. Childhood cancers of the urinary tract should be managed by multidisciplinary teams in specialist centres.

Further reading

D'Angio GJ. The treatment of Wilms' tumor. Results of the National Wilms' Tumor Study. *Cancer* 1976; **38**:633–46.

Dasgupta R, Rodeberg DA. Update on rhabdomyosarcoma. *Sem Pediatr Surg* 2012; **21**:68–78.

Hamilton TE, Shamberger RC. Wilms tumor: recent advances in clinical care and biology. *Sem Pediatr Surg* 2012; **21**:15–20.

Knudson AG, Strong LC. Mutation and cancer: a model for Wilms' tumor of the kidney. *J Natl Cancer Inst* 1972; **48**(2):313–24.

Metcalfe PD, Farivar-Mohseni H, Farhat W, McLorie G, Khoury A, Bagli DJ. Pediatric testicular tumors: contemporary incidence and efficacy of testicular preserving surgery. *J Urol* 2003; **170**:2412–5.

Pritchard-Jones K. Controversies and advances in the management of Wilms' tumour. *Arch Dis Child* 2002; **87**:241–4.

Rescorla FJ. Pediatric germ cell tumors. *Sem Pediatr Surg* 2012; **21**:51–60.

References

1. Stiller CA, Parkin DM. International variations in the incidence of childhood renal tumours. *Br J Cancer* 1990; **62**:1026–30.
2. D'Angio GJ. The treatment of Wilms' tumor. Results of the National Wilms' Tumor Study. *Cancer* 1976; **38**:633–46.
3. Wilms M. *Die Mischgeswulste der niere*. Leipzig, Germany: Verlag von Arthur Georgi. 1899.
4. Coppes-Zantinga AR, Coppes MJ. Max Wilms and "Die Mischgeswulste der Niere". *CMAJ* 1999; **160**:1196.
5. Miller RW, Fraumeni JF Jr, Manning MD. Association of Wilm's tumor with aniridia, Hemihypertrophy, and other congenital malformations. *N Eng J Med* 1964; **270**:922–7.
6. Olshan AF, Breslow NE, Falletta JM, *et al.* Risk factors for Wilms tumor. Report from the National Wilms Tumor Study. *Cancer* 1993; **72**:938–44.
7. Fischbach BV, Trout KL, Lewis J, Luis CA, Sika M. WAGR syndrome: a clinical review of 54 cases. *Pediatrics* 2005; **116**:984–8.
8. Wiedemann HR. Familial malformation complex with umbilical hernia and macroglossia—a "new syndrome"? (in French). *J génétique humaine* 1964; **13**:223–32.
9. Beckwith J. Macroglossia, omphalocoele, adrenal cytomegaly, gigantism and hyperplastic visceromegaly. *Birth Defects* 1969; **5**:188.
10. Porteus MH, Narkool P, Neuberg D, *et al.* Characteristics and outcome of children with Beckwith-Wiedemann syndrome and Wilms' tumor: a report from the National Wilms Tumor Study Group. *J Clin Oncol* 2000; **18**:2026–31.
11. Denys P, Malvaux P, Van Den Berghe H, Tanghe W, Proesmans W. Association of an anatomo-pathological syndrome of male pseudohermaphroditism, Wilms' tumor, parenchymatous nephropathy and XX/XY mosaicism (in French). *Arch Fr Pediatr* 1967; **24**:729–39.
12. Drash A, Sherman F, Hartmann WH, Blizzard RM. A syndrome of pseudohermaphroditism, Wilms' tumor, hypertension, and degenerative renal disease. *J Pediatr* 1970; **76**:585–93.
13. Choyke PL, Siegel MJ, Craft AW, Green DM, DeBaun MR. Screening for Wilms tumor in children with Beckwith-Wiedemann syndrome or idiopathic hemihypertrophy. *Med Pediatr Oncol* 1999; **32**:196–200.
14. Knudson AG, Strong LC. Mutation and cancer: a model for Wilms' tumor of the kidney. *J Natl Cancer Inst* 1972; **48**(2):313–24.
15. Mitchell JD, Baxter TJ, Blair-West JR, McCredie DA. Renin levels in nephroblastoma (Wilms' tumour). *Arch Dis Child* 1970; **45**:376–84.
16. Leckie BJ, Birnie G, Carachi R. Renin in Wilms' tumour: prorenin as an indicator. *J Clin Endocrinol Metab* 1994; **76**:1742–6.
17. Pritchard-Jones K. Controversies and advances in the management of Wilms' tumour. *Arch Dis Child* 2002; **87**:241–4.
18. Lamerle J, Voute PA, Tournade MF, *et al.* Preoperative versus postoperative radiotherapy, single versus multiple courses of Actinomycin D in the treatment of Wilms' tumor. Preliminary results of a controlled clinical trail conducted by the International Society of Paediatric Oncology (SIOP). *Cancer* 1976; **38**:647–54.
19. Lemerle J, Voute PA, Tournade MF, *et al.* Effectiveness of preoperative chemotherapy in Wilms tumor: results of an International Society of Paediatric Oncology (SIOP) clinical trial. *J Clin Oncol* 1983; **1**:604–9.
20. Mitchell C, Pritchard-Jones K, Shannon R, *et al.* Immediate nephrectomy versus preoperative chemotherapy in the management of non-metastatic Wilms' tumour: results of a randomised trail (UKW3) by the UK Children's Cancer Study Group. *Eur J Cancer* 2006; **42**:2554–62.
21. Pritchard-Jones K, Moroz V, Vujanic G, *et al.* Treatment and outcomes of Wilms' tumour patients: an analysis of all cases registered in the UKW3 trial. *Ann Oncol* 2012; **23**:2457–63.
22. Green DM, Breslow NE, Beckwith JB, *et al.* Treatment with nephrectomy only for small, stage I/favorable histology Wilms' tumor: a report from the National Wilms Tumor Study Group. *J Clin Oncol* 2001; **19**:3719–24.
23. Vujanic GM, Kelsey A, Mitchell C, Shannon RS, Gornall P. The role of biopsy in the diagnosis of renal tumours of childhood: results of the UKCCSG Wilms tumour study 3. *Med Pediatr Oncol* 2003; **40**:18–20.
24. D'Angio GJ, Evans A, Breslow N, *et al.* The treatment of Wilms' tumor: results of the second National Wilms' Tumor Study. *Cancer* 1981; **47**:2302–11.
25. D'Angio GJ, Breslow N, Beckwith B, *et al.* Treatment of Wilms' tumor. Results of the third National Wilms' Tumor Study. *Cancer* 1989; **64**:349–60.
26. Green DM, Breslow N, Beckwith B, *et al.* Effect of duration of treatment on treatment outcome and cost of treatment for Wilms' tumor: a report from the National Wilms' Tumor Study Group. *J Clin Oncol* 1998; **16**:3744–51.
27. Green DM, Breslow NE, Beckwith JB, *et al.* Comparison between single-dose and divided-dose administration of dactinomycin and doxorubicin for patients with Wilms' tumor: a report from the National Wilms' Tumor Study Group. *J Clin Oncol* 1998; **16**:23–45.
28. Ritchey M, Daley S, Shamberger RC, *et al.* Ureteral extension in Wilms' tumor: a report from the National Wilms' Tumor Study Group (NWTSG). *J Pediatr Surg* 2008; **43**:1625–9.
29. Ritchey ML, Shamberger RC, Haase G, Horwitz J, Bergemann T, Breslow NE. Surgical complications after primary nephrectomy for Wilms' tumor: report from the National Wilms' Tumor Study Group. *J Am Coll Surg* 2001; **192**:63–8.
30. Cotton CA, Peterson S, Norkool PA, *et al.* Early and late mortality after diagnosis of Wilms tumor. *J Clin Oncol* 2009; **27**:1304–9.
31. Green DM, Beckwith JB, Breslow NE, *et al.* Treatment of children with stages II to IV anaplastic Wilms' Tumor: a report from the National Wilms' Tumor Study Group. *J Clin Oncol* 1994; **12**:2126–31.
32. Ritchey ML, Green DM, Breslow NB, Moksness J, Norkool P. Accuracy of current imaging modalities in the diagnosis of synchronous bilateral Wilms' tumor. A report from the National Wilms Tumor Study Group. *Cancer* 1995; **75**:600–4.
33. Hamilton TE, Ritchey ML, Haase GM, *et al.* The management of synchronous bilateral Wilms tumor: a report from the National Wilms Tumor Study Group. *Ann Surg* 2011; **253**: 1004–10.
34. Lall A, Pritchard-Jones K, Walker J, *et al.* Wilms' tumor with intracaval thrombus in the UK Children's Cancer Study Group UKW3 trial. *J Pediatr Surg* 2006; **41**:382–7.
35. England RJ, Haider N, Vujanic GM, *et al.* Mesoblastic nephroma: a report of the United Kingdom Children's Cancer and Leukaemia Group (CCLG). *Pediatr Blood Cancer* 2011; **56**:744–8.
36. Leclair MD, El-Ghoneimi A, Audrey G, Ravasse P, Moscovici J, Heloury Y. The outcomes of prenatally diagnosed renal tumors. *J Urol* 2005;**173**:186–9.
37. Rousseau-Merck MF, Nogues C, Nezelof C, Martin-Cudraz B, Paulin D. Infantile renal tumors associated with hypercalcemia. *Arch Pathol Lab Med* 1983; **107**:311–4.
38. Howell CG, Othersen HB, Kiviat NE, Norkool P, Beckwith JB, D'Angio GJ. Therapy and outcome in 51 children with mesoblastic nephroma: a report of the National Wilms' Tumor Study. *J Pediatr Surg* 1982; **17**:826–31.
39. Breslow NE, Beckwith JB, Perlman EJ, Reeve AE. Age distributions, birth weights, nephrogenic rests, and heterogeneity in the pathogenesis of Wilms tumor. *Pediatr Blood Cancer* 2006; **47**:260–7.

40. Rohrschneider WK, Weirich A, Rieden K, Darge K, Troger J, Graf NUS. US, CT and MR imaging characteristics of nephroblastomatosis. *Pediatr Radiol* 1998; **28**:435–43.
41. Seibel NL, Li S, Breslow NE, *et al.* Effect of duration of treatment on treatment outcome for patients with clear-cell sarcoma of the kidney: a report from the National Wilms' Tumor Study Group. *J Clin Oncol* 2004; **22**:468–73.
42. Ognjanovic S, Linabery AM, Charbonneau B, Ross JA. Trends in childhood rhabdomyosarcoma incidence and survival in the United States, 1975–2005. *Cancer* 2009; **115**:4218–26.
43. Mazzoleni S, Bisogno G, Garaventa A, *et al.* Outcomes and prognostic factors after recurrence in children and adolescents with nonmetastatic rhabdomyosarcoma. *Cancer* 2005; **104**:183–90.
44. Punyko JA, Mertens AC, Baker KS, Ness KS, Robison LL, Gurney JG. Long-term survival probabilities for childhood rhabdomyosarcoma. A population-based evaluation. *Cancer* 2005; **103**:1475–83.
45. Perez EA, Kassira N, Cheung MC, Koniaris LG, Neville HL, Sola JE. Rhabdomyosarcoma in children: a SEER population based study. *J Surg Res* 2011; **170**:e243–51:
46. Turc-Carel C, Lizard-Nacol S, Justrabo E, Favrot M, Philip T, Tabone E. Consistent chromosomal translocation in alveolar rhabdomyosarcoma. *Cancer Genet Cytogenet* 1986; **19**:361–2.
47. Oberlin O, Rey A, Lyden E, *et al.* Prognostic factors in metastatic rhabdomyosarcomas: results of a pooled analysis from United States and European cooperative groups. *J Clin Oncol* 2008; **26**:2384–9.
48. De Corti F, Dall'Igna P, Bisogno G, *et al.* Sentinel node biopsy in pediatric soft tissue sarcomas of extremities. *Pediatr Blood Cancer* 2009; **52**:51–4.
49. Punyko JA, Mertens AC, Gurney JG, *et al.* Long-term medical effects of childhood and adolescent rhabdomyosarcoma: a report from the childhood cancer survivor study. *Pediatr Blood Cancer* 2005; **44**:643–53.
50. Raney B, Anderson J, Jenney M, *et al.* Late effects in 164 patients with rhabdomyosarcoma of the bladder/prostate region: a report from the international workshop. *J Urol* 2006; **176**:2194–5.
51. Rodary C, Gehan EA, Flamant F, *et al.* Prognostic factors in 951 non-metastatic rhabdomyosarcoma in children: a report of the Intergroup Rhabdomyosarcoma Workshop. *Med Pediatr Oncol* 1991; **19**:89–95.
52. Martelli H, Haie-Meder C, Branchereau S, *et al.* Conservative surgery plus brachytherapy treatment for boys with prostate and/or bladder neck rhabdomyosarcoma: a single team experience. *J Pediatr Surg* 2009; **44**:190–6.
53. Alanec S, Shukla AR. Bladder malignancies in children aged <18 years: results from the Surveillance, Epidemiology and End Results database. *Br J Urol* 2010; **106**:557–60.
54. Ahmed HU, Arya M, Muneer A, Mustaq I, Sebire NJ. Testicular and paratesticular tumors in the prepubertal population. *Lancet Oncol* 2010; **11**:476–83.
55. Lin HC, Clark JY. Testicular teratoma presenting as a transilluminating scrotal mass. *Urology* 2006; **67**:1290–5.
56. Metcalfe PD, Farivar-Mohseni H, Farhat W, McLorie G, Khoury A, Bagli DJ. Pediatric testicular tumors: contemporary incidence and efficacy of testicular preserving surgery. *J Urol* 2003; **170**:2412–5.
57. Haas RJ, Schmidt P, Göbel U, Harms D. Treatment of malignant testicular tumors in childhood: results of the German National Study 1982–1992. *Med Pediatr Oncol* 1994; **23**:400–5.
58. Schlatter M, Rescorla F, Giller R, *et al.* Excellent outcome in patients with stage I germ cell tumors of the testes: a study of the Children's Cancer Group/Pediatric Oncology Group. *J Pediatr Surg* 2003; **38**:319–24.
59. Mann JR, Raafat F, Robinson K, *et al.* The United Kingdom Children's Cancer Study Group's second germ cell tumor study: carboplatin, etoposide, and bleomycin are effective treatment for children with malignant extracranial germ cell tumors, with acceptable toxicity. *J Clin Oncol* 2000; **18**:3809–18.
60. Stewart RJ, Martelli H, Oberlin O, *et al.* Treatment of children with nonmetastatic paratesticular rhabdomyosarcoma: results of the Malignant Mesenchymal Tumors studies (MMT 84 and MMT 89) of the International Society of Pediatric Oncology. *J Clin Oncol* 2003; **21**:793–8.
61. Kaye JD, Levitt SB, Friedman SC, Franco I, Gitlin J, Palmer LS. Neonatal torsion: a 14-year experience and proposed algorithm for management. *J Urol* 2008; **179**:2377–83.
62. Rich MA, Keating MA. Leydig cell tumors and tumors associated with congenital adrenal hyperplasia. *Urol Clin North Am* 2000; **27**:519–28.

SECTION 9

Renal function

Section editor: Rutger Ploeg

CHAPTER 9.1

Renal function

Chris A. O'Callaghan

Introduction—an overview of renal physiology

The kidneys are major homeostatic organs and play a key role in the maintenance of an extracellular environment in which cells can survive. They do this primarily by regulating the composition of plasma, which indirectly influences the composition of the extracellular fluid in which cells are bathed. The red cell content of blood is also regulated by the kidneys through the secretion of erythropoietin. The kidneys are important endocrine organs and, in addition to erythropoietin, the other major endocrine products include renin and vitamin D.

Within the kidneys, the glomeruli filter plasma and the renal tubules adjust the composition of this filtered liquid, or filtrate, as it passes along them (Fig. 9.1.1). This adjustment arises from large scale reabsorption of most of the filtered water and soluble plasma components. In addition to filtration and reabsorption, the kidneys can also secrete plasma constituents into the filtrate, to promote the excretion of these substances.

The combination of the glomerulus, its tubules and associated blood vessels is referred to as a nephron (Fig. 9.1.1). Each kidney has around 400,000–800,000 nephrons, although the number of nephrons declines with age.

Glomerulus
Afferent arteriole
Efferent arteriole
Juxtaglomerular apparatus
Proximal tubule
Distal tubule
Collecting ducts
Loop of Henle

Fig. 9.1.1 The nephron. Filtrate is formed within the glomerulus and then passes along the tubular system where it is modified by reabsorption and secretion.

A range of different transport processes occur along the tubules to move ions or molecules (Fig. 9.1.2). Active transport requires the consumption of energy by the breakdown of adenosine triphosphate (ATP). Passive transport occurs when ions or molecules move because there is a gradient in concentration or electrical potential. Water molecules cannot be pumped but move by osmosis when there is an osmotic gradient across a semi-permeable membrane.

The kidneys have three major effects on extracellular fluid homeostasis.

- They adjust body water content by controlling the volume of urine produced.
- They adjust the ionic composition of extracellular fluid by controlling the excretion of plasma ions including sodium,

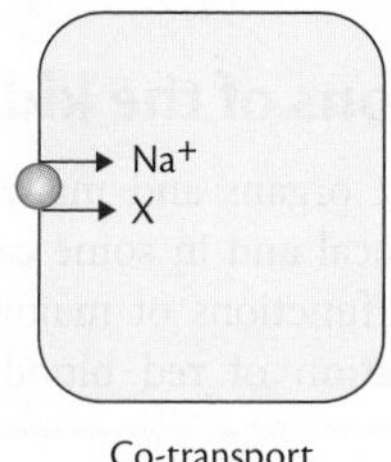

Co-transport

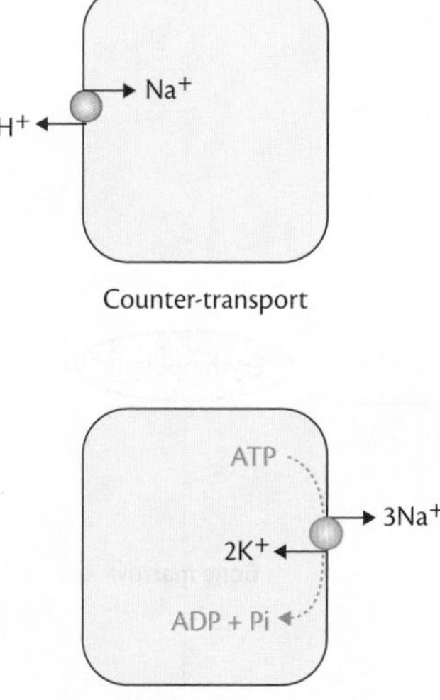

Fig. 9.1.2 Transport processes. Ions can move passively across membranes along concentration of electrical gradients by co-transport or counter-transport. Active transport can occur even against such gradients and is directly powered by adenosine triphosphate (ATP).

potassium, calcium, magnesium, and their associated anions, such as chloride and phosphate.

- They adjust acid-base status to maintain body pH by regulating the urinary excretion of acid.

The kidneys have a very high blood flow, most of which is channelled into specialized capillary bundles in the glomeruli. The blood vessels beyond the glomerular capillaries are arterioles rather than venules. These efferent arterioles are able to contract which produces a high pressure within the upstream glomerular capillaries and so promotes filtration in the glomerulus. The filtered fluid from each glomerulus passes along a tubule and along this course it is modified by reabsorption and secretion.

Despite their modest size, the combined blood flow to both kidneys is around 20% of the total cardiac output. Although the total volume of the circulating plasma is around three litres, the total extracellular volume is much higher at around 15 litres. Plasma and extravascular extracellular fluid are in equilibrium, so the kidneys needs to adjust plasma composition continuously to keep it within a tight range and so maintain a stable extracellular environment for cells. This homeostatic regulation occurs in such a way that there are no excessive changes in the levels of extracellular fluid constituents that might otherwise occur with metabolic activity. The high renal blood flow ensures that this is an efficient process, even on a minute-to-minute timescale. The net result is that plasma fluid composition remains remarkably stable even though the kidneys are removing very substantial amounts of excreted products from the plasma.

Endocrine functions of the kidney

The kidneys are complex organs and many soluble compounds are produced that have local and in some cases systemic actions. However, key endocrine functions of major recognized importance concern the regulation of red blood cell production by erythropoietin, of divalent ions and bone metabolism by vitamin D production and of the angiotensin axis by renin production (Fig. 9.1.3).

Erythropoietin is a protein produced by fibroblastoid cells located within the renal interstitium near to the tubules in the cortex and outer medulla of the kidney. There is a low basal level of erythropoietin production, which is upregulated if oxygen delivery is reduced by hypoxia or anaemia. Erythropoietin acts on an erythropoietin receptor on early erythroid precursor cells to promote their survival and development. In the absence of erythropoietin these cells die by apoptosis and red cell numbers decline which results in a fall in blood haemoglobin levels and haematocrit.

Vitamin D is produced by a multistep synthesis from cholesterol. The first step happens in the skin in a process requiring ultraviolet light and this is followed by a further step in the liver which produces 25-hydroxy vitamin D. The kidney is then responsible for the final step whereby a further hydroxyl group is added to produce the active form of vitamin D which is 1,25-dihydroxy vitamin D. This active form of vitamin D acts on receptors in the gut, kidneys, and bone to raise calcium and phosphate levels by promoting their absorption by the gut, their reabsorption by the kidneys and their release from bone.

Renin is produced by cells which form part of the juxtaglomerular apparatus of each glomerulus. Each juxtaglomerular apparatus is formed where the afferent and efferent arterioles of a glomerulus are in close proximity to a section of the tubule that drains the glomerulus (Fig. 9.1.1). Granular cells that exist within this structure release renin in response to a number of stimuli which can come about as a result of changes in renal perfusion pressure, sympathetic nervous system activity, and alterations in the sodium and chloride levels in the tubules. Renin promotes the production of angiotensin I which is converted to angiotensin II. Angiotensin II promotes vascular smooth muscle contraction and promotes sodium retention both directly and by acting on the adrenal gland to increase aldosterone production. These actions maintain blood pressure.

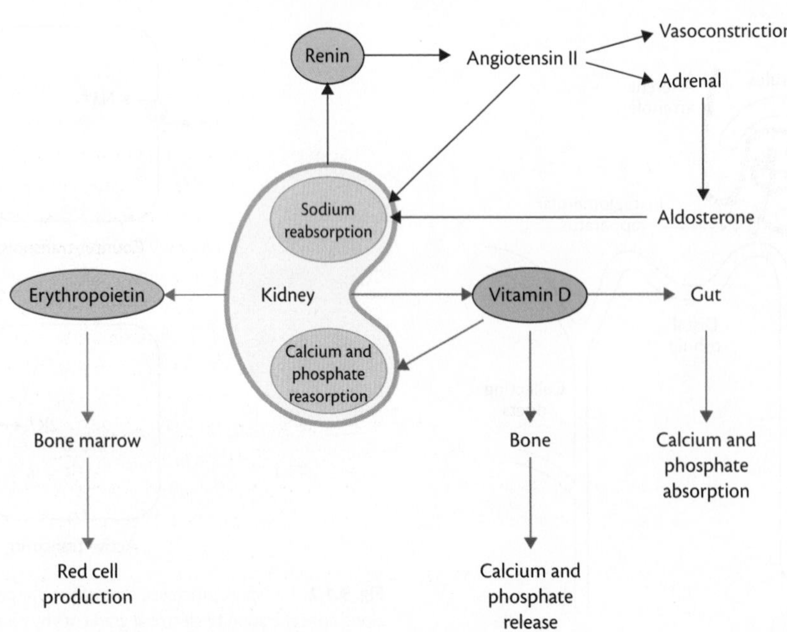

Fig. 9.1.3 Endocrine functions of the kidney. Key endocrine products of the kidney are renin, vitamin D, and erythropoietin—their key actions are illustrated here.

Endocrine influences on the kidney

The kidney is a key effector arm of endocrine organ function. In addition to those hormones produced by the kidney, major hormones acting on the kidney include vasopressin, angiotensin, aldosterone, parathyroid hormone, and the relatively recently characterized phosphatonin FGF-23.[1] Vasopressin promotes water reabsorption. Angiotensin II and aldosterone promotes sodium reabsorption. Parathyroid hormone promotes renal phosphate excretion, calcium reabsorption, and renal vitamin D production. FGF-23 reduces renal vitamin D production and promotes phosphate excretion.[1]

Renal blood flow

The kidneys are highly vascular organs and together they receive around 20% of the total cardiac output. Typically each kidney receives a single renal artery from the aorta, although there are many variations on this and it is common for more than one renal artery to supply a kidney. The renal artery usually divides within the kidney into several segmental arteries, which each give rise to interlobar arteries (Fig. 9.1.4). The interlobar arteries penetrate further into the kidney and divide into arcuate arteries that run parallel to the outer surface of the kidneys. From these arcuate arteries the smaller interlobular arteries arise and run radially outwards through the cortex of the kidney. Afferent arterioles arise from these interlobular arteries and supply the glomerular capillary bundles.

The capillary bundle of each glomerulus is drained by an efferent arteriole. The glomerulus is the only vascular bed that is both supplied and drained by arterioles. Beyond the efferent arteriole, there are two distinct patterns of vascular arrangement. In the outer cortex of the kidney efferent arterioles flow into a peritubular capillary network that is closely wrapped around the tubule that leads away from the glomerulus that the afferent arteriole supplied. This allows exchange between the tubule and the capillaries of reabsorbed or secreted ions or molecules. Those efferent arterioles that arise from nephrons in the juxtamedullary or deep cortex give rise to a capillary network that also incorporates the vasa recta which are small vessels that descend to form a capillary network and then rejoin to reascend with the loop of Henle before rejoining the capillary network around the remaining tubules in that nephron. The descending and ascending vasa recta are close to each other as they travel through the renal medulla and are the only blood supply that the renal medulla receives. They operate as a countercurrent transport system that plays a role in maintaining the high osmolality in the renal medulla that is required for the production of a concentrated urine. Beyond the tubular capillaries blood enters venules that then progressively join to form increasingly larger vessels. Eventually blood leaves the kidneys in the renal veins which drain into the inferior vena cava. As with renal arteries, variations in the number of renal veins are well recognized.

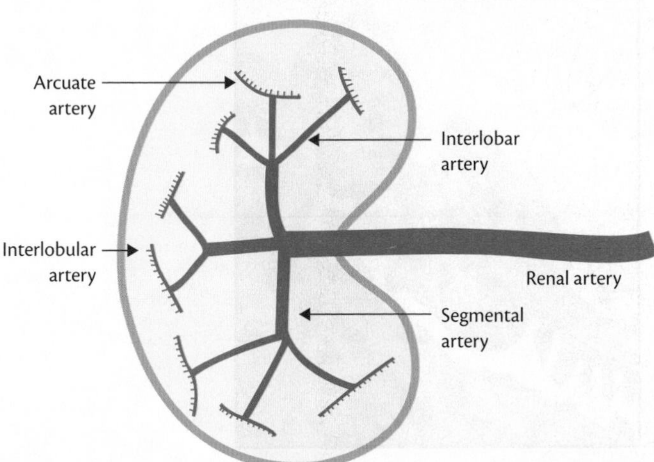

Fig. 9.1.4 Renal blood supply. The renal arteries subdivide progressively into interlobular arteries from which the afferent arterioles arise to supply the glomeruli.

Measurement of renal blood flow

Renal blood flow (RBF) can be measured in various ways. The standard physiological approach is to use a substance such as *p*-aminohippuric acid (PAH) which is fully removed from plasma after a single pass through the kidneys. Given this, the amount of PAH that is removed from plasma by the kidneys must equal the amount of PAH that is excreted in the urine over a given time. Therefore, if the renal arterial and venous plasma concentrations of PAH are determined and urine flow rate and urine concentration of PAH are determined, it is possible to calculate the renal plasma flow (RPF):

$$(\text{Arterial [PAH]} - \text{Venous [PAH]}) \times \text{RPF} = \text{Urine [PAH]} \times \text{Urine flow rate}$$

Renal blood flow can then be calculated from RPF because

$$\text{RBF} = \text{RPF}/\ (1 - \text{haematocrit})$$

In routine clinical practice it is not straightforward to undertake these measurements directly. However, ^{99m}Tc-labelled DTPA (diethylenetriaminepenta-acetic acid) and MAG3 (mercaptoactyltriglycine) are removed by the kidney and can be used to estimate renal blood flow. Flow in the renal arteries can also be assessed using transcutaneous Doppler studies.

Regulation of renal blood flow

Renal blood flow is affected by a wide range of influences and how these are integrated is incompletely understood. Within the nephron there is local regulation of the arterioles. In particular, tubuloglomerular feedback occurs such that a rise in glomerular pressure and so glomerular filtration rate (GFR) triggers the release of adenosine which acts on A1 receptors, causing afferent arteriolar vasoconstriction and thus lowering glomerular pressure and filtration rate. The input to this feedback mechanism is the sensing of tubular sodium and chloride by the macula densa cells in the distal tubule which are part of the juxtaglomerular apparatus (JGA) (Fig. 9.1.1). A rise in GFR reduces the time available for sodium and chloride reabsorption and so increases their concentration in the tubule.

The juxtaglomerular apparatus can also release renin in response to a fall in afferent arteriolar pressure, reduced sodium and chloride concentration at the macula densa and sympathetic nervous activity acting on beta 1 receptors within the JGA. The action of renin triggers angiotensin II production which will acts on AT1 receptors causing vasoconstriction of both afferent and efferent arterioles. However, as the effect is stronger on the efferent arterioles the effect is an increase in intraglomerular pressure and so a rise in GFR.

The sympathetic nervous system within the renal nerves mediates afferent and efferent arteriolar constriction through the action of noradrenaline on alpha 1 adrenergic receptors. A range of vasodilating prostaglandins such as PGE2 and PGI2 (prostacyclin) oppose the action of vasoconstrictors.

A variety of other compounds have effects on RBF. Well recognized effects include those of endothelin which acts on ETB receptors to cause renal vasoconstriction, vasopressin which acts on V1 receptors to cause vasoconstriction, adrenomedullin which causes renal vasodilation, nitric oxide which causes renal vasodilation and bradykinin which promotes prostaglandin synthesis and vasodilation.

Renal filtration

Following the branching subdivision of the renal arteries, blood passing through an afferent arteriole enters a glomerular capillary bed. This is a highly specialized capillary network that forms a ball-like structure or glomerulus. The glomerular capillary endothelial cells are relatively flat cells with the capillary lumen on one side and a specialized basement membrane known as the glomerular basement membrane on the other side.[2] On the opposite side of the glomerular basement membrane are epithelial cells that form the inner surface of Bowman's capsule. These tubular epithelial cells are highly specialized and are known as podocytes because of their 'foot processes' (Fig. 9.1.5). During the embryological development of the kidney, each glomerular capillary invaginates a developing tubule to form a glomerulus. The result is that each mature glomerular capillary is surrounded by the tubular collecting system. Filtration occurs within the glomerulus and fluid passes from the glomerular capillary lumen into the tubular system. The space immediately beyond the filtration barrier into which the filtered fluid passes is known as Bowman's space.

Blood which leaves the glomerular capillary network first passes through an efferent arteriole. The ability of this arteriole to contract allows the precise regulation of intraglomerular pressure. As efferent arteriolar constriction increases, the hydrostatic pressure within the glomerular capillary system rises and this drives the filtration process. The filtrate which is produced then passes down the tubule.

The filtration barrier

The filtration barrier itself consists of three principal components, the glomerular endothelial cell, the basement membrane and the tubular epithelial cell or podocyte (Fig. 9.1.5). The endothelial cells are very thin and are described as 'fenestrated' because they have multiple pores of around 70 nm in diameter which are filled with negatively charged glycoprotein.

The glomerular basement membrane is a complex network of glycoproteins which include a three-dimensional scaffold composed of helical strands of type IV collagen on which the other components are attached. These other proteins include heparan sulphate proteoglycan, laminin, podocalyxin, fibronectin, and entactin. The glomerular basement membrane is organized into three layers known, from the endothelial side to the epithelial side as the lamina densa, lamina rara interna, and lamina rara externa. The lamina densa is a relatively homogeneous dense layer, but the two lamina rara layers are less dense and have a significant negative charge.

The epithelial cells or podocytes lining Bowman's space have well-developed foot processes which are attached to the tubular side of the glomerular basement membrane. The foot processes from different podocytes interdigitate, but do not touch each other. Between these interdigitating foot processes are spaces known as a filtration slits which are around 25–65 nm across. A network of proteins associated with the podocytes foot processes forms 'slit pores' across these slits. Proteins involved in slit pores include podocalyxin, nephrin, NEPH1, P-cadherin, CD2AP, ZO-1, and podocin.[3] Within the glomerulus there are also mesangial cells which have both contractile and phagocytic properties and appear to serve a structural role in supporting the capillary loops.

The filtration process

Together these multiple layers of the filtration barrier provide a matrix through which size and charge selection occurs as plasma is filtered. The high pressure in the glomerulus forces water and solutes through the filtration barrier. The extent to which a substance is filtered depends to some extent upon its electrical charge and to a larger extent upon its size. There remains debate about the precise role of each layer of the barrier, but molecular defects in a range of

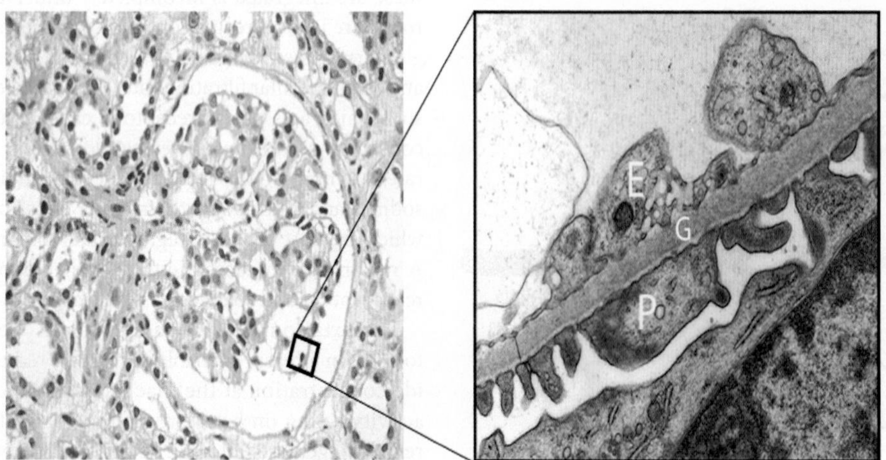

Fig. 9.1.5 The filtration barrier. The left panel shows a light microscopic image of a glomerulus and the right panel is an electron micrograph of the filtration barrier. (E) indicates the endothelial cell lining the glomerular capillary, while (G) is the glomerular basement membrane, and (P) is the podocyte with its foot processes lining Bowman's space.

Reproduced courtesy of Professor Ian SD Roberts, John Radcliffe Hospital, Oxford, UK.

the proteins that contribute to the barrier can disrupt the barrier function resulting in proteinuria.[4]

How is filtration measured

The physiological approach to the measurement of the rate of filtration is based on the clearance of a substance from plasma by the kidney. Clearance per minute is the volume of plasma from which the substance is removed in one minute. For studies of filtration an ideal substance would be freely filtered in the glomerulus and not secreted or reabsorbed in the tubules. The polysaccharide inulin has these properties, so following intravenous administration of inulin it is possible to calculate the clearance of inulin if urine flow rate and plasma and urine concentrations of inulin are measured. This is because the amount removed from the plasma in any given time period must be the same as the amount excreted in the urine in that time period.

$$\text{Clearance} = U[\text{inulin}]V / P[\text{inulin}]$$

Other approaches to estimating the rate of filtration in clinical practice are considered later in this chapter.

Tubular function

The filtration process occurring in the glomerulus produces a large volume of filtrate, which is then processed as it passes along the tubular system to produce a much smaller volume of the final urine. If an individual has a GFR of 120 mL/min/1.73m^2 which might be a typical figure for a young healthy adult, then the volume of filtrate produced per day would be around 172 litres per day. As the volume of urine produced per day is of the order of only a few litres there must be substantial reabsorption of fluid in the tubules. Substances such as sodium, potassium and glucose which are freely filtered in the glomerulus are present in the filtrate at the same concentration as their plasma concentration. Therefore, the filtrate produced during 24 hours contains very large amounts of these substances (e.g. 23 moles of sodium or over 1 kg of salt) so there must be substantial reabsorption of solutes from the filtrate. Such large scale reabsorption requires considerable energy expenditure and the kidney is a highly metabolic organ.

The tubular system is most generally divided into the proximal tubules and the distal tubules (Fig. 9.1.1). In nephrons that are deep within the cortex (juxtamedullary nephrons) the proximal tubule leads into a section of tubule known as the loop of Henle which can descend deep into the renal medulla before reascending to lead into the distal tubule. The distal tubule leads into the collecting duct which descends deep into the kidney. There are three sections of the collecting duct as it descends through the kidney, known as the cortical collecting duct, the outer medullary collecting duct and the inner medullary collecting duct. The inner medullary collecting duct eventually flows into a papillary duct which exits from a renal papilla into a minor calyx and so into the renal pelvis.

The tubular system of the nephron is lined with tubular epithelium which is only one cell thick. The tubular cells are generally columnar in type and are joined together by tight junctions at their luminal edges. These junctions allow transport processes to establish gradients across the tubular epithelial layer. Molecules can move through the tight junctions and this movement is controlled by transmembrane proteins known as claudins.[5]

In general terms, the bulk of the reabsorption of water and solutes takes place in the proximal tubules and then further fine tuning of this reabsorption takes place in the more distal tubular segments (Fig. 9.1.6). Within the proximal tubule key electrolytes, glucose, amino acids, other substances and water are absorbed and there is

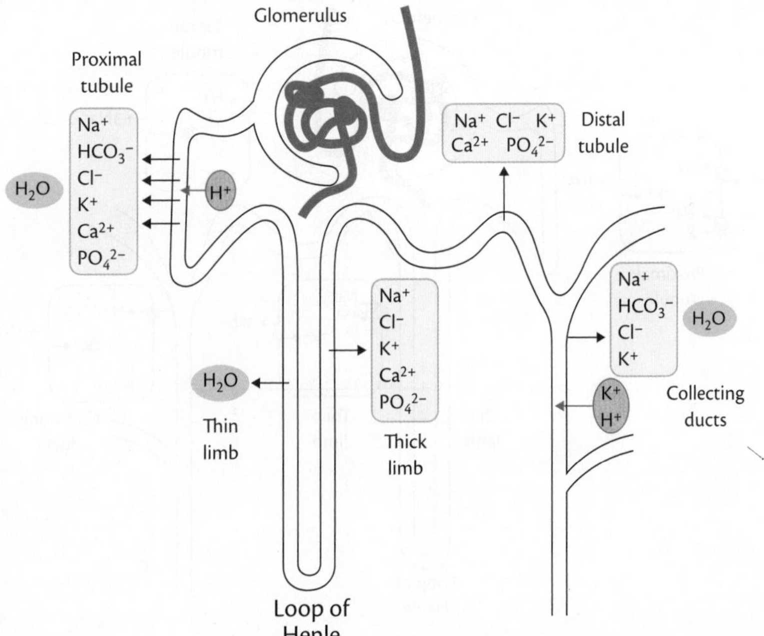

Fig. 9.1.6 Processing of filitrate along the nephron. The filtrate is formed in the urine and processed along the nephron as shown. The red arrows indicate secretion and the purple arrows indicate reabsorption. The bulk of the reabsorption of ions and water occurs in the proximal tubule and is refined along the nephron under endocrine influences.

endocytic uptake of filtered proteins which bind to the endocytic receptor megalin.[6] Much of the transport is active transport of solutes and there is concomitant movement of water by osmosis. However, although there is substantial reabsorption in this segment of the tubules, the filtrate remains iso-osmotic with plasma.

The loop of Henle plays a central role in the production of a concentrated urine.[7] Within the loop of Henle the descending limb has relatively flat cells which do not undertake active transport, whereas the ascending limb has thicker cells which are responsible for significant active transport. In the distal tubule there is significant endocrine regulation of tubular function, especially from vasopressin and aldosterone. The major active driving force for tubular solute transport is the activity of the Na^+/K^+ ATPase molecules which are predominantly localized to the lateral and basal membrane regions of the tubular cells. This activity establishes sodium and potassium gradients which can be used to drive the movement of other ions or molecules by co-transport or counter-transport with sodium or other ions.

Renal sodium handling

Sodium and chloride are freely filtered in the glomerulus. In each segment of the tubules where sodium reabsorption occurs, sodium is pumped out of the basolateral membrane of the tubular cells by the Na^+/K^+ ATPase (Fig. 9.1.7). This generates a sodium gradient that drives influx of sodium into the tubular cells. Different tubule segments employ different molecules to transport sodium across the apical membrane of the cells.[8–10] In some portions of the nephron there is also paracellular movement of sodium driven by the sodium gradient. Around 65% of the filtered sodium is reabsorbed in the proximal tubule. In the proximal tubule sodium movement at the apical luminal membrane is mediated by the NHE3 sodium-hydrogen exchanger, such that sodium enters the cell and H^+ leaves it. Sodium also enters proximal tubular cells using a set of co-transporter molecules which transport sodium together with other molecules including bicarbonate, glucose, amino acids, or other organic compounds. The sodium that leaves the cell is then removed at the basal surface by the Na^+/K^+ ATPase. The loop of Henle reabsorbs a further 25% of the filtered sodium. The thin-walled descending limb is impermeable to sodium, but sodium enters the cells of the thicker ascending limb using the NKCC2 transporter which is a co-transporter for sodium, potassium, and chloride ions and the target of action of the loop diuretics, such as furosemide. Within the distal tubule a further 5% of the filtered sodium is reabsorbed. Sodium crosses the apical portion of the distal tubular cells using the NCC which is a co-transporter for sodium and chloride and the target of action of the thiazide diuretics. Around 2–5% of the filtered sodium is reabsorbed in the collecting ducts in cells known as principal cells. Sodium crosses the apical portion of these cells using the ENaC channel which is the drug target of amiloride. Angiotensin II enhances proximal tubule sodium reabsorption and aldosterone has a major regulatory role whereby it enhances collecting duct sodium reabsorption.[11–13]

Renal potassium handling

Potassium is freely filtered in the glomerulus like sodium, but is handled very differently by the tubules (Fig. 9.1.6).[8–10] Sodium is reabsorbed along the tubules and the sodium that is excreted is that which has not been reabsorbed. In contrast, almost all filtered potassium is reabsorbed before the collecting duct and then the potassium that is to be excreted is secreted into the collecting duct. As with sodium, around 65% of the filtered potassium is reabsorbed in the proximal tubule. This reabsorption is largely paracellular as potassium moves by convection with water that follows sodium reabsorption by osmosis. This potassium movement

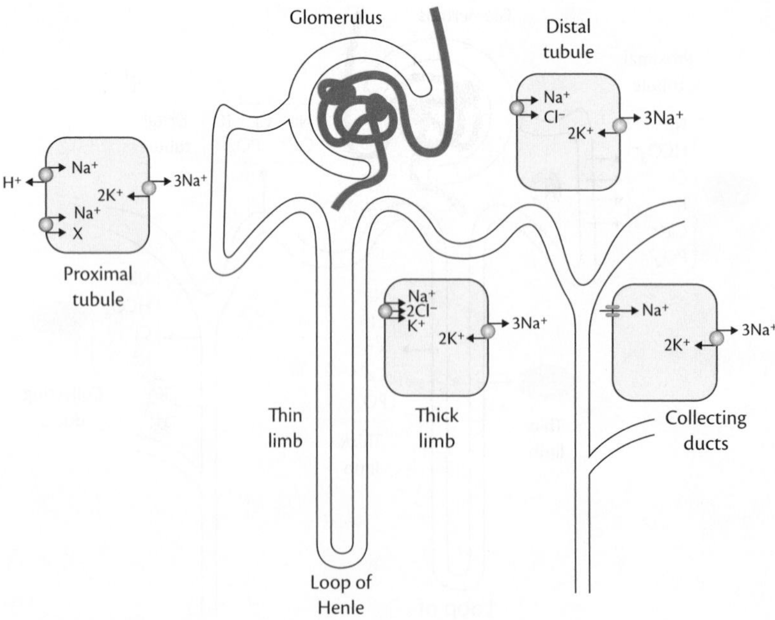

Fig. 9.1.7 Renal sodium handling. The typical sodium handling activity of tubular cells in different regions of the nephron is illustrated. In each case the tubular cell is coloured pale yellow and the tubular lumen is considered to be to the left of the cell. The bulk of the sodium is reabsorbed in the proximal tubule. In the early proximal tubule, this is predominantly by sodium-hydrogen exchange, but later in the proximal tubule there is substantial co-transport of sodium with other molecules (denoted by X) such as glucose.

is likely to be fuelled by the activity of Na^+/K^+ ATPase molecules which remove potassium from the intracellular spaces and by the electrical gradient in the later proximal tubule. A further 30% of the filtered potassium is removed in the thick ascending limb of the loop of Henle via the NKCC co-transporter and via the paracellular route. Further potassium reabsorption occurs in the distal tubule, but the key physiological control step is in the collecting ducts. Here the predominant feature of potassium handling is secretion of potassium by principal cells.[14] The Na^+/K^+ ATPase molecules at the basolateral surfaces pump potassium into the cells and this drives potassium out of the cells at the apical luminal membrane surface through KCC potassium-chloride co-transporter channels and through ROMK and BK channels.[15] At high urinary flow rates potassium secretion increases in part because the high flow rate maintains a high potassium gradient and in part because it triggers opening of BK channels. Aldosterone promotes potassium secretion in the principal cells.

Renal acid-base handling

The kidney plays a key role in maintaining acid-base status by excreting acid and to do this, adequate buffering capacity must be present in the urine.[16] Bicarbonate is freely filtered in the glomerulus and is mostly reabsorbed (Fig. 9.1.6). In the early nephron H^+ ions are secreted and combine with bicarbonate ions in a process which results in bicarbonate reabsorption. Further down the nephron secreted H^+ combines with buffers to contribute to net acid excretion.

H^+ are secreted along the tubule from the apical membranes of tubular cells via the NHE3 sodium-hydrogen exchanger in return for sodium which is moving along the sodium gradient generated by the Na^+/K^+ ATPase molecules in the basal membrane. 80% of filtered bicarbonate is reabsorbed in the proximal tubule as a result of H^+ secretion (Fig. 9.1.8). This process relies upon the enzyme carbonic anhydrase in the tubule which can be thought of as catalysing the interaction of H^+ and bicarbonate to form carbon dioxide and water and *vice versa*.[17] The carbon dioxide and water enter tubular cells and break down into H^+ and bicarbonate again. The H^+ is secreted again and so is recycled without contributing to net acid excretion. However, the bicarbonate leaves the basal membrane of the cell mainly through the NBC sodium bicarbonate co-transporter. Further bicarbonate is reabsorbed in this way in the ascending limb of the loop of Henle. In the distal tubule acid excretion begins with H^+ buffered principally by interactions with phosphate and ammonia. This H^+ is not reabsorbed or recycled and so is lost in the urine as excreted acid. In the collecting ducts, type A intercalated cells are the predominant cells involved in H^+ secretion and carbonic anhydrase in these cells catalyses the formation of H^+ and bicarbonate. An apical H^+ ATPase actively secretes H^+ into the lumen and the bicarbonate generated exits the cells at the basolateral surface via the AE1 bicarbonate/chloride transporter.

Ammonia plays an important role in acid-base handling by the kidney.[18] Proximal tubular cells, in particular, metabolize glutamine in a series of interactions which ultimately generate ammonia, bicarbonate, and glucose. The bicarbonate and glucose pass into the body via the basolateral route, but the ammonia enters the tubule where it can be protonated to form NH_4^+ ions which remain in the urine and contribute to the removal of H^+ from the body. NH_4^+ can

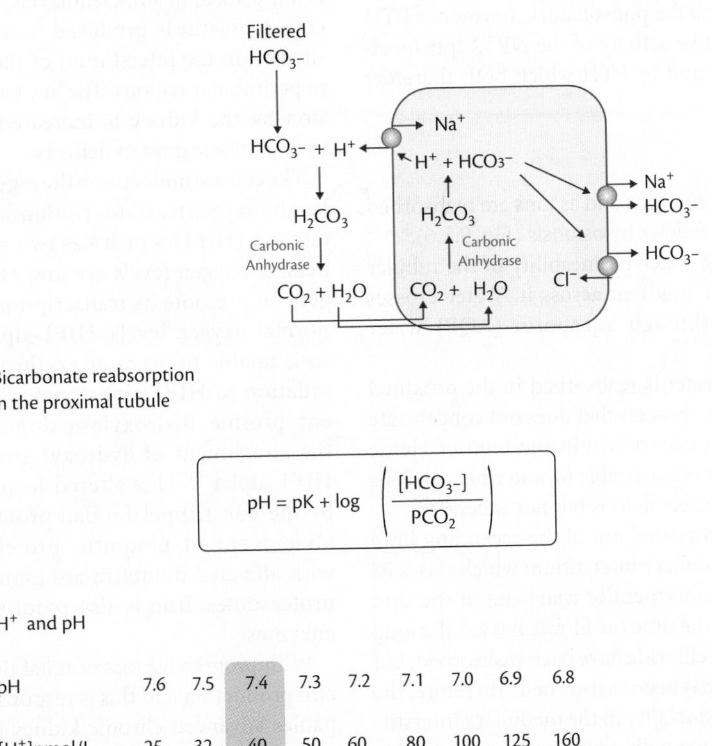

Fig. 9.1.8 Renal acid handling. The upper panel illustrates bicarbonate reabsorption in the proximal tubule. Carbonic anhydrase in the tubular cell and outside the cell play a key role in bicarbonate reabsorption. The tubular lumen is to the left of the cell. The middle panel illustrates the relationship between extracellular body fluid pH, bicarbonate, and PCO_2. The lower panel illustrates the relationship between pH and H^+ concentration.

also form within the tubular cell and be transported out of the cell in exchange for sodium at the apical membrane.

Renal calcium handling

The plasma calcium that is not bound to proteins is freely filtered in the glomerulus and around 90% of this is reabsorbed in the proximal tubule and thick ascending limb of the loop of Henle.[19] The route for this reabsorption is paracellular and the calcium moves with the water that is moving in these regions as a result of the actively established sodium gradient. An electrical gradient also contributes to this movement. In contrast, reabsorption in the distal tubule is transcellular. Calcium crosses the luminal apical membrane via the TRPV5 calcium channels and is transported within the cells by calcium-binding proteins including calbindin-D_{28K} which prevents major fluctuations in free intracellular calcium concentration.[20] At the basolateral surface calcium leaves via the PMCA Ca^{2+} ATPase and the NCX sodium-calcium exchanger. Parathyroid hormone activates TRPV5 channels and promotes PMCA activity, thus increasing calcium reabsorption. The effect of vitamin D is described below.[21]

Renal phosphate handling

Phosphate that is not protein bound is freely filtered in the glomerulus and reabsorbed along the tubules.[22] 80% of the phosphate is reabsorbed in the proximal tubules, by co-transport with sodium via the NPT2 family of sodium phosphate co-transporters. There is further reabsorption using the same mechanisms in the distal tubules and collecting ducts (Fig. 9.1.6). The kidneys have a limited capacity for phosphate reabsorption, so above a certain threshold level, (the Tm_{Pi}) excess filtered phosphate is excreted. Raised phosphate levels promote secretion of the phosphaturic hormones PTH and FGF-23.[21,23] The reabsorptive activity of the NPT2 transporters is inhibited by the FGF-23 and by PTH which both therefore increase phosphate excretion.

Renal water handling

Water is freely filtered in the glomerulus and as ions are reabsorbed along the tubular system water follows by osmosis (Fig. 9.1.6).[8,9,24] This movement depends on the water permeability of the tubular epithelium and on the osmotic gradient across it. Water crosses the tubular cell membranes through aquaporin (AQP) water channels.[25]

Around 65% of the filtered water is reabsorbed in the proximal tubules but this is an iso-osmotic process that does not concentrate the urine. Urine concentration occurs within the loop of Henle where the thin descending limb is permeable to water but not ions and the ascending limb is permeable to ions but not water.[26,27]

Sodium and chloride are transported out of the ascending limb of the loop of Henle into the medullary interstitium which raises its osmolality. This promotes the movement of water out of the thin descending limb of the loop. By the time the filtrate has left the loop a further 25% of the sodium and chloride have been reabsorbed, but only a further 10% of the water has been reabsorbed. Therefore, the loop serves to maintain a high osmolality in the medullary interstitium with the osmolality increasing with depth in the medulla. No significant water reabsorption occurs in the distal tubules, but in the collecting ducts water reabsorption occurs under regulation by vasopressin. Vasopressin binds V2 receptors on collecting duct cells which promotes the insertion of vesicles containing water channels, especially AQP2 channels into apical membrane, thus increasing water permeability and promoting water reabsorption.[25]

The medullary collecting ducts of all nephrons pass down through the high osmolality environment of the medulla and if the collecting duct cells are permeable to water then water will be reabsorbed, so leading to urinary concentration. As all collecting ducts descend through the medulla, even those without long loops of Henle can take advantage of the high medullary osmolality to concentrate the filtrate in their lumen. Urea also plays a role in water reabsorption and the reabsorption of urea in the collecting ducts contributes to the high osmolality of the medullary interstitium.[28,29]

The vasa recta are the only blood supply to the medulla and function as countercurrent exchangers to maintain the high medullary osmolality. In general terms, water diffuses out and solutes diffuse into the descending vessels, and solutes diffuse out of and water diffuses into the ascending vessels. This prevents blood flow from washing away the high osmolality of the deep medullary interstitium.

Endocrine function

The kidney produces a range of locally and systemically active substances and is a major endocrine organ (Fig. 9.1.3).

Erythropoietin

Erythropoietin is a 165 amino acid protein that binds to the erythropoietin receptor EpoR on red cell precursors.[30,31] The receptor is expressed on early erythroid progenitor cells and the levels of its expression increase during red cell development. If erythropoietin is not present at sufficient levels, these cells die by apoptosis. Most erythropoietin is produced by type 1 fibroblastoid cells that are situated in the interstitium of the renal cortex and outer medulla in peritubular regions. The low basal level of erythropoietin expression by the kidney is increased by hypoxia or anaemia which impairs tissue oxygen delivery.

The central molecule in the regulation of erythropoietin production by oxygen is a transcription factor known as hypoxia-inducible factor 1 (HIF1) which has two subunits, HIF1-alpha and HIF1-beta. If oxygen levels are low, HIF1 binds to the erythropoietin gene to promote its transcription.[32] However, in the presence of normal oxygen levels, HIF1-alpha undergoes degradation, and so is unable to promote erythropoietin transcription. The degradation of HIF1-alpha comes about because oxygen-dependent proline hydroxylase domain enzymes (PHDs) catalyse the attachment of hydroxyl groups to proline amino acids in HIF1-alpha.[33] This altered form of HIF1-alpha is then bound by the von Hippel-Lindau protein (VHL) which promotes the attachment of ubiquitin proteins to HIF1-alpha.[34] Proteins with attached ubiquitin are rapidly degraded within the cell by proteasomes. Iron is also required for efficient activity of PHD enzymes.

With progressive loss of renal tissue there is a fall in erythropoietin production and this is responsible for the anaemia that accompanies advanced chronic kidney disease. Although there may be some loss of erythropoietin producing cells, the principle problem is a failure of the cells to respond to hypoxia. In addition to this, in inflammatory diseases, cytokines such as TNF-alpha reduce erythropoietin production. Replacement therapy with recombinant erythropoietin or modified derivatives of erythropoietin is routine in the care of patients with advanced chronic kidney disease.

Renin and the angiotensin-aldosterone axis

Renin secretion is promoted by three key stimuli. Firstly a fall in renal perfusion pressure, secondly a fall in the delivery of sodium chloride to the macula densa region of the distal tubule and thirdly by increased sympathetic nervous activity which acts on beta1 adrenergic receptors.[9,35] Renin is produced within the juxtaglomerular apparatus (Fig. 9.1.1) and is an enzyme that catalyses the formation of angiotensin I. Angiotensin I is formed by renin-catalysed cleavage of the precursor protein angiotensinogen. Angiotensin I is itself further cleaved by angiotensin converting enzyme to form the short highly active peptide angiotensin II.

Angiotensin II exerts its key effects through binding to AT_1 receptors.[36] These receptors are present in a wide range of sites and mediate a series of different and important effects that generally act to maintain adequate blood pressure.[37] Angiotensin II causes potent vasoconstriction and this can elevate blood pressure. Within the kidneys angiotensin II acts directly on proximal tubular cells to promote the activity of the NHE3 sodium-hydrogen exchanger and so promote sodium reabsorption.[13,30] In addition, it causes vasoconstriction of both the afferent and efferent arterioles; the predominant effect is on the efferent vessels which increases intraglomerular pressure and so raises the glomerular filtration rate.[9] Other renal effects include sensitization of tubule-glomerular feedback and effects on glomerular mesangial cell contraction which may moderate the increase in GFR. It also acts on the brain to enhance thirst, promotes vasopressin release from the posterior pituitary and may have widespread influences on cellular activity which affect cardiac and vascular remodelling. A key action is the stimulation of aldosterone production by the adrenal cortex. Aldosterone is a mineralocorticoid hormone which acts on the distal tubule and collecting ducts to promote sodium reabsorption and potassium excretion. Key renal effects of aldosterone are promotion of basal membrane Na^+/K^+ ATPase activity and upregulation of apical ENaC activity.[4]

Vitamin D

Vitamin D can be made in the body from cholesterol which is converted to vitamin D3 (cholecalciferol) in a process in skin which requires ultraviolet light (Fig. 9.1.9).[21,38] Vitamin D3 can also be absorbed in the gut from dietary sources. The liver then converts vitamin D3 to 25-hydroxy vitamin D (25-hydroxycholecalciferol). Within the kidney 1 alpha-hydroxylase enzyme in proximal tubular cells converts 25-hydroxy vitamin D to 1,25-dihydroxy vitamin D (1,25-dihydroxycholecalciferol). This enzyme is itself regulated by 1,25-dihydroxy vitamin, PTH and FGF23 (21). 1,25-dihydroxy vitamin D is the highly active form of vitamin D and as renal function declines, so too does the capacity to produce 1,25-dihydroxy vitamin D, which may contribute to renal bone disease.[31]

Vitamin D binds to the nuclear vitamin D receptor which is expressed in many different tissues and acts as a transcription factor to promote expression of a wide range of genes.[39] The consequences of vitamin D action are widespread, but generally promote the maintenance of adequate calcium and phosphate levels. A major effect is to increase the absorption of both calcium and phosphate in the gut. In bone vitamin D acts to promote bone

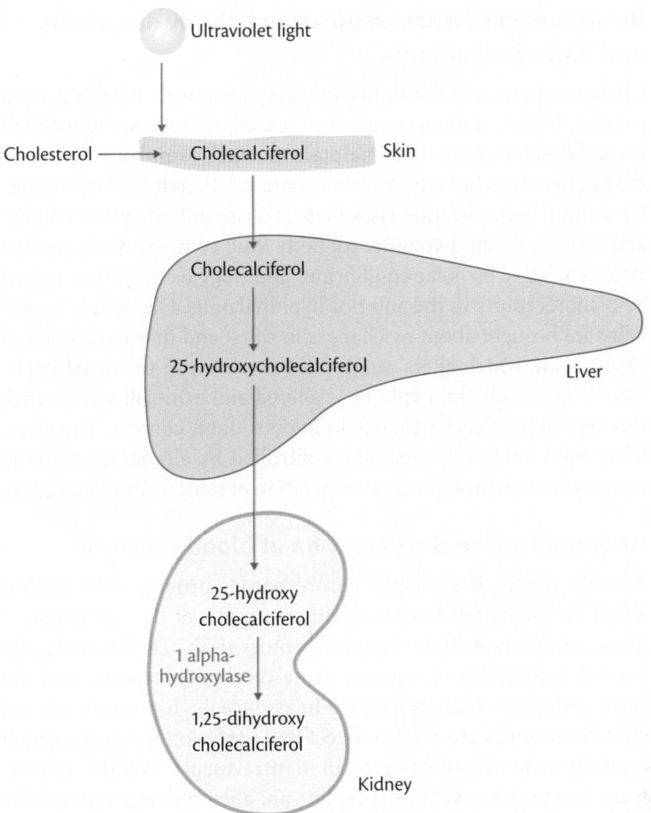

Fig. 9.1.9 Vitamin D metabolism. Cholecaliferol is produced in skin and metabolized to 25-hydroxycholecalciferol in the liver. The enzyme 1 alpha-hydroxylase in the kidney plays a key role by converting the 25-hydroxycholecalciferol to highly active 1,25- dihydroxycholecalciferol.

resorption and so release of calcium and phosphate into the circulation. In the kidney vitamin D acts to promote calcium and phosphate reabsorption. Vitamin D increases the activity of molecules involved in the transport of these ions including the PMCA Ca^{2+} ATPase and calbindin levels in the distal tubular cells.[19,39]

Blood pressure control

Blood pressure is influenced by the cardiac output, the systemic vascular resistance, and the circulatory volume.[35,40] The kidney plays a central role in blood pressure control by regulating circulatory volume and by endocrine effects on the state of vasoconstriction in the arterial tree, especially the systemic arterioles.[8,10] When kidney function is impaired, hypertension is common and may reflect impaired sodium and water excretion or alterations in the endocrine output of the kidney, especially the renin output from the juxtaglomerular apparatus. The influence of the kidney on blood pressure is well demonstrated in patients on dialysis who have little, if any, residual renal function. In this situation, the blood pressure is influence to a substantial effect by the amount of fluid which is removed by dialysis.[9,31] If fluid removal is inadequate the patient generally remains hypertensive. If it is excessive they generally remain hypotensive. In addition to this, alterations in vasoconstriction produced by drugs can also influence the blood pressure without altering body fluid volume.

Relationship between regulation of body osmolality and body fluid volume

Changes in extracellular fluid osmolality are poorly tolerated, so in general, if body sodium content is altered, there is an adjustment in body water content to maintain normal osmolality and so a change in extracellular body water content.[8] Therefore, if extracellular sodium concentration rises there is a rise in body water content and so in body fluid volume. All body fluid compartments are in a state of relative osmolar equilibrium and body osmolality is sensed by osmoreceptors in the anterior hypothalamus. Changes in osmolality are brought about by changes in thirst and in the secretion of vasopressin, which alters renal water excretion in the distal nephron.[8,10,40] If body fluid volume is altered and osmolality is normal, this typically reflects a change in body sodium content. Therefore, body fluid volume is generally controlled by alterations in body sodium content brought about regulation of renal sodium excretion.

Afferent arms in the detection of blood pressure

A wide range of systemic baroreceptors provide information about the state of distension of different parts of the circulation.[40] These receptors include stretch receptors in the cardiac atria, the carotid baroreceptors, various tissue mechanoreceptors, and the renal juxtaglomerular apparatus. In essence, high pressure arterial stretch receptors are able to detect low perfusion pressures which typically arise when there is a fall in intravascular volume. In contrast, low pressure venous receptors are able to detect venous distension which typically indicates raised intravascular volume.

Renal efferent arms in the regulation of blood

Sodium excretion is influenced by multiple factors, but a major influence is the renin-angiotensin-aldosterone axis. In the proximal tubule, angiotensin II promotes the activity of the NHE3 sodium-hydrogen exchanger and so increases sodium reabsorption.[13,33] In the principal cells of the collecting ducts in the distal nephron, aldosterone promotes the activity of the Na^+/K^+ ATPase and the apical ENaC sodium channels and so promotes sodium reabsorption.[4] Glucocorticoids typically display some mineralocorticoid activity and so can cause sodium retention and hypertension.

Other factors that influence sodium excretion include atrial natriuretic peptides produced by the cardiac atria upon distension.[41] A key action of these peptides is on NPR receptors in collecting duct cells to reduce the activity of the apical ENaC sodium channels and so inhibit sodium reabsorption. Catecholamines promote the activity of the NHE3 sodium-hydrogen exchanger to promote proximal tubular sodium reabsorption.

Renal factors in hypertension

Renal artery stenosis can cause a fall in renal blood flow and in the glomerular filtration rate. This promotes renin release from the juxtaglomerular apparatus and the production of angiotensin II and an increase in aldosterone release. Much has been learnt about the pathophysiology of hypertension from clinical disorders associated with hypertension.[9,31] Liddle's syndrome of pseudohyperaldosteronism is caused by a mutation in the gene encoding the ENaC sodium channels in the collecting duct.[42] The mutation causes the channels to stay open in an unreglated manner and so promotes the reabsorption of sodium with concomitant hypertension. Mutations of the WNK1 and WNK4 kinases can cause type 2 pseudohypoaldosteronism by promoting the activity of the NCC sodium chloride co-transporters in the distal tubule and so enhancing sodium reabsorption and hypertension.[43,44]

Acid-base homeostasis

The concentration of free acid in the body is very tightly controlled and the kidneys play a central role in this regulation.[16] Metabolic acid production and dietary acid intake must be balanced by acid excretion. While carbon dioxide itself can be excreted by the lungs, acids such as sulphuric and phosphoric acids are excreted by the kidneys. The concentration of free H^+ ions is very low at around 35–45 nmol/L in extracellular fluids. Buffers exist within the body and act to minimize the effects of changes in acid concentration on the concentration of free H^+ ions or pH (Fig. 9.1.8). Buffers are typically weak acids or bases that can donate or bind to H^+ ions to change from an acid to a base or *vice versa*. In doing this they can to some extent counterbalance the effects of the addition or loss of H^+ to the extracellular fluid. The acid and base forms of the buffer together constitute a buffer pair. The dominant extracellular buffer is the bicarbonate system, although sodium phosphate and proteins are important buffers in cells.

Renal acid excretion

Within the early tubular segments secreted H^+ is used to reabsorb bicarbonate (Fig. 9.1.8), but in the more distal nephron the secreted H^+ interacts with buffers and is excreted. Acid excretion by the kidney requires the presence of buffers in the urine to lower the urinary concentration of free acid. This is because there is a limit to the gradient of free H^+ concentration that the tubular mechanisms responsible for acid secretion into the tubules can generate. Consequently, the lowest urine pH that can be produced is around 4.4. However, substantial amounts of acid can be excreted in the urine in buffered form. Urinary sodium phosphate buffers some acid in the urine, but most acid excretion arises through the excretion of ammonium ions (NH_4^+).[18] Acid can be excreted in the form of ammonium (NH_4^+) ions which are produced in proximal tubule cells by the metabolic degradation of glutamine to ammonium and bicarbonate (HCO_3^-). The ammonium ions are secreted into the tubular fluid and the bicarbonate ions pass into the blood.

Role of carbonic anhydrase

The enzyme carbonic anhydrase plays a key role in acid-base regulation by catalysing the reaction $OH^- + CO_2 = HCO_3^-$. This is more usually written as $H_2O + CO_2 = H_2CO_3 = H^+ + HCO_3^-$ because water must first dissociate to form H^+ and OH^-.[17] Within the kidney, the enzyme exists in different forms within tubular cells and at the apical luminal membranes of the cells (Fig. 9.1.8). In essence, the equilibrium allows carbon dioxide and bicarbonate to function as a buffer pair. Carbon dioxide levels can be regulated by changes in ventilation and bicarbonate levels can be regulated by changes in renal bicarbonate excretion.

Renal responses to acid-base disturbances

As carbon dioxide levels rise, extracellular fluids become more acidic, whereas as bicarbonate levels rise they become more alkaline. If one member of the bicarbonate buffer pair rises, then the change in pH can be reduced by a rise in the other member of the pair. For example, a fall in pH due to inadequate respiration can be compensated to some extent by a rise in extracellular fluid HCO_3^-.

Role of the liver

The liver also plays a role in acid-base metabolism. The breakdown of proteins in the liver generates both HCO_3^- and NH_4^+ which combine together to form urea. However, a proportion of the NH_4^+ that is produced is used in the synthesis of glutamine. This glutamine is transported in the blood to the kidney where it is degraded in the proximal tubular cells to produce HCO_3^- and NH_4^+. For each of these NH_4^+ ions that is secreted into the tubule, a HCO_3^- ion is added to the blood.[18]

Acidosis

Acidosis promotes liver glutamine synthesis and renal glutamine breakdown and so increases the delivery of NH_4^+ into the tubules while supplying HCO_3^- to the blood. Bicarbonate reabsorption is increased along the tubule by upregulation of the apical NHE3 sodium-hydrogen exchangers and the basolateral NBC sodium bicarbonate co-transporters. The activity of the H^+ secreting H^+ ATPase in the distal nephron is increased by acidosis. Renin production increases with acidosis promoting angiotensin II production and increased aldosterone secretion from the adrenals. This in turn promotes H^+ secretion by the H^+ ATPases in the apical membrane of the type A intercalated cells in the distal nephron.

Alkalosis

Chloride plays an important role in the renal response to alkalosis and low chloride levels can be problematic.[45] Within the type A intercalated cell the active secretion of H^+ by the H^+ ATPase is linked to passive co-transport of chloride to maintain electroneutrality. If plasma chloride levels are low this results in low chloride levels in the tubular filtrate which enhances chloride movement into the tubule and so H^+ secretion. The effect is to worsen the alkalosis. In type B intercalated cells bicarbonate normally enters the cells from the tubular lumen in exchange for chloride and this process is reduced if plasma and so tubular chloride levels are low. High plasma bicarbonate levels inhibit the breakdown of glutamine to produce NH_4^+ in the proximal tubular cells.

Effects of potassium on renal acid-base metabolism

Hyperkalaemia promotes acidosis and hypokalaemia promotes alkalosis. Potassium inhibits glutamine breakdown in the proximal tubular cells and can compete with NH_4^+ for secretion into the tubules in the loop of Henle via the NKCC2 co-transporter. Low potassium levels can promote H^+ excretion along the nephron and in type A intercalated cells stimulate the H^+/K^+ ATPase which reabsorbs potassium from the filtrate and secretes H^+ into the tubule.

Assessment of renal function

The assessment of renal function generally focuses on the assessment of glomerular filtration rate and on the assessment of the integrity of the filtration barrier by measurement of protein or albumin levels in the urine. Nevertheless, other aspects of renal function may need investigation, particularly tubular function and endocrine function.[46]

Assessment of glomerular filtration rate

Glomerular filtration rate can be measured using the clearance method described earlier. However, for this approach to be reliable, the substance used for the measurement must be freely filtered and neither reabsorbed nor secreted along the nephron. Inulin fulfils these criteria and can be used for research purposes, but its use is not straightforward for routine purposes. A simple approximate substitute is creatinine clearance, but this has the inherent error that creatinine is secreted into the tubules and so creatinine clearance typically overestimates GFR. A further source of error is that the clearance technique requires collection of urine over a timed period, typically 24 hours, and this is prone to errors associated with incomplete collection of urine.

To address the issue of incomplete collection of urine, an alternative approach is to look at the rate of removal of a filtered substance from the blood by taking blood samples at different times following administration of the substance, typically by intravenous injection. If the rate of removal is only dependent upon GFR and this is relatively constant, then carefully timed measurements allow a good estimate of the GFR to be made. Both ^{51}Cr-EDTA (chromium-51-labelled ethylenediaminetetra-acetic acid), ^{99m}Tc-DTPA (technetium-99m-labelled diethlenetraminepetna-acetic acid) and ^{125}I-iothalamate (125-iodine-labelled iothalamate) are removed by glomerular filtration after intravenous administration. GFR can be estimated by measuring the levels of these substances in plasma following intravenous injection and techniques have been developed that use only a single blood sample. Approaches have also been developed that rely on imaging the isotopic activity over the kidney at time points following injections, although these are typically less accurate than those that rely on the clearance approach.

Given the difficulties involved for patients with all of the above techniques, approaches have been sought that use information about an individual patient to estimate GFR based on their plasma creatinine level. Creatinine is produced by muscle and muscle mass and creatinine production depend on a variety of factors including age, gender, and ethnicity. By taking these factors into account it is possible to improve the extent to which creatinine can be used to estimate renal function. A variety of algorithms have been produced to do this including the Cockcroft-Gault, the MDRD (modification of diet in renal disease) and the newer CKD-EPI (chronic kidney disease-epidemiology collaboration) algorithms. The MDRD algorithm has been widely adopted for routine reporting of eGFR (estimated GFR). The different stages of CKD (chronic kidney disease) are differentiated primarily on the basis of eGFR estimation.

The integrity of the filtration membrane is assessed in clinical practice by the analysis of the protein content of urine. Levels are normally low, but early damage to the filtration membrane results in micro-albuminuria and late damage results in substantial more generalized proteinuria.

Proteinuria

The level of proteinuria is strongly correlated with the rate of deterioration of renal function and so with progression to end stage renal disease and the requirement for renal replacement therapy. Proteinuria has traditionally been assessed using 24-hour urine collections, but results of spot urine protein:creatinine ratios correlate well with outcome. Urine albumin:creatinine ratios are used, especially in the monitoring of diabetes mellitus and have high sensitivity for early renal damage.

Tubular function

Detailed assessment of tubular function is seldom formally assessed, even by nephrologists, but tubular dysfunction can arise as a consequence of a range of renal disorders. Tubular dysfunction may be indicated by electrolyte abnormalities or as inadequate bicarbonate reabsorption which results in renal tubular acidosis.

Conclusion

Kidneys are complex organs and play a wide range of homeostatic roles. Disturbances of kidney function result in many diverse effects which can be understood in the light of these roles. Renal function is central to the normal control of extracellular fluid volume and composition. As well as being important effector organs, the kidneys also regulate other body functions and are key endocrine organs. Kidneys require a substantial blood flow and adequate blood pressure to sustain glomerular filtration and to supply the metabolic needs that arise from tubular activity, especially tubular reabsorption. There has been substantial progress in understanding renal function and this provides a firm platform for rational clinical management of clinical disorders involving the kidneys.

Further reading

Berne RM, Levy MN, Koeppen BM, Stanton BA. *Berne & Levy Physiology*, 6th edition. Philadelphia, PA: Mosby/Elsevier, 2008.

Brenner BM, Rector FC. Brenner & Rector's *The Kidney*, 8th edition. Philadelphia, PA: Saunders Elsevier, 2008.

Davison AM. *Oxford Textbook of Clinical Nephrology*, 3rd edition. Oxford, UK: Oxford University Press, 2005.

Hall JE, Guyton AC. *Textbook of Medical Physiology*, 12th edition. Philadelphia, PA: London, UK: Elsevier Saunders, 2011.

Koeppen BM, Stanton BA. *Renal Physiology*, 4th edition. Edinburgh, UK: Elsevier Mosby, 2007.

Lote CJ. *Principles of Renal Physiology*, 4th edition. Boston, MA: Kluwer Academic Publishers, 1999.

O'Callaghan CA. *The Renal System at a Glance*, 3rd edition. Chichester, UK: Wiley-Blackwell, 2009.

Valtin H, Schafer JA. *Renal Function: Mechanisms Preserving Fluid and Solute Balance in Health*, 3rd edition. London, UK: Little Brown, 1995.

References

1. Bergwitz C, Juppner H. FGF23 and syndromes of abnormal renal phosphate handling. *Adv Exp Med Biol* 2012; **728**:41–64.
2. Farquhar MG. The glomerular basement membrane: not gone, just forgotten. *J Clin Investig* 2006; **116**(8):2090–3.
3. Nielsen JS, McNagny KM. The role of podocalyxin in health and disease. *JASN* 2009; **20**(8):1669–76.
4. Haraldsson B, Nystrom J, Deen WM. Properties of the glomerular barrier and mechanisms of proteinuria. *Physiol Rev* 2008; **88**(2):451–87.
5. Van Itallie CM, Anderson JM. Claudins and epithelial paracellular transport. *Annu Rev Physiol* 2006; **68**:403–29.
6. Christensen EI, Verroust PJ, Nielsen R. Receptor-mediated endocytosis in renal proximal tubule. *Pflugers Arch* 2009; **458**(6):1039–48.
7. Layton AT, Layton HE, Dantzler WH, Pannabecker TL. The mammalian urine concentrating mechanism: hypotheses and uncertainties. *Physiology* 2009; **24**:250–6.
8. O'Callaghan CA. *The Renal System at a Glance*, 3rd edition. Chichester, UK: Wiley-Blackwell, 2009.
9. Brenner BM, Rector FC. *Brenner & Rector's The Kidney*, 8th edition. Philadelphia, PA: Saunders Elsevier, 2008.
10. Koeppen BM, Stanton BA. *Renal Physiology*, 4th edition. Edinburgh, UK: Elsevier Mosby, 2007.
11. Briet M, Schiffrin EL. Aldosterone: effects on the kidney and cardiovascular system. *Nat Rev Nephrol* 2010; **6**(5):261–73.
12. Riquier-Brison AD, Leong PK, Pihakaski-Maunsbach K, McDonough AA. Angiotensin II stimulates trafficking of NHE3, NaPi2, and associated proteins into the proximal tubule microvilli. *Am J Physiol Renal Physiol* 2010; **298**(1):F177–86.
13. Geibel J, Giebisch G, Boron WF. Angiotensin II stimulates both Na(+)-H+ exchange and Na+/HCO3- cotransport in the rabbit proximal tubule. *Proc Nat Acad Sci U S A* 1990; **87**(20):7917–20.
14. Rodan AR, Cheng CJ, Huang CL. Recent advances in distal tubular potassium handling. *Am J Physiol Renal Physiol* 2011; **300**(4):F821–7.
15. Grimm PR, Sansom SC. BK channels in the kidney. *Curr Opin Nephrol Hypertens* 2007; **16**(5):430–6.
16. Koeppen BM. The kidney and acid-base regulation. *Adv Physiol Educ* 2009; **33**(4):275–81.
17. Purkerson JM, Schwartz GJ. The role of carbonic anhydrases in renal physiology. *Kidney Int* 2007; **71**(2):103–15.
18. Weiner ID, Verlander JW. Role of NH_3 and NH_4^+ transporters in renal acid-base transport. *Am J Physiol Renal Physiol* 2011; **300**(1):F11–23.
19. Lambers TT, Bindels RJ, Hoenderop JG. Coordinated control of renal Ca2+ handling. *Kidney Int* 2006; **69**(4):650–4.
20. de Groot T, Bindels RJ, Hoenderop JG. TRPV5: an ingeniously controlled calcium channel. *Kidney Int* 2008; **74**(10):1241–6.
21. Perwad F, Portale AA. Vitamin D metabolism in the kidney: regulation by phosphorus and fibroblast growth factor 23. *Mol Cell Endocrinol* 2011; **347**(1–2):17–24.
22. Renkema KY, Alexander RT, Bindels RJ, Hoenderop JG. Calcium and phosphate homeostasis: concerted interplay of new regulators. *Ann Med* 2008; **40**(2):82–91.
23. Juppner H. Phosphate and FGF-23. *Kidney Int Suppl* 2011; **79**(Suppl 121):S24–7.
24. Valtin H, Schafer JA. *Renal Function: Mechanisms Preserving Fluid and Solute Balance in Health*, 3rd edtion. London, UK: Little Brown, 1995.
25. Moeller HB, Fenton RA. Cell biology of vasopressin-regulated aquaporin-2 trafficking. *Pflugers Arch* 2012; **464**(2):133–44.
26. Michel CC. Renal medullary microcirculation: architecture and exchange. *Microcirculation* 1995; **2**(2):125–39.
27. Pallone TL, Turner MR, Edwards A, Jamison RL. Countercurrent exchange in the renal medulla. *Am J Physiol Regul Integr Comp Physiol* 2003; **284**(5):R1153–75.
28. Sands JM, Layton HE. The physiology of urinary concentration: an update. *Semin Nephrol* 2009; **29**(3):178–95.
29. Fenton RA, Knepper MA. Urea and renal function in the 21st century: insights from knockout mice. *JASN* 2007; **18**(3):679–88.
30. Wojchowski DM, Sathyanarayana P, Dev A. Erythropoietin receptor response circuits. *Curr Opin Hematol* 2010; **17**(3):169–76.
31. Davison AM. *Oxford Textbook of Clinical Nephrology*, 3rd edition. Oxford, UK: Oxford University Press, 2005.
32. Ratcliffe PJ. From erythropoietin to oxygen: hypoxia-inducible factor hydroxylases and the hypoxia signal pathway. *Blood Purif* 2002; **20**(5):445–50.
33. Schofield CJ, Ratcliffe PJ. Oxygen sensing by HIF hydroxylases. *Nat Rev Mol Cell Biol* 2004; **5**(5):343–54.
34. Maxwell PH, Wiesener MS, Chang GW, *et al.* The tumour suppressor protein VHL targets hypoxia-inducible factors for oxygen-dependent proteolysis. Nature. 1999;**399**(6733):271–5.
35. Berne RM, Levy MN, Koeppen BM, Stanton BA. *Berne & Levy Physiology*, 6th edition. Philadelphia, PA: Mosby/Elsevier, 2008.
36. Hunyady L, Catt KJ. Pleiotropic AT1 receptor signaling pathways mediating physiological and pathogenic actions of angiotensin II. *Mol Endocrinol* 2006; **20**(5):953–70.
37. Siragy HM. AT1 and AT2 receptor in the kidney: role in health and disease. *Semin Nephrol* 2004; **24**(2):93–100.
38. Henry HL. Regulation of vitamin D metabolism. *Best Pract Res Clin Endocrinol Metab* 2011; **25**(4):531–41.
39. Pike JW, Zella LA, Meyer MB, Fretz JA, Kim S. Molecular actions of 1,25-dihydroxyvitamin D3 on genes involved in calcium homeostasis. *J Bone Miner Res* 2007; **22**(Suppl 2):V16–19.

40. Hall JE, Guyton AC. *Textbook of Medical Physiology*, 12th edition. Philadelphia, PA: London, UK: Elsevier Saunders, 2011.
41. Antunes-Rodrigues J, de Castro M, Elias LL, Valenca MM, McCann SM. Neuroendocrine control of body fluid metabolism. *Physiol Rev* 2004; **84**(1):169–208.
42. Warnock DG. Liddle syndrome: genetics and mechanisms of Na+ channel defects. *Am J Med Sci* 2001; **322**(6):302–7.
43. Uchida S. Pathophysiological roles of WNK kinases in the kidney. *Pflugers Arch* 2010; **460**(4):695–702.
44. Bergaya S, Vidal-Petiot E, Jeunemaitre X, Hadchouel J. Pathogenesis of pseudohypoaldosteronism type 2 by WNK1 mutations. *Curr Opin Nephrol Hypertens* 2012; **21**(1):39–45.
45. Gennari FJ. Pathophysiology of metabolic alkalosis: a new classification based on the centrality of stimulated collecting duct ion transport. *Am J Kidney Dis* 2011; **58**(4):626–36.
46. Lote CJ. *Principles of Renal Physiology*, 4th edition. Boston, MA: Kluwer Academic Publishers, 1999.

CHAPTER 9.2

Acute kidney injury

Edward Sharples

Definition of acute kidney injury

Acute kidney injury (AKI) is now the consensus term for the syndrome characterized by a significant decline in renal excretory function that occurs over a period of hours or days. It is typically diagnosed by the accumulation of end products of nitrogen metabolism or with oliguria, which is a frequent sign although not invariable, or both.

There have been a number of labels and terms used, but in the last couple of years a more rigorous approach towards a definition has led to the general uptake of two classifications—the Risk Injury Failure Loss and End-Stage Kidney Disease (RIFLE) classification of the Acute Dialysis Quality Initiative (ADQI) and the more recent AKI staging system (Table 9.2.1) derived from this by the Acute Kidney Injury Network (AKIN). There is a great deal of overlap between these two systems, but they have served the purpose of emphasizing that acute changes in renal function that lead to small changes in serum creatinine are associated with poorer patient outcome.

Epidemiology of acute kidney injury

The true incidence of AKI is difficult to determine from published reports, and estimates vary greatly depending on clinical setting, demographics of the patient population and, in particular, the definition of renal insufficiency utilized. Four large studies from the United Kingdom between 2001 and 2005 reported that the incidence of severe AKI in adults (creatinine >500 umol/l) was between 202 and 746 per million population per year. AKI is common in hospitalized patients. A large American study demonstrated an overall incidence of AKI of 5% in a hospitalized population, using a definition of AKI as an increase in serum creatinine of >44 µmol/L (0.5 mg/dl) above the measured baseline value. AKI was associated with decreased renal perfusion (42%) or major surgery (18%) in the majority of cases. The major predictors of poor prognosis included a reduced urine output (<400 mL/ 24 hr). The use of more stringent RIFLE classification has reduced the observed incidence of AKI. Data from the National Hospital Discharge survey, a nationally collected sample of approximately 330,000 inpatient admissions from 500 hospitals in the USA, demonstrated a 1.9% incidence of AKI in hospitalized patients. Patients with AKI were more likely to have the sepsis syndrome or other non-renal acute organ system dysfunction. Elderly patients are at higher risk of developing AKI, with increased risk of end-stage renal failure and death. The incidence of AKI in a large UK study rose from 17 per million in those under 50 years of age to 949 per million in those aged between 80 and 90. More severe AKI requiring dialysis treatment is increasing in incidence,

Table 9.2.1 Acute kidney injury defined by the RIFLE criteria and AKI stage

Criteria or stage	Urine output	Serum creatinine	GFR
RIFLE criteria			
Risk	<0.5 mL/kg body weight per hour for 6 hours	1.5-fold increase	25% decrease
Injury	<0.5 mL/kg body weight per hour for 12 hours	2-fold increase	50% decrease
Failure	<0.5 mL/kg body weight per hour for 24 hours; or anuria for 12 hours	3-fold increase	75% decrease
Loss	Complete loss of kidney function >4 weeks		
End-stage renal disease	Complete loss of kidney function >12 weeks		
AKI stage			
1	<0.5 mL/kg body weight per hour for 6 hours	Increase >0.3 mg/dl (26 umol/L) or 1.5–2-fold increase	
2	<0.5 mL/kg body weight per hour for 12 hours	2–3 fold increase	
3	<0.3 mL/kg body weight for 24 hrs or anuria for 12 hr	Increase to >4 mg/dl (354 umol/L) with acute increase >0.5 mg/dl (44 umol/L) or >3-fold increase	

RIFLE criteria adapted from R Bellomo *et al.*, 'Acute renal failure—definition, outcome measures, animal models, fluid therapy and information technology needs: the Second International Consensus Conference of the Acute Dialysis Quality Initiative (ADQI) Group,' *Critical Care*, Volume 8, Issue 4, pp. R204–R212, Copyright © 2004 Bellomo *et al.*; licensee BioMed Central Ltd, DOI:10.1186/cc2872. This is an Open Access article: verbatim copying and redistribution of this article are permitted in all media for any purpose. AKI stage adapted from RL Mehta *et al.*, 'Acute kidney injury network: report of an initiative to improve outcomes in acute kidney injury,' *Critical Care*, Volume 11, Issue 2, R31, Copyright © 2007 Mehta *et al.*; licensee BioMed Central Ltd, DOI:10.1186/cc5713. Reproduced under the Creative Commons Attribution 2.0 Generic Licence (CC BY 2.0). **Source:** data from 'American Society of Nephrology Renal Research Report,' *Journal of the American Society of Nephrology*, Volume 16, Number 7, pp. 1886–1903, Copyright © 2005 by the American Society of Nephrology.

particularly in the elderly, with a large population study in the US demonstrating an increase from 2002 with cases of 200 per million patient years increasing to over 500 per million patient years in 2010.

The severity of kidney injury may determine the natural history and patient outcome in AKI. Large population studies can only show an association between AKI and mortality, especially in intensive therapy unit-based studies, because it is often part of the spectrum of multiple organ failure. However, published observational studies have demonstrated a consistently elevated relative risk associated with AKI despite full adjustment for co-morbid conditions and severity of illness. This increased relative risk of death associated with small changes in serum creatinine (consistent with AKI stage 1) was shown in a large heterogeneous cohort of patients, in a study of 19,201 admissions to a large urban hospital. This demonstrated that even a 50% increase in serum creatinine above baseline was associated with an increased mortality adjusted odds ratio of 5.8 (4.6–7.5), with similar increases (odds ratio 4.1 (3.1–5.5) in mortality observed in patients with AKI stage 1 (28 μmol/L (0.3 mg/dl) increase in serum creatinine).

The question is why is even relatively mild AKI associated with high mortality? Firstly, the observed increase in mortality may be only indirectly related to AKI, as the risk factors for developing AKI are also well-known risk factors for cardiovascular disease and mortality, and AKI occurs much more commonly in those with higher co-morbidity, including pre-existing renal impairment. Patients with relatively early stage chronic kidney disease (CKD) (eGFR 30–45 mL/min) have a 5-fold increased odds ratio of AKI when compared to matched controls. Moreover, the increase in mortality associated with even quite small changes in renal function may be related to the distant systemic effects of hypovolaemia and ischaemia on other organ systems. Models of AKI have shown induction of a more general systemic inflammatory response, with apoptotic cell death in the myocardium and changes in cardiac function, vascular dysfunction, and neutrophil aggregation in the lungs with associated inflammation.

Causes of acute kidney injury

There are many possible causes of acute kidney injury (Table 9.2.2), but in any clinical context few of these are likely to require consideration. The frequency of a particular cause of AKI will vary depending on the population studied. Shock, with a sustained impairment of renal perfusion, is the most common factor that predisposes patients to ischaemia-induced tubular injury, and is implicated in approximately 70% of community acquired AKI, and 40% of hospital-related events. Intrinsic renal disease, including rapidly progressive glomerulonephritis and interstitial nephritis accounts for 10% of cases of AKI. Urinary obstruction typically accounts for 25% or more of cases of acute impairment of renal function. Hospital acquired cases are more often multifactorial, with an accumulation of multiple acute insults, including exposure to nephrotoxic agents such as radiocontrast agents, treatment with non-steroidal anti-inflammatory drugs (NSAIDs), and infection, often in the presence of co-morbidities including cardiac dysfunction and diabetes.

Table 9.2.2 Causes of AKI established in all cases (748) admitted to 13 tertiary care hospitals in Madrid, Spain, over a nine-month period

Cause	Proportion of patients (%)
Acute tubular necrosis	45
Pre-renal shock	21
Acute on chronic renal failure	13
Urinary tract obstruction	10
Glomerulonephritis/vasculitis	4
Acute interstitial nephritis	2
Atheroemboli	1

Adapted by permission from Macmillan Publishers Ltd: *Kidney International*, Liano F and Pascual J, 'Epidemiology of acute renal failure: a prospective multicentre, community based study. Madrid Acute Renal Failure Study group', Volume 50, Issue 3, pp 811–18, Copyright ©1996, Rights Managed by Nature Publishing Group.

Clinical approach to the patient with acute kidney injury

Diagnosis of acute kidney injury

A high clinical index of suspicion is essential to diagnose AKI, ideally at an early stage in its development. The consequences of reduced renal function, especially the accumulation of fluid, electrolytes, acid, and uraemic waste products, that cause the symptoms and signs associated with AKI are rarely apparent until late in the course of AKI. Furthermore, the signs may not be specific, as for example, hyperkalaemia may cause cardiac arrest before any symptoms. All patients admitted to hospital with acute illness, or for elective surgery, should be considered at risk for developing AKI. Those with pre-existing kidney disease are especially susceptible to acute exacerbations. This was highlighted in the UK NCEPOD report in 2009 'Acute Kidney Injury: Adding Insult to Injury', which recommended that all patients admitted as an emergency should have measurement of renal function, and that recognition of the acute deteriorating patient was essential to avoid hospital acquired AKI and the associated mortality.

It is recognized that serum creatinine represents a poor biomarker—an acute decline in kidney function may not be reflected by a rise in serum creatinine for many hours. A number of alternative biomarkers, which respond either specifically to renal injury or to a small decline in glomerular filtration rate (GFR) have been researched, and include neutrophil gelatinase associated lipoprotein, kidney injury molecule-1 (KIM-1), interleukin-18, and cystatin C. Changes in these biomarkers have been shown to predict AKI following cardiac or vascular surgery. Further work is required however before they can replace the use of serum creatinine in diagnosis of AKI.

The initial assessment of the patient with suspected acute kidney injury aims to determine whether the kidney dysfunction is acute, whether urinary obstruction is a possibility, and the likelihood of an inflammatory systemic condition. It is extremely important that a diagnosis of obstruction should not be missed, since most cases are readily treatable and delayed diagnosis and intervention may lead to permanent kidney damage. Initial assessment could include careful history and examination, evaluation of the urine for blood and protein, casts or signs of an inflammatory renal lesion, and ultrasound as first-line investigation to exclude obstruction.

Specific causes of acute kidney injury

Pre-renal and ischaemic acute kidney injury

The majority of cases of acute kidney injury are associated with renal hypoperfusion, where restoration of renal perfusion leads to recovery, and used to be described as 'acute tubular necrosis'. AKI can follow any episode of severe circulatory failure, but often requires a prior compromising insult, such as cardiac failure, sepsis, trauma, or major surgery. AKI is common after ruptured aortic aneurysm repair (20%) as compared to elective repair (3%), hepatobiliary surgery, cardiac surgery, pancreatitis and major burns (2–38%, depending on severity). The diagnosis of ischaemic AKI is based on the clinical situation, which often involves circulatory compromise, and exclusion of obstruction, or a renal inflammatory condition through appropriate imaging and investigations is required.

In health, the kidneys receive 25% of cardiac output, but renal blood flow is not uniformly distributed within the renal parenchyma, so that tissue perfusion and oxygen consumption are highly heterogeneous—resulting in areas susceptible to reduced oxygen tension. The anatomical arrangement of pre-glomerular arterial and corresponding post-capillary venous vessels which is necessary for the counter-current mechanism necessary for urinary concentration and dilution lead to the arterio-venous shunting of oxygen and areas of hypoxia. The kidney maintains GFR through the physiological autoregulation of glomerular blood flow in the face of haemodynamic compromise, but prolonged or severe ischaemic insults, alone or in synergistic combination with nephrotoxins, overcome these autoregulatory mechanisms, in part through failure to increase post-glomerular vascular resistance. This loss of perfusion initiates epithelial and vascular cell injury, resulting in an extremely rapid decrease in GFR, which has been appropriately referred to as the *initiation phase* of AKI. A variety of mechanisms of cellular injury are initiated, included calcium influx, ATP depletion, cytokine, and toll-like receptor activation, leading to both programmed cell death, apoptosis, and necrosis with associated local inflammatory reaction. Chemokines released by injury cells and necrotic areas lead to the infiltration of leukocytes and increased inflammation.

Restoration of haemodynamic stability and renal perfusion, initiates an immediate partial recovery of blood flow, or 'reperfusion', followed by a profound and sustained reduction in capillary blood flow. There is evidence of retrograde flow in some vessels, and temporary loss of vessel patency. The pattern of glomerular microcirculation is similar to that of the peritubular capillaries; initial brief recovery of flow is followed by 'no flow'. Restoration of flow in these capillary beds, however, is different. Glomerular circulation is re-established initially, while return of blood flow to peritubular capillaries is significantly delayed. This period of ischaemia is associated with endothelial and epithelial cell death through apoptosis, and sometimes necrosis.

The initiation phase is immediately followed by the *extension phase*, in which multiple interrelated events dependent on altered vascular function lead to worsening of epithelial and endothelial cell injury and subsequent cell death, primarily in the corticomedullary region of the kidney. Established ischaemic AKI is associated with a reduction in renal perfusion by 30–50%, and there is evidence of selective reduction in blood supply to the outer medulla. The *maintenance phase* represents a phase of stabilization of injury, and subsequent correcting events leading to cellular repair, division, and re-differentiation. This sets the stage for improved epithelial and endothelial cell function and recovery of GFR during the *recovery phase*. Correction of the initiating insult with appropriate therapy during the early initiation and extension phases of AKI may limit the degree of cellular injury and hence the duration of the maintenance phase, allowing more rapid onset of the recovery phase and hence preservation of kidney function.

Recovery from ischaemic AKI requires proliferation and differentiation of remaining surviving epithelium cells to repopulate the renal tubule structure. Although there is great interest in the role of circulating stem cells to this process, the majority of repopulating cells are locally derived, either from the epithelium, or local renal stem cell populations. Circulating mesenchymal stem cells may contribute to repair through paracrine mechanisms, through secretion of cytokines and growth factors.

Nephrotoxins

A wide variety of agents, including many therapeutically prescribed drugs, can cause acute kidney injury (Box 9.2.1). Certain drugs are particularly common in the management of patients in the intensive care or perioperative setting. Gentamicin is nephrotoxic, and the risk of AKI is increased by age, pre-existing CKD or AKI, high dosage or prolonged treatment, and when administration occurs in combination with other nephrotoxins. The typical picture is the development of non-oliguric AKI coming on after one week of treatment. The urine analysis shows proteinuria and hyaline casts. A proximal tubular defect with Fanconi syndrome, hypocalcaemia and hypokalaemia can complicate AKI. The risk of nephrotoxicity can be reduced by ensuring the patient is not volume depleted, using a one-daily dosing regime, adjusting the dose according to renal function and routine monitoring of drug levels to aid prescribing.

Box 9.2.1 Nephrotoxins that can cause acute kidney injury

- Antibiotics
  - Aminoglycosides
  - Tetracyclines
  - Amphoteracin
  - Pentamidine
  - Vancomycin
- Iodinated radiocontrast media
- Anaesthetic agents
  - Methoxyflurane
  - Enflurane
- Chemotherapeutic agents
  - Cicylosporin
  - Cisplatinium compounds
  - Methrotrexate
  - Organic solvents
  - Ethylene gycol
- Non-steroidal anti-inflammatory drugs
  - Ibuprofen
  - Diclofenac
  - Indomethacin

Contrast media

The incidence of AKI associated with the use of iodinated radiocontrast media varies greatly in the literature (0–50%). This variability probably reflects the differences in standard risk factors in the populations under examination, and the definition of AKI used. Risk factors known to be associated with a higher risk of contrast induced AKI are pre-existing CKD, diabetes mellitus, myeloma, volume depletion, and the incidence varies with the type of procedure and the volume of contrast administered. AKI typically develops 24–48 hours following the examination, is usually mild and recovery often is observed with five to seven days. Dialysis requiring AKI is relatively uncommon, and again generally reflects the overall risk burden of the patient rather than the contrast load in isolation.

Glomerulonephritis and vasculitis causes

A large number of glomerulonephritic and vasculitic causes can cause AKI, sometimes in association with pulmonary haemorrhage. They make up only 5–10% of cases of AKI, but early recognition and correct management is essential because of the management required.

As part of the initial assessment of the patient with AKI, the history and examination should consider the systemic symptoms and signs of vasculitis. Dipstick testing of the urine for blood and protein, and microscopy to look for the presence of red cell casts are required. Serological tests including measurement of anti-neutrophil cytoplasmic antibodies are usually positive in AKI associated with a rapidly progressive glomerulonephritis, and renal biopsy is the gold standard procedure to determine extent and severity of disease.

Obstructive nephropathy

Obstructive nephropathy can manifest as either a sudden or an insidious decline in renal function, which can be halted or even reversed by relief of obstruction; hence obstructive nephropathy is a potentially curable cause of AKI. Obstruction can be due to an anatomical or functional abnormality of the urethra, bladder, ureter, or renal pelvis, which may be congenital or acquired, and it can also be a consequence of diseases extrinsic to the urinary tract. Although dilatation of the outflow system proximal to the site of obstruction is a characteristic finding, widening of the ureter and pelvicalyceal system does not necessary indicate the presence of obstruction, and flow may be obstructed without such dilatation being present.

It is clear that complete or prolonged partial urinary tract obstruction can lead to tubular atrophy and eventually irreversible renal injury. The renal prognosis after relief of urinary tract obstruction is dependent upon the severity and duration of the obstruction. With total ureteral obstruction, for example, there is evidence that relatively complete recovery of GFR can be achieved within one week, while little or no recovery occurs after 12 weeks. In addition to the persistent reduction in GFR, tubular function may also be impaired by chronic obstruction. This may be manifested by polyuria due to decreased concentrating ability, because of decreased expression of water channels, mild sodium wasting, and by distal renal tubular acidosis with hyperkalaemia due to diminished distal hydrogen and potassium secretion.

Following the onset of obstruction, there is an initial increase in pressure proximal to the obstruction due to continued glomerular filtration. This rise in pressure is eventually responsible for the dilatation of the collecting systems that can be detected by renal ultrasonography or computed tomography (CT) scanning. The elevation in pressure is also transmitted back to the proximal tubule, lowering the GFR by counteracting the high intraglomerular pressure that normally drives glomerular filtration. However, the rise in intratubular pressure induces secondary renal vasoconstriction, resulting in a reduction in glomerular blood flow. This response is regulated locally by individual obstructed nephrons and is mediated in part by the release of angiotensin II and thromboxanes. The net effect is that the chronic reduction in GFR is due primarily to the decrease in renal perfusion, added to later by tubular atrophy induced by ischaemia and inflammation. The injury that is independent of pressure may be due both to ischaemia and to the influx of inflammatory cells, which contribute to development of fibrosis and atrophy.

Ultrasonography is used as first-line screening test to examine for urinary tract obstruction in patients with unexplained AKI. It has a high sensitivity and specificity, although approximately 5% of patients with obstruction will not have calyceal dilatation. In a patient with anuria or no other explanation for AKI and an apparently normal ultrasound appearance, unenhanced CT imaging is well-tolerated and more sensitive.

General aspects of management of acute kidney injury

The principle of management of established AKI is to treat or remove the precipitating factors, and maintain homeostasis while recovery takes place. Nutritional support should be started early and contain adequate calorie and protein intake. There is no evidence that specific renal nutritional interventions are useful or necessary, in contrast to chronic renal failure.

Hyperkalaemia

Hyperkalaemia is important in the context of acute kidney injury because it can cause cardiac arrthythmias and death. Patients may occasionally have symptoms of muscle weakness or paralysis, but the significance of these symptoms is rarely appreciated, and usually there are no symptoms at all. Hyperkalaemia is associated with typical changes in the electrocardiogram, which if present occur progressively:

(i) 'Tenting' of T waves

(ii) Reduction in the size of P waves, increase in P-R interval, and widening of the QRS complex

(iii) Disappearance of the P wave

(iv) Irregular 'sinusoidal' elctrocardiogram (ECG)

(v) Asystole

Treatment of hyperkalaemia is described in Table 9.2.3.

Pulmonary oedema

The most serious complication of salt and water retention in AKI is the development of pulmonary oedema. This can often be iatrogenic, caused by continued intravenous infusion of fluids into patients with established AKI and oliguria. Examination reveals cyanosis, tachypnoea, widespread wheeze, and inspiratory

Table 9.2.3 Treatment of hyperkalaemia

Treatment	Comment
(i) Intravenous calcium (10 mL of 10% calcium) gluconate, over 1 minute, repeated if required	Treatment to be given immediately if hyperkalaemia is associated with ECG changes. Acts to stabilize cardiac membrane. Does not alter plasma potassium
(ii) Intravenous insulin and glucose (10 units of rapidly acting insulin plus 50 mL 50% glucose, over 10 minutes)	Insulin stimulates Na K ATPase in muscle and liver, thus mobilizing potassium into cells. Plasma potassium falls 1–2 mmol/l over 30–60 minutes. Monitor blood glucose
(iii) Nebulized salbutamol (10–20 mg)	Beta 2 agonists stimulate Na K ATPase in muscle and liver, thus driving potassium into cells. Induces tremor and tachycardia
(iv) Intravenous bicarbonate (50–100 mL of 1.4% solution)	Only to be used if severe acidosis in fluid deplete that merits treatment in its own right. large sodium load
(v) Haemodialysis/haeomofiltration	Definitive management likely to be required except in rare cases where AKI resolves rapidly on medical therapy

crepitations throughout the chest. Investigation demonstrates arterial hypoxaemia, and the chest radiograph shows widespread interstitial shadowing. The patient should be sat up and given oxygen by facemask. In some situations, the patient may respond to furosemide as a venodilator, but the definitive treatment is the removal of fluid by haemodialysis or haemofiltration.

Bleeding

In severe AKI, as with advanced CKD, the bleeding time is prolonged, and this is in addition to any abnormality of haemostatis that be stimulataneously induced by the condition that precipitated AKI. The routine use of H_2-receptor antagonists and an awareness about haemorrhage risk has reduced the risk of upper-gastrointestinal bleeding, a previously frequent and often occult occurrence in patients with AKI, particularly in an intensive care unit (ITU). Practical management of haemostasis should include review of the use of prophylactic or therapeutic anticoagulation, review of dose of subcutaneous anticoagulation, particularly low-molecular weight heparins, and maintenance of an adequate haemoglobin concentration.

Sepsis

Overwhelming septicaemia is a common cause of AKI. Sepsis may also be the precipitating factor in a patient who is either postoperative or has been resuscitated from major trauma. The clinical index of suspicion must be set very high—especially in a patient with AKI who appears to be deteriorating in any way. Care must be taken with the management of intravenous lines and urinary catheters, and unused or unnecessary ones should be removed. There should be a low threshold for repeating microbiological investigations, and review of antibiotic therapy. All infections should be treated promptly and aggressively, with the most appropriate antimicrobial agent, with intelligent therapy based on the results of investigations and regular cultures.

Renal replacement therapy

In the absence of effective pharmacological therapies for AKI, the care of the patient with AKI is limited to supportive management, in which renal replacement therapy plays an essential role. Multiple modalities of renal replacement therapy (RRT) are available, including intermittent haemodialysis (IHD), continuous replacement therapies, and hybrid techniques such as slow low-efficiency dialysis (SLED). Despite these varied techniques, mortality in patients with AKI remain high, greater than 50% in severely ill patients. The main indications for initiation of RRT include severe volume overload, hyperkalaemia, metabolic acidosis, and overt uraemic manifestations such as pericarditis.

Although progress has been made with regard to renal replacement therapy prescription through large randomized controlled trials, the optimal timing of initiation of RRT and the preferred modality of therapy remains controversial. Two recent large studies have examined the role of early initiation of RRT in renal and patient outcomes. The PICARD study showed that there was an increased risk of death at 60 days for those patients who began on dialysis with high blood urea levels (>76 mg/dl). The BEST kidney study compared outcomes for patients with AKI in intensive care units with early or late initiation of dialysis. Patients were eligible for the trial if they presented with AKI defined as a BUN >84 mg/dl or a urine output <200 mL over 12 hours. Patients in the late group had a higher rate of dialysis dependence at hospital discharge, and longer inpatient stays. Overall, there was lower mortality in the early initiation group, and there was a correlation between length of stay on ITU prior to RRT and outcome. An analysis of RRT for AKI associated with cardiac surgery demonstrated higher survival in patients in whom continuous therapy was initiated in response to reduced urine output, when compared to patients in whom it was commenced only on reaching biochemical parameter threshold measurement.

Several observational studies have demonstrated an association between the severity of fluid overload at the time of initiation of RRT and mortality. Although fluid overload may contribute to organ dysfunction and contribute to mortality risk, the results of these observational studies cannot prove a causal relationship.

There is a paucity of high-quality evidence to demonstrate clinical superiority of either IHD or continuous therapies. The majority of studies comparing continuous renal replacement therapy (CRRT) and IHD have been observation or retrospective case series. After adjustment for severity of illness, there is no survival benefit associated with continuous therapy. Randomized controlled trials in an intensive care setting have also not demonstrated a benefit. The HemoDiafe study, a prospective multicentre study, randomly assigned 360 patients with AKI to IHD or CRRT. At 60 days, survival in both groups was similar, and both therapies were associated with similar rates of hypotension.

In summary, the initiation of RRT, by whichever technique is most suited to the individual patient circumstances, should occur prior to the development of overt symptoms and signs of renal failure, such as advanced uraemic encephalopathy. There is not, however, consensus of the threshold biochemical changes associated with AKI that are definitive markers for initiation. Volume status, and early signs of fluid overload may necessitate an earlier start to RRT than is merited by biochemical changes, and appropriate management of fluid replacement and nutrition are essential to renal recovery and minimization of AKI associated mortality.

Prognosis

Mortality from AKI remains high, particularly in the critically ill patient, in whom mortality was 53% in the large acute tubular necrosis (ATN) trial, and 44.7% in the RENAL trial of renal replacement therapies in intensive care. Several large epidemiology studies show that the mortality of AKI outside the intensive care setting is slowly reducing, but still remains close to 25% for a single episode of dialysis requiring AKI. AKI is also linked with a higher risk of CKD, development of end-stage renal failure and hence mortality. This suggests that even a short episode of AKI might contribute to long-term morbidity and mortality. The patients at higher risk for AKI are not surprisingly those with established classic risk factors for CKD and cardiovascular mortality. Early identification, careful and immaculate management and ideally the prevention of more severe stages of AKI must be the overwhelming priority in the management of these patients during medical illness or in the perioperative period.

Further reading

Bagshaw SM, Uchino S, Bellomo R, *et al.* Timing of renal replacement therapy and clinical outcomes in critically ill patients with severe acute kidney injury. *J Crit Care* 2009; **24**:129–40.

Bellomo R, Kellum JA, Ronco C. Acute kidney injury. *Lancet* 2012; **380**:756–66.

Borthwick E, Feguson A. Perioperative acute kidney injury: risk factors, recognition, management and outcomes. *BMJ* 2010; **341**:c3365.

Coca SG, Yusuf B, Shlipak MG, *et al.* Long-term risk of mortality and other adverse outcomes after acute kidney injury: a systematic review and meta-analysis. *Am J Kidney Dis* 2009; **53**:961–73.

Ftouh S, Lewington A; Acute Kidney Injury Guideline Development Group convened by the National Clinical Guidelines Centre and commissioned by the National Institute for Health and Care Excellence, in association with The Royal College of Physicians' Clini. Prevention, detection and management of acute kidney injury: concise guideline. *Clin Med* 2014; **14**:61–5.

Hsu R, McCulloch C, Adams Dudley R, Lo L, Hsu C-Y. Temporal changes in incidence of dialysis-requiring AKI. *J Am Soc Nephrol* 2012; **24**:1–6.

Levy EM, Viscoli CM, Horwitz RI. The effect of acute renal failure on mortality. A cohort analysis. *JAMA* 1996; **275**:1489–94.

Lo LJ, Go AS, Chertow GM, *et al.* Dialysis requiring acute renal failure increases the risk of progressive chronic kidney disease. *Kidney Int* 2009; **76**:893–9.

Mehta RL, Kellum JA, Shah S, *et al.* Acute Kidney Injury Network (AKIN): report of an initiative to improve outcomes in acute kidney injury. *Crit Care* 2007; **11**:R31.

Molitoris BA, Sutton TA. Endothelial injury and dysfunction: role in the extension phase of acute renal failure. *Kidney Int* 2004; **66**:496–9.

Palevsky PM, Zhanf, JH, O'Connor TZ, *et al.* Intensity of renal support in critically ill patients with acute kidney injury. *N Eng J Med* 2008; **359**:7–20.

CHAPTER 9.3

Chronic kidney disease and dialysis

Richard J. Haynes and James A. Gilbert

Introduction to chronic kidney disease

Chronic kidney disease (CKD) has replaced chronic renal failure as the term used to describe persistent (often progressive) kidney damage with or without a reduction in renal function. Glomerular filtration rate (GFR) is the standard measure of renal function and is usually estimated with equations based on serum creatinine concentration, age, sex, and other variables depending on the equation. Estimated GFR (eGFR) is a measure of the excretory function of the kidney, but the kidney also regulates blood pressure, red blood cell production, acid-base balance, and mineral bone metabolism. CKD when complicated by reduced renal function is therefore characterized by disturbances in a wide variety of basic physiological functions.

Definition

CKD is defined as 'kidney damage or GFR <60 mL/min/1.73m^2 for three months or more, irrespective of the cause'.[1] Kidney damage can be demonstrated by abnormal urinary constituents (proteinuria and/or haematuria), imaging (e.g. parenchymal scarring or cysts) or by histological examination of kidney tissue usually obtained by biopsy. A staging system was introduced in 2002 that was updated in 2012 and stages CKD by cause, eGFR and albuminuria (Table 9.3.1).[2]

All routinely-used formulae used to estimate GFR are based on serum creatinine concentration and are unreliable when renal function is normal or near-normal (as it is in the vast majority of people). Creatinine is a convenient but imperfect marker of renal function as the concentration is altered by diet (high-protein diets may increase creatinine) and drugs that alter creatinine secretion. End-stage renal disease (ESRD) is defined as eGFR <15 mL/min/1.73m^2 (i.e. stage 5 CKD) or treatment with dialysis or transplantation.

Table 9.3.1 Classification of chronic kidney disease (CKD) based on glomerular filtration rate (GFR) based on Kidney Disease Improving Global Outcomes (KDIGO) guidelines

		Albuminuria category		
		A1	A2	A3
GFR category	**GFR (mL/ min/1.73 m^2)**	**<3 mg/mmol**	**3–30 mg/mmol**	**>30 mg/mmol**
G1	≥90			
G2	60–89			
G3a	30–44			
G3b				
G4	15–29			
G5	<15			

Source: data from Kidney Disease: Improving Global Outcomes (KDIGO), KDIGO 2012 Clinical Practice Guideline for the Evaluation and Management of Chronic Kidney Disease, *Kidney International Supplement*, Volume 3, Issue 1, pp. 1–150, Copyright © 2013 KDIGO.

Aetiology

CKD is not a diagnosis in itself and the first consideration once CKD is recognized is to consider the underlying cause. These can be divided (like causes of acute renal failure) into pre-renal, renal, and post-renal causes (see Table 9.3.2). The cause of CKD is not actively pursued in most patients so the hierarchy of causative diseases has not been described. However, national registries of patients receiving renal replacement treatment (RRT) provide information of the causes of CKD that reach ESRD (which may differ from those that cause earlier CKD) due to 'survivor bias' (i.e. some causes may be associated with an increased risk of death prior to ESRD so have a lower prevalence in patients receiving RRT). Table 9.3.3 shows the estimates of the primary cause of ESRD in the incident RRT populations in 2008 in three different developed countries.

There are marked geographic variations in the cause of ESRD within Europe: more than 80% of patients with ESRD in Finland are classified as having chronic glomerulonephritis (compared to 12% in the United Kingdom). Amyloidosis is very common in the Mediterranean where it accounts for 30% of ESRD. Even within countries there can be marked racial differences: diabetic nephropathy is about 30% more common among African and Hispanic Americans than Caucasians.

Epidemiology

The incidence and prevalence of CKD are impossible to assess accurately because CKD is usually asymptomatic. The National Health and Nutrition Examination Survey (NHANES) in America has estimated the prevalence of the CKD stages 1, 2, 3, 4, and 5 (combined) to be 3.2%, 4.1%, 7.8%, and 0.5%, respectively (or

Table 9.3.2 Identifiable causes of chronic kidney disease

	Common	Less common
Pre-renal	Renal arterial disease	
Renal	Glomerular disease	Glomerular disease
	Diabetic nephropathy	Amyloidosis
	IgA nephropathy	Vasculitis
	Focal segmental glomerulosclerosis	Haemolytic-uraemic syndrome
	Tubulointerstitial disease	Tubulointerstitial disease
	Reflux nephropathy	Myeloma
	Polycystic kidney disease	Analgesic nephropathy
Post-renal	Obstruction	Obstruction
	Prostatic	Retroperitoneal fibrosis

15.6% overall). It is more common (as currently defined) in the elderly (odds ratio [OR] of about 6 for 60+ years versus <40 years), females (OR 1.5), ethnic minorities (OR 1.2) and in people with diabetes (OR 2.5), hypertension (OR 1.8), and cardiovascular disease (OR 2).[3]

Other studies have used albuminuria as a marker of kidney disease; this is again controversial when microalbuminuria (i.e. 30–300 mg/day) is assumed to indicate structural kidney disease. The PREVEND study in Groningen, Netherlands found a prevalence of microalbuminuria of 7.2% but only 0.7% for macroalbuminuria (i.e. >300 mg/day) in the 8,000 people who responded to their request for a urine sample.[4]

In the United Kingdom, the NEOERICA project analysed routinely-collected renal function results of over 130,000 individuals and found the age-standardized prevalence of CKD stages 3–5 to be 10.6% in females and 5.8% in males. Whereas such CKD was uncommon in those younger than 45 years, the prevalence rose steeply with age to over 40% in men and women aged over 83.[5] However, this survey did not apply the three month chronicity criterion (i.e. it was based on single measurements) so it overestimated the prevalence of CKD. In comparison, data from an American healthcare organization using a more stringent definition of CKD found the prevalence of CKD (stages 1–5) to be 2.16%.[6]

Table 9.3.3 Cause of end-stage renal disease: estimates from three national registries

Cause of ESRD	UK	USA	Australia
Diabetes	24%	44%	34%
Glomerulonephritis	12%	7%	22%
Polycystic disease	7%	2%	6%
Hypertension	6%	28%	15%
Renovascular	7%	*	*
Pyelonephritis	8%	*	3%
Other	15%	15%	12%
Unknown	21%	4%	8%

*included in the 'other' category for that country.

Pathology and pathogenesis

CKD classically progresses by two main mechanisms: those of the primary kidney disease and those of non-specific injury. Clearly those of the primary kidney disease are disease-specific, whereas 'natural progression' describes a common pathophysiological course once the initial insult has occurred. All chronic renal diseases cause a loss of functioning nephrons (the functional unit of the kidney). The remaining nephrons then compensate by increasing their intraglomerular pressure which allows 'hyper-filtering' to maintain GFR. However, the increased glomerular pressure is harmful and causes progressive endothelial injury, glomerular sclerosis, and eventually nephron loss. This is observed histologically as glomeruli which are either segmentally or globally sclerosed. The circulation through the glomerulus is reduced causing the tubule derived from that glomerulus to atrophy from ischaemia. The progression of CKD therefore becomes largely independent of the initial insult and renal function declines in a linear fashion (if GFR or reciprocal creatinine is plotted against time; see Fig. 9.3.1 for an example).

Not all patients have such a classical linear loss of renal function. Some patients remain stable for some time, and others may progress slowly but have marked 'step changes' in their renal function which coincide with renal insults such as episodes of sepsis, hypotension or treatment with nephrotoxic agents such as non-steroidal anti-inflammatory drugs or iodinated contrast medium (see Fig. 9.3.1).

Diagnosis

As explained above, the diagnosis of CKD depends on persistent abnormalities in laboratory measures of kidney function and or evidence of injury.

History

Symptoms develop late in CKD and generally only when ESRD is imminent (<20% of kidney function). However, a history of nocturia is a useful and reliable guide to the chronicity (see section on differential diagnosis below). A history of recurrent urinary tract infections in early childhood and/or enuresis may suggest reflux

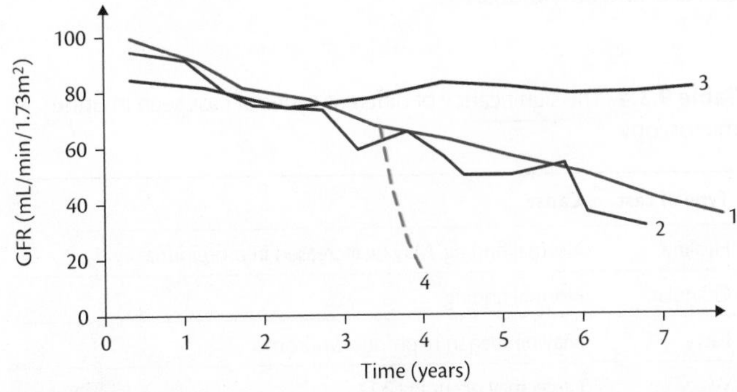

Fig. 9.3.1 Examples of progression of CKD. Line 1 (green) demonstrates the classical linear decline in GFR (or 1/Cr) with time. Line 2 (blue) demonstrates step-wise progression and line 3 (red) demonstrates stable kidney function. Line 4 (dashed green) demonstrates acute-on-chronic renal failure.

nephropathy as the cause of CKD. A careful systematic review is required to elicit pointers to systemic diseases such as diabetes or vasculitis. The drug history should be checked (including 'over the counter' medications such as analgesia or herbal remedies) and the social history should check for occupational exposures such as lead or hydrocarbons. A positive family history may suggest polycystic kidney disease, Alport's Syndrome, or other heritable causes of CKD.

Symptoms of uraemia include itching, muscle cramps, anorexia, nausea, and cognitive impairment or confusion. The presence of such symptoms—if attributable to CKD—is a relative indication that renal replacement therapy should be started.

Examination

A full physical examination is required including blood pressure measurement, abdominal examination looking for enlarged kidneys, bruits, or a distended bladder, fundoscopy, and urinalysis. A careful assessment of the volume status is critical because hypovolaemia may cause impaired renal function whereas hypervolaemia is a complication of CKD. Peripheral pulses should be assessed for bruits as this may suggest the presence of renal arterial disease (either stenosis or a source of cholesterol emboli) which is an increasingly recognized cause of CKD and ESRD.

Urinalysis is essential: the presence of significant proteinuria (≥2+) suggests a glomerular disease. Haematuria (i.e. the presence of red cells) on dipstick does not necessarily imply intrinsic renal disease, but if microscopy is available, dysmorphic red cells suggest glomerular bleeding (as does coexistent proteinuria). Casts may be seen with microscopy; the significance of these is outlined in Table 9.3.4.

Investigations

Investigations are performed to identify the cause of CKD and to identify any complications (see below). Immunological tests (e.g. serum and urine electrophoresis, autoantibodies including antinuclear and antineutrophil cytoplasm antibodies, complement levels, and viral serology) seldom identify an underlying cause of CKD, and are more helpful in acute kidney injury. They are performed to identify cases of indolent vasculitis, myeloma or primary (AL) amyloid.

Ultrasound gives an indication of renal size and can exclude hydronephrosis. Normal-sized kidneys do not exclude CKD as renal size is often preserved in diabetic nephropathy, polycystic disease, and amyloidosis.

Table 9.3.4 The significance of different types of cast seen in urine microscopy

Type of cast	Cause
Hyaline	Normal finding. May be increased in proteinuria
Granular	Normal finding
Fatty	May be seen in nephrotic syndrome
Waxy	Large; may occur in CKD
Red cell	Indicate glomerular bleeding due to active glomerulonephritis
White cell	Suggest acute (usually bacterial) infection

Differential diagnosis

The main differential diagnosis of CKD is acute renal failure (or acute kidney injury [AKI] as it has become known more recently). The definitive distinction between these two entities is evidence of persistently impaired renal function (i.e. the presence of historical measurements of abnormal renal function). However, these may not always be available (and indeed CKD and AKI can overlap in cases of acute-on-chronic renal failure).

There are no clinical, laboratory, or radiological tests that can 100% reliably distinguish AKI from CKD. For example, anaemia (which is a complication of CKD) can develop rapidly in AKI; similarly, hyperphosphataemia and hypocalcaemia may occur in rhabdomyolysis as well as advanced CKD. Small kidneys on ultrasound usually indicate chronicity but not invariably. The distinction therefore relies on the overall assessment of the patient (especially the history) and concerted effort to access any previous creatinine measurements.

Management

The management of a patient with suspected CKD includes:

(i) To exclude AKI (or acute-on-chronic renal failure);

(ii) To diagnose the cause of CKD and halt the pathology;

(iii) To retard 'natural progression' of CKD;

(iv) To identify and treat complications of CKD;

(v) To counsel the patient and prepare them for RRT (if appropriate) or palliative care.

The first two priorities are covered above. Retarding the progression of kidney disease is essential in order to both delay the associated complications (see section below) but also to delay the need for RRT. As discussed above, progression may be due to the underlying kidney disease or to natural progression.

Treating underlying kidney disease

Removal or amelioration of the underlying kidney disease may slow the progression of kidney disease. However, it seldom halts it entirely if the vicious cycle of intraglomerular hypertension and hyperfiltration has been set in motion as these can continue independently of the initial insult.

The history of treatments for primary renal diseases has been disappointing. Various immunosuppression strategies have been used for primary glomerulonephritides including membranous nephropathy, IgA disease, and focal segmental glomerular sclerosis. Renal artery stenosis is increasingly recognized as a cause of CKD in patients with other vascular disease, but trials of angioplasty and stenting have been disappointing in showing no benefit in terms of long-term kidney function. Relief of urinary tract obstruction has obviously never been formally tested but is mandated by the other potential complications of urinary stasis (including stones and infections). It is recognized that patients with CKD caused by obstruction that has been relieved progress slowly or not at all especially if they have not developed proteinuria indicating secondary glomerular damage. There is good evidence that strict blood glucose control is beneficial in early diabetic nephropathy so the development of this adds extra incentive to control blood sugars.[7] However, there is no evidence that tight glycaemic control delays the progession of established macroalbuminuric (>300 mg/day) diabetic nephropathy.

Slowing natural (non-disease-related) progression

The key intervention for slowing natural progression is blood pressure control. Higher levels of blood pressure are associated with more rapid decline in kidney function and randomized trials have demonstrated that stricter blood pressure control is more effective at slowing natural progression than standard treatment.[8] Current guidelines recommend blood pressure to be <130/80 mmHg in patients with CKD.

Inhibitors of the renin-angiotensin system (i.e. angiotensin converting enzyme inhibitors [ACEi] or angiotensin receptor blockers [ARBs]) are probably the first choice antihypertensive, especially if proteinuria is present.[9] ACEi and ARB therapy reduce proteinuria because of their renal haemodynamic effects: by reducing angiotensin II they cause efferent arteriolar vasodilatation and hence reduce intraglomerular pressure. This reduces proteinuria, but also reduces GFR acutely. Therefore a moderate (up to 25%) reduction in GFR can be expected when ACEi or ARB are introduced. Care should therefore be taken when such therapy is started to check renal function shortly afterwards and to ensure any acute decline in GFR is not progressive or severe which may imply critical bilateral or single kidney renal artery stenosis (a rare but much feared condition). However, once the acute decline has stabilized, the long-term benefits of the reduction in intraglomerular pressure accrue and if these treatments are introduced early enough in the course of CKD, the onset of ESRD can be delayed by many years (Fig. 9.3.2).

The anti-proteinuric effect of ACEi or ARB therapy is augmented by sodium restriction and/or diuretic therapy. In the later stages of CKD sodium retention (and resultant intravascular volume expansion) contributes to hypertension and hence diuretic therapy (in relatively high doses) can reduce blood pressure successfully. Patients with CKD often need multiple agents to control blood pressure. However, there is little evidence to guide the choice of add-on therapy after ACEi or ARB treatment and diuretics.

All patients should be advised to stop smoking (because smoking is associated with vascular disease and cancer) and avoid obesity. Certain medications have an adverse effect on renal haemodynamics and can precipitate acute-on-chronic renal failure (which may require dialysis and may not be reversible). The most common of these are non-steroid anti-inflammatory drugs (NSAIDs). Ideally these should be avoided altogether, especially once stage 4 CKD develops. Short courses in patients with earlier stages of CKD should be allowed (e.g. in patients with acute gout).

Other drugs can also be nephrotoxic (e.g. gentamicin) and should be avoided or—if mandated—have their dose reduced. Iodinated contrast media are also nephrotoxic and the benefit of the extra information that contrast enhancement provides should be weighed against the risks of nephrotoxicity. The risk of nephrotoxicity can be reduced by ensuring the patient is well hydrated; other measures (e.g. N-acetyl-cysteine and sodium bicarbonate) are of less-clear benefit. Gadolinium-based magnetic resonance contrast media should also be considered carefully in advanced CKD due to the risk of nephrogenic systemic fibrosis (a disabling scleroderma-like condition which can be fatal). All medications should be reviewed to ensure that the dosing is appropriate for the level of renal function.

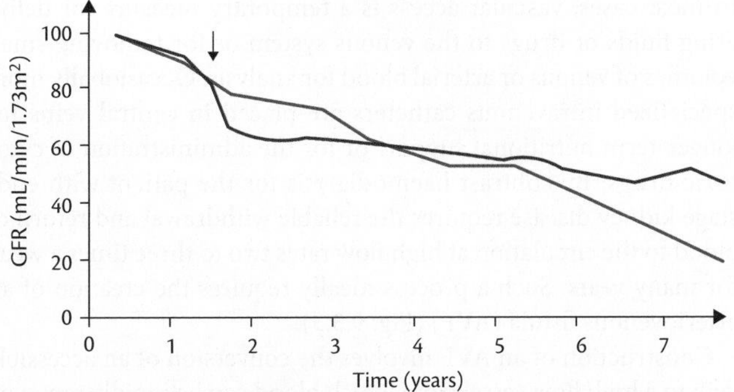

Fig. 9.3.2 Benefits of ACEi or ARB therapy in proteinuric nephropathy.The green line shows the natural progression associated with proteinuric nephropathy. The red line shows the acute decline in GFR caused by the introduction of a ACEi treatment (arrow) followed by a reduction in the rate of progression.

Complications and their management

CKD has numerous complications; the pathogenesis and management of the most common are outlined below.

Cardiovascular disease

Cardiovascular disease (CVD) is the single most common cause of death in patients with CKD (accounting for almost half of all mortality) and patients with late stage CKD (3B, 4 and 5) are at very high risk of cardiovascular events (e.g. a 40 year old dialysis patient has the same cardiovascular risk as an 80 year old patient without CKD). The reasons for this are multifactorial: there is both an increased burden of traditional risk factors (e.g. hypertension and diabetes) but also a constellation of novel risk factors (e.g. anaemia and mineral bone disease, see below). It appears that as CKD progresses, the associated CVD changes from typical atherosclerotic disease to a form of arterial stiffness accompanied by structural heart disease so that dialysis patients die of similar causes to patients with advanced heart failure. Reducing low-density lipoprotein (LDL) cholesterol has been shown to reduce atherosclerotic events and is therefore indicated in most patients with CKD.[10]

Anaemia

The kidneys (specifically interstitial fibroblasts) are the main source of erythropoietin. As CKD progresses, erythropoietin production declines, and anaemia develops. It typically manifests at or below a GFR of about 40 mL/min/1.73m^2 but the cause of CKD can modify this (it typically occurs earlier in diabetic nephropathy and later—if at all—in polycystic kidney disease). In addition, CKD confers a state of 'functional iron deficiency' in which the bone marrow is starved of iron because of inhibition by hepcidin of release of iron stores from the liver. Therefore the treatment of anaemia in CKD often involves iron repletion and supplementation and erythropoietin replacement in the form of an ESA (erythropoiesis stimulating agent).[11]

Renal anaemia has been linked to both cardiovascular disease and progression of CKD. The avoidance of blood transfusion (with its attendant risks of viral infection and sensitization to human leukocyte antigen (HLA) antigens which prejudice future transplantation) and a possible improvement in quality of life are major indications for correction of anaemia with erythropoietin, but the target haemoglobin is controversial as trials have suggested that attempts to normalize haemoglobin may be harmful.[12] Current guidelines therefore suggest a target of 11–12 g/dL.

Mineral bone disease

CKD induces a complex disturbance in mineral bone metabolism which is incompletely understood. As GFR falls, the kidney's ability to excrete the phosphate absorbed in the diet is exceeded and hence serum phosphate starts to rise. This—in conjunction with reducing renal 1α-hydroxylase activity (which converts 25-hydroxy-vitamin D to the highly active 1,25-dihydroxy-vitamin D)—leads to secondary hyperparathyroidism. Homeostatic parathyroid hormone (PTH) secretion is stimulated by high phosphate concentrations, low concentrations of calcium and 1–25-dihydroxy-vitamin D all attempting to normalize plasma calcium and phosphate. This is referred to as the 'trade-off hypothesis'. Although these biochemical changes may be evident in the later phases of stage 3 CKD, symptomatic bone disease (i.e. with pain or pathological fractures) does not develop until patients have been on dialysis for many years. However in children it has a significant effect on bone growth, mineralization, and maturation at earlier stages of CKD.

Currently, hyperphosphataemia is treated by dietary restriction and—when this is insufficient or unsuccessful—dietary phosphate binders which bind phosphate in the intestine and prevent is absorption. These may be calcium-based (e.g. calcium carbonate or acetate) or calcium-free (e.g. sevelamer or lanthanum). Hyperparathyroidism is treated with 1α-hydroxylated vitamin D initially. Calcimimetic agents (cinacalcet) which sensitize the calcium-sensing receptor on parathyroid tissue to the prevailing calcium concentration and thereby reduce PTH concentrations, have recently become available. If the hyperparathyroidism becomes autonomous (i.e. unresponsive to treatment) or the treatments have unacceptable side effects (e.g. hypercalcaemia from activated vitamin D) then surgical parathyroidectomy can be performed. All four parathyroid glands are removed so—if successful—patients have no detectable PTH following surgery.

Acidosis

As the kidneys are central to acid-base balance, a metabolic acidosis develops as their function deteriorates. Although this may initially have a normal anion gap, in the later stages it becomes a raised anion gap acidosis, due to the accumulation of acidic uraemic toxins. This acidosis can interact with other complications (e.g. worsen anaemia, mineral bone disease, and hyperkalaemia) and is treated with oral sodium bicarbonate which has to be taken four times a day. The sodium load of this treatment may worsen salt and water retention and hence hypertension—so acidosis is one indication for starting dialysis. However, a recent small randomized trial has suggested that bicarbonate supplementation may retard the progression of CKD.[13]

Other

CKD can also disturb the production, protein binding, catabolism, and tissue effects of other hormones. Plasma thyroxine levels may be low but this does not cause clinical hypothyroidism and thyroid-stimulating hormone remains a reliable diagnostic test. Insulin clearance is reduced, but this is counterbalanced by increased peripheral insulin resistance so again this is not clinically manifest. In men, hyperprolactinaemia and low testosterone levels may contribute to sexual dysfunction, including reduced fertility. Erectile dysfunction is also common and multifactorial, but often responds to phosphodiesterase type-5 inhibitors. In women with advanced CKD the menstrual cycle is impaired and cycles become irregular and anovulatory.

CKD is also known to cause a neuropathy which typically starts with sensory loss, paraesthesiae, and insensitivity to temperature but may progress to motor loss. An autonomic neuropathy is also common which can cause postural hypotension and may contribute to sudden cardiac death.

End-stage renal disease

In a small group of patients with CKD (about 100 per million population per year in the UK) renal function declines to a level that is not sufficient to maintain health and RRT is required (or a decision made to manage the symptoms conservatively). The options for RRT include dialysis or kidney transplantation.

Dialysis

Dialysis involves the removal of uraemic toxins, excess extracellular fluid and electrolytes (sodium and potassium) by artificial means. It requires the patient's blood to be approximated to dialysate fluid (the composition of which can be modified according to the individual's requirements) with a semi-permeable membrane in between.

Haemodialysis involves an extracorporeal blood circuit and an artificial membrane. The pores in the membrane are large enough to allow most small uraemic toxin molecules across but small enough to ensure essential proteins (e.g. albumin) are not removed. Dialysate fluid is passed in the opposite direction on the other side of the membrane so a diffusive gradient is maintained leading to toxin removal into the dialysate. The transmembrane pressure can be increased to force extra fluid across the membrane allowing the extracellular volume to be controlled and toxins to be removed by filtration.

The key element of successful haemodialysis is access to the patient's circulation.

Vascular access for haemodialysis

Access to the circulation is essential in many aspects of medicine. In most cases, vascular access is a temporary measure for delivering fluids or drugs to the venous system or for removing small volumes of venous or arterial blood for analysis. Occasionally more specialized intravenous catheters are placed in central veins for longer-term nutritional support or for the administration of cytotoxic drugs. By contrast haemodialysis for the patient with end-stage kidney disease requires the reliable withdrawal and return of blood to the circulation at high flow rates two to three times a week for many years. Such a process ideally requires the creation of an arteriovenous fistula (AVF) (Fig. 9.3.3).

Construction of an AVF involves the conversion of an accessible vein to a high flow vessel from which blood can be rapidly removed and returned via two needles during a dialysis session. Veins are low-pressure, low resistance capacitance vessels. Their relative lack of elastic recoil compared to that seen in arteries allows them to progressively increase in size if high-pressure flow passes through

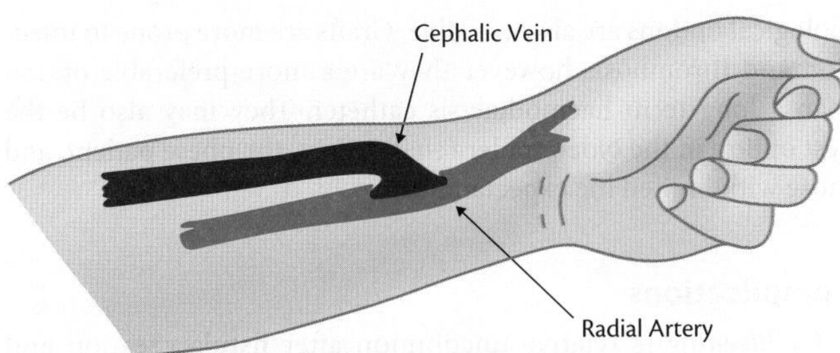

Fig. 9.3.3 Pictorial representation of left radiocephalic arteriovenous (AV) fistula.

them. This is essentially what happens when an AVF is created. After a vein has been anastomosed onto an artery, high-pressure arterial flow passes into the low-pressure capacitance vein. The subsequent increased turbulent flow gives rise to a palpable thrill and an audible bruit within the AVF. In addition, due to the capacitance nature of the vein, the fistula vein increases in size over time. It is this second feature that is crucial for needling and subsequent haemodialysis to take place. As a general rule, the fistula vein needs to be a minimum of 6 mm diameter and no more than 6 mm depth beneath the skin surface six weeks after creation of the fistula if needling is to be attempted and haemodialysis successful.

Timing of access

Given that there is a minimum of six weeks maturation time of a fistula from the point of its creation, the timing of fistula creation in relation to the predicted start of dialysis is critical. Permanent vascular access in the form of a fistula should be created well in advance to allow not only for maturation but also for further procedures should there be failure of the initial access procedure. Many guidelines exist regarding the timing of vascular access. In the US the NKF-DOQI guidelines[14] recommend:

- Patients with GFR <30 mL/min should be educated on all modalities of RRT including transplantation
- A fistula should be placed at least six months before the anticipated start of dialysis
- A new AVF should be allowed to mature for at least one month and preferably three to four months prior to cannulation
- Prosthetic grafts should be placed three to six weeks prior to the anticipated need for haemodialysis
- Never insert haemodialysis catheters until actually needed

In the United Kingdom, the Renal Association[15] and the joint working party of the Renal Association, the Vascular Society of Great Britain and Ireland and the British Society of Interventional Radiology[16] have produced the following standards:

- 60% of all patients presenting within three months of dialysis should start haemodialysis on a useable AVF
- 80% of all prevalent haemodialysis patients should be dialysed using a native AVF
- No patient requiring dialysis should wait more than 4 weeks for fistula construction
- Permanent access should be constructed 16 weeks and preferably 6 months before anticipated need for dialysis
- Preservation of arm veins is critical and unnecessary venepuncture must be avoided

The Vascular Access Society[17] recommendations are very similar and as with those of NKF-DOQI and the Renal Association state that arm veins must be preserved and that the planning of access should commence when a patients GFR reaches 20–25 mL/min. Patients should see an access surgeon when the GFR is 15 mL/min so that access can be created 6–12 months in advance of dialysis (or even sooner if progression is very rapid).

Emerging data suggest that AVF outcomes in terms of patency are significantly improved if access is constructed earlier rather than late on when the patient is on the brink of dialysis.[18] It is unclear why this may be so but it has been suggested that worsening uraemia affects vascular biology especially at the level of the AVF anastomosis.[19]

Early referral and planning are critical to avoid poor outcomes, if the near end-stage patient is to successfully move to RRT particularly in the form of haemodialysis.[20]

Patient assessment

When assessing patients for potential AVF a number of principles exist to increase the likelihood of a good outcome.

There should always be an attempt to try and use autologous (the patient's own) vein when constructing an AVF. This is because of the low infection rates and high patency rates associated with vein compared with a prosthetic graft.

As a general rule fistula creation begins in the non-dominant arm and at the level of the wrist if possible. If a patient has visible upper limb cephalic veins that distend with a tourniquet and arterial pulses are easily palpable then it is reasonable to proceed with surgery without any further tests or imaging. All patients should have an Allen test performed to check for ulnar circulation. If there is concern regarding the quality of the radial or brachial pulse, or if a previous fistula has been created and has failed then a pre-operative arterial duplex is required. If veins are poorly visible then a venous duplex in the presence of a tourniquet will also be required. Many centres routinely use pre-operative venous duplex to map all patients undergoing access creation although it appears that a selective policy is reasonable.[21] There are higher rates of early fistula failure if the artery is less than 2 mm and/or the vein diameter is less than 2.5mm with a tourniquet.[22,23] Such findings are common among older female and diabetic patients.

Most access surgery can be done under local anaesthetic and in the day case setting. When patients require more complex access surgery regional blockade or general anaesthetic will be needed and patients often require a brief 24–48 hour in-hospital stay. This is certainly the case with creation of a transposition fistula or insertion of a prosthetic graft.

Surgical options

The radiocephalic AVF is the primary access procedure of choice if at all possible. It was first described by Brescia and Cimino in 1966 and is constructed utilizing the cephalic vein and the radial artery at the level of the wrist. The fistula can be created under local anaesthetic. A 3–4 cm longitudinal incision is made between the cephalic vein and radial artery just proximal to the flexor retinaculum of the wrist. The vein is dissected out and divided distally. A dorsal slit is made in the vein to create a small hood and an end to side anastomosis with the artery is created. If the forearm cephalic vein is too small or non-existent or if there has been a previous failed attempt to create a radiocephalic fistula then a brachiocephalic AVF will be attempted. The procedure can also be done under local anaesthetic and in the day case setting. A transverse incision is made at the level of the antecubital fossa. The median cubital vein or cepahalic vein are dissected out and ligated as distally as possible. The vein is then swung medially across to the brachial artery where an end to side anastomosis is constructed.

It is usually possible to construct a radiocephalic and/or a brachiocephalic fistula in the majority of patients. Even if it is not possible to do so in the non-dominant arm, one or both options are likely to exist in the dominant arm and therefore every attempt should be made to construct either fistula in both arms in all patients before considering more complex secondary access procedures. There will of course be patients in whom there is no cephalic vein option and with more and more patients going onto dialysis there are an increasing number of patients who exhaust primary access options fairly rapidly. In such patients it is common practice to consider utilization of the basilic vein or insertion of a prosthetic graft.

The basilic vein lies in the medial aspect of the arm. It is relatively superficial in the forearm and if a good ulnar pulse exists than some surgeons will attempt to create an ulna-basilic AVF. Quite often however, it is the basilic vein in the upper arm that is utilized for fistula formation. The problem with the vein at this level is that it lies deep and has the median cutaneous nerves of the arm running across it. This makes needling potentially difficult and patients struggle to hold their arms out in supination for the 4-hour dialysis period. As a result the basilic vein has somehow to be brought into a position whereby it is easily accessible for dialysis. Fully mobilizing the vein from the antecubital fossa to the level of the axilla and then tunnelling it superficially under the skin of the anterior surface of the arm can achieve this. The vein comes to lie adjacent to the brachial artery as a result of the tunnelling process where an anastomosis can be created. This so called brachio-basilic transposition fistula provides an excellent autologous vein option in patients who will withstand a major upper limb operation and in whom all primary options have been exhausted. Some surgeons advocate this procedure in two stages and will look to do a primary brachio-basilic anastomosis under local anaesthetic and then secondarily transpose the arterialized vein at a later operation. The procedure ideally requires the patient to undergo a general anaesthetic. Such patients are invariable high anaesthetic risk and so regional blockade and sedation also enable the procedure to be successfully carried out.

When there is no longer an autologous vein option it is standard practice to consider a prosthetic graft for dialysis access. The principles of graft insertion are simple and involve ensuring there is a good inflow artery for take-off of the graft and a good outflow vein on which to 'land' the graft. The common sites to place a graft are the forearm, the upper arm, and the leg. The graft may be straight or looped and may take a variety of anatomical configurations such as the radio-basilic and brachio-basilic in the forearm, the brachio-axillary in the upper arm or the femoro-femoral thigh loop. Most grafts are easy to establish and require a brief period of incorporation (two weeks) before they are needled for dialysis. The usual prosthetic material is polytetrafluroethylene (PTFE) although biological options are also available. Grafts are more prone to infection and thrombosis however they are a more preferable option than a long-term haemodialysis catheter. They may also be the best option in the older, frailer renal patient, the obese patient, and those with limited life expectancy.

Complications

(i) *Bleeding* is relative uncommon after fistula creation and most bleeding that occurs is usually from the anastomotic line when clamps are removed. It usually settles or requires an extra suture. It is more likely to occur if intravenous heparin has been given and therefore its reversal may be required. If bleeding manifests as a postoperative haematoma it may compress the anastomosis, prevent dilatation of the vein and lead to infection or more commonly thrombosis of the fistula. Most significant haematomas should be evacuated.

(ii) *Wound infections* are infrequently seen and settle with a short course of antibiotics. Between 3–5% of autologous radiocephalic and brachiocphalic AV fistula develop a wound infection postoperatively and due to these low rates very few surgeons give prophylactic antibiotics. Infections overlying a prosthetic graft are more worrisome as the graft can become infected. Consequently most surgeons will give antibiotic prophylaxis at the time of surgery. If infection does occur it is advisable to give intravenous antibiotics. Sometimes there is redness and swelling along the line of the graft tunnel for a few days after surgery. This is often labelled as a postoperative infection when actually it is a direct response of the tunnelling process and settles conservatively.

(iii) *Thrombosis* is the most common complication. Approximately 10% of all autologous fistulae fail within the first six hours after creation. A further 10% fail to develop adequately or thrombose within the first six weeks. Thrombosis may be due to technical factors, poor selection of small or diseased vessels or a generalized thrombotic tendency. In the case of early thrombosis (within the first six hours) patients can return to theatre for exploration and thrombectomy. While this may result in a working fistula, re-thrombosis rates are high. In such a situation it is often best to create a new fistula at a higher level on the next available theatre list. General anaesthesia usually causes a drop in blood pressure, which can contribute to thrombosis. This is certainly the case with prosthetic grafts so the use of heparin may be warranted.

(iv) *Failure of maturation* is mainly seen in autologous fistulae. As most vein fistulae require six weeks maturation time it is standard practice to check all new fistulae at this time to look for signs of maturation. The fistula is usually checked for its size (ideally >6 mm diameter) and its patency. A dialysis nurse is the best person to do the check as they best placed to assess whether the fistula can be needled. Most fistulae that fail to mature because the artery or vein were too small or diseased to begin with. The non-maturing fistula can be investigated with duplex or a fistulogram and occasionally can be improved with surgical revision. More often than not however, a new fistula has to be created at a higher level in the arm.

(v) *Steal syndrome* is the clinical situation where flow through the fistula is greater than that getting to the hand (the fistula is stealing flow). The clinical consequence is that of distal ischaemia and may manifest with a range of symptoms from mild pins and needles in the fingers with a cool hand through to digital necrosis. Most patients with steal syndrome fall somewhere between the two extremes. Steal is extremely rare with the distal fistula especially if there is good flow down the ulnar artery (normal Allen test) but does occur when the AVF or graft insertion is at the level of the brachial artery. Ligation of the fistula cures the symptoms but then the access is lost. It is therefore important to ascertain whether the fistula is 'low flow' or 'high flow'. If the access flow is less than 600 mL/minute and is inducing a steal then ligation is the only option as such access flows are just about adequate to ensure dialysis adequacy. If however the fistula is high flow (anything in excess of two litres per minute), and this is the case with most steal syndrome, then reducing the inflow by banding the fistula just beyond the anastomosis may well be curative. Occasionally this is unsuccessful and more complex procedures involving a bypass to distally revascularize the hand—the DRIL procedure (distal revascularization interval ligation) are required.

(vi) *Aneurysm formation* can occur in a fistula over time. The aneurysm may be isolated and at the level of needling sites or may be uniform throughout the length of the fistula. Needle site aneurysms are common and result from poor needling technique where needles have been 'clustered' around the same site. This gives rise to progressive weakening of the fistula vein with subsequent dilatation. There is a classic 'dumbbell' or 'hour glass' appearance and over time there is a risk of rupture. The uniformly dilated and aneurysmal fistula develops over time and is the result of longstanding high flows through a fistula vein that has good compliance and distensibility; it may be unsightly for the patient. If there is an appearance of imminent rupture then urgent revision surgery or ligation is required.

(vii) *Venous hypertension* manifests with limb swelling and in severe cases prominent venous branches in the arm and across the chest. It is usually the result of a central stenosis in one of the main draining veins of the arm. There is a higher incidence of venous hypertension in patients who have a previous history of long-term central catheters. This leads to the swelling and a fistula that becomes noticeably more pulsatile. Treatment options include angioplasty of the stenotic lesion with or without stent placement. Occasionally the fistula will have to be tied off.

(viii) *High output cardiac failure* is an occasional problem and is more common in the elderly or those with known cardiac disease. The high flow nature of a fistula increases pre-load but there is not a resultant increase in contractility leading to progressive cardiac failure. Such fistulae usually require ligation.

Vascular access is associated with complications both in the short and long term. All fistulae and grafts have to therefore be under surveillance after their creation. Despite these potential problems, vascular access surgery remains vital and central to the life and the wellbeing of the renal patient on dialysis.

Peritoneal dialysis (PD) is an alternative modality of renal replacement therapy to haemodialysis. It uses the patient's own peritoneal membrane (which has a rich blood supply) as the semi-permeable membrane across which to dialyse. Dialysate is instilled into the peritoneal cavity via a catheter and is left to equilibrate with the blood before it is drained out and replaced with fresh fluid. The osmolality of the dialysate can be altered (usually be altering the glucose concentration) and this can control the amount of extra fluid that is drained out (the ultrafiltration volume). PD can be done manually (continuous ambulatory PD) or via machines to which the patient attaches overnight (continuous cycling PD or automated peritoneal dialysis (APD)).

PD is preferred in motivated patients or in those where haemodialysis will be a problem such as severe cardiac, arterial, and central venous occlusive disease. For patients who opt for PD as their modality of RRT, successful insertion of a catheter is essential. A variety of catheters are available for PD however, the standard, double cuff Tenckhoff catheter is still the most widely used access device. Each catheter consists of an extra-abdominal, intramural, and intraperitoneal segment. The extra-abdominal segment is the portion that protrudes from the exit site. The intramural component is the part of the catheter that runs from the peritoneum through the rectus sheath and subcutaneous tunnel to the exit site. This part of the catheter has two Dacron cuffs. The deep cuff is usually anchored to the peritoneum as this is closed after placement of the catheter. The superficial cuff (the one nearest the exit site) lies in the subcutaneous tunnel. There is usually a fibrous reaction that takes place around each cuff to hold them, and the catheter in place. The intraperitoneal portion of the catheter is the part that lies within the pelvis.

Any patient being considered for PD should be fully assessed to ensure there are no surgical contraindications to PD (see Table 9.3.5). Prior to insertion the exit site should be marked and bowel preparation with laxatives to avoid constipation should be considered. Administration of prophylactic antibiotics at the time of placement is standard practice to prevent subsequent catheter infection, peritonitis, and wound infection.

Catheters are placed under strict aseptic technique either as an open procedure and to date more often as a laparoscopic procedure under general anaesthesia. They may also be inserted blind using a Tenckhoff trocar or the Seldinger technique.

Complications of catheter insertion

(i) *Haemorrhage* may occur as a result of trauma to omental or mesenteric vessels as the catheter is inserted. This is more

Table 9.3.5 Surgical contraindications to continuous ambulatory peritoneal dialysis (CAPD)

Absolute contraindications	Relative contraindications
Extensive intra-abdominal adhesions	Peritoneal leaks
Sepsis of abdominal wall	Large polycystic kidneys
Encapsulating peritoneal sclerosis	Stomas
Non-reparable defects (e.g. hernia, omphalocele, gastroschisis)	Inflammatory, ischaemic bowel disease, or frequent episodes of diverticulitis

Table 9.3.6 Options for immunosuppression in kidney transplantation. Most patients receive induction therapy (usually anti-CD25) followed by maintenance therapy with a calcineurin inhibitor, an antimetabolite, and steroids (which may be withdrawn in the early postoperative phase)

Class	Drug names	Common side effects
Induction antibody		
Non-depleting		
Anti-CD25	Basiliximab, daclizumab	Rare
Depleting		
Monoclonal	Campath-1H (anti-CD52)	Lymphopenia
Polyclonal	Anti-thymocyte globulin (ATG)	Lymphopenia, infections, lymphoma
Calcineurin inhibitor	Ciclosporin	Nephrotoxicity, hypertension, hyperlipidaemia, gum hyperplasia, tremor
	Tacrolimus	Nephrotoxicity, tremor, hyperlipidaemia, glucose intolerance
Target of rapamycin inhibitor	Sirolimus, everolimus	Impaired wound healing, lymphocele, proteinuria, hyperlipidaemia, acne, rash, lung injury
Antimetabolite	Mycophenolate	Diarrhoea, leucopenia
	Azathioprine	Macrocytosis, leucopenia, myelodysplasia
Corticosteroids	Prednisolone	Hypertension, glucose intolerance, skin thinning, osteoporosis

common with blind insertion. Heavy bleeding particularly with hypotension will require a return to theatre.

(ii) *Perforated viscus* is a well-recognized hazard of blind and laparoscopic insertion. It is rare with open insertion. The commonest injuries are to the bowel and bladder.

(iii) *Wound infections* are relatively rare but if they happen are a serious complication as they may jeopardize the success of the catheter. Usual organisms include *Staphylococcus aureus* and *Pseudomonas* species. If the exit site and tunnel are infected then it is highly likely that the catheter will have to be removed.

(iv) *Catheter displacement* is probably the most common problem encountered after PD insertion. It manifests within the first few weeks after insertion and usually when peritoneal dialysis is commenced. Dialysate fluid runs into the cavity but drains out slowly or not at all. An abdominal X-ray usually confirms the diagnosis and plans have to be made to re-position the catheter surgically or radiologically.

The longer-term risk of PD is infection i.e. peritonitis caused by contamination of the fluid during the exchange procedure usually by staphylococcus species. This can present in many different ways, but the common finding is always a 'cloudy' bag (cloudy effluent because of the increased number of leucocytes). The patient may feel well, or have abdominal pain and peritonitis on examination. Very rarely they may present with septic shock. Alternative causes of peritonitis such as bowel perforation should be considered and excluded, especially if the PD fluid grows multiple bowel flora organisms (consistent with perforation) or the patient is very sick. However, intraperitoneal air is a common finding in PD and does not prove perforation.

A later complication of PD (which may develop after the technique is stopped for other reasons) is encapsulating peritoneal sclerosis. This presents typically with symptoms of sub-acute small bowel obstruction and intestinal failure. It is associated with prior recurrent peritonitis or high usage of high-strength dialysate, but there are no proven effective therapies once it develops except for radical peritonectomy and it is often eventually fatal.

Kidney transplantation

Transplantation has revolutionized the prognosis of patients with ESRD improving both the quantity and quality of life of recipients. Donors may be deceased (either heart beating or non-heart beating) or living (either related or unrelated). All recipients require lifelong immunosuppression (see Table 9.3.6) which has associated risks of infections and malignancy. Furthermore, the most commonly-used immunosuppressants (i.e. calcineurin inhibitors) are nephrotoxic so management of immunosuppression is a balance of avoiding rejection and prevention complications of immunosuppression. Specific urological aspects of transplantation are discussed elsewhere.

Conclusion

CKD (as currently defined) is common but frequently mild. However, CKD may progress and advanced CKD and ESRD have major implications for those affected. Priorities of management include cardiovascular risk reduction, retarding progression of kidney disease and preparing for renal replacement therapy.

Further reading

Levey AS, Eckardt KU, Tsukamoto Y, *et al.* Definition and classification of chronic kidney disease: a position statement from Kidney Disease: Improving Global Outcomes (KDIGO). *Kidney Int* 2005; **67**(6):2089–100.

References

1. Levey AS, Eckardt KU, Tsukamoto Y, *et al.* Definition and classification of chronic kidney disease: a position statement from Kidney Disease: Improving Global Outcomes (KDIGO). *Kidney Int* 2005; **67**(6):2089–100.
2. Kidney Disease: Improving Global Outcomes (KDIGO) CKD Work Group. KDIGO 2012 Clinical Practice Guideline for the Evaluation

and Management of Chronic Kidney Disease. *Kidney Int Suppl* 2012; **3**:1–150.

3. Coresh J, Selvin E, Stevens LA, *et al.* Prevalence of chronic kidney disease in the United States. *JAMA* 2007; **298**(17):2038–47.
4. Hillege HL, Janssen WM, Bak AA, *et al.* Microalbuminuria is common, also in a nondiabetic, nonhypertensive population, and an independent indicator of cardiovascular risk factors and cardiovascular morbidity. *J Int Med* 2001; **249**(6):519–26.
5. Stevens PE, O'Donoghue DJ, de Lusignan S, *et al.* Chronic kidney disease management in the United Kingdom: NEOERICA project results. *Kidney Int* 2007; **72**(1):92–9.
6. Rutkowski M, Mann W, Derose S, *et al.* Implementing KDOQI CKD Definition and Staging Guidelines in Southern California Kaiser Permanente. *Am J Kidney Dis* 2009; **53**(3 Suppl 3):S86–S99.
7. Effect of intensive therapy on the development and progression of diabetic nephropathy in the Diabetes Control and Complications Trial. The Diabetes Control and Complications (DCCT) Research Group. *Kidney Int* 1995; **47**(6):1703–20.
8. Klahr S, Levey AS, Beck GJ, *et al.* The effects of dietary protein restriction and blood-pressure control on the progression of chronic renal disease. Modification of Diet in Renal Disease Study Group. *New Engl J Med* 1994; **330**(13):877–84.
9. Jafar TH, Schmid CH, Landa M, *et al.* Angiotensin-converting enzyme inhibitors and progression of nondiabetic renal disease. A metaz analysis of patient-level data. *Ann Int Med* 2001; **135**(2):73–87.
10. Baigent C, Landray MJ, Reith C, *et al.* The effects of lowering LDL cholesterol with simvastatin plus ezetimibe in patients with chronic kidney disease (Study of Heart and Renal Protection): a randomised placebo-controlled trial. *Lancet* 2011; **377**(9784):2181–92.
11. Schaefer L, Schaefer RM. A primer on iron therapy. *Nephrol Dial Transplant* 2007; **22**(9):2429–31.
12. Pfeffer MA, Burdmann EA, Chen C-Y, *et al.* A trial of darbepoetin alfa in type 2 diabetes and chronic kidney disease. *New Engl J Med* 2009; **361**(21):2019–32.
13. de Brito-Ashurst I, Varagunam M, Raftery MJ, Yaqoob MM. Bicarbonate supplementation slows progression of CKD and improves nutritional status. *J Am Soc Nephrol* 2009; **20**(9):2075–84.
14. National Kidney Foundation. NKF-DOQI Clinical Practice Guidelines for Vascular Access. 2006. Available at: http://www.kidney.org
15. The Renal Association. *Treatment of Adults and Children with Renal Failure: Standards and Audit Measures*, 3rd edition. Available at: http://www.renal.org [Online].
16. Winearls CG, Fluck R, Mitchell DC, *et al.* The Organisation and Delivery of the Vascular Access Service for Maintenance Haemodialysis Patients. Report of a Joint Working Party, 2006. Available at: http://www.vascularsociety.org.uk/Docs/VASCULAR%20ACCESS%20JOINT%20WORKING%20PARTY%20REPORT.pdf [Online].
17. Vascular Access Society Guidelines. Available at: http://www.vascularacesssociety.com [Online].
18. Roy-Chaudhury P, Arend L, Zhang J, *et al.* Neointimal hyperplasia in early arteriovenous fistula failure. *Am J Kidney Dis* 2007; **50**(5):782–90.
19. Kokubo T, Ishikawa N, Uchida H, *et al.* CKD Accelerates Development of Neointimal Hyperplasia in Arteriovenous Fistulas. *J Am Soc Nephrol* 2009; **20**(6):1236–45.
20. National Kidney Care Audit: Vascular Access Report 2011. Available at: http://content.digital.nhs.uk/article/2021/Website-Search?productid=2411&q=National+Kidney+Care+Audit%3a+Vascular+Access+Report+2011&sort=Relevance&size=10&page=1&area=both#top [Online].
21. Wells AC, Fernando B, Butler A, *et al.* Selective use of ultrasonographic vascular mapping in the assessment of patients before haemodialysis access surgery. *Br J Surg* 2005; **92**(11):1439–43.
22. Lemson MS, Leunissen KM, Tordoir JH, Does pre-operative duplex examination improve patency rates of Brescio-Cimino fistulas? *Nephrol Dial Transplant* 1998; **13**(6):1360–1.
23. Tordoir JHM, Rooyens P, Dammers R, *et al.* Prospective evaluation of failure modes in autogenous radiocephalic wrist access for haemodialysis. *Neprol Dial Transplant* 2003; **18**(2):378–83.

CHAPTER 9.4

Kidney transplantation

Jeff A. Lafranca, Dennis A. Hesselink, and Frank J.M.F. Dor

Introduction to kidney transplantation

Chronic kidney disease (CKD) is an important clinical problem. In the United States, between 1988–1994 and 2005–2010, the overall prevalence estimate for CKD, defined by an eGFR <60 mL/min per 1.73 m^2 or an albumin/creatinine ratio ≥30 mg/g), rose from 12.3% to 14.0%.[1] In addition, in 2010, a total of 116,946 patients began renal replacement therapy (RRT) for end-stage renal disease (ESRD). In the United States, on 31 December 2010, the total prevalent population with treated ESRD was 593,086.[1]

Although patients with ESRD can be successfully treated with haemodialysis or peritoneal dialysis, kidney transplantation is by far the best therapeutic option for the majority of patients with ESRD.[2,3] Compared to other forms of RRT, kidney transplantation leads to superior survival, improved quality of life, enhanced psychosocial development and growth in children, and a reduction of societal costs.[4,5] Currently, over 86,000 patients in the United States are on the wait list for a donor kidney. However, in 2010, only 17,778 kidney transplants were performed. In Eurotransplant, on 31 December 2011, 10,622 patients were waitlisted for a kidney transplant; 3,633 kidneys were transplanted from a deceased donor, 1,339 from a living donor.[6] Only 3 out of 10 patients with ESRD are transplanted, the remaining group stays on dialysis and dies while on the wait list or is removed from the wait list because of a deteriorated clinical condition (Fig. 9.4.1).[1]

Regretfully, the shortage in donor organs prevails. The amount of donor kidneys retrieved by deceased donation still remains insufficient to meet the demand. One of the solutions to this problem is live kidney donation. The advantages of live donor kidney transplantation are numerous and include among others, that it is an elective operation with short ischaemia times. Transplantation with a kidney from a living donor shows superior outcome in comparison to deceased donation with a mean graft survival benefit of 10 years.[7] For those patients who cannot directly receive a kidney from their living donor, inventive alternative programmes for living kidney donation have been developed. Such programmes include paired-kidney exchange, blood group AB0-incompatible transplantation, and desensitization of the sensitized recipient. Furthermore, living kidney donation programmes also increase the chances of being transplanted for those patients who do not have a living donor by making the limited number of deceased donor kidneys available for fewer patients.

However, one must be aware that live donor nephrectomy is a major operation, especially because the donor is not a patient but a healthy person. Donor safety and ensuring an optimal condition of the donor kidney are therefore crucial requirements for the success of living donor kidney transplant programmes.

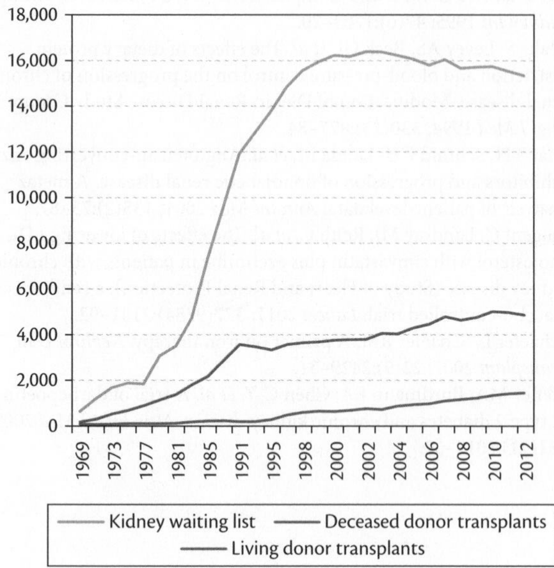

Fig. 9.4.1 Dynamics of the Eurotransplant kidney transplant waiting list and transplants between 1969 and 2012.

Source: data from Axel Rahmel (ed), *Eurotransplant International Foundation, Annual Report 2012*, Eurotransplant, The Netherlands, Copyright © 2012, available from https://www.eurotransplant.org/cms/mediaobject.php?file=AR2012.pdf

Deceased kidney donation

Deceased kidney donation can be divided in two types: donation after brain death (DBD); and donation after circulatory death (DCD). Formerly, these types were classified as heart-beating donation (HBD) and non-heart-beating donation (NHBD).[8]

Donation after brain death

The majority of organs of deceased donors are retrieved from DBD donors, although in the Netherlands, a trend towards more DCD is seen; in 2011, more than 50% of the deceased donor kidney transplants (KTXs) performed came from a DCD.[9] DBD can only be performed when a patient is declared brain death, which is based on strict neurological criteria (irreversible loss of all functions of the entire brain, including the brain stem). It can be further divided into 'standard criteria' and 'extended criteria' donation. Organ donors who meet the standard criteria for donation after brain death are 59 years of age or younger. The extended criteria for donation after brain death involve the use of organs from donors older than 60 and from donors between 50 and 59 years who have two or three of the following conditions: cerebrovascular accident as the cause of death, a serum creatinine concentration of more than 1.5 mg per decilitre (133 μmol/L), and a history of hypertension. In recent years, as a result of organ donor shortage, an increase has been observed in the use of extended criteria DBD donors, which are considered of inferior quality compared to standard criteria donors, resulting in worse patient and graft survival.[10]

After declaration of brain death and consent for donation, a DBD donor is transported to the operating room, with artificial circulation and respiratory support. Then, when dissection of the organs is finished, the major thoracic and abdominal vessels are cannulated. The start of the cold perfusion resembles the start of the cold ischaemia time. Hereafter, the procurement of the organs can be continued. After retrieval, the organs are prepared for travel (cold storage or machine perfusion).

Donation after circulatory death

DCD has been developed as a valuable addition to DBD as a means to expand the deceased donor organ pool. The major difference in this type of donors compared to DBD is the fact that the organs are no longer perfused after circulatory arrest (usually after a 'switch off' in the ICU or operating theatre), and therefore have an additional warm ischaemia time (from circulatory arrest until cold perfusion). A DCD donor must be rapidly transported to the operating room after a period of five minutes 'no touch', as the procedure is focused on minimizing the warm ischaemia time. Longer warm ischaemia time has always been associated with more and longer delayed graft function (DGF) and poorer graft survival. However, in recent years, outcome of transplantation with organs from DCD donors has proved to be more or less equal to DBD.[11–14] To classify DCD, the modified Maastricht classification is used (Table 9.4.1).[15] Categories I, II, and V describe organ retrieval that follows unexpected cardiac arrest (uncontrolled DCD). Categories III and IV refer to retrieval that follows death resulting from the planned withdrawal of life-sustaining cardiorespiratory support (controlled DCD).[16] New definitions and guidelines are underway following a recent consensus meeting.

Right or left?

In deceased donor kidney transplantation, in general, both kidneys are normally retrieved. Several studies report no significant differences regarding outcome of a right or left donor kidney.[17,18] However, Vacher-Coponat *et al.* report that receipt of a right kidney from a DBD donor, is a risk factor for inferior outcome, namely more DGF in the first year after transplantation and lower one-year survival of right-sided kidney grafts; this was attributed to the fact that a venous anastomosis may be more complicated in case of a short right vein.[19]

Live kidney donation

As pointed out above, increasing the donor pool is extremely important. Campaigns to stimulate people to register as a donor are propagated worldwide. Most countries have an 'opt-in' system (if you wish to be a donor, you should register as such), some use an 'opt-out' system (everyone is a presumed donor unless stated otherwise). Nonetheless, the amount of available organs retrieved from deceased donors is by far not sufficient for the rising need of donor kidneys. Furthermore, it is unlikely that these campaigns and regulations will ever lead to a sufficient amount of kidneys. Different strategies have been developed in order to increase the donor pool. Expanding criteria for deceased donation and modulation of these organs by new technology to improve quality, such as by machine perfusion,[20] as well as changing legal systems into 'opt-out' systems have been ventured. In our opinion, the promotion of living kidney donation has proved to be the most successful solution to this problem. In the authors' centre, currently about 75% of all transplanted kidneys come from live donors.

Types of live donation

The former most used classification of donation was divided in 'related' and 'unrelated' donation, which only refers to the fact whether the donor and recipient are genetically related or not. In 2011, the Living Organ Donation working group of 'Ethical, Legal, and Psychosocial Aspects of Transplantation (ELPAT)', a section of the European Society for Organ Transplantation, proposed a new type of classification regarding donors,[21] as it was noticed that many different (confusing) classifications of live organ donation were in practice internationally. This new classification is based on the degree of specificity with which donors identify intended recipients and to subsequently verify whether the donation to these recipients occurs directly or indirectly. The classification is divided in 'specified' and 'unspecified' donation. Specified donation includes direct donation to an intended recipient, donation to a genetically and/or emotionally (un)related recipient. It can be subdivided by direct donation, or indirect donation, which comprehends indirect donation to the intended donor, or donation through an exchange programme (Fig. 9.4.2). Unspecified donation is donation to an

Table 9.4.1 Modified Maastricht classification for types of DCD (TC = Transplant centre, ICU = intensive care unit)

Category (type of DCD)	Status of donor	Practiced
Category I (uncontrolled)	Dead on arrival	Emergency department (TC)
Category II (uncontrolled)	Unsuccessful resuscitation	Emergency department (TC)
Category III (controlled)	Anticipating cardiac arrest	Emergency department and ICU
Category IV (controlled)	Cardiac arrest while brain dead	Emergency department and ICU
Category V (uncontrolled)	Unexpected arrest in ICU-patient	ICU (TC)

Adapted from *Transplantation proceedings*, Volume 27, Number 5, Kootstra, G *et al.*, 'Categories of non-heart-beating donors', pp. 2893, Copyright © 1995, with permission from Elsevier, http://www.sciencedirect.com/science/journal/00411345. **Source:** data from Sánchez-Fructuoso *et al.*, 'Renal transplantation from non-heart beating donors: a promising alternative to enlarge the donor pool', *Journal of the American Society of Nephrology*, Volume 11, Number 2, pp. 350–358, Copyright © 2000 by the American Society of Nephrology.

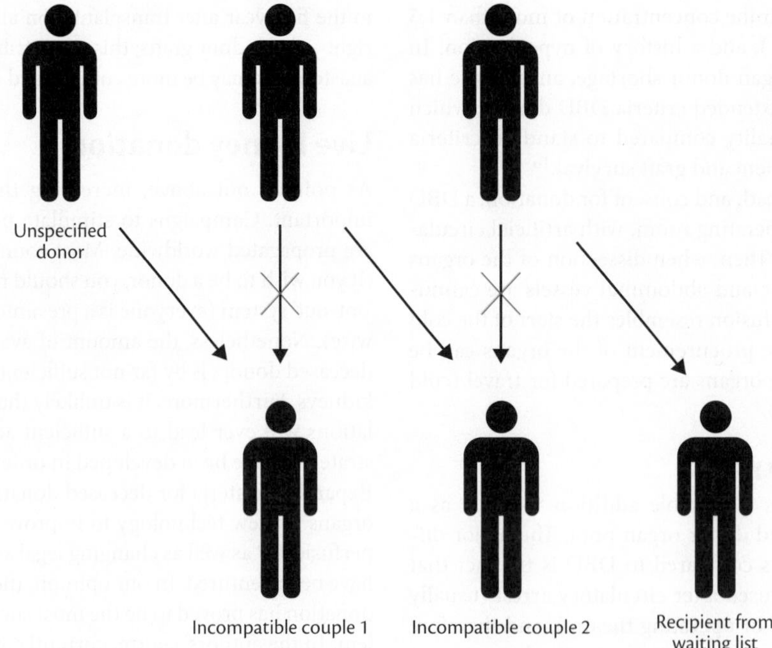

Fig. 9.4.2 Schematic illustration of the domino-paired exchange programme principle.

anonymous and unspecified recipient (e.g. donation to the waiting list or to the recipient of an exchange couple in the case of domino-paired exchange).

Selection and screening of living kidney donors

Obviously, not everyone can donate a kidney. Ideally, living donors are carefully screened by the transplant team, consisting of nephrologists, transplant surgeons, anaesthetists, psychologists, social workers, and nurse practitioners. In some conditions, the donor is also screened by a cardiologist. Donors are extensively screened for several viruses, blood type, human leukocyte antigen (HLA) type, kidney function, and risk factors for the future development of kidney disease. Prior to surgery, all donors undergo imaging (either a computed tomography (CT) scan or an MRI) to visualize the renal anatomy and parenchyma (to identify cysts or other anatomical variations). Based on this scan, a decision is made which kidney will be extracted. Factors that are assessed on the scan are renal vascular multiplicity, renal artery stenosis, and the size and aspect of the kidneys. In general, a potential living kidney donor is a healthy person with no co-morbidities.

In a recent European Union sponsored project, the 'Living Organ Donation in Europe' (EULOD) project, current European practices in live organ donation were investigated, and found to differ significantly within Europe (and compared to the United States).[22] The transplant community has established international guidelines for the living kidney donor (e.g. Amsterdam Forum 2004).[23] However, since the community is seeking for options to further expand the donor pool, there is a tendency towards accepting so called 'extended live kidney donors', which are discussed below.

Extended criteria living kidney donors

Extended live donors consist of potential kidney donors with one or more defined co-morbidities, such as overweight or obesity, hypertension, and advanced age. Some centres consider donors with more than one renal artery or vein as an extended donor as well. In most transplant centres, a BMI higher than 35 is considered a relative contraindication for donation. Because obesity increases the risk of complications after surgery, obese donors were also thought to be more prone for complications. However, in general, live donors consist of a highly selected group of healthy individuals and therefore cannot be compared to the general population regarding general health or co-morbidities. Furthermore, a recent meta-analysis revealed that, at least regarding short-term outcome, obesity is no contraindication for live kidney donation.[24] Long-term consequences of live kidney donation for this specific group are not yet fully clear. One can envisage a possible higher lifetime risk of hypertension, diabetes mellitus, or other morbidity. A possible solution for potential donors with morbid obesity could be bariatric surgery prior to donation. Several case reports have been published with good results.[25,26]

Increasing the maximum age for live kidney donation will provide more donors. However, using older donors for live kidney transplantation remains controversial. This specific group of donors is believed to have a higher chance on complications compared to 'younger' donors. No consensus is reached in current guidelines, however several studies show that older donors (e.g. above 65 years) have no higher postoperative complication rate, although kidneys from older donors tend to have inferior graft outcome.[27] In the centre of the authors from 1994 to 2006, 539 donors were followed, of which 117 donors were 60 years of age or older. Donor age did not influence graft survival. After kidney donation, the decline in eGFR of the donors themselves was not different in younger donors compared to the elderly. Therefore, live kidney donation by elderly is considered safe.[28,29]

In 2004, in 'the Consensus Statement of the Amsterdam Forum on the care of the live kidney donor', a guideline regarding donors with hypertension was adopted. Donors with a blood pressure >140/90 mmHg should generally not be accepted as donors. Some donors with easily controlled hypertension who meet other defined criteria (e.g. >50 years of age, GFR >80 mL/min per 1.73 m^2, and urinary albumin excretion <30 mg/day) may represent a low-risk group for development of kidney disease after donation and may be acceptable as kidney donors.[23] Little literature is available regarding these extended live kidney donors, although it seems that a hypertensive donor has no worse outcome after donor nephrectomy.[30–32] Recent data suggest that hypertensive living kidney donors have similar outcome in terms of blood pressure and renal function as donors without hypertension, early, and one and five years after donation.[33] Although practice in countries differs,[22] it is generally accepted that well-controlled hypertension, with a maximum of two antihypertensive drugs, is safe.

Recently, a systematic review is published, giving an overview of several extended donor criteria and outcome after live kidney donation.[34]

Alternative programmes for living kidney donation

Cross-over (exchange programme)

The cross-over programme is a useful addition to the live kidney donation programme. In certain cases, the problem arises that donor-recipient couples are incompatible because of blood group AB0 incompatibility or a positive cross-match. Donor and the recipient are then enrolled in the exchange programme and if a match is found, a cross-over donation/transplantation is executed. For example, if donor A and recipient A are incompatible, and the same holds true for donor B and recipient B, then donor A can donate to recipient B, and donor B to recipient A.[35,36] These inventive strategies to optimize the living donor kidney pool have been initiated in the Netherlands, where a national kidney exchange programme is successful. Since the start of this programme in 2004, 544 domino-recipient pairs have enrolled, 214 exchange transplantations have been carried out, and 198 pairs have been transplanted outside this specific programme (transplantation after unspecified donation or domino-paired exchange). Currently, there are 56 pairs still waiting. Four times a year, a computerized matching is performed, which ranks on six conditions: a maximum number of matched couples; blood group identical above blood group compatible matches; priority to patients with a low match probability; short chains (e.g. rather two doublets than one quartet); couples distributed over multiple centres and wait time calculated from the first day of dialysis.

In the Netherlands, the donor travels to the centre where the transplantation is performed. In other countries, such as the United States, the kidney is transported to the centre of the recipient after retrieval.

Another relatively new concept is the unbalanced exchange donation. This type of donation/transplantation can be organized if a compatible pair is willing to exchange and thereby facilitate transplantation for individuals with an incompatible live donor. With this programme, the number of kidney transplants can be increased even further.[37]

Unspecified donation

A relatively new and rapidly growing source of donor organs is established by unspecified donation. Former terminology used for this kind of donation was 'anonymous', 'altruistic' or 'Good Samaritan' donation. However, these terms might not entirely cover the meaning of an unspecified donation.[21] Two options of unspecified donation are possible; unspecified donation to one recipient on the waitlist or unspecified donation in the domino-paired exchange programme (explained below). A psychological assessment is performed in most transplant centres before donation to clarify the donor's motives. From 2000 to 2008, in the authors' centre, 51 unspecified donations have been performed, ultimately resulting in 85 transplantations.[38] Since 2008, an additional 39 unspecified donations have been performed, leading to 69 transplantations. In total, until September 2012, there have been 90 unspecified donations, leading to 154 transplantations in our centre (unpublished data).

Domino-paired (exchange programme)

Another type of cross-over donation is domino-paired donation. If an unspecified donor is willing to donate, the organ can be allocated to the best recipient match on the waiting list. By this, the donor's gift can initiate a chain of matches. In example, unspecified donor X, can donate to recipient A, which is incompatible with his donor A. However, donor A can now donate to recipient B and his incompatible donor B can donate to recipient C, and so on (Fig. 9.4.2).[38,39] The optimal chain length for living donor kidney exchange programmes is three. Longer chains with their inherent logistic burden do not lead to significantly more transplants.[36]

Blood group AB0-incompatible transplantation

One of the recent developments in successful alternative programmes is blood group AB0-incompatible kidney transplantation. The first attempt of this kind of transplantation was made in 1955.[40,41] However, due to poor graft survival as a result of anti-blood group antibodies, this technique was abandoned. For this reason AB0-incompatibility was, until recently, an absolute contraindication for donation and the only solution was a specified indirect donation through the national exchange programme. However, with the use of apheresis techniques, which allow for the (selective) removal of naturally-occurring anti-blood group AB0 antibodies and the use powerful specific immunosuppressive drugs (such as rituximab and intravenous immunoglobulin), this form of transplantation has become possible without the need for pre-transplant splenectomy.[35,42–45]

Desensitization prior to transplantation

Kidney recipients who have become sensitized to HLA as a result of previous transplantation, pregnancy, or blood transfusion have an increased likelihood of a positive cross-match, indicating the presence of donor-specific anti-HLA antibodies. This is associated with hyper-acute antibody-mediated rejection, and leads to a high rate of allograft loss. A way to enable this type of transplantation is to 'desensitize' the recipient. By using apheresis techniques and administering specific new immunosuppressive agents, the donor-specific anti-HLA antibodies are removed and their production decreased. Although initial results seem promising, this form of transplantation should be regarded as experimental and long-term outcomes are awaited, before this type of transplantation can become a fully accepted therapy.[46]

The above-mentioned alternative programmes for living kidney donation give an overview of the actual 'hierarchy'. Specified direct living donor kidney transplantation is the preferred option. If a recipient has an incompatible live donor or no live donor at all, he or she can enrol in one of the crossover programmes (specified indirect or unspecified). If no match is found, AB0-incompatible transplantation or desensitization become options (specified direct).

Operation techniques for live donor nephrectomy

Since the first live donor nephrectomy in 1954,[47] there has been a great development in operation methods and techniques, with an important shift towards more minimally invasive techniques. The latter has significantly contributed to the success of live donor KTx. Several techniques are available, open or endoscopic, with a trans- or retroperitoneal approach. Furthermore, hand- or robot-assisted techniques are optional in laparoscopic donor nephrectomy.

Open donor nephrectomy (lumbotomy)

The first commonly used open technique was carried out with a lumbotomy (flank incision) with the incision covering the rib cage (10–20 cm). The main disadvantage of this technique is that this incision is 'muscle-cutting' and is therefore more prone to complications and chronic pain.[48,49] Furthermore, in some centres, this technique is combined with a rib resection in order to create a wider operative field. After incision, the fat is dissected, and the peritoneum is mobilized. Gerota's fascia is opened and the perirenal fat is dissected in all directions, hereby exposing the kidney. After identification of the ureter, the renal hilum is dissected, and vessels identified. After dividing the ureter, the vessels are divided using a stapler or clamps (and later closed with sutures). After preparing the kidney on the bench, all anatomical layers of the donor wound are closed with appropriate sutures.

Anterior subcostal extraperitoneal donor nephrectomy

In 1981, the anterior subcostal extraperitoneal approach was described.[50] Similar to the lumbotomy, this extraperitoneal approach reduces the chance of damaging intra-abdominal organs to a minimum. However, the incision size is generally smaller (up to 15 cm). The rest of the operation is comparable to the lumbotomy approach.

Open transperitoneal donor nephrectomy

This approach is in essence comparable to the technique above; however, its transperitoneal aspect has a great risk of intra-abdominal injury.[51] Therefore, this technique is not widely used in transplant centres anymore.[22,52]

'Mini-open' donor nephrectomy

First described by Nadey Hakim,[53] this technique is essentially the same as the standard open nephrectomy, however with a smaller incision (4–10 cm) (Fig. 9.4.3). An advantage of this technique is shorter recovery time and less pain compared to the standard open technique.[54] Disadvantage is the limited exposure created with this incision. The donor is placed in the lateral decubitus position. When after incision Gerota's fascia is reached, the dissection of the fat is the same as for the lumbotomy approach. Dividing of the ureter and vessels is mostly performed with articulating staplers.

Endoscopic donor nephrectomy

In 1995, the first laparoscopic donor nephrectomy (LDN) was performed by Lloyd Ratner and Louis Kavoussi.[55] Over the years, this technique has become increasingly more adopted and proves to have superior donor and graft outcome above the open techniques.[22,52,56–58] The clearest advantage is the use of several small incisions (0.5–1 cm) for the trocars instead of a large incision (Figs 9.4.4 and 9.4.5). After positioning of the patient and insertion of the trocars, the colon is mobilized, thereby exposing the retroperitoneal space. Gerota's fascia is then opened and the perirenal fat is dissected away from the kidney. After dissection of the ureter, the renal artery and vein are prepared. Several techniques are available for ligation and stapling of the vessels.[59] Most transplant centres use a linear or reticulating stapler. For extraction of the kidney, a Pfannenstiel

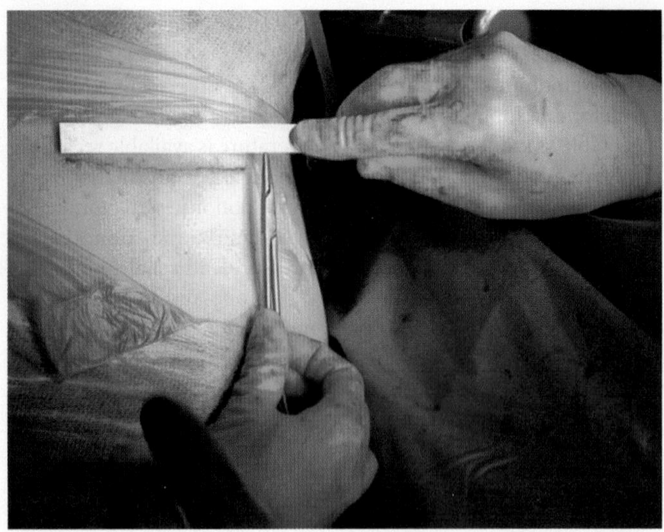

Fig. 9.4.3 Live donor nephrectomy, mini-open technique.

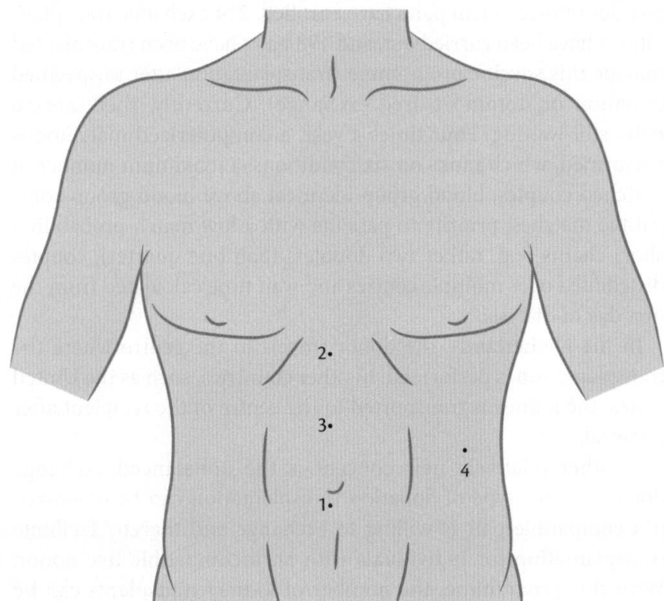

Fig. 9.4.4 Schematic illustration of the positions of the trocars placed during left-sided laparoscopic donor nephrectomy. (1) Infraumbilical open introduction of 10–12 mm blunt tip trocar; (2, 3) 5 mm and 10 mm trocar in epigastric region; and (4) 5 mm trocar laterally above the anterior superior iliac spine, inserted after mobilization large intestine and opening of Gerota's fascia; in small patients trocar 3 can be placed lateral to the umbilicus.

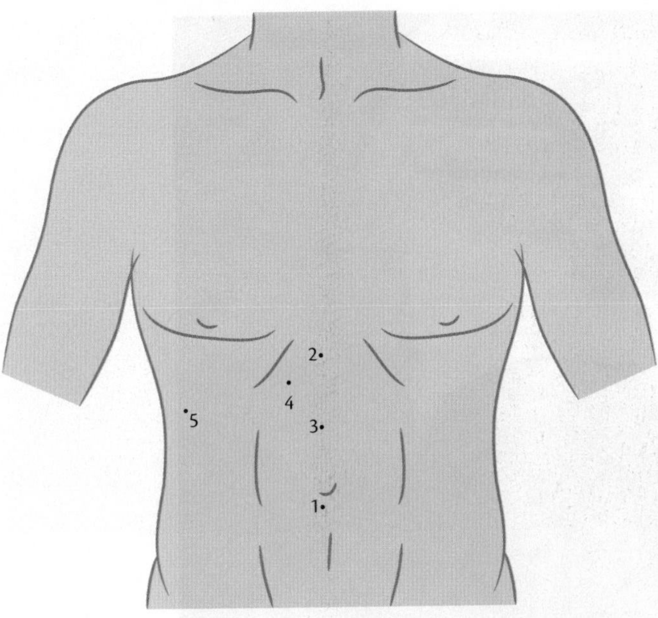

Fig. 9.4.5 Schematic illustration of the positions of the trocars placed during right-sided laparoscopic donor nephrectomy. (1) Infraumbilical open introduction of 10–12 mm blunt tip trocar; (2, 3) 5 mm and 10 mm trocar in epigastric region; (4) second 5 mm trocar in epigastric region, inserted after partial mobilization of the right liver lobe; and (5) 5 mm trocar laterally above the anterior superior iliac spine, inserted after mobilization large intestine and opening of Gerota's fascia.

(caesarian) incision is made of about 9–10 cm. Over the years, there has been an enormous increase in the use of a laparoscopic approach in live donor nephrectomy[22,52,60,61] and is considered as the golden standard in most transplant centres (Fig. 9.4.6).

Hand-assisted transperitoneal laparoscopic donor nephrectomy

In 1998, the hand-assisted laparoscopic donor nephrectomy (HALDN) was described by Wolf *et al.*[62] Using this technique, a port is mounted in the Pfannenstiel-incision through which the hand of a surgeon can be placed. The rest of the procedure is similar to the LDN. This approach enables more accuracy and immediate manual control of any possible bleeding, thus minimizing the possibility of conversion to open surgery. Furthermore, shorter warm ischaemia times (WIT) and shorter operative times are acquired because of the direct manual removal of the kidney after dissecting the vessels.[63–66] Disadvantages are the possible intra-abdominal damage that can occur by this transperitoneal approach and adhesions may be induced. Also, if the donor had previous abdominal surgery, adhesions can be present, and can cause difficulty during the nephrectomy. However, this poses a possible difficulty in all types of transperitoneal nephrectomies.

Hand-assisted retroperitoneoscopic donor nephrectomy

Several years after the introduction of HALDN, in 2002, the hand-assisted retroperitoneoscopic technique was introduced by Wadstrom.[67] In this approach, the surgeon manually dissects the peritoneum from the abdominal wall until a pneumoretroperitoneal space can be created. The kidney can then be visualized and freed from Gerota's fascia and perirenal fat. The other steps of the operation are similar to the (HALDN). The retroperitoneal approach also reduces the theoretical risk of intestinal injury and postoperative intestinal complications, with shorter hospital stay, shorter operative time, and shorter warm ischaemia time and

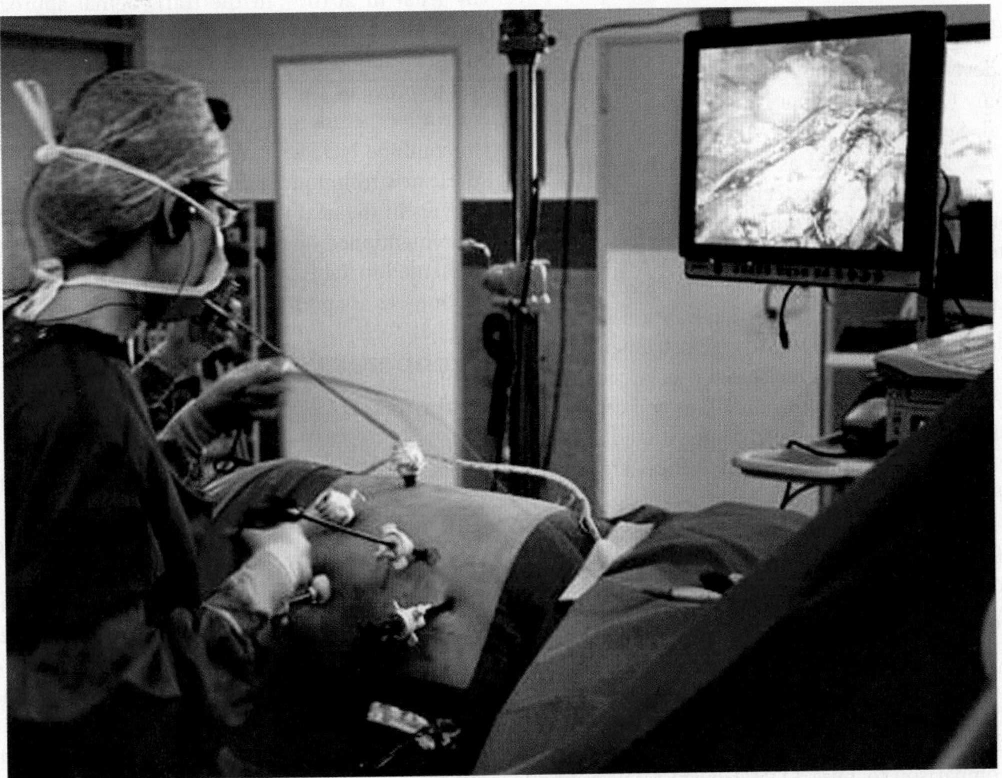

Fig. 9.4.6 Live donor nephrectomy, laparoscopic technique.

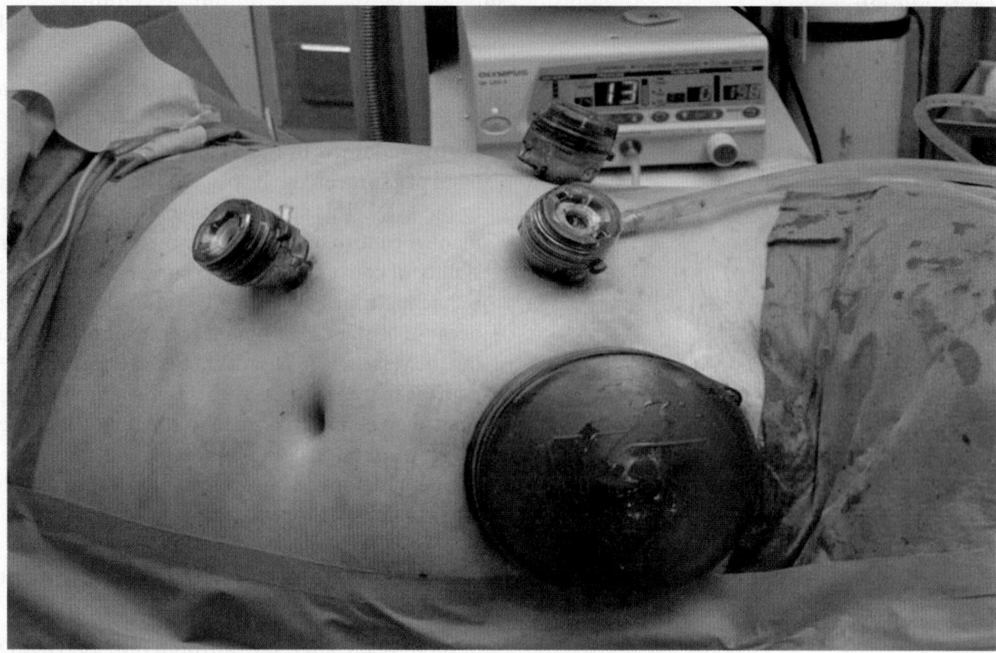

Fig. 9.4.7 Live donor nephrectomy, hand-assisted technique.

convalescence as a consequence.[68,69] One general disadvantage of the hand-assisted approaches is the generally uncomfortable position and the fact that that the surgeon's arm is inside the patient for a couple of hours (although with intervals), which can cause a numb hand. This may be explained by the narrow entrance that the hand port, placed in the Pfannenstiel-incision, and the fascia opening, offer (Fig. 9.4.7).

Robot-assisted laparoscopic donor nephrectomy

One of the latest developments is the robotic-assisted laparoscopic donor nephrectomy (RADN) with the Da Vinci Surgical System (Intuitive Surgical, Sunnyvale, CA, USA) and first described in 2002 by Horgan.[70,71] It can be used as in the 'laparoscopic only' approach or with hand assistance. This technique brings more comfort to the surgeon as he or she can sit while operating and does not necessarily have to be in the near proximity of the patient. Surgeons are provided with superior 3D visualization, enhanced dexterity because of an enhanced rotation angle of the robotic wrists (540 degrees vs. 180 degrees in case of laparoscopic instruments being moved by human hands), greater precision, an enlarged image, computerized correction of undesirable vibrations and ergonomic comfort. The feasibility and safety has been demonstrated in recent studies, however studies regarding cost-effectiveness are eagerly awaited (Fig. 9.4.8).[72–74]

Laparoendoscopic single site surgery donor nephrectomy

The first single-port umbilical donor nephrectomy was described by Gill.[75] Through an intra-umbilical incision a tri-lumen port is inserted in the abdomen. Advantage is that no extra-umbilical skin incisions have to be made. The kidney is also extracted transumbilically. Several studies have shown faster recovery time after donor nephrectomy in comparison to 'pure' LDN. However, this method is associated with a longer warm ischaemia time, not necessarily leading to impaired graft function.[76–78]

Natural orifice transluminal endoscopic surgery donor nephrectomy

This method comprehends several techniques using natural orifices. The first series of transvaginal natural orifice transluminal endoscopic surgery (NOTES)-assisted donor nephrectomy was described by Alcaraz in 2011.[79] The idea was originally described by Allaf in 2010.[80] In the transvaginal approach, the vagina is used as a working port during the whole procedure, and as kidney extraction site. Since this technique is relatively new, it has yet to prove its value. Importantly, this technique leads to a longer warm ischaemia time. A combination of the latest approaches is to combine NOTES with robotic-assistance.[81,82] Experience with these new techniques has yet to be expanded, but they could be key players in the next era of live kidney donation. An overview of all aforementioned operation techniques and their (dis)advantages is presented in Table 9.4.2 and available literature comparing several techniques are presented in Table 9.4.3.

Preoperative considerations

Right or left?

Since the introduction of the laparoscopic donor nephrectomy technique, left-sided nephrectomy was believed to be preferred, because the liver could pose a technical problem in right-sided nephrectomy.[83,84] However, in 2002, Lind *et al.* described no significant differences between sides regarding conversion rate, complications, hospital stay, thrombosis, graft function, and graft survival.[85] Furthermore, in 2009, Dols *et al.* described superior results of right-sided donations regarding blood loss and operative time.[86] Furthermore, although the left kidney has a longer renal vein, resulting in an easier venous anastomosis in the recipient, more veins drain into the left renal vein (adrenal vein, gonadal vein, lumbar veins), which may complicate dissection of the left renal vein. Recent data suggest comparable outcome of right-sided donor nephrectomy.[86,87] If both kidneys from a donor have the same size,

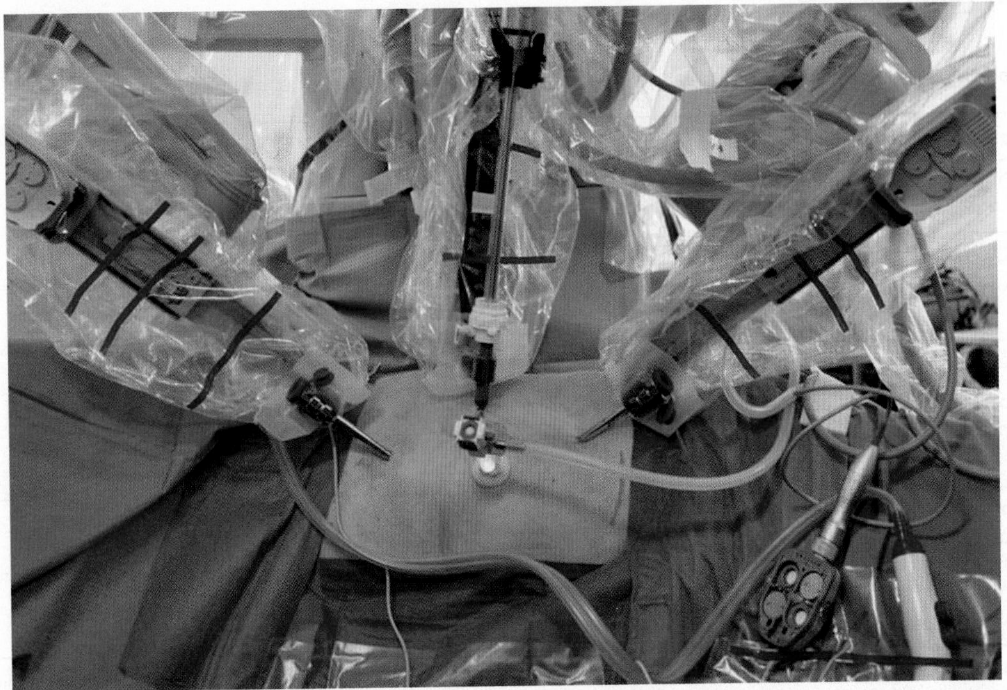

Fig. 9.4.8 Laparoscopic donor nephrectomy, robot-assisted technique.

Table 9.4.2 Overview of different operation techniques of live donor nephrectomy and their (dis)advantages

Operation technique	Advantages	Disadvantages
Open donor nephrectomy	◆ Manual control of bleeding if required	◆ Incision length ◆ Longer hospital stay ◆ Longer recovery time ◆ Rib resection (optional) ◆ Muscle-splitting -> chronic pain
Anterior subcostal extraperitoneal donor nephrectomy	◆ All benefits of the standard open approach ◆ Smaller incision size	◆ All disadvantages of the standard open approach
Open transperitoneal donor nephrectomy	◆ Large exposure	◆ Possible intra-abdominal damage
'Mini-open' donor nephrectomy	◆ Smaller incision size	◆ Limited exposure/view
Laparoscopic transperitoneal donor nephrectomy	◆ Small scars ◆ No muscle-splitting ◆ Faster recovery time ◆ Shorter hospital stay	◆ Little longer warm ischaemia time ◆ No manual control possible
Hand-assisted transperitoneal laparoscopic donor nephrectomy	◆ All benefits of the laparoscopic approach ◆ Shorter warm ischaemia time ◆ Manual control of bleeding if required	◆ Possible intra-abdominal damage ◆ Adhesions if prior surgery is present
Hand-assisted retroperitoneal donor nephrectomy	◆ All benefits of the laparoscopic approach ◆ All benefits of the hand assistance ◆ Minimal chance on intra-abdominal damage	◆ Relatively new technique ◆ New learning curve
Robot-assisted laparoscopic donor nephrectomy	◆ Enhanced rotation angle ◆ 3D-vision ◆ Correction of unnecessary vibration	◆ Cost-effectiveness ◆ Possible intra-abdominal damage ◆ Longer operative time due to set-up ◆ Learning curve
Laparoendoscopic single site surgery (LESS) donor nephrectomy	◆ Improved cosmesis ◆ Faster recovery	◆ Longer warm ischaemia time
Natural orifice translumenal endoscopic surgery (NOTES) donor nephrectomy	◆ Absence of abdominal scars	◆ Longer warm ischaemia time ◆ No manual/difficult control ◆ Possible intra-abdominal damage

Table 9.4.3 Overview of literature of several operation techniques of live donor nephrectomy

Operation technique	LoE	Literature	Ref	Outcome
CO versus MO donor nephrectomy	3	PS RS, historical controls	157, 160	MO > CO
MO versus LDN	1	RCT PS Meta-analysis	161,158,162	LDN > MO LDN + MO > CO LDN > MO
MO versus HA donor nephrectomy	2	RCT	163	MO
Laparoscopic versus HA donor nephrectomy	2	RCT PS RS historical controls	164–174	Equal outcome HA > LDN > CO HA > LDN
Laparoscopic versus HARP donor nephrectomy	3	PS RS	175–177	HA LS-HA = RS-HA
RA versus CO donor nephrectomy	3	RS, historical controls	178	RA = CO
RA versus LDN	3	PS	74	RA ~ LDN

LoE: level of evidence, CO: conventional open, MO: mini-incision, PS: prospective studies, RS: retrospective studies, LDN: laparoscopic donor nephrectomy, HA: hand-assisted, LS-HA: left-sided hand-assisted, RS-HA: right-sided hand-assisted, HARP: hand-assisted retroperitoneoscopic, RA: robot-assisted

Reproduced with permission from Dols LF *et al.*, 'Live donor nephrectomy: a review of evidence for surgical techniques', *Transplant International*, Volume 23, pp. 121–30, Copyright © 2009 The Authors. Journal compilation © 2009 European Society for Organ Transplantation.

most transplant surgeons nowadays choose a kidney with a single artery (if present) over a kidney with multiple renal arteries, irrespective of the side.

Vascular multiplicity

In order to perform a successful transplantation, careful preparation and extraction of the graft is of great importance. If there is more than one artery, the localization is very important. Donor kidneys with multiple renal vessels constitute 17.1% of the live donor kidneys transplanted over the world.[88–90] The presence of multiple renal arteries presents a challenge, because it may affect the safety of the donor. This, because having multiple renal arteries may lead to intraoperative technical difficulties and complications, such as increased operation time, and dissection or bleeding. Furthermore, arterial reconstructions may need to be made after the kidney has been extracted to enable single arterial anastomosis in the recipient, although others advocate multiple arterial anastomoses in the recipient (Papalois *et al.*, unpublished), sometimes combined with extracorporeal techniques.[91] Although a kidney with single anatomy is preferred, vascular multiplicity is no longer considered as a hard contraindication and has similar outcome both in the donor as in the recipient.[92–95] Usually, a small (capsular) artery that vascularizes a minor part of the upper pole of the kidney can be safely sacrificed. However, accessory lower pole arteries must be spared at all costs in order to prevent possible ischaemia of the ureter. Renal veins normally communicate, and (small) accessory renal veins can be safely sacrificed and do not require reconstructive bench surgery.[96]

Ureter

Ideally, the donor ureter length should be as long as possible, to create a ureteroneocystostomy without any tension. Furthermore, the distance between the transplanted kidney and the bladder is difficult to predict beforehand. In LDN, the ureter should be divided at the level crossing the iliac vessels. However, the lower part of the ureter is vascularized from the bladder, so if the ureter is left too long, ischaemia can occur, leading to related complications. In rare cases, the surgeon is forced to create a pyelo-cystostomy or uretero-ureterostomy. This is performed if the ureter is or has become ischaemic, or if the donor ureter is too short. However, based on the literature, in general the ureteroneocystostomy is to be preferred, because of shorter operative time and reduced potential additional morbidity.[97]

Parenchyma

Prior to donation and surgery, the parenchyma of the kidneys is screened for abnormalities. One of these possible abnormalities is a renal cyst, which is a common finding in live kidney donors. Rule *et al.* report that about 53% of 1948 analysed kidney donors between 2000–2008 had one or more cysts.[98] The Bosniak classification for renal cysts is instrumental to judge the risk for malignancy. In the authors' centre, all cysts up to a Bosniak type IIF (cysts with an increased number of hairline-thin septae, with possible minimal enhancement or thickening of the septae or wall) are accepted for donation after appropriate screening by CT-imaging.[99] Living donors from families with autosomal dominant polycystic kidney disease (ADPKD) are at risk for developing ADPKD and should be screened prior to donation. Although, in general, radiological imaging is adequate for diagnosis, it can be missed in donors younger than 40 since ADPKD develops with age. Huang *et al.* described a DNA-screening technique to rule out the diagnosis. They advocate this technique in donors younger than 30 with fewer than 3 (or no) cysts and in donors aged between 30 and 59 with a few non-diagnostic renal cysts.[100]

Selection and screening of recipients

As pointed out earlier, kidney transplantation provides great benefit for patients with ESRD. However, several important factors arise when selecting which patients will benefit and who will not. Obviously, any co-morbidity that may endanger anaesthesia and surgery in general is a relative contraindication. In most recipients, the technical feasibility poses no problem. Possible issues can be peripheral arterial occlusive disease, recurrent deep venous thrombosis, obesity, and previous abdominal surgery in general, or hernia surgery using a mesh. Also, previous urological surgery is not uncommon in kidney transplant recipients (i.e. urinary diversions, such as Bricker's ileal conduit, neobladder reconstructions, such as Studer's pouch, or other bladder reconstruction); in these cases, a urological presence is required if the kidney transplant surgeon is not a urologist.

An increasing problem is the recipient who has been transplanted more than twice. In these cases, a transplant nephrectomy has to be performed prior to a third transplantation. If a recipient has (poly)cystic native kidneys that compromise access to the iliac fossae due to their size, a native nephrectomy is warranted prior to transplantation. In case of suspected vascular pathology (atherosclerosis or deep venous thrombosis), a preoperative CT or MRI scan is used to ensure optimal conditions for vascular anastomosis during implantation. If necessary, a percutaneous transluminal angioplasty is performed, sometimes combined with a stent. In rare cases, an aorto-iliac bypass is necessary.

Another issue is that most renal transplant candidates have a high cardiovascular risk. Careful cardiac screening is mandatory to reduce perioperative risks. Dobutamine stress echocardiography is widely recognized as an accurate diagnostic method for use in the general population and studies have proved its diagnostic and prognostic value in patients with ESRD.[101]

Finally, every recipient requires lifelong immunosuppressive drug therapy and the associated increased risks of infection, malignancy, and specific drug-related toxicities. A recipient must know of these risks and be aware of the necessity to take his drugs regularly.[102,103]

Contraindications to kidney transplantation

There are only a few contraindications to kidney transplantation. Severe respiratory or neurological disease and active infections are considered an absolute barrier to transplant surgery. In general, (metastasized) malignancy is considered a contraindication. However, survivors of cancer can be transplanted after appropriate follow-up. Psychiatric conditions that may lead to impaired compliance are considered relative contraindications for transplantation. Morbid obesity is in most cases also considered a contraindication because the associated poorer long-term graft survival.[104] However, there is evidence that bariatric surgery prior to kidney transplantation may lead to good transplantation outcomes.[105–108]

Recipients

Implantation

Before implantation can be performed, the graft must be carefully prepared. Directly after removal, it is flushed with a cold preservation fluid (e.g. University of Wisconsin solution, which is now most commonly used).[109] Furthermore, in the case of multiple arteries, we recommend to perform a reconstruction 'on the bench' to minimize the number of anastomoses to be made during implantation and the associated longer warm ischaemia time during transplantation. This is to minimize the amount of anastomoses that has to be made during the implantation (and thus the second warm ischaemia time). Usually, if multiple veins are present, they can be safely sacrificed. In general, most right-handed transplant surgeons prefer the right iliac fossa for a first transplantation for an easy anastomosis, and because the iliac vessels are situated more superficially then on the left side.[110] A semi-lunar suprainguinal incision is made in the left or right lower quadrant of the abdomen. The fascia, external oblique, transversus abdominus, and internal oblique muscle are divided. The inferior epigastric vessels are divided to gain access to the pre-peritoneal space. In males, the spermatic cord evidently should be preserved, but in women the round ligament of the uterus is usually divided. When the iliac fossa is exposed and the external iliac artery and vein are prepared, the venous anastomosis (end-to-side) is created first. After creating the arterial end-to-side anastomosis, the perfusion is restored. The kidney should fully restore his former pink colour and turgor. If not, this indicates insufficient perfusion. If the kidney becomes purple, it may indicate an insufficient outflow. Both conditions necessitate immediate surgical correction.

Although the above-described technique of implantation is widely used, several other techniques exist. Modi *et al.* described a laparoscopic implantation technique.[111,112] However, this technique has a long warm ischaemia time. Some centres connect the renal artery and vein to the internal iliac artery and vein or the common iliac artery and vein. Both techniques show similar results regarding short-term as well as long-term outcomes.[113,114]

Ureterovesical anastomosis

After reperfusion, the ureterovesical anastomosis is created. Before surgery, a urine catheter is placed and the bladder is filled with warm saline solution. This enables a safe identification of the bladder before the ureteroneocystostomy is made. Several techniques of ureterovesical anastomosis are available; the most commonly practised are the intra and extravesical anastomoses. The first type of ureteroneocystostomy, was the intravesical technique described by Politano and Leadbetter (Fig. 9.4.9).[115] This is an anastomosis in which the ureter is first inserted in the bladder with the help of a second cystostomy. The ureter is then anastomosed inside of the bladder. However, since the vascularization of the ureter is thought to be inferior in the distal part, an extravesical technique is presently preferred in most centres. For this, a shorter ureter can be used, with better vascularization, leading to fewer complications such as stenosis and leakage.[116] The extravesical anastomosis was first described by Lich-Gregoir (Fig. 9.4.10).[117] The type of anastomosis used for each implantation is mostly depending on the surgeon's preference. Recent data show that the extravesical anastomoses have fewer postoperative complications after kidney transplantation.[118]

After the ureteroneocystostomy is made, a suprapubic catheter or JJ stent is placed with the proximal end of the stent placed in the donor ureter. This is done to prevent dehiscence of the anastomosis or stenosis. Also, with this method, a distinction can be made between diuresis from the graft and diuresis (if present) from the native kidneys. According to published literature, routine stenting of the ureteroneocystostomy is recommended.[119,120] Before closure of the fascia, muscles, and wound, a percutaneous drain is placed.

Splint versus JJ stent

The primary goal of a ureteral stent is to prevent urinary leakage and/or stricture of the ureter. Two types of stents tend to be used

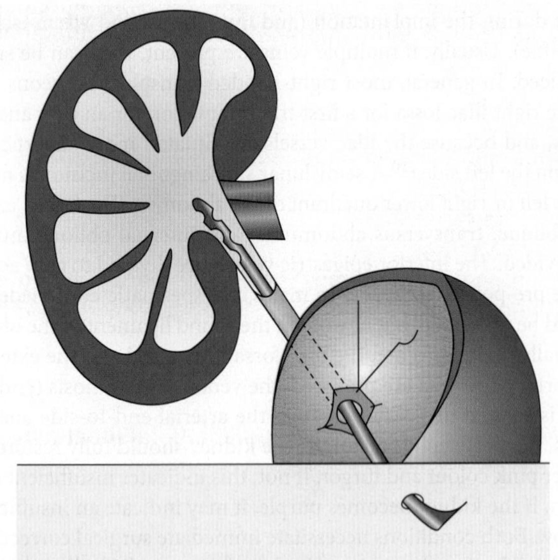

Fig. 9.4.9 Intravesical ureterovesical anastomosis, with a stent placed in the pelvis of the kidney and externalized as a suprapubic catheter.

Reprinted by permission from Macmillan Publishers Ltd: Kidney International, Slagt IKB *et al.*, 2013, 'A randomized controlled trial comparing intravesical to extravesical ureteroneocystostomy in living donor kidney transplantation recipients', *Kidney International*, Volume 85, Issue 2, pp. 471–477, Copyright © 2013.

in kidney transplantation: a 'conventional' suprapubic splint and a JJ stent (double J). The disadvantage of a JJ stent is that it must be removed with use of a cystoscopy, which is an uncomfortable procedure for the patient. A general suprapubic catheter (stent) can be removed manually. However, these catheters have a higher chance to dislocate. Several findings regarding a possible advantage of a ureteral stent have been published over the years. Some authors report no benefit of a stent, others show a significant decrease of urinary leakage and ureteral stenosis.[121,122] There is no published evidence in favour of either a suprapubic or a JJ stent.

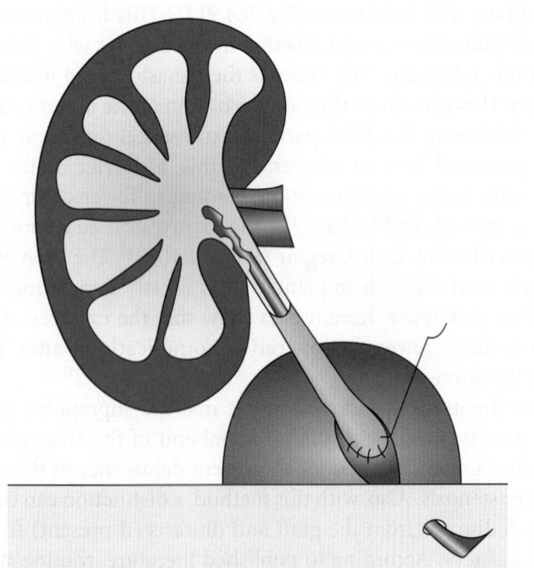

Fig. 9.4.10 Extravesical ureterovesical anastomosis with a stent placed in the pelvis of the kidney and externalized as a suprapubic catheter.

Reprinted by permission from Macmillan Publishers Ltd: Kidney International, Slagt IKB *et al.*, 2013, 'A randomized controlled trial comparing intravesical to extravesical ureteroneocystostomy in living donor kidney transplantation recipients', *Kidney International*, Volume 85, Issue 2, pp. 471–477, Copyright © 2013.

Surgical complication

Surgical complications after donation

Several general complications can occur after LDN. A division can be made between early and late complications.

Early complications

Early complications consist of peri/postoperative bleeding (estimated to occur in approximately 1.6% of cases),[123] wound infection, pulmonary embolism, and deep venous thrombosis. Although, often not scored as a complication, in approximately 1–2% of donor nephrectomies, a conversion to another type of technique has to be performed. By taking appropriate precautions complications can be minimized. In our opinion, all donors should wear stockings perioperatively (although no evidence exists) and thrombosis prophylaxis should be given. Segev *et al.* reported in 2010 that the mortality is approximately 3 per 10.000 donors.[30] In 2012, Friedman *et al.* strictly discouraged the use of hem-o-lock clips in donor nephrectomy, since at least eight donors died after use.[124] Other causes of death after LDN are reported due to haemorrhage and pulmonary embolism.[125,126]

Late complications

Late complications consist of hypertension, diabetes, proteinuria, and renal failure, with incidences of approximately 7.5%, 7%, 1.2% and 0.3%, respectively.[127] Reassuringly, these numbers are comparable to the general population.[127] However, transplant centres must remain cautious regarding extrapolating these results to specific donor groups.[128] Especially, in the extended donors careful considerations must be made, because this group is possibly more prone to late complications.[129]

Incisional hernias are a common surgical problem leading to significant morbidity, including pain, disability, and in some cases even intestinal obstruction and strangulation. An incidence of 1.5% of incisional hernias after donor nephrectomy is reported.[130] This rate is similar for the mini-open and laparoscopic approach.

Surgical complications after kidney transplantation

Surgical complications after KTx have reduced over time since the techniques have been refined. Reported rates of surgical complications are low (5–10%).[131]

Early complications

Haemorrhage following surgery mostly occurs as a result of bleeding from the arterial or venous anastomosis and is rare, with an average risk of 0.3%. A reoperation is only required when the bleeding does not stop spontaneously, which is usually the case.

Renal artery thrombosis, in contrast to renal artery stenosis, mostly occurs early after transplantation. Thrombosis is mostly due to a dissection of the intima or kinking of the renal artery. Diagnosis can be made with duplex ultrasound or with a radioisotope renography (MAG3-scan) or CT-angiography. However, in clinical practice, these examinations may take too long, as in the case of a suspected thrombosis, an immediate intervention is required in order to save the graft. When there is no urine production from the graft, and an emergency ultrasound reveals no perfusion, an emergency intervention should be undertaken. Possible interventions include reoperation with thrombectomy or percutaneous transluminal angioplasty. In case of a timely diagnosis, such procedures are fairly successful but long-term graft survival is diminished because of extensive warm ischaemia times.[132,133]

Renal vein thrombosis (RVT) can be caused by surgical problems and occurs in about 4% of transplantations and most often within the first 48 hours after surgery. Again, immediate surgery is required in order to salvage the graft and prevent bleeding. In addition, RVT may occur a few weeks after transplantation and is then mostly associated with hypercoagulable states such as may occur in patients with severe nephrotic syndrome or circulating anti-phospolipid antibodies. Furthermore, extension of a deep venous thrombosis may extend into the renal vein.[134] Since these are normally ambulant patients, the moment of a definite diagnosis by duplex may be too late to salvage the graft, although theoretically thrombolysis may be an option.

Renal artery dissection is a rare complication after transplantation and is mostly directly diagnosed during surgery. Mostly, the intima of the vessel wall is dissected, which can be immediately repaired by stitching/suturing the intimal flap and if necessary, with a (non-) or autologous patch or stentgraft.

Another rare complication is pseudoaneurysm formation after transplantation. This is caused by a dehiscence of the arterial anastomosis or localized infection.[135,136] This complication can be asymptomatic, or result in hypovolaemic shock. Diagnostic modalities consist of ultrasound and/or angiography.

Urinary leakage is mostly caused by a full or partial breakdown of the ureterovesical anastomosis. The recipient may present with pain, decreased urine output, leakage from the operation wound, delayed graft function, or worsening of renal function (as indicated by a rise in serum creatinine). Diagnosis is made with a MAG3-scan or (CT-)pyelography (Fig. 9.4.11). A percutaneous nephrostomy drain can be placed to release tension and divert the urine. In most cases, the ureterovesical anastomosis heals over time. If not, surgical intervention is required.[137]

The incidence of lymphoceles varies and is reported up to 18%.[138] Lymphoceles mostly occur several weeks after transplantation. Large lymphoceles can cause compression of the ureter. To diagnose a lymphocele, first an ultrasound should be performed and, ideally, a puncture of the fluid collection could be taken when discrimination between haematoma or urinoma is clinically relevant. Not all lymphoceles lead to symptoms, some resolve over time, and do not require an intervention. If symptomatic or in case of hydronephrosis, percutaneous drainage can be performed, although there is a risk of infection. If recurrent, a laparoscopic fenestration should be considered, with a high success rate up to 95%.[139] Others advocate sclerosis with ethanol.[140] A higher incidence of lymphoceles (OR 2.07) has been reported in association with the use of immunosuppressive agents belonging to the mTOR inhibitor class.[141]

The incidence of wound infections differs in the literature with reported incidences as high as 20–25%.[142,143] Most commonly, this complication is caused by wound haematomata, urine leakage, or lymphoceles. Fortunately, it rarely has a negative impact on the graft.[144] Wound infections can be superficial or deep. Superficial infections are mostly related to contamination from skin flora.

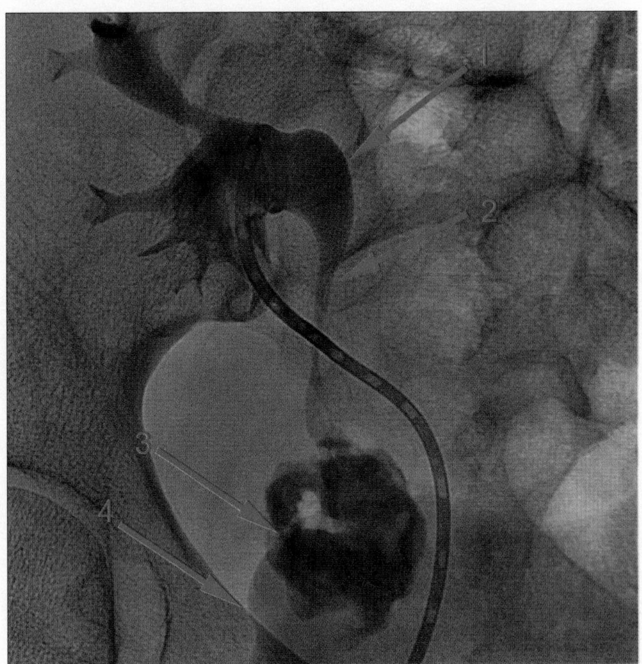

Fig. 9.4.11 Pyelography with leakage in the region of the ureterneocystostomy. (1) Pyelum; (2) ureter; (3) leakage; (4) bladder.

Factors that pose a risk to the incidence of wound infections are urine leakage, diabetes, obesity, and use of mTOR inhibitors.[141] Deep infections are rare and mostly caused by urine leakage. Superficial infections can in generally be treated by opening the wound. If necessary, antibiotics can be prescribed in more severe cases to prevent systemic infections. Deep infections are treated with drainage and usually antibiotics. In most kidney transplant protocols, perioperative antibiotic prophylaxis with cefazoline is included.

Incisional hernias occur in 3–5% of kidney transplantations. Risk factors include reoperation, obesity and immunosuppressive agents (steroids, mTORi).[110,131,145]

Late complications

Renal artery stenosis may occur post-transplantation and may lead to ischaemia of the kidney allograft and sometimes even loss of the graft. This is mostly a late complication occurring years after transplantation. Diagnostic options consist of a CT scan, or angiography. If a radiological intervention is not possible, surgery can be performed to restore vascularization.[146]

Despite the use of ureteral stents, stenosis or obstruction of the ureter may occur, and lead to hydronephrosis (about 25%) (Figs 9.4.12 and 9.4.13).[147] Patients present with a declining graft function or prolonged DGF. Ultrasound imaging is the best modality to determine whether there is hydronephrosis. Additionally, a (CT-) pyelography can be performed to reveal more specifically the position of the obstruction. In most cases it is necessary to place a percutaneous nephrostomy (PCN) to relieve the hydronephrosis. Reoperation (approximately 5%) with the construction of a new ureteroneocystostomy is the most common treatment with a high success rate.[148] Another treatment option is balloon-dilatation or laser endoureterotomy of the ureter.[149,150]

A rare, but serious complication after peritoneal dialysis is encapsulating peritoneal sclerosis (EPS). This complication is not unique

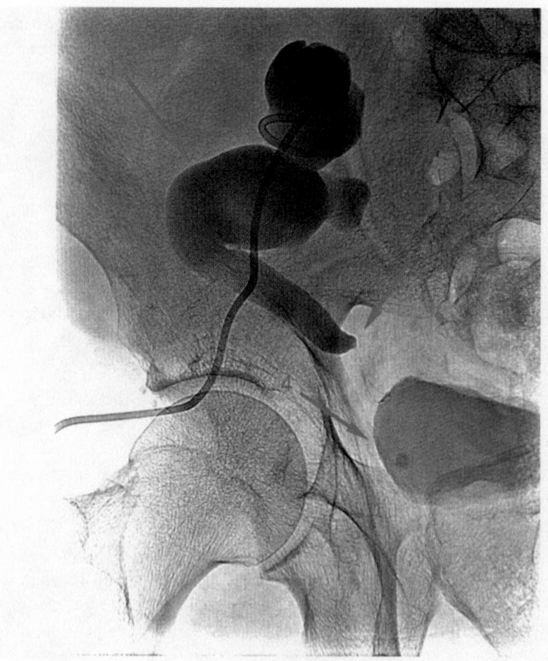

Fig. 9.4.12 Pyelography showing hydronephrosis and obstruction in the distal part of the ureter. (1) pyelum; (2) ureter; (3) distal obstruction; (4) bladder.

to peritoneal dialysis patients, and can occur in other clinical conditions as well (cirrhosis with ascites, generalized peritonitis, or even idiopathic). The incidence of EPS in patients after peritoneal dialysis is reported in a range of 0.7% to 3.7%.[151] The exact aetiology is yet unknown, although exposure time to peritoneal dialysis fluids seems to be a risk factor. Paradoxically, discontinuing peritoneal dialysis (PD) seems to have a correlation with EPS and this can explain why it frequently occurs after transplantation. EPS is characterized by diffuse peritoneal membrane fibrosis, which leads to partial or complete encapsulation of the bowel, and ultimately to intestinal obstruction. The consequences of EPS are devastating and mortality rates exceed 50%, most commonly because of complications related to persistent bowel obstruction (e.g. perforation) and prolonged parenteral feeding.[152] Therapeutic options consist

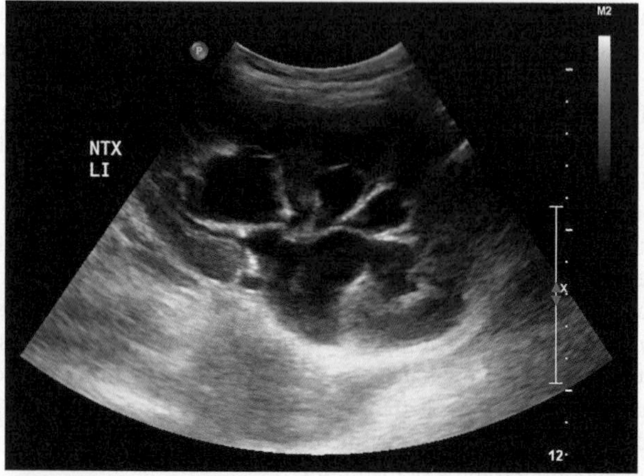

Fig. 9.4.13 Ultrasound showing distended renal calices in a patient with ureteral obstruction.

of immunosuppressors like steroids and tamoxifen. Surgical enterolysis and peritonectomy is an increasing successful therapeutic option for EPS.[153–155]

Conclusion

The incidence of ESRD continues to rise but the number of deceased kidney donors is by far not sufficient to meet demands. As a result, live kidney donation is increasingly performed. This can be attributed to the increasing awareness and the development of new donor-exchange programmes. Cross-over programmes may be further expanded and ideally a European living exchange programme is created. However, a programme of this magnitude will require extensive work and collaboration between transplant centres. Further future challenges lie in improving deceased donor organ quality (e.g. by machine perfusion[20] or ischaemic conditioning[156]), thereby increasing the numbers of organs suitable for transplantation. Also, legislation for a mandatory registration of being a donor (or not) could increase the number of available organs.

Acknowledgements

We hereby acknowledge the guidance and inspiration by Willem Weimar, MD PhD, and Jan N.M. IJzermans, MD PhD.

Further reading

Antcliffe D, Nanidis TG, Darzi AW, *et al.* A meta-analysis of mini-open versus standard open and laparoscopic living donor nephrectomy. *Transpl Int* 2009; **22**:463–74.

Augustine T, Brown PW, Davies SD, *et al.* Encapsulating peritoneal sclerosis: clinical significance and implications. *Nephron Clin Pract* 2009; **111**:c149–54; discussion c54.

Dasgupta P, Challacombe B, Compton F, *et al.* A systematic review of hand-assisted laparoscopic live donor nephrectomy. *Int J Clin Pract* 2004; **58**:474–8.

de Klerk M, Kal-van Gestel JA, Haase-Kromwijk BJ, *et al.* Eight years of outcomes of the Dutch Living Donor Kidney Exchange Program. *Clin Transpl* 2011; 287–90.

Dols LF, Weimar W, Ijzermans JN. Long-term consequences of kidney donation. *N Engl J Med* 2009; **360**:2371–2; author reply 2.

Dols LFC, Kok NFM, Tran TCK, *et al.* Hand-assisted retroperitoneoscopic versus standard laparoscopic donor nephrectomy: single blind, randomised controlled trial. *Transpl Int* 2011; **24**:25.

Friedman AL, Peters TG, Jones KW, *et al.* Fatal and nonfatal hemorrhagic complications of living kidney donation. *Ann Surg* 2006; **243**:126–30.

Gorodner V, Horgan S, Galvani C, *et al.* Routine left robotic-assisted laparoscopic donor nephrectomy is safe and effective regardless of the presence of vascular anomalies. *Transpl Int* 2006; **19**:636–40.

Hariharan S, Johnson CP, Bresnahan BA, *et al.* Improved graft survival after renal transplantation in the United States, 1988 to 1996. *N Engl J Med* 2000; **342**:605–12.

Kok NF, Lind MY, Hansson BM, *et al.* Comparison of laparoscopic and mini incision open donor nephrectomy: single blind, randomised controlled clinical trial. *BMJ* 2006; **333**:221.

Lennerling A, Loven C, Dor FJ, *et al.* Living organ donation practices in Europe—results from an online survey. *Transpl Int* 2013; **26**:145–53.

Modanlou KA, Muthyala U, Xiao H, *et al.* Bariatric surgery among kidney transplant candidates and recipients: analysis of the United States renal data system and literature review. *Transplantation* 2009; **87**:1167–73.

Moers C, Pirenne J, Paul A, *et al.* Machine perfusion or cold storage in deceased-donor kidney transplantation. *N Engl J Med* 2012; **366**:770–1.

O'Callaghan JM, Knight SR, Morgan RD, *et al.* Preservation solutions for static cold storage of kidney allografts: a systematic review and meta-analysis. *Am J Transplant* 2012; **12**:896–906.

Pascual J, Zamora J, Pirsch JD. A systematic review of kidney transplantation from expanded criteria donors. *Am J Kidney Dis* 2008; **52**:553–86.

Ratner LE, Ciseck LJ, Moore RG, *et al.* Laparoscopic live donor nephrectomy. *Transplantation* 1995; **60**:1047–9.

Roodnat JI, Zuidema W, van de Wetering J, *et al.* Altruistic donor triggered domino-paired kidney donation for unsuccessful couples from the kidney-exchange program. *Am J Transplant* 2010; **10**:821–7.

Segev DL, Muzaale AD, Caffo BS, *et al.* Perioperative mortality and long-term survival following live kidney donation. *JAMA* 2010; **303**:959–66.

Slagt IK, Klop KW, Ijzermans JN, *et al.* Intravesical versus extravesical ureteroneocystostomy in kidney transplantation: a systematic review and meta-analysis. *Transplantation* 2012; **94**:1179–84.

Tan JC, Chertow GM. Cautious optimism concerning long-term safety of kidney donation. *N Engl J Med* 2009; **360**:522–3.

van den Akker EK, Manintveld OC, Hesselink DA, *et al.* Protection against renal ischemia-reperfusion injury by ischemic postconditioning. *Transplantation* 2013; **95**:1299–305.

Wadstrom J, Lindstrom P. Hand-assisted retroperitoneoscopic living-donor nephrectomy: initial 10 cases. *Transplantation* 2002; **73**:1839–40.

Weber M, Dindo D, Demartines N, et al. Kidney transplantation from donors without a heartbeat. *N Engl J Med* 2002; **347**:248–55.

Wilson CH, Bhatti AA, Rix DA, Manas DM. Routine intraoperative ureteric stenting for kidney transplant recipients. *Cochrane Database Syst Rev* 2005; **19**(4):CD004925.

References

1. US Renal Data System. USRDS 2012 Annual Data Report: Atlas of Chronic Kidney Disease and End-Stage Renal Disease in the United States, National Institutes of Health, National Institute of Diabetes and Digestive and Kidney Diseases, Bethesda, MD, 2012.
2. Davis CL, Delmonico FL. Living-donor kidney transplantation: a review of the current practices for the live donor. *J Am Soc Nephrol* 2005; **16**: 2098–110.
3. Innocenti GR, Wadei HM, Prieto M, *et al.* Preemptive living donor kidney transplantation: do the benefits extend to all recipients? *Transplantation* 2007; **83**: 144–9.
4. Wolfe RA, Ashby VB, Milford EL, *et al.* Comparison of mortality in all patients on dialysis, patients on dialysis awaiting transplantation, and recipients of a first cadaveric transplant. *N Engl J Med* 1999; **341**:1725–30.
5. McDonald SP, Craig JC, Australian and New Zealand Paediatric Nephrology Association. Long-term survival of children with end-stage renal disease. *N Engl J Med* 2004; **350**:2654–62.
6. Oosterlee A, Rahmel A. Eurotransplant International Foundation: Annual Report 2011. Leiden: Eurotransplant International Foundation, 2012.
7. Hariharan S, Johnson CP, Bresnahan BA, *et al.* Improved graft survival after renal transplantation in the United States, 1988 to 1996. *N Engl J Med* 2000; **342**:605–12.
8. Rao PS, Ojo A. The alphabet soup of kidney transplantation: SCD, DCD, ECD—fundamentals for the practicing nephrologist. *Clin J Am Soc Nephrol* 2009; **4**:1827–31.
9. Dutch Transplantation Society: Annual Report 2011–2012.
10. Pascual J, Zamora J, Pirsch JD. A systematic review of kidney transplantation from expanded criteria donors. *Am J Kidney Dis* 2008; **52**:553–86.
11. Weber M, Dindo D, Demartines N, *et al.* Kidney transplantation from donors without a heartbeat. *N Engl J Med* 2002; **347**:248–55.
12. Summers DM, Johnson RJ, Allen J, *et al.* Analysis of factors that affect outcome after transplantation of kidneys donated after cardiac death in the UK: a cohort study. *Lancet* 2010; **376**:1303–11.
13. Thomas I, Caborn S, Manara AR. Experiences in the development of non-heart beating organ donation scheme in a regional neurosciences intensive care unit. *Br J Anaesth* 2008; **100**:820–6.
14. Akoh JA, Denton MD, Bradshaw SB, *et al.* Early results of a controlled non-heart-beating kidney donor programme. *Nephrol Dial Transplant* 2009; **24**:1992–6.
15. Kootstra G, Daemen JH, Oomen AP. Categories of non-heart-beating donors. *Transplant Proc* 1995; **27**:2893–4.
16. Manara AR, Murphy PG, O'Callaghan G. Donation after circulatory death. *Br J Anaesth* 2012; **108**(Suppl 1):i108–21.
17. Salehipour M, Bahador A, Jalaeian H, *et al.* Comparison of right and left grafts in renal transplantation. *Saudi J Kidney Dis Transpl* 2008; **19**:222–6.
18. Johnson DW, Mudge DW, Kaisar MO, *et al.* Deceased donor renal transplantation—does side matter? *Nephrol Dial Transplant* 2006; **21**:2583–8.
19. Vacher-Coponat H, McDonald S, Clayton P, *et al.* Inferior early posttransplant outcomes for recipients of right versus left deceased donor kidneys: An ANZDATA registry analysis. *Am J Transplant* 2013; **13**:399–405.
20. Moers C, Pirenne J, Paul A, *et al.* Machine perfusion or cold storage in deceased-donor kidney transplantation. *N Engl J Med* 2012; **366**:770–1.
21. Dor FJ, Massey EK, Frunza M, *et al.* New classification of ELPAT for living organ donation. *Transplantation* 2011; **91**:935–8.
22. Lennerling A, Loven C, Dor FJ, *et al.* Living organ donation practices in Europe—results from an online survey. *Transpl Int* 2013; **26**:145–53.
23. Ethics Committee of the Transplantation S. The consensus statement of the Amsterdam Forum on the Care of the Live Kidney Donor. *Transplantation* 2004; **78**:491–2.
24. Lafranca JA, Hagen SM, Dols LF, *et al.* Systematic review and meta-analysis of the relation between body mass index and short-term donor outcome of laparoscopic donor nephrectomy. *Kidney Int* 2013; **83**(5):931–9.
25. Branco AW, Branco Filho AJ, Kondo W. Laparoscopic live donor nephrectomy in patients surgically treated for morbid obesity. *Int Braz J Urol* 2007; **33**:377–9; discussion 9.
26. Koshy AN, Wilkinson S, Coombes JS, *et al.* Laparoscopic adjustable gastric band in an obese unrelated living donor prior to kidney transplantation: a case report. *J Med Case Rep* 2010; **4**:107.
27. Lim WH, Clayton P, Wong G, *et al.* Outcomes of kidney transplantation from older living donors. *Transplantation* 2013; **95**:106–13.
28. Dols LF, Kok NF, Roodnat JI, *et al.* Living kidney donors: impact of age on long-term safety. *Am J Transplant* 2011; **11**:737–42.
29. Dols LF, Weimar W, Ijzermans JN. Long-term consequences of kidney donation. *N Engl J Med* 2009; **360**:2371–2; author reply 2.
30. Segev DL, Muzaale AD, Caffo BS, *et al.* Perioperative mortality and long-term survival following live kidney donation. *JAMA* 2010; **303**:959–66.
31. Young A, Storsley L, Garg AX, *et al.* Health outcomes for living kidney donors with isolated medical abnormalities: a systematic review. *Am J Transplant* 2008; **8**:1878–90.
32. Textor SC, Taler SJ, Driscoll N, *et al.* Blood pressure and renal function after kidney donation from hypertensive living donors. *Transplantation* 2004; **78**:276–82.
33. Tent H, Sanders JS, Rook M, *et al.* Effects of preexistent hypertension on blood pressure and residual renal function after donor nephrectomy. *Transplantation* 2012; **93**:412–7.
34. Ahmadi AR, Lafranca JA, Claessens LA, *et al.* Shifting paradigms in eligibility criteria for live kidney donation: a systematic review. *Kidney Int* 2015; **87**(1):31–45.
35. de Klerk M, Kal-van Gestel JA, Haase-Kromwijk BJ, *et al.* Eight years of outcomes of the Dutch Living Donor Kidney Exchange Program. *Clin Transpl* 2011;287–90.
36. De Klerk M, Van Der Deijl WM, Witvliet MD, *et al.* The optimal chain length for kidney paired exchanges: an analysis of the Dutch program. *Transpl Int* 2010; **23**:1120–5.
37. Ratner LE, Rana A, Ratner ER, *et al.* The altruistic unbalanced paired kidney exchange: proof of concept and survey of potential donor and recipient attitudes. *Transplantation* 2010; **89**:15–22.

38. Roodnat JI, Zuidema W, van de Wetering J, *et al.* Altruistic donor triggered domino-paired kidney donation for unsuccessful couples from the kidney-exchange program. *Am J Transplant* 2010; **10**:821–7.
39. Rees MA, Kopke JE, Pelletier RP, *et al.* A nonsimultaneous, extended, altruistic-donor chain. *N Engl J Med* 2009; **360**:1096–101.
40. Hume DM, Merrill JP, Miller BF, *et al.* Experiences with renal homotransplantation in the human: report of nine cases. *J Clin Invest* 1955; **34**:327–82.
41. Starzl TE, Marchioro TL, Holmes JH, *et al.* Renal homografts in patients with major donor-recipient blood group incompatibilities. *Surgery* 1964; **55**:195–200.
42. Shin M, Kim SJ. ABO Incompatible kidney transplantation-current status and uncertainties. *J Transplant* 2011; **2011**:970421.
43. Magee CC. Transplantation across previously incompatible immunological barriers. *Transpl Int* 2006; **19**:87–97.
44. Tyden G, Kumlien G, Genberg H, *et al.* The Stockholm experience with ABO-incompatible kidney transplantations without splenectomy. *Xenotransplantation* 2006; **13**:105–7.
45. Genberg H, Kumlien G, Wennberg L, *et al.* ABO-incompatible kidney transplantation using antigen-specific immunoadsorption and rituximab: a 3-year follow-up. *Transplantation* 2008; **85**:1745–54.
46. Montgomery RA, Lonze BE, King KE, *et al.* Desensitization in HLA-incompatible kidney recipients and survival. *N Engl J Med* 2011; **365**:318–26.
47. Harrison JH, Merrill JP, Murray JE. Renal homotransplantation in identical twins. *Surg Forum* 1956; **6**:432–6.
48. Nicholson ML, Elwell R, Kaushik M, *et al.* Health-related quality of life after living donor nephrectomy: a randomized controlled trial of laparoscopic versus open nephrectomy. *Transplantation* 2011; **91**:457–61.
49. Dunn JF, Nylander WA, Jr., Richie RE, *et al.* Living related kidney donors. A 14-year experience. *Ann Surg* 1986; **203**:637–43.
50. Connor WT, Van Buren CT, Floyd M, *et al.* Anterior extraperitoneal donor nephrectomy. *J Urol* 1981; **126**:443–7.
51. Ruiz R, Novick AC, Braun WE, *et al.* Transperitoneal live donor nephrectomy. *J Urol* 1980; **123**:819–21.
52. Klop KW, Dols LF, Kok NF, *et al.* Attitudes among surgeons towards live-donor nephrectomy: a European update. *Transplantation* 2012; **94**:263–8.
53. Hakim N, Zarka ZA, El-Tayar A, *et al.* A fast and safe living donor nephrectomy technique. *Transplant Proc* 2003; **35**:2555–6.
54. Antcliffe D, Nanidis TG, Darzi AW, *et al.* A meta-analysis of mini-open versus standard open and laparoscopic living donor nephrectomy. *Transpl Int* 2009; **22**:463–74.
55. Ratner LE, Ciseck LJ, Moore RG, *et al.* Laparoscopic live donor nephrectomy. *Transplantation* 1995; **60**:1047–9.
56. Finelli FC, Gongora E, Sasaki TM, *et al.* A survey: the prevalence of laparoscopic donor nephrectomy at large U.S. transplant centers. *Transplantation* 2001; **71**:1862–4.
57. Nanidis TG, Antcliffe D, Kokkinos C, *et al.* Laparoscopic versus open live donor nephrectomy in renal transplantation: a meta-analysis. *Ann Surg* 2008; **247**: 58–70.
58. Greco F, Hoda MR, Alcaraz A, *et al.* Laparoscopic living-donor nephrectomy: analysis of the existing literature. *Eur Urol* 2010; **58**:498–509.
59. Sundaram CP, Bargman V, Bernie JE. Methods of vascular control during laparoscopic donor nephrectomy. *J Endourol* 2006; **20**:467–9; discussion 9–70.
60. Brook NR, Nicholson ML. An audit over 2 years' practice of open and laparoscopic live-donor nephrectomy at renal transplant centres in the UK and Ireland. *BJU Int* 2004; **93**:1027–31.
61. Axelrod DA, McCullough KP, Brewer ED, *et al.* Kidney and pancreas transplantation in the United States, 1999–2008: the changing face of living donation. *Am J Transplant* 2010; **10**:987–1002.
62. Wolf JS, Jr., Tchetgen MB, Merion RM. Hand-assisted laparoscopic live donor nephrectomy. *Urology* 1998; **52**:885–7.
63. Buell JF, Hanaway MJ, Potter SR, *et al.* Hand-assisted laparoscopic living-donor nephrectomy as an alternative to traditional laparoscopic living-donor nephrectomy. *Am J Transplant* 2002; **2**:983–8.
64. Gaston KE, Moore DT, Pruthi RS. Hand-assisted laparoscopic nephrectomy: prospective evaluation of the learning curve. *J Urol* 2004; **171**:63–7.
65. Dasgupta P, Challacombe B, Compton F, *et al.* A systematic review of hand-assisted laparoscopic live donor nephrectomy. *Int J Clin Pract* 2004; **58**:474–8.
66. Chandak P, Kessaris N, Challacombe B, *et al.* How safe is hand-assisted laparoscopic donor nephrectomy?—results of 200 live donor nephrectomies by two different techniques. *Nephrol Dial Transplant* 2009; **24**:293–7.
67. Wadstrom J, Lindstrom P. Hand-assisted retroperitoneoscopic living-donor nephrectomy: initial 10 cases. *Transplantation* 2002; **73**:1839–40.
68. Dols LFC, Kok NFM, d'Ancona FCH, *et al.* Randomized controlled trial comparing hand-assisted retroperitoneoscopic versus standard laparoscopic donor nephrectomy. *Transplantation* 2014; **97**:161–7.
69. Klop KWJ, Kok NFM, Dols LFC, *et al.* Can right-sided hand-assisted retroperitoneoscopic donor nephrectomy be advocated above standard laparoscopic donor nephrectomy: a randomized pilot study. *Transpl Int* 2014; **27**:162–9.
70. Horgan S, Vanuno D, Benedetti E. Early experience with robotically assisted laparoscopic donor nephrectomy. *Surg Laparosc Endosc Percutan Tech* 2002; **12**:64–70.
71. Horgan S, Vanuno D, Sileri P, *et al.* Robotic-assisted laparoscopic donor nephrectomy for kidney transplantation. *Transplantation* 2002; **73**:1474–9.
72. Janki S, Klop KW, Hagen SM, *et al.* Robotic surgery rapidly and successfully implemented in a high volume laparoscopic center on living kidney donation. *Int J Med Robot* 2016; Epub ahead of print.
73. Gorodner V, Horgan S, Galvani C, *et al.* Routine left robotic-assisted laparoscopic donor nephrectomy is safe and effective regardless of the presence of vascular anomalies. *Transpl Int* 2006; **19**:636–40.
74. Hagen SM, Dols LFC, Terkivatan T, *et al.* Robot-Assisted Live Kidney Donation: The Rotterdam Experience. *Transpl Int* 2011; **24**:340.
75. Gill IS, Canes D, Aron M, *et al.* Single port transumbilical (E-NOTES) donor nephrectomy. *J Urol* 2008; **180**:637–41; discussion 41.
76. Canes D, Berger A, Aron M, *et al.* Laparo-endoscopic single site (LESS) versus standard laparoscopic left donor nephrectomy: matched-pair comparison. *Eur Urol* 2010; **57**:95–101.
77. Kurien A, Rajapurkar S, Sinha L, *et al.* First prize: Standard laparoscopic donor nephrectomy versus laparoendoscopic single-site donor nephrectomy: a randomized comparative study. *J Endourol* 2011; **25**:365–70.
78. Lunsford KE, Harris MT, Nicoll KN, *et al.* Single-site laparoscopic living donor nephrectomy offers comparable perioperative outcomes to conventional laparoscopic living donor nephrectomy at a higher cost. *Transplantation* 2011; **91**:e16–7.
79. Alcaraz A, Musquera M, Peri L, *et al.* Feasibility of transvaginal natural orifice transluminal endoscopic surgery-assisted living donor nephrectomy: is kidney vaginal delivery the approach of the future? *Eur Urol* 2011; **59**:1019–25.
80. Allaf ME, Singer A, Shen W, *et al.* Laparoscopic live donor nephrectomy with vaginal extraction: initial report. *Am J Transplant* 2010; **10**:1473–7.
81. Kaouk JH, Khalifeh A, Laydner H, *et al.* Transvaginal hybrid natural orifice transluminal surgery robotic donor nephrectomy: first clinical application. *Urology* 2012; **80**:1171–5.
82. Pietrabissa A, Abelli M, Spinillo A, *et al.* Robotic-assisted laparoscopic donor nephrectomy with transvaginal extraction of the kidney. *Am J Transplant* 2010; **10**:2708–11.
83. Buell JF, Edye M, Johnson M, *et al.* Are concerns over right laparoscopic donor nephrectomy unwarranted? *Ann Surg* 2001; **233**:645–51.

84. Buell JF, Hanaway MJ, Potter SR, *et al.* Surgical techniques in right laparoscopic donor nephrectomy. *J Am Coll Surg* 2002; **195**:131–7.
85. Lind MY, Hazebroek EJ, Hop WC, *et al.* Right-sided laparoscopic live-donor nephrectomy: is reluctance still justified? *Transplantation* 2002; **74**:1045–8.
86. Dols LF, Kok NF, Alwayn IP, *et al.* Laparoscopic donor nephrectomy: a plea for the right-sided approach. *Transplantation* 2009; **87**:745–50.
87. Tsoulfas G, Agorastou P, Ko D, *et al.* Laparoscopic living donor nephrectomy: is there a difference between using a left or a right kidney? *Transplant Proc* 2012; **44**:2706–8.
88. Fettouh HA. Laparoscopic donor nephrectomy in the presence of vascular anomalies: evaluation of outcome. *J Endourol* 2008; **22**:77–82.
89. Desai MR, Ganpule AP, Gupta R, *et al.* Outcome of renal transplantation with multiple versus single renal arteries after laparoscopic live donor nephrectomy: a comparative study. *Urology* 2007; **69**:824–7.
90. Paragi PR, Klaassen Z, Fletcher HS, *et al.* Vascular constraints in laparoscopic renal allograft: comparative analysis of multiple and single renal arteries in 976 laparoscopic donor nephrectomies. *World J Surg* 2011; **35**:2159–66.
91. Firmin LC, Johari Y, Nicholson ML. Explantation of the recipient internal iliac artery for bench-surgery during live donor renal transplants with multiple renal arteries. *Ann R Coll Surg Engl* 2010; **92**:356.
92. Hsu TH, Su L, Ratner LE, *et al.* Impact of renal artery multiplicity on outcomes of renal donors and recipients in laparoscopic donor nephrectomy. *Urology* 2003; **61**:323–7.
93. Kok NF, Dols LF, Hunink MG, *et al.* Complex vascular anatomy in live kidney donation: imaging and consequences for clinical outcome. *Transplantation* 2008; **85**:1760–5.
94. Dols LF, Kok NF, Ijzermans JN. Live donor nephrectomy: a review of evidence for surgical techniques. *Transpl Int* 2010; **23**:121–30.
95. Kamali K, Abbasi MA, Ani A, *et al.* Renal transplantation in allografts with multiple versus single renal arteries. *Saudi J Kidney Dis Transpl* 2012; **23**:246–50.
96. Gerstenkorn C, Papalois VE, Thomusch O, *et al.* Surgical management of multiple donor veins in renal transplantation. *Int Surg* 2006; **91**:345–7.
97. Kayler L, Kang D, Molmenti E, *et al.* Kidney transplant ureteroneocystostomy techniques and complications: review of the literature. *Transplant Proc* 2010; **42**:1413–20.
98. Rule AD, Sasiwimonphan K, Lieske JC, *et al.* Characteristics of renal cystic and solid lesions based on contrast-enhanced computed tomography of potential kidney donors. *Am J Kidney Dis* 2012; **59**:611–8.
99. Bosniak MA. The Bosniak renal cyst classification: 25 years later. *Radiology* 2012; **262**:781–5.
100. Huang E, Samaniego-Picota M, McCune T, *et al.* DNA testing for live kidney donors at risk for autosomal dominant polycystic kidney disease. *Transplantation* 2009; **87**:133–7.
101. Feringa HH, Bax JJ, Schouten O, *et al.* Ischemic heart disease in renal transplant candidates: towards non-invasive approaches for preoperative risk stratification. *Eur J Echocardiogr* 2005; **6**:313–6.
102. Berben L, Dobbels F, Kugler C, *et al.* Interventions used by health care professionals to enhance medication adherence in transplant patients: a survey of current clinical practice. *Prog Transplant* 2011; **21**:322–31.
103. Ruppar TM, Russell CL. Medication adherence in successful kidney transplant recipients. *Prog Transplant* 2009; **19**:167–72.
104. Furriel F, Parada B, Campos L, *et al.* Pretransplantation overweight and obesity: does it really affect kidney transplantation outcomes? *Transplant Proc* 2011; **43**:95–9.
105. Newcombe V, Blanch A, Slater GH, *et al.* Laparoscopic adjustable gastric banding prior to renal transplantation. *Obes Surg* 2005; **15**:567–70.
106. Koshy AN, Coombes JS, Wilkinson S, *et al.* Laparoscopic gastric banding surgery performed in obese dialysis patients prior to kidney transplantation. *Am J Kidney Dis* 2008; **52**:e15–17.
107. Modanlou KA, Muthyala U, Xiao H, *et al.* Bariatric surgery among kidney transplant candidates and recipients: analysis of the United States renal data system and literature review. *Transplantation* 2009; **87**:1167–73.
108. Marszalek R, Ziemianski P, Lisik W, *et al.* Bariatric surgery as a bridge for kidney transplantation in obese subjects. Case report. *Ann Transplant* 2012; **17**:108–12.
109. O'Callaghan JM, Knight SR, Morgan RD, *et al.* Preservation solutions for static cold storage of kidney allografts: a systematic review and meta-analysis. *Am J Transplant* 2012; **12**:896–906.
110. Thiruchelvam PT, Willicombe M, Hakim N, *et al.* Renal transplantation. *BMJ* 2011; **343**:d7300.
111. Modi P, Rizvi J, Pal B, *et al.* Laparoscopic kidney transplantation: an initial experience. *Am J Transplant* 2011; **11**:1320–4.
112. Modi P, Thyagaraj K, Rizvi SJ, *et al.* Laparoscopic en bloc kidney transplantation. *Indian J Urol* 2012; **28**:362–5.
113. Matheus WE, Reis LO, Ferreira U, *et al.* Kidney transplant anastomosis: internal or external iliac artery? *Urol J* 2009; **6**:260–6.
114. Mohamed IH, Bagul A, Doughman T, *et al.* Use of internal iliac artery as a side-to-end anastomosis in renal transplantation. *Ann R Coll Surg Engl* 2012; **94**:e36–7.
115. Politano VA, Leadbetter WF. An operative technique for the correction of vesicoureteral reflux. 1958. *J Urol* 2002; **167**:1055–61; discussion 62.
116. Slagt IK, Klop KW, Ijzermans JN, *et al.* Intravesical versus extravesical ureteroneocystostomy in kidney transplantation: a systematic review and meta-analysis. *Transplantation* 2012; **94**:1179–84.
117. Gregoir W. [the Surgical Treatment of Congenital Vesico-Ureteral Reflux] Le Traitement Chirurgical Du Reflux V'esico-Ur'et'eral Cong'enital. *Acta Chir Belg* 1964; **63**:431–9.
118. Slagt IKB, Dor FJMF, Tran TCK, *et al.* A randomized controlled trial comparing intravesical to extravesical ureteroneocystostomy in living donor kidney transplantation recipients. *Kidney Int* 2014; **85**:471–7.
119. Wilson CH, Bhatti AA, Rix DA, Manas DM. Routine intraoperative ureteric stenting for kidney transplant recipients. *Cochrane Database Syst Rev* 2005; **19(4)**:CD004925.
120. Mangus RS, Haag BW. Stented versus nonstented extravesical ureteroneocystostomy in renal transplantation: a metaanalysis. *Am J Transplant* 2004; **4**:1889–96.
121. Dominguez J, Clase CM, Mahalati K, *et al.* Is routine ureteric stenting needed in kidney transplantation? A randomized trial. *Transplantation* 2000; **70**:597–601.
122. Tavakoli A, Surange RS, Pearson RC, *et al.* Impact of stents on urological complications and health care expenditure in renal transplant recipients: results of a prospective, randomized clinical trial. *J Urol* 2007; **177**:2260–4; discussion 4.
123. Mjoen G, Oyen O, Holdaas H, *et al.* Morbidity and mortality in 1022 consecutive living donor nephrectomies: benefits of a living donor registry. *Transplantation* 2009; **88**:1273–9.
124. Friedman AL, Peters TG, Ratner LE. Regulatory failure contributing to deaths of live kidney donors. *Am J Transplant* 2012; **12**:829–34.
125. Matas AJ, Bartlett ST, Leichtman AB, *et al.* Morbidity and mortality after living kidney donation, 1999–2001: survey of United States transplant centers. *Am J Transplant* 2003; **3**:830–4.
126. Friedman AL, Peters TG, Jones KW, *et al.* Fatal and nonfatal hemorrhagic complications of living kidney donation. *Ann Surg* 2006; **243**:126–30.
127. Ibrahim HN, Foley R, Tan L, *et al.* Long-term consequences of kidney donation. *N Engl J Med* 2009; **360**:459–69.
128. Tan JC, Chertow GM. Cautious optimism concerning long-term safety of kidney donation. *N Engl J Med* 2009; **360**:522–3.
129. Lin J, Kramer H, Chandraker AK. Mortality among living kidney donors and comparison populations. *N Engl J Med* 2010; **363**:797–8.

130. Klop KW, Hussain F, Karatepe O, Kok NF, Ijzermans JN, Dor FJ. Incision-related outcome after live donor nephrectomy: a single-center experience. *Surg Endosc* 2013; **27**(8):2801–6.
131. Humar A, Matas AJ. Surgical complications after kidney transplantation. *Semin Dial* 2005; **18**:505–10.
132. Sankari BR, Geisinger M, Zelch M, *et al.* Post-transplant renal artery stenosis: impact of therapy on long-term kidney function and blood pressure control. *J Urol* 1996; **155**:1860–4.
133. Osman Y, Shokeir A, Ali-el-Dein B, *et al.* Vascular complications after live donor renal transplantation: study of risk factors and effects on graft and patient survival. *J Urol* 2003; **169**:859–62.
134. Melamed ML, Kim HS, Jaar BG, *et al.* Combined percutaneous mechanical and chemical thrombectomy for renal vein thrombosis in kidney transplant recipients. *Am J Transplant* 2005; **5**:621–6.
135. Koo CK, Rodger S, Baxter GM. Extra-renal pseudoaneurysm: An uncommon complication following renal transplantation. *Clin Radiol* 1999; **54**:755–8.
136. Garrido J, Lerma JL, Heras M, *et al.* Pseudoaneurysm of the iliac artery secondary to Aspergillus infection in two recipients of kidney transplants from the same donor. *Am J Kidney Dis* 2003; **41**:488–92.
137. Fechner G, von Pezold C, Hauser S, *et al.* Impairment of long-term graft function after kidney transplantation by intraoperative vascular complications. *Int Urol Nephrol* 2008; **40**:869–73.
138. Khauli RB, Stoff JS, Lovewell T, *et al.* Post-transplant lymphoceles: a critical look into the risk factors, pathophysiology and management. *J Urol* 1993; **150**:22–6.
139. Bailey SH, Mone MC, Holman JM, *et al.* Laparoscopic treatment of post renal transplant lymphoceles. *Surg Endosc* 2003; **17**:1896–9.
140. Tasar M, Gulec B, Saglam M, *et al.* Posttransplant symptomatic lymphocele treatment with percutaneous drainage and ethanol sclerosis: long-term follow-up. *Clin Imaging* 2005; **29**:109–16.
141. Pengel LH, Liu LQ, Morris PJ. Do wound complications or lymphoceles occur more often in solid organ transplant recipients on mTOR inhibitors? A systematic review of randomized controlled trials. *Transpl Int* 2011; **24**:1216–30.
142. Mehrabi A, Fonouni H, Wente M, *et al.* Wound complications following kidney and liver transplantation. *Clin Transplant* 2006; **20**(Suppl 17):97–110.
143. Sousa SR, Galante NZ, Barbosa DA, *et al.* [Incidence of infectious complications and their risk factors in the first year after renal transplantation]. *J Bras Nefrol* 2010; **32**:75–82.
144. Menezes FG, Wey SB, Peres CA, *et al.* What is the impact of surgical site infection on graft function in kidney transplant recipients? *Transpl Infect Dis* 2010; **12**:392–6.
145. Humar A, Ramcharan T, Denny R, *et al.* Are wound complications after a kidney transplant more common with modern immunosuppression? *Transplantation* 2001; **72**:1920–3.
146. Etemadi J, Rahbar K, Haghighi AN, *et al.* Renal artery stenosis in kidney transplants: assessment of the risk factors. *Vasc Health Risk Manag* 2011; **7**:503–7.
147. Dols LF, Terkivatan T, Kok NF, *et al.* Use of stenting in living donor kidney transplantation: does it reduce vesicoureteral complications? *Transplant Proc* 2011; **43**:1623–6.
148. Baston C, Harza MC, Bogdan SI, *et al.* Urological complications after renal transplantation - therapeutical management: 2533. *Transplantation* 2012; **94**:603.
149. Asadpour A, Molaei M, Yaghoobi S. Management of ureteral complications in renal transplantation: prevention and treatment. *Saudi J Kidney Dis Transpl* 2011; **22**:72–4.
150. Gdor Y, Gabr AH, Faerber GJ, *et al.* Holmium:yttrium-aluminum-garnet laser endoureterotomy for the treatment of transplant kidney ureteral strictures. *Transplantation* 2008; **85**:1318–21.
151. de Sousa E, del Peso-Gilsanz G, Bajo-Rubio MA, *et al.* Encapsulating peritoneal sclerosis in peritoneal dialysis. a review and European initiative for approaching a serious and rare disease. *Nefrologia* 2012; **32**:707–14.
152. Habib SM, Betjes MG, Fieren MW, *et al.* Management of encapsulating peritoneal sclerosis: a guideline on optimal and uniform treatment. *Neth J Med* 2011; **69**:500–7.
153. Kawanishi H, Ide K, Yamashita M, *et al.* Surgical techniques for prevention of recurrence after total enterolysis in encapsulating peritoneal sclerosis. *Adv Perit Dial* 2008; **24**:51–5.
154. Habib SM, Hagen SM, Korte MR, *et al.* Localized encapsulating peritoneal sclerosis constricting the terminal ileum—an unusual appearance requiring surgical intervention. *Perit Dial Int* 2013; **33**:503–6.
155. Augustine T, Brown PW, Davies SD, *et al.* Encapsulating peritoneal sclerosis: clinical significance and implications. *Nephron Clin Pract* 2009; **111**:c149–54; discussion c54.
156. van den Akker EK, Manintveld OC, Hesselink DA, *et al.* Protection against renal ischemia-reperfusion injury by ischemic postconditioning. *Transplantation* 2013; **95**:1299–305.
157. Neipp M, Jackobs S, Becker T, *et al.* Living donor nephrectomy: flank incision versus anterior vertical mini-incision. *Transplantation* 2004; **78**:1356–61.
158. Lewis GR, Brook NR, Waller JR, *et al.* A comparison of traditional open, minimal-incision donor nephrectomy and laparoscopic donor nephrectomy. *Transpl Int* 2004; **17**:589–95.
159. Kok NF, Alwayn IP, Schouten O, *et al.* Mini-incision open donor nephrectomy as an alternative to classic lumbotomy: evolution of the open approach. *Transpl Int* 2006; **19**:500–5.
160. Schnitzbauer AA, Loss M, Hornung M, *et al.* Mini-incision for strictly retroperitoneal nephrectomy in living kidney donation vs flank incision. *Nephrol Dial Transplant* 2006; **21**:2948–52.
161. Kok NF, Lind MY, Hansson BM, *et al.* Comparison of laparoscopic and mini incision open donor nephrectomy: single blind, randomised controlled clinical trial. *BMJ* 2006; **333**:221.
162. Martin GL, Guise AI, Bernie JE, *et al.* Laparoscopic donor nephrectomy: effects of learning curve on surgical outcomes. *Transplant Proc* 2007; **39**:27–9.
163. Hofker HS, Nijboer WN, Niesing J, *et al.* A randomized clinical trial of living donor nephrectomy: a plea for a differentiated appraisal of mini-open muscle splitting incision and hand-assisted laparoscopic donor nephrectomy. *Transpl Int* 2012; **25**:976–86.
164. Bargman V, Sundaram CP, Bernie J, *et al.* Randomized trial of laparoscopic donor nephrectomy with and without hand assistance. *J Endourol* 2006; **20**:717–22.
165. Oyen O, Line PD, Pfeffer P, *et al.* Laparoscopic living donor nephrectomy: introduction of simple hand-assisted technique (without handport). *Transplant Proc* 2003; **35**:779–81.
166. El-Galley R, Hood N, Young CJ, *et al.* Donor nephrectomy: A comparison of techniques and results of open, hand assisted and full laparoscopic nephrectomy. *J Urol* 2004; **171**:40–3.
167. Gershbein AB, Fuchs GJ. Hand-assisted and conventional laparoscopic live donor nephrectomy: a comparison of two contemporary techniques. *J Endourol* 2002; **16**: 509–13.
168. Ruiz-Deya G, Cheng S, Palmer E, *et al.* Open donor, laparoscopic donor and hand assisted laparoscopic donor nephrectomy: a comparison of outcomes. *J Urol* 2001; **166**:1270–3; discussion 3–4.
169. Lindstrom P, Haggman M, Wadstrom J. Hand-assisted laparoscopic surgery (HALS) for live donor nephrectomy is more time- and cost-effective than standard laparoscopic nephrectomy. *Surg Endosc* 2002; **16**:422–5.
170. Velidedeoglu E, Williams N, Brayman KL, *et al.* Comparison of open, laparoscopic, and hand-assisted approaches to live-donor nephrectomy. *Transplantation* 2002; **74**:169–72.
171. Percegona LS, Bignelli AT, Adamy A, Jr., *et al.* Hand-assisted laparoscopic donor nephrectomy: comparison to pure laparoscopic donor nephrectomy. *Transplant Proc* 2008; **40**:687–8.
172. Ruszat R, Sulser T, Dickenmann M, *et al.* Retroperitoneoscopic donor nephrectomy: donor outcome and complication rate in comparison with three different techniques. *World J Urol* 2006; **24**:113–7.

173. Salazar A, Pelletier R, Yilmaz S, *et al.* Use of a minimally invasive donor nephrectomy program to select technique for live donor nephrectomy. *Am J Surg* 2005; **189**:558–62; discussion 62–3.
174. Wadstrom J, Lindstrom P, Engstrom BM. Hand-assisted retroperitoneoscopic living donor nephrectomy superior to laparoscopic nephrectomy. *Transplant Proc* 2003; **35**:782–3.
175. Dols LFC, Kok NFM, Tran TCK, *et al.* Hand-assisted retroperitoneoscopic versus standard laparoscopic donor nephrectomy: single blind, randomised controlled trial. *Transpl Int* 2011; **24**:25.
176. Gjertsen H, Sandberg AK, Wadstrom J, *et al.* Introduction of hand-assisted retroperitoneoscopic living donor nephrectomy at Karolinska University Hospital Huddinge. *Transplant Proc* 2006; **38**:2644–5.
177. Narita S, Inoue T, Matsuura S, *et al.* Outcome of right hand-assisted retroperitoneoscopic living donor nephrectomy. *Urology* 2006; **67**:496–500; discussion 500–1.
178. Renoult E, Hubert J, Ladriere M, *et al.* Robot-assisted laparoscopic and open live-donor nephrectomy: a comparison of donor morbidity and early renal allograft outcomes. *Nephrol Dial Transplant* 2006; **21**:472–7.

SECTION 10

Radiology

Section editor: Michael Weston

CHAPTER 10.1

Ionizing radiation and radiation protection

Jeannette Kathrin Kraft and Peter Howells

Introduction to ionizing radiation and radiation protection

In 1895 the German physicist Wilhelm Conrad Röntgen discovered X-rays when he noted that a fluorescent screen began to glow while he was experimenting with a vacuum tube. Soon after in 1896, Becquerel noted that photographic plates stored with uranium were fogged, discovering natural occurring radiation. By the early 1900s X-rays were used widely in medical imaging. However soon after discovery adverse health effects became apparent. Many early radiologists died of radiation-induced sickness and cancer.[1] In 1915 the British Roentgen Ray Society adopted radiation protection recommendations, probably representing the first joint effort at radiation protection. In the 1920s film badges were introduced for routine personnel monitoring and in 1925 the first exposure limits were set.

The study of biological effects continued with the long-term follow up of people exposed to radiation from atomic bombs in Japan in the 1950s and is still ongoing today.[2,3] Radiation accidents such as Chernobyl in 1986 and Fukushima in 2011 increased public awareness.

After the advent of computed tomography (CT) in the 1970s the use of ionizing radiation in medical imaging is steadily increasing. It is estimated that approximately 62 million CT examinations are performed yearly in the United States and approximately 4 billion radiological examinations are performed worldwide.[4,5] The first direct study of cancer risk in children who have undergone CT scanning has recently been published.[6] Although the risk for any individual may not be substantial; the increasing radiation exposure to the population may be a health risk in the future.[5] However, there is still a lack of awareness of radiation exposure and its associated risks among medical practitioners.[7]

Definition of ionizing radiation

Radiation is a form of energy transmitted through space. There are many types of radiation such as heat, light, radio waves, microwaves, X-rays, and gamma rays. The frequency of the waves describes its position in the electromagnetic spectrum. Low energy radio waves with low frequencies are at one end of the electromagnetic spectrum; high frequency, high energy waves such as X-rays or gamma rays at the other end. High frequency waves that carry a large amount of energy can penetrate material and transfer energy to an atom that may cause displacement of an electron from its orbit around the nucleus. This process is called ionization. Ionizing radiation can be electromagnetic radiation such as X-rays or gamma rays or particulate radiation such as alpha particles, beta particles, or neutrons. It can be produced in a generator such as an X-ray machine or come from radioactive material as used in nuclear medicine or radiotherapy.

Measuring radiation

Absorbed dose

When ionizing radiation passes through tissue, it deposits energy causing ionization and excitation of the matter. The amount of energy deposited divided by the mass of tissue exposed is called the absorbed dose. The unit of absorbed dose is joule per kilogram (J/kg) but for convenience it has been given a special name: gray [Gy]. This is an easy quantity to measure but is not a useful indicator of long-term risk.

Equivalent dose

Different kinds of radiation cause different biological effects for the same amount of energy deposited. For instance neutrons or alpha particles cause more damage per unit absorbed dose compared to X-rays or gamma rays. To allow for this a quality factor for radiation was introduced resulting in the equivalent dose. For X-rays and gamma rays, the absorbed dose equals the equivalent dose. The unit of equivalent dose is also joule per kilogram (J/kg) but to avoid confusion it has been given a different name: sievert [Sv].

Effective dose

In addition tissues have different sensitivity to radiation due to cell turnover rate and tissue specific characteristics. To account for this a tissue weighting factor was added to modify equivalent dose resulting in the effective dose. The unit for the effective dose stays the same: sievert [Sv]. Doses in medical imaging and radiation protection are usually organ specific and refer to effective doses. As they are often small, most are expressed as milli sievert [mSv].

Indicators of dose

In practice, it is not possible to measure effective dose directly. Within a procedure other indicators of dose are generally used, such as the dose area product (DAP) in radiography and fluoroscopy or dose length product (DLP) in CT. DAP measures the dose in air multiplied by the X-ray beam area at a point close to the X-ray unit. This quantity is a constant for any distance from the X-ray tube. DLP measures the dose per rotation of the CT scanner multiplied by the length of the patient included in the scan. Effective dose can be inferred from each of these values but only with knowledge of other parameters.

Sources of ionizing radiation

Radiation is a natural phenomenon which we are exposed to continuously from natural and artificial man-made sources. Low levels of radiation cannot be seen or felt, so people are not usually aware of it.

Natural background radiation

Natural background radiation is all around us and includes high energy cosmic rays, radioactive nuclides from the earth crust such as uranium and thorium and radon gas. The annual effective dose from natural background radiation varies substantially throughout the country and the world due to variation in altitude and the constituents of the soil. The average annual effective dose from natural sources in the world is estimated to be 2.4 mSv.[8] When describing radiation exposure from medical examinations we often compare the dose received from that examination to natural background radiation.

Man-made radiation

Radiation exposure may be increased in several ways due to human activity and technological processes, for example air travel (increased levels of cosmic radiation); nuclear testing and nuclear accidents such as Chernobyl 1986; nuclear power production; occupational exposure; and consumer products such as electronic equipment, fire alarms, and luminous numbers on watches and clocks. However the largest amount of man-made radiation exposure is through medical imaging procedures.

Medical exposures

Medical exposures account for 98% of the contribution from all artificial sources and are now the second largest contributor to the population dose worldwide, representing approximately 20% of the total from all sources. It is estimated that from 1997–2007 approximately 3.6 billion medical radiation procedures were performed annually worldwide, an increase of 40% on the last decade.[8] This increase is demonstrated particularly for high dose examinations, such as CT scanning which are increasing more rapidly than other techniques. Medical radiation procedures were 65 times more frequent in developed countries compared to underdeveloped countries reflecting an imbalance of radiation exposure and healthcare provision. In several countries medical radiation exposure is now larger than exposure from natural sources.[8]

Potential health effects of ionizing radiation

Biological effects

As previously described high energy ionizing radiation causes displacement of an electron from its orbit around the nucleus. This electron can cause direct damage when the electron hits a strand of DNA or indirect damage when the electron reacts with surrounding water molecules producing free radicals or ions. A free radical is a molecule with unpaired electrons that in turn avidly undergoes chemical reactions with surrounding molecules such as DNA. Damage to a cell's DNA may have several consequences. Single strand breaks may simply be repaired without detrimental effects to the cell. However double strand breaks could be repaired incorrectly which can potentially cause hereditary effects if occurring in gonadal cells or produce malignancy through activation of oncogenes.[4]

The amount of damage to an individual or organ depends on the type and amount of radiation and therefore the energy transferred to the tissues, the duration of exposure, the distance from the radiation source and whether the exposure was continuous or intermittent.

The probability of a tissue or organ to suffer effects from ionizing radiation is called radiosensitivity. Tissues with high rates of mitosis and undifferentiated cells are the most sensitive. Therefore bone marrow cells, gonads, lens cells, and bowel mucosal cells are highly sensitive whereas bone and neural cells are relatively less radiosensitive.

Tissue reactions (deterministic effects)

Ionizing radiation may cause acute effects which are largely due to cell death. They require a threshold dose of manifestation which is not the same for each individual or tissue. These are also known as deterministic or non-stochastic effects and are usually seen at high radiation doses such radiotherapy or radiation accidents. Because a threshold can be identified, radiation protection measures and occupational dose limits can eliminate such effects for workers. Deterministic effects include skin erythema, ulceration and burns, bone marrow depression, cataracts, acute radiation sickness, sterility, and foetal death.[9] Healing may occur but damage to tissues may result in fibrosis or necrosis. Although relatively rare such effects have been observed from medical imaging such as CT scanning and interventional procedures.[10–12]

Random (stochastic effects)

Damage to a cell's DNA increases the probability of cancer induction. If germ cells are affected, hereditary effects in dependents may be observed. Those effects are random and long-term, and also known as stochastic or non-deterministic effects. The first study investigating the direct risk of cancer induction from medical imaging was published in 2012. It has shown a small increased risk of leukaemia and brain cancer after cranial CT in children.[6] More recent studies also report a link between childhood CT scans and increased risk of cancer with some taking predisposing factors for cancer into consideration.[13–15] Lifespan studies on atomic bomb survivors indicate increased risk for development of leukaemia and solid cancers including stomach, lung, liver, colon, breast, gallbladder, oesophagus, bladder, and ovary after exposure to ionizing radiation.[2,3]

Estimating risk from medical examinations

Cancer risk

At the low radiation doses (effective doses less than 100–200 mSv) commonly used in medical imaging, statistical limitations make it difficult to accurately estimate cancer risk. Extraordinarily large numbers of patients would need to be followed up over a lifetime to quantify risk at low doses of radiation exposure.[16] Most of the available data on cancer induction was therefore extrapolated from high radiation doses received over a short time interval such as from the atomic bomb survivors and radiation accidents. The assumption that radiation risk continues in a linear fashion when extrapolated from high to low doses is termed the linear non-threshold model.[16,17] At present this model is the most widely accepted theory to describe radiation effects at low doses. It assumes that no level of radiation exposure is safe and that even the smallest dose of radiation has a potential to cause harm.

Data from atomic survivors and radiation accidents has been used to develop risk models and theories. Such models predict that for a radiation exposure of 0.1 Sv above background radiation one person in 100 would be expected to develop cancer. Similarly, for a radiation exposure of 10 mSv, which is approximately the effective dose that would be received from a CT scan of the abdomen, 1 in 1,000 people could be expected to develop cancer.[17] At present it is not possible to determine whether a cancer was induced by radiation or any other cause. In a population, radiation effects especially from low dose radiation can be obscured by the large number of non-radiation cancers occurring: 1 in 3 people will develop cancer from natural causes and 1 in 6 people are predicted to die of such cancer.[17]

There is also a considerable latent period between radiation exposure and the induction of cancer. The mean latent period for leukaemia is 7–10 years, for bone tumours 10–15 years, and approximately 20 years for most solid tumours.[18] This time lag of cancer induction explains the higher risk for younger patients and the relatively low risk for elderly patients.

Hereditary defects

Excess hereditary effects due to radiation exposure have not been demonstrated in humans and were not detected in atomic bomb survivors of Hiroshima and Nagasaki.[4,17] Minor effects are likely to be so small that current studies are unable to differentiate them from naturally occurring mutational effects. However radiation-induced mutations can theoretically occur in reproductive cells (egg and sperm) resulting in hereditable diseases. Such effects have been previously demonstrated in animal studies, mainly mice.[19]

Risks to the foetus

In utero radiation of the foetus can cause great anxiety. Radiation exposure very early on in a pre-implantation stage could lead to an all or nothing phenomenon of spontaneous abortion or normal pregnancy. High doses delivered during organogenesis may cause central nervous system (CNS) abnormalities inducing microcephaly or mental retardation. Malformations are thought to have a threshold of 100–200 mGy absorbed dose which is rarely reached in medical diagnostic imaging. During the third trimester the organs are developed and the risk of congenital malformations is low but there is a small risk of inducing cancer or leukaemia. However diagnostic radiological procedures should not normally exceed 50–100 mGy and with such an exposure there is a 99% chance that the child will not develop cancer or leukaemia.[20,21] Children and the foetus are more sensitive to ionizing radiation than adults due to the larger number of dividing cells and the longer lifespan available to develop cancer.

Absolute risk to a patient

An estimation of somebody's risk from a medical procedure can be made by applying the average effective dose of the procedure and taking the age of exposure, the organ irradiated, and the sex into account.[22] As risk from radiation exposure is cumulative, radiation doses from several procedures are added to calculate risk.

However, considering the benefits from imaging in diagnosing illness and injury, a medically indicated imaging study will almost always outweigh the risk associated with it. This is especially apparent when evaluating risks associated with common daily activities such as driving a car. Those activities carry a much higher risk of dying than the cancer risk of 1:1,000 associated with a single CT scan of abdomen delivering a dose of 10 mSv.[17,23,24] Therefore when assessing radiation exposure at very low radiation doses such as for instance for single exposure of a chest radiograph (0.01 mSv), the risk of radiation-induced cancer persists but in practice becomes negligible.[24]

Quantifying radiation in medical imaging

When describing radiation doses received by patients we often compare this to natural background radiation (2.4 mSv per year). Effective doses for most radiological examinations have been published.[25] Plain film radiographic examinations vary by a large factor from 0.001 mSv to 10 mSv, CT examinations have relatively high average effective doses between 2 and 20 mSv and interventional procedures can give effective doses between 5 and 70 mSv.[25] For comparison a round trip flight from London to New York will result in a radiation exposure due to increased cosmic radiation of about 0.1 mSv.[16]

From time to time, the Health Protection Agency (HPA), now Public Health England publishes the results of national patient dose surveys performed in the United Kingdom, for radiological examinations and for CT.[26,27] The doses are typically shown as entrance dose, DAP or DLP for CT, but effective doses can be estimated from tables published by the National Radiation Protection Board.[28] Doses of selected examinations are shown in Table 10.1.1 and Table 10.1.2.

Managing patient risk

Even though uncertainties remain about the absolute risk of low dose radiation, the risk is not entirely negligible. Concerns about radiation and induction of cancer are likely to be in the public focus for the foreseeable future. It is therefore the responsibility of all healthcare professionals to manage and control the risk to protect patients. This point is reinforced by government authority through legislation.

The Ionising Radiation (Medical Exposure) Regulations 2000

The Ionising Radiation (Medical Exposure) Regulations 2000 impose obligations on hospital authorities and clinicians to minimize radiation doses to patients.[29] The three principles governing patient protection in medical imaging are justification, optimization and dose reference levels (DLRs).

Table 10.1.1 Typical effective doses to adults from selected radiological procedures

Radiograph	3rd quartile dose area product (DAP) per radiograph (Gycm²)	Effective dose estimated from NRPB coefficients (mSv)
Chest PA	0.3	0.03
Abdomen AP	4.4	1.1
IVU	14	2.5

Source: data from Hart D *et al.*, *Doses to patients from radiographic and fluoroscopic X-ray imaging procedures in the UK-2010 Review*, Health Protection Agency, HPA-CRCE-034, Chilton, UK Copyright © 2012; and *Estimation of Effective Dose in Diagnostic Radiology from Entrance Surface Dose and Dose-Area Product Measurements*, NRPB-R262, National Radiological Protection Board, Chilton, UK, Copyright © 1994.

Table 10.1.2 Typical effective doses to adults from selected CT procedures

CT scan	Reference dose length product (DLP) per scan (Gycm)	Effective dose estimated from NRPB coefficients (mSv)
Chest (high resolution)	170	2.4
Abdomen	470	7.1
Chest, abdomen, and pelvis	940	14.1

Source: data from Shrimpton PC *et al., Doses from Computed Tomography (CT) Examinations in the UK-2003 Review*, NRPB-W67, National Radiological Protection Board Chilton, UK Copyright © 2005; and *Estimation of Effective Dose in Diagnostic Radiology from Entrance Surface Dose and Dose-Area Product Measurements*, NRPB-R262, National Radiological Protection Board, Chilton, UK, Copyright © 1994.

Imaging selection

Not all imaging modalities use harmful radiation. The same information might be acquired with an imaging modality that does not use ionizing radiation such as sonography or magnetic resonance imaging. Sometimes it can be beneficial just to observe the patient for a time period for symptoms to unmask. This is part of a decision process to justify the examination.

Justification

For each examination performed there should be careful risk/ benefit analysis. It is the responsibility of the clinician as the 'Referrer' (term under IRMER) to supply sufficient information for the radiology professional as the 'Practitioner' to decide whether the examination is justified. The *iRefer: Making the best use of clinical radiology* publication by the Royal College of Radiologists can help clinicians to select appropriate imaging.[30] For most examinations, the radiographer or 'Operator' working within departmental protocols will decide whether to proceed and perform the examination. This is not unique to the risk assessment associated with ionizing radiation. Similar consideration are made for instance when considering the risk of bleeding or infection from a diagnostic biopsy, the risk of general anaesthesia or simply whether it is safe for the patient to be transferred to a different department.

Technique selection and optimization

If imaging using ionizing radiation is necessary the radiology professional will aim to use the lowest possible radiation dose giving an accurate diagnosis. This attempt at optimization refers to the ALARA principle of reducing the radiation dose to 'as much as reasonably achievable or practicable'. This includes only scanning the area indicated (e.g. renal area rather than the whole abdomen), working under local protocols, adjusting scanning parameters for children and to avoid multiple phase scanning (e.g. non-contrast, arterial and portal venous phase CT scans) and controlling scan time in fluoroscopy. Optimization also includes quality assurance programmes, regular audits, and planned replacement of elderly or outdated equipment.

Repeat studies

Repeat studies can be avoided. Patients with chronic or long-term problems such as young patients (e.g. with nephrolithiasis) should be carefully managed as radiation dose is thought to be cumulative over time. These patients should not be repeatedly subjected to CT scans each time they present. Perhaps the clinical question can be answered with an ultrasound scan, reserving CT scanning for problem solving. Discussion with the radiology professional should be encouraged.

Diagnostic reference levels

Under IRMER, diagnostic reference levels (DRLs) should be established for each standard examination and type of equipment at each imaging department. These levels indicate the radiation dose a typical patient is likely to receive from a standard radiological examination. However DRLs are not strictly dose limits as the radiation dose received by a patient depends on factors such as patient size, the technique selected, and for fluoroscopic examinations the screening time. DRLs may be seen as action thresholds and are regularly audited. If they are regularly exceeded further optimization of technique, or particular justification is needed.

Radiation doses from interventional procedures can be high, particularly to the skin where the same area is persistently irradiated during an extended procedure. For such procedures, similar action thresholds, in terms of DAP or total screening time, can be used to inform the radiology professional of the possibility of tissue reactions and possible injury that would be likely to result if the same body area is continuously irradiated.

Communication and education

Communication between the clinician and the radiology professional is important and will help to tailor a radiological investigation to the patient's needs reducing the amount of radiation. Educating clinicians and patients about the risk of radiation exposure from medical procedures is the aim of campaigns such as 'Image gently' for children and 'Image wisely' for adults.[31,32]

Minimizing risk to staff

Principles

Any measures that reduce patient dose also reduce potential occupational dose to staff.[33] During fluoroscopy, dose can be reduced by reducing the beam size through collimation, using pulsed fluoroscopy, and last image hold instead of continuous screening and by keeping exposure times as short as possible.

While it is commonly known to stay away from the primary beam directed at the patient, a significant dose to the operator when performing fluoroscopic examinations in theatre is from scattered radiation. The inverse square law demonstrates that doubling the distance to the source reduces the dose by a factor of four. Therefore stepping back during exposure or using a remote control will significantly reduce staff doses. Structural shielding and protective clothing such as aprons, thyroid shields, and goggles reduce the dose received by staff. Local rules and procedures are in place to protect staff and should be regularly reinforced through continuous education and training.

Dose monitoring

Usually, employees working with ionizing radiation are regularly monitored. The International Commission on Radiological Protection (ICRP) has recommended dose limits for staff working with ionizing radiation and these are reiterated in UK radiation protection legislation.[34] For employees over 18 years of age the annual limit on effective dose is 20 mSv, for trainees and employees under 18 years, 6 mSv and 1 mSv per year for the general public.[33,34]

Additional annual limits on dose are set at 500 mSv equivalent dose for extremities, such as the fingers and hands of those involved in interventions, and for each 1 cm^2 skin. An annual limit on dose to the lens of the eye is set at 150 mSv, but is under review at the time of writing, with the expectation that it will be reduced to 20 mSv. In practice, occupational doses are constrained below these annual limits with a requirement to 'classify' radiation workers whose doses are expected, following risk assessment of their work, to exceed three-tenths of any annual limit.

Conclusion

Medical imaging using ionizing radiation has become invaluable in evaluating the sick patient. Radiation should not be feared, especially in emergency situations such as trauma imaging with a clear benefit from scanning. Radiation cannot be entirely avoided but it can be managed following the ALARA principle. Medical exposures should be justified, duplication of scans should be avoided and the lowest radiation dose consistent with the diagnostic objective should always be used.

Further reading

Brenner DJ, Doll R, Goodhead DT, *et al.* Cancer risks attributable to low doses of ionising radiation: assessing what we really know. *Proc Natl Acad Sci U S A*. 2003; **100**(24):13761–13766.

Brenner DJ, Hall EJ. Computed tomography—An increasing source of radiation exposure. *NEJM* 2007; **357**:2277–84.

Department of Health. The Ionising Radiation (Medical Exposure) Regulations 2000 (together with notes on good practice). Available at: http://webarchive.nationalarchives.gov.uk/20130107105354/http://www.dh.gov.uk/prod_consum_dh/groups/dh_digitalassets/@dh/@en/documents/digitalasset/dh_064707.pdf [Online].

Health Protection Agency. National Radiation Protection Board. X-rays—How safe are they? Patient information leaflet, 2001. Available at: http://webarchive.nationalarchives.gov.uk/20140714084352/http://www.hpa.org.uk/webc/HPAwebFile/HPAweb_C/1194947388410 [Online].

Image Gently. Available at: http://www.pedrad.org/associations/5364/ig/ [Online].

Image Wisely. Available at: http://www.imagewisely.org/ [Online].

iRefer: Making the Best Use of Clinical Radiology. London, UK: The Royal College of Radiologists, 2012.

Mettler FA, Huda W, Yoshizumi TT, Mahesh M. Effective doses in radiology and diagnostic nuclear medicine: A catalogue. *Radiology* 2008; **248**(1):254–63.

National Academy of Sciences. Health risk from exposure to low levels of ionising radiation: BEIR VII Phase 2 (Free Executive Summary) 2006. Available at: http://www.nap.edu/catalog/11340.html [Online].

Pearce MS, Salotti JA, Little MP, *et al.* Radiation exposure from CT scans in childhood and subsequent risk of leukaemia and brain tumours: a retrospective cohort study. *Lancet* 2012; **380**(9840):499–505.

References

1. Berry RJ. The radiologist as guinea pig: radiation hazards to man as demonstrated in early radiologists and their patients. *J Royal Soc Med* 1986; **79**:506–809.
2. Ozasa K, Shimizu Y, Suyama A, *et al.* Studies of the mortality of atomic bomb survivors, report14, 1950-2003: An overview of cancer and non-cancer diseases. *Radiat Res* 2012; **177**:229–43.
3. Richardson D, Sugiyama H, Nishi N, *et al.* Ionizing radiation and leukemia mortality among Japanese atomic bomb survivors, 1950-2000. *Radiat Res* 2009; **172**:368–82.
4. United Nations Scientific Committee on the Effects of Atomic Radiation (UNSCEAR). 2010 Report: Summery of low dose radiation effects on health, New York, 2011. Available at: http://www.unscear.org/docs/reports/2010/UNSCEAR_2010_Report_M.pdf [Online].
5. Brenner DJ, Hall EJ. Computed tomography—An increasing source of radiation exposure. *NEJM* 2007; **357**:2277–84.
6. Pearce MS, Salotti JA, Little MP, *et al.* Radiation exposure from CT scans in childhood and subsequent risk of leukaemia and brain tumours: a retrospective cohort study. *Lancet* 2012; **380**(9840):499–505.
7. Shiralkar S, Rennie A, Snow M, Galland RB, Lewis MH, Gower-Thomas K. Doctors' knowledge of radiation exposure: questionnaire study. *BMJ* 2003; **327**(7411):371–2.
8. United Nations Scientific Committee on the Effects of Atomic Radiation (UNSCEAR). 2008 Report: Sources of Ionising Radiation, Annex A: Medical radiation exposures, New York, 2010. Available at: http://www.unscear.org/docs/reports/2008/09-86753_Report_2008_Annex_A.pdf [Online].
9. Mettler FA, Upton AC. *Medical Effects of Ionising Radiation*, 3rd edition. Philadelphia: Saunders Elsevier, 2008: pp. 285–388.
10. Shope TB. Radiation-induced skin injury from fluoroscopy. *RadioGraphics* 1996; **16**:1195–9.
11. Bogdanich W. After stroke scans, patients face serious health risks. New York Times, 10 July 2010. Available at: http://www.nytimes.com/2010/08/01/health/01radiation.html?_r=4 [Online].
12. Banaag L de O, Carter ML. Radionecrosis induced by cardiac imaging procedures: a case study of a 66-year-old diabetic male with several comorbidities. *J Invasive Cardiol* 2005; **20**(8):E2336
13. Mathews JD, Forsythe AV, Brady Z, *et al.* Cancer risk in 680,000 people exposed to computed tomography scans in childhood and adolescence; data linkage study in 11 million Australians. *BMJ* 2013; 21; **346**:f2360. doi: 10.1136/bmj.f2360
14. Berrington de Gonzales A, Salotti JA, McHugh K, *et al.* Relationship between paediaitric CT scans and subsequent risk of leukaemia and brain tumours; assessment of the impact of underlying conditions. *British Journal of Cancer* 2016; **114**:338–94. doi: 10.1038/bjc.2015.415
15. Krille L, Dreger S, Schindel *et al.* Risk of cancer incidence before the age of 15 years after exposure to ionising radiation from computed tomography: results from a German cohort study. *Radiat Environ Biophys* 2015; **54**:1–12.
16. Brenner DJ, Doll R, Goodhead DT, *et al.* Cancer risks attributable to low doses of ionising radiation: assessing what we really know. *Proc Natl Acad Sci U S A* 2003; **100**(24):13761–13766.
17. National Academy of Sciences. Health risk from exposure to low levels of ionising radiation: BEIR VII Phase 2 (Free Executive Summary) 2006. Available at: http://www.nap.edu/catalog/11340.html [Online].
18. Mettler FA, Upton AC. *Medical Effects of Ionising Radiation*, 3rd edition. Philadelphia, PA: Saunders Elsevier, 2008: pp. 71–116.
19. United Nations Scientific Committee on the Effects of Atomic Radiation (UNSCEAR). 2001 Report: Hereditary effects of radiation, Annex, New York, 2001. Available at: http://www.unscear.org/docs/reports/2001/2001Annex_pages%208-160.pdf [Online].
20. International Commission on Radiological Protection (ICRP), Pregnancy and medical radiation. ICRP Publication 84. *Ann ICRP* 2000; **30**(1).
21. Brent RL. The effects of embryonic and fetal exposure to x-ray, microwave and ultrasound. *Clin Obstet Gynecol* 1984, **26**(2);484–510.
22. Wall BF, Haylock R, Jansen JTM, Hillier MC, Hart D, Shrimpton PC. Radiation risks from medical X-ray examinations as a function of age and sex of the patient. Health Protection Agency. HPA-CRCE-028, Chilton, 2011. Available at: http://www.hpa.org.uk/webc/HPAwebFile/HPAweb_C/1317131197532 [Online].
23. National Safety Council. Injury fact. Lifetime odds of death for selected causes, United States 2006. 2010 edition. Available at: http://www.nsc.org/news_resources/Documents/nscInjuryFacts2011_037.pdf [Online].

24. Health Protection Agency. National Radiation Protection Board. X-rays—How safe are they? Patient information leaflet, 2001. Available at: http://webarchive.nationalarchives.gov.uk/20140714084352/http://www.hpa.org.uk/webc/HPAwebFile/HPAweb_C/1194947388410 [Online].
25. Mettler FA, Huda W, Yoshizumi TT, Mahesh M. Effective doses in radiology and diagnostic nuclear medicine: A catalogue. *Radiology* 2008; **248**(1):254–63.
26. Hart D, Hillier MC, Shrimpton PC. Doses to patients from radiographic and fluoroscopic X-ray imaging procedures in the UK-2010 Review. Health Protection Agency. HPA-CRCE-034, Chilton, 2012. Available at: http://www.hpa.org.uk/webc/HPAwebFile/HPAweb_C/1317134577210 [Online].
27. Shrimpton PC, Hillier MC, Lewis MA, Dunn M. Doses from Computed Tomography (CT) Examinations in the UK—2003 Review. National Radiological Protection Board NRPB-W67, Chilton, 2005. Available at: http://webarchive.nationalarchives.gov.uk/20140714084352/http://www.hpa.org.uk/webc/HPAwebFile/HPAweb_C/1194947420292 [Online].
28. National Radiological Protection Board. NRPB-R262. Estimation of Effective Dose in Diagnostic Radiology from Entrance Surface Dose and Dose-Area Product Measurements, 1994.
29. Department of Health. The Ionising Radiation (Medical Exposure) Regulations 2000 (together with notes on good practice). Available at: http://webarchive.nationalarchives.gov.uk/20130107105354/http://www.dh.gov.uk/prod_consum_dh/groups/dh_digitalassets/@dh/@en/documents/digitalasset/dh_064707.pdf [Online].
30. iRefer: Making the Best Use of Clinical Radiology. London, UK: The Royal College of Radiologists, 2012.
31. Image Gently. Available at: http://www.pedrad.org/associations/5364/ig/ [Online].
32. Image Wisely. Available at: http://www.imagewisely.org/ [Online].
33. Heron JL, Padovani R, Smith I, Czarwinski R. Radiation protection of medical staff. *Eur J Radiol* 2010; **76**:20–3.
34. The Ionising Radiations Regulations 1999, SI 1999 N0. 3232. Available at: http://www.legislation.gov.uk/uksi/1999/3232/pdfs/uksi_19993232_en.pdf [Online].

CHAPTER 10.2

Ultrasound

Toby Wells and Simon J. Freeman

Ultrasound physics

Greyscale ultrasound

Ultrasound creates an image using short duration pulses of high frequency sound waves generated by electrically stimulating a piezoelectric crystal in a hand-held ultrasound transducer. The pressure wave generated is transmitted to the patient using a coupling gel between the transducer and skin surface. Returning echoes hit the same crystal and the vibrations induced are reconverted to an electrical signal which is then processed to create the image.

Different tissues reflect to varying degrees when exposed to the ultrasound beam; this behaviour is largely determined by tissue density and is expressed as the 'acoustic impedance'—at the boundaries between soft tissues of different acoustic impedance the sound wave is partially reflected. If the interface is close to perpendicular with the ultrasound beam (more than 60 degrees) the reflected echo will return to the transducer and be detected; its strength determines the brightness of the interface on the display. At soft tissue/air or soft tissue/bone interfaces the difference in acoustic impedance is so great that almost all the sound is reflected and none left to image deeper structures; the inability of ultrasound to penetrate gas-filled organs (such as bowel or lung) and bone can cause difficulty in obtaining a diagnostic ultrasound study. Other echoes are derived from tiny tissue structures that are similar in size to the ultrasound wavelength; rather than reflect the ultrasound beam these cause it to be scattered in all directions. This phenomenon is of particular importance in generating a Doppler signal from moving red blood cells. Ultrasound is assumed to have a constant velocity in soft tissue (about 1,540 m/s); therefore the time interval between transmission of the ultrasound pulse and reception of the returning echo can be used to calculate the distance of the reflecting interface from the transducer. The crystals within the transducer are fired sequentially and the returning reflected and backscattered echoes analysed for their strength and delay. This information is used to construct a real-time two-dimensional image, referred to as the greyscale or B (brightness)-mode.

Higher frequency sound produces images of higher resolution, but the sound is attenuated more quickly and so tissue penetration is reduced. This should be borne in mind when selecting the appropriate transducer for an ultrasound study; a high frequency transducer (7–11 MHz) gives better resolution and is ideal for imaging superficial structures such as the testes, or for endocavity use such as in transrectal ultrasound. A lower frequency transducer (3.5–5 MHz) is usually required to visualize abdominal structures such as the native kidneys. Selecting the appropriate transducer is therefore a trade-off between image quality and depth penetration. Resolution is optimized by ensuring that the focus of the beam is adjusted to the level of the region of interest. High frequency transducers usually have a flat surface (linear array) producing a parallel ultrasound beam of the width of the transducer (see 'Penile ultrasound' section). Lower frequency abdominal (see 'Paediatric urological ultrasound' section) and endocavity transducers (see 'Bladder ultrasound' section) usually have a curved surface producing a diverging ultrasound beam and a wide ultrasound sector.

Harmonic imaging and spatial compounding are techniques that are now routinely employed by most manufacturers to produce images with less artefact and greater resolution or clarity.

Doppler ultrasound

The Doppler effect is the change in frequency that occurs when a sound source or detector are moving relative to one another. This is a familiar phenomenon to us in our everyday lives; for example, the change in tone of a siren as an emergency vehicle passes a static observer. The same principle can be employed in diagnostic ultrasound to demonstrate and measure blood flow. The frequency shift of an ultrasound wave that has been scattered by cells in moving blood is proportional their velocity. Blood flowing towards the transducer will increase the frequency; conversely flow away from the transducer will decrease the frequency. The frequency shift that results is small in comparison with the transmitted frequency; usually in the audible range. The Doppler frequency shift also depends on the transmitted ultrasound frequency and the cosine of the angle between the ultrasound beam and the direction of blood flow. The greatest Doppler frequency shift is generated when blood is flowing directly towards or away from the transducer, and there is no Doppler signal if the vessel is parallel to the transducer. The ultrasound practitioner must therefore optimize probe positioning and, where possible, utilize electronic beam steering to ensure a satisfactory angle. If measurement of flow velocity is required the angle of blood flow relative to the ultrasound beam must be manually selected using angle correction which permits the flow velocity to be calculated from the Doppler frequency shift; in this situation the angle should be 60 degrees or less. Doppler information may be displayed as either a plot of velocity against time on a pulse wave (spectral) graph, or alternatively direction of flow and velocities, and may be translated into different colours on a colour flow map. Power Doppler is another mode that assigns colour to blood flow, but it uses the power of the Doppler signal rather than the frequency shift. It is more sensitive to low flow than colour Doppler but gives no information about velocity or direction of flow.

The normal spectral arterial renal Doppler trace has high velocity flow in systole but also persistent forward flow throughout diastole, with a trace likened to a 'ski slope' (see 'Renal transplants' section).

Various parameters have been described to quantify this pattern. One of these, the resistance index (RI), is described in the renal transplant ultrasound section.

Ultrasound contrast imaging

Ultrasound contrast agents are being increasingly used in many different areas of ultrasound practice. The most recent agents are based on stabilized microbubbles of perfluorocarbon gas in lipid shells. These have an excellent safety profile and no renal toxicity.[1] Ultrasound takes advantage of the resonant properties of the microbubbles in the sound beam, enhancing visualization of blood flow. Contrast-enhanced ultrasound (CEUS) studies are performed at very low power settings using harmonic techniques; this requires specific software which is now available on most mid and high range systems. There are many potential applications of ultrasound contrast agents in urology, including characterization of complex renal cysts, renal vascular disorders, infection, transplant assessment, differentiation between complex renal cysts and solid lesions and between renal pseudomasses and tumours.[2] There are further applications for CEUS in scrotal, bladder, and prostatic ultrasound.[3]

Safety

Ultrasound is a safe imaging technique which does not involve ionizing radiation. Despite the enormous number of ultrasound studies performed there are no confirmed deleterious medical side effects of this technique but it is good practice to minimize exposure by adjusting the power output to the lowest possible levels to obtain a diagnostic quality image, and minimizing scan time. This is of particular importance in obstetric imaging when scanning the foetus.

Energy is transmitted to the patient during ultrasound examinations and this may cause mechanical or thermal effects. The main mechanical concern is cavitation (the collapse of gas filled bubbles liberating energy) with a risk of local tissue damage. An estimate of the probability of cavitation occurring is displayed as the mechanical index (MI) on the ultrasound machine display. Cavitation is of particular concern when ultrasound contrast microbubble agents are used at high acoustic power settings and at gas/ tissue interfaces. The probability of tissue heating occurring is displayed as the thermal index (TI).

For a more comprehensive review of clinically based ultrasound principles and physics, the reader is directed towards Allan *et al.* (2011) in the suggested reading list.

Renal ultrasound

Introduction

Ultrasound is established as the primary imaging modality in many conditions affecting the kidney. It is usually the first choice investigation for renal functional impairment, haematuria,[4] and urinary tract infection. Although non-contrast computed tomography (CT) is the imaging investigation of choice in most patients presenting with loin pain, ultrasound is still used in certain circumstances such as pregnancy and in children. Ultrasound is also frequently used to characterize incidental lesions found on other imaging modalities as solid or cystic.

Technique and normal appearances

To achieve accurate diagnosis requires attention to good ultrasound technique. The kidneys are orientated such that their upper poles are situated posteromedially to the lower poles. This should be borne in mind when orientating the transducer to obtain a true long axis image of the kidneys. Close anatomical relation to the bowel means the lower poles are frequently obscured by bowel gas, and the upper poles may be obscured by ribs. Scanning usually begins with the patient in the supine position using a 3–5 MHz curvilinear transducer. Views of the right kidney can be facilitated by using the liver as an acoustic window. Scanning intercostally but angling down towards the feet may allow visualization of the lower poles when they would otherwise be obscured and compression can be used to displace gas. Rolling the patient into the lateral decubitus position and deep inspiration may also be of assistance. Fasting is generally not considered necessary preparation for renal ultrasound.

It should be noted that although the kidneys, adrenals, and perinephric fat are enclosed in Gerota's fascia, the two layers may not be fused inferiorly and medially to the kidneys. This can allow considerable mobility of the kidneys inferiorly and across the midline when rolling some patients onto their side.

The renal cortex, medulla, and sinus can be differentiated on ultrasound. The central renal sinus fat is usually echogenic and the medullary pyramids are echo poor. The cortex covers the bases of the pyramids, extends down between them in the columns of Bertin, and is of intermediate echogenicity (Fig.10.2.1). The relative reflectivity of the cortex is often compared to the adjacent liver or spleen, with the normal renal cortex being less echogenic (darker) than the normal liver and spleen.

Much of ultrasound assessment of the kidney is subjective, but a commonly used quantitative measurement is renal length. Normal adult renal length is 10–12 cm, typically slightly larger on the left side and in male patients. Renal length correlates with the patient's height and a decrease in size is seen in old age.[5] Other measurements such as renal parenchymal thickness can be performed (where a value of more than 10mm is normal).[6]

Direct visualization of renal arteries and veins can be achieved at the renal hila or by scanning the aorta and retroperitoneum from a variety of positions. Assessment of the spectral Doppler wave form in the main renal artery is often possible; a peak systolic flow velocity of greater than 180 cm/s is considered by many to be an indicator of haemodynamically significant renal artery stenosis,[7]

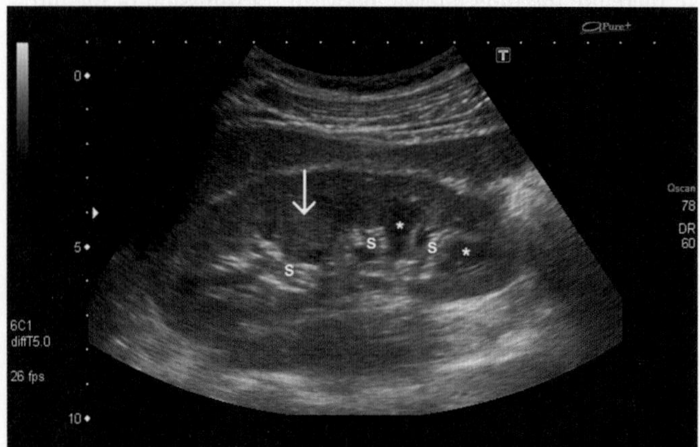

Fig. 10.2.1 Greyscale image of a normal kidney. There is a small hypertrophied column of Bertin (arrow). Echopoor medullary pyramids (*) and echogenic renal sinus fat (s) can be appreciated.

while other authors have found that the ratio of renal artery to aortic peak velocity more reliable.[8] Ultrasound assessment of native renal artery stenosis is however frequently technically difficult or impossible and CT or MRI angiography is now considered a more reliable technique.[9] Renal perfusion can usually be readily demonstrated by colour or power Doppler with vessels as small as the interlobular arteries frequently resolved in slim patients and transplant kidneys.

Congenital abnormalities and pseudomasses

Numerous congenital abnormalities and pseudomasses of the kidneys have been described and can be demonstrated with ultrasound.

Renal ectopia is most commonly due to incomplete ascent. Pelvic kidneys are found in between 1 in 2,200 and 1 in 3,000 patients, are more common on the left side and are prone to ureteropelvic junction obstruction and formation of calculi.[10] The pelvic kidney can usually be identified by ultrasound but will frequently be mal-rotated and hydronephrotic and may be misinterpreted as a pathological mass by the unwary ultrasound practitioner who fails to note the absence of a kidney in the ipsilateral renal fossa. The most common fusion abnormality is the horseshoe kidney, which occurs in 1 in 400 individuals. The isthmus of tissue joining the lower poles is not always visible on ultrasound as it may be very thin or obscured by bowel gas, and ultrasound diagnosis may be difficult.[11] This condition should be suspected if the kidneys have an abnormal orientation with medial displacement and poor visualization of the lower poles, anterior position of the renal pelvis and a curved renal shape. Crossed fused renal ectopia is occasionally also seen on ultrasound as an enlarged elongated unilateral kidney with two distinct renal sinus complexes, often with a different orientation.[12] Unilateral renal agenesis has an approximate incidence of 1 in 1,000, and is usually associated with compensatory hypertrophy of the contralateral kidney.

Duplex kidneys are one of the more common congenital abnormalities found in between 2.7–4.2% of patients on urographic series.[13] Although ultrasound cannot usually make a definitive diagnosis, the condition can be inferred when the kidney is large in comparison with the contralateral side with a band of renal cortex dividing the sinus in the interpolar region. The upper moiety may be hydronephrotic due to obstruction by a ureterocoele,[14] which should be sought on bladder scanning. The lower moiety may have a dilated collecting system or cortical scarring secondary to reflux.

Hypertrophied columns of Bertin represent a protrusion of normal parenchymal tissue into the renal sinus and are a regular finding on ultrasound, seen in almost half of kidneys in one study.[15] The column is isoechoic with adjacent renal cortex and there should be no contour abnormality of the overlying renal tissue (Fig. 10.2.1). Splenic (Dromedary) humps are a focal bulge of normal renal parenchyma arising from the interpolar region of the kidney, usually on the left side. Many patients also show regular indentations of the renal contour representing persistent foetal lobulation. These conditions need to be recognized as a normal variant rather than a renal mass or scarring.[16] Ultrasound contrast agents can be very helpful in confirming that pseudomasses are normal renal tissue (Fig. 10.2.2).[17]

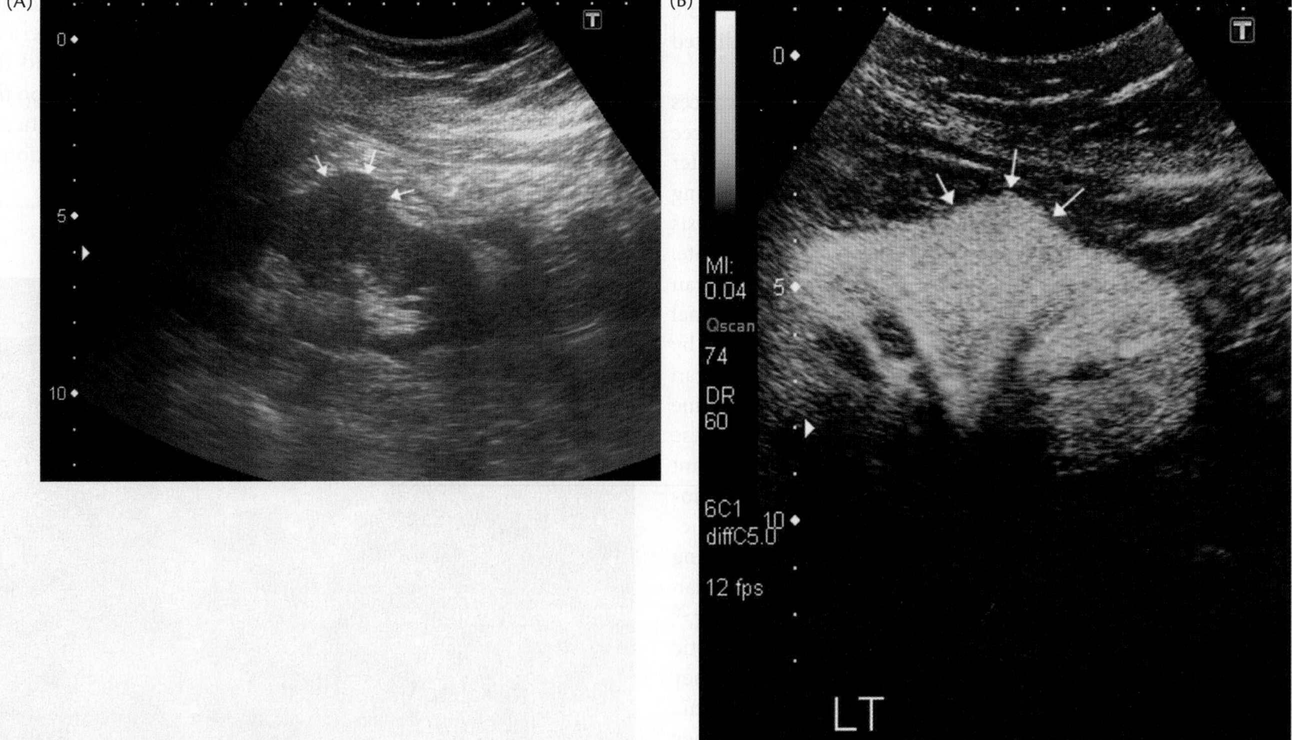

Fig. 10.2.2 Splenic (dromedary) hump. (A) Greyscale ultrasound shows a focal bulge (arrow) of the middle-third of the left kidney of concern for a pathological mass. (B) Following injection of ultrasound contrast microbubbles, the area of concern shows identical enhancement to normal renal parenchyma confirming that it represents normal renal tissue.

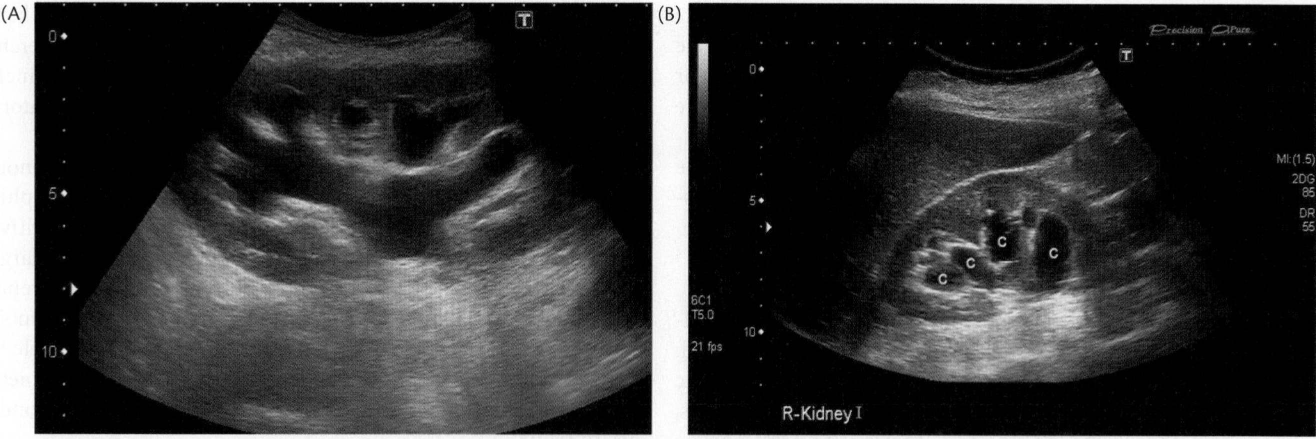

Fig. 10.2.3 Hydronephrosis and parapelvic cysts. (A) Hydronephrosis: there are interconnecting fluid-filled spaces in the renal sinus representing the dilated pelvicalyceal system. (B) Parapelvic cysts: cystic areas in the renal sinus (c) represent cysts rather than collecting system dilatation. Note the similarities between the two conditions; in difficult cases further imaging (IVU or CT urography) may be necessary to distinguish between the two.

Ureteric obstruction and renal stone disease

Ultrasound is frequently requested to rule out obstruction, either as a cause of renal functional impairment or in patients with flank pain. Ultrasound is extremely accurate in detecting hydronephrosis,[18] but it should be remembered that ultrasound demonstrates anatomical rather than functional changes.[19] Pelvicalyceal dilatation may occur in conditions other than obstruction, such as vesicoureteric reflux, and there may be no dilatation for several hours following the onset of ureteric obstruction.[20] Hydronephrosis is recognized when the echogenic renal sinus is replaced by communicating fluid-filled anechoic spaces, representing the dilated pelvicalyceal system (Fig. 10.2.3A). It is important to demonstrate this communication as parapelvic cysts can be mistaken for dilated calyces (Fig. 10.2.3B).

There is also a delay in the restoration of normal appearances after relief of an obstruction, often for several days, and a degree of pelvicalyceal dilatation may persist indefinitely, particularly after relief of longstanding or severe obstruction. A number of grading systems have been proposed for the severity of hydronephrosis but simply stating mild, moderate, or severe is usually adequate. The accuracy of ultrasound in diagnosing renal obstruction can be improved by the use of Doppler techniques. Elevated intrarenal vascular resistance in an obstructed kidney can be demonstrated by spectral Doppler examination.[21,22] Colour Doppler ultrasound can also be used to demonstrate absence or abnormality of jets of urine entering the bladder in patients with ureteric obstruction.[23] These techniques can be of particular value in the evaluation of pregnant patients with flank plain where differentiation between physiological hydronephrosis and hydronephrosis due to stone obstruction can be particularly difficult and where the use of imaging investigation using ionizing radiation is undesirable.[24,25] MRI can be very helpful in difficult cases and is safe after the first trimester.[26]

Renal stones appear as a bright echogenic focus with acoustic shadowing extending posteriorly (Fig. 10.2.4). Within the kidney it can be difficult to distinguish a small stone from the echogenic renal sinus. Sensitivity is improved by using a higher frequency transducer and ensuring the focus is located at the level of the suspected calculus. Ultrasound has a reported sensitivity of 96% and specificity of 89% for detection of stones in the pelvicalyceal system (with tomography as the gold standard),[27] but the figure is as low as 37% for ureteric calculi,[28] largely due to overlying bowel gas. In female patients transvaginal ultrasound can be used to demonstrate distal ureteric stones.[29] CT has now emerged as the investigation of choice for renal stone disease and should be the first line investigation for most patients with acute onset loin pain performing much better than ultrasound (and intravenous urography) in this situation.[30]

Solid and cystic renal masses

Ultrasound is excellent at differentiating solid from cystic lesions of the kidney. Simple cysts are very common and increase in incidence with age.[31] Sonographically cysts are anechoic, normally spherical, and have posterior acoustic enhancement—the area behind the cyst appears brighter than at the equivalent depth elsewhere on the image. They may be parapelvic, intraparenchymal or exophytic, in which case observing movement with the kidney on respiration is helpful in making the diagnosis.

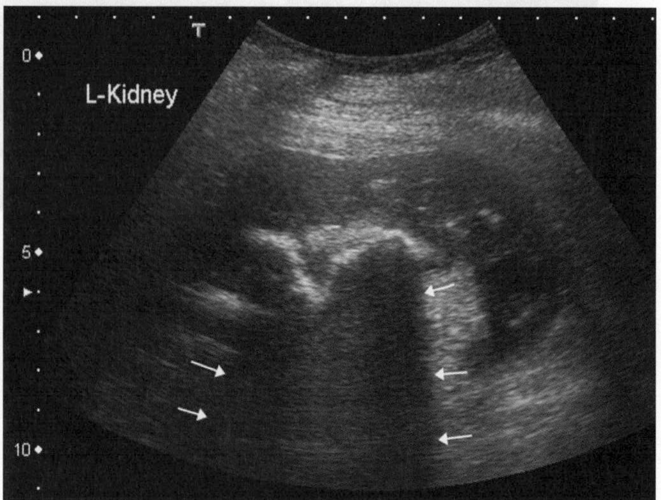

Fig. 10.2.4 Large renal stone showing an echogenic interface with dense posterior acoustic shadowing (arrows).

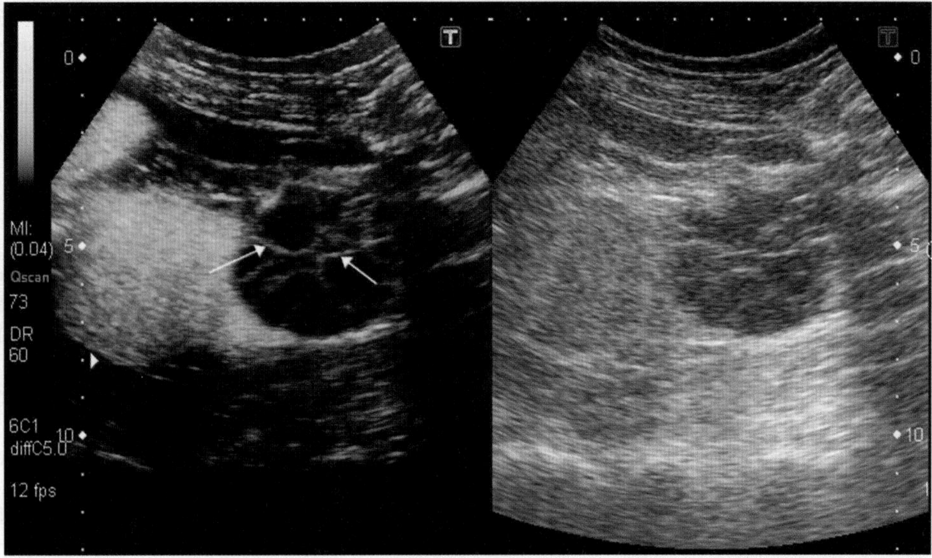

Fig. 10.2.5 Complex renal cyst. This split screen ultrasound image shows a conventional greyscale image to the reader's right and ultrasound contrast-enhanced image to the readers left. Note the multiple thickened and enhancing septa (examples arrowed) within the cyst raising concerns for a cystic malignancy.

Benign cysts must be distinguished from cystic malignancy; septations, loculations, or solid components increase the likelihood of malignancy. The Bosniak classification categorizes cystic lesions by complexity based on their appearances at CT and is used to guide management.[32] Central to this classification is the degree of enhancement following contrast medium administration. This is easily measured on CT, but only possible on ultrasound using microbubble contrast media (Fig. 10.2.5).[33] Caution should therefore be applied when extrapolating the Bosniak system to ultrasound practice and most complex cystic renal masses will require further evaluation with CT. A number of other non-malignant renal lesions may appear as complex cystic masses on ultrasound including multilocular cystic nephroma, hydatid disease, abscess, haematoma, and xanthogranulomatous pyelonephritis.

Hereditary renal cystic conditions may be encountered with ultrasound. The most common is autosomal dominant polycystic kidney disease (ADPKD) which results in enlarged kidneys with multiple cysts of varying size, randomly distributed throughout the kidney. Ultrasound is sometimes requested to screen a first order relative of a patient known to have ADPKD. Diagnostic criteria exist relating the number of cysts to the patient's age.[34,35] Screening ultrasound may give a false negative result if performed below 30 years of age.[36]

The ultrasound appearances of renal cell carcinoma are variable. Large tumours tend to be heterogenous but predominantly hypoechoic. Smaller tumours may be hyperechoic and impossible to distinguish from angiomyolipomas.[37] The presence of vascular invasion into the renal vein and inferior vena cava is readily assessed on ultrasound, although CT is required for complete staging (Fig.10.2.6).

Other solid renal masses include angiomyolipomata, which are usually brightly echogenic on ultrasound due to the presence of fat. Oncocytomas are usually impossible to distinguish from renal cell carcinoma on ultrasound, although a central scar is said to be characteristic and colour Doppler ultrasonography may show central radiating vessels.[38] Upper tract transitional cell carcinoma is unreliably visualized on ultrasound; the sensitivity of CT urography or intravenous urography is much greater.[39] Lymphoma has a variable appearance which includes diffuse infiltration and focal masses which are typically hypoechoic.

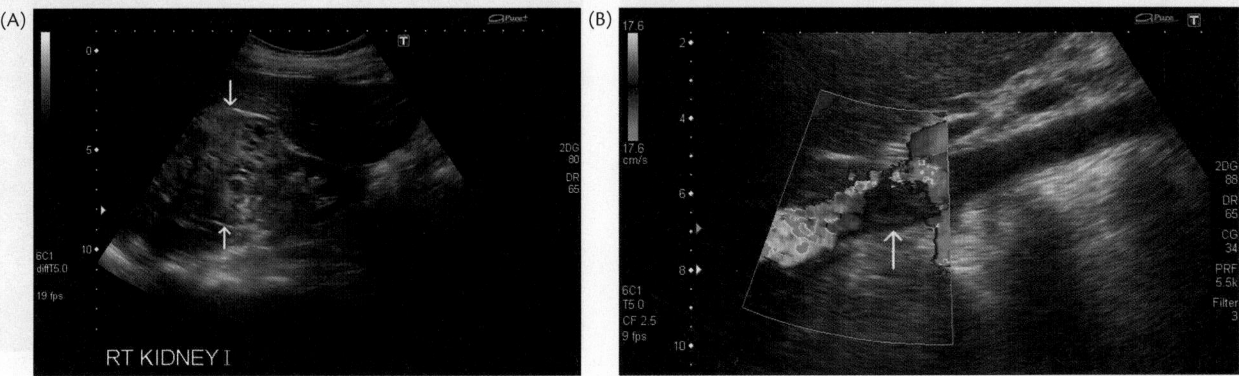

Fig. 10.2.6 Renal cell carcinoma with vascular invasion. (A) There is a large soft tissue mass arising from the right kidney (arrows). (B) Views of the inferior vena cava with colour Doppler show tumour extension into the lumen of the cava (arrow).

Infection

Ultrasound imaging is often requested for suspected pyelonephritis. The findings may include reduced parenchymal echogenicity and increase in renal size. Perfusion defects may be detected using colour or power Doppler; however the scan is frequently normal. In focal pyelonephritis (lobar nephronia) part of the kidney may be enlarged or of altered echogenicity, either increased, mixed, or decreased.[40] The principle role of ultrasound is to exclude pyonephrosis or abscess formation.

Emphysematous pyelonephritis has a characteristic appearance on ultrasound. The renal parenchyma contains gas which produces bright echoes with heterogeneous ('dirty') posterior acoustic shadowing. When the perinephric soft tissues are involved the entire kidney may be difficult to identify.

Chronic pyelonephritis secondary to vesico-ureteric reflux may cause renal scarring, seen on ultrasound as focal cortical thinning overlying a dilated or clubbed calyx. Renal cortical scintigraphy (DMSA) is used more frequently in this setting due to its greater sensitivity.[41] In xanthogranulomatous pyelonephritis chronic low grade infection is usually secondary to a central obstructing stone. There are no pathognomonic ultrasound features but stones may be identified in an enlarged kidney, with cystic spaces and fluid collections in the perinephric soft tissues.[42]

Trauma

Improved access to CT scanning with modern multi detector row machines has meant that ultrasound is now rarely used as the first line investigation for renal trauma. However, the portability of ultrasound means it is still occasionally useful in the emergency department, and it does have a role in follow up. The key findings are loss of continuity of the renal cortex, perinephric collections of blood or urine, and disruption of renal perfusion. The use of ultrasound contrast agents may improve accuracy but as they are not excreted in the urine cannot be used to detect collecting system injuries.

Medical renal disease

The various causes of medical renal disease have similar sonographic appearances—enlarged or normal size kidneys with increased echogenicity of the cortex. Frequently the medullary pyramids are unaffected giving increased cortico-medullary differentiation. If the process progresses to end-stage renal disease there is a reduction in renal size and the kidney often becomes uniformly highly reflective. The main role of ultrasound in this setting is to measure renal size, assess parenchymal thickness, exclude obstruction and, when appropriate, to guide biopsy.

Renal transplants

Transplantation is the treatment of choice for most patients with end-stage renal failure and its success is tempered only by the limited availability of organs. Ultrasound is vital in detection of the complications of renal transplantation, and is used both for regular surveillance and as the first line imaging investigation for graft dysfunction.

Renal transplants are typically placed in either iliac fossa, but the axis of the kidney is variable and the scan plane must be tailored to accommodate this. The superficial position of the transplant usually allows it to be easily assessed and a higher frequency transducer can often be used. The scan technique involves a thorough greyscale assessment of the transplant and evaluation of the surrounding soft tissues for fluid collections. Global renal perfusion is then assessed with colour Doppler followed by a spectral Doppler assessment of several interlobar arteries. Finally the main vascular pedicle and iliac vessels should be evaluated.

In the early postoperative period peritransplant collections may represent urinoma, haematoma, lymphocoele, or abscess formation; ultrasound guided needle aspiration may be necessary to differentiate between them. Renal artery thrombosis (global or segmental) is easily recognized by an absence of perfusion of all or part of the transplant. Renal vein thrombosis may be difficult to directly visualize but can be inferred when the normal low resistance intrarenal arterial spectral Doppler pattern is replaced by a high resistance pattern with reversal of diastolic flow (Fig. 10.2.7). Arteriovenous fistulae and pseudoaneurysms are usually related to biopsy and are readily identified with Doppler techniques. A mild degree of hydronephrosis is a common finding and does not necessarily indicate ureteric obstruction but progressive hydronephrosis in the face of deteriorating graft function may require antegrade pyelography to exclude obstruction or nephrostomy drainage. The early medical

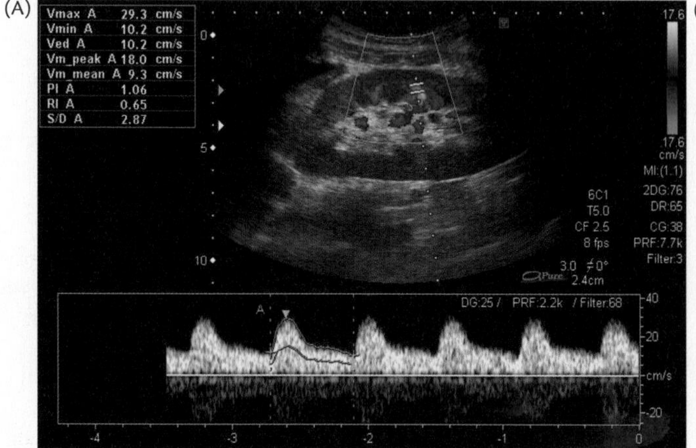

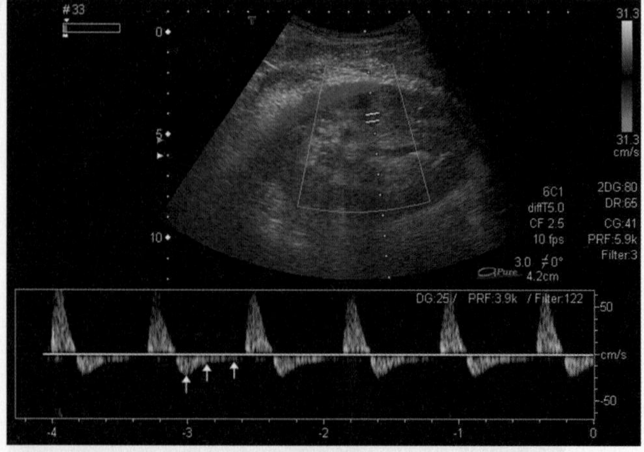

Fig. 10.2.7 Transplant renal vein thrombosis. (A) Normal transplant arterial spectral Doppler trace. Note the forward flow in diastole with a trace likened to a 'ski slope', and resistance index (RI) of 0.65. (B) The spectral arterial Doppler trace from this renal transplant demonstrates reversed diastolic flow (arrows) due to renal vein thrombosis.

complications of transplantation are mainly due to acute tubular necrosis (ATN) and rejection. Despite early optimism[43] ultrasound has been unsuccessful in accurately differentiating between acute rejection and ATN.[44,45] In both conditions the intrarenal vascular resistance increases[46] (usually measured by calculating the RI from a spectral Doppler trace of an interlobar artery; the upper limit of normal is <0.7). Ultrasound guided biopsy is usually required.

Ultrasound can also identify some of the causes of late transplant failure. Peak systolic flow velocities of >250 cm/s in the main transplant artery indicate a haemodynamically significant stenosis.[47] Increasing hydronephrosis suggests a ureteric stricture. Resistance index measurements are not useful in the diagnosis of chronic allograft nephropathy (chronic rejection) although CEUS shows some promise in this area.[48]

Scrotal ultrasound

Technique

The scrotum is ideally suited to ultrasound imaging. Its superficial position allows the use of high frequency transducers resulting in excellent resolution. Common indications for ultrasound include palpable scrotal masses, pain, hydroceles, varicoceles, and trauma, although almost any symptom or sign may be an indication, and only very rarely is any other imaging modality used.

To facilitate scanning, the scrotum may be stabilized using a folded sheet placed beneath it, over the patient's legs. It is useful to ask the patient to identify any lumps and ideally to stabilize the abnormality between their thumb and finger allowing it to be specifically scanned during the ultrasound study. Longitudinal and transverse views of both testes should be obtained; a transverse view of both testes on the same image is useful to allow comparison of echogenicity and size. Views of the epididymis often require oblique lateral orientation of the transducer.

Tumours

Ultrasound is extremely accurate in locating scrotal masses as intra or extratesticular. Focal testicular masses have a wide differential diagnosis including neoplasm, haematoma, focal orchitis, abscess, or infarction. Ultrasound is sometimes unable to reliably distinguish between these different possibilities; correlation with the history and laboratory data may be helpful, but any focal solid echopoor intratesticular lesion should be regarded as suspicious of malignancy.

The appearance of germ cell tumours (GCT) is variable, but these are usually solid and predominantly hypoechoic relative to the normal testis; internal blood flow can usually be demonstrated with colour or power Doppler. Cystic spaces and calcifications are more commonly seen in non-seminomatous GCT (Fig. 10.2.8). An irregular outline to the testis is a worrying feature. Non-germ cell tumours (Leydig and Sertoli cell) do not have ultrasound appearances that allow them to be differentiated from GCTs. Lymphoma is the commonest testicular malignancy in older men. It may appear as one or more focal lesions that are hypoechoic and usually highly vascular on colour Doppler assessment or as diffuse testicular infiltration.[49] Simple testicular cysts are often asymptomatic incidental findings; any complexity raises the suspicion of a cystic tumour.

Testicular microlithiasis (TM) is characterized by the presence of tiny (1–3 mm), non-shadowing, echogenic foci within the testicular parenchyma and can be subdivided into classical and limited forms.[50] This condition is associated with testicular GCT and intratubular germ cell neoplasia but there is a lack of consensus regarding its optimal management.[51] It is now thought TM may be a manifestation of the testicular dysgenesis syndrome and recommendations for management have been proposed which do not recommend ultrasound surveillance except for small specified high risk cohorts.[52,53] Ultrasound surveillance of all patients with TM is probably not cost-effective.[54] The incidence of TM may be higher in the paediatric than adult population.[55]

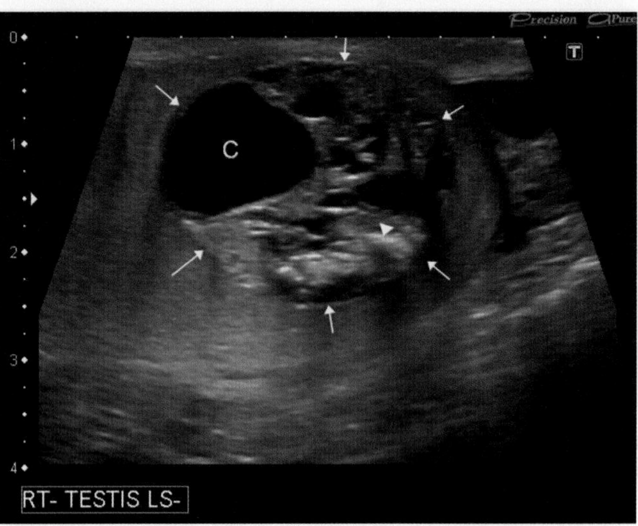

Fig. 10.2.8 Non-seminoma testicular germ cell tumour (arrows). Note the intratumoural cystic spaces (c) and calcifications (arrow head).

Infection

Acute epididymitis is the commonest cause of acute scrotal symptoms.[56] Ultrasound examination typically shows an enlarged, hypoechoic epididymis, often with a reactive hydrocele and scrotal skin thickening. If infection spreads to the testis it will also become globally or focally hypoechoic. Hyperaemia on colour Doppler examination facilitates the diagnosis.[57] Abscess formation occurs in 3–5% of cases[58] and should be suspected if there is a focal complex fluid collection. The presence of gas in the scrotal soft tissues, appearing as echogenic foci with acoustic shadowing, is a feature of Fournier's gangrene.[59]

Spermatic cord torsion

Ultrasound is occasionally requested if there is clinical doubt in a case of suspected spermatic cord torsion but should not delay surgical exploration in cases where the presentation is typical. The bell-clapper deformity, found in as many as 12% of adolescent males,[60] predisposes to this condition and may be identified on ultrasound, particularly when there is a hydrocele. In the early stages of torsion the greyscale appearances are often normal. Later the testis and epididymis may become swollen and hypoechoic and there may be a reactive hydrocele;[61] thus differentiation from epididymo-orchitis on greyscale images is often impossible. Ultrasound diagnosis is based on Doppler examination; absent or reduced intratesticular blood flow (in comparison with the asymptomatic side) is regarded as a positive study. Ultrasound practitioners and clinicians should be aware of the difficulties of diagnosing incomplete torsion,[62] the limitations of ultrasound in young boys[63] and the falsely reassuring Doppler appearances following spontaneous detorsion.

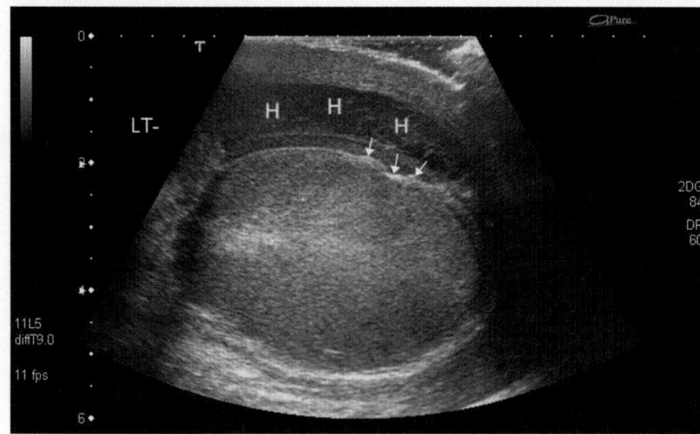

Fig. 10.2.9 Testicular rupture. Note the contour abnormality of the anterior testicular tunical surface (arrows) and the haematocoele (H).

Trauma

The role of ultrasound in scrotal trauma is to triage those patients requiring surgical exploration from those who can be managed conservatively.[64] Clinical examination is difficult in the presence of scrotal swelling and pain; ultrasound is accurate in the diagnosis of testicular rupture which should be suspected when there is a focal contour abnormality of the testis (Fig. 10.2.9) indicating protrusion of testicular parenchyma through a defect in the tunica albuginea,[65] particularly when there is an intratesticular haematoma.[66] Doppler ultrasound and CEUS are able to assess testicular perfusion in the setting of trauma and so determine testicular viability.[67]

Varicocele

Varicoceles represent dilatation of the pampiniform venous plexus which is located cephalad and posterior to the testis. Sonographically they appear as a serpentiform collection of tubules, measuring greater than 2 mm in diameter. Colour flow Doppler helps to make the diagnosis and a Valsalva manoeuvre can be used to confirm retrograde flow. If a varicocoele is identified many authorities advocate extending the examination to the abdomen to exclude a left renal or retroperitoneal tumour obstructing the testicular vein, although yield is likely to be very low in young patients.[68]

Extratesticular scrotal lesions

The vast majority of extratesticular scrotal masses are benign. The role of ultrasound is to differentiate solid from cystic masses and locate their position. Epididymal cysts and spermatocoeles are common benign lesions easily diagnosed with ultrasound. Solid lesions present a greater challenge. Small epididymal granulomata are common, particularly after trauma or vasectomy. Extratesticular tumours are rare; adenomatoid tumour of the epididymis is the least uncommon and may be seen on ultrasound as a solid epididymal mass with varying echogenicity. Excision biopsy is often recommended for large (>2 cm) solid masses or enlarging lesions as the rare malignant extratesticular masses frequently do not have characteristic sonographic features.[69]

Hydroceles

A small amount of fluid is normal in the scrotum, and the diagnosis of a small hydrocele is subjective. The role of ultrasound is to distinguish between simple and complicated hydroceles (which contain internal echoes representing blood or inflammatory cells) and to exclude an underlying testicular malignancy, particularly when the testis is impalpable.

Penile ultrasound

Penile ultrasound is performed with a high frequency linear transducer. The penis is placed on the patient's anterior abdominal wall and imaged in longitudinal and transverse plane systematically from base to glans. The root of the penis is scanned through the perineum.

The use of ultrasound in the diagnosis of erectile dysfunction has declined following the introduction of phosphodiesterase type-5 inhibitor medications but may still be required for cases refractory to drug treatment. The paired corpora cavernosa are seen as cylindrical low echogenicity structures, the dorsal corpus spongiosum is smaller and more echogenic. The cavernosal arteries can be identified and spectral flow waveforms can be traced before and after intracavernosal injection of vasoactive drugs[70] to give more information on vascular causes of erectile dysfunction—poor arterial inflow or failure of venous occlusion (venous leak).[71]

Other indications for penile ultrasound include evaluation of priapism (Fig. 10.2.10), penile and pelvic trauma, and Peyronie's disease.[72] Ultrasound can also be used for local staging in penile carcinoma, although MRI is now preferred for this indication.[73]

Prostatic ultrasound

Prostate ultrasound is most commonly performed to guide biopsy for cancer detection but may also be used in investigation of such conditions as infertility, prostatitis, and haematospermia. While the prostate can usually be visualized on transabdominal scanning this route provides very limited diagnostic potential. Better visualization and access for biopsy is achieved if the scan is performed transrectally (TRUS).

Limited prostatic zonal anatomy can be distinguished on TRUS, particularly in older patients with benign prostatic hyperplasia (BPH). The peripheral and central zones (outer gland) tend to be of higher echogenicity than the transition zone (inner gland). Appreciation of zonal anatomy allows targeted systematic multicore biopsies. TRUS is also valuable for examining the seminal vesicles and ejaculatory ducts and for estimating prostate volumes.

Fortunately for imaging, the majority of prostatic carcinomas arise in the outer gland and nodules of BPH in the inner gland. Prostatic carcinoma may sometimes be identified on TRUS, usually as hypoechoic nodules relative to normal prostatic parenchyma.[74] Any suspicious nodules should be specifically targeted in addition to the standard biopsy locations. Not all echopoor nodules are malignant and TRUS has a low sensitivity and specificity for cancer detection, therefore targeted biopsy cannot replace systematic biopsy.[75] Cancer detection can be improved by the use of Colour and Power Doppler,[76] CEUS,[77] (both of which also tend to identify more aggressive tumours), and ultrasound elastography.[78]

Calcification is frequently seen along the surgical capsule and multiple diffuse calcifications are an age related normal finding. Larger calculi may be symptomatic and act as a nidus for infection in prostatitis.

Cystic lesions of the prostate are commonly seen on TRUS. These may be congenital or acquired.[79] They are rarely clinically significant although may be associated with ejaculatory duct obstruction

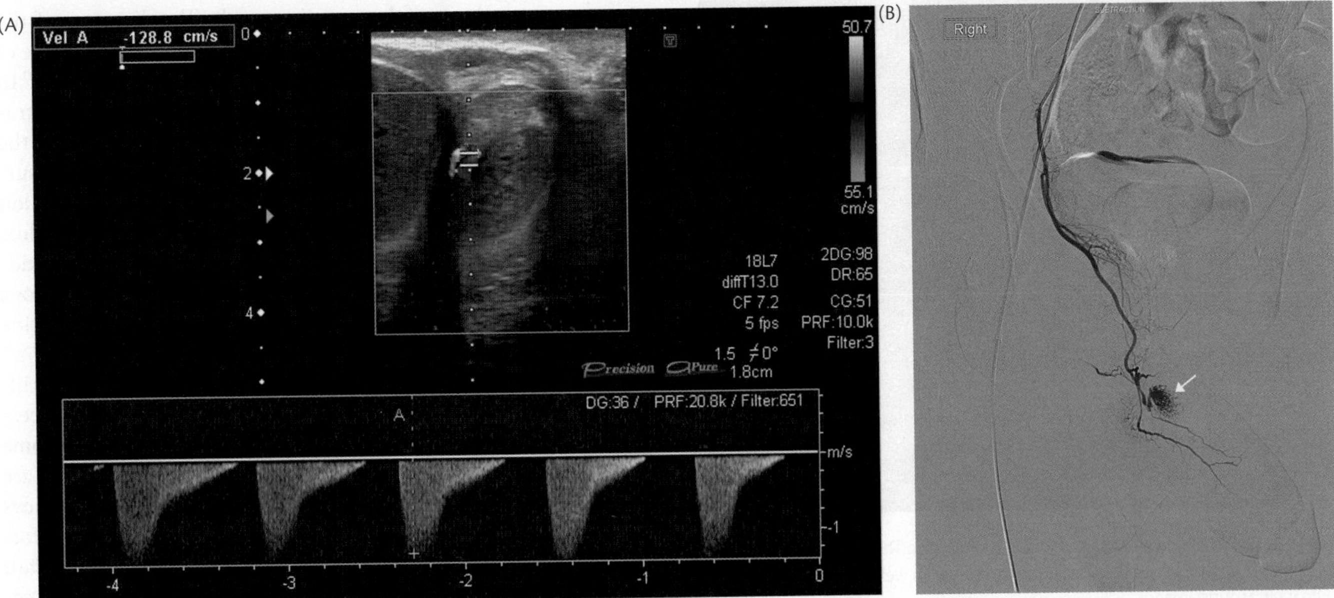

Fig. 10.2.10 High-flow priapism secondary to a traumatic arteriovenous fistula. (A) Ultrasound of the base of the penis shows an area of very high velocity flow arising from the corporal artery. (B) Subsequent digital subtraction angiography confirms the abnormality (arrow) which was successfully embolized.

in patients with infertility. Abscess formation should always be considered when a cystic lesion is seen in the appropriate clinical setting and ultrasound can be used to guide drainage.

Bladder ultrasound

The bladder is usually evaluated through a suprapubic approach with a standard abdominal curvilinear transducer. To achieve useful information requires the bladder to be well distended. The bladder can also be evaluated on trans-vaginal and TRUS studies.

Quantification of bladder volume is easily achieved and is of particular importance in patients with lower urinary tract symptoms. This requires measuring distances in both transverse and the longitudinal planes, and is often performed pre and post micturition. A commonly used formula for converting these linear measurements to an approximate volume is:

$$V = (H \times W \times L) \times 0.625$$

(V is volume, H is height, W is width, and L is length of the bladder).

Most ultrasound systems will automatically perform these calculations but the result tends to slightly underestimate bladder volume; accuracy is however acceptable for routine clinical use.[80] Three-dimensional ultrasound may give more accurate measurements[81] but it is not widely available. The normal bladder wall measures 3–5 mm in thickness which may be useful in predicting the severity of bladder outlet obstruction, but measurements depend on the degree of bladder distension and which part of the bladder wall is measured.[82]

Many bladder abnormalities can be identified and assessed by ultrasound including diverticula, urachal abnormalities, stones, and blood clots. In patients with cystitis bladder ultrasound is usually normal (but bladder emptying can be assessed). In chronic cystitis there may be bladder wall thickening. The presence of echogenic foci with acoustic shadowing (representing gas) in the bladder wall should alert the ultrasound practitioner to the possibility of emphysematous cystitis. Gas in the bladder lumen, in the absence of instrumentation, is suggestive of a vesicoenetric fistula. Ureterocoeles can be elegantly demonstrated on bladder ultrasound; they are seen as cystic structures projecting into the bladder lumen from the ureteric orifices and can frequently be observed to fill and empty on real-time scanning (Fig. 10.2.11). Detection of an ectopic ureteocoele arising from the upper moiety of a duplex kidney inserting below the bladder neck can be facilitated by scanning through the perineum.[83]

Transitional cell bladder cancer can frequently be identified on ultrasound as a soft tissue projection into the bladder lumen (Fig. 10.2.12); unsurprisingly polypoid tumours are much more reliably identified than sessile ones. Tumours smaller than 5mm in size and those located on the anterior wall or bladder neck are frequently more difficult to identify[84] and ultrasound cannot replace

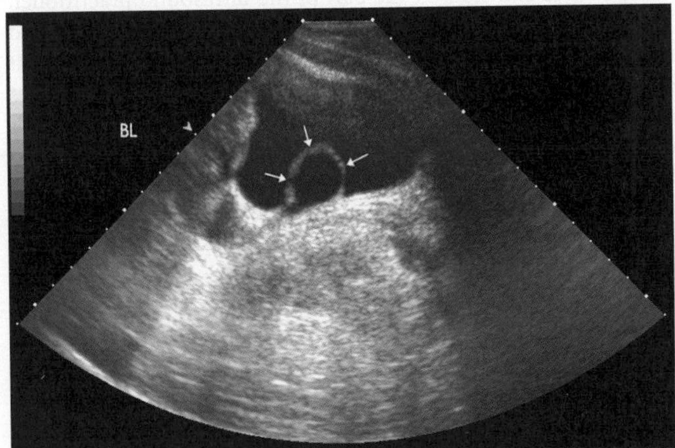

Fig. 10.2.11 Ureterocoele seen as a cystic structure projecting into the bladder lumen (arrows) from the ureteric orifice.

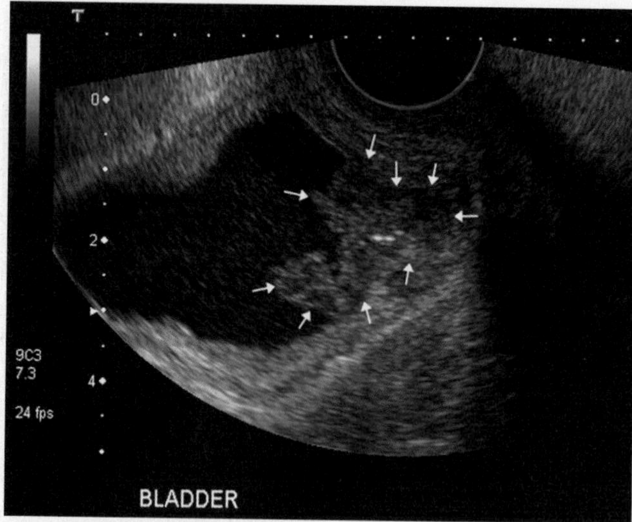

Fig. 10.2.12 Transitional cell carcinoma of the bladder. There is a polypoid soft tissue mass (arrows) projecting into the bladder lumen well seen on this transvaginal ultrasound image.

cystoscopy.[85] Ultrasound has a limited ability to differentiate transitional cell carcinoma from other bladder masses including other types of bladder tumour, invasive prostate carcinoma, adherent clots, and endometriosis—cystoscopic inspection and biopsy is required. The simple manoeuvre of rolling the patient onto their side will differentiate dependent debris and clot from posterior tumour. The presence of flow within a bladder mass on Doppler interrogation usually indicates a bladder tumour.

Transabdominal ultrasound has a limited role in assessing the depth of invasion by bladder tumours and particularly cannot usually definitively differentiate stage T2 from T3a tumours.[86] Local staging of bladder cancer remains predominantly the remit of histological evaluation of biopsy specimens, clinical examination, and MRI.[87]

Paediatric urological ultrasound

Ultrasound is the primary imaging modality in paediatric urology for almost all conditions, largely because it does not involve ionizing radiation. However, to obtain good images requires the cooperation of the child and parents, warm coupling gel, a relaxed atmosphere, and patience and skill on the part of the ultrasound practitioner. The use of higher frequency transducers is often possible and transducers with a smaller 'footprint' are often used. Urinary tract abnormalities diagnosed in infancy and childhood are sometimes associated with other extrarenal abnormalities or syndromes, for example the 'VACTERL' collection of non-randomly associated birth defects.

Neonatal kidneys are of greater relative size than adults, and charts are available to relate renal size to age.[88] The renal cortex is brighter than in adult kidneys, the medullary pyramids relatively large, corticomedullary differentiation greater, and there is little renal sinus fat.[89] By one year of age these morphological differences will have resolved and the kidneys resemble those of adults.

Antenatal detection of urological abnormalities by scans performed in pregnancy is relatively common. Postnatal imaging for antenatal detected hydronephrosis is optimally performed at 48–72 hours after birth, as relative dehydration in the early postnatal period may produce a false negative result. The diameter of the renal pelvis is often used as a reproducible measure of the degree of hydronephrosis and can be used to guide further management.[90] In most patients renal pelvic dilatation is due to an unobstructed extrarenal pelvis but postnatal ultrasound is required to identify the subgroup of patients with urological diseases that may require surgical intervention. These conditions include ureteropelvic junction obstruction (UPJO), congenital megaureter, vesicoureteric reflux, posterior urethral valves, duplex kidney, multicystic dysplastic kidney, and prune belly syndrome. Additional imaging investigations such as the micturating custourethrogram, and nuclear medicine diuretic isotope renogram are sometimes required.[91]

Autosomal recessive and autosomal dominant polycystic kidney (ADPKD) disease can both present in childhood. The recessive form also involves the liver leading to hepatic fibrosis in some patients. In young children with this condition the renal cysts are often tiny and impossible to resolve with ultrasound, the kidneys appearing enlarged and globally echogenic, but with time cyst formation may become apparent.[92] ADPKD typically presents in adult patients, but enlarged kidneys containing multiple cysts may occasionally be seen in older children. Renal cysts may also be seen in patients with tuberous sclerosis but characteristically these patients have multiple renal angiomyolipomas, appearing as echogenic nodules within the renal parenchyma. Multicystic dysplastic kidney is another cause of a unilateral cystic kidney; it is usually detected on prenatal ultrasound and may be associated with contralateral UPJO in some patients.

In paediatric renal infection an ultrasound study is usually performed to exclude structural urinary tract abnormality. In infants this is frequently accompanied by a micturating cystogram to exclude vesicoureteric reflux and a DMSA scan to detect renal scarring. The National Institute of Clinical Excellence (NICE) have produced comprehensive guidelines on the management of urinary tract infection in childhood.[93]

Wilm's tumour (nephroblastoma) is the commonest malignancy in childhood usually occurring in children aged between two to five years. The commonest presentation is with an abdominal mass. On ultrasound Wilm's tumour is seen as a solid mass replacing all or part of the kidney, often with hypoechoic areas of necrosis (Fig. 10.2.13).[94] 5–10% are bilateral and there are a number of associated urogenital abnormalities.[95] Staging requires CT or MRI. Wilm's tumour cannot be reliably differentiated from mesoblastic nephroma on ultrasound, a more benign entity.

Bladder abnormalities such as neurogenic bladder, stones, cystitis, urachal abnormalities, or rhabdomyosarcoma may be seen on ultrasound. Scanning with a full bladder is usually required.

The normal neonatal adrenal is usually seen on routine ultrasound, unlike adults, due to its larger relative size. There is progressive cortical involution in the first few weeks of life and tables are available for normal adrenal size in the newborn.[96] Adrenal masses such as neuroblastoma and adrenal haemorrhage may be identified on ultrasound and Doppler may help to differentiate between these two conditions.[97]

Ultrasound for procedures

In addition to its extensive diagnostic role in urology, ultrasound is ideally suited to guide urological interventions.[98] It allows the insertion of a needle under direct visualization, and if necessary

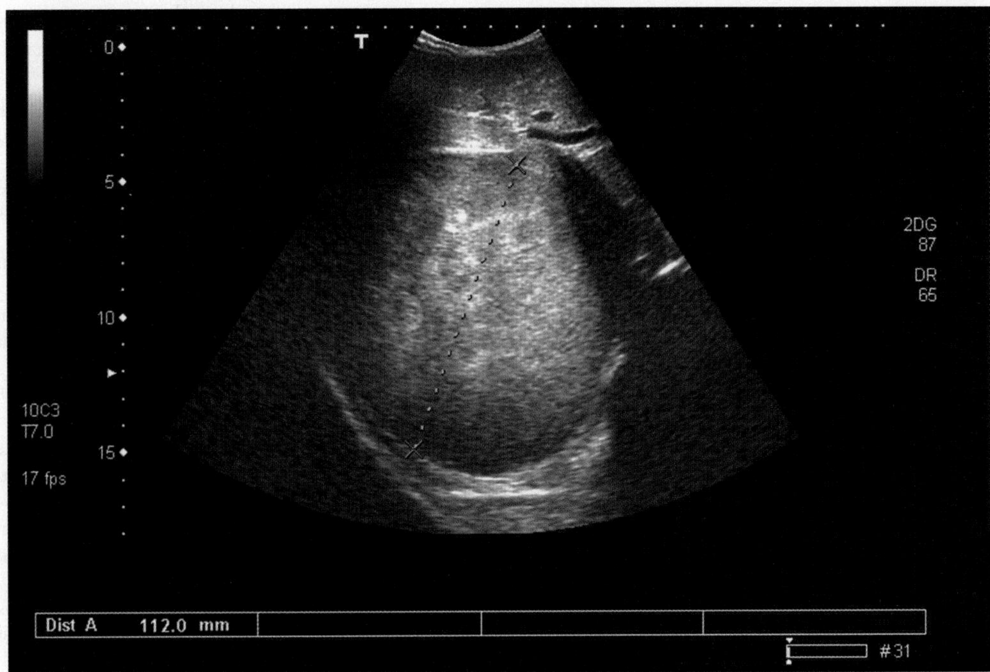

Fig. 10.2.13 Wilm's tumour—a large heterogeneous mass arising from, and replacing the kidney in a two-year-old child.
Image reproduced courtesy of Dr J Foster, Consultant Radiologist, Derriford Hospital, Plymouth, UK.

this can be performed in an operating theatre using a portable machine. Experience is required to keep the needle in the ultrasound sector and identify the position of the needle tip. Bowel is less easily visualized (and so avoided) than on CT.

Renal biopsy, biopsy of masses in the kidney, adrenal gland, or prostate, abscess drainage, and insertion of nephrostomy drains are examples of procedures commonly performed under ultrasound guidance. Ultrasound can also be used to guide needle placement for ablative procedures such as renal tumour radiofrequency ablation or cryotherapy. TRUS is used to allow precise seed placement in prostate cancer brachytherapy.

Conclusion

We have described many of the common indications for the use of ultrasound in modern urological practice. Its safety, portability, real-time imaging capacity, and relative low-cost are significant advantages. The limitations of ultrasound have also been described, and it is worth reiterating that it is most effectively used in conjunction with clinical assessment, often alongside other complementary imaging modalities.

Further reading

Allan PL, Baxter GM, Weston MJ (eds). *Clinical Ultrasound*, 3rd edition. London, UK: Churchill Livingstone, Elsevier, 2011.

Allan PL, Dubbins PA, Pozniak MA, McDicken WN (eds). *Clinical Doppler Ultrasound*, 2nd edition. London, UK; Elsevier, 2006.

Bosniak MA. The Bosniak Renal Cyst Classification: 25 years later. *Radiology* 2012; **262**(3):781–5.

Cochlin DLI, Dubbins PA, Goldberg BB, Halpern EJ (eds). *Urogenital Ultrasound: A Text Atlas*, 2nd edition. London, UK: Taylor and Francis, 2006.

Edwards TJ, Dickinson AJ, Natale S, Gosling J, McGrath JS. A prospective analysis of the diagnostic yield resulting from the attendance of 4020 patients at a protocol-driven haematuria clinic. *BJU Int* 2006; **97**:301–5.

McArthur C, Baxter GM. Current and potential renal applications of contrast-enhanced ultrasound. *Clin Radiol* 2012; **67**(9):909–22.

National Institute for Health and Clinical Excellence. CG54: Urinary tract infection: Diagnosis, treatment and long term management of urinary tract infection in children. Available at: www.nice.org.uk/CG54 [Online].

O'Connor OJ, Fitzgerald E, Maher MM. Imaging of hematuria. *AJR Am J Roentgenol* 2010; **195**(4):263–7.

Patel U, Rickards D. *Handbook of Transrectal Ultrasound & Biopsy of the Prostate*. London, UK: Martin Dunitz, 2002.

Piscaglia F, Nolsøe C, Dietrich CF, *et al.* The EFSUMB guidelines and recommendations on the clinical practice of contrast enhanced ultrasound (CEUS): Update 2011 on non-hepatic applications. *Ultraschall Med* 2012; **33**:33–59.

Webb JAW. Ultrasonography and Doppler studies in the diagnosis of renal obstruction. *BJU Int* 2000; **86**(s1):25–32.

References

1. Correas JM, Bridal L, Lesavre A, Méjean A, Claudon M, Hélénon O. Ultrasound contrast agents: properties, principles of action, tolerance, and artefacts. *Eur Radiol* 2001; **11**(8):1316–28.
2. McArthur C, Baxter GM. Current and potential renal applications of contrast-enhanced ultrasound. *Clin Radiol* 2012; **67**(9):909–22.
3. Piscaglia F, Nolsøe C, Dietrich CF, *et al.* The EFSUMB guidelines and recommendations on the clinical practice of contrast enhanced ultrasound (CEUS): Update 2011 on non-hepatic applications. *Ultraschall Med* 2012; **33**:33–59.
4. Edwards TJ, Dickinson AJ, Natale S, Gosling J, McGrath JS. A prospective analysis of the diagnostic yield resulting from the attendance of 4020 patients at a protocol-driven haematuria clinic. *BJU Int* 2006; **97**:301–5.

5. Emamian SA, Nielsen MB, Pedersen JF, Ytte L. Kidney dimensions at sonography: correlation with age, sex, and habitus in 665 adult volunteers. *AJR Am J Roentgenol* 1993; **160**(1):83–6.
6. Dubbins P. The kidney. (Chapter 1) In: Cochlin DLI, Dubbins PA, Goldberg BB, Halpern EJ (eds). *Urogenital Ultrasound: A Teaching Atlas*, 2nd edition. London, UK: Taylor and Francis, 2006.
7. Strandness DE Jr. Duplex imaging for the detection of renal artery stenosis. *Am J Kidney Dis* 1994; **24**(4):674–8.
8. Li J-C, Wang L, Jiang Y-X, Dai Q, Cai S, Lv K, Qi Z-H. Evaluation of renal artery stenosis with velocity parameters of doppler sonography. *J Ultrasound Med* 2006; **25**(6):735–42.
9. Halpern EJ, Rutter CM, Gardiner GA Jr, *et al.* Comparison of Doppler US and CT angiography for evaluation of renal artery stenosis. *Acad Radiol* 1998; **5**(8):524–32.
10. Cinman NM, Okeke Z, Smith AD. Pelvic kidney: associated diseases and treatment. *J Endourol* 2007; **21**(8):836–42.
11. Strauss S, Dushnitsky T, Peer A, Manor H, Lisbon E, Lebensart PD. Sonographic features of horseshoe kidney: review of 34 patients. *J Ultrasound Med* 2000; **19**(1):27–31.
12. Goodman, JD, Norton KI, Carr L, Yeh H-C. Crossed Fused Renal Ectopia: Sonographic Diagnosis. *Urol Radiol* 1986; **8**(1):13–16.
13. Mascatello VJ, Smith EH, Carrera GF, Berger M, Teele RL. Ultrasonic evaluation of the obstructed duplex kidney. *AJR Am J Roentgenol* 1997; **129**(1):113–12.
14. Nussbaum AR, Dorst JP, Jeffs RD, Gearhart JP, Sanders RC. Ectopic ureter and ureterocele: their varied sonographic manifestations. *Radiology* 1986: **159**:227–35.
15. Lafortune M, Constantin A, Breton G, Vallee C. Sonography of the hypertrophied column of bertin. *AJR Am J Roentgenol* 1986; **146**(1):53–6.
16. Bhatt S, MacLennan G, Dogra V. Renal pseudotumors. *AJR Am J Roentgenol* 2007; **188**(5):1380–7.
17. Mazziotti S, Zimbaro F, Pandolfo A, Racchiusa S, Settineri N, Ascenti G. Usefulness of contrast-enhanced ultrasounography in the diagnosis of renal pseudotumors. *Abdom Imaging* 2010; **35**(2):241–5.
18. Ellenbogen PH, Scheible FW, Talner LB, Leopold GR. Sensitivity of Grey Scale Ultrasound in Detecting Urinary Tract Obstruction. *AJR Am J Roentgenol* 1978; **130**(4):731–3.
19. Webb JAW. Ultrasonography and Doppler studies in the diagnosis of renal obstruction. *BJU Int* 2000; **86**(s1):25–32.
20. Laing FC, Jeffrey RB Jr,Wing VW. Ultrasound versus excretory urography in evaluating acute flank pain. *Radiology* 1985; **154**:613–16.
21. Platt JF, Rubin JM, Ellis JH. Distinction between obstructive and nonobstructive pyelocaliectasis with duplex Doppler sonography. *AJR Am J Roentgenol* 1989; **153**(5):997–1000.
22. Platt JF, Rubin JM, Ellis JH. Acute renal obstruction: evaluation with intrarenal duplex Doppler and conventional US. *Radiology* 1993; **186**:685–8.
23. Burge HJ, Middleton WD, McClennan BL, Hildebolt CF. Ureteral jets in healthy subjects and in patients with unilateral calculi: comparison with color Doppler US. *Radiology* 1991; **180**:437–42.
24. Hertzberg BS, Carroll BA, Bowie JD, *et al.* Doppler US assessment of maternal kidneys: analysis of intrarenal resistivity indexes in normal pregnancy and physiologic pelvicaliectasis. *Radiology* 1993; **186**:689–92.
25. Haddad MC, Abomelha MS, Riley PJ. Diagnosis of acute ureteral calculus obstruction in pregnant women using colour and pulsed doppler sonography. *Clin Radiol* 1995; **50**(12):864–6.
26. Spencer JA, Chahal R, Kelly A, Taylor K, Eardley I, Lloyd SN. Evaluation of painful hydronephrosis in pregnancy: magnetic resonance urographic patterns in physiological dilatation versus calculous obstruction. *J Urol* 2004; **171**(1):256–60.
27. Middleton WD, Dodds WJ, Lawson TL, Foley WD. Renal calculi: sensitivity for detection with US. *Radiology* 1988; **167**:239–44.
28. Aslaksen A. Göthlin JH. Ultrasonic diagnosis of ureteral calculi in patients with acute flank pain. *Eur J Radiol* 1990; **11**(2):87–90.
29. Laing FC, Benson CB, DiSalvo DN, Brown DL, Frates MC, Loughlin KR. Distal ureteric calculi: detection with vaginal US. *Radiology* 1994; **192**:545–8.
30. Yilmaz S, Sindel T, Arslan G, *et al.* Renal colic: comparison of spiral CT, US and IVU in the detection of ureteric calculi. *Eur Radiol* 1998; **8**(2):212–17.
31. Ravine D, Gibson RN, Donlan J, Sheffield LJ. An ultrasound renal cyst prevalence survey: Specificity data for inherited renal cystic diseases. *Am J Kidney Dis* 1993; **22**(6):803–7.
32. Bosniak MA. The Bosniak Renal Cyst Classification: 25 years later. *Radiology* 2012; **262**(3):781–5.
33. Tamai H, Takiguchi Y, Oka M, *et al.* Contrast-Enhanced Ultrasonography in the Diagnosis of Solid Renal Tumors. *J Ultrasound Med* 2005; **24**(12):1635–40.
34. Pei Y, Obaji J, Dupuis A, *et al.* Unified Criteria for Ultrasonographic Diagnosis of ADPKD. *JASN* 2009; **20**(1):205–12.
35. Ravine D, Sheffield LJ, Danks DM, Gibson RN, Walker RG, Kincaid-Smith P. Evaluation of ultrasonographic diagnostic criteria for autosomal dominant polycystic kidney disease 1. *Lancet* 1994; **343**:824–7.
36. Nicolau C, Torra R, Badenas C, *et al.* Autosomal dominant polycystic kidney disease types 1 and 2: Assessment of US sensitivity for diagnosis. *Radiology* 1999; **213**:273–6.
37. Vallancien G, Torres LO, Gurfinkel E, Veillon B, Brisset JM. Incidental detection of renal tumours by abdominal ultrasonography. *Eur Urol* 1990; **18**(2):94–6.
38. Fan L, Lianfang D, Jinfang X, Yijin S, Ying W. Diagnostic efficacy of contrast-enhanced ultrasonography in solid renal parenchymal lesions with maximum diameters of 5 cm. *J Ultrasound Med* 2008; **27**(6):875–85.
39. O'Connor OJ, Fitzgerald E, Maher MM. Imaging of hematuria. *AJR Am J Roentgenol* 2010; **195**(4):263–7.
40. Farmer KD, Gellett LR, Dubbins PA. The sonographic appearance of acute focal pyelonephritis 8 years experience. *Clin Radiol* 2002; **57**(6):483–7.
41. Roebuck DJ, Howard RG, Metreweli C. How sensitive is ultrasound in the detection of renal scars? *Br J Radiol* 1999; **72**(856):345–8.
42. Tiu C-M, Chou Y-H, Chiou H-J, *et al.* Sonographic features of xanthogranulomatous pyelonephritis. *J Clin Ultrasound* 2001; **29**(5):279–85.
43. Rifkin MD, Needleman L, Pasto ME, *et al.* Evaluation of renal transplant rejection by duplex doppler examination: value of the resistive index. *AJR Am J Roentgenol* 1987; **148**(4):759–62.
44. Kelcz F, Pozniak MA, Pirsch JD, Oberly TD. Pyramidal appearance and resistive index: insensitive and nonspecific sonographic indicators of renal transplant rejection. *AJR Am J Roentgenol* 1990; **155**(3):531–5.
45. Chow L, Sommer FG, Huang J, Li KCP. Power Doppler imaging and resistance index measurement in the evaluation of acute renal transplant rejection. *J Clin Ultrasound* 2001; **29**(9):483–90.
46. Saarinen O. Diagnostic value of resistive index of renal transplants in the early postoperative period. *Acta Radiologica* 1991; **32**(2):166–9.
47. Patel U, Khaw KK, Hughes NC. Doppler ultrasound for detection of renal transplant artery stenosis—threshold peak systolic velocity needs to be higher in a low-risk or surveillance population. *Clin Radiol* 2003; **58**(10):772–7.
48. Schwenger V, Zeier M. Contrast-enhanced sonography as early diagnostic tool of chronic allograft nephropathy. *Nephrol Dial Transplant* 2006; **21**(10):2694–6.
49. Mazzu D, Jeffrey RB Jr, Ralls PW. Lymphoma and leukemia involving the testicles: findings on grey-scale and color Doppler sonography. *AJR Am J Roentgenol* 1995; **164**(3):645–7.
50. Backus ML, Mack LA, Middleton WD, King BF, Winter TC 3rd, True LD. Testicular microlithiasis: imaging appearances and pathologic correlation. *Radiology* 1994; **192**:781–5.
51. Ravichandran S, Smith R, Cornford PA, Fordham MVP. Surveillance of testicular microlithiasis?: Results of a UK-based national questionnaire survey. *BMC Urol* 2006; **6**:8.

52. Tan M-H, Eng C. Testicular microlithiasis: recent advances in understanding and management. *Nat Rev Urol* 2011; **8**:153–63.
53. Richenberg J, Brejt N. Testicular microlithiasis: is there a need for surveillance in the absence of other risk factors? *Eur Radiol* June 2012; **22**(11):2540–6.
54. Cast JEI, Nelson WM, Early AS, Biyani S, Cooksey G, Warnock NG, Breen DJ. Testicular microlithiasis prevalence and tumor risk in a population referred for scrotal sonography. *AJR Am J Roentgenol* 2000; **175**(6):1703–6.
55. Deganello A, Svasti-Salee D, Allen P, Clarke JL, Sellars MEK, Sidhu PS. Scrotal calcification in a symptomatic paediatric population: prevalence, location, and appearance in a cohort of 516 patients. *Clin Radiol* 2012; **67**(9):862–7.
56. Dogra V, Bhatt S. Acute painful scrotum. *Radiol Clin North Am* 2004; **42**(2):349–63.
57. Horstman WG, Middleton WD, Melson GL. Scrotal inflammatory disease: color Doppler US findings. *Radiology* 1991; **179**:55–9.
58. Desai KM, Gingell JC, Haworth JM. Fate of the testis following epididymitis: A clinical and ultrasound study. *J Royal Soc Med* 1986; **79**(9):515–19.
59. Begley MG, Shawker TH, Robertson CN, Bock SN, Wei JP, Lotze MT. Fournier Gangrene: Diagnosis with Scrotal US. *Radiology* 1988; **169**:387–389.
60. Caesar RE, Kaplan GW. Incidence of the bell-clapper deformity in an autopsy series. *Urology* 1994; **44**(1):114–16.
61. Bird K, Rosenfield AT, Taylor KJW. Ultrasonography in testicular torsion. *Radiology* 1983; **147**:527–34.
62. Sanders LM, Haber S, Dembner A, Aquino A. Significance of reversal of diastolic flow in the acute scrotum. *J Ultrasound Med* 1994; **13**:137–9.
63. Bader TR, Kammerhuber F, Herneth AM. Testicular blood flow in boys as assessed at color doppler and power Doppler sonography. *Radiology* 1997; **202**:559–64.
64. Lynch TH, Martínez-Piñeiro L, Plas E, *et al.* EAU guidelines on urological trauma. *Eur Urol* 2005: **47**(1):1–15.
65. Kim SH, Park S, Choi SH, Jeong WK, Choi JH. Significant predictors for determination of testicular rupture on sonography: a prospective study. *J Ultrasound Med* 2007; **26**(12):1649–55.
66. Guichard G, El Ammari J, Del Coro C, *et al.* Accuracy of ultrasonography in diagnosis of testicular rupture after blunt scrotal trauma. *Urology* 2008; **71**(1):52–6.
67. Lobianco R, Regine R, De Siero M, Catalano O, Caiazzo C, Ragozzino A. Contrast-enhanced sonography in blunt scrotal trauma. *J Ultrasound* 2011; **14**(4):188–95.
68. El-Saeity NS, Sidhu PS. Scrotal varicocele, exclude a renal tumour. Is this evidence-based? *Clin Radiol* 2006;**61**(7):593–9.
69. Frates MC, Benson CB, DiSalvo DN, Brown DL, Laing FC, Doubilet PM. Solid extratesticular masses evaluated with sonography: pathologic correlation. *Radiology* 1997; **204**:43–6.
70. Schwartz AN, Wang KY, Mack LA, *et al.* Evaluation of normal erectile function with color flow Doppler sonography. *AJR Am J Roentgenol* 1989; **153**(6):1155–60.
71. Quam JP, King BF, James EM, *et al.* Duplex and color Doppler sonographic evaluation of vasculogenic impotence. *AJR Am J Roentgenol* 1989; **153**(6):1141–7.
72. Wilkins CJ, Sriprasad S, Sidhu PS. Colour Doppler ultrasound of the penis. *Clin Radiol* 2003; **58**(7):514–23.
73. Scardino E, Villa G, Bonomo G, *et al.* Magnetic resonance imaging combined with artificial erection for local staging of penile cancer. *Urology* 2004; **63**(6):1158–62.
74. Dähnert WF, Hamper UM, Eggleston JC, Walsh PC, Sanders RC. Prostatic evaluation by transrectal sonography with histopathologic correlation: the echopenic appearance of early carcinoma. *Radiology* 1986; **158**:97–102.
75. Onur R, Littrup PJ, Pontes JE, Bianco FJ Jr. Contemporary impact of transrectal ultrasound lesions for prostate cancer detection. *J Urol* 2004; **172**(2):512–14.
76. Kuligowska E, Barish MA, Fenlon HM, Blake M. Predictors of prostate carcinoma: Accuracy of grey-scale and color Doppler US and serum markers. *Radiology* 2001; **220**:757–64.
77. Mitterberger MJ, Aigner F, Horninger W, *et al.* Comparative efficiency of contrast-enhanced colour Doppler ultrasound versus systematic biopsy for prostate cancer detection. *Eur Radiol* 2010; **20**(12):2791–6.
78. Pallwein L, Mitterberger M, Struve P, *et al.* Comparison of sonoelastography guided biopsy with systematic biopsy: impact on prostate cancer detection. *Eur Radiol* 2007; **17**(9):2278–85.
79. Nghiem HT, Kellman GM, Sandberg SA, Craig BM. Cystic lesions of the prostate. *Radiographics* 1990; **10**:635–50.
80. Nwosu CR, Khan KS, Chien PFW, Honest MR. Is real-time ultrasonic bladder volume estimation reliable and valid? A systematic overview. *Scand J Urol Nephrol* 1998;**32**(5):325–330
81. Byun SS, Kim HH, Lee E, Paick JS, Kamg W, Oh SJ. accuracy of bladder volume determinations by ultrasonography: Are they accurate over entire bladder volume range? *Urology* 2003; **62**(4):656–60.
82. Oelke M, Höfner K, Jonas U, de la Rosette JJ, Ubbink DT, Wijkstra H. Diagnostic accuracy of noninvasive tests to evaluate bladder outlet obstruction in men: detrusor wall thickness, uroflowmetry, postvoid residual urine, and prostate volume. *Eur Urol* 2007; **52**(3):827–35.
83. Vijayaraghavan SB. Perineal sonography in diagnosis of an ectopic ureteric opening into the urethra. *J Ultrasound Med* 2002; **21**(9):1041–6.
84. Itzchak Y, Singer D, Fischelovitch Y. Ultrasonographic assessment of bladder tumors. 1. Tumor detection. *J Urol* 1981; **126**(1):31–3.
85. Ozden E, Turgut AT, Turkolmez K, Resorlu B, Safak M. Effect of bladder carcinoma location on detection rates by ultrasonography and computed tomography. *Urology* 2007; **69**(5):889–92.
86. Denkhaus H, Crone-Münzebrock W, Huland H. noninvasive ultrasound in detecting and staging bladder carcinoma. *Urol Radiol* 1985; **7**(1):121–31.
87. Tekes A, Kamel I, Imam K, *et al.* Dynamic MRI of bladder cancer: Evaluation of staging accuracy. *AJR Am J Roentgenol* 2005; **184**(1):121–7.
88. Rosenbaum DM, Korngold E, Teele RL. Sonographic assessment of renal length in normal children. *AJR Am J Roentgenol* 1984; **142**(3):467–9.
89. Hricak H, Slovis TL, Callen CW, Callen PW, Romanski RN. Neonatal kidneys: sonographic anatomic correlation. *Radiology* 1983; **147**:699–702.
90. Sidhu G, Beyene J, Rosenblum ND. Outcome of isolated antenatal hydronephrosis: A systematic review and meta-analysis. *Pediatr Nephrol* 2006; **21**(2):218–24.
91. Belarmino JM, Kogan BA. Management of neonatal hydronephrosis. *J Earlhumdev* 2006; **82**(1):9–14.
92. Blickman JG, Bramson RT, Herrin JT. autosomal recessive polycystic kidney disease: long-term sonographic findings in patients surviving the neonatal period. *AJR Am J Roentgenol* 1995; **164**(5):1247–50.
93. National Institute for Health and Clinical Excellence. CG54: Urinary tract infection: Diagnosis, treatment and long term management of urinary tract infection in children. Available at: www.nice.org.uk/CG54 [Online].
94. De Campo JF. Ultrasound of Wilms' tumor. *Pediatr Radiol* 1986; **16**(1):21–4.
95. Breslow N, Olshan A, Beckwith JB, Green DM. Epidemiology of Wilms tumor. *Med Pediatr Oncol* 1993; **21**(3):172–81.
96. Scott EM, Thomas A, McGarrigle HH, Lachelin GC. Serial adrenal ultrasonography in normal neonates. *J Ultrasound Med* 1990; **9**(5):279–83.
97. Deeg KH, Bettendorf U, Hofmann V. Differential diagnosis of neonatal adrenal haemorrhage and congenital neuroblastoma by colour coded Doppler sonography and power Doppler sonography. *Eur J Pediatr* 1998; **157**(4):294–7.
98. Frede T, Hatzinger M, Rassweiler J. Ultrasound in endourology. *J Endourol* 2001; **15**(1):3–16.

CHAPTER 10.3

Computed tomography

Eugene Teoh and Michael Weston

Basic theory and principles of computed tomography

Computed tomography (CT) is the most widely utilized cross-sectional imaging modality to date. Introduced in the 1970s, CT served as a means of generating images in the transverse plane (axial images) of the internal organs of the patient. It has since evolved to be used to obtain volumes of image data of the relevant body section, which may be manipulated with image processing software to view the internal organs on sub-millimetre sections in multiple planes, and a whole host of other applications including surface rendering.

The rudimentary construct of the CT scanner involves an X-ray tube and a row of detectors built into a rotatable gantry. The patient lies on a couch that can move longitudinally through the gantry and images are acquired from relevant sections of the patient's body when they are in position within the gantry (see Fig. 10.3.1). The gantry rotates around the patient and X-rays are exposed to acquire data from different angles, which are used to construct the image using image reconstruction algorithms.

In modern day helical CT scanners, this process is relatively rapid and seamless, with the gantry in constant rotation and constant exposure and image acquisition being performed as the body part of interest moves through the gantry. The speed of acquisition is also boosted by the use of multiple rows of detectors, allowing the whole body to be imaged in a matter of seconds.

The constructed CT image is laid out as a matrix of pixels, each designated its own CT number or Hounsfield unit (HU). The CT number corresponds to the average density of tissues (and thus level of grey) within the pixel, with a positive correlation between density and CT number. For example, air has a CT number of -1000, water of zero, and bone 500–1,500. This leads on to the concept of windowing, which is integral to the interpretation of CT studies.

A common CT number range produces over 4,000 levels of grey, which if all displayed on a single scale would result in a very flat image. Windowing an image narrows the scale according to the range of CT numbers most represented by the organ/tissue type of interest. For example, to evaluate bone, a window range set around the aforementioned limits would demonstrate bone in detail with all structures less dense than bone greyed out. There are normally preset window settings for different organs and tissue types on imaging workstations, with the function to fine-tune the range accordingly. The importance of windowing and CT numbers to evaluate areas of interest will be expanded on in the 'Interpretation' section.

Since the advent of multidetector CT (MDCT), its use in the evaluation of the urinary tract has expanded widely and is now considered to have replaced intravenous urography (IVU) and the plain radiograph. A variety of CT techniques exist for evaluation of the urinary tract and the choice of technique depends largely on the indication, taking into account other patient factors (e.g. age, contraindications to iodinated contrast).

Practical techniques (including contrast agents)

Unenhanced CT KUB

Unenhanced CT of the urinary tract (CT KUB) is the most accurate and now considered to be the primary investigation for suspected ureteric colic.[1] Accuracy rates for this technique are high with reported sensitivities of 96–100% and specificities of 95.5–100%.[2]

The patient is normally scanned in a prone position with images obtained from the top of the kidneys to the bladder base. The use of oral or intravenous contrast is not required with a full urinary bladder being the only pre-requisite to allow more sensitive detection of bladder calculi. Low dose techniques are routinely employed, having been demonstrated to maintain high rates of accuracy for detecting lithiasis despite the compromise in image quality of soft tissue structures. With MDCT, the images can be acquired in a single breath hold and reconstruction of thin-sections are essential to avoid missing small calculi, particularly those of low density.[3]

Renal CT

Renal CT is the first line investigation for the characterization of a renal mass[1] detected on a different imaging investigation (e.g. ultrasound, CT KUB). The examination requires the administration of intravenous contrast and routinely involves two phases, an unenhanced and nephrographic phase.

The unenhanced phase is acquired before contrast administration. It allows for baseline characterization of the density of the lesion to establish enhancement patterns (if any) and detection of high density components which may be otherwise obscured with the administration of contrast. The nephrographic phase is acquired 100 seconds after administration of intravenous contrast. It produces homogeneous enhancement of the renal parenchyma, allowing for reliable detection of renal masses.[4]

In appropriate cases, a corticomedullary phase of enhancement may be acquired before the nephrographic phase by imaging the kidneys 40 seconds after contrast administration. The corticomedullary phase of enhancement depicts the renal

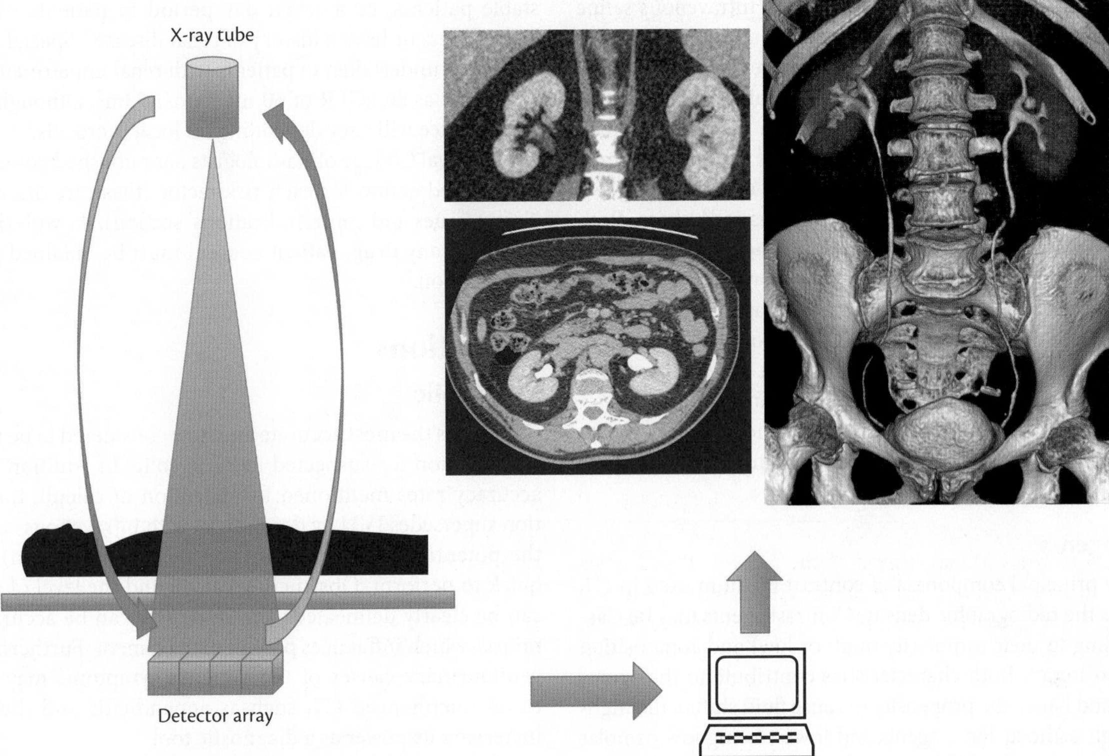

Fig. 10.3.1 Basic schematic of computed tomography (CT) scanning.

vasculature, which may be of use in pre-operative planning or where there is suspicion that the detected renal mass may be vascular in origin.[4,5]

CT urography

CT urography (CTU) is the best test for detecting renal calculi, renal masses and upper tract urothelial tumour[1] and thus may be considered as the one-stop imaging investigation of haematuria in the appropriate patient group (discussed in detail under the section 'Indications').

The technique involves imaging the urinary tract in three phases: unenhanced, nephrographic, and excretory, akin to the sequence of radiographs performed in IVU (see Fig. 10.3.2). The unenhanced phase is performed as a CT KUB. The nephrographic phase is acquired of the kidneys (as previously described) after administration of intravenous contrast, allowing for detection of renal masses.

The excretory phase of the study assesses the collecting systems, ureters and, to a lesser extent, the urinary bladder when optimal luminal opacification of these structures has taken place following contrast excretion by the kidneys. It is best acquired 10–12 minutes after intravenous contrast administration. Non-opacification of segments of ureter, particularly the distal ureter, is not an uncommon occurrence and several strategies have been described to optimize ureteric opacification with varying levels of evidence. These include prone positioning,[6] a further delayed acquisition,

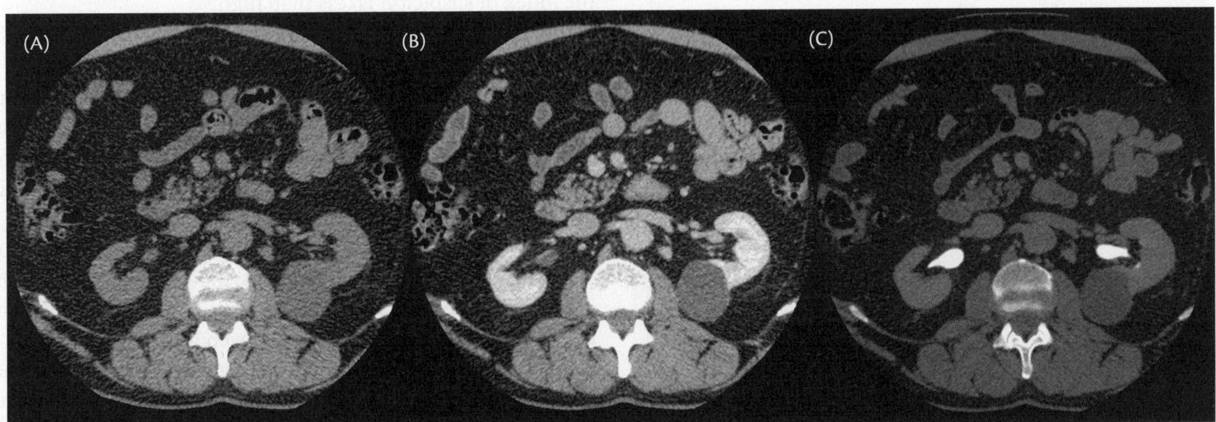

Fig. 10.3.2 The three phases of CTU: (A) unenhanced; (B) nephrographic; (C) excretory.

abdominal compression (as employed in IVU), intravenous saline bolus after contrast administration and diuretic administration.

The three phases can be imaged as three separate series, the nephrographic and excretory phases being obtained after a single dose of intravenous contrast, as was done with IVU. A described variation of the technique allows acquisition of both the nephrographic and excretory phase in a single series by administering two boluses of intravenous contrast after the unenhanced phase. Both doses are administered 10 minutes apart with image acquisition performed after a suitable nephrographic phase delay from the second dose. At this time point, the kidneys would be imaged in the nephrographic phase and contrast from the first dose would have begun to undergo renal excretion. This affords a radiation dose saving to the patient and improves workflow by reducing scanning time.

As with CT KUB, reconstruction of thin slices is essential to avoid missing small lesions, and allow data manipulation for producing multiplanar reformats.

Contrast agents

Iodine is the principal component of contrast medium used in CT, as it provides the radiographic density. Contrast agents may be classified according to their osmolarity (high or low) and composition (ionic or non-ionic). Both characteristics contribute to the agents osmolality (and hence the propensity to cause fluid shifts), the highest being high osmolar ionic agents and lowest being low osmolar non-ionic. In modern day CT, low osmolar non-ionic contrast agents are used, being 5–10 times safer than their ionic counterparts.[7]

Prior to the examination, checks for contraindications to contrast administration and risk factors for contrast-related adverse effects (drug reactions, nephrotoxicity and lactic acidosis) must be undertaken (see Box 10.3.1). Essential points to cover are a history of previous contrast reaction, asthma, renal disease, diabetes mellitus, allergies, and metformin therapy.[7] The renal function of the patient must be checked prior to the examination. This should be in the form of the estimated glomerular filtration rate (eGFR), taken within a three month period prior to the examination in clinically stable patients, or a seven day period in patients who have an acute illness or have a history of renal disease.[7] Special precautions should be undertaken in patients with renal impairment. This is set arbitrarily as an eGFR of 60 mL/min/1.73m^2, although thresholds and practice will vary depending on local protocols.[7]

The Royal College of Radiologists has published guidance on recommended action for each risk factor (these are discussed in the 'Safety issues and contraindications' section). As with the administration of any drug, patient consent must be obtained prior to the examination.[7]

Box 10.3.1 Risk factors for contrast-related adverse effects

Is there a history of:

- Previous contrast reaction
- Asthma
- Renal disease
- Diabetes mellitus
- Allergies
- Metformin therapy

Is the eGFR <60 mL/min/1.73m^2:

- In the last three months in clinically stable patients
- In the last seven days in patients with renal disease or an acute illness

Source: data from The Royal College of Radiologists, *Standards for Intravascular Contrast Administration to Adult Patients, Third Edition*, The Royal College of Radiologists (RCR), London, UK, Copyright © The Royal College of Radiologists 2015.

Indications

Renal colic

CT KUB is the most accurate and now considered to be the primary investigation for suspected ureteric colic. In addition to the high accuracy rates mentioned for detection of calculi, the investigation supersedes IVU by doing away with intravenous contrast (and the potential complications from its administration) and being quick to perform. Obstructing calculi and the level of obstruction can be clearly delineated. The stone size can be accurately determined, which influences patient management. Furthermore, extra-genitourinary causes of the patient's symptoms may be alluded to on unenhanced CT, such as appendicitis and diverticulitis,[2] increasing its power as a diagnostic tool.

While CT KUB has become well established for this clinical indication, added consideration should nonetheless be paid to young, particularly female, patients. Even with the use of a low dose technique, the potential carcinogenic effects of ionizing radiation in the long term cannot be ignored in this patient group. Patients should be triaged according to a stringent selection criteria, and where this raises doubt regarding the working diagnosis of renal colic, alternative imaging assessment should be contemplated.

This is of particular relevance to young female patients where an alternative gynaecological cause is prevalent. Published series have revealed that the detection rate of lithiasis is generally higher in males than females (55–61.6% vs. 18–27.5%),[8–11] with one of the series reporting detected gynaecological abnormality in 6% of females.[10] In the largest of these series (n = 1,357), the presence and absence of hydronephrosis in young female patients with significantly sized ureteric calculi (deemed to be >4 mm) was 83% vs. 17%, respectively.[8] This sets the premise for the use of ultrasound to assess for hydronephrosis in this patient group, particularly where the index of suspicion is less than high.

Haematuria

The utmost concern in the patient presenting with haematuria is that of urological malignancy. The choice of imaging investigation is dictated by the pre-test probability, which is influenced by two main factors: age and nature of haematuria. Other risk factors should also be taken into account (e.g. smoking and exposure to aniline dyes). While the presence of pain is of relevance in the clinical work-up (e.g. to exclude infection and guide symptom management), its role is limited in the choice of imaging due to the prevalence of alternative causes of haematuria despite proven lithiasis.[12]

CTU is indicated in older patients presenting with frank haematuria, where the risk of malignancy is high. There is no stipulated reference standard with regards to the age cut-off between high and low risk although evidence from large series support the age of 40 years as a suitable threshold for this indication. In all-age cohorts investigated for macroscopic haematuria, the prevalence of patients diagnosed with urological cancer and below 40 years has been reported to be 0.4–0.6% (overall cancer prevalence of 18.9–20.3%).[13,14] The detection rate for malignancy increases with age, exceeding 1 in every 10 patients with macroscopic haematuria above 50–60 years of age.[14]

Urolithiasis is the most common benign diagnosis made in patients presenting with haematuria and certainly in younger patients presenting with frank haematuria, CT KUB is indicated to evaluate for stone disease.

The choice of imaging investigation is somewhat less clear-cut in the context of microscopic haematuria. Most cases of upper tract cancers demonstrate persistent haematuria and in the older patient with microscopic haematuria, interval testing to establish persistence should inform the decision on the use of CTU.[14]

In the younger patient with microscopic haematuria, multiple factors should be considered prior to the use of CT. Apart from persistence of microscopic haematuria, the presence of pain in this context adds more weight, with the prevalence of urolithiasis in patients presenting with asymptomatic microscopic haematuria reported to be only 4–4.6% from large series data.[15] Awareness needs to be raised to the higher prevalence of renal parenchymal disease in this patient group and patients with associated risk factors, suggestive findings on clinical and urine dipstick examination, or abnormal renal function should be considered for referral to the nephrologists. It would thus be reasonable to perform an ultrasound in the younger patient with microscopic haematuria (to assess kidney size, look for hydronephrosis and ancillary signs of renal parenchymal disease). A CT KUB can be considered when there is a corroborating history of renal colic or if the ultrasound examination does not yield positive findings.

These guidelines, as with many aspects of clinical medicine, are by no means hard and fast rules, as they do not completely account for the small subgroup of young patients with urological malignancy, which may not necessarily be detected on unenhanced CT KUB even if they present with macroscopic haematuria. The decision on CT imaging has to be guided by the overall clinical assessment, particularly risk factors for (and against) malignancy, and cystoscopic findings. This must be balanced against the risk of ionizing radiation from CT and relatively lower sensitivity of other imaging investigations. Discussion with radiologists can be helpful in such cases and the patient's informed choice must be factored in.

Characterization of renal masses

Renal CT is the first line investigation for the characterization of a renal mass,[1] usually detected on a different imaging investigation. Based primarily on its enhancement characteristics and morphological features, renal CT should inform the clinician as to whether the mass is a surgical or non-surgical lesion, or if it exhibits characteristics warranting follow-up.[4]

Detection and characterization of urothelial lesions

CTU is now considered to have superseded IVU in terms of its ability to depict the upper urinary tract with increased sensitivity and specificity for urothelial abnormality.[16] As a cross-sectional technique, it depicts extraluminal pathology and where relevant, pathology within the urachus. It also has the advantage of revealing extra-genitourinary findings, which may be of direct relevance to the upper tract abnormality.

Detection and characterization of urinary tract injury

The excretory phase of CTU (+/– unenhanced phase depending on prior imaging) is a non-invasive means of evaluating selected cases with this indication, particularly in cases of suspected ureteric injury where a conventional cystogram might not yield the required information. An example is illustrated in Figure 10.3.3. Where there is suspicion of urinary tract injury in a patient who has undergone a trauma series CT, this can be performed with relative ease if the suspicion is raised early as the patient can be scanned after the appropriate excretory phase delay without having to receive a further dose of intravenous contrast (stressing the importance of the secondary survey in trauma).

With CT, a better spatial representation of the pattern and extent of injury can be depicted compared to cystography. In selected cases where this degree of detail is essential (e.g. for surgical planning), the excretory phase of CTU is also useful in depicting urinary tract fistulas.

Percutaneous nephrolithotomy planning

The excretory phase provides a clear road map for the approach to percutaneous nephrolithotomy by depicting the position and burden of calculi within the pelvicalyceal system, the anatomy of which can be complex. Clear demonstration of the spatial relations of the surrounding structures (e.g. pleura, vasculature) also help to plan a safe approach to accessing the pelvicalyceal system.[17,18]

Cancer staging

CT is widely used in cancer imaging to establish the presence and extent of distant disease, with urological cancer being no exception. Staging CT of the chest, abdomen and pelvis (if not already imaged) is used widely in renal cell carcinoma (RCC), where 28% of patients have disseminated disease at presentation. The incidence of metastatic disease is positively associated with tumour size with lung being the commonest site of spread. Lymph nodes, liver, and bone are other common sites of involvement.[19] In bladder cancer, MRI is the most accurate imaging modality for local staging. Staging CT is indicated for cases of confirmed muscle-invasive bladder cancer, including CTU for complete examination of the upper urinary tracts.[20] Lung and liver are common organs of involvement in bladder cancer.

There is no routine indication for the use of CT in the staging and follow-up of prostate cancer, with MRI being used for local staging and bone scan to assess for bone metastases. CT should be reserved for guiding further management in selected scenarios. These include biochemical failure after treatment with curative intent and where symptoms raise the possibility of extra-osseous metastatic disease.[21]

Interpretation and limitations

CT KUB

The study should be reviewed on an imaging workstation capable of producing multiplanar reformats. The thin slice axial images should be reviewed first, with close scrutiny of the renal parenchyma and collecting system for calculi, which would appear as high density foci. Both ureters should be traced down to their points of insertion into the urinary bladder. The urinary bladder should be reviewed for vesical calculi, particularly within the dependent part of the bladder.

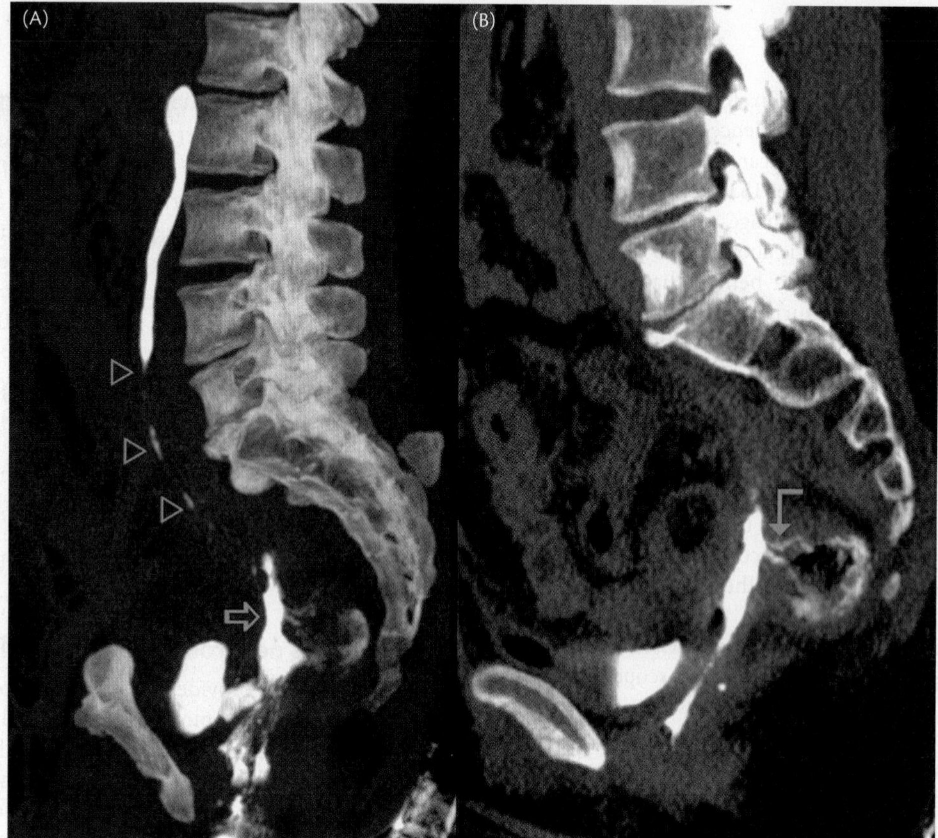

Fig. 10.3.3 An example of CTU delineating ureteric injury in a patient presenting with vaginal discharge of urine three weeks post pelvic surgery. (A) Contrast opacification of a blind-ending left distal ureter (arrowheads) with a fine track of contrast leading into the vaginal cavity (arrow) which is opacified. (B) A separate communication between the vagina and rectum (arrow) is also demonstrated.

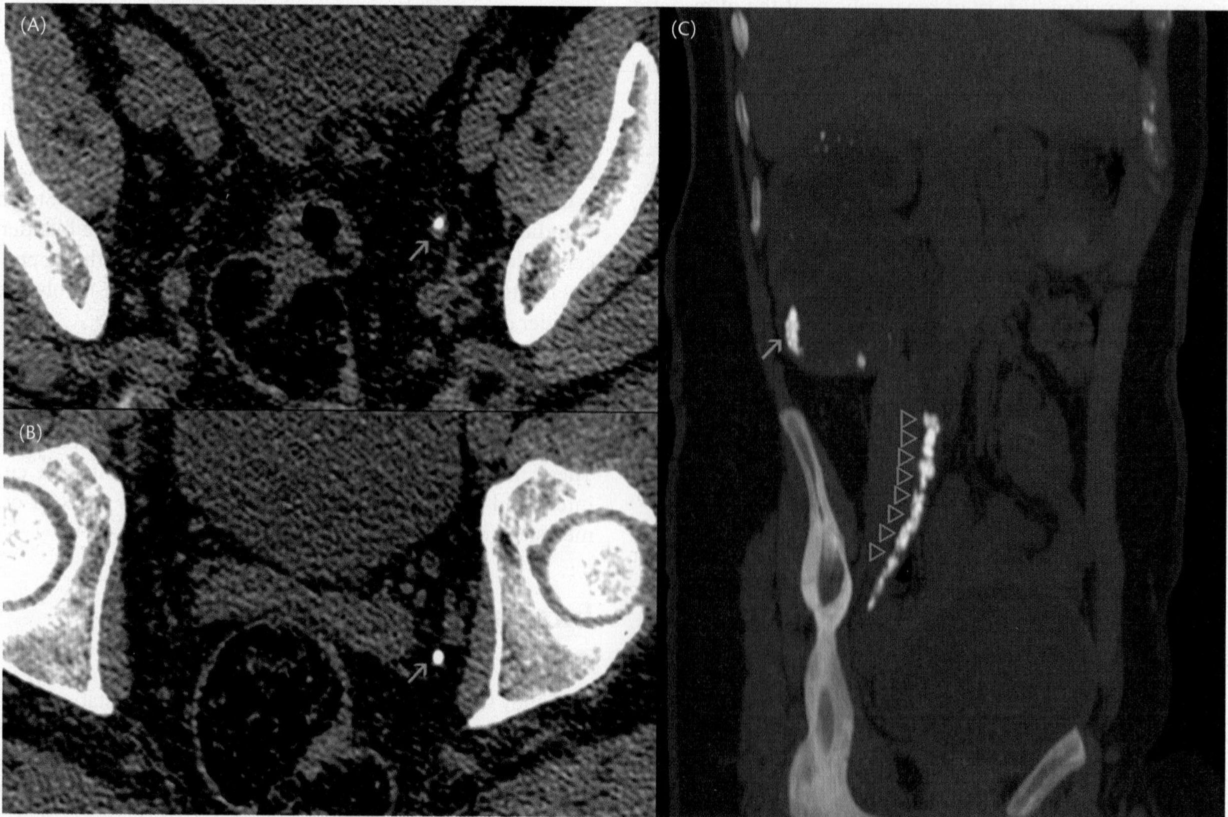

Fig. 10.3.4 (A) An example of a ureteric calculus with the typical multifaceted appearance exhibiting the soft tissue rim sign (arrow). This is compared to a phlebolith in the same patient (B—arrow). (C) Reformatted image of the right kidney in a patient with significant stone disease previously treated with extracorporeal shock wave lithotripsy. There is hydronephrosis and hydroureter secondary to the formation of 'steinstrasse' (street of stones) within the distal ureter (arrowheads). There are also residual renal calculi predominantly within the lower pole calyx (arrow).

Ancillary signs of urolithiasis should be actively sought. These include hydronephrosis and/or hydroureter caused by distal obstruction (see Fig. 10.3.4, Fig. 10.3.4C), and perinephric and/or periureteric fat stranding representative of inflammation. These features are of particular use when calculi are not detected on the study, to indicate recent stone passage or the presence of radiolucent calculi (particularly when there is a clear transition point of ureteric obstruction).[22]

The thin axial slices can be reformatted into sagittal and coronal images which should be reviewed routinely. This is of importance in assessing the maximum size of calculi, which may be underestimated on axial images, in turn influencing patient management. Anatomical relationships of areas of pathology can also be better represented on different projections, particularly coronal images, for pre-procedural planning.

The presence of phelboliths can occasionally make image interpretation difficult. While phleboliths can be reliably identified if they are extra-ureteric, this can be challenging in patients with a paucity of intra-abdominal fat which makes tracing the ureters difficult. In such indeterminate areas of calcification, a helpful feature to look out for is the soft tissue rim sign, characterized by a rim of soft tissue density around the calcification (see Fig. 10.3.4A). Where present, this is strongly suggestive of a ureteric calculus.[23] Other features of phleboliths include having a rounded morphology compared to calculi which tend to appear multifaceted (see Figs 10.3.4A and B). As with the general principles of image interpretation, one should use the clinical history, in particular side of the patient's symptoms, to guide interpretation.

Review of the other abdominal organs is essential, particularly when no urinary tract abnormalities are detected. Common extra-genitourinary findings on CT KUB include, appendicitis, diverticulitis, and gynaecological pathology. The bones and lung bases should be reviewed using appropriate windowing to detect abnormalities which may be of relevance to the patient's symptoms or genitourinary findings.

While additional stone compositions (cystine and uric acid) can be detected on CT compared to plain radiography, it is important to be aware of its limitations. The aforementioned stone compositions are of relatively lower density compared to their counterparts like calcium oxalate and struvite and small stones with a low attenuation value can be overlooked on helical CT.[3] Furthermore, indinavir (an antiretroviral drug associated with urolithiasis) and pure matrix calculi are radiolucent on CT.[24,25] Thus, additional scrutiny should be applied when ancillary signs of urolithiasis are present.

Renal CT

The nephrographic phase in renal CT should produce uniform enhancement of the renal parenchyma, allowing detection of small lesions, even in the absence of renal contour abnormality. The key to interpreting renal CT is establishing whether the lesion demonstrates enhancement, which in broad terms characterizes the lesion as surgical or non-surgical. This is established by comparing the density of the lesion on the unenhanced phase to the density on the nephrographic phase. A lesion is deemed to have unequivocal enhancement if the density rises by more than 20 HU, and indeterminate if it rises by 10–20 HU.[4] Benign cystic lesions will not enhance to these thresholds. The density is measured using a region-of-interest tool on the imaging workstation to interrogate the internal content of the lesion.

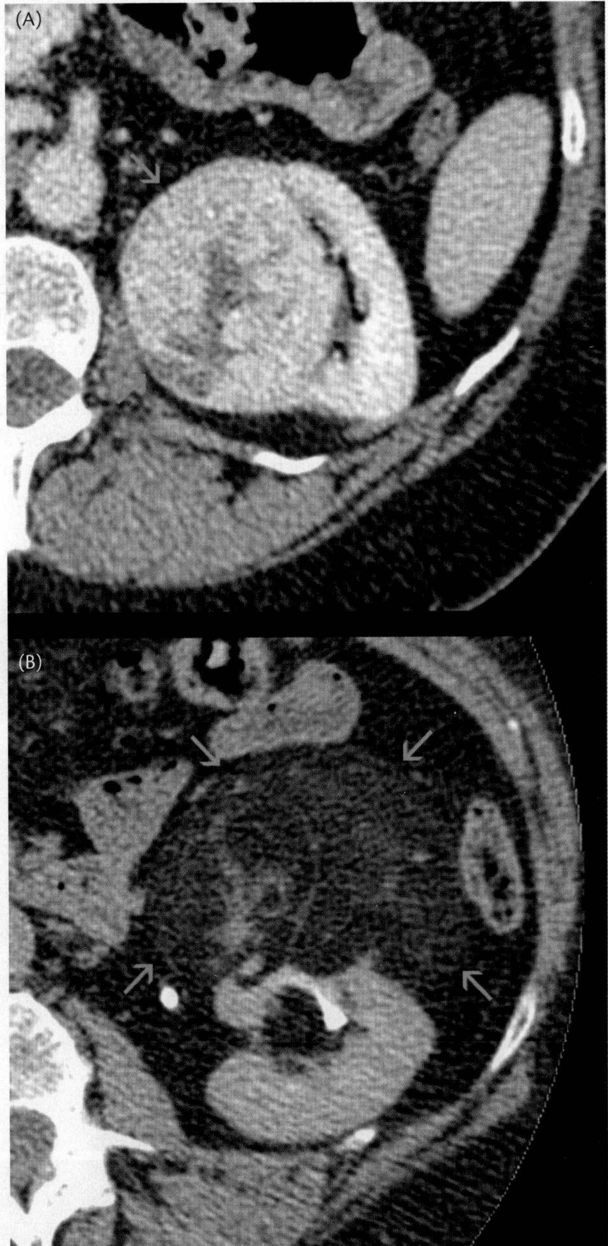

Fig. 10.3.5 (A) An example of an enhancing predominantly solid renal mass (arrows), subsequently diagnosed to be RCC. (B) A fat-containing mass with an average density of -69 HU (arrows), in keeping with an angiomyolipoma.

When evaluating a lesion, it is helpful to consider it as either solid or cystic. RCC is the commonest renal parenchymal tumour and are mostly solid (Fig. 10.3.5, Fig. 10.3.5A) although 2–5% are predominantly cystic. RCC varies widely in size, uniformity, and extent on CT, that is why it cannot be definitively diagnosed using this investigation. It also cannot be distinguished from oncocytoma on CT.

Other solid renal masses include angiomyolipoma, lymphoma, and metastases. Of these, an angiomyolipoma can be definitively diagnosed by the detection of fat within the mass (Fig. 10.3.5B). This is done by measuring the CT number of low density areas within the lesion (fat has a CT number of −60 to −150 HU). Lymphoma and metastatic disease typically feature as multiple bilateral solid masses.

In some cases (mostly in the context of known malignancy), a distinction between these two entities can be made based on the clinical history and additional imaging findings (e.g. lymphadenopathy, disseminated metastases). Where this distinction cannot be made, a definitive histological diagnosis should be obtained to dictate management, bearing in mind that RCC can also present with similar appearances.

When evaluating a cystic renal mass, the well-established Bosniak renal cyst classification is applied.[4] It allows the lesion to be categorized into one of five groups based on morphological characteristics and enhancement patterns, which dictate the probable nature of the lesion. These are described in Table 6.26.2 and Figure 10.3.6. Each category has accompanying clinical management recommendations which should never be adhered to strictly. They should serve as a guide to manage each individual case, taking into account clinical factors such as history, co-morbidity, and patient choice, particularly in patients with category III lesions.[4]

CTU

Due attention should be paid to all three phases of CTU. Using the same approach to CT KUB, the unenhanced phase should be reviewed for urinary tract calculi as a cause of the patient's symptoms. If stone disease is identified, the hunt for urinary tract pathology should not be prematurely called off, as a second source of haematuria coexists in a proportion of these patients.[12] Similarly, if a renal mass is detected on the nephrographic phase, the excretory phase should still be scrutinized for urothelial abnormality. It can be difficult to differentiate RCC from invasive transitional cell carcinoma (TCC) of the collecting system and in the context of the latter, multifocal disease can occur in up to 40% of patients.[16]

As one would do in reviewing a CT KUB, thin slice axial images should be reviewed on an imaging workstation capable of producing multiplanar reformats. The urinary tract should be scrutinized from the upper pole calyx down to the bladder base. The two pillars

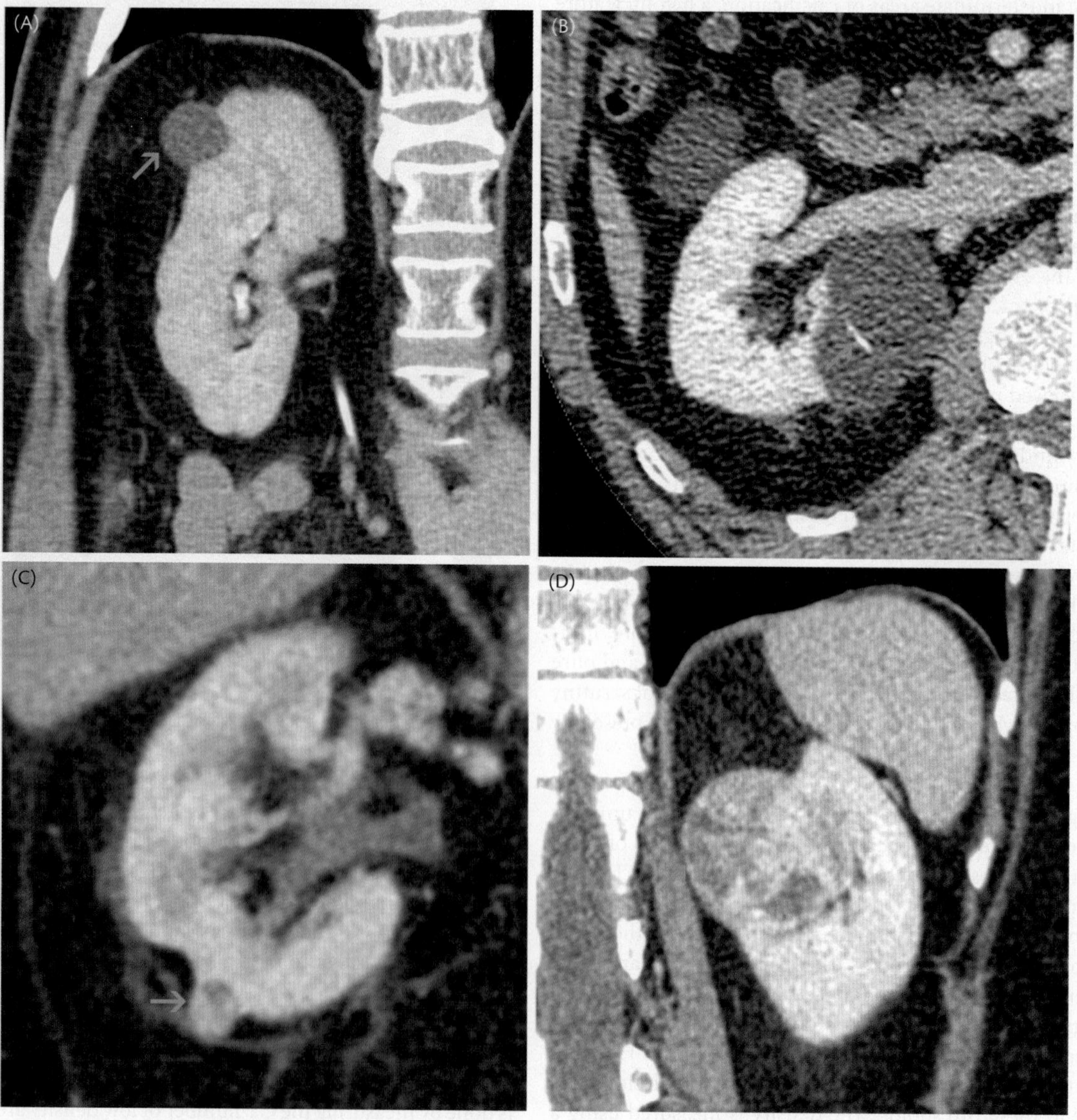

Fig. 10.3.6 (A) A Bosniak Category I simple cyst within the upper pole of the right kidney (arrow). (B) A Bosniak Category II cyst with a hairline thin calcified septa (arrow). (C) A Bosniak Category III cyst within the lower pole of the right kidney with an enhancing thickened and nodular inferior wall (arrow). (D) A Bosniak Category IV cystic mass with an enhancing soft tissue component independent of its enhancing thickened wall (arrow).

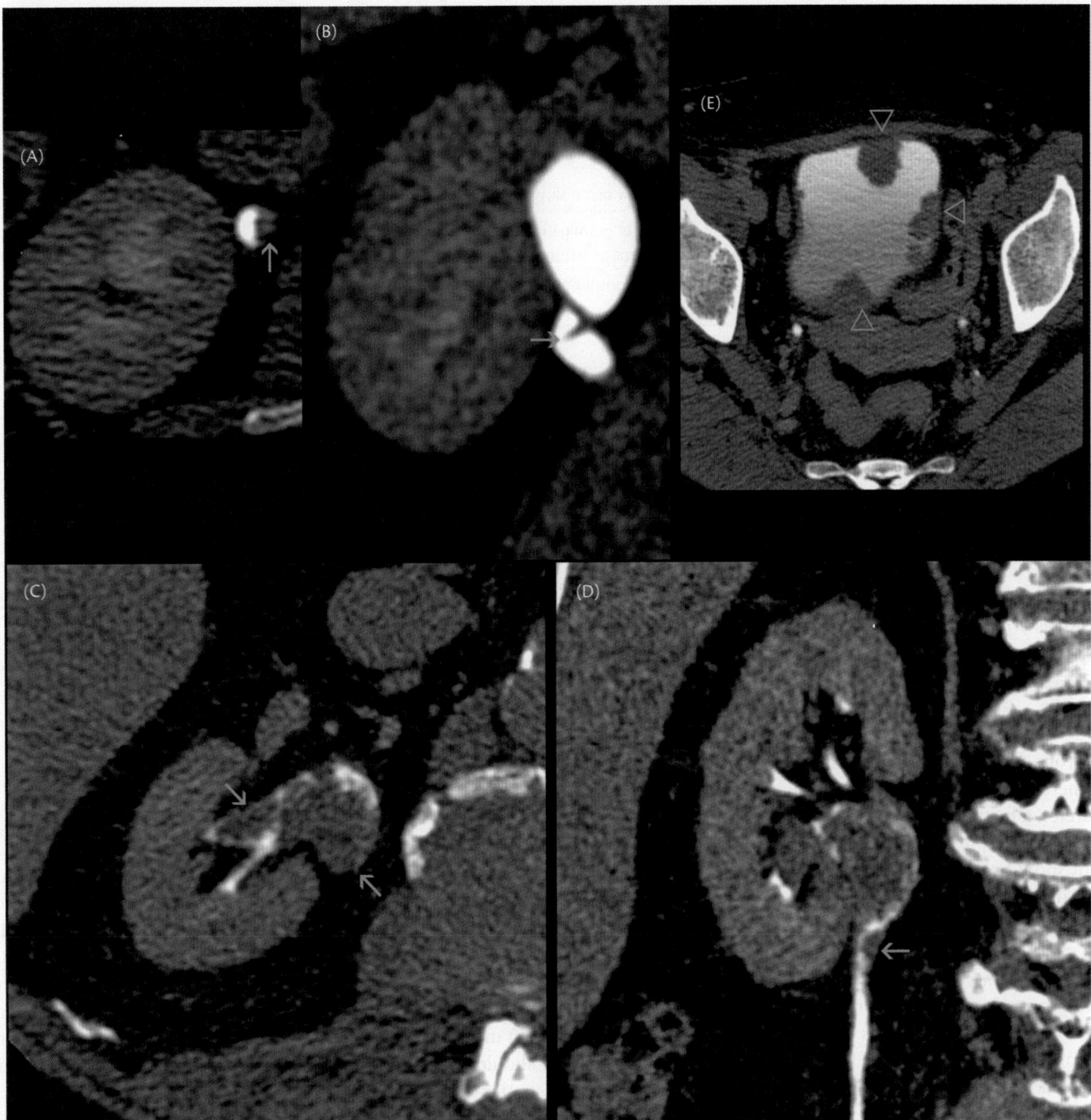

Fig. 10.3.7 (A) An apparent filling defect within the proximal ureter (arrow) which is confirmed to be a ureteric kink on the coronal images (B—arrow). (C) Axial image demonstrating multiple filling defects within the calyceal system (arrows), subsequently diagnosed to be TCC. (D) Coronal image on the same patient, demonstrating further disease in the proximal ureter (arrow). (E) Multiple filling defects within the bladder (arrowheads) confirmed to be multifocal bladder cancer.

of evaluating the excretory phase are adequate windowing and multiplanar review. Wide windowing is essential to avoid missing small urothelial lesions which might otherwise be obscured by contrast. Taking the time to review the urinary tract in three planes pays off as it can often depict abnormality not easily appreciated on axial images. These include carpet-like lesions along the dome of the bladder and small lesions within the upper pole calyces. Likewise, it is also helpful in resolving areas of concern, such as apparent filling defects on axial images due to tortuosities of the ureter (see Fig. 10.3.7, Fig. 10.3.7AB).

Upper urinary tract urothelial cell carcinoma (UUT-UCC) can be seen as enhancing soft tissue density masses and tend to cause filling defects within the opacified urinary tract (Fig. 10.3.7C and D). Some UUT-UCCs can manifest as circumferential wall thickening which may not even distort the lumen, stressing the importance of close evaluation of the wall, particularly in the absence of intraluminal abnormality.[16] Small lesions may manifest with more obvious secondary effects such as hydronephrosis and isolated calyceal dilatation.

In cases where the ureters are not well-opacified with contrast, measures should be taken to improve opacification using the previously discussed techniques (see the 'Practical techniques' section) as underlying UUT-UCC cannot otherwise be reliably detected. Of the various techniques, repeating the acquisition with the patient

Table 10.3.1 Recommended action in patients with increased risk of adverse effects

<table>
<tr><th>Risk factor</th><th colspan="2">Action</th></tr>
<tr><td>Previous reaction</td><td>◆ Establish nature of reaction and causative agent
◆ Reassess the need for contrast, risk-benefit of its use, and consider the use of other investigations
◆ If absolutely necessary, use a different low osmolality agent</td><td rowspan="3">If deemed necessary:
◆ proceed with a low osmolality agent
◆ maintain cloase medical supervision for 30 minutes with IV access maintained
◆ ensure all other safety measures are in place</td></tr>
<tr><td>Asthma</td><td>◆ If symptomatic/not well-controlled, defer examination if not urgent, subject to improved management of asthma
◆ If well-controlled, reassess the need for contrast and consider the use of alternative investigations</td></tr>
<tr><td>Multiple allergies/ single severe allergy</td><td>◆ Establish the nature and sensitivity of allergy
◆ Reassess the need for contrast, risk-benefit of its use, and consider the use of alternative investigations</td></tr>
<tr><td>Renal disease/Diabetes mellitus*</td><td colspan="2">◆ Considering the severity of renal impairment, reassess the need for contrast, risk-benefit of its use, and potential use of other investigations
◆ Use the smallest possible does of low osmolality agent
◆ Ensure the patient is optimally hydrated before and after contrast injection</td></tr>
<tr><td>Metformin</td><td colspan="2">◆ If renal function is normal, no further action is required
◆ If renal function is abnormal, cessation of metformin for 48 hours is recommended in consultation with the referring doctor</td></tr>
</table>

*Coexistent diabetes mellitus in patients with renal impairment carries significant risk.

Source: data from The Royal College of Radiologists, *Standards for Intravascular Contrast Administration to Adult Patients, Third Edition*, The Royal College of Radiologists (RCR), London, UK, Copyright © The Royal College of Radiologists 2015.

in the prone position is probably the most practical, although in cases where there is delayed excretion due to hydronephrosis and hydroureter, a further delayed series would yield a better result. In such scenarios despite poor ureteric opacification, a dilated ureteric segment should raise the suspicion of UUT-UCC regardless, particularly if it enhances.[16]

One should be aware of the potential mimics of UUT-UCC. Causes can be considered into three groups: urothelial, luminal, and extraurothelial.[26] Urothelial causes include ureteric injury, irritation by calculi/stent, fibroepithelial polyps, or nephrogenic adenoma.[26] Clot or debris can cause luminal filling defects. Extraurothelial causes include RCC and vascular indentation. Correlation with clinical history (e.g. previous urinary tract instrumentation), MPR review and assessment of enhancement is required to minimize/clarify false positive findings. Retrograde ureteropyelography (RUP) can aid in clarification where there are equivocal appearances or non-diagnostic studies.

Bladder tumours can manifest as filling defects within a contrast-opacified bladder (Fig. 10.3.7E), focal masses, or asymmetric wall thickening, whereas uniform wall thickening tends to represent benign disease.[27] In the specific context of suspected bladder cancer, CTU should act as an adjunct to cystoscopy, as opposed to being a replacement for evaluating the bladder.[28] Lesion detection is suboptimal where there is layering of contrast and non-contrast-opacified urine within the bladder, which is more often the case. Flat bladder tumours may produce little in the way of filling defects or focal wall thickening. In patients who have undergone local therapy to the bladder, areas of scarring and wall thickening post-therapy make detection of new malignancy difficult on CT.[27]

Finally, after studying the urinary tract, the remainder of the abdomen and pelvis should be reviewed in abdominal and bone windows for extra-genitourinary disease.

Safety issues and contraindications

Contrast administration

Several practical measures must be addressed prior to the administration of contrast.[7] An appropriately trained doctor should be immediately available to manage severe reactions. Within the confines of the radiology department, an appropriately trained individual should be immediately available to identify and manage severe contrast reactions. Resuscitation facilities should be readily available and be subject to regular checks. A patient should not be left unsupervised within 5 minutes of contrast administration, and should remain on the premises for 15 minutes after (30 minutes in patients with an increased risk of contrast reaction).[7]

Low osmolar iodinated contrast agents are generally associated with a low rate of adverse effects (0.153% in large series data),[29] the majority of which are mild and can be treated within the confines of the radiology department. Severe reactions (anaphylactic spectrum) are rare, constituting 3.3% of all adverse effects.[29] Nonetheless, where identified (see the 'Techniques' section), appropriate precautions need to be undertaken to reduce the risk of the adverse effects from contrast administration. These are summarized in Table 10.3.1. The responsibility for deciding on contrast use eventually lies with the supervising radiologist.[7]

Radiation protection

The main disadvantage of CT is the high ionizing radiation dose to the patient. The total effective dose of an optimized CTU protocol (low dose unenhanced scan, followed by a combined nephrographic and excretory phase) acquired by a modern 64-slice CT scanner is 20.1 mSv.[30] This is equivalent to just over nine years of UK background radiation or an added risk of fatal cancer of 1 in 1,000. Hence, despite its superior accuracy, CT examinations of the urinary tract should not be undertaken lightly and as with all diagnostic ionizing radiation examinations, should be justified in terms of the clinical benefit against the radiation risk.[1] As previously discussed, appropriate selection of patients with a high pre-test probability of disease is the key to this process, particularly in the context of haematuria. This requires clear referral guidelines to be established and adhered to by radiologists and the referrer to have a sound understanding of indications for each examination. Open discussion between both parties should always be maintained, particularly for deciding on the best imaging pathway for complex cases.

Further reading

Anderson EM, Murphy R, Rennie AT, Cowan NC. Multidetector computed tomography urography (MDCTU) for diagnosing urothelial malignancy. *Clin Radiol* 2007; **62**(4):324–32.

Cowan NC, Turney BW, Taylor NJ, McCarthy CL, Crew JP. Multidetector computed tomography urography for diagnosing upper urinary tract urothelial tumour. *BJU Int* 2007; **99**(6):1363–70.

Israel GM, Bosniak MA. How I do it: evaluating renal masses. *Radiology* 2005; **236**(2):441–50.

Royal College of Radiologists (Great Britain). Faculty of Clinical Radiology. Board. *Standards for Intravascular Contrast Agent Administration to Adult Patients*, 2nd edition. London, UK: Royal College of Radiologists, 2010.

Royal College of Radiologists (Great Britain). *iRefer: Making the Best Use of Clinical Radiology*. London, UK: Royal College of Radiologists, 2012.

Tamm EP, Silverman PM, Shuman WP. Evaluation of the patient with flank pain and possible ureteral calculus. *Radiology* 2003; **228**(2):319–29.

Van Der Molen AJ, Cowan NC, *et al.* CT urography: definition, indications and techniques. A guideline for clinical practice. *Eur Radiol* 2008; **18**(1):4–17.

References

1. Royal College of Radiologists (Great Britain). *iRefer: Making the Best Use of Clinical Radiology*. London, UK: Royal College of Radiologists, 2012.
2. Tamm EP, Silverman PM, Shuman WP. Evaluation of the patient with flank pain and possible ureteral calculus. *Radiology* 2003; **228**(2):319–29.
3. Saw KC, McAteer JA, Monga AG, Chua GT, Lingeman JE, Williams JC Jr. Helical CT of urinary calculi: effect of stone composition, stone size, and scan collimation. *AJR Am J Roentgenol* 2000; **175**(2):329–32.
4. Israel GM, Bosniak MA. How I do it: evaluating renal masses. *Radiology* 2005; **236**(2):441–50.
5. Yuh BI, Cohan RH. Different phases of renal enhancement: role in detecting and characterizing renal masses during helical CT. *AJR Am J Roentgenol* 1999; **173**(3):747–55.
6. McNicholas MM, Raptopoulos VD, Schwartz RK, *et al.* Excretory phase CT urography for opacification of the urinary collecting system. *AJR Am J Roentgenol* 1998; **170**(5):1261–7.
7. Royal College of Radiologists (Great Britain). Faculty of Clinical Radiology. Board. *Standards for Intravascular Contrast Agent Administration to Adult Patients*, 2nd edition. London, UK: Royal College of Radiologists, 2010.
8. Patatas K, Panditaratne N, Wah TM, Weston MJ, Irving HC. Emergency department imaging protocol for suspected acute renal colic: re-evaluating our service. *Br J Radiol* 2012; **85**(1016):1118–22.
9. Patatas K. Does the protocol for suspected renal colic lead to unnecessary radiation exposure of young female patients? *Emerg Med J* 2010; **27**(5):389–90.
10. Chowdhury FU, Kotwal S, Raghunathan G, Wah TM, Joyce A, Irving HC. Unenhanced multidetector CT (CT KUB) in the initial imaging of suspected acute renal colic: evaluating a new service. *Clin Radiol* 2007; **62**(10):970–7.
11. Yong AW. Review of the current use of CT KUB to diagnose renal colic in the Royal Infirmary of Edinburgh from December 2007–February 2008. *Scott Med J* 2009; **53**:54.
12. Song JH, Beland MD, Mayo-Smith WW. Hematuria evaluation with MDCT urography: is a contrast-enhanced phase needed when calculi are detected in the unenhanced phase? *AJR Am J Roentgenol* 2011; **197**(1):W84–9.
13. Khadra MH, Pickard RS, Charlton M, Powell PH, Neal DE. A prospective analysis of 1,930 patients with hematuria to evaluate current diagnostic practice. *J Urol* 2000; **163**(2):524–7.
14. Edwards TJ, Dickinson AJ, Natale S, Gosling J, McGrath JS. A prospective analysis of the diagnostic yield resulting from the attendance of 4020 patients at a protocol-driven haematuria clinic. *BJU Int* 2006; **97**(2):301–5; discussion 305.
15. Tomson C, Porter T. Asymptomatic microscopic or dipstick haematuria in adults: which investigations for which patients? A review of the evidence. *BJU Int* 2002; **90**(3):185–98.
16. Anderson EM, Murphy R, Rennie AT, Cowan NC. Multidetector computed tomography urography (MDCTU) for diagnosing urothelial malignancy. *Clin Radiol* 2007; **62**(4):324–32.
17. Thiruchelvam N, Mostafid H, Ubhayakar G. Planning percutaneous nephrolithotomy using multidetector computed tomography urography, multiplanar reconstruction and three-dimensional reformatting. *BJU Int* 2005; **95**(9):1280–4.
18. Van Der Molen AJ, Cowan NC, *et al.* CT urography: definition, indications and techniques. A guideline for clinical practice. *Eur Radiol* 2008; **18**(1):4–17.
19. Dèahnert W. *Radiology Review Manual*, 7th edition. Philadelphia, PA: Lippincott Williams and Wilkins, 2011.
20. Stenzl A, Cowan NC, De Santis M, *et al.* The updated EAU guidelines on muscle-invasive and metastatic bladder cancer. *Eur Urol* 2009; **55**(4):815–25.
21. Heidenreich A, Bellmunt J, Bolla M, *et al.* EAU guidelines on prostate cancer. Part 1: screening, diagnosis, and treatment of clinically localised disease. *Eur Urol* 2011; **59**(1):61–71.
22. Smith RC, Verga M, Dalrymple N, McCarthy S, Rosenfield AT. Acute ureteral obstruction: value of secondary signs of helical unenhanced CT. *AJR Am J Roentgenol* 1996; **167**(5):1109–13.
23. Heneghan JP, Dalrymple NC, Verga M, Rosenfield AT, Smith RC. Soft-tissue "rim" sign in the diagnosis of ureteral calculi with use of unenhanced helical CT. Radiology 1997; **202**(3):709–11.
24. Schwartz BF, Schenkman N, Armenakas NA, Stoller ML. Imaging characteristics of indinavir calculi. *J Urol* 1999; **161**(4):1085–7.
25. Quaia E. *Radiological Imaging of the Kidney*. Berlin, Germany: Springer, 2011.
26. Cowan NC, Turney BW, Taylor NJ, McCarthy CL, Crew JP. Multidetector computed tomography urography for diagnosing upper urinary tract urothelial tumour. *BJU Int* 2007; **99**(6):1363–70.
27. Cohan RH, Caoili EM, Cowan NC, Weizer AZ, Ellis JH. MDCT Urography: Exploring a new paradigm for imaging of bladder cancer. *AJR Am J Roentgenol* 2009; **192**(6):1501–8.
28. Blick CG, Nazir SA, Mallett S, *et al.* Evaluation of diagnostic strategies for bladder cancer using computed tomography (CT) urography, flexible cystoscopy and voided urine cytology: results for 778 patients from a hospital haematuria clinic. *BJU Int* 2012; **110**(1):84–94.
29. Hunt CH, Hartman RP, Hesley GK. Frequency and severity of adverse effects of iodinated and gadolinium contrast materials: retrospective review of 456,930 doses. *AJR Am J Roentgenol* 2009; **193**(4):1124–7.
30. Vrtiska TJ, Hartman RP, Kofler JM, Bruesewitz MR, King BF, McCollough CH. Spatial resolution and radiation dose of a 64-MDCT scanner compared with published CT urography protocols. *AJR Am J Roentgenol* 2009; **192**(4):941–8.

CHAPTER 10.4

Magnetic resonance imaging in urology

Raj Das, Susan Heenan, and Uday Patel

The physics and technical aspects of magnetic resonance imaging

Basic principles of magnetic resonance

Magnetic resonance imaging refers to a complex interplay between the laws of electromagnetic induction governing atomic nuclei and the application of external magnetic fields to produce an image.

An atomic nucleus contains both protons and neutrons which are constantly spinning about their axis while negatively charged electrons orbit the nucleus. The spinning of the nuclear particles creates an angular momentum. This is zero when there is an equal number of neutrons and protons but in the case of hydrogen, which as a constituent of water is present throughout the human body, a single proton is present within the nucleus. As a result, the hydrogen nucleus has a positive charge, which as it spins produces a small magnetic field and acts as a tiny bar magnet.

The external magnetic field and free precession

When the body is placed under a strong external magnetic field (B_0), the spinning hydrogen protons become aligned to the external field. However, they do not all align in the same direction. While the majority align in a parallel fashion at a lower energy level, some align antiparallel to this field which results in them gaining higher energy levels. This alignment generates a small net magnetic field (or net magnetic vector).

The hydrogen protons then start to 'wobble', a type of motion called precession. They start to spin around a central axis (similar to a spinning top), begin to tilt and move in a circular orbit (precess). For example, if the net magnetization is placed in the X-Y plane, then the proton will also rotate about the Z-plane. This occurs at a given frequency proportional to the strength of the external magnetic field (B_0) and is called the Larmor frequency (see Fig. 10.4.1, Fig. 10.4.1A).

Magnetic resonance and the radiofrequency pulse

Different nuclei have a natural frequency at which they tend to vibrate which is referred to as a resonant frequency. If energy is applied at a material's natural resonant frequency then the material will absorb the energy and subsequently increase the amplitude of its oscillations. The resonant frequency of the body's hydrogen nuclei lies within the radiofrequency wave bandwidth and this therefore allows manipulation of the electromagnetic field.

When the body is exposed to radiofrequency waves at the resonant frequency of the hydrogen nuclei, energy can be transmitted from the radiofrequency (RF) pulse to the hydrogen nuclei.

Without exposure to radiofrequency (RF) waves the net magnetic vector (NMV) lies parallel to the external magnetic field and cannot be detected. With exposure to RF pulse, the NMV can form in a plane perpendicular to the external magnetic field and this 'transverse magnetic vector' can be detected (Fig. 10.4.1B).

When the RF wave is stopped, the protons lose energy passing from the higher to the lower energy state to reach equilibrium, thereby causing precession of the transverse magnetic vector. This generates a small oscillating magnetic field and induction of an alternating current which can then be detected by the adjacent receiver coils in the MRI magnet.

Therefore, by applying different RF pulses, the differing currents allow spatial encoding and with amplification and computer processing this is able to produce the digital MR image.

Relaxation times and image weighting

Relaxation is the dynamic process by which the spinning protons return to equilibrium. There are two main components: (i) the recovery of longitudinal magnetization, aligned with B0, which follows an exponential curve characterized by time constant T1; (ii) the decay of transverse magnetization, according to an exponential curve characterized by time constant T2.

A spin echo sequence (most commonly used to produce standard T1 and T2 weighted imaging) requires an excitation pulse (90-degree RF pulse) and an 180-degree re-phasing pulse. The time elapsed between a 90-degree pulse and 180-degree pulse is TE/2.

An MR signal is acquired following an echo time (TE), when the signal of the echo is of greatest amplitude.

The 90–180-degree RF pulses sequence must be repeated as many times as the number of lines of pixels in the data matrix. The time elapsed between each 90-degree RF pulse (excitation pulse) is called the repetition time (TR) and can be altered according to the MRI controls.

With a spin echo sequence:

- TR modifies T1-weighting: i.e. long TR produces a more T1-weighted image
- TE modifies T2-weighting: i.e. a shorter TE produces a less T2-weighted image.

(A)

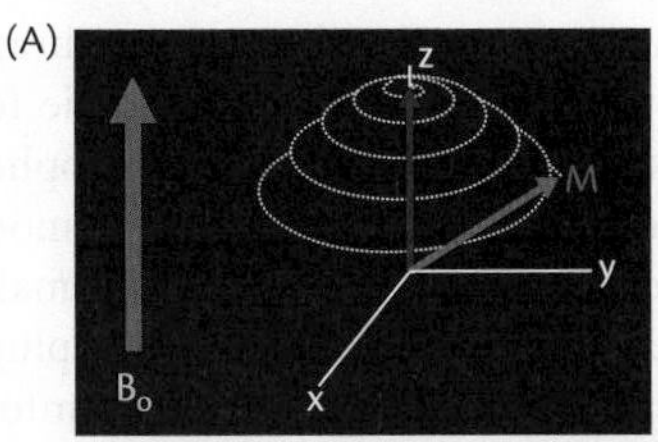

(B)

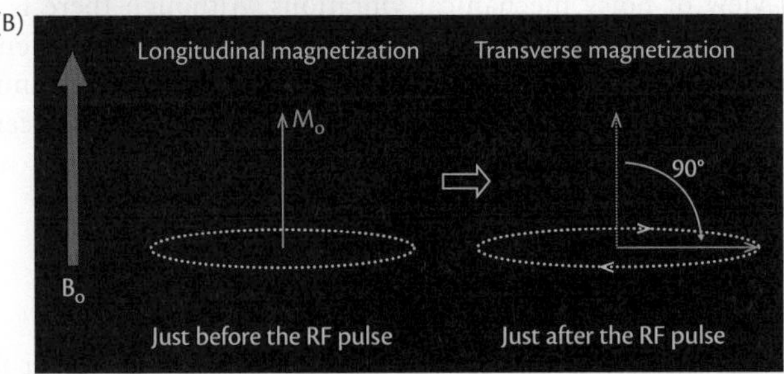

Fig. 10.4.1 (A) How an RF pulse affects the magnetization. The net magnetization vector M precesses about the time-varying magnetic field (not shown) induced by the RF pulse, as well as about the static magnetic field Bo (brown arrow) generated by the scanner magnet. As a result, the RF pulse causes the magnetization to spiral toward the transverse (x–y) plane. The white dotted line shows the path traced out by the tip of the net magnetization vector as it 'nutates' toward the x–y plane. The dark-purple vector on the z axis represents the position of the magnetization just before the RF pulse is applied. (B) A 90° RF pulse converts longitudinal magnetization into transverse magnetization. The thermal equilibrium magnetization (vertical solid green arrow, labeled Mo) is parallel to the static magnetic field Bo (solid brown arrow), and has only a longitudinal component just before the RF pulse is applied. The 90° RF pulse rotates the thermal equilibrium magnetization through 90° to become transverse magnetization (horizontal solid green arrow). Hence, just after the 90° RF pulse, the longitudinal component of the magnetization is zero (for reference, the original longitudinal component is indicated on the right by a thin dotted arrow), and the transverse magnetization generated by the RF pulse precesses (rotates) about the z axis at the resonant frequency. The magnitude of the transverse magnetization immediately after the RF pulse is equal to that of the longitudinal magnetization just before the RF pulse.
Credit line: (A) Adapted from Mugler JP III. Basic principles. In: Edelman RR, Hesselink JR, Zlatkin MB, Crues JV III, eds. Clinical Magnetic Resonance Imaging, 3rd ed. Philadelphia: Saunders Elsevier, 2006.

Therefore:

- A short TR and a short TE produces a T1-weighted image.
- A long TR and a long TE produces a T2-weighted image.

Image weighting and contrast

Different body tissues have different T1 and T2 times and therefore generate tissue contrast.

Generally T1 weighted images result in fat returning high signal and water/fluid corresponding to low signal. T1 weighted images are useful for characterization of masses and the presence of fat or haemorrhagic components, as well as assessment of pathology following intravenous contrast enhancement.

On T2 weighted images fluid containing tissues/structures are of high signal, whereas fat is of low signal. T2 weighted images are better at demonstrating pathology as most pathological conditions will result in increased water content in the tissues/oedema and will generate high signal on T2 weighted images.

Of note, haemorrhage has a complex appearance with variable T1 and T2 weighted signal characteristics due to the evolution of deoxyhaemoglobin and methaemoglobin and does not follow the characteristics of fluid.

Image saturation and specific sequences

In addition to T1 and T2 weighted sequences in orthogonal planes (which is the mainstay of standard MRI imaging) there are further sequences that are useful to be familiar with.

Inversion recovery sequences use a spin echo sequence that begins with an 180° inverting pulse thereby inverting the NMV through 180 degrees. Following a time interval TI or tau (time from inversion) a further 90-degree RF pulse is applied, followed by an 180-degree pulse producing an echo at time TE. By manipulating the TI, it is possible to form inversion recovery sequences. Short TI/tau inversion recovery (STIR) sequences coordinate the TI to coincide the 90-degree RF pulse with the time that the NMV of fat is passing through the transverse plane and thereby nulls the signal of fat, resulting in a fat-supressed, relatively T2 weighted image. STIR images are good at identifying pathology within fat-containing tissues and highlight oedema.

FLAIR (fluid attenuated inversion recovery) is a similar technique used in brain imaging to null the signal of cerebrospinal fluid (CSF).

Specific T1 fat-suppression sequences may be required for the assessment of pathology with high T1 signal and if post-contrast scans are required.

Heavily T2-weighted images can be produced to produce images which show static fluid as high signal with relative suppression of signal returned from other tissues. These are of use in MR urography resulting in an intravenous urography (IVU)-style image.

Diffusion-weighted imaging

Diffusion is the term applied to describe molecules moving due to random thermal motion. Free diffusion allows movement of molecules in all planes. In restricted diffusion, there is altered cell membrane permeability, cellular swelling, and absorption of extracellular water resulting in restricted motion.

In diffusion-weighted imaging (DWI), diffusion gradients are applied in differing direction with differing intensity according to a 'b-value'. A higher b-value is generated according to a higher intensity of diffusion gradients. Typical b-values range from 500 s/mm^2 to 1,000 s/mm^2.

DWI images are associated with an inherent T2-weighting. By performing the diffusion gradients at two different levels (e.g. b = 0 and b = 1,000) it is possible to subtract the T2-weighting which results in an apparent diffusion coefficient (ADC) map. This allows differentiation of 'T2 shine-through artefact' and true diffusion restriction.

Initial applications of DWI were in brain imaging in ischaemic stroke. Research has since demonstrated that cancers and malignant tissue also exhibit restricted diffusion due to altered cell membrane function and thereby allows improved cancer detection.

Cancerous tissue should therefore demonstrate high signal on DWI sequences and a corresponding low signal abnormality on the ADC map. Diffusion-weighted imaging has more recently become standard practice in oncological MRI such as in prostate cancer.

MRI specific contrast agents

Gadolinium is a T1 shortening agent that is the most widely used extracellular paramagnetic contrast agent in the form of various chelates. Its action to reduce the T1 relaxation times results in increased signal intensity on T1 weighted images and therefore results in T1 enhancement.

Gadolinium is excreted renally by glomerular filtration without tubular secretion or reabsorption.

The pattern and time frame of contrast enhancement is similar in pharmacokinetics to iodinated contrast in computed tomography (CT) scanning. Adverse reactions can occur but are much less common than experienced with iodinated contrast. These may include mild transient increase in bilirubin and blood iron, mild headaches, nausea, vomiting, hypotension.

Further cell specific MRI contrast agents are available for use in the hepatobiliary and reticulo-endothelial systems but are not routinely used for assessment of the urological system at present.

Intravenous administration of iron-oxide particles (SPIO) is generally used in the liver resulting in signal loss of the normal liver on heavily T2-weighted images. Iron oxides have been used to detect early lymph node metastases. This technique uses gradient-echo (T2*) imaging to detect susceptibility artefact occurring in normal lymph nodes (appear blacker) with no effect on malignant nodes, thereby allowing differentiation of abnormal nodes.

Nephrogenic systemic fibrosis

Gadolinium does not tend to cause contrast induced nephropathy, as is the case with iodinated contrast media but has been described in the aetiology of nephrogenic systemic fibrosis, previously called nephrogenic fibrosing dermopathy. The association is rare but is associated with use in patients with an eGFR <30 mL/minute. This is detailed in the European Society of Urogenital Radiology (ESUR)[1] and the Royal College of Radiologists guidelines.[2] The disease state involves the development of skin lesions than rapidly fibrose and can subsequently be associated with contractures and limb shortening. Systemic fibrosis of the lungs, liver, and heart can ensue and the condition is fatal in a proportion of cases. Cyclical gadolinium chelates, such as gadoteric acid, are thought to be of lower risk than the linear agents in patients with reduced renal function.

Dynamic contrast-enhanced MRI

Identification of malignant tissue is facilitated by the process of neovascularization, whereby cancers induce an angiogenic response. The rates of blood flow within tumours and surrounding tissues is altered in comparison to normal tissue and can be assessed by dynamic contrast-enhanced MRI (DCE-MRI). This involves the rapid acquisition of images following a bolus injection of gadolinium at different time points (e.g. 10–20 second intervals). The signal intensity can be plotted against time and by assessment of the gradient of the curve and time of onset of enhancement these findings can be matched to time-intensity curves. Specific features such as early enhancement and rapid washout are more strongly associated with malignant enhancement.

DCE-MRI has been used in breast cancer for the last decade and the technique is now gaining evidence for use in prostate cancer, improving sensitivity, and specificity in diagnosis.

Patient suitability for MRI

MRI safety is normally carried out by local MRI units but patients with pacemakers, ferromagnetic or electronically activated devices such as implantable cardiac defibrillators, ocular foreign bodies, cochlear implants, intracranial implants, shrapnel injury, or recent surgery/prostheses may be unsuitable for MRI. Up to 10% of patients experience a degree of claustrophobia and on occasion some patients refuse to proceed. More modern scanners have a wider bore and a shorter tunnel which make the experience more tolerable. All patients must wear earplugs or headphones while being scanned to mitigate any discomfort in view of noisy mechanical vibrations. Although there is no there is no specific evidence to the contrary, pregnant women in their first trimester are generally excluded from the MR scanner. Consultation with the MRI department if there are any concerns is essential.

MRI for kidneys and MR urography

Indications for MRI renal imaging

Renal MRI is generally used as a problem solving tool after initial renal investigations such as ultrasound or CT. Evaluation of the indeterminate renal lesion is the major indication. However, there are situations when this is used as the primary renal imaging modality, for example during pregnancy, in children, in patients on extended renal surveillance and those allergic to iodinated contrast media. This article will focus on MRI imaging as related to the renal parenchyma and collecting system. Renal arterial imaging, for example, for suspected renal artery disease or for pre-transplant donor work-up, will not be covered.

Technical aspects and specific MRI sequences

Motion artefact is a constant concern with renal imaging and fast imaging acquisition is necessary. Respiratory-gating or triggering may be necessary in some. Sequences will vary but at the least should include T1 and T2 weighted sequences in the axial and coronal planes, with some further post-contrast sequences. Each sequence can be uniquely informative. Most solid lesions are of low signal on T1. High T1 signal may be seen with haemorrhagic lesions, masses containing macroscopic fat or melanin, or cysts with highly proteinaceous content. T2 sequences are particularly useful for characterizing cysts and evaluation of hydronephrosis, as well as for better characterization of renal masses. T1 sequences acquired such that signal from fat is selectively suppressed; and can be used to confirm fat containing masses such as angiomyolipoma or retroperitoneal liposarcoma.

Post intravenous contrast studies can be timed for the arterial, nephrographic, or pyelographic phases. The arterial phase is useful for suspected renal artery stenosis and for vascular staging and planning of renal tumour surgery. The nephrographic phases are indispensable for the evaluation of renal masses, as the study of neo-vascularity is central for the radiological investigation of suspected renal malignancy. MR urographic phase is less commonly used compared to CT but has its place in the evaluation of hydronepherosis, especially during pregnancy and in childhood. Pyelographic images can be obtained without the use of contrast, as the T2 weighting of the scan be selectively boosted to the render the urine filled collecting system especially signal bright—so-called heavy T2 weighted scans, and this is especially useful scan in the pregnant woman with loin pain. Diffusion-weighted imaging has shown some promise regarding renal tumour grading.

Renal mass analysis and characterization

Evaluation of the content, morphology, and most importantly vascularity, the latter being a surrogate measure of the neo-vascularity in the case of malignancy, is central to the radiological assessment of renal masses.

(i) *Content*—the signal characteristics should differentiate a cyst from a solid mass, and the latter can be further characterized as fat containing or non-fatty. Broadly speaking, cysts are low T1, high T2; masses are low T1 and low T2, with fat containing masses being especially low signal on the fat-suppressed images. Non-fat-containing masses will not further change on fat-suppressed masses. There are exceptions. Hyperdense cysts will be high on T1 scans, as will haemorrhagic cysts; but in both cases will maintain their high T2 signal and this is used to differentiate them from renal tumours. Signal form blood products can also vary according to the time.

(ii) *Morphology*—this is used for characterization of complex cysts according to the Bosniak system, and is further discussed below.

(A)

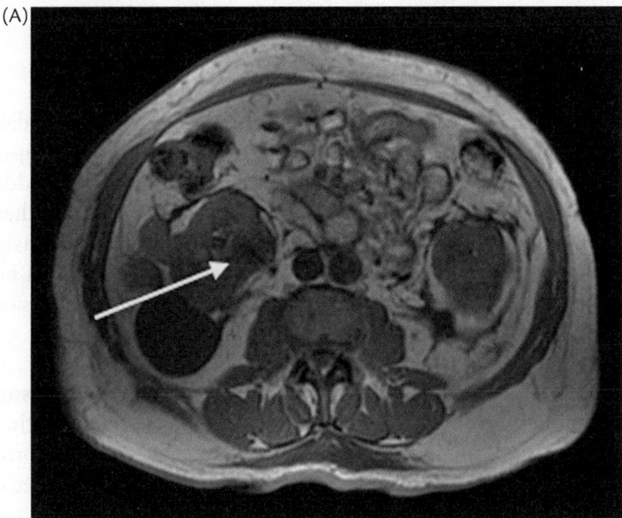

(B)

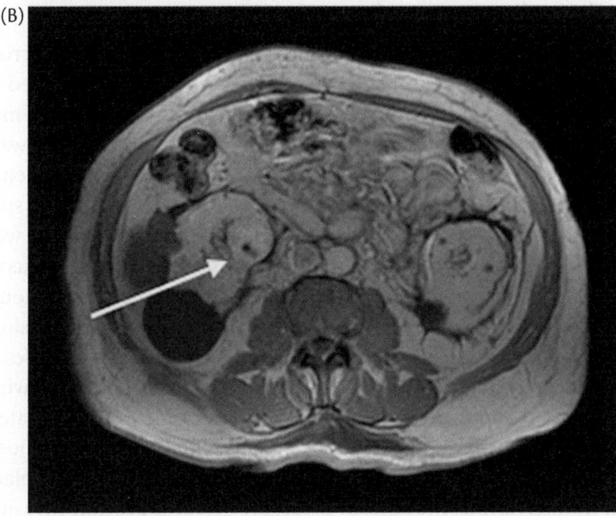

Fig. 10.4.2 Enhancing right mid-pole renal mass (white arrow) pre-contrast (A) and post-contrast axial T1-weighted images (B).

(iii) *Enhancement*—is the principal indicator of possible malignancy in a non-fat containing renal lesion (see Fig. 10.4.2). Unlike with CT, MRI does not easily allow quantitative measurement of enhancement as MR signals are not calibrated in the same way as CT attenuation values. The MR signal is dependent on multiple variables (e.g. tissue characteristics, the size of the patient, pulse sequence, gain setting of the MRI system, and the MRI coils used, none of which can be easily standardized). However, subjective assessment of enhancement in renal lesions has demonstrated accurate detection of renal cell carcinoma.[3,4] The pre-contrast images can be subtracted from the post-contrast images to produce a 'subtraction' series. This is excellent for determination of mass enhancement. The overall sensitivity of subtraction imaging was 99% for the diagnosis of a malignant lesion when compared to 95% using quantitative evaluation.[4] Caution must be applied with lesions that are T1 hyperintense on the pre-contrast scans, as this may obscure enhancement. Small lesions may also be difficult to assess accurately.[5]

MRI features to aid carcinoma subtyping

Clear cell carcinomas (80–90% of renal cell carcinomas) have been shown to demonstrate a greater degree of early enhancement on MRI (and CT).[6] Clear cell carcinomas are more likely to be necrotic (seen as moderate to high signal on T2 weighted images—indicator of the 'liquid' fraction due to necrosis) with lack of enhancement on post-contrast sequences in the necrotic regions. An irregular solid rim of enhancing tumour is often seen surrounding necrosis.

Fat content implies an angiomyolipoma, but very rarely fat can also be seen with clear cell carcinomas, either because the tumour has engulfed perinephric/sinus fat or secondary to metaplastic bone formation within malignant tissue. The presence of calcification may assist diagnosis as intralesional calcification is extremely rare in AML. A lesion with macroscopic fat content and calcification is therefore more suggestive of renal cell carcinoma. However, caution should be employed as there is no MRI signal from calcification, resulting in a signal void that may be easily overlooked. Other modalities such as ultrasound or CT should be reviewed.[7] Internal haemorrhage within the tumour can complicate appearances, seen as high T1 and T2 signal, but long-standing haemorrhage with haemosiderin deposition results in low T1 and T2 signal.

Papillary renal carcinomas account for up to 10–15% of renal cell carcinomas. Type 1 (basophilic) papillary tumours are associated with homogeneous low signal intensity on T2-weighted images and low-level enhancement, although can less commonly exhibit haemorrhage or necrosis. Type 2 (eosinophilic) papillary tumours tend to exhibit a more complex appearance with haemorrhage and necrosis and may demonstrate enhancing papillary projections at the periphery of the mass. A fibrous capsule (especially low T1 signal) can be associated with papillary renal carcinomas.

Cystic renal lesions

MRI is more sensitive than CT or ultrasound for the morphological evaluation of features such as the presence, thickness, and enhancement of septa; as well as wall or septal nodularity and soft tissue enhancement (see Fig. 10.4.3). In a comparative study, Bosniak

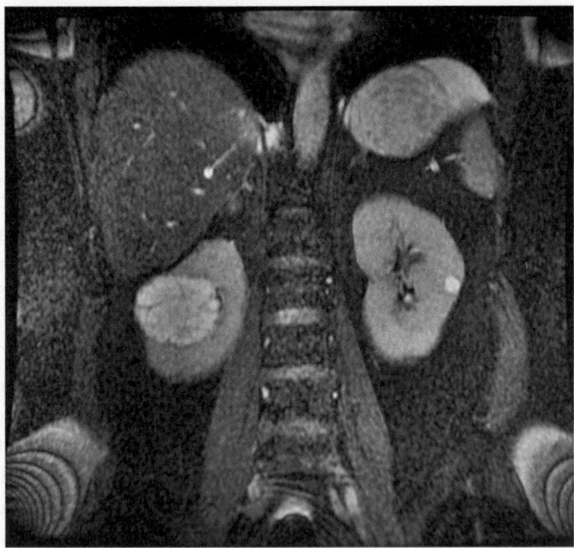

Fig. 10.4.3 Coronal FIESTA fat-saturated sequence demonstrating right complex renal cyst with multiple internal septations.

categorization on CT and MRI was similar in 81% of 69 complex cysts, but in the other 19%, MRI better demonstrated septa and enhancement, such that cysts were upstaged in 10% of cases.[8] MRI is especially suited for surveillance of complex cysts, as it is more accurate and of course safer.

MRI in staging of renal cell carcinoma

Staging by CT or MRI are of similar accuracy. Partial nephrectomy is increasingly performed for renal cell carcinoma (RCC) and by utilizing multiplanar reformats, maximal intensity projections can accurately portray the proximity of the tumour to the renal hilum or collecting system. The presence of a pseudocapsule, a hypointense rim on both T1 and T2 weighted images is detected with higher sensitivity on MRI than CT. The pseudocapsule is a rim of compressed renal and fibrous tissue and is a sign of lack of perinephric invasion and thereby a favourable indicator for partial nephrectomy.

Contrast-enhanced T1 weighted angiographic sequences will depict renal vein invasion (T3b disease) and the presence of tumour thrombus as a filling defect with high accuracy.[9] The cranial extent of tumour thrombus into the IVC (T3c disease) was better depicted on MRI than CT in some studies.[10] In the past, MRI was felt to be the modality of choice for the evaluation of venous invasion, but this advantage may no longer hold with the advent of multidetector, multiformat CT. The use of gadolinium contrast enhancement is also useful in differentiating tumour thrombus from bland thrombus, with enhancement of the thrombus indicating tumour thrombus.[11] MRI also has a role in detecting tumour invasion into the wall of the IVC (T3c disease) but accuracy is still to be fully evaluated.[3] It is possible that MRI is better than CT for the identification of bland thrombus and for evaluation of venous wall invasion but there are no comparative studies.

MR urography

This allows the visualization of the ureters and pelvicaliceal system. MR urography has a specific role in assessing painful hydronephrosis in pregnancy (see Fig. 10.4.4). There are two main techniques in acquiring MR urography:

(i) Heavily T2-weighted images (e.g. single shot fast spin echo—SSFSE) may clearly depict urine in the renal collecting system by virtue of the long T2 relaxation times.[12] Construction of a MIP (maximum intensity projection) results in an 'IVU' style image that readily illustrates the level of obstruction.

(ii) Contrast-enhanced T1 weighted delayed images can be used with delayed images obtained at five to eight minutes post injection. Many centres administer a diuretic, such as Furosemide, to dilute the contrast in the collecting system and enhance distension of the collecting system.

There are no established advantages of MR urography compared to CT urography, other than its relative safety, but it may better demonstrate periureteric oedema secondary to obstruction.[13] However, in MRI a ureteric filling defect appears as a non-specific signal void. The filling defect can be due to calculus or tumour, clot, gas, or sloughed papilla, and in this situation additional MR sequences or CT may be more specific.[12]

This highlights the significant disadvantage of MR. Compared to CT it is relative insensitivity to small calcified stones in the collecting system or ureters. Therefore in certain circumstances it may be prudent to obtain a plain radiograph or non-contrast CT to evaluate for nephrolithiasis.[13]

MRI of the bladder

Imaging of the urinary bladder is challenging and imaging modalities cannot displace direct cystoscopy for the evaluation of superficial tumours of the bladder. However, muscle invasive bladder cancer is difficult to visually assess and imaging has a role in these patients. CT urography has vastly facilitated the non-invasive assessment of the urothelial tract, including the bladder, but CT has limitations in differentiating depth of bladder wall muscle invasion.

Indications for bladder MRI

Common indications are to stage known bladder carcinoma, assess for bladder tumour recurrence, measure response to chemotherapy, to evaluate for secondary invasion from gynaecological, prostate, or rectal malignancy, and to assess congenital anomalies or anatomical variations

Technical aspects and specific MRI sequences

A moderately full bladder is optimal. A compression band across the abdomen and administration of antispasmodics can be used to minimize respiratory and peristaltic artefacts. Thin slices (4–5 mm thickness or less) are used for better definition of the bladder wall. Sequences will vary but usually include a T1 weighted axial sequence of the pelvis for nodal analysis and T1 and T2 weighted fast spin echo sequences in two planes (axial and coronal) for bladder wall analysis and tumour localization. An additional T2 weighted axial sequence taken in an oblique plane perpendicular to the tumour-bladder wall interface is helpful for analysis of muscle invasion. Post-contrast studies are not routine, but T1 weighted sequences at 20 seconds (arterial) and 70–115 seconds (venous phase) following gadolinium administration, with delayed images (at approximately five minutes) are of help—in particular, sagittal and coronal post-contrast sequences aid visualization of the bladder dome and bladder neck invasion. The latter is especially useful as prostate invasion will upstage the tumour. Diffusion-weighted imaging may also be used but its role has not been clearly established.

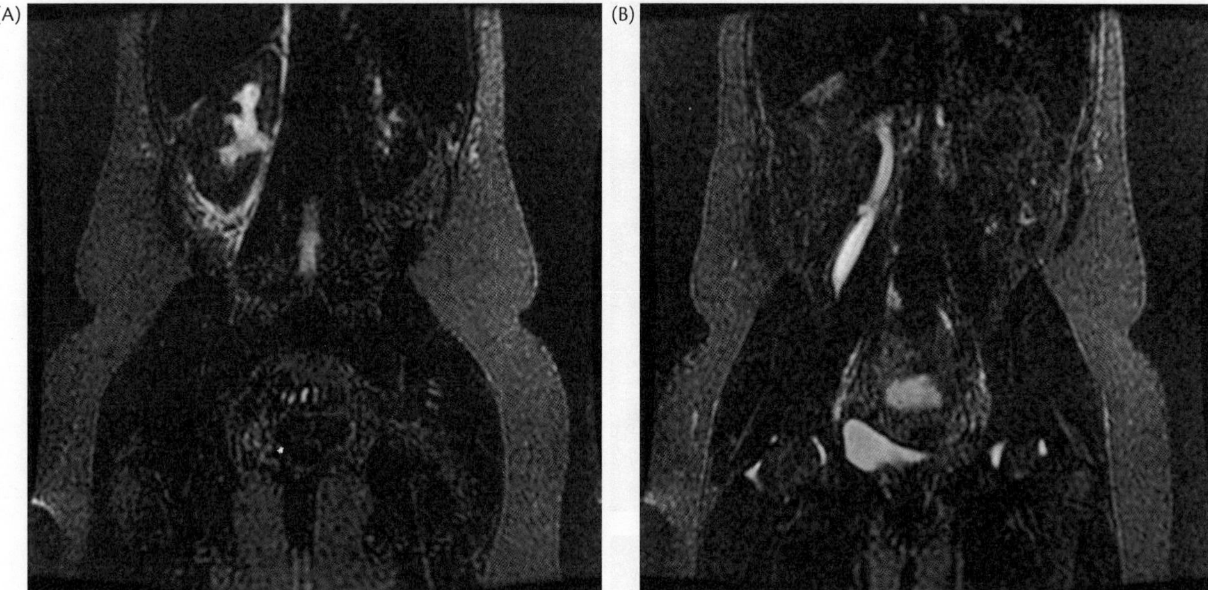

Fig. 10.4.4 MR urography performed in a 28-week gravid female with persistent right loin pain and hydronephrosis on ultrasound. (A) Right perinephric oedema suggest concomitant pyelonephritis. (B) The dilated right ureter tapers due to compression by the gravid uterus with no calculus present.

Signal characteristics of the normal bladder and tumour

The normal bladder wall is of low signal intensity on T1 and T2 weighted images. Normally there is a smooth contour between the low signal of bladder outer wall and high signal of the perivesical fat (unless fat-saturation has been used).[14] Urine is of especially high signal on T2 weighted images (Fig. 10.4.5, Fig. 10.4.5A). Signal characteristics of bladder tumour and bladder wall are variable. On T1-weighted images the tumour is of similar intensity to bladder wall, Higher signal than urine (urine is dark on T1 weighted images) but of lower signal than perivesical fat (Fig. 10.4.5B). On T2-weighted images the tumour is of intermediate to high signal intensity and of higher signal than bladder wall and muscle but lower signal than urine (on T2 weighted images, urine is high signal). On DWI studies, the tumour is of high signal but of restricted diffusion on the ADC maps (Figure 10.4.5C and 10.4.5D).

Staging local invasion (T stage)

The TNM staging classification is most widely used for this and is detailed in Section 6.

Analysing bladder MRI

Use the contrast-enhanced fat-saturated T1 weighted images in combination with T2w images to assess muscle invasion. Contrast administration especially aids differentiation between T2a and T2b tumours (superficial versus deep muscle invasion) and T3b tumours (extension through the bladder wall).[15] Tumour enhances much earlier than the bladder wall due to neovascularization. The normal bladder wall does not enhance significantly on the early enhanced images and in the arterial phase (20 seconds) bladder tumours enhance more than the adjacent bladder wall.[16] The bladder wall enhances later at about 60–90 seconds. On these early phase images, urine will remain low intensity on T1 but on delayed images (at five minutes) the urine within the bladder will become of high intensity.[17] The detrusor muscle is a low intensity line on T2w imaging and this line is interrupted in the presence muscle invasive disease.

Microscopic perivesical disease (T3a disease) cannot be reliably detected using MRI (or CT for that matter). Differentiation is especially challenging soon after deep bladder biopsies, in which case the perivesical planes will be ill-defined. A delay of 4 weeks after biopsy is recommended. A measurable extravesical mass designates T3b disease and invasion of the tumour into surrounding structures such as the uterus, vagina, prostate, or seminal vesicles further upstages it. Staging accuracy is reported as variable even using MRI with contrast and ranged between 52–93% although many studies are no longer contemporary.[16,18–20] Overall accuracy has been reported up to 92% when using T2 weighted, contrast-enhanced T1 and diffusion-weighted sequences, in combination.[21] The contribution of DWI has not yet been clearly defined.

Caveats regarding MRI of the bladder

It is very difficult to differentiate T2a (superficial muscle) from T2b (deep muscle) disease. Overstaging is a common pitfall in evaluating local extent of bladder malignancy due to the presence of post-biopsy inflammation, granulation tissue, and fibrosis which can be mistaken for invasion. Under or overdistension of the bladder can lead to misinterpretation of bladder wall muscle invasion. Small tumours may be undetected; and flat or sessile tumours may also be missed. Delayed contrast-enhanced images can result in gadolinium-enhanced urine layering within the bladder and obscuring small bladder lesions.[14]

Nodal disease

It is essential to review the images for enlarged perivesical, pelvic side wall or distant/para-aortic lymph nodes. Nodal staging is detailed in Section 6. The most common site for regional lymph node spread is to the obturator nodes.[17]

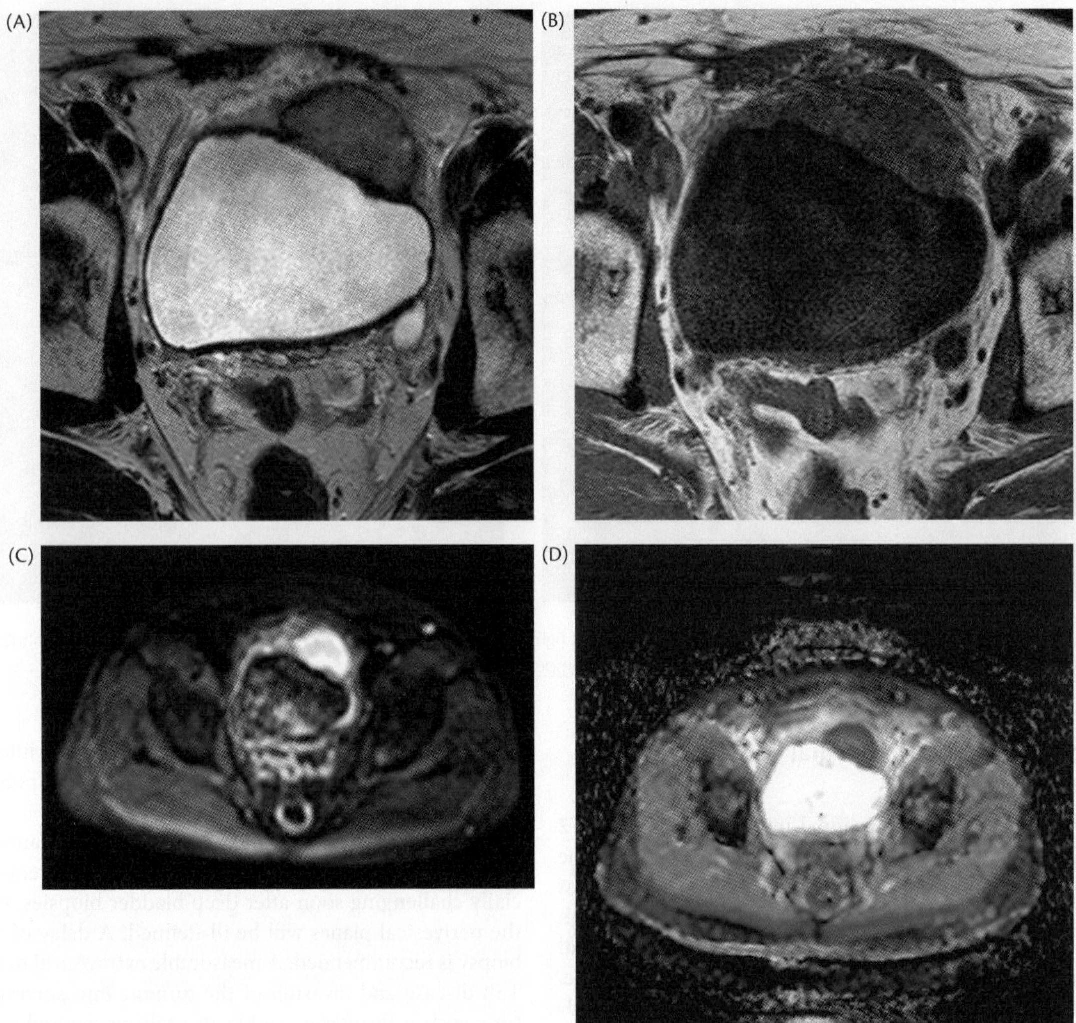

Fig. 10.4.5 (A) Axial T2 weighted image of low signal anterior bladder tumour (note the urine in the bladder is high signal on T2). (B) Axial T1 weighted image demonstrating the bladder tumour as a low signal lesion. (C) Axial diffusion-weighted image (DWI) of low signal anterior bladder tumour. High signal within the lesion confirms restricted diffusion. (D) The ADC map (apparent diffusion coefficient) confirms true restricted diffusion with low signal corresponding to the mass.

Detection of involved lymph nodes in transitional cell carcinoma (TCC) is challenging as measuring by size criteria (10mm short axis if ovoid and 8mm if round morphology) is not 100% reliable. Metastatic TCC can be present in normal-sized lymph nodes and both CT and MRI carry a false-negative rate. In addition, lymph node metastases may enhance to the same degree as the primary tumour and this may cause difficulty in discrimination from adjacent blood vessels. Round lymph nodes of the same signal as the bladder tumour are more likely to be malignant. Better results have been reported using intravenous administration of ultra-small iron-oxide particles (USPIO or ferrumoxtran-10) to detect early nodal metastases in both bladder and prostate cancer. This technique uses gradient-echo (T2*) imaging to detect susceptibility artefact within normal lymph nodes (i.e. they appear darker, almost black) with no effect on malignant nodes.[22]

MRI of the prostate

Indications for prostate MRI

Prostatitis, benign prostatic hyperplasia (BPH), and prostate abscess are better evaluated with ultrasound, as is suspected abnormalities of the ejaculatory ducts or seminal vesicles. The main indication for prostate MRI is for the staging of prostate cancer. Thus far MRI has been used in the staging of biopsy confirmed prostate cancer and to detect locoregional recurrence after definitive treatment for prostate cancer. Emerging indications are for the pre-biopsy risk stratification of the man with an elevated prostate-specific antigen (PSA), its use when prostate cancer is suspected despite negative biopsy, as part of an active surveillance policy and to assist in the selection and monitoring of focal ablative treatments. These emerging indications are not yet of proven value, but much research is active in this area.

Technical aspects and specific MRI sequences

MRI prostate should ideally be delayed for four to six weeks after prostate biopsy to prevent false positive diagnoses due to post-biopsy inflammation or haemorrhage. Studies have demonstrated a significant decrease in post-biopsy haemorrhage on MRI after six to eight weeks,[23] but other studies have shown that it can persist for up to four months.

Sequences will vary but usually include a T1w axial study of the pelvis for staging of nodes, local tumour invasion, and pelvic bone metastasis, followed by high definition focused T1 and T2w studies of the prostate gland and seminal vesicles. Ideally the T2w sequences should be in three orthogonal planes (axial, sagittal, coronal; but at the least axial and coronal). Diffusion-weighted imaging (with an ADC map) has been proven to aid tumour localization; but the value of MR spectroscopy or dynamic contrast-enhanced MRI is still debated. Nevertheless, the most recent published recommendations advocate the use of at least DWI—so-called multiparametric MRI of the prostate gland.

Normal anatomy

The zonal anatomy of the prostate is key to MRI interpretation. On T1-weighted imaging the normal prostate, seminal vesicles, and periprostatic veins are of uniform intermediate signal and the zonal anatomy cannot be distinguished. On T2 weighted imaging, the peripheral zone is of homogeneous high signal intensity, with a thin low signal rim of the prostate capsule, and the anterior (or inner) gland is of lower and heterogeneous signal comprising the inseparable central and transition zones. With increasing age and the development of BPH, the transition zone becomes even more heterogeneous with distinct, well-defined mixed signal adenomas, increases in size, and compresses the peripheral zone into a thin stripe. On T2-weighted images the seminal vesicles have a high signal multilocular cystic structure with thin low intensity walls. The lumen is clearly identifiable. The anterior fibromuscular stroma is of especial low intensity on both T1 and T2 weighted imaging. The neurovascular bundles pass posterolateral to the capsule at the 5 and 7 o'clock positions. At the apex and the base there are vessels penetrating the capsule and these are an important location to assess for extracapsular spread.[24,25]

The prostate can be divided into sextants in a similar fashion to transrectal ultrasound. Division in the craniocaudal plane into base, mid-gland, and apex and then a vertical division into left and right sides is the most common nomenclature; but more complex patterns have been described.

Imaging of prostate cancer and how to stage

Most prostate cancers arise from the peripheral zone and are of low signal on T2 weighted imaging. Post-biopsy haemorrhage is also of low signal on T2 weighted images, but can be differentiated by the presence of high signal on T1 weighted images (see Fig. 10.4.6).

On the DWI sequences, the tumour may of high signal on the long b-value DWI series and of low signal, in keeping with restricted diffusion, on the ADC maps. On the dynamic post-contrast series, cancer is seen as an area of early avid vascularity with rapid washout. Tumours arising in the anterior gland are not easily distinguishable from coexistent BPH and adenomas, but the commonest recognizable pattern is as a low signal, crescentic area, so-called brush stroke appearance. DWI and post-contrast studies are less helpful in the anterior gland. TNM or Jewett-Whitmore Staging systems can be used but TNM staging is most widely used (please see https://cancerstaging.org for further information of TNM staging).

Staging accuracy of prostate cancer

It is difficult to quote a precise staging accuracy as there is considerable diversity in reported sensitivity and specificity. Accuracy values for staging vary between approximately 55% to in excess 90% with standard techniques using pelvic coils. Techniques can vary with some centres using endorectal coils (ERC) and the advent of diffusion-weighted imaging and dynamic contrast enhanced techniques which are improving accuracy. There has been ongoing discussion regarding the value of endorectal coils (ERC) versus pelvic phased array (PPA) coils. Previously authors have stated that significant artefacts relating to endorectal coils can result in image degradation and non-diagnostic studies Experience with ERC coils has

(A)

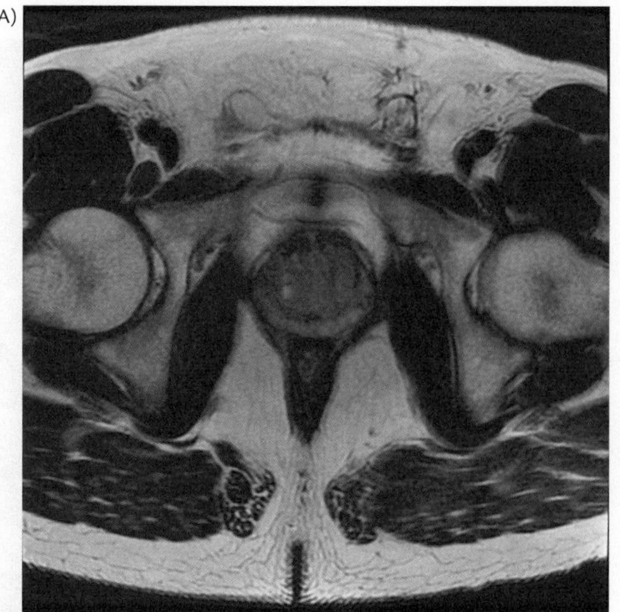

(B)

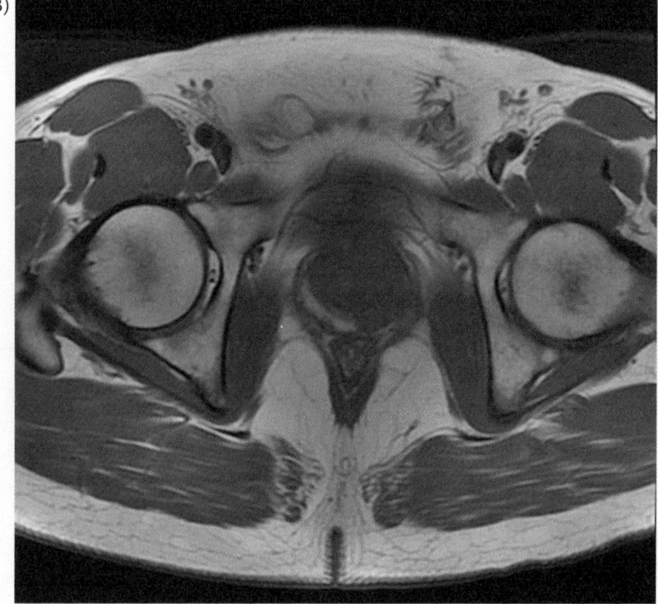

Fig. 10.4.6 (A) Axial T2MRI demonstrates intermediate to low signal change in the right peripheral zone at the 6 to 8 o'clock positions. (B) Axial T1 sequence in the same patient as (A) demonstrates high T1 signal in the corresponding 6 to 8 o'clock position confirming post-biopsy haemorrhage rather than tumour infiltration. The patient was recalled for repeat interval imaging.

reduced such artefacts, but parallel improvements of PPA coils and the advent of 3T magnets has also improved pelvic coil imaging.

Multiple studies in the last decade have reported a wide range of sensitivities and specificities (approximately between 49–97%) for the detection of extracapsular extension and seminal vesicle invasion.[26,27] In an MRI imaging/pathological correlation study using endorectal coils at 1.5 Tesla, a high overall specificity of 95% was reported, but the sensitivity of MR imaging was more limited for detection of occult T3 tumour.[28] Studies using 3T MRI have quoted accuracy of 94%, sensitivity of 88% and specificity of 96%. With high levels of radiological experience and new technologies, staging accuracy can be considered of a high standard.[29–31] However, these studies are form expert centres with experiences readers. The true accuracy of MRI in routine practice is still not thoroughly defined.

What to look for

Correlation with clinical findings (DRE, PSA level, family history, and so on) is essential. Review the T1w sequences for high signal within the prostate gland which may represent post-biopsy haemorrhage. Look closely at the peripheral zone on the T2-weighted images and identify areas of focal low signal which may reflect tumour. Correlate with the T1-weighted sequences to ensure these are not due to haemorrhage. Assess whether there is unilateral or bilateral tumour involvement. If available, review the diffusion-weighted images. Areas of tumour may be of high signal on DWI, however it is vital to look at the ADC map (apparent diffusion coefficient) as lesions with true restricted diffusion (i.e. tumour) will demonstrate a corresponding low signal on the ADC map. Signs of extracapsular invasion include[25] capsular breach, obliteration of the rectoprostatic angle, asymmetry of the neurovascular bundle, tumour encasement of the neurovascular bundle, asymmetric prostate capsular bulge with irregular margins or low signal or enlargement of the seminal vesicle (see Fig. 10.4.7 and Fig. 10.4.8).

Look at the adjacent rectum, bladder neck, and other pelvic structures for evidence of invasion into adjacent structures. Review the wider field of view T1 and T2 weighted images for any obturator, pelvic, iliac, or para-aortic lymphadenopathy. Look at the bony pelvis, femora, and visualized vertebrae for any evidence of bony metastatic disease. Bone metastases most often are low signal on both T1 and T2 weighted images.

There are some caveats to the diagnosis and staging of prostate cancer on MRI

Background prostatitis can result in an intermediate low T2w signal in the peripheral zone, and this can closely mimic cancer. DWI images should help as tumour is of restricted diffusion, but some restriction may also be seen with inflammation. This is a particular issue with differentiating low grade (Gleason 6 or less) tumour from inflammation. Furthermore, inflammation will also be of increased vascularity. Florid BPH changes can cause significant heterogeneity within the central and transition zones leading to difficulty in identifying tumour in these locations. Small anterior gland tumours are especially challenging, as some adenomas can be of homogenous, low T2 signal, and indistinguishable from cancer. Under or overstaging of extracapsular spread also occurs, and post-biopsy artefact is the usual culprit with the latter. All these issues are being extensively explored and further refinements can be expected.

Other MRI techniques

3T MRI and dynamic contrast-enhanced MRI prostate

These have already been alluded to above. 3T improves the signal to noise ratio with higher resolution T2W studies. Dynamic contrast enhanced MRI sequences can improve tumour detection and visualization of capsular penetration. This involves real-time analysis of increasing enhancement following intravenous gadolinium administration.

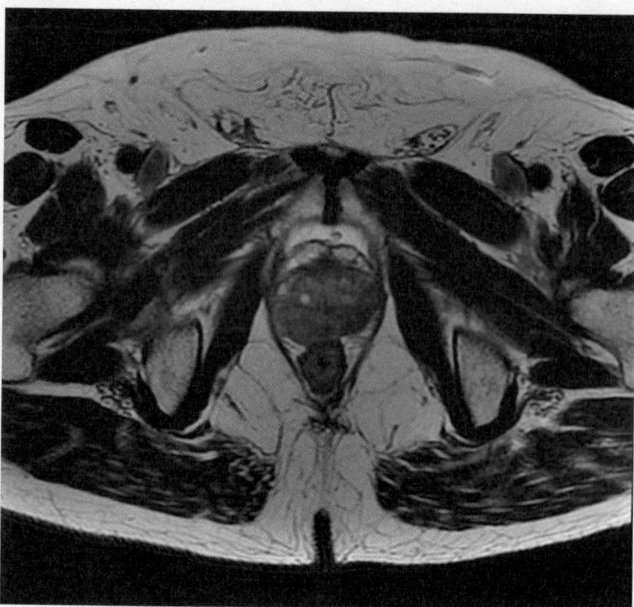

Fig. 10.4.7 Axial high resolution T2 weighted image. Asymmetric prostatic capsular bulge and obliteration of the rectoprostatic angle consistent with right peripheral zone extracapsular invasion (T3A staging).

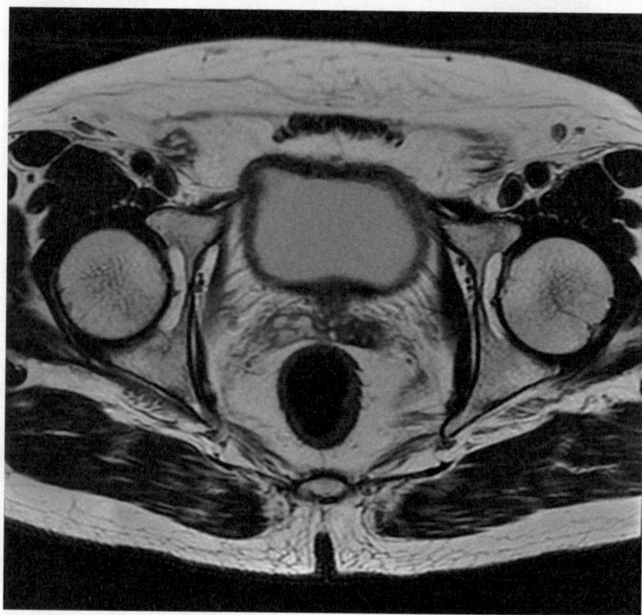

Fig. 10.4.8 Axial high resolution T2 weighted image. Low signal change within the medial left seminal vesicles indicates tumour invasion (T3B disease).

Tumours demonstrate more rapid washout of contrast than normal tissue due to malignant angiogenesis. Time-enhancement curves can be used to plot the contrast enhancement within a specified 'region-of-interest' to identify curves more specific for malignancy.

Overall the technique has not yet gained universal favour. A study evaluating the combination of T2-weighted imaging, DCE-MRI and DWI for the detection and localization of prostate cancer has assessed these techniques in combination also termed multiparametric MRI.[32] For peripheral zone tumours sensitivity of 80% and specificity of 97% (95% CI of 93–99%) was achieved for tumour identification to a given quadrant. For transitional zone tumours, T2 weighted imaging alone demonstrated sensitivity of 71% and specificity of 98% which was identical to that achieved using T2w and DWI in combination.

MR spectroscopy in prostate cancer

MR spectroscopy (MRS) is a functional study and assesses the concentration of specific metabolites. In prostate cancer three metabolites—citrate, creatine, and choline—are measured. Tumours have higher choline and lower citrate levels compared to normal tissue and BPH. MRS may assist in identifying cancers, especially within the transition zone, but the experience so far has been mixed.[33,34] It is used in only in some centres.

Problem solving with MRI

Testicular pathology

Although ultrasound is the most commonly used modality for the investigation of scrotal pathology, MRI can be a helpful adjunct in certain circumstances such as characterization of spermatic cord and extratesticular masses such as spermatic cord lipomas, haematomas, sarcomas, and fibrous pseudotumours. The added information provided by MRI may allow for a more conservative approach to patient management by accurate demonstration of the presence of a haematoma or fatty tissue.

The multiplanar capabilities, large field of view and lack of ionizing radiation make MRI the next best investigation after ultrasound for the localization of impalpable, undescended testes. Coronal sequences allow for the demonstration of the gubernaculum testes and spermatic cord which can be traced to the scrotum, while the pelvis and retroperitoneum can also be interrogated for ectopic testes. The addition of diffusion-weighted sequences can increase the sensitivity of the study as normal testicular tissue returns intense high signal against adjacent tissues.

Penile and urethral pathology

Once again a combination of clinical assessment and ultrasound are used in the vast majority of patients with penile pathology. However in selected patients with a history of trauma, MRI can help demonstrate subtle penile fractures given this modality's high sensitivity for the demonstration of haemorrhage and detection of tunical disruption (see Fig. 10.4.9). MRI may also demonstrate supplementary information not readily assessed on any other modalities, such as cavernosal avulsion from the ischium or damage to the suspensory ligaments. There may be some role in patients with priapism. Cavernosal ischaemia due to low flow priapism can be visualized on post-contrast MRI sequences and help assess the likelihood of recovery. With high flow priapism, the culprit fistula may be seen. Although there is no defined role for MRI in the staging of penile cancers, depth of invasion may be more accurately assessed using a combination of pre and post-contrast imaging to aid surgical planning. Meanwhile in women, MR imaging can elegantly delineate urethral diverticula, clearly differentiating these from other periurethral and perivaginal cysts.

(A)

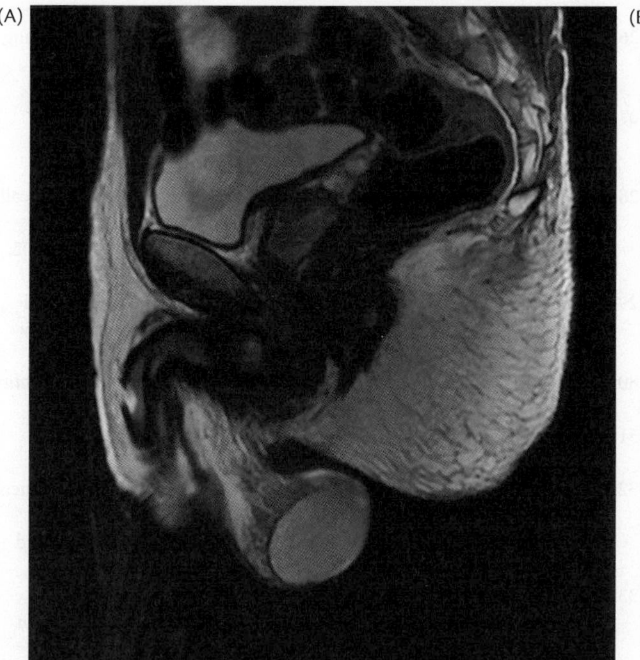

(B)

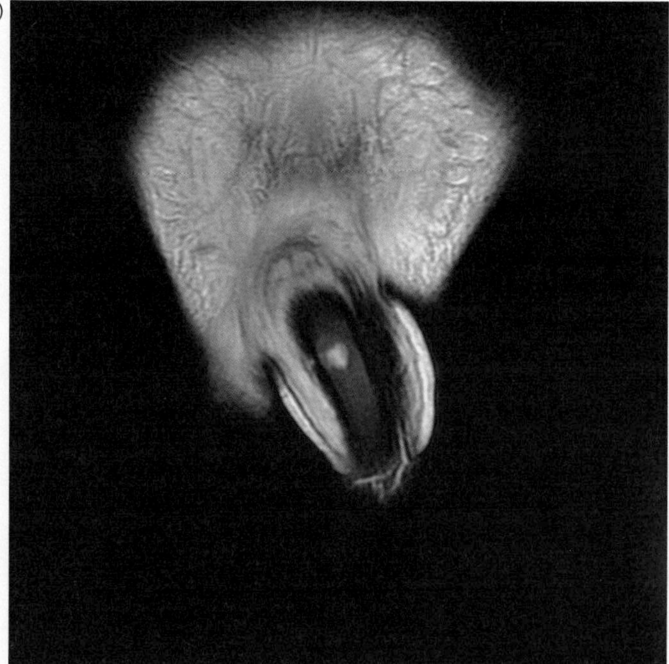

Fig. 10.4.9 (A) Sagittal T2 weighted MRI penis demonstrates small defect in the dorsolateral wall of the right corpus cavernosum diagnosing penile fracture. (B) Also demonstrates the penile fracture in coronal plane.

Chronic pelvic pain

This enigmatic and common condition, whereby pain is perceived in structures within the pelvis, can be difficult to manage but MRI of the pelvis and sacrum can be of use in excluding pathologies with more specific management options such as sacral spinal cord disease, perianal fistula, and endometriosis.

Further reading

Barentsz JO, Richenberg J, Clements R, *et al.* ESUR prostate MR guidelines 2012. *Eur Radiol* 2012; **22**(4):746–57.

Bonekamp D, Jacobs MA, El-Khouli R, Stoianovici D, Macura KJ. Advancements in MR imaging of the prostate: from diagnosis to interventions. *Radiographics* 2011; **31**(3):677–703.

Fütterer JJ. MR imaging in local staging of prostate cancer. *Eur J Radiol* 2007; **63**(3):328–34.

Hoeks CM, Barentsz JO, Hambrock T, *et al.* Prostate cancer: multiparametric MR imaging for detection, localization, and staging. *Radiology* 2011; **261**(1):46–66.

Kang SK, Kim D, Chandarana H. Contemporary imaging of the renal mass. *Curr Urol Rep* 2011; **12**(1):11–7.

Nikken JJ, Krestin GP. MRI of the kidney-state of the art. *Eur Radiol* 2007; **17**(11):2780–93.

Tekes A, Kamel I, Imam K, *et al.* Dynamic MRI of bladder cancer: evaluation of staging accuracy. *AJR Am J Roentgenol* 2005; **184**(1):121–7.

Verma S, Rajesh A, Prasad SR, *et al.* Urinary bladder cancer: Role of MR imaging. *Radiographics* 2012; **32**(2):371–87.

Verma S, Rajesh A. A clinically relevant approach to imaging prostate cancer: review. *AJR Am J Roentgenol* 2011; **196**(Suppl 3):S1–10.

Westbrook C. *MRI at a Glance*. Chichester, UK: Wiley-Blackwell Publishing, 2002.

References

1. RCR guidelines—Nephrogenic Systemic Fibrosis. Available at: https://www.rcr.ac.uk/system/files/publication/field_publication_files/BFCR0714_Gadolinium_NSF_guidanceNov07.pdf [Online].
2. ESUR guidelines—Nephrogenic Systemic Fibrosis. Available at: http://www.esur.org/guidelines/ [Online].
3. Ho VB, Choyke PL. MR evaluation of solid renal masses. *Magn Reson Imaging Clin N Am* 2004; **12**(3):413–27.
4. Hecht EM, Israel GM, Krinsky GA, *et al.* Renal masses: quantitative analysis of enhancement with signal intensity measurements versus qualitative analysis of enhancement with image subtraction for diagnosing malignancy at MR imaging. *Radiology* 2004; **232**(2):373–8.
5. Kang SK, Kim D, Chandarana H. Contemporary imaging of the renal mass. *Curr Urol Rep* 2011; **12**(1):11–7.
6. Sun MR, Ngo L, Genega EM, *et al.* Renal cell carcinoma: dynamic contrast-enhanced MR imaging for differentiation of tumor subtypes—correlation with pathologic findings. *Radiology* 2009, **250**:793–802.
7. Nikken JJ, Krestin GP. MRI of the kidney-state of the art. *Eur Radiol* 2007; **17**(11):2780–93.
8. Israel GM, Hindman N, Bosniak MA. Evaluation of cystic renal masses: comparison of CT and MR imaging by using the Bosniak classification system. *Radiology* 2004, **231**:365–71.
9. Choyke PL, Walther MM, Wagner JR, *et al.* Renal cancer: preoperative evaluation with dual phase three-dimensional MR angiography. *Radiology* 1997; **205**:767–71.
10. Hallscheidt PJ, Bock M, Riedasch G, *et al.* Diagnostic accuracy of staging renal cell carcinomas using multidetector-row computed tomography and magnetic resonance imaging: a prospective study with histopathologic correlation. *J Comput Assist Tomogr* 2004; **28**:333–9.
11. Laissy JP, Menegazzo D, Debray MP, *et al.* Renal carcinoma: diagnosis of venous invasion with Gd-enhanced MR venography. *Eur Radiol* 2000; **10**:1138–43.
12. Kawashima A, Glockner JF, King BF Jr. CT urography and MR urography. *Radiol Clin North Am* 2003; **41**:945–61.
13. Regan F, Kuszyk B, Bohlman ME, Jackman S. Acute ureteric calculus obstruction: unenhanced spiral CT versus HASTE MR urography and abdominal radiograph. *Br J Radiol* 2005; **78**:506–11.
14. Rockall A. Bladder tumors: The role of MRI in staging and treatment planning. Proc Intl Soc Mag Reson Med 2011; **19**.
15. Hamm B, Forstner R, Beinder E, Baert FRW. *MRI and CT of the Female Pelvis*. Berlin, Germany: Springer, 2007.
16. Tekes A, Kamel I, Imam K, *et al.* Dynamic MRI of bladder cancer: evaluation of staging accuracy. *AJR Am J Roentgenol* 2005; **184**(1):121–7.
17. Verma S, Rajesh A, Prasad SR, *et al.* Urinary bladder cancer: Role of MR imaging. *Radiographics* 2012; **32**(2):371–87.
18. Kim B, Semelka RC, Ascher SM, Chalpin DB, Carroll PR, Hricak H. Bladder tumor staging: comparison of contrast-enhanced CT, T1- and T2-weighted MR imaging, dynamic gadolinium-enhanced imaging, and late gadolinium-enhanced imaging. *Radiology* 1994; **193**(1):239–45.
19. Narumi Y, Kadota T, Inoue E, *et al.* Bladder tumors: staging with gadolinium-enhanced oblique MR imaging. *Radiology* 1993; **187**(1):145–50.
20. Tanimoto A, Yuasa Y, Imai Y, *et al.* Bladder tumor staging: comparison of conventional and gadolinium-enhanced dynamic MR imaging and CT. *Radiology* 1992; **185**(3):741–7.
21. Takeuchi M, Sasaki S, Ito M, *et al.* Urinary bladder cancer: diffusion-weighted MR imaging—accuracy for diagnosing T stage and estimating histologic grade. *Radiology* 2009; **251**(1):112–21.
22. Deserno WM, Harisinghani MG. Taupitz M, Jager GJ, Witjes JA, Mulders PF. Urinary bladder cancer: preoperative nodal staging with ferumoxtran-10-enhanced MR imaging. *Radiology* 2004; **233**:449–56.
23. Kim CK, Park BK, Kim B. Diffusion-weighted MRI at 3 T for the evaluation of prostate cancer. *AJR Am J Roentgenol* 2010; **194**(6):1461–9.
24. Heenan SD, Magnetic resonance imaging in prostate cancer. *Prostate Cancer Prostatic Dis* 2004; **7**(4):282–8.
25. Verma S, Rajesh A. A clinically relevant approach to imaging prostate cancer: review. *AJR Am J Roentgenol* 2011; **196**(3 Suppl): S1–10.
26. Hricak H, Choyke PL, Eberhardt SC, Leibel SA, Scardino PT. Imaging prostate cancer: a multidisciplinary perspective. *Radiology* 2007; **243**(1):28–53.
27. Bonekamp D, Jacobs MA, El-Khouli R, Stoianovici D, Macura KJ. Advancements in MR imaging of the prostate: from diagnosis to interventions. *Radiographics* 2011; **31**(3):677–703.
28. Cornud F, Flam T, Chauveinc L, *et al.* Extraprostatic spread of clinically localized prostate cancer: factors predictive of pT3 tumor and of positive endorectal MR imaging examination results. *Radiology* 2002; **224**(1):203–10.
29. Fütterer JJ, Heijmink SW, Scheenen TW, *et al.* Prostate cancer: local staging at 3-T endorectal MR imaging—early experience. *Radiology* 2006; **238**(1):184–91.
30. Fütterer JJ. MR imaging in local staging of prostate cancer. *Eur J Radiol* 2007; **63**(3):328–34.
31. Barentsz JO, Richenberg J, Clements R, *et al.* ESUR prostate MR guidelines 2012. *Eur Radiol* 2012; **22**(4):746–57.
32. Delongchamps NB, Rouanne M, Flam T, *et al.* Multiparametric magnetic resonance imaging for the detection and localization of prostate cancer: combination of T2-weighted, dynamic contrast-enhanced and diffusion-weighted imaging. *BJU Int* 2011; **107**(9):1411–8.
33. Mazaheri Y, Shukla-Dave A, Muellner A, Hricak H. MRI of the prostate: clinical relevance and emerging applications. *J Magn Reson Imaging* 2011; **33**(2):258–74.
34. Hoeks CM, Barentsz JO, Hambrock T, *et al.* Prostate cancer: multiparametric MR imaging for detection, localization, and staging. *Radiology* 2011; **261**(1):46–66.

CHAPTER 10.5

Interventional radiology

Steven Kennish

Introduction to interventional radiology

Although imaging technology and interventional techniques are being constantly improved and refined, the basic foundation procedure for interventional uroradiology; the percutaneous insertion of a nephrostomy drain, remains the most commonly performed intervention.

Natural extensions of this technique include both percutaneous stone removal and antegrade ureteric stenting. The urological surgeon must have a complete grasp of what these fundamental procedures entail, their indications, the techniques involved in performing them, and the recognized limitations and complications. The most commonly requested uroradiological interventions are given appropriate emphasis in the following pages.

Percutaneous nephrostomy

Introduction

Radiologically guided percutaneous drainage of the kidney has become a basic tenet for the management of renal tract obstruction, having been first described in 1955.[1]

Indications

Indications vary slightly depending on local expertise and preferences, but the main reasons for inserting a percutaneous nephrostomy (PCN) are detailed in Box 10.5.1.

Renal tract obstruction may be congenital, developmental, stone related, malignant, or iatrogenic. Chronic obstruction may present acutely if secondary infection develops.

An acutely obstructed kidney suffers ischaemic damage and a PCN is a quick and effective method of decompressing the collecting system, draining infected urine, and relieving pressure on the renal functional units.[2,3] Often the decision to proceed to PCN is made before the exact cause of obstruction has been diagnosed.

There is little evidence to indicate that a PCN is superior to a retrograde stent as the primary treatment for an infected obstructed collecting system, although it does avoid a general anaesthetic and ureteric manipulation.[4]

Box 10.5.1 Percutaneous nephrostomy (PCN) indications

- Relief of ureteric obstruction
- Drainage of infected urine
- Pain relief in ureteric colic
- Urinary diversion to facilitate the healing of leaks or fistulae
- Prerequisite to percutaneous renal tract surgery

The timing of PCN insertion should be commensurate with the patient's clinical status. Bilateral renal obstruction, obstruction of a single functioning kidney, systemic features of sepsis, or refractory hyperkalaemia necessitate an urgent PCN.

Malignant ureteric obstruction can be caused by infiltrative primary tumour, nodal enlargement, or other metastatic disease. PCN drainage of the kidneys has a dual role, preserving nephrons and preventing urosepsis, allowing for nephrotoxic and immunosuppressive chemotherapy where appropriate.

Iatrogenic ureteric occlusion or injury is an infrequent complication of major laparoscopic surgery.[5] Percutaneous urinary diversion allows healing of a leak at a site of injury, or a defective ureteroileal anastomosis. Fistulating disease within the pelvis, incontinence and irritative bladder symptoms post radiotherapy are also recognized indications for urinary diversion necessitating bilateral PCN insertion.

Techniques

PCN insertion techniques are very much tailored by individual radiologists. The basic principles of the procedure are outlined in Box 10.5.2.

The risks quoted for haemorrhage, infection and procedural failure should be based on individual operator audit data (see Table 10.5.1). Pre-procedural analgesia is recommended, and the

Box 10.5.2 Principles of percutaneous nephrostomy technique

Insertion of PCN

1. Aseptic skin preparation and draping
2. Infiltration of local anaesthetic down to the renal capsule
3. Ultrasound guided puncture of a target calyx
4. Aspiration of urine
5. Careful contrast administration under fluoroscopy guidance
6. Guidewire placement through the puncture sheath in to the pelvicalyceal system
7. Dilatation of a percutaneous track
8. PCN drain insertion and deployment in the pelvicalyceal system
9. Fixation of the PCN drain with dressings and connection to a drainage bag

Table 10.5.1 Complication rates associated with percutaneous nephrostomy (PCN) insertion

Complication	Rate
Haemorrhage	<4%
Urosepsis	<4%
Renal pelvic injury	<1%
PCN dislodgement	<15%

Source: data from Wah TM *et al.*, 'Percutaneous nephrostomy insertion: outcome data from a prospective multi-operator study at a UK training centre', *Clinical Radiology*, Volume 59, Issue 3, pp. 255–261, Copyright © 2004 The Royal College of Radiologists; and Lewis S *et al.*, 'Major complications after percutaneous nephrostomy—lessons from a department audit', *Clinical Radiology*, Volume 59, Issue 2, pp. 171–79, Copyright © 2004 The Royal College of Radiologists.

patient's coagulation profile should be normal. Antibiotics are administered if there is a clinical suspicion of infection or there are risk factors such as stone disease, recent instrumentation, or an indwelling foreign body.

Traditionally PCN insertion has been fluoroscopically guided and performed in the prone position, but ultrasound allows for safe supine/oblique PCN insertion. Supine positions are expedient for pregnant women and those patients with painful anterior abdominal wounds, stomas, spinal injuries, and tracheostomy tubes. A posterior axillary line approach allows a puncture along the avascular plain of Brödel, a natural watershed territory between the dorsal and ventral branches of the renal arteries, so as to minimize vascular injury.[6]

Ultrasound allows the visualization and avoidance of bowel, solid viscera and lung edge/pleura. The dark anechoic fluid-filled hydronephrotic pelvicalyceal system is very clearly demonstrated against the echo-bright renal sinus fat.

Intravenous contrast can be used to opacify the collecting system in non-obstructed cases. Fluoroscopy is then used to guide the needle puncture of a calyx by angling the C-arm and using parallax to correct the needle trajectory. Ileal conduits allow for retrograde opacification.

A subcostal approach avoids transgressing the pleura, which is painful and runs the risk of complications. Puncturing above the twelfth rib is commonly performed but venturing above the eleventh rib is not recommended due to a very high association with pleural complications.[7,8]

Most radiologists use ultrasound alone to guide the initial puncture.

Typically a thin 22 G trocar needle or a larger 19 G needle with a 15 G outer sheath can be used for calyceal puncture. The thinner needle is less traumatic and can be easily and safely repositioned, but it can be difficult to visualize with ultrasound because of its low acoustic impedance profile. The larger needles are better visualized and provide for more secure access but are a little more traumatic.

In expert hands the hydronephrotic pelvicalyceal system is usually accessed safely by a single puncture during suspended respiration. The non-hydronephrotic kidney is much more of a challenge.

Limitations

Spinal deformities and ectopic kidneys provide challenging anatomy, but it is uncommon for overlying pleura or bowel to completely preclude a percutaneous approach. The only absolute contraindication to PCN is an uncorrected bleeding diathesis. Haematology advice is valuable.

Extra long puncture needles have been developed to deal with the morbidly obese patient who is often diabetic, and typically presents with acute sepsis. Ultrasound transducer mounted needle guides are helpful in securing a trajectory predicted by an on screen pre-calibrated tramline target (Fig. 10.5.1). Larger sheathed puncture needles with crosshatched echo-bright tips improve visibility within the subcutaneous fat.

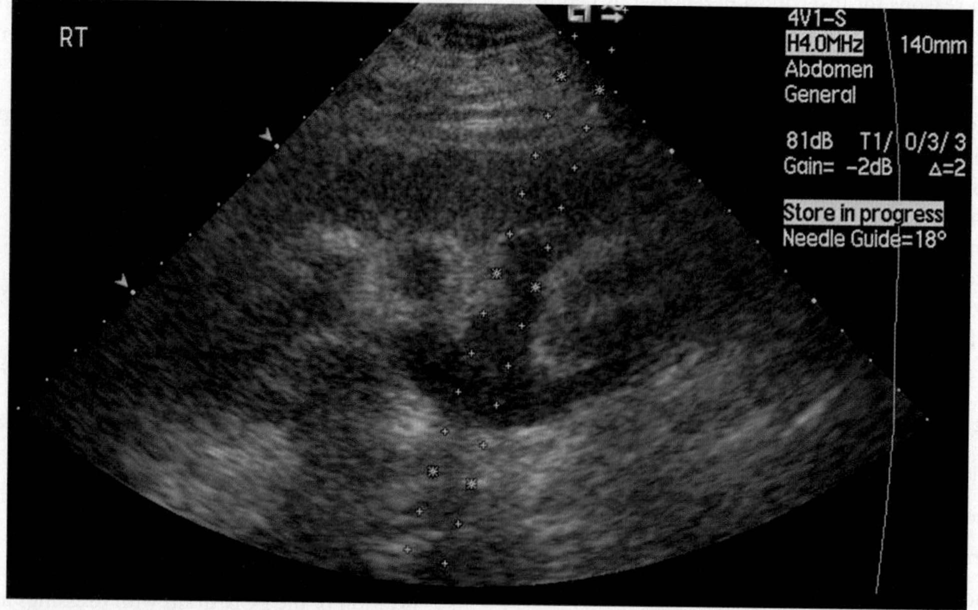

Fig. 10.5.1 The dark anechoic hydronephrotic pelvicalyceal system contrasts with bright hyperechoic renal sinus fat. The pre-calibrated needle guide tramlines can be used to assist renal puncture.

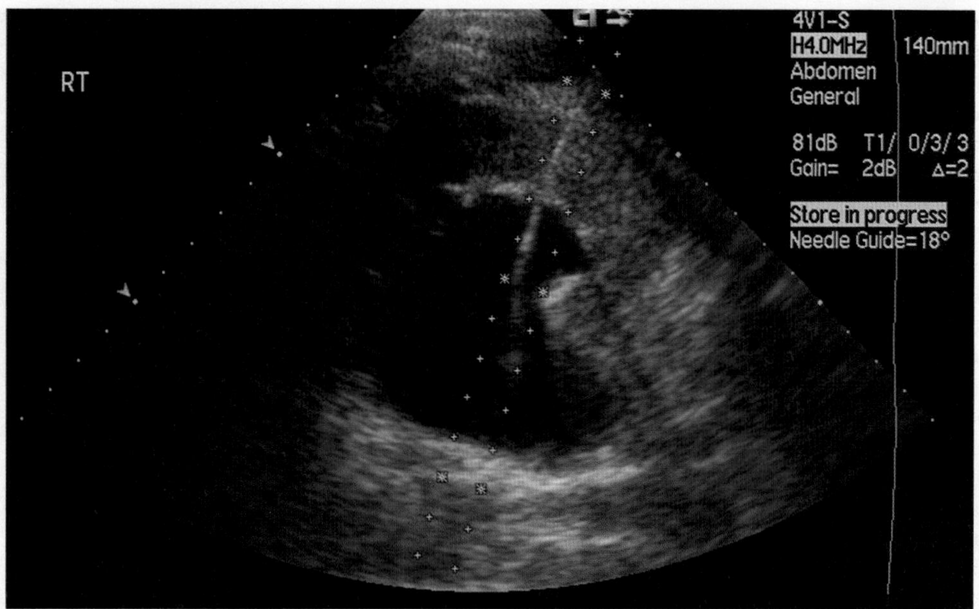

Fig. 10.5.2 The 0.038-inch wire can be easily visualized with ultrasound alone to confirm position.

A single-step 8 Fr needle trocar-mounted drain insertion may be appropriate in the grossly hydronephrotic infected kidney, reducing manipulation, and therefore the risk of bacteraemia.

A 0.038-inch J-tipped guidewire can be adequately visualized with ultrasound alone, if fluoroscopy is not immediately available, or undesirable, such as in the pregnant patient (Fig. 10.5.2). Often a retrograde ureteric stent is preferable. Children require general anaesthesia.

Complications

PCN is a safe procedure, far more commonly performed to ameliorate the complications of surgery than a source of surgically relevant complications. Nevertheless, as with any intervention, complications can and do arise. Procedures performed at night and by radiologists who do not normally perform PCN insertion may be subject to higher complication rates.[9,10]

Frank haematuria is normal post nephrostomy insertion. It usually clears within 24–48 hours, but often, reassuringly, as the patient leaves the radiology suite. Even large clots are lysed by urokinase within a day or two.

Persistent or worsening haematuria is an indication for a nephrostogram. If the nephrostomy tube has migrated and drain sideholes lie within the vascular renal parenchyma, then a replacement tube to tamponade the track is needed. Pseudoaneurysms and arteriovenous fistulae are rare, and embolization for bleeding post PCN is exceptionally uncommon (Table 10.5.1).[11]

Despite best efforts to avoid manipulation within, and overdistension of the infected collecting system, systemic urosepsis can arise due to pyelovenous backflow. Inadvertent enteric injury is rare and minimized by the use of ultrasound.[12]

PCN tubes have in-built fixation mechanisms, they do not 'fall out', but are often inadvertently pulled out. PCN tubes can encrust, block, kink, and migrate and interventional radiologists have a number of tips and tricks for dealing with these scenarios.

An external urine drainage bag is never popular with a patient, unless there is no other option, and the PCN is understood to be preserving or improving quality of life. Internalized drainage with a ureteric stent is always a more attractive option, but may not work, or cause side effects. There is little good evidence as to the effects of PCN on quality of life, but preserving renal function and prolonging life in the terminally ill patient is something that requires very careful consideration, and should ultimately be a decision taken by the patient.

Percutaneous nephrolithotomy

Introduction

Fernström and Johansson first described what is now known as percutaneous nephrolithotomy (PCNL) in 1976.[13]

PCNL has replaced open stone surgery, offering similar stone clearance rates with reduced morbidity. Nevertheless, PCNL remains a major undertaking, not least because extracorporeal shock wave lithotripsy (ESWL), modern endourological stone fragmentation techniques and flexible ureteroscopes are pushing the PCNL case mix in the direction of the most complex and challenging cases.

Indications

The main indications for PCNL are stones greater than 2.5 cm in diameter, obese patients with a poor response to ESWL, stones associated with distal renal tract obstruction, lower pole stones, and stones associated with indwelling foreign bodies, such as encrusted stents. Failed primary or repeated ESWL and/or ureteroscopy treatment are also common indications.

Techniques

Pre-procedural imaging should be carefully evaluated in a combined endourology meeting. A planning computed tomography (CT) scan should be used to evaluate all but the simplest of stones. An unenhanced phase demonstrates the stone burden and a delayed urographic phase details the pelvicalyceal anatomy, invaluable for planning access. Three-dimensional reconstructions are particularly helpful. Aberrant pelvicalyceal anatomy can be identified, and the pleural reflections and position of the colon can be taken into account when considering the approach.

Stones are colonized, and preoperative antibiotics mitigate against the worst consequences of procedure related bacteraemia.

A prone or supine approach is possible. It is intuitive to keep the patient supine if retrograde ureteric catheterization in the lithotomy position is undertaken, allowing for combined percutaneous and retrograde intrarenal stone surgery. The Galdakao-modified supine Valdivia position and other described supine and supine-oblique positions are now well accepted, and have been shown by some to be more time efficient.[14,15] Others have demonstrated a tendency to longer operative times and reduced stone free rates, but with lower rates of post procedural haemorrhage and fever.[16] At present there is no strong evidence to favour any one patient position for PCNL over any other, though your anaesthetist and theatre staff will prefer the supine approach.

Preoperative imaging should be displayed in theatre on a large screen, but the planned approach may be modified on the basis of real-time ultrasound and retrograde fluoroscopic assessment of the anatomy and stone burden. A radiologist is an expert at interpreting and cross-referencing CT, fluoroscopic, and ultrasound imaging to plan for the safest and best collecting system access.

The usual approach is to target a calyx, which is in line with the long axis of the stone. The aim is to create the fewest tracks possible to clear the maximum stone volume, see Table 10.5.2. Although flexible instruments and laser lithotripsy can be invaluable, an optimally placed track will allow for much more effective rigid ultrasonic or pneumatic lithotripsy. The kidney will only allow so much intrapelvicalyceal manoeuvring before the collecting system or parenchyma splits. Acute angles between the track and stone are to be avoided, and occasionally large staghorn stones require multiple tracks.

Parallel lower pole calyceal fragments are often inaccessible from a lower pole puncture. Techniques such as pulling the kidney in a caudad direction using either the sheath of an initial lower pole track, or an inflated ureteric occlusion catheter have been advocated to bring the upper pole calyx away from overlying pleura, but these methods should be adopted with caution.

A radiologist will bring expertise in renal pelvicalyceal access and antegrade guidewire manipulation to allow the rapid placement of a safety wire down the ureter and in to the bladder.

Tracks of between 24 and 30 Fr diameter can be created by telescopic metal dilators or serial fascial dilators, but there is a risk of kinking the heavy-duty access wire. The balloon dilatation system is preferred.

Once a 9 Fr track has been created with a fascial dilator, the balloon device with radio-opaque markers can be appropriately placed and inflated under fluoroscopic control. Contrast is used to fill the balloon up to 10 mm in diameter. A stiff 30 Fr sheath can then be advanced with a rotational force over the carefully supported balloon, until it too lies at an appropriate position. It has been suggested that the lateral (rather than shearing) forces created by balloon dilatation may reduce the risk of parenchymal tearing, but the UK PCNL audit demonstrates a nonsignificant trend towards a higher transfusion rate with this method.[17,18]

A guidewire placed all the way down to the bladder can offset the need for a separate safety wire, but this is not always possible. Losing a newly created track by inadvertent withdrawal of the sheath can lead to disaster if there is no facility for rescue (Fig. 10.5.3).

Occasionally intraoperative bleeding will halt progress. A large bore nephrostomy tube can be placed, and a second look procedure can be arranged once things have settled down. A post PCNL nephrostomy is not always necessary however (Table 10.5.3).

Recent data indicates that 76% of PCNL patients in the UK still have a covering nephrostomy tube placed.[18]

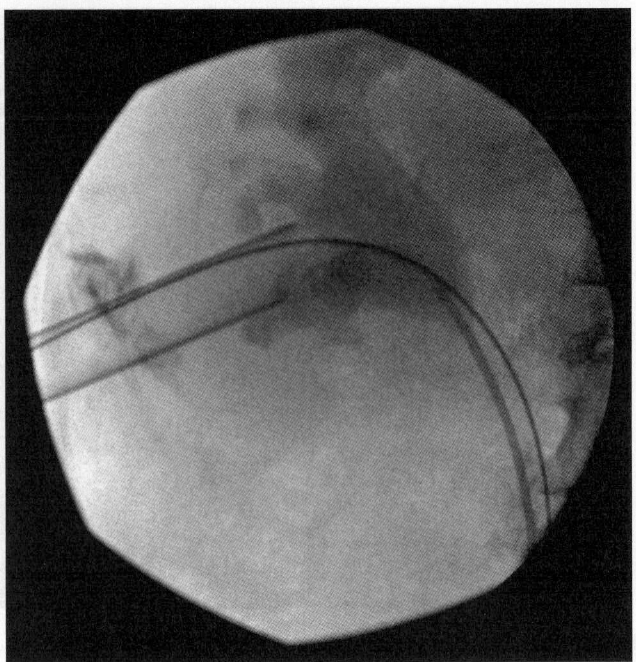

Fig. 10.5.3 A 30 Fr access sheath, safety wire, and retrograde catheter are required for percutaneous management of this staghorn stone.

Limitations and complications

Retrograde catheter placement is not always possible in patients with complex lower tract anatomy or urinary diversions. If the stone burden is large enough to warrant PCNL, a direct ultrasound guided puncture on to a calyx or calyceal stone is usually possible.

Table 10.5.2 Approach to pelvicalyceal stone burden

Stone location	Track
Isolated lower pole	Direct lower pole puncture
Multiple lower pole	Upper pole puncture
Isolated or multiple upper pole	Lower pole puncture
Staghorn	Lower pole +/− further tracks

Table 10.5.3 Advantages of post-percutaneous nephrolithotomy (PCNL) nephrostomy placement versus 'tubeless PCNL'

Post PCNL Nephrostomy	Tubeless
Allows drainage	Reduced post-op pain
Allows post-op nephrostogram	Reduced post-op hospital stay
Tamponades track	No increased risk of bleeding

Table 10.5.4 A UK PCNL audit based on 1,028 procedures documents complication rates

Complication	Rate
Haemorrhage requiring transfusion	2.5%
Haemorrhage requiring embolization	0.4%
Post procedural fever	16%
Post procedural sepsis	2.4%
Visceral injury	0.4%

Source: data from Armitage JN *et al.*, 'Percutaneous Nephrolithotomy in the United Kingdom: Results of a Prospective Data Registry', *European Urology*, Volume 61, Issue 6, pp. 1188–1193, Copyright © 2012 European Association of Urology. Published by Elsevier B.V. All rights reserved.

There is little agreement in the literature about how to assess for residual post PCNL fragments, and what constitutes a stone free state.[18] Comparison studies are limited by uncertainty over stratification of case mix and complexity, but the Guy's Stone Score has been shown to accurately predict post PCNL stone free rate, albeit so far, at a single centre.[19]

Complications are usually related to haemorrhage, urosepsis or urine leak, and have been classified by severity on the basis of the nature of further treatment required, using a modified Clavien grading system (Table 10.5.4).[20]

If there is clinical concern for significant postoperative bleeding, an urgent CT angiogram should be arranged after appropriate resuscitation.

Post PCNL imaging follow up should be tailored to the individual patient, with rapid staghorn formers, and those with underlying metabolic predispositions requiring a more intense schedule. Repeat unenhanced CT is a cumulative radiation hazard, and the combination of plain film and ultrasound is usually sufficient if recurrent stones are to be treated with ESWL in the first instance.

Less traumatic specially designed miniaturized dilators, sheaths and instruments are preferred in the paediatric population but are associated with longer operative times in the adult.[21] Fluid balance and prevention of hypothermia are particular concerns in the anaesthetised child.

Antegrade ureteric stent insertion

Introduction

The placement of a ureteric stent in an antegrade fashion is a natural extension of the PCN technique. Most patients find internal drainage more convenient and cosmetically acceptable.[22] A ureteric stent is less likely to be inadvertently displaced than a PCN drain, and usually has a lower morbidity.[23]

Indications

Ureteric stents drain the pelvicalyceal system in cases of ureteric obstruction (Table 10.5.5) and allow fistulae and leaks to resolve by providing a frame around which ureteral epithelialization is facilitated.

An antegrade (as opposed to a retrograde) approach to stenting offers a greater success rate, especially for distal ureteric strictures. Even if a contrast injection demonstrates complete occlusion, it is often still possible to negotiate the stricture in an antegrade fashion with a torque-controlled hydrophilic wire (Fig. 10.5.4). Antegrade ureteric stent placement requires percutaneous renal access, which can be secured in advance with a PCN, or gained at the same sitting.

Table 10.5.5 Causes of ureteric obstruction

Ureteric obstruction	
Non-malignant	**Malignant**
Stone disease	Bladder
Tuberculosis	Prostate
Post radiotherapy	Cervical
Retroperitoneal fibrosis	Breast
Pelviureteric junction obstruction	Retroperitoneal
Hydronephrosis of pregnancy	

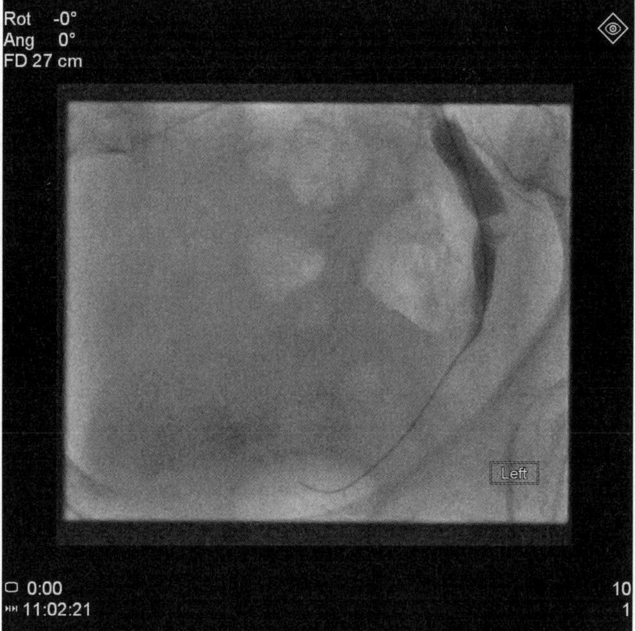

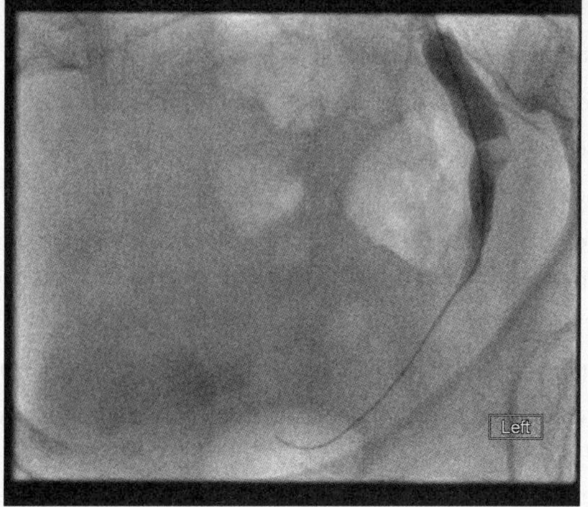

Fig. 10.5.4 Even very tight distal ureteric strictures can be easily crossed with a guidewire and catheter.

Techniques

See Box 10.5.3.

An upper pole or interpolar calyceal track provides the best angle of approach towards the pelviureteric junction. Lower pole calyceal nephrostomy tracks can be utilized, but there is a tendency for the intrapelvicalyceal portion of the guidewire, catheter, and stent to buckle in the renal pelvis when the tip of the device meets distal resistance. Vascular sheaths can be used to provide rigid outer support, preventing proximal loop coiling.

A mature PCN access track of 8 Fr aids the procedure immensely, but single-step percutaneous puncture and stent deployment can be undertaken.

Gentle continuous rotation of the hydrophilic wire is all that is often needed to allow passage through very tight strictures and in to the bladder. An acute sense of urinary urgency is often felt by the patient, which may be eased by distending the bladder with a saline-contrast mix to distance the guidewire tip from the trigone. The hydrophilic wire is exchanged for an 0.038-inch working wire via a catheter.

Occasionally a stricture cannot be crossed by the softer stent material, which may buckle. The stent then needs to be carefully withdrawn to allow balloon dilatation if appropriate.

The tip of the stiff wire is left within the pelvicalyceal system when the proximal stent pigtail is deployed, so as to facilitate the placement of a covering PCN tube. This can be used if there is early stent failure, which can occur if a percutaneous track has been created at the same sitting, due to fresh occlusive blood clots. Even if a covering PCN is not planned, keeping the guidewire within the track for a minute or two will allow monitoring for bleeding which could be tamponaded by a PCN.

Covering PCN tubes can be capped off to allow renal function monitoring. The use of non-locking tubes is advised as locking sutures can become entangled with the proximal stent pigtail. After several days, non-locking PCN drains can be removed on the ward, or under fluoroscopic guidance once a nephroureterogram confirms satisfactory drainage.

Box 10.5.3 The basic outline of an antegrade ureteric stent insertion

- Patient consent
- Preparation including antibiotics and sedo-analgesia
- Aseptic skin preparation and draping
- Local anaesthesia
- Creation of a percutaneous track or exchange of a pre-existing nephrostomy over a guidewire for an angiographic catheter
- Nephro-ureterogram to demonstrate the anatomy
- Guidewire and catheter manipulation through the obstruction
- Exchange of hydrophilic wire for stiff wire and removal of catheter
- Stent insertion and deployment
- Placement of a covering non-locking loop drain

Limitations and complications

Advances in the development of polyurethane and silicone copolymers have led to the creation of soft stents, which are relatively resistant to occlusion, fracture and migration, and are well tolerated. Nevertheless these factors remain problematic. Stent encrustation is a particular problem in a subset of patients whose risk factors include a long indwelling time, urinary sepsis, history of stone disease, and metabolic abnormalities.[24] Ureteric stents should not be placed in patients with an active urinary tract infection.

Co-polymer stent patency rates have been demonstrated to fall from 95% at 3 months post insertion, to 54% at six months.[25] Full-length metal stents provide increased patency rates for up to 12 months in patients with malignant ureteric strictures. Nevertheless, both co-polymer and metallic stents remain vulnerable to failure from extrinsic malignant compression of the ureter. Nephrostograms demonstrate that most flow occurs around, rather than through a ureteric stent. Vesicorenal reflux can be minimized by bladder catheterization.

Irritative bladder symptoms due to stimulation of the trigone by the distal stent pigtails can be minimized by careful stent positioning. Short thermoexpandable titanium-nickel stents, which do not contact the trigone, are an option in the patient with a short malignant stricture.

In the United Kingdom, registering a stent insertion with the British Association of Urological Surgeons (BAUS) national stent register has become best practice. The clinician is alerted by e-mail when stent exchange is required; avoiding the forgotten severely encrusted stent, which often requires both an endourological and percutaneous approach to retrieval.[26]

Drainage of collections

Introduction

Percutaneous imaging-guided drainage offers a rapid way of dealing with troublesome fluid collections. It is well tolerated by the patient, and avoids the risks of further surgery.

Indications

A renal or perirenal abscess may present acutely as a source of systemic sepsis. Specific postoperative collections include urinomas in the cystectomy patient, and lymphoceles in the radical prostatectomy patient. Collections associated with bowel injury are often best managed operatively.

If a fluid collection is believed to be infected, painful, or otherwise detrimental to the patients' progress it is appropriate to request drainage. The collection must be judged to be safely accessible by the radiologist.

Techniques

Radiologists often favour either ultrasound or CT based on expertise and familiarity. There are however specific factors which would favour using one modality over the other. It is vital to avoid iatrogenic injury to important overlying or adjacent structures such as large blood vessels and bowel.

If a safe percutaneous route is not available in an axial plane then ultrasound is favoured over CT as the modality of choice to guide drainage. The ultrasound probe can be angled steeply and used to

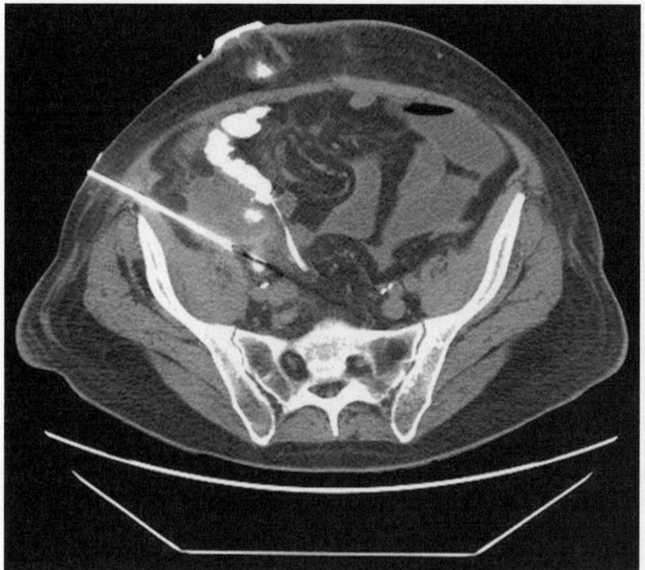

Fig. 10.5.5 A urinoma consequent to a ureteroileal anastomotic defect is drained percutaneously with CT guidance.

negotiate overlying structures. Ultrasound also allows safe continuous real-time imaging where the progress of the advancing needle tip can be followed. CT on the other hand involves ionizing radiation and even with CT fluoroscopy the radiologist has to advance the needle, pause and re-image (Fig. 10.5.5).

CT more accurately depicts a gas and liquid filled collection from gas and liquid filled adjacent bowel. It is often difficult to make this distinction with ultrasound as highly echogenic gas bubbles prevent the ultrasound beam from progressing to deeper tissues.

Discomfort, bleeding, and subsequent drain complications such as blockage and migration should be included in patient consent. Damage to adjacent organs is also a possibility. Pre-procedural antibiotics and a normal clotting profile are required.

Antiseptic skin preparation, draping, and local anaesthesia are the next steps. Local anaesthetic infiltration can be imaged with ultrasound or CT to ensure that sensitive structures such as the peritoneum are anaesthetised adequately, and that the needle trajectory is appropriate. Long 20 G needles can be used to infiltrate local anaesthetic and act as pathfinders down to the collection to guide subsequent trocar-mounted drain placement. A tandem technique can be used which allows for single-step track dilatation. An 8Fr drain is inserted alongside the long needle.[27] Final positioning is confirmed with CT before advancing the drain over the inner trocar and aspirating.

A modified Seldinger technique is more widely practised. A 15 G sheath mounted on a 19 G needle is inserted in to the collection. Withdrawing the inner needle allows fluid aspiration prior to inserting a 0.038 J-tipped wire. Positioning can be confirmed with ultrasound or CT prior to serial fascial dilatation and subsequently drain placement over the wire. The initial aspirate can be sent for analysis.

Special drain dressings can be supplemented with sutures for security. Tension on the drain should be avoided. Migration and eventually drain displacement leaves a partially drained collection, which is much more difficult to redrain.

Irrigation of an infected collection is not routinely advocated, as it has a tendency to drive bacteraemia. Once several doses of appropriate antibiotics have been administered the drain can be flushed if required.

Limitations and complications

Endo-cavity ultrasound guided aspiration may be an option for the patient with a deep pelvic collection which is otherwise inaccessible.

Haemorrhage, adjacent organ injury, sepsis, and infecting a previously sterile fluid collection are recognized complications. Drains can be painful and may kink, block, and be pulled out.

It is important when draining a urinoma that urinary diversion away from the leak is also considered.

Suprapubic catheterization

Introduction

Suprapubic catheterization (SPC) is a commonly performed intervention in urological practice. If a patient has a palpable bladder, no history of lower abdominal surgery and urine is readily aspirated using a needle inserted along the planned catheter track, the landmark technique can be used by a suitably experienced urologist. For patients who have had previous lower abdominal surgery or whose bladder is not palpable due to abdominal wall deformity or obesity, an ultrasound guided approach is recommended to avoid iatrogenic bowel injury.[28]

Indications

Suprapubic catheter insertion is an important means of managing acute or chronic urinary retention if urethral catheterization is not possible or desirable, or has become a source of complications. Patients with spinal pathology, urinary incontinence, and urethral trauma may also be managed by SPC insertion.

Technique

Ultrasound can be used to image the distended bladder and identify any interposing structures such as bowel loops. It is important that ultrasound be undertaken by someone who is appropriately trained.[29]

The patients' clotting profile should be within normal limits. Written consent, aseptic technique, and generous local anaesthetic administration are mandatory. Ultrasound can be used to guide the delivery of local anaesthesia down to and through the detrusor muscle. A skin incision appropriate to the size of the catheter insertion kit is made. It is helpful to make a reasonably deep incision to part the anterior detrusor muscle fibres, so as to facilitate trocar insertion and dilatation. The bladder should be distended where at all possible to provide an adequate non-mobile target. A variety of kits are available. The most appropriate equipment for an ultrasound guided procedure uses a modified Seldinger technique, where the initial puncture needle and guidewire can be visualized by ultrasound. This necessitates serial dilatation however, which may be uncomfortable for the patient.

A Foley catheter is placed and the balloon filled to secure placement, which can again be confirmed with ultrasound. Ultrasound can also be used to guide the needle puncture of a suprapubic or urethral catheter balloon which is stuck and cannot be deflated (Fig. 10.5.6).

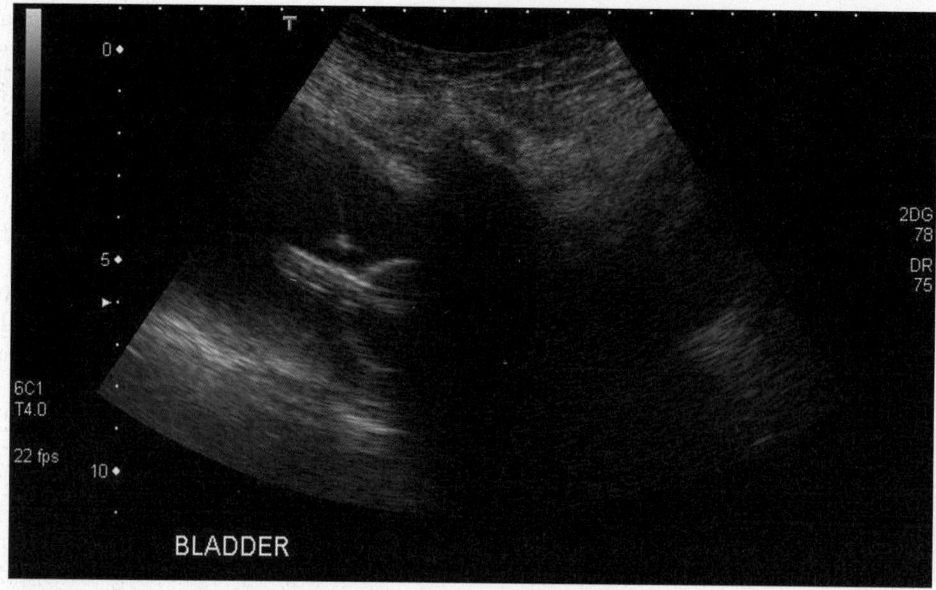

Fig. 10.5.6 A percutaneously inserted long needle approaches the catheter balloon under ultrasound guidance.

Limitations and complications

SPC insertion is contraindicated in bladder cancer, uncorrected coagulopathy, abdominal wall sepsis, and the presence of a subcutaneous suprapubic vascular (femoro-femoral cross-over) graft.

Ultrasound guided SPC insertion minimizes the risk of bowel injury, but a risk of haemorrhage, infection, loss of access, and longer term catheter problems remains.

Renal biopsy

Introduction

Real-time imaging is essential for a safe needle biopsy of the kidney. Ultrasound or CT can be utilized.

Indications

Non-focal renal parenchymal biopsy is utilized to diagnose a diffuse nephropathy or to exclude renal transplant rejection.

Targeted renal biopsy is being increasingly utilized for assessing the indeterminate small solid renal lesion, although its use remains somewhat controversial. Even relatively recently, many authorities argued that the imaging features of a small single renal mass are diagnostically more accurate than histological analysis of core biopsy specimens.[30] With modern advancements in histological techniques however the targeted biopsy of small renal lesions is gaining popularity as a way of avoiding the unnecessary morbidity of either surgery or ablation for benign lesions.[31]

Technique

Written informed consent and a normal patient clotting profile are again mandatory prerequisites. A posterior approach to the native kidney avoids transgressing the peritoneum. Ultrasound is preferred as it offers continuous real-time imaging and the flexibility to alter the planned trajectory at any time. An angled approach with the needle allows ribs, pleura, and bowel to be avoided.

Aseptic technique and draping are employed. A sterile ultrasound probe cover is utilized. Infiltration of local anaesthesia can be guided by ultrasound to anaesthetise a track down to the renal cortex. A small skin incision to allow the insertion of a spring loaded core biopsy needle is then made. Suspended patient respiration stabilizes the target kidney.

The goal of non-focal renal biopsy is to maximize the amount of cortex obtained while avoiding damage to the renal hilum. The fewest cores possible should be obtained to minimize bleeding complications. Immediate assessment with microscopy is useful.

Patients should have bed rest and regular assessment of blood pressure and heart rate for at least 8 hours post procedure. If there are any concerns for significant bleeding an unenhanced and post contrast arterial phase CT should be arranged in tandem with resuscitative measures. Renal angiography and embolization is the gold standard treatment for active bleeding.

The needle track for iliac fossa transplant kidneys should pass lateral to the incision scar to avoid transgressing the peritoneum.

Limitations and complications

It can be reasonably expected that 95% of patients undergoing non-focal renal biopsy have an adequate diagnostic sample taken at one visit. Targeted renal biopsy has the greatest sensitivity (97%) and negative predictive value (89%) for larger lesions of between 4–6 cm in size.[32,33]

Renal biopsy is a safe procedure but minor bleeding is very common. Small perinephric haematomas are seen in approximately 50% of patients and up to a third have frank haematuria post procedure. Severe bleeding is uncommon however, with transfusion rates of approximately 1% and embolization required in far fewer. Iatrogenic arteriovenous fistulae tend to be self limiting if small.

Tumour seeding of the renal biopsy needle track is very rare with only a handful of case reports in the literature.

Vascular radiology

Introduction

Endovascular coil embolization is now a well established safer alternative to open surgery for dealing with iatrogenic or traumatic renal haemorrhage.

Indications

A skilled vascular interventional radiologist can arrest haemorrhage, coil pseudoaneurysms, break up emboli, and stent arterial dissection in almost any organ in the body.

Diagnosis of significant haemorrhage is usually made by comparing unenhanced and arterial phase CT sequences. Traumatic lesions demonstrate abnormal intravenous contrast accumulation or extravasation and guide subsequent conventional angiography. It is when the patient demonstrates signs of haemodynamic instability (i.e. active bleeding, that the diagnostic CT is most sensitive). Patients who are haemodynamically unstable require aggressive resuscitation, the involvement of an intensivist and the early involvement of the radiology department.

Techniques

The basic technique for renal artery angiography is outlined in Box 10.5.4.

Traumatic lesions demonstrate abnormal patterns of perfusion with interrupted vessels, pseudoaneurysm sacs, and extravasation of contrast media. The goal of embolization is to arrest haemorrhage while preserving as much renal parenchyma as possible. Embolic materials include coils, particulate agents, and liquid embolic agents. Coils are often preferred because they are easier to use and are clearly visible with fluoroscopy.

Pseudoaneurysm formation is a recognized complication of nephron-sparing surgery with an incidence reported at 0.43% for open and 1.7% for laparoscopic partial nephrectomy.[34]

Box 10.5.4 Basic technique for renal artery angiography

Catheter angiography

1. Written informed consent
2. Aseptic skin preparation and draping with ideally a femoral artery approach
3. Local anaesthetic
4. Arterial access and guidewire insertion
5. Catheter deployment in the aorta at the L1 level
6. Aortography and renal artery cannalization
7. Microangiography and embolization if required

Endovascular embolization is a safe and effective alternative to conventional surgery, which carries the risks of additional partial or total nephrectomy (Fig. 10.5.7).

Limitations and complications

Not all hospitals have immediate 24-hour access to interventional vascular radiologists, although much work and further investment in this area is anticipated.

It is rare for embolization to result in further significant nephron loss. Iatrogenic vascular dissection is also uncommon and can usually be ballooned and stented when recognized.

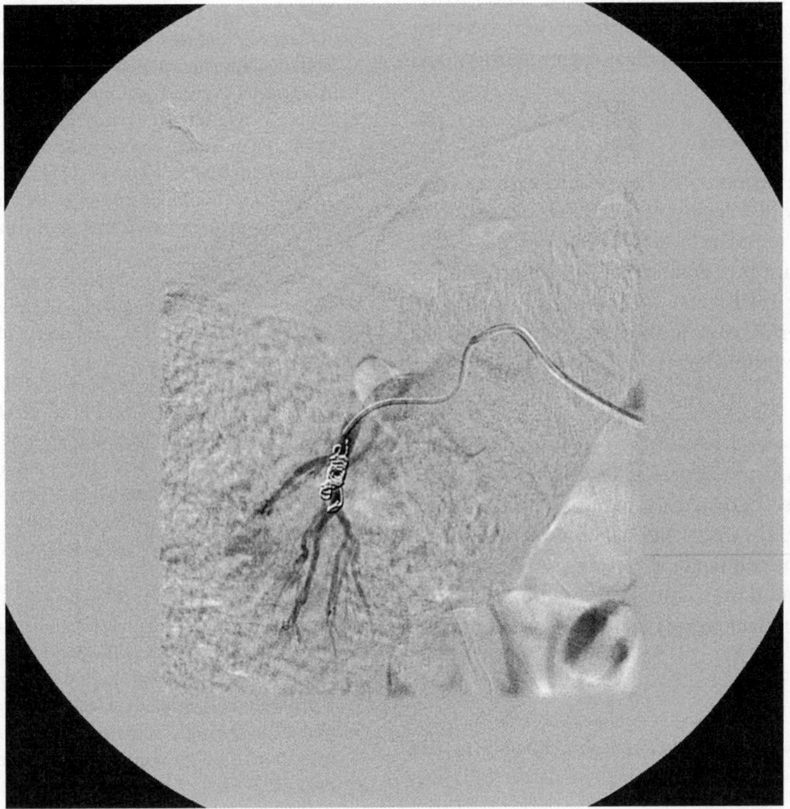

Fig. 10.5.7 Embolization coils are placed in to the feeding artery for a post nephrectomy bleeding pseudoaneurysm.

Prostate biopsy

Introduction

Prostate tissue is required to confirm the diagnosis of prostate cancer and to assign a Gleason score.

Indications

A raised prostate specific antigen (PSA) blood test or palpable prostatic abnormalities on digital rectal examination are the usual triggers to biopsy. Concern about PSA velocity, especially in a patient deemed to be at high risk is also a recognized indication.

Technique

Multiplanar transrectal probes with disposable biopsy guides and spring loaded core biopsy needle devices are utilized. Acoustic gel and probe covers are employed. Antibiotic prophylaxis is recommended and an example of a regime is 1 gram of oral Ciprofloxacin one hour prior to biopsy, then 160 mg gentamicin intravenously immediately prior to biopsy.

Written consent must include an explanation of the approximately 50% risk of haematuria, 10% risk of haematospermia, and less than 1% risk of precipitating urinary retention or prostatitis.

Local anaesthetic has been shown to reduce pain and the procedure is usually well tolerated. Nevertheless vaso-vagal episodes are not uncommon. The peripheral zone forms the main basis for needle sampling, although a pre-procedural MRI may have highlighted a specific area for attention. Conventional greyscale ultrasound used with colour and power Doppler may also demonstrate focal areas of concern. Nevertheless, the appearances are not sensitive enough to eliminate the need for additional standard systematic biopsy, usually 10 or 12 cores in total, as prostate cancer is often multifocal.

Contrast-enhanced ultrasound, elastography, and MRI-ultrasound fusion offer hope for better localization and targeting for biopsy. The role of focal treatments such as high intensity focal ultrasound is not fully established.

Limitations and complications

Repeat biopsy may become necessary in the patient with a raised PSA who lacks confirmatory histology. Anterior lesions are difficult to access, and transperineal template biopsy may be needed.

Severe haemorrhage is rare post transrectal ultrasound guided prostate biopsy, and brisk transrectal bleeding can usually be arrested with a gloved finger. Prostatitis and abscess formation are uncommon when antibiotic prophylaxis is employed.

Conclusions

Interventional uroradiological procedures have revolutionized the management of a wide range of urological conditions, and continue to evolve in modern practice. The interventional uroradiologist must have complete mastery of the full range of imaging modalities and interventional techniques. Good team work between urological surgeons and radiologists is essential for providing optimal patient care.

Further reading

Armitage JN, Irving SO, Burgess NA. percutaneous nephrolithotomy in the united kingdom: results of a prospective data registry. *Eur Urol* 2012; **61**:1188–93.

Dyer RB, Regan JD, Kavanagh PV, *et al.* Percutaneous nephrostomy with extensions of the technique: step by step. *Radiographics* 2002; **22**:503–25.

Harrison SC, Lawrence WT, Morley R, *et al.* British Association of Urological Surgeons' suprapubic catheter practice guidelines. *BJU Int* 2010; **107**:77–85.

Türk C, Knoll T, Petrik A, *et al.* Guidelines on Urolithiasis. European Association of Urology 2012. Available at: http://uroweb.org/wp-content/uploads/22-Urolithiasis_LR_full.pdf [Online].

Uppot RN, Harisinghani MG, Gervais DA. Imaging-guided percutaneous renal biopsy: rationale and approach. *AJR Am J Roentgenol* 2010; **194**:1443–9.

References

1. Goodwin WE, Casey WC, Woolf W. Percutaneous trocar (needle) nephrostomy in hydronephrosis. *JAMA* 1955; **157**:891–4.
2. Heyman SN, Fuchs S, Jaffe R, *et al.* Renal microcirculation and tissue damage during acute ureteral obstruction in the rat: effect of saline infusion, indomethacin and radiocontrast. *Kidney Int* 1997; **51**:653–63.
3. Rickards D, Jones S, Kellett M. Percutaneous nephrostomy. (pp. 23–33) In: Rickards D, Jones S, Thomson KR, Rifkin MD (eds). *Practical Interventional Radiology.* London, UK: Edward Arnold, 1993.
4. Türk C, Knoll T, Petrik A, *et al.* Guidelines on Urolithiasis. European Association of Urology 2012. Available at: http://uroweb.org/wp-content/uploads/22-Urolithiasis_LR_full.pdf [Online].
5. Palaniappa NC, Telem DA, Ranasinghe NE, *et al.* Incidence of iatrogenic ureteral injury after laparoscopic colectomy. *Arch Surg* 2012; **147**(3):267–71.
6. Dyer RB, Regan JD, Kavanagh PV, *et al.* Percutaneous nephrostomy with extensions of the technique: step by step. *Radiographics* 2002; **22**:503–25.
7. Picus D, Weyman PJ, Clayman RV, *et al.* Intercostal-space nephrostomy for percutaneous stone removal. *Am J Roentgenol AJR* 1986; **147**(2):393–7.
8. Radecka E, Brehmer M, Holmgren K, *et al.* Complications associated with percutaneous nephrolithotripsy: supra-versus subcostal access. A retrospective study. *Acta Radiol* 2003; **44**(4):447–51.
9. Wah TM, Weston MJ, Irving HC. Percutaneous nephrostomy insertion: outcome data from a prospective multi-operator study at a UK training centre. *Clin Rad* 2004; **59**:255–61.
10. Lewis S, Patel U. Major complications after percutaneous nephrostomy—lessons from a department audit. *Clin Rad* 2004; **59**:171–9.
11. Farrell TA, Hicks ME. A review of radiologically guided percutaneous nephrostomies in 303 patients. *J Vasc Interv Radiol* 1997; **8**(5):769–74.
12. Zagoria RJ, Dyer RB. Do's and don't's of percutaneous nephrostomy. *Acad Radiol* 1999; **6**(6):370–7.
13. Fernström I, Johansson B. Percutaneous pyelolithotomy. A new extraction technique. *Scand J Urol Nephrol* 1976; **10**(3):257–9.
14. Hoznek A, Rode J, Ouzaid I, *et al.* Modified supine percutaneous nephrolithotomy for large kidney and ureteral stones: technique and results. *Eur Urol* 2012; **61**(1):164–70.
15. Kumar P, Bach C, Kachrillas S, *et al.* Supine percutaneous nephrolithotomy (PCNL): 'in vogue' but in which position? *BJU Int* 2012; **110**(11):1118–21.
16. Valdivia JG, Scarpa RM, Duvdevani M, *et al.* Supine versus prone position during percutaneous nephrolithotomy: a report from the clinical research office of the endourological society percutaneous nephrolithotomy global study. *J Endourol* 2011; **25**(10):1619–25.
17. Tomaszewski JJ, Smaldone MC, Schuster T, *et al.* Factors affecting blood loss during percutaneous nephrolithotomy using balloon dilatation in a large contemporary series. *J Endourol* 2010; **24**(2):207–11.

18. Armitage JN, Irving SO, Burgess NA. percutaneous nephrolithotomy in the united kingdom: results of a prospective data registry. *Eur Urol* 2012; **61**:1188–93.
19. Thomas K, Smith NC, Hegarty N. The guy's stone score-grading the complexity of percutaneous nephrolithotomy procedures. *Urology* 2011; **78**(2):277–81.
20. Tefekli A, Ali Karadag M, Tepeler K, *et al.* Classification of percutaneous nephrolithotomy complications using the modified clavien grading system: looking for a standard. *Eur Urol* 2008; **53**(1):184–90.
21. Wah TM, Kidger L, Kennish S, *et al.* MINI PCNL in a pediatric population. *Cardiovasc Intervent Radiol* 2013; **36**(1):249–54.
22. Banner MP. Antegrade and retrograde ureteral stent placement. (pp. 96–127) In: Banner MP (ed). *Radiologic Interventions: Uroradiology.* Baltimore, MA: Williams and Wilkins, 1998.
23. Holmes SA, Christmas TJ, Rickards D. Ureteric stents. (pp. 53–65) In: Rickards D, Jones S, Thomson KR, Rifkin MD (eds). *Practical Interventional Radiology.* London, UK: Edward Arnold, 1993.
24. Ahallal Y, Khallouk A, El Fassi MJ. Risk factor analysis and management of ureteral double-j stent complications. *Rev Urol* 2010; **12**(2-3):147–51.
25. Lu DS, Papanicolaou N, Girard M. Percutaneous internal ureteral stent placement: review of technical issues and solutions in 50 consecutive cases. *Clin Rad* 1994; **49**(4):256–61.
26. British Association of Urological Surgeons (BAUS) Stent Registry. Available at: http://www.baus.org.uk/professionals/sections/endourology/stent_registry.aspx [Online].
27. Uppot RN. Nonvascular interventional radiology procedures. (pp. 271–87) In: Quaia E (ed). *Radiological Imaging of the Kidney.* Heidelberg, Germany: Springer, 2011.
28. Harrison SC, Lawrence WT, Morley R, *et al.* British Association of Urological Surgeons' suprapubic catheter practice guidelines. *BJU Int* 2010; **107**:77–85.
29. The Royal College of Radiologists. *Ultrasound Training Recommendations for Medical and Surgical Specialities,* 2nd edition. London, UK: The Royal College of Radiologists, 2012.
30. Zagoria RJ. Imaging of small renal masses: a medical success story. *AJR Am J Roentgenol* 2000; **175**:945–55.
31. Beland MD, Mayo-Smith WW, Dupuy DE, *et al.* Diagnostic yield of 58 consecutive imaging-guided biopsies of solid renal masses: should we biopsy all that are indeterminate? *AJR Am J Roentgenol* 2007; **188**:792–7.
32. Uppot RN, Harisinghani MG, Gervais DA. Imaging-Guided Percutaneous Renal Biopsy: Rationale and Approach. *AJR Am J Roentgenol* 2010; **194**:1443–9.
33. Rybicki FJ, Shu KM, Cibas ES, *et al.* Percutaneous biopsy of renal masses: sensitivity and negative predictive value stratified by clinical setting and size of masses. *AJR Am J Roentgenol* 2003; **180**:1281–7.
34. Albani JM, Novick AC. Renal artery pseudoaneurysm after partial nephrectomy: three case reports and literature review. *Urology* 2003; **62**:227–31.

CHAPTER 10.6

Radioisotopes in urology

Sobhan Vinjamuri

Introduction to radioactivity

Atoms of all elements are composed of known arrangements of protons, neutrons, and electrons which characterize them as individual nuclides. Nuclides containing the same number of protons have the same atomic number and have the same chemical properties, and are known as isotopes. The most prevalent isotopes are usually stable and comprise naturally occurring elements. Radioisotopes are unstable members of the group of isotopes of an element. The nuclei of radioisotopes undergo rearrangement and change to a stable form, emitting radiation in the process. A radionuclide is a specific radioactive atom, designated by indicating the element and its atomic mass number such as Iodine-131 or Tc-99m.

The radiation emitted by a radionuclide enables the detection of extremely small masses, below the limits of chemical detection. It is thus possible to use radionuclides as true tracers for substances without introducing disturbing amounts. The radiation emitted by radionuclides is characteristic and unique in terms of the rate of decay, type of radiation, and the energy of that radiation.

Radionuclides used in nuclear medicine may emit alpha particles, beta particles, or gamma radiation. Alpha particles are large particles that are emitted from the nucleus with high energy levels. It is a charged particle with a charge of +2 as it has lost two of its electrons and is essentially a helium ion. Beta particles are similar in terms of charge and other physical properties to electrons. While ordinary electrons are found in the electronic shells orbiting the nucleus, beta minus particles are emitted from nuclei. They have high kinetic energy. Gamma rays are analogous to energy packets emitted from the nucleus as part of its emissions to enable the achievement of a more stable physical state. Alpha and beta emitters are commonly used for radionuclide therapy.[1,2] Gamma rays are more readily transmitted through tissue and therefore the internal administration of gamma emitting radionuclides allows external measurements and imaging of patients using a gamma camera.

When the radionuclides are combined with a chemical or a pharmaceutical compound with particular physiological properties, the resultant compound is a radiopharmaceutical and this compound is subject to strict pharmaceutical controls as is every other medicine suitable for human use.

Clinical nuclear medicine usually involves the detection and quantification of ionizing radiation emitted from radioactive substances. A Gamma camera produces an image corresponding to the distribution of radioactive substances in the body. Computer display and enhancement of the images with numerical assessment is frequently employed.

Tc99m is the most commonly used radionuclide in nuclear medicine imaging. It has a half-life of 6.02 hours and this allows patients to attend for outpatient procedures and travel to home after the procedure without any strict radiation precautions. It has a gamma ray energy of 140keV, which is optimally primed for use with the modern gamma camera. The image quality is therefore of a very high quality. It can be readily complexed with a range of compounds to assess different physiological functions in the body and does not have any pharmacological action by itself. It is not toxic and does not elicit an immune response when injected into humans (see Table 10.6.1).

Radiation exposure and effective dose

Radiation is a property of matter that is all around us and is much more common than people realize. Radiation is analogous to the passing of energy through matter. Most of the radiation does not change the environment it passes through and is called non-ionizing radiation. However, when radiation interacts with the matter as it passes through, this is then termed 'ionizing radiation'.

When the energy associated with the radiation is deposited in a particular tissue it is termed as 'absorbed dose'. This property is useful when a therapeutic benefit is required, however, in most diagnostic settings, this is not helpful and the risk to the individual should be weighed against the benefit of a result that can have a substantial impact on patient management.

Effective dose is an estimate of the total radiation burden to the patient from the exposure to the radioactive compound. This is a useful term that also allows comparison of relative radiation exposure across all modalities involving exposure to different forms of ionizing radiation including X-rays, computed tomography (CT) scans, nuclear medicine procedures and Positron emission tomography (PET) scans.[3]

Absorbed organ doses in patients and effective doses are not measurable quantities but actually based on estimates. Most of what is known about the carcinogenic effects of radiation is derived from studies of atomic bomb survivors. There are additionally studies involving medical uses of radiation which have provided some epidemiological data.

Radiation exposure is commonly known to be associated with some dose-dependent toxicities such as hair loss, and acute radiation sickness. The development of cancer was believed to be a non-dose-dependent association of radiation. However, recent studies have strongly suggested a dose-dependent increase in cancer mortality. Additionally some cancers are passed on to a child when the exposure has happened during pregnancy (teratogenic); or passed on to other generations if the exposure has happened while the patient was not pregnant (genetic).

Table 10.6.1 Common radioisotopes and their common medical indications

Radioisotope	Common indication(s)	Comment
Cr51 EDTA	Glomerular function	Gold standard for estimation of renal function for research, oncology
Tc99m MDP bone scans	Staging of prostate cancer	Highly sensitive, but not very specific. May require correlative imaging and/or biopsy for solitary lesions
^{18}F-FDG PET-CT scans	Staging of cancers	Estimate of metabolically active metastases
Sr-89, Rh-168, Sm-153	Bone pain palliation	Systemic therapy useful for multiple metastatic lesions, not responsive to first line therapy
Ra-223	Bone pain palliation	Likely to be a better target for multiple bone metastases than beta emitters
Tc99m colloid	Sentinel lymph node biopsy	Status of sentinel lymph node usually indicates status of regional lymph node groups

Introduction to isotope renography

Since nuclear medicine uses functional techniques to assess different physiological processes, the early understanding of kidney function relied heavily on nuclear medicine techniques. Due to advances in other imaging techniques including ultrasound and MRI, some earlier indications for isotope renography are now covered by tests involving no exposure to ionizing radiation. However, there are some fundamental clinical questions that can be answered speedily and efficiently and conclusively by using isotopic techniques. Although the exposure to ionizing radiation is an important factor to consider, a detailed risk-benefit analysis in individual patients usually highlights the clinical value of a test result in the context of a small additional radiation burden.

Principles of imaging the renal tract using radionuclides

Although the kidney has many functions, three broad areas that can be assessed using radionuclides include glomerular filtration, tubular secretion and cortical function/ activity. Agents that are physiologically inert and cleared from the body exclusively by glomerular filtration are useful to assess the glomerular filtration rate. These agents include Cr51-EDTA and Tc99m-DTPA. Tc99m-MAG3 is a tubular agent that has a higher extraction efficiency from the blood and is easy to prepare. Tc99m-DMSA is predominantly a cortical agent that provides an index of cortical function or activity.[4]

Patient preparation

The most important prerequisite for the renogram is an adequate state of hydration of the patient which has to be maintained during the test. It is important to avoid an oliguric state since the result can mimic an obstructive pattern owing to sluggish urine flow. The bladder is emptied immediately before the examination and the patient is positioned in a sitting or prone position with the gamma camera against the patient's back. It is important to position the patient in a comfortable position as they need to maintain the same posture for 20–40 minutes. After intravenous injection of the appropriate dose of the radiopharmaceutical, images are acquired for 20 to 40 minutes. The patient is asked to empty his/her bladder at the end of the procedure to reduce the radiation dose to the pelvic organs.[5]

Interpretation: Studies are analysed by producing clear summed computer images and defining the regions of interest over each kidney and the urinary bladder. Curves are then obtained from the detected count rate against time for each region and the obtained curves are expressed as a percentage of injected dose. The normal renogram shows three classic phases. Immediately following the intravenous injection of the radiopharmaceutical, there is a rapid rise which reflects the vascular supply to the kidney. The second phase is a more gradual slope which corresponds to the renal handling of the tracer by the kidneys and is dependant on various factors such as supply rate, extraction efficiency, intraluminal transit, and excretion. In a normal kidney curve reaches a peak at two to five minutes and activity starts to leave the renal area which is the beginning of the third phase. At this point the tracer activity starts to appear in the bladder and this is now predominantly the excretory phase (see Fig. 10.6.1).[6,7]

DTPA vs. MAG3 renography

Tc99m labelled–diethylene triamine pentacetate (Tc99m-DTPA) is a physiologically inert compound that is predominantly excreted by the glomerular system (approximately 90% excreted by 4 hours). Upto 10% of the injected activity is bound by plasma proteins and is not available for excretion and therefore the net value may represent a slight underestimation. It does not get secreted or filtered by the tubules and also does not localize to the parenchyma/ cortex.

Tc99m labelled–mercapto acetyl triglycine (Tc99m-MAG3) is a predominantly tubular secretory agent (95% tubular secretion versus 5% glomerular clearance). Although we cannot measure glomerular filtration rate with this agent, another aspect of renal function ie effective renal plasma flow can be measured and this represents a surrogate marker of global renal function.

Due to the relative ease of preparation of Tc99m-MAG3, better visualization of the renal parenchyma; unpredictable nature of protein binding of Tc99m DTPA, better image quality, and the relative reproducibility of tubular function at poorer renal function, for most routine indications, most diagnostic departments offer Tc99m MAG3 renography rather than Tc99m DTPA renography.[8]

MAG3 or DMSA?

Tc99m DMSA scanning provides information on cortical or parenchymal activity predominantly. Tc99m DMSA renography has been widely considered a better test to estimate differential kidney

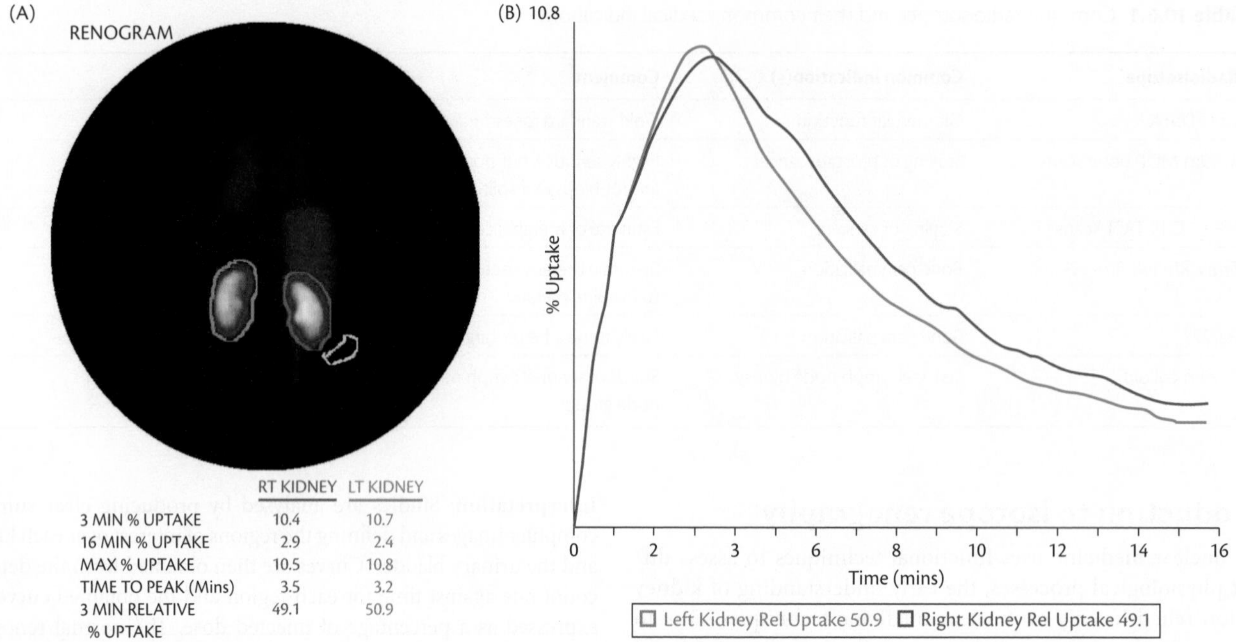

Fig. 10.6.1 (A) Good uptake in both kidneys (approx. 10% of injected activity), and good differential function (50:50%). (B) Activity–time curves for both the kidneys with symmetrical uptake by both kidneys and good excretion bilaterally.

function, mainly because it is a parenchmyal agent and routine views include anterior as well as the standard posterior views. This agent is particularly useful when both kidneys are not located at the same depth in the anteroposterior plane or if one kidney is rotated with respect to the other. Tc99m DMSA is also the preferred agent when one kidney is poorly functioning and there is a requirement to assess the differential function to a higher degree of accuracy.

Tc99m DMSA is the obvious agent of choice in suspected pyelonephritis and the degree of cortical damage or scarring needs assessment.

Tc99m MAG3 is the preferred agent of choice for any assessment of excretion or possible obstruction. The early phase of the Tc99m MAG3 renogram is the parenchymal phase and these first few set of images can be used to assess parenchymal integrity and differential function. In routine clinical practice, where there is an expectation that both kidneys are located at the same depth, and morphologically similar, Tc99m MAG3 does provide a good estimate of the differential renal function. Due to the higher radiation burden associated with Tc99m DMSA renography, and due to the fact that Tc99m MAG3 renography provides additional information about renal function, Tc99m MAG3 renography can be adequately used to provide an index of differential function in most situations (see Table 10.6.2).

Routine clinical indications for isotope renography

- Assessment of differential kidney function
- Assessment of possible pelviuteric obstruction
- Assessment of renal damage post pyelonephritis
- Renal transplant imaging
- Assessment of vesicoureteric reflux
- Assessment of renal artery stenosis

Differential renal function

While biochemical tests can provide a very good estimate of overall renal function, it is useful to know individual kidney function in selected indications such as in potential living kidney donors. Anatomical tests such as Ultrasound and Computed Tomography rely on symmetry of size between the two kidneys and in the vast majority of cases, this should be adequate. However, it is now well accepted that even if the two kidneys have the same size, they may actually contribute differently to the overall renal function. It is important to quantify this asymmetry and isotopic tests provide quick, easy and reproducible results (Fig. 10.6.2). All three of the commonly used isotopes (Tc99m DTPA, Tc99m MAG3 and Tc99m DMSA) can be used to provide an estimate of the differential function. However, in routine clinical practice Tc99m MAG3 is preferred and in patients with known asymmetry of depth of the kidneys, or rotated kidneys, Tc99m DMSA is recommended.

Obstructive nephropathy

Diuretic renograms provide a time-tested mechanism to assess the level and severity of any obstruction in the renal outflow tracts. Intravenous furosemide (0.5 mg/kg body weight) is administered during the excretory phase of the routine renogram (i.e. 15–20 minutes after injection of the radiotracer). Known renal patients with either unilateral or bilateral flank pain and/or patients with baggy renal pelves identified on ultrasound or CT scanning are best assessed with a diuretic renogram.

Broad categories of no response (renogram curve shows no change—see Fig. 10.6.3); partial response (some improvement in excretory pattern post-diuretic administration) and good response (significant improvement in excretion post diuretic, see Fig. 6.4) are recognized. Diuretic renograms also offera good functional tool to assess the effectiveness of pyeloplasty for an obstructed renal outflow tract.[9,10]

Table 10.6.2 Common clinical questions and suggested procedures

Clinical question(s)	Procedure to request	Comment
Need accurate estimate of relative renal function	DMSA renal scan	In situations where accuracy is paramount (e.g. prior to planned nephrectomy) or where renographic estimate is likely to be technically difficult (e.g. in certain infants). No information is provided on the status of the outflow tract
Suspected renal scarring	DMSA renal scan	Estimate of relative renal function will be routinely provided
Suspected PUJ (and/or ureteric) obstruction	Diuresis MAG3 renogram	Estimate of relative renal function will be routinely provided
Suspected renal scarring and suspected upper tract obstruction	Diuresis MAG3 renogram	Scarring may be apparent on the early MAG3 images. If not proceed to a DMSA scan
Suspected VUR (or UUR in duplicated systems)	Basic MAG3 renogram followed by Indirect radionuclide Cystogram	Estimate of relative renal function will be routinely provided
Suspected VUR and suspected upper tract obstruction	Diuresis MAG3 renogram followed by indirect cystogram	If indirect cystogram negative for reflux, repeat the test without furosemide
Need accurate estimate of absolute GFR in ml/min	GFR measurement (51Cr-EDTA)	Could also use 99mTc-DTPA
Need estimate of both relative and absolute GFR	Basic DTPA renogram with GFR	In principle, both can be measured by a single injection of 99mTc-DTPA. However, in children (or adults with compromised renal function) it is preferable to inject 99mTc-MAG3 and 51Cr-EDTA simultaneously. Absolute GFR is measured by blood sampling

Pyelonephritis

Tc99m DMSA scintigraphy is a highly sensitive and specific tool to detect and confirm renal involvement associated with lower urinary tract infections, especially in the paediatric population. Renal sequelae such as renal scarring secondary to vesicoureteric reflux can also be assessed in the post-acute or chronic phases. Tc99m DMSA scintigraphy is recommended for the evaluation of children with presumed acute pyelonephritis and is also recommended for the evaluation of extent of scarred tissue in both children and adults with chronic pyelonephritis (see Fig. 10.6.5).

Recently SPECT (single photon emission computed tomography)-CT scanning has been shown to increase the diagnostic confidence for detecting cortical defects associated with pyelonephritis.

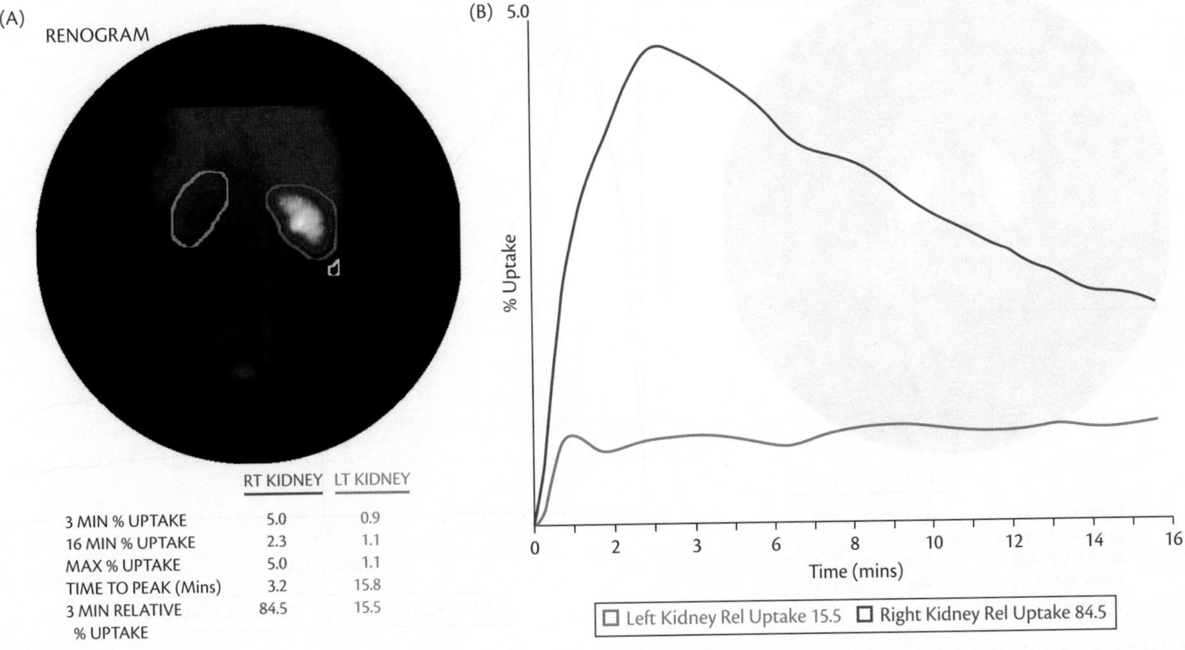

Fig. 10.6.2 (A) Poor uptake by the left kidney, and asymmetrical renal function (R: L; 85:15%). (B) Activity–time curves for both the kidneys with good uptake and excretion by the right kidney and poor uptake and excretion by the left kidney.

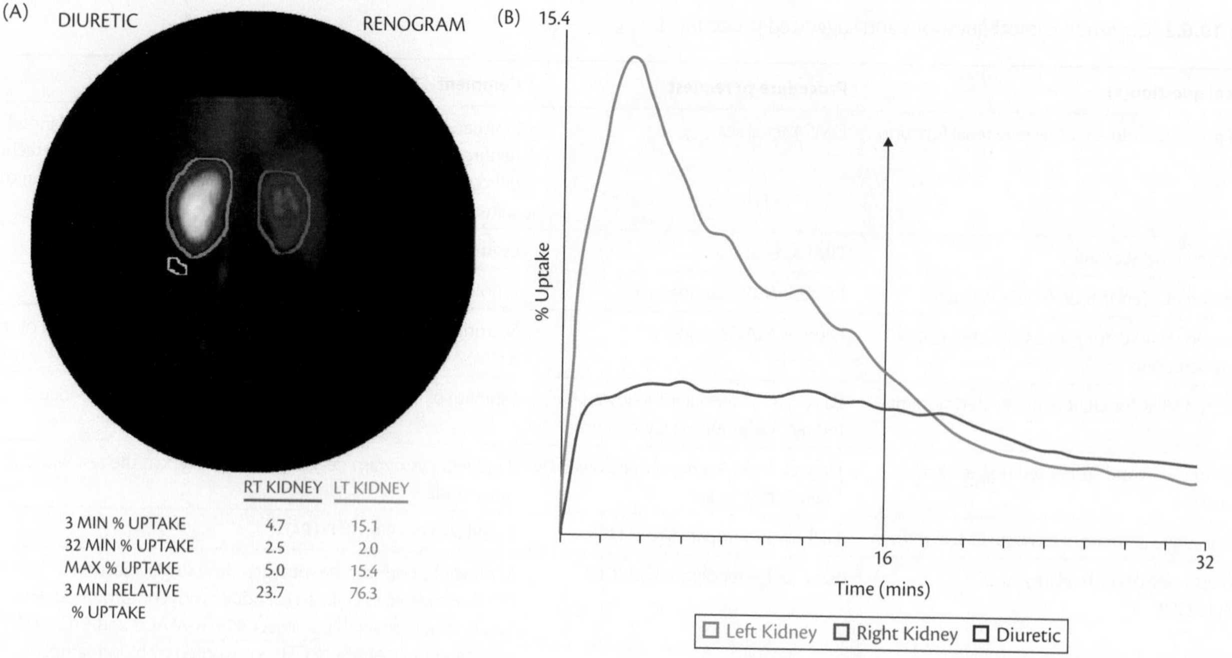

Fig. 10.6.3 (A) Poorer uptake by the right kidney (approx. 4.7% of injected activity), and asymmetrical renal function (R:L 24:76%). (B) Activity–time curves for both the kidneys with good uptake and excretion by the left kidney and poorer uptake and incomplete excretion pre and post diuretic by the right kidney.

Vesicoureteric reflux

Although the commonest presentation of vesicoureteric reflux is with a urinary tract infection, especially of the lower poles, sometimes it is useful to visualize the location and extent of the reflux. If visualization of vesicoureteric reflux is required, then there are two isotopic methods available. Direct cystography involves instilling some radioactive tracer directly into the urinary bladder and then visualizing any activity in the ureters or lower poles of the kidneys. Due to practical considerations however, the more commonly used protocol involves the addition of a micturating cystoureterogram phase to a normal renogram. After completion of the excretory phase of the normal renogram, the patient is encouraged to void urine while images are acquired and the resulting back-pressure in the ureters could identify any instances of reflux.[11]

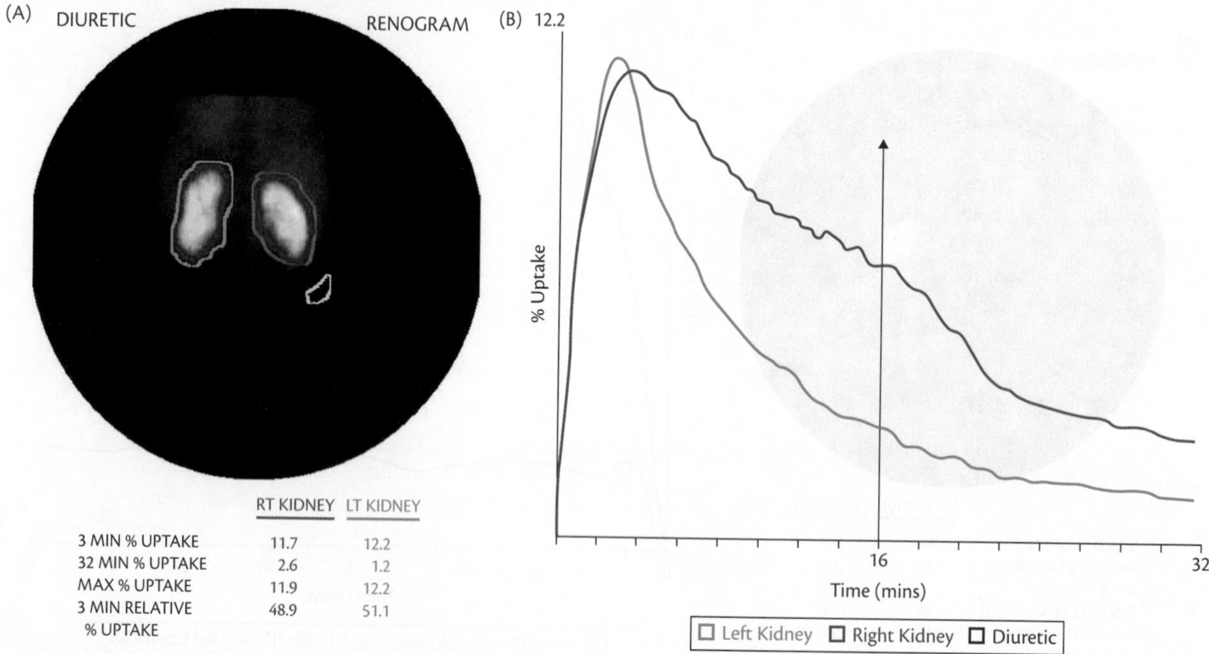

Fig. 10.6.4 (A) Good uptake by both kidneys and symmetrical renal function (R:L; 49:51%). (B) Activity–time curves for both the kidneys with good uptake and excretion by the left kidney. Right kidney shows incomplete excretion till 16 minutes and a good response to the diuretic.

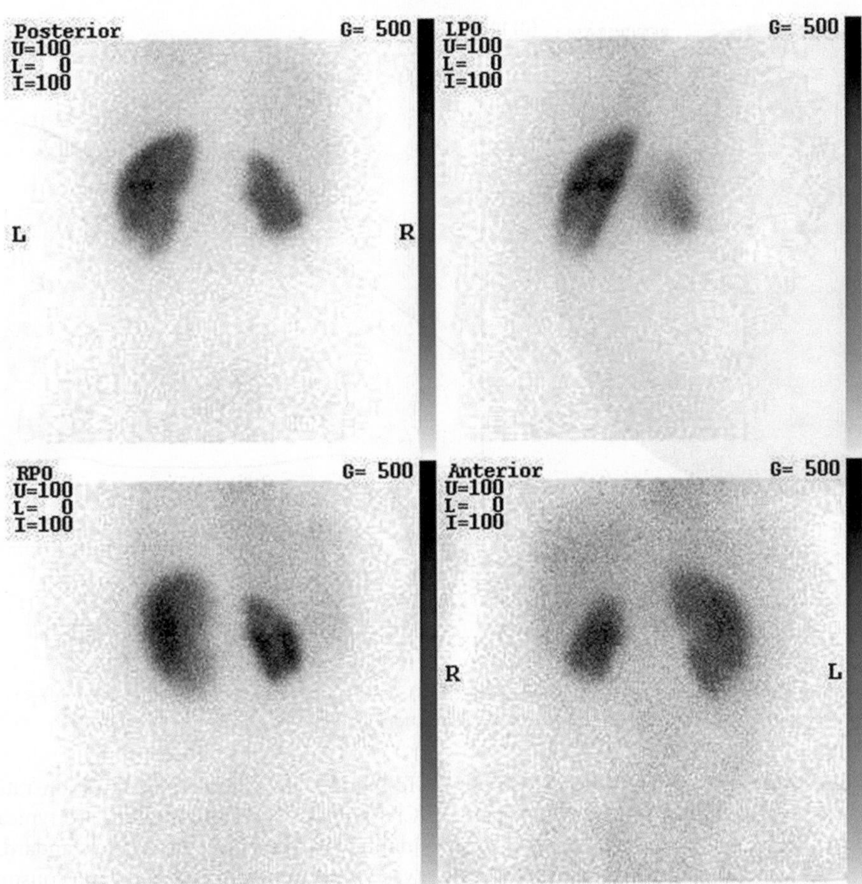

Fig. 10.6.5 This represents a DMSA renogram showing asymmetrical uptake in the kidneys (right smaller than left, probably scarred); with cortical defects at left lower pole and right upper and lower poles likely secondary to chronic pyelonephritis.

Transplant renography

The main indication for isotope renograms in post-transplant evaluation is the differentiation of rejection from acute tubular necrosis. Rejected kidneys have poor perfusion as well as poor tubular excretion. In acute tubular necrosis. There is normal perfusion/visualization of the transplanted kidney, but the excretory phase shows nil or minimum excretion, Urinary bladder is frequently not visualized in spite of the kidney being visualized. Unfortunately cyclosporin toxicity can also appear similarly on a functional aspect and this is a common differential diagnosis that needs exclusion when a transplant renogram is suggestive of acute tubular necrosis (Fig. 10.6.6).[12–16]

Captopril renography

Captopril renography has had proven value in the identification of renovascular hypertension in patients with high blood pressure. This test also has a value int he evaluation of asymmetrically sized kidneys and the confirmation or exclusion of functional impairment secondary to renal artery stenosis. The test has two phases. A baseline phase assesses the baseline differential function and excretory patterns, while a 'captopril phase' study is conducted another day after oral administration of captopril and repeating the renogram. A reduction in renal uptake (unilateral reduction by at least 10%) or prolonged retention of the radiotracer in the renal parenchyma after administration of captopril, and in comparison with the baseline study is considered a positive indicator of functional renal artery stenosis causing renovascular hypertension. The captopril phase can also be performed with other ACE (acetylcholinesterase) inhibitors such as enalapril or lisinopril and the longer acting medication does not need to be stopped for the 'captopril phase' (Fig. 10.6.7).[17–21]

Limitations of routine isotope renography

Although the use of radioactive tracers is considered a limitation by some, the value of assessing function and the physiology of the renal tract has been well tried and tested and the benefit of undergoing the procedures frequently outweighs the small radiation associated risks.

Due to the requirement to assess the dynamic phase of renal function, it is vital that the radiotracer or any related medication such as diuretics should not be extravasated into interstitial tissue at the site of intravenous injection.

Insufficient hydration which can either be self-induced or due to other co-morbidity can result in delayed uptake and excretion by one or both kidneys, and may be misinterpreted as poor function.

Significant Patient motion during the study may introduce errors in the activity-time curve analysis.

When conducting diuretic renograms, the diuretic should not be administered too early, before the maximum distension of the collecting system, as the response may not reflect true physiology.

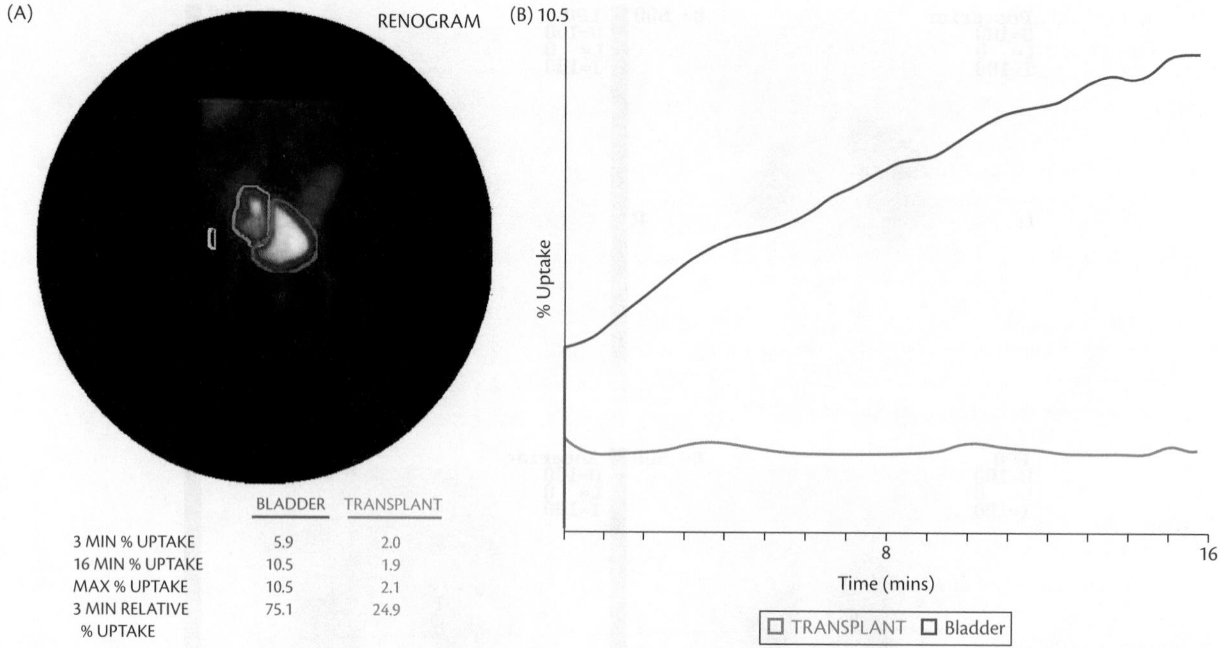

Fig. 10.6.6 (A) Good uptake by the transplant kidney. The bladder is also visualized. (B) Activity–time curves for the kidney and bladder with no obvious excretory pattern. However, the bladder activity shows progressive increase suggesting a well-functioning transplant kidney.

Also if the function in one kidney is so poor that there is poor uptake in the kidney, it is frequently difficult to comment on any possible obstruction.[22–24]

Chromium-51 EDTA estimation

Glomerular filtration rate is a commonly accepted standard measure of renal function.

It is routinely measured using tracers that are cleared exclusively by glomerular filtration, the most common being Cr-51 EDTA and Tc-99m DTPA. Glomerular filtration rate is best assessed using Cr-51 EDTA. Clearance values are typically 85% of those using inulin which is the accepted gold standard. Because this technique was found to be difficult and time consuming to perform, it was therefore considered inappropriate for routine clinical use. Since Cr-51 EDTA is expected to be excreted solely by the glomerular filtration route, it has been shown that the rate of disappearance of this compound from the blood is proportional to renal clearance. Hence there is no need to obtain urinary samples. The commonly used protocols involve at least two timed venous blood samples at

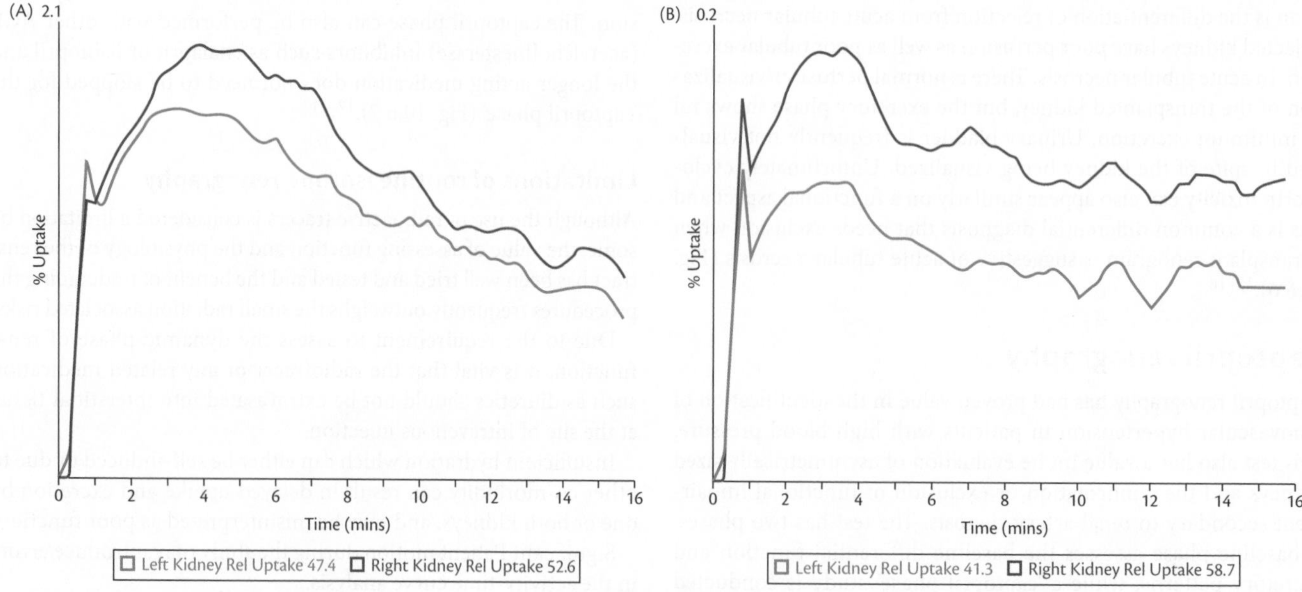

Fig. 10.6.7 (A) The baseline phase of a captopril renogram. There is good uptake in both kidneys; good excretory pattern, and good differential function (R:L: 53:47%). (B) The captopril phase of a captopril renogram. The left kidney shows relatively reduced tracer uptake (R:L: 59:41%) and there is bilaterally delayed excretion. Findings indicate bilateral renovascular disorder worse on the left side.

two to three hours after intravenous injection of the radiotracer. If more samples are obtained, there is higher mathematical accuracy.

It is commonly used for monitoring of drugs that might cause nephrotoxicity; calculation of dose in chemotherapy; detection of renal failure with inconclusive serum creatinine values; and in the assessment of potential live donors for transplantation.

However, the values should be interpreted with caution in patients with ascites, oedema or other expanded body space, and in patients receiving intravenous fluids, where the renal clearance value may be overestimated.

Final values may be corrected for body surface area rather than for weight, as in the paediatric population, the body surface area corrected GFR increases with age from birth up to two years of age and remains constant thereafter into adulthood.

Isotope bone scans

Bone seeking radiopharmaceuticals such as Tc99m Methylene diphosphonate have been used to identify sites of possible bony metastatic involvement. In the initial diagnostic work-up of patients with carcinoma of prostate, some protocols routinely incorporate an estimation of possible bony involvement. While serum prostate specific antigen levels can usually provide a good index on possible bone metastatic involvement, when these levels are elevated, it is useful to perform an isotope bone scan. Isotope bone scans are sensitive but not specific, therefore, a normal scan can exclude metastatic involvement with a high degree of accuracy, while an abnormal scan may not always represent metastases. Further confirmation by means of plain films, MRI scanning, or even direct bone biopsy may be required for solitary metastases. Generally, isotope bone scans have very low value if the serum PSA levels are less than 10 ng/mL (see Figs 10.6.8 and 10.6.9).

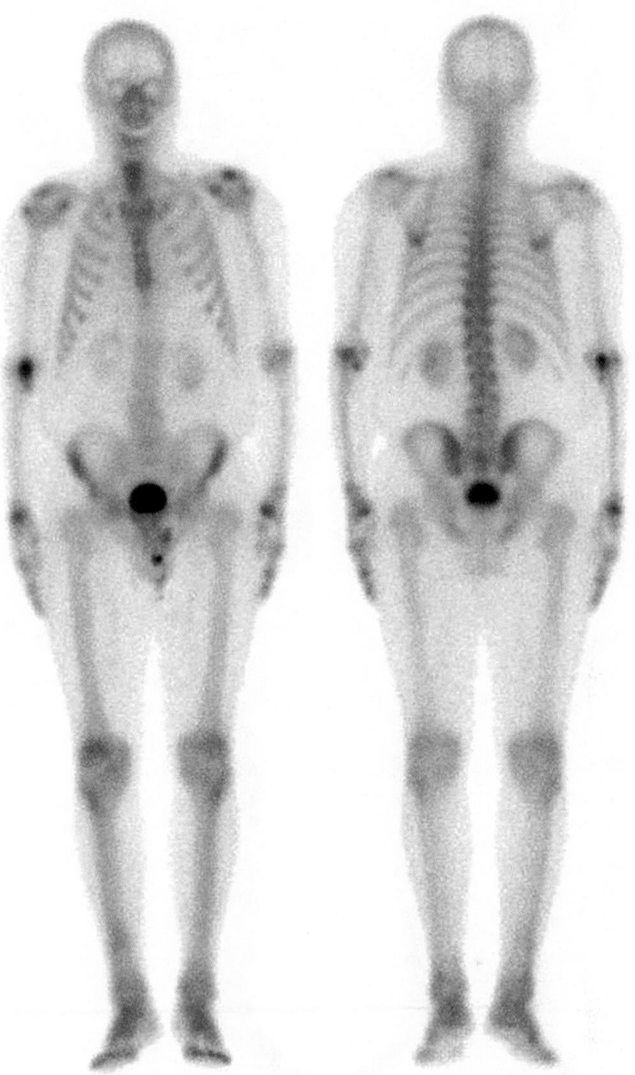

Fig. 10.6.8 A normal bone scan with no abnormal foci of increased osteoblastic activity.

PET-CT scans

Essentially, the procedure involves the injection of a known amount of positron emitting radiopharmaceuticals, and imaging of the whole body or specific organs using a PET scanner. The combination of a PET scanner with CT or MRI technology has enabled the addition of anatomical context to the functional scans.

Bone pain palliation

Due to rapid advances in diagnostic and therapeutic options available for patients with common cancers including prostate cancer, there are an increasing number of patients presenting with cancer related bone pain. Bone pain is usually caused by bony infiltration by the tumour cells and expansion of periosteal membranes, which have a high density of pain receptors. Some patients also have mechanical instability due to weakening of weight bearing bones such as the pelvis and femur. Although there are now very effective treatment approaches to pain management including the use of stronger analgesics, radiation therapy and nerve blocks, frequently the scale of the metastatic involvement renders any local approaches ineffective and systemic approaches are preferred.[25]

The intravenous administration of bone seeking radiopharmaceuticals provides one more approach to pain management. Due to the close relationship between bone marrow and the bone matrix, any tracer that localizes to the bone matrix has the potential to deposit energy in the marrow as well, leading to haematological complications.

The ideal radiopharmaceutical for treating bone metastases is a pure beta emitter that localizes to bone metastases in preference to the skeleton. A small amount of gamma emission may assist in imaging, and this property has obvious advantages. The energy of the beta emission should be high, and it should have a relatively short half-life, so that the energy would be deposited in bone over a short period of time.

Commonly used agents include Strontium-89 which is a calcium analogue and bone precursor. The greater the osteoblastic activity, the greater the concentration of therapeutic agents in and around the tumour. Sr89 has a half-life of 50.5 days and an energy of 1.43 MeV. Samarium153 EDTMP (ethylene diamine tetra methylene phosphonic acid) has a short half-life of 46.8 hours, while Rhenium 168 HEDP (hydroxy ethylidine diphosphonate) has a half-life of 3.8 days, and also has a 137 keV gamma emission which is suitable for imaging.

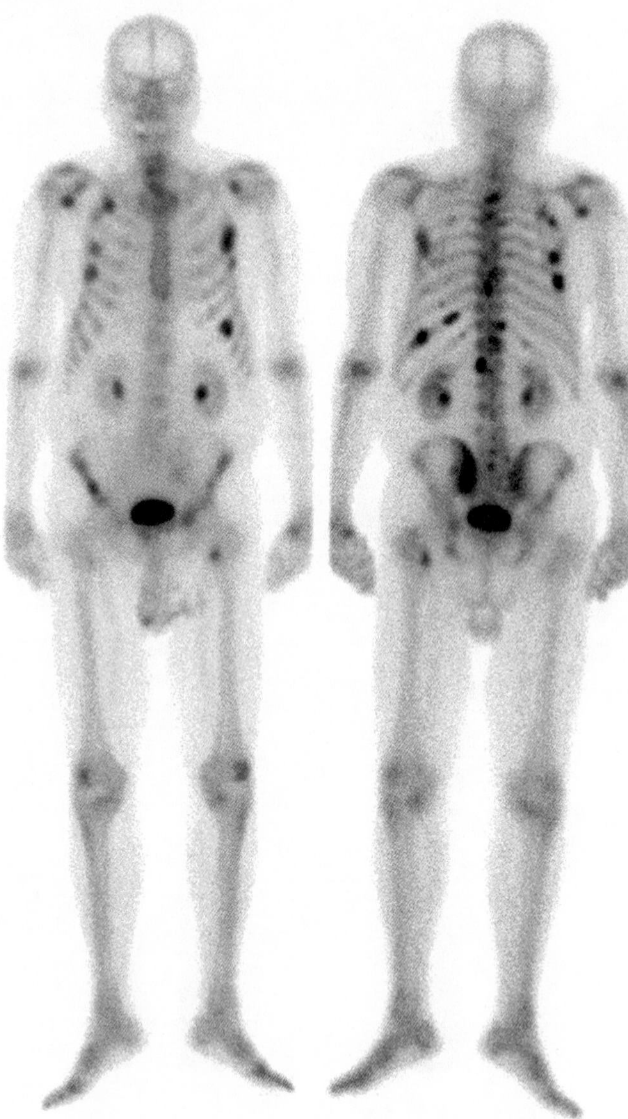

Fig. 10.6.9 A patient with several sites of abnormal osteoblastic activity in the axial and appendicular skeleton, highly suggestive of multiple skeletal metastases.

Alpha emitters

The current justification for targeted radionuclide therapy is based on the preferential targeting of abnormal cells by the internal localization of the radioactive tracer. Unfortunately, this is still not very efficient and some energy is also spent on irradiation of normal tissue. The use of alpha particle emitters has been suggested to further improve the target to non-target irradiation of tumour cells. Alpha particles travel smaller distances and are able to deposit higher energy in comparison with beta particles. The toxic potency is believed to be of the order of 100 times more than beta particles and thus these constitute some of the most cytotoxic compounds known. They are also easy to manufacture, ship, and administer. Radium-223 has been recently undergoing advanced evaluation for the treatment of skeletal metastases from prostate carcinoma. It has a half-life of 11.4 days and has an intrinsic affinity for bone metastases. Use of Ra-223 has been associated with reduced bone alkaline phosphatase levels, markers of bone turnover, and improved prostate specific antigen response. Other alpha emitters under medical evaluation include thorium 227, actinium 225, astatine 211, and bismuth 212.

Sentinel lymph node imaging

Within surgical oncological practice, the sentinel lymph node is recognized as the first node that drains the tumour. The fundamental premise is that when cancers spread via the lymphatic route, they do so in a step-wise manner, with local lymph nodes being involved first in this process. By identifying the sentinel lymph node and removing it and analysing it further, it is possible to decide whether the regional and distant lymph nodes are involved.

A combination of preoperative imaging and/or intraoperative localization of the sentinel lymph node using a gamma probe with or without blue dye is used to identify the sentinel lymph node, and then this node is sent for further histological scrutiny.

If the sentinel lymph node is not involved in the malignant process, then it is highly unlikely that the patient has disseminated nodal metastases, and relatively conservative treatment approaches can be adopted. If the sentinel lymph node has malignant tissue, this is usually an indication for regional lymph node dissection.

Sentinel Lymph node biopsy has been well established for breast carcinoma. Other tumours where sentinel lymph node biopsy has been considered and is under evaluation include penile cancer, urinary bladder cancer, prostate cancer, testicular cancer, and renal cell cancer.

Principles of PET imaging

PET scanning is a nuclear medicine imaging modality that detects high energy gamma rays produced by positrons when they collide with electrons. Patients are injected with positron emitting radionuclides, and the pharmaceutical components of these compounds are used to localize the combined tracer to a particular function within a defined site. For instance, in a cancer patient, the injection of the positron emitting radiopharmaceutical ^{18}F-fluorodeoxyglucose results in the production of a metabolic map of all tumour-related activity both within the primary tumour and additionally in any possible sites of metastatic involvement. The positron emitters usually have a short half-life and include 11C (20 min), 13N (10 min), 15O (2 min), and 18F (110 min), among others.

At the site of localization, as the positrons travel through matter, after a very short distance, they interact with electrons, resulting in an annihilation reaction that produces two pairs of 511-keV gamma rays emitted simultaneously in nearly 180 degrees opposing directions. The PET scanners are used to detect these 511 keV photons. Inside the PET scanner, there are hundreds of detector blocks made of scintillating materials such as bismuth germanium oxide, lutetium oxyorthosilicate, or gadolinium oxyorthosilicate arranged in consecutive full or half rings surrounding the patient cylindrically, enabling the detection of many slices of coincidence data emerging from the patient at one time. The detectors are paired with the opposing side at 180 degrees. Each pair of detectors in the ring defines a possible emission path. Any signal that approaches each of the paired detectors simultaneously or within 12–15 nanoseconds of each other is considered a true event, while those coincidence events that fall outside this range consist usually of undesired random and scatter data and are rejected by the coincidence timing circuitry. All the true events are then summed and analysed and a probability map of the true location of the event along this path between the two detectors is generated.

Some modern, fast scintillators can accurately estimate the location of an annihilation event along this path by measuring the difference in the arrival times of the annihilation photons at the opposing detectors (time-of-flight PET systems). With time-of-flight (TOF) information, the annihilation point can be localized to a limited range within the line of response (LOR), whereas without time-of-flight information, annihilation is assumed to be located with equal probability along the entire LOR. In the latter case, many intersecting LORs are needed for the precise 3-dimensional localization of the activity, whereas in the former detector types, this information is identified both within the LOR and by the intersecting LORs.

When the 511-keV photons strike the scintillation crystal, they are absorbed within the crystal lattice and produce light photons that strike the photocathode of a photomultiplier tube coupled to the crystal. A pulse is generated at the photomultiplier tube and then increased by an amplifier. The energy and spatial position of the signal are determined, and finally a count is recorded. When two such events are detected by a pair of opposing detectors simultaneously within the time window, a coincidence event is recorded.

Corrections are then required for the attenuation of photons in the body tissue or reduction in the final signal to facilitate their inclusion as true coincidence events.

The most commonly used radiopharmaceutical using a PET tracer is ^{18}F-fluorodeoxyglucose (FDG). It has been widely recognized as a metabolic marker and is a useful staging tool for many cancers such as lung cancer, colorectal cancer, lymphomas, etc. It has also been widely used in neurological practice to identify metabolic patterns associated with dementias; and in cardiological practice for the assessment of cardiac patients and their suitability for surgery.[26,27]

Basics of PET-CT and PET-MRI imaging

Due to the need for anatomical localization of sites of abnormal tracer activity on PET scans, there was recognition of the need to develop fusion imaging whereby anatomical context can also be provided. Initial efforts were focused on registering PET and CT data obtained separately and using advanced computer software to merge or fuse the two scans. However, this approach was superseded by combining the PET and CT technologies into one scanner. The patient therefore undergoes one examination at one sitting, and there is minimal patient motion and other technical problems. More recently combined PET-MRI imaging has been introduced into clinical practice with the added advantage of reducing radiation exposure.

PET-CT scanners now form the main bulk of functional scanners, with manufacturers slowly phasing out PET only scanners and promoting advances in PET-CT and PET-MRI scanning.

One limitation of current PET/CT technology is that data are acquired sequentially rather than simultaneously. This then limits the ability to study functional processes that change between the two scans. Another factor for consideration is the radiation dose to patients. Artefacts caused by patient motion or organ motion between the two sets of images coupled with different breathing protocols for PET and CT can result in problems for data interpretation. Mis-registration between the two sets of images is a recognized disadvantage which is factored in while reporting PET-CT scans.

Data acquisition with new hybrid PET/MRI scanners provides the option of real-time simultaneous studies. MRI offers better soft tissue contrast and the challenge of developing viable PET-MRI systems focused on addressing apparent technical incompatibilities such as the fact that PET detectors are based on scintillation crystal blocks which are highly sensitive to even small magnetic fields; and space constraints of fitting in two technologies in one ergonomic system suitable for patient use and convenience. Therefore the type of sequential imaging performed with PET-CT is not a viable option for PET-MRI and the way forward was to combine both systems into one gantry system.

The use of optical fibres coupled to the PET detector's scintillation crystals enables the x-ray and gamma ray detection elements to remain in the magnetic field while the scintillations are conveyed out of the magnetic field by the light fibres. Another method relies on the replacement of photomultiplier tubes with solid-state scintillation detectors which are insensitive to magnetic fields, and can be directly connected to the scintillation crystal block within the magnetic field. Light loss is minimized and the conversion of light to electronic signals occurs inside the MR subsystem, making the use of fragile and bulky optical fibres unnecessary. These detectors are also smaller than photomultiplier tubes and contribute to a smaller overall size. The disadvantage is that they have a lower gain and are more sensitive to temperature variations.[28]

PET-CT imaging in urological cancer

Functional imaging with radioisotopes including PET tracers has a key and established role in the management of cancers such as lung carcinoma, lymphomas, and colorectal cancers. Within the field of urological cancer, there is increasing recognition of the role of newer imaging technologies such as PET-CT scanning for the early detection, more accurate staging, surveillance, and assessment of treatment response.[29,30]

Prostate malignancy

Early detection and identification or confirmation of prostate malignancy is frequently based on non-invasive screening tests with high sensitivity and confirmatory tests such as image-guided biopsy with high specificity. The role for functional imaging within this context is not well established and is not perhaps required.

Functional imaging has an increasing role in identifying the nodal status of prostate carcinoma. Unfortunately, the routine work-horse of PET-CT scanners (i.e. ^{18}F-fluorodeoxyglucose (^{18}F-FDG)) has been shown to have poor accuracy. This is primarily because of the low metabolic rate of prostate tumours; and also because there is high background activity in the region from urinary bladder and the ureters. The use of C11 labelled choline or acetate has been shown to be useful because these tracers map different aspects of metabolism such as increased lipid metabolism or cell membrane integrity and the reported sensitivity and specificity is of the order of 80–95%.

Radioimmunoscintigraphy with prosta-scint has a reported sensitivity of 60–70% in the accurate identification of nodal disease.

While routine bone scanning with Tc99m MDP has a recognized role in the identification of skeletal metastases, there is an increasing recognition for the role of newer hybrid imaging techniques such as SPECT-CT (single photon emission computed tomography-computed tomography) or PET-CT using ^{18}F-fluoride. There is recognition that these techniques have a high sensitivity and high negative predictive value but low specificity and positive predictive value for solitary metastases.

Bone scanning also has a role in the confirmation or exclusion of bony recurrence in the context of a rising serum PSA value.

Renal cell cancer

Most renal cell cancers are incidentally detected when patients undergo cross-sectional imaging for other indications. Since these patients are usually asymptomatic, the bladder tumours detected in this manner are usually smaller, not metastatic, and more amenable to curative treatment.

Nuclear medicine procedures and PET tracers are not specific enough for routine use in the detection and diagnosis of renal cell cancers. However, when the abnormalities are marked, such as very high levels of glucose metabolism, then there is a higher likelihood of malignancy. PET scanning with ^{18}F-FDG has been shown to be effective in the detection of distant metastases thereby influencing therapeutic decisions for staging, assessment of recurrent disease, or new metastases after initial therapy.

Urinary bladder carcinoma

Most nuclear medicine and PET procedures involve the injection of radiotracers that are excreted by the urinary tract and bladder. Hence, there is an inherently low sensitivity for picking up bladder cancers. However, recent approaches to image the patients after bladder catheterization and forced diuresis have been shown to increase the sensitivity. Imaging with C-11 methionine has been shown to further increase the sensitivity.[31]

Testicular tumours

^{18}F-FDG PET has been shown to have low sensitivity and specificity in the assessment of testicular cancers. In addition to increased uptake in testicular tumours, inflammatory and granulomatous tissues also show extensive ^{18}F-FDG uptake, lesions of <1 cm are often not detected, and mature teratomas are frequently indistinguishable from normal and necrotic tissue.

^{18}F-FDG may be used as a standard tool in evaluating residual seminomatous tissue post-chemotherapy.[32]

PET-CT in radiotherapy treatment planning

The concurrent advances in the fields of PET-CT and in radiotherapy have resulted in a renewed assessment of the role of functional imaging in radiotherapy planning for large cancers.

Radiotherapy treatment plans incorporate a range of information from diagnostic and staging tests. The target volume for the radiotherapy needs to be specified as also the shapes and orientations of the treatment beams. The use of PET-CT scans using ^{18}F-FDG has been routinely incorporated into radiotherapy treatment plans for patients with non-small cell lung cancer and oesophageal as well as head and neck cancers.

Additional functional information can be provided to indicate viable tumour tissue using the glycolytic pathway with ^{18}F-FDG or amino acid metabolism with C-11 methionine. ^{18}F-fluorothymidine provides information on cell proliferation based on its incorporation into DNA. ^{18}F-misonidazole can provide a map of hypoxia.

PET scan based tumour volumes have the risk of increasing the radiation field to include some non-neoplastic tissue when the scan shows possible positive tissue extending beyond an anatomically identified lesion on CT or MRI only. Conversely, a non-functional tumour on PET runs the risk of excluding neoplastic tissue from the radiotherapy field. There is therefore a requirement to give due and appropriate weight to all the imaging information available for radiotherapy treatment planning.

There are some additional considerations while using PET-CT images for radiotherapy planning purposes. Images for use in radiotherapy planning have to be acquired in the standard treatment position, using a flat couch rather than a concave bed, and appropriate immobilization devices. Skin markers in standard positions are used to identify key anatomical landmarks for appropriate registration of diagnostic and treatment planning scans. Software used to register the different data sets needs to be of an appropriate standard so that there is high confidence when deciding on target tumour volume for radiotherapy. Additional efforts to reduce the effects of internal motion due to breathing, peristalsis, bladder filling etc are also required.

The additional value of PET-CT scanning to normal radiotherapy planning is being evaluated and the ultimate aim of ensuring an improvement in patient outcomes by optimizing target tumour volumes is yet to be proved conclusively.[33]

^{18}F-fluoride

^{18}F-labelled sodium fluoride imaging has had a resurgence for imaging bones and bone metastases in patients with breast and prostate cancers. The added value of superior quality of images and the full body anatomical survey at the same time have resulted in the increased usage of ^{18}F-fluoride PET-CT scans rather than the traditional isotope bone scans. While there is an element of improved diagnostic certainty in most patients, solitary metastatic foci can still remain a challenge and further confirmatory imaging and/or biopsy may still be required in selected cases. Figure 10.6.10 shows an abnormal ^{18}F-fluoride scan showing metastatic lesions. Figure 10.6.11 shows an abnormal ^{18}F-fluoride scan with multiple levels of spinal involvement consistent with arthropathy.

^{18}F-fluorocholine

Choline is a vital component of lipid metabolism in cell membranes, and the identification of changes in choline metabolism is known to correlate with proliferative changes seen in cancer cells. Choline uptake by cancer cells is also known to be associated with alterations in choline transport and the activity of choline kinase. PET Imaging with C-11 choline or C-11 acetate and ^{18}F-labelled choline analogues have been shown to be vastly superior to ^{18}F-FDG imaging for the detection of primary lesions, regional nodal status, and distant bone metastases.

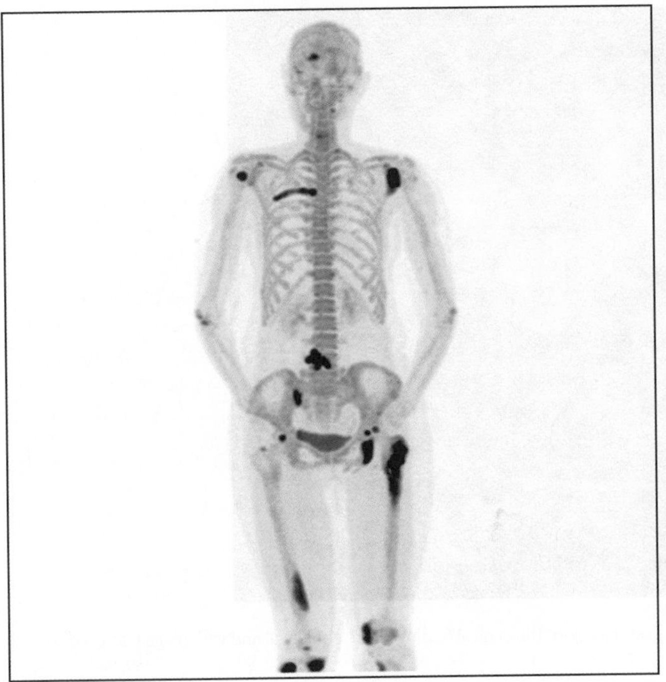

Fig. 10.6.10 An abnormal ^{18}F-fluoride PET-CT study with several areas of increased tracer uptake compatible with multiple bone metastases.

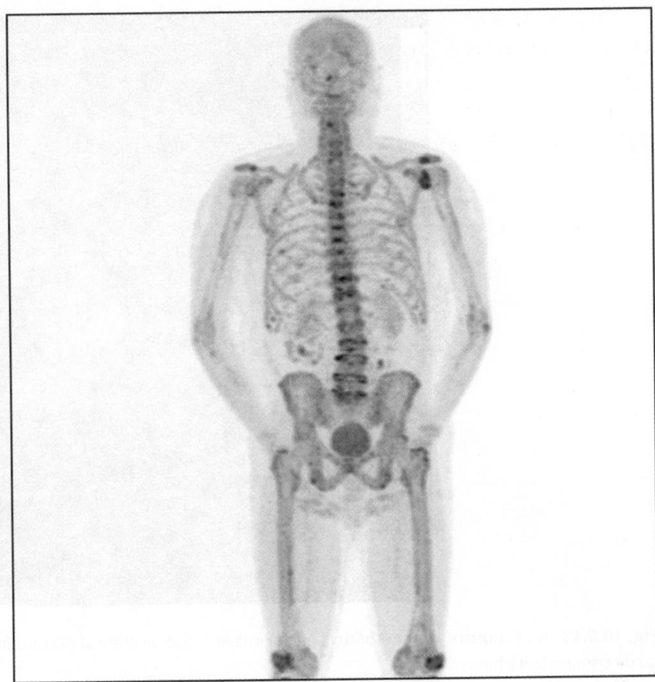

Fig. 10.6.11 An abnormal tracer activity of ^{18}F-fluoride in several spinal levels compatible with multiple joint arthropathy.

There is sufficient evidence with ^{18}F-choline analogues to recommend their use in

(a) targeting biopsy site in high-risk men with persistently elevated PSA and repeatedly negative biopsies;

(b) initial staging among intermediate to high-risk populations;

(c) restaging of recurrent disease and castrate-resistant disease;

(d) selection of men for salvage radiotherapy with suspected local recurrence, but adverse features;

(e) definition of dominant intraprostatic foci or limited lymph node recurrence for focal therapy planning such as radiotherapy planning;

(f) treatment monitoring of hormone therapy or radiation therapy.

Figure 10.6.12 shows an abnormal ^{18}F-fluoroethyl choline scan showing inhomogenous tracer uptake in the prostate gland. Gold seed implanted for marking purposes also noted.

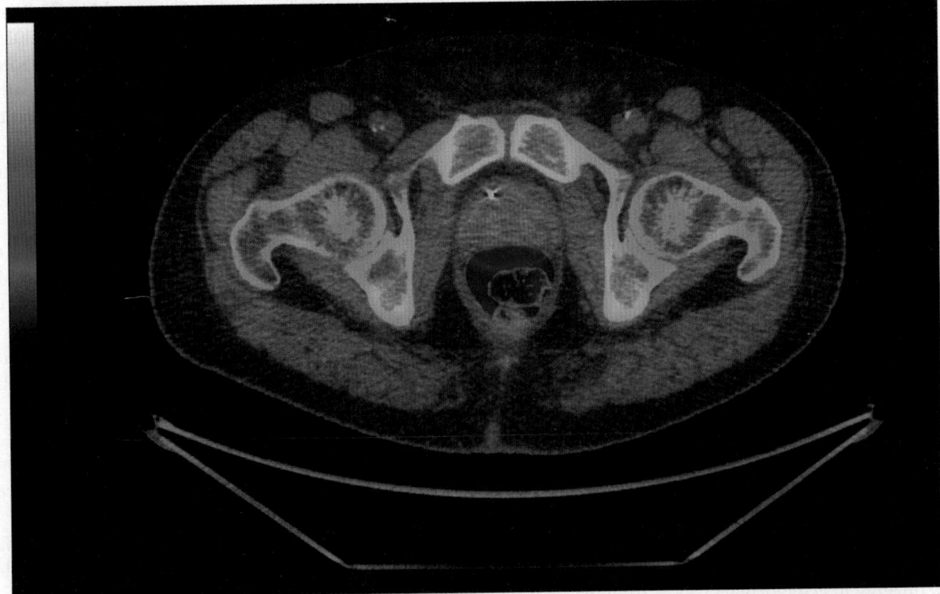

Fig. 10.6.12 An abnormal ^{18}F-fluoroethylcholine uptake in the prostate at 90 minutes post injection. Images are useful for radiotherapy treatment planning. Incidental gold seed noted for marking purposes.

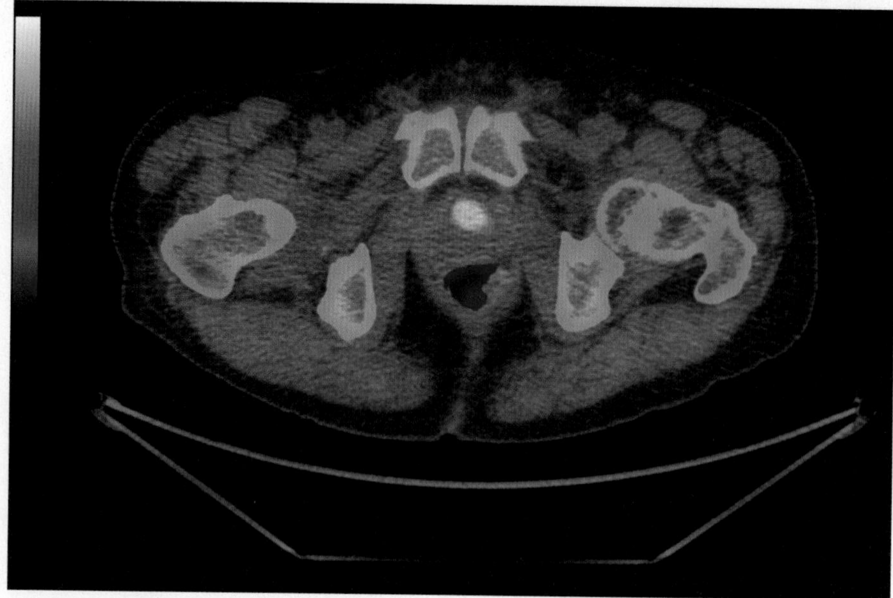

Fig. 10.6.13 An abnormal ^{18}F-fluoroethylcholine image in the prostate at 60 minutes post injection. The clinical findings were equivocal and this image was used to guide confirmatory biopsy.

Figure 10.6.13 shows abnormal focal uptake of ^{18}F-fluoroethyl choline in the prostate gland.[34]

PET scanning in non-cancer urological practice

Since PET scanning of the brain can map functional changes in response to motor activity and other neuronal activity, there have been some early studies on central control of bladder function, detrusor overactivity, and the pelvic floor.

Conclusion

Nuclear medicine techniques provide a range of diagnostic and therapeutic options in urological practice.

Further reading

Bauman G, Belhocine T, Kovacs M, Ward A, Beheshti M, Rachinsky I. ^{18}F-fluorocholine for prostate cancer imaging: a systematic review of the literature. *Prostate Cancer Prostatic Dis* 2012; **15**(1):45–55.

De Jong IJ, Breeuwsma AJ, Pruim J. Positron emission tomography in Urology. *EAU-EBU Update Series 5* 2007:93–104.

Jarritt PH, Carson Kj, Hounsell AR, Visvikis D. The role of PET/CT scanning in radiotherapy planning. *Br J Radiol* 2006;**79**:S27–35.

Mettler FA, Guiberteau MJ. *Essentials of Nuclear Medicine Imaging*, 5th edition. Philadelphia, PA: Saunders Elsevier, 2006.

Murray IPC, Ell PJ. *Nuclear Medicine in Clinical Diagnosis and Treatment*. London, UK: Churchill Livingstone 1994.

Robinson RG, Preston DF, Spicer JA, Baxter KG. Radionuclide therapy of intractable bone pain. *Semin Nucl Med* 1992; **22**:28–32.

Sandler MP, Coleman RE, Wackers FJT, Patton JA, Gottschalk A, Hoffer PB. *Diagnostic Nuclear Medicine*. Baltimore, MD: Williams and Wilkins, 1996.

Tsakiris P, de la Rosette J. Imaging in genitourinary cancer from the urologists' perspective. *Cancer Imaging* 2007; 7:84–92.

Wagner RH, Karesh SM, Halama JR (eds). *Questions and Answers in Nuclear Medicine*. St Louis, MI: Mosby, 1999.

References

1. Ramdahl T, Larsen R. Targeted alpha emitters in tumour therapy. *IPT* 2006; **20**:36–8.
2. Campa JA, Payne R. The management of intractable bone pain: A clinician's perspective. *Semin Nucl Med* 1992; **22**:3–10.
3. Karesh SM. Principles of radiation. In: Wagner RH, Karesh SM, Halama JR, (eds). *Questions and Answers in Nuclear Medicine*. St Louis, MI: Mosby, 1999.
4. Piepsz A, Colarinha P, Gordon I, Hahn K, Olivier P, Sixt R, van Velzen J. Guidelines for glomerular filtration determination in children, 2000. Available at: www.eanm.org/publications/guidelines/gl_paed_gfrd.pdf [Online].
5. Achong DM, Tenorio LE. Abnormal MAG3 Renal scintigraphy resulting from dehydration. *Clin Nucl Med* 2003; **28**:683–4.
6. Oh S-J, Moon DH, Kang W, Park YS, Park T, Kim KS. Supranormal differential renal function is real but may be pathological: Assessment by 99mTechnetium MAG3 renal scan of congenital unilateral hydronephrosis. *J Urol* 2001: **165**:2300–4.
7. Chertin B, Pollack A, Koulikov D, *et al.* Long term follow up of antenatally diagnosed megaureters. *J Ped Urol* 2008; **4**:188–91.
8. Esteves FP, Taylor A, Maantunga A, Folks RD, Krishnana M, Garcia EV. 99Tcm MAG3 Renography: Normal values for MAG3 clearance and curve parameters, excretory parmameters, and residual urine volume. *AJR* 2006; **187**:W610–W617.
9. Koff SA, Peller PA. Diagnostic criteria for assessing obstruction in the newborn with unilateral hydronephrosis using the renal growth-renal function chart. *J Urol* 1995; **154**:662–6.
10. Sfakianikis GN, Sfakianaki E, Georgiou M, *et al.* A renal protocol for all ages and all indications: MAG3 with simultaneous injection of frusemide (MAG3-F0): A 17 year experience. *Semin Nucl Med* 2009; **39**:156–73.
11. Dineen MD, Duffy PG, Lythgoe MF, Ransley PG, Gordon I. MAG3 renography and indirect radionuclide cystography in posterior urethral valves. *Br J Urol* 1994; **74**:785–9.
12. Nankivell BJ, Cohn DA, Spicer ST, Evans SG, Chapman JR, Gruenwald SM. Diagnosis of kidney transplant obstruction using MAG3 diuretic renography. *Clin Transplant* 2001; **15**:11–18.

13. Kocabas B, Aktas A, Aras M, Isiklar I, Gencoglu A. Renal scintigraphy findings in allograft recipients with increased resistance index on doppler sonography. *Transplantation Proceedings* 2008; **40**:100–3.
14. Palmer MR, Donohue KJ, Francis JM, Mandelbrot DA. Evaluation of relative renal function for patients who had undergone simultaneous liver-kidney transplants using Tc99m-MAG3 scintigraphy with attenuation correction from anatomical images and SPECT/CT. *Nucl Med Commun* 2011; **32**:738–44.
15. Aktas A, Aras A, Colak T, Gencoglu A, Karakayali H. Comparison of Tc99m DTPA and Tc99m MAG3 perfusion time-activity curves in patients with renal allograft dysfunction. *Transplantation Proceedings* 2006; **38**:449–53.
16. Majima T, Hattori Y, Funahashi Y, *et al.* 99Tcm MAG3 renography to monitor renal transplant function among kidneys from donors after cardiac death. *Transplantation Proceedings* 2012: **44**:49–53.
17. Broekuezen-de Gast HS, Tiel-van Buul MMC, Van Beek EJ. Severe hypertension in children with renovascular disease. *Clin Nucl Med* 2001; **26**:606–9.
18. Schreij G, van Es PN, van Kroonenburgh MJPG, Kemerink GJ, Heidendal GAK, de Leeuw PW. Baseline and postcaptopril renal blood flow measurements suspected of renal artery stenosis. *J Nucl Med* 1996; **37**:1652–5.
19. Dondi M, Monetti N, Fanti S, *et al.* Use of technetium-99m-MAG3 for renal scintigraphy after angiotensin converting enzyme inhibition. *J Nucl Med* 1991; **32**:424–8.
20. Kahn D, Ben-Haim S, Bushnell DL, Madsen MT, Kirchner PT. Captopril enhanced Tc99m MAG3 renal scintigraphy in subjects with suspected renovascular hypertension. *Nucl Med Commun* 1994: **15**:515–28.
21. Dondi M, Fanti S, de Fabritis A, *et al.* Prognostic value of captopril renal scintigraphy in renovascular hypertension. *J Nucl Med* 1992; **33**:2040–4.
22. Kiratli PO, Caner B, Altun B, Cekirge S. Superiority of Tc99m MAG3 to Tc99m DTPA in treating a patient with mild renal artery stenosis. *Annals of Nucl Med* 2001: **15**:45–8.
23. Fanti S, Dondi M, Corbelli C, *et al.* Evaluation of hypertensive patients with a solitary kidney using captopril renal scintigraphy with Tc99m-MAG3. *Nucl Med Commun* 1993; **14**:969–75.
24. Caglar M, Moretti JL, Buchet P, *et al.* Enalapril plus frusemide MAG3 scinitgraphy in hypertensive patients with atherosclerosis and moderate renal insufficiency. *Nucl Med Commun* 1998; **19**:1135–40.
25. Hosain F, Spencer RP. Radiopharmaceuticals for palliation of metastatic osseous lesions: biologic and physical background. *Semin Nucl Med* 1992; **22**:11–16.
26. Alavi A, Mavi A, Basu S, *et al.* Is PET-CT the only option? *Eur J Nucl Med Mol Imaging* 2007; **34**:819–21.
27. Mankoff DA, Muzi M, Zaidi H. Quantitative analysis in nuclear oncologic imaging. (pp. 494–536) In: Zaidi H (ed). *Quantitative Analysis of Nuclear Medicine Images*. New York, NY: Springer, 2006.
28. Shao Y, Cherry SR, Farahani K, *et al.* Simultaneous PET and MR imaging. *Phys Med Biol* 1997; **42**:1965–70.
29. Sanz G, Rioja J, Zudaire JJ, Berin JM, Richter JA. PET and prostate cancer. *World J Urol* 2004; **22**: 351–2
30. Heidenreich A, Aus G, Bolla M, *et al.* EAU guidelines on prostate cancer. *Eur Urol* 2008; **53**:68–80.
31. Jana S, Blaufox MD. Nuclear medicine studies of the prostate, testes, and bladder. *Semin Nucl Med* 2006; **36**:51–72.
32. Becherer A, De Santis M, Karanikas G, *et al.* FDG PET is superior to CT in the prediction of viable tumour in postchemotherapy seminoma residuals. *Eur J Radiol* 2005; **54**:284–8.
33. de Jong IJ, Pruim J, Elsinga PH, Jongen MM, Mensink HJ, Vaalburg W. Visualisation of bladder cancer using (11)C-choline PET: first clinical experience. *Eur J Nucl Med Mol Imaging* 2002; **29**:1283–8
34. Gofrit ON, Mishani E, Orevi M, *et al.* Contribution of 11C-choline positron emission tomography/computerized tomography to preoperative staging of advanced transitional cell carcinoma. *J Urol* 2006; **176**:940–4.

CHAPTER 10.7

Plain radiography, excretion radiography, and contrast radiography

Robert P. Hartman, Akira Kawashima, and Andrew J. LeRoy

Essentials

Plain radiography is both a primary abdominal examination technique and an initial component of subsequent excretion and contrast radiographic studies. Excretion radiography is performed by means of antegrade opacification of the renal collecting systems, ureters, and bladder following intravenous contrast administration. Contrast radiography is obtained following direct injection of contrast media into the urinary tracts in an antegrade or retrograde fashion.

Although ultrasound, computed tomography, and magnetic resonance imaging are increasingly used to compensate for the limitations of excretion radiography, conventional urographic examinations remain important in the diagnosis of some urinary tract conditions.

Introduction to radiology

Radiology is an essential component in the evaluation of the urinary tract. For decades, excretion radiography following intravenous (IV) administration of iodinated contrast media (also referred to as intravenous urography (IVU), intravenous pyelography (IVP), and excretory urography (EXU)), has been the primary imaging modality of the urinary tracts. In recent years, other imaging modalities such as ultrasonography (US), computed tomography (CT), and magnetic resonance imaging (MRI) have superseded excretion radiography. However, these cross-sectional imaging examinations also have their limitations. Plain radiography, contrast radiography, and EXU still remain important in the diagnosis of some urinary tract diseases (Table 10.7.1).

Plain radiography is both a primary abdominal examination technique and an essential initial component of subsequent excretion and contrast radiographic studies. Contrast radiography is obtained following direct injection of contrast material into the urinary tracts in an antegrade or retrograde fashion. The urographic imaging sequence with IV contrast material or direct contrast injection is designed to optimize depiction of specific portions of the urinary tract during maximal contrast opacification, and a tailored urographic study may provide diagnostic detail beyond the current capabilities of other imaging modalities.[1–3]

This chapter will outline basic uroradiologic imaging with each subsection providing information on technique, indications, complications, and normal anatomical findings.

Plain radiography

Plain radiography of the abdomen and pelvis is most often referred to as a KUB (*K*idneys, *U*reters, and *B*ladder) film or an abdominal 'flat plate' (Fig. 10.7.1), and can provide important information about radio-opaque urinary calculi (Figs 10.7.2 and 10.7.3), calcifications, renal masses (Fig. 10.7.2), and renal size and contour.[4,5] A combination of projection radiographs and non-contrast coronal tomography is valuable in outlining the kidneys and visualizing calculi. An anteroposterior (AP) projection radiograph of the abdomen in supine position may also be referred to as a scout (preliminary) image prior to IV or direct contrast injection for conventional urography. This scout radiograph helps establish appropriate radiographic exposure technique factors, evaluate the patient's positioning, and confirms that residual oral contrast material from previous studies has been eliminated from the gut. The indications for the examinations and patient risk factors should be reviewed carefully. A menstrual history should be obtained in women of childbearing age. Radiation exposure should always be limited appropriately. The presence of a foetal skeleton on the scout image justifies postponing the planned contrast study. A scout image is imperative prior to contrast studies because stones and calcifications can be obscured by contrast material in the urinary tract on subsequent images.

Anatomical landmarks

Several abdominal and pelvic organs can be identified on plain radiographic images. Organs such as the liver, spleen, kidneys, and bladder can be outlined on the image based on the contrasting densities of the organs themselves compared to surrounding retroperitoneal or mesenteric fat. The outline of the kidneys is helpful for assessing renal size, focal cortical scarring or mass, and for delineating intrarenal calcifications. The psoas muscle margins usually can be seen on the plain radiograph (see Fig. 10.7.1), but may be obscured by retroperitoneal fluid or mass.

This chapter previously published as Chapter 11 in the Oxford Textbook of Clinical Nephrology 4e.

Table 10.7.1 Glossary of terminology in uroradiography

Terms (abbreviation)	Definitions
Plain abdominal radiography, KUB, plain film, conventional radiograph, flat plate, scout	Film-screen or digital projection radiograph without use of iodinated contrast medium
Excretion radiography, excretory urography (EXU), intravenous urography (IVU), intravenous pyelography (IVP)	Imaging of the kidneys and urinary tracts before and after the IV administration of iodinated contrast medium
Contrast radiography	
Retrograde pyelography	Imaging of the upper urinary tracts before and after the direct retrograde injection of contrast medium
Antegrade pyelography	Imaging of the upper urinary tracts before and after the direct antegrade injection of contrast media with percutaneous needle puncture of a calyx
Cystography	
Static cystography	Imaging of the bladder before, during, and after the direct contrast administration either in a retrograde fashion through a transurethral Foley catheter or in an antegrade manner through a suprapubic tube
Voiding cystourethrography (VCUG)	Imaging of the bladder and urethra during micturition after the direct administration of contrast medium into the bladder. The procedure is monitored under fluoroscopy and recorded with spot films or video recording
Retrograde urethrography (RUG)	Imaging of the urethra before, during, and after contrast injection in a retrograde manner through a catheter in the anterior urethra (e.g. fossa navicularis).
Loopography ileal conduit study	Opacification of the ileal loop before, during, and after the direct injection of contrast medium with reflux into the upper urinary tracts. The procedure is monitored under fluoroscopy and recorded with spot and overhead films
Pouchgraphy	Imaging of the pouch before, during, and after contrast injection via the stoma or urethra.

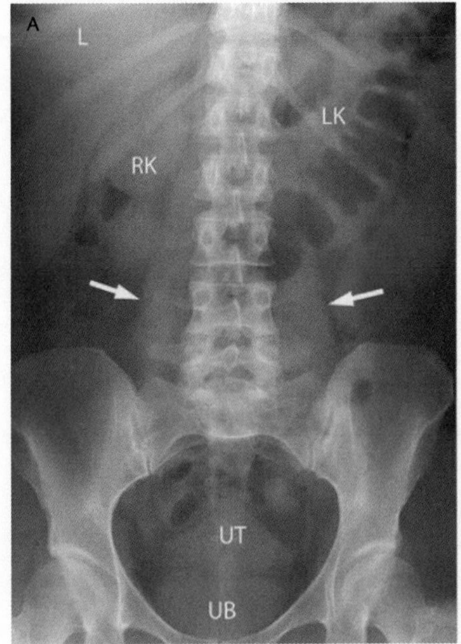

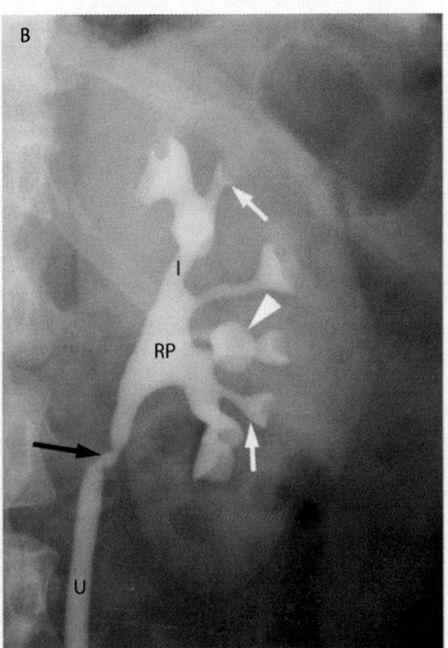

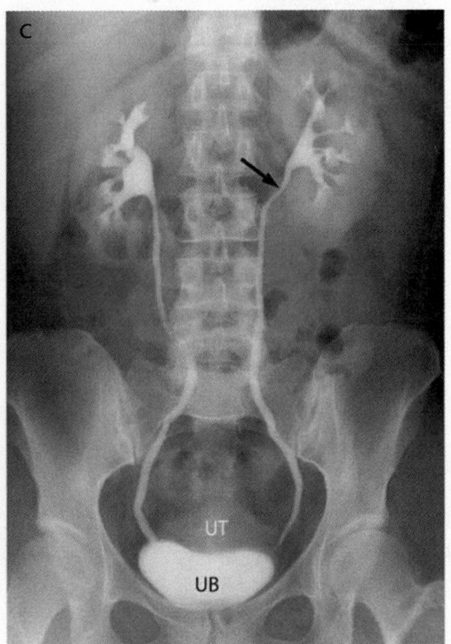

Fig. 10.7.1 Plain radiography and excretion radiography. (A) Plain radiograph of the abdomen and pelvis reveals normal contour of the kidneys and the medial margin of the psoas muscles (arrows). L = liver; LK = left kidney; RK = right kidney; UB = urinary bladder; UT = uterus. (B) Magnified view of the left kidney with abdominal compression 8 minutes after IV contrast material administration. Calyx (white arrows), infundibulum (I), renal pelvis (RP), proximal ureter (U). The calyx which project posteriorly is seen en face (white arrowhead). Normal fold of the ureter at the ureteropelvic junction (black arrow). (C) Abdominal radiograph after release of ureteral compression reveals normal ureters and urinary bladder (UB). The left ureter at the ureteropelvic junction (arrow) is better distended and straight. UT = uterus.

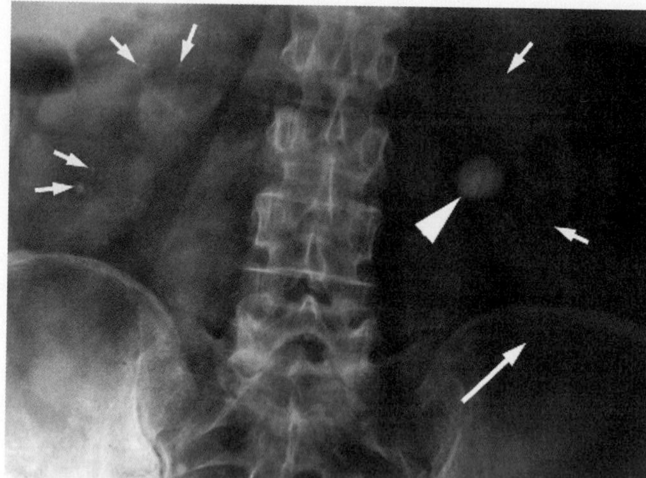

Fig. 10.7.2 Patient with renal stones and renal cell carcinoma. Plain radiograph demonstrates bilateral renal calculi (short arrows) with the largest over the left renal hilum (arrowhead). A round mass is projected over the lower pole of the left kidney (long arrow).

Plain films can demonstrate abnormalities of the bowel gas pattern (e.g. ileus, bowel obstruction, and faecal impaction) and also allow for evaluation of skeletal anomalies, such as sacral agenesis and spinal dysraphism.

Excretion radiography

Excretion radiography is frequently used as a non-invasive screening procedure for the entire urinary tract because it provides both anatomic and functional information.[6]

Patient preparation

A thorough pre-examination 'bowel prep' with a mild laxative (e.g. 10 ounces (28 g) of magnesium citrate solution) the night before the procedure is advisable to rid the colon of stool, which may interfere with clear visualization of the urinary tract. Withholding of fluid and solid food overnight improves renal concentration and excretion of the contrast medium. An empty stomach also decreases the possibility of aspiration of solid food by a patient vomiting after IV contrast administration.

Filming procedure

A plain abdominal radiograph prior to the administration of IV contrast media is essential. After contrast medium is injected, lower abdominal compression is applied anteriorly. Approximately two to three minutes after the contrast material has been administered, nephrotomograms (usually three) are obtained to visualize the renal parenchyma (nephrographic phase).[1] Radiographs obtained 8–10 minutes after the contrast injection demonstrate the calyces, pelves, and proximal ureters (pyelographic phase) (Fig. 10.7.1). The ureters are generally well visualized on the 10-minute radiograph after release of external compression. Films of the bladder (often including a post-void film) conclude the examination.

Diuretic excretion radiography

This modification of excretion radiography is reserved for those patients suspected of having volume-dependent hydronephrosis in whom the initial (dehydrated) excretion radiography revealed no obstruction. With a brisk diuresis after furosemide injection (Lasix®, 20 mg IV), a borderline ureteropelvic junction or ureteral narrowing may become inadequate to allow free flow of the increased urine volume and may reveal in hydronephrosis, and even reproduce or worsen the pain associated with obstruction.

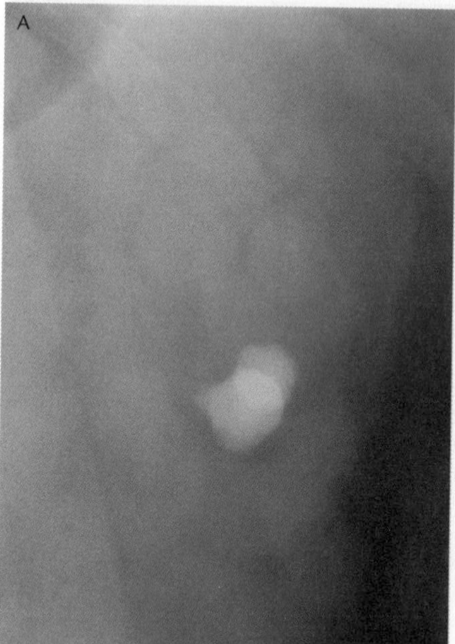

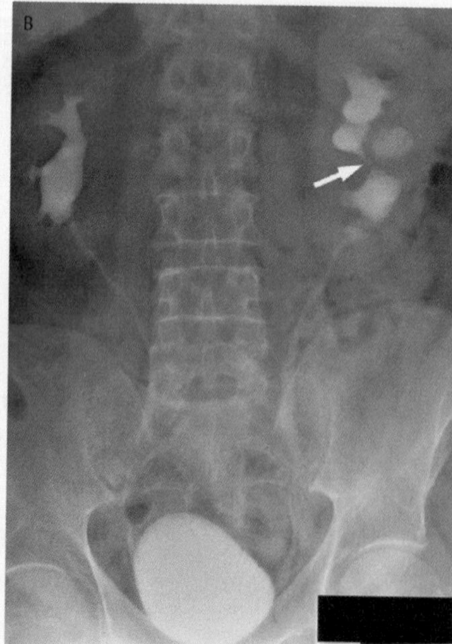

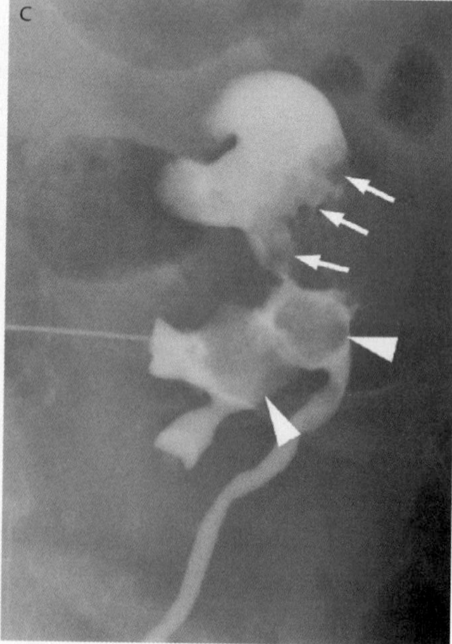

Fig. 10.7.3 Patient with renal stones and transitional cell carcinoma. (A) Magnified view of plain radiograph demonstrates two adjacent stones projected over the lower pole of the left kidney. (B) Excretory radiograph shows the left renal stones in the lower intrarenal collecting system. Note the irregular narrowing of the left renal pelvis (arrow) with associated caliectasis. Kidneys are congenitally malrotated bilaterally. (C) Magnified view of antegrade pyelogram following a percutaneous needle puncture of a lower pole calyx shows a large filling defect in the mid to upper left renal pelvis with urothelial irregularity (arrows), characteristics of urothelial tumour. The two stones (arrowheads) lie in the lower left collecting system.

Contrast media

IV iodinated contrast material is excreted by glomerular filtration with little or no tubular secretion, with subsequent concentration in the tubules and collecting ducts and then progressive opacification of the urinary tract. Urine concentrations are determined by the dose administered, the glomerular filtration rate, and the renal tubular function. As the urine is concentrated in the renal collecting ducts, the relative concentration of the contrast media is enhanced 50–100-fold.

Contrast dosage

Contrast medium can be administered either as a bolus injection or as a drip infusion. The bolus injection allows for a rapid and dense nephrogram when images are obtained two to three minutes after the injection. In the average-size adult, 60–100 mL of contrast medium is usually administered.

Adverse effects

The majority of adverse effects of iodinated contrast media are mild or moderate and only observation, reassurance, and support are required. However, the more severe adverse effects are often preceded by mild or moderate symptoms or prodrome. Reactions to contrast agents usually occur within 20 minutes following IV injection. The most threatening contrast reactions are those unanticipated events that result in sudden compromise of critical body functions, particularly systemic anaphylactic reactions or profound cardiovascular collapse. The widely used newer non-ionic, low-osmolar contrast media (LOCM) offer a slightly more comfortable, safer examination to patients who are sensitive to the older high-osmolar contrast media (HOCM) and produce fewer adverse effects. The risk of rare life-threatening reactions is not, however, eliminated by the use of these LOCM.[7,8] Appropriate training and vigilance by healthcare workers are therefore necessary in clinical areas where contrast media are administered.

Anaphylactoid (idiosyncratic) reactions are generally classified as (i) mild, (ii) moderate, and (iii) severe.[9] Minor side effects do not usually require therapy. Nausea and vomiting are the most common adverse reactions. Other minor reactions include rash, itching, hives (asymptomatic), swelling, headache, dizziness, shaking, nasal congestion, pallor, flushing, chills, sweats, and anxiety. These symptoms are usually self-limiting, but observation is required to confirm resolution and lack of progression. Only supportive treatment is necessary. Patient reassurance is usually helpful. Moderate reactions include tachycardia, bradycardia, hypertension, mild hypotension, vasovagal reactions, dyspnoea, bronchospasm, wheezing, and pronounced cutaneous reaction such as extensive hives (symptomatic) or diffuse erythema. The observed clinical signs and symptoms of moderate reactions should be considered as indications for immediate treatment (Table 10.7.2). These situations require close, careful observation of possible progression into a life-threatening event. Patients with moderate symptoms such as systemic urticaria or facial oedema are treated with antihistamines and subcutaneous adrenaline. Severe types of reactions include laryngeal oedema, and/or, severe hypotension, require small doses of 1:10,000 dilution of adrenaline IV. The most severe reactions include convulsions, arrhythmias, unresponsiveness, and cardiopulmonary arrest.

Prophylactic corticosteroids are strongly recommended for 'at-risk' patients who require contrast media.[10,11] They should also receive LOCM. However, no regimen has eliminated repeat reactions completely. Pre-testing is not predictive, and may itself be dangerous, so is not recommended.[12] Alternative means of imaging to obtain the required information should be considered before embarking on this potentially dangerous path.

Contrast-induced acute kidney injury

IV contrast media may aggravate pre-existing renal dysfunction in a small percentage of patients. The mechanism is not known. There is no standard definition for reporting contrast media-induced nephrotoxicity. The definition of 'significant' changes varies considerably among studies. Acute contrast-induced nephrotoxicity has been defined as an increase in the baseline creatinine values of 20–50% or an absolute increase from 0.5 mg/dL to 1.0 mg/dL.[13] Most cases of contrast media-induced nephrotoxicity are unrecognized because the serum creatinine concentration is not systematically checked after procedures. This nephrotoxicity is usually self-limiting. Serum creatinine usually peaks within 3–5 days, and usually returns to baseline within 10–14 days.[13] Nephrotoxicity is extremely rare when kidney function is normal.

Patients with chronic kidney disease appear to be the most at risk of developing contrast-induced nephropathy. They are more susceptible when dehydrated and when exposed to relatively large volumes of contrast agents. Therefore, in high-risk patients, hydration is advised. Because treatment options are limited once oliguric renal failure has developed, most clinical effort has been aimed at prevention of contrast-induced acute kidney injury. Alternatively, CT urography with oral or IV hydration and with reduced contrast dose could be performed. In addition to active hydration, several studies have suggested various pharmacologic agent administrative regimens may be of benefit in preventing contrast-induced acute kidney injury, including *N*-acetylcysteine.[14]

In patients with underlying chronic renal failure who undergo regular dialysis, contrast media is readily cleared by dialysis because contrast media molecules are not protein bound. Unless there is significant underlying cardiac dysfunction, or very large volumes of contrast media have been administered, there is no need for urgent dialysis.

In diabetic patients with normal renal function taking the oral agent metformin (Glucophage®), discontinuing metformin is advised for at least 48 hours after administration of IV contrast material to minimize the risk of developing metformin-associated lactic acidosis.

Inadvertent subcutaneous extravasation of IV administered contrast medium is not uncommon. Such extravasation may result in local pain, erythema, and swelling. These symptoms usually resolve with local therapy including both warm and cold compression and elevation of the affected extremity.[9] An immediate surgical consultation is indicated when patients develop increased swelling or pain after two to four hours, altered tissue perfusion, changes in sensation in the affected extremity, or skin ulceration.

The normal excretion urogram

The renal parenchyma is best assessed during the nephrographic phase of urography. The normal kidney may range from 9 to 13 cm in cephalocaudal dimension depending on sex and age. The left kidney is frequently larger that the right kidney by approximately 0.5 cm. The kidneys have sharp margins and a smooth contour. Congenital fetal lobulation, a common normal variant, can be differentiated

Table 10.7.2 Reactions to iodinated contrast material and treatment

Type of reactions	Treatment
Hives	Contrast injection discontinued if not completed. Minimal (less than four): observation If diffuse or symptomatic, diphenhydramine PO/IV 25–50 mg If severe, adrenaline IV (1:10,000) 0.1 mL/kg slow push over 2–5 min
Angio-oedema	Closely monitor the airway, O_2 by mask Isotonic IV fluid, 0.9% normal saline, or lactated Ringer's Adrenaline SQ: (1:1000) 0.1–0.3 mL(0.1–0.3 mg) If severe or associated with hypotension or airway compromise, adrenaline IV (1:10,000) 0.1 mL/kg slow push over 2–5 min, up to 3 mL/dose. Repeat as needed
Diffuse erythema	Isotonic IV fluid, 0.9% normal saline or lactated Ringer's 1–2 L rapidly If hypotensive: adrenaline IV (1:10,000), 0.1 mg (1 mL) slowly. Repeat up to 1 mg Hydrocortisone (Solu-Cortef®) IV 200–300 mg push over 1–2 min
Bronchospasm	O_2 10 L/min by mask Isotonic IV fluids Beta-agonist inhalers, metaproterenol (Alupent®) and albuterol (Proventil®), two puffs and inhale. Repeat as necessary Adrenaline SQ (1:1000), up to 0.3 mL. Repeat up to 1 mg total. If hypotensive, add adrenaline (1:10,000), slowly IV 0.1 mg (1 mL) slowly Repeat up to 1 mg total
Laryngeal oedema	O_2 6–10 L/min by mask Isotonic IV fluid, 0.9% normal saline, or lactated Ringer's Adrenaline IV (1:10,000), 0.1 mg (1 mL) slowly. Repeat up to 1 mg total
Pulmonary oedema	Elevate torso O_2 10 L/min by mask Furosemide (Lasix®) 10–40 mg IV over 2 min Morphine 1–3 mg IV Hydrocortisone (Solu-Cortef®) IV 200–300 mg push over 1–2 min Transfer to intensive care unit or emergency department
Hypotension with tachycardia (anaphylactic shock)	Legs elevated 60 degrees or more, or Trendelenburg position O_2 by mask Isotonic IV fluid, 0.9% normal saline, or lactated Ringer's 1– 2 L rapidly Adrenaline IV (1:10,000) 0.1 mg (1 mL) slowly. Repeat up to 1 mg total Transfer to intensive care unit or emergency department
Hypotension with bradycardia (vagal reaction)	Legs elevated 60 degrees or more, or Trendelenburg position O_2 by mask Isotonic IV fluid, 0.9% normal saline, or lactated Ringer's Atropine 0.5–1.0 mg IV push slowly. Repeat up to 3 mg
Hypertensive crisis	O_2 10 L/min by mask Secure IV access Furosemide (Lasix®) 40 mg slowly over 2 min. Nitroglycerine 0.4 mg tablet sublingual. Repeat every 5–10 min Transfer to intensive care unit or emergency department
Seizures/convulsions	O_2 6–10 L/min by mask Lorazepan (Ativan®) 2–4 mg IV Transfer to emergency room for further evaluation and workup

Source: data from Cohan, R. H., Jafri, S., Choyke, L.P., et al. (2010). Manual on Contrast Media, Version 7. Reston, VA: American College of Radiology.

from scars, prior renal infarction or inflammation by their smooth contour and regular spacing and relationship to normal calyces and is often bilateral. Renal parenchyma measures 3–3.5 cm in thickness in the polar regions and 2–2.5 cm in the interpolar regions. The number of the calyces varies considerably. Each calyx (minor calyx) is deeply cupped and surrounds one papilla. The peripheral portion of the calyx is called the fornix. A group of calyces, termed compound calyces, drains two to four papillae and is frequently seen in the polar regions. Two or more infundibula (major calyces), each leading to single or multiple calyces, arise separately from the renal pelvis. Conventionally, all branches from the renal pelvis, whether single or multiple, are termed infundibula. Normal infundibula are straight without bowing or displacement. The renal pelvis sometimes appears to be outside of the confines of the kidneys, where it often has a distended appearance (the extrarenal pelvis).

The upper ureter usually begins as a smooth extension from the renal pelvis and descends lateral to the transverse processes of the upper lumbar vertebrae. The middle third of the ureter is usually superimposed on the transverse processes of the lower lumbar vertebrae. The ureter crosses anterior to the iliac vessels at a slightly higher position on the right than the left. The distal ureter courses posterolaterally and then anteromedially to enter the bladder. Peristaltic activity may change the size and shape of the calyces, pelvis, and ureter from image to image. When the bladder is progressively distended, it is smoothly marginated, and appears roughly spherical. On a post-void image, the mucosal pattern of the bladder is frequently identified.

Computed tomography urography

Cross-sectional imaging studies including US, CT, and MRI are now used more often to assess the renal parenchyma because it has been shown that the sensitivity of detection of small renal masses with excretory urography is greatly decreased. With introduction of helical CT, CT urography has been increasingly used as a more definitive study for the evaluation of the urinary tract. The renal parenchyma is evaluated with CT scans before and after IV contrast administration, and then the collecting system is visualized by reformatted images generated from thin-section multidetector helical CT images obtained during excretory phase of contrast enhancement.[15-17] CT urography has replaced standard excretion radiography in the majority of patient evaluations with urologic indications.

Contrast radiography

Retrograde pyelography

Retrograde pyelography is the opacification of the ureter and pelvicaliceal system by the direct retrograde injection of contrast media at the time of cystoscopy (Fig. 10.7.4).[18] The examination may be done in a cystoscopic suite, or the ureter may be cannulated and the patient may be subsequently brought to the radiology department for the examination. The examination is best performed with fluoroscopy and appropriate spot and overhead images. When a urothelial lesion is suspected, subsequent endoscopy with brushing or biopsy of the lesion for a histological diagnosis is performed under fluoroscopic control.

Retrograde pyelography is performed to investigate lesions of the ureter and renal collecting system that cannot be defined adequately by less invasive imaging, or to visualize the collecting systems and ureters when IV iodinated contrast media is contraindicated.

The procedure is performed with a sterile technique and is contraindicated in a patient with a urinary tract infection. Retrograde pyelography cannot be performed when patients cannot or should not undergo cystoscopy (e.g. patients recovering from recent bladder or urethral surgery). The procedure may be impossible or incomplete when it is difficult to cannulate the ureter (e.g. patients with very large prostates).

Delayed images can be obtained after retrograde pyelography to evaluate drainage of the collecting system. If significant obstruction is identified during retrograde pyelography, then ureteral stent placement should be considered to avoid the risk of bacterial spread into the upper tract above the obstruction.

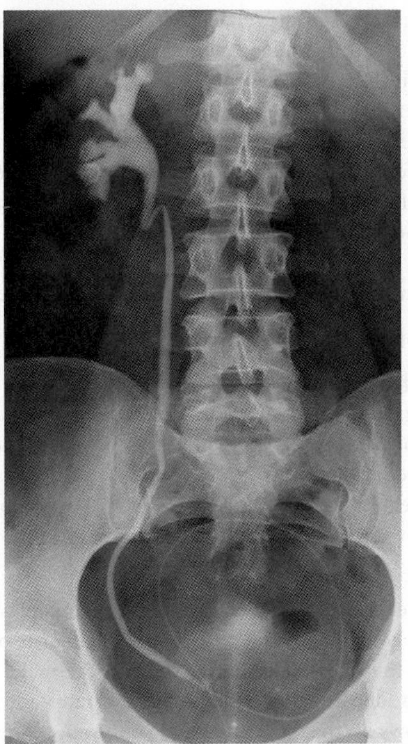

Fig. 10.7.4 Retrograde pyelogram reveals normal contrast filling of the right ureter and intrarenal collecting system.

Other complications of retrograde pyelography include ureteral perforation and contrast reaction. The most common ureteral injury during retrograde pyelography is perforation, occurring during advancement of the catheter or guidewire. These injuries are usually managed with either observation or stent placement depending upon the extent of the injury. Up to 10–15% of contrast media can be absorbed during retrograde pyelography. Caution is therefore advised in patients with a known contrast allergy. Fluoroscopic monitoring of retrograde pyelography is helpful to avoid excess contrast volume injection, reducing the amount of extravasation from the distended upper collecting system.

Antegrade pyelography

Antegrade pyelography is performed to visualize the upper tracts and to delineate the site or nature of upper urinary tract obstruction when excretion radiography is unsatisfactory, retrograde pyelography cannot be performed (e.g. ureteral diversion), or alternative imaging techniques (US, CT, and MRI) are not definitive. This technique is indicated to determine whether a dilated collecting system is obstructed or not when there is renal dysfunction after kidney transplantation. Pyelography is an essential component of upper urinary tract urodynamic testing (Whitaker test).

Antegrade pyelography is contraindicated in patients with uncorrectable bleeding diatheses, diffuse skin infection over the puncture site, or anatomic anomalies which preclude safe renal puncture. Non-dilated collecting systems are not a contraindication, but it is much more difficult to puncture a non-dilated collecting system percutaneously.

A peripheral calyx or the renal pelvis is punctured percutaneously with a 21-gauge, thin-walled needle from a posterior or posterolateral approach (Fig. 10.7.3). Renal localization is provided by means of contrast excreted after an IV injection or, in the event of a non-visualizing kidney, with ultrasound guidance. The procedure is carried out under fluoroscopic control and spot images are obtained.

The side effect of this procedure is inadvertent puncture of adjacent intraabdominal structures. Although puncture of the renal vein, kidney parenchyma, liver, spleen, or colon is possible, few complications ensue because of the small size of the needle.

Cystography

Static cystography

Static cystography provides information on bladder volume, contour, position, and integrity. Static cystography is performed to assess suspected bladder rupture, to demonstrate bladder diverticula, delineate vesicoenteric fistulae, and to assess postoperative healing following bladder or distal ureteral surgery.

The normal cystogram

The distended bladder is a smooth-walled organ with either a round or an oval shape. The oval-shaped bladder is often aligned vertically in the female and horizontally in the male. In the newborn, the bladder lies above the symphysis pubis and descends as the child grows. In the older child and young adult, the bladder lies at or below the level of the symphysis pubis.

Voiding cystourethrography

Voiding cystourethrography (VCUG) provides anatomic information about the lower urinary tract during the physiologic act of micturition. VCUG is performed to diagnose vesicoureteral reflux, to assess bladder emptying, and to evaluate the urethra for posterior urethral valves in the infant male, urethral stricture disease, and urethral diverticula in female patients. VCUG is useful in assessing certain types of voiding dysfunction (e.g. detrusor-external sphincter dyssynergia and neuropathic bladder) and demonstrating reflux into an ectopic ureter which inserts into the urethra.

The bladder is filled with contrast material using a transurethral catheter as for a static cystogram. Once filled, the older child or adult patient is asked to void in the upright position. The procedure is monitored with videofluoroscopy and recorded with either spot images or video recording. In male patients, the voiding images should be obtained with the pelvis in a 45-degree oblique position similar to retrograde urethrography (RUG), so that the entire length of urethra is better demonstrated (Fig. 10.7.5).

Retrograde urethrography

RUG provides detailed visualization of the anterior urethra in the male. Unlike a voiding cystourethrogram, RUG often incompletely visualizes the posterior urethra because of the resistance to retrograde flow provided by the external urethral sphincter. Complete evaluation of the entire urethra often requires both procedures, which may be performed at separate intervals. RUG is rarely indicated in female patients.

RUG is most frequently indicated to assess suspected or known urethral stricture disease, suspected urethral trauma, and to demonstrate urethral diverticula, fistulae, and neoplasms.[19] Retrograde urethrograms should be performed in all patients with pelvic trauma prior to cystography in order to minimize further urethral injury with planned bladder drainage catheter insertion.

Loopography and pouchography

After cystectomy, anastomoses of the ureters to an isolated intact segment (loop) of ileum, transverse colon, or a detubularized large or small bowel segment (pouch) is the most common method of

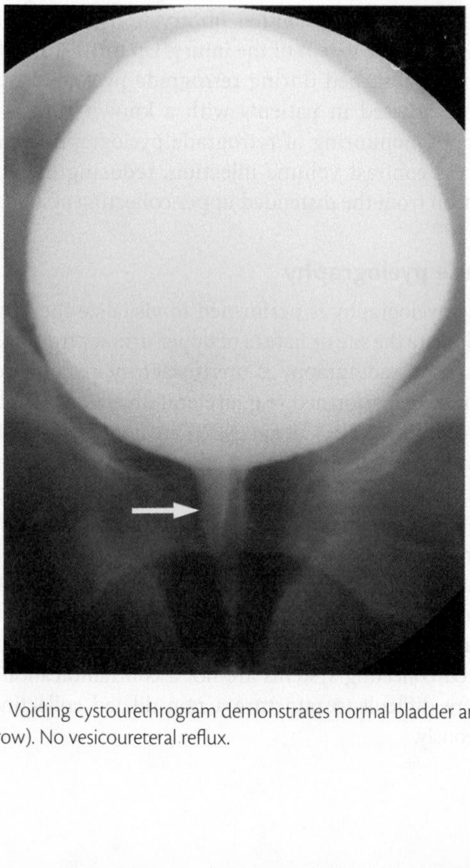

Fig. 10.7.5 Voiding cystourethrogram demonstrates normal bladder and female urethra (arrow). No vesicoureteral reflux.

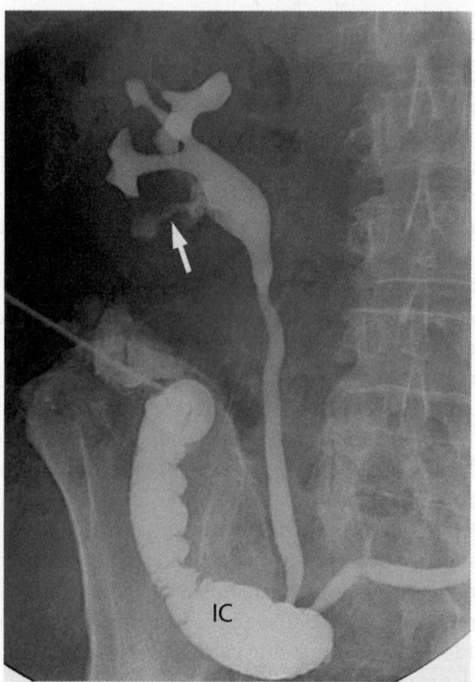

Fig. 10.7.6 Loopogram shows contrast filling of the ileal conduit (IC) with reflux into the distal ureters bilaterally. A large filling defect in the right lower intrarenal collecting system with urothelial irregularity (arrow) is characteristic of urothelial tumour.

establishing permanent urinary diversion.[2,20] The isolated but otherwise intact bowel loop serves as a simple conduit for urinary flow, transporting urine outward toward the stoma in a continuous, rhythmic, isoperistaltic manner. The detubularized pouch, on the other hand, lacks the contractivity to propel urine to the outside, thus becoming a reservoir (e.g. neobladder, continent diversion) rather than a conduit. Radiographic examination of loops or pouches is referred to as loopography or pouchgraphy, respectively.

A loopogram is performed to visualize the bowel conduit and subsequently the upper urinary tracts by reflux of injected contrast media (Fig. 10.7.6). This procedure is utilized in postoperative patients with progressive renal failure to assess conduit integrity and to exclude ureteral obstruction. In such patients, the absence of reflux may indicate ureteral anastomotic obstruction. Alternatively, neobladder and continent diversion ureteral anastomoses are often created with antirefluxing techniques. Therefore, the absence of reflux into the ureters on pouchograms may not indicate urinary obstruction. Loopography is essential to delineate the anatomy of a urinary diversion and probable site of ureteral implantation prior to any planned endourologic or interventional procedures on the diverted ureters.

References

1. Hattery RR, Williamson B Jr, Hartman GW, *et al.* Intravenous urographic technique. *Radiology* 1988; **167**:593–9.
2. Banner MP. Diagnostic uroradiology. In: Hanno P, Malkowicz SB, Wein AJ (eds). *Clinical Manual of Urology*, pp. 87–133. New York, NY: McGraw-Hill, 2001.
3. Dyer RB, Chen MY, Zagoria RJ. Intravenous urography: technique and interpretation. *Radiographics* 2001; **21**:799–821.
4. Dyer RB, Chen MY, Zagoria RJ. (1998). Abnormal calcifications in the urinary tract. *Radiographics* 1998; **18**:1405–24.
5. Barbaric ZL, Pollack HM. Abdominal plain radiography. In Pollack HM, McClennon BL (eds). *Clinical Urography* (Vol. **1**), pp. 67–146. Philadelphia, PA: W.B. Sanders, 2000.
6. Friedenberg RM, Harris RD. Excretory urography. In: Pollack HM, McClennon BL (eds). *Clinical Urography* (Vol. **1**), pp. 147–281. Philadelphia, PA: W.B. Sanders, 2000.
7. Palmer FJ. The RACR survey of intravenous contrast media reactions. Final report. *Australas Radiol* 1988; **32**:426–8.
8. Katayama H, Yamaguchi K, Kozuka T, *et al.* Adverse reactions to ionic and nonionic contrast media. A report from the Japanese Committee on the Safety of Contrast Media. *Radiology* 1990; **175**:621–8.
9. Cohan RH, Jafri S, Choyke LP, *et al. Manual on Contrast Media, Version 7*. Reston, VA: American College of Radiology, 2010.
10. Lasser EC. Pretreatment with corticosteroids to prevent reactions to i.v. contrast material: overview and implications. *AJR Am J Roentgenol* 1988; **150**:257–9.
11. Greenberger PA, Patterson R. The prevention of immediate generalized reactions to radiocontrast media in high-risk patients. *J Allergy Clin Immunol* 1991; **87**:867–72.
12. Yamaguchi K, Katayama H, Takashima T, *et al.* Prediction of severe adverse reactions to ionic and nonionic contrast media in Japan: evaluation of pretesting. A report from the Japanese Committee on the Safety of Contrast Media. *Radiology* 1991; **178**:363–7.
13. Katzberg RW. Urography into the 21st century: new contrast media, renal handling, imaging characteristics, and nephrotoxicity. *Radiology* 1997; **204**:297–312.
14. Tepel M, van der Giet M, Schwarzfeld C, *et al.* Prevention of radiographic-contrast-agent-induced reductions in renal function by acetylcysteine. *N Engl J Med* 2000; **343**:180–4.
15. Chow LC, Sommer FG. Multidetector CT urography with abdominal compression and three-dimensional reconstruction. *AJR Am J Roentgenol* 2001; **177**:849–55.
16. Caoili EM, Cohan RH, Korobkin M, *et al.* Urinary tract abnormalities: initial experience with multi-detector row CT urography. *Radiology* 2002; **222**:353–60.
17. Kawashima A, Vrtiska TJ, LeRoy AJ, *et al.* CT urography. *Radiographics* 2004; **24**(Suppl. 1):S35–54
18. Imray TJ, Lieberman RP, Pollack HM. Retrograde pyelography. In: Pollack HM, McClennon BL (eds). *Clinical Urography* (Vol. **1**), pp. 282–302. Philadelphia, PA: W. B. Sanders, 2000.
19. Kawashima A, Sandler CM, Wasserman NF, *et al.* Imaging of urethral disease: a pictorial review. *Radiographics* 2004; **24**(Suppl. 1):S195–216.
20. Spring DB, Deshon GE, Jr. Radiology of vesical and supravesical urinary diversions and orthotopic bladder replacements. In: Pollack HM, McClennon BL (eds). *Clinical Urography* (Vol. **1**), pp. 357–77. Philadelphia, PA: W.B. Sanders, 2000.

Index

Tables, figures, and boxes are indicated by an italic *t*, *f*, and *b* following the page number.

Q

R

V

W

X

Y